PFENNINGER AND FOWLER'S

Procedures
for Primary Care

PFENNINGER AND FOWLER'S

Procedures for Primary Care

Edited by

John L. Pfenninger, MD
Director
The National Procedures Institute
Midland Michigan
Clinical Professor
Department of Family Practice
Michigan State College of Human Medicine
East Lansing, Michigan

Grant C. Fowler, MD
Professor and Vice Chair
Department of Family Practice and Community Medicine
University of Texas Houston Health Science Center Medical School
Houston, Texas

SECOND EDITION

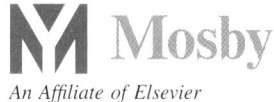
Mosby
An Affiliate of Elsevier

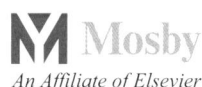

An Affiliate of Elsevier

11830 Westline Industrial Drive
St. Louis, MO 63146

PFENNINGER AND FOWLER'S PROCEDURES FOR PRIMARY CARE, 2ND EDITION

Notice

Medicine is an ever-changing field. Standard safety precautions must be followed, but as new research and clinical experience broaden our knowledge, changes in treatment and drug therapy may become necessary or appropriate. Readers are advised to check the most current product information provided by the manufacturer of each drug to be administered to verify the recommended dose, the method and duration of administration, and contraindications. It is the responsibility of the treating physician, relying on experience and knowledge of the patient, to determine dosages and the best treatment for each individual patient. Neither the publisher nor the editor assumes any liability for any injury and/or damage to persons or property arising from this publication.

Previous edition copyrighted 1994

Library of Congress Cataloging-in-Publication Data

Pfenninger and Fowler's procedures for primary care / edited by John L. Pfenninger, Grant
  C. Fowler.—2nd ed.
        p. ; cm.
      Rev. ed. of: Procedures for primary care physicians. c1994.
      Includes bibliographical references and index.
      ISBN-13: 978–0–323–00506–7 (alk. paper)   ISBN-10: 0–323–00506–3 (alk. paper)
      1. Primary care (Medicine) 2. Surgery, Minor. I. Title: Procedures for primary care. II.
  Pfenninger, John L. III. Fowler, Grant C. IV. Procedures for primary care physicians.
        [DNLM: 1. Primary Health Care—methods. 2. Diagnostic Techniques and Procedures. 3.
  Surgical Procedures, Operative—methods. W 84.6 P528 2004]
  RC48.P76 2004
  616—dc21
                                                                    2003056227

Acquisitions Editor: Thomas Moore
Senior Managing Editor: Kathy Falk
Publishing Services Manager: Patricia Tannian
Project Manager: Richard Hund
Book Design Manager: Gail Morey Hudson
Cover Designer: Teresa Breckwoldt

ISBN-13: 978–0–323–00506–7
ISBN-10: 0–323–00506–3

Printed in China

Last digit is the print number: 9   8   7   6   5

Contributors

OLASUNKANMI W. ADEYINKA, MD
Assistant Professor and Medical Director
Department of Family Practice and Community Medicine
University of Texas, Houston Health Science Center
  Medical School
Houston, Texas

PAULINE M. AHAM-NEZE, MD, MPH
Private Practice
Houston, Texas

PHILIP J. ALIOTTA, MD, MHA, FACS
Instructor in Urology, Assistant Clinical Professor
Department of Neurosciences
State University of New York at Buffalo School of Medicine
  and Biomedical Sciences;
Medical Director
The Center for Urologic Research of
  Western New York, LLC
Main Urology Associates, PC, Attending Urologist
Catholic Health System and Kaleida Health System
Williamsville, New York

MICHAEL ALTMAN, MD
Assistant Professor
Department of Family Practice and Community Medicine
University of Texas, Houston Health Science Center
  Medical School
Houston, Texas

BARBARA S. APGAR, MD, MS
Clinical Professor, Department of Family Medicine
University of Michigan Medical School
Ann Arbor, Michigan

BARRY I. AUSTER, MD
Clinical Instructor, Department of Dermatology
Wayne State University School of Medicine
Head, Division of Dermatology, DMC Grace—Sinai Hospital
Detroit, Michigan

DENNIS E. BABEL, PhD, HCLD
Clinical Mycologist, Drug Trial Division
Midwest Cutaneous Research Corporation
Clinton Township, Michigan

JOSÉ BAYONA, MD, MPH
Director, Urban Family Medicine
Department of Family Practice and Community Medicine
University of Texas, Houston Health Science Center
  Medical School
Lyndon B. Johnson Hospital
Houston, Texas

ROBERT K. BECK, MD
Private Practice, Otolaryngology
Terrecula, California

FRANCIE BERNIER, RNC, MSN
Clinical Education Specialist, Hollister Incorporated
Libertyville, Illinois

CHRISTOPHER J. BIGELOW, MD
Chairman, Department of Ophthalmology, Otolaryngology,
  and Oral Surgery
MidMichigan Medical Center
Midland, Michigan

DEXTER W. BLOME, MD, PhD
Clinical Faculty
Department of Plastic Surgery
Ohio State University School of Medicine;
Riverside Methodist Hospital, Mount Carmel East Hospital
Columbus, Ohio

DAVID T. BORTEL, MD
Chairman
Department of Orthopedics
MidMichigan Medical Center
Midland, Michigan

DAVID B. BOSSCHER, DO, FAAFP
Staff Physician
Dayspring Family Health Center, Jellico, Tennessee;
Clinical Professor, Department of Family Medicine
University of Tennessee
Knoxville, Tennessee

GREGORY L. BROTZMAN, MD
Professor, Department of Family and Community Medicine
Medical College of Wisconsin
Milwaukee, Wisconsin

RICHARD E.A. BRUNADER, MD
Associate Professor of Family Medicine
Department of Family Practice
University of California—Davis
University of California Davis Medical Center
Sacramento, California

THOMAS A. BZOSKIE, MD
Associate Professor of Family Practice
University of California—Los Angeles
Associate Physician
Family Medicine and Urgent Care Center
Woodland Hills Medical Center, Kaiser Permanente
Los Angeles, California

RICHARD C. CHERKIS, MD
Clinical Associate Professor
Department of Obstetrics and Gynecology
University of Rochester, School of Medicine;
Director, Cervical Screening Center
Department of Obstetrics and Gynecology
Unity Health System
Rochester, New York

BETH A. CHOBY, MD
Assistant Professor, Department of Family Medicine
Area Health Education Center
University of Arkansas for Medical Sciences
Fort Smith, Arkansas

ASHLEY K. CHRISTIANI, MD
Clinical Instructor, Department of Family Practice
University of California—Los Angeles School of Medicine
Los Angeles, California;
Associate Physician, Department of Family Practice
Santa Monica—UCLA Medical Center
Santa Monica, California

WENDY C. COATES, MD
Associate Professor, Department of Medicine
University of California—Los Angeles School of Medicine
Los Angeles, California;
Director of Education
Department of Emergency Medicine
Harbor—UCLA Medical Center
Torrance, California

ANDREW S. COCO, MD
Assistant Clinical Professor, Department of Family Practice
Penn State Medical School, Hershey, Pennsylvania
Associate Residency Director
Department of Family & Community Medicine
Lancaster General Hospital
Lancaster, Pennsylvania

J. FINTAN COOPER, MD, BCH, BAO
General and Vascular Surgeon
Department of General Surgery
MidMichigan Medical Center
Midland, Michigan

THOMAS H. CORBETT, MD, MPH
Staff Anesthesiologist, Department of Anesthesiology
St. Luke's Hospital
Maumee, Ohio

SCOTT A. COTA, MD
Lieutenant Commander, Medical Corps
United States Navy, Naval Hospital
Camp Pendleton, California

RAFAEL F. CRUZ, MD
Resident, Department of Anesthesiology
University of Louisville Hospital
Louisville, Kentucky

JAMES A. DAITCH, MD
Subspecialist, Male Infertility, Urology Associates, Ltd.
Phoenix, Arizona

GEORGE C. DENNISTON, MD
Clinical Assistant Professor, Department of Family Medicine
University of Washington
Seattle, Washington

DANIEL J. DERKSEN, MD
Associate Professor
Department of Family and Community Medicine
University of New Mexico School of Medicine
University of New Mexico Hospital
University of New Mexico Health Sciences Center
Albuquerque, New Mexico

WILLIAM DERY, MD
Associate Professor, Department of Family Practice
Michigan State University, East Lansing, Michigan;
Director, Midland Family Practice Residency
MidMichigan Medical Center
Midland, Michigan

KATHLEEN T. DOR, MD
Associate Physician, Clinical Faculty
Department of Family Medicine
Kaiser Permanente Medical Center
Woodland Hills, California

TIMOTHY J. DOWNS, MD, FAAFP
Private Practice
Muskegon, Michigan

DAVID M. DUSH, PhD
Director, Psychological Training and Consultation Center
Central Michigan University, Mount Pleasant, Michigan;
Behavioral Science Director
Midland Family Practice Residency
MidMichigan Medical Center
Midland, Michigan

SCOTT W. EATHORNE, MD
Program Director, Providence Athletic Medicine
Providence Hospital and Medical Center
Novi, Michigan

STEVEN H. EISINGER, MD
Professor of Family Medicine
Associate Professor of Obstetrics and Gynecology
Department of Family Medicine
University of Rochester School of Medicine and Dentistry
Rochester, New York

COLIN ELLIOTT, MD
Procedural Lecturer, Department of Family Practice
Wayne State University
Detroit, Michigan

WILLIAM JACKSON EPPERSON, MD, MBA
Private Practice, Inlet Medical Associates, PA
Murrells Inlet, South Carolina

WILLIAM C. EVERTS, DO
Private Practice
Zephyr Cove, Nevada

DAVID B. FELLER, MD
Assistant Professor
Department of Community Health and Family Medicine
University of Florida College of Medicine
Gainesville, Florida

STEVEN FETTINGER, MD
Associate Clinical Professor
Department of Reproductive Biology and Human Medicine
Michigan State University, East Lansing, Michigan;
Vice Chief of Staff, Covenant Health Center
Saginaw, Michigan

LES B. FORGOSH, MD, FACC, FACP
Clinical Assistant Professor, Department of Family Practice
University of Minnesota, Minneapolis, Minnesota
St. Paul Cardiology
St. Paul, Minnesota

GREGORY J. FORZLEY, MD
Medical Director, Systems Development, Advantage Health
Grand Rapids, Michigan

GRANT C. FOWLER, MD
Professor and Vice Chair
Department of Family Practice and Community Medicine
University of Texas, Health Science Center, Houston
    Medical School
Houston, Texas

VICTOR F. FROELICHER, MD
Professor of Medicine, Department of Cardiology
Stanford University, Stanford, California;
Director, ECG/Exercise Lab
Veteran's Affairs Health Care System
Palo Alto, California

JOSÉ RAMÓN GARCÍA, MD
Private Practice
Odessa, Texas

JEFFREY A. GERMAN, MD
Assistant Professor, Department of Family Medicine
Louisiana State University Health Sciences Center
Shreveport, Louisiana

REBECCA H. GLADU, MD
Associate Professor and Residency Program Director
Department of Family Practice and Community Health
University of Hawaii, John A. Burns School of Medicine
Honolulu, Hawaii

KEN GRAUER, MD
Professor, Associate Residency Director
Department of Community Health and Family Medicine
University of Florida College of Medicine
Gainesville, Florida

LEE A. GREEN, MD, MPH
Associate Professor, Department of Family Medicine
University of Michigan;
University of Michigan Health System
Ann Arbor, Michigan

JESSICA Y. HACKMAN, DMD
Resident
Oral and Maxillofacial Surgery Department
University of California—Los Angeles
Los Angeles, California

MATS HAGSTROM, MD
Attending Physician
St. Joseph Hospital
Orange, California

FRED M. HANKIN, M.D.
Staff Physician
Section of Orthopedic Surgery
St. Joseph Mercy Hospital
Ypsilanti, Michigan

DEBRA KAY HARVEY, MD
Assistant Professor
Department of Family Practice and Community Medicine
University of Texas, Houston Health Science Center
  Medical School
Houston, Texas

ANDREW THOMAS HAYNES, MD
Staff Physician
Department of Emergency Medicine
Willis Knighton Medical Center
Shreveport, Louisiana

JOHN HARLAN HAYNES III, MD
Clinical Professor, Department of Family Practice
University of Texas—Southwestern, Dallas, Texas;
Medical Director, Med Alliance Health Center
Fort Worth, Texas

HAROLD H. HEDGES III, MD
Assistant Clinical Professor
Department of Family & Community Medicine
University of Arkansas School of Medicine;
Little Rock Family Practice Clinic
Little Rock, Arkansas

SCOTT T. HENDERSON, MD
Associate Professor Family Practice
Family Practice Residency Program at Cheyenne
University of Wyoming
Cheyenne, Wyoming

STANLEY A. HIRSCH, MD
Active Staff, Department of Surgery
University of Pittsburgh Medical Center
Pittsburgh, Pennsylvania

JERRY W. HIZON, MD
Assistant Clinical Professor
Department of Community and Preventive Medicine
University of California, San Diego, San Diego, California;
Medical Director, O.U.C.H. Sports Medical Group
Muvvièha, California

JOHN E. HOCUTT, Jr., MD
Clinical Assistant Professor of Family Medicine
Department of Family Medicine
Thomas Jefferson University, Philadelphia, Pennsylvania;
Department of Family Medicine
Christiana Care Health System—St. Francis Hospital;
Private Practice, AI DuPont Institute
Wilmington, Delaware

JOHN R. HOLMAN, MD, MPH, CDR, MC, USN
Clinical Faculty, Department of Family Medicine
University of Washington, Seattle, Washington
Faculty Development Specialist
Department of Family Medicine, Naval Hospital
Camp Pendleton, California

THOMAS E. HOWARD, MD
Formerly, Department of Family Practice, Duluth Clinic —
  Deer River
Deer River, Minnesota

KENNETH HU, MD
Lead Physician, Internal Medicine Department
Kaiser Permanente
Camp Springs Medical Center
Temple Hills, Maryland

KARL S. HUBACH, MD
Family Practitioner, Inlet Medical Associates, PA
Murrells Inlet, South Carolina

ERIC M. HUGHES, MD
Private Practice
Gallipolis, Ohio

DOUGLAS R. JACKSON, MD
Orthopedic Surgeon, Department of Orthopedic Surgery
MidMichigan Medical Center
Midland, Michigan

JAMES L. JACKSON, MD, FACS
Ophthalmologist, MidMichigan Medical Center
Midland, Michigan

ROBERT E. JAMES, MD, FACS
Clinical Instructor, Department of Urology
University of California—San Francisco
San Francisco, California;
Department of Urology and Renal Transplantation
Santa Rosa Memorial Hospital
Santa Rosa, California

RAYMOND F. JARRIS, Jr., MD
Emergency Department Physician
Swedish Medical Center/Ballard
Seattle, Washington

PENNY JENKINS, RN, NP
Nurse Practitioner
Department of Gynecology and Urogynecology
Cleveland Clinic Florida
Westin, Florida

ROBERT H. JOHR, MD
Associate Clinical Professor of Dermatology and Pediatrics
Director, Pigmented Lesion Clinic
University of Miami School of Medicine
Sylvester Comprehensive Care Center
Miami, Florida

ROBERT L. KALB, MD
Adjunct Professor, University of Toledo
Clinical Instructor—Orthopedics
Private Practice, Bone, Joint, and Spine Surgeons
Toledo, Ohio

LEE A. KAPLAN, MD
Private Practice, Dermatology, La Jolla, California;
Associate Clinical Professor
Department of Medicine and Dermatology (Voluntary)
University of California—San Diego
San Diego, California

NEERAJ KOHLI, MD
Assistant Professor
Department of Obstetrics and Gynecology
Harvard Medical School;
Director, Division of Urogynecology
Mount Auburn Hospital
Beth Israel Deaconess Medical Center
Boston, Massachusetts

JEFFREY R. KOVAN, DO
Director of Sports Medicine
Department of Physical Medicine and Rehabilitation
Michigan State University College of Osteopathic Medicine
East Lansing, Michigan

CHANTAL LEMOINE, MD
Associate Clinical Professor
Department of Internal Medicine
Division of Rheumatology and Clinical Immunology
University of Southern California School of Medicine
Los Angeles, California

MADELINE R. LEWIS, DO
Clinical Assistant Professor
Department of Family Medicine
Indiana University School of Medicine;
Associate Director
Memorial Family Practice Residency Program
Memorial Hospital
South Bend, Indiana

JOHN THOMAS LITTELL, MD
Medical Consultant and Instructor, Natural Family Planning
Kissimmee, Florida

NEAL M. LONKY, MD, MPH
Assistant Chief, Department of Obstetrics and Gynecology
Kaiser Permanente, Anaheim, California;
Director of Medical Education and Research
Clinical Professor of Obstetrics and Gynecology
University of California, Irvine School of Medicine
Irvine, California

BRIAN D. MADDEN, MD
Informatics Director, Department of Family Practice
UCLA School of Medicine, Los Angeles, California;
Attending Staff Physician, Department of Family Practice
Santa Monica—UCLA Medical Center
St. John's Hospital and Health Center
Santa Monica, California

GREGORY A. MAROLF, MD
Family Physician, CAQ Sports Medicine
Bayfront Convenient Care Clinics
St. Petersburg, Florida

DONALD N. MARQUARDT, MD, PhD
Staff Physician
Department of Family Medicine
Yukon Kuskokwim Delta Regional Hospital
Yukon Kuskokwim Health Corporation
Bethel, Alaska

EDWARD. J. MAYEAUX, Jr., MD, FAAFP
Professor of Family Medicine and Obstetrics and
    Gynecology
Department of Family Medicine
Louisiana State University Health Sciences Center
Shreveport, Louisiana

WILLIAM L. McDANIEL, Jr., MD
Clinical Associate Professor of Community Science Program
Department of Family Practice
Mercer University School of Medicine, Macon, Georgia;
Staff Physician, Department of Family Practice
Hamilton Medical Center
Dalton, Georgia (Whitfield)

CARLOS A. MORENO, MD, MSPH
Vice President of Community and Educational Outreach
Professor and Chair
Department of Family Practice and Community Medicine
University of Texas, Health Science Center Houston Medical
    School;
Chief of Family Practice, Memorial Hermann and Lyndon B.
    Johnson Hospitals
Houston, Texas

REX E. MOULTON-BARRETT, MD, FACS
Clinical Instructor, Department of Surgery
Contra WSTA Regional Medical Center—U.C. Davis
Active Staff, Department of Surgery
Contra WSTA Regional Medical Center, Martinez, California;
Alameda Hospital, Alameda, California;
Oakland Children's Hospital
Oakland, California

JULIE GRAVES MOY, MD, MPH
Faculty Physician
Austin Medical Education Programs
Family Practice Residency
Austin, Texas

SUSAN E. MURPHEY, MD
Assistant Professor
Clinical Cancer Prevention
University of Texas M.D. Anderson Cancer Center
Houston, Texas

ROGER Y. MURRAY, MD
Private Practice
The Murray Center for Veins, Aesthetics & Anti-Aging
Altamonte Springs, Florida

JUDY WYNNE NEFF, RN, BSN
Clinical Nurse
Department of Urogynecology
Good Samaritan Hospital
Cincinnati, Ohio

GARY R. NEWKIRK, MD
Clinical Professor, Department of Family Medicine
University of Washington School of Medicine;
Director, Family Medicine Spokane Residency and Rural
    Training Tracts
Spokane, Washington

JOHN O'BRIEN, MD
Clinical Associate Professor
Department of Family Medicine
University of Michigan Medical School
Ann Arbor, Michigan

THEODORE X. O'CONNELL, MD
Associate Physician, Clinical Faculty
Department of Family Medicine
Kaiser Permanente Medical Center
Woodland Hills, California

KATHLEEN M. O'HANLON, MD
Professor, Department of Family and Community Health
Marshall University
Huntington, West Virginia

CAROL OSBORN, MD
Assistant Professor Clinical Medicine
Department of Family Preventive Medicine
University of Utah School of Medicine
Salt Lake City, Utah

NELLY A. OTERO, MD, FAAFP
Associate Professor and Medical Director
Department of Family and Community Medicine
Texas Tech University Health Sciences Center
Odessa, Texas

JAMES R. PALLESCHI, MD
Chair, Section of Renal Transplantation
Department of Surgery, Santa Rosa Memorial Hospital
Santa Rosa, California

SCOTT A. PALUSKA, MD
Assistant Professor, Department of Family Medicine
University of Washington
Seattle, Washington

HELEN A. PASS, MD
Director, Breast Care Center
William Beaumont Hospital
Royal Oak, Michigan

PAUL M. PAULMAN, MD
Professor and Predoctoral Director
Department of Family Medicine
University of Nebraska Medical Center
Omaha, Nebraska

JAMES F. PEGGS, MD
Clinical Associate Professor
Department of Family Medicine
University of Michigan
Ann Arbor, Michigan

JOHN L. PFENNINGER, MD, FAAFP
President and Director
The National Procedures Institute, Midland, Michigan;
Clinical Professor, Department of Family Practice
Michigan State College of Human Medicine
East Lansing, Michigan;
Director, The Medical Procedures Center, PC
Midland, Michigan

MADELYN POLLOCK, MD
Clinical Assistant Professor
Department of Family and Community Medicine
University of Texas Health Science Center
San Antonio, Texas

JOHN BARTELS POPE, MD
Associate Professor of Clinical Family Medicine
Department of Family Medicine and Comprehensive Care
Louisiana State University Health Sciences Center
Shreveport, Louisiana

DAVID V. POWER, MB, MPH
Associate Director, Medical Student Education
Department of Family Practice and Community Health;
Course Director, Primary Care Clerkship
University of Minnesota Medical School
Minneapolis, Minnesota

CHRISTIAN RAIGOSA, MD
Physician, Santa Monica—University of California—
    Los Angeles Family Practice Residency
Santa Monica—University of California—
    Los Angeles Medical Center
Santa Monica, California

ARNOLD M. RAMIREZ, MD
Assistant Professor, Department of Family Medicine
University of South Florida College of Medicine
Tampa, Florida

STEPHEN F. RAMIREZ, MD
Chief of Family Practice, North Central Baptist Hospital;
President, Stone Oak Family Practice
San Antonio, Texas

STEPHEN RATCLIFFE, MD, MSPH
Professor and Program Director
Department of Family and Preventive Medicine
University of Utah
Salt Lake City, Utah

SUMANA REDDY, MD, FAAFP
Private Practice
Acacia Family Medical Group
Salinas, California

RONALD D. REYNOLDS, MD
Private Practice
New Richmond Family Practice, New Richmond, Ohio;
Volunteer Associate Professor
Department of Family Medicine, University of Cincinnati
Cincinnati, Ohio

TERRY REYNOLDS, BS RDCS
Director, School of Cardiac Ultrasound
Arizona Heart Institute
Phoenix, Arizona

RALPH M. RICHART, MD
Vice Chairman for Anatomic Pathology
Professor of Pathology in Obstetrics and Gynecology
Columbia University College of Physicians and Surgeons;
Attending Pathologist, Department of Pathology
New York Presbyterian Hospital
New York, New York

DAVID RODEN, MD, FACS
Department of Otolaryngology
MidMichigan Medical Center
Midland, Michigan

EDWARD A. ROSE, MB, MSA, FAAFP
Assistant Professor, Department of Family Medicine
Wayne State University, Detroit, Michigan;
Director of Clinical Information Management
University Family Physicians
Royal Oak, Michigan

TERRY S. RUHL, MD
Associate Director
Altoona Family Physicians Residency
Altoona, Pennsylvania

GARY E. RUOFF, MD, FAAFP
Clinical Professor, Department of Family Practice
Michigan State University College of Medicine
East Lansing, Michigan; Borgess Hospital; Bronson Hospital;
Director of Clinical Research
Westside Family Medical Center
Kalamazoo, Michigan

RAMIRO SANCHEZ, MD
Medical Director, Outpatient Clinical Care
Houston, Texas

LEN SCARPINATO, DO, MS, FACP, FCCP, FAAFP, FCCM
Professor and Program Director
Medical College of Wisconsin's Racine Family Practice
   Residency;
Chair, Department of Family Medicine
All Saints Healthcare
Racine, Wisconsin

MARY BETH SHAW, MSPT, ATC
Physical Therapist, Athletic Trainer
Outpatient Rehabilitation, St. Anthony's Healthcare
St. Petersburg, Florida

TODD M. SHEPERD, MD
Sports Medicine Fellow, Providence Athletic Medicine
Providence Hospital and Medical Centers
Novi, Michigan

JAMES R. SHEPICH, MD
MidMichigan Medical Center (Staff)
Department of General Surgery
MidMichigan Medical Center
Midland, Michigan

VICTOR S. SIERPINA, MD
Assistant Professor, Clinic Medical Director
Department of Family Medicine
University of Texas Medical Branch
Galveston, Texas

LARRY SKOCZYLAS, DDS, MS
Oral and Maxillofacial Surgeon
Department of Ophthalmology, Otolaryngology, Oral &
   Maxillofacial Surgery, MidMichigan Medical Center
Midland, Michigan

CHAD J. SMITH, DO
Adjunct Assistant Professor of Family Medicine
Uniformed Services University of Health Sciences
Bethesda, Maryland;
Staff Physician, Department of Family Medicine
Naval Hospital
Camp Pendleton, California

CLARK B. SMITH, MD
Associate Professor, Department of Family Medicine
University of Tennessee College of Medicine;
Active Staff, Department of Family Practice, Obstetrics, and
   Gynecology
St. Francis Hospital
Memphis, Tennessee

DAVID W. SNIDER, DPM
Director, International Diabetes Center Foot Clinic
Department of Podiatry, MidMichigan Medical Center
Midland, Michigan

GARY L. SNYDER, DPM, RVT
Chief Medical Officer, Vein Institute at Vail Inc.
Lakewood, Colorado

ANDREW C. STEELE, MD
Residency Program Director, OB/GYN
Division of Urogynecology and Reconstructive Pelvic
   Surgery, David Grant USAF Medical Center
Travis AFB, California

JAMES A. SURRELL, MD
Associate Clinical Professor, College of Human Medicine
Michigan State University, East Lansing, Michigan;
Staff Surgeon, Department of Colon and Rectal Surgery
Spectrum Health and Ferguson Clinic
Grand Rapids, Michigan

LYNN L. SWAN, MD
Assistant Clinical Professor
Michigan State University College of Human Medicine
Munson Medical Center
Traverse City, Michigan

ROBERT S. TAN, MD, MBA
Associate Professor (Geriatrics)
Department of Family Practice and Community Medicine
University of Texas, Health Science Center Houston
   Medical School;
Medical Director, Garden Terrace Alzheimer's Center
Houston, Texas

SUSAN TAYLOR, MD
Clinical Instructor, Department of Medicine
University of California—Los Angeles
Los Angeles, California;
Department of Family Medicine
Santa Monica—UCLA Medical Center
Santa Monica, California

JAMES L. TELFER, MD
Staff Physician
Section of Orthopedic Surgery
St. Joseph Mercy Hospital
Ypsilanti, Michigan

ANTHONY J. THOMAS, Jr., MD
Head, Section of Male Infertility
Urological Institute, Cleveland Clinic Foundation
Cleveland, Ohio

SHEILA THOMAS, MD
Assistant Director of Clinical Affairs
Department of Family Medicine
University of Tennessee/Baptist HealthPlex Family Practice
   Center
Memphis, Tennessee

STEPHEN K. TOADVINE, MD, MPH
Associate Professor, Voluntary Faculty
Department of Family Practice
University of Kentucky, Lexington, Kentucky;
Site Director, Baptist Regional Medical Center
University of Kentucky, Family Practice Residency Program
Corbin, Kentucky

THOMAS N. TOLD, DO
Clinical Professor of Family Medicine, Colorado Springs
   Osteopathic Foundation
Family Medicine Residency
Director Rural Residency Training, Craig Medical Center
Craig, Colorado

DUANE E. TOWNSEND, MD, FACOG
Private Practice
Park City, Utah

MICHAEL L. TUGGY, MD
Clinical Associate Professor, Department of Family Medicine
University of Washington
Director, Swedish Family Medicine
Swedish Medical Center
Seattle, Washington

GERALDINE N. URSE, DO
Residency Director
Doctors Hospital Family Practice, Ohio Health
Grove City, Ohio

RICHARD USATINE, MD
Associate Dean of Medical Education
Department of Family Medicine, Florida State University
Tallahassee, Florida

DEEPA VASUDEVAN, MD
Assistant Professor and Medical Director
Department of Family Practice and Community Medicine
University of Texas, Houston Health Science Center
   Medical School
Houston, Texas

ROGER K. WAAGE, MD
Associate Program Director
Duluth Family Practice Residency
Duluth, Minnesota

BRIANA WALTON, MD
Director, Benign Gynecology
Division of Urogynecology and Female Pelvic Medicine
Washington Hospital Center
Washington, DC

JOHN J. WARD, MD
Assistant Professor, Department of Orthopedic Surgery
Louisiana State University Health Sciences Center
Shreveport, Louisiana

LYDIA A. WATSON, MD
Assistant Clinical Professor
Department of Obstetrics and Gynecology
Michigan State University College of Human Medicine
East Lansing, Michigan;
Staff Physician, Department of Obstetrics & Gynecology
Midland Hospital
Midland, Michigan

DAVID GLENN WEISMILLER, MD, SCM
Assistant Professor of Family Medicine
Director of Women's Health
Department of Family Medicine
The Brody School of Medicine at East Carolina University;
Attending Physician, Pit County Memorial Hospital
Greenville, North Carolina

CHARLES E. WERNER, Jr., MD
Attending Staff, Department of Obstetrics and Gynecology
MidMichigan Medical Center
Midland, Michigan

STEPHEN J. WETMORE, MCISC, MD, FCFP
Assistant Professor, Department of Family Medicine
University of Western Ontario
London, Ontario, Canada

BRETT WHITE, MD
Formerly, Resident
Department of Family Medicine
Santa Monica—University of California—Los Angeles
    Medical Center
Santa Monica, California

RUSSELL D. WHITE, MD
Clinical Associate Professor, Department of Family Medicine
University of South Florida College of Medicine
Tampa, Florida;
Associate Director, Family Practice Residency
Director, Sports Medicine Fellowship Program
Department of Family Practice, Bayfront Medical Center
St. Petersburg, Florida

J. MARK WIEDEMANN, MD, MS
Emergency Room Staff Physician, Mad River Community
    Hospital
Arcata, California

TOLBERT S. WILKINSON, MD
Director, Cosmetic Surgery Center and Spa;
Department of Plastic Surgery
University of Texas Health Science Center
San Antonio, Texas

ROBERT WILLIAMS, MD, MPH
Associate Professor
Department of Family and Community Medicine
University of New Mexico School of Medicine
Albuquerque, New Mexico

VERNEETA L. WILLIAMS, MD
Associate Director, Department of Family Practice
Riverside Regional Medical Center
Newport News, Virginia

KAREN E. WILSON, MD
Attending Physician, Voluntary Faculty
Department of Family Medicine, Wayne State University
Detroit, Michigan

THOMAS C. WRIGHT, Jr., MD
Associate Professor
Department of Pathology
College of Physicians and Surgeons of Columbia University
New York, New York

GEORGE G. ZAINEA, MD, FASCRS
Surgeon
Colon and Rectal Surgery
Surgical Associates of MidMichigan, P.C.
Midland, Michigan

DANIEL A. ZELLING, MD, FAAFP
Private Practice
Ohio Institute of Medical Hypnosis, Inc.
Akron, Ohio

EDWARD M. ZIMMERMAN, MD
Private Practice, Aesthetic Medicine
Las Vegas, Nevada

STEWART L. ZUCKERBROD, MD
Clinical Associate Professor
Department of Ophthalmology
University of Texas, Houston Health Science Center
    Medical School
Houston, Texas

EDWARD G. ZURAD, MD
Clinical Assistant Professor
Department of Family and Community Medicine
Temple University School of Medicine
Philadelphia, Pennsylvania;
Chairman, Department of Family Medicine
Tyler Memorial Hospital, Tunkhannock, Pennsylvania;
Local Medical Director, Procter and Gamble Paper Products
Mehoopany, Pennsylvania

Dedication

The dedication of the first edition of this text was to our families, and rightly so. However, as we have so aptly learned, sometimes "it takes a village. . . ."

To promote the procedural skills field, it has taken the support of many colleagues. The travel associated with teaching procedures makes it impossible for me to continue the emergency room "on call" needed to maintain privileges at MidMichigan Medical Center. In 1991, the physicians in our Family Practice Department voted unanimously to share my "on call" coverage obligations. This is truly magnanimous support.

Subsequently, during the past 12 years, many family physicians have awakened to answer a phone call or handle an admission in the middle of the night on my behalf. For those who have never had to experience "emergency room on call," there is no way to explain what a difficult service it is to provide. There is no sufficient way to say how much I appreciate their help.

So, I am dedicating my portion of this second edition to all of those family physicians listed below who have covered for me over the past 14 years. Know that, although you were in the background and others do not know who you are, you have helped to compile this text, to teach others, and to be a role model of a supportive colleague. Thank you.

Finally, as this text was being completed, Daniel Vincenzo Maura was born to Stacey and Romolo Maura. Stacey is my daughter and Daniel is my first grandchild. May all of Daniel's dreams and those of his parents be fulfilled.

MidMichigan Medical Center—Midland, Michigan

Jennifer R. Aloff, MD	Alan A. Fantuzzo, MD
Michael G. Beaulieu, MD	Jerry L. Ferrell, MD
Thomas M. Bellinger, MD	James H. Frye, MD
Wendy S. Biggs, MD	Sharron P. Grannis, MD
Andrew P. Bone, MD	Kelly J. Hill, MD
Kirk J. Bortel, MD	Frederick R. Holland, MD
David B. Bosscher, DO	Caroline K. Hosapple, MD
William R. Brooks, Jr., MD	J. Christopher Hough, MD
Pauline Po Chiu, MD	Charles C. Johnson, DO
Sheree Clark, MD	David W. Jordahl, MD
J.D. Cline, MD	Paula J. Klose, MD
William H. Dery, MD	Timothy J. Kosinski, MD
David M. Easton, DO	Robert J. Lachance, MD
Jeffrey C. Eschbach, MD	Carl W. Lovell, MD

Kenneth M. MacKinnon, MD	Stephen D. Redman, MD
Elizabeth S. Neal, MD	Terry S. Ruhl, MD
Christopher J. Noah, MD	Marciso D. Santiago, MD
Lisa L. Olson, MD	Gary S. Smith, MD
Mark S. Ostahowski, MD	Craig R. Sonke, MD
Rebecca C. Phillips, MD	M. David Sutton, MD
Tammy S. Phillips, MD	David W. Torkelson, MD
Jack T. Pinney, MD	Dawn R. West, DO
Jamie A. Poliskey, MD	A. Frederic Youn, MD
Gary A. Posner, MD	Thomas J. Zuber, MD

John L. Pfenninger, MD

To our friends, families and colleagues who continue to be supportive and cover for us either when we are not completely present or when we are outright absent.

To Grandmother Nona Mae Fowler Betts, who raised four children with little money, few doctors, lots of prayers, and a bedside medicine textbook, *Domestic Medical Practice,* published in 1927. To Grandmother Harriet Wilson Fowler, who provided spiritual guidance. To Grandfathers Marion King Betts and Joseph P. Fowler, Jr., who brought their families to Texas.

To my father, Joseph P. (Jack) Fowler III, for his vision and willingness to try something new and for being the role model for a generalist in all aspects of life. He taught me how to do it yourself, think outside the box, try something new, and be good at more than one thing. To my mother, Frances Betts Fowler, for her spiritual guidance, which often keeps things on track, her persistence, her willingness to sacrifice, and her unwillingness to accept anything less than the best.

To Mathew Pfenninger, a miracle of modern science and spirituality who proved many doctors wrong, overcame his cancer, never gave up, and serves as a role model for us in many areas beyond illness.

To primary care clinicians everywhere who continue to provide patient education along with the procedures they perform. Also, to primary care clinicians willing to learn new procedures or to continue to improve their skills with established procedures to provide better care for their patients. This book is dedicated to you!

Grant C. Fowler, MD

Foreword

As a comprehensive guide to performing medical and surgical procedures in the office, hospital, or emergency department, *Pfenninger and Fowler's Procedures for Primary Care* might be considered an antidote to the evils that originated from Pandora's box. According to Greek mythology, Pandora (whose name means "rich in gifts") found a buried box and impulsively removed its lid. Out of the box, scattering in every direction, came disease, death, and all the other evils that afflict humankind. Like Eve in the Christian scriptures, Pandora introduced mortality into our world. However, her box also contained an antidote—hope—and she closed the lid just in time to prevent this quality from escaping.

In combating the myriad diseases that Pandora supposedly unleashed, primary care clinicians have long been powerful agents for hope and healing. Because of advances in treatment options, including minimally invasive outpatient surgical techniques, many procedures that previously would have necessitated hospitalization or consultation now can be performed by primary care clinicians in the office, hospital, or emergency room. This arrangement allows continuity of care, hopefully provides excellent patient education, and, by moving some procedures out of the hospital, may offer significant economic advantages. However, as their role expands, these clinicians must continue to use sound judgment and keep the patient's welfare uppermost. They should avoid procedures beyond their expertise, they should avoid procedures that might necessitate repetition, and they should avoid procedures that might cause them medicolegal problems.

Like Pandora, *Pfenninger and Fowler's Procedures for Primary Care* is rich in gifts, but these are of the life-affirming kind. More than 200 chapters provide up-to-date information for a continually evolving specialty. The book includes practical, step-by-step instructions for performing an extensive array of medical and surgical procedures, as illustrated by line drawings and clear photographs. It also covers indications and contraindications, equipment and suppliers, complications, billing codes, and other practical topics. In the literature for primary care clinicians, few other books cover such a wide range of topics. Indeed, I know of no other volume that is likely to be more useful to its intended audience.

Some readers may wonder why this foreword is being written by a cardiovascular surgeon and not by a primary care clinician. Perhaps they will allow heart disease to serve as an example for many other diseases. Primary care clinicians are at the leading edge of the battle against many diseases—not only in treatment but also in prevention. In heart disease, their advice is often the deciding factor in convincing patients to make positive changes with respect to fat intake, physical activity, cigarette smoking, and other lifestyle factors. An example from the recent literature supports this premise: in a study involving patients with coronary artery disease at Creighton University, recommendations from primary care clinicians concerning the assessment of lipid profiles and use of statin therapy significantly reduced the number of adverse cardiovascular outcomes. As the average age of the population continues to increase and congestive heart failure becomes increasingly prevalent, primary care clinicians can be expected to play an even greater role in diagnosing and treating this disorder. If primary care clinicians can do this with heart disease, it is my hope that they can use their abilities in many other areas of medicine.

The book also contains patient education handouts. When primary care clinicians perform a procedure, they must know the disease well. In so doing, they also have a golden opportunity to teach some prevention principles. I hope that they will never miss the opportunity to treat the whole patient and potentially change the course of the disease by educating the patient before, during, and after performing the procedure.

In conclusion, I congratulate Drs. Pfenninger and Fowler on producing such an excellent volume. It should help improve the quality of care in many aspects of medical practice, and I highly recommend it for every primary care clinician and trainee. There are some who consider me a pioneer in heart disease; I hope that this book encourages medical pioneers everywhere to prevent and treat early the diseases that Pandora supposedly released.

Denton A. Cooley, MD
Surgeon-in-Chief
Texas Heart Institute;
Clinical Professor of Surgery
University of Texas Medical School
Houston, Texas

Foreword to the First Edition

In 1930, more than 80% of the physicians in the United States were general family doctors, providing comprehensive health care at a reasonable cost. By 1980, the self-reported percentage of family doctors in the United States was 15%. Along with this trend of dwindling numbers has been a gradual decline of diagnostic and therapeutic skills held by those physicians who do practice general family medicine.

One definition of a generalist physician (formerly a general practitioner) is a family physician who can provide a breadth and continuity of commonly needed health care services. These physicians care for children, deliver babies, manage simple fractures, counsel single parents, go to the hospital, maintain an office, and, when all else fails, comfort the dying. Their goal is to provide health care from the nursery to the nursing home, without taking the patient to the poor house along the way

Today, of the 625,000 physicians in the United States, fewer than 10% comprehensively wield the clinical skills needed to provide such care. The headlong rush to subspecialize in medicine has left family physicians in the minority. Still, they are an important minority whose number is now growing in response to the projected needs of the twenty-first century American health care system.

Since 1983, a group of family physicians, supported by the American Academy of Family Physicians (AAFP), has constructed a series of demonstration projects to propagate diagnostic and therapeutic skills in family medicine. Many of the procedural pioneers in family practice have quietly and unselfishly contributed their professional energies to the resuscitation of full-service family practice within a medical education system gone far, far astray. This book stands as a contribution to that effort. Although some may view the teaching and learning of clinical skills as "proceduralism," the skills that are depicted in this book represent the desire of physicians to remain clinically excellent. No amount of psychosocial expertise can overcome the credibility lost when a physician cannot perform basic clinical services on behalf of his or her patient.

Recently a prominent dean of a well-known medical school asked me why the residency programs at my institution, the University of Tennessee, persisted in reaching a comprehensive set of procedural clinical skills when, in his opinion, managed care organizations and health maintenance organizations would effectively amputate these skills from the day-to-day practice of family physicians. I disagree with this vision of the future, but it is true that some family physicians voluntarily relinquish many of the clinical skills described in this book. It is my hope that the skills described in its pages will become required curriculum, nor only for residents, but, particularly, for faculty. One of the major challenges for the success of this book (and the specialty of family practice) is the development of accountability in a health care system that has become overly fragmented, costly, and inaccessible.

Are these skills needed? During the past 20 years, family physicians have been manipulated, exploited, and oppressed in a variety of ways that makes study of their actual needs very complex. For example, a lack of reported interest in obstetrical care cannot be used to justify the tremendous void that exists in women's health care as provided by family physicians. Residents are not likely to acquire clinical skills that family physician faculty members cannot themselves demonstrate in their positions as role models. A lack of procedural skill among family practice faculty and practitioners is particularly troubling in rural and underserved communities. These communities cannot afford platoons of various subspecialized physicians.

Although excellent health care is available from a combination of obstetricians, pediatricians, and internists, a well-trained, comprehensive-care family physician should be able to deliver continuing health care unrestricted by age, sex, organ system, and pregnancy. The physician should be skilled in many of the procedures described here to screen for, prevent, and treat common disease entities. If family practice simply becomes synonymous with "generic primary care," there will be very little need for many of the skills described in this book. My compliments to the editors and the authors for executing a labor of love in an outstanding fashion. They have chosen the road less traveled.

Wm. MacMillian Rodney, MD, FAAFP, FACEP
Meharry/Vanderbilt Professor and Chair
Department of Family and Community Medicine
Professor Surgery/Emergency Medicine
Meharry Medical College
Nashville, Tennessee

Preface

Six years after signing of the authors' contract, this second edition of *Pfenninger and Fowler's Procedures for Primary Care* is finally coming to fruition. The title has been changed slightly, the content has increased 30%, there are improved illustrations and more comprehensive patient education handouts, and billing information has been added. We are trying to live up to the *JAMA* review of our first edition, that "this is the most comprehensive source of information on primary care procedures available anywhere!"

Feedback on the first edition has been rewarding and interesting. One Navy physician described performing a procedure on a ship. He had our book open and would frequently refer to it. The patient asked if he (the doctor) had ever done the procedure before and the physician replied, "Only once or twice, but this is a great book. However, if you want to wait for 2 months until we get back to port, someone else can do it then!" Others wrote telling of the excitement they experienced after completing a procedure and being able to diagnose a melanoma in an early curable stage, or doing a fine needle biopsy of the breast to diagnose a cancer while it was still localized.

Countless students and residents have told us how this book aided their education. Some have said it helped them realize that the choice of primary care as a specialty offers much more than just taking care of sore throats and earaches. Faculty members have commented on how much time the book saved them when teaching procedures and writing curriculum.

When primary care clinicians perform procedures, it truly does enhance the overall care and practice of medicine. If someone comes to the office with an unusual lesion on the arm that is growing rapidly, the knee jerk response is to refer him or her to a dermatologist. Perhaps the patient is seen 4 to 6 weeks later and a letter finally returns a few weeks after that, stating "it was a keratoacanthoma and we took care of it." By that time, the primary care clinician has forgotten what the lesion even looked like. A few months later a patient with a similar lesion comes in and the cycle repeats itself. The clinician rarely gains the clinical acumen to make the diagnosis, and the patient loses the benefit of continuity of care. However, if the diagnosis is unknown and the clinician immediately performs a biopsy, the patient benefits from management by someone familiar with the whole person, not just his or her problem, and the feedback from histology becomes a timely educational experience. There is an additional benefit: On the second observation of a similar lesion, the clinician may wonder if it too is a keratoacanthoma, which the biopsy subsequently confirms. By the third time, the clinician becomes comfortable and basically says, "Oh, just another keratoacanthoma!" Being a part of the diagnostic process is different from just sending the patient off for a consultation.

Similarly, by performing a fiberoptic examination of the upper GI tract, the clinician can see the pathology firsthand and differentiate the histories that are associated with reflux, gastritis, duodenal ulcers, etc. At my (JLP) courses I often ask the attendees to describe the smell of a rose so that someone else who cannot smell knows what it is like. It's impossible. And it is sometimes impossible to really know a disease without examining it from all angles, close up. Doing procedures allows you to smell, feel, and see the disease in a different perspective.[1]

As we write this preface, we note that most of the Foreword and the Preface from the first edition still apply, so we have included them in this edition. Since the first edition, certain pressures have persisted in our society. Healthcare costs continue to spiral out of control, patients continue to have fast-paced lifestyles with their time still at a premium, and they continue to prefer one-stop shopping with their clinicians. Medicine seems to be in more of a crisis. HMOs, PPOs, Medicare cuts, litigation, and increased legislation all contribute to the hassle factor that takes the fun out of medicine. Financial survival in a practice is not guaranteed, as is seen by the number of clinicians who are filing for bankruptcy. The future does not always look bright. However, the data support the advisability of comprehensive care by the primary care clinician, which includes procedures. Rodney[2] has shown that even in the worst case scenario, with a 40% reimbursement of charges, procedures still pay off financially in a primary care office.

But, for most physicians, medicine is about more than financial return—it is about taking care of people. Dr. Rodney was reinforcing this when he said, "Most physicians do not enter medical practice with the sole purpose of maximizing revenue by any legal means available to them."[2] If money was their primary interest, there are other professions in which its accumulation can be accomplished more easily. If this book helps you to be the best proceduralist in the world, but you forget about the patient, we have failed. We are physicians and clinicians, not technicians; we have a noble calling and must remember how privileged we are to be able to care for patients.

Money matters are not totally irrelevant, though. We must be responsible stewards for patients', insurance providers', and society's funds. Doing procedures in the office reduces the cost of healthcare markedly—sometimes by 70% to 80%! Medicare and some insurance providers are finally recognizing this by reimbursing physicians more for doing procedures in the office (e.g., colonoscopy, EGD) rather than in the healthcare facilities. We must consider costs of healthcare in everything we do.

In the Preface and Foreword to the first edition, we presented our vision of the role procedures should play in primary care medicine. If you haven't had the chance, read them—or read them again; as Dr. Rodney noted in his Foreword to that first edition, we remain committed to the view that primary care physicians provide a breadth and continuity of healthcare services; the skill sets required to provide such a breadth of services must include cognitive, interpretive, and procedural skills. This second edition is another step on that journey we envisioned down "the road less traveled." We are encouraged and heartened that primary care clinicians are performing these procedures to maximize the healthcare of their patients. We prefer to teach what can be done, not what can't be. We want physicians and practitioners of all sorts to enjoy the practice of medicine. We want patients to be happy and to enjoy a high quality of life as long as possible.

These dreams have supported and enabled the past 6 years of labor on this second edition. As planning for the third edition begins, we need your feedback. Help us help you to help your patients.

John L. Pfenninger, MD
Grant C. Fowler, MD

REFERENCES

1. Pfenninger JL, Colposcopy, LEEP, and other procedures: the role for family physicians, *Fam Med* 28:505, 1996.
2. Rodney WM, Impact of the limited generalist (no hospital, no procedures) model on the viability of family practice training, *J Am Board Fam Pract* 15:191, 2002.

Preface to the First Edition

The inspiration for this text came from busy primary care physicians across the country. Medicine in the 1990s is changing rapidly. The high cost of hospital care, emergency room visits, and even the expenses of freestanding day surgery centers have created a forceful impetus for physicians to perform previous hospital-based procedures and surgeries in the office. Fast-paced lifestyles have added performance pressure: the patient's time is at a premium. No longer will they accept referrals for simple procedures or the subsequent inconvenience. Patients expect their physician to perform most routine procedures. In certain areas of the country, competition for patients has increased, resulting in the need for physicians to master certain procedural skills to enhance their status and desirability. Overwhelmed with paperwork and other responsibilities, primary care physicians have little time to spend preparing for or performing a procedure (much less orienting their staff), and yet some procedures in the office are becoming more complex. Thus, among other things, physicians are pressured from patients, health care plans, greater competition, paperwork, and their own staff. It was at the urge and cry of these pressured physicians for a concise and yet all-encompassing reference for procedures that this book was created.

Coupled with these pressures, there has been a parallel explosion in new technology. There has also been a clarification and refinement in techniques and indications for older technology. Safer medications and monitoring units are also available to facilitate performing procedures in the office. However, few primary care physicians have the time to stay up-to-date with the changes in technology. New technology or new applications of old technology allow definitive care for conditions in a simpler fashion with less risk and expense than ever before. Radio-frequency loop cervical conization, which is now done in the office setting, has or will soon replace the majority of in-hospital cervical conizations. This procedure may cost as little as 20% of in-hospital costs. Fiberoptic diagnoses allow for a more comprehensive evaluation and earlier diagnosis of cancer. More importantly, these diagnoses can now be made by the same physician who cares for the patient most of the time.

These technological advances save lives, add to the quality of life, are cost effective, and decrease liability.

Interestingly, there is a wide variety of procedures currently being performed by primary care physicians. However, there is a large individual and geographic variation. These variations will no doubt diminish with the advent of managed care. It is well known that it is very cost effective to keep procedures in the hands of primary care physicians, yet there is no comprehensive text detailing the performance of these procedures. With our first attempt, this text is not yet perfect. We relied on authors from all over the country and more than 80 authors contributed.

There is a wide range of style and practicality. The intent of the text is to give direction and to serve as a resource and brief review for a particular procedure—not to be all-inclusive in a single text.

The chapters in this book in no way intend to make the reader an expert at any procedure. It is a rare procedure that can be safely "learned from the book." The majority of procedures will be mastered by attending courses and then followed by a preceptor arrangement. The text merely combines and lists those procedures that primary care physicians perform, sometimes on a daily basis. The text may serve as a review for physicians and staff on those procedures that are not performed on a day-to-day basis.

Procedures for Primary Care Physicians is not a static document. It will grow and change with time. The chapters will be refined and the contents revised to be more concise and direct. This can only happen through feedback from the readers. Suggestions from you, the reader, would be most appreciated. Submissions of new or even alternatives to current chapters are most welcome.

As the title states, this text is directed to primary care physicians—family and general practitioners, emergency physicians, pediatricians, obstetricians, internists, house officers, medical students, military medics, paramedics, nurse practitioners, and all other "primary care providers." It is hoped that the contents will enhance the performance of procedures, improve patient care and satisfaction, and lead to greater physician self-fulfillment.

John L. Pfenninger, MD
Grant C. Fowler, MD

Acknowledgments

The editors would like to give special acknowledgment to Timothy J. Downs, MD. Tim is a family physician who was very helpful and supportive in the initial editing of this text. We, the editors, want to express our special gratitude to him. Thanks, Tim.

Pat Wolfgram, the medical librarian at MidMichigan Medical Center, has been invaluable in finding various articles, references, and illustrations to help us complete this text. Pat is special and helped make the task of editing much easier.

My wife, Kay, filled in wherever she was needed. When slides had to be duplicated or created, when help was needed with grammatical phrases, when we were short on typing—whatever—she was willing to pitch in. She too lost weekends, vacation days, and holidays while the book was worked on—and there was never a complaint.

And lastly, Linda Hallmann, my office manager, typed, mailed, corresponded, found, and did whatever was necessary to complete the book.

A special thanks goes out to each and every one of these people.

John L. Pfenninger, MD

I would also like to acknowledge Glenda Thurman, in the Department of Family Practice and Community Medicine at UT Houston Medical School, for her tireless corresponding, mailing, and copying whenever it was needed.

Special thanks are due to the staff, residents, and faculty of the Department of Family Practice and Community Medicine at UT Houston Medical School for not only writing many of the chapters, but also being very supportive throughout this lengthy project.

Special acknowledgments are due to Pamela Promecene, MD, and Pamela Berens, MD, faculty in the Department of Obstetrics, Gynecology, and Reproductive Medicine at UT Houston Medical School, for answering endless questions about the latest approach to many women's health topics.

Grant C. Fowler, MD

Acknowledgments to the First Edition

The number of people to be thanked in a text of this magnitude is too great to allow mention of them all. Each, in his or her own way, has added greatly to its value. The special people who provided their support and encouragement include: Grant Fowler, MD, for giving large blocks of his time and expertise—without his assistance, the text would be nowhere near completion; Len Scarpinato, DO, for his editorial assistance; Barbara Apgar, MD, for the moral support needed when the "going got rough"; Don DeWitt, MD, for encouraging the vision; Pat Wolfgram, the hospital librarian, for retrieving the voluminous number of reference articles; Joan Haddix, Joi Henton, and Shirley Marsh, for their typing assistance; and Beth Moe, Denise Willard, and Linda Hallman for their secretarial skills. To Ted Huff, I give my sincere thanks for developing educational diagrams out of what were sometimes mere scratchings of the pen. A sincere thanks goes to Cindy Trickel of Carlisle Publishers Services, who provided invaluable editorial guidance in converting thoughts into words.

A special thanks also goes to all the family physicians in Midland, Michigan. They not only provided after-hours coverage for me, but also provided the encouragement to continue on through many personal crises. My office staff and nurses also deserve my gratitude.

Each and every author of this book also deserves special recognition. There were many refusals to assist in this project because of over-commitment and lack of belief in the project. For those authors who did contribute, it meant extra sacrifice and dedication. They participated in a dream that has now come to fruition.

To all of these, a sincere thank-you.

John L. Pfenninger, MD

A special thanks to the residents, faculty, and staff of the Hermann/LBJ Family Practice Program and the Department of Family Practice and Community Medicine at the University of Texas Houston Health Science Center—Medical School for their contributions, patience, and encouragement—without which this book might not have happened.

Grant C. Fowler, MD

Table of Contents

PART ONE

Anesthesia

CHAPTER 1

Bier Block

Robert Williams

Intravenous (IV) regional anesthesia, also known as a *Bier block,* is a useful method of providing operative anesthesia to wide areas of the distal portion of an extremity. When executed with proper technique, the Bier block is a safe alternative to local or hematoma infiltration, and it provides anesthesia superior to these other methods. At the same time, it has the advantage of being technically simpler to perform than other regional alternatives (e.g., axillary or brachial plexus infiltration).

INDICATIONS

Although the technique of IV regional anesthesia has been used on the lower extremity, it is most often used in applications involving the upper extremity. Some experts suggest that one not consider a block of the lower extremity until sufficient experience with upper-extremity blocks is obtained. Any condition of the distal extremity requiring more than just local anesthesia would be an indication for a Bier block. Examples include reductions of fractures or dislocations, repair of extensive lacerations, drainage of large abscesses, and tendon repair.

CONTRAINDICATIONS

Documented sensitivity to local anesthetics is an absolute contraindication (see Chapter 4, Local Anesthesia, and Chapter 5, Local and Topical Anesthetic Complications). Relative contraindications include the following:
- Injuries to the proximal extremity that would be adversely affected by application of a tourniquet (e.g., crush injury)
- Conditions predisposing to arterial thrombosis
- Difficulty in maintaining arterial occlusion with a tourniquet (e.g., inadequate cuff size in a massively obese patient)

EQUIPMENT

- Double-cuff automatic pneumatic tourniquet that can individually or simultaneously inflate or deflate both cuffs to preset pressures. (As an alternative, ordinary blood pressure cuffs can be used if the dimensions of the arm can accommodate two appropriately sized cuffs between the axilla and the elbow without overlap.)
- Lidocaine (without epinephrine), 1 ml/kg of the 0.5% solution for upper-extremity blocks, 2 ml/kg of the 0.25% solution for lower-extremity blocks
- Intravenous needle-cannula
- Sterile skin preparation solution (povidone-iodine)
- Tape
- Elastic bandage of sufficient size to wrap the entire extremity distal to the tourniquet

Although the risk of serious adverse reaction is very small when the procedure is followed correctly, it should be conducted only in facilities capable of managing serious local anesthetic toxicities. (See the "Complications" section.)

PREPROCEDURE
PATIENT PREPARATION

Advise the patient that 95% of patients experience good or complete anesthesia with a Bier block; the remainder require additional analgesics or sedatives. Explain the potential for complications to the patient. Anesthesia will resolve within 30 minutes of tourniquet release.

TECHNIQUE

1. Measure the patient's blood pressure.
2. Test the pneumatic tourniquet or blood pressure cuffs for accuracy and maintenance of pressure, and

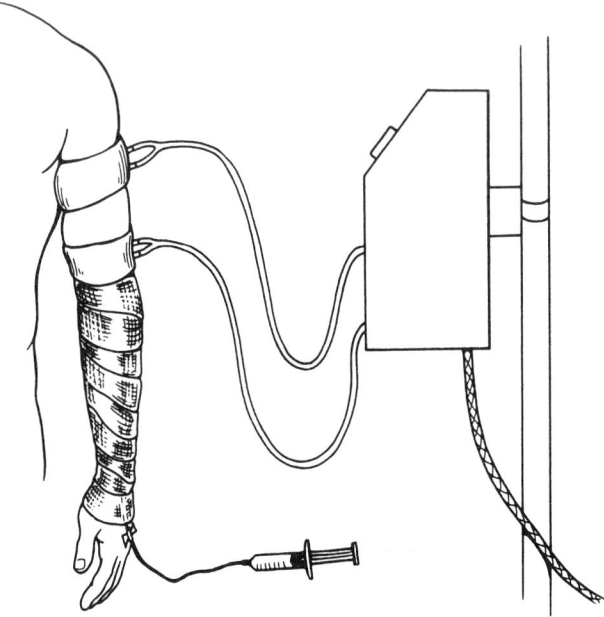

Fig. 1-1
Bier block procedure, before removal of elastic bandage and injection of lidocaine, showing inflation of proximal cuff.

then place them on the proximal portion of the extremity.

3. After skin prep, place the IV needle-cannula in a vein in the distal portion of the extremity, preferably distal to the operative site. Attach the syringe with lidocaine and tape in place.

4. Have an assistant elevate the extremity above the heart while you wrap the elastic bandage around it, wrapping from distal to proximal (from fingers or toes up to the distal cuff).

5. Rapidly inflate the proximal cuff to 50 mm Hg above the systolic blood pressure for upper-extremity blocks and twice the systolic blood pressure for lower-extremity blocks. Assign an assistant to be responsible for continuously monitoring the maintenance of cuff pressures throughout the remainder of the procedure (Fig. 1-1).

6. Lower the extremity, remove the elastic bandage, and check the distal pulses. If no pulse is palpable, inject the appropriate dose of lidocaine. The IV may be removed.

7. After approximately 10 to 15 minutes, check the adequacy of anesthesia by gently manipulating the operative site. Additional time may be required to achieve full effect, although if after 20 to 30 minutes the anesthesia still is inadequate, supplementary analgesia or sedation is advised.

8. After the initial 10 to 15 minutes, inflate the distal cuff to the same pressure as the proximal cuff, and then deflate the proximal cuff. This use of two cuffs reduces the pain associated with the occlusive tourniquet by allowing infusion of anesthetic under the proximal cuff before it is inflated.

9. When anesthesia is deemed adequate, the operation may proceed up to a maximum inflation time of 2 hours. Periodically monitor the blood pressure on the contralateral side to ensure proper tourniquet pressure. The tourniquet may remain inflated during the process of taking intraoperative x-ray films.

10. At completion of the procedure, but no sooner than 20 minutes after lidocaine injection (to permit diffusion of some of the lidocaine out of the vascular system), deflate and remove the cuffs. Some physicians recommend cycles of deflation and inflation, but this has no advantage in lowering systemic plasma lidocaine levels.

11. Observe the patient for 10 to 15 minutes for signs of toxicity.

COMPLICATIONS

Minor adverse reactions to the lidocaine (dizziness, tinnitus, bradycardia, etc.) occur in less than 2% of patients after cuff deflation. Serious reactions (including seizures, cardiovascular collapse, and death) occur almost exclusively when the lidocaine is injected with the cuffs deflated—because of operator error or equipment malfunction—and are rare.

SUPPLIERS

Double-cuff pneumatic tourniquet

Zimmer, Inc.
727 North Detroit Street
Warsaw, IN 46580
Phone: 1-800-613-6131
Website: www.zimmer.com

VBM Medical, Inc.
15013 Herriman Boulevard
Noblesville, IN 46060
Phone: 1-800-580-7117
Website: www.vbm-medical.de/set2.html

Thomas Medical, Inc.
4100-C Nine McFarland Drive
Alpharetta, GA 30004
Phone: 1-800-556-0349
Website: www.thomasmedical.com/vbmproducts2.htm

CPT/BILLING CODE

01995   Regional IV administration of local anesthetic agent (upper or lower extremity)

BIBLIOGRAPHY

Blasier RD, White R: Intravenous regional anesthesia for management of children's extremity fractures in the emergency department, *Pediatr Emerg Care* 12(6):404, 1996.

Bolte RG, Stevens PM, Scott SM, Schunk JE: Mini-dose Bier block intravenous regional anesthesia in the emergency department treatment of upper-extremity injuries, *J Pediatr Orthop* 14(4):534, 1994.

Brown EM, McGriff JT, Malinowski RW: Intravenous regional anesthesia (Bier block): review of 20 years' experience, *Can J Anaesth* 36(3):307, 1989.

Farrell RG, Swanson SL, Walter JR: Safe and effective IV regional anesthesia for use in the emergency department, *Ann Emerg Med* 14(4):288, 1985.

Lowen R, Taylor J: Bier's block—the experience of Australian emergency departments, *Med J Aust* 160(3):108, 1994.

Salo M, Kanto J, Jalonen J, Laurikainen E: Plasma lidocaine concentrations after different methods of releasing the tourniquet during intravenous regional anaesthesia, *Ann Clin Res* 11:164, 1979.

CHAPTER 2

Conscious Sedation (Sedation and Analgesia)

Thomas H. Corbett

Conscious sedation, also called "sedation and analgesia," is a useful technique to alleviate or reduce pain and anxiety during medical, surgical, diagnostic, or therapeutic procedures. It is achieved by the IV administration of sedative, amnesic, and analgesic drugs, singly or in combination. The goal of conscious sedation is to produce a patient who is conscious but relaxed, and comfortable yet cooperative.

Conscious sedation is intended to achieve minimal depression of consciousness and to allow the patient to retain complete control of reflexes and vital functions, particularly with regard to respiration. Patients should also remain able to respond appropriately to verbal commands. Inadequate sedation or analgesia may lead to unacceptable patient discomfort or injury because of excessive movement, lack of cooperation, or adverse response to stress. Deeper levels of sedation also incur considerable risk, including loss of the airway with resultant hypoxia and the potential for cardiac arrest. When required, only qualified anesthesia personnel should perform purposeful deep sedation or general anesthesia.

Nonanesthesiologist physicians who perform conscious sedation must have adequate personnel and necessary equipment available during the procedure. They must also be knowledgeable in proper patient selection, monitoring procedures, drug administration, and postsedation care. Deficiency in any of these requirements can lead to serious complications and death. Guidelines for the administration of safe conscious sedation are available from the American Society of Anesthesiologists (ASA). Before using conscious sedation, the nonanesthesiologist physician must become familiar with practice guidelines. All applicable codes and regulations, guidelines, clinical practice protocols, and official recommendations should be followed, including ongoing quality assessment and improvement.

INDICATIONS

Conscious sedation is frequently used to supplement local anesthesia for certain painful diagnostic or therapeutic procedures. Other procedures may require only conscious sedation. Procedures for which conscious sedation can be useful include the following:
- Biopsy procedures
- Bone marrow aspiration or biopsy
- Bronchoscopy
- Cardioversion
- Cervical dilation
- Dental procedures
- Dressing changes
- Endometrial biopsy
- GI endoscopy
- Hysterosalpingogram
- Lumbar puncture
- MRI or CT scan
- Orthopedic procedures (certain fracture reductions, joint dislocation reductions)
- Plastic surgery procedures
- Phlebectomy procedures

CONTRAINDICATIONS

- Severe systemic disease (ASA Class 3 or higher)
- Nonfasting patient
- Pregnancy for elective procedures
- Patients with difficult-to-manage airway

Careful patient selection is critical to performing safe conscious sedation. A thorough history and physical examination should be performed preoperatively. The ASA has developed a preoperative risk classification system for patients undergoing anesthesia. This system is ideal for selecting patients for conscious sedation in an office setting. The ASA system is based on physical status and is divided into five risk categories:

Class 1: Healthy patient

Class 2: Mild systemic disease

Class 3: Severe systemic disease

Class 4: Severe systemic disease that is a constant threat to life

Class 5: Moribund, not expected to live 24 hours respective of operation

Class 2 patients include those with well-controlled hypertension, controlled noninsulin-dependent diabetes, and minimal cardiac or respiratory disease. Class 3 patients include those with insulin-dependent diabetes mellitus, poorly controlled hypertension, significant cardiac or respiratory disease, and significant renal or hepatic disease. Based on individual experience and skill in administering conscious sedation, practitioners may decide to limit the amount of patient risk they are willing to accept, using the ASA guidelines. Preprocedure consultation with an anesthesiologist is recommended for high-risk patients.

To avoid the possibility of vomiting with aspiration, patients should fast before receiving conscious sedation. A preoperative pregnancy test should be considered on reproductive-age female patients. Elective procedures for pregnant patients might best be deferred until after delivery. Patients with difficult airway access are not suitable candidates for the office setting.

EQUIPMENT

- A single unit with BP and ECG measurements, variable-pitch beep pulse oximeter, and automatic recording device is the ideal monitor for conscious sedation. Individual units are acceptable but require repeated manual recording of the readings on the patient's chart.
- IV solution, tubing and stand
- Medications for sedation
- Reversal medications
- Suction apparatus
- Crash cart or Banyan kit with equipment and medications for basic and advanced cardiac life support (ACLS)
- Defibrillator
- Oxygen source

Basic monitoring equipment includes a pulse oximeter for oxygen saturation in arterial blood (Sao_2) and pulse rate, and a BP monitor. ECG monitoring is optional but recommended for Class 1 patients. It is required for older patients and those with a history of cardiac disease. Optional monitoring equipment includes temperature and end-tidal CO_2 monitors.

An oxygen source and delivery system is essential and should be considered on every patient undergoing conscious sedation. Suction must always be immediately available, as must all necessary equipment for basic life support and ACLS, including a defibrillator and "crash cart" or Banyan kit.

Airway management equipment, including laryngoscopes, endotracheal tubes, oral-nasal airways, and bag-valve masks must be immediately available.

PERSONNEL

Conscious sedation requires two specially trained, experienced, and competent providers with appropriate credentials, privileges, and necessary authorization to perform the assigned functions. The ordering physician performs the medical procedure and dispenses the medication or prescribes the medications to be administered. The professional clinical assistant (usually a registered nurse with special training and experience in conscious sedation) is responsible for medicating and monitoring the patient. Both providers require training in the relevant pharmacology, monitoring, and airway management. At least one of the two providers present must remain with the patient from the beginning of sedation until recovery is complete. One provider must be capable of emergency management, including establishing an open airway, use of oral and nasopharyngeal airways, bag-valve-mask ventilation, and basic life support. At least one clinician capable of definitive airway management (endotracheal intubation) and ACLS must be immediately available in the facility.

Adequate back-up support must be obtainable through a well-marked call system to assist in cases of unexpected developments such as malignant hyperthermia, seizures, myocardial ischemia, severe allergic reaction, respiratory arrest, or cardiac arrest. A plan for rapid transfer to a full-service medical facility should be in effect.

The clinician should consult the conscious sedation guidelines applicable to the office, clinic, hospital, and state as well as Joint Commission on Accreditation of Healthcare Organizations' mandates for precise requirements for training, credentials, privileges, and authority.

PREPROCEDURE PATIENT ASSESSMENT

- Perform and document a careful history and physical examination and obtain appropriate laboratory results. Then classify the patient according to the ASA Physical Classification Guidelines. Accept for office-based conscious sedation only ASA Class 1 and 2 patients.

- Discuss plans and alternatives as well as risks with the patient or guardian and obtain documented informed consent.

PREPROCEDURE PATIENT PREPARATION

- If the initial assessment was performed at an earlier date, confirm the healthy status of the patient.
- Confirm that gastrointestinal disease–free patients have fasted for at least 6 hours for solid foods and nonclear liquids, and at least 3 hours for clear liquids. Patients with a history of gastroesophageal reflux disease, esophageal motility disorder, or diabetes mellitus should fast for at least 8 hours and be pretreated with Zantac 150 mg PO (or equivalent) with sips of water 2 to 4 hours before the procedure and with Reglan 10 mg PO 30 to 60 minutes before the procedure to minimize the possibility of vomiting with aspiration.
- Confirm that the patient has arranged for an escort to drive home and that home care has been arranged.
- Have the patient void, if needed, before the procedure.
- Start and secure IV fluid line, and ensure it is functioning properly.
- Check availability of both routine and emergency equipment, medications, and personnel.
- Confirm patient allergies and drug sensitivities.
- Apply monitors to the patient. Obtain and document baseline vital sign measurements of BP, pulse rate, Sao_2, respiratory rate, and ECG (if indicated). Begin supplemental oxygen and note any increase in Sao_2.
- Instruct the patient to relate any symptoms he or she may experience during the procedure, including pain,

anxiety, discomfort, nausea, shortness of breath or other breathing difficulty, itching, muscle symptoms, or other urgent symptomatology.
- Prepare a documentation sheet or form to document time, monitoring used, medications and dosages administered during the procedure, and any significant changes in the patient's condition. If there were no changes or problems, document it.

TECHNIQUE

These guidelines apply to healthy adult patients. For pediatric, geriatric, and other special cases, appropriate adjustments must be made. Recommendations for drugs and healthy adult dosages are listed in Table 2-1. Practitioners of conscious sedation must be thoroughly familiar with drug profiles, warnings, and manufacturers' prescribing directions before beginning the procedure.

1. Position the patient as comfortably as possible for the procedure, using warm blankets and placing pillows under the head and/or knees.
2. For painful procedures, begin IV administration with an initial dose of a rapid-onset, short-acting narcotic followed by a small bolus of IV fluid to ensure the medication enters the circulation. Maintain verbal contact with the patient. Observe the patient for slurred speech, droopy eyelids, and calm affect. The patient should stir to verbal commands and be able to follow them. Remember that the effects should start within several minutes but may not peak for up to 7 minutes.
3. If the patient is not sedated adequately after a modest dose of narcotic, administer a small dose of a short-acting benzodiazepine and continue to ob-

TABLE 2-1

Commonly Used Medications for Sedation and Analgesia in Healthy Adults

Medication	Class	Description	Initial IV Dose	Repeat Dose	Minimum Interval
Midazolam (Versed)	Benzodiazepine	Short acting sedation/amnesia	1-2 mg	0.5-1 mg to 5 mg max* with narcotics	5 min
Diazepam (Valium)	Benzodiazepine	Long acting sedation	5.0 mg	2.5-5.0 mg	5 min
Sublimaze (Fentanyl)	Opiate	Short acting	50-100 mg	25-50 mg	5 min
Meperidine (Demerol)	Opiate	Medium acting	25-50 mg	25 mg	5 min
Flumazenil (Romazicon)	Benzodiazepine antagonist	Reversal agent for benzodiazepine	0.2 mg	0.2 mg up to 1.0 mg	1 min
Naloxone (Narcan)	Opiate antagonist	Reversal agent for opiates	0.2-0.4 mg	0.2 mg	2-3 min
Propofol	Sedative/Hypnotic	Rapid onset	0.4-0.5 mg/kg	10-20 mg	Prn repeat

Lower doses of benzodiazepines and opiates are generally used in older patients. Patients with psychiatric disorders (e.g., schizophrenia) or who drink alcohol on a daily basis may require greater than the maximal recommended doses. *For pediatric doses, consult product literature.*
*Other authorities recommend 7.5 mg maximum dose of midazolam.

serve for effects. Recall the synergistic effects of these drugs.

- Once the patient is adequately sedated, begin the procedure. For longer procedures, additional increments of medications will probably be necessary as the procedure progresses.
- Continually observe the effects as additional increment doses of narcotic or benzodiazepine are administered. Ensure that the IV fluid flow rate is adequate to add the incremental doses to the circulation.

4. From the beginning of sedation, the patient monitors must continuously be observed audibly and visually, and the patient must be monitored continually for head position, level of consciousness, airway patency, and adequacy of respiration and oxygenation. Observation of ventilation is essential, especially when using supplemental oxygen, which will delay the detection of apnea by pulse oximetry.

5. Heart rate, oxygen saturation, BP, and respiratory rate should be recorded initially and every 2 to 5 minutes during the procedure. Recording strips from a single unit monitor with BP, EKG, and pulse oximeter readings are efficient for this purpose. Along with the monitoring data, drug dosages with times administered should be documented on the permanent record for the patient's chart.

6. For painful procedures, narcotic administration should be emphasized. For painless but anxiety-producing procedures, there should be more emphasis on benzodiazepine administration.

7. At all times, consider the potential side effects and overdose effects, as well as their synergistic effects, of all medications administered.

8. An appropriate level of analgesia and sedation should be in effect before initiating the procedure. Be sure to inform the patient of what is happening and why as you proceed.

9. The monitoring assistant can be helpful in allaying anxiety and providing reassurance by maintaining verbal contact and handholding.

COMPLICATIONS

Common Complications of Conscious Sedation

- Excessive discomfort from inadequate sedation
- Respiratory compromise
- Nausea or vomiting
- Loss of consciousness
- Aspiration
- Bradycardia (may progress to asystole)
- Other arrhythmias

Less Common Complications of Conscious Sedation

- Paradoxical reaction to benzodiazepines, including hallucinations and agitation
- Myocardial infarction
- Malignant hyperthermia
- Allergic reactions

If at any time the monitoring assistant becomes aware of a significant change in the patient's status, the operating physician must be notified immediately and corrective action must be taken. Attending personnel must be qualified to handle all of the above complications, as well as any other emergent conditions resulting from the administration of conscious sedation or from the procedure being performed. Appropriate equipment and medications must also be immediately available.

Respiratory compromise is one of the most common complications of conscious sedation, and it may require assisted ventilation. The usual cause of respiratory compromise is medication overdose leading to hypoventilation, obstruction, atelectasis, aspiration, and/or cardiac malfunction.

It is important to observe the patient's respiratory efforts because hypoventilation can be masked by the use of supplemental oxygen. If the minute volume is decreased, $Paco_2$ will increase and respiratory acidosis will develop. It is therefore important to make sure adequate ventilation is maintained.

If the patient fails to respond to loud verbal commands to breathe deeply, and the Sao_2 continues to deteriorate, ventilation with an Ambu-bag connected to oxygen is required immediately. If assisted ventilation proves difficult, and if the patient is unconscious, attempt to insert an oral or a nasal airway and resume assisted ventilation. Endotracheal intubation may be necessary.

Reversal agents (Narcan [Naloxone] or equivalent and Romazicon [Flumazenil]) must be available for overdose treatment of narcotics and benzodiazepines respectively. These reversal agents should be used judiciously, since they occasionally produce unwanted side effects. Both reversal drugs have shorter half-lives than the drugs they are meant to reverse, and repeated doses may be necessary. Narcotic- or benzodiazepine-overdosed patients often require observation for several hours after use of reversal agents.

Nausea occurs occasionally during and after conscious sedation, especially when larger doses of narcotics are used. Antiemetic therapy (e.g., Zofran) should be administered intravenously.

Arrhythmias may arise during conscious sedation. Vasovagal stimulation may lead to bradycardia, which may progress to asystole. For most patients, bradycardia below 50 bpm must be treated promptly with atropine 0.4 to 0.8 mg (IV). Exceptions are athletes or other patients who normally maintain a slow pulse rate. In these patients, treatment should commence when a significant drop (20% or more) from the initial pulse rate is noted. Tachyarrhythmias and other rhythm disturbances may also occur, and appropriate drugs for treatment must be readily available. Patients with undiagnosed severe coronary artery disease may show ischemic changes. Skeletal muscle rigidity has been reported from use of narcotic agents. Its occurrence is rare to infrequent but may require the use of muscle relaxants and positive pressure ventilation.

Most complications can be avoided by maintaining a safe environment; careful patient selection; detailed preparation; and an attentive, vigilant staff with adequate training, continuous monitoring, and slow administration of drugs.

POSTPROCEDURE PATIENT EDUCATION

A provider specially trained and experienced in postsedation complications and recovery should closely observe patients during the recovery phase of conscious sedation. Continuous pulse-oximetry should be maintained after the procedure, and vital signs monitored every 5 minutes for the first half hour of recovery. Respiratory compromise or other complications can still occur during this phase, and patients may require verbal or tactile stimulation during the initial phases of recovery. A clinician trained in airway management must be present during the recovery phase and should be notified immediately if the patient's level of consciousness, vital signs, ventilation, or oxygen saturation falls outside criteria assigned for the specific patient. The patient will be ready for discharge when a set of criteria for recovery is met, including return to baseline for vital signs, respiration, oxygen saturation on room air, and gross level of consciousness. Swallowing, coughing, and gag reflexes should be intact. Patients should be able to stand, walk, void, and ingest fluids. Dressings and wounds should be checked. Nausea and vomiting should be controlled. Patients should be given explicit written discharge instructions, including 24-hour contacts for an emergency, before being discharged to the care of a responsible adult. Discharge instructions should include the following:

- Do not drive a car or operate hazardous equipment until the next day.
- Do not make important decisions or sign legal documents for 24 hours.
- Do not take medications unless your physician has prescribed them specifically for the next 24 hours.
- Avoid alcohol, sedatives, and other depressant drugs for 24 hours.
- Notify your health care provider of pain, severe nausea, difficulty breathing, difficulty voiding, bleeding, or other new symptoms.

CPT/BILLING CODES

99141   Sedation with or without analgesia (conscious sedation); IV, IM, or inhalation.
94761   Pulse oximetry, multiple determinations (time and measurement must be recorded for permanent record to be reimbursable)
36000   Introduction of needle or intracatheter, vein

SUPPLIERS

Vital signs monitors
Welch Allyn
4341 State Street Road
P.O. Box 220
Skaneatles Falls, NY 13153-4100
Phone: 1-800-535-6663
Website: www.welchallyn.com

Heartstream semiautomatic defibrillator
Philips Medical Systems
Heartstream Operation
2401 4th Ave, Suite 500
Seattle, WA 98121-1436
Phone: 1-800-263-3342
Website: www3.medical.philips.com

Banyan kits
Banyan International Corp.
2118 E. Interstate 20
P.O. Box 1779
Abilene, TX 79604-9963
Phone: 1-800-351-4530
Website: www.statkit.com/banyanhome.asp

ADDITIONAL RESOURCES

- See the sample patient education handout titled "Conscious Sedation" on page 1740 of Appendix G.
- See the sample patient consent form titled "Conscious Sedation" on page 1741 of Appendix G.

BIBLIOGRAPHY

Avramov MN, White PF: Methods for monitoring the level of sedation, *Crit Care Clin* 11(4):803, 1995.
Christian M, Yeung L, Williams R, et al: Conscious sedation in dermatologic surgery, *Am Soc Dermatol Surg* 26:923, 2000.

Higgins TL, Hearn CJ, Maurer WG: Conscious sedation: what an internist needs to know, *Cleve Clin J Med* 63(6):355, 1996.

Practice Guidelines for Sedation and Analgesia by Non-Anesthesiologists, *Anesthesiology* 84(2):459, 1996. (This article is available from the American Society of Anesthesiologists, Park Ridge, Ill.)

Proudfoot J: Analgesia, anesthesia, and conscious sedation, *Emerg Med Clin North Am* 13:357, 1995.

Trytko RL: Office-based sedation and monitoring. In Kaminer MS, Dover JS, Arndt KA, editors: *Atlas of cosmetic surgery,* Philadelphia, 2002, WB Saunders.

CHAPTER 3

Epidural Anesthesia and Analgesia

Thomas H. Corbett

Epidural anesthesia (i.e., complete relief of pain and significant motor block) and analgesia (i.e., the relief of pain only, with as little motor block as possible) can be accomplished by injecting opiates, local anesthetics, or a combination of these medications into the epidural space. An epidural is an extremely versatile procedure; it may be used to enhance the birthing experience or to provide anesthesia or analgesia during or after surgical procedures. For prolonged analgesia, a catheter may be left in the epidural space for several days to allow additional medication to be injected by repeated bolus, patient-controlled epidural anesthesia (PCEA) pump, or controlled continuous infusion.

From an anesthetic perspective, the *level* of anesthesia refers to an anatomic level or segment of effect (e.g., up to the level of the umbilicus [T10] or the level of the xyphoid [T8]), whereas *depth* refers to the amount of sensation or motor activity remaining. Depth of blockade is determined by choice of drugs and concentrations. Segmental level of anesthesia or analgesia can be controlled by the level of the injection, the volume of solution injected, as well as other factors (see the note after the "Technique" section), and the level can be increased or decreased as the clinical situation dictates. Such control is one of the advantages of epidural anesthesia over other forms of regional anesthesia.

Clinicians administering epidural anesthesia must have a good understanding of not only the anatomy involved and needle placement techniques, but also the pharmacology and physiology involved. They must be familiar and experienced with the diagnosis and management of possible complications. Epidural anesthesia or analgesia should be performed only in a hospital, surgery center, or facility where equipment and adequately trained personnel are available to manage any and all possible complications.

Editor's note: Although there is general agreement that epidural anesthesia is safe and is the most effective method of pain relief in labor, there has been some controversy regarding possible side effects. Metaanalyses attempting to determine whether epidurals increase the risk for cesarean section are conflicting. However, there is consensus among studies that epidurals prolong labor, especially the second stage. There is also consensus that epidurals increase the need for assisted delivery and the likelihood of maternal fever. (The cause of epidural-associated maternal fever is unknown.) Fetal heart rate changes are also common with epidurals during labor. Whereas the cause of heart rate changes is not known, one theory suggests reduced uterine blood flow from maternal hypotension as the mechanism. Intravenous (IV) fluid preloading (volume expansion) may help reduce the risk of maternal hypotension. However, IV fluid preloading must be performed cautiously or slowly in patients with pregnancy-induced hypertension.

ANATOMIC CONSIDERATIONS

The spinal canal contains the spinal cord, its coverings (i.e., pia mater, arachnoid mater, dura mater), and spinal fluid. The pia mater is closely attached or adherent to the spinal cord. The dura mater is the separate, toughest, and outermost covering of the spinal cord. The arachnoid membrane is a delicate membrane interposed between the dura and the pia. It is separated from the pia by the subarachnoid space, which contains the spinal fluid.

The epidural space is a potential space, external to the dura mater and located between the dura and the ligamentum flavum (connective tissue covering the vertebrae) (Fig. 3-1). Although the epidural space is a potential space, it is filled with spongy connective tissue, fat, and blood vessels. This allows for solutions injected into the space to flow freely in all directions and to bathe the nerve roots as they exit the spinal canal.

PHYSIOLOGIC CONSIDERATIONS

When an epidural is used in labor and delivery, it is important to remember that visceral pain from uterine contractions is partly conducted through the sympathetic nervous system. Impulses travel through the inferior, middle, and superior hypogastric plexuses to the sympathetic chain. This chain then connects to the spinal cord through the tenth, eleventh, and twelfth thoracic nerves.

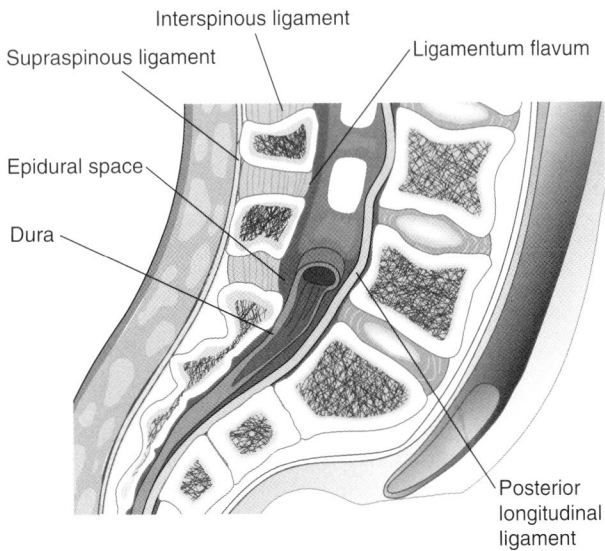

Fig. 3-1
Anatomy of the vertebral column and its contents in the lower lumbar and upper sacral regions. (Redrawn from Moore DC: *Regional block,* ed 4, Springfield, Ill, 1979, Charles C Thomas.)

Any effective analgesic solution must spread cephalad enough to affect these levels.

INDICATIONS

- As an alternative to general or spinal anesthesia for selected surgical procedures
- Requested by patient or suggested by clinician (e.g., to avoid maternal fatigue) for labor and delivery
- Postoperative analgesia

Note: Continuous epidural analgesia is being used more and more for obstetrics and postoperative analgesia; however, spinal anesthesia is still the most commonly used regional technique for surgical procedures.

CONTRAINDICATIONS

- Patient declines
- Localized infection at the puncture site
- Severe, uncorrected hypovolemia
- Blood dyscrasias; coagulopathy; prolonged international normalized ratio (INR), prothrombin time (PT), or activated partial thromboplastin time (APTT)
- Anticoagulant therapy (e.g., heparin, warfarin, enoxaparin [Lovenox], clopidogrel [Plavix])
- Allergy to specific epidural agents
- Spinal abnormalities, including scoliosis and other structural abnormalities
- Active systemic infection

- Lack of proper resuscitative equipment, skills, or trained staff
- Preexisting neurologic diseases (amyotrophic lateral sclerosis [ALS], other degenerative nerve diseases, polio)
- Preoperative headache
- Aortic stenosis
- Anemia

EQUIPMENT

- Disposable sterile gloves
- Equipment for the clinician to observe universal blood and body fluid precautions
- Disposable epidural tray containing the following:
  1. Appropriate prep solutions, swabs, and sterile 4 × 4 gauze pads
  2. Disposable drapes
  3. Epidural catheter, threading assist guide, and syringe adapter attachment
  4. Syringes:
     a. Plastic Luer-Lok (3 ml) for local infiltration of lidocaine 1%
     b. Plastic syringe (20 ml) for administration of epidural agent
     c. Glass Luer-Lok procedural syringe (5 ml) filled with saline for loss of resistance technique (see Fig. 3-2)
  5. Needles:
     a. Skin puncture needle (18 gauge)
     b. Tuohy epidural needle (18 gauge) or other epidural needle
     c. Filter needle (19 gauge) for drawing solutions into the syringes
     d. Skin wheal needle (25 or 27 gauge)
  6. Filter (0.2 μm) and filter straw (4 inch)
  7. Medications:
     a. Lidocaine 1% (5-ml vial) for local infiltration
     b. Sodium chloride 0.9% injectable (10-ml ampule)
     c. Test dose lidocaine 1.5% injectable, with epinephrine 1:200,000 (5-ml vial)
     d. Epinephrine injectable 1:1000 (1-ml vial)
- Epidural medications (Table 3-1)
- Patient-monitoring equipment (e.g., automated blood pressure [BP] device, continuous electrocardiogram [ECG] monitor, pulse oximeter, fetal monitor [if used for obstetrics])
- Emergency and resuscitative equipment (e.g., suction, Ambu-bag, oxygen, defibrillator) as well as an anesthesia machine
- Emergency and other drugs not included in the epidural kit:
  1. Ephedrine 5% (1 ml) for use if hypotension develops (usual dose to treat hypotension is 10 mg [0.2 ml] IV)

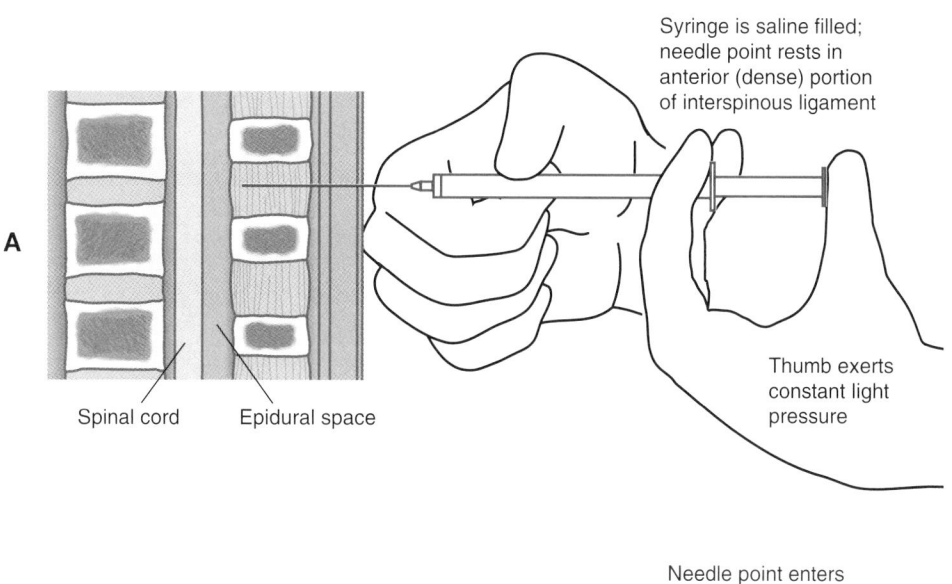

Syringe is saline filled; needle point rests in anterior (dense) portion of interspinous ligament

Thumb exerts constant light pressure

Spinal cord   Epidural space

A

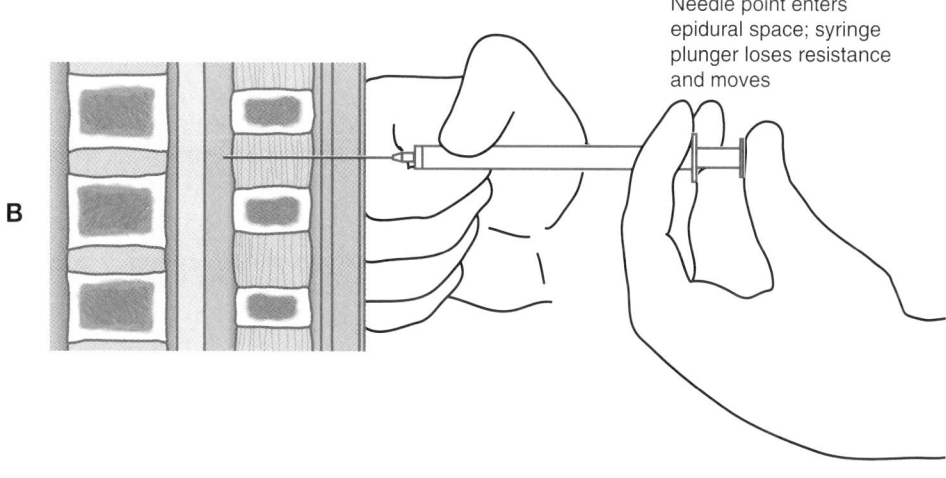

Needle point enters epidural space; syringe plunger loses resistance and moves

B

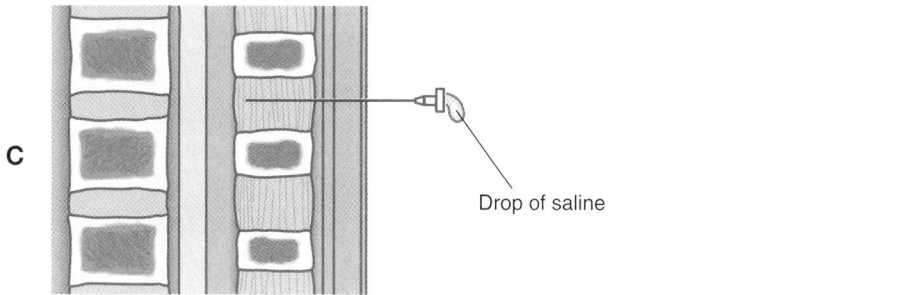

Drop of saline

C

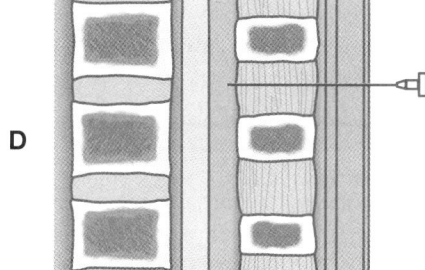

D

Fig. 3-2
Loss of resistance and hanging drop methods of ascertaining when the point of the needle rests in the epidural space. **A,** Needle rests in interspinous ligament. **B,** Syringe plunger loses resistance when needle enters epidural space. **C,** Saline-filled syringe has been removed, leaving a hanging drop. **D,** Hanging drop disappears when needle enters epidural space. (**A-B,** Redrawn from Moore DC: *Regional block,* ed 4, Springfield, Ill, 1979, Charles C Thomas.)

TABLE 3-1

Local Anesthetics Commonly Used for Epidural Anesthesia

Agent	Concentration	Dose (ml)	Dose (mg)	Onset (min)	Duration (hr)	Sensory Block	Motor Block
Lidocaine	2%	10-20	100-400	5-15	1-2	Good	Good
Bupivicaine	0.5%	10-20	50-100	10-20	2-4	Good	Good
Levobupivicaine	0.5%	10-20	50-150	10-15	4-6	Good	Good
Ropivacaine	0.5%	15-30	75-150	15-30	2-4	Good	Good
Ropivacaine	0.75%	15-25	113-188	10-20	3-5	Good	Excellent

TABLE 3-2

Local Anesthetics Commonly Used for Epidural Analgesia

Agent	Concentration	Dose (ml)	Dose (mg)	Onset (min)	Duration (hr)	Sensory Block	Motor Block
Lidocaine	2%	10-20	100-200	5-15	1-2	Good	Good
Bupivicaine	0.125%-0.25%	10-20	25-50	15-20	1-3	Good	Minimal
Chirocaine	0.125%-0.25%	10-20	25-50	15-20	1-2	Good	Minimal
Ropivacaine	0.2%	10-20	20-40	10-15	0.5-1.5	Good	Minimal

2. Neo-Synephrine
3. Atropine
4. Diphenhydramine (Benadryl)
5. Metoclopramide (Reglan), ranitidine (Zantac), and Bicitra
6. Diazepam or Midazolam

Note: A 1% solution equals 10 mg/ml.

EPIDURAL AGENTS: LOCAL ANESTHETICS

The two most commonly used local anesthetics for epidural anesthesia are lidocaine and bupivicaine (Table 3-1). Lidocaine has a rapid onset (5 to 15 minutes) and lasts 1 to 2 hours, whereas bupivicaine has a slower onset of action (10 to 20 minutes) and a longer duration of action, lasting 2 to 4 hours. In general, increasing the concentration of the drug while maintaining the same volume decreases the latency (time to onset of anesthesia). The addition of epinephrine to lidocaine (available premixed 1:200,000 with lidocaine) or to 0.25% (or less) bupivicaine appears to increase the duration of action.

Bupivicaine is widely used for both obstetric and surgical epidural anesthesia and analgesia. Bupivicaine 0.25% provides adequate sensory analgesia with minimal motor blockade for 1 to 3 hours, and it is well suited for both obstetrics and postoperative analgesia (Table 3-2). When used at 0.5% concentration, bupivicaine produces significant motor blockade. Because of toxicity at higher levels, bupivicaine 0.75% is not recommended for use in obstetrics.

Levobupivicaine (Chirocaine) is a newer agent that is similar to bupivicaine in duration and action but with less central nervous system (CNS) and cardiac toxicity. Another agent, ropivacaine (Naropin), has less cardio-toxicity than bupivicaine but more than lidocaine. In addition, ropivacaine has a significantly higher threshold for CNS toxicity than bupivicaine. In studies, 15 to 30 ml ropivacaine 0.5% provided epidural anesthesia comparable to bupivicaine 0.5% for cesarean section; however, the duration of motor blockade was shorter with ropivacaine.

When lumbar epidural anesthesia is used for surgical procedures, initial volumes of 10 to 20 ml are recommended in adult patients, depending on the concentration of anesthetic and the desired level of anesthesia. Sensory levels are then checked, and the dose adjusted accordingly. Additional incremental doses are administered through the epidural catheter as needed. Lower initial volumes (6 to 10 ml) are usually adequate for analgesia in the obstetric patient.

Note: The clinician should always use preservative-free local anesthetics and narcotic agents specifically formulated for spinal or epidural anesthesia.

EPIDURAL AGENTS: OPIATES

Anesthetic agents tend to cause motor blockade. Although they do not cause motor blockade, epidural opioids alone are not as effective as dilute concentrations of local anesthetics for anesthesia or analgesia. However, when opiates are used in combination with local anesthetic agents, they allow for a reduction in the necessary concentration of the anesthetic agents, thereby minimizing motor blockade. This makes epidural opioids particularly useful in situations where motor blockade is undesirable (e.g., labor, control of postoperative pain). Table 3-3 shows doses and effects of combining bupivicaine and opioids for control of labor pain.

TABLE 3-3

Concentrations of Bupivacaine With or Without Opioids for Labor Analgesia (Bolus Injection)

Bupivicaine Concentration	Dose (ml)	Opioid	Result
0.5%	5-10	None	Both sensory and motor blockade
0.25%	10-15	None	Sensory and partial motor blockade
0.125%	10-15	Fentanyl 1-3 µg/ml	Sensory and minimal motor blockade
0.06%	10-15	Sufentanil 0.5 µg/ml	Analgesia and no motor blockade

PREPROCEDURE PATIENT PREPARATION

A thorough medical history and physical examination should be performed to rule out contraindications to epidural anesthesia. Laboratory studies should be performed if indicated. The medical history should include questions about any history of spine trauma, neurologic or cardiopulmonary disease, blood dyscrasias, coagulopathies, headache (recent), and whether the patient is currently taking any medications. Physical examination should include careful observation of the back to rule out anatomic deformities or other physical problems that might make epidural anesthesia difficult. Laboratory studies should include a coagulation profile if indicated.

The patient should be informed of the available anesthesia and analgesia options. A fact sheet can be given to the patient to read before surgery or before the procedure is performed (see the sample patient education handout titled "Epidural Anesthesia" on page 1742 of Appendix G) or, for obstetric patients, before the onset of labor. For obstetric care, patients should be informed that any anesthetic procedure is optional and that there are associated risks. Preferably the fact sheet is given to the patient as a part of the prenatal care. Desired anesthesia or analgesia should be included in the patient's birth plan.

Shortly before performing an epidural, the clinician should answer any questions, review the options again with the patient including the benefits and specific risks, and obtain signed informed consent. The patient should have nothing to eat or drink for 8 hours before the scheduled procedure.

TECHNIQUE

1. Informed consent and permission forms should be signed and in order.
2. Establish IV access with a 20-gauge or larger catheter and give a bolus of 500 to 1000 ml of IV fluids. The patient should be well hydrated before the procedure to minimize the risk of hypotension.

Note: Administer the IV fluids slowly in patients with pregnancy-induced hypertension.

3. Secure the continuous BP, ECG, and pulse oximetry monitors on the patient and record the initial values. Cycle the BP monitor to observe carefully for hypotension by measuring the BP every 2.5 minutes. Vital signs should be recorded on the anesthesia chart at least every 5 minutes. All medications, doses, routes, and times administered must be recorded on the record. For obstetric patients, fetal monitoring should be used.
4. Open the disposable epidural kit and mix the appropriate solutions. Use the filtered needle to draw the solutions that will be administered epidurally. All epidural medications must be preservative free.
5. Place the patient in either the sitting or the lateral position, with the back and neck flexed and the spine straight and not rotated. An assistant should stand in front of the patient during the procedure, helping the patient to remain in that position.
6. Locate the appropriate interspace. Perform the sterile prep and drape the area.
7. A midline approach through the L2 to L3, L3 to L4, or L4 to L5 interspace is most commonly employed for epidural anesthesia. Administer local anesthesia (lidocaine 1%) to the interspace area by first making a skin wheal, then injecting into the deeper tissues at the angle the epidural needle will follow.
8. Preliminarily puncture just the skin with an 18-gauge needle to allow for later easy passage of the epidural needle.
9. Pass the Tuohy epidural needle through the skin, angling it appropriately to pass directly toward the spinal canal, until it has firmly passed into the interspinous ligament. Using either the loss-of-resistance technique or the hanging-drop method (Fig. 3-2), the needle is now advanced into the epidural space.

Note: The proper angle to direct the tip depends on which interspace is used. The proper angle is almost perpendicular at the L4 to L5 interspace (90 degrees), although it decreases to about 70 degrees at the L2 to L3 interspace. The proper location is usually just below the inferior border of the spinous processes. For epidural anesthesia, insertion angle and location are identical to those used for saddle block anesthesia; however, the depth of insertion is unique to each procedure.

10. Single-shot epidural injections may be employed for surgical procedures of short duration. If a longer duration procedure is anticipated and/or if postoperative pain relief is desired, place an epidural catheter. Catheter placement must be performed very carefully, since improper placement can cause life-

threatening complications (e.g., intravascular injection, or total spinal anesthesia if in the subarachnoid space). Rotate the needle so that the catheter will pass either cephalad or caudally as it exits the needle. Note the markings toward the hub of the epidural catheter that are usually 1 cm apart after the first mark. In most cases, the first mark is the same distance from the tip of the catheter as the needle is long. In other words, when inserting the catheter, after the first mark has passed into the needle hub, for every centimeter mark further that the catheter is advanced, the tip advances a centimeter into the spinal canal.

11. Place the tip of the catheter through the hub of the Tuohy epidural needle and advance it slowly through the needle and into the epidural space. A slight resistance is usually encountered as the catheter tip passes through the needle into the epidural space. Advance the catheter no more than 2 to 3 cm into the epidural space. The needle is then slowly withdrawn over the catheter, and the catheter secured at the puncture site and along the back with tape.

Note: The clinician should *never* attempt to withdraw the catheter while the needle is in place. The catheter may shear off, leaving the distal segment in the epidural space. Never readvance the needle after the catheter is in place, for the same reason.

12. Secure the catheter hub so that it is easily accessible for injections from the head of the operating table. Fasten the syringe adapter filter to the proximal end of the catheter.

13. Administer the test dose through the catheter or through the needle hub if not using a catheter. The test dose is performed to detect either intravascular or subdural placement of the catheter or needle. Begin by aspirating to check for presence of blood or spinal fluid. If either is present, the needle has been inserted improperly and must be corrected. Next, administer 2 to 4 ml of 1.5% lidocaine with 1:200,000 epinephrine. If the needle is intravascular, a noticeable increase in heart rate, BP, or both will usually be detected within 3 minutes after the injection. Sensory and motor function of the lower extremities will be affected if the catheter or needle is in the subdural space. If abnormal placement is detected, the catheter or needle should be removed and the procedure repeated at a different interspace.

14. After the test dose has confirmed proper placement, the patient is ready for the epidural injection. Aspirate to check for the presence of blood or spinal fluid before each injection or before placing the patient on an infusion pump or PCEA pump. (Use of infusion pumps or PCEA pumps is beyond the scope of this chapter. Please refer to standard anesthesia textbooks for this information.) Check and record the level of analgesia after the injection. A sharp object (e.g., a needle) can be used to do this.

Note: The factors affecting the level of epidural analgesia include the level of the epidural injection; the volume and concentration of anesthetic solution used; the rate of injection; the addition of a vasoconstrictor; patient age, height, and physical condition; and the position of the patient.

COMPLICATIONS

- Hypotension:
  - It is the most common cardiovascular complication of epidural anesthesia.
  - It is caused by widespread sympathetic block.
  - Hypovolemic patients are more susceptible to hypotension.
  - The clinician should treat significant hypotension with positioning, IV fluids, and an IV vasopressor if needed.

Note: Significant bradycardia may be treated with atropine.

- Subarachnoid injection: Injection of large volumes of anesthetic solution into the subdural or subarachnoid space may result in a high or total spinal, with respiratory arrest, severe hypotension, and possibly cardiac arrest. These conditions must be recognized and treated immediately.
- Postspinal headache: Subdural puncture, always a risk when performing epidural anesthesia, carries a high risk for spinal headache, particularly in younger and pregnant patients. For severe or persistent headache, a blood patch may be necessary.
- Toxicity from anesthetic agents:
  - Accidental injection of local anesthetic into the bloodstream or anesthetic overdose may lead to systemic toxic reactions, including (1) *CNS toxicity* (which begins with numbness of tongue, lightheadedness, dizziness, tinnitus, blurred vision, disorientation, drowsiness, muscle twitching, and tremors, possibly progressing to convulsions), and (2) *cardiovascular toxicity* (initially a mild increase in BP and heart rate is observed, followed by hypotension). The clinician should treat initial hypotension with ephedrine. In severe cases the patient may experience an irreversible state of cardiovascular depression.

Note: For CNS toxicity, treat convulsions by (1) maintaining a patent airway and assisted or controlled ventilation and (2) administering IV sodium Pentothal, midazolam, or diazepam. Intubation may be required.

— Local tissue toxicity is also possible (but it is rare when preservative-free anesthetic solutions are used).

• Respiratory complications, which can be caused by paralysis of intercostal muscles, and hypoxia or hypercarbia can occur, especially in patients with underlying respiratory disease (e.g., chronic obstructive pulmonary disease [COPD]).

• Neurologic damage: Postepidural neurologic sequelae are due to (1) trauma, (2) anterior spinal artery syndrome (i.e., a syndrome resulting from damage or thrombosis of the anterior spinal artery caused by trauma from the epidural needle), which is almost always avoided by using a midline approach when inserting the needle, and (3) hematoma.

Note: Because of decreased peripheral sensation, the patient is at increased risk of lower extremity injury as long as the epidural is in place. Risk of neural injury in the operating room can be kept to a minimum through careful patient positioning. Postoperatively, patients must be followed closely to detect potentially treatable sources of neurologic injury, including expanding spinal hematoma or epidural abscess, constrictive dressings, improperly applied casts, and increased pressure on neurologically vulnerable sites. A neurologist or a neurosurgeon should evaluate new neurologic deficits promptly to formally document the patient's evolving neurologic status, to arrange further testing or intervention, and to provide long-term follow-up.

• Catheter complications:
— Epidural catheters may be inadvertently inserted into a blood vessel or into the subarachnoid space. The test dose is used to avoid this possibility and to prevent placing a large dose of anesthetic into either the circulation or the subarachnoid space.
— The distal portion of the catheter may break off in the epidural space. This may occur if an attempt is made to withdraw the catheter through the epidural needle. It may also occur if the needle is readvanced after the catheter is deployed. If the catheter will not advance through the needle, remove the needle and catheter together and repeat the procedure at another interspace.

SUPPLIERS

Disposable trays, infusion pumps, etc.

B. Braun Medical, Inc.
824 12th Avenue
Bethlehem, PA 18018
Phone: 1-800-854-6851
Website: www.bbraunusa.com

Anesthesia and critical care pharmaceuticals

Baxter Healthcare Corp.
95 Spring Street
New Providence, NJ 07974
Phone: 1-800-667-0959
Website: www.baxter.com

Becton, Dickinson and Co.
1 Becton Drive
Franklin Lakes, NJ 07417
Phone: 1-888-237-2762
Website: www.bd.com/surgical/anesthesia/
epidural.asp

Rusch, Inc
2450 Meadowbrook Parkway
Duluth, GA 30096
Phone: 1-800-553-5214
Website: www.ruschinc.com

Sims Portex Inc
10 Bowman Drive
Keene, NH 03431
Phone: 1-800-258-5361
Website: www.portexusa.com

Epidural and saddle block needles

Kendall Company
15 Hampshire Street
Mansfield, MA 02048
Phone: 1-800-962-9888
Website: www.kendallhq.com

CPT/BILLING CODES

62273	Injection, lumbar epidural, of blood or clot patch
62278	Injection of diagnostic or therapeutic anesthetic or antispasmodic substance (including narcotics); epidural, lumbar or caudal, single
62279	Injection of diagnostic or therapeutic anesthetic or antispasmodic substance (including narcotics); epidural, lumbar or caudal, continuous

ICD-9-CM DIAGNOSTIC CODES

For ICD-9-CM codes for other surgical procedures, see the appropriate chapter.

| V22.2 | Pregnant state, NOS |
| 650 | Spontaneous vaginal deliveries |

A fifth digit (represented by the * symbol in the following codes) is used to denote the current episode of care for codes 640 to 648 and 651 to 669. Following are the digits used and the episodes of care they represent:

0	Unspecified
1	Delivered with or without mention of antepartum condition
2	Delivered with mention of postpartum complication
3	Antepartum condition or complication
4	Postpartum condition or complication

652.2*	Breech presentation
653.5*	Unusually large fetus causing disproportion
660.4*	Shoulder dystocia
644.2*	Premature labor with delivery (less than 37 weeks)

The following are codes related to deliveries with forceps or vacuum:

662.2*	Prolonged second stage of labor
659.7*	Abnormality in fetal heart rate or fetal distress

The following are codes related to episiotomy, episiotomy repair, and repair of low vaginal lacerations:

664.0*	First-degree perineal laceration
664.1*	Second-degree perineal laceration
664.2*	Third-degree perineal laceration
664.3*	Fourth-degree perineal laceration
664.4*	Unspecified perineal laceration

The following are codes that relate to pain:

724.5	Back pain
719.4	Joint pain
729.5	Limb or leg pain

Note: More specific locations will usually reimburse at higher levels.

307.80	Psychogenic pain, site unspecified
307.89	Psychogenic pain, other (This code can be used to indicate pain in most areas.)

ADDITIONAL RESOURCES

- See the sample patient education handout titled "Epidural Anesthesia" on page 1742 of Appendix G.

BIBLIOGRAPHY

Echt M, Begneaud W, Montgomery D: Effect of epidural analgesia on the primary cesarean section and forceps delivery rates, *J Reprod Med* 45:557, 2000.

Hofmeyr GJ: Prophylactic intravenous preloading for regional analgesia in labour, *Cochrane Database Syst Rev* (2): CD000175, 2000.

Horlocker TT: Complications of spinal and epidural anesthesia, *Anesthesiol Clin North America* 18(2):461, 2000.

McClellan KJ, Faulds D: Ropivacaine: an update of its use in regional anesthesia, *Drugs* 60(5):1065, 2000.

Thorp JA: Epidural analgesia during labor, *Clin Obstet Gynecol* 42(4):785, 1999.

CHAPTER 4

Local Anesthesia

Daniel J. Derksen

Local anesthetics are extremely useful in a wide variety of clinical settings. From simple laceration repair to abscess incision and drainage, local anesthetics are critical to patient comfort and physician ability to perform the necessary procedure. Local anesthetics prevent the generation and conduction of nerve impulses by several mechanisms: they increase the electrical excitation threshold, slow the propagation of nerve impulses, and disrupt the action potential and sodium permeability of nerve fibers. For the practicing physician, it is important to know that the progression and the duration of a local anesthetic is related to many factors, including the size of the area to be anesthetized; the nerve fiber diameter, myelination, and conduction velocity; the presence of infection; the blood supply in the area; the presence of chronic disease (e.g., diabetes); and the patient's pain threshold and anxiety level. Local anesthesia includes the use of injectable or topical agents. (Also see Chapter 11, Topical Anesthesia.)

INDICATIONS

- Relief of pain caused by a clinical procedure (e.g., excisions)
- Diagnostic nerve blocks
- Relief of pain from local trauma, fractures, etc.

See Tables 4-1 and 4-2 for a selection of local anesthetics and their characteristics. See Box 4-1 for selection criteria for local anesthetics.

CONTRAINDICATIONS

Local anesthetics should not be used in patients with a *known sensitivity*. However, this is very uncommon with the injectable amide anesthetics (lidocaine [Xylocaine], mepivacaine [Carbocaine], bupivacaine [Marcaine], and prilocaine [Citanest]). The older injectable anesthetics were esters (procaine [Novocaine] and tetracaine [pontocaine]) and caused more allergic reactions. The two groups do not cross-react, so a patient reporting an allergy to procaine can use lidocaine successfully. However, multidose vials also include parabens preservatives, which are chemically similar to ester anesthetics, and may induce an allergic response in sensitive patients. Single-dose vials do not contain preservatives and may be indicated for the patient reporting allergy.

The use of vasoconstrictors (i.e., epinephrine) with local injectable anesthetics decreases bleeding, reduces systemic absorption, and prolongs the duration of action, but it is contraindicated in several circumstances. Local anesthetics with vasoconstrictors should be used only with extreme caution when vasoconstriction could cause permanent destruction of tissue. In general, vasoconstrictors should not be used on the extremities—the nose, ear, penis, or ends of digits (fingers and toes). In addition, patients with known peripheral vascular disease may have an exaggerated vasoconstrictor response. Extreme care should be taken if local anesthetics with vasoconstrictors are used in patients with diabetes, hypertension, arteriosclerosis, thyrotoxicosis, heart block, or cerebral vascular disease. If a skin flap has marginal viability or if blood flow to a flap is compromised, epinephrine should not be used. Likewise, if the wound is contaminated, epinephrine will increase the likelihood of infection because of the diminished blood flow.

TABLE 4-1

Commonly Used Injectable Local Anesthetics in the Office Setting (also see Table 8-1)

Local Anesthetic	Onset (min)	Duration (hr)	Equivalent Concentration (%)
Lidocaine (Xylocaine)	1	0.5-1	1
Lidocaine w/epinephrine	1	2-6	1
Mepivacaine (Carbocaine)	3-5	0.75-1.5	1
Bupivacaine (Marcaine)	5	2-4	0.25
Bupivacaine w/epinephrine	5	3-7	0.25
Etidocaine (Duranest)	3-5	3-7	0.5

Modified from Cada DJ et al, editors: *Drug facts and comparisons,* St Louis, 2000, Wolters Kluwer.

TABLE 4-2

Maximum Dosages of Commonly Used Injectable Local Anesthetics (also see Table 8-1)

Anesthetic	Concentration	Maximum Adult Dose
Lidocaine (Xylocaine)	1%	4.5 mg/kg not to exceed 300 mg (30 ml in adult)
Lidocaine (Xylocaine) w/epinephrine	1%	7 mg/kg not to exceed 500 mg (50 ml in adult)
Bupivacaine (Marcaine) w/epinephrine	0.25%	3 mg/kg not to exceed 175 mg (50 ml per average adult)
Bupivacaine (Marcaine)	0.25%	3 mg/kg not to exceed 225 mg

From McEvoy GK, editor: *AHFS drug information,* Bethesda, 1999, American Society of Health-System Pharmacists.

BOX 4-1

Selection of Local Anesthetics and Effects

Lidocaine (Xylocaine) Without Epinephrine (1% to 2%)
Can cause vasodilation
Can last 30 to 60 minutes depending on site or vascularity
Use in contaminated wounds
Use in fingers, nose, penis, toes, earlobes
Use if vascular disease is present or if patient is immunocompromised
Use if there are cerebrovascular or cardiovascular risks
Use for nerve block

Lidocaine (Xylocaine) with Epinephrine (1% to 2%)
Causes vasoconstriction
Has longer duration
Use in highly vascular areas to improve visualization of field
Use in clean wounds
In general, do not use on fingers, nose, penis, toes, and earlobes

Bupivacaine (Marcaine)
For longer duration
For nerve blocks

APPROACHES FOR ALLERGIC PATIENTS

• Use a cooling agent (ice cube, ethyl chloride, etc.).
• For small lesions, use no anesthetic.
• Use single-dose vials instead of multidose vials.
• Use bacteriostatic saline.
• Substitute an amide for an ester (if offending agent can be identified).
• Use diphenhydramine (Benadryl). Inject 10 to 50 mg in the usual fashion (50 mg/ml diphenhydramine mixed with 4 ml of normal saline).

EQUIPMENT

• Sodium bicarbonate 7% to 10% in 5-ml vials
• 18-gauge needle to draw up solution
• 27- to 30-gauge needle for injection (various lengths)
• Alcohol swabs
• Various size syringes
• Anesthetic of choice

PREPROCEDURE PATIENT PREPARATION

A standard consent form is used for whatever procedure is to be performed. The risks include allergic reaction to the anesthetic, infection, bleeding, damage to the area resulting from ischemia (if epinephrine or other vasoconstrictors are used), and systemic absorption of the local anesthetic.

TECHNIQUE FOR INJECTABLE LOCAL ANESTHESIA

1. Using an alcohol swab, wipe the top of the vial of local anesthetic. Draw up the anesthetic with a large-bore needle (e.g., 18 gauge) into an appropriately sized syringe (most office procedures require less than 5 ml of local anesthetic). For the common shave or biopsy excisions, 1 ml is sufficient. Discard the large-bore needle in an appropriate container (avoid recapping any needle, even if "sterile").

2. Depending on the tissue to be infiltrated, choose an appropriately sized needle. For most skin surgeries, a 1-inch, 27- to 30-gauge needle provides the necessary rigidity and causes minimal discomfort.

3. Inject either intradermally (creating a wheal) or subcutaneously (subdermal, into the adipose tissue), depending on the lesion and surgery intended. (It takes longer for subcutaneous injections to take effect, but they are less painful.) Before infiltration, draw back the syringe plunger. If there is blood return, do not infiltrate; this will prevent systemic injection. Reposition the needle and draw back the plunger. If there is no blood return, infiltrate as the needle is withdrawn. Never infiltrate as the needle is advanced; this also helps to prevent systemic injection. Before any digital or other block, a review of the related anatomy is recommended. In the case of digital blocks, it is important to remember the location and number of nerves supplying each digit (Fig. 4-1). See Chapter 8, Peripheral Nerve Blocks and Field Blocks. *Inability to obtain adequate pain elimination is usually due to a failure to wait the necessary time for the local anesthetic to work.*

4. If a cancer is suspected, do not go through the abnormality. Although cancer supposedly does not

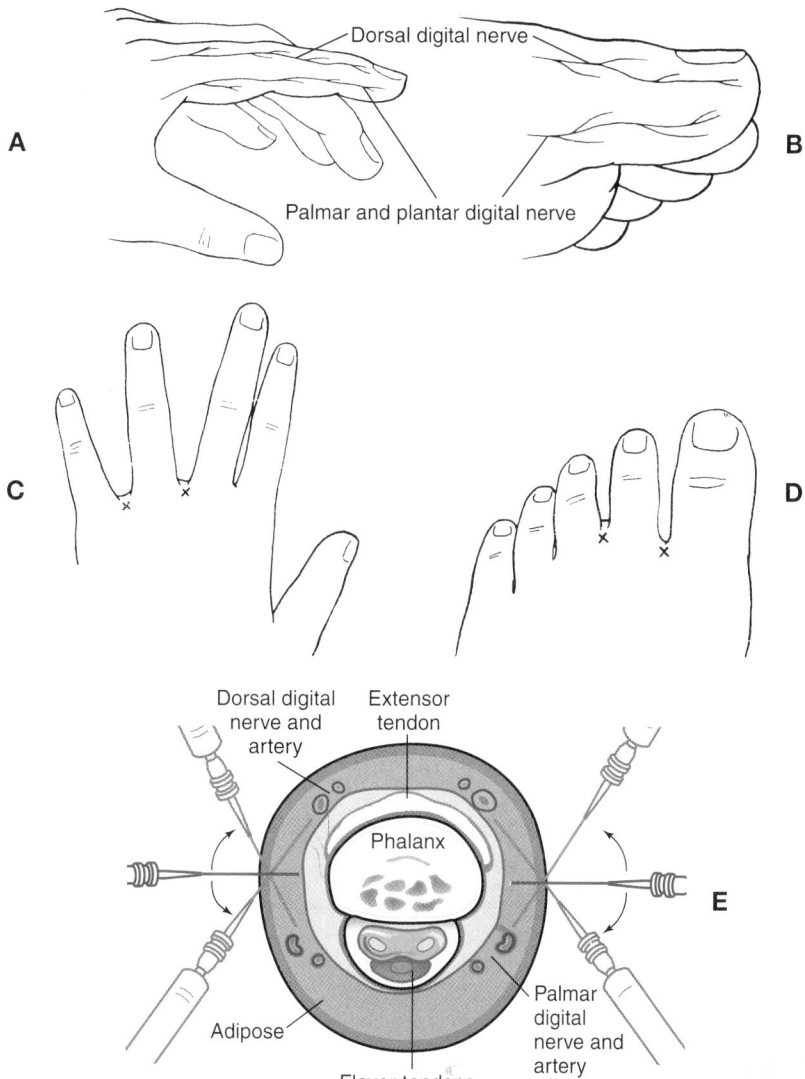

Fig. 4-1
The anatomy of a **digital block.** In the, **A,** finger and, **B,** toe, there are four nerves to block in order to obtain a successful digital block. A dorsal and palmar branch on each side of the digit needs to be blocked. If the proper sites of infiltration are chosen (**C,** finger or, **D,** toe), the four nerves should be well anesthetized. First, the web space on both sides of each digit is injected. Insert the needle parallel to the digits, directed toward the hand or foot. Insert 1 to 2 cm and inject 1 to 2 ml of anesthetic. Repeat on the other side. After the web space is infiltrated, insert the needle perpendicular to the base of the digit on each side of the digit. Insert until the needle touches bone. Withdraw a few millimeters and inject 1 ml of anesthetic (red needle and syringe). It is also helpful to then perform a "ring block" **(E).** Inject from the midline on top to the midline on the bottom from both sides to complete a "ring" around the entire digit (gray needle and syringe). A digital block may take several minutes to take effect because there is so much accessory innervation. In the case of a severely inflamed paronychia, or an ingrown toenail in which the nail must be partially or entirely removed, additional local anesthetic may still be necessary just proximal to the site of inflammation to eliminate pain and to allow the removal. It is best to avoid vasoconstrictor agents in local anesthetics for digital blocks. In addition, care should be taken to avoid systemic injection. See Fig. 8-2 for more details.

travel down needle tracks, do not take the chance. Also, do not inject through an area of infection.

5. Injection over a subcutaneous lesion may obscure it from further palpation. Use a field block technique and inject around the area to be anesthetized (Fig. 4-2). This allows the lesion to remain palpable after injection.

6. For adverse reactions and concerns about toxic doses, see Chapter 5, Local and Topical Anesthetic Complications.

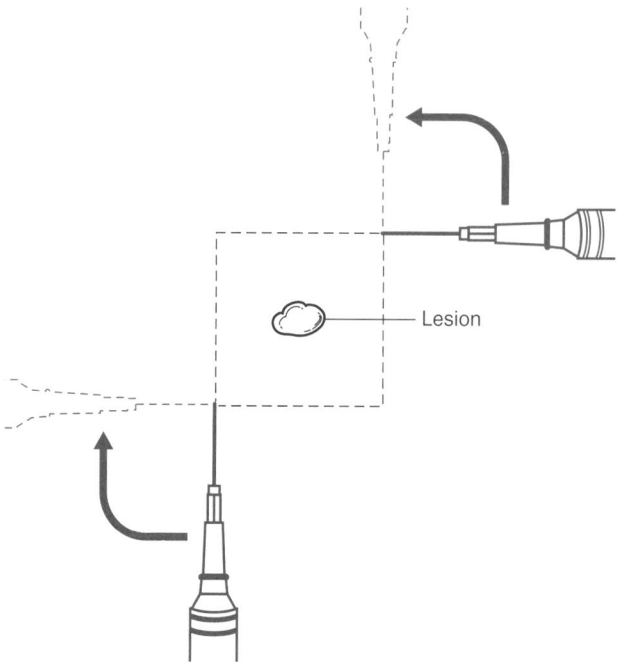

Fig. 4-2
Field block. Inject at 90-degree angles on both sides of the skin lesion to be excised. Usually only two injection sites are necessary. After injecting in one direction, withdraw the needle, rotate it 90 degrees, and inject again. This avoids distortion of the central area around the lesion to be excised.

REDUCTION OF PAIN OF INJECTION

Injection of local anesthetics can cause pain, which is related to the size of the needle, the rapidity of injection, and the temperature. The acidity of the solution (pH 4.05 to 6.49) also causes a significant burning sensation. This short-lived pain can be reduced by using a small needle, pinching up the skin, injecting slowly, warming the solution, and adding 1 ml of sodium bicarbonate solution (7% to 10%) to 9 ml of anesthetic. Patients, especially children, will note remarkable improvement in comfort. Infiltration with unbuffered solution has been found to be 2.8 to 5.7 times more painful than infiltration with buffered counterparts. There has been no significant difference detected in the time of onset or duration of anesthesia or in the surface area of skin anesthetized. Occasionally, the addition of bicarbonate can make the solution cloudy, but there are no known adverse effects from this.

Previously, it was recommended that the buffered solution be discarded after 24 hours. Buffered lidocaine is stable for 1 week at room temperature. Refrigeration may nearly double that time. Warming the buffered solution to above room temperature may also decrease the discomfort of injection (Box 4-2).

TOPICAL ANESTHETICS

Certain clinical situations favor the use of a topical anesthetic. Examples include combative children too large for the papoose board and too small to reason with, and patients with nosebleeds, eye injuries, corneal abrasions, or lesions on mucous membranes that need to be treated with painful modalities, such as liquid nitrogen or electrodiathermy. Mucous membranes (nose, mouth, throat, esophagus, and genitourinary tract) can be anesthetized successfully with many of the local anesthetics by direct topical application. Care must be taken to avoid excess systemic absorption of the topical anesthetic near mucous membranes (see Chapter 5, Local and Topical Anesthetic Complications, and Chapter 11, Topical Anesthesia).

COMPLICATIONS

When a local anesthetic is used properly, complications are rare. Allergic reactions may occur (see Chapter 203, Anaphylaxis). Other complications are related to systemic absorption of the local anesthetic, toxic doses, or to the effect of vasoconstriction when local anesthetics with epinephrine are used (see Chapter 5, Local and Topical Anesthetic Complications). Although rare, the use of epinephrine may cause arrhythmias or other cardiovascular or cerebrovascular changes. Warm compresses to increase peripheral circulation can be used when excess vasoconstriction is observed (such as cyanosis, decreased pulse, or decreased capillary refill).

POSTPROCEDURE PATIENT EDUCATION

Instruct patients to watch for signs of infection or local reaction to the local anesthetic. Redness, pus, increased pain, red streaks up the extremity, or other problems should prompt a phone call or return visit to the physician.

SUPPLIER

Sodium bicarbonate 7% to 10% (Abbott or Astra), or sodium bicarbonate (Neutracaine) in 5-ml vials
MD, Inc.
408 State of Franklin Road, Suite 43
Johnson City, TN 37604
Phone: 1-615-461-6185 or 1-800-35-MDINC

CPT/BILLING CODES

Administration of local anesthesia is included in the CPT code for most procedures, and no extra fee is allowed.

BIBLIOGRAPHY

Achar S, Kundu S: Principles of office anesthesia: part 1, infiltrative anesthesia, *Am Fam Physician* 66(1):91, 2002.

Bartfield JM, Homer PJ, Ford DT, Sternklar P: Buffered lidocaine as a local anesthetic: an investigation of shelf life, *Ann Emerg Med* 21:16, 1992.

Cada DJ et al, editors: *Drug facts and comparisons,* St Louis, 2000, Wolters Kluwer.

Doyle DJ: A closer look at local anesthetics, *Emerg Med* 23:147, 1991.

Ernst AA, Marvez-Valls E, Nick TG, Wahle M: Comparison trial of four injectable anesthetics for laceration repair, *Acad Emerg Med* 3(3):228, 1996.

Holmes HS: Options for painless local anesthesia, *Postgrad Med J* 89:71, 1991.

McKay W, Morris R, Mushlin P: Sodium bicarbonate alleviates pain on skin infiltration with lidocaine, with or without epinephrine, *Anesth Analg* 66:572, 1987.

Moy RL, Pfenninger JL: Taking the sting out of local anesthesia, *Patient Care* March 15:61, 2000.

Scarfone RJ, Jasani M, Gracely EJ: Pain of local anesthetics: rate of administration and buffering, *Ann Emerg Med* 31:36, 1998.

Sectish TC: Use of sedation and local anesthesia to prepare children for procedures, *Am Fam Physician* 55(3):909, 1997.

Trott AT: *Wounds and lacerations: emergency care and closure,* St Louis, 1991, Mosby.

Usatine RP, May RL: *Anesthesia in skin surgery: a practical guide,* St Louis, 1998, Mosby.

Zempsky WT, Karasic RB: EMLA versus TAC for topical anesthesia of extremity wounds in children, *Ann Emerg Med* 30(2):162, 1997.

CHAPTER 5

Local and Topical Anesthetic Complications

William L. McDaniel, Jr.

Many in-office surgical procedures require the use of local or topical anesthetics. Topical anesthetics are used more frequently in children for dermatologic procedures and in persons having nasopharyngoscopy and esophagogastroduodenoscopy (EGD).

The primary care physician must have an understanding of the types of complications that may be encountered when using these anesthetics and must be equipped to diagnose and deal with them. **For maximum recommended dosages, see Chapter 4, Local Anesthesia.**

ALLERGIC REACTIONS

- Low incidence (less than 1%).
- Older agents such as procaine and tetracaine (esters) are more likely to cause allergic reactions, because they are derivatives of para-aminobenzoic acid, a known allergen.
- There are no reported allergic reactions to lidocaine (an amide).
- In known or suspected local anesthetic allergy, avoid *multi-dose vials* of an amide such as lidocaine. Many contain methylparaben preservatives, which have a structure similar to para-aminobenzoic acid.
- True allergic reactions may vary from mild to life threatening with anaphylaxis and circulatory collapse.
- Plasma losses may equal 35% of circulating blood volume within minutes.
- Rapid replacement of volume with colloid and administration of epinephrine are indicated. (See Chapter 203, Anaphylaxis.)
- If epinephrine fails, norepinephrine infusion may be lifesaving.

ALTERNATIVES TO OBTAIN PAIN RELIEF

- Use single-dose vials of lidocaine, which lack preservative.
- A small local anesthetic effect can be obtained by injecting sterile normal saline into tissue.
- Dilute 1 ml of 50 mg of diphenhydramine with 4 ml sterile normal saline and inject 10 to 50 mg locally for anesthetic effect.
- Use ice cubes, Frigiderm, liquid nitrogen (sparingly), or hypnosis to obtain topical anesthesia.

OVERDOSE REACTIONS

Central Nervous System Toxicity

Local anesthetics reach the central nervous system after slow absorption or by direct intravenous injection. An inadvertent direct intravenous injection may create a transient high local central nervous system level of anesthetic, which can cause *convulsions*. Most convulsions created in this way terminate within minutes, provided the administration of the drug has stopped.

A warning of less serious central nervous system effects may include *circumoral numbness, lightheadedness, tinnitus, visual disturbance, muscular twitching,* and *irrational behavior.*

If high serum levels persist, *grand mal seizures, apnea, unconsciousness,* and *death* may occur. An alert patient, in most cases, tells the physician before a seizure develops. This would be absent in the case of rapid inadvertent intravenous injection.

Acidosis and *hypercarbia* increase the likelihood of central nervous system toxicity. Pulse oximetry monitoring during the procedure may be an invaluable tool to alert the clinician to some of the effects of toxicity.

With serious central nervous system toxicity, stop the offending agent and begin *oxygen and support ventilation* if needed. Alert patients can be asked to hyperventilate. This may temporarily alleviate twitching. Seizures can usually be stopped with *IV midazolam (Versed), diazepam (Valium),* or *lorazepam (Ativan).* Lorazepam and diazepam are inconsistently absorbed in the IM route. Midazolam (Versed) may be used IM if an IV line is not available. Flumazenil (Romazicon) should be available as an antagonist for benzodiazepines in case of respiratory depression from the drugs.

Cardiovascular Toxicity

Cardiovascular toxicity can occur with any of the local anesthetic drugs. Local anesthetics prolong conduction through the Purkinje fibers and heart muscle. *Prolonga-*

tion of PR interval and *widening of the QRS* may be observed. Higher concentrations decrease heart muscle contractility. *Hypotension, respiratory depression,* and *bradycardia* are observed with lidocaine.

If cardiovascular toxic effects are suspected, discontinue or *remove the agent* when possible. *Basic cardiopulmonary resuscitation is the cornerstone* of immediate management. There is no clear-cut medical management of ventricular ectopy, ventricular fibrillation, or arrest. Various studies indicate cardiotoxicity of bupivacaine is more severe and difficult to treat than that associated with lidocaine. Cardiovascular and anesthesiology consults should be obtained as soon as available.

METHEMOGLOBINEMIA (See Chapter 216, Venous Methylene Blue Therapy)

Methemoglobinemia is a rare but serious complication of topical and local anesthetic agents. It is of particular importance because it can be clinically suspected and diagnosed. Early diagnosis and treatment can prevent the serious complications of brain damage and death.

The best way to illustrate the point is with a case history. A 27-year-old white male underwent outpatient EGD and developed unexplained cyanosis. During his recovery phase the nurse noted cyanosis, which did not resolve on high flow oxygen. Vital signs and arterial blood gases were within the normal range. Diagnoses such as pulmonary thromboembolic phenomenon and allergic reactions to Demerol or Valium were considered.

An astute respiratory technician saved the day by reporting that the arterial blood drawn for the arterial blood gases was brown. The diagnosis of methemoglobinemia was suspected and confirmed by discovering a methemoglobin level of 14%.

The patient involved had received Cetacaine spray four or five times before the EGD procedure. The endoscopist had requested that the patient swallow the material each time. This spray contains about 14% benzocaine, which was the culprit in this case. Physicians may be lulled into a false sense of security in using this spray, since the 2001 *Physicians' Desk Reference* does not list methemoglobinemia as a potentially adverse effect of Cetacaine.

Normal hemoglobin contains iron in the ferrous (+2) state. Methemoglobinemia contains iron that has been oxidized to the abnormal ferric (+3) state. Normal levels of methemoglobin range up to 3%.

Prevent methemoglobinemia by avoiding overdose of benzocaine, prilocaine, and lidocaine. Prilocaine and lidocaine in an eutectic mixture of 2.5% each (EMLA) is considered safe when used as recommended. EMLA is applied topically and is often used in infants and children. One case of methemoglobinemia has been reported with its use over large areas for a long period.

BOX 5-1

Consideration for Acquired Methemoglobinemia

A local anesthetic agent was used.
A larger than usual dose was needed.
Environmental predisposition present (nitrates) or other predisposing drugs such as sulfonamides, Dilantin, amyl nitrate, dapsones, sodium nitroprusside, quinones, and nitroglycerin.
Cyanosis does not respond to usual O_2.
Arterial blood appears chocolate brown; usually 15% to 20% levels of methemoglobin present. Administer 1% methylene blue over about 5 minutes for treatment.
Infants and the elderly seem more susceptible to developing methemoglobinemia.

Other drug causes of methemoglobinemia include sulfonamides, Dilantin, amyl nitrate, dapsones, sodium nitroprusside, quinones, and nitroglycerin.

The following signs are noted at the various levels:
- Up to 15%: graying of skin
- 15% to 20%: cyanosis becomes apparent and chocolate-brown blood
- 20% to 50%: weakness, dizziness
- 50% to 70%: arrhythmias, acidosis, convulsions, and coma may occur
- Over 70%: death and cerebral anoxia may occur

Nitrates, foods, and contaminated well water may predispose to methemoglobinemia and may lower the threshold for local anesthetics.

Treatment varies with the level of methemoglobin present and the condition of the patient. Methylene blue 1% administered over 5 minutes should result in improvement. (See Chapter 216, Venous Methylene Blue Injection.) A second dose can be given within about an hour if the response was inadequate.

Hyperbaric oxygen may help by increasing the amount of dissolved oxygen in the blood. Consider exchange transfusions in the most severely affected patients. This may require a tertiary center.

Successful treatment will not be available unless the astute clinician considers the diagnosis of methemoglobinemia (Box 5-1).

BIBLIOGRAPHY

Greenberg MJ: Diagnosing acquired methemoglobinemia can be confusing at best, *EMS News* January 8, 1995.

Lee JJ, Rubin AP: Emla cream and its current uses, *Br J Hosp Med* 50(8):463, 1993.

McCaughey W: Adverse effects of local anaesthetics, *Drug Safety* 7(3):178, 1992.

Physicians' Desk Reference: Cetacaine, Oradell, NJ, 2001, Medical Economics.

Rodriguez LF, Smolik LM, Zbehlik AJ: Benzocaine-induced methemoglobinemia, *Ann Pharmacother* 28(5):643, 1994.

Smith C: Pharmacology of local anaesthetic agents, *Br J Hosp Med* 52(9):455, 1994.

CHAPTER 6

Nitrous Oxide Sedation

Jessica Y. Hackman
Thomas A. Bzoskie

Nitrous oxide (N_2O) sedation can be considered as an alternative to IV sedation. First used as an anesthetic agent in 1844, it is now used by approximately 85% of pediatric dentists and is growing in popularity in general dental and medical offices. N_2O is a rapidly effective sedative with onset of effects within 2 to 3 minutes of administration and peak effects within 5 minutes. Dosing can be adjusted easily and rapidly to increase or decrease depth of sedation during the procedure. Recovery time is short, since elimination through the lungs occurs as rapidly as absorption. The drug is not metabolized within the body to any significant extent and therefore can be used safely on most patients. Patients remain conscious and reflexes are intact so there is minimal risk of aspiration or over sedation. Gaining experience with N_2O sedation can be achieved by observing an experienced practitioner and performing the sedation under supervision. Continuing education courses are available and practitioners who are not familiar with the technique are encouraged to participate. Oral surgery residents begin using this technique independently very early (first month) in their training, and it is not necessary to have extensive experience with IV sedation to be able to perform N_2O sedation safely. Again, the patient remains conscious with intact reflexes throughout the sedation. In addition, N_2O does not cause respiratory depression, making it safer than fentanyl, Versed, or chloral hydrate. Technically, it is easier to perform than IV sedation. There is no need to gain venous access; a face mask or nasal hood is simply placed on the patient.

INDICATIONS

- Anxious patients undergoing minor office surgical or dental procedures to reduce fear and apprehension
- Patients needing increased pain reaction threshold
- Patients who are unable to tolerate other sedatives

CONTRAINDICATIONS

- Pregnancy (first trimester)
- Airway obstruction and severe asthmatic conditions
- Severe psychiatric disorders (N_2O can cause dreaming and hallucinations)
- Pulmonary hypertension
- Pneumothorax
- Severe cardiac disease
- Hyperthyroidism
- Sickle cell anemia
- Chronic bronchitis/emphysema
   N_2O should not be used to replace local anesthesia or to control defiant or uncontrolled behavior.

ADVANTAGES

- Recovery is rapid and monitoring time during recovery is brief.
- A driver is not needed once the patient has recovered (patients should be monitored for approximately 30 minutes after the use of N_2O before release to full functional status), unlike IV sedation in which limited activity is advised for long periods of time after administration of the drug.

LIMITATIONS

- Lack of potency
- Expense of equipment

EQUIPMENT

- Inhalation sedation machine (Fig. 6-1)
- Breathing circuit
- Reservoir bag
- Scavenging system

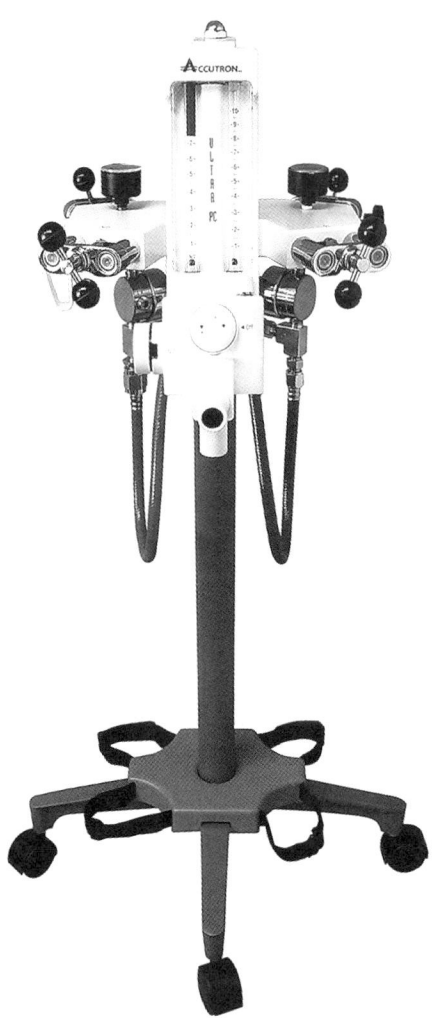

Fig. 6-1
Accutron 4-Cylinder Portable Manifold. (Courtesy Accutron, Inc., Phoenix, Ariz.)

- Nasal hood or facial mask
- Oxygen and N_2O supply (N_2O is stored in compressed form as a liquid in cylinders)
- Pulse oximeter
- Oral pharyngeal airway available
- Emergency cart with appropriate drugs (consider the Banyan kit; see Chapter 203, Anaphylaxis)

PRESEDATION ASSESSMENT AND CONCERNS

- A complete medical history should be obtained from the patient. Relevant information includes history of cardiac or respiratory disease, medications, allergies, prior surgeries and complications from anesthesia, history of tobacco use, and history of substance abuse.

- Evaluation of the airway. The oropharynx should be evaluated for any abnormalities or evidence of obstruction. A history of sleep apnea can indicate airway abnormalities such as narrow airways and tonsillar hypertrophy. Obesity, especially involving the face and neck, may lead to difficulties in spontaneous ventilation under sedation.
- N_2O will potentiate drugs that depress the respiratory system.
- Sensations and the procedure should be described to the patient in advance. N_2O can produce a feeling of euphoria, dreaminess, and detachment. It can also cause numbness and tingling of the extremities. It may cause nausea and confusion in higher doses.

PREPROCEDURE PATIENT PREPARATION

- Always have a specially trained, experienced and competent assistant present.
- Confirm that the patient has fasted for at least 6 hours for solid foods and nonclear liquids and at least 3 hours for clear liquids.
- Perform a full check of the inhalation sedation machine to ensure that it is safe to use and that it has an adequate supply of gasses to allow the procedure to be completed. The scavenging system should also be checked for proper functioning.

DOCUMENTATION

- Informed consent should be obtained for both the planned procedure and the N_2O sedation.
- The patient's blood pressure, heart rate, and oxygen saturation by pulse oximetry should be recorded at regular intervals throughout the procedure and during recovery.
- For documentation, any standardized anesthesia form can be used; alternatively, vitals, level of sedation, and concentration of N_2O being used at 5-minute intervals can simply be recorded (see Chapter 2, Conscious Sedation).
- All written and verbal instructions, including consent with risks, benefits, alternatives and contraindications, should be documented.

TECHNIQUE

1. Always have an assistant present.
2. Begin the inhalation sedation session with a full check of the inhalation sedation machine to ensure that it is safe to use and that it has an adequate

supply of gasses to allow the procedure to be completed. Also check the scavenging system for proper functioning.

3. Once the presedation check has been completed, position the patient properly for the procedure to be performed. Record vital signs, including continuous pulse oximetry. The gas flow rate should be initially set to 6 L/min of 100% oxygen only.

4. Place a nasal hood or facial mask and titrate the flow rate to the patient's requirement. Adjust the flow rate so that the reservoir bag can be seen moving during each breath without completely emptying.

5. Once the patient has been positioned and the flow rate adjusted to the proper level, introduce the N_2O. Patient tolerance and nitrous requirement varies significantly for each person; therefore it is important to titrate the dose slowly. Initially 10% nitrous is introduced and the patient is allowed to breathe this mixture for 1 minute. If this dose provides adequate sedation, the operative or dental procedure can begin. If it is not sufficient, provide an additional 10% N_2O and allow the patient to breathe the mixture for 1 minute before reassessment. This cycle can be repeated to a maximum mixture of 70% N_2O: 30% O_2. Overdose should be avoided because it can result in unpleasant feelings for the patient.

Note: Minimum dose is 10% N_2O: 90% O_2. Maximum concentration is 70% N_2O: 30% O_2. Average maintenance dose is typically between 20% N_2O: 80% O_2 and 40% N_2O: 60% O_2. Document the levels and length in the chart.

6. Signs of adequate sedation include reduction in anxiety (patient will appear more relaxed and comfortable), slowing of the blink reflex, decreased response to painful stimuli, and general decrease in movements.

7. Reduce the N_2O concentration with the first sign of overdose. *Signs of overdose* include agitation, sweating, nausea, vomiting, lack of cooperation or response to questions, and unconsciousness. The patient may also complain of unpleasant feelings such as intense tingling or detachment from reality.

8. With lengthy administration (greater than 30 minutes), reduce N_2O concentration. The duration of exposure to an anesthetic can have an effect on recovery time. Accumulation of anesthetics in tissues such as muscle, skin, and fat increases with continuous inhalation and can delay recovery time. This is especially true of the more soluble anesthetics, but it can also occur to some degree with low solubility anesthetics.

9. Once the procedure is complete, the N_2O can be reduced and the patient returned to breathing 100% O_2. This should be achieved by reducing the inspired concentration of N_2O by 20% per minute until it is reduced to nothing.

10. The patient should breathe 100% O_2 for a minimum of 2 minutes (preferably 3 to 5 minutes) after the procedure and ideally 3 to 5 minutes to prevent diffusion hypoxia (see the "Postsedation Procedure and Concerns" section).

COMPLICATIONS

- *Oversedation* or prolonged administration *can lead to* agitation, sweating, nausea, vomiting, and feelings of detachment, confusion, hallucinations and unconsciousness.
- N_2O can cause myocardial and respiratory depression in high doses (greater than 70%).
- *Chronic* effects of N_2O exposure can include bone marrow suppression, mostly because of oxidation of vitamin B_{12}. Central nervous system degeneration is common among those who abuse N_2O. Chronic exposure to N_2O has also been linked with an increased rate of miscarriages. Scavenging of waste gases is therefore crucial to protect office staff. The National Institute for Occupational Safety and Health (NIOSH) recommends limiting the room concentration of N_2O to 25 ppm.

POSTSEDATION PROCEDURE AND CONCERNS

- The patient should breathe 100% O_2 for 3 to 5 minutes after the procedure to prevent diffusion hypoxia.
- Diffusion hypoxia is a condition caused by the rapid release of N_2O from the blood. Since N_2O is insoluble, it leaves the bloodstream rapidly once the inspired concentration is reduced. If the inspired concentration of nitrous oxide is high, then a large amount of gas will quickly emerge from solution into the alveoli, displacing oxygen. Room air does not have an O_2 concentration high enough to compensate for high N_2O concentration released from the alveoli following the procedure; thus hypoxia can occur if supplemental O_2 is not given.
- Symptoms of diffusion hypoxia include disorientation and severe headache. Diffusion hypoxia can be avoided by having the patient breathe 100% O_2 for at least 2 minutes and ideally 3 to 5 minutes until the N_2O has washed out of the alveoli.
- Vital signs along with pulse oximetery should be monitored during recovery, and the patient should be alert and oriented before discharge.
- All written and verbal instructions that were given should be documented.

- Postoperative instructions are more relevant to the actual procedure that was performed; therefore there are no specific postoperative instructions for N_2O sedation.
- Unlike IV sedation, the patient may drive himself or herself home.

CPT/BILLING CODES

99141   Sedation with or without analgesia (conscious sedation); intravenous, intramuscular or inhalation.

Note: 94760-94762 may not be reported in addition to 99141.

BIBLIOGRAPHY

Katzung BG: *Basic and clinical pharmacology,* ed 7, New York, 1998, Appleton & Lange.

Meechan JG, Robb, ND, Seymour RA: *Pain and anxiety control for the conscious dental patient,* Oxford, 1998, Oxford University Press.

Morgan GE, Mikhail MS: *Clinical anesthesiology,* ed 2, New York, 1996, Appleton & Lange.

Trojan J, Saunders B, Woloshynowych M, et al: Immediate recovery of psychomotor function after patient administered nitrous oxide/oxygen inhalation for colonoscopy, *Endoscopy* 29(1):17, 1997.

Wiener-Kronish JP, Gropper MA: *Conscious sedation,* Philadelphia, 2001, Hanley & Belfus.

CHAPTER 7

Pediatric Sedation

David B. Bosscher

Anyone who performs minor procedures on pediatric patients knows the value of being able to safely and predictably sedate them. Children, especially preschool children, are often fearful of painful or unfamiliar techniques. When verbal reassurance does not allow the physician to perform the needed procedure safely, sedation is required. Sedation does not anesthetize the child sufficiently to perform a painful procedure, but it promotes cooperation of the child, allowing proper anesthetics to be administered.

INDICATIONS

Any necessary, minor procedure for which the cooperation of the child cannot be obtained with verbal reassurance

CONTRAINDICATIONS

• A medical condition that would cause respiratory compromise during sedation
• Sensitivity to one of the agents being used

EQUIPMENT

• The medication and the means to administer it. (In most cases, this will mean a syringe and needle.)
• The means to support respiration if necessary. (A bag and mask, an oral airway tube, and the equipment to administer oxygen are minimum respiratory support equipment required. Although intubation is rarely needed, appropriately sized endotracheal tubes and a laryngoscope should be available for emergency use.)

PRESEDATION CONCERNS

• Pediatric sedation does not relieve the practitioner of the need to explain the anticipated procedure to both the child (when appropriate) and the parent or guardian. Informed consent for both the sedation and the procedure should be obtained and documented.
• A trained nurse or other similar person can help to monitor the child and to assist with the procedure.

The physician should be aware of the duration of action of the agent used for sedation. On one hand, the duration of action should be sufficient to complete the procedure comfortably. On the other hand, if the duration of action is prolonged, the physician needs to ensure that the child will be properly monitored after the procedure is completed.

An assessment should be performed before initiating any sedation. The pertinent points are outlined in Box 7-1.

BOX 7-1
Presedation Assessment

History
Reschedule or use extra caution in the following situations:
  Ingestion of milk or solids in previous 6 hr
  Ingestion of clear liquids in previous 3 hr
  History of:
    Apnea
    Seizures
    Tolerance to previous sedation medications or methods
    Airway compromise
    Cardiac or pulmonary disease
    Bleeding disorders
  Concurrent medications with potential sedative drug interactions
  Caregiver is either not available or fully competent

Physical
Blood pressure, temperature, pulse, respiratory rate, pulse oximetry
Evidence of:
  Acute respiratory illness
  Cardiac abnormalities
  Neuromuscular problems
  Craniofacial abnormalities

Adapted from Sectish TC: *Am Fam Physician* 55(3):909, 1997.

DOCUMENTATION

Documentation of any procedure should be scrupulous and complete. Obtain informed consent for both the contemplated sedation technique and the procedure itself. Document the issues discussed in obtaining informed consent in the patient record. Some medicolegal experts also recommend asking a parent or guardian to sign a form listing each procedure that the physician might perform. With regard to pediatric sedation, the physician should document how well the patient tolerated the method used. If side effects from the medication occur, document your approach to dealing with them. Time-based recordings of assessments and monitoring must be made until the patient is fully recovered. Finally, the physician should document that written instructions were provided that cover the care of the child after discharge from the office or hospital.

TECHNIQUE

Many pediatric procedures can be done by simply gaining the child's confidence, offering basic information regarding the procedure, and then talking him or her through it. The physician should be honest about when it might hurt. This strategy is most effective in children 6 years old or older.

With the preschool-aged child, when "verbal sedation" is not likely to be sufficient, several pediatric sedation techniques are available:

1. The *"Lytic Cocktail."* This time-honored mixture of chlorpromazine (Thorazine), promethazine (Phenergan), and meperidine (Demerol) is given intramuscularly according to weight of the child: chlorpromazine 0.5 mg/kg, promethazine 0.5 mg/kg, and meperidine 0.7 mg/kg. It is **not recommended** because (1) the physician must deal with the side effects of three medications instead of one, and (2) its effect can be erratic and unpredictable.

2. *Chloral Hydrate (Noctec).* The wide margin of safety of this oral liquid has earned it a place among those who perform pediatric procedures. The dosage for the child is 50 to 100 mg/kg (maximum 2 g). Chloral hydrate has an unpleasant smell and taste, making it difficult to entice a child to take much of it. After oral administration, it has an onset of action of around 60 minutes, making it relatively impractical for unplanned use. In addition, its sedative effects can be difficult to predict. Duration of action is 4 to 8 hours. An hour after ingesting chloral hydrate, the patient can be wide-awake and unwilling to submit to the procedure.

Chloral hydrate can be given intramuscularly or by rectal suppository, but these forms of the medication are often unavailable and have other disadvantages. Major toxicity is respiratory depression.

3. *Intranasal Midazolam (Versed).* This rapidly acting benzodiazepine is widely used by anesthesiologists who like its predictable onset of action, its low side-effect profile, and its amnestic effect. It is also now reversible. The medication causes children to become very cooperative, although it does not appear to sedate them. Intranasal midazolam dosage is 0.1 to 0.2 mg/kg of the injectable formulation. (Some researchers have used these dosages in subjects up to 18 years of age.) The solution is drawn up into a tuberculin syringe, the needle removed, and the drug then instilled in the child's nasal cavity. The onset of action is typically 10 to 15 minutes, and the duration of action is generally 15 to 20 minutes, with some effects lasting up to several hours. Midazolam can be used as a back-up strategy in instances in which the physician unsuccessfully attempts to perform the procedure under "verbal anesthesia."

Oral midazolam has also been used because of its longer duration of action but inducing sedation also takes longer through this route. Dosage for oral midazolam is 0.5 to 0.75 mg/kg (maximum 25 mg). The IV dose is 0.05 to 0.10 mg/kg (maximum 5 mg).

With all administration routes, side effects are rare and are typical of benzodiazepines in general (occasional agitation, euphoria). Neither excessive drowsiness nor respiratory depression was seen in studies using these dosages.

4. *Intramuscular Ketamine.* This medication induces predictable sedation, which generally lasts longer than midazolam. At an IM dose of 2 to 4 mg/kg, ketamine has both sedative, anesthetic, and pain-relieving properties lasting 15 to 60 minutes. The use of IM ketamine requires presedation administration of atropine (0.01 mg/kg IV) to reduce the flow of saliva. Intranasal midazolam administered at the same time as the IM ketamine also reduces unpleasant emergence reactions.

Before ketamine is administered, the medical provider should thoroughly explain to parents the postsedation hallucinations and emesis as well as the prolonged recovery time (up to 2 hours). Respiratory depression has been described only rarely with this medication.

5. *Nitrous Oxide.* This is safe and effective for children older than 8 years (see Chapter 6, Nitrous Oxide Sedation).

POSTSEDATION CONCERNS

Respiratory depression is rare with any of these medications, but if it occurs, it is a significant problem. Flumazenil (Romazicon) (0.002 to 0.02 mg/kg IV) is an injectable antagonist of midazolam and can reverse any respiratory depression midazolam causes. Alert the parent or guardian to possible breathing problems. Naloxone (Narcan) (0.01 mg/kg IM or IV) can be used to reverse narcotic suppression.

All of these medications can cause atypical or unexpected behaviors, ranging from acting drunk to making nonsensical statements or even agitation. Parents must be aware of the need to supervise the child constantly for several hours after the procedure. In addition, they should be prepared to protect the child and to reorient him or her as necessary until the medication effects wear off.

COMPLICATIONS

- Respiratory compromise is the most common complication. The physician must remain alert for this possibility and be prepared to respond with appropriate measures.
- Children can experience unpredictable reactions to medications. The physician should be familiar with the most common idiosyncratic reactions of the agent being used. *AMA Drug Evaluations* or a similar text offers more pertinent help than either the *Physicians' Desk Reference* or the drug package insert.
- The usual doses of medications will not always properly sedate some pediatric patients. At times, it may be impossible to perform the anticipated procedure.

CPT/BILLING CODE

99142   Sedation with or without analgesia (conscious sedation), oral, rectal, and/or intranasal.

ADDITIONAL RESOURCES

- See the sample patient education handout titled "Pediatric Sedation" on page 1743 of Appendix G.

BIBLIOGRAPHY

American Academy of Pediatrics Committee on Drugs: Guidelines for monitoring and management of pediatric patients during and after sedation for diagnostic and therapeutic procedures, *Pediatrics* 89(6 Pt 1):1110, 1992.

Pediatric Committee of American College of Emergency Physicians: Pediatric analgesia and sedation, *Ann Emerg Med* 23:237, 1994.

Pediatric Sedation Project. Available at an.hitchcock.org/PediSedation (accessed August 16, 2001).

Proudfoot J: Analgesia, anesthesia, and conscious sedation, *Emerg Med Clin North Am* 13(2):357, 1995.

Sectish TC: Use of sedation and local anesthesia to prepare children for procedures, *Am Fam Physician* 55(3):909, 1997.

Wilton NC, Leigh J, Rosen DR, Pandit UA: Preanesthetic sedation of preschool children using intranasal midazolam, *Anesthesiology* 69:972, 1988.

CHAPTER 8

Peripheral Nerve Blocks and Field Blocks

Julie Graves Moy

John L. Pfenninger

Many ambulatory procedures lend themselves well to local anesthesia with a field block or a peripheral nerve block. A *field block* is a method of providing anesthesia to a relatively small area by injecting a "wall" of anesthetic solution across the path of the nerves supplying the operative field (Fig. 8-1). Instead of the injection being made directly into the area of the procedure, it is made into the soft tissue some distance away, where the nerves are situated. Advantages include longer duration of anesthesia and no distortion of the operative field.

A *nerve block* is the infiltration of a local anesthetic near the nerve branch supplying sensation to a particular area. Blocking a nerve provides longer duration of anesthesia than that obtained with local cutaneous infiltration. Knowledge of the anatomy of peripheral nerves and a scrupulous sterile technique are important for successful peripheral nerve blocks. Use of this technique may reduce the amount of anesthetic needed, reduce distortion of tissues, and allow palpation of pathology to be excised.

In some sites (e.g., the breast) a nerve block cannot be obtained, and thus the field block is the only reasonable alternative. However, where possible, the nerve block may be the procedure of choice. Also see Chapter 9, Oral/Facial Anesthesia.

INDICATIONS

- Local anesthetic at the site of incision may not be effective (e.g., with infected tissue)
- When the edema from the local anesthetic injection would distort anatomic landmarks and make approximation and repair difficult.
- To palpate the deep tissue to be excised.
- When repairs or excisions are quite large and prohibit the use of large amounts of anesthetic.
- For fracture and dislocation care.
- For nail removal.

CONTRAINDICATIONS

Absolute Contradictions

- Need to inject through infected tissue
- Presence of septicemia
- Profound bleeding tendencies
- History of allergy to local anesthetics would also contraindicate injections (see Chapter 4, Local Anesthesia, and Chapter 5, Local and Topical Anesthetic Complications).

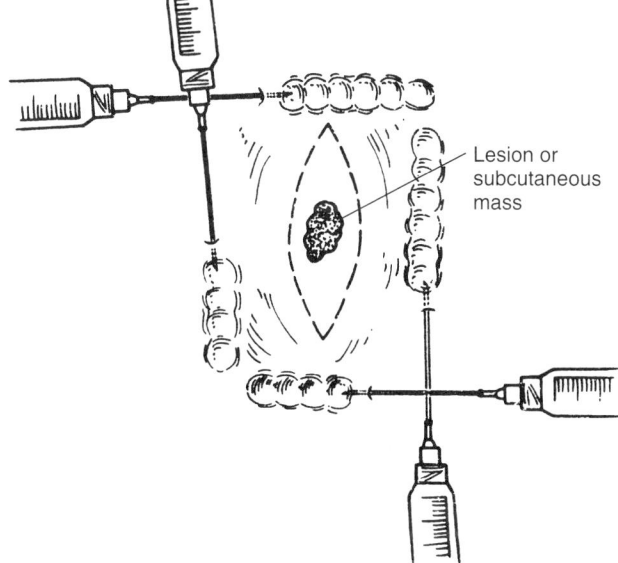

Fig. 8-1
Field block technique. This method of injecting around the lesion prevents distortion of the anatomy and allows any deeper central lesion to remain palpable.

Lesion or subcutaneous mass

Relative Contraindications

- Any neurologic damage existing before the procedure. Document findings before injection.
- In general, epinephrine-containing solutions should not be used in the hand, foot, penis, nose, or earlobes, nor should epinephrine be used in areas with poor vascular supply.

EQUIPMENT

- Sterile field and agent for sterile preparation of skin
- Local anesthetic agent (see Table 8-1 and Chapter 4, Local Anesthesia)
- 18-gauge needle to draw up solution
- 25- to 30-gauge needle for injection and appropriate size syringes (1 to 10 ml)
- Syringe
- Gloves

PREPROCEDURE PATIENT PREPARATION

There are few complications with field and nerve blocks. The benefits of the blocks versus the other alternatives (such as general anesthesia, no anesthesia, and Bier block) may be explained. Depending on the agent used, the duration of anesthesia may be prolonged and the patient should be informed of the expected length of action. In rare instances a nerve could be traumatized, but long-term consequences are rare. Any precautionary advice such as avoidance of heat or cold after the procedure should be given to the patient. The possibility of paresthesia during the injection should be explained.

TECHNIQUE

Field Block

The technique of administering a field block is similar to the technique discussed for local anesthetics (Chapter 4). In this instance, however, the area to be incised is spared from the injection. Rather, the area around the site is injected (Fig. 8-1). Repeat injections are made until the entire border of the field has been infiltrated. Allowing 5 to 10 minutes for the block to take effect improves the resulting anesthesia.

Nerve Block

1. Before beginning any peripheral nerve block, perform a neurologic examination of the area to be anesthetized and document the results in the medical record. If any neurologic defect is present, include a description of it in the document of informed consent for the procedure, and have the patient sign a statement agreeing that the defect was present before the administration of the anesthetic.
2. Identify the appropriate nerve(s) and site to block.
3. Obtain informed consent.
4. Carefully clean and prepare the skin over the injection site in a sterile fashion.

TABLE 8-1

Local Anesthetic Agents (Also See Tables 4-1 and 4-2)

Type	Name	Equivalent Concentration	Onset	Duration	Maximum Dose
Amino esters	Procaine (Novocaine)	2%	Slow	15-30 min plain 30-90 min w/epi	600 mg
	Tetracaine (Pontocaine)	0.25%	Slow	120-240 min plain 240-480 min w/epi	100 mg plain 200 mg w/epi
	Chloroprocaine (Nesacaine)	2%	Fast	15-30 min plain 30-90 min w/epi	800 mg plain 1000 mg w/epi
Amino amides	Lidocaine (Xylocaine)	0.5%-2%	Fast	30-120 min plain 60-400 min w/epi	300 mg plain 500 mg w/epi
	Etidocaine (Duranest)	0.5%	Fast	120-240 min plain	300 mg plain 400 mg w/epi
	Mepivacaine (Carbocaine)	1%	Moderate	30-120 min plain 60-400 min w/epi	300 mg plain 500 mg w/epi
	Bupivacaine (Marcaine)	0.25%	Slow	120-240 min plain 240-480 min w/epi	175 mg plain 225 mg w/epi

Note: Duration of action for adults and older children; prolonged duration of action in neonates and young children possible.
epi, Epinephrine.

5. Draw up the anesthetic. Usually a 25- to 30-gauge needle can be used to inject the anesthetic. The amount of anesthetic used varies depending on the location of the nerve.

6. Insert the needle into the site, withdrawing the plunger slightly to test for intravascular placement of the needle and moving the needle if necessary to avoid intravascular injection. If the patient experiences paresthesia, withdraw the needle slightly, since it is probably within the nerve. The goal is to inject perineurally, not into the nerve itself. If no paresthesia is noted at the expected site, confirm that there is no potential for intravascular injection and slowly inject the anesthetic. If the proper site has been identified, often as little as 1 or 2 ml will provide an excellent anesthetic field.

7. Allow 5 to 15 minutes for the block to take effect. Confirm anesthesia to pinprick before making an incision.

Common Nerve Blocks (Also See Chapter 9, Oral/ Facial Anesthesia)

1. Digital Block of Finger or Toe. Use 4 to 6 ml of 1% to 2% lidocaine *without* epinephrine for each finger, and 6 to 8 ml of the same for toes. Insert the 25- to 30-gauge, ½-inch needle fully into the skin at the base of the finger or toe in the web space and inject 1 ml. Repeat this on the other side unless it is the first or fifth digit. For those toes, 2 ml can be used. Then insert the needle perpendicular to the bone at the base of the digit, touch the bone, and pull back a little. Inject 1 ml into the lateral aspect, then 1 ml across the dorsal and ventral surfaces in the subcutaneous space. Repeat this on the contralateral side of the digit. The dorsal digital nerves in both instances lie close to bone. As the bone is touched with the needle tip, withdraw 1 or 2 mm and inject the solution (Fig. 8-2).

2. Median Nerve Block. The median nerve supplies sensation to the palmar aspect of the thumb and index and middle fingers. In addition, the radial half of the palm is supplied by the median nerve. A nerve block may be indicated for extensive lacerations and incisions in these areas. The median nerve lies between the flexor carpi radialis and the palmaris longus. With slight flexion of the wrist and simultaneous flexion of the middle finger only at the metacarpal phalangeal joint, the palmaris longus stands out. The injection should be made at the flexor crease of the wrist just radial to the palmaris longus. Use 3 to 5 ml of 1% lidocaine *without* epinephrine (Figs. 8-3 and 8-6).

3. Ulnar Nerve Block. The ulnar nerve innervates the dorsal and palmar aspects on the ulnar side of the hand (fifth finger and ulnar side of the fourth finger). There are actually two branches of the ulnar nerve, which divides 4 to 5 cm proximal to the wrist. Therefore the easiest way to obtain an ulnar block is to inject the ulnar nerve at the elbow where the nerve lies only 0.5 cm below the skin, between the medial epicondyle and the olecranon (Figs. 8-4 and 8-6). For all nerve blocks, it is best not to inject directly into the nerve but around it; 2 to 3 ml of 1% lidocaine should be sufficient here.

4. Radial Nerve Block. The radial nerve innervates the dorsum of the thumb, the index and middle fingers, and the radial portion of the dorsum of the hand. Because of multiple divisions of the radial nerve, 10 ml of anesthetic is often required to obtain good results. Inject 3 ml of solution along the lateral border of the radial artery two finger breadths above the wrist. Then lay a superficial ring of solution from this point extending dorsally over the border of the wrist and into the snuffbox area created by the tendons of the abductor pollicis longus and extensor pollicis brevis muscles. The nerve is in the superficial fascia just deep to the skin (Figs. 8-5 and 8-6).

5. Supraorbital and Supratrochlear Nerve Blocks (Forehead Block) (Also See Chapter 9, Oral/Facial Anesthesia). The supraorbital and supratrochlear nerves innervate the forehead and anterior scalp. The nerves exit at the supraorbital ridge. To ensure that both nerves have been injected, infiltrate just above the bone beneath the entire medial two thirds of the eyebrow (Fig. 8-7, *A-B*).

6. Infraorbital Nerve Block. Palpate a notch in the infraorbital rim. The infraorbital nerve exits just beneath this small notch. Infiltrate through the skin directly over the infraorbital area, or use an intraoral technique. The latter approach requires a 1½-inch needle, ideally 27 gauge. Introduce the needle at the gingival-buccal margin over the maxillary canine tooth. Advance it under the skin until the infraorbital foramen is reached. Use approximately 2 ml of anesthetic. This block is used especially to repair upper lip lacerations so that the vermilion border can be approximated appropriately. It can also be used for lacerations of the lower lateral nose and the lower eyelid (Fig. 8-7, *A-C*).

7. Mental Nerve Block. The mental nerve innervates the lower half of the lip. To avoid distortion that is inevitable with local injection around the vermilion border, inject the mental nerve. In adults the nerve exits the mandible just inferior to the second mandibular bicuspid, midway between the upper and lower edges of the mandible, and 2.5 cm from the midline of the jaw. As with the infraorbital nerve injection, introduce the needle at the gingival buccal margin inferior to the

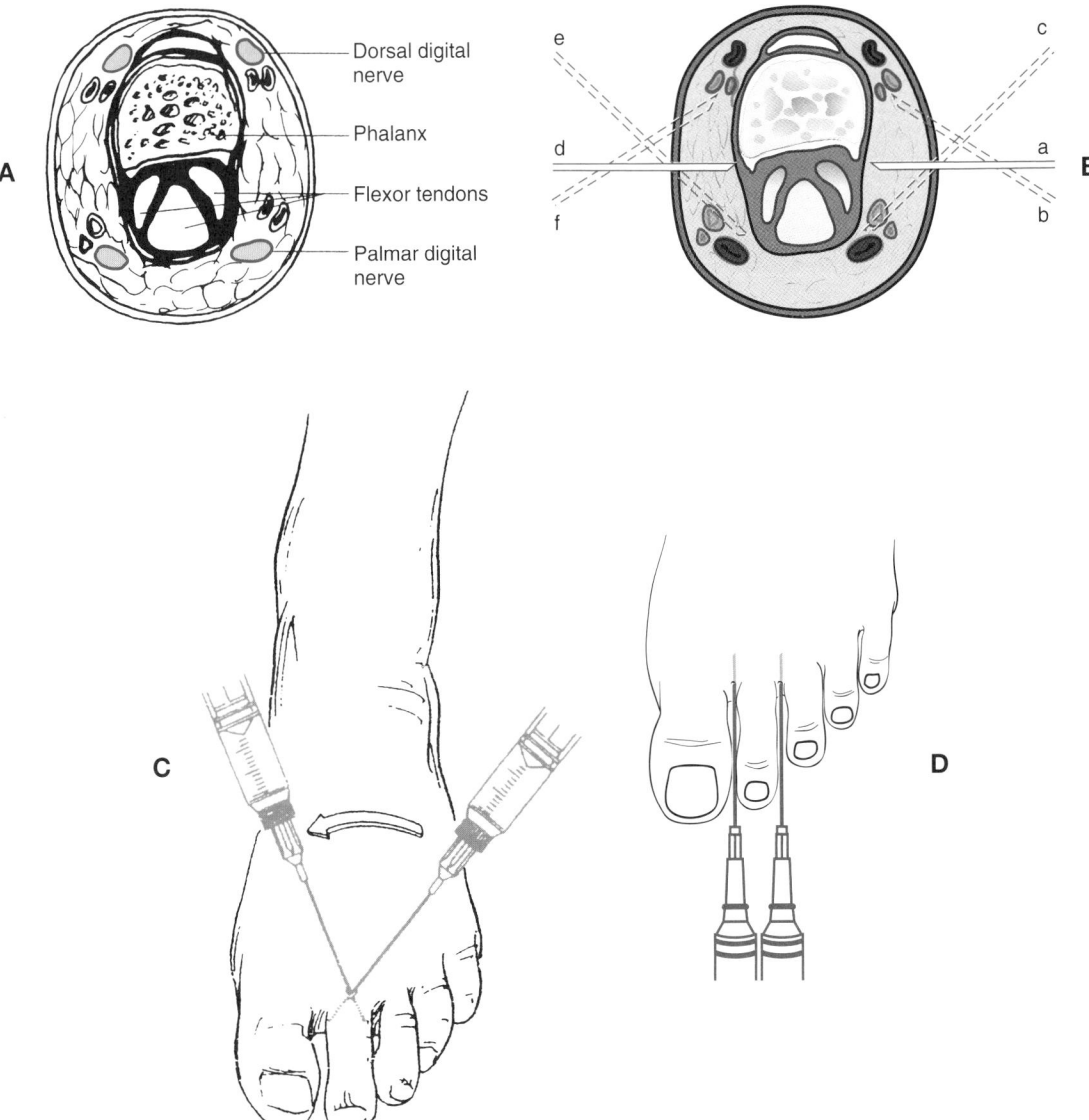

A, Dorsal digital nerve

Phalanx

Flexor tendons

Palmar digital nerve

Fig. 8-2
Anatomy and injection technique for digital nerve block. **A,** Four digital nerves of the digit. The bone is used as a landmark to find the proper plane of the dorsal digital nerve. **B,** Digital nerve block of the finger. The sites of the nerves are injected bilaterally. Insert the needle, and after touching bone, withdraw slightly and then inject 0.5 ml of anesthetic *(a)*. Direct the needle superiorly to the midline, and inject 0.5 to 1 ml from the midline down *(b)*. Do the same inferiorly *(c)*. Repeat the same technique on the contralateral side *(d-f)*. This "ring block" effectively anesthetizes the entire digit. **C,** Digital nerve block of the toe, showing an alternative method of injection from the dorsal aspect. This is followed by a ventral injection in the same manner. **D,** Site of injection in web space. When removing a toenail, an additional 1 ml of local can be placed just proximal to the nail. See Fig. 4-1 for alternative method. (**A** and **C,** Modified from Trott A: *Wounds and lacerations: emergency care and closure,* ed 2, St Louis, 1998, Mosby.)

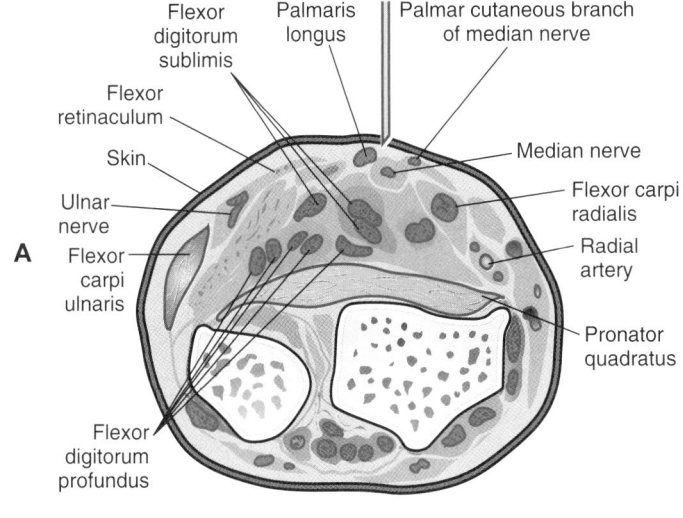

A

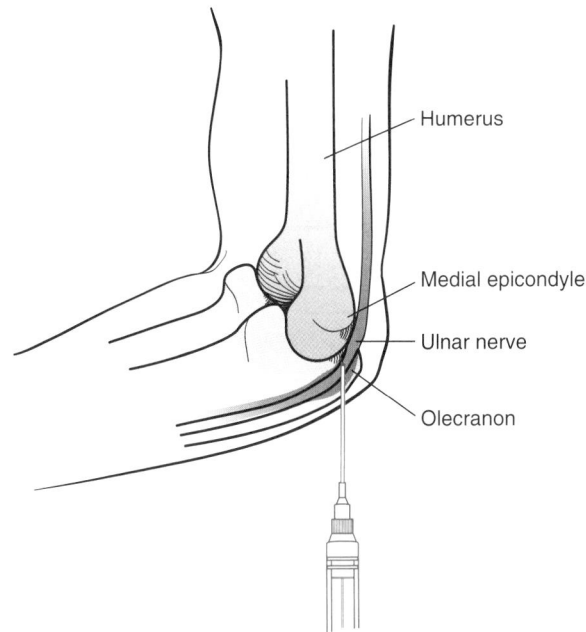

Fig. 8-4
Site of an ulnar nerve block. (Modified from Trott A: *Wounds and lacerations: emergency care and closure,* ed 3, St Louis, 1997, Mosby.)

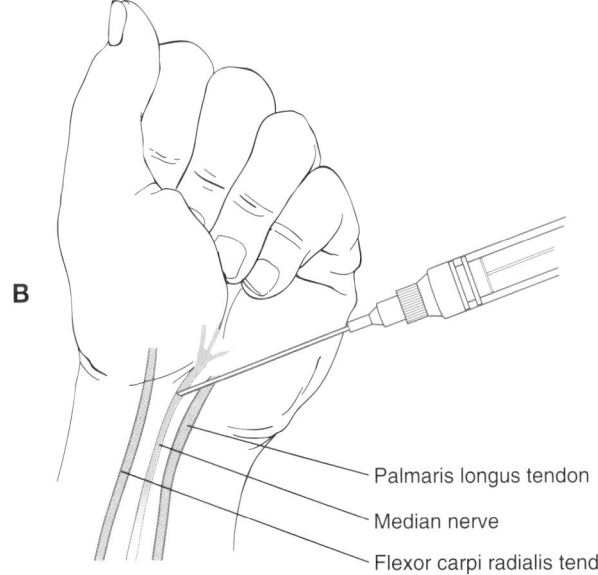

B

Palmaris longus tendon

Median nerve

Flexor carpi radialis tendon

Fig. 8-3
Median nerve block. **A,** Cross-sectional anatomy of the wrist (left wrist, palm up). **B,** Location of injection. (Adapted from Trott A: *Wounds and lacerations: emergency care and closure,* ed 3, St Louis, 1997, Mosby.)

second bicuspid. After aspiration, inject 2 ml of anesthetic (Fig. 8-7, *A-D*).

8. Ear Block. Because of complex nerve innervations of the ear, it is impossible to infiltrate a solitary nerve. In addition, it is difficult to infiltrate *over* the cartilage, since the skin here is so thin. A complete block of the auricle can be obtained by infiltrating completely around the ear with approximately 10 ml of 1% lidocaine *without* epinephrine (Fig. 8-8). This block will not numb the concha or the ear canal.

9. Foot Block. Foot blocks are indicated not so much to prevent distortion but rather to limit discomfort. The

sole of the foot is exquisitely sensitive to injection, and it is often subject to puncture wounds, lacerations, and foreign bodies. Nerve blocks can actually be more comfortable than direct infiltration. The sural nerve runs behind the fibula and lateral malleolus to supply the heel and lateral aspect of the foot. The *tibial nerve* is found between the Achilles tendon and the medial malleolus, and its course is along the posterior tibial artery. The tibial nerve supplies the medial portion of the sole and the medial side of the foot. The two nerves do overlap innervation along the middle of the foot (Fig. 8-9). To block the sural nerve, insert the needle lateral to the Achilles tendon 1 to 2 cm proximal to the level of the distal tip of the lateral malleolus. To ensure that the entire nerve is infiltrated, introduce the needle several times in a fan-shaped motion, directing it to the posterior medial aspect of the fibula (Fig. 8-10).

To obtain a tibial nerve block, identify the posterior tibial pulsation. Pass the needle medial to the Achilles tendon toward the posterior tibial artery behind the medial malleolus. Infiltration is around the artery, and careful aspiration must be carried out to prevent intraarterial injection (Fig. 8-11). Other regional nerve blocks are dealt with in other chapters, for pudendal nerve (Chapter 175, Pudendal Anesthesia), paracervical (Chapter 174, Paracervical Block), penile (Chapter 119, Adult Circumcision), oral-facial and nose (Chapter 9, Oral/Facial Anesthesia).

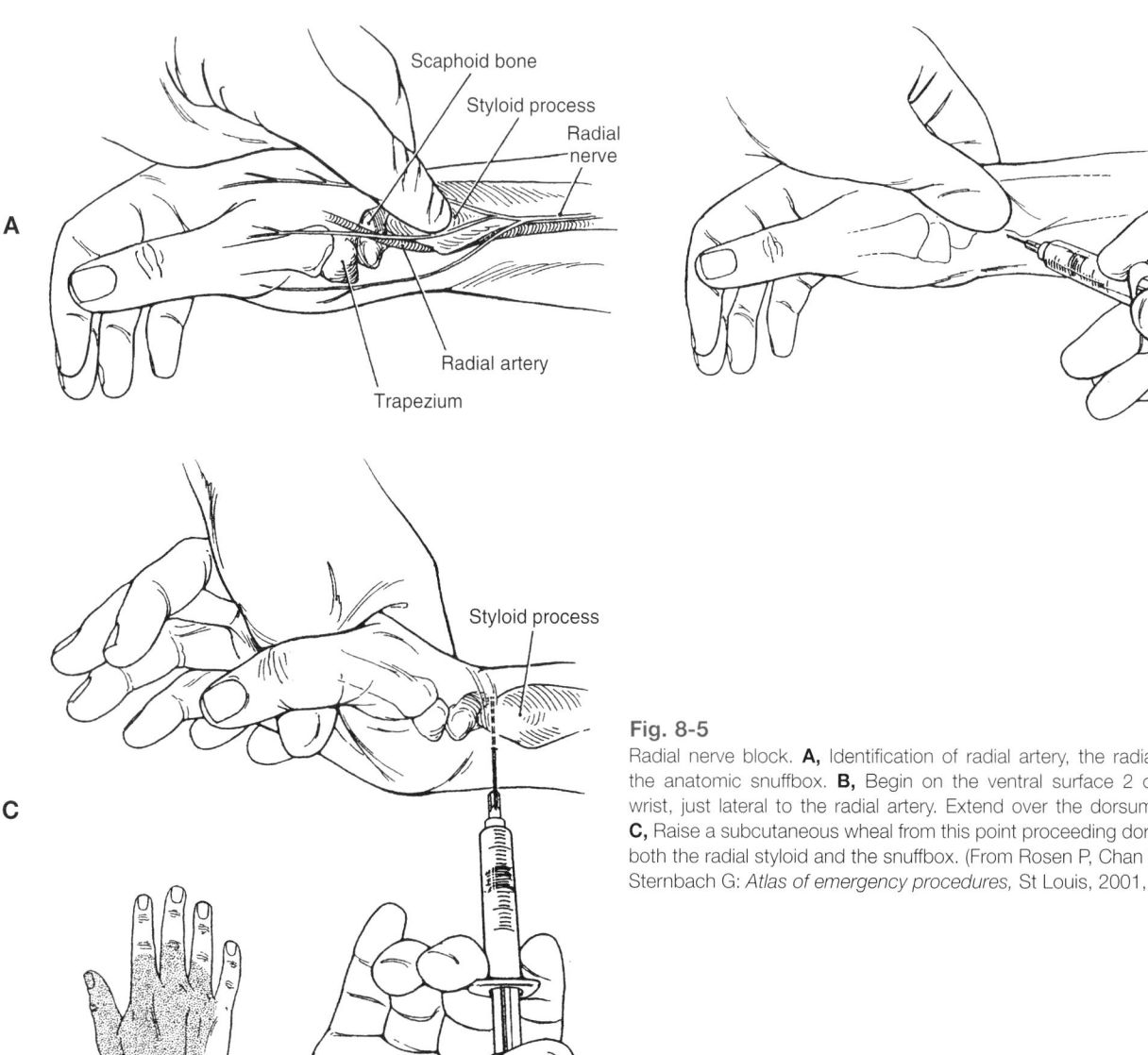

Fig. 8-5

Radial nerve block. **A,** Identification of radial artery, the radial styloid, and the anatomic snuffbox. **B,** Begin on the ventral surface 2 cm above the wrist, just lateral to the radial artery. Extend over the dorsum of the wrist. **C,** Raise a subcutaneous wheal from this point proceeding dorsally, crossing both the radial styloid and the snuffbox. (From Rosen P, Chan TC, Vilke GM, Sternbach G: *Atlas of emergency procedures,* St Louis, 2001, Mosby.)

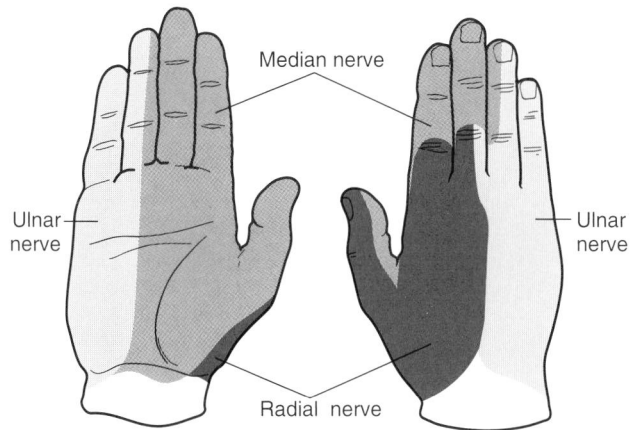

Fig. 8-6
Distribution of cutaneous sensation by the radial, ulnar, and median nerves of the hand.

CPT/BILLING CODE

64450   Introduction/injection of anesthetic agent (nerve block), diagnostic or therapeutic

Be sure to document both the diagnostic and procedural code for the local anesthesia. The CPT system allows separate billing for local anesthetic if it is administered by a physician different than the surgeon, but the CPT code includes local anesthesia for the surgical procedure in most cases. A code for the instrument tray is allowed if the procedure requires more than basic instruments. If the nerve blocks are performed for diagnostic reasons, they can be billed separately.

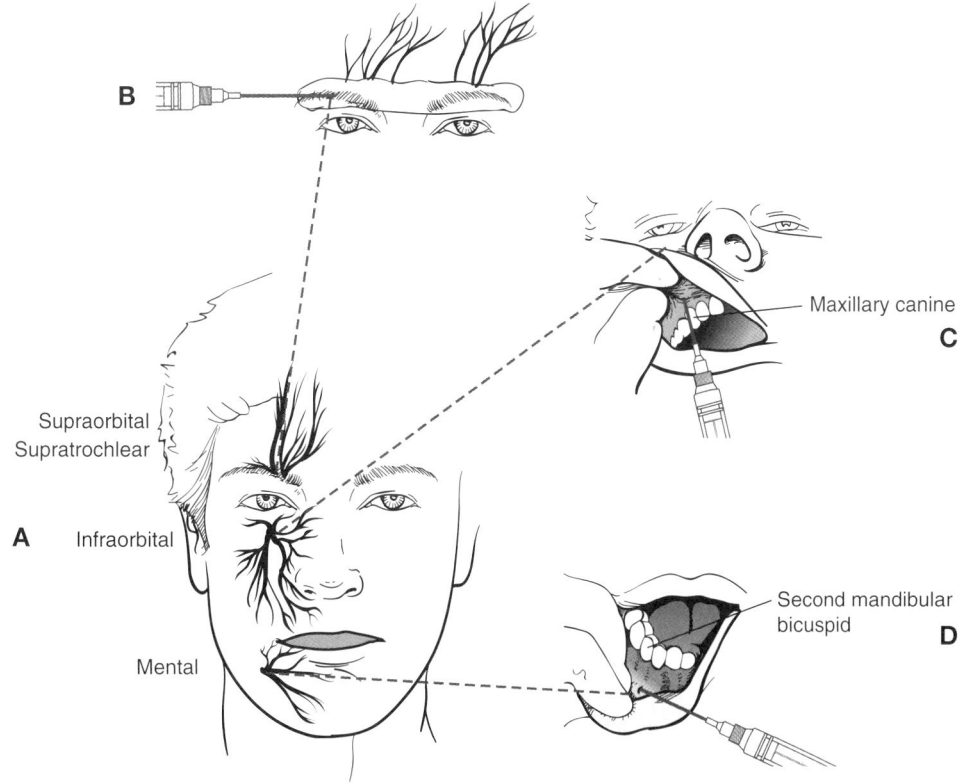

Fig. 8-7
Locations of various nerves of the face and methods to obtain a nerve block. **A,** Position and course of the supraorbital, supratrochlear, infraorbital, and mental nerves. **B,** Technique for deposition of the anesthetic to accomplish a supratrochlear and supraorbital (forehead) nerve block. **C,** Intraoral technique to anesthetize the infraorbital nerve. **D,** Intraoral technique to anesthetize the mental nerve. Also see Chapter 9, Oral/Facial Anesthesia. (Adapted from Trott A: *Wounds and lacerations: emergency care and closure,* ed 3, St Louis, 1997, Mosby.)

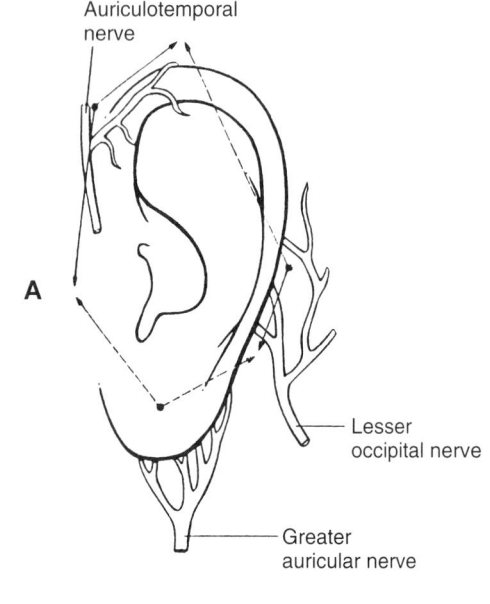

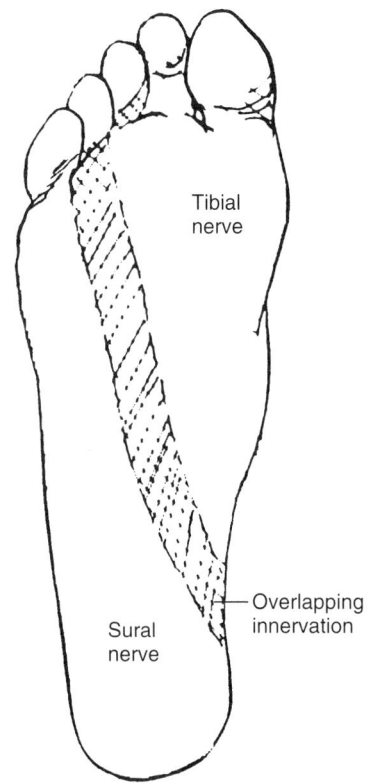

Fig. 8-9
Distribution of sensory innervation to the foot. (From Trott A: *Wounds and lacerations: emergency care and closure,* ed 3, St Louis, 1997, Mosby.)

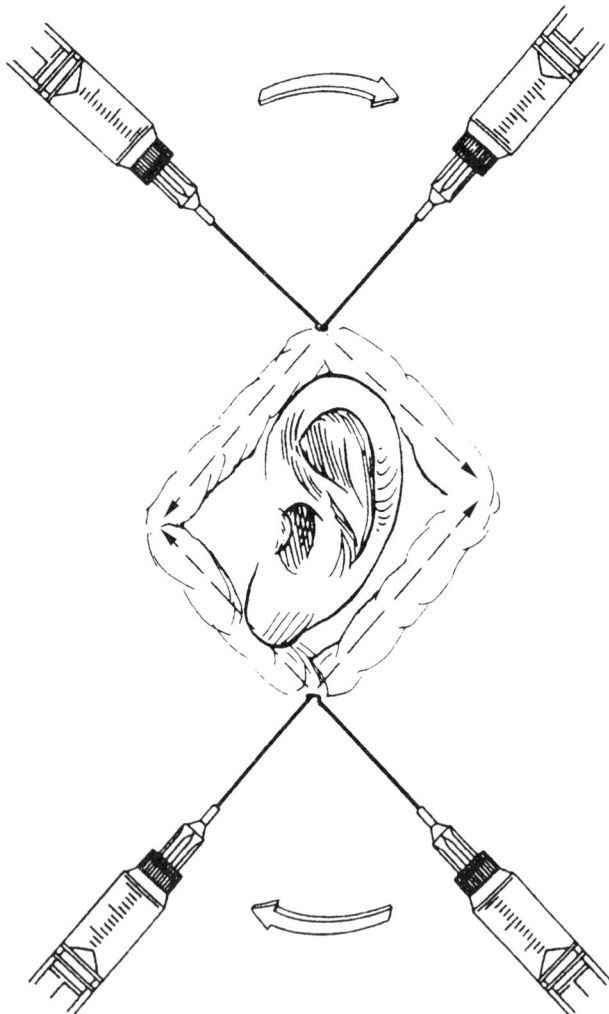

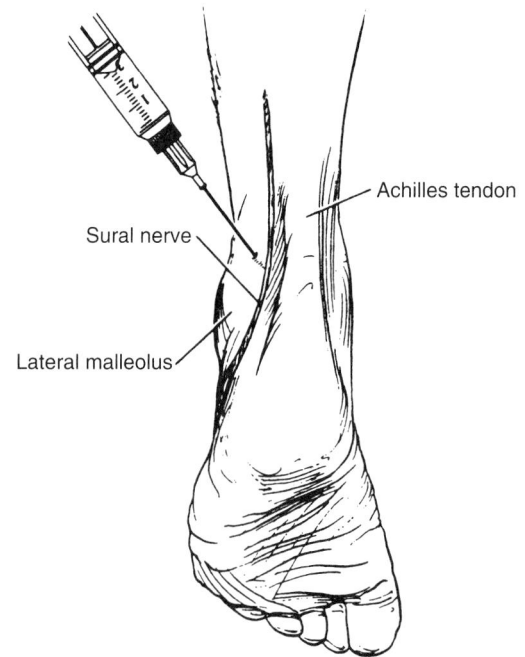

Fig. 8-8
A, Ear block. Dots show insertion sites of needles. Arrows show direction of needles injecting anesthetic. (Modified from Robinson JK: *Atlas of cutaneous surgery,* Philadelphia, 1996, WB Saunders.)
B, Alternative technique to achieve field anesthesia of the ear. (From Trott A: *Wounds and lacerations: emergency care and closure,* ed 3, St Louis, 1997, Mosby.)

Fig. 8-10
Location of the sural nerve block. (From Trott A: *Wounds and lacerations: emergency care and closure,* ed 3, St Louis, 1997, Mosby.)

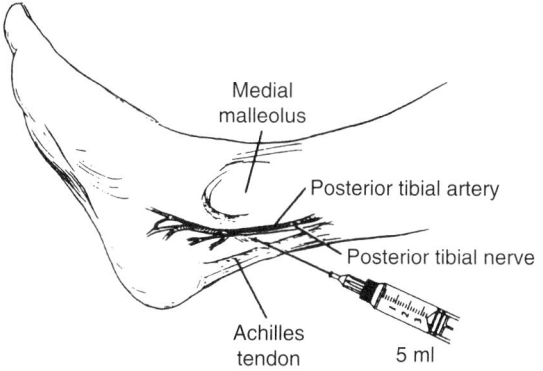

Fig. 8-11
Location of the tibial nerve block. (From, Trott A: *Wounds and lacerations: emergency care and closure,* ed 3, St Louis, 1997, Mosby.)

ICD-9-CM DIAGNOSTIC CODES

ICD-9-CM codes are variable depending on the diagnosis.

ADDITIONAL RESOURCES

- See the sample patient education handout titled "Peripheral Nerve Blocks and Field Blocks" on page 1744 of Appendix G.
- See the sample patient consent form titled "Peripheral Nerve Blocks and Field Blocks" on page 1745 of Appendix G.

BIBLIOGRAPHY

Gillette RD: *Procedures in ambulatory care,* New York, 1987, McGraw-Hill.

Hahn MB, McQuillan PM, Sheplock GJ, editors: *Regional anesthesia,* St Louis, 1996, Mosby.

Homes HS: Options for painless local anesthesia, *Postgrad Med J* 89(30):71, 1991.

Lebowitz PW, Newberg LA, Gilette MT, editors: *Clinical anesthesia procedures of the Massachusetts General Hospital,* Boston, 1982, Little, Brown & Co.

Mulroy MF: *Regional anesthesia: an illustrated procedural guide,* Boston, 1989, Little, Brown.

Robinson JK, Arndt KA, LeBoit PE, Wintroub BU, editors: *Atlas of cutaneous surgery,* Philadelphia, 1996, WB Saunders.

Simon RR, Brenner BE: *Anesthesia and regional blocks in emergency procedures and techniques,* ed 3, Baltimore, 1994, William & Wilkins. *(Editorial note: This is an excellent resource.)*

Trott A: *Wounds and lacerations: emergency care and closure,* ed 3, St Louis, 1997, Mosby.

Wolcott MW, editor: *Ambulatory surgery and the basics of emergency surgical care,* ed 2, Philadelphia, 1988, JB Lippincott.

WEBSITES

www.sambahq.org (Society for Ambulatory Anesthesia)
www.soba.org (Society for Office Based Anesthesia)

CHAPTER 9

Oral/Facial Anesthesia

Larry Skoczylas

The ability to perform site specific and facial regional nerve blocks is an important adjunct to almost any medical practice. Physicians are often the first practitioners to evaluate facial pain. This pain may be due to trauma, localized swelling and infection, or even facial neuralgias and tics. Properly infiltrated local anesthetic can eliminate discomfort when closing wounds, can provide pain control to a patient with a tooth abscess until he or she can be treated, or can be used as a diagnostic test to see if a suspected neuralgia is due to a peripheral or a central source. If peripheral, pain should be eliminated by the anesthesia. If central, it may not be.

This discussion involves both intraoral and extraoral anesthetic techniques. Therefore an understanding of regional anatomy is crucial to properly perform these infiltrations and nerve blocks. The sensory innervation of the face and oral cavity is primarily from the trigeminal nerve (fifth cranial nerve). This nerve is divided into ophthalmic (V_1), maxillary (V_2), and mandibular branches (V_3) (Figs. 9-1 and 9-2).

The *ophthalmic division* is purely sensory and supplies the eyeball, conjunctiva, lacrimal gland, parts of the mucous membrane of the nose, paranasal sinuses, and the skin of the forehead, eyes, and nose. When this nerve is paralyzed, the ocular conjunctiva becomes insensitive to touch. Sensory anesthesia of V_1 is usually obtained by local infiltration with a supraperiosteal extraoral block.

The *maxillary division,* like the ophthalmic division, is purely sensory. It supplies innervation to the skin of the middle portion of the face, lower eyelid, side of the nose, upper lip, maxillary teeth, and periodontal tissues. In addition, this nerve is sensory to the mucous membrane of the nasopharynx, maxillary sinus, tonsils, and hard and soft palate. This nerve can be blocked by both intraoral and extraoral injection.

The *mandibular division* has a large sensory as well as a small motor component. Blockage of the motor division can lead to decreased muscle function of the masseter, temporalis, pterygoid, mylohyoid, digastric, and soft palate elevators. Sensory innervation is to the temporal region and ear, cheek, lower lip and chin, parotid gland, TMJ and mastoid area. Orally, the mandibular teeth and periosteal tissues, bone of the mandible, anterior two thirds of the tongue, and all intraoral mucosa are affected. The majority of anesthetic given for the mandibular division is intraoral, although some extraoral blocks may be indicated.

GENERAL CONSIDERATIONS
INDICATIONS

- Whenever anesthesia is desired in a fairly large anatomic area
- To limit the amount of medication given
- For laceration repair or lesion removal
- Around infection sites for incision and drainage
- To limit distortion of tissues and allow a better repair
- To anesthetize periosteum before more painful subperiosteal procedures such as tooth removal
- As a diagnostic block to determine cause or site of pain
- To control pain

CONTRAINDICATIONS

- History of allergy or reaction to local anesthetics (or bisulfite preservatives).
- Risk of hematoma (e.g., in hemophiliacs or with anticoagulant use). Trauma to vascular bundles can increase risk of bleeding and hematoma *(relative contraindication).*
- Uncooperative patients (e.g., pediatric or mentally retarded may require sedation before local anesthetic) *(relative contraindication).*

COMPLICATIONS

See Chapter 5, Local and Topical Anesthetic Complications.

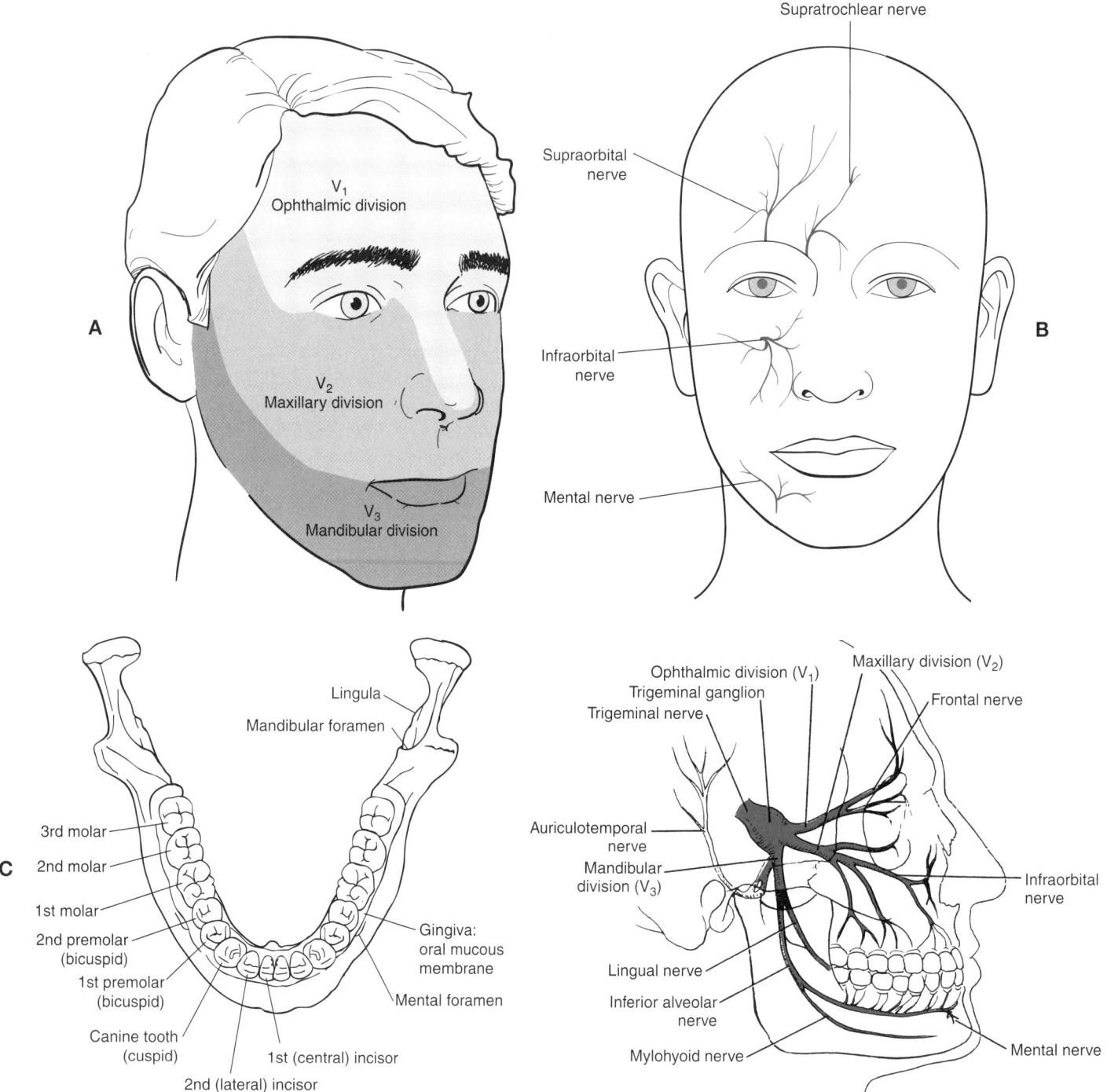

Fig. 9-1

Sensory innervation of the face and oral cavity is primarily from the trigeminal nerve. **A,** The trigeminal nerve is divided into three branches: the ophthalmic branch (V$_1$), the maxillary branch (V$_2$), and the mandibular branch (V$_3$). **B,** Sensory distribution of the terminal branches of the trigeminal nerve. Supratrochlear nerve (ST), supraorbital nerve (SO), infraorbital nerve (IO), and mental nerve (M). **C,** Anatomy of the mandibular arch and the lower teeth. **D,** Distribution of the trigeminal nerve. (**D,** Modified from Roberts JR, Hedges JR: *Clinical procedures in emergency medicine,* ed 2, Philadelphia, 1991, WB Saunders.)

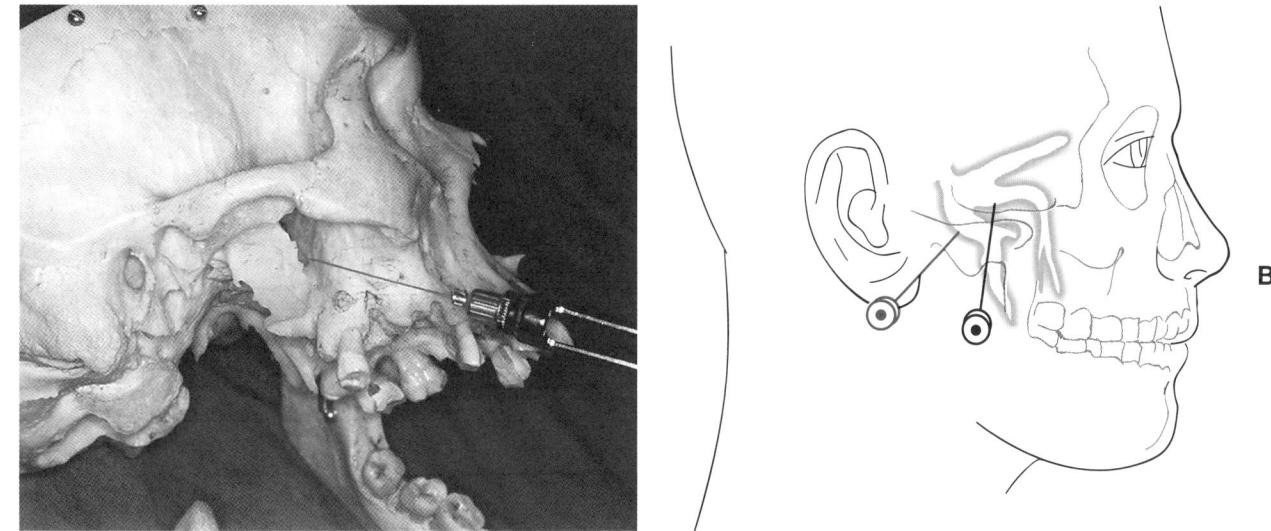

Fig. 9-2
A, Maxillary nerve block. Angle of needle to obtain intraoral maxillary (V₂) block. **B,** Location of needles for extraoral block (not described). The black needle is shown blocking the maxillary branch; the red needle is shown blocking the mandibular branch. Note that needles are not injected directly into the nerve.

- *Syncope:* Most common untoward reaction to anesthetic injections, often resulting from pain during the injection. A semisupine or supine position and slow injection technique are recommended.
- *Broken needle:* Very rare, but it is best to always leave some needle showing and to not "bury" to the hub when injecting.
- *Hematoma:* Rare, often resulting from torn capillaries or vessels that are punctured during injection.
- *Persistent paresthesia:* Occurs after the anesthetic should have worn off. Indicates damage to the nerve from physical or local chemical trauma. Can be temporary or permanent.
- *Ischemic ulcer:* Usually resulting from vasoconstrictor use in relatively *avascular* tissue (e.g., subperiosteally in the hard palate). Skin is very vascular and ischemia is extremely rare when local anesthetic with epinephrine of a low concentration (1/100,000 or 1/200,000) is used.
- *Blanching:* Occurs at the site of injection because of pressure of anesthetic and vasoconstriction. If remote from the injection site, then it is probably due to inadvertent intravascular injection. No treatment is needed.
- *Tachycardia:* Can occur from pain of injection, but it is most likely due to intravascular injection of or rapid absorption of local anesthetic with epinephrine.
- *Paralysis:* Results from inadvertent anesthesia of facial nerve (seventh cranial nerve). It is usually temporary. If longer-acting anesthetics such as bupivacaine are used and patient cannot close the eyelid, the lid can be

taped down (to avoid dryness of the eye) until the anesthetic wears off.
- *Visual disturbance:* Rare, probably due to vascular spasm or intraarterial injection. Normal vision usually returns in about 30 minutes.
- *Overdosage:* Seizures and cardiac arrhythmias

EQUIPMENT

- 10-ml syringe with Luer-Lok hub (for aspiration)
- 1- or 1½-inch (25 to 30 gauge) needle
- Local anesthetic, such as 2% lidocaine with or without 1:100,000 epinephrine, or 0.5% bupivacaine with or without 1:200,000 epinephrine
- Mepivacaine (pka 7.6) (may give better anesthesia in infected tissue, which usually has an acidic environment [pka <7.5])
- Dental aspirating syringe (a good alternative; would need specific anesthetic carpules and needles for this system)

SPECIFIC INJECTION TECHNIQUES
TECHNIQUE (GENERAL)

1. Anesthetic solution is usually deposited just above the bone around the nerve trunks in the submucosa or subcutaneous tissue, where the nerves exit from the bone itself (e.g., supraorbital, infraorbital, or mental nerves). This technique is known as a

supraperiosteal injection. It may be approached from either an intraoral or extraoral route, depending on the nerve block desired.

2. If going through facial skin, clean the skin with alcohol. If giving local anesthetic to repair traumatic lacerations, clean thoroughly with normal saline. Tent or support the tissue and slowly infiltrate (for 30 to 60 seconds) into the area to be addressed. Identify landmarks before infiltration; they can become "ballooned" and hard to appreciate after local anesthetic is given.

3. If going through the oral mucosa, tissues are rarely scrubbed before injection. Cleaning any obvious debris in a trauma site with normal saline is indicated prior to closure. Lift up and tent lips or cheek. The target of the injection should be the procedure site.

INTRAORAL APPROACHES

MAXILLARY (V₂) NERVE BLOCK: INTRAORAL (Figs. 9-1 and 9-2)

Indications

- Anesthesia of the entire hemimaxilla for trauma repair or pathological surgery
- For diagnostic blocks of the second division of the trigeminal nerve to evaluate neuralgias and tics
- To aid in anesthetizing infected sites or areas of tooth removal

Advantage

- Decreases the amount of anesthetic solution used and the number of injection sites needed for maxillary anesthesia

Technique

1. Place patient in a semi-supine position. Partially open the patient's mouth and pull mandible toward side of injection (mandible to right for upper right injection).
2. Pull taut and retract cheek with index finger to gain visibility.
3. Aim for the area posterior and lateral to back of upper jaw (pterygopalatine fossa area). The area of insertion is the height of the mucobuccal fold above the distal aspect of the upper wisdom tooth area (lateral to the approximate junction of the hard and soft palate). Orient the bevel of the needle toward the bone.
4. Advance the needle slowly in the superomedial

direction to a depth of about 30 mm (if necessary, measure on the needle beforehand to get an idea of the length).

5. No resistance should be felt. If resistance is noted, the angle of the needle toward the midline is too great.
6. Aspirate and deposit the local anesthetic (2 to 3 ml); continue to aspirate intermittently throughout the course of injection.

MANDIBULAR (V₃) INTRAORAL INFERIOR ALVEOLAR NERVE BLOCK (Figs. 9-1 and 9-3)

Indications

- For anesthesia of entire hemimandible. Can be achieved bilaterally if anesthesia of entire mandible or anterior mandible is needed.
- For fracture repair, bone biopsy, removal of teeth, or pain control resulting from tooth infection or swelling.

Disadvantages

- Not 100% successful (80% to 85%).
- Blind technique (by palpating landmarks). Intraoral swelling can make palpation of landmarks difficult.
- Intraoral landmarks are different in children than in adults. The lingula (a small bony bump) of the inner ramus of the mandible (where the nerve enters the jaw) is at a lower level in children.

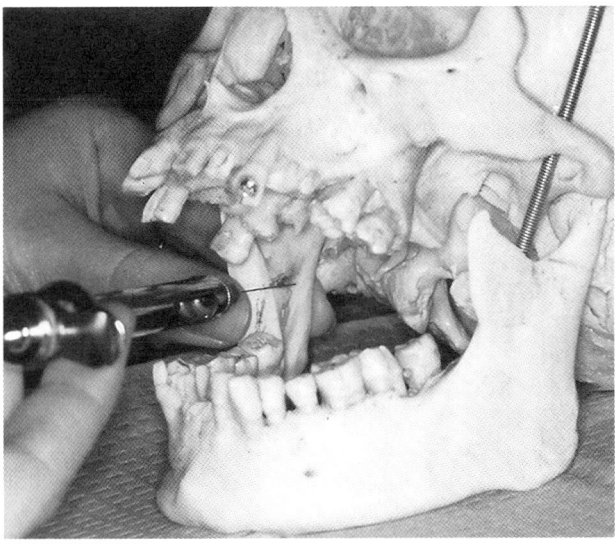

Fig. 9-3
Site of intraoral mandibular (V₃) inferior alveolar block.

Technique

1. Place the patient in a semi-supine position and instruct him or her to keep the mouth open.
2. The target site is the lingula, a small bony bump about half way back on the inner ramus of the mandible, where the inferior alveolar nerve enters the jaw.
3. Place the *thumb* of the noninjecting hand over the pterygomandibular raphe (the band of tissue in the posterior cheek between the upper and lower wisdom teeth). Use the thumb to pull the tissue laterally until the *deepest* depression in the anterior border of the ramus is felt. This creates a tense area for needle penetration.
4. Gently grasp the posterior border of the mandible with the middle finger of the noninjecting hand, as high superiorly as the ear allows. The line between the thumb and finger establishes the vertical height of the target area on the inner aspect of the ramus. The lingula should always be on or just below this line (and will always be below this line in children).
5. The anterior-posterior position of the nerve (the target site) is located midway between the thumb and middle fingers. The line of needle insertion is an oblique angle estimated by placing the barrel of the syringe over the bicuspid teeth (or midmandibular body region) of the opposite side.
6. The needle is inserted to the target site until bone is gently contacted. Depth of penetration is 1 to 2 cm. Always leave part of the needle showing to identify direction. Correct length should be about one half to three fourths of a 1½-inch needle.
7. If bone is contacted before half the length of the needle is inserted, the angle of penetration is usually too anterior. If no bone is contacted, the angle is too parallel to the inner aspect of the ramus of the mandible. In these instances it is best to withdraw the needle and start again.
8. Aspirate and slowly inject over 60 seconds. Continue to aspirate intermittently while injecting.

AKINOSI INTRAORAL CLOSED MOUTH MANDIBULAR (V₃) BLOCK
(Fig. 9-4)

Indications

- For mandibular V₃ anesthesia
- When the patient is unable to open his or her mouth because of pain, swelling, trismus, or infection
- For an uncooperative patient
- When conventional mandibular block has failed

Technique

1. Place the patient in the same position as that for the V₃ block.
2. Place the noninjecting finger (the thumb may be too big) at the greatest depression of the anterior ramus, as previously described for the V₃ block.
3. Identify the maxillary tuberosity—essentially a rounded area of bone just past the upper wisdom tooth area intraorally, which is the end of the maxillary bone.
4. Hold the barrel of the syringe parallel to the plane of upper teeth, with the bevel of the needle toward the midline of the upper jaw.
5. The needle is inserted at the gingival (gum) level, about 0.5 cm superior to the tooth-gum interface.
6. Advance the needle between your finger and the maxillary tuberosity about 25 mm into the tissue, directing the needle slightly laterally to stay parallel to the plane of upper teeth.
7. Aspirate and inject 2 to 3 ml of local anesthetic slowly over 60 seconds. Motor nerve paralysis of the masseter and lateral pterygoid muscles often occurs and can help decrease trismus. There can also be a facial nerve palsy if injection is through the sigmoid notch of the mandibular ramus and into the parotid gland. Maintaining the correct depth of penetration will help decrease this complication.

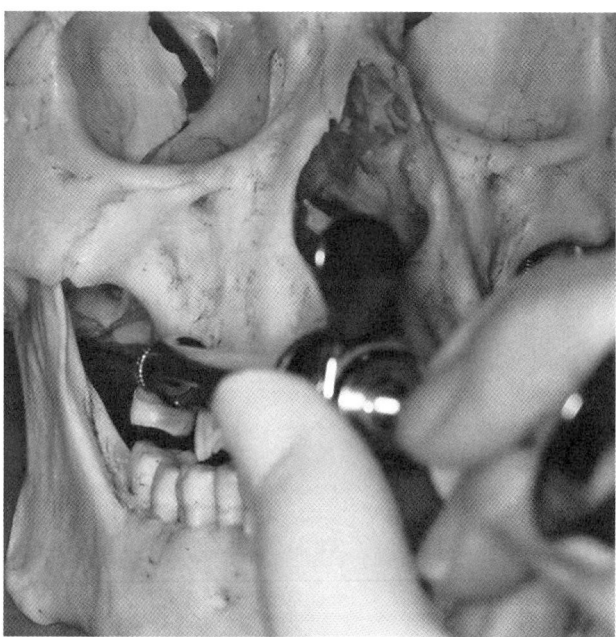

Fig. 9-4
Position of needle for closed mouth Akinosi intraoral mandibular (V₃) block.

EXTRAORAL TECHNIQUES

EXTRAORAL BLOCK OF INFRAORBITAL NERVE (Figs. 9-1 and 9-5)

Indications

- To anesthetize upper face, lips, or nose for trauma repair or excision.
- To provide local anesthetic effect when infection intraorally causes too much pain to tolerate intraoral injection.
- For diagnostic nerve block for neuralgias or tics.

This is an easy block to administer, whether the intraoral or extraoral approach is used. It is also frequently employed since it avoids the distortion created by direct local injection when lip repair and fine approximation are needed to avoid unsightly scars.

Disadvantage

- Technique performed by blind palpation of infraorbital foramen.

Technique

1. Palpate the infraorbital foramen just below the lowest level of the infraorbital rim, on a line between the pupil and the corner of the mouth.
2. Approach the infraorbital nerve from 1 cm below the bony rim and slightly medial to the palpated foramen. It is *not* necessary to enter the infraorbital foramen.
3. Slowly deposit 1 to 3 ml of local anesthetic. Paresthesia of the upper lip is sometimes (but not always) noted when the nerve is touched by the needle before injection.

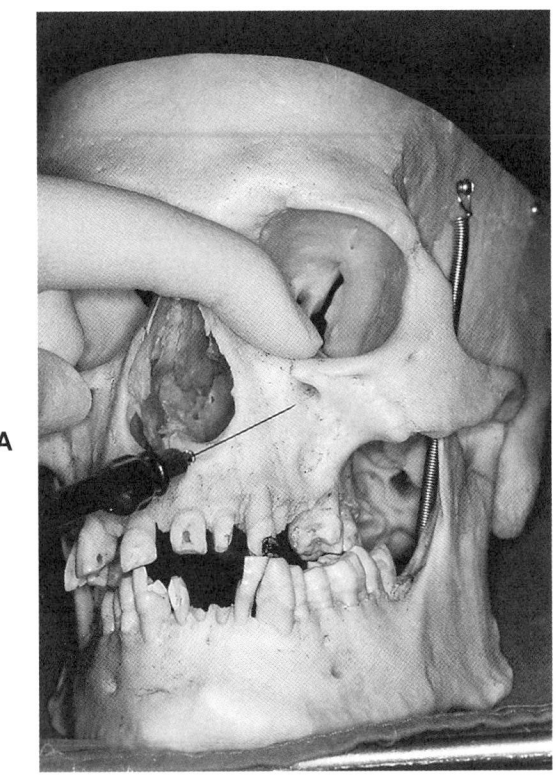

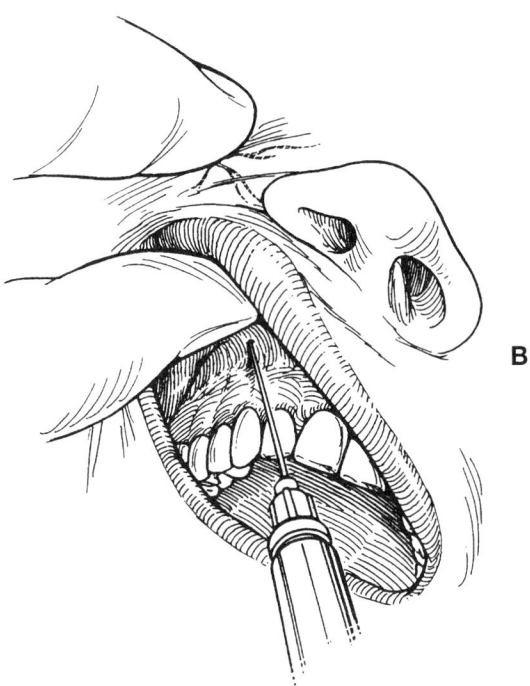

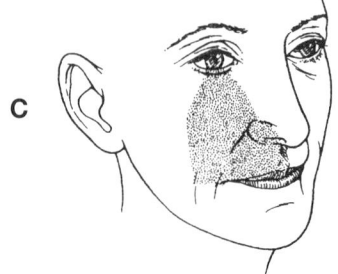

Fig. 9-5
A, Proper location for an extraoral infraorbital nerve block. **B,** Intraoral infraorbital nerve block (see text). **C,** Area of anesthesia obtained with infraorbital blocks. (**B** and **C,** From Rosen P, Chan TC, Vilke GM, Sternbach G, editors: *Atlas of emergency procedures,* St Louis, 2001, Mosby.)

4. For an intraoral approach, use the same anatomic landmarks, and approach the nerve through the mucobuccal fold over the maxillary second bicuspid, aiming at the infraorbital foramen. A long needle will be needed.

MAXILLARY EXTRAORAL BLOCK OF SUPRAORBITAL AND SUPRATROCHLEAR NERVES (Fig. 9-6)

Indications

- To anesthetize the forehead (supraorbital nerve lateral, supratrochlear nerve medial)
- Use with infraorbital block to anesthetize periorbital tissues

Technique

1. Palpate the supraorbital foramen, which lies just superior to the supraorbital notch. This lies on a vertical line with the pupil when the eye is focused forward.
2. Insert the needle just above the notch and inject 2 to 4 ml of anesthetic. You do *not* need to be injecting directly into the foramen to block the supraorbital nerve.
3. The supratrochlear nerve can be blocked by redirect-

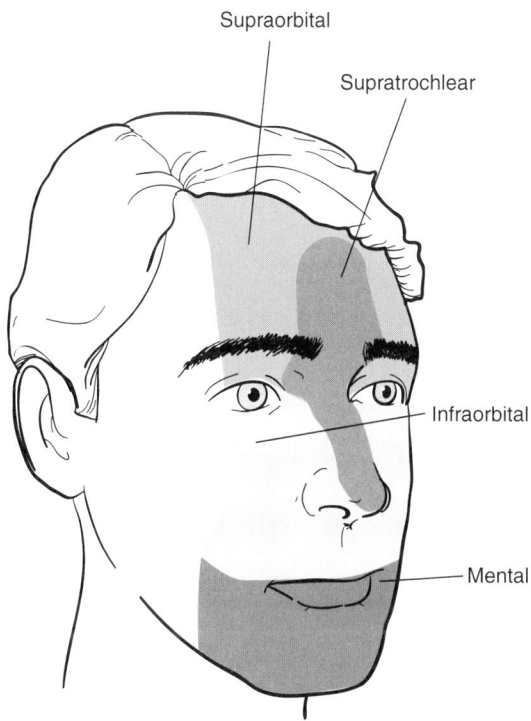

Supraorbital

Supratrochlear

Infraorbital

Mental

Fig. 9-6
Sensory distribution of the terminal branches.

ing the needle to 1 cm below and medial to the supraorbital foramen, staying on the bony rim, and injecting another 2 ml.

MANDIBULAR EXTRAORAL MENTAL NERVE BLOCK (Figs. 9-1 and 9-7)

Indications

- To anesthetize lower lip and chin area for trauma repair or excision
- To provide local anesthetic effect when infection intraorally causes too much pain to tolerate intraoral injection
- For diagnostic nerve blocks for lower face neuralgias and tics

Disadvantage

- Technique performed by blind approximation of the mental nerve position in the mandible.

Technique

1. Approach the mandible extraorally from a position below the bicuspid teeth. The mental nerve foramen is located in the middle of the lower jaw on a line exactly vertically down from the previously described infraorbital nerve foramen. (This area can also be approached vertically from the inferior border of the mandible.)
2. Enter the skin with the needle perpendicular to the bone. Advance the needle until bone is touched, then back off 2 to 3 mm. It is *not* necessary to enter the mental foramen.
3. Deposit 1 to 3 ml of local anesthetic. Paresthesia of the lower lip is sometimes (but not always) noted when the nerve is touched by the needle.
4. The mental nerve can also be approached intraorally. The needle is inserted in front of the teeth at the junction of the gum and lip mucosa at the level of the premolar/molar teeth (fifth tooth from the midline). Direct the needle inferiorly just above bone for approximately 1 cm and inject 2 to 3 ml of anesthetic.

NOSE: SKIN AND NASAL MUCOSA (Fig. 9-8)

Indications

- For paranasal biopsy, or repair of bony or soft tissue nasal trauma (anesthesia for elective rhinoplasty is quite specific and will not be covered)

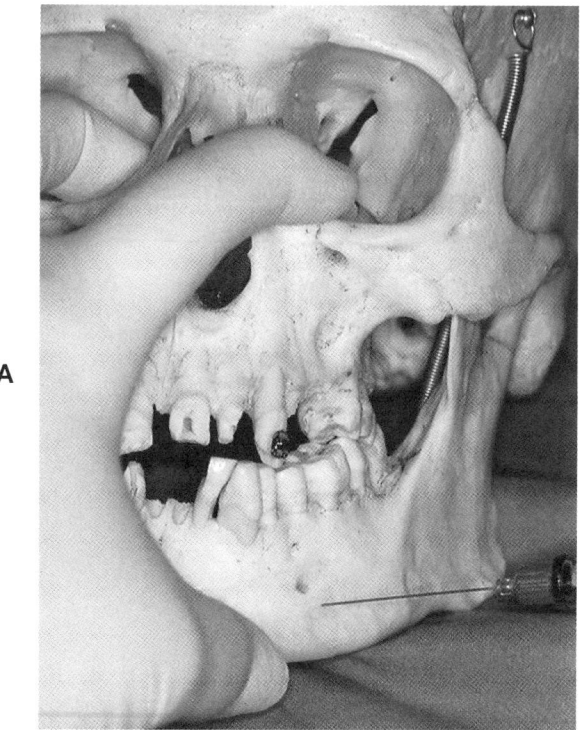

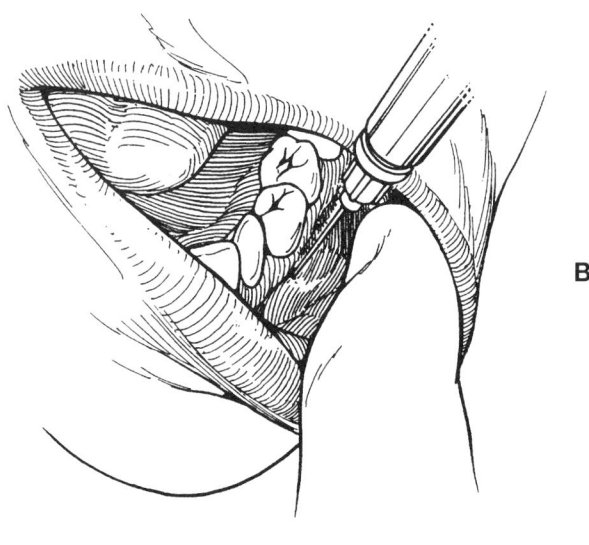

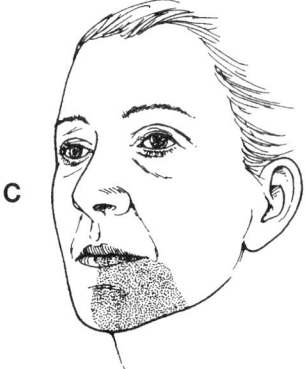

Fig. 9-7
A, Site of extraoral mental nerve block. **B,** Intraoral approach. **C,** Area of anesthesia obtained with mental nerve block. (**B** and **C,** From Rosen P, Chan TC, Vilke GM, Sternbach G, editors: *Atlas of emergency procedures,* St Louis, 2001, Mosby.)

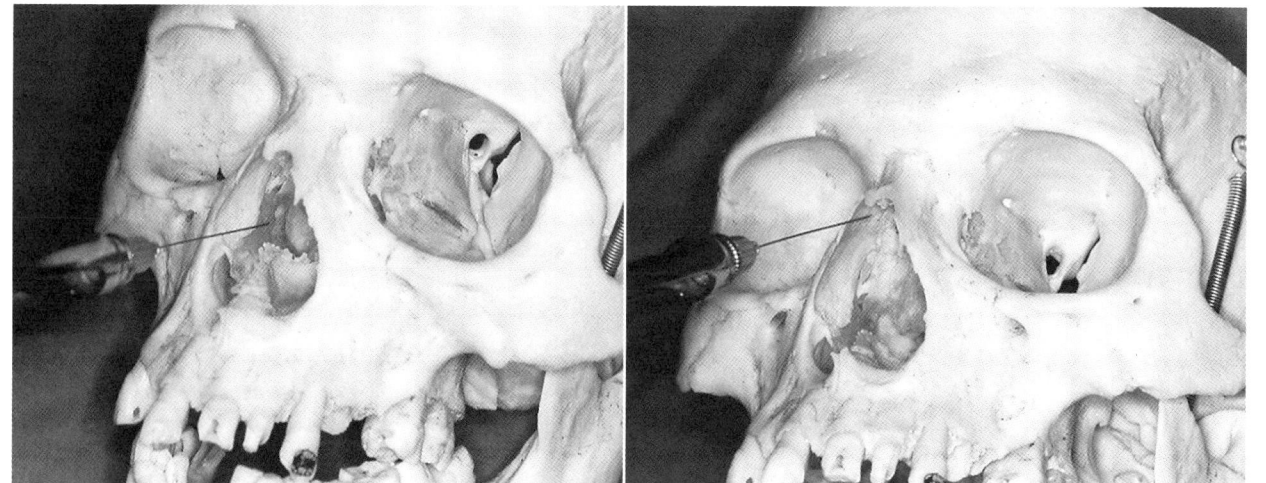

Fig. 9-8
Obtaining nasal septal anesthesia. **A,** Area of septal infiltration. **B,** Area of nasal bones subperiosteally.

• Often used in conjunction with extraoral infraorbital nerve block for nasal procedures

Disadvantage

• Can be painful to administer in awake patient.

Technique

1. Apply topical spray anesthetic to each nostril.
2. Q-Tips with 4% cocaine solution are used to paint the nasal mucosa. Leave in place for 5 minutes. This may be contraindicated in cardiac patients.
3. Perform bilateral infraorbital nerve blocks, extraoral technique (see above).
4. Infiltrate the skin along the base of the nares, and continue as subcutaneous infiltration up the nasal-facial crease.
5. Inject the septal mucosa with local anesthetic containing vasoconstrictor to help decrease bleeding, especially in nasal or septal fractures. Use 1½-inch needle and inject from posterior to anterior. Now inject subperiosteally between the nasal bones and the tissue, and along the lateral nasal region.

CPT/BILLING CODE

64400   Injection, anesthetic agent; trigeminal nerve, any division or branch

BIBLIOGRAPHY

Allen GD: *Dental anesthesia and analgesia (local and general),* Baltimore, 1984, Williams & Wilkins.

Bramhall J: Regional anesthesia for aesthetic surgery. In Kaminer MS, Dover JS, Arndt KA, editors: *Atlas of cosmetic surgery,* Philadelphia, 2002, WB Saunders.

Edlich EF, Rodeheaver GT, Thacker JG: Local and regional anesthesia for wound repair. In Tintinalli JE, Krome RL, Ruiz E, editors: *Emergency medicine: a comprehensive study guide,* ed 5, New York, 1996, McGraw-Hill.

Katz, J: *Atlas of regional anesthesia,* Norwalk, 1985, Appleton-Century-Crofts.

Malamed, SF: *Handbook of local anesthesia,* St Louis, 1990, Mosby.

Roberts GJ, Rosenbaum NL: *Color atlas of dental anesthesia and sedation,* Alesbury, England, 1991, Hazell Books.

CHAPTER 10

Trigger-Point Injection

Gary E. Ruoff

Both myofascial pain syndromes and fibromyalgia demonstrate trigger-point involvement. Trigger points are tender spots or muscle hardenings located in different muscle groups, often near bony attachments (Fig. 10-1). Interruption of the pain cycle by trigger-point injection as well as spray-and-stretch maneuvers might produce prolonged relief. Also, passive stretching after trigger-point therapy might provide additional benefit.

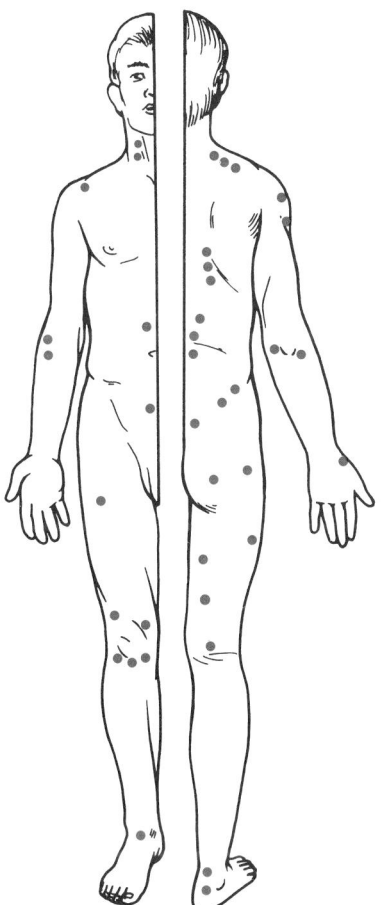

Fig. 10-1
Common points of maximal tenderness. Note predominant locations at moving parts and sliding surfaces.

Adjunctive therapies include acupressure, heat or ice massage, and electrical stimulation. The mechanism of action of injecting these points is not known, since saline solution injection alone often relieves the discomfort.

INDICATIONS

- Focal tender area identifiable by palpation without other identifiable neurologic or musculoskeletal findings or pathology. May be caused by trauma, muscle tension, or repetitive motion activities.

CONTRAINDICATIONS

- Infection at the site of the needle insertion
- Concomitant use of an anticoagulant
- Hemorrhagic syndrome
- Septicemia
- Resuscitation equipment not available
- Significant psychiatric disturbance
- Untreated, underlying endocrinopathy if diffuse and multiple trigger points are present (hypothyroidism, estrogen deficiency, hypoparathyroidism and hyperparathyroidism, pituitary disorders, and Cushing's disease)

PREPROCEDURE PATIENT PREPARATION AND EVALUATION

- Provide the patient with a detailed explanation about the procedure and obtain informed consent. A signed (written) form is generally not necessary.
- Explain to the patient that the "area of pain reference" is caused by irritation of an area known as a "trigger point," and at times it may be somewhat distant from the site of pain.
- Palpate the various muscle groups to locate the trigger point and the corresponding "area of pain reference" (point of maximal tenderness [PMT]).

- Explain to the patient that the periods of immediate relief resulting from the treatment can be followed by pain greater than the original pain, and that follow-up injections may be necessary.

EQUIPMENT

- Alcohol wipes.
- Gloves.
- Several gauze pads.
- Skin-marking pencil.
- Antiseptic solution.
- Lidocaine (0.25% to 1% *without* epinephrine) or bupivacaine (0.125% to 0.25%); steroid can also be used along with the local anesthetic. (Dosage varies, depending on agent used, but generally a very small amount is needed.)
- 22-, 25-, or 27-gauge needles of varying lengths, depending on site to be injected.
- 3-, 5-, or 10-ml syringes.
- Resuscitation equipment (as for any injection).

TECHNIQUE

1. Place the patient in a comfortable or recumbent position to protect the patient in the event of a vasovagal reaction, such as syncope.
2. Identify the trigger point or PMT by systematically palpating the area to localize the area of pain. If necessary, grasp the area between the thumb and forefinger to stabilize. (Often, muscle spasms or a nodule can be palpated.)
3. Mark the precise site with a marking pencil.
4. Prepare the skin with an antiseptic solution or alcohol.
5. Use a 25-gauge needle—or a 27-gauge needle when possible—for superficial muscle injections.
6. Begin with 5 ml of lidocaine (0.25% to 1%) or bupivacaine (0.125% or 0.25%).
7. Inject 0.25 to 0.50 ml of local anesthetic into the skin to produce a weal *(optional)*.
8. Slowly advance the needle perpendicular to the skin until the trigger point is identified.
9. Aspirate through the needle to determine if a blood vessel has been punctured.
10. Inject 0.5 to 2 ml of solution once the trigger point is located. The patient should experience immediate relief if the injection is properly located.
11. Withdraw the needle slightly and reinject the site two or three times (Fig. 10-2).
12. Remove the needle, and wipe the skin clean with a disinfectant.
13. After withdrawing the needle, massage the entire

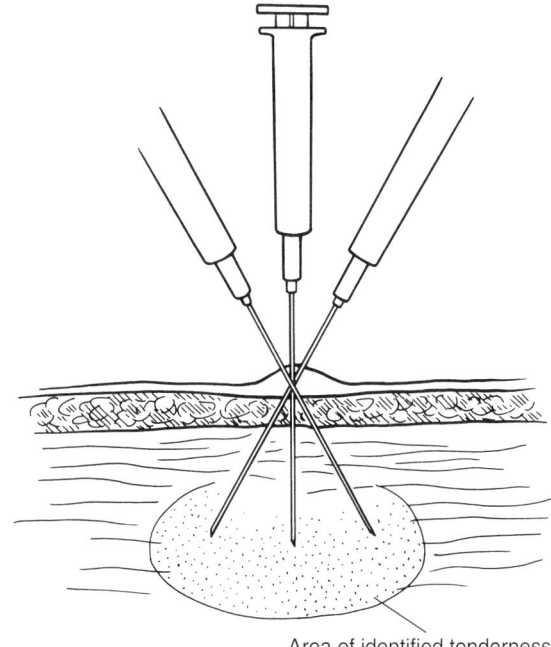

Area of identified tenderness

Fig. 10-2
Injection of a trigger point.

area to diffuse the anesthetic and check for pain relief. It might be necessary to reinject or expand the pattern to relieve all pain. Pain relief should be evident within minutes.

Note: Never inject more than 10 ml of solution into any one trigger-point area. No more than 4.5 mg/kg of lidocaine, or 300 mg maximum for all sites, is to be used at any one time (1% lidocaine = 10 mg/ml). Trigger-point injection may be repeated as frequently as needed if no steroids are used. To break the cycle of pain, an injection may be required every 3 to 4 days.

POSTPROCEDURE CARE

- Observe for a decrease in the patient's pain, which should be almost immediate.
- Observe for signs and symptoms such as lightheadedness, tinnitus, peripheral numbness, slurring of speech, drowsiness, or evidence of seizure activity. These may indicate a toxic reaction to the local anesthetic.
- Observe for any bleeding into skin or muscle compartment.
- Assign stretching exercises, physical therapy, or rest as indicated.
- Warn the patient that pain may recur and actually may worsen for 1 to 2 days.
- See the patient in 3 to 4 days to check for compliance with stretching exercises and to evaluate the need for

another injection. Four to five injections may be necessary per site over a fairly short period.

- Advise that steroids can be added if needed and that antidepressants often provide additional relief.
- Consider physical or massage therapy.

COMPLICATIONS

- Vasovagal syncope.
- Skin infection.
- Toxic reactions to the local anesthetic.
- Hematoma formation.
- Neuritis.
- Rebound pain.
- Pneumothorax (if injecting over thorax). Avoid this if possible by positioning the injection area over the top of a rib. Point the needle tangentially instead of vertically. Have the patient hold his or her breath during the injection.
- Compartment syndrome.

CPT/BILLING CODES

J code	As appropriate for the steroid used
20552	Injection; single or multiple trigger point(s), one or two muscle group(s)
20553	Injection; single or multiple trigger point(s), three or more muscle groups

ICD-9-CM DIAGNOSTIC CODES

729.1	Fibromyalgia, myositis (also see "Pain" and specific sites)

ADDITIONAL RESOURCES

- See the sample patient consent form titled "Trigger-Point Injection" on page 1746 of Appendix G.

BIBLIOGRAPHY

Alvarez DJ, Rockwell PG: Trigger points: diagnosis and management, *Am Fam Physician* 65(4):653, 2002.

Andres E, Sola AE, Bonica JJ: Myofascial pain syndromes. In Bonica JJ, editor: *The management of pain,* ed 2, Philadelphia, 1990, Lea & Febiger.

Bonica JJ: Management of myofascial pain syndromes in general practice, *JAMA* 146:732, 1957.

Christiani AK, Wallis D: Trigger point injection. In *Clinics atlas of office procedures,* Philadelphia, 2002, WB Saunders.

Driscoll CE, Rakel RF: *"Trigger point injection" in patient care: procedures for your practice,* ed 2, Los Angeles, 1991, Practice Management Information.

Simons DG, Travell JG: Myofascial origins of low back pain, *Postgrad Med* 73(2):68, 1983.

Sola AE: Trigger point therapy. In Roberts JR, Hedges JR, editors: *Clinical procedures in emergency medicine,* Philadelphia, 1985, WB Saunders.

CHAPTER 11

Topical Anesthesia

William Dery

Topical anesthesia offers patients an alternative to local injectable anesthetics. The ideal topical anesthetic should provide 100% anesthesia on intact skin with rapid onset of action, have prolonged duration, and have no local or systemic side effects. To date the perfect topical agent has not been developed. Newer formulations have improved efficacy and application options for topical anesthetics. Various preparations are listed in Table 11-1. (Also see Chapter 215, Transcutaneous Electrical Nerve Stimulation, Phonophoresis, and Iontophoresis; Chapter 4, Local Anesthesia; and Chapter 5, Local and Topical Anesthetic Complications.)

Much has changed with topical anesthetics in recent years. TAC (tetracaine, adrenalin, and cocaine) used to be the workhorse. LET/LAT (lidocaine, epinephrine/adrenalin, tetracaine) solution-gel has been found to be equally efficacious when compared with TAC. LET eliminates cocaine (thus lessening the risk for toxicity-seizure), avoids documentation issues, and lowers the cost. Liposomes are man-made biological membranes that are composed of lipid layers surrounding aqueous layers. Liposomes are a new drug delivery system that allows medications to penetrate the stratum corneum more readily and is used in the liposomal lidocaine 4% cream (ELA-Max) preparation. In addition to shortening the onset of action, liposomes do not cause local irritation, can control the release of the drug delivered, and allow for a longer duration of action. ELA-Max can replace or augment local anesthetics. EMLA (eutectic, mixture of local anesthetics) and liposomal lidocaine are the future workhorses as topical anesthetics.

Iontophoresis is an advanced method of delivering topical anesthetics and is discussed in Chapter 215.

INDICATIONS

LET/LAT

Scalp and facial lacerations.

TAC/Half TAC

Replaced by safer medications.

EMLA/EMLA Disc

Food and Drug Administration (FDA): For use on normal *intact* skin for local anesthesia.

ELA-Max

FDA: Temporary relief of pain associated with minor cuts, abrasions, minor burns, skin irritation, and insect bites.

Literature-supported uses: venipuncture, venous cannulation, arterial puncture, suture removal, shave biopsy, punch biopsy, chemical peels, curettage of molluscum contagiosum, cryotherapy of venereal warts, intracutaneous allergy testing, epilation, debridement of otitis media with an intact tympanic membrane, removal of an embedded foreign body, circumcision at more than a 37-week gestation, skin grafting, debridement of ulcers, lumbar puncture.

Adjunct to: vasectomy, dermabrasion, laser resurfacing, postsurgical discomfort.

Nonsurgical uses: postherpetic neuralgia, meralgia paresthetica.

Lidocaine Acid

Lidocaine in acid mantle uses compounds to hydrate skin to increase absorption. Not studied as well as EMLA and may not be as effective when used in laser procedures. Intact skin only.

Lidoderm Patch

FDA: Relief of pain associated with postherpetic neuralgia.

TABLE 11-1

Summary of Topical Anesthetics

Agents	Concentration	Status	Maximum Dose or Area*	Onset of Action	Duration	Pregnancy Category†
Skin						
EMLA cream or anesthetic disc	2.5% Lidocaine/ 2.5% Prilocaine	Rx Rx	20 g/200 cm² for 7-12 y/o and >20 kg (A) and (C)*	60-120 min	180 min	B
ELA-Max cream	4% Lidocaine plus vitamin E, propyleneglycol, benzyl alcohol, lecithum, cholesterol, carborner-940, triethanolamine, polysorbate 80	OTC	100 cm² (A)	‡	‡	B
Amethocaine gel	4% Tetracaine	Europe	50 mg (A)	40 min	240 min	C
Lidocaine acid mantle (Novartis)	30%-40% Lidocaine	Rx		20 min	30-60 min	—
Ethyl chloride spray	Skin refrigerant	OTC		<1 min	Transient	—
Dermal						
TAC	0.5% Tetracaine/1:1000 epinephrine/11.8% cocaine	Compounded		10-20 min	30-60 min	C
"Half-strength" TAC	0.25% Tetracaine/1:2000 epinephrine/5.9% cocaine	Compounded				
LAT	4% Lidocaine/1:2000 epinephrine/1% tetracaine	Compounded				
Mucous Membrane						
Xylocaine		Rx	300 mg (A)/ 100 mg (C)	2-5 min	15-45 min	B
Viscous solution	2% Lidocaine			1-2 min	15-20 min	
Liquid	5% Lidocaine			2 min		
Ointment	2.5%, 5% Lidocaine					
Patch (Lidoderm)	5% Lidocaine					
Benzocaine						
Cetacaine						
spray	14% Benzocaine	Rx				
liquid	2% Tetracaine	Rx				
gel						
ointment						
Hurricane						
liquid	20% Benzocaine	OTC		<5 min	15-45 min	C
gel						
spray						
Cocaine solution	4% and 10%	C-II§	200 mg (A)	1-5 min	30-60 min	C
Ophthalmic						
Alcaine solution	0.5% Proparacaine	Rx		20 sec	15-20 min	C
Pontocaine solution	0.5% Tetracaine	Rx	50 mg (A)	20 sec	15-20 min	C

Adapted from Huang W, Vidimos A: *J Am Acad Dermatol* 43:286, 2000.
ELA-Max, Liposomal lidocaine 4% cream; *EMLA,* eutectic, mixture of local anesthetics; *LAT,* lidocaine, adrenalin, tetracaine; *OTC,* over the counter; *Rx,* prescription; *TAC,* tetracaine, adrenalin, cocaine.
*A, Adults; C, children.
†Pregnancy category B: Animal studies have not shown a fetal risk but there are no controlled studies in pregnant women. Pregnancy category C: Animal studies are not available. Safety for use during pregnancy has not been established. Use only when potential benefits outweigh potential hazards to the fetus.
‡No clinical studies.
§C-II: Controlled substances schedule II drug (Controlled Substances Act of 1970). Cocaine must be stored in a locked cabinet; and separate written records must be maintained for a period of 2 years after the drug is dispensed.

Thermal (Ice/Ethyl Chloride Spray) (Gebauer Co.)

Skin tag clipping, incision and drainage of simple abscess, and injections (blood draws, skin grafting, sports injuries).

Iontocaine

Iontophoretic procedures (80% to 100% effective): venipuncture, venous cannulation, arterial line, skin biopsy, fine needle biopsy, laser surgery, incision, superficial dermatologic procedures.

Xylocaine, Benzocaine (Mucous Membranes)

Painful, irritated, inflamed mucous membranes; anesthesia before minor surgical procedure and esophagogastroduodenoscopy; 2% viscous lidocaine for aphthous ulcers and mucositis in immunosuppressed patients.

Ophthalmic Preparations

Removal of foreign bodies, short eyelid procedures (e.g., chalazion removal), and placement of eyeshields.

CONTRAINDICATIONS

LET/LAT

Sensitivity to tetracaine, adrenaline, cocaine, and lidocaine.

TAC/Half TAC

- Contact with mucous membranes, compromised skin (denuded, infected, burned)
- Impaired circulation, end arterial locations (finger, nose, penis, toes), skin flap
- Cocaine: toxicity/seizure risks, arrhythmias
- Sites other than face/scalp: less efficacious

EMLA

- Advanced liver disease (hepatic metabolism)
- Methemoglobinemia risks (see Chapter 216, Venous Methylene Blue Therapy)

EMLA Disc

Sensitivity to lidocaine, prilocaine (rare).

ELA-Max

Avoid mucous membranes: absorption increases toxicity risks.

Efficacy diminishes as the skin thickness (lack of absorption) and vascularity (rapid clearance) increases. Physician should avoid palms and soles since they are ineffective even if occluded for hours.

Lidocaine

In acid mantle: creams contain parabens preservatives, and some patients are allergic. Use only on intact skin.

Lidoderm Patch

Sensitivity to lidocaine (rare); denuded skin; mucous membranes. Do not use more than 12 hours out of a 24-hour period to avoid toxicity.

Do not use in infants younger than 12 months of age with methemoglobin-inducing agents (Box 11-1).

Use with caution in infants under 3 months (maximum dose of 1 g for 1-hour application if term).

Thermal Ice/Ethyl Chloride Spray

Raynaud's phenomenon, cryoglobulinemia; not effective for skin biopsy, and alters specimen.

Iontocaine

Sensitivity to lidocaine, sulfite, and denuded skin.

Ophthalmic Preparations

- Not to be used to control pain long term.
- Inhibits healing and since no sensation, may lead to inadvertent trauma.
- May also eliminate blinking, leading to drying of cornea.

BOX 11-1
Agents Associated with Methemoglobinemia*

Acetaminophen	Nitroprusside
Acetanilid	Pamaquine
Aniline dyes	Para-aminosalicylic acid
Benzocaine	Phenacetin
Chloroquine	Phenobarbital
Dapsone	Phenytoin
Naphthalene	Primaquine
Nitrates and nitrites	Quinine
Nitrofurantoin	Sulfonamides
Nitroglycerin	

From Huang W, Vidimos A: *J Am Acad Dermatol* 43:286, 2000.
*Used with caution with eutectic, mixture of local anesthetics (EMLA).

TECHNIQUE

LET/LAT

Apply 1.5 to 3.0 ml of LET to a soaked gauze and wipe in and over a facial or scalp laceration, being careful to avoid mucous membranes. Contact with the wound should be a minimum of 10 minutes and a maximum of 30 minutes.

Watch for blanching, which correlates with anesthesia.

EMLA/EMLA Disc

EMLA cream is a eutectic mixture of 2.5% lidocaine and 2.5% prilocaine. A eutectic mixture is one that melts at a lower temperature than do any of its ingredients. Therefore both anesthetics exist in a liquid form.

Remove oil from skin with an alcohol swab. Consider thinning the stratum corneum through tape stripping of superficial cells. Apply the disc or 1 to 2 g per 10 cm^2 of the cream. Cover with an occlusive dressing (Tegaderm, OpSite, or Band-Aid) for 60 minutes for a 3-mm depth. Every additional 30 minutes provide 1 mm of more depth; a 2-hour maximum time is equivalent to 5 mm. Cream should still be visible when the dressing is removed. If it is not visible, an inadequate amount was used (Table 11-2).

ELA-Max

Current use is determined by the experience of the physician because clinical studies of the pharmacodynamic variables are lacking. In general, a thick layer of cream is applied under an occlusive dressing (Tegaderm, OpSite, or Saran Wrap) as with EMLA (however, the onset of action is shortened to approximately 30 minutes).

Lidoderm 5% Patch

Apply up to 3 patches at one time to cover the most painful area (postherpetic neuralgia) for a maximum of 12 hours within a 24-hour period. Patches may be cut to

TABLE 11-2

Recommended Maximum Dose and Application Area of Eutectic, Mixture of Local Anesthetics (EMLA)

Age	Body Weight	Max Total Dose and Time	Max Application Area (cm^2)
1-3 mo	<5 kg	1 g (1 hr)	10
4-12 mo	>5 kg	2 g (4 hr)	20
1-6 yr	>10 kg	10 g (4 hr)	100
7-12 yr	>20 kg	20 g (4 hr)	200

Adapted from Huang W, Vidimos A: *J Am Acad Dermatol* 43:286, 2000.

smaller sizes for smaller lesions or impaired elimination (hepatic disease).

Iontocaine

Lidocaine 2%, epinephrine 1:100,000; lidocaine iontophoresis involves the use of direct current to transfer the charged molecules into the dermis. Limit the iontophoretic treatment in children to 40 mA-min.

$$\text{Time (min)} \times \text{Current (mA)} = \text{Total dose (mA-min)}$$

One study suggested this technique may be more effective than EMLA. (See Chapter 215, TENS Unit, Phonophoresis, Iontophoresis.)

Benzocaine and Lidocaine–Mucous Membrane Use

Wolfe et al (2000) recently reported that atomized lidocaine 4% solution decreased the discomfort of nasogastric tube placement. The combination of 1.5-ml atomized intranasal plus 3.0-ml oropharyngeal plus 5 ml of 2% lidocaine jelly intranasal is superior to jelly alone. Caution should be used because of impaired swallowing after use. Patients should expectorate excess anesthetic to avoid systemic absorption and toxicity. Plasma levels are similar to IV injection. For viscous solution, do not exceed 1 tablespoon (15 ml) every 3 hours or 1 teaspoon (5 ml) of 5% liquid in an adult (see Chapter 4, Local Anesthesia, and Chapter 5, Local and Topical Anesthetic Complications, for maximum doses). Ingestion of food should be avoided for at least 1 hour after oral use to prevent aspiration.

Thermal-Ice Ethyl Chloride

Hold ice in direct contact for 10 seconds and clip tag immediately.

Spray the vaporized coolant 1 to 2 seconds until the dermis turns white and immediately clip the tag or incise and drain the abscess. Caution: overapplication causes blistering.

Ophthalmic Use

Apply one or two drops in the eye. The effects of anesthetic are rapid in 30 seconds and persist up to 15 minutes. An additional drop can be placed every 5 to 10 minutes for a total of 7 to 10 drops.

CONCLUSION

In the past, topical anesthetic options for dermatologic procedures were limited to ice and coolant sprays. At the time of the first edition of this textbook, EMLA was just entering the marketplace. Now ELA-Max is entering the market and these two agents will be the topical workhorses for the near future. Since studies suggest that LET is equally efficacious when compared with TAC, LET seems to be replacing TAC for safety, cost, and documentation advantages.

BIBLIOGRAPHY

Ernst AA, Marvez E, Nick TG, et al: Lidocaine adrenaline tetracaine gel versus tetracaine adrenaline cocaine gel for topical anesthesia in linear scalp and facial lacerations in children aged 5 to 17 years, *Pediatrics* 95:255, 1995.

Huang W, Vidimos A: Topical anesthetics in dermatology: clinical review, *J Am Acad Dermatol* 43(2 Pt 1):286, 2000.

Lander J, Brady-Fryer B, Metcalfe JB, et al: Comparison of the ring block, dorsal penile nerve block, and topical anesthesia for neonatal circumcision: a randomized controlled trial, *JAMA* 278:2157, 1997.

Lerner EV, Bucalo BD, Kist DA, Moy RL: Topical anesthetic agents in dermatologic surgery: a review, *Dermatol Surg* 23:673, 1997.

Moy RL, Pfenninger JL: Taking the sting out of local anesthesia, *Pat Care* March 15:61, 2000.

Package Insert: EMLA, Westborough, Mass, Astra USA.

Package Insert: Iontocaine, North Chicago, Ill, Abbott Lab, USA.

Wolfe TR, Fosnocht DE, Linscott MS: Atomized lidocaine as topical anesthesia for nasogastric tube placement: a randomized, double blind, placebo-controlled trial, *Ann Emerg Med* 35:421, 2000.

PART TWO

Dermatology

CHAPTER 12

Acne Therapy: Surgical Approaches*

Michael Altman

Acne is the most common skin disease of adolescents and is estimated to affect 80 percent of individuals between 11 and 30 years of age. It is a disease of the pilosebaceous unit. Acne involves increased sebum production, obstruction of the pilosebaceous glands with keratinization of the canal, bacterial proliferation, and inflammation. Many topical and systemic medications have been developed to treat acne. When these medications fail to control the disease, or when significant lesions develop, several procedures may be used to intervene. This chapter focuses on the procedures a primary care physician might consider in the office treatment of acne.

COMEDO REMOVAL

The removal of open comedones (black heads, noninflamed plugged pores) enhances the patient's appearance while preventing the development of inflamed acne lesions (with its complications). Instruments such as the round loop (or oval loop) extractor (Fig. 12-1) or the Schamberg extractor effectively extract the plug by allowing uniform, smooth pressure to encircle the pore (Fig. 12-2). They can be obtained from any medical supply provider, and some are even sold over the counter. Cystic acne can be worsened by attempted treatment with a comedo extractor.

Open comedones that offer resistance can be loosened with one of two techniques:

1. Application of tretinoin (Retin-A), a topical keratolytic, for 1 month prior to comedo extraction.
2. Use of a no. 11 blade, tip of a needle, or the pointed end of a comedo extractor to stretch the walls of the pore opening without cutting into tissue. The physician should insert the scalpel point 1 mm into the comedo, following the angle of the follicle opening, and angle the tip to bring the plug upward through the enlarged pore opening.

*This chapter was originally published in the first edition by Thomas J. Zuber, MD, and John L. Pfenninger, MD. Dr. Altman has updated it for this edition.

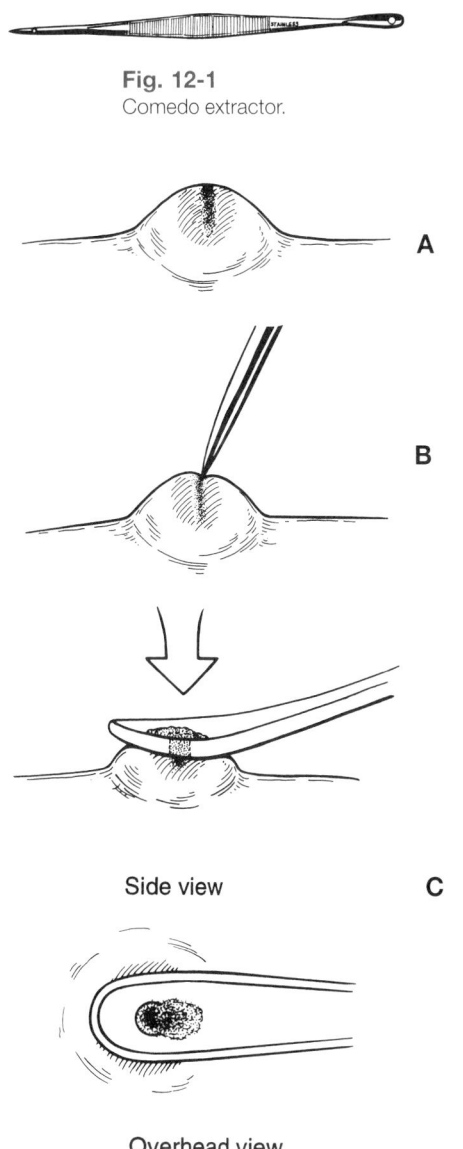

Fig. 12-1
Comedo extractor.

A

B

Side view **C**

Overhead view

Fig. 12-2
Use of comedo extractor to express cystic contents. **A,** Comedo. **B,** Incising lesion with sharp point. **C,** Expressing contents through central hole. Using an extractor forces the contents out through the central opening, preventing material from being forced into normal tissue.

If there is still resistance, the comedo extractor should be held in the other hand and lateral pressure applied with the blunted end to the base of the canals as the blade lifts the plug through the center of the extractor. A large amount of sebaceous material may be found beneath the plug and should be removed.

ACNE SURGERY FOR PUSTULES AND CYSTS

The surgical drainage of acne pustules and cysts, when performed correctly, speeds resolution of the lesions, prevents subdermal rupture, and enhances cosmetic appearance. Closed comedones can also be opened to prevent their progression to inflammatory lesions.

Enter the head of a white pustule with a small (25-gauge) needle, with the tip (tiny nick) of a no. 11 blade, or the pointed end of the comedo extractor. Drain the pustule with lateral pressure or with the assistance of an extractor. Superficial cysts that have thin roofs, and easily palpated fluid can be drained by making a small incision less than 4 mm long. Some physicians advocate that the base of a drained superficial cyst be gently curetted to dislodge any necrotic debris. Nodules and cysts are best treated by intralesional corticosteroid injection.

INTRALESIONAL CORTICOSTEROID INJECTION

Individual nodular or cystic acne lesions often dramatically decrease in size after an intralesional injection of a corticosteroid. It is reassuring to patients to know that a fast, relatively painless procedure is available when lesions arise. Patients with severe acne often require repeated injections every 2 to 3 weeks. Multiple cysts can be treated in one session.

The steroid preparation triamcinolone acetonide 10 mg/ml (e.g., Kenalog-10) is a preferred agent and should be diluted to about 2.5 mg/ml with saline or local anesthetic (e.g., 1% xylocaine). Saline is the preferred diluent because injections of local anesthetics are painful. Triamcinolone acetonide is particularly useful in that it is insoluble and therefore can remain deposited for months at the injection site, achieving its desired local effect without risk for adrenal suppression.

When preparing for an injection, shake the steroid vial to disperse the suspension. First draw the saline into a tuberculin syringe, followed by an appropriate amount of triamcinolone. (If xylocaine is the diluent, use only single-dose vials to prevent precipitation of the steroid.) An air bubble can be aspirated into the syringe to mix the two. Then insert a 30-gauge needle through the thinnest portion of the cyst roof and deliver 0.05 to 0.3 ml of the resulting 2.5-mg/ml triamcinolone acetonide mixture. Some physicians advocate using a maximum volume of 0.2 ml to reduce the risk of skin atrophy. The injection usually blanches the cyst.

Inject directly into the cyst, not the skin. Skin atrophy can follow injections if the steroid is deposited into the skin, below the cyst, or if the steroid concentration is too high. One session of injections should not exceed 10 to 20 mg total to avoid systemic effects. It may be necessary to repeat intralesional injections at 2-week intervals, not to exceed three total sessions.

Fluctuant lesions can be aspirated first with a large-bore needle attached to a 1- or 3-ml syringe before steroid injection. Skin atrophy remains unlikely, but the patient should be forewarned that atrophy still might take place independent of the injection because of underlying inflammation involving the collagen bed. Secondary bacterial infections do not occur. Avoid injecting the periorbital and perinasal areas as inadvertent injection of steroid crystals into vessels may drain into the cerebral venous sinuses or central retinal artery.

Finally, counsel patients that skin depression may occur, but in most cases it is temporary and gradually resolves in 4 to 6 months.

ALPHA-HYDROXY ACID PEELS

α-Hydroxy acid peels have no place in acne management. No benefit is achieved, and their use only causes skin irritation.

CRYOTHERAPY

Cryotherapy involves painting the skin with a slush prepared with acetone and mixed with solid carbon dioxide. This cold slush is thinly applied on nodules and cysts just long enough to cause erythema and superficial desquamation. It is no longer advocated because it frequently causes hypopigmentation or hyperpigmentation. Some physicians have tried to soften scars, but its effects are only temporary.

SCAR REVISON

A variety of procedures can be used to remove or revise acne scars. Deep, "ice-pick" scars can be excised, through the use of a punch biopsy, and immediately replaced with a full-thickness punch graft of normal skin. Another technique, punch-graft elevation, uses a punch just slightly larger than the pitted scar. A cylindrical incision is made into the dermis, allowing the core to "pop-out" above the skin surface. A Steri-Strip secures this skin core just above the surrounding skin. Dermabrasion of the remaining treatment site may be required at a later date. Results are unpredictable. Collagen injections can also be used to smooth the skin surface.

Dermabrasion involves the use of a high-speed hand drill with a diamond-studded steel sander under local anesthesia to smooth out scars. Microdermabrasion (see Chapter 52) can also be used. It is less aggressive and there is little recovery time, but many (six to eight) visits may be needed. It is best reserved for more superficial scars. Carbon dioxide and neodymium: yttrium-aluminum-garnet lasers are sometimes used to treat pitted or depressed acne scars.

COMPLICATIONS

Complications include adverse pigmentary changes, deeper and longer scars, and increased skin sensitivity to sunlight.

CPT/BILLING CODES

10040	Acne surgery, opening of multiple cysts, comedones, or pustules
10060	Incision and drainage of abscess
11900	Intralesional injection of up to 7 lesions
11901	Intralesional injection of more than 7 lesions
15780-87	Dermabrasion
15790-91	Chemical peel
17340	Cryotherapy (CO_2 slush)
17360	Chemical exfoliation for acne

ICD-9-CM DIAGNOSTIC CODES

| 706.1 | Acne |
| 695.3 | Acne rosacea |

BIBLIOGRAPHY

Berson DS, Shalita AR: The treatment of acne: the role of combination therapies, *J Am Acad Dermatol* 32:S31, 1995.

Habif TP, editor: Clinical dermatology, St Louis, 1996, Mosby.

Kligman AM, Plewig G: *Acne and rosacea,* Berlin, 1993, Springer-Verlag.

Nguyen QH, Kim YA, Schwartz RA: Management of acne vulgaris, *Am Fam Physician* 50(1):89, 1994.

Zuber T, Pfenninger JL: Acne therapy. In Pfenninger JL, Fowler GC, editors: *Procedures for primary care physicians,* St Louis, 1994, Mosby.

CHAPTER 13

Approach to Various Skin Lesions

John L. Pfenninger

This chapter provides guidelines for the diagnosis and treatment of common skin lesions. Table 13-1 can be used as a guide for proper biopsy and treatment techniques. Many of the techniques are reviewed elsewhere in this textbook. These guidelines are not intended to be all-inclusive, but they do provide a framework for the approach to common skin lesions.

All excised skin lesions are best sent to the pathologist for definitive diagnosis. With selected lesions, such as skin tags or sebaceous cysts, many physicians will rely on their clinical judgment and avoid the added laboratory expense. However, in today's litigious society, the physician must be absolutely certain of the diagnosis when deciding not to send tissue to the pathologist for evaluation. Numerous benign lesions can be placed in a single formalin container (e.g., skin tags, obviously benign nevi, etc.) to basically cover the legal aspects. Each bottle sent to pathology costs approximately $160 to $200 to process!

ANGIOMA (HEMANGIOMA)

If the angiomas are small, the physician should use a ball electrode to cauterize them lightly. Tissue should be wiped away and the process repeated until no vessel is seen. Focal cryotherapy or sclerotherapy will also work. If the angiomas are large, the physician should perform a light shave excision followed by cautery of the base.

ACROCHORDON (SKIN TAG)

Although many physicians prefer to use electrosurgery or cryotherapy to remove acrochordons, the most direct and simple approach is to elevate the tag with pickups and excise it with sharp tissue scissors at the level of the surrounding skin. If it has a broad base, a local anesthetic may be required. Monsel's solution (ferric subsulfate) or aluminum chloride may be used for hemostasis. It is essential to have good quality scissors so the lesion is "cut," not "pinched."

If the tag is small enough, a ball electrode can be used to lightly and quickly cauterize the tag. It is then simply "wiped away."

Cryocautery can be effective, but it is difficult to limit the freeze solely to the tag. A unique method with liquid nitrogen is to use the Styrofoam cup method, dipping the flat pickups in the liquid, and then grasping the tag with the cooled metal. The tag usually necroses off. The tag should be frozen twice in the same visit.

ACTINIC KERATOSES

Actinic keratoses are sun-induced, premalignant lesions. Single lesions can be shaved, cauterized, or more commonly treated with cryotherapy. When multiple lesions are present, they can be treated with fluorouracil (Efudex) or masoprocol (Actinex). Lesions that do not resolve require surgical sampling for biopsy. The risk that actinic keratoses will progress to SCC is probably less than 1% in early lesions, and as high as 10% to 20% for persistent hypertrophic lesions. The patient should be counseled that both fluorouracil and masoprocol cause significant erythema and tenderness in the areas treated. The medication is applied twice a day for 3 to 4 weeks to the face and three to four times per day on the arms. Steroid creams may be used to reduce the inflammatory response. Alternatively, daily application of retinoic acid (Retin-A) 0.025% or 0.05% may resolve early lesions and prevent new ones. Protection from the sun is essential.

BASAL CELL CARCINOMA

Basal cell carcinomas (BCCs) characteristically have small, central ulcerated depressions and raised, pearly borders (*nodular-cystic type*). However, their actual appearance can vary markedly from the classic description. *Sclerosing* (or morpheaform) BCCs may manifest as flat lesions with nondescript borders. Others are non-healing ulcerations that never do become elevated. Some

TABLE 13-1

Surgical Diagnosis and Management of Common Skin Lesions

Lesion	Punch Biopsy	Shave Biopsy	Shave Removal	Fusiform Excision	Incisional Biopsy	Curettement Alone	Cautery/Curettement (ED&C)	Cryotherapy	Electrosurgery (Radiofrequency)	85% Trichloroacetic Acid	Laser Ablation	Radiation	Fluorouracil 5% or Masoprocol 10%	Incision and Drainage	Other
Acrochordon (skin tags)		X*	X*					X	X						
Angiomas															
Cherry	X	X	X			X	X*	X	X*		X				
Spider									X†		X				X†
Bowen's disease (SCC in situ)	X	X	X	X	X		X*	X*			X				
Cancer, basal cell	X	X		X	X		X*	X			X	X	X		
Cancer, squamous cell	X			X*	X			X			X	X	X		
Condyloma acuminata‡	X	X	X	X§				X	X	X	X		X‖		X‡
Dermatofibroma	X	X	X*	X*	X		X*	X			X				
Hemangiomas, cherry	X	X	X			X	X*	X	X*		X				
Keratoacanthoma	X	X		X*	X		X*	X			X		X		
Keratosis, actinic	X	X	X*	X	X		X*	X*	X	X	X		X*		
Keratosis, seborrheic	X	X	X*	X§	X	X	X	X*	X		X				
Lentigo	X	X	X		X			X*	X	X	X				
Lentigo maligna	X			X*	X										
Lipomas				X											X* (see text)
Melanoma	X			X*	X										X
Milia	X	X	X				X*		X					X*	
Molluscum contagiosum	X§	X	X				X*	X	X		X				X
Mucoceles				X					X		X				
Neurofibroma	X	X	X¶	X	X		X#		X						
Nevi, acquired	X		X**	X	X				X**		X**				
Nevi, atypical	X		X††	X*	X										
Nevi, giant congenital	X			X	X						X**				
Paronychia††														X*	X
Pyogenic granuloma	X	X		X			X*	X	X		X				
Rashes	X														X
Sebaceous cysts				X										X*	X
Sebaceous hyperplasia	X	X	X	X§		X	X*	X	X						
Skin tags		X*	X*					X	X						
Telangiectasias									X†		X				X†
Warts (verruca vulgaris); see Chapter 42, Wart (Verruca) Treatment	X	X	X		X§		X*	X*	X	X	X				X*‡‡
Warts, plantar	X	X					X	X*	X	X	X				X‡‡
Warts, planar	X	X	X			X*	X	X	X	X	X				X§§
Xanthelasma		X	X	X					X		X				X

*Procedure of choice.
†Face only; legs require sclerotherapy or laser.
‡Aldara, Condylox, Interferon; see Chapter 157, Treatment of Noncervical Condyloma Acuminata.
§Used only if cancer is a possibility or nature of lesion unknown.
‖Not approved by the Food and Drug Administration.
¶Followed by cautery and curettement.
#Preceded by shave removal.
**An exception; used only if certain that lesion is benign.
††If used here, must be sure to use deep saucerlike shape and that entire lesion removed in initial sample (*do not* use if suspect melanoma).
‡‡*Candida* antigen; bleomycin; see Chapter 42, Wart (Verruca) Treatment.
§§Retin-A.

are *pigmented* and may be confused with seborrheic keratoses (SKs), nevi, or even melanomas. They may appear erythematous and bleed easily, mimicking a pyogenic granuloma. *Superficial* BCCs commonly occur on the back and are flat and scaly. They may look like a squamous cell carcinoma (SCC), actinics, eczema, or even tinea. A biopsy should be taken of all nonhealing, changing, or enlarging skin lesions. Once a diagnosis is made, the proper approach for treatment can be planned.

When a biopsy is taken of a suspected basal cell carcinoma, almost any area of the lesion is appropriate for sampling. Biopsy of ulcerated lesions is best obtained at the border, which may not be involved in the ulceration process (normal skin is not needed). Chronic sun exposure and human papillomavirus appear to be the causative factors.

BCCs can be aggressive in the nasolabial folds and in the preauricular areas. The inner canthal area can be an especially difficult area to excise and treat because of tear duct involvement. In these locations, if size is greater than 5 mm, Mohs' chemosurgery may be indicated as a primary excisional method because it ensures complete removal. Careful follow-up is needed to detect early recurrences. Any lesion that is less than 5 to 6 mm in any location generally has an excellent response to almost any treatment modality.

There are many approaches to the treatment of BCCs. *Radiation* therapy is rarely used, but it may be necessary when the lesions are located in areas such as the lid margins or the inner canthal areas, and in large lesions found on elderly patients.

BCCs generally involve the upper portions of the skin and very rarely metastasize. Deaths are extremely rare and reportable. For the majority of lesions that are smaller than 1 cm, treatment with *cautery and curettement (electrodesiccation and curettage [ED&C])* is a rapid and effective solution. Cure rates approach 95% to 98%, and scarring is usually minimal (Figs. 13-1 and 13-2).

1. After local anesthesia, with the *cautery and curettement* method, scoop out the lesion with a large dermal curette. Scrape the base of the lesion until a gritty feeling is encountered.
2. Then fulgurate or cauterize the entire base to destroy remaining cells and to control bleeding.
3. After the first cauterization, again vigorously curette the site to remove any of the char. Again, scrape until "grittiness" is palpable.
4. Perform fulguration or cauterization a second time, as before.
5. Carry out the third and final curettement with a smaller dermal curette that more easily enters any tiny crevices in the wound site. Be careful not to penetrate

too deeply and pass through the entire dermis. If this should happen, a small window of fatty tissue will be visible in the bottom of the wound. If this should happen, formal excision is indicated because the tumor most likely went quite deep.

6. After the third curettement, fulgurate or cauterize the lesion for the final time. Place a dressing. Although the wound appears significantly ulcerated at this point, the long-term cosmetic results of this procedure are very acceptable if patients follow moist healing practices (see the sample patient education handout titled "Moist Healing After Skin Surgery" on page 1747 of Appendix G).

Encourage the patient to wash the area three or four times a day with soap and water to prevent an eschar from forming. Immediately after washing, have the patient apply an antibiotic ointment to keep the area moist. The ointment can be applied six or eight times a day, not so much to prevent infection, but rather to aid the reepithelialization of the wound. Vaseline may work as well. Cover the wound only at night if it is on a nonclothed area. Otherwise a dressing will be needed all the time.

Lesions in younger patients, larger-sized (over 1 cm) lesions, lesions in more aggressive locations (nasolabial folds, preauricular areas, eyelids), sclerosing-type BCC lesions, and lesions with ill-defined margins may require *complete excision* to enable the pathologist to examine the margins. Remove 3 to 4 mm of normal skin around all edges. Margins can be marked to aid in the histologic evaluation. Some physicians believe that excision is more cosmetically acceptable than cautery and curettement. An advantage of ED&C over cryotherapy is that the necrotic lesion can be "felt" with the curette, so the surgeon knows how far and deep to proceed with the scraping. All the various clinical factors should be weighed when selecting the method of lesion removal.

Laser therapy can be used to oblate the lesions. *Topical 5-fluorouracil* has been approved to treat superficial basal cells. *Cryotherapy* has excellent results for lesions less than 1 cm wide. A good freeze 5 mm past the lesion is required, followed by thawing, then a repeat freeze (see Chapter 15, Cryosurgery). Cure rates of 98% are reported.

After being treated for a BCC, the patient must be observed closely, because 30% of patients will develop new BCCs within 3 years.

Mohs' chemosurgery is not indicated for routine treatment of BCCs. Consider it for recurrent, morpheaform-type, or very large lesions. It may also be used for larger lesions in high-risk sites. The cost simply does not justify routine use, since cure rates are so good with the other methods too.

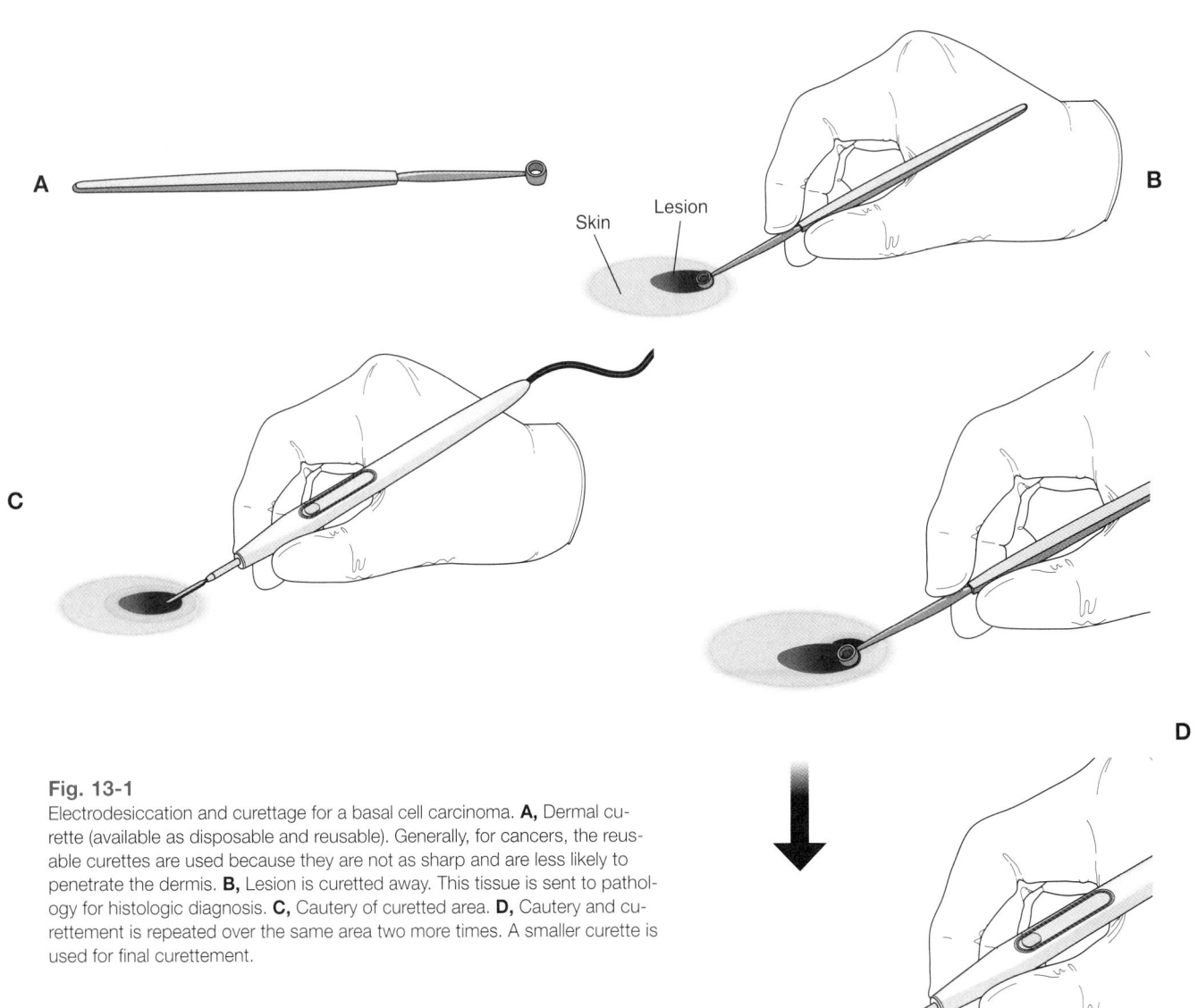

Fig. 13-1
Electrodesiccation and curettage for a basal cell carcinoma. **A,** Dermal curette (available as disposable and reusable). Generally, for cancers, the reusable curettes are used because they are not as sharp and are less likely to penetrate the dermis. **B,** Lesion is curetted away. This tissue is sent to pathology for histologic diagnosis. **C,** Cautery of curetted area. **D,** Cautery and curettement is repeated over the same area two more times. A smaller curette is used for final curettement.

SQUAMOUS CELL CARCINOMA

SCC often appears as a diffuse, nonhealing, crusted lesion. It frequently occurs at the base of an actinic keratosis or a keratoacanthoma. The lesions may be multifocal in origin and, as with actinic lesions, are due to solar damage. SCCs are more aggressive than BCCs and can metastasize. Because the margins of these lesions are not very clear, many clinicians prefer to excise all SCCs. If 5-fluorouracil (Efudex) or masoprocol (Actinex) is used to treat diffuse actinic changes, any posttreatment residual lesions (after 2 months) should be removed for biopsy to rule out SCC. When a biopsy is performed on a suspected SCC, try to include portions of the central area. A deep punch biopsy into subcutaneous fat is preferred by many pathologists. Early or small lesions can be treated with cautery and curettement (Figs. 13-1 and 13-2) or with cryotherapy with excellent results (see above). If excised, remove at least 5 mm of normal tissue to be sure all margins are clear.

Coding for skin cancer treatment is complicated. The biller must know the size, location, and method of removal to bill correctly. Lesions should be reevaluated in 3 and 9 months to document the cure. (See Appendix I.)

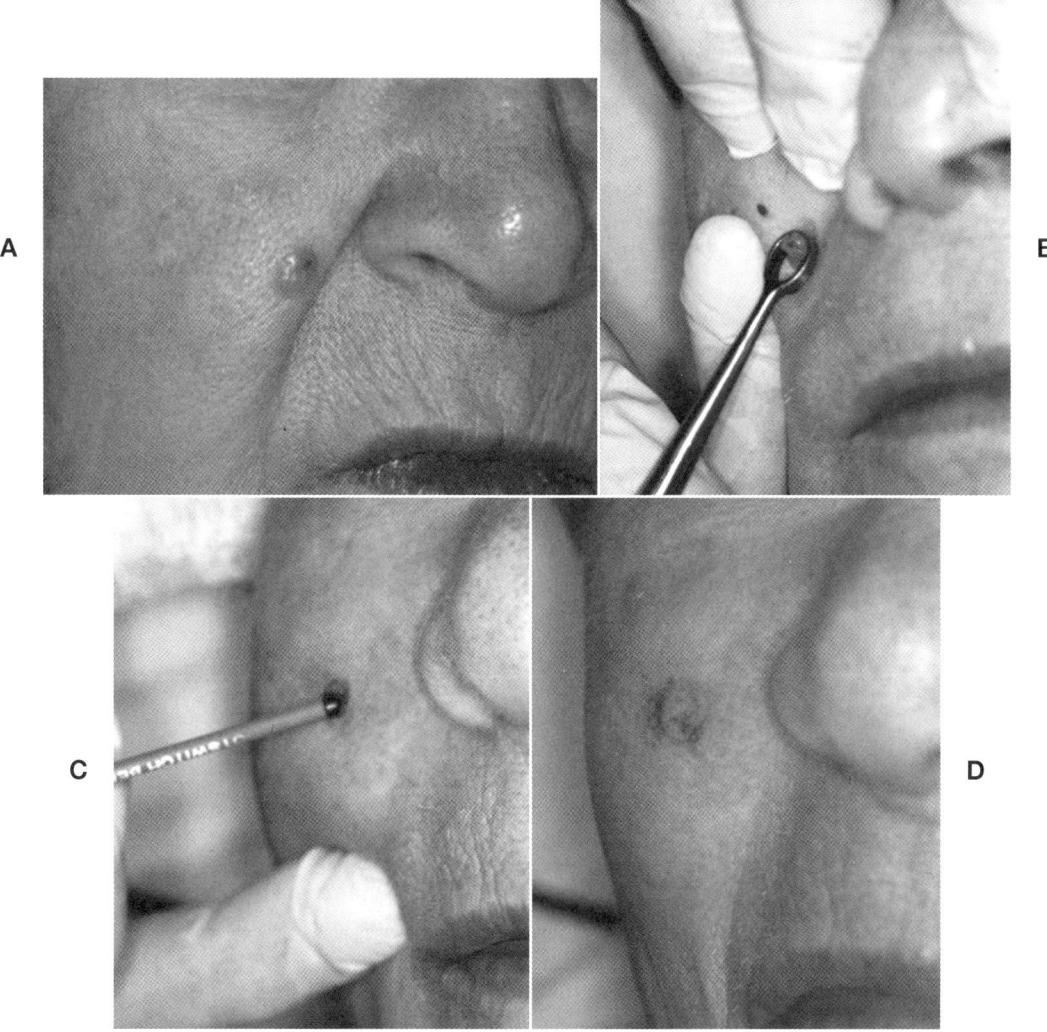

Fig. 13-2
A, Basal cell carcinoma of right cheek. **B,** After administration of local anesthetic, the lesion is curetted.
C, Cautery of the base with a ball electrode. Repeat curette and cautery for a total of three times.
D, Appearance of wound after completion of treatment. (Courtesy The National Procedures Institute, Midland, Mich.)

CONDYLOMA ACUMINATA

Many therapeutic interventions are available to treat condyloma acuminata. See Chapter 157, Treatment of Noncervical Condyloma Acuminata.

DERMATOFIBROMA

Dermatofibromas often occur on the anterior surface of the lower leg. The etiology is unknown, but dermatofibromas may represent a fibrous reaction to trauma, viral infection, or insect bites. They are often confused with verrucae or nevi. Dermatofibromas do not pro-gress to cancers, and once the diagnosis of dermatofibroma is confirmed, the physician often can merely observe the lesions. However, until the lesion is biopsied, only an educated guess is possible. Many BCCs of the lower extremities mimic dermatofibromas. Dermatofibromas are generally deep-seated and will require excision if complete removal is desired. Cryotherapy can be attempted, but dermatofibromas are generally quite cryoresistant. Since the lesions are often on the legs and are cut while shaving, the most judicious approach is to shave the lesion flat, which both provides tissue for confirmatory diagnosis and reduces the likelihood of further trauma. A pigmented spot may remain, but at least it will be flat. If final results are not satisfactory, they can still be excised or cryotherapy can be attempted.

KERATOACANTHOMA

Keratoacanthoma is a common, benign epithelial tumor found in elderly patients. This lesion may have a viral etiology. Keratoacanthoma often is confused with SCC, but it is a distinct entity.

The lesion begins as a dome-shaped papule that continues to enlarge rapidly. A fully developed tumor is a round, dome-shaped mass with a central keratin-filled crater. The lesion may stop growing after 6 weeks, and then it may slowly regress over the next 12 months. These lesions often occur on the dorsum of the hands, ears, and neck.

Because these lesions grow rapidly, most physicians do not advocate simple observation. Cryotherapy, a deep saucer-type shave, ED&C, or conventional excision provides acceptable results. Keratoacanthomas can recur, and patients should be followed closely during and after treatment. The major differential diagnoses for the clinician include basal and squamous cell cancer. Because of the rapid growth and high numbers of mitotic cells, even the pathologists experience difficulty and often will report that they "cannot rule out SCC" at the base.

SEBORRHEIC KERATOSES

SKs are benign, hyperkeratinized, superficial epidermal lesions that are common with aging. Their size ranges from 2 mm to 3 cm. They have no malignant potential. The typical lesion has the appearance that it can be easily lifted off with a fingernail. Patients often say that they have removed the lesion or rubbed it off with a towel, only to have it recur. SKs are occasionally confused with BCCs, SCCs, nevi, and verrucous lesions.

Most SKs can be easily removed, after anesthesia, with radiofrequency (electrosurgery) technique. Alternatively, shave excision with mild curetting of the base can be performed. Hemostasis can be accomplished with Monsel's solution or aluminum chloride. Minimal scarring should result because the lesion is superficial. Some physicians prefer cryotherapy; however, this treatment may cause more discomfort, results in significant watery discharge, precludes histologic assessment, and requires multiple treatments. It is essential that the clinician be absolutely sure of the diagnosis if cryotherapy is to be used. One study showed a correct preoperative diagnosis in only 49% of cases (Stern, 1989).

If many seborrheics occur all at once, consider an internal malignancy (Lesar-Trélat sign).

Medicare does not reimburse for removal of SKs unless they are markedly irritated or rapidly growing, or if the diagnosis is uncertain.

LENTIGO

Lentigos, or liver spots, are common brownish or tan macules that occur on the sun-exposed areas of the face, shoulders, arms, and hands. Lentigos increase in number during childhood and adult life, and occasionally they fade. Biopsy of lesions with irregular borders should be performed to rule out malignant melanoma. Cryotherapy is the treatment of choice, although bleaching and depigmenting creams may be used. Superficial ablation techniques with laser, radiofrequency, or trichloroacetic acid also may work.

LENTIGO MALIGNA (MELANOMA IN SITU)

Lentigo maligna is a sun-associated precursor of lentigo maligna melanoma, a type of invasive melanoma. These lesions can grow to be several centimeters in diameter and usually occur on the face. They are slow-growing macules with irregular borders and pigmentation. These lesions often are confused with liver spots, which are smaller, have a homogeneous color, and appear mainly over the dorsa of the hands and forearms. The estimated lifetime risk of transformation to melanoma is only 4.7%, and some physicians prefer close observation as the treatment of choice. Unless absolutely sure of the diagnosis, a biopsy should be done. Removal is probably best done with complete surgical excision.

LIPOMAS

Lipomas present as a palpable mass under the skin. Most lesions are nontender, move freely, and have a soft, irregular consistency. The differential is usually whether the lesion is a sebaceous cyst; cysts have pores; lipomas do not. Lipomas generally do not progress to malignancy, but rapidly growing or changing lesions should be removed. Removal also may be necessary when lipomas occur in areas of pressure or when they cause pain or discomfort. Lesions on the lower extremities have a higher likelihood of malignant degeneration. Lesions are removed by making a 1- to 2-cm incision through the dermis after as little as 1 ml of 2% xylocaine with epinephrine. The clinician should make the incision in line with the skin lines and use hemostats or curved

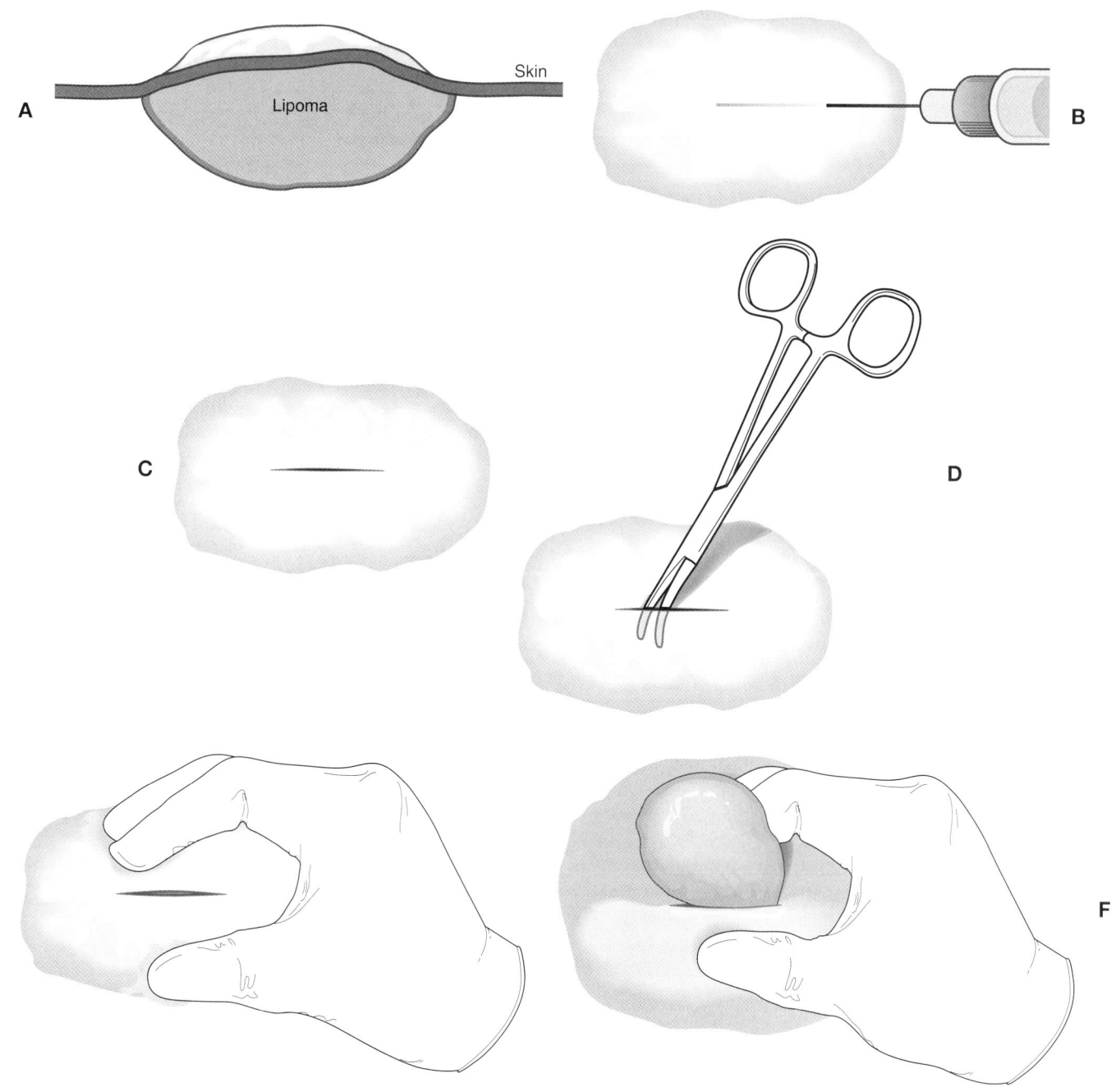

Fig. 13-3
Simple method for lipoma removal. **A,** Lipoma often will tent up the skin (cross-section view). **B,** Inject 3 to 4 ml of 2% lidocaine with epinephrine superficially into skin and deep around the palpable mass. **C,** Make a 1.0- to 1.5-cm incision over the mass with a no. 15 blade. **D,** Insert small curved hemostats into the wound and bluntly dissect around the mass, freeing it from surrounding tissue and the skin. **E,** Squeeze around the mass as if trying to express a pustule. **F,** The lipoma will literally "pop" out, and the base can be excised. Close with a Steri-Strip or tissue glue.

tissue scissors to dissect the lesion from the surrounding adhering tissue. Pressure on the base of the lesion often will extrude the lipoma through the small incision (Fig. 13-3). Some lipomas are encapsulated, but often the edges are obscure; it may be difficult to determine whether all of the lesion has been removed. Any apparent redundant fatty tissue should be removed. Closure usually can be obtained with Steri-Strips or tissue glue. Once the diagnosis of lipoma has been made in one area, other similar lesions do not necessarily require removal unless they are symptomatic. (Lesions that are larger than 4 to 5 cm may require formal excision with sterile technique and suture closure.) There are special CPT codes for removal of these lesions under "Excision of Benign Tumors" in the CPT code book.

MELANOMA

The major caveat regarding melanomas is that the *depth of lesion is very important in determining appropriate definitive treatment*. Primary care physicians should not feel uncomfortable about performing a biopsy of any lesion with characteristics that may be consistent with a melanoma. This does not spread the lesion or limit life expectancy in any way. On the contrary, early diagnosis may save the patient's life. The mnemonic *"A, B, C, D, E, F, G"* can be used as an aid for remembering the clinical features of malignant melanoma:

> *A*symmetry
> *B*order irregularity
> *C*olor variegation
> *D*iameter more than 6 mm
> *E*levation above skin surface
> *F*eeling different
> *G*rowth or change

Because it is so important to determine the depth of the lesion, *never* perform a shave biopsy or shave removal if melanoma is a consideration. When choosing a site for punch or incisional biopsy within a pigmented lesion, choose the area that is most nodular or atypical (darkest in color, inflamed, or irregular). Recent National Institutes of Health (NIH) guidelines indicate that with lesions that penetrate less than 1 mm, 1-cm clear excisional margins around the lesion should be adequate. An extensive work-up for metastases is not indicated for the minimal-depth lesions (Table 13-2).

MOLLUSCUM CONTAGIOSUM

Molluscums are small, 2- to 3-mm, papular, wartlike excrescences with central umbilication. They usually appear as a crop of multiple lesions. Expectant observation is certainly acceptable, but many patients desire to have these viral lesions removed. Table 13-1 describes the treatments that are possible. Curettement with a small dermal curette is the treatment of choice, and it rarely requires anesthesia. These lesions often occur in children; a topical anesthetic such as 20% benzocaine (Hurricaine gel) or EMLA cream (eutectic mixture of local anesthetic, a mixture of lidocaine and prilocaine) may increase patient cooperation during treatment. See Chapter 11, Topical Anesthesia.

NEUROFIBROMAS

These lesions are soft, nodular lesions that often appear to be minimally pigmented nevi. When a shave incision is performed, soft jellylike material is seen at the base. This is the "pathognomonic" sign of a neurofibroma. The soft tissue is curetted and the base cauterized. A significant cavity may exist, but with moist healing techniques, the results are excellent.

PYOGENIC GRANULOMAS

Pyogenic granulomas are small, rapidly growing, nodular, friable, vascular lesions that often bleed when

---

TABLE 13-2

Treatment of Suspicious Pigmented Lesions and Melanomas

Stage	Recommended Treatment	Survival
Suspicious pigmented lesion	Punch, incisional, or excisional biopsy down to subcutaneous fat	Not affected by biopsy procedure
Suspected positive lymph node with melanoma	Fine-needle aspiration/biopsy	Not affected by biopsy procedure
Early melanoma		
Melanoma in situ (limited to epidermis)	Excision with margin of 0.5 cm normal skin and layer of subcutaneous tissue	Not affected
Depth <1 mm	Excision with margin of 1 cm normal skin and subcutaneous tissue down to fascia	95% (8 yr)
Intermediate melanoma		
Depth 1-4 mm	After diagnostic biopsy, wide-margin excision and adjunctive therapy should be considered (Refer)	Poor
High-risk melanomas		
Depth >4 mm	After diagnostic biopsy, wide-margin excision and adjunctive therapy should be considered (Refer)	Poor

Modified from National Institutes of Health Consensus Conference: *JAMA* 268(10):1314, 1992.

touched. They occur at sites of trauma or previous surgery. Because of their vascular nature, pyogenic granulomas are best treated with curettement followed by cautery of the base. These lesions will recur if any tissue remains, and some physicians advocate complete excision.

ACQUIRED NEVI

Acquired nevi are benign, melanocytic nevi that are absent at birth and first appear in early childhood. The lesions become more numerous until middle age, and the majority of white adults have several acquired nevi. Lesions are often found on sun-exposed areas.

Common acquired nevi follow a predictable developmental progression. The earliest lesions are junctional nevi, with the nevus cells at the junction between the dermis and epidermis. By late adolescence, the growths develop into compound nevi, with nevus cells in both the dermis and epidermis. Compound nevi may develop hairs. By late adulthood, the lesions regress into intradermal nevi and appear nonpigmented.

If the lesions lose their pigment, they may turn pink or flesh-colored. At all stages, common benign acquired nevi have smooth, distinct, symmetric borders. Patients with large numbers of acquired nevi should be monitored closely, because they are at higher risk for developing melanoma.

Raised or pedunculated benign nevi often can best be excised with a shave removal technique (often radio-frequency technique is used [see Chapter 31, Radiofrequency Surgery]). There should be no suspicion whatsoever of melanoma if a shave technique is used. If malignancy is even a rare possibility, either a full-thickness biopsy of the lesion should be performed before removal, or the lesion should be treated by complete excisional removal rather than shave removal. Treatment of melanomas is based solely on the depth of the lesion. Superficial lesions generally do not recur, but the deeper compound nevi often do recur unless the full depth of the lesion is excised. It is difficult to determine when the entire lesion has been removed using a shave technique. The deeper dermal lesions are generally flat, whereas the superficial epidermal lesions are raised or pedunculated.

DYSPLASTIC NEVI

Dysplastic nevi (a histologic diagnosis), or atypical moles (a clinical diagnosis), are acquired nevi that become dysplastic over time. The lesions are generally larger than common acquired nevi, and may have irregular margins, variable pigmentation, and irregular surface contour. Because the risk for melanoma is increased in patients with atypical moles, and because melanoma can develop from an atypical lesion, some physicians advocate full excision of suspicious lesions. Shave excisions, if done, must be a deep, saucerlike shape to be sure the entire depth of the lesion is removed. Patients *often* can have numerous atypical nevi precluding the practicality of excising all of them. These patients need to be followed closely, as do their family members. Sun protection is a must.

Should the pathologist report that the "margins are positive," it behooves the surgeon to remove more tissue to ensure that the entire lesion has indeed been removed.

CONGENITAL NEVI

The approach to congenital nevi is based on three factors: size, color, and family history. Congenital nevi *larger than 20 cm²* often extend over large portions of the body. The lesions grow proportionally with the anatomic site, their surfaces may be irregular, and they may contain coarse hairs. Their management is very controversial, since excision is difficult and deforming. The lifetime risk of these nevi developing into melanoma is 5% to 20%; therefore some physicians advocate early removal and grafting. Others advocate close monitoring. Melanoma can develop at any site within the lesion, and biopsies of the most irregular portions of the lesions may not detect malignant change. Efforts to completely eradicate these lesions must be tempered by the potential for treatment-induced scarring and disfigurement. A recent study by Raeve et al (1998) suggests that vigorous curettement in the first weeks of life may be the best alternative.

Lesions between 1.5 and 20 cm² are easier to excise, and this is generally recommended. Lesions *less than 1.5 cm²* are the easiest to excise but also have the lowest malignant potential. Certainly those that are located in areas that are difficult to observe (scalp, buttocks, etc.) should be removed. Shave excisions are not adequate because congenital nevi are deep lesions.

Another factor to consider is the degree of pigmentation. Very light moles are less likely to degenerate into a cancer, do so in later years (after age 20), and allow early detection of changes. Dark, almost black, lesions are more likely to transform into a melanoma, do so earlier (teens), and are difficult to monitor, making their removal more appropriate.

PARONYCHIA

Paronychia are infections of the distal phalanx along the proximal and lateral edges of the nail. Paronychia produce signs of local infection including redness, tender-

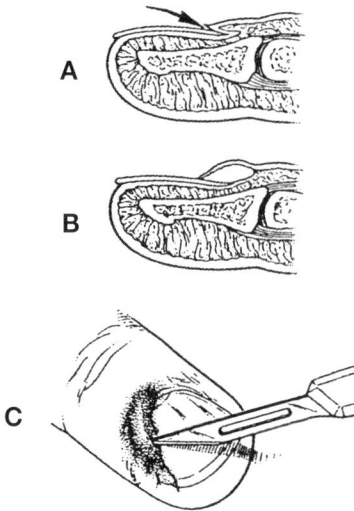

Fig. 13-4
Separation of the cuticle from the nail *(arrow)* **(A)** can lead to a paronychia **(B)**. In acute paronychia, drain any pus and consider a culture. A simple nick **(C)** through the most translucent area of the abscess is usually all that is required. (From Steck W: *Mod Mede* 55:51, 1987.)

ness, and swelling. Mild paronychia can be treated with soaks and antibiotics. More significant infections may develop into abscesses. As with all abscesses, it is best to incise and drain (I&D) them. A digital block often is needed. The incision technique is described in Fig. 13-4. Occasionally packing may be used to keep the abscess from reaccumulating. Chronic paronychia may be secondary to fungal infection.

RASHES (EXANTHEMS, DERMATOSES)

In many cases, biopsy of a "rash" or ill-defined dermatologic lesion is not very helpful. Unless the clinical diagnosis is fairly clear, the primary care physician may be wise to obtain a dermatology consultation. Biopsies of these lesions may be indicated for clarification of a fairly discrete differential diagnosis (as with inflammatory dermatoses) or for ruling out a cutaneous neoplasm.

When multiple sites are involved, the following simple guidelines may be followed for selecting a lesion for a biopsy specimen: It is best to select those areas that have the primary inflammatory changes but are free from secondary changes such as crusting, fissuring, erosion, ulceration, and infection. Choose sites where the scars will not be obvious and where hypertrophic scarring is generally not a problem.

If the primary lesion is a *macule,* select a "fresh" lesion that is more abnormal in color. Generally, perform a punch biopsy, advancing the punch into the subcutaneous fat. *Papules* should be removed completely, if possible. Select a mature lesion without sec-

ondary changes. If the lesion is a *plaque,* the biopsy specimen should consist of the thickest area through the full depth into the subcutaneous fat. The same technique is used for *nodular* lesions and *suspected neoplastic* lesions. Alternatively, a fine needle aspiration biopsy could be performed. For *vesicles and bullae,* choose an intact lesion whenever possible. Rupturing a sac makes histologic interpretation more difficult. Sample these lesions at the margin where the blister roof is attached to the remainder of the specimen and include normal skin.

SEBACEOUS HYPERPLASIA (ADENOSUM SEBACEUM)

Sebaceous adenosum, or senile sebaceous hyperplasia, are small growths composed of enlarged sebaceous glands. These very small, 2- to 5-mm lesions often can mimic early BCC. If numerous lesions are present in the temporal and forehead areas, they are very unlikely to be cancerous. (BCCs are more often solitary.) Treatment consists of removal of the elevated portions of the papule with shave or electrosurgical technique. Often the lesion is deep-seated and may require curettement to remove all of it. Unlike a soft necrotic cancer, these lesions are very dense and fibrotic. Biopsy is indicated if the nature of the lesion is uncertain. However, treatment can generally be carried out on the basis of the clinical diagnosis.

SEBACEOUS CYSTS

The *epidermal cyst,* or *sebaceous cyst,* is a round, tense, keratinizing cyst that is freely mobile and very superficial. When located in the scalp, they are called *tricholemmal cysts* or *wens.* Most patients present with a slowly growing lesion, which on physical examination is subcutaneous, smooth, and nontender. A history of drainage or inflammation with purulent discharge may or may not be present, but it does help solidify the diagnosis. A small central punctum (pore) or opening helps differentiate it from a lipoma.

In the past, a surgeon's adeptness was often judged by whether he or she could remove the lesion intact without rupturing the capsule. This required sterile technique and a fairly generous incision over the area and judicious removal of the *entire* sac, to decrease the likelihood of any recurrence. The cavity is then irrigated and closed with sutures

Another simpler technique is preferred by patient and physician alike. Maintaining an intact sac during removal is no longer felt to be required. After anesthesia, a small 5- to 6-mm incision is made directly into the cyst using a no. 11 blade. All contents are expressed using external

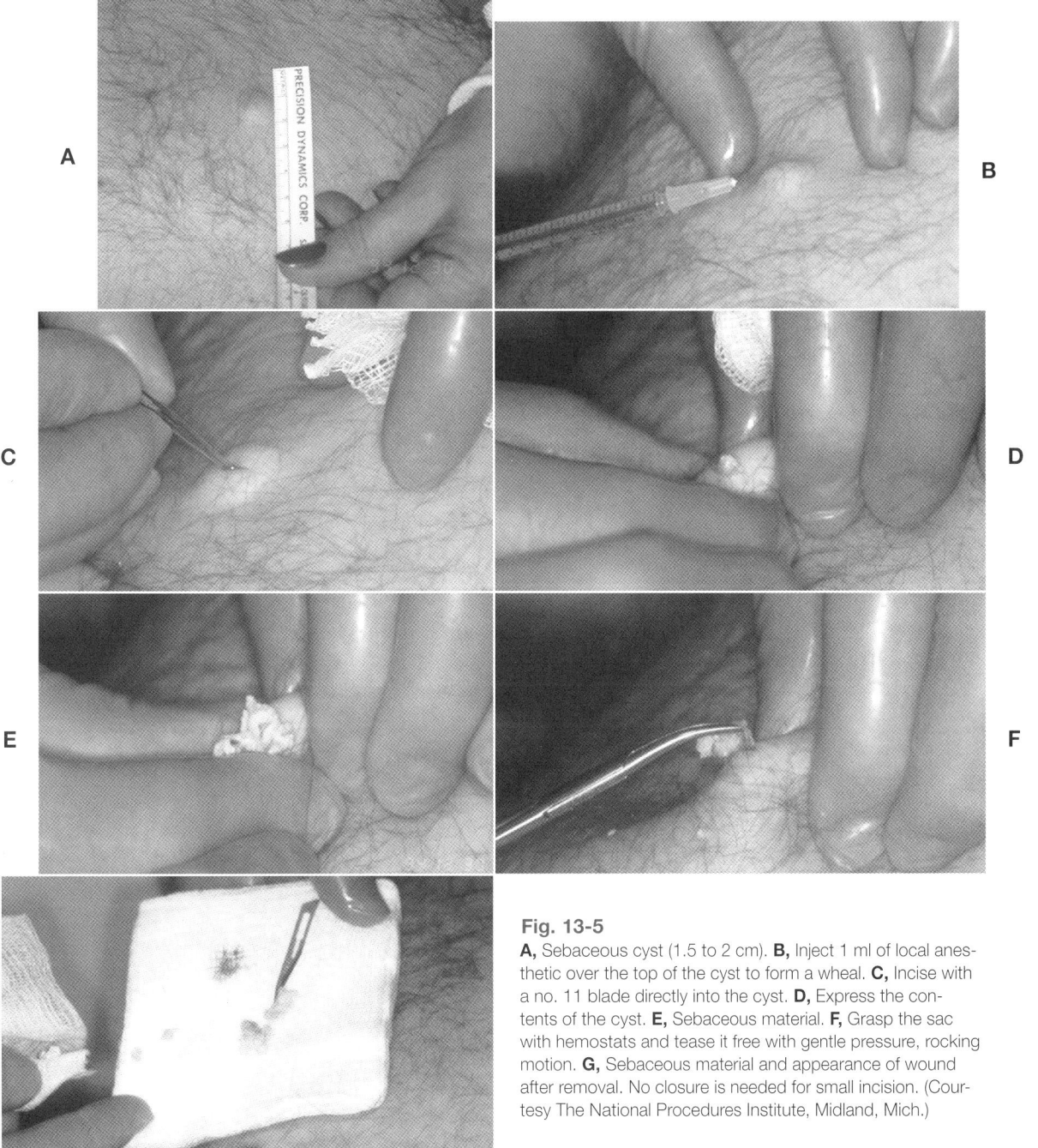

Fig. 13-5
A, Sebaceous cyst (1.5 to 2 cm). **B,** Inject 1 ml of local anesthetic over the top of the cyst to form a wheal. **C,** Incise with a no. 11 blade directly into the cyst. **D,** Express the contents of the cyst. **E,** Sebaceous material. **F,** Grasp the sac with hemostats and tease it free with gentle pressure, rocking motion. **G,** Sebaceous material and appearance of wound after removal. No closure is needed for small incision. (Courtesy The National Procedures Institute, Midland, Mich.)

pressure. Frequently (especially in scalp cysts where the sac is thick and firm), this external pressure will not only extrude the sebaceous material of the cyst but also the sac itself. If the sac is not produced, then curved hemostats are inserted into the wound and repeated attempts are made to grasp the sac and gently tug it out in its entirety. No suture closure is indicated so sterile technique (draping, etc.) is not indicated. If blood accumulates or the wound gets infected (both very rare), the patient just expresses it. Should some of the sac be left behind and the cyst reform, then formal excision will be required (Fig. 13-5).

Removal of the sac is usually successful unless it is quite large (over 2 cm), it has been infected previously, a previous attempt at removal has been made (causing surrounding scarring), or it is deep in the skin tissue. Wens, large and small, are almost always treated successfully in this fashion even with prior infection. The sacs are much thicker—almost like ping-pong balls! Three to four wens can readily be removed in a 15-minute visit.

Up to 95% of all sebaceous cysts can be treated with this simple method without recurrence.

A variation on the technique just described is to insert two large iodine crystals (iodine crystals USP) into the sac after expression of the contents. The sac for some reason contracts around the crystals in 48 to 72 hours; the clinician then easily expresses the entire complex through the incision. This technique can also be used if it appears that the entire sac has not been removed using the simple technique described above.

If infected, sebaceous cysts pose a bigger problem. *The treatment for an abscess is to I&D it!* Antibiotics are costly and many times there is not really an infection. Rather the cyst has ruptured, causing an inflammatory response. Treatment is the same: I&D. Formal excision is ill-advised, since infection is likely to occur if sutures are placed.

Technique

1. Prep with alcohol. Use 2 ml 2% xylocaine with epinephrine over the top of the lesion.
2. Use a no. 11 blade to incise the lesion. Be careful because the contents are often under pressure and come "flying out." All sebaceous material must be removed.
3. Insert hemostats to break up any pockets. Try to remove the sac as noted above, but it is usually too friable. Use a dermal curette and curette the inside, which may remove the sac.
4. Place ¼-inch iodoform gauze into the wound. Leave a small tail on the outside.
5. Cover with ointment so the dressing does not stick. Change the dressings two to three times per day. Change the gauze in 1 week and replace with clean gauze. Remove the new gauze in 3 weeks and let the wound heal.

Usually the cyst will not recur but rather scar down. If it recurs, formal excision is necessary, but not until the infection has resolved. No antibiotics are necessary after an I&D (see Chapter 21, Incision and Drainage of an Abscess).

TELANGIECTASIAS

Small cherry hemangiomas, a type of telangiectasia, are benign, small, red, vascular lesions that do not require treatment. If irritated or bleeding, they can be lightly cauterized and wiped off with a gauze. Malignancy is not a consideration. Spider veins, another type of telangiectasia, are best treated with sclerotherapy or laser if on the legs. Radiosurgery with a 30-gauge needle works extremely well on the face (see Chapter 31, Radiofrequency Surgery). Spider veins on the leg can produce

significant pain and paresthesias if left untreated. See Chapter 90, Sclerotherapy: Injection, and Chapter 91, Sclerotherapy: Radiofrequency.

WARTS (VERRUCA VULGARIS AND PLANTARIS)

The recurrence rates associated with all treatments of common warts are 30% or higher. Most over-the-counter and prescription preparations are acidic, caustic solutions. In time, 60% of warts will resolve spontaneously. Vitamins enhance the immune system and may aid wart resolution. Numerous treatment methods are used and noted in Table 13-1. (See Chapter 44, Wart [Verruca] Treatment.)

Plantar warts are treated with methods similar to those used with common warts. Physicians should avoid surgical excisions on the bottom of the feet because the scar tissue often remains painful after healing. A patient may suffer with the irritated scar, which produces an effect not unlike a pebble in a shoe. Soaking followed by paring of callous tissue will improve the efficacy of any treatment. Cryotherapy is effective without resulting in scarring. Treatment with *Candida* antigen has become the first line approach in all but simple cases of verruca.

WARTS (CONDYLOMA ACUMINATA)

See Chapter 157, Treatment of Noncervical Condyloma Acuminata.

WENS

See the previous section on sebaceous cysts.

XANTHELASMA

Xanthelasma, the most common form of xanthoma, is a yellow-white plaque on the eyelids. The diagnosis of xanthelasma can be made clinically. The goal of all treatments is to stay very superficial. Light fulguration or cauterization is often sufficient. With radiofrequency ablation, it is easier to control depth. Use the large loop at pure cutting and lightly vaporize the lesions until no residual white material exists. Often, if small, an incision can be made with an 18-gauge needle, and the lesion can be expressed. Surgically removing the abnormal tissue with a curvilinear elliptical excision provides excellent results when repaired using a 6-0 suture. Recurrences, because of the nature of the lesion, are common.

CPT/BILLING CODES

11200	Skin tag removal by excision or destruction: 1-15
11201	Each additional 10 or portion thereof
10060	I&D cyst/abscess, simple
10061	I&D cyst/abscess, complex or multiple

Note: If the sac is removed or gauze is placed, this is considered "complex."

Coding and billing of lesion removal and destruction is very complex. There are excision codes with simple and intermediate closures. Shave excisions are another whole section in the CPT code book. Destruction of lesions depends on whether they are benign or malignant, what their size is, and where they are located. For genital and anal lesions, it also depends on how they are "destroyed." It is of utmost importance that the clinician differentiate the methods for coding and billing for the treatment of these lesions. Clinicians should consider obtaining the current year's edition of *The Reimbursement Manual for Office Procedures* (Pfenninger JL, editor, The National Procedures Institute, 4909 Hedgewood Drive, Midland, Mich., 48642; 1-800-462-2492). This book not only lists appropriate procedure codes but provides a comparison and suggested fee for each code commonly used by primary care clinicians.

ADDITIONAL RESOURCES

- See the sample patient education handout titled "Moist Healing After Skin Surgery" on page 1747 of Appendix G.

BIBLIOGRAPHY

De Raeve LE, De Coninck AL, Dierickx PR, *Arch Fam Med* 134:114, 1998.

De Raeve LE, De Coninck AL, Dierickx PR, Roseeuw DI: Neonatal curettage of giant congenital melanocytic nevi, *Arch Dermatol* 132(1):20, 1996.

Guidelines of care for cutaneous squamous cell carcinoma: Committee on Guidelines of Care. Task Force on Cutaneous Squamous Cell Carcinoma, *J Am Acad Dermatol* 28(4):628, 1993.

Guidelines of care for malignant melanomas: Committee on Guidelines of Care: Task Force on Malignant Melanoma, *J Am Acad Dermatol* 28(4):638, 1993.

Habif TP: *Clinical dermatology,* ed 2, St Louis, 1990, Mosby.

Klin B, Ashkenazi M: Sebaceous cyst excision with minimal surgery, *Am Fam Physician* 41:1746, 1990.

Kuflik AS, Janniger CK: Basal cell carcinoma, *Am Fam Physician* 48(7):1273, 1993.

Kurban RS, Kurban AL: Skin disorders of aging: diagnosis and treatment, *Geriatrics* 48:30, 1993.

Lask G, Moyr ED: *Principles and techniques of cutaneous surgery,* New York, 1996, McGraw-Hill.

NIH Consensus Conference: Diagnosis and treatment of early melanoma, *JAMA* 268:1314, 1992.

Pariser RJ: Skin biopsy: lesion selection and optimal technique, *Modern Med* 57:82, 1989.

Pfenninger JL: *The reimbursement manual for office procedures,* Midland, Mich, 2002, The National Procedures Institute.

Roenigk RK, Roenigk HH: *Dermatologic surgery: principles and practice,* ed 2, New York, 1996, Marcel Dekker.

Stern RS, Boudreaux C, Arndt K: Diagnostic accuracy and appropriateness of care for seborrheic keratoses, *JAMA* 265:74, 1989.

Usatine RP, Moy RL, Tobinick EL, Siegel DM: *Skin surgery: a practical guide,* St Louis, 1998, Mosby.

CHAPTER 14

Burn Treatment

J. Fintan Cooper
Timothy J. Downs

More than 1.1 million burns are reported each year in the United States, according to the latest National Health Information Survey. Burns in the United States account for 700,000 emergency department visits, 45,000 hospitalizations, and 4500 fire- and burn-related deaths per year. Burn injuries can cause both severe psychological and physical disability. Early resuscitation and aggressive surgical intervention of burn injuries can reduce mortality and limit long-term morbidity.

BURN COMPLICATIONS REQUIRING RESUSCITATION

Inherent to burn injuries are a number of potential complications. Burn research has shown that the causes of early mortality are not the burns themselves, but complications related to hypoxia, hypoventilation, and circulation disorders, including hypovolemia and hypothermia. Complications requiring early resuscitation are as follows:

- Airway injury
  — Airway edema from thermal or chemical burns
- Inhalation injury/hypoxia
  — Chemical fumes are the most common cause of pneumonitis/pulmonary edema.
  — Smoke or other particulate material causes pneumonitis.
  — Carbon monoxide poisoning is common with fires in enclosed spaces.
- Hypothermia from loss of skin integrity and evaporative losses
- Hypovolemia or shock resulting from intravascular to extravascular fluid shifts and pain-vasoconstriction
- Cardiac asystole and arrhythmias (especially with high-voltage burns)

RESUSCITATION FOR EARLY BURN COMPLICATIONS

Advanced Trauma Life Support (ATLS) guidelines have helped focus resuscitation efforts to the most critical patient needs by using a simple-to-remember alphabetic pneumonic: A = Airway, B = Breathing, C = Circulation, D = Disability, E = Exposure, F = Fluids. Advanced Burn Life Support courses are available that help focus these guidelines even more specifically for burn injuries (see the "Websites" section at the end of chapter).

A = Airway

Airway management is the crucial first step in resuscitating a severe burn victim. Early endotracheal intubation is recommended when an injured airway is first diagnosed. Although airway edema normally stays above the vocal cords, delayed intubation can be much more difficult or traumatic. The manifestations of airway injury are often subtle and may not appear for 24 hours. A history of the victim being confined in a burning building (or closed space) or of having impaired mentation is suggestive of acute inhalational injury. With this history, a search for clinical evidence of inhalation injury should be undertaken carefully. Clinical clues to acute inhalation injury include facial burns, singed eyebrow or nasal hairs, oropharyngeal carbon deposits, or acute inflammation and carbonaceous sputum. If hoarseness, a brassy cough, or stridor develops, immediately intubate the patient. Intubation is also required before transport if transportation time will be prolonged. Airway injuries indicate major burn severity.

B = Breathing

Evaluate patient for spontaneous respirations. Check for stridor, wheezing, or rales. Administer 100% O_2 as soon

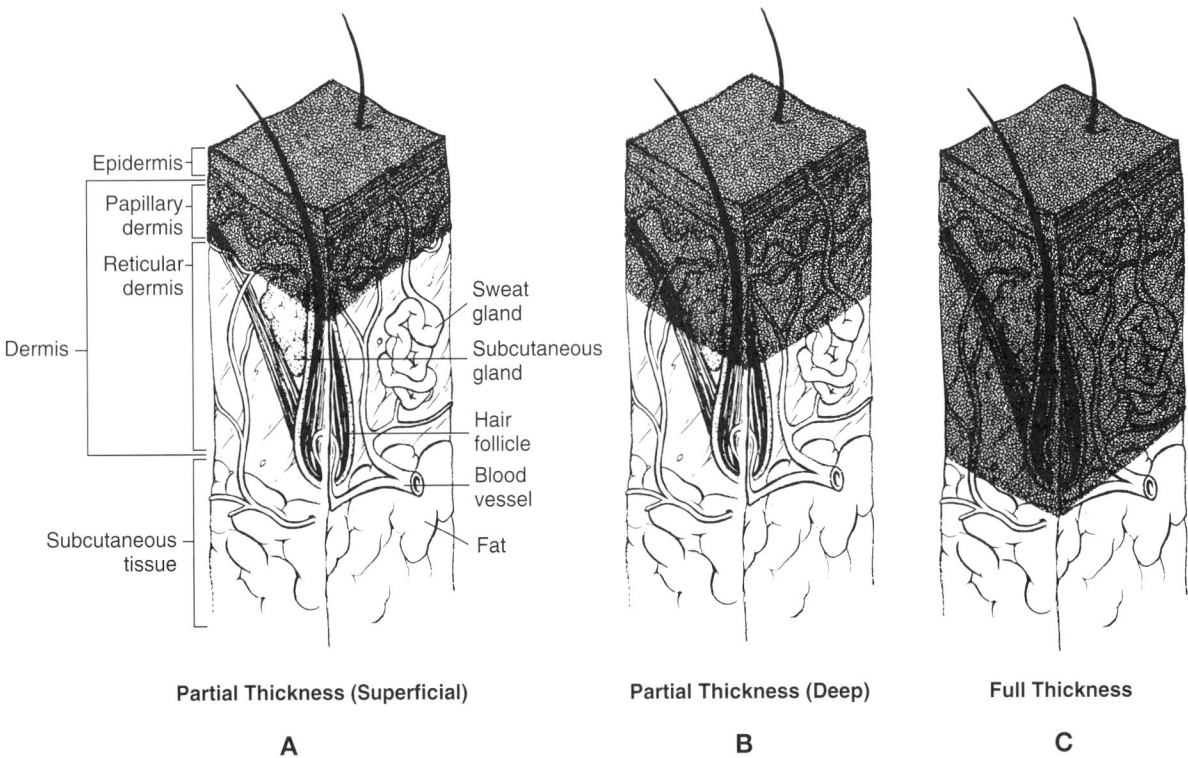

Partial Thickness (Superficial)

A

Partial Thickness (Deep)

B

Full Thickness

C

Fig. 14-1
A, Superficial partial-thickness burn. **B,** Deep partial-thickness burn. **C,** Full-thickness burn. Stippled area denotes depth of burn injuries. (Reproduced from Edlich RF et al: Thermal burns. In Marx JA et al: *Rosen's emergency medicine: concepts and clinical practice,* ed 5, St Louis, 2002, Mosby.)

as it is available. Carbon monoxide (CO) poisoning should be assumed if the burn victim was trapped in an enclosed space.

C = Circulation

Rapid shifts in intravascular fluid occur in burns of greater than 20% to 25% total body surface area (TBSA). Hypovolemia resulting from capillary leak and evaporative losses should be anticipated and corrected (see "F = Fluids" section). High-voltage burns can cause cardiac standstill. Lower voltage injuries may cause delayed arrhythmias. After removing the electrical source with a nonconducting piece of equipment or turning off the power source, begin basic life support in the pulseless victim. Advanced cardiac life support measures should be initiated as soon as appropriate equipment is available.

D = Disability

Remember to stabilize the cervical spine to prevent further disability. High-voltage injuries can cause tetanic muscle contractions severe enough to fracture the cervi-

cal spine, lumbar spine, or limbs. Jumps from burning buildings can also cause fractures.

E = Exposure

- Expose the patient by removing any nonadherent clothing, especially chemically contaminated or smoldering clothing.
- Examine for associated injuries. Document these injuries and list them on the problem list to be addressed after the patient is stabilized.
- Cover the patient with a clean, dry blanket to prevent hypothermia.

Estimating Burn Severity

The burn depth, burn size, and locations on the body must be assessed in order to determine the burn severity.

Fig. 14-1 and Table 14-1 describe the appearance and other characteristics of these four burn categories. Burn depth terminology no longer includes the use of "first-, second-, and third-degree burns." Note that superficial and superficial partial-thickness burns have minimal to no risk of scarring, are painful, and heal spontaneously by 3 weeks. Deep-partial thickness and

TABLE 14-1

Classification of Burns Based on Depth

Burn Classification	Definition and Characteristics
Superficial burn	Involves epidermis; local pain and erythema without blister formation
Superficial partial-thickness burn	Involves the epidermis and superficial papillary dermis; burn is painful, warm, moist with blister formation
Deep partial-thickness burn	Extends into reticular dermis; skin is mottled, waxy-white in appearance, with ruptured blisters; pain sensation is absent, but pressure sensation is intact
Full-thickness burn	Involves entire epidermis and dermis, entire capillary network is destroyed; burned skin has a white or leathery appearance with underlying clotted vessels, wound contracture, insensate with loss of pressure sensation and two-point discrimination

full-thickness burns have severe to very severe risk of scarring, decreased sensation, and delayed healing of greater than 3 weeks.

Initial estimates of the depth of the burn are crucial to timely triage. The final depth of injury cannot always be predicted at the initial evaluation; therefore sequential evaluations may be needed to revise the depth of the burn over the days and weeks following the injury.

Burn Size: Percent of Total Body Surface Area

Burn size is an important determinant of burn healing. Healing occurs from the fibroblasts migrating in from the burn margins and the oil glands and hair follicles (skin appendages). The skin appendages penetrate deep into the dermis and, except for full-thickness burns, are spared from destruction.

The adult body surface area can be divided into percentages of nine and multiples or fractions of nine: the "Rule of Nines" (Fig. 14-2). *Infants have greater proportion of TBSA on the head and neck and less on the legs. The posterior torso, including buttocks, still equals 18%, with each buttock equalling 2.5%. Palms are 1.25%.*

Burn Treatment Locations

The determination of whether a particular burn injury should be treated as an ambulatory case, a local hospital admission, or a direct admission to a regional burn center depends on burn involvement to some highly critical areas.

The American Burn Association (ABA) has set up criteria for referral to a burn center for treatment (see Box 14-1). The ABA's grading system recommends disposition to a burn center for these critical conditions because of the significantly increased risk of morbidity.

Certain burn locations or other potential injuries lead to automatic classification as *moderate burn severity.* The aforementioned fractures in association with burns increases the severity index.

F = Fluids

Aggressive fluid resuscitation is required in burn patients with more than 25% TBSA to prevent hypovolemia

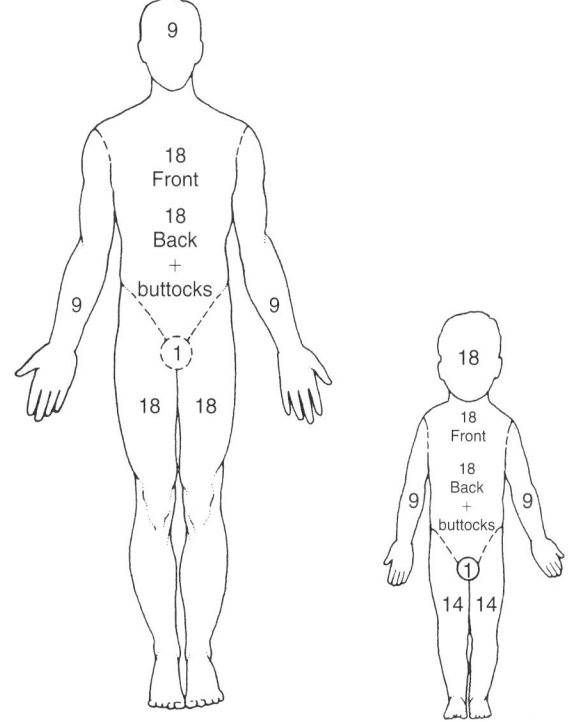

Fig. 14-2
Rule of Nines. (Modified from Krisanda TJ, Bethel CA: Burn care procedures. In Roberts JR, Hedges JR: *Clinical procedures in emergency medicine,* ed 3, Philadelphia, 1998, WB Saunders.)

and shock resulting from capillary leak and evaporative losses.

Intravenous Access

Insert two large-bore IVs, avoiding burned skin if possible. Central venous access may be needed.

Parkland Formula

The most widely accepted formula for fluid resuscitation is the Parkland Formula. The greatest intravascular to extravascular fluid shifts occur in the first 8 hours. Significant but slower fluid shifts continue for the next 16 hours. All fluid resuscitation formulas are designed to replace the intravascular volume as it is lost, most rapidly in the first 8 hours, then the next 16 hours.

> I. Second- and third-degree burns involving more than 10% of the body surface area in patients younger than 10 or older than 50 years of age.
> II. Second- and third-degree burns involving more than 20% of the body surface area in other age-groups.
> III. Significant burns of the face, hands, feet, genitalia, perineum, or the skin overlying major joints.
> IV. Full-thickness burns that involve more than 5% of the total body surface area in patients of any age.
> V. Significant electrical injury, including lightning injury.
> VI. Significant chemical injury.
> VII. Lesser burn injuries with associated inhalation injury, concomitant mechanical trauma, or significant preexisting medical disorders.
> VIII. Burn injury in patients who will require special social, emotional, or long-term rehabilitation, including cases of suspected or actual child abuse and neglect.

- *First 24 hours:* lactated Ringer's 4 ml/kg/% of burn (first half given in first 8 hours, second half given in next 16 hours).
- *Second 24 hours:* colloid 0.5 ml/kg/% burn + 2000 ml of 5% dextrose in water (D_5W) (given over second 24 hours).
- *Example:* 70-kg adult with 50% TBSA partial- and full-thickness burns requires 14 L of lactated Ringer's over the first 24 hours (4 ml × 70 kg × 50% burn = 14,000 ml/24 hr). Seven liters are given in the first 8 hours (875 ml/hr) and 7 L given in the next 16 hours (437.5 ml/hr).
- Evaluation of fluid resuscitation efforts is best gauged by *urine output* (see "Inpatient Management for Primary Provider" section).

Note: The time in which the fluids should be administered is measured from the time of the onset of the burn. If it takes 4 hours for a patient to begin receiving adequate fluid resuscitation, then all of the required replacement fluid must be administered within 20 hours instead of 24 hours. An accurate time of injury should be noted.

OTHER INITIAL BURN CARE

- Remove *nonadherent* burned clothing, constricting clothing, and jewelry.
- *Adherent* materials (clothing, tar, molten metal) should be cooled but not removed.
- Remove contaminated clothing. Brush away residual dry chemicals.
- Irrigate liquid residual chemicals copiously with water. Alkalies may require forceful irrigation (such as a shower) for up to an hour.
- Splash injuries to the eye require copious irrigation with tap water or saline. A Morgan lens can be both more effective and comfortable than an eye safety station or IV tubing dripping in one corner of the eye. Avoid contaminating an unaffected eye with the irrigation runoff.

DISPOSITION OF PATIENT BASED ON BURN SEVERITY AMERICAN BURN ASSOCIATION GUIDELINES

The ABA guidelines for disposition of burn patients is based on burn severity, which is based on depth, size, and location of the burn.

- Major burns: burn center (50% of burn hospitalizations were to burn center hospitals, up from 13% in 1971)
- Moderate burns: hospitalization
- Minor burns: outpatient management
  - Involve less than 10% TBSA of adults, 5% TBSA of young and old
  - Involve less than 2% TBSA full-thickness burns
  - Do not involve face, hands, feet, genitalia, or respiratory tract
  - Are not circumferential
  - No associated injuries or comorbidities

COMPLICATIONS ENCOUNTERED DURING BURN MANAGEMENT

Additional complications are encountered during the treatment of burns, whether in the hospital or as an outpatient. Any life-threatening complications encountered during the resuscitation phase of burn care require continued attention after the patient is stabilized and disposition has been determined. Burn centers have expertise in wound management and vigilance in late complications. Other complications that must be prevented if possible and addressed if they occur despite all preventive efforts include the following:

- Airway injury
  - Hypoxia
  - Airway edema
  - CO poisoning: PO_2 levels on blood gases may be normal even in the presence of CO poisoning. Carboxyhemoglobin levels should be measured. The presence of 100% O_2 provides appropriate supplementation and reduces CO levels. ($T_{1/2}$ of carboxyhemoglobin converting back to hemoglobin is reduced from 250 minutes on room air to 40 minutes on 100% O_2.) Severe cases of CO poisoning should receive hyperbaric oxygen therapy, which can be lifesaving.
  - CO poisoning symptoms related to percentage of carboxyhemoglobin: CO levels less than 20% are usually asymptomatic. At CO levels of 20% to 30%,

headache and nausea occur. At CO levels of 30% to 40%, confusion occurs and coma ensues when CO levels reach between 40% and 60%. Levels over 60% cause death.

- Cardiac arrhythmias: can occur for up to 3 days after high-voltage injury
- Pain
- Infection
  - Bacterial
  - Tetanus
  - Smoke inhalation/pneumonitis
  - Pneumonia
- Hypothermia
- Intravascular to extravascular fluid shifts
  - Hypovolemia/shock
  - Edema
  - Compartment syndrome
- Hypertrophic scars/contractures
  - Loss of function of hands, feet, eyes, joints, genitalia
  - Permanent disfigurement
- Pigmentary changes
  - Hypopigmentation for 6 to 24 months
  - Hyperpigmentation if not protected from ultraviolet damage
- Sensory dysfunction (sensory nerve damage)
  - Hypesthesias
  - Pruritus
- Xerosis (damaged sweat glands)
- Psychological
  - Depression
  - Anxiety disorders
  - Carcinoma in burn scars

INPATIENT MANAGEMENT FOR PRIMARY PROVIDER

According to the ABA's grading system for burn severity and disposition of patients, moderate and major burn injuries require hospitalization either locally or in a burn center. The primary provider may be the admitting provider for moderate and even severe burns if stabilization is needed before transfer to a burn center. The ABA's website (accessible at www.ameriburn.org) has search capability to assist in locating burn centers throughout the United States. Inpatient management of patients with moderate burn severity should include consideration of the following:

- History of burn injury
  - When? Initial time of burn important for fluid resuscitation.
  - How? Fire, steam, chemical, electrical, hot material.
  - Where? Enclosed space (inhalation injury)?
- Medical history

- Medical problems: diabetes and chronic steroid use increase risk of infection. Cardiopulmonary disease decreases physical reserves. Other medical problems will need to be addressed.
  - Medications: steroid use, blood thinners, diabetic medications, etc.
  - Allergies: sulfa allergy (use bacitracin ointment).
  - Last tetanus: boost if not received in last 12 months.
- Airway: suspected airway injury may need intubation if oropharyngeal edema develops during the 12 to 24 hours after injury. Observe for raspy cough, hoarseness, or stridor.
- Breathing: monitor for hypoxia
  - CO poisoning: 100% O_2 and/or hyperbaric oxygen therapy.
  - Pneumonitis or pulmonary edema: ventilation with high O_2 and positive end expiratory pressures may be needed.
  - Pneumonia: treat with appropriate systemic antibiotics.
- Circulation
  - Monitor urine output for adequate rehydration.
  - Monitor for cardiac arrhythmias with telemetry. Patients with high-voltage (greater than 440 volts) injuries can develop ventricular arrhythmias up to 3 days after the injury. The most common EKG finding of cardiac injury after electrical burn is nonspecific ST-T wave abnormalities. These patients should be admitted to the telemetry unit for cardiac monitoring until EKG normalizes. Treat with appropriate antiarrhythmics.
  - Compartment syndrome for circumferential wounds or if excessive rehydration.
    - Clinical diagnostic signs: delayed capillary refill, distal anesthesia, increasing limb pain, and decrease or loss of distal pulses. Clinical signs are only 60% sensitive (they miss 40% of true compartment syndromes).
    - Measure direct compartment pressures (see Chapter 189, Compartment Syndrome Evaluation).
    - Surgical consultation and escharotomy of affected limb including across joints. Rarely needed for circumferential burns of trunk.
    - Fasciotomy if escharotomy is not effective.
- Disability: obtain an x-ray skeletal survey for high-voltage burn or other suspected bone injury. Tetanic convulsion can cause fracture of cervical spine, lumbar spine, or limbs. A cross-table lateral of the cervical spine should be obtained before removal of full cervical spine precautions. Monitor the level of consciousness; mental alertness confirms adequate circulation.
- Exposure: avoid hypothermia, which can increase peripheral vasoconstriction. Evaporative fluid loss and loss of barrier to infection resulting from partial- and

full-thickness burns. Consider early excision of eschar and skin grafting or artificial covering.

- Fluids: continue rehydration per urine output. For adults, adequate urine output is 0.5 ml/kg/hr; for children, 1.0 ml of urine/kg/hr is needed. A Foley catheter is required. Excessive fluid administration can lead to increased edema, increased rate of compartment syndrome, and unnecessary faciotomies. Higher urine output and osmotic diuretics are normally required for high-voltage burns to prevent acute renal failure from rhabdomyolysis.
- Requirements decrease as the capillary leakage decreases over 2 to 7 days.
  — Admission weight and daily patient weights are required. Increased insensible losses through open wounds make patient weight invaluable.
  — Inputs and outputs: hourly fluid input and output required to monitor massive amounts of fluid used for resuscitation.
- Give tetanus prophylaxis for burns deeper than superficial partial thickness (if last tetanus greater than 12 months).
- Early nutrition first 12 to 24 hours, enteral if possible: burn injuries have increased metabolism from 1.3× to 2× baseline. Enteral feedings decrease gastrointestinal ulceration. Parenteral feedings may be required but significantly increase risk of sepsis at IV sites. Catheters should be replaced every 48 to 72 hours.
- Infection: common sources of infection in burn patients include the burn wounds, pneumonia, IV line sepsis, and urinary tract sepsis resulting from indwelling catheters. Burn wound infections usually require full-thickness biopsy and tissue culture to differentiate bacterial colonization from bacterial tissue invasion. Systemic antibiotics are required. Excision of infected burn tissue and grafting are often required. Culturing of central line catheter tips upon replacement is recommended. Worsening pulmonary status should prompt a chest x-ray examination.
- Pain: baseline pain medication with augmentation of pain relief by rescue medications is recommended. Some authorities recommend treatment of baseline pain with methadone and augmentation with morphine prior to dressing changes or activities such as physical therapy.

WOUND CARE

Burn Debridement

- Devitalized tissue removal is important to prevent bacterial colonization. Mild soaps such as chlorhexidine are recommended. Avoid Betadine, alcohol, and

hydrogen peroxide, which inhibit fibroblasts along with bacteria.

- Remove ruptured blisters, those blisters prone to break (e.g., over joints), and those with cloudy fluid that could be infected.
- Removal of small intact blisters is controversial. Some authorities recommend debridement of all blisters, whereas other authorities recommend leaving them undisturbed as a natural sterile barrier to infection.

Note: Delayed blister resolution longer than 2 weeks may indicate deep partial-thickness burn. Consider consultation for excision and skin grafting.

- Removal of adherent tar or clothing can be facilitated by application of petroleum jelly or bacitracin ointment for softening and removal during washing at dressing changes. Whirlpool baths are well tolerated for wound debridement.

Dressing Changes

- Standard dressings are changed twice a day. After dressing removal, the wounds are washed, inspected for healing or onset of infection, patted dry, treated with topical antibiotics, and covered with nonadherent dressings (Telfa) and gauze or stockinet.
- Consider Unna paste dressings. Advocates cite benefits such as decreased scarring, discomfort, and cost without increased infection rate. Dressings are changed every 3 to 7 days. Concerns include delayed detection of infection and overlooking of early scarring or other complications because of infrequent wound observation.

Topical Antibiotics

Topical antibiotics are used to decrease bacterial colonization of open blisters and deep burns. Their use significantly decreases wound infections. No single agents can be used in all cases. Several choices include the following:

- *Silver sulfadiazine (Silvadene 1% cream).* Silver sulfadiazine has intermediate eschar penetration and broad spectrum of antibacterial and anticandidal activity. It is easy to apply but should not be used on the face because of staining or in patients with sulfa allergy or glucose-6-phosphate dehydrogenase (G6PD) deficiency. It is expensive.
- *Mafenide acetate (Sulfamylon 8.5% cream).* Mafenide acetate has excellent eschar penetration and is the best antibacterial spectrum. It should be used on ears for prevention of chondritis. Some authorities recommend it on all full-thickness burns. Mafenide is painful after it is applied and expensive. Sleep disturbance is fairly

common after evening application. It is a carbonic anhydrase inhibitor; metabolic alkalosis may occur.

- *Silver nitrate 0.5% solution.* Silver nitrate has broad-spectrum antibacterial activity. The negatives include the need for frequent application (every 2 hours to moisten the dressings) and black stains on tissue, clothing, dressings, and bedding. It can also cause electrolyte imbalances and methemoglobinemia (see Chapter 216, Venous Methylene Blue Therapy).
- *Bacitracin zinc ointment 1%.* Bacitracin is best used for facial burns, around mucous membranes, in patients with sulfa allergy, and for loosening adherent tar or clothing before removal. Advocates note that it is inexpensive, readily available without prescription, and often effective. Bacitracin does not have good eschar penetration, has a narrower spectrum of antibacterial action, and can cause topical sensitization. It has no activity against *Candida albicans*. Controlled trials are needed comparing bacitracin to silver sulfadiazine.
- *Combination.* Some authorities recommend Sulfamylon for morning dressing change and Silvadene for the evening dressing change. The latter is considered painless with less sleep disturbance.

Excision and Skin Grafting

- Benefits of excision of the eschar and skin grafting include prevention of hypertrophic scarring and contractures as well as protection of deep tissues such as muscles and tendons (see Chapter 34, Skin Grafting). Decreases in evaporative fluid loss, pain, and susceptibility to infection are noted. Reduced time for rehabilitation and reduced time in hospital are also significant.
- Negative aspect of early excision and grafting is significant blood loss in a critically ill patient. Decreased blood loss occurs if excision is performed one day and grafting the following day.
- Options for skin grafting with the patient's own skin (autograft) include full-thickness versus split-thickness grafts as well as sheet grafts versus mesh grafts.
- Other grafting materials include allografts (cadaver), xenografts (usually porcine), cultured skin cells, and dermal substitutes such as collagen and bilayer substitutes (both dermal and epidermal components).

Prevention of Contractures or Hypertrophic Scarring

- Early consultation with burn specialist or surgeon with burn experience is recommended. Hypertrophic scarring and contractures are best prevented and, once started, are more difficult to treat.

- Hypertrophic scarring can occur up to 2 years after the burn injury.
- Increased risk of contracture in deep partial-thickness burns and full-thickness burns, black patients and at extremes of age range both young and old.
- Late excision (after 2 weeks) of eschar and skin grafting for deep partial-thickness or full-thickness burns masked by blisters. Non-resorption of blister by 2 weeks is a diagnostic clue.
- Early involvement with physical therapy and occupational therapy decreases contractures. Active range of motion (ROM) and stretching is superior to passive ROM in decreasing the risk of contracture. Avoid splinting of extremity burns if at all possible.
- Pressure dressings decrease hypertrophic scarring, even if initiated as late as 12 months after the burn injury. Early pressure dressing use is superior.

AMBULATORY MANAGEMENT FOR PRIMARY PROVIDER

Management of the majority of the 1.1 million burns per year in the United States occurs in an ambulatory setting. Of the 700,000 emergency room visits per year, the average visit frequency is only 1.2 visits per patient. The primary provider is well equipped to manage the initial burn care and follow-up burn care for minor burns. Minor burns involve less than 10% TBSA of adults, less than 5% TBSA of young and old patients, and less than 2% TBSA full-thickness burn; they do not involve the face, hands, feet, genitalia, or respiratory tract. They are not circumferential. These patients do not have significant associated injuries or comorbidities that predispose to infection.

Initial Ambulatory Visit

- Evaluation of burn severity and inclusion of only minor burns.
- Tetanus prophylaxis, if indicated.
- Burn debridement. (Give field block or regional anesthesia for discomfort; remove devitalized tissue, ruptured blisters, and blisters likely to rupture.*)
- Wound washed with soap (chlorhexidine) and warm water. (This is a clean but not sterile procedure.*)
- Wound dressing changes twice a day.*
- Early referral for excision of eschar and skin grafting as outpatient, if indicated.†

---

*The "Inpatient Management for Primary Provider" section includes more extensive discussion of this topic.
†See the "Indications for Referral to Burn Specialist/Surgeon" section.

- Pain control: nonsteroidal antiinflammatory drugs or acetaminophen recommended for baseline pain. (Prescribe oral narcotic pain relievers [e.g., acetaminophen with codeine] for before-dressing changes, for breakthrough pain, and at bedtime for pain during sleep.)
- Avoidance of splinting and encouragement of active ROM and stretching.
- Full-thickness burns less than 3 cm in diameter in a nonfunctional, noncosmetic area with normal-thickness skin may be allowed to heal by contracture.
- Patient teaching guide (see the sample patient education handout titled "Home Burn Care" on page 1748 of Appendix G).
- Follow-up appointment scheduled for the day after the burn injury.

Second Ambulatory Visit

- During the dressing change, reevaluation of burn severity (location, size, and depth), evaluation of pain control, and possible further wound debridement.
- Teaching wound care and dressing changes at this visit.
- Teaching patient to observe for infection, scarring, or other complication.
- Patient referral to physical and/or occupational therapy for burns involving the hands, feet, or joints.

Subsequent Visits

- Follow-up weekly until the wound is epithelialized. Continue daily follow-up if compliance of patient or communication with provider is not optimal.
- Epithelialized wounds no longer need antibiotic ointments or dressings, but they do need daily sunblock (SPF 15 or higher) for 6 to 24 months to prevent hyperpigmentation. Once repigmentation is complete and the wound no longer blanches from red-pink to white with pressure, additional sunblock is not needed.
- Subsequent follow-up for at least 6 months and reevaluation every 4 to 6 weeks to check for hypertrophic scarring.
- Hypoallergenic, unscented moisturizing creams for pruritus and xerosis. Antihistamines such as diphenhydramine or hydroxyzine pamoate (Vistaril).
- Patient education handout for home care. (See the sample patient education handout for "Home Burn Care" on page 1748 of Appendix G.)

Considerations for Referral to Burn Specialist or Surgeon

- Blacks, who have increased risk of hypertrophic scars (if not healed at 10 days)
- Children and elderly (if not healed at 2 weeks)
- Adults (if not healed at 3 weeks)
- Wound infection
- Early hypertrophic scarring

PREVENTION

- Encourage installation of smoke detectors on each floor of domestic dwellings, particularly at prenatal visits or well-child visits.
- Encourage parents to teach their children about the proper fire safety precautions, fire escapes, and the hazards of matches and fireworks.
- Encourage families to know and practice fire-escape routes. Purchase rope-escape ladders for bedrooms on the second floor.
- Advise smokers not to smoke in bed.

CONCLUSION

Burns are a common problem. Most burns are managed in an ambulatory setting. An understanding of burn depth, high-risk burn locations, and how to estimate the burned percentage of TBSA is necessary for appropriate patient disposition. Understanding the potential complications and management principles for burn injuries permits early and appropriate medical and surgical therapy. Helping patients to understand how to care for their burn injuries and what complications to look for will further decrease the complication rates. For slowly healing wounds, surgical referral for excision and skin grafting can reduce healing time, contractures, and infection. Encourage good prevention practices.

CPT/BILLING CODES

16000	Burns, initial treatment
16010-16042	Burns, debridement
16010-16030	Burns, dressings
16035	Burns, escharotomy
16040-16042	Burns, excision

See Chapter 34, Skin Grafting, for procedural coding for skin grafts.

ICD-9-CM DIAGNOSTIC CODES

940–947.X	Burns by specific site. Fourth digit of the code (0 to 5) indicates depth or severity.
948.XX	Burns classified according to extent of body surface involved. Fourth digit of

the code indicates percentage of TBSA involved (0 = <10%, 1 = 10% to 19%, and so on up to 9 = 90% or more involved). Fifth digit of the code indicates percentage of TBSA involved in full-thickness burns.

ADDITIONAL RESOURCES

• See the sample patient education handout titled "Home Burn Care" on page 1748 of Appendix G.

BIBLIOGRAPHY

Cameron JL, editor: *Current surgical therapy,* ed 6, St Louis, 1998, Mosby.

Lewis DP: Burns: Initial management and outpatient follow-up, *Fam Pract Recert* 23(2):19, 2001.

Monafo WW: Initial management of burns, *N Engl J Med* 335(21):1581, 1996.

Morgan ED, Bledsoe SC, Barker J: Ambulatory Management of Burns, *Am Fam Physician* 62:2015, 2000.

WEBSITES

www.ameriburn.org (American Burn Association, listing regional burn centers by state)

www.dmrti.army.mil (under "Courses We Offer," select "Advance Burn Life Support [ABLS]")

www.drkoop.com (health advice on a variety of medical conditions for the layman, including first aid advice under "burns")

CHAPTER 15

Cryosurgery

John E. Hocutt, Jr.
John L. Pfenninger

Cryosurgery is the deliberate destruction of diseased tissue by freezing in a controlled manner. It is critically important that all primary care physicians master the art and technique of cryosurgery. The procedure is often a better alternative than surgical excision, especially when convenience, healing, disability during healing, infectious disease risk (HIV, hepatitis), discomfort, and scar formation are considered. (Also see Chapter 141, Cryotherapy of the Cervix.)

GENERAL CONSIDERATIONS

- Lesions treated with cryosurgery usually heal with minimal or no scar formation. Even if inadvertent excessive freezing is done, scarring is rarely significant.
- Complete healing may take more than 6 to 8 weeks in extreme cases, but the results are usually excellent. Selective destruction of cells occurs during the freeze. However, the collagen and fibroelastic structural framework is preserved, so the epithelial cells grow back in an organized fashion within the preserved matrix.
- The procedure is safe, simple, and easy to learn. It usually takes less time than conventional surgery.
- Patients may prefer to avoid injections of local anesthetic, which is usually possible with cryotherapy.
- The freezing itself has an anesthetic effect, although a burning sensation is experienced initially and again on thawing. Explain to patients that the freezing will feel like an ice cube stuck to the skin. This often reassures them enough to cope with the minimal amount of pain experienced. However, very young children often will not accept the procedure without crying. Their fear of the unknown increases when the unpleasant cold sensation starts. They have difficulty trusting that the burning feeling will actually improve in a very short time instead of continually getting worse. In children and in some adults, a local anesthetic will be helpful, especially when freezing multiple or large lesions

and when attempting a deep freeze for malignant lesions.
- Other than keeping the lesions clean and protected, patients can essentially ignore the cryotreated lesion between treatments. They appreciate the omission of suture insertion and removal. Patients also welcome being able to bathe and swim while the lesion is healing.
- Secondary infection generally is not a significant problem. Even with overfreezing and with cryosensitive patients who overreact with excessive tissue destruction, infection occurs rarely. Excessive freezing may result in wound weeping for longer than 4 to 6 weeks, but infection should not be expected unless the area receives repetitive friction or poor skin care.
- Occasionally, most common in elderly patients, a profuse watery discharge may persist more than 3 to 4 days after treatment. Applying Monsel's solution often alleviates the discharge.
- Two theoretical concerns have arisen recently regarding cryosurgery and use of the nitrous oxide closed system. One is the spread of infectious agents by the equipment. Cryoprobes should be cleaned between procedures. Cidex soaking is accepted whereas some companies make their probes safe for autoclaves. Second, at least one state (South Carolina) requires nitrous oxide gas to be vented outside of the examination/treatment room. Female dental assistants exposed to high levels of nitrous oxide for more than 5 hours per week had an increased incidence of miscarriages. Therefore until more data are available on time and quantity of exposure, venting of the nitrous oxide gas is recommended by some. This can be accomplished by simply extending the exhaust tube on the unit under the door or out a window or by installing vents in an outside wall. The likelihood of a patient receiving enough exposure to do harm is very small and has not yet been reported. If laws become overly restrictive, carbon dioxide (which is an agent nearly as cold)

can be substituted for nitrous oxide, if a closed system is desired.

ADVANTAGES OF CRYOTHERAPY (CRYOSURGERY)

- Local anesthetic is optional, so needles can be avoided.
- Freezing produces minimal pain.
- Final healing is cosmetically excellent, with minimal or no scarring.
- Minimal physician time is required, and the procedure is easy to learn.
- Preoperative skin preparation is not required.
- Multiple lesions can be treated quickly in one setting.
- Postoperative infection is rare; cases are reportable.
- No significant postprocedure care is needed.
- No significant disruption of postprocedure activity is required.
- The procedure is ideal for patients with light-complexioned skin.
- The procedure is inexpensive and cost-effective.
- A wide variety of lesions can be treated without significant exposure to blood-borne pathogens.
- Units are portable and can be taken to nursing home facilities when needed.
- Units are inexpensive and start-up costs are minimal.
- Units take up little space in the office.

DISADVANTAGES OF CRYOTHERAPY

- Use is limited in patients with darker skin because of pigment changes. Even with brief partial-thickness freeze technique, some melanocytes are destroyed and the healed cryolesion may be slightly lighter in color than the surrounding skin, even in fair-skinned individuals.
- Cryotherapy is not recommended in areas of hair growth, such as around the eyebrows and eyelashes, and on scalps with thin hair, because even brief freezing tends to destroy hair follicles.
- Healed cryolesions may not tan sufficiently, often are more susceptible to sunburn, and may require added sunscreen protection.
- Tissue is not available for histopathologic diagnosis, so certainty of complete removal is lacking.
- Exposure to nitrous oxide gas if closed units are used (see above).

AGENTS USED FOR CRYOSURGERY

There are three basic methods of cryotherapy (Table 15-1).
- Closed systems (freezing is carried out with a cooled probe as opposed to the application of the agent itself)
  — Nitrous oxide
  — Carbon dioxide
- Liquid nitrogen
  — Thermos bottle/spray unit (Brymill, Wallach)
  — Cotton-tipped applicators and Styrofoam cup
- Aerosol canister
  — Tetrafluoroethane (Verruca-Freeze, Medi-Frig)
  — Ether/propane (Histofreezer)

Nitrous oxide is quite unstable, and once it is released into the probe, it immediately breaks down to molecular nitrogen and oxygen. The physical characteristics of the nitrous oxide gas enable the cryotip's temperature to be easily lowered to −89° C. A *carbon dioxide*–powered tip is not as cold, and it will take longer to achieve a quality freeze (−78° C).

TABLE 15-1
Cryogenic Agents

	Characteristics				
	Liquid Nitrogen	N_2O_2	CO_2	Tetrafluoroethane	Ether/Propane
Boiling Point	−196° C	−89° C	−78° C	−47° C	−29° C
Eff. Treatment Temp	−196° C	−89° C	−78° C	−70° C	−55° C
Use	Thermos-type guns Cotton-tip applicator Stored in large dewars	Cylinders with applicator gun (cryoprobe)	Cylinders with applicator gun (cryoprobe); dry ice slush	Aerosol canister	Aerosol canister
Method/system	Open	Closed	Closed; open	Open (spray/cones, buds)	Open (buds)
Shelf-Life	1 yr max with best dewars	Indefinite	Indefinite	5 yr	5 yr +
Flammable	—	—	—	—	+
Trade Name	Cryogun (Brymill) UltraFreezer (Wallach)	—	—	Verruca Freeze (CryoSurgery, Inc.) MediFrig (Ellman)	Histofreezer (STC Tech, Inc.)
Indications	All	All	All	Superficial only (no cancers)	Superficial only (no cancers)

Nitrous oxide comes in a closed gas cylinder (blue tank, versus brown for carbon dioxide and green for oxygen). The handheld cryogun, which is connected to the tank with tubing, is structured differently from the liquid nitrogen guns. It is designed to allow a controlled rapid evaporation of nitrous oxide on the cryoprobe tip, taking its temperature to −89° C. The storage tanks preserve nitrous oxide virtually "forever" by keeping the gas under pressure with no port for evaporation (except for cryogun activation). The tanks are moved from storage to use on small carts. The cryoprobes (tips) come in numerous shapes and sizes to match the lesion to be treated. The hemorrhoid probe; rounded, pointed tip; and the slanted flat tip are popular for dermatologic applications (Fig. 15-1). (The "hemorrhoid tip" is rarely, if ever, used for hemorrhoids, but its shape allows use for multiple dermatologic lesions.) The flat and slightly conical 19- and 25-mm tips are used for cryotherapy of the cervix.

Because nitrous oxide does not achieve a probe temperature as low as liquid nitrogen (−89° C versus −196° C), it is significantly slower at freezing tissue. This is especially important when treating multiple lesions. However, with nitrous oxide it is easier to control the extent of freeze because the area being frozen is more defined and the progress is slower. Both nitrous oxide and liquid nitrogen are effective for treating malignancies. Overlapping treatment areas for larger lesions using large probes ensures efficacy. Nitrous oxide units have an active defrost mode that rapidly frees the cryotip from frozen tissue.

Liquid nitrogen is the coldest cryogen effecting a rapid, deep freeze (−196° C). A storage dewar is needed. Newer dewars can store the nitrogen for up to 1 year. Liquid nitrogen is relatively inexpensive, but if not used, it will evaporate. The level of liquid nitrogen in the dewar must be monitored to be sure ample supply is present whenever a patient arrives for treatment. Liquid nitrogen may be applied by cotton-tipped applicators or a Thermos-type unit (Brymill Cryogun/CRY-AC3 or Wallach Ultrafreezer). The various apertures of the cryogun tips allow a variable amount of gas to cover a lesion,

giving some control as to the extent of freezing. A reusable plastic shield is now available to limit gas spread. Use of these units allows an efficient and rapid treatment of multiple lesions in a single clinical setting and enables a deeper freeze than cotton-tipped applicators. A tip is available that allows the Thermos to be used as a closed system, but there is no active defrost. Subsequently, the tip remains "stuck" to the tissue for a significant length of time before it thaws and detaches.

Canister refrigerants are the least expensive agents used for cryotherapy. They come prepackaged in small handheld canisters the size of a soda can, making them portable for use in nursing homes, satellite clinics, and multiple examination rooms. They have a very long shelf life. Unfortunately they do not achieve tissue temperature lowering sufficient enough to treat very many lesions. These agents are not indicated for malignancies, deep lesions, and large lesions. *Tetrafluoroethane* (Cryosurgery's Verruca-Freeze, Ellman's Medi-Frig) is a compressed gas that freezes tissue on vaporization (effective temperature of −70° C). *Ether/propane* (Histofreezer, −50° C) also comes in a canister but is not as cold and is flammable, as compared with the tetrafluoroethane.

TISSUE EFFECTS: PRINCIPLES FOR TREATMENT

It is important to recognize that at −2.2° C, cells begin to freeze. At −5° C, cells will super cool, but they recover. Tissue destruction only begins when the temperature is between −10° and −20° C. A deeper freeze with temperatures between −40° and −50° C ensures that malignant cells are completely destroyed.

The size of the ice ball that forms around the lesion provides a good estimate of the depth of the freeze. The *lethal zone* (tissue temperature less than −20° C) is 2 to 3 mm *inward* from the outer margin of the ice ball. This is especially crucial to remember in cases of premalignant or malignant lesions, which are deeper in the skin. *The size of the ice ball beyond the lesion is the most important criterion in determining how long to freeze.* Factors prolonging the freeze time include low tank pressure, increased tissue vascularity, excessive keratin covering (needs to be removed or moistened), and poor tip-to-lesion contact. The use of different systems (nitrous oxide, liquid nitrogen, carbon dioxide, canister gases, etc.) dramatically affects the rapidity and depth of freeze. Likewise, the method of applying liquid nitrogen (with the cotton-tipped applicator or in a spray fashion) affects freezing parameters. Similarly, it is important to observe *the time it takes for the area to thaw from the outer edge of the ice ball to the lesion edge ("halo thaw time")* and *the time for all the tissue to thaw (total thaw*

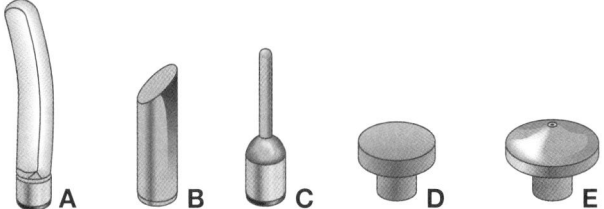

Fig. 15-1
Sample of varying shapes of cryoprobe tips. Most come in variable sizes. **A,** Hemorrhoid tip. **B,** Slanted flat tip. **C,** Pointed tip. **D,** Flat cervical tip. **E,** Slight conical cervical tip.

BOX 15-1

Freezing Guidelines for Skin

Benign Lesions
- Ice ball 2-3 mm beyond lesions.
- Correlate with thaw times below.
- Consider double freeze for difficult or premalignant lesions.

Malignant and Most Premalignant Lesions
- Ice ball 5 mm beyond lesion
- Double freeze (freeze, thaw, refreeze, using same parameters)

Freeze Time
- Variable, depending on cryogen, pressure applied, size of lesion, type of lesion, size of nozzle/tip, expertise of operator.
- Second freeze is faster.

Halo Thaw Time
- 1 minute (benign)
- 2-4 minutes (malignant)

Total Thaw Time
- 2-3 minutes (benign)
- 3-5 minutes (malignant)

Liquid Nitrogen
- Small swab (small lesions) and large swab (large lesions)
  - 10-second freeze
  - Total thaw time: 60 sec (superficial lesions)
- Spray: as noted above for other applications

See text for details and for specific lesions.

TABLE 15-2

Freeze Time Guidelines for Nitrous Oxide Technique*

Tissue	Lesion	Freeze Time†
Skin	Full-thickness benign	1-1.5 min
	Full-thickness, malignant	1.5-3 min‡
	Plantar warts (after debridement)	40 sec
	Condyloma	20-45 sec
	Verrucae	1-1.5 min
	Vascular lesions (with pressure)	1-1.5 min
	Seborrheic keratoses (2 mm margin)	30 sec‡
	Actinic keratoses (3 mm margin)	1-1.5 min‡
	Basal cell cancer (3-5 mm margin)	1.5 min‡
Hemorrhoids	Cryoligation	2 min
	Cryo without ligation	2-3 min‡
Cervix	Cervicitis	3 min
	Cervical intraepithelial neoplasia I, II, III	3 min‡
	Cervical intraepithelial neoplasia I, II (alternative method)	5 min

*The treatment times for liquid nitrogen spray are much shorter than those of nitrous oxide.
†Freeze times are approximate guidelines and should be adjusted to the size of the ice ball, which is far more important than the time.
‡Freeze-thaw-refreeze.

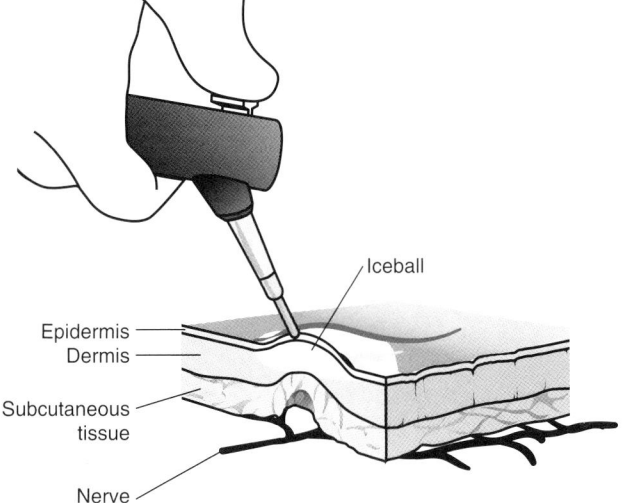

Fig. 15-2
With nitrous oxide, once cryotip is frozen to the skin, the probe can be retracted to avoid freezing nontarget underlying structures.

time) (Box 15-1). A brief freeze can turn tissue white, providing the ice ball desired; however, if it remains frozen only momentarily, it will have little effect.

Freeze times should be adjusted according to patient sensitivity, type and size of the lesion, presence of malignancy, and lesion vascularity (Table 15-2). Age, vascular flow, amount of pigment, depth of lesion, amount of keratin, location on the body, and cell type of the lesion all affect the amount of freezing required to destroy pathologic tissue. Adjust your freeze times accordingly. Applying pressure to the lesion with the fixed probes will increase the depth of freeze. Vascular lesions will require longer freezing times, and pressure from the probe will need to be applied to squeeze as much blood as possible out of the lesion prior to freezing. Any active bleeding will need to be controlled.

For *benign lesions,* a single freeze/thaw cycle is sufficient. The ice ball should extend 2 to 3 mm beyond the lesion margin. Resistant lesions such as warts often require a freeze/thaw/freeze cycle.

For *malignant or premalignant lesions,* a freeze/thaw/freeze cycle is recommended. The ice ball should extend 5 mm beyond the lesion margin each time the tissue is frozen. The second freeze is usually quicker and less painful.

Dry, keratinized tissue will not freeze easily and will insulate the lesion underneath from freezing. Remove as much keratin as possible before freezing, especially with nitrous oxide or the canister agents.

With the nitrous oxide cryotips, once the tip is "frozen" and fixed to the skin, the probe can be retracted to reduce the depth of freeze, thereby sparing critical structures (such as nerves) from exposure to freezing (Fig. 15-2).

Bandages are not necessary unless the lesion is continually irritated (i.e., by clothing) or begins to weep.

POSTTREATMENT PHYSIOLOGIC EFFECTS

Erythema and hyperemia are immediate responses to effective freezing. Edema and exudation (blister formation) peak within 24 to 48 hours and usually subside after 72 hours. Blood may accumulate under the blister. The extracellular collagen structures are more resistant to freezing than the cells themselves. The lesion becomes bloodless 72 hours after freezing. Crust formation begins, and this crust will slowly wither away over the next several days. Reepithelialization occurs from the outer margin inward. Fibroblasts lay down minimal new collagen along the preserved, well-formed collagen matrix, ensuring the lack of scar formation. If the collagen matrix had been destroyed, fibroblasts would produce collagen randomly, leading to scar formation. Cartilage (such as in the ear) is preserved.

If the patient or physician desires, the treated lesion can be surgically débrided in 24 to 48 hours. During this time, the dermis and epidermis separate, lifting the lesion to the top of the blister. Removal of the prepared lesion with iris scissors is painless. After 72 hours, however, the lesion may stick like a graft and may bleed on attempts at removal. If completely left alone, the lesion will eventually slough spontaneously. (Surgical debridement 1 or 2 days after freezing effectively removes the lesion and satisfies some patients sooner. However, many patients are quite happy to avoid the early return visit and are willing to wait to see how much of the lesion sloughs before returning for another treatment.) A disadvantage of this technique is that a second office visit is needed for the 24- to 48-hour debridement procedure.

The healed cryolesion is soft, with minimal to no scarring. This allows erections if penile lesions are to be frozen. Pigment is often decreased, and hair and sweat glands may be destroyed in the area of freezing. It is best to caution the patient *in advance* that although the area that was frozen is unlikely to develop much of a scar, the skin is often lighter. The inflammatory response may result in the development of a transient halo of hyperpigmentation. This will usually clear completely over several months.

INDICATIONS

- Abscesses, incision and drainage (I&D) (to anesthetize before incision, use a very light freeze)
- Actinic keratoses (full-thickness freeze)
- Angiomas or hemangiomas including congenital strawberry hemangiomas (more difficult)
- Basal cell cancer (full-thickness destructive double-freeze)
- Bowen's disease (squamous cell carcinoma in-situ)
- Cervical intraepithelial neoplasia (CIN, dysplasia), "cryoconization" (see Chapter 135, Cervical Conization)
- Chondrodermatitis nodularis helicis
- Condyloma acuminata
- Dermatofibromas (difficult)
- Freckles (lentigines)
- Granulation tissue
- Hemorrhoids (rarely done)
- Hypertrophic scars (multiple treatments over time)
- Keloids (as above)
- Molluscum contagiosum
- Mucocele
- Myxoid cysts
- Papular nevi (full-thickness freeze)
- Pyogenic granuloma
- Sebaceous cell cancers (full-thickness destructive double-freeze)
- Seborrheic keratoses
- Skin tags and polyps
- Verrucae (including plantar)
- Xanthoma

CONTRAINDICATIONS

Absolute Contraindications

- Proven sensitivity or adverse reaction to cryosurgery
- Patient nonacceptance of the possibility of skin pigment changes
- Melanoma
- Areas of end-stage compromised circulation
- Lesions in which identification of tissue pathology is required
- Sclerosing (morpheaform) or recurrent basal cell or squamous cell carcinoma

Relative Contraindications

- Any condition with high levels of cryoglobulins (most noted below)
- Immunoproliferative neoplasms (e.g., myeloma, lymphoma)
- Macroglobulinemia
- Active severe collagen vascular diseases
- Severe active ulcerative colitis
- Acute poststreptococcal glomerulonephritis (almost 100% of these patients have high levels of cryoglobulins)
- Active subacute bacterial endocarditis, syphilis, Epstein-Barr infection, cytomegalovirus infection
- Chronic severe hepatitis B
- High-dose steroid therapy

Note: Patients with the above conditions are likely to have an exaggerated response to cryosurgery because they have high levels of circulating cryoglobulins. If cryosurgery is appropriate or necessary for any of these patients, be sure to obtain informed consent and perform a pretest in the axilla or thigh area before treating a more prominent or cosmetically sensitive area. Proceed with caution and greatly shorten the freezing times until the response can be predicted. You may be able to freeze lesions effectively and safely with a much shorter freeze time. With overfreezing, the risk of tissue slough and marked hypopigmentation increase. Therefore start slowly and advise patients that extra visits and treatment sessions may be necessary. A conservative approach is best in light of their clinical situation.

- Basal cell or squamous cell cancers more than 1 cm in diameter

LESIONS DIFFICULT TO TREAT WITH CRYOSURGERY

- Dermatofibroma (these lesions require a longer freeze time)
- Hidradenitis
- Flat nevi (must be absolutely sure lesion in not a melanoma)
- Squamous cell cancer (usually reserved for practitioners who treat this cancer often)
- Most vascular lesions (especially if extensive)

AREAS NOT RECOMMENDED FOR CRYOSURGERY

- Areas where hair loss is critical to the patient
- Areas where pigment changes are critical to the patient
- Feet, ankles, and lower legs, when circulation is in question (especially diabetics)
- Over superficial cutaneous nerves (unless adequate skin traction to pull the skin away from the nerve is possible, usually with nitrous oxide technique)
- Basal cell cancers in nasolabial fold, in preauricular areas, and on lips (often more extensive and tend to recur)
- Any cancer that has not had histologic confirmation
- Periorbital area (may induce immediate and severe swelling)
- Port-wine stain (use laser)

EQUIPMENT

For all methods listed, consider local anesthesia for patient comfort and the ability to freeze long enough to obtain effect desired. The need for anesthesia will depend on the size of the lesion, number of lesions, patient age, and so forth.

Liquid Nitrogen

- Storage dewar (Fig. 15-3, *B*)
- Cryogun/Thermos unit (Fig. 15-3)
- Assorted various-sized nozzles
- Protective neoprene shield with assorted opening sizes (Fig. 15-4)
- Styrofoam cups
- Cotton-tipped applicators (small and large)

Nitrous Oxide (Fig. 15-5)

- Two 20-lb tanks (the "short, fat, blue one"; have two to ensure that a full one is always ready)
- Mobile storage cart
- Cryoprobe regulator with gun
- Cryoprobe tip assortment (Fig. 15-6)
- K-Y Jelly or CryoGel

Canister Gas Refrigerants

- Can of Verruca-Freeze or Medi-Frig with various sizes of ear speculums or cotton tips (Fig. 15-7)
- Can of Histofreeze with cotton tips

PREPROCEDURE PATIENT PREPARATION

Before the procedure, the patient should be advised of the basic technique, the expected sensation during treatment, and the possible complications. (See the sample patient education handouts titled "Wart Removal," "Cryotherapy [Freezing]" and "Wound Care After Cryosurgery" on pages 1749, 1750, and 1753, respectively, of Appendix G.) The advantages of and rationale for using cryosurgery also should be reviewed with the patient.

TECHNIQUE

Liquid Nitrogen: Thermos Gun Technique

Spray Technique Using Cryogun/CryAC-3 (Brymill) or Ultrafreezer (Wallach)

1. *Select the nozzle size.* The "C" tip is the one chosen most commonly for use with the Brymill; this size is a starting point. The "B" tip has a larger orifice and can treat large lesions faster. The "A" tip is larger still.
2. *Spray the lesion.* The spray can be continuous or, for a little better control, intermittent. Perpendicular spray is faster (Fig. 15-8). Hold the unit 3 to 4 cm from the

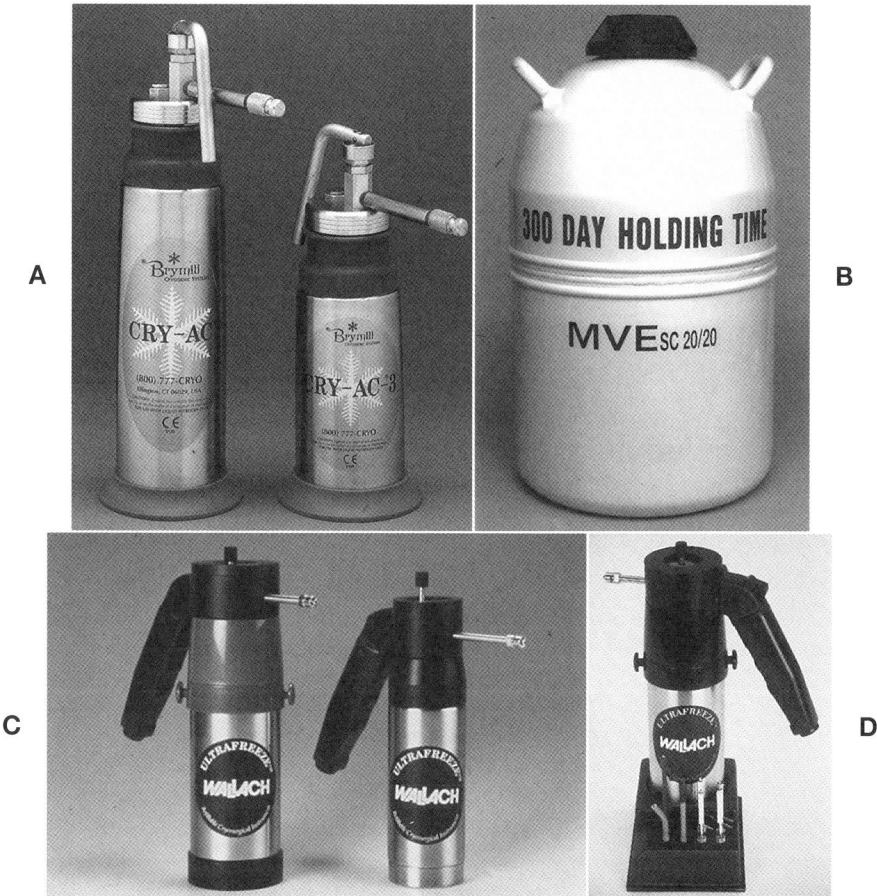

Fig. 15-3
A, Brymill Cryogun is refillable with liquid nitrogen. **B,** Brymill Dewar. **C,** Wallach Ultrafreezer. **D,** Wallach Ultrafreezer with stand. (**A-B,** Courtesy Brymill Corp., Ellington, Conn. **C-D,** Courtesy Wallach Surgical Devices, Orange, Conn.)

target. Tangential spray is somewhat slower but allows a more controlled freeze.

3. *Little movement of the gun is needed* unless the lesion is large. Usually it is a "point and shoot" technique, although some prefer an enlarging circular spray or side-to-side "brush stroke" application. Most lesions will be small, so freeze a central portion and allow expansion of the ice ball outward until the desired effect is obtained (Box 15-1).

4. *Using an ear speculum* (Fig. 15-9) or other available neoprene cone or the plate with variable-sized openings (Fig. 15-4) is recommended in most smaller lesions because it focuses the spray onto the area desired and limits destruction of normal tissue. Hold it tight against the skin to prevent leakage. Select the cone size to give the desired size of ice ball. The ice ball will still usually spread 1 to 2 mm beyond the size of the opening. Use freezing guidelines (Box 15-1) for desired effect.

Liquid nitrogen spray techniques achieve desired freezing levels eight to ten times faster than nitrous oxide.

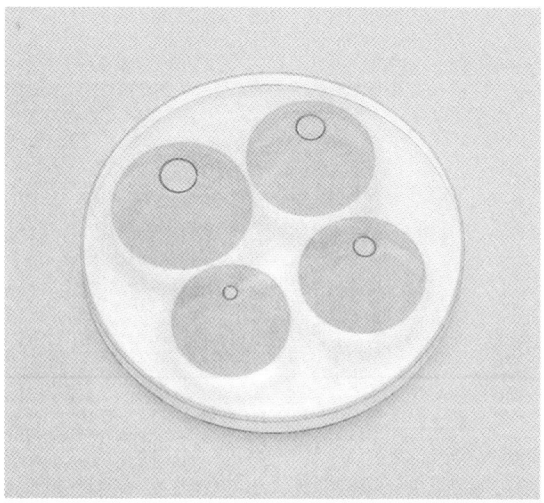

Fig. 15-4
Protective shield with various sized orifices, which limits spread of liquid nitrogen and protects surrounding skin.

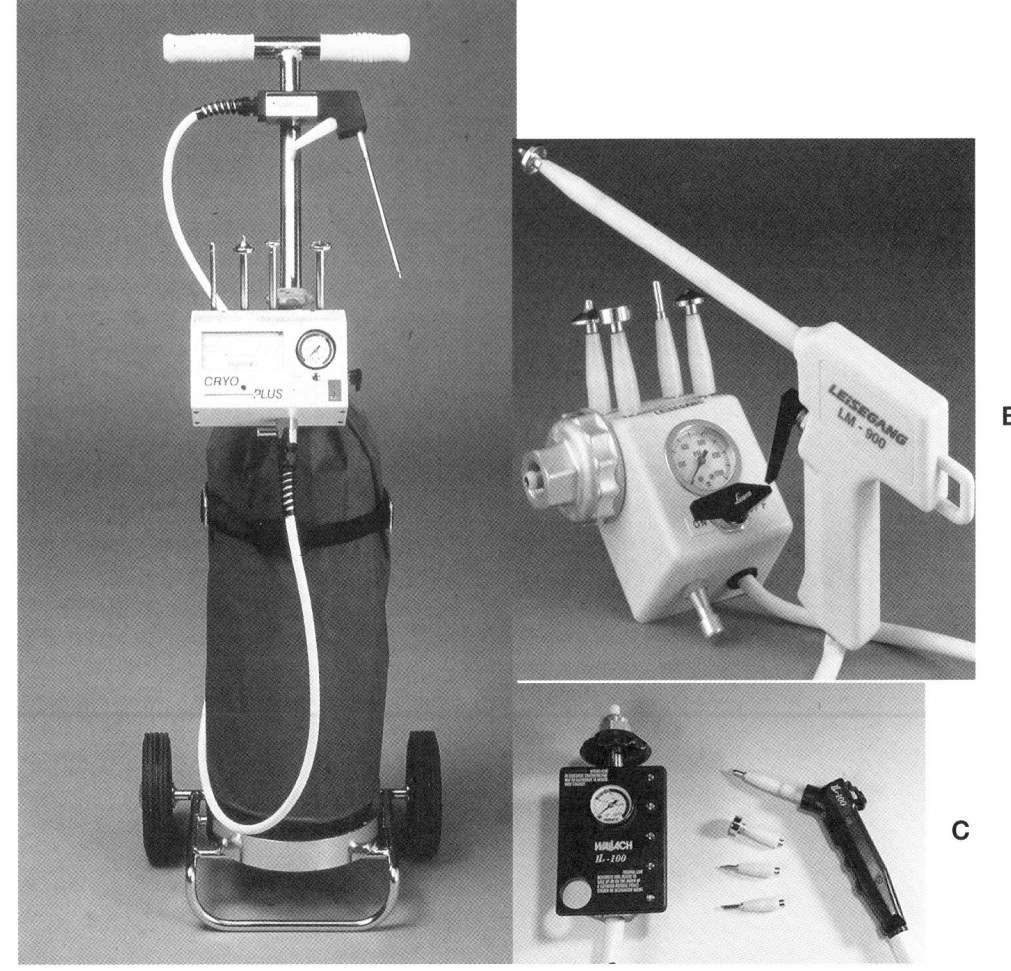

Fig. 15-5

A, Nitrous oxide cryosurgical unit. Handpiece is placed in holder, and connected to a 20-lb tank. **B,** Leisegang cryosurgical hand gun. **C,** *Left,* Wallach nitrous oxide yoke adapter with pressure gauge. *Right,* nitrous oxide cryogun for skin applications with various tips. Note the short shank on the gun for dermatologic uses. (**A-B,** Courtesy CooperSurgical, Trumbull, Conn. **C,** Courtesy Bruno Ratensperger, MD.)

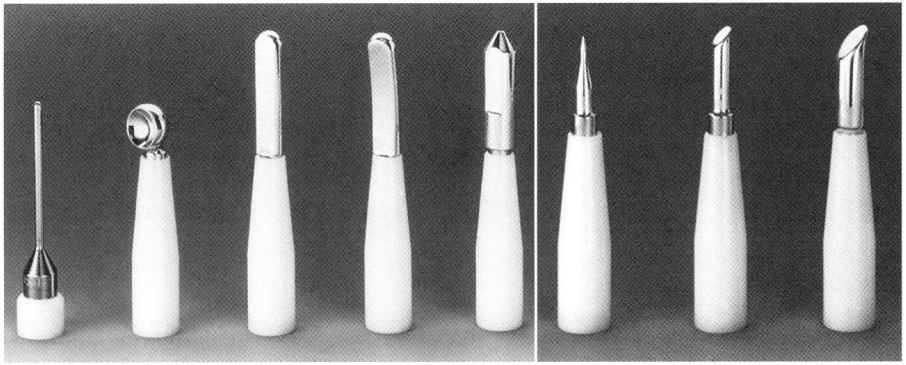

Fig. 15-6

Various cryosurgical tips for treatment of a variety of dermatological lesions with nitrous oxide (left to right): Fine point, small cup, round tip, hemorrhoid tip, slightly coned tip, another fine point, small slanted tip, and large slanted flat tip. (Also see Chapter 141, Cryotherapy of the Cervix.)

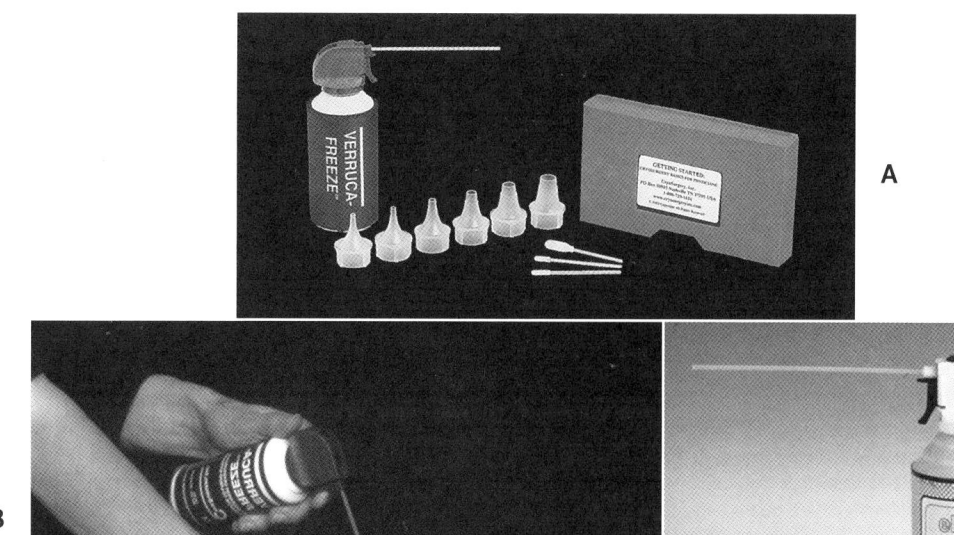

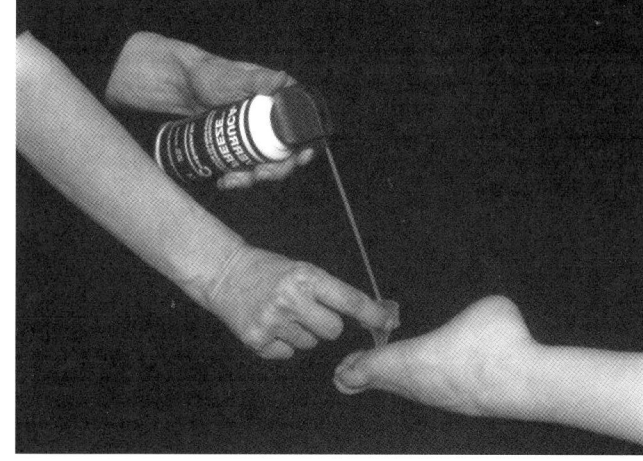

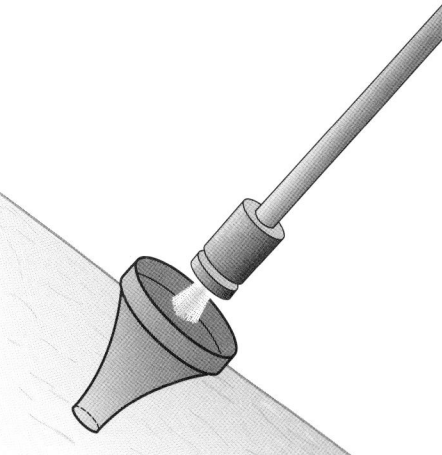

Fig. 15-7
A, Self-contained Verruca-Freeze unit with various sizes of specula. **B,** Application of Verruca-Freeze. **C,** Medi-Frig. (**A-B,** Courtesy CryoSurgery, Inc. **C,** Courtesy Ellman Corp.)

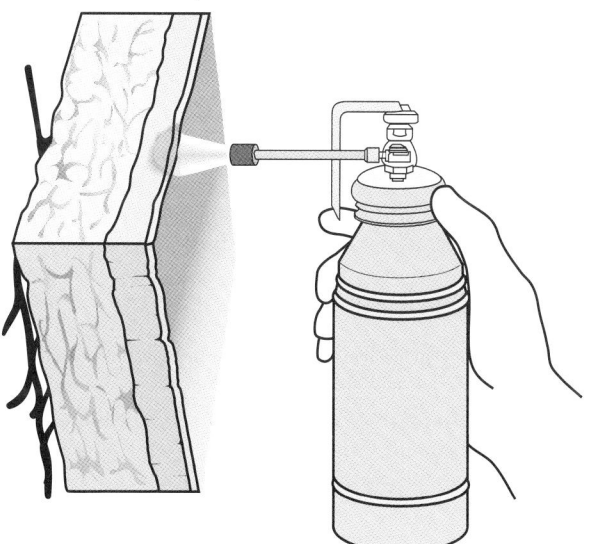

Fig. 15-8
Perpendicular spray technique using liquid nitrogen in a cryogun.

Fig. 15-9
Precise freezing may be obtained with either spray liquid nitrogen or the aerosol canisters using an ear speculum.

Liquid Nitrogen: Contact Probes

Small, solid tips much like the nitrous oxide tips also can be used with the thermos guns, but the diameter is only 2 to 4 mm.

1. Select the appropriate size and apply the probe tip directly to the skin or lesion.

2. Obtain the rim of ice ball size desired.
3. Allow to thaw.

The advantage of these tips is that the ice ball is well controlled and occurs much faster than with nitrous oxide. They can be used in areas such as around the eyes where it is necessary to avoid a wider spray. The major

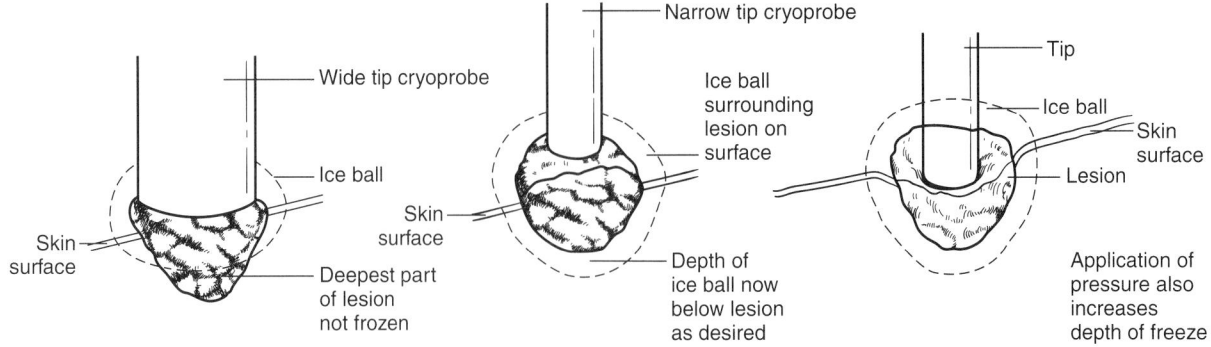

Fig. 15-10
Cryosurgery of a deep but narrow lesion. **A,** If a wide cryoprobe tip is used, the deepest part of the lesion will not be frozen even though a 3- to 5-mm margin of ice ball is obtained. **B,** To ensure that the entire lesion is frozen, a tip smaller than the lesion may be used, thereby limiting the rapid lateral spread of the ice ball. **C,** Alternatively, the cryoprobe tip may be pressed down until the top of the lesion is below the skin surface. The cold will penetrate deeper before too much normal tissue is frozen by lateral spread.

disadvantage of using these probes is that the thawing is passive and can take a long time. Although large cervical tips of this type are available, they should not be used for cervical dysplasia because studies providing efficacy are lacking.

Liquid Nitrogen: Cup/Cotton-Tipped Applicator Technique

1. Dispense a small amount of liquid nitrogen into a Styrofoam cup to prevent contaminating the primary source of liquid nitrogen.
2. Choose the size of the cotton-tipped applicator to match lesion.
3. Dip a clean cotton-tipped applicator into the cup and then touch the lesion with the applicator.
4. Keep the applicator cold by dipping it into the cup every several seconds and reapplying to the lesion to obtain the desired size of ice ball. Do not place a cotton-tipped applicator that has touched the patient, or the treatment cup supply, into the primary source of liquid nitrogen because contamination can occur. Likewise, do not return any unused liquid into the dewar. Viruses often are not killed when placed directly into liquid nitrogen and may be spread to others if contamination of the source occurs.
5. The size of the applicator and amount of pressure applied affect rapidity and depth of freeze.
6. Freezing times are markedly shortened with liquid nitrogen. The Q-Tip/cup method is not as fast as the cryogun, but it is still significantly faster than nitrous oxide.

A variant of the above method can be used for pedunculated lesions. Metal pickups are dipped into the cup, then pedunculated lesions are grasped with them. This limits the spread of the freeze and can be very effective.

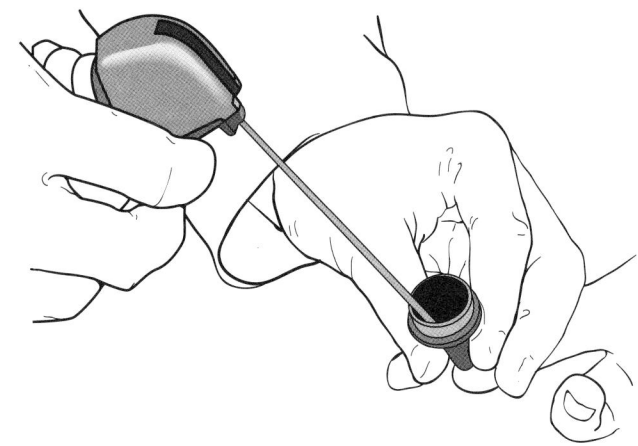

Fig. 15-11
Cannister gas being used to freeze a wart.

Nitrous Oxide Unit

1. *Debride* any keratin you can beforehand (e.g., plantar wart).
2. *Place a thin layer of water-soluble gel* on the lesion to hydrate the lesion and to enhance even contact with the cryoprobe. Alternatively, soak the lesion well with a wet 4 × 4 gauze pad.
3. *Select a probe* with a size and shape that corresponds to the lesion size (Fig. 15-10).
4. Hold the handpiece ("gun") with trigger in one hand, and *guide the probe tip* to a point over the site of freezing.
5. *Activate the gun* and quickly place it on the lesion. The tip will stick to the skin within 3 to 5 seconds.
6. *Freeze until desired ice ball is obtained.*
7. *Thaw.* This will be an active process. Some units will thaw automatically when the freeze trigger or button is released, whereas others require that a second

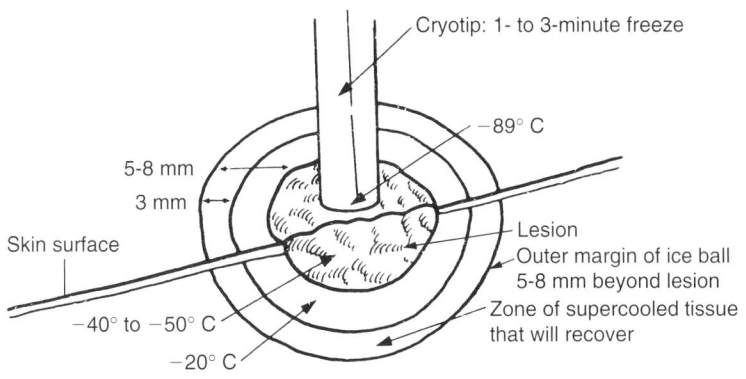

Cryotip: 1- to 3-minute freeze

−89° C

5-8 mm

3 mm

Skin surface

Lesion

Outer margin of ice ball 5-8 mm beyond lesion

Zone of supercooled tissue that will recover

−40° to −50° C

−20° C

Fig. 15-12
Nitrous oxide full-thickness destruction freeze technique (malignant lesions). Halo thaw time should be at least 1 minute for all methods.

button be pushed. *The gas to the handpiece must be turned on for this to occur!* The tip will "release" from the skin within seconds. The frozen skin will then thaw passively.

Verruca-Freeze/Medi-Frig (Fig. 15-7)

1. *Select a cone speculum size* that will completely encompass the lesion (which must be benign) plus 2 mm of normal tissue.
2. *Hold the speculum securely* against the skin to prevent leakage (essential!) (Fig. 15-11).
3. Dispense enough liquid from the canister to *fill the speculum approximately ⅛ to ¼ inch.* Avoid splattering; use a gentle spray.
4. *Allow the fluid to evaporate* (30 to 60 seconds).
5. *Remove* the cone speculum.
6. *Repeat,* if needed.

TECHNIQUE FOR SPECIFIC LESIONS

Keratin Removal

Lesions with dense keratin coverings (plantar warts, seborrheics) are very resistant to cryosurgery (especially to nitrous oxide and cannister gases). The patient can help prepare the wart with 2 weeks of salicylic acid application: After bathing and cleaning the area, the patient should apply a 17% solution (Compound W) to the wart(s). A piece of Mediplast (40% salicylic acid), or Trans-Ver-Sal, cut just a little larger than the wart can also be used. This is left in place 24 hours until the next day's application. (If the pad migrates significantly during the day, it may be used at night only.) After 2 weeks, a soft white layer of keratin can be peeled away revealing the base or root of the plantar wart lesion. Freezing time for the lesion should be shortened once the keratin layer and outer epidermis have been removed.

Alternatively, in lesions with significant keratin, a no. 10 or 15 blade can be used to shave off the keratin in thin layers until the first red punctate vasculature is seen

(verruca). Stop debridement at this point (punctate bleeding) to minimize bleeding.

Actinics

Usually actinic keratoses are quite superficial. If numerous, liquid nitrogen is much quicker to use than nitrous oxide. Anesthesia is rarely needed. Because these lesions are premalignant, however, a full-thickness freeze is suggested. Whichever technique is used, be sure to obtain at least a 3-mm ice ball. It may be best to freeze a second time. Moisten the lesion first (with K-Y Jelly), if nitrous oxide is used.

Malignancy

This technique is used for treating malignant lesions such as *basal cell carcinomas* less than 1 cm. Be sure to confirm the diagnosis by obtaining a punch biopsy specimen before treatment. Many physicians do not use cryosurgery on malignancies other than basal cells although studies would support treating smaller (less than 1 cm) squamous cells too. Melanomas should be excised to be certain of depth, which defines proper treatment. Most physicians prefer to have documented clear excisional margins for melanomas and squamous cell carcinomas. If cryosurgery is the chosen method of destruction for basal cells, follow the steps as shown above for the technique used and continue the freeze until the ice ball is 5 to 8 mm beyond the margins of the lesion (Fig. 15-12). When freezing is complete, activate the rapid thaw. Do not attempt to detach the cryoprobe until the rapid thaw has released the tip. Because a malignancy is being treated, it is especially wise to document the time *and* the extent of the freeze.

The probe can be applied directly to the lesion. Alternatively, shave (debulk) off most of the lesion and freeze the now thinned-out residual.

Allow 5 to 7 minutes for complete thawing, then *repeat the freeze.* Malignant cells are more cryoresistant, and destruction requires temperatures of −40° to −50° C.

Use only nitrous oxide probe or liquid nitrogen spray or probe methods. The freeze/thaw/refreeze technique is recommended in all malignancy cases and should be documented.

Full-Thickness Freeze Technique for Anatomically Large or Irregular Skin Lesions

Some lesions are too large to be completely frozen by a cryoprobe in a single freeze. Examples would be Bowen's disease, keloids, vascular lesions, or mosaic warts. In such cases, note the central location of the cryoprobe. This spot will be the lateral margin of the cryoprobe placement for the next adjacent freeze (after thawing occurs). This allows for the 50% overlap that is desired. Freezing of extremely large lesions can begin on one side, then the opposite side can be frozen while the first is thawing. Progressing from opposite sides to the center will save time and still allow for a 40% to 50% freeze overlap.

With liquid nitrogen, the spray can be focused in a general area and gradually extended. It is important that a good freeze be obtained over the entire lesion.

Hypertrophic Scars and Keloids

The hyperemia and edema that immediately follows freezing and thawing softens the hypertrophic scar or keloid and allows easy penetration by a needle and a more even distribution of intralesional steroid. Cryosurgery alone, without steroids, will reduce the size of large keloids, but numerous treatments may be needed. (Also see Chapter 39, Hypertrophic Scars and Keloids.)

1. For nitrous oxide select a cryotip slightly narrower than the scar. You do *not* want the ice ball to extend more than 1 mm beyond the scar.
2. Apply a thin coat of water-soluble gel to the scar only. (Do not cover any of the surrounding skin.)
3. Moisten and warm the cryotip. Freeze until the ice ball progresses just to the edge of the scar, usually for 20 seconds to 1 minute, occasionally longer if necessary.
4. Wait approximately 10 to 15 minutes for mild tissue swelling, then proceed with intralesional injection of a steroid (such as triamcinolone diacetate [Aristocort] or triamcinolone acetonide [Kenalog 10 mg/ml]) using a small 30-gauge needle. Use very dilute solutions (0.1 ml diluted with 0.5 to 0.9 ml of 1% lidocaine *without* epinephrine) and a sufficient volume to infiltrate the entire scar. (Increase the concentration on successive visits as necessary.)
5. For large scars, 4 to 5 treatments may be necessary at 6- to 8-week intervals to achieve optimal success.
6. Liquid nitrogen can also be used, but it may be difficult to limit the size of the freeze with smaller

lesions. Treatment may produce a copious discharge during the first few postoperative days.

Anesthesia for Incision and Drainage of Abscesses

The acid tissue around an abscess can prevent a local anesthetic from working. Cryotherapy provides momentary anesthesia to allow painless incision with a no. 11 blade.

1. For nitrous oxide, select a cryotip that will cover the intended area of incision. Apply a thin coat of water-soluble gel to the most dependent portion of the abscess.
2. Moisten and warm the nitrous oxide cryotip. Make firm contact with the tissue and activate the gun.
3. Freeze until the ice ball covers an area slightly larger than the area that is to be opened. Make the incision through the ice ball along the skin tension lines. As the tissue is thawing, insert a hemostat and spread the tissue to promote drainage.
4. Obtain cultures of purulent drainage, if desired, after thawing has occurred.
5. Insert sterile iodoform gauze or a small Penrose drain if needed. Apply a bulky gauze dressing to absorb drainage. Arrange for a follow-up visit.
6. Remember that the cryoprobe has anesthetized only the skin and thus probing or debridement inside the abscess will be painful. Cryosurgery for abscesses is used to obtain quick drainage, not for extensive probing.
7. If other agents are used, spray sufficiently to obtain a superficial ice ball.

Condyloma Acuminata

(See also Chapter 141, Cryotherapy of the Cervix, and Chapter 157, Treatment of Noncervical Condyloma Acuminata.)

1. Penile, perianal, and vulvar areas are sensitive. Individual lesions and small groups of condyloma can be frozen without anesthetic. Topical anesthetics can also be applied before freezing. In some situations, 20% topical benzocaine (Hurricane), 5% lidocaine, EMLA cream, or ELA-Max may be appropriate. Topical applications may require 30 to 60 minutes to achieve maximum effectiveness. ELA-Max is now available over-the-counter. Large or multiple lesions may require injections of local anesthetic or, rarely, general anesthetic. Such extensive lesions may best be left to those who treat them often.
2. Find all the lesions. For women, examine the genitalia and the cervix with a colposcope to look for very small lesions, particularly in the vaginal introitus, on the vaginal side walls, the vulva, and the rectum. (A

cryocone of the cervix is necessary if dysplastic lesions extend onto the cervix. A thorough colposcopic work-up is necessary and criteria must be met before treating any lesion on the cervix. Women with external condyloma have a high incidence of cervical dysplasia. See Chapter 139, Colposcopic Examination, and Chapter 141, Cryotherapy of the Cervix.)

3. If nitrous oxide is used, moisten the skin lesions with a water-soluble gel. Touch the lesion(s) with a small-tipped probe (or a large-tipped probe if the lesions are large). Activate the nitrous oxide–powered tip, and effect adherence after 3 to 5 seconds. Then apply gentle traction. Do not pull too hard, or you may tear the tissue being treated or the surrounding skin. Freeze for approximately 20 to 45 seconds. Judge actual freezing time by the size of the lesion and the ice ball, which should extend 2 mm beyond the margin of the lesion(s) (Fig. 15-13). Within minutes after freezing, the condylomata darken and then will turn black; they should slough within a few days. If they do not turn dark, refreezing may be necessary.

4. Liquid nitrogen in either form (spray or cotton-tipped applicator) is quicker for treating multiple lesions. Pickups dipped into a cup of liquid nitrogen will also work.

5. A combination of electrosurgery and cryosurgery may speed the treatment of extensive perianal, vulvar, or penile lesions. The cryosurgery component will allow preservation of the elastic tissue matrix and expandability of the anal canal, penis, and vulva after healing. The electrosurgery component is used for tissue debridement. First, superficially electrocoagulate multiple lesions, then debride with scissors or curette, and then freeze the base for 20 to 30 seconds. Be sure not to cut too deep. Alternatively, you may use an electrosurgical loop to excise the condyloma, and then freeze the base for 20 to 30

seconds. This can be used for treatment of large areas of condyloma often seen on the genitalia. However, any disruption of wart tissue can cause significant bleeding.

Molluscum Contagiosum

Freezing is often an excellent, nearly painless treatment for molluscum contagiosum. Advise your patients, particularly children, to protect the healing crust to decrease the chance of scar formation.

1. If using nitrous oxide, prepare each lesion with a small amount of water-soluble gel. Freeze each lesion for 30 seconds to 1 minute. Use very fine-tipped probes to avoid freezing normal skin.

2. With liquid nitrogen, only brief freezes of several seconds are necessary.

3. Advise the patient and parent that the lesions should fall completely off within 2 weeks or less. If they do not, the patient should return soon for retreatment to prevent their spread.

Vascular Lesions (Hemangiomas and Strawberry Hemangiomas)

As with malignant lesions, vascular lesions are more cryoresistant, and a freeze/thaw/refreeze technique is recommended (Fig. 15-14). Nitrous oxide is the preferred method both to control the extent of the freeze and to be able to compress the lesion to remove the blood.

1. Moisten and warm the cryotip in warm water, and apply water-soluble gel to the lesion.

2. Make contact with the probe on the hemangioma and *exert firm pressure* to squeeze the blood out of the vascular channels.

3. Activate the cryogun, and hold pressure against the lesion throughout the freeze. Begin timing when the

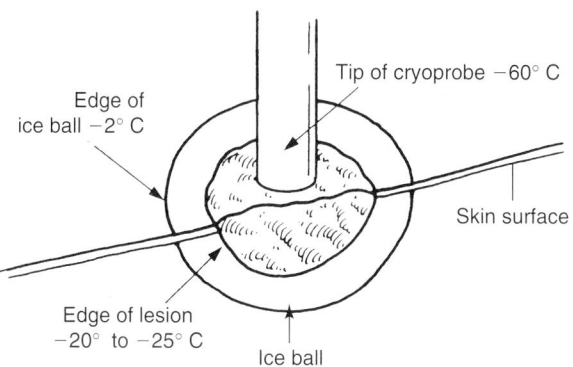

Fig. 15-13
Treatment of benign lesions. To ensure that all of the tissue of the lesion reaches the −20° to −25° C necessary for destruction, the outer edge of the frozen area (the "ice ball") should extend at least 2.0 to 3.5 mm in all directions beyond the lesion.

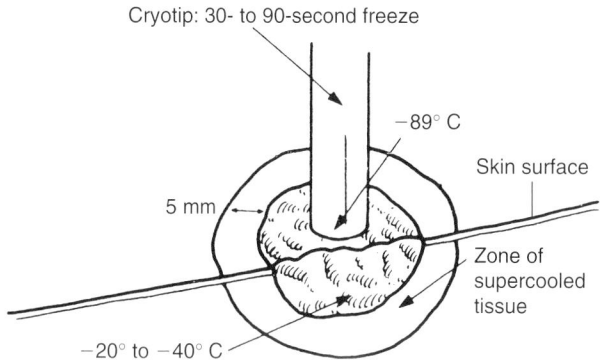

Fig. 15-14
Full-thickness destructive freeze of vascular lesion. Pressure is applied to the tip to express as much blood as possible.

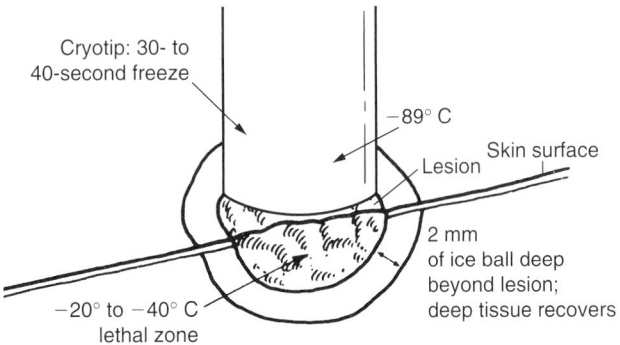

Fig. 15-15
Nitrous oxide partial-thickness freeze used for removal of superficial lesions (e.g., seborrheic keratoses). Cryotip should cover or nearly cover entire lesion to limit depth of freeze. Halo thaw time should be approximately 30 to 45 seconds for all methods.

ice ball becomes visible. For larger lesions, freeze for 1½ minutes or until the ice ball extends out 3 mm. Allow 5 to 7 minutes for thawing, and then repeat the freeze.

Skin Verrucae

Liquid nitrogen spray is the most effective and most rapid. Use a freeze-thaw-refreeze technique and obtain a 1- to 2-mm margin for each treated wart. Repeat the treatments every 1 to 3 weeks based on response.

Seborrheic Keratoses

Seborrheic keratoses are usually quite superficial. If N_2O_2 is used, the lesions need to be softened first with K-Y Jelly. A 2- to 3-mm ice ball margin should be sufficient for treatment (Fig. 15-15).

Cervical Cryotherapy for CIN

See Chapter 141, Cryotherapy of the Cervix.

COMPLICATIONS AND SHORTCOMINGS

- Pigment cells and hair cells may be destroyed by cryosurgery.
- Vascular lesions are quite resistant to treatment and may recur.
- Areas of poor circulation may be susceptible to *prolonged ulcer formation*, especially in elderly diabetic patients (e.g., anterior tibial compartment).
- Tissue pathology *documentation* and verification of *adequate destruction* of malignant lesions is *not possible* with cryosurgery. Pretreatment biopsy is recommended for basal cell carcinomas. A presumed "benign lesion" may be indeed malignant and thus insufficiently treated with cryosurgery alone. So, if there is doubt concerning a possible melanoma or squamous cell cancer, biopsy is recommended first.
- Cryosurgery in the periorbital area may cause *excessive swelling*, in which the eyelid may be shut for several hours or days. However, cryosurgery of small, well-localized lesions on the eyelids is usually well tolerated. Be conservative on the freeze time until the individual patient's reaction is documented.
- *Peripheral neuropathy* (the ulnar nerve at the elbow or peripheral nerves on the lateral aspect of the digits) can result when areas adjacent to nerves are frozen. The nerve sheath is cryoresistant, but the nerve tissue is more susceptible to damage. This side effect can be minimized by pulling the skin outward, away from the nerve, once good contact is achieved. If the nerve is affected, recovery occurs within 4 to 6 weeks, although 3 to 6 months may occasionally be required. Sensory nerves are more likely to be affected.
- In general, the skin of *infants and the elderly*, as well as previously damaged skin, is more susceptible to necrosis and blistering than normal skin. Skin may be damaged as a result of sun exposure, radiation, and chronic topical steroid application. Reduce freeze times until the reaction of a damaged area is known. Written informed consent is suggested when treating sensitive skin.

POSTPROCEDURE PATIENT EDUCATION

The patient should be informed of the additional healing time, the anticipated excellent results, and the need to call the office when there is an overreaction to freezing. (See the sample patient education handout titled "Wound Care After Cryosurgery" on page 1753 of Appendix G.) Document that the patient was told of permanent pigment changes, possible nerve involvement, and hair loss. Placing a copy of the handout that was given to the patient in the chart provides excellent medical-legal documentation as well as an excellent medical reference for staff and physician alike.

SUPPLIERS

ACMI Corp.*
136 Turnpike Road
Southborough, MA 01772
Phone: 1-866-879-0640
Website: www.acmicorp.com

---

*Nitrous oxide closed units.

Brymill Corp. (Cryogun/CRYAC-3)*
105 Windmere Avenue
Ellington, CT 06029
Phone: 1-800-777-2796
Website: www.brymill.com

CooperSurgical[†]
95 Corporate Drive
Trumball, CT 06611
Phone: 1-800-243-2974
Website: www.coopersurgical.com

Ellman International (Medi-Frig)[‡]
1135 Railroad Avenue
Hewlett, NY 11557
Phone: 1-800-835-5355
Website: www.ellman.com

Histofreezer[‡]
OraSure Technologies
150 Webster Street
Bethlehem, PA 18015
Phone: 1-800-869-3538
Website: www.stctech.com

Verruca-Freeze[‡]
CryoSurgery, Inc.
P.O. Box 50035
Nashville, TN 37205
Phone: 1-800-729-1624
Website: www.cryosurgeryinc.com

Wallach Surgical Devices, Inc.*[†]
235 Edison Road
Orange, CT 06477
Phone: 1-800-243-2463
Website: www.wallachsurgical.com

For companies supplying nitrous oxide units, also see Chapter 141, Cryotherapy of the Cervix. Liquid nitrogen dewars are available from most local oxygen and nitrogen supply firms, but they may not be the improved dewars that are available from Brymill. Try contacting a local veterinary supplier to rent/borrow a dewar flask, and arrange for a constant supply of liquid nitrogen. It is generally less expensive than medical grade but performs equally well.

*Liquid nitrogen cryoguns.
[†]Nitrous oxide closed units.
[‡]Canister kits.

CPT/BILLING CODES

Cryosurgery is billed out as "destruction of lesions." Certain areas require specific codes.

Destruction (Cryocautery, Electrocautery, Laser, Chemical, or Curettement)

Benign Lesions

(Site and size not needed, except for locations noted below)

17000	First lesion
17003	Lesions 2 to 14 (charge for each additional lesion treated)
17004	15 or more lesions (charge only this code if 15 or more lesions were frozen)
67850	Eyelid, lid margin
68135	Eyelid, conjunctiva
57511	Cervix
11200	Skin tags, 1 to 15 lesions
11201	Skin tags, additional 10 lesions
56501	Genitals (female), perineum, simple destruction
56501	Genitals (female), vulva/introitus, simple destruction
56515	Genitals (female), vulva/introitus, extensive destruction
57061	Genitals (female), vagina, simple destruction
57065	Genitals (female), vagina, extensive destruction
54056	Genitals (male), penis, cryotherapy, simple destruction
54065	Genitals (male), penis, cryotherapy, extensive destruction
46916	Anal (perianal), benign lesion, simple destruction
46924	Anal (perianal), benign lesion, extensive destruction
46614	Anal (perianal), with anoscopy
46934	Anal (perianal), internal hemorrhoid
46937	Anal (perianal), benign rectal tumor
17110	Flat warts/molluscum, up to 14 lesions
17111	Flat warts/molluscum, 15 or more lesions

Malignant Lesions

See codes 17260 to 17286 as follows.

Note: All of these codes have a 10-day global fee surgical period. Destruction by any method, with or without curettement, includes local anesthesia and ablation, and usually does not require closure. Sizes listed describe *lesion* diameter, not the width of the skin area destroyed.

17260	Trunk, arm, or leg (TAL): <0.5 cm
17261	TAL: 0.6-1.0 cm
17262	TAL: 1.1-2.0 cm
17263	TAL: 2.1-3.0 cm
17264	TAL: 3.1-4.0 cm
17266	TAL: >4.0 cm
17270	Scalp, neck, hand, foot, or genitalia (SNHFG): <0.5 cm
17271	SNHFG: 0.6-1.0 cm
17272	SNHFG: 1.1-2.0 cm
17273	SNHFG: 2.1-3.0 cm
17274	SNHFG: 3.1-4.0 cm
17276	SNHFG: >4.0 cm
17280	Face, eyelid, ear, nose, lip, or mucous membrane (Face mm): <0.5 cm
17281	Face mm: 0.6-1.0 cm
17282	Face mm: 1.1-2.0 cm
17283	Face mm: 2.1-3.0 cm
17284	Face mm: 3.1-4.0 cm
17286	Face mm: >4.0 cm

ICD-9-CM DIAGNOSTIC CODES

See ICD-9-CM Code Book under "neoplasm, skin." Then identify anatomic site and whether lesion is benign, malignant (primary or secondary), ca-in-situ, or uncertain. Also see Appendix H, Skin ICD-9 Codes.

ADDITIONAL RESOURCES

- See the sample patient education handouts titled "Wart Removal" on page 1749, "Cryotherapy (Freezing)" on page 1750, "What to Expect After Cryosurgery" on page 1752, and "Wound Care After Cryosurgery" on page 1753 of Appendix G.

BIBLIOGRAPHY

American Academy of Dermatology Committee on Guidelines of Care: Guidelines of care for cryosurgery, *J Am Acad Dermatol* 31:648, 1994.

Arnold H, Odom RB, James WD: *Cryotherapy: Andrew's diseases of the skin,* ed 8, Philadelphia, 1990, WB Saunders.

Burke WA, Baden TJ, Wheeler CE, Bowdre JH: Survival of herpes simplex virus during cryosurgery with liquid nitrogen, *J Dermatol Surg Oncol* 12(10):1033, 1986.

Dawber R, Colver G, Jackson A: *Cutaneous cryosurgery: principles and practice,* United Kingdom, 1992, Martin Duntiz Ltd.*

Elton RF: The appropriate use of liquid nitrogen, *Prim Care* 10(3):459, 1983.

Felmar E, Payton CE, Smietanka M: Primary care office procedures: treatment of genital lesions via cryocautery, *Prim Care* June 1988.

Ferris DG, Ho JJ: Cryosurgical equipment: a critical review, *J Fam Pract* 35:185, 1992.

Fewkes JL, Cheney MC, Pollack SV: *Illustrated atlas of cutaneous surgery,* Philadelphia, 1992, Lippincott.

Grealish RJ: Cryosurgery for benign skin lesions, *Fam Pract Recertification* 11(10):21, 1989.

Heidenheim M, Jemec GB: Side effects of cryotherapy, *J Am Acad Dermatol* 24:653, 1991.

Hocutt JE: Cryosurgery (parts 1, 2, 3), *Fam Pract Bulletin* 1(12):67, 1988; 1(16):91, 1989; 1(18):103, 1989.

Hocutt JE: Skin cryosurgery for the family physician, *Am Fam Physician* 48(3):445, 1993.

Jones SK, Darville JM: Transmission of virus particles by cryotherapy and multi-use caustic pencils: a problem to dermatologists? *Br J Dermatol* 121:481, 1989.

Kuflik EG: Cryosurgical treatment of cutaneous lesions. In Roenigle RK, Roenigle HH, editors: *Dermatologic surgery: principles and practice,* ed 2, New York, 1996, Marcel Dekker.

Kuflik EG: Cryosurgery updated, *J Am Acad Dermatol* 31(6) 925, 1994.

Kuflik EG, Gage AA, Lubritz RR, Graham GF: History of dermatologic cryosurgery, *Dermatol Surg* 26:715, 2000.

Kuwahara RT, Craig SR, Amonette RA: Forceps and cotton applicator method of freezing benign lesions, *Dermatol Surg* 27(2):183, 2001.

Mallon E, Dawber R: Cryosurgery in the treatment of basal cell carcinoma, *Dermatol Surg* 22:854, 1996.

Pfenninger JL: Good things still come in old packages: cryosurgery vs. LEEP, *J Am Board Fam Pract* 12:416, 1999.

Rowland AS, Baird DD, Weinberg CR, et al: Reduced fertility among women employed as dental assistants exposed to high levels of nitrous oxide, *N Engl J Med* 327:993, 1992.

Torre D: Cutaneous cryosurgery: current state of the art, *J Dermatol Surg Oncol* 11(3):293, 1985.

Torre D, Lubritz R, Kuflik E: *Practical cutaneous cryosurgery,* Norwalk, Conn, 1988, Appleton & Lange.

Usatine RP, Tobinick EL: Cryosurgical techniques in skin surgery: a practical guide. In Usatine RP, Moy RL, Tobinick EL, Siegel DM, editors: *Skin surgery: a practical guide,* St Louis, 1998, Mosby.*

Van Der Horst CM et al: Effect of the timing of the treatment of port-wine stains with the flash lamp pumped pulsed-dye laser, *N Engl J Med* 338:1028, 1998.

Yliskoski M, Saarikoski S, Syrjanen K, et al: Cryotherapy and CO_2-laser vaporization in the treatment of cervical and vaginal human papillomavirus (HPV) infections, *Acta Obstet Gynecol Scand* 68:619, 1989.

---

*An excellent reference and atlas for primary care physicians, and excellent for explaining cryosurgery to patients.

CHAPTER 16

Dermoscopy (Epiluminescence Microscopy)

Robert H. Johr

A serious problem exists for the clinician using the popular "ABCD" criteria (described in this chapter) to recognize early melanomas with the naked eye. Simply stated, millions of dysplastic nevi exist in our population that demonstrate the same clinical characteristics as melanoma. If a patient has a few atypically pigmented skin lesions, they can simply be excised. However, that strategy does not work on patients with multiple lesions. The answer to this common clinical dilemma is to evaluate them with dermoscopy. This approach is the standard of care in Europe, where it is used not only by dermatologists but also by family physicians, internists, and pediatricians. However, only 23% of U.S. dermatologists and even fewer primary care physicians make dermoscopy part of their standard of care.

Dermoscopy (also known as epiluminescence microscopy [or ELM], skin surface microscopy, and dermatoscopy) is an in vivo, noninvasive technique during which the skin is evaluated under magnification (10×), usually after a lotion or mineral oil is applied to the surface to make the epidermis more transparent. The color and structure in the epidermis, dermoepidermal junction, and papillary dermis thereby become more visible. These features cannot be seen with the naked eye or with the typical magnification that clinicians use. The proper analysis of these extra criteria has been shown to significantly increase the diagnostic accuracy of melanoma and other pigmented lesions, both melanocytic and nonmelanocytic (Box 16-1).

No special patient preparation or complications are associated with dermoscopy. It is cutting edge technology to evaluate pigmented skin lesions.

BOX 16-1
Benefits of Dermoscopy

Differentiation of melanocytic from nonmelanocytic skin lesions
Differentiation of benign from malignant skin lesions
Earlier diagnosis of melanoma
Helps to plan surgery
Helps avoid unnecessary surgery
Aids in following patients with dysplastic nevi
Provides patient reassurance

TECHNIQUE

Two instrument options are available: the relatively inexpensive handheld dermatoscope (Heine USA) (Fig. 16-1) or expensive digital computer system. With the dermatoscope, some type of oil or fluid (mineral oil, immersion oil, K-Y Jelly, alcohol, or water) is placed over the lesion to be examined. The liquid eliminates surface light reflection and renders the stratum corneum transparent, allowing visualization of subsurface color and structure. The dermatoscope is then placed directly over the lesion (Fig. 16-2). Variations on the theme of the dermatoscope are now available (e.g., DermLite, 3Gen), and fluid is no longer necessary to perform the technique.

There are three approaches to the analysis of criteria found with this handheld technique: *pattern analysis,* the *ABCD rule of dermatoscopy,* and the *seven-point checklist.*

Pattern Analysis

With pattern analysis, eight criteria and at least 28 variables of those criteria must be identified. The criteria

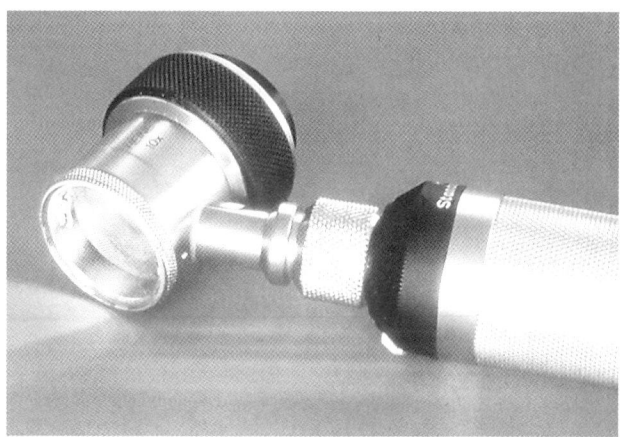

Fig. 16-1
Handheld dermatoscope.

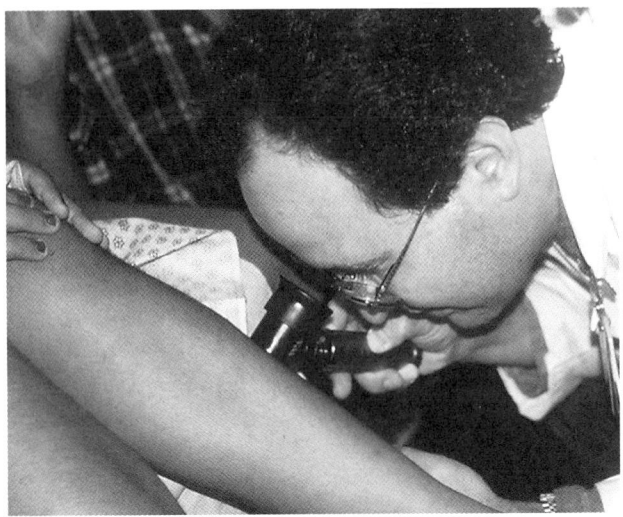

Fig. 16-2
After oil or fluid is placed on the lesion, the glass contact plate of the dermatoscope is placed directly on the skin over the lesion.

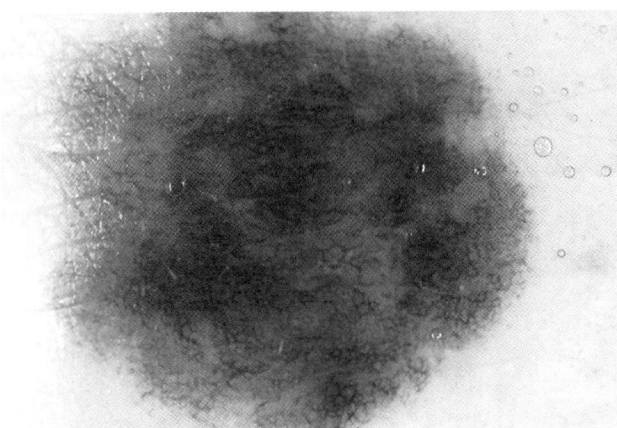

Fig. 16-3
Irregular and prominent pigment network in a superficial spreading melanoma.

are put into patterns, and the patterns correlate with specific pathology. There are patterns suggestive of the different types of melanoma (superficial spreading, nodular, lentigo maligna, and lentigo maligna melanoma), different types of melanocytic nevi (common, blue, dysplastic, and Spitz), hemangiomas, seborrheic keratosis, ink spot lentigo, dermatofibroma, and basal cell carcinoma.

The dermoscopic criteria that are evaluated include the following:
- *Pigment network:* honeycomb-like pattern of line segments; usually brown and reticulated (for those who perform colposcopy, similar to mosaicism); represents pigment in epidermal basal cells.
- *Diffuse pigmentation:* unstructured, diffuse, brown or black pigmentation; represents melanin in all levels of epidermis and/or upper dermis; some resemble ink spots.
- *Depigmentation:* regions (regression areas) of less pigmentation than the surrounding skin.
- *Brown globules:* globular (circular to oval) pigment aggregations; indicative of nests, melanocytes, or melanophages at the dermoepidermal junction or upper dermis.
- *Black dots:* punctate, discrete black pigment concentrations (in the stratum corneum).
- *Pseudopods:* fingerlike projections at periphery of the lesion; suggestive of radial growth phase of a melanoma.
- *Radial streaming:* radially oriented linear structures; brown to black streaks going from the border of a pigmented lesion into surrounding skin.
- *Blue-gray veil:* areas with the appearance of ground glass; melanoma is deep in dermis and appears blue.

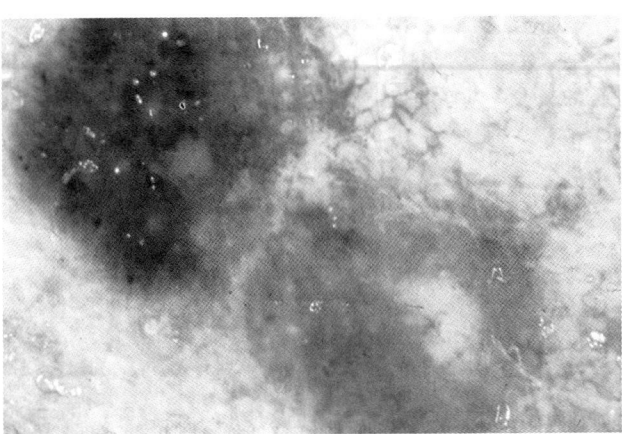

Fig. 16-4
Irregular (size and shape) black and brown dots and globules in an invasive melanoma.

With pattern analysis, if the physician can see the pigment network, he or she must determine if it is regular or irregular, prominent or subtle, and thins gradually at the periphery or ends abruptly. The more prominent and irregular the network, the greater the chance the lesion is malignant (Fig. 16-3).

If dots and globules are present, are they regular or irregular in size, shape, and distribution in the lesion (Fig. 16-4)? Symmetrical and uniform criteria favor a benign diagnosis. Asymmetry of color and structure plus the presence of high-risk criteria such as pseudopods, radial streaming, and blue-gray veil are patterns suggestive of melanoma (Box 16-2). No criterion by itself is 100% diagnostic of melanoma, and the physician should identify and analyze all of the criteria present before coming to a tentative dermoscopic diagnosis.

BOX 16-2
Melanoma Specific Criteria (Trunk, Extremities)

Multicomponent global pattern (three or more distinct dermo-
  scopic areas)
Atypical pigment network
Irregular pigmentation
Atypical vascular patterns
Five or six colors
Irregular dots or globules
Irregular streaks (pseudopods or radial streaming)
Regression areas (white and/or bluish-white)
Blue-whitish veil

Benign nevi have the following:
- Regular, netlike pigment network
- Regular, homogenous, diffuse pigmentation that grad-
ually thins at the periphery
- Uniform, regularly distributed globules and dots
- Uniform and homogeneous hypopigmented and
depigmented areas

Malignant melanomas are more likely to have the
following:
- Irregular, wide pigment network that just abruptly
ends at the periphery
- Heavy, dark, irregular, abruptly ending pigmentation
- Globules and dots are varied in size and shape and are
unevenly distributed throughout the lesion
- Depigmented areas irregularly present
- Pseudopods or radial streaming that projects into
normal skin
- Possible white areas of no pigment *within* the lesion
(in contrast to a halo nevus, where there is decreased
pigment in the surrounding skin that is totally benign)
- Grey-blue areas that are dense and ill defined

ABCD Rule

There is a great deal of subjectivity with pattern analysis,
and for that reason it is difficult to teach and learn. The
ABCD rule of dermatoscopy was developed in an attempt to simplify the process. Four criteria were found to
be significant cofactors for diagnosing melanoma: asymmetry (A), borders (B), colors (C), and the presence of
different structural components (D). The ABCD rule of
dermatoscopy is a semiquantitative mathematical approach that gives points for the criteria identified in a
lesion and a formula to determine the total dermatoscopy score (TDS) for each lesion. A TDS less than 4.75 in
most cases would be benign, a TDS of 4.75 to 5.45 is
suggestive of melanoma, and a TDS greater than 5.45 is
highly suspicious for melanoma. Lesions with a high TDS
should be considered for excision. One caveat with this
system is that you can get false high TDSs with benign
melanocytic lesions. With experience, less of these le-

BOX 16-3
Primary Dermoscopic Criteria

Criteria for Melanocytic Lesion
Pigment network
Aggregated globules
Streaks (branched pigment network)

Criteria for Seborrheic Keratosis
Milia-like cysts
Comedo-like openings
Fissures and ridges

Criteria of Basal Cell Carcinoma
Absence criteria for melanocytic lesion
Arborizing blood vessels
Grey globules of pigmentation

Criteria for Vascular Lesion
Red lacunas
Red-bluish homogeneous areas

Criteria for Dermatofibroma
Central white patch

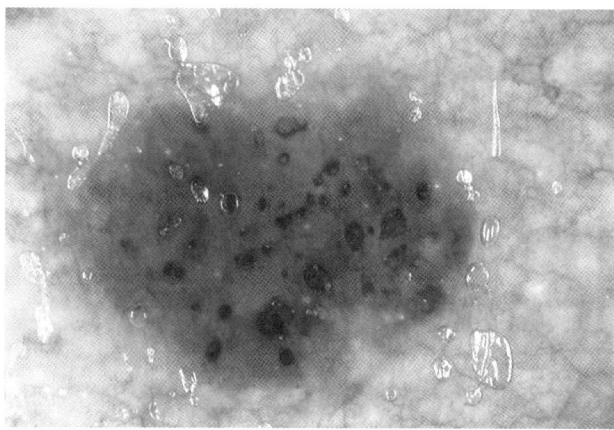

Fig. 16-5
Follicular openings (irregular dark circles) and milia-like cysts (yellow
pinpoint dots) in a seborrheic keratosis.

sions need to be excised, and now they can be followed
with digital systems.

Step one in the evaluation of a pigmented lesion with
dermoscopy is to determine if it is melanocytic or
nonmelanocytic. If a pigment network, branched streaks
(which are thickened branched pigment network), or
aggregated globules can be identified, this indicates a
melanocytic lesion. On the other hand, the lesion being
examined might not be melanocytic. There are primary
criteria to help diagnose other pigmented lesions that
are not melanocytic as well (e.g., seborrheic keratosis)
(Box 16-3 and Fig. 16-5). There are also dermoscopic
clues before the ABCD rule is applied that suggest
melanoma, including vascular patterns such as "milky

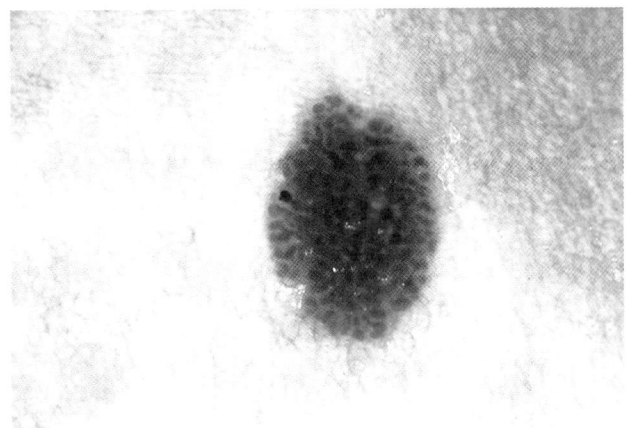

Fig. 16-6
Regular brown globules forming the "globular" pattern in a low-risk melanocytic nevus.

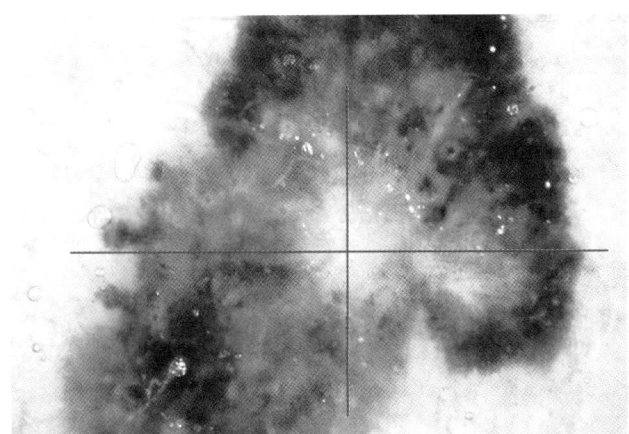

Fig. 16-8
Superficial spreading melanoma clearly asymmetrical in two axes for contour, color, and structure.

asymmetrical in one axis, and a maximum of two points for a lesion that is asymmetrical in both axes. One of the greatest benefits of the technique would be observation of a perfectly symmetrical lesion clinically, but with a great deal of asymmetry of color and structure becoming apparent when viewed with dermoscopy. These could be the early thin melanomas that might be dismissed as being benign if the technique was not used.

Border (B)

The lesion is visually divided into eight pie-shaped segments, and the number of segments is counted in which there is an abrupt cutoff at the margins (edge) anywhere in the pigment pattern (pigment network, branched streaks, dots and/or globules, and diffuse pigmentation). The score can range from zero to eight. Well-demarcated criteria (e.g., pigment net, dots, globules) at the edges are highly suggestive of melanoma.

Color (C)

Colors to look for are red, white, light brown, dark brown, blue-gray, and black. Each color gets a point, and the total score ranges from one to six. The presence of five or six colors, especially if they are bright and well defined, is considered one of the melanoma specific criteria.

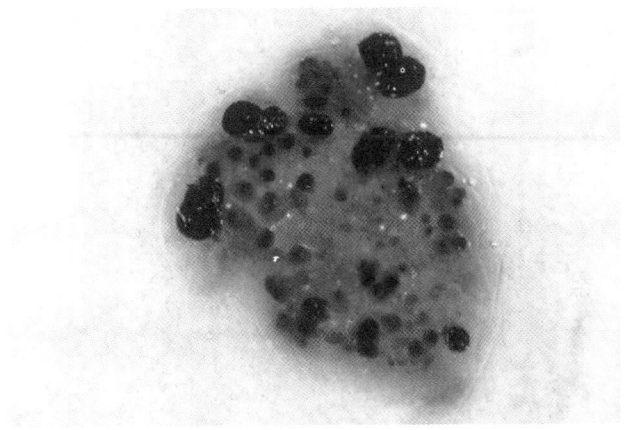

Fig. 16-7
"Saccular" pattern of a hemangioma. Clinically this lesion was dark and asymmetrical with irregular borders, which is highly suspicious for melanoma.

Different Structural Components (D)

A pigment network, branched streaks, structureless areas (color, but no structures such as pigment network, branched streaks, dots or globules), dots, and globules indicate different structural components. Each criterion that is identified gets a point; the range is 1 to 5 points.

red" areas, the polymorphous vascular pattern, and the presence of white or purple colors.

A few pigmented lesions will always have a pattern recognition diagnosis, and the ABCD rule should not be applied. The presence of the globular pattern seen with melanocytic nevi (the classic compound nevus) (Fig. 16-6), the starburst or targetoid pattern seen with Spitz nevi, and the saccular pattern of common hemangiomas (Fig. 16-7) are examples of this principle.

Step two would be to apply the ABCD rule once a melanocytic lesion has been confirmed and to calculate the TDS (Table 16-1).

Asymmetry (A) of Contour, Color, or Structural Components

The lesion is visually divided into two 90-degree, right-angle axes (Fig. 16-8). A score is then assigned, ranging from "zero" for a lesion that is completely symmetrical in contour, color, or structure, to "one" for a lesion that is

After all of the criteria are identified, it is time to calculate the total dermatoscopy score. The points are multiplied by conversion factors ([A × 1.3] + [B × 0.1] + [C × 0.5] + [D × 0.5]) to determine the TDS (Table 16-1).

TABLE 16-1

Calculation of ABCD Rule of Dermoscopy

Parameter	Range of Scores
Asymmetry × 1.3 +	(0-2)
Borders × 0.1 +	(0-8)
Colors × 0.5 +	(1-6)
Different structural components × 0.5 =	(1-5)
Total dermoscopy score	

<4.75: Benign
4.8-5.45: Suspicious for melanoma
>5.45: Highly suspicious for melanoma

TABLE 16-2

Seven-Point Checklist

Criteria	Seven-Point Score
Major Criteria	
1. Atypical pigment network	2
2. Atypical vascular pattern	2
3. Blue-whitish veil	2
Minor Criteria	
4. Irregular streaks (pseudopods/radial streaming)	1
5. Irregular pigmentation	1
6. Irregular dots or globules	1
7. Regression areas	1
Seven-point total score	<3: nonmelanoma >3: melanoma

Seven-Point Checklist

The newest approach to the analysis of criteria is called the seven-point checklist. Whereas the pattern analysis requires expert qualitative assessment of numerous individual criteria, and the ABCD rule of dermatoscopy is a semiquantitative analysis of only four criteria, the seven-point checklist is based on a blind study of 342 melanocytic lesions (117 melanomas and 342 melanocytic lesions). Major and minor criteria are identified. A major criterion receives two points each, and a minor criterion receives one point. A score of three or greater has a 95 percent sensitivity of being a melanoma (Fig. 16-9 and Table 16-2). Not included in the seven-point checklist are criteria not significantly associated with melanoma and criteria used for the diagnosis of nonmelanocytic lesions.

CONCLUSION

Formal training is needed in dermoscopy to increase accuracy. Be a purist and learn the proper vocabulary for each approach, and do not interchange them. If pattern analysis is preferred, learn that vocabulary and approach and do not use it and confuse it with the vocabulary and evaluation of the ABCD rule of dermatoscopy or with the seven-point checklist. For example, terms such as *blue-gray veil* and *radial streaming* are associated with

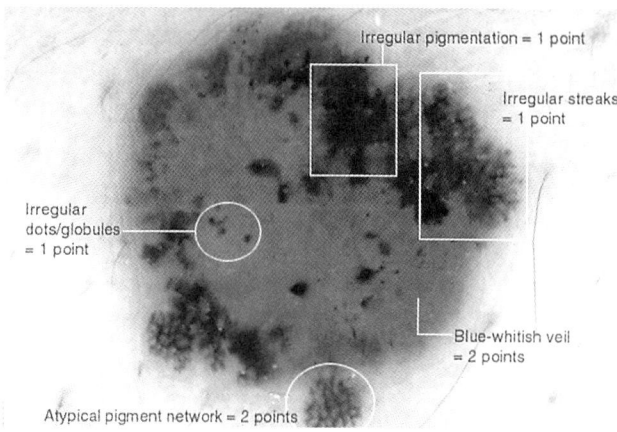

Fig. 16-9
Melanoma with seven points based on the seven-point checklist. (Courtesy Giuseppe Argenziano, MD, Naples, Italy.)

pattern analysis and should not be used in evaluation of a lesion with the ABCD rule of dermatoscopy.

Dermascopy, with all of the extra criteria evaluated, should be combined with the patient's personal and family history, clinical appearance, and history of the lesion before deciding for or against excision.

Experienced clinicians can diagnose melanoma clinically 60% to 70% of the time. With training and experience, the extra criteria seen with dermoscopy increase the diagnostics of melanoma into the 90% range. The most important point when examining pigmented skin lesions is not to miss a melanoma!

SUPPLIERS

Dermatoscope
Heine USA
1 Washington Street, Suite 555
Dover, NH 03820-3851
Phone: 1-800-367-4872
Website: www.heine.com

DermLite
3Gen
23801 Salvador Bay
Dana Point, CA 92629
Phone: 1-949-481-6384
Website: www.3genllc.com

EpiScope
Welch Allyn
4341 State Street Road
P.O. Box 220
Skaneatles Falls, NY 13153-0220
Phone: 1-800-535-6663
Website: www.welchallyn.com

BIBLIOGRAPHY

Argenziano G, Fabbrocini G, Carli P, et al: Epiluminescence microscopy for the diagnosis of doubtful melanocytic skin lesions: comparison of the ABCD rule of Dermatoscopy and a new 7-point checklist based on pattern analysis, *Arch Dermatol* 134(12):1563, 1998.

Argenziano G, Soyer HP, De Giorgi V, et al: *Interactive atlas of dermoscopy* [book on CD-ROM], Milan, 2000, EDRA Medical Publishing and New Media. Available at www.dermoscopy.com (accessed June 13, 2001).

Ascierto PA, Satriano RA, Palmieri G, et al: Epiluminescence microscopy as a useful approach in the early diagnosis of cutaneous malignant melanoma, *Melanoma Res* 8:529, 1998.

Binder M, Puespoeck-Schwarz M, Steiner A, et al: Epiluminescence microscopy of small pigmented skin lesions: short-term training improves the diagnostic performance of dermatologists, *J Am Acad Dermatol* 36:197, 1997.

Grin OM, Kopf AW, et al: Accuracy of the clinical diagnosis of malignant melanoma, *Arch Dermatol* 126:763, 1990.

Habif TP, editor: *Clinical dermatology*, St Louis, 1996, Mosby.

Johr R, Izakovic J: Should you be using epiluminescence microscopy? *Skin Aging*, March:28, 2000.

Nachbar F, Stolz W, Merkle T, et al: The ABCD rule of dermatoscopy: high prospective value in the diagnosis of doubtful melanocytic skin lesions, *J Am Acad Dermatol* 30:551, 1994.

Steiner A, Binder M, Schemper M, et al: Statistical evaluation of epiluminescence microscopy criteria for melanocytic pigmented skin lesions, *J Am Acad Dermatol* 29:581, 1993.

Stolz W, Braun-Falco O, Bilek P, et al: *Color atlas of dermatoscopy*, Oxford, England, 1994, Blackwell Scientific.

CHAPTER 17

Fishhook Removal

John Harlan Haynes III

Fishhook injuries are relatively common. Confidence in their management is paramount to successful outcomes. The method used to remove a fishhook depends on the anatomical location of the injury and the conditions under which the removal is to take place. The first and least harmful method described is the *string-yank* method, which may be used without anesthesia by anglers on the water. It is best used on the more resilient skin surfaces with underlying bone and muscle. For more embedded hooks, or for hooks in flaccid areas such as the earlobe, the needle cover *"barb-sheath"* or the *pull-through* technique may be more applicable. Local anesthesia with 1% lidocaine is well received by the anxious patient in an emergency setting. If the shank has already been clipped by a well-meaning first-aider, a strong needle driver or hemostat may be clamped over the exposed shank tip to facilitate removal.

Occasionally, radiographs may help in determining type of fishhook and depth of penetration. Assess proximity to underlying neurovascular or tendon structures and the potential for damage.

INDICATIONS

• Fishhook embedded in subcutaneous tissue

CONTRAINDICATIONS

• Penetration into the eye with scleral perforation (dictates ophthalmology referral)

ANGLER'S STRING-YANK METHOD

Equipment

• Silk suture (0 or larger diameter), umbilical tape, or ordinary string, 2 to 3 feet in length
• 2 to 3 ml of 1% lidocaine in syringe, 30-gauge needle

Technique

1. Cleanse the skin with an iodinated soap or similar antiseptic solution.
2. Inject 2 to 3 ml of 1% local anesthetic around the hook.
3. Tie the midpoint of the string or suture around the curve of the fishhook. Securely wrap the other ends several times around your index and middle finger (Fig. 17-1, *A*).
4. Place the involved extremity on a flat surface to provide stabilization. Depress the shank of the hook against the skin with the index finger of your non-dominant free hand until it meets resistance. The shaft of the hook is then lifted approximately parallel to the underlying skin by grasping the eye with the thumb and middle fingers (Fig. 17-1, *B*). This ma-

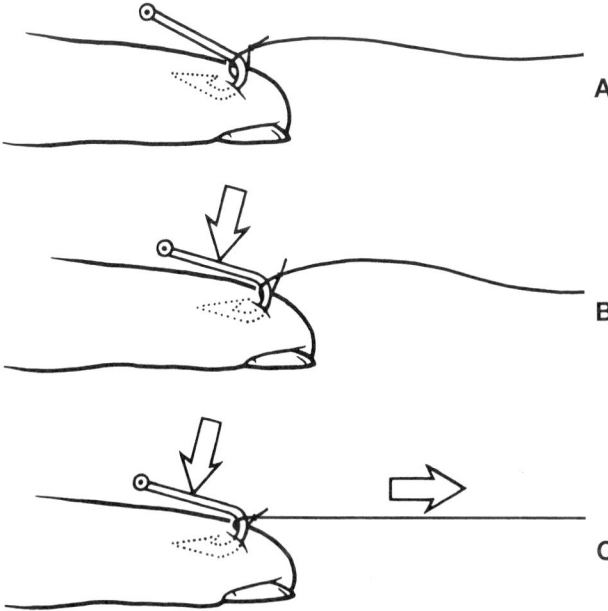

Fig. 17-1
A-C, Angler's string-yank method of fishhook removal. See text for details.

neuver disengages the barb from the subcutaneous tissue.

5. With the shank depressed and the barb disengaged, grasp the string 12 inches from the hook and firmly and quickly jerk the string, with follow-through, in one forceful move parallel to the shank (Fig. 17-1, *C*). Bystanders should stand clear from the flight path. This method is effective and produces no additional wounds.

NEEDLE COVER OF "BARB-SHEATH" METHOD

Equipment

- 0.5 ml lidocaine 1% in a syringe with a 30-gauge needle
- 18-gauge needle

Technique

1. After local anesthesia is injected, introduce the 18-gauge needle through the entrance track along the inside curvature of the hook, parallel to the shank, with the bevel toward the inside of the curve so that the needle opening can engage the barb (Fig. 17-2, *A-B*).
2. Advance the hook slightly to dislodge the barb from the tissue. Gently pull and twist the hook so that the barb is firmly sheathed by the lumen of the 18-gauge needle.
3. Back the hook and needle out together as a unit (Fig. 17-2, *C*).

TRADITIONAL PULL-THROUGH METHOD

Equipment

- 0.5 ml lidocaine 1% in syringe with 27-gauge needle
- Wire clipper

Technique

1. Provide local anesthesia over the point of the hook (Fig. 17-3, *A*).
2. Force the point through the anesthetized skin (Fig. 17-3, *B*).
3. When the barb tip is fully exposed, clip it off (Fig. 17-3, *C*).
4. Back the hook out along the direction of entry (Fig. 17-3, *D*).

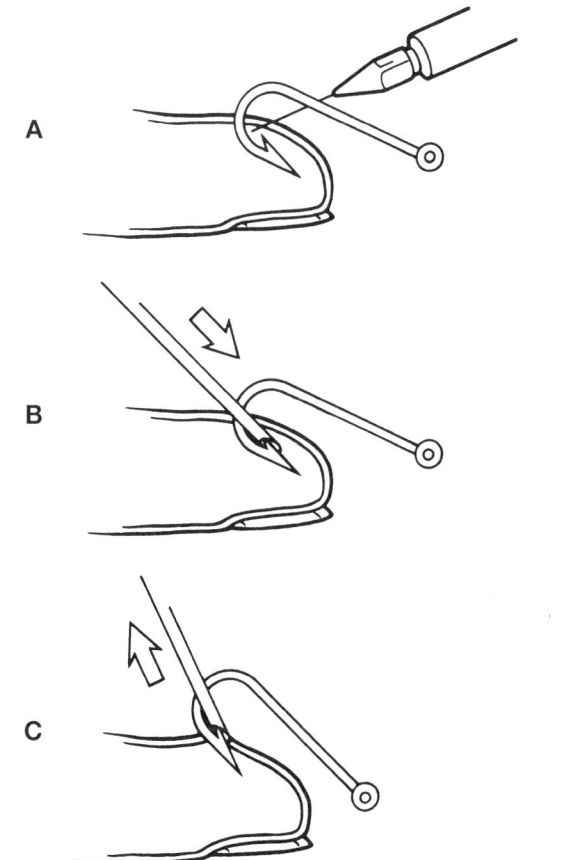

Fig. 17-2
A-C, Removal of a fishhook with anesthetic when the hook is large and not too deep in the skin. See text for details.

5. Alternatively, if the shank has multiple barbs, clip off the eye of the hook and pull on the sharp end of the hook until the entire hook is removed (Fig. 17-4).

POSTPROCEDURE CARE

- Explore the wound for possible foreign bodies and debride.
- Administer tetanus toxoid if more than 5 years have elapsed since its last administration.
- Prophylactic antibiotic therapy may be considered for persons who are immunosuppressed or have diabetes or peripheral vascular disease. Prophylactic antibiotics may also be used for deeper or contaminated wounds.
- Dress the wound with a sterile adhesive bandage and antibiotic ointment.
- Wash the area well with soap and water four to six times a day for 2 days.
- Warn the patient of the possibility of infection.

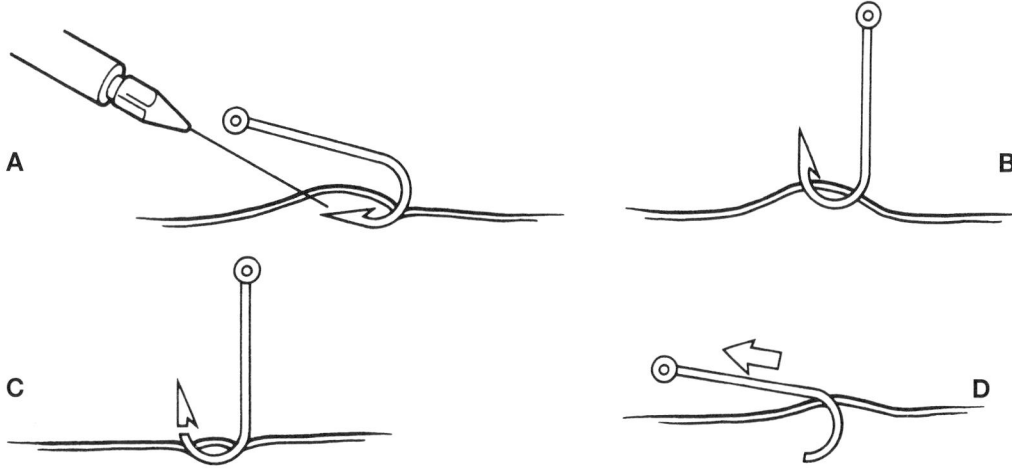

Fig. 17-3
A-D, Traditional pull-through method for removing a small fishhook. See text for details.

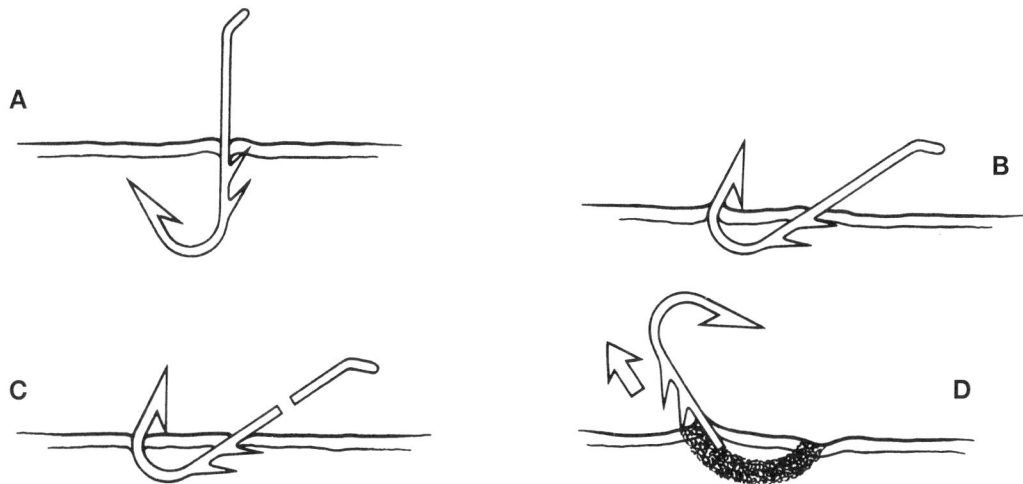

Fig. 17-4
Removal of a barbed fishhook. **A,** The hook embedded in soft tissue. **B,** Twist the hook forward until the sharp end is visible. **C,** Cut off the eye of the hook. **D,** Pull on the sharp end to remove.

CPT/BILLING CODES

10120	Removal of subcutaneous foreign body, simple
10121	Incisional removal, foreign body, complex

Removal of foreign body from the following:

20520	Muscle or tendon sheath, simple
23330	Shoulder subcutaneous
24200	Upper arm/elbow subcutaneous
27086	Pelvis/hip subcutaneous
28190	Foot subcutaneous
67938	Embedded eyelid

ICD-9-CM DIAGNOSTIC CODES

Foreign body in the following:

729.6	Soft tissue
919.6	Superficial without major open wound
930.1	Eyelid
931	Auricle
931	Ear
932	Nose
932	Nostril
935	Mouth
955.4	Musculocutaneous

BIBLIOGRAPHY

Gammons M, Jackson E: Fishhook removal, *Am Fam Physician* 63(11):2231, 2001.

Roberts JR, Hedges JR: *Clinical procedures in emergency medicine,* Philadelphia, 1985, WB Saunders.

Simon RR, Brenner BE: *Emergency procedures and techniques,* Baltimore, 1984, William & Wilkins.

Snider, RK, editor: Fishhook removal. In *Essentials of Musculoskeletal Care,* Rosemont, Ill, 1997, American Academy of Orthopedic Surgeons.

CHAPTER 18

Flaps and Plasties

Ashley K. Christiani
Mats Hagstrom

Appropriate wound closure following excision is essential in achieving a cosmetically pleasing result. Although many elliptical defects can be repaired with a basic side-to-side closure, large or complex defects may require more advanced techniques. Several techniques for wound closure and scar revision are described in this chapter, including advancement and rotation flaps, V-Y plasties, and the management of dog-ears. The specific flaps and plastic surgery closures described are chosen for their utility, reliability, and predictability of aesthetic result.

INDICATIONS

- A soft tissue defect is so large that a simple primary closure is not possible. If an elliptical defect may not be pinched together easily between the fingers with minimal tension, a simple side-to-side closure will likely be insufficient.
- There is excessive skin tension with simple closure techniques, and simple closure would yield a poor cosmetic result.
- Surgical skin remodeling techniques, or "plasties," may be indicated when dealing with dog-ears, complex wounds, or other defects that would cause an undesirable scar.

CONTRAINDICATIONS

When performed correctly, the closure techniques described in this chapter generally achieve good results. However, certain risk factors may lead to poor outcomes. Contraindications to complex skin closures and flaps include the following:
- Diabetes (relative)
- Impaired wound healing
- Vascular compromise to region
- Keloid or hypertrophic scar formation
- Prior radiation to region
- Coagulopathy (intrinsic or induced through anticoagulants such as warfarin)
- Wound location on lower extremity, especially the feet (due to slow healing) (relative)

It is particularly important to ask the patient about any history of abnormal scarring, keloids, or poor healing. Certain areas of the body are especially prone to hypertrophic scar and keloid formation, such as the chest, earlobes, and shoulders. Children also tend to scar more. Any patient at high risk for keloid formation should receive thorough preoperative counseling before proceeding with any skin surgery. These patients should be followed closely after surgery, since early keloid development may be curtailed by the judicious use of steroid injections and silicone gel sheeting. As a general rule, the physician should avoid the temptation to excise keloids, which may cause further keloid formation.

EQUIPMENT

Most skin excisions and closures can be performed with fairly simple equipment (as shown in the following list). Electrocautery and suction are not always necessary but are strongly recommended for meticulous control of bleeding. Adequate hemostasis is critical in preventing hematomas, wound dehiscence, and infection. Typical equipment should include the following:
- Topical antiseptic wash: povidone-iodine (Betadine) or chlorhexidine gluconate (Hibiclens).
- 5-ml syringe with needles (16 to 20 gauge to draw up anesthetic and 27 to 30 gauge for tissue injection).
- Injectable local anesthetic: 1% to 2% lidocaine with epinephrine for most areas; use without epinephrine in fingers, toes, genitals, and nose.
- Sterile drape.
- Sterile gloves.
- Sterile gauze pads.
- Telfa pad and Tegaderm for wound dressing.
- Skin-marking pen.
- Nylon suture (4-0, 5-0, or 6-0, depending on location).

- 4-0, 5-0, or 6-0 absorbable suture such as Vicryl or Dexon if deep sutures are indicated.
- Adson forceps.
- Needle holder (smooth).
- No. 15 scalpel.
- Suture scissors.
- Two skin hooks.
- Good lighting.

Strongly Recommended Equipment

- Electrocautery unit
- Suction device
- Injectable diphenhydramine and epinephrine available for anaphylactic reactions to anesthesia, latex, or other agent
- Crash cart including defibrillator, oxygen, and intubation equipment on site for emergencies (see Chapter 203, Anaphylaxis)

PREPROCEDURE PATIENT PREPARATION

History and Physical

On the preoperative history, topics of discussion should include the following:

- Medications, including herbal supplements, that the patient has taken in the past 6 weeks
- Allergies or adverse reactions to medications including iodine and local anesthetics, suture material, bandages, or latex
- Past surgical history and any history of keloid formation, hypertrophic scars, or poor wound healing
- Past medical history, including cardiac disease, diabetes, HIV, hepatitis, bleeding disorders, immunosuppression
- Whether the patient has a pacemaker or other implanted electronic device that may preclude the use of electrocautery
- Whether the patient has a history of valvular disease, rheumatic fever, joint replacement, or other indication for antibiotic prophylaxis
- Pregnancy (in reproductive age women)

Informed Consent

Before the procedure, the patient must give informed consent to undergo surgery. This includes a full description of the risks, benefits, and alternatives to the procedure. The patient must have the opportunity to ask questions regarding the procedure and have the answers provided to his or her satisfaction to constitute informed consent.

Risks

The risks of the procedure to be discussed with the patient include, but are not limited to, the following:

- Suboptimal result including the possibility of a worse scar after wound healing
- Infection
- Wound dehiscence
- Hypertrophic scar, keloid formation, or other poor scar result
- Swelling or bruising of the tissue
- Bleeding
- Pain
- Damage to nerves
- Allergic reaction to sutures, dressing, anesthetic, or other medications
- Recurrence of lesion and possible need for further surgery

Benefits

Benefits of the procedure may include, but are not limited to, the following:

- Improved cosmetic result
- Improved wound healing
- Improved overall results compared with conventional side-to-side closure

Alternatives

Alternatives to the cosmetic surgical closures listed above may include the following:

- Leaving the wound open to heal by secondary intention
- Side-to-side closure
- Performance of a skin graft
- Referral to a plastic surgeon

ANTIBIOTIC PROPHYLAXIS

Antibiotic prophylaxis should be used more liberally when flaps and plasties are performed, since the blood supply is often compromised with these closures, increasing the risk of infection. Antibiotic prophylaxis should be strongly considered in the following cases:

- When the surgical site involves an extremity, axilla, ear, the perineum, or genitalia because of an increased risk of wound infection in these areas
- Diabetes or immunosuppression
- If the wound is dirty or open more than 1 hour, or aseptic technique was not ideal
- If patient follow-up is difficult, or the patient is otherwise at increased risk of infection
- History of previously infected wounds for no apparent reason

PREOPERATIVE MEDICATIONS AND ANESTHESIA

The decision on whether to use sedation should be based on personal philosophy, patient desire, and the availability of proper monitoring. When performed correctly, most minor surgical procedures can be completed with minimal discomfort to the patient. However, some sedation may be indicated in anxious patients when the procedure is extensive or if significant discomfort is anticipated. (See Chapter 2, Conscious Sedation [Sedation and Analgesia].)

The use of local anesthetic warrants discussion. Lidocaine with epinephrine is preferable to lidocaine alone for nearly all cutaneous procedures, with the exception of regions involving terminal arteries such as fingers, toes, nose, and the tip of the penis. In the doses administered in local anesthesia, epinephrine is generally safe and its vasoconstrictive properties are important in controlling bleeding. Since epinephrine takes 7 to 10 minutes to achieve full effect, it is advisable to anesthetize the surgical site before prepping and draping the patient. The addition of 1 ml of sodium bicarbonate to every 9 ml of lidocaine with epinephrine helps neutralize the acidity of the solution and thus cause less pain with injection. Plain lidocaine does not benefit to the same extent with the addition of sodium bicarbonate because it is not as acidified. Bupivacaine (Marcaine) precipitates at a neutral pH and should never be used with sodium bicarbonate. When the longer-acting properties of bupivacaine are desired, it may be helpful to anesthetize the region using lidocaine with epinephrine (buffered with sodium bicarbonate) before injecting bupivacaine.

Additional techniques to minimize discomfort include the use of EMLA cream, cryoanesthesia (such as topical ethyl chloride), slow injections, and initiation of the anesthesia injection on the subdermal plane. It is advisable to draw up all injectable medications in advance and to keep scalpels, needles, and syringes out of the patient's view, particularly when working with pediatric patients.

PREPARATION OF SKIN AND HAIR

Hair removal at the surgical site may be accomplished by shaving or by cutting the hair with scissors (to minimize microabrasions that may increase the risk of infection). On the scalp, ointment can be used to spread the hair away from the operative site and to minimize the need to cut the hair. The skin is prepared with a povidone-iodine (Betadine) or chlorhexidine (Hibiclens) solution with gentle scrubbing. Note that Betadine must be allowed to dry before it is considered effective, and Hibiclens should be avoided on the face, since it is extremely toxic

to the eye. Skin markings may be made before or after prepping the patient. An overzealous scrub or an alcohol wipe, however, may remove preoperative markings, and a pen used before the skin preparation is no longer sterile.

DRAPES

Sterile drapes should be used with any skin procedures that require suturing to protect the suture material from becoming contaminated and introducing bacteria into the subdermal tissue. Fenestrated drapes that have adhesive around the opening to affix the hole securely over the surgical site are especially helpful. However, you may need to extend the aperture or design your own by cutting a hole in a sterile surgical drape. Sterile technique is particularly important with flaps and plasties because blood supply may be compromised, predisposing the wound to infection.

TECHNIQUE (Also see Chapters 22 through 26)

Tissue excision should be completed before committing to any particular flap or closure method. It is best to cut the shape of the defect, as well as the flap design, on a cotton towel before cutting the skin. This helps to prevent the common pitfall of creating flaps that are too short. The practitioner need not be limited to the following techniques. Some wounds may even heal best through secondary intention.

It is often preferable to convert a nonelliptical defect, such as a large punch biopsy site, to an ellipse along skin tension lines before closure. On occasion, a nonelliptical defect such as a triangle or rectangle may lend itself to a flap closure by advancement or rotation. Regardless of the shape of the defect, the base must be on an even plane in the subcutaneous tissue to allow for a good result.

The key to good wound closure is to provide optimal alignment of the skin edges under minimal tension. This is best accomplished by a *layered closure* with the majority of the strength of the closure provided by the dermal sutures, leaving little to no tension on the skin edges. All *buried sutures* should have the knot inverted (placed away from the skin side). Most skin sutures should be removed within 7 days to prevent the formation of "railroad track" scars.

Flaps are composed of skin and subcutaneous tissue that is cut from the donor site and moved a small distance to a recipient site without removing it from its vascular supply. Local skin flaps consist of rotation flaps that pivot into place and advancement flaps that move

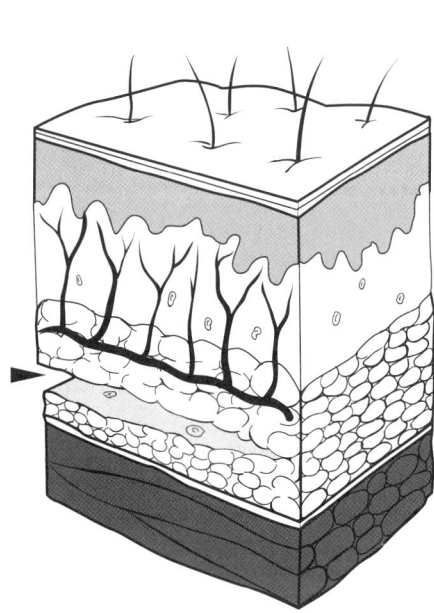

Fig. 18-1
Skin flap *(arrow)*, with proper level of undermining in subcutaneous adipose layer. This can be performed with a blade or sharp tissue scissors. It is important to maintain integrity of vessels and not create a flap that is too thin.

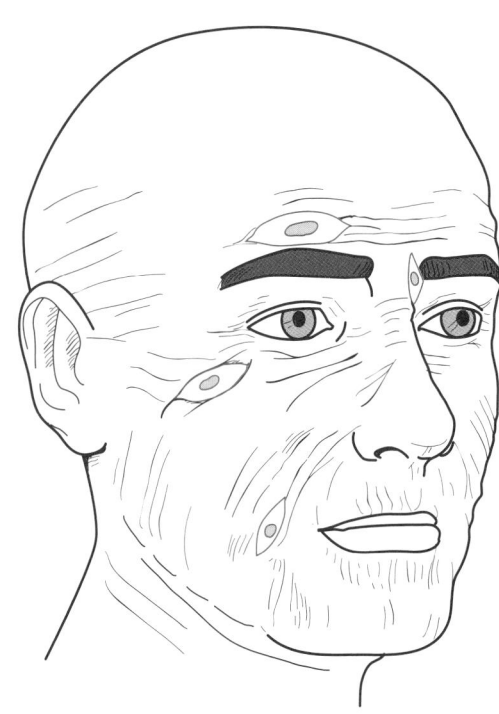

Fig. 18-2
It is essential to place elliptical excisions in relaxed skin tension lines.

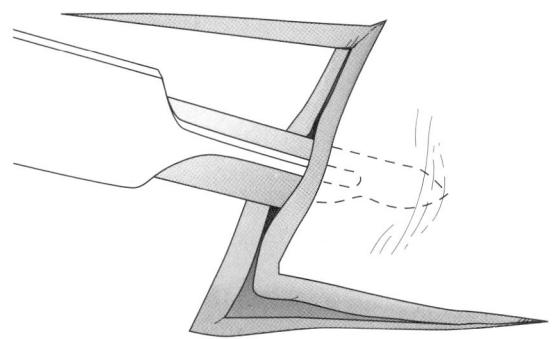

Fig. 18-3
Undermining of a flap using a no. 15 scalpel.

laterally. *Rotation flaps* maintain a base of intact skin, whereas some *advancement flaps* are completely incised with blood being supplied only from the subcutaneous tissues. Because flaps carry their own blood supply, it is important to avoid damaging the subdermal vascular plexus or cutting potential nutrient vessels. Flaps created with parallel incisions are at increased risk for necrosis because of limited blood supply, but they are sometimes unavoidable. Fig. 18-1 illustrates the proper level for undermining the flap tissue.

Tissue handling techniques are important for flap success. It is crucial to handle skin gently with minimal trauma. Lifting the skin gently with skin hooks is preferable to manipulation with forceps or pickups. When using skin forceps, do not apply more force than is absolutely necessary. Skin forceps are capable of exerting forces of greater than 400 lb per square inch. When grasping skin, take hold of the deep dermis and avoid the fragile epidermis.

Elliptical Excisions

The elliptical excision technique is appropriate for the vast majority of lesions requiring tissue removal, and it generally facilitates wound closure. Length/width ratios should be greater than 3:1, and the terminal angles should be less than 30 degrees to avoid dog-ears. The

long axis of the ellipse should run along wrinkle lines or, in younger patients, relaxed skin tension lines (Fig. 18-2). See Chapter 22, Incisions: Planning the Direction of the Cut.

If the closure is tight, gentle undermining may create more laxity. With flaps and plasties, some undermining will almost always be necessary. Undermining should be performed subdermally (between the skin and subcutaneous adipose tissue) to avoid injury to the vascular plexus (Figs. 18-1 and 18-3). (See Chapter 23, Laceration and Incision Repair.)

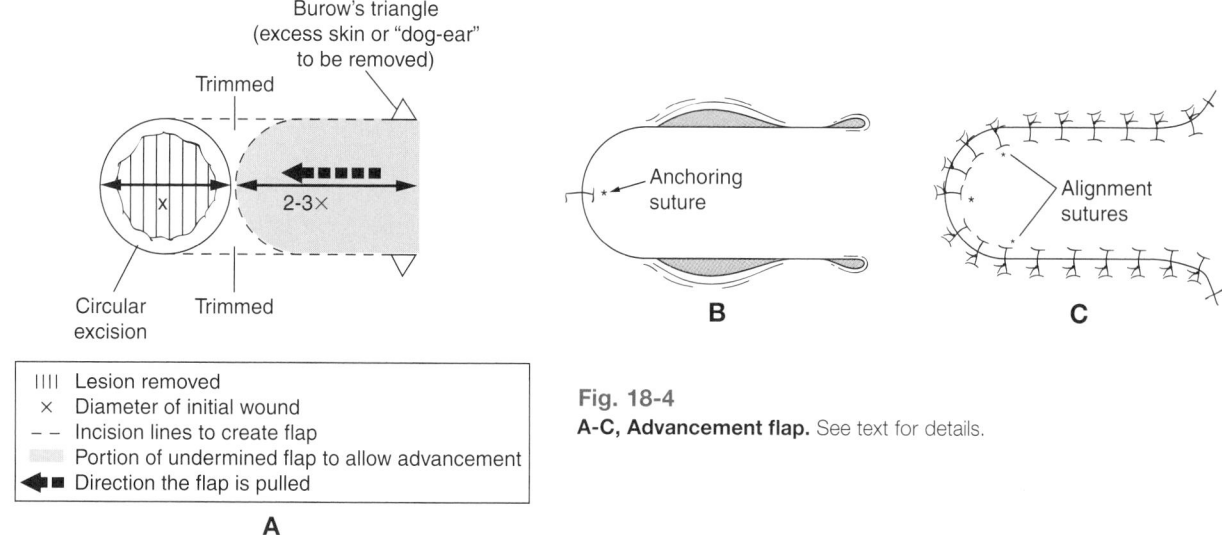

IIII   Lesion removed
×   Diameter of initial wound
– –   Incision lines to create flap
▨   Portion of undermined flap to allow advancement
◄■■   Direction the flap is pulled

A

Fig. 18-4
A-C, Advancement flap. See text for details.

When side-to-side closure is difficult due to skin tension, a variety of flaps can be used to close the defect, depending on skin availability and anatomic location.

Advancement Flap

Advancement flaps are conceptually simple but have limited application because of the parallel incisions required, as well as the increased skin tension created. The single pedicle advancement flap, with or without Burow's triangles, may be useful in highly vascular, elastic areas. All advancement flaps are moved laterally without any rotation. In planning the flap, remember that *the length of a simple advancement flap should be two to three times the length of the defect to be closed,* depending on skin laxity. On the face, flaps should not exceed a 3:1 length/width ratio. If a double advancement flap is to be used (advancing a flap from two sides), the length of each flap should generally be one to two times the length of the defect. As with the planning of all flaps, it may be helpful to cut the defect as well as the planned flap design on a surgical drape or other material before cutting skin.

1. Use a skin-marking pen to draw the desired flap on the patient's skin. In the case of a simple advancement flap, it is often preferable cosmetically to round the advancing edge creating a U-shaped closure. Remember to make the base of the pedicle long and wide enough to avoid closing the skin under tension.
2. Undermine the intended flap at the level shown in Fig. 18-1, and pull the flap into place.
3. Burow's triangles may be used to facilitate tissue movement (Fig. 18-4, *A*). See the "Dog-Ears" section.
4. Using the skin hook, advance the flap and place an anchoring suture (Fig. 18-4, *B*).

5. Place the next sutures as shown in Fig. 18-4, *C,* to ensure proper alignment of the flap, then complete the closure.

Double Advancement Flap

For the double advancement flap, perform the following:
1. Excise lesions with appropriate margins.
2. Draw out the anticipated repair with the skin-marking pen and create the incisions as shown. Trim the excess tissue to create a square defect (Fig. 18-5, *A*).
3. Undermine areas to be advanced.
4. Advance the opposing flaps toward each other and place the anchoring (tension-bearing) suture subcutaneously (Fig. 18-5, *B*).
5. Place a half-buried mattress ("V-flap" stitch) suture at each of the lateral flap edges (Fig. 18-5, *C*)
6. Close the remainder of the wound site with simple interrupted sutures (Fig. 18-5, *D*)

V-Y Plasty or Island Advancement Flap

The V-Y plasty or flap is an advancement flap that may be used in closing a circular defect. The technique should be limited to skin that is highly mobile and has an excellent blood supply. The technique may be *useful when* a vital structure prevents the standard elliptical excision or when an elliptical excision is too large to be closed without excessive tension. For larger lesions the V-Y flap may be advanced from both sides as a *double V-Y advancement* flap. The *disadvantage* of the V-Y flap is that the entire perimeter of the triangle is incised, which severely reduces the blood supply to only the vessels beneath the flap and thus limits the distance the flap can travel.

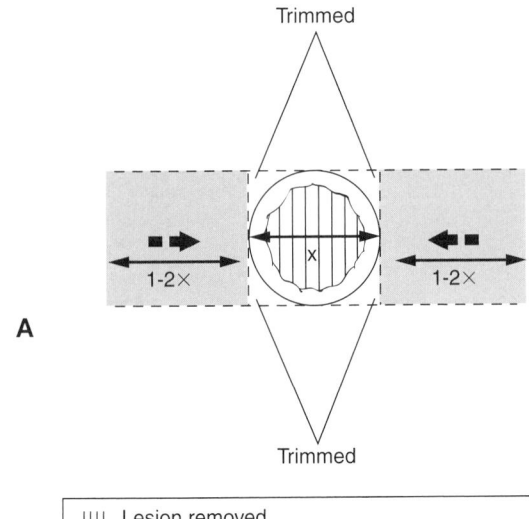

A

Trimmed

Trimmed

IIII	Lesion removed
×	Diameter of initial wound
– –	Incision lines to create flap
▧	Portion of undermined flap to allow advancement
◀■	Direction the flap is pulled

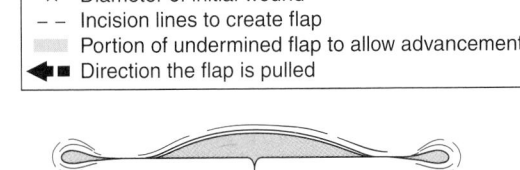

B

Tension-bearing suture is subcutaneous

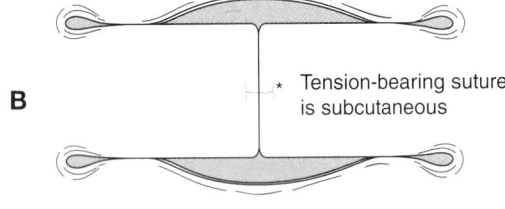

Half-buried mattress V-flap stitch

C

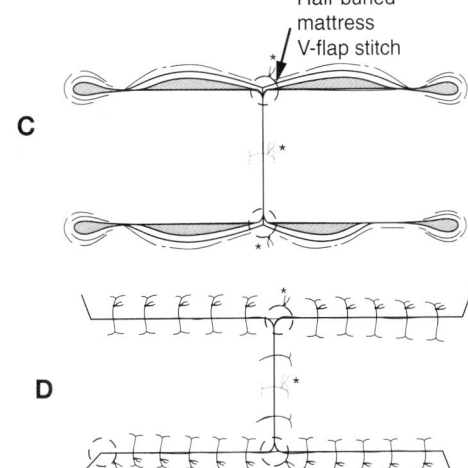

D

Fig. 18-5
A-D, Double advancement flap. For further information, see Chapter 23, Laceration and Incision Repair. See text for details.

Use of the V-Y flap to close a circular defect is demonstrated as follows (Fig. 18-6):
1. Excise the defect (Fig. 18-6, *A-B*).
2. Plan a triangle with a base approximately the diameter of the circular defect and an apical angle of 30 to 45 degrees (Fig. 18-6, *C*).

3. Incise the triangle and undermine laterally to allow eventual closure of the sides. *Do not* undermine under the flap itself, since the blood supply to the "island" is provided by the subcutaneous vessels (Fig. 18-6, *D*).
4. Trim the angles at the base of the triangle to fill the defect (Fig. 18-6, *E*).
5. Using your skin hooks, advance the flap into the defect and suture the top together (Fig. 18-6, *F*).
6. Close the remainder of the incisions with simple interrupted sutures to create a Y-shaped scar (Fig. 18-6, *G*).

Another method of creating a V-Y repair to close a wound under tension is as follows:
1. Create an elliptical excision large enough to remove the lesion (Fig. 18-6, *H*).
2. A V-shaped incision is made, then undermined to reduce skin tension (Fig. 18-6, *I*).
3. Close the ellipse first. When the V is closed, there will be a "dog-ear" that will need to be excised. Closing this area will form the vertical portion of the Y (Fig. 18-6, *J*).

The *double V-Y advancement flap* is performed in the same manner but with mirror image triangular flaps that are advanced toward each other. This technique may be helpful for larger lesions.
1. Create an elliptical excision around the lesion and excise (Fig. 18-7, *A*).
2. Incise the triangular flaps as described above. Undermine laterally. Using skin hooks, gently advance the two flaps toward each other and place the anchoring suture (Fig. 18-7, *B*).
3. Place the next sutures as shown to provide good alignment, followed by corner sutures. The closure may then be completed with subcutaneous or simple interrupted sutures (Fig. 18-7, *C*).

Rotation Flaps

The design of a rotation flap should be planned only after the original tissue has been excised completely. The flap should be generous in length (generally with *an arc length of four to five times the base of the defect to be closed*) to allow adequate tissue movement. The *advantages* of a rotation flap include the provision of good blood supply by avoiding parallel incisions, the ability to undermine the mobilized tissue if needed, and the ability to create a contralateral flap if more tissue is needed. The major *disadvantage* is that the final result may not blend into natural skin lines.
1. The illustrated lesion lends itself to an excision that may be trimmed to create a triangular defect (Fig. 18-8, *A*).
2. Draw the desired arc down to the "pivot point," according to the above guidelines (flap edge four to five times the length of the base of the triangular

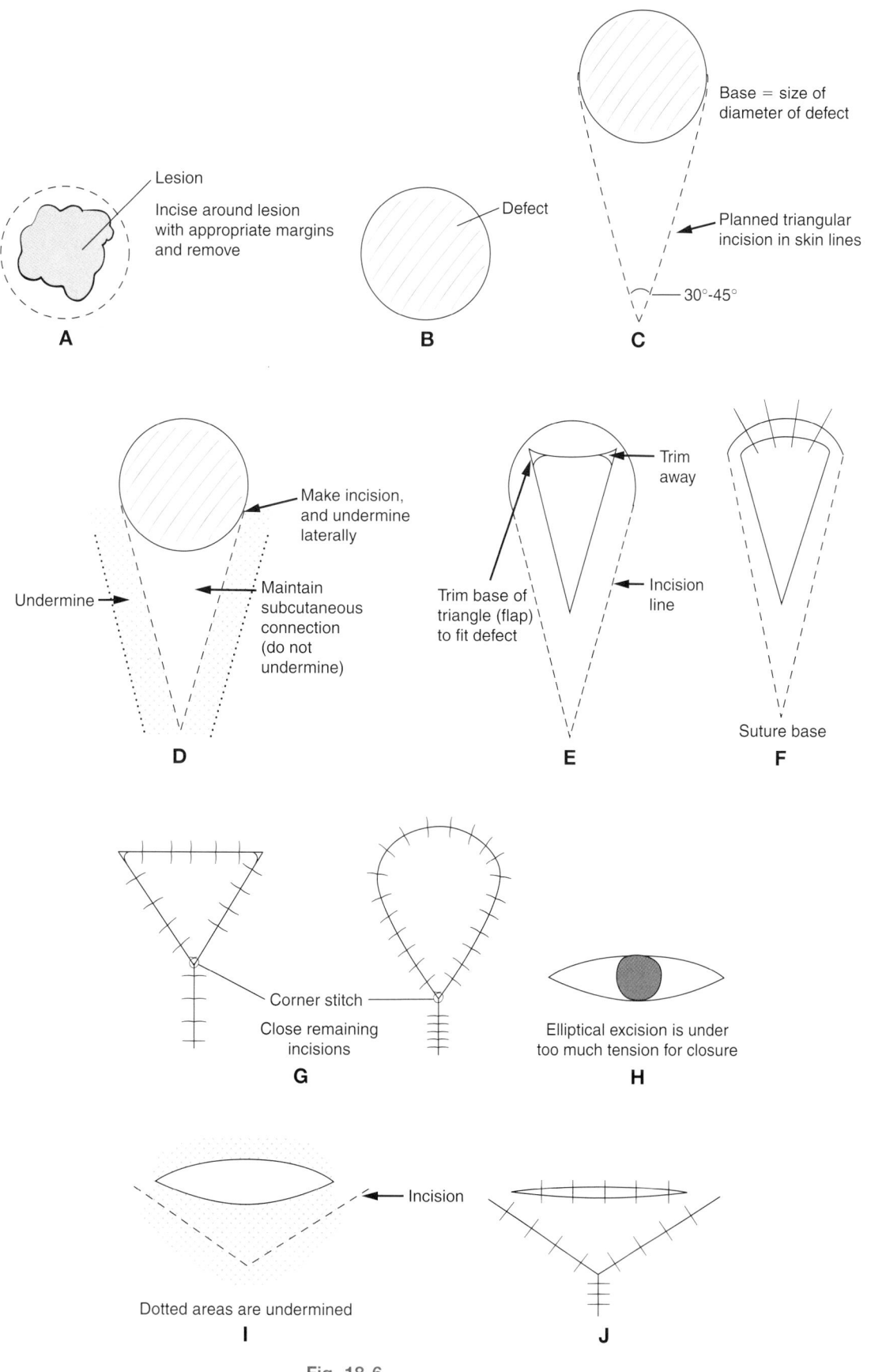

Fig. 18-6
A-J, V-Y flap. See text for details.

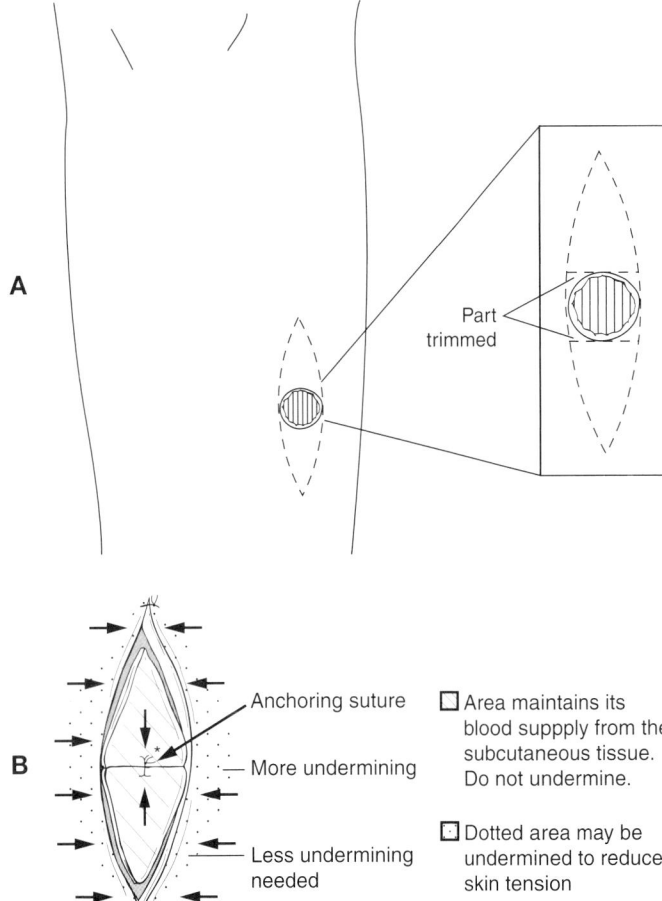

Anchoring suture

More undermining

□ Area maintains its blood supply from the subcutaneous tissue. Do not undermine.

Less undermining needed

□ Dotted area may be undermined to reduce skin tension

Part trimmed

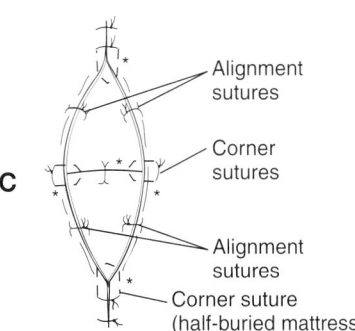

Alignment sutures

Corner sutures

Alignment sutures

Corner suture (half-buried mattress)

Fig. 18-7
A-C, Double V-Y advancement. See text for details.

defect). Be sure to allow recruitment of sufficient tissue. Some tissues like the face rotate easily. The scalp, however, is quite difficult. Again, it may be helpful to cut the defect in a surgical drape, along with the proposed repair flap design, before incising the skin and committing to a particular repair (Fig. 18-8, *B*).

3. Undermine the flap and surrounding tissue (Fig. 18-8, *C*).

4. Rotate the flap into place to fill defect. The tension-bearing sutures are placed first and are subcutaneous (one at the advancing edge and one at the point of maximal tension along the arc) (Fig. 18-8, *D*).

5. Suture into place with simple interrupted sutures (Fig. 18-8, *E*).

6. If more skin needs to be freed up for flap mobilization, or if a "dog-ear" is present, create a back-cut at the pivot point or excise a small "Burow's triangle." Although a larger triangle or back-cut provides more mobility, it also increases the risk of blood supply compromise by creating a circumferential incision (Fig. 18-8, *F*).

Z Plasty

The **Z** plasty is a particularly useful technique *for scar revision to redirect a scar into skin tension lines— making it less visible—or to release scar contractures.* Scar contracture is apt to occur when a laceration is perpendicular to skin creases as in the case of a vertical laceration on the finger (Fig. 18-9, *A*). Healing often contracts the scar, pulling the finger into a flexed position. Redirection of the scar can release skin tension. The *major drawback* to the technique is that the length of the scar is increased. In some areas, such as the face, it may be better to use a string of tiny **Z**'s to create a better visual effect.

1. Excise the linear scar or lesion in a narrow ellipse along its axis (Fig. 18-9, *B*).

2. Create the limbs of the **Z** at 60-degree angles from this axis. The length of each limb should equal the length of the defect (Fig. 18-9, *C*).

3. Using skin hooks, advance the two triangles as shown, by crossing them over one another (Fig. 18-9, *D*). Undermine the flaps as needed.

4. Place a "corner stitch" at each of the flap tips, as shown in Fig. 18-9, *E*. Then complete the wound closure with simple interrupted sutures. The new scar will now lie within the axis of the skin tension lines.

Dog-Ears

Dog-ears are caused by excess skin left at the end of the suture line. They commonly occur when skin edges are rotated or pulled, when interrupted sutures are not placed evenly, or when one side of a wound is longer than the other. Dog-ears can be avoided by closing the ends of an elliptical defect first and distributing the "extra skin" throughout the wound, keeping ellipse incision angles 30 degrees or less and maintaining 3:1 length/width ratios. Two techniques for repair are demonstrated below. *In either repair, the wound will be lengthened and excess tissue must be removed.*

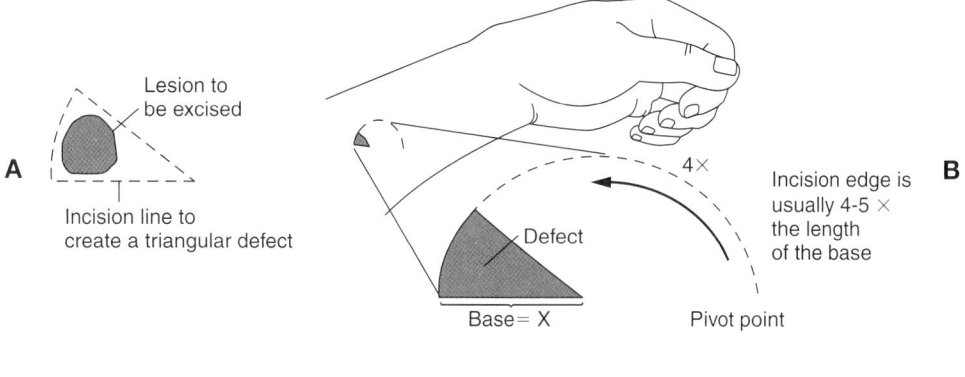

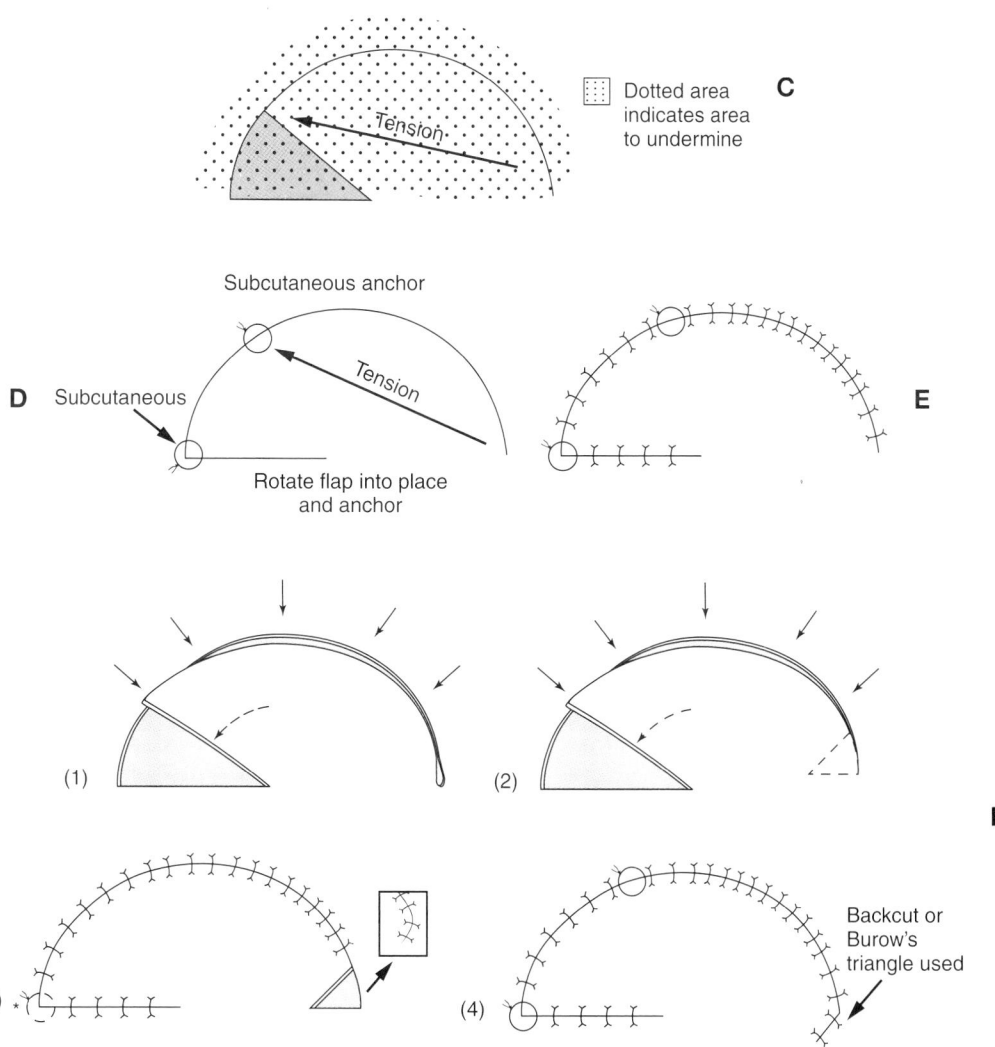

Fig. 18-8
A-F, Rotation flap. See text for details.

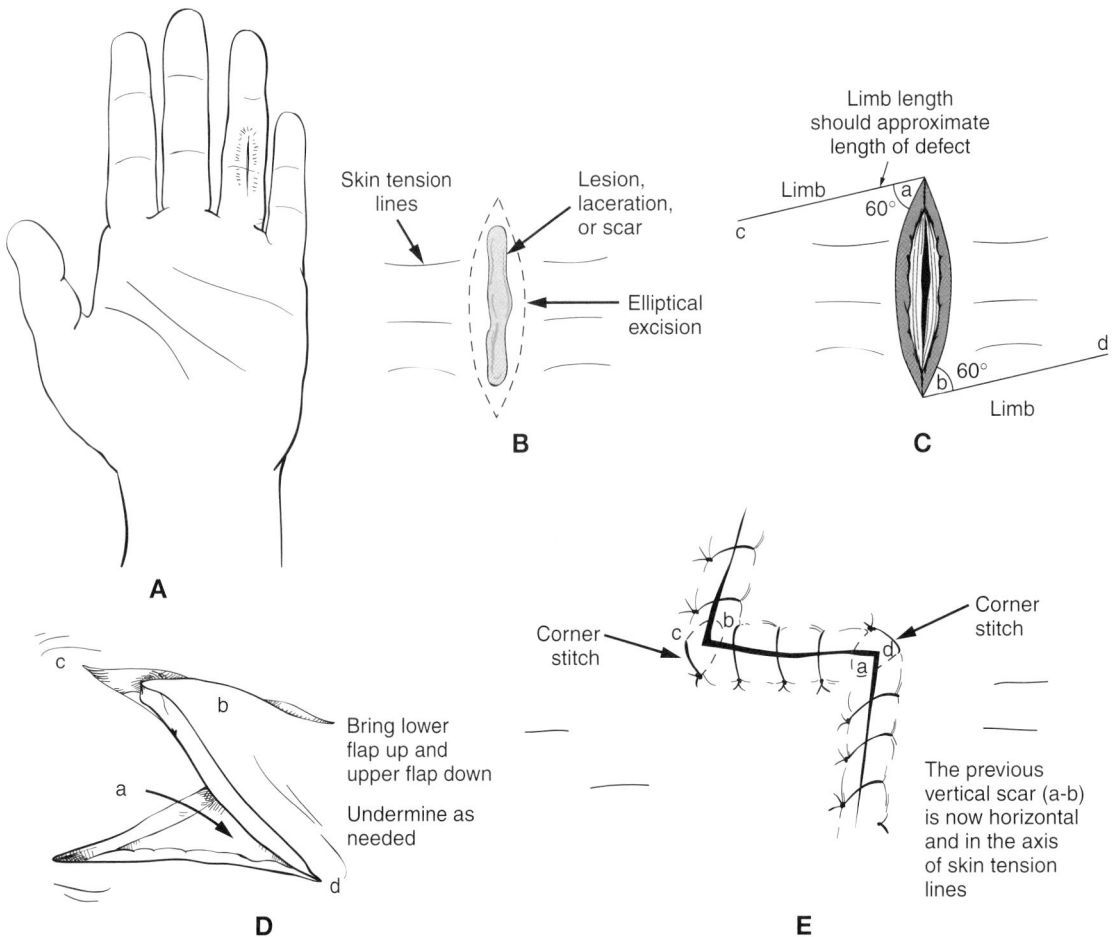

Skin tension lines

Lesion, laceration, or scar

Elliptical excision

B

Limb length should approximate length of defect

Limb

a 60°

c

b 60° d

Limb

C

A

Bring lower flap up and upper flap down

Undermine as needed

D

Corner stitch

Corner stitch

The previous vertical scar (a-b) is now horizontal and in the axis of skin tension lines

E

Fig. 18-9
A-E, Z plasty. See text for details.

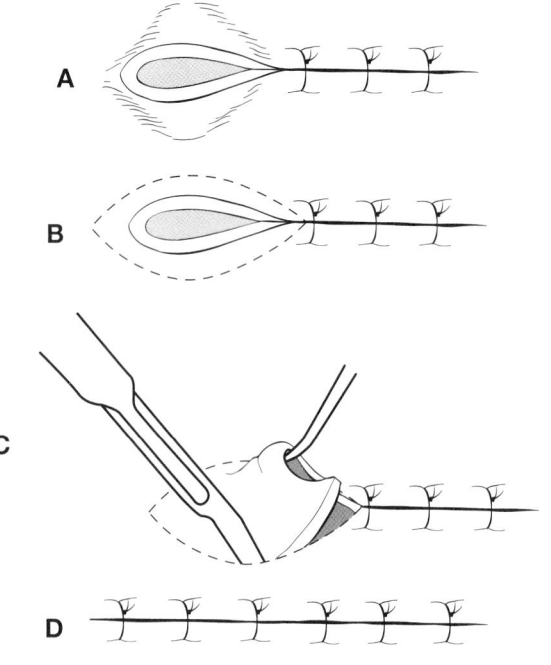

Fig. 18-10
Dog-ear repair: technique I.

Technique I

1. Excess skin "puckers up" at the end of the wound (a "dog-ear") (Fig. 18-10, *A*).
2. Make an elliptical excision as shown (Fig. 18-10, *B*).
3. Remove the excess skin. Note that the wound is extended in this repair and additional tissue removed (Fig. 18-10, *C*).
4. Close the wound (Fig. 18-10, *D*).

It is sometimes difficult with this technique to judge how much tissue should be removed.

Technique II

1. Excess tissue on one side of the wound closure creates a dog-ear (Fig. 18-11, *A*).
2. At the apex of the wound, incise the tissue at 150-degree angle to the wound. The length depends on the amount of excess tissue (Fig. 18-11, *B*).
3. Using the skin hook, pull the apex of the dog-ear over the extended incision line and excise the excess tissue with a blade or tissue scissors (Fig. 18-11, *C*).
4. Close the suture as shown (Fig. 18-11, *D*).

It is easier with this technique to judge the amount of tissue that must be removed.

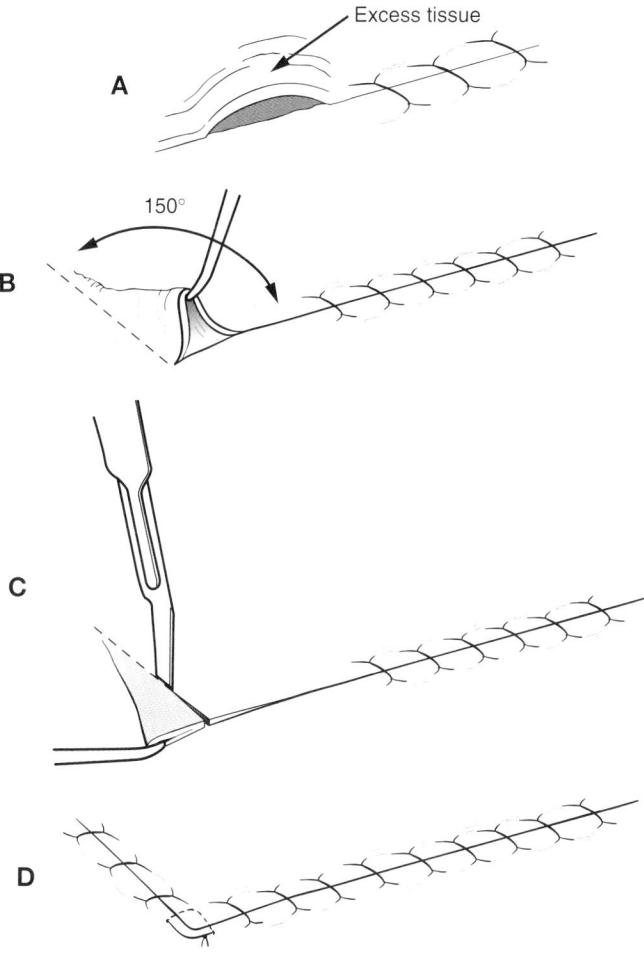

Fig. 18-11
Dog-ear repair: technique II.

COMPLICATIONS

Acute (Within 2 Weeks)

- Bleeding
- Bruising
- Swelling
- Hematoma
- Pain
- Infection
- Wound dehiscence

Chronic or Permanent

- Scarring/contractures
- "Railroad tracks" from delayed suture removal
- Hypertrophic scars
- Keloid
- Hyperpigmentation
- Hypopigmentation
- Nerve damage
- Ectropion and entropion of eyelid

- Disruption of vermilion border of upper lip
- Skin atrophy
- Hair loss
- Recurrence of excised lesion

Additional Considerations

In the excision of potentially malignant lesions, tumor-free margins must always be obtained before committing to any flap closure. If a later pathology report indicates incomplete excision of a malignant lesion, the appropriate area around the previous closure area will need to be resected. If this involves a flap technique, there may already be significant skin tension and/or little skin may be available for further repairs. The patient requiring more extensive repairs or grafting may be left with a large defect.

POSTPROCEDURE PATIENT EDUCATION

Proper postoperative care is more critical with skin flaps and plasties than with simple closures. For the first 24 hours after surgery, the patient must rest and avoid exertion. Instruct the patient to refrain from bending, heavy lifting, and exercising until the sutures are removed. The wound should be kept clean and dry for 24 hours. The patient should refrain from alcohol and aspirin-containing medicines for at least the first 24 hours after surgery. The wound should be dressed with a small piece of Telfa, covered by Tegaderm. If subcuticular sutures are used, Steri-Strips are placed, followed by the Telfa and Tegaderm dressing. A thick outer dressing of 4 × 4–inch gauze or other bandage is then placed.

After 24 hours the thick outer bandage may be removed. Instruct the patient to leave the thin inner dressing (Tegaderm) in place until the sutures are removed. At this time it is acceptable to shower and wash around the wound. It is generally safe to allow clean shower water to wash over the wound area, but the area should not be scrubbed. If the wound bleeds at any time, the patient should apply firm pressure for 15 minutes. If the thin dressing becomes wet from wound drainage, it should not be removed but covered with a second dressing. If the inner dressing begins to come off on its own, reinforce it with bandages or skin tape.

Instruct the patient to call the office or go to the emergency room if the wound bleeds significantly despite 15 minutes of firm pressure, if any signs of infection (e.g., purulence, redness, increased pain, swelling, or fever) are noted, or if there is any breakdown in wound or suture integrity.

In the case of surgery on the face, instruct the patient to sleep with his or her head slightly elevated for the first two nights after the procedure and to avoid sleeping on the same side as the wound. The patient should also avoid bending down (head below the heart) for the first 48 hours after the surgery. Arrange for office follow-up based on personal discretion, depending on the complexity of the procedure, the cleanliness of the wound, and patient factors. Sutures on the face are usually taken out within 4 days (3 to 6 days, depending on tension). Sutures on the neck are generally left in place for 4 to 7 days. On the trunk, groin, extremities, and scalp, sutures are left in longer, usually 10 to 14 days.

CONCLUSION

Achievement of a durable repair with a good cosmetic result after skin surgery is important. To obtain predictable quality outcomes, focus on simplicity. An ellipse excision with primary closure often gives the best results with the highest chance of successful healing. When wounds are difficult to close, flaps, skin grafts, and healing by secondary intention are always options.

SUPPLIERS

Acuderm, Inc.
5370 NW 35 Terrace
Fort Lauderdale, FL 33309
Phone: 1-800-327-0015
Website: www.acuderm.com

Delasco
608 13th Avenue
Council Bluffs, IA 51501-6401
Phone: 1-800-831-6273
Website: www.delasco.com

Miltex Instrument Company, Inc.
700 Hicksville Road
Bethpage, NY 11714
Phone: 1-800-645-8000
Website: www.miltex.com

Moore Medical Corp.
P.O. Box 1500
New Britain, CT 06050-1500
Phone: 1-800-234-1464
Website: www.mooremedical.com

SSR Surgical Instruments
P.O. Box 537, 5 Shore Avenue
Oyster Bay, NY 11771
Phone: 1-800-932-7364
Website: www.ssrsurgical.com

CPT/BILLING CODES

Excision and/or repair by adjacent tissue transfer or rearrangement, including Z plasty, V-Y plasty, rotation flap, and advancement flaps:

14000   Trunk <10 sq cm
14001   Trunk 10-30 sq cm
14020   Scalp, arms, legs <10 sq cm
14021   Scalp, arms, legs 10-30 sq cm
14060   Eyelids, nose, ears, lips <10 sq cm
14061   Eyelids, nose, ears, lips 10-30 sq cm
14040   Forehead, chin, cheek, mouth, neck, axilla, genitalia, hands, feet <10 cm
14041   Forehead, chin, cheek, mouth, neck, axilla, genitalia, hands, feet 10-30 cm
14300   Any area, unusual, or complicated repair

Note: These codes generally apply to full-thickness excision and repair by adjacent tissue mobilization. For reporting laceration repairs, the procedure must be created by the surgeon and not by the incidental shape of the laceration. Refer to the CPT book for further description.

ICD-9-CM DIAGNOSTIC CODES

See Appendix H, Neoplasm, Skin: ICD-9 Codes.

ADDITIONAL RESOURCES

- See the sample patient education handout "Home Wound Care Instructions" on page 1755 of Appendix G.
- See the sample patient consent form titled "Skin Surgery" on page 1756 of Appendix G.

BIBLIOGRAPHY

Brown JS: *Minor surgery: a text and atlas*, ed 4, London, 2001, Edward Arnold.

Fewkes JL, Pollack S, Cheney MC: *Illustrated atlas of cutaneous surgery*, Philadelphia, 1991, Gower Medical.

Georgiade GS, Riefkohl R, Levin LS, et al: *Plastic, maxillofacial and reconstructive surgery*, ed 3, Baltimore, 1997, Williams & Wilkins.

Grabb WC, Smith JW: *Plastic surgery*, ed 5, Philadelphia, 1997, Lippincott-Raven.

Grossman JA: *Minor injuries and repair*, New York, Gower Medical, 1993.

Hass AF, Grekin RC: Antibiotic prophylaxis in dermatologic surgery, *J Am Acad Dermatol* 32:155, 1995.

Jackson EA: The V-Y plasty in the treatment of fingertip amputations, *Am Fam Physician* 64(3):455, 2001.

Robinson JK, Arndt KA, LeBoit PE, Wintroub BU: *Atlas of cutaneous surgery*, Philadelphia, 1996, WB Saunders.

Usatine RP, Moy RL: *Skin surgery: a practical guide*, St Louis, 1998, Mosby.

CHAPTER 19

Foreign Body Removal from Skin and Soft Tissue

Grant C. Fowler

Patients frequently seek care from a primary care clinician for a foreign body in the skin or soft tissue. In fact, foreign bodies are present in 3% of wounds. In certain situations, removal may cause more trauma than leaving the object in place; hence, the patient may only require information or reassurance. However, the presence of a foreign body increases the risk of infection in most wounds, even if only slightly. A foreign body can also cause pain. Fortunately, removal is often accomplished with minimal trauma, resulting in considerable patient appreciation.

A foreign body should be suspected in all wounds caused by a high-velocity missile or a sharp fragile object. All wounds should be probed manually for the presence of foreign bodies. The most common error in the management of soft tissue foreign bodies is the failure to detect their presence. Failure to diagnose soft-tissue foreign bodies and manage them correctly is a common cause of malpractice in emergency medicine. With the techniques discussed below, attempts at removal may be simplified and the results maximized.

INDICATIONS

- Known foreign body in skin, subcutaneous or soft tissue
- Pain from foreign body or persistent inflammation
- Foreign body with toxic, infectious, or allergic potential
- Impairment of neurovascular or mechanical function
- Proximity to fractured bone or open joint
- Cosmetic deformity

Note: A general rule of thumb is that if one end of the foreign body can be palpated by hand or an instrument, it can be removed. Another rule is that although the foreign body may be palpable, removal will occasionally be more difficult than expected; therefore adequate time should be set aside for evaluation, exploration, planning, and removal. However, to minimize tissue damage, some authorities say that clinicians

should spend no more than 15 to 20 minutes exploring. Avoid causing damage by looking for a "needle in a haystack" and probing for too long. The final rule of thumb is that if a patient complains of a foreign body sensation, the clinician should assume the patient has one, even in the face of negative x-ray films.

CONTRAINDICATIONS

- Lack of knowledge of anatomic structures surrounding the foreign body
- Proximity of foreign body to a vital structure such as a nerve or artery
- An uncooperative patient who cannot be sedated (see Chapter 7, Pediatric Sedation) or anesthetized (see Chapter 4, Local Anesthesia)

Note: Consider referral for foreign bodies in the soft tissue of the face, the deep spaces of the hands or feet, or for broken glass if there are multiple shards. Deeply imbedded objects and those in joints may best be removed by a surgeon with the patient receiving general anesthetic.

EQUIPMENT

- Blunt-tipped, stiff, sterile metal probe
- Sterile tweezers (splinter forceps are very helpful)
- Adson pickup forceps with teeth
- Two mosquito hemostats
- Bright light that can be directed or focused (use of a headlamp allows both hands to be free for the procedure)
- Clear plastic tape
- Skin-marking pen
- Paper clips or BBs to be used as markers
- Scalpel (no. 11 or 15)
- Suture, if necessary for closure
- Topical and/or local anesthetic materials (see Chapter 11, Topical Anesthesia)

- Irrigant, such as saline
- Syringe for irrigation (5 ml for small wounds, 10 to 30 ml for larger wounds) with optional 18-gauge needle
- Magnifying glass or loupes
- Povidone-iodine solution (Betadine)
- Powerful magnet
- Sterile adhesive bandage
- Skin hook (optional)
- 3-mm skin punch for biopsy (optional)

PREPROCEDURE PATIENT PREPARATION

The clinician should explain to the patient that, although it may take days, weeks, or decades, it is safe for certain objects in the skin to be left to work their way to the surface. In some cases, it is safe for even lead and other metal objects to "rest" in the skin indefinitely. Their removal, especially if deeply imbedded, may cause more trauma than leaving the object in place, especially if the patient is not experiencing symptoms and has no signs of infection. The body tends to wall off nonporous materials and smooth objects such as bullets, glass, and metal, and even shrapnel. One exception is for objects made of wood or other organic material, which are likely to cause an inflammatory reaction or infection and usually have to be removed. The same is true for any object with toxic or allergic potential.

Patients should be aware that in some situations, removal may be impossible or unsuccessful and it may be necessary to leave the object in the tissue until it forms a cyst or localizes. If an infection develops, it will be treated with an antibiotic and the small pocket of fluid that develops may help with later removal. Inform the patient that if removal is attempted, a simple technique will be used to locate and remove the foreign body. To avoid more damage, the search will not extend beyond 15 to 20 minutes.

If removal is being considered, the patient should be informed that there is a possibility of infection after the procedure. There will also be minor trauma. Such trauma may be associated with discomfort during the procedure or some bleeding during or after the procedure. In certain situations, minimal or no anesthesia is used at first in order to better localize or grasp the object. A patient's intact sensation is usually much more accurate for locating an object than a clinician probing blindly under anesthetized skin, especially if the skin is distorted from the local anesthetic. For small or difficult-to-locate objects, the patient's intact sensation may be the only way possible to find the object. As soon as the object is grasped, stabilized, or removed, the discomfort is usually decreased or eliminated. After the object is grasped, local anesthetic can be used in some cases to minimize further discomfort.

The patient should be aware that most glass objects are difficult to visualize on x-ray film and that there may be multiple shards. For various reasons, glass is probably the most difficult object to remove. If the clinician is not comfortable that all of the foreign object(s) has been removed, referral may be required.

If the decision is made to attempt to remove the object(s), the patient should be aware that the procedure may be time consuming, although not more than 15 to 20 minutes will be spent exploring. He or she should be in a comfortable position that can be maintained for this amount of time. The patient should also be aware of the importance of remaining immobile during the procedure.

TECHNIQUE

1. Before removal, obtain as much history as possible regarding the foreign body. Knowledge of the material and method of injury may help decide which technique to use and whether a diagnostic study such as an x-ray film would be helpful. Knowledge of the angle of entry, whether tangential or perpendicular to the skin surface, may be helpful for localization. Information regarding the speed and force of entry may also be helpful.
2. Most superficially embedded, visible objects can be magnified and removed from soft tissue with a sterile needle and tweezers. Toothpicks and splinters usually enter tangentially and often their track can be envisioned based on the history. If no object is visible, various methods of localization are available.
3. If the object is not visible to the eye, consider radiographs for documentation if glass is involved to make sure there are not multiple shards. Only a small percentage of glass contains lead and is completely radiopaque; however, if the object is more than 2 mm in diameter, a slight shadow is usually seen on x-ray even with nonleaded glass. Metal, bone, gravel, teeth, glass, and some plastics usually produce at least a slight shadow on x-ray films. Painted wood can also sometimes be seen on x-ray films. Routine lateral anterior-posterior (AP) views may suffice. By ordering "soft-tissue" x-rays, slightly underpenetrated films are provided, which enhance visibility and localization efforts. Oblique and tangential views may also be helpful if the object is obscured by underlying bone. Xeromammograms and high-frequency ultrasound are alternatives for localizing nonradiopaque objects. (See Chapter 209, Emergency Department Ultrasound.) Computed to-

mography scanning and magnetic resonance imaging are helpful for diagnosis of foreign bodies, but they are rarely used because of the expense. For objects that must be removed, needle localization under fluoroscopy may remain the final option.

4. Attempt to localize the object before incising the skin. Measure and record the exact size and location of the externally visible entry wound. Examine the wound entrance to determine the angle of penetration and possibly the depth of penetration. Palpate the object, determine the exact orientation and approximate depth, and measure and record it. For larger metal objects, use a powerful magnet to draw the object to the skin surface in order to tent it up. If the skin tents, mark the outline of the object with the skin-marking pen. Glass is the most common foreign body, yet it is one of the more difficult substances to remove because it is transparent and slippery, and the size and outline of the pieces are unpredictable. If glass is suspected, to avoid cutting yourself do not probe with your finger. An unknown number of shards may be involved, and if there is uncertainty about whether all of the shards have been removed, referral should be considered.

5. If the object is not visible at the entrance wound, after palpation for orientation and depth, prep the skin with povidone-iodine and carefully use a sterile probe or mosquito hemostat to enter the wound. Gently follow the apparent track of the wound to locate the nearest edge. Use small, light, deliberate probing motions, gradually fanning in all directions, until contact is made with the probe. This may be felt or heard as a clicking sound between the probe and the foreign body. Excessive or unnecessary blind probing may conceal the foreign body further with blood and edema, or push it deeper into the tissue. For small objects, before using local anesthetic, attempt to use the patient's sensation as a guide. It may be more accurate than using a probe. In this situation, avoidance of local anesthetic not only minimizes local skin distortion but also the tissue destruction that may occur by cutting or exploring blindly under anesthesia. After the object is removed, if the patient is not anesthetized and their symptoms are completely abated, it is somewhat reassuring that everything was removed. If the patient continues to have a foreign body sensation, there may have been more than one foreign body and the exploration may need to continue.

6. After the object is located, fixate the probe in place in the clinician's nondominant hand. Rest this hand on a firm surface. Administer or inject local anesthetic with the dominant hand. Occasionally, the injection of anesthetic beyond the foreign body or on each side of the entry wound will force the foreign body out. After excluding the presence of a neurovascular bundle, tendon or other important structure, without moving the probe, cut down along the probe with a no. 11 or 15 scalpel blade until the foreign body is reached. Do not remove the probe. Reach into the incision and remove the foreign body with a pair of Adson forceps. Alternatively, if the entrance track is fairly long, and if the foreign body is very superficial and easily palpable beneath the skin, it may be advantageous to simply cut down through the skin directly over the object to remove it without the use of a probe.

7. As another alternative, if an edge of the object is easily located with the probe and the entrance wound is large, simply enlarge it further with mosquito forceps. This may allow the clinician to grasp the object firmly enough with another mosquito forceps to remove it. If the object has been in place for long enough to form a cyst, occasionally the cyst wall will need to be dissected or incised. This may be performed by the use of very small, deliberate strokes with the scalpel while the object is held by one set of mosquito forceps. The other set of mosquito forceps can be used to bluntly dissect down to the object by spreading anything that was incised with the scalpel. If the object is visible after incision and dissection of the cyst wall, it should be grasped through the incision with the second set of forceps. The first set of forceps can then be relaxed and the object removed. If the object is not visible, which is often the case when a foreign body has been in place for a long time, constant traction on the object with the first set of forceps may cause one end of the cyst to tent up. Continue dissection through this tent with the scalpel until the object is freed.

Note: Do not blindly grab something in a wound with a hemostat. Blind grasping can cause damage to an important or vital anatomic structure.

8. Yet another alternative, if the object is not visible yet readily palpable, is to perform a punch biopsy (see Chapter 33, Skin Biopsy). When the punch biopsy is performed, a hard "click" may reveal the position of the foreign body. Localization of the foreign body with a punch may prevent the need to make a larger incision. After the biopsy is performed, tease apart the tissue removed to identify the foreign body. If the foreign body cannot be found in the tissue, palpate or probe the wound to make sure the foreign body is not still beneath the biopsy site. If it is beneath the site, the decision can be made as to whether to deepen the site with the punch or to cut down with a no. 11 scalpel. Neither procedure should be per-

formed if the object is located close to an underlying vital structure (nerve, artery, or significant vein). In the same manner, a simple excision of a block of overlying skin can be used to remove a foreign body. Close the resultant wounds with sutures.

9. If the object is not palpable through the skin and able to be located by probing through the entry wound (yet is visible on x-ray films), paper clips or BBs may be used for localization with an x-ray film. Bend the paper clips in various shapes and tape them to the skin with clear plastic tape, or tape the BBs over the skin above and beside the approximate location of the object. With lateral and AP radiographs taken at precisely 90 degrees, the location of the foreign body can be predicted by measuring the distance from the paper clips or BBs on the film. Transfer this measurement to the skin with a marking pen. Next, remove the tape and clips, apply povidone iodine and local anesthetic. An incision can be made in the correct location to the depth measured on the x-ray film in order to remove the object. A punch biopsy may also be used in this manner if the measurements from the x-ray film are very accurate; however, if there is any error in the measurement, an incision may need to be made to expand the search for the object.

Note: It is very important to have true lateral and AP views in order to use x-ray film measurements for incising; otherwise the variances in the angle and x-ray beam to the film lead to the apparent location of the foreign body being significantly different than it actually is. This is especially true for small metal flakes.

10. After removal, irrigate the wound first with remaining anesthetic. Follow this irrigation with sterile saline irrigation pulsated from a syringe. Irrigation is helpful for removing any small fragments or debris that may be remaining. A jetted irrigation can be performed by attaching an 18-gauge needle to the syringe.

11. If a significant incision was made or punch biopsy performed, reapproximate the skin with suture. Cover the wound with a sterile adhesive bandage and give the patient postoperative instructions. See the patient in 2 days to assess for infection and prescribe antibiotics if necessary, and in 7 days (or whatever is appropriate, depending on location) for suture removal.

COMPLICATIONS

- Trauma to local vital structures, such as arteries, nerves, or tendons.
- Infection or bleeding.

- Scarring from the original wound, or the incision and sutures that were necessary to locate the object and close the wound.
- Failure to remove the object, partially or completely. Again, for those objects that must be removed, needle localization under fluoroscopy may remain the final option.

POSTPROCEDURE PATIENT EDUCATION

After removal, a dull ache or stretching sensation is normal for up to a day, especially if sutures were placed. Instruct the patient to watch for signs of infection. Itching is a normal sign of healing. The patient should follow up with the clinician in 2 days and again in the appropriate number of days (7 days in most cases) for suture removal if sutures were placed. A topical antibiotic may be applied, and the dressing should remain over the wound for 48 hours. It should be changed if it gets wet during that time. After the first 48 hours, a dressing should only be applied if the wound continues to drain or if it could get dirty. After the first 48 hours, the wound may be washed with soap and water. Tetanus prophylaxis should be provided if appropriate.

CPT/BILLING CODES

Note: As with all coding, the reimbursement is usually greater if there is a more descriptive code that includes the location (for example, 23330 is approximately twice the RVUs as 10120, whereas 28192 is approximately four times that of 10120.)

10120	Incision and removal of foreign body, subcutaneous tissues; simple
10121	Incision and removal of foreign body, subcutaneous tissues; complicated
20520	Muscle or tendon sheath; simple
20525	Muscle or tendon sheath; complicated
23330	Subcutaneous tissues; shoulder
24200	Subcutaneous tissues; upper arm, elbow
27086	Subcutaneous tissues; pelvis, hip
28190	Subcutaneous tissues; foot
28192	Foot; deep
28193	Foot; complicated

ICD-9-CM DIAGNOSTIC CODES

729.6	Residual foreign body in soft tissue
709.4	Foreign body granuloma of skin or subcutaneous tissue

ADDITIONAL RESOURCES

- See the sample patient education handout titled "Foreign Body Removal from Skin and Soft Tissue" on page 1757 of Appendix G.
- See the sample patient consent form titled "Foreign Body Removal from Skin and Soft Tissue" on page 1758 of Appendix G.

BIBLIOGRAPHY

Buttaravoli P, Stair T: *Minor emergencies*, St Louis, 2000, Mosby.

Friedman EM, Munter DW, Richards JR, Selbst SM: When and how to retrieve foreign bodies, *Pat Care* 15:186, 1997.

Howell JM, Altiere M, Jagoda AS, et al: *Emergency medicine*, Philadelphia, 1998, WB Saunders.

Singer AJ, Burstein JL, Schiavone FM: *Emergency medicine pearls*, Philadelphia, 1996, FA Davis.

CHAPTER 20

Fungal Studies: Collection Procedures and Tests

Dennis E. Babel

DIAGNOSTIC METHODS

The three basic methods used to diagnose fungal infections include direct microscopy (e.g., potassium hydroxide [KOH] method), fungal culture, and biopsy with histopathology.

Direct Microscopy

Early diagnosis of cutaneous mycoses can be made in the physician's office by direct microscopy of infected tissue or lesion exudate. A number of different clearing solutions can be applied to collected material to assist in direct microscopy. These agents help distribute the specimen so the clinician can more readily visualize any fungal structure. They can include solutions such as simple saline, potassium, or sodium hydroxide in various formulations and preparations, and various coloring agents.

Fungal Culture

The ultimate identification of fungal pathogens requires their isolation on fungal culture medium. This may be accomplished within the physician's office using fungal media such as Sabouraud's dextrose agar with cycloheximide (to inhibit fungal contaminants) and with chloramphenicol (to inhibit bacterial contaminants). These are commercially available as Mycosel Agar (BBL Corp.), or Mycobiotic Agar (Difco Corp.). Inoculation of an appropriate patient specimen on this agar should allow only the growth of the true causative fungal organism.

Biopsy and Histopathology

Biopsy specimens obtained from fungal lesions can reveal the in vivo morphology of the infectious agent as well as the host response to this invasive presence. The appropriately stained histopathology section can provide the clinician the proof of the presence of a fungal pathogen, clues to its identity, the extent of infection, and the patient's ability to respond to this invasion. Although this procedure might be considered the "gold standard" for the diagnosis of human mycoses, it is an invasive procedure, is somewhat costly, and is seldom required for the identification of cutaneous mycoses. A 3-mm punch biopsy is generally sufficient. The pathologist must be alerted if a fungal infection in the differential is considered.

EQUIPMENT

This equipment can be used for specimen collection of cutaneous mycoses. It includes materials for doing all of the methods described in the text, although not every item is needed for each collection method.
- Alcohol swabs
- 3 × 3–inch gauze squares
- Scalpel blade (no. 15)
- Toothbrush
- Cotton-tipped applicator
- Disposable biopsy punch (3 mm)
- Glass microscope slide (1 × 3 in)
- Coverglass (22 × 22 mm)
- 20% KOH with dimethyl sulfoxide solution
- Chlorazol Black E solution
- Microscope with 10× and 40× objectives
- Fungal culture media in tubes, vials, or plates

CUTANEOUS SPECIMEN COLLECTION PROCEDURE (FOR KOH PREPS AND FUNGAL CULTURES)

Hair

- Clean the area of alopecia thoroughly with alcohol.
- Collect a specimen with a scalpel, glass slide edge, new toothbrush, 3 × 3 gauze square, or cotton-tipped applicator.

- Appropriate specimen could include black dots (hair stubs) or scalp scale from the area of active infection. (Long hairs and hair clippings are unacceptable, since they are seldom actually infected and are frequently contaminated with bacteria.)

Skin

- For annular or serpiginous lesions of the skin, clean the advancing lesional edge with alcohol and obtain the scaling epithelium (avoid collecting scale from the center or oldest portion of the lesion, since it is unlikely that the fungal pathogen is still present in that "healed" area). Scrape over the area firmly with the side of a scalpel blade to prevent bleeding. Loosened epithelial debris may be scraped directly onto a glass microscope slide for KOH examination and directly onto the fungal media surface for culture.
- For intertriginous mycoses, once again clean and collect material from the dry scaling edge. (Avoid any central, moist, macerated material, since it is usually devoid of any viable fungi and is frequently contaminated with bacteria.)
- For vesicular mycoses of the skin, collect a portion of the vesicle roof by removing with a sterile scissors or scalpel blade. (Vesicle fluid and epithelium from the vesicle base are usually devoid of any fungi.)

Nail

- For distal subungual onychomycosis, trim back the nail to the leading edge of infection (edge closest to the proximal nail fold) and discard. Collect keratinaceous debris from beneath the trimmed nail plate edge.
- For proximal subungual onychomycosis, reverse this process and collect material from the active edge closest to the distal end.
- For white superficial onychomycosis, clean and collect material by simply scraping the surface area of involvement.

Note: Less-than-ideal specimens are nail clippings and whole-removed nail plate, since the true fungal reservoir is actually the nailbed (the exception being nail plate surface material from white superficial onychomycosis).

TECHNIQUE FOR KOH PREPARATION

1. Place appropriate specimen (collected as previously described) on a clean glass microscope slide.
2. Add one drop of 20% KOH with dimethyl sulfoxide solution*

---

*These solutions are commercially available (see the "Suppliers" section).

3. Add one drop of Chlorazol black E solution.*
4. Place a coverglass on top of the slide preparation and press down to eliminated air bubbles.
5. Blot excess solution from the finished slide preparation.
6. Place the preparation on the microscope stage and examine it with the *low* power (10×) objective.
7. To enhance contrast, reduce the microscope illumination by lowering the condenser until epithelial cells are clearly visible.
8. *Screen* the slide preparation under low power (10×) for the presence of fungal structures, such as hyphae or yeast (Fig. 20-1).
9. Examine suspicious structures with the 40× setting (high-dry objective) to confirm the presence of fungi (oil immersion objective is *not* needed).
10. The observation of hyphae or budding yeast and pseudohyphae constitutes a "positive" KOH preparation for fungus.

TECHNIQUE FOR A FUNGAL CULTURE (OFFICE PROCEDURE)

The greatest recovery of mycotic pathogens by fungal culture can be achieved through the inoculation of lesion material directly onto fungal media by the examining physician. (Alternatively, the patient specimen that will be sent to an outside laboratory for inoculation should be packaged carefully and delivered in a timely fashion.)

1. The patient specimen should be gently pressed onto the agar surface. Minimize the "stabbing" and avoid "slashing" of the agar, since these techniques may lead to a premature drying out of the culture system.
2. Fungal cultures from most cutaneous specimens should be incubated at room temperature (22° to 27° C) in a draft-free location and out of direct sunlight.
3. Presumptive pathogen media such as dermatophyte test media, which rely on a color change from orange to red when a fungal pathogen is present, should be observed for the first 10 days. The development of a red agar color after this period should be considered a false-positive result.

TECHNIQUE FOR BIOPSY FOR THE IDENTIFICATION OF CUTANEOUS MYCOSES

Biopsy specimens can be obtained for both the fungal culture as well as the histopathologic confirmation of the organism's presence in vivo.

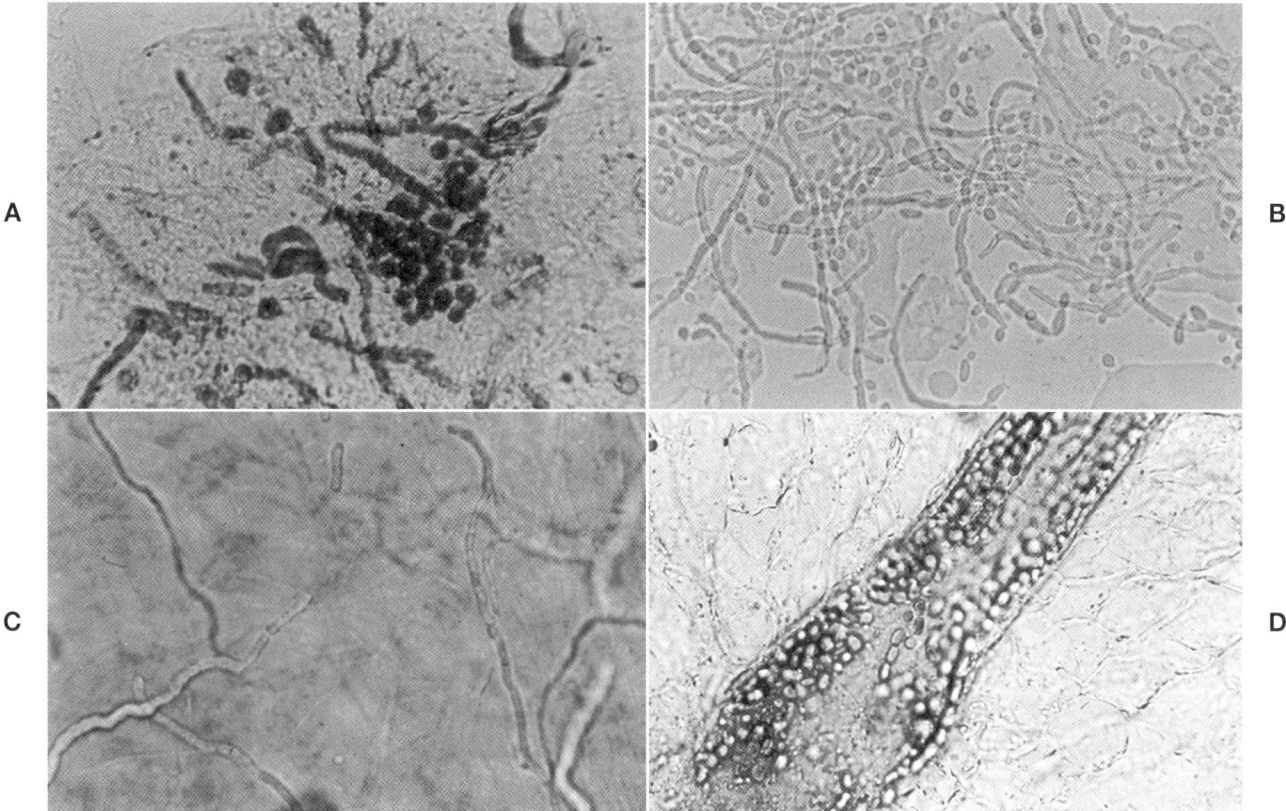

Fig. 20-1
KOH preparations of common cutaneous mycoses. **A,** Pityriasis versicolor: short hyphae and yeast. **B,** Candidiasis: pseudohyphae and budding yeast. **C,** Tinea corporis: branching, septate hyphae. **D,** Tinea capitis: hair with arthroconidia.

1. A 3-mm punch biopsy obtained from the lesional edge is usually sufficient for both purposes. (See Chapter 33, Skin Biopsy.)
2. The biopsy material should be divided longitudinally into two equal parts.
3. One biopsy portion should be placed into *formalin* and sent to the pathology laboratory with a request for "fungal stains."
4. The second biopsy portion should be placed in *sterile saline* and sent to the microbiology laboratory for "fungal culture."

SUPPLIERS

Instrument for Trimming Nail Plate
Henry Schein Co.
135 Duryea Road
Melville, NY 11747
Phone: 1-800-772-4346
Website: www.henryschein.com

KOH Solutions for KOH Micro Preps (20% KOH with Dimethyl Sulfoxide; Chlorazol Black E Fungal Stain)
Delasco
608 13th Avenue
Council Bluffs, IA 51501
Phone: 1-800-831-6273
Website: www.delasco.com

Mycosel Fungal Culture Media (Tight-Seal Petri Dishes)
Physicians Office Lab Supplies (POLS)
1913 East Lincoln Road
Royal Oak, MI 48067
Phone: 1-248-336-8075

REFERENCES

Aly R, Beutner KR, Malbach H, editors: *Cutaneous infection and therapy,* New York, 1997, Marcel Dekker.

Babel DE: Fungi. In Lesher J: *Manual of cutaneous micro-biology for the office laboratory,* Pearl River, NY, 2000, Parthenon Publishing.

Babel DE, Rogers AL: Dermatophytes: their contribution to infectious disease in North America, *Clin Microbiol New* 5:81, 1983.

Babel DE, Rogers AL, Beneke ES: Dermatophytes of the scalp: incidence, immune response, and epidemiology, *Myco-pathologia* 109:69, 1990.

Belsey RE, Skeels MR, Baer DM, Koneman EW: *Basic office microbiology,* Oradell, NJ, 1990, Medical Economics Books.

Daniel CR III, Elewski BE: The diagnosis of nail fungus revisited, *Arch Dermatol* 136:1162, 2000.

Krull EA, Babel DE: Diagnostic procedures of the skin: Part 1, *J Fam Pract* 3(3):309, 1976.

Krull EA, Babel DE: Diagnostic procedures of the skin: Part 2, *J Fam Pract* 3(4):427, 1976.

Sauer GC, Hall JC, editors: *Manual of skin diseases,* ed 7, Philadelphia, 1996, Lippincott-Raven.

Sinski JT: *Dermatophytes in human skin, hair, and nails,* Springfield, Ill, 1974, Charles C Thomas.

CHAPTER 21

Incision and Drainage of an Abscess

Daniel J. Derksen

An abscess is a localized infection characterized by a collection of pus surrounded by inflamed tissue. When a sweat gland or hair follicle infection forms an abscess, it is called a *furuncle,* or *boil.* If multiple follicles are involved with abscesses, it is referred to as a *carbuncle.* *Paronychia* is an abscess that involves the nail. A *felon* is an abscess in the tuft of soft tissue in the distal phalanx of the finger. A *hordeolum* is an abscess on the eyelid margin, whereas a *chalazion* is a chronic abscess of the eyelid itself in the meibomian glands beneath the tarsal plate (see Chapter 55, Chalazion and Hordeolum). *Hidradenitis suppurativa* is a chronic condition in the axilla and groin with recurrent abscess formation. *Pilonidal abscesses* are discussed in Chapter 111, Pilonidal Cyst and Abscess: Current Management; *perianal abscesses* in Chapter 109, Perianal Abscess Incision and Drainage; and *Bartholin's abscesses* in Chapter 132, Bartholin's Cyst/Abscess: Word Catheter Insertion, Marsupialization. For *olecranon* and *prepatellar* bursitis, see Chapter 194, Joint and Soft Tissue Aspiration and Injection.

Most often, *Staphylococcus aureus* is the causative agent in abscesses, but some abscesses are due to *Streptococcus* sp. or a combination of microorganisms, including gram-negative and anaerobic bacteria. Perianal abscesses are usually caused by a mix of aerobic and anaerobic enteric organisms. Abscesses can occur in any location, but they are commonly found on the extremities, buttocks, and breast or in hair follicles.

A small abscess may respond to warm compresses or antibiotics and drain spontaneously. As the abscess enlarges, the inflammation, collection of pus, and walling off of the abscess cavity render such conservative treatments ineffectual. **The treatment of choice for an abscess is incision and drainage (I & D),** and if this treatment is done properly, antibiotics are usually unnecessary. In a nonlactating woman, a *breast abscess* that is not subareolar is rare. If an abscess occurs away from the areola, it should prompt a biopsy in addition to I & D and raise the clinician's suspicion of a malignant tumor.

Patients with diabetes, debilitating disease, or compromised immunity should be observed closely after I &

D of an abscess. Although usually not necessary, consider a culture obtained by aspiration or swab of the abscess cavity, because the abscess may have been caused by unusual organisms in these compromised patients. The infection may also warrant the administration of antibiotics that cover *Staphylococcus* infection.

INDICATIONS

- A localized collection of pus that is tender and not spontaneously resolving. If the lesion is not "pointing" and localized, a trial of antibiotics may be indicated. However, antibiotics are inadequate once a collection of pus is present.

CONTRAINDICATIONS

- Facial furuncles should not be incised or drained if they are located within the triangle formed by the bridge of the nose and the corners of the mouth. These infections should be treated with antibiotics and warm compresses, since the risk of septic phlebitis with intracranial extension can follow I & D of a furuncle in this area.

EQUIPMENT

- Local anesthetic (1% to 2% lidocaine), sodium bicarbonate 7.5%, or diphenhydramine (Benadryl) 50 mg/ml
- Syringe with 25- to 30-gauge needle, usually ½ to 1 inch, since only the skin over the abscess is anesthetized
- Possibly a cryosurgery unit or ethyl chloride for anesthesia (to avoid a needle poke)
- Alcohol or povidone-iodine (Betadine) wipe
- 4 × 4–inch gauze
- No. 11 blade
- Curved hemostats

- Possibly iodoform gauze (¼- to ½-inch width, and up to 24 inches long depending on abscess size)
- Possibly culture materials
- Bandage scissors
- Dressing of choice

TECHNIQUE

Protective eyewear should be worn.

1. Prep the abscess area with povidone-iodine or alcohol.
2. Administer a field block with local anesthetic (see Chapter 8, Peripheral Nerve Blocks and Field Blocks) to allow an adequate incision to be made. Avoid infiltration of the abscess cavity; rather, concentrate on anesthetizing the perimeter of the tissue around the abscess. Local anesthetics usually work poorly in the acidic milieu of an abscess. More anesthetic than usual may be needed to relieve pain. Alternatively, diphenhydramine 10 to 25 mg can be injected into the area for anesthesia. Dilute a 50-mg (1-ml) vial in a syringe with 4 ml of normal saline (Fig. 21-1, *A*). Cryocautery can also be used to freeze the roof of the abscess. This can be performed with a nitrous oxide unit, liquid nitrogen, or ethyl chloride. The incision is then made through the cooled skin, which is now anesthetized.
3. Make a sufficiently wide incision with a pointed no. 11 blade to allow drainage of the abscess cavity and to prevent premature closure of the incision. If a large abscess is present, a 1-cm incision is generally large enough. Make the incision in the skin lines. Recurrence of the abscess is most often due to an inadequate incision and premature closure of the incision (Fig. 21-1, *B*).
4. If a culture is obtained, it should be from the abscess cavity and not from the superficial skin over the abscess. Alternatively, the abscess cavity can be aspirated with a large-bore (18-gauge) needle before the incision is made. The aspirated contents can then be sent for the appropriate cultures in more complicated cases. This is rarely helpful in the routine superficial abscesses.
5. Apply external pressure to express all pus. The abscess cavity should also be thoroughly explored with a sterile cotton-tipped applicator or with hemostats. Attempts should be made to break down any walled-off pockets or possible septa (Fig. 21-1, *C*). If the lesion began as a cyst (e.g., sebaceous cyst), a small derm curette can be used to curette the cavity in hopes of removing all of the sac. A residual sac can lead to a recurrent cyst. The cavity can be packed with a rubber drain or with packing material, preferably iodoform gauze (Fig. 21-1, *D* and *E*). The length and width depends on abscess size. A small "tail" of gauze should be left protruding from the wound for drainage. Apply an ointment over the wound to prevent the gauze from sticking to the overlying dressing and being inadvertently removed when the dressing is changed.
6. Depending on the location and the size of the abscess, the gauze can be advanced slowly over several weeks. The packing material can be changed daily, but it is painful and there is no real advantage to changing it. There may be some advantage to changing it after 5 to 7 days to reduce the purulence and recheck the wound. Leave the "wick" in for 4 weeks so that the abscess scars down from the inside. The patient can advance the drain every few days and cut off 2 inches.
7. A sterile dressing can be applied over the area to collect discharge. This should be changed several times daily. Healing should progress from the inside out; that is, epithelialization of the abscess cavity should occur before healing of the incision site to minimize the chance of recurrence.
8. In patients with hidradenitis, incision and drainage may traumatize the area and cause more long-term abscesses. However, the pain is usually so severe and acute with an abscess that incision and drainage is necessary. Most patients with hidradenitis require long-term antibiotics, similar to those patients with chronic acne. Some patients may require resection of all axillary or groin tissue involved.
9. A felon is an abscess in the distal tuft of the phalanx (Fig. 21-2, *A*). A digital block will best serve to anesthetize the area. Prep with alcohol or povidone-iodine. Incise the abscess in the midline parallel with the digit (Fig. 21-2, *B*). The large bilateral incisions of the past are now generally avoided. A small wick of iodoform gauze can be place in the cavity for 24 hours. Many physicians use antibiotics in patients with felons to cover for *Staphylococcus*.

Usually incision and drainage is sufficient to resolve an abscess. If cellulitis is present or the patient is at high risk for infections, an antibiotic can be used. It should cover *Staphylococcus*.

COMPLICATIONS

If the packing is tight in the abscess cavity, the pain can be sufficient to warrant the use of acetaminophen or nonsteroidal antiinflammatory drugs (NSAIDs). Narcot-

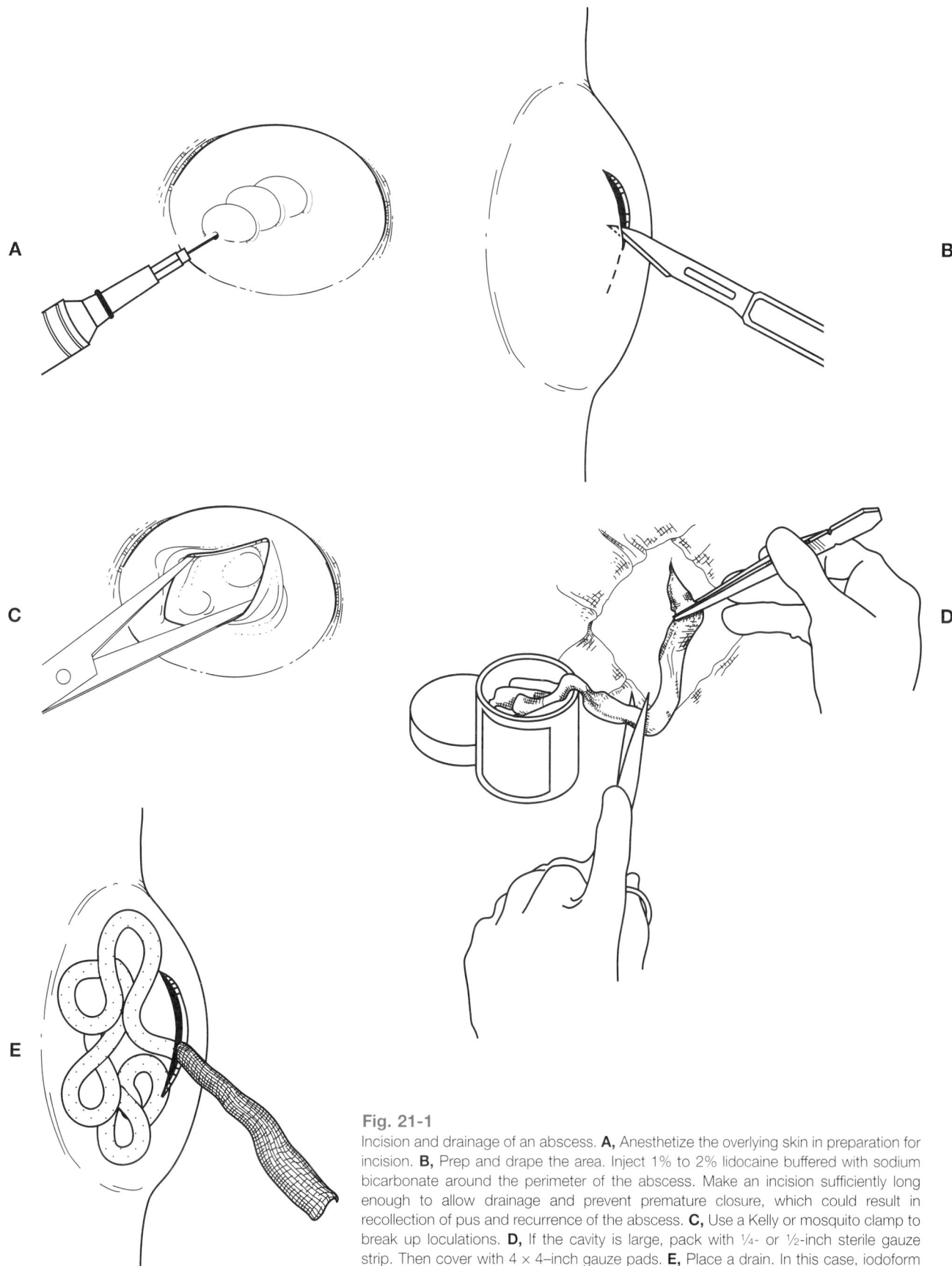

Fig. 21-1

Incision and drainage of an abscess. **A,** Anesthetize the overlying skin in preparation for incision. **B,** Prep and drape the area. Inject 1% to 2% lidocaine buffered with sodium bicarbonate around the perimeter of the abscess. Make an incision sufficiently long enough to allow drainage and prevent premature closure, which could result in recollection of pus and recurrence of the abscess. **C,** Use a Kelly or mosquito clamp to break up loculations. **D,** If the cavity is large, pack with ¼- or ½-inch sterile gauze strip. Then cover with 4 × 4–inch gauze pads. **E,** Place a drain. In this case, iodoform gauze is used.

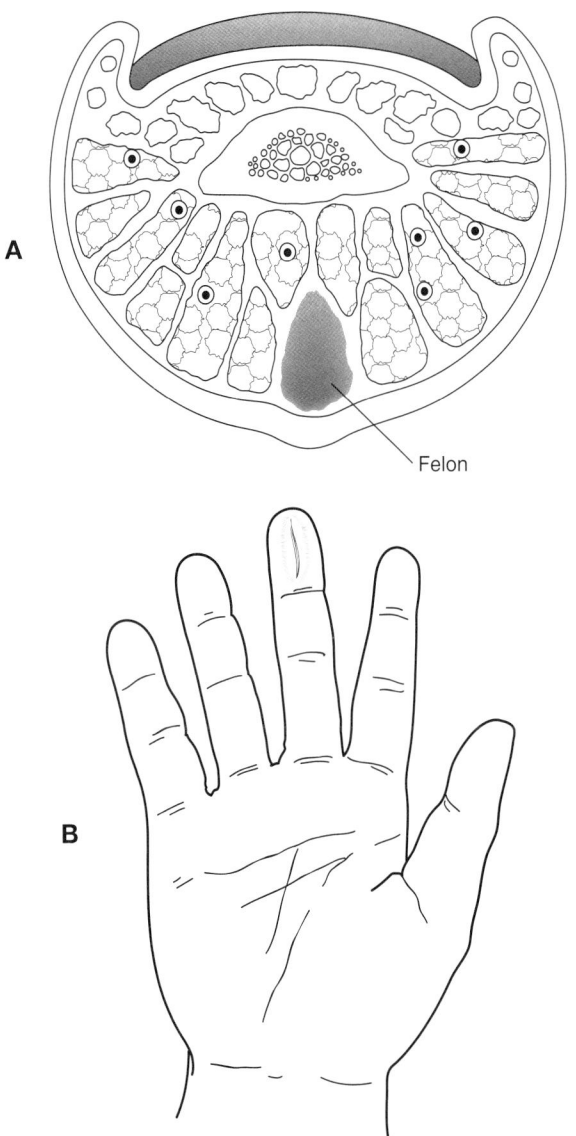

Fig. 21-2
A, Cross section of anatomy of the distal phalanx, showing the numerous fascial septa and a felon. **B,** Incision of a felon. Incision should be in the longitudinal digital midline and should not cross a flexor crease.

ics are rarely needed. The I & D alone may provide sufficient pain relief from a tense abscess such that no pain medication is needed. Complications include the following:

- Recurrence
- Scar or keloid
- Failure to resolve, causing a cellulitis, or progression to septicemia
- Formation of a fistula
- Osteomyelitis

An abscess in the palmar aspect of the hand can extend from superficial to deep tissue through the palmar fascia. Deep infection is suspected when the simple I & D fails to reduce the erythema, pain, pus, or swelling. More extensive surgical debridement, hospitalization, and intravenous antibiotics may be necessary in a patient with a deep palmar abscess, which is a surgical emergency.

A recurrent paronychia may require removal of the nail to resolve the infection (see Chapter 40, Ingrown Toenails). Also, consider treatment for *Candida* infection in such cases.

POSTPROCEDURE PATIENT PREPARATION

Some patients can be taught to change their own packing, replace the dressings, and advance the drain. Other patients may require a family member or home nurse visits or may have to return to the office to have this done. Patients should be instructed to watch for signs of recurrence of the abscess or for evidence of further infection such as cellulitis and to notify the clinician immediately if any of the following occur:

- Recollection of pus in the abscess
- Fever and chills
- Increased pain or redness
- Red streaks near the abscess
- Increased swelling in the area

Generally, bathing and frequent changes of the overlying dressing are encouraged.

CPT/BILLING CODES

Incision and drainage CPT codes vary by complexity and site.

10040	Acne surgery
10060	I & D one abscess
10061	I & D multiple/complex abscess
10080	I & D pilonidal cyst, simple
10081	I & D complicated pilonidal cyst
10140	I & D hematoma
10160	Aspirate abscess/cyst
10180	I & D complex/postoperative infection
19020	I & D deep abscess
21501	I & D deep, neck
23030	I & D deep, shoulder
23930	I & D deep, arm/elbow
23931	I & D infected olecranon bursa
25028	I & D deep, forearm
26010	I & D simple, abscess finger
26011	I & D complex, finger (felon)
26990	I & D deep, hip area
26991	I & D infected bursa, hip area
27301	I & D deep abscess/bursa knee
27603	I & D deep, leg/ankle

28001	I & D bursa, foot
28002	I & D deep, foot
30000	I & D inside
30020	I & D nasal septum (abscess hematoma)
40800	I & D vestibule mouth
40801	I & D complicated, mouth
41000	I & D lingual
41005	I & D sublingual (superficial)
41006	I & D sublingual, deep
41800	I & D gums
45005	I & D submucosal rect abscess
46040	I & D perirectal abscess
46050	I & D superficial perianal abscess
46083	I & D hemorrhoid, external
54015	I & D deep, penis
54700	I & D epididymis
55000	Aspirate hydrocele
55100	I & D scrotal wall abscess
56405	I & D vulva
56420	I & D Bartholin's abscess
67700	I & D eyelid abscess
69000	I & D abscess pinna
69005	I & D abscess, pinna, complicated
69020	I & D ear canal abscess

ICD-9-CM DIAGNOSTIC CODES

For ICD-9-CM diagnostic codes, look under "abscess" for specific site.

BIBLIOGRAPHY

Bobrow BJ, Pollack CV Jr, Gamble S, Seligson RA: Incision and drainage of cutaneous abscesses is not associated with bacteremia in afebrile adults, *Ann Emerg Med* 29(3): 404, 1997.

Brooks I, Frazier EH: The aerobic and anaerobic bacteriology of perirectal abscesses, *J Clin Microbiol* 35(11):2974, 1997.

Nagle D, Rolandelli RH: Primary care office management of perianal and anal disease, *Prim Care* 23(3):609, 1996.

Usatine RP: Incision and drainage. In Usatine RP, May RL, editors: *Skin surgery: a practical guide,* St Louis, 1998, Mosby.

CHAPTER 22

Incisions: Planning the Direction of the Cut

Stephen K. Toadvine*

Although generally considered minor procedures, skin incisions are invasive. They cause permanent change in skin architecture and carry the potential for deleterious patient outcomes in terms of cosmesis and function. No skin incision should be made without careful, thoughtful consideration and advance planning.

Several general issues should be addressed before deciding to perform an incision:

- Overall health status of the patient including assessment of risk for:
  - Significant bleeding (bleeding dyscrasias, medications including herbs)
  - Potential for delayed wound healing (e.g., diabetes, obesity, immunosuppression, steroid use, malnutrition, and peripheral vascular disease)
  - Allergy to any substance being used in conjunction with the procedure, including latex
- Need for antibiotic prophylaxis (dirty wounds, bites, infection, puncture, immunosuppression, diabetes, etc.)
- Ability of the patient or caregivers to properly care for the surgical wound
- Expected benefits versus risks of the procedure
- Physician must obtain an informed consent and assure that the patient knows the basic complications of pain, bleeding, infection, scarring, and distortion of the anatomy.

The physician must always consider the patient as a whole being and not simply focus on "the lesion." Many pitfalls are avoidable if this is kept in mind.

Technical factors to be considered include the following:

- Avoidance of damage to any underlying vital structures
- Proper orientation of incision lines
- Correct design and size of the excision
- Avoidance of significant anatomic distortion

AVOIDING DAMAGE TO UNDERLYING STRUCTURES

Simple full-thickness skin excisions performed with care generally do not pose a threat to underlying structures. The plane of removal should be at the junction of the adipose tissue and the dermis (Fig. 22-1). Nonetheless, familiarity with the anatomy of the proposed surgical site in regard to underlying nerves, vessels, tendons, bursae, and bony structures is essential. Of special concern are two nerves that lie superficially within the subdermal fat layer: the temporal branch of the facial nerve and the spinal accessory nerve (Figs. 22-2 and 22-3). Injury to the temporal branch of the facial nerve may cause inability to wrinkle the forehead and drooping of the eyebrow on the affected side. Damage to the spinal accessory nerve can lead to loss of use of the trapezius muscle. When performing excisions in these regions, physicians should

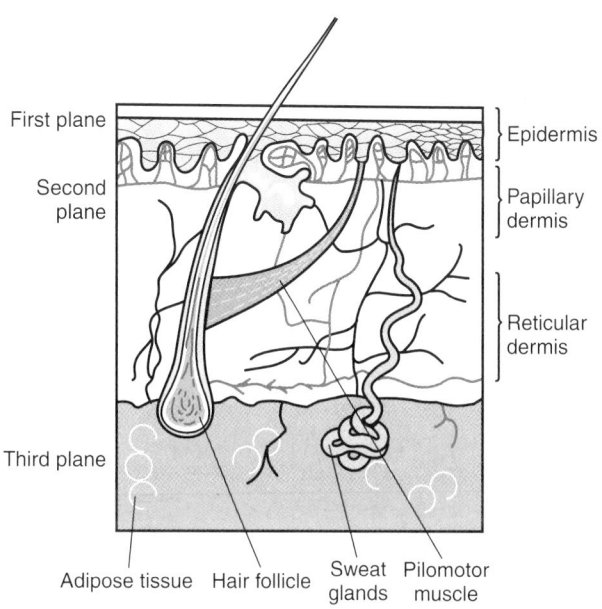

Fig. 22-1
Skin anatomy.

---

*Dr. Toadvine contributes to this edition with the understanding that he objects to the inclusion of Chapter 130 (Abortion) in this edition.

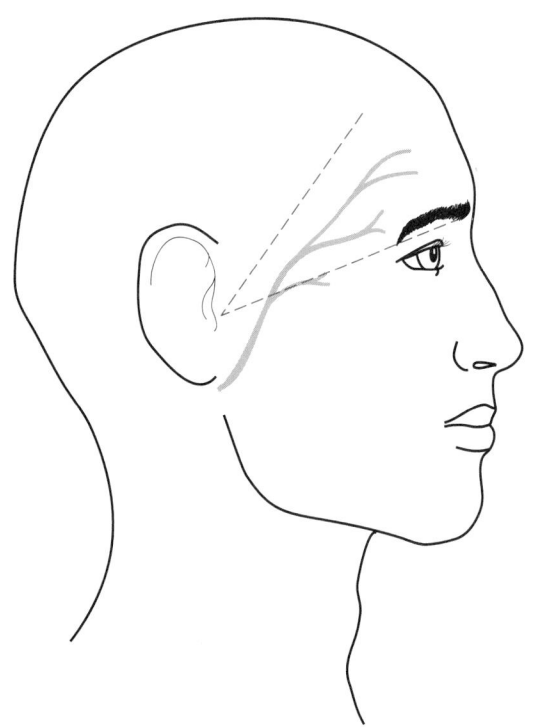

Fig. 22-2
Temporal branch of facial nerve. The nerve lies superficial within a triangle, created by a line extending from the tragus to the upper forehead wrinkle area and a line extending from the tragus to the lateral aspect of the eyebrow.

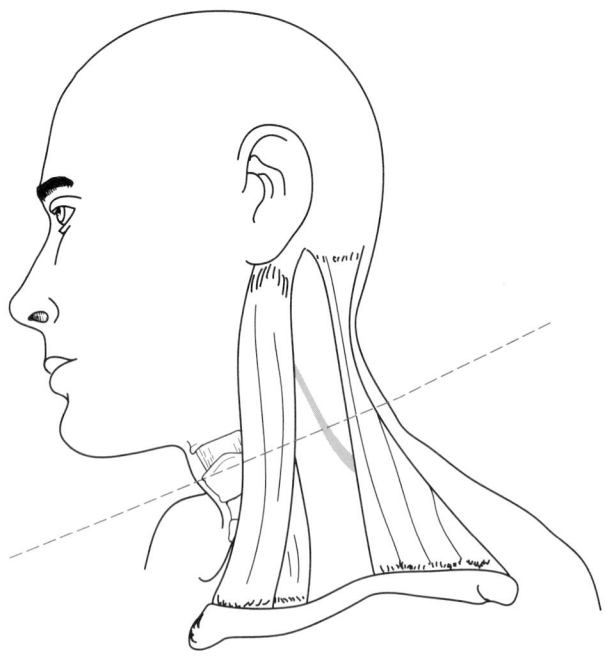

Fig. 22-3
Spinal accessory nerve. The nerve lies superficially within the posterior triangle of the neck at the level of the notch in the superior thyroid cartilage.

consider less invasive alternative methods for treating the particular lesion. If an incisional approach must be used, the patient should be advised of the potential complications. If the practitioner is not sufficiently experienced in dermatologic surgery, referral should be considered.

ORIENTATION OF THE INCISION

Skin incisions and excisions should be oriented in such a way as to minimize scarring and maximize function. Langer, in the nineteenth century, described lines of minimal skin tension. These lines, in general, lie perpendicular to the long axis of underlying musculature and can usually be demonstrated by pinching together a local area of skin. On the face, wrinkles form along these lines as a result of repeated contraction of the facial musculature. Linear incisions (e.g., for removal of underlying lesions such as lipomas or for incision and drainage) should be oriented along or parallel to wrinkle lines when possible (parallel to the lines of minimal skin tension). With an elliptical excision, in which a section of overlying skin is removed, the long axis of the ellipse should lie parallel to the lines of minimal skin tension. Standard depictions of Langer's lines (Fig. 22-4) assist in planning incisions, but lines of minimal tension should be evaluated on each patient individually before a procedure. For the face, the patient's simulating various facial expressions will aid in demonstrating natural wrinkle lines. It should also be noted that for certain elliptical excisions (especially on the face), the long axis of the excision may need to curve or angle instead of lying entirely in a straight line (Fig. 22-5). Cutting incisions along lines of minimal tension decreases transverse traction on the wound, thereby reducing scar potential. Certain areas, especially deltoid and sternum, are invariably prone to experiencing transverse traction, with a subsequent wider scar, and a higher propensity for keloid formation. Children also have an increased tendency to develop hypertrophic or keloid scars.

When lines of minimal tension are not apparent, even after the patient performs maneuvers to accentuate them, it may be helpful to first perform a circular excision, undermine the wound circumferentially, and then allow natural skin tension to orient the wound, usually into a more oval shape. At that point the resulting oval can be converted to an ellipse and the wound closed (Fig. 22-6).

Incisions across joint surfaces should be made transversely (or obliquely if necessary). Perpendicular lacerations or incisions across joint space lines have a tendency to contract, thus limiting range of motion. Chapter 18, Flaps and Plasties, includes a review of Z-plasty, an example of a situation in which a laceration extending across a joint is converted to a transverse wound to maximize joint function and minimize contracture.

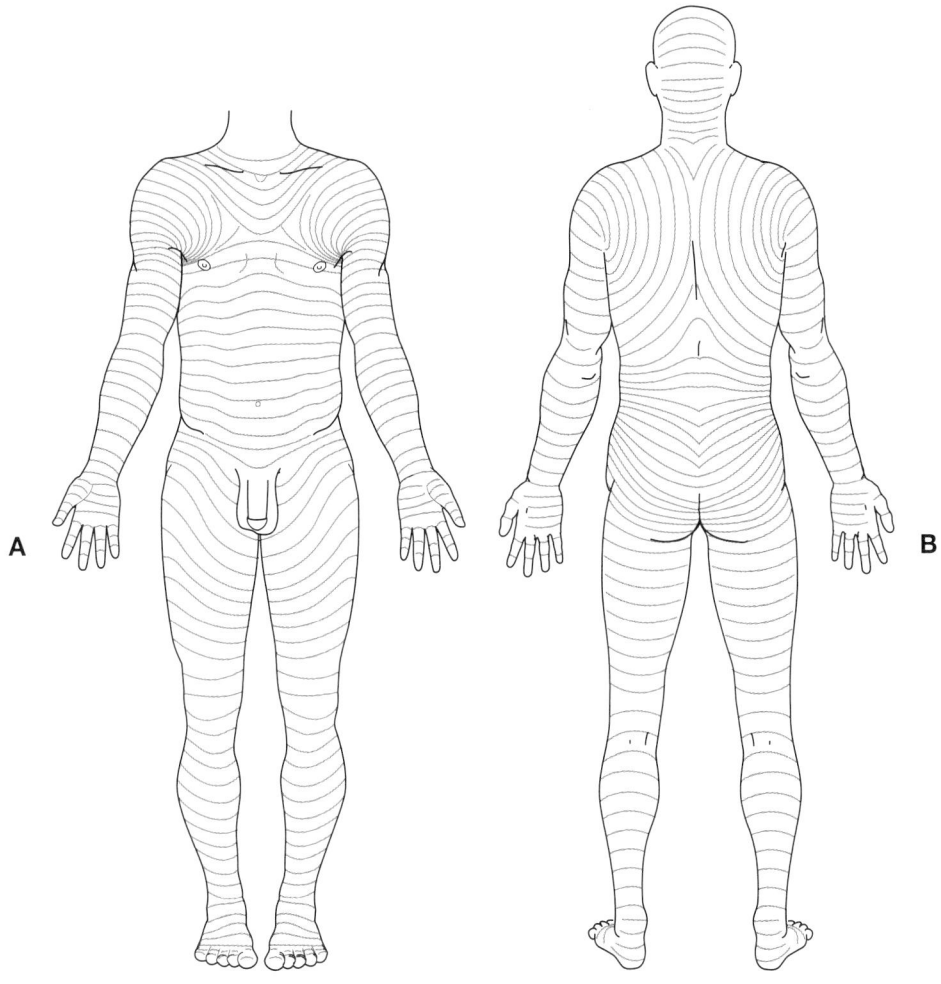

Fig. 22-4
Lines of minimal skin tension. **A,** Anterior body. **B,** Posterior view.

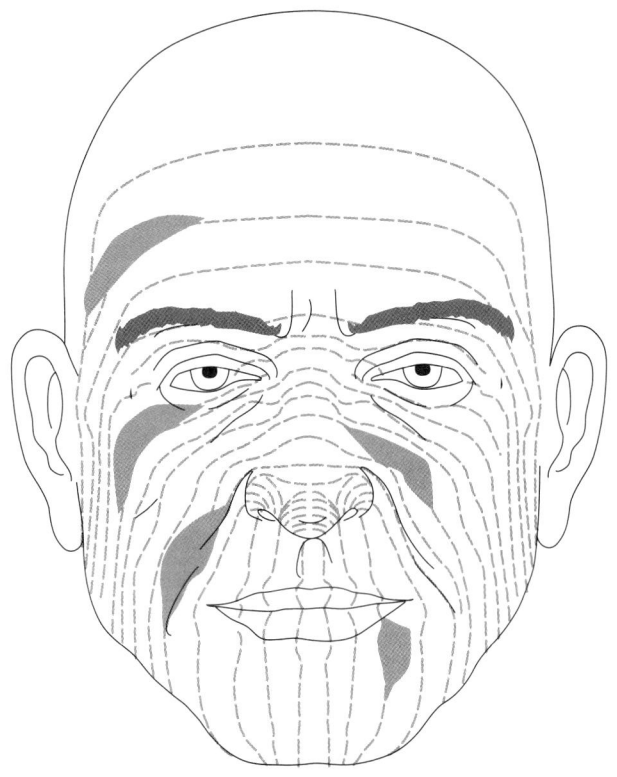

Fig. 22-5
Skin tension lines on the face and proper excision shapes.

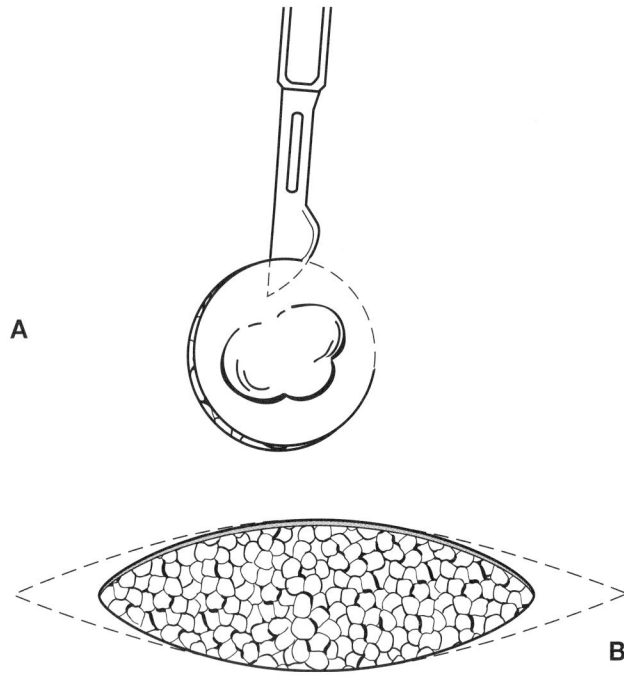

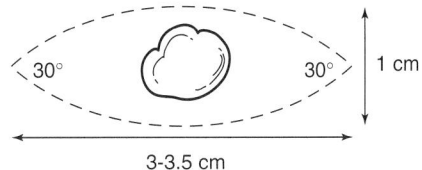

Fig. 22-6
A, Creating a circular wound, with conversion to an ellipse. **B,** Creating an ellipse.

Fig. 22-7
Creating an ellipse (proper dimensions).

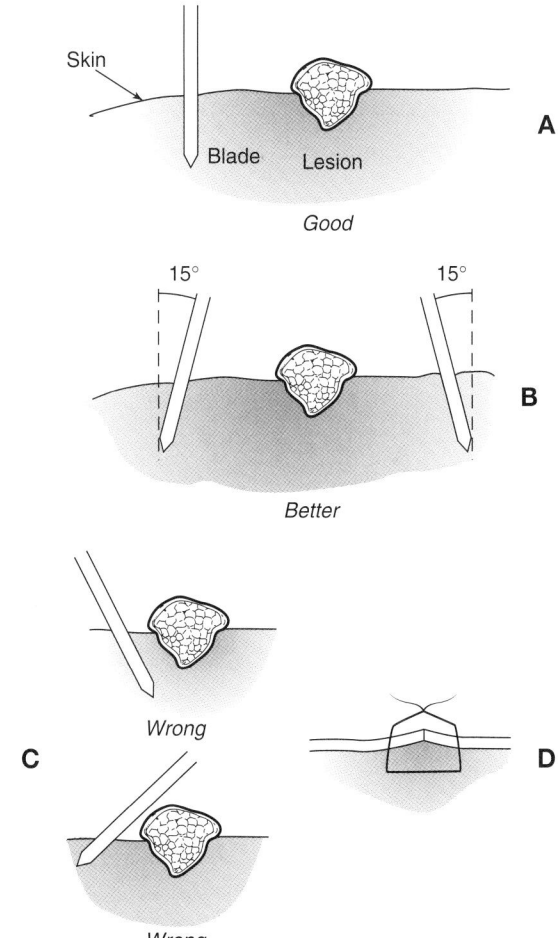

Fig. 22-8
Angles of scalpel blade when creating an ellipse. **A,** Good angle. **B,** Better angle. **C,** Wrong angles. **D,** Proper shapes of suture and skin margins on completion of closure.

DESIGN AND SIZE OF THE EXCISION

Surgical marking pens should be used freely in designing incisions. Planning, measuring, and marking are essential steps toward an optimal result. The majority of skin excisions are elliptical in shape. The wound should be three times as long as it is wide (Fig. 22-7). A wound that is not long enough will create dog ears when repaired. Because alcohol will remove most marking-pen inks, first use an alcohol wipe and anesthetize the wound, then mark and the measure the planned excision. Now prep the site with Betadine, which will not remove the ink, and then drape the patient.

When incising with the scalpel, a no. 15 blade is used and should be held perpendicular to the skin or angled up to 15% with the cutting edge angled away from the

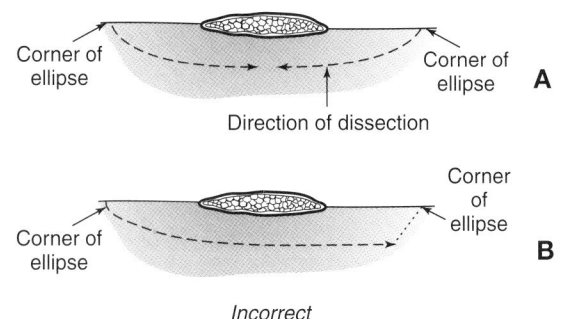

Fig. 22-9
Method of dissecting tissue free after the ellipse is incised. **A,** Going from each end to center. **B,** Going from one end to the opposite end (incorrect) leads to too deep of a dissection at the terminal end.

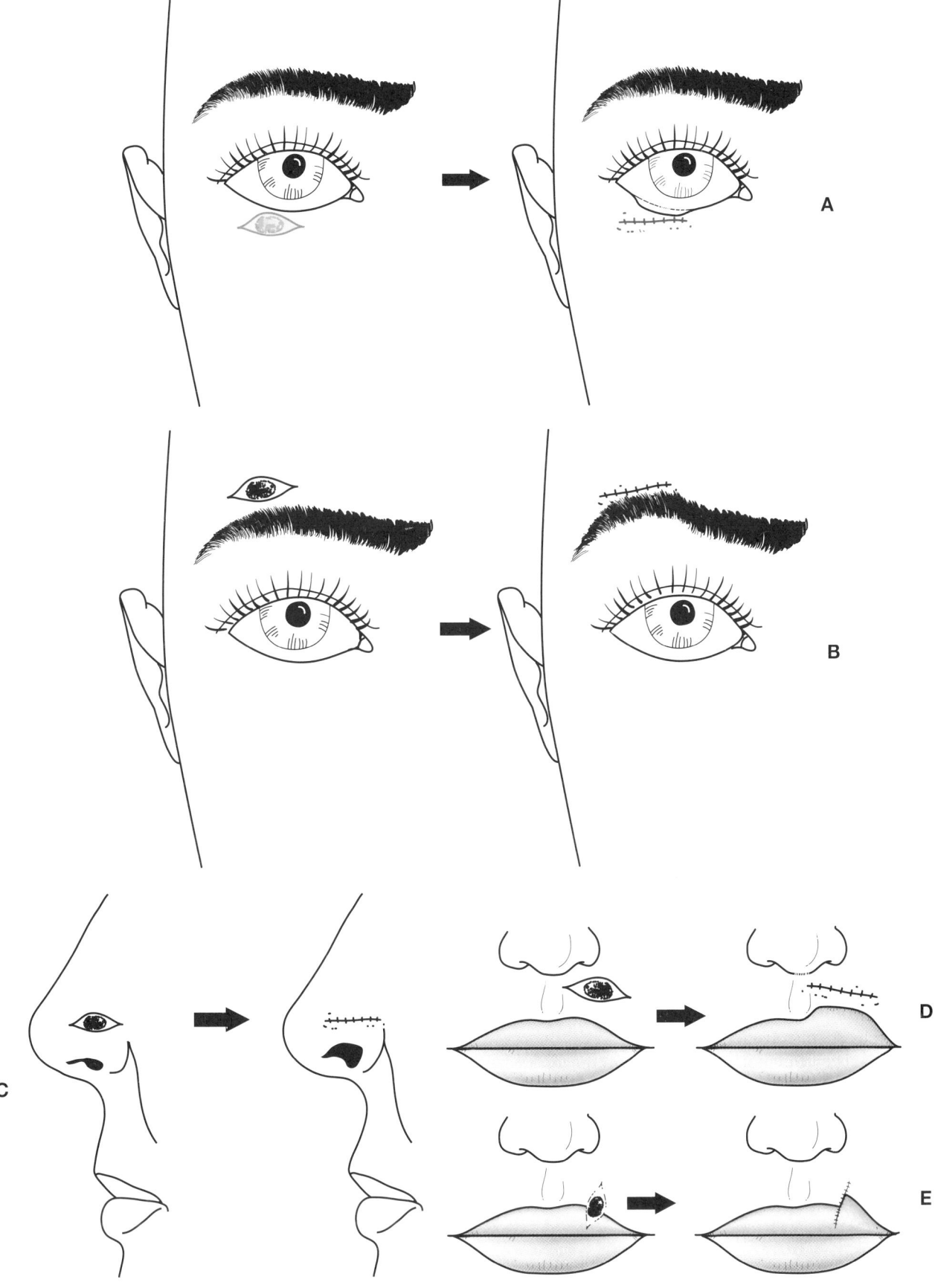

Fig. 22-10
Possible pitfalls in closing facial incisions/lacerations. **A,** Closing the defect on the lower lid causes an unsightly eversion of the lid. **B,** The lateral eyebrow is pulled upward. **C,** Nasal ala is flared resulting from too much tension on the wound. **D,** The upper lip is distorted and raised up laterally after closure of the excision site. **E,** The vermilion borders do not match.

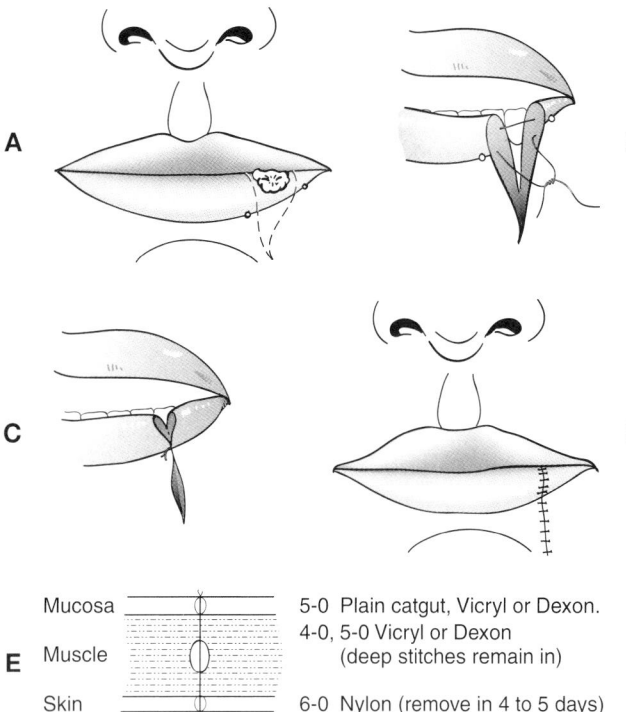

Mucosa — 5-0 Plain catgut, Vicryl or Dexon.
4-0, 5-0 Vicryl or Dexon
E Muscle — (deep stitches remain in)
Skin — 6-0 Nylon (remove in 4 to 5 days)

Fig. 22-11
Proper excision and repair of a lip lesion. **A,** Dashed lines show planned excision. Mark vermilion border. **B,** Muscle approximation with deep stitch. **C,** Vermilion alignment. **D,** Final results. **E,** Suture material. Vicryl or Dexon inside the mouth will need to be removed. Catgut will absorb in 3 to 4 days.

lesion (Fig. 22-8). Remember that slight eversion during the repair is desirable (Fig. 22-8, *D*). Slanting the blade in the opposite direction makes this difficult to accomplish. Remember to "build pyramids, not dig ditches" when incising. Angling the blade more than 15 degrees creates a very thin "slice" of tissue on the remaining skin, which may necrose and lead to more scar formation.

Margins of normal tissue that should be removed vary for *melanomas* (see Chapter 13, Approach to Various Skin Lesions). Generally a 5-mm margin is needed for superficial or in situ melanomas. A 1-cm margin is needed for any invasive lesions less than 1 mm. If greater than 1 mm deep, consider referral.

For basal cell carcinomas, a 3- to 5-mm rim of normal tissue, and for squamous cell carcinomas, at least a 5-mm band of normal tissue around the lesion should be removed.

After the ellipse is made, the tissue specimen is freed by cutting with the scalpel in the plane between dermis and adipose tissue. Using Adson pickups with teeth, grasp the end of the ellipse and dissect from end to center. Then grasp the other end and do the same. This technique avoids the tendency to travel too deep with the excision (Fig. 22-9).

AVOIDING DISTORTION OF SURFACE ANATOMY

The physician should always attempt to estimate the change in surface anatomy that results from an excision. Pinching together the two sides of a planned ellipse assists in demonstrating whether a defect can be closed in a direct side-to-side fashion and whether significant distortion will occur. The presternal and pretibial regions can be potentially quite difficult to close after a skin excision, as can wider excisions in any location. Excisions necessitating removal of a significant amount of tissue on the forehead, upper lip, and around the eyes often cause distortion of facial appearance (Fig. 22-10). Proper planning creates excellent cosmetic results (Fig. 22-11). Situations involving potentially significant cosmetic distortion or need for skin flaps or grafts should be managed by practitioners with appropriate expertise.

BIBLIOGRAPHY

Mackay GJ et al, Plastic and maxillofacial surgery. In Sabiston DC, editor: *Textbook of surgery,* Philadelphia, 1997, WB Saunders.

Moy RL, Usatine RP: Elliptical excision. In Usatine RP, Moy RL, Tobinick EL, Siegel DM, editors: *Skin surgery: a practical guide,* St Louis, 1998, Mosby.

Woods LK, Dellinger P: Current guidelines for antibiotic wound prophylaxis of surgery wounds. *Am Fam Physician* 57: 2731, 1998.

CHAPTER 23

Laceration and Incision Repair

Richard Usatine
Wendy C. Coates

LACERATION REPAIR

Lacerations are a commonly seen problem in physicians' offices, urgent-care centers, and hospital emergency departments. Lacerations can be repaired with sutures, wound-closure tapes, staples (see Chapter 35, Skin Stapling), or tissue adhesive (see Chapter 38, Tissue Adhesives).

The goals of laceration and incision repair are as follows:

1. Achieve hemostasis
2. Prevent infection
3. Preserve function
4. Restore appearance
5. Minimize patient discomfort

In repairing skin, it is helpful to understand the three phases of wound healing. These phases are listed in Box 23-1. Nonabsorbable skin sutures or staples are used to give the wound strength during the first two phases. After the nonabsorbable skin sutures are removed, wound-closure tapes or previously placed deep absorbable sutures may play an important role in the final phases of wound healing.

BOX 23-1

Three Phases of Wound Healing

Phase 1 (Initial Lag Phase, Days 0 to 5)
No gain in wound strength

Phase 2 (Fibroplasia Phase, Days 5 to 14)
Rapid increase in wound strength occurs
At 2 weeks, the wound has achieved only 7% of its final strength

Phase 3 (Final Maturation Phase, Day 14 Until Healing Is Complete)
Further connective tissue remodeling
Up to 80% of normal skin strength

INDICATIONS

- Lacerations that are open and less than 12 hours old (less than 24 hours old on the face)
- Some bite wounds in cosmetically important areas (close follow-up recommended)
- Repair of sites where a lesion has been surgically removed

CONTRAINDICATIONS

- Wounds more than 12 hours old (more than 24 hours old on the face)
- Animal and human bite wounds (exceptions: facial wounds, large dog bite wounds)
- Puncture wounds

EQUIPMENT

- Surgical prep (Betadine, Hibiclens); alcohol swabs (not to be used inside the wound)
- Ruler in centimeters
- Irrigation device for contaminated wounds: 30-ml syringe with 18-gauge angiocatheter or commercially manufactured splash shield device (Fig. 23-1) and sterile saline
- Appropriate anesthetic (see Chapter 4, Local Anesthesia)
- 1- to 10-ml syringe
- 27-gauge, 1¼-inch needle (small gauge needles are preferred to administer anesthesia)
- Sterile drapes; fenestrated drape (applied over the lesion)
- 4 × 4–inch gauze sponges; sterile cotton applicators are useful for hemostasis
- Sterile pack containing: 4½-inch needle holder; curved

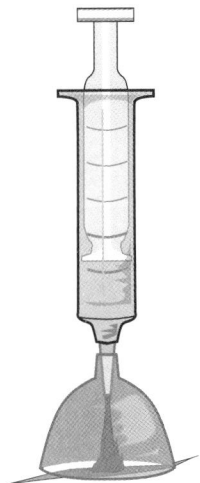

Fig. 23-1
Irrigation of a dirty wound using a syringe and plastic shield (Klenzalac).

dissecting scissors; one mosquito hemostat; suture scissors; Adson forceps with teeth; skin hook *(optional)*
- No. 15 blade for excisions with blade handle (single disposable unit also available)
- Appropriate suture (see Chapter 25, Laceration and Incision Repair: Suture Selection)
- Allis forceps for removal of deeper masses *(optional)*
- Skin-marking pen (for excision, if wound revision is needed)
- Electrosurgical unit should be available for cautery
- Specimen jar (when lesions are being excised)
- Sterile gloves
- Mask
- Protective glasses with shields

PREPROCEDURE PATIENT PREPARATION

The patient should be informed of the nature of his or her lacerations. If the laceration is in a cosmetically important area, consider offering the option of a plastic surgeon for the repair. Advise the patient about the risks of pain, bleeding, dehiscence, infection, and scarring. In the cases of lesion removals, warn that it is not always possible to be sure that the entire lesion is removed so it could recur. Inform the patient that most repairs cause some permanent scarring, although attempts will be made to optimize the appearance. Hyperpigmentation or hypopigmentation, hypertrophic scars, keloids, nerve damage, alopecia, and distortion of the original anatomy are all possible outcomes. It is advisable to have the patient sign a consent form (see the sample patient

TABLE 23-1
Essentials of Wound Assessment

Parameters	Factors to Consider
Mechanism of injury	Sharp vs. blunt trauma, bite
Dirty vs. clean	Outdoors vs. kitchen sink
Time since injury	Suture up to 12 hr; 24 hr on face
Foreign body	Explore and obtain radiograph for metal or glass
Functional examination	Neurovascular, muscular, tendons
Need for prophylactic antibiotics	If needed, give ASAP and cover *Staphylococcus aureus*; irrigate well

consent form titled "Skin Lesion Excision (Elective)" on page 1760 of Appendix G.

Initial Assessment

The initial evaluation before anesthesia should include an assessment of peripheral neurovascular status.

In elective excisions, see Chapter 22 to plan the direction of the incision. If a traumatic laceration is to be repaired, see Table 23-1 for essentials of wound assessment.

In general, antibiotics are not needed for either wound or subacute bacterial endocarditis (SBE) prophylaxis for cutaneous procedures. For SBE prophylaxis guidelines, see Chapter 204, Antibiotic Prophylaxis. Consideration should be given to coverage for *Staphylococcus aureus* infection in several situations (Box 23-2).

The following are major goals for prescribing antibiotics before or after skin surgery:
1. Prevention of bacterial endocarditis
2. Prevention of a new wound infection
3. Prevention of the spread of an existing local infection
4. Treatment of an existing infection

The clinical decision-making process of whether or not to use antibiotics before or after skin surgery is complex. The physician must consider host factors, the anatomic location of the surgery, the sources that might contaminate the wound, and method of wound injury. Because this topic concerns wound repair after multiple types of trauma and elective procedures, the full complexity of the decision-making process is beyond the scope of this chapter. Box 23-1 lists the multiple factors to be considered when making a decision about antibiotic prophylaxis for skin procedures.

The recommendations of the American Heart Association (AHA) for the prevention of bacterial endocarditis were last published in 1997. These guidelines state that endocarditis prophylaxis is not recommended for incision or biopsy of surgically scrubbed skin. However, they also acknowledge that "incision and drainage or other procedures involving infected tissues may result in bacteremia with the same organism causing the infection."

BOX 23-2

Possible Antibiotic Prophylaxis Situations or When to Consider Antibiotic Prophylaxis

Coexisting Conditions
Diabetes mellitus
Peripheral vascular disease
Elderly
Immunocompromised
Previous radiation to the site
Malnutrition (e.g., alcoholism, chemotherapy)
History of previous infection or slow healing
Chronic steroid use
Obesity

Locations
Increased bacteria
   Axilla, mouth, anogenital areas
End arterial locations (fingers, toes) with diseases of vascular
   compromise
Over joint spaces where there is a possibility of entering joint (e.g.,
   metacarpal-phalangeal joints)

Contamination
Dirty wounds, especially barnyards, meatpacking plants, etc.
Less than optimal sterile technique (should be rare)
Deep puncture wounds
Bites (especially human and cat bites)
Presence of a foreign body

Method of Wound Injury
Crush injury (tenfold increase in infection) with devitalized skin
Penetrating injury

For individuals at high or moderate risk for endocarditis (see Chapter 204, Antibiotic Prophylaxis), it is advisable to administer antimicrobial prophylaxis before the procedure. Specifically, for incision and drainage of an abscess, the guidelines recommend giving an antistaphylococcal penicillin or first-generation cephalosporin 1 hour before the procedure. Clindamycin is an acceptable alternative for those patients allergic to penicillin. In the current guidelines, the AHA no longer recommends antibiotics after the procedure.

Cummings and associates performed a metaanalysis of randomized studies on the use of antibiotics to prevent infection of simple wounds. They concluded that there is no evidence in published trials that prophylactic antibiotics offer protection against infection of nonbite wounds in patients treated in emergency departments. Cummings also performed a metaanalysis of randomized trials for antibiotics to prevent infection in patients with dog-bite wounds. He found that prophylactic antibiotics reduce the incidence of infection in patients with dog-bite wounds.

Antibiotics have a role in the treatment of many established skin infections. However, most skin abscesses are better treated with incision and drainage rather than with antibiotics. For skin procedures, there is not a consensus on when to give an antibiotic and the

appropriate timing for the administration. Recommendations for timing before the procedure vary from 1 hour (which is typical timing for bacterial endocarditis prophylaxis) to within 30 minutes of the procedure. While a single second dose 6 hours later was the standard in the past, it is no longer currently recommended for bacterial endocarditis prophylaxis but may be advocated for other reasons.

Controversy exists over which bite injuries should be treated with prophylactic antibiotics. Cat- and dog-bite injuries carry the risk of infection with *Pasteurella multocida,* and human-bite injuries carry the risk of infection with *Eikenella corrodens* and *S. aureus.* Based on the microbiology of these wounds, Augmentin often provides adequate prophylactic coverage for the bacteria affecting most bite injuries.

The best method for prevention of wound infections is to clean and irrigate traumatic wounds well, rather than using prophylactic antibiotics. The physician needs to weigh the benefits and the risks of antibiotic use based on the individual patient and the circumstances of the wound repair or skin surgery. The factors in Box 23-1 and the references at the end of this chapter should provide guidance for the physician making decisions about antibiotic prophylaxis for skin surgery.

Local Anesthesia

In traumatic wounds, after neurological function is assessed, the wound should be fully anesthetized to allow for painless examination of the tissue damage, thorough irrigation, and adequate closure. (See Chapter 4, Local Anesthesia, and Chapter 8, Peripheral Nerve Blocks and Field Blocks.)

Perform the following to minimize the pain of injecting local anesthetic:
* Use a small gauge needle (27 gauge or smaller)
* Inject slowly
* Inject directly into the dermis through the open wound (not through intact skin)
* Warm anesthetic to body temperature
* Buffer the anesthetic with sodium bicarbonate (10 ml to 1 ml) *(optional)*

Wound Preparation

After the initial assessment and administration of local or regional anesthetic, and antibiotics if indicated, wounds should be inspected thoroughly for foreign bodies, deep tissue layer damage, and injury to nerve, vessel, or tendon. A radiograph should be obtained to look for remaining glass or metal in wounds sustained with broken glass or metal. Complex wounds or those in cosmetically important areas should be closed by a practitioner with the appropriate expertise.

Cleansing

After the wound is anesthetized, cleansing of the wound should be performed by irrigation with normal saline at approximately 15 psi of pressure. This can be accomplished by attaching an 18-gauge angiocatheter or a commercially available splash shield to a 30-ml syringe (Fig. 23-1). At least 200 ml of irrigation is recommended. Chemical compounds such as hexachlorophene (pHiso-Hex), chlorhexidine gluconate (Hibiclens), or povidone-iodine (Betadine) should not be used inside wounds but may be applied to external, intact skin if desired. Greasy contaminants can be removed with any petroleum-based product, such as bacitracin ointment. To prevent a road rash tattoo, wrap Vaseline gauze around the fingers and wipe off the asphalt and other foreign material embedded in the skin.

Debridement

After the cleansing process, wounds should be examined for devitalized tissue that needs removal or debridement. This debridement may convert a jagged, contaminated wound into a clean surgical one and can be accomplished with a scalpel or sharp tissue scissors (Fig. 23-2). As much tissue as possible should be preserved in case future scar revision is necessary. After debridement, wound edges should be held together to see if they are under any tension. Wounds under significant tension are best repaired by a two-layer closure. In dirty wounds, however, this may increase the incidence of infection.

Undermining

Undermining can significantly reduce skin tension when there is a gap to be closed (Fig. 23-3). Undermining may increase the risk of infection and thus should be avoided in dirty wounds. Extreme care is also needed when undermining around vital structures. Approximately one third to half of the undermined tissue is freed up to be brought into the defect. Undermine bilaterally as far back as the wound is wide.

TECHNIQUE

Ideally, four principles should be incorporated in the process of closing any wound:
1. *Control all bleeding before closure.* This can be accomplished with electrocoagulation or by tying off bleeders with absorbable sutures.
2. *Eliminate "dead space"* where tissue fluid and blood can accumulate (Fig. 23-4).
3. *Accurately approximate tissue layers* to each other. Scars are most visible when shadows are created by depressed or elevated tissue. Also be sure that anatomic areas match on each side in critical areas such as the vermilion border of the lip.
4. *Approximate the wound with minimal skin tension.* If there will be significant tension, undermining and deep, inverted, buried sutures are used to decrease the tension on the skin margin. Ideally when the repair is completed the wound will be tented up slightly.

Lacerations and incisions are approximated using a variety of techniques:
1. *Simple interrupted suture* (Fig. 23-5). On completion, the skin margins should be slightly everted (Fig. 23-6). The needle should enter the skin

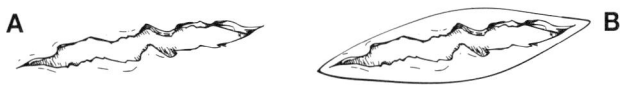

Fig. 23-2
Debridement. **A,** Irregular jagged wound. **B,** Excise a jagged wound or crush injury to create a more readily reparable wound.

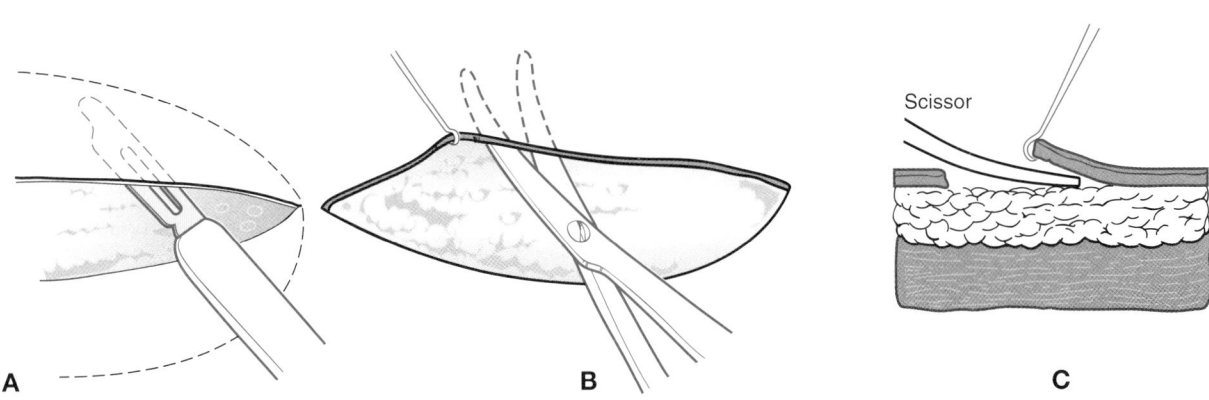

Fig. 23-3
When skin margins approximate with tension, this can be relieved by undermining the margins through the use of a blade **(A)** or scissors **(B** and **C)**. The usual plane is at the dermal-adipose junction. Undermine twice as far back as the wound is wide, if possible.

surface at a 90-degree angle (Fig. 23-7). The stitch should be as wide as it is deep. The suture on both sides of the wound should be equal distance from the wound margin and of equal depth. The final shape should appear like an Erlenmeyer flask (Fig. 23-8). As a general rule, these sutures need to be no closer than 2 mm in a fine plastic closure and can be substantially farther apart in other types of closures. The distance between sutures should equal half the total distance of the sutures across

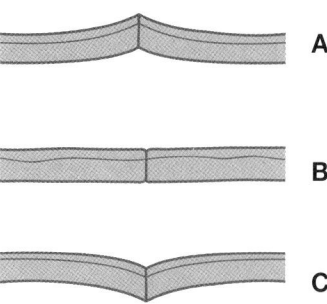

Fig. 23-6
Wound margin appearance after closure. **A,** Proper eversion of the skin edges on closure ("Build pyramids, not ditches"). **B,** Acceptable, but not optimal, closure. **C,** Improper closure, since healing will lead to further contraction and scar depression.

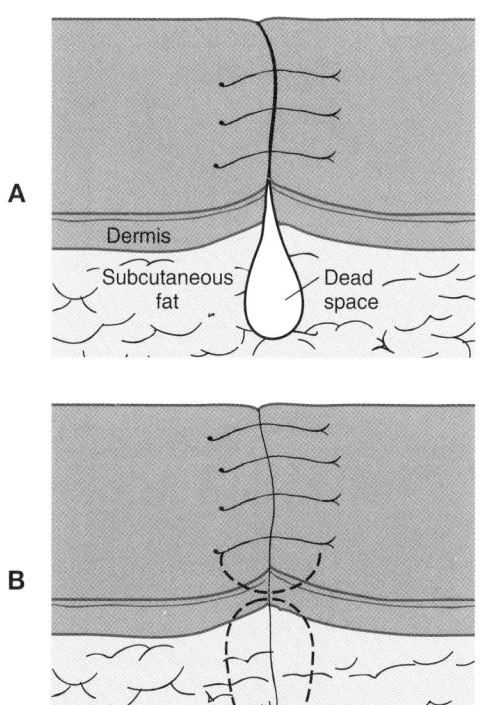

Fig. 23-4
Closing the dead space. **A,** Improper closure with dead space not closed. **B,** Proper closure with dead space closed by deep sutures.

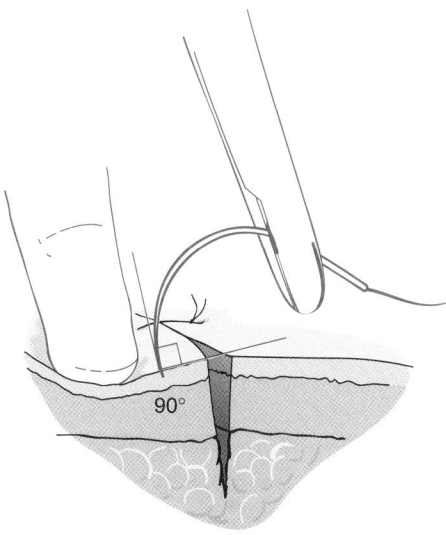

Fig. 23-7
Needle should enter the skin surface at a 90-degree angle. (Revised from Usatine RP, Moy RL, Tobinick EL, and Siegel DM: *Skin surgery: a practical guide,* St Louis, 1998, Mosby.)

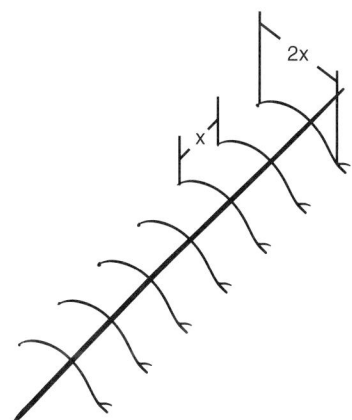

Fig. 23-5
Simple interrupted suture.

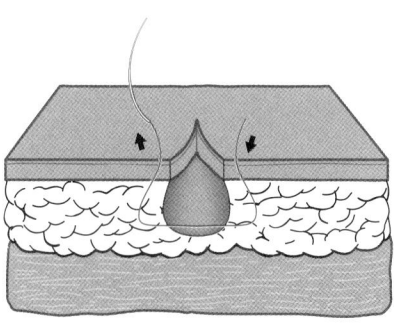

Fig. 23-8
Use the Erlenmeyer flask–shaped pathway to promote eversion of skin edges. (Revised from Usatine RP, Moy RL, Tobinick EL, and Siegel DM: *Skin surgery: a practical guide,* St Louis, 1998, Mosby.)

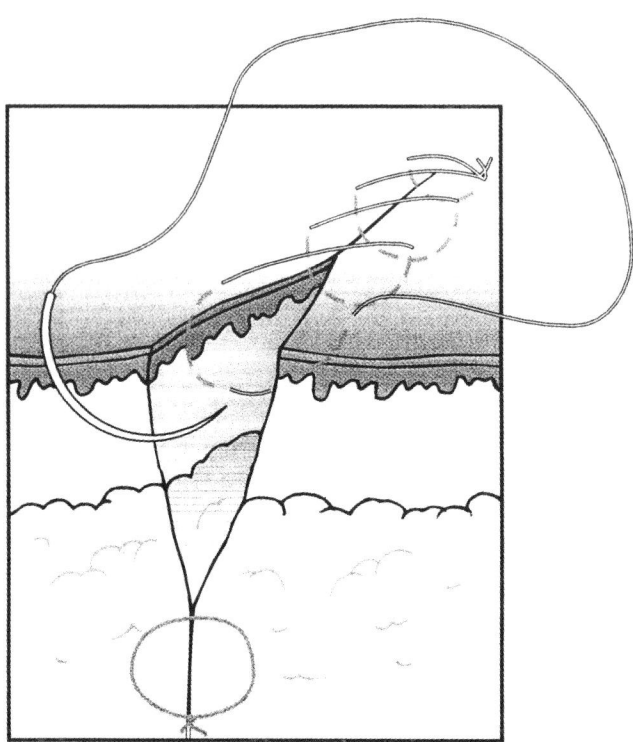

Fig. 23-9
Running stitch. Always keep the depth of the suture placement the same on each side. (From Usatine RP, Moy RL, Tobinick EL, and Siegel DM: *Skin surgery: a practical guide,* St Louis, 1998, Mosby.)

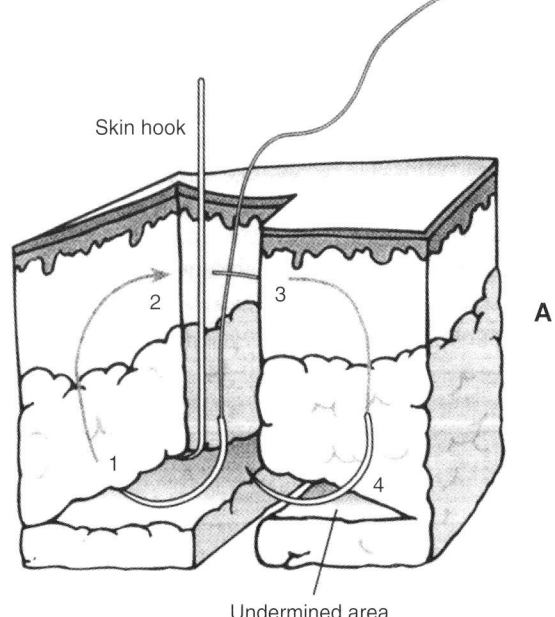

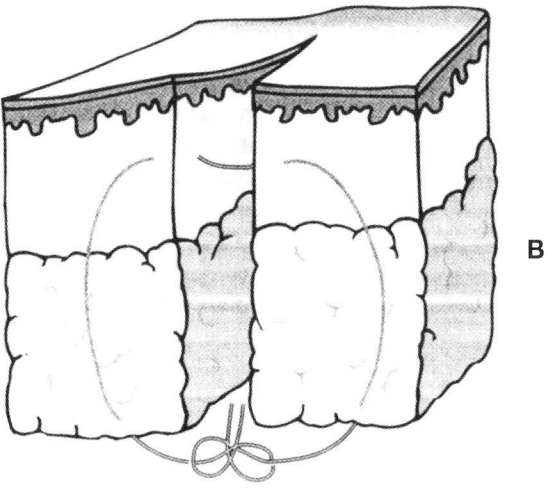

Fig. 23-10
Deep stitch with absorbable suture material. A, Needle should enter deep in the skin below the dermis where the undermining was accomplished *(1)* and exit in the upper dermis *(2).* The needle enters in the upper dermis *(3)* and exits below the dermis where the undermining was accomplished *(4).* **B,** The deep inverted buried stitch is tied at the bottom of the wound to avoid having the knot stick out of the incision. (From Usatine RP, Moy RL, Tobinick EL, and Siegel DM: *Skin surgery: a practical guide,* St Louis, 1998, Mosby.)

the incision. Avoid tying the knots too tight. The knots should be lined up on one side of the wound. The finer the suture, the closer the stitch needs to be. See Chapter 24 (Laceration and Incision Repair: Needle Selection) and Chapter 25 (Laceration and Incision Repair: Suture Selection) for needle and suture selection, respectively. See Chapter 26 (Laceration and Incision Repair: Suture Tying) for tying techniques.

2. *Simple running stitch* (Fig. 23-9). The advantages of the simple running stitch are that it is quick and distributes tension evenly. Cosmetic results are excellent if there is little skin tension. If there is significant gaping of the wound, other interrupted suture methods should be used. The relative disadvantage is that the entire stitch must be removed at once; with interrupted techniques, some sutures may be removed early for better cosmesis whereas a few remaining ones can be left for prevention of dehiscence and removed at a later date. This stitch is ideal in the scalp and is the one generally used for episiotomy repairs.

3. *Deep suture with inverted knot or "buried stitch"* (Fig. 23-10). Deeper wounds or wounds under tension are best closed by not relying solely on nonabsorbable superficial sutures. Well-placed

deep absorbable sutures can do much to aid in closing a wound, remove tension from the superficial skin sutures, and decrease scarring. The inverted knot technique places the bulk of the knot as far below the skin margins as possible to avoid suture spitting (migration of deep sutures to the skin surface). It also keeps the ends of the cut suture from protruding through the wound mar-

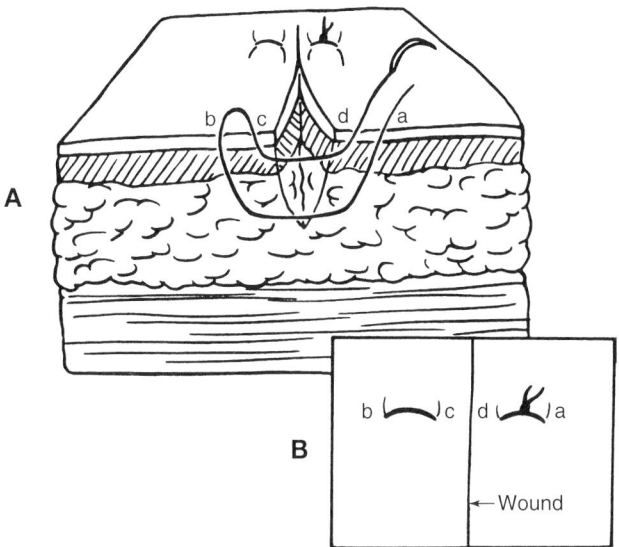

Fig. 23-11
Vertical mattress suture. A, Cross-section. **B,** Overhead view. Begin at *a,* and go under skin to *b.* Come out, go in at *c,* and exit at *d.*

gin. To start the stitch, begin at the bottom of the wound and come up usually just below the epidermal-dermal junction (remember, "Bottoms up!"). Go straight across the incision, enter at the same level at the opposite side, then go down to the base once again and tie. Care should be taken to achieve symmetry of depth and width on both sides of the laceration. Occasionally a second, more superficial, buried layer of sutures is required for deeper wounds. The surface (skin) is then fully closed with the closure of choice.

4. *Vertical mattress suture* (Fig. 23-11). This suture promotes eversion of the skin. It is also useful when the natural tendency of loose skin is to create inversion of the wound margins, which is to be avoided. A good example is the loose, flabby skin under the triceps muscle and thin skin in older people. The stitch is also appropriate when the skin is very thin and interrupted sutures have a tendency to pull through.

5. *Horizontal mattress suture* (Fig. 23-12). This suture is helpful in wounds under a moderate amount of tension and promotes wound edge eversion. It is especially useful on palms or soles and in patients who are poor candidates for deep sutures because of susceptibility to wound infections.

6. *Subcuticular running suture* (Fig. 23-13). This suture is used to close linear wounds that are not under much tension; it yields an excellent cosmetic result. The ends of the suture do not need to be tied; taping under slight tension preserves approximation. If desired, the two ends

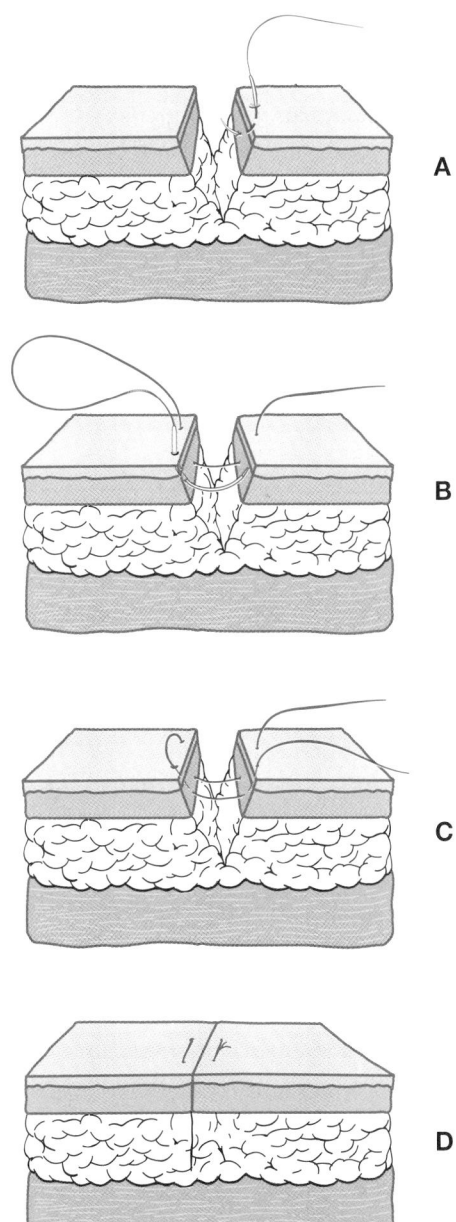

Fig. 23-12
Horizontal mattress suture. A, Needle is passed 0.5 to 1 cm away from wound edge deeply into the wound. **B,** Needle is passed through the opposite side and reenters the wound parallel to the initial suture. **C,** Reenter the skin perpendicularly to provide some eversion of the wound edges. Enter and exit both the wound and skin at the same depth, otherwise "buckling" and irregularities occur in the wound margin. **D,** Suture is then tied as shown.

can be tied over the wound, or a knot can be placed at each end to prevent slippage. Usually a polypropylene-coated nylon works best. Steri-Strips, tapes, or tissue glue can be used to supplement this type of stitch. Special care must be taken to avoid pressure on the wound, since this stitch separates easily.

7. *Three-point or half-buried mattress suture* (Fig. 23-14). This suture is designed to permit closure of the acute corner tip of a laceration without impairing blood flow to the tip. It is an intradermal stitch in which the needle is inserted initially into the intact skin on the nonflap portion of the wound and passed through the skin at the middermis level; at the same level, the suture is then passed transversely through the tip of the

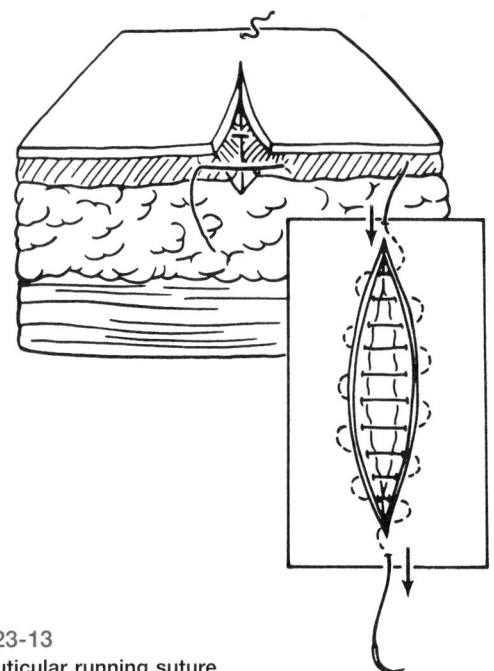

Fig. 23-13
Subcuticular running suture.

flap, returned on the opposite side of the wound, and brought through the skin, paralleling the point of entrance. The suture is tied by drawing the tip snugly into place in good approximation. Care should be taken not to have the knot tied over the point of the flap. This same approach can be used in closing a stellate laceration, drawing the tips together in a purse-string fashion. Repair of a "T" laceration also uses this technique (Fig. 23-15).

8. Repair of a *dog ear* or management of excess tissue can be performed as shown in Fig. 23-16 (see Chapter 186, Flaps and Plasties). Fig. 23-17 reviews the steps in the repair of a *C-flap* laceration.

Wound-Closure Tapes and Strips (Fig. 23-18)

Wound-closure tapes may be used alone for small, superficial wounds (especially in young children). When these tapes suffice to close a wound, they are easily placed without physical or psychological trauma to the patient. Wounds closed with tape are more resistant to infection than are sutured wounds. Tape cannot provide adequate skin-edge eversion or deep-tissue approximation when used alone. Thus tape is most commonly used as an adjunct to sutures or staples. Tape can help reinforce wounds closed subcuticularly or with conventional suturing techniques. Adhesion is enhanced by the application of a sticky substance to the skin surface. Traditionally, tincture of benzoin has been used for this purpose, but a preparation containing gum mastic (Mastisol) has been shown to provide stronger adhesion. Wound-closure tapes are especially helpful after suture

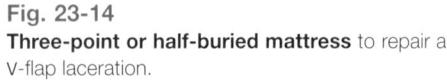

Fig. 23-14
Three-point or half-buried mattress to repair a V-flap laceration.

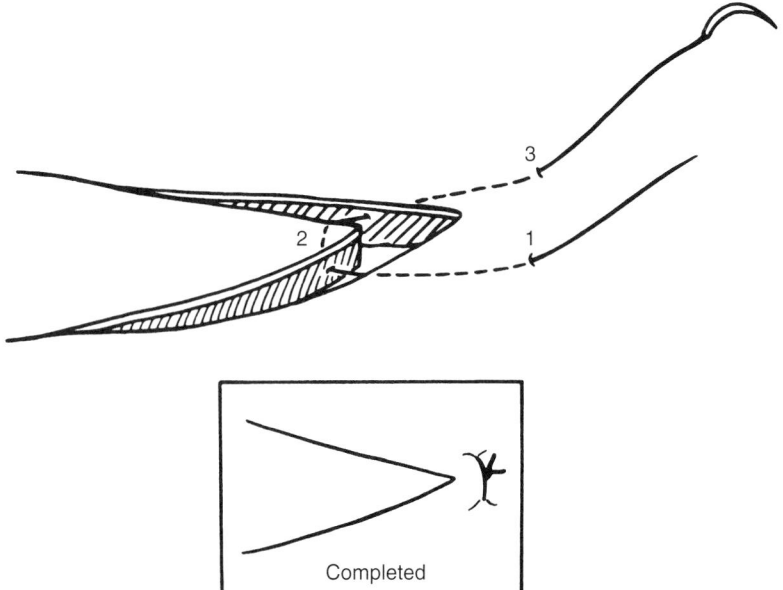

Completed

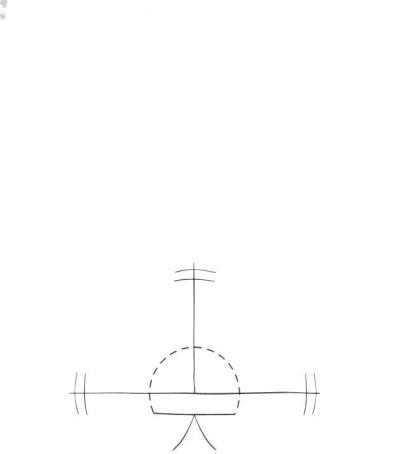

Fig. 23-15
T-laceration repair, using half-buried mattress suture technique.

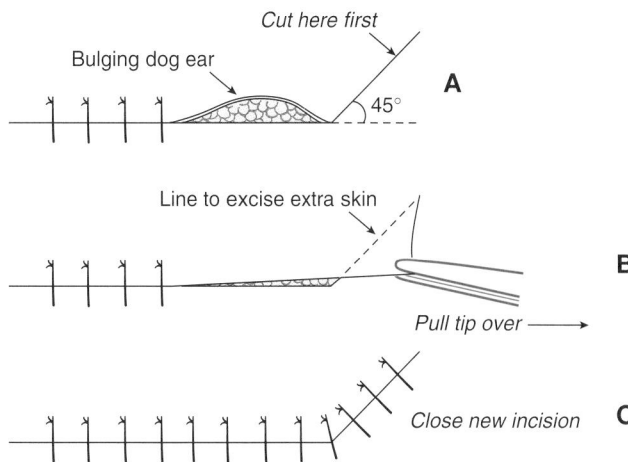

Fig. 23-16
Dog-ear repair. A, Note site of initial incision of bulging dog ear. **B,** Pull the tip over and excise. **C,** Close the new incision for skin to lie flat.

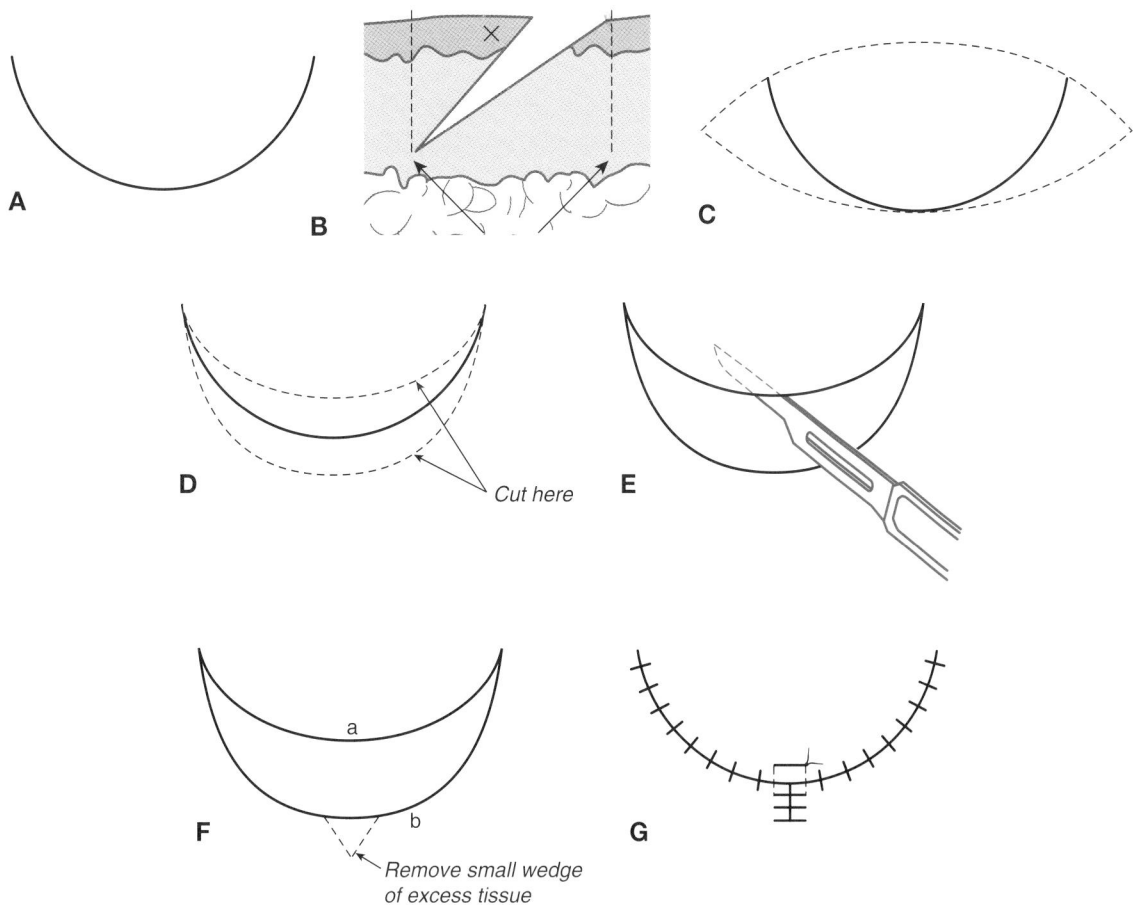

Fig. 23-17
C-flap repair. A, Laceration. **B,** The problem: the point X is often very thin and may necrose. Even if it does not, contracture will occur after healing and the slim margin along the X will be depressed, causing a more visible scar. **C,** If small enough, convert the wound to an ellipse for easier repair. **D,** Alternatively, excise the angled margins of skin to obtain "square" borders. **E,** Undermine. **F,** Close with interrupted sutures. Since side *a* is smaller than side *b,* a small wedge of tissue may need to be removed. **G,** Complete closure.

removal to prevent dehiscence and may be left on until they fall off. Patients may shower with them on.

The proper method of applying the strips is to apply Mastisol over the entire area, then place the strips in a parallel fashion without overlapping and without "tacking" strips (Fig. 23-18).

Tissue Adhesive

Tissue adhesives may be used to close certain wounds (see Chapter 38, Tissue Glues).

Delayed Primary Closure

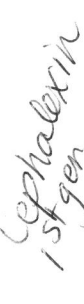

Wounds that are greater than 12 hours old (24 hours for facial lacerations) should not be closed immediately. To maximize the cosmetic result in this situation, the wound can be repaired by delayed primary closure. After cleansing the wound, insert a small piece of petroleum gauze between the wound edges and place the patient on an antibiotic, such as cephalexin, for 5 days. On the third day, the patient should return. The wound is then reirrigated and closed primarily with nonabsorbable sutures (i.e., no deep sutures because they increase the chance of infection). This is called *healing by secondary intent.*

In some instances of grossly contaminated or infected wounds, it is best to leave the wound open until it is healed on its own *(tertiary intent).* Frequent dressing changes and antibiotics are needed. Scarring and granulation tissue can be significant. Scar revision may be undertaken to improve the appearance of the site.

A summary of key points for suture repair is included in Box 23-3.

COMPLICATIONS

Possible Complications of Laceration Repair

The following complications may occur within the first 2 weeks:*

- Infection
- Pain
- Bleeding
- Dehiscence
- Hematoma
- Bruising and swelling
- Suture spitting

*Adapted from Usatine R, Moy R, Tobinick E, Siegel D: *Skin surgery: a practical guide,* St Louis, 1998, Mosby.

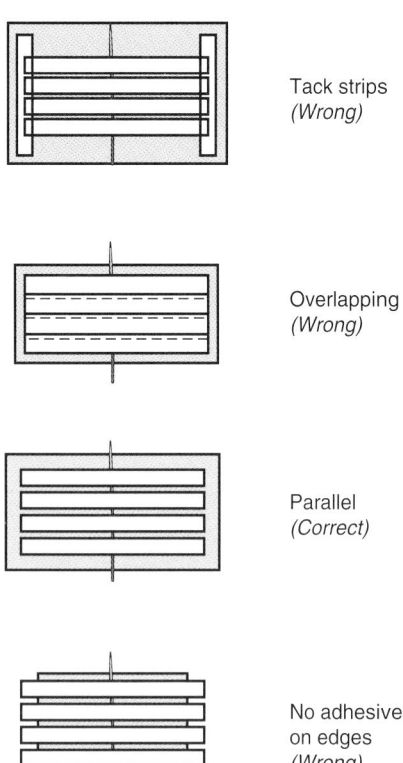

Tack strips
(Wrong)

Overlapping
(Wrong)

Parallel
(Correct)

No adhesive
on edges
(Wrong)

Fig. 23-18
The red rectangles illustrate where the Mastisol was applied to the skin.

BOX 23-3
Pearls of Suturing

Use 27- to 30-gauge needle for anesthesia; slow injection; warm solution.
Use 1% to 2% lidocaine (epinephrine is helpful to achieve hemostasis, except in fingers, toes, nose, and penis).
Make elliptical excision three times as long as wide.
Follow Langer's lines.
Undermine. Undermine. Undermine. Double the width of the wound on each side.
Eliminate all dead space.
Use deep inverted buried absorbable sutures to reduce skin tension ("Bottoms up").
Evert skin edges slightly ("Build pyramids, not ditches"). Inversion of wound edges results in 300% increase in time for epithelial bridging.
Place interrupted sutures half as far apart as they are across. The more tension, the more sutures needed. Follow the Erlenmeyer flask shape. The finer the suture, the more sutures needed, but the less scarring.
Edema occurs after closure. Only approximate tissues; do not strangulate.
Begin gentle washing of wound after 12-24 hr; if Steri-Strips and/or tissue glues are not used, apply an ointment to keep the wound moist to speed healing.
Apply Steri-Strips after suture removal.

Prolonged or permanent complications may include the following:

- Scarring
- Hypertrophic scars
- Keloid
- Hyperpigmentation
- Hypopigmentation
- Nerve damage
- Imperfect cosmetic alignment (e.g., the vermilion border)
- Recurrence of an incompletely excised lesion

POSTPROCEDURE PATIENT EDUCATION

Most wounds are best protected with some sort of dressing during the first 24 to 48 hours after closure. Continued oozing might be expected or pressure might be needed. For hemostasis, a pressure dressing should be applied over a nonstick type of gauze dressing. Trade names for such dressings include Xeroform, Adaptic, and Telfa. It is not usually necessary to keep a wound dry until the time of suture removal. Patients may shower after 24 hours. Moist healing (application of some type of ointment after gentle washing four times a day) aids in quicker healing. Suggestions for the timing for skin suture removal are listed in Table 23-2.

See Fig. 23-19 for proper suture removal techniques.

Wounds on the face or scalp may be dressed with a thin layer of antibiotic ointment in lieu of a mechanical dressing. It is best to cover them at night to avoid drying. Instruct patients to return if there are signs of wound infection. A routine wound check is not necessary for patients who understand the importance of monitoring the wound for signs of infection. An instructional handout can be given (see the sample patient education handout titled "Suture Care" on page 1759 of Appendix G).

TABLE 23-2

Timing for Suture Removal

Anatomic Area	Days Until Removal	External Suture Size	Buried Absorbable Suture Size
Face	3-5	5-0 or 6-0	5-0
Scalp	10	4-0, staples	3-0
Upper body	7-10	4-0	4-0
Hand	7-10	4-0	4-0
Lower body	10-14	4-0	3-0
Over joint (splint recommended)	14-21	4-0	3-0

Adapted from Coates WC, Lacerations to the face. In Tintinalli JE, Kellen GD, Stapczynski JS: *Emergency medicine, a comprehensive study guide,* ed 5, New York, 2000, McGraw-Hill.

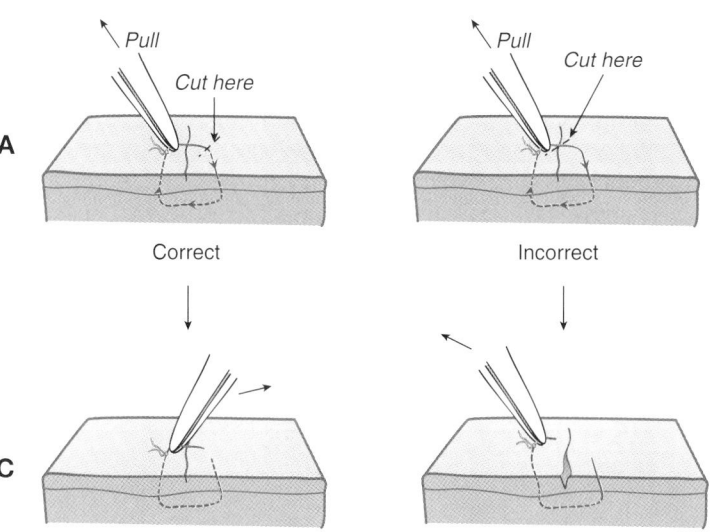

Fig. 23-19
Suture removal. A, Cut where the suture enters the skin. **B,** Cutting suture near knot leaves length of suture that is "dirty" and pulled into the tissue. **C,** Pull the forceps over the wound, which approximates wound edges. **D,** Pulling suture out this way tends to pull wound edges apart. Also, note dirty length of suture being pulled through wound.

TABLE 23-3

Centers for Disease Control and Prevention Recommendations for Tetanus Prophylaxis in Wound Management

	Clean, Minor Wounds		All Other Wounds*	
Vaccination History	Td[†]	TIG	Td[†]	TIG
Unknown or less than three doses	Yes	No	Yes	Yes
Three or more doses[‡]	No[§]	No	No[‖]	No

From Diphtheria, tetanus, and pertussis: recommendations for vaccine use and other preventive measures: recommendations of the Immunization Practices Advisory committee (ACIP): *MMWR Morb Mortal Wkly Rep* 40(RR-10):1-28, 1991.
TIG, Tetanus immune globulin.
*Such as, but not limited to, wounds contaminated with dirt, feces, soil, and saliva; puncture wounds; avulsions; and wounds resulting from missiles, crushing, burns, and frostbite.
[†]For children less than 7 years old, DTaP or DTP (DT, if pertussis vaccine is contraindicated) is preferred to tetanus toxoid alone. For patients older than 7 years old, Td is preferred to tetanus toxoid alone.
[‡]If only three doses of *fluid* toxoid have been received, a fourth dose of toxoid, preferably an absorbed toxoid, should be given.
[§]Yes, if more than 10 years since last dose.
[‖]Yes, if more than 5 years since last dose. (More frequent boosters are not needed and can accentuate side effects.)

CONCURRENT TREATMENT

Tetanus Prophylaxis

Table 23-3 is based on the current Centers for Disease Control and Prevention recommendations for tetanus prophylaxis in wound management.

Analgesic Medication

Analgesic medication may need to be administered for a few days depending on the extent of the trauma, the pain threshold of the patient, and the concerns of the family. If antibiotics are needed, refer to earlier discussion under initial assessment.

CONCLUSION

In the treatment of lacerations, careful inspection, adequate irrigation, skilled closure, and appropriate wound care can produce the best functional and cosmetic results. The principles and steps covered in this chapter show how lacerations can be repaired with maximal skill and minimal discomfort to the patient. More advanced skills and knowledge can be developed through experience and by reading Chapter 186 (Flaps and Plasties) and the sources listed in the bibliography.

SUPPLIER

Zerowet Splash Shields and Klenzalac Wound Irrigation Systems

Zerowet
P.O. Box 4375
Palos Verdes Peninsula, CA 90274
Phone: 1-800-438-0938

The remainder of the equipment can be obtained from any medical supplier.

CPT/BILLING CODES AND ICD-9-CM DIAGNOSTIC CODES

Coding and billing becomes very complex for laceration repair and excisions. Important factors to list for billing personnel are as follows:
- Location
- Size of lesion
- Length of closure or excision
- Simple or intermediate repair (intermediate includes either undermining or placement of deep buried sutures)
- Benign or malignant status
- Whether a true skin lesion or subcutaneous tumor or deep tumor was excised
- Method of removal (shave, excision, destruction)

Suture removal is included in the initial charge if the original sutures were placed by the same group of physicians. Suture removal can be billed if performed by an unassociated physician or group. Anesthetic, materials, and supplies are customarily also included in the reimbursement fees. If a lesion is excised and repaired in a simple fashion (no undermining, deep sutures, flaps, or plasties), the fee for excision includes repair and suture removal.

For CPT/billing codes, see Table 23-4. For ICD-9-CM diagnostic codes, see Appendix H.

ADDITIONAL RESOURCES

- See the sample patient education handout titled "Suture Care" on page 1759 of Appendix G.
- See the sample patient consent form titled "Skin Lesion Excision (Elective)" on page 1760 of Appendix G.

TABLE 23-4
CPT/Billing Codes

Benign Skin Excision	
11200	Tags, up to/including 15 lesions
11201	Tags, each additional 10 lesions
11400	TAL <0.6 cm
11401	TAL 0.6-1.0 cm
11402	TAL 1.1-2.0 cm
11403	TAL 2.1-3.0 cm
11404	TAL 3.1-4.0 cm
11406	TAL >4.0 cm
11420	SNHFG <0.6 cm
11421	SNHFG 0.60-1.0 cm
11422	SNHFG 1.1-2.0 cm
11423	SNHFG 2.1-3.0 cm
11424	SNHFG 3.1-4.0 cm
11426	SNHFG >4.0 cm
11440	Face <0.6 cm
11441	Face 0.6-1.0 cm
11442	Face 1.1-2.0 cm
11443	Face 2.1-3.0 cm
11444	Face 3.1-4.0 cm
11446	Face >4.0 cm

Malignant Skin Excision	
11600	TAL <0.6 cm
11601	TAL 0.6-1.0 cm
11602	TAL 1.1-2.0 cm
11603	TAL 2.1-3.0 cm
11604	TAL 3.1-4.0 cm
11606	TAL >4.0 cm
11620	SNHFG <0.6 cm
11621	SNHFG 0.6-1.0 cm
11622	SNHFG 1.1-2.0 cm
11623	SNHFG 2.1-3.0 cm
11624	SNHFG 3.1-4.0 cm
11626	SNHFG >4.0 cm
11640	Face <0.6 cm
11641	Face 0.6-1.0 cm
11642	Face 1.1-2.0 cm
11643	Face 2.1-3.0 cm
11644	Face 3.1-4.0 cm
11646	Face 4.0 cm

Simple Skin Repairs	
12001	SNAGTE <2.6 cm
12002	SNAGTE 2.6-7.5 cm
12004	SNAGTE 7.6-12.5 cm
12005	SNAGTE 12.6-20.0 cm
12006	SNAGTE 20.1-30.0 cm
12007	SNAGTE >30.0 cm
12011	FEENLMM <2.6 cm
12013	FEENLMM 2.6-5.0 cm
12014	FEENLMM 5.1-7.5 cm
12015	FEENLMM 7.6-12.5 cm
12016	FEENLMM 12.6-20.0 cm
12017	FEENLMM 20.1-30.0 cm
12018	FEENLMM >30.0 cm
12020	Superficial wound dehiscence

Intermediate Skin Repairs	
12031	SATAL <2.6 cm
12032	SATAL 2.6-7.5 cm
12034	SATAL 7.6-12.5 cm
12035	SATAL 12.6-20.0 cm
12036	SATAL 20.1-30.0 cm
12037	SATAL >30.0 cm
12041	NHFG < 2.6 cm
12042	NHFG 2.6-7.5 cm
12044	NHFG 7.6-12.5 cm
12045	NHFG 12.6-20.0 cm
12046	NHFG 20.1-30.0 cm
12047	NHFG >30.0 cm
12051	FEENLMM <2.6 cm
12052	FEENLMM 2.6-5.0 cm
12053	FEENLMM 5.1-7.5 cm
12054	FEENLMM 7.6-12.5 cm
12055	FEENLMM 12.6-20.0 cm
12056	FEENLMM 20.130.0 cm
12057	FEENLMM >30.0 cm

Benign Tumor Excisions (e.g., lipoma)	
21550	Bx, soft tissue, neck/thorax
21555	Neck/thorax SQ*
21556	Neck/thorax deep*†
21930	Back/flank*
22900	Abdominal wall deep*†
23075	Shoulder SQ
23076	Shoulder deep*†
24075	Upper arm/elbow SQ*
24076	Upper arm/elbow deep*†
25075	Forearm/wrist SQ*
25076	Forearm/wrist deep*†
26115	Hand/finger SQ*
26116	Hand/finger deep*†
27047	Pelvis/hip SQ*
27048	Pelvis/hip deep*
27327	Thigh/knee SQ*
27328	Thigh/knee deep*†
27618	Leg/ankle SQ*
27619	Leg/ankle deep*†
28043	Foot SQ*
28045	Foot deep*
38500	Exc/bx lymph node, superficial
41825	Gum/alveolar, no repair
41826	Gum/alveolar, simple rep

Face:	Face, ear, eyelid, nose, lip, or mucous membrane
FEENLMM:	Face, ear, eyelid, nose, lip, or mucous membrane
NHFG:	Neck, hand, foot, or external genitalia
SATAL:	Scalp, axilla, trunk, arm, or leg
SNAGTE:	Scalp, neck, axilla, genitalia, trunk, or extremity
SNHFG:	Scalp, neck, hand, foot, or genitalia
SQ:	Subcutaneous
TAL:	Trunk, arm, or leg.

Codes in bold have a 10-day global fee surgical period.
The sizes listed in codes 11400 to 11646 describe lesion diameter, not the length of the skin excised.
*90-Day global fee surgical period.
†Deep excision includes subfascial or intramuscular lesions.

BIBLIOGRAPHY

Coates WC: Lacerations to the face. In Tintinalli J, Kelen GD, Stapczynski JS, editors: *Emergency medicine: a comprehensive study guide,* ed 5, New York, 2000, McGraw-Hill.

Cummings, P: Antibiotics to prevent infection in patients with dog bite wounds: a meta-analysis of randomized trials, *Ann Emerg Med* 23(3):535, 1994.

Cummings P, Del Beccaro MA: Antibiotics to prevent infection of simple wounds: a meta-analysis of randomized studies, *Am J Emerg Med* 13(4):396, 1995.

Edlich RF, London SD: Wound repair: from ritual practice to scientific discipline, *J Trauma* 40(2):326, 1996.

Fernandez M, Coates WC: Lacerations to the extremities and joints. In Tintinalli J, Kelen GD, Stapczynski JS, editors: *Emergency medicine: a comprehensive study guide,* ed 5, New York, 2000, McGraw-Hill.

Haas AF, Grekin RC: Antibiotic prophylaxis in dermatologic surgery, *J Am Acad Dermatol* 32:155, 1995.

Howell JM, Chisholm CD: Wound care, *Emerg Med Clin North Am* 15(2):417, 1997.

Katz KH, Desciak EB, Maloney ME: The optimal application of surgical adhesive tape strips, *Dermatol Surg* 25:686, 1999.

Singer AJ, Hollander JE, Quinn JV: Evaluation and management of traumatic lacerations, *N Engl J Med* 337(16):1142, 1997.

Smack DP, Harrington AC, Dunn C, et al: Infection and allergy incidence in ambulatory surgery patients using white petrolatum vs bacitracin ointment: a randomized controlled trial, *JAMA* 276:972, 1996.

Usatine R, Moy R, Tobinick E, Siegel D: *Skin surgery: a practical guide,* St Louis, 1998, Mosby.

Woods RK, Dellinger EP: Current guidelines for antibiotic prophylaxis of surgical wounds, *Am Fam Physician* 57(11):2731, 1998.

CHAPTER 24

Laceration and Incision Repair: Needle Selection

William Jackson Epperson

Dozens of needle types have been developed for specific surgical needs. The needle facilitates the appropriate placement of suture. Inappropriate needle selection can damage the tissues, causing poor results and delayed healing. For example, a tapered point is needed in suturing the bowel, where prevention of leakage is imperative. A cutting needle would never be appropriate in the reanastomosis of bowel or blood vessels.

Most needles are made of noncorrosive stainless steel. Through a process of heating the metal, maximal strength and ductility (the ability to bend under pressure without breaking) are achieved. Each needle type is sharpened to a varying degree depending on its use. Also, to assist with passage through tissue, most needles receive a thin silicone coat.

NEEDLE DESIGN

The surgical needle is composed of an eye, a body, and a point (Fig. 24-1). There are three types of needle eyes: the closed eye, the French (split or spring) eye, and the swaged eye. The *closed eye* is commonly seen in the sewing needle. The closed-eye needle may be round, square, or oval. *French-eyed* needles have a longitudinal slit at the eye with internal ridges that catch and hold the suture in place. Both closed-eye and French-eye needles must be threaded. This threading is time consuming, and the unthreading of needles may often occur at an inopportune moment during a procedure. Tying the suture to a closed-eye needle increases the diameter of the eye being pulled through tissue, which can lead to unwanted results (Fig. 24-2). A *swaged eye,* in which the metal is literally molded around the suture, alleviates most needle-to-suture problems and prevents the repeated use of a dull or contaminated needle.

The *body* of the needle is important for both strength and grasping by the needle holder. Various shapes of the body are important for added strength as well as for matching the flow of the needle through the tissues as directed by the point. A flattened body with concave or convex surfaces helps to reduce unwanted needle rota-

tion when suturing. The shape of the body of the needle allows for a variety of uses (Fig. 24-3).

Needle *points* are the most important needle consideration. The basic types include cutting, tapered, and blunt, and most needles have a mixed variety of these features (Fig. 24-4).

The two opposing edges of a cutting needle allow for easy passage through tough tissues. This makes cutting needles ideal for suturing skin, with its dense supporting structures. However, these cutting edges have their drawbacks when it comes to tendons and oral mucous membranes, which are easily damaged by overcutting.

The *conventional cutting* needle has a cutting edge on its inside or concave curvature. The inside cutting in the direction of force is a negative characteristic of this needle. The suture force tends to concentrate at the apex of the triangle, and tissues outside of the desired suture channel are cut. For this reason, it is used less frequently than the reverse cutting needle (Fig. 24-4).

The *reverse cutting* needle has its cutting edge on the outer curvature of the needle. This gives a flat surface along the inner edge, thereby reducing the incidence of suture pulling through tissues into the margin of the

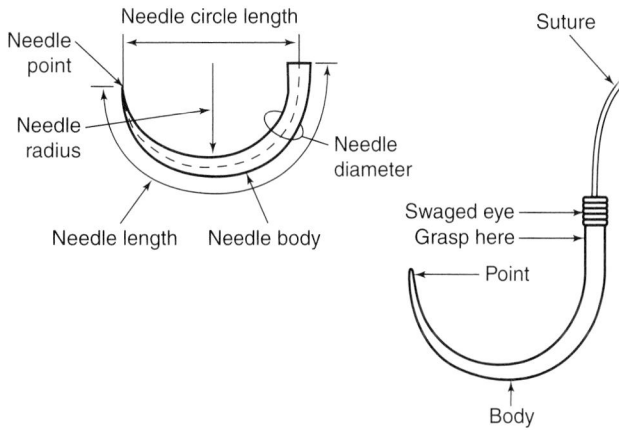

Fig. 24-1
Anatomy of a surgical needle.

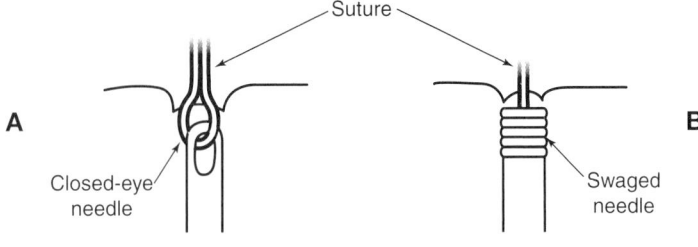

Fig. 24-2
A, Tissue disruption can be caused by double-suture strand with closed-eyed needle. **B,** Tissue disruption is minimized by a single-suture strand swaged to needle.

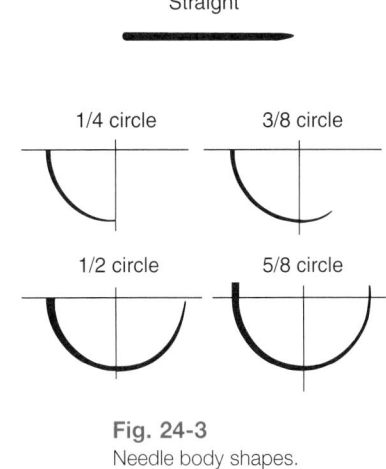

Fig. 24-3
Needle body shapes.

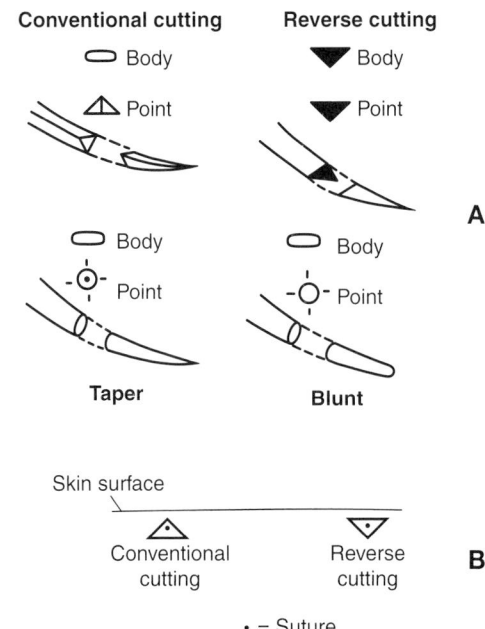

Fig. 24-4
A, Needle points and body shapes. **B,** In conventional cutting needles, the pressure is concentrated on the apex of the triangle and thereby has a tendency to tear through tissue. In reverse cutting, the advantage of piercing through tissue still exists, but the pressure from the suture is distributed over the whole base so unwanted tearing is reduced.

wound. Unless specified otherwise, a "cutting needle" now refers to a "reverse cutting" design.

Taper cut or *round* needles have an oval body to reduce twisting in the needle holder. These points are useful in less dense tissues that require small holes and minimal tissue injury, such as in fascia and bowel.

The *blunt point* needle is used in friable parenchymal tissue, such as tissues of the liver and kidney. This point allows for dissection through tissue, avoiding the trauma of cutting.

Many terms have been developed by suture manufacturers to categorize their products for different purposes and to denote their size. Unfortunately, there is no standard nomenclature. On thick skin, for skin (FS) and cutting (CE) needles should be used. On cosmetic areas, plastic (P), plastic skin (PS), premium (PRE), or precision cosmetic (PC) needles are recommended. Generally, a three-eighths curvature is adequate for most cutaneous procedures (Fig. 24-5). (FS and CE needles offer a significant cost savings and are sufficient in most cases, except in fine work with 6-0 sutures.)

Generally, a larger needle is used for deep buried sutures, whereas a smaller needle can be used to close the skin. Location of closure is also important. For instance, facial closures are often done with a P-3 needle, whereas other areas with thicker skin require an FS-2 or

FS-3. It is important to review the descriptions on the suture packet. Oftentimes, a picture of the needle can aid in proper selection.

Needles should be handled only with needle holders, otherwise damage to the needles may occur. The needle holder size must match that of the needle. The needle should be grasped below the swaged eye, but beyond the middle body region (Fig. 24-1). The swaged metal must be sufficiently soft to wrap around the suture; therefore, if it is grasped here, it bends easily. The body of the needle is firm, not malleable, and less likely to bend. The tip of the needle holder should just cover the needle, and the handle should be closed only to the first or second ratchet. During needle placement the force must be advanced in the direction of the curvature of the needle. The wrist must be everted out and supinated as the needle goes through tissue to avoid undue pressure and bending.

CONCLUSION

Often, an ordinary suturing procedure becomes more difficult than expected. This difficulty can often be improved by reassessing the appropriateness of the instruments being used. Needle selection is often a key factor in facilitating the ease of the operation and ultimate good surgical results.

Ethicon
Precision point needles

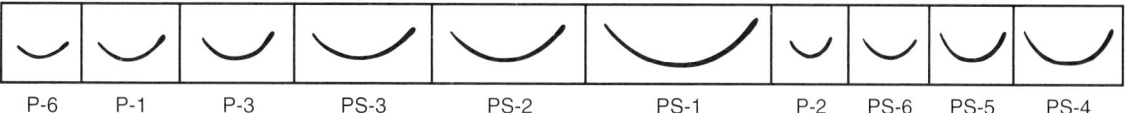

P-6   P-1   P-3   PS-3   PS-2   PS-1   P-2   PS-6   PS-5   PS-4

Precision cosmetic needles

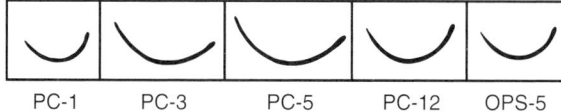

PC-1   PC-3   PC-5   PC-12   OPS-5

Davis & Geck

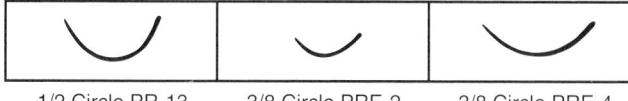

1/2 Circle PR-13   3/8 Circle PRE-2   3/8 Circle PRE-4

Fig. 24-5
Ethicon and Davis & Geck (Kendall) needle nomenclature for facial closures (actual sizes).

SUPPLIERS

Kendall Company (Ethicon and Davis & Geck)
15 Hampshire Street
Mansfield, MA 02048
Phone: 1-800-962-9888
Website: www.kendallhq.com

Ethicon/Johnson & Johnson
Phone: 1-800-255-2500

Most medical supply firms carry any suture material needed.

BIBLIOGRAPHY

Moy RL: Suture material in skin surgery, a practical guide. In Usatine R, Moy R, Tobinick E, Siegel D: *Skin surgery: a practical guide,* St Louis, 1998, Mosby.

Moy RL, Waldman B, Hein DW: A review of sutures and suturing techniques, *J Dermatol Surg Oncol* 18:785, 1992.

Schwartz SI, Shires GT, Spencer FC, Storer EH, editors: *Principles of surgery,* ed 7, New York, 1999, McGraw-Hill.

Tier WC: Considerations in the choice of surgical needles, *Surg Gynecol Obstet* 149:84, 1979.

Way LW: *Current surgical diagnosis & treatment,* ed 9, Norwalk, Conn, 1991, Appleton & Lange.

Wound closure manual, Somerville, NJ, 1985, Ethicon.

CHAPTER 25

Laceration and Incision Repair: Suture Selection

William Jackson Epperson

Numerous suture types have been developed that are best suited for a variety of tissue properties in the body. The qualities most important for suture include flexibility, strength, secure knotting, and low propensity for contribution to infection. The goal of suturing is to maintain the approximation of tissues securely until healing allows for tissue strength to be maintained alone.

The two main categories of suture are *absorbable* and *nonabsorbable*. All types of suture are foreign to the body; therefore the degree to which the body reacts against the suture is an important consideration in suture choice.

Suture size is indicated by use of a "0," with the more "0s" designating smaller sutures (e.g., 4-0 is smaller than 3-0). Suture materials are standardized by specific regulations, which assures consistent width and tensile strength.

Absorbable suture is a sterile strand of synthetic polymer or mammalian-derived collagen. The rate of absorption and the duration of tensile strength are important considerations. For example, the suture may lose effective strength long before it has been absorbed. Various coatings and materials have been developed to prolong the tensile-strength retention of absorbable suture. These coatings also aid in the passage of suture through tissue by decreasing friction.

The *natural absorbable suture (mammalian collagen or "gut" sutures)* are derived mainly from the submucosa of sheep intestine, the serosa of beef intestine, or the flexor tendons of beef. They are available in plain or chromic (coated with chromic salts to help delay reabsorption). Tensile strength is determined by the percent of collagen in the gut suture. Any noncollagen materials within the gut suture can cause severe tissue reactions, so purity of the protein is very important.

Common *synthetic absorbable* suture materials include polyglactic acid (Vicryl), polyglycolic acid (Dexon), and polydioxanone (PDS). These materials have the desirable property of extended time of tensile strength (Fig. 25-1).

Nonabsorbable suture is used for skin and for permanent internal placement such as in cardiovascular, orthopedic, and plastic surgery. Many raw materials are used, including silk, cotton, stainless steel, nylon, polyester, and polypropylene (Table 25-1). Table 25-2 reviews the various features of each of these sutures.

Nonabsorbable sutures are removed from the skin when no longer needed. With vascular and orthopedic applications there is often a need for more permanent materials that retain their tensile strength for a longer time. Tendon repair requires prolonged healing time and needs long-term tensile strength to give adequate time for self repair. Vascular grafts must have the support of suture for an indefinite period. The anastomosis of the graft and a blood vessel is never secured by the fibroblast and collagen of the body alone.

Braided suture adds strength and helps to secure the knotting, but it is more likely to harbor infection. *Monofilament* is better to use in the presence of infection, but its knots are less dependable. Tissue reaction is important in delicate tissues in which scar and

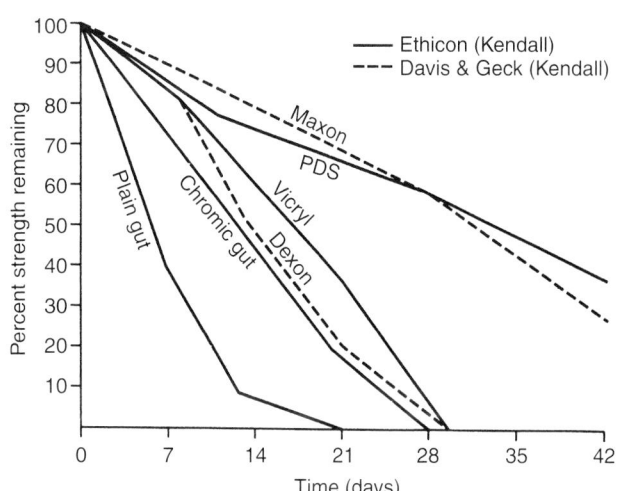

Fig. 25-1
In vivo strength retention of absorbable sutures.

TABLE 25-1
Nonabsorbable Sutures

Material	Type	Tensile Strength	Tissue Reaction	Cost
Silk	Braided	Poor	High	Low
Nylon (Ethilon, Dermalon)	Mono	Good	Minimal	Low
Polypropylene (Prolene, Surgilene)	Mono	Excellent	Minimal	High
Braided polyester (Mersilene)	Braided	Good	Minimal	High
Polybutester (Novafil)	Mono	Good	Minimal	Moderate

fissure formation may be a problem, which is why gut suture may not be a good choice for use on the face.

Knots are an important consideration in terms of whether they remain tied and, therefore, do not cause a significant reduction in the strength of the suture material. The knot is the weakest part of the completed suture ligature. Proper knotting technique requires the application of a square knot or double loop followed by a square knot tie. Oftentimes knots are accomplished as half-hitches that are weak and do not remain secure. The more friction a suture has, the less likely it is to incur slippage and loss of the knot's integrity. Braided suture knots rarely slip, whereas monofilament often comes untied in the absence of proper knotting technique. For proper tying techniques, see Chapter 26, Laceration and Incision Repair: Suture Tying.

TABLE 25-2
Common Suture Materials

Suture	Types	Make-Up	Usage	Tissue Reaction	Absorption Rate	Tensile Strength Retention
Absorbable Sutures						
Gut	Plain	Mammalian collagen	Superficial vessels and quick healing subcutaneous tissues	Moderate	70 days	2-4 days
Gut	Chromic	Mammalian collagen	Versatile; also good in the presence of infection; do not use on skin because of reaction	Moderate	90 days	7-10 days
Polyglycolic acid (Dexon)*	Mono	Synthetic polymer	Buried sutures; good tensile and knot strength	Mild	40% 7 days	20% in 15 days 5% in 28 days
Polydioxanone (PDS)†	Mono	Polyester polymer	Versatile; body cavity closure, bowel	Mild	210 days	70% in 14 days 50% in 28 days
Polyglactic acid (Vicryl)†	Braided	Coated polymer	Subcutaneous skin; buried sutures	Mild	60 to 90 days	60% in 14 days 30% in 21 days
Polyglyconate (Maxon)	Mono	Polyester	Smoother knot and excellent first-throw holding	Mild	180 to 210 days	81% in 14 days 59% in 28 days
Nonabsorbable Sutures						
Cotton	Twisted fibers	Cotton fiber	Ligating, some skin but generally too reactive	Minimal	Never; encapsulated in the body	50% in 6 months 30% in 2 years
Silk	Braided	Silkworm spun fiber	Ligating, some skin but rarely used	Moderate	2 years	Gone in one year
Steel	Mono	Alloy Fe-Ni-Cr	Tendons, sternum, abdominal wall	Low	Never; encapsulated in the body	Indefinite
Nylon (Ethilon, Dermalon)	Mono	Synthetic polymer	Skin	Very low	20% a year	Loses 20% a year
Polyester (Mersilene)	Braided	Polyester	Cardiovascular, general, and plastic surgery	Minimal	Never; encapsulated in the body	Indefinite
Polypropylene (Prolene)†	Mono	Synthetic polymer	Skin, vascular, plastic surgery	Minimal	Never; encapsulated in the body	Indefinite

*Dexon Plus has a synthetic coating to facilitate knot tying and passage through tissue.
†Vicryl, Prolene, and PDS are registered trademarks of Ethicon, Inc.

TABLE 25-3

Common Sutures for Cutaneous Surgery

	Skin (Interrupted)	Skin (Subcuticular)	Buried
Face	5-0 or 6-0 Nylon	4-0 or 5-0 Prolene	4-0 or 5-0 Synthetic absorbable or 6-0 clear nylon
Extremities, trunk	4-0 or 5-0 Nylon	3-0 or 4-0 Synthetic absorbable	4-0 Prolene or 3-0 or 4-0 synthetic absorbable

Each surgeon has his or her own choice of suture based on training and individual preferences. No one type of suture choice is always correct. Through application of the appropriate suture characteristics to the various applications in the body's tissues, the ease of operation will lead to an acceptable result.

Table 25-3 generalizes some recommendations for suture commonly used in an office setting. In general, the smaller the suture, the less tensile strength; thus more sutures will be needed, but the cosmetic result will be better. Physicians vary in their preferences, which proves that no one suture is satisfactory for all occasions. Nylon is a good, all-around, inexpensive material for surface skin suturing. It is not quite as strong or slippery as Prolene, but it ties easier and takes fewer knots. Prolene is stronger and glides through tissue easily but requires at least three, if not four, knots and still may not remain tight. Prolene works well for subcuticular stitches, and often, since it is stronger, a smaller size can be used for interrupted sutures.

BIBLIOGRAPHY

Bennett RG: Selection of wound closure materials, *J Am Acad Dermatol* 18(4):619, 1998.

Moy RL, Lee A, Zolka A: Commonly used suture materials in skin surgery, *Am Fam Physician* 4(6):2123, 1991.

Moy RL, Waldman B, Hein DW: A review of sutures and suturing techniques, *J Dermatol Surg Oncol* 18:785, 1992.

Postlethwait RW, Willigan DA, Ulin AW: Human tissue reaction to sutures, *Ann Surg* 181(2):144, 1975.

Schwartz SI, Shires GT, Spencer FC, Storer EH, editors: *Principles of surgery,* ed 7, New York, 1999, McGraw-Hill.

Usatine RP, Moy RL: *Skin surgery: a practical guide,* St Louis, 1998, Mosby.

Van Winkle W, Hastings JC: Considerations in the choice of suture materials for various tissues, *Surg Gynecol Obstet* 135:114, 1972.

Way LW: *Current surgical diagnosis and treatment,* ed 9, Norwalk, Conn, 1991, Appleton & Lange.

Wound closure manual, Somerville, NJ, 1985, Ethicon.

CHAPTER 26

Laceration and Incision Repair: Suture Tying

Ronald D. Reynolds

The knot is the weakest point of any suture. Even when properly tied, the knot is less than half the strength of the suture material that it is tied with and will always be the point at which a suture fails if it does so. Knots will slip apart if not correctly constructed. If excessive tension is applied, even to a properly tied suture loop, it will break at the knot because of internal shearing forces.

It is incumbent on the physician to know what suture material and size to use for each type of tissue that is to be approximated (see Chapter 25, Laceration and Incision Repair: Suture Selection). Once a suture is placed, it must be tied in an appropriate manner—not too tight or too loose and with a knot that will not fail before the tissue has healed. The knot must not be excessively large, because inflammation and infection are directly correlated with knot volume within tissue.

GENERAL PRINCIPLES OF KNOT TYING

A few generalities can be made about all knot tying. The suture material must always be treated with respect. Grasping the suture with an instrument will weaken it and thus should be avoided—except when holding a tail that will be cut away after an instrument tie. Shearing forces created by sawing two strands upon one another will weaken the strands. The first throw of a knot should just approximate the tissue, but subsequent throws must be tied firmly for knot security. Ideally, knots should be tied with equal tension on both strands. Tension should be applied parallel to the loop being closed and along the axis of the knot being tightened. Excessive throws do not add to knot security; they only add time and bulk.

KNOT MECHANICS

Suture knots are at the mercy of a number of factors. If the knot is tied in a *monofilament* material such as gut, nylon, polypropylene (Prolene), or polydioxanone (PDS), the *coefficient of friction* within the knot will be low, leading to a tendency to slip. These materials also

have *memory,* a tendency to maintain the shape in which they were manufactured, giving a straightening tendency that can lead to untying. The *pliability,* or ability to form a tight loop, of nylon is higher than that of the other monofilament materials. Braided *multifilament* suture materials such as silk, polyester (Mersilene, Ethibond), polyglactin (Vicryl), and polyglycolic acid (Dexon) have a higher coefficient of friction and less memory, making them easier to tie and less prone to slippage. The absorbability of a suture does not have a direct influence on its tying characteristics.

When knots are tied, great care must be taken as to the details. The *square knot* (Fig. 26-1, *A*) is the prototype suture knot because it is easy to tie, is strong, and does not loosen easily. Each twisting layer of the knot is called a *throw.* A square knot is constructed of one helical twist for the first throw, followed by one helical twist in the opposite direction for the second throw. If both helices are in the same direction, a *granny knot* (Fig. 26-1, *B*) results. Granny knots slip much more easily than square knots and therefore should be avoided when tying sutures.

After a helix for a knot throw is made with two suture strands, it must be kept in a helical configuration as the knot is tightened. If too much tension is applied to one strand, that strand will straighten and a *half hitch* (Fig. 26-1, *C*) in the other strand will result. As is obvious by its appearance, half hitches will slip on the straightened member of the suture and, therefore, are also to be avoided. It is unfortunately common for a physician who thinks that square knots are being laid down to instead make a series of slipping half hitches (Fig. 26-1, *D*). This is due to too much tension being applied to one strand during the tightening phase of tying.

If there is excess tension on wound edges when a square knot is being tied, the first throw of the knot may loosen before the second throw is placed and allow the edges to gape apart. The *surgeon's knot* (Fig. 26-l, *E*) is an adaptation of the square knot with two helical twists in the first throw. This additional twist increases the friction within the first throw and helps to hold it tight while the second throw is made. Whenever a surgeon's

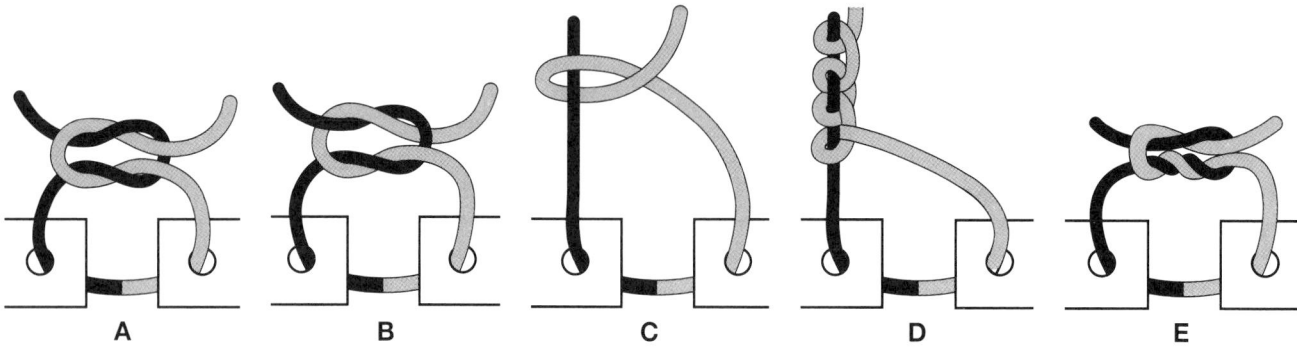

Fig. 26-1
Suture knots. **A,** Square knot. **B,** Granny knot. **C,** Half hitch. **D,** Series of "square" half hitches. **E,** Surgeon's knot. (Redrawn from Zimmer CA, Thacker JG, Powell DM, et al: *J Emerg Med* 9(3):107, 1991.)

knot seems necessary, the physician should give consideration to the need for a deep suture to approximate wound edges and take tension off the closure.

CHOOSING A SUTURE TYING TECHNIQUE

All physicians learn knot tying skills during medical school. Everyone is familiar with one-handed and two-handed ties, as well as instrument ties. There are some important points to consider when you decide which of these tying techniques to use.

Most procedures performed by primary care physicians are office procedures done on the skin. Physicians cannot afford to waste excess suture material just for the sake of knot tying. Studies of the economics of suture tying show that at least two to four times as many sutures can be constructed in a given length of suture material with an *instrument tie* than with a *hand tie*. While instrument tying is slightly slower than hand tying, it is much more economical and is the preferred technique for all skin procedures.

If a hand tie is to be done, the preferred method is the two-handed tie. Although the one-handed tie may be slightly faster than a two-handed tie, it is difficult to do well. One-handed ties are prone to creating a series of half hitches, because it is common to keep too much tension on one strand during tying. Also, because most wounds are sutured with the needle movement directed toward the physician and it is this closest strand (with its needle attached) that is primarily manipulated during a one-handed tie, there is a possibility of needlestick injury during a one-handed tie. Therefore one-handed tying is not covered in this chapter.

HOW TIGHT TO TIE THE LOOP

To appropriately approximate tissue, sutures must bring wound edges into apposition, but not place excessive force on the tissues ("approximate but don't strangulate"). If a suture loop is tied too loosely, a gap persists and the wound will not heal by primary intention but, instead, must heal by secondary intention from deeper within the defect. If tied too tightly, a suture loop will strangulate the tissue within, creating ischemia and poor wound healing. A too-tight skin suture will cut into the skin surface across the wound, creating a permanent "railroad track" scar.

Whether incised by accidental laceration or by an intentional surgical wound, all tissue will swell somewhat from the inflammation that is attendant in the healing process. Some allowance must be made for this anticipated swelling when tying each suture. It is the tension of the first throw, and maintenance of this tension while the second throw locks it in place, that is critical. Additional throws beyond these do not change the tension within the original loop.

As tension is applied to the first throw of a knot, the tissue edges should just barely touch together. If the edges are bunched together initially, subsequent swelling will make the loop too tight. With skin sutures, two subtle indications of excess loop tension include (1) a puckering effect of each suture that makes the wound mound up slightly between each loop and (2) a pale color of the skin underneath the suture. *It is far better to remove and replace an improperly tied suture than to leave it and hope for the best.*

HOW MANY THROWS TO PLACE

How many additional throws to place on top of the basic square or surgeon's knot for knot security is a slippery question, but one that needs an answer. Suture manufacturers will only say "additional throws as indicated by the surgical circumstance and the experience of the surgeon." (Believe me, they won't give a real answer, even when pressed. I've tried. Medicolegal concerns keep them from committing themselves.)

For a knot to be secure, additional throws are needed

beyond the basic two throws. Without added throws, the knot will slip loose when tension is applied to the loop. Any loosely tied knot will slip, so all throws past the first must be tied quite firmly, but without excessive force that will damage the integrity of the suture material.

Placing more throws than needed will unnecessarily add operative time and increase the bulk of the knot, without adding strength to the knot. Extra throws in a skin suture knot add operative time but have no consequence for the tissue because they are not buried. If the knot is buried, as in a subcuticular suture, additional bulk adds to the tissue reaction and can increase the infection risk. It is therefore necessary to know the minimum number of throws to tie to secure a knot in a variety of suture materials.

As a general rule, studies have shown that when 3- to 4-mm tails are left, monofilament materials need a total of four firm square throws to be secure, and braided materials need three. Obviously, if the knot is not tied squarely (alternating throws with helices in different directions), is tied loosely, or consists of half hitches rather than square throws, even the recommended number of throws will not suffice.

There are two exceptions to this general rule. First, nylon is pliable enough that it holds with three firm square throws. Second, when the suture is cut on the knot and no tails are left, one additional throw is required for knot security.

TECHNIQUES

Instrument Tie

An instrument tie uses the needle holder to form the twists in each throw. Directions are for a right-handed physician. Left-handed physicians can reverse the handedness in the directions and look at the figure in a mirror.
1. Place the suture moving toward yourself, and pull it through until just 2 to 3 cm of the tail is left outside the entry hole. Drop the needle beside the wound to minimize needlestick risk. Pick up the long end of the suture with your left thumb and index finger about 8 cm from its exit, and hold it above the wound.
2. Create the first throw by making a single twist (for a square knot) or double twist (for a surgeon's knot) around the tip of the needle holder with the long strand. To do this, the needle holder is held closed, but not locked, facing towards the left. The instrument tip approaches the long strand moving towards the physician. Both it and the long strand are moved in a clockwise motion to wrap the strand around the tip (Fig. 26-2, *A*), while being careful not to pull the suture through the wound. Grasp the short end with the very tip of the needle holder. Pull the short end through the loops around the needle holder's tip (Fig.

26-2, *B*). Keep even tension on both strands as you pull the short strand towards you with the needle holder and the long strand away from you with your left hand (Fig. 26-2, *C*). The sutures should maintain a helical configuration all the way down to the wound. Apply enough tension to just appose the wound. Release the short end.
3. The second throw is created by reversing the rotation of the long strand around the needle holder tip. While still holding the long strand in the left hand, bring it toward you while moving the needle holder away from yourself. As the needle holder tip touches the long strand, wrap counterclockwise around it (Fig. 26-2, *D*). Again grasp the short end in the needle holder tips (Fig. 26-2, *E*), and pull the short strand away from yourself while pulling the long strand toward you (Fig. 26-2, *F*). Carefully pull the throw down square to lock the knot.
4. Additional throws must be made, with the number depending on the suture material and circumstances. Repeat the cycle of clockwise-counterclockwise throws, being careful to lay each throw down with opposite rotation to the last throw. Tie each throw square (not half-hitched) with firm and even tension on both ends as the knot is snugged tight. When the knot is completed, excess material is cut away, either on the knot if it is to be buried or leaving 3- to 4-mm tails if it is a skin suture.

Two-Handed Tie

This version of the two-handed tie presumes that the suture to be tied has been sewn toward you, with the needle on your side of the wound. Following this sequence prevents you from having to cross your hands over the top of the wound, a motion that blocks your vision of the knot being formed.
1. The two-handed tie starts like the instrument tie with the suture being placed in the tissue and being pulled through, but leaving about 10 cm of the tail outside the wound. Grasp the tail in your right hand and the long end in your left hand. Palms are up when initially grasping the strands, which are held between the last three fingers and the palm. To start the knot, grasp the short end between your right index finger and thumb. Use the back of your left thumb to hold the long end as shown. Lay the short end across the side of your left thumb to form a loop (Fig. 26-3, *A*).
2. Drop your left index finger to contact the pad of your left thumb and hold the loop open. Maintaining the pinch, drop the loop off your thumb and move down to pinch the short end (Fig. 26-3, *B*), leaving your left index finger inside the loop. Push the free end up through the loop with the left thumb by extending your left wrist (Fig. 26-3, *C*). Release the free end

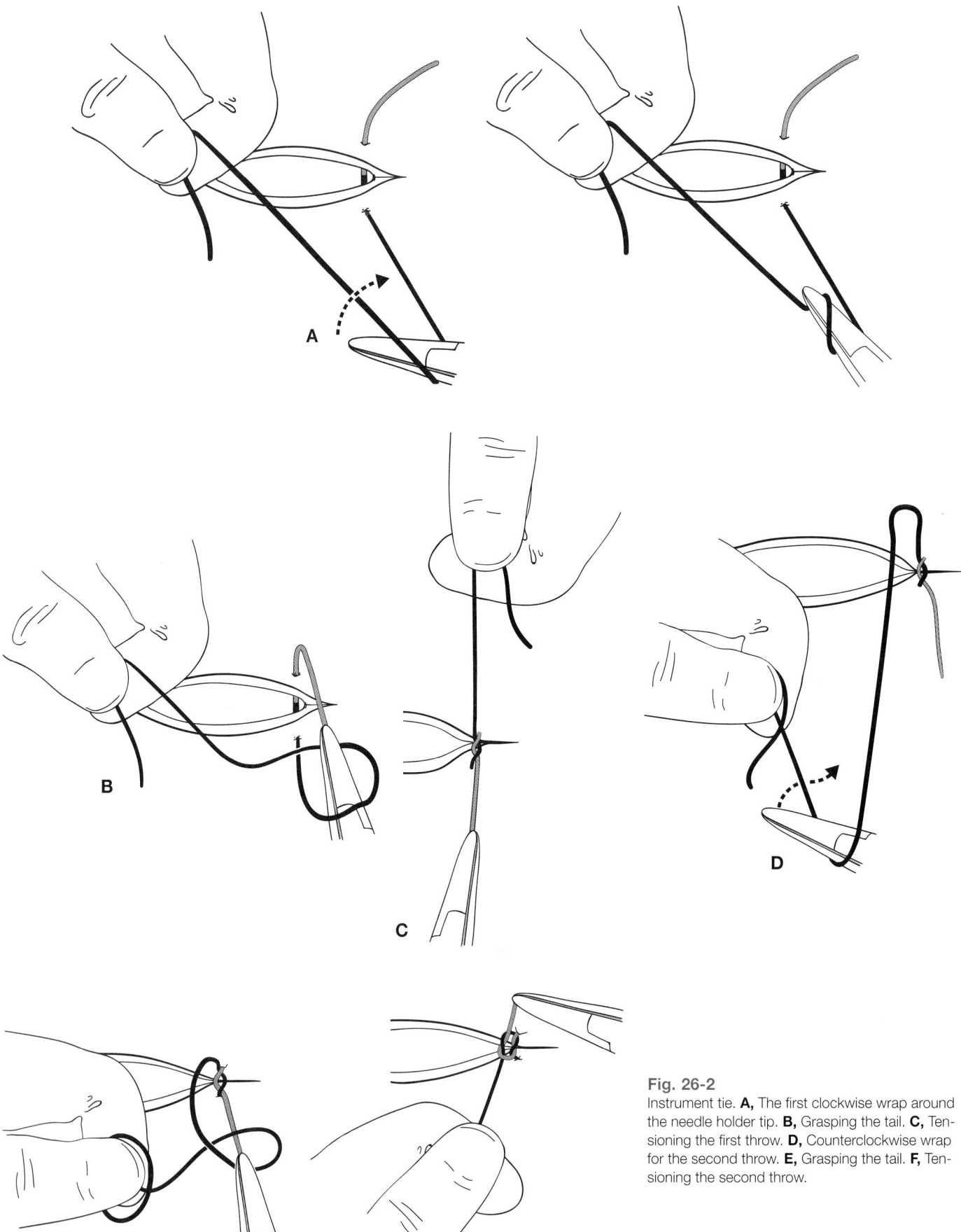

Fig. 26-2
Instrument tie. **A,** The first clockwise wrap around the needle holder tip. **B,** Grasping the tail. **C,** Tensioning the first throw. **D,** Counterclockwise wrap for the second throw. **E,** Grasping the tail. **F,** Tensioning the second throw.

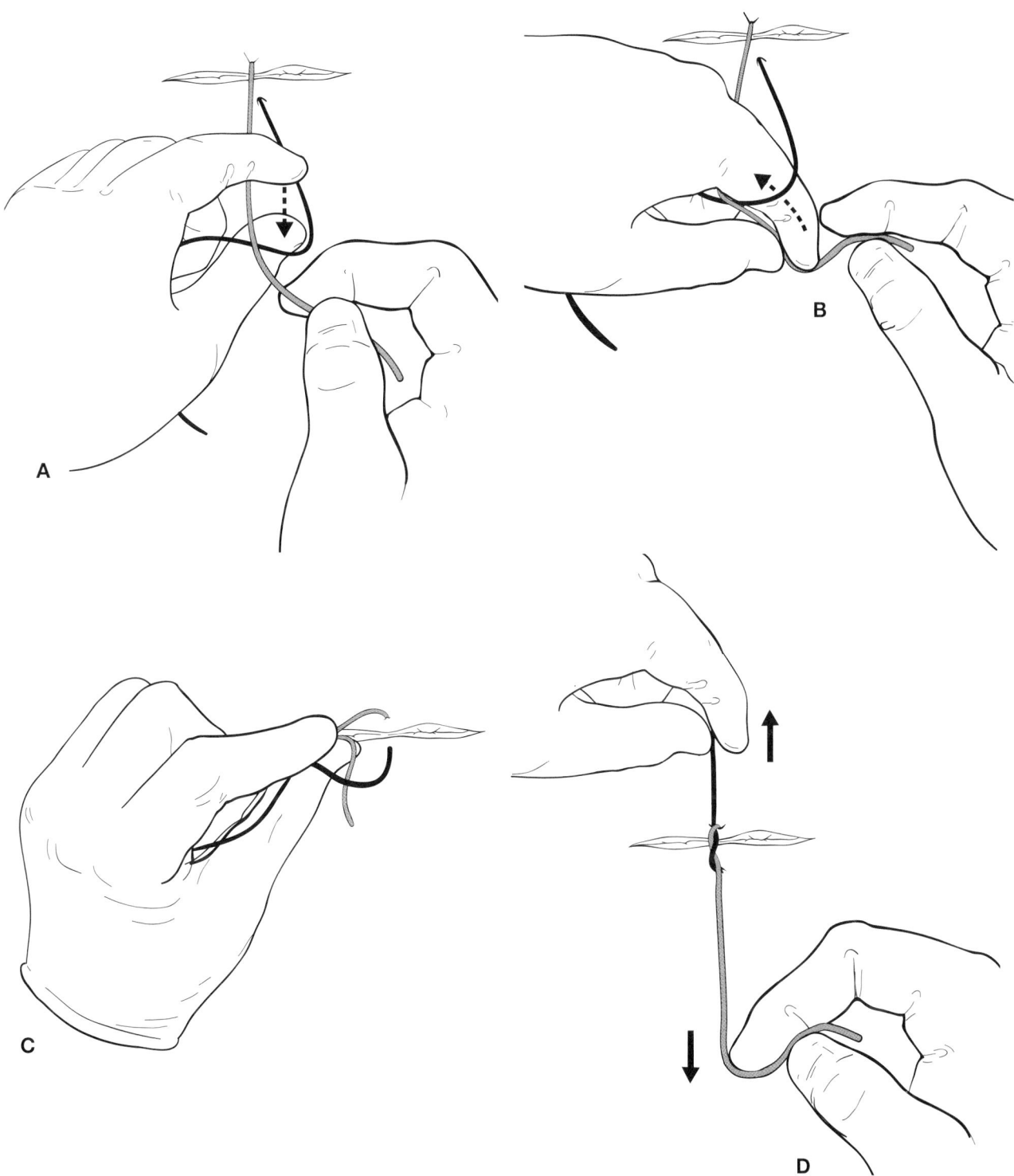

Fig. 26-3
Two-handed tie. **A,** Starting position. **B** and **C,** Creating the first throw. **D,** Tensioning the first throw.
(Redrawn from James JD, Wu MM, Batra EK, et al: *J Emerg Med* 10:469, 1992.)   *Continued*

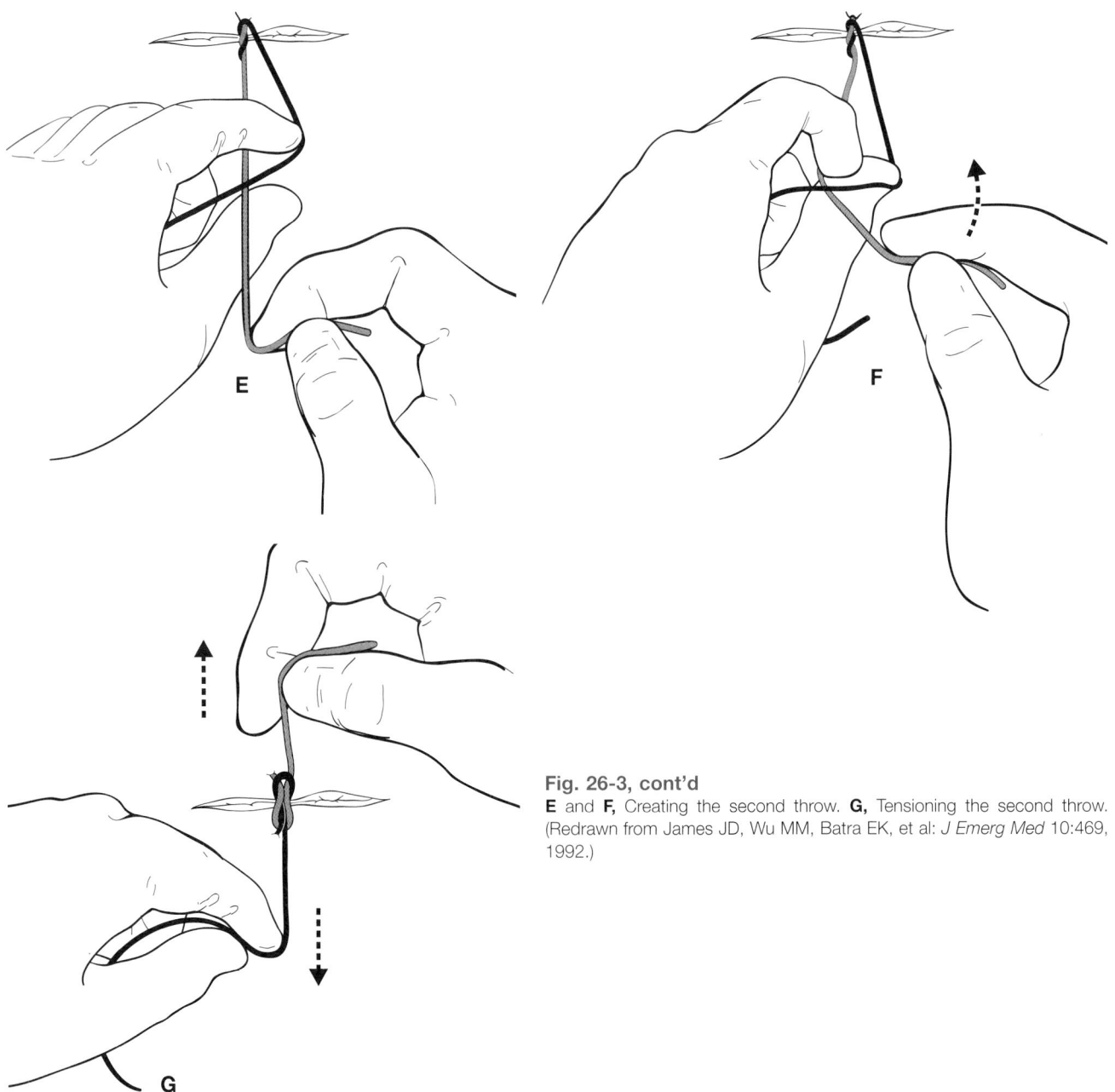

Fig. 26-3, cont'd
E and **F,** Creating the second throw. **G,** Tensioning the second throw. (Redrawn from James JD, Wu MM, Batra EK, et al: *J Emerg Med* 10:469, 1992.)

from your right hand and regrasp it as it is pulled through the loop. This same maneuver can be redone to make the second twist needed for a surgeon's knot. Draw down the first throw and tighten evenly by bringing your left hand away from and your right hand towards yourself (Fig. 26-3, *D*).

3. The second square throw is created by reversing these maneuvers. As you draw the long end back towards yourself with your left hand, use your left index finger to begin to create a loop. Reach under the short end with your left thumb (Fig. 26-3, *E*), and push your thumb up to hold the side of the loop. Bring your left thumb and index finger together

inside the loop (Fig. 26-3, *F*). Lift the short end in your right hand, and place it in the pinch of your left thumb and index finger. Push the short end down through the loop with your left index finger, release it from the right hand, and then regrasp. The second throw is then brought down by bringing the right hand away and the left hand toward yourself (Fig. 26-3, *G*).

4. Additional throws are added as needed by alternating the same process of the first and second throws. When the knot is completed, excess material is cut away, either on the knot if it is to be buried or leaving 3- to 4-mm tails if it is a skin suture.

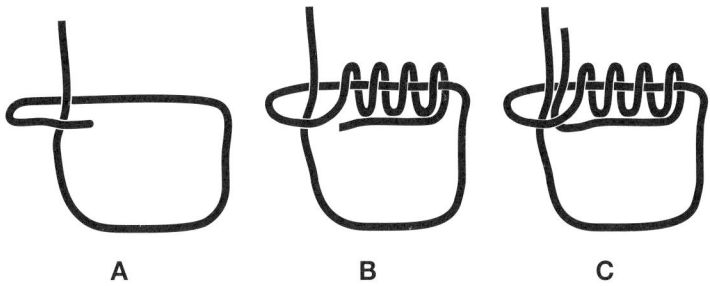

Fig. 26-4
Half blood knot. **A,** Tail passed around the long strand. **B,** Four loops around itself. **C,** Tail put through first loop. (Redrawn from Wattchow DA, Watts JM: *Br J Surg* 71:333, 1984.)

Half Blood Knot

It is useful to know one additional knot for tying suture—the half blood knot. Fishermen use this slipping knot to tie lures onto the end of fishing line. It is a very strong knot, retaining almost all of the strength of the suture material. The half blood knot is the best knot for securing the beginning of a running suture, particularly with monofilament material. General surgeons commonly use it to secure the beginning of a running suture in the linea alba when closing the abdomen, but it also works well to start a running cuticular or subcuticular suture.

After the suture is placed in the tissue, the tail is passed around the working strand of the suture (Fig. 26-4, *A*). Four twists of the tail around itself are made (Fig. 26-4, *B*). More than four twists do not add to the strength of the knot. The tail is then passed up through the first loop, parallel to the working strand (Fig. 26-4, *C*). The knot is tightened by pulling on the tail with a needle holder, then is slipped down to secure the tissue. The working end continues on to construct a running suture line.

CONCLUSION

Suture tying is an art that develops with experience. Close attention to detail is necessary when approximating tissue. The goal is to bring tissue edges into apposition without causing strangulation inside the loop as postoperative swelling develops. The instrument tie is preferred for skin sutures. If a hand tie is to be done, the two-hand technique is preferred. The physician must tie firm square throws by using even tension on each end and must know how many throws to place in each type of suture material to ensure knot security.

SUPPLIER

A useful *Knot Tying Manual* and practice board are available free of charge from the following manufacturer:

Ethicon, Inc.
P.O. Box 151
Sommerville, NJ 08876-0151
Phone: 1-800-255-2500
Website: www.ethiconinc.com

BIBLIOGRAPHY

Fewkes JL, Cheney ML, Pollack SV: *Illustrated atlas of cutaneous surgery,* Philadelphia, 1992, JB Lippincott.
James JD, Wu MM, Batra EK, et al: Technical considerations in manual and instrument tying techniques, *J Emerg Med* 10:469, 1992.
Knot tying manual, Sommerville, NJ, 1996, Ethicon, Inc.
Revington P, Bowyer RC: Sutures: the economics of knot tying techniques, *Ann R Coll Surg Engl* 76:281, 1994.
Rosin E, Robinson GM: Knot security of suture materials, *Vet Surg* 18:269, 1989.

CHAPTER 27

Laser Therapy

Edward M. Zimmerman

Ablating tissue, skin lesions, blood vessels, hair, and pigment with laser (*l*ight *a*mplification by *s*imulated *e*mission of *r*adiation) and intense, noncoherent, pulsed light (IPL) devices is an increasingly common area of in-office surgery. This chapter is primarily an introduction to lasers and covers safety, biophysics, and useful wavelengths.

Briefly, a laser beam is made of a group of massless particles of light energy called *photons*. It is generated when an external energy force is applied to a tube containing an excitable medium (gas, liquid, or solid). A population of photons is energized, and these photons bounce back and forth between the fully and partially reflecting mirrors at each end of the laser tube until a small number of them are released as a focused laser beam. These photons travel together in parallel, collimated paths. These photons are in coherent phase spatially and temporally and all share the same monochromatic wavelength.

Each laser is primarily one wavelength occupying a particular part of the electromagnetic spectrum, of which only some is visible light (Fig. 27-1). The different wavelengths are measured in nanometers or billionths of a meter. The energy of each particular wavelength is optimally absorbed by a specific-color target or *chromophore*. An *absorption curve* is the percentage of energy absorbed by chromophores (e.g., hemoglobin or melanin) by the various wavelengths across the electromagnetic spectrum. Therefore, if the objective is to ablate certain tissues, it makes sense to pick a wavelength with energies that are optimally absorbed by that given target. This accomplishes destruction of that target with the fewest side effects.

The energy of the 10,600-nm wavelength CO_2 laser is absorbed completely by water or anything containing water. CO_2 lasers with lower power and cost are generally adequate for ablating benign lesions, excising skin tumors and cysts, and performing minor cosmetic procedures. Skin resurfacing (laser dermabrasion) requires more expensive, high-powered, short-pulsed (Superpulse/Ultrapulse [with or without computer pat-

tern generators] or erbium:YAG) lasers that instantly vaporize tissue while minimizing thermal damage to adjacent areas.

Skin resurfacing is a procedure fraught with potential side effects and complications and has a significant learning curve compared with other, less invasive methods of skin rejuvenation, such as 1320 nm Nd:YAG use, superficial radiofrequency ablation, and microdermabrasion. All of these can be coupled with tissue fillers and Botox. (See Chapter 48, Botox [Botulinum A Exotoxin]; Chapter 49, Collagen Injections; and Chapter 52, Microdermabrasion.)

Lasers with wavelengths that are absorbed mainly by melanin pigment in benign skin lesions and hair follicles, and by hemoglobin in vascular lesions, have dropped in price and yet have increased in dependability, portability, power, and speed over the past decade. These machines are used primarily for cosmetic procedures.

IPL (PhotoDerm [Lumenis], Prolite [Alderm], etc.) produces intense flashes of visible light from 500 to 1200 nm. Depending on the pigment or pigments targeted, filters are used to block out unwanted wavelengths. Power, pulse duration, and delays between pulses are programmable. This proprietary equipment is still fairly expensive ($60,000 to $160,000 plus $5000 to $10,000 a year for the service contract). However, it offers a minimally invasive single-unit instrument for treating multiple vascular and pigmented lesions, including darker hair, and for performing superficial nonablative facial rejuvenation.

Decreases in insurance reimbursements have frustrated many physicians. However, the amount a patient is willing to pay and the demand for aesthetic procedures have grown, especially when the procedures are based in the office. It is now possible for some physicians to be trained and to maintain the proficiency necessary to operate lasers of various wavelengths in their offices, whether the lasers are owned, leased, or rented.

Lasers are expensive. The price of adding any equipment to the office should be analyzed carefully

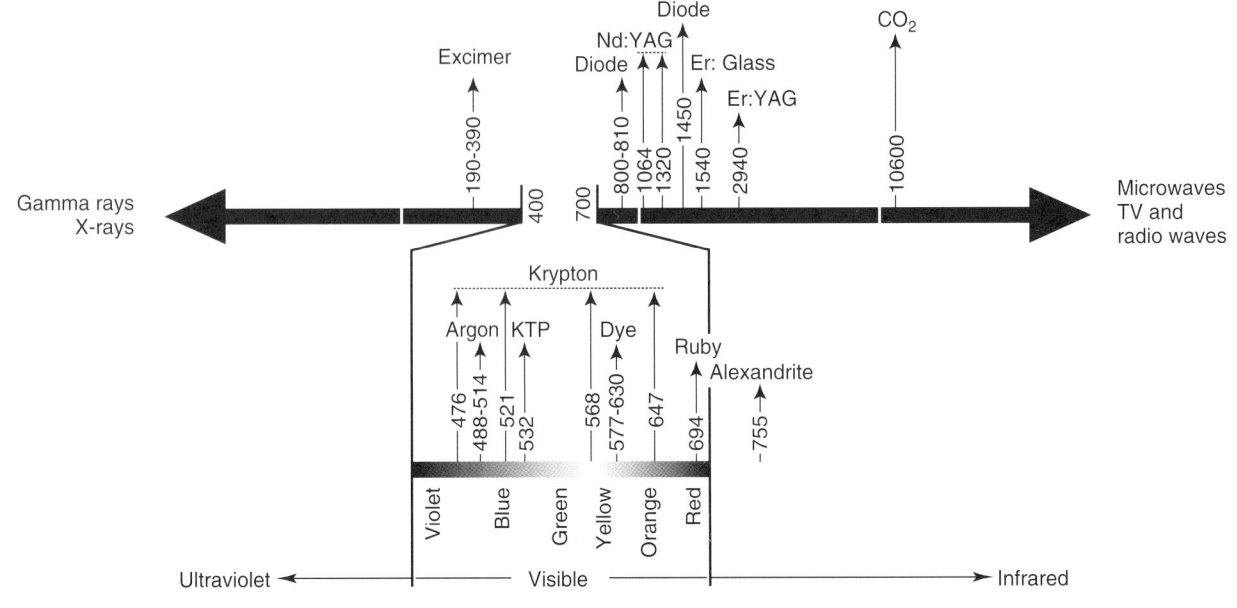

Fig. 27-1
Electromagnetic spectrum.

and justified conservatively before buying or renting it. In the cost analysis, the expense of continuing medical education courses, disposables (e.g., wave guides, handpieces, smoke evacuator filters, tips, laser-safe masks, eye protection), service contracts, office staff, taxes, insurance, and advertising must be considered. A good smoke evacuator is necessary for use with CO_2 or erbium lasers and costs $1500 to $4000 new.

Many primary care physicians (and even veterinarians) now own or share CO_2 lasers for office procedures because the prices of current solid state units have dropped on both the new and the secondary market. However, many of these units sit unused, are underused, or were returned to leasing companies following payment default because the physicians and staffs lacked good planning and follow-through. Most malpractice carriers and hospital credentialing committees currently evaluate training and proficiency on a case-by-case basis. The American Society for Laser Medicine and Surgery and The American Board of Laser Surgery are rich educational resources that are interested in furthering the growth and integrity of this field for all specialties.

INVASIVE LASERS

Table 27-1 provides a list of lasers. There are two types that can readily cut and ablate tissue: CO_2 and erbium:YAG lasers. (Erbium:YAG lasers are primarily for cosmetic skin resurfacing and beyond the scope of this chapter.)

CO_2 LASERS

Indications and Uses of CO_2 Lasers

- When there is a need for excellent surgical precision and bloodless field
- To ablate superficial skin lesions anywhere on the body (e.g., traumatized lesions, lesions rubbed by clothing, cosmetic reasons)
- To excise cysts, lipomas, and benign lumps under or in skin that bother patients because of irritation or cosmesis, and wide excision/biopsies of lesions suspicious for cancer
- To precisely undermine and revise scars and keloids
- To destroy periungual or extensive verrucae
- To ablate extensive condyloma (especially vaginal and perianal)
- To destroy actinic cheilitis
- To reduce rhinophyma
- For laser-assisted uvulopalatoplasty and laser-assisted tonsillar ablation
- To remove external hemorrhoids, skin tags, and grade 4 internal hemorrhoids (an infrared coagulator may be better for grades 1 to 2)
- To excise bowenoid papulosis, dysplasia, or squamous cell carcinoma (SCC) of the penis
- To excise SCC in situ of the vulva (VIN III)
- To treat cervical dysplasia (both ablation and conization)
- To obliterate syringomas and xanthelasma
- To treat ingrown and fungal nails (partial lateral and total matrixectomy)

TABLE 27-1

Laser Wavelengths and Uses

Type of Laser/ Cost (New)	Major Wavelength (nm)	Applications
Alexandrite $60,000-$80,000	755	Pigmented lesions/hair, black and green tattoo ink (Q-switched)
Argon, KTP, Krypton $20,000-$60,000	488/514, 532, 476/521/568/647	Photocoagulation in the eye, small vascular (1-3 mm) and pigmented lesions
CO$_2$ $20,000-$65,000	10,600	Cutting, drilling, and vaporizing any tissue except bone
Copper:Bromide $45,000-$60,000	511/578	Pigmented/vascular lesions
Diode $30,000-$130,000	800-810 1450	Pigmented lesions, small veins, and hair ablation Nonablative dermal remodeling and skin tightening
Dye (Pulsed) $90,000-$130,000	300 to 1000 (tunable); mainly 585-595	Vascular and pigmented lesions, lithotripsy, and red tattoo ink
Erbium:Glass $60,000-$75,000	1540	Nonablative, dermal remodeling/skin tightening
Erbium-YAG $42,000-$85,000	2940	Skin vaporization: no cautery or coagulation with 300-msec pulsewidth; less ablation and more subdermal heating/cautery with longer (750-1000 msec) pulsewidth
Gold Vapor N/A	628	Photodynamic cancer therapy
Helium-Neon N/A	633	Aiming beam, laser pointer, bar code and scanners
Holmium:YAG $80,000	2100	Endoscopic surgery
Neodymium:YAG $70,000-$90,000	1064 (veins and tattoos) 1320 (skin tightening)	Veins <5 mm, red tattoo ink (frequency doubled, Q-switched), skin tightening through induction of dermal collagenosis
Ruby $45,000-$90,000	694	Pigmented, vascular lesions/hair, black and green tattoo ink (Q-switched)

- When electrosurgery is contraindicated or other techniques have failed
- To remove tattoos (Q-switched laser, infrared coagulator, or PhotoDerm is better)
- To enable laser (cosmetic) skin resurfacing/facial rejuvenation

The laser can be used on a myriad of other lesions as well. The previous list of indications is narrowed to include only those clinical situations in which the CO$_2$ laser often produces better outcomes than other modalities.

Contraindications for Excision or Skin Resurfacing with CO$_2$ Lasers

- Large vascular lesions (other laser modalities or sclerotherapy are preferred)
- Known HIV-positive status *(relative contraindication)* because the virus has been found in the smoke (use a smoke evacuator with viral filter)
- Bleeding disorders *(relative contraindication)*
- Tendency to hyperpigment or hypopigment or form keloids *(relative contraindication)*

Advantages

- Cutting, vaporizing, and coagulation of tissue are precise.
- Better hemostasis provides a clean, dry surgical

field, which improves visibility and decreases surgical time.
- Scarring is reduced (in most instances).
- Infection is rare (CO$_2$ laser sterilizes as it cuts and vaporizes).
- Possibly, there is less pain and swelling because sensory nerve endings and lymphatics are cauterized.
- Procedure can be performed in the office with no special electrical or cooling requirements.
- Patients equate "high tech" with physician competence, providing an improved image and higher patient confidence.

Disadvantages

- There is a costly initial investment or long-term lease until the investment becomes profitable.
- Equipment requires significant space.
- There is a variable, often steep, learning curve.
- Incisions made with continuous wave CO$_2$ lasers take slightly longer to heal than scalpel or UltraPulsed CO$_2$ incisions.
- Need to be aware of safety issues (e.g., use nonreflective instruments, protect adjacent tissues, use eye protection).
- Smoke production requires a smoke evacuator to remove odors and possible viral and organic particles.

- The many nonvascular, skin lesions (e.g., skin tags, moles, and cysts) can be treated with less expensive modalities that are effective and safe and produce acceptable cosmetic results in the right hands.

Techniques for CO_2 Laser Use

Anything containing water absorbs the energy of the CO_2 laser wavelength (1060 nm). This makes the CO_2 laser particularly useful for cutting, sculpting, and precisely vaporizing tissue when the laser is focused perpendicular to the target so that a high-power density is achieved in a small (0.25- to 1-mm) spot. When the laser tip is defocused (pulled away from the tissue) so that the spot size enlarges and the power density decreases, the CO_2 laser cauterizes small vessels precisely.

The energy beam is actually not visible, but it is linked with a visible light so that the operator knows where it is aimed (active). This invisible laser functions like a scalpel or Bovie, but the tissue is not touched directly by any instrument. Everyone in the room must wear clear, wavelength-specific eye protection (the patient wears stainless steel corneal covers). A medical-grade smoke evacuator must be used to limit the resultant plume during surgery. Standard surgical techniques and closures are followed.

Complications

- Hypertrophic scarring (especially with tattoos)
- Postoperative skin texture and pigment (hyperpigmentation and hypopigmentation) changes
- Prolonged erythema and skin fragility
- Reactivation of herpes infections
- Eye injury to personnel or patients if their eyes are not properly protected *(rare)*
- Risk of fire or explosion *(very rare)* if combustible materials or oxygen is in the surgical field
- Unintentional burns to patients, personnel, or operator *(rare)*
- Unrealistic patient or physician expectations

NONINVASIVE LASERS (also see Chapter 51, Laser Hair Removal: Photoepilation)

A variety of lasers have been used to treat flat, vascular lesions (port-wine stains and telangiectatic vessels) since the late 1970s. Early lasers used an argon lasing medium, and hemoglobin and melanin were the pigmented targets (chromophores) for this wavelength. These machines were difficult to use because the spot size was limited to 1 to 2 mm, and the relatively long pulse duration did not allow selective photothermolysis.

Much more useful lasers like the pulsed tunable dye and other lasers listed in Table 27-1 became available later. These machines have larger treatment spot sizes and short or variable pulse durations, which allow the interior of small blood vessels to be destroyed without much heating of the surrounding tissue. Consequently, blood vessels are destroyed in preference to the surrounding dermis. This reduces the incidence of scarring to nearly zero. Superficial pigmented lesions (solar lentigines, or age spots) are treated in similar fashion.

Currently available lasers with wavelengths in the 500- to 700-nm range with larger spot sizes and the IPL devices penetrate up to 5 mm into the dermis.

Indications (please see Table 27-1)

- Flat and nearly flat vascular lesions such as port-wine stains, spider telangiectasias, and small hemangiomas (e.g., cherry angiomas, pyogenic granulomas)
- Larger hemangiomas (e.g., strawberry hemangiomas, cavernous hemangiomas, small [up to 3 mm] superficial vessels)
- Benign, flat, pigmented lesions like lentigines and melasma
- Hair removal

Diode (800 nm) and Nd:YAG (1064 nm) are also able to penetrate 3 to 5 mm into the dermis and are useful for treating the following:

- Blue, reticular vessels that are less than 5 mm in diameter
- Dark hair

Injection sclerotherapy and ambulatory phlebectomy are still the gold standard for larger leg veins. IPL is useful, not only for hair removal, but for treating the pigmentary and vascular changes of solar aging on the hands, chest, neck and face.

In the quest for reduced recovery periods and less side effects, several wavelengths have been found to cause "nonablative, dermal remodeling." These lasers (1320-, 1450-, and 1540-nm wavelengths) use scatter and absorption of energy by intracellular water and collagen to cause modest damage to the dermal and subcutaneous tissues with minimal epidermal trauma. Most of these units use some system of epidermal cooling. Healing causes new collagen and fibrin to be formed and a gradual, mild "rejuvenation appearance" ensues. Three to ten treatments, 3 to 6 weeks apart, followed by periodic maintenance treatments are required to decrease superficial wrinkles and acne scars 20% to 50% in all skin types. Younger patients usually respond better to these treatments. One pulsed dye laser (N-Lite) has been marketed aggressively to physicians for this purpose. However, it has been variably effective in double-blinded studies performed independently.

Tattoo Removal

Before the introduction of pulsed lasers, tattoos were removed by dermabrasion, CO_2 laser ablation, or excision, with obliteration and scarring being the usual result. Use of the infrared coagulator (see Chapter 54, Tattoo Removal: Infrared Light Obliteration Method) has been successful for some. Because different color tattoo inks optimally absorb the energy of different wavelengths, tattoo treatment requires several wavelengths of nanosecond-pulsed, Q-switched lasers over 6 to 12 treatments to decrease tattoo visibility.

In theory, the extremely short pulses of laser energy rupture the pigment molecules into smaller bits, allowing them to be extruded with the scab as the area heals or to be absorbed by macrophages. Scarring (sometimes hypertrophic) also helps obscure deeper pigment. Temporary pigment changes of the surrounding skin are not unusual. IPL has been used to soften and improve dark green, blue, and black tattoos, but it rarely eradicates them entirely without hypopigmenting the surrounding skin. No lasers currently treat yellow, white, and light blues. Some physicians perform erbium resurfacing first, in hopes of improving Q-switched laser penetration. There are no studies documenting additional success using this method.

Treatment of some light colors can result in irreversible and unpredictable darkening by changing ferric oxide (rust) to ferrous oxide (black). There are several reports of allergic reactions (even anaphylaxis) from laser-induced release of tattoo antigens. For these reasons, small test spots are always appropriate. It is wise to wait months between treatments to let the body rid itself of as much ink as possible and to heal from previous laser trauma before inducing more injury. Q-switched lasers can safely and effectively "remove" some tattoos containing dark greens, blues, and reds amazingly well. However, after a number of expensive and uncomfortable laser or IPL treatments, 30% of patients still have visible, laser-altered tattoos.

New and previously untreated tattoos of all colors may respond better—with less cost, side effects, and scarring—to a new technique by Rejuvi Laboratory. This system uses inorganic salts, driven into the skin by tattooing, to bind tattoo inks that are then expelled more easily by the body. All skin types can be treated. Previously treated tattoos do not seem to respond as well, and some hypertrophic scarring has been observed in initial trials (see Cheng, 2001).

Contraindications

- Inappropriate wavelength, spot size, and fluence for the application
- Active skin infection in the treatment area
- Darker skin types or recently tanned skin require conservative treatment or pretreatment with sunblocks and bleaches
- Imminent sun exposure (2 to 4 weeks after treatment) gives high risk for hyperpigmentation
- Recurrent herpetic infections; prophylactic medications should be given before and after treatment
- Unrealistic expectation for a "perfect" result

Advantages

- Appropriate wavelength, spot size and fluence gives better cosmesis in less treatments
- Performed in office
- Performed by staff if allowed by state regulations and malpractice (frees up physician)
- Only local or topical anesthesia required (if any, many new lasers use chill tips or spray cooling)
- Convenient for patients: short visits, weeks or months apart, little or no time required for patient to recuperate
- Perception of state-of-the-art practice is beneficial for attracting and retaining patients
- Most of these procedures are considered "cosmetic," not covered by insurance and thus paid for by the patient at the time of service

Disadvantages

- Costly, space-occupying equipment is required. (The newest units are compact, elegant, wheeled, and expensive. Older units are larger, still useful, and discounted substantially.)
- Safety issues are pressing: for example, wavelength-specific eye protection is required for everyone in the treatment room.
- Burnt hair smell is strong. (A smoke evacuator can be used, or the room can be vented with an exhaust fan.)
- Some systems require messy coupling gel (ultrasound gel).
- Multiple treatments are required (6 to 12 or more for tattoos).
- No one laser wavelength does everything well; therefore multiple lasers may be needed for some pathologies.
- Equipment is evolving so rapidly that it is difficult and expensive to maintain technology leadership.

Equipment

- Appropriate wavelength and pulse-width vascular/ pigment targeting laser (Table 27-1)
- Eye protection for patient, observers, medical assistants, and operator
- Pretreatment and posttreatment cooling of treatment area with "chillers," if necessary

- Clear ultrasound gel for some lasers and all IPL devices (refrigerated)
- Topical anesthesia gel or cream

PREPROCEDURE PATIENT PREPARATION

Patients must be thoroughly educated about the results, side effects, and cost of therapy per unit area; this cost varies depending on the laser system. Patients must realize that successful therapy may require multiple treatment sessions for each specific site. Insurance rarely covers cosmetic procedures. Treatments usually cost $400 to $600 per hour or are sold in packages for treatment of a given area to a certain result. Treatment is often given in quarter and half-hour sessions of 200 to 450 pulses. It helps to show patients representative photographs of preprocedure appearance, immediate postprocedure appearance, and results at 2- to 4-month intervals so that they appreciate what to expect along the course of treatment. Videotapes are also useful to enhance patient education. Most companies supply these for their particular products.

Performing a small test spot or patch in an inconspicuous area that the patient can easily watch is beneficial. It teaches the patient what the treatment feels like and what to expect when further treatments are done. Laser pulses feel like the sharp snap of a hot rubber band against the skin. The sensation gradually subsides, and treated areas feel sunburned for several days. Purpura and bruising can take several days to weeks to subside. Tattoos take months between treatments to eject pigment or absorb it through macrophage digestion. Patient discomfort varies with the level of patient anxiety (premedicating may be appropriate), the type of cooling provided, and the use of topical, local, or tumescent anesthesia.

Technique for Noninvasive Lasers

Laser procedures are painful, but they can be tolerated by most adults who are motivated to achieve the end result. After showing the patient the appropriate photographs and answering all questions, perform a test patch on several sites. Try to pick those areas most sensitive and least sensitive to the laser. Specific techniques of test patching vary. Some physicians prefer to use four separate energy levels within a single test patch. Others prefer to fill an area of about 1 cm^2 on a certain body site with laser pulses at a certain energy level, and then increase or decrease the energy levels on other body sites as needed. In general, all laser and IPL handpieces should be kept perpendicular to the treatment surface at the distance and parameters specified by the manufacturer for treating the particular lesion. Warn the patient that you are about to fire the instrument, and, after several pulses, examine the test patch for initial result.

Oral sedation or anesthesia helps some patients. Eutectic mixture of local anesthetic (EMLA) or similar creams and gels help reduce skin pain by 25% to 75%, depending on the patient and the degree of anxiety (see Chapter 11, Topical Anesthesia). For oral sedation and analgesia, try diazepam 10 mg or alprazolam 2 mg orally or sublingually for adults, and chloral hydrate 50 to 100 mg/kg orally for very young children (maximum 1 g). Versed also comes in syrup form and works well (see Chapter 7, Pediatric Sedation). A small piece of candy helps mask the bitter flavor of the sublingual medications. The advantage of sublingual medications is that the dose can be titrated during the procedure.

Endpoints of treatment are similar regardless of the system used. Parameters for each system are based on manufacturer guidelines, patient pathology, skin color, and lesion depth. Vascular lesions should blanch briefly, contract, and have delayed filling after compression. Purpura indicates that small vessels in the dermis have been ruptured. Pigmented lesions should darken or even turn slightly gray and contract. Epidermal dehiscence is not uncommon. Tattoos may erupt vigorously and become raised with punctate bleeding and appear (temporarily) more vibrant than before treatment. Hairs should develop a perifollicular elevation (like tiny hives) within minutes after treatment, and about 30% of the hairs should slide out easily when the ideal parameters are attained. Appropriate cleansing, topical applications, and dressings or sunblocks are applied after the treatment areas are cooled. The patient is given a written explanation of the treatment, and postoperative care and follow-up is scheduled. The patient should receive a phone call from the office a few days after the first treatment for reassurance and reinforcement of postoperative care.

The patient is seen again after 1 to 4 months, a sufficient amount of time for complete healing. On the patient's subsequent visits, treat larger areas with the laser parameters and postoperative care that have produced the best results with the fewest side effects. Each interaction that sunscreens and protective clothing should be emphasized as an important part of the protocol for successful, uneventful treatment.

Complications

- Same as for CO_2 lasers. Minimize complications by using the right wavelength, spot size, pulse width, and fluence (energy) for the job and treating the patient conservatively. More can always be performed later.

- Hyperpigmentation caused by trauma resolves over months. Skin bleaches, protective clothing, and sunblocks help the patient avoid long-term pigmentation. Postinflammatory pigmentation is part of normal healing.
- Temporary purpura, bruising, and histamine response are common.
- Unpredictable darkening of, hypertrophic scarring of, or allergic reactions to tattoo pigments during laser treatment can be lessened by performing small test patches with different parameters (wavelength, pulse width, fluence, hertz, etc.) to see which ones work best.
- Patients must understand that the treatment endpoint is improvement, not perfection. Some pigment, vessels or fine, light hairs are likely to remain or recur over time, despite best efforts.

POSTPROCEDURE PATIENT EDUCATION

Laser-treated skin is fragile, like newborn skin. It is crucial that the patient keep the area lubricated with a topical antibiotic ointment if the skin blisters or breaks down. (See the sample patient education handout titled "Skin Care Instructions After Laser Treatment" on page 1763 of Appendix G.) In addition, the patient must avoid sun exposure and local trauma. He or she should refrain from contact sports for the first 5 to 10 days.

Sunblocks should be often and liberally used for several months after treatment to decrease the risk of hyperpigmentation. Topical retinoids and fruit acids should be avoided for several weeks until the skin recovers. Makeup may be applied gently to intact skin. Patients should be reminded that the absorption curves of hemoglobin and melanin are similar enough of wavelengths that some damage to one is inevitable when treating the other. Transient erythema and variations in pigmentation are common, despite appropriate precautions and treatment parameters. Postinflammatory hyperpigmentation is a normal part of healing. It resolves with time, often 2 to 8 months. Textural changes, evidence of hypertrophic healing, and other symptoms should be treated as they arise on an individual basis. Patients must understand that they should be seen if there is any question or potential complication.

DOCUMENTATION

The surgical note should list the sites of treatment, wavelengths, anesthesia, treatment parameters, number of pulses delivered, initial response to treatment, whether analgesia was adequate, and patient condition on discharge. This is particularly important when treating children. A checklist can document that American National Standards Institute safety protocols were followed. These include documentation or checklist of signed consent, door signage, eye protection for patient and staff, smoke evacuation used (for ablative lasers), and windows and mirrors covered. Photographs taken immediately before and after the procedure are very helpful and become part of the patient's record. The photo log can double as a personal laser case log.

TRAINING

Training in use of lasers is just becoming available in residencies. Continuing medical education meetings and preceptorships are available by contacting the following organizations:

The American Society for Laser Medicine and Surgery
2404 Stewart Square
Wausau, WI 54401
Phone: 1-715-845-9283
Website: www.aslms.org

The Laser Institute of America
13501 Ingenuity Drive, Suite 128
Orlando, FL 32826
Phone: 1-407-380-1553
Website: www.laserinstitute.org

The National Procedures Institute
4909 Hedgewood Drive
Midland, MI 48640
Phone: 1-800-462-2492
Website: www.npinstitute.com

Fellowships for physicians with board eligibility in dermatology or surgical specialties are available through the following:
American Academy of Cosmetic Surgery
401 N. Michigan Ave.
Chicago, IL 60611-4267
Phone: 1-312-527-6713
Website: www.cosmeticsurgery.org

Also, many laser manufacturers and distributors offer education and preceptorships for the equipment they sell.

CONCLUSION

The arena of outpatient laser and IPL procedures is rapidly expanding and evolving. It is owned by no specialty at this time, but many regulatory bodies will try to enforce standards soon. It is in everyone's best interest to avidly train each other and ourselves so that all patients may reap maximal benefit from these new tools and so that sensible standards of care are developed.

SUPPLIERS

Laser manufacturers and distributors are numerous. In addition, many companies now sell refurbished lasers. Carefully weigh the age, dependability, and warranty on the unit as well as the reputation and longevity of the company.

Alderm N.A., LLC
17951 Skypark Circle, Suite G
Irvine, CA 92614
Phone: 1-800-254-8505
Website: www.aldermna.com

Altus Medical
821 Cowan Road
Burlingame, CA 94010
Phone: 1-650-552-9700
Website: www.altusmedical.com

Asclepion-Meditec AG
Goeschwitzer Strasse 51-52
07745 Jena
Germany
Phone: +49 (0) 36 41 / 2 20 — 0
Website: www.asclepion.com

Candela Corporation
530 Boston Post Road
Wayland, MA 01778
Phone: 1-800-654-6027
www.clzr.com

Convergent Laser Technologies
900 Alice Street
Oakland, CA 94607
Phone: 1-510-832-2130
Website: www.convergentlaser.com

Cosmos Medical Technologies, Inc.
42230 Zevo Drive
Temecula, CA 92590
Phone: 1-800-634-7921
Website: www.cosmosmed.com

Cynosure Inc.
10 Elizabeth Drive
Chelmsford, MA 01824
Phone: 1-800-886-2966
Website: www.cynosurelaser.com

Diomed Inc.
1 Dundee Park
Andover, MA 01810
Phone: 1-978-475-7771
Website: www.diomed-lasers.com

Focus Medical LLC (makes NaturaLase)
23 Francis J. Clarke Circle
Bethel, CT 06801
Phone: 1-866-633-5273
Website: www.focusmedical.com

ICN Pharmaceuticals, Inc. (bought CoolTouch)
3300 Hyland Avenue
Costa Mesa, CA 92626
Phone: 1-714-545-0100
Website: www.icnpharm.com

Iriderm
1212 Terra Bella Avenue
Mountain View, CA 94043
Phone: 1-650-940-4700
Website: www.iriderm.com

Laserscope
3070 Orchard Drive
San Jose, CA 95134-2011
Phone: 1-800-356-7600
Website: www.laserscope.com

Lumenis
2400 Condensa Street
Santa Clara, CA, 95051
Phone: 1-800-635-1313
Website: www.lumenis.com

Palomar
82 Cambridge Street
Burlington, MA 01803
Phone: 1-800-725-6627
Website: www.palmed.com

Saratoga Diagnostics
12619 Paseo Olivos
Saratoga, CA 95070
Phone: 1-800-998-1555
Website: www.saratogadiagnostics.com

Eye protection, books, supplies

Bernsco
25 Plant Avenue
Hauppauge, NY 11788-3804
Phone: 1-800-843-6266
Website: www.bernsco.com

Biodermis
3078 East Sunset Road, Suite #1
Las Vegas, NV 89120
Phone: 1-800-322-3729
Website: www.biodermis.com

Delasco
608 13th Avenue
Council Bluffs, IA 51501-6401
Phone: 1-800-831-6273
Website: www.delasco.com

Moore Medical Corp.
P.O. Box 1500
New Britain, CT 06050-1500
Phone: 1-800-234-1464
Website: www.mooremedical.com

Oculo-Plastik
200 Sauve West
Montreal (Quebec) Canada
H3L 1YD
Phone: 1-888-381-3292
Website: www.oculoplastik.com

Alternative tattoo removal system

Rejuvi Laboratory Inc.
360 Swift Avenue, Suite 38
South San Francisco, CA 94080
Phone: 1-800-588-2279
Website: www.rejuvilab.com

Patient education handouts

Patient education handouts are available from laser companies for specific procedures using their lasers. MJD Patient Communications makes customizable brochures for many cosmetic procedures.
MJD Patient Communications
7605 Leesburg Drive
Bethesda, MD 20817
Phone: 1-800-326-4869
Website: www.mjdpc.com

LASER CERTIFICATION

The American Board of Laser Surgery was chartered in 1984. It was developed to establish acceptable levels of training and competence for those people who want to use lasers for the care of patient's health. Examinations and peer review of applicants seeking certification of their competence to use lasers are available.
American Board of Laser Surgery
417 Palmtree Drive
Bradenton, FL 34210
Phone: 1-914-756-2316

CPT/BILLING CODES

Billing codes for laser therapy are generally the same as any other modality used for destruction or excision:

17000-17286　　Destruction by any method

Treatment of vascular lesions depend on the size of the area being treated:

17106　　Destruction of cutaneous vascular proliferative lesions <10 cm^2
17107　　Destruction of cutaneous vascular proliferative lesions 10 to 50 cm^2
17108　　Destruction of cutaneous vascular proliferative lesions >50 cm^2
57520　　Conization of the cervix
57513　　Laser ablation of the cervix

ADDITIONAL RESOURCES

See the sample patient education handouts titled "CoolTouch Laser Skin Rejuvenation" and "Skin Care Instructions After Laser Treatment" on pages 1761 and 1763, respectively, of Appendix G.

See the sample patient consent forms titled "Carbon Dioxide Laser Treatment" and "Intense Pulsed Light Treatment" on pages 1764 and 1765, respectively, of Appendix G.

Note: The patient education handout for the CoolTouch laser procedures is included. This sheet can be modified to better fit the procedure and wavelengths being used. Educational and postprocedural care handouts should be made for each procedure performed. The IPL consent form may be modified for pigment, hair, and vascular treatment by particular wavelengths of lasers.

BIBLIOGRAPHY

Aghassi D, Carpo B, Eng K: Complications of aesthetic laser surgery, *Ann Plast Surg* 43:560, 1999.
Alora MB, Anderson RR: Recent developments in cutaneous lasers, *Lasers Surg Med* 26:108, 2000.

Avram M: *Program Book of the Ninth International Symposium on Cosmetic Laser Surgery,* Schaumburg, Ill, 2000, The International Society of Cosmetic Laser Surgeons.

Cheng W: A non-laser method to reverse permanent makeup and tattoos, *Cosmet Dermatol* 14:47, 2001.

Dover J, Arndt K: *Illustrated cutaneous and aesthetic laser surgery,* ed 2, Norwalk, Conn, 2000, Appleton & Lange. (This has good chapters on laser parameters, laser selection, and each major type of laser and treatment protocols.)

Dover J: Roundtable discussion on laser skin resurfacing (review article), *Dermatol Surg* 25:639, 1999.

Dover J, Sadick N, Goldman M: The role of lasers and light sources in the treatment of leg veins, *Dermatol Surg* 25:328, 1999.

Fitzpatrick R, Goldman M: Cosmetic laser surgery, St Louis, 2000, Mosby. (This has good chapters on laser-tissue interactions, wound healing, CO_2 resurfacing of the face, nonablative laser treatment of facial rhytids, and laser treatment of leg veins.)

Lask G, Lowe N: *J Cutan Laser Ther* 1(3), 1999. (This entire issue is devoted to invasive and noninvasive laser procedures.)

Liew S: Unwanted body hair and its removal: a review, *Dermatol Surg* 25:431, 1999.

Nanni C, Alster T: Complications of cutaneous laser surgery, *Dermatol Surg* 24:209, 1998.

Negishi K, Tezuka Y, Kushikata N, et al: Photorejuvenation for Asian skin by intense pulsed light, *Dermatol Surg* 27:627, 2001.

CHAPTER 28

Mucocele Removal

Stephen K. Toadvine*

Oral mucous cysts form as a result of obstruction or trauma involving the ducts of minor salivary glands. Although these glands are found throughout the oral mucosa, mucoceles occur most frequently in the mucosa of the lower lip. Mucoceles appear as soft, compressible lesions with a bluish tinge. Typical size ranges from a few millimeters up to 1 cm, but occasionally much larger lesions occur. Mucoceles may rupture and not recur, but usually they remain persistent or recurrent and should be treated.

EQUIPMENT

- Lidocaine with epinephrine
- Scalpel with no. 11 blade and possibly a no. 15 blade
- Cryocautery or electrocautery unit

PREPROCEDURE PATIENT PREPARATION

See the sample patient education handout titled "Mucocele Treatment" on page 1767 of Appendix G for information to present the patient before the procedure.

TECHNIQUE

Lesions that are not excessively large can be treated effectively with cryotherapy, after the cyst is drained. An injection of lidocaine with epinephrine is given into the mucocele to produce anesthesia and to minimize bleeding by inducing vasoconstriction. With a no. 11 blade, a small stab wound is made in the cyst laterally and the seromucinous contents are expressed. Then a freeze of the lesion (see Chapter 15, Cryosurgery) is performed to produce a 2- to 3-mm rim of ice around the lesion. Cryotherapy without anesthesia and without decompression of the mucocele has been described, but much more effective freezing will be accomplished if the mucinous contents are first evacuated.

As an alternative to cryotherapy, electrocautery may be used to lightly desiccate the lesion after incision and drainage. For larger, or significantly protuberant lesions, shaving away the roof of the lesion with a no. 15 blade before proceeding to cryotherapy or electrodesiccation may improve results (Fig. 28-1). If cryotherapy is chosen, hemostasis should be obtained before the freeze. A chemical coagulant, such as Monsel's solution, is useful here.

Recurrent lesions may be retreated as above. Persistently recurrent lesions or cysts located more deeply in the submucosa may need to be completely excised.

CPT/BILLING CODE

40810   Excision/destruction, lesion of mucosa and submucosa, vestibule of mouth

ICD-9-CM DIAGNOSTIC CODE

527.6   Oral mucocele

ADDITIONAL RESOURCES

- See the sample patient education handout titled "Mucocele Treatment" on page 1767 of Appendix G.

---

*Dr. Toadvine contributes to this edition with the understanding that he objects to the inclusion of Chapter 130 (Abortion) in this edition.

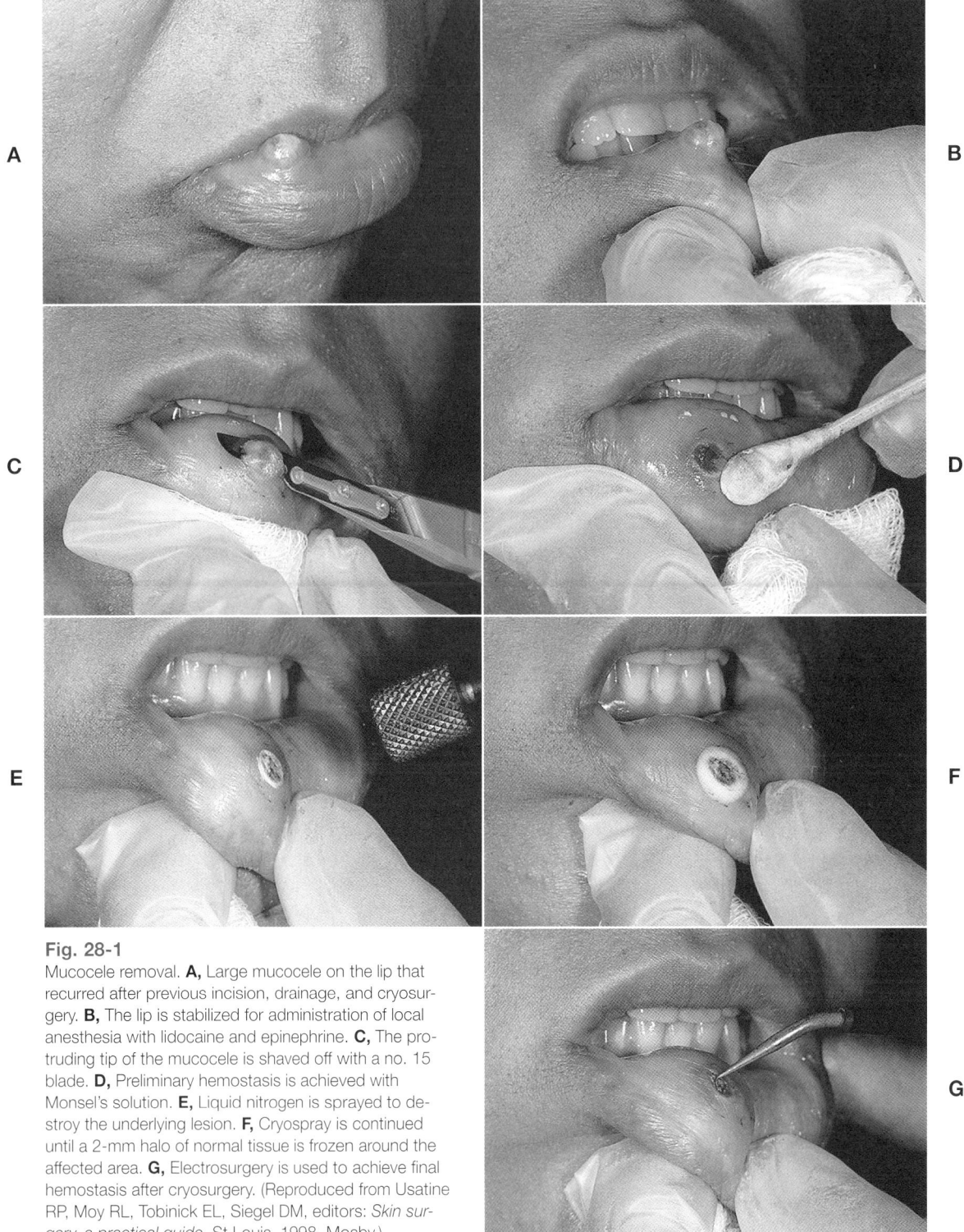

Fig. 28-1

Mucocele removal. **A,** Large mucocele on the lip that recurred after previous incision, drainage, and cryosurgery. **B,** The lip is stabilized for administration of local anesthesia with lidocaine and epinephrine. **C,** The protruding tip of the mucocele is shaved off with a no. 15 blade. **D,** Preliminary hemostasis is achieved with Monsel's solution. **E,** Liquid nitrogen is sprayed to destroy the underlying lesion. **F,** Cryospray is continued until a 2-mm halo of normal tissue is frozen around the affected area. **G,** Electrosurgery is used to achieve final hemostasis after cryosurgery. (Reproduced from Usatine RP, Moy RL, Tobinick EL, Siegel DM, editors: *Skin surgery, a practical guide,* St Louis, 1998, Mosby.)

BIBLIOGRAPHY

Allen CM, Blozia GG: Oral mucosal lesions. In Cummings CW, Harker LA, Krause CJ, et al, editors: *Otolaryngology: head and neck surgery*, ed 3, St Louis, 1998, Mosby.

Gill D: Two simple treatments for lower lip mucocoeles, *Australas J Dermatol* 37:220, 1996.

Granick MS et al., Benign and malignant tumors of the oral cavity. In Georgiade GS, Riefkohl R, Levin LS, editors: *Plastic, maxillofacial and reconstructive surgery*, ed 3, Baltimore, 1997, Williams & Wilkins.

Tobinick EL: Diagnosis and treatment of benign and premalignant lesions. In Usatine RP, Moy RL, Tobinick EL, Siegel DM, editors: *Skin surgery: a practical guide*, St Louis, 1998, Mosby.

Usatine RP: Electrosurgery. In Usatine RP, Moy RL, Tobinick EL, Siegel DM, editors: *Skin surgery: a practical guide*, St Louis, 1998, Mosby.

CHAPTER 29

Nail Bed Repair

Douglas R. Jackson

The fingernail is a highly evolved structure designed to enhance the functions of the distal finger. The fingernail functions to (1) protect the distal phalanx, (2) enhance the fine touch and fine digital movements, (3) facilitate scratching and grooming, and (4) provide esthetics and cosmetic considerations.

The appearance of the fingernails has long provided a clue to past history of local or systemic disease as well as events of previous trauma. The appearance of the fingernails is often regarded as a key indicator of personal hygiene. A severely deformed fingernail can be a source of embarrassment. The fingernail may be the first site of a benign or malignant tumor, which may manifest itself only as an area of "slow healing" or deformed or discolored nail plate. A good primary repair of the injured nail bed yields a high percentage of good results. Meanwhile the results of excessively delayed repairs and revisions of faulty repairs have a much poorer prognosis.

Consideration for repair includes (1) a thorough anatomic knowledge of the structure to be restored, (2) availability of all the sterile equipment required (including excellent lighting and loupe magnification), (3) the ability to counsel the patient on what to expect over the 6 to 12 months of follow-up that will be required to see the final nail growth, and (4) the ability to recognize those injuries that may exceed the physician's training and experience, requiring referral to a hand surgeon.

Informing the patient *before* any repair effort that the resultant fingernail may be deformed or absent in spite of your best efforts spares the physician and the patient much grief in the end. Preoperative (close-up) photographs are a strong document. Patients sometimes forget exactly what the physician had to start with and instead recall only how wonderful the fingernail looked before the injury, expecting the physician to replicate the preinjury status.

INDICATIONS

Any disruption of the normal anatomy distal to the tendinous insertions of the extensor and deep flexor tendons on the finger or the thumb may adversely influence the growth, configuration, quality, and function of the nail plate unit. Sometimes a crushing injury with no penetration of the nail may cause more disfigurement than a sharp penetration, which may extend through the nail to the underlying phalanx.

ANATOMY

The nail unit is composed of four distinct epithelial structures: the proximal nail fold, the nail matrix, the nail bed, and the hyponychium (Fig. 29-1). The lateral nail folds (Fig. 29-2) are adjacent normal epidermal folds that border the nail unit laterally. The proximal nail fits into a grove of tissue called the "proximal nail fold." The skin over the dorsum of the nail fold is the *nail wall*. The *eponychium* is the thin membrane extending from the nail wall onto the dorsum of the nail. The *lunula* is the curved, white opacity in the nail, just distal to the *eponychium*. It is the indicator of the junction between the germinal and sterile matrix. The matrix is the most important component of the nail unit, since it is responsible for the formation of the nail plate. Detailed anatomic understanding of the perionychial components of the nail area are required for consideration of nail repairs. They are as follows:

1. *Nail plate (nail)*. Formation begins in the germinal matrix under the proximal nail fold. It is made up of desiccated, keratinized, squamous cells. Note how the nail plate fits into the groove of the proximal nail fold (Fig. 29-1).

2. *Nail bed*. This lies under the nail plate, beginning at the distal edge of the nail matrix and continuing until the hyponychium. It is very vascular and thus appears pink. The space between the nail bed and underlying bony structure is very thin (1 to 3 mm) without any subcutaneous tissue.

3. *Eponychium*. Dorsal roof of the proximal fold that serves as protection for the underlying germinal matrix. It is a part of the germinal matrix providing a thin layer of cells and producing the shiny dorsal nail surface.

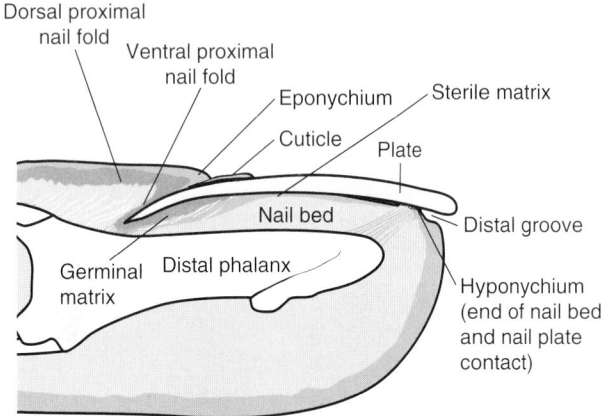

Fig. 29-1
Sagittal view of the nail and distal phalanx.

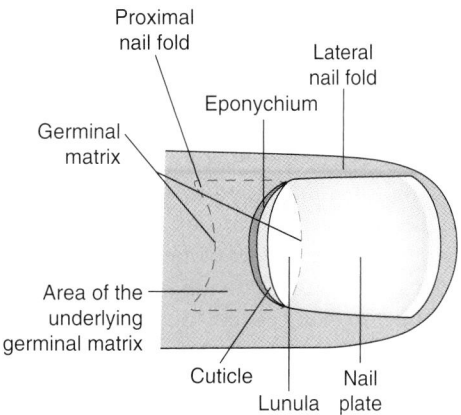

Fig. 29-2
Dorsal view of the nail. The sterile matrix underlies the nail plate distal to the lunula (proximal to the lunula is the germinal matrix) under the nail plate.

4. *Germinal matrix*. Site where nail production begins and extends distally just beyond the eponychium to end at the distal border of the lunula.
5. *Sterile matrix*. Described by some observers as the "road bed" for the advancing nail. It adds squamous cells to thicken the nail and enhance adherence of it to the nail bed. (Note: The sterile matrix is the distal portion of the nail bed, beyond the germinal matrix. The germinal matrix serves as the nail origin; the sterile matrix only adds to the nail thickness.)
6. *Hyponychium*. The distal site where the nail separates from the nail matrix. This area allows the nail to become independent of the nail matrix.
7. *Paronychium*. Consists of the lateral nail folds and adjacent cutaneous portions of the lateral nail borders.
8. *Lateral nail folds*. Epithelium bordering the nail laterally.
9. *Cuticle*. The translucent vein of tissue that extends out to the surface of the nail where it emerges from

beneath the proximal nail fold. It acts as a barrier or seal to protect the nail unit from external irritants and seals the proximal nail fold to the nail.

PHYSIOLOGY

Nail formation occurs in three layers. The *dorsal* layer arises from the dorsal roof of the nail fold, the *intermediate* layer from the ventral floor and the lateral walls of the proximal nail, and the *ventral* layer from the sterile matrix of the nail bed. The ventral layer provides adherence and enhances the nail thickness to compensate for wearing away on the dorsal surface. The nail grows distally as a resultant force of the pressure placed on the growing cell mass beneath the proximal nail fold. The resultant nail advances distally, hugging the underlying nail bed. Any distortion of these anatomic templates (e.g., proximal nail fold, nail matrix contour and composition) can lead to a deformed and unattractive nail.

Full-length fingernail growth takes 4 to 6 months and is frequently suspended completely for 3 weeks after an acute traumatic event. Fingernails reportedly grow four times as rapidly as toenails. Peak nail growth rate occurs at about age 30. The material produced by the roof of the nail fold is responsible for the shiny surface of the nail.

FRACTURES

An x-ray examination must be performed on any injury with possible involvement of the bone to avoid missing a fracture that may deform the nail bed if left unreduced and unstable. These fractures, when coupled with a drained subungual hematoma, automatically become open fractures and must be treated with the appropriate caution.

SUBUNGUAL HEMATOMA

(See Chapter 36, Subungual Hematoma Evacuation.)

The nail bed is a highly vascular area subject to bleeding with either sharp or nonpenetrating blunt trauma. If the trauma produces a hematoma occupying more than 30% of the visible nail space, the nail should be removed to facilitate meticulous magnified inspection and careful repair of the nail bed. The prerequisites for inspection include (1) good anesthesia, (2) good light and loupe magnification, (3) essential sterile equipment, (4) sterile saline for irrigation, and (5) adequate retraction assistance to carefully investigate the area deep to the proximal and lateral nail folds. To release the painful hematoma, first cleanse the finger with Betadine solution for several minutes (no anesthesia is required if the nail plate does not need to be removed). Use of a heated red-hot paper clip, drill, or microcautery releases the underlying pressure with minimal discomfort. The heated tip passes through the nail with minimal pressure and is cooled by the hematoma, thus not causing injury to the nail bed. The hole should be at least 2 mm in diameter to allow drainage to continue and not seal up when clot forms. If the nail is to be removed to inspect and possibly repair the nail bed, do not place the hole in the nail until the location of the repair site is known. After nail bed repair the vent hole should *not* overlay the repair site directly in order to achieve maximal contouring effect from the replaced nail plate.

EQUIPMENT

- Surgical loupes (preferably 2.5× magnification or greater)
- Freer septum elevator
- Kutz periosteal elevator
- Small periosteal Key elevator
- English nail splitter
- Double-action bone rongeur
- Double-action bone forceps
- Single- and double-pronged skin hooks
- No. 11 or 15 surgical blade and handles
- Small cuticle scissors
- Needle holders
- Suture scissors
- ⅜-inch Penrose drain
- Small hemostats (2)
- 6-0 and 7-0 absorbable suture (gut or white Vicryl)
- Silicone sheeting (0.020-inch thick)
- Vaseline gauze
- Antibiotic ointment (e.g., Neosporin)
- Small syringe and 30-gauge needle
- Xylocaine 1% plain (no adrenaline in the fingers)
- Adson pickups, with and without teeth
- Finger dressing material, small metal splints, and arm sling for postoperative elevation

NAIL PLATE AVULSION (SURGICAL)

The nail must be removed when the subungual hematoma exceeds 30% of the visible nail bed area and/or when the nail bed injury is directly visualized or strongly suspected (e.g., there is avulsion of the distal nail from the hyponychium or proximally from the eponychium). (See the editor's note following the bibliography.) Verify at this time if there is (1) displaced, unstable phalangeal fractures (requiring fixation), (2) large nail bed avulsions (with missing tissue requiring nail bed grafts), or (3) significant distal amputation of tissue (requiring some type of graft for closure). Consider early referral of this injury if its nature exceeds personal training, experience, and comfort level.

When the nail is removed (by the trauma or the surgeon), carefully cleanse the area and examine it with the loupes. Make an adequate record of the status of the entire nail bed, the proximal and lateral nail folds, and the hyponychium. Record these findings as part of the operative findings of the distal phalanx.

Anesthesia

Exploration of the nail bed can be completed under general, scalene block, axillary block, Bier block, or digital block (see Chapters 1 [Bier Block] and 8 [Peripheral Nerve Blocks and Field Blocks]). The first four can be used with an arm tourniquet and additional sedation as required for longer procedures in which multiple digits are involved. Uncooperative adults and restless children may be managed better by the use of a more formal type of anesthetic setting. Practitioners prefer to save the patients any additional anesthetic charges if possible, but their desires to economize should not compromise the examination or repair in any way when the patient is being uncooperative and moving about during a delicate repair under magnification.

After anesthesia the surgical field is prepped and draped in the usual manner to ensure sterility of the surgical field. At this time, if no other form of tourniquet is in use, a digital tourniquet can be established by use of a sterile, ⅜-inch Penrose drain, placed smoothly around the finger and secured with a small hemostat to occlude flow through the digital vessels. Depending on the site of the injury and personal preferences, there are two techniques to remove the nail and visualize the nail bed.

Distal Technique

The Freer elevator is placed under the free edge of the nail (Fig. 29-3) and advanced proximally, following the plane of cleavage between the nail plate and the nail bed. Substantial resistance is encountered along the nail bed until the germinal matrix is reached, where the progress becomes easier. Be careful to avoid advancing the elevator excessively into the proximal nail groove. Now gently work the elevator medially and laterally to free up the last of the soft tissue attachments deep to the nail plate. Place the elevator under the cuticle (on the dorsum of the nail) (Fig. 29-4) and dissect under the ventral portion of the proximal nail fold. Continue the dissection laterally on both sides to release any remaining soft tissue attachment while a hemostat is used to apply gentle distal traction, pulling distally. (The goal is

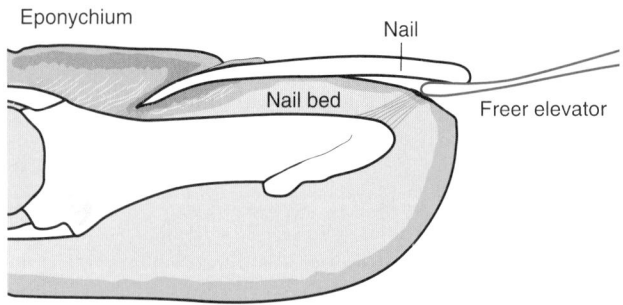

Fig. 29-3
Freer elevator placed under the nail. The nail bed is made up of the germinal matrix proximal to the lunula and the sterile matrix distally.

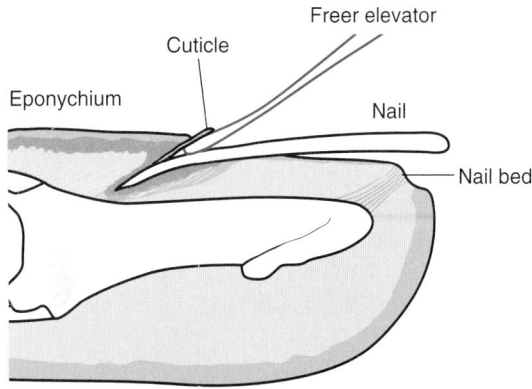

Fig. 29-4
Freer elevator placed under the cuticle.

to free the nail from any residual soft tissue attachments while not digging too deeply into either the proximal or lateral folds and not worsening any existing trauma.)

Proximal Technique

The proximal approach is often used when a distal cleavage plane cannot be identified because trauma or other pathology (such as onychomycosis) exists. The Freer elevator is placed under the cuticle and advanced to the proximal nail fold and worked to free the proximal and lateral gutters while avoiding damage to the cells in the depth of the folds. Proximal relaxing incisions (Fig. 29-5) facilitate exposure. Advance the elevator to locate the proximal edge of the nail plate. The skin hooks are now used to hold the eponychium folded proximally while the elevator comes over the top, then directed distally just deep to the nail plate as it dissects the plane between the nail plate and the nail bed. Keep the plane of the elevator turned so that the blade conforms as well as possible to the exact curvature of the nail plate in all areas.

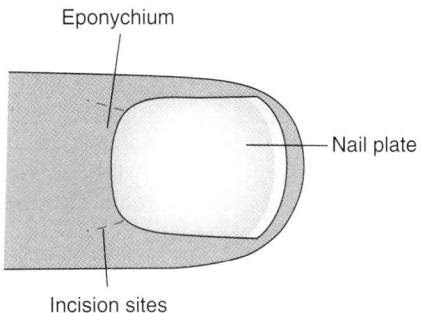

Fig. 29-5
Proximal relaxing incisions are used to facilitate exposure.

GENERAL CONSIDERATIONS FOR REPAIR

Injuries are often associated with subungual hematoma or avulsion of the nail from the paronychium or the proximal nail fold. After anesthesia is provided, perform a surgical preparation on the finger and remove the nail as previously described. Carefully scrape any residual nail bed tissue off the nail undersurface, and place it in the antibiotic solution to soak while the nail bed is examined. With the tourniquet inflated, cleanse and lavage the nail bed. With excellent light and loupes, the defects can be identified and any gross irregularities trimmed while leaving all the tissue that can be repaired and contoured. (Use of the nail plate itself or a naillike substance such as a postoperative splint helps with this.)

Best sutures for the nail bed repair are absorbable 6-0 or 7-0 chromic or Vicryl. (Zook et al [1980] have recommended 7-0 chromic on a micropoint spatula, double-armed, GS-9, ophthalmic needle [Ethicon].) Either a 5-0 or 6-0 monofilament suture is used to repair lacerations in the skin and to anchor an avulsed nail or avulsed nail bed matrix.

After repair of the nail bed, replace the nail (with the drain hole perforation at a point not directly over the repaired site). The nail serves as a stint to keep the nail folds open and to approximate the edges of the repair. The nail is well stabilized by the placement of a 5-0 or 6-0 monofilament suture through the nail into the fingertip area.

If the nail is not available or is damaged too badly to use as a splint, alternative materials may be used to provide contouring and protection to the nail bed. Materials such as medical-grade silicone sheeting (0.02 inch), Vaseline gauze, or Xeroform can be shaped to approximate the original nail (Fig. 29-6). They must be placed carefully so that they occupy the space of the proximal and lateral nail folds to prevent them from permanently scarring down. These stints must be anchored by a 6-0 monofilament or similar suture through

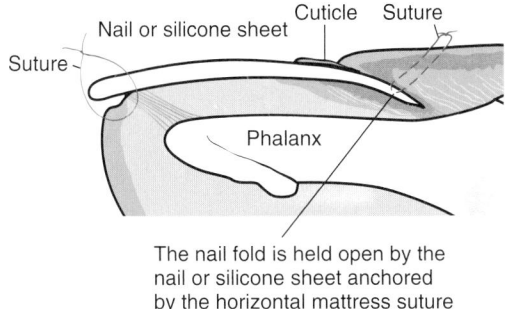

Suture

Nail or silicone sheet

Cuticle   Suture

Suture

Phalanx

The nail fold is held open by the
nail or silicone sheet anchored
by the horizontal mattress suture

Fig. 29-6
Replacement of the nail or alternative. The nail fold is held open to
prevent it from scarring down when the nail bed has been avulsed or
severely damaged. The nail itself or a silicone sheet is anchored by the
horizontal mattress suture.

the proximal portion of the nail folds to ensure their
position. These splints will (1) protect the nail while
healing, (2) maintain the contour of the nail plate, and
(3) prevent adherence of the proximal nail fold to the
matrix.

Sometimes the germinal matrix and nail bed may be
avulsed from its proximal origin below the proximal
fold. When this occurs, use of a monofilament (5-0 or
6-0) horizontal mattress suture (Fig. 29-7) restores the
anatomy. Be certain to replace the nail plate or use a
substitute to hold open the proximal and lateral nail
folds.

Avoid making the postoperative dressing too tight.
Use a sling to elevate the hand and provide enhanced
patient comfort. If nonadherent gauze is used as a stint
on the nail bed to hold open the nail folds, it should be
changed in 7 to 10 days. If the nail plate has been
replaced, it will usually come off in about 21 days.
Explain to the patient that the fingernail will require 6 to
12 months to grow out and to allow its final status to be
determined. Trim the advancing rough edges to prevent
accidental snags.

CLASSIFICATION
OF NAIL BED INJURIES

The **Type I** nail bed injury shown in Fig. 29-8, *A,* is
a small hematoma (less than 30% of visible nail) with
no major matrix injury. Any injury that produces a
subungual hematoma can be classified as a Type I
injury, including superficial lacerations of the nail bed.

The **Type II** injury shown in Fig. 29-8, *B,* is a large
hematoma (over 30% of visible nail) with a likely matrix
injury (e.g., a severe crushing injury). These injuries
have a poor prognosis, since the fragments are much
more difficult to reassemble anatomically and the
viability of this tissue is severely reduced from that of the

simple or stellate lacerations. The need for radiographs
to visualize fracture patterns and stability is increasingly
important in these more complex injuries. The same
general techniques as described above are used but
more time is spent informing the patient of the poor
prognosis and informing them of the likely need for
further surgery and possible partial or complete loss of
the nail.

A **Type III** nail bed injury (Fig. 29-8, *C*) with or
without a hematoma has a phalangeal fracture that may
or may not be reduced (distal phalangeal fracture—nail
bed lacerations). These fractures may be nondisplaced
or displaced and, more importantly, stable or unstable.

A **Type IV** nail bed injury has extensive matrix
fragmentation, but the bone is intact. The proximal nail
plate may or may not be avulsed from the proximal
nail fold.

A **Type V** nail bed injury, involving matrix avulsion,
can be categorized as follows:
1. Avulsed segment available for repair (Fig. 29-8, *E*).
2. Small avulsion (less than 2 mm width).
3. Large avulsion that requires a split- or full-thickness
   graft from adjacent finger or toe donor site.

TREATMENT GUIDELINES

Type I injuries often go untreated or may benefit from
decompression if throbbing pain occurs when the
hematoma is small.

Type II injuries involve nail removal (with a decompression hole) and suture repair of the nail matrix.
Replace the vented nail plate as a template into the
proximal and lateral nail folds, and anchor with 5-0 nylon
sutures through the distal nail and hyponychium to
prevent accidental removal (Fig. 29-9).

A careful search of the nail fragments should be
undertaken to find segments of nail bed that can then be
removed carefully with a small elevator and reattached
to the nail bed as a free graft to reapproximate the
original undamaged nail bed. Again, the intact nail plate
or the silicone sheet is used to contour and protect the
nail bed during the healing stage.

With **Type III** injuries, remove the nail. Repair the
viable matrix with absorbable suture, stabilize the fracture with 0.028 K-wire if required, and replace the nail for
splint (Fig. 29-10). If the nail is unavailable or unusable,
create a template from sterile silicone sheeting (0.02
inch) and secure in the place of the nail plate.

If the fracture is nondisplaced at the time of the x-ray
examination but is so unstable when examined surgically that it cannot be trusted to remain in anatomic
position, it must be stabilized with K-wire fixation. Any
inadvertent displacement of the dorsal phalangeal cortex
during the healing leads to nail bed irregularities and

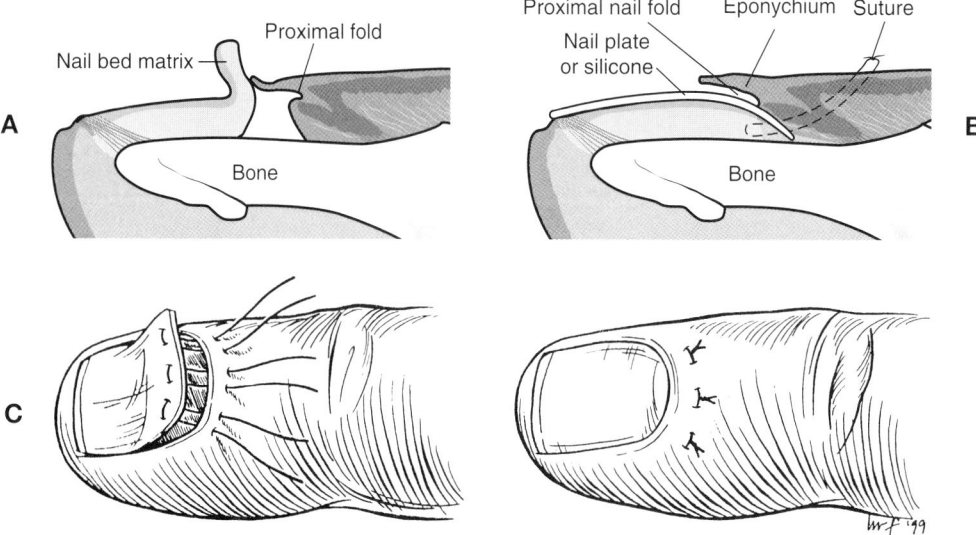

Fig. 29-7
Proximal nail bed avulsion. The nail plate has been removed. The *nail bed* consists of the germinal and the sterile matrix. The *matrix* extends from a point just distal to the insertion of the extensor tendon to the end of the fingernail attachment. The *germinal matrix,* which produces most of the nail, begins just 3 to 5 mm proximal and deep to the *eponychium* and extends distally to the lunula. The *lunula* is the white portion of the germinal matrix just beyond the *cuticle.* It marks the end of that portion of the germinal matrix that produces the fingernail. The *sterile matrix* begins proximally at the distal edge of the lunula and extends distally to the *hyponychium.* It also plays some role in production of the nail. The *eponychium* is the flap or tuft of skin that covers over the proximal nail. **A,** Nail bed has been avulsed from its normal location and displaced dorsally. **B,** Horizontal mattress suture through the nail wall is used to anchor the nail bed into proper site for healing. Proximal nail fold must be held open (with fingernail or substitute) to prevent scarring down and closure of nail fold. The nail plate or silicone sheet has been placed and anchored (with suture) to hold the proximal nail fold open. **C,** Appearance of wound after suturing. Sutures are removed from the nail in 3 weeks. The replaced nail or silicone sheet will dislodge in 1 to 3 months. (**C,** From Chudnofsky CR, Sebastian S, *Emerg Med Clinics North Am* 10:808, 1992.)

resultant deformed fingernails. The previous principles of repair apply, and serial radiographs are required to verify position of bone fragments and to observe for indication of osteomyelitis. As in other open fractures, prophylactic antibiotics are required until indication of proper wound healing is demonstrated.

With **Type IV** injuries, remove the nail and carefully repair the epithelial fragments. This may involve trimming some severely traumatized fragments with very minimal debridement, since the nail plate will hold the fragments down into a vascular bed and contour them to heal with the nail bed.

With **Type V** injuries, perform the following:
1. With an available avulsed segment, carefully remove it from the nail plate and reattach to nail bed with a 6-0 or 7-0 absorbable suture.
2. Small avulsions (less then 2 mm wide) may be closed primarily if the nail bed can be undermined with a small elevator and the tissue closed without

tension through the use of a 6-0 or 7-0 absorbable suture.
3. Larger avulsions require split- or full-thickness grafts from adjacent fingers or toes (See Shepard, 1990a,b).

As mentioned previously, with an avulsed nail bed, look carefully for remnants of the nail bed on large pieces of the nail plate that may accompany the patient. Ask family members or co-workers to look for any amputated fingertips, which may provide needed tissue for the nail bed reconstruction. Sometimes a fingernail and part of the nail bed may still be inside of a glove that was worn at the time of injury. If an adjacent finger was amputated or is otherwise unrepairable, it may serve as a donor for a full- or partial-thickness nail bed graft for the defect in question. A small defect may be repaired with a small split-thickness graft from an undamaged segment of the involved nail. In larger defects a split-thickness graft from the sterile matrix (do not include the germinal matrix) of the great toe can be used. After

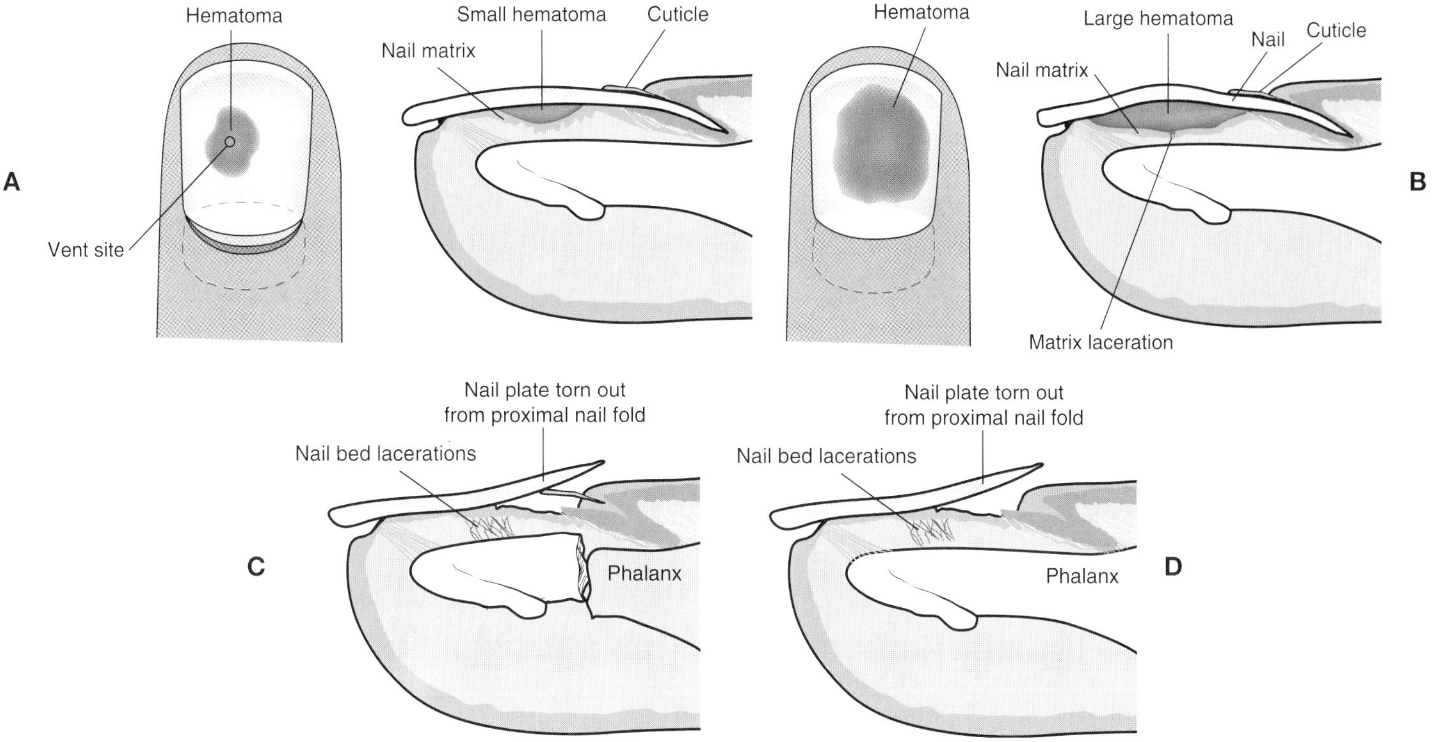

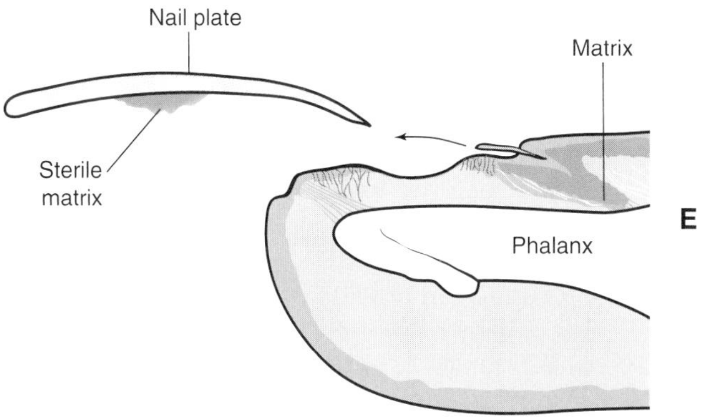

A

Hematoma

Vent site

Small hematoma

Nail matrix

Cuticle

Hematoma

Large hematoma

Nail matrix

Nail

Cuticle

Matrix laceration

B

Nail bed lacerations

Nail plate torn out
from proximal nail fold

Phalanx

C

Nail bed lacerations

Nail plate torn out
from proximal nail fold

Phalanx

D

Nail plate

Sterile
matrix

Matrix

Phalanx

E

Fig. 29-8

A, Type I nail bed injury: small hematoma. **B,** Type II nail bed injury: large hematoma (over 30%) with likely matrix injury. **C,** Type III nail bed injury with phalangeal fracture. **D,** Type IV nail bed injury: extensive matrix injury with intact phalanx. **E,** Type V nail bed injury with matrix avulsion. This particular matrix avulsion shows an avulsed segment available for repair.

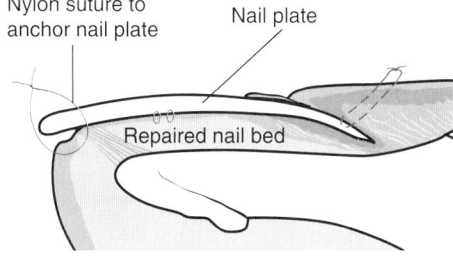

Nylon suture to
anchor nail plate

Nail plate

Repaired nail bed

Fig. 29-9

Repair of Type II injury with nail reattached. The nail bed is repaired, and the nail plate or substitute is anchored proximally and distally.

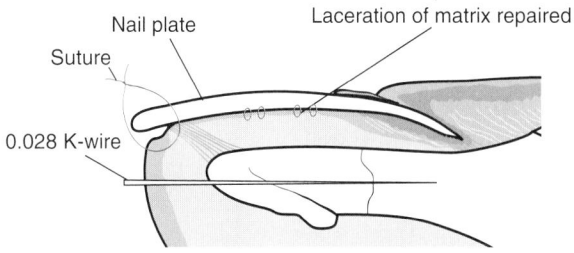

Nail plate

Laceration of matrix repaired

Suture

0.028 K-wire

Fig. 29-10

Repair of Type III injury. The unstable fracture is stabilized, the matrix repaired, and the nail plate secured by nylon suture.

removal of the great toenail, use a sterile surgical blade, with a thick graft sawing motion to shave approximately 0.014 inch from the nail bed (it is preferable to cut too thin than too thick). Carefully sew the graft in place with fine absorbable sutures, reapply the vented nail or other template, and secure in place when properly positioned to maintain the proximal and lateral folds in an open position.

In general, consider perioperative antibiotic use for Type III, IV, and V injuries, including distal amputations. Verify that tetanus status is up-to-date, since many of these wounds are grossly contaminated.

LATE RECONSTRUCTION OF THE NAIL MATRIX

Delayed reconstruction efforts are frequently associated with disappointment for the patients and the physicians. Patients must know up front that odds of a major improvement after surgery are very guarded, and it is possible for the nail to look even worse regardless of best efforts and surgical technique.

1. *Nail ridges* can result from either a scar below the nail bed or a fracture healing with a prominence of the dorsal phalangeal surface. Correction requires smoothing of the healed bone surface and removal of the scar tissue. The defect created by the scar removal must be closed either by undermining and direct approximation or by grafting as mentioned above.

2. *Split nails* can result from a ridge or longitudinal scar in the germinal or sterile matrix. Resection of the scar in the sterile matrix and use of a free graft, if primary closure is impossible, may be helpful. Use of the proximal eponychial incisions to visualize and graft the germinal matrix may provide some improvement. Some authors advocate use of the second toe as a donor rather than the great toe to avoid cosmetic alteration of the larger great toenail. Use a germinal matrix graft of similar size and shape to fill the resected scar site, as a free graft.

3. *Nonadherence* of the nail is caused from scars in the sterile matrix. Resection of the scar and replacement with a free split- or full-thickness matrix graft provides the best results.

CPT/BILLING CODES

11760   Repair of nail bed
11762   Reconstruction of nail bed with graft

ICD-9-CM DIAGNOSTIC CODES

883.0   Wound, open, nail, finger(s), thumb
883.1   Complicated
893.0   Wound, open, nail, toe(s)
893.1   Complicated

BIBLIOGRAPHY

Fleckman P, Christopher A: Surgical anatomy of the nail unit, *Dermatol Surg* 27(3):257, 2001.

Moossavi M, Scher RK: Complications of nail surgery: a review of the literature, *Dermatol Surg* 27(3):225, 2001.

Reardon CM, McArthur PA, Survana SK, Brotherston TM: The surface anatomy of the germinal matrix of the nail bed in the finger, *J Hand Surg (Br)* 24(5):531, 1999.

Rich P: Nail biopsy: indications and methods, *Dermatol Surg* 27(3):229, 2001.

Scher RK, Daniel CR III, editors: *Nails: therapy, diagnosis, surgery,* Philadelphia, 1990, WB Saunders.

Shepard GH: Management of acute nail bed avulsions, *Hand Clin* 6(1):39, 1990a.

Shepard GH: Nail grafts for reconstruction, *Hand Clin* 6(1): 79, 1990b.

Van Beek AL, Kassan MA, Adson MH, Dale V: Management of acute fingernail injuries, *Hand Clin* 6(1):23, 1990.

Zook EG, Van Beek AL, Russell RC, Beatty ME: Anatomy and physiology of the perionychium: a review of the literature and anatomic study, *J Hand Surg [Am]* 5:528, 1980.

Editor's note: There is some controversy regarding the necessity to remove the nail regardless of the hematoma size. Traditional teaching recommended removal. The study by Roser and Gellman (1999) and others questions this practice. Consult the following sources:

Fieg EL: Letter to the editor, *Am Fam Physician* 65(10):1997, 2002.

Lammes RL, Trott AT: Methods of wound closure. In Roberts JR, Hedges JR, editors: *Clinical procedures in emergency medicine,* ed 2, Philadelphia, 1998, WB Saunders.

Roser SE, Gellman H: Comparison of nail bed repair versus nail trephination for subungual hematomas in children, *J Hand Surg* 24:1166, 1999.

Selbst SM, Magdy A: Minor trauma: lacerations. In Fleisher GR, Ludwig S, editors: *Textbook of pediatric emergency medicine,* ed 4, Philadelphia, 2001, Lippincott, Williams & Wilkins.

Wang QC, Johnson BA: Fingertip injuries, *Am Fam Physician* 63:1961, 2001.

CHAPTER 30

Nail Plate and Nail Bed Biopsy

James F. Peggs

The presence of melanocytes in the germinal tissue of the nail matrix makes this a possible site for development of malignant melanomas. Primary subungual malignant melanomas frequently appear as pigmented bands or streaks in the nail plate, and they account for up to 3.5% of all cutaneous malignant melanomas (15% to 20% in blacks). Distinction between the numerous benign causes of pigmented streaks (trauma, malnutrition, and normal occurrence in many blacks and Asians) and malignant lesions is frequently difficult. Biopsy is often recommended to confirm the diagnosis.

The *nail plate* is the hard structure composed of keratinized squamous cells, which is commonly called the nail itself. The *nail bed* refers to the softer tissue beneath the nail that provides germinal tissue for the nail plate and to which the nail plate is attached (Fig. 30-1).

INDICATIONS

- Thickened, distorted nail plate with a negative evaluation for fungal infection (potassium hydroxide [KOH] scraping, culture)
- Longitudinal pigmented linear streak in the nail plate suspicious for malignancy

CONTRAINDICATIONS

- Allergy or sensitivity to local anesthetics (see Chapter 4, Local Anesthesia)
- Bleeding diathesis

EQUIPMENT

- 3-mm disposable skin biopsy punch
- Local anesthetic (e.g., 2% xylocaine) *without* epinephrine
- Sterile scissors with straight blades (or a narrow Locke periosteal elevator)
- Sterile rubber band, small Penrose drain, or Ellman disposable digit tourniquet
- Two sterile, straight hemostats
- Sterile gauze and tubular gauze dressing
- Antibiotic ointment (Mycitracin, Bactroban)
- 5-0 or 6-0 nylon sutures
- Needle holders
- Suture scissors

TECHNIQUE

Nail Plate (Nail) Biopsy

1. With steady pressure, hold the punch perpendicular to the nail; rotation of the punch will produce a round biopsy specimen without pain. No anesthetic is required.
2. Elevate the biopsy sample and lyse the underlying nail bed tissue with the scissors or scalpel.

Nail Bed Biopsy

1. Perform a digital block using xylocaine without epinephrine (Fig. 30-2).
2. Apply a tourniquet to decrease bleeding at the site and allow easier removal of specimen.
3. Partially remove the nail plate according to the procedure in Chapter 40, Ingrown Toenails.
4. When the affected nail bed has been exposed, use a 3- or 4-mm punch to obtain the biopsy specimen as close as possible to the proximal origin of the pigmentation. However, there is a higher chance of a deformed nail if the biopsy is obtained from the root portion of the nail under the proximal nail fold. The biopsy specimen should be 2 to 3 mm in thickness. Alternatively, small elliptical excisions can be made (Fig. 30-1). (See Chapter 33, Skin Biopsy.)
5. Close the biopsy site with one or two 5-0 or 6-0 nylon sutures oriented along the longitudinal plate (Fig. 30-3). Also see Chapter 29, Nail Bed Repair.
6. Remove the tourniquet.

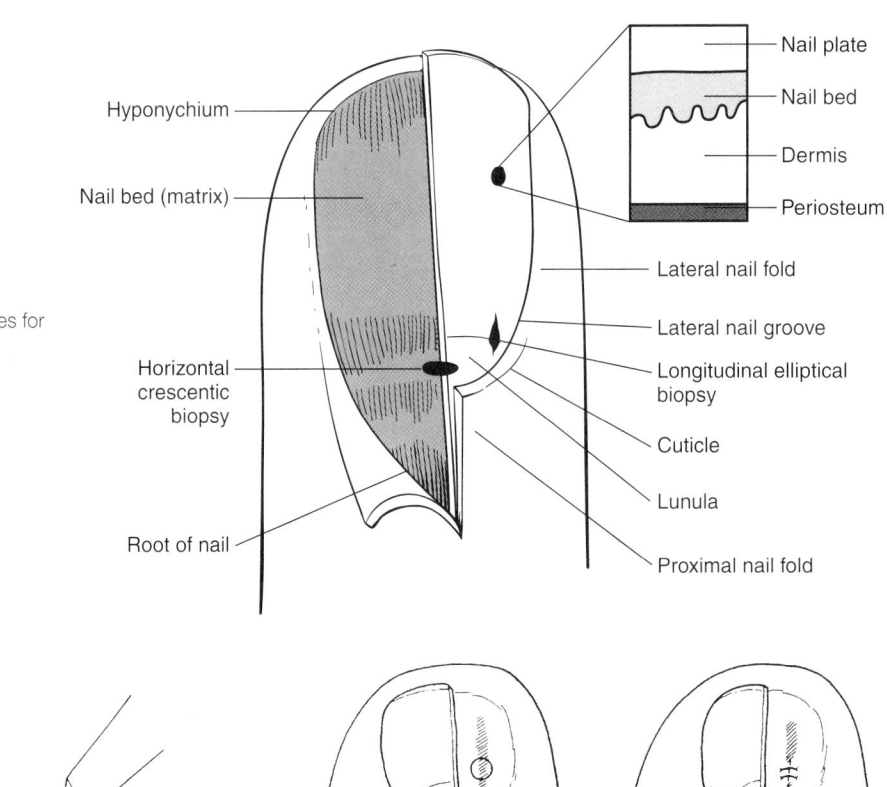

Fig. 30-1
Nail anatomy and possible sites and shapes for obtaining a nail biopsy.

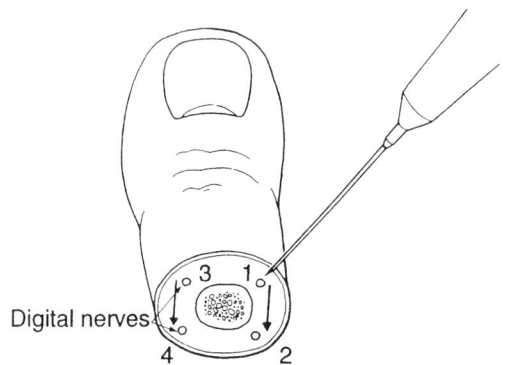

Fig. 30-2
Ring-block technique for digital nerve block. *1,* Raise a wheal at the dorsal surface of the base of the digit. *2,* Direct the needle toward the plantar surface, delivering 1 ml of anesthetic to the extensor and 1 ml to the plantar branches of the digital nerve. *3,* Perform a second puncture at the corresponding site of the other side, and, *4,* advance the needle in the plantar direction to allow delivery of 1 ml of anesthetic to each branch of the digital nerve. A minimum of 4 ml of anesthesia is used. Also see Chapter 8, Peripheral Nerve Blocks and Field Blocks.

7. Apply a dressing of antibiotic ointment and sterile gauze.

COMPLICATIONS

- Bleeding
- Infection
- Distortion of nail with regrowth

CPT/BILLING CODE

11755   Biopsy nail unit

Fig. 30-3
Nail bed biopsy. **A,** 3-mm Biopsy specimen obtained. **B,** Sutured nail bed.

ICD-9-CM DIAGNOSTIC CODES

1736   Finger lesion malignant
2166   Finger lesion benign
2382   Finger lesion uncertain

ADDITIONAL RESOURCES

- See the sample patient education handout titled "Nail Plate and Nail Bed Biopsy" on page 1768 of Appendix G.
- See the sample patient consent form titled "Nail Plate and Nail Bed Biopsy" on page 1769 of Appendix G.

BIBLIOGRAPHY

Baran R, Kechijian P: Longitudinal melanonychia, *J Am Acad Dermatol* 21:1165, 1989.

Daniel CR III, editor: Symposium on the nail, *Dermatol Clin* 3:371, 1985.

Fleckman P, Christopher A: Surgical anatomy of the nail unit, *Dermatol Surg* 27(3):257, 2001.

Moossavi M, Scher RK: Complications of nail surgery: a review of the literature, *Dermatol Surg* 27(3):225, 2001.

Reardon CM, McArthur PA, Survana SK, Brotherston TM: The surface anatomy of the germinal matrix of the nail bed in the finger, *J Hand Surg (Br)* 24(5):531, 1999.

Rich P: Nail biopsy: indications and methods, *Dermatol Surg* 27(3):229, 2001.

Stone OJ, Barr RJ, Herten RJ: Biopsy of the nail area, *Cutis* 21:257, 1978.

Tom DW, Scher RK: Biopsies of nails: melanonychia striata in longitudinem, *Am J Dermatopathol* 7(suppl):161, 1985.

CHAPTER 31

Radiofrequency Surgery (Modern Electrosurgery)

John L. Pfenninger
Donald E. DeWitt*

Radiofrequency surgery (RF)—modern electrosurgery—has become a versatile tool for the primary care physician in dermatological, surgical, and gynecological applications. It is both time- and cost-effective, and it provides efficacious treatment for a multitude of lesions. Appropriate selection of waveform and current intensity allows excision (cutting), cutting and coagulation (blend), pure coagulation (hemostasis), or fulguration. Tissue either can be removed delicately with excellent cosmetic results or can be totally ablated. The electrosurgical unit (ESU) can be used for treatment of both benign and malignant lesions.

This chapter is based on the Ellman Surgitron, a portable generator that creates high-frequency current of 3.8 to 4.0 MHz, which is comparable to radiowave frequency for broadcasting (Figs. 31-1, *A,B* and 31-2). Many other units have recently been introduced into the market, and most have focused on the performance of the large loop electrosurgical excision procedure (LEEP) (see Chapter 150, Loop Electrosurgical Excision Procedure [LEEP] for Treating Cervical Intraepithelial Neoplasia). Wave frequency can vary from 500,000 to 4 million cycles per second. The Surgitron has a long and successful history and can be used with a multitude of electrode tips for a large variety of applications. Although initially introduced into the dental field, it quickly became adapted to many dermatologic applications in the medical field. With the advent of LEEP in the 90s, it was a simple matter of developing new loops to accommodate this innovative procedure. The other unit that has been used as much in the dermatologic field as

the gynecologic field is the Wallach unit (Fig. 31-1, *B*). Unless otherwise noted, discussion here will be in reference to the Ellman Surgitron, but the reader can generalize the discussion to most other units quite readily.

There is a choice of three waveforms plus a fulguration current (four modes). By changing waveforms, practitioners obtain different effects. The settings of the Ellman unit are described as *filtered fully rectified, fully rectified,* and *partially rectified.* These correspond with a *pure cutting* effect (90% cutting, 10% coagulation), a *blended* current to allow 50% cut and 50% coagulation, and a 90% *coagulation* (hemostasis) effect, respectively. A separate outlet also provides a spark-gap fulgurating current (referred to as *hyfercation*) for very superficial cautery (Fig. 31-3).

Advantages of using radiofrequency technique include rapidity of treatment, a nearly bloodless field, minimal postoperative pain, and rapid healing. Local anesthetic is used except in rare instances. Since the frequency is so high, the current from this unit passes through the body without causing painful muscle contractions or nerve stimulation (Faraday effects). Radiosurgery using the *cutting wave* cuts without pressure, needing only a featherlike touch, and thus minimizes tissue damage. The tissue damage that does occur is very superficial and comparable with that of proper laser use. This is in contrast to true cautery, which causes damage similar to third-degree burns. In addition, radiosurgery avoids the risk of electrical burns to the patient. Instead of a ground plate, an *antenna* is used to focus the "radio waves." In contrast to electrical units, this antenna does not have to be in contact with a patient's skin; instead, it only needs to be under the patient near the operating field. (Most ESUs, however, do require true grounding pads or plates, so manufacturer's recommendations must be followed.)

The high-frequency energy of this unit is concentrated at the tip of each electrode. During each

*This chapter was initially written by Donald E. DeWitt, MD. Don introduced me to electrosurgery and was one of the first champions in the struggle advocating that primary care physicians perform procedures. He seemed to have no end to his energy and excitement for teaching procedures. Just before his death, he rode an Amigo motorized cart to go from presentation to presentation at the American Academy of Family Physicians Scientific Assembly. This chapter is dedicated to Don's memory.

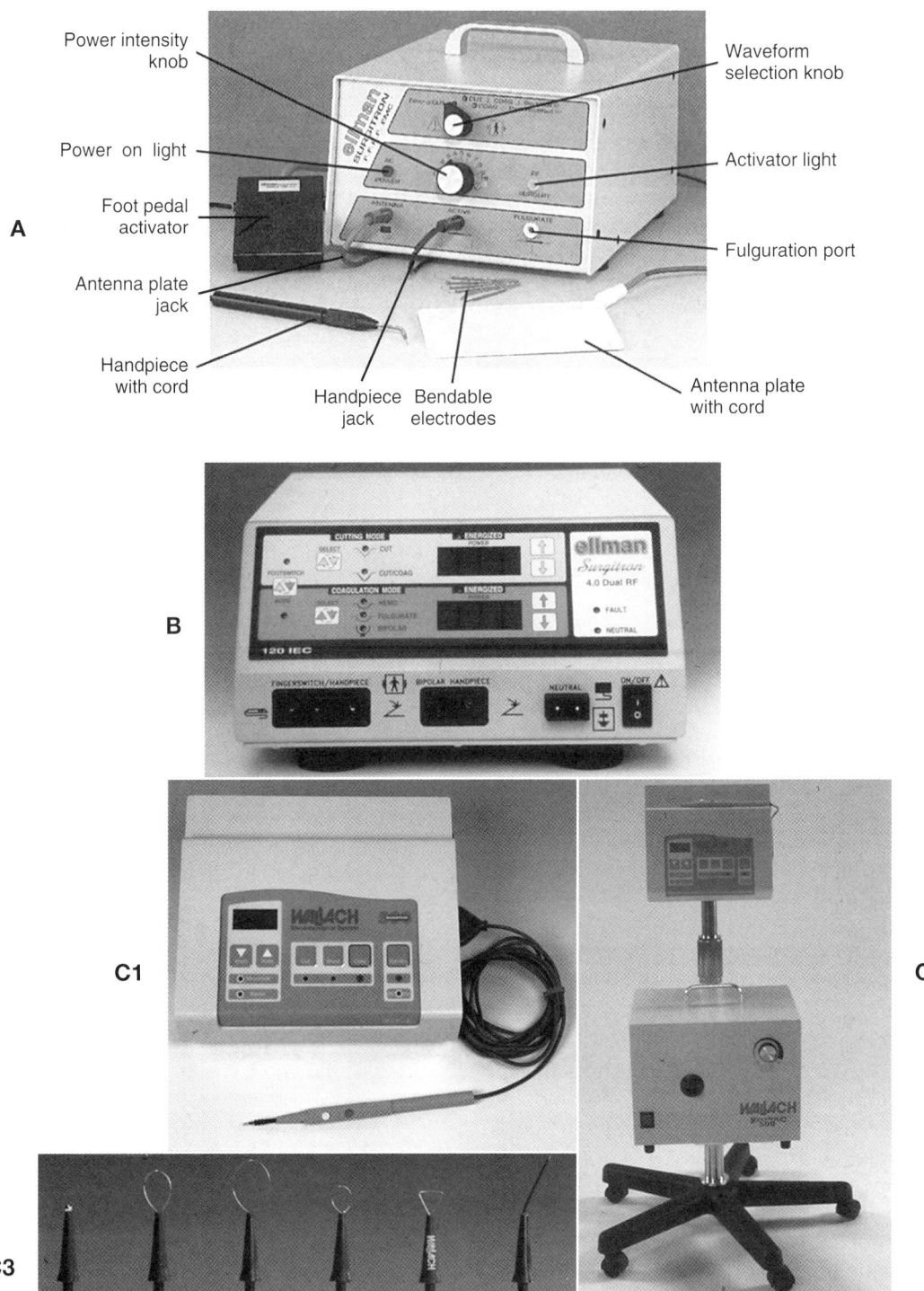

Power intensity knob

Power on light

Foot pedal activator

Antenna plate jack

Handpiece with cord

Waveform selection knob

Activator light

Fulguration port

Handpiece jack   Bendable electrodes

Antenna plate with cord

A

B

C1   **C2**

C3

Fig. 31-1
A, Ellman Surgitron radiofrequency unit with foot pedal, antenna plate, and hand wand tip holder. A variety of electrode tips are lying above the white antenna plate. **B,** Ellman Dual Frequency IEC II. **C,** The Wallach Q500 electrosurgical unit. *1,* ESU with finger control handpiece. *2,* ESU combined with smoke evacuator. The smoke evacuator activates when the ESU is activated and turns off a few seconds afterwards. *3,* The Wallach dermatologic tips. (**A-B,** Courtesy Ellman International, Inc., Hewlett, NY. **C,** Courtesy Bruno Ratensberger.)

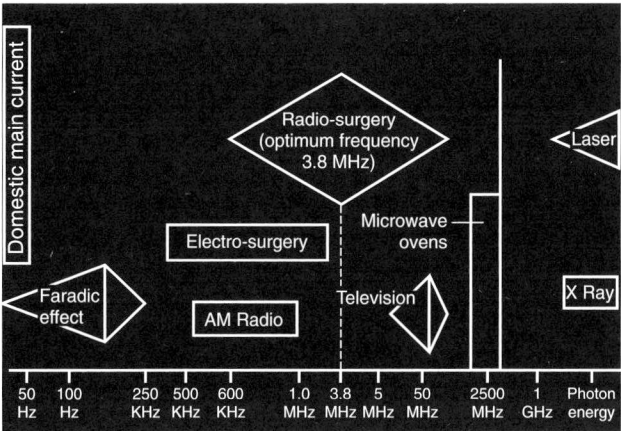

Fig. 31-2
Comparison of uses and effects of various electrical frequencies. (Courtesy Ellman International, Inc., Hewlett, NY.)

Mode or function	Waveform	Configuration
Electrocoagulation Hemostasis Cautery	Partially rectified	
Blend Cut and coag	Fully rectified	
Cutting Electrosection	Fully filtered and fully rectified	
Fulgeration Electrodessication	Markedly damped	

Fig. 31-3
Common terminology for various modes, waveform characterization, and waveform configuration for the outputs of the radiofrequency unit.

procedure, the electrode itself remains cold; however, the highly concentrated electrical energy creates molecular energy inside each cell it contacts, thereby creating intracellular heat and actually vaporizing the cell much the same as a laser does. The *amount of heat generated* is dependent on the amount of *time* the tip is in contact with the tissue, the *size* of the electrode, the *power setting*, the *type of waveform* selected, and the radiowave *frequency*. Higher frequency means less contact time, finer wire, less power, a more "cutting" waveform, and less tissue damage.

High-frequency electrosurgery is now replacing many laser applications because of the minimal tissue damage, low cost of equipment, minimal maintenance, ease of treatment, and excellent long-term results. As noted, it has mostly replaced laser in the gynecologic treatment of dysplasia (conization) and condyloma. It is now also being used for blepharoplasties, radio-assisted uvulo-

BOX 31-1
Common Uses and Lesions Treated with Radiofrequency Surgery

Incisions
Excisions
Shave removals
Electroepilation
Cauterization of "bleeders"
Nail plate ablation*
Skin tags
Verruca
Cervical conizations (LETZ, LEEP)†
Curettement and cautery (e.g., warts)
Telangiectasias (spider veins): face (not recommended for legs)
Pyogenic granulomas
Hemorrhoid tags
Mucosal lesions
Xanthelasma
Hemangiomas
Blepharoplasties
Basal cell cancers
Squamous cell carcinomas
Actinic keratoses
Sebaceous gland hyperplasia
Syringomas
Cervical biopsies
Chalazions
Condyloma
Varicosities‡
Nevi (benign)
Rhinophyma
Seborrheic keratoses
Hair transplants
Radio-assisted uvulopalatoplasties (RAUP)

*See Chapter 40, Ingrown Toenails.
†See Chapter 150, Loop Electrosurgical Excision Procedure (LEEP) for Treating Cervical Intraepithelial Neoplasia.
‡See Chapter 91, Radiofrequency Sclerotherapy: New Technique for Varicose Vein Treatment.

palatoplasty (RAUP) for snoring, spinal procedures, and many more applications.

INDICATIONS

Radiofrequency surgery can be used for a variety of skin and mucosal lesions. It is especially helpful when good cosmetic results are essential. It is also very helpful in well-perfused areas like mucosa and the anal area because the "cut and coag" setting can be used to control the bleeding. Common uses and lesions treated are listed in Box 31-1.

CONTRAINDICATIONS

• Cardiac pacemakers *(relative contraindication)*
• Uncooperative patient
It is best to avoid direct application of electrode tips around a cardiac pacer. The pacers are purportedly

"shielded" and the current in the electrosurgical units (ESUs) should not affect them, but all things are not perfect! Therefore caution is needed when the patient has a pacemaker. Asystole and tachycardias are potential adverse outcomes. Clinicians must apply the antenna plate or grounding pad near the lesion, use only short bursts of low intensity, and avoid the "cutting" setting when possible.

EQUIPMENT

- Alcohol wipe
- Local anesthetic (i.e., 2% xylocaine with or without epinephrine)
- 1-ml syringe with 30-gauge needle
- ESU
- Electrode tips (depending on procedure performed): reusable or disposable
- No. 15 scalpel blade
- Antenna (or grounding) plate
- Handpiece for tips (unit can be finger activated from this handpiece if desired)
- Foot pedal to activate handpiece (or use handpiece as above); foot pedal preferred for delicate surgeries
- Smoke evacuator (HIV and HPV have been found in smoke plume)
- Room air purifier (removes residual odor)
- Moveable cart to hold the ESU, smoker evacuator, tips, and all equipment for the procedures
- Mask
- Nonsterile gloves
- Monsel's or aluminum chloride for topical control of bleeders
- Antibiotic ointment
- Band-Aid
- Patient education handout on moist healing (which is essential to obtain optimal results) (See the sample patient education handout titled "Moist Healing After Skin Surgery" on page 1747 of Appendix G.)

(For LEEP procedure, see Chapter 150, Loop Electrosurgical Excision Procedure [LEEP] for Treating Cervical Intraepithelial Neoplasia.)

The *most common tips* used for removal of skin lesions are the large and small loops. The ball electrode is used frequently for coagulation and for ablation of lesions. Special tips are available for matrixectomy (see below and Chapter 40, Ingrown Toenails).

Disposable tips are convenient but can be costly. *Reusable tips* must be free of carbon buildup and shiny to obtain best results. After cleaning and sterilizing, and before repeat use, the tip must be examined. If it is not shiny, the carbon can be removed in several ways: (1) Use a 2 × 2–inch piece of fine sandpaper and, using the index finger to support the back side of the loop, rub it over the sandpaper. Turn it over and do the reverse side. Be sure to clean the entire wire loop. (2) Purchase the cleaning "blocks" available. (3) Place the units in an ultrasonic cleaner. Or (4) use a moistened piece of 4 × 4 gauze, insert the tip into the folded material and activate it on the cutting setting, level 5. When complete, the wire should be shiny (like new). One of the most *common reasons for poor cutting and "stalls"* during RF surgery is "dirty" (carbon-covered) loops.

Most ESUs have digital readouts for the watts (power intensity). The Ellman simply has an intensity dial labeled 1-10. Each unit roughly corresponds to 10 W. For skin surgery a setting of 2 to 4 (20 to 40 W) is usually needed. (As a "default," remember "pure cutting on level 2.")

Use of a smoke evacuator is a must. Not only have HPV and HIV been found in smoke plume (no infections have been documented), but the smell of burning flesh is very offensive and the examination room and office can smell for hours afterwards.

Ellman has recently introduced the dual frequency unit (Ellman Surgitron DF IEC II, Fig. 31-1, *B*). It is being used with increasing frequency for plastic surgery and neurosurgery applications. The coagulation potential is much better and it can coagulate in a "wet" (bloody) field using bipolar modality. This is achieved through the "dual frequencies" of 4 MHz for cutting but 1.7 MHz for bipolar coagulation. This unit will not interfere with any nearby electronics or electrical circuits. Other benefits include a higher frequency (4.0 versus 3.8 million cycles per second) than the original equipment; therefore there is still minimal thermal damage when cutting. It meets national safety codes for operating room use, and it is more user friendly because there is a two-pedal footswitch for cutting or coagulation and a three-button finger switch (for each modality). It has a memory for the most recent settings when turned off, digital power settings, and an audible sound when activated. This unit is significantly more expensive, and whether the benefits warrant the extra cost for the average practitioner remains to be seen.

TECHNIQUE

Proper technique is accomplished when the loop electrodes pass through the tissue smoothly, like cutting through soft butter. Generally, a motion of 5 to 8 mm/sec is appropriate. *If there is excess sparking and smoke,* the power setting is too high. *If the flow is not smooth,* the operator is going too fast, the power setting is too low, the skin is too dry or hyperkeratotic, or the electrode is dirty (debris or carbon buildup). It is important to remember that the least tissue damage occurs with the

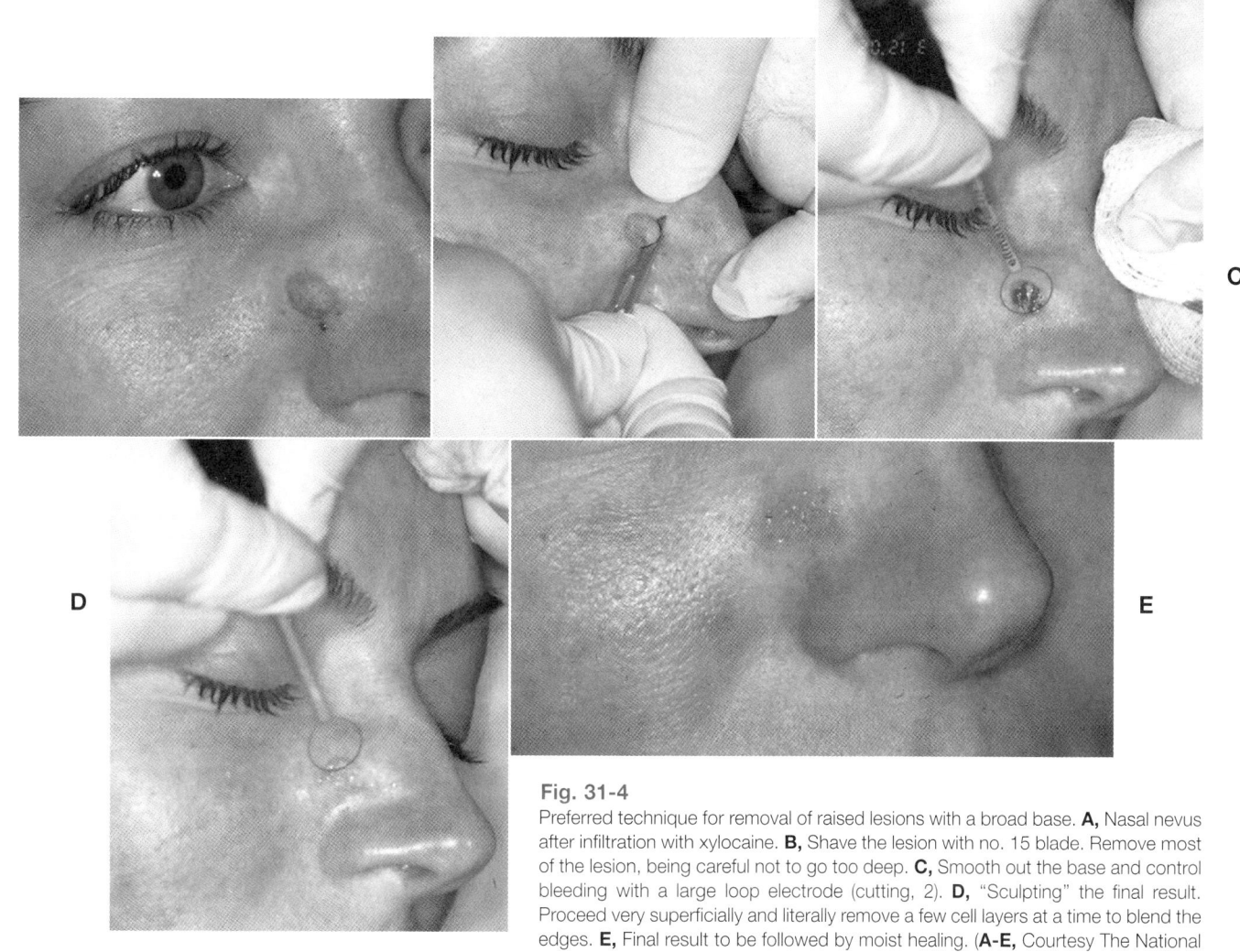

Fig. 31-4
Preferred technique for removal of raised lesions with a broad base. **A,** Nasal nevus after infiltration with xylocaine. **B,** Shave the lesion with no. 15 blade. Remove most of the lesion, being careful not to go too deep. **C,** Smooth out the base and control bleeding with a large loop electrode (cutting, 2). **D,** "Sculpting" the final result. Proceed very superficially and literally remove a few cell layers at a time to blend the edges. **E,** Final result to be followed by moist healing. (**A-E,** Courtesy The National Procedures Institute, Midland, Mich.)

pure cutting setting. Coagulation causes the most tissue destruction. If cosmetic results are desirable, judicious use of the coagulation setting and using as little power (watts) as possible is important.

The most common use for the RF unit in primary care is removal of elevated skin lesions such as nevi and seborrheics. Commonly, when using a blade to shave off a benign nevus, two things happen: bleeding and an irregular surface. As the surgeon tries to smooth out the "highs" in the base of the wound, blood obscures the area. Then, as the blade is used to shave off these highs, too much tissue is removed, leaving "dips." The "lows" (too much) and the "highs" (too little tissue removed) will leave adverse outcomes with undesirable scarring. Using the RF technique, both bleeding and an uneven wound base can be avoided.

The most successful technique of removing these elevated lesions appears to be to first "debulk" the majority of the lesion with a no. 15 blade in a shave fashion leaving some tissue behind (See Chapter 33, Skin Biopsy). Then, use the loop electrode on a pure cutting setting of 2 (20 W) to smooth out or vaporize any of the elevated areas. Pinch the skin around the area to control bleeding, activate the loop, and very superficially pass the tip through the tissue, gradually going down until the lesion is smoothed out adequately (Fig. 31-4). This "smoothing out" of the base provides an excellent outcome with rapid healing. The "cutting" setting has 10% coagulation so bleeding is nicely controlled. The tissue is literally vaporized "cell layer by cell layer." Healing results are excellent. Another advantage with the method described is that the tissue sent to pathology has no burn artifact.

Some advocate the removal of lesions primarily with the loop only (as opposed to using the blade). *Extreme caution is needed!* The loop cuts so quickly that it often goes too deep. Even in experienced hands too much tissue may be removed unless the process is very slow

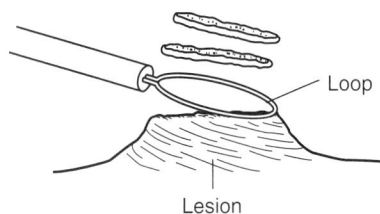

Fig. 31-5

"Feathering" technique for lesion removal. Rather than removing the entire lesion in one pass, it is removed a small amount at a time. This avoids removing too much and going too deep, causing scarring.

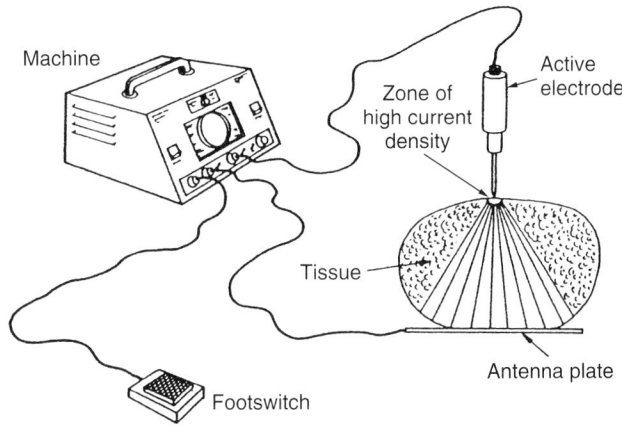

Fig. 31-6

Diagrammatic illustration of radiosurgery showing the distribution of energy. (Courtesy Ellman International, Inc., Hewlett, NY.)

and meticulous with only a small amount of tissue removed each time. *Do not try to remove all of the lesion with the first pass!* The only time the "layered" or "feathering" removal technique is recommended is for larger condyloma (Figs. 31-4 and 31-5).

Another advantage of shaving the lesion first with a blade is that a good specimen is available for pathology. If the total vaporization or the coagulation technique is used, minimal (if any) tissue can be sent. It is best that all pigmented lesions be sent for histology, since this is a very litigious area of medicine.

The Ellman unit does have a "fulguration port." This setting provides a very intense but superficial burn/coagulation. It can be used in place of the coagulation mode in many instances, but in general it has little benefit over the coagulation setting and is rarely used.

Novices are most concerned about the proper choice of settings when beginning electrosurgery. **Here are some pointers:**

- For removal of tissue, use pure cutting mode.
- For cutting on the skin, or the shave technique noted previously, usually an intensity of 2 (20 W or less) is sufficient. For removing large areas (i.e., cervical conization) or if the skin is hyperkeratotic, the intensity will need to be increased but rarely over 4 (40 W). *Remember the default setting:* cutting, level 2. The larger and drier the piece of tissue, the higher the power will need to be.
- When tissue destruction (matrixectomy, epilation, telangiectasias) or bleeding control is needed, turn to the coagulation mode. Most applications will require a level 3 (30 W). When small areas are treated without anesthesia (epilation, telangiectasias of the face), reduce the power level to 1.
- Use the cut/coagulation mode when bleeding is likely (inner lip, buccal mucosa, etc.) or where scarring is not so much of an issue (external hemorrhoidal tags). The setting will need to be a little higher (3, or 30 W).

Note: For removal of cervical tissue, the goal is to limit tissue artifact so the pathologist can readily read the specimen and discern if the entire lesion was removed. Use a pure cutting

mode; although scarring is not a concern, bleeding still is. Amazingly, however, there is generally very little bleeding, even with pure cutting, and the pathologist will be able to read to the margins of the excision, since the cutting mode leaves little burn artifact. (See Chapter 150, Loop Electrosurgical Excision Procedure [LEEP] for Treating Cervical Intraepithelial Neoplasia.)

- All electrosurgery will be accomplished easier at lower power (therefore causing less tissue destruction) if the tissue is moist and hyperkeratotic material has been removed. Just use a moistened 4 × 4 gauze pad and wipe it across the tissue after each pass or two.
- Most lesions will have to be anesthetized before removal with the RF unit.
- In general, place the antenna plate or grounding pad as close to the lesion as possible to limit the spread of the current and increase the intensity at the desired site (Fig. 31-6).

The proper electrode tips and power settings are summarized in Table 31-1.

Specific Approaches for Various Lesions

There are a multitude of applications possible with the variety of tips available (Fig. 31-7). There are loop and straight wire electrodes for excising, incising, or shaping tissue; ball electrodes for coagulation; and pointed rod electrodes for fulguration and desiccation. More specific electrodes are available for nail matrixectomies and large-loop electrical excision procedures of the cervix. The tips are changed much like the bits are changed in an ordinary drill. Most applications are accomplished with simple local anesthesia, regional field blocks, or digital blocks. Radiosurgery is relatively atraumatic when correctly applied; consequently, the risks of scar tissue formation are minimal compared with those associated with scalpel surgery.

TABLE 31-1

Proper Electrode Tips and Power Setting

Procedure	Mode	Power (Ellman/Watts)	Electrode
Condyloma	Cutting	2/20	Large or small round loop
Ear piercing	Cutting or cut/coag	2/20	Narrow, pointed tip
Electrodesiccation and curettage	Coag	3/25-30	Ball
Epilation	Coag	1/10	Vari-tip, 33-gauge needle on hub adaptors, or insulated needle
Epistaxis	Coag	3/30	Ball electrode
Hemorrhoid tags	Cut/Coag	3/25-30	Large loop or vari-tip
Hemostasis skin	Coag	2-3/20-30	Ball electrode
Incisions	Cutting	2-3/20-30	Vari-tip, fine needle, blade
LEEP	Cutting	4/35-40	Long, special LEEP electrodes
LEEP	Coag base/ hemostasis	6/40-60	Long, special LEEP ball
Matrixectomy	Coag	2-3/20-30	Special insulated matrixectomy electrodes (use the wider one), raise up on the eponychium, do not overcoagulate
Rhinophyma	Cutting	2/20	Large loop or rounded surgical blade (no. 10A)
Shave excision/smoothing	Cutting	2/20	Large or small loop
Skin tags/small condyloma	Coag	3/25-30	Pickups with ball electrode, bipolar pickups
Telangiectasias	Coag	1/10	Vari-tip, 33-gauge needle on hub adaptors, or insulated needle
Undermining	Cutting or cut/coag	2-3/20-30	Vari-tip, blade
Vasectomy			
Cauterizing vas ends	Coag	3/30	Narrow, pointed tip
Verruca	Cutting	3/25-30	Large loop, special cutting curette
Verruca	Coag	3/30	Ball electrode
Xanthelasma	Cutting	2/20-25	Large loop

LEEP, Loop electrosurgical excision procedure.

For the majority of cases, the handpiece is inserted into the color-coordinated "handpiece" port to enable the selection of various output modes. (If inserted into "fulguration port," that will be the only output.)

Biopsies or excisions of lesions may be accomplished with the standard ellipse technique using the *vari-tip electrode* (Fig. 31-8), or a scalpel blade inserted into a *chuck adaptor* (Fig. 31-9). The vari-tip has a fine wire that can be pulled out at variable distances to cut from 1 to 2 mm up to 1.5 cm deep. The unit is set at cutting mode. The proper power is usually between 2 and 3. The thickness and dryness of skin may cause some variation in this latter setting. Remove any hyperkeratinized tissue first, and be sure the skin is moist. In addition to incising and excising, these two electrodes are often used to undermine skin, since bleeding will be controlled if the cut/coag (blend) mode is used.

If the lesion to be removed is large and elevated, a biopsy specimen may be obtained by simply using the loop electrodes to remove the sample (Fig. 31-10). (See precautions above.) However, with smaller, flatter lesions, using the loop to obtain a shave biopsy specimen may cause sufficient artifact in the tissue specimen to obscure pathology. For smaller lesions,

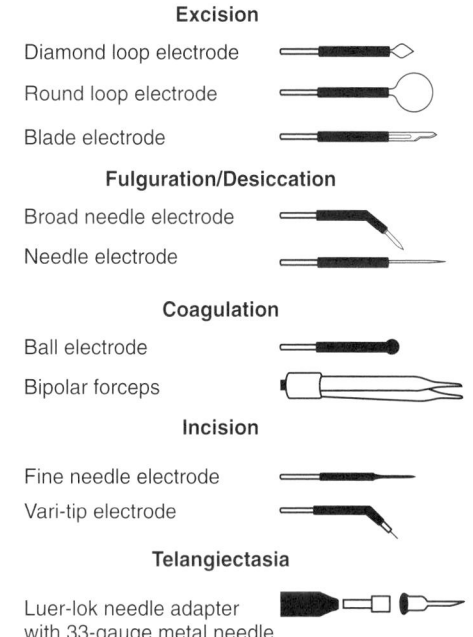

Excision
Diamond loop electrode
Round loop electrode
Blade electrode

Fulguration/Desiccation
Broad needle electrode
Needle electrode

Coagulation
Ball electrode
Bipolar forceps

Incision
Fine needle electrode
Vari-tip electrode

Telangiectasia
Luer-lok needle adapter with 33-gauge metal needle

Fig. 31-7

Multiple electrode tips available for the Ellman Surgitron radiofrequency unit.

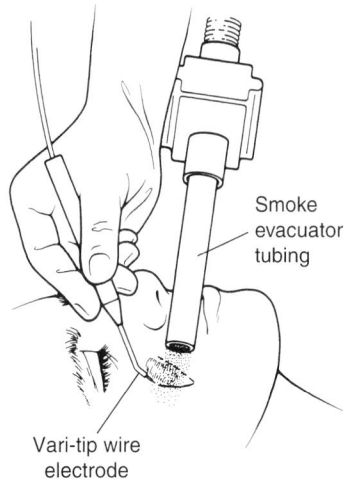

Fig. 31-8
Use of the vari-tip wire electrode to carry out an elliptical excision.

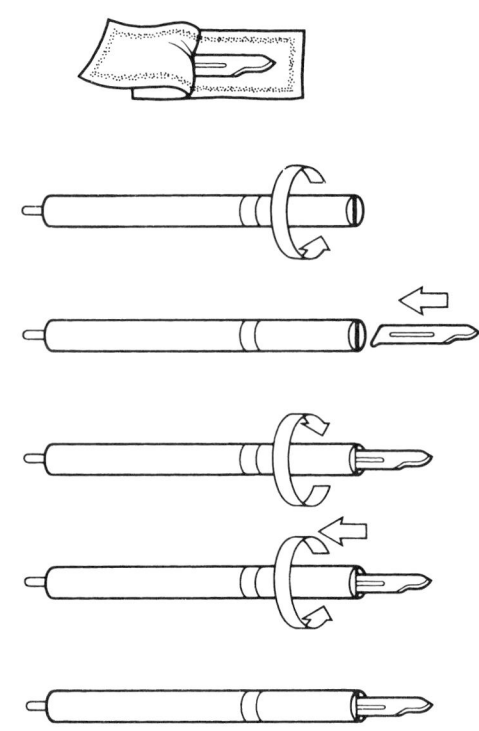

Fig. 31-9
Technique of inserting scalpel blade into handle for radiofrequency surgery. Most surgery is carried out with the loop electrodes or vari-tip wire. The scalpel is used most frequently for "bloodless" undermining.

then, use a regular scalpel blade (without current) to obtain a shave biopsy specimen. Follow this with the loop electrode to smooth out the base and control bleeding. Remember, when obtaining a biopsy sample for suspected melanoma, the depth of lesion penetrations is *very important*. Do *not* perform shave biopsies of pigmented lesions unless certain it is not a melanoma. (See Chapter 33, Skin Biopsy.)

Basal cell cancers may be treated using a combination of curettement and cautery (or fulguration). A *ball electrode* is used in the handpiece with a coagulation mode and the power set at approximately 3 to 4. After curetting the lesion, the base of the wound is cauterized. Cautery and curettement is generally carried out three times on the same visit. The tissue from the first curettement is sent for histology to confirm the clinical diagnosis. (See Chapter 13, Approach to Various Skin Lesions, and Chapter 33, Skin Biopsy.)

Condyloma acuminata may be excised using a loop electrode with the unit set at cutting (most commonly) or at *cut/coag* and power set at approximately 2 to 3. For larger lesions, "debulk" them with the initial pass, then successively remove more tissue and finally feather out the edges with a very light touch. Be very careful not to go too deep and remove too much tissue with the first pass! (Alternatively, any residual after the initial pass may be removed with coagulation of the bases.) *Small warts* on all parts of the body may be destroyed easily using a fine needle or ball electrode and the unit set at coagulation and a power setting just strong enough to "cook" the lesions (1 to 2). The smaller lesions can also be grasped with metal pickups and the electrode applied to the pickups while lifting the lesion. Apply enough current so that the lesion can be wiped off with moist gauze after coagulating them.

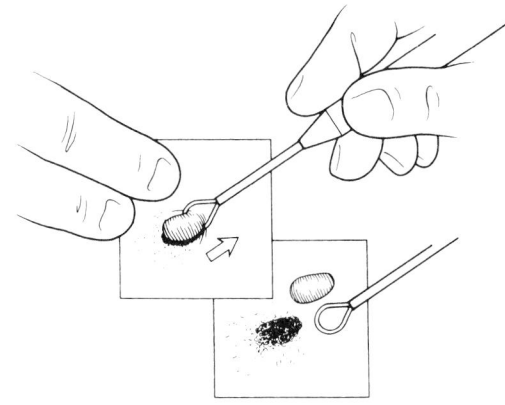

Fig. 31-10
Another technique of removing a raised skin lesion with a broad base.

Xanthelasma may be destroyed easily using a large loop and setting 2 with a cutting mode. Use very superficial passes over the lesion until all white material is removed. Use ophthalmic ointment to keep the wound moist until it is healed.

Fibroepithelial skin tags may be removed simply, usually without anesthesia, with the loop electrode, the cut (or cut/coag) setting, and power setting at slightly less than 2 (Fig. 31-11). They can also be treated like small condyloma as noted above.

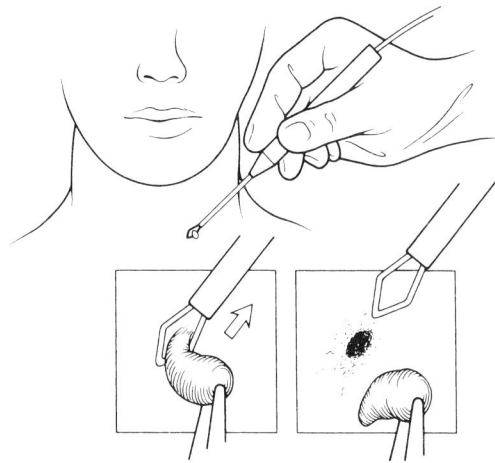

Fig. 31-11
Technique of removing a lesion with a pedunculated base.

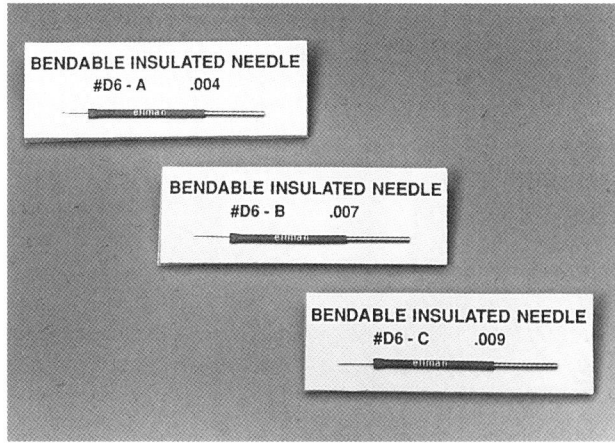

Fig. 31-12
Insulated needles available for treatment of telangiectasia. (Courtesy Ellman International, Inc., Hewlett, NY.)

Hemorrhoidal tags can be removed similar to skin tags. Be careful that the local anesthesia does not distort the base of the tag, which can create a false sense that more tissue has to be removed. This could leave a larger wound than needed. The cut/coag mode at level 3 to 4 works best. Usually the wound is left open.

Seborrheic keratoses are successfully treated using the technique described previously for shave excisions. Remember, the lesion is very superficial, so deep removal is not necessary. This will minimize scarring. Use a blade to shave off the bulk of the lesion and follow it with a large loop, cutting mode, and setting of 2, using the "feathering" technique.

Sebaceous cysts may be uncovered for intact removal or extraction of the capsule by using a small ellipse around the central pore. The cutting mode is selected and the power dial is set at no more than 2. The length and depth of the ellipse obviously depends on the size of the cyst and thickness of the skin. The vari-tip electrode is set at skin thickness (estimate). With an Allis clamp, put slight traction on the ellipsed area over the cyst wall itself. The lesion is bluntly dissected and removed.

Telangiectasias (face only) are effectively treated with the electrocoagulation technique. Use the coagulation (hemostasis) setting with the power set at 1, and a fine needle. A hypodermic needle adaptor is available for the handpiece; a short 33-gauge hypodermic needle with metal hub is then attached to the adaptor for this procedure (Fig. 31-7). Insulated needles can also be purchased from the manufacturer as well (Fig. 31-12). The special needles are active only at the very tip. Generally, only topical anesthetic is used (see Chapter 11, Topical Anesthesia). Treatment lasts a fraction of a second. The unit is activated before touching the telangiectasias. Vessels should be penetrated minimally at approximately 1- to 2-mm intervals. Begin distally and work proximal. (Doing the opposite—proximal to distal—causes the vessels to go into spasm, making them hard to locate.) Facial lesions respond the best, whereas spider veins on the lower extremity do not respond well. There is often prolonged pigmentation and recurrence of leg lesions. Sclerotherapy is the procedure of choice for the lower extremities (see Chapter 90, Sclerotherapy). *Spider angiomas* can be treated similarly. Occasionally all that is needed is coagulation of one central vessel. *Cherry hemangiomas* are best treated using light ball electrode desiccation, then wiped away.

Epilation of isolated hairs deploys a similar technique and needle. Choose the coag setting at level 1, grasp the hair with pickups, and slide the needle down the shaft. Activate the electrode; as the hair follicle is "cooked," the hair comes out easily. For large areas of unwanted hair, use the modern techniques of removal. (See Chapter 51, Laser Hair Removal: Photoepilation, and Chapter 41, Epilation of Isolated Hairs [Including Trichiasis].)

Actinic keratoses are easily treated with a desiccation technique; however, those lesions that do not respond appropriately should be studied further to rule out neoplastic changes. If there is any doubt, obtain a shave biopsy sample before treatment. Most commonly actinic keratoses are treated with cryotherapy or a shave followed by coagulation.

Plantar warts are treated in a multitude of ways (see Chapter 44, Wart [Verruca] Treatment). When other methods fail (candida injections, cryotherapy, bleomycin, etc.), the wart may have to be removed with curettement and coagulation. Perform this carefully because scarring on the bottom of the feet can cause painful nodules. Also, hyperpigmentation and some residual scarring are the norm rather than the exception.

After anesthesia, curette the lesions and follow it with coagulation. Curette again to ensure all wart tissue has been removed. Do not penetrate the dermis; warts are epithelial. Alternatively, a loop can be used to excise the lesion, but it frequently goes too deep (see precautions discussed previously). The new electrified curette works very well, but it too can go too deep, too fast, and too easily. Be careful and go slow.

For ingrown toenail surgery, where ablation of part or all of the growth center is desired, the *matrixectomy* electrodes perform superbly (Fig. 31-13). (See Chapter 40, Ingrown Toenails.)

Ear piercing: Use the thin, pointed electrode at the cutting or cut/coag setting, 2-3 or 25-30 watts. Identify the sites bilaterally and mark them. Stabilize the ear lobe then advance the tip through the anesthetized tissue. Remove the tip and insert the earring stud.

Cervical dysplasia: For those trained in colposcopy and treatment of cervical intraepithelial neoplasia (CIN), this unit can be adapted to the LLETZ (large loop excision of the transformation zone) procedure with a special set of electrodes designed for this specific purpose (Fig. 31-14). This office procedure allows a "tailored" cervical conization (see Chapter 150, Loop Electrosurgical Excision Procedure [LEEP] for Treating Cervical Intraepithelial Neoplasia).

Rhinophyma: Extra tissue is removed using the large round electrode and sculpting the nose back to the original form (Fig. 31-15). Use pure cutting, level 2.

Other lesions: *tattoos, sebaceous hyperplasia, eccrine hydrocystomas, milia, verrucae plana, verrucae vulgaris, venous lakes,* and *trichoepitheliomas.* For those performing laparoscopy, radiosurgical techniques can

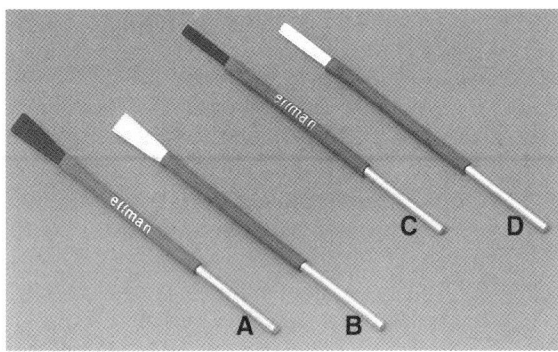

Fig. 31-13
Toenail matrixectomy electrodes. **A,** Wide blade, coated Teflon side up. **B,** Wide blade, brass uncoated side up. **C-D,** Similar with narrower sized electrode. Generally the wide one is used. The brass side goes down facing the matrix. The Teflon (coated side) faces and lifts up against the eponychium as it is slowly withdrawn.

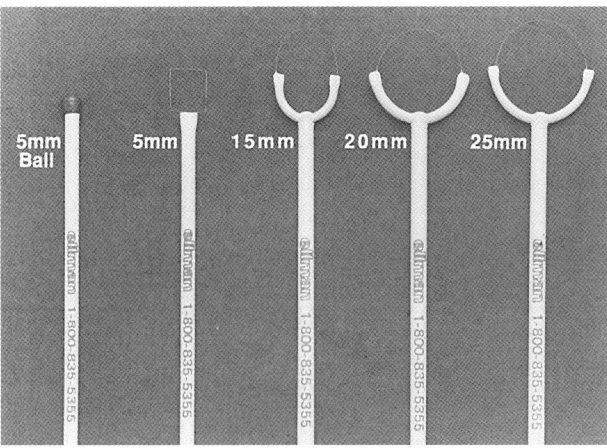

Fig. 31-14
LLETZ (large loop excision of the transformation zone) electrodes used to perform office cervical conizations. (Courtesy Ellman International, Inc., Hewlett, NY.)

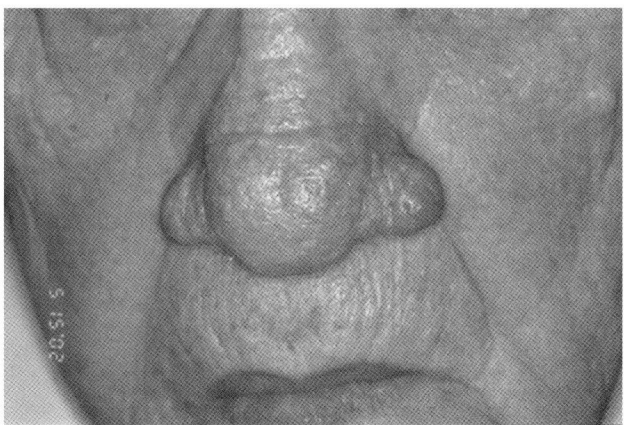

A

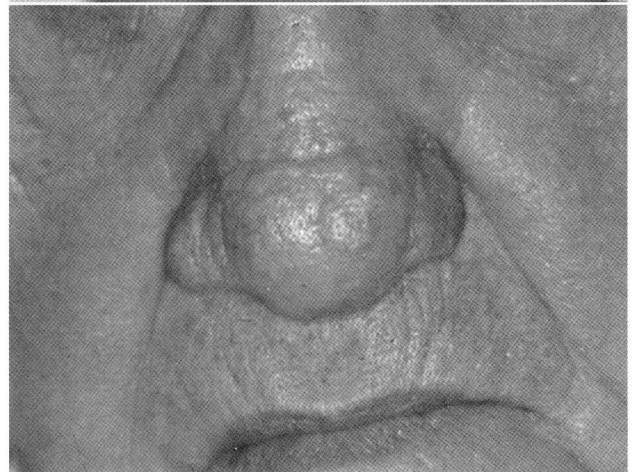

B

Fig. 31-15
Rhinophyma. **A,** Asymmetric rhinophyma on the left. Patient was only concerned about the appearance on the left. **B,** Postoperative appearance after using the large loop removal technique. (**A-B,** Courtesy The National Procedures Institute, Midland, Mich.)

be used for *endometriosis, pelvic inflammatory disease, myomectomy,* and, in skilled hands, ectopic pregnancy. The vari-tip has also been used for *blepharoplasties.* The larger pointed tips can be used for *body piercing. Uvuloplasties* are quite simple using excision or ablation techniques.

Warning: As with laser, vaporization of viral particles (HPV and HIV) in the smoke plume that accompanies destruction and/or excision of tissues with these techniques has been documented. Those present in the room should wear protective masks, and a smoke-evacuation system is mandatory (Fig. 31-16). The suction should be no further than 2 cm from the operative site. Proper vacuums have a viral filter as well as a charcoal filter to limit the offensive odor. Some physicians have created their own vacuum exhaust systems leading to the exterior of the building. Compact portable units are available from manufacturers that supply the electrosurgical units.

Modern electrosurgery (radiofrequency) techniques are easily mastered and are best accomplished by attending a workshop on radiosurgery or by following the instructions given in *Pollock's Electrosurgery of the Skin.* These instructions can be practiced at home on a piece of beefsteak. Simplicity, economy, and versatility are unique to this instrument. The lesions that can be removed are myriad, depending on the practitioner's scope of practice and versatility.

Key Points

- If adjusted to the *correct settings,* the tissue will cut like soft butter.
- If the power is too low, the stroke too fast, or the electrodes not totally clean; the *electrode will stick or catch.*
- If the power is *too high,* there will be excessive sparking and smoke.

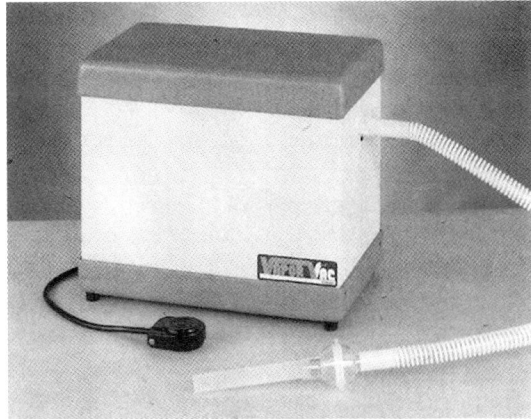

Fig. 31-16
Smoke evacuator with both viral and charcoal filters. (Courtesy Ellman International, Inc., Hewlett, NY.)

- The principle is to *minimize* the lateral heat. Less tissue damage occurs with the finer the tip, the less energy used, the less time the electrode stays in one spot, the more moist the tissue, use of a cutting mode, and use of a higher-frequency unit.

$$H = \frac{T \times I \times W \times S \times R}{F}$$

where heat (H) depends on time (T), intensity of current (I), waveform (W), area of surface contact or electrode size (S) and resistance of tissue (R) divided by frequency (F).

- Once the lesion has been removed, any remaining bleeding can be controlled with topical astringents. Monsel's or aluminum chloride work best (see Chapter 42, Topical Hemostatic Agents).

COMPLICATIONS

- Broken wire causing laceration (discard worn tips).
- Too deep an excision, causing excessive scarring and trauma to undesired tissue.
- Destruction of tissue for pathologic review, caused by improper technique.
- Handpiece in wrong port or unit in wrong mode to obtain desired effect.
- Pacemaker dysfunction.
- Inadvertent burns, either on the patient or operator, resulting from unintended activation of handpiece.
- Poor healing.
- Pain, bleeding, and infection (extremely rare).
- Scarring (usually very minimal, but could result in a depression, hypopigmentation or hyperpigmentation).
- Incomplete removal of a lesion.
- Recurrence of the lesion.
- Inadvertent shaving of a pigmented lesion that turns out to be a melanoma.
- Spreading infection between patients.
- Explosion of colonic gas (methane) if exposed to a spark (if the patient is asleep, a moist gauze should be placed in the anus to reduce the chance of a burn if working in that area).
- Sparks can cause explosions should alcohol or other agents be nearby.

Although some of these complications can be avoided, they still do occur on occasion. Removing a lesion on someone who is on aspirin or anticoagulant therapy may be accompanied by increased bleeding, necessitating heavier use of the coagulation waveform. Another complication that may be seen in diabetic patients or in older patients with thin, poorly perfused skin is slow or delayed healing. In this case, patients can often be instructed in self-care of the wound, with periodic inspections by the physician. Performing any procedures with these techniques on the lower extremities of diabetics can certainly be fraught with problems related to healing delay and possibly secondary infection. Scarring must also be considered a complication; however, once proper technique is established, a scar by this method of treatment is often less pronounced than those produced by other surgical and excisional techniques. Excising too deeply increases the likelihood of scars.

POSTPROCEDURE PATIENT CARE

Several approaches are acceptable in the postprocedure care of these lesions. Generally, the areas that were treated should be washed lightly four times per day with mild soap and water. The patient can use a washcloth for light debridement to prevent eschar formation. A topical antibiotic ointment is then applied as frequently as necessary to keep the lesion moist (even Vaseline will work). A dressing is not needed except at bedtime (or if under clothing) to ensure that the area stays moist. (See the sample patient education handout titled "Moist Healing After Skin Surgery" on page 1747 of Appendix G). Moist healing and prevention of eschar (scab) formation are essential to decrease the likelihood of scarring.

Moist healing can also occur when the lesion is simply covered with a small piece of synthetic material (Op-Site, Tegaderm, etc.) or the new Johnson & Johnson OTC product called "Advanced Healing" (see Chapter 46, Wound Dressings). A wound check in 3 to 4 days may be advised. The covering should be left in place for 1 week, providing there is not an excessive accumulation of serum. If serum does accumulate, the dressing should be changed. Usually, after 7 days, the wound can be left open to continue its healing process without any covering, unless it is in an area that may be irritated by clothing. This method is not practical in hair-bearing sites or if multiple lesions are removed.

SUPPLIERS

Ellman International, Inc.
1135 Railroad Avenue
Hewlett, NY 11557
Phone: 1-800-835-5355
Website: www.ellman.com

Wallach Surgical Devices, Inc.
235 Edison Road
Orange, CT 06477
Phone: 1-800-243-2463
Website: www.wallachsurgical.com

For other suppliers, see Chapter 150, Loop Electrosurgical Excision Procedure (LEEP) for Treating Cervical Intraepithelial Neoplasia.

CPT/BILLING CODES

Billing codes for radiofrequency surgery are very complex; codes vary with the lesion size, benign or malignant characteristics, location, and type of removal. Some lesions would be billed out as true "excision." Others would be billed as "shave excision," and still others would be termed "destruction" or "biopsy." The reader is advised to consult the most recent CPT coding manuals and other sections of this text.

ADDITIONAL RESOURCES

- See the sample patient education handout titled "Moist Healing After Skin Surgery" on page 1747 of Appendix G.

BIBLIOGRAPHY

Brown JS: *Minor surgery: a text and atlas*, ed 4, Arnold Publishers, New York, 2000, Oxford University (Ch. 16).

Chiarello S: Controlled radio-vaporization of tumor tissue utilizing 4.0 MHz radiofrequency cutting current through a patented radiofrequency blade, *Dermatol Surg* 27:157, 2001.

El-Gamal HM, Dufresne RG, Saddler K: Electrosurgery, pacemakers and ICDS: A survey of precautions and complications experienced by cutaneous surgeons, *Dermatol Surg* 27:385, 2001.

Hainer BL: Fundamentals of electrosurgery, *J Fam Practice* 4:419, 1991.

Hainer BL, Usatine RB: Electrosurgery for the skin, *Am Fam Physician* 66:1259, 2002.

Kannon GA: Moist wound healing with occlusive dressings: a clinical review, *Dermatol Surg* 21:583, 1995.

O'Grady KF, Easty AC: Electrosurgery smoke: hazards and protection, *J Clin Eng* 21:149, 1996.

Pollack SV: *Electrosurgery of the skin*, New York, 1991, Churchill Livingstone.

Editor's note: This is a comprehensive, concise, small text that provides a thorough practical review of radiosurgery.

Rex J, Ribera M, Bielsa I, et al: Surgical management of rhinophyma: report of eight patients treated with electrosection, *Dermatol Surg* 28:347, 2002.

Usatine RP: Electrosurgery. In Usatine RP, Moy RC, editors: *Skin surgery: a practical guide*, St Louis, 1998, Mosby.

Wedman J, Miljeteig H: Treatment of simple snoring using radio waves for ablation of uvula and soft palate: a day-case surgery procedure, *Laryngoscope* 112:1256, 2002.

Ring Removal from an Edematous Finger

John Harlan Haynes III
Andrew Thomas Haynes

Soft tissue swelling of a finger occurs with trauma, fluid retention, weight gain, arthritis, allergic reaction, infection, or iatrogenic infusion infiltration. When the finger is constricted by circumferential banding, such as with ring jewelry, venous outflow from the finger may be restricted, which can lead to nerve damage, ischemia, and digital gangrene if the ring is not removed promptly.

The involved finger should be evaluated initially for any lacerations or neurovascular compromise. This can be accomplished by testing for sensory deficits through the use of two-point discrimination to the distal fingertip and assessment of distal digital pulses with a doppler flow meter. In the absence of any signs of neurovascular compromise, ring sparing techniques may be attempted initially; however, if signs of compromise are present, ring cutting is indicated.

If ring removal is not accomplished by a trial of elevation, lubrication, and circular traction, the clinician may use the string-wrap method without harm to the patient or the ring. Alternatively, a conventional hand-operated circular saw or Steinmann pin cutter may be used to cut the ring. However, this damages jewelry and could injure the patient. Care should be taken to avoid implantation of metal filings, which may lead to foreign body granuloma and synovitis if the ring is cut.

After ring removal by any of these methods, a neurovascular examination should be performed as mentioned above. If any deficits in sensation or vascular flow are noted, prompt consultation with a hand specialist is required.

INDICATIONS

- Acute or chronic finger edema with proximal band constriction

RELATIVE CONTRAINDICATIONS

- Open wound or fracture
- Deeply embedded ring erosion
- Lack of patient cooperation

STRING-WRAP METHOD

Equipment

- Between 2 and 3 yards of string, braided suture of 0 gauge or larger, or umbilical tape—preferably on a spool
- Adhesive tape
- Small hemostat
- 1.5 ml 1% lidocaine *without* epinephrine *(optional)*
- 5-ml syringe with 27-gauge needle for digital nerve block *(optional)*
- Lubricating K-Y Jelly

Technique

1. Some patients may require a digital block in case the pain increases from the compression and unwinding. If needed, 0.5 to 0.75 ml of 1% lidocaine is infiltrated deep into the neurovascular bundle on the proximal volar aspect of the affected finger bilaterally.
2. Lightly lubricate the finger near the ring. Pass the hemostat from distal to proximal under the ring, grasp the end of the string, and thread it beneath the ring, pulling several inches of string through (Fig. 32-1, *A*). Tape the proximal end to the hand (Fig. 32-1, *B*).
3. Wrap the string circumferentially around the finger, beginning just adjacent to the ring margin. Care should be taken to not wrap the string so tight as to

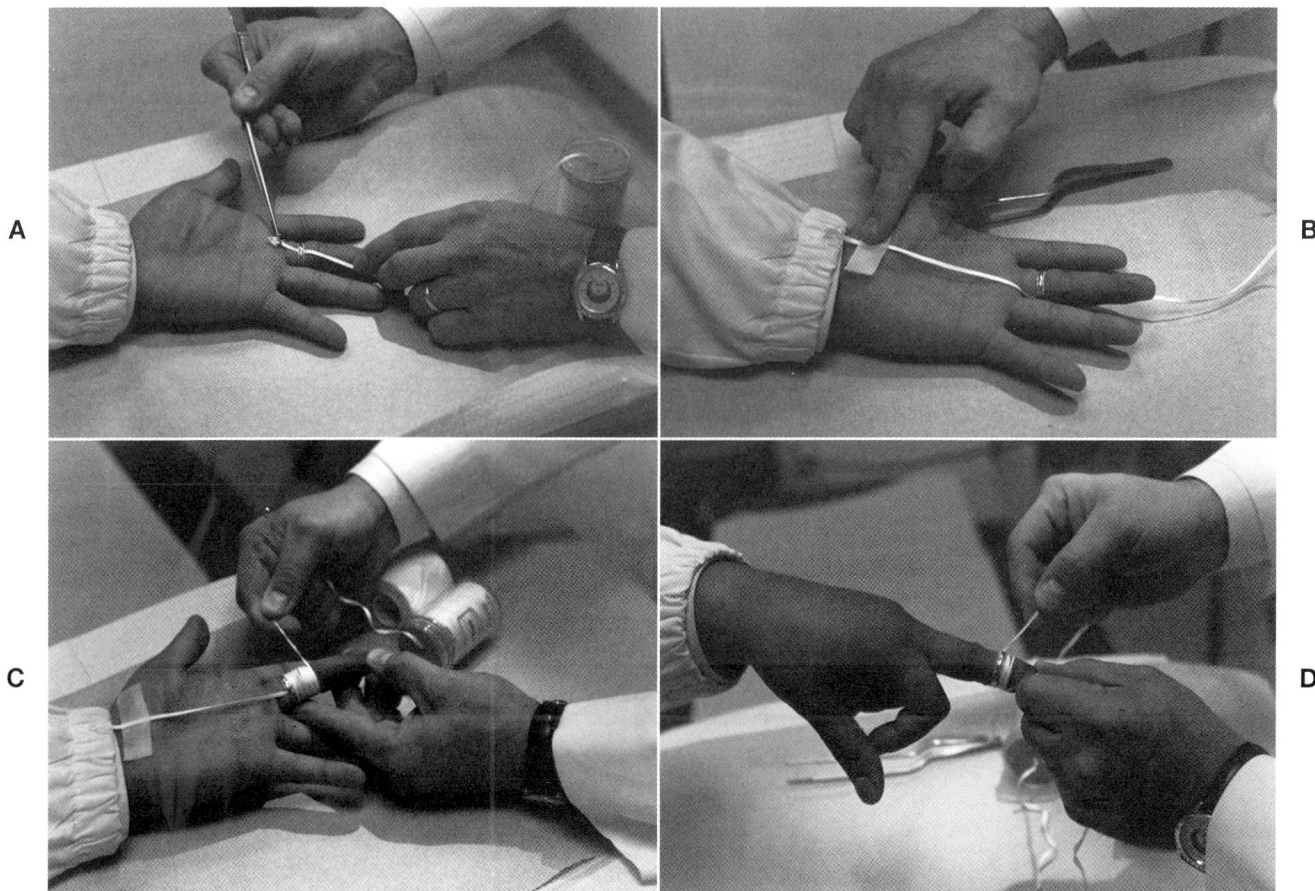

Fig. 32-1
A-D, String-wrap method of removing ring from a swollen finger. See text for details.

obstruct arterial flow. Wind the string in a smooth single layer going distally, using moderate tension until it encompasses the point of greatest swelling (Fig. 32-1, *C*).

4. Untape the proximal end of the string and pull distally toward the fingertip. Maintain tension along the long axis of the finger, moving the ring distally as the string unwinds beneath it. Force the ring over that portion of the finger that has been compressed by the wrap (Fig. 32-1, *D*). Once past the area of largest diameter, usually the proximal interphalangeal joint, the ring will slide off easily.

CIRCULAR SAW OR STEINMANN PIN CUTTER METHOD

Equipment

- Handheld circular-blade ring cutter (e.g., Beaver) or Steinmann pin cutter with a McDonald elevator

- Large hemostats (e.g., Kelly clamps)
- 20-ml syringe filled with saline and 20-gauge Intracath sheath

Technique

1. Slip the small hook of the ring cutter or elevator under the ring on the palmar surface to serve as a guide and barrier (Fig. 32-2). If elevation of this section is necessary for application of the ring cutter, the ring may be bent outward by using pliers with the jaws placed at 90 degrees from the cutting site.
2. Firmly grip the saw handle, and, using a 180-degree twisting motion, grind through the ring. Using the pin cutter, cut through the ring over the elevator.
3. The cut ends of the ring may be spread through the use of hemostats with steady opposing forces.
4. Rinse the area with high-pressure saline to ensure evacuation of all metal filings.

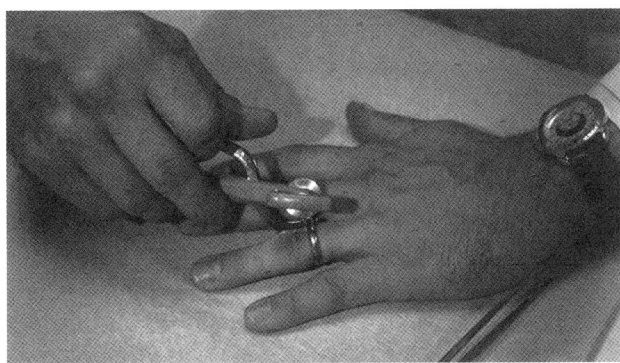

Fig. 32-2
Hook of the ring cutter serves as a guide and barrier.

CPT/BILLING CODES

20670   Superficial removal of constricting metal band

20680   Deep removal of constricting metal band

ICD-9-CM DIAGNOSTIC CODES

782.3   Traumatic edema NEC
719.04   Joint effusion, hand

BIBLIOGRAPHY

Clarke AC, Spencer RF: Ring removal from the injured or swollen finger, *Postgrad Med* 89:190, 1991.

Fasano FJ, Hansen RH: Foreign body granuloma and synovitis of the finger: a hazard of ring removal by the sawing technique, *J Hand Surg* 12A:621, 1987

Frary T: A few brief tips: ring removal, *J Am Acad Physician Assist* 3:156, 1990.

Huss CD: Removing a ring from a swollen finger. In Driscoll CE, Rakel RE, editors: *Patient care: procedures for your practice,* Oradell, NJ, 1988, Medical Economics Books.

Mizrahi S, Lunski I: A simplified method for ring removal from an edematous finger, *Am J Surg* 151:412, 1986.

Roberts JR, Hedges JR: *Clinical procedures in emergency medicine,* Philadelphia, 1985, WB Saunders.

Tintinalli JE, Ruiz E, Krome RL: *Emergency medicine: a comprehensive study guide,* New York, 1996, McGraw-Hill.

CHAPTER 33

Skin Biopsy

Stephen K. Toadvine*
John L. Pfenninger

Examination and appropriate history suffice to establish most dermatologic diagnoses. At times, however, invasive biopsies are necessary. A skin biopsy is typically performed to make or confirm a diagnosis and to guide definitive treatment. In many instances, a biopsy serves as the means of both diagnosis and treatment if it removes the entire lesion. Needle aspiration biopsy (Chapter 210, Fine-Needle Aspiration Cytology and Biopsy) is usually reserved for deeper lesions but at times can also be used to diagnose skin lesions.

Skin biopsies are generally quick, simple, and cost-effective. Diagnoses obtained by biopsy also serve to build a physician's experience and skill in dermatologic diagnosis, perhaps reducing need for future biopsies of similar lesions.

To enable the pathologist to provide the most information possible, provide a good history with each specimen submitted. Include aspects of the "seven Ds":
- *Demographics* (e.g., patient's age, history of travel, location of lesion)
- *Diseases* (other diseases the patient has [e.g., lupus])
- *Duration* (how long it has been present)
- *Drugs* applied to the lesion or taken by the patient that could be the cause or change the appearance of the lesion (e.g., topical or oral steroids)
- *Description* (e.g., papular, vesicular, hyperkeratotic)
- *Diameter*
- *Diagnosis* suspected

Skin biopsies are either partial or full thickness. Partial-thickness biopsies include shave excision and curettage. Full-thickness biopsies include standard excisional and incisional biopsies and the "punch" biopsy. Punch biopsies take only 5 to 7 minutes to complete; excisional or incisional types take longer. All of these may readily be incorporated in a primary care setting.

Priorities to be kept in mind when performing skin biopsies are (1) maintaining patient comfort and safety,

(2) obtaining an appropriate tissue sample for pathologic diagnosis, and (3) producing the best cosmetic and functional result possible.

INDICATIONS

- To obtain a tissue sample for histopathology, electron-microscopy, or immunofluorescence testing
- To obtain a deep culture (bacterial or fungal) and to avoid superficial contamination of wounds (e.g., decubiti)

Note: Lyme disease can be confirmed through cultures, which are usually sent to the health department.

- To perform an excision for curative or cosmetic purposes

In general, the main reasons to do a skin biopsy are to rule out cancer and to determine the disease process present. If the physician's answer to the question "What is it?" is "I don't know," that may be an indication for biopsy (not necessarily referral). The next question should be, "Could this be a melanoma?" If the answer is "yes," then a full-thickness biopsy (punch, incision, or excision) is indicated.

CONTRAINDICATIONS

- Significant coagulopathy
- Preparations, anesthetics, preservatives, or other materials to which the patient is allergic
- Partial-thickness biopsies are contraindicated if melanoma is suspected (must "biopsy for depth")

A biopsy does *not* spread disease, distort a future diagnosis of a melanoma, or compromise future care (unless a melanoma is shaved and transected!). The only real error that can be made in biopsying a lesion is to shave a melanoma and not remove the entire lesion. If the entire lesion is removed so depth of the lesion can be assessed, there is no consequence. However, if part

---

*Dr. Toadvine contributes to this edition with the understanding that he objects to the inclusion of Chapter 130, First-Trimester Abortion and Emergency Oral Contraceptives, in this text.

of the lesion is left behind thereby making it impossible to determine prebiopsy depth, it could compromise appropriate care. Melanoma treatment and prognosis are dependent on depth of the neoplasm. Thus, if there is a possibility of melanoma, it is best to "biopsy for depth."

EQUIPMENT

- Nonsterile gloves (sterile if sutures are to be placed)
- Alcohol wipes
- Local anesthetic (0.5 to 1.0 ml of 1% to 2% lidocaine with or without epinephrine)
- Hemostatic agents (see Chapter 42, Topical Hemostatic Agents)
- Antibiotic ointment
- Adhesive bandage
- Specimen container, usually containing formalin

For Punch Biopsy

- 3- or 4-mm punch biopsy tool (Fig. 33-1); disposable biopsy punches are convenient and inexpensive, and it is not necessary to clean, sterilize, or sharpen them; 2-mm punch to be used only for areas where scarring is to be avoided, because such a small amount of tissue may lead to a missed diagnosis or the tissue can become inappropriately crushed.
- Pickups.
- Sharp fine-tissue scissors.
- Suture kit or Steri-Strips (only if the biopsy site is 4 mm or larger).

For Curettage

A dermal curette (Fig. 33-2) is used. Disposable curettes are recommended, unless a cancer is suspected. Disposables are sharp but have a tendency to bend. When a cancer is treated, the tissue is necrotic, so sharp instruments are not as essential and reusables are less likely to cut into the normal skin. Curettes of 3-, 4-, 5-, and 6-mm should be available. The size used depends on the size of the lesion.

For Shave Excisions

A single edge flexible razor blade or scalpel blade (no. 10 or 15) is used (Fig. 33-3). A scalpel handle is not needed; not only does it take time to insert and remove but also medical personnel can be injured during removal of the blade from the handle. The blade itself or a radiofrequency unit may be used to smooth out the surface after use of a blade. (See Chapter 31, Radiofrequency Surgery,

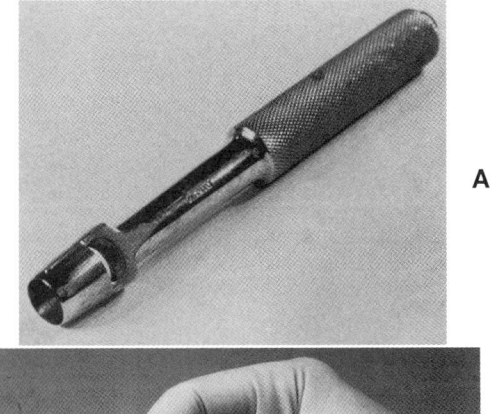
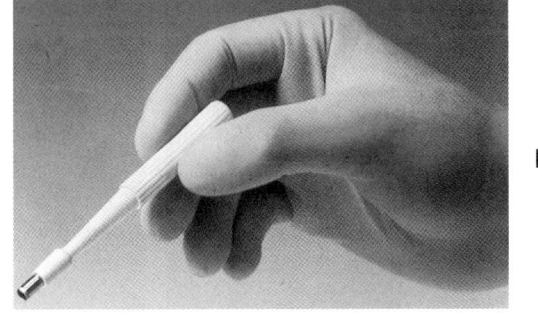

Fig. 33-1
Reusable (**A**) and disposable (**B**) punch biopsy instruments. (**B,** Courtesy CooperSurgical, Trumbull, Conn.)

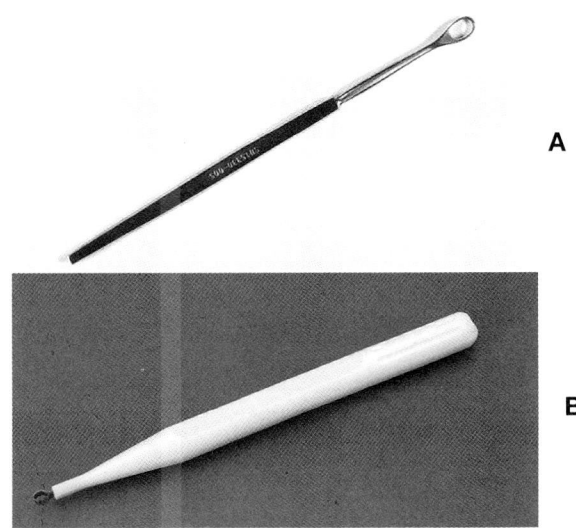

Fig. 33-2
A, Fox dermal curette (reusable). **B,** Acuderm disposable curette. (**B,** Courtesy Acuderm, Inc., Ft Lauderdale, Fla.)

to review the technique.) Sharp tissue scissors (Metzenbaum) can also be used to perform the "shave."

For Incisions and Excisions

- Minor surgical or laceration tray with scalpel, skin hooks, pickups, tissue scissors, and suture (see Chapter

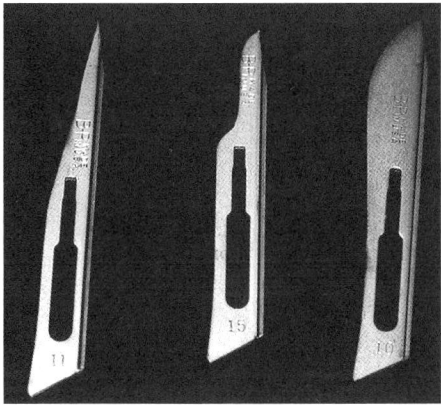

Fig. 33-3
No. 11, 15, and 10 scalpel blades used for shave excisions.

22, Incisions: Planning the Direction of the Cut; Chapter 23, Laceration and Incision Repair; and Chapter 25, Laceration and Incision Repair: Suture Selection).
- Radiofrequency unit if desired (see Chapter 31, Radiofrequency Surgery)

Note: Tissue for culture may need to be placed in saline, whereas immunofluorescent studies may require that the tissue be placed in dry ice. Check with the pathologist or health department to determine the proper handling to diagnose Lyme disease.

TECHNIQUE

Choosing a Biopsy Site

When there are multiple lesions that could be biopsied, **avoid** the following areas:
- Cosmetically important areas
- Upper chest and deltoid regions, where hypertrophic scarring is more common
- Fingers, toes, and areas overlying joints
- Regions in which secondary infection (e.g., axillae and groin) or delayed healing (e.g., pretibial) are common
- Areas that compromise underlying structures, including superficial nerves and vessels
- Old lesions (choose well-developed but "fresh" lesions free of excoriation or excessive inflammation)
- Ulcerated lesions (if the only available lesion is ulcerated, include a border of the lesion in the specimen)
- Areas of poor circulation

Although any skin area can be biopsied, being selective improves final outcome. See Table 33-1 for recommendations specific to particular lesions and Table 33-2 for anatomic sites.

It is *not* necessary to include normal tissue in the sample, except when biopsying a vesicular-bullous lesion. It is then necessary to biopsy (usually a punch) right

TABLE 33-1
Selection of Biopsy Site Based on Lesion Type

Lesion Suspected	Where to Biopsy
Basal cell carcinoma	Raised, nonulcerated area
Squamous cell carcinoma	Central, thickened area
Melanoma	Darkest, raised portion
Vesicular-bullous disease	Fresh lesion at the margin; include some normal tissue (see Fig. 33-4)
Rashes	Primary lesion without secondary excoriation or infection

Notes:
1. Normal tissue is not needed in most instances (only with vesicular-bullous lesions)
2. A biopsy does not spread cancer.
3. In biopsying a suspected melanoma, go for depth (i.e., a punch instead of a shave).
4. Most chronic dermatitis is nonspecific on biopsy. A dermatologic consult may be indicated and be more beneficial.

TABLE 33-2
Site-Specific Biopsy Guidelines

Location	Comments
Breast	Punch or shave
Cervix	Mini-Townsend or baby Tischler forceps (see Chapter 139, Colposcopic Examination)
Eyelid	Sharp tissue scissors for shave removal
Gingiva	Shave; consider radiofrequency unit to limit bleeding if lesion is elevated
Intraanal	Cervical biopsy forceps or flexible sigmoidoscopy "wire" biopsy forceps
Lip	Punch (bloody; heals quickly) or shave
Muscle	See Chapter 214, Muscle Biopsy
Nail bed	Remove portion of nail; use small punch; see Chapter 29, Nail Bed Repair
Penis	Thin skin; use shave technique; stay superficial; scissors work best
Perianal	Sharp tissue scissors
Pinna	Shave or superficial punch
Tongue	Punch; bloody; use suture
Trunk	Any method
Vagina	Cervical biopsy forceps
Vulva	Hair-bearing area: use punch Non-hair-bearing area: shave biopsy (see Chapter 161, Vulvar Biopsy)

at the margin where the skin is being lifted from the underlying tissue (Fig. 33-4). If small, a deep shave removing the entire lesion is also acceptable.

Punch Biopsy

The punch biopsy instrument is used to obtain a full-thickness cylindrical specimen. Punch biopsy is a good choice for complete removal of small lesions (less than 5 mm) or when there is doubt as to the diagnosis or optimal treatment for a particular lesion.

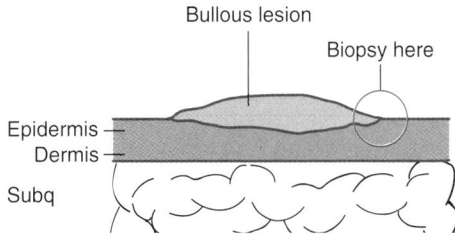

Fig. 33-4
Obtaining a skin biopsy when a vesicle or bulla is present. Normal tissue should be included in the specimen. "Fresh" lesions that have not ruptured and are not crusted should be chosen.

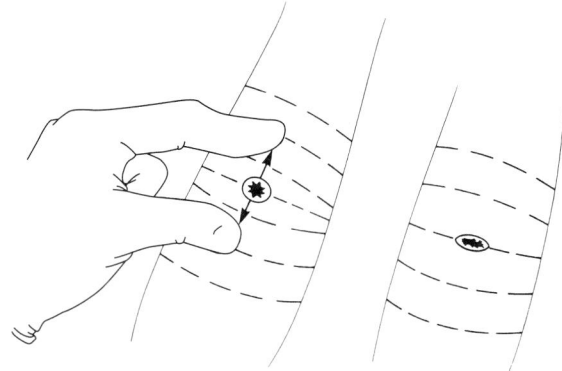

Fig. 33-5
Proper stretching of skin tension lines before punch biopsy. Upon release, the tendency of the skin is to make the circular biopsy become more elliptical and thus more cosmetically pleasing when healed.

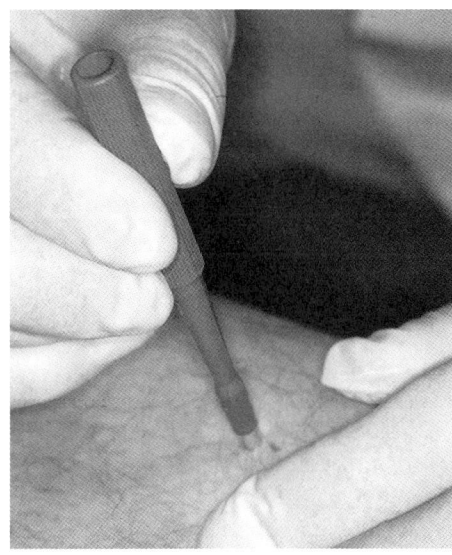

Fig. 33-6
Applying the punch for a skin biopsy. (Courtesy The National Procedures Institute, Midland, Mich.)

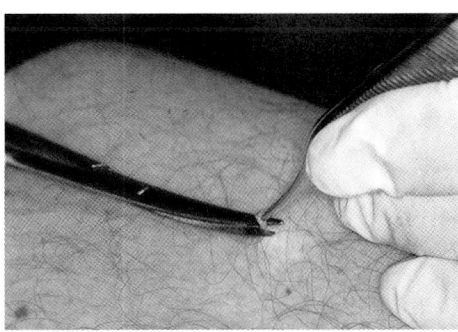

Fig. 33-7
Excising the tissue freed by the punch. (Courtesy The National Procedures Institute, Midland, Mich.)

1. Prepare the selected site with alcohol. Sterile technique should be followed if sutures are intended; otherwise, nonsterile gloves can be used. Biopsies of 2 or 3 mm do not need to be closed with sutures. A 4-mm biopsy on the face may need to be sutured, and a 5-mm biopsy nearly always requires suturing.

2. Place a ring of anesthesia around the lesion (field block) or deep to the lesion.

3. Choose the appropriate sized punch unit (2 to 5 mm). Remember that 2-mm biopsies may not provide adequate tissue for diagnosis. To minimize scarring, stretch the skin on both sides of the planned biopsy site away from the site, perpendicular to the lines of minimal skin tension, using the thumb and index finger of the nondominant hand (Fig. 33-5). Then push the unit vertically into the skin and rotate it to cut through the skin to the subcutaneous fat (Fig. 33-6). A decrease in resistance should be felt at the point where the dermis is completely penetrated (much like doing a lumbar puncture).

4. Withdraw the punch. Push down with the fingers on each side of the biopsy. If the "plug" goes down with the skin, the biopsy has not gone deep enough. If the plug pops up instead of going down, then the adipose tissue has been entered and the tissue has been freed adequately. Gently grasp the specimen with forceps or a skin hook. Lift the specimen and free it by cutting the subcutaneous base with sharp tissue scissors (Figs. 33-7 and 33-8). Apply pressure for hemostasis. Avoid chemical astringents in punch sites if the wound is to be closed with sutures, SteriStrips, or glues; otherwise, apply Monsel's, aluminum chloride, or gel foam to control the bleeding. (Biopsies 3 mm or less rarely, if ever, need closure.)

5. Large punch instruments (larger than 5 mm) are available, but closure of these wounds may require conversion of the circular defect into an ellipse because closure would otherwise cause "dog ears."

6. Use of absorbable sutures provides the same outcome cosmetically as does the use of nonabsorbable sutures.

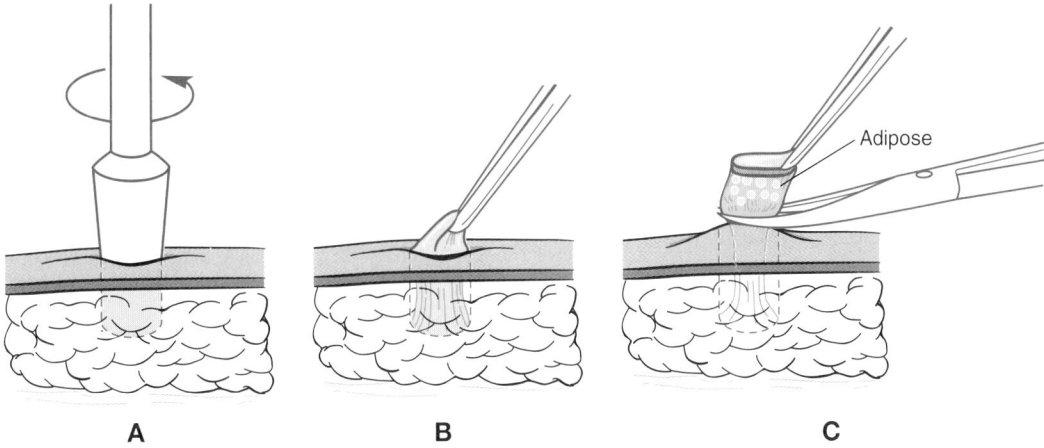

Fig. 33-8
Graphic representation of the punch biopsy technique. **A,** Twisting the punch with gentle pressure. **B,** Picking up the loosened piece. **C,** Cutting with scissors or a blade.

Curettage

Curettage is a partial-thickness technique and is particularly well suited for removal of basal cell carcinomas and hyperkeratotic epidermal lesions such as warts, molluscum, seborrheic keratoses, and actinic keratoses (see Chapter 13, Approach to Various Skin Lesions). A potential disadvantage of curettage in terms of obtaining a laboratory specimen is that, usually, multiple fragments of specimen are produced and the presence of disease-free margins cannot be determined. The physician performing the procedure decides if the removal is adequate.

Note: With benign lesions, it is clinically apparent when abnormal tissue has been removed. For malignant lesions, the curettement goes down to "gritty" tissue and is then followed by cautery. This process of curettement and cautery is done three times to ensure complete removal of any foci of neoplastic tissue.

1. Prepare the area with alcohol and obtain an anesthetic wheal. Use the curette to literally scrape away or scoop out a lesion, typically in multiple fragments. Send the curretted tissue to pathology.
2. Continue the curettage until only normal tissue remains at the margins. Usually, this is the upper aspect of the dermis, which feels "gritty" or "sandy" under the curette and demonstrates punctate surface bleeding. Use hemostasis as needed with topical hemostatic agents or light ball cautery. Carcinomas and severely dysplastic lesions generally feel soft and scrape out easily. Remember, when using curettage to treat a carcinoma, repeat a process of curettage and cautery three times (Fig. 33-9) (see Chapter 13, Approach to Various Skin Lesions).
3. If, in the case of cancer, curettage (or shave excision)

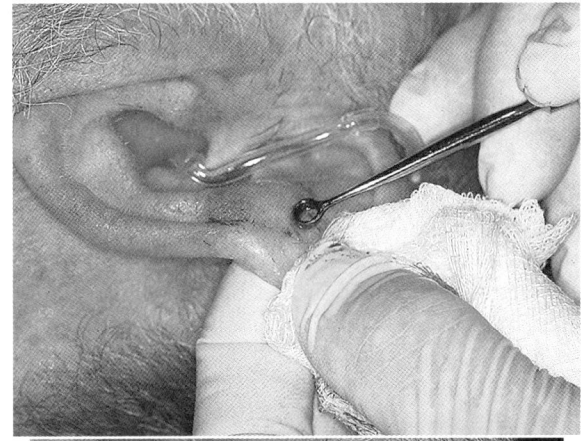

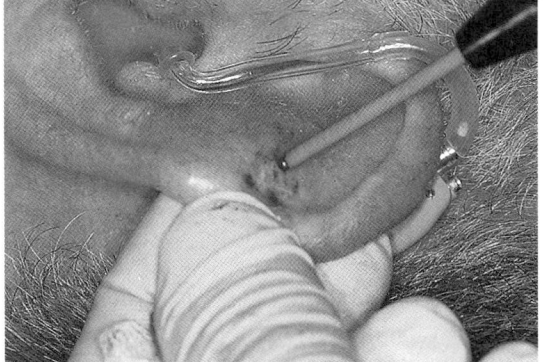

Fig. 33-9
A, Skin biopsy using curettement. **B,** Cautery after curettement. (Courtesy The National Procedures Institute, Midland, Mich.)

produces a full-thickness skin wound and adipose tissue is entered, this indicates that the tumor has probably invaded below the dermis. Set up a sterile field, excise the area, and close the wound with suture.

Shave Biopsy

Shave biopsy is used to remove the protruding portion of a raised skin lesion when a full-thickness sample is not required. *Shave excisions should not be performed if a melanoma is suspected* because they may interfere with the pathologist's ability to grade the depth of the invasion.

A melanoma is treated based on the depth of the invasion, and a difference of 0.1 mm or even 0.01 mm could be the difference between little further treatment and a radical resection. Lesions most amenable to shave excision include compound or intradermal nevi, skin tags, seborrheic keratoses, actinic keratoses, lentigines, and small basal-cell carcinomas.

Advantages of shave excision include minimal time requirement, simple equipment, lack of need for reapproximation and suturing, and generally good cosmetic results. Also, the pathologist can determine if the entire lesion has been removed.

1. Prepare the area with alcohol and use clean technique; sterile gloves are not necessary. Reserve full sterile setup for full-thickness skin excisions. Instill a local anesthetic within the dermis underneath the lesion to elevate the lesion slightly, facilitating removal.

2. Excise the lesion by shaving with a slightly bowed, flexible single-edge razor blade or with a scalpel blade kept parallel to the skin (Figs. 33-10 and 33-11). The resulting defect should be essentially level, or minimally depressed, in relation to the surrounding skin. The greater the depth of the invaded dermis, the more likely there will be resultant scarring. Apply simple pressure, pinpoint electrodesiccation, radiofrequency coagulation, or topical agents such as aluminum chloride or Monsel's solution to achieve hemostasis. Topical applications theoretically may inhibit healing. Monsel's (and silver nitrate) carry the risk of temporary staining.

3. Shave excision can be performed using a radiofrequency loop. Heat artifact may occur at the margins of the excision, hindering histopathologic evaluation, or in the case of a very thin lesion, obliterating the lesion entirely. Also, because of the ease of cutting with the radiofrequency unit, the novice user may inadvertently go too deep with the loop, causing excessive and unnecessary scarring. Many practitioners perform a shave biopsy with a scalpel blade then use a radiofrequency loop to "feather out" the edges of the defect created to complete the procedure (see Chapter 31, Radiofrequency Surgery).

4. Sharp tissue scissors can be used, especially for pedunculated lesions, to effectively shave off the abnormality.

5. A variation of the shave biopsy is the **"saucer excision."** With this technique, the central aspect of

the biopsy, instead of being flat, is more depressed than the periphery. One might use this technique for actinic lesions, nevi, or dermatofibromas. In cases of suspected dysplastic nevi (but not a melanoma), one may cautiously perform a "deep saucer shave"

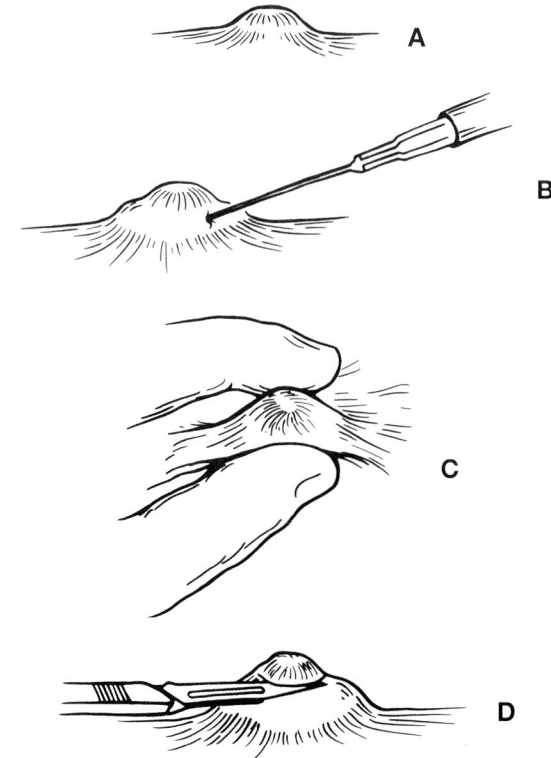

Fig. 33-10
One technique of shave biopsy. **A,** The lesion. **B,** Inject a local anesthetic to elevate the lesion. **C,** Roll the skin between the thumb and forefinger to create a flat cutting surface and a tamponade effect on the surrounding blood vessels. **D,** Holding a no. 15 blade parallel to the skin or at a slight downward angle, shave the lesion flush with or slightly below the surrounding skin.

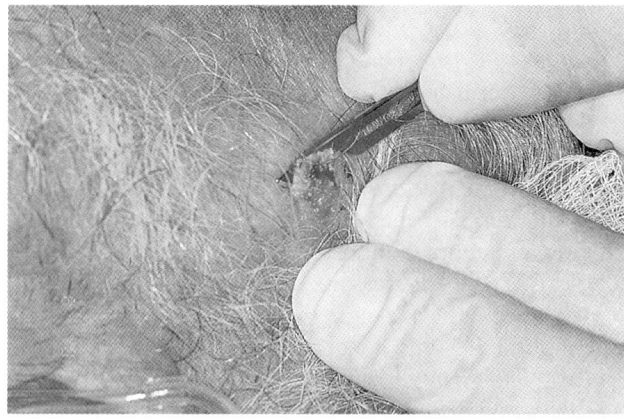

Fig. 33-11
Shave technique using a no. 15 blade. Note: No scalpel handle is necessary. (Courtesy The National Procedures Institute, Midland, Mich.)

because it allows histopathologic review of the tissue to ensure everything has been removed. Be sure, however, not to partially transect a melanoma; this is a very fine line. When in doubt, perform a deep punch biopsy first to confirm the lesion is benign.

Excisional or Incisional Biopsy

An **excisional biopsy** is used to remove an entire lesion in a manner that obtains a full-thickness specimen of skin. Diagnosis and treatment are carried out at the same time. Excisional biopsy is ideal for removal of malignant, or suspected malignant, skin lesions because margins can be assessed. An **incisional biopsy** removes only a portion of a larger lesion, but residual abnormal tissue remains. Generally, a single punch biopsy (or more, if the lesion is very large) would be quicker and more acceptable.

1. In performing an excision, use sterile technique. Establish anesthesia, preferably in a field block pattern. Use a surgical marking pen to outline the planned margins of excision and orient the long axis of the excision parallel to the lines of minimal skin tension (see Chapters 22 to 26). Form the planned excision in the shape of an ellipse with a length that measures three times its width. The corners of the ellipse should measure approximately 30 degrees (Fig. 33-12). See Chapter 13, Approach to Various Skin Lesions, for a discussion on appropriate margins for various lesions.

2. With the scalpel, make the initial incision along the outlined excision, then free up one corner of the ellipse, excising the full thickness of skin. Excise from one end to the center, then from the opposite end to the center, obtaining a specimen of uniform thickness. (A common error is to perform only a partial-thickness excision in the corners or lateral aspects of the wound.)

3. After the specimen is freed, undermine the edges on each side of the wound to a distance measuring one third to one half the width of the original wound (Fig. 33-13). Undermine between the dermis and subcutaneous tissue with a scalpel blade, tissue scissors, or a radiofrequency unit employing a vari-tip or fine needle with the unit set on the cut and coagulation setting.

4. A simple single layer closure suffices for wounds with minimal tension. Otherwise, absorbable subcutane-

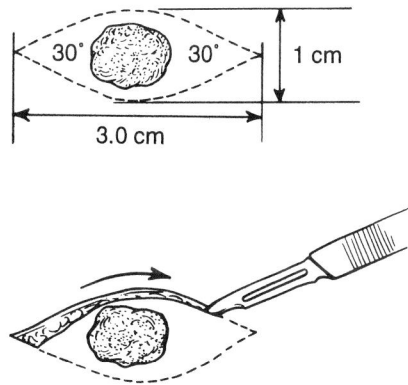

Fig. 33-12
Elliptical excision biopsy technique. See text for details.

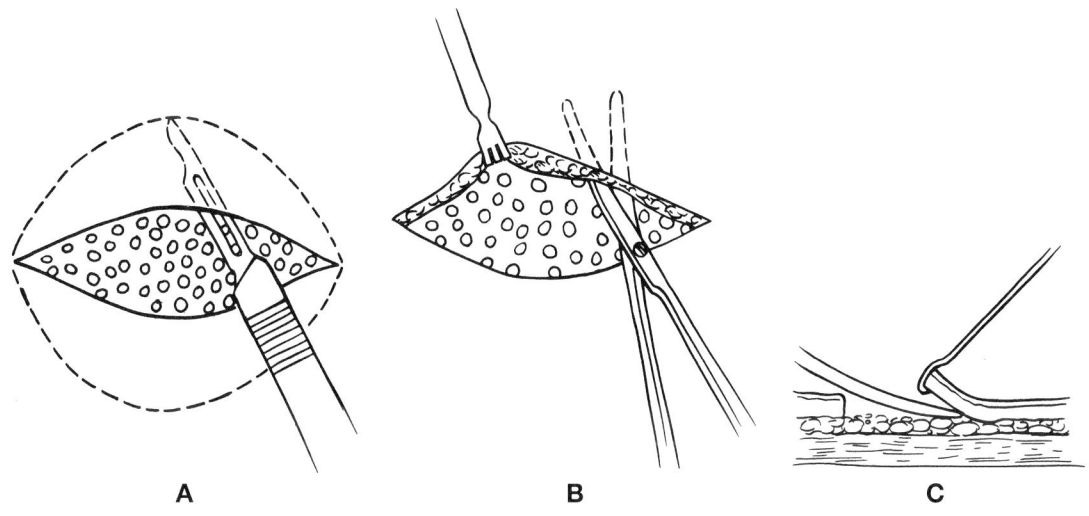

Fig. 33-13
Subcutaneous undermining to release tension on wound margins with, **A,** scalpel and, **B,** scissors. **C,** Proper level for undermining within subcutaneous fat.

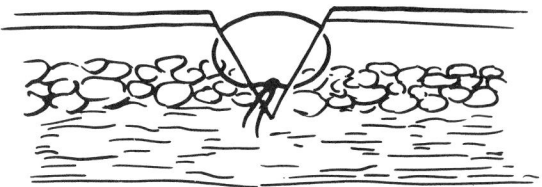

Fig. 33-14
Deep inverted absorbable sutures to close dead space after excision.

ous sutures (e.g., Dexon, Vicryl) placed with an inverted knot can be used to reduce tension on the skin edges before final closure is completed (Fig. 33-14; see also Chapter 23, Laceration and Incision Repair).

Note: The following topics can be found in their respective chapters: planning the excisional site (Chapter 22), choosing and administering the anesthetic (Chapter 4), selecting the suture (Chapter 25), performing proper closures (Chapter 26), and choosing dressings (Chapter 46).

COMPLICATIONS

- *Pain:* generally insignificant.
- *Infection:* If the patient washes the area three to four times per day with soap and water and applies ointment (antibiotic or otherwise) to keep it moist, there is rarely an infection.
- *Excessive bleeding:* almost nonexistent.
- *Scarring:* always a possibility. With punch biopsies, there may be an "acne-like" pock mark. Obviously, excision and incision leaves a line and possibly suture tracks. All methods can leave hypopigmentation. Some topical hemostatic agents (Monsel's and especially silver nitrate) can leave prolonged hyperpigmentation.
- *Missing the correct diagnosis:* A lesion may be sent for biopsy, but unless it is totally removed, the worst area could be missed. (Likewise, the practitioner could unknowingly shave and transect through a melanoma; therefore if there is any doubt, biopsy for depth.)
- *Allergic reactions:* To topical antibiotics, the anesthetic, dressings, and other agents (usually indicated by redness and itching).

POSTPROCEDURE PATIENT EDUCATION

Shave excisions and curettage require moist healing, as described for radiofrequency shave excisions in Chapter 31, Radiofrequency Surgery. Care for sutured full-thickness wounds is like that for primary clean lacerations and incisions described in Chapter 23, Laceration and Incision Repair.

SUPPLIERS

Disposable and reusable punches and curettes*
Acuderm
5370 NW 35 Terrace
Ft Lauderdale, FL 33309
Phone: 1-800-327-0015
Website: www.acuderm.com

Miltex
700 Hicksville Road
Bethpage, NY 11714-3490
Phone: 1-800-645-8000
Website: www.miltex.com

CooperSurgical
95 Corporate Drive
Trumbull, CT 06611
Phone: 1-800-645-3760
Website: www.coopersurgical.com

CPT/BILLING CODES

11100	Skin biopsy, one lesion
11101	Biopsy, each additional lesion
11755	Biopsy nail unit
30100	Biopsy intranasal
38500	Biopsy/excision lymph node, superficial
38505	Biopsy lymph node, by needle
45100	Biopsy anorectal wall
54100	Biopsy penis, cutaneous
54105	Biopsy penis, deep
56605	Biopsy lesion, vulva
57100	Biopsy vagina, simple
57105	Biopsy vagina, extensive
57500	Biopsy cervix
67810	Biopsy eyelid
68100	Biopsy of conjunctiva
69100	Biopsy pinna
69105	Biopsy ear canal

ICD-9-CM DIAGNOSTIC CODES

See Appendix H for a listing of ICD-9-CM codes for the skin.

ADDITIONAL RESOURCES

- See the sample consent form titled "Skin Lesion Excision (Elective)" on page 1760 of Appendix G.

---

*Any office medical supplier provides reusable instruments.

BIBLIOGRAPHY

Achar S: Principles of skin biopsies for the primary care physician, *Am Fam Physician* 54:2411, 1996.

Bergfield WF, Pfenninger JL, Weinstock MA: Skin biopsy: selecting an optimal technique, *Patient Care* March 30:11, 2001.

Boyd AS, Neldner KH: How to submit a specimen for cutaneous pathology analyses, *Arch Fam Med* 6:64, 1997.

Gabel EA, Jimenez GP, Eaglstein WH, et al: Performance of nylon and an absorbable suture material (Polyglactin 910) in the closure of punch biopsy sites, *Dermatol Surg* 26:750, 2000.

Moy RL, Usatine RP: Elliptical excision. In Usatine RP, Moy RL, Tobinick EL, Siegel DM, editors: *Skin surgery: a practical guide,* St Louis, 1998, Mosby.

Moy RL, Lee A, Zalka A: Commonly used suturing techniques in skin surgery, *Am Fam Physician* 44:1625, 1991.

Salasche SJ, Grabski WJ: Transverse sectioning of a pigmented lesion, *Dermatol Surg* 23:578, 1997.

Siegel MS, Usatine RP: The punch biopsy. In Usatine RP, Moy RL, Tobinick EL, Siegel DM, editors: *Skin surgery: a practical guide,* St Louis, 1998, Mosby.

Siegel MS, Usatine RP: The shave biopsy. In Usatine RP, Moy RL, Tobinick EL, Siegel DM, editors: *Skin surgery: a practical guide,* St Louis, 1998, Mosby.

Snell GF: Skin biopsy. In Pfenninger JL, Fowler GC, editors: *Procedures for primary care physicians,* St Louis, 1994, Mosby.

Tobinick EL, Usatine RP: Choosing the type of biopsy. In Usatine RP, Moy RL, Tobinick EL, Siegel DM, editors: *Skin surgery: a practical guide,* St Louis, 1998, Mosby.

CHAPTER 34

Skin Grafting

Paul M. Paulman
Thomas N. Told

PINCH (PATCH) GRAFTING

Pinch grafting (also known as patch grafting) is a method of treating leg ulcers by grafting small pieces of full thickness skin, usually harvested from the patient's medial thigh, to the ulcer site. First described in 1872, pinch grafting leads to a leg ulcer healing rate of 20% to 50%, depending on the cause of the ulcer. Pinch grafting should be considered as an adjunct to conservative therapy and a therapeutic alternative for the inpatient or ambulatory management of leg ulcers. (Chapter 43, Unna Paste Boot, describes another method for treating lower extremity venous ulcers using the Unna Boot.) Pinch grafting requires no special training and no specialized equipment or supplies, but it does require a prolonged period of leg elevation and bed rest following the procedure.

INDICATIONS

Pinch grafting can be used to treat any leg ulcer. Success rates for pinch grafting are highest for arterial ulcers (50%) and lowest for venous ulcers (20% to 40%). Compared with patients treated with conservative therapy, patients treated with pinch grafting have a shorter time to healing (reepithelialization) and a longer time until ulcer recurrence.

CONTRAINDICATIONS

- Allergy to anesthetic or antiseptic agents
- Skin infection at potential donor sites
- Lack of granulation base in ulcer (*relative contraindication*)
- Patient unwillingness or inability to comply with postprocedure instructions

EQUIPMENT

- Syringe and needle for anesthetic injection
- 1% or 2% xylocaine *without* epinephrine
- Antiseptic agent for donor site preparation (e.g., povidone-iodine)
- Sterile drape for donor site
- Sterile gloves
- Tissue forceps with teeth
- Scalpel with no. 15 blade
- Ruler
- Dressings for grafted ulcer (petrolatum [Vaseline] gauze, saline-soaked gauze, and pressure bandage)
- Normal saline gauze for transport of grafts
- Vaseline gauze dressing for donor site
- Vaseline impregnated stockinette

PREPROCEDURE PATIENT PREPARATION

The relative risks and benefits of pinch grafting should be explained to the patient. The patient must be willing and able to comply with postprocedure activity restrictions. The leg ulcer(s) must be clean and must have a granulation base. All supplies and equipment should be gathered at bedside or in the examination-treatment room. The ulcers should be measured to provide an estimate of the number of grafts needed. The donor site (the proximal medial thigh is the preferred donor site) should be prepped and draped in a sterile manner. The skin around the ulcer(s) should be prepped in a sterile manner. The ulcer base can be debrided with wet-to-dry saline gauze dressings for 3 to 4 days before the procedure. Pinch grafting should be performed under sterile conditions.

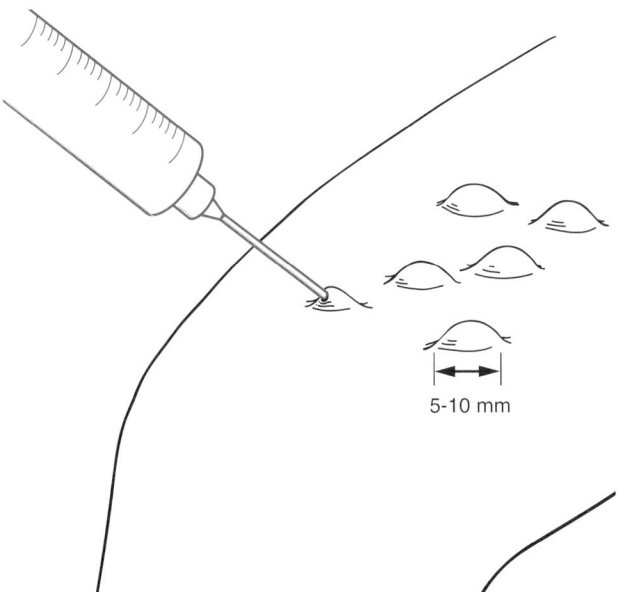

Fig. 34-1
Local anesthetic (without epinephrine) is injected into the donor site, forming wheals of 5 to 10 mm in diameter.

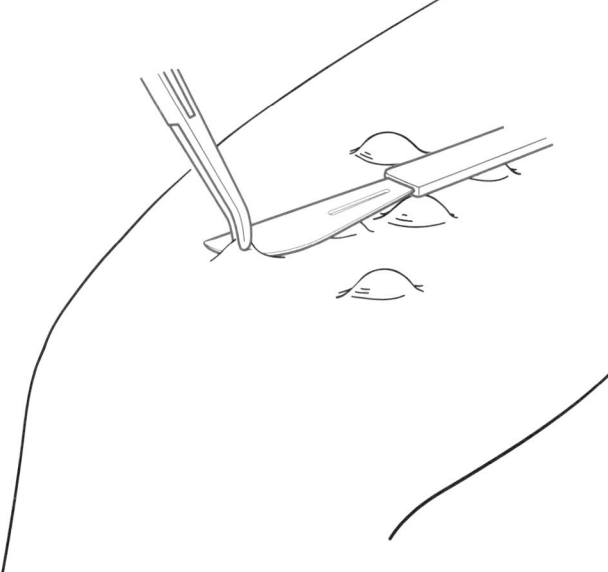

Fig. 34-2
Anesthetized skin is grasped with the tissue forceps, and full-thickness skin pieces 3 to 5 mm in diameter are removed.

TECHNIQUE

1. Prepare and drape both donor sites and ulcer(s).
2. Measure the ulcer(s).
3. Inject local anesthetic (without epinephrine) into the donor site to form wheals of 5 to 10 mm in diameter (the number of wheals should equal the number of grafts needed) (Fig. 34-1).
4. Grasp the anesthetized skin with the tissue forceps and remove full-thickness skin pieces 3 to 5 mm in diameter, avoiding subcutaneous fat (Fig. 34-2). Trim off any fat that may be adherent.
5. Store the graft pieces on a piece of sterile gauze soaked with normal saline.
6. Place the skin pieces on the leg ulcer. Leave 2- to 5-mm spaces between grafts as well as between grafts and the ulcer edge to allow drainage of wound secretions (Fig. 34-3).
7. Dress the ulcer with petrolatum gauze to cover the whole ulcer, followed by an occlusive dressing with saline gauze and a pressure bandage (e.g., Ace wrap, Coban).
8. Dress the donor site with petrolatum gauze, followed by dry gauze.
9. See below for postoperative care.

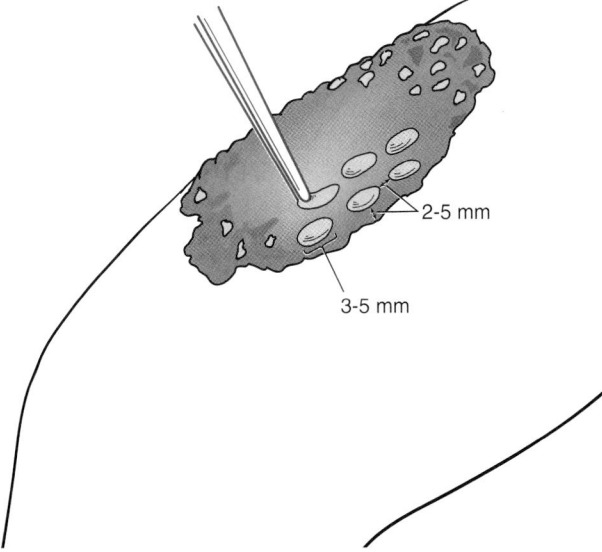

Fig. 34-3
Skin pieces are placed on the leg ulcer, with 2- to 5-mm spaces left between grafts as well as between grafts and the ulcer edge to allow drainage of wound secretions.

COMPLICATIONS

The most common complication is *graft failure. Infections* at both the donor site and the ulcer are rarely reported. *Deep venous thrombosis* is a possible complication of this procedure because of immobilization. *Bleeding* at the donor site occurs frequently but is almost always minor and easily controlled with local pressure.

POSTPROCEDURE PATIENT EDUCATION AND CARE

- Give the patient a teaching guide. (See the sample patient education handout titled "Pinch [Patch] Grafting" on page 1771 of Appendix G.)
- Patients must be placed on bed rest, with toilet privileges, with the grafted leg elevated for 7 days.
- The donor site dressing can be removed and replaced two to three times a day as needed. Wash gently with soap and water. Cover with petrolatum or antibiotic ointment, followed by the dressing.
- At 7 days after the procedure, the petrolatum gauze covering the ulcer is removed (if wound secretions are profuse, the saline compresses covering the petrolatum gauze are changed daily). After the petrolatum gauze is removed, an ointment-impregnated stockinette is applied and held in place with an elastic bandage.
- At 7 days after the procedure, the patient is allowed to ambulate.
- At 14 days after the procedure, the stockinette is removed and the ulcer dressed with gauze as needed.
- Some authorities recommend that low-molecular-weight heparin, or other clot prophylaxis, be given to patients at high risk of venous thrombosis for 7 to 10 days after pinch grafting.
- Prophylactic antibiotics have generally not been used but could be considered in high-risk situations.

CONCLUSION

Pinch grafting is a simple therapeutic procedure that may hasten and improve the healing of leg ulcers. The technique is relatively simple, can be performed at the bedside, and requires no special equipment or supplies. This procedure does require a prolonged period of postgraft ambulation restriction. Patients should know about and be prepared for this restricted ambulation. Clinicians should consider pinch grafting as an adjunct to conservative therapy for treatment of leg ulcers.

FULL-THICKNESS AND SPLIT-THICKNESS SKIN GRAFTS

Every primary care physician who manages wounds will encounter full-thickness skin loss that cannot be closed by conventional suturing techniques. One of the best ways to solve these full-thickness skin loss problems is through the use of skin grafting techniques. The cutaneous surgeon possessing the basic skills of skin closure can easily master this most useful technique. Donor skin reduces the size of the defect and speeds healing time. A properly selected and applied graft creates a minimal donor site defect and contributes to good function and cosmetic results.

INDICATIONS

- Full-thickness abrasions and burns where skin loss creates defects 1 cm or more in width between viable skin edges
- Full-thickness skin loss on areas that have tight skin that cannot be advanced or undermined (e.g., tip of the nose, fingers and toes)
- Large areas of skin loss that need to be reduced in size for better function
- Covering of surgical defects that cannot be closed (e.g., large skin excision sites, full-thickness skin flap donor sites, tendons, cartilage, and bone)
- Where excessive scarring of secondary granulation tissue may impair function or create adverse cosmetic results

CONTRAINDICATIONS

- Infection at the donor site
- Infection at the recipient site
- Excessive bleeding at the recipient site
- Contamination of the recipient site with imbedded foreign material
- Excessive edema at the recipient site
- Inadequate blood supply to sustain a graft

Note: Defects that are smaller than the size of a dime (1 cm in diameter) will heal well on their own without need for grafting. If wounds are contaminated with foreign material or infected, a delay of the grafting procedure will allow for the recipient site to establish granulation tissue that will better support the graft.

SKIN GRAFT TYPES

- Skin grafts are divided into two categories: *split thickness* and *full thickness* (Fig. 34-4).
- *Full-thickness grafts* consist of the epidermis and full-thickness dermis. *Split-thickness grafts* consist of the epidermis but only variable quantities of dermis. Full-thickness grafts are harvested by sharp dissection with a scalpel, and the thickness of the graft is determined by the region of the body where the donor skin originates.
- *Split-thickness grafts* require taking only a part of the dermis while leaving the rest of the dermis at the donor site to regenerate. There are three grades of thickness: thin, medium, and thick. The downward pressure, or a steeper angle applied to the cutting blade by the

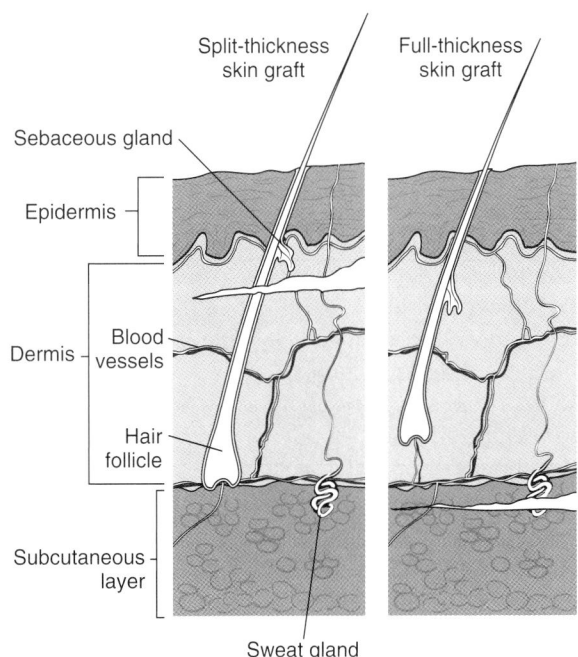

Fig. 34-4
Free skin grafts are divided into two main types: split-thickness and full-thickness skin grafts.

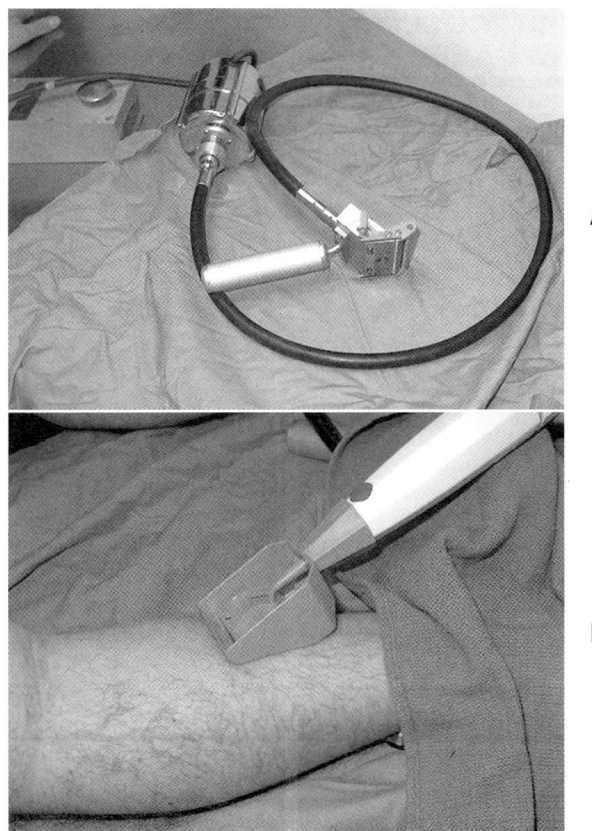

Fig. 34-5
A, Adjustable thickness motorized dermatome. **B,** Duval battery powered dermatome with disposable fixed depth and fixed width attachable head.

operator at the time of removal, determines the thickness of this graft. Mechanical dermatomes have an adjustable gate, or a preset thickness setting, that also determines graft thickness (Fig. 34-5).

• Whether the primary care skin surgeon uses a free hand shave technique or a preset dermatome, these techniques take practice to produce skin grafts of appropriate thickness.

Note: The tendency of the novice operator is to produce thicker split-thickness grafts than intended, even with the mechanical dermatomes set on the thinnest settings.

SPLIT-THICKNESS GRAFT ADVANTAGES

• Can be "meshed" and made to cover large areas of skin loss. In this technique small slits are cut in the graft similar to the holes in a piecrust allowing the sides of the graft to be stretched an expansion ratio of 1 to 1½ times (Fig. 34-6).

• Extensive "meshing" promotes drainage of blood and serum from under the graft and improves success of revascularization of the donor skin.

• Very thin split-thickness grafts (0.010 to 0.015 inch) vascularize quickly and heal much more rapidly.

• Tend to contract as they heal, thus drawing down the size of the original defect.

• Donor sites of split thickness grafts heal more rapidly.

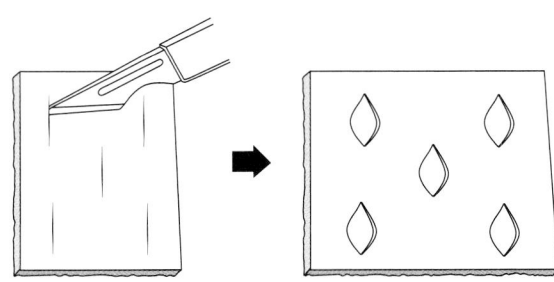

Fig. 34-6
Split thickness grafts can be expanded by "pie crusting" or cutting small slits in places that need expansion. This can expand a graft 50% over the original size.

• Require less blood supply to survive and may be the best choice for sites where vascularization is less than optimal.

The thickness of the graft can vary to satisfy the need for wear, appearance, hair growth, and speed of healing. Thin grafts (0.005 to 0.010 inch) heal rapidly but are not cosmetically pleasing. Grafts over 0.015 inch look better and resist wear better but heal more slowly.

SPLIT-THICKNESS GRAFTS DISADVANTAGES

- Not as resistant to trauma and can be injured easily in areas of friction and wear.
- Less like normal skin in color, texture, suppleness, and hair growth.
- "Meshing," or "pie crusting," causes additional scarring and skin hypertrophy.
- Do not germinate over bone without periosteum, or cartilage without perichondrium.
- Require the use of a dermatome, operating suite for large grafts.
- Free hand technique produces only postage stamp–sized grafts.
- Do not work well over joints, because they are more likely for cause contracture and restriction of the joint.

FULL-THICKNESS GRAFTS ADVANTAGES

- Match normal skin contours better than any other form of graft.
- Match color and texture better than other forms of repair and are more aesthetically pleasing over time.
- Have less postoperative contracture and will not influence the size of the defect.
- Will resist friction and wear better than the thinner grafts.
- Can be used to cover bone without periosteum and cartilage without perichondrium.

FULL-THICKNESS GRAFTS DISADVANTAGES

- Cannot be used to cover large areas without carrying their own blood supply.
- Large full-thickness donor sites must be covered with split-thickness grafts to heal.
- Need a good supply of blood at the recipient site to survive.
- Take the longest time of any graft to vascularize.
- The size of the donor site is determined by the defect size, and the graft cannot be meshed to expand its surface coverage.

EQUIPMENT

- Dermatome
  - Adjustable type with thickness settings, flexible shaft, and external power (Fig. 34-5, *A*)
  - Battery powered disposable head type (Fig. 34-5, *B*)
- Sterile tongue blade
- 5 to 10 ml sterile mineral oil
- Vaseline gauze, Tegaderm, or fine mesh gauze
- Minor surgical tray
- 5-0 suture (polyethylene or Vicryl)
- Skin stapler if sutures not used
- Steri-Strips
- Kerlix roll
- Ace wrap, Coban or elastic stockinette
- No. 10 or larger blade or a razor blade
- Two Adson tissue forceps
- 5-inch Halsey needle holder
- 4-inch curved Iris scissors
- 6-0 or 5-0 nylon sutures (monofilament, not braided)

FULL-THICKNESS GRAFT DONOR SITES
(Fig. 34-7)

- Postauricular area
- Supraclavicular area
- Suprapalpebral area
- Antecubital area
- Volar wrist area
- Lower abdominal area
- Inguinal area

SPLIT-THICKNESS GRAFT DONOR SITES
(Fig. 34-8)

- Posterior lateral thigh
- Superior buttocks
- Anterior abdomen
- Anterior thigh
- Inner surface of the upper arm for hairless skin
- Flexor surface of the forearm

Note: Facial defects should be handled with full-thickness grafts because these grafts cause less cosmetic disruption. Never use skin for the face from areas below the clavicle because these grafts do not match in color or texture, and they contain hair follicles, giving lifelong deformity.

TECHNIQUES

Full-Thickness Grafts (Fig. 34-9)

1. Make sure no active folliculitis exists close to the donor site.
2. Prepare the skin for surgery using aseptic technique.
3. Drape the donor site.
4. Infiltrate the skin to be transferred with lidocaine anesthesia.
5. Remove a fusiform piece of skin large enough

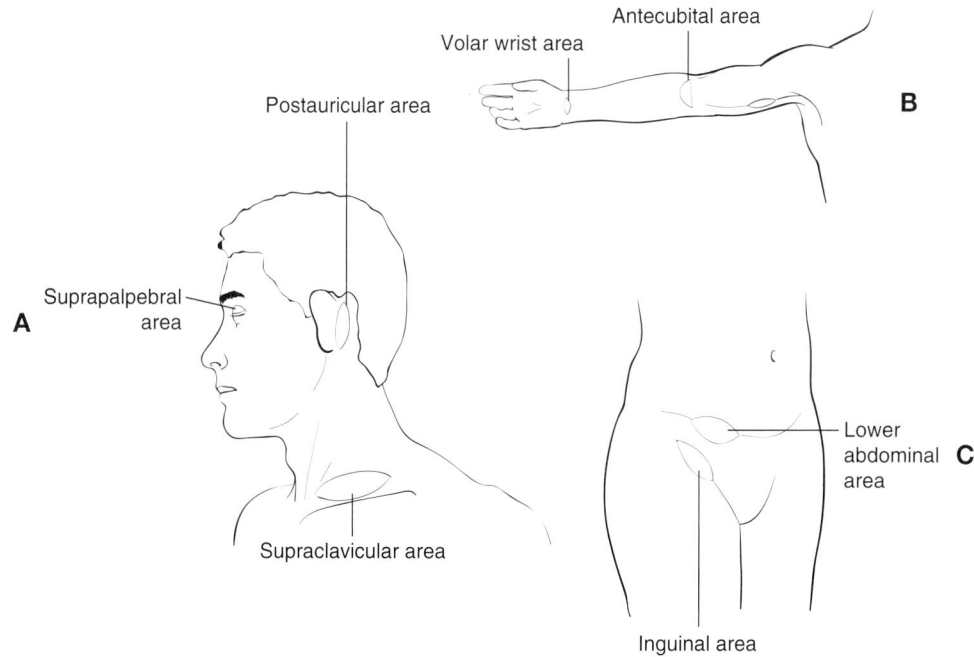

Fig. 34-7
Potential harvest areas for full-thickness grafts. **A,** Head. **B,** Arm. **C,** Lower abdomen and inguinal areas.
Note: Do not use grafts from areas shown in **B** and **C** to graft the face, head, and neck **(A).** The color will
never match and a permanent defect will remain.

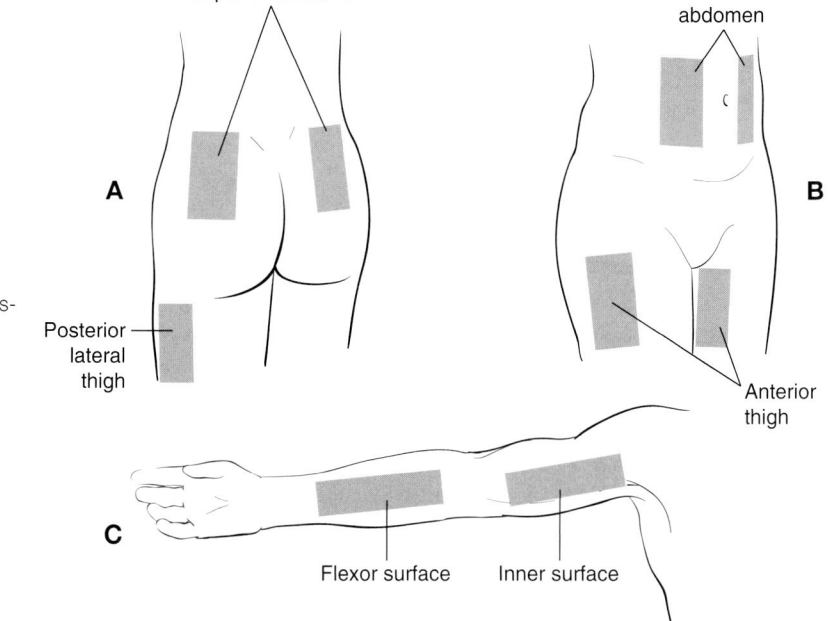

Fig. 34-8
Potential harvest areas for split-thickness grafts. **A,** Posterior buttocks and lateral thigh. **B,** Anterior abdomen
and thighs. **C,** Hairless areas of the arm.

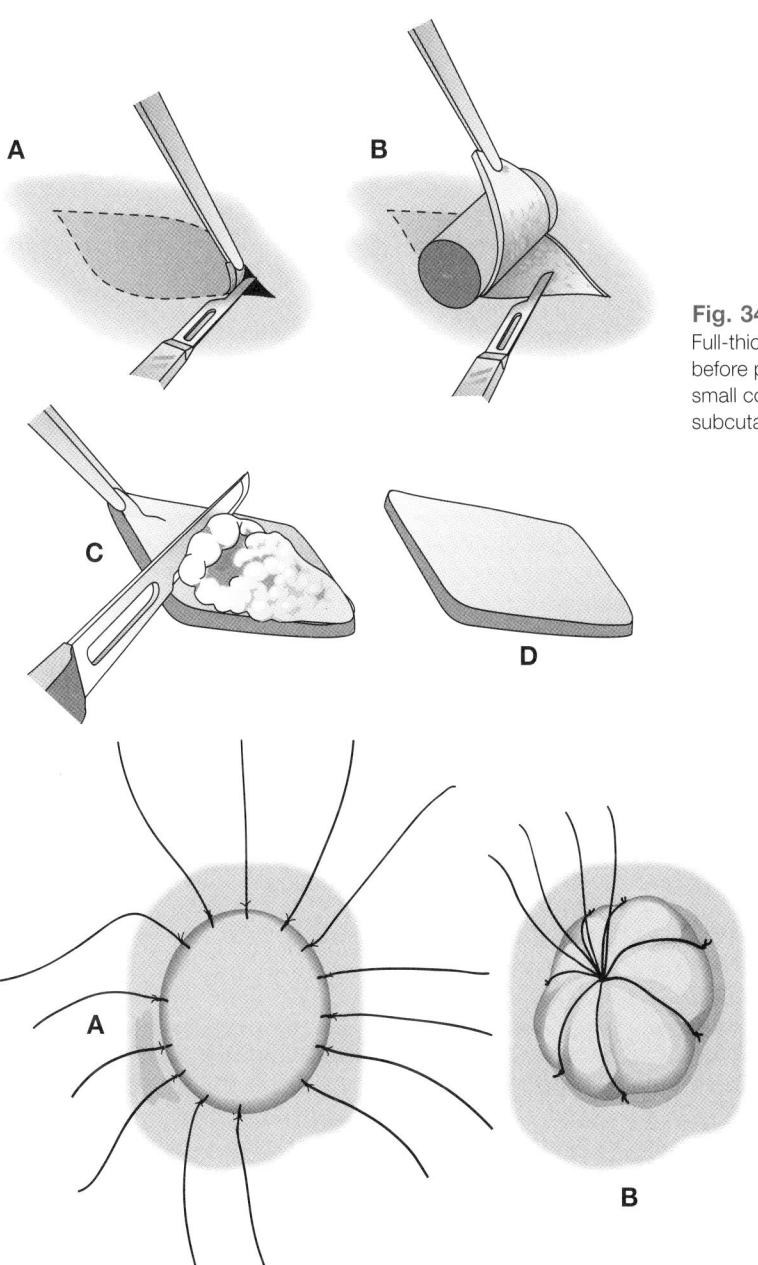

Fig. 34-9
Full-thickness grafts should have all the subcutaneous fat removed before placing it on the graft site. **A,** Excising the graft. **B,** Using a small cotton roll to aid in keeping the graft flat. **C,** Removing the subcutaneous fat from donor skin. **D,** Graft skin ready to be applied.

Fig. 34-10
Grafts can be secured best by using a stent. **A,** Suture tails are left long at the time of attachment of the graft, then tied over the dressing **(B)** to provide pressure and anchor the graft in place. An initial layer of nonadherent material is applied or the graft may be lubricated with antibiotic ointment to prevent the gauze stent from sticking.

to cover the defect without creating tension (Fig. 34-9, *A, B*).

6. Remove as much subcutaneous fat as possible without button holing the graft (Fig. 34-9, *C, D*).
7. Place the graft dermis side down on a saline-soaked gaze pad till ready for transfer.
8. Trim the graft to fit the defect.
9. Suture the graft into the defect, taking care to notice the skin lines and skin edges (Fig. 34-10, *A*).
10. Use polyethylene suture, staples and/or Steri-Strips.
11. Horizontal mattress sutures are less hemostatic and will protect the graft edges.
12. Close the donor site with sutures or staples. If the

donor site cannot be closed, a split-thickness graft can be used to cover the donor site.to cover the defect without creating tension (Fig. 34-9, *A, B*).

13. Place a nonadherent dressing on the donor site and treat as a laceration.
14. A stent dressing will best secure the graft (Fig. 34-10, *B*).

Harvesting Split-Thickness Grafts

Dermatome Technique
1. Make sure no active infection or atrophic skin diseases exist on or near the donor site or recipient site.

2. Prep and drape the area with surgical scrub and drapes.

3. Ready the dermatome by setting the desired thickness on the gauge. Usually the best intermediate thickness is the thickness of a scalpel blade. Thin grafts should transmit light like frosted glass. Disposable dermatome heads are set to produce thin grafts; the operator simply needs to decide on the blade width, since various heads have various widths.

4. Anesthetize the skin to be harvested with local or regional anesthesia for small grafts. General anesthesia can be used when the areas to be grafted are large.

5. Place a thin film of sterile mineral oil on the skin that will be run through the dermatome. This lubricates the surfaces and produces uniform thickness.

6. Have an assistant use the sterile tongue blade to depress the skin in front of the dermatome and provide countertraction to straighten out any wrinkles in the skin.

7. Start the dermatome and approach the skin at a fairly steep angle until the blade catches the skin and begins cutting. When this happens, flatten the angle so the undersurface of the dermatome is aligned perfectly parallel with the skin surface. Downward pressure on the handle will deepen the blade into the dermis and produce a thicker graft (Fig. 34-11).

8. The split-thickness graft will bunch up behind the blade, and an assistant will need to grasp the leading edges of the graft and gently lift them straight up (the way a thin slice of cheese is lifted from a cheese cutter to keep it from bunching up). The total length of the graft can be determined easily as it is lifted off the blade.

9. When the desired graft length is reached, release downward pressure on the dermatome handle and point the blade in a steep upward angle, severing the graft.

10. The graft is carefully spread out, with the dermis side down, on a saline-soaked gauze. In the case of extremely thin grafts the skin can be floated on the surface of sterile saline in a basin before being transferred to the recipient site.

    Note: The shiny side is always the dermis side and must go next to the vascular surface of the recipient site; otherwise it would be like laying grass sod upside down.

11. The donor site is dressed with Tegaderm, fine mesh gauze, or petrolatum-based antibiotic gauze, and left in place until it falls off in about 2 weeks. A gauze wrap and an Ace bandage can further protect the wound and reduce scar hypertrophy.

Free Hand Split-Thickness Grafts

1. This technique is well suited to the outpatient setting or emergency room, where small areas of skin loss elude conventional closure and require grafting.

2. A half-dollar sized (3 × 3 cm) area on the forearm or

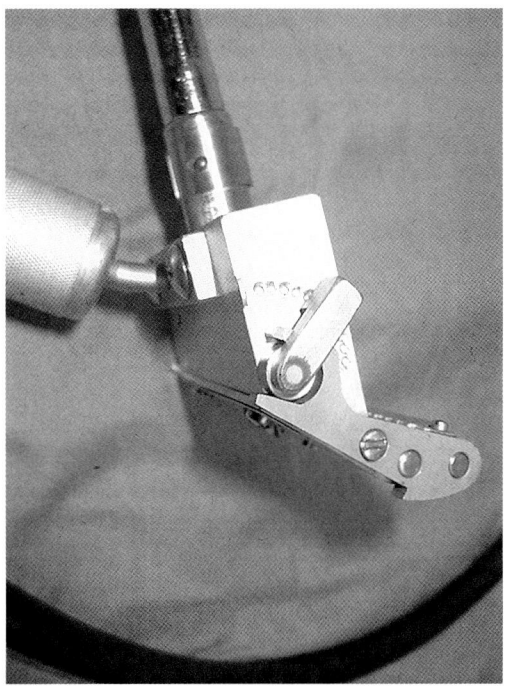

Fig. 34-11
Battery-powered dermatome at the correct cutting angle.

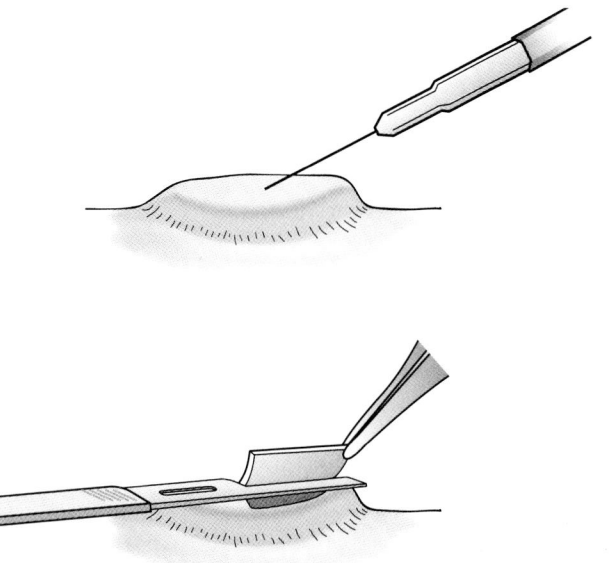

Fig. 34-12
Free hand split-thickness graft. **A,** Infiltration with local anesthesia will slightly raise the skin, making cutting easier. **B,** The large scalpel blade is held at a shallow angle to the skin, and the graft is shaved off to a desired length.

thigh is infiltrated with 2% plain xylocaine, prepped with antiseptic solution, and draped for surgery (Fig. 34-12, *A*).

3. Using a no. 20, no. 21, or no. 22 scalpel blade and handle, shave the skin at the desired thickness with a gentle slicing motion (Fig. 34-12, *B*).
4. Skin the width of a postage stamp can be removed to the desired length needed.
5. The skin can be transferred directly to the defect and sutured in place like any other split-thickness graft.

Recipient Site Preparation and Graft Stabilization

1. In the case of full-thickness grafts, meticulous homeostasis is the key to graft survival. Bipolar cautery is the best way to achieve homeostasis with very little thermal damage.
2. The full-thickness graft must be tailored precisely to the defect at the time of placement, whereas split-thickness grafts may overlap the margins.
3. The survival of split-thickness grafts depends on the growth of capillary beds into the raw undersurface of the graft. This may take several weeks of preparation to allow granulation tissue to develop. Try to use more natural methods of debridement and capillary bed enhancement, since enzyme debriding agents will attack the graft as well.
4. The graft must not move during the period of revascularization. The grafts can be secured with a 6-0 or 5-0 monofilament suture. One tail to the suture is intentionally left twice as long as the diameter of the defect so a stent dressing can be tied over the graft (see Fig. 34-10). The dressing will stay in place for 7 to 10 days. Avoid the temptation to look under the dressing during the healing processes.
5. Use as few sutures as necessary. Simple interrupted suture with monofilament material is the best tolerated. Do not put too much tension on the graft or the sutures. If more stabilization is needed, Steri-Strips can be used. Some surgeons report good success with Steri-Strips alone.
6. In the case of large split-thickness grafts, skin staples can be used. This is a more rapid method of attachment and is relatively atraumatic.
7. Large skin grafts may require a "piecrust" maneuver to vent bubbles or blood from under the graft itself. Small holes can be cut in the graft with fine scissors or scalpel to let out the fluid (see Fig. 34-6).
8. Nonadherent material is best used over the graft and firm pressure with gauze or Tegaderm over the nonadherent material.
9. The graft must be protected from trauma and from loss of contact with the vascular bed. Some cutaneous surgeons prefer to roll a cotton-tip applicator over the surface of the new graft, rolling from the middle of the newly applied skin to the outside. This serves to express unwanted blood, fluids, or air bubbles that will lift the healing graft away from the recipient bed.

COMPLICATIONS

The major complication of skin grafting is infection at the donor site (causing it to become a full-thickness defect) and loss of the graft at the recipient site (causing another full-thickness defect). The use of prophylactic antibiotics cannot make up for poor planning and bad surgical technique; therefore it is important to approach full-thickness skin loss with good preparation.

POSTPROCEDURE PATIENT EDUCATION

See the sample patient education handout titled "Skin Graft Postprocedure Instructions" on page 1770 of Appendix G.

SUPPLIERS

Adjustable dermatomes
Zimmer Orthopaedic Surgical Products
P.O. Box 10
200 West Ohio Avenue
Dover, OH 44622
Phone: 1-330-343-8801

Medical and surgical supplies
Bergen Brunswig Medical Corp.
5301 Peoria, Unit B
Denver, CO 80239
Phone: 1-800-411-9022

Surgical instruments
Miltex Instrument Co.
700 Hicksville Road
Bethpage, NY 11714
Phone: 1-800-645-8000

CPT/BILLING CODES

15100	Split graft, trunk, arms, legs, first 100 cm^2
15120	Split graft, face, scalp, eyelids, mouth, neck, ears, orbits, genitalia, hands, feet, first 100 cm^2
15200	Full-thickness graft, including direct closure of the donor site, trunk, 20 cm^2 or less

15220   Full-thickness graft including closure of the donor site, including scalp, arms, legs, 20 cm^2 or less

15240   Full-thickness graft including donor site closure forehead, cheeks, chin, mouth, neck, axillae, genitalia, hands and feet, 20 cm^2 or less

15260   Full-thickness, free, including closure of the donor site, nose, ears, eyelids, and/or lips, 20 cm^2 or less

ICD-9-CM DIAGNOSTIC CODES

Split-Thickness Grafts

709.2	Scar
707.0	Ulcers
942.32 to 945.59	Burns
879.0 to 881.2	Wounds

Full-Thickness Grafts

709.2	Scar
707.8	Ulcers
942.31 to 944.58	Burns
876.0 to 876.1 and 879.0 to 879.5	Open wounds

ADDITIONAL RESOURCES

- See the sample patient education handouts titled "Skin Graft Postprocedure Instructions" and "Pinch (Patch) Grafting" on pages 1770 and 1771, respectively, of Appendix G.
- See the sample patient consent form titled "Pinch (Patch) Grafting" on page 1772 of Appendix G.

BIBLIOGRAPHY

Ahnlide I, Bjellerup M: Efficacy of pinch grafting in leg ulcers of different aetiologies, *Acta Derm Venereol* 77(2):144, 1997.

Christiansen J, Ek L, Tegner E: Pinch grafting of leg ulcers: a retrospective study of 412 treated ulcers in 146 patients, *Acta Derm Venereol* 77:471, 1997.

Fewkes JL, Pollack S, Cheney ML: Grafts. In Fewkes JL, Pollack S, Cheney ML: *Illustrated atlas of cutaneous surgery,* New York, 1992, Gower Medical Publishing.

Gilmore WA, Wheeland RG: Treatment of ulcers on legs by pinch grafts and a supportive dressing of polyurethane, *J Dermatol Surg Oncol* 8(3):177, 1982.

Grossman JA: Principles of wound treatment and closure. In Grossman JA: *Minor injuries and repairs,* New York, 1993, Gower Medical Publishing.

Haas AF, Glogan RG: Composite graft. In Robinson JK, Arndt KA, LeBoit PE, Wintroub BU: *Atlas of cutaneous surgery,* Philadelphia, 1996, WB Saunders.

Leffell DJ: Split-thickness skin grafts. In Robinson JK, Arndt KA, LeBoit PE, Wintroub BU: *Atlas of cutaneous surgery,* Philadelphia, 1996, WB Saunders.

Lin TW: The algebraic viewpoint in microskin grafting in burned patients, *Burns* 20(4):347, 1994.

Oien RF, Hansen BU, Hahansson A: Pinch grafting of leg ulcers in primary care, *Acta Derm Venereol* 78(6):438, 1998.

Ongenal KC, Phillips T: Cultured epidermal grafts. In Robinson JK, Arndt KA, LeBoit PE, Wintroub BU: *Atlas of cutaneous surgery,* Philadelphia, 1996, WB Saunders.

Phillips TJ: Current approaches to venous ulcers and compression, *Dermatol Surg* 27:611, 2001.

Roenigk RK, Zalla MJ: Full-thickness skin grafts. In Robinson JK, Arndt KA, LeBoit PE, Wintroub BU: *Atlas of cutaneous surgery,* Philadelphia, 1996, WB Saunders.

Schwartz S (ed): *Principles of surgery,* ed 6, New York, 1994, McGraw-Hill.

Way LW: *Current surgical diagnosis & treatment,* ed 10, Norwalk, Conn., 1994, Appleton & Lange.

CHAPTER 35

Skin Stapling

J. Mark Wiedemann

Skin stapling is a satisfactory alternative to other methods of skin closure and wound repair. Experience with stapling now spans decades, and improvements are being introduced constantly, such as absorbable staples. A number of different staplers are now available, many with unique features. Some, for small lacerations, hold as few as 5 staples, whereas larger models can contain 35 or more. Disposable and reusable devices are available.

ADVANTAGES

Outcomes seem to be related to practitioners' experience. Most studies found cosmetic results equal to or superior to sutures as well as a slightly lower incidence of infection. They are generally well accepted by patients. Stapling, according to some articles, is about 80% faster than suturing and is usually less expensive when equipment costs alone are considered—almost always so when physician time is a factor. The longer the laceration, the more cost-benefit there is to stapling. Staples nicely evert wound edges and may create less tension on tissues than do sutures. Surgical stainless steel staples are less "reactive" than sutures, leading to less inflammation and infection. Staple ends do not completely communicate within the tissue (unlike sutures), which is another factor in the lower incidence of infection.

DISADVANTAGES

Some studies have found cosmetic results slightly inferior to suturing (may leave larger puncture scars, proportional to the amount of time they remain in tissue) and costs may be slightly higher, especially in smaller lacerations. Recycling of the spent devices is problematic.

INDICATIONS

- Useful in securing skin grafts and in wound repair and tissue closure where edges are easily reapproximated. Some surgeons have used skin staplers to repair traumatic lacerations to the myocardium.
- Especially appropriate in long wounds and in areas where cosmesis is not a concern.

CONTRAINDICATIONS

- Use on facial and neck tissue is relatively contraindicated, as there may be poorer cosmesis.
- Staples should not be used in areas of large tissue loss unless wound edges can be apposed easily (usually after appropriate undermining and use of layered, buried sutures).
- Relatively contraindicated in the soles of the feet or in areas of the body where they interfere with function.

EQUIPMENT

- Skin hooks or pick-ups. Traumatic or crushing type forceps should not be used.
- Skin stapler.
- Staple remover (usually given to patient if another practitioner will be removing the staples).
- Incision and laceration supplies may be needed. For a traumatic wound repair with staples, many practitioners do not use sterile drapes or sterile gloves.

PREPROCEDURE PATIENT PREPARATION

Generally, consent forms are not required, but community standards should dictate. The patient should be informed about the procedure, the intent to use staples, their advantages, disadvantages, possible complications, how to care for the repair, when to return for recheck and when to have staples removed.

TECHNIQUE

1. An operator and an assistant or the operator alone may perform stapling (Fig. 35-1).
2. The wound is prepped and (sometimes) draped in sterile fashion.
3. Topical anesthetics (usually a solution of lidocaine, epinephrine, and tetracaine) generally suffice for analgesia. Children and many adults greatly prefer this to local (injected) anesthetics, but preparation time is usually longer, and time or other considerations may mandate injection. In areas where injectable anesthetics with epinephrine are contraindicated (e.g., fingers, nose, penis, toes, ears), topical anesthetics that contain epinephrine also should not be used.
4. If there is tissue loss or if the wound is gaping, undermining and buried absorbable sutures may first be required to approximate wound edges. There should be no free space beneath the edges of the skin closure.
5. An assistant uses one or two pick-up forceps or skin hooks to approximate wound edges. The edges should not overlap, and some staplers perform better if a small gap is left, which the stapler will draw together. The operator staples the area, and a subsequent area is addressed. The distance between staple placement depends on the operator and his or her experience, but the wound margins should be approximated without gaps when complete. Some clinicians prefer to start closing at the middle of a wound, lessening the chance of "dog ears." Sometimes a "basting" or "helper" stitch in the center is required to temporarily hold the wound edges together. This is removed after all the staples are placed.
6. A lone operator may approximate the wound edges with a single pick-up, or with the fingers of the nondominant, sterile-gloved hand while stapling with the other. The tissue should be dry for good traction (Fig. 35-1, A).
7. The wound is then recleansed and dressed with antibiotic ointment. Except for some scalp lacerations, a gauze dressing is placed. Many wounds are prone to inflammation and edema and do much better if a snug compressive bandage is also applied. Oral narcotics are only rarely indicated.
8. In general, staples are removed after the same amount of time indicated for sutures in the same area. Staples are most easily removed with staple removers (some-times with a slight pinching sensation), but needle drivers or hemostats may also be used (Fig. 35-2).
9. After completion of the repair, the stapler should be considered a contaminated "sharp" and disposed of accordingly.

COMPLICATIONS

Complications, although rarely reported, include dehiscence, poor cosmesis, infection, and hematoma. These are all similar to a sutured wound (see Chapter 23, Laceration and Incision Repair).

POSTPROCEDURE PATIENT EDUCATION

See the sample patient education handout titled "Suture Care" on page 1759 of Appendix G.

CONCLUSION

Skin stapling offers an excellent alternative to suturing, especially in a busy emergency department or office. It proceeds far more quickly and is virtually always less expensive. There is good patient acceptance, and infection and other complication rates are lower.

SUPPLIERS

3M Product Information Center
3M Center Building 304-1-01
St. Paul, MN 55144-1000
Phone: 1-800-364-3577

Weck Closure Systems
One Weck Drive
Research Triangle Park, NC 27709
Phone: 1-800-234-9325

Minogue Medical
180 Dundas Street West
Suite 1507
Toronto, Ontario, Canada M5G 1Z8

Any good Internet search engine for "skin staplers" can find a myriad of websites selling the devices.

CPT/BILLING CODES

Coding is the same as for suture repairs. See Chapter 23, Laceration and Incision Repair.

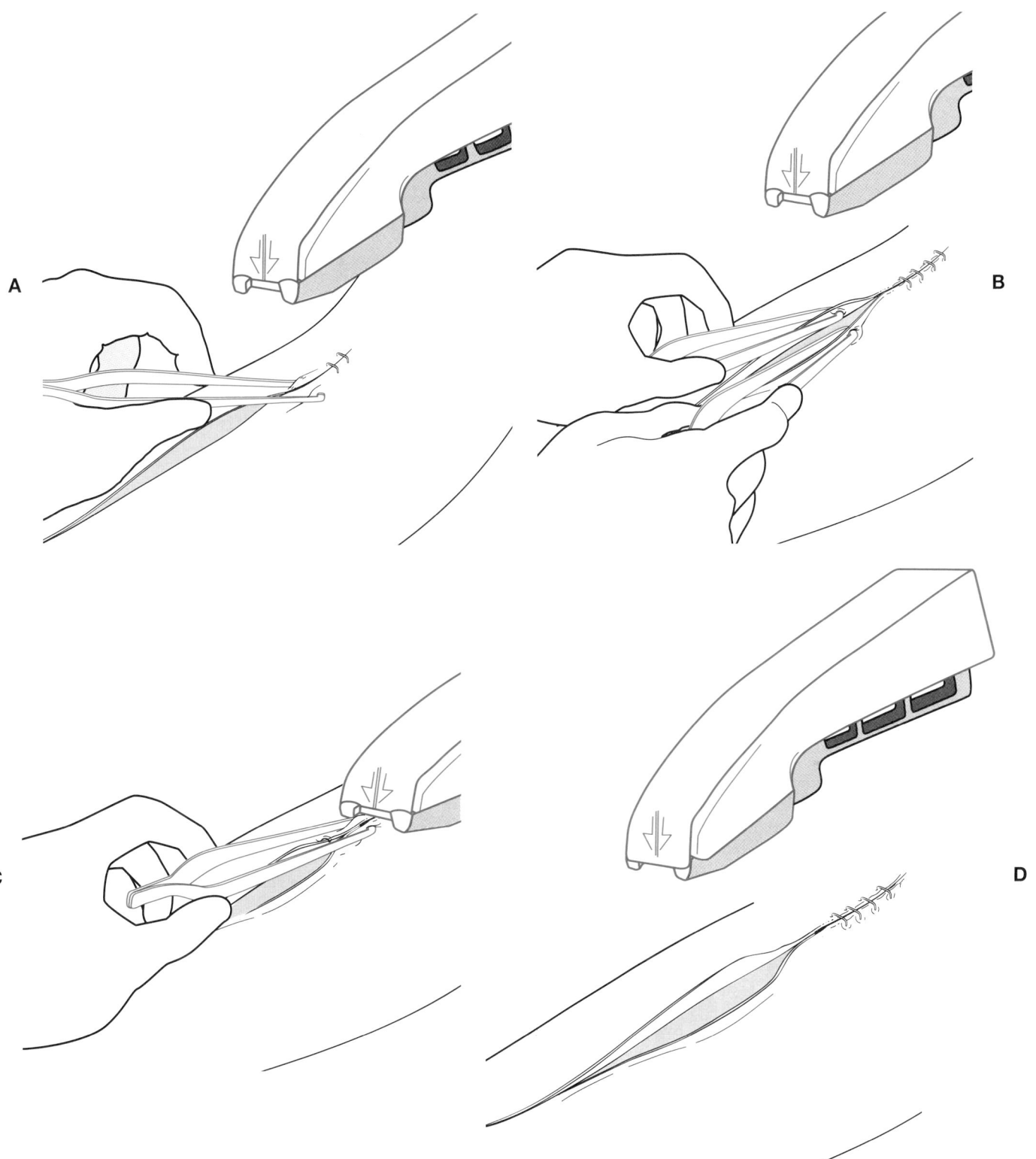

Fig. 35-1
Use of a skin stapler. Approximate skin edges so they are slightly everted with, **A,** one forceps or, **B,** two forceps. **C,** Position the instrument lightly over the everted skin edges, aligning the stapler arrow with the incision. Pressing down on the instrument too heavily may make staple removal difficult. **D,** Squeeze the trigger quickly and firmly until the trigger motion is halted. Release the trigger and back the instrument off the staple.

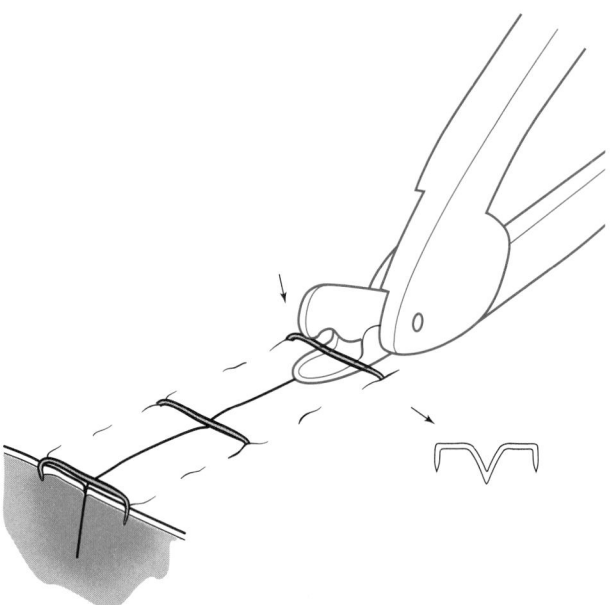

Fig. 35-2
Use of a stapler remover.

BIBLIOGRAPHY

dos Santos LR, Freitas CA, Hojaij FC, et al: Prospective study using skin staplers in head and neck surgery, *Am J Surg* 170(5):451, 1995.

Orlinsky M, Goldberg RM, Chan L, et al: Cost analysis of stapling versus suturing for skin closures, *Am J Emerg Med* 13(1):77, 1995.

Pories WJ, Thomas FT: *Office surgery for family physicians,* Boston, 1985, Butterworth.

Wolcott MW, editor: *Ambulatory surgery and the basics of emergency surgical care,* Philadelphia, 1988, Lippincott.

Subungual Hematoma Evacuation

James F. Peggs

Injuries to the nail bed and fingertip are the most common injuries to the upper extremity. Most common among these is a subungual hematoma, which results from a direct blow to the fingernail, causing bleeding into the space between the nail bed and the fingernail itself. Intense pain can result from the pressure generated by such a hematoma. Evacuation of the hematoma can produce significant relief and can be performed safely in the outpatient setting. Toenails can be treated in the same fashion.

INDICATIONS

• Visible, painful hematoma beneath the involved nail

CONTRAINDICATIONS

• Crushed or fractured nail bed.
• Hematomas involving greater than 50% of the nail *may* indicate laceration of the underlying nail bed. (Removal of the nail and repair of the laceration is recommended by some experts to avoid a posttraumatic nail deformity. Others recommend leaving the nail in place as a splint. The patient should be warned that the nail *may* be deformed unless the nail bed is examined and treated.)

EQUIPMENT

• Alcohol lamp or Bunsen burner, metal paper clip, and forceps or hemostat
• *Or* battery-operated cautery unit
• *Or* radiofrequency or electrocautery unit with needle or pointed electrode

TECHNIQUE

1. Wash the digit as thoroughly as possible with an antibacterial soap to decrease the possibility of contamination of the hematoma and subsequent infection.
2. Create a hole in the nail directly over the hematoma to allow decompression.
   Paper-clip method. Partially straighten a metal paper clip, grasp it with the forceps, and heat it over the lamp. Place the heated clip firmly on the nail, allowing it to melt the tissue for a few seconds until the nail is completely perforated (Fig. 36-1).
   Cautery method. In similar fashion, apply an electric (or better yet, battery) cautery tip to the nail and create a hole in the nail bed (Fig. 36-2).
   In both of the procedures just mentioned, the heated tip is cooled by the hematoma upon perforation of the nail, thereby preventing injury to the nail bed. The hole created in the nail should be of sufficient size so as not to self-close within a few hours (adequate size is 1 to 2 mm). Elevation of the finger, cool compresses, and a simple bandage are recommended during the first 12 hours.

COMPLICATIONS

• Infection of the remaining hematoma

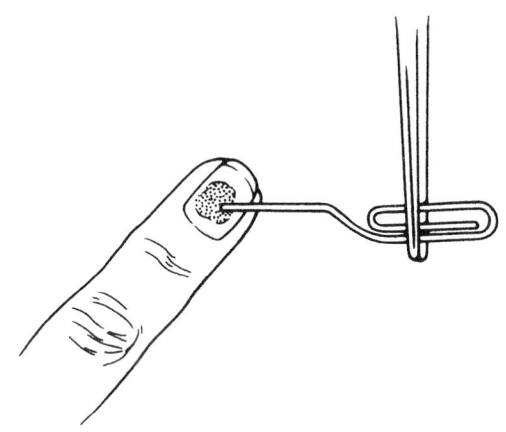

Fig. 36-1
Heated paper clip is placed directly over the hematoma to create a perforation of the nail.

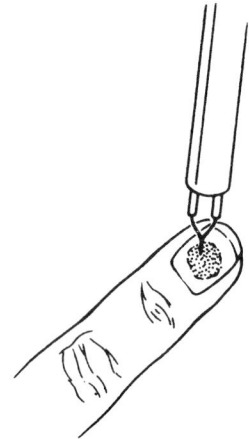

Fig. 36-2
Cautery unit may be used to perforate the nail and evacuate the subungual hematoma.

SUPPLIERS

Ellman Surgitron and Battery Unit
Ellman International, Inc.
1135 Railroad Avenue
Hewlett, NY 11557-2316
Phone: 1-800-835-5355
Website: www.ellman.com

AMI Battery Cautery
Advanced Meditech International, Inc. (AMI)
86-38 53rd Avenue
Flushing, NY 11373
Phone: 1-800-635-2452
Website: www.ameditech.com

Hyfrecator Plus
Birtcher Medical Systems, Inc.
1435 Henry Brennan Drive, #J
El Paso, TX 79936
Phone: 1-915-858-1895

CPT/BILLING CODE

11740   Subungual hematoma evacuation

ICD-9-CM DIAGNOSTIC CODES

959.5   Injury fingernail
923.3   Contusion finger(s) (nail) (subungual)

ADDITIONAL RESOURCES

* See the sample patient education handout titled "Subungual Hematoma Evacuation" on page 1773 of Appendix G.
* See the sample patient consent form titled "Subungual Hematoma Evacuation" on page 1774 of Appendix G.

BIBLIOGRAPHY

Simon RR, Wolgin M: Subungual hematoma: association with occult laceration requiring repair, *Am J Emerg Med* 5:302, 1986.
Van Beek AL: Management of acute fingernail injuries, *Hand Clin* 1:23, 1990.
Zook EG: Nail bed injuries, *Hand Clin* 1(4):701, 1985.

CHAPTER 37

Tick Removal and Prevention of Infection

John Harlan Haynes III

Outdoor work and recreation in wooded areas is often accompanied by tick exposure. Although most bites are harmless, severe illness may result from microorganisms and/or toxins transmitted by the tick. The physician should carefully check the entire skin surface for ticks following any outdoor activity. Several hours of tick attachment are thought to be required for transmission of most tickborne diseases; therefore expedient and effective tick removal is necessary to prevent illness.

Ticks are members of the class Arachnida. Two families of ticks—soft (argasid) ticks and hard (ixodid) ticks—transmit disease to humans. The hard (ixodid) ticks, Dermacentor and Ixodes, are most likely to be encountered by humans, and these ticks may transmit microorganisms hematogenously during all phases of development. Pathogens in the gut of the tick migrate to their salivary glands and are then transmitted to the host.

Ticks are vectors of infectious human diseases, such as Rocky Mountain spotted fever, Q fever, and typhus *(Rickettsia);* human granulocytic and monocytic ehrlichiosis *(Ehrlichia);* tick fever *(Flavivirus);* tularemia *(Francisella tularensis* coccobacillus); babesiosis (protozoa); and Lyme disease (spirochete). Also, envenomation of a neurotoxin secreted in the saliva of certain gravid Dermacentor ticks may cause a progressive ascending neuromuscular paralysis, much like Guillain-Barré syndrome. Tick bites can cause generalized allergic reactions as well as local infection and induration (Table 37-1).

Lyme disease, caused by the spirochete *Borrelia burgdorferi,* is transmitted to humans by hard *Ixodes* ticks. White-footed mice and white-tailed deer are the major reservoirs for *B. burgdorferi.* Enzyme-linked immunosorbent assay is preferred in laboratory tests to detect specific antibodies to *B. burgdorferi,* because it is more sensitive and specific than indirect immunofluorescence assay. A Lyme disease vaccine (LYMErix) is now commercially available for use in those at risk, and has been shown to be 76% to 92% effective at preventing symptomatic infections. Treatment should be given de-

pending on the clinical findings of the disease. If patients have symptoms of fever, chills, headaches, or myalgias, blood testing including a complete blood count, electrolytes, hepatic function studies, and serology should be performed. Skin biopsies can also be obtained and sent to the public health department in special media for the detection of the organism.

Hard adult ticks are best removed mechanically (note below an explanation for such tick removal). Care must be taken to remove the mouthpart and its surrounding, fleshlike "cement." If the "head" (mouthpart) is retained, it may be necessary to perform a punch biopsy in order to remove the surrounding skin and remnants. Empiric therapy with broad-spectrum antibiotics effective against tickborne diseases (e.g., tetracycline or doxycycline) is a good prophylactic measure.

A study of prevention of borreliosis (Lyme disease) in persons bitten by infected ticks was performed in Russia from 1992 to 1994. Adult Ixodes ticks were removed from the study subjects and live preparations made from the material obtained from the gut of each tick. Persons were divided into experimental and control groups. The experimental group received doxycycline (100 mg twice daily) for 3 to 5 days after the tick bite. The untreated group had a morbidity rate 11 times that of the treated group. The study concluded that the identification of *Borrelia* in ticks by microscopic analysis, followed by a short-term treatment with antibiotics according to microbiologic indications, is an efficient method for preventing persons from contracting borreliosis.

In the past, home remedies involved placement of oil on the tick, which in effect would smother it, or use of a hot match or cautery to get the tick to release itself. Both methods tend to cause the tick to regurgitate into the site and may promote disease transmission. Neither of these archaic techniques is recommended.

EQUIPMENT

- Blunt curved forceps or tweezers
- Rubber gloves

TABLE 37-1

Tickborne Diseases

Disease and Agent	Geographic Distribution	Common Presenting Symptoms	Initial Laboratory Findings	Treatment
Lyme disease *Borrelia burgdorferi*	Northeast and upper Midwest	Erythema migrans, fatigue, myalgias, arthralgias, headache, fever, chills	Initial tests are nonspecific; serology can confirm at 4-6 weeks	Amoxicillin Doxycycline (Vibramycin)
Human monocytic ehrlichiosis *Ehrlichia chaffeensis* *Ehrlichia ewingii*	South, Southeast, and Midwest	Fever, chills, headache, myalgias	Leukopenia, thrombocytopenia, elevated liver transaminases; serology can confirm at 1-2 weeks	Doxycycline Chloramphenicol (Chloromycetin) Rifampin (Rifadin)
Human granulocytic ehrlichiosis *Ehrlichia phagocytophila/ equi*	Northeast and upper Midwest	Fever, chills, headache, myalgias	Leukopenia, thrombocytopenia, elevated liver transaminases; serology can confirm at 1-2 weeks	Doxycycline Chloramphenicol Rifampin
Rocky Mountain spotted fever *Rickettsia rickettsii*	Southeast Atlantic coast states, and Midwest	Fever, headache, myalgias, malaise, vomiting, rash	Mild leukopenia, thrombocytopenia, elevated liver transaminases, hyponatremia; serology can confirm at 7-10 days	Tetracycline Chloramphenicol Doxycycline
Tularemia *Francisella tularensis*	South and Midwest	Fever, chills, headache, malaise, fatigue, cough, myalgias, vomiting, sore throat, abdominal pain, diarrhea, skin ulcers, lymphadenopathy	Normal or slightly elevated white blood cell count and erythrocyte sedimentation rate; serology can confirm at about 2 weeks	Streptomycin Gentamicin Tetracycline Chloramphenicol Fluoroquinolones

From Gayle A, Ringdahl E: *Am Fam Physician* 64(3):461, 2001.

- Povidone-iodine scrub and solution
- Normal saline specimen container or culture medium *(optional)*
- Gauze and bandage

In addition, for difficult removal or retained mouthparts:
- Punch biopsy equipment for 3- to 6-mm punch as appropriate
- Iris scissors
- Lidocaine 0.5 ml in syringe with 30-gauge needle
- Aluminum chloride solution 6.25% on a cotton-tip swab *(optional)*
- 5-0 Nylon suture *(optional)*

TECHNIQUE

1. Gently paint the surrounding area with povidone-iodine solution.
2. With blunt forceps, tweezers, or gloved fingers, grasp the tick as close to the skin surface as possible and pull upward and perpendicular with steady even pressure.
3. Do not twist or jerk the tick, since this may break off mouthparts.

4. *Never* squeeze, crush, or puncture the body of the tick, because its fluids may contain infectious agents.
5. The tick may be sent for microscopic analysis of the *Borrelia* spirochete or cultured for other organisms.
6. Disinfect the bite site with povidone-iodine scrub or antibacterial soap.

In cases of a particularly tenacious tick, retained mouthparts, or high-risk endemic areas, perform the following technique:
1. Disinfect the area with antibacterial soap. Infiltrate the area beneath the bite with lidocaine.
2. Apply the punch biopsy instrument perpendicular to the skin so that it encompasses the tick. Stretch the skin on each side of the lesion. Advance the biopsy punch downward with moderate pressure, using a clockwise-counterclockwise twisting motion. Penetration through the epidermis and dermis is confirmed with a marked decrease in resistance. (See Chapter 33, Skin Biopsy.)
3. Remove the punch. Lift the biopsy specimen with forceps, and cut the pedicle with iris scissors. Submit the tissue for histologic study.
4. Disinfect the area again, and apply pressure with gauze. If adequate hemostasis is not accomplished,

cauterize with aluminum chloride solution or close with suture. Apply bandage.

COMPLICATIONS

Patients should be advised of the possibility of local or systemic infection. Excessive bleeding may be encountered but should be stopped effectively with pressure, cauterization, or suture.

CPT/BILLING CODES

10120   Removal of superficial foreign body, skin
10121   Incisional removal of foreign body, complex

ICD-9-CM DIAGNOSTIC CODES

919.4   Injury, superficial, insect bite, without infection
919.5   Injury, superficial, insect bite, with infection or see specific site 910.4 to 919.4 without infection or 910.5 to 919.5 with infection

ADDITIONAL RESOURCES

- See the sample patient education handout titled "Tick Removal and Prevention of Infection" and "Tickborne Diseases: What You Should Know" on pages 1775 and 1776, respectively, of Appendix G.

BIBLIOGRAPHY

Berger BW, Johnson RC, Kodner C, Coleman L: Cultivation of *Borrelia burgdorferi* from human tick bites: a guide to the risk of infection, *J Am Acad Dermatol* 32(2 Pt 1):184, 1995.

Gayle A, Ringdahl E: Tick-borne diseases, *Am Fam Physician* 64(3):461, 2001.

Goodman JL: Ehrlichiosis: ticks, dogs, and doxycycline, *N Engl J Med* 341(3):195, 1999.

Jones BE: Human "seed tick" infestation, *Amblyomma americanum* larvae, *Arch Dermatol* 117:812, 1981.

Korenberg EI, Vorobyeva NN, Moskvitina HG, Gorban' LYa: Prevention of borreliosis in persons bitten by infected ticks, *Infection* 24(2):187, 1996.

Munns R: Punch biopsy of the skin. In Driscoll CE, Rakel RE, editors: *Patient care: procedures for your practice*, Oradell, NJ, 1988, Medical Economics.

Needham G: Evaluation of five popular methods for tick removal, *Pediatrics* 75(6):997, 1985.

Patterson J, Fitzwater J, Connell J: Localized tick bite reaction, *Cutis* 24(8):168, 1979.

Pearn J: Neuromuscular paralysis caused by tick envenomation, *J Neurol Sci* 34:37, 1977.

Spach DH, Liles WC, Campbell GL, et al: Tick-borne diseases in the US, *N Engl J Med* 329:936, 1993.

CHAPTER 38

Tissue Glues

J. Mark Wiedemann
John L. Pfenninger

Cyanoacrylates have been in widespread use outside of the United States for years, and the Food and Drug Administration approved their use for incision and laceration repair in 1998. The agents combine cyanoacrylates and formaldehyde. Some have added plasticizers for extra strength and flexibility. Dermabond (2-octylcyanoacrylate) (Ethicon Corp.) is available in single-use, small glass vacuum vials, and it forms a polymeric bond across apposed tissue edges on contact with moisture or air. The Ellman Corporation provides a less-expensive multiuse system. It is an isobutyl cyanoacrylate (IsoDent) and comes with four 2-ml vials of glue. Cosmesis is comparable or superior to sutures, and there is much greater acceptance, especially with children. The products have antimicrobial properties and negligible tissue toxicity and are easily applied. They significantly decrease wound repair time.

INDICATIONS

- Nonmucosal laceration or incision repairs
- Facial, scalp, torso, or extremity wounds
- After deep suture placement if skin tension is minimal
- Wounds less than 8 cm (gap less than 0.5 cm)
- Instead of 5-0 or smaller suture
- Removal of foreign bodies in ear or nose (physicians can apply a small drop of glue on wooden end of cotton swab, touch the object for 30 seconds, and remove)
- Repair of lacerated nails or nail beds

CONTRAINDICATIONS

- Mucosal lesions
- Significant wound margin tension
- Noncompliant patients
- Heavily contaminated wounds requiring debridement
- Human or animal bite or scratch wounds
- Puncture wounds

- Stellate, jagged, or crush wounds
- Axillae, perineum, and feet
- Hand or joint lacerations (in which repetitive movement or washing can weaken bond)

ADVANTAGES

- Faster than suturing or stapling
- Less painful
- Less need for painful, injectable anesthetic
- As effective as suturing in appropriately selected patients
- Some studies show a lower infection rate compared with staples and sutures
- No need for suture removal
- Low cost
- Reduces risk of needlestick injury

DISADVANTAGES

- Bond reaches strength equivalent to naturally healed tissue at 7 days after repair.
- Early dehiscence is the most common complaint. Wound strength on the first day is significantly less than with suture.
- Glue is very liquid, and inadvertent spillage or excessive application can cause adherence to gloves or other tissues.
- Dermabond is single use and is double or triple the cost of a single pack of nylon suture.

EQUIPMENT

- Dermabond single-use vials (Fig. 38-1, *A*) or IsoDent System multiuse vials consisting of 100 applicators, four 2-ml vials of glue, and four autoclavable dishes with various size wells (Fig. 38-1, *B*)
- Gloves

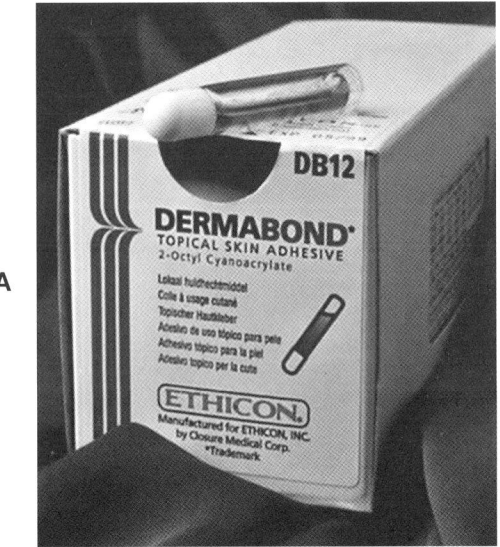

Dish with
variable-sized
wells to hold glue

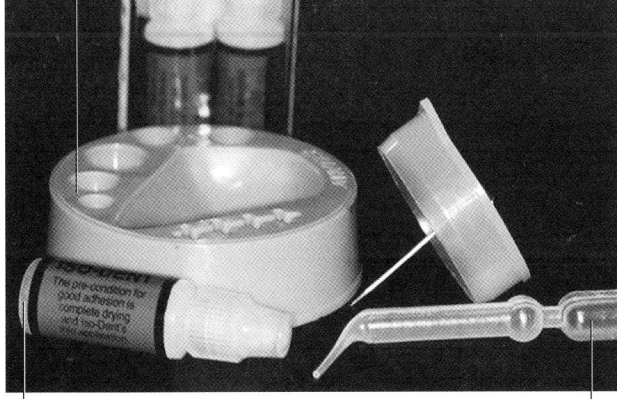

Vial of glue

Single-use disposable
aspirator/applicator

Fig. 38-1
A, Dermabond single-use vials. **B,** Ellman IsoDent System. (**A,** Courtesy Ethicon, Inc., Norwood, Mass. **B,** Courtesy Ellman International Inc., Hewlett, NY.)

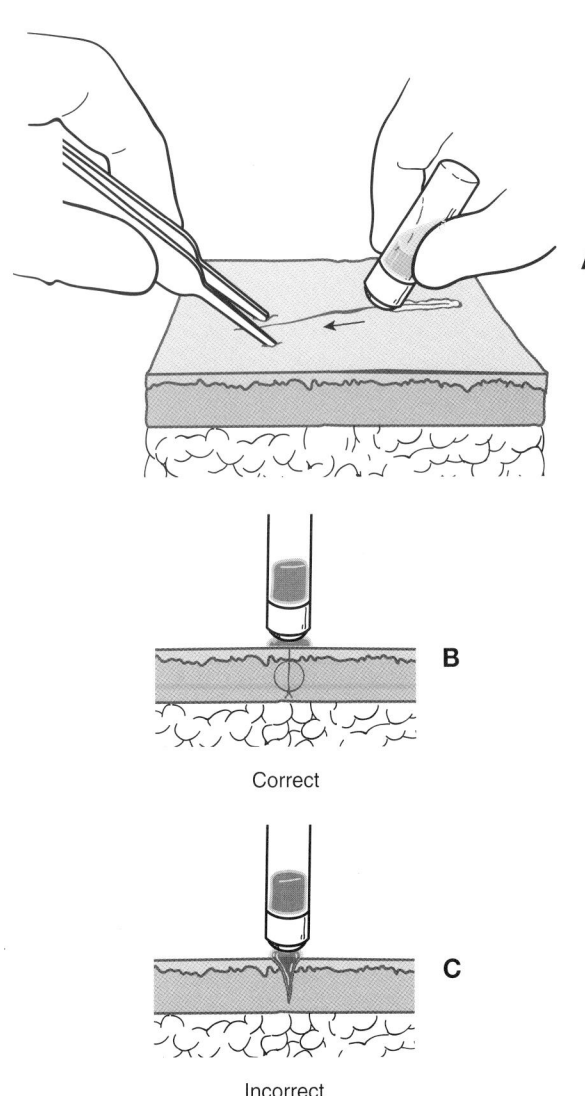

Correct

Incorrect

Fig. 38-2
A, Approximate margins and apply glue. **B,** Correct application. **C,** Incorrect application into the wound itself.

• Single-use tissue approximators (Bionix Corp.), gauze, or forceps (see Fig. 38-3, *A*) *(optional)*
• Super Glue remover *(optional)*

PREPROCEDURE PATIENT PREPARATION

Obtain verbal informed consent for the procedure. Explain that the wound will be cleansed and prepared, possibly involving analgesia. Some children may need to be restrained. Explain the procedure, and warn the patient there may be a slight sensation of heat or stinging.

TECHNIQUE (FIG. 38-2)

1. Meticulous wound preparation is essential and may require topical or infiltrated anesthetics. Good hemostasis must be achieved before application.
2. The patient should be positioned so that the fluid glue does not run off the wound to other areas.

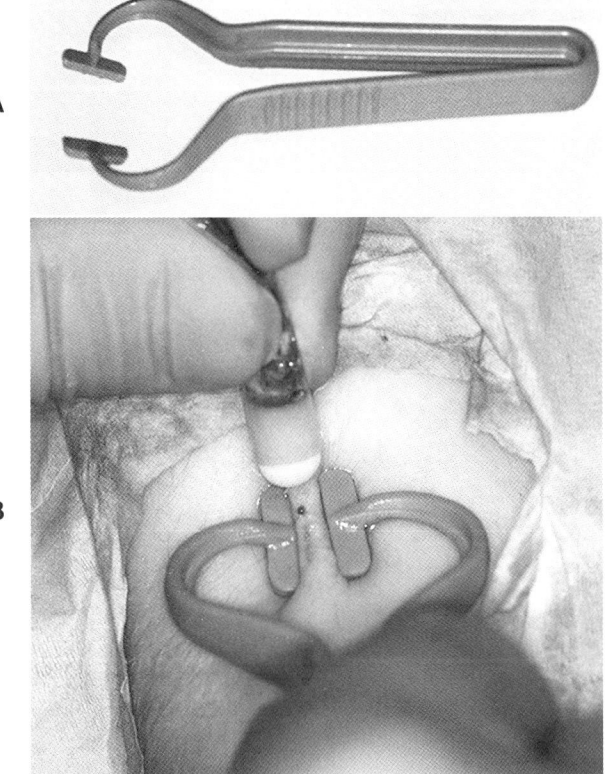

Fig. 38-3
A, Plastic tissue approximators for the application of tissue glue.
B, Application of tissue glue with the aid of plastic approximators.

3. The edges of the laceration are manually apposed. Clean, not sterile, gloves are acceptable for use, provided the wound is not inadvertently contaminated. For better traction, gauze, forceps, or disposable plastic tissue approximators may be used (Fig. 38-3).

4. The Dermabond vial is crushed and the glue touched to the wound edges. Dermabond has introduced a "chisel-tip" applicator, which purportedly also improves accuracy. With IsoDent, first the glue is placed in the wells of the disk. The various-sized wells hold variable amounts of glue, depending on the size of the wound. The glue is then aspirated from the small well in the dish with disposable small pipettes. Some practitioners have advocated aspirating the glue into a syringe, then attaching an angiocath for more accurate delivery.

5. The glue is gently painted over the wound. Care should be taken to keep the glue from entering into the wound, which can impair healing and precipitate a foreign body reaction. If there is doubt that the tissue edges can be reapproximated completely and evenly, suturing or stapling should be considered.

6. The glue should be applied in an ovoid area (the wound being central) for best adhesive strength.

7. The manufacturer recommends a minimum of three separate coats. Each layer should be allowed to dry. The first will dry in about 2½ minutes. The surface, when dry, looks slightly rougher and more undulant than when it is wet. Subsequent layers dry more rapidly. Excess adhesive may be wiped off within 10 seconds.

8. Steri-Strips, applied after drying, can help prevent dehiscence.

POSTPROCEDURE PATIENT EDUCATION

The adhesive is water resistant, and further dressing is not needed. The patient may wet the area but should pat it dry. Soaking is not recommended. Antibiotic ointment should be avoided because it can weaken the bond. A bandage may be appropriate for active people, for children, or for those inclined to pick or pull at the wound. The adhesive spontaneously sloughs in 5 to 14 days. Infections are unusual but can be detected early because the wound is visible, and purulent exudate normally "unroofs" the adhesive. In these cases, the adhesive should be gently removed and standard wound infection treatment, possibly including systemic antibiotics, implemented. Reclosure with cyanoacrylate is not recommended.

COMPLICATIONS

- Early dehiscence.
- If the practitioner's instruments, gauze, or gloves accidentally adhere to the wound or patient, pressure is placed adjacent to the area and the object is "rolled off" in a way that does not place traction on the repair.
- Adhesive that inadvertently binds the eyelids should be covered with generous amounts of ophthalmic antibiotic ointment and not pried open. The bond usually weakens and separates in 1 or 2 days. Cyanoacrylates are not harmful to the eye, and they are used routinely in ophthalmologic practice. Appropriate placement of a gauze during repairs can prevent spillage into the eyes.
- Petroleum jelly, antibiotic ointment, or a commercially available "Super Glue remover" can be used on dried run-off areas.
- Adhesive may insinuate itself between wound edges, resulting in unacceptable healing.

SUPPLIERS

Dermabond
Ethicon Inc.
249 Vanderbilt Avenue
Norwood, MA 02062
Phone: 1-800-356-4835
Website: www.ethicon.com

IsoDent
Ellman International, Inc.
1135 Railroad Avenue
Hewlett, NY 11557
Phone: 1-800-835-5355
Website: www.ellman.com

Wound Closure Forceps
Bionix Development Corp.
5154 Enterprise Boulevard
Toledo, OH 43612
Phone: 1-419-727-8421

COST

As of 2001, Dermabond is about $35 per vial and comes in boxes of 12. IsoDent is $96 for four 2-ml multiuse vials, which provide a minimum of 20 applications each (cost per use about $1). Less physician time is also a factor. Many institutions and offices are also now allowing other assistants to apply the adhesive.

CPT/BILLING CODES

See Table 23-4 for wound closure codes.

ICD-9-CM DIAGNOSTIC CODES

See Appendix H for wound closure codes.

ADDITIONAL RESOURCES

- See the sample patient education handout titled "Wound Care After Treatment with Topical Skin Adhesive (Tissue Glue)" on page 1777 of Appendix G.

BIBLIOGRAPHY

Bruns TB, Worthington JM: Using tissue adhesive for wound repair: a practical guide to Dermabond, *Am Fam Physician* 61:1383, 2000.

Pfenninger JL: Use of tissue glues (cyanoacrylate tissue adhesives). In Rakel R, editor: *Saunders manual of medical practice,* Philadelphia, 2000, WB Saunders.

Quinn J, Wells G, Sutcliffe T, et al: A randomized trial comparing octylcyanoacrylate tissue adhesive and sutures in the management of lacerations, *JAMA* 277:1527, 1997.

Simon HK, McLario DJ, Bruns TB, et al: Long-term appearance of lacerations repaired using a tissue adhesive, *Pediatrics* 99:193, 1997.

Singer AJ, Hollander JE, Valentine SM, et al: Prospective, randomized, controlled trial of tissue adhesive vs. standard wound closure techniques for laceration repair, *Acad Emerg Med* 5:94, 1998.

CHAPTER 39

Hypertrophic Scars and Keloids*

Edward M. Zimmerman

The skin of predisposed individuals may respond to injury or surgery by developing excessive growths known as hypertrophic scars or keloids. Common locations for these lesions are the head, neck, upper trunk, and proximal upper extremities. *Hypertrophic scars* are self-limited growths that enlarge within the boundaries of a wound and then often regress over time. Many hypertrophic scars spontaneously involute within 2 years. *Keloids* are benign, hard, fibrous proliferations of collagen that expand, either slowly or rapidly, beyond the original size and shape of a wound. They tend to persist and often invade surrounding tissue. They may become painful or pruritic as well as unsightly.

Hypertrophic scars and keloids represent abnormalities in the synthesis and degradation of collagen and extracellular matrix components. Hypertrophic scars have a threefold increase in collagen-synthesis enzymes over normal scars, whereas keloids may exhibit 20 times the normal levels. Hypertrophic scars can occur at any site of skin injury. Those following surgical incisions usually remain linear. Burns frequently produce unsightly, pink, hypertrophic scars that may contract. The scars may itch, but generally they do not produce the pain and hyperesthesia seen with keloids. The incidence of keloids in dark-skinned individuals is 15 to 20 times that found in light-skinned people, with an equal incidence of lesions in males and females. Keloids appear frequently in anatomic sites that are subject to motion, overlie bony prominences or areas of increased skin tension or recurrent stretch, such as the shoulders, upper back, and presternal areas. Keloids may develop on the face and scalp after acne, or on the earlobe after ear piercing. Children are also more likely to experience both problems.

This chapter focuses on office techniques used in the treatment of hypertrophic scars and keloids. Because of the natural regression of hypertrophic scars, therapy for these lesions is generally limited to topical application or injection of steroids and compression. Keloids are considered by some clinicians to be low-grade, benign, cutaneous tumors, and radiation therapy has been advocated. This therapy is not reviewed here. The malignancy potential of radiation in the treatment of a benign disease as well as its expense make radiation therapy a last resort. Location, size, and duration are factors in choosing the most appropriate therapy. Cryotherapy, corticosteroid injection, surgical excision, pressure therapy, and irradiation—or a combination of these modalities—may be chosen for the treatment of keloids.

CRYOTHERAPY

Tissue-destruction techniques used for treating keloids can incite further keloid formation. Cryotherapy, however, has been used with good results, with "good" reported in 65% to 75% of cases. Both liquid nitrogen and nitrous oxide methods can be efficacious (see Chapter 15, Cryosurgery). The younger the keloid, the better the response to cryotherapy. A 10- to 15-second freeze with *liquid nitrogen* (−189° C) is usually required for earlobe keloids and keloids on most sites other than the midsternal region. Freezing for more than 25 seconds with liquid nitrogen frequently produces persistent posttreatment hypopigmentation. A 30- to 45-second freeze is usually adequate for most keloids when *nitrous oxide* (−89° C) or similar instrument is used. A better guide is to continue the freeze until 1 to 2 mm of normal tissue is involved and the complete thaw time is 1.5 to 2 minutes. During each treatment visit, the entire lesion must be treated with two to three freeze-thaw cycles.

After cryotherapy, tissue edema will develop in 20 to 60 minutes. Within hours a significant bulla (blister) will develop. A rather copious serous discharge may follow. A moist environment (semiocclusive dressing) will aid healing. Depending on the size of the lesion, five to eight treatments may be needed at 6-week intervals. Start conservatively and increase the freeze times if there are no untoward adverse effects. (See the sample patient education handout titled "Wound Care After Cryosurgery" on

---

*This is the original chapter written by Thomas J. Zuber and John L. Pfenninger; Edward M. Zimmerman updated and edited the chapter for this edition.

page 1753 of Appendix G.) Cryotherapy can also be used to soften hard keloids immediately before injection of steroids. Edema of the skin allows better dispersal of the steroid and minimizes its deposition into the subcutaneous or surrounding normal tissue. Light cryotherapy (liq N_2 spray for 3- to 5-second burst[s]) improves keloid regression, allows for lower injection pressures, and decreases the pain associated with injections. Allow 20 to 60 minutes for the edema to occur before proceeding with the injection.

CORTICOSTEROID INJECTIONS

Once a scar is palpable, topical corticosteroids even under occlusion (e.g., Cordran tape) are rarely beneficial. Raised hypertrophic scars and keloids may be softened and flattened by intralesional corticosteroid therapy. Corticosteroids represent effective monotherapy for some hypertrophic scars and small keloids, and they are frequently used as the initial therapy for large keloids.

Early, small, or narrow lesions are initially treated with intralesional injection every 4 weeks. Early keloids are softer and more responsive to injection than older inactive lesions. Avoid injecting into surrounding normal skin to prevent perilesional subcutaneous atrophy and telangiectasia formation. When a lesion flattens to nearly the level of the skin surface, decrease the frequency and concentration of the injections. Overaggressive therapy can lead to hypopigmentation and a depression resulting from the atrophy.

Injections are frequently performed with a 27- or 30-gauge needle and a Luer-Lok syringe. Locked syringes help to prevent needle disengagement when injecting under pressure. Consider using cryotherapy immediately beforehand (see the previous section) to ease injection and the spread of the steroid.

Many steroid regimens have been developed, and there is considerable variation in guidelines and recommendations for dosages and drugs. No clear advantage has been shown for any one type of corticosteroid. Triamcinolone acetonide 10 mg/ml (Kenalog-10) is a popular choice because of its 4- to 6-week duration of action. Although undiluted steroid can be used for unresponsive or dense lesions, many physicians prefer to dilute the triamcinolone 1:3 with physiologic saline or 1% lidocaine to create a 2.5 mg/ml solution. This dilute concentration limits postinjection hypopigmentation and atrophy. Injecting only lidocaine around the lesion using a 27- to 31-gauge needle before steroid injection improves patient comfort. Once the response is known, the concentration of triamcinolone acetonide can be increased to 40 mg/ml, which can be diluted 1:2 or 1:1 with lidocaine if necessary for future injections to increase the effect. Some physicians add 150 mg of hyaluronidase to help disperse the steroid.

Administer the corticosteroid as the needle passes through the lesion. Keep the bevel of the needle pointed down. The scar may blanch temporarily with the injection. Try to keep the injection within the confines of the lesion to prevent side effects in the adjacent tissue. Firm lesions may practically limit the amount of medication that can be administered. Total amount will vary significantly depending on the size of the lesion. When the lesion is too dense to inject, consider treating with cryotherapy first as previously discussed.

Another method of injecting steroids is to use the MadaJet Injector (see Pearl no. 35 in Appendix I, Pearls of Practice). The same concentration is used. The spring-loaded "gun" fires (dispenses) the solution, which is under pressure, into the lesion. No needles are involved, and there is less pain. Injections may need to be repeated every 3 weeks to gain maximum benefit.

Systemic effects from the corticosteroids are rare, but possible with repeated injections of higher concentrations. Local effects include hypopigmentation, hyperpigmentation, perilesional atrophy, perilymphatic linear atrophy, and local telangiectasia. These effects often improve over time. This therapy is generally considered safe and effective.

SURGICAL EXCISION

Therapy of keloids limited to traditional surgical excision with primary closure leads to a recurrence rate of greater than 50%. Corticosteroids mixed with the local anesthetic at the time of surgical removal provide better results. The corticosteroid therapy may be initiated 2 months before surgery, at the time of surgery, or 2 to 4 weeks after surgery.

Proper surgical technique during the excision reduces the recurrence of keloids. Because tissue trauma may incite excessive growth, the wound bed and surrounding tissues must be handled gently. Avoid the use of instruments that crush tissue as well as overly aggressive cautery. Superpulse carbon dioxide lasers allow precise excision and cautery and cause minimal thermal damage to surrounding tissue. This makes them useful in excising some keloids, despite their relative expense. Radiofrequency surgery has similar results.

When an excision is performed, close the skin under minimal tension. Consider gentle undermining to decrease wound tension. Some surgeons avoid subcuticular absorbable sutures, which may increase tissue reaction. Skin closure should be accomplished with a very fine nonabsorbable suture material, such as 6-0 nylon. Topical adhesives ("tissue glues") and wound closure strips help close the wound with the least possible trauma and reduce tension on wound edges. They may also reduce the total number of sutures needed.

Some surgeons advocate removal of every vestige of

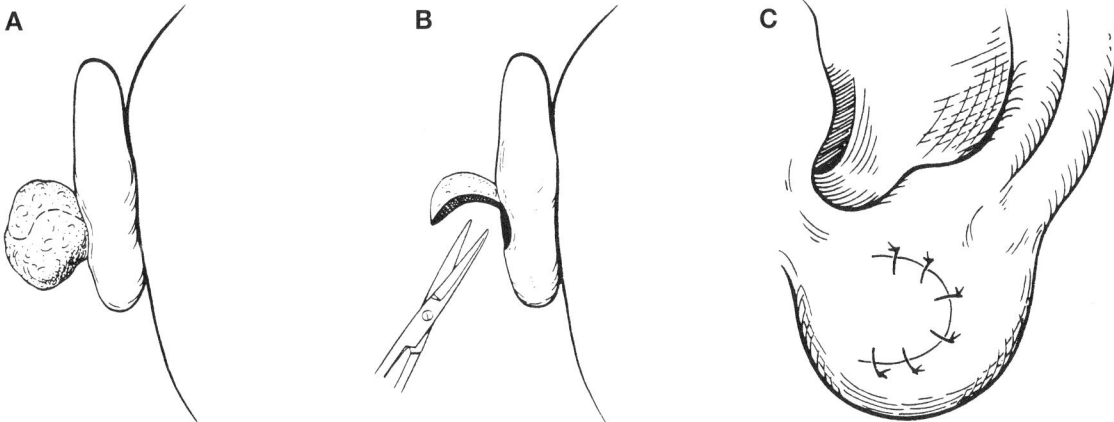

Fig. 39-1
Resection of a keloid on an ear lobe. The skin overlying a keloid can be used to create a low-tension wound closure. **A,** Half the skin is selected for the flap. **B,** The skin is sharply dissected from the underlying keloid, and the subcutaneous keloid is totally excised. **C,** The wound is closed with simple, interrupted, nonabsorbable, 6-0 nylon suture.

a keloid; however, wide excision of normal skin around keloids does not reduce the rate of recurrence. Other surgeons advocate leaving a rim of incompletely excised keloid in place to serve as a barrier to further keloid growth. It is unclear whether this technique provides significant benefit over standard excisions.

Local advancement flaps can be used to limit the wound tension after excision. Fig. 39-1 shows a low-tension flap created after the removal of a globular earlobe keloid. Although some practitioners advocate skin grafting to provide low-tension skin closure, large donor-site keloids can also develop. Evidence suggests using Silastic-silicone preparations (Mederma, ReJuveness, Biodermis, Mepiform, Kelokote) immediately after surgery may reduce the occurrence of keloids in those prone to excessive scarring.

Before attempting surgical excision of keloids, counsel the patient well. Patients with current or previous hypertrophic scars or keloids have the ability to form these types of scars after most surgical procedures, including dermabrasion. However, sculpting hypertrophic scars with traditional dermabrasion or carbon dioxide laser is usually beneficial and generally does not lead to recurrence of hypertrophic scars. It is more common in cases that are complicated by other factors such as previous isotretinoin therapy, infection, or patient noncompliance with postoperative therapy. A detailed informed consent is useful in creating appropriate patient expectations.

Postoperative results vary widely, and patients must understand that keloids may recur regardless of the treatment methods used. Warn patients that pigment variations may take several months following surgery to resolve and that skin bleaches are sometimes required.

Sunscreens are essential. Patients should be seen at monthly intervals to identify any recurrence, and steroid injections or silicone treatments should be initiated or reintroduced early before the lesion becomes mature and large.

PRESSURE THERAPY

Pressure applied to burn sites can prevent hypertrophic scar formation or induce regression of early hypertrophic scars. Similarly, pressure dressings and garments after keloid surgery reduce their rate of recurrence. Pressure bandaging is used until the scar is no longer red; however, patient compliance may be poor when months or years of therapy are required. Many physicians prefer to use postoperative injections to ensure adequate therapy. However, when wounds are large or numerous, fitted pressure garments may be the best alternative.

After earlobe keloid excision, a pressure earring can be worn as soon as the skin sutures are removed (usually 5 to 7 days). A spring-loaded, light-pressure earring prevents the complication of skin necrosis. Hypoallergenic pressure earrings with a self-adjusting clasp are available from Padgett Instruments (1-800-842-1029) and many other medical supply companies. These earrings cost about $40 and are available in a variety of styles and colors that encourage prolonged use. A less-expensive alternative is to use large, flat, back-clip earrings lined with Silastic sheeting cut to fit inside them. Silastic sheeting alone has been therapeutic in reducing keloids and hypertrophic scars but is best combined with repetitive intralesional steroid injections and compression to hold it in place.

LIGHT THERAPY (LASER AND OTHERS)

Continuous-wave, carbon dioxide laser used in the cutting mode has been shown to be effective for some refractory keloids. All possible keloid tissue is excised with the laser and the wound is allowed to heal by secondary intention or is closed with minimal tension as noted previously. Concurrent intralesional steroids, compression dressings, or silicone treatments may be helpful. Depending on the size, depth, and location of the wound, as well as the patient's health, healing may take as long as 3 months. Transient hypertrophic scars develop in up to 30% of cases; unfortunately, as with other treatments, recurrences are high. Superpulse carbon dioxide laser may prove to be better, but long-term studies are pending. Flashlamp-pumped pulsed-dye lasers (585 nm) and intense, pulsed-light lasers (e.g., PhotoDerm) are used to treat relatively flat hypertrophic scars and keloids. The advantage of using lasers relates to the precision with which the light energy can be delivered to the target rather than the surrounding tissue and the absorption of specific wavelengths of light by the vascular components of the target. Multiple sessions are required and cost may be a factor for some patients, but results are frequently impressive.

ALTERNATIVE METHODS

Some investigators inject *hyaluronidase* with steroids after cryotherapy with improved results. Although the mechanism of action is unknown, *topical silicone* gel and *silicone* sheeting is used with success. The gel's impermeability to water is thought to minimize evaporation and provide a semiocclusive dressing that accelerates healing and shortens the inflammatory phase. Topical Silastic gels and Mederma gel (a vegetable oil extract) have proved to be beneficial in reducing both volume and redness of lesions. The silicone sheets (Mederma, ReJuveness, Biodermis, Mepiform, Kelokote) must be worn 12 to 24 hours per day for 3 months or more. They are applied under tape or a pressure garment. The sheet is 3.5 mm thick and applied over the scar only. It is held in place with paper tape and removed and washed daily. Its effect is unrelated to pressure. Perioperative injection with *interferon* is a promising new therapy. One study of 12 patients showed a recurrence rate of less than 10% after traditional excision, interferon injection, and follow-up of nearly 15 months. Intralesional *bleomycin* has also been tried with some success. Also, *5-fluorouracil* 50 mg/ml mixed with Kenalog 1 mg/ml injected one to three times weekly into hypertrophic scars may be efficacious in decreasing scar tissue.

CONCLUSION

Stepwise treatment as well as combination of modalities may prove to be the most effective manner to treat keloids. If initial topical (or injected, high-potency) steroids and compression do not provide complete relief of the lesion, then cryotherapy may soften the lesion and allow improved injectability. Next, excision or careful vaporization of the bulk of a lesion with carbon dioxide superpulse laser may be indicated. Regardless of how the lesion is resected, careful and low-tension closure with minimal sutures or healing by secondary intention is recommended. Next, consider excision followed by several sessions of 500- to 600-nm pulsed light or laser and/or low-dose radiation. Application of topical gels and pressure dressings combined with various modalities seem to produce acceptable results with even difficult lesions.

SUPPLIERS

Madajet injector
Delasco Dermatologic Lab and Supply Co.
608 13th Avenue
Council Bluffs, IA 57501-6401
Phone: 1-800-831-6273
Website: www.delasco.com

Pressure earrings
Padgett Instruments, Inc.
1520 Grand Street
Kansas City, MO 64108-1404
Phone: 1-800-842-1029
Website: www.padgetinst.com

ReJuveness silicone sheets
ReJuveness, Inc.
Phone: 1-800-588-7455
Website: www.rejuveness.com

Mederma gel
Merz Pharmaceuticals
4215 Tudor Lane
Greensboro, NC 27410
Phone: 1-888-925-8989
Website: www.mederma.com

Silastic gel sheeting and topical products
Biodermis
3078 East Sunset Road, Suite #1
Las Vegas, NV 89120
Phone: 1-800-322-3729
Website: www.biodermis.com

Silastic topical gel (Kelokote)
Allied Biomedical Corp.
3850 Ramada Drive, C-2
Paso Robles, CA 93446
Phone: 1-800-276-1322
Website: www.alliedbiomedical.com

Mepiform (self-adherent silicone dressing)
Byron Medical
602 West Rillito
Tucson, AZ 85705
Phone: 1-800-777-3434
Website: www.byronmedical.com

PhotoDerm and lasers of all wavelengths
Lumenis (formerly ESC Medical Systems)
100 Morse Street
Norwood, MA 02062
Phone: 1-800-562-5916
Website: www.lumenis.com

CPT/BILLING CODES

There are no specific codes for treatment or excision of hypertrophic scars or keloids.

ICD-9-CM DIAGNOSTIC CODE

701.4   Keloid or scar

ADDITIONAL RESOURCES

- See the sample patient education handout titled "Wound Care After Cryosurgery" on page 1753 of Appendix G.

BIBLIOGRAPHY

Alster TS, Willims CM: Treatment of keloid sternotomy scars with 585 nm flashlamp-pumped pulsed-dye laser, *Lancet* 345:1198, 1995.

Berman B, Bieley HC: Keloids, *J Am Acad Dermatol* 33:117, 1995.

Berman B, Bieley HC: Adjunct therapy to surgical management of keloids, *Dermatol Surg* 22:126, 1996.

Coleman WP, Hanke CW, Alt TH, Asken S: *Cosmetic surgery of the skin,* ed 2, St Louis, 1997, Mosby.

de Oliveira GV, Nunes TA, Magna LA, et al: Silicone versus nonsilicone gel dressings: a controlled trial, *Dermatol Surg* 27(8):721, 2001.

English RS, Shenefelt PD: Keloids and hypertropic scars, *Dermatol Surg* 25:631, 1999

Espana A, Solario T, Quintarilla E: Bleomycin in the treatment of keloids and hypertropic scars by multiple needle punctures, *Dermatol Surg* 27:23, 2001.

Fitzpatrick RE: Treatment of inflamed hypertrophic scars using intralesional 5-FU, *Dermatol Surg* 25(3):224, 1999.

Fitzpatrick TB, Wolff K, Johnson RA: *Color atlas and synopsis of clinical dermatology,* ed 3, New York, 1997, McGraw-Hill.

Gold MH: Topical silicone gel sheeting in the treatment of hypertrophic scars and keloids, *J Dermatol Surg Oncol* 19:912, 1993.

Gold MH, Foster TD, Adair MA, et al: Prevention of hypertrophic scars and keloids by the prophylactic use of topical silicone gel sheets following a surgical procedure in an office setting, *Dermatol Surg* 27:641, 2001.

Habif TP: *Clinical dermatology,* ed 3, St Louis, 1996, Mosby.

Kantor GR, Wheeland RG, Bailin PL, et al: Treatment of earlobe keloids with carbon dioxide laser excision: a report of 16 cases, *J Dermatol Surg Oncol* 11:1063, 1985.

Murray JC: Keloids and hypertrophic scars, *Clin Dermatol* 12:27, 1994.

Nemeth AJ: Keloids and hypertrophic scars, *J Dermatol Surg Oncol* 19:738, 1993.

Niessen FB, Spauwen PH, Schalkwijk J, Kon M: On the nature of hypertrophic scars and keloids: a review, *Plast Reconstr Surg* 104(5):1435, 1999.

Rusciani L, Rossi G, Bono R: Use of cryotherapy in the treatment of keloids, *J Dermatol Surg Oncol* 19:529, 1993.

Stucker FJ, Shaw GY: An approach to management of keloids, *Arch Otolaryngol Head Neck Surg* 118:63, 1992.

WEBSITE ADDRESSES

For updated references, search "keloid treatment" at www.elibrary.com.

CHAPTER 40

Ingrown Toenails

James F. Peggs

An ingrown toenail is a common affliction that can result from a variety of conditions and that can produce a good deal of discomfort and disability. The great toe is virtually the only toe involved, and either the medial or lateral border of the nail may be affected.

Several palliative measures are available to relieve painful symptoms of ingrown toenails. These include elevation of the involved nail edge with a small cotton wick; selective trimming of the affected nail edge (although this usually provides only temporary relief at best); frequent soaking; and use of loose footwear. Unfortunately, resolution of the problem is rare without an operative approach.

Removal of the toenail, either partial or total, remains the definitive treatment for bothersome ingrown nails. For recurrent episodes, ablation of the germinal matrix tissue can be used to prevent regrowth of the nail. Permanent destruction can be effected by surgical excision (Winograd procedure) or by more conservative and equally successful measures using chemicals or radiofrequency energy.

INDICATIONS

- Onychocryptosis (ingrown nail)
- Onychomycosis (fungal infection of the nail)
- Chronic, recurrent paronychia (inflammation of the nail fold)
- Onychogryposis (deformed, curved nail)

The basic idea is to try to correct all offending practices, just remove the offending portion of the nail initially and allow regrowth. If all else fails, permanently ablate the portion of nail matrix causing the problem if it recurs.

CONTRAINDICATIONS

- Allergy to local anesthetics (see Chapter 5, Local and Topical Anesthetic Complications).
- Bleeding diathesis.

- More caution needs to be taken when diabetes mellitus or peripheral vascular disease is present.
- Phenol should not be used in pregnancy.

EQUIPMENT

- 5- or 10-ml syringe with long (1½-inch) needle (25 or 27 gauge)
- Local anesthetic *without* epinephrine (see Chapter 4, Local Anesthesia)
- Narrow Locke periosteal elevator (nail elevator)
- Sterile scissors with straight blades (or an English nail splitter)
- Rubber band, small Penrose drain, or donut digital tourniquet (Ellman Corp.)
- Two straight hemostats
- Alcohol swabs
- Betadine solution
- Sterile gauze and tubular gauze dressing
- Antibiotic ointment (Polysporin, Bactroban)
- Phenol solution (88%) and isopropyl alcohol for permanent ablation of the nail, if desired
- As an alternative to phenol, the Ellman Surgitron (radiofrequency unit) with specially designed, Teflon-insulated matrix tip (less inflammation and excellent results) (see Chapter 31, Radiofrequency Surgery)

TECHNIQUE

Removal of Partial or Full Nail

1. With the patient supine, scrub the toe with Betadine.
2. Administer a digital block as described in Chapter 8, Peripheral Nerve Blocks and Field Blocks.
3. Apply tourniquet.
4. Use a straight hemostat to firmly secure a wide rubber band or Penrose drain around the base of the toe. Alternatively, use the donut tourniquet made specifically for this purpose. When anesthesia is achieved

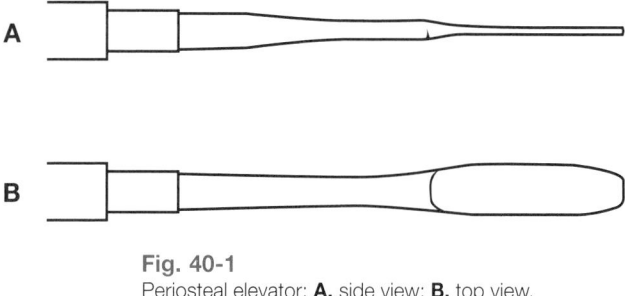

Fig. 40-1
Periosteal elevator: **A,** side view; **B,** top view.

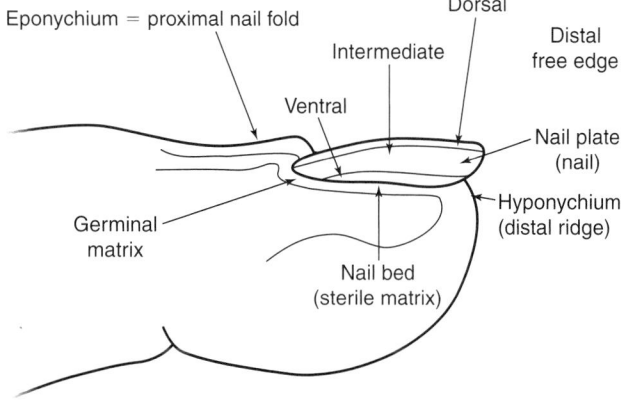

Fig. 40-2
Nail bed anatomy and terminology. Also see more details in Chapter 29, Nail Bed Repair.

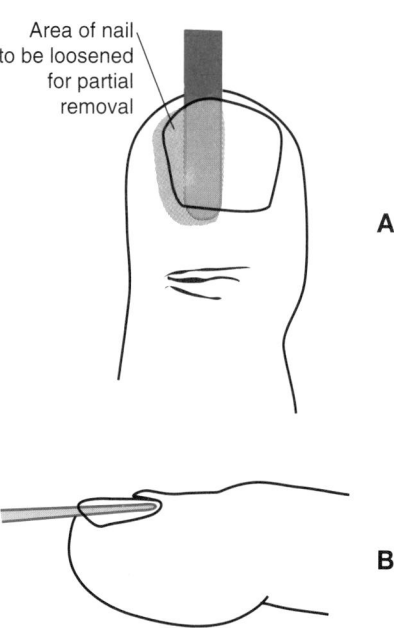

Fig. 40-3
A, Periosteal elevator advanced all the way under the proximal nail fold. **B,** Lateral view. Advance with upward pressure on the nail with forward motion until more pressure is felt under the nail fold.

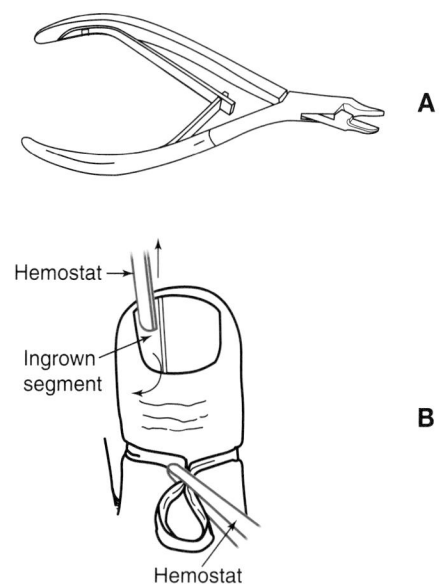

Fig. 40-4
A, Nail splitter. **B,** Technique for nail removal after nail has been elevated and split. Grasp that portion of the nail to be removed lengthwise with a straight hemostat, and remove it using a steady pulling motion with a simultaneous upward twist of the hand toward the affected side.

(5 to 10 minutes), loosen and lift the nail (at least 25% of the nail for partial removal) from the nail bed by using the flat, pointed blade of the scissors, a single jaw of a straight hemostat, or a narrow periosteal elevator. The elevator works best to decrease the likelihood of injury to nail bed (Fig. 40-1). Introduce and advance the instrument with continued upward pressure against the nail and away from the nail bed to minimize injury and bleeding (Figs. 40-2 and 40-3). It is important to completely free the proximal nail at its base under the nail fold to allow removal and to expose the germinal tissue of the nail bed. Loosen the entire nail in this fashion if the entire nail is to be removed.

5. For a partial nail removal, scissors or a nail splitter (better) should be used to completely split the nail 5 to 6 mm in from the lateral or medial margin in a longitudinal direction. Include the base of the nail that rests beneath the nail fold. Grasp that portion of the nail to be removed lengthwise with a straight hemostat and remove it, using a steady pulling motion with a simultaneous upward twist of the hand toward the affected side (Fig. 40-4). This twisting action ensures that the nail will be rolled out from beneath the affected nail margin instead of rolling over it. If the entire nail is to be removed, the nail

may be removed in two halves or in its entirety after a thorough loosening and lifting of the nail. In removing the entire nail, the forceps should produce lifting and distal traction on the nail as it separates from the nail bed.

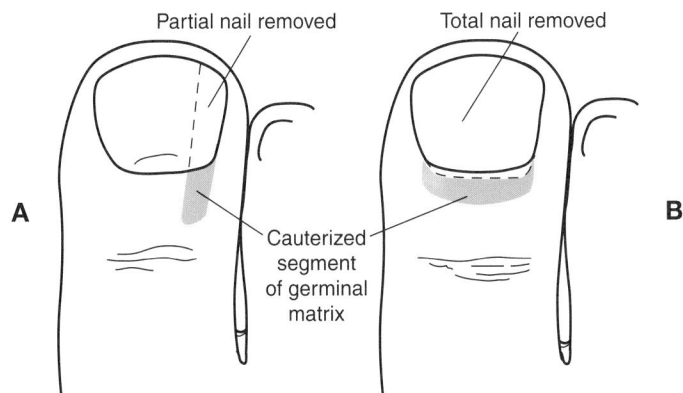

Fig. 40-5
Area of nail bed to be cauterized in, **A,** partial and, **B,** total nail removal.

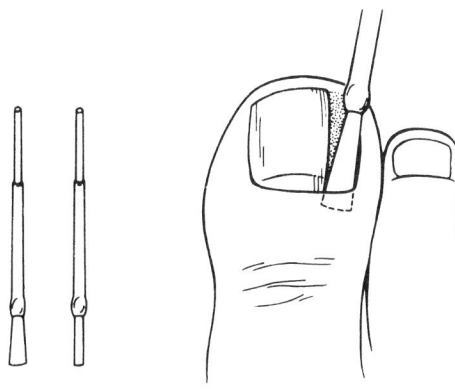

Fig. 40-6
Application of nail matrixectomy electrode with Teflon-coated side up. The medial 25% of the nail has been removed.

6. Remove all granulation tissue by grasping with hemostats and pulling. Light curettement with a dermal curette removes any residual tissue from the nail groove. Without a tourniquet there will be significant bleeding.

7. It may take 6 to 12 months for nail regrowth.

Nail Plate Ablation

In the case of recurrent problems with the regrowing toenail (pain or infection), permanent ablation of the germinal tissue is recommended.

1. Remove total or partial nail as described previously. The area must be dry and not bleeding. Remove all granulation tissue.

2. Sponge the exposed nail bed dry with cotton swabs, and then cauterize the germinal tissue, including that under the nail fold, by application of phenol on a cotton swab to the nail bed tissues (Fig. 40-5). Use caution to avoid phenol contact with normal skin. A skin hook can be helpful in elevating the skin fold from the nail matrix. Hold the phenol-dampened cotton swab in place for 3 minutes.

3. After 3 minutes, drip 70% isopropyl alcohol into the nail groove and swab the area to neutralize the phenol.

Alternatively, the Ellman Surgitron radiofrequency unit (see Chapter 31, Radiofrequency Surgery) can be used. The inflammatory response is markedly reduced.

1. Remove whole or partial nail as described previously.

2. Place antenna lead under the heel of foot.

3. Turn unit to "Hemo-part rect" (hemostasis/coagulation setting) and set the power at 2 to 3.

4. Insert wide or narrow (wide is more common) insulated matrixectomy tip over nail matrix, under the eponychium as far as it will go, insulated side up (Fig. 40-6). These electrodes are insulated with Teflon on one surface to prevent damage to the undersurface of the proximal nail fold while ablating the nail matrix with the uninsulated surface beneath. A slight upward pressure should be exerted against the undersurface of the nail fold to ensure that no pressure is exerted on the underlying matrix. The field must be free of blood. For proper effect, there should be a slight gap between electrode and matrix.

5. Apply power and slowly withdraw the electrode. Contact should be for only 5 to 6 seconds, and a sizzling sound should be heard. This step can be repeated once or twice over the same area after a 15-second cooling period. Multiple applications are necessary to ablate the entire germinal matrix of the toe; slight overlapping should not be a problem. Caution: two to three passes over the same tissue area are sufficient. Avoid overtreatment. The matrix is very thin, and bone lies immediately beneath it.

When either partial or complete ablation is completed, apply antibiotic ointment to the nail bed, cover with a sterile gauze pressure dressing, remove the tourniquet, and wrap with tubular gauze dressing.

COMPLICATIONS

- Infections (treat with soaks and appropriate antibiotics)
- Regrowth of nail and return of symptoms (regrowth rate following phenol cauterization is 4% to 25%; for radiofrequency, less than 5%)
- Excessive tissue destruction with radiofrequency unit, leading to prolonged healing and possible osteomyelitis

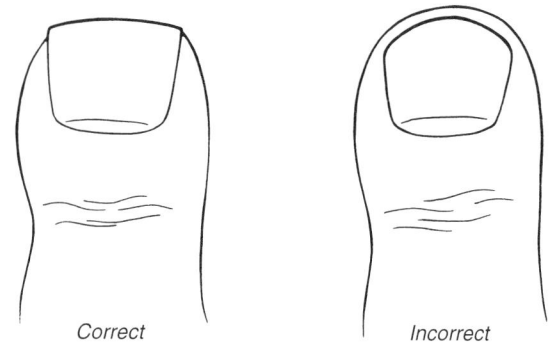

Correct *Incorrect*

Fig. 40-7
Proper nail care prophylaxis. Trim the nail flat and not too short.

POSTPROCEDURE PATIENT EDUCATION

The foot should be rested and preferably elevated during the first 12 to 24 hours. Because phenol ablates the nerve endings of the nail plate, pain should be absent when it is used. There is minimal pain with the radiofrequency unit. Nonsteroidal antiinflammatory drugs may be used for discomfort.

The dressing should be changed in 12 hours, at which point ambulation can be encouraged. The toe should be washed with soap and water three to four times a day for 4 days. Some physicians recommend topical antibiotics. Tell the patient to expect a sterile exudate from the nail bed for several weeks. Emphasize proper nail hygiene to prevent further recurrences (Fig. 40-7).

SUPPLIERS

Ellman Surgitron radiofrequency unit (see Chapter 31, Radiofrequency Surgery).

CPT/BILLING CODES

11730   Nail removal, partial or complete
11750   Permanent nail removal (matrixectomy), partial or complete

ICD-9-CM DIAGNOSTIC CODES

703.0   Ingrown toenail
110.1   Onychomycosis
703.8   Onychogryposis

BIBLIOGRAPHY

Freiberg A, Dougherty S: A review of management of ingrown toenails and onychogryposis, *Can Fam Physician* 34:2675, 1988.

Hettinger DF, Valinsky MS, Nuccio G, Lim R: Nail matrixectomies using radio wave technique, *J Am Podiatr Med Assoc* 81(6):317, 1991.

Hill GJ: *Outpatient surgery,* ed 2, Philadelphia, 1980, WB Saunders.

Mori H, Umeda T, Nishioka K, et al: Ingrown nails: a comparison of the nail matrix phenolization method with the elevation of the nail bed–periosteal flap procedure, *J Dermatol* 25(1):1, 1998.

Robb JE, Murray WR: Phenol cauterization in the management of ingrowing toenails, *Scott Med J* 27(3):236, 1982.

Zuber T, Pfenninger J: Management of ingrown toenails, *Am Fam Physician* 52(1):181, 1995.

CHAPTER 41

Epilation of Isolated Hairs (Including Trichiasis)

Kathleen M. O'Hanlon

The method used to remove problem hairs or permanently destroy hair follicles depends on the anatomic location, presence, or absence of ingrown hairs and the condition of the surrounding skin. The simplest approach, typically used by electrologists but increasingly by primary care physicians, applies current to cause follicular destruction. In the presence of ingrown hairs, a more comprehensive skin care program should be used first to decrease the density of inflammatory papules and pustules. After this, a more aggressive epilation technique, also described here, will be necessary. Ingrown or misdirected eyelashes pose a range of problems and may respond to simple tweezing or electrolysis.

INDICATIONS

- Hirsutism
- Pseudofolliculitis barbae and related disorders
- Trichiasis

CONTRAINDICATIONS

- Inflammatory skin condition
- Active herpetic outbreak

RELATIVE CONTRAINDICATIONS

- History of recurrent herpes (premedicate prior to epilation)

EQUIPMENT

- Electrosurgery unit *or* Epilator (electrolysis unit)
- 33-gauge needle (insulated types available)
- Small tweezers
- Alcohol wipe
- Loupes or magnification lamp *(optional)*

TECHNIQUE FOR EPILATION

The most direct approach uses electrolysis equipment to deliver a small current through a needle-like probe placed into the hair follicle. The Ellman Surgitron radiofrequency unit can also be used with either the "insulated needle" electrodes or 33-gauge regular needle on a hub-tip adapter (Figs. 41-1 and 41-2). The usual setting is 10 watts or less (level 1, coagulation setting for the Ellman). Identify the exposed end of the hair, pull the shaft gently with tweezers, insert the probe into the follicle until resistance is met, and activate the unit. Remove the hair with tweezers. The treatment lasts a fraction of a second and generally does not require anesthesia. For unusually sensitive clients or large areas of the body, prior application of a topical anesthetic may be helpful (e.g., EMLA, ELA-Max, Hurricaine gel). (See Chapter 11, Topical Anesthesia.)

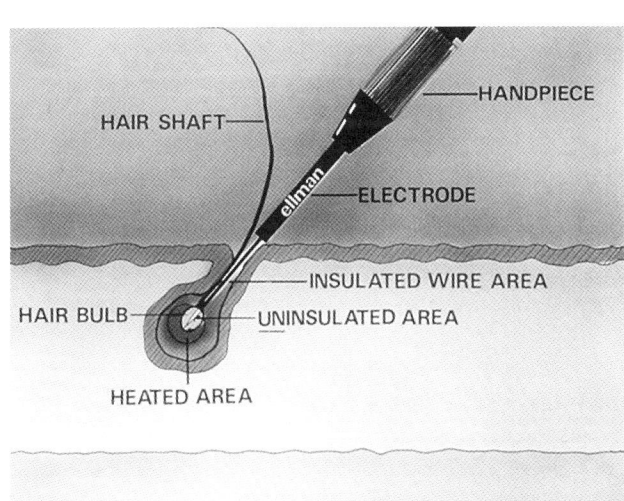

Fig. 41-1
Using a fine needle electrode for epilation. (Courtesy Ellman International, Hewlett, NY.)

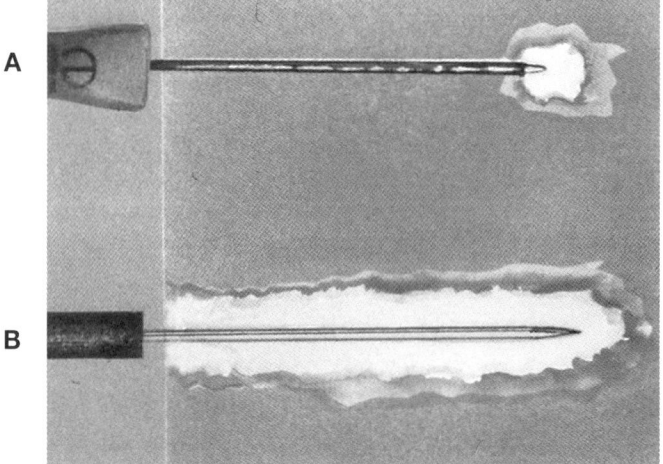

Fig. 41-2
Two common needles used for epilation. **A,** Coated with only the tip active. **B,** Uncoated with entire needle active. (Courtesy Ellman International, Hewlett, NY.)

TECHNIQUE FOR INGROWN HAIRS

Ingrown hairs, *pili incarnati,* originate from a variety of causes. Razor-shaved hair ends have very sharp tips that may curve back toward the skin surface and reenter the epidermis a short distance from the mouth of the follicle (common in blacks or people with curly hair). Double-edged razors, in which the hair is pulled out of the follicle by the first razor and cut by the second razor, leaves the resultant hair tip recoiled in the follicle below the surface of the skin. The curved hair may then grow into the follicular wall. As the hair tips pierce the epidermis or penetrate the dermis, a foreign body inflammatory reaction ensues. Usually the ingrown hairs are completely buried but may have an identifiable recurving loop. In treating such hairs, the unattached end of the hair must be exposed above the surface of the skin using sharp forceps. Impacted hairs, which cannot be freed, should be left in place until a subsequent visit. The shaft should be pulled gently to indicate the direction of the follicle, and a preferably flexible probe should be inserted for epilation. Probes that do not conform to the curvature of the hair may not reach the hair root. Incomplete electrolysis may create an ingrown hair if a distorted follicle is sealed off by the current.

TECHNIQUE FOR EYELASHES

Abnormal eyelashes may be congenital, may result from trauma, or may be caused by chronic disease, allergies, medication use, or even the aging process. *Cilia inver-*

sum is a rare finding in which a lash originates in the tarsal conjunctiva. *Cilia incarnata,* an anomaly akin to the ingrown hair, develops when a lash is entrapped beneath the skin near the lid margin. True trichiasis, an acquired condition in which one or more lashes is misdirected posteriorly toward the conjunctiva or cornea, may pose a range of problems from irritation to corneal abrasion or ulceration. Localized large hairs may be suitable for tweezing, followed by electrolysis if they recur. *Cilia incarnata* requires freeing of the lash, tweezing, and then electrolysis in the case of recurrence. Lanugo hairs or widespread trichiasis may require more specialized surgical procedures and should be referred to an ophthalmologist.

For more extensive hair removal, see Chapter 51, Laser Hair Removal: Photoepilation.

CPT BILLING/CODES

17380	Electrolysis epilation; each ½ hour
67820	Correction of trichiasis; epilation by forceps only
67825	Correction of trichiasis epilation by electro-surgery
67830	Correction of trichiasis by incision of lid margin

ICD-9-CM DIAGNOSTIC CODES

7041	Hirsutism
7041	Hypertrichosis (excessive growth of hair)
374.54	of eyelid
7042	Trichiasis
374.05	eyelid
374.00	eyelid with entropion

BIBLIOGRAPHY

Blackwell G: Cosmetic dermatology: ingrown hairs, shaving, and electrolysis, *Cutis* 19:172, 1977.
Brown LA: Pathogenesis and treatment of pseudofolliculitis barbae, *Cutis* 32:373, 1983.
Crutchfield CE: The causes and treatment of pseudofolliculitis barbae, *Cutis* 61:351, 1998.
Jones W: Ingrown eyelashes, *Am J Optom Physiol Opt* 57:265, 1979.

Note: Special assistance was provided by: Michael Krasnow, D.O., Ophthalmologist, and Judy Lafferty, Electrologist.

CHAPTER 42

Topical Hemostatic Agents

Jerry W. Hizon
Lee A. Kaplan

GENERAL CONSIDERATIONS

In medical training there is a cynical phrase quoted to novice medical students on a surgery rotation: "All bleeding ultimately stops." Although this is true, the lesson to learn is that usually the best amount of bleeding is the least amount of bleeding. Effective, rapid hemostasis is the goal of physicians' performing cutaneous surgery. Many methods are available, and this chapter covers the most useful (Table 42-1).

The various methods range from physical techniques, such as simple pressure with an index finger and gauze pad, to chemical, electrical, and even laser techniques.

The method used depends on the specifics of the surgery being performed, the experience of the office surgeon, and the availability of the agents or equipment.

Each method has its own benefits and drawbacks, and the astute clinician will match the method that best fits the needs of the particular patient. The older chemical agents (the so-called vasoconstrictive, vaso-occlusive, or denaturing agents) cause an eschar and actually cause some tissue damage. Newer, so-called physiologic agents, facilitate the clotting mechanism but can be exorbitantly expensive (e.g., $30 or more for a single pack of Gelfoam). It is therefore important for the physician or healthcare provider to be familiar and

TABLE 42-1

Topical Hemostatic Agents

Generic/Product Name	Effectiveness	Difficulty of Preparation/Application	Undesired Tissue Destruction	Chance of Pigment Stain	Cost
Vasoocclusive/Denaturing Agents					
Silver nitrate sticks	+++	+	++	++++	++
Ferric subsulfate solution (20%) (Monsel's solution)	+++	++	+	++	++
Aluminum chloride (30%)	+++	++	+	−	++
Trichloroacetic acid (50% to 85%)	++	+++	+++	−	++
Zinc chloride paste	++	++	+	−	++
Phenol 50%	++	++	+++	−	++
Hydrogen peroxide	+	+	+	−	+
Agents Producing a Physical Meshwork					
Absorbable gelatin sponge (Gelfoam)	+++	++	−	−	++++
Oxidized cellulose (Surgicel)	++++	+++	−	−	++++
Microfibrillar collagen (Avitene)	+++++	+++++	−	−	+++++
Physiologic Hemostatic Agents					
Cocaine hydrochloride	+++	++++	−	−	+++
Epinephrine	+++	+	−	−	+
Thrombin (Thrombostat)	+++++	++++	−	−	+++++
Fibrin sealant	+++++	++++	−	−	++++

Agents rated from:
+ Mildly effective   to   +++++   Highly effective
+ Easy to prepare/apply to   +++++   Difficult to prepare/apply
+ Minimal damage   to   +++++   Significant destruction
+ Low pigment stain   to   +++++   High chance of pigment stain
+ Low cost   to   +++++   High cost
(− indicates no effect)

accomplished with multiple methods to ensure the best chance of a positive outcome.

INDICATIONS

- For bleeding after cutaneous surgery such as a shave biopsy.
- To treat abrasions or denuded skin.
- To treat the nail bed after removal of either partial or full nail.
- To cauterize excess granulation tissue.
- To treat cuts or open wounds that cannot or will not be primarily closed.
- To close small wounds of the face, primarily with skin adhesive.
- For topical agents to be effective, the bleeding must not be profuse. These topical agents will not control briskly bleeding vessels ("pumpers").

CONTRAINDICATIONS

- Allergy to the hemostatic agent utilized
- Large, deep wounds that require primary surgical closure with suture
- Select medical conditions
- Cardiac pacemaker may preclude use of electrosurgery (Bovie, Hyfrecator, etc.)

Note: "Cautery" technically refers to a hot wire (most often, a battery-powered unit). These are generally safe for pacemaker patients. On the other hand, "electrocautery" (Bovie, Hyfrecator, Ellman Surgitron, etc.) produces a low amperage current (causing electrofulguration, electrodessication, or electrocoagulation) that may pose a risk to pacemaker users. Most new pacemakers are shielded. Use of these units should not be a problem, but why take the chance?

HEMOSTATIC AGENTS

Vasoocclusive Denaturing Agents

- Ferric subsulfate solution (20%) (Monsel's solution)
- Aluminum chloride (30% solution) (Drysol)
- Silver nitrate sticks or 20% to 50% solution
- Trichloroacetic acid (50% to 85% solution)
- Zinc chloride paste
- Phenol 50% solution
- Hydrogen peroxide 3% solution

Agents Producing a Physical Meshwork

- Absorbable gelatin sponge (Gelfoam)
- Oxidized cellulose (Surgicel)

- Microfibrillar collagen (Avitene); *note:* requires dry instruments
- Cyanoacrylates (Dermabond, IsoDent) (see Chapter 38, Tissue Glues)

Physiologic Hemostatic Agents

- Epinephrine or lidocaine with epinephrine
- Thrombin (Thrombostat)
- Fibrin sealant
- Cocaine hydrochloride solution

MECHANICAL METHODS

- Electrocautery ("hot-wire," battery-operated unit)
- Electrosurgery (Bovie, Hyfrecator, Ellman Surgitron, etc.)
- Hemoclips
- Laser (carbon dioxide)
- Shaw scapel (Teflon-coated scalpel blade with heating element)
- Application of ice

EQUIPMENT

- Cotton-tipped swabs
- 4 × 4–inch sterile gauze
- Eye protection (goggles)
- Gloves
- Protective chux pads
- Final dressings (nonadherent)

PREPROCEDURE PATIENT PREPARATION

Determine if the patient is known to be allergic to any of the agents. Discuss the procedure, including the rare but possible risks of further bleeding, infection, nerve damage, pigmentary changes ("tattooing," which is usually temporary), and scarring. Position the patient, usually supine, on the examination or procedure table.

AGENTS AND TECHNIQUES

Vasoocclusive Denaturing Agents

These agents are applied topically and are *not* used if a wound is to be closed surgically. Monsel's solution and aluminum chloride are the most commonly used agents.

Ferric Subsulfate Solution (20%) (Monsel's Solution)

First described by Leon Monsel in 1856, this liquid is perhaps the most commonly used topical hemostatic agent. The solution is dark brown and almost black. If the bottle is left open, evaporation allows a precipitate and a pasty supernatant solution results. Since it is more concentrated, it is more effective. Do not let it become too thick. Virtually all dermatologists use the overlying supernatant. Hemostasis is effective with only rare staining, which can last up to 3 months. Application of Monsel's solution to a relatively dry wound bed (achieved by stretching and blotting the skin) controls oozing effectively.

Monsel's solution is applied with a cotton-tipped swab after drying and stretching the skin with the other hand. The swab is applied with light pressure. The low pH and the subsulfate group denature protein and occlude blood vessels. The practitioner cannot use too much. Once in contact with blood, the black, coagulated mixture can be wiped away. Monsel's is used after cervical biopsies, loop electrosurgical excision procedures, or anorectal biopsies because it works so well. It is also commonly used after shave excision and punch biopsies except in very fair-skinned individuals.

Monsel's solution is inexpensive, easily applied, easily stored, and readily available. However, there is a rare risk of "tattooing," so some physicians do not recommend it for the face, especially in light skin. In clinical practice there is often a compromise in which Monsel's, given its superior hemostatic properties, is still used for the face and on patients with a very light complexion. (Aluminum chloride is nonstaining and should be tried first in these cases.) The tattooing can last several months. Monsel's may also cause temporary artefactual changes in skin and cervical biopsies, confounding the histologic evaluation of reexcisions for a few weeks thereafter. It also stains clothing. Stains on lab coats can be removed with dilute hydrochloric acid, such as that often found in toilet bowl cleaners or by using Iron-Out. Monsel's stains need to be treated before washing in hot water or drying with heat, since each seems to set the stain permanently.

Aluminum Chloride (30%)

Aluminum chloride is usually applied topically to a wound as a 30% solution (Drysol, Lumicaine, etc.) on a swab with light pressure. It is colorless and forms a thin coagulum over the wound. Although not as effective as Monsel's, it does not cause tattooing. This solution is commonly used after surgical shave biopsies.

Silver Nitrate

Silver nitrate is available as a 20% to 50% solution and as a solid on a wooden stick. The sticks are more conve-

nient and are consequently more popular. The silver nitrate on the end is activated when the tip is placed on a moist wound bed. Silver ions cause proteins to precipitate, causing the occlusion of blood vessels. The eschar that forms in the wound bed prevents deeper tissue penetration by the hemostatic agent. Silver salts stain the tissue black because of the deposition of reduced silver. Although most of the stain disappears spontaneously within a few weeks, there is a modest possibility of permanently tattooing the treated site. Care must be used with silver nitrate to avoid damaging normal tissue surrounding a wound. Because of these concerns, silver nitrate is most often restricted to cauterization of excess granulation tissue or for use in nonvisible areas (cervix, rectum, etc.).

Trichloroacetic Acid (50% to 85%)

Trichloroacetic acid is a topically applied agent that also forms an eschar at the wound bed. When it touches the tissue, the acid also causes superficial tissue destruction, and subsequently is rarely used for hemostatic purposes. Without anesthesia it can be painful, so application should be precise and rapid.

Other Agents

Zinc chloride paste is an effective hemostatic agent that was used in the original fixed-tissue Mohs' micrographic surgery, and it is still occasionally used today. *Phenol 50%* is effective, but the severe caustic effects on normal tissue may enlarge a wound. *Hydrogen peroxide* is readily available and is a weak hemostatic agent. It has obvious germicidal action, is inexpensive, and is easy to apply. Hydrogen peroxide is commonly applied directly to the wound in saturated gauze with direct pressure. It too causes some degree of tissue destruction and is rarely used for hemostasis alone.

Agents Producing a Physical Meshwork

Surgical wound closure is acceptable after use of most of the following agents.

Absorbable Gelatin Sponge (Gelfoam)

Gelatin powder is applied dry to the wound bed with light pressure. Absorbable gelatin sponges are manufactured in various forms from purified gelatin solution. Gelatin sponges can be applied dry or moistened with saline or thrombin. Absorbable gelatin holds blood and provides a matrix for clot formation and granulation tissue to form. The sponges are costly for a private office but are convenient and easy to handle. The gelatin powder can be difficult to handle and may be less effective than other meshwork agents.

Side effects can be excessive granuloma formation and fibrosis. Care should be taken if these sponges are used near tendons, since they have been known to cause excessive fibrosis, especially in these areas.

Oxidized Cellulose (Surgicel)

Oxidized cellulose consists of absorbable fibers prepared from cellulose. Woven strips or sheets of cellulose can be cut and held with firm pressure on the wound bed. Oxidized cellulose provides a meshwork for coagulation and causes local vasoconstriction. This preparation is moderately priced, easy to handle, and mildly bactericidal.

Foreign-body reaction is possible if excessive amounts of cellulose are left in a wound. Cellulose should not be used under grafts or flaps because it separates the graft from the blood supply. Some experts feel that the removal of oxidized cellulose after obtaining hemostatis frequently produces rebleeding.

Microfibrillar Collagen (Avitene)

Microfibrillar collagen is prepared by mechanically breaking down bovine collagen into fibrils. It is available in a fibrous (granular) form or a web form. The fibrous form is applied directly to the wound and held in place. The highly effective collagen products aggregate platelets on their surface. Collagen matrix applied to skin biopsy sites produces fewer infections, faster healing, and better cosmetic results than Monsel's solution.

Microfibrillar collagen adheres to wet gloves or surfaces, and it must be applied with dry instruments. Although the collagen is eventually absorbed, *it cannot be used at skin closure sites because it impedes the healing of wound edges.* The high cost and difficulty in handling make this agent impractical for most office dermatologic surgery.

Cyanoacrilates (Dermabond, IsoDent)

Tissue glues can seal wound edges and halt bleeding. See Chapter 38, Tissue Glues.

Physiologic Hemostatic Agents

Epinephrine

Epinephrine is a potent activator of adrenergic receptors, and the activation of alpha receptors produces vasoconstriction in the skin. Epinephrine is available in local anesthetics such as lidocaine with epinephrine or as adrenaline chloride solutions. Epinephrine is inexpensive and readily available, and it does not harm normal tissue at the base of the wound. It can be applied topically to control bleeding (e.g., the nose) or injected into a bleeding site (e.g., cervical biopsy). Effects are temporary (about 2 hours). Control of the bleeding, however, allows electrocoagulation or application of other topical agents if necessary.

Complications are actually quite rare. The precaution is always to avoid it in end arterial areas (finger, nose, penis, toes) for fear of causing gangrene of the digits. This rarely occurs. However, caution is advised in the vascular compromised patient. Rebound vasodilation can potentially cause delayed bleeding. Cardiac arrhythmias and neurologic symptoms have been reported with the use of epinephrine in dermatologic procedures.

Thrombin (Thrombostat)

Thrombin is a potent physiologic clotting agent produced by the activation of bovine prothrombin. This freeze-dried powder either can be mixed with isotonic saline and sponged or sprayed on the wound bed or can be applied directly as powder. The wound should be sponged free of excess blood before thrombin is applied. For superficial surgery or plastic surgery involving flaps, dilute solutions of 100 units/ml may be effective.

Thrombin does not injure tissue or produce residue on the tissue bed. Once the solution is prepared, it must be used within 6 hours. Thrombin is expensive and prohibits the routine use of this agent for office procedures.

Fibrin Sealant

Fibrin sealant is produced by making two components of human clotting factors immediately before application. Fibrin clot forms in about 30 seconds; the sealant can be applied with a special spraying device that mixes the components as they are delivered into the wound. Fibrin glue is one of the most effective agents available for hemostasis. The cost, the risk in the use of human blood products, and the cumbersome administration make this therapy undesirable for routine dermatologic surgery.

Cocaine Hydrochloride

Cocaine hydrochloride is useful as a powerful vasoconstrictor, but the potential for abuse, the cost, and the need for locked storage makes its use problematic.

Mechanical Methods

- *Cautery (electrosurgical or battery-operated unit):* For hemostasis, use the coagulation or fulguration settings and set at a very low power. Gently "tap" the area, being careful to avoid excessive tissue damage. Larger vessels (over 3 mm) should be tied off rather than coagulated.
- *Laser (carbon dioxide):* Rarely used for this purpose.
- *Shaw scapel* (Teflon-coated scalpel blade with heating element).
- *Ice packs:* Cause vasoconstriction and reduce bleeding and swelling.

COMPLICATIONS

- Rebound bleeding
- Infection
- Nerve damage
- Scarring or tattooing
- Swelling
- Excessive tissue damage

POSTPROCEDURE PATIENT EDUCATION

Instruct the patient on the following:

- Keep the area clean and moist, but avoid maceration. Any ointment including those with antibiotics aids healing.
- Change the dressing at least two to three times a day (preferably four) and wash gently with soap and water.
- Follow up as directed; do so sooner if there is an increase in redness, swelling, pain, fever, nightsweats or chills, or other signs of infection such as purulent drainage.
- Avoid cleansing with hydrogen peroxide since it kills fibroblasts.

CONCLUSION

Hemostatic agents are useful during cutaneous surgery or when faced with an open wound that cannot be primarily closed with sutures. Topical hemostatic agents are not a substitute for meticulous surgical technique, and many cannot be used inside a wound to be sutured. Physical measures such as direct pressure, cold application, or suture ligatures should also be considered when trying to control bleeding. The various agents have benefits and limitations. It is important to become familiar with several, such as Monsel's solution, aluminum chloride, absorbable gelatin sponge (Gelfoam), and oxidized cellulose (Surgicel).

CPT/BILLING CODES

Application of topical hemostatics is included in the biopsy charge and should not be "unbundled."

ICD-9-CM DIAGNOSTIC CODES

ICD-9-CM codes are indicated for the particular lesion being addressed.

BIBLIOGRAPHY

Grabski WJ, Salasche ST: Hemostatic techniques and materials. Wheeland RJ, editor: *Cutaneous surgery*, Philadelphia, 1994, WB Saunders.

Kuwahara RT, Ammonette RA: A novel method to remove Monsel's stain, *Dermatol Surg* 26:507, 2000.

Spitzer M, Chernys AE: Monsel's solution-induced artifact in the uterine cervix, *Am J Obstet Gynecol* 175:1204, 1996.

Stegman SJ, Tromovitch TA, Glogau RG: Hemostasis. In *Basics of dermatologic surgery*, Chicago, 1982, Year Book Medical Publishers.

CHAPTER 43

Unna Paste Boot: Treatment of Venous Stasis Ulcers and Other Disorders

Timothy J. Downs

The Unna paste boot is used primarily when a semiimmobilizing soft-pressure dressing or gradient-pressure dressing over a joint, extremity, or even the scalp is needed. It is commonly available in a 4-inch roll or bandage that is impregnated with a calamine–gelatin–zinc oxide compound. Unna paste dressings are soothing and antipruritic and require less frequent dressing changes than conventional dressings. When dressing changes can be scheduled from 3 to 11 days, instead of one to three times per day, savings in healthcare cost and patient convenience can be realized.

INDICATIONS

- Phlebitis and thrombophlebitis of the lower extremity
- Venous stasis ulcers
- Postphlebitic syndrome
- Lymphedema
- Split and full-thickness skin graft sites
- Split and full-thickness skin graft donor sites
- Acute and chronic tendonitis
- Acute ankle sprains without fracture

Use of the Unna paste dressing has varied over the years. With the advent of air cushion or foam splints, use for ankle sprains has diminished. Unna paste dressings continue as a therapeutic mainstay for chronic venous disease, with or without venous stasis ulcers. Without some type of dressing, healing-associated pruritus can lead to scratching of and then enlargement of the ulcers. The Unna boot can be used as a symmetrical gradient pressure dressing for venous stasis ulcers to help reduce venous hypertension, control edema, and prevent delayed venous return. It is an effective part of overall therapy. Debridement should be carried out first (if indicated), and then the ulcer should be covered with a permeable dressing, such as Tegaderm (pouched or regular).

Recent studies have advocated Unna paste dressings over split or full-thickness skin grafting of burns on extremities. The advantages of using the Unna paste dressing compared with conventional dressing changes two to three times per day include early hospital discharge, patient comfort (because of fewer painful dressing changes), and higher graft acceptance rate (near 100% in some studies), probably due to less graft disturbance during the critical microcirculation formation.

Unna paste dressings have been used over the skin graft donor sites on the scalp. Use on scalp donor sites led to a significant reduction in a complication called "concrete scalp" (thick exudative crusting over the hair-bearing scalp, which tends to scar).

When pediatric patients excoriated their lower extremity skin grafts because of pruritus, the Unna paste dressings allowed healing and higher percentage skin graft acceptance. Parents spent less time changing the dressings (15 minutes versus 3.5 hours per week), and the children had fewer play and sleep time disturbances when compared with conventional three-times-per-day dressing changes and use of antihistamines.

When Unna paste dressings were used over skin-grafted, molten metal burns of the lower extremity, the benefits included early ambulation, hospital discharge, and return to work (44 versus 84 days).

In acute and chronic tendonitis, the Unna boot acts as a soft immobilizer.

CONTRAINDICATIONS

- Acute sprains with fractures
- Significant arterial insufficiency when used with compression covering
- Venous stasis ulcers that are infected and need debridement and cleaning (e.g., ulcers with heavy exudate and crusted ulcers with associated cellulitis)
- Active superficial phlebitis if infection is a major concern
- Sensitivity to any of the dressing components

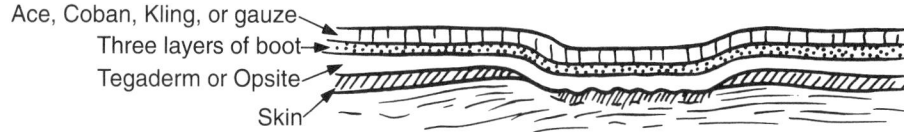

Fig. 43-1
Layered method of applying Unna paste boot for a decubitus ulcer.

Acute fractures can continue to swell. Because the gauze in the Unna paste dressing is nondistendible, pressure sores or compartment syndrome could occur with marked swelling.

Circulatory compromise and necrosis have been reported when a compression dressing is used in the presence of arterial insufficiency. Use a handheld Doppler and blood pressure cuff to compare the ankle-brachial pressures. The ratio of the systolic pressure at the posterior tibial or dorsalis pedis divided by the brachial pressure should be equal to or greater than 1. If the ratio is 0.7 or less, significant arterial insufficiency is present and compression is contraindicated. If infection is a concern, use of a dressing that is not changed for 3 to 11 days may mask progressive infection and postpone appropriate treatment.

TECHNIQUE

1. Cleanse the skin with slightly warm water or saline. If the skin is dry, petroleum jelly can be used as a moisturizer. Avoid topical antibiotics, povidone, and hexachlorophene, which can be topically sensitizing and cause a contact dermatitis. Topical steroids can be applied after washing if dermatitis is present.
2. For venous stasis ulcers, debride the ulcer. Hydrocolloid dressings such as DuoDerm can aid in healing. Some experts recommend extending the DuoDerm 1 inch past the edge of the ulcer. It is normal for these moist dressings to develop an anaerobic odor that does not necessarily indicate an infection. Alternatively the ulcer can be covered with a permeable dressing like Tegaderm.
3. A smooth snug layer of Kling or Kerlex can be used as an underwrap if desired. This may prevent chafing of the skin as the Unna paste dries.
4. For the lower extremity, keep the ankle at a right angle. Start wrapping at the metatarsal heads and roll proximally with a 50% overlap. It is important to avoid ridges, which can cause discomfort.
5. Cover the heel completely. Alternate a horizontal wrap to cover the Achilles tendon with an oblique turn to cover the posterior aspect of the heel. Cut the dressing and start another wrap around the heel. Wrap snugly and cut the dressing frequently during

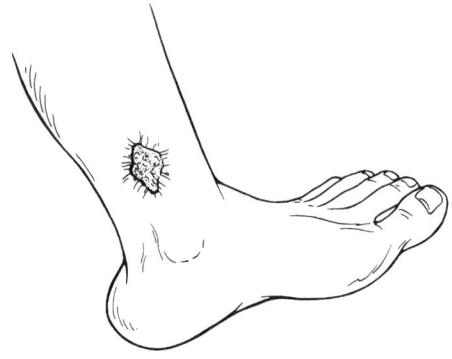

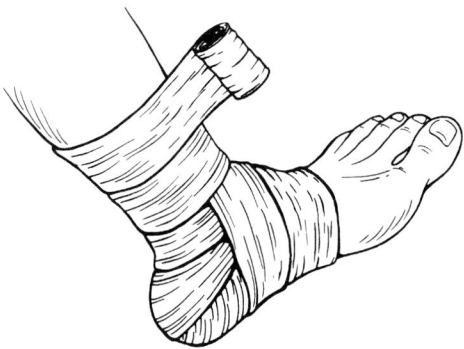

Fig. 43-2
Technique of rolling on the Unna paste boot.

the wrap. This helps prevent constriction bands and their tourniquet effect. Do not reverse directions as with plaster casting material; wrap only in one direction (clockwise or counterclockwise) to prevent ridges (Figs. 43-1 and 43-2).
6. Wrap the Unna paste dressing in three layers and proceed all the way to the tibial tuberosity.
7. Several options for covering the Unna paste dressing include elastic bandage, Coban, Kling, or stockinet. Both the elastic bandage and Coban dressing help with needed compression.
8. For wounds that are very moist, the dressing should be changed in 3 days. If moist discharge is minimal, the dressing can be changed in 7 days.
9. The Unna "cap" for a skin graft donor site on the scalp is applied with an initial layer of Aquaphor gauze

followed with an Unna paste dressing. Excellent results with no "concrete scalp" complications were achieved with dressing changes every 3 days in one small study.

COMPLICATIONS

- Occasional contact dermatitis
- Neurovascular compromise if dressing is applied too tightly or in the presence of arterial insufficiency
- Masking of cellulitis developing in a stasis ulcer under the dressing

POSTPROCEDURE PATIENT EDUCATION

- The dressing must be kept dry.
- Patients should cover the entire dressing with a plastic bag or other impermeable covering to bathe.
- Remove the boot with a large bandage scissors. Lifting the bandage and use of petroleum jelly on the scissors can prevent discomfort or inadvertent injury during removal.
- Cleanse and dry the skin thoroughly. When the boot is used for stasis ulcers, inspect the area carefully for the presence of infection and debride again if necessary before applying a second boot. Venous stasis ulcers can take 2 to 3 months to heal.
- For good results, the patient must comply with all other aspects of medical therapy.
- As the swelling subsides in sprains, the compression advantage will be lost. Instruct the patient to return in 2 or 3 days or when the Unna paste dressing becomes loose or develops wrinkles (which can cause pressure sores). A second boot will have to be applied, or else more appropriate therapy, such as an inflated splint, must be utilized.
- Teach the patient to check for signs of impaired circulation and to report any paresthesia or unusual discomfort promptly.

SUPPLIERS

Unna Boot Paste dressing is a trade name, and more than 25 companies make these dressings. Check with your local medical supply company or contact.

Unna-Flex bandage
Convatec (division of Bristol-Myers Squibb)
P.O. Box 5254
Princeton, NJ 08543-5254
Phone: 1-800-422-8811
Website: www.convatec.com

Dome-Paste medicated bandage (4-inch × 10-yard)
Miles Inc. (Pharmaceutical Division)
1127 Myrtle Street
Elkhart, IN 46514
Phone: 1-800-800-4793

Aquaphor gauze
Beiersdorf
P.O. Box 5529
Norwalk, CT 06856-5529
Phone: 1-203-853-8008
Website: www.beiersdorf

Medicopaste bandage
Graham-Field, Inc.
400 Rabro Drive
East Hauppauge, NY 11788
Phone: 1-516-582-5900

CPT/BILLING CODE

29580   Unna paste boot application
(Or use a specific code for joint immobilization [e.g., ankle: 29540].)

ICD-9-CM DIAGNOSTIC CODES

451.0   Phlebitis or thrombophlebitis, superficial vessels of lower extremities
451.19   Phlebitis or thrombophlebitis, deep vessels of lower extremities
454.0   Varicose veins of the lower extremities with ulcers
454.2   Varicose veins of the lower extremities with inflammation
457.0   Lymphedema, idiopathic hereditary
457.1   Lymphedema, acquired
459.1   Postphlebitic syndrome
459.2   Phlebitis or thrombophlebitis, leg
707.0   Decubitus ulcers
782.3   Edema, legs
825.25   Metatarsal fractures

BIBLIOGRAPHY

Barone CM, Mastropieri CJ, Peebles R, Mitra A: Evaluation of the Unna Boot for lower-extremity autograft burn wounds excoriated by pruritus in pediatric patients, *J Burn Care Rehabil* 14(3):348, 1993.

Carter YM, Summer GJ, Engrav LH, et al: Incidence of the concrete scalp deformity associated with deep scalp donor sites and management with the Unna cap, *J Burn Care Rehabil* 20(2):141, 1999.

Cullum N, Nelson EA, Fletcher AW, Sheldon TA: Compression for venous leg ulcers (abstract of Cochrane Review). Available at www.cochrane.org/cochrane/revabstr/ab000265.htm. Accessed September 7, 2001.

Grube BJ, Heimbach DM, Engrav LH: Molten metal burns to the lower extremity, *J Burn Care Rehabil* 8(5):403, 1987.

O'Donoghue JM, O'Sullivan ST, Beausang ES, et al: Calcium alginate dressings promote healing of split skin graft donor sites, *Acta Chir Plast* 39(2):53, 1997.

Phillips TJ: Current approaches to venous ulcers and compression, *Dermatol Surg* 27:611, 2001.

Sanford S, Gore D: Unna's boot dressings facilitate outpatient skin grafting of hands, *J Burn Care Rehabil* 17(4):323, 1996.

Summer GJ, Hansen FL, Costa BA, et al: The Unna "cap" as a scalp donor site dressing, *J Burn Care Rehabil* 20(2):183, 1999, discussion 182.

Wells NJ, Boyle JC, Snelling CF, et al: Lower extremity burns and Unna paste: can we decrease health care costs without compromising patient care? *Can J Surg* 38(6):533, 1995.

CHAPTER 44

Wart (Verruca) Treatment

John L. Pfenninger
William C. Everts

Warts are a disease of antiquity. They have no regard for class or social status. They do not discriminate by race or color. There is an equal political distribution between Republicans and Democrats. They are annoying, sometimes disfiguring and painful, and due to the angst of patient and physician, they recur. With ardent attempts to rid the pest by heating, freezing, burning, cutting and electrifying, treatment has induced as much anxiety as the disease itself. But the physician persists.

William C. Everts

Warts are caused by the human papilloma virus (HPV). There are over 100 individually numbered types. Common warts are caused by types 1, 2, 4, and 7; flat warts, types 3 and 10; and plantar warts, types 1, 2, and 4. Genital condyloma acuminata are generally caused by types 6 and 11.

HPV causes numerous epithelial cancers. Cervical dysplasia and cervical cancer is the most commonly recognized type. However, 31% of squamous cell carcinomas and 36% of basal cell carcinomas of the skin contain HPV in nonimmunosuppressed patients. In immunosuppressed patients 65% of squamous cell carcinomas and 60% of basal cell carcinomas contain HPV! Subsequently, treatment becomes more than just a cosmetic issue.

Warts have the following various presentations:
- Flat warts
- Mosaic wart, or a cluster of warts that fuse together
- Verruca vulgaris including periungual ("common wart")
- Plantar wart
- Genital/anal wart (condyloma acuminata)
- Laryngeal papillomatosis

The treatment of condyloma is dealt with in Chapter 157, Treatment of Noncervical Condyloma Acuminata. Laryngeal papillomatosis is not addressed in this textbook.

DIFFERENTIAL DIAGNOSIS

- Actinic keratosis
- Seborrheic keratosis
- Nevus
- Molluscum contagiosum
- Calluses
- Corns (clavi)
- Nonspecific papules
- Cutaneous dysplasias

Plantar lesions are the most difficult to differentiate. Hypertrophic callus buildup makes identification of the primary pathology confusing. The telltale signs of a plantar wart is that, as the callus is pared away, the practitioner sees small punctate sites of bleeding. This is nearly pathognomonic for HPV disease.

INDICATIONS FOR TREATMENT

- Pain
- Bleeding
- Recurrent trauma
- Lack of spontaneous resolution
- Psychosocial sequelae
- Employment repercussions (e.g., waitress)
- Rapid growth or multiplication
- Concerns regarding transmission
- Persistence as a cause for possible malignancy

A large number of verruca do not resolve spontaneously. HPV can remain dormant for long periods, then suddenly grow rapidly or multiply. With any treatment the role of the immune system should not be underestimated. With induced inflammation from whatever treatment modality is used, the immune system may finally be triggered into activity to recognize and then resolve the virus.

The virus itself is never totally eliminated. Rather, the immune system merely keeps it in remission, much like herpes. The virus can recur with any immunosuppressed state at any time during the patient's life. The goal of treatment is to reduce visible disease, not to eliminate the virus.

CONTRAINDICATIONS

- Lack of compliance
- Cellulitis
- Allergy to treatment modality
- Ambiguous diagnosis

TREATMENT (BOX 44-1)

General

It is important to enhance the immune system as much as possible during the treatment of all wart manifestations. Smoking is known to increase the growth potential and the persistence of warts on the cervix. Smoking reduces the cells of Langerhans' in the skin in general and subsequently decreases all immunity. It is best if the patient does not smoke. Illicit drugs have been known to suppress the immune system, and they, too, should be avoided. Various vitamins (e.g., folic acid) have been shown to play an important role in suppressing HPV. Subsequently, consider using a good multivitamin with minerals to maximize the immune system capabilities. Finally, the patient should be instructed to eat a diet that includes five helpings of fruits and vegetables a day.

Medications such as steroids that suppress immunity should be limited if at all possible.

The physician's job becomes difficult in the treatment of verrucae in patients who have organ transplants or are immunosuppressed as a result of diseases such as AIDS. Patients should be made aware that the success rate in such cases is poor.

Research into the efficacy of various treatments for warts is difficult, since studies have shown that even hypnosis can resolve them. Many folktales carry the belief that banana peels, raw potatoes, cerumen, spider webs, and other items resolve warts. Spontaneous resolution is always possible and often occurs for no apparent reason.

Many physicians recommend expectant observation. An old maxim states that "wart" patients should not be referred to a physician friend for treatment, since it will generally make them look bad! Anyone who has treated warts can become frustrated in dealing with them. Not only can they persist, but they may indeed multiply.

BOX 44-1

Modalities for Treating Human Papilloma Virus (Warts, Verruca Vulgaris)

General (maintaining healthy immune system)
    Eating a diet high in fruits and vegetables
    Taking vitamins with folic acid
    Avoiding smoking and secondhand smoke
    Avoiding immunosuppression when possible
Expectant observation
Hypnosis
Chemicals: topical
    Over-the-counter medication (usually an acid preparation)
    Topical salicylic acid 15%-40%
    Formalin
    Cantharidin (Cantherone) 0.7% coloidian solution
    Trichloroacetic acid
    Bichloroacetic acid
    Tretinoin (Retin-A 0.05% solution, or 0.025%, 0.05%, or 0.1% cream)
    5-Fluorouracil (Efudex, Fluoroplex), 5% cream
    Imiquimod (Aldara)
    Podofilox (Condylox)
    Silver nitrate
Chemicals: oral
    Cimetidine (Tagamet) 20-40 mg/kg/day (especially in pediatric patients)
Chemicals: injection
    Candida antigen (Candin) 1:500 solution
    Bleomycin
    Interferon
Contact immunotherapy
    Dinitrochlorobenzene
    Candida antigen (Candin) 1:500 solution
Mechanical
    Tape occlusion
    Cryotherapy
        Liquid nitrogen (−196° C)
        Nitrous oxide (−89° C)
        Carbon dioxide (−78° C)
        Tetrafluoroethane (−47°/−70° C): MediFrig, Verruca Freeze
        Ether/propane (−29°/−55° C): Histofreezer
    Electrodesiccation and curettage
    Electrocautery
    Laser
    Infrared coagulator (IRC)
    Excision

Also see Chapter 157, Treatment of Noncervical Condyloma Acuminata.

Frequently, treatment of a single wart with a modality such as cryotherapy or cautery will result in a ring of warts around the area that was frozen or burned. The simple common wart has indeed humbled the best clinicians. Subsequently, many again recommend simple observation.

Warts have "no roots" and are totally epidermal lesions. Treatment ideally should not cause scarring. There is no communication between warts—no "mother wart"! However, treatment of a single wart or some of the warts can lead to resolution of all the warts because of an immune activation.

Chemicals

Over-the-Counter Medications

Numerous over-the-counter (OTC) medications are available for the treatment of warts, such as Compound-W, Mediplast, Trans-Ver-Sal, Occlusal, Duofilm, and Duoplant.

Method: Pare away callus and/or soak lesions in warm water. Hydrating the keratin allows better penetration of the liquid or agent being applied. Apply medication as directed by supplier and cover. Repeat each day, being sure to remove the dead tissue with paring or with a pumice stone. Treatment is nonscarring and generally effective but requires compulsive and persistence of daily treatments, often for 4 to 6 weeks.

Bichloroacetic or Trichloroacetic Acid (50% to 85%)

These are potent chemicals and should not be provided for home treatment.

Method: Prepare the lesion as described above for OTC medications. Apply the acid, being careful to avoid normal skin. If the lesion is raised and convoluted, work the acid into the lesion with a toothpick. Cover. Repeat weekly.

Cantharidin (Cantharone, Verr-Canth)

Cantharidin causes blistering at the dermoepidermal junction.

Method: Apply the chemical directly on the wart and cover it with tape for 48 hours. Evaluate the patient weekly and remove any residual blister. Then reapply the cantharidin. Repeat until wart has resolved.

Silver Nitrate

Method: Silver nitrate is available on the end of sticks. Apply after paring as above for OTC medications. Repeat weekly.

Formalin

Formalin is used in resistant cases, large mosaic warts, or for treatment of large areas.

Method: Soak daily for 30 minutes in 3% to 4% formalin solution. Lazerformaldehyde solution (10%) can be applied directly to warts. Both methods can cause sensitization to formalin.

Tretinoin Cream (Retin A)

Method: 0.025%, 0.05%, or 0.1% cream or solution is rubbed in thoroughly at bedtime. This is frequently used with diffuse flat warts on the legs or face, so it is rubbed over the entire area. The application may be repeated daily. The goal is to have a mild erythema with fine scaling. It is not uncommon to take months to resolve the warts. It can be used in combination with 5-fluorouracil or imiquimod.

5-Fluorouracil (Efudex, Fluoroplex)

5-Fluorouracil is a second line treatment for truly resistant warts. There is no Food and Drug Administration (FDA) approval for this indication.

Method: 2% solution or 5% cream is applied as for Tretinoin. It is important to rub in thoroughly. 5-Fluorouracil can be used for condyloma (see Chapter 84, Treatment of Noncervical Condyloma Acuminata).

Imiquimod (Aldara)

Imiquimod is not a caustic agent but rather a new approach and an immune enhancer. It is not approved by the FDA for verruca (only for condyloma) but is frequently used as a sole treatment or an adjunct in combination with other treatment therapies. It is essential to pare down the callus (especially on a plantar wart) and to rub in the imiquimod thoroughly. For verruca, it is applied daily.

Podofilox (Condylox)

Podofilox is generally used for condyloma.

Oral Tagamet

Method: Studies in children have shown resolution of verruca with dosages of 20 to 40 mg per kg per day for 2 months maximum. Controlled studies have been small, but it does work in some cases. It can be used in addition to other caustic modalities to accentuate efforts.

Chemicals: Injected

Candida *antigen*

Editor's note: After OTC topicals, this method is my absolute first choice to treat all but the simplest verruca. I have not tried it on condyloma. It can be used on single large warts, mosaics, or to treat patients with 80 to 100 lesions! I have used it for 11 years now, and results are excellent with few adverse reactions.

Candida antigen is used for verruca vulgaris (hands and feet). It has not been tried on condyloma acuminata. The FDA has not approved this indication, although it has been used for over 40 years as the control for tuberculosis testing. Subsequently, it is covered by malpractice policies.

Pfenninger Protocol

- *Candida* antigen is available as Candin and as a generic.
- Mix 1:1 Candin and xylocaine without epinephrine, or, 1 part generic candida antigen with 4 parts xylocaine.
- Inject 0.1 to 0.3 ml per wart (depending on size), using a 30 g needle and tuberculin 1-ml Luer-Lok syringe.

- Try for an *intradermal* injection to create an immune response; it can also be injected *intralesionally*. If the solution goes in easily, it is in too deep. Create a bleb if possible. Wear protective glasses, since the material often "squirts" out through a verruca pore.
- Limit the *total amount* to 1 ml at any one visit. If there are numerous warts, this may mean injecting only minute amounts into each one. Even if all the warts are not injected individually, the immune response may generalize and all warts may disappear.
- Repeat injection in 1 month if residual tissue.
- Limit the injections to three at 1-month intervals; if the injections have not worked by then, they probably will not. However, when warts are extensive, there are not many other options, and five to six total monthly injections can be tried.
- Expect 65% to 75% effectiveness with the first injection. Of the remainder, 50% respond with each succeeding injection.
- Expect pruritus, drying of the lesion, and peeling of dead tissue. The lesion may turn black, regress spontaneously without any outward signs, or become erythematous (localized).
- *Adverse reactions* include rash (allergy), adenopathy, and persistence of the lesion.

The *advantages* of the *Candida* injection are that allergic reactions are extremely rare. There is usually none of the scarring or hyperpigmentation or hypopigmentation that can occur more frequently after some of the other modalities of treatment. There is no "downtime"; patients can exercise, play sports, go back to work, and do whatever they want immediately after treatment. There is minimal pain. The pain at the time of injection has been reduced through the use of MadaJet to inject the solution (see Appendix I, Pearls of Practice). However, a lot of expensive solution is lost just to prime the "gun." The real advantage to using *Candida* antigen is that, unlike many of the other modalities, the immune system is induced into responding and resolving the lesion(s). Recurrences are rare, and efficacy is 80% to 85% after three treatments at monthly intervals.

Candida antigen is expensive, but a generic form is now available. Physicians can provide the antigen for the first visit but write a prescription for the patient to bring it in at subsequent visits. This markedly reduces costs. Insurance companies generally do not reimburse the physician, but they will commonly pay for the patient's prescription.

The most critical aspect of treatment is to inject the solution into the lesion itself. Do not go below the dermis. The injection should be difficult; if the solution goes in easily, the placement is too deep. Fig. 44-1 shows appropriate needle placement.

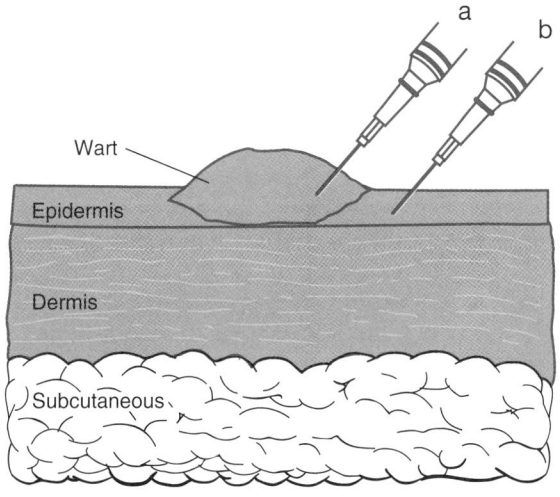

Fig. 44-1
Injecting *Candida* antigen for the treatment of warts. *a*, Intralesional injection. *b*, Intradermal injection creating a wheal. If injected into the subcutaneous tissue, the level is too deep.

For a more complete review of the entire procedure, go to www.altoonafp.org/wartstudy.

Bleomycin

When all other methods fail, intralesional bleomycin can be considered. Pregnancy must be excluded.

Method: A 15-U vial of bleomycin sulfate (Blenoxane, Bristol-Myers) is diluted with 5 ml of bacteriostatic water or 0.9% sodium chloride to form a 3-U/ml solution. When stored at 4° C, the solution can be used for up to 4 months. Mix 2 ml of this solution with 10 ml of 1% lidocaine without epinephrine. This provides 12 ml of solution with 0.5 U bleomycin/ml. Use a 30-gauge needle. Inject directly into the wart as follows:

Wart Size	Amount of Solution (0.5 U bleomycin/ml)
Less than 5 mm	0.2 ml
5 to 10 mm	0.2 to 0.5 ml
Greater than 10 mm	1 ml
Multiple warts	Up to 3 ml (1.5 U)/visit

Warts will initially appear hemorrhagic, then clear (48% to 92%). Repeat injection can be performed in 2 to 4 weeks. Three to four treatments are often required. Alternatively, the drug can be "dropped" onto the wart and "pricked" into the lesion using a Monolet needle.

Bleomycin is expensive unless all the initial vial of drug is used up treating several patients. It is also quite painful. The main mode of action of bleomycin is the inhibition of DNA synthesis with some evidence of RNA inhibition. When injected locally, this causes vascular microthrombosis.

Interferon

Alfa interferon is approved by the FDA for treatment of condyloma in patients over 18 years of age. Two preparations are available:

- Alferon N injection (Interferon alfa-n3): 1 ml vial, 0.05 ml/wart injected two to three times per week for up to 8 weeks.
- Intron-A (Interferon alfa-2b): 10 million IU/vial, 0.1 ml (reconstituted) per wart three times per week for 3 weeks.

Some practitioners use interferon for verruca as well. It is expensive and can often be followed by flulike symptoms for 24 hours. Subsequently, its use is quite limited.

Contact Immunotherapy

Candida

See the "*Candida* Antigen" section.

Dinitrochlorobenzene

Dinitrochlorobenzene has documented carcinogenicity and is no longer used. Diphenylcyclopropenone may eventually be a safer alternative but has not yet been proven.

MECHANICAL METHODS

Tape Occlusion

For young children or for those who are afraid of needles, tape occlusion can be tried, although no controlled studies have been reported on efficacy. The wart is simply covered with tape (some practitioners have used duct tape!) for a week. Tape is removed for 12 hours and then reapplied. The patient is seen 1 week later, and macerated tissue is removed. Any of the previously discussed topical medications can be applied. The cycle is repeated until the wart(s) resolves. Obviously there can only be a limited number of lesions.

Cryotherapy

The real advantage to cryotherapy is that there is little disability and generally no scarring. Some persistent hypopigmentation may occur. See Chapter 15, Cryosurgery.

Electrodesiccation and Curettage/ Electrocautery

Warts can be treated readily with electrocautery. Small ones can be touched with the battery-powered "hot wires" and wiped away. Similarly, electrical units can be placed on fulguration or coagulation settings and the warts coagulated with the ball tips. It helps to have them moistened first. Smaller lesions can be grasped with metal pick-ups, with the current transferred to the wart by touching the cautery tip to the forceps.

All lesions need to be anesthetized. Keratin (such as in plantar warts) must be pared away, since it has little moisture and does not coagulate readily. That is why many practitioners curette the wart first and then coagulate the base. Bleeding from the curettement is controlled with digital pressure.

The major complication from electrodestruction is extensive scarring, which occurs to some degree in all areas treated this way. The physicians must be especially careful on the plantar surface of the feet not to create a hypertrophic scar. This can become a persistently painful area analogous to walking on a stone in a shoe.

The greatest advantage of using curettement before electrocautery is that the abnormal tissue will separate from normal skin. Cautery is then applied, and repeat light curettement is performed. This limits excessive removal of normal tissue and scarring. Alternatively, large warts can be shaved off to debulk them before cautery.

Primary excision using radiofrequency loop removal (see Chapter 31, Radiofrequency Surgery) is to be discouraged, since the loop cuts so rapidly that it is easy to overexcise the lesion and leave a large pit and subsequent scarring. Tendons, nerves, and periosteal tissue can be injured inadvertently even by the experienced practitioner. It is more critical to be familiar with the relevant anatomy when using any of the electrocautery techniques.

Of all methods, the electrocautery technique is one of the most effective, but it has the disadvantage of scarring.

Laser Method

The laser method is expensive but offers the advantage of precise control of depth and removal of "just the right amount" of tissue. When properly used, results are excellent and scarring is minimal. (See Chapter 27, Laser Therapy.)

Infrared Coagulation (Redfield)

The latest treatment for warts—another method of destruction—is the use of the infrared coagulator. It is quick and effective. Much of the research has been done on condyloma. The probe is placed on the wart for 0.75 to 1 second, and the trigger is pulled. Local anesthesia is necessary. Blistering followed by sloughing and then superficial ulceration can be expected. Scarring is possible.

TABLE 44-1

Treatments of Choice

	Primary	Secondary
Filiform wart	STS excision	Electrocautery/ cryotherapy
Flat warts (planar)	*Candida* antigen	Tretinoin, 5-FU
Verruca		
Single or few	Cryocautery	Electrocautery
Multiple	*Candida* antigen	Cryocautery
Mosaic	*Candida* antigen	Cryocautery
Plantar	*Candida* antigen	Cryocautery
Periungual	*Candida* antigen	Cryocautery
Resistant to *Candida* × 3	Cryocautery	Electrocautery/IRC
Condyloma*	85% TCA	Radiofrequency loop excision, IRC
Urethral meatus*	5-FU	STS excision/ electrocautery
Vaginal*		
Few	85% TCA	Electrocautery
Multiple	5-FU	Laser
Anal, vulvar*	85% TCA	Radiofrequency excision/ cryocautery
Rectal*	85% TCA	Electrocautery/ cryocautery
Laryngeal papillomatosis	Laser	Mumps antigen

5-FU, 5-Fluorouracil; *IRC,* infrared coagulator; *STS,* sharp tissue scissor; *TCA,* trichloroacetic acid.
*Also see Chapter 157, Treatment of Noncervical Condyloma Acuminata.

Excision

Many pedunculated and filiform warts can be grasped with pick-ups and quickly excised with sharp tissue scissors or a blade. Often the base is lightly cauterized, not only to control the bleeding but also to destroy any residual injected tissue. It is only in the extremely rare case of an isolated wart or two that has resisted everything that frank formal excision with suture placement is necessary. This is especially discouraged on the plantar surface of the feet, since painful scarring can be a significant complication.

Table 44-1 shows the optimal methods of treating various wart presentations. OTC medications are often tried first.

COMPLICATIONS

• Scarring
• Persistence
• Pain
• Bleeding
• Traumatic seeding and increase in number of warts

SUPPLIERS

Candida antigen (Candin)
Allermed Laboratories
7203 Convoy Court
San Diego, CA 92111
Phone: 1-800-221-2748

Candida antigen (generic)
Antigen Laboratories, Inc.
P.O. Box 123
Liberty, MO 64069
Phone: 1-800-821-7013
Website: www.antigenlab.com

Hollister-Stier Labs
3525 North Regal
Spokane, WA 99220-3145

MadaJet
MADA Medical Products
625 Washington Avenue
Carlstadt, NJ 07072
Phone: 1-800-526-6370
Website: www.madamedical.com

For cryotherapy, radiofrequency, and electrocautery units, see the appropriate chapters mentioned throughout this chapter. For the infrared coagulator, see Chapter 108, Office Treatment of Hemorrhoids.

CPT/BILLING CODES

Intralesional injection
11900   Up to and including 7
11901   Over 7
(Plus charge for medication used—there is no code for *Candida* antigen)

Destruction (electrocautery, cryotherapy, laser, chemicals, curettement)
17000   Benign—first
17003 (each)   2-14
17004   15 or more
17110   Flat warts, destruction any method, less than 15
17111   Over 14

ICD-9-CM DIAGNOSTIC CODES

07810   Verruca vulgaris
07811   Condyloma acuminata

ADDITIONAL RESOURCES

• See the sample patient education handout titled "Wart (Verruca) Treatment" on page 1780 of Appendix G.

BIBLIOGRAPHY

Amer M, Diab N, Ramadan A, et al: Therapeutic evaluation for intralesional injection of bleomycin sulfate in 143 resistant warts, *J Am Acad Dermatol* 18:1313, 1988.

Cordro AA, Guglielmi HA, Woscoff A: The common wart: intralesional treatment with bleomycin sulfate, *Cutis* 26:319, 1980.

Epstein E: Immunotherapy of warts with masoprocol cream, *Cutis* 59:287, 1997.

Eriksen K: Treatment of the common wart by induced allergic inflammation, *Dermatologica* 160:161, 1980.

Fleischer AB Jr, Feldman SR, McConnell RC: The most common dermatologic problems identified by family physicians, 1990-1994, *Fam Med* 29:648, 1997.

Habif TP: *Warts, herpes simplex and other viral infections: clinical dermatology,* ed 3, St Louis, 1996, Mosby.

Haller KH: *Candida* antigen injection proves effective treatment for warts, *Am Fam Physician* 61(2):478, 2000.

Johnson SM, Roberson PK, Horn TD: Intralesional injection of mumps or *Candida* skin test antigens: a novel immunotherapy for warts, *Arch Dermatol* 137:451, 2001.

Marchese-Johnson S, Kincannon JM, Horn TD: *A novel treatment for warts: immunotherapy using mumps and* Candida *antigen. Poster abstracts,* Scientific Poster Session, 58th Annual American Academy of Dermatology, March 13, 2000, San Francisco.

Marchese-Johnson S, Roberson PK, Horn TD: Intralesional injection of mumps or *Candida* skin test antigens: a novel immunotherapy for warts, *Arch Dermatol* 137:451, 2001.

Miller OM, Brodell RT: Human papillomavirus infection: treatment options for warts, *Am Fam Physician* 53:135, 1996.

Munn SE, Higgins E, Marshall M, Clement M: A new method of intralesional bleomycin therapy in the treatment of recalcitrant warts, *Br J Dermatol* 135:969, 1996.

Naylor MF, Neldner KH, Yarbrough GK, et al: Contact immunotherapy of resistant warts, *J Am Acad Dermatol* 19:679, 1988.

Phillips RC, Ruhl TS, Pfenninger JL, Garber MR: Treatment of warts with *Candida* antigen injection, *Arch Dermatol* 136:1274, 2000.

Shamanin V, zur Hausen H, Lavergne D, et al: Human papillomavirus infections in nonmelanoma skin cancers from renal transplant recipients and nonimmunosuppressed patients, *J Natl Cancer Inst* 88:801, 1996.

Signore R, Gillis K: Candida *albicans intralesional injection immunotherapy of warts: a novel therapeutic approach.* The 58th Annual American Academy of Dermatology, Scientific Poster Discussion Session, March 13, 2000, San Francisco.

Sollitto RJ, Pizzano DM: Bleomycin sulfate in the treatment of mosaic plantar verrucae: a follow-up study, *J Foot Ankle Surg* 35(2):169, 1996.

Tosti A, Piraccini BM: The nail unit: surgical and non-surgical approaches, *Dermatol Surg* 27:235, 2001.

Usantine RP, Moy RL: *Skin surgery: a practical guide,* St Louis, 1998, Mosby.

CHAPTER 45

Wood's Light Examination

Stephen K. Toadvine*

The Wood's lamp (black light) produces ultraviolet rays with a wavelength of 365 nm and above by projecting a beam of light through a filter of glass containing nickel oxide. Invisible light in the long-wave ultraviolet range and visible blue-white light is created. The fluorescence produced as the light hits objects varies in color depending on qualities of the surface itself. Characteristic appearances have been described for several dermatologic conditions. The Wood's light examination provides a quick, inexpensive, and useful adjunct in their diagnosis (Fig. 45-1).

Diagnostic uses for the examination include the following:

- Tinea capitis
- Erythrasma
- Vitiligo, albinism, tuberous sclerosis, and other pigmentary conditions
- *Pseudomonas* infections
- Porphyria cutanea tarda
- Tinea versicolor
- Detection of some chemicals that are applied to the skin or taken systemically
- Adjunct in finding corneal abrasions or herpetic corneal lesion

INDICATIONS

- Any dermatitis in body folds such as the inguinal, perianal, interdigital, axillary, or inframammary areas (e.g., erythrasma, *Pseudomonas* infections)
- Patches of scalp scaling and partial hair loss, especially when the hairs are broken or shorter than normal (tinea capitis)
- Pigmentary conditions
- Blisters or punctated erosions on the exposed portions of the hands and forearms, with follow-up urine examination (porphyria cutanea tarda)

*Dr. Toadvine contributes to this edition with the understanding that he objects to the inclusion of Chapter 130 (Abortion).

- Patches of scaling and altered pigmentation of the skin (tinea versicolor)

TECHNIQUE

Let the light warm for a few minutes. From a distance of approximately 8 inches, focus the Wood's light on the area of interest. Darken the room to improve visualization of the resultant fluorescence. Observe and record findings carefully. It is crucial to observe the specific color of fluorescence, not simply its presence. Soaps, lotions, cosmetics, other chemicals, and fragments of scaling skin may themselves yield fluorescence. In addition, patients should not bathe 24 hours before the examination. Otherwise the examination may show little or no fluorescence.

COMMON FINDINGS

- *Tinea capitis:* The majority of cases in the United States are caused by *Trichophyton tonsurans,* which *does*

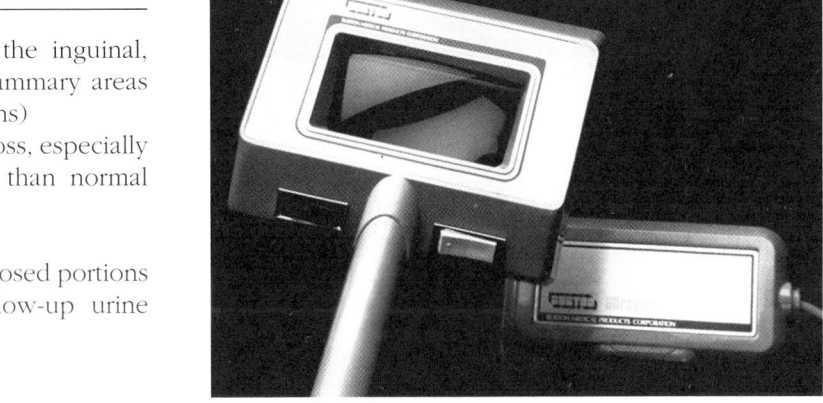

Fig. 45-1
Wood's lamp (ultraviolet light).

not fluoresce. Also, *Trichophyton verrucosum* does not fluoresce. Hair, but not the skin of the scalp, may fluoresce yellow-green if infected with *Microsporum canis* or *Microsporum audouinii,* or a pale white-green in the rare event of *Trichophyton Schoenleinii.* In these cases, sensitivity may be relatively low. Sensitivity of approximately 50% has been reported for *M. canis* (Kefalidou et al, 1997). Fluorescence of affected hair should be sought, particularly in the follicular portion of the hair. Potentially infected, broken-off hair may be plucked and the subepidermal portion then viewed under the Wood's light.

- *Tinea corpora:* Fungal infections of the skin do not fluoresce, except for tinea versicolor (usually a golden yellow).
- *Erythrasma:* This produces a brilliant coral-red fluorescence. Erythrasma, frequently confused with tinea, is not fungal in origin but is caused by *Corynebacterium minutissimum.* Treatment is with erythromycin.
- Pseudomonas *infection:* This fluoresces aqua-green or white-green. Wood's light examination can be used to screen burn patients, since infection fluoresces before it becomes clinically apparent. *Pseudomonas* can also be found in ear discharge, intertrigo pedis, and secondary pseudomonal infection of the scrotum.
- *Vitiligo:* Wood's light accentuates hypopigmented areas and is particularly useful for examining patients with fair complexions.
- *Tuberous sclerosis:* Wood's light is helpful in highlighting characteristic hypopigmented skin lesions, exhibiting the shape of a mountain ash leaf
- *Tinea versicolor:* This produces a pale yellow-gold fluorescence. In this case Wood's lamp helps to differentiate skin lesions such as vitiligo.
- *Porphyria cutanea tarda:* Urine fluoresce a bright pink-orange. This may be accentuated by acidifying the urine, adding an equal volume of 1.5 N HCl.
- *Tetracycline:* In patients taking tetracycline systemically, some inflammatory lesions (including acne papules) may exhibit a yellow fluorescence under the Wood's lamp. This same fluorescence may be observed in dried or concentrated urine containing the drug.
- *Fluorescein:* The dye is used topically by moistening a small strip of impregnated paper (available commercially) and allowing a drop to then fall in the conjunctival sac. Any areas of denudation (trauma, herpes, etc.) on the cornea then fluoresces when viewed through the Wood's lamp.
- *Miscellaneous:* Many cosmetics, topical medications, and industrial chemicals may be detected on the skin by their fluorescence.

PRECAUTIONS

- Not all tinea fluoresces.
- Washing before the examination may yield a false-negative result.
- Do not confuse pathology with other substances, such as lint, sulfur laden scales of skin, serum exudate, ointment, deodorants, soaps, or tetracycline.

SUPPLIER

Burton Medical Products
21100 Lassen Street
Chatsworth, CA 91311
Phone: 1-800-444-9909

CPT/BILLING CODES

Use standard "Evaluation and Management" codes.

ICD-9-CM DIAGNOSTIC CODES

111.0	Tinea capitis
039.0	Erythrasma
709.01	Vitiligo
111.0	Tinea versicolor
277.1	Porphyria cutanea tarda

BIBLIOGRAPHY

Cwach NL, Driscoll CE: Wood's light examination. In Driscoll CE, Rakel RE, editors: *Patient care procedures for your practice,* ed 2, Los Angeles, 1991, Practice Management Information.

Dewitt DE: Wood's light exam. In Pfenninger JL, Fowler GC, editors: *Procedures for primary care physicians,* St Louis, 1994, Mosby.

Habif TP: *Clinical dermatology,* St Louis, 1996, Mosby.

Kefalidou S, Odia S, Gruseck E, et al: Wood's light in *Microsporum canis* positive patients, *Mycoses* 40:461, 1997.

Krull ED, Babel DE. Diagnostic procedures of the skin: Part one: Wood's light, KOH slide, Gram's stain, and cultures, *J Fam Pract* 3(3):309, 1976.

CHAPTER 46

Wound Dressing

Ramiro Sanchez

Occlusive dressings have become increasingly popular in the management of wounds. Although the causes of wounds are different, they can be classified into groups according to their physical condition and appearance. Box 46-1 depicts the Wagner classification of nonpressure ulcers. The development of the notion of moist wound healing has lead to hundreds of different dressings. To choose an appropriate dressing, clinicians must consider several factors.

The ideal dressing should help to do the following:
- Remove excess exudate and toxic components
- Maintain high-humidity environment at the wound-to-dressing interface
- Allow gaseous exchange across the dressing
- Maintain thermal insulation
- Protect from wound contamination and secondary infection
- Protect wound against toxic contaminants
- Simplify dressing removal without trauma to the peri-wound area

In a landmark study in 1962, Winter and associates discovered that wounds reepithelialize faster under occlusion. Before this study it was thought that wounds would heal faster if kept dry and open.

Today moist wound care is the standard of care. Among its many advantages is the reduction of wound necrosis and desiccation, growth factor stimulation, and activation of enzymes needed for debridement. Occlusive dressings decrease the pH of the wound, stimulate angiogenesis, and decrease bacterial proliferation by enhancing phagocytic and lysosomal function. These dressings also increase neutrophilic inflammatory response.

Air exposure causes wound desiccation, creating more surface necrosis. The formation of eschar prevents epithelial cell migration because cells must migrate from the wound edges and need to travel underneath the base of the eschar.

An occlusive dressing maintains lower moisture vaporization rates, thus promoting faster healing rates. Occlusive dressings increase reepithelialization. Moist dressings stimulate the proliferation of fibroblast and endothelial cells; furthermore they increase proliferation and migration of keratinocytes.

Many factors (e.g., bacterial infection, oxygen tension, wound bleeding) can influence any part of the healing process. The mental and physical condition of the patient may also influence wound healing.

It is impossible to completely sterilize skin; consequently all wounds quickly become colonized. Devitalized tissue, poor patient health, and foreign bodies (even buried sutures) increase the likelihood for infection.

PRIMARY CLOSED WOUNDS

Surgical wounds and clean lacerations heal faster when they are closed with proper tissue alignment and their borders maintained without tension with sutures or staples. They should be covered with woven gauze (in several layers with cotton pads) to absorb any secretion or exudate from the incision; this wick mechanism will avoid accumulation of blood and serum around sutures, which creates an excellent medium for bacterial growth (Tables 46-1 and 46-2). A layer of antibiotic ointment or a sterile nonadherent dressing material is applied between the wound and gauze to prevent the dressing from sticking to the wound surface.

Superficial wounds that are left open to heal by secondary intent (e.g., shave biopsies) should be kept moist. Washing with a mild soap and water three to four

---

BOX 46-1

Wagner Classification on Nonpressure Ulcers

Grade 0: Preulcerative lesion, healed ulcers, presence of bony deformity
Grade 1: Superficial ulcer without subcutaneous tissue involvement
Grade 2: Penetration through the subcutaneous tissue (may expose bone, tendon, ligament, or joint capsule)
Grade 3: Osteitis, abscess, or osteomyelitis
Grade 4: Gangrene of the forefoot
Grade 5: Gangrene of the entire foot

TABLE 46-1

Wound Dressing and Application: Gauze

Types of Wounds and Indications	Dressing Description	Contraindications	Examples
• Protection of surgical wounds • Mechanical debridement of a yellow slough (wet-to-dry) • Autolytic debridement (saline-moistened gauze) • Absorption of minimal to heavy exudates in wounds • Infected wound (impregnated or moistened with topical antibiotics) • Filler for packing dead space in large, deep wound cavities	Absorbent, made of 100% meshed cotton fabric, woven into squares, rolls, and packing strips; available in sterile and nonsterile packages	• May adhere to healthy tissue and cause injury on removal • Some products may shed, leaving lint in wound	• Curity gauze sponges by Kendall • Super Sponge by Kendall • Kling gauze rolls by Kendall • NuGauze packing strips by Johnson & Johnson

TABLE 46-2

Wound Dressing and Application: Films (Polyurethane or Copolyester with Adhesive Backing)

Types of Wounds and Indications	Dressing Description	Contraindications	Examples
• Nondraining primary closed wounds • Acute partial-thickness wound with minimal exudates • Protection of high-friction areas (e.g., heels, Stage I ulcers) • IV sites • Split-thickness skin graft donor sites • Retention of primary dressing	Permeable to moisture and other gases but impermeable to liquids Transparency allows for wound inspections	• Infected wounds • Heavy-exudate wounds (fluid retention leads to fluid collection) • Macerated wounds (can cause skin tears) • Dressing wet wounds may promote yeast colonization • Some newer films designed to keep IV sites dry (these have higher moisture vapor permeability [MVP]; should not be used for open wounds)	• Bioclusive by Johnson & Johnson • Omiderm by CanDerm • Op-Site by Smith + Nephew, Inc, Wound Management Division • Tegaderm by 3M

Usual dressing change is up to three times per week.

times a day and then applying an ointment will enhance healing. Wounds should not be "scrubbed," nor should toxic agents (e.g., hydrogen peroxide, iodine, mercurochrome) be used. (See the patient education handout titled "Moist Healing after Skin Surgery" on page 1747 of Appendix G.)

Although most clinicians use an antibiotic ointment to enhance wound healing (e.g., Bacitracin, Polysporin, Neosporin, gentamicin, erythromycin, Bactroban), there is no real evidence to show that the antibiotic is the effective ingredient. A study by Smack et al (1996) showed that white petrolatum was just as effective, cheaper, did not select out resistant bacteria, and was not a potential allergen. If wounds are infected, antibiotics do make a difference and Bactroban may be as effective topically as oral antibiotics.

The dressing is left in place for 24 to 72 hours (depending on the surgeon's preference) to allow the dermis to regenerate under sterile conditions. This sterility barrier can be broken if the outer dressing becomes moist with wound secretions, and the dressing can be changed as often as necessary (e.g., if it becomes saturated with secretions). When changing the dressing, the clinician should always use a sterile or do-not-touch technique. Subsequent dressing changes are dependent on the patient's condition (Table 46-1).

With many wounds, adhesive dressings (e.g., Band-Aids) can be used. With larger wounds, nonstick dressings, such as Telfa or one of the film coverings are helpful (Table 46-2). Alternatively, 4 × 4 gauze bandages can be used and will not stick if ointment is applied over the wound. Many wounds can be left open during the day but must be covered at night so that they do not dry on bedding material.

OPEN WOUNDS

Dehisced surgical wounds, traumatic injuries, and chronic ulcers are often left open and allowed to heal by secondary intention. These wounds take much longer to heal and will have microorganisms colonizing the surface. Calcium alginate or hydrocolloid (DuoDerm) dressings can be selected.

TABLE 46-3

Wound Dressing and Application: Hydrogel

Types of Wounds and Indications	Dressing Description	Contraindications	Examples
• Dry sloughy wounds • Necrotic wounds • Infected surgical wounds • Sinuses • Pain relief in radiation and damaged tissue • Superficial burns • Dermabrasion • Chemical peels • Filler for deep wounds	Semipermeable hydrophilic polymers composed of 80% water, 20% glycerin, available in both gel and sheet forms. Gel can absorb or donate liquid according to the tissue to which it is applied. When applied to dry and necrotic wound, it promotes autolytic debridement. Wound gels are excellent for helping to create or maintain a moist environment. Some hydrogels provide absorption, desloughing and debriding capacities to necrotic and fibrotic tissue.	• Heavily exuding wounds	• Nu-Gel by Johnson & Johnson • IntraSite Gel by Smith + Nephew, Inc, Wound Management Division • SAF-Gel by ConvaTec • Tegagel by 3M

Method of use: A liberal layer of gel is applied to the surface of the wound and covered with perforated plastic film such as Telfa. If the wound is too dry, use a more occlusive dressing such as Op-Site or Tegaderm to reduce water vapor loss and to prevent drying of the gel. In very dry wounds the dressing needs to be changed at least once a day. Hydrogel wound cover (gauze or sheet) is usually changed once per day. If it has an adhesive border, it is usually changed up to three times per week. Hydrogel wound filler is usually changed once daily. No more than 3 oz of filler is typically medically necessary per wound in a 30-day period.

TABLE 46-4

Wound Dressing and Application: Hydrocolloids

Types of Wounds and Indications	Dressing Description	Contraindications	Examples
• Light, moderately exuding wounds • Chronic venous stasis ulcers • Grade 2-3 pressure sores • Necrotic or dry slough • Prevention and treatment of friction blisters in athletes • Prophylaxis of friction area of diabetic neuropathies • Psoriatic plaques • Dystrophic epidermolysis bullosa	Material self-adhesive with gelatin, pectin and carboxymethylcellulose, applied to a thin polyurethane film or foam sheet; usually do not cause pain on removal, giving good use in pediatric wounds; hydrocolloid sheets help promote autolytic débridement by keeping wound exudate in contact with necrotic tissue (slough and eschar)	• Greater than grade 3 pressure ulcers • Diabetic neurotropic ulcers • Infected wounds	• DuoDerm by ConvaTec • Restore by Hollister • Tegasorb by 3M • DermAssist by AssisTec Medical

Method of use: This is an easy dressing to use. The clinician should choose an appropriate size (the dressing should extend 1 inch over the edge of the wound to avoid leakage). The backing of the dressing is removed, and the dressing is applied over the wound. Usual dressing change for a hydrocolloid is up to three times per week. The dressing can be left for a maximum of 5 to 7 days.

To select appropriate dressings the clinician should consider the wound's color, the presence of infection, the amount of the exudate produced, the depth, and the condition of the periwound skin.

WOUND COLOR

When performing assessment of an open wound, the clinician should assess for the presence of either black eschar, yellow devitalized tissue, or red granulating tissue. The color of the wound is determined by the presence of necrotic tissue and new scar formation. A wound with healthy progress has a red or pink color, with little formation of eschar or necrotic tissue.

A black eschar represents full-thickness destruction. Stage 3 or 4 pressure ulcer lesions are black, 2° to gangrene from vascular disease. Surgical debridement of the eschar is necessary to control infection and promote healing, but many physicians prefer conservative treatment to manage small, black necrotic wounds. Uninfected wounds with a dry eschar may be left undisturbed if a dry environment is maintained (Table 46-3). Another approach for active patients is the use of chemical enzymatic agents for debridement (see Table 46-4).

Devitalized tissue in a moist environment causes a

soft yellow, cream-colored, or gray necrotic slough with a thick purulent wound exudate.

The difference between an open wound covered with yellow slough, and necrotic tissue from another wound that is truly infected, is very small; therefore care should be taken to minimize the progression to an infected wound. Wound infection factors include the size of the wound, local tissue perfusion, and the resistance of the host.

For patients at low risk for infection, the use of moisture-retentive dressings enhances debridement of yellow wounds through an autolysis (hydrocolloids or alginates) (see Tables 46-4 and 46-5). When using dressing materials for autolytic debridement, the need for dressing change increases. Bacteria that is present under the occlusive dressing releases proteolytic enzymes that liquefy necrotic tissue, thereby increasing the amounts of exudates. Changing the dressing when it becomes saturated with exudates is important. To extend the usable period of the dressing, an absorbing material should be used.

One method to debride wounds that is used less frequently is the wet-to-dry technique. To apply wet-to-dry dressings, the wound must be cleaned with saline solution; the saline-moistened 4 × 4 gauzes are extended into two layers and applied directly to the entire wound surface. Next, several fluffed and moistened gauzes are placed on top of the contact layer (Table 46-1).

When the contact layer begins to dry it shrinks, thereby trapping debris within its fibers. When the dressing is removed dry, entrapped dead tissue is removed with the dressing.

Removal of dry dressing is painful, and the patient should be given pain medication at least 30 minutes

TABLE 46-5

Wound Dressing and Application: Alginates

Types of Wounds and Indications	Dressing Description	Contraindication	Examples
• Open wounds with moderate to heavy exudates • Superficial granulating wounds • Full-thickness wounds • Postoperative wound needing hemostasis • Decubitus and chronic ulcers • Partial and full-thickness burns • Sinuses • Split-thickness grafts • Mohs' surgery defects	Derived from fibers formed from ion exchanges of alginate salts (e.g., kelp and algae with calcium) Ion exchange forms soluble non-adherent gel with limited hemostatic properties Soluble in 0.9% saline solution Does not physically inhibit wound contractions as would gauze	• Third-degree burns	• AlgiDERM by Bard • Curasob by Kendall • Kaltostat by ConvaTec • Sorbsan by Dow Hickman

Method of use: The clinician should choose a good size dressing and apply it directly to the wound. The makers of Kaltostat recommend that their dressing be cut to conform to wound size and shape. The dressing is then covered with a secondary layer of dressing, such as perforated plastic film (e.g., Telfa) or semipermeable film (e.g., Op-Site, Tegaderm, Uniflex), depending on the amount of the exudate produced by the wound. Sorbsan is soluble in 0.9% sodium chloride and easily removed by saline irrigation. Kaltostat is less soluble; therefore it can be removed from the wound intact. Alginate wound cover is usually changed once daily.

TABLE 46-6

Wound Dressing and Applications: Foams

Types of Wounds and Indications	Dressing Description	Contraindications	Examples
• Weeping ulcers, such as a venous stasis • Acute or chronic partial-thickness exudate wounds that require mechanical débridement • Deep cavity wounds (as packing to prevent premature closure while absorbing the exudate and maintaining a moist environment) • Protection of friable periwound skin (nonadhesive pads) • Infected wounds (after appropriate intervention and close monitoring) • Autolytic debridement of yellow slough • Padding of tracheostomy sites	Semipermeable polyurethane foams, moisture retentive; foams that absorb exudate will decrease maceration to surrounding tissue; comfortable, nonocclusive; highly absorbent foams may allow caregiver to change dressings less often; available in pads and pillows for filling wound cavities; available in adhesive and nonadhesive; some products need tape to cover and secure dressing	• Sinus tracts • Wounds with a minimal exudate	• Allevyn by Smith + Nephew, Inc, Wound Management Division • CURAFOAM by Kendall • LYOfoam by ConvaTec

Usual dressing change is up to three times per week. Usual dressing change in foam fillers is once a day.

before the dressing change. If bleeding occurs, it suggests that healthy tissue is being injured and the method of dressing system used should be changed (Table 46-6). Drying out of the tissue could actually impair healing.

When a slough is removed from the wound surface, granulation tissue should be visible as a red color. These wounds should be dressed with material that maintains a clean and moist wound environment to minimize damage to healing tissue. Lists of available dressing types are explained further in Tables 46-4 to 46-6; namely, alginate dressing, foam dressing, hydrocolloid dressing, and low-adherent dressings.

INFECTED WOUNDS

Prevention of infection requires an equilibrium between local tissue resistance, bacterial invasion, and the level of the virulence of microorganisms. The absence of necrotic tissue does not preclude the possibility of wound infection. In older and immune-compromised patients, local control of bacterial proliferation can be the deciding factor in patient outcomes.

Local management of infected wounds requires removal of necrotic tissue, drainage of deep abscesses, and employment of systemic antibiotics. In weak and elderly patients, the use of nonocclusive and absorbent dressings helps to soak up purulent exudates from the wound to assist control of infection (Tables 46-4, 46-5, and 46-7).

EXUDATE

To select an appropriate dressing, viscosity and amount of exudate must be considered. Using nonabsorbent dressings would cause accumulation of the exudate and contribute to periwound maceration as well as bacterial and yeast growth. On the other hand, the use of a dressing that is highly absorptive would desiccate granulation tissue, thus increasing the depth of the wound (Tables 46-4 to 46-7).

The autolysis of necrotic tissue will augment wound drainage and will decrease gradually as granulation tissue fills the wound. If a grade 4 decubitus ulcer has large quantities of the exudate without infection present, the clinician should suspect osteomyelitis and treat accordingly.

WOUND DEPTH

Superficial wounds can be managed with sheet or wafer dressings. Deep wounds require dressing fillers. Wound fillers maintain direct contact with the wound and fill up dead space (Tables 46-4 and 46-6); therefore fillers avoid the accumulation of secretion and formation of soft-tissue abscesses. The best and most economic choice for wound depth is moist gauze packing (Table 46-7).

PERIWOUND SKIN

The condition of the periwound skin is another factor that needs to be considered in the wound dressing system. Adhesive material can have strong adhesive that can strip or tear skin in an elderly patient. Therefore the clinician should avoid adhesive material when possible, especially if the patient's skin is irritated or damaged (Table 46-6). When their use is necessary, the clinician should paint undamaged skin with protective skin sealants to facilitate nontraumatic removal.

Macerated skin, such as around venous ulcers, requires more absorptive material (see Tables 46-5 and 46-6). Accumulation of secretions can lead to skin lesions, especially with occlusive dressings. Allergies to adhesive material are another common problem. Use of mild local steroids and a change of dressing system are necessary.

TABLE 46-7

Wound Dressing and Application: Absorptive Fillers

Types of Wounds and Indications	Dressing Description	Contraindications	Examples
• Absorption in full-thickness wound with moderate to heavy exudates • Autolytic debridement of yellow slough in deep wounds with an uneven wound surface • Odor control	Several product types: absorptive powders, pastes, and beads; highly absorptive, oxygen permeable; hydrophilic cleansing action and reduction of bacterial count	• Sinus wound • Deep wound with tunneling	• Bard absorption dressing by Bard • DuoDerm paste and granules by ConvaTec

Usual dressing change is once a day for a dressing without an adhesive border and up to every other day for a dressing with an adhesive border.

As shown in the tables throughout this chapter, many different wound care products and categories are available, namely absorptive dressings, alginates, enzymatic debriders, fillers, foam dressings, hydrocolloids, hydrofiber, hydrogel, hydrogel-impregnated gauze, hydrogel sheets, transparent films, and cotton gauze. See the "Suppliers" section for further detail on manufacturers.

CONCLUSION

Occlusive dressings are now the standard of care, but choosing the appropriate one is a challenge. Different types of dressing can be used in the same type of wound. It is the clinician's duty to choose the dressing that will give the fastest wound healing at the lowest possible cost to the patient. To do this it is advisable to know what types of dressings are available at local hospitals and managed care system pharmacies. The physician should also obtain support from rehabilitation services to offer patients the best comprehensive care available. In the setting of chronic wound care, clinicians must pay attention to the psychological needs of these patients and offer referral to wound support groups.

SUPPLIERS

Bard
730 Central Avenue
Murray Hill, NJ 07974
Phone: 1-800-367-2273
Website: www.bard.com

CanDerm Pharma Inc.
5353 Thimens
St. Laurent, Quebec, Canada
H4R 2H4
Phone: 1-877-278-3265
Website: www.canderm.com

ConvaTec
P.O. Box 5254
Princeton, NJ 08543-5254
Phone: 1-800-631-5244
Website: www.convatec.com

Johnson & Johnson Medical Inc.
2500 East Arbrook Boulevard
Arlington, TX 76014-3631
Phone: 1-800-255-2500
Website: www.johnsonandjohnson.com

Kendall
15 Hampshire Street
Mansfield, MA 02048
Phone: 1-800-962-9888
Website: www.kendallhq.com

Smith + Nephew, Inc.
Wound Management Division
11775 Starkey Road
P.O. Box 1970
Largo, FL 33779-1970
Phone: 1-800-876-1261
Website: www.snwmd.com

3M Corporation
3M Center Bldg. 275-4E-01
P.O. Box 33275
St. Paul, MN 55133-3275
Phone: 1-800-228-3957
Website: www.3m.com

CPT/BILLING CODES

Procedures 16000 to 16030 refer to local treatment of burned surface only.

16000   Initial treatment, first-degree burn, when no more than local treatment is required

16010   Dressing and/or debridement, initial or subsequent, under anesthesia, small

16015   Under anesthesia, medium or large, or with major debridement

16020   Without anesthesia, office or hospital, small

16025   Without anesthesia, medium (e.g., whole face or whole extremity)

16030   Without anesthesia, large (e.g., more than one extremity)

15852   Dressing change (for other than burns) under anesthesia (other than local)

ICD-9-CM DIAGNOSTIC CODES

707.0   Decubitus

For abrasions, see the ICD-9 book under "Injury, superficial" for listing of sites.

For burns, see the ICD-9 book under "Burn" for specific locations and degree of injury.

BIBLIOGRAPHY

Brown CD, Zitelli JA: Choice of wound dressings and ointments, *Otolaryngol Clin North Am* 28(5):1081, 1995.

Cuzzell J: Choosing a wound dressing, *Geriatr Nurs* 18(6):260, 1997.

Freedline A: The wound care information network: 1995-98 (on-line). Available at www.medicaledu.com (accessed November 18, 2002).

Hastings B, Roth A, Nolan D, Miller S: Wound coverage: is there a difference? *J Burn Care Rehabil* 17(5):416, 1996.

Higgins KR: Wound dressing and topical agents, *Clin Podiatr Med Surg* 12(1):31, 1995.

Kannon GA, Garrett AB: Moist wound healing with occlusive dressings: a clinical review, *Dermatol Surg* 21(7):583, 1995.

Smack DP, Harrington AC, Dunn C, et al: Infection and allergy incidence in ambulatory surgery patients using white petrolatum vs. bacitracin ointment: a randomized control trial, *JAMA* 276:972, 1996.

Song C: Infection and the impact on cost-effectiveness in wound care, *Adv Wound Care* 8(5):58, 1995.

Surgical Materials Testing Laboratories (SMTL): Welsh Office Health Department, Wound Management Practice Resource Center (WMPRC): *Review of wound management materials*, 1996, Bridgend General Hospital, Mid Glamorgan. Available at www.smtl.co.uk/WMPRC/VFM-report/VFM-Chapter4-l.html (accessed November 18, 2002).

Tallon RW: Wound care dressings, *Nurs Manage* 27(10):68, 1996.

Winter GD: Formation of a scab and the rate of epithelialization of superficial wounds in the skin of the young domestic pig, *Nature* 193:293, 1962.

PART THREE

Aesthetics

CHAPTER 47

Body Piercing

John J. Ward
Brian D. Madden
Thomas A. Bzoskie

Modification of the body in the form of piercing and skin art has been demonstrated in virtually every culture dating back to at least 2000 BC. Egyptian pharaohs pierced their navels, and Roman soldiers pierced their nipples. Perhaps better known are the piercings and body art of African and Native American communities. The popularity of ear piercing has steadily increased since the 1950s in the United States, and since the 1990s, piercing other areas of the body has become popular. Primary care physicians may decide to offer this service to their patients.

Physicians have the advantage of being trained in anatomy, physiology, and aseptic technique. This background is necessary to perform safe piercings. In addition, physicians can recognize potential complications and have the capacity to therapeutically intervene early and effectively. As their knowledge about body modification increases, physicians' rapport with and trust among pierced patients can improve. At the very least, all primary care physicians need to be familiar with the techniques and complications that are unique to body piercing.

Commonly pierced areas of the body include the ears, eyebrows, tongue, nose (i.e., ala, septum, and bridge), umbilicus, nipples, lips, and genitals. Each site carries unique risks. The physician needs to be cognizant of these risks when evaluating whether to pierce a specific location and needs to counsel the patient accordingly.

INDICATIONS

- Cosmetic procedure
- No traditional medical indications
- The clitoral hood piercing may improve the sexual experience for women who have lost sensitivity

CONTRAINDICATIONS

- External skin and systemic disorders

Medical contraindications to body piercing are related to external factors involving the skin and to systemic conditions. Local skin infection, a cyst, severe eczema, or any other significant skin disorder at the site is a contraindication to piercing. A history of keloid formation, not necessarily hypertrophic scarring, is also a condition that warns against piercing.

- Steroid use and coagulation disorders

In addition, chronic steroid use or a coagulation disorder also precludes the procedure.

- Immunodeficiency syndromes

Patients with an immunodeficiency disorder, such as AIDS, present unique difficulties. For many of these patients, body modification is an important part of life, and the piercing would benefit their overall sense of well-being. Although, theoretically, AIDS might be considered a contraindication to piercing, realistically, unless the patient's T-cell levels are significantly compromised, piercing can be successfully accomplished in the patient with AIDS.

- Pregnancy

Clinicians should discuss pregnancy intentions with women seeking nipple or navel piercings. Controversy exists regarding whether a nipple piercing affects lactation. There are 15 to 20 milk ducts in the nipple. Although scar tissue may occlude some ducts, a properly placed piercing with appropriate jewelry should not adversely affect breast function. Excessive scarring may lead to duct occlusion, which could cause decreased or absent milk expression, persistent breast engorgement, and increased risk of infection or abscess formation during lactation. Women interested in nipple piercings should be aware of the unknown and potentially adverse effects on the ability to breastfeed. Also, because the infant may aspirate the jewelry or develop metal allergies, the jewelry is removed during actual breastfeeding.

Navel piercings can take 6 to 10 months to heal. This should be taken into consideration if a pregnancy is being considered. Navel piercings also tend to migrate. Tissue distortion that occurs during pregnancy can exacerbate this problem, and it may be necessary to remove the jewelry as gestation progresses.

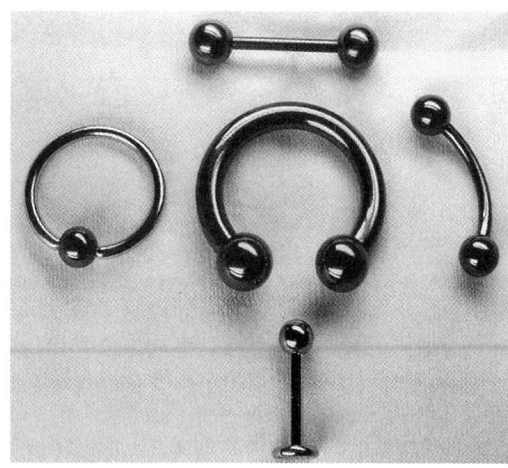

Fig. 47-1
Jewelry styles: straight barbell (*top*), captive ring (*left*), circular barbell (*center*), curved barbell (*right*), and labret stud (*bottom*).

EQUIPMENT

Jewelry

It is important to use the proper jewelry to avoid complications. Patients should wear only jewelry made of surgical grade stainless steel (316 L [low carbon], 316 LVM [low carbon, volume melt]), titanium, niobium, platinum, solid white or yellow gold (14K or 18K), or Tygon. Gold-plated jewelry contains reactive metals such as nickel and can cause allergic reactions. Silver will tarnish in the moist environment of a new piercing or in contact with any mucosal surface.

The most common types of jewelry are bead ring, captive bead ring, straight barbell, circular barbell, and curved barbell (Fig. 47-1). Size is defined in terms of gauge and either diameter or length. If the jewelry is not provided by the physician's office, patients should be advised to purchase the jewelry that is appropriate for the piercing they desire and bring it with them. Table 47-1 summarizes the initial jewelry commonly used for each location.

The bead ring and captive bead ring are opened and closed either by hand or with specialized ring-opening, ring-closing pliers. The use of other pliers may distort the shape of the ring. It is important to maintain the integrity and shape when opening and closing the ring.

TABLE 47-1

Jewelry Selection*

Location	Type and Size	Gauges	Comments
Ear lobe	BR, CBR, or LB; ⅜-½ inch	18-10 gauge	Avoid ear studs; occlusive and difficult to clean
Ear cartilage (outer)	BR, CBR, or LB; 5/16-7/16 inch	18-14 gauge	Choose jewelry least likely to be uncomfortable during sleep
Ear cartilage (tragus)	BR, CBR, or BB; 5/16-⅜ inch	18 or 16 gauge	Choose jewelry least likely to be uncomfortable during sleep
Eyebrow	BR, CBR, BB, or LB; ⅜-7/16 inch	18 or 16 gauge	Risk of tearing with smaller gauges; risk of migration with larger gauges
Nostril	Nostril screw; BR, CBR; 5/16-7/16 inch	20 gauge; 18 gauge	Nostril screw has small loop at right angle to hold it in place
Nasal septum	BR, CBR, BB or CB; ⅜-½ inch	16-10 gauge	Use a needle-receiving tube
Tongue	BB; ¾-1 inch	14-10 gauge	Length accounts for initial edema; downsize jewelry in 2-3 weeks; minimum ball size is 6 mm.
Labret	Labret stud; ⅜-½ inch	14 gauge	Minimum ball size is 5 mm; can downsize later
Nipple (female)	BR, CBR, BB or CB; ⅝-¾ inch	14-10 gauge	Consider future breastfeeding plans; postpone piercing if pregnancy is in the near future
Nipple (male)	BR, CBR, BB or CB; 9/16 inch	14 or 12 gauge	
Navel	BR, CBR, or LB; 7/16-⅝ inch	14 or 12 gauge	Pierce navel fold; avoid small jewelry that can constrict skin
Clitoral hood (vertical)	BR, CBR, or LB; 7/16-9/16 inch	14 or 12 gauge	Position jewelry so that ball rests on the clitoris
Penis (Prince Albert)	BR, CBR, LB or CB; 9/16-1 inch	12 or 10 gauge	Use a needle-receiving tube

BB, Straight barbell; *BR,* bead ring; *CB,* circular barbell; *CBR,* captive bead ring; *LB,* curved barbell.
*When using gauge readings, the size actually decreases as the gauge number gets larger.

Piercing Equipment

- Appropriate jewelry: sterilize in an autoclave.
- Antiseptic cleanser: use povidone-iodine (Betadine), Techni-Care, or ethyl alcohol.
- Ring-closing pliers: use with captive or bead rings; usually not needed if jewelry is annealed. (The annealing process allows jewelry to be manipulated more easily, particularly by hand.)
- Piercing needles: have various sizes available, including 10, 12, 14, 16, and 18 gauge. (For most piercings, the needle size should match the gauge of the jewelry being inserted [Fig. 47-2].)
- Needle-receiving tube: use for piercings involving the nostril, septum, penis, clitoral hood, and some parts of the ear cartilage (Fig. 47-3).
- Rubber bands: use to provide tension for piercing clamps.
- Insertion taper: a solid metal rod that is larger at one end and gradually becomes smaller at the other end; gauge measurement is based on size of larger end; use to help transfer jewelry or for stretching; in a fresh piercing the tapers gauge will be the same as the jewelry gauge. "Transfer" means to place the tip of the jewelry into the needle or taper and pass it into place in the hole previously made by the needle.
- Needle pusher/acrylic needle holder: helps pass the needle through skin.
- Tissue forceps: use Pennington, Mini-Pennington, or ring forceps; slotted-style optional. (The forceps is tensioned with two rubber bands; this helps avoid clamping skin too tightly.)
- Surgical marking pen: use very fine point. (Sharpie Fine Point pens can be used.)
- Gentian violet: to mark tongue and oral cavity piercings.
- Toothpicks: to apply gentian violet.
- Cotton applicators: use to adjust the size or site of insertion marks at the piercing site; erase or fine-tune the marks with alcohol-soaked applicators.
- Gauze: to cleanse the site after piercing.
- Gauge wheel: confirm gauge of needle or jewelry.
- Caliper: confirm size of jewelry.
- Sterile barrier field: cover instrument tray.
- Cork: cover needle tip after insertion. (Protects against needle injury.)
- Ethyl alcohol (70%): can use as a skin cleanser. (Removes excess ink marks.)

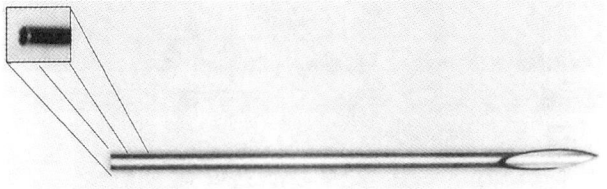

Fig. 47-2
Piercing needle. This is a hollow tri-beveled needle. Jewelry is held against the nonpointed end of the needle for passage through the skin. After passage, a cork can be placed on the needle tip to prevent needlestick injuries.

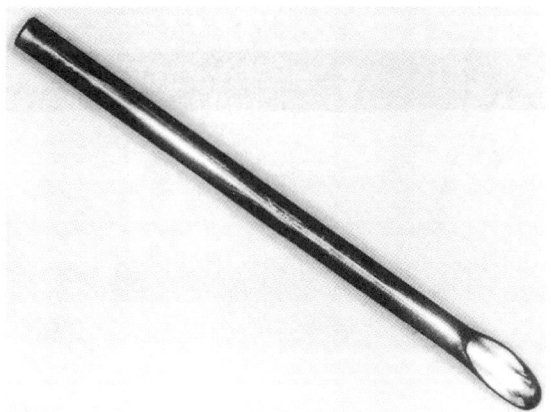

Fig. 47-3
Needle-receiving tube. This is a hollow tube that is used in ear cartilage, nostril, and genital piercings. The needle is passed through the area being pierced into the tube. The tube protects adjacent structures from inadvertent injury.

STERILIZATION

Most piercing equipment can be sterilized in a steam autoclave. Items that are reusable should be cleansed in an ultrasonic cleaner before sterilization. Those items that are heat sensitive can be cleansed with a broad-spectrum, environmentally safe germicidal that kills such organisms as human immunodeficiency virus, hepatitis (particularly B), and tuberculosis.

PREPROCEDURE PATIENT PREPARATION

Inform the patient of all possible complications of piercing in general and those specific to the location requested. Thorough documentation of the informed consent is mandatory. All patients under 18 years of age need legal guardian consent. Patients should anticipate the average healing time depending on the location of the piercing (Table 47-2). (See the sample patient education handout titled "Body Piercing" on page 1782 of Appendix G and the sample patient consent form titled "Body Piercing" on page 1783 of Appendix G.)

TECHNIQUE

Universal precautions should always be followed. Instruments and jewelry need to be appropriately sterilized. In rare circumstances, certain jewelry will need to be soaked in an antiseptic solution for 30 minutes. This solution is removed with alcohol before insertion.

Navel Piercing

1. Prepare the sterile instrument tray (Fig. 47-4).
2. Clean the navel and the surrounding abdominal wall with an antiseptic solution (sterile preparation).
3. Mark entry and exit points with the surgical marker (Fig. 47-5). Confirm acceptability of location with the patient before proceeding. Use the crest of the navel fold as a guide. On the abdominal wall, mark the entrance site at a distance half the length of the curved barbell or the diameter of the ring from the edge of the skin fold. On the undersurface of the navel skin fold, mark the exit site at the same distance from the edge of the fold as the entrance site. This is above the deep, flat base of the umbilicus. Have the patient lie, sit, stand, protrude, and retract the abdomen to evaluate placement of the markings as they vary with each position. Make adjustments in the markings if needed. If an umbilical hernia or other anatomic variants are present, a navel piercing should be avoided.

Note: Our preferred method is to start with the patient in a supine position, and mark the exit hole within the fold of skin over the navel. Have the patient stand, and evaluate tissue above the navel fold for a natural indentation. Mark this site as the entrance hole. Choose the appropriate jewelry size ($7/16$, $1/2$, $9/16$, or $5/8$) to match the navel's anatomy as determined by the placement of the markings.

4. Place rubber bands on the forceps and adjust the tension. Grasp and tent the skin with traction. Avoid actually clamping the forceps because this will crush the skin (Fig. 47-6).
5. Position the piercing needle perpendicular to the tented skin and parallel to the floor and the markings (Fig. 47-7).
6. Pass the needle through the skin. Remove the forceps. Attach the jewelry to the nonpointed end

TABLE 47-2

Average Healing Times for Piercing Locations

Location	Healing Times
Ear lobe	4-6 wk
Ear cartilage	2-3 mo
Eyebrow	6-8 wk
Nostril	2-3 mo
Nasal septum	4-6 wk
Tongue	4-6 wk
Labret	6-8 wk
Nipple (female)	2-3 mo
Nipple (male)	2-3 mo
Navel	6-10 mo
Clitoral hood	4-6 wk
Penis (Prince Albert)	4-6 wk

(Fig. 47-2) of the needle, then pass the jewelry into the piercing. For a captive ring, the ring needs to be twisted back and forth to allow easy transfer (Fig. 47-8). After the ring is in place, straighten the ring and insert the ball (Fig. 47-9).

7. Remove the antiseptic cleansing agent with sterile saline.

Other Piercings

Ear Lobe

1. Cleanse the front and back of the lobe.
2. Mark the front and back in the center of the lobe.
3. Use the Pennington forceps to stabilize the lobe when passing the needle. Do not ratchet down the forceps.
4. Pierce perpendicular to the plane of the lobe.

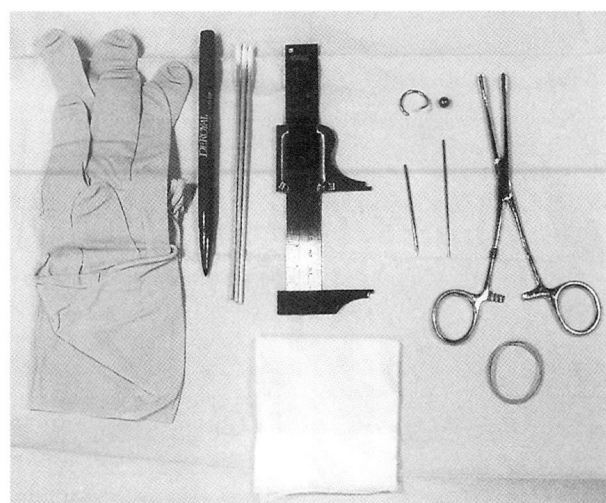

Fig. 47-4
Instrument tray. Items shown *(left to right):* gloves, marking pen, cotton applicators, caliper, gauze, captive bead ring, piercing needle, insertion taper, Pennington forceps, and rubber bands. All items are appropriately sterilized.

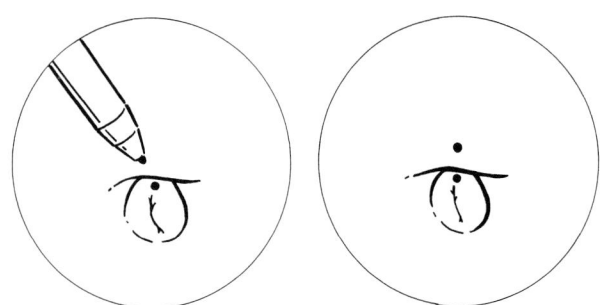

Fig. 47-5
Schematic representation of the skin markings for umbilical piercing. The longitudinal line in the circular area represents the base of the umbilicus. The transverse line represents the navel skin fold. The area between the longitudinal and transverse lines represents the undersurface of the skin fold. The markings are usually equal distances from the edge of the fold.

Ear Cartilage

1. Clamping is not recommended for cartilage because of potential crushing and increased risk of complication.
2. Use a free hand technique or a needle-receiving tube.
3. Pierce perpendicular to the plane of the cartilage.

Eyebrow

1. Can be performed similar to the navel technique.
2. The piercing is placed over the lateral third of the eyebrow to avoid the supraorbital nerve.

3. Slant the piercing toward the nose with the lower mark made medial to the upper mark.
4. Avoid a shallow piercing because this can lead to migration.

Nostril

1. The entrance point is at the natural indentation of the alar fold; the direction of the piercing is external to internal.
2. Use a needle-receiving tube placed inside the nostril to avoid tissue damage.

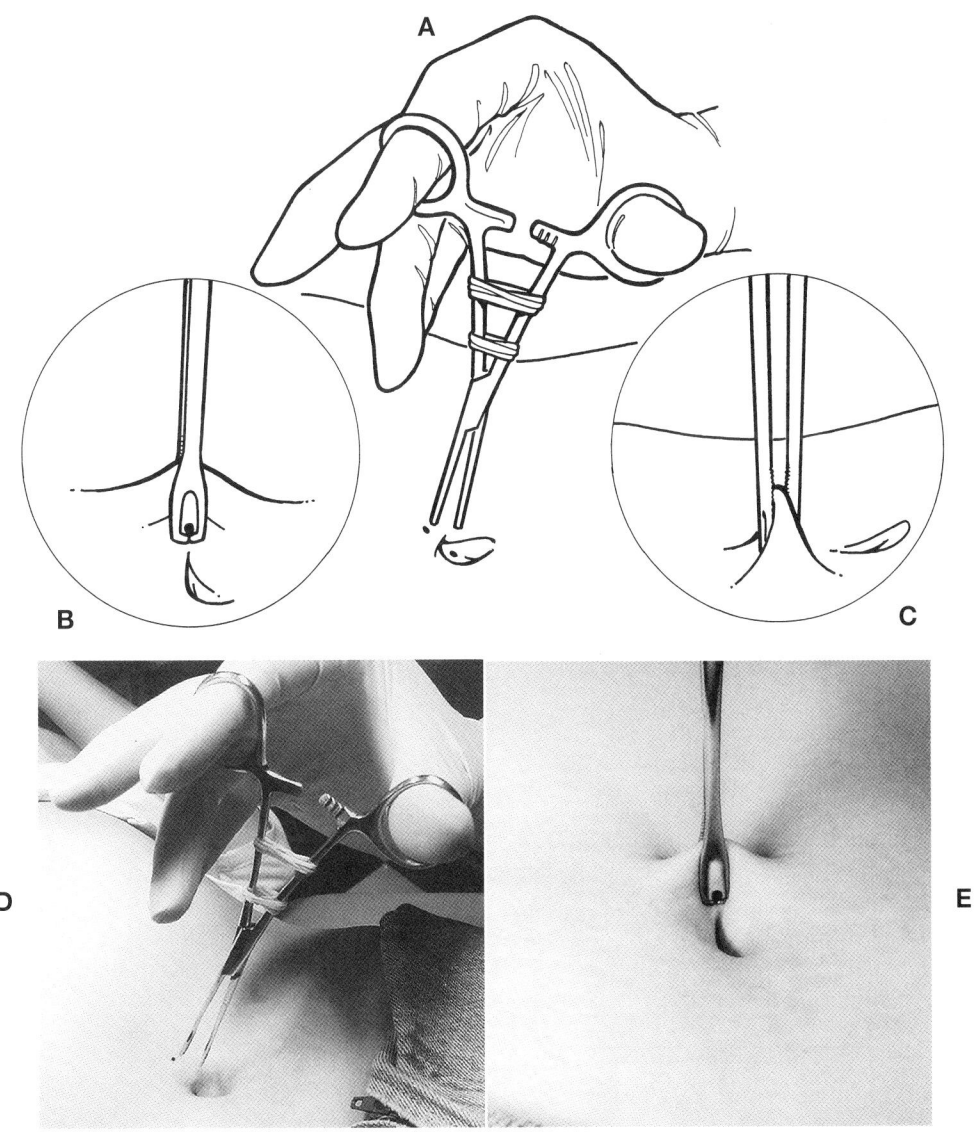

Fig. 47-6

Schematic representation of forceps application for umbilical piercing. The patient is supine. **A,** The navel skin fold has been marked (*center*). (Note markings above and below the marked skin fold.) The forceps have two rubber bands in place for tensioning. The skin fold will be gently held by the forceps. **B,** The markings are positioned at the edge of the clamp opening. The skin fold is then gently tented and held perpendicular to the floor. It is important *not* to engage the clamp's ratchets. **C,** Forceps application. Skin fold is gently tented and held perpendicular to the floor. Note the deep aspect of the umbilicus is *not* involved in the piercing. **D,** Photograph of step **A. E,** Photograph of step **B.**

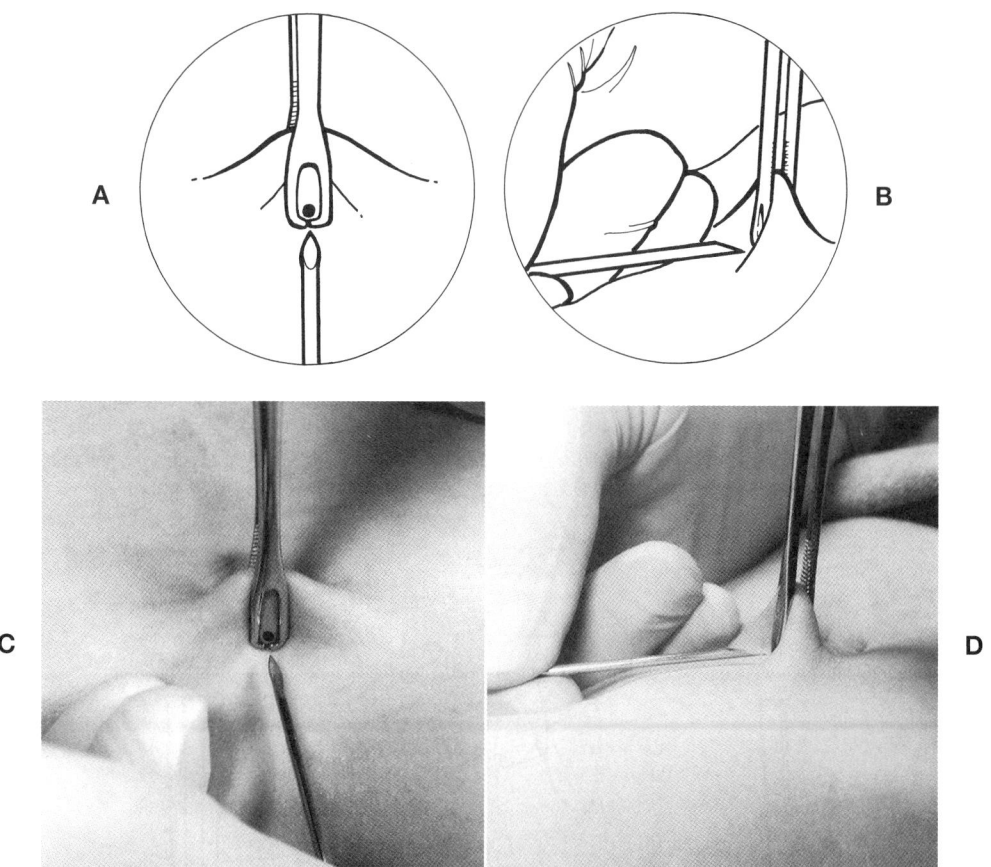

Fig. 47-7
Schematic representation of the needle position for umbilical piercing. A, With the skin gently tented, the needle is positioned perpendicular to the skin and parallel to the floor. The direction of the piercing is cephalad to caudad (i.e., the needle is pointing toward the foot). **B,** The needle is positioned perpendicular to the skin fold and parallel to the floor. The needle is aligned with the markings and is pointing cephalad to caudad (i.e., toward the foot). **C,** Photograph of step **A. D,** Photograph of step **B.**

3. Avoid using a clamp on the ala because this will crush the cartilage.

Nasal Septum
1. Piercing is done through the soft membrane inferior to the nasal cartilage.
2. The piercing is located ¾ inch from the external tip of the nose and ⅛ inch below cartilaginous edge.
3. Use a needle-receiving tube to stabilize the septum.

Labret or Lip
1. These are unique piercings, since they involve two different tissue surfaces, facial skin, and the mucosa of the oral cavity.
2. The piercing site in the skin is usually placed below the vermillion border of the lip.
3. On the mucosal surface, the site is positioned so the jewelry does not rest on the gums.
4. Appropriate jewelry for these piercings are rings or labret studs (see Fig. 47-1). Jewelry size is ⅜ to ½ inch.

Cheek
1. Prior to the piercing, use a pen light to identify vascular structures, particularly the branches of the facial artery and vein. This will help avoid the branches of the facial nerve.
2. Pierce through the facial skin anterior to the laugh line into the oral cavity.
3. Inside the oral cavity, the hole should avoid the parotid duct.

Tongue
1. Choose a central and midline location in the natural bend of the tongue. Have the patient cup the tongue to find this indentation.
2. The exit site is anterior to the frenulum. Avoid the veins that are easily visualized on the underside of the tongue.

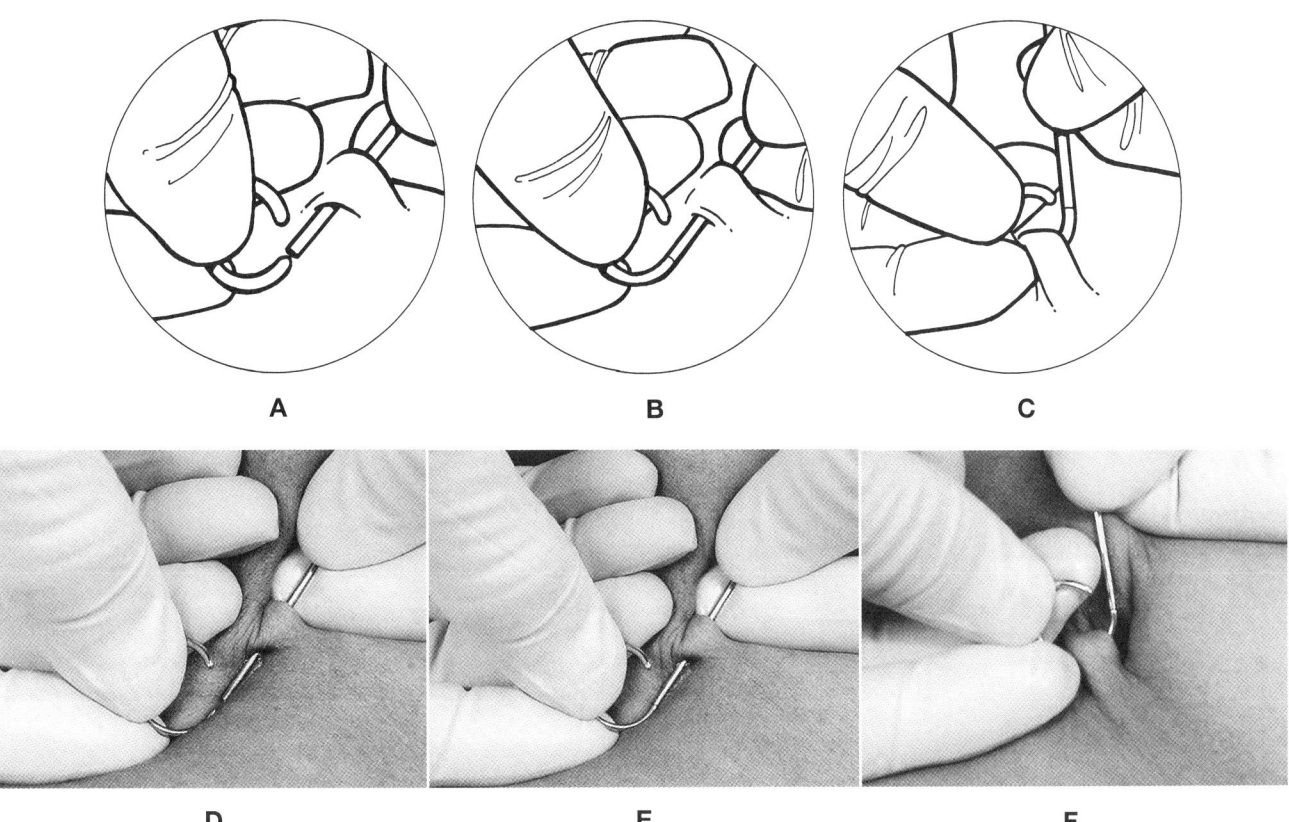

Fig. 47-8

Schematic representation of jewelry transfer for umbilical piercing. A, The sharp end of the needle is held with the fingers of one hand. The point can be protected with a cork. **B,** The jewelry is positioned against the nonpointed end. **C,** The skin fold is stabilized against the finger during transfer. The jewelry is gently twisted to help clear the skin fold. **D,** Photograph of step **A** showing jewelry positioning. The sharp end of the jewelry is held with the fingers of one hand. The jewelry is being placed on the nonpointed end of the needle. The jewelry is gently twisted to help clear the skin fold. **E,** Photograph of step **B**. The jewelry abuts the nonpointed end of the needle. The skin fold is stabilized against the finger holding the sharp end. **F,** Photograph of step **C** showing jewelry transfer. The jewelry has been transferred through the skin fold. During the transfer, the jewelry is held against the nonpointed end of the needle. The jewelry is gently twisted to help clear the skin fold.

3. Use gentian violet to mark the entrance and exit sites. With the tongue in an extended position, the entrance and exit sites should be perpendicular. This allows for a slightly angulated position when the tongue is retracted.
4. During the piercing, hold the tongue in an extended position with gauze or a sponge forceps.

Nipple

1. The horizontal axis is preferred for women, but they may prefer the piercing to be vertical. The horizontal or vertical axis can be used for men.
2. For women, the piercing is placed through the base of the nipple at or just below the midline. In men, placement is at the junction of the nipple with the areola at or just above the midline.

Clitoral Hood

Actual clitoral piercings are rare, and they depend on the size of the clitoris. Damage to the neural tissue can occur. Most patients who request a clitoral piercing actually desire the clitoral hood piercing.

Vertical Piercing

1. Find the apex of the hood at the base of the clitoris.
2. Mark the outer skin of the hood at this site.
3. Measure the distance to the edge of the hood and to the head of the clitoris. Choose a jewelry size ($\frac{7}{16}$ to $\frac{9}{16}$ inch) that allows the ball to rest on the head. Typically the jewelry will be a $\frac{7}{16}$- or $\frac{1}{2}$-inch curved barbell.
4. Insert the jewelry; the preferred jewelry is a curved barbell.

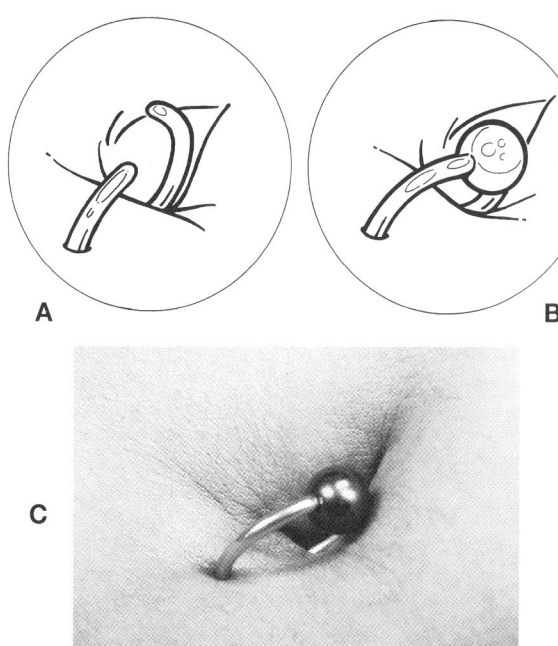

Fig. 47-9
Schematic representation of jewelry for umbilical piercing.
A, The ring has a gentle twist and must be untwisted for bead placement. **B,** The bead has indentations, and these are positioned between the ends of the ring. **C,** The captive bead ring is positioned in the navel's skin fold.

Horizontal Piercing

1. Pierce through the clitoral hood tissue at a similar distance from the clitoris as in the vertical piercing.
2. Avoid the veins that pass down the hood; use a penlight to identify the veins.
3. Use lightweight jewelry because the weight of the jewelry can pull the hood beyond the clitoris, and the desired effect will be lost.

Penis (Prince Albert)

1. This is the most commonly requested penile piercing.
2. Place the piercing in the thin soft triangular tissue that lies between the corona of the glans at the frenulum.
3. Evaluate the penis in both a flaccid and an erect state to locate the entrance site that accommodates an erection.
4. Choose the jewelry size based on the erect state of the penis; the jewelry is generally ⅝ to ¾ inches long.
5. Mark the entrance site at the frenulum.
6. Place a needle-receiving tube through the meatus into the urethra. Position the end of the tube (which is now inside the urethra) at the entrance site.
7. Pass the needle through the skin into the receiving tube.

8. Remove the tube and protect the sharp end of the needle with a cork.
9. Position the jewelry on the needle and transfer.

Note: The Prince Albert has a tendency to bleed for several days following the piercing.

COMPLICATIONS

General Complications

Some complications are inherent in all piercing procedures and include the following.
- Pain
- Bleeding
- Infection: Tuberculosis, tetanus, hepatitis, HIV, and toxic shock syndrome have been attributed to contamination at the time of piercing. Genital piercings increase the risk of hepatitis and HIV infections due to the open wounds and associated trauma.
- Hypertrophic scarring
- Keloid formation
- Granuloma or cyst formation
- Migration or expulsion of jewelry
- Contact dermatitis or other skin reaction
- Possible negative social stigma

Specific Complications by Location

Navel
- Migration
- Scar formation

Ear Cartilage
- Infection from *Lactobacillus, Pseudomonas*
- Toxic shock syndrome (very rare)
- In one study, 34% of ear piercings experienced complications such as mild infection, pain, allergic reaction, etc.

Ear Lobe
- Keloids, especially in black individuals
- Enlargement of the opening and traumatic lacerations tearing through the lobe
- Lack of symmetry between the two sides

Eyebrow
- Periorbital infection
- Damage to supraorbital nerve

Nostril
- Damage to cartilage
- Infection (staphylococcal)

Nasal Septum
- Pressure necrosis of cartilaginous border and alae

Tongue
- Damage to dentition and gums
- Loss of bone supporting the teeth
- Lingual nerve damage
- Hematoma
- Aspiration of jewelry

Labret and Lips
- Damage to dentition and gums

Cheek
- Damage to parotid duct branches of the facial artery, vein, and nerve
- Uncontrolled drooling

Nipple
- Interference with lactation
- Mastitis and abscess formation

POSTPROCEDURE PATIENT EDUCATION

Advise the following:
- Always wash hands thoroughly before touching the piercing.
- Avoid tight clothing that can cause increased friction at the piercing site.
- Expect serosanguineous fluid to ooze and crust around the entrance and exit sites. This crusting will last until the piercing has completely healed. Only when the crusting has stopped can jewelry exchange or a stretching procedure be considered. The crusted material harbors bacteria and needs to be removed. Soak the piercing site with a warm sea salt solution (¼ teaspoon of sea salt in 8 oz of distilled water) using a soft cloth, gauze, or an inverted glass for 5 to 10 minutes. Then remove the crusted material with a clean, damp cloth or cotton applicators before carefully twisting the jewelry in the moistened area to ensure it is not trapped.
- Use a mild antibacterial soap that does not contain fragrances. We prefer Provon (GOJO Laboratories) and Septicare (Sage Laboratories). If using soap, lather the area and the jewelry, then rinse well with water. Allow to air dry. If using Septicare, allow it to dry without rinsing.
- If redness and swelling develop, use warm compresses four times a day for 24 hours. If the redness and swelling do not go away or if a purulent discharge (pus) develops, see a physician.
- For tongue piercings, use an antibacterial mouthwash that does not contain alcohol or a saline solution after meals and smoking. Gargle for 30 to 60 seconds. It is preferable to avoid smoking. Use a new toothbrush and change it every 30 days. Brush the jewelry with the toothbrush to remove plaque.
- Do not use antibacterial ointments such as polymyxin B sulfate, neomycin sulfate, bacitracin (Neosporin); bacitracin; or polymyxin B sulfate, bacitracin zinc (Polysporin). These ointments are petroleum-based and can occlude the piercing. Occlusion will trap serosanguineous fluid and dead cells, delay healing, and promote possible infections. Prolonged use of antibacterial ointments can also irritate the skin. If necessary, prescribe mupirocin (Bactroban) ointment for the first 24 to 48 hours if mild redness or swelling develop. Rub the ointment gently on the jewelry and the surrounding skin until a thin, nonvisible layer is present.
- Avoid using alcohol, which can dry the skin and the cells involved in healing the piercing.
- Avoid using hydrogen peroxide and povidone-iodine, which are toxic to healing tissues.

CONCLUSION

Body piercing is an elective procedure that patients may be surprised to learn a physician understands and can perform. Anatomic evaluation, aseptic technique, appropriate aftercare, and proper selection of jewelry to fit the location are keys to a successful piercing procedure. Understanding the patient who requests a piercing is necessary to obtain an excellent result.

SUPPLIERS

Anatometal
411 Ingalls Street
Santa Cruz, CA 95060
Phone: 1-888-262-8663
Website: www.anatometal.com

Body Circle Designs
P.O. Box 68249
Seattle, WA 98168
Phone: 1-800-244-8430
Website: www.bodycircle.com

Body Vision
220 West Fifth Street
Suite 802
Los Angeles, CA 90013
Phone: 1-888-991-2639

Cold Steel
45-46 Millmead Industrial Centre
Tottenham Hale N17 9QU
London, England
Phone: +44 (020) 8880 3334
Website: www.coldsteel.co.uk

Custom Steel
13 Custom Steel Drive
Paguate, NM 87040
Phone: 1-800-877-5855
Website: www.customsteel.com

Good Art, LLC
1420 Fourth Street
Santa Monica, CA 90401
Phone: 1-310-395-4663
Website: www.goodart.com

Industrial Strength
1945 Martin Luther King, Jr. Way
Berkeley, CA 94704
Phone: 1-510-644-0968
Website: www.isbodyjewelry.com

ONYX Body Jewelry
22817 Ventura Boulevard, #495
Woodland Hills, CA 91364
Phone: 1-818-999-2540
Website: www.onyxbodyjewelry.com

Unimax Supply Company
365 Canal Street
New York, NY 10013
Phone: 1-800-986-4629
Website: www.unimaxsupply.com

ADDITIONAL RESOURCES

- See the sample patient education handout titled "Body Piercing" on page 1782 of Appendix G.
- See the sample patient consent form titled "Body Piercing" on page 1783 of Appendix G.

BIBLIOGRAPHY

Angel E: The worst piercing story, *The Point* 23:15, 2002.

Campbell A, Moore A, Williams E, et al: Tongue piercing: impact of time and barbell stem length on lingual gingival recession and tooth chipping, *J Periodontol* 73(3): 289, 2002.

Gawkrodger DJ: Nickel dermatitis: how much nickel is safe, *Contact Derm* 35:267, 1996.

Geronemus RG, Mertz PM, Eaglstein WH: Wound healing—the effects of topical antimicrobial agents, *Arch Dermatol* 115:1311, 1979.

Haudrechy P, Foussereau J, Mantout B, Baroux B: Nickel release from nickel-plated metals and stainless steels, *Contact Derm* 31:249, 1994.

Jia W, Beatty MW, Reinhardt RA, et al: Nickel release from orthodontic arch wires and cellular immune response to various nickel concentrations, John Wiley and Sons, Inc. *J Biomed Mater Res (Appl Biomater)* 48:488, 1999.

Khanna R, Kumar SS, Srinivasa Raju B, Kumar AV: Body piercing in the accident and emergency department, *J Accid Emerg Med* 16:418, 1999.

Kretchmer MC, Moriarity JD: Metal piercing through the tongue and localized loss of attachment: a case report, *J Periodontol* 72(6):831, 2001.

Landeck A, Newman N, Breadon J, Zahner S: A simple technique for ear piercing, *J Am Acad Dermatol* 39:795, 1998.

Liden C, Menne T, Burrows D: Nickel-containing alloys and platings and their ability to cause dermatitis, *Br J Dermatol* 134:193, 1996.

McDonagh AJG, Wright AL, Cork MJ, Gawkrodger DJ: Nickel sensitivity: the influence of ear piercing and atopy, *Br J Dermatol* 126:16, 1992.

Meuer C, Bredberg M, Fischer T, Widstrom L: Ear piercing, and nickel and cobalt sensitization, in 520 young Swedish men dosing compulsory military service, *Contact Derm* 32:147, 1993.

More DR, Seidel JS, Bryan PA: Ear-piercing techniques as a cause of auricular chondritis, *Pediatr Emerg Care* 15(3):189, 1999.

Meyer D: Body piercing: old traditions creating new challenges, *J Emerg Nurs* 26:612, 2000.

Nielsen NH, Menne' T: Nickel sensitization and ear piercing in an unselected Danish population, *Contact Derm* 29:18, 1993.

Er N, Ozkavaf A, Berberoglu A, Yamalik N: An unusual cause of gingival recession: oral piercing, *J Periodontol* 71(11): 1767, 2000.

Samantha S, Tweeten M, Rickman LS: Infectious complications of body piercing, *Clin Infect Dis* 26:735, 1998.

Scully C, Chen M: Tongue piercing (oral body art), *Br J Oral Maxillofac Surg* 32:37, 1994.

Simplot TC, Hoffman HT: Comparison between cartilage and soft tissue ear piercing complications, *Am J Otolaryngol* 19(5):305, 1998.

Smith-Sivertsen T, Dotterud LK, Lund E: Nickel allergy and its relationship with local nickel pollution, ear piercing and atopic dermatitis: a population-based study from Norway, *J Am Acad Dermatol* 40:726, 1999.

EDUCATIONAL RESOURCES

The following brochures are available from the Association of Professional Piercers (APP) (Website: www.safepiercing.org). The APP has also written the *APP Procedural Manual*.

- *Picking Your Piercer*
- *Aftercare Guidelines for Facial and Body Piercings*
- *Aftercare Guidelines for Oral Piercings*
- *Body Piercing Troubleshooting: For You and Your Healthcare Professional*

WEBSITES

www.safepiercing.org (Association of Professional Piercers)

www.piercinglinks.com (Almost Complete Body Piercing Links)

www.bme.freeq.com/index.html (BME: Body Modification Ezine)

www.cs.uu.nl/wais/html/na-dir/bodyart/piercing-faq/.html (Bodyart Newsgroup FAQ on Piercing)

www.tribalectic.com (Tribalectic Piercing Community)

www.bodyworkprod.com (Body Work Productions)

www.ringsofdesire.com (Rings of Desire)

dir.yahoo.com/Arts/Visual_Arts/Body_Art/ (Yahoo! Body Art)

CHAPTER 48

Uses of Botulinum Exotoxin

Edward M. Zimmerman

The Food and Drug Administration (FDA) approved the first batch of botulinum A exotoxin (BTX-A) in 1989 for the treatment of strabismus and blepharospasm associated with dystonia, benign essential blepharospasm, and facial nerve (CN VII) disorders in patients 12 years or older. This chapter discusses the cosmetic uses of Botox, which include the temporary alleviation of dynamic wrinkles of the upper face, lips, and neck. It is also used for blepharospasm, focal hyperhidrosis of the axillae, palms, and soles; and recently, pain control of muscular-tension headaches. In 2002, the FDA approved Botox Cosmetic for temporary alleviation of dynamic wrinkles of the glabellar area.

BTX-A is available in two forms: *Botox* is a purified neurotoxin complex produced by Allergan of Irvine, California. It is available in 100 unit vials. Speywood Pharmaceuticals, Ltd. in Maidenhead, England makes *Dysport* in 500-unit vials. Botox is more readily available in the United States and is four to five times stronger than Dysport.

There are seven serotypes of BTX, named A through G. Type A is the most potent, and it was the first one commercially available. BTX-A appears to work at the level of the neuromuscular junction of striated muscle, where it irreversibly binds and then inhibits the release of acetylcholine. This causes paralysis of that muscle until a new neuromuscular junction is sprouted by the nerve ending, a process that can take weeks to months depending on the density of innervation and on the site, amount, and concentration of the solution injected. The onset of muscle paralysis, reduced sweating, or pain control varies from site to site and patient to patient. Most patients notice a gradual increasing response in 3 to 7 days that plateaus and lasts for 2 to 11 months, with a gradual redevelopment of wrinkles, sweating, or pain. Some patients respond more quickly and completely to the injections. A small percentage of patients are minimally responsive, even to large amounts of Botox. Some become resistant to injections. Resistance has not been documented in patients treated with less than 100 U per session for either blepharospasm or aesthetic purposes. Patients who become resistant to BTX-A because of

antibody development after repeated, large doses or laboratory workers who are specifically immunized, may respond to BTX-B and BTX-F, which are currently undergoing clinical trials. BTX-B was approved by the FDA in December, 2000, for treatment of patients with cervical dystonia. It is produced by Elan Pharmaceuticals and is undergoing further trials at this time to determine appropriate dosages for cosmetic uses as well. Initial opinion is that BTX-A is about 50 times as potent as BTX-B.

SAFETY OF BOTOX

The Botox LD 50 for humans is estimated to be 2500 to 3000 U of toxin for a 70-kg human, or approximately 40 U/kg. For cosmetic purposes, doses of Botox are limited to 100 U; therefore Botox can be considered a safe and useful chemical. No irreversible clinical effects have been reported.

INDICATIONS

FDA-Approved Indications

- Strabismus
- Blepharospasm with dystonia
- Benign essential blepharospasm
- Cervical dystonia (spasmodic torticollis)
- Dynamic glabellar rhytids

Other Indications

- Cosmetic reduction of wrinkles in upper face, lips, and neck
- Hyperhidrosis of the axillae, palms, and soles
- Anal fissures resulting from an increase in rectal sphincter tone
- Asymmetric face, acquired (e.g., Bell's palsy, hemifacial spasm, or, after facial trauma, the unaffected side causes reduced movement or unopposed muscle tension)

CONTRAINDICATIONS

- Pregnancy
- Preexisting neuromuscular diseases (this is a relative contraindication; obtain neurologist's opinion before initiating BTX-A for cosmetic reasons in these patients)
- Sensitivity or allergy to any of the constituents of reconstituted Botox, including BTX-A, human albumin, and saline
- Aminoglycosides may potentiate the effect of large doses of BTX-A (generally not a problem for the small doses used for cosmetic procedures)
- Concurrent treatment with other injections (tissue fillers) or procedures

EQUIPMENT

- One vial of Botox (100 U frozen)
- Sterile normal saline *without preservatives* (single-dose vials) (Although not recommended by the company, using multidose vials *with* preservatives is acceptable and the reconstituted mixture stores safely in a refrigerator for several weeks.)
- 20-gauge needle to reconstitute the vial of Botox with saline and load syringes of diluted toxin
- Two to ten 1-ml syringes for storage of reconstituted toxin
- 30-gauge, ½-inch needles for injection syringes
- Alcohol wipes to cleanse injection sites
- Facial tissues or clean gauze to hold pressure on injection sites
- Nonsterile gloves to wear during injection
- Ice packs or small bags of ice to topically anesthetize the skin and constrict blood vessels at injection sites before injection
- Small tray to store syringes of reconstituted BTX-A in refrigerator
- Electromyogram (EMG) and metal needles for electromyographic guidance *(optional)*

PREPROCEDURE PATIENT PREPARATION

A vial of Botox purchased directly from Allergan costs about $425 at this time.

Note: Batching several patients on the same day can reduce overhead costs because of Botox's brief shelf life once reconstituted.

Botox is delivered by overnight transport in a thick Styrofoam container packed with dry ice in order to keep the potent but fragile toxin stable. Allergan recommends storage of the unmixed toxin at –5° C or lower (frozen). Potency of the toxin is measured in units (U) where one unit is the amount of toxin that kills 50% (LD50) of a standardized mouse model when injected intraperitoneally. Each vial of Botox contains at least 100 U of toxin, plus 0.5 mg of human albumin and 0.9 mg of sodium chloride. The toxin is lyophilized and sealed in the vial under negative pressure.

BTX-B (Myobloc) is delivered premixed in several quantities: 2500 U in 0.5 ml, 5000 U in 1 ml, and 10,000 U in 2 ml. (BTX-B may be stored undiluted in the refrigerator at 2° to 8° C for up to 21 months. If diluted, it should be used promptly as it contains no preservatives.)

An injection site record (Fig. 48-1) should be available before the procedure begins.

Reconstitution and Handling of Botox

Alcohol used to cleanse the rubber stoppers and injection sites can inactivate the toxin. Allow it to evaporate completely before proceeding. Allergen recommends that from 1 to 10 ml of sterile saline *without preservatives* (single-dose vials to not contain preservatives) be mixed in the vial of Botox using the large needle to reconstitute it. A vial that does not demonstrate a vacuum should not be used. The reconstituted Botox should be mixed by gently rolling or swirling the vial. Shaking the vial (i.e., causing foaming) denatures the Botox, leading to decreased potency of the solution. Once reconstituted, the toxin should be kept at 2° to 8° C (refrigerated) and used as quickly as possible. The package insert recommends using the toxin within 4 hours when mixed with sterile saline without preservatives. Some studies have shown little loss of potency at 30 days. However, other authors have raised concerns about decreased potency and prolonged refrigerated storage of a solution without preservatives. Freezing the reconstituted toxin in the 1-ml syringes for 7 to 10 days does not appear to alter its potency. There appears to be little difference in potency or longevity of response when bacteriostatic saline with preservatives is used.

Dilution varies by use and personal preference. More concentrated dilutions seem to cause effects sooner, which last longer but may be more difficult for the clinician to inject accurately. Most clinicians dilute 100 U of lyophilized Botox with 1 to 6 ml of saline. Dilutions of 100 U/1 ml (10 U/0.1 ml) or 100 U/2 ml (5 U/0.1 ml) are commonly used for hyperhidrosis. Dilutions of 100 U/3 ml (3.3 U/0.1 ml) to 100 U/6 ml (1.67 U/0.1 ml) are often used for cosmetic or frontal headache treatments. The area of effect associated with each injection point can be up to 2 to 3 cm in diameter.

BOTOX Cosmetic Injection Site Record

Patient Name:_____
Chart#/Ident.:_____

<u>Notes</u>

		Area 1	Area 2	Area 3	Area 4
Location					
Botox Lot Number					
Botox Expiration Date					
Treatment Date					
	Dilution (cc)				
	Units/0.1 cc				
Total Units/Site					
	Site A				
	Site B				
	Site C				
	Site D				
Total Units Used					

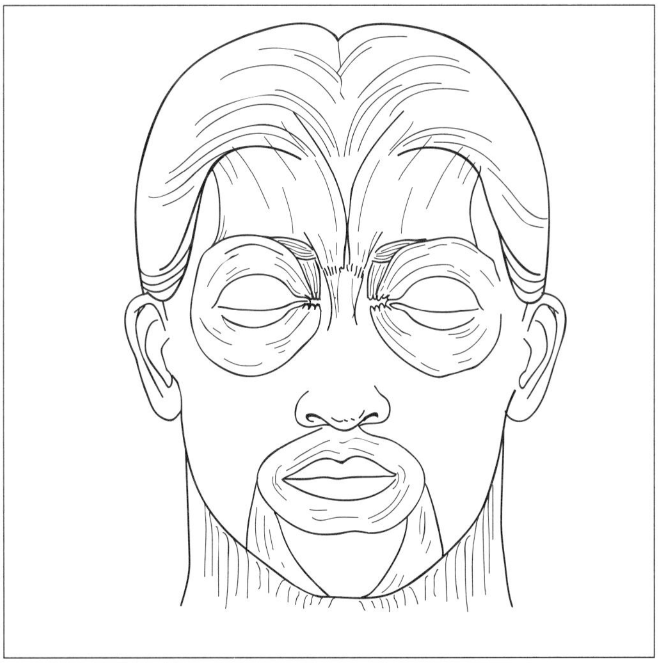

Fig. 48-1
Sample record of injection sites.

Patient Education

Before injection, the patient should review and sign the informed consent. They should appreciate that the treatment produces temporary results and that some wrinkles may not be totally eradicated. Efficacy and duration of action vary from patient to patient, but both generally increase with serial injections as a result of muscle atrophy.

Caution the patient against prior use of aspirin, large doses of vitamin E, garlic, and diet pills, which increase the risk of bruising. Cosmetics covering treatment areas can be removed just before injection and reapplied immediately after, provided the patient *does not rub the treatment areas afterward*. Rubbing the treatment areas can spread the Botox into areas not intended for treatment, increasing the risk of complications such as ptosis.

TECHNIQUE

Cosmetic Uses

Botox has been used to treat *forehead wrinkles* caused by frontalis muscle contraction; *glabellar (frown) lines* and ridges across the *bridge of the nose* caused principally by corrugator and procerus contraction; lateral *"crow's-feet"* and *inferior eyelid wrinkles* from orbicularis oculi tension; *lipstick lines* from orbicularis oris contraction; *chin clefting* from overactive mentalis muscles; depressed lateral commissures from overactive depressor anguli, and even *neck bands* from overactive platysma (Fig. 48-2). Treatment of any site starts with appropriate patient education and consent:

- Take pretreatment photos of the patient frowning, smiling, puckering, and with the brows raised for later evaluation of treatment efficacy and duration.
- Cleanse the area to be injected with alcohol and allow to dry completely.
- Topically applied anesthesia (e.g., Betacaine) may be used at injection sites.
- Apply a cold gel pack or glove with ice or water to the proposed injection site to decrease injection discomfort and to cause vasoconstriction.
- After injection, apply a dry 4 × 4 gauze or tissue and ask the patient to hold pressure for a few minutes to reduce bruising.
- Injections are most effective and comfortable when made into the subcutaneous or muscle tissue rather than at the level of the periosteum or intradermally.

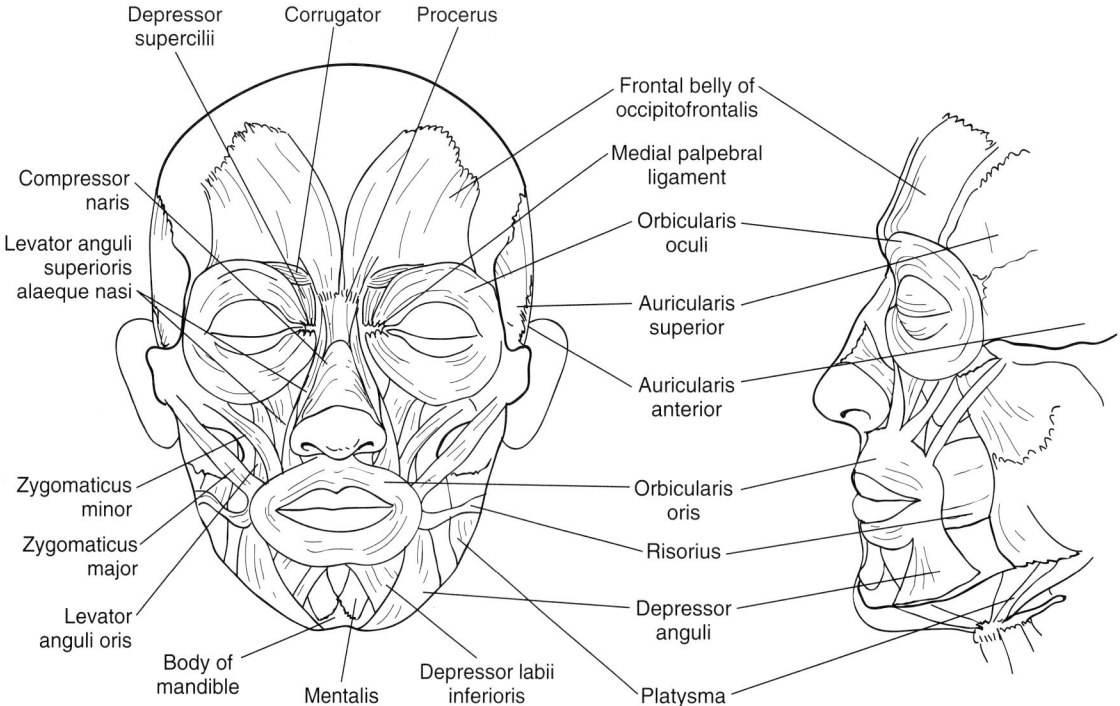

Fig. 48-2
Anatomy of the face with muscles noted.

Note: If the patient has a history of becoming vasovagal with injections, lay him or her supine first.

Treatment of Forehead Wrinkles and Frontalis Muscle Contraction Headaches

Horizontal forehead wrinkles and some "stress" headaches are caused by contraction of the frontalis muscle. This muscle usually runs in two bands from the upper margin of the orbits to the scalp. Mid-forehead creases are usually "sympathy" wrinkles, but this area occasionally requires injection as well, which can be performed at the follow-up session if needed.

- Take pretreatment photos of the patient.
- Cleanse the injection sites with alcohol and allow to dry.
- Have the patient raise the eyebrows to delineate the muscles. Keep muscles tensed during the injection.
- Inject a total of 10 to 20 U of Botox *subcutaneously* (Fig. 48-3) into the *ridges* between the wrinkles (furrows) at indicated sites (1.25 to 2.5 U per site). Intramuscular injections tend to bleed more and are more uncomfortable but do not provide any better of a response. Avoid the area between the eyebrows and 1 cm above the superior edge of the orbit lateral to the midpupillary line (or the lowest frontal wrinkle) to decrease the risk of iatrogenic ptosis. Eyebrow or upper lid ptosis can last several weeks before fading.

Treatment of Glabellar Wrinkles (Frown Lines)

Frown lines are mainly caused by the contraction of several muscles; the corrugator runs diagonally from the skin of the medial brow to the bony bridge of the nose. The procerus is a Y-shaped muscle that runs up the bridge of the nose to the forehead, and the orbicularis oculi courses around the orbit of the eye. The depressor supercilii muscle is between them. It adds to the depression of the medial brow. Have the patient frown and scrunch his or her nose to identify the dynamic wrinkles, and inject a total of 12 to 40 U of Botox (Allergan currently recommends at least 20 U) into these areas after each site is cleansed with alcohol, thoroughly dried, and chilled. A 1-ml syringe with a ½-inch, 30-gauge needle works well to precisely instill 2 to 5 U of toxin into each of the five to seven injection sites. The injection sites are as follows (Fig. 48-4):

- *Site 1:* The bridge of the nose at the level of the lower margin of the upper lid with the eye normally open (5 to 6 U; 0.25 to 0.3 ml of 2 U/0.1 ml).
- *Sites 2 and 3:* Directly above *each* medial canthus *at or above* the level of the medial orbital bone (2 to 4 U; 0.1 to 0.2 ml of 2 U/0.1 ml) (injecting below the edge of the orbit may cause lid ptosis).

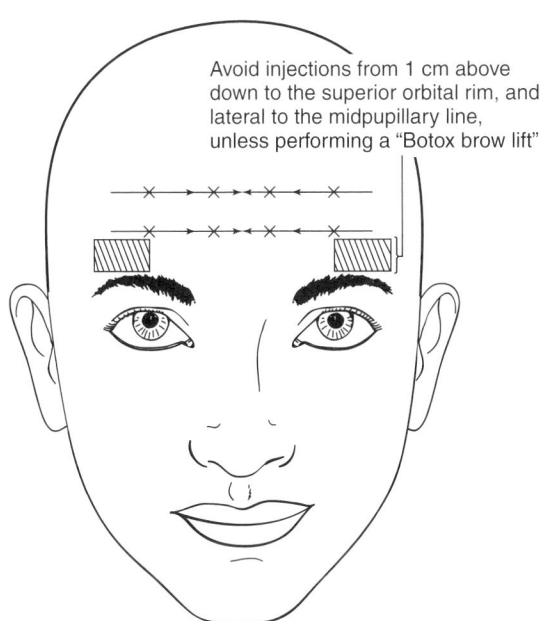

Fig. 48-3
Treatment of frontalis muscle (forehead wrinkles). See text for details.

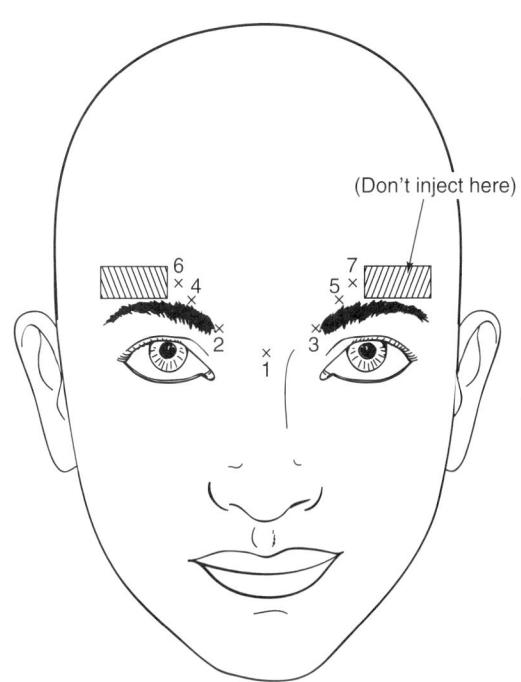

Fig. 48-4
Treatment of frown lines (glabellar muscle). Direct the needle into the bulk of the contracted muscle for corrugator, procerus, and lip injections. All others are directed subcutaneously. See text for details.

- *Sites 4 and 5:* About 1 cm above that and slightly laterally following the direction of the corrugator on each side (2 to 4 U; 0.1 to 0.2 ml of 2 U/0.1 ml); (look for the concavity creating an arrow-shaped valley pointing toward the bridge of the nose on each side).
- *Sites 6 and 7:* About 1 cm above the brow at each midpupillary line, if necessary (2 to 4 U; 0.1 to 0.2 ml) (Fig. 48-4).

An example of Botox dilution for Site 1 is as follows: with Botox at 100 U/vial, add 5 ml of saline.

$$100 \text{ U}/5 \text{ ml} = 20 \text{ U/ml} = 2.0 \text{ U}/0.1 \text{ ml}$$

This could then be drawn into five 1-ml syringes (20 U/syringe).

Variations in muscular anatomy should be appreciated and treated accordingly in terms of dose and injection location. Do not inject below the edge of the orbit, even if the patient has preexisting brow ptosis; this can result in brow and upper lid ptosis (droop).

Treatment of Lateral Orbital Wrinkles (Crow's Feet)

Lateral orbital creases are created by contraction of the orbicularis oculi and photoaging. Photoaging and lateral brow ptosis cause static wrinkles, which may not be removed by Botox injections alone. Therefore, in older patients who have significant photoaging, the object of treatment is to minimize rather than abolish the wrinkles entirely. A total of 4 to 15 U of Botox are injected in a fanlike pattern into two to five sites on each side, running in vertical fashion 1 cm lateral to the edge of the orbit (Fig. 48-5). Injections made too close to the lower lid margin may cause temporary lower eyelid droop or scleral show or may worsen infraorbital festoons. Laser treatments to the static wrinkles complement the use of Botox in this area. Hypertrophic orbicularis oculi under the eyes are treated with 1 to 2 U injected at the inferior orbital edge and massaged across while the patient gazes upward.

Insert the needle from a lateral approach, perpendicular to the skin. Start superiorly and inject 2 to 3 U of Botox into each furrow (two to five wrinkles) by partially withdrawing the needle and reangling it into the next furrow. Alternatively, make one insertion centrally, inject, withdraw until the bevel is just under the skin, and reposition to inject sites above or below.

Botox "Brow Lift"

The Botox "brow lift" relaxes the lateral brow depressors and medial aspect or corrugator so that the action of the frontalis is unopposed. Inject 3 to 5 U of Botox at or above the lateral orbit into the brow where you feel the suture line between the frontal and temporal bones on each side. Then inject 3 to 5 U into the corrugator above the medial canthus on each side. Do not inject frontalis, or little effect will be achieved.

Treatment of Perioral Lines

Contraction of the orbicularis oris can cause vertical lines through and above the vermilion margin, which worsen with smoking and photoaging. Careful injection of 1 to 2 U of Botox into the valley of the wrinkle at one or two sites per side into the orbicularis oris muscle helps alleviate contraction (Fig. 48-6). This helps decrease a "gummy" smile in select patients, but they must be warned about the risk of temporary lip droop, which leads to drooling, or lessened or asymmetric smiles.

After injections, have the patient remain vertical for 2 to 4 hours and avoid rubbing the injection sites to decrease the risk of migration of the toxin to adjacent muscles.

Treatment of Depressed Commissures

Inject 3 to 5 U of Botox along the margin of the jaw directly below each corner of the mouth. Check results in 2 weeks. Reinforce with further injections if needed.

Treatment of Wrinkle ("Walnut") Chin

Inject 5 U of Botox centrally into the lower part of the chin. Too high of an injection can cause lower lip droop. Check results in 2 weeks. Reinforce with further Botox as needed.

Treatment of Focal Hyperhydrosis

Excessive sweat production of the hands and armpits are common conditions that are often treated with topical applications of aluminum salts, iontophoresis, and local and systemic anticholinergic medications. When such treatments fail or give unacceptable side effects, several small trials have shown that Botox injections may inhibit sweating for 1 to 8 months without muscle weakness or other side effects. The exact mechanism of action is not well documented at this time. Clinicians are referred to the bibliography for further details on this subject.

COMPLICATIONS

- Ptosis of the upper eyelid
- Temporary discomfort
- Swelling
- Bruising

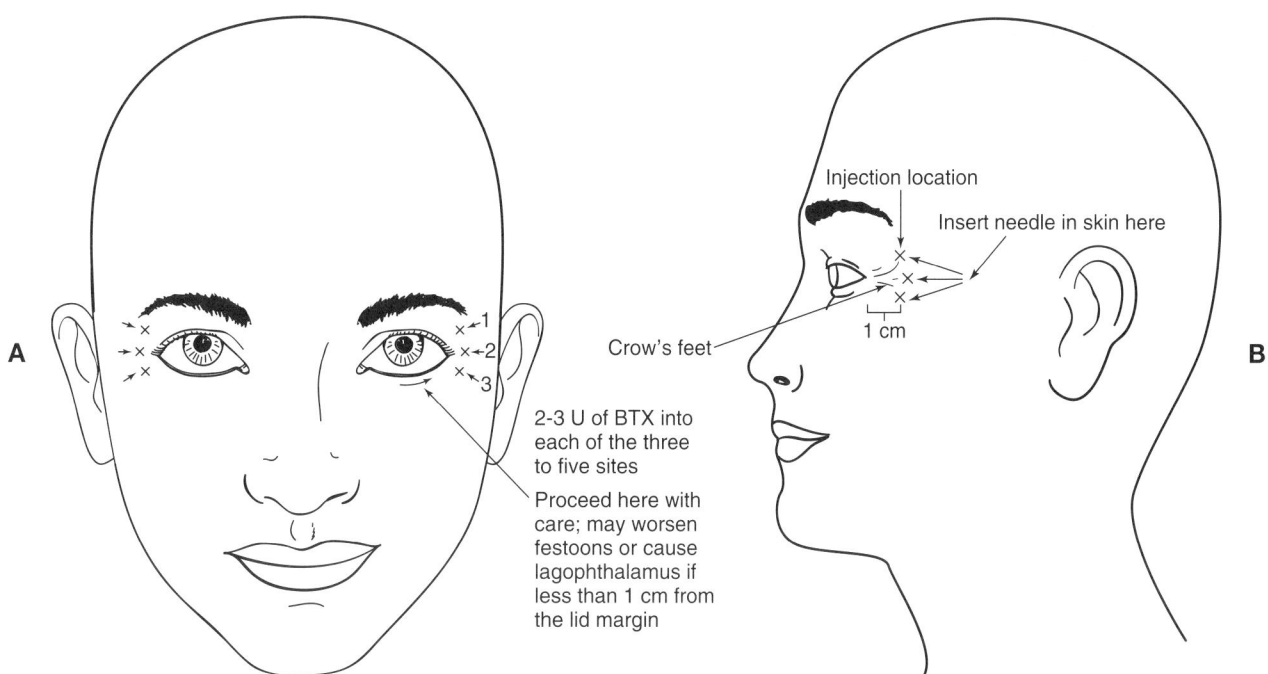

Fig. 48-5
Treatment of lateral orbital wrinkles (crow's feet). In this case, three crow's feet wrinkles are treated with three injections. **A,** Frontal view. **B,** Lateral view.

- Lip droop and drooling
- Temporary facial asymmetry
- Dry mouth (reported after Myobloc injections)

There have been no long-term adverse effects or health hazards related to the use of Botox. Little if any allergy or hypersensitivity has been documented. Repetitive doses of greater than 300 U may lead to blocking antibodies making the patient resistant to further treatment. However, it is rare that more than 40 to 100 U of Botox are used at any one time for cosmetic uses or greater than 200 U used at one sitting for the treatment of hyperhydrosis. Ptosis of the upper eyelid is infrequent (1% to 2%). This temporary side effect of Botox injection that can be treated with apraclonidine 0.5% (Iopidine, Alcon) ophthalmic drops (2 drops tid to affected eyes). Some patients find injections uncomfortable, which can be minimized by the use of topical anesthetic or ice before injection. The risk of bruising and swelling at injection sites is minimized by preinjection chilling and postinjection direct pressure, as described previously. Aspirin and other antiplatelet medications should be avoided for 2 weeks before treatment if possible. Keep injection volumes low. **Do not inject below or less than 1 cm above the superior orbital margin lateral to the midpupillary line in order to prevent brow and upper-lid ptosis.**

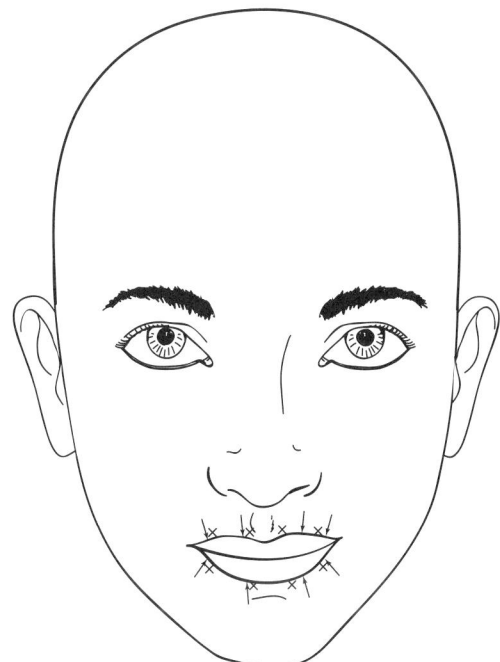

Fig. 48-6
Treatment of perioral lines. Inject up to 2 U of botulinum toxin into each valley caused by orbicularis oris contraction.

POSTPROCEDURE PATIENT EDUCATION

It is important that the patient understands that Botox may not entirely alleviate all dynamic wrinkles every time and that the results of the treatment are temporary. Most patients achieve a 60% to 90% improvement 3 to 14 days after their injections. Recheck the patient in about 2 weeks. Review the preinjection photographs, and reinject the areas that have not responded satisfactorily. If an area is still resistant, EMG-guided injection should be considered. Otherwise the patient may be resistant to the effect of Botox.

CONCLUSION

Botulinum toxin has been used safely in humans since 1984. The FDA has now approved Botox for cosmetic uses, which is a logical extension of the previous FDA-approved uses. Botox has been demonstrated to be a safe and effective therapy in a number of studies. It is well accepted in the medical community as a valuable adjunct for the treatment of dynamic wrinkles of the face and neck, control of frontal or muscle contraction headaches, and treatment of hyperhydrosis. The effects of the injections generally last from 3 to 5 months and then fade gradually.

SUPPLIERS

Betacaine LA and Betacaine Plus
Medical Center Pharmacy
4600 North Habana Avenue
Tampa, FL 33614
Phone: 1-800-226-7094

Botox (and information on it)
Allergan, Inc.
2525 Dupont Drive
P.O. Box 19534
Irvine, CA 92623-9534
Phone: 1-800-433-8871
    1-800-44BOTOX (for information on off-label uses, storage and handling, reconstitution, injection site information, and package inserts)
    1-800-BOTOXMD (physician and consumer information)
Website: www.allergan.com
    www.botoxcosmetic.net (physician and consumer information)
    www.facialenhance.org (CME accredited website; injection techniques)

Teaching Videos for Clinicians and Patients
Bernsco Surgical Supply, Inc. (now a subsidiary of George Tiemann & Co.)
4055 23rd Avenue W
Seattle, WA 98199-1208
Phone: 1-800-231-8409
Website: www.bernsco.com
Bernsco supplies two VHS videos narrated by John Arlette, MD: a 3½-minute one for patient information and a 20-minute one for physician training

Dr. Auster and Jean Carruthers, MD, offer a new set of videos at their website: www.carruthers.net.

Customizable patient education brochures
Contemporary Health Communications
167 Lamp and Lantern Village, Suite 291
Chesterfield, MO 63017
Phone: 1-800-234-1742

MJD Patient Communications
7605 Leesburg Drive
Bethesda, MD 20817
Phone: 1-800-326-4869
Website: www.mjdpc.com

George Tiemann and Co.
25 Plant Avenue
Hauppauge, NY 11788-3804
Phone: 1-800-843-6266
Website: www.georgetiemann.com

ADDITIONAL RESOURCES

- See the sample patient education handout titled "Botox Injections: Cosmetic Denervation of Frown, Forehead, and Eye Expression Lines" on page 1784 of Appendix G.
- See the sample patient consent form titled "Botulinum Toxin Type A (Botox Cosmetic)" on page 1786 of Appendix G.

BIBLIOGRAPHY

Arndt KA, LeBoit PE, Robinson JK, Wintroub BU: Botox, *Sem Cutan Med Surg* 20(2):69, 2001.

Binder WJ, Blitzer A, Brin MF: Treatment of hyperfunctional lines of the face with botulinum toxin A, *Dermatol Surg* 24(11):1198, 1998.

Botulinum toxin (Botox Cosmetic) for frown lines, *Med Lett Drugs Ther* 44:47, 2002.

Carruthers A, Carruthers J: Cosmetic uses of botulinum A exotoxin, *Adv Dermatol* 12:325, 1997.

Carruthers A, Carruthers J: Clinical indications and injection technique for the cosmetic use of botulinum A exotoxin, *Dermatol Surg* 24(11):1189, 1998.

Draelos ZD: Performing a dermatologic cosmetic office examination. In Merli GJ: *The clinics atlas of office procedures: basic cosmetic procedures,* Philadelphia, 2000, WB Saunders.

Flynn TC, Carruthers JA, Carruthers JA: Botulinum-A toxin treatment of the lower eyelid improves infraorbital rhytides and widens the eye, *Am Soc Dermatol Surg* 27:703, 2001.

Foster JA, Wule AE: Cosmetic use of botulinum A toxin, *Facial Plast Surg Clin North Am* 6(1):79, 1998.

Garcia A, Fulton JE: Cosmetic denervation of the muscles of facial expression with botulinum toxin: a dose-response study, *Dermatol Surg* 22:39, 1996.

Glogau RG: Botulinum A neurotoxin for axillary hyperhidrosis, *Dermatol Surg* 24(11):817, 1998.

Kaminer MS, Hruza GJ: Botulinum A exotoxin injections for photoaging and hyperhidrosis. In Kaminer MS, Dover JS, Arndt KA, editors: *Atlas of cosmetic surgery,* Philadelphia, 2002, WB Saunders.

Klein AW: Botulinum toxin and collagen for the aging face, *Cosmet Dermatol* August:23, 1998.

Kaminer MS, Hruza GJ: Botulinum A exotoxin injections for photoaging and hyperhidrosis. In Kaminer MS, Dover JS, Arndt KA, editors: *Atlas of cosmetic surgery,* Philadelphia, 2002, WB Saunders.

Naver H, Aquilonius SM: The treatment of focal hyperhidrosis with botulinum toxin, *Eur J Neurol* 4(Suppl 2):S75, 1997.

Note: The entire November 1998 issue of *Dermatologic Surgery* is devoted to Botox.

CHAPTER 49

Collagen Injections

Colin Elliott

Collagen has been used for soft tissue augmentation since the early 1980s. Its simplicity, ease of use, and excellent results make it ideal for small procedures. Collagen's main drawback is its short life. In addition, a small percentage (3%) may be allergic to bovine collagen. Thus preprocedure testing is mandatory.

Three types of Collagen Replacement Therapy® (CRT) are currently in use, and they differ in their concentrations of collagen and the processing of material. All three use pepsin digestion to decrease anti-genicity of bovine collagen. Zyderm® 1 and 2 contain 35 and 65 mg/ml, respectively, of type I (95%) and type III (5%) collagen. They are injected into the papillary dermis. Zyplast® has the same concentration as Zyderm 1 but has been cross-linked with glutaraldehyde for more stability. It is injected into the deeper reticular dermis. A "Collagen Public Meeting" held by the Food and Drug Administration (1991) found no biologic or statistical evidence of increased risk of connective tissue disease in these patients receiving collagen.

INDICATIONS

There are 10 to 12 sites on the face that can be treated with collagen. The indication is basically cosmetic. It can also be used to diminish pitting from acne or other scars. Different anatomic areas require different products, have varied durations of effect, and necessitate different methods for injection (especially the vermilion border of the lip). An injection into a relatively immobile area such as an acne scar will last much longer than one in the nasolabial line. An overview of the application site, duration of correction, type of collagen, etc., is given in Table 49-1. Figs. 49-1 to 49-5 show a variety of anatomic areas before and after collagen replacement.

CONTRAINDICATIONS

A thorough medical history is important for patient selection. Fig. 49-6 shows an initial encounter form that can be used to discuss any issues with the patient.

Absolute Contraindications

- Allergy to bovine collagen products.
- Previous anaphylactic response.
- Multiple drug/food allergies.
- Zyplast for frown lines and crow's feet.

TABLE 49-1

Overview of Collagen Injection

Site	Agent(s)	Duration (mo)	Typical Amounts Used (ml)	Filling
Frown/glabellar lines	Zyplast	6-8	<0.5	Overcorrect 150%
Acne scar	Zyplast	8-12	<0.5	Little or none
Cheek depression	Zyplast	8-12	<0.5	Little or none
Vertical lip lines	Zyderm I & II	6	<0.5	Overcorrect 150%
Perioral lines				
Marionette lines	Zyplast; Zyderm I	4-6	1.0 on each side	Little or none
Forehead lines			<0.5	
Worry lines	Zyderm I & II	4-6	<0.5	Overcorrect 150%
Deep smile lines	Zyplast	4	<0.5	Little or none
Smile lines	Zyplast; layered with Zyderm I	4-6	<0.5	Little or none
Periorbital lines			<0.5	Do not inject inside orbital rim
Crow's feet	Zyderm I	4-6	<0.5	Little or none

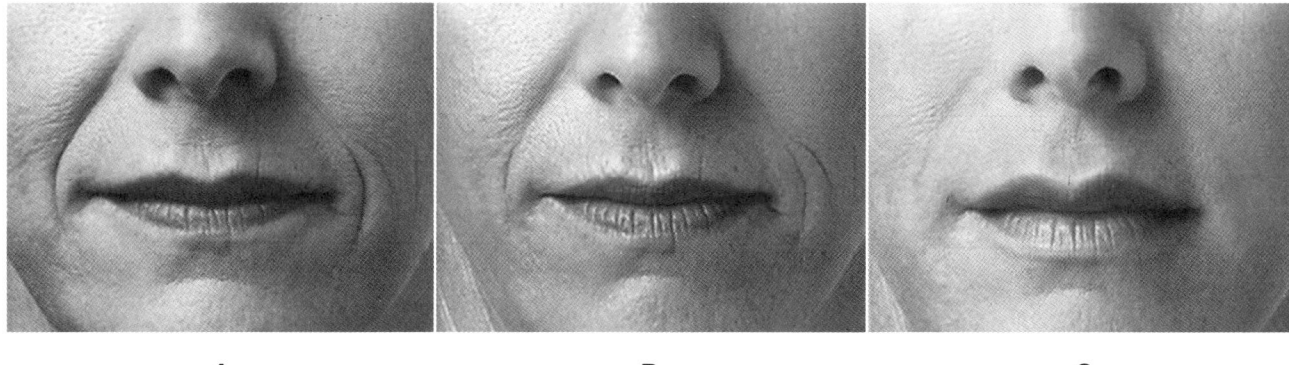

A   B   C

Fig. 49-1
Marionette lines. **A,** Before collagen replacement. **B,** Partial treatment (after 1.5 ml). **C,** After treatment (3 ml). (Courtesy Inamed Aesthetics, Santa Barbara, Calif.)

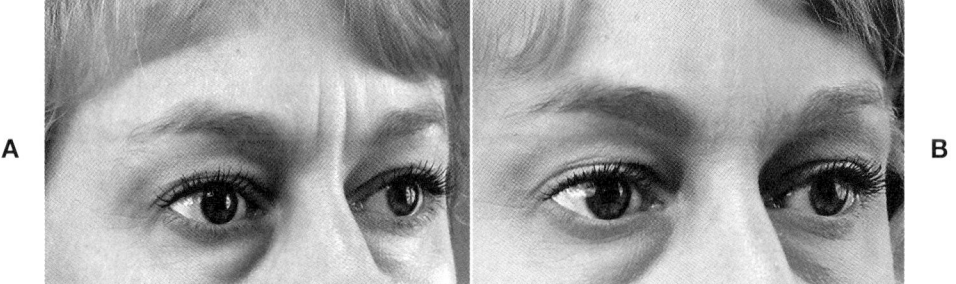

A   B

Fig. 49-2
Frown lines. **A,** Before and, **B,** after collagen replacement. (Courtesy Inamed Aesthetics, Santa Barbara, Calif.)

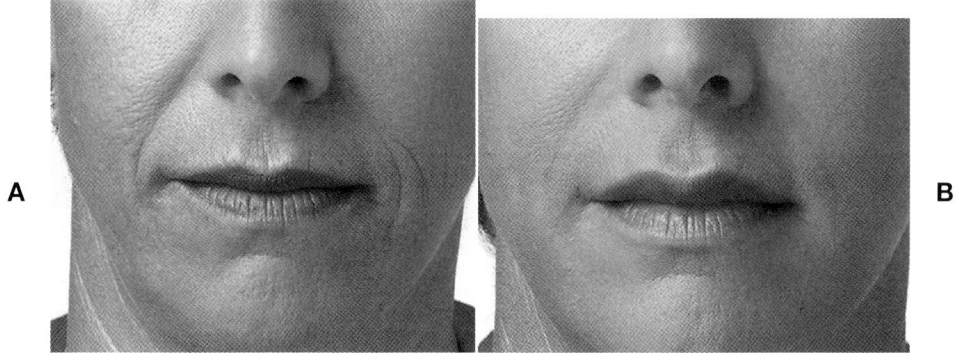

A   B

Fig. 49-3
Lip edges. **A,** Before and, **B,** after collagen replacement. (Courtesy Inamed Aesthetics, Santa Barbara, Calif.)

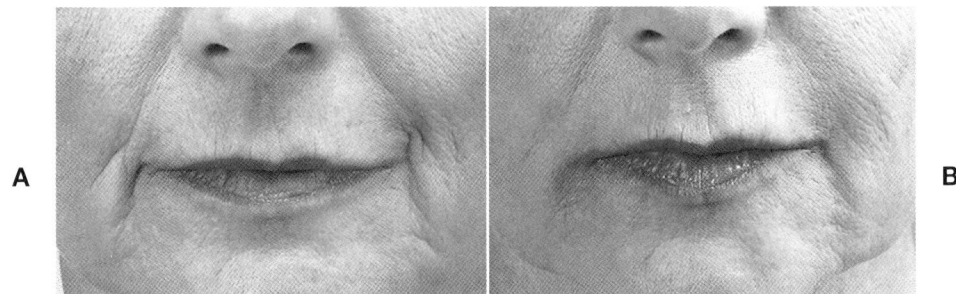

Fig. 49-4
Marionette lines. **A,** Before and, **B,** after collagen replacement. (Courtesy Inamed Aesthetics, Santa Barbara, Calif.)

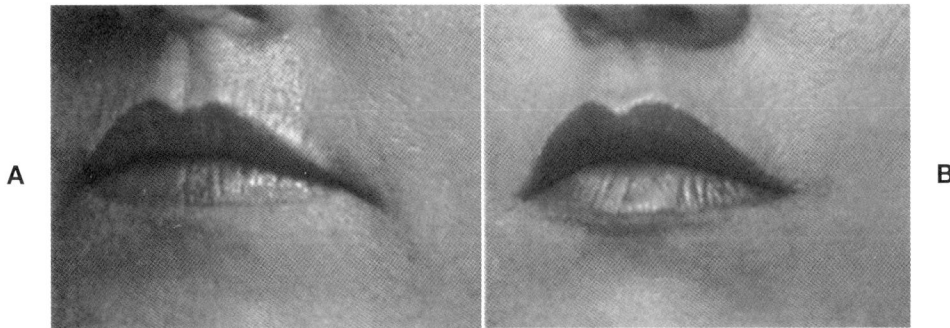

Fig. 49-5
Vermillion border of the lip. **A,** Before and, **B,** after collagen replacement. (Courtesy Inamed Aesthetics, Santa Barbara, Calif.)

Initial Encounter Form

Skin is your body's largest and most visible organ. Your skin is composed of two layers. The uppermost layer of skin, the epidermis, acts as a protective barrier. The epidermis regulates loss of water from cells and tissues. Beneath the epidermis is the dermis, which is composed primarily of a protein called collagen. Collagen forms a network of fibers with two purposes: (1) it provides a framework for the growth of cells and blood vessels, and (2) it is a support structure for the skin.

Lines appear on skin as you get older. Younger skin is elastic and moist because the collagen framework is intact. The skin is also resilient, so that a smile or frown disappears when you stop smiling or frowning. With age, that framework weakens and causes skin to lose its elasticity. Facial lines no longer disappear after a smile or frown because older skin is less resilient.

1. Do you understand that collagen injections cause only temporary changes?   Y   N
2. Do you have or have you ever had a diagnosis of an autoimmune disease such as systemic lupus, rheumatoid arthritis, or collagen vascular disease?   Y   N
3. Have you ever had an allergic/anaphylactic reaction?   Y   N
4. Are you allergic to bovine collagen products? (This is not the same as a lactose deficiency.)   Y   N
5. Do you have multiple drug/food allergies?   Y   N
6. Are you allergic to any local anesthetics (e.g., novocaine)?   Y   N

Fig. 49-6
Sample initial encounter form.

- Zyderm 1 for periocular injection.
- Zyderm collagen implant therapy must not be initiated if the patient has an untoward response to the required test implantation.
- Zyderm collagen implant must not be used in patients with severe allergies manifested by a history of anaphylaxis or history or presence of multiple severe allergies.
- Zyderm collagen implant contains lidocaine and must not be used in patients with known lidocaine hypersensitivity.
- Zyderm collagen implant must not be used in patients with a history of allergies to any bovine collagen product, including but not limited to collagen injectables, collagen implants, hemostatic sponges, and collagen-based sutures, because these patients are likely to have hypersensitivity to Zyderm collagen implant.
- Zyderm collagen implant must not be used in patients undergoing or planning to undergo desensitization injections to meat products, as these injections can contain bovine allergan.
- Zyderm collagen implant is contraindicated for use in breast augmentation, and for implantation into bone, tendon, ligament, or muscle.

Relative Contraindications*

- Rheumatoid arthritis, systemic lupus erythematosus, and other collagen-vascular disorders
- Psoriasis
- Undergoing desensitization to meat products

EQUIPMENT AND MATERIALS

- Zyderm 1: various-sized syringes and assist devices (collar)
- Zyderm 2: various-sized syringes and assist devices (collar)
- Zyplast
- Zyderm collagen implant test syringe (0.1 ml)
- Alcohol wipes
- Fine gauge needles (30 gauge)
- Adjustable depth gauge needles (ADG® needle)
- Topical anesthetic *(optional)*
- Oral benzodiazepam *(optional)*

The material comes premixed (including the lidocaine in the collagen) and must be refrigerated. It has a shelf-life of 2 to 3 years. A starter pack is recommended for first-time users.

PREPROCEDURE
PATIENT PREPARATION

Inamed Aesthetics (previously McGhan Medical) provides a brochure and consent form. The patient must understand that the effects are not permanent and must have a realistic expectation for the duration of the change accomplished. Touch-ups may be needed near the end of the expected duration of correction.

After verifying no contraindications exist, a 0.1-ml test dose is injected intradermally into a test site (four finger breadths proximal to the flexural crease in the nondominant hand or behind the ear near the hairline). The area should be monitored over the 4-week waiting period for a positive response—defined as erythema of any degree, induration, tenderness, or swelling at the test site with or without pruritus that persists more than 6 hours and appears more than 24 hours after the test implantation. It is advisable to perform a second test to further decrease the possibility of adverse events in those patients at higher risk of a reaction. Even so, adverse events have occurred in a small fraction (1% to 2%) of patients receiving CRT.

TECHNIQUE

1. Have the patient sit upright or slightly reclined so gravitational effects are normalized. Decide what areas are to be corrected, what type(s) of collagen is (are) to be used, and whether a full or partial correction is desired. For example, a full correction in the nasolabial furrow of an older patient may look artificial. The patient may be better served with a partial correction, especially on the first visit.

2. Most areas use the serial (multiple) puncture technique (Fig. 49-7). For Zyderm 1 and 2, the angle of insertion is about 10 to 25 degrees and the insertion depth is about 1 mm (into the papillary dermis). An immediate blanch will be observed with proper placement. If no blanch is seen, withdraw completely and reinsert. Partial withdrawal simply lets the injectant escape below the proper plane thus wasting material. The Zyderm products are used for shallow defects such as crow's feet and periorbital lines. Deeper impressions are best corrected by a layered approach in which Zyplast is injected first for foundation, overlaid by Zyderm 1 or 2.

3. Although lidocaine is premixed with the collagen, a useful method to decrease injection pain is to cover the area with an ice water–filled glove for cryoanesthesia. (See Chapter 11, Topical Anesthesia.) Even so, some patients may require local anesthetic in very sensitive areas (nasolabial folds, vermilion border). If a local is administered, use a 1¼-inch needle to place

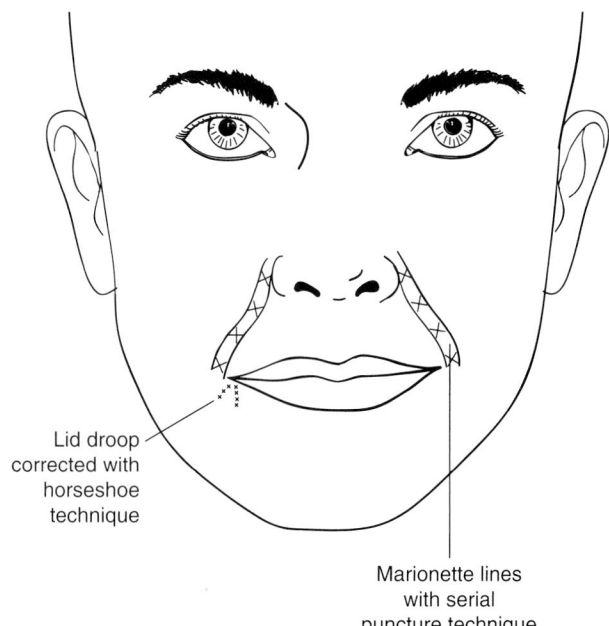

Lid droop corrected with horseshoe technique

Marionette lines with serial puncture technique

Fig. 49-7
Collagen injection sites. The *Xs* represent injection sites.

a line parallel to the surface, near the line of correction. Little if any epinephrine should be in the local, otherwise a camouflaging blanch would be seen making it impossible to identify when enough collagen has been injected. Because of Zyderm's greater lability (and water content), areas treated with Zyderm 1 and 2 (except crow's feet) should be overcorrected by 200% and 150%, respectively.

4. Inject Zyplast into deeper (reticular) dermis at a 45-degree angle. Zyplast placed too superficially can cause a beaded appearance, which can be partially corrected by massaging the area. Areas solely injected with Zyplast, such as the vermilion border of the lip, should have little or no overcorrection. This is also the only area where a threading technique is generally used. A longer needle is injected parallel to the lip edge and the injectant is placed as the needle is withdrawn. A horseshoe pattern of Zyplast provides very good structural support for lid droop (Fig. 49-7).

COMPLICATIONS

Complications include occasional superficial bruising, rare hypersensitizations (urticaria and erythema) that occur following unrecognized or unreported positive skin tests, and one case of blindness.

Local necrosis is a rare event that has been observed after collagen implantation. Most necroses reported through post-marketing surveillance have occurred in the glabella. It is thought to result from the injury, obstruction, or compromise of blood vessels. Zyplast collagen implant is more often injected deeper into the dermis closer to the local vascular supply than is Zyderm collagen implant. In addition, Zyplast collagen implant does not undergo synthesis after injection. Therefore interruption of the local blood supply may occur more likely with Zyplast collagen implant. It is recommended that correction in the glabellar region be performed using Zyderm collagen implant rather than Zyplast collagen implant.

No sloughing of skin nor any infection has been reported. Overcorrection corrects itself with time; undercorrection requires a touch-up of an area.

POSTPROCEDURE PATIENT EDUCATION

- Moisturizer with sun screen
- Retin-A
- Smoking cessation
- Regularly scheduled touch-ups (two to four times per year after a good initial foundation)

CRT is an effective, simple way of correcting some skin damage and age effects. With an adequate history and pretesting, it provides a quick, effective, and patient-friendly way of helping patients look their best.

CPT/BILLING AND ICD-9-CM DIAGNOSTIC CODES

There are no pertinent CPT or ICD-9 codes. Collagen injection is essentially always a cosmetic procedure.

SUPPLIERS

Inamed Aesthetics (formerly McGhan Medical)
5540 Ekwill Street
Santa Barbara, CA 93111
Phone: 1-800-766-0171
Website: www.inamedaesthetics.com

ADDITIONAL RESOURCES

- See the sample patient education handout titled "Collagen Replacement Therapy" on page 1789 of Appendix G.

BIBLIOGRAPHY

Alster TS, West TB: Human-derived and new synthetic injectable materials for soft-tissue augmentation: current status and role in cosmetic surgery, *Plast Reconstr Surg* 105(7):2515, 2000.

Fagien S: Autologous collagen injections to treat deep glabellar furrows, *Plast Reconstr Surg* 93(3):642, 1994.

Fagien S: Facial soft-tissue augmentation with injectable autologous and allogeneic human tissue collagen matrix (autologen and dermalogen), *Plast Reconstr Surg* 105(1):362, 2000.

Hanke CW, Higley HR, Jolivette DM, et al: Abscess formation and local necrosis after treatment with Zyderm or Zyplast collagen implant, *J Am Acad Dermatol* 25:319, 1991.

Klein AW: Skin filling: collagen and other injectables of the skin, *Dermatol Clin* 19(3):491, 2001.

Maas CS, Papel ID, Greene D, Stoker DA: Complications of injectable synthetic polymers in facial augmentation, *Dermatol Surg* 23(10):871, 1997.

Melton J, Hanke CW: Soft tissue augmentation: new techniques and recent controversies. In Roenik RK, Roenik HR: *Surgical dermatology*, St Louis, 1993, Mosby.

Robinson JK, Hanke CW: Injectable collagen implant: histopathologic identification and longevity of correction, *J Dermatol Surg Oncol* 11(2):124, 1985.

WEBSITE

www.inamed.com

CHAPTER 50

Dermasanding (Manual Dermabrasion)

Theodore X. O'Connell

Manual dermabrasion is a technique that has been used to treat a variety of problems, including acne scars, hypertrophic and traumatic scars, and skin with actinic damage. Although motor-driven dermabrasion has been more widely used, studied, and publicized than manual dermabrasion, it requires a significant amount of training and skill. For certain indications, motor-driven dermabrasion may also be more of an intervention than is needed. For other indications, results are not always superior to manual dermabrasion, also known as dermasanding. In addition, since motor-driven dermabrasion is a more aggressive procedure, it has a higher risk of complications (e.g., it frequently produces sharp lines of demarcation) than dermasanding. The splatter associated with motor-driven devices also increases the risk of transmitting infectious diseases.

With proper supervision, dermasanding is easily mastered and, if used carefully, only lightly abrades the skin. When healed, the area that has been abraded blends in softly with the surrounding skin. Dermasanding is excellent for the correction of scars, especially new ones. Superficial, sharply demarcated scars are often completely removed (Fig. 50-1). Uneven scars or saucerlike depressions can also usually be improved, if not eliminated completely. Deeper scars may require scar revision, excision, or punch elevation before the procedure is performed; however, following proper preparation, deeper scars also usually respond well to dermasanding.

INDICATIONS

- Hypertrophic scars (see Chapter 39, Hypertrophic Scars and Keloids)
- Traumatic scars
- Acne scars
- Skin with actinic damage
- Dyschromia

Note: Scars from excisional surgery or trauma heal best when they are dermasanded 6 to 8 weeks after sutures are removed. In general, older wounds do not respond as well to dermasanding unless they are reexcised and then dermasanded.

CONTRAINDICATIONS

- History of abnormal wound healing
- History of keloids or severe hypertrophic scarring
- Treatment with isotretinoin (Accutane) within the last year
- Treatment with a topical retinoid (e.g., Retin-A) for more than a month in the last year
- Active infection (herpes simplex, human papilloma virus, cellulitis, acute acne pustule)
- Burn scars
- Possible melanoma or squamous cell carcinoma in region to be treated
- Xeroderma pigmentosum
- Pyoderma
- Psychosis or significant psychoneurosis
- Alcoholism
- Poorly controlled diabetes mellitus

Note: Patients with a history of herpes simplex (cold sores or fever blisters) should be approached with caution. Avoid dermabrasion in areas of frequent recurrence. For patients with

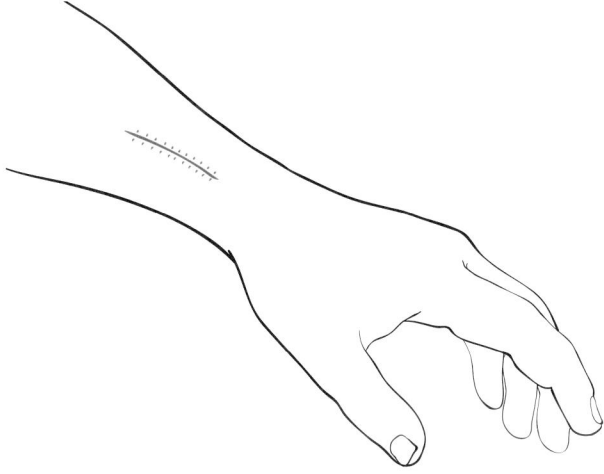

Fig. 50-1
Linear scar. This is an excellent example for use as a trial for the patient; it can be covered by clothing until the erythema resolves, which may take 3 or 4 months.

frequent recurrence, appropriate oral antiviral medications should be given prophylactically for 3 days before the procedure and continued until the skin has healed.

PREPROCEDURE PATIENT PREPARATION

Emphasize to the patient that improvement is expected, but do not promise to completely eliminate scars. They should also be aware that whenever the skin is wounded, there is a risk of further scarring and infection. There is also a risk of pigmentary augmentation that is both short term, which almost always resolves, and long term. There is a slight risk of permanent pigmentary augmentation. Although rare, persistent hyperpigmentation is often treatable with prescribed bleaching agents. (See the "Complications" section for a formula.)

Patients should be counseled about the other potential complications as outlined below. They should be aware that with dermasanding the effects will be quite obvious to friends and colleagues. (For less dramatic treatments, see Chapter 53, Skin Peels.) Patients should avoid aspirin, nonsteroidal antiinflammatory drugs, and high doses (>400 U) of vitamin E for 2 weeks before the procedure.

The patient's emotional stability must be carefully assessed during the initial consultation. If there is any question about the patient's stability, consultation from a psychiatrist is recommended, just as it would be before any cosmetic procedure. Informed consent should be carefully obtained and documented in writing.

EQUIPMENT

- Silicone carbide paper (320 or 400 grit, 400 to 600 grit) cut into 2 × 3–inch pieces and autoclaved. Attachments used for microdermabrasion (fraises) can often be used as a handheld device for dermasanding. Special handles are made for this purpose. In addition, fine mesh metal screens with abrasives attached are available.

Editor's Note: To our knowledge, none of this equipment has been approved by the Food and Drug Administration for this application. However, in the majority of the literature regarding dermasanding, clinicians used over-the-counter silicon carbide sandpaper.

- Povidone-iodine (Betadine) or chlorhexidine (Hibiclens)
- Alcohol swabs

- Gentian violet skin marker
- Sterile gauze and three pairs of sterile gloves
- 5-ml syringe or rolled gauze to wrap sandpaper around
- 5-ml syringe for anesthesia
- 30-gauge needle
- 1% lidocaine with epinephrine
- 500 ml of normal saline if tumescent anesthesia is to be used
- Topical antibiotic ointment (bacitracin, Polysporin, or polymyxin)*
- Telfa pads
- Kerlix dressing
- Excellent lighting
- Magnification and goggles or eye protection for the clinician

TECHNIQUE

1. Administer 75 mg Demerol or 60 mg Toradol IM approximately 30 minutes before the procedure. Anxiolytic premedication may be considered in appropriate cases.
2. Clean the skin with povidone-iodine, followed by alcohol wipes. Alternatively, Hibiclens may be used.
3. Preprocedure photography of the affected area is recommended for the purpose of documentation.
4. Mark the area to be sanded with a gentian violet skin marker.
5. Anesthetize the area to be sanded with regional nerve blocks or tumescent anesthesia. (See the following chapters: Chapter 4, Local Anesthesia; Chapter 5, Local and Topical Anesthetic Reactions; Chapter 9, Oral/Facial Anesthesia; and Chapter 11, Topical Anesthesia.)
6. Wear three pair of sterile gloves and make sure that magnification and an excellent light source are available. Wet the silicon carbide paper with Hibiclens or 1% lidocaine with epinephrine. Wrap it around a syringe or rolled gauze (or a comparable abrading instrument), stretch the area of skin to be sanded (Fig. 50-2), and gently abrade the skin. Use both back-and-forth and circular motions.
7. At first, the abrasive will glide over moistened skin. In a short time it will become gritty; the paper can actually be heard scratching the skin. With magnification the glistening skin will turn to a dull, rougher skin. Eventually it will appear beefy and red,

---

*Neomycin and neomycin-containing preparations (Neosporin) should be avoided after the procedure because they may delay reepithelialization. For the same reason, povidone-iodine should not be applied after abrading.

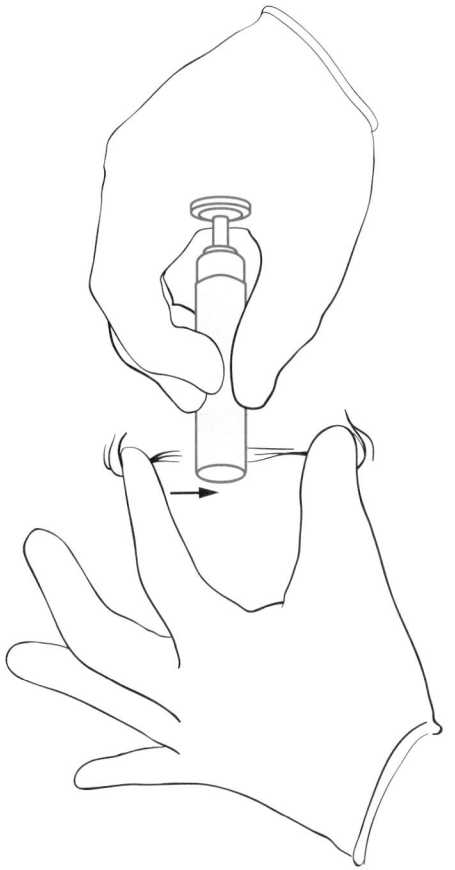

Fig. 50-2
While the clinician applies traction with the nondominant hand, the sandpaper-wrapped instrument is used to gently abrade the skin with back-and-forth, circular motions.

without bleeding. Abrade the skin further and stop when bleeding points appear. Under magnification, bleeding points tend to appear as the tissue begins to fray and the smooth texture of the connective tissue begins to roughen.

8. Under magnification, inspect the entire abraded area. Make sure that the dermabrasion is even and that the appropriate depth has been achieved for the degree of skin involvement.

9. Be careful around the mid-upper lip, especially above the upper lateral incisors on each side. This area is more prone to scarring. Avoid oversanding this area and the use of any pressure from the fingers while sanding.

10. If sanding near the lip, sand right up to the vermilion border; otherwise, an unsightly "ledge" will form. For stubborn, deeper wrinkles, 320 to 400 grit paper should be used.

11. After all areas have been sanded and the stubborn

areas have had repeated sanding, the final sand should be with 400 to 600 grit paper. This should be used to even out the entire area.

12. Inevitably after sanding, some carbide particles will have become attached to the skin. Cleanse these away with Aquanil or Cetaphil and a 4 × 4–inch gauze. Rub the skin firmly but gently for about a minute. Next, coat the affected area with a topical antibiotic ointment (e.g., Bactroban [avoid Neomycin]).

13. The affected area is then covered with Telfa pads and a Kerlix dressing. The goal is to keep the skin moist during the entire healing process.

Note: Clinicians should be very conservative when dermasanding until they obtain considerable experience. Be conservative not only in the choice of patients, but also in the application and depth of dermasanding. Initial supervision by a dermatologist, dermatologic surgeon, or cosmetic surgeon may be prudent.

For patients new to the procedure, it may be prudent to perform it on a very small test area at first. The remainder of the procedure can be performed several days to weeks later. Test an area that can be covered with clothing. Testing lets both the patient and the clinician see how well the procedure is tolerated and whether the initial skin damage is too disfiguring for the patient to tolerate. It also allows the clinician to determine how aggressive they can be.

COMPLICATIONS

- Bleeding
- Infection
- Hyperpigmentation
- Hypopigmentation
- Milia
- Keloid formation
- Hypertrophic scarring
- Persistent erythema

To minimize risk of persistent erythema after the procedure, for Native Americans or patients allergic to parabens (the most common preservative in over-the-counter sunblocks) or perfumes, prescribe oral steroids for 10 to 14 days following the procedure. After oral steroids, use a topical, paraben-free corticosteroid cream until healing is complete. Many dermatologists suspect that hypererythema is the result of a reaction to the preservatives or perfumes in topical treatments as opposed to the procedure. However, preservatives and perfumes may be difficult to avoid, so oral and topical steroids should be considered.

Persistent hyperpigmentation in any patient is often treatable with bleaching agents. Prescribe a compound of 30-g paraben-free corticosteroid cream combined with 15-g 4% hydroquinone. This should be applied daily starting at 4 weeks following the procedure if hyperpigmentation is developing.

Note: Patients with as little as 1/32 Native American heritage may be at increased risk of persistent erythema as well as subsequent hyperpigmentation after dermasanding. Special precautions should be taken to prevent exposure to topical allergens or irritants.

POSTPROCEDURE PATIENT EDUCATION

- Postprocedure care and precautions should be very similar to those for a second-degree burn.
- A mild pain medication may be prescribed to relieve any tingling or throbbing.
- The patient must clean the area several times daily with a soap-free cleanser (e.g., Aquanil, Cetaphil). After cleansing, the antibiotic ointment is reapplied.
- For the first several days, oozing, edema, and crusting of the area will occur. This crust usually sheds within 10 days. At this point, new skin will be apparent, and the patient can return to normal activities while avoiding the sun. After the crust has been shed, most patients note some degree of erythema, which may take up to 3 or 4 months to resolve.
- After dermasanding, the skin is more susceptible to sun damage and sunburn (indefinitely) because it is thinner. Sunburn may occur at lower doses of sunlight and lead to hyperpigmentation or hypopigmentation. A sunblock should be applied every day to avoid sun damage. Preservatives, scents, or any chemicals may provoke a sensitivity reaction and cause persistent erythema; therefore a hypoallergenic, unscented, complete sunblock for sensitive skin should be used.
- Thinner or irritated skin is also more susceptible to dessication, so a moisturizer should be applied daily.
- Patients should be informed about any postprocedure medications (e.g., bleaching agents, oral steroids, or steroid creams) that they will need to use or apply.

SUPPLIERS

Aquanil
Person and Covey Dermatologicals
616 Allen Avenue
Glendale, CA 91221-5018
Phone: 1-800-423-2341

Cetaphil
Galderma Laboratories, L.P.
14501 North Freeway
Fort Worth, TX 76177
Phone: 1-817-961-5000
Website: www.galderma.com

Silicone carbide Wetordry sandpaper
3M Abrasive Systems Division
3M Center, Building 223-6N-01
St. Paul, MN 55144-1000
Phone: 1-800-742-9546
Website: www.3m.com

Norton silicon carbide paper
Norton Construction Products (Construction Products Division, North America)
P.O. Box 2898
Gainesville, GA 30503-2898
Phone: 1-770-967-3954
Website: www.nortonabrasive.com

CPT/BILLING CODES

15780 Dermabrasion, total face (e.g., for acne scarring, fine wrinkling, rhytids, general keratosis)
15781 Segmental, face
15782 Regional, other than face
15783 Superficial, any site (e.g., tattoo removal)
15786 Abrasion, single lesion (e.g., keratosis, scar)
15787 Each additional four lesions or less (list separately in addition to code for primary procedure)

ICD-9-CM DIAGNOSTIC CODES

Although most insurers consider dermasanding a cosmetic procedure, they occasionally reimburse for treatment of acne or actinic keratoses.

706.1 Acne
702.0 Actinic keratosis
709.2 Disfigurement due to scar
709.00 Dyschromia, unspecified
701.4 Hypertrophic scar
709.09 Lentigo
709.3 Senile dermatosis

BIBLIOGRAPHY

Chiarello SE: Tumescent dermasanding with cryospraying: a new wrinkle on the treatment of rhytids, *Dermatol Surg* 22(7):601, 1996.

Chiarello SE: Regarding the use of topical retinoid acid after dermasanding, *Dermatol Surg* 26(2):170, 2000.

Harris DR, Noodleman FR: Combining manual dermasanding with low strength trichloroacetic acid to improve actinically injured skin, *J Dermatol Surg Oncol* 20:436, 1994.

Lawrence N, Mandy S, Yarborough J, Alt T: History of dermabrasion, *Dermatol Surg* 26(2):95, 2000.

Matarasso SL, Hanke CW, Alster TS: Cutaneous resurfacing, *Dermatol Clin* 15(4):569, 1997.

Moschella SL, Hurley HJ, editors: *Dermatology,* Philadelphia, 1985, WB Saunders.

Moy RL, Usatine RP: *Complications and their prevention in skin surgery: a practical guide,* St Louis, 1998, Mosby.

Roenigk RK, Roenigk HH, editors: *Surgical dermatology: advances in current practice,* St Louis, 1993, Mosby.

CHAPTER 51

Laser Hair Removal: Photoepilation

Barry I. Auster

The process of laser hair removal has rapidly evolved in the last 3 years. Numerous Food and Drug Administration (FDA)–approved laser or intense pulsed light (IPL) sources are available for hair removal. The current technology evolved from the clinical observation of hair reduction in laser-treated congenital (pigmented) hairy nevi. Nearly $2 billion a year is spent in the United States on either electrolysis or other methods of hair removal such as epilation, depilatories, or waxing. The potential market for laser hair removal is even larger. This chapter describes the principles of laser photoepilation.

Physician interest in laser hair removal has increased not only because the technology has progressed and the equipment is becoming more affordable (although each machine represents a significant monetary outlay), but also because cosmetic treatments like this are generally on a cash payment basis. Medical insurance billing and the problems with the referral approval process, delayed payments, discounted payments, and nonpayments are all moot points. New sets of problems do arise with adding a cosmetic component to a medical practice, such as determining the market audience and potential market share; advertising ethics, strategies, and costs; obtaining training and experience with the selected equipment; and patient-client expectations (which are based more on satisfying the perceptions of a cash-paying customer than on achieving a desired state of health or, for example, normalizing a blood pressure measurement). Discussion of these topics, which are different in a cosmetic practice compared with a medical practice, is beyond the scope of this chapter. Obtaining professional consultation in marketing and advertising is advised if the practitioner is not already experienced with this type of cosmetic practice.

Initial training and experience with laser devices can be obtained from most companies that sell these devices (at various costs). Conservative claims for efficacy and documenting results with pretreatment and posttreatment photographs can be helpful tools for satisfying client expectations.

PRINCIPLES OF PHOTOEPILATION

Light energy from the laser or an IPL source is absorbed by a pigmented object (in this case, hair) and turned into heat energy. The heat energy destroys the hair follicle and hopefully causes a long-term reduction in hair growth. This process of using light energy to heat and destroy specifically targeted pigmented tissue is called *photothermolysis*.

Melanin is the pigmented object in the hair that preferentially absorbs the light energy and is called a *chromophore*. Hemoglobin is another example of a chromophore that, when targeted, can destroy vascular lesions. Each chromophore has a spectral absorption pattern that determines the wavelengths of light that are most absorbed and converted to thermal energy. Lasers are monochromatic, which means the light is a single wavelength or color. Each type of laser has a different wavelength. It is important to match the wavelength of the laser with the specific chromophore for targeted destruction and to avoid damage to adjacent tissues. For this reason, certain types of laser are more effective at destroying the hair follicles without causing excessive damage to the surrounding tissue, which could lead to burns or scarring.

The lasers used for epilation fall into four categories: Alexandrite (755 nm), Nd:YAG (1064 nm), ruby (694 nm), and diode (810 nm). Spot sizes vary from 2 to 15 mm, and pulse widths vary from 10 to 100 msec. In addition, the repetition rate (in Hertz) varies from 1 to 10 pulses per second. Faster repetition rates improve efficiency in treating large truncal areas such as the back.

The amount of energy needed to destroy the hair follicle is usually not much different from the energy level where damage to the skin occurs. Determining the treatment energy level for a particular patient is generally the most clinically demanding task. Lasers and IPL machines most often measure *fluence*, or the energy level delivered to the skin in joules per square centimeter (J/cm^2). The size of the treatment area (spot size) is variable from machine to machine and from laser tip to laser tip. Generally the larger the spot size, the

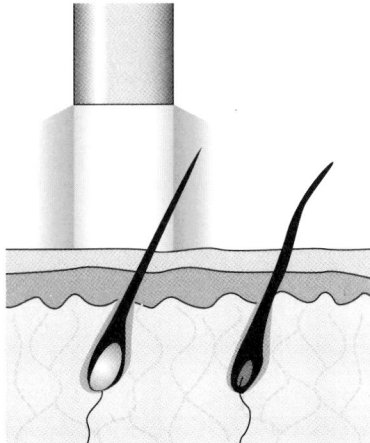

Fig. 51-1
Three principles of selective photothermolysis: (1) Penetrating wavelength of light should be absorbed selectively by target tissue, (2) pulse duration should match thermal relaxation time of target tissue, and (3) sufficient fluence (J/cm²) should be applied to damage target tissue. (Redrawn from Brian Zelicksen, MD, ASLMS Meeting 4/02.)

greater the depth of light penetration at the same energy level.

The concept of selective photothermolysis was first presented by Anderson and Parrish in 1983. This is the process by which thermal damage is confined to the particular target media. It is based on two important factors. The first is that the chromophores are colored bodies that preferentially absorb light of specific wavelengths. The second is thermal relaxation time (TRT), which is defined as the time required for an object to cool to 50% of the temperature resulting from laser exposure. When the target tissue absorbs the laser light, energy is changed to heat, which causes thermal damage. A laser with a pulse width less than the TRT of the target conducts very little heat to the surrounding tissues. Consequently it is possible to confine the laser's destructive effect to a specific area of tissue (e.g., hair follicle, blood vessels, melanosome) (Fig. 51-1).

The IPL source (EpiLight [Fig. 51-2]) is a unique device that emits light over the entire visual spectrum and, therefore, is not coherent like a laser. Specificity for different hair colors and skin types may be achieved with various cutoff filters.

The ideal patient to treat is someone with light skin and dark hair, so all thermal energy is focused on the pigmented area (i.e., the hair).

INDICATIONS

- Hypertrichosis
- Hirsutism
- Cosmetic (e.g., bikini lines)

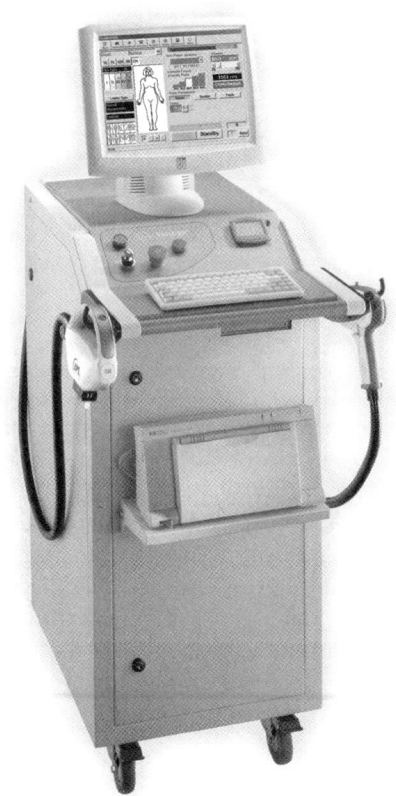

Fig. 51-2
VascuLight Hair Removal System. (Courtesy Lumenis, Inc., Santa Clara, Calif.)

Hypertrichosis (excessive vellus or lanugo hair) may be localized or generalized and may occur in both men and women. It is not related to excess testosterone. Hirsutism involves development of coarse terminal hair in children or women resulting from increased levels of male hormone (e.g., on the face). The most common clinical cause in women is congenital adrenal hyperplasia and polycystic ovaries. Screening serum levels of testosterone and dehydroepiandrosterone sulfate may be indicated, and, if elevated, referral to an endocrinologist may be necessary.

Pseudofolliculitis barbae resulting from ingrowing hairs is improved dramatically by photoepilation. By reducing the number of hairs the severe infection may be significantly diminished and markedly improve the patient's symptoms. Although there may be some pigmentary changes, they may improve over time and the risks may be outweighed by the benefit to the patient's quality of life.

CONTRAINDICATIONS

- History of keloids
- Accutane use in past 6 months
- Herpes simplex (active)
- Photosensitizing medications (St. John's Wort, tetracycline, thiazides, Capoten, etc.)
- Recent plucking, waxing, or electrolysis
- Pregnancy
- White hair
- Recently tanned skin

There are certain relative contraindications to laser phototricholysis: history of keloids, the use of oral isotretinoin (Accutane) within the last 6 months, and active herpes simplex at the treatment site. Individuals with a history of herpes simplex should be treated prophylactically with antivirals. Individuals who have been on Accutane within 6 months tend to have adverse healing and susceptibility to hypertrophic scarring. In addition, patients on photosensitizing medications may be treated, but treatment dosages should be conservative. St. John's Wort is a common herbal medication that is particularly photosensitizing. In addition, because the hair itself provides the major chromophore for the laser, patients may need to avoid waxing, electrolysis, plucking, depilatories, or shaving before treatment. For effective treatment, approximately 1 mm of hair protruding above the skin surface is necessary. For female patients with hypertrichosis who have plucked hair on a daily basis, the latter requirement may be a hardship and the treating physician should be sensitive to this. Between treatments patients are allowed to continue their own hair-removal methods.

SAFETY ISSUES WITH LASER USE

Physicians who use lasers for hair removal should be acutely aware of the potential for ocular damage. All of the devices are Class I (except for the EpiLight, which is Class II) and may cause blindness if accidentally fired through the ocular pupil. Eye protection for both the practitioner and the patient is paramount; many physicians employ technicians to perform laser hair removal, so this must be strongly stressed to the practitioners. The handpiece must be carefully guarded, and those using it should be conscious that it is pointed away from the eyes at all times. Some office practices have assigned the safety duties to one of the clinical personnel (often a nurse). This person is designated the "laser safety officer" and is in charge of ensuring that eye protection is worn by all in the treatment room and that warning signs are posted outside the door when the laser is in operation. The warning sign should be taken

Depth as a Result of Wavelength

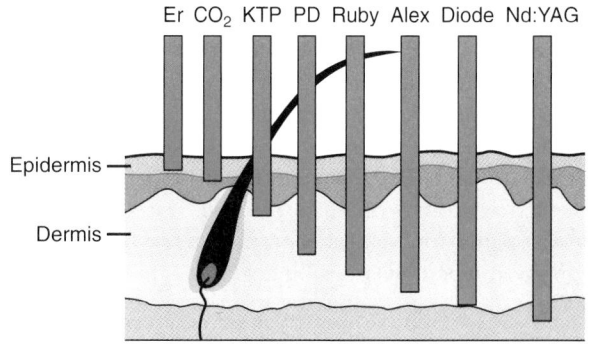

Fig. 51-3
Depth of penetration of various cutaneous lasers.

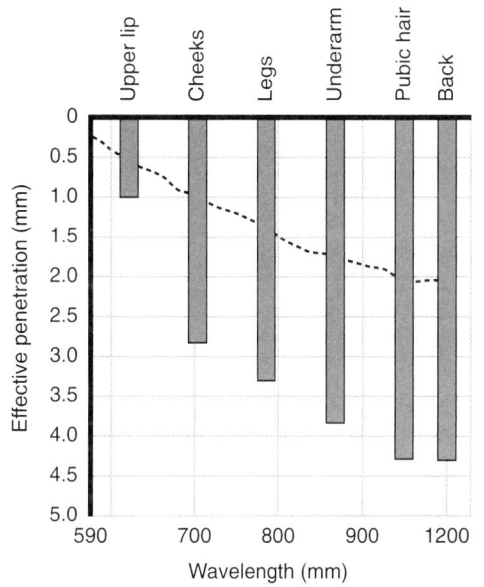

Fig. 51-4
Depth of hair follicles in different body locations.

down when the laser is not in use, or the sign will soon be ignored. (See Chapter 27, Laser Therapy.)

HAIR GROWTH PHASES AND TREATMENT IMPLICATIONS

Intrinsically, hair follicles have been difficult to treat with lasers. There is a wide variation in depth at different anatomic sites, with the deepest follicular bulbs at 5 mm in depth. This is beyond the range of penetration of most lasers (Figs. 51-3 and 51-4). Upper lip hairs range from 1.0 to 2.5 mm in depth, whereas pubic hair and axillary hairs may be as much as 5.0 mm in depth. In addition, most authorities agree that only the anagen phase of follicular growth is responsive to laser energy. The percentage of follicles in anagen at any one anatomic site very from 30% (truncal) to 80% (scalp). Therefore, to understand laser hair removal more fully, a better knowledge of hair anatomy and development is crucial.

Hair is composed of keratinous fibers that grow from follicles over the entire body surface except from the palms and soles. The number of follicles is finite at birth. The active growth phase is *anagen*, during which the hair contains abundant melanin. *Catagen* is a period of regression when cell division terminates in the long part of the follicle and the lower part of the follicle begins to involute. The final resting phase is *telogen*, during which the old hair is emitted before the development of a new

hair. During telogen there is very little or no melanin *in the follicle*. The length of the three individual phases varies widely with the anatomic site. Because of this, patients must be advised that 100% hair reduction may be impossible because of the relative unresponsiveness of the telogen follicle to laser irradiation. Hairs, particularly on the trunk, may remain in telogen for longer than 3 months. Therefore patients need to be advised that follow-up treatments may be needed up to 1 year after initiation of therapy in order to allow for conversion of telogen hairs to anagen.

Hairs are of two types: terminal hairs are thick, long, and pigmented with melanin and found throughout the body surface, whereas vellus hairs are small in diameter, short, and depigmented. In Fig. 51-5, the structure of a

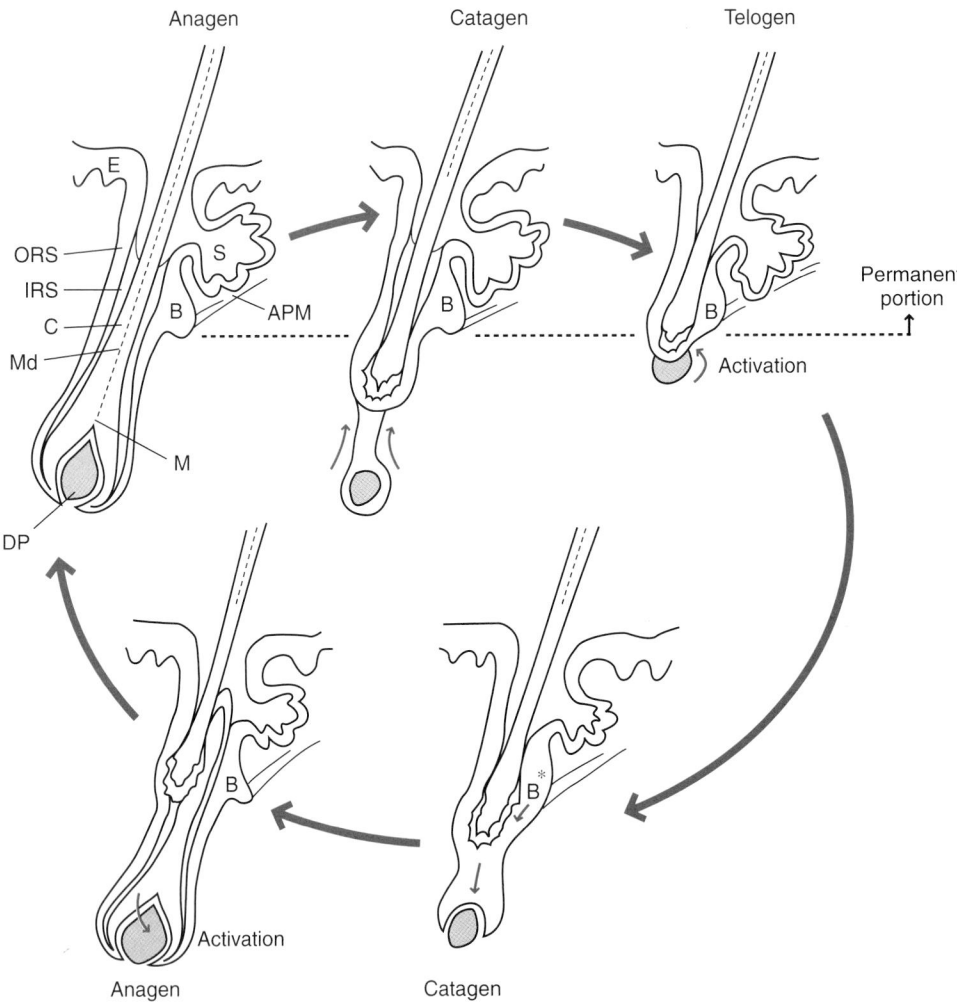

Fig. 51-5
Hair cycle. Illustrated are different phases of the hair cycle including anagen, catagen, and telogen. Different structures are labeled, including arrector pili muscle *(APM)*, bulge *(B)*, cortex *(C)*, dermal papilla *(DP)*, epidermis *(E)*, inner root sheath *(IRS)*, matrix *(M)*, medulla *(Md)*, outer root sheath *(ORS)*, and sebaceous gland *(S)*. B and B* denote quiescent and activated bulge cells, respectively. Follicular structures above the dotted line form the permanent portion of the follicle; keratinocytes below the bulge degenerate during catagen and telogen. (Redrawn from Cotsarelis G, Sun Tung-Tien, Lavker RM: *Cell* 61:1333, 1990.)

typical hair is demonstrated. The hair itself grows from the bulb, which consists of the hair matrix and the dermal papilla. The papilla is an area of highly vascularized connective tissue and provides the nutrients for the rapidly dividing cells of the matrix. During periods of active growth, matrical cells divide every 24 to 72 hours and migrate upwards to become keratinized and packed into layers that compose the hair shaft.

The "bulge," which is a protrusion near the attachment of the arrector pili muscle, has recently been determined to consist of stem cells important in hair regeneration. The bulge is generally located 1.0 to 1.5 mm below the cutaneous surface. Therefore the target of laser thermolysis is twofold: the bulge and the papilla. As mentioned previously, hairs grow in recurrent cycles (Table 51-1).

FITZPATRICK SKIN TYPES AND TREATMENT IMPLICATIONS

It has become clear as the hair removal technique has developed that proper patient selection ensures success. The two preeminent factors are skin type and hair color. Skin types are based on the Fitzpatrick Classification System:

Type I	Always burns, never tans
Type II	Always burns, sometimes tans
Type III	Sometimes burns, always tans
Type IV	Rarely burns, always tans
Type V	Moderately pigmented
Type VI	Black skin

Fitzpatrick grouped patients into the six different skin types based on the amount of pigmentation found in the skin. Skin Type I has the least pigment and Type VI has the most. The lower skin types are most sensitive to ultraviolet (UV) radiation ("sunburn") and to development of solar damage in the way of actinic changes and skin cancer. More freckles are also found in the skin Types I and II and fewer after Type III. The higher the number of the skin type, the more melanin is found and the more resistant the skin is to sunburning. Hair color is an independent variable in determining resistance to sunburn and the amount of pigmentation in the skin. Laser hair treatment is easier in patients who are most sensitive to UV radiation because they have less melanin in their skin to absorb the light. More light energy passes through to the hair follicles, and there is less risk of photothermal damage to the skin.

Generally skin Types I and II are most easily treated. Tanned Types III, IV, and V are more difficult to treat. Skin Type VI may only be treated in certain circumstances. Because of increased epidermal melanin, there is a risk of thermal damage to the skin in Types V and VI. This may cause scarring or, at the very least, pigmentary alterations such as hypopigmentation or postinflammatory hyperpigmentation. Only some units have received FDA approval to treat Type VI skin.

PREPROCEDURE PATIENT PREPARATION

Many practices perform a physician counseling session and perform test patches on the patient at an initial visit. The power settings are determined and safety of the treatment is determined at this setting. For the darker skin type (Fitzpatrick Types IV and V), adverse reactions such as edema and crusting may be noted up to 2 days after treatment. Some practitioners treat the ideal patient (Fitzpatrick Type I or II with dark brown or black hair) at this initial appointment.

FACTORS INFLUENCING TYPE OF EQUIPMENT

- Reliability
- Purchase price
- Technical support

TABLE 51-1

Hair Depth and Hair Cycle

Body Area	Telogen Hair (%)	Anagen Hair (%)	Telogen Duration	Follicles Density (1/cm^2)	Depth of Follicle (mm)
Scalp	13	85	3-4 mo	350	3-5
Beard	30	70	10 wk	500	2-4
Upper lip	35	65	6 wk	500	1-2.5
Axillae	70	30	3 mo	65	3.5-4.5
Trunk				70	2-4.5
Pubic area	70	30	12 wk	70	3.5-4.5
Arms	80	20	18 wk	80	
Legs and thighs	80	20	24 wk	60	2.5-4
Breasts	70	30		65	3-4.5

Skin Typing

For successful hair removal, it is necessary to determine the correct typing of your skin. Your doctor will consider your skin type when planning your treatment program.

Skin type is categorized by the Fitzpatrick skin type scale, which ranges from Type I (fair) to Type VI (black). The main factors that influence skin type are genetic disposition and reaction to sun exposure and tanning habits.

Skin type is determined genetically and is one of the many aspects of overall appearance. Genetics also determines the eye color, hair color, and the way skin pigments react to light. The way your skin reacts to sun exposure is important in correctly assessing your skin type. Sunbathing or artificial tanning (e.g., tanning creams) affects the evaluation of your skin color.

Please take a few minutes and fill out this questionnaire to help us determine your skin type and treat you properly.

Genetic Disposition

	0	1	2	3	4	Score
What color are your eyes?	Light blue, gray, green	Blue, gray, green	Blue	Dark brown	Brownish black	
What is the natural color of your hair?	Sandy red	Blond	Chestnut/dark blonde	Dark brown	Black	
What color is your skin (unexposed areas)?	Reddish	Very pale	Pale with beige tint	Light brown	Dark brown	
Do you have freckles on unexposed areas?	Many	Several	Few	Incidental	None	
					Genetic Disposition Total	

Reaction to Sun Exposure

	0	1	2	3	4	Score
What happens when you stay too long in the sun?	Painful redness, blistering, peeling	Blistering followed by peeling	Burns sometimes followed by peeling	Rare burns	Never had burns	
To what degree do you turn brown?	Hardly or not at all	Light tan	Reasonable tan	Tan very easy	Turn dark brown quickly	
Do you turn brown with several hours of sun exposure?	Never	Seldom	Sometimes	Often	Always	
How does your face react to the sun?	Very sensitive	Sensitive	Normal	Very resistant	Never had a problem	
					Reaction to Sun Exposure Total	

Fig. 51-6
Sample form to determine skin type. (Courtesy The National Procedures Institute, Midland, Mich.)
Continued

- Warranty program including cost
- Available training
- Physician advisors experienced with particular equipment

Purchase of a specific hair removal device is a difficult decision. It is important to ascertain the reliability of said device. Appropriate technical support is important because these units are mechanically complicated and do break down, so the cost of a warranty program should be considered. Even more important is educational support. All units have a learning curve, and training seminars with on-site education on an ongoing basis is crucial. It is also important to find out if there is a charge for upgrades to the unit. Many companies

Tanning Habits

	1	2	3	4	5	Score
When did you last expose your body to sun (or artificial sunlamp/tanning cream)?	More than 3 months ago	2-3 months ago	1-2 months ago	Less than a month ago	Less than 2 weeks ago	
Did you expose the area to be treated to the sun?	Never	Hardly ever	Sometimes	Often	Always	
					Tanning Habits Total	

Add up the total scores for each of the three sections for your Skin Type Score. This will give you a better evaluation of your skin type.

Summary

Genetic Disposition Total	
Reaction to Sun Exposure Total	
Tanning Habits Total	
Skin Type Score	

Your Fitzpatrick Skin Type

Skin Type Score	Fitzpatrick Skin Type
0-7	I
8-16	II
17-24	III
25-30	IV
Over 30	V-VI

Note: This questionnaire is intended as a guideline for skin typing. Final evaluation of skin type should be determined by your doctor.

Fig. 51-6, cont'd

periodically alter the machines to improve efficacy. Finally, discussions with physicians who have experience with a certain device are vital.

TECHNIQUE OF HAIR REMOVAL

1. The patient's skin type is determined on the Fitzpatrick skin type scale (Fig. 51-6).
2. Proper settings are selected (individualized with each unit).
3. The hair is clipped to 1 mm of length. Topical anesthetics can be used (e.g., EMLA [eutectic mixture of local anesthetics] cream). (See Chapter 11, Topical Anesthesia.)
4. The cooling gel is applied for the IPL device only; other lasers have integrated cooling systems.
5. Eye protection is provided to the practitioner and the patient.
6. Photoepilation is performed.
7. Observe for the proper tissue reaction (see below).
8. Ice packs or chilled Aloe gel are applied.
9. Follow-up sessions are scheduled.

At the treatment session, hairs are clipped to 1 mm in length. If long hairs are left on the skin surface, there is a risk that they will act as a heat sink and singe the underlying epidermis. Protective goggles are placed on the patient. Proximity of the treatment spots vary from one device to another, but in general should either be abutted or slightly overlapped (10% to 20%). *Observation of clinical response during the treatment is crucial.* If either obvious burning of the skin or no effect to hairs is noted, then energy fluences should be adjusted accordingly. Look for shearing or fracture of about 20% to 30% of the hairs during the treatment session, and note the "sulfur" smell of thermally damaged hair. The ideal cutaneous response is discrete perifollicular erythema and edema without coalescence into solid erythema. Patients should be advised that further hairs will fall out over the ensuing 2 to 3 weeks and will be variable depending on the site.

COMPLICATIONS

- Discomfort
- Ocular burns and blindness
- Second-degree burns
- Hypopigmentation
- Hyperpigmentation (postinflammatory)
- Scarring
- Lack of satisfactory response with regrowth

POSTPROCEDURE PATIENT EDUCATION

- Sunscreen (SPF 30 or greater) should be used between sessions.
- Multiple treatments will be needed at all anatomic sites, but the number varies.
- Treatment intervals every 3 to 4 weeks for five to six sessions, then every 3 months for a year.

Discomfort associated with photoepilation is generally mild and transient and has been described as similar to a large rubber band snapping against the skin when a light pulse is triggered. Topical anesthetics like EMLA cream may be used before treatment. On occasion, patients experience blistering, which causes crusting. This usually does not occur until the following day. If this does happen, the patient can apply warm compresses and a topical antibiotic ointment (bacitracin, etc.). Cool compresses can be applied for 2 to 3 hours after treatment but are usually not needed after this time. Like any laser procedure there is always potential for complications. Postinflammatory hyperpigmentation may be treated with bleaching creams (e.g., Hydroquinone), light chemical peeling, or even pigment specific lasers. Hypopigmentation is a much more difficult problem to treat, but it usually improves on its own over a longer period. Hypertrophic scarring or keloids should be treated with acceptable modalities (intralesional steroids, silicone-gel sheeting, pulsed dye laser).

CONCLUSION

Laser hair removal is a developing technology in the cosmetic medical field. In comparison with electrolysis, treatments are more rapid, more comfortable, and at least as efficacious. As the understanding and experience with this technology continue in the future, improved responses will result.

SUPPLIERS

Patient education materials

MJD Patient Communications
4641 Montgomery Avenue, Suite 350
Bethesda, MD 20814
Phone: 1-800-326-4869
Website: www.mjdpc.com

Laser/hair removal equipment companies

Aesculap-Meditec
2323 McGaw Avenue
Irvine, CA 92623
Phone: 1-949-660-2770
Website: www.asclepion.com

Candela Corp.
530 Boston Post Road
Wayland, MA 01778
Phone: 1-508-358-7637
Website: www.clzr.com

Continuum Biomedical
3150 Central Expressway
Santa Clara, CA 95051
Phone: 1-800-956-7757
Website: www.continuumlasers.com/mainswf.html

Convergent Laser Technologies
900 Alice Street
Oakland, CA 94607
Phone: 1-510-832-2130
Website: www.convergentlaser.com

Crystal Focus
19 rue Ampere
91302 Massy, France
Phone: +33-1-69-20-84-54

Cynosure, Inc.
10 Elizabeth Drive
Chelmsford, MA 01824
Phone: 1-800-886-2966
Website: www.cynosurelaser.com

Diomed, Inc.
1 Dundee Park
Andover, MA 01810
Phone: 1-978-475-7771
Website: www.diomed-lasers.com

Iriderm
1212 Terra Bella Avenue
Mountain View, CA 94043
Phone: 1-650-940-4700
Website: www.iriderm.com

Laserscope
3070 Orchard Drive
San Jose, CA 95134-2011
Phone: 1-408-943-0636
Website: www.laserscope.com

Lumenis, Inc.
2400 Condensa Street
Santa Clara, CA 95051
Phone: 1-800-562-5916
Website: www.lumenis.com

Palomar Medical Technologies, Inc.
82 Cambridge Street
Burlington, MA 01803
Phone: 1-800-725-6627
Website: www.palmed.com

Thermolase Corp. (Thermo Electron Corp.)
81 Wyman Street
Waltham, MA 02454-9046
Phone: 1-781-622-1000
Website: www.thermo.com

CPT/BILLING CODE

17380   Electrolysis, epilation each half-hour

ICD-9-CM DIAGNOSTIC CODES

704.1   Hypertrichosis
704.1   Hirsutism

CHARGES

A wide variation in charges for photoepilation exists between practices and within a practice. Variables determining the pricing include local competition, cost of equipment, and size of the area being treated. The larger the area being treated, the more provider or technician time is needed and the more wear and tear to the equipment.

ADDITIONAL RESOURCES

• See the sample patient education handout titled "Photoepilation/Laser Hair Removal" on page 1791 of Appendix G.
• See the sample patient consent form titled "Photoepilation/Laser Hair Removal" page 1793 of Appendix G.

BIBLIOGRAPHY

Anderson RR, Parrish JA: Selective photothermolysis: precise microsurgery by selective absorption of pulsed radiation, *Science* 220:534, 1983.
Draelos ZD: Hair removal techniques. In Merli GJ: *The clinics atlas of office procedures: basic cosmetic procedures,* Philadelphia, December 2000, WB Saunders.
Eremia S, Li C, Newman N: Laser hair removal with alexandrite versus diode laser using four treatment sessions: 1-year results, *Dermatol Surg* 27:925, 2001.
Eremia S, Li CY, Umar SH, Newman N: Laser hair removal: long-term results with a 755 nm Alexandrite laser, *Dermatol Surg* 27:920, 2001.
Grossman MC, Diereckx C, Farinelli W, et al: Damage to hair follicles by normal-mode ruby laser pulses, *J Am Acad Dermatol* 35:889, 1996.
Ort RJ, Dierickx C: Laser hair removal. In Kaminer MS, Dover JS, Arndt KA, editors: *Atlas of cosmetic surgery,* Philadelphia, 2002, WB Saunders.
Sun T, Cotsarelis G, Lavker RM: Hair follicular stem cells: the bulge-activation hypothesis, *J Invest Dermatol* 96(suppl 5):77S, 1991.
Tope WD, Hordinsky M: A hair's breadth closer (editorial), *Arch Dermatol* 134:867, 1998.
Wagner RF, Tomich JM, Grande DJ: Electrolysis and thermolysis for permanent hair removal, *J Am Acad Dermatol* 12:441, 1985.

CHAPTER 52

Microdermabrasion

Dexter W. Blome

The concept of smoothing the skin by removing, or abrading, the upper layers can be dated as far back as 1500 BC, when Egyptian physicians used a type of "sandpaper" to treat scars. Modern dermabrasion was developed in Germany in the early 1900s by Kromayer, who used human-powered rotating wheels and rasps as a means of removing the epidermis and superficial portions of the dermis. This new technology was mainly used to treat scars, hyperpigmentation and keratoses; however, acceptance was not forthcoming. It was not until Kurtin, Burks, and others began using motorized wire brushes in the early to mid 1950s that the power of the technology was realized. In spite of the great benefits possible with dermabrasion, there are many potential negatives: need for anesthesia, scarring, prolonged downtime, wound care, infection, and contaminated operative field with aerosolized particles that endanger the practitioner and staff. (Many of these problems are also encountered with other techniques, such as laser resurfacing and deep chemical peels.) These factors, as well as economic considerations, have pushed for development of a new technology that is initially less debilitating, safer, and more affordable: microdermabrasion (MDA).

MDA was developed in Italy in 1985 and introduced to the American market during the mid 1990s. MDA has spread at an explosive rate; currently, nearly 30 companies manufacture similar units.

MECHANISM OF ACTION

The most superficial layer of the skin is the *stratum corneum,* which is a lifeless accumulation of flattened keratinocytes that forms a barrier to protect the skin from a myriad of invasive insults. From the time a keratinocyte is formed in younger skin, it takes approximately 28 days to mature, die, and flake off the skin surface as dander. As humans age, keratinocyte transit times dramatically increase, trapping pigment and debris in the superficial epidermal layers to give the characteristic stained appearance of aging or actinic damage. Another skin cell of major importance is the fibroblast, which lies within the dermis and synthesizes collagen, a function that decreases with aging and actinic damage. The process of MDA addresses both the stained, debris-ridden epidermis and the sluggish collagen production of dermal fibroblasts.

Epidermal Effects of Microdermabrasion

The micrographs (Fig. 52-1) exhibit the immediate sequential thinning and smoothing of epidermal structures as a result of the abrasive effect of the aluminum oxide crystals moving rapidly across the skin surface. The gentle planing of the upper layers of the skin removes pigmentary impurities and debris held within the stratum corneum and yields a smoother, softer skin surface. Each pass of the MDA handpiece is estimated to ablate approximately 15 µm of skin, roughly equal to one pass of the erbium laser. In addition to the immediate smoothing of the skin, the abrasive process over the long term seems to stimulate keratinocyte turnover. Larson and Shehadi have shown increases in epidermal thickness in porcine skin by 9% with MDA.

Dermal Effects of Microdermabrasion

Most MDA machines are quite simple in principle, having a crystal reservoir that supplies abrasive crystals through a flexible tube to a handpiece that is moved across the skin by the operator. The skin is "tented up" by the negative pressure generated in the machine, and abrasive crystals, usually aluminum oxide (corundum), are simultaneously blown and "sucked" across the skin to remove the upper layers of the epidermis. This can be compared with a fine "sandblasting" technique. Other types of particulate materials are occasionally used for the abrasion process, such as sodium chloride crystals, sodium bicarbonate (baking soda), and magnesium oxide crystals. However, aluminum oxide seems ideal because it is widely available, is inert, is very hard, has multiple sharp edges, does not readily absorb liquid, and is nontoxic even if inadvertently inhaled. Used crystals

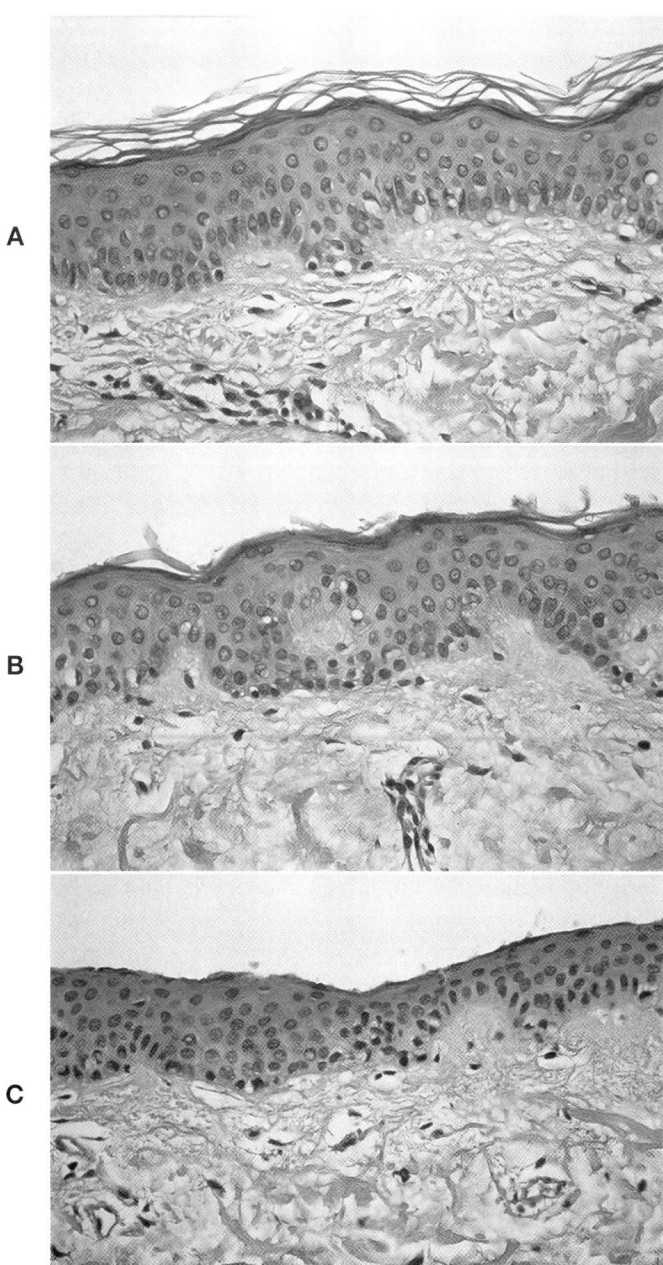

Fig. 52-1
A, Pretreatment photomicrograph of human skin of the upper back showing fully intact stratum corneum and stratum granulosum. **B,** Upper back skin on same patient after two passes. Note that the stratum corneum has been markedly ablated. **C,** Upper back skin after four passes; same region of the back as **A** and **B,** but separated by 20 minutes. Exhibits total removal of the stratum corneum and most of the stratum granulosum. (Courtesy Dr. Rick Wilson, Dallas, Tex.)

and cutaneous debris are removed through suction and collected in a separate waste container, thus creating a closed-loop system that avoids the airborne contaminants of open dermabrasion. The handpieces usually can be fitted with reusable metal tips or disposable plastic tips. The metal tips must be sterilized before use with different patients.

Treatments are superficial enough that they do not cause bleeding or "serum ooze." Some patients with very sensitive skin may experience slight discomfort, but treatments are certainly not painful and are generally well tolerated. After each pass, the bulk of crystals should be removed before continuing. The *second pass* should be at right angles, or perpendicular, to the direction of the first pass. A *third pass,* if made, is usually done with a swirling or circular motion, making sure that the skin is taut and the handpiece tip is moving and not stationary over a single skin point.

Skin changes are cumulative and treatment sessions are recommended at 7- to 10-day intervals. Depending on the type and severity of the skin problem(s), usually between 6 and 15 treatments are offered on an "as-needed" basis between 1 and 3 months. The patient is usually able to return to most normal activities immediately, unless the skin is extremely sensitive, which may exhibit mild erythema for 12 to 24 hours.

Depth of penetration is controlled by four separate factors that can be varied according to the patient's unique circumstance and requirements. This gives the operator great flexibility in treating patients and improves outcomes. These four factors are straightforward and easily controlled:
- Density of crystal flow
- Number of passes completed by the operator
- Vacuum pressure
- Speed with which the operator moves the handpiece over the skin surface

High vacuum settings (anything above 20 cm Hg) may be required in some instances (e.g., acne scarring), but this is not the norm. Vacuum settings and crystal flow will definitely vary with different machines.

INDICATIONS

- Minor acne scarring
- Postoperative-traumatic scarring
- Fine lines and wrinkles
- Lentigines
- Superficial pigmentation
- Blending post-laser pigmentation
- Skin texture irregularities
- Actinic keratoses
- Enlarged pores
- Clogged pores and blackheads
- Whiteheads
- Some mild forms of acne

Patients with stage I, II, or III *acne* have done well when MDA is combined with topical retinoid therapy (Fig. 52-2). In this instance, MDA's action on the

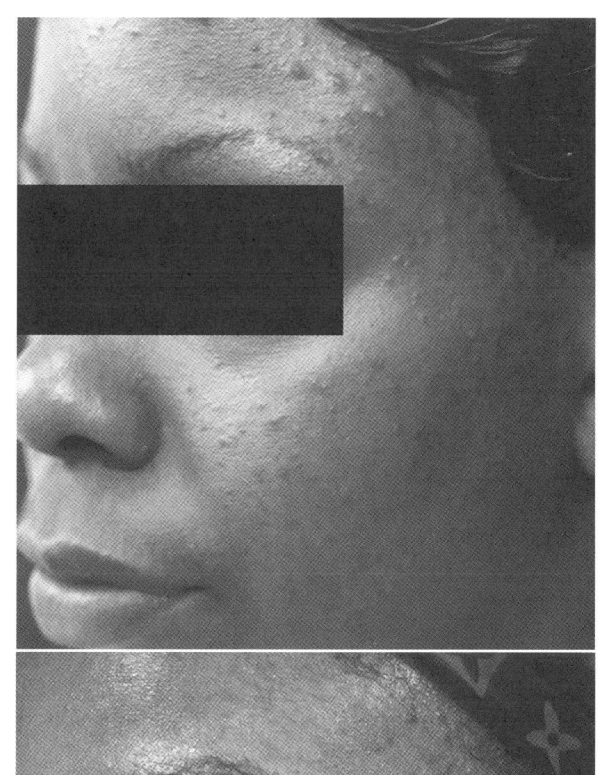

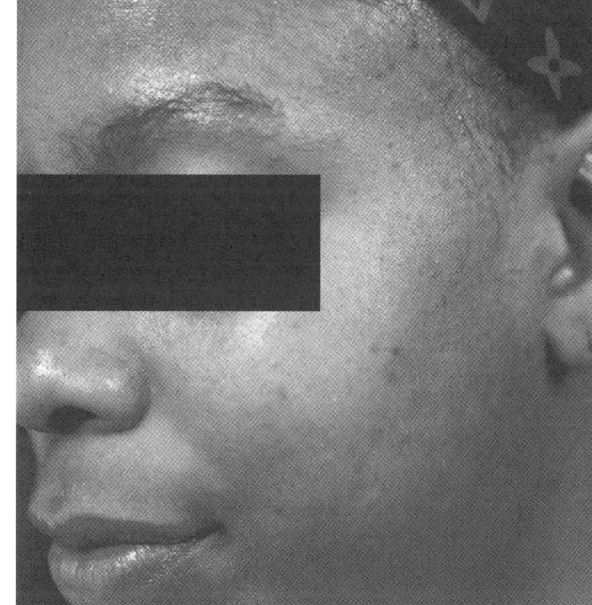

Fig. 52-2
A, Black female with stage II acne prior to treatment. **B,** Same patient after six microdermabrasion treatments with simultaneous use of daily topical retinoids.

stratum corneum allows for better absorption of topical medications.

Although many practitioners are claiming success treating *stretch marks*, I have not had success in this area and cannot recommend MDA for this purpose at present. I have had some minimal diminution in the appearance of abdominal stria with repeated MDA sessions, but progress has not been gratifying. Perhaps

new protocols will be established in the near future for effective treatment of stria.

CONTRAINDICATIONS

- Pregnancy
- Accutane use within the last 12 months
- Presence of skin malignancy
- Presence of herpetic lesion(s)

PATIENT SELECTION

MDA is safe and effective; however, proper patient selection is essential. Poor patient selection will cause patient dissatisfaction, staff frustration, and ultimate failure of the MDA program in any given practice.

MDA is an excellent modality for all skin types, even those patients with Fitzpatrick skin Types V and VI (see Chapter 51, Laser Hair Removal: Photoepilation). These patients are especially vulnerable to hyperpigmentation or hypopigmentation by administration of more aggressive skin resurfacing techniques. MDA is safe in these patients because the depth of penetration is usually limited to the superficial epidermis. *Elderly patients* with thin skin are not good candidates for MDA unless pretreated with other modalities to improve skin quality.

INITIAL EVALUATION

Every patient must be seen and evaluated by the physician before initiation of a treatment protocol. Unfortunately, some offices turn the MDA practice over to an esthetician and the process runs independent of physician input. This situation is more apropos of a beauty salon and, in my view, does not meet the standards of a professional medical practice. A physician has the responsibility of seeing and evaluating every patient who is treated in his or her practice. Anything less than this shortchanges the patient and puts the physician on tenuous medical-legal ground should complications arise.

After filling out the usual history form, with special notice to current medications, the physician sees the patient and the skin is evaluated with references to the following factors:

- Fitzpatrick skin typing (see Chapter 51, Laser Hair Removal: Photoepilation)
- Thickness
- Skin tone
- Site-specific rhytids
- Depth and severity of rhytids

- Dryness
- Acne
- Acne scarring
- Other scarring
- Vascular anomalies
- Telangiectasias
- Ecchymosis
- Nevi
- Pigmentation problems
- Skin malignancies
- General actinic damage
- Actinic keratoses
- Current tanning status
- Poikiloderma
- Open sores
- Herpetic lesions

Once these and other individual factors are considered, a treatment protocol can be determined for the patient. Instructions should be written or checked off on a patient paradigm sheet and communication with the MDA technician concerning the patient's treatments completed (Figs. 52-3 and 52-4).

Pretreatment and posttreatment photos are recommended and are a part of the patient's permanent record. They will allow the physician and staff to evaluate the results. However, do not expect miracles on every patient. I have found it extremely difficult to photographically document improvement in patients who initially had good skin and just wanted "freshening." Certainly, those patients with major pigment problems, acne scarring, and other extreme conditions yield documentable photographic improvement.

COMPLICATIONS

Complications can result from any type of treatment regardless of how innocuous the technology may seem. Certainly, MDA is no different. However, the very factor that has contributed to MDA's widespread success is that it has very few, if any, long-term complications. The physician and staff should receive bona fide training before embarking on patient treatments and know the potential complications and treatment options to provide a good outcome.

Erythema is the most common side effect of MDA and has a nearly linear relationship with the aggressiveness of the treatment. Some patients have very sensitive skin and will exhibit some erythema no matter how mild the treatment settings. Most erythema will resolve spontaneously within a few hours. Inform the patient to avoid the sun or tanning bed exposure during the time of his or her treatment sessions, since this will surely increase skin irritation. All patients must use sunblock to protect their skin.

Most patients experience a mild amount of *tingling,* which is very tolerable. However, a few patients will complain of *burning and skin discomfort* for up to 24 hours after the peel. These patients can be treated effectively with moisturizers.

Purpura, ecchymosis, and petechial hemorrhages are all a function of vacuum settings that are too aggressive. Apply ice to the area when first noticed and decrease the vacuum setting to minimize the problem. If one of these complications should occur, do not return to the affected area for peeling at that same treatment session. Skin should return to normal appearance in most patients below age 50 within 10 to 14 days. Older patients may take longer to resolve these problems.

Scarring is almost unheard of with MDA, but is possible in the following unusual situations:
- Patient circumstance demands aggressive therapy (e.g., treatment of mild to moderate acne scarring on the cheeks, which requires deep planning).
- Aggressive treatments administered to patients currently using Accutane or patients who have been on Accutane within 1 year of initiating MDA.
- Mild skin abrasion in a noncompliant patient or a patient who has compromised immune function and suffers wound contamination and subsequent infection.
- MDA technician treatment error in being too aggressive or in allowing the handpiece to stop or dwell on specific skin areas for too long.

Minor skin abrasions can easily occur. Simply having the patient clean these areas and keep antibiotic ointment applied until reepithelialization has occurred should alleviate the situation.

Ocular damage is a potential. Protection of the eyes for both the patient and practitioner is an absolute "must." Tsai and associates (1995) discussed development of ocular pain, photophobia, epiphora, and conjunctival congestion with crystal adherence to the cornea and punctuate keratopathy resulting from ophthalmologic crystal contamination during MDA. Ocular contamination can be prevented by placing moist folded 4×4 gauze pads over the eyes and holding them in place with suntanning goggles. Alternatively, the special eye shields noted can be used alone. After treatment, the technician must meticulously remove crystals from the periorbital region before allowing the patient to get off the treatment table and wash.

EQUIPMENT

- MDA unit with tips (sterile, reusable metal; plastic disposable) (see Fig. 52-6)
- Power examination table and adjustable stool for the technician
- Alcohol wipes

AESTHETIC SERVICES PATIENT PROFILE

Name: _____ DOB:_____ Age:_____ Sex:_____

Are you pregnant? Yes____ No____
Do you wear contact lenses? Yes____ No____

Do you currently have a sunburn/windburn/red face? Yes____ Why? _____ No____
Are you in the habit of going to tanning booths? Yes____ No____

Do you currently get facial waxing/undergo electrolysis/use depilatories? Yes____ No____
Are you currently using Biore/snore strips? Yes____ No____

Are you currently using Retin-A/Renova/Differin? Yes____ No____ What strength? _____
For how long? ____ How frequently? ____ Where applied? _____
Are you now or have you ever used Accutane? Yes____ No____ How long? _____ When? _____

Are you currently having microdermabrasion? Yes____ No____ How long? _____
Do you have regular collagen injections? Yes____ No____
Do you have regular Botox injections? Yes____ No____
Have you ever had a peel? Yes____ No____ Within the last 14 days? Yes____ No____
What kind?_____ Describe your reaction:_____
Have you recently had facial surgery? Yes____ No____ Describe: _____ When? _____
Have you recently had laser resurfacing? Yes____ No____ When? _____ What kind? _____

What type of work do you do? _____ Airline travel? Yes____ How often? _____ No____
Do you participate in vigorous aerobic activity or sports? Yes____ No____ What type? _____

Do you smoke? Yes____ No____
Do you develop cold sores/fever blisters? Yes____ No____ Last breakout? _____

Are you allergic/sensitive to: (check all that apply) milk____ apples____ citrus____ grapes____
aloe vera____ aspirin____ perfumes____ latex____ hydroquinone____
Other allergies (if so, what)? _____
Are you sensitive to alcohol-based products? Yes____ No____
Please list all medications you take, including thyroid supplements, hormone replacement therapy, birth control
    pills, Accutane, and Coumadin: _____

How would you describe your skin? (check all that apply) Thick____ Thin____ Saggy____ Firm____ Normal____
    Dry____ T-zone/Combination____ Oily____ Acne____ Comedones____ Milia____ Cysts____ Breakouts____
    Acne scarred____ Large pores____ Small pores____ Florid____ Rosacea____ Eczema____ Freckled____
    Sun-damaged____ Uneven/blotchy____ Mature____ Wrinkled____ Patchy dryness on_____ Sallow____
    Melasma____ Perfume-stained____ Hypopigmented____ Hyperpigmented____ Psoriasis____
    Dehydrated (lacking moisture)____ Asphyxiated____ Telangiectasia/broken surface capillaries____
Do you consider your skin SENSITIVE____ RESILIENT____ NOT SURE____

Eye color: Blue____ Green____ Hazel____ Gray____ Lt Brown____ Med Brown____ Dk Brown____
Hair color: Blonde____ Red____ Lt Brown____ Med Brown____ Dk Brown____ Black____ Gray/Silver/White____
Skin tone: Pale/White____ Light____ Medium____ Reddish____ Freckled____ Lt Olive____ Med Olive____
    Dark Olive____ Lt Brown____ Med Brown____ Dk Brown____ Soft Black____ Black____
What is your hereditary makeup? _____

Are you using glycolic/AHA home care products? Yes____ No____ If so, which one(s)? _____
How does your skin react to them? _____
Have you ever used any products that caused a bad reaction? Yes____ No____ Describe_____
What is your daily home care regimen? _____
What are the cosmetic improvements you would like to see in your skin? _____
_____

Patient/Client Signature: _____

Treatment recommendations: _____
Patch test: Date_____ Solution_____ Test area_____ Result_____
Physician/Esthetician Signature_____

Fig. 52-3

Sample form: Aesthetic services patient profile. (Courtesy The Medical Procedures Center, Midland, Mich.
Adapted from various sources.)

- Crystals (usually aluminum chloride); approximately one-half of a cup (30 to 35 ml) for the face and more for larger areas
- Nonsterile gloves
- Moist 4×4–inch gauzes
- Surgical cap for patient
- Suntanning goggles for patient (Alternatively, Derm-Aid Non-Laser Disposable Eye Shields [GPT Glendale, Inc., Lakeland, Fla.] work very well.)
- Saline eye wash
- Towel or gown to drape around patient's neck
- Protective glasses with shields for operator
- Mask for operator (to reduce inhalation)
- Postoperative moisturizer (e.g., Theraplex, aloe, Kinerase)
- Flow sheet to record settings and progress
- Close-up camera (ideal but optional)

Crystals vary widely in quality and cost. Cheaper materials contain multiple-sized particles and may not be pure. Fine powdery substances are not only less effective but aerosolize when the containers are emptied. Not only do these substances cause a sediment in the room, but they may be irritating to the patient or clinician. The lower limits of size should be 20 μm. Crystals should also be prepared in a "medically clean" way to avoid any type of contamination.

The aperture holes that the crystals traverse eventually wear larger from the crystal passage. Check to see if the tip needs repair/replacement by observing a wider crystal flow that lacks uniformity.

Handpiece tips must be replaced or sterilized (cold or hot) for each patient. Angled handpieces are somewhat more comfortable for the operator to use.

PREPROCEDURE PATIENT PREPARATION

- Have the patient wash his or her face to remove all make-up and lotions.
- The patient must wear eye protection and a surgical cap to keep crystals from getting into the hair. Should crystals get into the eye, they can be very irritating and must be washed out with saline.

**CHEMICAL PEEL/MICRODERMABRASION
NEW PATIENT CONSULTATION CHEKLIST**

Name: _____   Date: _____

Analyze the Skin: **Initial Photographs:**
____Visually
____Patient Profile Form
____Consent Form signed (copy to patient)
____Fee Schedule Form signed (copy to patient)
____Photos Taken

Discuss Peel Treatments with Patient:
____Expectations
____Possible Reactions and Side Effects
____Sunblock Use

Home Care Program:
____Sample Kit
____Instructions
____Home Care Regimen
____Post Peel Tip Sheet

Peel Appointment:
____Preparation for Peel Treatment
____Date of First Treatment

Fig. 52-4
Sample form: Chemical peel/microdermabrasion new patient consultation checklist. (Courtesy The Medical Procedures Center, Midland, Mich. Adapted from various sources.)

- The patient is placed in the supine position on the treatment table. The technician is seated at the head with clear three-sided access to the patient.
- Place a towel, or gown, around the patient's neck to keep crystals from getting on the clothing.
- Cleanse the face with isopropyl alcohol to remove any lingering skin oils, make-up, and lotions.
- Examine the skin in the areas to be treated. Open sores should be avoided. Also, be attentive for any type of herpetic outbreak. If the patient does exhibit a herpetic lesion, cancel the treatment for at least 2 weeks and make sure the patient is treated with the appropriate antiviral medication(s) (Valtrex, Zovirax, etc.). Prophylaxis for patients with frequent herpetic outbreaks is not inappropriate; however, it should be individualized to each patient's circumstance.

TECHNIQUE

1. The usual power setting for initial treatment starts at 12 to 14 cm Hg and works up to 18 to 20 cm Hg for most patients (those with special problems such as acne scarring may require 20 to 35 cm Hg). The practitioner can make a good estimate of correct suction level by applying the handpiece to a colored page from a magazine for 3 to 4 seconds. If all color is removed, the power is too high. If most is removed, it is just right. If most color is left, it is too low.
2. With a nonsterile gloved hand, spread the skin between the thumb and index or middle finger with a moderate amount of tension. Place the MDA treatment head on the skin and move the handpiece parallel to the direction of tension between the two fingers (Fig. 52-5, *A*). *Keep the handpiece head moving, and definitely avoid stopping and holding it in contact with one area* of the skin; this could cause deep penetration and seriously damage the skin and cause scarring. Hold the handpiece perpendicular (90 degrees) to the skin.
3. After completing a small area of skin with parallel strokes, move the handpiece for a second pass perpendicular to the direction of movement of the first pass (Fig. 52-2, *B*). This crosshatches the area and decreases any streaking or linear erythematous markings.
4. If a third pass is to be made, use a circular or swirling motion. When initiating MDA with a new patient, it may be prudent to see how two passes are tolerated before making a third.
5. After two or more passes, some patients exhibit a darkened or grayish hue to the skin because of the crystal interaction with skin oils. Do not be alarmed,

since this will be removed completely with posttreatment cleansing.

6. When the treatment is completed, the technician should remove the crystals from the face while the patient is still in the supine position, taking great care to remove all crystal remnants from the periorbital region by suction or gentle removal with a moist cloth.
7. Have the patient cleanse with mild soap and water.
8. A light moisturizer, such as aloe, Theraplex, or Kinerase, will decrease any mild irritation.

After treatments, it is important to leave the crystal container heater on whenever the machine is not in use to prevent moisturization of the crystals, which

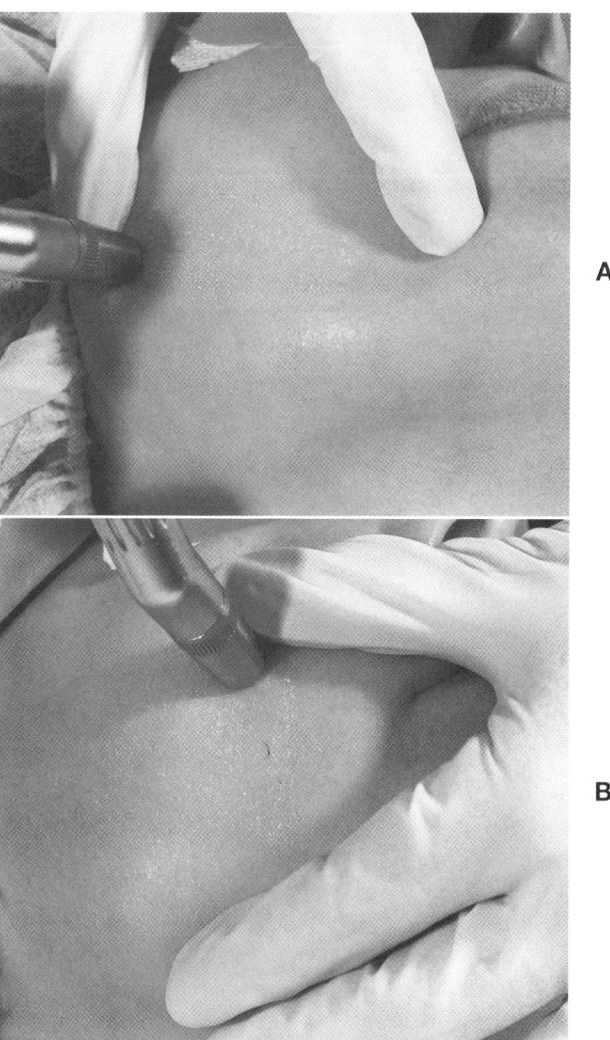

A

B

Fig. 52-5
A, First MDA pass on the patient's right cheek. The technician's fingers are tensing the skin in a horizontal direction while using parallel movements of the handpiece. **B,** A second pass in the right cheek with the skin tensed in a more vertical orientation perpendicular to the direction of the first pass seen in **A.** Note crystal residue on skin.

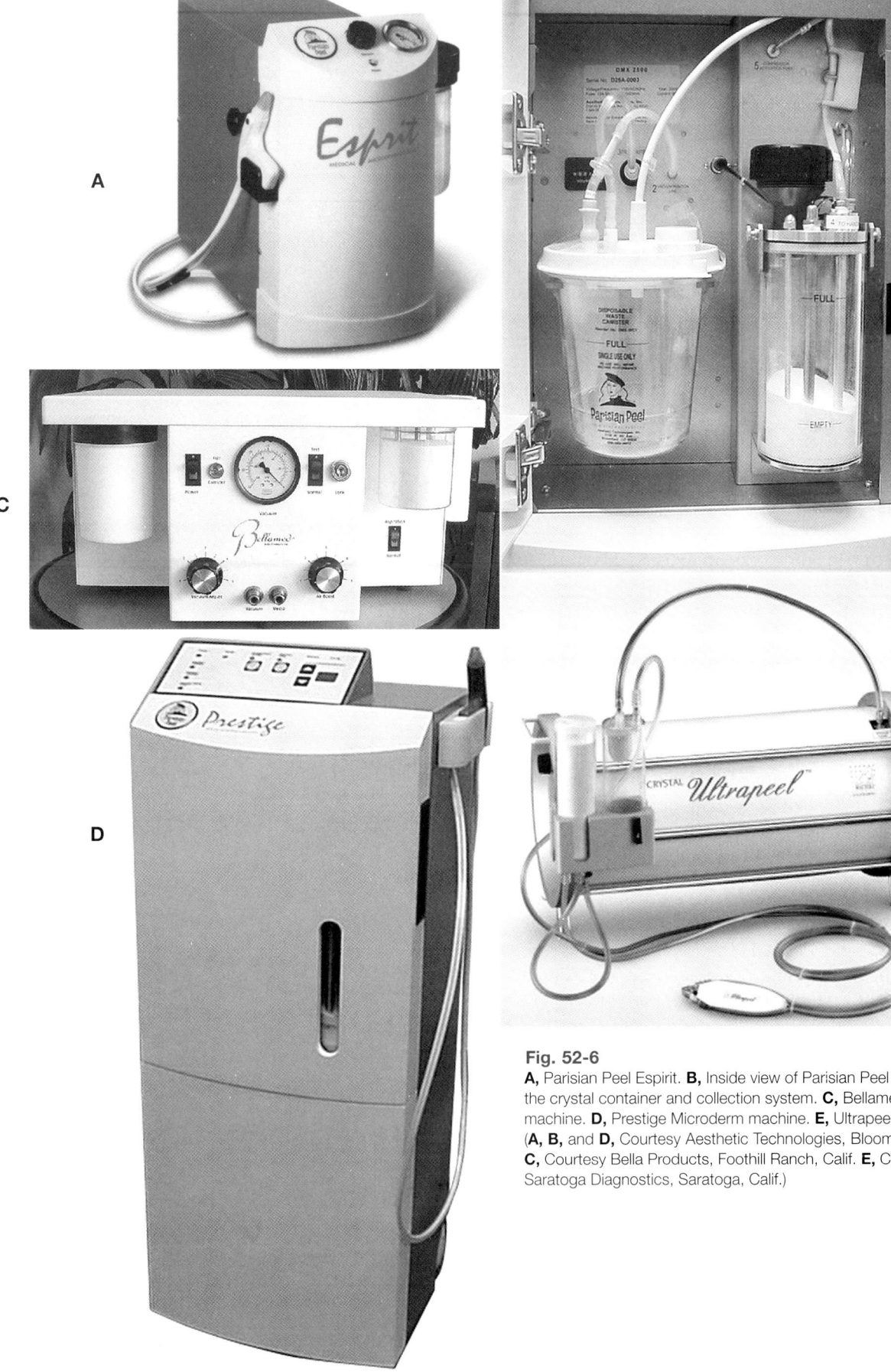

Fig. 52-6
A, Parisian Peel Espirit. **B,** Inside view of Parisian Peel unit showing the crystal container and collection system. **C,** Bellamed Microderm machine. **D,** Prestige Microderm machine. **E,** Ultrapeel Crystal. (**A, B,** and **D,** Courtesy Aesthetic Technologies, Bloomfield, Colo. **C,** Courtesy Bella Products, Foothill Ranch, Calif. **E,** Courtesy Saratoga Diagnostics, Saratoga, Calif.)

would result in poor crystal flow and possible malfunction.

POSTPROCEDURE PATIENT EDUCATION

Instruct the patient to avoid applying make-up, if possible, for the next 12 to 18 hours and to avoid significant sun exposure for 3 to 4 days after each treatment. The patient must wear sunblock whenever going out. See the sample patient education handout for "Chemical Peel/Microdermabrasion Posttreatment Instructions" on page 1795 of Appendix G.

PURCHASING A MICRODERMABRASION SYSTEM

Before purchasing an MDA machine (Fig. 52-6 shows some examples), consider several factors:

- Do you currently have access to a patient base that is appropriate to the use of this technology?
- Can ancillary treatments or therapies be offered to enhance the patient's results and to generate additional income (e.g., skin care products)?
- Do you have the personnel to support these new activities?
- Make sure the local region is not saturated with machines. Is there a realistic market potential?
- Evaluate machine functions such as crystal flow, vacuum capacity, and the operator's ability to vary treatment parameters. Machine flexibility is important in treating a variety of skin types, conditions, and problems.
- Evaluate the propensity of the machine to clog, which may occur in a humid, moist environment. Most machines have a crystal heater that maintains dry crystals. The heater is left on continually.
- In today's market, warranty coverage, technical support, and possible shared marketing arrangements have become increasingly important factors in determining purchase decisions.
- Along with designated staff, attend a course that covers the essentials of MDA. These courses are usually sponsored by the equipment manufacturer or physician experts in the field.

SUPPLIERS

Parisian Peel
Aesthetic Technologies, Inc.
2150 W. Sixth Avenue
Bloomfield, CO 80020
Phone: 1-800-262-4412
Website: www.parisianpeel.com

Bellamed
Bella Products, Inc.
27136 Burbank
Foothill Ranch, CA 92610
Phone: 1-877-550-5655
Website: www.bellaproducts.com

MicroDelivery Peel II
BioMedic
4602 East Hammond Lane
Phoenix, AZ 85034
Phone: 1-800-736-5155
Website: www.biomedic.com

EuroPeel
Cosmos Medical Technology, Inc.
42230 Zevo Drive
Temecula, CA 92590
Phone: 1-800-634-7921
Website: www.cosmosmed.com

MegaPeel
DermaMed, Inc.
394 Parkmount Rd.
P.O. Box 198
Lenni, PA 19052-0198
Phone: 1-877-789-MEGA
Website: www.megapeel.com

Diamond Peel
Diamond Medical Aesthetics
One Madison St., Building C
East Rutherford, NJ 07073
Phone: 1-877-754-6749
Website: www.slimtoneusa.com

MD Peel
Emed, Inc.
31320 Via Colinas, Suite 112
Westlake Village, CA 91362
Phone: 1-888-848-3633
Website: www.4emed.com

Power Peel
Power Peel
530 College Parkway
Annapolis, MD 21401
Phone: 1-800-925-5022
Website: www.powerpeel.com

Ultrapeel Crystal
Saratoga Diagnostics
12619 Paseo Olivos
Saratoga, CA 95070
Phone: 1-800-998-1555
Website: www.saratogadiagnostics.com

SmartPeel
SoundSkin Corp.
429 S. Main Street
Oswego, IL 60543
Phone: 1-888-596-5277
Website: www.soundskin.com

Derm-Aid Non-Laser Disposable Eye Shields
GPT Glendale, Inc.
5300 Region Court
Lakeland, FL 33815
Phone: 1-800-500-4739
Website: www.glendale-laser.com

CPT/BILLING CODES

15780   Dermabrasion,* total face (e.g., for acne scarring, fine wrinkling, rhytids, general keratosis)
15781   Dermabrasion,* segmental, face
15782   Dermabrasion,* regional, other than face
15783   Dermabrasion,* superficial, any site (e.g., tattoo removal)
15786†   Abrasion, single lesion (e.g., keratosis, scar)
15787†   Abrasion, each additional four lesions or less (list separately in addition to code for primary procedure)

---

*No code is available for microdermabrasion as of publication of the 2003 CPT codes. "Dermabrasion" here refers to the traditional, deeper abrasion techniques.
†Service includes surgical procedure only.

ICD-9-CM DIAGNOSTIC CODES

706.1   Acne vulgaris
702.0   Actinic keratosis
695.3   Rosacea
709.09   Melasma
709.2   Scarring
701.8   Wrinkling of skin; rhytids facialis
709.0   Dyschromia, unspecified

ADDITIONAL RESOURCES

- See the sample patient education handouts for "Microdermabrasion Preparation" and "Chemical Peel/Microdermabrasion Posttreatment Instructions" on pages 1794 and 1795, respectively, of Appendix G.
- See the sample patient consent form for "Microdermabrasion" on page 1796 of Appendix G.

BIBLIOGRAPHY

Fields KA: Skin breakthroughs in the year 2000, *Int J Fertil Womens Med* 45(2):179, 2000.

Hernandez-Perez E, Ibiett EV: Gross and microscopic findings in patients undergoing microdermabrasion for facial rejuvenation, *Dermatol Surg* 27:637, 2001.

Larson D: Personal communication, 2001.

Lawrence N, Mandy S, Yarborough J, Alt T: History of dermabrasion, *Dermatol Surg* 26:95, 2000.

Root LL: *A complete guide to microdermabrasion: treatment, techniques, and technology 2001,* Scottsdale, Ariz, 2001, Esthetic Education Resource.

Root LL: *Microdermabrasion: technique for the medical skin care clinic 2001,* Scottsdale, Ariz, 2001, Esthetic Education Resource.

Tan MH, Spencer JM, Pires LM, et al: The evaluation of aluminum oxide crystal microdermabrasion for photodamage, *Dermatol Surg* 27:943, 2001.

Tsai RY, Wang CN, Chan HL: Aluminum oxide crystal microdermabrasion: a new technique for treating facial scarring, *Dermatol Surg* 21(6):542, 1995.

CHAPTER 53

Skin Peels

Grant C. Fowler
Stephen F. Ramirez

With America's population aging, more patients are requesting treatment for photo-damaged or aging skin. In fact, it has become one of the most common reasons for patients to consult a dermatologist. In addition, although oral isotretinoin (Accutane) now prevents much of the deep scarring from acne, occasionally patients request treatment for minor scarring or post-inflammatory hyperpigmentation. Chemical peels and certain topical medications are among the growing number of aesthetic techniques used to rejuvenate skin damaged by all of these conditions. Superficial-depth peels have become so common and are deemed so safe that nonclinicians now perform them in health spas and salons. However, many patients would prefer to have even superficial-depth peels performed under the trusted supervision of their primary care clinician if it were available.

Although skin aging is both intrinsic (Table 53-1) and extrinsic (Table 53-2), the majority of damage is from extrinsic causes. Intrinsically, chronic use of the muscles of expression, dermal thinning, and loss of fibers produce some wrinkles and skin lines. Most intrinsic aging, such as that associated with hormonal changes, is the result of both chronologic and genetic causes.

Extrinsic aging is caused by environmental hazards, such as ultraviolet radiation, wind, smoking, and chemical exposure. Years of sun exposure can produce wrinkles and pigmentary or surface changes. The stratum corneum thickens, and the granulosum and spinosum layers become thinner. Atypical cells develop, the skin becomes less translucent, and pigmentation becomes markedly irregular. Lentigines (freckles) and actinic precancerous lesions develop (Fig. 53-1), the papillary dermis thins, and the skin loses elasticity while developing a sallow color. Extrinsic aging causes blood vessels to dilate, telangiectasias to proliferate, and collagen to become sparse (clumping in bundles). In turn, the reticular dermis fills with abnormal elastin fibers. Eventually, hair follicles and pores dilate and become filled with desquamated debris.

TOPICAL TREATMENTS AND ADJUNCTS TO PEELS

Considerable improvements in sun-damaged skin can be achieved with topical therapy alone if the patient is willing to apply it consistently. Topical retinoids, such as tretinoin (Retin-A or the petrolatum emollient form Renova) or tazarotene (Tazorac), have been shown to clinically and histologically reverse sun damage. In fact, the more severely damaged the skin, the better the

TABLE 53-1

Intrinsic (Chronologic and Genetic) Aging of the Skin

Cause	Effect
Decreased vascularity	Yellow skin
Dermal thinning	Atrophy
Decreased dermal cellularity	Irregular texture
Loss of elastic fibers	Fine lines or wrinkles
Decreased mechanical properties with decreased elastic recoil after stretching	Laxity

Adapted from Lewis AB, Gendler EC: *Semin Cutan Med Surg* 15:139, 1996.

TABLE 53-2

Extrinsic (Solar and Environmental) Aging of the Skin

Cause	Effect
Altered cell maturation	Dry, coarse texture, actinic keratoses
Melanocyte alteration (overstimulated or destroyed)	Solar lentigos, mottled pigmentation
Decreased collagen fiber number and strength; elastic fiber curling, branching, and thickening; degeneration into solar elastoses	Fine wrinkling
Loss of collagen support of vessels	Solar (senile) purpura
Alteration of vascular network	Yellow hue, loss of pink color

Adapted from Lewis AB, Gendler EC: *Semin Cutan Med Surg* 15:139, 1996.

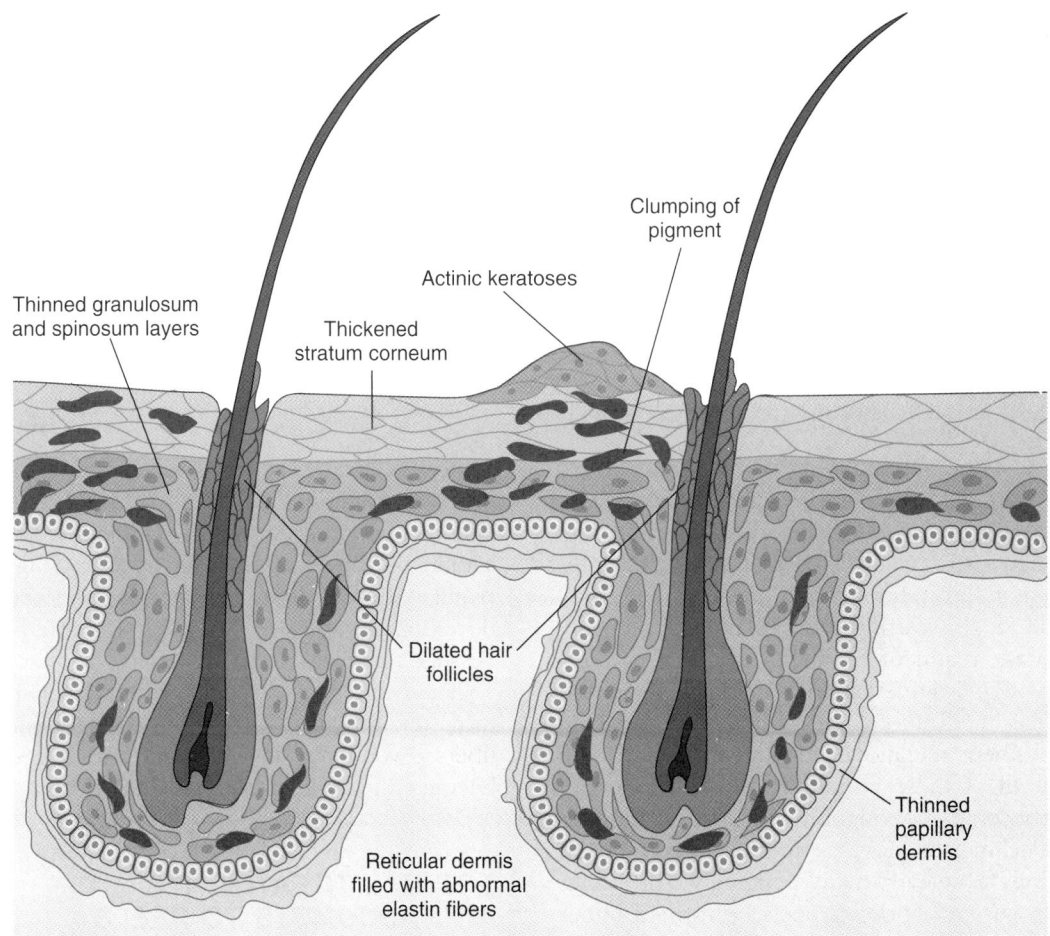

Thinned granulosum
and spinosum layers

Thickened
stratum corneum

Actinic keratoses

Clumping of
pigment

Dilated hair
follicles

Thinned
papillary
dermis

Reticular dermis
filled with abnormal
elastin fibers

Fig. 53-1
Skin damage from years of sun exposure. (Redrawn from Edwards L, Maibach HI, Roenigk HH: *Patient Care* 30(14):68, 1996.)

response to therapy. Renova is becoming the more popular form of tretinoin because of its emollient base, which has less of a tendency to irritate, especially at the 0.05% strength. Third-generation retinoids, with even fewer side effects, may soon be available. Following the use of topical retinoids, biopsies demonstrate deposition of new dermal collagen, formation of new blood vessels, and normalization of epidermal atypia. Accumulated melanin in the basal layer is transported to the surface and shed, improving pigmentation. Epidermal cell turnover is stimulated, producing a proliferation of new cells and improving skin texture. Improved blood supply to the dermis enhances both skin color and the transportation of nutrients to the skin. However, a minimum of 24 weeks is necessary to manifest visible signs of improvement. Unfortunately, these treatments must also be used forever to maintain any improvements. Fortunately, retinoids are now available generically, so the cost has decreased; however, some dermatologists insist that the generic preparations have a higher risk of skin irritation because of their preservatives. Those likely to benefit the most from retinoids are fair-skinned individuals in their

30s and 40s, who have blotchy pigmentation, sunspots, or fine lines around their eyes.

Lustra is another popular antiaging cream that contains 2% glycolic acid (GA), antioxidants, and hydroquinone (a bleaching agent). It is also available in a preparation that contains a complete sunblock (Lustra AF). Such a preparation can be used in combination with topical retinoids to treat areas of hyperpigmentation, such as melasma. Because the combination of preparations can be slightly irritating to the skin, they should be used every other day for the first 2 weeks and then daily. A mild steroid cream or ointment (triamcinolone 0.1%) applied sparingly and concomitantly, once a day, may reduce the associated erythema and flaking.

α-Hydroxy acids (AHAs) can be applied at low strength (2% to 20%) by the patient to improve collagen and elastin synthesis and to promote protein regeneration. Studies have indicated that both the papillary dermis and the epidermis can be thickened, elastic fibers improved, and melanin dispersed with the use of AHAs. Fine wrinkles and lines may be eliminated, and skin color and contour can be improved. At low doses this occurs without inflammation. Because AHAs do not cause angiogenesis (as opposed to retinoids), they are preferred for the treatment of patients with telangiectasias from rosacea photodamaged skin. In addition, because AHAs work by a different mechanism, they can be used concurrently with retinoids. Retinoids are usually applied at night, whereas AHAs can be used during the day. Skin texture, and to some degree skin pigmentation, may benefit at any age from retinoids, AHAs, or both. Bleaching agents may be added to treat irregular or abnormal pigmentation.

There are many AHA preparations available, buffered to various pH levels. It has been theorized that the beneficial or antiaging effects of AHAs are due to activation of transforming growth factor β (TGF-β) that is increasingly activated at cutaneous pH levels below 5. The prolonged application of "acid" AHAs may reduce the cutaneous pH and activate this growth factor. Most unbuffered AHAs have a low pH; however, a low pH also increases the risk of local skin irritation. Buffered preparations with pH levels above 2 are available and may be preferred. They eventually achieve the same effect with less irritation. In addition, using a low-strength AHA before a chemical peel will allow the clinician to not only judge patient tolerance, it will also enhance the penetration of the peel.

CHEMICAL PEELS AND ALTERNATIVE PROCEDURES

If topical treatment alone is not satisfactory, AHAs can be used at higher strengths (20% to 70%) or with other agents to cause an inflammatory response or a skin peel. Chemical peeling relies on penetration of an irritating exfoliate into the dermal level to produce a wound that results in sloughing of the superficial skin layers. The injury also evokes a nonspecific tissue regeneration that produces a smoother and more youthful appearing skin. A peel can be used after the skin has been prepared over time with retinoids, AHAs, or both, or it can be used as an alternative to the continuous application of these topicals. Individuals likely to benefit the most from superficial-depth skin peels for photodamage are from 25 to 50 years of age. (Significant photodamage is unusual before 25 years of age; after 50 years of age, intrinsic aging mechanisms may prevent optimal outcomes.) Fair-skinned, light-eyed individuals with a lot of sun damage or wrinkles at rest also benefit the most from peels. Fine wrinkles with skin motion, such as with smiling, may respond to a peel but often not as well as wrinkles at rest. Deep wrinkles at rest, such as those seen with intrinsically aged skin, may require deeper peels or plastic interventions. Periodic Botox injections may also improve wrinkles with motion in the upper face and the perioral areas (see Chapter 48, Uses of Botulinum Exotoxin). Deeper wrinkles that are muscle or motion induced will probably not respond to any peeling or resurfacing technique.

It is not surprising that AHAs improve the skin; fermented food products that contain them have long been used to exfoliate the skin. Ancient Egyptians used the "hemayet" fruit, Greeks used facial masks, and Romans applied various combinations of salts and plants for this purpose. In America, from the early 1900s until the 1950s, chemical peels were popular for skin rejuvenation. When dermabrasion was developed in the 1950s, it soon became the favored technique. With newer commercial preparations available and America's "baby boomers" aging, yet able to afford cosmetic treatments, chemical peels have become popular again. Recent developments with cryotherapy and laser have also become available for more complex interventions. In addition to describing various types of peels, the advantages and disadvantages of the alternatives to chemical peels are discussed briefly in the following paragraphs.

Four levels of chemical peels are available: (1) superficial, (2) superficial to medium, (3) medium, and (4) deep (Table 53-3). The deeper the peel, the higher the risk of complications, patient inconvenience, and discomfort. With deeper peels, it is usually obvious to the patient's friends and colleagues that a cosmetic procedure has been performed. On the other hand, most superficial-depth peels can be performed on a Thursday if the patient is not working on the weekend, and the patient can return to work the following Monday with little noticeable skin damage. Superficial-depth peels are the procedure of choice for individuals with ethnic skin, such as blacks, and glycolic acid (GA) is often the first choice of the experts.

Note: With the ability to achieve many of the effects of deep peels by repeated superficial-depth peels combined with retinoid preparation, the need for deep peels has somewhat diminished. For these and other reasons, including a higher risk of permanent skin damage and scarring with deep peels, deep peels should be performed by someone formally trained or significantly experienced in this area. Properly trained dermatologists, dermatologic surgeons, or plastic surgeons usually perform deep peels. For this chapter, deep peels are discussed only for the sake of completeness and to provide the clinician with an understanding of older, alternative techniques.

Although chemical peels are the least complex of the cosmetic procedures discussed here, they should not be taken lightly or performed without the proper experience, skills, and knowledge. With chemical peels, there is less control of the depth of skin penetration and damage than with other skin procedures; therefore in unskilled hands it is wise to start with very superficial-depth peels. Deeper peels should not be performed until the clinician has significant experience.

Of the alternatives to chemical peels, cryopeels are the most similar in effect (see Chapter 15, Cryosurgery).

TABLE 53-3

Levels of Chemical Peeling

Type of Peel	Chemical Formula	Indications
Superficial, stratum granulosum/papillary dermis (up to 0.06 mm)	AHA (GA 20%-70%) BHA (SA 20%-30%)	Fine rhytides (wrinkles)
	5-Fluorouracil TCA (10%-20%)	Bad skin texture

	Jessner's solution:
	  14 g resorcinol
	  14 g SA
	  14 g lactic acid
		Acne vulgaris (comedonal/inflammatory, papular-pustular)

	95% ethanol (quantity sufficient to add up to 100 ml)	Acne rosacea (papular-pustular)
	Unna's paste	Pigmentary changes (especially postinflammatory)
	Carbon dioxide (solid)	Superficial actinic keratoses
Superficial to medium (0.06-0.45 mm)	20%-30% TCA Series of AHA (GA 20%-70%) or BHA (SA 20%-30%) peels (see Table 53-4)	Persistent fine rhytides or bad skin texture Persistent acne vulgaris or rosacea Persistent mild pigmentary changes Isolated but deeper actinic keratoses
Medium, upper reticular dermis (0.45-0.6 mm)	50% TCA or 35% TCA plus initial keratolytics Initial keratolytics: Jessner's solution, carbon dioxide (solid), or 70% GA	Moderate rhytides (wrinkles) Chronic photo damage Multiple epidermal/premalignant lesions Pigmentary changes and solar lentigos Multiple actinic keratoses Multiple flat warts

Deep, midreticular dermis (0.6-0.8 mm)	Baker-Gordon formula:
	  3 ml 88% phenol
	  Three drops croton oil
	  Eight drops hexachlorophene
	  2 ml distilled water
		Severe rhytides (wrinkles)
		Epidermal lesions
		Superficial neoplasms
		Deep pigmentary changes

AHA, α-Hydroxy acid; *BHA,* β-hydroxy acid; *GA,* glycolic acid; *SA,* salicylic acid; *TCA,* trichloroacetic acid.

Many primary care clinicians already use liquid nitrogen for spot freezing or for cryotherapy of warts, actinic keratoses, seborrheic keratoses, or angiomas. With considerable experience, and often aided by a special attachment, the clinician can treat the entire face with cryotherapy to produce a cryopeel. It is less expensive than a deep chemical peel and results last for 1 to 2 years. Although a cryopeel may result in more swelling initially, it may also remove more wrinkles and result in smoother skin than a chemical peel.

Originally designed to remove acne scars, surgical skin planing or dermaplaning was soon found to be useful for scarring from other causes such as photodamage. After freezing, the skin layers are removed mechanically. Although postoperative healing is slower with dermaplaning and the cost is much higher than a peel (as much as $4000 for a full-face dermaplane), more severe lesions can be treated and the results of the skin resurfacing last longer (usually for 10 years or more). While chemical peels are the procedure of choice for fine wrinkles, and the effects may have a more prolonged effect than dermaplaning; dermaplaning is superior for deep acne scars. Dermabrasion is similar to dermaplaning (preparations, indications, etc.) and most often used to improve the look of facial scars caused by accidents or previous surgery or to smooth out fine facial wrinkles. The patient should be aware that following dermaplaning or dermabrasion, the effects on the face will be quite obvious to friends and colleagues.

A variant of dermabrasion is "microdermabrasion," in which the skin is "sandblasted" with silicon or aluminum crystals. This method is much less expensive than dermabrasion (about $100 to $150 per treatment), but three to six treatments are needed at weekly intervals for significant results. Among cosmetic surgeons this is the most equivalent to facial chemical peels; however, this procedure is not often attractive to primary care clinicians because of the $8000 to $50,000 cost of equipment. Another variant of dermabrasion, similar to microdermabrasion but with less equipment cost, is dermasanding (see Chapter 50, Dermasanding [Manual Dermabrasion]).

Carbon dioxide laser resurfacing is another option, but it often requires general or tumescent anesthesia and costs as much as $5000. Although studies have not been published comparing laser surgery with dermabrasion, anecdotal evidence indicates it to be as effective as dermabrasion for removing deep wrinkles around the mouth. There have been no comparative studies showing advantages of laser resurfacing of the whole face over dermabrasion or chemical peeling. Long-pulse (i.e., 1000 msec) erbium-YAG lasers are now being used to achieve results similar to superficial-depth and medium-depth chemical peels. They can be used anywhere on the body with only topical anesthesia and some oral sedation (see Chapter 27, Laser Therapy).

Intense pulsed light (IPL) therapy is a new option for skin rejuvenation. It seems to work best for redness, flushing, or dilated capillaries but can also be used for overall skin rejuvenation. There is no downtime for patients and minimal discomfort during the four to six required treatments. Unfortunately, the cost of equipment ($75,000 to $150,000) again prevents many primary care clinicians from offering this procedure. Certain brands of this equipment can also be used for hair removal. Office laser equipment can even be used for myringotomy (see Chapter 65, Myringotomy and Tympanocentesis).

Various chemicals have been used for skin peels, also known as chemexfoliation or chemabrasion. These include phenol, trichloroacetic acid (TCA), AHAs (e.g., GA, lactic acid, citric acid, malic acid, mandelic acid, tartaric acid), and β-hydroxy acids (i.e., salicylic acid [SA]). Combinations are also used. For single agents, lactic acid, GA, and SAs are used most frequently. Weaker chemicals such as resorcinol have been used and are relatively free of side effects; however, except in combination with AHAs, they are rarely used at prescription strength anymore. Advantages of chemical peels over dermabrasion and laser include the lower cost of equipment and less of a need for formal training, especially for superficial-depth peels. Again, the effects of a light peel are so subtle that friends and colleagues may not realize that a cosmetic procedure has been performed.

Among the benefits of using GA, TCA, and SA preparations are the fact that they are stable and water soluble. In addition, GA is colorless, odorless, and nontoxic if ingested. Some controversy exists, but many experts consider GA to be safer for ethnically darker skin. Disadvantages to GA include the fact that the peels are somewhat variable: some patients have a brisk inflammatory response to only 30% GA, whereas others have only a slight response to as high as 70% GA. There is also some dispute concerning the degree of buffering to be used for GA and how best to neutralize it after application.

One benefit of SA over GA or any other AHA is that the precipitate is visible, or "frosts," after application. This allows the clinician to verify that the application is even. SA also has less of a need for neutralization after application. If not clearly visible after application and drying, SA fluoresces under a Wood's light, which can be used to ensure complete application. These characteristics may be important when clinicians are first learning the procedure. Because it penetrates the epidermal lipids of the skin more deeply than GA, SA usually causes more desquamation (allowing patients to see the peeling and note the changes). In addition, SA is comedolytic; therefore it is perhaps the best preparation to use with acne rosacea. With these differences, it would appear that SA is superior to the AHAs; however, in reality most experts do not use these differences to make their choice, but rather their own personal experience.

TCA, AHAs, and SA (at the listed strengths) are not as deeply absorbed through the skin and do not burn the skin as deeply as phenol. Therefore using only these preparations avoids most of the long-term sequelae associated with deep phenol peels (e.g., total loss of pigmentation, irregular pigmentation, hypertrophic scars). As a result of these risks and a theoretic risk of toxicity if absorbed, phenol peels are used much less frequently these days. With such safe and effective AHA and SA peels available, there is a question as to whether primary care clinicians should use even TCA. Both phenol and TCA work by coagulating skin proteins; decreasing the concentration of TCA toward 20% decreases the depth of exfoliation, perhaps making it safer. Before the advent of AHAs and SA, TCA was found to be safer than phenol for treating transition zones, such as the area between the face and neck. It was also found to be excellent for treating the thin skin of the hands. In both of these areas, a deeper burn might increase the risk of scar formation. With AHAs, application of a series of superficial-depth peels, especially if the skin has been prepared by the use of topical retinoids for many weeks, may produce the same effects as one medium peel or even some of the effects of a deep peel. With experience, AHAs allow you to customize the treatment to the area of the body.

INDICATIONS (see Table 53-3)

- Minor to-moderate photodamaged skin, especially in 25- to 50-year-old patients
- Failure of topical therapy or the patient is unsatisfied with results
- Irregular skin texture
- Actinic keratoses
- Acne vulgaris (comedonal and inflammatory, papular and pustular)
- Acne rosacea (papular and pustular)

- Irregular pigmentation (e.g., melasma, freckles, lentigines)
- Superficial acne scars or hyperpigmentation
- Fine wrinkles
- Multiple fat warts

Note: If peels are used to treat acne or the complications of acne, the acne should be approximately 75% resolved with whatever primary treatment is being used (e.g., oral antibiotics or topical treatments) before using a peel. In addition, SA is probably the chemical of choice for acne rosacea.

CONTRAINDICATIONS

- Concurrent hormone therapy.
- Concurrent isotretinoin (Accutane) therapy. (This should be discontinued for 6 months before undergoing a chemical peel.)
- Concurrent radiation therapy.
- Patients with known allergies or hypersensitivities to agents used for chemical peels.
- Possible melanoma, squamous cell carcinoma, or basal cell carcinoma in the region to be treated.
- Recurrent labial herpes. (They should receive prophylactic antiherpetic medications before undergoing a chemical peel.)
- Hemangiomas and nevi flammeus (which do not respond to chemical peels).
- Inflammatory lesions (e.g., herpes simplex, acute acne papule, cellulitis, severe seborrheic dermatitis) should be avoided during chemical peels. More peeling occurs in the areas of inflammation and hyperpigmentation can result. Dermatitis or infection should be controlled before peels; otherwise the chemicals will penetrate more deeply.
- Peels are futile in alcoholics or if the patient will not commit to reduced or stopping smoking. Heavy alcohol use impairs healing. The changes induced by peels will not counteract the damage to the skin from heavy smoking.
- Medium and deep chemical peels of the neck should be approached with caution. In this area there is difficulty controlling the depth of the peel, thus increasing the risk of hypertrophic scarring.

Note: Although peels are not contraindicated, patients with as little as ¹/₃₂ Native American heritage may be at increased risk of persistent erythema and subsequent hyperpigmentation after a peel. This may be due in part to a reaction to chemicals. Patients with a history of an allergy to parabens or perfumes may be at the same risk; therefore, for both groups, every precaution should be taken to prevent an allergic reaction to any agents, preservatives, or perfumes (see the "Technique" section). Oral and topical steroids should be considered. If this fails, bleaching agents may also be used (see the "Complications" section

for a formula or the "Suppliers" section to order Bleacheze from Medical Center Pharmacy).

EQUIPMENT

- Petroleum jelly (Vaseline).
- Cotton-tipped swabs.
- Benzoyl peroxide 5% to 10% wash. (Sebum pads are available, but benzoyl peroxide seems more effective at removing skin oils and debris.)
- Moisturizer and sunblock to apply immediately after the peel. (Theraplex brand has been found to be very effective, especially if applied before the patient leaves the office.)

Superficial-Depth Peels

Kits are available for superficial chemical peels, ranging in price from $4 to $10 per peel. The patient is charged from $65 to $100 per peel. Treatment for photodamage usually obtains optimal benefit after four to six peels, each 1 month apart.

- TCA 10% to 20%
- GA 20% to 70%
- SA 20% to 30%
- Other AHAs 20% to 70% (e.g., lactic acid, citric acid, malic acid, mandelic acid, tartaric acid)

Note: Although lower-pH (i.e., pH below 2) GA (50% to 70%) solutions create more necrosis, there is no evidence that this leads to a more favorable peel. Additional necrosis produces additional crusting, making it more obvious that the patient has had a procedure performed as well as increasing the risk of complications. Therefore, partially buffered or neutralized GA solutions (i.e., pH above 2) are recommended.

Superficial- to Medium-Depth Peels

- TCA 20% to 30%
- A series of AHA or BHA peels (Table 53-4)

Medium-Depth Peels

- TCA 50% or TCA 35% plus initial keratolytics

Note: For patient safety and standardization, TCA should be compounded by a weight-to-volume method (i.e., 15% TCA is made by diluting 15 g of TCA crystals in distilled water up to a total volume of 100 ml).

Optional Topical Anesthetic for Medium-Depth Peels

- Lidocaine 2.5% and prilocaine 2.5% (EMLA) mixture
- Lidocaine 4% (ELA-Max)

TABLE 53-4
Protocols for Serial Glycolic Acid Peels (Performed 2 to 4 Weeks Apart)

Indication	I. Conc (%)	Time (min)	II. Conc (%)	Time (min)	III. Conc (%)	Time (min)
Acne	70	2	35	3	50-70	1-3
Melasma	70	3	35	4	50-70	2-4
Actinic keratoses	70	4	50	3	70	5-7
Fine wrinkles	70	5	50	4	70	4-8
Solar lentigines	70	6	70	3	70	4-8
Back or chest (any indication)	70	7	70	4	70	5-10

Modified from Gendler EC: *Dermatol Clin* 15(4):561, 1997.

PREPROCEDURE PATIENT PREPARATION

Patients can be informed that applying the chemicals to produce most peels takes very little time. After the face is prepped with petrolatum, it usually takes less than 1 minute to apply the solution for superficial- to medium-depth peels. However, deep peels require several hours to prepare the face, apply the chemical, and complete the peel.

Native Americans need to inform the clinician of their heritage, and anyone with allergies to parabens, perfumes, or other skin preparations needs to inform the clinician so that they can use precautions against hypererythema (see the "Technique" section). He or she needs to receive a patient teaching guide and must inform the clinician of any other possible contraindication. (See the sample patient education handout titled "Skin Peels" on page 1797 of Appendix G.)

For superficial-depth peels, patients may experience a stinging or burning sensation during application of the peel. This increases for 2 minutes after application, reaches a peak at 3 minutes, and then goes away over the following minute. The chemicals themselves cause superficial anesthesia; giving patients this information may be psychologically reassuring. In addition, patients usually report a slight tightness and smoothness of the skin immediately after superficial-depth peels. Within several days, some patients will experience slight skin crusting, swelling, and possibly purpura in the lower eyelid areas, which resolve rapidly.

Whenever the skin is peeled or wounded, there is a risk of scarring and infection. Also, pigmentary augmentation is both a short-term (which almost always resolves) and a long-term risk. There is a slight risk of permanent pigmentary augmentation. The deeper the peel, the higher the risk of all of these side effects and complications. Superficial peels very rarely cause complications; medium and deep peels are higher risks.

Patients should be aware that their postoperative appearance has the risk of being frightening, especially for medium or deep peels. This is rare for superficial-depth peels. Clinicians should use hypoallergenic, non-scented, complete sunblock (skin protection factor [SPF] 20 or greater). Erythema almost always resolves in a few weeks.

In many cases patients will be asked to pretreat the skin with topical retinoids for 3 to 5 weeks before the peel. Benefits of pretreatment include the fact that it accelerates the epidermal turnover, which will reduce healing time. If the topical retinoids cause bothersome or severe desquamation, they should be discontinued for several days and then resumed on alternate days.

For superficial-depth peels, the patient can wear makeup the day of the peel. It will be removed in the clinician's office. Topical retinoids should be stopped 3 days before the procedure. For medium and deep peels, the skin should be washed the evening before the procedure to remove all cosmetics and again the next morning to ensure smooth, even skin penetration.

Note: Disappointment from a chemical peel is often the result of overly high expectations, by either the clinician or the patient. Patients should be given a patient teaching guide and made aware that superficial-depth peels yield only modest clinical effects. Following multiple peels they should be able to better appreciate the benefits. Patients should also be reminded that the effect of a medium-depth peel is not comparable to a face-lift.

TECHNIQUE

Note: Patients with a history of allergy to parabens (the most common preservative in over-the-counter sunblocks) or with a history of allergy to perfumes should be treated with oral steroids for 10 to 14 days after the procedure. This is followed by the use of a topical, parabens-free corticosteroid cream until healed. It may also be prudent to use this treatment in all individuals of Native American heritage to minimize the risk of complications.

Superficial-Depth Peels

1. Choose the proper mixture or concentration for the patient. AHA 20% to 70%, β-hydroxy acid 20% to 30% (i.e., SA), and TCA 10% to 20% cause detachment of keratinocytes at the lower concentrations and epidermolysis at the higher concentrations.
2. Cleanse skin of residual debris, makeup, and body surface oils with benzoyl peroxide 5% to 10%. Alcohol and acetone can also be used to remove skin oils.
3. Using cotton-tipped applicators, apply petroleum jelly around the edges of the eyes, the mouth corners, and the edges of the nose (i.e., nasoalar junction). These are typically dry areas of the face and therefore need protection. Any inflamed lesion, such as an active acne lesion, should be avoided. Ask the patient if there are any other dry areas of the face that need protection from the peel. Patients usually know which areas of their nose and face are the driest.
4. Apply the mixture evenly to the entire face. Gentle stretching of the skin will allow the fluid to coat the depths of wrinkles evenly. Peels usually do not need to be extended below the line of the jaw, and the fluid should not be applied closer than a couple of millimeters to the eyelid margin. Feather the solution into the hairline and along the chin to prevent a line of demarcation between the treated and untreated areas. Also apply to desired areas of the chest, neck, arms, and hands.
5. Allow to remain in place for the appropriate time (usually 3 to 5 minutes).
6. Dilute and wash with either water or sodium bicarbonate solution if it needs neutralizing.
7. A hypoallergenic, nonscented moisturizer and complete sunblock (e.g., Theraplex) should be applied immediately after the peel.
8. These peels may make low-strength topical (not peeling strength) GA or other AHA solutions more effective to use later at home.

Superficial- to Medium-Depth Peels

1. As for superficial-depth peels, choose the proper mixture technique to obtain a superficial- to medium-depth peel. A single agent can be used (TCA 20% to 30%) or superficial-depth peels may be repeated every 2 to 4 weeks for a deeper peel effect or until the desired results are obtained. For AHAs or TCA, three or four treatments may be adequate (Table 53-4); however, often six to eight SA peels are performed. In most cases, the best results are obtained if the patient waits 1 month between peels.
2. If TCA 20% to 30% is chosen, the skin to be peeled must first be dekeratinized to ensure uniform TCA penetration. AHA or β-hydroxy acid superficial-depth peels in the office a few days before the procedure can be used for this purpose. Dekeratinization can also be performed by the patient before arrival by applying topical retinoids to the skin surface daily for 3 to 5 weeks.
3. Although anesthesia is not necessary, intravenous conscious sedation or topical anesthetic (see below) may be used.
4. Protect the necessary areas of the face with petroleum jelly in the same manner as for superficial-depth peels.
5. Using a cotton-tipped applicator with the tip wrung out well to avoid dripping or splashing, apply the TCA to the entire face. It should be applied evenly to produce a smooth, white surface. Greater penetration in certain areas may be achieved by rubbing the applicator vigorously. Gently stretching the skin will allow the fluid to coat the depths of wrinkles evenly. The peel should not be extended below the jaw line. Desired areas of the hands and arms may also be treated.
6. Treatments may be repeated, if necessary, in 1- to 3-month intervals to achieve the desired effect.

Medium-Depth Peels

Note: Pretreatment with 0.1% tretinoin (Retin-A) daily for at least 2 weeks will enhance wound healing from medium-depth peels.

Using a Combination of 70% Glycolic Acid and 35% Trichloroacetic Acid

1. After protecting areas of the face with petroleum jelly in the same manner as for superficial-depth peels, apply a 70% GA mixture to the entire face.
2. Allow to remain in place for 2 minutes. A fan in the room may ease patient discomfort from the stinging associated with the peel.
3. Wash with water.
4. Optional but effective: Apply a topical anesthetic (EMLA, ELA-Max, or Betacaine) for 30 minutes without occlusion.
5. Remove the topical anesthetic and apply 35% TCA to the entire face as previously described.
6. If successful and there are no complications, this technique can be extended to the hands, arms, and chest during the next peel.
7. A cool compress applied to the area after a peel may ease patient discomfort.

Note: A study comparing two topical anesthetics (EMLA and ELA-Max) with each other and with a placebo found a statistically significant decrease in pain with both topical anesthetics and no difference in efficacy between the two anesthetics. Neither anesthetic affected the depth of penetration of the peel. Betacaine can be used in the same manner (see the "Suppliers" section).

Trichloroacetic Acid 50%

The technique is the same as for a superficial- to medium-depth peel with TCA as described above.

COMPLICATIONS

Persistent hyperpigmentation is a slight risk, but it is often adequately treated with bleaching agents. One published formula combines 30 g of paraben-free corticosteroid cream, 15 g of 4% hydroquinone, and 20 g of Retin-A 0.1% into a cream to be applied starting 2 weeks after the procedure if hyperpigmentation is developing. Another option is Bleacheze (see the "Suppliers" section).

The use of oral corticosteroids for 2 weeks postprocedure followed by a steroid cream may prevent persistent hyperpigmentation (see the note at the beginning of the "Technique" section).

POSTPROCEDURE PATIENT EDUCATION

For superficial-depth peels, the effect is maximal at 48 hours, so the patient should attempt to avoid the sun completely for at least 3 days. The skin is most vulnerable to damage during this time and sun exposure can cause many problems, including a deepening of the peel or postinflammatory hyperpigmentation.

Actual peeling usually begins 2 days after the peel and can last for up to 7 days. Most patients peel in the central part of the face more heavily than peripherally and only lightly on the forehead. Some patients peel in fine sheets, but most peel in flakes.

As stated previously, patients usually report a slight tightness and smoothness of their skin immediately after superficial-depth peels and some patients experience slight skin crusting. Occasionally, swelling will occur as well as purpura in the lower eyelid areas. These symptoms resolve rapidly. The deeper the peel, the more likely the patient will have these side effects.

The effect of a medium-depth peel is maximal at 48 hours, usually subsides within the first week, and is gone by the third month after the procedure. Crusts or scabs usually appear and some swelling may occur. Prescribing a mild pain medication may relieve any tingling or throbbing. In about 7 to 10 days, new skin will be apparent and the patient should be healed sufficiently to return to normal activities. They should continue to avoid the sun for several months.

After all peels, sunburn may occur at lower doses of sunlight and lead to hyperpigmentation or hypopigmentation. Preservatives, scents, or the chemicals used may also provoke a sensitivity reaction and cause persistent erythema; therefore a hypoallergenic, nonscented, complete sunblock (SPF 20 or greater) for sensitive skin should be used. Even after healing, the skin is thinner after a peel and is more susceptible to sun damage and sunburn. The patient should learn to wear a complete sunblock every day and to avoid the sun.

Thinner or irritated skin is also more susceptible to desiccation, so a moisturizer should be applied daily.

SUPPLIERS

Salicylic acid
Beta lift 2-0 (20%) and 3-0 (30%)
Bioglan
7 Great Valley Parkway
Malvern, PA 19355
Phone: 1-888-246-4526
Website: www.bioglan.com

Note: Theraplex, an excellent postpeel emollient and sunblock, is also available from Bioglan.

Betacaine and Bleacheze
Medical Center Pharmacy
4600 N. Habana Avenue
Tampa, FL 33614
Phone: 1-800-226-7094

Trichloroacetic acid (TCA), glycolic acid (GA) and other supplies
Delasco/Dermatologic Lab and Supply, Inc.
608 13th Avenue
Council Bluffs, IA 51501
Phone: 1-800-831-6273
Website: www.delasco.com

Dermatopics or Pharmatopix
Pharmagen, Inc.
155 Knickerbocker Avenue
Bohemia, NY 11716
Phone: 1-800-445-2595

Glycolic acid
Gly-derm
ICN Pharmaceuticals
3300 Hyland Drive
Costa Mesa, CA 92626
Phone: 1-800-556-1937
Website: www.icnpharm.com

MD Forte
Allergan, Inc.
P.O. Box 19534
Irvine, CA 92623-9534
Phone: 1-800-553-6783
Website: www.allergan.com/profpath/js_ind.htm

CPT/BILLING CODES

15788	Chemical peel, facial; epidermal
15789	Chemical peel, facial; dermal
15792	Chemical peel, nonfacial; epidermal
15793	Chemical peel, nonfacial; dermal

ICD-9-CM DIAGNOSTIC CODES

Although most insurers consider chemical peels a cosmetic procedure, occasionally they reimburse for treatment of acne, actinic keratoses, or acne rosacea.

706.1	Acne
695.3	Acne rosacea
702.0	Actinic keratosis
709.2	Disfigurement because of scar
709.00	Dyschromia, unspecified
709.09	Lentigo
709.09	Melasma
709.3	Senile dermatosis

ADDITIONAL RESOURCES

- See the sample patient education handout titled "Skin Peels" on page 1797 of Appendix G.

BIBLIOGRAPHY

Arndt KA, Kaminer M, Wheeland RG: The promises and limits of cosmetic dermatology, *Patient Care* 33(9):97, 1999.

Bernstein EF: Chemical peels. In Kaminer MS, Dover JS, Arndt KA, editors: *Atlas of cosmetic surgery,* Philadelphia, 2002, WB Saunders.

Brody HJ: *Chemical peeling and resurfacing,* ed 2, St Louis, 1997, Mosby.

Coleman III WP, Coleman KM: Techniques for peeling of the face. In Merli GJ: *The clinics atlas of office procedures: basic cosmetic procedures,* Philadelphia, December 2000, WB Saunders.

Edwards L, Maibach HI, Roenigk HH: What can be done for photoaged skin? *Patient Care* 30(14):68, 1996.

Farber GA: Prolonged erythema after chemical peel, *Dermatol Surg* 24:933, 1998.

Gendler EC: Topical treatment of the aging face, *Clin Dermatol* 15(4):561, 1997.

Kligman D, Kligman AM: Salicylic acid peels for the treatment of photoaging, *Dermatol Surg* 24:325, 1998.

Koppel RA, Coleman KM, Coleman WP: The efficacy of EMLA versus ELA-Max for pain relief in medium-depth chemical peeling: a clinical and histopathologic evaluation, *Dermatol Surg* 26(1):61, 2000.

Matarasso SL, Hanke CW, Alster TS: Cutaneous resurfacing, *Clin Dermatol* 15(4):569, 1997.

Rees TD: Chemabrasion and dermabrasion. In Rees TD, LaTrenta GS, editors: *Aesthetic plastic surgery,* ed 2, Philadelphia, 1994, WB Saunders.

WEBSITES

www.plasticsurgery.org/surgery/chempeel.htm
www.plastic-surgery.net (Plastic Surgery Network)
www.plastic-surgery.net/procedures/chemical.html
(Plastic Surgery Network: Chemical peels)
www.plastic-surgery.net/procedures/dermabrasion.html
(Plastic Surgery Network: Dermabrasion and dermaplaning)

CHAPTER 54

Tattoo Removal: Infrared Light Obliteration Method

Tolbert S. Wilkinson

Tattoos cannot be "removed" but can be obliterated with varying degrees of scar formation. Scarring is related to the amount of depth and density of pigment within the dermis and the technique involved in removing it. The infrared coagulator (IRC) is an inexpensive tool for tattoo obliteration with fewer treatments and less cost than alternatives including dermabrasion, salabrasion, excision with tissue expansion, and a variety of lasers. In an effort to provide a less costly, less time-consuming program, the Gang-X Tattoo Removal protocol was developed to remove tattoos from gang members and as a continuation of an evaluation project for the Innovative Procedures Committee of the American Society for Aesthetic Plastic Surgery.

The Redfield IRC has been cleared by the U.S. Food and Drug Administration (FDA) for the treatment of various cutaneous problems, including warts, hemorrhoids, angiomas, and for the treatment of tattoos. Although the infrared light delivers more heat to the dermis than standard laser techniques, treating the site afterwards as a superficial second-degree burn with appropriate burn therapy has minimized scar formation with over 5000 patients. Individuals who followed the aftercare protocol have "blurs" that are equal to or are occasionally preferable to those obtained with the laser (Fig. 54-1). Tattoo obliteration is often completed in one or two sessions under local anesthesia. The clinician can treat all colors and all varieties of tattoos in a matter of minutes. This makes the technique applicable for individuals who do not have the financial resources nor the time for laser surgery, but who must remove tattoos for emotional or career reasons.

The energy source for the inexpensive portable IRC is a 15-V tungsten halogen lamp that provides a range of wavelengths of light from 400 to 2500 nm in each pulse. The energy is delivered directly to the tattoo through a quartz rod with a sapphire tip (see Fig. 108-9). Tissue damage as well as obliteration of the tattoo is directly related to time of application. The longer the light is activated, the deeper the damage.

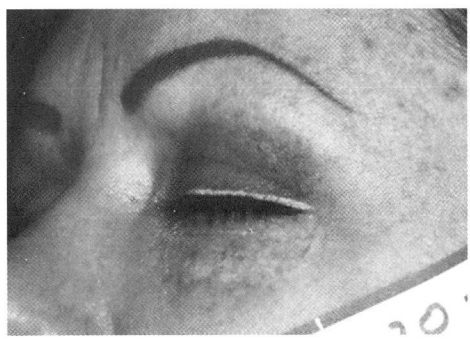

Fig. 54-1
Typical patient appearance after treatment with the infrared coagulator for "double teardrop" on the left malar area. It has a lighter skin color and will not tan, but it is otherwise acceptable in appearance.

Through a period of trial and error, the Tattoo Obliteration by Infrared Light (TOBIL) protocol was developed, which eliminates the majority of complications, such as tissue loss and hypertrophic scarring, that occur with all tattoo obliteration modalities. Training sessions are available for all practitioners.

INDICATIONS

Professional and amateur tattoos may be treated. Best results are obtained with tattoos of letters or lines. Solid figures must be treated in a "polka-dot" or "striped" pattern with skip areas to avoid disruption of blood supply to the overlying skin (Fig. 54-2). "High scar areas," such as the shoulder or between the breasts, must be approached with caution (Fig. 54-3).

After patients are shown before-and-after and healing phase photographs, a decision is made on whether to proceed based on the history of scar formation in that individual, the scar location, the depth of penetration of pigment, and the patient's personal feelings about scarring.

The decision to obliterate a tattoo is an emotional

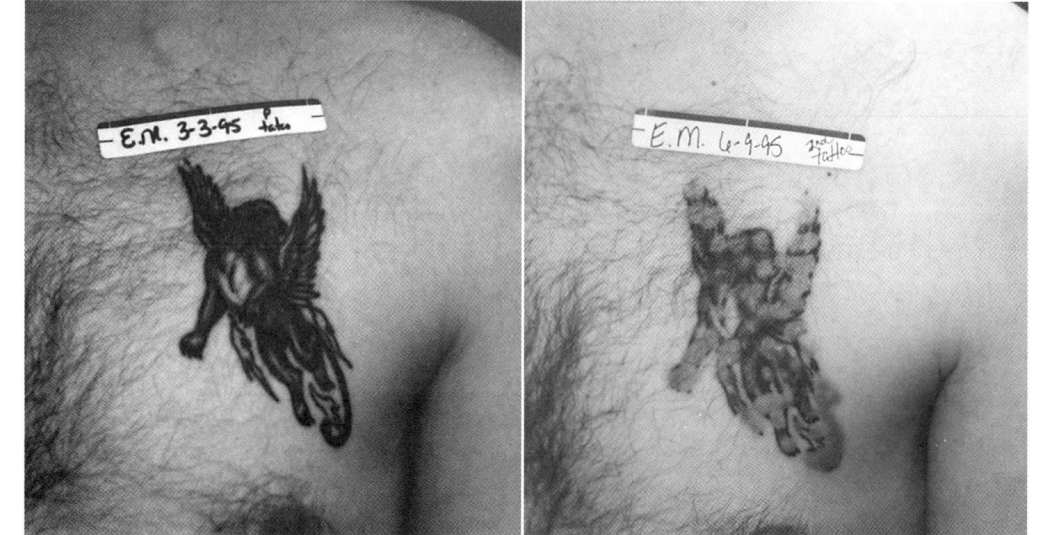

Fig. 54-2
A, Typical professional tattoo may vary in the depth of ink placement, but the hazard is that blood supply will be compromised if the entire tattoo is treated at one session. **B,** "Polka-dot" pattern of application of half-second bursts of energy led to this improvement. A second session may be scheduled as early as 30 days after resolution to this point. Note that this patient has rigorously followed the guidelines to prevent infection and reduce scarring in one of the most scar-vulnerable areas on the body.

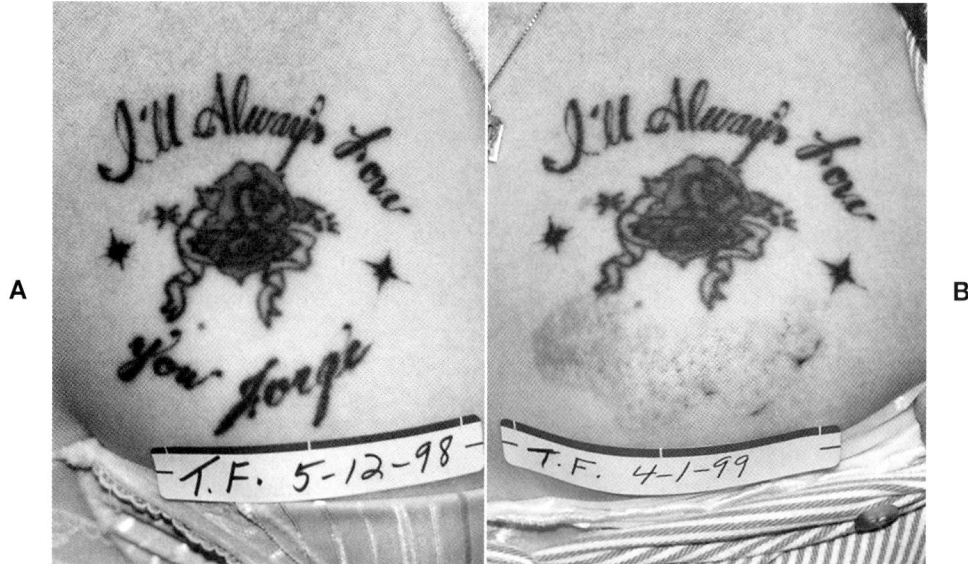

Fig. 54-3
A, Tattoos that cover a palm-sized area and tattoos in the most scar-vulnerable areas of the body (the shoulder and between the breasts) should be approached with caution, or not treated at all. Removal of a tattoo by laser or infrared coagulator leaves scarring in the deep dermis. If a tattoo covers the entire shoulder, it would be best not to attempt any method of tattoo removal because the resultant scar limits mobility and will be vulnerable to trauma. This tattoo is located on the left upper breast area. The area was treated was less risky because the script areas are not a compact mass of pigment. If we had attempted to treat the central rose area, a less pleasing scar and even central skin loss would have likely resulted.
B, Resolution of the tattoo pigment with "wash-up" areas at the edges. This is tattoo pigment that has been fragmented but has drifted to the edge of the tattoo. Many patients prefer to leave this untouched, but it can certainly be treated with additional bursts of infrared energy.

and/or social decision. Some individuals obtain tattoos to promote self-esteem or affiliation. Yet the presence of the tattoo renders them unsuitable for employment in fast-food outlets, the military, airlines, and other establishments.

CONTRAINDICATIONS

- Closely tattooed circular patterns of the wrist and ankle
- Wide patterns covering the center of the chest or shoulder
- Heavily pigmented circular patterns of the fingers or toes

EQUIPMENT

- The IRC (see Fig. 108-9). The small unit is extremely easy to use. It is simply turned on and the tuner is set for the length of light pulse desired. With newer models, a new plastic disposable sheath is used to cover the tip for each session.
- 0.5% Xylocaine with or without epinephrine.
- Antiseptic solutions.
- 20-gauge spinal and 25-gauge, 1½-inch injection needles.
- Telfa pads.
- Coban or Vetrap.
- Topical antibiotic.
- Nonsterile gloves.
- Basin with alcohol sponges.
- Prescription for topical steroids (Hytone 2.5%).
- Topical refrigerant spray.

The light intensity with the IRC is constant. The variables in the treatment are the length of time of application, the tip size of the probe, the amount of overlap of treatment, and the character of the tattoo itself.

PREPROCEDURE PATIENT PREPARATION

Each patient is counseled extensively regarding scarring, recovery, and his or her responsibility in caring for what should be described as the equivalent of "a cigarette burn." Most tattoos are obliterated in a single procedure, but the patient must be aware that several procedures may be necessary for complete removal of all pigment. Large tattoo removal may also be tolerated better if done in stages. Although complications may occur and cause expensive problems, they are rare.

Since many individuals seeking tattoo obliteration wish to abandon gang affiliations, care must be taken to document the original and postoperative appearance of the scar for law-enforcement agencies. The Texas Program, which assists youths in abandoning gangs, requires fingerprints and tattoo photographs, as well as complete and detailed permit forms. These permit forms must include documentation of counseling with the treatment physician before treatment, the awareness of complications, etc.

Costs must also be discussed since insurance companies will not pay for these procedures. It is best to have the patient pay before treatment.

TECHNIQUE

The IRC does not require special glasses or a protective environment, but the light is bright and it is best to look away as the unit is activated. Experience in burn therapy is essential. The planning of the program for each individual must take into account the pattern of the tattoo, the operator's assessment of each obliteration session, and the individual's response to antibiotics and pressure in the recovery phase.

Darker pigments in the tattoo necessitate a longer time of application than do lighter colors. Overlap of the applicator tip may ensure smooth obliteration, but, to maintain a good blood supply in solid tattoos that cover more than 1 cm square of skin, a "striping" or "polka-dot" pattern is used. All tattoos are initially treated with 0.5-second bursts of infrared energy (Figs. 54-4 and 54-5). This is easily dialed into the machine. Secondary procedures are determined by the depth of the pigment as well as individual skin thickness, tattoo location, and skin pigmentation. Secondary sessions may be at the same interval or more commonly at 0.75 second (or even at 1.0 second), but increasing "power" (time on tissue) poses a greater risk of skin destruction and scarring.

1. Use ethyl chloride spray to "freeze" the skin proximal to each tattoo (optional).
2. Use 1% xylocaine with or without epinephrine for anesthesia. For large lesions, dilute the 1% Xylocaine with saline to give 0.5% Xylocaine with 1:400,000 epinephrine. Also in large lesions, use a 20-gauge spinal needle passed centrally, then moved in a radial pattern beneath the dermis until the entire area is anesthetized. This allows for just one penetration of the skin with a needle. When going beneath the dermis, it will take longer for the anesthetic to take effect, so wait approximately 5 minutes.
3. Determine the setting of the unit based on the appearance, design, and color of the tattoo. Darker colors require more time than lighter colors. Begin with the time frame of 0.5 second per burst with a minimal overlap of each delivery spot. Amateur

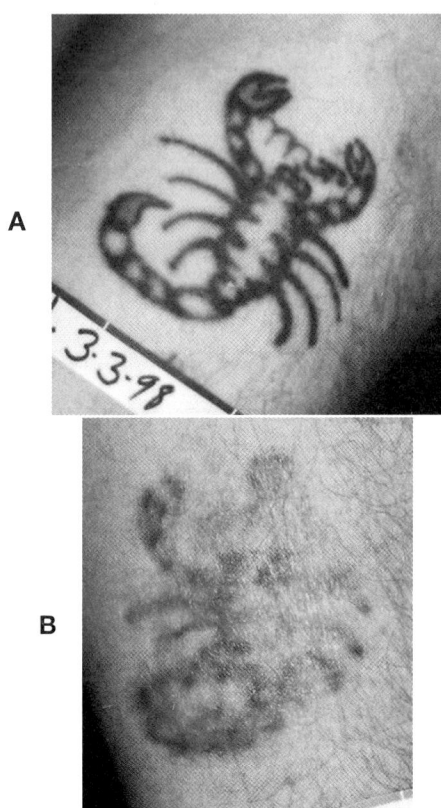

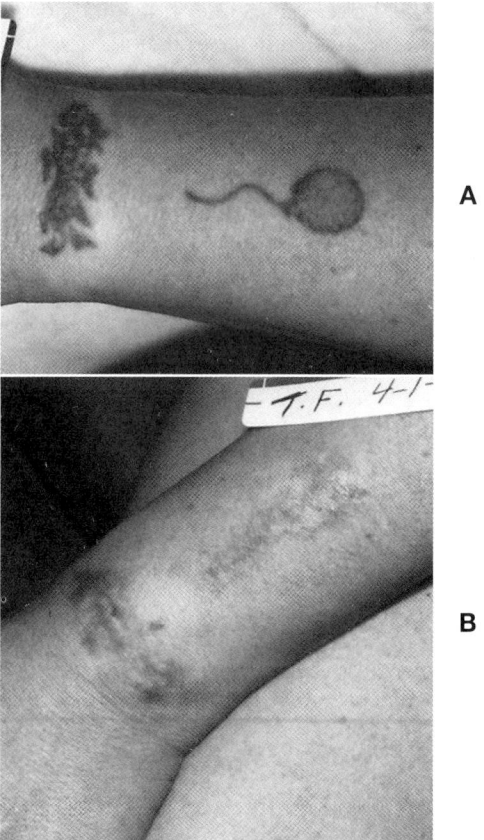

Fig. 54-4
A, Typical professional tattoo of the forearm responds well to the infrared light obliteration program because pressure can be applied for as long as 3 months after the initial and secondary sessions. In this patient the area has been infiltrated with 0.25% Xylocaine with epinephrine through a single entry point above the tattoo, using a 22-gauge spinal needle to fill the subcutaneous tissue. After 10 to 15 minutes, the entire area is anesthetized with little pain. **B,** Single application to this widely spaced tattoo, leaving only certain areas for "skip zones," led to this degree of resolution. A similar pattern may occur when certain areas of the tattoo pigment are placed deeper in the dermis. However, it is wiser to treat initially at half-second bursts of energy, as in this patient.

Fig. 54-5
A, Professional and amateur tattoos in the extremities respond well to the half-second bursts. Protection is necessary not only to prevent scar hypertrophy, but also to prevent accidental trauma during the healing phase. **B,** Resolution of these tattoos after one session of treatment. Small areas of hypertrophic scar are treated with Cordran tape and/or steroid injections, as well as a reapplication of pressure.

tattoos also often go deeper and may require longer application.

4. Place the tip of the wand directly on the tattooed skin and pull the trigger. The unit automatically shuts off at the time selected. Only minimal pressure is needed on the skin. A "pop" is often heard as the tip is activated.

5. Allow a few seconds for the tip to cool between applications.

6. Treatment releases a lot of heat. For better healing with widely spaced "line" tattoos, use minimal energy to obliterate the actual outline of the figure or the wording. Individual judgment is required whether overlapping should be performed at the initial session, at a second session, or never. For dense tattoos,

it is best to leave a significant gap between each application of the tip.

7. Continue treatment until the entire tattoo pattern has been covered in the fashion desired.

COMPLICATIONS AND AFTEREFFECTS

- Depigmentation (common)
- Hypertrophic or keloid scarring
- Failure to remove all pigment (more likely in amateur tattoos)
- Secondary infection
- Pain
- Prolonged healing

Treatment effectively causes a second-degree burn. Just as with burns, depigmentation and scarring to some degree is common. Thick scars may require aggressive treatment, including Cordran tape, intralesional steroid injections, or prolonged application of Silastic materials.

(See Chapter 39, Hypertrophic Scars and Keloids.) Residual pigment may need further treatment sessions or actual excision of pigment beneath the dermis, which may further require complex techniques. A second application with the IRC is usually delayed 4 to 8 weeks to allow for complete healing.

It is extremely important to follow postoperational directions to reduce adverse outcomes. Even after doing this, the wound may take 4 to 6 weeks to heal and then several months for the inflammation and erythema to resolve.

After the first few days, pain is generally minimal.

It is rare for the treated area to regain normal pigment, and rarely will it tan synchronously with the other skin.

POSTPROCEDURE PATIENT EDUCATION

- Topical antibiotics, a telfa pad, and pressure wraps are applied over the treated area and are to remain in place for 36 hours.
- Blisters usually form and break leading to significant oozing. The wound should be washed three to four times per day and fresh antibiotic ointment and dressings applied.
- Late postoperative care is designed to prevent hypertrophic scarring. Topical steroids and pressure are continued for a minimum of 3 months, beginning when the blisters appear to be "healed."
- Pigment will not begin to leave the area until 2 to 3 weeks. The treated skin is also more vulnerable to trauma and infection. If this occurs, it will inevitably lead to excessive skin loss or hypertrophic scarring.
- It may be best to reexamine the patient in 1 to 2 weeks just to evaluate how well he or she is doing.
- The second procedure is scheduled between 30 and 60 days to allow full healing and revascularization at the initial treatment site.

CONCLUSION

Infrared coagulation is an alternative to laser obliteration. There are advantages of portability, cost-effectiveness, rapidity of the treatment, and patient satisfaction with outcomes and degree of scarring comparable to other techniques. The technique is easy to learn. It is often easier to explain a "blur" than it is to exhibit an unwanted tattoo.

SUPPLIERS

TOBIL System
Cosmetic Surgery Center and Spa
109 Gallery Circle #127
San Antonio, TX 78528
Phone: 210-495-8825

Byron Medical Corp.
602 W. Rillito
Tucson, AZ 85705
Phone: 1-800-777-3434
Website: www.byronmedical.com

Redfield Corp.
336 West Passaic Street
Rochelle Park, NJ 07662
Phone: 1-800-678-4472
Website: www.redfieldcorp.com

CPT/BILLING CODE AND ICD-9-CM DIAGNOSTIC CODE

This is a cosmetic procedure, and no codes are applicable. The practitioner could consider using skin lesion destruction codes.

ADDITIONAL RESOURCES

- See the sample patient consent form titled "Tattoo Treatment Using the Infrared Light Obliteration Method" on page 1800 of Appendix G.

BIBLIOGRAPHY

Wilkinson TS: *Practical procedures in aesthetic plastic surgery: tips and traps,* New York, 1994, Springer Verlag.
Wilkinson TS: Infrared coagulator for tattoos: technical forum, *Bull Int Soc Clin Plast Surg,* April:6, 1995.
Wilkinson TS: The infrared coagulator and the Gang-X tattoos program: technical forum, *Bull Int Soc Clin Plast Surg* Sept:2, 1998.
Wilkinson TS: Affordable tattoo removal, *Assoc Plast Surg Assist Netw Pub* 13(4):20, 1999.

PART FOUR

Eyes, Ears, Nose, and Throat

CHAPTER 55

Chalazion and Hordeolum

James L. Jackson

Chalazions and hordeola are common inflammatory conditions of the eyelids encountered in primary care practice. Patients invariably complain of a "stye." Both conditions may be treated cautiously by the prudent non-ophthalmologist. However, care must be taken not to injure the eye or sensitive components of the eyelids, particularly the lacrimal drainage system ("tear ducts") and eyelid margin.

A *chalazion* is an acute or chronic granulomatous inflammation of a meibomian gland within the eyelid. A *hordeolum* is an acute abscess of a meibomian or Zeis gland. An *internal hordeolum* is on the conjunctival surface of the lid, whereas an *external hordeolum* is on its external surface of the skin at the edge of the lid.

The meibomian glands are located deep within the upper and lower eyelids (Fig. 55-1). They constantly produce a lipid material that drains through long ducts and emerges from orifices at the eyelid margin to enter the tear film. This lipid material helps keep the surface of the eye well lubricated and slows evaporation of the tears.

PATHOPHYSIOLOGY

Meibomian secretions are naturally somewhat viscous, but under certain conditions the meibomian secretions become thicker than normal and may plug the duct of a gland. The gland continues to produce secretions, which eventually leak between the cells of the gland into the surrounding tissue of the eyelid. Here, the lipid in the secretions causes a chronic granulomatous inflammation (a *chalazion*). As more secretions are produced, the inflammation worsens and may smolder chronically, sometimes for more than a year.

Clinically, the inflammation causes a localized swelling within the lid, sometimes with associated erythema and mild (usually) tenderness. The chalazion may be located immediately at the lid margin or within the lid some distance from the margin. At times a chalazion may be prominent externally, but at other times it may be visualized only from the inner (palpebral conjunctiva)

surface of the lid. The inflammation may cause a soft or even liquid center, and patients may report spontaneous drainage from the chalazion, either internally, externally, or through the lid margin. Spontaneous drainage may or may not lead to clinical improvement. The chalazion may wax and wane and may spontaneously resolve.

Some people tend to experience multiple chalazia over time or even concurrently. This is more common in people with rosacea or with chronic blepharitis, a bacterial colonization of the eyelids characterized by crusting at the base of the eyelashes and thickening and erythema of the eyelid margins. (The findings of chronic blepharitis, usually requiring a slitlamp examination to diagnose, are often fairly subtle and not easily detected by the non-ophthalmologist.)

A *hordeolum,* in contrast to a chalazion, is an acute bacterial abscess of a meibomian gland. Hordeola are classified as internal or external, based on the primary anatomic focus of the inflammation, which is generally clinically obvious. A hordeolum is typically characterized by an acute tender mass within the eyelid, with associated erythema and often the obvious presence of a collection of pus. Hordeola are commonly accompanied by acute preseptal cellulitis of the eyelid, characterized by erythema, edema, and tenderness of the surrounding skin. (Preseptal eyelid cellulitis is a different entity than the much less common orbital cellulitis, a vision and life-threatening inflammation of the orbit usually caused by extension of sinusitis and not caused by hordeola.) A hordeolum frequently drains spontaneously, which often relieves the condition.

DIFFERENTIAL DIAGNOSIS

Differentiation of a chalazion from a hordeolum may be a clinical challenge. A hordeolum is usually more tender and tense, often with obvious fluctuance. (Although a chalazion may have a liquefied center, it is not a collection of pus.) The presence of significant preseptal eyelid cellulitis suggests a hordeolum, but a chalazion may be associated with surrounding erythema and

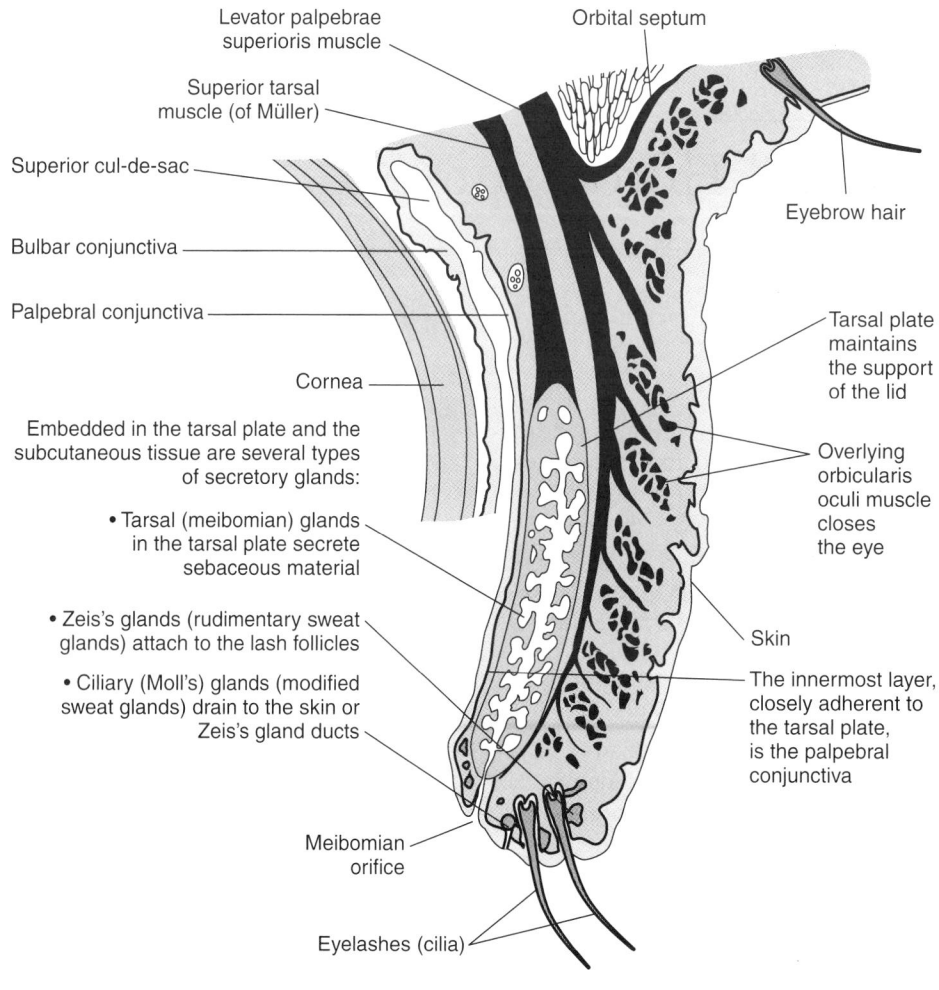

Levator palpebrae
superioris muscle

Orbital septum

Superior tarsal
muscle (of Müller)

Superior cul-de-sac

Bulbar conjunctiva

Palpebral conjunctiva

Cornea

Embedded in the tarsal plate and the
subcutaneous tissue are several types
of secretory glands:

• Tarsal (meibomian) glands
in the tarsal plate secrete
sebaceous material

• Zeis's glands (rudimentary sweat
glands) attach to the lash follicles

• Ciliary (Moll's) glands (modified
sweat glands) drain to the skin or
Zeis's gland ducts

Eyebrow hair

Tarsal plate
maintains
the support
of the lid

Overlying
orbicularis
oculi muscle
closes
the eye

Skin

The innermost layer,
closely adherent to
the tarsal plate,
is the palpebral
conjunctiva

Meibomian
orifice

Eyelashes (cilia)

Fig. 55-1
Anatomy of the eyelid.

edema. However, the level of tenderness of the surrounding skin is usually much less with a chalazion, as compared with a hordeolum with acute preseptal eyelid cellulitis, in which the skin is markedly tender. The natural history of a hordeolum is often more acute, but a chalazion can present acutely as well. If the swelling is located nasal to the medial canthus (inner corner of the eyelids) rather than in the eyelid itself, the patient likely has *dacryocystitis* rather than a hordeolum. Consider a prompt referral to an ophthalmologist, since dacryocystitis is a potentially life-threatening infection.

CHALAZION

Nonoperative Management

A chalazion may respond to medical treatment. Treatment may consist of one or more of the following:
• Warm compresses to the eyelid (four times a day if possible)

• Eyelid scrubs of the lid margins at bedtime each night (at base of eyelashes) with the use of diluted baby shampoo (diluted to half strength with water, applied with a cotton swab or washcloth) or commercially available ocular cleansing pads
• Application of antibiotic ointment (usually erythromycin) to eyelid margin after washing
• Oral doxycycline
• Intralesional steroid injection (triamcinolone acetonide) 40 mg/ml, 0.2 to 0.4 ml, 30-gauge needle through the conjunctival (inner) surface of the eyelid, with the use of topical anesthesia with Tetracaine drops. However, steroid injection carries the risk of skin hypopigmentation, especially in dark-skinned individuals.

Indications for Chalazion Excision

A chalazion is a nuisance rather than a harmful disorder, but it can certainly cause cosmetic concerns; large chalazia can even induce astigmatism, causing blurred vision. If the chalazion does not respond to medical treatment, if it is of substantial size (large enough to easily palpate), and if the patient wishes to be rid of it, excision is an effective option. Chalazion excision is a minor surgical procedure that can be performed in the office setting.

Contraindications to Chalazion Excision

Chalazion excision is relatively contraindicated if the chalazion has recently drained through the skin or if the skin appears crusted or markedly inflamed. If excision (which is performed from the inner surface of the eyelid) is attempted under these circumstances, a through-and-through defect of the eyelid may easily result, leading to a visible scar and prolonged healing time. Chalazion excision is also relatively contraindicated in an anticoagulated patient.

Chalazion excision by a non-ophthalmologist is contraindicated if near the lacrimal punctum, as damage to the lacrimal drainage system may easily result. The lacrimal punctum is a tiny opening in the nasal aspect of each eyelid margin. Tears drain through the punctum into the canaliculus, which runs just beneath the skin toward the nose. Damage to the punctum or canaliculus may lead to chronic tearing and the need for a complicated surgical repair. If the chalazion is close enough to the punctum that the punctum has any chance of being damaged, the patient should be referred to an ophthalmologist for excision of the chalazion.

Beware of recurrent or multiple chalazia in older patients, especially with associated ocular inflammation. This could represent sebaceous cell carcinoma, which is very aggressive and not always noted on pathology examination of an excised chalazion. If a presumed chalazion does not behave as expected, particularly in an elderly patient, tissue should be sent for pathology testing, and sebaceous cell carcinoma should be highly suspected even if the initial pathology report is negative.

Equipment for Chalazion Excision (Fig. 55-2)

- Sterile tray-top
- Skin-marking pen
- Tetracaine eyedrops
- Alcohol pads
- Local anesthetic for injection, 2% lidocaine with epinephrine, 3-ml, 30-gauge needle
- Betadine swabs
- Sterile gloves
- Sterile drape, fenestrated
- Chalazion clamps (two or three sizes)
- Scalpel (no. 15 or no. 11 blade)
- Chalazion curettes (two sizes)
- Cotton swabs
- Ocular tissue forceps, 0.2 tips
- Westcott scissors

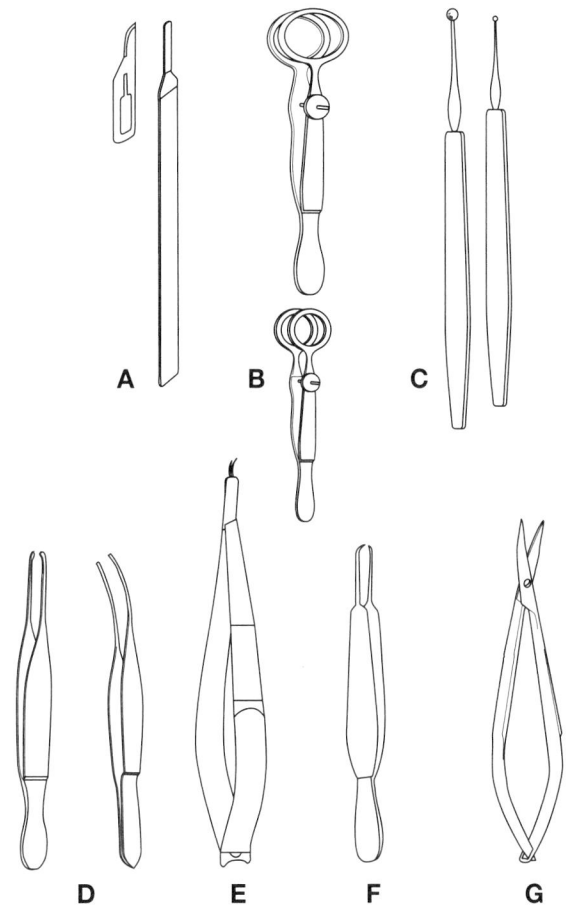

Fig. 55-2
Instruments for chalazion excision. **A,** Scalpel (no. 15 blade). **B,** Chalazion clamps. **C,** Chalazion curettes. **D,** Ocular tissue forceps. **E,** Needle holder. **F,** Suturing forceps. **G,** Westcott scissors.

- 4 × 4–inch gauze pads
- Antibiotic-steroid combination ophthalmic ointment (such as Maxitrol or TobraDex)
- Eyepatches (two or three) and medical tape
- Suture (6-0 nylon, silk, or chromic)
- Needle holder

Preprocedure Patient Preparation for Chalazion Excision

The patient should discontinue aspirin for 1 week and anticoagulants for 4 days before the procedure. The patient should be counseled on the risks of: scarring; possible need for sutures; recurrence; need for repeat excision; short-term swelling/bruising of eyelid; excessive bleeding; infection; and, rarely, damage to the lacrimal drainage system, causing chronic tearing.

Technique for Chalazion Excision

The physician can achieve good access to the eye by sitting near the top of the head. The patient should lie supine. Good lighting is essential. Injection of the local anesthetic may make palpation of the chalazion difficult, so it is helpful to use a skin marker to mark it before the injection.

Administer several drops of topical Tetracaine. Then administer 2% lidocaine with epinephrine through the skin, infiltrating the area where the chalazion clamp is to be applied (Fig. 55-3, *A*).

Place a chalazion clamp over the chalazion, with the open side inside the eyelid (Fig. 55-3, *B*). Tighten the clamp to achieve a firm grip on the eyelid, which also maintains hemostasis during the procedure. Do not overtighten. Evert the eyelid using the clamp as a lever. The chalazion should now be evident and bulging through the opening of the clamp.

With a no. 15 blade, make two incisions in the form of a cross, taking care not to go through the eyelid skin but only into the substance of the chalazion (Fig. 55-3, *C*). Some soft material may be released, confirming that the

incision is in the correct location. Use the curettes and cotton swabs to remove as much soft inflamed material as possible (Fig. 55-3, *D*). Then, using the Westcott scissors and tissue forceps, remove a small amount of the inflamed tarsal plate (the cartilage underneath), if necessary (Fig. 55-3, *E*). Take care not to tent the deeper tissue, which can lead to inadvertent incision of the underlying skin and cause a "buttonhole." Also, avoid damaging the eyelid margin.

Remove the chalazion clamp, which will likely lead to significant bleeding because of the excellent vascularity of the eyelid. Apply direct pressure with cotton swabs and/or gauze pads to achieve hemostasis. This may take 5 to 10 minutes. Once hemostasis has definitely been achieved, apply an antibiotic-steroid eye ointment and place a pressure patch on the eye.

If a full-thickness eyelid defect is present, suture the outer skin while taking care that the suture does not include the conjunctival (inner) surface of the eyelid;

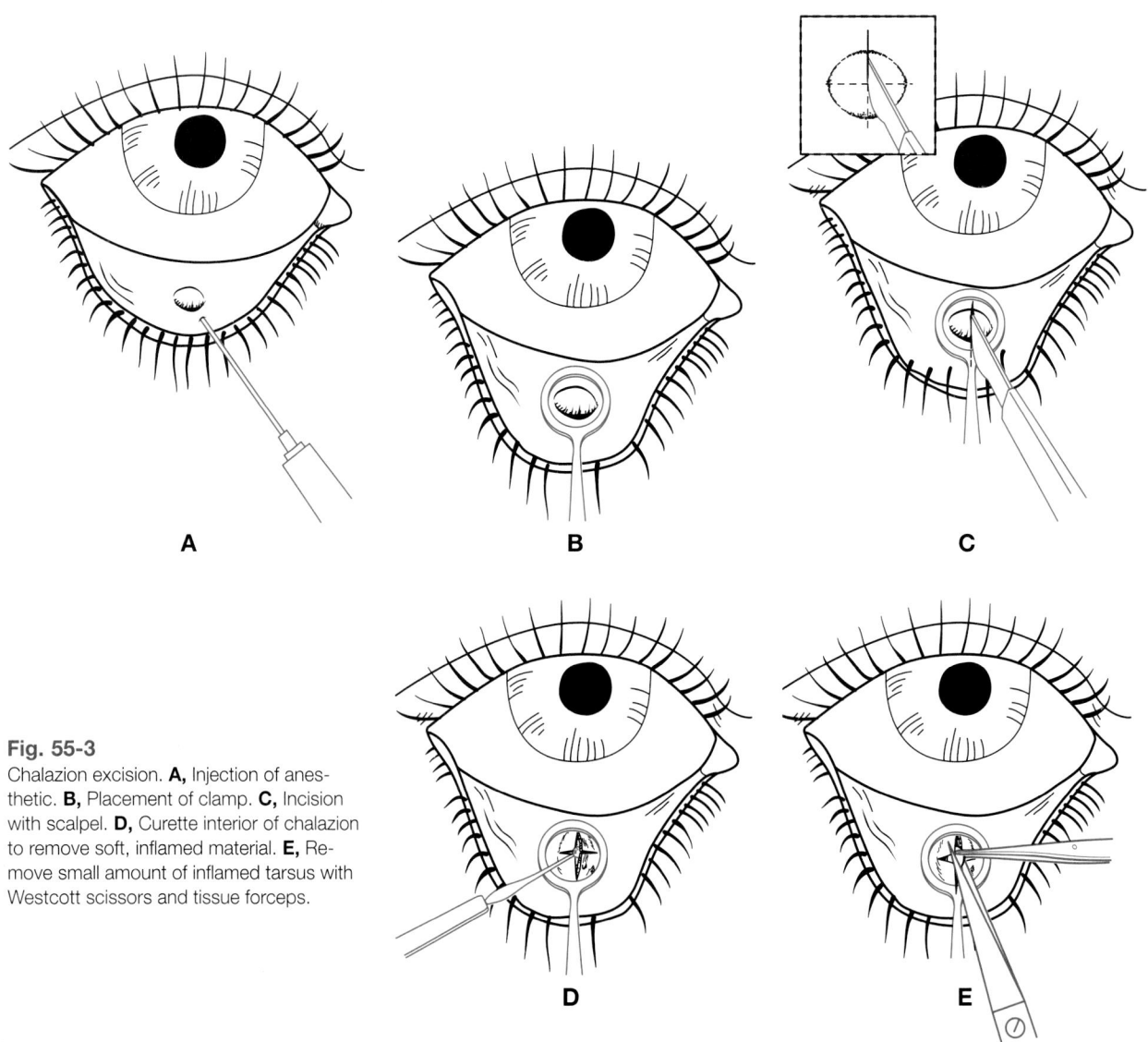

Fig. 55-3
Chalazion excision. **A,** Injection of anesthetic. **B,** Placement of clamp. **C,** Incision with scalpel. **D,** Curette interior of chalazion to remove soft, inflamed material. **E,** Remove small amount of inflamed tarsus with Westcott scissors and tissue forceps.

A   **B**   **C**

D   **E**

this would cause a great deal of irritation and possibly a corneal abrasion.

Postprocedure Patient Education After Chalazion Excision

The patient may remove the patch the evening after the procedure. Tell the patient that he or she can expect a large amount of clotted blood and mattering of the eye. The patient should then begin to apply an antibiotic eye ointment (such as erythromycin) in the eye twice a day until judged "back to normal." If the eyelid begins to bleed again, the patient should apply pressure until it stops, and should seek medical attention if the bleeding does not stop.

The patient can be seen in the first several days following the excision and 2 or 3 weeks after the procedure in order to assess healing. It may take several weeks for the swelling and tissue distortion to return to normal.

HORDEOLUM

Indications for Hordeolum Incision and Drainage

If a significant localized accumulation of pus is evident, particularly if the patient is in pain or significant eyelid cellulitis is present, the hordeolum should be incised and drained. If less severe and not yet "pointing," the hordeolum may be treated with frequent warm compresses and an oral antibiotic active against staphylococcus. However, if the patient is being treated medically, he or she should be watched closely in case the need for incision and drainage develops.

Contraindications to Hordeolum Incision and Drainage

If the hordeolum is located near the lacrimal punctum, refer the patient to an ophthalmologist because of the risk of damaging the lacrimal drainage system. If the swelling is located nasal to the medial canthus (inner corner of the eyelids), the patient likely has dacryocystitis rather than a hordeolum and should be referred promptly to an ophthalmologist.

Equipment for Incision and Drainage of Hordeolum

- Tetracaine eyedrops
- Alcohol pads
- Local anesthetic for injection, 2% lidocaine with epinephrine, 3-ml, 30-gauge needle
- Nonsterile gloves
- Scalpel (no. 11 blade)
- Cotton swabs
- Some 4 × 4–inch gauze pads

Preprocedure Patient Preparation for Incision and Drainage of Hordeolum

The patient should discontinue aspirin and anticoagulants before the procedure if possible, although it is usually necessary to perform the procedure without much advanced planning. The patient should be counseled on the risks of scarring; recurrence; need for repeat incision and drainage; short-term swelling/bruising of eyelid; excessive bleeding; spread of infection; and, rarely, damage to the lacrimal drainage system, causing chronic tearing.

Technique for Hordeolum Incision and Drainage

Prepare the patient as for chalazion treatment.

The hordeolum typically points either internally or externally and should be incised from whichever surface allows the best access to the collection of pus (Fig. 55-4, *A*). Use the scalpel blade to make an incision into the

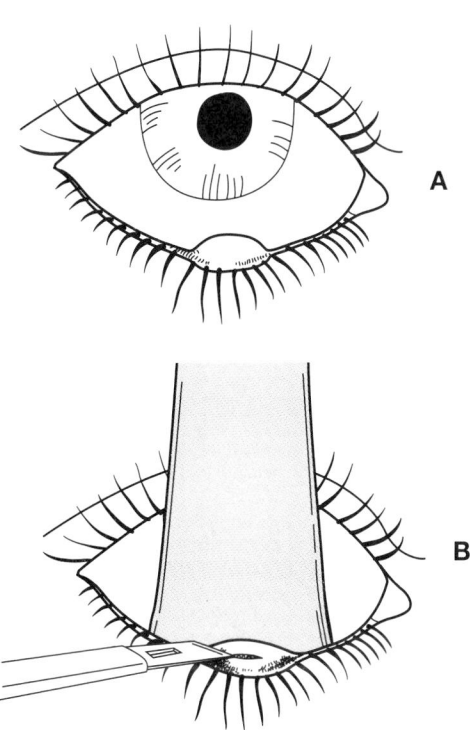

Fig. 55-4
Hordeolum excision. **A,** Hordeolum pointing externally. **B,** Incision and drainage of external hordeolum with a tongue blade or metal elevator protecting the eye.

hordeolum until pus is obtained, taking care to avoid a through-and-through eyelid defect or injury to the eye or eyelid margin (Fig. 55-4, *B*). If significant cellulitis is present, it may be prudent to send a sample of the pus for culture and sensitivity testing.

Apply direct pressure with gauze pads to achieve hemostasis. This may take 5 to 10 minutes. An eyepatch is not necessary.

If a full-thickness eyelid defect is present, do not suture the skin because of the presence of acute infection.

Postprocedure Patient Education After Hordeolum Incision and Drainage

The patient should be given an oral antibiotic with good coverage for staphylococcus. If the eyelid begins to bleed again, the patient should apply pressure until it stops and should seek medical attention if the bleeding does not stop.

The patient should be seen on the first day after the excision, and again daily if necessary until it is clear that any cellulitis is resolving and the pus is not reaccumulating.

SUPPLIERS

Any medical instrument supplier can provide the necessary equipment.

CPT/BILLING CODES

67800	Excision of chalazion, single
67801	Excision of chalazion, multiple, same lid
67805	Excision of chalazion, multiple, different lids
67700	Blepharotomy: drainage of abscess, eyelid

ICD-9-CM DIAGNOSTIC CODES

373.2	Chalazion
373.11	Hordeolum, external
373.12	Hordeolum, internal

ADDITIONAL RESOURCES

- See the sample patient education handout titled "Chalazion/Hordeolum" on page 1803 of Appendix G.
- See the sample patient consent form titled "Chalazion/Hordeolum (Stye) Excision" on page 1806 of Appendix G.

BIBLIOGRAPHY

Berens C, King JH: *An atlas of ophthalmic surgery,* Philadelphia, 1982, JB Lippincott.

Clayman HM, editor: *Atlas of contemporary ophthalmic surgery,* St Louis, 1990, Mosby.

Easty DL, Smolin G: *External eye disease,* Stoneham, Mass, 1988, Butterworth.

Griffith DG, Salasche SJ, Clemons DE: *Cutaneous abnormalities of the eyelid and face: an atlas with histopathology,* New York, 1987, McGraw-Hill.

Jacobs PM, Thaller VT, Wong D: Intralesional corticosteroid therapy of chalazion: a comparison with incision and curettage, *Br J Ophthalmol* 68:836, 1984.

King JH, Wadsworth JAC: *An atlas of ophthalmic surgery,* ed 2, Philadelphia, 1988, JB Lippincott.

WEBSITES

www.emedicine.com/EMERG/topic94.htm
www.emedicine.com/EMERG/topic755.htm
www.eyenet.org
www.inform.umd.edu/UHC/Library/Handouts/chalaz.html
www.rxmed.com/illnesses/chalazion.html
www.vh.org/Providers/ClinRef/FPHandbook/Chapter12/04-12.html

CHAPTER 56

Corneal Abrasions and Removal of Corneal or Conjunctival Foreign Bodies

Grant C. Fowler

A complaint of "something in the eye," and corneal or conjunctival abrasions or foreign bodies, are common problems for primary care clinicians. In most cases the management is uncomplicated and can be completed in the clinician's office, but important guidelines are available for preventing impaired vision or blindness.

A detailed history is important, especially what the patient was doing when he or she first noticed a problem. The clinician should ask if the patient was wearing any eye protection, was around hammered metal, or came into contact with a high-velocity foreign body.

Note: Since the first edition of this textbook was published, considerable scientific evidence has become available that questions the need to patch an eye after corneal trauma. New medications (ophthalmic nonsteroidal antiinflammatory drugs) are available as an alternative to the analgesia provided by patching. However, the decision whether to patch or treat is still between the clinician and the patient. Some of the evidence is discussed further under the "Technique" section and may be helpful for the patient when making a decision. Also, with this edition, please note Chapter 57, Slit Lamp Examination. If a slit lamp is available, a more thorough evaluation of the eye may be performed for a corneal abrasion or foreign body. In the absence of a slit lamp, this chapter indicates when a slit lamp referral is required.

FLUORESCEIN EXAMINATION OF THE CORNEA AND CONJUNCTIVA

INDICATIONS

- Unilateral foreign body sensation, hypersensitivity to light, excess tearing, or pain—especially on opening or closing the eye
- Red eye
- Eye trauma
- Unilateral, persistent eye irritation in contact lens wearers
- History of exposure to ultraviolet (UV) light from such sources as a welding torch, sunlight, or a tanning bed (UV light can penetrate the cornea even when the patient's eyes are closed if protective lenses are not being worn)
- Mild chemical exposure to eye
- Neonates or infants with persistent crying, unilateral tearing, hypersensitivity to light, or conjunctival inflammation

CONTRAINDICATIONS

Patients with the following should be referred to an ophthalmologist after urgent care:

- Suspected high-velocity injury to the eye (e.g., patients exposed to metal hammering or heavy machinery). High-speed metallic or nonmetallic fragments may produce minimal symptoms and penetrate the globe with unnoticed damage to the cornea. As a result, significant internal damage must be excluded.
- A hyphema, lens opacification, scleral tear, abnormal anterior chamber examination, or irregularity of the pupil may suggest that the globe has been penetrated. Orbital x-ray films may confirm a metal foreign body. An ophthalmologist needs to be involved.
- Long-standing (>24 hours) inflammation as evidenced by iritis, photophobia, or ciliary blush suggests the presence of an intraocular foreign body or a more serious injury. This requires slit-lamp examination or evaluation by an ophthalmologist.

Note: A pressure patch is contraindicated in a penetration injury of the globe. For such an injury or a complex lid laceration, a nonpressure protective eyeshield should be applied before referral. Metal shields are manufactured for this purpose, or a nonpressure shield can be fashioned from a paper cup (Fig. 56-1). All patches and shields should be taped in the same direction, from the medial forehead across the eye toward the ear.

- Exposure to caustic or acidic media: immediate management includes copious irrigation that should con-

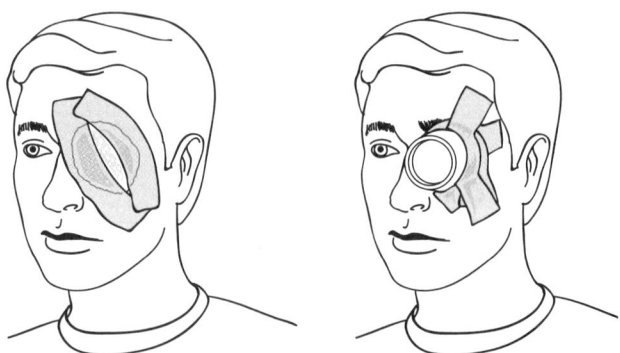

Fig. 56-1
Nonpressure patch to protect ruptured globe. A metal shield or a paper cup can be used.

tinue for at least 15 minutes. (It can begin at home with tap water from a shower or hose.)
- Mild chemical exposure if the clinician is not knowledgeable about the management of the specific chemical after contacting a Poison Control Center.
- Ruptured globe.
- Uncooperative patient. (Infants may have to be sedated; see Chapter 7, Pediatric Sedation.)

EQUIPMENT

- Snellen's chart at 6 meters (20 feet), or an equivalent visual acuity chart. (If a chart is unavailable, ask the patient to read a magazine at arm's length. If the patient cannot do so, measure and record the distance at which the patient can count fingers.)
- Topical ophthalmic anesthetic such as 0.5% proparacaine (Alcaine or Ophthaine) or 0.5% tetracaine (Pontocaine), unless contraindicated (e.g., ruptured globe or allergy to local anesthetics)
- Fluor-I-Strip, sterile fluorescein sodium strips. (Since fluorescein is incompatible with preservatives effective against *Pseudomonas* and *Proteus,* multidose dropper bottles of fluorescein solution should not be used. An inoculation of abraded corneal epithelium with either bacteria could cause infection, permanent scarring, or blindness.)
- Bright white light source (a single point source such as a penlight is preferable).
- Cobalt-blue light source (Wood's lamp is adequate).
- An 8- to 10-power magnification lens (loupes, a magnifying glass, a colposcope, or an ophthalmoscope on the +20 to +40 diopter setting).
- Sterile cotton-tipped applicators.
- Isotonic ophthalmic irrigant (sterile saline, Dacriose).
- Facial tissues (Kleenex).

PREPROCEDURE PATIENT PREPARATION

Emphasize the need for the patient to follow up daily with the clinician until the abrasion is completely healed. This will detect early complications such as infection. Instruct the patient to call the office if persistent or recurrent symptoms occur. Soft contact lenses should be removed before the eye is stained. Before instilling the topical anesthetic, tell the patient that it may cause a burning sensation until the eye becomes numb.

TECHNIQUE

1. Check and document visual acuity in both eyes *before* instilling topical anesthetic. Documentation of baseline visual acuity *before* anesthetic is important because initial anesthetic discomfort (burning) may later be suspected by the patient as having caused impaired vision. Baseline acuity documentation helps counter such misperceptions as well as any misperceptions that a preexisting visual impairment may have been caused by this procedure.

    If the patient normally uses corrective lenses for refractive error, check visual acuity with refraction. After the acuity check, the patient will probably be most comfortable in the supine position for the remainder of the examination.

Note: If the patient's corrective lenses are not available, pinhole myopia correctors can be used. These are commercially available, but they are also easy to make. With an 18-gauge needle, punch eight to ten holes within a 5-cm (2-inch) circle on an index card. Have the patient select the hole that provides the best vision for viewing the Snellen chart. This effectively corrects the patient's vision.

2. Hand the patient a tissue and instill one to two drops of topical anesthetic into his or her affected eye. (This is not mandatory but does facilitate patient cooperation and comfort.)
3. Inspect the affected eye with a bright white light source, and compare it with the opposite eye. The sclera should be intact. The anterior chamber should be free of pus or blood. The iris should be normal in size and shape. The pupil should be normal in size, shape, and reactivity, and it should be symmetric with the other pupil unless there is already a history of asymmetry. *If all of these conditions are not met, the patient should be referred to an ophthalmologist.* (In the follow-up examination the next day, pupil dilation from the cycloplegic may persist. In this case, uneven pupil size should correlate with the half-life of the cycloplegic agent.)

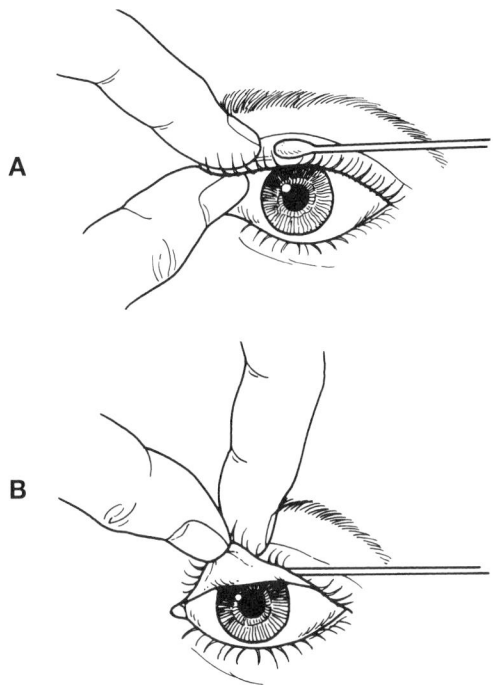

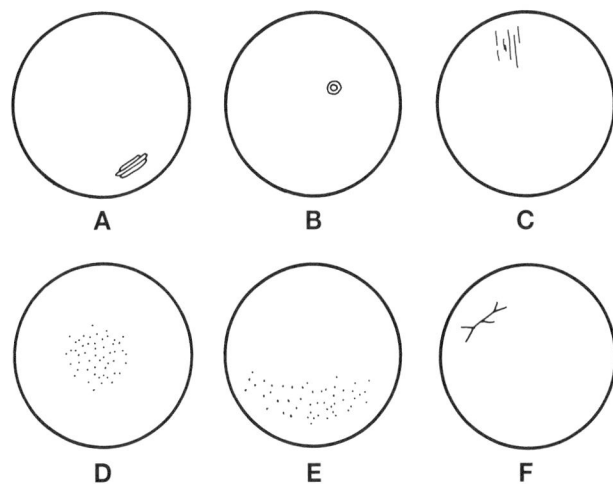

Fig. 56-3
Corneal defect staining patterns for specific injuries. **A,** Typical abrasion. **B,** Abrasion around a corneal foreign body. **C,** Abrasion from a conjunctival foreign body under the upper lid. **D,** Abrasion from excessive wearing of a contact lens. **E,** Ultraviolet exposure (resulting from sunlamp exposure, welding, or snow blindness). **F,** Herpetic dendritic keratitis.

Fig. 56-2
A, Grasp the upper eyelashes between the thumb and index finger. With the tip of the other index finger or a cotton-tipped applicator, press down gently on the skin of the upper lid. **B,** Pull outward on the lashes and rotate the tarsal plate upward until it forms a right angle with the eyeball. A gentle tug upward should flip the plate into eversion, clearly exposing the conjunctival surface of the upper lid.

4. Eversion of the upper lid is usually necessary to examine the entire conjunctiva (Fig. 56-2). Inspect the entire bulbar and palpebral conjunctiva for trauma, foreign bodies, or other sources of symptoms, such as a hordeolum or an ingrown or inverted eyelash. Examine carefully the groove about 2 mm from the lash margin of the everted lid. Tiny objects frequently lodge there and may not be immediately visible. Use the ophthalmoscope for magnification if necessary. For a foreign body, refer to the "Corneal or Conjunctival Foreign Body Removal" section later in this chapter. Older patients often have ingrown hairs, or trichiasis, causing a foreign body sensation. (See Chapter 41, Epilation of Isolated Hairs [Including Trichiasis].) These sensations most frequently involve the lower lid. If there are only a few hairs, they can be plucked out with fine forceps. The patient with many hairs should be referred for electrolysis of the roots.

5. Instill fluorescein dye by moistening a fluorescein strip with one or two drops of sterile saline or topical anesthetic, asking the patient to look up, and gently touching the lower conjunctival sac for 3 to 5 seconds. When wetting the strip, use a minimal amount of solution so that only the defect will be stained, not the entire eye. Try not to touch the cornea directly with the strip because this may cause iatrogenic staining. After instilling the dye, have the patient blink a few times to remove excess tears, and blot them with the tissue. This is helpful to distinguish true staining from fluorescein saturation of the tear film.

6. Inspect the cornea with magnification under a cobalt-blue light source. If the entire cornea is stained, irrigate the eye again and reexamine. Abraded areas of the cornea should remain highlighted with fluorescein. Make a drawing of the cornea for later reference, detailing the areas of abnormality. If no source of symptoms is found or if vertical streaking is found on the cornea, suspect an embedded conjunctival foreign body in the eyelid and examine the entire conjunctiva under cobalt-blue light. Keep in mind that fluorescein is taken up by mucus on the conjunctiva; therefore dye uptake in conjunctival injuries is less specific than with corneal injuries. If still no source of symptoms can be found, the eye should be examined under a slit lamp. A slit lamp is helpful when a plain fluorescein examination is nondiagnostic. For deep, dendritic, or central ulcerations or for ulcerations in which infection is suspected (i.e., if there is clouding of the cornea or a purulent discharge), the patient should be referred to an ophthalmologist (Fig. 56-3).

TREATMENT OF UNCOMPLICATED CORNEAL ABRASIONS

CONSIDERATIONS

Some emergency department clinicians send all patients with abrasions to ophthalmologists for follow-up. However, risk for permanent visual impairment can be stratified based on the number and magnitude of certain factors: abrasion depth, size, location, and susceptibility to infection. With minimal magnification, the depth of the abrasion is often difficult to assess; referral should be considered for suspected deep or large lesions or for those centrally located in the line of vision. One way to assess a borderline case is to wait until the follow-up examination the next day. The corneal epithelium is one of the fastest-healing areas of the body, and if considerable progress toward healing has not been made by the next day or if there are signs of infection (cloudiness of cornea or pus), refer the patient immediately.

EQUIPMENT

- Topical ophthalmic anesthetic
- Isotonic irrigant (sterile saline or Dacriose)
- Sterile eye patches and 1-inch (preferably nonallergenic) paper tape
- Ophthalmic antibiotics: tobramycin (3 mg per gram of ointment) or sulfacetamide (10% ointment)
- Cycloplegic drops, such as 1% mydriacil (Opticyl, Tropicacyl) or 1% to 2% cyclopentolate HCl (Cyclogyl, Pentolair), are useful for pain control. Their duration of action ranges from hours to a day. For a longer duration of cycloplegia (often needed for patients with darkly pigmented irises that absorb cyclopentolate and shorten the duration of the drops), 0.25% scopolamine HBr (Isopto Hyoscine) can be considered.

TECHNIQUE

1. Irrigate copiously with ophthalmic irrigant, with the patient's head turned laterally toward the affected side.
2. Instill one to two additional drops of local anesthetic.
3. For significant pain, consider a cycloplegic. Trauma often leads to spasm of the iris with resulting pain.
4. Apply an antibiotic ointment. Even under the best of conditions, infection is a possibility because of the avascular nature of the cornea. Prophylaxis with antibiotics is important.
5. This is where there is some controversy (see Note below). For all but very minor abrasions, a double patch (pressure patch) can be used and may be prudent. The first patch is folded and the fold placed immediately under the brow (this adds padding and prevents opening of the eye). This patch is covered with the second patch.
6. With three to five strips of paper tape, secure the patches by taping from the middle of the forehead, across the eye, and toward the ear (Fig. 56-4).

Note: In 1997, a survey with a response from 83% of the ophthalmic units in the United Kingdom revealed that patching, cycloplegic, and antibiotics were still considered the mainstay of treatment for corneal abrasions. However, topical antibiotics alone and antibiotics together with a cycloplegic were the most common immediate treatments. The most common treatment over the next few days was topical antibiotics. Interestingly, 4% of their units' management decisions were made by the nursing staff alone!

Also in 1997, a study of 46 randomized patients compared patching with no patching. It found no significant acceleration of reepithelialization, no reduction in the incidence and severity of inflammation, and no improved pain relief in patched patients.

Another important study was published in 1997. With no patches being used, a randomized, double-masked, placebo-controlled study compared treatment with either ophthalmic 0.5% ketorolac or placebo in 100 patients. These patients had noninfected corneal abrasions that were not traumatic, not related to contact lens, and not related to foreign body removal. Abrasions were less than 36 hours in duration, and a cycloplegic was used in all patients. Ophthalmic ketorolac significantly reduced pain, photophobia, and foreign body sensation compared with placebo.

As a result of these and other studies, many clinicians no longer use eye patching. Another option that has been studied, for the busy individual who *must* have continuous use of both

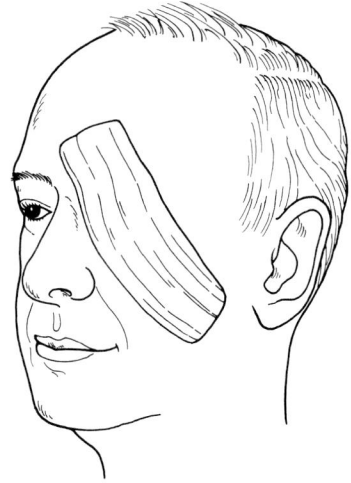

Fig. 56-4
Pressure eye patch.

eyes, is a soft contact lens. A soft contact usually increases comfort and protection and should not impair healing. However, if a contact lens is used, the patient should be followed closely and warned for signs of infection.

7. Do not use eyepatches on young children. There is the theoretical risk of permanently affecting the use of one eye or of making amblyopia worse. Very young children typically remove the patch anyway.

8. Pain medication should be prescribed in an amount appropriate to the symptoms. However, additional local anesthetic should not be prescribed because it may retard corneal healing and cause corneal scarring. As noted above in one of the studies, topical ophthalmic nonsteroidal antiinflammatory drops can be prescribed if the patient is not patched.

9. Reexamine in 24 hours using fluorescein and magnification. If the abrasion has healed, antibiotic drops should be used for an additional 3 days. If the defect is smaller, instill a cycloplegic and the antibiotic ointment, and examine again in 24 hours. If patched, consider repatching. If at any time during the follow-up; a cloudiness of the cornea or suppuration is seen, refer the patient to an ophthalmologist.

10. The visual acuity test should be repeated and documented just before the patient is discharged from care.

11. Tetanus immunity should be verified or provided.

Note: If infection is suspected, an eyepatch is contraindicated. Also note that abrasions resulting from fingernails or plant matter are notoriously slow to heal. Their progress should be followed patiently, just like any other abrasion, while observing for any signs of early infection.

COMPLICATIONS

- Infection
- Scarring (the highest morbidity occurs when the abrasion is near the central line of vision)
- Permanent visual impairment

POSTPROCEDURE PATIENT EDUCATION

Instruct the patient not to rub his or her eyes, especially on awakening. Rubbing may disrupt the new layers of epithelializing cornea. Reepithelialization can take weeks to complete. Inform the patient that the local anesthetic wears off in a few minutes to hours and that additional pain medication may be necessary. Topical ophthalmic nonsteroidal antiinflammatories have been found to be safe and effective. Moist compresses may be applied for some relief of discomfort if the patient's eye has not been patched. Instruct the patient to return to the office daily until healed and if persistent or recurrent symptoms develop. If cycloplegics were used, inform the patient. Also inform the patient to tell the clinician if he or she will be seen in another center or referred. Instruct the patient not to overuse the unpatched eye, such as by watching television or reading for prolonged periods. This is especially true for children or anyone with a history of amblyopia. It is important to document the degree of healing observed during the discharge examination. Safety goggles or protective glasses should be emphasized if the abrasion was an occupational or exposure injury.

CORNEAL OR CONJUNCTIVAL FOREIGN BODY REMOVAL

INDICATIONS

- Noninfected, small, recent corneal or conjunctival foreign bodies

CONTRAINDICATIONS

The contraindications are the same as those for "Fluorescein Examination of the Cornea and Conjunctiva," as well as the following (which also require referral):

- Signs or symptoms that suggest infection, such as edema and clouding of the cornea surrounding the foreign body, ulceration exceeding the size of the foreign body, or purulent discharge (If infection is suspected, patching is contraindicated.)
- Large metal foreign bodies or those with potential to cause a large rust ring (i.e., those that have been embedded in the cornea for longer than 24 hours)
- Apparently deeply or centrally embedded foreign bodies

EQUIPMENT

- Topical ophthalmic anesthetic
- Sterile fluorescein sodium strips
- Sterile cotton-tipped applicators
- Bright white light source and cobalt-blue light source
- Magnification as previously listed (it may be necessary to have an assistant hold the magnifier to allow the operator to use both hands)
- Isotonic ophthalmic irrigant, such as sterile saline or Dacriose

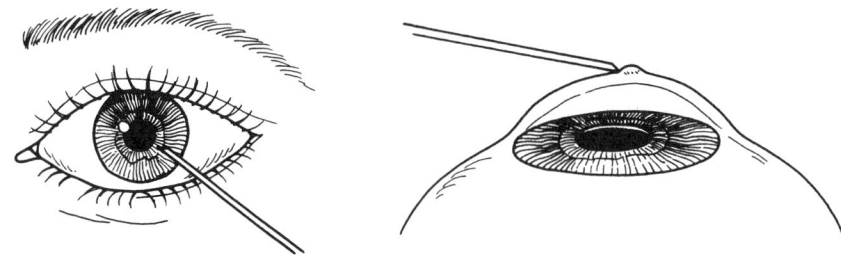

Fig. 56-5
Removal of a superficial corneal foreign body. Side view illustrates the thickness of the cornea relative to the beveled needle edge. The needle or eye spud should be held tangential to the cornea, and the object should be gently scraped off of the cornea.

- Snellen chart or equivalent visual acuity chart
- Sterile 18-gauge needle with small syringe
- Sterile dental burr or cornea drill (optional)

Note: Instead of an 18-gauge needle, a tuberculin syringe with a 26-gauge needle, a sterile eye spud, or a small, sterile chalazion curette may be substituted, depending on user experience

PREPROCEDURE PATIENT PREPARATION

Instruct the patient that it will be important to fix his or her gaze on a distant object, maintain that focus, and hold the head motionless, regardless of what is seen or experienced. The patient will have the urge to blink, but it will be important to keep the eye open. Inform the patient that the eye will be numb from the local anesthetic, but that he or she may feel pressure during the procedure. The patient should know that you will need to touch them.

Advise the patient of possible complications and that referral may be necessary regardless of outcome. Some clinicians obtain signed informed consent.

TECHNIQUE

Controversy exists about using a swab or spud to remove a corneal foreign body and whether this causes more damage. Only experienced users should consider a swab or spud, and they should only use them for small foreign bodies. The swab is more successful with very recent, superficial foreign bodies. Irrigation alone is not usually successful unless the foreign object is very recent, consists of carbon, or is water soluble. The patient's tears would normally have already washed away anything that irrigation would remove.
1. Record the patient's visual acuity.

2. With the patient supine, hold the eyelids apart with your thumb and index finger, and position the patient's head so that the foreign object is at the highest point on the eyeball. The patient should fix his or her gaze. For conjunctival foreign bodies, the head should be positioned for maximal access.
3. Make an attempt to dislodge the object. Noting the controversy regarding swab or spud use, try to lift the object by lightly touching it with a cotton swab moistened with local anesthetic. This occasionally dislodges the particle. Never use any force to rub the cornea, as this will dislodge the epithelium and cause a larger abrasion. The same maneuver can be attempted for a conjunctival foreign body.
4. To use a sterile needle, approach the object from a direction tangential to the eyeball, with the needle bevel upwards and the syringe held with a pencil grip (Fig. 56-5). Rest your hand on the patient's zygoma so that if the patient moves, your hand will move with the patient. Use the needle tip to lift the object gently from its bed. Several attempts may have to be made, but use of a slit lamp (see Chapter 57, Slit Lamp Examination) or referral should be considered if further corneal damage is anticipated. If several attempts with a needle are unsuccessful (noting the controversy discussed), a spud or chalazion curette may be considered. For conjunctival foreign bodies, the technique is the same: attempt to lift them from their bed with the same instruments. More vigorous force, if controlled, may be used on the conjunctiva.
5. After removal of the foreign body, if a residual corneal rust ring is found under magnification, it can occasionally be removed with the sterile needle alone. A cornea drill may also be considered. It should have a pressure-sensitive automatic shutoff to minimize corneal damage. Another published technique involves the use of a sterile dental burr held between the thumb and forefinger to approach the rust ring vertically (Fig. 56-6). After the burr has made one gentle rotation, reexamine the eye under magnifica-

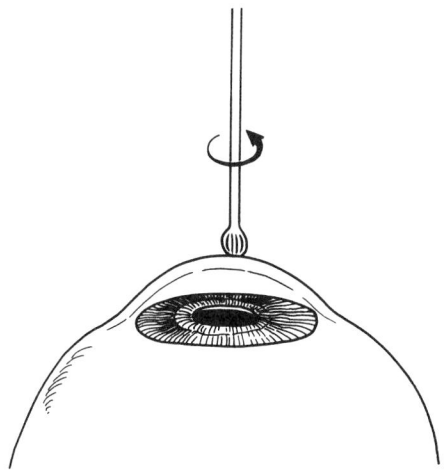

Fig. 56-6
Dental burr rotated once. Note vertical approach.

tion to verify complete removal of the ring. Rust is toxic to corneal epithelium and prevents healing; it may also cause nighttime visual defects. If attempts to remove the rust ring are unsuccessful or if they will cause further damage to corneal epithelium, referral should be made for management under slit lamp magnification.

6. Retest and record the patient's visual acuity.

POSTPROCEDURE PATIENT EDUCATION

Follow the guidelines for treatment of an uncomplicated corneal abrasion. If the object cannot be removed, the resultant rust ring is too large, or the patient is referred to an ophthalmologist for any other reason, the ophthalmologist should provide further patient education.

COMPLICATIONS

- Same as the complications associated with treatment of a routine corneal abrasion, except the risk of corneal scarring is greater
- Perforation of the cornea or globe
- Incomplete removal of a foreign body
- Failure to heal because of a retained rust ring, infection, or other causes

CPT/BILLING CODES

65205   Removal of foreign body, external eye; conjunctival superficial
65210   Removal of foreign body, external eye; conjunctival embedded (includes concretions), subconjunctival, or scleral nonperforating
65220   Removal of foreign body, external eye; corneal without slit lamp
99070   Eye tray: supplies and materials (except spectacles) provided by physician over and above those that are usually included with the office visit or other services rendered (list drugs, trays, supplies, or materials provided)
99173   Screening test of visual acuity, quantitative, bilateral

ICD-9-CM DIAGNOSTIC CODES

364.70   Adhesions of iris, unspecified
364.00   Acute iritis
918.1   Corneal abrasion
371.82   Corneal injury due to contact lens
930.0   Corneal foreign body
930.1   Foreign body in conjunctival sac
918.2   Superficial injury of conjunctiva
361.00   Retinal detachment with retinal defect, unspecified
370.20   Superficial corneal keratitis without conjunctivitis
370.24   photokeratitis
360.60   Intraocular foreign body

BIBLIOGRAPHY

Arbour JD, Brunette I, Boisjoly HM, et al: Should we patch corneal erosions? *Arch Ophthalmol* 115(12):1607, 1997.

Kaiser PK, Pineda R II: A study of topical nonsteroidal anti-inflammatory drops and no pressure patching in the treatment of corneal abrasions, *Ophthalmology* 104(8):1353, 1997.

Murtagh J: Removal of corneal foreign body. In *Practice tips,* Sydney, 1991, McGraw-Hill.

Sabri K, Pandit JC, Thaller VT, et al: National survey of corneal abrasion treatment, *Eye* 12(2):278, 1998.

CHAPTER 57

Slit Lamp Examination

Christopher J. Bigelow

The slit lamp biomicroscope is used for a thorough evaluation of the eye as well as for diagnosis of various eye conditions. As with any instrument, repeated use facilitates comfort with the scope as well as the ability to obtain the desired or necessary information. With its many levers and knobs (Fig. 57-1), the slit lamp can be somewhat intimidating at first. However, after learning a few simple techniques, even the infrequent user should feel comfortable. Granted, not every primary care clinician's office has a slit lamp. However, if one is available, it can be an invaluable diagnostic opportunity that should not be missed because of lack of experience. The goal of this chapter is to provide even the novice user with guidance for performing a useful and reproducible slit lamp examination.

A slit lamp consists of both an illumination and an observation system (Fig. 57-1). Since the cornea is very clear and most light passes right through it, a bright light and condenser system are necessary to get light to backscatter and illuminate faint corneal nuances or abnormalities. The light source is an incandescent lamp contained within the body of the instrument. The light passes through a condenser, the slit mechanism, and an objective lens and is then reflected by an inclined mirror onto the patient's eye. When projected onto the globe, the slit beam of incandescent light creates an optical cross section of the eye. The height and width of the beam (Fig. 57-2) can be adjusted with controls (often different on each slit lamp). It can be changed from a small pinpoint spot to a slit beam or made even wider for broad illumination. As the beam is narrowed, the scattered light from adjacent tissue is minimized, allowing greater detail to be seen in the cross section. Beam sizes, their widths, and their usefulness are discussed

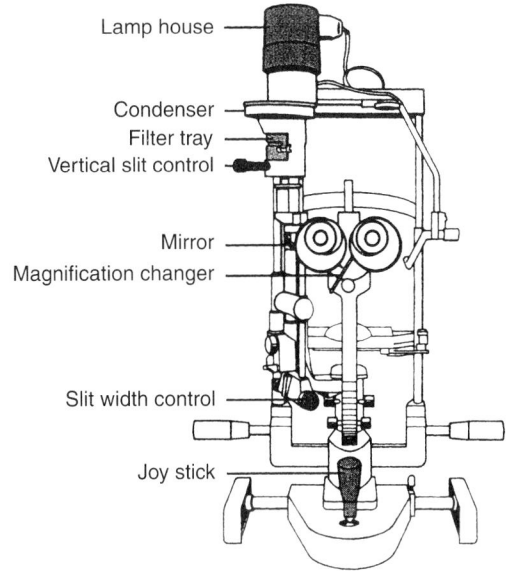

Fig. 57-1
A slit lamp and its optics. (From Solley WA, Broocker G: General eye exam. In Palay DA, Krachmer JH: *Ophthalmology for the primary care physician,* St Louis, 1997, Mosby.)

Lamp house
Condenser
Filter tray
Vertical slit control
Mirror
Magnification changer
Slit width control
Joy stick

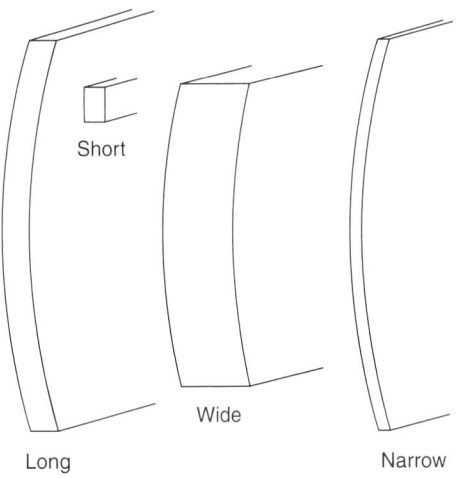

Fig. 57-2
Different dimensions of the slit lamp beam.

Short
Long
Wide
Narrow

under the "Technique" section. Light intensity can also be adjusted. The observation system is a microscope with a long working distance. Most slit lamps offer a choice of magnification between 5× and 50×. The necessary degree of magnification depends on the tissue being examined.

Use of the slit lamp biomicroscope is indicated in any situation where brighter illumination and increased magnification of the anterior segment structures (eyelids, cornea, iris, lens) would be helpful. With increased magnification, oblique illumination, and a stereoscopic view, a much better evaluation of lesions can be obtained. Such evaluation of lesions includes a more accurate estimation of lesion depth. In addition, high-powered lenses are available for most slit lamps to allow visualization of the posterior structures such as the fundus.

INDICATIONS

- Need for bright illumination of anterior segment structures (e.g., corneal abrasion, keratitis).
- Need for magnification of anterior segment structures (e.g., corneal foreign body, iritis).
- Need for a thorough evaluation of the posterior eye.
- Patient with a foreign body sensation and normal routine fluorescein examination, or when the routine fluorescein examination is inconclusive or unsuccessful
- Suspected deep or large abrasions or those centrally located in the line of vision on fluorescein examination. Such lesions increase the risk of vision loss and should be evaluated thoroughly and followed clinically with a slit lamp.
- After several unsuccessful attempts at removing a corneal foreign body in the standard fashion, before additional trauma is inflicted on the cornea, the foreign body and cornea should be evaluated under a slit lamp. It may also be necessary to remove the foreign body with slit lamp guidance.
- When routine fluorescein examination is relatively contraindicated (e.g., when there is long-standing [more than 24 hours] inflammation). The presence of iritis, photophobia, or ciliary blush may indicate long-standing inflammation, or it may be the result of an intraocular foreign body or a more serious injury. If the etiology is not evident with a slit lamp examination, the patient should be referred to an ophthalmologist.
- Same indications as for routine fluorescein examination or for foreign body removal (see Chapter 56, Corneal Abrasions and Removal of Corneal or Conjunctival Foreign Bodies). If a slit lamp is available, it will enhance the techniques found in that chapter.

CONTRAINDICATIONS

After urgent care has been provided, patients with the following should be referred to an ophthalmologist:
- Suspected high-velocity injury to the eye (e.g., patients exposed to metal hammering or heavy machinery): high-speed metallic or nonmetallic fragments may penetrate the globe with unnoticeable damage to the cornea. Although they may produce minimal symptoms, significant internal damage may have occurred. A hyphema, lens opacification, an abnormal anterior chamber examination, or an irregularity of the pupil may suggest that the globe has been penetrated. Orbital x-ray films can confirm a metal foreign body.

Note: A pressure patch is contraindicated in a penetration injury of the globe. Also, for complex lid lacerations, a nonpressure protective eye shield should be applied before referral (see Fig. 56-1).

- Exposure to caustic or acidic media: urgent management includes copious irrigation, which should continue for at least 15 minutes. (It can begin at home with tap water from a shower or hose.)
- Other chemical exposure if the clinician is not knowledgeable about its management after contacting a Poison Control Center.
- Ruptured globe.
- An uncooperative patient. (Mild sedation for infants may be helpful; see Chapter 7, Pediatric Sedation.)
- Foreign body removal if there are signs or symptoms that suggest infection (e.g., edema and clouding of the cornea surrounding the foreign body, ulceration exceeding the size of the foreign body, or purulent discharge). If infection is suspected, patching is contraindicated and referral is necessary.
- Large metal foreign bodies or those with potential to cause a large rust ring (i.e., those that have been embedded in the cornea for longer than 24 hours).
- Apparently deeply or centrally embedded foreign bodies.

Note: For the final three contraindications, although the slit lamp may be helpful for a primary care clinician, an ophthalmologist usually manages these situations.

EQUIPMENT

- Topical ophthalmic anesthetic, such as 0.5% proparacaine (Alcaine or Ophthaine) or 0.5% tetracaine (Pontocaine), unless contraindicated (e.g., ruptured globe or allergy to local anesthetics).
- Fluor-I-Strip, sterile fluorescein sodium strips. (Since fluorescein is incompatible with preservatives effective

against *Pseudomonas* or *Proteus,* multidose dropper bottles of fluorescein solution should not be used. An inoculation of abraded corneal epithelium with either of these bacteria could cause infection, scarring, or permanent blindness.)

- Sterile cotton-tipped applicators.
- Isotonic ophthalmic irrigant (sterile saline, Dacriose).
- Slit lamp: the two most common slit lamps in use are manufactured by Haag-Streit and Zeiss (see "Suppliers" section).

PREPROCEDURE PATIENT PREPARATION

Patients should be informed about the indication(s) for the slit lamp examination. Once positioned on the scope, patients should be asked to get into a comfortable position that can be maintained for a while. They should be instructed to breathe normally and, especially children, asked to remain still once comfortable. Children may need assistance to help them hold still. Patients should know to blink normally unless their eye is being held open by the examiner or they are asked to hold their eye open. They should be aware of the need for the examiner to touch their face and even to pull on their eyelids. It should be explained that the room is going to be darkened and that a bright light can be expected, especially if the pupil is dilated. Reassurance that this bright light will not cause permanent visual damage is usually appreciated. In fact, patients should be assured that the reason for using this bright light (in most cases) is to *prevent* permanent damage to their vision.

The patient needs to know that he or she will be asked to direct vision to certain locations and that eyedrops or dye may be necessary to enhance the examination. Before instilling fluorescein, warn the patient that objects in his or her vision may temporarily appear yellow. Tears may also remain yellow for a short while after the examination. Before topical anesthetic is instilled, the patient should be warned that it may cause a burning sensation until the eye becomes numb.

TECHNIQUE

1. Proper patient positioning is absolutely essential for a satisfactory examination. Both the patient and the examiner should be comfortable. An improperly positioned patient is more likely to move backwards and out of focus. They are also less likely to maintain positioning for extended periods of time.

    The patient is seated during the examination. The examination chair height should be such that the patient can easily place his or her chin in the adjustable chin rest and forehead against the headrest. Some slit lamps have an eye level marker to assist in gauging head positioning. If the patient is unable to place his or her forehead against the headrest, either elevate the chair or lower the chin rest. If the patient is not positioned against the headrest, it will be difficult to focus on deeper ocular structures. This common mistake often causes a great deal of frustration for the novice slit lamp user. After the patient is positioned, loss of focus may indicate that he or she has moved his or her head backward. It should be repositioned. Small children should sit in the chair on their knees, stand up on the footrest, or sit in their parent's lap.

2. Examiner positioning is also important. He or she should be able to reach the patient's eye comfortably and to easily rest an elbow on the slit lamp table. Such a position is important if the eyelids need to be manipulated and for holding instruments used in foreign body removal. The examiner should also be seated comfortably in the chair so that his or her eyes easily reach the eyepiece without leaning forward. This description may seem overly simplistic, but many a novice slit lamp examiner looks like a baseball catcher coming up from a crouch. This is not a position that can be maintained for long.

3. Turn on the power to the lamp selecting the next-to-highest power setting. The eyepieces can be adjusted to correct your refractive error, although it is often simpler to set the eyepieces at zero (1×) and wear your spectacles or contact lenses. Once the eyepieces are adjusted, the interpupillary distance is set. After this adjustment, no further manipulation of the eyepieces should be necessary. Magnification can be changed with a knob, anterior to the eyepieces on some slit lamps, or by shifting a lever found below the eyepieces on models such as the Haag-Streit 900.

4. After positioning and eyepiece adjustment, darken the examination room as much as possible. The eyepieces (and thus the examiner) should remain perpendicular to the chin rest throughout the examination. The light source, not the oculars, should be moved to facilitate viewing. Move the light source vertically by using the control lever located at the base of the slit lamp. Horizontal movement is accomplished by moving the swing arm with the examiner's other hand. Position the slit beam at an oblique angle, starting at the temporal side of each eye and moving the light nasally. Beware when moving the light source from the temporal side of the eye: From this position, if the examiner is not careful, the patient's nose is often struck by the mirror or light

source. To view the nasal portion of an eye, have the patient gaze temporally in that eye. This should bring the desired area into focus.

5. The depth of focus is adjusted by moving the slit lamp backward and forward. Focusing is typically accomplished at the same time as vertical positioning with the joystick. Remember to examine both eyes, even if the symptoms are monocular. The "normal" eye can be used for comparison if there is pathology in the other eye.

6. At the start of the examination, the patient should be instructed to look toward the examiner's ear opposite to the eye being examined (i.e., the patient looks at the examiner's left ear while the right eye is being examined). Some slit lamps have a fixation light to direct the patient's gaze, but it is often simpler to instruct the patient to focus on a larger, nonmoving object such as the examiner's ear.

7. Evaluation of the ocular structures has already begun with a focused history, the measurement of visual acuity in both eyes, and a gross handlight examination of the eyelid skin and surrounding structures. The slit lamp examination should then proceed in a systematic manner from external (lids and lashes) to internal (vitreous). Failing to be systematic can cause the examiner to get caught up in the fine detail that the slit lamp provides. In this manner, the examiner can miss the "forest for the trees."

8. Choose the white light beam filter lens. A long, wide beam is useful for scanning tissues such as the lids and lashes. Observe the general appearance of the lid margin; the lid's color, position, and vascularity; and any meibomian gland openings. Examine the lashes and eyebrows for the presence of inflammation, scaling, or elevated or ulcerated lesions. Also examine the lashes for evidence of lid debris and for missing or additional lashes. Scan for the misdirection of lashes (trichiasis; see Chapter 41, Trichiasis), which can cause a severe foreign body sensation in an otherwise normally positioned lid. If there are only a few misdirected eyelashes, pluck them with fine forceps. If there are many, the patient should be referred for electrolysis of the roots. Also evaluate lid position for being turned in (entropion) or out (ectropion). Note discrete changes in lid pigmentation.

Examination of the lower lid is aided by having the patient look up while pulling the lower lid down with your index finger. This exposure provides a good view of the posterior lid margin and the lower palpebral conjunctiva. Eversion of the upper lid is necessary to properly examine the upper palpebral conjunctiva and to localize foreign bodies. Lid eversion can be performed by having the patient close his or her eyes and look down. Grasp the

upper lid margin gently between thumb and index finger. A cotton-tipped swab is then placed about 15 mm from the lid margin. The lid is then moved out, up, and over the cotton-tipped swab. A drop of local anesthetic often enhances patient comfort with this procedure. Examine very carefully the few millimeters proximal to the lid margin. This is a common location for small foreign bodies missed on the routine examination.

9. A long wide beam is also used to examine the conjunctiva. The examiner gently separates the eyelids with the opposite hand while the patient is asked to look in all directions of gaze. The conjunctiva is normally a transparent tissue with the white sclera visible beneath. Occasionally, there are slightly elevated, yellow lesions at the three- and nine-o'clock positions at the limbus (edge of cornea) called *pinguecula*. These benign lesions are more common with advancing age. Areas of pigmentation of the conjunctiva can also be seen. These are commonly benign nevi, most often translucent and flat. For irregularly shaped or pigmented lesions suspicious of melanoma, the patient should be referred to an ophthalmologist.

10. Usually a long, narrow beam is used to examine the cornea; this produces an optical cross section. Within the optical cross section, the epithelium or tear film is seen as the most anterior band. The stroma can be seen as the large middle layer and the posterior band represents the endothelium (Fig. 57-3). The slit lamp beam is brought across the cornea from the temporal to nasal limbus with attention paid to the regularity of the corneal surface. Any disruption in the corneal surface such as an abrasion should be easily noted as an irregular, distorted, or dulled light reflex. When the light is shone from a lateral position, it produces greater shadows and provides an excellent appreciation of the depth and texture of corneal lesions.

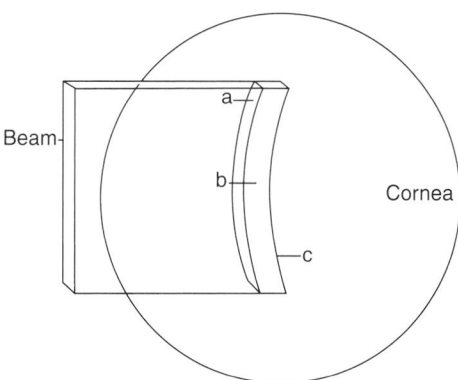

Fig. 57-3
Optical cross section of the cornea. *a,* Corneal epithelium; *b,* corneal stroma; *c,* corneal endothelium.

If a corneal abrasion is suspected, a fluorescein strip should be used. It will stain areas of absent epithelium bright green when viewed with a cobalt blue light filter. (For instilling fluorescein, see Chapter 56, Corneal Abrasion and Removal of Corneal or Conjunctival Foreign Body.) Be careful to use minimal amounts of fluorescein to avoid flooding the eye with dye, obscuring the abnormal epithelium. Avoid touching the cornea directly with a fluorescein strip because this may result in an iatrogenically stained cornea. If either of these occurs, have the patient blink, blot the excess fluorescein away and then reexamine. If the eye is still flooded, flush it with ophthalmic saline and again have the patient blot away the excess.

Another technique useful to screen for a corneal lesion or foreign object uses limbal scatter. If the scope is placed laterally and light is directed at the closest portion of the limbus, the cornea simulates a fiberoptic element. Light is transmitted medially through the cornea to the limbus on the other side. A lesion or foreign body in the cornea should cause light to backscatter and should be seen clearly against the dark pupillary background.

By focusing deeper than the surface epithelium, the clinician can examine the corneal stroma, which makes up 90% of the corneal tissue. A narrow slit beam will allow for accurate determination of the depth of either a foreign body or penetrating injury. Opacities or haze may be noted, which are indicative of previous trauma, infection, or inflammation. Old lesions tend to be more circumscribed, whereas an active keratitis usually produces a diffuse pattern of corneal haze.

The endothelium is visible as the posterior line in the optical section. Abnormalities may present either as folds in the endothelium or as changes that resemble the surface of a golf ball called *corneal guttae*. Both of these changes may be indicative of endothelial cell loss.

11. The anterior chamber is the space between the corneal endothelium and the iris. Gauge the anterior chamber depth by estimating the distance between the corneal endothelium and the front surface of the iris. This distance is normally 3 mm or more. The aqueous humor is examined with a short, narrow beam with bright illumination and high magnification for the presence of cells or flare. Cells in the aqueous humor may indicate inflammation (iritis) or hemorrhage (hyphema). Cells appear against the dark pupillary background as white specks when iritis occurs and as red specks when hyphema occurs. The aqueous humor is normally clear, with light passing through it without change. Protein in the aqueous humor, seen with intraocular inflamma-

tion, causes a visible flare (Tyndall effect). This effect is similar to that seen when shining a flashlight through smoke (Fig. 57-4).

12. The iris has numerous crypts that should be plainly visible with the slit lamp. Nevi, surgical openings, neovascularization, atrophy, tears, or abnormally pigmented lesions may be seen with magnification. If the iris is scarred to the lens (posterior synechiae) or cornea (anterior synechiae), it should be noted. Of interest in those patients who have undergone cataract extraction, a tremulousness of the iris called *iridodonesis* is often seen. It is caused by removal of the support usually provided by the lens.

13. Next, use a long, narrow slit beam to examine the layers of the lens. Dilating the pupil allows for the most thorough evaluation of the lens. Any opacity in the crystalline lens is called a *cataract*. The slit beam passes through multiple layers in the lens from anterior to posterior: anterior capsule, anterior cortex, nucleus, posterior cortex, and posterior capsule (Fig. 57-5). Cortical cataracts resemble spokes radiating from the lens equator. Nuclear cataracts are central and are often seen as a yellow or amber hue discoloring the normally clear lens. Posterior subcapsular cataracts often appear as clustered punctate vacuoles. These can be seen either directly or with retroillumination.

Retroillumination uses the red reflex and often provides a striking view of lens opacities through a dilated pupil. The slit beam is directed parallel to the visual axis to either the nasal or temporal side of the lens. The examiner then views the red reflex, which is the light reflected off the retina and back through the lens. Against this red background, lens opacities such as capsular cataracts are prominently displayed.

14. After examining the posterior lens capsule, next examine the anterior vitreous humor. Normally, the vitreous humor is a relatively clear fluid with minimal cellular material. If cellular material is noted, refer

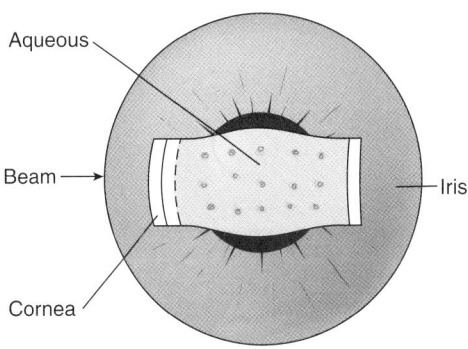

Fig. 57-4
Optical cross section of the anterior chamber showing cell and flare.

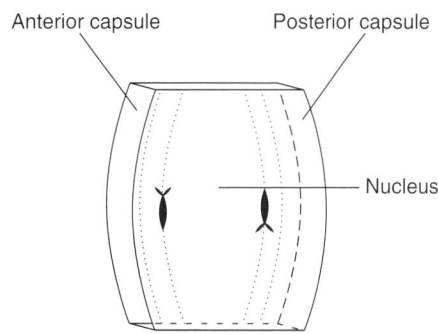

Fig. 57-5
Optical cross section of the lens.

the patient. Gross vitreous opacities, such as floaters, can also be seen with the slit beam.

15. Special lenses can be used to increase the capabilities of a slit lamp examination. The vitreous body and fundus can be viewed by using a lens (Hruby) attached to the slit lamp, or by using a handheld lens positioned in front of the eye. With the Hruby lens, the examiner must insert the lens spindle into the groove of the lens guide plate on the slit lamp. With any of the lenses, the slit beam is positioned parallel to the visual axis. Distracting light reflections off the lenses can often be resolved by slightly tilting the lens.

POSTPROCEDURE PATIENT EDUCATION

The findings should be discussed with the patient, as well as any postprocedure care. Any necessary referrals should be made. For corneal foreign bodies or abrasions, see Chapter 56, Corneal Abrasions and Removal of Corneal or Conjunctival Foreign Bodies, for management and postprocedure patient information.

SUPPLIERS

Zeiss
One Zeiss Drive
Thornwood, NY 10594
Phone: 1-914-747-1800
Website: www.zeiss.de

CPT/BILLING CODES

65222	Removal of foreign body, external eye; corneal with slit lamp
92002	Ophthalmologic services: medical examination and evaluation with initiation of diagnostic and treatment program; intermediate, new patient
92012	Intermediate, established patient

Note: Intermediate examination includes biomicroscopy.

99070	Eye tray: supplies and materials (except spectacles) provided by physician over and above those that are usually included with the office visit or other services rendered (list drugs, trays, supplies, or materials provided)

ICD-9-CM DIAGNOSTIC CODES

364.70	Adhesions of iris, unspecified
364.00	Acute iritis
918.1	Corneal abrasion
371.82	Corneal injury due to contact lens
930.0	Corneal foreign body
930.1	Foreign body in conjunctival sac
361.00	Retinal detachment with retinal defect, unspecified
918.2	Superficial injury of conjunctiva
	Superficial corneal keratitis without conjunctivitis
370.20	unspecified
370.24	photokeratitis
360.60	Intraocular foreign body

BIBLIOGRAPHY

Coles WH: *Ophthalmology: a diagnostic text,* Baltimore, 1989, Williams & Wilkins.

Miller D, Greiner JV: Corneal measures and tests. In Albert DA, Jakobiec FA, editors: *Principles and practice of ophthalmology,* ed 2, Philadelphia, 2000, WB Saunders.

CHAPTER 58

Tonometry

Deepa Vasudevan

Tonometry is used to detect increased intraocular pressure, which is common in patients at risk for glaucoma. Glaucoma is actually caused by a group of conditions, all of which can lead to optic nerve damage and a loss of visual function. More than 1.6 million persons in the United States are estimated to have some degree of blindness caused by glaucoma. It is the third most common cause of blindness, and incidence increases with age. Despite the fact that most blindness caused by glaucoma is preventable, or at least able to be delayed, there are estimates that less than half of patients with glaucoma have been diagnosed. Tonometry remains one of the easiest methods of screening for glaucoma, although it is true that patients with glaucoma can have normal intraocular pressures, and at the same time not all patients with increased intraocular pressures have glaucoma. Currently researchers are pursuing other risk factors associated with glaucomatous changes in the eye in order to develop additional practical screening techniques. When these risk factors are found, glaucoma will be more readily diagnosed in those with normal intraocular pressure. Until then, tonometry, when used in combination with funduscopic examination and visual field testing, is very sensitive and specific in the early detection of glaucomatous changes in the eye. Patients at high risk for glaucoma should be screened with all three.

There are two types of tonometry. *Impression tonometry* measures the depth of the impression produced on the ocular wall by a given force. The Schiøtz tonometer uses this technique. *Applanation tonometry* measures the force necessary to flatten an area of the cornea. Applanation tonometry is more accurate than Schiøtz tonometry, provided the examiner has the necessary skills. However, the Schiøtz tonometer is less expensive and can be used with ease in the office of a well-trained primary care clinician. The clinician may recommend other tests or a referral if the initial test is abnormal. This chapter discusses the technique used in Schiøtz tonometry.

INDICATIONS

- Age over 45 years
- Family history of glaucoma
- Black race (fourfold to sixfold higher risk than whites)
- Diabetes mellitus
- Decreased visual acuity (myopia or hyperopia)
- Ocular pain
- History of visual field loss
- Iatrogenic causes: Use of corticosteroids, mydriatics, phenothiazines, and sympathomimetics can precipitate glaucoma.

CONTRAINDICATIONS

- Eye infection
- Recent eye trauma
- Patients who cannot keep their eyes still

EQUIPMENT

- Schiøtz tonometer kit (each kit contains the tonometer, three plunger weights, a concave test block, conversion tables, pipe cleaners, and instructions for care)
- Topical ophthalmic anesthetic, such as proparacaine hydrochloride 0.5%

PREPROCEDURE PATIENT PREPARATION

Explain the reason for measuring the intraocular pressure with the tonometer (e.g., presence of risk factors or positive physical findings). Briefly explain the procedure as well as the fact that this test only detects increased intraocular pressure. Explain that the presence of a normal intraocular pressure does not completely exclude glaucoma. If glaucoma is suspected, even with a normal intraocular pressure, tonometry should be combined with the other tests mentioned above.

TECHNIQUE

1. Check and record the patient's visual acuity. Immediately following the funduscopic examination, place two drops of anesthetic in each eye. (The anesthetic will take effect while you prepare the tonometer.)
2. Assemble the tonometer with the 5.5-g weight in place, and test for accuracy on the convex metal test block (Fig. 58-1). The Schiøtz tonometer is precalibrated by the manufacturer and must be returned for repair if it does not read "0" when resting on the test block.
3. Have the patient lie on a table in the supine position.
4. Ask the patient to relax and fix his or her gaze on a spot on the ceiling, with the line of vision perpendicular to the table. Retract the lids of the eye against the bony margin of the orbit with one hand and hold the tonometer by its handles with the thumb and middle finger of the other hand. Center the foot plate of the tonometer over the cornea and gently lower the tonometer until it is resting on the cornea (Fig. 58-2). The indicator will come to rest at a position to the right of 0. The tonometer should be perpendicular to the cornea in a vertical position.

Note: To assist the patient in fixing his or her gaze, ask him or her to extend an arm straight upward and to stare at the thumbnail.

5. Record the scale reading. If it is less than 4, repeat the reading because this indicates an elevated intraocular pressure. Perform another reading after adding the 7.5- or 10-g weight, as necessary, to obtain a scale reading between 4 and 8. Convert the scale reading to millimeters of mercury (mm Hg), using the calibration scale included with the kit (Table 58-1). Record this in the chart. Recommend a consultation with an ophthalmologist if the pressure in either eye is greater than 20 mm Hg.
6. Carefully clean the tonometer after each use to prevent transmission of disease. It can then be soaked in a special stand that only soaks the tip. A sterilizing solution that can eliminate HIV should be used. Rinse carefully and allow to dry before use. Alternatively, set the tonometer in an ultraviolet sterilizer stand. The tonometer should be disassembled at the end of each day, and a pipe cleaner with sterilizing solution should be run through the barrel to remove any debris, which could interfere with the motion of the plunger. Next, another pipe cleaner should be

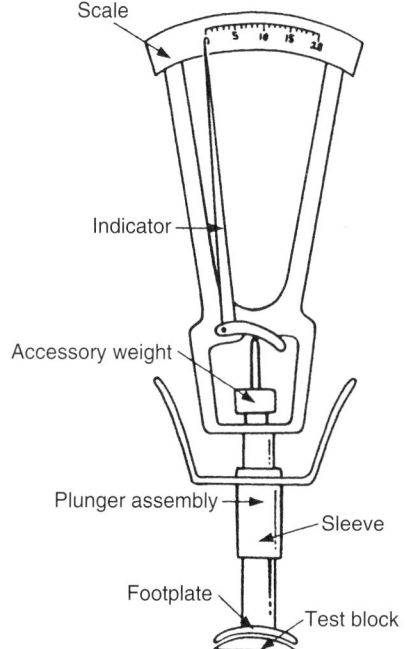

Fig. 58-1
Tonometer.

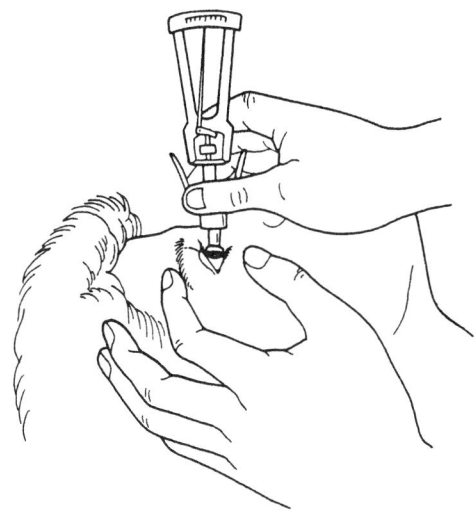

Fig. 58-2
Examination with the tonometer.

used to dry the barrel. The tonometer should not be oiled.

POSTPROCEDURE PATIENT EDUCATION

Routine prophylactic topical antibiotics are no longer prescribed after the procedure. The patient should be instructed to avoid rubbing, touching, or traumatizing

TABLE 58-1
Sample Calibration Scale for Schiøtz Tonometer

Scale Reading	Intraocular Pressure (mm Hg) by Plunger Load			
	5.5 g	7.5 g	10.0 g	15.0 g
0	41	59	82	127
0.5	38	54	75	118
1.0	35	50	70	109
1.5	32	46	64	101
2.0	29	42	59	94
2.5	27	39	55	88
3.0	24	36	51	82
3.5	22	33	47	76
4.0	21	30	43	71
4.5	19	28	40	66
5.0	17	26	37	62
5.5	16	24	34	58
6.0	15	22	32	54
6.5	13	20	29	50
7.0	12	19	27	46
7.5	11	17	25	43
8.0	10	16	23	40
8.5	9	14	21	38
9.0	9	13	20	35
9.5	8	12	18	32
10.0	7	11	16	30
10.5	6	10	15	27
11.0	6	9	14	25
11.5	5	8	13	23
12.0		8	11	21
12.5		7	10	20
13.0		6	10	18
13.5		6	9	17
14.0		5	8	15
14.5			7	14
15.0			6	13
15.5			6	11
16.0			5	10
16.5				9
17.0				8
17.5				8
18.0				7

(From Schiøtz Tonometer Kit literature, courtesy of Gulden Ophthalmics, Elkins Park, Penn.)

the eyes for 1 or 2 hours after the test to avoid injuring the cornea. Contact lens should not be worn until the eye regains sensation. Patients should be warned that an anesthetized eye is easily traumatized and should be told to call their clinician's office immediately if symptoms of a corneal abrasion occur.

If the result is abnormal (increased intraoccular pressure), follow-up care should be discussed. The patient needs to know the importance of follow-up; however, he or she should be aware that increased intraocular pressure does not always mean that they have glaucoma.

COMPLICATIONS

- Trauma to the cornea during Schiøtz tonometry is uncommon; however, a corneal abrasion can occur after the procedure while the cornea is still anesthetized.
- Infection can usually be avoided by properly cleaning the tonometer.

LIMITATIONS

Falsely elevated intraocular pressure readings can be a normal variant, or they can be the result of an inflamed cornea, a scarred cornea, or pressure placed on the globe during the procedure. They can also occur with a thick or steeply curved cornea. Falsely low measurements can be a normal variant, or they can result from high-grade myopia or rapidly repeated measurements.

SUPPLIERS

Schiøtz Tonometer Kit
Gulden Ophthalmics
225 Cadwalader Avenue
Elkins Park, PA 19027
Phone: 1-215-884-8105
Website: www.guldenindustries.com

CPT/BILLING CODES

Ophthalmological services constitute integrated services. Itemization of tonometry is not applicable.

92002   Ophthalmologic services: medical examination and evaluation with initiation of diagnostic and treatment program; intermediate, new patient

92012   Ophthalmologic services: medical examination and evaluation with initiation of diagnostic and treatment program; intermediate, established patient

99173   Screening test of visual acuity, quantitative, bilateral (cannot be used with 92002 or 92012)

ADDITIONAL RESOURCES

- See the sample patient education handout titled "Tonometry" on page 1807 of Appendix G.

• See the sample patient consent form titled "Tonometry" on page 1809 of Appendix G.

BIBLIOGRAPHY

Berson FG, editor: *Ophthalmology study guide,* San Francisco, 1987, American Academy of Ophthalmology.

Chatterjee BM: Glaucoma and intraocular pressure. In *Handbook of ophthalmology,* ed 6, New Delhi, India, 1997, CBS Publishers.

Kanski J: *Clinical ophthalmology,* ed 3, Boston, 1994, Butterworth Heinemann.

Krachmer J, Palay D: *Ophthalmology for the primary care physician,* St Louis, 1998, Mosby.

Morse RM, Heffron WA: Preventive health care in family practice. In Rakel RE, editor: *Textbook of family practice,* ed 6, Philadelphia, 2002, WB Saunders.

WEBSITES

www.eyecare.org (New Jersey's Eyecare Organization)
www.glaucoma.com (Glaucoma Research Foundation)

CHAPTER 59

Visual Function Evaluation

Michael Altman

Stewart L. Zuckerbrod

Of the senses, vision may be the most vital; however, evaluation of the eyes and visual system is often overlooked or is performed in a perfunctory manner. This may be due to the perception that the examination is difficult or requires specialized equipment. Although parts of the examination require specific instruments, much can be done with equipment available in most offices.

Warning: It is vital to identify children at risk for amblyopia. If not identified early, this condition causes permanent loss of vision as a result of interruption of normal visual pathway development. Causes include tumor, cataract, strabismus, or uncorrected refractive error during the first 5 or 6 years of life. Screening is accomplished by checking visual acuity and motility (see the "Technique" section).

Ophthalmologists evaluate the eyes in a systematic manner called the "8-point examination." These "points" include: (1) external examination, (2) visual acuity, (3) pupillary examination, (4) visual fields, (5) motility, (6) pressure testing, (7) slit lamp examination, and (8) fundus examination. Most of these points are included under the "Technique" section. Many aspects of the slit lamp examination can be achieved with a careful external examination. For a more detailed description of the slit lamp examination, see Chapter 57.

Every visual function evaluation should consider preventable causes of blindness. Although quantitative assessment of intraocular pressure requires specialized equipment and practice, qualitative techniques are also available to screen for glaucoma (see Chapter 58, Tonometry). Observation of children's eyes sometimes reveals evidence of elevated intraocular pressures (large corneas, cloudy corneas, and asymmetric ocular size), but in adults this is rarely obvious. Other potentially preventable or reversible causes of loss of vision include diabetic or hypertensive retinopathy, cataract, pituitary adenoma, choroiditis, creeping inferior retinal detachment, and choroidal melanoma. In addition, glaucoma, retinitis pigmentosa, intracerebral tumors, and detached retina (or hysteria if the size of the field loss is independent of distance) can appear as an insidious loss of visual fields.

INDICATIONS

1. History (or suspicion) of visual loss, or any patient being evaluated for ocular pain, ocular trauma, or visual complaint
2. All newborns, infants, and school-age children
3. All children, as soon after the third birthday as possible, should be screened for asymmetry in visual acuity
4. Redness or discoloration of eyes or periorbital structures
5. Suspicion of glaucoma from history or physical findings, or patient at risk of glaucoma
6. Misalignment of the eyes or complaint of diplopia
7. Suspicion of intracranial process involving the visual system
8. Suspicion of ocular involvement of systemic disease
9. Commercial aircraft pilots and people who operate heavy equipment (color vision should also be tested)

CONTRAINDICATIONS

There are no contraindications.

EQUIPMENT

1. Bright penlight for testing response to light and eliciting corneal light reflex (infants and children).
2. Snellen and *Illiterate E* charts (Fig. 59-1). The latter, also called *Tumbling E,* consists of the letter *E* in various sizes and positions. A well-lit, 20-foot hallway is usually necessary to administer the test unless otherwise specified. (Reverse Snellen charts are available for use with mirrors if a 20-foot hallway is not available.)

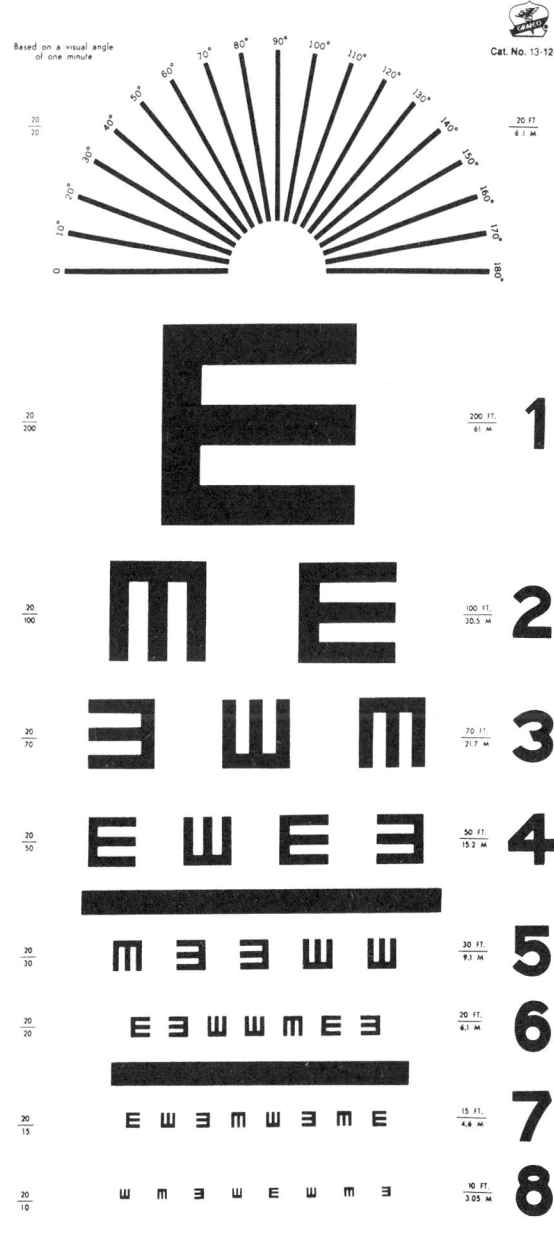

Fig. 59-1
Illiterate E chart.

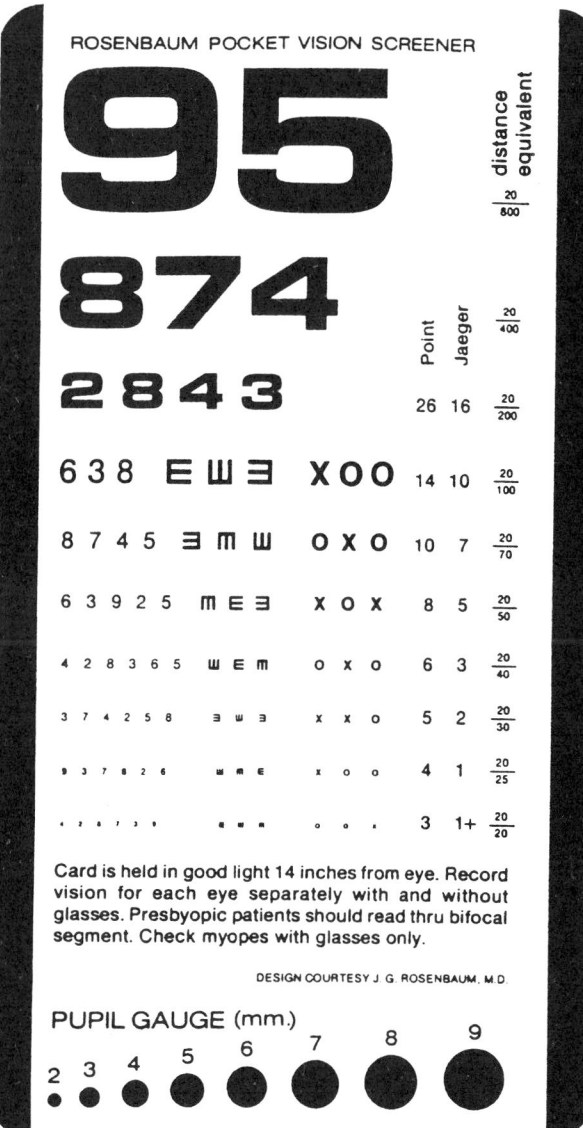

Fig. 59-2
Near vision chart.

3. Pinhole cards (or pinhole test; see Fig. 59-4) for those with severely impaired vision.
4. Ishihara's or Hardy-Rand-Rittler pseudoisochromatic plates for color-vision testing. These are a series of numbers or figures presented against a background of colored dots, arranged in such a way as to present a confusing and thus unreadable pattern to the person who has abnormal color discrimination.
5. Standard near vision chart for adults (e.g., Rosenbaum Pocket Vision Screener) (Fig. 59-2).

TECHNIQUE

1. External Examination

Look for asymmetry between the eyes (proptosis or "bulging," ptosis or "lid droop," unilateral redness or discoloration), patterns of redness (ciliary flush in iritis, solid red areas in subconjunctival hemorrhage), and obvious opacification of the cornea (ulcer, scar) or lens (leukocorea or "white pupil," suggestive of cataract or intraocular tumor).

Use of the "shadow test" can identify individuals at risk for narrow angle and angle closure glaucoma.

Simply shine a light lateromedially across the anterior chamber. The light should illuminate both the lateral and medial portion of the iris; if the medial portion is shadowed, the anterior chamber is shallow. Use of mydriatics and other medications that can cause pupillary dilation (such as Neosynephrine) are relatively contraindicated in such patients.

2. Visual Acuity
3. Pupillary Examination
4. Visual Fields
5. Motility

Infants and Newborns

a. Test eye fixation on an object and the tracking of a moving object (opticokinetic testing) to demonstrate an intact visual pathway to the visual cerebral cortex.

Step 1. Hold the infant upright and slowly move your face in front of the infant's face. The normal response is for the eyes to follow your facial movement briefly. If the test is abnormal, ask the parent to perform the same maneuver.

Step 2. Hold three of your fingers together, palm toward you, in front of one of the infant's eyes to block vision. Simultaneously test the uncovered eye as in Step 1. Repeat for the opposite eye. (The standard visual occluder is not necessary and is more likely to be rejected by children.)

Step 3. If any one of these tests is abnormal in patients aged 3 to 4 months, refer the patient to an ophthalmologist.

b. Next, test for intact third cranial nerves by looking for the expected positive reflex of pupillary constriction to light.

c. Visual field testing is performed by shining the light at the periphery of vision; expect the infant to turn its head in that direction.

Distractions need to be minimized for these three tests, and the nursery lights need to be dimmed for the latter two.

Note: Gross retinal examination should be performed on all newborns by eliciting the *red reflex,* normally a symmetric orange-red light reflected by both fundi. Hold the ophthalmoscope 1 to 2 feet from each eye and observe the color in the pupil. Asymmetry in color might indicate toxoplasmosis or a retinoblastoma and should be evaluated further.

Young Children (under 3 years old)

a. Confirm that there is vision in each eye and screen for visual field deficits using an object, such as a favorite toy, to attract the patient's attention.

Step 1. Cover one eye and pass the object successively from the periphery into each of the visual fields.

Obvious facial brightening or verbal acknowledgement confirms detection of the object. The child's eye should follow the object.

Step 2. Repeat Step 1 with the other eye. If one eye is abnormal, the child may cry when the normal eye is covered. Likewise, the inability to fixate or follow indicates a visual deficit in the same-sided eye.

Note: Do not touch the child's face during fixation testing. They will not like it!

b. Test for strabismus. Shine a penlight or similar point light source toward the eyes from about 3 or 4 feet while having the patient gaze at a distant object. The reflection of light from each cornea should be located symmetrically (Fig. 59-3). If symmetric, it is usually centered over the pupils. (Momentary eye wandering in infancy is common up to 3 or 4 months of age.)

Older Children

a. Test visual acuity. By the time they are 3 to 4 years of age, children should be tested for standard acuity using an Illiterate E chart (Fig. 59-1). It is especially important to detect asymmetry in visual acuity.

Step 1. Show the child the chart at a distance from which it can be seen easily. Explain that he or she is to point in the direction that the "legs" of the "E" point. Demonstrate this activity. Allow the child to practice reading the letters to help overcome confusion and anxiety.

Step 2. With the child 20 feet from the chart, cover one of his or her eyes (use a patch if necessary) and test from the largest to the smallest readable letters. Record the lowest line on which the patient can correctly identify at least half the total number of letters. Repeat for the other eye, and then for both simultaneously.

Step 3. If the child cannot read any line at 20 feet, walk him or her toward the chart, and record as the numerator the distance at which the top line can be read. (For example, if the child can read the top line—which normally can be read at 200 feet—at a maximum of 10 feet, record this as 10/200 vision.)

Step 4. If the patient is unable to see the top line at 3 feet, have him or her count your fingers. Record the maximal distance at which the patient can count fingers as "CF/[insert the maximal distance]."

Step 5. If the patient is unable to count fingers at 1 foot, have them determine the direction of hand motion. Record as "HM/[the maximal distance]."

Step 6. For a patient with even poorer vision, have him or her attempt to determine the position of a light ("LP with projection"), the presence of light without

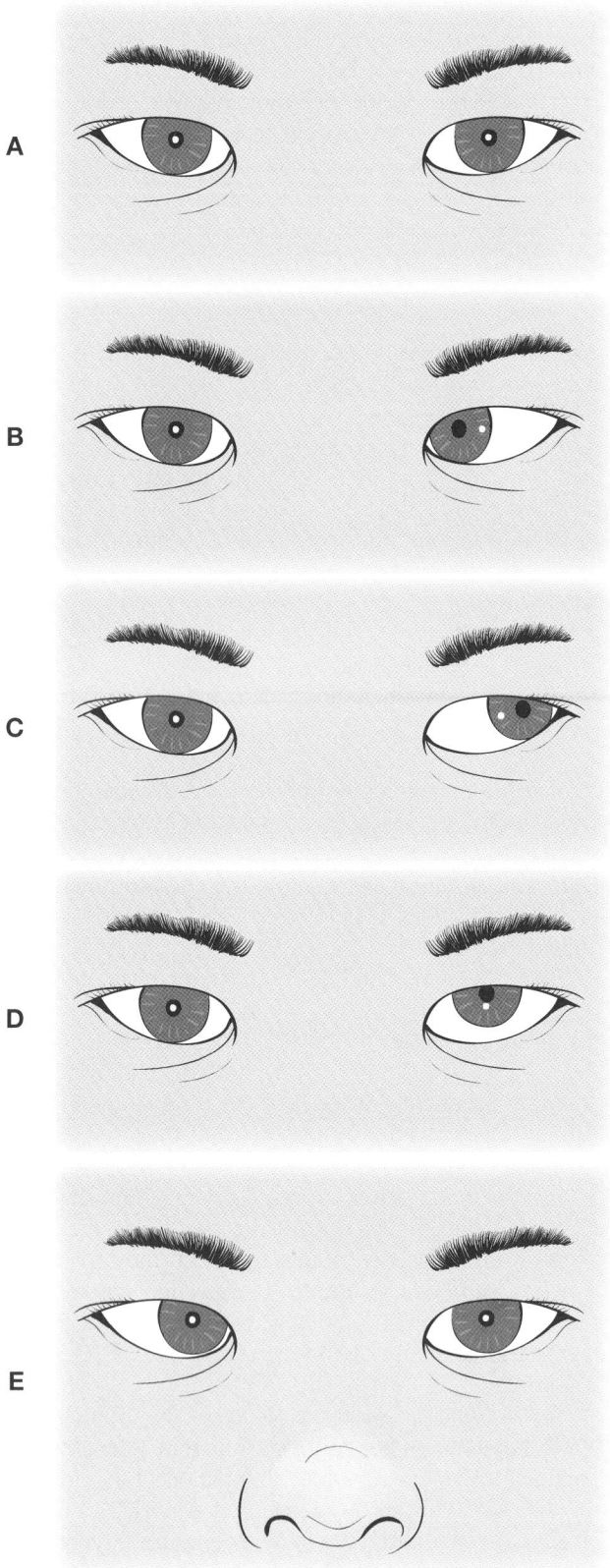

the ability to determine its position ("LP/no projection"), or no light perception ("NLP").

Step 7. Test any person who scores less than 20/20 vision by having him or her look through a pinhole (Fig. 59-4; adult used for demonstration). If the vision is improved, this suggests that corrective lenses will improve the vision.

Step 8. A difference in acuity between the two eyes of two or more levels is suggestive of amblyopia. Refer such patients to an ophthalmologist, who can evaluate for additional disease and assist with management. Appropriate management may be as simple as temporary occlusion of vision in the stronger eye to strengthen the weaker one.

b. Examine pupils

Step 1. Pupillary size. Have the patient look at (or imagine looking at) a distant object in order to eliminate accommodation. Measure the pupillary size with a millimeter ruler or by comparing to a pupillary gauge. Anisocoria (pupillary asymmetry of greater than 1 mm) should be noted and, if new, investigated further. Check pupillary response to light to determine which pupil is abnormal. Fixed, unilateral pupillary dilation may signify syphilis, Adie's pupil, or prior trauma; fixed constriction is suggestive of Horner's syndrome. Horner's syndrome is the triad of anhidrosis (decreased sweating), constricted pupil, and ipsilateral ptosis, although anhidrosis is inconsistent. Brainstem stroke, carotid dissection, or neoplasm impinging on the sympathetic chain are occa-

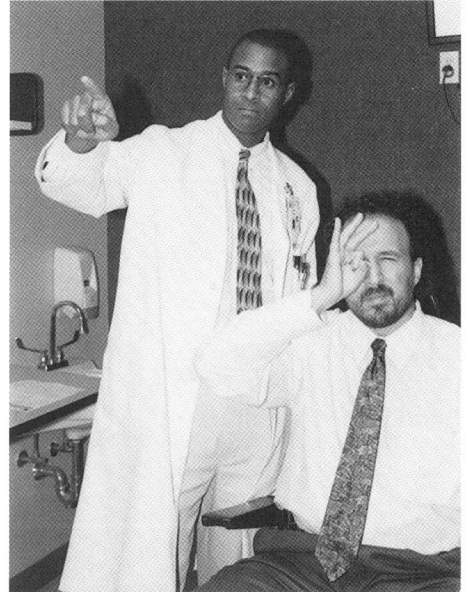

Fig. 59-3
Findings during corneal light reflection. **A,** Normal alignment; **B,** left esotropia; **C,** left exotropia; **D,** left hypertropia; **E,** pseudostrabismus resulting from a flat nasal bridge, wide epicanthal folds, and closely placed eyes.

Fig. 59-4
Pinhole test. Have the patient roll the forefinger and hold it with the thumb. He or she should read the eye chart while looking through the small "pinhole" created by this maneuver. This approximates the vision that can be achieved by correcting any refractive error.

sionally identified as the cause of Horner's, but most are idiopathic.

Step 2. Pupillary function: Once again, have the patient look at a large, distant object in a dimly lit room. Shine a penlight at each eye. There should be a brisk contraction (Fig. 59-5; adult used for demonstration) as the normal light response. If there is quick constriction, there is no need to check accommodation. Unilateral poor contraction is suggestive of one of the problems mentioned in Step 1. Bilateral poor contraction should be investigated further by checking the near or accommodative response. Have the patient gaze alternately between a distant object and his or her fingertip held about 14 inches from the face. Observe this pupillary response under dim light. An accommodative response greater than the previous response to bright light is considered "light – near disassociation" and is suggestive of diabetes, neurosyphilis, lesions of the dorsal midbrain (obstructive hydrocephalus, pineal region tumors), or the result of nerve regeneration (oculomotor nerve palsy, Adie's tonic pupil).

Finally, check for a relative afferent pupillary defect (Marcus Gunn pupil) by rapidly moving a bright light from one eye to the other; both pupils should constrict (consensual usually less direct) when the light is shone in one eye. Dilation of one of the pupils when the light is swung to that eye (consensual more direct) is abnormal, and suggests a significant deficit of the anterior visual pathway on that side (retina or optic nerve damage from retinal disease, advanced glaucoma, tumor, aneurysm, etc.)

c. Test visual fields. Elicit cooperation from the older child in actively reporting when he or she detects an object in each successive visual field. Sit facing the patient at arm's length. Cover your right eye and ask the patient to cover his or her left eye. Ask the patient to look at your left eye with his or her right eye. Making sure the patient's eye maintains its gaze, extend your left arm to your left, move your first two fingers, and slowly bring your hand inward toward you (Fig. 59-6; adult used for demonstration). Ask the patient to indicate when he or she can see your fingers moving; compare this with your own response. Do this from all directions (use the right hand as well), then switch eyes. Deficits of a peripheral visual field can be due to a vast array of ocular and intracranial disorders. Discussion of patterns of field loss is beyond the scope of this chapter. Use this technique as a screening procedure; formal visual field testing should be performed to quantify suspected field deficits.

d. Test for strabismus.

Step 1. Observe for obvious deviation of one eye. A permanent nasal or inward deviation is designated *esotropia;* a temporal or lateral deviation is *exotropia.* Tropias produce permanently deviated lines of vision where phorias are latent or tending toward deviation. Primary strabismus in children is most often esotropia. Exotropia is often a result of another cause. Both should be evaluated further if symptoms are persistent. If there is a misalignment, have the child look up, down, right, and left to determine if the deviation is the same in all fields (comitant) or is significantly varied (neurologically significant paralytic strabismus).

Step 2. If Step 1 was negative, as for young children, observe the corneal light reflection in each eye, screening for a more subtle degree of deviation (Fig. 59-3).

Step 3. If still unable to detect strabismus, perform maximally sensitive "cover/uncover" and "alternate cover" tests (Fig. 59-7). Have the child stare at a light source approximately 12 inches (33 cm)

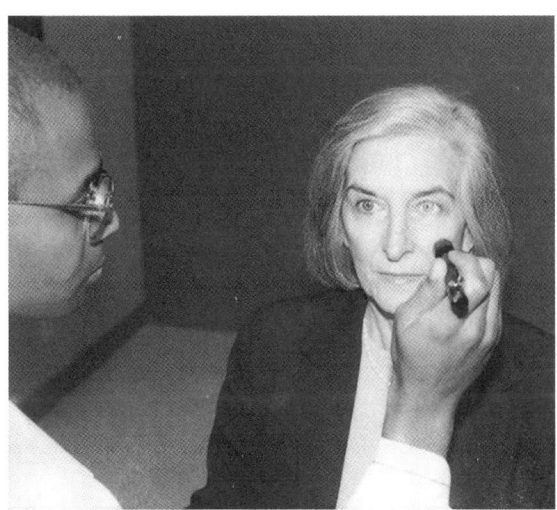

Fig. 59-5
Pupil examination.

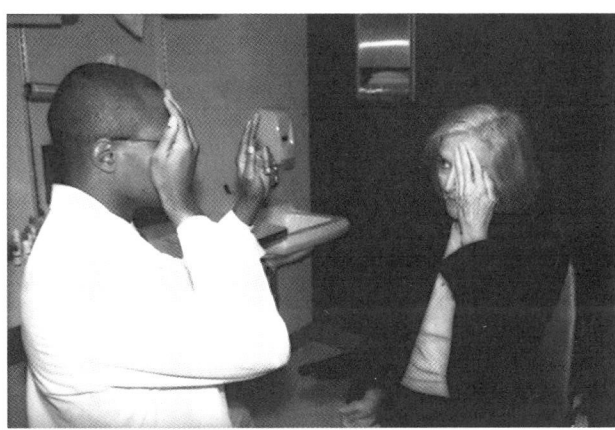

Fig. 59-6
Confrontation visual field testing.

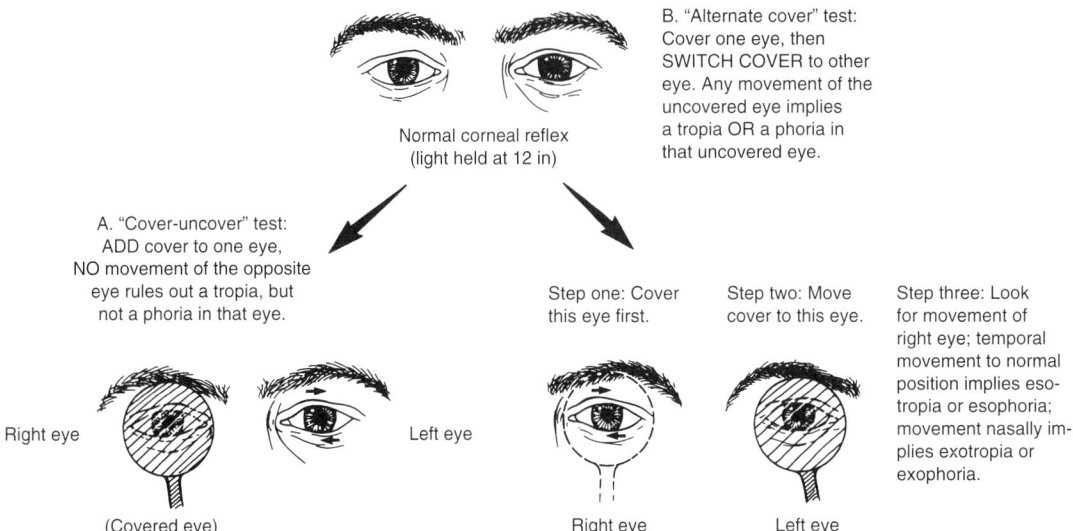

Fig. 59-7

Tropia and phoria screening. For the "cover-uncover" test, esotropia, or inward eye deviation, is suspected when the eye was originally deviated inward and moved temporally to achieve a normal, fixated position. Exotropia, or external (temporal) eye deviation, is suspected when the eye was originally deviated outward (before the good eye was covered) and moved nasally to achieve a normal, fixated position. For the "alternate cover" test, movement in the previously covered eye must be monitored.

away, occlude the vision from the right eye with one hand, and observe for any movement (which indicates tropia) of the left eye (cover-uncover).

Step 4. Watch for movement of the until-now occluded right eye as the cover is moved to the opposite eye (alternate cover). Any right eye movement, especially if there was none from the left eye in Steps 1 through 3, suggests that the right eye requires a constant visual stimulus to remain fixated. This indicates that there is a latent deviation, or phoria.

Step 5. Repeat Steps 3 and 4, covering and uncovering the left eye.

Step 6. Cardinal gaze should also be evaluated with a penlight at a distance of 18 to 24 inches. Have the child follow the light as you move it in the six cardinal positions (right, then up and down, next left, then up and down). Check the light reflex in each position; the light reflection should remain centered in both pupils in all gaze positions. Abnormal light reflections in one or more positions indicate disturbances of motility and should be further investigated.

Step 7. Refer to an ophthalmologist for a previously unevaluated strabismus.

Adults

a. Test for distant acuity with the standard Snellen chart. With encouragement, patients will often read one line smaller to provide a more accurate assessment.

Note: The Snellen chart is used in a fashion similar to the Illiterate E. Test adults and record results, as described for older children.

b. Test for near vision with a standard near-vision card (Fig. 59-2). If not available, use printed text and record the font size. Near vision should be checked if distant vision needs to be corrected or if the patient has a complaint.

c. Test pupillary function (Fig. 59-4) and visual fields, and test for strabismus, as for older children.

d. Test for color vision, if indicated, using appropriate charts such as the Ishihara or Hardy-Rand-Rittler set. Ensure good illumination, and have the patient wear corrective lenses if they are normally used for near vision. Record the numbers of the charts that cannot be read. Refer to the specific instructions for the chosen set to interpret the specific type of color vision defect, if any.

6. Pressure Testing Without Equipment (Ballotment)

Although not terribly accurate, ballotment will give some indication of intraocular pressure (also see Chapter 58, Tonometry). Gently place both forefingers side by side on top of the closed upper lid (Fig. 59-8). Ballot the eye; repeat on the other side. Highly elevated pressure (as in angle closure glaucoma) is demonstrated by unilateral firmness of the globe; with experience, more subtle variations can be detected.

Remember that glaucoma is present in nearly 1% of the American population; nearly 50% of affected individuals do not know they have the disease. Be sure to screen all individuals with known risk factors (family history, African-American heritage, old age, etc.).

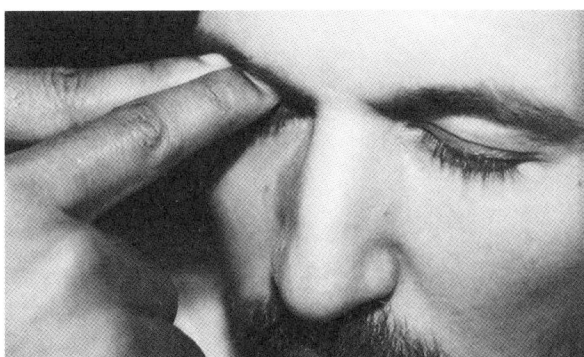

Fig. 59-8
Ballotment.

7. Slit Lamp Examination

See Chapter 57, Slit Lamp Examination.

8. Fundus Examination

Use of the direct ophthalmoscope is an acquired skill. Evaluating the eye with the pupil dilated simplifies the process, but patients often object to the loss of accommodation and the sensitivity to light after the use of mydriatics. Fortunately, it is quite possible to perform a good fundus examination on a nondilated eye.

Seat the patient in a dimly lit room and have him or her gaze at a distant object. To examine the patient's right eye, use your right eye, and examine their left eye with your left eye.

Turn on the ophthalmoscope light (round, white beam) and set the diopter setting to "0." Shine the light at the patient's eye and locate the red reflex as you look through the aperture. Following the reflex, come in closer to the patient until you are 4 to 5 inches from the eye. You should be able to see the retinal vessels on the disc. Adjust the diopter setting until these are in focus.

Note: Focusing the ophthalmoscope on your own hand, until the fingerprints come sharply into view, may help you estimate the proper distances necessary to visualize the fundus.

Examine the ocular structures systematically. First examine the nerve. Check to be sure the disc margins are sharp and distinct; blurring may indicate a swelling of the nerve head. (Papilledema is due to increased intracranial pressure, possibly associated with tumor or hemorrhage. Papillitis is an inflammatory process due to ischemia or infection.) Determine the size of the optic cup (the depression in the center of the nerve where the vessels originate). The normal cup is circular, and less than or equal to three tenths of the total disc diameter. Enlargement of the cup or asymmetry of the cups in the two eyes is suggestive of neurologic loss such as that found with glaucoma.

Follow the vessels; look for abnormal reflections from the arterioles ("silver wire" changes typical for hypertension or collagen vascular disease), arteriovenous nicking (hypertension), or leakage of blood or serum (hemorrhage or exudates, typical of diabetes mellitus). Abnormal nets of blood vessels (neovascularization) indicate advanced ischemic processes such as those associated with diabetes mellitus, vein occlusion, and sickle cell anemia. Finally, examine the fovea by having the patient look directly at the light. You should see a light reflection off the indented fovea and a slightly yellowish coloration. Abnormal foveal appearance may be indicative of macular degeneration (discoloration or elevation of the fovea), diabetic maculopathy (elevation, or presence of hemorrhage or exudate), or other conditions that may have profound effects on the vision.

CPT/BILLING CODES

Visual function evaluation cannot be billed separately. It is considered part of a routine office visit with the complexity of the visit incorporated into the E/M coding.

ICD-9-CM DIAGNOSTIC CODES

365.22	Acute angle closure glaucoma
368.00	Amblyopia
379.41	Anisocoria
743.46	congenital
369.60	Blindness, one eye
366.10	Cataract, senile, unspecified
368.2	Diplopia
367.1	Myopia
379.93	Red eye
368.8	Blurred vision
379.91	Eye pain
368.40	Visual field defect, unspecified
369.70	Vision low, one eye

BIBLIOGRAPHY

Abramson DH, Frank CM, Susman M, et al: Presenting signs of retinoblastoma, *J Pediatr* 132:505, 1998.

Broderick P: Pediatric vision screening for the family physician, *Am Fam Physician* 58:691, 1998.

Butler RN, Faye GE, Kupfer C: Keeping an eye on vision: primary care of eye related ocular disease, *Geriatrics* 52:30, 1997.

Jackson C, Glasson W: Prevention of visual loss: screening in general practice, *Aust Fam Physician* 27:150, 1998.

Taylor D, Hoyt C: *Paediatric ophthalmology,* Malden, Mass, 1997, Blackwell Science.

CHAPTER 60

Audiometry

Gregory J. Forzley

Audiometry quantifies an individual's ability to hear sound through a range of intensities and frequencies. It can be helpful for diagnosing hearing disorders as well as for assessing the degree of impairment. Audiometry is most commonly used for young children and elderly patients, who are most at risk for hearing disorders. However, audiometry may be needed or useful at any age.

Tuning forks that use the C-notes of the musical scale from low to high frequencies are commonly used to screen for hearing loss. The pure-tone audiometer (PTA) is another method of evaluating the auditory system, and it does so electronically. In the tradition of tuning forks, it also samples the octave series of the C-scale. A PTA may be used either to screen for hearing deficits by spot checking certain frequencies or to evaluate deficits more completely and formally. The tones of the audiometer are "pure" in that they are relatively free of noise or overtones. During audiometric testing, the tone can be interrupted when desired, or the intensity (in decibels [dB]) can be varied. The PTA is made up of a variable-frequency oscillator that produces electrical impulses to be converted into sound, an attenuator that permits variations of intensity (often in 5-dB steps), and a transducer, such as an earphone, to convert electrical energy into acoustic energy. With earphones held snugly to the head, each ear is tested separately and the results are then graphed as the *air-conduction audiogram*. An air-conduction audiogram evaluates both the sensorineural and conductive hearing mechanisms.

A separate test can be performed using a bone-conduction oscillator or vibrator, held against the mastoid or forehead by a headband, to evaluate for isolated sensorineural hearing loss. Sensorineural hearing refers to that produced by the cochlea of the inner ear, the auditory nerve, and the cochlear nuclei of the brain (see below for the differential diagnosis of cochlear loss). The vibrator sets the skull into oscillation, producing a disturbance of the fluid in the cochlea. This disturbance is sensed by the cochlea, transmitted down the auditory nerve, and perceived through the cochlear

nuclei. Results are graphed as the *bone-conduction audiogram*. With sensorineural hearing loss, both the air- and bone-conduction impairments are significant but about the same. With air-conductive hearing loss, the bone conduction is normal and the air conduction is impaired. The differences between the air- and bone-conduction thresholds, or the air-bone gap, should not exceed 10 dB. A gap larger than this indicates an air-conduction problem (middle or outer ear) as the source of hearing loss.

The goal of audiometry is to determine the lowest decibel intensity that can be heard for each frequency tested. This is defined as the threshold for that frequency for that person. The individual's threshold is compared with the *audiometric zero,* or 0 dB. Audiometric zero is defined as "normal" by the American National Standards Institute and is derived from sampling a large population of ear-disease–free young adults. As an example, if a person's threshold at a given frequency is 20 dB, it means that the individual can only hear sound at that frequency when it is 20 dB louder than that needed for an average disease-free young adult.

The notations used to record the graphic results of the audiograms have been standardized by the American Speech-Language Hearing Association (ASHA). The audiogram grid reflects the frequency in hertz (Hz) logarithmically on the horizontal axis, and the hearing level in decibels linearly on the vertical axis. The symbols used are noted in Fig. 60-1. In the past, the results were color coded in red for the right ear and in blue for the left ear. This is no longer recommended because color is lost when the results are photocopied.

Note: Approximately 1 in 1000 newborns have severe sensorineural hearing loss. The Joint Committee on Infant Hearing and the National Institutes of Health Consensus Statement recommend screening all infants for hearing loss, preferably during the newborn period. For abnormal screening test results in the very young, options for further evaluation include behavioral observation audiometry, auditory brainstem response, otoacoustic emissions testing, visual reinforcement audiometry, and conditioned play audiometry. These evaluations are beyond the scope of this text.

Response*

Modality	Ear		
	Left	Unspecified	Right
Air conduction: earphones			
Unmasked	X		O
Masked	□		△
Bone conduction: mastoid			
Unmasked	>	∧	<
Masked	]		[
Bone conduction: forehead			
Unmasked	L	v	⌐
Masked	Γ		⌐
Air conduction: sound field	χ	s	∅

Fig. 60-1
Standardized symbols for recording audiogram results. *For "no response," use a downward 45-degree arrow pointing to the left for the right ear symbols, and to the right for left ear symbols (e.g., ↙O for no response in the right ear unmasked).

In addition to PTA, certain audiograms evaluate speech-recognition thresholds (SRT). Similar to pure-tone thresholds, an SRT represents the lowest level of intensity at which the speech stimulus can be repeated back. Performing SRT during initial testing may further validate the resultant air-conduction thresholds. Air conduction thresholds are considered confirmed if there are only small decibel differences between the SRT and PTA. SRT also provides the ability to test hearing aids before purchase and to further evaluate them after use. In the absence of technical difficulties and patient misunderstanding of instructions, if the results from the SRT are significantly better than from PTA, a functional etiology should be considered. Although these evaluations are beyond the scope of this text, referral should be considered.

INDICATIONS

- Subjective complaints of hearing loss, unilateral or bilateral
- Persistent serous otitis media, especially bilateral in children
- Anyone undergoing tympanometry with suspected sensorineural hearing loss (an abnormal tympanogram usually implies conductive hearing loss; however, sensorineural hearing loss may also be present)
- Formal evaluation of a failed screening test

Note: There are estimates that 5% of school age children will have fluctuating hearing loss during the school year because of middle ear effusions. Retesting is imperative.

- General screening in children at the earliest age possible and in the elderly during geriatric assessment
- Patient complaints of tinnitus, dizziness, or vertigo
- Speech delay in children
- Persistent behavioral problems or changes in children or the elderly
- Occupational screening and follow-up for individuals with noisy work environments
- Following severe head trauma
- Following use of ototoxic drugs
- Following meningitis, encephalitis, or other serious viral or bacterial infections that could affect hearing

CONTRAINDICATIONS

- Inexperienced technician
- Acute otitis media
- Local pinna infection that would cause pain from the earphone application
- Uncooperative patient
- Uncontrollable background noise in the room when testing

EQUIPMENT

- PTA. (Options range from screening instruments used to test only selected tones and decibel levels through multiple-frequency, pure-tone, air-and-bone conduction audiometers. The comprehensive instruments generally include frequencies of 125, 250, 500, 750, 1000, 1500, 2000, 3000, 4000, 6000, and 8000 Hz in tone amplitudes ranging from 0 to 100 dB.)
- An individual trained in proper techniques for obtaining reliable, reproducible, and valid test results. (For industrial screening, the individual should be certified by the Council for Accreditation of Occupational Hearing Conservationists.)
- Quiet or sound-treated room, preferably tested (by an outside company) for acceptable ambient noise levels. If ambient noise levels are too high, thresholds may be artificially elevated, particularly in the lower frequencies.

TECHNIQUE

1. Seat the patient comfortably in such a way that they are looking neither at the examiner nor at the control panel. Usually, patients are seated in a position that provides a side profile view to the examiner.
2. Large earrings, glasses, hats, and other items that may interfere with earphone application should be removed.
3. Instruct the patient to respond to the faintest detectable sound at each frequency. The lowest level

of sound (in decibels) heard for each frequency is defined as the threshold. Responses can consist of raising a hand or finger or pressing a test button when sound is first heard. The patient should continue to signal for the duration of audible sound. Having the patient indicate the entire duration of audible sound allows the examiner to determine if the responses are reproducible. If reproducible, the threshold should be the same at the beginning and at the end for a particular frequency at least 50% of the time. Patients should be tested from low to high decibels and back to low. This step helps the examiner exclude false-positive responses.

Note: For small children above age 2, the use of play-conditioned audiometry often provides a reliable test with at least six thresholds tested. Perform this test by having the child place colored rings on pegs when tones are heard. Practicing with a loudspeaker before headphone testing may be helpful. Children from 16 months to 2 years may respond to the same methods, but the number of successes or thresholds determined will be decreased.

4. Place the earphone speaker over the opening of the auditory canal. Check the tragus to make sure it is not covering the opening.
5. Threshold testing is then initiated in the better ear (or the right ear if hearing is equal in both) with the following recommended sequence of frequencies: 1000, 2000, 4000, 8000, 1000 (repeat), 500, and 250 Hz. Start with 0-dB hearing levels and produce the tones for 1 to 2 seconds unless the patient responds.
6. Increase the tone by 5 dB, and, if the patient responds, reduce it by 10-dB increments until it is inaudible.
7. Continue repeated ascents in 5-dB increments and descents in 10-dB increments until a 50% reproducible response is obtained. Generally this requires three to four repetitions, with the patient attaining the same response at least half of the time. This result is then entered with the appropriate symbol on the audiogram.
8. Test the frequencies sequentially as previously noted, starting 15 to 20 dB below the threshold of the previously tested frequency. Continue testing until all frequencies have been tested.
9. If bone-conduction testing is planned, this same sequence can be applied and the results recorded with the appropriate symbols.
10. It may be necessary to mask or obscure one sound by another when the difference in hearing loss between ears is great (e.g., a 50-dB difference). In that situation, crossover of sound to the better ear may occur and artificially lower the threshold of the

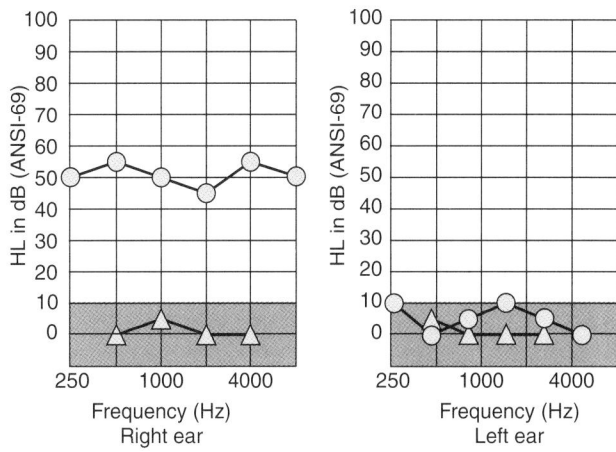

Fig. 60-2
Nine-year-old boy with right acute otitis media with effusion. Using masking, the curves would probably appear the same; however, there would be slightly more assurance of the accuracy of the study. (The corresponding tympanogram would be Type B.) (Redrawn from Jacobsen JT, Northern JL, editors: *Diagnostic audiology,* Austin, Tex, 1991, Pro-Ed.)

impaired ear. For more information on this technique, refer to Adams, Boies, and Hilger (1989).

INTERPRETATION

Air-conduction testing alone can approximate the degree of hearing loss. However, conductive, sensorineural, or mixed (both) hearing loss can often be differentiated by performing both air- and bone-conduction testing.

A threshold of up to 20 dB is considered normal. Above that, hearing can be divided into degrees of hearing loss as follows: mild, 21 to 40 dB; moderate, 41 to 55 dB; moderately severe, 56 to 70 dB; severe, 71 to 90 dB; and profound, 91 dB or greater. Others have suggested slightly different ranges, but the degrees are quite similar.

Certain patterns of hearing loss, especially unilateral, can indicate disease. Hearing asymmetry of more than 20 dB may indicate a retrocochlear lesion or mass. Such patients should be evaluated further or referred. Additional interpretation of results is beyond the scope of this text.

Figs. 60-2 through 60-11 illustrate classic patterns of hearing loss. In the examples, hearing thresholds have been converted to hearing loss (HL). In addition, since each ear was recorded separately, the standardized symbols were not necessary to distinguish left from right.

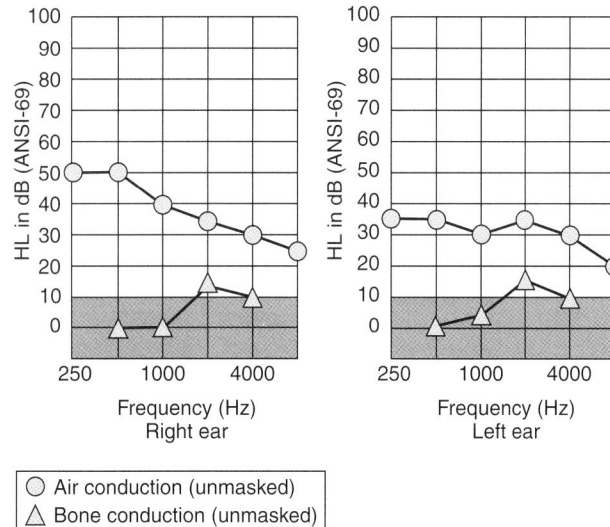

Fig. 60-3

Forty-year-old woman with bilateral otosclerosis. (The corresponding tympanograms would be Type A or A$_S$.) This disorder is autosomal dominantly inherited with about 40% penetrance. (Redrawn from Jacobsen JT, Northern JL, editors: *Diagnostic audiology,* Austin, Tex, 1991, Pro-Ed.)

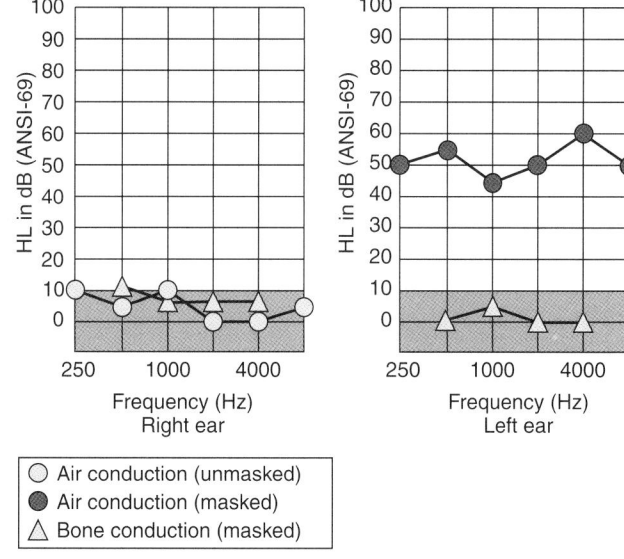

Fig. 60-4

Twenty-year-old man with ocular disruption on the left after mild head trauma. (The corresponding left ear tympanogram would be Type A$_D$.) (Redrawn from Jacobsen JT, Northern JL, editors: *Diagnostic audiology,* Austin, Tex, 1991, Pro-Ed.)

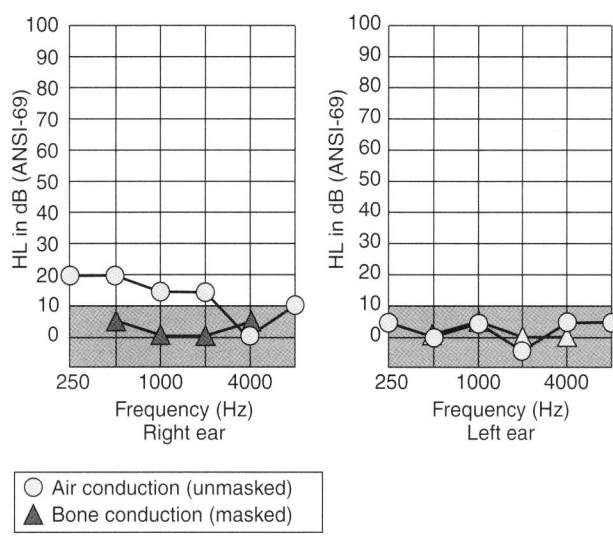

Fig. 60-5

Fifteen-year-old girl with right tympanic membrane perforation. (The corresponding right ear tympanogram would be Type B.) (Redrawn from Jacobsen JT, Northern JL, editors: *Diagnostic audiology,* Austin, Tex, 1991, Pro-Ed.)

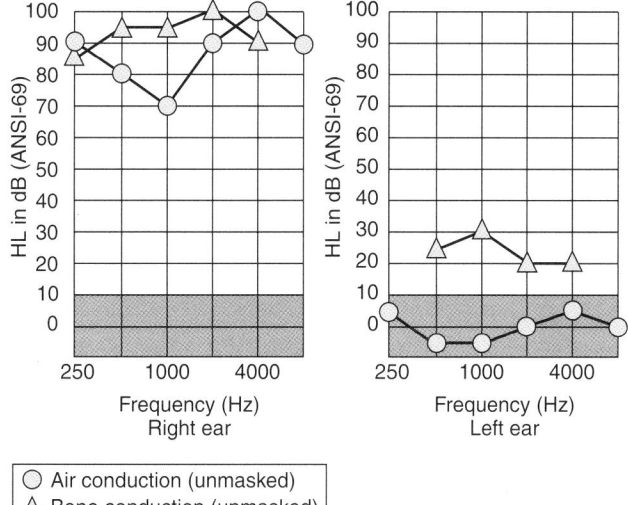

Fig. 60-6

Forty-year-old man with suspected functional hearing loss after industrial accident with a single exposure to high-intensity noise (e.g., an explosion). Bone conduction should be intact following a single exposure. (The corresponding tympanograms would be Type A or normal.) (Redrawn from Jacobsen JT, Northern JL, editors: *Diagnostic audiology,* Austin, Tex, 1991, Pro-Ed.)

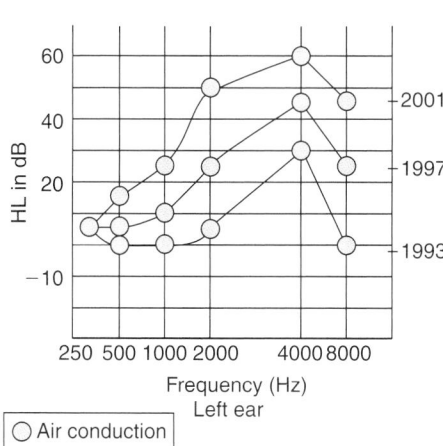

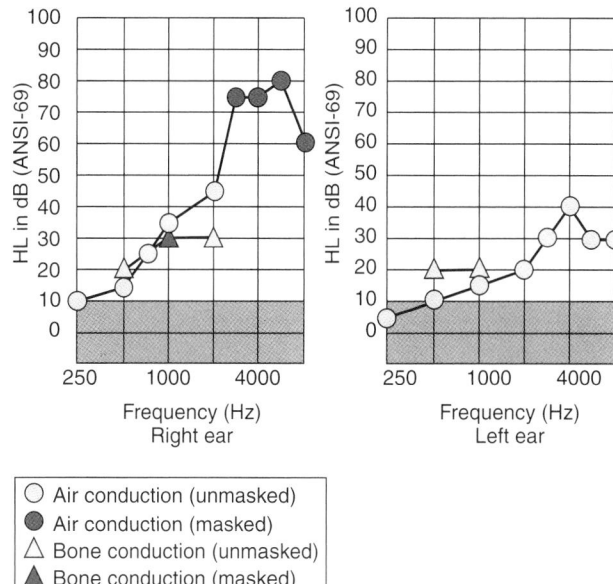

Fig. 60-7

Fifty-five-year-old man with gradually progressive left neurosensory hearing loss over several years. Such a hearing loss can be seen in an individual that hunts and shoots left-handed. In most such cases, the audiogram differs from that of presbycusis because it spares the upper frequencies (8000 Hz). (The corresponding tympanogram would be Type A or normal.) (Redrawn from Jacobsen JT, Northern JL, editors: *Diagnostic audiology,* Austin, Tex, 1991, Pro-Ed.)

Fig. 60-8

Sixty-year-old man with suspected right acoustic neuroma. Note the unilateral hearing loss. (The corresponding tympanograms would be Type A or normal.) (Redrawn from Jacobsen JT, Northern JL, editors: *Diagnostic audiology,* Austin, Tex, 1991, Pro-Ed.)

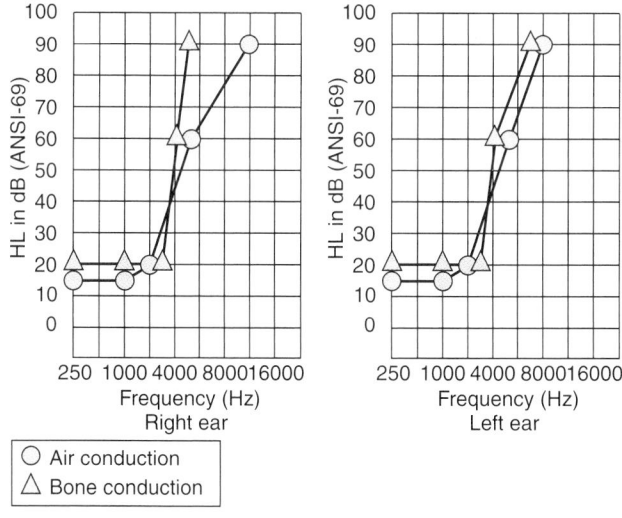

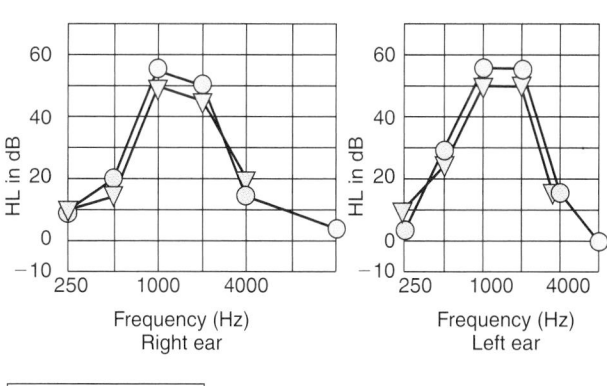

Fig. 60-9

Eighty-year-old man with presbycusis, or hearing loss caused by advancing age. It is usually bilateral, and in males it often affects the higher frequencies more severely. In women, in addition to symmetric high frequency loss, there may be hearing loss in the lower frequencies. (The corresponding tympanograms would be Type A or normal.) (Redrawn from Jacobsen JT, Northern JL, editors: *Diagnostic audiology,* Austin, Tex, 1991, Pro-Ed.)

Fig. 60-10

Fifty-year-old woman with long-term exposure to loud occupational noise, which could include loud music. Note the speech frequencies are more affected than the higher frequencies. (The corresponding tympanogram would be Type A or normal.) (Redrawn from Jacobsen JT, Northern JL, editors: *Diagnostic audiology,* Austin, Tex, 1991, Pro-Ed.)

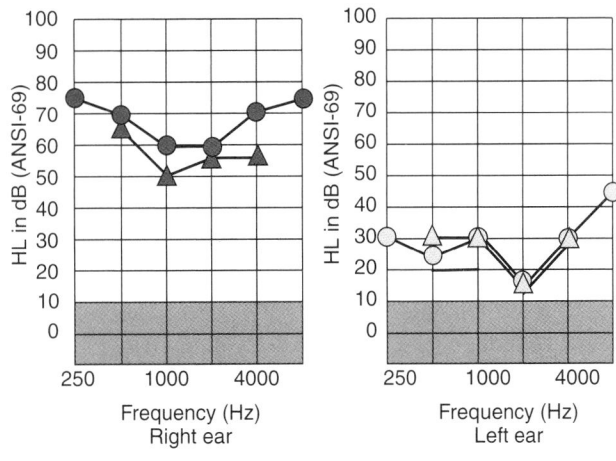

Fig. 60-11

Fifty-two-year-old man with Meniere's disease. This hearing loss is often associated with episodes of tinnitus and vertigo, frequently at the same time. Remission can occur as well as exacerbation. Over time, the hearing loss typically progresses to moderate or moderately severe and persistent. (The corresponding tympanograms would be Type A or normal.) (Redrawn from Jacobsen JT, Northern JL, editors: *Diagnostic audiology,* Austin, Tex, 1991, Pro-Ed.)

CAUSES OF SENSORINEURAL HEARING LOSS

Newborn

- Birth trauma
- Prematurity
- Hyperbilirubinemia requiring exchange transfusion
- Anoxia, asphyxia, hypoxia
- Genetic causes, expressed at birth
- Bacterial infections
- TORCH syndrome (toxoplasmosis, maternal rubella, cytomegalovirus, herpes simplex)
- Congenital syphilis

Acquired Causes

- Bacterial meningitis
- Congenital or acquired syphilis
- Ototoxic medications
- Excessive noise levels
- Measles
- Mumps
- Herpes zoster

- Human immunodeficiency virus/acquired immunodeficiency syndrome
- Meniere's disease
- Head trauma (temporal bone fractures or labyrinthine concussion)
- Perilymphatic fistula
- Lyme disease
- Glomus tumors
- Vascular disorders
- Autoimmune inner ear disorders
- Labyrinthitis
- Cranial radiation therapy
- Genetic

SUPPLIERS

Grason-Stadler, Inc.
1 Westchester Drive
Milford, NH 03055-3056
Phone: 1-800-700-2282
Website: www.grasonstadler.com

Handtronix
P.O. Box 21081
Salt Lake City, UT 84121
Phone: 1-800-832-7715
Website: www.handtronix.com

Maico Diagnostics
9675 W. 76th Street
Eden Prairie, MN 55344
Phone: 1-888-941-4201
Website: www.maico-diagnostics.com

Micro Audiometrics
655 Keller Road
Murphy, NC 28906
Phone: 1-800-729-9509
Website: www.microaud.com

Welch Allyn, Inc.
4341 State Street Road
P.O. Box 220
Skaneateles Falls, NY 13153-0220
Phone: 1-800-535-6663
Website: www.welchallyn.com

Note: Handtronix and Welch Allyn produce handheld, air-conduction screening devices even more portable than the portable traditional audiometer. These are very useful for screenings, such as those done in schools or in geriatric assessment. Their results are fairly reproducible by pure-tone audiometry.

CPT/BILLING CODES

92551   Screening test, pure-tone air only (e.g., single-decibel-level device with selected frequencies)

92552   Pure-tone audiometry (threshold); air only

92553   Pure-tone audiometry, air and bone

ICD-9-CM DIAGNOSTIC CODES

Selected codes:

389.0   Conductive hearing loss

389.2   with sensorineural loss

389.9   Deafness

951.5   Traumatic deafness

BIBLIOGRAPHY

Adams GL, Boies LR Jr, Hilger PA: *Boies' fundamentals of otolaryngology,* Philadelphia, 1989, WB Saunders.

American Speech-Language Hearing Association: Guidelines for audiometric symbols, *ASHA* 32(suppl 2):25, 1990.

Buttross SL, Gearhart JG, Peck JE: Early identification and management of hearing impairment, *Am Fam Physician* 51(6):1437, 1995.

Joint Committee on Infant Hearing 1994 position statement, *Audiol Today* 6:6, 1994.

Mannina J: Finding an effective hearing testing protocol to identify hearing loss and middle ear disease in school-aged children, *J Sch Nurs* 13(5):23, 1997.

Nielsen SE, Olsen SO: Validation of play-conditioned audiometry in a clinical setting, *Scand Audiol* 26(3):187, 1997.

Silverman CA: Audiologic assessment and amplification, *Prim Care* 25(3):545, 1998.

Smith PA, Evans PIP: Hearing assessment in general practice, schools and health clinics: guidelines for professionals who are not qualified audiologists, *Br J Audiol* 34:57, 2000.

CHAPTER 61

Auricular Hematoma Evacuation

Gregory J. Forzley

An auricular hematoma can result from a direct or indirect blow to the external ear, as commonly seen in wrestling and boxing. Since the posterior surface of the auricle has a cushion of subcutaneous fat to dissipate direct force, skin can slide over the underlying cartilage. However, the skin of the anterior surface is tightly adherent to the underlying perichondrium and cartilage. With blunt force, the anterior surface of the auricle tends to shear the perichondrium from the underlying cartilage and tear the blood vessels within the perichondrium, forming a hematoma.

Swelling may occur immediately or several hours after trauma. Auricular hematomas can also occur spontaneously in older patients. As blood, serum, or a hematoma accumulates between the perichondrium and auricular cartilage, local pressure is produced and interferes with the blood supply to the cartilage. The goal of treatment is to remove the fluid collection and to maintain compression in the area in order to prevent reaccumulation of fluid. Early treatment helps to prevent aseptic necrosis, loss of cartilage, and resultant distortion of the ear. With an auricular hematoma, there are also risks of secondary infection, perichondritis, and ultimately "cauliflower ear." Cauliflower ear may develop if the clot organizes with deposition of fibrin. Primary care clinicians, especially those involved in sports medicine, should know how to evacuate an auricular hematoma.

Note: Patients presenting 10 days or more after the time of injury need extensive management. By this time, there is newly formed cartilage and perichondrium; these patients are beyond the scope of this chapter.

INDICATIONS

- Auricular hematoma: Red, reddish purple, or bluish, fluctulant swelling, usually involving the entire auricle. It is usually exquisitely tender.

CONTRAINDICATIONS

- Hematoma accompanied by auricular laceration
- Injury beyond the abilities of the clinician

EQUIPMENT

- Topical antiseptic, such as povidone-iodine (Betadine)
- For aspiration, 20-gauge needle and syringe
- Adhesive plastic ear drape or fenestrated drape
- Sterile gloves
- No. 15 scalpel blade and holder
- Curved hemostat
- Forceps
- For anesthesia, 30-gauge needle and syringe
- Local anesthetic such as lidocaine 1% with 1:100,000 epinephrine
- Small suction catheter or curette
- Penrose drain or sterile rubber band and scissors
- Gauze dressing
- Petrolatum gauze or cotton balls soaked with petroleum jelly
- For alternate compression techniques: (1) cotton dental roll or tightly folded gauze, and silk or Vicryl suture (3-0) with needle and a needle holder, or (2) ENT silicone putty
- Antibiotic ointment (Polysporin or Bactroban)
- Eye protection

PREPROCEDURE PATIENT PREPARATION

Explain the indications and possible complications. The possible complications from not performing the procedure should also be explained to the patient. Obtain informed consent, if possible. Also explain the discomfort of injected local anesthetic and the necessity for the patient to remain very still during the procedure. The patient should be prepared for some mild discomfort during hematoma removal, even with use of the local anesthetic.

TECHNIQUE

1. Position the patient comfortably in the supine position with the injured ear accessible.
2. Cleanse the helix with antiseptic solution. Examine for associated lacerations.

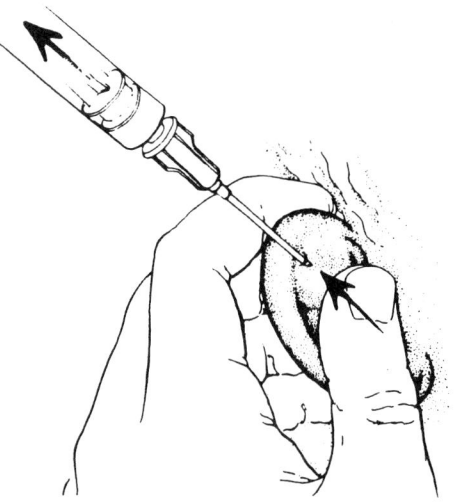

Fig. 61-1
While stabilizing the pinna with the thumb and fingers, puncture the most fluctulant part of the hematoma. Use the thumb to "milk" the hematoma into the syringe. From Roberts JR, Hedges JR, editors: *Clinical procedures in emergency medicine,* ed 3, Philadelphia, 1998, WB Saunders.

3. Following universal blood and body fluid precautions, attempt aspiration of the hematoma (Fig. 61-1). This may be all that is necessary to evacuate the hematoma, especially if the injury is quite recent. If so, proceed to step 9 or to the "Alternative Compression Techniques" section.

Note: If the hematoma has been present for 6 to 8 hours, it is likely an organized clot. This will be difficult to aspirate, and incision and drainage will probably be required.

4. If aspiration does not completely evacuate the hematoma, instill a small volume of local anesthetic anteriorly and posteriorly. Inject both into the skin overlying the hematoma and the hematoma itself. If necessary, the entire pinna can be anesthetized with several small injections into the soft tissue in the sulcus behind the ear. In this case, 1% lidocaine *without* epinephrine must be used. (See Chapter 8, Peripheral Nerve Blocks and Field Blocks.)
5. While waiting for the anesthetic to take effect, drape the patient in a manner that keeps his or her hair away from the involved area.
6. Note the anatomy of the external ear (Fig. 61-2).

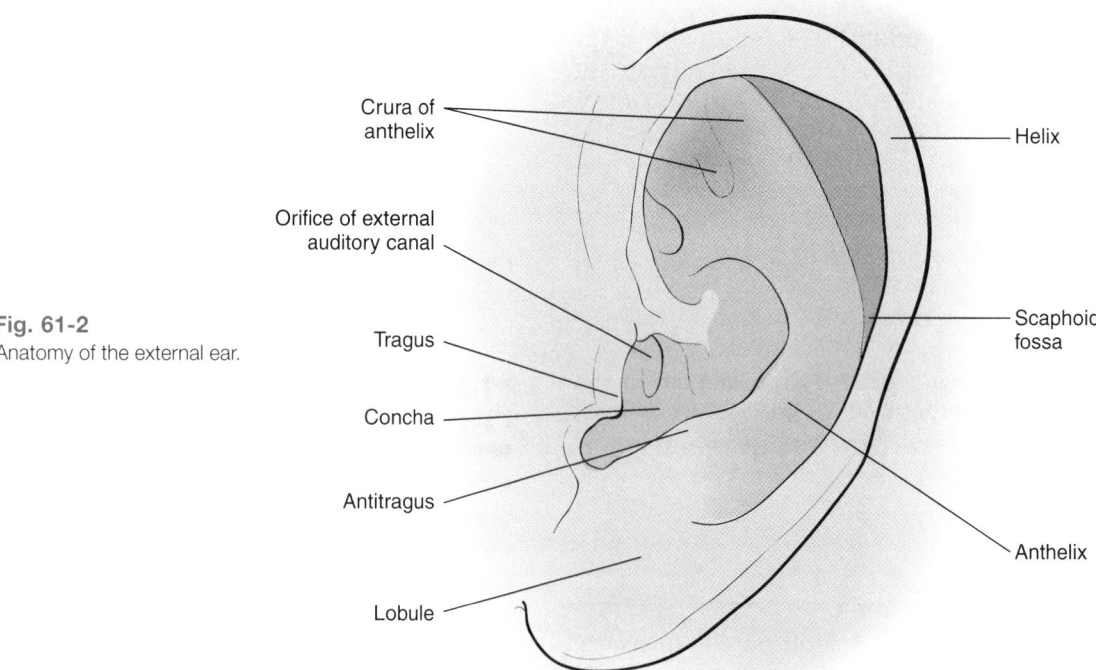

Fig. 61-2
Anatomy of the external ear.

Crura of anthelix

Orifice of external auditory canal

Tragus

Concha

Antitragus

Lobule

Helix

Scaphoid fossa

Anthelix

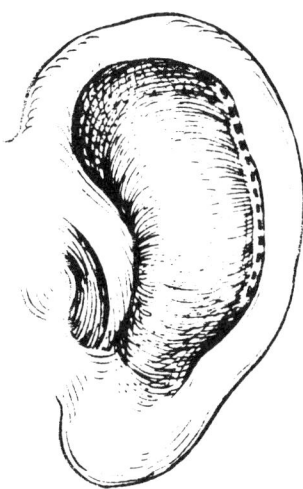

Fig. 61-3
Curvilinear incision is made. From Cummings CW, editor: *Otolaryngology: head and neck surgery,* ed 2, St Louis, 1993, Mosby.

With the no. 15 scalpel, make a curvilinear incision over the hematoma, usually 4 to 5 mm in length. For the best cosmetic result, the incision should follow the natural recessions of the ear between the helix and antihelix, or the antihelix and the concha (Fig. 61-3). Multiple incisions may be needed. The hematoma may then be expressed or removed by using the forceps, by gentle suctioning, or by curettage.

7. Probe the cavity with the hemostat to ensure complete evacuation. Additional manipulation can be performed, if necessary, with digital pressure applied to assist with complete evacuation. Apply pressure until hemostasis is obtained.
8. Insert a piece of the Penrose drain or rubber band into the incision.
9. Apply antibiotic ointment to the area of the incision.
10. Fit the petroleum jelly–treated cotton externally to the contours of the ear. Apply a gauze compression dressing to the ear (Fig. 61-4).
11. Prescribe prophylactic oral antibiotics and appropriate analgesia. Antibiotics are important if the hematoma has been present for more than 24 hours, if the hematoma recurs and requires repeated incison and drainage, or if there are signs of cellulitis. They should cover *Staphylococcus aureus, Pseudomonas aeruginosa,* and a variety of other gram-negative bacteria.
12. Instruct the patient to return in 48 hours for dressing removal and a reevaluation. Redrain the ear or reapply the dressing as needed to maintain ear compression for 2 weeks.

ALTERNATIVE COMPRESSION TECHNIQUES

Cotton Dental Rolls

The alternative compression technique uses cotton dental rolls for compression after evacuation. First, follow steps 1 through 7 described previously.
8. Next, cut a dental roll to fit over most of the hematoma. The smaller remnant of the cut roll will be stitched posteriorly. (Two tightly packed pieces of gauze can be stitched in a similar manner, with similar effects.)
9. After slightly straightening the suture needle, pass it through one end of the cut dental roll.
10. Pass the needle through the most cephalad end of the hematoma from anterior to posterior. In order to use the smaller remaining piece of dental roll as posterior compression, pass the needle back and forth through the smaller roll (Fig. 61-5).
11. Next, pass the needle through the inferior portion of the hematoma from posterior to anterior and then through the other end of the anterior dental roll. If necessary, multiple rolls can be used (Fig. 61-6).
12. Tie the suture securely. This creates both front and back compression of the hematoma.
13. Apply antibacterial ointment liberally over the dental rolls and the ear. Next apply a gauze dressing. Oral antibiotics are given as in Step 11 above.
14. Ask the patient to return in 24 hours, at which time the gauze dressing is removed. Instruct the patient to continue applying antibacterial ointment until the dental roll dressing is removed in 2 weeks.

ENT Silicone Putty

The technique using ENT silicone putty is the same as that for steps 1 through 7 described previously.
8. Next, mold ENT silicone putty to fit the anterior ear just lateral to the external auditory meatus. Wrap the putty posteriorly to match the pinna (Fig. 61-7). The putty contains a hardener, causing it to solidify in a few minutes.
9. A head bandage is then applied for 2 days. The mold should be left in place for a week. Use oral antibiotics as above. Instruct the patient to return in 48 hours for reevaluation.

POSTPROCEDURE PATIENT EDUCATION

The patient should be aware of the importance of maintaining compression for 2 weeks. He or she should understand the risk of complications, regardless of management, and should see a clinician if there are signs

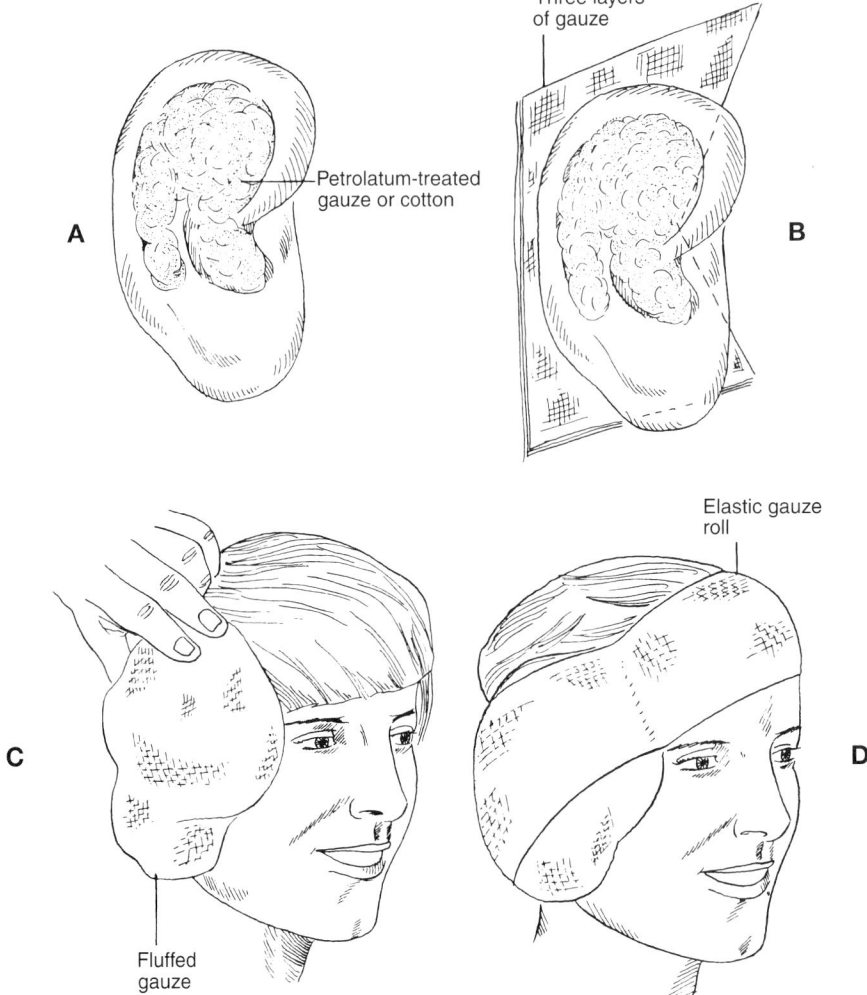

Fig. 61-4
External gauze compression dressing. **A,** Dry cotton is first placed into the ear canal. A conforming material is then carefully molded into all the convolutions of the auricle. **B,** When the convolutions are fully packed, a posterior gauze pack is placed behind the ear. A V-shaped section has been cut from the gauze to allow it to easily fit behind the ear. **C,** Multiple layers of fluffed gauze are placed over the packed ear, and, **D,** the entire dressing is held in place with Kling or an elastic gauze roll. The ear is thus compressed between two layers of gauze, and the packing ensures even distribution of pressure to all parts of the auricle. From Roberts JR, Hedges JR, editors: *Clinical procedures in emergency medicine,* ed 3, Philadelphia, 1998, WB Saunders.

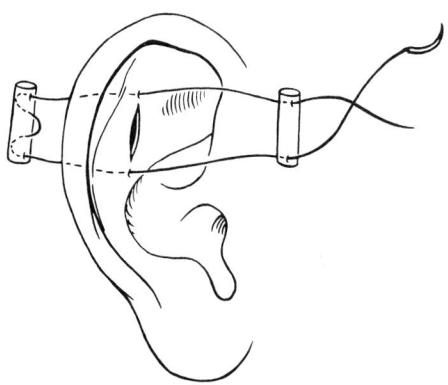

Fig. 61-5
Alternative technique using cotton dental roll for compression.

of infection. He or she should know when to return to the clinician's office and what possible complications to report.

COMPLICATIONS

- Bleeding
- Scar at the site of the incision
- Perichondritis (risk minimized by prophylactic oral antibiotics)
- Auricular deformity, either in spite of appropriate treatment, or if the treatment of the hematoma is inadequate

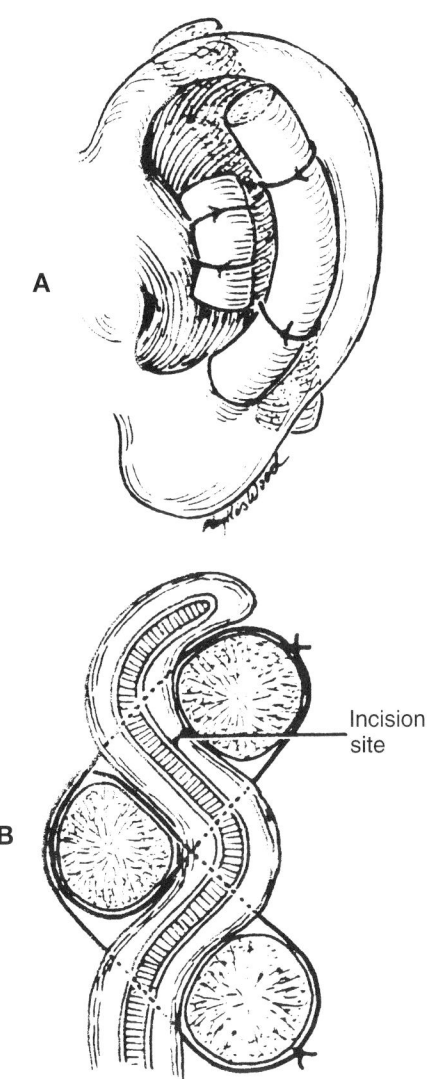

Fig. 61-6
Multiple dental rolls used for compression following evacuation of a large hematoma. **A,** Posterior auricular. **B,** Anterior auricular. From Cummings CW, editor: *Otolaryngology: head and neck surgery,* ed 2, St Louis, 1993, Mosby.

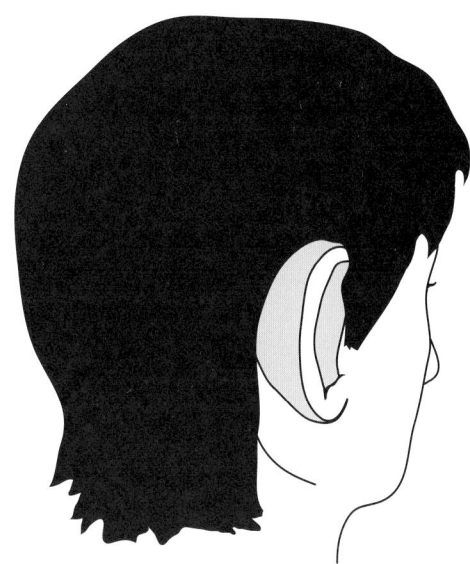

Fig. 61-7
ENT putty used for compression. The putty is molded to fit the ear, and an external compression dressing is used for 2 days. By then the putty is hardened and can be left open to air.

ICD-9-CM DIAGNOSTIC CODE

380.31   Auricular hematoma

BIBLIOGRAPHY

James DM: Management of auricular hematoma. In James DM, editor: *Field guide to urgent and ambulatory care procedures,* Philadelphia, 2001, Lippincott, Williams & Wilkins.

Lee D, Sperling N: Initial management of auricular trauma, *Am Fam Physician* 53(7):2339, 1996.

Quine SM, Roblin DG, Cuddihy PJ, Tomkinson A: Treatment of acute auricular hematoma, *J Laryngol Otol* 110(9):862, 1996.

Roberts JR, Hedges JR, editors: *Clinical procedures in emergency medicine,* ed 3, Philadelphia, 1998, WB Saunders.

Schuller DE, Dankle SD, Strauss RH: A technique to treat wrestlers' auricular hematoma without interrupting training or competition, *Arc Otolaryngol Head Neck Surg* 115(2): 202, 1989.

CPT/BILLING CODES

69000   Drainage external ear, abscess or hematoma; simple
69005   Complicated

CHAPTER 62

Bifid Earlobe Repair

Stephen K. Toadvine*

Repetitive traction on jewelry worn in a typical pierced earlobe may eventually cause a large elongated hole. This condition usually occurs over time. Eventually the defect may extend completely through the tip of the lobe, creating a bifid lobe that is completely reepithelialized (Fig. 62-1). Trauma can also cause the earring to tear through the lobe. The results are an unacceptable appearance for many patients, and it is impossible to wear a standard earring in that site. Some patients may opt for piercing at an adjacent site and wear large earrings to cover the defect, or some may try to place clip-on earrings over the defect to hide it.

Primary care physicians can successfully repair the earlobe in the office, and it can often bring great satisfaction to a patient in terms of improved cosmetic appearance and convenience in wearing jewelry.

EQUIPMENT

- Sterile prep and setup
- Lidocaine with or without epinephrine (usually a young person tolerates epinephrine)
- Laceration repair kit including skin hooks, 5-0 Vicryl or Dexon suture, and 6-0 Nylon
- Scalpel with a no. 15 or 15c blade, and possibly a no. 11 blade
- Sterile dressing
- If available, an electrosurgical unit (e.g., Ellman Surgitron) with a fine cutting needle or wire works well to excise the tissue (see Chapter 31, Radiofrequency Surgery)

TECHNIQUE

1. Sterile technique is used.
2. A wheal of lidocaine *without epinephrine* placed circumferentially around the entire base of the ear

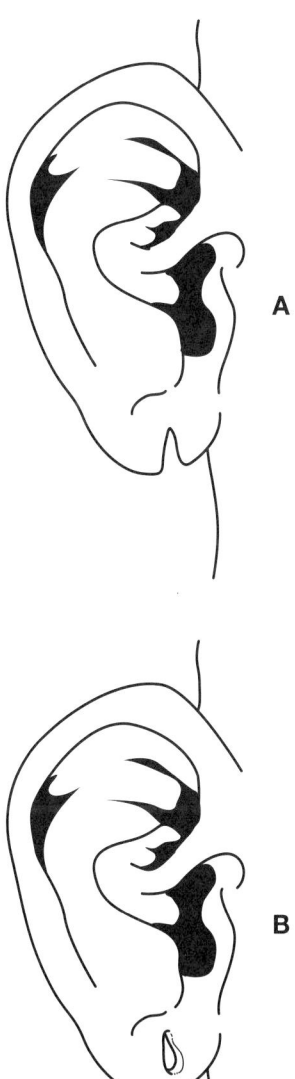

Fig. 62-1
The torn earlobe defect. **A,** Complete tear. **B,** Incomplete tear with resulting large hole defect.

---

*Dr. Toadvine contributes to this edition with the understanding that he objects to the inclusion of Chapter 130 (Abortion).

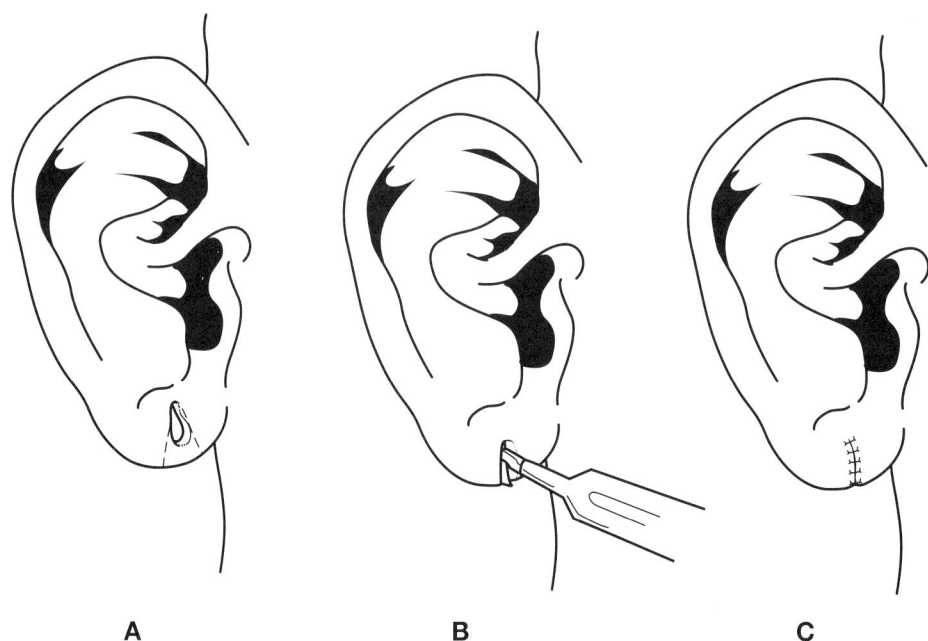

A   **B**   **C**

Fig. 62-2
Excising reepithelialized skin within the defect using a no. 11 blade. **A,** Area to be excised. In this case, an enlarged opening is being converted into a "V." Alternatively, a small elliptical excision could be made around the hole to preserve the lower margin of the lobe. **B,** Making the excision. **C,** Appearance after closure.

will provide good anesthesia (ear block) (see Chapter 8, Peripheral Nerve Blocks and Field Blocks). The concha and ear canal retain sensation. Use of the circumferential block as opposed to injection directly into the lobe avoids distortion of the anatomy of the lobe.

3. Excise defects with a no. 15 or 15c blade, a no. 11 pointed blade, or with the electrosurgical unit (e.g., Ellman Surgitron) (level 2, pure cut, Varitip or fine needle) (Fig. 62-2). If the defect is a large hole, it is often easier just to excise all the way through the lobe to create a "V." Various sterilized objects with a flat surface have been used to support the lobe during the excision since it is so flaccid, but with gentle traction by the nondominant hand, the lobe should remain stable. The radiofrequency unit makes this step easier, especially if the defect is a hole and you are trying to preserve the lower intact rim of tissue. Care should be taken to excise a smooth line and to treat the exposed subcutaneous tissue and wound edges extremely gently. If needed, skin hooks should be used. At all costs avoid grasping skin edges with forceps. This delivers a crushing type force, induces unnecessary trauma, and increases scarring.

4. Control bleeding with pressure.

5. Reapproximate the edges with one or two 5-0 Vicryl or Dexon sutures placed subcutaneously.

6. Close the skin edges anteriorly to posteriorly with interrupted 6-0 Nylon (Fig. 62-3). It is wise to begin suturing anteriorly first so that any malalignment is confined to the posterior aspect. Also, sutures may be placed first intermittently with gaps filled in to conclude the repair. Proper approximation at the tip of the lobe is important. The wound edges may invert, and a vertical mattress stitch may be helpful to prevent this.

7. Apply an antibacterial ointment.

8. Place a pack behind the earlobe and against the mastoid to secure the lobe and ensure that it will not suffer trauma or excessive motion. Cover the wound with sterile pressure dressing.

POSTOPERATIVE CARE

1. For the first few hours, have the patient lie on that side to compress the area and to reduce bleeding.

2. Have the patient remove the dressing in 12 to 24 hours and wash the area gently three times a day with soap and water and keep moist with ointment.

3. Remove sutures in 5 days. Some physicians use Steri-Strips to give additional support for several days.

4. Repiercing of the ear may be performed after 6 to 8 weeks in a location off of the wound line.

5. Instruct the patient to avoid heavy, dangling, or large loop earrings in the future to avoid repeated, undue traction on the lobe.

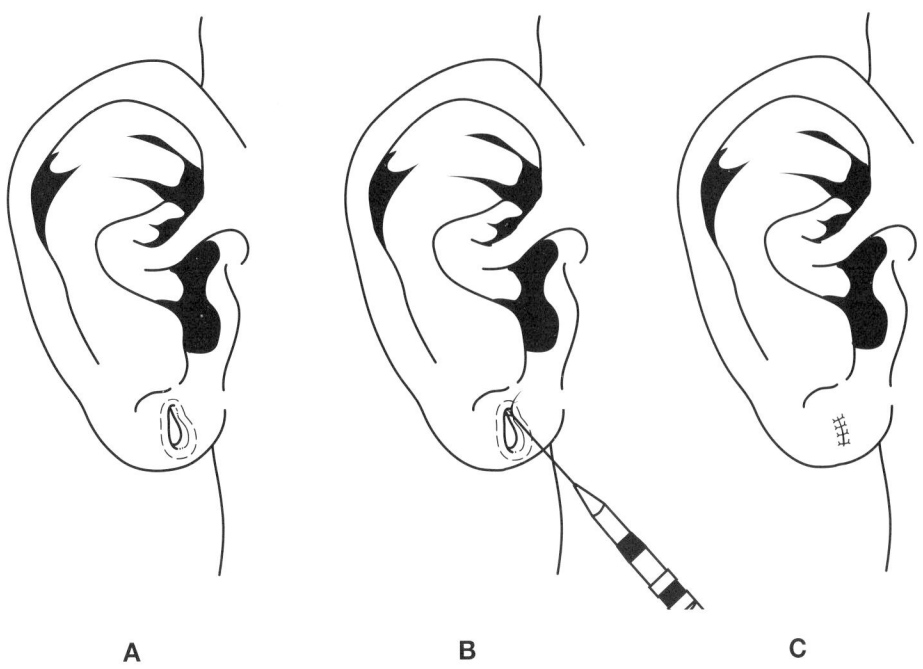

A   **B**   **C**

Fig. 62-3
Excising reepithelialized skin within the defect using a radiofrequency unit and a fine needle to maintain integrity of the lower rim. This can be carried out with a no. 11 blade but is more difficult. **A,** Area to be excised. **B,** Making the excision. **C,** Appearance after closure.

CPT/BILLING CODE

12051   Repair, intermediate ear (<2.6 cm)

ICD-9-CM DIAGNOSTIC CODES

906.0   Late effect of open wound, head, neck, trunk
872.01   Laceration, external ear without mention of complication
873.40   Wound, face

ADDITIONAL RESOURCES

• See the sample patient education handout titled "Bifid Earlobe Repair" on page 1810 of Appendix G.

BIBLIOGRAPHY

Agarwal R: Repair of cleft earlobe using double opposing Z-plasty, *Plast Reconstr Surg* 102:1759, 1998.
Nikko A, Hsu S, Quan LT, Greenbaum SS: Surgical pearl: repair of partially torn earlobes—punch technique versus conversion to complete tear, *J Am Acad Dermatol* 43:99, 2000.
Smith C, Glaser DA: Surgical pearl: repair of split or deformed ear lobe with tongue blade for stabilization during surgery, *J Am Acad Dermatol* 38(6 pt 1):990, 1998.

CHAPTER 63

Cerumen Impaction Removal

Gregory J. Forzley

Cerumen impaction is the most common otologic problem encountered by primary care clinicians. Cerumen is a naturally occurring lubricant and protectant of the external auditory canal. The predominant form is a wet, sticky, honey-colored wax that can darken, but a dry scaly form occurs in some patients. Normally cerumen is carried from inside the canal to the outside by tiny cilia. Accumulation of cerumen can cause hearing loss, tinnitus, vertigo, infection, or a sensation of increased pressure. Accumulation is common in elderly patients and in patients working in dusty environments. Patients often do a poor job of removing cerumen with cotton-tipped sticks or over-the-counter preparations, leaving the clinician to complete the procedure. In fact, overzealous use of these applicators frequently disrupts the natural ciliary cleaning process. For removal by the clinician, anesthesia may be desired; foreign bodies may also need to be removed (see Chapter 68, Removal of Foreign Bodies from the Ear and Nose). The overall goal of this procedure is to remove cerumen under direct visualization or by irrigation without causing injury.

INDICATIONS

- Tympanic membrane or ear canal obscured by cerumen
- Patient complaint of decreased hearing on the side with a cerumen accumulation
- Patient complaint of otalgia associated with cerumen
- External otitis associated with cerumen

CONTRAINDICATIONS

- Uncooperative patient or infant who cannot be adequately restrained.
- Operator unfamiliar with or unable to define anatomy of the external auditory canal.
- Patient with distorted anatomy (e.g., prior or current injury obscuring normal anatomy).

- Previous ear surgery with resultant scarring and increased risk of perforation.
- Known or suspected cholesteatoma.
- The affected ear is the only hearing ear (referral should be considered).
- For irrigation, acute otitis media or known/suspected perforation of the tympanic membrane are contraindications. In these situations, the curette or suction catheter should be used under direct visualization.

EQUIPMENT

- Ear curette.
  —Metal: *rigid,* Buck, Shapleigh, or Yankauer; *flexible,* Billeau flexible earloop.
  —Plastic: Flex-loop ear curette or infant ear scoop, both produced by Bionix Corporation.
- Ear syringe (large stainless steel syringe with irrigant deflector), *or* a commercially available jet irrigator (on "ENT table units," or an oral Water-Pik), *or* a 22-gauge butterfly intravenous catheter tubing (with needle and butterfly removed) and a 20- to 50-ml syringe. An 18-gauge Angiocath type IV catheter can also be used with a syringe.

Note: Hollow ear candles have not been found to be effective.

- Operating-head otoscope, or ear speculum and light source.
- Ear forceps.

The following are used for irrigation:
- Lukewarm tap water ("lukewarm" is confirmed when a drop placed on the inner forearm of the examiner is comfortable, similar to testing baby formula).
- Towels or plastic drape.
- Cotton gauze strip.
- Emesis or ear basin to collect irrigant.
- Aqueous-based cerumenolytics, in contrast to the traditional organic or oil-based preparations, have been found to be most effective with in vitro studies. Distilled water could be used, but 5% to 10% sodium

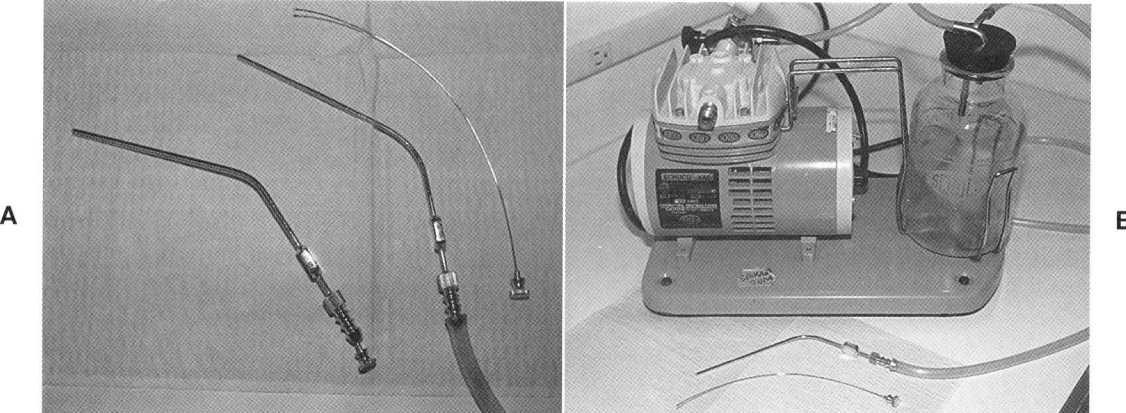

Fig. 63-1
A, Suction catheters and, **B,** basic suction pump can assist in managing ear canal obstruction.

bicarbonate or 3% hydrogen peroxide were superior in studies. Sialic acid took twice as long as distilled water to dissolve cerumen.
- Various auditory suction catheters with suction source *(optional)* (Fig. 63-1).

PREPROCEDURE PATIENT PREPARATION

- For curette removal, discuss the chance of perforation and minor trauma to the ear canal associated with pain.
- For irrigation removal, discuss the risk of perforation and potential dizziness with the irrigation. Local discomfort may also be experienced, especially when the ear syringe is used.
- Stress the importance of remaining still during the procedure.
- The patient should expect to hear occasional loud noises while the clinician is working in the ear, especially if suction is used.
- Patients should be aware that firmly adherent cerumen frequently tears the skin lining of the canal when removed, regardless of the technique used. As a result, there may be some bleeding. Slight bleeding does not indicate perforation. There is also a slightly increased risk of external otitis after cerumen removal. For this reason, antibiotic ear drops are frequently prescribed.

TECHNIQUE

Curette or Suction Technique

A curette is usually the fastest way to remove cerumen and may be preferred for small amounts of easily visible and reachable wax. It is also usually the easiest method to use with children who may find it difficult to remain still for irrigation. In adults, suction can be used for deeper or slightly more adherent impactions. Young children are often frightened by the noise that suction makes. For children and adults, irrigation will be necessary for dense, adherent, or circumferential impactions.

1. Seat the patient on the examination table. If available, a neck rest, such as those on a dental or ENT (otolaryngology) chair, may help adults remain immobile. Children often tolerate the procedure better supine, with the parent or assistant stabilizing the head.
2. With the operating otoscope, first visualize the opposite canal to become familiar with the patient's normal anatomy. Next, visualize the cerumen in the affected canal using posterior traction on the helix as necessary.
3. Using the selected curette or suction catheter, reach through the partially open magnifying posterior shield of the operating otoscope and gently remove the impacted cerumen. Take care to avoid traumatizing the bony ear canal. Work either through the scope (Fig. 63-2, *A*) or, after identifying the location of the cerumen, by direct visualization (Fig. 63-2, *B*). Suction catheters (Fig. 63-1) are quite loud when used in the external canal, so the patient should be warned and instructed not to pull away from the noise.
4. If hard wax is encountered, installation of 8 to 10 drops of 3% hydrogen peroxide for 5 to 10 minutes should facilitate removal. For wax adherent to the tympanic membrane, irrigation or suction may be necessary.
5. Firmly adherent cerumen frequently tears epithelium as it is removed. Consider prescribing topical otic antibiotics if epithelium is disrupted.

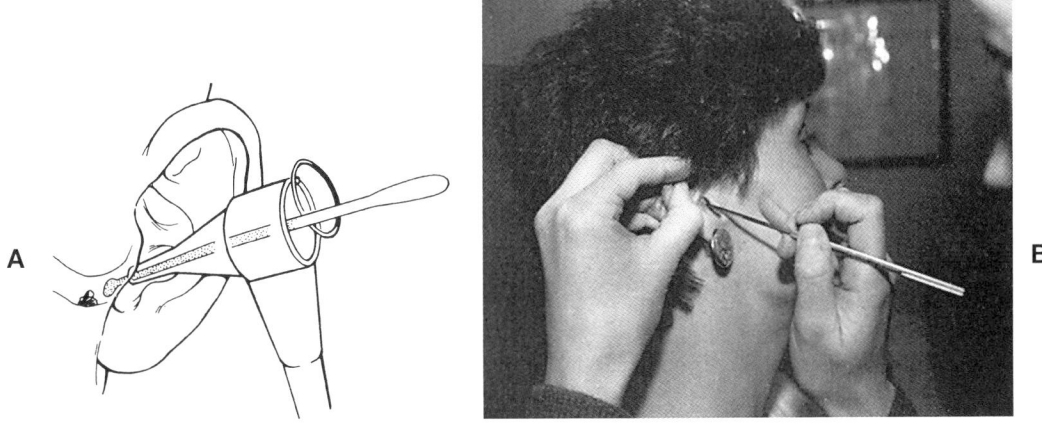

Fig. 63-2
A, Removal through the scope. **B,** Often, foreign bodies or cerumen in the ear canal can be removed with direct visualization once careful, magnified, otoscopic examination is completed. Notice how the patient's head is supported and the clinician's hand rests on the face.

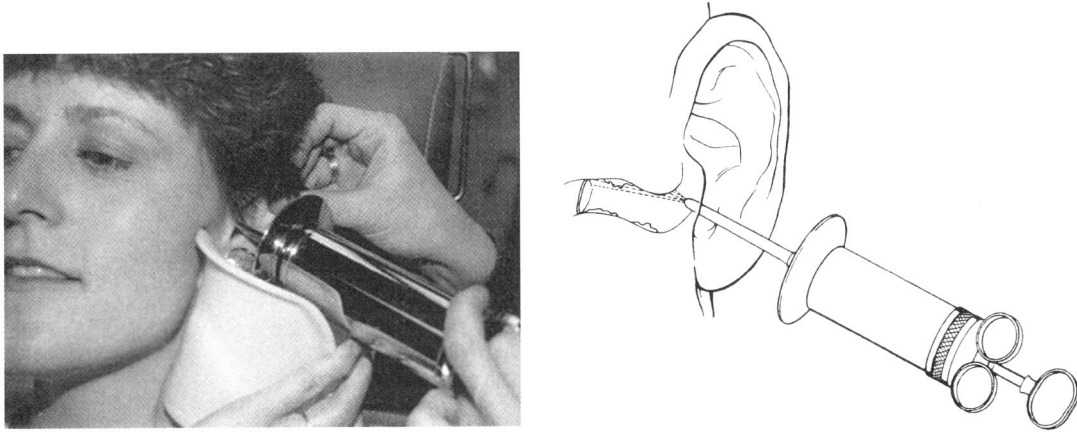

Fig. 63-3
Typical commercial ear canal irrigation setup. The water should be at body temperature. The initial stream should be directed toward the superior canal. Patients often feel reassured when allowed to help hold the basin. Cover the upper torso with a splash bib.

Irrigation Technique (Figs. 63-3 through 63-5)

The irrigation technique takes longer than the curette or suction technique and is often used when other techniques have failed or caused pain. Irrigation rarely fails.

1. Fill the irrigator (syringe) with *body temperature* tap water. This reduces the chance for stimulation of the vestibular reflex, causing nystagmus and nausea. Test the water temperature by placing a drop on the inner forearm of the examiner. It should feel neither warm nor cold to touch.

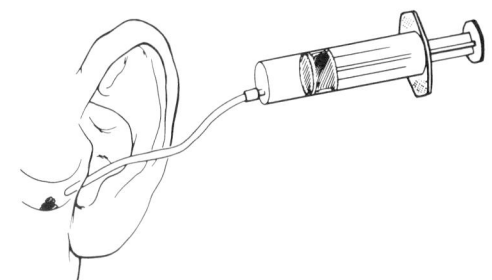

Fig. 63-4
Alternative irrigation setup. Butterfly tubing with needle and butterfly removed or 18-gauge plastic IV catheter.

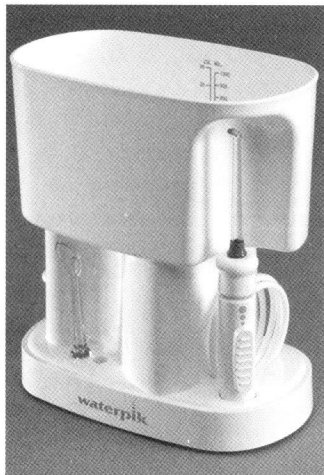

Fig. 63-5
Waterpik oral cleaning system (not marketed by the company for cerumen impaction removal). (Courtesy Waterpik Technologies.)

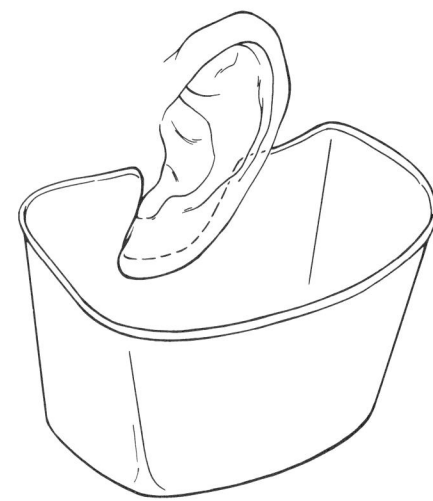

Fig. 63-6
Basin cup that fits under ear.

Note: If the jet irrigator is used, adjust the pressure to the *lowest* setting to reduce the risk of perforation or acoustic trauma. Higher-pressure settings produce-peak wave pressures strong enough to rupture the tympanic membrane.

2. Protect the patient with a towel or plastic sheet to collect excess water.
3. Have the patient tilt their head to the side being irrigated, and hold the ear basin (Fig. 63-6) below the patient's earlobe. Advise the patient not to pull his or her head away from the irrigating tip.
4. Using the selected device, direct the water jet superiorly toward the occiput, allowing space for the return of the water and cerumen. Directed in this manner, water circulates first above and then behind the cerumen. It then pushes it out of the ear. The irrigation should *not* be directed onto the tympanic membrane. No device should be inserted more than 1 cm into the canal.

   If the ear syringe is used, fairly vigorous force may be needed. The use of large (25- to 50-ml) syringes prevents excessive pressure. Be sure that air bubbles are removed from the syringe before use.

   If the jet irrigator or catheter-syringe unit is used, direct the flow superiorly and rotate the tip back and forth to change the direction of spray.
5. Often the cerumen washes out in one or two large pieces in a few seconds, at which point the canal is reexamined. If the canal is clear, stop the irrigation and dry the canal by inserting and removing a small length of cotton gauze.
6. Occasionally the impacted cerumen will need to be prodded with an ear curette. If irrigation is still unsuccessful after a few moments, terminate the procedure and send the patient home to use a liquid ear wax softener. Have the patient return in a few days for a repeat irrigation.
7. Consider prescribing topical otic antibiotics if the epithelium was disrupted to provide prophylaxis against external otitis.

COMPLICATIONS

- Tympanic membrane perforation and damage to ossicles with theoretical decreased hearing or loss of hearing
- Otitis externa
- Vertigo and/or nausea and vomiting
- Minor canal wall abrasions—as mentioned above, some bleeding may occur if hard wax is adherent to the epithelium and causes desquamation with removal (if noted, antibiotic otic drops should be used for a few days)
- Tinnitus

POSTPROCEDURE PATIENT EDUCATION

Instruct the patient to contact the clinician's office if decreased hearing, purulent drainage, or pain occurs in the affected ear. The patient should also notify the clinician for persistent vertigo or fever. Slight bleeding from the affected ear may be expected if the skin was disrupted. Diabetics and other immunocompromised patients should be especially observant for signs of infection, since they are prone to developing malignant otitis externa.

Unless contraindicated, inform the patient to perform

monthly or bimonthly ear cleansing using peroxide or distilled water and a squeeze bulb syringe. Advise the patient to avoid self-instrumentation of the ear canal with cotton-tipped applicators or any other instruments. It may be helpful to explain to the patient that cotton-tipped applicators or other instruments may disrupt the natural ear cleansing mechanisms, often causing an accumulation of cerumen. Cotton-tipped applicators should only be used on the external ear and never inserted into the canal.

SUPPLIERS

Plastic curettes
Bionix Corporation
757 Warehouse Road
Toledo, OH 43615
Phone: 1-800-551-7096
Website: www.bionix.com

CPT/BILLING CODE

69210   Removal of impacted cerumen (separate procedure), one or both ears

ICD-9-CM DIAGNOSTIC CODES

380.4   Cerumen impaction
380.10   Otitis externa (secondary diagnosis)

BIBLIOGRAPHY

Dinsdale RC, Roland PS, Manning SC, Meyerhoff WL: Catastrophic otologic injury from oral jet irrigation of the external auditory canal, *Laryngoscopy* 101:75, 1991.

Jabor MA, Amedee RG: Cerumen impaction, *J La State Med Soc* 149(10):358, 1997.

Kelly KE, Mohs DC: The external auditory canal: anatomy and physiology, *Otolaryngol Clin North Am* 29(5):725, 1996.

Murtagh J: Ear wax and syringing. In Murtagh J, *Practice tips*, Sydney, 1991, McGraw-Hill.

Robinson AC, Hawke M: The efficacy of cerumenolytics: everything old is new again, *J Otolaryngol* 18:263, 1989.

CHAPTER 64

Ear Piercing

Gregory J. Forzley

For various reasons, primary care clinicians may be asked to pierce ears. The mother of a young child may not only wish to maintain longitudinal, comprehensive care, but may also trust the clinician's ability to handle a particular child. Perhaps a patient or parent trusts that licensed clinicians use a more aseptic approach and have more knowledge of potential problems than do others who pierce ears. At the very least, ear piercing is a procedure with which the primary care clinician should be familiar.

The current popularity of body piercing has heightened questions and concerns from patients and parents. Body piercing other than the ear is beyond the scope of this chapter, but the primary care clinician may be asked to evaluate and treat some of the complications from self-piercing or piercing of various body parts. Patients and clinicians should know that certain instruments for ear piercing (e.g., ear-piercing guns) are designed specifically for ears and should not be used to pierce other body parts.

INDICATIONS

- Either the patient or parent requests ear piercing

CONTRAINDICATIONS

- Local skin infection, severe eczema, a cyst, or any other significant skin disorder
- History of keloid formation
- Immunodeficiency
- Coagulation disorder

EQUIPMENT

- Commercial ear-piercing kit, including gun, piercing earrings, and backings (disposable kits are generally not as reliable as professional models)

Equipment for Alternative Technique

- Two 18-gauge, 1½-inch and two 21-gauge, 1½-inch hypodermic needles or two 20-gauge Angiocaths and scissors
- Surgical skin-marking pencil
- Cold-sterilizer basin and solution, such as cetyldimethylethylammonium bromide (Cetylcide)
- Sterile forceps
- Povidone-iodine (Betadine) wash or 70% isopropyl alcohol
- Ice cubes for topical anesthesia *(optional)*

PREPROCEDURE PATIENT PREPARATION

Inform the patient or parent of the possible complications. If high ear piercing is requested (and it is currently popular), the complications of auricular cartilage infection should be discussed. The patient should be encouraged to expect a realistic rather than a minimal amount of pain. This is especially important in children.

TECHNIQUE

1. Cold-sterilize the gun, piercing earrings, and backings for 20 minutes.
2. Have the patient or family member mark the anterior surface of the earlobe with the skin-marking pencil at the exact location desired for the earrings. Again, it is recommended that the auricular cartilage be avoided to reduce the risk of complications.
3. Using the sterile forceps and sterile technique, load the ear piercer (proximally with the piercing earring, and distally with the backing in the stop plate of the piercing gun [Fig. 64-1, *A*]).
4. Generally, no anesthetic is required. If the patient desires some surface anesthetic, the earlobe may be held between two ice cubes for a minute or two, or

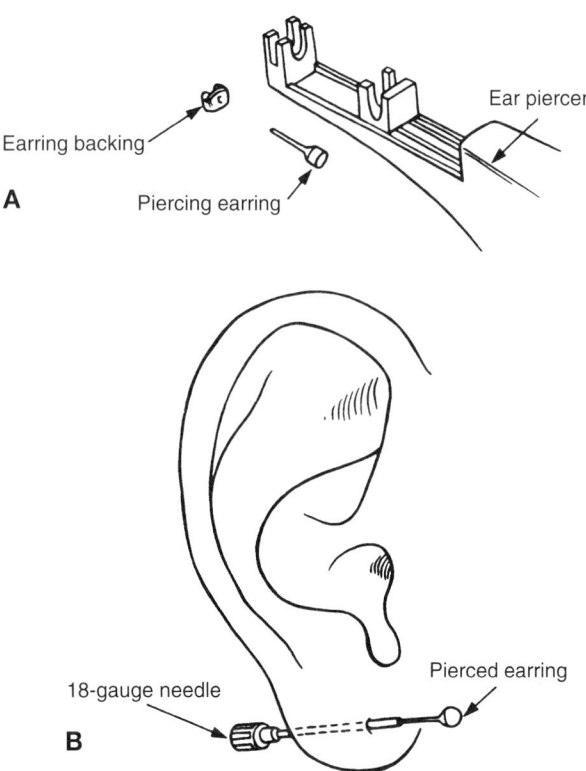

Fig. 64-1
A, Ear-piercing gun. **B,** Ear-piercing technique using needles.

the earlobe may be squeezed between the clinician's thumb and index finger for 30 seconds.
5. Cleanse the earlobe with topical antiseptic, then pierce the earlobe at the marked site from anterior to posterior using the spring-loaded ear-piercer. Follow universal blood and body fluid precautions.
6. If necessary, after removing the piercer, attach the backing more firmly to the piercing earring. Repeat the process for the other ear.

Alternative Technique

1. Using the patient's own earrings requires a modified technique. In place of the ear-piercing kit, the necessary equipment includes two 21-gauge and two 18-gauge, 1½-inch needles (one of each for each ear), or two 20-gauge Angiocaths and a pair of scissors. The patient's earrings (preferably stainless-steel posts to minimize the risk of contact dermatitis and infection) are used.
2. After following Steps 1, 2, and 4 in the previous section, cleanse the earlobe with topical antiseptic, then pierce the earlobe from anterior to posterior at the marked site with either the 21-gauge needle or a 20-gauge Angiocath. Follow universal blood and body fluid precautions.
3. If the needles are used, the 21-gauge needle already

inserted at the marked site serves as a guide. The 18-gauge needle is then applied over the 21-gauge needle and inserted through the ear from posterior to anterior. Remove the 21-gauge needle from the lumen of the 18-gauge, and in its place, insert the earring post (Fig. 64-1, *B*). Then withdraw the 18-gauge needle posteriorly through the earlobe, pulling the earring post with it. Remove the 18-gauge needle and apply the backing to anchor the earring in place.
4. If the Angiocath is used, insert approximately half the length, from anterior to posterior. Remove the needle introducer, leaving the plastic cannula in the earlobe, and cut off the hub. Place the earring into the cut end of the cannula using the forceps. With the earring inside, pull the cannula through the back of the earlobe, leaving the earring inserted in the earlobe. Discard the cannula and apply the backing to anchor the earring.
5. Repeat the procedure for the other ear, using the same technique.

POSTPROCEDURE PATIENT EDUCATION

Instruct the patient to do the following:
- Cleanse the earring post and backing daily with a cotton swab and 70% isopropyl alcohol.
- Rotate the earring several times daily (to help prevent it from becoming embedded).
- To help avoid allergic reactions or skin sensitization, avoid exposure to strong soaps, hair spray, or cosmetics.
- Check the earlobe daily for redness or other signs of infection. If any is noted, apply moist, warm compresses to the lobe four times daily. If the problem has not cleared after 24 hours, call the clinician's office for further instructions.
- Leave the earring in place for 6 weeks, at which time it may be removed and another one inserted. Again, stainless-steel posts minimize the chance of a local skin reaction.

COMPLICATIONS

- Poor cosmetic result, usually as a result of a poor choice of location by patient or parent
- Local infection or sepsis
- Keloid formation (See Chapter 39, Hypertrophic Scars and Keloids, for treatment of keloids, or use pressure earrings as listed in the "Suppliers" section.)
- Granuloma or cyst formation
- Bifid earlobe deformity if earring pulls down through the earlobe

- Auricular hematoma (see Chapter 61, Auricular Hematoma Evacuation)
- Nickel or gold dermatitis

Note: A recent study suggests that becoming sensitized to gold as a result of ear piercing is second in frequency to nickel.

- Embedded earring stud or backing

SUPPLIERS

Professional ear piercing kit

J. Hewitt Incorporated
6 Faraday, Unit B
Irvine, CA 92618
Phone: 1-800-543-9488
Website: www.medi-system.com

Hypoallergenic jewelry (nickel-free and surgical stainless-steel jewelry)

Roman Research, Inc.
430 Court Street
Plymouth, MA 02360
Phone: 1-800-451-5700
Website: www.romanresearch.com

Pressure earrings for those at risk of developing keloids

Padgett Instruments, Inc.
1730 Walnut Street
Kansas City, MO 64108-1384
Phone: 1-800-842-1029

Disposable ear piercer (not recommended)

Available through many piercing shops and online stores.

CPT/BILLING CODE

69090   Ear piercing

ICD-9-CM DIAGNOSTIC CODES

V50.3   Ear piercing
692.83   Metal or jewelry dermatitis

BIBLIOGRAPHY

Driscoll CE: Procedures for your practice: ear piercing, *Patient Care* August:194, 1990.

Muntz HR, Pa-C DJ, Asher BF: Embedded earrings: a complication of the ear-piercing gun, *Int J Pediatr Otorhinolaryngol* 19:73, 1990.

Nakada T, Iijima M, Nakayama H, Maibach HI: Role of ear piercing in metal allergic contact dermatitis, *Contact Dermatitis* 36(5):233, 1997.

Staley R, Fitzgibbon JJ, Anderson C: Auricular infections caused by high ear piercing in adolescents, *Pediatrics* 99(4):610, 1997.

Von Baeyer CL, Carlson G, Webb L: Underprediction of pain in children undergoing ear piercing, *Behav Res Ther* 35(5):399, 1997.

Zachowski DA: An IV cannula stent for ear piercing, *Plast Reconstr Surg* 80(5):751, 1987.

CHAPTER 65

Myringotomy and Tympanocentesis

Gregory J. Forzley

Tympanocentesis is needle aspiration of the middle ear contents for diagnostic purposes, and myringotomy is an incision of the tympanic membrane to allow ventilation of the middle ear or to permit drainage of middle ear fluid. Myringotomy is often indicated after tympanocentesis. If myringotomy is performed without tympanocentesis, it may also be used to obtain cultures from an infected middle ear; however, there is a higher risk of contamination from external canal flora. In children, these procedures are generally performed in the outpatient setting under general anesthesia in conjunction with tympanostomy tube placement. In a cooperative older child or adult, or in an infant who is appropriately restrained, it is possible to perform these procedures with local anesthesia. Although usually performed by an otolaryngologist, it may also be appropriate for the experienced surgeon or primary care clinician to perform diagnostic tympanocentesis or myringotomy. Recent national educational programs have been prepared for primary care clinicians to learn how to perform tympanocentesis. (Visit the Outcomes Management Educational Workshops' website at www.omew.com.)

INDICATIONS

Tympanocentesis

- To culture middle ear fluid for otitis media that is failing to respond to appropriate antimicrobial therapy, especially if there is persistent or recurrent otalgia and/or fever
- To culture middle ear fluid in a critically ill child with suspected otitis media
- To culture middle ear fluid for otitis media occurring during the course of antimicrobial therapy given for another infection, when that agent should be effective against the most common organisms causing otitis media
- As an emergency procedure when otitis media is complicated by mastoiditis, meningitis, paralysis of the facial nerve, or any other serious condition

- To culture middle ear fluid for otitis media in an immunocompromised patient, including a neonate

Note: Carbon dioxide lasers are available that can be used not only for skin ablation, wart removal, pediatric applications, etc., but also for performing OtoLAM, which is probably the fastest, least painful technique for tympanocentesis. However, the cost of equipment ($25,000 to $35,000) is prohibitive for most primary care clinicians.

Myringotomy

- For alleviation of conductive hearing loss from chronic middle ear effusion. (Outcomes data indicate that myringotomy with a tympanostomy tube is more effective than myringotomy alone in children who have chronic otitis media with effusion unresponsive to antimicrobial therapy.)
- For immediate relief of pain and pressure from middle ear effusion, otitis media, or barotrauma with fluid. (Relief may be temporary unless a tympanostomy tube is placed.)
- As an emergency procedure after tympanocentesis when otitis media is complicated by mastoiditis, meningitis, paralysis of the facial nerve, or any other serious condition.
- Whenever diagnostic tympanocentesis is indicated, myringotomy may be useful for further, prolonged drainage following aspiration. Myringotomy is especially helpful when there is a copious amount of middle ear fluid obtained by tympanocentesis.

CONTRAINDICATIONS

- Known anomalous positioning of the jugular bulb
- Uncooperative patient
- Permanent hearing loss in the opposite ear (in this situation, the procedure should be performed by an otolaryngologist, if possible)
- Acute external otitis
- Possible contraindication: effusion associated with rheumatoid arthritis, although the current literature is vague in this situation

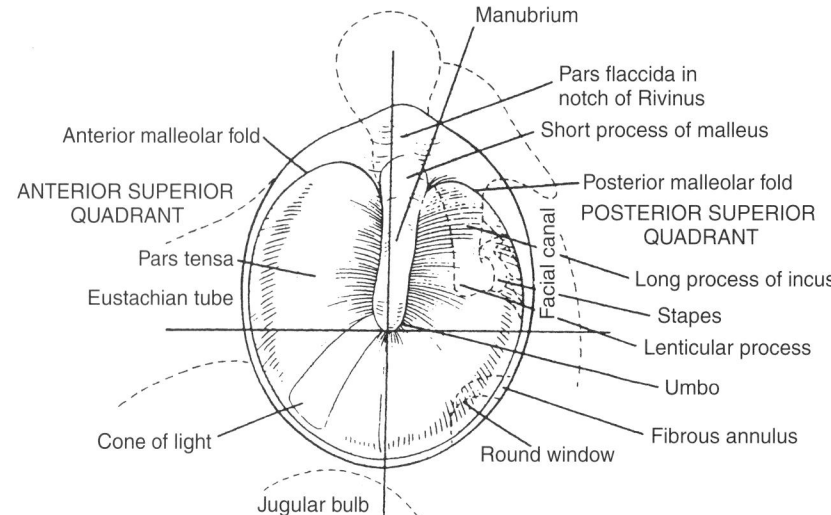

Fig. 65-1
Anatomy of the middle ear.
From Miglets AW,
Paparella MM, Saunders
MH: *Atlas of ear surgery,*
ed 4, St Louis, 1986,
Mosby.

EQUIPMENT

- For myringotomy: a myringotomy knife; for tympanocentesis: a 20-gauge spinal needle, or equivalent, along with a collection device
- Phenol solution (or, if local anesthesia is preferred, 1% lidocaine with a 27-gauge needle and syringe)
- Light source with magnification, such as an otoscope with an operating head or an operating microscope and ear speculum (a head mirror can be used, but magnification is advantageous)
- Sterile, small ear forceps or bayonet forceps
- Sterile, small cotton-tipped applicator
- Lidocaine 4% mixed 1:1 with neomycin/polymixin B sulfate/hydrocortisone eardrops or a sulfa-based topical ophthalmic (sulfacetamide and prednisolone acetate)
- Baron suction tube (3 or 5 French) with finger cut-off, if middle ear suctioning is desired (*optional*)
- Eye protection

PREPROCEDURE PATIENT PREPARATION

As in all surgical cases, explain the indications, possible complications, and overall procedure(s) to the patient. Obtain signed informed consent and document it in the chart. Preoperative oral analgesia with ibuprofen or acetaminophen has not been found to be effective.

TECHNIQUE

1. Position the patient comfortably, either in the sitting position or supine, with the head turned to one side. For the young infant, mild sedation, a restraining board, and an able assistant are often helpful (see Chapter 7, Pediatric Sedation). Universal blood and body fluid precautions should be observed.

2. Using the operating otoscope, gently clean the ear canal of obstructing debris. (Although it is not as commonly available, an operating microscope, when used with an ear speculum, may provide superior binocular vision.)

3. With a small cotton-tipped applicator, carefully apply phenol to the exact location on the tympanic membrane for tympanocentesis or myringotomy. To minimize discomfort, avoid touching any other tissue with the phenol. Most clinicians perform the procedure(s) at some point on an imaginary horizontal line through the inferior tip of the manubrium (Fig. 65-1). The best location is usually limited to one quadrant, either the anterior inferior or posterior inferior quadrant. However, in some cases it may be necessary for the myringotomy to extend into both lower quadrants.

Note: Although technically more difficult, anesthesia may be obtained by injecting the cartilaginous external auditory canal with the 27-gauge needle and 1% lidocaine at three or four points around the canal. The anesthetic is allowed to dissect down and blanch the ear canal and drum during the injection (see the "Anesthesia for Auditory Canal Foreign Body Removal" section in Chapter 68, Removal of Foreign Bodies from the Ear and Nose).

4. With the sharp myringotomy knife or tympanocentesis needle (Fig. 65-2), incise or puncture the eardrum through the white spot produced by the phenol to a depth of no more than 2 mm. A small opening is generally sufficient for thin mucoid or serous material. However, a larger circumlinear incision encompassing both inferior quadrants may be necessary for suctioning purulent fluid or if an opening is needed for a longer time (Fig. 65-3). If suction is available,

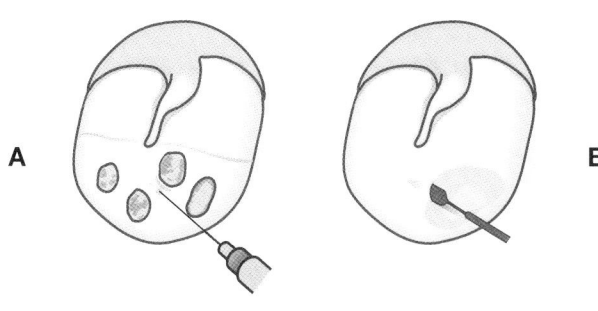

Fig. 65-2
A, Tympanocentesis. **B,** Myringotomy.

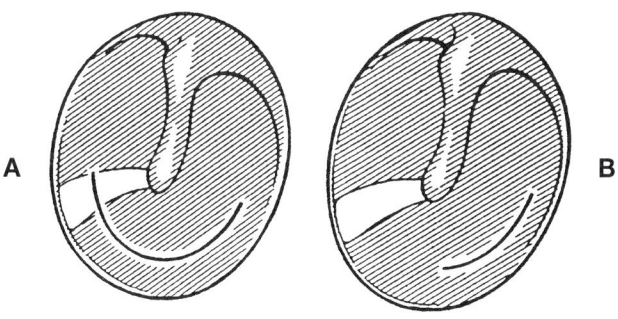

Fig. 65-3
Tympanocentesis and myringotomy incisions locations. A tympanocentesis could precede either of these myringotomy incisions in the same location. **A,** Wide myringotomy incision through the drumhead might be used in a patient with refractory purulent otitis media or for prolonged drainage of pus if necessary. **B,** More limited myringotomy incision is used for the same purpose or for inspection of the middle ear. From Miglets AW, Paparella MM, Saunders MH: *Atlas of ear surgery,* ed 4, St Louis, 1986, Mosby.

attempt to aspirate as much of the middle-ear effusion as possible. Insertion of the suction tip through the incision enhances removal of the effusion and provides a larger opening, hopefully helping the incision to remain open longer.

5. Instill 4% lidocaine/antibiotic drops, in a 1:1 mixture, to cover the tympanic membrane.

COMPLICATIONS

• Chronic perforation of the tympanic membrane.
• Persistent otorrhea causing eczema (can be treated with otic drops containing antibiotics and hydrocortisone).
• Pain and bleeding resulting from injury of the mucosal covering of the medial wall of the middle ear (promontory). This may result if the incision is greater than 2 mm in depth.

• Injury to a high-lying jugular bulb, dislocation of the incudostapedial joint, or injury to the facial nerve (rare).
• Atrophic scar at the site of the incision.
• Possible permanent damage to or loss of hearing (rare). (A recent study has suggested that, because there is such a low incidence of sensorineural or conductive hearing loss after myringotomy, preoperative screening audiometry may not be necessary.)
• For myringotomy alone, no instances of chronic perforation or tympanosclerosis were found in long-term follow-up studies.

POSTPROCEDURE PATIENT EDUCATION

• Instruct the patient to avoid water in the external auditory canal until the incision is closed (generally 2 to 4 weeks) and the patient is reevaluated.
• Instruct the patient to contact a clinician if the ear canal becomes inflamed or painful or if drainage persists.

CPT/BILLING CODE

69420   Myringotomy including aspiration and/or eustachian tube inflation

ICD-9-CM DIAGNOSTIC CODES

Some commonly used codes:

381.01   Acute serous otitis
382.90   Chronic serous otitis
381.30   with effusion
382.90   Acute otitis media
381.00   with effusion
388.70   Otalgia

ADDITIONAL RESOURCES

• See the sample patient consent form titled "Myringectomy/Tympanocentesis" on page 1811 of Appendix G.

BIBLIOGRAPHY

Bennie RE, Boehringer LA, McMahon S, et al: Postoperative analgesia with preoperative oral ibuprofen or acetaminophen in children undergoing myringotomy, *Paediatr Anaesth* 7(5):399, 1997.

Culpepper L: Tympanocentesis: to tap or not to tap, *Am Fam Physician* 61:1987, 2000.

Derkay CS, Wadsworth JT, Darrow DH, et al: Tube placement: a prospective, randomized double-blind study, *Laryngoscope* 108:97, 1998.

Emery M, Weber PC: Hearing loss due to myringotomy and tube placement and the role of preoperative audiograms, *Arch Otolaryngol Head Neck Surg* 124(4):421, 1998.

Lawhorn CD, Bower CM, Brown RE Jr, et al: Topical lidocaine for postoperative analgesia following myringotomy and tube placement, *Int J Pediatr Otorhinolaryngol* 35(1):19, 1996.

Riley DN, Herberger S, McBride G, Law K: Myringotomy and ventilation tube insertion: a ten-year follow-up, *J Laryngol Otol* 111(3):257, 1997.

WEBSITES

www.omew.com (offers workshops nationally for primary care clinicians to learn tympanocentesis)

www.earinfections.org (OtoLAM)

CHAPTER 66

Reduction of Dislocated Temporomandibular Joint (with TMJ Syndrome Exercises)

Robert S. Tan
Grant C. Fowler

Although anyone may be affected, dislocation of the temporomandibular joint (TMJ) is more common in older patients. The cause is often uncertain, but it may be related to either rheumatoid arthritis or osteoarthritis. Excessive laughter or yawning may cause a luxation of the TMJ. Trauma can also cause a TMJ dislocation; the history often reveals a blow to the chin while the mouth is slightly open. Dislocation occurs when the muscles and ligaments supporting the mandible are relaxed enough to allow the condyle to jump anteriorly or posteriorly over the articular eminence of the fossa. The luxation of the joint is exhibited by an open mouth that cannot be closed. Swallowing and talking are difficult for the patient. Unilateral dislocation causes a deviation away from the affected side. Once the dislocation occurs, trismus and muscle spasm prevent the joint from returning to its natural position.

For clicking or tender TMJs, splinting by a dentist or oral surgeon is a common treatment. In the "Postprocedure Patient Education" section, three published alternatives to splint therapy are described.

INDICATIONS

• Unilateral or bilateral TMJ dislocation(s) without fractures. (The dislocation should be confirmed with a radiograph, which also rules out a fracture.)

CONTRAINDICATIONS

• Fractured condyles. (Patient should be referred to a maxillofacial surgeon.)

EQUIPMENT

• Gloves
• Parenteral muscle relaxation may be helpful (e.g., diazepam, lorazepam)
• Examination chair with firm neck rest
• 5 ml of 2% lidocaine in a 10-ml syringe with a 25-gauge needle, povidone-iodine (Betadine) solution *(optional)*

PREPROCEDURE PATIENT PREPARATION

Inform patients that while the joint is being reduced, they may experience considerable pressure on the molars. They may also experience some referred pain to the neck, face, or ear, as well as mild, aching TMJ arthralgia after the reduction. Stress the importance of remaining relaxed and not moving while their jaw is being reduced.

TECHNIQUE

Passive Reduction

Muscle spasms may be severe enough to inhibit simple reduction of the dislocated TMJ. Administration of appropriate titrating doses of a muscle-relaxing drug such as diazepam IV is one possible approach to the problem. Often, as the muscle relaxant is titrated, the reduction of the joint occurs spontaneously. Alternatively, after preparing the site with povidone-iodine, an injection of 3 to 5 ml of lidocaine into the TMJ may allow for spontaneous reduction (Fig. 66-1). One theory suggests that the

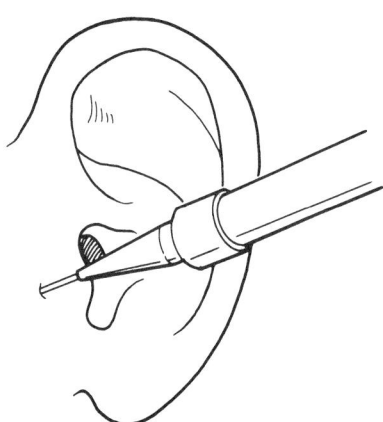

Fig. 66-1
Injection of lidocaine into the joint.

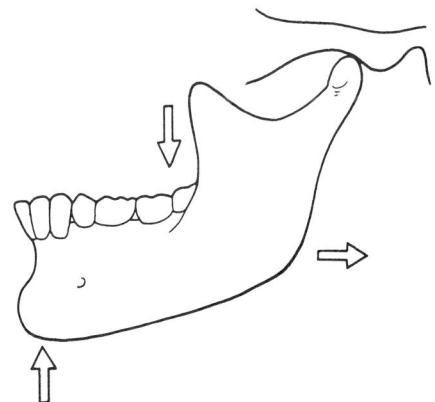

Fig. 66-2
Direction of combined forces necessary for reduction.

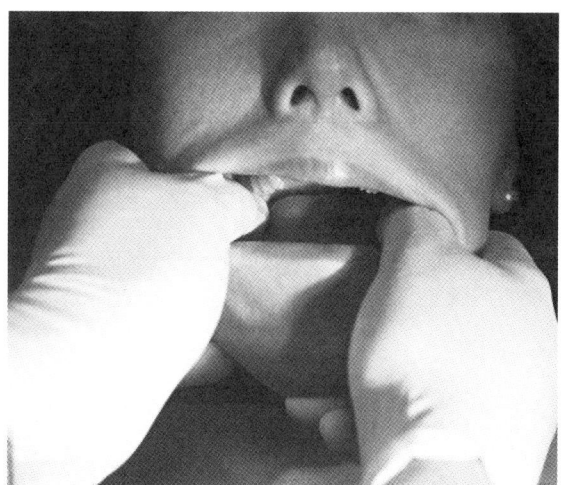

Fig. 66-3
Reduction of a dislocated mandible from a position in front of the patient.

dislocation is maintained by muscle spasm caused by painful stimuli arising from the capsule. A few minutes after localized unilateral injection, even with bilateral dislocation, the patient might be able to close his or her mouth and retract the mandible into its normal position. If passive reduction by muscle relaxation is not successful, active reduction may be necessary.

Active Reduction

While standing in front of the patient, place your thumbs on the occlusal surfaces of their posterior lower teeth. The patient's head should be against a high headrest or the wall. Firmly grasp the mandible on the outside with your fingertips. Exert downward force on the molars (Fig. 66-2). After 30 to 60 seconds of downward pressure, apply very light pressure in a posterior direction and elevate the chin. This light pressure and chin elevation

can be accomplished by rotating the posterior or inferior mandible with your fingertips. At this point, the condyles should clear the articular eminence and allow the mandible to slide into its normal closed position (Fig. 66-3). Take care to protect your thumbs since the mandible may snap sharply back into place. Gauze can be wrapped over the thumbs to protect them. Should these procedures fail, reduce the TMJ under conscious sedation or general anesthesia.

If the patient can swing his or her jaw from side to side, the reduction has been successful. If the jaw immediately dislocates after successful reduction, a Kerlix-type gauze should be wrapped around the jaw and over the top of the head, producing a pressure-type dressing to keep the jaw closed.

Note: For recurrent dislocations, search for possible causes (e.g., occlusal disharmony causing muscle spasm, phenothiazine-induced trismus, or rheumatoid arthritis).

POSTPROCEDURE PATIENT EDUCATION

The patient should not yawn widely, take large bites of food, or laugh excessively for several days. In some instances, immobilization of the jaw is needed after reduction. For immobilization, refer the patient to a dentist. Some dentists immobilize the jaw for up to 2 weeks to give the stretched muscles and ligaments an opportunity to heal. This also allows the edema to subside. Inadequate immobilization may lead to recurrence of dislocation. If the dislocation was not traumatic, inform the patient that repeating the action that caused the dislocation will again cause dislocation. This is particularly true in the 4 to 6 weeks after a dislocation when the ligaments are not fully healed. Also warn the patient that recurrent dislocations may lead to permanent TMJ arthritis. In recurrent TMJ dislocation, the patient should be referred and the jaw should remain immobilized for 4 to 6 weeks.

COMPLICATIONS (ALL RARE)

- Posterior dislocation of TMJ from reduction of anterior dislocation
- Anesthesia complications (e.g., allergic reaction to lidocaine)
- Nerve damage
- Permanent TMJ arthritis related to an improperly managed or undiagnosed condylar fracture. This is particularly a risk if the fracture extends into the articular surface. Prolonged disarticulation (several days) or recurrent disarticulation are also associated with TMJ arthritis.

THREE ALTERNATIVES TO SPLINT THERAPY FOR A TENDER AND/OR CLICKING TEMPOROMANDIBULAR JOINT*

Method A

1. Have the patient obtain a soft wooden or plastic rod, approximately 15 cm long and 1.5 cm in diameter (e.g., a wooden dowel or large carpenter's pencil).
2. The patient should thrust the mandible forward and grasp this rod with his or her back molars.
3. At least three times a day, for 2 to 3 minutes, the patient should then rhythmically bite on the object with a grinding movement (Fig. 66-4).

Method B

1. Although it may be initially uncomfortable, this exercise should eventually lead to relief in uncomplicated TMJ.
2. At least four to five times a day, for 15 repetitions, the patient should rhythmically thrust the lower jaw forward and backward, in an anterior-posterior direction. The mouth should be slightly open, and when performed correctly, the patient will look like a cheeky schoolchild exposing the bottom lip (Fig. 66-5).

*As published in Murtagh, 1991.

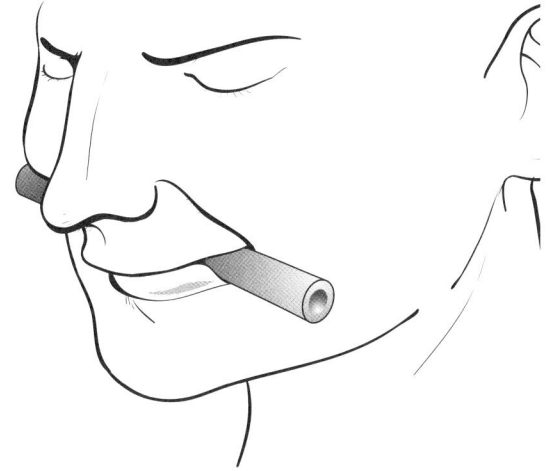

Fig. 66-4
Chewing the wooden rod exercise.

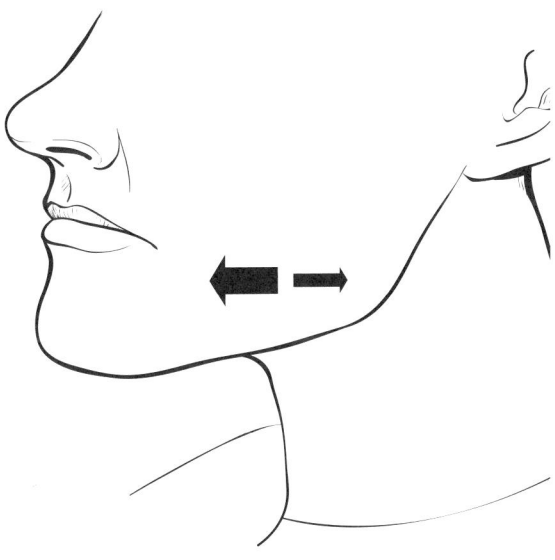

Fig. 66-5
The lower jaw-thrust exercise.

Method C (Six Exercises to be Repeated Six Times per Day, or Six by Six)

Note: These exercises were recommended by an oral surgeon and should be performed without causing pain. If they are uncomfortable when performed, the intensity should be reduced as opposed to reducing the number and frequency of repetitions.

1. Have the patient hold the front third of their tongue to the roof of his or her mouth and take six deep breaths.
2. Next, have the patient hold his or her tongue to the roof of the mouth and open the mouth six times. The jaw should not click.

3. Have the patient hold the chin with both hands, keeping the chin still. *Without* actually letting it move, the patient should *attempt* to move their chin up, down, and to each side.

4. Next, with the chin between the heels of both hands, and the fingertips behind the neck, have the patient pull his or her chin toward the neck. Hold for 6 seconds.

5. Next, have the patient push his or her upper lip back *as if* to push the head straight back while using the neck muscles to *prevent* the head from being pushed back. Hold for 6 seconds.

6. To finish the exercises, have the patient pull the shoulders back, as if to touch the shoulder blades together, and hold for 6 seconds.

CPT/BILLING CODES

21480   Closed uncomplicated treatment of temporo-mandibular dislocation, initial or subsequent

21485   Closed complicated treatment of temporo-mandibular dislocation, initial or subsequent

ICD-9-CM DIAGNOSTIC CODES

830.0   Dislocation temporomandibular joint, closed
624.69   Dislocation temporomandibular joint, recurrent

BIBLIOGRAPHY

James DM: Reduction of a dislocated mandible. In James DM, editor: *Field guide to urgent and ambulatory care procedures,* Philadelphia, 2001, Lippincott Williams & Wilkins.

Murtagh J: Temporomandibular joint. In Murtagh J, editor: *Practice tips,* Sydney, 1991, McGraw-Hill.

Rowe NL, Williams JL: *Maxillofacial injuries,* ed 2, vol 1, New York, 1994, Churchill Livingstone.

Upton GL: Management of injuries to the temporo-mandibular joint. In Fonsceca RJ, editor: *Oral and maxillofacial trauma,* Philadelphia, 1991, WB Saunders.

CHAPTER 67

Tympanometry

Gregory J. Forzley

Several methods are available to evaluate the middle ear and eardrum for dysfunctions that could either affect the hearing ability of the patient or put him or her at risk for repeated infections. These modalities include pneumatic otoscopy, tympanometry, static immittance, and acoustic reflectometry. Primary care clinicians are most familiar with tympanometry and pneumatic otoscopy. Tympanometry, routinely performed since the 1970s, provides reproducible measurements of the compliance or mobility of the tympanic membrane as well as the pressure within the middle-ear system. In addition to evaluating tympanic membrane function, these measurements aid in assessing eustachian tube function and in demonstrating the continuity and mobility of the ossicular chain, even in a fairly uncooperative child. With guidelines changing for management of otitis media with effusion (OME), it is more important than ever to obtain objective evidence of an effusion. Tympanometry continues to be a proven method of accurately documenting OME.

The goal of tympanometry is to evaluate the *immittance* of the tympanic membrane, which reflects the performance of the middle-ear transmission system. Immittance is a hybrid term (derived from combining *impedance* and *admittance*) and is descriptive of the transfer of acoustic energy. It is measured as either the acoustic *admittance* (flow of energy into the middle-ear system), or as the reciprocal of the acoustic admittance—the acoustic *impedance* (opposition to the flow of energy into the middle ear).

A tympanometer consists of hardware and a probe. The probe is inserted into the patient's ear and must maintain an airtight seal against the canal wall. Within the probe are three small openings. Through one, an oscillator- and loudspeaker-generated tone (226 Hz) is directed toward the tympanic membrane. A microphone is located in another probe opening to pick up reflected sound waves. Air is pumped through the third opening to vary the air pressure in the canal, creating positive or negative (relative to atmospheric) air pressure in the space between the probe tip and the tympanic membrane (Fig. 67-1).

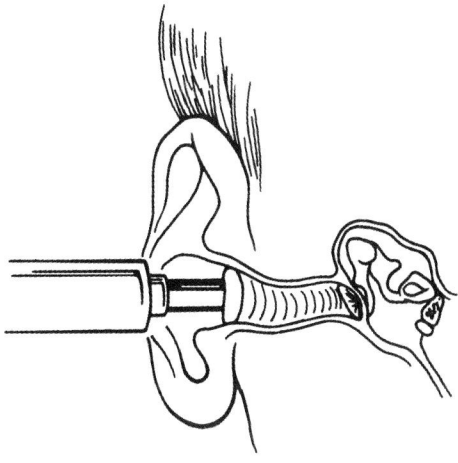

Fig. 67-1
Tympanometry is performed with a probe inserted into the external ear canal. A 226-Hz tone is transmitted through the probe. Movement of the tympanic membrane in response to the tone is measured while the air pressure in the external canal is varied. The pressure at which peak movement (compliance) occurs is recorded.

At the core of the hardware is an electroacoustic impedance bridge to translate the input received from the microphone in the probe. Another part of the hardware, the oscillator, produces the tone transmitted through the speaker. The remaining hardware consists of the pump, recorder, and manometer. Parameters measured by the hardware include the *compliance* of the tympanic membrane as well as the *change in impedance* as the canal pressure varies. Devices that measure the acoustic *admittance* rather than the impedance obtain similar results but also produce a *tympanometric gradient* (curve width).

INDICATIONS

- To verify middle-ear abnormalities suspected by clinical otoscopy
- To check for eustachian tube patency when there is

suspected dysfunction, even when the tympanic membrane appears normal
- To evaluate hearing loss or ear pain, especially in the young
- To detect or follow tympanic membrane perforations
- To evaluate patency of pressure-equalization (PE) tubes
- To assist in evaluation of suspected fixation of the ossicular chain
- To help assess middle-ear function in a young child who cannot cooperate with audiometry
- To document or follow persistent middle-ear effusions (MEE) or OME
- To quantify middle ear abnormalities suspected by pneumatic otoscopy

Note: An abnormal tympanogram usually implies some degree of conductive hearing loss. However, a sensorineural hearing loss may also be present. If the clinician has any reason to suspect sensorineural involvement, audiometry should also be performed (see Chapter 60, Audiometry).

CONTRAINDICATIONS

- Ear canal totally occluded by cerumen or an object
- Fulminant external otitis

A relative contraindication is age less than 7 months. Before 7 months, the auditory canal itself is elastic and may act like a compliant tympanic membrane. Even in the presence of an effusion, results may yield a misleading Type A_D or C curve. However, clinicians should not completely forego tympanometry in this age range because negative results are occasionally useful. Positive results may also be useful based on likely diagnoses (e.g., a low-compliance tympanogram [Type B] probably indicates an effusion.) Multifrequency tympanometry is emerging as a new option for evaluating middle ear function in infants.

EQUIPMENT

Tympanometry equipment is quite varied in size and features available. Some features to consider include the following:
- 220-Hz probe tone is preferred; most probes supply 226-Hz probe tones.
- Air-pressure range of −400 to +100 mm H_2O is preferable; however, a range of −300 to +100 is acceptable. It should be noted that many instruments measure air pressure in decaPascals (daPa) (i.e., 1.02 mm H_2O = 1.0 daPa).
- Results should be rapidly obtainable and easy to read.
- Results should be easily printable for documentation.

PREPROCEDURE PATIENT PREPARATION

Explain the indications for the procedure and that the patient will need to remain immobile for a brief period. It is especially important for the patient to remain immobile after a seal has been obtained while taking measurements. Reassure the patient (or parents) that this is a painless procedure.

TECHNIQUE

1. Check the ear canal for at least partial patency.
2. Have the patient sit, either independently or, in the case of a young child, in the parent's lap.
3. With the older child and adult, apply gentle traction to the helix in the posterior upward direction to straighten the auditory canal. With young children, posterior downward traction on the inferior helix is needed to straighten the canal.
4. Select the appropriate size of soft probe tip to occlude the ear canal adequately without entering it deeply.
5. Once a seal has been obtained, the tympanometer will automatically deliver the sound, vary the air pressures, and record the various parameters. Parameters measured include the tympanic membrane compliance, the canal pressure and volume, and, in instruments so equipped, the acoustic reflex.

INTERPRETATION

The resultant tympanogram is a graph of the compliance of the middle-ear system on the vertical axis and the pressure in the ear canal (in mm H_2O or daPa) on the horizontal axis. The graph may vary with the instrument, but the classically described types of tympanogram results are shown in Fig. 67-2. For corresponding audiogram results, see Chapter 60, Audiometry.

Tympanogram Curve Results

Type A. Since the maximum tympanic membrane compliance occurs when air pressure is equal on both sides of it, the peak of the *normal tympanogram tracing* ("A" in Fig. 67-2) occurs at approximately 0 mm H_2O on the horizontal axis.

Type A_S. The Type A_S pattern shows a shorter peak, but with maximum compliance still occurring at or near zero pressure. It indicates conditions such as ossicular fixation or stiffening, thickening of the tympanic membrane, or a middle-ear effusion.

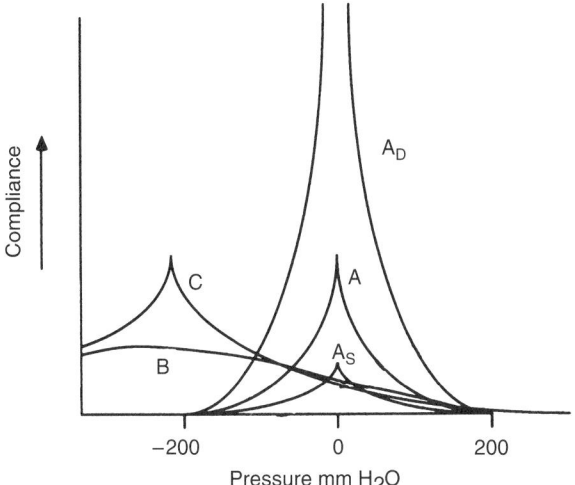

Fig. 67-2
Tympanogram results. See text for details.

Type A_D. The Type A_D tympanogram has a very high peak that exceeds or goes off of the compliance scale. It may indicate ossicular disruption, a flaccid tympanic membrane, or a monomeric tympanic membrane (a single layer of membrane covering an old eardrum perforation).

Type B. If the tympanogram is flat with no distinct peak, it represents a Type B pattern, which is highly specific and sensitive for the presence of middle-ear fluid. Other conditions associated with a Type B tympanogram include cerumen impaction, perforation of the tympanic membrane, stenosis of the ear canal, a thickened eardrum, or an open, functioning PE tube; these possibilities can often be eliminated by measuring the canal volume. A normal canal volume is 0.2 to 2.0 ml but varies widely according to the patient's age and bone structure. An excessive volume may indicate perforation or a functioning PE tube, whereas decreased volume indicates obstruction or debris, such as cerumen.

Type C. A Type C tympanogram is indicative of normal compliance; however, occurs with a negative pressure of more than -100 mm H_2O. Type C is associated with eustachian tube dysfunction, with or without accompanying middle-ear fluid. Negative middle-ear pressures are generally considered clinically significant if they exceed -180 to -200 mm H_2O.

A peaked result in either a Type A or Type C tympanogram generally excludes middle ear fluid. The results are most reliable in a cooperative patient.

When interpreting tympanograms, the examiner should be aware that a localized abnormality (e.g., perforation) of the tympanic membrane may obscure the ability to evaluate the rest of the middle-ear system.

When a perforation is suspected, unfortunately, pneumatic otoscopy may elicit movement of a tympanic membrane despite a pinpoint perforation. As a result, tympanometry may diagnose a perforation missed by pneumatic otoscopy. In contrast, middle ear mucosal edema may be sufficient to mask even a large perforation when evaluated by tympanometry.

Newer devices are often equipped to measure auditory reflex (AR) and tympanometric width (TW). As more studies become available comparing accuracy and outcomes using these measurements, they may become more useful for primary care clinicians.

POSTPROCEDURE PATIENT EDUCATION

Based on the patient's results, discuss the diagnosis as well as the management that he or she should follow. If applicable, the need for further evaluation should also be discussed.

SUPPLIERS

Tympanometers
Grason-Stadler, Inc.
1 Westchester Drive
Milford, NH 03055-3056
Phone: 1-800-700-2282
Website: www.grasonstadler.com

Maico Diagnostics
9675 W. 76th Street
Eden Prairie, MN 55344
Phone: 1-888-941-4201
Website: www.maico-diagnostics.com

Micro Audiometrics
655 Keller Road
Murphy, NC 28906
Phone: 1-800-729-9509
Website: www.microaud.com

Welch Allyn, Inc.
4341 State Street Road
P.O. Box 220
Skaneateles Falls, NY 13153-0220
Phone: 1-800-535-6663
Website: www.welchallyn.com

CPT/BILLING CODES

92567   Tympanometry (impedance testing)
92568   Acoustic reflex testing

ICD-9-CM DIAGNOSTIC CODES

381.01	Acute serous otitis
382.90	Chronic serous otitis
381.30	with effusion
382.90	Acute otitis media
381.00	with effusion
384.20	Perforation tympanic membrane
384.81	Healed tympanic membrane perforation
872.61	Perforation: traumatic

BIBLIOGRAPHY

Brookhouser PE: Use of tympanometry in office practice for diagnosis of otitis media, *Pediatr Infect Dis J* 17(6):544, 1998.

Buttross SL, Gearhart JG, Peck JE: Early identification and management of hearing impairment, *Am Fam Physician* 51(6):1437, 1995.

Hunter LL, Margolis RH: Effects of tympanic membrane abnormalities on auditory function, *J Am Acad Audiol* 8(6):431, 1997.

Palmu A, Puhakka H, Rahko T, Takala AK: Diagnostic value of tympanometry in infants in clinical practice, *Int J Pediatr Otorhinolaryngol* 49:207, 1999.

Shahnaz N, Polka L: Standard and multifrequency tympanometry in normal and otosclerotic ears, *Ear Hear* 18(4):326, 1997.

Silverman CA: Audiologic assessment and amplification, *Prim Care* 25(3):545, 1998.

Van Balen FAM, Aarts AM, DeMelker RA: Tympanometry by general practitioners: reliable? *Int J Pediatr Otorhinolaryngol* 48:117, 1999.

Waters GWR, Jones JE, Freeland AP: The predictive value of tympanometry in the diagnosis of middle ear effusion, *Clin Otolaryngol* 22:343, 1997.

CHAPTER 68

Removal of Foreign Bodies from the Ear and Nose

John Harlan Haynes III
Gary R. Newkirk

The external auditory canal and nasal orifices occasionally collect small objects such as beads, insects, peanuts, pebbles, or beans. Foreign bodies in this area are especially common in pediatric patients and mentally impaired individuals. Various instrument techniques are available for removing foreign bodies and are discussed below; however, simple attempts at removal should be pursued before instrumentation.

In children with nasal foreign bodies, nebulized epinephrine can be used to assist expulsion with simple nose blowing. A positive-pressure technique (as in mouth-to-mouth resuscitation) using a pediatric Ambu bag may be used in young children and infants. Block the unaffected nostril and, while not exceeding recommended maximal pressure with the Ambu bag (cardiopulmonary resuscitation guidelines), force air briskly through the oropharynx and out the obstructed nostril to dislodge the object. In older children and adults, vasoconstrictive nasal solutions (e.g., Afrin or Neo-Synephrine) may be used to reduce mucosal edema. Wait 10 minutes after application and have the patient blow forcefully to dislodge the object. Even if the object does not come out, the relaxed and decongested mucosa gives the clinician more room to work.

In the external ear canal, pulsating saline irrigation through an 18-gauge (Intracath) catheter and directing it posteriorly may dislodge the impacted object. If tympanic membrane perforation is suspected, however, irrigation is contraindicated. Knowledge of the type of foreign body and how long it has been lodged in the orifice is very helpful. If an expanding material is suspected (e.g., organic materials, beans, seeds), irrigation with saline may be contraindicated because it may cause additional expansion of the object. Timeliness may be a priority because the object may become more firmly lodged in place as the canal swells. Reactive debris may accumulate as a local response to the irritation. These principles also apply to nasal foreign bodies that are composed of expanding materials. Manual removal or suction may be required to remove these objects.

The use of strong acrylic glue (cyanoacrylate or Dermabond) has recently been advocated for removing beads from either the external canal or the nose. The ultimate goal when removing a foreign body with this technique, as well as with all techniques, is to remove the object with as little trauma as possible and to avoid pushing it further toward the tympanic membrane or posterior nasal passage.

Both reassurance and immobilization are important in manual removal of nasal or external canal foreign bodies. In addition, the proper tools and an adequate light source are necessary. Attempts should be made to remove foreign bodies under direct visualization if at all possible. Referral to an ear, nose, and throat (ENT) specialist may be prudent (1) if the examiner is dealing with expanding materials (unless there is a high probability of successful removal), (2) when the nasal passage or external ear canal is completely occluded and surrounded by marked edema and inflammation, (3) if the object is adherent or adjacent to the tympanic membrane, or (4) if attempts to remove the object will worsen the scenario. For such difficult removals, local or even general anesthesia may be necessary. If an ENT agrees and if the patient is in considerable pain, the patient may appreciate instillation of topical anesthetic before transportation.

Note: Miniature disc or button batteries are increasingly used in watches, calculators, cameras, hearing aids, travel clocks, and even greeting cards that play music. Because they are becoming more common and smaller, they are more frequently seen as foreign objects in ears and noses. Removal is a high priority because permanent damage to the ear can result if they are allowed to remain for more than a short time. Although button batteries contain toxic heavy metals such as mercury and other poisonous substances, their greater danger lies in the fact that they can produce electrochemical current. They should be promptly removed; irrigation, nose drops, or eardrops are strictly contraindicated.

Also note: If a recent foreign body turns out to be a moth, take the patient into a dark room and shine a flashlight into the ear or nose. It will likely fly out toward the light.

INDICATIONS

• Known foreign body

Note: A general rule of thumb for the ear is that if the object is in the outer two thirds of the canal and is easily accessible, it can generally be removed. If it is closer to the eardrum and cannot be removed by irrigation, referral should be considered.

CONTRAINDICATIONS

• Lack of knowledge of normal anatomy of external ear canal or nasal passage.
• External ear canal or nasal passage is obscured because of trauma.
• An uncooperative patient who cannot be sedated (see Chapter 7, Pediatric Sedation) or anesthetized (see the "Anesthesia for Auditory Canal Foreign Body Removal" section and Chapter 4, Local Anesthesia).
• For a button battery, do not use nose or ear drops.
• For organic or expanding materials, unless the clinician is fairly certain of a successful removal, saline flushing is contraindicated. Flushing can hasten or enhance the swelling.
• For other contraindications to removal from ear, see Chapter 63, Cerumen Impaction Removal.

EQUIPMENT

• Traditional foreign-body extraction tools such as suction tips, alligator or bayonet forceps, ear curettes, or wire loop curettes (Fig. 68-1)
• Cotton-tipped swabs
• Ear speculum or nasal speculum (select the largest that will fit the canal or orifice)
• Magnification, either in the form of an otoscope with an operating head or a loupe
• Bright light that can be directed or focused. If a headlamp is available, both hands will be freed to perform the procedure
• Topical anesthetic (see below for techniques of topical and local anesthesia of the external canal or see Chapter 11, Topical Anesthesia)
• Irrigant such as saline
• Wall or portable suction unit
• Strong magnet and magnetizable nail

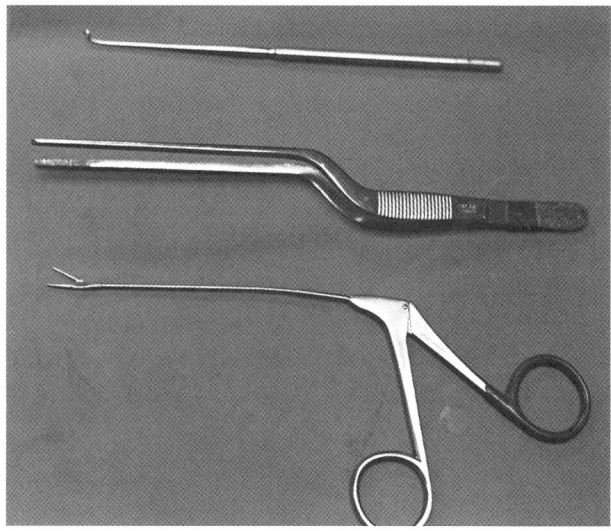

Fig. 68-1
Traditional instruments used for foreign-body extraction. *Top to bottom:* ear curette, nasal forceps, and alligator forceps.

• For ear, irrigation equipment as noted in Chapter 63, Cerumen Impaction Removal
• *Optional:* No. 4 Fogarty/Foley or Swan-Ganz catheter
• *Optional for "Alternative Technique: Glue":* Dacron-tipped applicator or plastic ear curette and Acrylic glue (cyanoacrylate or Dermabond)
• *Optional for "Alternative Technique: Suction":* 30-inch plastic intravenous extension tubing or 10-French suction catheter, heat source (burner, alcohol lamp, or lighter), blunt end of metal ear curette handle or atomizer tip, and hemostat

PREPROCEDURE PATIENT PREPARATION

• Stress the importance of remaining immobile during the procedure.
• For ear irrigation or instrument removal, discuss the risk of perforation and dizziness.
• For ear or nasal foreign body removal, discuss the chance of minor trauma. This may be associated with discomfort during the procedure or some bleeding after the procedure.
• For nasal foreign bodies, the risk of aspiration should be discussed.

TECHNIQUE: NASAL FOREIGN BODY

1. Topical anesthesia and vasoconstriction can be applied as a spray or with drops, using a mixture of 4% lidocaine and 0.25% phenylephrine hydrochlo-

ride. After waiting a few minutes for the decongestant to work, carefully examine the nostril and determine the best instrument or technique. Extend the patient's head. Apply pressure on the tip of the nose in a superior and posterior direction to help visualize the nasal canal. Irrigation should not be used in the nasal cavity because it may push the object into the oropharynx or larynx, causing aspiration.

2. Smooth, round objects can be removed using suction or right-angle hooks. For the right-angle hook, slide it past the object with the tip parallel to the nasal sidewall. Once it has passed the object, turn it 90 degrees and gently pull the object out.

3. An alligator or bayonet forceps may be used to grasp an object that has a small leading edge.

4. A no. 4 Fogarty/Foley or Swan-Ganz catheter can be passed beyond the foreign body. After inflating the balloon, gentle traction will either facilitate removal or stabilize the foreign body to prevent oropharyngeal aspiration.

5. In all cases, instruments introduced into the nasal passage require a steady hand resting on the patient's head in case of sudden movements, which can be involuntary if pain is elicited.

6. After removal, examine the orifice closely to make sure that another foreign body was not behind the first and that all debris has been removed. Any particles left behind can lead to irritation, inflammation, drainage, or chronic granulation. Also check the unaffected nasal and ear orifices for any other surprises.

TECHNIQUE: OTIC FOREIGN BODY

1. Small children may need to be sedated. Instill a topical anesthetic. After several minutes, use suction for pus, topical anesthetics, or blood as necessary to visualize the object. Small children need to be warned that suction can be very loud (see Chapter 7, Pediatric Sedation). With adults, visualization of the external ear is aided by pulling the auricle upward and backward to straighten the canal. In small children, the auricle is pulled downward.

2. The depth and surface qualities of the object usually suggest which tool(s) to use. Grasp fibrous objects (cotton, plant matter) with the alligator forceps (Fig. 68-2). Smooth objects (e.g., beans, seeds, or popcorn kernels) that are blocking no more than half of the diameter of the canal might be dragged out by passing an ear curette or wire loop beyond the object and gently withdrawing it. Larger, smooth, and hard items such as small batteries and BBs may be teased out with a fine, 1-mm, right-angle hook (Fig. 68-3). Slide the right-angle hook past the object with the tip parallel to the canal sidewall. Once it has passed the

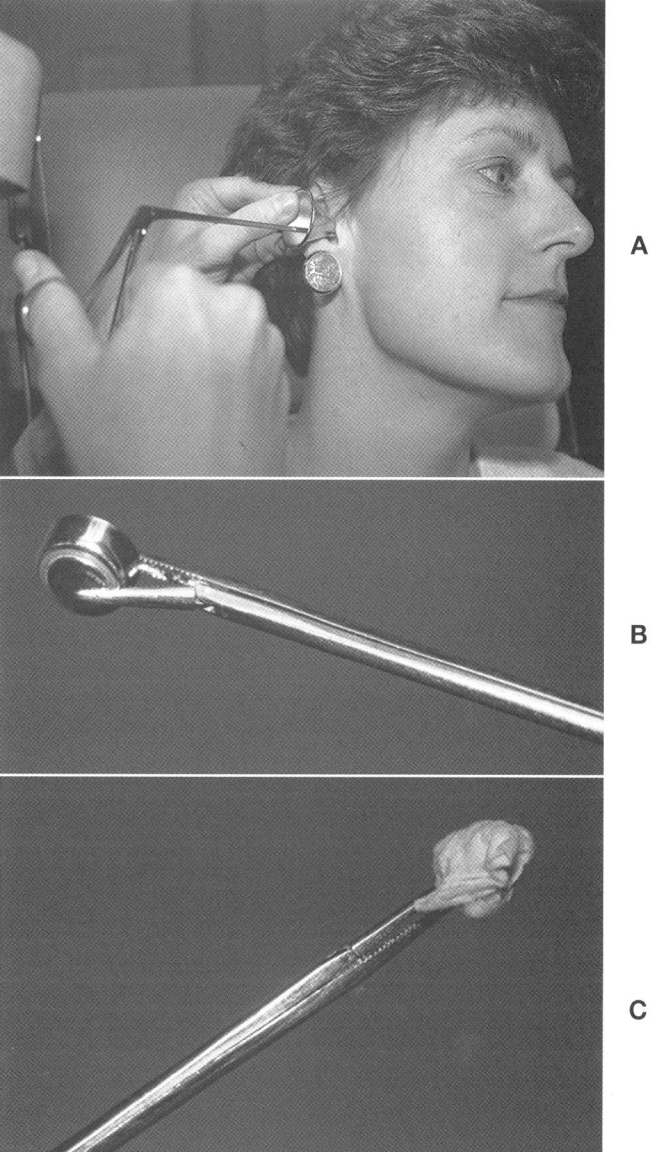

A

B

C

Fig. 68-2
A, Alligator forceps for retrieving small batteries (**B**) and paper balls (**C**) from auditory canal.

object, turn it 90 degrees and pull the object out. Objects with sharp projections, such as earrings and screws, may need to be grasped with cup forceps to avoid laceration of sensitive membranes.

3. Irrigation may move a foreign body far enough away from the eardrum to increase the chance of extraction.

4. Occasionally, iron-containing items such as a BB can be removed with a small magnet probe. A probe can be fashioned from a nail that has been blunted and magnetized by drawing it across any strong perma-

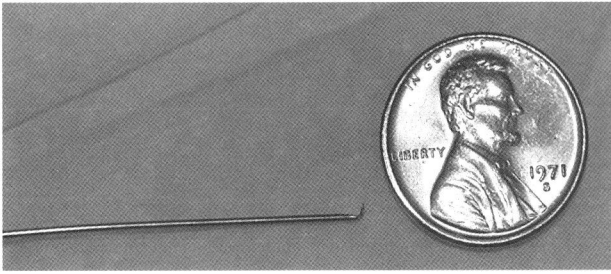

Fig. 68-3
Precise right-angle hook made from bending a 1½-inch, 21-gauge needle tip at a right angle is an excellent tool for removing smooth objects, such as beans and corn kernels.

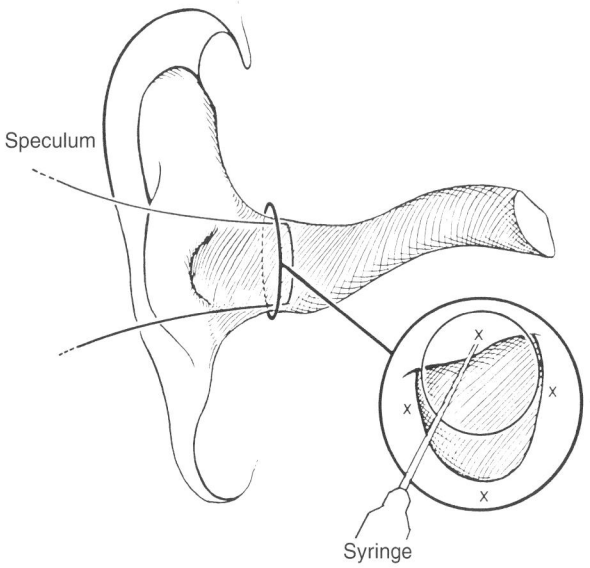

Fig. 68-4
Four-quadrant field block anesthesia of the external auditory canal. Local anesthetic is injected subcutaneously in the four quadrants of the lateral portion of the ear canal. The largest speculum that will fit is used to guide the injections. The speculum is withdrawn slightly, tilted toward each of the four quadrants, and the needle is inserted subcutaneously (x). A very small amount of anesthetic (0.25 to 0.5 ml) is injected to produce a slight bulge in the soft tissue. A total of 1.5 to 2 ml of anesthetic is usually sufficient to anesthetize the ear canal and permit painless removal of a foreign body. (From Roberts JR, Hedges JR, editors: *Clinical procedures in emergency medicine,* ed 3, Philadelphia, 1998, WB Saunders.)

nent magnet. Permanent magnets are available in hardware stores or can be found in the rear of stereo speaker cones.

5. Irrigation may be useful in certain instances after object removal, such as when small fragments of debris remain.

6. Insects in the auditory canal should be drowned or smothered by instilling oil, lidocaine, or a benzo-

caine solution. The liquid kills the insect, and an alligator forceps can then be used to grasp and remove the insect. Suction can also be used to remove both the insect and the liquid.

7. In all situations, instruments introduced into the auditory canal require a steady hand resting on the patient's head in case of sudden movements, which can be involuntary if pain is elicited.

8. Light, general (such as intramuscular or intravenous) anesthesia is mandatory to remove foreign bodies in individuals who cannot tolerate instrumentation with or without local agents. Field block anesthesia of the external auditory canal may be helpful if tolerated (Fig. 68-4).

9. After removal, make sure that another foreign body is not behind the first and that all debris has been removed. Any particles left behind can lead to irritation, inflammation, drainage, or chronic granulation. Also check the unaffected nasal and ear orifices for any other surprises.

ALTERNATIVE TECHNIQUE: SUCTION

This technique is a safe, reliable, and nontraumatic method of removing spherical foreign bodies from the ear and nasal cavity.

1. Cut off the tip of the tubing or suction catheter (Fig. 68-5, *A*). Heat the end of the curette handle or metal atomizer tip (Fig. 68-5, *B*). Flange the cut tube end with the preheated handle or tip so that it molds to the blunt rounded metal (Fig. 68-5, *C* and *D*).

2. Clamp the tubing and attach the opposite end to the suction unit (Fig. 68-5, *E*).

3. Gently insert the flanged end into the orifice containing the foreign body under direct visualization and advance it to the object.

4. When the flange is in contact with the object, quickly unclamp the suction catheter tubing (Fig. 68-5, *F*) and apply full suction immediately through the suction cup onto the foreign object.

5. While suctioning, gently extract the tubing and the suction-attached foreign body (Fig. 68-5, *G*).

ALTERNATIVE TECHNIQUE: GLUE

This technique is safe, reliable, nontraumatic, and especially effective for removing plastic beads from the ear or nasal cavity.

1. Place a small drop of acrylic glue (cyanoacrylate or Dermabond) on the blunt end of an applicator or curette.

2. Quickly, but carefully, touch the glue on the end of

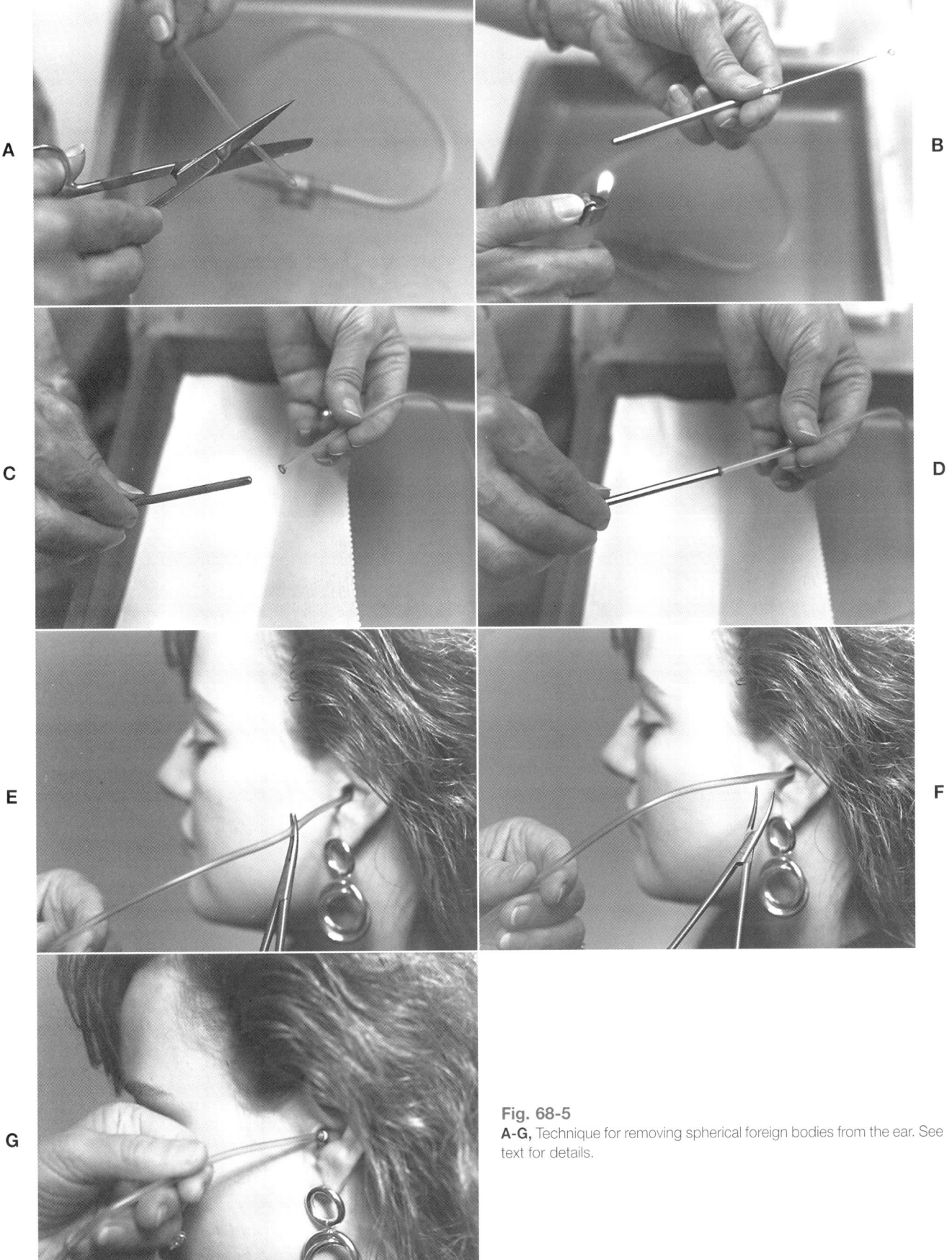

Fig. 68-5
A-G, Technique for removing spherical foreign bodies from the ear. See text for details.

the applicator to the foreign body. Establish and maintain contact. Avoid contacting the mucosa en route or pushing the object any farther inward. Hold the applicator still and maintain contact for 30 seconds until the glue hardens.
3. Gently pull the applicator out of the orifice with the foreign body stuck to it.

ANESTHESIA FOR AUDITORY CANAL FOREIGN BODY REMOVAL

For local anesthesia, instill 5 drops of sterile 4% lidocaine or 20% benzocaine into the canal and allow it to remain for 10 minutes. Suction to remove fluid and canal debris before injection of a local anesthetic (if needed) under direct visualization. If tympanic membrane rupture is suspected, eardrops and irrigation are contraindicated.

For local field anesthesia of the external half of the auditory canal, inject small amounts (usually less than 2 ml total) of 1% lidocaine with epinephrine at three or four sites equally spaced along the exterior verge of the canal (Fig. 86-4). For deeper canal anesthesia (much more sensitive area), subcutaneous injections (0.5 to 1 ml) of plain 1% lidocaine can be used within the canal just external to the junction of the cartilaginous and bony canal (approximately halfway into the canal). Beginning at the posterior and superior aspect of the canal, use a 27-gauge, 1½-inch needle to slowly infiltrate lidocaine. Repeat this at two or three spots equally spaced around the canal. Allow the lidocaine to dissect down, "blanching" the ear canal and drum, if visible. Topical lidocaine or benzocaine applied to the auditory canal before an injection is often useful. Wait 5 to 10 minutes before instrumentation.

COMPLICATIONS

- Trauma to mucous membranes with the possibility of trauma-related infection or bleeding.
- Injury to the canal, tympanic membrane, middle ear, or nasal passages.
- Deeper progression of the object leading to the inability to extract in the office.
- Aspiration (nasal passage foreign bodies).
- With delayed or incomplete removal of nasal foreign bodies, the patient may be at risk of obstructive sinusitis and even meningitis from local extension of the sinusitis.
- With foreign bodies of the ear, acute otitis externa is common and may result from injury caused by the foreign body itself or by its removal. Also, when instruments are placed in the ear, the patient may experience nausea or vomiting (or both).

POSTPROCEDURE PATIENT EDUCATION

Inform the patient to watch for signs of infection (see Chapter 63, Cerumen Impaction Removal). The patient should follow up with the clinician in 1 to 2 days. He or she should report headache, fever, or drainage after removal of a foreign body. These symptoms could indicate sinusitis or meningitis or other serious infection. After removal of nasal foreign bodies, the patient should use saline irrigation, two to three times a day for 2 or 3 days.

CPT/BILLING CODES

30300   Removal foreign body, intranasal; office type procedure
30310   Removal foreign body, intranasal; requiring general anesthesia
69200   Removal foreign body from external auditory canal; without general anesthesia
69205   Removal foreign body from external auditory canal; with general anesthesia

ICD-9-CM DIAGNOSTIC CODES

932   Foreign body, nostril
931   Foreign body, external ear

ADDITIONAL RESOURCES

- See the sample patient education handout titled "Foreign Body Removal from Nose or Ear" on page 1812 of Appendix G.
- See the sample patient consent form titled "Foreign Body Removal from Nose or Ear" on page 1813 of Appendix G.

BIBLIOGRAPHY

Backlin SA: Positive-pressure technique for nasal foreign body removal in children, *Ann Emerg Med* 25:554, 1995.

Douglas AR: Use of nebulized epinephrine to aid expulsion of intra nasal foreign bodies in children, *J Laryngol Otol* 110(6):559, 1996.

Finkelstein JA: Oral Ambu-bag insufflation to remove unilateral nasal foreign bodies, *Am J Emerg Med* 14(1):57, 1996.

Friedman EM, Munter DW, Richards JR, Selbst SM: When and how to retrieve foreign bodies, *Pat Care* 15:186, 1997.

Hanson RM, Stephens M: Cyanoacrylate-assisted foreign body removal from the ear and nose in children, *J Paediatr Child Health* 30(1):77, 1994.

Jensen JH: Technique for removing a spherical foreign body from the nose or ear, *Ear Nose Throat J* 55:46, 1976.

Kadish HA, Corneli HM: Removal of nasal foreign bodies in the pediatric population, *Am J Emerg Med* 15(1):54, 1997.

Roberts JR, Hedges JR, editors: *Clinical procedures in emergency medicine*, ed 3, Philadelphia, 1998, WB Saunders.

CHAPTER 69

Flexible Fiberoptic Nasolaryngoscopy

Grant C. Fowler

Although the incidence of cancer of the oral cavity and pharynx has declined slightly over the last 20 years, the overall survival rate for cancer of the larynx has also declined. Fortunately, with early diagnosis, the cure rate continues to improve for all of these cancers. In primary care clinicians' offices, the number of nasopharyngeal complaints also continues to increase. For example, sinusitis is now the most common chronic disease in the United States. These facts—combined with the fact that many primary care clinicians admit to having difficulty visualizing the nasal passages, oropharynx and larynx— has led many practitioners to seek alternatives. Fiberoptic nasolaryngoscopy has now been used for over 30 years. The ease of learning the technique (especially for clinicians already performing endoscopic procedures), its low risk, the rapidity of the procedure (most procedures are completed in 5 to 10 minutes), and the relatively low cost of equipment ($3500 to $6000) has resulted in increased numbers of primary care clinicians using this valuable diagnostic tool. In addition, patients appreciate the immediate diagnostic results that this procedure provides, especially when performed in the familiar and comfortable environment of their primary care clinicians' office.

The primary indications for nasolaryngoscopy, especially in smokers or those with unilateral conditions, are chronic upper-respiratory complaints. It is also helpful in certain acute disorders (e.g., one study found nasolaryngoscopy more effective than sinus films for diagnosing acute maxillary sinusitis).

INDICATIONS

Chronic Conditions

- Chronic hoarseness (more than 3 weeks)
- Chronic acid (reflux) laryngitis
- Chronic sinusitis or sinus discomfort, especially unilateral
- Chronic serous otitis media or eustachian tube dysfunction in an adult, especially unilateral
- Recurrent otalgia

- Suspected neoplasia
- Chronic cough
- Chronic nasal obstruction or postnasal drip
- Chronic rhinorrhea
- Chronic pharyngeal pain
- Halitosis
- History of previous head and neck cancer
- History of conservative treatment of laryngeal polyps
- Head or neck masses or adenopathy
- Recurrent epistaxis
- Dysphagia
- Globus hystericus
- Foreign-body sensation in pharynx
- Evaluation of snoring
- Vocal cord paralysis
- Further reassurance against serious disease in any chronic upper-respiratory condition, especially in smokers

Acute Conditions

- Hemoptysis
- Acute sinusitis
- Acute epistaxis (without profuse hemorrhage)
- Suspected nasal foreign body
- Suspected laryngeal foreign body
- Acute onset of hoarseness after straining voice

CONTRAINDICATIONS

- Acute epiglottitis (may precipitate complete airway obstruction)
- Acute epistaxis (bleeding source may be difficult to visualize with profuse hemorrhage)
- Uncooperative patient

EQUIPMENT

- Flexible fiberoptic nasolaryngoscope with light source (Newer scopes are completely immersible, which simplifies cleaning and disinfection. Frequently, light sources used for other endoscopes in the office may be adaptable to a nasolaryngoscope. This might be an important consideration when purchasing a flexible sigmoidoscope or gastroscope.)

- Nasal speculum
- Sterilizing solution, such as glutaraldehyde (Cidex)
- Decongestant*: phenylephrine (0.25% to 2%) spray (Neo-Synephrine) or epinephrine 1:50,000 (Adrenalin) or oxymetazoline hydrochloride 0.05% spray (Afrin)
- Anesthetic: lidocaine (2% to 4%) solution (Xylocaine)† in an atomizer spray bottle or benzocaine spray (14%) (Cetacaine)†
- Optional supplies include cotton balls or pledgets soaked in either a decongestant or anesthetic. Three ear, nose, and throat spuds with soaked cotton applicators are another option. Cocaine solution (4% to 10%) can be used for both decongestion and anesthesia. At this strength, it does not produce a euphoric effect; however, many clinicians choose not to stock cocaine because of the mandatory record keeping and the risk of burglary. If cocaine is considered for the anesthetic, the risk of metabolites being found in their urine should be explained to patients in case they have on-the-job drug screening.

PREPROCEDURE PATIENT PREPARATION AND EVALUATION

After a thorough head and neck history and examination, as well as the remainder of a complete history and physical examination, explain the procedure to the patient. The procedure is brief enough to be performed on the initial visit. If the procedure cannot be performed on the initial visit, when the patient returns, obtain the interval history, examine the head and neck, and explain the procedure again.

Inform the patient that he or she may experience an intense tickling sensation upon insertion of the scope. Warning the patient beforehand can minimize his or her response. The objectives of the procedure should be described carefully. Explain to the patient that he or she may speak during the procedure, and that you should be told of any significant discomfort other than pressure. The patient will be asked to say certain words or sounds and may be asked either to swallow or to avoid swallowing at different stages.

Although nasolaryngoscopy can be performed without anesthesia, visualization and patient tolerance is usually improved by using a topical decongestant fol-

lowed by an anesthetic spray. This may be especially helpful with inexperienced operators or anxious patients.

Ask the patient to gently blow his or her nose to clear the nasal passage. Give the patient some tissues to hold in one hand and a plastic emesis basin to hold in the other. The patient should be draped over the shoulders with an absorbent sheet that is then tucked inside the collar. With the patient sitting up, apply decongestant with a generous spray of atomized solution to both nostrils. If the same spray nozzle is to be used with another patient, it should not touch him or her. One spray should be directed superiorly and a second posteriorly. After spraying, have the patient tilt his or her head back to allow the liquid to drain as far back as possible. The patient should then swallow any residual. Unless both nares need to be intubated, determine by visual inspection which nostril is the least obstructed. After decongestion, this is the nostril that should be anesthetized for scope insertion.

After waiting 5 to 10 minutes for the decongestant to take effect, anesthetize the nostril(s) chosen for scope insertion. Spray liberal amounts of lidocaine or benzocaine aerosol spray; direct the spray superiorly for 1 second and then posteriorly for about 1 second with the patient tilting his or her head back and again swallowing any residual. The patient should be warned that lidocaine has a sour taste. Swallowing the anesthetic assists with suppression of the gag reflex. For patients with a hyperactive gag reflex, gargles with lidocaine solution or a generous spraying of the pharynx with benzocaine may be helpful. The patient is ready for the procedure when he or she reports a lack of sensation at the back of his or her throat.

To use soaked cotton balls or pledgets, with offset or bayonet forceps, insert them through the nasal speculum. One cotton ball (or pledget) should be inserted superiorly. Another one should be inserted in the middle meatus, and a third posteriorly. They should remain for 5 to 10 minutes and be removed before insertion of the scope. Three ENT spuds with cotton applicators can be used in the same manner. If pledgets or spuds are used, the back of the pharynx should also be sprayed with anesthetic to suppress the gag reflex.

TECHNIQUE

1. Before insertion and while waiting for the anesthesia to take effect in the patient, the operator should become reacquainted with the scope (for those who do not regularly perform endoscopic procedures). Deflect the tip both ways to observe which direction and how far it moves for a given movement of the deflector. The focal length on most scopes is about

---

*Should be used with caution in those who are severely hypertensive or have a history of sensitivity to the agent.
†Should be used with caution in those who have a history of an allergy or sensitivity to the agent.

5 mm or greater, so view an external object through the scope for a sense of distance and magnification. In general, as it is advanced, the tip of the scope moves toward whatever structure is directly in the center of the field of view. For these very small scopes, a slight deflection of the tip can cause a marked change in direction of the scope.

It should be noted that the most difficult aspect of nasolaryngoscopy is not scope manipulation, but maintaining familiarity with the complex anatomy of the nose and throat. Clinicians who do not frequently perform the procedure may benefit from a brief review of the anatomy before each procedure. Atlases and videotapes are available for such reviews (see the "Bibliography" section).

2. Place the patient in either an erect (sitting) or supine position. Both examiner and patient should be in a position that they can maintain comfortably for 20 minutes. The patient is protected from injury caused by his or her own sudden movements or by jumping away from the scope if in the supine position. Patients who are sitting can be protected by placing their head all the way back against a high, firm headrest. A small child may want to sit in a parent's lap; the parent should hold the child firmly, especially the head, since protection from injury resulting from involuntary movements.

3. Rest the hand used for guiding the endoscope on the patient's cheek. Your middle, ring, and little fingers should form a tripod to support the index finger and thumb while handling and guiding the tip of the scope. As you gain more experience, you may wish to rest this tripod on the patient's forehead to sense for tensing of the frontalis muscle, which is often the first indication that the patient is experiencing significant discomfort. Turn on the light source. Tell the patient to close his or her eyes and to expect a bright light and possibly a tickling sensation. Insert the tip through the least-obstructed nostril, past the nasal hairs at the vestibule, and rest it against the nasal septum to warm it. Warming the scope usually defogs it.

4. The floor of the nasal cavity, which is within the inferior meatus, usually offers the most open channel and the best passage for intubations (Fig. 69-1). The meatus is the space below each turbinate. Advance the scope only toward visualized objects and avoid advancing the scope blindly or against significant resistance. As with other endoscopic procedures, if only white is visible (a "whiteout"), the scope is probably resting against mucosa and should be withdrawn until the actual structure that the mucosa is covering is visualized. A deviated septum or large maxillary ridge may impede advancement of the endoscope along the floor. In this situation, make an

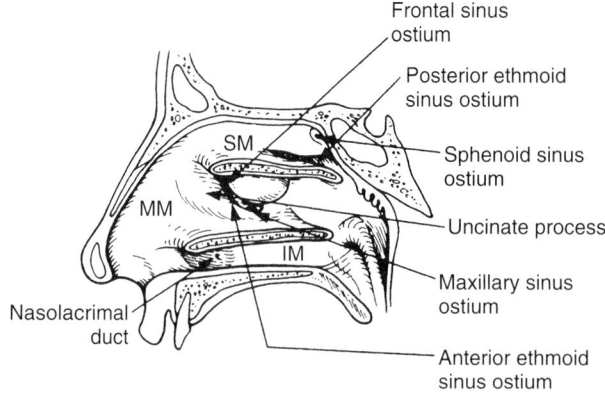

Fig. 69-1
Sagittal section of the head with the turbinates removed to demonstrate ostia of the paranasal sinuses and the nasolacrimal duct. *IM,* Inferior meatus; *MM,* middle meatus; *SM,* superior meatus.

attempt to pass the scope through the middle meatus, keeping in mind that the patient usually experiences more discomfort whenever the scope is directed or advanced superiorly. If this is unsuccessful, withdraw the scope and intubate the other nostril.

5. As the scope is advanced along the floor, the feet of the medial crura (of the lower lateral septal cartilages) can frequently be seen protruding from the medial aspect of the nasal passage. The inferior turbinate is visualized about 1 cm into the passage. Note the texture and size of the inferior turbinate, as well as any polypoid degeneration or swelling of the covering mucosal membranes. Flexion of the scope slightly upward often illuminates the middle turbinate in the distance and its meatus. The nasolacrimal duct drains into the inferior meatus and is usually not seen; however, purulent fluid draining from it is evidence of a nasolacrimal gland infection. If the patient has had surgical antral windows made into the maxillary sinus, the openings are frequently located in the inferior meatus. These openings can often be entered with a scope (Fig. 69-2). The condition of the mucosa should be noted.

6. Next, pass the scope posteriorly about 4 to 5 cm until the choana comes into view. The choana is the junction between the nasal fossa and the nasopharynx, and it looks just like a posterior "nostril." It should form a halo in front of adenoid tissue. If desired, move the scope laterally and superiorly to allow entry into the middle meatus. However, since superior reflection of the scope may result in discomfort to the patient, it may be prudent to examine the middle meatus on the way out after visualizing the larynx. Again, if the nasal floor is obstructed, there may be no choice but to attempt passage of the scope through the middle meatus.

7. Upon entering the choana, the adenoid pad appears on the posterior wall of the pharynx. Star-shaped scarring may be all that is seen if the patient has had an adenoidectomy. Advance the endoscope into the nasopharynx, and when the posterior margin of the septum is passed (when it is no longer seen), slightly flex the tip of the endoscope and rotate 90 degrees laterally to observe the torus tubarius. The torus is the valve at the opening of the eustachian tube (Fig. 69-3). Ask the patient to say "key, key, key" while you observe valve function. The eustachian tube should open and close slightly. Adenoid or lymphoid hyperplasia may be noted in this area or elsewhere throughout the procedure. It may actually block the torus tubarius. By advancing the scope slightly and rotating 180 degrees while making sure to avoid the septum, the opposite torus is illuminated. Its function should also be observed. Purulent fluid may be seen draining from a eustachian tube and should be noted. Posterior to both tori and anterior to the adenoid pad lie the clefts of Rosenmüller, each of which should be carefully inspected. Most nasopharyngeal malignancies are found in this area.

8. Next, advance the scope inferiorly and toward the posterior wall of the oropharynx (Fig. 69-4).

Note: If possible, avoid touching the posterior pharynx, which may elicit the gag reflex.

Instruct the patient to breathe through the nose to keep the soft palate from obstructing the view. As the patient swallows or talks, the normal movement of the soft palate can be seen. Downward flexion and slight rotation of the scope as it nears the posterior wall will allow for inspection of the uvula, the soft palate, and the lateral and posterior walls of the pharynx. The epiglottis should be seen in the distance. Note the presence of any masses, scarring, inflammation, exudate, mucosal irregularities, or pulsations. In some cases, dysphagia may be explained by lymphoid hyperplasia in this area, especially if the hyperplasia is associated with enlarged palatine tonsils and an exudate.

9. When the scope has passed the soft palate, it enters the oropharynx. Again, for the remainder of the procedure, attempt to avoid touching the posterior pharynx while keeping the scope as close as possible to it. If the scope becomes fogged, tell the patient to swallow; this often clears the scope. With slight flexion and rotation, examine the posterior tongue, lingual tonsils, palatine tonsils, epiglottis, and medial and lateral glossoepiglottic folds. Examine the valleculae from above (Figs. 69-5 and 69-6). Ask the patient to stick out his or her tongue to improve visualization of the valleculae.

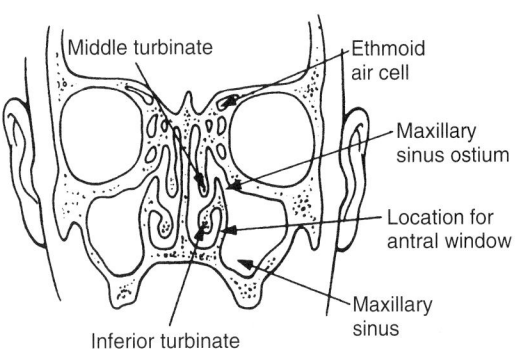

Fig. 69-2
Frontal section of the head. In this section, eight ethmoid air cells (four on each side) are shown in their location medial to the orbit. A rather large maxillary sinus ostium is demonstrated, as well as the location in the inferior meatus for surgical placement of antral windows.

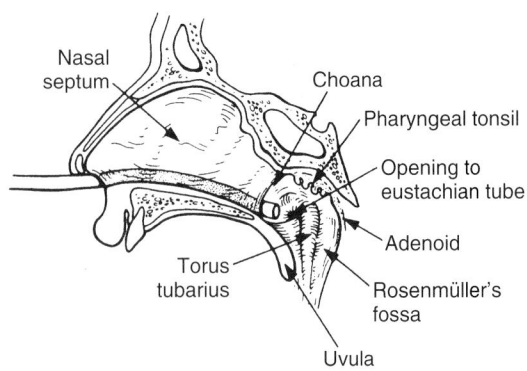

Fig. 69-3
Anatomy of nasopharynx and oropharynx.

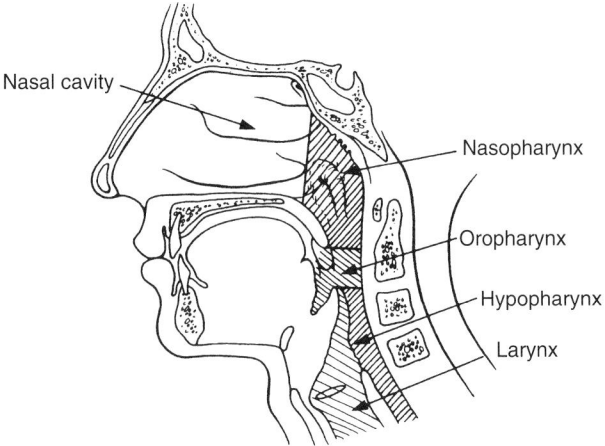

Fig. 69-4
Anatomic divisions of the upper airway. All five divisions may be inspected with a fiberoptic nasolaryngoscope.

10. When the scope has passed the epiglottis, it enters the hypopharynx (Fig. 69-4). Ask the patient to refrain from swallowing; at this level, swallowing can induce an unusual foreign-body sensation or provoke coughing. Assure the patient that if it is unavoidable, it is all right to swallow; however, he or she may experience the sensation of swallowing the scope. If this sensation becomes too strong, the scope may be withdrawn until the sensation passes. The arytenoid cartilages, the corniculate and cuneiform cartilages, and the aryepiglottic folds can be visualized at this level. The piriform sinuses posterior to the cords should be at least partially inspected. Closely examine the false and true vocal cords and the ventricles during quiet respiration (Fig. 69-6). Tell the patient to hold a prolonged high "eee" sound while you watch for symmetry of cord mobility as well as edema, hemorrhages, erythema, nodules, or masses of the cords or surrounding structures. Record any mucosal or structural abnormalities.

Note: The scope should *never* touch or pass below the cords. When nearing the cords, if the patient accidentally swallows, the operator should be prepared to quickly withdraw the scope enough to avoid touching them. If the cords are touched, severe laryngospasm can occur with resultant patient asphyxia.

11. Next, withdraw the scope to a position just anterior to the choana and direct it very superiorly, almost inverted on itself (Fig. 69-7). With the tip in this position, carefully withdraw the scope slightly again, and the sphenoid bone should appear. (The sphenoid bone will appear in what was previously an anterior position in scope orientation, before inversion.) The superior turbinate may be seen, as might an anatomical variant, the supreme turbinate. The ostia of the sphenoid sinus—medial to the superior turbinate—should be visible. The sphenoid sinus, which can be thought of as a large posterior ethmoid air cell (Fig. 69-8), is usually the only sinus in the posterior ethmoid group with a visible ostium (Fig. 69-1). Again, care is necessary when directing the scope superiorly. This is an area where anesthesia is

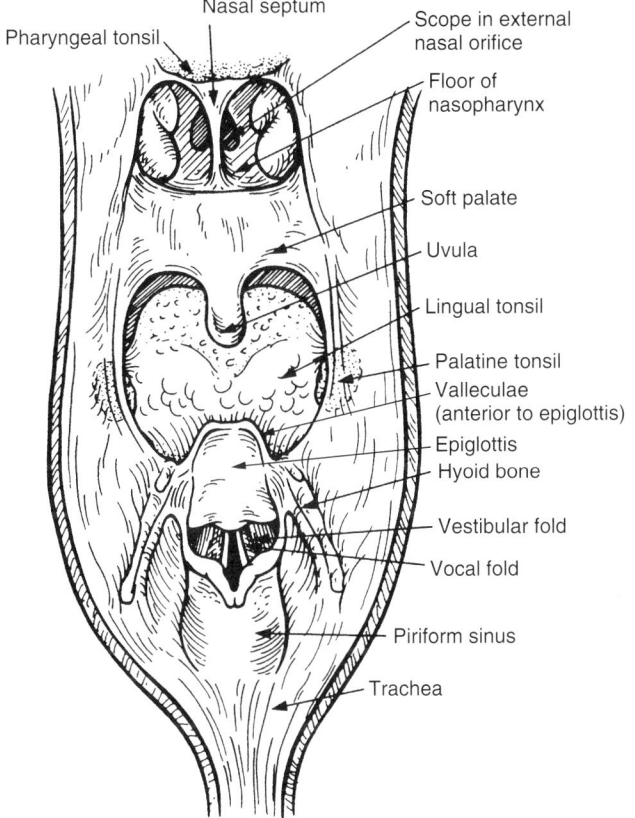

Fig. 69-5
Oropharyngeal and laryngeal areas, viewed from posterior.

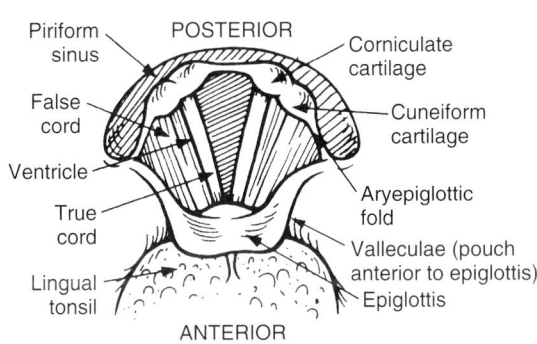

Fig. 69-6
Larynx viewed from above and oriented as it would be seen with a fiberoptic nasolaryngoscope.

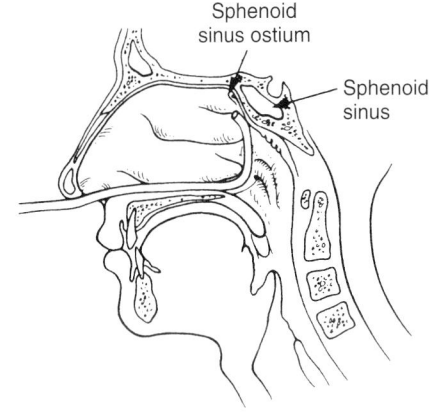

Fig. 69-7
Nasolaryngoscope is withdrawn to a position just anterior to the choana and retroflexed.

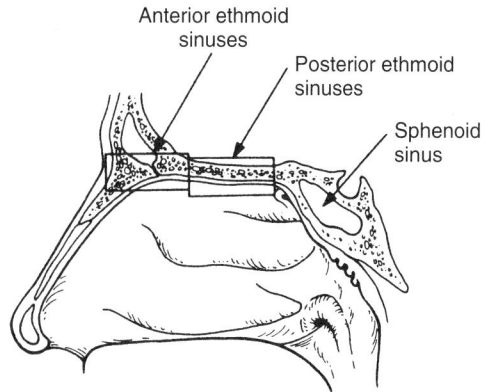

Fig. 69-8
Parasagittal section of the head showing the relationship of the anterior and posterior ethmoid sinuses. The bone in this area is eggshell thin.

frequently incomplete, and this maneuver may cause the patient some discomfort.

12. Straighten the scope and withdraw to the level where the complete choana comes into view. Move the scope in a superior and lateral direction to allow examination of the middle meatus. In most cases it is easier to examine the middle meatus from posterior to anterior. The frontal sinus, anterior ethmoid cells, and maxillary sinus ostia are located in the middle meatus, with the maxillary sinus ostia the most likely to be visualized. Observe for any drainage from ostia.

Note: Drainage of pus from an ostium is diagnostic of acute sinusitis, with accuracy possibly greater than x-ray films.

Inflammation should be recorded, and attempts should be made to identify the source of any purulent fluid or polyps protruding from or occluding the ostia. The majority of polyps are seen in the middle meatus, originating from the anterior ethmoid cells. Typical polyps are slightly yellow, translucent, and relatively avascular. They can originate from nasal mucosa (most common) or they can result from polypoid degeneration of a turbinate. Polyps can be filled with mucus or fluid. Frequently they have a stalk, or extension of mucosa, that can be traced back to their sinus of origin. Through air drying and subsequent keratinization, polyps can develop benign squamous metaplastic changes, becoming more opacified and whiter or grayer in appearance.

13. On completion of the examination, withdraw the scope and explore the opposite nasal cavity, if indicated.

Note: As with any endoscopic procedure, the natural tendency during nasolaryngoscopy is for the examiner to move toward whatever is being visualized. This action may form a tight loop in the scope outside the patient's nose. Such a tight loop may actually break fibers in the scope. To prevent this tendency,

remember to relax and maintain the same distance from the patient throughout the procedure. If you straighten the scope at the end of the procedure before removing it from the patient's nose, the patient is usually grateful.

CARE OF EQUIPMENT AND CLEANING

Although nasolaryngoscopes are fairly indestructible, they are composed of fibers and lenses that can both be broken; hence avoid bending the scope into tight angles or traumatizing the tip. Wash the scope with soap and water between procedures, followed by a 10-minute soak in glutaraldehyde. Make sure the glutaraldehyde is thoroughly rinsed from the scope, before air drying, to avoid irritating the next patient's mucosa. Clean the lens with lens cleaner and paper.

COMPLICATIONS

- Adverse reaction to anesthetic or decongestant (most common)
- Sneezing and gagging severe enough to prevent completion of the examination
- Laryngospasm with possible asphyxia; prevented by remaining above the level of the vocal cords
- Blood pressure elevation (very rare and usually related to an adverse drug reaction)
- Vasovagal reaction (rare)
- Epistaxis (it is possible to dislodge eschar or to traumatize a tumor)
- Vomiting with possible aspiration

SUPPLIERS

Flexible fiberoptic nasolaryngoscope with light source
Fujinon Medical
10 High Point Drive
Wayne, NJ 07470
Phone: 1-800-872-0196
Website: www.fujinon.com

Olympus America Corp.
2 Corporate Center Drive
Melville, NY 11747
Phone: 1-800-548-5515
Website: www.olympusamerica.com

Pentax Precision Instruments Corporation
30 Ramland Road
Orangeburg, NY 10962-2699
Phone: 1-800-431-5880
Website: www.pentaxmedical.com

Welch Allyn Corporation
4341 State Street Road
P.O. Box 220
Skaneateles Falls, NY 13153-0220
Phone: 1-800-535-6663
Website: www.welchallyn.com

Vision-Sciences, Inc.
(Manufactures a scope as well as disposable sheath covers for various brands of scopes)
9 Strathmore Road
Natick, MA 01760
Phone: 1-800-874-9975
Website: www.visionsciences.com

CPT/BILLING CODES

31231   Nasal endoscopy, diagnostic, unilateral or bilateral (separate procedure)
31505   Laryngoscopy, indirect; diagnostic (separate procedure)
31575   Laryngoscopy, flexible fiberoptic; diagnostic (separate procedure)
92511   Nasopharyngoscopy with endoscope
99070   Supplies and materials (except spectacles) provided by the physician over and above those usually included with the office visit or other services rendered (list drugs, trays, supplies or materials provided)

ICD-9-CM DIAGNOSTIC CODES

784.41   Aphonia
786.05   Chronic dyspnea
382.4   Chronic otitis media, suppurative
382.9   unspecified
786.2   Cough, chronic
491.0   smokers
787.2   Dysphagia
388.7   Earache
784.7   Epistaxis
933.0   Foreign body in pharynx
933.0   hypopharynx
933.1   larynx

300.11   Globus hystericus
784.9   Halitosis
786.3   Hemoptysis
784.49   Hoarseness
V16.2   Laryngeal cancer, history
161.9   Laryngeal cancer, NEC
478.4   Laryngeal polyp
471.0   Nasal polyp
784.2   Neck mass
472.1   Pharyngitis, chronic
306.1   Psychogenic dysphonia
472.0   Rhinitis, chronic
           Sinusitis, chronic-
473.0   maxillary
473.1   frontal
473.2   ethmoidal
471.8   Sinus polyp
786.09   Snoring
786.1   Stridor
478.30   Vocal cord paralysis

BIBLIOGRAPHY

American Academy of Family Physicians: Nasolaryngoscopy for the family physician, East Carolina University School of Medicine, Greenville, NC, 1998, Center for Medical Communications (videotape).

Corey GA, Hocutt JE, Rodney WM: Preliminary study of rhinolaryngoscopy by family physicians, *Fam Med* 20(4): 262, 1988.

Hocutt JE, Corey GA, Rodney WM: Nasolaryngoscopy for family physicians, *Am Fam Physician* 42(5):1257, 1990.

Olympus Corporation: Fiberoptic examination of the pharynx and larynx, Melville, NY, 1994 (videotape).

Olympus Corporation: Nasolaryngoscopy: the inside view, East Carolina University School of Medicine, Greenville, NC, 1988, Center for Medical Communications (videotape).

Patton D, DeWitt DE: Flexible nasolaryngoscopy: a procedure for primary care, *Prim Care Cancer* 12(5):13, 1992.

Pentax Corporation: Current concepts in examination of the nasopharynx and larynx, New York, 1995 (videotape).

Tenenbaum DJ: A buyer's guide to nasopharyngoscopes, *Fam Pract Mgmt* 2:43, 1995.

Welch Allyn Corporation: Rhinolaryngoscope exam, Skaneateles Falls, NY, 1992 (videotape).

Zuber TJ: Flexible nasolaryngoscopy. In *Office procedures,* Baltimore, 1999, Williams & Wilkins.

CHAPTER 70

Management of Epistaxis

Robert K. Beck
Jerry W. Hizon

Patients with nosebleeds are common in the offices of primary care clinicians. Fortunately, approximately 90% of nosebleeds stop without treatment. Patients simply need to compress their nose between the thumb and index finger (Fig. 70-1) or with a Kleenex under their nose until the bleeding stops. An ice pack applied to the bridge of the nose (Fig. 70-2) may also be helpful.

Epistaxis is most common in low humidity environments that dry the nasal mucosa (e.g., in the desert, or in cold climates when heating is necessary). Patients with allergic rhinitis are also susceptible to nosebleeds. The majority of epistaxis is self limited, but this chapter discusses the 10% of nosebleeds that require cautery, packing, or ligation. With advancements in technology and new kits available, the treatment of epistaxis has been simplified. Treatment is usually straightforward unless the nosebleed is due to systemic illness, coagulopathy, cancer, or trauma.

Patients under 40 years of age or those with recent trauma or an upper respiratory tract infection should lead the clinician to suspect an anterior bleed. Anterior epistaxis is frequently associated with a local cause and can often be managed with digital pressure or simple cautery. Although a teenage boy with marked intermittent nosebleeds may well have a juvenile angiofibroma in the posterior nasopharynx, it would be very unusual. Posterior epistaxis is usually seen in patients over 40 years of age and can be associated with systemic disease (Box 70-1). Posterior bleeding can be life threatening, requiring posterior packing with subsequent hospitalization. It can be especially troublesome to treat.

Note: Although clinicians are trained and patients are educated to suspect severe or uncontrolled hypertension when epistaxis is seen, hypertension is rarely the cause. However, it is not unusual for the patient to have an elevated blood pressure when epistaxis occurs. Often this is due to the patient's anxiety from the nosebleed. Since elevated blood pressure may hinder hemostasis, treatment of the anxiety and hypertension should be considered.

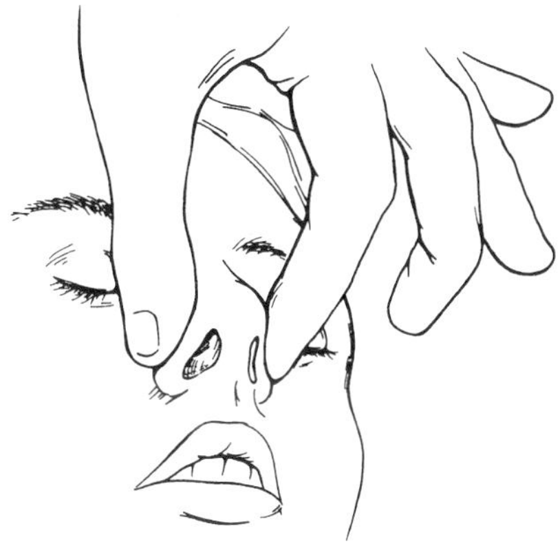

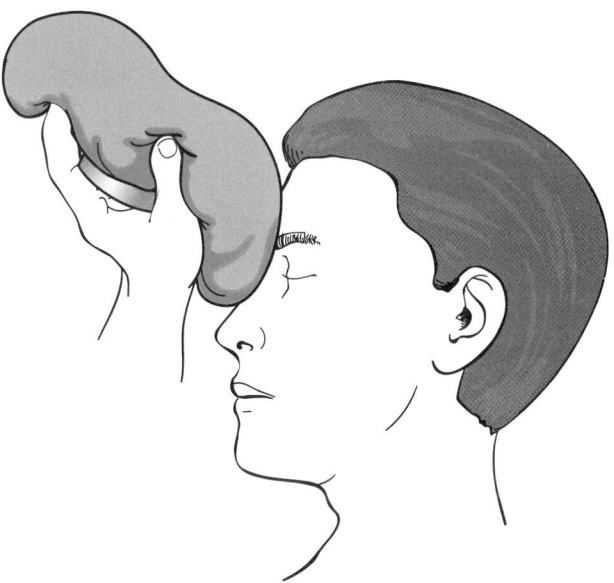

Fig. 70-1
Apply pressure by pinching the nose to stop the bleeding.

Fig. 70-2
Ice pack can be applied to the bridge of the nose.

BOX 70-1
Local and Systemic Factors Associated with Epistaxis

Local	Systemic
Nose picking and other trauma	Hypertension
Dry mucosa (from environment or medication)	Rendu-Osler-Weber disease (hereditary hemorrhagic telangiectasia)
Infection	Coagulation deficiencies (Factors VIII and IX, and von Willebrand)
Foreign bodies	
Septal perforation or deformity (spur)	
Vascular friability	Leukemia
Angiofibroma	Medications: aspirin, warfarin, heparin, clopidogrel, dipyridamole
Neoplasm	
Churg-Strauss syndrome	
	Sarcoidosis
	Thrombocytopenia
	Wegener's granulomatosis

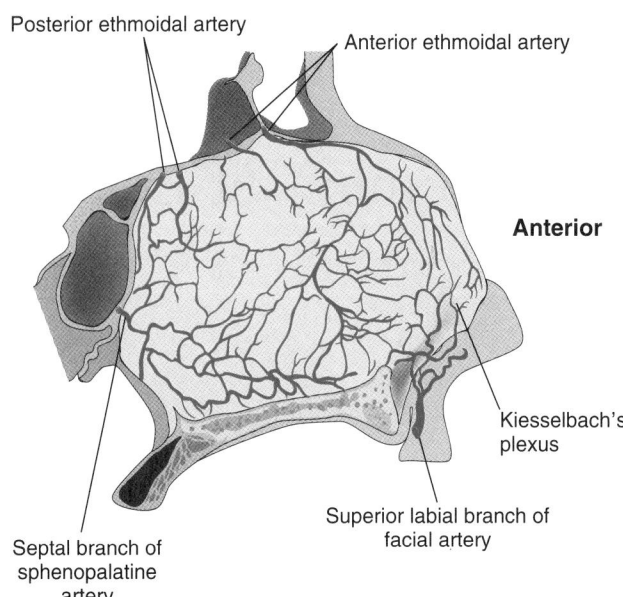

Fig. 70-3
Anatomy of the septal blood supply.

ANATOMY AND NASAL BLOOD SUPPLY

The nasal blood supply has three primary sources with multiple anastomoses (Fig. 70-3). The primary artery is the septal branch of the sphenopalatine artery. It is a terminal branch of the internal maxillary artery, which originates from the external carotid artery. In addition, the ethmoidal arteries (anterior and posterior) provide blood superiorly. They originate from the ophthalmic branch of the internal carotid artery. The superior labial branch of the facial artery provides blood to the septum anteriorly and inferiorly.

Over 90% of nosebleeds are anterior and involve the nasal septum in Kiesselbach's plexus (Fig. 70-3). An occasional source of anterior bleeding is an exposed edge from a perforated nasal septum. Anterior bleeding from the lateral nasal cavity is rare and is usually due to trauma caused by an inexperienced clinician. Another source of lateral bleeding, albeit rare, is hereditary hemorrhagic telangiectasia (Rendu-Osler-Weber disease).

The clinician treating epistaxis must understand the normal anatomy of the nose and must be familiar with the nasal septum and its appropriate midline position. Clinicians should be able to identify the inferior and middle turbinates. With an understanding of normal anatomy, when a patient has a nosebleed, the examiner should quickly notice if there are any anatomic abnormalities (e.g., a deviated nasal septum, a nasal polyp, or a mass). With a deviated nasal septum, bleeding is not unusual at either the convexity or the concavity of the deformity.

INDICATIONS

- Epistaxis that persists despite continuous external pressure or application of ice for at least 10 minutes
- Recurrent epistaxis
- Epistaxis from trauma with a suspected nasal fracture
- Epistaxis from a septal perforation or other anatomical abnormality
- Epistaxis in high-risk medical patients (e.g., severe or uncontrolled hypertension, a coagulopathy, congestive heart failure, respiratory disorders, chronic anemia, or dehydration)

CONTRAINDICATIONS (RELATIVE)

- Clotting abnormalities: Aggressive nasal packing, especially posterior packing, may cause further bleeding. Attempts should be made to normalize clotting (e.g., transfuse with fresh frozen plasma) before packing (or before removing nasal packs if already packed).
- Chronic obstructive pulmonary disease (COPD) or heart disease: Nasal packing may invoke the nasopulmonary reflex, causing a drop in the arterial oxygen pressure of about 15 mm Hg. In patients with COPD or severe heart disease, this drop may be critical. These patients should be given supplemental oxygen and monitored closely.
- Massive trauma with airway compromise: The airway should be secured first.
- Known or suspected cerebrospinal fluid leak (clear fluid that is positive for glucose), such as with a fracture of the cribriform plate (otolaryngology consult should be obtained)

EQUIPMENT

Keep either a Merocel Pak, Pope Pak, Epistat II, Rhino Rocket or equivalent available at all times. Also, keep a tray available labeled "nosebleed tray" containing all the other essential materials. Trying to assemble such a tray during an emergency is not always convenient.

Anterior Pack

- Emesis basin
- Gowns for patient and clinician
- Chux or towel for covering the patient's lap; additional Chux may also be useful for protecting the examination table and floor
- Surgical mask and goggles (or protective glasses) for clinician
- Gloves
- Head lamp for a good light source
- Nasal speculum
- Bayonet forceps
- Suction with no. 5 Frazier tip
- Cotton pledgets or cotton balls
- 4% topical lidocaine mixed 1:1 with oxymetazoline, *or* 2% tetracaine (Pontocaine) mixed 1:1 with 1% phenyl-ephrine (Neo-Synephrine) or 1% pseudoephedrine, or epinephrine 1:1000
- Silver nitrate sticks
- Electric cautery (ophthalmic tips are useful)
- Bacitracin or petrolatum ointment
- Merocel Pak, Pope Pak, Rhino Rocket, or similar packing (½ × 5–inch sticks of foam or compressed cellulose that expand when wet and conform to the nose; the Rhino Rocket is contained in a syringe for ease of insertion)
- Suture scissors
- Alternative: anterior balloons are available (Epistat I)
- Alternative: petrolatum (Vaseline) gauze packing (½ × 72 inch)

Posterior Pack

Equipment for the posterior pack is the same as that for the anterior pack, plus the following:
- Soft rubber Foley catheter, 12 to 14 French (or commercial epistaxis balloon kit)
- Tongue depressor
- Benzocaine (Cetacaine) spray
- Supplemental oxygen
- Pulse oximeter
- Umbilical clamp with gauze padding *(optional)*
- Alternative: a soft in-and-out catheter with a rolled petrolatum (3 × 36 inch) gauze pack attached (use two 18-inch pieces of umbilical tape or heavy silk–nonabsorbable suture to attach)

PREPROCEDURE PATIENT PREPARATION

Any allergy to local anesthetics should be determined. Describe the risks of packing to the patient as listed under the "Complications" section. Anterior packing is possibly painful, and posterior packing is usually painful. A mild sedative or narcotic may be helpful for posterior packing if the patient is stable. Warn the patient about the discomfort, yet remind them of the importance of remaining as still as possible. Consider offering the patient a gown to minimize the splatter of blood on their clothes, especially if they are not already bloodied. Place a protective Chux on the patient's lap, examination table, and floor to facilitate postprocedural cleanup. Be sure to document the patient's preprocedural vital signs. A pulse oximeter in place, with available supplemental oxygen, may be useful.

TECHNIQUE: BASIC MANAGEMENT OF RECURRENT EPISTAXIS

1. While the patient is applying pressure or ice, obtain a brief history and attempt to determine the cause and perhaps the site of bleeding.
2. For recurrent nosebleeds that stop spontaneously, often as soon as the patient walks through the clinic door, the most common site of bleeding is Kiesselbach's plexus. This is a frequent site in young children, and the most common cause is nose picking. Attempt to visualize excoriations of the septal mucosa near Kiesselbach's plexus to confirm the diagnosis. Parents should trim the child's nails short in order to minimize this trauma. They may want the child to wear mittens or socks over their hands at night to protect the nose during sleep.
3. For all other recurrent anterior bleeds that stop spontaneously, moisturizing the mucous membrane with ointment (e.g., A & D ointment) is the initial primary treatment. Examination of Kiesselbach's plexus usually reveals tissue overexposed to dry air with resulting cracking and bleeding. This is also common in children. Ointment can be supplemented with normal saline nose sprays.
4. Adults with recurrent nosebleeds from an unidentified site occasionally respond to a trial of decongestant nasal spray, applied twice a day to the affected side. After spraying, the patient should keep the nostril occluded with a small piece of cotton so that no air passes through the nasal cavity to cause dryness or irritation.
5. Instruct patients (or parents) to apply extra ointment to Kiesselbach's plexus at night. A vaporizer or hu-

midifier in the bedroom at night can help counteract the drying effect of heated air.

TECHNIQUE: PROCEDURAL MANAGEMENT OF EPISTAXIS

If the patient is pale, hypotensive, or orthostatic, start an IV with normal saline. A severely hypertensive patient should be treated (systolic > 210, diastolic > 110). If the patient is anxious, a sedative (hydroxyzine [Vistaril], lorazepam [Ativan], or midazolam [Versed]) may slow the bleeding. The only contraindication to procedural management is if the treatment could turn a non-life-threatening condition into a life-threatening one. For example, if there is minor blood flow and the physical examination reveals a mass in the nasal cavity, it would be wise to treat this situation conservatively, initially, and to then refer the patient. Use of instruments to stop the bleeding in this situation might uncover a vascular lesion, cause a hemorrhage and turn a controlled situation into a life-threatening one. Another example would be an older patient with multiple medical problems, especially COPD or severe heart disease, who may not tolerate a posterior pack. Posterior packing may induce the nasopulmonary reflex, causing severe oxygen desaturation.

Note: If the clinician is at all uncomfortable with the severity of the nosebleed or the patient's underlying condition, especially if attempting to manage these in the office, it is best to contact an otolaryngologist or to transfer the patient to the emergency department. In the emergency department, the clinician has the advantage of treating the patient in a controlled environment. It is also important for the clinician to remain calm to help the patient remain calm, to enhance their confidence, and to minimize hyperventilation, discomfort, and anxiety.

Anterior Epistaxis

1. The patient should be given an emesis basin and a gown to use as needed for bleeding. He or she should be sitting upright and facing you. Continue to apply ice and/or pressure while the equipment is being assembled. Before spraying any medication in the nasal cavity, attempt to locate the site of bleeding. Next, and before spraying any type of vasoconstrictive spray, spray with local anesthetic. With topical anesthetic applied, the patient is less prone to move, thereby simplifying the examination.
2. If large clots are present, cotton pledgets soaked with anesthetic and decongestant should be available before attempting to remove the clots.
3. Clots should be removed manually, if possible, with suction or forceps. If not removable, have the patient gently blow their nose. A clot itself may be keeping the offending blood vessel open; once the clot is removed, the vessel may stop bleeding spontaneously. It is also impossible to apply adequate local anesthetic or decongestant when clots are in the way.
4. If bleeding does not stop after clot removal, application of a decongestant-soaked cotton pledget(s) or cotton ball(s) may stop or reduce the bleeding. If the general source of bleeding can be localized to one area of the nasal cavity, direct a pledget to that area. If there is no discernable source of bleeding, but it is unilateral, the pledgets may have to be applied blindly to that entire side. Direct one pledget superiorly, one posteriorly, and one inferiorly.
5. After 10 minutes, remove the pledgets. Using the nasal speculum—if the bleeding site cannot be located because of bleeding—suction gently with the Frazier tip. Proceed slowly and posteriorly until the tip is located posterior to the bleeding site (i.e., blood no longer returns through the suction tip). If you are able to get behind the source of the bleeding, it can be managed in the office. At this point you may even consider applying electrocautery down the Frazier tip. If the bleeding is reduced, attempt again with the nasal speculum to identify the bleeding site. The site will usually be marked by an erosion in the mucosa or a lingering drop of blood. If it cannot be located, brush the area lightly with a cotton-tipped applicator. Next, choose the best treatment plan for the patient while attempting to minimize trauma to the nasal cavity.
6. Small areas (less than 1 cm in diameter) may be cauterized with silver nitrate or electrocautery. Silver nitrate is especially useful for children. Dry the mucosa as much as possible with a cotton-tipped applicator to minimize the spread of the silver nitrate. For best results, the topical anesthetic should have been in place for a minimum of 15 minutes. Apply silver nitrate peripherally (approximately 0.5 cm from site) and in a circular motion around the offending vessel. Gradually move toward the center of the site until the bleeding stops. Electrocautery should be applied in the same manner. Again, as mentioned above, it can also be applied down the suction tip. If the cautery is successful, ointment should then be applied to keep the mucosa lubricated. Observe for 30 minutes for any rebleeding. If there is no further bleeding, the patient may return home with instructions to keep the mucosa lubricated and to not blow or pick his or her nose for a week. The patient should also attempt to avoid straining or bending over during that time.

Note: Bilateral cautery must be avoided because it may disrupt the blood supply on both sides of the cartilage, leading to necrotic cartilage and an eventual perforation. Even unilateral cautery may result in a perforation if it is used too aggressively. The clinician should always inquire about previous trauma, cauterizations, or septal surgery. Any of these may have resulted in a compromised blood supply on one side of the septum, and subsequent cautery on the opposite side could result in a necrotic septum.

7. If the patient is bleeding from anticoagulation or thrombocytopenia, apply a clot-promoting dressing of gelatin (Gelfoam), collagen (Avitene), or cellulose (Surgicel, Oxycel) in place of cautery. For severe bleeding or for patients at risk, attempt to correct their bleeding problem intravenously.

8. For large areas or heavy bleeding, an anterior pack should be inserted. One should also be inserted if the source of the bleeding cannot be located or if the bleeding does not stop after cautery or a dressing is applied. Cautery is usually attempted before packing because packing is not focused on the actual source of the bleeding. However, with the development of new kits and materials (Merocel Pak, Pope Pak, Rhino Rocket), packs have become much more effective. They also cause less trauma to the nasal mucosa than prior techniques. The Rhino Rocket uses a syringe to simplify the insertion of compressed foam. Some clinicians use the packs first.

9. To insert a cellulose pack, first coat it with an antibiotic ointment to minimize the absorption of fluid or blood until it is fully in place. However, leave one area of the cellulose uncoated so it can absorb water to expand the pack. Grasp the end (the end with the string attached) with fingers or forceps. Gently and quickly insert the other end along the floor of the nasal cavity until the packing is completely inserted (up to where the string begins). If the

packing has not expanded in 30 seconds, irrigate with 10 ml of saline or water. Tape the string to the nose and trim the ends.

10. An anterior pack can also be put together from half-inch petroleum gauze ($\frac{1}{2} \times 72$ inch). Coat the petrolatum gauze with antibiotic ointment and fold it in half (making it 36 inches long). Using bayonet forceps, insert the doubled end first to prevent the free end from entering the pharynx (Fig. 70-4). Fold layers onto the floor of the nose (Fig. 70-5), like an accordion, as far posterior as possible. Press down on the layers with the forceps to pack them down, and fold additional layers on top. Continue to add layers from the floor to the turbinates. Approximately 3 to 5 feet of gauze will be needed per nostril. If the bleeding is from one side and the septum is intact, the patient will be able to breath from the other nostril. The pack should be left in place for 48 hours. If the bleeding is anterior and markedly reduced by packing but not completely stopped, packing the opposite side can increase the pressure. (Packing both sides increases the pressure by preventing the septum from bowing over into the side of the nose that is not packed.)

11. If the bleeding site is seen or known to be slightly more posterior, a large Merocel Pak may be placed and expanded over the site. In this situation, it is necessary to place the patient on systemic antibiotics. Merocel packing should be removed within 48 hours and the patient reevaluated.

12. To remove a cellulose pack, rehydrate with 10 ml of saline or water until saturated. Waiting 5 to 10 minutes for the pack to soften will reduce trauma, pain, and rebleeding. Grasp the drawstring or the proximal end of the packing and gently withdraw.

13. Balloon tamponade is another effective treatment for anterior bleeding, although it causes some discomfort. Devices such as the Xomed Epistat I anterior and posterior nasal balloon can be used. In this

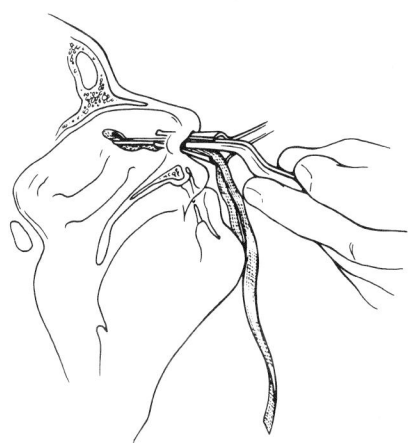

Fig. 70-4
Insert anterior pack with folded end inserted first.

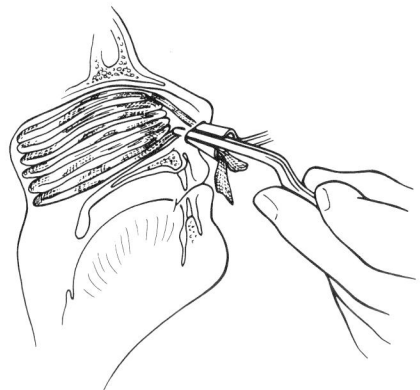

Fig. 70-5
Pack folded gauze in layers, from nasal floor to turbinates.

situation, only the anterior balloon should be inflated. It should be filled gently with normal saline until the bleeding has subsided. Due to the discomfort, pain management may be needed. Also, obstruction of the nasal cavity may incite the nasopulmonary reflex, leading to oxygen desaturation. If there is any doubt about cardiovascular stability, admit the patient for observation and monitoring.

14. After anterior epistaxis is controlled, observe for posterior epistaxis. Look again in 30 minutes before discharging the patient. Posterior epistaxis can be intermittent and may recur after sedation, antihypertensive treatment, or topical therapy wears off.

15. Taping a small, folded gauze pad beneath the nose before discharging the patient may catch minor drainage. The patient should also be placed on antibiotics before discharge.

16. For patients with a severely deviated septum, it may be impossible for the clinician to reach the bleeding site. In such a case, it is best to immediately refer the patient to the local otolaryngologist. Surgical repair of the septum may be necessary.

Posterior Epistaxis

1. A posterior source of bleeding should be suspected when an anterior pack fails to stop the bleeding or if the patient complains of blood in the throat when sitting upright. Again, attempts should be made to identify the primary source of the bleeding. If the bleeding appears posterior in origin, or the source is unable to be visualized directly, and there is a steady flow, a posterior pack may be considered initially. A posterior pack may also be considered in addition to an anterior pack. If this decision is made, the anterior pack needs to be removed and the nasal cavity anesthetized again.

Note: Placement of a posterior pack is uncomfortable and stressful to the already anxious patient. Before placing the packing, the procedure should be explained thoroughly to the patient. Continuous reassurance may keep the patient calm. It is also important for the clinician to remain calm. If the situation appears futile or outside of your comfort zone, transfer the patient immediately to the emergency department and/or notify an otolaryngologist. If you do not know how to manage posterior epistaxis appropriately or how to insert the packing, this is not the time to learn.

2. After topical anesthetic had been applied, the easiest method to manage posterior epistaxis is to gently insert a Foley catheter through the affected side. Before insertion, use scissors to remove and discard the tip of the Foley that is distal to the balloon. Lubricate the catheter with antibiotic ointment, and insert it through the bleeding nostril and past the

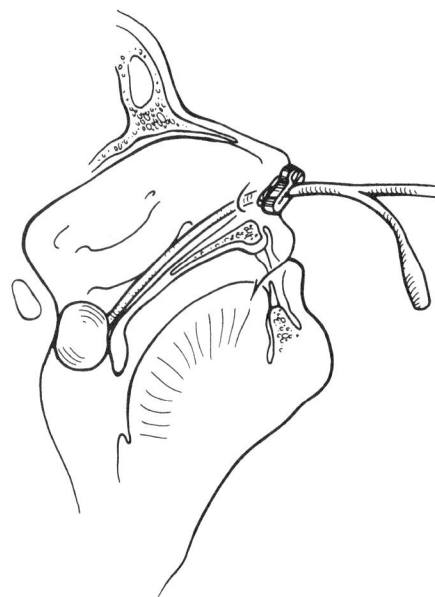

Fig. 70-6
Foley catheter as posterior pack.

choana. Using the tongue depressor and headlight, watch through the patient's mouth for the tip of the catheter. It should fall just below and behind the free edge of the soft palate.

3. Next, inflate the balloon with 5 ml normal saline and gently pull back on the catheter until it comes into contact with the soft tissue surrounding the posterior choana (Fig. 70-6). Repeat on the other side if necessary to stop the bleeding.

4. If the bleeding stops, to keep the balloon from sliding back into the nose, fix the catheter(s) anteriorly with an umbilical clamp. Padding should also be placed between the clamp and the nose. If the bleeding ceases entirely, the balloon may be deflated after several hours. However, leave the catheter in place for 12 hours in case of rebleeding.

5. Commercial balloons are available with channels for the patient to breathe through. These balloons are inserted in the same manner as the Foley.

6. Alternatively, if balloons are not available, a posterior pack can be made from a 3 × 36–inch petrolatum gauze rolled into a tight, cylindrical, 3-inch-long pack (Fig. 70-7). The pack should be impregnated with antibiotic ointment. Two 18-inch pieces of umbilical tape should be tied around the middle of the pack.

7. Before inserting this pack, spray the posterior pharynx with benzocaine (Cetacaine) spray.

8. Next, insert a soft rubber catheter through the bleeding nostril. Visualize the catheter tip through the patient's open mouth as it passes behind the

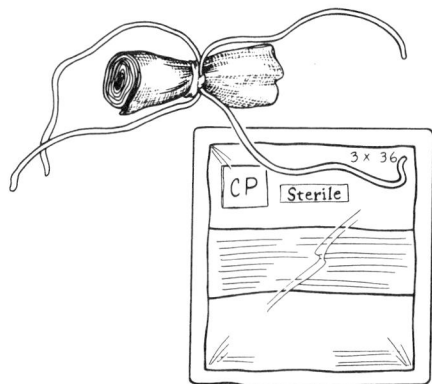

Fig. 70-7
Prepare posterior pack.

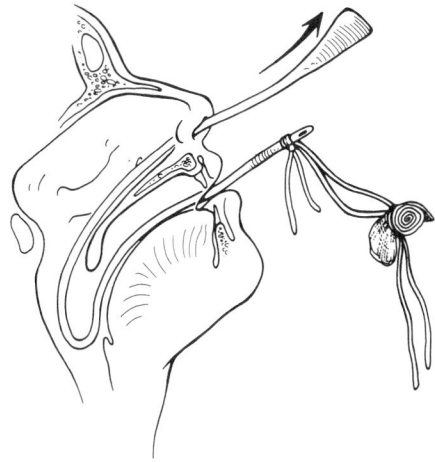

Fig. 70-8
Tie or suture posterior pack to catheter.

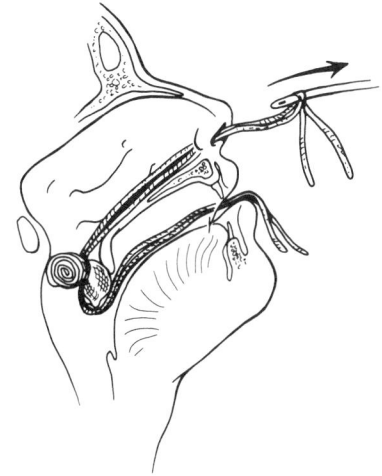

Fig. 70-9
Pull pack into position.

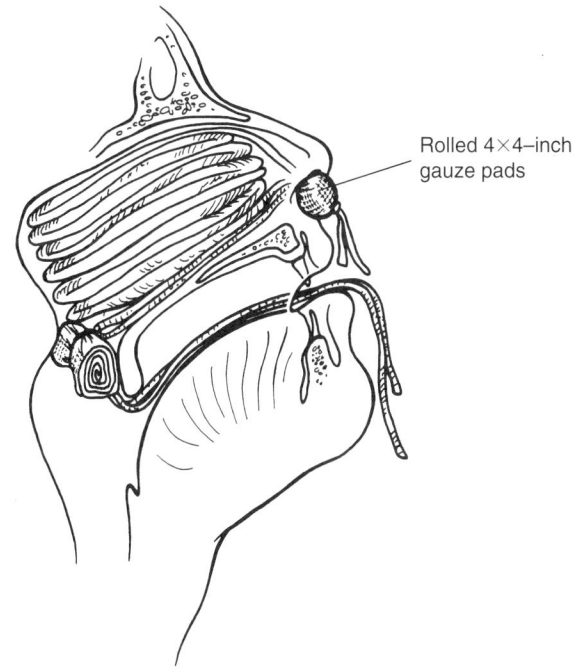

Rolled 4×4–inch gauze pads

Fig. 70-10
Securing posterior pack after placing anterior pack.

palate. Pull the tip from the pharynx and out of the patient's mouth with forceps.

9. Tie both ends of one piece of umbilical tape (or heavy nonabsorbable suture) around the catheter (Fig. 70-8). Pull the catheter back through the nose and the roll of gauze against the posterior aspect of the choana. Guide the pack into the posterior nose after pushing it around the soft palate with your finger. Leave the second piece of umbilical tape hanging from the mouth for pack removal in the future (Fig. 70-9).

10. Secure the posterior pack by tying the piece of umbilical tape that is in the patient's nose around rolled 4 × 4–inch gauze pads. These rolls should be fitted flush, but not too firmly, against the nares (Fig. 70-10).

11. If the bleeding slows but does not subside with balloon tamponade or posterior packing, it will be necessary to inflate the anterior balloon or place (or replace) a large anterior pack such as a Merocel

Pak, Pope Pak, Rhino Rocket, or Vaseline gauze (Fig. 70-10).

Note: If bleeding does not subside with these techniques, otolaryngology consult is indicated. With advancements in technology, new instruments and techniques are available and the treatment of posterior nosebleeds has become more precise. In fact, the use of instrumentation should always be weighed against the possible complications of antero-posterior packing. Sinus endoscopes can now be used to locate the site of bleeding and to cauterize it. Ligation of the anterior ethmoid artery or the internal maxillary artery may be another option. These procedures are especially helpful in patients for whom packing has failed or is contraindicated. Once the patient is stabilized, it may also be possible to embolize the appropriate artery with a minimally invasive technique.

12. After these steps are complete, the patient should be transferred to the hospital for observation and monitoring. He or she should be at bed rest with the head elevated. Oxygen therapy and IV antibiotics should be used, if necessary. The patient is at high risk for stasis sinusitis, and antibiotic coverage should be adequate for the usual pathogenic bacteria of the sinus. Serial blood counts and coagulation studies should be considered for profuse bleeding.

13. Packing should be removed after 2 to 3 days. If the alternative, rolled petrolatum posterior pack was used, extract it through the mouth after cutting the umbilical tapes around the gauze rolls at the nares. For balloons catheters, simply aspirate the entire balloon contents and slowly withdraw the catheter.

14. Nasal packing fails to stop epistaxis in up to 25% of cases. If bleeding reoccurs or if there is persistent oozing of blood around the packing, obtain an otolaryngology consult. If necessary, anticoagulants, aspirin, ibuprofen or other therapies that affect hemostasis should be discontinued.

COMPLICATIONS

- Rhinitis
- Otitis media
- Sinusitis
- Hemotympanum
- Bacteremia
- Oxygen desaturation and/or respiratory distress, especially in those with underlying, serious cardiac or lung disorders
- Cardiac arrhythmias
- Pressure necrosis of nasal ala or mucous membranes
- Rupture of balloon with aspiration of saline (if Foley catheter or balloon was used for the posterior pack)
- Allergic reaction to local anesthetic

POSTPROCEDURE PATIENT EDUCATION

If cautery was used, have the patient (or parent) apply Bacitracin or A & D ointment three times a day for a minimum of 1 week. Continue applying A & D ointment

twice a day thereafter. Instruct patients to not blow orpick their nose for the following week. They should also try to avoid bending over, sneezing, and straining. If they must sneeze, they should try and sneeze with their mouth open.

If an anterior pack has been used, tell the patient that the pack will be left in place for 48 hours and that he or she may go home. The patient should be covered for sinus and nasal pathogens with prophylactic antibiotics, such as a cephalosporin or amoxicillin-clavulanic acid. With the pack in place, ask the patient to report any fever or recurrent bleeding and to return for removal in 2 days.

The patient with a posterior pack requires hospitalization for observation while the pack is in place. Risks include those outlined in the "Complications" section. After either an anterior or posterior pack is removed, caution the patient to notify you for fever, facial or ear pain, or recurrent bleeding. Instruct the patient to return to the office in 1 week for reexamination or sooner if problems develop.

CPT/BILLING CODES

30901	Control nasal hemorrhage, anterior, simple (limited cautery and/or packing) any method
30901-50	(use modifier "-50" for bilateral)
30903	Control nasal hemorrhage, anterior, complex (limited cautery and/or packing) any method
30903-50	(bilateral)
30905	Control nasal hemorrhage, posterior, with posterior nasal packs and/or cauterization, any method, initial
30906	(subsequent)

ICD-9-CM DIAGNOSTIC CODES

784.7	Epistaxis (acute)
478.1	Nasal septal perforation, nontraumatic

SUPPLIERS

Rhino Rocket
Shippert Medical Technologies (also manufactures nasal packing kits and balloons, with and without airways)
7002 South Revere Parkway, Suite 60
Englewood, CO 80112-6703
Phone: 1-800-888-8663
Website: www.shippertmedical.com

The **Xomed Epistat I** is a double (anterior and posterior) balloon catheter. The **Epistat II** is a posterior balloon catheter with anterior packing attached. It also contains an airway and can be used for bleeding from an indeterminate site, whether posterior, anterior, or both. If posterior bleeding stops, the balloon catheter and airway can be removed, leaving the anterior packing in place.

Medtronic Xomed Surgical Products, Inc.
(Manufacturer of nasal balloons and packing kits, including the Epistat, Merocel Pak, and Pope Pak)
6743 Southpoint Drive North
Jacksonville, FL 32216-0980
Phone: 1-800-874-5797
Website: www.xomed.com

ADDITIONAL RESOURCES

- See the sample patient education handout titled "Epistaxis (Nosebleed)" on page 1814 of Appendix G.
- See the sample patient consent form titled "Treatment of Epistaxis (Nosebleed)" on page 1816 of Appendix G.

BIBLIOGRAPHY

Barton CA: *Management of office emergencies,* New York, 1999, McGraw-Hill.
Buttaravoli P, Stair T: *Minor emergencies,* St Louis, 2000, Mosby.
Howell JM, Altiere M, Jagoda AS, et al: *Emergency medicine,* Philadelphia, 1998, WB Saunders.
Murtagh J: Treatments for epistaxis. In Murtagh J: *Practice tips,* Sydney, 1991, McGraw-Hill.

CHAPTER 71

Nasal Turbinate Injection and Reduction

Rex E. Moulton-Barrett

Although turbinates are useful for warming, cooling, and filtering air, significant turbinate hypertrophy can be a problem. Inferior turbinate hypertrophy is the most common cause of nasal obstruction in patients with chronic rhinitis. This chapter reviews the evaluation and treatment options for inferior turbinate hypertrophy including surgery, laser injection, cryotherapy, electrocautery, and the newer method of infrared coagulation (IRC). Many primary care clinicians are becoming adept with IRC in their office, having become familiar with the technology when treating hemorrhoids (see Chapter 108, Office Treatment of Hemorrhoids).

Rhinitis is chronic when symptoms of nasal obstruction, sneezing, itchy nose, or rhinorrhea persist for more than 3 months each year. Chronic rhinitis is designated infective, as opposed to noninfective, if more than five polymorphonuclear leukocytes per high-power field appear on a nasal smear. Infective chronic rhinitis is usually caused by sinusitis. One in every four households is afflicted with noninfective chronic rhinitis, of which most (48%) is allergic; 15% is nonallergic eosinophilic and 37% is vasomotor in origin. Allergic rhinitis alone affects 24 million Americans, resulting in 2.5% of all office visits. It is the single most common chronic disease treated in the United States. Overall, noninfective chronic rhinitis affects even more individuals and it often goes untreated.

Nasal obstruction is the most common symptom associated with noninfective chronic rhinitis, and, unfortunately, it is the least responsive to medical therapy. Intranasal steroids relieve nasal obstruction in approximately 50% of patients with chronic rhinitis of allergic or eosinophilic origin. Unfortunately, intranasal steroids do not help much for vasomotor rhinitis, and poor long-term patient compliance limits their efficacy for any disorder. Ipratropium bromide, antihistamines, and cromolyn sodium have little treatment benefit, if any, over placebo. Although most patients obtain relief of nasal obstruction with oral sympathomimetics, long-term use may lead to associated side effects. As a result of the limitations of medical therapy, half of those with nasal obstruction from noninfective chronic rhinitis become candidates for a procedural intervention.

A persistent finding in obstructive noninfective chronic rhinitis is engorgement of the membranous head of the inferior turbinate. In normal noses the isthmus nasi or "nasal valve" is the site of maximal nasal airflow resistance. In this area, a normal amount of resistance usually does not cause nasal obstruction symptoms. However, in the presence of inferior turbinate hypertrophy, the head of the inferior turbinate (termed "Area IV" by Cottle), which lies immediately posterior to the nasal valve and attic (Areas II and III, respectively), becomes the site of maximal airflow resistance. This resistance can cause symptoms of nasal obstruction. Steroid injection of the turbinate may provide results within a few days; however, the results are usually temporary, lasting only 8 to 10 weeks. Turbinate reduction by cryotherapy, electrocautery, or IRC decreases this airflow resistance and subsequent symptoms. Although the "Technique" section of this chapter is limited to these procedures, alternative techniques are also discussed below. It is the author's experience that cryotherapy and electrocautery are not well tolerated under local anesthesia in the office.

Turbinectomy

Many rhinologists still believe that the gold standard for symptomatic relief of turbinate hypertrophy is turbinectomy. Excision may be confined to the anterior third (partial) as opposed to the traditional total turbinectomy. Contrary to earlier reports, turbinectomy is no longer associated with the development of atrophic rhinitis. Most often the procedure is performed under general anesthesia and in conjunction with septorhinoplasty. Most patients require postoperative nasal packing for 3 to 5 days. Discomfort, pain, and crusting are significant for up to 10 weeks. Significant bleeding occurs in 3% to 5% of patients and may require hospitalization.

Outfracture

Outfracture is also usually performed under general anesthesia in the operating room. It is often performed during septoplasty, nasal reconstruction, or partial turbinectomy. After adequate decongestion (usually an injection), the inferior turbinate is clamped and rotated outward. In this way, the "fracture" is achieved. The advantages to this procedure include the small amount of bleeding and the ease of performing it. However, turbinate outfracture does not address the membranous portion of the turbinate head. For this reason, 25% of patients show no improvement.

Submucosal Resection

Submucosal resection consists of removing the inner bony portion of the inferior turbinate. In this procedure, usually performed under general anesthesia, an anterior incision is made over the head of the inferior turbinate. The anterior third is resected with curved scissors. This procedure is useful for uncontrolled perennial inferior turbinate symptoms. It is easy to perform and causes little bleeding or postoperative crusting. Results are similar to cryotherapy because submucosal resection preserves the mucosa. The disadvantages to this procedure include the need for general anesthesia and postoperative packing.

Lasers

The carbon dioxide laser has been used in a defocused beam to treat turbinate hypertrophy. At a setting of 10 W, the laser is applied continuously in a cross-hatching pattern. When applied to the anterior third of the inferior turbinate, it is purported to cause less bleeding and pain and to produce faster healing than standard turbinectomy. The major disadvantages associated with laser treatment are the cost of the equipment rental or purchase and the small risk of injury to the surrounding mucosa with subsequent synechiae formation. Similarly, the KTP laser (532 Laserscope) has been used to treat the inferior turbinate in a 1-mm wide, 1-mm deep, cross-hatching pattern. At a setting of 8 W, the laser is applied continuously. Teflon-coated splints are placed after the procedure. An 85% improvement in symptoms has been reported at 2-year follow-up. No packing is required, and it is almost never complicated by bleeding. The major disadvantage, again, is the requirement for specialized equipment. Patients may also experience up to 2 weeks of postoperative rhinorrhea and 8 weeks of crusting. It is also the author's experience that laser is not well tolerated in the office under local anesthesia.

Infrared Coagulation

The Redfield infrared coagulator generates a narrow band of infrared light by reflecting tungsten light off a gold-plated mirror (Fig. 71-1). The light is channeled within a solid quartz column to a Teflon-coated tip. The photothermal effect, on tissue contact, produces a

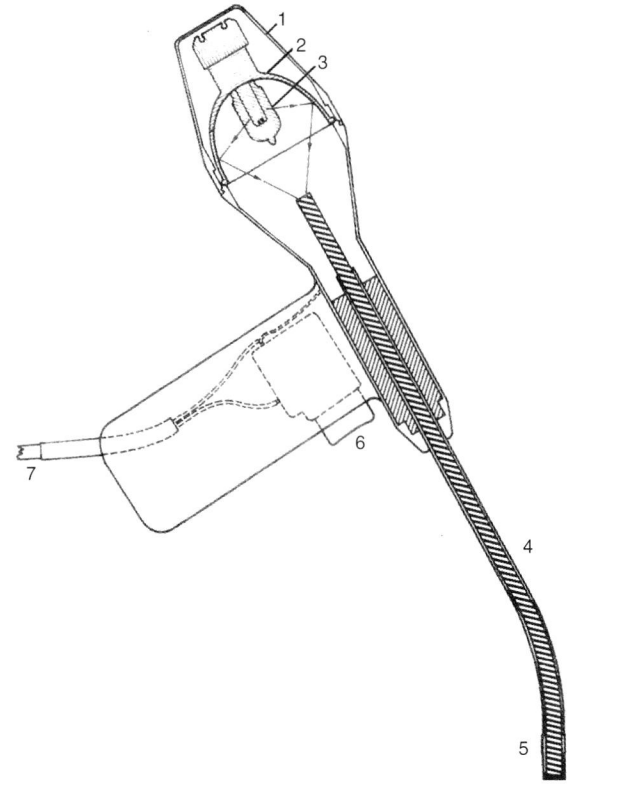

A

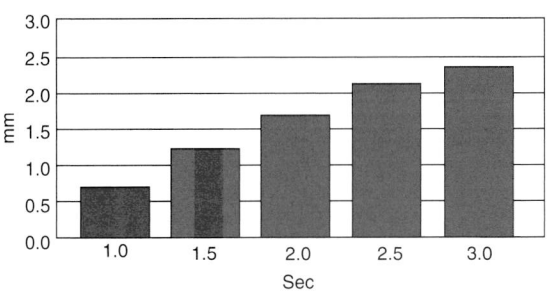

B

Fig. 71-1

A, Schematic drawing of the hand applicator portion of an infrared coagulator. *1,* Light housing; *2,* gold-coated reflector; *3,* halogen tungsten lamp; *4,* interchangeable light guide; *5,* Teflon-covered tip; *6,* switch; *7,* Flexible lead via transformer and timer to main current. **B,** Graph showing relationship between depth of coagulation and duration of exposure for hemorrhoidal tissue.

sharply demarcated tissue injury at 100° C. The depth of injury is reproducibly controlled by the duration of exposure. Studies on fresh cadaveric turbinates indicate that a 1.5-second exposure produces three-quarter thickness coagulation without injury to the periosteum of the turbinate and with little scatter to the surrounding tissue. Sparking does not occur, no electrical current is transferred to the patient, there is no surface adhesion, and no protective eyewear is required. These features allow use in patients with demand pacemakers, during pregnancy, near the eye, and with high oxygen flow. It is the author's experience that IRC provides the most rapid, safe, easily learned, and effective method for inferior turbinate reduction in the office.

INDICATIONS

- Noninfected, symptomatic inferior nasal turbinate hypertrophy
- Chronic noninfective obstructive symptoms, resulting from hypertrophy, that have failed medical therapy

CONTRAINDICATIONS

- Infective chronic rhinitis (sinusitis)
- Uncontrolled bleeding disorders or patients on anticoagulants (e.g., Lovenox, clopidogrel)
- Operator not familiar with the procedure or anatomy

Relative Contraindications (Techniques Will not Work)

- Patients with obstruction because of a collapse of Cottle's area II or III
- Patients with a partial choanal obstruction (posterior mulberry hypertrophy or a nasopharyngeal mass)

EQUIPMENT

- Nasal smear (see the "Suppliers" section for kit from Arlington Scientific that provides the clinician with a fixative and a mail-in package)
- Topical decongestion/anesthesia and injected local anesthesia

The author recommends a combination of equal parts oxymetazoline and 2% pontocaine or 0.05% oxymetazoline, and 4% lidocaine for topical decongestion/anesthesia. Five percent topical cocaine pledgets can also be used. Note that at this percentage, cocaine does not have a euphoric effect. However, the presence of cocaine in a clinician's office may increase the risk of theft. Also, patients with employers that use random drug testing may wish to avoid the use of cocaine.

After topical decongestion/anesthesia, local anesthesia is produced by injection of 0.2 to 0.5 ml of 1% or 2% lidocaine with 1:100,000 epinephrine to the head of each inferior turbinate. Patients with heart problems should receive lidocaine without epinephrine.

For Turbinate Steroid Injection

- 25-gauge spinal needle
- 3- to 5-ml syringe
- Triamcinolone (Kenalog) injectable, 40 mg/ml

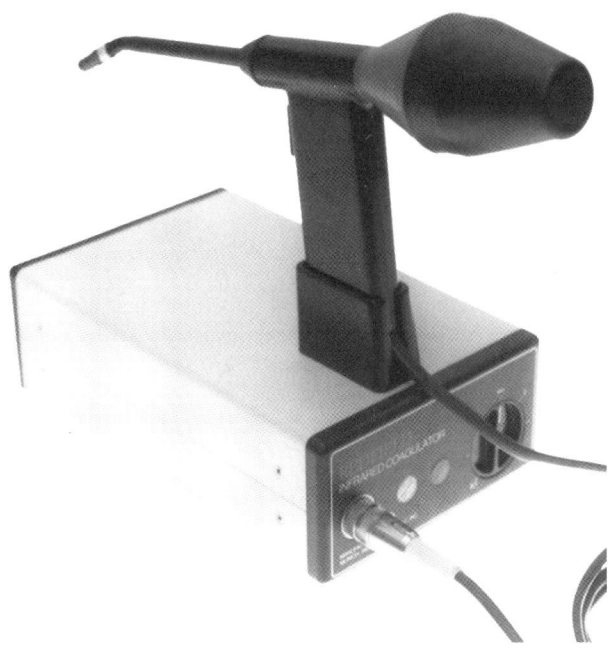

Fig. 71-2
Infrared coagulator (Redfield) with a 6-mm tip.

For Cryotherapy

- Nitrous oxide cryogun (−40° C)

For Soft Tissue Electrocautery

- 25-gauge spinal needle and standard office electrocautery unit, *or*
- Radiofrequency cautery unit with two-point bipolar attachment (Ellman)

For Infrared Coagulation

- Sterile Teflon-coated, 4- to 6-mm IRC tip
- Infrared coagulator (Redfield) (Fig. 71-2)

PREPROCEDURE PATIENT PREPARATION

Informed consent should be obtained prior to any of the procedures just described. Risks and benefits to each should be explained. Patients should avoid antiplatelet medications, if possible, following these procedures and until crusting and bleeding has stopped.

The patient should be informed that although steroid injection is the least invasive technique, there is a 5% risk of facial flushing and even a slight risk of blindness. There are 11 cases of blindness following injection reported in the literature.

Patients should be aware that for cryotherapy or electrocautery techniques, they will experience some discomfort if performed in the office under local anesthesia. These procedures may cause persistent rhinorrhea and a worsening of nasal obstruction from edema and crusting for up to 4 weeks. There is also a risk of injury to the inferior turbinate with these procedures. Following vidian nerve cryotherapy, 25% of patients will experience dry eyes.

For IRC, patients will develop nonobstructing crusts that usually resolve within 2 weeks of the surgery. Frontal headaches may occur but should last less than 5 hours after treatment. Bloody nasal discharge occurs infrequently soon after surgery but should cease by 4 days after the procedure.

TECHNIQUE

Evaluation: History, Examination, and Diagnostics

History

1. The workup for nasal airway obstruction should include a detailed history of personal or familial allergies, current medications, and duration or precipitating events related to the symptoms. In addition to obstruction, inferior turbinate hypertrophy may be associated with symptoms of headache or facial pressure. A common misperception is that these latter symptoms are always due to sinusitis. Symptoms of nasal obstruction may occur when upright or only when supine, and they may affect the patient unilaterally or bilaterally. Diminished nasal airflow should be graded from mild to complete. The clinician must be aware of the "nasal cycle." The nasal cycle is a spontaneous variation in nasal congestion as a result of variations in parasympathetic tone, which occur every 4 to 8 hours. Obstruction requiring a procedural intervention will not vary significantly with the nasal cycle.

Examination and Diagnostics

2a. *An inferior turbinate size:* Size can be assessed with a nasal speculum and can be graded subjectively from mildly enlarged to complete occlusion. Topical decongestion with oxymetazoline allows the examiner to distinguish between membranous hypertrophy and a prominent bony architecture. As it turns out, prominent bony architecture of the inferior turbinate is quite rare. Ideally, all patients with nasal obstruction should undergo nasolaryngoscopy (see Chapter 69, Flexible Fiberoptic Nasolaryngoscopy) to exclude posterior nasal obstruction or nasopharyngeal masses.

2b. *Nasal smear:* With some experience, harvesting a representative sample for a nasal smear (cytology) requires little time and effort. The swab should be obtained from the lateral nasal wall, as superior and as far posterior from the inferior turbinate as possible. In fact, if possible, it is preferable to obtain the smear at the head of the middle turbinate. A kit for this purpose is now commercially available. (See the "Suppliers" section.) The kit provides the clinician with a fixative and a mail-in package for microscopic evaluation.

2c. *Distinguishing allergic from nonallergic eosinophilic chronic rhinitis:* Patients with allergic chronic rhinitis usually have a history of positive skin testing and/or a personal and family history strongly suggestive of atopy. The history is the main distinguishing factor because both of these conditions may have eosinophils on the nasal smear. Both are also usually responsive to intranasal steroids, which should be instituted as primary therapy. Patients should undergo a trial of therapy for at least 8 to 12 weeks.

2d. *Vasomotor rhinitis:* In the absence of atopy, a patient with symptomatic inferior turbinate hypertrophy probably has vasomotor rhinitis, which is confirmed if no eosinophils are noted on the nasal smear. Typically these patients complain of nasal congestion at mealtime or with a change in room temperature. Vasomotor rhinitis shows a variable response to topical ipratropium bromide. Apart from topical decongestants, which are contraindicated for chronic use, and oral decongestants, there are no current pharmacologic agents that lack significant side effects.

2e. *Infective chronic rhinitis or sinusitis:* A nasal smear demonstrating more than five polymorphonuclear leukocytes per high power field is suggestive of chronic sinusitis. Sinusitis failing antibiotic therapy may require further diagnostic evaluation, including a sterile nasal wash culture (see below) or radiologic studies. Computed tomography (CT) limited to the sinuses best defines the situation and, in many centers, is as cost effective as plain radiographs. If a sterile nasal wash culture does not reveal antibiotic-resistant bacteria that may be treated with a change of antibiotics, referral should be considered. Sinus CT films are also useful to the otolaryngologist preparing for surgery.

2f. *Sterile nasal wash/culture:* This is performed for therapeutic as well as diagnostic reasons. First, decongest the patient in one nostril with oxymetazoline. After waiting a minute, while the patient is leaning over a sterile bowl in a sink, inject body temperature sterile saline (IV normal saline or ¼ teaspoon of salt in 8 oz of boiled/sterile water) into the decongested nostril from a filled, sterile squeeze bulb or ear bulb syringe. Any runoff from the injected saline should be collected in the sterile bowl. After the runoff has ceased with the patient holding the opposite nostril closed, have him or her blow forcefully through the injected nostril into the sterile bowl. To obtain a culture, dip a sterile culture swab into the saline in the bowl. This technique effectively washes the sinuses while obtaining a sample for culture. In patients with chronic sinusitis unresponsive to antibiotic therapy, these cultures frequently reveal bacteria resistant to standard antibiotics, yet sensitive to second- or third-line antibiotics. The patient can repeat the irrigation technique at home, without a sterile bowl, for symptomatic relief as needed.

Procedure: Steroid Injection

1. Topically decongest and anesthetize one or both inferior turbinate(s).
2. Using a 25-gauge spinal needle, slowly *(over several minutes)* inject the anterior half of the inferior turbinate with 0.5-ml triamcinolone (40 mg/ml).
3. Repeat the procedure on the opposite side, if indicated.

Procedure: Cryotherapy

1. Topically decongest and anesthetize, and then inject anesthetic locally, into one or both inferior turbinate(s). The injection should elevate mucosa from bone. Not only does injection of local anesthesia produce some hydrodissection of the turbinate tissue, but it also somewhat protects the turbinate bone from damage by separating the tissue from bone.
2. Apply the cryo gun for 60 to 75 seconds to four places on the superior and anterior head of the inferior turbinate.
3. Cryotherapy can also be used to provide parasympathetic denervation to the nasal cavity by applying it to the vidian nerve. The vidian nerve lies immediately posterior to the sphenopalatine ganglion, 1 cm superior to the lateral border of the choana and 5 mm posterior to this point. See the "Complications" section.
4. Repeat the procedure on the opposite side, if indicated.

Procedure: Soft Tissue Electrocautery

1. Topically decongest and anesthetize, and then inject anesthetic locally, into one or both inferior turbinate(s). Again, by using injected local anesthetic the turbinate bone is partially protected from cautery damage.
2. Insert a 25-gauge spinal needle submucosally into the inferior half of the head of the inferior turbinate for 3 to 4 cm posteriorly.

3. As the needle is withdrawn, a handheld cautery is applied to the needle using 15 W in the coagulation mode. One- to two-second spurts of current are used until visual blanching occurs.
4. Repeat the insertion, in a parallel direction, and apply cautery with withdrawal twice again on the medial convex surface of the inferior half of the turbinate (total of three applications of cautery).
5. Repeat the entire procedure for the opposite turbinate, if indicated.
6. Alternatively, a double-needle, two-point bipolar cautery unit can be used (Fig. 71-3). The needles should be applied to the turbinate(s) in a similar fashion. Before cautery, insert the needles approximately 2 mm into the turbinate tissue, and try a test dose to ensure that the machine is working and the current is being delivered properly. After the correct setting is established with a test dose, the needles are then inserted submucosally and longitudinally, the full length of the turbinate, in the inferior half of the turbinate. One- to two-second spurts of current are used until visual blanching occurs. After blanching occurs, the probes are removed. The same procedure can be performed on both sides, if needed. In most cases, the nose opens immediately and the postoperative edema is not enough to completely obstruct the airway again.

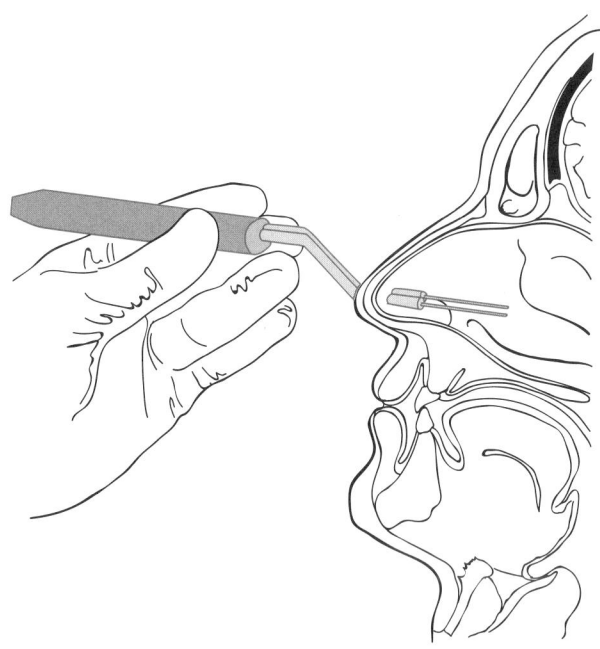

Fig. 71-3
Application of bipolar probe to inferior turbinate. (Redrawn from Ellman, Hewlett, NY.)

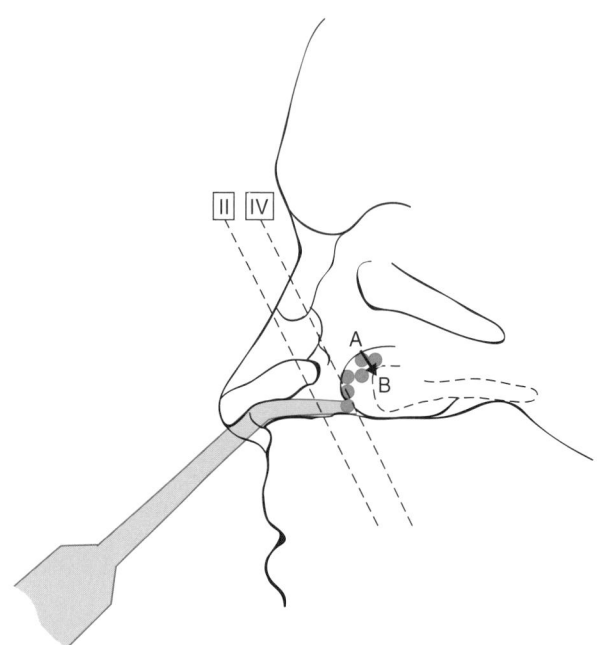

Fig. 71-4
Diagram showing infrared reduction of a hypertrophic inferior turbinate along the anterosuperior portion, leading to a reduction in turbinate size (as outlined) from A to B. Treatment of inferior turbinate hypertrophy causes the site of maximal intranasal resistance to shift from Cottle's area IV (head of inferior turbinate) back to the normal site (Cottle's area II).

Procedure: Infrared Coagulation

1. Decongest and anesthetize topically, and inject local anesthetic into one or both inferior turbinate(s).
2. With the coagulator in the dominant hand, place the sterile, Teflon-coated, 4- to 6-mm IRC tip along the anterior-superior edge of the head of the inferior turbinate. Use a setting of 1.5 seconds for a total of six to ten exposures (Fig. 71-4) in this area.
3. Use of nonoverlapping (nonconfluent) eschars (burns) from less than 2 seconds of exposure, whenever possible, should facilitate early remucosalization and hopefully avoid bony injury.
4. Repeat the procedure on the opposite side, if indicated.
5. If the patient continues to complain of nasal obstruction and there is persistent engorgement of the head of the turbinate, the entire procedure can be repeated one to two times within 6 weeks.

Note: For IRC, the author has found that the duration of exposure required is best judged by the quality of tissue contact. When the tissue contact is firm and complete, a 1-second exposure time is adequate. When the tissue contact is incomplete, a 1.5-second exposure is better.

COMPLICATIONS

Steroid Injection

There is a 5% risk of facial flushing, and there are at least 11 reports of blindness in the literature. The latter is considered avoidable through slow injection (over a period of several minutes).

Cryotherapy

Rhinorrhea is a troublesome complication for many weeks after treatment and often provides inferior results when compared with turbinectomy. Vidian neurectomy is complicated by dry eye in 25% of patients.

Soft Tissue Electrocautery

During this procedure, it is difficult to determine the degree of thermal injury. Pain may also be difficult to control with local anesthesia. If there is too much thermal injury, mucosal loss and remucosalization can be prolonged (i.e., crusting and rhinorrhea are prolonged). There is also a small risk of bony sequestrum and persistent swelling, fetor, rhinorrhea, and crusting.

With the bipolar unit, there is approximately a 3% risk of bleeding for 2 to 3 weeks after the procedure. This can be treated with cottonballs saturated with oxymetazoline nose drops and external pressure. Postprocedure bleeding is associated with turbinates that have been cauterized too vigorously. To minimize the risk of this complication, discontinue cautery immediately after blanching is observed.

Infrared Coagulation

Complications are infrequent and include bloody nasal discharge, usually for less than 4 days, and frontal headaches, usually for less than 5 hours. Nonobstructing crusts are observed in all patients, and they usually resolve within 2 weeks.

POSTPROCEDURE PATIENT EDUCATION

The appropriate information provided earlier in the "Preprocedure Patient Preparation" section should be repeated. Patients should be encouraged to apply saline solution (¼ teaspoon of salt in 8 oz of sterile water), or to wash with saline solution in a squeeze- or ear-bulb syringe, for at least 3 weeks following cryocautery, electrocautery, or IRC. Patients should report high fever, significant bloody nasal discharge, or worsening of symptoms (after the first week) to the clinician's office.

After cryotherapy or electrocautery, the patient should return to the office in 2 weeks to have the final crust removed.

For IRC, most patients initially report a worsening of symptoms, especially during the first day after the procedure. Improvement in nasal obstruction is most often reported by the fourth day, and maximal improvement is found in less than 4 weeks. Symptomatic improvement continues for over 18 months in most patients.

SUPPLIERS

Nasal smear kit
Arlington Scientific, Inc (ASI)
1840 North Technology Drive
Springville, UT 84663
Phone: 1-800-654-0146
Website: www.arlingtonscientific.com

Electrocautery or radiofrequency cautery unit
Ellman, Inc.
1135 Railroad Ave.
Hewlett, NY 11557
Phone: 1-800-835-5355
Website: www.ellman.com

Infrared coagulator
Redfield Corp.
336 West Passaic Street
Rochelle Park, NJ 07662
Phone: 1-201-845-3990
Website: www.redfieldcorp.com

CPT/BILLING CODES

Note: For IRC, use 30140 with 52 Modifier

30140   Submucous resection of turbinate, partial or complete, any method
30200   Injection into turbinate(s), therapeutic
30801   Cauterization and/or ablation, mucosa of turbinates, unilateral or bilateral, any method, separate procedure; superficial
30802   Cauterization and/or ablation, mucosa of turbinates, unilateral or bilateral, any method, separate procedure; intramural

ICD-9-CM DIAGNOSTIC CODE

478.0   Hypertrophy of nasal turbinate(s)

BIBLIOGRAPHY

Elwany S, Harrison R: Inferior turbinectomy: comparison of four techniques, *J Laryngol Otol* 104:206, 1990.

Levine H: The potassium-titanyl phosphate laser for treatment of turbinate dysfunction, *Otolaryngol Head Neck Surg* 104(2):247, 1991.

Mabry RL: Visual loss following intra-nasal corticosteroid injection: incidence causes and prevention, *Arch Otolaryngol* 107:484, 1981.

Moulton-Barrett RE, Passy V, Horlick D, Branuel G: Infra-red coagulation of the inferior turbinate: a new treatment for refractory chronic rhinitis, *Otolaryngol Head Neck Surg* 111:674, 1994.

Ophir D: Long-term follow-up of the effectiveness and safety of interior turbinectomy, *Plast Reconstr Surg* 90(6):985, 1992.

Ozenberger J: Cryotherapy for the treatment of chronic rhinitis, *Laryngoscope* 83:508, 1973.

el Shazly M: Endoscopic surgery of the vidian nerve: preliminary report, *Ann Otol Rhinol Laryngol* 100:536, 1991.

Williams H, Fisher E, Golding-Wood D: Two-stage turbinectomy: sequestration of the inferior turbinate following submucosal diathermy, *J Laryngol Otol* 105(1):14, 1991.

Cricothyroidotomy, Transtracheal Catheter Insertion and Tracheostomy

David Roden

Cricothyroidotomy and its alternatives are usually performed in emergencies, whereas tracheostomy is usually performed under stable conditions. All are used to provide an airway when nonsurgical approaches such as endotracheal intubation are contraindicated or have failed. Nonsurgical emergency personnel usually use cricothyroidotomy as a temporary lifesaving maneuver. One advantage of this procedure is the speed with which it can be performed. In addition, the airway is most superficial at the level of the cricothyroid membrane. Landmarks are easily identifiable, making this an ideal location for even the untrained clinician to create an airway. Serious bleeding and perforation of other structures can also usually be avoided at this site.

If the necessary high-pressure (30 to 60 psi) oxygen equipment is available, an alternative to cricothyroidotomy when respiratory arrest is imminent is transtracheal catheter ventilation. It may be performed even more rapidly than cricothyroidotomy or intubation and perhaps prevent respiratory arrest. Special kits are available to simplify this technique (see the "Suppliers" section). However, this technique is usually a more temporary method of managing airway obstruction than cricothyroidotomy. In addition, this technique may not provide enough ventilation to prevent carbon dioxide accumulation, so the catheter airway may need to be rapidly converted to a more definitive airway. There may also be a higher risk of producing a pneumothorax, since oxygen is delivered at high pressure. Without adequate ventilation this oxygen can also become entrapped, again raising the risk of pneumothorax.

Another alternative to cricothyroidotomy is the insertion of an 11-gauge needle through the cricothyroid membrane. This procedure can be performed rapidly, supporting a patient's spontaneous respirations for a few minutes. However, if oxygenation is needed for more than a few minutes, the needle airway will need to be converted to a transtracheal catheter or cricothy-

roidotomy. The goal of this procedure is to simply provide the precious minutes of oxygenation or ventilation necessary to prevent a respiratory arrest.

The final option to be mentioned for emergencies is percutaneous dilational cricothyroidotomy. In this procedure, a small vertical incision is made and a cricothyroidotomy tube is advanced over a guidewire device and dilator. Equipment is now commercially available for this procedure. Again, the goal is to rapidly provide a temporary airway.

Standard tracheostomy is performed two tracheal rings below the cricothyroid membrane. Since this site is farther removed from the larynx, the incidence of laryngeal injury is much lower with this procedure, especially if used for several weeks. However, since there are overlying structures at this site, the clinician must be familiar with the local anatomy to minimize risk. Tracheostomy is associated with two to five times the complication rate when performed as an emergency procedure; therefore it is rarely performed except under controlled circumstances in the operating room. In addition, the complete procedure usually takes too long to be useful for emergency airway management and can be difficult for the untrained clinician to perform. The only situation in which emergency tracheostomy is preferred is when the specific location of the pathology (e.g., subglottic tumor or thyroid cartilage fracture) precludes alternatives.

CRICOTHYROIDOTOMY
INDICATIONS

- Upper airway obstruction, usually resulting from infection, neoplasm, edema, or trauma.
- When endotracheal or nasotracheal intubation has failed, is contraindicated, or is unavailable.
- For patients with a cervical spine fracture (recommended by some authorities instead of intubation)

- As a lifesaving maneuver, if the patient is in extreme respiratory distress or is cyanotic, or after a single failed attempt at intubation in such a patient
- Transtracheal catheter or needle cricothyroidotomy complicated by carbon dioxide retention or air entrapment

CONTRAINDICATIONS

- Intact, functioning nonsurgical airway
- Subglottic obstruction
- Thyroid cartilage fracture
- Patient less than 12 years old (needle cricothyroidotomy is the preferred procedure for this age group; see the note below)

EQUIPMENT

- No. 15 scalpel blade with handle
- Size 4 to 6 endotracheal tubes or size 4 to 6 Shiley cuffed tracheostomy tubes
- Adhesive tape
- Umbilical tape and 2-0 monofilament nylon suture and needle holder (if a tracheostomy tube is used)
- Sterile 4 × 4–inch gauze sponges
- Self-refilling bag-valve-mask unit (Ambu-Bag), with tubing and oxygen source
- Suction and suction catheters
- Goggles or eye protection

If time allows:
- Povidone-iodine (Betadine) or other surgical skin preparation
- Mask, cap, and sterile gloves
- Sterile fenestrated drape
- Lidocaine 1% with epinephrine in 10-ml syringe with 22-gauge, ⅝-inch needle

If a tracheostomy tray is available:
- Mosquito clamps (2)
- Kelly clamps (2)
- Tracheal dilator (Delaborde)
- Curved scissors

Note: An 11-gauge needle inserted through the cricothyroid membrane may maintain spontaneous respirations for a few minutes. This is the procedure of choice for children under 12 years old. Therefore keeping such a needle in tracheostomy or cricothyroidotomy trays or in areas (emergency or urgent care departments) where airway obstruction is likely to be treated may be useful. If available, equipment for percutaneous dilational cricothyroidotomy may be helpful in the same manner.

PREPROCEDURE PATIENT PREPARATION

No patient education is needed in the emergency setting. Risks include intraoperative bleeding, aspiration, infection, subsequent tracheal stenosis at the cuff site, or permanent damage to the larynx. Short-term changes in the voice may also occur. Documentation should be made in the patient's chart that an explanation of the procedure was given, if time allowed. If time did not allow an explanation, the emergent need should be documented.

TECHNIQUE

Note: In extremely urgent situations, the goal is to save a life, so some concerns about sterile technique should be postponed. There should be no hesitancy if the exact anatomy or the particular steps of the procedure cannot be recalled precisely. If no equipment is available, an 11-gauge needle or an ink pen with the cartridge removed can be inserted through the cricothyroid membrane in the same area as described below. This may keep the patient alive. A more formal description of the location for needle cricothyroidotomy is found in the note following Step 4.

1. Position the patient in the supine position with the chin directly midline and maximally extended (if no cervical spine trauma). If a cervical fracture is suspected, the neck should remain immobilized in a neutral position.
2. Clean the neck with povidone-iodine solution, if time allows.
3. Observe universal blood and body fluid precautions. Observe sterile technique (cap, gloves, mask, and drapes), if time allows.
4. Use the nondominant hand to identify the cricothyroid membrane, which is located immediately caudal to the prominent thyroid cartilage (Adam's apple). It is the first small depression or indentation inferior to the hard thyroid cartilage, between the cricoid and thyroid cartilages. It should be easily palpable even in obese individuals.

Note: The cricothyroid membrane averages 9 mm in the cephalad-caudad dimension and 30 mm in the left-to-right dimension in adults. It should be easily palpable and accessible. However, it is much smaller in children under 12 years of age, which is why cricothyroidotomy is contraindicated in children and needle cricothyroidotomy is preferred.

5. If the patient is awake, and time allows, use the 10-ml syringe with the 22-gauge needle to infiltrate lidocaine in a large subcutaneous wheal encompass-

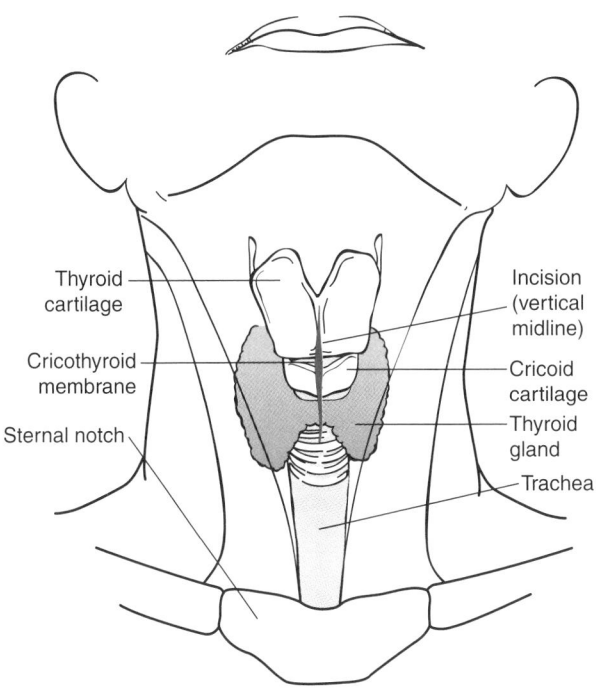

Fig. 72-1
Neck extended, with cricothyroid membrane identified.

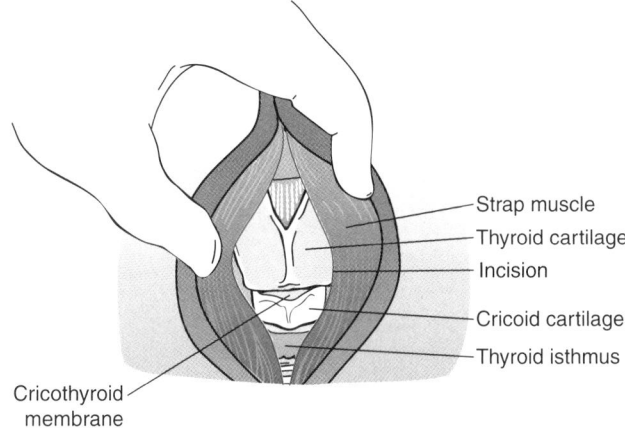

Fig. 72-2
After a vertical skin incision, soft tissue structures are retracted laterally with the nondominant hand.

ing the future vertical skin incision. Next, infuse lidocaine in a transverse line across the membrane.
6. With the nondominant hand, immobilize the thyroid cartilage and hold the skin taut over the cricothyroid membrane. Using the no. 15 blade, make a 3-cm vertical (longitudinal) skin incision centered over the cricothyroid membrane (Fig. 72-1).

Note: Certain authorities recommend a transverse skin incision; however, if the transverse skin incision is accidentally extended too far laterally (e.g., when the procedure is performed under duress), the anterior jugular veins may be injured.

7. Use the finger and thumb of the nondominant hand to retract the incision edges laterally (Fig. 72-2).
8. Divide the neck fascia and strap muscles vertically in the midline with the scalpel until the thyroid and cricoid cartilages are encountered. These structures provide considerable resistance to the scalpel and are not easily injured.
9. Retracting soft tissue structures laterally, locate the cricothyroid membrane by palpation with the dominant hand and use the scalpel to create a 1 to 2 cm transverse incision centered in the midline, immediately above the cricoid cartilage. Be aware that at this point any respiratory effort by the patient will expel sputum, blood, and air into the wound. A low

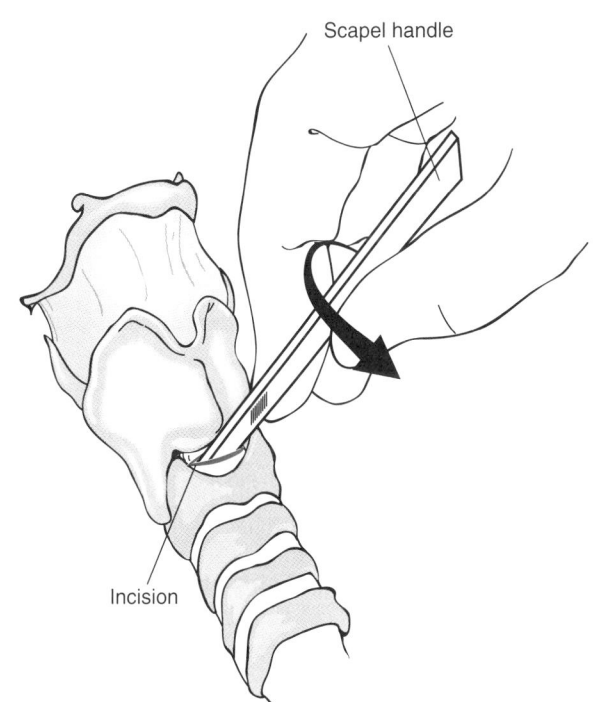

Fig. 72-3
Knife handle inserted into incision and twisted vertically to open it.

incision should avoid vocal cord injury and the cricothyroid arteries. The posterior aspect of the cricoid cartilage should be avoided, but even if the knife goes too deep, the cricoid cartilage should stop the progression of the knife.
10. Reverse the scalpel, placing the handle into the cricothyroidotomy incision horizontally. Rotate the handle 90 degrees to open the incision (Fig. 72-3).

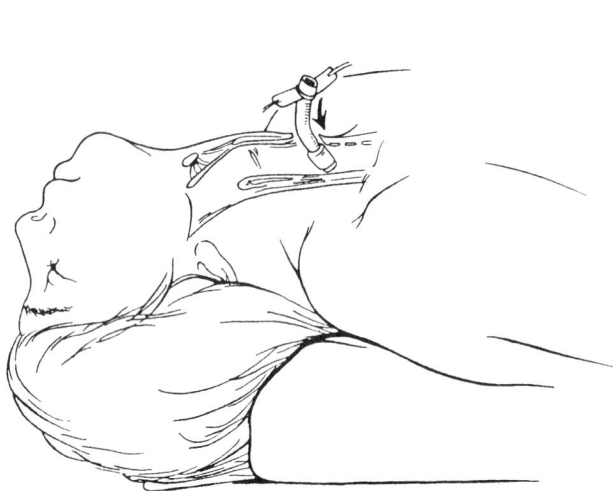

Fig. 72-4
Tube is inserted into the incision. Scalpel handle is still in cricothyroid membrane (not shown for clarity).

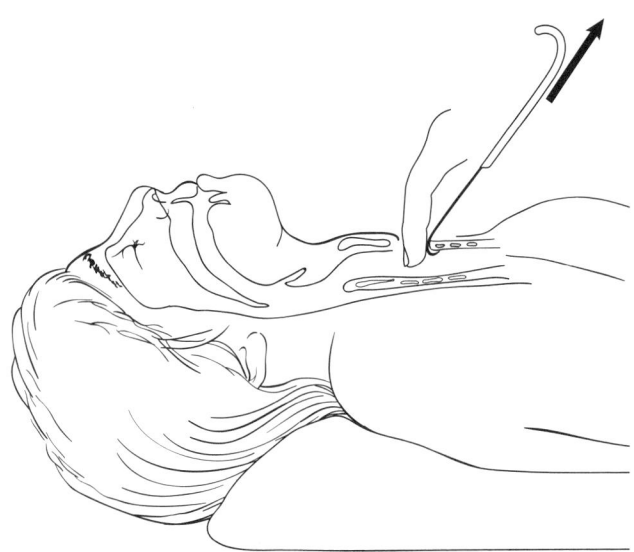

Fig. 72-5
Index finger dissects downward while upward traction is applied on the hook.

11. Use the nondominant hand to place the largest possible endotracheal tube or, preferably, tracheostomy tube into the incision. The scalpel handle can be used as both a retractor and a guide. Direct the tube tip toward the patient's feet and attempt to visualize its insertion into the trachea (Fig. 72-4).
12. Connect the bag-valve unit to the tube and ventilate with 100% oxygen. Check for bilateral breath sounds to ensure that the tube is properly placed above the carina.
13. Inflate the cuff with enough air to stop any audible air leaks.
14. Secure the tube and then apply a dressing. If an endotracheal tube is being used, secure the tube in place using tape. If a tracheostomy tube is being used, secure the tube with umbilical tape around the patient's neck. Place four interrupted sutures with 2-0 nylon through the tube's flange to secure it to the skin.
15. Suction the trachea.
16. Obtain arterial blood gases and a chest radiograph immediately. The radiograph should demonstrate tube position above the carina and should ensure the absence of a pneumothorax.

If a tracheostomy tray is available, alternatives to Steps 9 and 10 are as follows:

9. After using the scalpel to make a transverse midline incision in the cricothyroid membrane, insert a mosquito or Kelly clamp with the points downward into the incision and spread. A rush of air indicates patency of the airway.

10. Extend the incision laterally with a tracheal dilator. The dilator should be used for blunt extension to approximately 1 cm on each side of the midline.

Note: An alternative technique being tested by Rafael Cruz, MD, uses a horizontal stab wound through skin, tissue, and the localized/stabilized cricothyroid membrane. A tracheal hook is then inserted through the stab wound and attached to the cricoid cartilage. Upward traction is applied with the hook while the back of the hook is used to guide the index finger for blunt dissection down to the opening in the cricothyroid membrane. The index finger is then used to guide the endotracheal tube for insertion (Fig. 72-5).

COMPLICATIONS

- Intraoperative and postoperative bleeding (direct pressure will usually stop bleeding after the airway is established)
- Improper tube placement with asphyxia
- Tube displacement or obstruction
- Subcutaneous or mediastinal emphysema
- Vocal cord injury
- Voice changes, such as hoarseness
- Infection
- Subglottic stenosis
- Perforated esophagus
- Creation of a false passage

To prevent subcutaneous or mediastinal emphysema or infection, the skin incision should not be closed around the tube. If the cricothyroidotomy is only necessary for 48 to 72 hours (e.g., resolving infection, angioedema of tongue); the patient can be decannulated without converting to a tracheostomy. If a longer period of intubation is required (see the "Tracheostomy" section for a discussion of the controversies of timing), the procedure should be revised to a tracheostomy to prevent subglottic stenosis.

POSTPROCEDURE PATIENT EDUCATION

If prolonged airway management is needed, convert the cricothyroidotomy to a tracheostomy and provide the appropriate patient education. If the cricothyroidotomy is able to be removed within 48 to 72 hours, give the patient instructions for the routine care of a skin laceration. The patient should be aware that the fistula will close spontaneously. He or she should have a follow-up appointment within a week and should call or go to the emergency room for signs of severe hemorrhage, hemoptysis infection, or subcutaneous emphysema.

TRANSTRACHEAL CATHETER VENTILATION

INDICATIONS

- Temporary need for an airway.
- Imminent respiratory arrest.
- Same indications as for cricothyroidotomy, except that this procedure is predominantly indicated when equipment is not available for cricothyroidotomy, or if it is certain that there will only be temporary airway obstruction.

CONTRAINDICATIONS

- Intact nonsurgical airway
- Subglottic obstruction
- Thyroid cartilage fracture

EQUIPMENT

- 14- or 16-gauge over-the-needle catheter
- 5- or 10-ml syringe
- Lidocaine 1% with epinephrine in 10-ml syringe with 22-gauge, ⅝-inch needle
- Skin-sterilizing supplies (if time allows)
- High-pressure oxygen supply (30 to 60 psi) with a pressure gauge and a pressure-regulating valve
- Relief valve connected in-line with tubing to the catheter
- Hand-operated release valve

Note: A very small, permanent indwelling transtracheal catheter is available for continuous oxygen therapy (Transtracheal Systems, Englewood, Colo). It is inserted under elective conditions below the cricothyroid membrane.

PREPROCEDURE PATIENT PREPARATION

Instructions are the same as those for cricothyroidotomy.

TECHNIQUE

1. Follow Steps 1 through 4 for cricothyroidotomy. Positioning, skin preparation, precautions, and defining anatomy are the same.
2. If the patient is awake, and time allows, infiltrate lidocaine as a wheal and then down to the membrane in the desired location using the 10-ml syringe with the 22-gauge needle.
3. With the nondominant hand, immobilize the thyroid cartilage and hold the skin taut over the cricothyroid membrane.
4. Direct the catheter-over-needle attached to the syringe downward in the midline and caudally at an angle of 45 degrees (Fig. 72-6). Aspirate with the syringe during insertion. When air is obtained with aspiration, the needle has entered the trachea.

Note: This is the same location and technique that should be used for needle cricothyroidotomy or percutaneous dilational cricothyroidotomy.

5. Advance the catheter over the needle, withdraw the needle and syringe, and attach the distal end of the high-pressure tubing to the catheter.
6. Open the hand-operated release valve to deliver pressurized oxygen to the trachea. As soon as the chest rises, assume that the patient has been oxygenated; the release valve should be closed. Open the valve, watch the chest rise, and close the valve—in a rhythmic pattern—to approximate actual breathing. Adjust the overall pressure level to allow adequate lung expansion.
7. Most upper airway obstructions are incomplete and allow some ventilation to occur with forced exhalations. If the chest remains inflated during the exhalation phase, a complete proximal airway obstruction may be present. In this case, a second large-bore over-the-needle catheter can be inserted next to the original catheter. If the chest still remains distended, cricothyroidotomy should be performed.

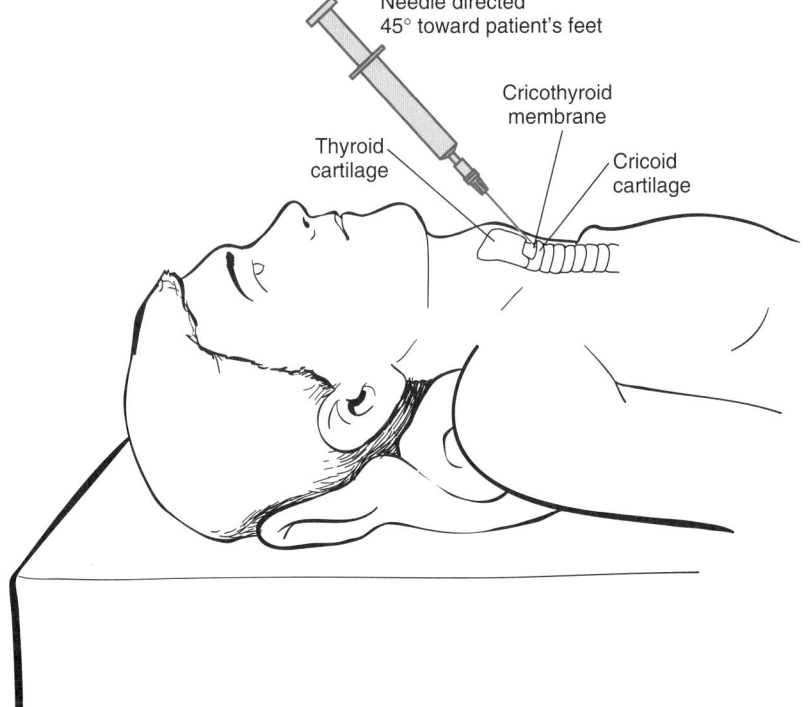

Fig. 72-6
Over-the-needle catheter is inserted through cricothyroid membrane with syringe attached. The clinician should aspirate while inserting the needle.

TRACHEOSTOMY

INDICATIONS

- Chronic ventilatory failure (most common indication)
- Upper airway obstruction (e.g., infection, neoplasm, edema, or trauma) with or without temporary airway established by needle, catheter, or surgical cricothyroidotomy
- Anticipated prolonged endotracheal intubation
- Facial trauma with compromised airway
- Tracheal trauma
- Fractured larynx or subglottic obstruction (cricothyroidotomy contraindicated)
- Chronic impaired pulmonary toilet
- Management of chronic aspiration

Note: Management of bronchial secretions is much easier with a tracheostomy tube than with an endotracheal tube. Risk of endotracheal tube complications (e.g., sinusitis, tube kinking) is also reduced with conversion to a tracheostomy. However, the recommended timing for conversion has been debated extensively. Supporters for early conversion (7 days) suggest that laryngeal complication rates and patient comfort are improved with early conversion. Advocates for delayed placement of tracheostomy (14 to 21 days) state that unnecessary procedures will be avoided, reducing local wound and other complications. Most experts have adopted an intermediate approach that is individualized to the patient. If the patient is expected to be intubated for considerably longer than 7 days, a tracheostomy is placed early. However, if the patient's course cannot be predicted, the conversion can be delayed until prolonged need becomes evident.

CONTRAINDICATIONS

- Lack of familiarity with the procedure
- Known preexisting severe tracheal pathology
- Uncontrolled coagulopathy

EQUIPMENT

- Povidone-iodine solution
- 4 × 4–inch sterile gauze sponges
- Sterile gown, gloves, and fenestrated drape
- Cap, mask and eye protection
- Electrocautery
- 10- and 50-ml syringes
- 22- and 25-gauge, ⅝-inch needles
- No. 15 scalpel blade with handle
- Mosquito hemostats (4)
- Large hemostats (2)
- Subcutaneous or Army-Navy retractors (2)
- Trousseau (tracheal) dilator
- Allis clamps (2)
- Tracheal hook
- Sizes 4, 6, and 8 cuffed Shiley tracheotomy tubes
- Needle holder
- Umbilical tape and 2-0 monofilament nylon suture

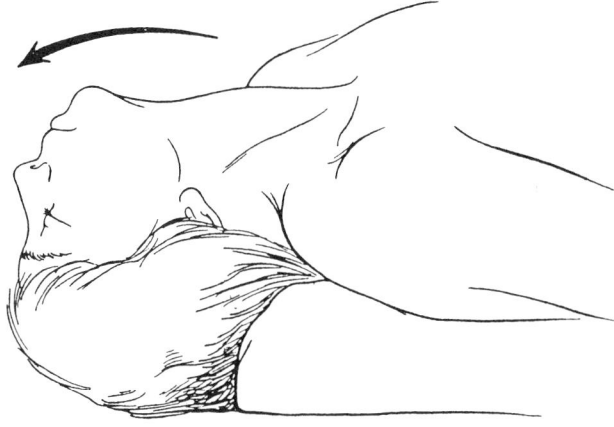

Fig. 72-7
Patient is positioned.

- Suction apparatus, tubing, and catheters
- Ventilation equipment: bag-valve-mask unit (Ambu-Bag) with tubing and 100% oxygen available
- 3-0 Dexon or chromic absorbable suture on a cutting needle

PREPROCEDURE PATIENT PREPARATION

Education of the patient and family should include the indication for tracheostomy and possible complications. Benefits of the procedure, as well as the risks of not performing it, should be explained to the patient and family. Informed consent should be obtained in non-emergent situations.

TECHNIQUE

1. Tracheostomy can be performed under local anesthesia on a spontaneously breathing patient, or under general anesthesia on a previously intubated patient. Exercise caution in administrating sedation to a nonintubated patient with a compromised airway.

2. Position the patient in the supine position with a roll under the shoulders and, if there is no cervical spine trauma, with the neck maximally extended (Fig. 72-7). (This position may be contraindicated in patients with epiglottitis or croup.) Placement of an endotracheal tube before elective tracheostomy (or leaving an existing tube) allows for better airway control and minimizes complications, especially in children. The anesthetist should stand above the patient's head for better access to the endotracheal tube, if present.

3. Prep the neck with povidone-iodine solution, from

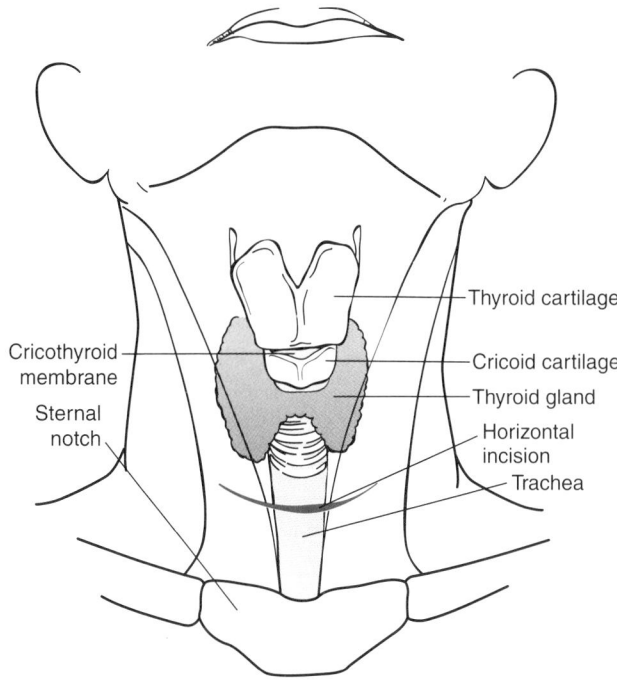

Fig. 72-8
Horizontal incision is made through the skin.

sternal notch to chin, and laterally to the sterno-cleidomastoid muscles. Apply the fenestrated drape.

4. Check the tracheostomy tube cuff for leaks. A second tube should be tested and available, if possible.

5. Palpate landmarks: the sternal notch, cricoid cartilage, and inferior border of the thyroid cartilage. Outline a horizontal incision two fingerbreadths above the sternal notch, centered in the midline over the trachea.

6. For conscious patients, inject lidocaine subcutaneously around the intended incision site. Lidocaine can then be injected down to the anterior tracheal wall beneath the incision.

7. Using the scalpel, make a horizontal incision through skin and subcutaneous tissue down to the strap muscles (pink color), approximately 1 to 2 cm superior to the sternal notch (Fig. 72-8). Alternatively, once the skin has been incised, electrocautery can be used to divide the subcutaneous tissue horizontally, deepening the incision until the strap muscles are encountered.

8. Clamp the subcutaneous tissue with Allis clamps and retract superiorly and inferiorly. Next, incise the fascia vertically in the midline, in the raphe between the strap muscles. Incise down to the pretracheal fascia (Fig. 72-9).

Note: Often the strap muscles are fused in the midline and covered by a network of troublesome veins. Attempts should be made to cauterize or ligate these veins.

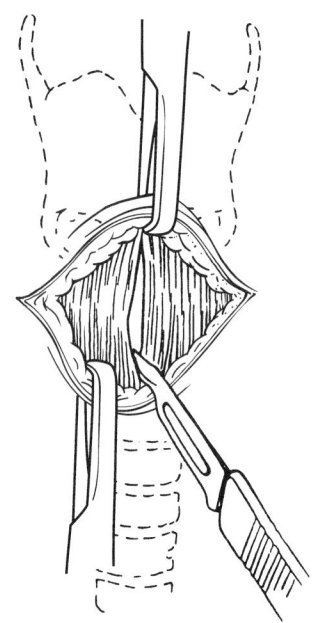

Fig. 72-9
Fascia and strap muscles are divided in the midline.

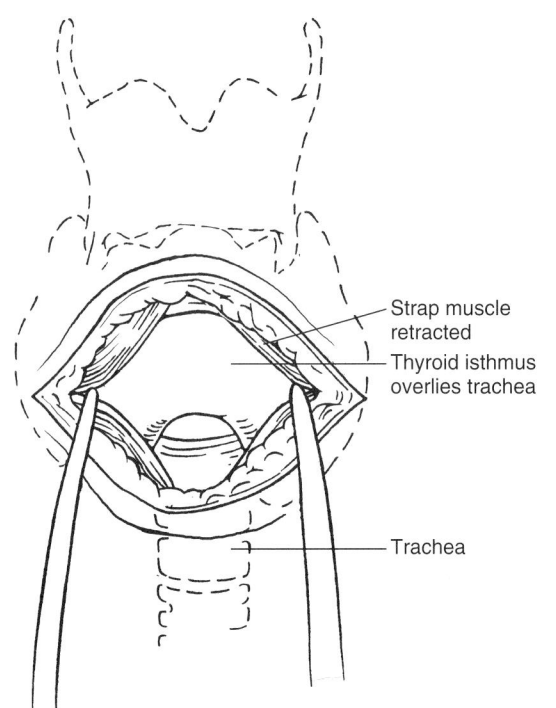

Strap muscle
retracted

Thyroid isthmus
overlies trachea

Trachea

Fig. 72-10
Strap muscles are retracted laterally to expose the thyroid isthmus.

9. Place retractor(s) beneath the strap muscles and apply traction laterally. Incise the pretracheal fascia to expose the thyroid isthmus and tracheal ring (Fig. 72-10).

10. Retract the thyroid isthmus superiorly, if possible, to increase visibility. If exposure is inadequate, horizontally incise the fascia immediately caudal to the lower border of the cricoid cartilage. Insert a hemostat through this incision pointed toward the patient's feet, parallel to the trachea. Bluntly dissect the thyroid isthmus off the anterior wall of the trachea. After an additional attempt at superior or inferior retraction, if visibility is still inadequate, it may be necessary to divide the thyroid isthmus with clamps and suture the ligated edges (Fig. 72-11). A 3-0 chromic suture is used to oversew each edge for hemostasis.

Note: It is important to remain in the midline with this procedure to minimize complications, especially in children.

11. If unsure that the object visualized is the trachea, aspirate for air with a small-bore needle to confirm before proceeding. Next, place a tracheal hook beneath the cricoid cartilage and elevate it anteriorly and toward the patient's head. If using local anesthesia, 1 to 2 ml should be injected beneath the second tracheal ring into the tracheal lumen. This should stimulate the nonanesthetized patient to cough.

12. Make a transverse incision between the second and third ring (Fig. 72-12). Be prepared for a spurt of blood, air, or sputum, and have suction ready. Take care not to puncture the endotracheal tube cuff, if present.

13. Insert a Trousseau dilator into the trachea and dilate (Fig. 72-13).

14. Withdraw the endotracheal tube (if one is in place) until the tip is just above the tracheostomy. Under direct visualization, insert the appropriately sized tracheostomy tube through the dilated incision, with the tube tip directed downward (Fig. 72-14). Inflate the tracheostomy tube cuff. Check the tube placement by suctioning with a flexible suction catheter through the tube.

15. Attach the tube to the Ambu-Bag device and check for bilateral breath sounds with ventilation.

16. Remove the retractors and the cricoid hook when the tube is adequately positioned. Secure the tracheostomy tube around the neck with umbilical tape. Secure the flange to the patient's skin with four interrupted 2-0 nylon sutures.

17. Apply a sterile dressing around the tube.

18. A chest radiograph should be taken immediately to assess placement and to ensure absence of iatrogenic pneumothorax.

To prevent infection, pneumothorax, pneumomediastinum, or subcutaneous emphysema, do not close the skin incision around the tracheostomy tube. A tracheostomy provides access to the trachea for an unlimited amount of time. Once the indication for the tube has

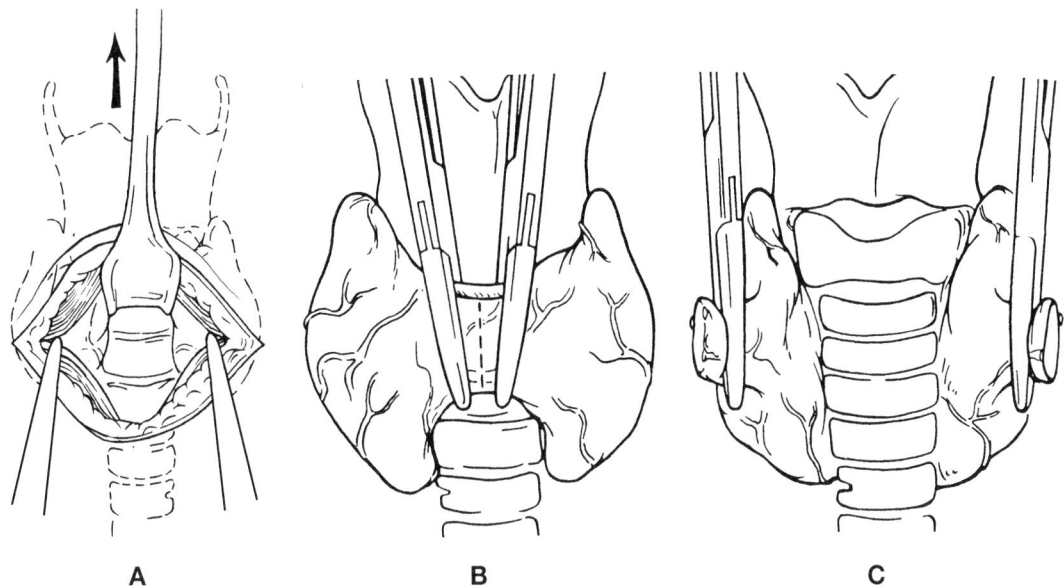

Fig. 72-11
A, Thyroid isthmus is retracted. If exposure is inadequate, the thyroid isthmus should be clamped **(B)** and divided **(C).**

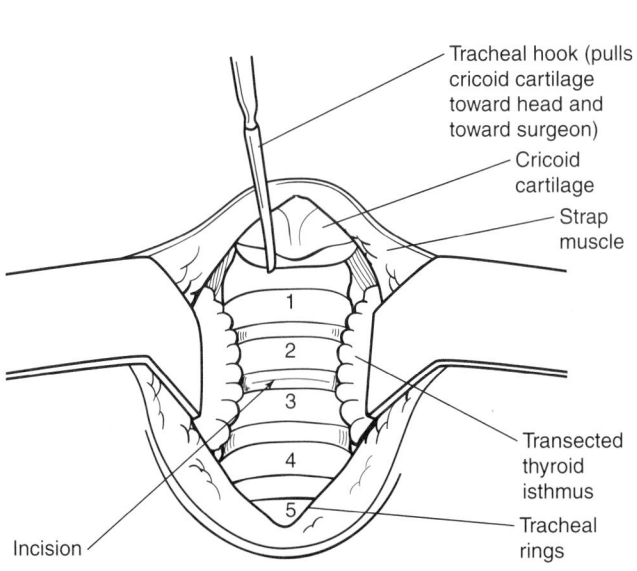

Tracheal hook (pulls cricoid cartilage toward head and toward surgeon)

Cricoid cartilage

Strap muscle

1
2
3
4
5

Incision

Transected thyroid isthmus

Tracheal rings

Fig. 72-12
Tracheal hook is placed in the cricoid cartilage and elevated anteriorly. The incision is made between the second and third ring.

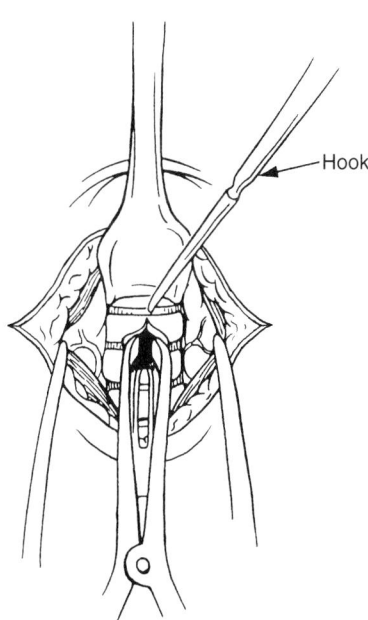

Hook

Fig. 72-13
Insert the dilator into the trachea.

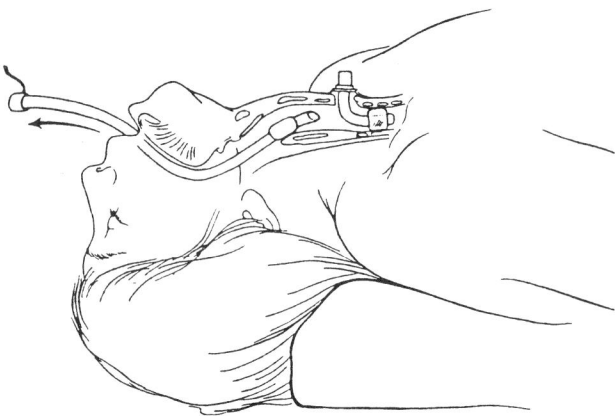

Fig. 72-14
Remove the endotracheal tube after inserting the tracheostomy tube.

resolved, it is removed to allow the tracheocutaneous fistula to close spontaneously.

COMPLICATIONS

In some studies of tracheostomy in children, mortality has been very high from the complications listed below, as well as from such complications as torn carotid arteries and completely severed tracheas.
- Bleeding
- Subcutaneous emphysema
- Wound infection
- Pneumomediastinum
- Pneumothorax
- Tracheoesophageal fistula
- Tracheoinnominate artery fistula
- Recurrent laryngeal nerve damage
- Aspiration
- Tube obstruction
- Malpositioned or displaced tube
- Tracheal stenosis
- Dysphagia
- Sepsis

Note: Placement of tracheostomies can be technically difficult, especially in children, obese patients, and patients with deformed or fixed cervical spines. For these individuals, tracheostomies should definitely be avoided in emergency situations and performed at a later date under more controlled circumstances.

POSTPROCEDURE PATIENT EDUCATION

The patient will be cared for initially in the hospital, and no postprocedure education will be necessary. If the patient is discharged with a tracheostomy, he or she will need someone trained to care for them.

SUPPLIERS

Indwelling transtracheal catheter
Transtracheal Systems
109 Inverness Drive East, Suite J
Englewood, CO 80112-5105
Phone: 1-800-527-2667
Website: www.TTO2.com

Shiley tracheostomy products
Mallinckrodt Medical
675 McDonnell Boulevard
Hazelwood, MO 63042
Phone: 1-800-635-5267 or 1-888-744-1414
Website: www.mallinckrodt.com

Bivona Medical Technologies
5700 West 23rd Avenue
Gary, IN 46406
Phone: 1-800-348-6064
Website: www.bivona.com

CPT/BILLING CODES

31500   Intubation, endotracheal, emergency procedure
31600   Tracheostomy, planned (separate procedure)
31603   Tracheostomy, emergency procedure; transtracheal
31605   Tracheostomy, emergency procedure; cricothyroid membrane
31612   Tracheal puncture, percutaneous with transtracheal aspiration and/or injection

ICD-9-CM DIAGNOSTIC CODES

478.79   Other diseases of larynx, not elsewhere classified (abscess, obstruction, necrosis)
518.81   Acute respiratory failure
518.82   Acute respiratory distress
518.83   Chronic respiratory failure
518.5   Pulmonary insufficiency following trauma or surgery
519.8   Obstruction airway, NEC
807.5   Fracture larynx, closed

ADDITIONAL RESOURCES

- See the sample patient education handout titled "Tracheostomy" on page 1817 of Appendix G.
- See the sample patient consent form titled "Tracheostomy" on page 1818 of Appendix G.

BIBLIOGRAPHY

Cummins RO, editor: *Advanced Cardiac Life Support handbook,* Dallas, 1997, American Heart Association.

Florete OG, Airway management. In Civetta JM, Taylor RW, Kirby RR, editors: *Critical care,* ed 2, Philadelphia, 1992, JB Lippincott.

Futran ND, Dutcher PO, Roberts JK: The safety and efficacy of bedside tracheotomy, *Otolaryngol Head Neck Surg* 109:707, 1993.

Kozol RA, Fromm D, Konen JC: *When to call the surgeon: decision making for primary care providers,* Philadelphia, 1999, FA Davis.

Lewis R: Tracheostomies, indications, timing and complications, *Clin Chest Med* 13(1):137, 1992.

Subcommittee on Advanced Trauma Life Support: *ATLS Team student booklet,* Chicago, 1999, American College of Surgeons Committee on Trauma.

Weissler M: Tracheotomy and intubation. In Bailey B, editor: *Head and neck surgery: otolaryngology,* Philadelphia, 1993, JB Lippincott.

CHAPTER 73

Indirect Mirror Laryngoscopy

Grant C. Fowler

Even though fiberoptic laryngoscopy is often available for visualization of the upper respiratory tract, indirect mirror laryngoscopy remains the simplest, fastest, least expensive, and often most helpful diagnostic method of examining the upper tracheal rings, vocal cords, epiglottis, larynx, and hypopharynx. In certain instances, combining mirror laryngoscopy with an adequate history will complete the diagnosis. For those comfortable with performing the procedure, it requires very little preparation, only a few inexpensive instruments, and very little time and care of equipment; it is successful in most adults and children over the ages of 6 or 7 years. Mirror laryngoscopy may be especially useful when nasolaryngoscopy is not available, for patients at low risk of malignancy, and during follow-up for a known lesion after complete nasolaryngoscopy has excluded other lesions. It may also be useful as a preliminary examination before nasolaryngoscopy. It should be noted that since a mirror is used, everything visualized will be in reverse.

Note: When not used on a regular basis, the required coordination of instruments for mirror laryngoscopy often makes it difficult, and occasionally impossible, to examine patients—even for expert laryngologists. This fact was highlighted when a survey in the 1980s reported that less than 30% of practicing primary care physicians in Ohio were able to visualize a larynx, and that less than 4% included inspection of the larynx as part of their complete physical examination. Primary care clinicians in Ohio are probably representative of those elsewhere, and a few commented anonymously that they had never visualized a larynx!

INDICATIONS

- Chronic hoarseness (more than 3 weeks)
- Suspected or previous neoplasia
- Chronic cough
- Chronic dyspnea
- Halitosis
- Head or neck masses
- Dysphagia
- Phonation disturbance such as vocal weakness in the elderly or psychogenic dysphonia
- Chronic foreign-body sensation in pharynx
- Hemoptysis
- Suspected laryngeal foreign body
- Acute onset of hoarseness after straining voice
- Stridor, particularly inspiratory stridor
- Posttraumatic evaluation
- Any unilateral upper respiratory complaint in a smoker
- Any clinical situation in which visualization of the hypopharynx and larynx will aid in diagnosis or therapy

CONTRAINDICATIONS

- Acute epiglottitis. (Patient has a toxic appearance, leans forward, drools secretions, and may not be able to talk.) Laryngoscopy may precipitate complete airway obstruction.
- Infants and very young children who are unable to cooperate (not suitable candidates).
- Acute inflammation or infection of the throat *(relative contraindication)*.
- Patients who cannot adequately open their mouth *(relative contraindication)*.

EQUIPMENT

- Bright headlight or head mirror with external light source
- No. 4 and no. 5 laryngeal mirrors; smaller sizes for children
- 4 × 4–inch gauze sponges
- Local anesthetic: lidocaine* spray (2% to 4%) or benzocaine* spray (14%)

---

*Should be used with caution in those who have a history of an allergy or sensitivity to the agent (see Chapter 4, Local Anesthesia).

• Goggles
• Alcohol lamp or bowl of hot water to warm mirrors *(optional)*

PREPROCEDURE PATIENT PREPARATION AND EVALUATION

After performing a thorough head and neck history and examination, as well as the remainder of a complete history and physical examination, explain the indications, alternatives, and the procedure itself. Inform the patient that it is important to relax and that the mirror will be placed in the top of the back of his or her mouth, avoiding the throat. The patient should know that in most cases, if performed properly or if anesthetic is used, this procedure should not stimulate the gag reflex. Possible complications should be explained. Dentures should be removed.

TECHNIQUE

1. The patient should sit upright with the body straight, preferably in a high-backed chair with a headrest. Tell the patient to lean slightly forward. The head and jaw should jut forward in a "sniffing" position (Fig. 73-1). The chin should be up.
2. Sit slightly to the side of the patient. Sitting slightly higher than the patient should also facilitate visualization of the laryngeal structures. Position the light source or mirror so that light is directed parallel to your visual axis and focused on the patient's posterior pharynx. The examiner should be comfortable and understand that the use of a hurried approach can make this procedure more difficult.
3. Spray the patient's pharynx with anesthetic and have him or her gargle and spit it out.
4. Select the largest mirror that will fit comfortably in the back of the throat, and warm it over the alcohol lamp, in the warm water, or inside the patient's cheek. If the mirror is externally warmed, check its temperature on the back of your hand to make sure it is not too hot before insertion. Warming the mirror should prevent fogging.
5. Cover the patient's protruded tongue with gauze, and grasp it firmly between the thumb and middle finger of your nondominant hand. Do not pull so hard as to cause discomfort. Use your index finger to retract the patient's upper lip.
6. Ask the patient to breathe in and out through the mouth or to "pant like a puppy." This opens the space between the soft palate and the tongue. Have the patient focus on your forehead or headband to serve as a distraction.
7. With the warm mirror in the dominant hand and the glass surface pointing downward, slowly introduce the mirror and visualize the epiglottis. Next, slowly and gently apply the posterior aspect of the mirror to the uvula and a portion of the soft palate. With a smooth, gentle movement, slowly lift them upward and backward out of the way. Avoid touching either the posterior pharyngeal wall or the base of the tongue. Touching these might stimulate the gag reflex (Fig. 73-2).

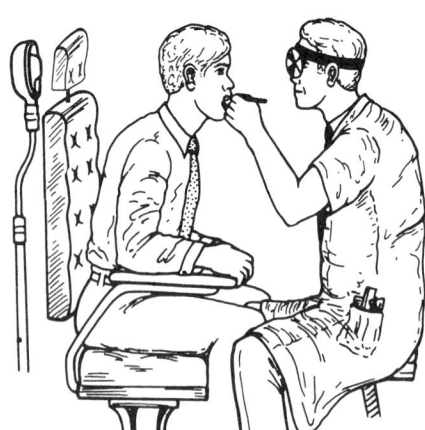

Fig. 73-1
Proper positioning of the patient is essential for successful visualization of the larynx.

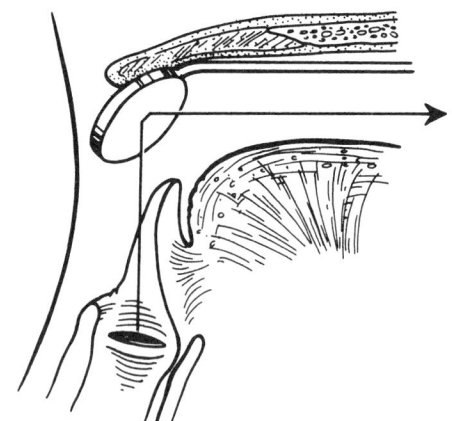

Fig. 73-2
Laryngeal mirror is inserted into the pharynx, lifting the uvula but avoiding contact with the posterior pharyngeal wall.

Note: In certain patients, adequate anesthesia is not attainable for this portion of the procedure. In those cases, nasolaryngoscopy should be performed.

8. With the mirror gently lifting the uvula and soft palate out of the way, tilt it in various directions to visualize the larynx, the hypopharynx, and the anterior oropharynx, including the base of the tongue. Move your head toward and away from the mirror to focus the light source maximally on visualized objects (Fig. 73-3). Continue to encourage the patient to breathe gently in and out through the mouth. If the structures are not adequately visualized after lifting the soft palate and uvula out of the way, check the positioning of the patient's chin and neck. Reposition if necessary.

9. With the larynx visualized, observe vocal cord activity during quiet respiration. Next, observe cord activity while the patient holds a prolonged high "eee" sound. Observe for symmetry of cord mobility and for edema, hemorrhages, erythema, nodules, or masses of the cords or surrounding structures. Note any other mucosal or structural abnormalities (see Fig. 69-6 in Chapter 69, Flexible Fiberoptic Nasolaryngoscopy).

Note: All structures viewed will be seen in mirror image (upside-down and backwards).

10. If the mirror fogs up during the procedure, it needs to be reheated. If externally heated, it needs to be tested again before use. For those patients whose pharynx is not suitably visualized by this technique, or for those in which a closer evaluation of an

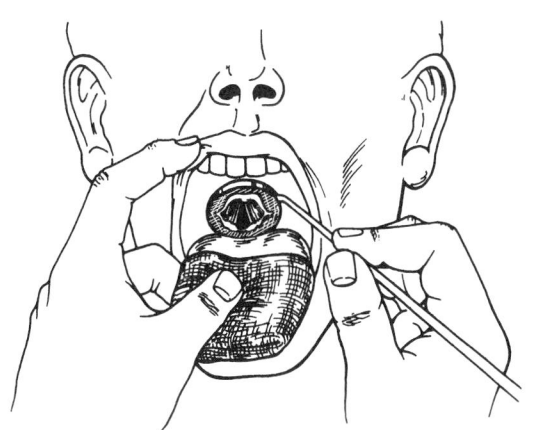

Fig. 73-3
The tongue is pulled forward with gauze, and the mirror is tilted in various directions to visualize the larynx, the hypopharynx, and the anterior oropharynx.

abnormality is indicated, fiberoptic nasolaryngoscopy should be performed or referral to an otolaryngologist considered.

FINDINGS

- Epiglottis: usually has a slightly curved and regular upper edge but is sometimes acutely curved and conical ("infantile type"). It may hang backwards and obscure the view of the cords in the relaxed state or hang forward to hide the valleculae. It rises upwards and forwards during phonation.
- Aryepiglottic folds: may have swelling or ulceration.
- Interarytenoid area: may be thickened or covered with papilla.
- False cords: may show swelling or ulceration.
- Vocal cords must be examined for the following:
  Color: normal color is pearly white.
  Movement: may be restricted by paresis or by infiltration of tumor. Arthritis of cricoarytenoid joint also limits movement.
  Surface: may be intact or ulcerated.
  Edge: may be irregular.
  Anterior commissure: not always seen.
- Subglottic space: difficult to examine but swellings may be seen below the level of the vocal cords.

COMPLICATIONS

- Possible laceration of the undersurface of the tongue from stretching the tongue over the teeth
- Possible adverse reaction to anesthetic
- Vomiting—with possible aspiration
- Failure to diagnose an abnormality because of inadequate visualization

CPT/BILLING CODE

No separate code is available for this procedure. Consider using a more comprehensive E/M code.

ICD-9-CM DIAGNOSTIC CODES

784.41	Aphonia
786.05	Chronic dyspnea
786.2	Cough, chronic
491.0	smokers
787.2	Dysphagia
933.0	Foreign body in pharynx
933.0	hypopharynx

933.1	larynx
784.9	Halitosis
786.3	Hemoptysis
784.49	Hoarseness
161.9	Laryngeal cancer, NEC
784.2	Neck mass
306.1	Psychogenic dysphonia
786.1	Stridor

BIBLIOGRAPHY

Benjamin BNP, *Diagnostic laryngology,* Philadelphia, 1990, WB Saunders.

Gray RF, Hawthorne M, *Synopsis of otolaryngology,* ed 5, Oxford, 1992, Butterworth-Heinemann.

CHAPTER 74

Peritonsillar Abscess Drainage

Roger K. Waage

Peritonsillar abscess, an infection in the space between the tonsil and the pharyngeal constrictors, is the most common deep infection of the head and neck. Historically, it was thought that peritonsillar abscess developed as a progression of acute exudative tonsillitis. Currently, peritonsillar abscess is thought to originate in Weber's salivary glands in the supratonsillar fossa. Weber's salivary glands are a group of 20 to 25 mucous salivary glands located in the space just above the tonsil that are connected by a duct to the surface of the tonsil. They assist with digestion of food particles trapped in the tonsillar crypts. The fact that a peritonsillar abscess can occur despite tonsillectomy supports the theory that Weber's glands are involved in the pathogenesis.

Peritonsillar abscess is usually polymicrobial in nature. The most common organisms are *Streptococcus pyogenes, Staphylococcus aureus,* and *Bacteroides.* Herzon (1995) has shown that outcomes are the same regardless of which antibiotic is used (appropriate for these organisms) and which of these organisms is involved.

Peritonsillar abscess commonly occurs in the second and third decade and rarely occurs in young children. Symptoms include fever, malaise, severe sore throat, and dysphagia with drooling and trismus. Pain is often referred to the ear, and the patient may have a "hot potato" voice. Signs of peritonsillar abscess include marked edema, a fluctuant fullness of the soft palate, and a shiny membrane superior to the tonsils. The classic sign is deflection of the swollen uvula to the opposite side. There is often inferior and medial displacement of the affected tonsil. Tender cervical adenopathy is often present.

The differential diagnosis of peritonsillar abscess includes peritonsillar cellulitis, neoplasm, retropharyngeal abscess, herpes simplex tonsillitis, infectious mononucleosis, and retromolar abscess. It is important to differentiate because peritonsillar cellulitis has nearly identical symptoms but markedly different treatments. One basic difference is that pus cannot be aspirated or drained from cellulitis. Therefore diagnosis of peritonsillar cellulitis is often made after peritonsillar abscess has been excluded. Intraoral ultrasonography may be another diagnostic option, but it requires a skilled and experienced ultrasonographer. If the diagnosis is made early, treatment of cellulitis does not require drainage, but rather IV antibiotics.

The treatment of peritonsillar abscess has traditionally been either tonsillectomy or incision and drainage (I&D). If untreated, the abscess can rupture, possibly causing aspiration, pneumonia, sepsis, or death. An untreated abscess can also spread locally or hematogenously with resultant extensive local infection or meningitis. Patients with a peritonsillar abscess and a history of three episodes of tonsillitis in the past year should probably be sent for an abscess/tonsillectomy. However, for those patients without recurrent tonsillitis, there is growing evidence that needle aspiration may be the treatment of choice. Needle aspiration has been shown to have a 94% success rate. Of those patients who initially respond, 10% will have a recurrence. A second needle aspiration should again have a 94% success rate. Patients who fail a second or third needle aspiration should probably have an abscess/tonsillectomy. The 6% who fail to resolve with a needle aspiration on their initial presentation should probably have an I&D or be referred to an otolaryngologist to rule out a possible pterygomaxillary space abscess. An algorithm for the management of peritonsillar abscess is shown in Fig. 74-1.

Needle aspiration does have some drawbacks. It is painful, invasive, and performed blindly. A recent series of 12 patients evaluated by Haeggstrom and associates demonstrated that abscesses were located within 4 to 25 mm of the carotid artery. Needle aspiration also only samples one area in the tonsillar fossa and may require repeated attempts. However, it is relatively simple to perform, even by those who are not ear, nose, and throat specialists, and does not require expensive or specialized equipment. Herzon's (1980) study on the efficacy of needle aspiration showed that 80% of aspirations were performed by interns and 20% by emergency medicine specialists.

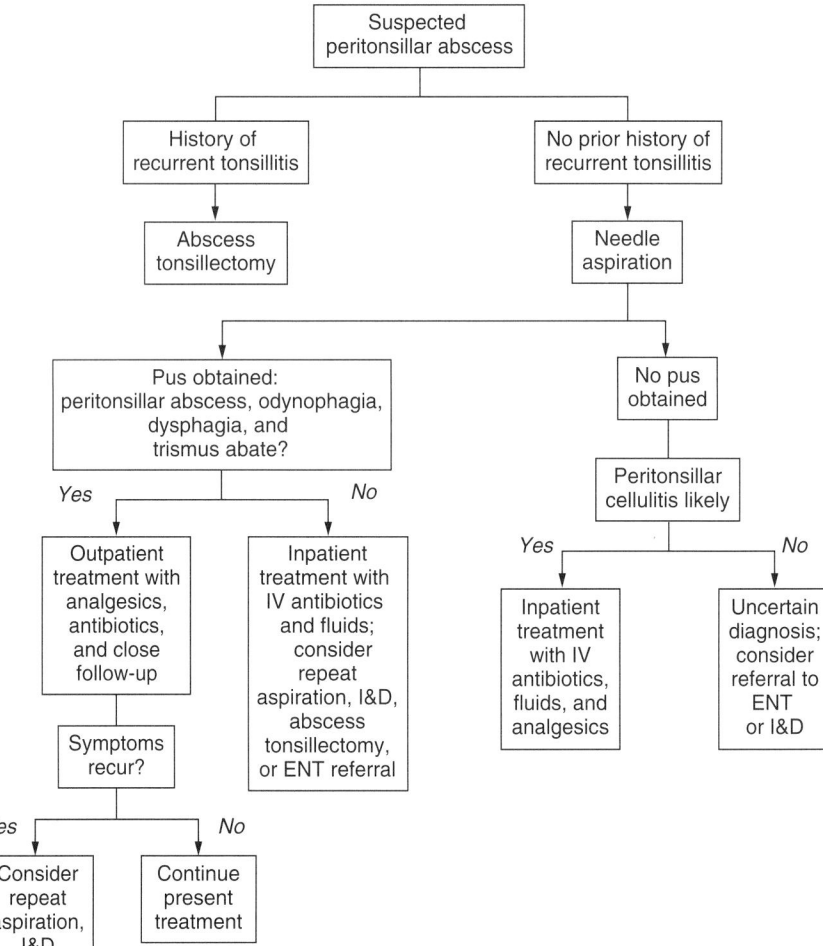

Fig. 74-1
Algorithm for management of peritonsillar abscess. *ENT,* Ear, nose, and throat; *I&D,* incision and drainage.

INDICATIONS

- Peritonsillar abscess in a patient who is not indicated for abscess/tonsillectomy

CONTRAINDICATIONS

- Septic shock or impending respiratory compromise (patient should first be stabilized)
- Uncooperative patients
- Operator unfamiliar with anatomy
- Inadequate equipment

EQUIPMENT

For needle aspiration:
- Cetacaine spray (or 4% cocaine)
- 2% lidocaine with epinephrine 1:100,000 with a 25-gauge, 1½-inch needle
- 18-gauge spinal needle on a 10-ml syringe or Cameco syringe pistol

(*Note:* As a guide to keep from going too deep, place a Steri-Strip 8 mm proximal to the needle tip or cut the end off of the needle cover, leaving 8 mm of needle exposed.)
- Suction: Tonsillar or no. 8 Frazier
- Good lighting: headlight or head mirror with gooseneck lamp
- Kidney basin
- Tongue depressor
- Surgical assistant

For I&D:
- All of the above, plus a curved tonsil or Kelly clamp and a no. 15 scalpel blade

PREPROCEDURE PATIENT PREPARATION

The procedure of choice for most patients is needle aspiration. Advise the patient that the pus can usually be aspirated successfully and, if so, the symptoms will improve dramatically. If this is successful, the patient can be treated with oral antibiotics and analgesics, and hospitalization can be avoided. If the abscess is not successfully drained or if the symptoms do not resolve, further treatment and hospitalization may be required. The patient should also be told that there is a 10% chance of recurrence. Other potential risks and complications should be discussed.

TECHNIQUE

1. Seat the patient leaning slightly forward, at a level at which he or she is eye to eye with the operator. A kidney basin should be available for the patient to expectorate. Suction must be readily available with either a tonsillar or no. 8 Frazier. Good lighting is necessary, provided either by a headlight or a head mirror with a bright light source behind the patient.

2. Have the patient open his or her mouth as wide as possible. If trismus restricts jaw motion, the patient may need some encouragement to open more widely. Mild pressure on the lower jaw may also be necessary to help open the mouth. Palpate the soft palate to localize the fluctuant area, and administer topical Cetacaine or spray 4% cocaine to the affected side. When the topical anesthetic has taken effect, inject 2% lidocaine with epinephrine (using a 25-gauge, 1½-inch needle or tonsil needle) into the mucosa, just above and lateral to the tonsil.

3. After a few minutes, attempt aspiration. Hold the tongue depressor in your nondominant hand and the aspirating syringe in your dominant hand. You may need to ask your assistant to create suction with the syringe. Insert the 18-gauge spinal needle on a 10-ml syringe, and attempt aspiration (Fig. 74-2). The Cameco syringe pistol allows both injection and aspiration with one hand. The needle should not be inserted more than 8 mm. If you aspirate pus, continue until no more pus returns. Scientific evidence suggests there is no reason to culture the aspirated fluid, which is usually between 2 and 14 ml of pus.

4. If you do not aspirate any pus, withdraw the needle slightly and redirect inferiorly. When performing this procedure, be aware that the carotid artery lies approximately 2 cm posterior and lateral to the tonsillar pillars. In fact, the more the needle is directed toward the lower pole of the tonsil, the more likely it is to enter the carotid artery. Never aspirate lateral to the molar or to a depth greater than 1 cm. If blood returns on aspiration, the procedure should be stopped, the needle should be removed, and direct pressure should be applied to the puncture site. An otolaryngologist should be consulted immediately.

5. If the aspiration is unsuccessful and the diagnosis of peritonsillar abscess is certain, an immediate I&D can be performed. With a no. 15 scalpel, make an incision

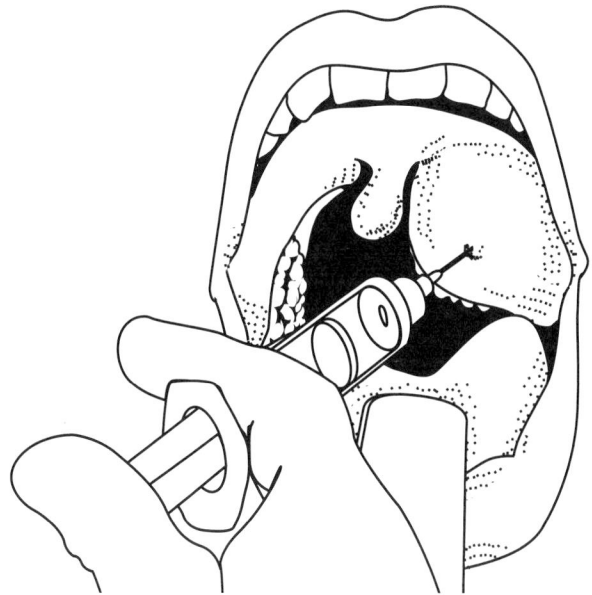

Fig. 74-2
Classic appearance of a peritonsillar abscess. This should be anesthetized topically with Cetacaine, injected with 2% lidocaine with epinephrine, and then aspirated with an 18-gauge spinal needle at the point of maximal fluctuance.

just through the mucosa above the upper pole of the tonsil at the point of maximum prominence (Fig. 74-3). Maximum prominence is usually demonstrated as a shiny membrane over the abscess. After an incision is made through this membrane, there is often prompt expression of pus. Immediate and aggressive suction is required. Having the surgical assistant ready with the suction placed at the incision site—before the incision is made—often provides the patient with the most comfort.

6. Sometimes the incision needs to be widened with a tonsillar clamp. Any loculations that are apparent should be opened. Loculations are especially common inferiorly. Any remaining pus or blood should be suctioned before the procedure is finished.

7. All patients successfully treated by needle aspiration or I&D may be sent home with penicillin (or erythromycin if they are allergic to penicillin). Liquid elixirs are much easier for the patient to swallow. Anaerobic coverage with metronidazole or clindamycin is probably not necessary.

COMPLICATIONS

- Hemorrhage
- Tracheal aspiration of purulent material
- Respiratory distress
- Pneumonia
- Failed aspiration or I&D, cellulitis, or recurrence

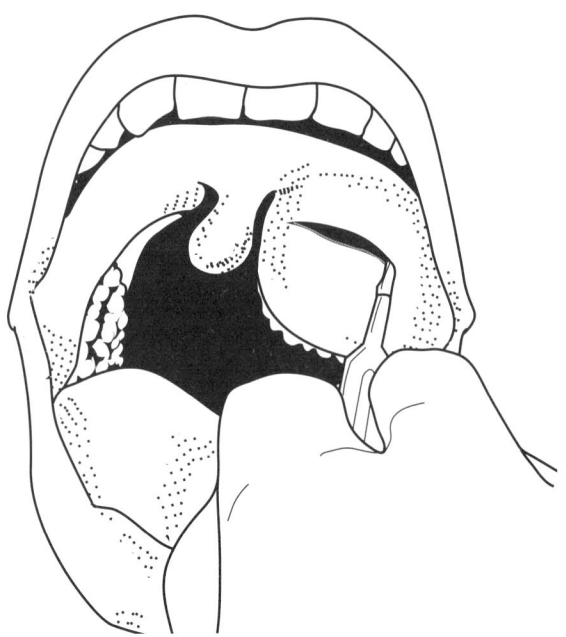

Fig. 74-3
If incision and drainage is the preferred treatment, the incision should be made above the upper pole of the tonsil at the point of maximal fluctuance. The incision may need to be probed or widened with a curved Kelly or tonsillar clamp.

INTERPRETATION OF FINDINGS

Most patients can be managed by following the algorithm in Fig. 74-1. If the trismus and odynophagia subside, the patient may be treated as an outpatient and followed closely. If no pus is obtained even after the needle is redirected, the diagnosis of peritonsillar abscess is questionable. Many of these patients have peritonsillar cellulitis that responds to IV antibiotics. If there is uncertainty, referral to an otolaryngologist is indicated.

POSTPROCEDURE PATIENT EDUCATION

All patients who have been treated for a peritonsillar abscess need adequate antibiotics and analgesia, preferably liquid. Salt-water gargles help, along with following a soft diet. Patients should be instructed to return if they experience a recurrence of symptoms, fever greater than 101° F, or trouble breathing or swallowing. A follow-up appointment within 48 hours should be scheduled.

SUPPLIERS

Cameco Syringe Pistol
Precision Dynamics Corporation
13880 Del Sur Street
San Fernando, CA 91340-3490
Phone: 1-800-847-0670

CPT BILLING CODES

42700   Incision and drainage of peritonsillar abscess
88170   Needle aspiration (send location in remark area of insurance billing)

ICD-9-CM DIAGNOSTIC CODE

475   Peritonsillar abscess, quinsy, peritonsillar cellulitis

ADDITIONAL RESOURCES

- See the sample patient education handout titled "Peritonsillar Abscess Drainage" on page 1819 of Appendix G.
- See the sample patient consent form titled "Peritonsillar Abscess Drainage" on page 1820 of Appendix G.

BIBLIOGRAPHY

Epperly T, Wood T: New trends in the management of peritonsillar abscess, *Am Fam Physician* 42:102, 1990.

Haeggstrom A, Gustafsson O, Engquist S, et al: Intraoral ultrasoundography in the diagnosis of peritonsillar abscess, *Otolaryngol Head Neck Surg* 108:243, 1993.

Herzon F: Peritonsillar abscess: incidence, current management practices, and a proposal for treatment guidelines, *Laryngoscope* 105:1, 1995.

Herzon F, Aldridge J: Peritonsillar abscess: needle aspiration, *Otolaryngol Head Neck Surg* 89:910, 1980.

Passy LV: Pathogenesis of peritonsillar abscess, *Laryngoscope* 104:185, 1994.

Strong E, Woodward P, Johnson L: Intraoral ultrasound evaluation of peritonsillar abscess, *Laryngoscope* 105:779, 1995.

CHAPTER 75

Management of Tooth Fracture and Reimplantation of an Avulsed Tooth

Grant C. Fowler

Traumatic damage to a tooth, ranging from a slight enamel chip to avulsion, is one of the most common injuries to the face. It occurs 3 million times annually in the United States. Often, the primary care clinician is the first person to evaluate such an injury. Occasionally, the clinician will receive a phone call from a patient requesting guidance after an avulsion or fracture. Knowledge of proper storage and treatment of an avulsed tooth is important to optimize the chances of successful replantation (reimplantation). Proper management of a fracture may minimize pain and disfigurement.

Management of a dental fracture is based on the extent of the fracture (Fig. 75-1) and the age of the patient. An Ellis I fracture only involves the enamel of the tooth. It may be a mere "chip" off of the tooth. Management is only necessary if a resultant sharp edge is disturbing the adjacent soft tissues. In that case, a nail file can be used to file down the edge. Referral can made to a general dentist for cosmetic restoration.

An Ellis II fracture involves not only the enamel, but also exposes the dentin layer. Patients should be warned that any trauma to a tooth may lead to pulpal necrosis or tooth resorption, regardless of management. Dental referral is required within 24 hours. Patients under 12 years of age have less dentin, so there is usually less discomfort. Regardless of age, the exposed dentin should be covered with calcium hydroxide paste or toothpaste and then with a dry gauze. Patients over 12 years of age should be advised to avoid extremes of intraoral temperatures. A piece of tinfoil over the paste and gauze may protect the patient further from temperature extremes.

Ellis III fractures expose the pulp of the tooth. Dentin can be distinguished from pulp in that dentin produces a red blush whereas exposed pulp will yield a drop of blood. These fractures are a dental emergency. Significant delay in care can lead to long-term pain and abscess formation. The clinician should not attempt to probe the pulp or remove any material; he or she should cover the affected area with tinfoil, provide adequate analgesia, and consider oral antibiotics to cover mouth flora. The patient should consult a dentist immediately.

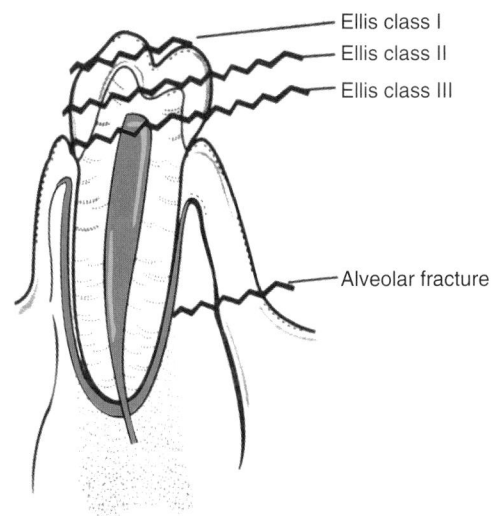

Fig. 75-1
Ellis classification for fractures of anterior teeth. (From James DM: Immediate management of tooth fracture and avulsion. In James DM, editor: *Field guide to urgent and ambulatory care procedures,* Philadelphia, 2001, Lippincott, Williams & Wilkins.)

Teeth are held in place by surrounding periodontal membrane fibers and ligaments (Fig. 75-2). With trauma, these fibers may be concussed (Fig. 75-3), a tooth may be subluxated (ligaments damaged), or an entire tooth may be avulsed (Fig. 75-4). If examination of the surrounding gingiva reveals blood, there has usually been ligamentous damage. If the tooth can be wiggled, it confirms such damage. Minimally mobile teeth will "firm up" over a week or two. The patient should maintain a soft diet and avoid undue pressure on the affected teeth.

In the event of avulsion, the neurovascular supply is disrupted. The more rapidly the tooth is replanted, the more likely the tooth will remain viable. If the tooth can be replanted within 5 minutes, there is a greater than 80% chance that the tooth will remain vital. Given this urgency, bystanders or clinicians should not be overly

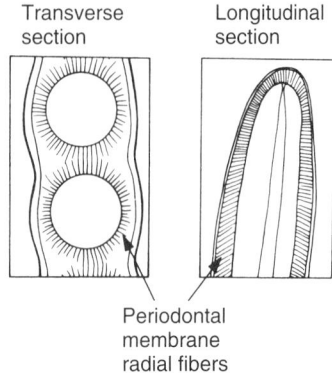

Fig. 75-2
Arrangement of periodontal fibers.

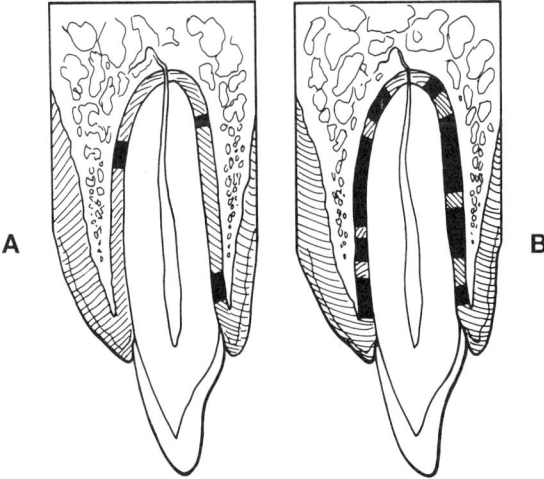

Fig. 75-3
A, Slightly and, **B,** moderately concussed tooth.

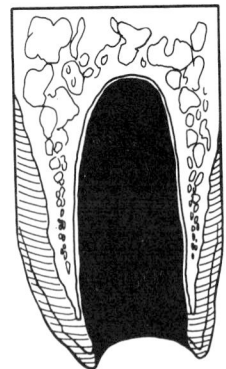

Fig. 75-4
Avulsed tooth.

concerned about cleaning or flushing the socket or tooth before replanting. To prepare for reimplantation, while avoiding touching the root, debris and large clots should merely be brushed off. Small clots or dirt can be removed by having the patient place the tooth under his or her tongue for just a few seconds. Then immediate replantation with follow-up by a dentist is all that is necessary.

However, for the tooth that is not immediately replanted, proper storage is a crucial factor for later success. Prognosis deteriorates rapidly—within minutes—as the tooth dries out, causing pulpal and periodontal damage. Storage media available to prevent drying, in order from most to less successful, are milk, physiologic (normal) saline, and saliva. An egg white may also be used. These fluids have an osmotic pressure similar to those of the pulp and periodontal tissues and help preserve these structures. Tap water is an inappropriate storage media because of its hypotonicity.

Although milk is superior to saliva as a storage media, the prevention of dessication is much more important than waiting until milk is available. If milk is not *immediately* available, the tooth can be stored in saliva. When it becomes available, perhaps the best and most readily available preservative is milk on ice (between 4° and 20° C).

INDICATIONS

- Avulsed permanent tooth with minimal pulpal and periodontal damage, especially a tooth from the front of the mouth
- Tooth out of its socket for only a brief period
- Tooth stored in the proper physiologic medium

Note: One readily available source of saliva is the mouth; therefore the tooth can be stored in the patient's mouth (under the tongue), or in the mouth of a relative if the patient is unconscious, until replantation. If stored in the patient's mouth, he or she needs to concentrate on not swallowing the tooth! Universal blood and body fluid precautions should be remembered if stored in someone else's mouth.

CONTRAINDICATIONS

- Deciduous (milk or temporary) teeth should not be reimplanted. (Reimplanting these teeth may result in their fusion to the supporting bone and possible facial deformity.)
- Gross caries or fractures in an avulsed tooth.
- Significant loss of periodontal support before traumatic incident (periodontitis).
- Nonvital periodontal ligament (tooth has dried for 1 hour or more).

EQUIPMENT

- Adequate light
- Sterile normal saline
- Irrigation syringe
- Local anesthetic and syringe
- Cotton gauze or tooth forceps
- Tinfoil
- Dental radiograph equipment and supplies
- Penicillin VK 500 mg tablets (18 to 26 tablets) and parenteral antibiotics (for those at risk, see Chapter 204, Antibiotic Prophylaxis for Bacterial Endocarditis)
- Cyanoacrylate glue *(optional)*

PREPROCEDURE PATIENT PREPARATION

Explain the possible complications and the need for follow-up to the patient. They will need to remain still but should experience minimal discomfort.

Note: Immediate replantation (within 5 minutes) is one of the most critical factors related to periodontal healing. If the interval is more than 30 minutes before replantation, the success rate falls to less than 20%. If the patient or family member calls and is more than 5 minutes away from clinical care, an attempt to replant the tooth immediately provides the best outcome. Have the patient rinse the tooth under cold water or place it under his or her tongue for a few seconds, and then reimplant it at once. Instructions or words of encouragement may be needed. However, accident-associated factors such as the person's emotional state, a lack of knowledge of proper first aid, a lack of confidence by the bystanders, or informed consent issues are often obstacles at the accident site. If these obstacles cannot be overcome, the only choice may be to store the tooth in the best available medium and to transport the patient to the clinic.

TECHNIQUE

1. If the tooth is stored in milk upon arrival, leave it in the milk. If it is stored in saliva or no media, place the avulsed tooth in normal saline as soon as possible.
2. If the patient is at risk for bacteremia, administer parenteral antibiotics.
3. Conduct a rapid medical history and systematic evaluation of the traumatized individual:
   - Where, how, and when did the trauma occur? Are there fractures?
   - Is there any neurologic damage? Unconsciousness? Amnesia? Headache? Nausea?
   - Are there any underlying medical conditions? Immunocompromise? Diabetes? Prostheses or severe mitral valve prolapse? Heart murmurs? If any of

these are life- or limb-threatening, they should be managed first. If not, make mental notes of other problems while rapidly preparing to reimplant the tooth.
4. When the patient is stable, administer local anesthetic to the socket area if necessary.
5. Perform a brief clinical examination:
   - Are there any other intraoral lacerations or disturbances?
   - Is the bite disturbed by other displaced teeth?
   - Make mental notes of these findings while rapidly preparing to reimplant the tooth.
6. Examine the tooth socket and flush with normal saline. Remove all clot material.
7. Rinse the root and apex of the tooth with normal saline while being careful not to handle the root surface.

Note: Although flushing the socket and rinsing the tooth are commonly suggested in practice guidelines, there is little scientific evidence to support these activities. That is why replanting the tooth at the scene of the accident, if it can be accomplished within 5 to 10 minutes, is much more important than waiting to flush the socket or tooth.

8. Hold the tooth with gauze or tooth forceps, and replant the tooth as close as possible to its normal position using finger pressure. *Do not touch the root.* Make sure the alignment is anatomic (remember that the curved side faces the tongue!).
9. Take a radiograph of the area, if possible.
10. Refer to a dentist for semi-rigid splinting and follow-up. If a dentist is not available, aluminum foil can be wrapped over the tooth, and the neighboring teeth to act as a splint. A small paper clip can also be bent to conform to the buccal side of the neighboring teeth. Glue the paper clip to the reimplanted tooth as well as two or three neighboring teeth with cyanoacrylate glue. The dentist can later remove glue with a dental pick.
11. Administer penicillin VK 1 g immediately (for those not already given parenteral dose), then 500 mg four times a day for 4 to 6 days (for those not allergic to penicillin).
12. Administer tetanus toxoid if the patient has not had a booster within 5 years.

POSTPROCEDURE PATIENT EDUCATION

Patients should be warned that any trauma to a tooth may cause pulpal necrosis or tooth resorption, regardless of management. For an Ellis II fracture, dental referral should occur within 24 hours. An Ellis III fracture is an emergency.

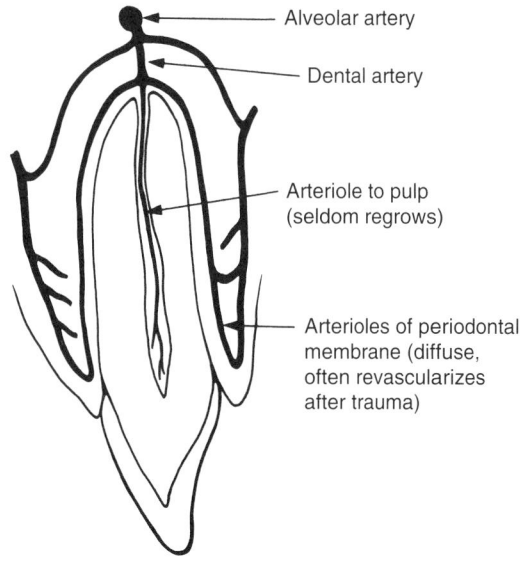

Alveolar artery

Dental artery

Arteriole to pulp
(seldom regrows)

Arterioles of periodontal
membrane (diffuse,
often revascularizes
after trauma)

Fig. 75-5
Blood supply to tooth.

For an avulsed tooth, inform the patient that the prognosis depends on the length of time the tooth was out of the socket and the medium in which it was stored. Fortunately, a tooth has two sources of blood supply (Fig. 75-5). However, pulpal revascularization of the pulpal arterioles is almost nonexistent in teeth after complete root development (adult teeth). It is unusual even with immature root development. Periodontal ligament preservation is also infrequent, depending on the length of drying time to which the tooth was exposed. Fortunately, the periodontal ligament has a more diffuse blood supply and revascularizes more readily than the pulp. However, the importance of consulting a dentist for the appropriate follow-up care should be stressed, especially if further splinting is necessary.

COMPLICATIONS

- Necrosis of the pulp or periodontal ligament or complete loss of the tooth can occur. (Necrotic pulp tissue necessitates subsequent endodontic work.)

- With a nonvital periodontal ligament, ankylosis or osteoclastic root resorption can occur. This result requires a root canal.
- Localized infection or bacteremia can occur, but it is very rare.

CPT/BILLING CODE

D7270   Tooth reimplantation and/or stabilization of accidentally avulsed or displaced tooth and/or alveolus (HCPCS Code)

ICD-9-CM DIAGNOSTIC CODE

525.11   Loss of teeth due to trauma
873.63   Avulsed tooth or open fracture of tooth

BIBLIOGRAPHY

Barrett EJ, Kenny DJ: Avulsed permanent teeth: a review of the literature and treatment guidelines, *Endod Dent Traumatol* 13:153, 1997.
James DM: Immediate management of tooth fracture and avulsion. In James DM, editor: *Field guide to urgent and ambulatory care procedures,* Philadelphia, 2001, Lippincott, Williams & Wilkins.
Layug ML, Barrett EJ, Kenny DJ: Interim storage of avulsed permanent teeth, *J Can Dent Assoc* 64(5):357, 365, 1998.
Protocols for clinical pediatric dentistry, ed 3, Boston, 1995, The Journal of Pedodontics.
Treatment of the avulsed permanent tooth: recommended guidelines of the American Association of Endodontists, American Association of Endodontists, *Dent Clin North Am* 39(1):221, 1995.

CHAPTER 76

Tongue-Tie Snipping (Frenotomy) for Ankyloglossia

Gary R. Newkirk

"Tongue-tie," or ankyloglossia, can be maxillary or mandibular. Maxillary ankyloglossia occurs when the tongue is ankylosed to the hard palate or the alveolar ridge, or, if cleft palate coexists, the tongue can be ankylosed to the lower edge of the nasal septum. Mandibular ankyloglossia results from underdevelopment of the lingual frenulum. In this situation the frenulum is attached from the midline near the tip of the tongue, along the floor of the mouth to the lower gingiva.

Infants differ substantially in the degree to which their frenulum attaches to the tongue. Most cases of tongue-tie are thought to resolve spontaneously by adulthood with little likelihood of feeding or speech-development problems. Usually parents are the first to notice tongue-tie in their infant or child and bring this to the clinician's attention (Fig. 76-1). The condition can easily be overlooked during the newborn examination, because infants typically retract the tongue when their mouth is open. A retracted tongue covers up a short frenulum. Furthermore, a newborn rarely sticks out their tongue, so no one notices if the tongue cannot be protruded because of ankyloglossia.

Since tongue-tie is a rare condition that lacks a precise definition, there have been no formal outcome studies comparing infants who have and who have not undergone frenotomy. However, problems with sucking, breastfeeding, chewing, swallowing, dentofacial growth and development, gingival hygiene, and speech have been attributed to tongue-tie. Some researchers feel that the parents, not the child, have the problem. Others feel that simple frenotomy, also referred to as tongue-tie snipping, remains a quick, easy, and safe procedure with benefits. Even if the benefits are only cosmetic, they may in some instances outweigh the family anxiety generated by this condition.

The best method and timing for reducing partial ankyloglossia remains debatable. When ankyloglossia *severely* interferes with lingual function (e.g., "frozen tongue"), few would argue the need for reduction; but in this case, Z-plasty is necessary. The patient should be referred to a surgeon, since this procedure requires general anesthesia. Some clinicians feel that frenotomy should be attempted if partial ankyloglossia contributes to poor infant sucking and other breastfeeding problems such as insufficient infant weight gain, sore nipples, or recurrent mastitis in the mother. Simple frenotomy for infants and small children who have partial ankyloglossia can be performed in the clinic or outpatient setting.

INDICATIONS

- Clinical evidence of short lingual frenulum inhibiting tongue protrusion, feeding, swallowing, or speech

CONTRAINDICATIONS

- Lack of clinical evidence or suspicion that ankyloglossia is a problem for the infant or child.
- Unstable medical conditions, such as bleeding disorders or diabetes mellitus.
- The procedure should be postponed if there is evidence of dental or oral infection, until the infection is adequately treated or resolves.
- Severe ankyloglossia, which requires frenectomy under general anesthesia. (Usually this procedure involves Z-plasty or a similar plastics procedure.)

EQUIPMENT

- Tongue retractor
- Small Metzenbaum scissors
- Small mosquito clip or hemostat
- Topical benzocaine 20% (e.g., Hurricane syrup)
- Lidocaine 1% with epinephrine
- Cotton-tipped swabs
- Ice cubes *(optional)*

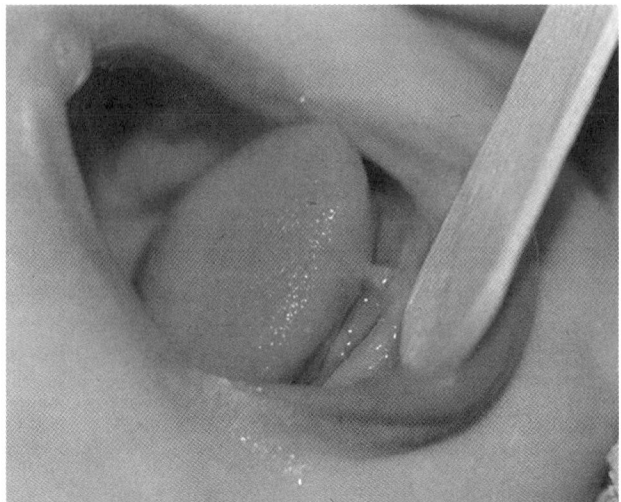

Fig. 76-1
Eight-week old infant with ankyloglossia (tongue-tie) noticed by the parents. This finding was not identified at the time of the newborn examination.

PREPROCEDURE PATIENT PREPARATION

Describe the risks to the parents, including possible medication reaction (if used), injury, infection, or bleeding. For children, parents may help by holding them in their lap and holding the child's head still. They may also help hold the child's mouth open. However, for newborns and infants—for the same reasons as for a circumcision—parents may want to leave the room. After examining the child, if more than one technique is possible, the clinician should explain the various techniques to the parents. Attempt to obtain their input on the desired technique.

TECHNIQUE

1. With assistance as necessary, position or hold small infants or children in such a way that they will remain still.

Note: Crying often improves exposure of the frenulum.

2. Identify the frenulum and the necessary degree of surgical lysis. A limited "snipping" of the lucent, membranous portion of the distal frenulum is usually all that is required.

3. Many clinicians snip a lucent membranous or very thin fibrinous distal frenulum without topical agents or the use of a hemostat. This technique may increase local bleeding; however, for a thin membrane, there should be no more bleeding than when a child falls

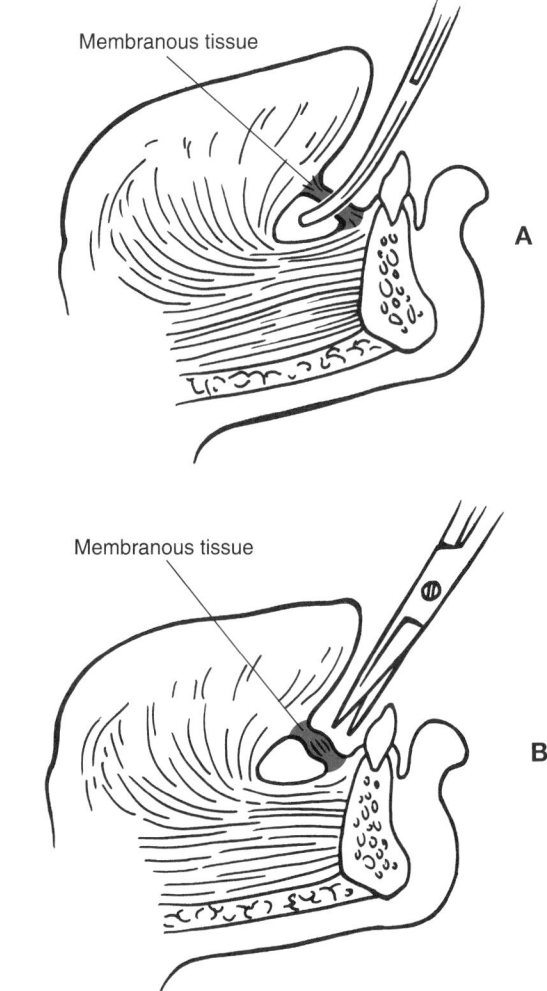

Fig. 76-2
Tongue-tie snipping technique. **A,** Crush the frenulum where the snip is to be made. **B,** Cut through the crushed area.

and bites a lip or tongue. This technique may cause less overall trauma than with the use of a hemostat. If the child is old enough not to aspirate, have him or her suck on ice, ice chips, or a Popsicle before and after the procedure for a certain degree of anesthesia and to minimize bleeding. Younger children may use a frozen teething ring.

4. For a thicker or coarser frenulum, anesthesia may be beneficial. Dip a cotton-tipped swab in Hurricaine syrup, and apply it to the lower mouth and bottom of the tongue for excellent local anesthesia. Mild sedation may also be beneficial (see Chapter 7, Pediatric Sedation).

5. If necessary, retract the tongue. A small spoon or wooden tongue blade with a slit fashioned in the end may be helpful.

6. With the tip of the mosquito clamp, grab and crush

the frenulum to the depth and at the position where the scissor snip will be made (Fig. 76-2, *A*). After the discomfort from crushing the tissue has resolved, a certain degree of anesthesia is experienced in the crushed area.

7. Snip the crushed portion of the frenulum (Fig. 76-2, *B*). *Warning:* If tissue is snipped outside or beyond the crushed area of the frenulum, more bleeding and pain results.

Note: Although crushed tissue is somewhat anesthetized, a patient experiences some discomfort at the time of the crush. A child's immediate memory of pain as the result of an instrument being placed in the mouth may make it difficult to open the mouth again to snip the crushed frenulum. This is why some clinicians perform the procedure by simply snipping without using a hemostat when the frenulum is very thin. However, for a thicker and coarser frenulum, crushing the tissue with a hemostat is necessary. For older children, there is value in telling them that the painful part of the procedure is over after the hemostat has been applied and removed.

8. Use a dry cotton-tipped swab, or one soaked in 1% lidocaine with epinephrine, to control any bleeding or oozing. Ice, a teething ring, or a Popsicle may also help control oozing.

COMPLICATIONS

- Bleeding
- Infection
- Injury to tongue or sublingual mucosa or tissue

POSTPROCEDURE PATIENT EDUCATION

- Ask the patient (or parent) to report significant bleeding or signs of infection.
- Instruct parent(s) to allow infants and children to resume normal feeding habits immediately.
- Ice chips, an ice cube, or a Popsicle for children old enough to not aspirate—or a frozen teething ring for infants—may help stop any later bleeding or oozing.

- Ask the patient (or parent) to report any feeding difficulties or significant swelling.
- Inform the patient to return for follow-up in 2 weeks, or sooner if complications arise.

SUPPLIERS

Hurricaine Syrup
Beutlich LP Pharmaceuticals
1541 Shields Drive
Waukegan, IL 60085
Phone: 1-800-238-8542
Website: www.beutlich.com

CPT/BILLING CODE

41010   Incision of lingual frenulum (frenotomy)

ICD-9-CM DIAGNOSTIC CODE

750.0   Ankyloglossia

BIBLIOGRAPHY

Conway A: Ankyloglossia—to snip or not to snip: is that the question? *J Hum Lact* 6(3):101, 1990.

Marmet C, Shell E, Marmet R: Neonatal frenotomy may be necessary to correct breastfeeding problems, *J Hum Lact* 6(3):117, 1990.

Messner AH, Lalakea ML, Aby J, et al: Ankyloglossia: incidence and associated feeding difficulties, *Arch Otolaryngol Head Neck Surg* 126(1):36, 2000.

Paradise JL: Evaluation and treatment for ankyloglossia, *JAMA* 263:2371, 1990.

Wright JE: Tongue-tie, *J Paediatr Child Health* 31(4):276, 1995.

PART FIVE

Cardiovascular and Respiratory System Procedures

CHAPTER 77

Ambulatory Blood Pressure Monitoring

Russell D. White

GENERAL CONSIDERATIONS

Definition

Ambulatory blood pressure monitoring (ABPM) is an automated, noninvasive technique in which blood pressure measurements are obtained at predetermined intervals over an extended period (usually 24 hours or greater). The process involves application of a measuring and recording device to a patient. These devices are lightweight and use auscultatory and/or oscillometric methods to determine blood pressure. The auscultatory method works better during periods with patient movement and low noise, whereas the oscillometric method works better with high environmental noise and resting conditions. The recordings can be downloaded for analysis.

Principle

Hypertension is usually defined as systolic blood pressure of 140 mm Hg or greater and diastolic blood pressure of 90 mm Hg or greater. Hypertension is a major risk factor for such common diseases as cardiovascular disease, stroke, aortic aneurysm rupture, renal failure, and retinopathy.

Over 50 million Americans are thought to be hypertensive. Since some patients are hypertensive only during specific hours of the day, documentation of adequate blood pressure control over 24 hours is imperative to prevent sequelae. Studies have shown that hypertension during ABPM correlates with end-organ damage better than sporadic blood pressure measurements in a clinical setting. In addition, overtreatment of hypertension has led to complications such as transient hypotension, dizziness, and myocardial ischemia. Finally, as many as 21% of patients with mild blood pressure elevation in the office are *incorrectly* diagnosed with and treated for hypertension. ABPM facilitates appropriate diagnosis and management.

INDICATIONS

Routine sporadic blood pressure measurements in the clinical setting remain the recommended method to screen for and monitor hypertension. ABPM should not be used indiscriminately as a screening device. However, since clinical blood pressure measurements have led to false positive and false negative results, ABPM can be useful. Indications may include the following:

- Normal or borderline office hypertension with end-organ damage
- Persistent office hypertension without end-organ damage
- Discrepancy between office and home blood pressure measurements
- Episodic hypertensive measurements
- Episodic angina or pulmonary congestion *unrelated* to exercise
- Determination of the duration or efficacy of antihypertensive medications during the 24-hour treatment cycle
- Dosage adjustment of antihypertensive medications
- Documented hypertension unresponsive to treatment ("drug resistance")
- Suspected pressor ("white coat") hypertension
- Autonomic dysfunction
- Hypotensive symptoms while on antihypertensive medication
- Evaluation of syncope or pacemaker syndromes
- Scientific research

CONTRAINDICATIONS/LIMITATIONS

- Cost: some insurance companies may not reimburse for ABPM
- Irregular, rapid heart rate: limits blood pressure measurement
- Severe obesity: limits blood pressure measurement
- Severe patient anxiety to instrument

METHODOLOGY

Consent

Obtain either verbal or written consent.

Equipment-Technique

1. Place the microphone over the brachial artery proximal to the elbow of the *nondominant* arm (Fig. 77-1). *Proper positioning of the microphone is critical.*
2. Select the appropriate cuff size. The bladder inside the cuff should encircle 80% of the upper arm circumference without overlap.
3. Attach and secure the automatic cuff to the upper arm. To prevent shifting of the cuff on the arm, an adhesive-backed snap is placed on the arm. The cuff is then placed around the arm and secured to the adhesive-backed snap.
4. Connect the cuff-microphone to the monitor.
5. Calibrate the monitor for each patient in the lying, sitting, and standing positions. Measure blood pressure simultaneously with a manual cuff or with a mercury sphygmomanometer attached to the monitor through a T-tube device. (Three consecutive

measurements should be within 3 to 5 mm Hg of each other).
6. If Holter monitoring is performed simultaneously, attach the electrodes to the indicated sites (see Chapter 84, Holter Monitoring). Shave hair, clean body oils, and remove desquamated cells with light abrasion.
7. Secure the hose and microphone cable to minimize patient discomfort.
8. Set the frequency of recordings. (Typical is three to four times per hour during waking hours and one to two times per hour during sleeping hours.)
9. Instruct the patient to record any symptoms or events during the monitoring period.
10. Instruct the patient to not speak or move during cuff deflation (recording phase).
11. Instruct the patient to avoid strenuous activity (e.g., running or racquet sports) during study.
12. Remove monitoring and recording device at end of study period and retrieve recorded data.

COMPLICATIONS

- Interference with normal sleep patterns
- Inconvenience related to device
- Petechiae at measurement site
- Arm edema distal to cuff
- Transient arm discomfort
- Dermatitis
- Ulnar nerve palsy (rare)

INTERPRETATION OF RESULTS

Information acquired from ABPM includes (1) *average* level of blood pressure, (2) *diurnal fluctuations* in blood pressure, and (3) *short-term variability* of blood pressure.

Most normotensive individuals exhibit a circadian pattern of blood pressure readings. This pattern shows a peak during the daytime hours and reaches a nadir after midnight. (Nocturnal blood pressure decreases by 10% to 20% in most individuals.) With awakening and increased activity, recordings increase in the early morning. Staessen et al (1991) reviewed several studies and summarized diurnal blood pressures found in Table 77-1.

With the recent criteria of the JNC-VI report from the National Institutes of Health (Joint National Committee, 1997), the following diagnostic criteria are suggested:
- Hypertension is suggested if more than 30% of the 24-hour diastolic recordings are over 90 mm Hg.
- A *blood pressure load* (percent of elevated systolic and diastolic pressures during a 24-hour period) of

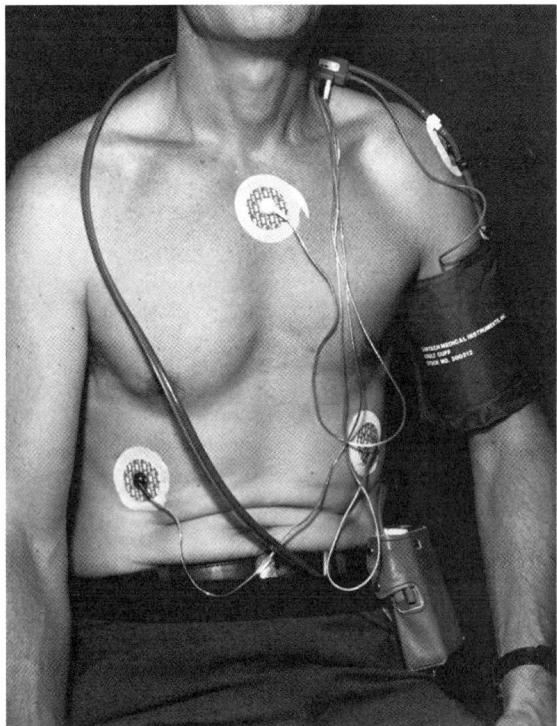

Fig. 77-1
Placement of ambulatory blood pressure monitoring unit.

30% or greater is correlated with the diagnosis of hypertension.
- Finally, patients whose blood pressure recordings vary widely during the 24-hour study period may require medication changes to provide control during the entire 24-hour day (Fig. 77-2).

In summary, most ABPM recordings have the following properties:
- Lower than office readings during waking hours (below 135/85)
- Lower while patients are asleep (below 120/75)
- A measure of systolic and diastolic blood pressure load
- Correlates better than office readings with target organ damage, especially echocardiographically determined left ventricular hypertrophy.

SUPPLIERS

Advanced Medical Products, Inc.
111 Research Drive
Columbia, SC 29203
Phone: 1-800-443-3816

Suntech Medical Instruments, Inc.
8917 Glenwood Avenue
Raleigh, NC 27612
Phone: 1-919-782-3005
Website: www.suntechmed.com

CPT/BILLING CODES

93784　Ambulatory blood pressure monitoring, for 24 hours or longer, including recording, scanning analysis, interpretation, and report
93786　Recording only
93788　Scanning analysis with report
93790　Physician review with interpretation and report

ICD-9-CM DIAGNOSTIC CODES

425.4　Cardiomyopathy, cardiac (idiopathic)
796.2　Elevated blood pressure (incidental without diagnosis)
401.XX　Hypertension (includes essential, labile, uncontrolled)
402.XX　Hypertension (includes cardiac)
403.XX　Hypertension (includes renal)
404.XX　Hypertension (cardiorenal)
Hypotension
458.9　Constitutional
458.2　Iatrogenic
458.0　Orthostatic
Syncope (near)
780.2　Cardiac, pre, near
337.0　Carotid sinus
337.9　Autonomic dysfunction

TABLE 77-1

Average Ambulatory Blood Pressure Monitoring Values

	Daytime	Nighttime	24-Hour
Normal Blood Pressure			
Average blood pressure	123/76	106/64	118/72
Range (Systolic)	(101-146)	(86-127)	(97-139)
Range (Diastolic)	(61-91)	(48-79)	(57-87)
Probable Hypertension			
Average blood pressure	>140/90	>125/80	>135/85
Blood Pressure Load (percent of elevated systolic and diastolic pressures/24 hr)			
Systolic load	>30% elevated/24 hr	>30% elevated	>30%
Diastolic load	>30%	>30%	>30%

Data compiled from Staessen JA, Fagard RH, Lijnen PJ, et al: *Am J Cardiol* 67:723, 1991; and Pickering T: *Am J Hypertens* 9:1, 1996.

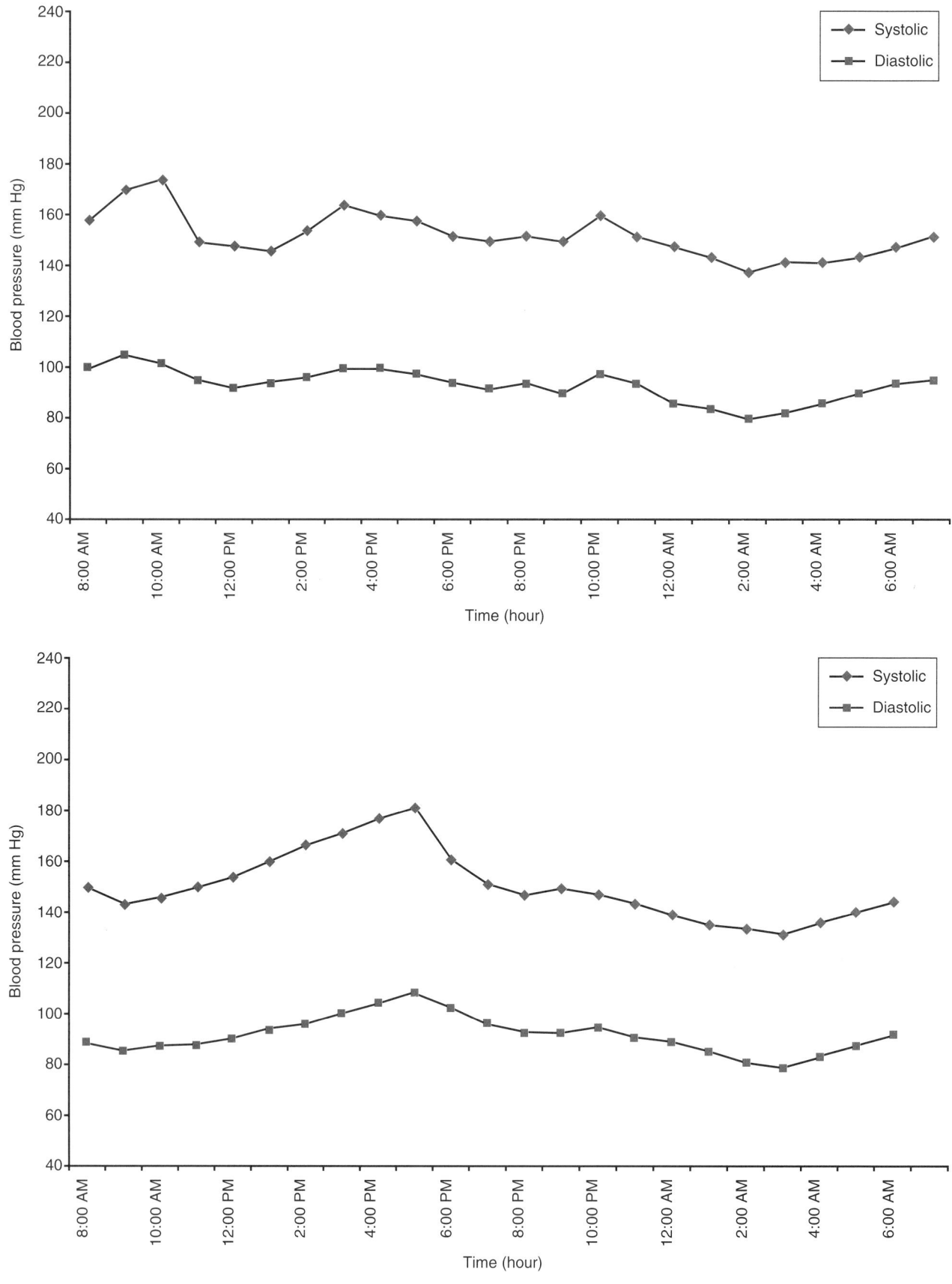

Fig. 77-2
Two examples of 24-hour ambulatory blood pressure monitoring (ABPM) recordings in a patient.

ADDITIONAL RESOURCES

• See the sample patient education handout titled "Ambulatory Blood Pressure Monitoring" on page 1821 of Appendix G.

BIBLIOGRAPHY

Audet AM: Position paper: automated ambulatory blood pressure and self-measured blood pressure monitoring devices: their role in the diagnosis and management of hypertension, *Ann Int Med* 118:889, 1993.

Gardner SF, Schneider EF: 24-hour ambulatory blood pressure monitoring in primary care, *J Am Board Fam Pract* 14:166, 2001.

Grin JM, McCabe EJ, White WB: Management of hypertension after ambulatory blood pressure monitoring, *Ann Int Med* 118:833, 1993.

Hornsby JL, Mongan PF, Taylor AT: Ambulatory blood pressure monitoring in hypertension, *Am Fam Physician* 43:1631, 1991.

Joint National Committee on Prevention, Detection, Evaluation, and Treatment of High Blood Pressure: The sixth report of the Joint National Committee on Prevention, Detection, Evaluation, and Treatment of High Blood Pressure, *Arch Intern Med* 157:2413, 1997.

National High Blood Pressure Education Program Coordinating Committee: National high blood pressure education program working group report on ambulatory blood pressure monitoring, *Arch Intern Med* 150:2270, 1990.

Pearce KA, Evans GW, Summerson J, Rao JS: Comparisons of ambulatory blood pressure monitoring and repeated office measurements in primary care, *J Fam Pract* 45:426, 1997.

Pickering T: Recommendations for the use of home (self) and ambulatory blood pressure monitoring, *Am J Hypertens* 9:1, 1996.

Rogers MAM, Small D, Buchan DA, et al: Home monitoring service improves mean arterial pressure in patients with essential hypertension, *Ann Intern Med* 134:1024, 2001.

Sheps SG, Clement DL, Pickering TG, et al: Ambulatory blood pressure monitoring. Hypertensive Diseases Committee, American College of Cardiology, *J Am Coll Cardiol* 23:1511, 1994.

Staessen JA, Byttebier G, Buntinx F, et al: Antihypertensive treatment based on conventional or ambulatory blood pressure measurement: a randomized control trial, *JAMA* 278:1065, 1997.

Staessen JA, Fagard RH, Lijnen PJ, et al: Mean and range of the ambulatory pressure in normotensive subjects from a meta-analysis of 23 studies, *Am J Cardiol* 67:723, 1991.

White WB, Berson AS, Robbins C, et al: National standard for measurement of resting and ambulatory blood pressures with automated sphygmomanometers, *Hypertension* 21:504, 1993.

White WB, Schulman P, McCabe EJ, Dey HM: Average daily blood pressure, not office blood pressure, determines cardiac function in patients with hypertension, *JAMA* 261:873, 1989.

Yarows SA: Ambulatory blood pressure monitoring, *JAMA* 279:196, 1998.

WEBSITES

www.australianprescriber.com (Carney S: 24-hour blood pressure monitoring: what are the benefits? 20:1, 1997)

www.nevdgp.org.au/geninf/heart_f/professional/Ambulatory%20blood.htm (Heart Foundation of Australia: Ambulatory blood pressure monitoring)

CHAPTER 78

Ambulatory Phlebectomy

Karl S. Hubach
Roger Y. Murray

The treatment of venous disease has undergone considerable change in the past decade. Ambulatory phlebectomy (AP) is growing in popularity as a surgical means of removing large varicose veins. This chapter introduces the basic techniques and ideas behind AP, which is an in-office surgical technique used to remove varicose veins through multiple small incisions. It is performed with local anesthetic and provides excellent cosmetic and functional results. It also allows the patient immediate ambulation with a compression bandage.

INDICATIONS

- To remove virtually any size vein for symptomatic or cosmetic reasons.
- Primarily used for the removal of symptomatic, visible varicose veins of the lower extremity. Since AP must be used along with correction of the highest point of reflux in the venous system, junctional ligation, ultrasound-guided sclerotherapy, or venous stripping may also be required.

CONTRAINDICATIONS

- Known metastatic carcinoma
- Allergy to the local anesthetic
- Hypercoagulable or hypocoagulable state
- Severe arterial occlusive diseases
- Hemodynamically important secondary varicosities
- Poor general health
- Incapacitated elderly patient
- CREST (calcinosis, Raynaud phenomenon, esophageal involvement, sclerodactyly, and telangiectasia) involving the lower extremities

Relative Contraindications

- Superficial thrombophlebitis
- Certain bloodborne infectious diseases
- Pregnancy
- Coagulopathies
- Keloid formers
- Significant fibrosis of the vein
- Acute deep venous thrombosis
- Overlying infection
- Deep venous insufficiency

EQUIPMENT

- Camera
- Surgical marking pen
- 10-ml syringe with a 25-gauge, 1½-inch needle
- 0.5% lidocaine with epinephrine
- Betadine prep
- Sterile draping
- Sterile gloves and Occupational Safety and Health Administration (OSHA)–approved attire
- Set of phlebectomy hooks
- Curved iris scissors
- Minimum of six curved, micro mosquito forceps
- Four towel clamps
- Needle holder (to hold the blade at desired depth and size of incision)
- No. 11 blade
- 4 × 4–inch gauze
- Steri-Strips (plain or saturated with Betadine)
- Benzoin spray
- 4-inch web roll (as an absorbent wrap over the 4 × 4–inch dressing)
- Non-stretch compression dressing (e.g., Comprilan)
- Class II thigh-high compression stockings
- Shower bag to cover dressing, when needed

- Written postoperative instructions
- Consent form

ANATOMY AND PATHOLOGY OF VENOUS DISEASE

Before proper treatment options can be determined, the physician must have a clear understanding of the underlying anatomy and the disease process. The physician should also have undergone an advanced study of the lower extremity venous system before performing AP. This section serves only as a brief overview and is far from comprehensive. (The reader is also referred to Chapter 90, Sclerotherapy, and Chapter 85, Noninvasive Venous and Arterial Studies of the Lower Extremities.)

There are primarily three venous components in the leg. They are comprised of the superficial venous system, which lies above the deep fascia; the deep venous system, which lies under the deep fascia; and the perforator vein system, which connects the superficial with the deep systems (Fig. 78-1). The muscular pump of the leg produces a distal to proximal compression,

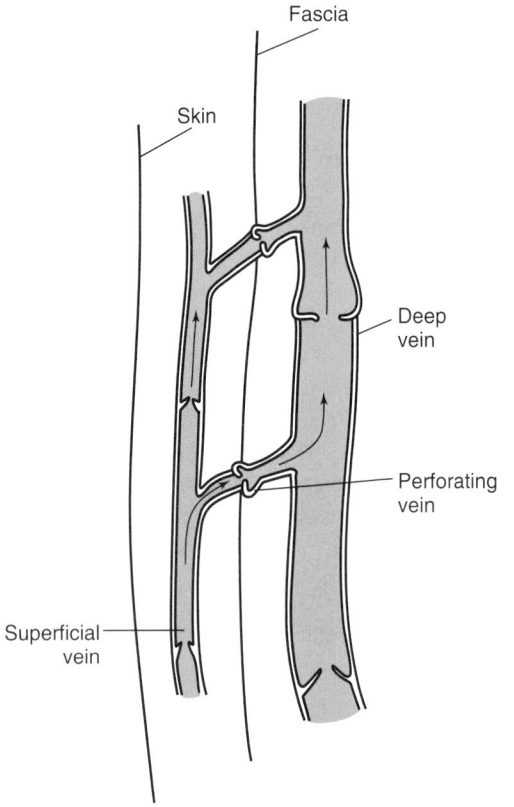

Fig. 78-1
Venous compartments of the leg consist of superficial venous system, the deep venous system, and the perforator vein system.

facilitating blood flow back to the cardiopulmonary system. Normal veins usually allow unidirectional flow by using a valvular system along the course of the vein.

The superficial veins consist of a network of veins that feed two primary vessels: the greater saphenous vein and the lesser saphenous vein. The greater saphenous vein terminates at the saphenofemoral junction as it courses from the dorsal arch vein of the foot along the medial leg and medial thigh. The lesser saphenous vein also begins with the dorsal arch vein but travels behind the lateral malleolus along the lateral leg. Once reaching the region of the popliteal fossa it has a variable termination point to the popliteal vein of the deep venous system at the saphenopopliteal junction. (See Figs. 90-2 and 90-3.)

Perforator veins allow blood to flow from the superficial to the deep system. By doing so, more than 90% of the blood travels through the deep venous systems, back to the heart. The importance of competent venous valves to enforce unidirectional flow in such a low-pressure system is often unappreciated. Once venous reflux occurs through incompetent valves, normal blood flow is altered, intraluminal pressures increase, and the disease process worsened. The increased flow and pressure to the superficial system leads to dilated vessels and varicose development. As chronic venous insufficiency develops, approximately one third goes on to develop problems with superficial thrombophlebitis, dermatitis, lipodermatosclerosis, or ulceration.

It is important for the phlebologist to have a clear understanding of the sensory nerves and lymphatic vessels of the leg. Both of these systems lie in close proximity to the superficial veins. Consequently, potential complications can develop from damage to these structures. The most frequent nerve damage occurs along the distal portion of the greater saphenous vein close to the dorsal foot veins and along the short saphenous vein with the accompanying sural nerve (Fig. 78-2). Damage to the lymphatic vessels most commonly occurs below the medial knee in the anterior tibial region near the Boyd's perforators.

PREPROCEDURE PATIENT PREPARATION

An accurate patient history and examination allows the physician to formulate a better diagnosis and treatment that will best suit the patient's needs. The examination must also be conducted to unveil any potential contraindications. Additional studies, such as an EKG, complete blood count, bleeding studies, and SMA-7 may be required. Fig. 78-3 shows a general history form with a focus on venous-related history.

The venous examination accurately maps the veins of the lower extremity. The physician should also note if chronic changes are present. Dermatitis, edema, and lipodermatosclerosis or ulcerative disease may raise a suspicion for potential deep venous disease or long-standing chronic venous insufficiency.

The handheld Doppler is often referred to as the phlebologist's stethoscope. It is an invaluable instrument to examine the patient for venous reflux. The Doppler examination is performed with the patient in the standing position, bearing his or her weight on the opposite leg. The Doppler probe is placed at a 45-degree angle over the vein to be examined. Compression of the calf muscle distal to the probe induces blood flow in a proximal direction. In a diseased vein, reflux is heard as a loud rumbling sound after a sudden release of compression of the calf muscle. A normal vein has only a monophasic signal. By performing this simple maneuver, the examiner can locate the most proximal source of reflux. (See Chapter 85, Noninvasive Venous and Arterial Studies of the Lower Extremities.)

Duplex ultrasound examination allows the addition of important details to provide an even better venous mapping. The examination is typically performed with a 7.5-MHz linear probe and the patient in a standing position. Areas of venous dilation and large perforators can reveal sources of proximal venous reflux. The deep venous system can also be visualized to assess for thrombus or incompetence. Areas of reflux in the superficial system, which may be difficult to visualize or palpate, can be studied easily. Duplex scanning also allows a hard copy documentation of the venous disease before and after treatment.

Many phlebologists evaluate the leg function with an additional test, photoplethysmography. This is most helpful to document normal or correctable deep venous function in those patients with evidence of stasis changes. (See Chapter 90, Sclerotherapy.)

Once a complete understanding of the underlying disease is obtained, an accurate treatment plan can be formulated. It needs to be emphasized that the highest point of reflux must be corrected. This often requires a junctional (saphenofemoral and saphenopopliteal) ligation in addition to AP. Other techniques, such as ultrasound-guided sclerotherapy and a partial stripping of the greater saphenous or ligation of the short saphenous vein, may also be used in conjunction with AP. When a higher level of venous incompetence is identi-

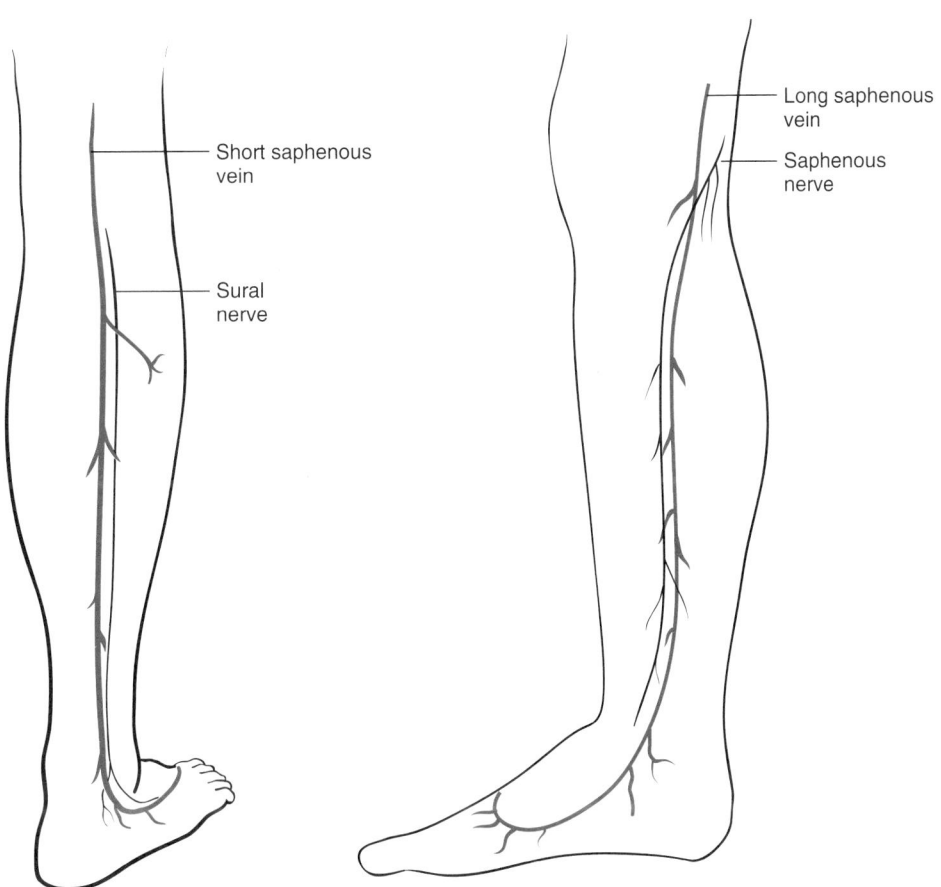

Fig. 78-2
Sensory nerves and location relative to vessels of the leg.

Name:_____ Date:_____ Age:_____ Ht:_____ Wt:_____

When did you first notice your enlarged or discolored veins? _____

Which leg bothers you the most?　　　　　Right _____ Left _____ Both _____

What symptoms are you having?

1. Sharp pain.............Yes　No	8. Burning.................Yes　No
2. Dull pain................Yes　No	9. Heaviness.............Yes　No
3. Aching legs...........Yes　No	10. Cramps...............Yes　No
4. Swelling................Yes　No	11. Throbbing...........Yes　No
5. Itching...................Yes　No	12. Restless legs.......Yes　No
6. Leg ulcers.............Yes　No	13. Appearance.........Yes　No
7. Tiredness..............Yes　No	

Have you ever had any of the following:

　*　1. Phlebitis (clots in legs) ....Yes_____ No_____ When _____
　*　2. Deep vein thrombosis ....Yes_____ No_____ When _____
　　　3. Pulmonary embolus (blood clot in lung) .... Yes_____ No_____ When _____
　*　4. Leg or ankle ulcers ....Yes_____ No_____ When _____
　*　5. Painful varicose veins ....Yes_____ No_____ When _____
　　　6. Venogram (vein x-rays) ....Yes_____ No_____ When _____

Have you ever been pregnant?　　Yes_____ No_____
How many times?　　　　　　　　_____
How many deliveries?　　　　　　_____
Are you currently pregnant?　　　Yes_____ No_____

List all medicines you are currently taking (including aspirin, if applicable):

_____　　_____　　_____
_____　　_____　　_____

List any hormones you are taking:

_____　　_____　　_____

Birth control pills:　Yes_____ No_____

List all allergies:

_____　　_____　　_____
_____　　_____　　_____

Have you ever had any adverse reactions with scars?　　Yes_____ No_____

Have you ever had any of the following:

AIDS or HIV positive ....Yes　　　　　No
Diabetes ....Yes　　　　　No
Thyroid disease..Yes　　　　　No
High blood pressure ....Yes　　　　　No
Heart disease ....Yes　　　　　No
Jaundice or hepatitis ....Yes　　　　　No
Cancer ....Yes　　　　　No
Recent weight change ....Yes　　　　　No
Major injury or surgery in your legs...................................Yes　　　　　No
Leg pain at night ....Yes　　　　　No
Leg pain caused by walking..Yes　　　　　No
Leg pain caused by standing ....Yes　　　　　No
Clotting or blood problems..Yes　　　　　No

Continued

Fig. 78-3
Sample general patient history form with a focus on venous-related history.

Have you ever used prescription compression hose for your legs?   Yes _____ No _____ When _____

Have you ever had sclerotherapy before?   Yes _____ No _____ When _____

Have you ever smoked?   Yes _____ No _____ Packs/day ____ Number of years _____

Are you currently smoking?   Yes _____ No _____ Packs/day × years _____

List any and all family members with vein problems:

_____   _____   _____

_____   _____   _____

Who can we thank for referring you to our office? _____

FOR DOCTOR USE ONLY

Movie seen: Yes _____   No _____
Telangiectasias: Right _____   Left _____   Severity _____
Reticulars: Right _____   Left _____   Severity _____
Varicose veins: Right _____   Left _____   Severity _____
*V. V.:   Size: _____ mm
*SFJ Reflux: Right _____   Left _____
*SPJ Reflux: Right _____   Left _____
PPG: Yes _____ No _____ Right _____ Left _____ Ven _____ Art _____ Both _____
U.S.:   Yes _____ No _____ Right _____ Left _____
Appt. for sclero: Yes _____ No _____

Fig. 78-3, cont'd

fied, the physician may choose to consult another surgeon. Many physicians use a team approach to ensure that all areas of incompetence are corrected. This helps to ensure a lower reoccurrence rate and better relief of symptoms resulting from venous insufficiency.

See the sample patient education handout titled "Ambulatory Phlebectomy (Preprocedure)" on page 1822 of Appendix G.

TECHNIQUE

1. On the night before surgery the patient should shave his or her legs carefully, minimizing any areas of nicking. Males may find the use of "Magic Hair Removal" or a depilatory to be helpful in place of shaving.

2. Preoperative pictures are highly recommended.

3. Just before surgery, have the patient stand for venous marking with a surgical marking pen. Proper lighting in a warm room with a period of standing before marking will maximize venous dilation and visibility. Some physicians mark the most superficial, easily palpable, portion of vein with a crosshatch.

4. Once the visible veins have been marked, use a focused Duplex examination to locate and mark perforator veins and large branches along the vein to be excised (Fig. 78-4).

5. Place the patient in a 10- to 15-degree Trendelenburg's position to empty the veins during surgery. The foot can be propped on a pillow or cushion.

6. Prep the area with a 5-minute Betadine or Hibiclens scrub and sterile draping of the area.

7. Perform perivascular injection of 0.5% lidocaine with epinephrine on each side of the marked veins using a 25-gauge, 1½-inch needle. Many physicians use a tumescent technique, originally developed for use in liposuction surgery. This uses large amounts of a very dilute 0.2% Lidocaine with a 1:500,000 concentration of epinephrine instilled with a 22-gauge spinal needle. Some physicians believe the larger volumes instilled in the perivascular space provide additional local compression to further minimize bleeding.

8. Starting proximally, make a small 2- to 3-mm vertical incision over or adjacent to the marked vein. A no. 11 blade or an 18-gauge needle may be used for the incisions. A no. 11 blade can be placed in a needle holder at the desired depth and size of the incision (Fig. 78-5).

9. Gently insert a phlebectomy hook through the incision (Fig. 78-6). It may be necessary to break up

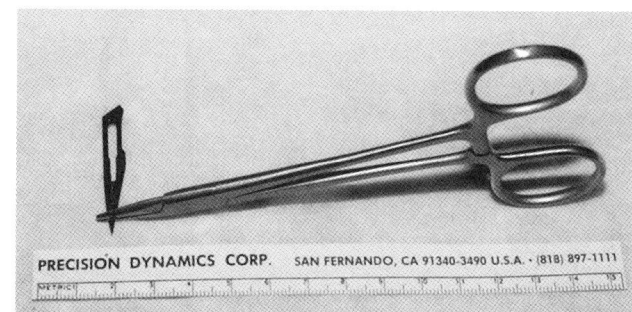

Fig. 78-5
No. 11 blade placed in needle holder in preparation for incision.

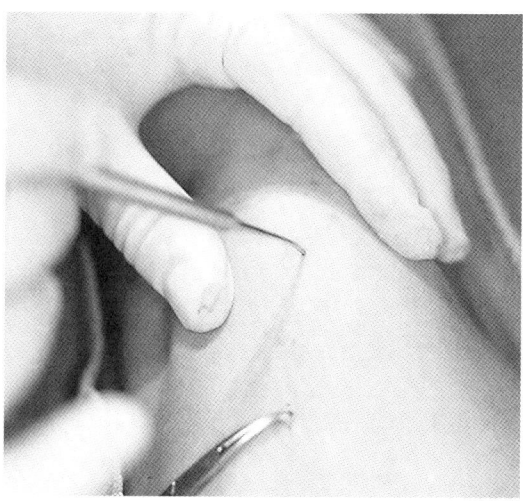

Fig. 78-6
Phlebectomy hook gently inserted through incision.

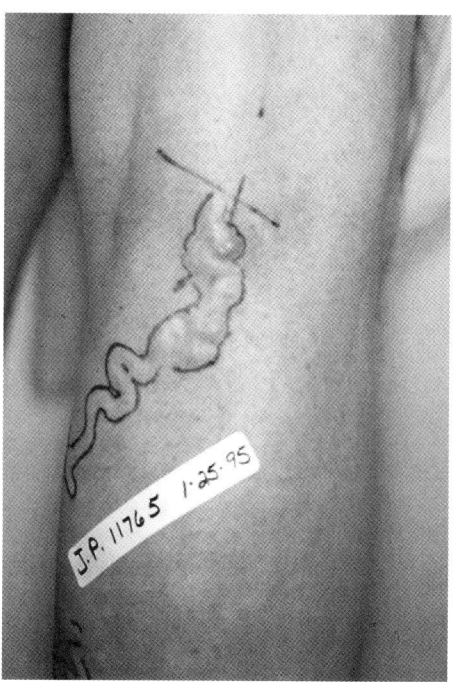

Fig. 78-4
Venous marking with surgical marking pen.

adhesions and fibrous attachments to the vein before extraction by undermining with the stem of the phlebectomy hook.

10. Hook the vein with a gentle rotation and retraction technique. When the vein is pulled through the incision, it will be identified by its distinguishing pearly white appearance (Fig. 78-7).

11. The vein is grasped with a set of fine curved mosquito hemostats. As the vein is exteriorized, the tension on the vein will produce a palpable cord under the skin. The next incision is made at the distal point of the palpable cord, or the next crosshatch.

12. The most proximal end of the vein being excised is tied off with 3-0 Vicryl. The authors also choose to tie off as many perforators as possible, which are located easily with the Duplex-guided marking done prior to surgery. Many phlebologists choose to simply tear the vein loose from the perforator and have an assistant apply constant pressure to the area for 5 to 10 minutes.

13. The vein is sequentially pulled through successive distal incisions until it is totally excised. When removed in pieces, they can be laid out along the course to ensure total removal of the vein (Fig. 78-8).

14. With extensive varicosities, the surgeon may choose to perform the AP in stages, separated by 7 to 14 days for each surgery. The procedure, when performed in stages, typically begins on the distal part of the limb. With experience it will take the surgeon less time to remove the same length of vein. Several hours should be allowed for each surgery, and one leg should be done at a time.

15. Clean the limb with sterile water and pat dry. Benzoin spray is used to increase the adhesion of the Steri-Strips applied over the incisions.

16. Apply gauze or an absorbent padding along the course of the excised vein.

17. Wrap the leg in a distal-to-proximal direction with a nonstretch compression bandage (e.g., Comprilan). Coban may also be used.

18. Place a thigh-high, Class II compression stocking over the dressing.

COMPLICATIONS

Box 78-1 shows a complete list of complications seen in a review of the literature done by Dr. Albert-Adrien Ramelet. Transient, patient-perceived complications might be as high as 5% to 10% and include such

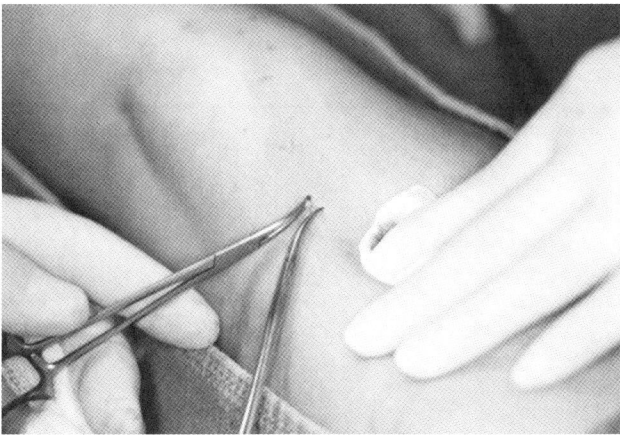

Fig. 78-7
Vein pulled through incision.

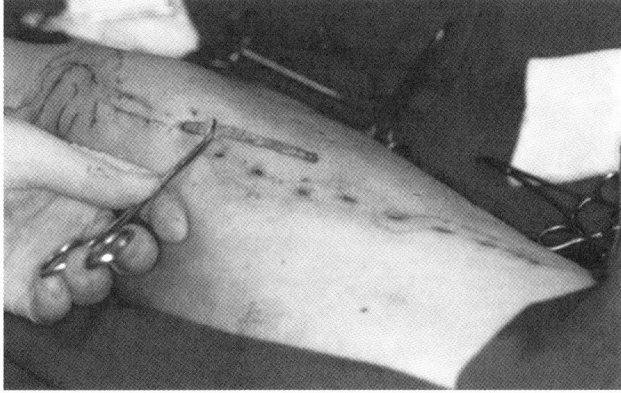

Fig. 78-8
Vein is sequentially pulled through successive distal incisions.

BOX 78-1
Complications of Ambulatory Phlebectomy

Cutaneous Complications
Skin blisters from dressing
Transitory hyperpigmentation
Visible scars
Contact dermatitis
Infections
Keloid and hypertrophic scars
Tattooing with pen
Koebner's phenomena
Skin necrosis

Neurologic Complications
Postoperative pain
Paresthesia

Vascular Complications
Hematomas
Postoperative hemorrhage
Superficial phlebitis
Matting
Lymphatic pseudocyst
Lymphorrhea
Persistent edema
Deep venous thrombosis with potential pulmonary embolus

Data from Ramelet A: *Dermatol Surg* 23:947, 1997.

TABLE 78-1
Frequency of Complications of Ambulatory Phlebectomy

Rank	Type	No. of Events/ Phlebectomy	Percentage/ Phlebectomy
1	Blister formation	214	5.4%
2	Pigmentation (transitory)	183	4.6%
3	Telangiectasia matting	145	3.6%
4	Localized superficial phlebitis	110	2.8%
5	Temporary dysesthesia	15	0.4%
6	Lymphocele	6	0.2%
7	Extensive superficial phlebitis	5	0.1%
8	Delayed bleeding	4	0.1%
9	Hematoma	4	0.1%
10	Dimpling	3	0.07%
11	Skin necrosis	3	0.07%
12	Tattooing	3	0.07%
13	Wound infection	3	0.07%
14	Allergic reaction to wrappings	3	0.07%
15	Keloid	3	0.07%
16	Local anesthetic overload	2	0.05%
17	Deep vein thrombosis	1	0.02%
	Totals	**707**	**17.79%**

Data from Olivencia JA: *Am J Cosmet Surg* 17:3, 2000.

things as skin blisters, hyperpigmentation, and contact dermatitis (Table 78-1). True complications that may require professional attention or that have long-term sequela are quite rare.

Complications can be divided into cutaneous, vascular, and neurological. Most *cutaneous complications* can be avoided with the proper use and application of the postoperative dressing. The size and type of vessels operated on, the anatomical location of the surgery, and the individual patient's history of previous sclerotherapy, phlebitis, or lipodermatosclerosis affects vascular complications. Many of the *vascular complications* are avoidable by applying adequate compression and stressing the importance of postoperative ambulating. *Neurologic complications* can occur from the local anesthetic, directly from the phlebectomy, or from the postoperative dressing. The most problematic nerve injury of the sural nerve must be carefully avoided when dealing with the short saphenous vein. Many sensory nerves can be avoided because the patient will complain of pain, allowing the surgeon to prevent destruction of the nerve. Excessive compression to the dorsal foot can induce a painful tarsal syndrome.

The primary care physician does not require special training to handle the complications that occur with AP. Emphasis must be placed, however, on adequate training to perform AP and on the proper understanding of the underlying pathophysiology.

POSTPROCEDURE PATIENT EDUCATION

Written and oral postoperative instructions should be provided to the patient (see the sample patient education handout titled "Ambulatory Phlebectomy (Postprocedure)" on page 1824 of Appendix G). All patients should be encouraged to walk approximately one half mile immediately after surgery, then 1 to 3 miles per day for the next 2 weeks. They should start taking one aspirin every day for 2 weeks, starting 12 to 16 hours after surgery. Strenuous workouts, heavy lifting, and long standing should be avoided for 2 weeks. Over-the-counter ibuprofen should be sufficient for any discomfort that may occur after surgery. The dressing is to remain in place and dry until the follow-up appointment 1 week later. At that time the dressing will be removed and the incisions inspected. The compression stocking alone is worn during the day for an additional week. The Steri-Strips will be removed 2 weeks after surgery, and then any further surgeries or required therapy can be scheduled.

CONCLUSION

Outpatient AP is a convenient, safe and cost-effective treatment for varicose veins. The patient is able to walk out of the office with little to no change in his or her level of activity. The rate of complications is extremely low. Because the procedure can be performed without hospitalization or general anesthesia, and because it allows for a return to normal activity, the expense to the patient and the healthcare system is markedly reduced. AP provides an excellent addition to the total care and treatment of varicose veins and venous disease.

SUPPLIERS

An excellent general resource for all sclerotherapy and phlebotomy instruments and equipment:
Wagner Medical
P.O. Box 431
202 Dodd Street
Middlebourne, WV 26149
Phone: 1-304-758-2370

Phlebectomy hooks
Venoscan
1617 N. Fayetteville Street
Asheboro, NC 27203
Phone: 1-910-672-6062

Aesculap
3773 Corporate Parkway
Center Valley, PA 18034
Phone: 1-800-282-9000
Website: www.aesculap-usa.com

Compression stockings
Beiersdorf-Jobst, Inc.
Wilton Corporate Center
187 Danbury Road
Wilton, CT 06897
Phone: 1-203-563-5800

Sigvaris
1119 Highway 74
Peachtree City, GA 30269
Phone: 1-770-631-1778
Website: www.sigvaris.com

Medi USA
76 West Seegers Road
Arlington Heights, IL 60005
Phone: 1-800-633-6334
Website: www.mediusa.com

Juzo, Inc
80 Chart Road
P.O. Box 1088
Cuyahoga Falls, OH 44223
Phone: 1-800-222-4999
Website: www.juzo.com

Venosan
718 Industrial Park Avenue
P.O. Box 106
Asheboro, NC 27204-1067
Phone: 1-888-250-7617
Website: www.venosanonline.com

Shower bag cover
Gill Podiatry Supply
7803 Freeway Circle
Middleburg Heights, OH 44130-6399
Phone: 1-800-321-1348

Compression wrap
STD Pharmaceutical
Fields Yard, Plough Lane
Hereford, HR4 0EL, England
Phone: +44 (0)1432 353684
Website: www.stdpharm.co.uk

PHLEBOLOGY SOCIETIES

American College of Phlebology
100 Webster Street, Suite 101
Oakland, CA 94607-3724
Phone: 510-834-6500
Website: www.phlebology.org

TRAINING COURSES

The National Procedures Institute
4909 Hedgewood Drive
Midland, MI 48640
Phone: 1-800-462-2492
Website: www.npinstitute.com

CPT/BILLING CODES

37700	Ligation and division of greater saphenous vein
37785	Ligation of secondary varicose veins
37799	Unlisted vascular procedure
76986	Ultrasonic guidance, intraoperative
37785	"Mini" phlebectomy, one leg; ligation, division, and/or excision of recurrent or secondary varicose vein (clusters), one leg; modify for bilateral use

ICD-9-CM DIAGNOSTIC CODES

459.81	Venous insufficiency
454	Varicose veins of the lower extremities

ADDITIONAL RESOURCES

- See the sample patient education handouts titled "Ambulatory Phlebectomy (Preprocedure)" on page 1822 and "Ambulatory Phlebectomy (Postprocedure)" on page 1824 of Appendix G.
- See the sample patient consent form titled "Ambulatory Phlebectomy" on page 1825 of Appendix G.

BIBLIOGRAPHY

Brown JS: Stab-avulsion varicose veins. In Brown JS: *Minor surgery: a text and atlas*, ed 4, New York, 2001, Oxford University Press.
Flynn JC: *Procedures in phlebotomy*, ed 2, Philadelphia, 1999, WB Saunders.

Goldman M, Bergan J: *Ambulatory treatment of venous disease: an illustration guide,* St Louis, 1995, Mosby.

Olivencia JA: Maneuver to facilitate ambulatory phlebectomy, *Dermatol Surg* 22(7):654, 1996.

Ouriel K: *Lower extremity vascular disease,* Philadelphia, 1995, WB Saunders.

Ramelet A: Complications of ambulatory phlebectomy, *Dermatol Surg* 23:947, 1997.

Ricci S, Georgiev M, Goldman M: *A practical guide for treating varicose veins,* St Louis, 1995, Mosby.

Sadick NS: *Manual of sclerotherapy,* Philadelphia, 2000, Lippincott.

Tibbs D, Sabiston D, Davis M, et al: *Varicose veins, venous disorders, and lymphatic problems in the lower limbs,* Oxford, 1997, Oxford University Press.

Weiss R, Weiss M: *Ambulatory phlebectomy compared to sclerotherapy for varicose and telangiectatic veins: indications and complications, vol 2, Advances in dermatology,* St Louis, 1996, Mosby.

Weiss RA, Dover JS: Leg vein management: sclerotherapy, ambulatory phlebectomy, and laser surgery. In Kaminer MS, Dover JS, Arndt KA, editors: *Atlas of cosmetic surgery,* Philadelphia, 2002, WB Saunders.

CHAPTER 79

Arterial Puncture and Percutaneous Arterial Line Placement

Grant C. Fowler
Debra Kay Harvey

ARTERIAL PUNCTURE

An arterial puncture can be useful in urgent, acute, and some chronic conditions, or whenever an arterial blood sample is needed. If frequent sampling will be required or intraarterial blood pressure monitoring is necessary, placement of an intraarterial line should be considered. With proper technique and equipment, an arterial puncture is a safe and simple procedure. However, advancements in technology for noninvasive monitoring may eventually make this procedure obsolete. Use of oxygen saturation (O_2 sat) monitoring has already markedly decreased the need for arterial punctures. In most cases, an arterial puncture is now used to assess and confirm hypoxia only when indicated by a low O_2 sat.

INDICATIONS

- To confirm a clinically suspected acute problem with carbon dioxide or oxygen exchange, or with acid-base balance, such as patients with severe asthma, pulmonary thromboembolism, diabetic ketoacidosis, refractory cardiac dysrhythmias, or patients who are newly comatose.
- To confirm the clinical status in a patient with a chronic condition that affects gas exchange or acid-base balance, such as chronic obstructive pulmonary disease.
- To confirm hypoxia, when O_2 sats are not available.
- To confirm the need for home oxygen therapy. (By Medicare rules, the company providing the oxygen cannot be the same company that does the blood gas testing. Medicare now accepts low O_2 sats as confirmation of hypoxia.)
- To obtain arterial blood for certain laboratory tests (lactate, ammonia, or carbon monoxide levels, although some laboratories can use venous blood).

- To obtain a blood sample in an emergent situation when phlebotomy cannot be performed or when there are no venous sites.

CONTRAINDICATIONS

- Inability to palpate arterial pulsation.
- Known or suspected severe arterial disease of aneurysmal, atherosclerotic, inflammatory, or vasospastic nature.
- Previous surgery in the area may have caused scarring, thereby complicating the procedure.
- Poor collateral perfusion from the ulnar artery when the radial artery is the intended puncture site.
- When a functional indwelling arterial line is present.
- Relative contraindications: bleeding dyscrasias, anticoagulant therapy, or possible later thrombolytic therapy. These patients should be monitored carefully after arterial puncture to prevent complications.

Note: If continuous pressure monitoring is indicated or frequent arterial specimens are required, an arterial line should be inserted.

EQUIPMENT

- 3- to 5-ml sterile plastic or glass syringe with a freely movable plunger. (Kits are made in which the preheparinized syringe plunger should not be moved. These kits also contain the needle and rubber stopper.)
- 25-gauge, ⅝-inch (1.6-cm) needle for radial, brachial, dorsalis pedis, and femoral puncture. For femoral puncture in obese patients, a 22-gauge, 1½-inch (3.8-cm) needle may be helpful.
- Heparin 1000 U/ml.

- Antiseptic skin preparation, such as povidone-iodine (Betadine) or 70% isopropyl alcohol.
- 1% lidocaine *without* epinephrine.
- 3-ml syringe with 25-gauge, ⅝-inch (1.6-cm) needle for lidocaine.
- Plug for syringe or rubber stopper for end of needle.
- Sterile 4 × 4–inch gauze pads.
- Container of crushed ice for sample transport (plastic bag, emesis basin, cup, etc.).
- Sterile gloves.
- Goggles or eye protection for the clinician.

ARTERIAL SITE SELECTION

Each site for arterial puncture has its own risks and benefits. Because of its proximity to the skin surface, the radial artery is the most commonly preferred site, especially on the nondominant hand. It is an excellent location if there is adequate ulnar artery collateral circulation (see the following section) and if the clinical situation is stable. In severely hypotensive patients or during cardiopulmonary resuscitation, the femoral artery is usually the most readily palpable and most conveniently located artery, in spite of its association with a higher risk of complications. Alternative sites in decreasing order of preference include the brachial, superficial temporal, and dorsalis pedis arteries. The brachial artery should be reserved for use when radial artery puncture cannot be performed or is contraindicated. Although the dorsalis pedis artery is absent, usually bilaterally, in 12% of the population, it is another option for puncture. Before dorsalis pedis artery puncture is performed, collateral flow should be demonstrated in a manner similar to the Allen test. Superficial temporal artery puncture will not be discussed. Ultimately, operator experience and local anatomy are the deciding factors in choice of sites. The operator should avoid an artery where the overlying cutaneous defenses are not intact, such as sites of infection, burn, or other skin damage.

ASSESSMENT OF ULNAR COLLATERAL CIRCULATION

Radial artery puncture can lead to thrombosis of the distal artery. To minimize the risk of permanent ischemic damage to the hand, collateral circulation should be assessed prior to puncture. This is especially important because up to 12% of hands have either poor or no collateral flow because of an incomplete palmar arch (Fig. 79-1). Even if there is excellent collateral flow, the nondominant hand should be used, if possible.

The Allen test, used to evaluate ulnar collateral flow, was first described in 1929. It has since been modified to

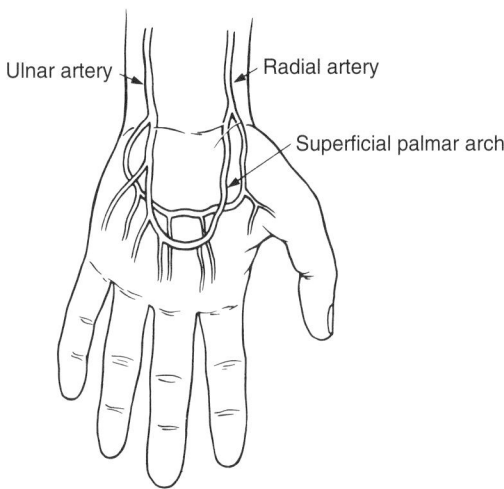

Fig. 79-1
Anatomy of radial and ulnar arteries at wrist and superficial palmar arch.

minimize falsely abnormal results. The modified Allen test is performed as follows:

1. Have the patient hold his or her arm above heart level, and then open and close the hand several times to exsanguinate it. Next, have the patient clench the fist tightly. The clinician then compresses both the radial and ulnar arteries (Fig. 79-2, *A*). About a minute should be allowed for blood to drain from the hand. In a comatose or anesthetized patient, the hand can be elevated and clenched passively by an assistant. The hand should be at least room temperature (more than 70° F). It can be warmed in water, if necessary.
2. Next, the fist should be lowered below the level of the heart and unclenched (Fig. 79-2, *B*) while pressure is released on the ulnar artery (Fig. 79-2, *C*). Care should be taken to avoid hyperextension of the wrist or fingers, which can lead to a falsely abnormal test. When the pressure on the ulnar artery is released, the cadaveric color of the entire hand should return to normal color within 6 seconds (Fig. 79-2, *D*). Color usually returns to the palm first, and then to the entire hand. If any area of the hand does not rapidly return to its normal color within 6 seconds, this is a positive test for abnormal ulnar collateral flow. Further tests or another location should be considered before arterial puncture or any arterial procedure is performed on the radial artery. The thumb, index finger, and thenar eminence are the areas most commonly involved in a positive test. These areas often have an inadequate collateral blood supply and are entirely dependent on the radial artery for perfusion.

When there is an abnormal or equivocal modified Allen test, various types of noninvasive studies can be used to further evaluate the situation. If available, a handheld Doppler can be used to rapidly evaluate collateral

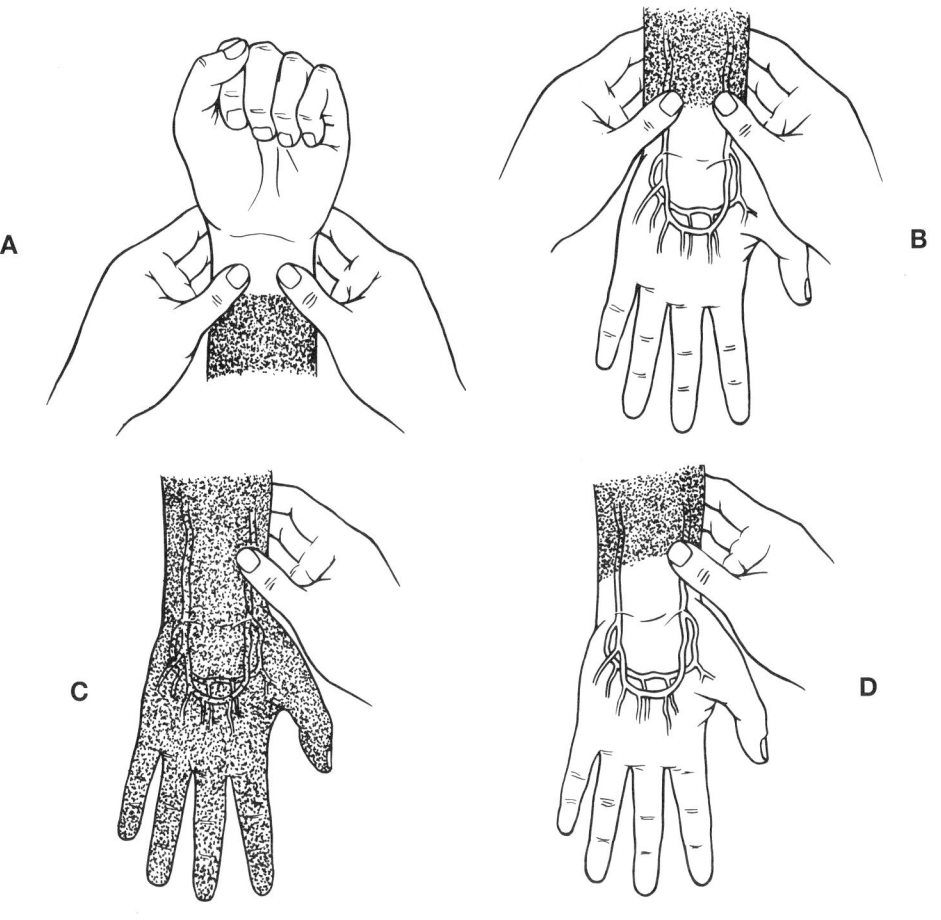

Fig. 79-2
Modified Allen test. **A,** Hand is elevated and fist clenched while radial and ulnar arteries are occluded for 1 minute. **B,** Hand is lowered and fist is unclenched. Hand is cadaveric. **C,** Ulnar artery compression is released while radial artery compression is continued. In a negative test, the entire hand regains color in less than 6 seconds. **D,** Positive test. With inadequate collateral perfusion from the ulnar artery, the hand remains cadaveric as long as radial artery compression is maintained. When inadequate collateral perfusion is demonstrated, another puncture site should be considered.

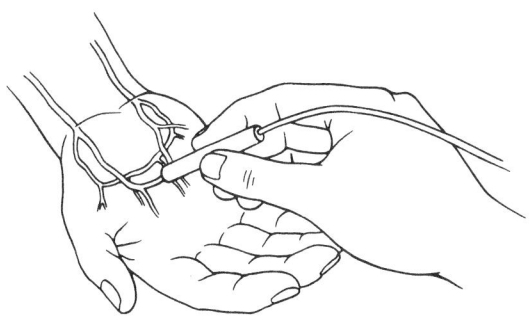

Fig. 79-3
Assessment of the superficial palmar arch with Doppler instrument.

circulation with a technique more sensitive and specific than the Allen test. If time allows, formal Dopplers, either portable or in the radiology department, can be used to confirm the absence or presence of collateral flow.

Performing a Doppler Evaluation

1. After placing the probe between the heads of the third and fourth metacarpals on the palm, angulate the probe and advance it proximally until maximal auditory signal is obtained (Fig. 79-3).
2. With the palmar arch identified and maximal signal obtained, compression of the radial artery should not cause a change of the signal if the palmar arch is complete and supplied by collateral ulnar circulation. A decrease in signal indicates poor collateral flow. This is a much more sensitive and specific test than the Allen test.

ASSESSMENT OF DORSALIS PEDIS COLLATERAL CIRCULATION

To minimize the risk of permanent ischemic damage to the distal foot, collateral circulation should be assessed before dorsalis pedis artery puncture is attempted.

1. The foot should be at least room temperature (more than 70° F). It can be warmed in water, if necessary.
2. After locating and palpating the dorsalis pedis artery (Fig. 79-4), occlude it with compression.
3. Blanch the great toenail by compressing for several minutes.

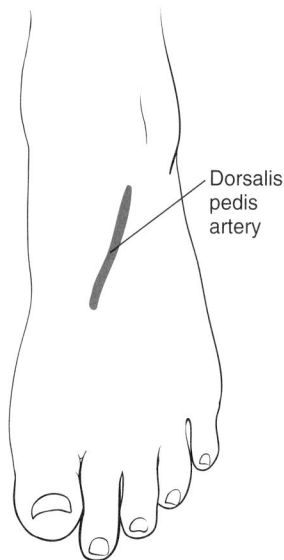

Fig. 79-4
Location of the dorsalis pedis artery.

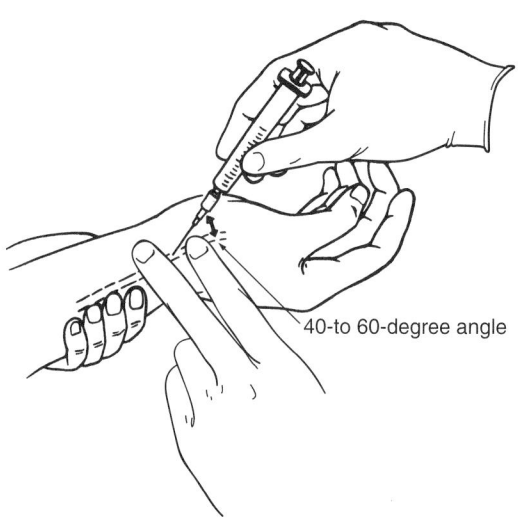

Fig. 79-5
This patient is left-hand dominant. Palpate the patient's radial pulse with your left hand. While holding the heparinized syringe with your right hand (reverse hands if left-handed), puncture the skin at approximately a 60-degree angle, directing the needle toward the radial pulsation.

4. Release pressure on the nail and observe for flushing. A rapid return of color indicates adequate collateral flow.

Note: In most persons, collateral circulation of the foot is provided by a branch of the posterior tibial artery. A handheld Doppler can be used to assess collateral flow between the dorsalis pedis and posterior tibial arteries in a manner similar to that used to test collateral flow in the palmar arch.

PREPROCEDURE PATIENT PREPARATION

The clinician and patient should be in a comfortable position that can be maintained up to 10 to 15 minutes, if necessary. The procedure and its necessity should be explained to the alert patient. In nonemergent situations, informed consent should be obtained (see the sample patient consent form titled "Arterial Puncture" on page 1829 in Appendix G). The patient should be prepared to expect some discomfort, and the clinician should observe universal blood and body fluid precautions.

TECHNIQUE

1. Rinse the syringe with a small amount (1 or 2 ml) of heparin and then empty it through the needle. For glass syringes, this step not only coats the syringe with heparin, but it also eliminates the dead space in the syringe and needle. Although heparin does not adhere to plastic syringes, performing this step with

plastic syringes will displace any air and fill the dead space.

Note: Certain kits contain syringes that are already heparinized, and the plunger should not be moved.

2. Prep the skin in an aseptic manner and put on gloves.
3. Palpate the selected artery with the balls of two or three fingers, and immobilize it with these fingers along its course. Use the nondominant hand of the clinician to immobilize the artery.
4. *Optional:* Local anesthetic (lidocaine) can be injected for a particularly anxious patient to minimize hyperventilation artifact. However, use minimal amounts to avoid anatomic distortion, which could make it difficult to palpate and puncture the pulse.
5. Wearing gloves and holding the barrel of the syringe like a pencil in the dominant hand, keep the needle bevel up.
6a. *For radial artery puncture.* Dorsiflex about 30 degrees, and slightly rotate the supine wrist of (preferably) the patient's nondominant hand. It should be supported by a firm surface, such as an assistant's hand, a rolled towel, washcloth, or 500-ml IV bag. Insert the needle where the pulse is most prominent—½ to 1 inch proximal to the wrist crease—at a 40- to 60-degree angle. Direct it slowly along the long axis of the artery toward the pulsation (Fig. 79-5).

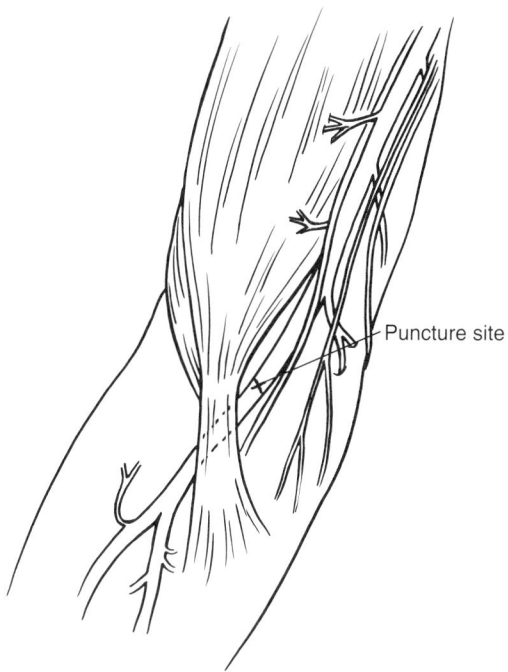

Fig. 79-6
Right brachial artery, its branches, and the anatomic site for brachial artery puncture.

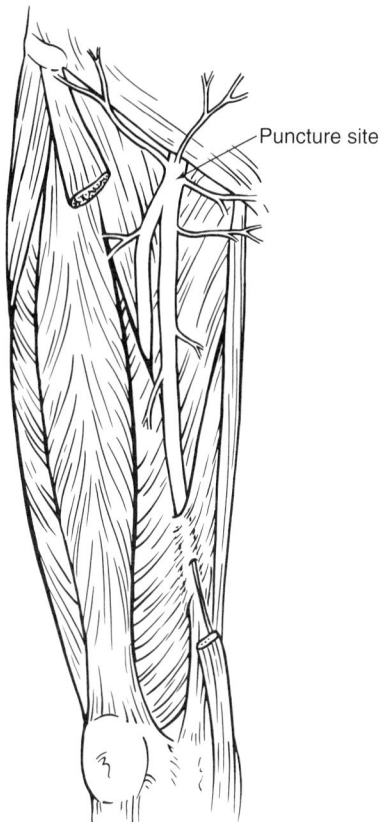

Fig. 79-7
Right femoral artery and branches.

Note: Avoid "spearing" or going through the artery. Osteomyelitis and large hematomas have resulted from "spearing" through the artery.

6b. *For brachial artery puncture:* Place the patient's elbow on a rolled towel or washcloth. Slightly hyperextend and supinate the arm (palm up) with the patient's wrist in the anatomic position (palm up) but rotated slightly outward. Insert the needle at about a 45- to 60-degree angle, slightly above the elbow crease. Aim along the long axis of the artery toward the pulsation, which should be palpable in the median aspect of the antecubital fossa (Fig. 79-6).

6c. *For femoral artery puncture* (Fig. 79-7): With the patient in a supine position and legs straight, rotated slightly outward, insert the needle 1 to 1½ inches distal to the inguinal ligament at about the inguinal crease. It should be angled 60 to 90 degrees and aimed toward the pulsation (Fig. 79-8). Avoid puncturing lateral to the pulsation because the femoral nerve could be damaged.

6d. *For dorsalis pedis artery puncture* (Fig. 79-9): With the patient in a supine position, insert the needle where the pulse is most prominent, at a 45- to 60-degree angle. Aim toward the pulsation.

7. Although penetration into the artery can occasionally be sensed, puncture is usually detected when blood enters the syringe. It should enter the syringe spon-

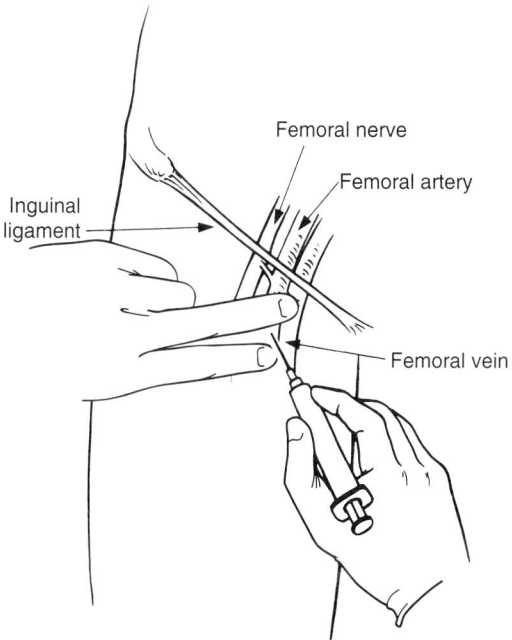

Fig. 79-8
Technique of femoral artery puncture. The first two fingers of the free hand are used to palpate the femoral artery.

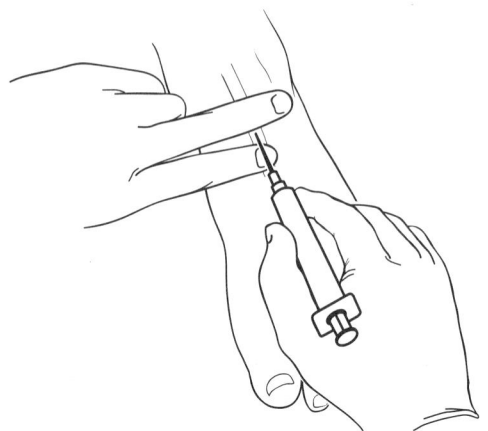

Fig. 79-9
Technique of dorsalis pedis artery puncture.

taneously without withdrawing the plunger if the syringe is specifically designed for arterial punctures. With plastic syringes or in severely hypotensive patients, slight aspiration may be necessary. Otherwise, attempt to avoid aspiration in order to decrease the chance of obtaining venous blood. If blood is not obtained during the insertion, slowly withdraw the needle and stop if blood appears.

8. If no blood appears, withdraw the needle completely and start again. For additional attempts, advance the needle without changing the angle of approach but with the needle directed ⅛ inch to either side of the previous attempt.

9. When blood appears, collect 3 ml of blood and remove the needle from the artery with a smooth swift motion while applying pressure to the site. Steady pressure should be maintained for at least 5 to 10 minutes (longer in hypertensive patients and patients on anticoagulant therapy).

10. While applying pressure at the site with one hand, use the other hand to hold the syringe with the needle tip upright and expel any air bubbles. Tapping the syringe may help expel bubbles clinging to the sides.

11. Secure the needle tip by impaling it on a rubber stopper or remove the needle and cap the syringe securely. Special rubber caps are available for this purpose. Do not allow any room air to get into the syringe or any air bubbles to remain.

12. Roll the syringe between the palms of the hands four or five times to mix the blood uniformly with the heparin.

13. Label the syringe appropriately with the patient's name and number(s), and place the syringe on ice. Immediately transport the syringe to the laboratory.

14. Return in 15 minutes and check the puncture site for hematoma formation and for adequate distal perfusion.

COMPLICATIONS

- Repeated punctures at the same site increases the risk of all complications.
- Hemorrhage or hematoma, the most common complications, can be minimized by prompt, continuous application (for 5 to 10 minutes) of pressure after the procedure, and by using a small-gauge (25-gauge) needle.
- Thrombosis is a possible complication of any arterial puncture. It more commonly results from puncture of the radial artery and those arteries with occlusive disease. The risk increases with repeated punctures. For a diminshed pulse after puncture, prompt vascular surgical consultation should be obtained. Ischemia and resulting gangrene are additional possible complications.
- Nerve damage can occur either from direct needle insertion into the nerve or from the pressure of a resultant hematoma. This is more common with brachial and femoral artery punctures.
- Infection is a possible complication including septic arthritis with femoral artery puncture. Try to avoid puncturing down to the bone with either a femoral artery puncture or any other puncture.
- Pseudoaneurysms have been reported, especially with femoral artery punctures. A pseudoaneurysm appears as a "pulsating tumor" with a bruit anterior to the artery. These occur more often following resolution of a large hematoma. Treatment is surgical removal of the pseudoaneurysm.
- An arteriovenous fistula may form after femoral puncture. In part, this is why the radial artery is a preferred site because there is no accompanying large vein.
- Spurious lab results are most often the consequence of mixing venous blood with the arterial sample, but they can also be due to an excessive quantity of heparin in the syringe. Heparin has a very low pH; therefore mixing with too much can cause not only a falsely low partial pressure of carbon dioxide (Pco_2), but also a low pH. Delay in analyzing the specimen or improper chilling can cause the blood to metabolize the oxygen, or for the oxygen to dissociate from hemoglobin. This will falsely lower the oxygen and pH and falsely elevate the Pco_2. Air in the syringe may markedly lower the Pco_2, since room air contains little carbon dioxide. Depending on whether the initial partial pressure of oxygen (Po_2) was greater or less than room air, mixing the sample with air may either falsely lower or elevate the Po_2. Vacutainers should not be used to draw arterial blood, because even though they are filled with nitrogen, they contain measurable

amounts of oxygen. Even this small amount of oxygen will significantly alter the arterial P_{O_2}.

POSTPROCEDURE PATIENT EDUCATION

The patient should be instructed not to rub the site. He or she should report any bleeding, pain, swelling, numbness, or tingling after the arterial puncture. If the extremity turns cold or blue, the patient should inform the nurse or clinician. If the patient is awake and alert, he or she can help hold pressure on the site while the clinician is delivering the specimen to the laboratory.

CPT/BILLING CODE

36600   Arterial puncture; withdrawal of blood for diagnosis

ICD-9-CM DIAGNOSTIC CODES

276.4   Acid-base mixed disorder
276.2   Acidosis
276.2   Acidosis, lactic
276.3   Alkalosis
493.01   Asthma, extrinsic with status asthmaticus
493.90   Asthma, unspecified with status asthmaticus
986.0   Carbon monoxide, toxic effect
427.5   Cardiac or cardiorespiratory arrest
491.2   Chronic obstructive bronchitis
491.20   Chronic obstructive bronchitis with emphysema
780.01   Coma
250.1   Diabetic ketoacidosis
493.9   Dyspnea, asthma
428.1   Dyspnea, cardiac
492.8   Emphysema, NOS
491.2   Emphysema, with chronic bronchitis
786.09   Hypercapnia
799.0   Hypoxia
428.1   Pulmonary edema (left heart failure)
415.1   Pulmonary embolism
518.5   Pulmonary insufficiency after trauma and surgery
799.1   Respiratory arrest
518.82   Respiratory distress: acute
786.09   Respiratory distress: NOS or respiratory insufficiency
518.81   Respiratory failure, NOS
518.83   Respiratory failure, chronic
518.84   Respiratory failure, acute and chronic
785.50   Shock, unspecified
785.51   Shock, cardiogenic
785.59   Shock, other (hypovolemic, septic)

ADDITIONAL RESOURCES

- See the sample patient education handout titled "Arterial Puncture" on page 1827 of Appendix G.
- See the sample patient consent form titled "Arterial Puncture" on page 1829 of Appendix G.

BIBLIOGRAPHY

Allen EV: Thromboangiitis obliterans: methods of diagnosis of chronic occlusive arterial lesions distal to the wrist with illustrative cases, *Am J Med Sci* 178:237, 1929.

American Heart Association: *Textbook of advanced cardiac life support,* Dallas, 1997, American Heart Association.

Baskett JF, Dow A, Nolan J, et al: *Practical procedures in anesthesia and critical care,* London, 1995, Mosby.

Kamienski RW, Barnes RW: Critique of the Allen test for continuity of the palmar arch assessed by Doppler ultrasound, *Surg Gynecol Obstet* 142:861, 1976.

Simon RR, Brenner BE: *Emergency procedures and techniques,* ed 3, Baltimore, 1994, Williams & Wilkins.

Slabach R: Arterial puncture. In Proehl JA, editor: *Emergency nursing procedures,* ed 2, Philadelphia, 1999, WB Saunders.

PERCUTANEOUS ARTERIAL LINE PLACEMENT

Intraarterial procedures are now common, with arterial dye studies and angioplasty even being performed by noncardiologists and nonsurgeons, such as interventional radiologists. The most common intraarterial procedures are arterial puncture and arterial cannulation. If arterial cannulation is to be performed, support staff and facilities must be properly trained and prepared to deal with the complications, which can be more frequent and more severe than with intravenous cannulation or arterial puncture. The site (radial, femoral, or dorsalis pedis artery) should be chosen according to the risks and priorities established in the "Arterial Puncture" section. Benefits of arterial cannulation include the following: arterial pressure measurements are more accurate, discomfort and injury from frequent arterial punctures are avoided, and arterial samples are obtained without disturbing the steady state (e.g., pain induced with arterial puncture can cause hyperventilation, resulting in falsely low P_{CO_2} measurements).

Note: For noninvasive monitoring of arterial pressure, Korotkoff's sounds are commonly used. With increased wall tension (e.g., in vasoconstricted patients, such as those with increased systemic vascular resistance from shock) the ability of the arterial walls to produce the Korotkoff's sounds may be altered. Therefore, in these patients, low cuff pressure does not necessarily indicate hypotension. Relying on Korotkoff's sounds alone in such patients can result in dangerous errors in therapy. Stiff walls from atherosclerosis can also alter Korotkoff's sounds as can using the wrong cuff size.

INDICATIONS

- When there is difficulty obtaining or risk of inaccuracy of cuff blood pressure in a critically ill patient
- When continuous monitoring of arterial blood pressure is needed, especially in patients in shock, patients with resultant increased systemic vascular resistance, patients who have the potential to become hemodynamically unstable, and during major surgery or administration of parenteral vasopressor or dilator medications
- With labile or accelerated hypertension and evidence of progressive vascular damage (Mean arterial pressure [MAP] is a much more consistent blood pressure monitoring parameter for accelerated hypertension than the systolic or diastolic pressure alone.)
- To monitor MAP in patients in whom it is necessary to maintain MAP at 50 mm Hg or higher to maintain cerebral perfusion pressure
- When continuous access to arterial blood is needed (to avoid repeated arterial punctures)
- To measure cardiac output by the dye dilution method

CONTRAINDICATIONS

- Inadequate collateral blood flow distal to where the arterial line will be placed (e.g., positive Allen test or dorsalis pedis collateral flow test, or the Doppler ultrasound examination reveals inadequacy of the collateral arterial circulation; see the "Arterial Puncture" section)
- Patients with a significant injury to the same extremity, especially if it may compromise distal perfusion
- Severe atherosclerotic or vasospastic arterial disease
- Hypercoagulable states

Relative Contraindications

The following are relative contraindications; in life threatening or certain other situations, the benefits of arterial cannulation may outweigh the risks of bleeding. In some patients, arterial cannulation will decrease the risks of bleeding from multiple punctures.
- Local skin compromise, such as with infection or a burn
- Anticoagulation from bleeding disorders, anticoagulant therapy, or potential future thrombolytic therapy

Note: Cannulation of the brachial artery is no longer recommended because of the potential for thrombosis and ischemia of the lower arm and hand.

EQUIPMENT

- Sterile gloves, drapes, and 4 × 4–inch gauze sponges
- Equipment for the clinician to observe universal blood and body fluid precautions
- Antiseptic skin preparation, such as povidone-iodine
- In the alert patient *(optional),* 1% lidocaine without epinephrine and a 3-ml syringe with 25-gauge, ⅝-inch (1.6-cm) needle
- Short arm board and a rolled gauze, towel, or washrag, about 3 inches in diameter, for radial artery cannulation
- For radial or dorsalis pedis artery cannulation, a 20-gauge, 1¼- to 2-inch (3.2- to 5.1-cm) Teflon catheter-over-needle with a nontapered shaft (Deseret Angiocath, Becton-Dickinson IV Cath, etc.)
- For femoral artery cannulation, a 19- or 20-gauge, 16-cm cannula
- For the Seldinger or wire-guided technique, a flexible guidewire small enough to pass through the catheter and needle
- Fluid-filled connector tubing attached to a transducer (using a stiff, low-capacitance tubing will minimize the artifact; also, attempt to minimize the length of tubing)
- Antibiotic ointment, such as povidone-iodine ointment
- Silk or nylon 4-0 suture, preferably on a skin needle
- Hypoallergenic adhesive tape
- Suture scissors
- Sterile three-way stopcock
- Bag of sterile dextrose water (D_5W) intravenous fluid mixed with heparin to make a 1-U/ml solution for flushing (this should be in-line with the connector tubing)
- Scissors for clipping hair for femoral insertion
- Handheld Doppler *(optional)*

PREPROCEDURE PATIENT PREPARATION

Explain the indications, complications, and necessity of the procedure to the patient if they are alert and awake. If they are unconscious, explain this to the next of kin. If there are alternatives available, discuss them as well as the benefits of this procedure. Discuss the importance of immobilization while the procedure is being performed, and warn the patient of the discomfort that will be felt with the insertion. Inform the patient that this catheter is more dangerous than an intravenous catheter and that care must be taken with the catheter after insertion. Obtain written consent for the procedure or document implied consent in the chart if they are unconscious.

TECHNIQUE

1. The clinician and the patient should be in a comfortable position that can be maintained as long as necessary. When using nonclosed systems, observe universal blood and body fluid precautions.

2. Palpate the artery selected and immobilize it along its course with two or three fingers of your nondominant hand.

3. Prep the skin in an aseptic manner. For femoral cannulation, use scissors to clip any long hairs in the area of the cannulation.

4. Local anesthetic (lidocaine) can be injected for a particularly anxious patient. It may also prevent arterial spasm when the artery is punctured. Use minimal amounts to prevent anatomic distortion with resultant difficulty in palpating the pulse. If the anatomy does get distorted from the anesthetic injection, attempt to massage it into the surrounding skin and soft tissue.

5. Drape the area with sterile towels.

6. Wearing sterile gloves, hold the catheter needle hub like a pencil in your dominant hand with the needle bevel up.

7a. *For radial artery cannulation:* On the patient's selected hand (preferably their nondominant hand if not contraindicated), slightly dorsiflex (about 30 degrees) and immobilize the wrist by taping a gauze roll between the supinated wrist and the dorsally applied arm board (Fig. 79-10, *A*). The 3-inch roll should be between the arm and the board. Apply tape over the proximal interphalangeal joints (excluding the thumb) and around the armboard. Also apply tape more proximally, securing the forearm to the armboard. Insert the needle ½ to 1 inch proximal to the wrist crease, at about a 30-degree angle. Direct it slowly along the long axis of the artery toward the pulsation (Fig. 79-10, *B*).

7b. *For femoral artery cannulation:* With the patient in the supine position and legs straight, rotated slightly outward, insert the needle at a 45-degree angle and direct it toward the patient's head. Also, direct it toward the femoral artery pulsation, 2 to 5 cm distal to the inguinal ligament at the inguinal crease. After the flash of blood, the angle can be lowered to 20 or 30 degrees relative to the leg. Large hematomas are not uncommon in this area because of the surrounding soft tissue. Femoral artery cannulation also carries the risk of more serious complications. A puncture proximal to the inguinal ligament could produce a retroperitoneal hematoma. The proximity of this location to the groin may increase the risk of infection. This location is also less popular for patients if they are awake and mobile (see Fig. 79-7).

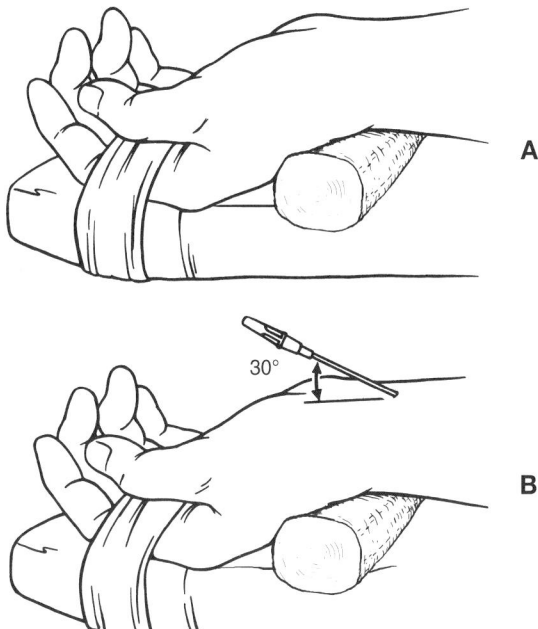

Fig. 79-10
A, Position for radial artery cannulation. **B,** Catheter is directed along the long axis of the artery.

7c. *For dorsalis pedis artery cannulation:* With the patient in the supine position, the foot plantar-flexed and stabilized on a firm surface, such as the bed, the dorsalis pedis artery should be palpated and stabilized using sterile technique (Fig. 79-11). Direct the needle tip and catheter slowly towards the arterial pulsation at a 20- to 30-degree angle.

Note: Because collateral circulation in the foot is usually good, dorsalis pedis arterial cannulation should be considered when radial artery cannulation is not an option. In patients with good cardiac output and palpable dorsalis pedis and posterior tibial pulses, dorsalis pedis arterial cannulation by experienced personnel has been demonstrated to have minimal risk of adverse events such as ischemia and thrombosis. It also allows the patient to be less movement restricted compared to sites other than the radial artery.

8. Puncture is detected when blood appears in the needle hub. For radial and dorsalis pedis artery cannulation, while holding the needle fixed, advance the catheter-over-needle·into the artery (Fig. 79-12). For femoral artery cannulation, do the same unless the Seldinger technique is desired. With the Seldinger technique, insert the wire through the needle into the artery, remove the needle, insert the catheter over the wire, and remove the wire. A modified Seldinger technique can be used for radial artery cannulation. Although the Seldinger technique

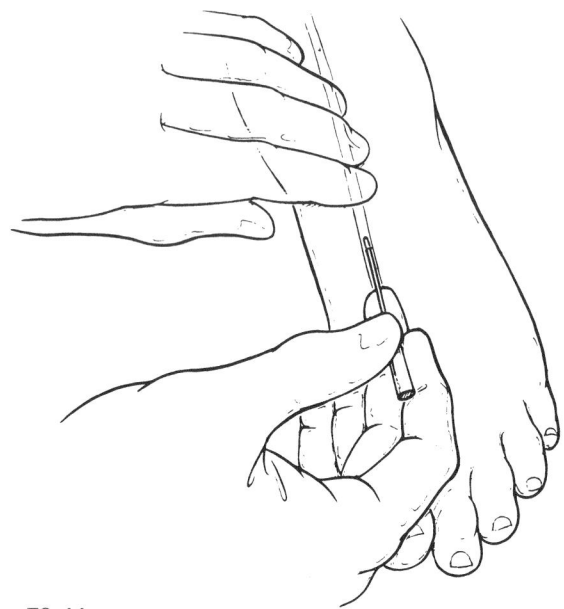

Fig. 79-11
Dorsalis pedis artery cannulation. (From American Heart Association: *Textbook of advanced cardiac life support,* Dallas, 1997, AHA.)

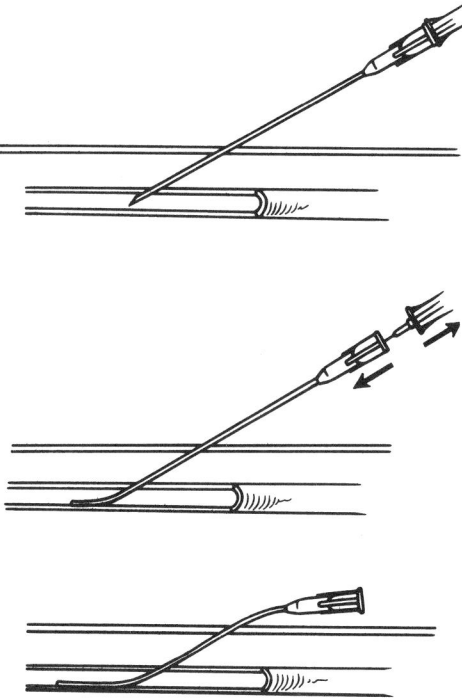

Fig. 79-12
Insert the angiocatheter through the skin and cannulate the artery.

is useful, an ordinary cannula is usually quicker and easier.

Note: The wire-guided technique may be more successful for arterial cannulation when the pulse is either weak or absent, especially in females.

9. If the artery cannot be cannulated after the flash of blood has appeared, the posterior artery wall has probably been penetrated. Remove the needle entirely, slowly withdraw the catheter until blood flows into it, and readvance the catheter.
10. For the Seldinger technique, to minimize the chance of intramural insertion or dissection, make sure the wire passes without *any* resistance.
11. If after three attempts the artery has not been entered, discontinue the procedure on that side and attempt on the other side or at another site; a cutdown might also be considered. Pressure should be applied to the unsuccessful site for at least 10 minutes, followed by a pressure dressing.
12. After insertion, advance the catheter until the hub is in contact with the skin, and attach it to the connector tubing (Fig. 79-13). Flush the catheter and zero the transducer system by opening the three-way stopcock to atmosphere and pushing the zero button on the pressure monitor. Return the three-way stopcock to the patient position and observe the arterial tracing. It should be sharp and clean. If it is not, reposition the catheter. If successful, securely stitch the catheter into position, apply antibiotic ointment, and cover with a sterile

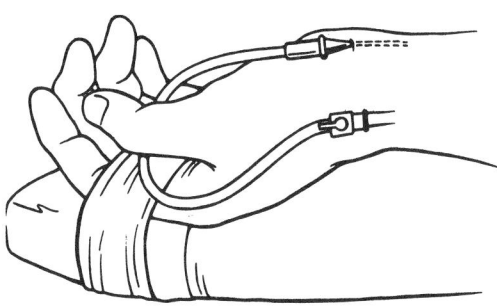

Fig. 79-13
Attach connector tubing to the catheter and fix in position.

dressing. For radial artery cannulation, remove the 3-inch roll.
13. Staff should check the extremity every 4 hours for perfusion, and the site for signs of a hematoma or early cellulitis. The dressing should be changed daily along with regular flushing of the line while cannulated and following catheter removal, observe the patient for bleeding, extremity pain, numbness, swelling, or discoloration.

Note: If the Seldinger technique is not used, the "liquid stylet" method may be useful. If a flash of blood is seen in the hub and the artery cannot be cannulated, fill a 10-ml syringe with 5 ml of sterile normal

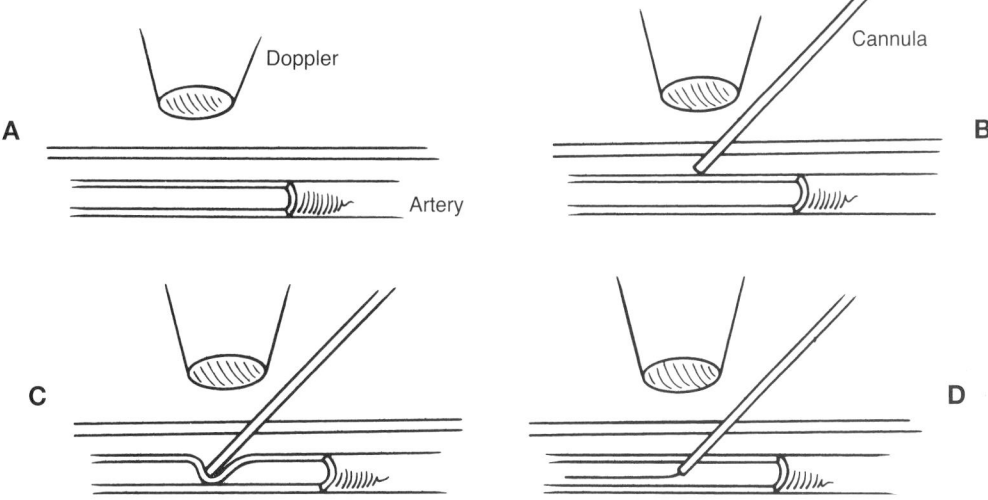

Fig. 79-14
Radial artery cannulation is being guided by Doppler ultrasound. **A-B,** The Doppler locates the artery and helps in guiding the cannula. **C-D,** The catheter occludes the artery temporarily and then punctures the arterial wall and is placed intraluminally.

saline. Attach the syringe to the catheter hub, and aspirate 1 to 2-ml of blood to verify intraluminal position. The blood should be very easy to aspirate. Slowly inject the fluid from the syringe and advance the catheter behind the fluid wave.

Alternative Method for Radial Artery Cannulation: Doppler Ultrasound Guided

1. Position the wrist in a slightly extended position and prep as previously described.
2. Using antiseptic ointment (such as povidone-iodine) as transmission gel, have an assistant align the handheld Doppler with the radial artery, at a site slightly proximal to the puncture site. The assistant should pass it back and forth medial to lateral over the artery and determine the point of maximal flow. He or she should then hold the Doppler in place at the point of maximal volume.
3. Insert and advance the catheter-over-needle slowly and with constant pressure, at a 45-degree angle to the skin and directed toward the point of maximal flow (Fig. 79-14, *A-B*).
4. Contact with the artery is discerned by a slight decrease in arterial flow sound.
5. As the needle compresses the artery before puncture, the flow sound may transiently cease (Fig. 79-14, *C-D*).
6. The characteristic sound of arterial blood flow should resume as the artery is punctured and a flash of bright red blood is seen in the needle hub.
7. Advance the cannula, and secure and calibrate it as described previously.

Troubleshooting for a Variance Between Cuff and Intraarterial Pressure and Preventive Maintenance for Accurate Readings

A variance or disparity of 5 to 20 mm Hg between measured cuff (indirect) and intraarterial (direct) pressures is normal and expected. If the intraarterial pressure is higher than cuff pressure, possible causes include improper cuff size or placement and improper calibration or zeroing of the transducer.

If cuff pressure is recorded as greater than intraarterial pressure, either equipment malfunction or technical error is likely. Damping of the arterial waveform suggests a problem with the intraarterial measurement. Air bubbles or blood in the line or transducer dome, a clot at the catheter tip, mechanical occlusion of the catheter or tubing, and loose or open connections are all possibilities. If the arterial waveform is not dampened, other causes include improper cuff size and placement, failure to calibrate the sphygmomanometer and the transducer, and an error in electrically or mechanically zeroing the transducer.

The variance of 5 to 20 mm Hg may be physiologic because the arterial pulse wave is transformed as it travels peripherally. As a result, the systolic pressure may become higher and the diastolic pressure lower. MAP, however, is unchanged.

If the disparity is 20 to 30 mm Hg, severe vasoconstriction (e.g., patient in shock or hypothermia) may be the cause, and inevitably the auscultated cuff pressure is lower. With occlusive atherosclerotic peripheral disease, if the radial or dorsalis pedis artery has been cannulated, cuff pressures are frequently higher than the directly measured pressures due to the more distal location of cannulation.

If the disparity is greater than 30 mm Hg, the most common cause is resonance in the catheter system. This can be minimized by using stiff tubing that is kept as short as possible. Directly measured pressure may be significantly higher than cuff pressure when a single-end-hole catheter is used in a narrow artery with high flow. If the hole faces the flow, the direct blood pressure may be falsely elevated.

To minimize disparities and to maximize accurate readings, the following 10 preventive steps should be followed or considered:

1. Allow the transducer and the amplifier to warm up for at least 10 minutes before zeroing and calibrating the system.
2. Purge all air from the pressure system; always observe for bubbles in the line and attempt to remove them if seen.
3. Use stiff, noncompliant extension tubing of the shortest possible length. Avoid the use of more than one stopcock between the catheter and the transducer. Place the extension tube near the patient to prevent a pulsating line.
4. Electrically zero and calibrate the system with a mercury manometer or a water column.
5. Mechanically zero the transducer.
6. At least once a shift, staff should check all fittings for tightness, check the zero setting (both electrically and mechanically), and check the calibration.
7. Avoid draining blood samples from the full length of the plumbing system.
8. Maintain a continuous low-flow flushing system to avoid clotting.
9. When the level of the patient is changed, recheck the mechanical and electrical zero positions and recalibrate the system if necessary.
10. Avoid making adjustments to the amplifier except at the time of calibration.

COMPLICATIONS

- Significant blood loss can occur if the tubing becomes disconnected.
- Arterial thrombosis (risk minimized by reducing the duration of cannulation, by choosing larger arteries, and by flushing properly). The risk of thrombosis increases if the cannula is left in place for longer than 72 hours.
- Embolism, usually distal. Retrograde arterial embolism can also occur from retrograde flushing of the cannula, and may enter the cerebral circulation. This danger is greater with smaller patients. For this rea-

son, with smaller patients either maintain a slow continuous flushing system or use volumes of heparinized solution smaller than 3 ml to avoid dislodging thrombi.
- Ischemia or necrosis distal to the site of arterial thrombosis, embolism stenosis, or occlusion.
- Hemorrhage or local hematoma.
- Aneurysm or pseudoaneurysm. The patient will present with a pulsatile mass. Management is surgical removal.
- Arterial occlusion. With the Seldinger technique, it is possible to cause a small dissection and arterial occlusion by passing the guide wire between the intima and the media.
- Local infection or sepsis, particularly after about 4 days.
- Arteriovenous fistula. This is more common with femoral artery cannulation, because of the proximity of the large vein.
- Neurologic complications, same as with arterial puncture.
- Vasovagal reactions.
- Permanent radial dorsalis pedis, or femoral artery stenosis or occlusion.

Note: A vascular surgeon should be consulted immediately if arterial flow is compromised in any way.

POSTPROCEDURE PATIENT EDUCATION

Explain to the alert patient and family the greater danger of a disconnected arterial line compared with a normal IV line. Instruct the patient not to rub or manipulate the site, line, or connectors. The patient should report any local pain, swelling, discoloration, or numbness at the site, or any bubbles in the line. He or she should also report any blood or dampness near the site. After catheter removal, the patient should also report bleeding, extremity pain, numbness, swelling, or discoloration.

CPT/BILLING CODE

36620   Arterial catheterization or cannulation for sampling, monitoring, or transfusion (separate procedure); percutaneous

ICD-9-CM DIAGNOSTIC CODES

In addition to ICD-9-CM diagnostic codes used for arterial puncture, the following are commonly used for arterial lines:

401.0   Hypertension, accelerated, malignant
411.1   Angina, unstable
410.9   Myocardial infarction, acute

ADDITIONAL RESOURCES

- See the sample patient education handout titled "Arterial Line" on page 1826 of Appendix G.
- See the sample patient consent form titled "Arterial Line (Cannulation)" on page 1828 of Appendix G.

BIBLIOGRAPHY

American Heart Association: Invasive monitoring techniques. In *Textbook of advanced cardiac life support*, Dallas, 1997, AHA.

Anderson JS: Arterial cannulation: how to do it, *Br J Hosp Med* 57(10):497, 1997.

Chapin JD: Section 14, Procedure 88/Section 3, Procedure 20. In Proehl JA, editor: *Emergency nursing procedures*, ed 2, Philadelphia, 1999, WB Saunders.

Franklin CM: The technique of dorsalis pedis cannulation, *J Crit Illn* 10(7):493, 1995.

Gerber DR, Zeifman CW, Khouli HI, et al: Comparison of wire-guided and non-wire-guided radial artery catheters, *Chest* 109(3):761, 1996.

Maher JJ, Dougherty JM: Radial artery cannulation guided by Doppler ultrasound, *Am J Emerg Med* 7:260, May 1989.

Mangar D, Thrush DN, Connell GR, Downs JB: Direct or modified Seldinger guide wire–directed technique for arterial catheter insertion, *Anesth Analg* 76(4):714, 1993.

CHAPTER 80

Electrical Cardioversion

Les B. Forgosh
David V. Power

Transthoracic direct-current electrical shock, or electrical cardioversion, is a safe and effective procedure for terminating most sustained tachyarrhythmias. It is useful for converting acute arrhythmias that are causing acute deterioration of the patient's condition, and for chronic arrhythmias that are symptomatic, carry a poor prognosis, or are unresponsive to drug therapy. Cardiac arrhythmias often can be converted to sinus rhythm with medications (chemical cardioversion), but electrical cardioversion refers to the direct application of electrical current.

CARDIOVERSION VERSUS DEFIBRILLATION

Cardioversion differs from defibrillation in that, with electrical cardioversion, the electrical discharge is synchronized with the R wave of ventricular depolarization in order to minimize the risk of triggering ventricular fibrillation. External paddles or patches are used to apply the electrical current, which causes total depolarization of the atria and ventricles. This depolarization frequently causes the instantaneous conversion of an arrhythmia to sinus rhythm. Electrical defibrillation is a procedure in which nonsynchronized electrical current is applied to convert chaotic fibrillation, or other rhythms that lead to unstable clinical conditions, to a normal sinus rhythm. Defibrillation is warranted in an unconscious, pulseless, and apneic patient once ventricular fibrillation (VF) is identified. Patients in VF or *pulseless* ventricular tachycardia (VT) should receive immediate defibrillation at 200 joules (J). Defibrillation should be repeated at 200, 300, and then 360 J if the rhythm does not convert. Defibrillation is an emergency procedure. One of the most generally accepted protocols for defibrillation is available through Advanced Cardiac Life Support (ACLS) courses given by many local hospitals and registered through the American Heart Association.

INDICATIONS

- Atrial fibrillation (AF)
- Atrial flutter
- Hemodynamically stable VT unresponsive to pharmacologic therapy
- Hemodynamically unstable VT
- Hemodynamically unstable supraventricular (SVT) arrhythmias
- Certain SVT arrhythmias unresponsive to pharmacologic therapy, including bypass tract SVT (e.g., Wolff-Parkinson-White syndrome)

CONTRAINDICATIONS

Absolute Contraindications

- Absent pulse (patient needs Basic Life Support measures and/or defibrillation)
- Severely unstable patients (patient needs resuscitation)
- Severe electrolyte disturbances
- Digitalis toxicity
- Left atrial or atrial appendage thrombus (for elective cardioversion)

Relative Contraindications

- Large left atrial diameter greater than 4.5 cm in AF.
- Sick sinus syndrome
- Multifocal atrial tachycardia
- Sinus tachycardia
- Minimal hemodynamic or clinical improvement while in sinus rhythm
- Inadequate anticoagulation and more than 48 hours duration of AF (unless transesophageal echo [TEE] negative)

A left atrial diameter greater than 4.5 cm in patients with AF is associated with a low likelihood of maintaining sinus rhythm. Patients with sick sinus syndrome or sinoatrial node block should not undergo cardioversion until a pacemaker has been placed. Multifocal atrial tachycardia and sinus tachycardia do not normally respond to cardioversion. Patients with a history of minimal hemodynamic or symptomatic improvement while in sinus rhythm may not need cardioversion because of an increased risk-to-benefit ratio. Inadequately anticoagulated patients with AF of longer than 48 hours duration have an increased risk of thromboembolic stoke or arterial embolization (5% rate in the first 2 weeks after cardioversion).

EQUIPMENT

- Handheld paddle electrodes, or 8- to 12-cm diameter, self-adherent pad electrodes or posterior paddle adapter
- Electrode gel or patches
- ACLS equipment:
  - Oxygen, nasal cannula
  - Airways and intubation equipment
  - Suction equipment
  - Emergency drug kit, including IVs
  - Medication to follow ACLS protocols
- ECG electrodes and ECG monitoring capabilities
- Direct current defibrillator-cardioversion unit, with synchronization capabilities and optional "quick look" paddles
- Sedatives for elective cardioversion

PREPROCEDURE PATIENT PREPARATION

Urgent cardioversion is indicated when the patient is unstable. Examples include symptomatic hypotension with central nervous system changes or syncope resulting from decreased perfusion. If the patient is alert, briefly explain the procedure while connecting the equipment. Informed consent is not necessary for a life-threatening situation. Document the indications and risks to the patient as time permits. The following preparation for elective cardioversion is not required for urgent cardioversion (if the clinical status of the patient is so tenuous that they would not survive).

Echocardiography

Echocardiography is helpful before elective cardioversion to estimate left atrial diameter (see Chapter 87, Echocardiography). Transesophageal echocardiography has been suggested as a method to identify small atrial thrombi, especially in the left auricular appendage, that are not visible with transthoracic echocardiography in

patients for whom anticoagulation with coumadin poses high risk.

Anticoagulation and Antiarrhythmics

All patients with AF for more than 48 hours should be anticoagulated adequately for 3 weeks before elective cardioversion because of the risk of embolizing intra-atrial thrombi when sinus rhythm (and atrial contractions) are reestablished. The incidence of emboli may be up to 5% for the first 2 weeks after cardioversion in nonanticoagulated patients. Recent trials indicate the benefits of anticoagulation in all chronic nonrheumatic AF patients. The international normalized ratio for anticoagulation should be maintained between 2.0 and 3.0 for at least 3 weeks before and 4 weeks after the procedure. The routine use of anticoagulation in arrhythmias other than AF is controversial.

Editor's note: A TEE is much more sensitive than a transthoracic echocardiogram for detecting thrombi, especially in the atrial appendage. Although the absence of a detectable thrombus does not preclude thromboembolism after cardioversion, a TEE-guided strategy (Klein, 2000) for elective cardioversion of AF has been reported that results in comparable outcomes compared with conventional anticoagulation.

There is some evidence suggesting that having the patient already therapeutic on antiarrhythmics before cardioversion may prevent recurrence. In the event that they might chemically convert, they should have been adequately anticoagulated or the TEE negative for thrombus before starting antiarrhythmics.

Fasting and Informed Consent

Instruct the patient to fast after midnight or for at least 4 to 6 hours before the procedure. Explain the indications for the procedure and the risk of complications to the patient. Explain that sedation will be used, but the patient may experience some achy discomfort in the arms and chest after the procedure. ECG monitoring for at least several hours will be necessary due to the risk of a recurrent or new arrhythmia. In addition, a minor skin irritation or burn may occur. Document the informed consent discussion and obtain the patient's signature on the consent form (see the sample patient consent form titled "Cardiac Procedure–Cardioversion" on page 1830 of Appendix G).

TECHNICAL CONSIDERATIONS FOR ELECTIVE CARDIOVERSION

Paddle-Electrode Selection and Placement

Apply the electrodes in either the standard paddle position (right upper parasternal and left apical) (Fig. 80-1, *A*) or alternative anterior-posterior paddle posi-

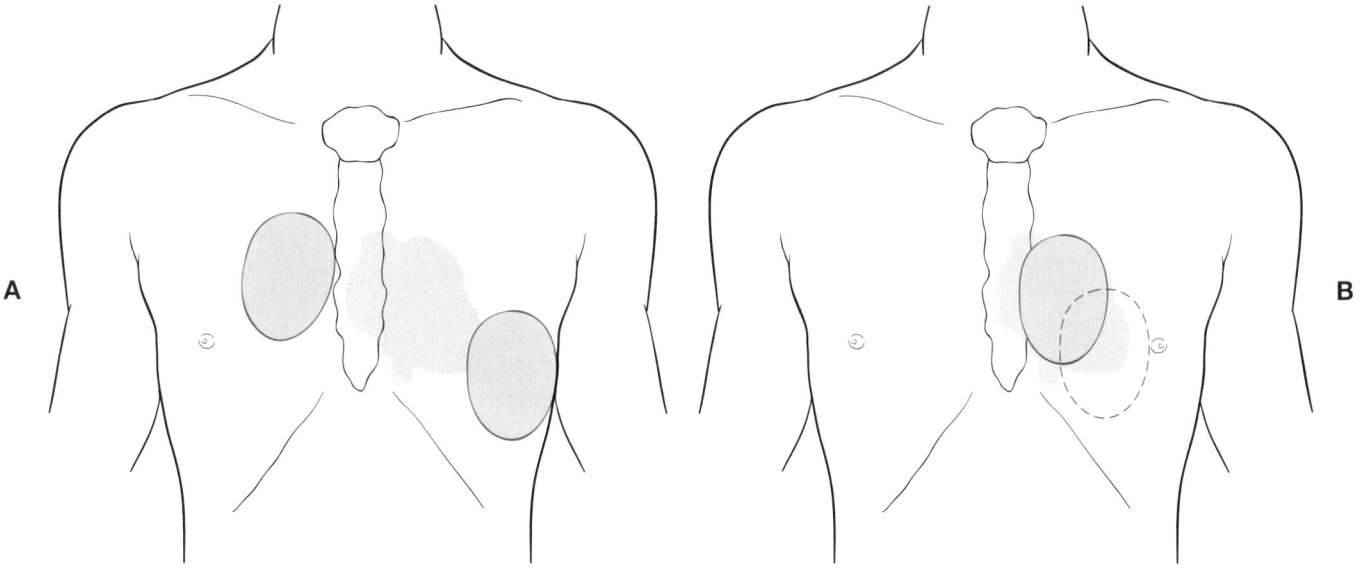

Fig. 80-1
A, Standard electrode position. **B,** Alternative electrode position.

tion (Fig. 80-1, *B*). Handheld paddle electrodes or self-adherent pad electrodes 8 to 12 cm in diameter deliver adequate energy for cardioversion. To maximize the current flow to the heart, correct paddle or electrode placement is crucial. Either positioning technique is acceptable, but anterior-posterior positioning may reduce energy requirements for cardioversion (through reduced electrical resistance) by up to 50%. In a large patient, this may increase cardioversion success. Self-adherent electrodes are available that can be used in place of the standard paddles. These electrodes are well suited to the anterior-posterior positioning. Alternatively, a posterior paddle adapter is available in which the paddle adapter is placed below the left scapula while the sternal paddle is applied directly to the patient's left anterior precordium. Either paddles or electrodes must be positioned far enough apart so that electrical current travels through the heart. Avoid paste or gel smeared on the skin between electrodes, which might allow the current to travel along the external chest wall. Electrodes should also be placed far enough away from a pacemaker generator to prevent damage to its electrical components.

ECG Monitoring

A set of ECG electrode patches should be placed on the patient, which are connected to the defibrillator, so that the shock can be synchronized. An additional set of ECG patches can be used to connect to a telemetry monitor.

Synchronization

Synchronization refers to the delivery of electrical current to the myocardium during a nonrefractory period (e.g., not when repolarization of the entire myocardium is occurring). Shocking the myocardium during the relative refractory period (the T wave) can simulate the "R on T" phenomenon and induce VF. In synchronized mode the energy is delivered at the peak of the QRS complex, the R wave. Synchronized administration reduces the energy requirements and complication rates of elective cardioversion.

Most defibrillators indicate when active synchronization is selected by highlighting the QRS peak. The practitioner can simply select and press the synchronization button for most cases of elective cardioversion. In cases with rapid ventricular response, the defibrillator in a synchronized mode may not be able to distinguish between the peak of the QRS complex and the peak of a T wave. As a safety feature, the defibrillator will not discharge if QRS complex and T waves cannot be distinguished. In this case, the provider should switch off the synchronization switch and perform unsynchronized defibrillation, realizing the increased risk of precipitating VT or VF. Alternatively, medications may be added to reduce the rapid ventricular response.

Energy Selection

Cardioversion is accomplished by passing an electrical current of sufficient magnitude through the heart to depolarize the myocardial tissues. Current flow is determined by the energy flow as measured in joules and by the resistance of the thoracic wall tissues as measured in ohms. The transthoracic resistance in an average adult is 70 to 80 ohms. If the transthoracic resistance is too high, the energy may fail to accomplish cardiac depolarization.

TABLE 80-1

Recommended Initial Energy Settings for Electrical Cardioversion

	Initial Energy Settings (J)
Atrial flutter	50
Atrial fibrillation	100*
Paroxysmal supraventricular tachycardia	50
Monomorphic ventricular tachycardia	100
Polymorphic ventricular tachycardia	200

*See text for details.

Some *SVT arrhythmias* are very sensitive to electrical current. Low energy settings may depolarize the myocardium in atrial flutter and allow the heart to resume a sinus rhythm. Recommended initial energy settings for cardioversion of various arrhythmias are listed in Table 80-1. For AF, the usual recommended initial energy setting is 100 J. However, recent evidence suggests that higher initial energy settings are more effective at achieving cardioversion, and some authors currently recommend an initial energy setting of 360 J.

Cardioversion energy for *VT* depends on the rate and morphologic features of the electrical activity. Monomorphic VT presents with a regular ECG form and rate, and it is generally responsive to cardioversion beginning at energies of 100 J. Polymorphic VT has an irregular form and rate and is less responsive to electroshock therapy. Polymorphic VT behaves like VF, and the initial defibrillator shock energy should be 200 J (unsynchronized).

If the first shock fails to cardiovert any arrhythmia, repeated attempts should be undertaken with stepwise energy increases. The transthoracic resistance increases after each shock, so the energy must be increased to overcome that resistance. The standard sequence for synchronized cardioversion is 100, 200, 300, and 360 J; the energies used depend on the initial energy selected. For example, after starting with 200 J, the second attempt to convert polymorphic VT should be with an energy of 300 J. Patients with large thoraces, chest wall deformities, or large amounts of adipose tissue may require higher initial settings.

Environment and Personnel

Elective cardioversion should be performed in a prepared environment, generally in a cardiac care unit with telemetry capabilities. The American College of Cardiology/American Heart Association guidelines (November, 2000) review the cognitive and technical skills necessary to perform external DC cardioversion and suggest a minimum requirement of eight prior supervised electrical cardioversions. Sedation or anesthesia is typically used with elective cardioversion, requiring appropriate personnel and monitoring. (See Chapter 2, Conscious Sedation [Sedation and Analgesia].)

TECHNIQUE

1. Review laboratory values and echocardiogram results or perform an echocardiogram (see Chapter 87, Echocardiography). Confirm that adequate levels of anticoagulation, normal electrolyte values (particularly potassium), and serum digoxin (if indicated) are in the normal range. If indicated, patients should already be therapeutic on an antiarrhythmic medication. Review echocardiogram findings, noting the absence of intraatrial thrombi (if appropriate) and an atrial diameter less than 4.5 cm.
2. Ensure that the patient has fasted.
3. Obtain a resting 12-lead ECG, and confirm the persistence of the rhythm disturbance.
4. Obtain informed consent (see the sample patient consent form titled "Cardiac Procedure–Cardioversion" on page 1830 of Appendix G).
5. Premedicate the patient with a sedative. Many experts recommend anesthesia standby if this service is available. Administration of a sedative (e.g., diazepam, midazolam) or a barbiturate can be combined with an analgesic (e.g., meperidine, fentanyl) to improve patient comfort.
6. The patient should be lying on a flat, dry surface.
7. Monitor the patient's ECG, pulse oximetry, and blood pressure throughout the procedure.
8. Initiate intravenous access. Apply supplemental oxygen.
9. Have suction, resuscitation equipment, and support staff immediately available.
10. Apply conductive material and electrodes.
11. Turn on the defibrillator.
12. Select the appropriate energy level for the dysrrhythmia, body habitus, and electrode positioning.
13. Turn on the synchronizer circuit.
14. Charge the capacitors to the preselected energy level.
15. Position the paddles or electrodes.
16. Call "All clear!" to indicate all personnel should move away from the patient's bed to avoid receiving a shock. Double-check by visually confirming all personnel (including yourself) have moved back and have no physical contact with the patient or the bed.
17. Deliver electrical energy by depressing appropriate discharge buttons on both paddles. (Keep buttons depressed until the shock is delivered.)
18. Assess the cardiac rhythm on the monitor.
19. Assess the patient and administer more sedation if needed.

20. If necessary, repeat cardioversion process (steps 12 through 17) at a higher energy setting.
21. Remember to reset the synchronization switch, if necessary. Some defibrillators reset the switch to the "off" position after a shock is delivered.
22. If cardioversion is unsuccessful after a shock at 360 J, abort the procedure and consider additional antiarrhythmic medications.

COMPLICATIONS

- Unsuccessful cardioversion
- Transient mild arrhythmias
- Conversion to VT or VF
- Bradycardia
- Elevated cardiac enzymes (up to three times normal values)
- Localized cutaneous burns
- Accidental shock to attending personnel because of contact with the patient or bed
- Damage to electrical equipment in contact with the patient or bed
- Thromboembolic events
- Recurrence of original arrhythmia

If the original arrhythmia persists after more than three shocks and up to 360 J, the cardioversion is considered unsuccessful. In this case, the procedure should be aborted. Allow the patient to waken. Explain that the cardioversion was unsuccessful despite maximal safe efforts, and list the various options available to the patient and anyone else present. Options include internal cardioversion, antiarrhythmic medications, devices such as pacemakers, or no further treatment. Catheter ablation techniques are now also becoming available. In a significant number of patients with unresponsive AF, internal cardioversion with intracardiac electrode catheters has been successful. In this case, anticoagulation needs to be withheld temporarily because of the risk of bleeding at the catheter site. Alternatively, additional, more specific antiarrhythmic medications could be considered. The cardioversion may be reattempted after therapeutic blood levels are achieved (usually a few days). The patient may decide that further attempts are not worth the perceived risks.

Other complications following cardioversion are uncommon in the absence of digitalis toxicity or hypokalemia and with a properly delivered shock. Bradycardia is sometimes noted immediately after cardioversion in patients with a history of inferior myocardial infarction. If symptomatic, atropine may be used. Transient mild arrhythmias or creatine kinase elevations of less than three times normal may be noted, but they are generally inconsequential.

With any cardioversion, especially with rapid heart rates, there is a risk of producing a worse rhythm, such as VT or VF. Any attempted cardioversion that results in VF should be *defibrillated (synchronization off)* immediately, starting with 200 J of energy. On some defibrillators, the synchronization must be shut off manually to administer a nonsynchronized shock.

Application of adequate amounts of electrode paste to the paddles can minimize cutaneous burns. Electrical shock is a possibility for anyone in contact with the patient or the patient's bed. Any attached electrical equipment can be damaged. Systemic emboli may develop if the patient is not adequately anticoagulated, causing neurological deficit or occlusion of a peripheral artery. The original arrhythmia may recur, despite successful cardioversion.

POSTPROCEDURE MONITORING

- Monitor the patient for 2 to 4 hours. An example of monitoring orders includes vital signs with neurological checks every 15 minutes for 1 hour, then every hour for 2 hours. Provide continuous ECG telemetry during this time. Atrial or ventricular ectopy and bradycardia are not uncommon in the first 15 to 30 minutes after cardioversion.

CONCLUSION

Elective external cardioversion is usually a safe procedure. However, serious complications can occur, and basic competence and training, with maintenance of that competency, is recommended for clinicians who perform cardioversion. The clinician should be ACLS certified. New developments continue to occur in this field with the arrival of defibrillators that provide a biphasic shock, which may replace the monophasic shocks of current units. Newer units permit lower energy use and convert more patients on the first shock. Low-energy internal cardioversion is now a safe and effective alternative for failed external cardioversion. Increasingly, implanted cardioverter-defibrillators are recommended for patients at high risk of serious arrhythmia, and these are likely to become a routine outpatient procedure. However, external cardioversion presently remains a common and effective procedure, particularly for patients in AF.

SUPPLIERS

Most hospitals have this equipment. Familiarize yourself with the equipment available in your particular setting.

CPT/BILLING CODES

92950   Cardiopulmonary resuscitation
92960   Cardioversion, elective; electrical conversion of arrhythmia, external

ADDITIONAL RESOURCES

- See the sample patient consent form titled "Cardiac Procedure–Cardioversion" on page 1830 of Appendix G.

BIBLIOGRAPHY

Catherwood E, Fitzpatrick WD, Greenberg ML, et al: Cost-effectiveness of cardioversion and antiarrhythmic therapy in nonvalvular atrial fibrillation [see comments], *Ann Intern Med* 130(8):625, 1999.

DeSilva RA, Graboys TB, Podrid PJ, Lown B: Cardioversion and defibrillation, *Am Heart J* 100(6):881, 1980.

Joglar JA, Hamdan MH, Ramaswamy K, et al: Initial energy for elective external cardioversion of persistent atrial fibrillation, *Am J Cardiol* 86(3):348, 2000.

Klein EA: Assessment of cardioversion using transesophageal echocardiography (TEE) multicenter study (ACUTE I): clinical outcomes at eight weeks, *J Am Coll Cardiol* 36:324, 2000.

Mathew TP, Moore A, McIntyre M, et al: Randomised comparison of electrode positions for cardioversion of atrial fibrillation, *Heart* 81(6):576, 1999.

Reuter D, Ayers GM: Future directions of electrotherapy for atrial fibrillation, *J Cardiovasc Electrophysiol* 9(8 Suppl):S202, 1998.

Stroke Prevention in Atrial Fibrillation Investigators: Stroke prevention in atrial fibrillation study, *Circulation* 84(2):527, 1991.

Tracy CM: American College of Cardiology/American Heart Association clinical competence statement on invasive electrophysiology studies, catheter ablation, and cardioversion, *J Am Coll Cardiol* 36:1725, 2000.

Truong JH, Rosen P: Current concepts in electrical defibrillation, *J Emerg Med* 15(3):331, 1997.

Walker JR: Anesthesia for cardioversion, *J Perianesth Nurs* 14(1):35, 1999.

CHAPTER 81

Central Venous Catheter Insertion*

Thomas A. Bzoskie
Brian D. Madden

Approximately 3 million central venous (CV) catheters are placed annually in the United States. As a result, if clinicians are managing hospitalized patients, it is very likely that some of their patients will require central venous catheterization. It is important for clinicians to know how to properly insert a CV catheter as well as the indications and complications, whether they personally insert the catheter or choose to consult another clinician.

INDICATIONS

- CV pressure measurement and monitoring
- For venous access when peripheral veins are inadequate (burn patients may require CV catheterization)
- Emergency venous access needed
- Access for hyperalimentation and administration of hyperosmolar or irritant solutions (especially those associated with soft tissue necrosis with extravasation)
- Administration of cardiac medication during cardiopulmonary resuscitation (CPR)
- Hemodialysis or plasmapheresis
- As an alternative to repetitive venous cannulations
- Before pulmonary artery (Swan-Ganz) catheter placement
- Access for temporary transvenous pacemaker, cardiac catheterization, or pulmonary angiography

CONTRAINDICATIONS

- Distortion of local anatomy or landmarks
- For subclavian, moderate to severe chest wall deformities that distort local anatomy
- Suspected injury to the superior vena cava (e.g., superior vena cava syndrome; in that situation, venous access below the diaphragm is preferable)
- Bleeding diathesis or anticoagulation therapy (unless emergent catheterization is required, antecubital venous cutdown is preferred)
- Full-thickness burn, cellulitis, or other infection over the anticipated insertion site
- Pneumothorax or hemothorax on the contralateral side
- Inability to tolerate pneumothorax on ipsilateral side

RELATIVE CONTRAINDICATIONS

- Suspected prior injury to the vein intended for insertion.
- Morbid or marked obesity.
- Marked cachexia.
- Vasculitis that predisposes to sclerosis or thrombosis of the veins.
- Previous long-term central catheterization, injection of hyperosmotic or irritant solution, or recently discontinued catheter in the same vein.
- Surgery is proposed in the area and on the side of catheter insertion.
- Patients receiving ventilatory support with high end–expiratory pressures (e.g., positive end–expiratory pressure; if possible, ventilation should be interrupted briefly while attempting to locate the vein with the catheter or introducing needle).
- Intraclavicular subclavian insertion during CPR. (If CPR can be halted briefly, insertion is easier and safer; jugular access can usually be obtained without stopping CPR. Otherwise peripheral access may be preferable; see Chapter 96, Venous Cutdown.)
- Children less than 2 years old due to high risk of complications (the internal jugular vein is the best route for central access, if it must be obtained).
- Severe hypovolemia, if peripheral access can be used or provided with a large-bore catheter (16-gauge or larger).

Note: A large volume of fluid can actually be infused more rapidly through a large-bore peripheral catheter than through a small-bore central catheter.

---

*This chapter was modified from the chapter written for the first edition by John F. Donnelly and John M. Passmore, Jr.

- Additional contraindications specific to *internal jugular vein* cannulation include significant carotid artery disease, distorted cervical anatomy, and recent, unsuccessful contralateral cannulation (to prevent bilateral neck hematomas that could compromise the patient's airway).

EQUIPMENT

- Sterile prep solution (povidone-iodine, or hexachlorophene if the patient is iodine-allergic)
- Sterile swabs
- Sterile gloves and drapes (mask and sterile gown if CV catheter will be used for pulmonary artery catheterization)
- Goggles or eye protection
- Prep razor
- Lidocaine 1%
- Needle (25 gauge) for anesthetic
- 3- to 5-ml syringe for anesthetic
- 10-ml syringe
- Intravenous solution and connector tubing, flushed and ready
- CV catheter and insertion set (review the contents to ensure that it contains the appropriate catheter and to anticipate any other items that may be needed)
- Bath towel
- 4 × 4–inch sterile gauze pads
- Needle holder (can be excluded if a Keith needle is used)
- Silk or nylon sutures (3-0 or 4-0) on a cutting needle
- Suture scissors
- Topical antimicrobial ointment
- Tincture of benzoin or dressing adhesive
- Adhesive or cloth tape in precut lengths

Use the following equipment for the optional Seldinger technique:
- Introducing needle (typically 20 gauge)
- Guidewire or J-wire (flexible wire 35 cm long, 0.089 cm in diameter with a 3-mm radius of curvature)
- Catheter/sheath and dilator/introducer
- No. 11 blade scalpel

Note: Dedicated ultrasound units are available for insertion of central lines and are often available in intensive care units (see Chapter 209, Emergency Department and Office Ultrasound).

PREPROCEDURE PATIENT PREPARATION

Since CV catheterization is often an emergency procedure, written informed consent may not be available. However, explain the indications, risks, and benefits of the procedure to the patient and the family, if possible. The implied consent should be documented.

If the procedure is performed in a controlled situation, obtain informed consent. This includes a review of the risks, benefits, alternatives, and contraindications. Review the major complications that may require a chest tube placement, surgery, or cardioversion along with the general risks of pain, infection, bleeding, and scar formation. Explain the major steps of the procedure, including positioning (Trendelenburg) and sterile draping. Inform the patient that he or she will experience some discomfort. If a ventilator is being used, discuss temporary interruption during introducer needle insertion. Document your informed consent before the procedure.

OVERVIEW

1. Before attempting to place a CV catheter, the clinician should consider whether the situation actually requires CV access. Patients who require volume resuscitation can often be managed with large-bore peripheral lines.

Note: Again, a large volume of fluid can actually be infused more rapidly through a large-bore peripheral catheter than through a small-bore central catheter.

2. The clinician should obtain central access through the route with which they are most comfortable and most experienced if the patient's anatomy is amenable. Knowledge of the regional anatomy is important for successful cannulation and for minimizing the risk of complications. Keep in mind that each case is different, and always maintain a healthy respect for the possible severe complications that can occur.
3. Strict adherence to sterile technique is necessary to prevent infectious complications. This will be especially important if the central line must remain in place longer than 3 days or may be converted to a pulmonary artery catheter. Since optimal observation of aseptic technique is difficult during CPR, at the earliest opportunity consider replacing central lines placed during resuscitative efforts. Until then, consider prophylactic intravenous antibiotics to decrease the possibility of infection with skin pathogens. This may be accomplished with one dose of cefazolin (1 g) or vancomycin (500 mg).
4. Excluding intrinsic thoracic disease or other contraindications, the *right* subclavian vein is preferred over the left because (1) the lung apex is slightly lower, (2) there is a linear relationship between the right internal jugular vein and the superior vena cava, and (3) the left-sided thoracic duct cannot be injured.
5. With unilateral chest trauma, the insertion should be attempted on the injured side. This protects the

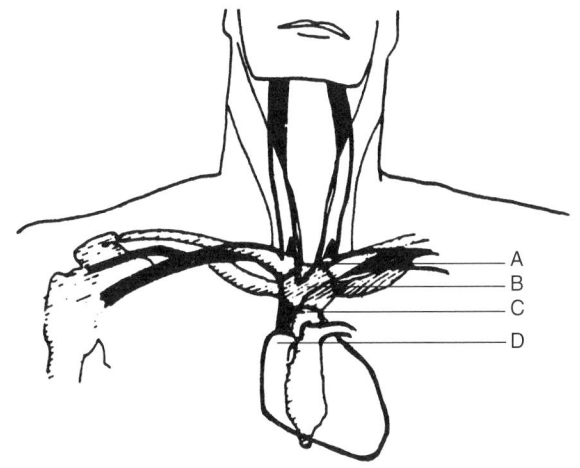

Fig. 81-1
Surface markers on chest wall to determine length of catheter placement. *A*, Sternoclavicular joint, subclavian vein; *B*, midmanubrial area, brachiocephalic vein; *C*, manubrial-sternal junction, superior vena cava; *D*, 5 cm below manubrial-sternal junction, right atrium. (From American Heart Association: *Textbook of advanced cardiac life support*, Dallas, 1997, American Heart Association.)

uninjured hemithorax in the event that there are complications from the procedure. If attempted catheterization is unsuccessful, consider the ipsilateral internal jugular or supraclavicular subclavian approach before trying the contralateral infraclavicular subclavian. This reduces the risk of bilateral complications.

6. The desired final position of the catheter is with the tip in the superior vena cava near the right atrium. This distance can be estimated by holding the catheter above and parallel to the chest wall before insertion. The catheter will be threaded until the tip is approximately 2 to 3 cm below the manubrial-sternal junction. Use this surface anatomy correlation to estimate the desired catheter length (Fig. 81-1).

7. Universal blood and body fluid precautions should be followed throughout the procedure.

8. A chest radiograph should be completed and read immediately after insertion (or failed insertion) to verify correct catheter position or to rule out complications from the procedure.

SUBCLAVIAN VEIN CATHETERIZATION (INFRACLAVICULAR APPROACH)

The key to this technique is an appreciation of the anatomic relationship between the clavicle and the subclavian vein.

Anatomy

The subclavian vein begins as a continuation of the axillary vein at the lateral border of the first rib, and it

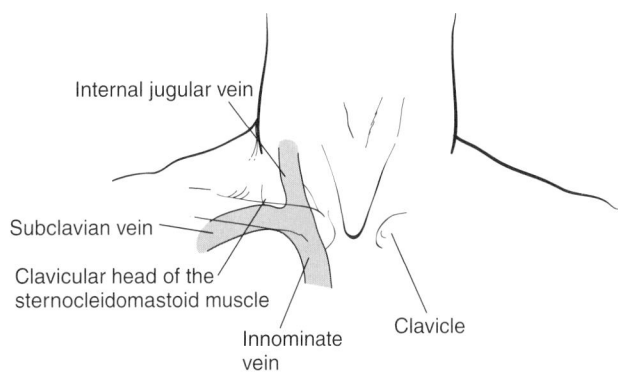

Fig. 81-2
Anatomic relationships of the subclavian vein.

joins the internal jugular vein to form the innominate (braciocephalic) vein (Fig. 81-2). As it crosses behind the first rib, the subclavian vein lies posterior to the medial third of the clavicle; it is only in this region that an intimate anatomic relationship exists between the subclavian vein and the clavicle. The subclavian vein is valveless and has a diameter of 1 to 2 cm. The costoclavicular ligament lies anterior and inferior to the subclavian vein. The subclavian artery is superior and posterior to the vein; the anterior scalene muscle separates the subclavian vein from the artery. Nearby structures of significance include the phrenic nerve; the thoracic duct (on the left side); and the lymphatic duct (on the right side), which enters the subclavian vein near its juncture with the internal jugular. The dome of the pleura of the lung is also nearby and may extend above the first rib on the left side. It rarely extends this far cephalad on the right.

Patient Position

Proper positioning of the patient is crucial for successful cannulation and to minimize risk of complications.

1. Place the patient in Trendelenburg's position at an angle of 15 to 30 degrees (or as much as the patient can tolerate). As it turns out, this position does not cause vein engorgement in euvolemic patients, but it does decrease the risk of air embolism by creating positive pressure inside the vein. Raise the bed to a comfortable level for the operator.

2. Turn the patient's head to the opposite side, but less than 45 degrees. This position may decrease the risk of contamination of the insertion site and minimize the patient's anxiety during the procedure. However, turning the head to the opposite side has not been proven to influence vessel diameter or the relationship of the subclavian vein to the clavicle. Turning beyond 45 degrees may increase the risk of catheter malposition.

3. Consider placing a rolled bath towel between the patient's scapulae to allow the shoulders to assume a

neutral position in slight retraction. This is one of the key elements to a successful subclavian catheterization. However, if the clavicles are more prominent with the towel in place, the towel should be removed. Such positioning decreases the space between the clavicle and first rib, making the subclavian vein less accessible.

4. Both arms should be at the patient's sides, restrained if necessary, to prevent interference with the procedure.

Procedure

1. Position the patient in at least 15 degrees of Trendelenburg, with the head turned to the opposite side, as described above.
2. Observe sterile technique and use sterile gloves. Again, some experts recommend use of a facemask, cap, and gown, especially if the central line may be converted into a pulmonary artery catheter.
3. Scrub, shave, and prepare a wide area over the insertion site. In a sterile fashion, drape the infraclavicular and supraclavicular areas.
4. Assemble the introducing needle and a 3-ml syringe, with the bevel of the needle aligned with the markings of the syringe. This alignment allows awareness of the bevel direction after the skin is punctured.
5. Note important anatomic landmarks. Palpate the region that is inferior to the clavicle to locate the costoclavicular ligament connecting the first rib to the clavicle. This ligament lies at the junction of the medial third and middle third of the clavicle at the point where the clavicle bends posteriorly. Place

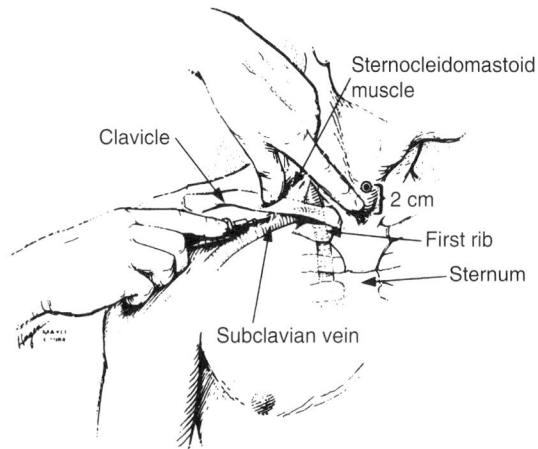

Fig. 81-3
Technique of subclavian vein catheterization. With the index finger in the suprasternal notch and the thumb marking the costoclavicular ligament, insert the needle just medial to the thumb. (From Schwartz RS et al: Cardiac catheterization and angiography. In Giuliani ER, Fuster V, Gersh BJ, et al: *Cardiology: fundamentals and practice,* ed 2, St Louis, 1991, Mosby.)

your thumb over the costoclavicular ligament and your index finger in the suprasternal notch (Fig. 81-3). The subclavian vein traverses the imaginary line connecting these two points. For an alternate landmark for puncture, note the location of the lateral aspect of the clavicular head of the sternocleidomastoid muscle.

6. In the alert, conscious patient, anesthetize the skin at the puncture site with several milliliters of 1% lidocaine, using the 10-ml syringe and 25-gauge, 1½-inch needle. Anesthetize the subcutaneous tissue and periosteum of the clavicle along the anticipated route of cannulation. As the needle is advanced and before injecting lidocaine, make sure that the needle is not in the vein by aspirating.
7. It is helpful to have several milliliters of local anesthetic in the introducing syringe so that during insertion, the subcutaneous tissue can be further anesthetized, as needed. This also allows for the needle to be continuously flushed of any skin plugs.
8. With your thumb over the costoclavicular ligament and index finger in the suprasternal notch, insert the introductory needle caudal to the clavicle and just medial to the thumb. Aim slightly cephalad and posterior to the index finger in the suprasternal notch. An alternative description of the puncture site below the clavicle is 1 cm lateral, 1 cm inferior (below clavicle), 1 cm posterior to the lateral border of the clavicular head of the sternocleidomastoid muscle.
9. If the patient is being ventilated with positive pressure, it is advisable to temporarily stop the ventilator as the needle punctures the chest wall. Ventilation should not be interrupted longer than 30 seconds. A respiratory therapist should be available to assist, if necessary.
10. While gently aspirating, advance the needle at a 5- to 10-degree angle relative to the patient's chest wall until the needle contacts the patient's clavicle. The needle bevel should be facing medially, facilitating later passage of the guidewire or catheter down the brachiocephalic vein. At this point, decrease the angle of the needle so that it is parallel to the patient's chest wall. Carefully advance it under the clavicle while still directing it slightly cephalad. Aim toward your finger in the suprasternal notch. Maintain continuous negative pressure on the syringe as you advance the needle, slowly, while keeping the needle shaft parallel to the patient's chest wall (Fig. 81-4).

Entry of the vein is indicated by a flash of dark venous blood, which usually occurs at a depth of 1 to 2 cm. Blood return should flow freely if the needle is truly intraluminal and not lodged against the vessel wall.

Note: Some authorities recommend locating the vein first with a smaller needle, such as a 22-gauge needle attached to a 3-ml syringe. When the vein is located, the smaller needle is removed and the introductory needle assembly is directed in the same manner at the same location and angle.

11. Pulsatile, bright red blood indicates inadvertent puncture of the subclavian artery. Withdraw the needle and apply firm pressure for 10 minutes over the puncture site.
12. If no flash of blood is observed at a depth of 3 cm, slowly withdraw the needle while maintaining negative pressure on the syringe. A flash may be encountered while the needle is being withdrawn.
13. If the first attempt is unsuccessful, completely withdraw the needle and flush it with air to remove any tissue plugs. Repeat the process as described previously, but direct the needle approximately 5 degrees cephalad to the finger in the suprasternal notch and slightly more posteriorly.

Note: We recommend changing the direction of the needle only after totally withdrawing it, to minimize the risk of lacerating the vein or puncturing neighboring structures. Seek assistance after three to four attempts, or consider venipuncture of the ipsilateral internal jugular vein or contralateral subclavian vein (after the chest radiograph rules out pneumothorax).

14. When the vein has been entered successfully, rotate the needle so that the bevel (which is still aligned with the syringe markings) faces caudally. Verify that blood flows freely with aspiration; rotation of the

needle may have placed its tip against the vessel wall. If blood does not flow freely, carefully withdraw or advance the needle 1 to 2 mm while aspirating slightly.

15. When the needle is positioned properly, stabilize it by grasping it with your thumb and index finger. Hold it firmly against the chest while detaching the syringe. Immediately occlude the needle hub with your thumb to prevent an air embolus. During this step, ask the alert patient to perform a Valsalva's maneuver or to exhale, which raises intrathoracic pressure. If the syringe is firmly affixed to the needle, a hemostat may be useful to grasp and anchor the needle during removal of the syringe; this may minimize the risk of needle displacement from the vessel lumen. Do not draw blood specimens until the catheter is securely threaded into the vessel. Drawing blood through the needle increases the chance of displacing the needle tip from the vessel lumen.

Catheter-through-the-needle devices

a. Quickly thread the catheter through the needle while stabilizing the needle with the other hand (Fig. 81-5). The catheter should advance without resistance. If resistance occurs, *do not force the catheter;* rather, recheck for blood return by aspirating before advancing the catheter again. Gently twisting and advancing the catheter may free it if it has become trapped against the opposite vessel wall or advanced past the junction of the subclavian vein and internal jugular veins. It may also

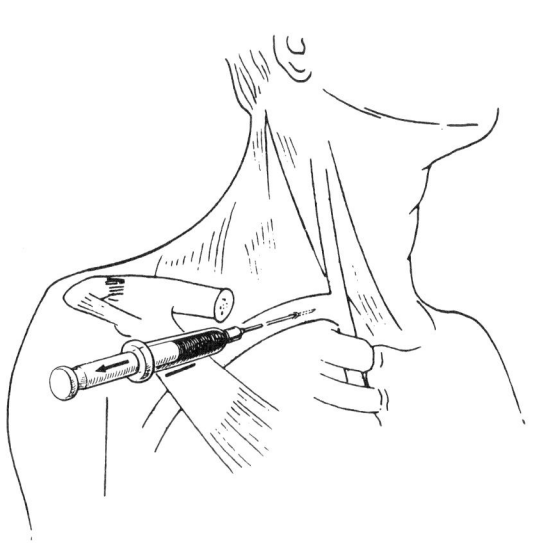

Fig. 81-4
Proper needle advancement. See text for details.

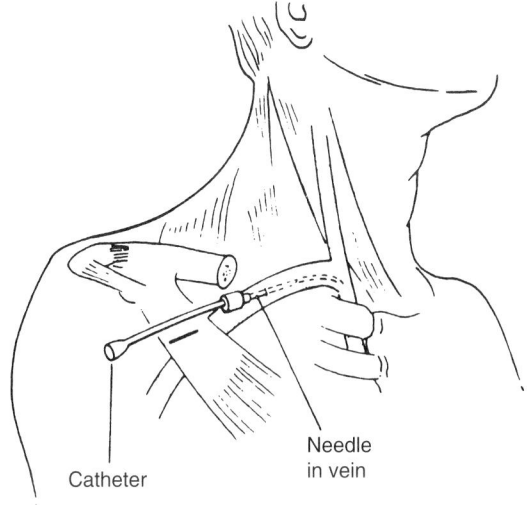

Fig. 81-5
Catheter threading. After removal of the syringe, thread the catheter fully into the needle. (From Roberts JR, Hedges JR, editors: *Clinical procedures in emergency medicine,* ed 3, Philadelphia, 1998, WB Saunders.)

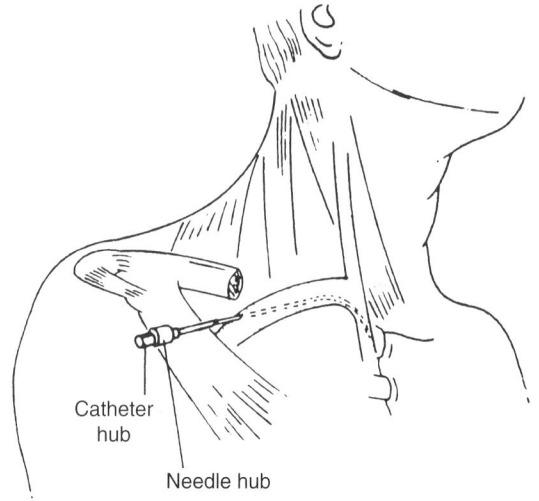

Fig. 81-6
Withdrawal of the needle and the catheter hub, slightly, leaves only the catheter beneath the skin and in the vein.

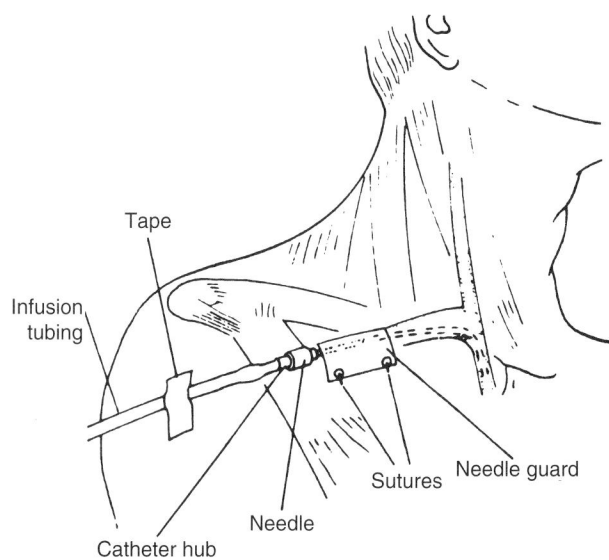

Fig. 81-7
Place the guard and suture it to the skin below the clavicle.

help unwind a kinked catheter. If the catheter cannot be advanced despite these measures, withdraw the catheter and needle as a unit. *Do not withdraw the catheter alone, through the needle, since this may transect the catheter and cause a catheter fragment embolus. For the same reason, never advance the needle after the catheter has been deployed past the needle tip.*

b. When the catheter threads smoothly, advance it fully into the needle hub and toward its desired final position in the superior vena cava. If the patient is being continuously monitored (by an electrocardiogram), the operator or assistant should watch the monitor for arrhythmias while the catheter is being advanced. Withdraw, slightly, for PVCs or arrhythmias.

c. After the catheter is inserted, withdraw the needle from the vein over the catheter (and then with the catheter hub) until the needle is just outside the skin (Fig. 81-6).

d. Immediately attach the guard over the needle (Fig. 81-7).

e. Attach the syringe to the catheter hub and attempt to aspirate blood. Free blood return is presumptive, but not definitive, evidence of intravascular positioning of the catheter. (Blood return may also occur from a hematoma or hemothorax, with the catheter not residing in the vessel lumen.)

f. If blood return is obtained, remove the syringe and connect the intravenous tubing to the catheter hub. Before infusing intravenous fluids, lower the intravenous solution bag beside the bed to a level below the patient, and observe for backflow of

blood. This further confirms the intravascular catheter position.

Note: Do not infuse intravenous fluids or medications until a chest radiograph confirms that the CV catheter is in the proper position.

g. Secure the catheter at the insertion site by placing a 3-0 or 4-0 silk or nylon suture through the skin, tying it, looping it around the catheter hub three to four times, and tying the suture again. Ensure that the suture does not constrict the catheter lumen. Alternatively, the needle guard may be affixed to the chest wall at two points parallel and caudal to the clavicle by placing silk suture through the skin and then through the two holes of the needle guard.

h. Apply antimicrobial ointment to the insertion site. Cover it with a sterile transparent cover, to facilitate routine inspection, followed by a 4 × 4–inch gauze sponge. Tape the dressing in place. Consider incorporating the catheter hub within the tape to minimize the risk of accidental disconnection (Fig. 81-8).

i. Again, make sure that the catheter is neither kinked nor sharply angulated, and check the integrity and patency of all connections. Tape all of the connections.

j. Take the patient out of Trendelenburg's position.

k. Confirm breath sounds bilaterally by auscultation to exclude the possibility of a pneumothorax.

l. Order an immediate postprocedure chest radiograph (preferably with the patient in the erect or semierect position) to verify catheter position

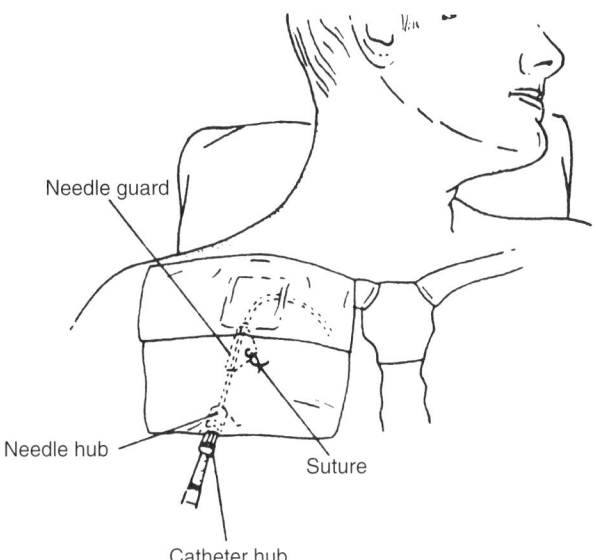

Needle guard

Needle hub

Suture

Catheter hub

Fig. 81-8
Alternative method of securing the subclavian catheter to allow free use of the arm. (From Vander Salm TJ, Cutler BS, Wheeler HB: *Atlas of bedside procedures,* ed 2, Boston, 1988, Little, Brown.)

and to check for a possible pneumothorax or hemothorax. Reposition inadequately placed catheters. Again, chest radiographs should be obtained even after unsuccessful attempts to exclude a pneumothorax.

Catheter-over-Needle Devices

Advance the needle as described previously in Step 10 until venous backflow is observed. At this point, the needle tip, but not necessarily the catheter, is in the vessel lumen.

a. Advance the needle 1 to 2 mm, then advance the catheter over the needle into the vessel lumen.
b. Once the catheter is successfully threaded, withdraw the needle and syringe.
c. Immediately place your thumb over the catheter hub to prevent an air embolus, and connect the intravenous tubing after flushing it with fluids. *Never withdraw the catheter over the needle, since this may cause a catheter fragment embolus. For the same reason, never advance the needle after the catheter has been deployed past the needle tip.*
d. Demonstrate backflow of blood by lowering the IV bag below the patient. Secure and dress the catheter, and obtain an immediate chest radiograph.

Seldinger Technique

Advance an introducing needle (large enough to accommodate the guidewire) as previously described in Step 10 until venous backflow is noted.

a. Remove the syringe; occlude the needle hub with

your thumb (Fig. 81-9, *A*), and thread the flexible end of the guidewire through the needle (Fig. 81-9, *B*). The guidewire should advance smoothly. If resistance occurs, gently rotate the needle and guidewire. If this maneuver is unsuccessful, withdraw the guidewire, reattach the syringe, and aspirate to determine if the needle is still positioned within the vessel lumen. Thread the guidewire until at least one fourth of its length is within the vessel lumen. If the patient is undergoing cardiac monitoring, watch the cardiac monitor for arrhythmias that may result as the guidewire is advanced.
b. While holding the guidewire to prevent it from moving, remove the introducing needle so that only the guidewire remains in the vessel (Fig. 81-9, *C*).
c. Using a no. 11 mounted scalpel blade, make a small skin incision approximately the diameter of the catheter at the site of entry of the guidewire (Fig. 81-9, *D*).
d. Thread the catheter sheath and dilator over the guidewire until the tip of the dilator is 1 to 2 cm from the skin surface (Fig. 81-9, *E*). It is critical to ensure, at this point, that the guidewire is protruding through the proximal end of the sheath dilator unit enough to be grasped; otherwise, the guidewire may be lost in the vessel. If the guidewire is not visible, carefully withdraw the guidewire, passing it through the introducer unit until it is visible (Fig. 81-9, *F*).
e. Grasp the guidewire and advance the sheath-dilator introducer unit over the guidewire. Advance the dilator alone for several centimeters down to the vessel, then withdraw it to advance the sheath with the dilator to its full length in the vessel. As described above, the sheath should advance without resistance. Never force the sheath against resistance; rather, gently twist and push the sheath to advance it (Fig. 81-9, *G*). Remove the dilator and guidewire together, leaving the sheath in the selected vessel (Fig. 81-9, *H*). Withdraw the guidewire slowly and gently to avoid dissecting the vein or the sheath.
f. Confirm that the catheter is positioned within the vein: connect the flushed intravenous tubing, confirm blood return by lowering the IV bag below the level of the patient, and obtain an immediate chest radiograph. Secure and dress the sheath.

Supraclavicular Approach

With the supraclavicular approach, the intent is to enter the subclavian vein in the superior aspect near its junction with the internal jugular vein (Fig. 81-2). Advantages of the supraclavicular approach include the ability to cannulate without interrupting chest compressions during CPR, little interference with airway management, and a relatively low complication rate. Again, the right side is preferred for the same reasons as cited previously.

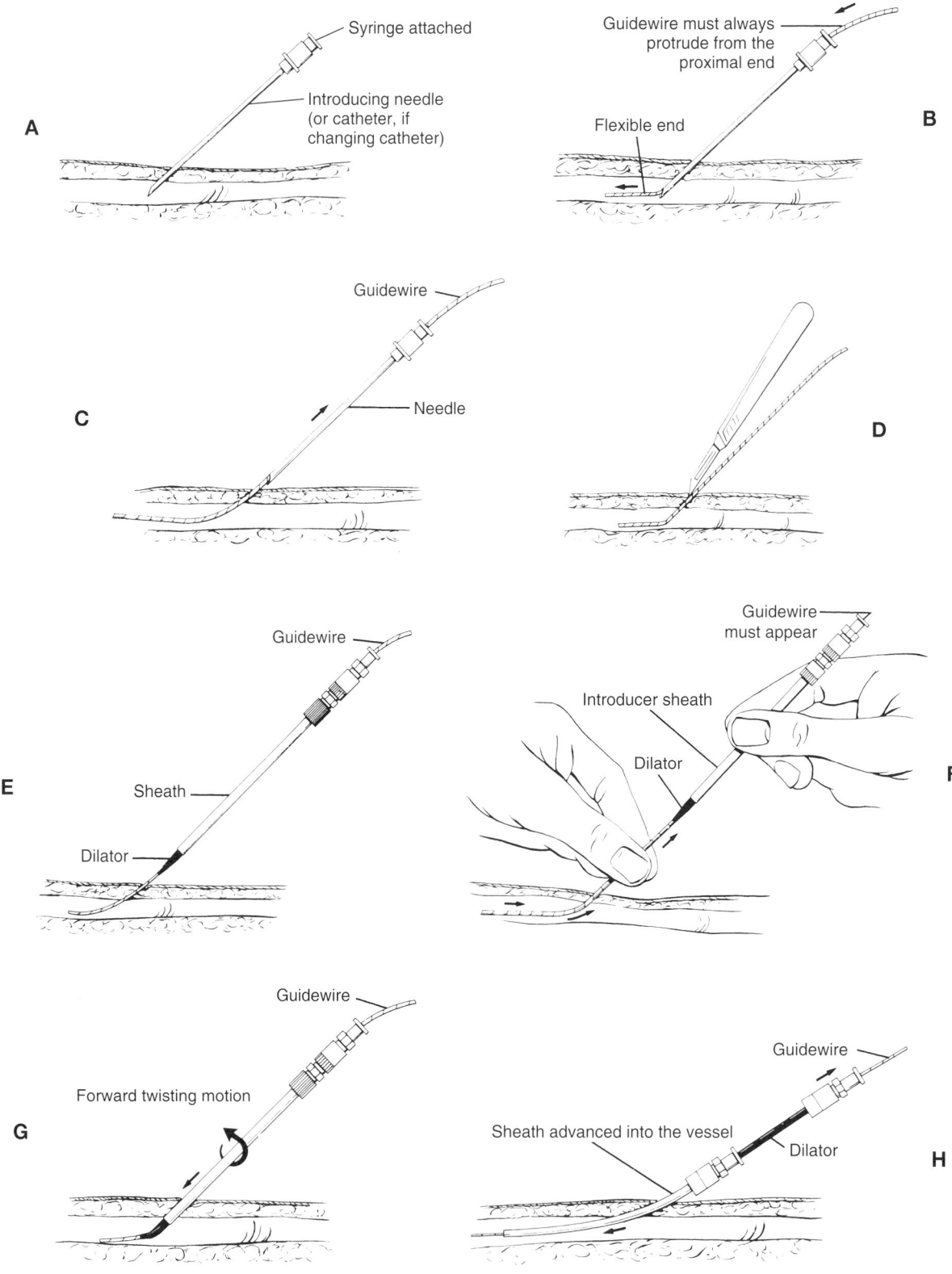

Fig. 81-9
Placement of Seldinger-type guidewire and catheter. **A,** Introducing needle with tip in lumen. **B,** Advance guidewire into vein. **C,** Remove introducing needle over guidewire. **D,** Make small skin incision. **E,** Advance dilator and sheath until tip is near skin. Grasp guidewire. **F,** If guidewire tip cannot be grasped, withdraw it slightly from the vein by grasping below the dilator tip. **G,** Advance dilator and sheath along guidewire and into vein. **H,** After sheath is fully advanced, slowly withdraw dilator and then guidewire. Immediately cover catheter hub with finger or attach to IV tubing. Also see text for details. (From Roberts JR, Hedges JR, editors: *Clinical procedures in emergency medicine,* ed 3, Philadelphia, 1998, WB Saunders.)

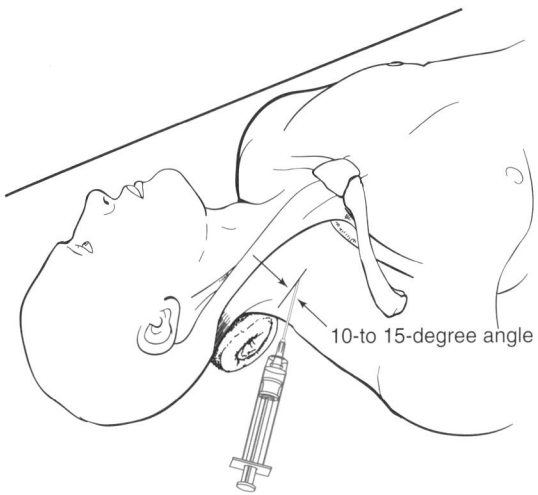

Fig. 81-10
Inserting a needle in the supraclavicular approach. Correct angle is 10 to 15 degrees above the horizontal plane.

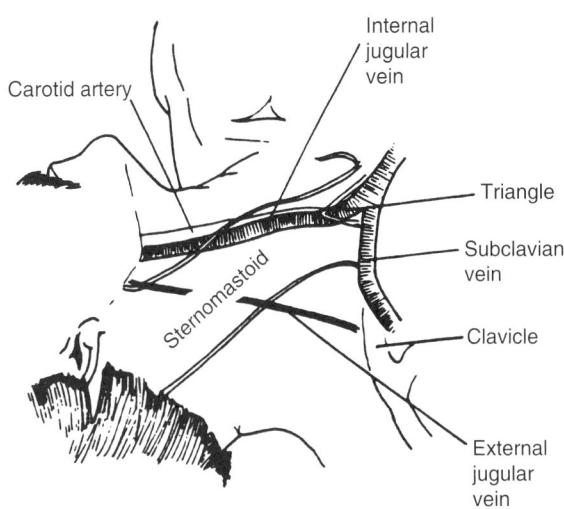

Fig. 81-11
Anatomy of the internal jugular vein. (From American Heart Association: *Textbook of advanced cardiac life support,* Dallas, 1997, American Heart Association.)

Procedure

1. Position, prepare, and drape the patient as described previously for the infraclavicular approach.
2. Anesthetize with 1% lidocaine at a point 1 cm lateral to the clavicular head of the sternocleidomastoid muscle and 1 cm cephalad to the clavicle. The needle may also be used to locate the vein.
3. While gently aspirating with a 3-ml syringe attached to a 14-gauge needle, advance the needle through the anesthetized site. Direct the needle toward the contralateral nipple in the male patient or the fifth intercostal space in the midclavicular line for a female. The needle shaft should be approximately 10 to 15 degrees above the patient's chest wall. Successful venipuncture is evidenced by freely flowing venous blood return, which usually occurs at a depth of 2 to 3 cm (Fig. 81-10).
4. The methods of insertion, securing, dressing, and evaluation of the catheter position are identical to those described for the infraclavicular subclavian approach.

INTERNAL JUGULAR VEIN CATHETERIZATION (CENTRAL APPROACH)

Advantages of the internal jugular technique include the ability to cannulate the vessel without interrupting chest compressions during CPR and a relatively low complication rate. In addition, bleeding complications from attempted cannulation are more easily detected and local compression can be applied more readily. As a result, the internal jugular approach is preferred over the subclavian approach for patients with coagulopathies. However, antecubital cutdown is probably the optimal approach for serious bleeding disorders in nonemergent situations. Disadvantages of the internal jugular approach include limited neck motion after insertion (especially troublesome for the conscious patient), interference with airway management, and increased neurologic complications (the recurrent laryngeal nerve, phrenic nerve, and brachial plexus can be injured in this procedure).

Anatomy

Like the subclavian vein, the internal jugular vein has relatively constant, predictable anatomic relationships. The internal jugular vein drains the intracranial region, and then travels with the carotid artery and vagus nerve in the carotid sheath. It lies lateral and slightly anterior to the carotid artery near its termination into the innominate vein; therefore palpation of the carotid pulse may be helpful when attempting to locate the internal jugular vein. The internal jugular vein travels under the apex of the triangle formed by the sternal and clavicular heads of the sternocleidomastoid muscle and the clavicle (Fig. 81-11), and it courses inferomedially until it joins the subclavian vein cephalad to the clavicle (Fig. 81-12).

Patient Position

Proper positioning of the patient is crucial and is similar to that described for subclavian vein cannulation. It is not necessary to place a towel between the patient's scapulae. Trendelenburg's position may slightly distend the internal jugular vein and will create positive pressure within the vein to minimize the risk of an air embolism. The internal jugular vein may also be distended by having the conscious patient perform a Valsalva maneu-

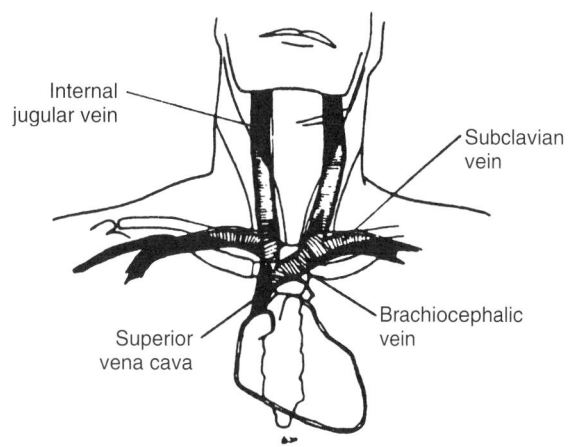

Fig. 81-12
Anatomy of the subclavian vein. (From American Heart Association: *Textbook of advanced cardiac life support,* Dallas, 1997, American Heart Association.)

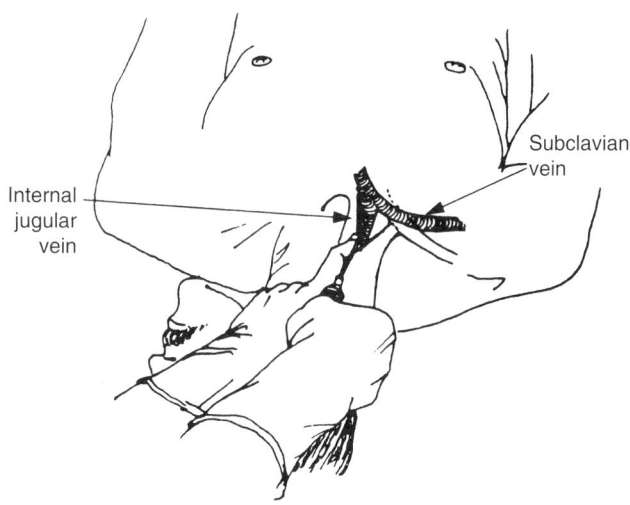

Fig. 81-13
Central approach for internal jugular venipuncture. (From American Heart Association: *Textbook of advanced cardiac life support,* Dallas, 1997, American Heart Association.)

ver or by having an assistant compress the patient's epigastrium.

Overview of the Procedure
The same principles described for the subclavian route of access apply to the internal jugular approach.

Central Approach to the Internal Jugular Vein (Procedure)
1. Prepare the patient and equipment in a sterile fashion as described for subclavian catheterization infraclavicular approach, Steps 1 to 4.
2. Note important anatomic landmarks. With the left index finger, identify and palpate the triangle formed by the clavicle and the two heads of the sternocleidomastoid muscle (Fig. 81-13). Briefly palpate the carotid artery, which runs posteromedially to the jugular vein. Prolonged palpation of the carotid artery may decrease the caliber of the jugular vein; therefore it should be avoided.
3. For the alert patient, use 1% lidocaine to anesthetize the skin at the catheter puncture site just caudal to the apex of the triangle formed by the two heads of the sternocleidomastoid muscle. Anesthetize the subcutaneous tissue, directing the needle toward the ipsilateral nipple and the junction of the medial third and middle thirds of the clavicle. This direction courses parallel to the carotid artery. The angle of the needle shaft should be approximately 30 to 45 degrees above the horizontal plane of the patient. Aspirate before injecting to prevent injection of lidocaine intravenously.
4. Some clinicians initially attempt to cannulate with the catheter device, whereas others recommend using a smaller needle (e.g., 22 gauge) to locate the vein, thereby minimizing injury to neighboring structures.

5. Puncture the skin at the anesthetized site with the catheter device, and direct the needle caudally toward the ipsilateral nipple, as noted in Step 2. Palpate the carotid artery pulsation with your free hand. Some clinicians recommend retracting the carotid artery medially and away from the internal jugular vein, but others feel that prolonged palpation of the carotid artery decreases the diameter of the internal jugular vein.
6. While aspirating with the syringe, slowly advance the needle while observing for dark venous blood return. Puncture of the vein usually occurs at a depth of 2 cm or less. If the vessel has not been entered at a depth of 4 cm, slowly withdraw the needle, maintaining negative pressure. If the attempt is unsuccessful, withdraw the needle completely and reinsert it, angling 5 to 10 degrees lateral to the initial landmarks.
7. Return of bright red or pulsatile blood signifies inadvertent carotid artery penetration. In an elective situation, withdraw the needle and apply firm pressure for 10 to 20 minutes. In an emergency situation, withdraw the needle and immediately attempt to cannulate again, remembering, however, that a soft tissue hematoma may compromise an unprotected airway.
8. When blood returns, rotate the needle 360 degrees to confirm that the bevel is completely within the vein. If blood flow is interrupted during this maneuver, slowly advance or withdraw the needle to bring the needle tip away from the vessel wall.
9. When the needle tip is properly positioned in the vessel lumen, disconnect the syringe in the same fashion as described for the subclavian approach

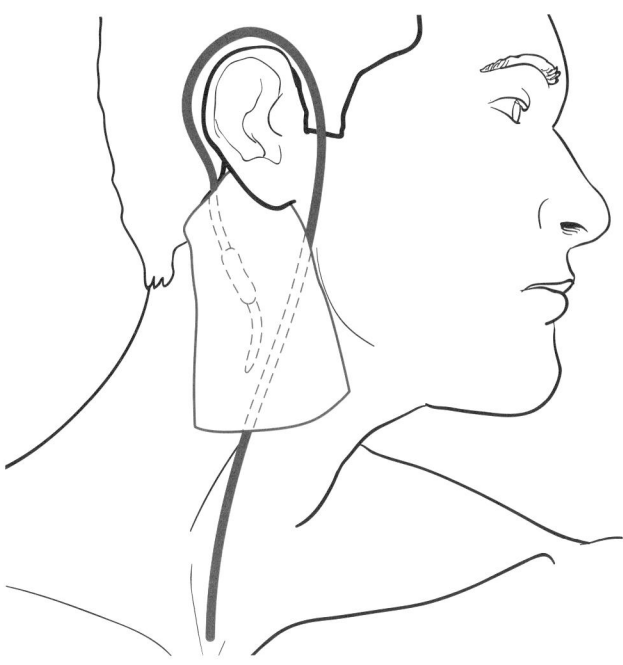

Fig. 81-14
Internal jugular line secured by looping the catheter around the ipsilateral ear.

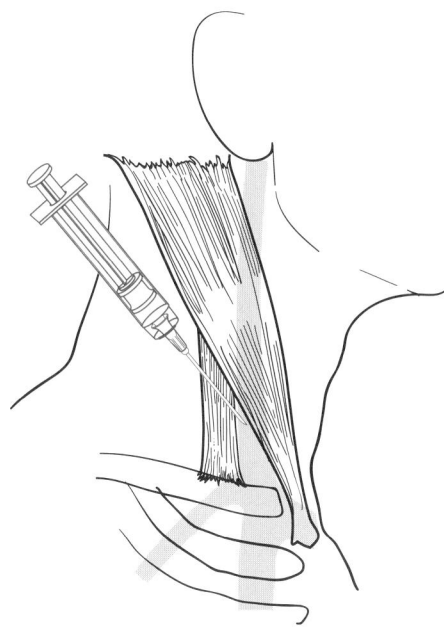

Fig. 81-15
Posterior approach for internal jugular vein catheterization. (Redrawn from Dunphy JE, Way LW, editors: *Current surgical diagnosis and treatment,* ed 5, New York, 1981, Appleton & Lange.)

and immediately occlude the needle hub with your thumb to prevent an air embolus. If the patient is cooperative, ask him or her to exhale or to perform a Valsalva maneuver to increase pressure in the vein during this portion of the procedure.

10. Pass the catheter through the introducing needle; advance the catheter over the needle, or pass a guidewire through the needle, depending on the catheter device being used, as outlined for subclavian venipuncture. Use the same precautions as discussed in the subclavian approach for each of these methods.

11. Confirm intravascular position of the catheter as previously described for the subclavian approach.

12. Secure the catheter as described for subclavian by placing a 3-0 or 4-0 silk or nylon suture through the skin, tying three square knots, looping the suture around the catheter hub three to four times, and again tying the suture. Check the catheter to make sure that the lumen is not constricted. Apply an antimicrobial ointment in a sterile dressing. Consider looping the catheter around the ipsilateral ear to reduce the risk of catheter kinking (Fig. 81-14).

13. Take the patient out of Trendelenburg's position.

14. Order an immediate chest radiograph to confirm the catheter position and to detect possible pneumothorax or hemothorax. Reposition inadequately placed catheters.

Posterior Approach to the Internal Jugular Vein

1. Insert the needle under the sternocleidomastoid muscle near the junction of the middle and caudal thirds of the lateral muscle border (Fig. 81-15). This point is approximately 5 cm above the clavicle, or just above where the external jugular vein crosses the sternocleidomastoid muscle.

2. While aspirating with the syringe, direct the needle under the sternocleidomastoid muscle toward the suprasternal notch at an angle of 45 degrees above the horizontal plane.

3. The vein is usually entered at a depth of 5 to 7 cm.

4. Follow the steps previously outlined for the central approach.

COMPLICATIONS

- Hemorrhage, hematoma, or thrombosis (risk of hemorrhage is increased with the use of three-way stopcocks or extension tubes; risk of thrombosis is especially common with prolonged catheterization and may extend to the superior vena cava and lead to vena caval obstruction or even a pulmonary thromboembolism).
- Pneumothorax.
- Local and systemic infection (the risk of infection, both local and systemic, increases significantly for catheters left in place more than 3 days).
- Hydrothorax or hydromediastinum (results from infu-

sion of intravenous fluids into the pleural space), hemothorax, and chylothorax.

- Perforation of the trachea.
- Perforation of an endotracheal tube cuff.
- Air embolus: detected when "squishy" heart sounds are heard and a sharp fall in blood pressure occurs. (The patient should be placed immediately in a steep, head-down position with the right side elevated.)
- Catheter fragment embolus (especially with catheter-through-the-needle devices).
- Laceration of the subclavian or carotid artery.
- With subclavian placement, laceration of the thoracic duct (on the left side) or lymphatic duct (on the right side).
- Arteriovenous fistula.
- Pericardial tamponade.
- Injury to neighboring nerves (phrenic, recurrent laryngeal, brachial plexus).
- Cardiac dysrhythmias.
- Catheter kinking.
- Guidewire-catheter malposition.
- Soft tissue hematomas in the neck, which may compromise the airway.

Complications may be minimized by proper patient selection, by having a thorough knowledge of the anatomy and by adhering to sterile technique. In addition, complications may be prevented by having an experienced or supervised operator perform the procedure and by changing lines that were inserted under less than sterile conditions (e.g., during CPR), or that are suspected of causing infection, as soon as feasible. It may be prudent for an individual or institution to use only one brand of CV catheter kit to ensure familiarity with its use.

POSTPROCEDURE PATIENT EDUCATION

Instruct the patient with an indwelling catheter (or his or her caregiver) to report symptoms or signs of local or systemic infection or swelling, and explain the risks of hemorrhage. The patient should undergo formal training for management of the catheter unless another trained individual is going to provide the catheter care. When a central catheter is removed, the patient should be informed to notify a nurse or clinician if pain, swelling, or signs of infection occur at the insertion site. The patient should also notify the nurse or clinician for any related chest symptoms, such as chest pain (pleuritic or other), dyspnea, or hemoptysis.

SUPPLIERS

Arrow International
2400 Bernville Road

Reading, PA 19605
Phone: 1-800-233-3187
Website: www.arrowintl.com

Bard Access Systems, Inc.
5425 West Amelia Earhart Drive
Salt Lake City, UT 84116
Phone: 1-800-545-0890
Website: www.bardaccess.com

Cook, Inc.
925 South Curry Pike
P.O. Box 489
Bloomington, IN 47402-0489
Phone: 1-800-457-4500
Website: www.cookincorporated.com

Weslee Medical, Inc.
1187 Wilmette Ave. PMB 149
Wilmette, IL 60091-2719
Phone: 1-877-624-6681
Website: www.wesleemedical.com

CPT/BILLING CODES

36010   Introduction of catheter, superior or inferior vena cava
36011   Selective catheter placement, venous system; first-order branch (e.g., renal vein, jugular vein)

ICD-9-CM DIAGNOSTIC CODES

(See also ICD-9-CM Codes for Chapter 93, Swan-Ganz Catheterization, and Chapter 94, Temporary Pacing)

260.0   Protein calorie malnutrition
276.5   Dehydration
276.5   Hypovolemia
415.0   Cor pulmonale, acute
423.9   Pericardial effusion, tamponade heart, or unspecified disease of pericardium
427.1   Paroxysmal ventricular tachycardia
427.5   Cardiac or cardiorespiratory arrest
428.0   Right heart failure, secondary to left
428.0   Heart failure, congestive
428.1   Pulmonary edema (left heart failure)
585.0   Chronic renal failure
785.50 Shock, unspecified
785.51 Shock, cardiogenic
785.59 Shock, other (hypovolemic, septic)
998.0   Surgical shock
958.4   Traumatic shock

ADDITIONAL RESOURCES

- See the sample patient education handout titled "Central Venous Catheter Insertion" on page 1833 of Appendix G.
- See the sample patient consent form titled "Central Venous Catheter Insertion" on page 1834 of Appendix G.

BIBLIOGRAPHY

American Heart Association: *Textbook of advanced cardiac life support,* Dallas, 1997, American Heart Association.

American Heart Association Staff: *2000 Handbook of emergency cardiovascular care for healthcare providers,* Dallas, 2000, The American Heart Association.

Tan BK, Hong SW, Huang MH, Lee ST: Anatomic basis of safe percutaneous subclavian venous catheterization, *J Trauma* January 48:82, 2000.

Saunders CE, Ho MT: *Current emergency diagnosis and treatment,* ed 5, Norwalk, Conn, 1996, Appleton & Lange.

Schug CB, Culhane DE, Knopp RK: Subclavian vein catheterization in the emergency department: a comparison of guide wire and nonguide wire techniques, *Ann Emerg Med* 15:769, 1986.

Tintinalli JE, Ruiz E, Krome RL: *Emergency medicine: a comprehensive study guide,* ed 4, 1996, McGraw-Hill.

Teaching and training videotapes are available from Arrow International, 2400 Bernville Road, Reading, PA 19605. Available at www.arrowintl.com.

WEBSITES

www.vh.org/Providers/ClinRef/FPHandbook/FPContents.html

www.vh.org/Providers/ClinRef/FPHandbook/Chapter17/06-17.html

www.hsc.virginia.edu/medicine/clinical/anesth/education/bfssm96.htm

www.cookgroup.com/cook_critical_care/cvc.html

CHAPTER 82

Chest Tube Insertion and Removal

Nelly A. Otero

José Ramón García

Chest tube placement is a common therapeutic procedure, frequently performed in the hospital, operating room, or emergency department. The first known chest tube with sealed drainage was developed and placed by Bulan in 1875. The objective of this procedure is to evacuate an abnormal collection of air or fluid from the pleural space. The procedure can also be used for diagnostic purposes if a sample of collected fluid is sent for analysis to determine the cause of the fluid accumulation.

INDICATIONS

- Pneumothorax: iatrogenic, spontaneous, tension, or traumatic
- Hemothorax
- Chylothorax
- Empyema
- Drainage of recurrent pleural effusion
- After thoracotomy

Note: A moderate spontaneous pneumothorax may be managed by simple aspiration (See the "Alternative Technique Using Aspiration or Catheter in Needle Thoracentesis Tray" section). Chest tube placement should be used more aggressively in a traumatic pneumothorax, since the associated injuries are more predictable. Consider surgical consultation in all cases of traumatic pneumothorax or hemothorax because these conditions can rapidly deteriorate into life-threatening situations. An exception to this rule is a pneumothorax occurring after central line placement or a thoracentesis. These iatrogenic pneumothoraces usually respond to conservative management.

CONTRAINDICATIONS

- Systemic anticoagulation therapy or bleeding dyscrasia
- Small, stable pneumothorax (this may resolve spontaneously)

- Empyema caused by acid-fast organisms
- Loculated hydrothorax or pneumothorax
- Previous chest tube insertion, thoracic surgery, or pleurodesis in the same area may have caused the pleura to become scarred down or stuck together, preventing chest tube insertion

EQUIPMENT

- Sterile gloves and gown
- Surgical mask, cap, and goggles
- Antiseptic solution (povidone-iodine [Betadine])
- Local anesthetic (usually included in the tray)
- White petrolatum-impregnated gauze
- Adhesive tape (hypoallergenic)
- Chest tubes: 22 to 36 French for adults (32 French is average); 16, 20, 24 French for children
- Appropriate suction-drainage system (a three-bottle system or a commercial model such as the Pleur-Evac or Aqua Seal) (Fig. 82-1)
- Properly working wall suction unit
- Clear plastic tubing (6-foot length, ½-inch diameter)
- Thoracostomy tray (Box 82-1)
- Sterile towels or paper drapes (if not included in the thoracostomy tray)
- Sterile Y-connector
- Thoracentesis tray if using method described in the "Alternative Technique Using Aspiration or Catheter in Needle Thoracentesis Tray" section

PREPROCEDURE PATIENT PREPARATION

Explain the procedure and its indications to the patient, and obtain written informed consent if possible. Patients should be aware of the risks and potential complications of the procedure. They should also be aware that, although a local anesthetic will be used, they will experience discomfort during the procedure.

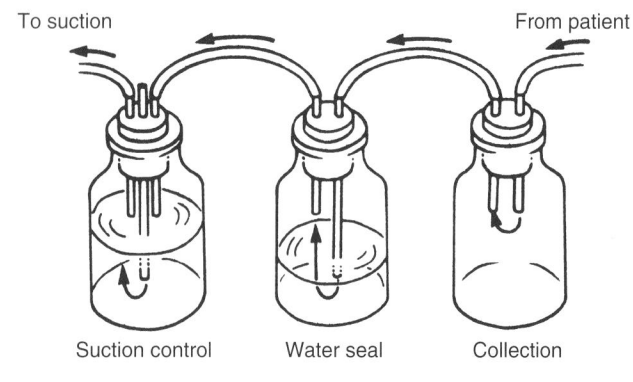

To suction   From patient

A

Suction control   Water seal   Collection

B

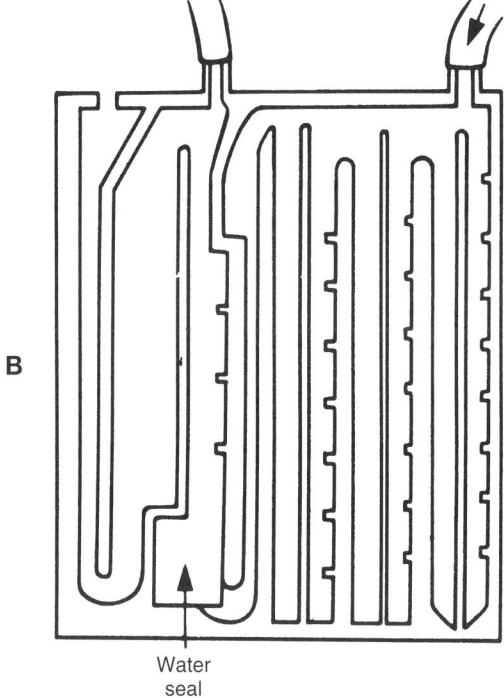

Water
seal
chamber

Fig. 82-1
A, Three-bottle system: first bottle, the collection chamber; second bottle, the water seal; third bottle (closest to wall suction), the suction control chamber. **B,** Disposable suction unit.

BOX 82-1

Thoracostomy Tray

Lidocaine 1% with 10-ml syringe and 22- and 25-gauge needles
Sterile towels (4)
Basin for antiseptic solution
Sterile 4 × 4–inch gauze pads
Towel clips (optional)
Large straight scissors
Large curved (Mayo) scissors
Large clamps (Kelly) (2)
Medium clamps (2 to 4)
Needle holder
Nonabsorbable sutures (1-0 or 2-0) on large cutting needles (2)
No. 10 or no. 11 mounted scalpel blades
Forceps

Since this procedure is rather painful, sedate the patient if he or she is not in severe respiratory distress. Demerol 25 mg with Phenergan 12.5 mg IV can be used for pain and to relax the patient.

If possible, obtain a prothrombin time, partial thromboplastin time, and platelet count (or simply a bleeding time) before performing the procedure. A chest x-ray or ultrasound (see Chapter 209, Emergency Department and Office Ultrasound) may be helpful for localizing the air or fluid levels and for excluding any anatomic variants that could place the patient at risk.

TECHNIQUE

1. Observe sterile technique by using a facemask and sterile gown. Universal blood and body fluid precautions should also be observed. Prepare all the necessary equipment under sterile conditions.
2. Select the proper chest tube. For a pure pneumothorax, an 18- to 20-French catheter should be large enough. Alternatively, for a small pneumothorax, a thoracentesis tray may be used. For a fluid accumulation or hemothorax, a 32- to 36-French catheter is suggested. Some clinicians use a 38- to 40-French catheter in trauma patients.
3. Assemble the suction-drain system according to the manufacturer's recommendations.
4. Connect the suction system to a wall suction outlet. Adjust the suction as needed until a steady stream of bubbles is produced in the water column.
5. Position the patient properly for the chosen insertion location. Three common locations for insertion are the anterior axillary line, anterior chest, and posterior chest. The anterior approach is better for removing air, whereas the anterior axillary line and posterior approaches are better for removing fluid. For axillary line insertion, with the patient supine, elevate the head of the bed 30 to 60 degrees and place the arm on the affected side over the patient's head. It is advisable to restrain the patient's arm in this position. For posterior insertion, the patient can straddle a chair or sit on the edge of the bed and lean forward on a pillow. For anterior insertion, the patient can be sitting up in bed.
6. Determine the insertion site and mark it with a fingernail indentation or skin marker. The most common site is the lateral thorax at the anterior axillary line, lateral to the nipple in males, or lateral and about two fingerbreadths above the sternoxiphoid junction in females. At this site, the tube will be in the fourth or fifth intercostal space, above the diaphragm. In the posterior approach, the 7th, 8th, or 9th intercostal space between the posterior axillary line and midline may be used (approximately 5 to 10

cm lateral to spine). It is best to use the interspace below the upper limit of fluid collection. For the anterior approach, use the 2nd or 3rd intercostal space in the midclavicular line.

Warning: The liver or spleen can be lacerated during anterior axillary and posterior insertions if the patient is not properly positioned or if the tube is inserted below the appropriately designated rib level. The diaphragm and liver or spleen may shift superiorly with certain chest abnormalities, and a prior chest x-ray or ultrasound may be helpful for excluding anomalies. Also, with the anterior approach, the aorta or diaphragm can be punctured.

7. While wearing sterile gloves, open the thoracostomy tray, observing sterile technique. Arrange the instruments, and verify the tray's inventory.

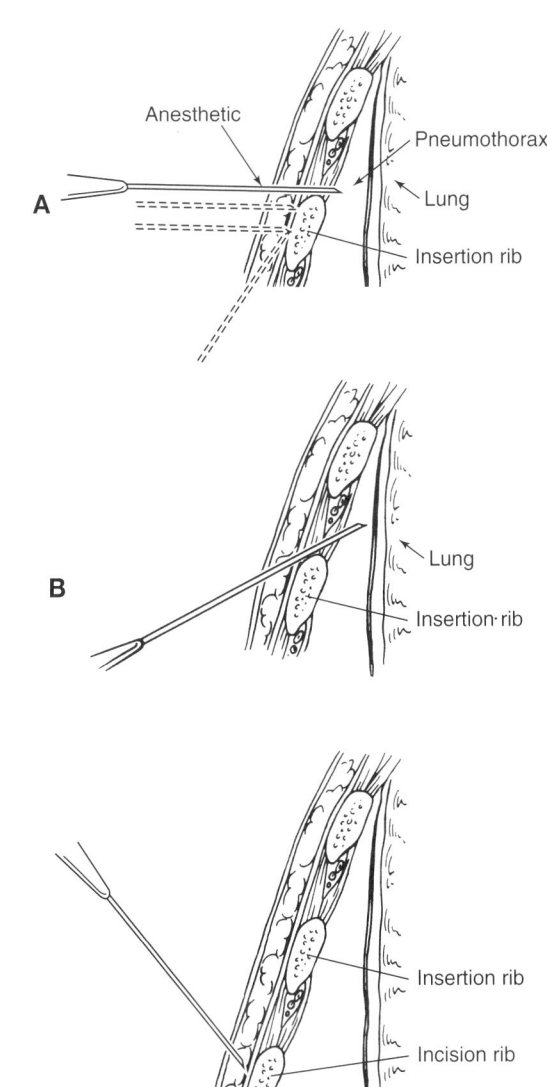

Fig. 82-2
Infiltration of **A,** subcutaneous tissue, muscle, and rib, **B,** pleura, and, **C,** skin incision site with local anesthetic.

8. Sterilize the skin with antiseptic solution, covering a wide area.

9. Proper application of local anesthetic minimizes discomfort. At the rib chosen for the pleural *insertion* site, through a skin wheal, anesthetize the skin over the middle to superior aspect of the rib with 1% lidocaine, using the 10-ml syringe and 25-gauge needle. Be careful to remain near the superior border of the rib. With the anesthetic needle and syringe, infiltrate the subcutaneous tissue, the muscle, the periosteum, and down to the parietal pleura with the 22-gauge needle (Fig. 82-2, *A*). Inject and aspirate into the pleural cavity and check for the presence of fluid or air (Fig. 82-2, *B*). If none is obtained, repeat the procedure or change the insertion site. Through a skin wheal at the *incision* area (the rib below the rib chosen for pleural insertion), infiltrate anesthetic for a skin incision (Fig. 82-2, *C*). Anesthetic can also be injected upward along the track that the chest tube will follow.

At this point, the procedure varies depending on the chosen location for insertion and the type of equipment used. See the following sections for traditional and alternative techniques.

Traditional Technique Using Incision and Kelly Clamp

10. After anesthetizing the skin at the incision area, make a 2- to 4-cm transverse incision through the skin and the tissues overlying the rib. Direct the incision toward the intercostal space above (Fig. 82-3). Using a Kelly clamp, extend the incision by blunt dissection down to the fascia overlying the intercostal muscle.

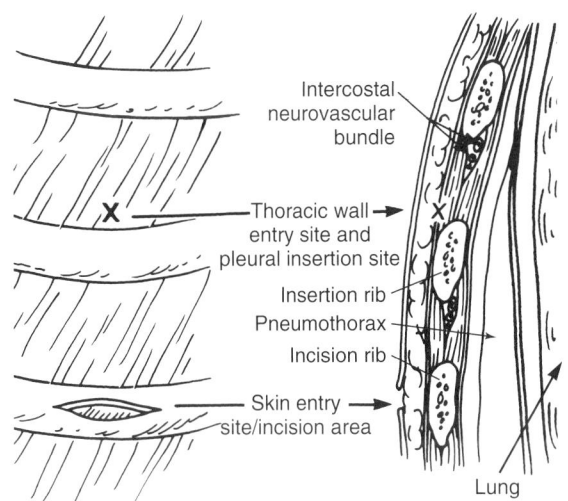

Fig. 82-3
Skin incision is made one rib below the rib over which the tube will pass. Location of the intercostal neurovascular bundle is shown.

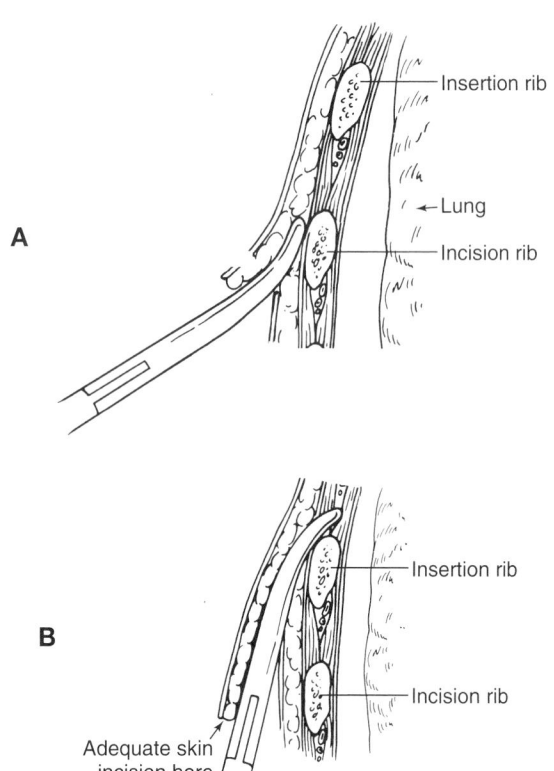

Fig. 82-4
A-B, Tunneling procedure diagram. See text for details.

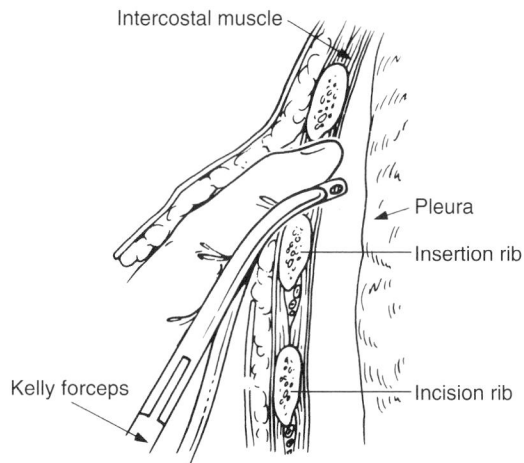

Fig. 82-5
Tip placement in the pleural cavity, using the finger as a guide.

Bluntly dissecting between planes, continue tunneling toward the superior aspect of the rib above (Fig. 82-4, *A*).

11. Once the previously anesthetized superior border of the rib above is reached, close and turn the Kelly clamp and push it through the parietal pleura with steady, firm, and even pressure (Fig. 82-4, *B*).

12. Once inside the pleural cavity, open the clamps widely and withdraw. Either air or fluid will rush out when the pleura is opened.

13. *Important:* Insert a gloved index finger to verify that the pleural space has been entered rather than the potential space between the pleura and chest wall. Also, with your finger, confirm that there are no pleural adhesions. Check for unanticipated findings, such as the diaphragm.

14. Now grasp the chest tube with a curved clamp so that the tip of the tube protrudes beyond the jaws of the clamp. Clamp the opposite, free distal end of the tube with a separate clamp, and cut the beveled distal end so that it is square and fits the suction connector better. Guide the proximal end of the tube into the pleural space using your finger, which should still be inside the pleural space (Fig. 82-5). Direct the tip of the tube superiorly, medially, and *posteriorly* for fluid drainage. Smaller tubes may be directed *anteriorly* and superiorly for pneumotho-

rax evacuation. Regardless of direction, all the ventilation holes in the chest tube must finally rest within the pleural space.

Note: Chest tubes equipped with an intraluminal trocar are not recommended. Trocars are associated with a higher incidence of intrathoracic complications.

Alternative Technique Using Aspiration or Catheter in Needle Thoracentesis Tray

10. An alternative for managing a moderate spontaneous pneumothorax is by simple aspiration. First, estimate the volume of the pneumothorax from the chest x-ray or ultrasound. After anesthetizing the skin at the site, pass a 21-gauge needle attached to a 30- to 50-ml syringe, while aspirating slowly, over the superior aspect of the rib. When air returns with aspiration, the needle is in the proper location. Aspirate the amount of air that was estimated from the x-ray or ultrasound. Repeat the x-ray examination after the aspiration in order to verify the effect. Use of a blunt-tipped needle or other protective catheter for aspiration may minimize the risk of puncturing lung or visceral pleura.

11. For catheter insertion, anesthetize the skin at the incision area. While aspirating, pass a 14-gauge needle, bevel down, over the superior aspect of the rib. When fluid (or air from a pneumothorax) is obtained or "flashes," the pleural space has been entered. The catheter is then advanced completely and the needle withdrawn. The catheter should advance easily. Use of the round-tipped, modified Husted needle will improve outcomes (Fig. 82-6). Many of the new thoracentesis trays also come equipped with catheter tips specially designed to avoid puncturing the pleura or other structures.

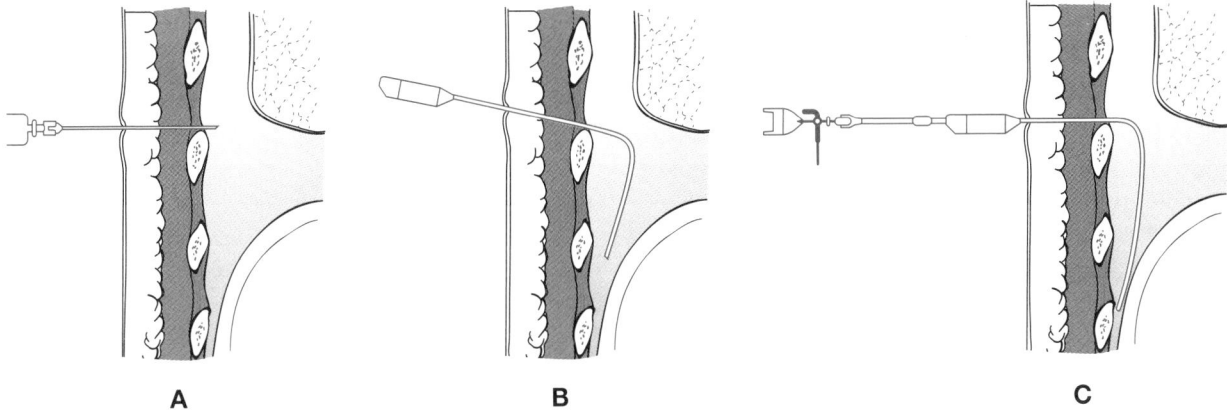

A   **B**   **C**

Fig. 82-6
Placement of a catheter within a needle. **A,** Insert the needle slightly above the rib. **B,** When air or fluid returns, attempt to advance the catheter while directing the needle downward for fluid or superiorly for pneumothorax. **C,** The catheter can be attached directly to a syringe for aspiration or through a three-way stopcock. (Redrawn from Quigley RL: *Crit Care Clin* 11:121, 1995.)

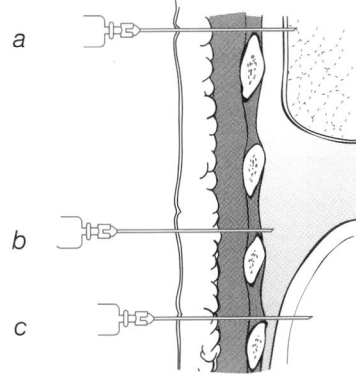

a

b

c

Fig. 82-7
Technique showing correct versus incorrect placement. If the needle is inserted too high or too low, the lung *(a)* or diaphragm *(c)* may be punctured. Air is returned with *(a)*, but blood (or nothing) is returned with *(c)*. Correct placement *(b)* avoids the neurovascular bundle on the inferior edge of the ribs. Redrawn from Quigley RL: *Crit Care Clin* 11:121, 1995.

Puncturing the lung or visceral pleura can cause a persistent pneumothorax.

12. Once the catheter is completely inserted, pleural fluid or air can be aspirated into a large (usually 50-ml) syringe. Fluid should be sent for analysis. If the catheter is not in the pleural space, or if it is too high above the fluid level, no fluid or air will be collected (Fig. 82-7). In that situation, the procedure should be repeated at a different, lower rib level.

13. Step 10 can be repeated several times, if necessary, and the fluid or air aspirated manually. For fluid aspiration, the catheter can also be attached to connecting tubing for suction drainage.

14. This technique is not very good for removing large volumes of fluid, for a large pneumothorax, or for prolonged periods of use.

Note: Never pull the catheter back while holding the needle in place or advance the needle into the catheter after it has been extended. Such maneuvers can shear off the end of the catheter tip with devastating consequences. Unless the catheter is being advanced with the needle held in place, both the needle and catheter should be inserted or pulled back together as a unit.

Additional note: If the patient is in respiratory distress, or if the pneumothorax enlarges or recurs after aspiration, a chest tube should be placed.

Connecting Chest Tube to Drainage System

1. Attach the tube to the previously assembled suction-drainage system. If no underwater seal is available, a Penrose drain can be temporarily attached in line with the tube temporarily to act as a one-way valve. Air will exit through the Penrose but not enter the chest. When the underwater seal is available, release the distal clamp. Ask the patient to cough, and observe if bubbles form at the water seal level. This confirms the patency of the system. (There are several types of suction-drainage systems, so be sure you understand the mechanics and the proper use of your particular system before performing the procedure.)

2. If the tube has not been properly inserted in the pleural space, no fluid will drain and the level in the water column will not vary with respiration.

3. To suture the tube in place, use 1-0 or 2-0 silk or nonabsorbable suture material. Place the first suture next to the tube and tie firmly (Fig. 82-8). Leave the ends long. Wind both suture ends around the tube, starting at the bottom and working toward the top. Tie the ends of the suture tightly around the tube and cut the ends. With a second suture, place a horizontal mattress suture or purse-string suture

around the tube at the skin incision site (Fig. 82-9); this will be used to close the incision when the tube is removed. Pull both ends of this suture together, and close the skin tight around the tube with a surgeon's knot. Wind the loose ends tightly around the chest tube, and make a bow for the final knot. This bow identifies the suture to be used to close the skin when the tube is removed.

4. Wrap the petrolatum-impregnated gauze around the tube where it enters the skin. Cover the tube and petrolatum gauze with two or more sterile 4 × 4–inch gauze pads into which Y-shaped cuts have made for them to fit around the tube. Tape the gauze and tube in place. Tape together the connection between the chest tube and the suction tube, and tape the chest tube to the patient's side.

5. After the chest tube has been placed, observe for any evidence of air leaks. The presence of an air leak may predict recurrence once the tube is removed. For recurrent episodes, administration of a sclerosing agent through the chest tube may be necessary before removal of the tube.

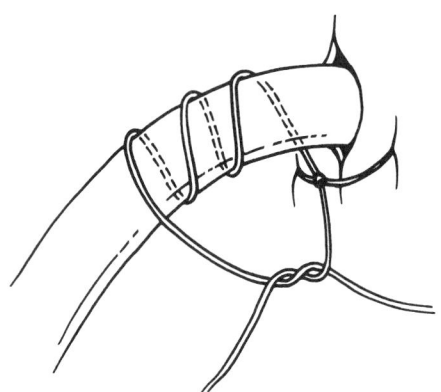

Fig. 82-8
Chest tube is fastened with a stay suture.

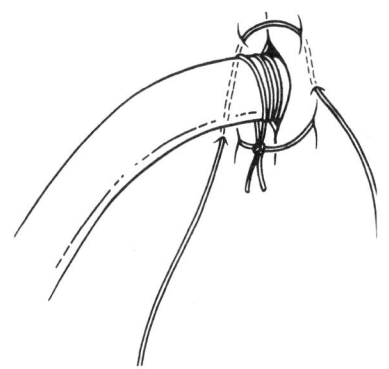

Fig. 82-9
Purse-string suture is placed to ensure a seal when the chest tube is withdrawn.

6. Change the chest tube dressing according to hospital protocols, preferably every 48 to 72 hours.

7. Obtain an erect posteroanterior and lateral chest x-ray to confirm tube placement. Document the degree of resolution of the initial condition for which the chest tube was inserted.

8. Chest tubes are generally removed when there is less than 150 ml of drainage per 24 hours (usually 3 to 4 days after insertion). If inserted to remove air, tubes can be removed when there is no drainage for more than 24 hours (anywhere from 2 to 10 days after insertion).

Note: For a pneumothorax that does not resolve or seal, some institutions have successfully used thoracoscopy to locate, evaluate, and occasionally treat the leak. Usually performed by cardiothoracic surgeons, thoracoscopy involves insertion of a scope into the pleural cavity, often through the chest tube, to make the evaluation. Bleb resection and pleural abrasion by thoracoscopy are quite effective as definitive therapy.

CHEST TUBE REMOVAL

1. Place the patient in the same position as when the tube was inserted.

2. Using sterile technique, prepare the area. Remove the suture holding the tube, loosen the purse-string suture, and prepare the suture for tying.

3. Clamp the chest tube and disconnect the suction system.

4. Ask the patient (if awake) to hold his or her breath, and remove the tube with a swift motion. If the patient is receiving ventilator support, pause the ventilator.

5. Tie the purse-string suture. (If a purse-string suture was not used or provided, the tract and skin opening can be occluded with petroleum-impregnated gauze and secured in place with a pressure dressing and tape.)

6. Apply an occlusive dressing (gauze impregnated with petrolatum or antibiotic ointment) and tape securely.

7. Observe for any new symptoms or complications after the chest tube is removed. Repeat the chest x-ray examination. After 48 hours, the dressing can be removed. The patient should follow routine wound care instructions.

COMPLICATIONS

- Injury to the heart, great vessels, lung, diaphragm, liver, spleen, or even the intestines
- Subdiaphragmatic placement of tube
- Open pneumothorax

- Tension pneumothorax
- Dislodgment of the tube
- Subcutaneous emphysema
- Unexplained or persistent air leakage
- Hemorrhage from an injured intercostal artery
- Local or more generalized infection

SUPPLIERS

Atrium Ocean Water Seal Chest Drain System and Thoracostomy Tubes
Atrium Medical Corporation
5 Wentworth Drive
Hudson, NH 03051
Phone: 1-800-528-7486
Website: www.atriummed.com

Pleur-Evac Water Seal Chest Drain System and Thoracostomy Tubes
Genzyme Biosurgery
One Kendall Square
Cambridge, MA 02139
Phone: 1-800-367-7874
Website: www.genzymebiosurgery.com

Water Seal Chest Drain Systems, Thoracostomy Tubes, Thoracentesis Trays, and Pneumothorax Tray with 8-French Catheter
Argyle Aqua Seal Systems
Argyle Turkel Safety Thoracentesis and Pneumothorax Tray
The Kendall Company
15 Hampshire Street
Mansfield, MA 02048
Phone: 1-800-962-9888
www.kendallhq.com

Emergency pneumothorax kits
Cook, Inc.
925 South Curry Pike
P.O. Box 489
Bloomington, IN 47402-0489
Phone: 1-800-457-4500
Website: www.cookcriticalcare.com

Thoracentesis tray with catheter in needle
Allegiance Healthcare Company
1430 Waukegan Road
McGaw Park, IL 60085-6787
Phone: 1-800-964-5227
www.allegiance.net

CPT/BILLING CODES

32020   Tube thoracostomy with or without water seal (e.g., for abscess, hemothorax, empyema)
32002   Thoracentesis with insertion of tube with or without water seal (e.g., for pneumothorax)

ICD-9-CM DIAGNOSIS CODES

457.8   Chylous hydrothorax
510.9   Empyema
012.0   Empyema, tuberculous
511.8   Hemothorax
511.1   Hemothorax, bacterial
860.2   Hemothorax, traumatic
772.8   Hemothorax, newborn
511.9   Pleural effusion
197.2   Pleural effusion, malignant
511.1   Bacterial, nontuberculous
012.0   Tuberculous
862.29   Traumatic
512.1   Pneumothorax, due to operative injury of chest wall or lung
512.8   Pneumothorax, spontaneous
512.0   Pneumothorax, tension
860.0   Pneumothorax, traumatic
860.4   Pneumothorax, traumatic, with hemothorax
0111.7   Pneumothorax, tuberculous

BIBLIOGRAPHY

Ho MT, Saunders CE, editors: *Current emergency diagnosis and treatment,* Norwalk, Conn, 1990, Appleton & Lange.
Kozol RA, Fromm D, Konen JC, editors: *When to call the surgeon,* Philadelphia, 1999, FA Davis.
Quigley RL: Thoracentesis and chest tube drainage, *Crit Care Clin* 11(1):111, 1995.

WEBSITES

www.cme101.com (Medicine, surgery, diagnostic and interventional radiology online)
www.int-med.uiowa.edu/michael-peterson/iceland/gross/sld031.htm (PowerPoint slides)
www.merck.com/pubs/mmanual/section6/chapter65/65f.htm (Tube thoracostomy)
www.pepid.com (Portable Emergency and Primary Care Information Database)

CHAPTER 83

Tracheal (Endotracheal and Nasotracheal) Intubation

Len Scarpinato

In an emergency, primary care clinicians may be called on to perform endotracheal intubation as a life-saving procedure. Occasionally primary care clinicians also perform intubation under controlled circumstances. Primary care clinicians may be needed to perform intubation in a large university hospital intensive care unit when no subspecialist is available, on code teams in any hospital, in emergency departments staffed by primary care clinicians, or in small rural hospitals where they may be the only caregivers.

There are many options for insertion of an endotracheal tube: through the mouth or through the nose, with direct visualization or blindly, with the patient awake or unconscious, through a cricothyroidotomy, or with the assistance of bronchoscopy. It is important not to forget the concomitant medical problems during this procedure; arrhythmias, congestive heart failure, coronary artery disease, chronic obstructive pulmonary disease (COPD), or other conditions may be affected. A respiratory therapist and a trained assistant should be present, if possible, throughout the procedure.

The first method described in this chapter (endotracheal) is used primarily for emergent direct intubation in the unconscious patient. This method causes minimal nasal bleeding and sinusitis, leads to easier suctioning, and can be learned relatively quickly. Nasotracheal intubation is also described in this chapter. Although beyond the scope of this chapter, other techniques for stabilizing the airway include: the use of a lighted stylet to guide intubation by transillumination of the neck, the use of a bougie to guide intubation, retrograde intubation guided by a wire placed through the cricothyroid, and tactile intubation guided by two of the clinician's fingers placed in the patient's pharynx.

Note: Reading this chapter alone is not sufficient for mastering the skill. Manikins are available for practice and should be used. They are often owned by hospitals for use in advanced cardiac life support (ACLS) classes. Reading some of the references at the end of this chapter, reviewing pertinent anatomy, and taking an ACLS course can be instructional.

Observation of trained anesthesiologists in the operating room under controlled circumstances can add to the practitioner's experience. Observing an actual cardiopulmonary resuscitation or a "code" can help the practitioner truly appreciate that conditions are not always optimal for intubation. A mentor should be used while this skill is learned. Trained personnel should supervise initial attempts. The more times intubation has been performed, the greater the probability of success with fewer complications.

INDICATIONS

Endotracheal Intubation

- Respiratory failure: Hypoxia (consider when Pao_2 <60 with Fio_2 >0.5), hypercapnia, tachypnea, or apnea from such causes as adult respiratory distress syndrome (ARDS), asthma, pulmonary edema, infection, COPD exacerbation, etc.
- Inability to ventilate unconscious patient with conventional methods
- Maintenance or protection of an intact airway: to assist the collection and removal of bronchopulmonary secretions, to prevent aspiration of gastric contents, or to bypass oropharyngeal trauma or obstruction
- Cardiac arrest with ongoing chest compressions
- Medication administration

Note: If indicated in an unconscious patient, intubation should be performed as soon as possible by trained personnel. Attempts to provide adequate lung inflations without intubation may cause gastric distention, increasing the risk for regurgitation and aspiration of gastric contents.

Nasotracheal Intubation

Indications are the same as for endotracheal intubation, except nasotracheal intubation requires slightly more skill and experience and occasionally takes longer to perform. However, it is especially useful in conscious patients with respiratory distress, a fractured mandible, or trismus. For patients with cervical spine disorders or cervical trauma, a single attempt at nasotracheal intubation (with an assistant stabilizing the spine) may be reasonable. Meanwhile, another assistant should be assembling the equipment necessary to perform cricothyroidotomy in case intubation is unsuccessful.

CONTRAINDICATIONS

Endotracheal Intubation

- Inability of patient to extend the head (e.g., severe degenerative cervical spine disorders or severe rheumatoid arthritis involving the cervical spine)
- Moderate to severe trauma to the cervical spine or anterior neck (patients with gunshot wounds to this area are candidates for cricothyroidotomy)
- Infection in the epiglottal area
- Mandibular fracture or trismus
- Mild hypoxia (relative contraindication: administer 100% oxygen through a bag-mask assembly first, then observe oxygen SATs or redraw arterial blood to determine if the Po_2 has risen to a normal level)
- Uncontrolled oropharyngeal hemorrhage (e.g., inability to visualize larynx, so cricothyroidotomy or other airway should be considered)
- Intact tracheostomy (relative contraindication: endotracheal intubation can be performed if a tracheostomy

tube falls out; however, obviously the best action is to replace the tracheostomy tube)

Nasotracheal Intubation

In addition to some of the orotracheal contraindications, nasotracheal intubation is contraindicated in patients with apnea because spontaneous breathing efforts are required for blind intubation. Significant midface traumas, such as fractures of the base of the skull or ethmoid sinus, are contraindications because they could lead to intubation of the cranial vault. Coagulopathies are also contraindications because epistaxis could be life threatening.

EQUIPMENT (FIG. 83-1)

- Laryngoscope.
- Blades: curved (MacIntosh) *and* straight (Miller, Wisconsin, Flagg, etc.). (Inexperienced clinicians find the curved blades easier to use. For pediatric patients the straight blade is usually better.)
- Endotracheal tubes of various sizes:
  - For neonates and full-term infants, no. 0 and 1; for adult women, 7.0 to 8.0 mm i.d. tube; for adult men, 8.0 to 8.5 mm i.d. Suppliers include Mallinckrodt, Portex, and Rusch. Preference should be for a high-flow, low-cuff-pressure tube. (Minimum cuff pres-

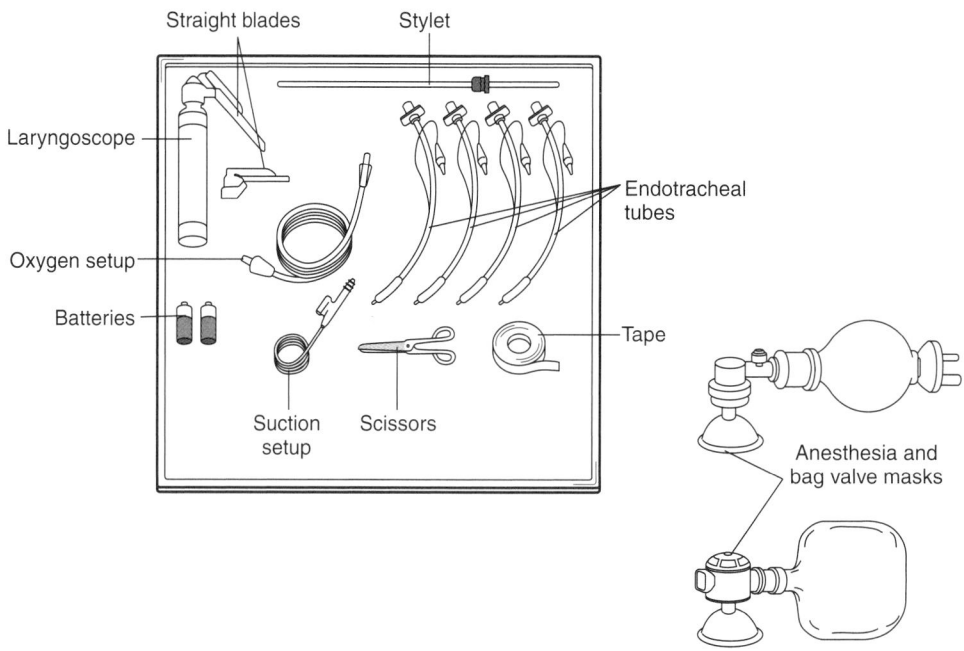

Fig. 83-1
Suggested intubation equipment.

sure to prevent aspiration is 25 cm H_2O; risk of tracheal ischemia increases at pressures greater than 40 cm H_2O.)

Note: To approximate tube size for pediatric patients:

$$i.d. = (age\ in\ years/4) + 4$$

Another rough estimate for tube size is that it should equal the width of the fingernail of the fifth digit of the patient's hand.

- Nasotracheal: At least 0.5 mm smaller than the size used for endotracheal intubation.
- Lubricant (sterile and water soluble).
- 10-ml syringe (to inflate endotracheal tube cuff).
- Adhesive tape in ½- and ¾-inch rolls.
- Tincture of benzoin.
- Oxygen (100%) supply and tubing.
- Manual resuscitation bag with mask (anesthesia or bag valve mask).
- Pulse oximeter.
- Ventilator.
- Suction apparatus.
- Rigid suction catheter (Yankauer, 10 to 12 French).
- Tracheal suction catheter.
- Cardiac monitor.
- Defibrillator.
- Clock or watch with a second hand.
- Stethoscope.
- Local anesthetic (benzocaine spray [Cetacaine], lidocaine); intravenous skeletal muscle relaxant (vecuronium, atracurium, or succinylcholine); benzodiazepine (midazolam or diazepam); short-acting barbiturate (thiopental) or narcotic.
- Sterile gloves and goggles or other eye protection.
- Oropharyngeal airway, especially for endotracheal intubation.
- Vasoconstrictor nasal spray (Neo-Synephrine), for nasotracheal intubation.

Note: All equipment should be checked before attempting to intubate.

Optional Equipment

- Suction tube trap to catch the first intubated specimen for Gram stain and culture.
- Malleable stylet, preferably plastic coated.
- Whistles are available that fit endotracheal tubes to confirm the flow of exhaled air. Carbon dioxide detectors, including inexpensive purple-yellow detectors, are also available. Neither carbon dioxide nor exhaled air will be detected if the esophagus is intubated.
- Magill forceps (for nasotracheal intubation or for removing foreign material).
- Scissors.

- Bite block.
- Bed with removable headboard and lockable wheels.

PREPROCEDURE PATIENT PREPARATION

Endotracheal intubation is often an emergency procedure, and there is usually no time for written informed consent. Talk to the patient and family, explain the situation, and document an implied consent. Complications of the procedure should be mentioned, as well as what might happen to the patient if the procedure is not performed. For nasotracheal intubation, there is often time to obtain signed informed consent.

TECHNIQUE

Endotracheal Intubation

1. Obtain informed consent, if possible.
2. Decide whether to use a local anesthetic, or a combination of a skeletal muscle relaxant, a benzodiazepine, and thiopental. In most emergent situations, muscle relaxants and general anesthetics are not necessary. If needed, consider using intravenous midazolam or diazepam, a short-acting barbiturate (thiopental), and a skeletal muscle relaxant (vecuronium, atracurium, or succinylcholine). Be prepared to take over all respirations once the patient is paralyzed. After paralysis, if you cannot intubate, a cricothyroidotomy or tracheostomy is indicated.
3. With the patient supine, use a chin lift and, if necessary, a jaw thrust (Fig. 83-2) to allow the patient to maintain spontaneous respirations during the procedure. Place padding or a towel(s) under the occiput, and arrange the patient's head and body so

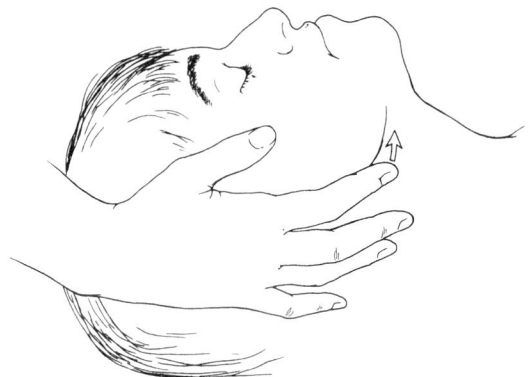

Fig. 83-2
Jaw thrust. Rotate mandible forward with index fingers. Arrow indicates motion to bring soft tissues forward to relieve airway obstruction.

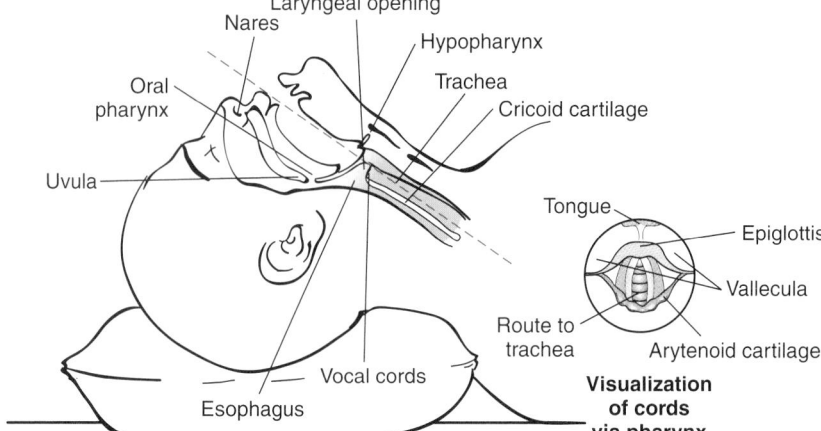

Fig. 83-3
Anatomic landmarks of the head and neck.

that the mouth, pharynx, and trachea are all in a line (Figs. 83-3 and 83-4). The patient should be in the "sniffing" position, with the head extended and neck flexed. Remove full or partial dentures, or any foreign bodies in the mouth.

4. Stand behind the patient's head. Remove the headboard if possible, and raise the bed to a comfortable working height. Although this is a good position at which to obtain leverage, do not let the patient's head hang over the end of the bed.

5. Verify that all equipment and personnel are present, working, and in the right location. Arrange the equipment in order of need. Attach the pulse oximeter to the patient and turn it on.

6. Select and attach the appropriate blade. The curved blade is easy to use; however, the straight blade is the anesthesiologist's favorite (Fig. 83-5) and is probably the best blade to use in children.

7. Verify that the light on the laryngoscope is working (usually by flipping the blade down or open to about 90 degrees).

8. Select the appropriate tube size, noting that in an emergency a 7.5-mm i.d. is usually good for both women and men. Check the cuff by filling the syringe with air and injecting it into the cuff. If the cuff loses air, it is leaking and the tube needs to be replaced. After checking for leaks, deflate the cuff.

9. Check the length of the endotracheal tube by placing it next to the patient's neck. The tube should extend from the mouth to beyond the sternal notch.

10. Wear eye protection and sterile gloves. Remove the endotracheal tube from its package, lubricate the outside with a water-soluble lubricant, and, if it is going to be used, insert the stylet. It may be also preferable to lubricate the stylet with the same lubricant before inserting it into the tube. After insertion, the end of the stylet should be recessed at least 1 to 1.5 cm within the tube.

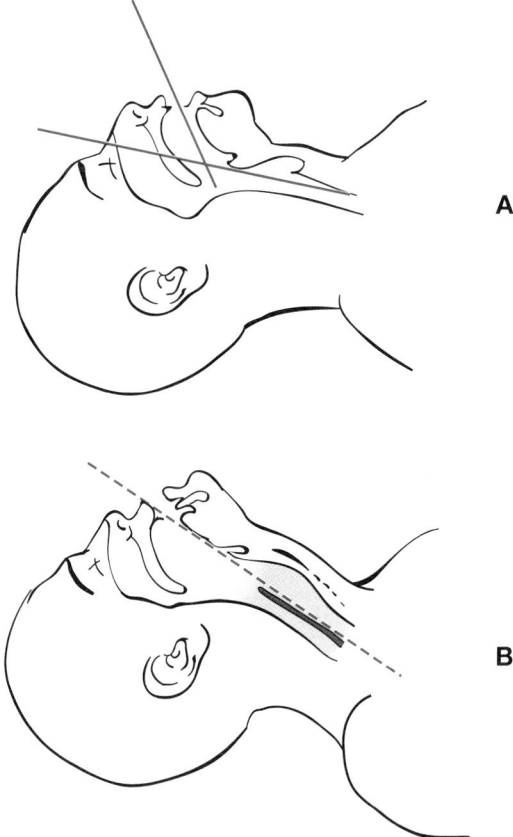

Fig. 83-4
Proper head position is important for successful endotracheal intubation. Axes of the mouth, pharynx, and larynx need to be aligned. **A,** Divergent axes. **B,** Axes in line, or "sniffing position."

11. Administer 100% oxygen through the mask for 1 minute.

12. Begin a 20-second count, because intubation must be completed within that time. If it is not, the oxygen must be reapplied.

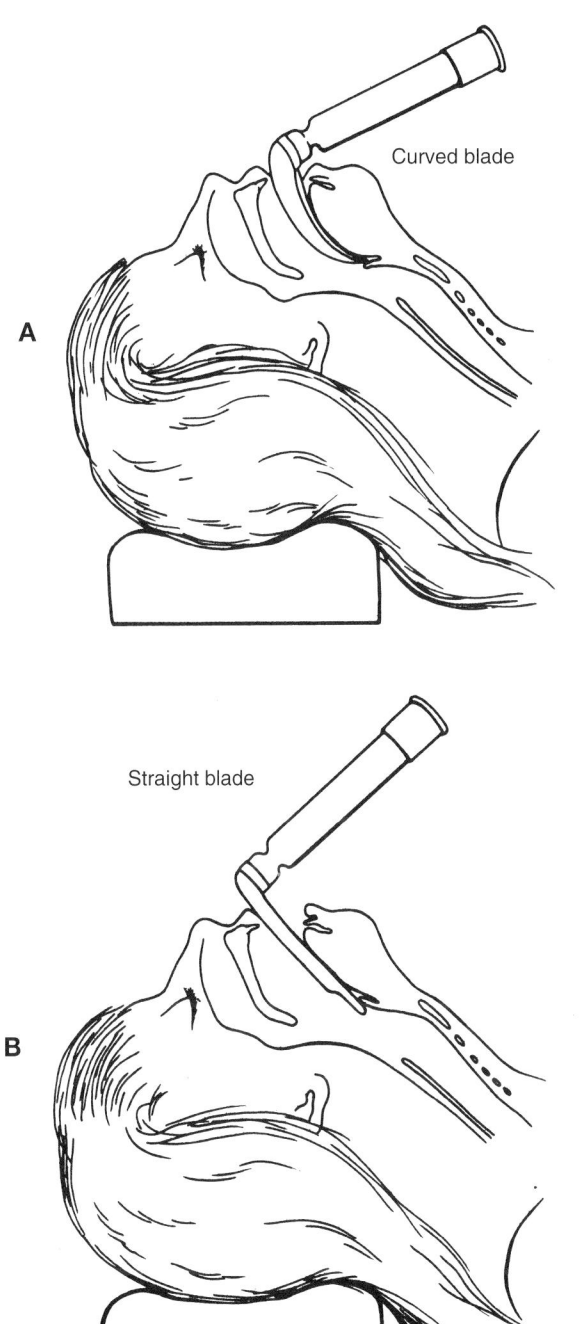

Fig. 83-5
Blade placements. **A,** Curved blade (Macintosh) may be less traumatic and less reflex stimulating because it avoids the larynx (tip of blade is in vallecula). **B,** Laryngoscopic technique with straight blade (Miller). This is mechanically easier if patient has no large central incisors.

13. Remove the patient's mask, and open the patient's mouth. Recheck for dentures and other possible obstructions, and remove them if found.
14. Regardless of your "handedness," pick up the laryngoscope with your left hand, and turn it on by

flipping down the blade (opening it to 90 degrees). Place the suction catheter near your right hand. Opening the mouth with the fingers of your right hand, place the scope in the patient's mouth. If you are using a straight blade, insert the scope on the right side and push the tongue to the left side. If you are using a curved blade, insert the scope in the center of the mouth and pass it up into the vallecula (Fig. 83-5).
15. While keeping the blade in the midline, push the blade posteriorly to the correct position (in which no part of the tongue can be visualized distally). Your right index finger should be used to keep the patient's lower lip away from the blade.
16. It may be necessary to use suction (or McGill forceps) to remove secretions and fluids that are in the posterior pharynx; however, if proper procedure is followed, this is often unnecessary. Always keep suction nearby. (If the patient still exhibits a gag reflex, reconsider the use of topical lidocaine or Cetacaine spray. Intravenous general anesthetics or benzodiazepines might also be appropriate.)
17. Lift the whole blade assembly and laryngoscope forward and toward the ceiling. The best position for the handle of the laryngoscope is at a 30- to 45-degree angle above and toward the patient's feet. Avoid fulcrum movement, which you can feel in your biceps (Fig. 83-6). Especially avoid using the upper teeth as a fulcrum.
18. Watch for the vocal cords (Fig. 83-7). In adults, if the vocal cords are not visible, have an assistant gently press the cricoid cartilage using the Sellick maneuver (Fig. 83-7), which also helps prevent aspiration of gastric contents. This is especially important when the timing of the last meal is unknown. If cords still cannot be seen, modify the patient's position. If more than 20 seconds have elapsed, stop the attempt, administer 100% oxygen through bag ventilation for 1 minute, and then retry intubation.

Note: Some authorities recommend the Sellick maneuver throughout the procedure to prevent aspiration in adults. Pressure should be applied to the anterolateral aspects of the cricoid cartilage with the thumb and index finger. Avoid overzealous pressure, and maintain the pressure until the cuff is inflated and proper tube position is verified.

19. Once the vocal cords have been visualized, pick up the endotracheal tube in your right hand *without looking away from the scope* (Fig. 83-8). Move the distal end of the tube past the right side of the patient's mouth, into their posterior pharynx, and *through* the vocal cords. An assistant can help by retracting the right corner of the patient's mouth. Visualization of the tube going through the cords is crucial for proper tracheal intubation—otherwise,

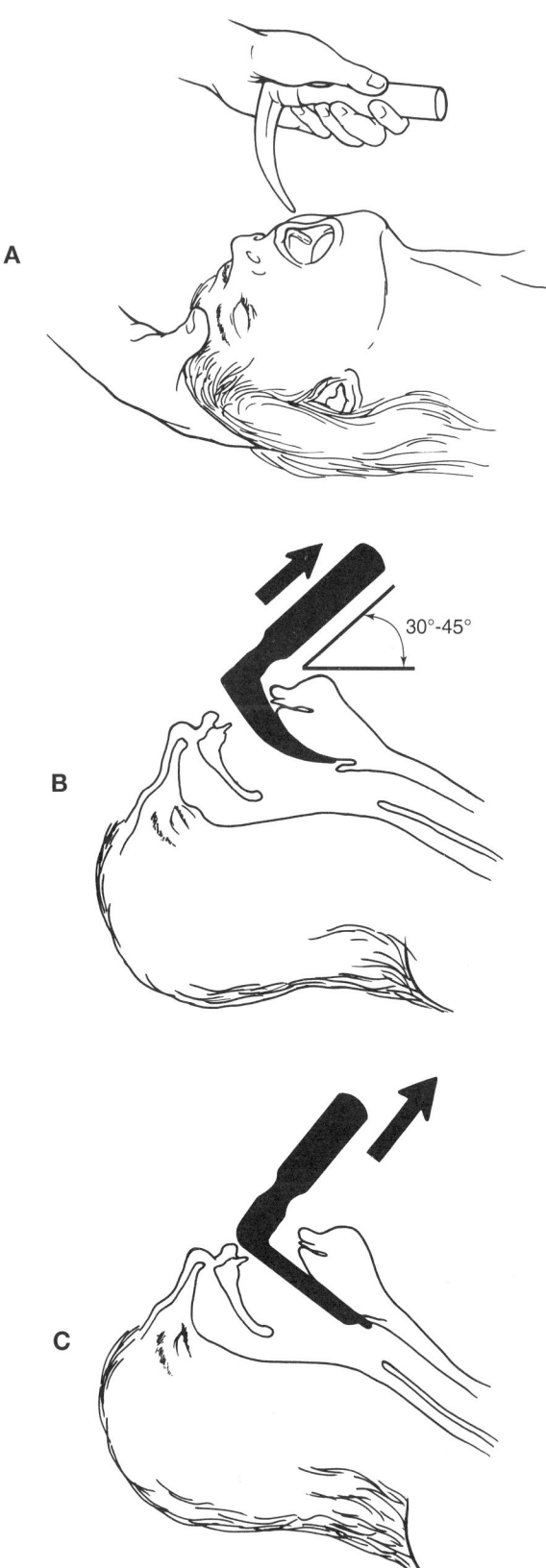

Fig. 83-6
A, Insertion of laryngoscope. **B,** Correct nonfulcrum movement of curved laryngoscope blade. **C,** Straight blade.

the tube may enter the esophagus. Insert the tube just far enough for the cuff to rest slightly below the vocal cords, or about ½ to 1 inch below the vocal cords. This correlates to about where the mark on the tube would rest in the corner of the mouth, which is 23 cm in men and 21 cm in women (distal tip will be 2 cm above the carina). In children, the distance from the teeth to the midportion of the trachea (in centimeters) is approximately (age in years/2) + 12.

20. Keep holding the endotracheal tube in your right hand and stabilize it against the patient's face. Remove the laryngoscope.

21. Have the assistant remove the stylet from the endotracheal tube while you continue to stabilize the tube. If there is no assistant, use your left hand to remove the stylet while you stabilize the tube with your right hand.

22. Ventilate oxygen through the bag and observe the chest wall for evidence of bilateral, symmetric thoracic inflation. Auscultate over the lungs for air flow to check for symmetry, and auscultate over the stomach to be sure there are no air sounds (Fig. 83-9). If there are air sounds in the stomach, the esophagus has been intubated, and the tube should be removed and oxygen supplemented. If lung sounds are asymmetric (with asymmetry, the right side is usually the louder side), the endotracheal tube is too deep and the right lung has been intubated because it has a straighter path. Mark the tube and pull it back 1 to 2 cm. Auscultate again. Air excursion should be symmetric and effective. The tube needs to rest just above the carina.

23. Using the syringe, inflate the endotracheal tube cuff with enough air to occlude the airway (usually about 10 to 20 ml). Fullness is indicated by a senescent bag; do not overinflate or it will feel *hard* to compress. Minimum cuff pressure to prevent aspiration is 25 cm H_2O; risk of tracheal ischemia increases at pressures >40 cm H_2O.

24. Attach the oxygen source (bag valve mask or ventilator).

25. Apply tincture of benzoin to the skin, place the bite block on the endotracheal tube, and tape the tube. If desired, obtain a specimen for Gram stain and culture.

26. Obtain a chest radiograph to verify tube location and check for complications.

27. An oropharyngeal airway can be placed instead of or in addition to the bite block. Consider insertion of a nasogastric or feeding tube to deflate the stomach and act as a reminder to supplement nutrition early.

28. Order the ventilatory parameters for respiratory therapy: rate (usually 12 to 16 inhalations per minute), tidal volume (usually 10 to 14 ml/kg), and 100%

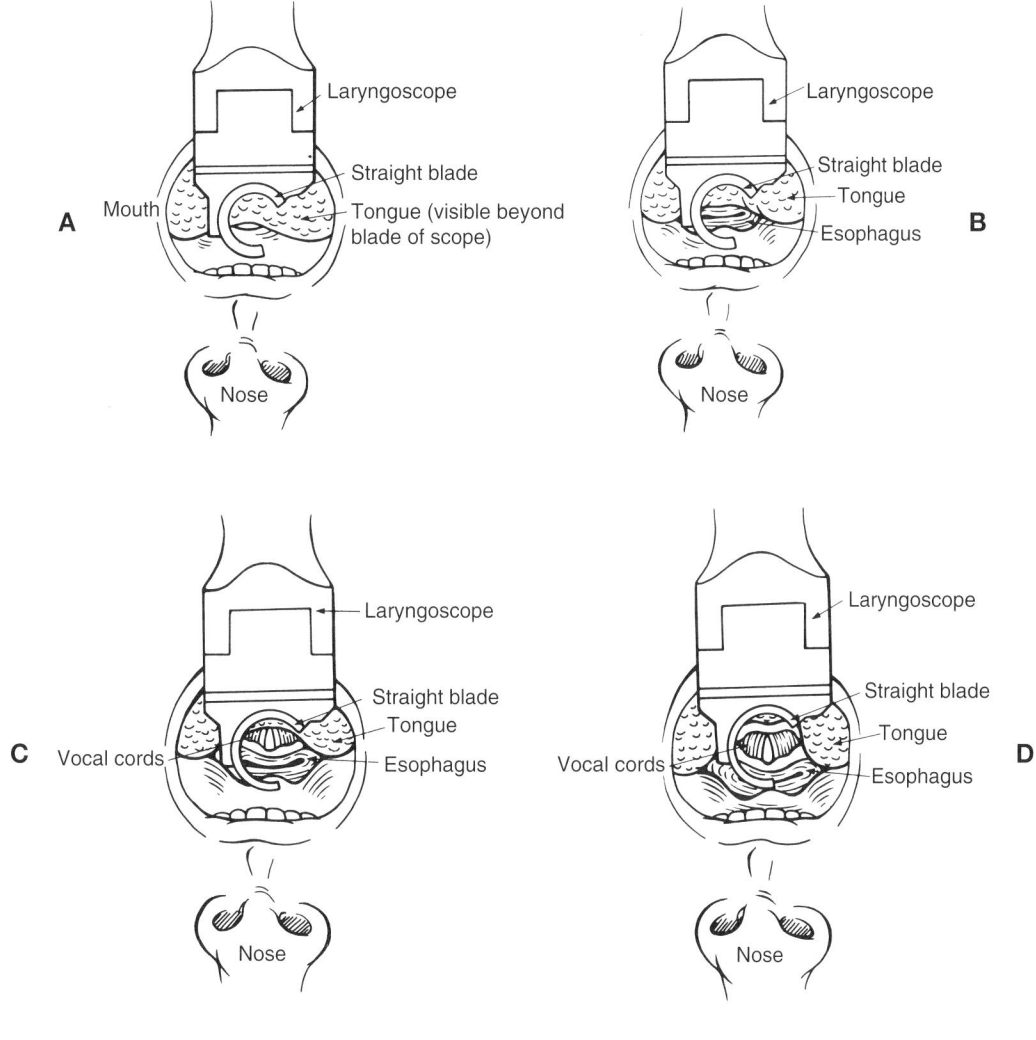

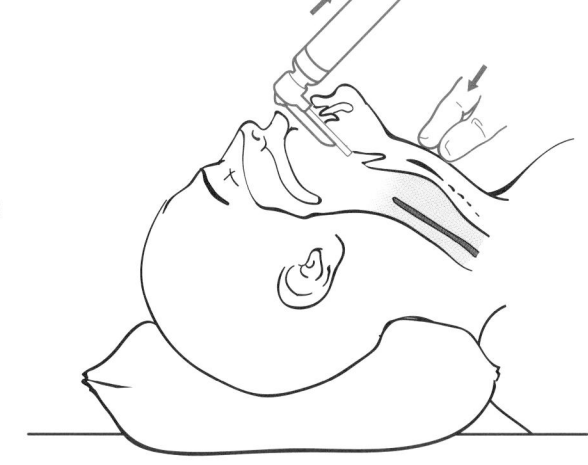

Fig. 83-7
Different views with correct and incorrect placement of laryngoscope. **A,** Blade is not inserted far enough, only the tongue is visible. Push blade in further. **B,** Blade is in too far; the esophagus is visible, but the vocal cords are not visible. Pull the blade out. **C,** Correct position with partial view of vocal cords. Lift the blade in a nonfulcrum movement (see Fig. 83-6). **D,** Correct view for intubation. **E,** Sellick maneuver. Either the operator or an assistant uses the thumb and index finger to provide posterior pressure and bring the larynx into view. (Some suggest performing this in adults with every intubation attempt to also avoid aspiration.)

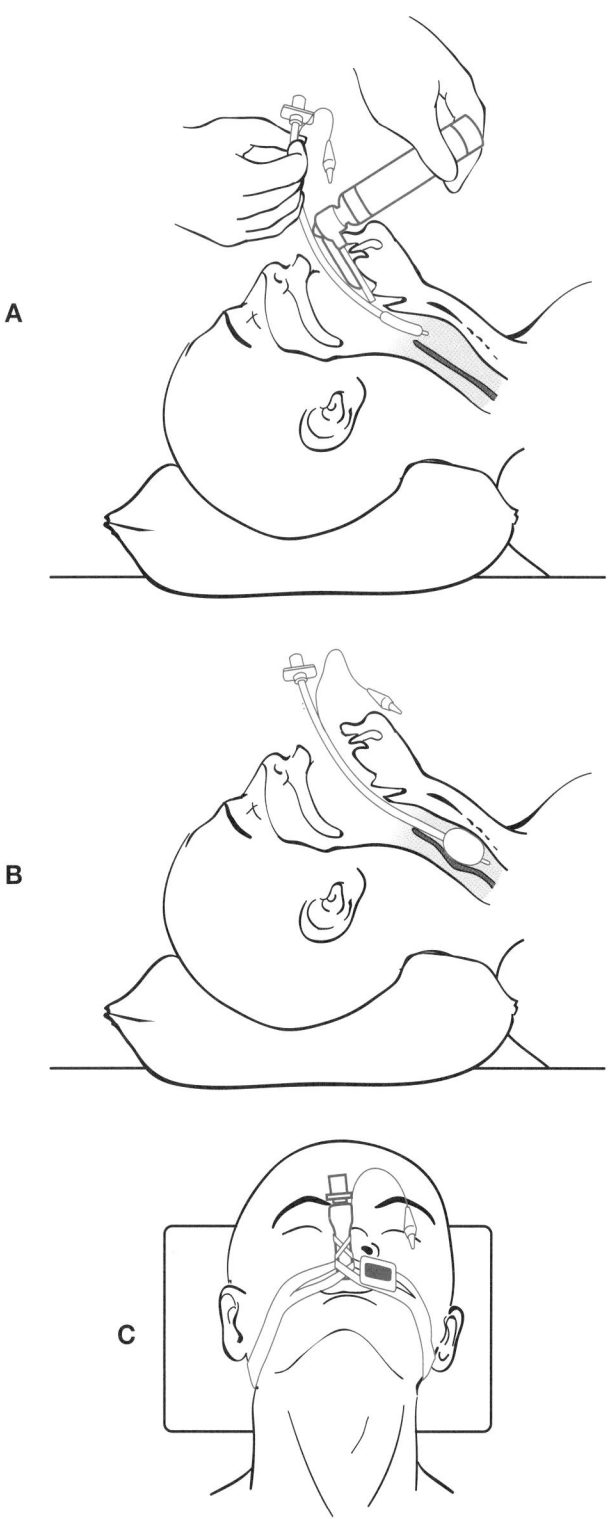

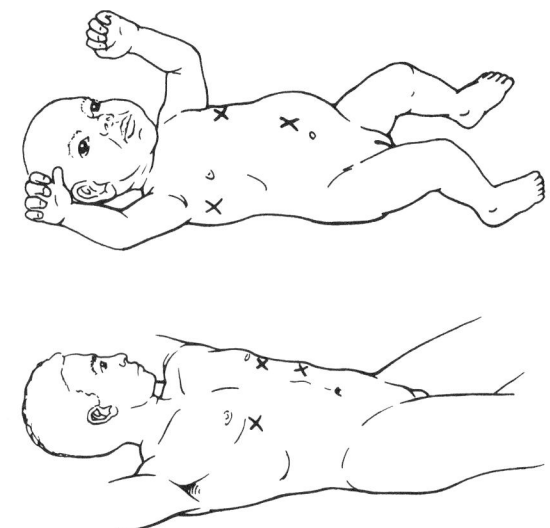

Fig. 83-9
Auscultation points of right and left chest for respiratory movement and over stomach for lack of sound.

oxygen or Fio_2 = 1.0. When in doubt, start with 100% oxygen and rapidly reduce the percentage, depending on the readings from a pulse oximeter and/or results of judiciously timed arterial blood gases.

Remember the Following:

- If intubation requires more than 20 seconds, abort the attempt, ventilate the patient with 100% oxygen (bag valve mask or mouth-to-mask), and then try again. Consider continuous positive airway pressure (CPAP) with the use of a tight-fitting mask. CPAP can improve oxygenation if a routine mask is not sufficient while awaiting intubation.
- Check tube position and reposition as needed. Suction excess debris.
- The stylet can be bent to whatever angle is needed by pushing it against the hard palate.
- Prior placement of a nasogastric tube will show you where *not* to go.
- With obstructive lung disease, lower respiratory rates should be used to allow for more complete exhalation. Care must be taken in these patients, as well as asthmatics, to prevent air trapping that may result in a positive end-expiratory pressure effect.

Further questions and considerations: Does the patient have an anteriorly displaced larynx? Need the Sellick maneuver? Is pharyngeal anatomy such that you need more extension? Flexion? Do you need to make a blind passage through arytenoids (not desirable, but sometimes necessary)?

Fig. 83-8
Insertion of endotracheal tube with laryngoscope in place. **A,** Insert the tube just lateral to the path of the laryngoscope so a clear view can be maintained at all times. Watch the tube pass through cords. **B,** The tube is correctly positioned when the proximal end of the tube cuff is just below the vocal cords. When the tube is in place, remove the laryngoscope and carefully withdraw the stylet. **C,** Secure the tube to minimize patient discomfort while maintaining correct positioning.

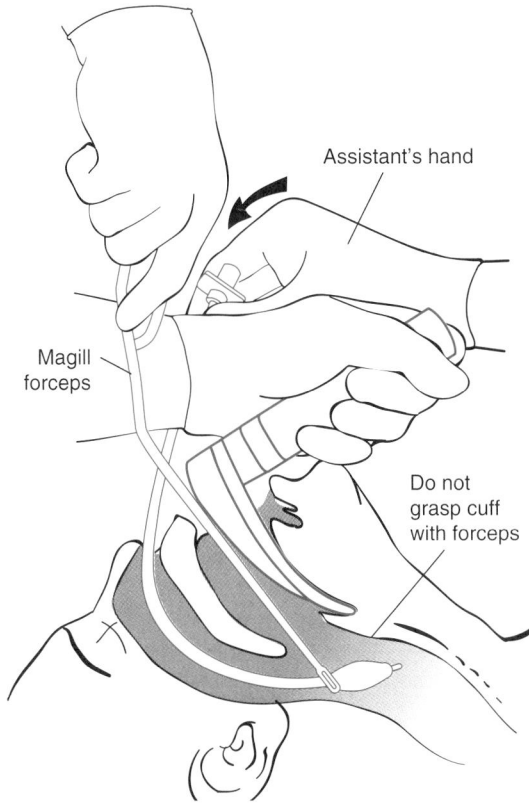

Fig. 83-10
Nasotracheal intubation with use of a laryngoscope and Magill forceps. The forceps do not pull the tube but only serve to guide the tip of the tube through the vocal cords while an assistant advances the tube. The cuff is frequently damaged if it is grasped. (Modified from Roberts JR, Hedges JR, editors: Clinical procedures in emergency medicine, ed 3, Philadelphia, 1998, WB Saunders.)

Nasotracheal Intubation

1. Obtain informed consent, if possible. Position the patient in the sniffing position, which may be sitting up. Spray both nares with vasoconstricting spray and topical anesthetic.
2. Gently insert the tube into a naris with the bevel facing toward the septum to avoid Kiesselbach's plexus. As the tube passes posteriorly, gently rotate the tube into the anteroposterior plane. There should be a decrease in resistance as the tube passes through the choana. As the tube passes down the posterior pharynx, listen for movement of air through the tube. The use of an endotracheal tube whistle may enhance the detection of air movement.
3. Air flow through the tube should be at its maximum just proximal to the glottis. If air movement decreases, withdraw the tube slightly and rotate it either left or right until maximal air flow is noted.
4. Advance the tube forward during inspiration. As the tube passes through the vocal cords, it should fog

from exhaled warm air. When the tube fogs, it confirms placement.
5. Secure the tube as with endotracheal intubation.
6. Direct visualization can also be used to place a nasotracheal tube. With the patient supine, use the laryngoscope in the same manner as for endotracheal intubation. While visualizing the cords, use the Magill forceps to grasp the tube already inserted through the nasopharynx, and pass it through the cords (Fig. 83-10). Avoid tearing the cuff when grasping the tube with the forceps.

POSTPROCEDURE CARE

- Order daily chest x-ray films to verify tube placement.
- The respiratory services department of the hospital usually supplies the ventilator, tape, and other equipment as well as provides care; however, the clinician is ultimately responsible.
- Check the patient and the respiratory setup frequently. Carbon dioxide detectors and whistles can be used to confirm expiratory efforts.

COMPLICATIONS

- Short-term laryngeal edema: sore throat occurs in almost every patient after extubation (repeated attempts at intubation by unskilled personnel may cause enough edema to preclude intubation by highly skilled clinicians)
- Trauma:
  - Broken teeth
  - Oral lacerations or ulcerations (lip, tongue, pharynx, esophagus, or trachea)
  - Bleeding, hematoma, or abscess formation as a result of trauma
  - Avulsion of arytenoid cartilage
- Hypoxia resulting from the following:
  - Long duration of procedure
  - Esophageal intubation (most commonly results from not visualizing the vocal cords)
  - Intubation of a bronchus
  - Failure to recognize esophageal or bronchus intubation
  - Pneumothorax
  - Failure to secure the placement
  - Failure to recognize misplacement of the tube
  - Aspiration of vomited material, especially in conscious or semiconscious patient
  - Laryngospasm
- Hypertension-hypotension
- Bradycardia
- Tachycardia with or without arrhythmias

- Sequelae (of long-term endotracheal tube placement):
  - Nosocomial infection
  - Pneumothorax
  - Corneal abrasions
  - Epistaxis
  - Sinusitis
  - Vocal cord paralysis (left cord more frequently involved than right)
  - Tracheomalacia and stenosis (occurs more frequently in males; more common with older tubes that use higher cuff pressures)
  - Tracheoesophageal fistula
  - Innominate artery erosion by endotracheal cuff

Note: Rarely are teeth broken with nasotracheal intubation. However, acute epistaxis and nasal trauma can result. Pulmonary infection can also be caused by nasal flora introduced through the nasotracheal tube.

SUPPLIERS

Mallinckrodt
675 McDonnell Boulevard
Hazelwood, MO 63042
Phone: 1-800-635-5267
Website:www.mallinckrodt.com/respiratory/resp/index.html

Cook, Inc.
925 South Curry Pike
P.O. Box 489
Bloomington, IN 47402-0489
Phone: 1-800-457-4500
Website: www.cookcriticalcare.com

Rusch
2450 Meadowbrook Parkway
Duluth, GA 30096
Phone: 1-770-623-0816
Website: www.ruschinc.com

Sims Portex
Hythe, Kent CT21 6JL
United Kingdom
Phone: +44(0) 1303 260551
Website: www.portex.com

CPT/BILLING CODE

31500   Intubation, endotracheal; emergency procedure

ICD-9-CM DIAGNOSTIC CODES

276.4	Acid-base mixed disorder
276.2	Acidosis
276.3	Alkalosis
493.01	Asthma, extrinsic with status asthmaticus
493.90	Asthma, unspecified with status asthmaticus
427.5	Cardiac or cardiorespiratory arrest
491.2	Chronic obstructive bronchitis
491.2	Chronic obstructive bronchitis with emphysema
780.01	Coma
492.8	Emphysema, NOS
491.2	Emphysema, with chronic bronchitis
786.09	Hypercapnia
799.0	Hypoxia
428.1	Pulmonary edema (left heart failure)
518.5	Pulmonary insufficiency following trauma and surgery
799.1	Respiratory arrest
518.82	Respiratory distress: acute
786.09	Respiratory distress: NOS or respiratory insufficiency
518.81	Respiratory failure, NOS
518.83	Respiratory failure, chronic
785.50	Shock, unspecified
785.51	Shock, cardiogenic
785.59	Shock, other (hypovolemic, septic)

ADDITIONAL RESOURCES

- See the sample patient education handout titled "Endotracheal Intubation" on page 1835 of Appendix G.

BIBLIOGRAPHY

American Heart Association: *Textbook of advanced cardiac life support,* Dallas, 1997, American Heart Association.

Baskett P, editor: International Guidelines 2000 for CPR, ECC: A consensus on Science; Part 6: advanced cardiovascular life support. Section 3: adjuncts for oxygenation, ventilation, and airway control, *Resuscitation* 46(1-3):115, 2000.

Gallagher TJ: Endotracheal intubation, *Crit Care Clinics* 8(4):665, 1992.

Howell JM, editor: *Emergency medicine,* Philadelphia, 1998, WB Saunders.

Hubmayer RD, Irwin RS: Mechanical ventilation. In Irwin RS, Cerra FB, Rippe JM, editors: *Irwin and Rippe's intensive care medicine,* ed 4, Philadelphia, 1999, Lippincott-Raven.

Roberts JR, Hedges JR, editors: *Clinical procedures in emergency medicine,* ed 3, Philadelphia, 1998, WB Saunders.

CHAPTER 84

Ambulatory Electrocardiography: Holter and Event Monitoring

David B. Feller
Ken Grauer

There are approximately 350,000 sudden cardiac deaths per year in the United States, and most are probably due to ventricular fibrillation (VF) or ventricular tachycardia (VT). Patients who survive VF or sustained VT are likely to have recurrences, and many of these are fatal. Although pharmacologic therapy has been disappointing in certain aspects of the management of ventricular arrhythmias, fortunately the outlook is improving because of increased knowledge of which antiarrhythmics to use, and when, and because of the development of implantable cardioverter-defibrillators (ICDs). As our knowledge and treatment of arrhythmias continues to improve, accurate diagnosis becomes even more important.

Approximately 1 to 2 million middle-aged American men have silent myocardial ischemia (SMI). The number of postmenopausal women with SMI is not as well known. Although exercise testing (ET) may be a more effective method of determining the clinical significance of SMI, ambulatory electrocardiography is often used to make the diagnosis. For treatment of significant ischemic heart disease, outcome studies have indicated that the goal should be to reduce as much ischemia as possible. However, as discussed in this chapter, it is important to know the statistics related to ambulatory electrocardiography before attempting to document a reduction in the number of ischemic episodes for a particular patient.

Norman Holter developed ambulatory electrocardiography in the form of Holter monitoring in the early 1960s. The first device weighed about 85 pounds. Although in the past Holter recordings were almost exclusively the domain of cardiologists and internists, this procedure as well as other forms of ambulatory monitoring have become increasingly popular among all primary care clinicians. Holter monitoring is helpful not only in the diagnosis and management of ventricular arrhythmias, but also with atrial arrhythmias. For arrhythmias that occur only occasionally or sporadically, event monitoring can be used for weeks or months and may be more useful. In fact, partly due to the frustration with arrhythmias not occurring during the typical 24-hour Holter tracing, certain clinicians now use event monitors more frequently than Holters.

As primary care clinicians have increased their competence in interpreting and/or managing the results, they have become more comfortable providing Holter and event monitoring in their offices. Benefits include more readily, and perhaps more rapidly, available data for their patients. These data allow for more complete and definitive care for many patients. If a referral is necessary, it is usually more appropriate (e.g., directly to the electrophysiologic [EP] cardiologist as opposed to the general cardiologist).

Ambulatory electrocardiography is attractive because it requires little of the clinician's time to interpret the results and is therefore a time-efficient, income-generating test. With more widespread use the cost of equipment has also decreased. However, acquisition of an office monitoring system is not a decision to be taken lightly. Although it is relatively easy to interpret the results, it is considerably more difficult to apply them clinically. The clinician must have a clear interest in cardiac arrhythmias and be willing to invest the time needed to learn the system. The clinician must also make the commitment to promptly interpret the results of all tests performed. Realistically, with training and a modicum of practice clinicians can interpret and dictate the results of most Holter reports within 5 to 15 minutes. Interpretation of event monitoring usually takes even less time.

Despite being more readily available, ambulatory monitoring should not be considered a routine procedure. From the patient's and insurer's perspective, it is expensive and time consuming. It should be reserved for specific indications.

COMPARISON OF AVAILABLE METHODS OF EVALUATION AND ARRHYTHMIA MONITORING

Patient History

- Unreliable in subjects who are unaware of an arrhythmia or ectopic beats.
- Potentially valuable for subjects who *can* accurately sense the occurrence of a documented arrhythmia (i.e., "poor person's Holter monitor").
- Symptoms that strongly suggest a patient is having a VT, VF, or a hemodynamically compromising arrhythmia include palpitations, a sensation in the chest of rapid or irregular cardiac rhythm, dizziness, and unexplained syncope.

Combined History, Physical Examination, and Cardiac Auscultation

- Unreliable for distinguishing between premature supraventricular beats and premature ventricular beats (PVCs), and for diagnosis of rhythm abnormalities. However, the history and physical may suggest a reduced ventricular ejection fraction, which is important information for the management and prognosis of a ventricular arrhythmia.

12-Lead ECG and Rhythm Strip

- Only monitors cardiac rhythm for a short period.
- Prolongation of the QT interval or a right bundle-branch block with ST-segment elevation may be associated with VT, but rarely is VT observed on an isolated ECG.

24-Hour Holter Monitor

- Gold standard for arrhythmia monitoring when arrhythmias are frequent.
- Subject's diary enables a correlation of symptoms to the timing of arrhythmias.
- Expensive ($250 to $500 test in most institutions).
- May not identify subjects with infrequent but potentially lethal arrhythmias.
- Can identify subjects with silent ischemia and dangerous arrhythmias as well as quantify the amount; however, the interpreter must be aware of the tremendous spontaneous variability in frequency of not only ectopy, but also ST segment changes indicating ischemia.

Event or Loop Transtelephonic Monitoring

- In certain centers, more widely used than Holter.
- Helpful for documenting arrhythmias that occur infrequently (better than Holter for this) or when symptoms are very transient.
- The patient must be aware of arrhythmias when they occur and must maintain consciousness long enough to touch a button and/or freeze the monitor, and/or to transmit the arrhythmia over the telephone.
- With loop monitors, up to 45 minutes of prior ECG data are captured or "frozen" when the patient pushes a button at the time of an event. The data are then transmitted over the telephone to a center for analysis. If the button is not pushed, the ECG loop starts over every 45 minutes and the data are replaced. Technicians are on call 24 hours a day to interpret the data when transmitted. If necessary, they can coordinate a trip to the emergency department or call for emergency medical services.
- Other developments in this area include finger and wrist electrodes. They may replace the need for patients to wear chest or limb electrodes for a month. For extremely infrequent arrhythmias, devices are also now available that can be implanted subcutaneously for 24 to 36 months. They also record on 40- to 45-minute continuous ECG loops, and results are transmitted telephonically. For the future, systems are under development to use wireless transmission through the Internet. Electrodes are being designed to be worn like a watch, and with Internet connectivity, continuous ambulatory telemetry may become available.

Signal Averaged ECG

- Used widely in the past, it is now known that the positive predictive value of signal averaged ECG (SAECG) is no more than 20%. As a result, it is rarely used anymore.
- Used almost exclusively after myocardial infarction (MI).
- May only be of value in symptomatic patients.
- Negative values on this test are more useful.

Electrophysiology Studies

- For post-MI patients at high risk of a life-threatening arrhythmia.
- Helpful in patients with a low ejection fraction, documented ischemic disease, and a history of syncope or near syncope.
- Can determine whether an arrhythmia is inducible.
- Although this is an invasive procedure, it is particularly helpful when Holter or event monitoring results are equivocal.

Exercise (Stress) Testing

- Especially helpful as a screening test for the presence of underlying ischemia or coronary artery disease (CAD).
- May confirm ischemia as the etiology of an arrhythmia or document its association with an arrhythmia.
- Demonstrates the effect of activity on ventricular arrhythmias.
- May detect some forms of complex ventricular ectopy not detected by Holter monitoring.
- ST-segment depression in the absence of chest pain may alert the clinician to silent ischemia.
- Not nearly as sensitive as Holter monitoring for detection of PVCs.
- Systems are now available to check for T-wave alternans, a possible risk factor for VT and VF. Although the data on T-wave alternans as a risk factor are promising, they are not yet clear.

Echocardiography or Gated Ventriculograms

- Useful for determining the ejection fraction in patients with myopathy, ischemic heart disease, or previous MI.
- Most helpful for choice of medications: an asymptomatic post-MI patient with an ejection fraction (EF) greater than 50% rarely needs an antiarrhythmic treatment of any kind.
- For an EF greater than 40%, but less than 50%, treatment decisions are less clear-cut. Definitely treat if symptomatic, even if symptoms are mild.
- For an EF less than 40%, aggressive management of arrhythmias should be considered.

BENEFITS AND DRAWBACKS OF AVAILABLE MONITORING METHODS

Physical examination and cardiac auscultation are unreliable for distinguishing supraventricular from ventricular premature beats. The least expensive yet reliable method to document these arrhythmias is a standard 12-lead ECG with a short rhythm strip. Unfortunately, with an ECG the cardiac rhythm is monitored only for a short period. Considering that the commonly accepted definition of "frequent" ventricular ectopy is more than 10 to 30 PVCs an hour, it becomes easy to see how even "frequent" PVCs can be overlooked by this method. On the other hand, if any PVCs are noted on a short rhythm strip, it is likely that the patient has both frequent and complex ventricular ectopy. Both would probably be detected during a longer period of monitoring.

In the past, Holter recordings of only a few hours' duration were used for arrhythmia detection. Although practical and economical, such brief recordings do not accurately reflect the severity of cardiac arrhythmias in many individuals. This point is best illustrated by reviewing what is known about the frequency of ventricular arrhythmias over the course of a 24-hour period. Simply stated, even with the same patient, a tremendous amount of spontaneous variability in PVC frequency exists between one Holter recording and the next. For example, in a study by Winkle et al (1981) of 57 patients who had three consecutive 24-hour Holter recordings performed during the late phase of acute myocardial infarction, 12 had VT. In those patients who were found to have VT, this arrhythmia occurred very sporadically during the 72-hour monitoring period. VT was seen on all three 24-hour recordings of only one of the 12 patients and was not detected at all on 2 of the 3 days of monitoring in 9 of the 12 patients.

Marked variability in PVC frequency also occurs in ambulatory patients with chronic ventricular arrhythmias. As demonstrated by Morganroth et al (1978), PVC frequency varies greatly from one day to the next, between successive 8-hour monitoring periods, and even from hour to hour within a single day. Certain individuals exhibit PVCs primarily during the day; others manifest them principally at night. As might be expected, PVC frequency often varies with physical activity and emotional state. However, in many individuals marked spontaneous variability in PVC frequency persists even when monitoring conditions are kept absolutely constant.

Because of such fluctuations in PVC frequency, a monitoring period of at least 24 hours is usually recommended for adequate characterization of an arrhythmia. For most individuals, 24-hour monitoring not only permits recognition of diurnal variations in arrhythmias, but it also allows detection of the maximal grade of ectopy.

A review of the statistics behind spontaneous variability in PVC frequency is essential if the practitioner is to use Holter recordings to evaluate the effectiveness of antiarrhythmic therapy, especially now that nonrepetitive ventricular ectopy is treated much less often than it was in the past.

For example, reduction in PVC frequency from 5000 to 2500 PVCs per day after institution of an antiarrhythmic agent would seem to suggest drug efficacy; however, the practitioner cannot *statistically* exclude spontaneous variation by this response. To do so, a reduction in PVC frequency of at least 80% between Holter recordings is required. In this case the number of PVCs would have to be decreased from 5000 to less than 1000 before the practitioner could confidently and *statistically* conclude that the reduction was truly a response to the medication and not simply due to chance.

Assessment of drug efficacy by follow-up Holter monitoring is also made more difficult because antiarrhythmic agents themselves have a proarrhythmic effect. Between 5% and 10% of all antiarrhythmic drugs paradoxically worsen the very arrhythmia that the clinician is trying to treat. Even more alarming, current data indicate that antiarrhythmics can actually increase mortality. In the Cardiac Arrhythmia Suppression Trials (CAST in 1989 and CAST-II in 1992), although certain Class I antiarrhythmics prevented ventricular arrhythmias, their use nonetheless increased mortality. Consequently, both studies were terminated prematurely. Most clinicians are now reluctant to treat patients, especially with any degree of ischemia, with sodium channel blocking agents. Encainide has been withdrawn from the U.S. market as a result of these trials. Therefore, although it may be challenging, assessment of drug efficacy with Holter is more important than ever.

Proarrhythmic effects are most commonly seen in patients with impaired left ventricular function or other structural heart disease, in those who have malignant ventricular arrhythmias, and in those treated with antiarrhythmic agents that reduce conduction velocity, such as class I.a. or I.c. drugs and moricizine. In addition, agents that prolong refractoriness, such as amiodarone or sotalol, can also be arrhythmogenic. However, these proarrhythmic effects can occur in patients who have simple ventricular ectopy (i.e., without couplets, salvos, or longer runs of PVCs), in those who do not have underlying heart disease, and in those treated with beta-blockers or class I.b. antiarrhythmic agents. Spontaneous variability in PVC frequency and the possibility of a proarrhythmic effect can make it very difficult to determine whether a particular drug is making the patient better or worse.

In general, subjects with frequent ventricular ectopy almost always develop complex forms. However, the converse is not always true. Certain individuals with potentially lethal ventricular arrhythmias have very infrequent episodes of ventricular ectopy between periods of serious arrhythmias (e.g., VT). Malignant ventricular arrhythmias can therefore remain undetected if they do not produce symptoms and do not occur on the day of monitoring.

As another example, consider the case of a man with CAD who has fewer than 100 PVCs during 24 hours of monitoring but who does demonstrate an asymptomatic 20-beat run of VT. Making an empiric treatment decision on the basis of this finding could be problematic for several reasons. First, antiarrhythmic treatment of *asymptomatic* nonsustained VT has not been shown to improve prognosis, especially if the patient has a normal ejection fraction. On the contrary, empiric antiarrhythmic treatment of such patients could be deleterious. Furthermore, short of invasive EP testing, there is no reliable way to monitor the success of such treatment. Even a follow-up Holter that fails to detect VT cannot be taken as assurance that this infrequent but potentially lethal arrhythmia is no longer occurring!

A key caveat of 24-hour Holter monitoring is that no conclusions can be reached about whether a symptomatic arrhythmia exists or not unless symptoms occur on the day of monitoring. As noted previously, a patient may even have a malignant symptomatic ventricular arrhythmia that occurs only intermittently, sometimes as infrequently as every few weeks. To exclude this possibility, the practitioner would have to either extend the period of Holter monitoring or consider another method for arrhythmia detection. Performing Holters for 2 or more consecutive days until symptoms occur is both cumbersome to the patient and extremely expensive. A far more effective method for documenting the occurrence of a sporadic ventricular arrhythmia is to use a form of event monitoring.

Although many variations of event monitoring exist, patients are generally issued a set of electrode leads and a device that transmits the patient's rhythm over the telephone. Usually the equipment remains with the patient for a few days or weeks. Implantable units are also now available that may be used for months. The principal weaknesses to event monitoring are that patients must be aware of arrhythmias when they occur, and they must maintain consciousness long enough to capture or transmit the rhythm.

In the past, most clinicians began with full 24-hour Holter monitoring and proceeded to event monitoring only for those cases when symptoms persisted despite negative Holter findings. However, this trend has changed. Since asymptomatic Holter results are often complicated and confusing, and there is often a low yield of positive findings on Holter when arrhythmias are not frequent, many clinicians use event monitoring first. Overall, event monitoring is at least as effective as Holter monitoring for detection of symptomatic arrhythmias with the advantage of not revealing asymptomatic background arrhythmias that need not be treated (Kinlay, 1996). For these reasons, among others, event monitoring is now ordered more frequently in the United States than Holter monitoring.

When Holter or event monitoring results are equivocal, EP studies may be helpful. Although this is an invasive study, the information obtained may be critical. Patients in whom a clinically relevant arrhythmia can be induced during EP testing usually have a worse prognosis, even if asymptomatic, than patients in whom an arrhythmia cannot be induced.

Although patients with CAD and negative EP testing have a better prognosis, it is important to realize that the technique has a small but significant false-negative rate. Results in patients with nonischemic cardiomyopathy are also difficult to interpret. Approximately 20% to 40% of these patients with negative EP studies in fact have serious arrhythmias.

An all-too-often-ignored adjunct for monitoring is

the patient's history (perception) of arrhythmia occurrence. Although many individuals are totally unaware of their arrhythmias, others are able to sense each and every ectopic beat. For individuals with non-life-threatening arrhythmias who have this awareness—and in whom electrocardiography has confirmed a temporal relation between symptoms and the occurrence of their arrhythmias—the *patient's account of symptoms* may serve as a fairly reliable and cost-effective adjunct for long-term monitoring. As such (the "poor person's Holter monitor"), it may greatly reduce the need for (and expense of) repeated Holter recordings for judging the effect of treatment.

Consider the case of a patient who is markedly symptomatic from extremely frequent ventricular ectopy. Baseline Holter monitoring reveals several thousand PVCs during the day of monitoring but no runs of VT. The patient's diary confirms a definite relationship between symptoms and periods of greatest ectopy. Treatment with a beta-blocker (or a reduction in stimulants such as caffeine) leads to complete resolution of symptoms. Does the Holter need to be repeated?

The key question is whether repeating the Holter would alter treatment. Or will the patient's account of symptoms (i.e., the "poor person's Holter") be adequate for guiding management? In many instances, such as this particular case, it is adequate.

SAECG is a noninvasive test that has been advocated as a screening test for malignant ventricular arrhythmias after myocardial infarction. By computer averaging signals for several hundred recorded beats, background "noise" can be filtered out to allow detection of low-amplitude, high-frequency late potentials after the QRS. These late potentials are suggestive of areas of slower conduction that may facilitate development of ventricular reentry. Unfortunately, the positive predictive accuracy of late potentials on SAECG following MI is less than optimal, being no greater than 20% for prediction of VT or VF. However, negative findings on this test are more useful, so the test may be of some value as a screening technique. SAECG may also be of value for evaluating the patient with unexplained syncope, especially in the setting of impaired ventricular function or other structural heart disease. However, in reality, SAECG is seldom used anymore and most of the equipment owned by hospitals is currently gathering dust.

ET is the final office-based method for evaluating PVCs and certain other arrhythmias. It serves as a convenient, noninvasive screening tool for underlying CAD. If CAD is diagnosed, ET can also evaluate the severity and assist with the management. It also demonstrates what effect exercise has on arrhythmias. In general, PVCs that diminish with progressively increasing degrees of activity are less worrisome and tend to be associated with a better prognosis than those brought on by low levels of exercise. Although not nearly as accurate as Holter monitoring for quantitative or qualitative assessment of PVCs, complex ventricular arrhythmias (including VT) and symptoms are sometimes elicited only by vigorous exercise. Holter monitoring and exercise testing may thus be complementary procedures that provide different information, and both tests should sometimes be considered for the complete evaluation of patients with ventricular arrhythmias.

It should be emphasized that detection of PVCs per se on ET is not indicative of an ischemic response. However, PVCs are cause for more concern when they occur in association with evidence of ischemia, such as ST-segment depression or substernal chest pain in patients who are likely to have CAD. Thus it is not advisable to allow a middle-aged individual who has coronary risk factors to exercise in an unsupervised manner if ET produces frequent PVCs and ST-segment depression or symptoms. Instead, further evaluation, including cardiac catheterization, is warranted.

On the other hand, many clinicians are much more comfortable allowing healthy young adults who have frequent PVCs to exercise vigorously if ET does not produce ST-segment depression or if PVCs resolve with exercise. When these younger, asymptomatic, and otherwise healthy adults go out and exercise, their PVCs and symptoms will probably resolve with activity in a manner similar to what happened on the treadmill. Moreover, such individuals are much less likely to have underlying heart disease. Rare, life-threatening complex arrhythmias, seen only at peak exercise, will also be excluded with ET; therefore it is ideal as an evaluative method for the younger individual wishing to exercise vigorously.

ET systems are becoming available that screen for T-wave alternans with exercise. The research studies are not completed, but a combination of this test with SAECG may approximate the results of an EP study and do it noninvasively. These data appear most useful in those patients at risk of sudden cardiac death after MI and with prolonged QT syndrome.

SILENT MYOCARDIAL ISCHEMIA

In recent years, increasing importance has been attached to managing not only angina, but also SMI. This diagnosis is made when objective documentation of transient myocardial ischemia occurs in the absence of chest pain or anginal equivalents.

SMI is considered much more prevalent than is generally appreciated, perhaps affecting as many as 2 million American males. The number of women afflicted is unknown, but it may be as high in postmenopausal women. It occurs in asymptomatic individuals as well as in those with known CAD. Among the latter group, it is thought that silent ischemic episodes are actually far more common than painful ischemic episodes. Because episodes of SMI are not alarming to the patient, they frequently go undetected and are left untreated.

The two modalities most commonly used for diagnosing SMI are Holter monitoring and ET. At the present state of technology, detection by Holter monitoring is still problematic, especially when transient ST-segment depression is noted in an otherwise asymptomatic individual without cardiac risk factors. It appears that in most such cases, this abnormality reflects a false-positive result. In contrast, when episodes of transient ST-segment depression are detected on Holter monitoring or during ET of an individual with multiple risk factors or known CAD, such findings are much more likely to represent true disease.

The reason that detection of SMI is important in patients with ventricular ectopy is that ischemia may be the underlying or exacerbating cause of the arrhythmia. In such cases, treatment with nitroglycerin (NTG) or calcium channel blockers may be far more appropriate than antiarrhythmic therapy. Among the antiarrhythmic agents, beta-blockers offer the advantage of potentially benefiting both the ischemia and the arrhythmia.

Reservations about the use of Holter monitoring as a routine procedure for detection and evaluation of SMI include the following:

- Right-sided monitoring leads (such as lead V_1) that are commonly used for detection of cardiac arrhythmias only rarely demonstrate ST-segment depression.
- Special attention must be directed at ensuring optimal lead placement to rule out position-induced ST-segment deviations.
- Relatively long period of monitoring (48 to 72 hours) may be needed to assess the true frequency and duration of ischemic episodes in many patients.
- Follow-up of patients identified as having SMI is both expensive and problematic.

Intuitively, it would seem logical to treat patients with CAD who are identified as having significant SMI with NTG, beta-blockers, or calcium channel blockers. It would seem logical that follow-up Holter monitoring should be performed to demonstrate the efficacy of such treatment (i.e., to document a decrease in the number and duration of silent ischemia episodes with treatment). Unfortunately, spontaneous variability of both the frequency and duration of SMI detected on Holter is even greater than that of PVC frequency. Nabel et al (1988) showed that in order to statistically exclude spontaneous variability, virtually *all* episodes of silent ischemia must be eliminated on the follow-up Holter. Obviously, this is an almost impossible task.

Fortunately, we now have outcome studies for treatment of SMI. From one moderate-sized study of 600 patients with significant CAD (of such significance that

they would benefit from revascularization), those found to have SMI on Holter had improved outcomes if treated to relieve as much ischemia as possible as opposed to just treating to relieve angina (ACIP study).

HIGH-RISK PATIENTS

Conditions associated with VT include CAD, dilated or hypertrophic cardiomyopathy, right ventricular dysplasia, long QT syndrome, electrolyte abnormalities, use of antiarrhythmic drugs, and valvular heart disease.

In general, patients with ischemic heart disease, especially those with a history of MI, have a very high risk for a serious or fatal arrhythmic event. Patients in whom VT developed in the immediate postinfarction period have a mortality rate as high as 75% at 12 months. In all groups, individuals with higher ejection fractions (EFs greater than 50%) have better prognoses than those with low EFs (less than 35% to 40%). A low EF, especially in patients with PVCs, nonsustained VT (usually defined as three or more consecutive PVCs, but less than 30 seconds duration, or inducible ventricular arrhythmia(s), has a poor prognosis, even in the absence of CAD. The arrhythmia recurrence rate is 20% to 30% per year.

INDICATIONS

Evaluation of Patients with Symptoms of Suspected Cardiac Origin

Symptoms of patients with VT or VF include palpitations, a sensation in the chest of rapid or irregular cardiac rhythm, dizziness, and unexplained syncope. These symptoms strongly suggest a hemodynamically compromising arrhythmia.

However, not all patients with symptoms such as palpitations, dizziness, and syncope need Holter event monitoring. An occasional episode of skipped, dropped, or racing beats is not suggestive of VT or VF. Symptom duration and severity, the likelihood of underlying cardiac disease, the existence and effect of potentially reversible extracardiac factors (e.g., caffeine, alcohol, sleep deprivation, viral illness, electrolyte abnormalities, and nonessential medications), the patient's or clinician's "need to know," and cost concerns should all be considered. Therefore, on a patient's first visit, do *not* routinely order Holter monitoring for patients who lack underlying heart disease or risk factors, especially if symptoms are of recent onset and are not particularly bothersome to the patient. On the other hand, you probably should consider some form of ambulatory monitoring for a patient with activity-limiting symptoms, especially when the symptoms are persistent, and especially when the patient has multiple risk factors or underlying heart disease.

Evaluation of palpitations is a special case, with insight provided in a study by Weber (1996) in which fully one third of patients coming to an emergency facility with palpitations as their chief complaint had a psychological cause for this symptom (either generalized anxiety or panic disorders). Four factors were found in this study to be independently predictive of a cardiac (arrhythmia) cause: male gender, a history of heart disease, subjective sensation of an irregular heart beat, and symptom duration (palpitations) of more than 5 minutes.

Awareness of these findings may help in the decision of when to order an objective form of arrhythmia detection.

Evaluation of Heart Disease When the Presence of Symptomatic (or Asymptomatic) Arrhythmias Is Felt to Be of Prognostic Significance

The more impaired the EF, the more significant the ventricular arrhythmia.

The dilemma in using Holter or event monitoring to evaluate patients with ventricular arrhythmias is highlighted by the lack of evidence that treatment of PVCs per se improves prognosis. However, if PVCs are associated with ischemia, treatment of the ischemia can improve the prognosis. Also, clinical trials have demonstrated benefits of implantable cardiac defibrillators (ICDs) that have exceeded the expectations of even the most optimistic investigators. In fact, ICDs are fast replacing pharmacologic therapy as the treatment of choice for ventricular arrhythmias in certain clinical situations.

One of the most common indications for Holter monitoring in the elderly is sick sinus syndrome. Holter is the procedure of choice for diagnosing and evaluating this disorder, especially if the patient is symptomatic; as it turns out, pacemaker implantation in asymptomatic individuals has not been shown to prolong life.

Evaluation of Antiarrhythmic Drug Therapy

Although it makes intuitive sense to evaluate the efficacy of antiarrhythmic treatment with follow-up Holter monitoring, doing so is not only expensive but problematic. Drug-induced phenomena (e.g., proarrhythmia effects) or spontaneous variability in baseline PVC frequency often make it exceedingly difficult to assess the degree of efficacy (if any) of a particular drug. Moreover, even when antiarrhythmic therapy leads to near-total abolishment of arrhythmic events, prognosis may not be improved because the precipitating cause of

the arrhythmia—heart disease—remains. Surprisingly, monitoring *after* discontinuation of antiarrhythmic medications is sometimes more useful.

Evaluation of Patients for Silent Myocardial Ischemia

SMI remains a somewhat controversial indication for Holter monitoring. Unfortunately, use of Holter monitoring to analyze ST-segment changes and their clinical implications (possible ischemia) in an unselected population is often more problematic than using the procedure to evaluate and manage patients with ventricular arrhythmias. Diagnosing SMI in patients for which the Holter has been ordered for another indication is also problematic. Practically speaking, in patients *without known coronary disease* undergoing Holter monitoring for evaluation of possible cardiac arrhythmias, most ST-segment shifts are *not* the result of silent ischemia.

As mentioned earlier, for patients with significant CAD (disease of such severity that they would benefit from revascularization), evaluation for SMI has been shown to improve outcomes. Those treated to minimize ischemia, as documented by Holter, have better outcomes than those treated to just minimize symptoms. This would seem to be the major indication for Holter in those with SMI.

Overall Clinical Perspective

Although awareness of the relative frequency and complexity of ventricular arrhythmias in different populations is important, especially for those patients with an impaired EF, practically speaking the indications for treating nonsustained ventricular arrhythmias are greatly reduced from what they were in the past. This is because treatment with antiarrhythmic drugs is not benign, and it has never been shown that treating such patients prolongs life. As a result, the presence of symptoms has become an even more important determinant of whether or not to obtain some form of ambulatory monitoring. As might be expected, event monitoring (rather than 24-hour Holter monitoring) is increasingly used for this purpose.

In contrast, assessment of the patient with bradycardia remains a major indication for 24-hour Holter monitoring. For that patient, a Holter should assess the severity of the bradycardia and whether there is need for permanent pacing. It should be noted that short pauses (of up to 2 seconds) are common and not necessarily abnormal. Pauses become more of a clinical concern when they are frequent and of longer duration (3 seconds or more). If frequent or longer pauses are accompanied by symptoms, and are not the result of recent infarction or rate-slowing drugs, permanent pacing should be considered.

PREPROCEDURE PATIENT EDUCATION AND PREPARATION

- Explain to the patient why Holter or event monitoring is necessary.
- Explain to the patient the need for, as well as how to keep, a symptom diary.

An essential part of the Holter recording is the patient's symptom diary. Considering how often supraventricular and ventricular ectopy are found in the general population as well as how frequently patients come to a clinician with symptoms suggestive of cardiac arrhythmias, the importance of establishing a cause-and-effect relationship between the two should be evident. For example, if symptoms are noted at 10 am, 2 pm, 5 pm, and 11 pm, but no cardiac arrhythmias are seen at these times, it is unlikely that the symptoms are cardiac related. Therefore much useful information may be obtained from Holter recordings even if no arrhythmias occur—provided the diary is completed carefully.

In symptomatic individuals who actually demonstrate cardiac arrhythmias on Holter monitoring, one can determine whether the arrhythmias are likely to be the cause of their symptoms by the temporal relationship in the diary. For example, if long runs of ventricular bigeminy occur while the patient is relaxed and totally unaware of the arrhythmia—and palpitations or chest discomfort are noted only during periods of sinus rhythm—ventricular bigeminy is probably not related to the patient's symptoms.

Unfortunately, in clinical practice, completion of the diary is all too often neglected. As a result, consider the following:

- Emphasize the importance of filling out the diary to your patient.
- Be sure that the patient can read and write before providing the diary. If the patient is unable to do so, see if someone can help the patient fill out the diary.
- For hospitalized patients, consider actively involving the nursing staff to ensure accurate completion of the patient diary.

Note: Use of event monitoring is much more conducive to correlating symptoms with arrhythmias. The occurrence of symptoms is what prompts the patient to initiate recording.

EQUIPMENT

- Holter or event monitor with desired capabilities (check for cracked or broken wires, dead batteries, or damage to the carrying case)

- Printer paper, ink, extra cassettes (for the Holter report to be printed out for interpretation)
- Razor
- Rubbing alcohol
- Electrodes
- Electrode cream, if disposable electrodes are not used
- Lead attachment kit

Most of the time, hospitals and commercial Holter or event laboratories employ trained technicians to scan Holter recordings for the interpreting clinician. This is a tremendous timesaving feature because the technician can highlight the principal findings, thus sparing the clinician the need to meticulously scan each of the full-disclosure printouts.

On the other hand, the luxury of having a trained technician to scan full-disclosure tracings is not available to many clinicians in private practice who have purchased their own Holter monitoring system. Options include the following:

- Having the hard copy of the Holter recording processed and scanned by a commercial laboratory—an expensive option!
- Hiring or training a technician to scan, which may be the most cost-effective solution for the busy practitioner who has a nurse or technician with interest and expertise in arrhythmia interpretation.
- Not printing 24-hour full disclosure. Depending on the area's third-party payment regulations, the practitioner may not receive full reimbursement unless 24-hour full disclosure is printed out.
- Printing but ignoring 24-hour full disclosure, or looking only at those portions of the printout that seem relevant to the clinical problem (i.e., looking at full disclosure only at times when symptoms are noted on the diary, or at times of densest ectopy as suggested on the hourly summary). This saves time, but if something is missed, it will be documented.
- Printing 24-hour full disclosure and scanning the printout yourself. Although this takes a greater amount of time to accomplish, it may be time well spent.
- Purchasing a Holter system that does not provide full disclosure. If reimbursement for this modality in your area is comparable to that for full-disclosure systems, this alternative may be both cost and time effective, especially if the practitioner does not have great interest or expertise in arrhythmia interpretation. Realize, however, that such systems are more likely to yield equivocal findings, and that they may overlook potentially important arrhythmias. Personal interpretation of Holters recorded on such systems is only as good as the system's computer software.

Note: The authors feel that full 24-hour disclosure is indispensable for optimal Holter interpretation. In their experience, it is essential for someone to scan the entire recording, even when trend analyses, hourly summaries, and selected rhythm strips are normal. At the very least, the first 10 to 20 Holters performed on a system in an office should be scanned meticulously, as a quality control measure; that is, when the Holter printout says "no runs of tachycardia," there should be confidence in its accuracy. The authors have been "burned" more than once for not manually scanning the 24 hours of full disclosure.

Systems that offer data compression are not providing full disclosure. Using signal averaging to evaluate "compressed" data, and then reexpanding it, does not allow every QRS complex to be reproduced.

TECHNIQUE

1. The patient's report form should be completed with relevant patient information such as cardiac risk factors, medications, activity level, and other medical problems that may assist in interpretation.
2. Monitoring parameters on the equipment should be set.
3. Attach the ECG electrodes in the locations indicated for the particular model of Holter or event monitor (see the operating instructions or illustrations provided by the monitor manufacturer). In general, place the limb leads more centrally than with an office ECG.

Equipment Settings

Most Holter systems provide the operator some flexibility in selecting the parameters used to scan for abnormalities. Some routine settings are shown in Table 84-1. In this example, the computer will record a full-size rhythm strip for those tachycardias that are faster than 120 beats per minute (automatic high rate); for bradycardias slower than 40 beats per minute (automatic low rate); and for pauses longer than 2 seconds (automatic pause). Since automatic abnormal is set at 3, the machine should record the first three incidents of tachycardia that occur during any given hour, to a maximum of 5 strips per hour for any

TABLE 84-1

Equipment Settings

Automatic high rate	120 beats/min
Automatic low rate	40 beats/min
Automatic pause	2.00 sec
Automatic supraventricular ectopic	25%
Automatic ST level	2 mm
Automatic abnormal	3/hr
Periodic storage	2 hr
Strips per hour	5

reason—which may still yield a total of 60 pages of rhythm strips to wade through (up to 5 strips per hour × 24 hours = 120 strips/2, since two rhythm strips are displayed per page).

Since periodic storage is set at 2 hours, the computer should record at least one rhythm strip every 2 hours, even if no abnormalities occur. This guarantees that the interpreter will have at least 12 rhythm strips to view, even if the Holter is completely normal.

Note: The authors are generally not comfortable accepting the computer's reading of "normal" unless a certain minimal number of normal full-size rhythm strips are displayed.

One reason for favoring 120 beats per minute as the upper rate limit is that lower numbers (i.e., 100 or 110 beats per minute) are more likely to produce an excessive number of benign sinus tachycardia strips, whereas higher numbers (i.e., 130 or 140 beats per minute) might prevent the detection of significant tachycardias with relatively slow rates, such as VT at 125 beats per minute.

Note: Selection of equipment settings always involves a compromise, and the setting of 120 beats per minute may occasionally yield a monotonous deluge of sinus tachycardia strips at 120 to 125 beats per minute.

For similar reasons, a lower rate limit of 40 beats per minute is favored. For example, selecting a lower rate limit of 50 beats per minute might result in a deluge of benign sinus bradycardia strips if the Holter was performed on an otherwise healthy individual who happened to have a slow resting heart rate.

Pauses of up to 2 seconds are common, especially in the elderly, and are usually benign. Longer pauses, especially those accompanied by frequent episodes of bradycardia with rates of less than 40 beats per minute, suggest the possibility of sick sinus syndrome.

The automatic supraventricular ectopic (SVE) setting of 25% should record rhythm strips demonstrating a greater than 25% variation in R-R interval. This is how SVEs such as premature atrial contractions (PACs) are picked up. Setting the SVE lower (i.e., at 10%) would detect many more PACs but would also pick up sinus arrhythmia. Higher settings might miss too many PACs. But even with a setting of 25%, imagine the number of strips that would result when the underlying rhythm is atrial fibrillation!

The most controversial parameter is the automatic ST level, which is usually set at 2 mm, unless the reason for performing the Holter is to "seek and search for" silent ischemia. Resolution of ST-segment images may be less than ideal, and in an otherwise unselected population, a majority of individuals with episodes of ST-segment depression between 1 and 2 mm will be false positives; that is, they will not have true silent ischemia. Setting the

ST-segment parameter at 2 mm greatly increases the specificity of this finding for true silent ischemia. The tradeoff is that some patients with CAD may have frequent episodes of silent ischemia with lesser degrees of ST-segment depression. Although the ST-segment trend analysis (see Fig. 84-4) should reflect this, it is important to document the phenomenon by recording at least a few full-size strips that demonstrate definite ST-segment depression. This is one benefit of lowering the ST-segment parameter to 1 mm when the principal reason for performing the Holter is to evaluate the patient with probable CAD for silent ischemia.

Note: The technique and equipment settings for event monitors are usually similar to those for Holter monitors.

INTERPRETATION

Appreciation of the wide range of normal is essential for meaningful interpretation of ambulatory ECG recordings. Premature supraventricular and ventricular contractions, as well as certain other cardiac arrhythmias, are common in otherwise healthy, asymptomatic individuals who are not in need of costly evaluation or treatment (which can be associated with unpleasant side effects or even be harmful).

Although a detailed description of all of the variants of "normal" is beyond the scope of this review, a brief discussion of the prevalence of ventricular arrhythmias and then an overview of the clinical perspective of the process may be helpful.

Prevalence of Premature Ventricular Contractions in the General Population

PVCs are common; they are found in up to 50% of otherwise healthy, asymptomatic young adults. Their frequency increases with age; thus most adults over 60 have some ventricular ectopy during a 24-hour period of monitoring. Less well appreciated is the fact that in the absence of underlying heart disease, complex forms of ventricular ectopy (e.g., multiform PVCs, ventricular couplets, salvos, or longer runs of VT) are uncommon. In contrast, both frequent and complex ventricular ectopy are common when underlying heart disease is present.

The term *frequent* when used to quantify ventricular ectopy is subject to interpretation. In a population of middle-aged individuals with underlying heart disease, frequent ventricular ectopy is most often defined as an average of more than 10 to 30 PVCs per hour over 24 hours of monitoring (i.e., at least 240 PVCs per day). In contrast, among otherwise healthy, asymptomatic young adults, a much lower number to define *frequent* should probably be used. As noted above, although up to half of these individuals have some PVCs during 24 hours of monitoring, it is unusual for them to have as many as 100 PVCs per day.

A notable exception to the generalities just described is in the small subset of patients with primary electrical disease. These individuals have extremely frequent and complex ventricular ectopy despite an apparent absence of underlying heart disease. Kennedy et al (1985) studied 73 such subjects (with a mean age of 46) and followed them for a period of up to 10 years. Holter monitoring initially demonstrated a mean frequency of 566 PVCs per hour (range of 78 to 1994 PVCs per hour) for the group. Multiform PVCs were present in 63%, ventricular couplets in 60%, and VT in 26%. Extensive noninvasive cardiac evaluation failed to reveal underlying heart disease in these asymptomatic individuals, although subsequent cardiac catheterization did disclose CAD in a small percentage of them. Survival data for the group showed a significantly lower mortality rate than would be expected for age-matched controls. Thus even individuals with exceedingly frequent and complex ventricular ectopy can have a relatively benign clinical course in the absence of underlying heart disease.

Clinical Significance of Premature Ventricular Contractions

The significance of ventricular ectopy depends on the clinical setting in which it occurs. Patients with PVCs who do not have underlying heart disease tend to have a benign prognosis. Even among individuals with primary electrical disease and frequent, complex PVCs (as noted above), treatment is probably not indicated in the absence of both symptoms and underlying heart disease. In contrast, in the setting of acute ischemia, especially if associated with angina, any ventricular ectopy at all must be viewed as significant and as a potential trigger of VF.

Although left ventricular function is the most important predictive factor of mortality during the year after acute myocardial infarction, PVCs are also an independent risk factor. Mortality in this year is related to the frequency of ventricular ectopy, as detected by Holter monitoring before discharge from the hospital. Patients with less than one PVC per hour tend to have a low (less than 10%) mortality. The figure rises sharply as a function of PVC frequency. About half of the total PVC-associated mortality happens at PVC frequencies as low as three per hour. A mortality plateau (20% to 30% for the ensuing year) is reached above PVC frequencies of 10 per hour. Thus a predischarge Holter monitor recording obtained on a myocardial infarction patient needs to be interpreted in a different light than that of one obtained on a patient with chronic ventricular ectopy. The definition of "frequent" ventricular ectopy should probably be adjusted downward even further in post-MI patients.

The frequency of ventricular arrhythmias detected in the postinfarction period is time dependent. PVCs are infrequent for 3 to 5 days following infarction. They tend to increase in frequency over the next 6 to 12 weeks, and then the frequency levels off. Despite the tendency of PVC frequency to increase after discharge from the hospital, it may be more practical to obtain a baseline Holter monitor in selected patients *before* they go home.

Repetitive forms of ventricular ectopy (e.g., ventricular couplets, and especially salvos and longer runs of VT) are additional cause for concern. Their presence more than doubles the first-year mortality risk over that of patients who do not demonstrate repetitive forms. In contrast to previous thinking, multiform PVCs and R-on-T complexes are considered much less worrisome than repetitive forms.

Much less can be said about the clinical benefit of drug treatment for PVCs in postinfarction patients. In the absence of extremely frequent and complex forms, many clinicians consider beta-blocker therapy first. Beta-blockers are favored because they are generally well tolerated, have a low proarrhythmia effect, and may reduce both postinfarction mortality *and* ventricular ectopy.

Despite acknowledgment of the increased risk that postinfarction ventricular arrhythmias confer, data showing benefit of pharmacologic treatment of such arrhythmias is still lacking. On the contrary, the CAST studies demonstrated a twofold to threefold *increase* in mortality when postinfarction patients with ventricular arrhythmias were routinely treated with flecainide or encainide. As a result, encainide was withdrawn from the U.S. market. Treatment of such patients with a class I.a., I.b., or I.c. antiarrhythmic agent when beta-blockers cannot be used is therefore not indicated. In view of the potential for these antiarrhythmic drugs to be proarrhythmic and to increase the risk of mortality, the decision to initiate empiric pharmacologic antiarrhythmic therapy should never be taken lightly. Fortunately, implantable cardioverter-defibrillators may offer an alternative to pharmacologic therapy in certain cases.

SAMPLE HOLTER MONITOR

Many types of Holter monitor systems are on the market. Each has its own advantages and disadvantages. The field continues to evolve at an amazingly rapid pace, so that current drawbacks of a particular system may be corrected by the next edition of that system. It behooves the interested clinician to become familiar, at least in general terms, with the pros and cons of several types of Holter systems. This should assist them in selecting those operative features that are likely to be most applicable for a particular practice setting.

On the following pages, the information provided by one particular full-disclosure Holter system is illustrated. Although resolution quality of P-wave and ST-segment morphology is admittedly less than optimal with this system, it should still be adequate for office monitoring. The general principles illustrated by this Holter system are applicable to other systems, as well as to many of the principles involved in event monitoring. The main difference with event monitoring is that 24-hour full disclosure is not included.

CASE STUDY

A 60-year-old man has dyspnea on exertion, which has been increasing for 1 month. He had a myocardial infarction in the distant past, but he has been active for years and otherwise doing well without the need for cardiac medications. He did not complain of chest pain or palpitations but recently described frequent episodes of intense dyspnea, weakness, and dizziness, most often associated with activity. Physical examination was unremarkable, and a resting ECG revealed normal sinus rhythm without any acute changes. Because of the frequent occurrence of symptoms with activities of daily living, the practitioner decided to obtain a Holter before exercise testing.

Patient Diary

It is important for patients to keep a diary to aid in interpreting the results of Holter monitoring. As mentioned earlier, symptoms of potential cardiac etiology and arrhythmias are common in the general population. The only way to prove that symptoms are cardiac related is to document a temporal correlation between their occurrence and the occurrence of arrhythmias on a Holter.

As emphasized earlier, completion of a diary can provide the clinician with much useful information, even if the Holter is entirely normal. Thus, if multiple symptoms are noted on the day of monitoring and no arrhythmias are detected on the Holter, the patient can be reassured that symptoms are unlikely to be cardiac in origin. The diary is especially helpful in this case (Fig. 84-1) because it indicates eight symptomatic episodes of weakness, dizziness, and/or shortness of breath.

12-Lead Electrocardiogram

Many clinicians obtain a preprocedure 12-lead ECG on all patients scheduled for Holter monitoring to screen for baseline artifact. If there is significant artifact on the 12-

Time	Activity	Symptoms
1PM	Lunch, relax	
2PM	Rake leaves	Weak, dizziness
4PM	Sitting, resting	Weak, dizziness
6PM	Resting	Weak
7PM	Watching TV	Dizziness
9PM	Went to bed	Dizziness
7AM	Breakfast	Short of breath
8AM	Resting	Short of breath, dizzy
9AM	Drove to doctor's office	Weak, dizziness

Fig. 84-1
Patient diary for Holter monitoring.

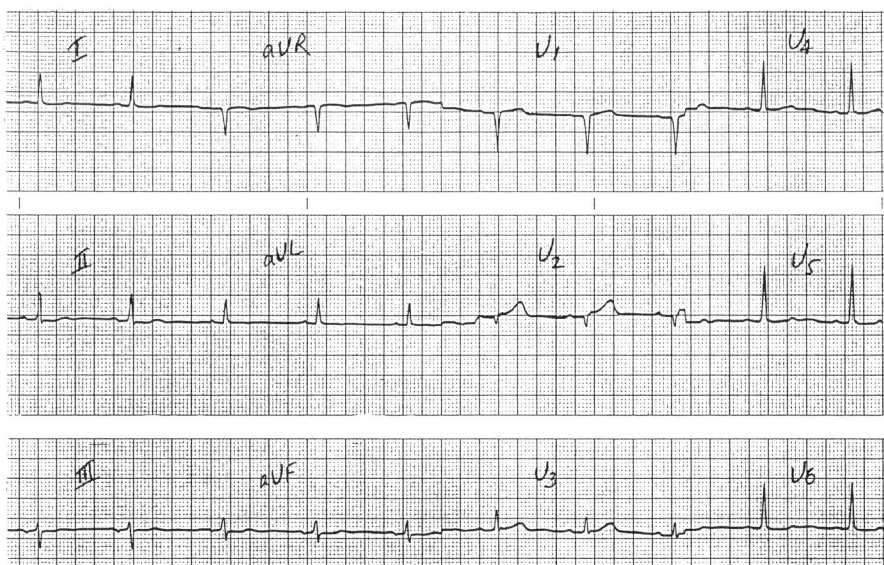

Fig. 84-2
Baseline 12-lead electrocardiogram.

lead, such artifact will likely be seen on the Holter and might preclude accurate assessment of the P-wave morphology. However, this additional step may be considered unnecessary and time consuming by technicians since the patient has usually undergone a 12-lead ECG at a recent clinical visit. In most cases, proper attention to lead placement precludes baseline artifact.

If there has been a frequent problem with the quality of Holter results, certain systems offer the ability to test the three or five leads of a Holter through a 12-lead ECG at the time of lead attachment. Others require the use of a "block," a conversion device available from the manufacturer, to connect the Holter to a 12-lead ECG for testing.

In the case example, despite the fact that the P-wave amplitude is small on the patient's 12-lead ECG (Fig. 84-2), fortunately the underlying rhythm turns out to be clearly identified as sinus on the eventual Holter (since the P wave is upright in lead II). Although this overall Holter is interpretable, on many of the selected rhythm strips, as predicted by the 12-lead, a sinus rhythm is harder to identify with certainty.

Other benefits of obtaining a baseline 12-lead ECG include accurate determination of intervals (PR, QRS, and QT), and a much better appreciation of the baseline ST segment. As a result, determination of ST-segment shifts (i.e., silent ischemia) is greatly facilitated. In this Holter example, all intervals are normal. There is some

BOX 84-1
Narrative Summary of Holter Recording

The patient was monitored for a period of 23:36 hours and minutes.

During this period the average heart rate was 75 bpm with a maximum heart rate of 160 bpm at 16:45 and a minimum heart rate of 36 bpm at 03:38.

There were 29 tachy episodes detected during the monitoring period.

These episodes ranged from 120 bpm to 160 bpm.

There were seven brady episodes detected during the monitoring period.

These episodes ranged from 36 bpm to 39 bpm.

There were 57 pause episodes detected during the monitoring period.

These episodes ranged from 2.14 sec to 3.29 sec.

There were 25 SVE episodes detected during the monitoring period.

The patient pressed the event button two times during the monitoring period.

There were no ST episodes detected during the monitoring period.

During the monitoring period there were 1151 abnormal beats detected.

There were two successive abnormal episodes detected during the monitoring period.

nonspecific ST-T wave flattening in the inferolateral leads, but no significant ST-segment depression and no acute changes.

Narrative Summary

Most Holters produce a narrative summary (Box 84-1) that consolidates the principal findings detected by the computer. Practically speaking, the main task of the interpreter is to verify that this computerized summary of pertinent findings is accurate.

In this case example, the narrative summary indicates a number of abnormal findings. The interpreter will certainly want to see representative samples of the following:

• Episodes of tachycardia (with a heart rate of up to 160 beats per minute)
• Episodes of bradycardia (with a heart rate between 36 to 39 beats per minute)
• Pauses (between 2.14 and 3.29 seconds in duration)
• Rhythm strips at the time the patient activated the event button (which occurred on two occasions)
• "Abnormal beats" (1151 were detected), including the two episodes of "successive abnormal episodes"

The clinician-interpreter does not need to find each of the 1151 abnormal beats. Nevertheless, he or she should verify that the beats are truly abnormal (not artifactual), whether the "abnormal" beats are truly PVCs, and whether these PVCs seem to be occurring frequently enough to explain the computer count. Practically speak-

ing, it matters little if there are 1151 abnormal beats or 1100 abnormal beats—or 800 or 500, for that matter—since the difference between 1151 and 800, or 500, is still well within the range for spontaneous variability. Clinically, it is unlikely that treatment would differ for a patient who has 1151 PVCs or 500 PVCs. In both situations, it is probably sufficient to say that there are "frequent" PVCs.

Remember: To evaluate any intervention, a reduction of at least 80% of the PVCs from one Holter to the next must be demonstrated to rule out the possibility of spontaneous variation. Therefore, in this particular case, the number of PVCs would have to be reduced from 1151 to *less than* 230 to eliminate this possibility.

Finally, this particular Holter system does not indicate whether the PVCs are uniform or multiform; it simply gives the sum of all "abnormal" beats. Once again, practically speaking, this really does not matter in view of the following facts:

• The prognostic implications of multiformity are not nearly as ominous as previously thought. Much more important than multiform PVCs are *repetitive* PVCs (e.g., couplets, salvos, and longer runs of VT).
• Almost all individuals with frequent ventricular ectopy over a 24-hour period demonstrate at least some degree of multiformity.

Trend Analysis of Abnormal Beats

The trend analysis of abnormal beats allows the interpreter, at a glance, to see what time of day PVC frequency peaks. In this case example, minimal ventricular ectopy occurs at night and maximal ectopy occurs during the daytime and evening hours (e.g., between noon and midnight) when the patient is active (Fig. 84-3).

Note: In the authors' experience, PVCs are most often distributed throughout the entire 24-hour period of monitoring. However, some patients manifest a distinct diurnal variation in which ventricular ectopy is minimal at night and peaks in the early morning hours (6 to 7 AM)—shortly before awakening. A second, less-well-defined peak is occasionally seen in the early evening hours.

Identifiable periods of peak ventricular ectopic activity may suggest a specific approach to treatment. For example, patients who manifest diurnal variation or increased ectopic activity during the hours of maximal daily activity often have an increase in sympathetic tone as part of their etiology. Therefore these patients are optimal candidates for beta-blocker therapy. Patients on antiarrhythmic therapy who demonstrate a peak in ectopic activity 6 to 10 hours after the last dose of their medication may benefit from an increased dosing frequency or by use of a sustained-release product.

Trend Analysis of Heart Rate and ST-Segment Level

The heart rate trend analysis demonstrates, at a glance, heart rate variations throughout the day. In this case example, it is easy to see that a tachycardia of approximately 150 beats per minute was sustained for most of the period between 16:00 and 17:00 (Fig. 84-4). The ST-level trend analysis shows that 1 mm of ST-segment depression was sustained throughout much of this same period *(arrow),* suggesting that the ST-segment depression is likely to be at least partially rate related.

The ST-level trend analysis may facilitate quantitative assessment of the type and duration of ST-segment depression in patients with silent ischemia.

Hourly Summary

Most Holter systems produce an hourly summary in some type of tabular format. Although it usually takes some time and practice to become familiar with this type of format, doing so tremendously facilitates interpretation. The hourly summary shows exactly where to look on the full-disclosure tracings to verify abnormal findings.

The hourly summary in this case example (Fig. 84-5) indicates the following:

- The lowest heart rate (36 beats per minute) was recorded between 03:00 and 04:00. The fastest heart rate (160 beats per minute) was recorded between 16:00 and 17:00. The greatest hourly frequency of PVCs, or "isolated abnormalities" (235) occurred, between 16:00 and 17:00.
- The event button was activated twice (once between 15:00 and 16:00, and once between 09:00 and 10:00).
- All 57 pause episodes (38 + 19) occurred between 19:00 and 21:00.

Selected (Full-Size) Rhythm Strips

Inspection of selected representative full-size rhythm strips is essential for verifying pertinent computer findings. Thus, in this case example, the patient had a 10-beat run of paroxysmal atrial fibrillation at 13:03:20 (Fig. 84-6). He was in a regular, presumably sinus rhythm of 80 beats per minute at 15:03:20 (Fig. 84-7). An ever-so-slightly irregular supraventricular tachycardia (rapid atrial fibrillation) is evident at 15:51:09 (Fig. 84-8). This strip was "patient activated," which means that the patient was symptomatic at that time and activated the event button to record the strip.

Another rhythm strip was automatically recorded at 15:55:53 (Fig. 84-9), presumably because of the rapid, irregular rhythm and associated ectopic activity. Finally, a rhythm strip is shown at 21:56:13 (Fig. 84-10) when the computer probably interpreted the tracing, mistakenly,

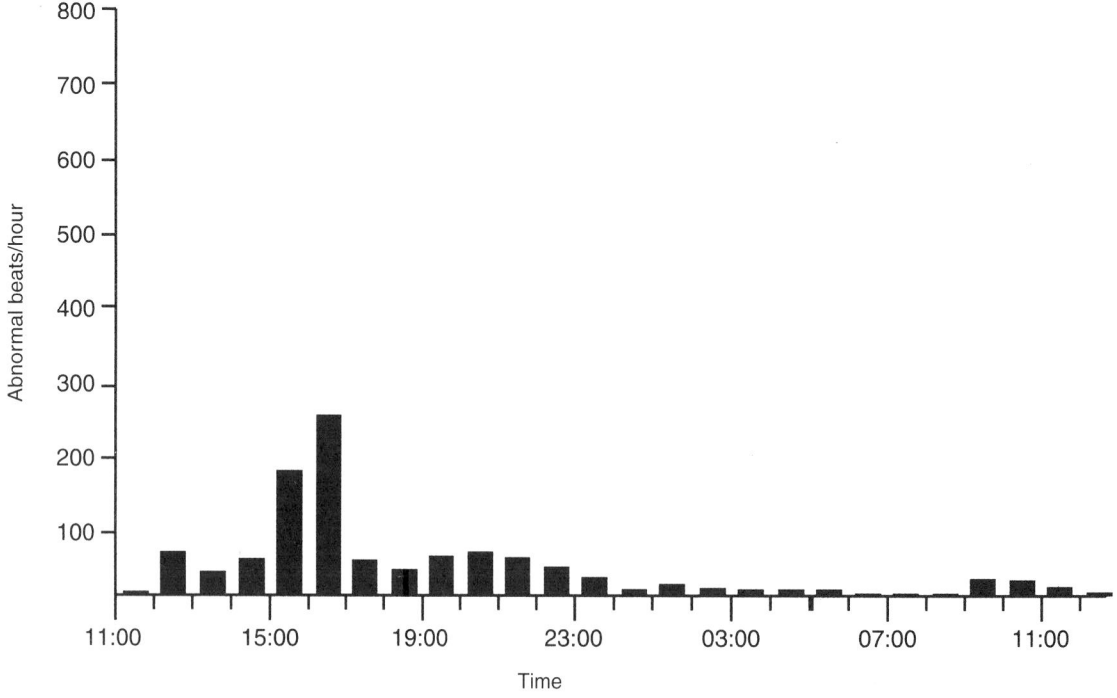

Fig. 84-3
Trend analysis of abnormal beats during 24-hour Holter monitoring.

as representing ventricular ectopic beats. Close inspection suggests that the baseline irregularity is really due to artifact.

Full-Disclosure Strips

Many states and carriers now require full (that is, 24-hour) disclosure as a prerequisite for maximal financial compensation. The obvious benefit of having this miniaturized recording of the entire 24 hours is to enable the interpreter to later review any or all events of the day. The interpreter can also print out a full-size rhythm strip of any abnormality not initially recognized by the computer. Interpretation of full-disclosure tracings probably seems like an overwhelming task to the uninitiated. This need not be the case.

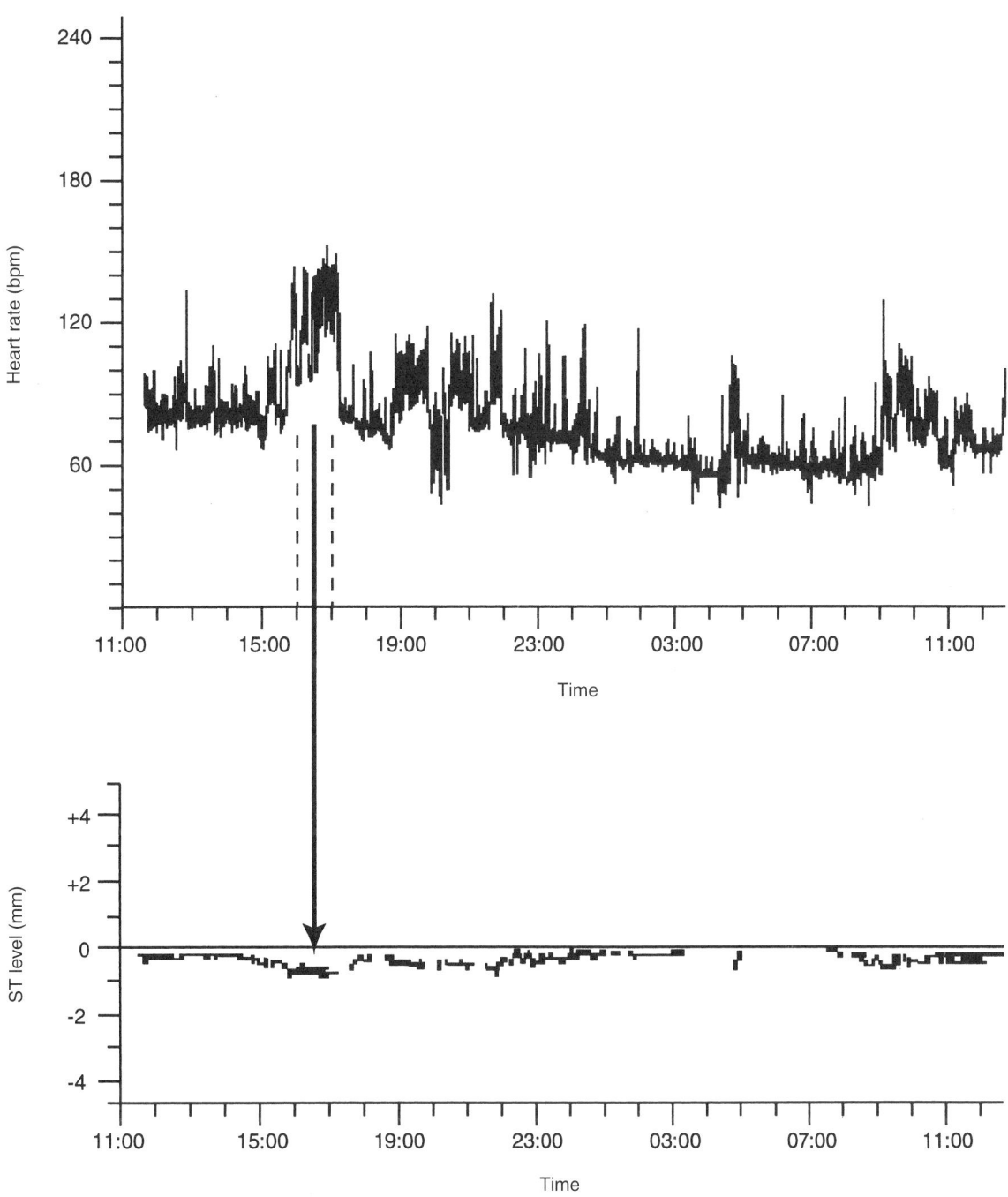

Fig. 84-4
Heart rate and ST trend analysis during Holter monitoring.

TIME	HEART RATE AVG	MAX	MIN	S/T LEV	SLP	TACHY EPS	BRADY EPS	PAUSE EPS	SVE	ISO ABN	COUP.	SUCC. ABN	PAT. EVENT
11:00	87	105	70	-0.4	-02	0	0	0	0	5	0	0	0
12:00	82	105	62	-0.4	-02	0	0	0	0	64	0	0	0
13:00	80	139	63	-0.4	-01	0	0	0	1	40	0	0	0
14:00	81	114	68	-0.4	-02	0	0	0	0	67	0	0	0
15:00	94	153	63	-0.8	-09	3	0	0	2	176	0	0	1
16:00	129	160	89	-1.0	-17	8	0	0	10	235	0	0	0
17:00	83	159	67	-0.4	-04	4	0	0	3	71	0	0	0
18:00	82	136	63	-0.2	-01	2	0	0	0	57	0	0	0
19:00	85	141	37	-0.4	-01	4	3	38	1	79	0	0	0
20:00	87	129	44	-0.4	-02	4	0	19	0	86	0	0	0
21:00	84	144	50	-0.4	-06	4	0	0	1	62	0	0	0
22:00	73	126	51	-0.2	-03	0	0	0	1	51	0	0	0
23:00	73	124	56	-0.2	-03	0	0	0	0	32	0	0	0
00:00	62	94	43	0.0	-04	0	0	0	0	9	0	0	0
01:00	61	122	53	0.0	-05	0	0	0	0	16	0	0	0
02:00	58	81	39	0.0	-04	0	1	0	2	9	0	0	0
03:00	58	110	36	0.0	-05	0	1	0	0	6	0	1	0
04:00	63	105	42	0.0	-03	0	0	0	0	7	0	1	0
05:00	58	91	50	0.0	-03	0	0	0	1	4	0	0	0
06:00	56	91	39	0.0	-03	0	1	0	0	3	0	0	0
07:00	56	99	38	0.0	-03	0	1	0	1	4	0	0	0
08:00	87	137	53	-0.4	-01	0	0	0	1	23	0	0	0
09:00	72	101	55	-0.2	-01	0	0	0	0	20	0	0	1
10:00	70	93	48	-0.2	-01	0	0	0	1	13	0	0	0
11:00	70	105	55	-0.2	-03	0	0	0	0	5	0	0	0
AVG	75			-0.2	-04	1	0	2	1	48	0	0	0
TOTAL						29	7	57	25	1144	0	2	2

Fig. 84-5
Hourly summary for 24-hour Holter study.

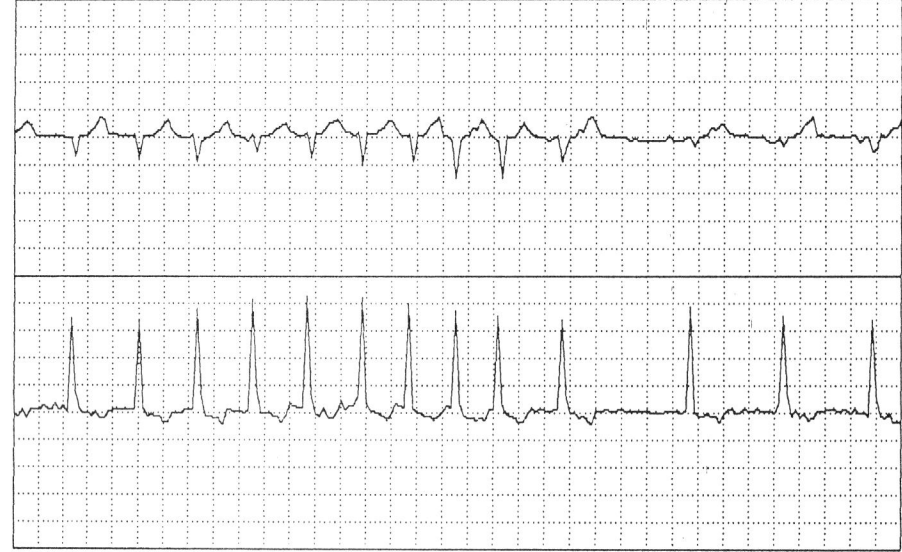

Fig. 84-6
Selected rhythm strip at 13:03:20.

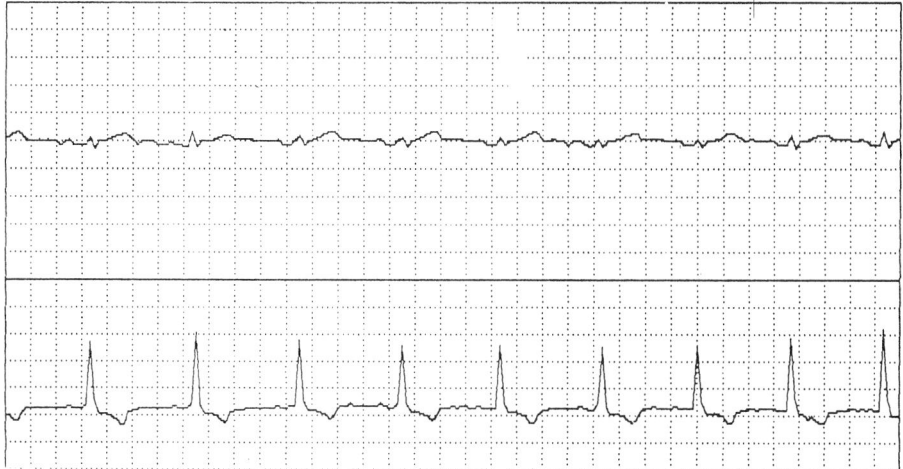

Fig. 84-7
Selected rhythm strip at 15:03:20.

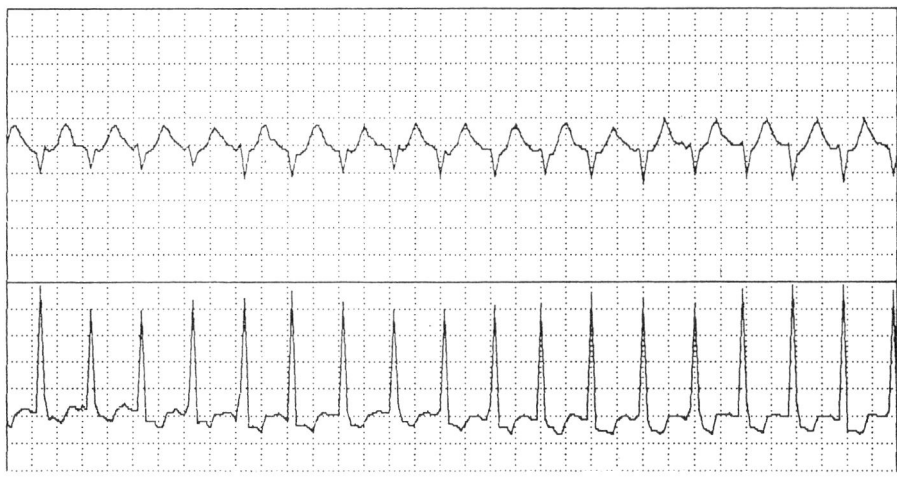

Fig. 84-8
Selected rhythm strip at 15:51:09.

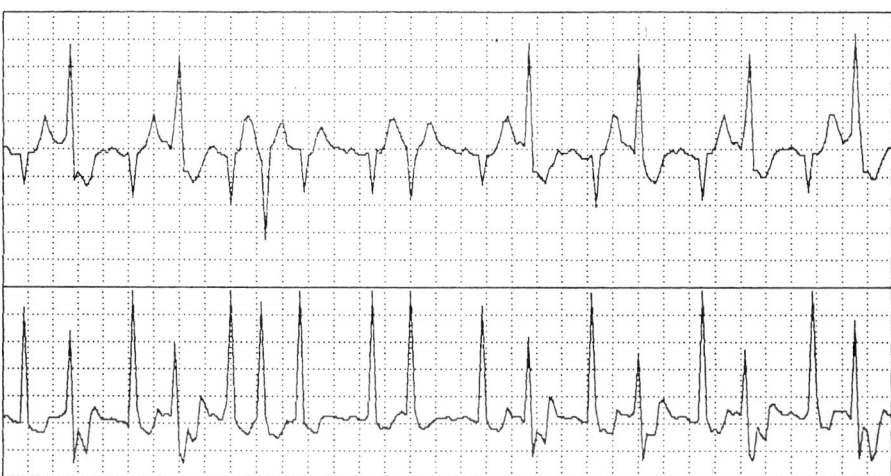

Fig. 84-9
Selected rhythm strip at 15:55:53.

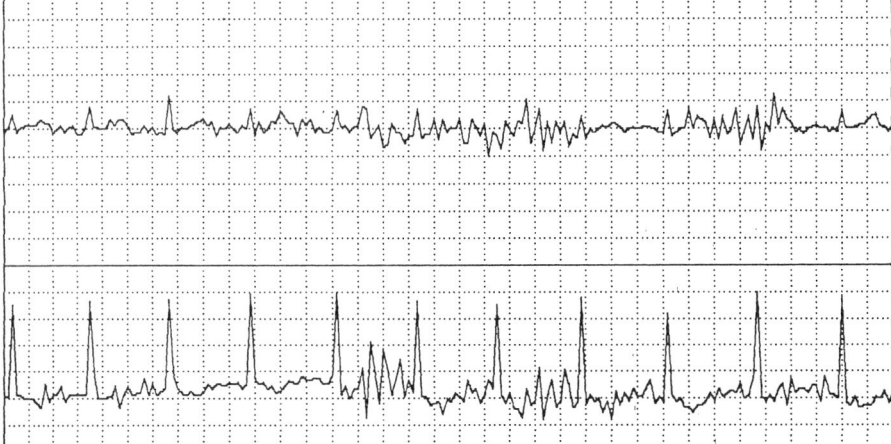

Fig. 84-10
Selected rhythm strip at 21:56:13.

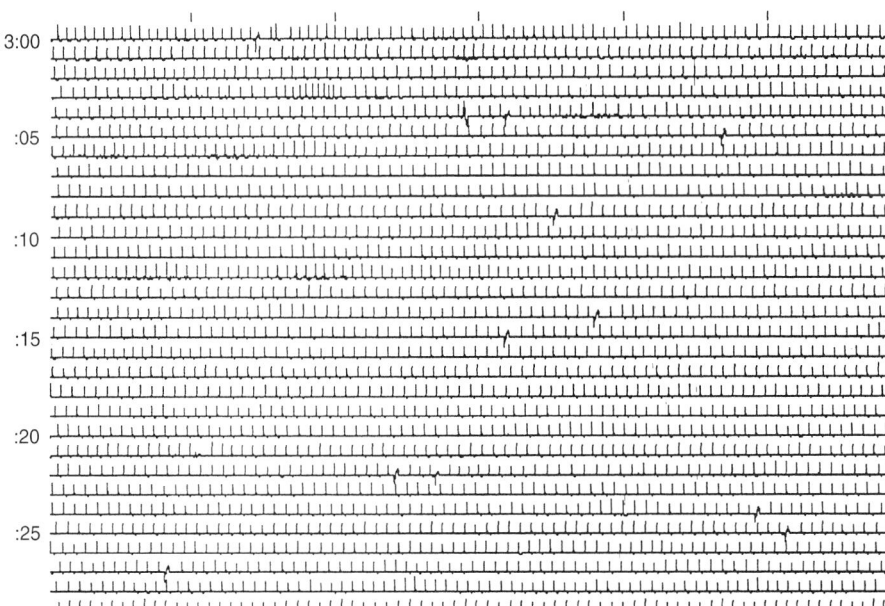

Fig. 84-11
Full-disclosure strip between 13:00 and 13:29.

For orientation to full-disclosure tracings, portions of three pages from the case example Holter are displayed. Normally, each page contains a miniaturized account of a full hour of Holter from a single monitoring lead. One minute of recording is represented by each of the 60 lines on the page. Because of space constraints for this chapter, only half of a page (30 minutes) is used for each demonstration. Thus the period from 13:00 to 13:29 is shown on Fig. 84-11; from 15:30 to 15:59 on Fig. 84-12; and from 16:00 to 16:29 on Fig. 84-13.

A scan of the first few lines of Fig. 84-11 shows how deceptively easy it is to identify the short run of supraventricular tachycardia that occurs between 13:03:10 and 13:03:20. (Fig. 84-6 demonstrates the full-size recording of this short burst of tachycardia.) Also note how easy it is to both spot the "different looking" (i.e., abnormal) beats, which are PVCs, and to

see that the baseline undulation on the 13:06 and 13:12 lines is likely due to artifact.

With practice, self-discipline, and diligent concentration, the interpreter should be able to rapidly scan each page (i.e., each hour of recording) in less than 10 seconds and still be able to identify most major abnormalities on the page.

Now look at Fig. 84-12. The selected full-size rhythm strips previously reviewed demonstrated rapid atrial fibrillation at 15:51:09 (Fig. 84-8) and rapid atrial fibrillation with frequent ventricular ectopy at 15:55:53 (Fig. 84-9). Find these arrhythmias on the full-disclosure tracing.

Once a particular abnormality has been seen on the miniaturized full-disclosure tracing, it becomes relatively easy to spot other episodes of that abnormality. Thus other short runs of frequent ventricular ectopy on lines

15:30

:35

:40

:45

:50

:55

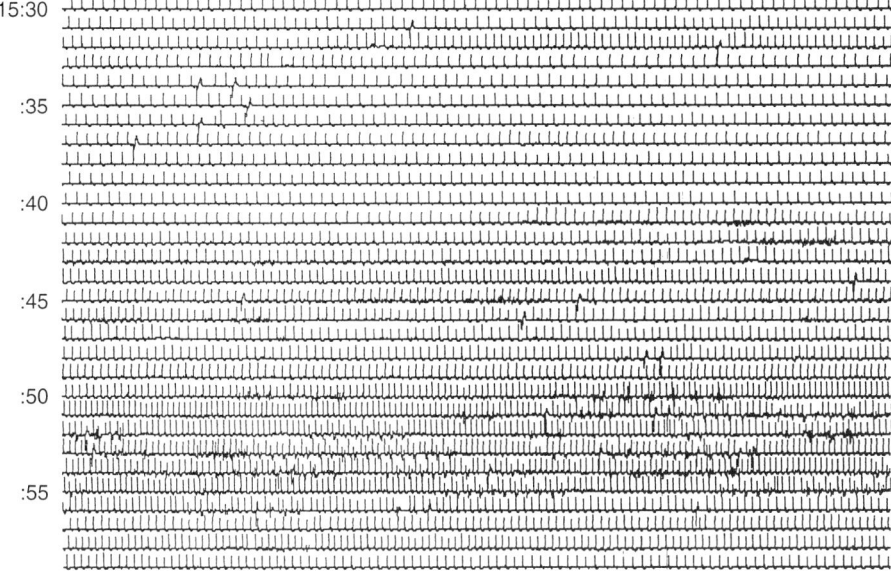

Fig. 84-12
Full-disclosure strip between 15:30 and
15:59.

16:00

:05

:10

:15

:20

:25

Fig. 84-13
Full-disclosure strip between 16:00 and
16:29.

15:52, 15:53, 15:54, and 15:56 are easily noticed. Finally, look at Fig. 84-13. Note how the patient has a sustained tachycardia for a substantial portion of this monitoring period. Actual-size rhythm strips reveal persistence of rapid atrial fibrillation during much of the hour.

INTERPRETATION OF CASE STUDY

This case study is an excellent example of how to use a Holter to determine the cause of a patient's symptoms. In this case, the patient's symptoms were not well defined; they included increasing dyspnea, weakness, and dizziness over the previous month. There were no palpitations, and apart from some nonspecific ST-T wave changes, the patient's baseline ECG was unremarkable. With this history, although most clinicians would include a cardiac arrhythmia in the differential diagnosis, other entities would merit equal attention. However, after combining the results of this Holter with the diary, there is little doubt as to the final diagnosis.

Final Interpretation

- Sinus rhythm with periods of sinus bradycardia down to 36 to 40 beats per minute
- Several episodes of rapid, paroxysmal atrial fibrillation lasting minutes, with heart rates up to 160 beats per minute
- Normal intervals

Holter Interpretation Form

Name of patient _____ Name of clinician _____ Date _____

Baseline ECG Interpretation _____

_____

PR interval _____ QRS duration _____ QTc: Normal ☐ Borderline ☐ Long ☐

Trend Analysis:

The heart rate varies from ____ to ____, with an average rate of ____/min.

ST Segment Shifts?   Yes ☐   *No significant ST segment shifts* ☐

ST elevation? ☐   ST depression? ☐ with Sx? ☐ without Sx? ☐

Estimated duration of ST segment depression over 24 hours _____.

Rhythm:

Selected strips show the rhythm to be _____.

Arrhythmias:

Number of **PVCs** *counted* by computer _____.

Probable *accuracy* of computer **PVCs count**

```
 |-------------|-------------|-------------|-------------|-------------|
 Poor                      Moderate                     Excellent
(PVCs are rare;                                    (Computer count
much artifact present)                            is probably accurate)
```

True **PVCs appear to be:** Common ☐ Occ ☐ Rare/absent ☐   Multiform? ☐

Number of ventricular couplets _____. Couplets are: Common ☐ Occ ☐ Rare/absent ☐

Number of runs of VT (≥ 3 PVCs) _____. VT runs are: Common ☐ Occ ☐ Rare/absent ☐

Number of **PACs/PJCs** counted by computer _____.

PACs/PJCs are: Common ☐ Occ ☐ Rare/absent ☐

Longest tachyarrhythmia (type) _____. *No significant tachyarrhythmias* ☐

Duration of run _____. Time _____ with Sx? ☐ without Sx? ☐

Longest bradyarrhythmia (type) _____. *No significant bradyarrhythmias* ☐

Duration of run _____. Time _____ with Sx? ☐ without Sx? ☐

Longest pause (type) _____. *No significant pauses* ☐

Number of pauses >2.0 sec _____ at _____. with Sx? ☐ without Sx? ☐

Continued

Fig. 84-14
Standardized interpretation form. (Modified from Grauer K, Leytem B: *Am Fam Physician* 45:1641, 1992.)

- No significant ST-segment shifts
- Frequent PVCs (1151 recorded), especially during the waking hours—but virtually no repetitive forms
- Diary indicates eight symptomatic episodes of weakness, dizziness, and dyspnea that correlate precisely with episodes of rapid, paroxysmal atrial fibrillation. These findings strongly suggest that the patient's symptoms are cardiac related (and should be treated)

Despite notation on the narrative summary of 57 pause episodes of up to 3.29 seconds, close inspection of full-disclosure tracings did not reveal any sustained pauses, suggesting that this count may reflect computer error.

Standard Interpretation Form

Use of a standardized form greatly facilitates the task of Holter interpretation. The two-sided form that the authors have developed (Fig. 84-14) organizes the key components of an ambulatory ECG study. In so doing, it not only saves time, but also ensures consistency in interpretation, provides clear documentation of findings, and facilitates the reporting of information in an easily understood, clinically relevant manner.

Several components of this form deserve special mention. Because artifact is often misread by the computer as ventricular ectopy, a boxed commentary (under "Arrhythmias") is included on the form to reflect

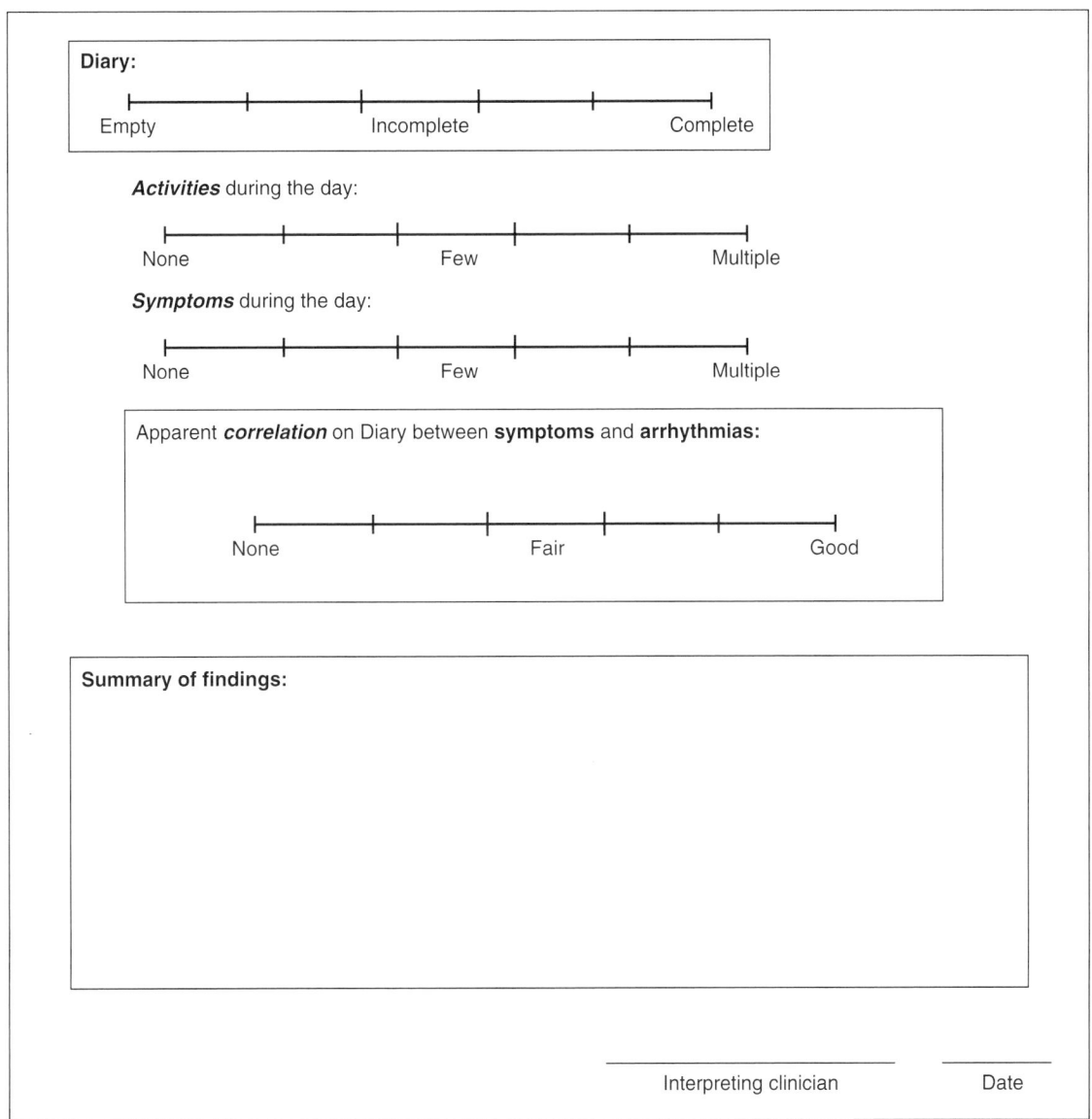

Fig. 84-14, cont'd

the interpreter's assessment of the computer's PVC count. The interpreter should indicate whether the count is likely to be accurate or a distortion produced by artifact. Rather than focusing exclusively on the number of ectopic beats, a greater emphasis is placed on whether the occurrence of premature atrial, junctional, and ventricular contractions (including couplets and runs of VT) is "common," "occasional," or "rare/absent."

Finally, it is occasionally difficult to convey the clinical relevance of a patient's diary, especially when attempting to correlate it with the ambulatory ECG recording. The relative scales on the back of the interpretation form help resolve this problem. They attempt to clarify the interpreter's assessment of the validity of the patient's diary and the correlation (if any) between patient symptoms and the arrhythmias that are noted.

SUPPLIERS

Del Mar Medical Systems
1621 Alton Parkway
Irvine, CA 92606-4878
Phone: 1-949-250-3200
Website: www.delmarmedical.com

Space Labs Burdick
500 Burdick Parkway
Deerfield, WI 53531
Phone: 1-800-777-1777
Website: www.burdick.com

Philips Medical Systems
Cardiac and Monitoring Systems Headquarters
3000 Minuteman Road
Andover, MA 01810
Phone: 1-800-934-7372
Website: www.medical.philips.com

Note: The editors recommend a Holter system from a company with a proven track record. Many companies have come and gone over the years. Often, the companies with a proven track record also produce equipment for other procedures, such as exercise testing. Choosing such a company may simplify service contracts.

CPT/BILLING CODES

93224   Electrocardiographic monitoring for 24 hours by continuous original ECG waveform recording and storage, with visual superimposition scanning; includes recording, scanning analysis with report, physician review, and interpretation
93225   Recording (includes hook-up, recording, and disconnection)
93226   Scanning analysis with report
93227   Physician review and interpretation
93230   Electrocardiographic monitoring for 24 hours by continuous original ECG waveform recording and storage, without superimposition scanning using a device capable of producing a full miniaturized printout; includes recording, microprocessor-based analysis with report, physician review, and interpretation
93235   Electrocardiographic monitoring for 24 hours by continuous computerized monitoring and noncontinuous recording, and real-time data analysis using a device capable of producing intermittent full-size waveform tracings, possibly patient activated; includes monitoring and real-time data analysis with report, physician review, and interpretation
93268   Patient demand single or multiple event recording with presymptom memory loop, per 30-day period; includes transmission, physician review, and interpretation

BIBLIOGRAPHY

Bigger JT, Coromilas J: Identification of patients at risk for arrhythmic death: role of Holter ECG recording, *Cardiovasc Clin* 15:131, 1985.
Brodsky M, Wu D, Denes P, et al: Arrhythmias documented by 24-hour continuous electrocardiographic monitoring in 50 male medical students without apparent heart disease, *Am J Cardiol* 39:390, 1977.
The Cardiac Arrhythmia Suppression Trial (CAST) Investigators: Preliminary report: effect of encainide or flecainide in a randomized trial of arrhythmia suppression after myocardial infarction, *N Engl J Med* 321:406, 1989.
Conti CR, Geller NL, Knatterud GL, et al: Anginal status and prediction of cardiac events in patients enrolled in the asymptomatic cardiac ischemia pilot (ACIP) study: ACIP investigators, *Am J Cardiol* 79:889, 1997.
Grauer K: Silent myocardial ischemia: dilemma or blessing? *Am Fam Physician* 42(suppl):13S, 1990.
Grauer K, Cavallaro D: *ACLS: certification preparation,* vol I, ed 3, St Louis, 1993, Mosby.
Grauer K, Leytem B: A systematic approach to Holter monitor interpretation, *Am Fam Physician* 45:1641, 1992.
Hatch R, Grauer K, Gums J: Cardiac arrhythmias. In Taylor RB, editor: *Family medicine: principles and practice,* ed 4, New York, 1993, Springer-Verlag.
Kennedy HL, Whitlock JA, Sprague MK, et al: Long-term follow-up of asymptomatic healthy subjects with frequent and complex ventricular ectopy, *N Engl J Med* 312:193, 1985.
Kinlay S, Leitch JW, Neil A, et al: Cardiac event recorders yield more diagnoses and are more cost-effective than 48-hour Holter monitoring in patients with palpitations: a controlled clinical trial, *Ann Intern Med* 124:16, 1996.
Morganroth J, Michelson EL, Horowitz LN, et al: Limitations of routine long-term electrocardiographic monitoring to assess ventricular ectopic frequency, *Circulation* 58:404, 1978.
Nabel EG, Barry J, Rocco MB, et al: Variability of transient myocardial ischemia in ambulatory patients with coronary artery disease, *Circulation* 78:60, 1988.
Weber B, Kapoor W: Evaluation and outcomes of patients with palpitations, *Am J Med* 100:138, 1996.
Winkle RA, Peters F, Hall R: Characterization of ventricular tachyarrhythmias on ambulatory ECG recordings in post-myocardial infarction patients: arrhythmia detection and duration of recording, relationship between arrhythmia frequency and complexity, and day-to-day reproducibility, *Am Heart J* 102:162, 1981.

SUGGESTED READING ON ELECTROCARDIOGRAPHIC INTERPRETATION AND CARDIAC ARRYTHMIAS

Grauer K, Cavallaro D: *Arrhythmia interpretation,* St Louis, 1997, Mosby.
Grauer K: *12-Lead ECGs: a "pocket brain" for easy interpretation,* Gainesville, Fla, 1998, KG/EKG Press.
Grauer K: *A practical guide to ECG interpretation,* St Louis, 1998, Mosby.

CHAPTER 85

Noninvasive Venous and Arterial Studies of the Lower Extremities

Grant C. Fowler

The accuracy of noninvasive vascular studies is *very* dependent on the skills of the operator and the interpreter, and somewhat on the quality of the equipment. However, with state-of-the-art equipment and clinician confidence, some vascular surgeons perform arterial surgery without preoperative arteriography, and clinicians may initiate anticoagulation therapy on the basis of unequivocal noninvasive venous studies alone.

The literature has clearly demonstrated the accuracy and benefit of plain ultrasound scanning, or duplex scanning if it is available, in the emergency department. This is often performed by emergency medicine clinicians to exclude deep venous thrombosis (DVT). As a result, ultrasound has basically become the standard of care for excluding DVT in emergency departments at larger hospitals (see Chapter 209, Emergency Department and Office Ultrasound). As more emergency medicine clinicians become comfortable with duplex scanning, there is little doubt that their use of duplex scanning will be extended into arterial and other studies.

In the remainder of the hospital or in vascular laboratories, during normal working hours, duplex or color Doppler ultrasound has basically become the standard for evaluation of lower extremity arteries and veins. This has especially been noted since the publication of the first edition of this textbook. Not only have older noninvasive techniques been replaced, but newer noninvasive studies have essentially replaced contrast venography, and in many cases preoperative arteriography. Therefore the risk of complications from contrast dye has been decreased. However, it should also be noted that most vascular labs continue to use older noninvasive techniques because duplex or color Doppler ultrasound is not always available. Most centers can only afford one or two units, and they are often busy. In many settings the cost of equipment for even one duplex or color Doppler ultrasound unit is prohibitive. As a result, older alternative techniques are included in this chapter for those locations and for the office setting of primary care clinicians with this equipment. Despite not being as "high-tech," the data obtained may be very useful clinically. Older, alternative techniques may yet see a further resurgence in popularity because they are very cost-effective, less operator dependent, and often available at all hours. In fact, they may find permanent use as a preliminary screening test to determine who should undergo Doppler testing.

Regarding venous studies, an *algorithm* (Barloon and Bergus, 1997; Wells et al, 1995) has been developed and studied for accuracy using plain ultrasound: (1) symptomatic patients with an abnormal study can be treated without any further testing, (2) if the patient has a low pretest probability of DVT (Box 85-1) and the study is negative, no further testing is required, or (3) if the patient has a negative study, yet a moderate or high pretest probability of DVT, ultrasound or duplex scanning should be used. This algorithm provides a safe and cost-effective manner of excluding DVT. The evidence (Kearon et al, 1998) indicates that impedance plethysmography (IPG) can be used in the same manner, especially for the diagnosis of a first symptomatic proximal DVT.

BOX 85-1

Probability of Deep Venous Thrombosis (DVT) Based on Clinical Predictors (see Box 85-2)

High Probability (85%)
Has no alternative diagnosis with three or more major factors or two or more major factors and two or more minor factors

Medium Probability (33%)
Includes all patients without a high or low probability of DVT

Low Probability (5%)
Has no alternative diagnosis with one major factor and one or no minor factors, or no major factors and two or fewer minor factors
Has alternative diagnosis with one major factor and two or fewer minor factors or no major factors and three or fewer minor factors

Adapted from Wells PS, Hirsch J, Anderson DR, et al: *Lancet* 345:1326, 1995.

NONINVASIVE VENOUS STUDIES

Each year in the United States, approximately 200,000 patients die as a result of a pulmonary embolus. DVT can be found in about 80% of patients with a pulmonary embolus. The incidence of DVT increases with age and is more common in women than men. One third to half of patients over 40 years of age experiencing an acute myocardial infarction, a hip fracture, major surgery (especially orthopedic, pelvic, or urologic), or a stroke develop venous thrombi. For traditional risk factors in hospitalized patients, see Box 85-3. Lower limb DVT affects 1% to 2% of hospitalized patients. In addition, as a result of previous DVT, the prevalence of postphlebitic sequelae in the adult population has been estimated to be 5%.

Early diagnosis of DVT is important to minimize long-term complications, such as venous stasis or ulceration from chronic venous insufficiency. Accurate diagnosis is also crucial for limiting anticoagulation therapy to those who need it, thereby minimizing risk. Venous thrombi arise at bifurcations and in valve cusps (Fig. 85-1). The aging thrombus adheres to the vein wall, and nearby valves can be damaged or destroyed. The two most important valves for controlling venous hydrostatic pressure are the valve of the proximal superficial femoral vein and the valve of the distal popliteal vein. Destruction of those valves is more likely to lead to sequelae. Hopefully diagnosis of DVT can be made before the thrombus becomes extensive and causes permanent damage to valves.

Clinical diagnosis of acute DVT, without the benefit of radiographic or noninvasive techniques, has been reported for years to have an accuracy rate of only about 50%. However, this accuracy rate was probably underestimated because it was based upon older studies per-

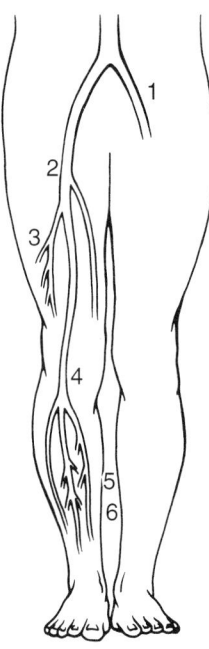

Fig. 85-1
Six most common sites of deep venous thrombosis in the lower body. *1,* Left iliac vein; *2,* common femoral vein; *3,* termination of deep femoral vein; *4,* popliteal vein at adductor canal; *5,* posterior tibial vein; *6,* intramuscular veins of calf.

formed on seriously ill, hospitalized patients. Recent data are helpful, especially when determining clinical probability of DVT in ambulatory patients (Boxes 85-1 and 85-2). These data should be combined with further diagnostic studies or the previously mentioned algorithm to confirm or exclude DVT.

In the attempt to diagnose DVT, various techniques are available. Although both invasive and noninvasive techniques are available, only noninvasive methods are covered in the "Technique" section.

1. *Contrast venography* is regarded as the "gold standard" for diagnosis of DVT; however, it is not without its own risks—including allergic reactions, congestive heart failure, acute renal insufficiency, and postvenography syndrome. (Between 10% and 20% of patients experience transient discomfort in the calf for 24 to 48 hours after contrast venography; most cases resolve without treatment, but some may progress to actual DVT.) In addition, venography is not easily repeated, and it is usually only performed in one limb. Venography may be impossible to perform in those patients with poor venous access, especially obese patients and those with severe edema or cellulitis. It may also be difficult to perform in urgent situations without proper support staff. Furthermore, contrast venography cannot be performed in 20% to 25% of patients because of previous thrombosis. For these reasons, as well as the fact that they have become more readily available, color Doppler or duplex ultrasonography has basically replaced contrast venography.

2. *Electrical IPG* was previously the most extensively studied and commonly used noninvasive technique. It remains the least expensive and least operator-dependent alternative to venography. IPG provides a functional evaluation of the venous system for outflow obstruction. High false-positive rates are found with obesity, congestive heart failure, external venous compression (e.g., gravid uterus in pregnancy), and chronic DVT. It is inaccurate in the diagnosis of thrombi in calf veins (rarely of clinical significance), profunda femoris, or internal iliac veins. IPG is also limited for diagnosing postoperative asymptomatic DVT nonocclusive thrombi, diagnosing clots in paired veins, or determining the progression of disease or clot lysis. For these reasons, duplex or color Doppler imaging has mostly replaced IPG.

3. *Standard or plain ultrasound imaging (hi-frequency, B-mode, real-time)* may also have limitations with obese and asymptomatic postoperative patients. Ultrasound's ability to visualize the venous system above the inguinal ligament (the iliac veins) or distal to the popliteal vein is also limited. However, if venography is not being used, ultrasound is the primary technique for scanning for DVT. Since it is less operator dependent than duplex scanning, ultrasound is also the most common technique used in large urgent-emergent care settings and after hours. However, since this is a less expensive technique, it may have a resurgence. In fact, most centers have only one Doppler or duplex ultrasound machine, and with the algorithm noted in the beginning of this chapter, plain ultrasound may be used in certain patients as a screen to determine whether or not Doppler is needed. It may also provide useful data when the Doppler ultrasound is not available. This algorithm shows that, although approximately 10% of isolated calf DVT will be missed, calf DVT by itself is not life threatening and may even be of questionable clinical significance. Benefits of this technique include the ability to actually visualize the veins, valves, and thrombus. Compressibility of the vein, normal valve motion, and absence of visualized thrombi may help exclude the possibility of DVT. Standard ultrasound may be necessary in special cases in which (other than obesity) IPG has unclear results or limitations. Standard ultrasound is also usually used to locate veins and scan them briefly before duplex scanning.

4. *Duplex scanning* is the combination of velocity measurements by Doppler technology and ultrasound imaging. Studies have shown that color enhancement of the Doppler velocities improves accuracy, especially in smaller vessels. Duplex scanning may be used to confirm findings from standard ultrasound imaging. IPG combined with duplex studies yields results essentially as accurate as venography.

5. *Plain Doppler* (handheld or with recorded velocities, without images) may also add information to IPG studies. In particular, plain Doppler can add information about the calf veins. Handheld Doppler was included in the protocols of many of the original noninvasive venous studies.

6. *Radionuclide scintigraphy or magnetic resonance imaging* may be useful in selected patients. Scintigraphy uses radio-labeled albumin or tagged red blood cells as the contrast for venography. However, it may be unreliable in the calf and not helpful in those with previous DVT. Radio-labeled autologous platelets or peptides can also be used to detect active thrombus formation. These techniques may be helpful in symptomatic patients with a previous history of DVT. MRI is particularly useful in the diagnosis of pelvic and calf vein DVT. However, MRI is highly operator dependent, expensive, and not always available in urgent situations. It should probably be reserved for cases in which scintigraphy is contraindicated. Both radionuclide scintigraphy and magnetic resonance imaging are beyond the scope of this textbook.

7. D-*dimer* testing is complementary to ultrasound and IPG, especially in symptomatic patients with a suspected first episode of DVT.

INDICATIONS

Nongravid

- Verification of clinically suspected acute DVT. (This may require serial studies if calf thrombosis is suspected, and especially if IPG or plain ultrasound imaging is the diagnostic study used. Neither of these techniques is highly sensitive for calf thrombosis, and serial studies are recommended to monitor for more proximal progression of a thrombus.)

- Diagnosis of recurrent DVT.
- Evaluation before discontinuation of anticoagulation for DVT. (The IPG should be repeated every 4 to 6 weeks after discharge from the hospital until the results return to normal.)
- Venous evaluation of patient with pulmonary embolism.
- Preoperative study before saphenous vein stripping.
- Preoperative study before venous sclerotherapy.
- Venous insufficiency.

Gravid

- Gravid patients with superficial venous thrombosis should be evaluated thoroughly because up to 17% will also have DVT. DVT in a gravid patient places them at very high risk of pulmonary thromboembolism. (One review of maternal deaths revealed that pulmonary embolism was the second leading cause of death.)

Considerations

- Unilateral or unexplained edema of the lower extremity
- Screening of certain groups of high-risk patients (e.g., postoperative, especially with multiple risk factors [Box 85-2])

ELECTRICAL IMPEDANCE PLETHYSMOGRAPHY

Various plethysmography techniques are available to study a change in physical function as a result of a change in volume (e.g., strain gauge, air, and IPG). Electrical IPG records the impedance (the inverse of conductivity) of the lower extremity as the blood volume varies. When venous return is restricted in the lower extremity by a cuff, venous volume in the lower extremity increases. Because blood is a good conductor of electricity, conductivity in the lower extremity also increases (i.e., resistance or impedance decreases). This is evaluated by administering a weak electrical current that is imperceptible to the patient, and then measuring the current's strength after it passes through the area. When the cuff is released, conductivity should rapidly decrease if the deep venous system is patent. In patients with a thrombus, the rate of change of electrical conductivity is reduced, especially if the thrombus is in the popliteal or more proximal vein. IPG has been proved to be safe, painless, reliable, and

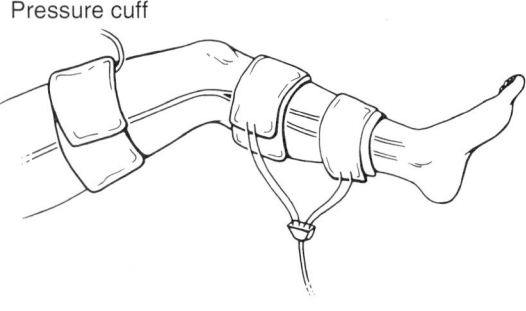

Pressure cuff

Area measured

Fig. 85-2
For impedance plethysmography testing, elevate the leg 25 to 30 degrees. Apply electrodes around the calf, and place a pressure cuff around the thigh.

cost-effective (cost to the patient is about the same as an ECG, usually $50 to $100). With proper patient selection (Box 85-1), accuracy approaches 98% for detection of proximal DVT, and treatment decisions can be based on unequivocal IPG studies alone.

Relative Contraindications

- Significant pain or the inability to relax (may result in false-positive results).
- Patients with any potential risk of false-positive test results (e.g., patients with congestive heart failure, external vein occlusion [including that resulting from pregnancy], obesity, or chronic DVT). In these patients, the risk of a false-positive result and initiation of anticoagulation should be weighed against the risks of waiting for the availability of other venous studies.
- Patients who are unable to remain supine, such as those with severe orthopnea.

Personnel and Equipment

- A clinician or technician trained to perform and record IPG
- A clinician trained to interpret IPG
- IPG recorder
- Appropriate 8-inch cuff and electrodes

Technique

1. Place the patient in the supine position, with the leg to be examined elevated 25 to 30 degrees (Fig. 85-2). This can be accomplished by placing a pillow under the calf and heel. All tight garments should be removed, and the leg to be studied should be well exposed. To relax the patient, the leg is allowed to rotate externally at the hip. The knee is slightly flexed—10 to 20 degrees—to prevent compression of the popliteal vein.

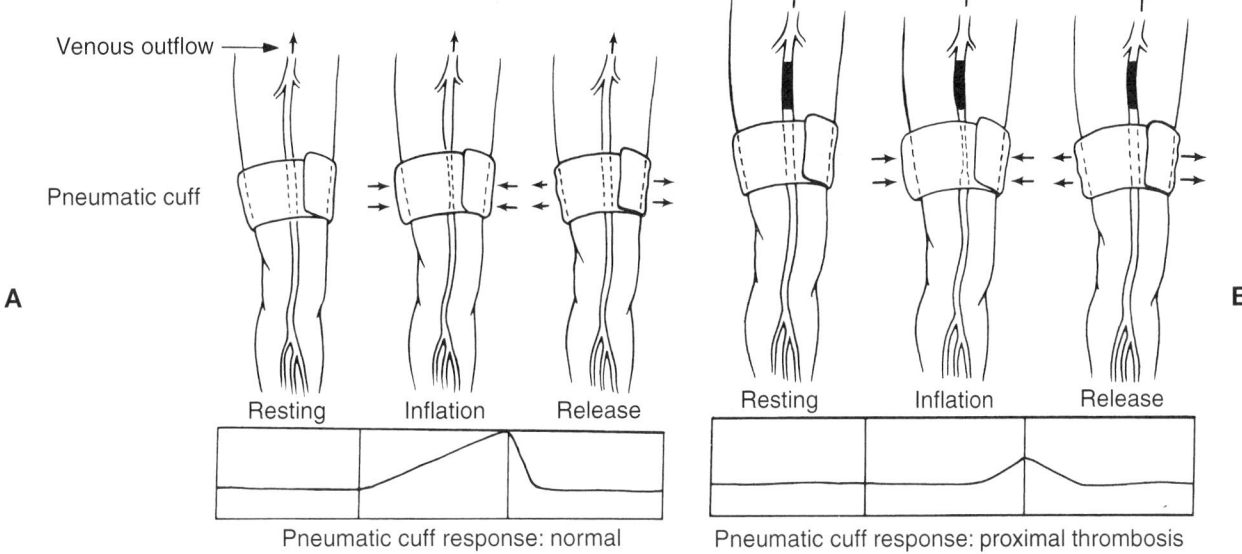

Fig. 85-3
A, Normal and, **B,** abnormal impedance plethysmography tracings.

2. Place an 8-inch-wide pneumatic cuff around the thigh, and place electrodes circumferentially around the calf.
3. After the instrument has been electrically balanced and a stable baseline has been obtained, inflate the cuff to the manufacturer's specifications, which is usually 50 mm Hg. This blocks the venous outflow but does not impair arterial inflow.
4. After the cuff has been inflated for 2 minutes, and the pressure tracing has reached a stable plateau, suddenly release the pressure in the compression cuff.
5. The total rise of the IPG tracing during cuff occlusion and the fall during the first 3 seconds of deflation is now plotted on a two-way graph (Fig. 85-3 shows normal and abnormal IPG tracings, and Fig. 85-4 shows plotting).

Interpretation and Sources of Error

Overall, the major shortcoming of IPG is a false-positive rate of approximately 5%. Sensitivity increases in the symptomatic patient and is slightly reduced during evaluation for silent proximal thrombosis, such as with postoperative screening. The error rate can be minimized by a clinician with experience who takes into consideration the following factors:

• Positive predictive accuracy is improved for those with a high pretest likelihood of DVT (Box 85-1).
• If the first result falls below the discriminant line, it is not necessarily abnormal. With repeated testing, the values may fall above the discriminant line, where they are considered normal. In the presence of true outflow

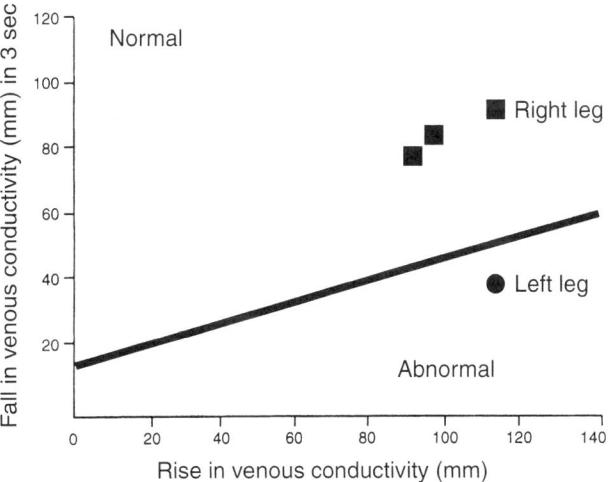

Fig. 85-4
Typical result of impedance plethysmography. This reading suggests deep venous obstruction in the left leg, with normal venous function in the right leg.

obstruction, the result remains fixed. To improve the accuracy of IPG, a five-test sequence can be used with occlusion times of 45, 45, 120, 45, and 120 seconds.
• The closer the result falls to the discriminant line on either side, the more likely that it is abnormal. Such test results (close to the line) should be confirmed with either venography or duplex scanning.
• Some references suggest that if abnormal results are found with both lower extremities, they are likely false-positive results; therefore the patient should be evaluated further with another technique.

- Excessive tightness of the cuff, particularly in obese patients, may cause tension on the skin during cuff occlusion and thus a false-positive result.
- Patients who are unable to relax (such as those who are apprehensive or in pain) may impede venous return with involuntary muscle restriction, which may lead to a false-positive test.
- A full bladder, particularly in the elderly patient, may cause muscle tension.
- False-positive results may be seen from extrinsic compression in patients with popliteal cysts or masses and in patients with elevated central venous pressure (e.g., congestive heart failure).
- Any systemic disease limiting arterial inflow or venous outflow will interfere with results.

ULTRASOUND IMAGING

Real-time, B-mode sonography in the higher frequency ranges (5 to 10 MHz) allows direct "visualization" (imaging) of the venous system, and it allows the technician or clinician to search for a thrombus. Sound waves are best transmitted in fluid; therefore large veins and arteries are easily visualized with the proper probe and adequate acoustic gel interface. Arteries are differentiated from veins by their thicker walls and pulsatile nature. They are also not as easily compressible when pressure is applied on the leg with the probe. In addition,

arteries do not engorge with a Valsalva maneuver or vary with respiration.

In some situations, such as after 5 PM in certain emergency departments, ultrasound may be the only diagnostic modality available. Studies of such situations have indicated that accuracy of diagnosis of DVT by ultrasound approaches the accuracy of venography. In many cases, the ultrasound scanning was performed by the emergency medicine clinicians themselves.

Personnel and Equipment

- A clinician or technician familiar with venous anatomy (Fig. 85-5) as well as ultrasound technology
- 5- to 10-MHz probe (transducer) and scanner
- Acoustic gel

Technique

1. Place the patient in the supine position with the lower extremities lowered about 20 or 30 degrees (reverse Trendelenburg), slightly separated and externally rotated. This position increases the fluid volume in the veins and facilitates scanning. The patient should be relaxed and comfortable to avoid venous compression by tense muscles.
2. Apply ample acoustic gel. With the probe perpendicular to the vessel and beginning at the groin, scan the common femoral and superficial femoral veins distally

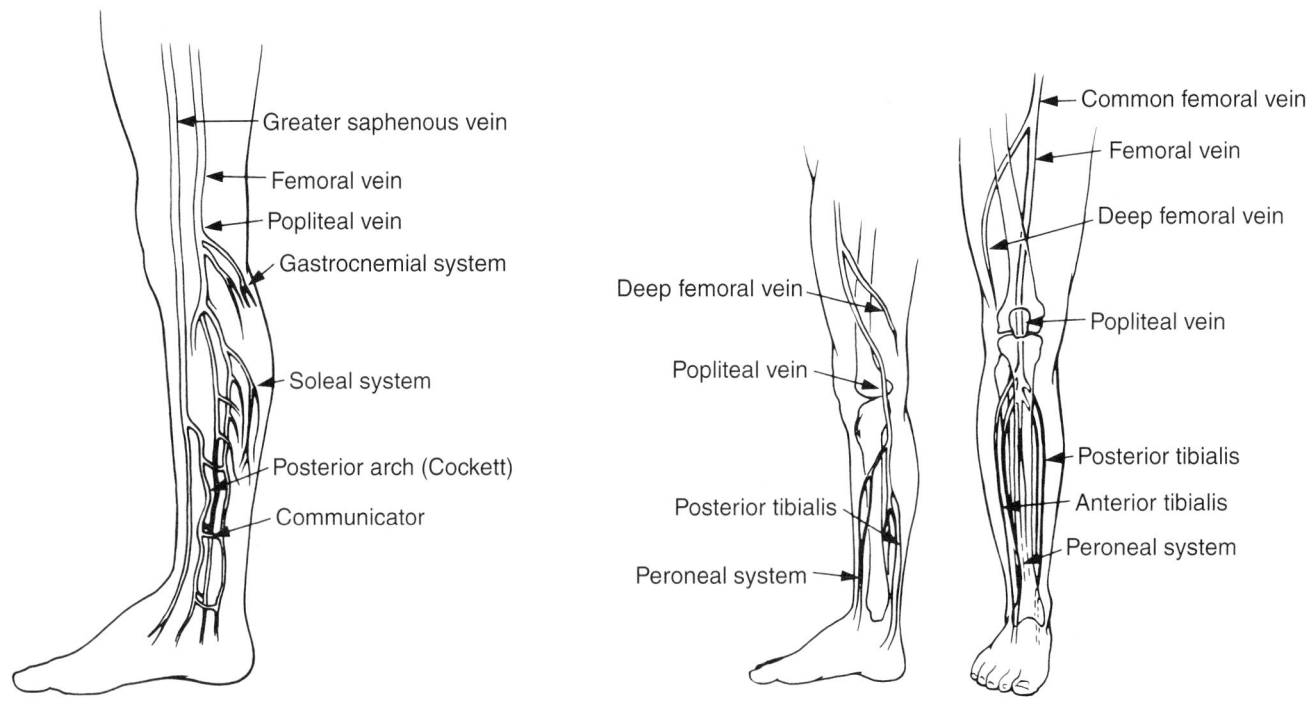

Fig. 85-5
Venous system of the lower extremity.

in the longitudinal and transverse dimensions. Longitudinal scanning is usually used to localize the vein, and transverse scanning is used to check compressibility. Having the patient perform a Valsalva usually expands the veins, enhancing visualization as distal as the popliteal veins. *Echogenic* matter (which appears white) within the vessels should be studied carefully to exclude a possible thrombus. Presence or absence of thrombus should be recorded. Partially obstructing thrombi may be confused with scarred, thickened venous walls; therefore it is important to record and comment about wall thickness.

3. If no thrombus is visualized, turn the probe transversely and apply gentle pressure in order to compress the vessel walls. If the vessel walls are not compressible, an early thrombus may be preventing compression, but it may not have become organized or dense enough to be visualized. Compressibility of the vessel walls should be recorded. Compressibility alone was the diagnostic criterion used for the prospective study for the Wells and Barloon algorithm.

4. Proceed distally and continue scanning vessels in the longitudinal and transverse dimensions to the medial thigh. Fascial planes at the adductor hiatus may obscure visualization of the superficial femoral vein at that level.

5. Scan the popliteal vein either with the patient in this position or by rotating the patient to a prone position with the knees flexed 20 or 30 degrees. A pillow placed under the feet may facilitate this position while enhancing patient comfort.

6. In about 30% of patients, infrapopliteal vessels can be scanned, with the anterior and posterior tibial veins visualized more easily than peroneal veins.

7. Valve thickness and motion should be recorded when observed.

8. Vein response to Valsalva's maneuver and deep inspiration should be recorded at the level of the common femoral, superficial femoral, and popliteal veins.

Interpretation

• Visualization of an intraluminal thrombus is diagnostic. A thrombus is usually white or echogenic. This is further confirmed when the Valsalva's maneuver produces minimal changes in vein diameter and when the vessel wall is incompressible. Early studies indicate that these diagnostic criteria are superior to all other techniques, except venography, for diagnosing DVT. In a symptomatic patient, treatment (anticoagulation) can be initiated with the visualization of a thrombus alone. Ultrasonography is also a superior diagnostic technique for screening for silent DVT, which is occasionally seen in the postoperative patient. Again, absence of a visible thrombus does not completely rule out the presence of a *new* (acute) thrombus, which may have the same density as flowing blood. Before treatment is withheld, other indirect signs or Doppler studies should be used in suspicious cases in which a thrombus is not visualized.

• A *possible positive* study is one in which the veins are incompressible or do not distend with Valsalva's maneuver. Consider duplex scanning for confirmation if a thrombus is not visualized by ultrasonography. The accuracy and outcomes of duplex scanning have been studied extensively, producing diagnostic results similar to venography in cases in which a thrombus is not visualized.

• Occasionally, an acute thrombus can be differentiated from a chronic thrombus. Acute thrombi have a homogenous texture, can be free floating, and are somewhat compressible. They often lead to distal dilation of the vein. Chronic thrombi usually are not compressible, have heterogeneous echogenicity, and are firmly attached to the walls with a normal-sized or slightly contracted distal vessel.

• Increased wall thickness can be due to previous or chronic DVT or to a partially obstructing thrombus. All of these possibilities should be strongly considered in a symptomatic patient, since all of these scenarios also place the patient at risk for DVT.

• At least one published study indicates safety in withholding treatment with a completely negative ultrasound study. This result should be weighed against the availability of duplex scanning.

DUPLEX SCANNING

Duplex scanning adds another parameter—venous blood velocity—to the data obtained from a routine ultrasound study. With duplex scanning, Doppler technology is incorporated into the probe of an ultrasound scanner. Duplex scanning is accurate and reproducible, and compared with venography, the sensitivity and specificity for DVT are more than 90%. Both the positive and negative predictive values, or the ability to predict the presence or absence of DVT, are in the 90% to 95% range. The drawbacks to duplex scanning include its cost to the patient (averaging $300 to $600 per study), the cost and nonportability of equipment, the time required for a complete examination, and the experience required for the technician and clinician to perform and interpret the study. In many centers, it is not available at all hours or in urgent situations. As with ultrasound, the ability to study the venous system above the inguinal ligament, and occasionally the superficial femoral and tibial veins at the adductor hiatus, is poor compared with IPG.

Normal venous physiology provides spontaneous

blood return to the heart, which can be heard in the area of the vein with a handheld auditory Doppler or can be recorded with a Doppler velocity instrument. This spontaneous flow should be phasic (i.e., vary with respirations) and decrease with a Valsalva maneuver. In addition, compression of the limb distal to the probe should augment the flow toward the heart.

Duplex scanning has special advantages over routine ultrasound in areas where compressibility of the vein cannot be determined because of physical restrictions, such as with smaller vessels (infrapopliteal) or with a suspected thrombus. With duplex scanning, other measurable or demonstrable parameters of venous function can be evaluated if a suspected thrombus is not clearly visualized with routine sonography. Even with a thrombus that is clearly visualized, confirmation by these four factors can be comforting before anticoagulation therapy is initiated.

Technique

The technique of duplex scanning is the same as for ultrasound, except that there are three additional criteria for a positive result: (1) the absence of phasicity during quiet respiration, (2) the absence of spontaneous blood flow, and (3) the absence of augmentation of flow when the limb is compressed distal to the site of probe placement. The effect of the Valsalva's maneuver should also be observed. In addition, valve function can be assessed by compressing the limb proximal to the site of probe placement. Functional valves should not allow augmentation of reverse flow with proximal compression. The extent of valve function at the level of the common femoral, femoral, and popliteal veins should be routinely recorded. They should also be evaluated and recorded as far distally as possible.

Interpretation

Treatment decisions in most large centers are based on duplex scans alone. Occasionally, venography and duplex results differ. If clearly abnormal findings on a duplex scan are contradicted by normal findings on venography, it may be due to the presence of a duplicate vein (up to 20% of patients). Also, thrombosis of a superficial femoral or popliteal vein can be missed by a venogram. For a patient with a normal venogram, significant symptoms, and a clearly abnormal duplex scan, treatment is not out of the question.

VENOUS DOPPLERS

Plain Doppler studies (without ultrasound imaging), such as those obtained with a handheld Doppler, can be used to qualitatively assess the venous system. The plain Doppler probe translates the velocity of venous blood into an audible signal or onto a chart recorder. Velocities are evaluated while the patient undergoes various maneuvers. This technology has not been studied as extensively as IPG or duplex scanning. Advantages to plain Doppler studies include inexpensive equipment and, in most cases, more portable equipment. The safety of withholding anticoagulant treatment in patients with normal plain Doppler results has never been evaluated formally. For anyone performing noninvasive venous studies, a working knowledge of this technique is important to understand basic venous physiology.

Indications

Practical indications are slightly different than those previously discussed; for example, Dopplers may be used alone when other diagnostic methods are unavailable for confirming proximal DVT in a symptomatic patient, or they may be used to diagnose postphlebitic syndrome. This technique can also be used for screening patients to decide if duplex scanning or IPG is indicated, especially if those studies are not readily available. If the screening test is positive, the additional cost or effort of obtaining a duplex or IPG study may be warranted. A Doppler is more reliable than IPG for the diagnosis of DVT in patients with severe arterial insufficiency or with a leg in traction. Used alone, a Doppler provides mainly qualitative evidence of venous function.

Relative Contraindications

Obese patients and patients with massive leg swelling may be difficult to study.

Personnel and Equipment

- A clinician or technician familiar with venous anatomy and Doppler ultrasound technology. (Since the vein cannot be visualized with this technique, a better knowledge of anatomy may be required than with ultrasound [Fig. 85-5]. Experience significantly increases the accuracy of this examination.)
- 5- to 10-MHz probe (transducer). It can often be used for listening to fetal heart tones as well.
- Acoustic gel.

Technique

1. Prepare the room and patient. The room temperature should be warmer than 70° F to prevent vasoconstriction. Place the patient in the supine position with the head slightly elevated. All tight garments should be removed and the leg well exposed. (Tight-fitting

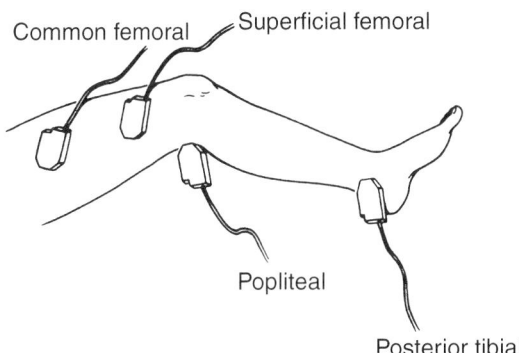

Fig. 85-6
Doppler sonographic examination. The patient is supine with the head slightly elevated. Examine the common femoral, superficial femoral, popliteal, and posterior tibial veins sequentially.

garments may interfere with venous return.) The leg should be slightly abducted, externally rotated, and slightly flexed at the knee. It should also be relaxed to prevent compression of the deep veins. Support the knee with a pillow for better muscle relaxation.

2. Locate the common femoral vein by first finding the artery and then moving the probe medially until the characteristic venous flow or tone is found. The best tone is usually obtained with the probe angled toward the heart (in the direction of venous flow). Use minimal probe pressure to keep from compressing the vein. Arterial flow is characterized by a high-pitched, usually abrupt, tone. Venous flow is usually lower pitched and more continuous.

3. Evaluate the patient with the Doppler from the level of the common femoral vein distally to the superficial femoral, popliteal, and posterior tibial veins (Fig. 85-6). When the level of the popliteal vein is reached, the patient may be turned to a prone position with knees slightly flexed. Rest the patient's feet on two pillows.

4. Compare the sound or tracing from one leg with that of the other leg at each level of the examination and record the results.

Interpretation

Four characteristics describe normal venous flow:
• It is *patent* if flow is heard at the anatomic level of the vein.
• It is *spontaneous* if it can be heard at all levels of the vein.
• It varies with respiration, or is *phasic*.
• It is *augmented* by distal compression of the limb or by release of proximal compression.

Patent. Rarely does the flow completely disappear with DVT, because some flow is usually preserved around a thrombus or through collateral vessels. Differences between one side and the other may be more important, and DVT is frequently associated with a continuous, high-pitched signal. A pulsatile tone that varies with the cardiac cycle is not normal and indicates increased venous pressure.

Spontaneous. DVT causes loss of spontaneous flow. Other causes of loss of spontaneity include anything leading to vasoconstriction. As previously stated, low ambient room temperature can cause patient anxiety or vasoconstriction. The posterior tibial vein may not have a spontaneous signal in normal individuals. Presence of spontaneity is usually found when venous flow is phasic.

Phasic. This characteristic variation of flow with respiration may be lost with DVT. A Valsalva's maneuver should decrease the signal, and a deep breath should augment the signal with normal veins.

Augmented. Firm, gentle compression of the limb for a few seconds distal to the vein should cause augmentation of the flow. When proximal compression is released, it should also demonstrate augmentation. DVT causes a more abrupt and shorter augmentation—if augmentation remains present at all—compared with that of a normal leg. Reverse augmentation produced by proximal compression, or after releasing distal compression indicates valvular incompetence. Presence of augmentation provides support that the vein is patent.

False-negative results may occur in patients with incomplete venous obstruction by thrombi, and false-positive results may be caused by extrinsic venous compression. When treatment decisions are made, the fact that no good outcome studies are available using plain Doppler alone must be weighed against the availability of duplex, IPG, or contrast studies. Abnormal Doppler results are frequently confirmed with another technique. It should be noted that inexpensive, portable plain Doppler equipment is available, the same as with various types of plethysmography. Either can be used alone, but in combination they may complement each other and provide additional types of quantitative data. These supplementary studies may be helpful to the clinician when determining which patients need further evaluation.

NONINVASIVE ARTERIAL STUDIES

Peripheral artery disease (PAD) affects 12% to 15% of the population who are more than 50 years old. Although only a small proportion of individuals with PAD and intermittent claudication develop skin breakdown or limb loss, the associated pain and disability from PAD often restrict ambulation and the overall quality of life. PAD can progress to pain at rest, ulceration, and gangrene. Men are affected nine times more frequently than women. Diabetics also develop this disease more frequently and at an earlier age; the prognosis, unlike that in nondiabetics, is grave because the disease almost always progresses. Diabetics also have a greater incidence of vessel involvement between the knee and ankle. Diabetic PAD is responsible for about half of all amputations.

A history of intermittent claudication or absent/diminished peripheral pulses are unreliable signs and symptoms of PAD. PAD most frequently involves the superficial femoral and popliteal arteries, followed by the distal aorta and iliac arteries in order of decreasing frequency. The absence of a posterior tibial pulse is a more useful finding on examination than the absence of a dorsalis pedis pulse; 10% to 15% of persons have congenitally absent dorsalis pedis pulses. However, neither finding is overly accurate.

Multiple noninvasive techniques are available for *diagnosis* of lower-extremity PAD. A comprehensive history and physical examination and a combination of at least two noninvasive tests should be performed to confirm both the diagnosis and the location of the lesion. If the location of a hemodynamically significant lesion is known, the risks associated with tests involving contrast dye can be minimized; and this knowledge can also guide the radiologist's approach for optimal contrast visualization. Different and sometimes more useful information can be gained from noninvasive studies than with contrast studies; as a result, some surgeons operate without subjecting the patient to preoperative contrast studies. Although it can be very operator dependent for an artery as small as a renal artery, accuracy of magnetic resonance angiography (MRA) is similar to that of a contrast study. Contrast studies may also be avoided if noninvasive studies fail to demonstrate a hemodynamically significant lesion consistent with the patient's symptoms.

Note: The clinician must always consider the possibility of cardiac and cerebrovascular disease in patients with PAD. Intermittent claudication is often the first symptom of generalized arteriosclerotic disease, and these patients most frequently succumb to myocardial infarctions (MIs) or cerebrovascular accidents (CVAs). As many as 28% of patients with PAD have concomitant coronary artery disease, and at least 10% have cerebrovascular disease. Treatment should be targeted to prevent MI or CVA as much as to prevent complications of PAD.

Regarding *screening,* although noninvasive studies are more accurate than physical examination, the literature does not demonstrate a benefit to early detection of PAD. Additional data are needed before noninvasive testing should be considered for routine screening.

Risk Factors for Peripheral Artery Disease

- Diabetes
- Hypertension
- Cigarette smoking
- Family history
- Hyperlipidemia

INDICATIONS (ESPECIALLY IN DIABETICS)

- Intermittent claudication
- Nonhealing foot ulcer
- Exertional leg pain of unknown etiology
- Possible trauma to an artery

Considerations

- To screen before lower extremity surgery in a diabetic patient
- To screen patients with a neuropathy who may have ischemia without symptoms (numbness from neuropathy)
- To follow a patient after reconstructive arterial surgery or angioplasty or for whom nonoperative therapy is selected

It has been said that an experienced clinician can diagnose PAD in most patients by using history and examination alone. However, many clinicians see patients with extremity pain and are neither experienced nor current in the management of vascular disease. Noninvasive studies allow for an objective, definitive diagnosis so that the clinician can either rule in PAD or exclude it and search for other causes.

SEGMENTAL PRESSURE MEASUREMENT

The segmental pressure study is the most generally accepted and widely applied noninvasive arterial test. Segmental pressures are often the initial study for arterial abnormalities.

Personnel and Equipment

- A clinician or technician familiar with arterial anatomy of the foot and Doppler ultrasound technology
- 5- to 10-MHz plain Doppler probe (transducer) with audio
- Acoustic gel

- Aneroid (gauge) manometer
- Four cuffs for each leg (they can be of the same diameter; if eight are available, study time is considerably reduced)

With arterial stenosis and especially with collateral flow, arterial resistance is significantly increased. This increased resistance leads to a large or asymmetric drop in arterial blood pressure, compared with the other leg, over the particular arterial segment with obstruction. The brachial pressure can also be used as a standardized reference for the pressures of the lower extremity. At a minimum, brachial pressure should always be recorded along with its ratio to the pressure at the ankle (ankle-arm pressure index [API] or ankle-brachial index [ABI]).

Since an aneroid manometer is more mobile, faster, and more convenient than a mercury manometer, it is used by most technicians for studying segmental blood pressure measurements. Artifact is not a concern if the same gauge is used throughout the study, since ratios and gradients are the values obtained as opposed to absolute blood pressure measurements.

Likewise, the same cuff widths can be used throughout the lower extremities without concern for cuff artifact. Interpretation has taken into account cuff artifact. In most cases this technique produces a high-thigh systolic pressure greater than brachial artery pressure, which is acceptable for calculating ratios.

Technique

1. With the patient in the supine position, measure systolic pressure in both arms with the aneroid manometer and record them.
2. Apply four lower-limb segmental cuffs (Fig. 85-7). The systolic values recorded refer to the cuff level rather than the artery studied.
3. Using the Doppler, evaluate each of the three major arteries of the foot (dorsalis pedis, posterior tibial, and peroneal) for the strongest signal. For the remainder of the study, use the artery that has the strongest signal. When determining pressures, hold the Doppler probe consistently over the artery at the angle and in the direction that produces the strongest signal.
4. Use the same aneroid manometer throughout. Attach it to a cuff, and inflate the cuff until the Doppler signal in the foot disappears.
5. Deflate the cuff slowly until the first signal is audible in the foot, and record this systolic value for that cuff level.
6. Sequentially inflate and deflate and record the systolic values for each cuff level throughout both lower extremities.
7. Calculate the API (ABI) for both ankles, which is the ankle systolic pressure divided by the arm systolic pressure.

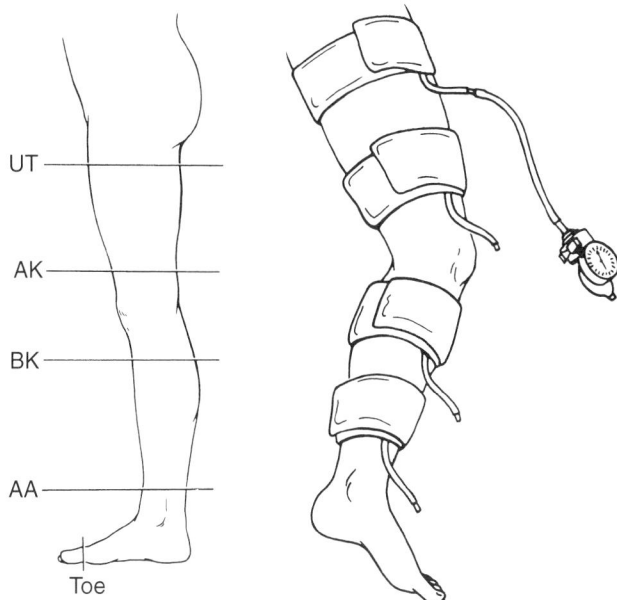

Fig. 85-7
Segmental arterial pressure measurement. Cuff positions: *AA,* Above ankle; *AK,* above knee; *BK,* below knee; *UT,* upper thigh.

Sources of Error

Most errors arise when the examiner moves the probe off the artery while inflating the cuff. One limitation with this technique is that although it is fairly sensitive for diagnosing PAD, it is not a very good study for localizing lesions.

Vessel calcification, such as that found in patients with diabetes and chronic renal failure, may lead to an arterial segment that is only compressible at very high pressures and may produce unusual results. In fact, segmental pressures may appear to follow a reverse gradient.

With an API (ABI) less than 1.0, always consider the possibility of an obstructed aorta or bilaterally obstructed iliac arteries. Because of cuff artifact, high-thigh pressures may be greater than brachial pressures and mask aortic or iliac obstruction.

With an abnormal study, consider comparing the systolic pressures in all the arteries of the foot. This prevents the artifact that might be produced if there is localized obstruction of just one pedal artery.

Interpretation

The single best method of quantitative screening for PAD is an API (ABI) determined by Doppler ultrasound. Normally, the ankle pressure is equal to or slightly greater than the arm pressure. Any API (ABI) less than 0.95 is abnormal. Typically, patients with rest claudication or gangrene have APIs (ABIs) less than 0.5, which often indicates multisegmental disease. Patients with intermittent claudication usually have APIs between 0.5 and 0.9, generally associated with single-segment disease.

During a follow-up evaluation, a change in the API (ABI) of more than 0.15 is considered clinically significant. A decrease in this amount usually indicates disease progression or a problem with a reconstructive procedure. An increase suggests improvement in circulation resulting from development of collaterals. It should be noted that there is no current consensus on how often studies should be repeated.

A high-thigh pressure less than the arm pressure, any pressure drop of 30 mm Hg or more from one segment to the next, or a difference of 30 mm Hg or more between extremities at the same segmental level signifies a probable obstruction in that segment. Some asymmetry of results in the lower extremities is normal. Remember that pressure drops may represent the sum of more than one lesion.

WAVEFORM ANALYSIS

Velocity or *pulse volume* waveform analysis is indicated whenever there is an abnormal API (ABI) or segmental pressure study. These studies can confirm each other and assist in localization of the obstruction.

Velocity Waveform Analysis

Personnel and Equipment
- A clinician or technician familiar with arterial anatomy of the lower extremity and Doppler ultrasound technology
- 5- to 10-MHz probe (transducer) with audio and chart recorder
- Acoustic gel

Note: This same equipment can be used for venous Doppler studies.

Technique
1. Prepare the room and patient. The room temperature should be greater than 70° F to prevent vasoconstriction. The patient should rest in the supine position for at least 10 minutes. The leg should be well exposed, slightly abducted, externally rotated, and slightly flexed at the knee. Supporting the knee with a pillow may increase patient comfort.
2. Beginning at the common femoral artery, apply acoustic gel and auscultate with the probe for maximal tone and amplitude on the recorder. The best tone is usually obtained with the probe pointed away from the heart in the direction of arterial flow. Arterial flow is characterized by a high-pitched, usually abrupt, tone. This should be differentiated from the sound of venous flow, which is usually lower pitched and more continuous.
3. Obtain tracings from common femoral, popliteal, and posterior tibial arteries. For the popliteal arteries, the patient may be turned to a prone position with knees slightly flexed and feet resting on two pillows if this position is more comfortable.
4. Compare the sound or tracing from one leg with the other leg at each level of the examination and record.

Sources of Error
- Dense objects or tissue (e.g., such as local excess fat, hematoma, scar tissue, or plaque on the anterior wall of the vessel) may significantly interfere with ultrasound transmission, making it more difficult to obtain a tracing.
- Prosthetic vessels are almost impossible to study.
- In severe disease, tracings may be unobtainable in spite of being able to hear a tone, especially in distal extremities.
- With an incorrect probe angle, the multiphasic components of a tracing can be missed or lost.

Interpretation
The normal arterial velocity signal is multiphasic, characterized by one systolic and one or more diastolic components. With a directional Doppler study, the diastolic component at first may be briefly negative followed by a positively directed diastolic flow component (Fig. 85-8). The diastolic component may be decreased in a vasodilated individual and increased in a vasoconstricted individual.

The arterial velocity signal produced *just proximal* to an occlusion is usually of low amplitude and short duration (Fig. 85-9, *A*). The arterial velocity signal pro-

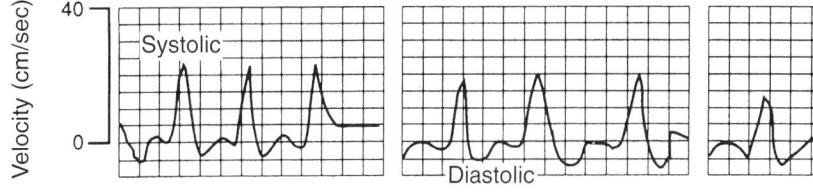

Fig. 85-8
Normal arterial Doppler velocity tracings.

duced *over* a stenotic segment is characteristically high pitched with less prominent diastolic components (Fig. 85-9, *B*). The arterial velocity signal produced *distal* to a stenotic segment usually lacks a diastolic component and has a dampened systolic signal. It is not as high pitched as the stenotic signal (Fig. 85-9, *C*). The arterial signal *far distal* to a stenotic segment is like the post-stenotic segment but is likely to have an even lower amplitude. *Collateral* signals are high pitched and nearly continuous.

To differentiate the contour of normal arterial signals from the contour of obstructed arterial signals, clinicians often describe them as "teepees" and "igloos." "Teepees" refer to the shape of the velocity tracing of a normal artery with its rapid upstroke and resultant high amplitude. The sluggish upstroke tracing with minimal amplitude, as seen with the typical postobstructed artery, might well be described as an "igloo."

A rule of thumb: the presence of a *multiphasic* Doppler signal in a distal vessel, such as that of the foot, strongly suggests that the proximal artery is normal.

Pulse Volume Waveform Analysis

Pulse volume recordings (PVRs) are less operator dependent, are not limited by calcification of the vessel walls, and are readily and rapidly obtained using the same cuffs already in place for segmental pressure measurements. This is a quantitative measurement that allows reasonably accurate localization of a lesion or lesions.

Personnel and Equipment
- A clinician or technician familiar with PVR technology
- Pulse volume recorder

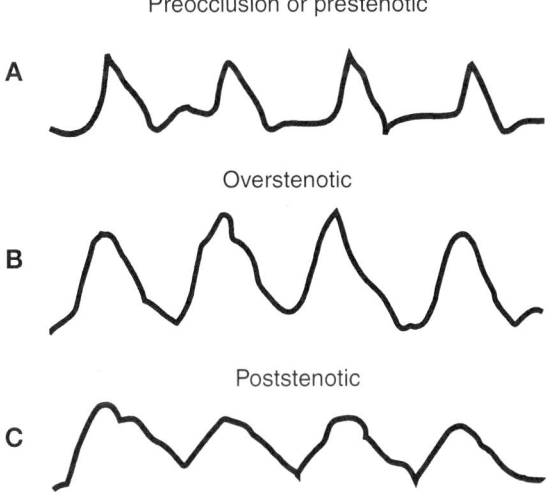

Preocclusion or prestenotic

A

Overstenotic

B

Poststenotic

C

Fig. 85-9
Examples of, **A,** prestenotic, **B,** overstenotic, and, **C,** poststenotic tracings.

- Four cuffs for each leg (they can be of the same diameter; if eight are available, the study time is greatly reduced)

Technique
1. Place the patient in the supine position. Cuffs are placed in the same locations as for segmental pressure determinations and are inflated to 65 mm Hg.
2. Record the PVR at each level.

Interpretation
Changes in waveforms with progression of PAD are seen in Fig. 85-10, *A*. First noted is the loss of the reflected diastolic wave. Next, with more progressive disease, a decrease is seen in the rate of fall of the catacrotic limb, or the downsloping portion. Finally, a further delay in the rise of the anacrotic limb, or the upsloping initial portion of the wave, is noted. With moderate to severe disease, an "igloo" is the predominant feature.

Source of Error
With severe proximal disease it may be difficult to assess the degree of distal disease because the PVRs are often flat throughout the extremity.

OTHER STUDIES

For the patient with a history compatible with claudication or intermittent claudication, and yet the studies are normal, additional studies are available.

1. Vascular stress testing is probably the next most commonly used study. Because of the cost of equipment, a referral to a vascular laboratory may be necessary. For those with a treadmill, after recording ankle systolic pressures, have the patient walk at a speed of 2 mph with a 12-degree grade until pain begins or 5 minutes elapses. Patients over 50 years of age should have continuous ECG monitoring. The time it takes to induce pain is noted as the maximal walking time. Once the pain begins, or 5 minutes has elapsed, the patient is placed in a supine position and the ankle systolic pressure is again recorded. In healthy individuals, strenuous exercise causes a transient fall in ankle systolic pressure, which quickly returns to baseline at rest. In contrast, when a patient with PAD exercises, pain usually commences before 5 minutes and the ankle pressure falls precipitously, often to unrecordable levels. It usually does not recover for several minutes. A fall of more than 20 mm Hg from baseline and a recovery time of more than 3 minutes are considered abnormal.

2. MRA—although sometimes a long, complex, and expensive procedure—is slowly replacing contrast angiography as the definitive diagnostic procedure.

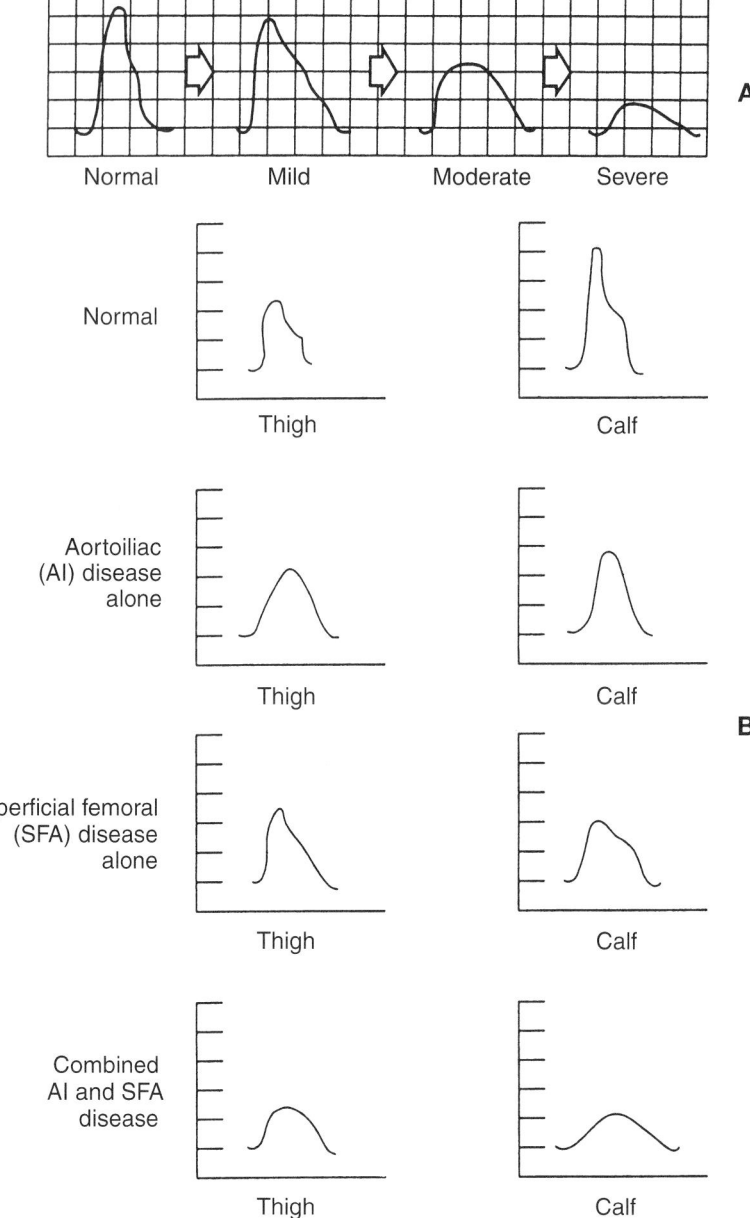

Fig. 85-10
A, Alterations seen in pulse volume waveform as arterial occlusive disease progresses from mild to moderate to severe. **B,** Various thigh and calf waveform patterns characteristic of aortoiliac and superficial femoral arterial occlusive disease. In the normal example, notice the contour of both the thigh and calf waveforms as well as the characteristic increase in amplitude of the calf pulse volume recordings.

SUPPLIERS

For plain ultrasound suppliers and equipment, see Chapter 209, Emergency Department and Office Ultrasound.

Portable Vascular Equipment, Including Duplex
BioMedix
4205 White Bear Parkway
Vadnais Heights, MN 55110
Phone: 1-877-854-0012
Website: www.biomedix.com

Nicolet Vascular
6355 Joyce Drive
Golden, CO 80403
Phone: 1-800-525-2519
Website: www.nicoletvascular.com

Vascular Equipment, Including Duplex (also Pocket Dopplers)
Parks Medical Electronics
19460 SW Shaw
Aloha, OR 97006
Phone: 1-800-547-6427
Website: www.parksmed.com

Pocket Dopplers

Medasonics (Cooper Surgical)

38875 Cherry Street

Newark, CA 94560

Phone: 1-800-227-8076

Website: www.coopersurgical.com

CPT/BILLING CODES

93922   Noninvasive physiologic studies of upper or lower extremity arteries, single level, bilateral

93923   Noninvasive physiologic studies of upper or lower extremity arteries, multiple levels or with provocative functional maneuvers, complete bilateral study (e.g., segmental blood pressure measurements, segmental Doppler waveform analysis, segmental volume plethysmography)

93924   Noninvasive physiologic studies of lower extremity arteries, at rest and following treadmill stress testing, complete bilateral study

93925   Duplex scan of lower extremity arteries or arterial bypass grafts, complete bilateral study

93926   Duplex scan of lower extremity arteries or bypass graft, unilateral or limited study

93965   Noninvasive physiologic studies of extremity veins, complete bilateral study

93970   Duplex scan of extremity veins including responses to compression and other maneuvers; complete bilateral study

93971   Duplex scan of extremity veins including responses to compression and other maneuvers; unilateral or limited study

ICD-9-CM DIAGNOSTIC CODES

415.11   Pulmonary embolism, iatrogenic

415.19   Pulmonary embolism, other

440.20   Atherosclerosis of native arteries of the extremities, unspecified

440.21   with intermittent claudication

440.22   with rest pain

440.23   with ulceration

440.30   of unspecified graft

440.31   of autologous vein bypass graft

451.0   Phlebitis and thrombophlebitis, superficial vessels, lower extremity

451.11   femoral vein (deep or superficial)

451.19   other

451.81   iliac vein

459.1   Postphlebitic syndrome

459.2   Edema, leg resulting from venous obstruction

459.81   Venous (peripheral) insufficiency, unspecified

707.1   Chronic ulcer of skin, lower extremity

729.5   Pain, leg

782.3   Edema, legs

BIBLIOGRAPHY

AbuRahma AF, Bergan JJ, editors: *Noninvasive vascular diagnosis,* London, 2000, Springer.

Barloon TJ, Bergus GR: Diagnostic imaging of lower limb deep venous thrombosis, *Am Fam Physician* 56(3):791, 1997.

Bernstein EF, editor: *Vascular diagnosis,* ed 4, St Louis, 1993, Mosby.

Brodksy CM, Martin R: Ultrasound and Doppler examination of veins and arteries, *Atlas Off Proced* 3(3):421, 2000.

Chance JF, Abbitt PL, Tegtmeyer CJ, Powers RD: Real-time ultrasound for the detection of deep venous thrombosis, *Ann Emerg Med* 20(5):494, 1991.

Heller M, Jehle D: *Ultrasound in emergency medicine,* Philadelphia, 1995, WB Saunders.

Kearon C, Julian JA, Newman TE, Ginsberg JS: Noninvasive diagnosis of deep venous thrombosis. McMaster Diagnostic Imaging Practice Guidelines Initiatives, *Ann Intern Med* 129(5):425, 1998.

Moneta GL, Porter JM, Peripheral vascular ultrasonography. Lanzer P, Rosch J, editors: *Vascular diagnostics: noninvasive and invasive techniques: periinterventional evaluations,* New York, 1994, Springer-Verlag.

Wells PS, Hirsh J, Anderson DR, et al: Accuracy of clinical assessment of deep-vein thrombosis, *Lancet* 345:1326, 1995.

Zafar MU, Farkouh ME, Chesebro JH: A practical approach to lower-extremity arterial disease, *Patient Care* 30:96, 2000.

CHAPTER 86

Office Electrocardiograms

Jerry W. Hizon
Victor F. Froelicher

The resting electrocardiogram (ECG) is the most widely used cardiovascular diagnostic test. Approximately 75 million are performed each year in the United States and probably twice that number around the world. Current estimates are that half are performed or interpreted by clinicians without fellowship training in cardiology. The clinician supervising, performing, or interpreting ECGs must be familiar with the proper use of the machine and electrode placement. In addition, guidelines and clinical competency statements are available (see the Bibliography).

The validity of using the resting 12-lead ECG as a screening test for cardiovascular disease in asymptomatic individuals has never been demonstrated convincingly. One reason is the relatively low prevalence of ECG abnormalities in the general population. Such a low prevalence limits the ECG's sensitivity for screening, its predictive accuracy, and its usefulness (Fig. 86-1).

INDICATIONS

In the office the following situations are the most common to warrant an ECG:

- Chest pain of suspected cardiac origin
- Dysrhythmia recognition and management
- Baseline or longitudinal data for patients with hypertension or diabetes
- Preoperative screen for patients with known coronary artery disease (CAD) or who are at high risk for adverse cardiac events

Patients can be classified into three major groups when undergoing an ECG: (1) patients with known cardiovascular disease or dysfunction, (2) patients who are suspected of having or who are at increased risk of developing cardiovascular disease or dysfunction, and (3) patients with no apparent or suspected heart disease or dysfunction. For patients in the first two groups, an ECG is indicated if there has been a change in symptoms or if the therapy may change the ECG. The last group (group 3) represents a large proportion of the patients treated in the usual office practice. The following guide-

lines regarding indications are more specific for this group, but they may apply to any group, especially for diabetic patients.

Baseline

- As part of the physical examination of those over 40 years of age
- Before administration of pharmacologic agents that are known to have a high incidence of cardiovascular effects (e.g., cancer chemotherapy or medications causing a QT prolongation)
- Before exercise testing
- Those in special occupations that require high cardiovascular performance

Response to Therapy

- Patients prescribed therapy known to produce cardiovascular effects (e.g., cancer chemotherapy or medications causing QT prolongation)

Follow-up

- Asymptomatic persons over 40 years of age with cardiac risk factors

Before Surgery

- Patients over 40 years old (or younger if the surgery involves organ transplantation).

Note: The routine use of a resting ECG to screen for CAD in asymptomatic adults is not recommended by the American College of Physicians, the American Academy of Family Physicians, or the Canadian Task Force on the Periodic Health Examination. The U.S. Preventive Services Task Force says there is insufficient evidence to recommend for or against screening ECGs.

Although the American Heart Association does not recommend routine or repeated ECGs for risk assessment,

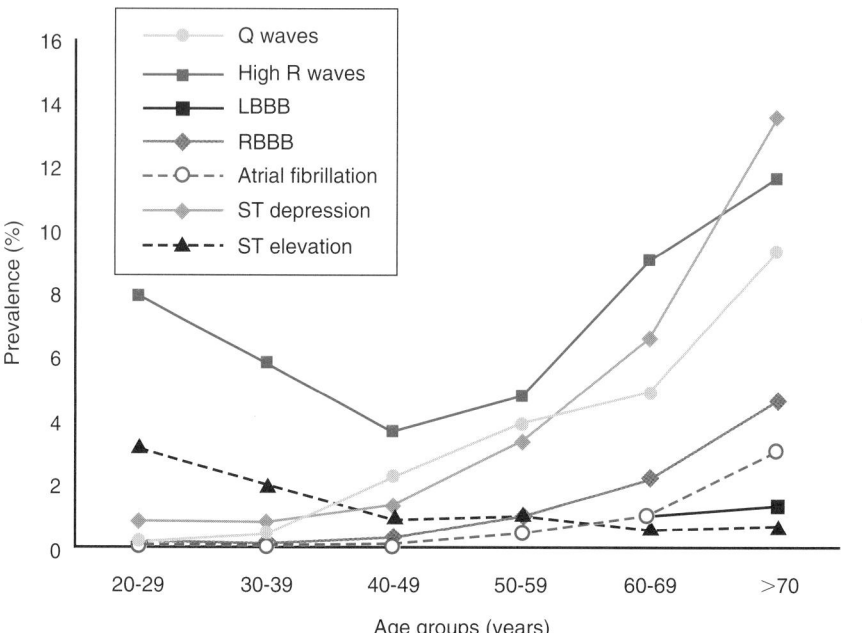

A

Fig. 86-1
Prevalence of electrocardiogram abnormalities
in, **A,** males and, **B,** females.

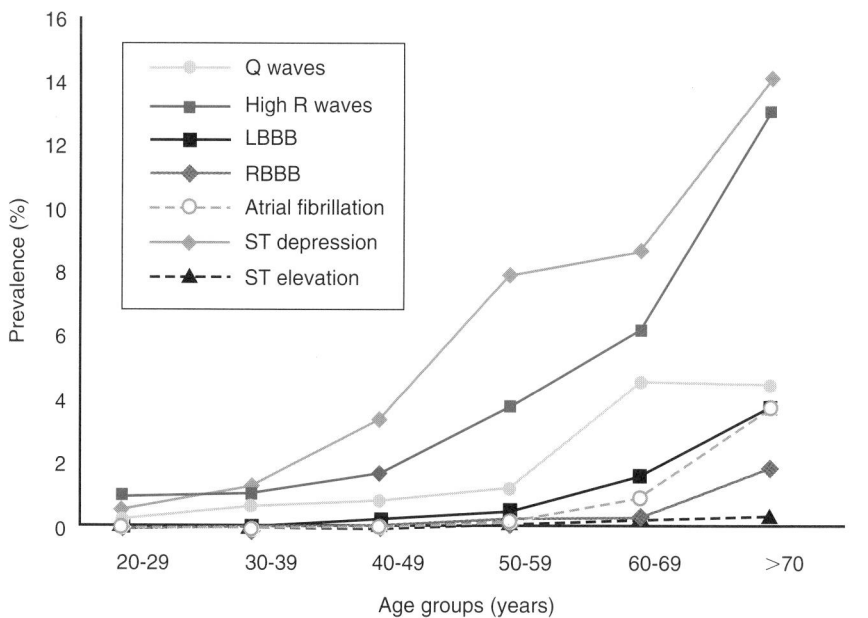

B

various ECG abnormalities have been reported to have predictive power. For example, ST-segment depression, nonspecific T-wave abnormalities, left ventricular hypertrophy (LVH), bundle-branch blocks, and ischemic findings on the resting ECG have been found to have independent predictive power for both coronary mortality and total cardiovascular mortality. In some studies, patients with one or more of these abnormalities were associated with two to four times increased risk (i.e., multivariate-adjusted relative risks between 2.0 and 4.0), suggesting that these findings alone might signify intermediate to high risk. Such risk may deserve intensive

further investigation or risk reduction. Persistent abnormalities on the resting ECG on serial tracings are associated with higher risk than transient findings alone.

CONTRAINDICATIONS

- Patient phobia, refusal, or inability to remain still or in one position
- Emergent need for airway maintenance or management of breathing or circulation (these needs should be addressed before an ECG procedure is performed)

- Skin conditions (e.g., burns or infections) that interfere with electrode placement

EQUIPMENT

- Electrodes with appropriate conductive material or gel
- ECG machine with appropriate patient cables and paper
- If computerized storage is expected, a floppy disk (or other digital media) should be inserted or a connection made to the Internet, Intranet, or telephone line

In the United States, $200 million worth of ECG recorders are sold yearly and most of the current models include a computerized interpretive program at an inclusive price as low as $2000. (See Chapter 92, Exercise [Stress] Testing, for a list of manufacturers.)

PREPROCEDURE PATIENT PREPARATION

Explain the procedure to the patient and discuss why the patient needs to remain as immobile as possible, maintain normal respiration, and not talk during the procedure. Occasionally, there is a need to assure the patient that the procedure is safe and will not cause an electrical shock (e.g., "It takes electricity out of you and does not put it in"). The patient should be aware that further cardiac workup may be necessary regardless of the outcome of the ECG. The patient should also be aware that a normal ECG does not eliminate the possibility of CAD or significant heart disease. Moreover, abnormal ECGs do not always indicate significant disease.

TECHNIQUE

Most modern ECG machines are so simple that an operator's manual is not needed. Standardization is accurate with digital machines, which often automatically adjust for excessive voltage. Perform the ECG procedure in a room away from powerful electrical equipment (electric motors, x-ray equipment, etc.), if possible. Electrode placement remains the biggest challenge.

1. Place the patient in the supine position on the table. Arms should rest at the sides of the torso. Legs should be flat, apart, and not touching each other. If the patient is in a position other than lying flat (e.g., resulting from orthopnea), the heart's electrical axis is altered, possibly an issue when comparing serial tracings. In such cases, a note should be made on the ECG strip of degree or angle of patient elevation so that future ECG procedures can be performed at the same angle for comparison. While the patient's chest

and distal extremities are exposed, keep the rest of the body covered. This should prevent shivering, which can cause a tremor artifact on the ECG tracing.
2. Bring the ECG machine near the table, and turn it on. The usual paper speed is 25 mm per second and the amplitude 1 mV per 10 mm.

Note: Older equipment, especially analog equipment, occasionally needs to be standardized. If available, review the operator's manual regarding standardization. Standardize the machine when it is tracing at 25 mm per second by briefly depressing the standardization button. One mV should deflect exactly 10 mm, and full standardization should be used if possible. If standardization is not performed or is allowed to vary, evaluation of serial tracings is less accurate.

3. Wipe the areas for electrode placement with an alcohol swab. It may be necessary to shave some areas so that the electrodes stick. We recommend shaving *after* using the alcohol swab to avoid applying alcohol to any abrasions resulting from shaving. We also recommend using adhesive electrodes with a tab for fastening the alligator clip from the cable lead.
4. Place the limb electrodes. The red electrode is for the left leg and is labeled "left leg." The electrode for the right leg is universally green and is labeled "right leg." The electrode for the right arm is often banded in white and labeled "RA." The electrode for the left arm is banded in black and labeled "LA."
5. Place the chest electrodes in the following order (Fig. 86-2):
   a. V_1 (red): Fourth intercostal space at right sternal border
   b. V_2 (yellow): Fourth intercostal space at left sternal border
   c. V_4 (blue): Fifth intercostal space at the midclavicular line
   d. V_3 (green): Halfway between V_2 and V_4
   e. V_5 (tan): Anterior axillary line at the same level as V_4 (directly lateral, in the same transverse plane)
   f. V_6 (violet): Midaxillary line at the same level as V_4 and V_5 (again, directly lateral to V_5)

   For approximate landmarks, the nipples are in the midclavicular line; on men they usually overlie the fourth intercostal space. For consistent placement, use only bony landmarks for precordial electrodes. The sternal angle, usually palpated between the manubrium and body of the sternum, is immediately above the second intercostal space. V_4 through V_6 are placed in the same horizontal plane as V_4.
6. Perform the ECG procedure with the electrodes in their proper locations. For dysrhythmias, an extended rhythm strip or another attempt at a 12-lead ECG may be indicated for improved technical quality. Multichannel machines are superior to single-channel machines for rhythm strips. When a second channel is available, it is best to display lead II for rhythm and

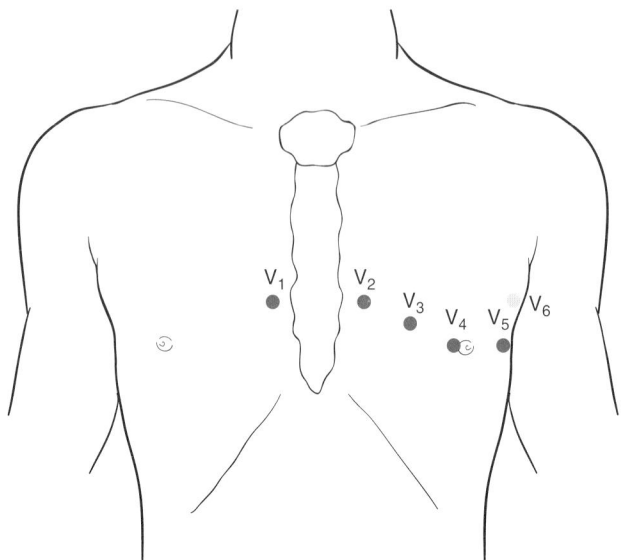

Fig. 86-2
Placement of electrodes. Note that V_6 is in the same horizontal plane as V_4 and V_5, but more lateral, in the midaxillary line.

V_5 for ischemia. If three channels are available, it is best to display leads AVF, V_2, and V_5.

Note: For continuous monitoring (telemetry), any lead can be used; however, most coronary care units use a modified bipolar chest lead. The negative electrode is near the left shoulder and the positive is the traditional V_1. A third is placed at a more remote area of the chest and serves as a ground. However, of all leads, V_5 is the most sensitive for diagnosis of ischemia. Ventricular arrhythmias are more ominous when ischemia is present (see Chapter 84, Ambulatory Electrocardiography: Holter and Event Monitoring). If a single channel is all that is available and ischemia is a concern, V_5 should be used.

7. Remove the electrodes from the patient, dispose of them, and clean the areas on the patient where the electrodes were attached. Modern adhesive electrodes are dry and leave very little residue.

INTERPRETATION

Although computer interpretive programs provide the noncardiologist with a quick and convenient second opinion, they do not provide advice on what to do with an abnormality. The following discussion is aimed at supplementing the available interpretive programs with a suggested course of management including troubleshooting for errors.

Limb Lead Reversal

Limb lead reversal is the most common noticeable error involving the frontal leads. It usually occurs between the right and left arm electrodes, probably because these leads are usually grouped, bundled, or connected together. Lead reversal has become more common as non-experienced personnel replace ECG technicians. Fortunately, the right and left leg electrodes can be switched without affecting the recorded ECG. The clinician should consider this possibility whenever the computer interpretation is *marked right axis deviation,* especially if it is new when compared with a previous tracing, or when precordial leads do not exhibit the normal R wave progression. When every tracing from an ECG machine exhibits this pattern, the ECG leads may be mislabeled.

The second most common placement error is reversal of V_1 and V_3 (again, frequently in the same group or bundle of leads). This should be considered a possibility when R wave amplitude does not increase from V_1 to V_3 and there is T wave inversion in V_3.

Management includes repeating the ECG procedure after checking previous ECGs from the patient, checking the ECG machine, and verifying lead placement. If limb lead reversal is excluded and the finding is still not explained, check the precordial leads for normal R wave progression. If the R waves do not progress normally, move the precordial leads to the patient's right side and record for the possibility of dextra-cardia. If dextra-cardia is confirmed, correlation with a chest x-ray is the next step.

Wolff-Parkinson-White

Wolff-Parkinson-White (WPW) is an ECG pattern characterized by a short PR interval followed by a delta wave and a prolonged QRS duration. The QRS duration may be longer than 120 ms, but it may also be shorter, depending on the degree of fusion of conduction. These characteristics are due to aberrant conduction of ventricular activation through an accessory pathway. WPW occurs in 1 out of 10,000 individuals and can be entirely asymptomatic, or it can be associated with tachycardia and palpitations. When WPW is present, the ST segments cannot be used to identify ischemia. Q waves are actually negative delta waves and are not due to infarction. Individuals who are incidentally found to have this ECG finding are usually otherwise normal. However, they should be questioned about symptoms of palpitations or syncope. Also, a family history of syncope or sudden death could have significance. If either of these symptoms have occurred or the family history is positive, referral to an electrophysiology cardiologist is appropriate.

Right Atrial Abnormality (not Present on Prior ECGs)

If the right atrial abnormality (RAA) or P-pulmonale is new when compared with previous ECGs, consider the clinical possibilities of a pulmonary embolus (tachycardia, pleuritic chest pain, cough, fever, hypoxia, presence of cancer or immobilization) versus an exacerbation of lung disease.

Right Atrial Abnormality on Prior ECGs

If the RAA is a consistent finding, examine the patient for chronic lung disease (prolonged expiration, hyperresonance, rhonchi and distant breath sounds, lowered diaphragms) and consider the overall history including possible exposure to asbestos, coal dust, or cigarette smoke. Pulmonary function testing may be indicated.

Left Atrial Abnormality (not Present on Prior ECGs)

If the left atrial abnormality (LAA) or P-mitrale is new when compared with previous tracings, consider the clinical possibilities of new congestive heart failure (CHF) and/or mitral valvular insufficiency. Mitral valvular insufficiency is confirmed by a holosystolic murmur radiating into the axilla and, if necessary, by echocardiography.

Left Atrial Abnormality on Prior ECGs

If the LAA or P-mitrale is consistent when compared with previous tracings, evaluate the ECG for additional LVH criteria. LVH plus LAA can be an ominous marker for future events such as CHF, stroke, or death. Physical examination and an echocardiogram can confirm the findings.

Right Axis Deviation (not Present on Prior ECGs)

When right axis deviation (RAD) is a new finding, it can be due to an exacerbation of lung disease, a pulmonary embolus, or simply a tachycardia. If RAD is a change from previous ECGs, question the patient for symptoms consistent with an exacerbation of lung disease or a pulmonary embolus. If the patient has findings consistent with embolus, a nuclear ventilation/perfusion (VQ) scan or CT angiogram is usually indicated. If a VQ mismatch or thrombus is noted, anticoagulation is appropriate.

Right Axis Deviation on Prior ECGs

Chronic RAD is normal in those less than 21 years of age and in athletes. It can also be a chronic finding in patients with lung disease and right ventricular hypertrophy (RVH).

Left Axis Deviation

Left axis deviation (LAD) is the most common "abnormality" in adults, occurring in over 8% of patients. It can

be part of the criteria for LVH, but in isolation it has little significance. Marked LAD (45% or more) is called *left anterior hemiblock* or *left anterior fascicular block*. If LAD is present and the patient is not known to be hypertensive, it may be worth efforts to exclude the diagnosis of hypertension with frequent blood pressure checks or ambulatory blood pressure monitoring.

Right Bundle Branch Block

Right bundle branch block (RBBB) can be normal (occurring without underlying disease) or due to trauma, increased right ventricular pressure, ischemia, or infarction. An incomplete RBBB has a QRS duration of less than 120 msec and an rsr' pattern in V_1 and V_2 without an R wave greater than the amplitude of the S wave. It sometimes is simply called an *Rsr' pattern* and usually is a normal finding. Very rarely, it can be associated with an atrial septal defect. Incomplete RBBB or right ventricular conduction delay (RVCD) is not necessarily a precursor of RBBB or any conduction abnormality. Such atypical right ventricular conduction patterns are seen more frequently in people less than 21 years of age and in athletes, and they can also be normal variants. Although wide splitting of the second heart sound is a very common finding among normal patients, fixed splitting of the second heart sound can also be associated with an atrial septal defect. Remember that the abnormalities of the second heart sound must be heard in the sitting position, since splitting is often wide in normal individuals when supine. If present, an echocardiographic air contrast ("bubble") study is indicated. Any pulmonary disease process can be associated with RVCD, and RVCD can occur acutely with exacerbation of lung disease or a pulmonary embolus. Clinical correlation is necessary; either treatment of the lung disease or a VQ scan/CT angiogram might be indicated.

Left Bundle Branch Block

Left bundle branch block (LBBB) can result from severe trauma (car accident), ischemia, or infarction. It is often associated with LVH or dilation. LBBB can also result from fibrosis of the conduction system. LBBB has a weak predictive power in a young asymptomatic population (consistent with Bayes' rule) but is quite ominous in an older population as a marker for an increased risk of death, stroke, and CHF. Incomplete LBBB and the hemiblocks are usually not associated with cardiac disease. Clinical correlates including the cardiac examination should direct any further studies in response to a new LBBB. If the patient has an enlarged heart with signs or symptoms of CHF, an echocardiogram is usually indicated. If a patient with LBBB has chest pain, unfortunately neither the resting nor the exercise ECG can be used as a diagnostic tool. Cardiac enzymes, stress echocardiogram, or a nuclear perfusion test is required. When LBBB is new and noted in the patient with prolonged anginal pain, thrombolysis is indicated.

Right Ventricular Hypertrophy

RVH can be a normal finding in people under 21 and in athletes. It can be associated with chronic obstructive pulmonary disease (COPD), primary and secondary pulmonary hypertension, pulmonary embolus, and CHF. Clinical correlation is indicated. If the RVH is new when compared with previous tracings, consider the clinical presentation for pulmonary embolus or exacerbation of lung disease. The patient may require hospitalization and treatment with heparin for pulmonary embolism, or bronchodilators, antibiotics, and steroids for COPD. If the pulmonary disease ECG criterion is not a new finding, examine the patient for chronic lung disease (prolonged expiration, hyperresonance, rhonchi and distant breath sounds, lowered diaphragms) and consider the overall medical history, including possible exposure to asbestos, coal dust, or cigarette smoke. Pulmonary function testing as well as an echocardiogram may be indicated.

Left Ventricular Hypertrophy

LVH requires clinical correlation beginning with blood pressure measurement and physical examination for cardiac size and murmurs or morbid obesity. A complete medical history should be obtained with emphasis on symptoms of aortic valve disease (angina, syncope) and CHF. If aortic stenosis is suspected after the history or examination, an echocardiogram is indicated. In patients without known heart disease, a lipid panel should be obtained so that the Framingham point system can be used to predict the risk of cardiac events. If the blood pressure is elevated, therapy should be begun with diuretics, followed by an added beta-blocker if the blood pressure does not normalize. If there is a history of CHF or an abnormal cardiac exam, an echocardiogram is indicated. LVH is one of the most ominous ECG indicators of risk for future cardiovascular events in patients over 30 years of age.

Acute ST Depression

Acute ST depression can be associated with ischemia, non-Q wave infarction (acute coronary syndrome), electrolyte abnormalities, osmolality changes, hyperventilation, standing up, and certain drugs. An ECG should be obtained in any patient with chest pain of uncertain etiology because an acute ST shift can confirm that it is due to ischemia. ST depression may also be associated with subendocardial damage, as opposed to Q waves, which are associated with transmural damage from

infarction. Although *chronic ST depression* is nonspecific as a marker for cardiac disease, it is associated with a poor outcome. It can be due to electrolyte abnormalities and drugs, particularly digoxin. The patient should be questioned about a past or present history of cardiac ischemic pain. Blood chemistries including electrolytes, glucose, calcium, magnesium, blood urea nitrogen (BUN), and creatinine should be obtained. All medications should be recorded carefully, and any nonprescription drugs that the patient may be taking should be noted. Many nonprescription drugs, especially from other countries, contain diuretics and even digoxin.

Prolonged QT Interval

Diagnosis of prolonged QT interval is complicated by the inherent difficulty in identifying T wave end and the inaccuracy of Bazett's formula for correcting for heart rate. It may be preferable to judge the QT interval prolonged when it changes in length or when it exceeds 50% of the R-R interval. QT prolongation can be due to multiple causes, but its importance is its association with premature ventricular contractions, ventricular tachycardia, and ventricular fibrillation; in other words, it is associated with vulnerability to lethal arrhythmia. The following is a list of conditions that can cause QT prolongation: hereditary syndromes (rare), electrolyte-metabolic abnormalities, medications (e.g., type Ia antiarrhythmics such as quinidine and Norpace; tricyclic antidepressants, antihistamines, anticholinergic drugs, antibiotics [e.g., macrolides], and antifungals), central nervous system disorders, systemic illnesses, and myocardial infarction. Obtain blood chemistries including electrolytes, glucose, calcium, magnesium, BUN, and creatinine. Take a careful medication history including noncardiac drugs such as decongestants, anti-GERDs (gastroesophageal reflux disease), and antibiotics. Ask specifically about any family history of syncope or sudden death.

Troubleshooting

- Older ECG machines use thermal-head printers that automatically adjust for tracing intensity. Some newer machines use laser printers that actually write the grid. They use regular paper rather than the more expensive, heat-sensitive, grid papers. Extra paper, styluses, or printer cartridges should always be available.
- For a wandering baseline, there is either poor electrode contact, a bad cable, or the patient is slowly moving or breathing deeply. For older equipment, especially analog equipment, the machine may not be warmed up adequately.
- A jagged baseline is from wall current (AC) interference, a broken wire, improper grounding, or other electrical interference.
- For older equipment with heat-sensitive paper, if the

baseline is too light or thin, the stylus is not hot enough. If the baseline is too thick, the stylus is too hot (refer to the operating manual). Improper stylus pressure is detected by using the standardization pulse. With proper pressure, the standardization pulse should produce a tracing with sharp corners. Rounded or exaggerated angles indicate improper pressure.

COMPLICATIONS

- Local skin irritation or allergic reaction to electrode placement or adhesive
- Patient distress over abnormal ECG
- Incorrect interpretation because of improper lead placement, ECG performance, or computer or clinician error
- Unnecessary diagnostic workup because of no prior ECG tracing with which to compare, an inadequate clinical correlation, or a normal ECG variant

POSTPROCEDURE PATIENT EDUCATION

For persistent symptoms, the patient should schedule a follow-up visit with his or her clinician, regardless of the ECG result. The patient should be given the results of the ECG, as well as instructions for medications, follow-up, or further workup, as necessary. The clinician may wish to give the patient a copy of the ECG or ECG interpretation for his or her personal records.

CPT/BILLING CODES

93000	Electrocardiogram, routine, with at least 12 leads; with interpretation and report
93005	Tracing only, without interpretation and report
93010	Interpretation and report only

Note: An ECG is usually needed to rule out a contraindication for exercise testing; however, Medicare will not reimburse for an ECG on the same day as an exercise test. For this and other reasons, it is usually better to bring the patient back on another day for an exercise test. Before every exercise test, another comparison ECG is performed; it is just not reimbursable by Medicare.

ICD-9-CM DIAGNOSTIC CODES

410.91	Acute myocardial infarction, NOS, initial
410.92	Acute myocardial infarction, NOS, subsequent care
413.9	Angina pectoris, NOS
414.00	Arteriosclerotic heart disease

427.31	Atrial fibrillation
427.9	Cardiac arrhythmia
429.3	Cardiomegaly
786.50	Chest pain, unspecified
786.51	Chest pain, precordial
786.52	Chest wall pain, anterior
414.00	Coronary heart disease
V81.0	Coronary heart disease, screening
428.0	Heart failure, congestive
401.9	Hypertension, NOS
401.1	Hypertension, benign
402.10	Hypertensive heart disease, benign, without CHF
402.11	Hypertensive heart disease, benign, with CHF
426.3	Left bundle branch block
402.90	Left ventricular hypertrophy, hypertensive, without CHF
402.91	Left ventricular hypertrophy, hypertensive, with CHF
412	Myocardial infarction, old
785.1	Palpitations
427.69	Premature beats, other, including ventricular
426.4	Right bundle branch block
414.9	Ischemic heart disease, chronic, NOS
785.0	Tachycardia, NOS

ADDITIONAL RESOURCES

- See the sample patient education handout titled "Office Electrocardiograms (ECG or EKG)" on page 1836 of Appendix G.

BIBLIOGRAPHY

American Academy of Family Physicians: *Age charts for periodic health examination (reprint no 510)*, Kansas City, MO, 1994, American Academy of Family Physicians.

Ashley EA, Raxwal VK, Froelicher VF: The prevalence and prognostic significance of electrocardiographic abnormalities, *Curr Probl Cardiol* 25:1, 2000.

Canadian Task Force on Preventive Health Care: *Current recommendations: 2001 review.* Available at www.ctfphc.org (accessed December 6, 2001).

Eddy DM, editor: *Common screening tests,* Philadelphia, 1991, American College of Physicians.

Fisch C: Clinical competence in electrocardiography: a statement for physicians from the ACP/ACC/AHA Task Force on clinical privileges in cardiology, *J Am Coll Cardiol* 25(6): 1465, 1995.

Froelicher V, Quaglietti S: *Handbook of ambulatory cardiology,* Philadelphia, 1997, Lippincott, Williams & Wilkins.

Grauer K: *12-Lead ECGs: a 'pocket brain' for easy interpretation,* Gainesville, 1998, KG EKG Press.

Grauer K: *A practical guide to ECG interpretation,* ed 2, St Louis, 1998, Mosby.

Grundy SM, Bazzarre T, Cleeman J, D'Agostino RB Sr, et al: Prevention Conference V: Beyond secondary prevention: identifying the high-risk patient for primary prevention: medical office assessment: Writing Group I, *Circulation* 101(1):E3, 2000.

Schlant RC, Adolph RJ, DiMarco JP, et al: Guidelines for electrocardiography: a report of the American College of Cardiology/American Heart Association Task Force on Assessment of Diagnostic and Therapeutic Cardiovascular Procedures (Committee on Electrocardiography), *J Am Coll Cardiol* 19(3):473, 1992.

U.S. Preventive Service Task Force: *Guide to clinical preventive services,* ed 2, Baltimore, 1996, Williams & Wilkins.

WEBSITES

www.americanheart.org

www.cardiology.org (examples of ECG abnormalities and what to do about them)

www.ctfphc.org (Canadian Task Force on Preventive Health Care)

CHAPTER 87

Echocardiography

Grant C. Fowler
Terry Reynolds

With the population of older Americans increasing, the prevalence of heart disease will continue to increase. The amount of heart disease managed by primary care clinicians will also continue to increase. In many cases, both the management and the prognosis of heart disease is based upon the amount of remaining viable myocardium. This is especially true for patients with congestive heart failure (CHF), cardiomyopathy, ventricular arrhythmias, and ischemic heart disease. One method of quantitatively assessing the amount of viable myocardium is to determine the ejection fraction. In fact, the most common reason echocardiography is currently performed is to determine the ejection fraction.

Many common symptoms, signs, or diagnoses (e.g., palpitations, cardiomegaly on ECG or chest x-ray, atrial fibrillation, CHF) are evaluated or managed based upon data from echocardiography (Table 87-1). In certain situations, the more readily available the echocardiogram, the better the management. Acute chest pain is managed differently when echocardiography is immediately available. For example, even extracardiac causes for acute chest pain can be diagnosed with echocardiography, some of which can be life threatening (e.g., pulmonary embolus or aortic dissection). If an acute myocardial infarction (MI) is diagnosed, risk stratification can be performed immediately. Complications from an acute MI can also be diagnosed early.

Other common diagnoses that can be made in the primary care clinician's office with echocardiography include mitral valve prolapse, dilated left atrium (important for patients with atrial fibrillation), left ventricular hypertrophy, and ischemic heart disease. Whether in the clinician's office or in the emergency department, a rapid diagnosis of pericardial tamponade or a pericardial effusion may be life saving. Furthermore, if pericardiocentesis is needed, the risk of complications is significantly reduced if it is performed under ultrasonic guidance.

Improvements in image quality, portability, and affordability for real-time sonography have allowed it to become a valuable adjunct for the clinician in their office

or in the emergency department. For those clinicians with a large number of adult patients, two-dimensional (2D) and M-mode echocardiography may be a welcome addition to their practice. If the primary care clinician is not comfortable performing echocardiography, contractors are available to provide sonographers. Overreading services are also available (see the "Suppliers" section). This chapter predominately describes the performance of a 2D/M-mode echocardiogram with a brief summary of common findings. Since color and Doppler flow imaging are helpful for almost all echocardiograms, especially for those assessing the hemodynamic severity of an abnormality, they will also be discussed briefly. For a discussion of ultrasound principles and concepts, and for information regarding limited echocardiography, see Chapter 209, Emergency Department and Office Ultrasound. Electromechanical dissociation, pericardial effusion, and pericardial tamponade are discussed in that chapter.

2D echocardiography provides the clinician with cross-sectional, real-time images of various cardiac structures. In this manner, cardiac chambers, walls, valves, and other structures can be observed as they move through the cardiac cycle. Freeze-framing and the use of calipers allow the clinician to measure certain structures, if needed, at various points during the cardiac cycle.

M-mode echocardiography produces graphic images in which time makes up the horizontal axis and the structures in motion being scanned compose the vertical axis. In other words, wherever the cursor is placed on the image, a linear beam of ultrasound is directed through the corresponding tissue and movement of the structures is graphically imaged over time. The resultant M-mode tracing can then be used to look at excursion and contraction patterns as well as to precisely measure distances from the various horizontal structures over time. Chamber dimensions, wall thicknesses, and valve excursions can be measured precisely throughout the cardiac cycle. From chamber dimensions, an ejection fraction can be estimated.

Doppler flow imaging is used to measure the velocity of blood flowing over certain structures. Using the

TABLE 87-1

Common Symptoms and Differential Diagnosis
for Echocardiography

Reason for Echocardiography	Differential Diagnosis
Chest pain	Coronary artery disease: acute myocardial infarction or angina
	Aortic dissection
	Pericarditis
	Pulmonary embolism
	Valvular stenosis
	Hypertrophic cardiomyopathy
Heart failure	Left ventricular systolic dysfunction (global or segmental)
	Valvular heart disease
	Left ventricular diastolic dysfunction
	Pericardial disease
	Right ventricular dysfunction
Palpitations	Left ventricular systolic dysfunction
	Mitral valve disease
	Congenital heart disease (e.g., atrial septal defect, Ebstein's anomaly)
	Pericarditis
	No structural cardiac disease
Murmur: systolic	Flow murmur (no valve abnormality)
	Aortic stenosis, subaortic obstruction, hypertrophic obstructive cardiomyopathy
	Mitral regurgitation
	Ventricular septal defect
	Pulmonic stenosis
	Tricuspid regurgitation
Murmur: diastolic	Mitral stenosis
	Aortic regurgitation
	Pulmonic regurgitation
	Tricuspid stenosis
Cardiomegaly on chest x-ray	Pericardial effusion
	Dilated cardiomyopathy
	Specific chamber enlargement (e.g., left ventricle in chronic aortic regurgitation)
Systemic embolic event	Left ventricular systolic function and segmental wall motion abnormalities (aneurysms)
	Left ventricular thrombus
	Aortic valve disease
	Mitral valve disease
	Left atrial thrombus (only diagnostic if seen, otherwise transesophageal echo needed)
	Patent foramen ovale

Adapted from Otto CM: *Textbook of clinical echocardiography,* ed 2, Philadelphia, 2000, WB Saunders.

Bernoulli equation, pressure gradients (e.g., across a valve) can also be determined. As with M-mode, time and the cardiac cycle are graphed along the horizontal axis while the vertical axis consists of blood velocity in meters per second. By convention, flow toward the transducer is depicted (above the baseline) and flow away from the transducer is depicted below the baseline. Pulsed wave (PW) technology and measurements utilize tiny, three-dimensional sample volumes to detect the exact location of any abnormalities. However,

PW Doppler is limited when there is high velocity flow. Continuous wave (CW) technology utilizes two crystals (one continuously emitting sound waves, the other continuously listening for echoes) and can measure high velocities (e.g., stenotic valves). However, it is of limited use for localizing abnormalities. As a result of these limitations, both PW and CW should be utilized with every valve. Color flow Doppler is a special adaptation of PW technology. It uses thousands of sampling volumes to produce a color image of velocities. Flow away from the transducer is blue, by convention, and flow toward the transducer is depicted in red. The intensity of the color increases with the velocity.

INDICATIONS

- Determine ejection fraction (most common indication)
- Acute chest pain
- Acute myocardial infarction
- Atrial fibrillation
- Cardioversion preparation
- Cardiomegaly on chest x-ray
- Congestive heart failure
- Embolus (systemic or pulmonary)
- Hypertensive heart disease
- Ischemic heart disease
- Mitral valve prolapse
- Murmur
- Palpitations
- Pericardial effusion, electromechanical dissociation, or suspected pericardial tamponade
- Suspected cardiomyopathy
- Suspected left ventricular hypertrophy (e.g., LVH on ECG)
- Transient ischemic attack
- Valvular stenosis or insufficiency
- Ventricular arrhythmias (with suspected cardiac structural abnormality)

CONTRAINDICATIONS

- Patient too unstable or too uncooperative to be scanned
- Patient needs Doppler flow imaging or a color Doppler scan, and the equipment does not have this capability

PREPROCEDURE PATIENT PREPARATION

Indications for the study and possible findings should be explained to the patient. The patient should be prepared to change positions, if possible, while being scanned.

They should be prepared for adequate gel to be applied to the parasternal, apical, suprasternal, and possibly subxiphoid areas of the chest wall. The patient should be gowned and in the supine or left-lateral decubitus position.

EQUIPMENT

- For best images, an ultrasound machine with several probes of varying frequency should be available. Among these probes, a low frequency (e.g., 2.5 MHz) probe with 2D, M-mode, and cardiac Doppler capabilities is necessary. An ultrasound machine with harmonic imaging ensures high-quality images. A method of recording the examination (e.g., VCR, disk) is also needed for documentation. For limited scans in emergency situations, a machine without Doppler capability can be used.
- Ultrasonic jelly and towels to cleans up after scanning.
- Patient gown.

TECHNIQUE

Two-Dimensional Echocardiography

Viewing the front of the chest, if the 12 o'clock position is considered cephalad and the 6 o'clock direction caudal, the axis of the heart is usually located in a line drawn between the 10 o'clock and the 4 o'clock positions. Placing the marker dot of the transducer at about the 4 o'clock position usually produces the long-axis view of the heart, especially if the probe is located parasternally. A line drawn between the patient's right shoulder and the left hip also approximates the long-axis of the heart. The long-axis view is essentially the longitudinal view of the heart if described in the conventional terminology of ultrasound for the remainder of the body. Rotating the marker dot almost 90 degrees or perpendicular to the long-axis, to the 8 o'clock position, produces the short-axis view of the heart. This is essentially a transverse view of the heart (Fig. 87-1). A line drawn between the left shoulder and the right hip also approximates this axis.

Since the patient is usually lying on his or her back while being scanned and the transducer is placed on the anterior chest wall (or abdominal wall for the subxiphoid view), the transducer edge will be noted at the top of the image. Posterior cardiac structures will be located at the bottom (inferior aspect) of the image. With the usual orientation, if the directional marker is noted on the left side of the image, objects to the left of the screen will correspond to objects near the marker dot on the transducer.

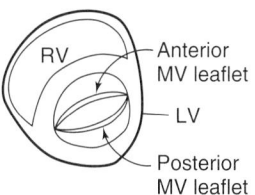

Fig. 87-1
Parasternal short-axis view at the level of the mitral valve *(MV)*. *LV,* Left ventricle; *RV,* right ventricle. (From Reynolds T: *The echocardiographer's pocket reference,* ed 2, Phoenix, 2000, School of Cardiac Ultrasound at Arizona Heart Institute.)

1. With the patient in the supine position, attempt to scan by first placing the transducer in the parasternal location (third to fourth intercostal space, next to the sternum) or the apical location (inferolateral to the left nipple at the point of palpated maximal cardiac impulse [PMI]). These are the same two traditional auscultatory points used for a stethoscope. If the best window is found at the apical location, skip to no. 12.
2. When scanning parasternally, the probe will be rotated so that the marker dot is either in the 4 o'clock (long axis) or the 8 o'clock (short axis) position. The short-axis view at the level of the mitral valve is often a good view for assessing the adequacy of the window, since the mitral valve is usually prominent and easily located (Fig. 87-1).

Note: Some ultrasound equipment places the marker dot 180 degrees away from this standard orientation (that is, the 10 o'clock position is what should be the 4 o'clock position). To determine the orientation of the probe, the directional marker on the image should be found. It corresponds with the marker dot on the probe.

3. If you can change the patient's position easily, place the patient on his or her left side. This causes the lingula of the lung to fall away from the heart and often provides a better window.
4. For unresponsive patients, those who cannot be moved, patients with chronic obstructive pulmonary disease, or other technical difficulties impairing the use of ultrasound in the parasternal positions, the subxiphoid position will often provide a good window. Place the transducer directly below the xiphoid and angle it toward the patient's head with the marker dot toward the patient's left side. If this is the only location where an adequate window can be obtained, skip to no. 16.
5. If a good window can be found at the parasternal short-axis view, rotate the transducer 90 degrees to the parasternal long-axis view (Fig. 87-2). With this view, observe the anterior and posterior leaflets of the mitral valve as it is scanned lengthwise. With prolapse, the leaflets will close beyond 90 degrees

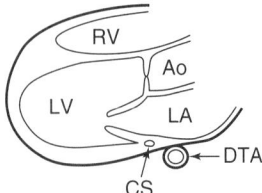

Fig. 87-2
Parasternal long-axis view. *Ao,* Aortic root; *DTA,* descending thoracic aorta; *LA,* left atrium; *LV,* left ventricle; *RV,* right ventricle; *CS,* coronary sinus. (From Reynolds T: *The echocardiographer's pocket reference,* ed 2, Phoenix, 2000, School of Cardiac Ultrasound at Arizona Heart Institute.)

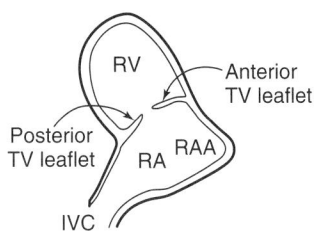

Fig. 87-3
Parasternal long-axis view of the right ventricular inflow tract (RVIT view). *IVC,* Inferior vena cava; *RA,* right atrium; *RAA,* right atrial appendage; *RV,* right ventricle, *TV,* tricuspid valve. (From Reynolds T: *The echocardiographer's pocket reference,* ed 2, Phoenix, 2000, School of Cardiac Ultrasound at Arizona Heart Institute.)

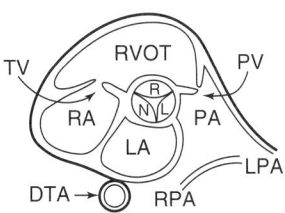

Fig. 87-4
Parasternal short-axis view at the level of the aortic valve. *DTA,* Descending thoracic aorta; *L,* left coronary cusp; *LA,* left atrium; *LPA,* left pulmonary artery; *N,* noncoronary cusp; *PA,* pulmonary artery; *PV,* pulmonic valve; *R,* right coronary cusp; *RA,* right atrium; *RPA,* right pulmonary artery; *RVOT,* right ventricular outflow tract; *TV,* tricuspid valve. (From Reynolds T: *The echocardiographer's pocket reference,* ed 2, Phoenix, 2000, School of Cardiac Ultrasound at Arizona Heart Institute.)

or cross the plane of the mitral annulus. True prolapse is often associated with thickened valves. Also with this view, the right ventricle is seen at the superior portion of the image and the interventricular septum is noted as the inferior border of the right ventricle. Beneath the interventricular septum to the left of the image is the left ventricular chamber bordered by its posterior wall. Note that the ventricular walls thicken during systole, reducing the size of the ventricular cavity. Very little of the apex can be visualized with this view, since it is beyond the left side of the image. The left atrium is to the right side of the image, immediately inferior to the aortic root. The left atrial diameter should be about the same as the aortic root diameter. If either is markedly larger than the other or more than 4 cm in their anteroposterior diameter, they are considered dilated. The descending thoracic aorta is noted behind the left atrium. Rotate the transducer slightly clockwise if a better longitudinal view of the aorta is desired.

6. To obtain the long-axis view of the right ventricular inflow tract (RVIT view), from the parasternal long-axis view, tilt the transducer inferomedially or toward the right hip. This is a good view in which to study the tricuspid valve and the right ventricle (Fig. 87-3). The posterior and anterior tricuspid leaflets separate the right atrium from the right ventricle. In fact, this is about the only view where the posterior leaflet of the tricuspid valve can be seen. Liver tissue is usually noted adjacent to the diaphragmatic wall of the right ventricle.

7. After angling the probe back again to the parasternal long-axis view, rotate the transducer 90 degrees so that the marker dot is at the 8 o'clock position. This will produce the parasternal short-axis view again (Fig. 87-1). Note the appearance in real-time of the opening and closing mitral valve. Some have likened this image to that of a "fish-mouth" opening and closing, especially if there is any stenosis. Without stenosis, the lateral and medial commissures of the valve are easy to distinguish. At this

level, the ventricular wall can be divided into six segments and the contractility of all of the segments should be observed (see no. 10). In the normal heart, the segments should be contracting uniformly and symmetrically. The tricuspid valve may be seen to the left of the mitral valve.

8. Next, without actually moving or rotating the transducer, merely angle it more cephalad toward the base of the heart to observe the aortic valve (Fig. 87-4). In this transverse view of the aortic valve, it produces a characteristic "Y sign" when the leaflets are closed. If the valve itself is viewed as the face of a clock, the commissures are noted in the 2, 6, and 10 o'clock positions at the edges of the "Y." When the valve is open in systole, it should produce a triangular shape. If it produces an oval shape with opening, the aortic valve is bicuspid. This is one of the most common abnormal findings on adult echocardiography, occurring in 1% to 2% of the population. If it is found, the patient should also be scanned for coarctation of the aorta, seen in 50% to 80% of those with bicuspid aortic valves (see the suprasternal notch view, no. 21). At this level of the parasternal short-axis view, the right ventricular

outflow tract (RVOT) can be seen curving above and around the aortic valve. The tricuspid valve is noted to the left of the aortic valve and the pulmonic valve is located superiorly and to the right. The right ventricle is located between the two. The right atrium is located in the inferior portion of the image to the left of the aortic valve. The left atrial appendage can often be seen to the far right of the aortic valve, and the left atrium is noted inferior or posterior to the aortic valve. Part of the atrial septum can be noted between the atria. The three cusps of the aortic valve are labeled the right, left and noncoronary cusps. The right cusp is located next to the right ventricular outflow tract, the noncoronary cusp closest to the right atrium, and the left coronary cusp next to left atrium. In a normal heart, the corresponding right or left coronary arteries originate from the same-labeled cusps.

9. Tilting the transducer yet more superiorly, beyond the aortic valve, the aortic root can be visualized in its short axis (transversely). At this level, on the right side of the image of the aortic root, the pulmonary artery can often be noted to bifurcate into the right and left pulmonary arteries.

10. Next, angle the probe back through the mitral valve down to the level of the papillary muscles (Fig. 87-5). This level provides an excellent view for assessing left ventricular wall motion and the severity of left ventricular hypertrophy if it is present. At this level, the left ventricular wall can again be divided into six segments—the anterior, anteroseptal, anterolateral, inferolateral (posterolateral), inferoseptal (posteroseptal), and inferior (posterior) segments—which are all visualized. This same segmentation system can be used on the parasternal short-axis view at the level of the mitral valve. Each of the segments should contract in a uniform manner. With coronary artery disease, determining which wall becomes hypokinetic with ischemia may predict which coronary artery is obstructed (see "Findings and Interpretation" section). Usually there are two papillary muscles visualized at this level, one located anterolaterally and the other posteromedially. At this level, only part of the right ventricle can usually be visualized and it will be to the left of the image.

11. Next, slide the transducer slightly toward the apex and obtain a short-axis view of the ventricles at the apex (Fig. 87-6). The interventricular septum at the apex separates the right from the left ventricle. The right ventricle is heavily trabeculated at this level. By convention, the left ventricular wall is only divided into four segments (anterior, lateral, septal, and inferior [posterior]) at this level. In the normal heart, all four segments will contract uniformly.

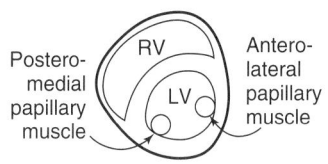

Fig. 87-5
Parasternal short-axis view of the left ventricle at the level of the papillary muscles. *LV,* Left ventricle; *RV,* right ventricle. (From Reynolds T: *The echocardiographer's pocket reference,* ed 2, Phoenix, 2000, School of Cardiac Ultrasound at Arizona Heart Institute.)

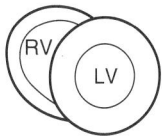

Fig. 87-6
Parasternal short-axis view at the level of the apex. *LV,* Left ventricle; *RV,* right ventricle. (From Reynolds T: *The echocardiographer's pocket reference,* ed 2, Phoenix, 2000, School of Cardiac Ultrasound at Arizona Heart Institute.)

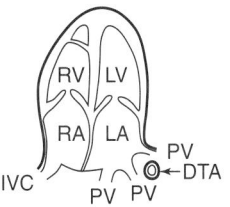

Fig. 87-7
Apical four-chamber view. *DTA,* Descending thoracic aorta; *IVC,* inferior vena cava; *LA,* left atrium; *LV,* left ventricle; *PV,* pulmonary vein; *RA,* right atrium; *RV,* right ventricle. (From Reynolds T: *The echocardiographer's pocket reference,* ed 2, Phoenix, 2000, School of Cardiac Ultrasound at Arizona Heart Institute.)

12. By moving the transducer to the apex, which can be located by palpating the PMI inferolateral to the left nipple, the apical four-chamber view can be obtained (Fig. 87-7). At this position, the majority of scanning is usually performed with the marker dot at the 4 o'clock position. Angle the transducer back up toward the base of the heart to obtain the best possible four-chamber image. To confirm the orientation while scanning, note that the septal leaflet of the tricuspid valve is closer to the apex than the anterior leaflet of the mitral valve. By convention, the tricuspid valve and the right ventricle should be on the left side of the image. If the orientation of the probe is 180 degrees from this, the mitral valve and the left ventricle will be on the left side of the image. The right ventricle can also usually be distinguished from the left ventricle because the right ventricle has the echogenic

moderator band extending from the apex to the septal wall. Again, the right ventricular wall is more trabeculated than the left ventricular wall. With this view, again observe the ventricular wall motion for uniformity of contraction. From this transducer position, observe the valves again for abnormalities.

13. Tilt the transducer slightly anteriorly, toward the anterior chest wall (tail of transducer is tilted downward slightly), from the apical four-chamber view to obtain the apical five-chamber view (Fig. 87-8). This view provides an excellent image of the left ventricular outflow tract as well as an excellent view to exclude hypertrophic obstructive cardiomyopathy.

14. Rotate the transducer ¼ turn counterclockwise and tip it slightly laterally to obtain the apical two-chamber view (Fig. 87-9). The left ventricle and atrium will be visualized, separated by the mitral valve. With this image, the full length of the inferior wall of the left ventricle can be visualized. Observe this wall, along with the anterior wall of the left ventricle, for uniform contractility.

15. Rotate the transducer counterclockwise so that the sector plane passes through the long axis of the heart to obtain the apical long-axis view (Fig. 87-10). The aortic root can be evaluated, while the aortic valve is noted to be contiguous with the base of the anterior mitral leaflet. This view is very similar to the parasternal long-axis view, but the apex is visualized from this position. With this image, the anterior interventricular septum and the inferolateral ventricular wall can be inspected for uniform contractility.

16. Moving the transducer to below the xiphoid, the subxiphoid (subcostal) four-chamber view (Fig. 87-11) can be obtained with the marker dot to the patient's left side. Usually a portion of the liver is used as a window. With this view, the apex of the heart is usually not visualized. The ventricles will be to the left side of the image and the atria to the right side. The left ventricle and atrium will be located behind (below) the right ventricle and atrium. Inspect both the mitral valve and the tricuspid valve, and observe wall motion for uniformity of contraction.

17. From the subxiphoid four-chamber view, by tilting the transducer anteriorly, visualize the aortic valve lengthwise. This will provide an image similar to that seen with the parasternal long-axis view. This technique of imaging may be very valuable if the standard parasternal long-axis image cannot be obtained because of technical difficulties.

18. From the subxiphoid four-chamber view, it is also possible to angle the transducer to visualize the entire atrial septum. This position is the most reliable for evaluating patients for atrial septal defects.

19. From the subxiphoid view, the inferior vena cava (IVC) can be imaged (Fig. 87-12) and its diameters

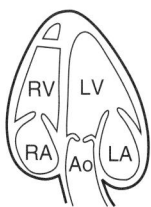

Fig. 87-8
Apical five-chamber view. *Ao,* Aortic root; *LA,* left atrium; *LV,* left ventricle; *RA,* right atrium; *RV,* right ventricle. (From Reynolds T: *The echocardiographer's pocket reference,* ed 2, Phoenix, 2000, School of Cardiac Ultrasound at Arizona Heart Institute.)

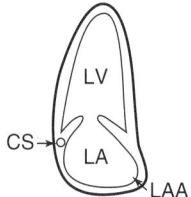

Fig. 87-9
Apical two-chamber view. *CS,* Coronary sinus; *LA,* Left atrium; *LAA,* left atrial appendage; *LV,* left ventricle. (From Reynolds T: *The echocardiographer's pocket reference,* ed 2, Phoenix, 2000, School of Cardiac Ultrasound at Arizona Heart Institute.)

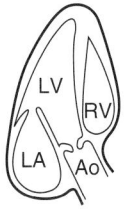

Fig. 87-10
Apical long-axis view. *Ao,* Aortic root; *LA,* left atrium; *LV,* left ventricle; *RV,* right ventricle. (From Reynolds T: *The echocardiographer's pocket reference,* ed 2, Phoenix, 2000, School of Cardiac Ultrasound at Arizona Heart Institute.)

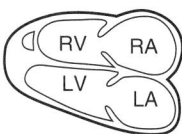

Fig. 87-11
Subxiphoid four-chamber view. *LA,* Left atrium; *LV,* left ventricle; *RA,* right atrium; *RV,* right ventricle. (From Reynolds T: *The echocardiographer's pocket reference,* ed 2, Phoenix, 2000, School of Cardiac Ultrasound at Arizona Heart Institute.)

measured. The diameter of the IVC can be used to estimate right atrial pressure (RAP). With the marker dot toward the patient's head and the transducer located in the midline, the long-axis view of the IVC can be obtained by angling slightly to the patient's right side. Normally the IVC is less than 2.0 cm in diameter and collapses more than 50% with inspiration. It will also normally collapse with pressure from the transducer. If it does not, the formula in the "Findings and Interpretation" section can be used to estimate RAP. The IVC is thin walled compared with the aorta, and it may appear to pulsate as a result of pulsations transmitted through solid tissue from the aorta. When it collapses with inspiration, these pulsations will be minimized.

20. In addition to what has been described, almost all of the parasternal short-axis views can be obtained with scanning from the subxiphoid position. However, because of the depth of tissue necessary to scan from this position, there is usually some loss of resolution. This is especially true when compared with scanning from the parasternal position.

21. Placing the transducer in the suprasternal notch with the marker dot to the patient's right side, scan the aortic arch in its long axis (Fig. 87-13) to provide what some call the "candy cane" view. With this image, the ascending aorta, its horizontal arch, and the proximal descending thoracic aorta can be visualized. The origins of the left subclavian and left carotid arteries off of the aorta can usually be visualized, and occasionally the origin of the brachiocephalic artery can be seen. The right pulmonary artery is usually noted in short-axis view beneath the arch. This is the best view for excluding coarctation of the aorta.

22. From the suprasternal view, by angling the transducer anteriorly and to the patient's right, the aortic root can often be visualized.

23. Further clockwise rotation can be used to obtain short axis views from the suprasternal notch (Fig. 87-14). The right pulmonary artery can often be visualized in this manner. The right pulmonary artery is located between the aorta and the left atrium. It may be possible to visualize where the pulmonary veins drain into the left atrium.

Note: With the incidence of abdominal aortic aneurysm (AAA) increasing (5% to 7% of individuals over the age of 60), there is a strong correlation between individuals having an AAA and having an echocardiogram for other indications. With the patient already gowned and covered with jelly, it may be an excellent opportunity to screen for an AAA, even if no one is charged for the service.

M-Mode Echocardiography

From the parasternal position, with either the long-axis or the short-axis view, M-mode images are usually obtained at three different levels: the level of the aortic valve, the level of the mitral valve and the level of the papillary muscles in the left ventricle (Fig. 87-15). The subxiphoid transducer position can also be used for M-mode scanning when there is difficulty obtaining the standard parasternal images.

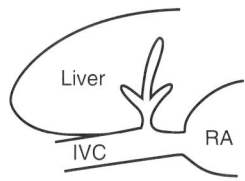

Fig. 87-12
Subxiphoid long axis of inferior vena cava. *IVC,* Inferior vena cava; *RA,* right atrium. (From Reynolds T: *The echocardiographer's pocket reference,* ed 2, Phoenix, 2000, School of Cardiac Ultrasound at Arizona Heart Institute.)

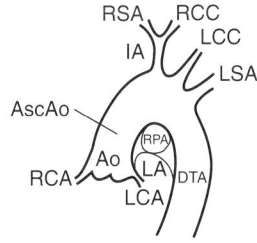

Fig. 87-13
Suprasternal notch long-axis view of aortic arch. *Ao,* Aortic root; *AscAo,* ascending aorta; *DTA,* descending thoracic aorta; *IA,* innominate artery; *LA,* left atrium; *LCA,* left coronary artery; *LCC,* left common carotid; *LSA,* left subclavian artery; *RCA,* right coronary artery; *RCC,* right common carotid; *RPA,* right pulmonary artery; *RSA,* right subclavian artery. (From Reynolds T: *The echocardiographer's pocket reference,* ed 2, Phoenix, 2000, School of Cardiac Ultrasound at Arizona Heart Institute.)

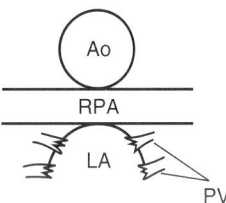

Fig. 87-14
Suprasternal notch short-axis view of aortic arch. *Ao,* Aortic root; *LA,* left atrium; *PV,* pulmonary veins; *RPA,* right pulmonary artery. (From Reynolds T: *The echocardiographer's pocket reference,* ed 2, Phoenix, 2000, School of Cardiac Ultrasound at Arizona Heart Institute.)

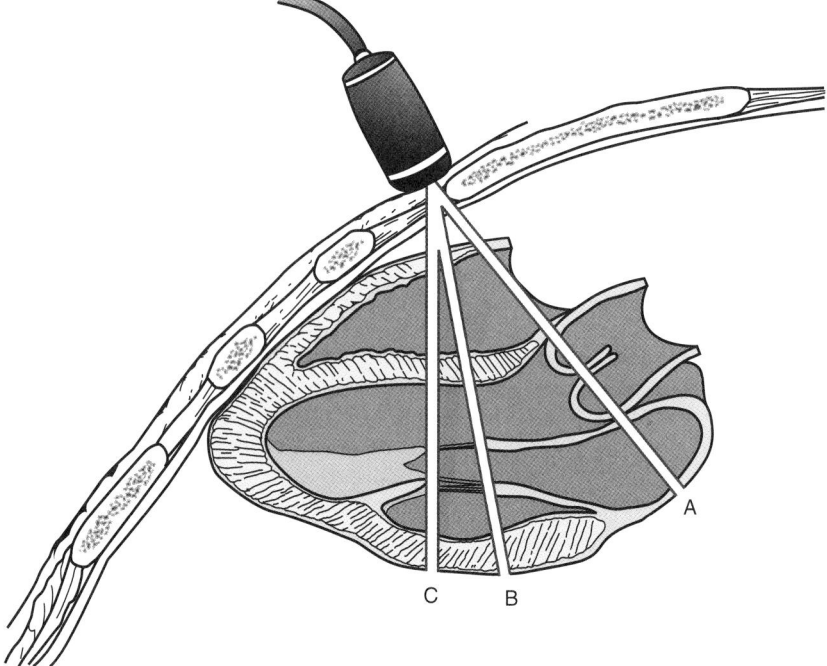

Fig. 87-15
Levels to obtain M-mode images. *A,* level of aortic valve; *B,* level of mitral valve; *C,* level of the papillary muscle. (From Reynolds T: *The echocardiographer's pocket reference,* ed 2, Phoenix, 2000, School of Cardiac Ultrasound at Arizona Heart Institute.)

1. At the mitral valve level, the anterior mitral leaflet makes an "M"-shaped pattern. The posterior leaflet moves as its mirror image to make a "W"-shaped pattern. The point of maximal early opening excursion is labeled E (Fig. 87-16). Next, the rapid filling phase of early diastole occurs, and then the valve closes partially. While it is closing partially, the valve moves along the E to F slope. Note that this slope will be flatter if there is any condition impairing left ventricular filling. The E to F slope is followed by the remainder of diastole. During this phase, the A point indicates atrial systole. After atrial systole, the valve moves to the fully closed position labeled C. The closed leaflets then move together in systole until they separate at the D point. The B point is labeled but does not exist for normal patients. It only occurs if the A to C line is interrupted due to elevated left end-diastolic pressure or diastolic dysfunction (Fig. 87-16).

   To determine the E to F slope, first draw diagonal Line 4 through Line 1 (i.e., basically a continuation of Line 1). Draw a horizontal line (Line 5) near the bottom of the tracing where Line 4 intersects one of the time lines on the tracing. Draw line 5 horizontal to the left for a distance corresponding to exactly one second on the tracing. Next, draw a vertical line (Line 6) from line 5 to where it intersects Line 4. Line 6 should be perpendicular to Line 5. The length of Line 6 in mm is the E to F slope of the anterior leaflet in mm/sec (normal range 70 to 150 mm/sec).

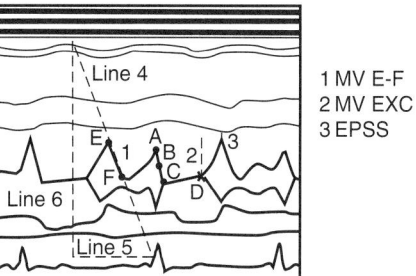

Fig. 87-16
M-mode at the level of the mitral valve. *E,* E-point (point of anterior leaflet maximal early opening); Line 1, *MV E-F* (mitral valve, E to F slope); Line 2, *MV EXC,* vertical distance, mitral valve excursion (normal range 18 to 28 mm) Line 3, EPSS [E-point septal separation (normal range 2 to 7 mm)]; *A,* atrial systole; *C,* valve fully closed; *D,* leaflets separate (valve opens). See text for explanation of lines 4, 5, and 6 and how to calculate E to F slope. (From Reynolds T: *The echocardiographer's pocket reference,* ed 2, Phoenix, 2000, School of Cardiac Ultrasound at Arizona Heart Institute.)

   The EPSS is the vertical distance between the E-point and the septal wall. It is enlarged for dilated cardiomyopathy.

2. With M-mode imaging at the aortic valve level (Fig. 87-17), typically only two aortic cusps are identified. At the onset of systole, they separate abruptly; at the end of systole they close abruptly, producing a "square box" on the image. Since normal aortic valves are very thin and often difficult to follow throughout the M-mode tracing, if the cusps are easily visualized, they may in fact be thickened. Following closure of the valve, the

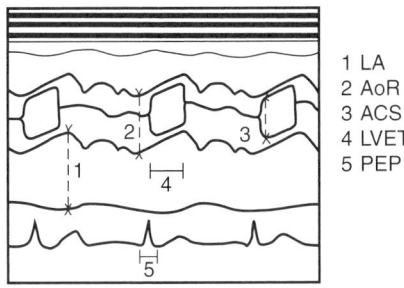

1 LA
2 AoR
3 ACS
4 LVET
5 PEP

Fig. 87-17
M-mode at the level of the aortic valve. *AoR,* aortic root end-diastolic diameter (normal range 2 to 3.7 cm); *ACS,* aortic cusps separation in systole (normal range 1.5 to 2.6 cm); *LA,* left atrium end-systolic dimension (normal range 1.9 to 4.0 cm); *LVET,* left ventricular ejection time; *PEP,* preejection period. (From Reynolds T: *The echocardiographer's pocket reference,* ed 2, Phoenix, 2000, School of Cardiac Ultrasound at Arizona Heart Institute.)

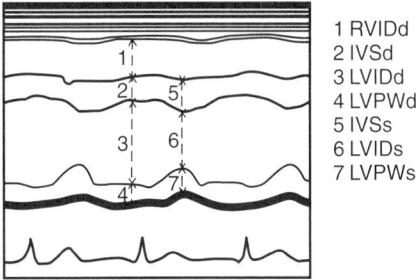

1 RVIDd
2 IVSd
3 LVIDd
4 LVPWd
5 IVSs
6 LVIDs
7 LVPWs

Fig. 87-18
M-mode at the level of the mitral valve chordae tendineae. *IVSd,* Interventricular septum thickness in diastole; *IVSs,* interventricular septum thickness in systole; *LVIDd,* left ventricular internal diameter, diastole; *LVIDs,* left ventricular internal diameter, systole; *LVPWd,* left ventricular posterior wall thickness in diastole; *LVPWs,* left ventricular posterior wall thickness in systole; *RVIDd,* right ventricular internal diameter in diastole. (From Reynolds T: *The echocardiographer's pocket reference,* ed 2, Phoenix, 2000, School of Cardiac Ultrasound at Arizona Heart Institute.)

cusps remain opposed (closed) throughout diastole. The image at the level of the aortic valve is the most difficult to obtain with M-mode. Measurements of the left atrium, the aorta and the valve cusp separation (opening diameter) are also taken at this level.

3. To obtain measurements of systolic time intervals, calipers can be used. The ejection time (LVET) is the time from the opening of the aortic valve until it closes. The preejection period (PEP) is the time from the onset of the QRS to the onset of aortic valve opening (Fig. 87-17).

4. Left ventricular measurements are best made slightly above the level of the papillary muscles, at the level of the chordae tendineae (Fig. 87-18). This is an excellent view and level for obtaining right ventricular internal dimensions as well as left ventricular systolic and diastolic dimensions. Precise measurements of the thickness of all walls can also be made, in both diastole and systole.

5. For tricuspid valves, usually only one leaflet is traced with the M-mode for normal individuals. The RVIT view is an excellent view for tracing this single tricuspid leaflet. The pattern of motion for a single leaflet is similar to that of a mitral leaflet.

6. For pulmonic valve M-mode tracings, the parasternal short axis view at the level of the aortic valve can be used. Once again, usually only one leaflet is traced for normal individuals. Since normal tricuspid cusps are very thin, it is often difficult to follow the leaflet motion throughout the cycle.

Color and Doppler Flow Echocardiography

Multiple views can be used for this application, but inevitably the apical four-chamber view provides the best view for evaluating three of the valves. The parasternal short axis view is often utilized to complete the evaluation of the valves. As each valve is being studied, the transducer should be placed so that it is as close as possible to being in line with the maximal flow across the valve. This can be guided by the 2D image, by the maximal velocity on graphic image, by maximizing the sound, or by all three. Each operator develops their own technique for performing a complete examination and he or she should follow this technique with every evaluation (Fig. 87-19). A sample technique is provided here.

1. From the apical position, evaluate the left ventricular inflow tract with PW. Next, evaluate the left ventricular outflow tract.

2. The right ventricular or tricuspid inflow tract should then be evaluated. Next, either continuing to use the apical four-chamber view or shifting to the parasternal short axis view at the level above the aortic valve, the right ventricular/pulmonic outflow tract should be evaluated.

3. Repeat the evaluation with CW.

4. If available, repeat the evaluation with color Doppler.

FINDINGS AND INTERPRETATION

A. Two-Dimensional (2D)/M-Mode

Overview of Study. The quality of every study should be described in the report (e.g., good, fair, poor). This often depends on the quality of the window, the equipment used, and the body habitus of the patient. Every report should also have at least a *qualitative* comment about the ejection fraction and segmental wall motion (e.g., normal, moderately impaired, severely impaired). These can also be measured *quantitatively:*

1. Ejection Fraction — With 2D, the ejection fraction can be calculated by summing a series of discs, if the equipment software is capable of tracing the ventricular cavity. It can also be calculated using M-mode measurements applied to Table 87-2.

$$\text{Ejection fraction} = [(EDV - ESV)/EDV] \times 100$$

End-diastolic volume (EDV) and end-systolic volume (ESV) are both obtained from Table 87-2 using the left ventricular internal diameter in diastole (LVIDd) and then the left ventricular internal diameter in systole (LVIDs) as the dimension in the table. LVIDs is measured at the lowest vertical point of the septum. (See Table 87-3 for normal ranges.)

Note: At the Arizona Heart Institute, M-mode echocardiography is no longer used for determining the ejection fraction. Instead, at the end of every 2D study, the ejection fraction is either quantitatively measured using calipers or cavity tracings or estimated as normal (60%), moderately impaired (40%), or severely impaired (20%). As it turns out, various studies have compared qualitative estimates of ejection fraction with calculated ejection fractions, especially for those patients with suboptimal imaging. Qualitative estimates have been found to be fairly accurate.

2. Segmental Wall Motion — The American Society of Echocardiography has established the convention of dividing the heart into 17 segments (see Fig. 87-20). These segments are distributed across three levels. Anything above the level of the head of the papillary muscle, where it joins the mitral leaflet, is defined as the basal level of the heart. The mid-level of the heart is defined by the entire length of the papillary muscle. Anything below the level of the base of the papillary muscle, where it attaches to the ventricular wall, is designated the apical level.

Each wall segment has a corresponding coronary artery that perfuses it. In general, the anterior and anteroseptal walls and the entire apex are supplied by the left anterior descending coronary artery (LAD). Therefore, even though the apex is divided into four segments—anterior, lateral, septal and inferior (posterior) segments—all of these segments are usually perfused by the LAD. Both the mid-level of the heart and the basal level are divided into six segments. The inferior (posterior) wall and the inferoseptal (posteroseptal) walls at the basal and mid-levels are supplied by septal perforators (posterior descending artery [PDA]) from the dominant coronary artery on the inferior (posterior) surface of the heart. The lateral walls of the ventricle (anterolateral and inferolateral [posterolateral]) above the apex are supplied by the left circumflex artery.

Wall motion in each segment is scored based on the recommendations of the American Society of Echocardiography:

> Normally contracting segment (or hyperkinetic segment) = 1
> Hypokinesia = 2
> Akinesis = 3
> Dyskinesis = 4
> Aneurysmal segment (i.e., deformed during diastole) = 5

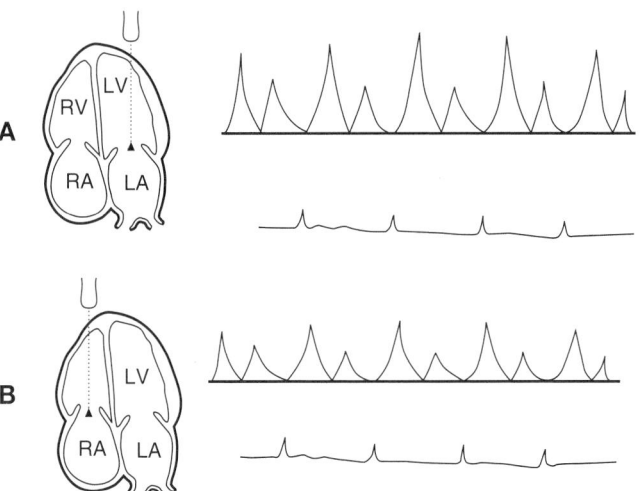

Fig. 87-19
Normal Doppler tracings. **A,** Left ventricular inflow tract (mitral valve). **B,** Right ventricular inflow tract (tricuspid valve). *LA,* Left atrium; *LV,* left ventricle; *RA,* right atrium; *RV,* right ventricle. (From Reynolds T: *The echocardiographer's pocket reference,* ed 2, Phoenix, 2000, School of Cardiac Ultrasound at Arizona Heart Institute.)

Fig. 87-20
American Society of Echocardiography 17-segment model of heart. *RV,* right ventricle; *A,* anterior; *AS,* anteroseptal; *AL,* anterolateral; *IS,* inferoseptal; *PS,* posteroseptal; *I,* inferior; *P,* posterior; *S,* septal; *L,* lateral; *LAX,* long axis. (From Reynolds T: *The echocardiographer's pocket reference,* ed 2, Phoenix, 2000, School of Cardiac Ultrasound at Arizona Heart Institute.)

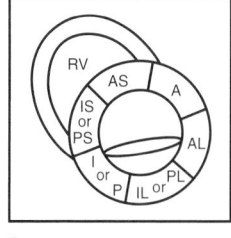

Base

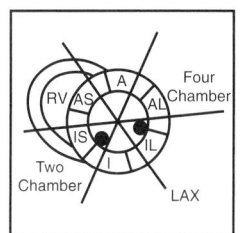

Mid

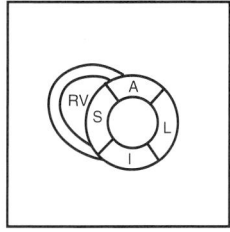

Apex

The wall motion score index is derived from the sum of all scores divided by the number of segments visualized. A normally contracting left ventricle has a wall motion score index (WMSI) of 1 (i.e., each of the 17 segments receives a wall motion score of 1; thus the total score is 17 and the WMSI is 17/17 = 1). Patients at increased risk for future cardiac events after an acute MI can be identified in part by a high WMSI (greater than or equal to 1.7).

Multiple views should be obtained with 2D to compare the wall motion between various segments and to obtain the wall motion scores. Hypokinesis is defined as a less than 30% increase in wall thickening during systole and akinesis is defined as a less than 10% increase in thickening. Dyskinesis is present when the wall moves paradoxically outward when systolic thickening should be occurring. Comments should be made about wall motion, but more importantly the walls should be scanned carefully for systolic thickening, which can be blunted by ischemia or infarction. Although wall motion scores may slightly overdiagnose the severity of an acute MI (e.g., severe ischemia can mimic an infarction), echocardiography is still much more accurate than an ECG. Of note, M-mode has limited value when scanning for ischemia.

Acute MI. In the setting of acute MI, 2D is very helpful because it provides immediate information, is noninvasive, and can be performed at the bedside. It can usually determine not only the location of the infarct, but also the extent of the infarct. Since 2D is noninvasive, serial scans can be performed to track progression. An abnormal wall motion score or evidence of a complication on 2D is valuable prognostic data. These patients should be triaged for aggressive therapy as opposed to those patients who can be safely discharged early. In comparison, when using an ECG to determine risk (either high or low), the severity or the location of the lesion cannot be predicted by ECG changes. While an ECG may be helpful for diagnosing the acuity of an infarct, 2D is usually much more helpful overall because it can be used to actually stratify the patient's risk.

Mechanical complications of an acute MI that can be diagnosed early with 2D include pericarditis, pericardial effusion, pericardial tamponade, electromechanical dissociation, ventricular aneurysm, acute ischemic cardiomyopathy, mural thrombus, rupture of a papillary muscle (posteromedial much more commonly than anterolateral), or rupture of the ventricular free wall or septum.

TABLE 87-2

Ventricular Volumes for Calculating Ejection Fraction

Ventricular volumes (EDV and ESV) calculated from ventricular dimensions (LVIDd and LVIDs, respectively), using the formula of Teichholz: $\text{Volume} = \dfrac{7}{2.4 + D} \times D^3$

Dim.	Vol.	Dim.	Vol.	Dim.	Vol.
2.0	13	4.0	70	7.0	254
2.1	14	4.1	74	7.1	265
2.2	16	4.2	79	7.2	272
2.3	18	4.3	83	7.3	280
2.4	20	4.4	88	7.4	288
2.5	22	4.5	92	7.5	300
2.6	25	4.6	97	7.6	307
2.7	27	4.7	103	7.7	315
2.8	30	4.8	107	7.8	327
2.9	31	4.9	113	7.9	336
3.0	35	5.0	118	8.0	343
3.1	38	5.1	123	8.1	356
3.2	41	5.2	129	8.2	364
3.3	44	5.3	135	8.3	372
3.4	47	5.4	142	8.4	385
3.5	51	5.5	148	8.5	393
3.6	55	5.6	155	8.6	407
3.7	59	5.7	159	8.7	415
3.8	62	5.8	166	8.8	429
3.9	66	5.9	174	8.9	439
		6.0	180		
		6.1	187		
		6.2	194		
		6.3	202		
		6.4	209		
		6.5	216		
		6.6	224		
		6.7	232		
		6.8	240		
		6.9	246		

From Teichholz LE, Cohen MV, Sonnenblick EH, Gorlin R: *N Engl J Med* 291:1220, 1974.
EDV, End-diastolic volume; *ESV,* end-systolic volume; *LVIDd,* left ventricular internal diameter in diastole; *LVIDs,* left ventricular internal diameter in systole.

Atrial Fibrillation. A left atrial dimension of greater than 4.5 cm indicates an increased risk of developing atrial fibrillation as well as a high probability of unsuccessful cardioversion. For more than twenty years, left atrial dilation in conjunction with mitral stenosis and atrial fibrillation has been associated with an increased risk of peripheral embolism and stroke. Such a finding should be managed aggressively with anticoagulate (if not contraindicated).

Note: Atrial appendage thrombi are best excluded by transesophageal echo.

Cardiac Tumors. Cardiac tumors are seen as echogenic masses and the majority (75% to 80%) of primary cardiac tumors are benign and curable. Thirty percent of benign tumors are myxomas, and they are usually attached by a stalk to the interatrial septum. They often partially or completely prolapse into the left ventricle during diastole.

Cardiac Tamponade and Pericardial Effusion. These, as well as electromechanical dissociation (EMD), are discussed in Chapter 209, Emergency Department and Office Ultrasound.

Cardiomyopathy, Dilated. Cardiomyopathy is defined as a primary disease of the myocardium and, by definition, is not due to ischemia or valvular disease. Dilated cardiomyopathy is by far the most common type of cardiomyopathy. It is characterized by dilation of all four chambers and reduced systolic function in both ventricles. Left ventricular dimensions (end-diastolic and end-systolic) and volumes are increased, whereas wall thicknesses are usually normal or slightly decreased. There will be a spherical configuration to the left ventricle with decreased left ventricular posterior wall and interventricular septal wall systolic thickening. As a result, there will be a decreased left ventricular ejection fraction. On M-Mode, the left ventricular ejection time will be shortened with a resultant prolonged PEP/LVET ratio (greater than 0.40). The distance of the anterior mitral leaflet from the septal wall (EPSS) is increased. The presence of a B-bump on the mitral valve tracing indicates increased left ventricular end-diastolic pressure (greater than 15 mm Hg). There may be pulmonary hypertension, and for an ejection fraction less than 35%, an echogenic mural thrombus (in either ventricle) must be excluded. Mitral regurgitation is present to some degree in most patients with dilated cardiomyopathy.

Cardiomyopathy, Hypertrophic. This is much less common than dilated cardiomyopathy, and is an autosomal dominantly inherited disease with variable penetrance. The hypertrophy is usually asymmetric and the interventricular septum is often involved (asymmetric septal hypertrophy [ASH]). Less commonly, the left ventricular free wall or the apex can be asymmetrically involved. ASH can also be associated with obstruction of the left ventricular outflow tract, frequently as a result of the proximity of the anterior mitral leaflet to the septal wall (hypertrophic obstructive cardiomyopathy [HOCM]). Anterior motion of this leaflet during systole (systolic anterior motion [SAM]) can be noted on real-time or M-mode to obstruct the outflow tract. Ventricular chambers are usually small. Most patients have mitral regurgitation as a result of SAM. On M-mode, midsystolic closure of the aortic valve can also be noted.

Cardiomyopathy, Restrictive (nondilated/nonhypertrophic). This is rare and is characterized by normal ventricular wall thicknesses and cavity size at initial presentation. The systolic function is normal and the heart failure is due to a stiff, hypertrophied ventricle with resultant impaired diastolic function. Biatrial enlargement is usually noted. The etiology is usually a fibrotic or infiltrative process such as hemochromatosis, sarcoidosis, of hypereosinophilic syndrome. As the disease progresses, the patient can develop a dilated cardiomyopathy. Although amyloid heart has a separate definition than fibrotic or restrictive, it can appear very similar on echocardiography. It is common to find an associated pericardial effusion with amyloid heart.

Ischemic Heart Disease. Ischemic heart disease is assessed by looking at (1) global ventricular function (quantified with an ejection fraction) and (2) segmental wall function. Both should be assessed because both ischemia and infarction can cause significant segmental wall dysfunction without markedly impacting the ejection fraction.

Left Ventricular Hypertrophy (LVH). A common cause is hypertensive heart disease, initially with concentric hypertrophy, increased left ventricular mass, impaired diastolic function and normal systolic function. As LVH progresses toward end stage heart disease, systolic dysfunction develops and the left ventricle dilates. The left atrium will eventually dilate because of decreased left ventricular compliance and possibly mitral regurgitation. (A left atrial dimension greater than 4.5 cm indicates an increased risk of developing atrial fibrillation.) Frequently, the aortic root will dilate and there will be associated aortic valve sclerosis. There may also be mitral annular calcification.

Concentric Hypertrophy. There is an equally distributed (uniform or globular) increase in ventricular wall thicknesses with normal ventricular dimensions (e.g., patients with valvular aortic stenosis or systemic hypertension). Left ventricular mass can be calculated to follow progression of LVH (Table 87-3).

Eccentric Hypertrophy. Commonly seen with aortic or mitral regurgitation, there is a spherical configuration to the left ventricle with normal wall thicknesses.

Mitral Valve Prolapse (MVP). In past years, MVP was over-diagnosed with echocardiography. As a result, a more formal definition was developed. Since the mitral valve, when closed, bulges normally or is "saddle-shaped" in the plane of the mitral annulus, true prolapse should only be diagnosed if a portion of the anterior leaflet prolapses beyond this plane. By new criteria, it must prolapse more than 2 mm beyond the mitral annular plane on the parasternal long-axis view or more than 1 cm on the apical four-chamber view. Posterior

TABLE 87-3

Normal M-Mode Measurements

	Mean	Range
Mitral Valve		
E-F slope	80 mm/sec	70-150 mm/sec
D-E excursion	20 mm	18-28 mm
EPSS	5 mm	2-7 mm
Aortic Root and Valve		
Root diameter	2.7 cm	2.0-3.7 cm
Root index	1.5 cm/m^2	1.2-2.2 cm/m^2
Valve systolic separation	1.9 cm	1.5-2.6 cm
Left Atrium (LA)		
LA diameter	2.9 cm	1.9-4.0 cm
LA index	1.6 cm/m^2	1.2-2.2 cm/m^2
LA/Ao ratio	1.0	0.87-1.11
Left Ventricle		
LVIDd	4.7 cm	3.7-5.6 cm
LVIDd index	2.6 cm/m^2	1.9-3.2 cm/m^2
LVIDs	3.1 cm	2.0-3.8 cm
LVIDs index	1.6 cm/m^2	1.3-1.9 cm/m^2
Interventricular Septum (IVS) and Left Ventricular Posterior Wall (LVPW)		
IVS diastolic thickness	0.9 cm	0.6-1.1 cm
IVS excursion	0.7 cm	0.44-1.2 cm
LVPW diastolic thickness	0.9 cm	0.6-1.1 cm
LVPW excursion	1.2 cm	0.9-1.4 cm
Maximum velocity of LVPW excursion	61 mm/sec	40-78 mm/sec
IVS/LVPW ratio	<1.3:1.0	<1.5:1.0 hypertensive patient
Right Ventricle (RV)		
RVIDd (left lateral)	1.7 cm	0.9-2.6 cm
RVIDd index	0.9 cm/m^3	0.4-2.5 cm/m^2
RVIDs	1.8 cm	1.5-2.2 cm
RVIDs index	0.9 cm/m^2	0.7-1.1 cm/m^2
RV free wall excursion	0.9 cm	0.7-1.0 cm
RV free wall systolic thickening	50	30-38
RV velocity of systolic free wall excursion	41 mm/sec	36-55 mm/sec
RV wall thickness		0.5-0.8 cm
Pulmonary Valve		
"a" dip		2-7 mm
E-F slope		6-115 mm/sec
Left Ventricular Systolic Function		
IVS % thickening [a]	46%	27%-70%
LVPW % thickening[b]	45%	25%-80%
Fractional shortening [c]	33%	28%-41%
Ejection fraction [d]	62%	45%-90%
Mean circumferential fiber shortening [e]	1.2 circ/sec	1.0-1.9 circ/sec
Relative wall thickness [f]	37	30-45

[a] IVS % thickening = [(IVSs − IVSd) + IVSd] × 100
[b] LVPW % thickening = [(LVPWs − LVPWd) + LVPWd] × 100
[c] Fractional shortening = [(LVIDd − LVIDs) + LVIDd] × 100
[d] Ejection fraction = [(EDV − ESV) / EDV] × 100
[e] Mean Vcf = (LVIDd − LVIDs) + (LVIDd × LVET)
[f] Relative wall thickness = 2 × LVPWd + LVIDd or IVSd + LVPWd + LVIDd

Left Ventricular Mass

American Society of Echocardiography

$$1.04\,[(LVIDd + IVSd + LVPWd)^2 - (LVIDd^2)] \times 0.8 + 0.6\ g$$

Penn Convention

$$1.04\,[(LVIDd + IVSd + LVPWd)^2 - (LVIDd^2)] - 13.6\ g$$

From Reynolds T: *The echocardiographer's pocket reference,* ed 2, Phoenix, 2000, School of Cardiac Ultrasound at Arizona Heart Institute.
Ao, Aortic root; *EDV,* end-diastolic volume; *EPSS,* E-point septal separation; *ESV,* end-systolic volume; *IVS,* interventricular septum; *LA,* left atria; *LVIDd,* left ventricular internal diameter in diastole; *LVIDs,* left ventricular internal diameter in systole; *LVPW,* left ventricular posterior wall; *RVIDd,* right ventricular internal diameter in diastole; *RVIDs,* right ventricular internal diameter in systole.

leaflet prolapse is diagnosed if any of the leaflet prolapses beyond the mitral annular plane in the parasternal long-axis view, the apical four-chamber view, or by more than 2 mm on the apical two-chamber view. The mitral annular plane is defined by drawing an imaginary line from the base of the anterior leaflet to the base of the posterior leaflet.

Myxomatous degeneration is the result of an increase in the middle layer of the valve, the spongiosa. With proliferation, the spongiosa replaces part of the fibrosa layer and the valve is weakened. Eventually, the valve becomes thickened, redundant, and elongated. In fact, it can develop the physical appearance of a hemorrhoid in its short-axis view. Myxomatous degeneration is usually diagnosed with 2D echocardiography; however, the thickness of the valve can be measured with either 2D or M-mode. The leaflets are considered redundant if they are 5 mm or more thick on the parasternal long-axis view during diastole, or more than 1.4 times the wall thickness of the posterior wall of the aorta during diastole. On M-mode, the thickness is considered abnormal if 5 mm or greater.

B. Preliminary 2D/M-Mode Scanning Before Using Color and Doppler Flow

Diastolic function is best determined with color and Doppler flow imaging. As mentioned previously, color and Doppler flow imaging also assist with determining the hemodynamic severity of lesions and are therefore helpful for assessing valvular abnormalities. Color-flow Doppler also produces jets that are characteristic for certain abnormalities. Eccentric jets are very helpful for aligning continuous wave (CW) Doppler when attempting to optimize the spectrum. Such spectrum analysis is helpful for further quantifying regurgitant lesions.

Note: When assessing tricuspid valve regurgitation (TR) with color and Doppler flow imaging, note that TR is very common (90% of population). As a result, the regurgitation itself does not always need to be assessed. More importantly, the severity of the tricuspid regurgitation can be used to determine right-sided atrial and ventricular pressures. Pulmonary valve regurgitation is less common than TR and mitral regurgitation is much less common. Aortic valve regurgitation is somewhat rare and its presence is always considered pathological.

Despite the fact that the disorders below are best scanned with color and Doppler flow imaging, some information is usually obtained with preliminary 2D/M-mode scanning before using Doppler.

Aortic Stenosis. Aortic stenosis (AS) is usually the result of either rheumatic heart disease or a bicuspid valve. With *rheumatic/degenerative aortic stenosis,* the aortic cusps are usually thickened and there is associated concentric left ventricular hypertrophy, a dilated aortic root, a dilated left atrium, mitral annular calcification (50%), and a decreased mitral valve E-F slope.

As discussed earlier, the most common abnormality in adult echocardiography is a bicuspid aortic valve. With AS resulting from a *bicuspid valve,* thickened leaflets are often noted as well as the characteristic oval shape to the valve opening. All of the findings of rheumatic/degenerative AS are also seen except for the mitral annular calcification.

Aortic Regurgitation. With aortic regurgitation, all of the findings of bicuspid aortic stenosis can be seen except that the aortic root may not be dilated. Additional findings include premature closure of the mitral valve and premature opening of the aortic valve. Ventricular hypertrophy may be noted, either the eccentric or the globular type. There may also be an anatomic reason for the regurgitation (e.g., ascending aortic aneurysm, bicuspid aortic valve, valvular vegetation).

Mitral Stenosis. Mitral stenosis causes a decreased E-F slope and a decreased A wave on the M-mode tracing. The mitral leaflets may be thickened or they may be noted to have decreased mobility. In addition, the mitral valve opening orifice may be decreased, giving it the appearance of a "fish mouth" on 2D. The clinician should attempt to determine the degree of commissural and subvalvular involvement with the stenosis and scan for calcification of either the valve or the annulus. Possible associated findings include atrial dilation, a steep A-C slope, pulmonary hypertension, or an atrial septal defect. If the atrium is dilated, the clinician should scan for the presence of an echogenic thrombus. There may be right ventricular hypertrophy or dilation and evidence of right-sided volume overload. Clinicians should also scan for involvement of other valves. Doppler is needed to determine the orifice opening diameter when the leaflets are densely calcified, when there is an inadequate parasternal short axis image, when there has been a surgical commissurotomy, or when there is extensive subvalvular involvement (e.g., a secondary orifice located below the valve).

Mitral Regurgitation. With mitral regurgitation, there is usually echocardiographic evidence of left atrial and left ventricular volume overload patterns, as well as an associated right-sided overload pattern. Pulmonary hypertension may be noted. LVH may be present, and serial scans may be needed to monitor the progression of LVH. In addition, the mitral annulus may be dilated (normal 2.3 ± 0.5 cm) on the apical four-chamber view. There may be an anatomic basis for the regurgitation; myxomatous degeneration of the valve with subsequent prolapse is the leading cause for regurgitation in

TABLE 87-4
Normal Echo Measurements

Measurement	TTE
A. Normal Values of the Right Heart Chambers by TTE	
RV anteroposterior, diastole (cm)	2.5-3.8
RV anteroposterior, systole (cm)	2.0-3.4
RV mediolateral, diastole (cm)	2.1-4.2
RV mediolateral, systole (cm)	1.9-3.1
RV area, diastole (cm^2)	11-36
RV area, systole (cm^2)	5-20
RV ejection fraction (%)	> 40
RV free-wall thickness (mm)	2-5
RV outflow tract, systole (cm)	1.8-3.4
RA anteroposterior, systole (cm)	—
RA mediolateral, systole (cm)	2.9-4.6
RA volume (mL)	15-58 in men, 14-44 in women
RA area (cm^2)	8.3-19.5
B. Normal Measurements of the Left Heart Valves and Great Vessels	
Mitral valve area (cm^2)	4-6
Mitral annulus, diastole (cm)	2.0-3.4
Mitral leaflets thickness (mm)	≤ 4
Mitral regurgitation (overall %)	38-45
Pulmonary veins (mm)	8-15
Aortic valve area (cm^2)	3-5
Aortic annulus, systole (cm)	1.4-2.6
Aortic regurgitation (overall %)	0-2
Aortic root sinuses, diastole (cm)	2.1-3.5
Aortic root tubule, diastole (cm)	1.7-3.4
Aortic arch (cm)	2.0-3.6
Descending aorta (cm)	2.0-2.5
C. Normal Measurements of the Right Heart Valves and Great Vessels	
Tricuspid valve area (cm^2)	4-6
Tricuspid annulus, diastole (cm)	2.0-4.0
Tricuspid leaflet thickness (cm)	≤ 4
Tricuspid regurgitation (overall %)	15-78
Superior vena cava (cm)—	
Proximal inferior vena cava (cm)	1.2-2.3
Hepatic vein (cm)	0.5-1.1
Coronary sinus (cm)	—
Pulmonic valve area (cm^2)	3-5
Pulmonic valve annulus (cm)	1.0-2.2
Pulmonic regurgitation (overall %)	28-88
Right ventricular outflow tract, systole	1.8-3.4
Main pulmonary artery	1.0-2.9
Right or left pulmonary artery	0.7-1.7
D. Normal Values of the Left Heart Chambers by TTE	
LV anteroposterior, diastole (cm)	3.5-5.7
LV anteroposterior, systole (cm)	2.5-4.3
LV mediolateral, diastole (cm)	3.7-5.6
LV mediolateral, systole (cm)	2.5-4.8
LV volume, diastole (mL)	59-157
LV volume, systole (mL)	16-68
LV area, diastole (cm^2)	18-47
LV area, systole (cm^2)	8-32
LV fractional shortening (%)	30-35
LV ejection fraction (%)	≥ 55
LV interventricular septal thickness, diastole (cm)	0.6-1.1
LV posterior wall thickness, diastole (cm)	0.6-1.0
LV mass (g)	< 294 in men, < 198 in women
LV outflow tract, systole (cm)	1.8-3.4
LA anteroposterior, systole (cm)	2.2-4.1
LA mediolateral, systole (cm)	2.5-4.5
LA volume (mL)	20-77 in men, 15-59 in women
LA area (cm^2)	9-23
LA appendage length (cm)	—
LA appendage diameter (cm)	—

From Reynolds T: The Echocardiographer's Pocket Reference, ed. 2. School of Cardiac Ultrasound at Arizona Heart Institute, Phoenix, 2000.
LA, Left atrial; *LV*, left ventricular; *RA*, right atrial; *RV*, right ventricular; *TTE*, transthoracic echocardiography.

the United States, but flail leaflets, annular calcification, or LV dysfunction (e.g., from ischemia) can be noted. The clinician should scan carefully to exclude flail leaflets.

Pulmonary Hypertension. With pulmonary hypertension, right atrial pressure (RAP) will be elevated. The dimensions of the IVC can be used to estimate RAP.

	RAP (mm Hg)
IVC <2.0 cm diameter and collapses >50% with inspiration	5
IVC <2.0 cm diameter and collapses <50% with inspiration	10
IVC >2.0 cm diameter and collapses <50% with inspiration	15
IVC >2.0 cm diameter and does not collapse with inspiration	20

With pulmonary hypertension, there will also usually be evidence of right ventricular hypertrophy (>8 mm thickness), especially if it is chronic. This hypertrophy may cause impingement on the left ventricle, resulting in a D-shaped left ventricle. The right atria and pulmonary artery may also be dilated. The interatrial septum may be deviated toward the left atrium.

On M-mode, mitral valve disease may be diagnosed. Paradoxical septal motion as well as an increased septal wall thickness may be noted. There will also be abnormalities of the pulmonic valve cusp motion.

Tricuspid Regurgitation. With TR, there is usually evidence of a right ventricular volume overload pattern, including right atrial dilation. A "B bump" of the anterior tricuspid leaflet is often noted on M-mode. The tricuspid valve annulus may be dilated (≥3.4 cm diameter in systole, ≥3.2 cm in diastole). There may be signs of pulmonary hypertension. For regurgitation, there may be an anatomic etiology (e.g., valvular vegetation, ruptured chordae tendineae).

Tricuspid Stenosis. With tricuspid stenosis, thickened valve leaflets may be noted. The right atrium is usually dilated as well as the IVC (normal 1.2 to 2.3 cm) on M-mode. There will be decreased tricuspid valve excursion (D-E) and a decreased or absent A wave of the anterior leaflet.

C. Color & Doppler Flow

A complete listing of all of the possible findings and interpretation with color and Doppler flow imaging is beyond the scope of this book. However, there are some rules of thumb:
1. Any velocity greater than 2 m/sec in the heart must be explained. Something as simple as a hyperdynamic

heart from anemia can cause it; however, pathologic causes should be excluded.
2. The Bernoulli equation can be used to determine pressure drops across values

$$\Delta P \text{ mm Hg} = 4 \times [\text{velocity (M/sec)}]^2$$

3. An approximation for right ventricular systolic pressure (RVSP) is

$$\text{RVSP (mm Hg)} = \Delta P \text{ [tricuspid valve (mm Hg)]} + 10 \text{ mm Hg}$$

The actual method of calculating RSVP is

$$\text{RSVP (mm Hg)} = 4 \times (\text{TR peak velocity})^2 + \text{RAP}$$

TR = tricuspid regurgitation
RAP = right arterial pressure (estimated in the "Pulmonary Hypertension" section); for most patients, RAP ≅ 10 mm Hg
4. Normal aortic and pulmonic valves produce a "bullet-shaped" pattern on spectral analysis. Normal mitral and tricuspid valves produce an "M-shaped" pattern on spectral analysis.
5. Laminar flow produces linear spectral analyses but turbulent flow fills in the area under the curve. Regurgitant flow is always turbulent.
6. With color Doppler, a green hue indicates turbulent flow. Highly turbulent flow is mosaic in appearance.

COMPLICATIONS

- Failure to provide an adequate scan
- Failure to diagnose

SUPPLIERS

There are several manufacturers with a range of products from the very sophisticated to the very basic. Small hand-held machines are now available. Biosound Esaote, General Electric Medical, Medison, Phillips, Acuson Siemens, and Toshiba all offer a range of devices from hand-held to research oriented (see the "Suppliers" section in Chapter 173, Obstetric Ultrasound, for the internet and mailing addresses as well as the phone numbers for many manufacturers). An excellent way to review the equipment is to visit the company websites. Used equipment is also available, but the cost and inconvenience of service and repairs is often a disadvantage.

Overreading services
Overread.com
Pleasanton, CA
Phone: 1-925-426-3111
Website: www.overread.com

CPT/BILLING CODES

93307	Echocardiography, transthoracic, real-time with image documentation (2D) with or without M-mode recording; complete
93308	Follow-up or limited study

ICD-9-CM DIAGNOSTIC CODES

427.31	Atrial fibrillation
441.09	Aortic dissection- thoracic
424.1	Aortic stenosis
402.11	Hypertension, benign, with CHF
429.3	Cardiomegaly
425.4	Cardiomyopathy, NOS
425.5	Cardiomyopathy, alcoholic
429.1	Cardiomyopathy, arteriosclerotic
434.1	Cerebral embolism
435.8	Cerebral ischemia, transient
786.50	Chest pain, unspecified
428.0	Congestive heart failure, acute
428.1	Congestive heart failure, left
414.00	Coronary atherosclerosis
402.1	Heart disease or hypertensive LVH due to benign hypertension
423.0	Hemopericardium
424.0	Mitral valve prolapse
394.0	Mitral stenosis
429.79	Mural thrombus (atrial, ventricular) acquired following myocardial infarction
410.90	Myocardial infarction, acute, unspecified site and episode
214.2	Myxolipoma, intrathoracic organs
785.1	Palpitations
423.9	Pericardial effusion, tamponade heart, or unspecified disease of pericardium
420.90	Pericardial effusion, acute
420.99	Pericarditis, acute, purulent
420.91	Pericarditis, acute, idiopathic
416.0	Pulmonary hypertension, primary, chronic
416.8	Pulmonary hypertension, secondary, chronic
435.9	Transient ischemic attack

BIBLIOGRAPHY

Otto CM: *Textbook of clinical echocardiography,* ed 2, Philadelphia, 2000, WB Saunders.

Reynolds T: *The echocardiographer's pocket reference,* ed 2, Phoenix, 2000, School of Cardiac Ultrasound at Arizona Heart Institute.

CHAPTER 88

Pericardiocentesis

Edward A. Rose
Karen E. Wilson

Pericardiocentesis is a procedure performed to extract fluid from the pericardial space for diagnostic or therapeutic purposes. It was first described in 1840, and a blind-approach technique with a trocar was used. By the end of the nineteenth century, the trocar-and-cannula method was commonly used. Currently, the most common method involves puncture with a 2- to 5-inch needle under ultrasonic guidance, followed by introduction of a pigtail catheter over a Seldinger wire. Although sedation may be helpful, the procedure can be performed in the conscious patient.

It must be emphasized that when performed on an elective basis, pericardiocentesis is best performed under ultrasonic guidance. The use of ultrasound (see Chapter 209, Emergency Department and Office Ultrasound), or alternatively fluoroscopy, can reduce the complication rate from between 15% and 20% to between 0.5% and 3.7%. In the case of emergent pericardiocentesis (if the clinician anticipates a delay before ultrasound is available and the patient is too unstable to transport or to wait for the pericardiocentesis), puncture should be performed using a spinal needle under the guidance of an electrocardiogram (ECG).

Whereas a small amount of serous fluid is normally present within the pericardium, pericardial effusions result from the accumulation of a significant amount of blood (usually resulting from trauma) or other fluid (e.g., infection, neoplasm). Hemopericardium is usually an acute process resulting from blunt or penetrating trauma, but it may also result from coagulopathies, ventricular rupture, aortic dissection, treatment of pericarditis (misdiagnosed as myocardial infarction) with anticoagulants or thrombolytics, or insertion or removal of an epicardial pacemaker or defibrillator wires. Acute hemopericardium can result in rapid cardiac tamponade followed by death if the diagnosis is not made rapidly and treated emergently. Nonhemorrhagic effusions have a number of causes, including uremia, neoplasm, and infectious agents. Because these effusions often accumulate slowly, the relatively stiff pericardium has time to stretch its capacity from the normal 25 to 35 ml to hold as much as 2000 ml of fluid. In this situation, the need for performance of pericardiocentesis may not be as urgent.

The degree of urgency for pericardiocentesis is usually dependent upon whether there is tamponade. Symptoms of cardiac tamponade include dyspnea or orthopnea, altered mental status from decreased perfusion, diaphoresis, chest pain sometimes referred to the intrascapular area, and right upper quadrant pain from hepatic congestion. Possible findings on the physical examination include distended jugular veins, tachypnea, tachycardia, muffled heart sounds (although these can also be normal), a weak or dull apical pulse, lateral displacement of the cardiac apex, hepatojugular reflux or hepatomegaly from venous congestion, narrowed pulse pressure, pulsus paradoxus (greater than 10 mm Hg). There may be decreased voltage or electrical alternans on an ECG. A chest radiograph may reveal an increased cardiac silhouette, even when compared with a very recent x-ray film.

Diagnostic pericardiocentesis is elective and should be performed with ultrasonic guidance. Therapeutic pericardiocentesis is usually more urgent and may be performed blind with ECG assistance. Pericardiocentesis is not a definitive treatment for acute hemopericardium but rather a temporizing modality, because the blood usually reaccumulates rapidly. Thoracotomy with pericardiectomy is usually required for definitive diagnosis and treatment. An unstable clinical status and some or all of the findings from above are indications for emergent pericardiocentesis.

INDICATIONS

Diagnostic Indication

- To determine the cause or to confirm the presence of a pericardial effusion. Possible causes include autoimmune disorders (lupus), tuberculosis or other bacterial infections, hemopericardium, malignancy, etc. Pericardiocentesis may also help differentiate between radiation and metastatic pericarditis.

Therapeutic Indication

• Relief of cardiac tamponade

CONTRAINDICATIONS

• None: Although there are no absolute contraindications to pericardiocentesis, it should be avoided (given its high complication rate) if better, safer alternatives exist.

Relative Contraindication

• Ultrasound or fluoroscopy unavailable for an elective procedure, because the complication rate increases dramatically for blind procedures.

EQUIPMENT

• 10% povidone-iodine solution
• Sterile gloves
• Sterile fenestrated drape
• Sterile gown
• Mask and any needed equipment for universal blood and body fluid precautions
• Intravenous (IV) line in place
• Cardiac monitoring
• 5 ml 1% plain Lidocaine with at least a 1½-inch needle
• Sterile ECG monitoring cord with alligator clip (attached to any single precordial [V_1 to V_6] lead, although V_5 is best)
• Aspirating syringes (10 to 20 ml and 60 ml)
• 7.5- to 12.5-cm, 16- to 18-gauge spinal needle with obturator, *or* 7.5- to 12.5-cm, 18-gauge, Teflon-sheathed intracatheter needle
• Sterile dressings and antiseptic ointment
• Specimen-collecting tubes for fluid analysis and cultures
• Prepackaged pericardiocentesis set that includes the following:
  — Needle for puncture
  — Seldinger wire
  — Dilator
  — Catheter guide
  — Pigtail catheter

PREPROCEDURE EVALUATION

For a clinically stable patient with a slowly accumulating pericardial effusion, an echocardiogram may confirm the diagnosis of pericardial effusion (see Chapter 209, Emergency Department and Office Ultrasound); however, the cause of that effusion may need to be established. Preprocedure laboratory studies may include the following:

• Complete blood count (CBC) with platelet count
• Sedimentation rate or C-reactive protein
• Blood urea nitrogen (BUN), creatinine, TSH
• Antinuclear antibodies (ANA) and skin testing for tuberculosis, blood cultures
• Prothrombin time, partial thromboplastin time, and international normalized ratio

If a cause can be identified noninvasively for a pericardial effusion that is not life threatening, a treatment trial is usually indicated. Inflammatory pericarditis with effusion usually responds to antiinflammatories, either IV Decadron or oral steroids, or for mild cases, nonsteroidal antiinflammatory drugs (NSAIDs). If the cause cannot be determined, diagnostic pericardiocentesis under ultrasonic guidance should be performed. Ultrasound can identify the area of greatest fluid accumulation, guiding the selection of the puncture site. It can also guide the angle and depth of puncture. An ECG before the procedure can rule out arrhythmias and be helpful for comparison with tracings made during and after the procedure tracings. Assessment of vital signs is critical to ensure that this is indeed an elective rather than an urgent or emergent procedure. Conscious sedation may be indicated for the alert patient.

Efforts to stabilize patients with cardiac tamponade include aggressive treatment with IV fluids and parenteral inotropic medications to increase ventricular-filling pressures. Preload-reducing agents, such as nitrates and diuretics, will worsen this condition and are contraindicated. They may even be fatal.

PREPROCEDURE PATIENT PREPARATION

In the emergent or urgent situation, there may be little or no time to educate the patient. In fact, attempts to educate the patient may delay this much-needed procedure. However, the patient who is awake and undergoing the procedure on an elective, diagnostic basis warrants informed consent. (See the sample patient consent form titled "Pericardiocentesis" on page 1839 of Appendix G.) This patient should be told that there are risks associated with this procedure, even the risk of serious injury or death (see the "Complications" section). Alternatives, if there are any, should be discussed with the patient. Signed, informed consent should be obtained. Antiplatelet and anticoagulant medications should be discontinued for an appropriate time preoperatively. During the procedure, every attempt should be made to maintain a sterile environment and to monitor cardiac function diligently.

The patient should strive to remain as still as possible, because the sharp needle will be advanced toward a target that is constantly in motion. There may be pain at the initial puncture and a sharper chest pain when the pericardium is pierced. Any other unusual symptoms should be reported immediately during the procedure. (See the sample patient education handout titled "Pericardiocentesis" on page 1837 of Appendix G.)

TECHNIQUE

1. Elevate the head of the bed to 45 degrees if the patient's clinical condition allows. If the abdomen is distended, decompress with nasogastric suctioning.
2. The sterile ECG cord with an alligator clip should be attached to any one of the precordial (V_1 to V_6, although V_5 is best) leads by the nonalligator clip end. The rest of the cord, including the alligator clip, is then placed on the sterile field to clip to the pericardiocentesis needle.
3. Prepare the entire lower chest and epigastric area with Betadine.
4. Select the best approach:
   - *Parasternal:* Needle is inserted perpendicular to the skin in the left fifth intercostal space medial to the border of cardiac dullness. Penetration immediately lateral to the sternum minimizes the risk of laceration of the internal mammary artery.
   - *Subxiphoid:* Needle is inserted between the xiphoid process and the left lower costal margin at a 30- to 45-degree angle to the skin. To minimize the risk of injury to the right atrium, aim toward the left shoulder (Fig. 88-1, *A*)
5. Anesthetize the skin at the puncture site and along the planned needle track. Because the pericardium is very sensitive, it too should be anesthetized.
6. When using the spinal needle, the obturator is left in place during skin puncture. The obturator is then removed and an aspirating syringe attached.
7. Begin ECG monitoring by attaching the alligator clip of the sterile ECG cord to the metal hub of the needle. Select the appropriate precordial lead channel on the ECG machine and monitor for current of injury (sudden ST and T wave elevation, PR elevation, or premature ventricular contractions).
8. Slowly advance the needle and syringe while gently aspirating with the syringe. The needle will penetrate the pericardium at a depth of about 6 to 8 cm below the skin (in adults) (Fig. 88-1, *B*). Sometimes a discrete *pop* may be felt as the needle enters the pericardial space. The patient who is awake may complain of a sharp chest pain as this occurs.
9. When pericardial fluid is obtained, the needle should not be advanced further (Fig. 88-1, *C*).
10. If a current of injury is noted on the ECG, the needle should be withdrawn a few millimeters until the injury pattern resolves.
11. Pericardial fluid can be withdrawn using the needle-and-syringe combination, or an indwelling catheter can be placed. To place the catheter, while continuously monitoring the ECG, a guidewire is passed through the needle; then a dilator is passed over the wire to expand the tract. A pigtail catheter can then be passed over the guide wire (Fig. 88-1, *D*) and into the pericardial space. Fluoroscopy can be very helpful during this step.
12. Secure the catheter to the chest wall in the preferred manner. Apply a sterile dressing.
13. Aspirate as much fluid as possible, then connect the catheter to continuous or intermittent drainage (Fig. 88-1, *E*).
14. Fluid should be sent to the laboratory for chemical, cytologic, and microbiologic analysis. Testing of the fluid is similar to testing pleural fluid: cell count and differential, glucose, total protein (i.e., body fluid/serum ratio), lactate dehydrogenase, pH, appearance (i.e., clear or cloudy), color, Gram's stain and culture, acid-fast bacillus stain and culture, fungal culture, and cytology.
15. For tamponade, successful aspiration of fluid (even the first, relatively small aliquot) should result in rapid improvement in blood pressure and cardiac output, with a decrease in atrial and pericardial pressures, a simultaneous decrease in the degree of any paradoxic pulse, and a decrease or disappearance of electrical alternans. Regardless of indication for pericardiocentesis, obtain a portable chest radiograph immediately after the procedure to rule out a pneumothorax. A repeat ultrasound at 24 hours may help to diagnose reaccumulation of fluid.

COMPLICATIONS

- Pneumothorax, hemothorax, or both
- Myocardial laceration
- Coronary artery laceration
- Liver laceration
- Dysrhythmias
- Air embolism
- Vasovagal reaction from pericardial irritation leading to bradycardia and rarely to asystole

The clinician should be aware that the pericardiocentesis needle can injure anything within its reach, causing a pneumothorax, a myocardial laceration, a coronary artery laceration, a liver laceration, etc. Air embolism can occur, as well as arrhythmias related to epicardial injury. Ultrasonic and fluoroscopic guidance have reduced the

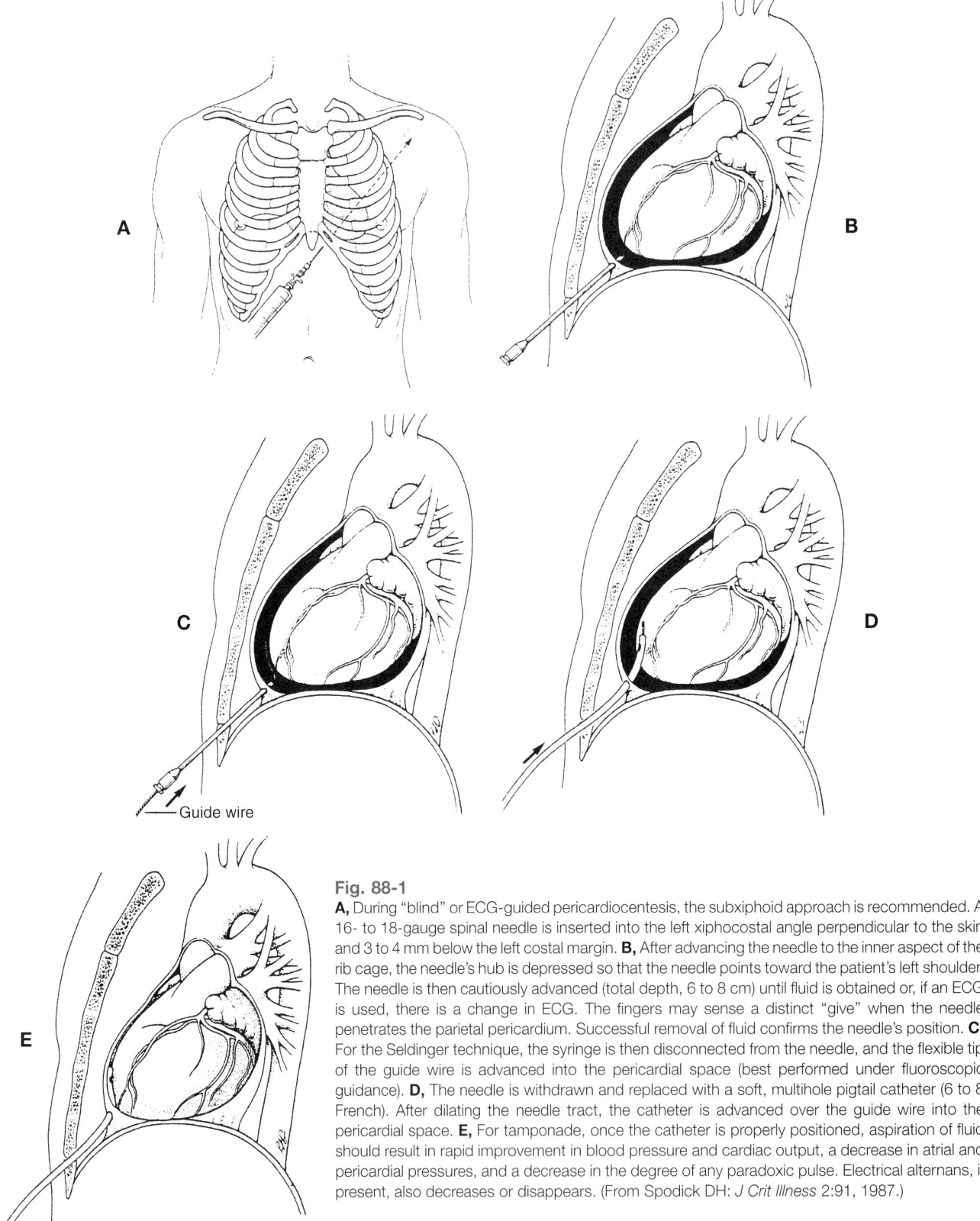

Fig. 88-1
A, During "blind" or ECG-guided pericardiocentesis, the subxiphoid approach is recommended. A 16- to 18-gauge spinal needle is inserted into the left xiphocostal angle perpendicular to the skin and 3 to 4 mm below the left costal margin. **B,** After advancing the needle to the inner aspect of the rib cage, the needle's hub is depressed so that the needle points toward the patient's left shoulder. The needle is then cautiously advanced (total depth, 6 to 8 cm) until fluid is obtained or, if an ECG is used, there is a change in ECG. The fingers may sense a distinct "give" when the needle penetrates the parietal pericardium. Successful removal of fluid confirms the needle's position. **C,** For the Seldinger technique, the syringe is then disconnected from the needle, and the flexible tip of the guide wire is advanced into the pericardial space (best performed under fluoroscopic guidance). **D,** The needle is withdrawn and replaced with a soft, multihole pigtail catheter (6 to 8 French). After dilating the needle tract, the catheter is advanced over the guide wire into the pericardial space. **E,** For tamponade, once the catheter is properly positioned, aspiration of fluid should result in rapid improvement in blood pressure and cardiac output, a decrease in atrial and pericardial pressures, and a decrease in the degree of any paradoxic pulse. Electrical alternans, if present, also decreases or disappears. (From Spodick DH: *J Crit Illness* 2:91, 1987.)

incidence of complications significantly. Even with such aids available, ultrasound is highly operator dependent, with the complication rate being predicted by the experience of the ultrasonographer. However, in most published series that studied complication rates, patients were often moribund and critically ill, casting a bias on death rates. Regardless, pericardiocentesis should not be performed casually.

Cardiac arrest and death are the most dreaded complications, and they occur in up to 2% of patients. Lacerations of the heart wall, coronary vessels, and lung occur in up to 9% of patients, even in the hands of experienced clinicians. Such a laceration may cause an acute hemopericardium, necessitating emergent thoracotomy. Serious dysrhythmias are rare, whereas premature ventricular contractions are relatively common and benign. Sudden pulmonary edema and circulatory collapse are reported, presumably because of dramatic changes in pump function and intravascular volume from removal of large amounts of fluid. Preprocedure treatment with atropine has been advocated to prevent the vasovagal reaction.

POSTPROCEDURE PATIENT EDUCATION

Given the known complications (described previously), it is prudent to maintain continuous cardiac monitoring (along with frequent vital signs) while awaiting the results of the postprocedure chest radiograph. The patient should be counseled about the signs and symptoms of infection, pulmonary edema, or reaccumulation of the pericardial effusion with possible cardiac tamponade. The patient should know when to notify the clinician.

CPT/BILLING CODES

33010	Pericardiocentesis, initial
33011	Pericardiocentesis, subsequent
76930	Ultrasonic guidance for pericardiocentesis, radiologic supervision and interpretation

93000	ECG, routine with at least 12 leads; with interpretation and report

ICD-9-CM DIAGNOSTIC CODES

017.9	Pericarditis, tuberculous
391.00	Pericarditis, rheumatic with effusion
420.90	Effusion, pericardial (acute)
420.99	Pericarditis, septic (acute)
423.00	Hemopericardium
423.90	Effusion, pericardial

ADDITIONAL RESOURCES

- See the sample patient education handout titled "Pericardiocentesis" on page 1837 of Appendix G.
- See the sample patient consent form titled "Pericardiocentesis" on page 1839 of Appendix G.

BIBLIOGRAPHY

Harper RJ, Callaham ML: Pericardiocentesis and intracardiac injections. In Roberts JR, Hedges JR, editors: *Clinical procedures in emergency medicine,* ed 3, Philadelphia, 1998, WB Saunders.

Palacios IF: Pericardial effusion and tamponade, *Curr Treat Options Cardiovasc Med* 1:79, 1999.

Shields TW, Lo Cicero J, Ponn RB, editors: *General thoracic surgery,* ed 5, Philadelphia, 2000, Lippincott, Williams & Wilkins.

Tintinalli JE, Kelen GD, Stapczynski JS, editors: *Emergency medicine: a comprehensive study guide,* ed 5, New York, 2000, McGraw-Hill.

Tsang TS, Seward JB, Barnes ME, et al: Outcomes of primary and secondary treatment of pericardial effusion in patients with malignancy, *Mayo Clin Proc* 75:248, 2000.

Tsang TSM, Oh JK, Seward JB: Diagnosis and management of cardiac tamponade in the era of echocardiography, *Clin Cardiol* 22:446, 1999.

CHAPTER 89

Pulmonary Function Testing

José Bayona

Pulmonary function testing is an important tool used by clinicians to evaluate individuals for lung disease. The parameters commonly measured include lung volume, airflow (timed volume), and airway reactivity. As it turns out, clinicians cannot reliably identify obstructive or restrictive patterns from history taking and physical examination alone. In one study, when clinicians ordering lung function tests were asked to predict the results, they correctly predicted an obstructive pattern 83% of the time. However, when predicting a normal or restrictive pattern, they were correct only about half of the time. Besides identifying abnormalities, lung function tests allow the severity of an abnormality to be quantified and the amount of reversibility to be determined. This ability to quantify also allows a clinician to follow treatment results in an objective manner.

A spirogram is a recording of exhaled volume over time. Spirometric examination is the most widely used tool to assess pulmonary function in office practice. It can be used to evaluate patients suspected of having disease on the basis of clinical findings or to monitor changes in a patient over time. Although full pulmonary function tests (PFTs) are more comprehensive and, if necessary, can provide an objective measure of impairment, spirometry is all that is needed in many cases.

In fact, spirometry is underused. Such examinations should be readily available in most medical offices. The Spirometry Subcommittee of the National Lung Health Education Program would like to see spirometry used as commonly as the sphygmomanometer is used to measure blood pressure. The National Asthma Education Program recommends an objective measurement of lung function (either spirometry or PFTs) whenever diagnosing or managing asthma. Without an objective measurement, there is evidence that both patients and clinicians have inaccurate perceptions of the severity of asthma, thereby increasing the risk of mortality.

Note: Although useful information can be obtained from spirometry or PFTs, these physiologic tools alone do not establish a diagnosis. The test results must be carefully correlated with clinical and chest x-ray findings.

Definitions and Pathology

Common lung volumes measured by spirometry are illustrated in Fig. 89-1. The simplest test of lung function is based on a forced expiration. It is also one of the most informative tests, and it requires minimal equipment and calculations. The *vital capacity* is the total volume of gas that can be exhaled after a full inspiration. The vital capacity measured with a forced expiration may be less than that measured with a slower exhalation, so the term *forced vital capacity (FVC)* is generally used.

Any reduction in FVC affects the ventilatory capacity. The FVC can be affected by conditions affecting the thoracic cage (kyphoscoliosis), diseases affecting the nerve supply to the thoracic muscles, intrinsic diseases of the muscles, abnormalities of the pleural cavity, space-occupying lesions, pathology of the lung tissue, or stagnation of blood flow in the lungs as seen in heart failure. In addition, diseases of the airways such as asthma and chronic bronchitis cause peripheral small airways to close prematurely during expiration. This limits the volume that can be exhaled rapidly.

Forced expiratory flow (FEF$_{25\%-75\%}$) is the flow over the middle half of the FVC, the average flow from the point at which 25% of the FVC has been exhaled to the point at which 75% has been exhaled. It is measured in volume (liters) divided by time (seconds). It is the most sensitive office measurement of small airway obstruction or disease. *Forced expiratory volume (FEV$_1$)* is the volume of gas exhaled in 1 second by a forced expiration from full inspiration. The forced expiratory volume (FEV$_1$) and related indices (such as the FEF$_{25\%-75\%}$) are affected by the airway resistance during forced expiration. Any increase in resistance reduces the ventilatory capacity. Possible causes include bronchoconstriction (e.g., asthma or the inhalation of irritants such as cigarette smoke); structural changes in the airways (e.g., chronic bronchitis); obstructions within the airways (e.g., inhaled foreign body or excess bronchial secretions); and destructive processes in the lung parenchyma, which impair the support needed to keep the lumen open.

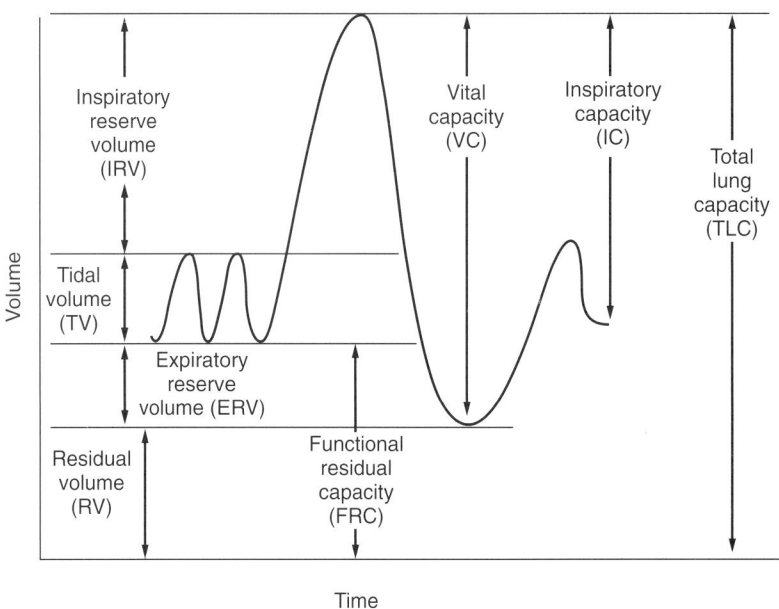

Fig. 89-1

Spirogram showing tidal breathing and the divisions of total lung capacity. The residual volume is measured by indirect techniques. (From Muller G, Eigen H: Pulmonary function testing in pediatric practice, *Pediatr Rev* 15(10):403, 1994.)

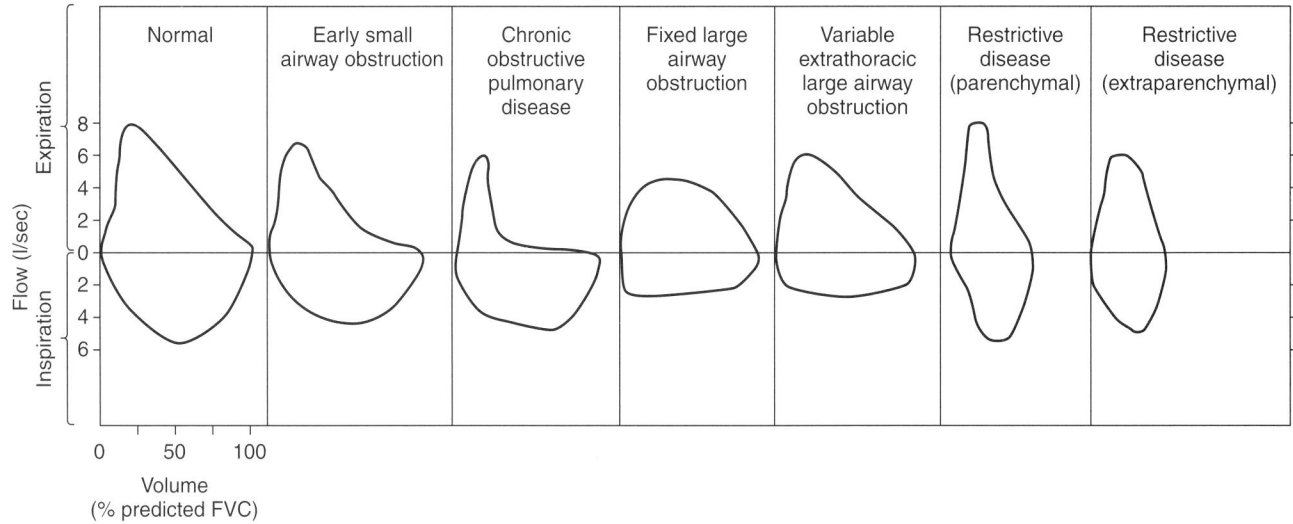

Fig. 89-2

Characteristic flow-volume curves of restrictive disease and various types of obstructive diseases compared with normal. The top part of the curve represents maximal forced expiration while the bottom represents maximal inspiration. (*FVC,* Forced vital capacity.)

The inspiratory *flow-volume curve* allows the clinician to determine when the peak flow rate occurs during inspiration and how high it is (Fig. 89-2). This curve is not affected by anything causing dynamic compression of the airways because the pressures during inspiration always expand the bronchi. However, a large (fixed or variable) airway obstruction will cause flattening of the curve because maximal flow is limited. The expiratory flow-volume curve will also be flattened by a fixed large airway obstruction. With restrictive airway diseases the flow-volume curve will be smaller or narrower.

INDICATIONS*

Diagnostic Indications

- To evaluate symptoms, signs, or abnormal results of other diagnostic tests
  a. Symptoms: cough, dyspnea, wheezing, orthopnea, or chest pain
  b. Signs: overinflation, expiratory slowing, cyanosis, chest deformity, wheezing, or unexplained crackles
  c. Abnormal results of diagnostic tests: hypoxemia, hypercapnia, polycythemia, or abnormal chest radiographs
- To measure the effect of disease on pulmonary function
- To screen persons at risk for pulmonary disease (e.g., smokers; persons with occupational exposure to injurious substances, some persons at the time of a routine physical examination)
- To assess preoperative risk
- To assess prognosis for lung disease

Monitoring Indications

- To assess effectiveness of a therapeutic intervention (e.g., bronchodilatory therapy, steroid treatment for asthma or interstitial lung disease, management of congestive heart failure)
- To track the course of a disease affecting lung function (e.g., pulmonary disease, such as obstructive airways disease or interstitial lung disease; cardiac disease, such as congestive heart failure; neuromuscular disease, such as Guillain-Barré syndrome)
- To assess current status of persons with occupational exposure to injurious substances
- To detect adverse reactions to drugs with known pulmonary toxicity

Evaluation of Disability or Impairment

- To assess patients as part of a rehabilitation program (e.g., medical, industrial, vocational)
- To assess risks for an insurance evaluation
- To assess the condition of persons for legal reasons (e.g., social security or other program involving government compensation, personal-injury lawsuits)

Public Health

- Epidemiologic surveys
- Derivation of normal values for PFTs

---

*From Crapo R: Pulmonary-function testing, *N Engl J Med* 331:25, 1994.

CONTRAINDICATIONS

- Severe debilitation and excessive tiring (patients who cannot expend the required effort for testing)
- Severe or moderately severe respiratory distress
- Patients not motivated or desiring to take the test
- Patients taking a medication that might affect the respiratory cycle or the function of the chest muscles (not a contraindication, but must be taken into account)

EQUIPMENT

- Pulmonary function testing machine/spirometer
- Comfortable chair and private area of office for testing (avoids patient embarrassment)
- Nose clips (soft clips are preferred and recommended to prevent air leaks)
- Various inhalants for testing response to bronchodilators (if indicated)

The office spirometer should conform to minimal requirements or specifications established by the American Thoracic Society (ATS) (Table 89-1). Not all commercially available spirometers meet these standards. Ideally, the computerized spirometer should have software that allows formulas and algorithms to be modified. Routine preventive maintenance, cleaning, and quality control measures are necessary to ensure accurate results in spirometric testing. Daily calibration according to manufacturer's instructions is highly recommended. The spirometer should also be evaluated daily for leaks. Instructions for maintenance, as well as how to perform tests for quality control, should be provided by the manufacturer. The clinician is responsible for ensuring that the office personnel are trained to carry out the recommended maintenance.

Note: Peak flow meters are advantageous for patients to use at home but do not provide the documentation needed in the office.

PREPROCEDURE PATIENT PREPARATION

Before performing a PFT, review the patient's respiratory history, including any medications the patient may be taking for respiratory problems. A clear explanation of the test and what is to be expected is essential to the patient's performance. The PFT has both an effort dependent and an effort independent portion. The best overall result is obtained when the patient gives a maximal effort. Patients not previously experienced in performing a PFT should make two to three practice

TABLE 89-1

Minimal Recommendations (Specifications) for Diagnostic Spirometry*

Test	Range/Accuracy (BTPS) (at body temperature [37° C] and ambient pressure)	Flow Range (L/s)	Time (sec)	Resistance and Back Pressure	Test Signal
VC	0.5 to 8 L ± 3% of reading or ± 0.050 L, whichever is greater	0 to 14	30		3-L Cal syringe
FVC	0.5 to 8 L ± 3% of reading or ± 0.050 L, whichever is greater	0 to 14	15	Less than 1.5 cm $H_2O/L/s$	24 standard waveforms 3-L Cal syringe
FEV_1	0.5 to 8 L ± 3% of reading or ± 0.050 L, whichever is greater	0 to 14	1	Less than 1.5 cm $H_2O/L/s$	24 standard waveforms
Time zero	The time point from which all FEV_1 measurements are taken			Back extrapolation	
PEF	Accuracy: ± 10% of reading or ± 0.400 L/s, whichever is greater Precision: ± 5% of reading or ± 0.200 L/s, whichever is greater	0 to 14		Same as FEV_1	26 standard waveforms
$FEF_{25\%-75\%}$	7.0 L/s ± 5% of reading or ± 0.200 L/s, whichever is greater	± 14	15	Same as FEV_1	24 standard waveforms
$\dot{V}$	± 14 L/s ± 5% of reading or ± 0.200 L/s, whichever is greater	0 to 14	15	Same as FEV_1	Proof from manufacturer
MVV	250 L/min at TV of 2 L within ± 10% of reading or ± 15 L/min, whichever is greater	± 14 ± 3%	12 to 15	Pressure less than ± 10 cm H_2O at 2-L TV at 2.0 Hz	Sine wave pump

From American Thoracic Society: Standardization of spirometry: 1994 update, *Am J Resp Crit Care Med* 152:1107, 1995.
FEF, Forced expiratory flow; *FEV_1,* forced expiratory volume; *FVC,* forced vital capacity; *L/s,* liters per second; *MVV,* maximal voluntary ventilation; *PEF,* peak expiratory flow; *TV,* tidal volume; *$\dot{V}$,* volume; *VC,* vital capacity.
*Unless specifically stated, precision requirements are the same as the accuracy requirements.

attempts until a maximal effort is obtained. A demonstration of the test may be helpful.

Usually the patient is seated to perform the test. The thorax should be erect and the head should be in a neutral position. Explain that this test measures lung function and that the best results are obtained when the patient takes a deep breath and then blows out as hard and as fast as possible for as long as possible. Smokers should try to abstain from smoking for at least 1 hour before testing.

TECHNIQUE

1. Prepare the equipment to test for FVC. Machine calibration and parameter setups vary between spirometers. See the individual instructions pertaining to the particular instrument for this portion of the procedure.
2. Document the patient's position (usually seated). If for some reason the patient is standing, it will increase FVC.
3. Have the patient breath in and out several times with the nose clips in place, to become comfortable.
4. Ask the patient to take in as deep a breath as possible, to completely fill their lungs.

5. Then have the patient quickly insert the mouthpiece. It should be between the teeth, making a seal with the lips.
6. Next, have the patient blow out as hard and as fast as possible, for as long as possible (try for at least 6 seconds) (Fig. 89-3). Enthusiastically coach the patient to breathe out until the forced vital curve flattens out (usually 5 to 6 seconds).
7. When the lungs are completely emptied, have the patient breathe in as deeply as possible, to obtain the inspiratory parameter and complete the evaluation. To follow the diagram (Fig. 89-1), the patient first takes several normal (tidal) breaths, after which he or she will perform a maximal inspiration to total lung capacity (TLC). They then exhale fast and hard, as much as they can (FVC).
8. Repeat the test three times. A minimum of three and a maximum of eight maneuvers are performed until three acceptable curves are obtained. Two or three maneuvers that have values within a 5% difference of each other indicate reproducibility. The best effort is then saved and reported. Acceptability and reproducibility criteria are summarized in Box 89-1.
9. If prebronchodilator and postbronchodilator comparison PFTs are needed, administer a β-agonist or a bronchodilator through a handheld inhaler.

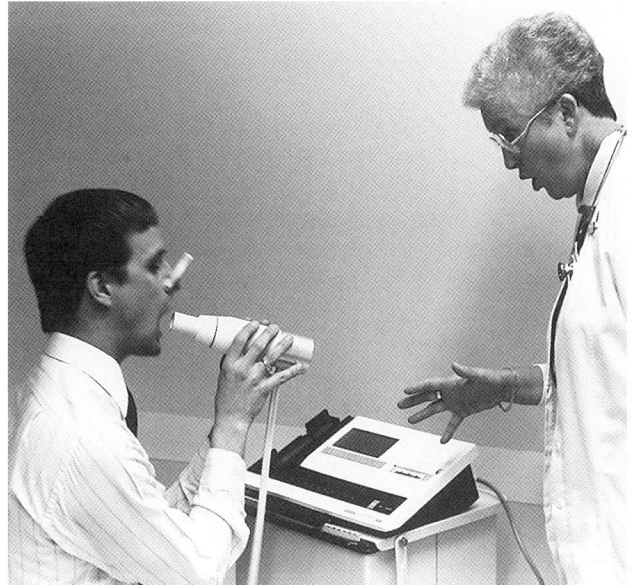

Fig. 89-3
Patient takes a deep breath, inserts the mouthpiece, and blows out as fast and as hard as possible.

10. Wait about 20 minutes for bronchodilation to occur. Then repeat the FVC maneuver for the postbronchodilation measurements, as in steps 1 through 8.

INTERPRETATION

Some of the factors that influence the normal values of PFTs include the formula used to predict the normal values, test quality, height, age, weight, gender, ethnicity, posture, effort, smoking, and even circadian rhythm. The results and interpretation depend on the clinician paying careful attention to the characteristics of the equipment used, the patient's performance and clinical condition, and the reference values chosen. A patient's own baseline values will provide the best reference data for assessing a patient over time with chronic pulmonary disease.

Interpretation of PFTs can be categorized into three basic patterns: normal function, obstructive, and restricted (Fig. 89-4). A diagnosis is then made by correlating the test result with the clinical findings from the history, physical examination, and radiology films.

An obstructive process, such as asthma or chronic bronchitis, is characterized by flow that is low relative to lung volume. Characteristically, timed volume (FEV_1) and flow ($FEF_{25\%-75\%}$) are decreased. A decrease in $FEF_{25\%-75\%}$ may detect obstruction in the smaller airways early in the course of the disease, before a change in FEV_1 is evident. This is especially common in smokers, and may be their best early warning before permanent

BOX 89-1
Acceptability and Reproducibility Criteria: Summary

Acceptability Criteria
Individual spirograms are "acceptable" if:
1. They are free from artifacts, such as:
   - Cough or glottis closure during the first second of exhalation
   - Early termination or cutoff
   - Variable effort
   - Leak
   - Obstructed mouthpiece
2. They have good starts
   - Extrapolated volume less than 5% of FVC or 0.15 L, whichever is greater; or
   - Time-to-PEF of less than 120 msec (optional until further information is available)
3. They have a satisfactory exhalation
   - Six sec of exhalation and/or a plateau in the volume-time curve; or
   - Reasonable duration or a plateau in the volume-time curve; or
   - If the subject cannot or should not continue to exhale

Reproducibility Criteria
After three acceptable spirograms have been obtained, apply the following tests:
   - Are the two largest FVC within 0.2 L of each other?
   - Are the two largest FEV_1 within 0.2 L of each other?
If both of these criteria are met, the test session may be concluded.
If both of these criteria are not met, continue testing until:
   - Both of the criteria are met with analysis of additional acceptable spirograms; or
   - A total of eight tests have been performed; or
   - The patient/subject cannot or should not continue
Save at a minimum the three best maneuvers.

From American Thoracic Society: Standardization of spirometry: 1994 update, *Am J Resp Crit Care Med* 152:1107, 1994.

lung damage. A reduction in $FEF_{25\%-75\%}$ from small-airway obstruction gives the flow-volume curve a characteristic concave shape. Other causes of obstructive patterns include cystic fibrosis, bronchiolitis, and bronchiectasis.

Low volumes and normal flows characterize a restrictive lung process. The primary criterion for this diagnosis is a reduction in TLC; however, the presence of restriction is commonly inferred from a decreased FVC. It should be kept in mind that a decreased FVC only infers a restrictive process because FVC can also be reduced in the presence of airflow obstruction. Significant decreases in FEV_1 and the FEV_1/FVC ratio are key findings that will help differentiate an obstructive from a restrictive pattern when FVC is reduced (Fig. 89-4, *A*). In addition, when there is both airflow obstruction and reduced FVC, the possibility of restriction can usually be eliminated with evidence of overinflation on the physical examination or a chest radiograph.

When there is any question about the cause of a reduced FVC, TLC should be measured. Measuring TLC

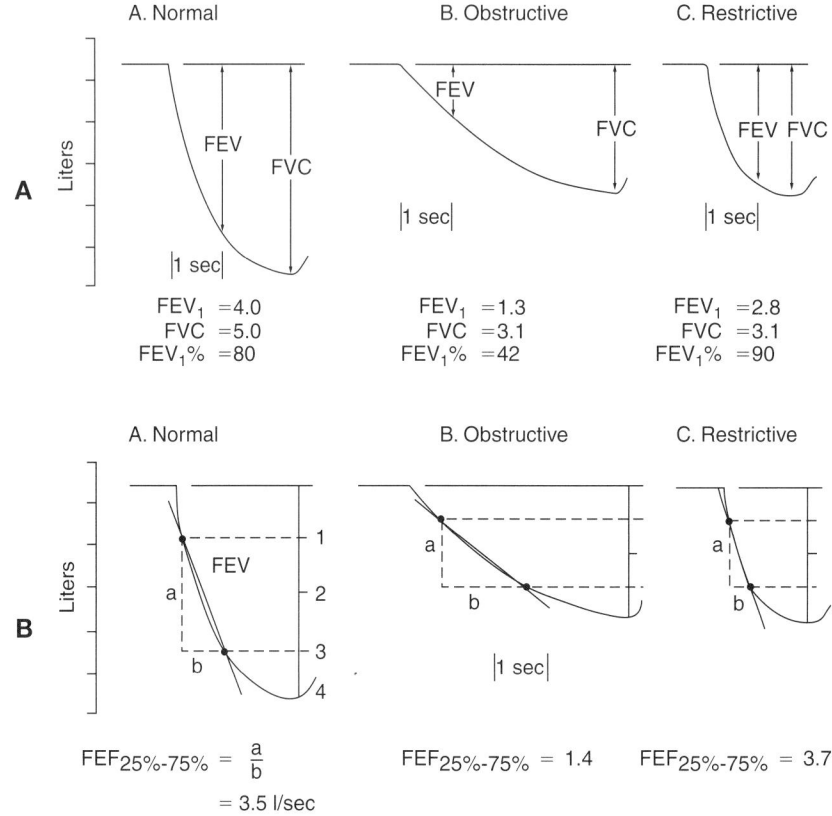

Fig. 89-4

A, Normal, obstructive, and restrictive patterns of a forced expiration. **B,** Calculation of forced expiratory flow between 25% and 75% of the FVC *(FEF$_{25\%-75\%}$)*. *FEV$_1$*, forced expiratory volume at one second; *FVC*, forced vital capacity. FEV$_1$% = (FEV$_1$/FVC) × 100. (From West JB: Pulmonary pathophysiology. In West JB, editor: *Respiratory physiology: the essentials,* ed 6, Baltimore, 2000, Williams & Wilkins.

requires referral to a pulmonary function laboratory. Measurement of lung volume by helium dilution, nitrogen washout, or body plethysmography can definitively confirm a diagnosis of a restrictive lung condition. Although a reduced TLC defines restriction, measuring FVC has frequently been demonstrated to be more useful for following the course of restrictive chest disease. Restrictive disease can be divided into parenchymal and extraparenchymal based on etiology. Parenchymal causes include silicosis, pneumoconiosis, idiopathic pulmonary fibrosis, sarcoidosis, and drug- or radiation-induced interstitial lung disease. Extraparenchymal disease can be due to loss of lung volume (e.g., pleural effusion, pneumothorax), chest wall deformity, extrathoracic compression (e.g., ankylosing spondylitis, ascites, kyphoscoliosis, obesity), or neuromuscular problems (e.g., Guillain-Barré, myasthenia gravis, muscular dystrophy, cervical spine injury, or diaphragmatic weakness or paralysis). Suspicion of restrictive disease warrants referral. Table 89-2 summarizes the characteristic patterns of obstructive and restrictive lung diseases as measured by spirometry.

Many systems are available to quantify the severity of

TABLE 89-2

Characteristic Patterns of Obstructive and Restrictive Lung Disease as Measured by Spirometry*

	Obstruction	Restriction
FVC	Normal or ↓	↓
FEV$_1$	↓	Normal or ↓
FEV$_1$/FVC	Normal (early) or ↓	↑
FEF$_{25\%-75\%}$	↓	Normal, ↑ or ↓

From Muller G, Eigen H: Pulmonary function testing in pediatric practice, *Pediatr Rev* 15(10):403, 1994.
FEF, Forced expiratory flow; *FEV$_1$,* forced expiratory volume; *FVC,* forced vital capacity.
*Low flows with normal volumes characterize obstructive disease, whereas normal flows with low volumes characterize restrictive disease. In severe obstruction, gas trapping reduces forced vital capacity because of an increased residual volume.

pulmonary impairment; however, there is currently no universal standard. In practice, severity is usually described as a percentage of either predicted FEV$_1$ for obstructive conditions or predicted TLC for restrictive conditions. ("Normal" predicted test values are obtained by testing a large group of people who have been determined to be free of lung disease.) The test results for a given patient are then expressed as a percentage of the predicted value for age, height, sex, and race. In reality, no one set of equations will be entirely accurate for every person in a given population. For the final report, the ATS recommends that clinicians define the lower limits of normal by using calculations of the lower 95th percentiles (from the specific set of prediction equations that have been selected as standard reference values); these should be recorded, rather than just the percentages of predicted function (e.g., 80% for $FEV_1/FVC\%$). The patient should be comparable in age, race, and sex to the reference population. In computerized equipment, it is essential for population standards to be defined in the software.

Although using percentage of predicted function to evaluate results may not be recommended, below are some guidelines the clinician can use to get a general clinical picture of pulmonary function:

Vital Capacity
FVC

80% to 120% of predicted value	Normal
70% to 79% of predicted value	Mild reduction
50% to 69% of predicted value	Moderate reduction
<50% of predicted value	Severe reduction

Again, *restrictive* lung disease is characterized by reduced vital capacity and relatively normal airflow rates. If obstruction is present (see the "Flow Rates" section), the reduction in vital capacity may only be reported as "probably secondary to obstruction" if the severity of the reduced vital capacity and that of the obstructive findings are approximately equal. In comparing vital capacities obtained at different times (including those obtained before and after bronchodilator administration), the expiratory time must be considered and compared. The raw curves should also be compared.

Flow Rates
FEV_1 can be plotted as the percentage of vital capacity [$(FEV_1/FVC \times 100)$ or $FEV_{1\%}$.].

FEV₁ %

>75%	Normal
60% to 75%	Mild obstruction
50% to 59%	Moderate obstruction
<49%	Severe obstruction

Note: For patients less than 25 years old, add 5% to these figures; for those more than 60 years old, subtract 5%.

FEF₂₅%₋₇₅%

>79% of predicted value	Normal
60% to 79% of predicted value	Mild obstruction
40% to 59% of predicted value	Moderate obstruction
<40% of predicted value	Severe obstruction

In most cases of *obstructive* lung disease, the percentage of the predicted value of the $FEF_{25\%-75\%}$ will be "worse" than the percentage of the predicted value of the FEV_1. However, the modifier used to describe the type of *obstruction* (as mild, moderate, or severe) should be that associated with the value of the FEV_1, not the $FEF_{25\%-75\%}$. The $FEF_{25\%-75\%}$ may be separately referred to with such statements as ". . . particularly affecting small airways, as reflected in the $FEF_{25\%-75\%}$." Should the $FEF_{25\%-75\%}$ *alone* be abnormal, the diagnosis of obstructive lung disease should not be assumed; rather, the reduction should be interpreted as compatible with "early small airways disease." Again, for comparison over time, the raw curves should be examined to determine adequacy of effort.

Therefore an $FEV_{1\%}$ less than 75% indicates some loss of elastic recoil (e.g., emphysema) or obstructive disease (e.g., asthma), whereas reduced FVC and FEV_1 (but $FEV_{1\%}$ greater than 75%) indicates restrictive disease. Again, suspicion of restrictive disease warrants referral.

For the final interpretation, the flow-volume loops can be useful in conjunction with the volume-time spirogram. A flow-volume loop can help determine whether an obstruction is in the larger or the smaller airways. They can also help determine whether a restrictive pattern is due to a parenchymal or an extraparenchymal cause. The most useful information obtained from flow-volume loops is usually in the expiratory portion of the flow loop (Fig. 89-2). However, flow-volume loops may only be derived if the spirometer is accurate in displacement and time.

ERRORS AND RULES OF THUMB IN PULMONARY FUNCTION TESTING

Some technical errors and their effects in pulmonary function testing include the following:
- An air leak due to a poorly fitting noseclip or mouthpiece can result in a wandering baseline, which can lead to underestimation of many spirometric measurements.
- An incomplete expiration may give a falsely low reading of FVC and a spurious increase in $FEF_{25\%-75\%}$.
- Poor initial expiratory effort may give a falsely low reading of the FEV_1 and $FEF_{25\%-75\%}$.

PFTs have a false-positive rate of approximately 5%. Borderline values should be interpreted cautiously. In addition to the ranges listed in Table 89-3, the changes in spirometric results over time for an individual can affect the interpretation of the results. The coefficient of variation relates the standard deviation to the main value and is a measure of test-to-test variability in a given individual. The interval between tests, the intrinsic variability of the test, and the presence of disease are among the factors that determine the coefficient of variation.

TABLE 89-3

Change in Spirometric Indexes Over Time

	Percent Changes Required to be Significant		
	FVC	FEV$_1$	FEF$_{25\%-75\%}$
Within a Day			
Normal subjects	≥5%	≥5%	≥13%
Patients with COPD	≥11%	≥13%	≥23%
Week to Week			
Normal subjects	≥11%	≥12%	≥21%
Patients with COPD	≥20%	≥20%	≥30%
Year to Year			
Normal subjects	≥15%	≥15%	
Patients with COPD	≥15%	≥15%	

Adapted from American Thoracic Society: Lung function testing: selection of reference value and interpretive strategies, *Am Rev Respir Dis* 144:1202, 1991. *COPD,* Chronic obstructive pulmonary disease.

Lung function declines with age. It is estimated that vital capacity decreases 60 ml per year after peaking during young adulthood. Differentiating "real" decline in lung function from expected test variability across time can be difficult. Recommended requirements for significant spirometric changes (normal variability) have been calculated and are listed in Table 89-3.

Adolescents should not be compared with adult standards until growth and puberty are complete. This recommendation is necessary because leg length, thorax height, and total body height proportions change throughout puberty.

Other sources of error include inadequate preventive maintenance of the equipment, inadequate training of the staff, inadequate patient motivation, not correlating the results with the entire clinical picture (e.g., history, physical examination, x-ray findings), and not ordering more definitive tests when the results are unclear (e.g., obtaining a formal TLC measurement when both FVC and flow are reduced).

In the past, when managing patients with chronic obstructive pulmonary disease (COPD), if FEV$_1$ went below 1.0, the prognosis was thought to worsen dramatically (similar to a cardiac ejection fraction <20%). We now know that patients occasionally can survive for years with an FEV$_1$ <1.0 if they stop smoking and have a good exercise capacity (e.g., can walk several blocks).

For final values that are confusing or do not make sense (e.g., hyperinflation on chest x-ray and abnormal PFTs, yet no history of smoking and no other risk factors for COPD), cardiopulmonary exercise testing (expired gas exercise testing) may be helpful. Also, one of the most common causes of emphysema (or premature emphysema in smokers) is α-1 antitrypsin deficiency. This tends to run in families and can be excluded by a simple blood test that many laboratories perform.

SUPPLIERS

Medical Systems International Corp.
6414 Northwest 82nd Avenue
Miami, FL 33166
Phone: 1-305-597-0322
Website: www.medicalsystems.com

Puritan Bennett (Tyco Healthcare)
4280 Hacienda Drive
Pleasanton, CA 94588
Phone: 1-800-635-5267
Website: www.puritanbennett.com

SB Office Diagnostics, Inc.
10 Hampden Drive
Easton, MA 02375
Phone: 1-800-678-5782

Vitalograph
8347 Quivira
Lenexa, KS 66215
Phone: 1-800-255-6626
Website: www.vitalograph.com

Welch Allyn
4341 State Street Road
P.O. Box 220
Skaneateles Falls, NY 13153
Phone: 1-800-535-6663
Website: www.welchallyn.com

CPT/BILLING CODES

94010   Spirometry, including graphic record, total and timed vital capacity, expiratory flow rate measurement(s), with or without maximal voluntary ventilation

94060   Bronchospasm evaluation: spirometry as in 94010, before and after bronchodilator (aerosol or parenteral)

94375   Respiratory flow volume loop

ICM-9-CM DIAGNOSTIC CODES

493.00   Asthma, extrinsic, without mention status asthmaticus

493.90   Asthma, unspecified, without mention status asthmaticus

491.0   Chronic bronchitis, simple

491.2   Chronic bronchitis, obstructive

491.9   Chronic bronchitis, unspecified

492   Emphysema

514   Pulmonary edema

BIBLIOGRAPHY

American Thoracic Society: Lung function testing: selection of reference value and interpretative strategies, *Am Rev Respir Dis* 144:1202, 1991.

American Thoracic Society: Standardization of spirometry: 1994 update, *Am J Respir Crit Care Med* 152:1107, 1995.

Crapo R: Pulmonary function testing, *N Engl J Med,* 331:25, 1994.

Ferguson G, Petty TL: Screening and early intervention for COPD, *Hosp Pract (Off Ed)* 33:67, 1998.

Ferguson GT, Enright PL, Buist AS, et al: Office spirometry for lung health assessment in adults: a consensus statement from the National Lung Health Education Program, *Chest* 117:1146, 2000.

Margolis M: PFT principles and bronchodilator testing in clinical practice: a guide for primary care physicians, *Comp Ther* 24(9):441, 1998.

McIvor RA, Taskin DP: Underdiagnosis of chronic obstructive pulmonary disease: a rationale for spirometry as a screening tool, *Can Respir J* 8(3):153, 2001.

Mueller G, Eigen H: Pulmonary function testing in pediatric practice, *Pediatr Rev* 15(10):403, 1994.

National Asthma Education Program: Expert panel report. In *Guidelines for the Diagnosis and Management of Asthma,* Bethesda, Md, 1991, Department of Health and Human Services.

Petty TL: Simple office spirometry, *Clin Chest Med* 22(4):845, 2001.

Sly M: Decreases in asthma mortality in the United States, *Ann Allergy Asthma Immunol* 85:121, 2000.

West JB: Pulmonary pathophysiology. In West JB, editor: *Respiratory physiology: the essentials,* ed 6, Baltimore, 2000, Williams & Wilkins.

CHAPTER 90

Sclerotherapy

Stanley A. Hirsch
John L. Pfenninger

Sclerotherapy is a technique used to eliminate unwanted veins (both varicosities and spider veins). This is accomplished by injecting a noxious agent into the lumen of the vein, which causes destruction of the endothelium with an inflammatory response. When used with compression, it results in obliteration of the vessel. The goal of treatment is to eradicate abnormal veins while preserving healthy veins.

BACKGROUND

Ancient physicians and scholars, including Hippocrates and Homer, recognized varicose veins. Improvements in syringes and needles and the development of more effective and safe sclerosing solutions allowed sclerotherapy to become a modern and effective method of treatment. Clinicians now use sclerosants developed in the twentieth century (e.g., hypertonic glucose, hypertonic saline,

sodium morrhuate, chromated glycerin, ethanolamine oleate, and stabilized polyiodide iodine). However, the most popular agents used in sclerotherapy are sodium tetradecyl sulfate (STS, Sotradecol), polidocanol (POL, Aethoxysklerol), and hypertonic saline (HS) (Table 90-1).

Organizations worldwide—including the American College of Phlebology and the American Venous Forum in the United States—have been formed to further research and education in venous disease. Currently there is a petition before the American Medical Association to create the subspecialty of phlebology.

ANATOMY

The venous system is divided into three levels: *deep, perforating,* and *superficial* veins. The veins treated with sclerotherapy are the perforating and the superficial veins.

TABLE 90-1
Most Common Sclerosing Agents in the United States

Agent	Food and Drug Administration Approval	Supply	Maximum Dose Per Visit	Indications	Companies	Comments
Sodium tetradecyl sulfate (Sotradecol, STS)	Yes	2 ml ampules (1%, 3%)	10 ml 3% solution	0.1%-0.25% up to 2 mm; 0.25%-0.5% reticular; 0.5%-1% <4 mm; 1%-3% >4 mm	Elkin-Sinn, Inc, Cherry Hill, NJ; Wyeth-Ayerst, Philadelphia, PA	Painless; can cause extravascular necrosis
Hypertonic saline	Yes, as abortifacient	30 ml ampules (23.4%); dilute as needed with lidocaine 1% (may be stored dilute for up to 12 weeks)	10 ml; more can cause leg cramps, significant salt load	11.7% <2 mm (especially for matting); 23.4% >2 mm (many use the 18.7% solution for all vessels; see text)		Major advantages: no anaphylaxis and inexpensive; some discomfort on injection
Polidocanol (Aethoxyskerol)	No	2 ml & 30 ml ampules (0.5%, 1%, 2%, 3%)	2 mg/kg	0.25%-1% telangiectasias and reticulars <4 mm	Kreussler & Co, D6200, Wiesboden-Bielsrich, Germany	Painless; less extravascular necrosis; need to have compounded or obtain out of USA

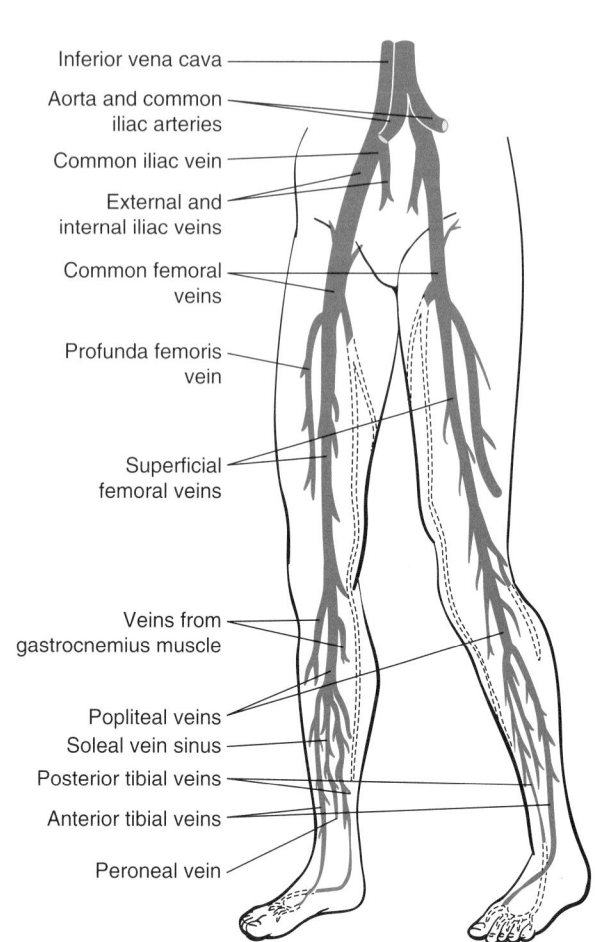

Fig. 90-1
Main venous conduits formed by the deep veins of the lower limbs; numerous branch veins join these.

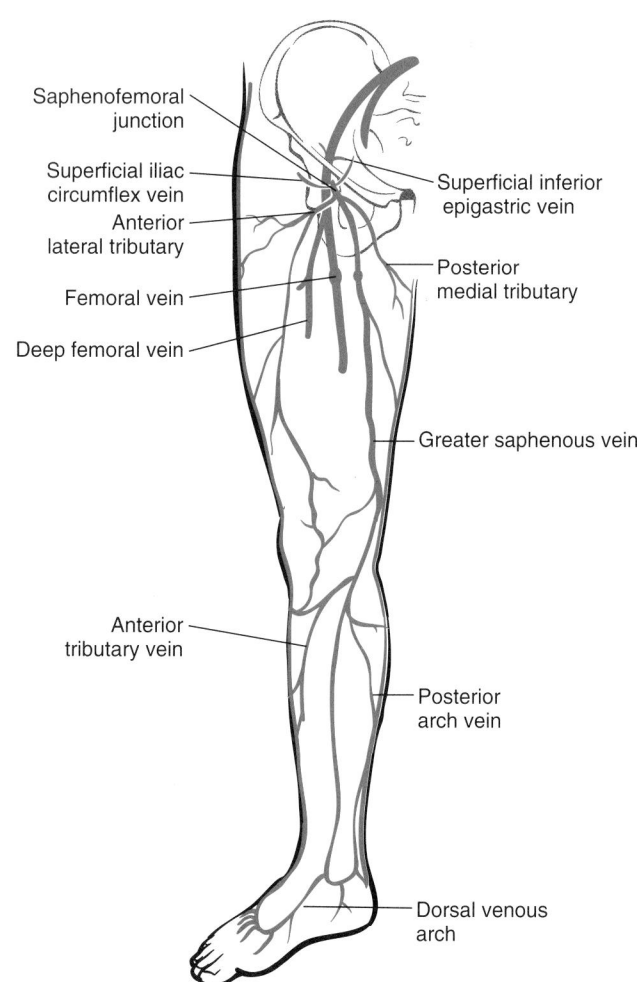

Fig. 90-2
Normal anteromedial superficial venous anatomy is depicted. The greater saphenous vein ascends from the dorsal venous arch and dominates the anteromedial superficial drainage system. It receives the posterior arch vein (vein of Michelangelo). It also receives variable anterior and posterior tributary veins in the anteromedial calf just below the knee. As the saphenous vein reaches its termination, it receives important tributaries medially and laterally. These tributaries are commonly visualized in duplex ultrasound examinations, which may identify reflux in one or both of these vessels.

Deep veins are encased in fascia and muscle. In ascending order, they are the *anterior* and *posterior tibial veins,* the *peroneal vein,* the *tibioperoneal trunk,* the *popliteal vein,* the *superficial femoral vein,* the *deep femoral vein,* the *common femoral vein,* and *the iliac vein.* These veins convey blood from the lower limb back to the heart (Fig. 90-1).

The *superficial venous system* is confined to the veins above the fascia in the subcutaneous tissue and involves the greater and lesser saphenous veins and their tributaries, in addition to the lateral subdermal veins (of Albanese) around the knee (Figs. 90-2 and 90-3).

Approximately 150 *perforating veins* connect the superficial and deep systems. Many of these veins have eponyms for the anatomists who demonstrated them (Fig. 90-4).

In the middle area of the thigh are the Hunterian perforators, and in the distal thigh are the Dodd perforators. These veins connect the thigh portion of the greater saphenous vein to the superficial femoral vein.

Below the knee is Boyd's perforator, connecting the greater saphenous vein to the popliteal vein. The perforating veins of the medial aspect of the leg below the knee do not connect the saphenous vein to the deep system; instead they connect a major branch known as the posterior arch vein or the vein of Leonardo to the posterior tibial vein.

There are also perforating veins of importance on the posterior aspect of the calf, connecting the lesser saphenous system to the tibial venous system, and perforators at the lateral aspect of the knee that connect the lateral subdermal plexus of Albanese to the deep system. Another important posterior vein (recently described) is the posterior thigh perforator that connects

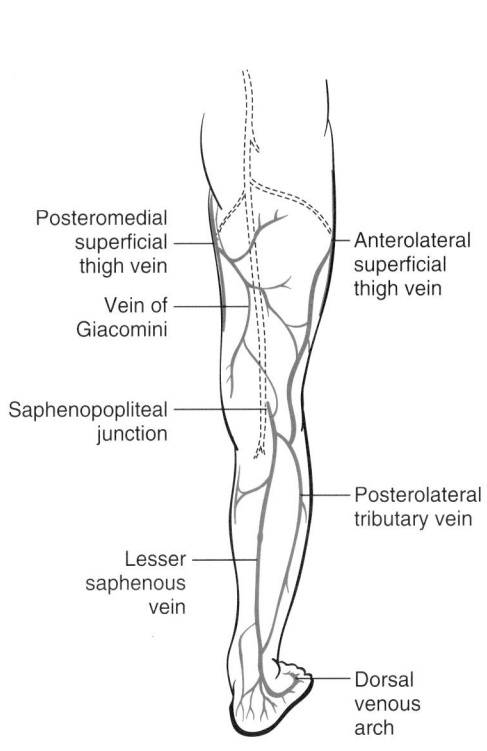

Fig. 90-3

Lesser saphenous vein dominates the posterolateral superficial venous drainage. It originates in the dorsal venous arch; at the posterolateral ankle, it is intimately associated with the sural nerve. Note the important posterolateral tributary vein and the posterior thigh vein, which ascends and connects the lesser saphenous venous system with the greater saphenous venous system. The anterolateral superficial thigh vein and the posterolateral tributary vein can be very important in congenital venous anomalies, such as Klippel-Trénaunay syndrome.

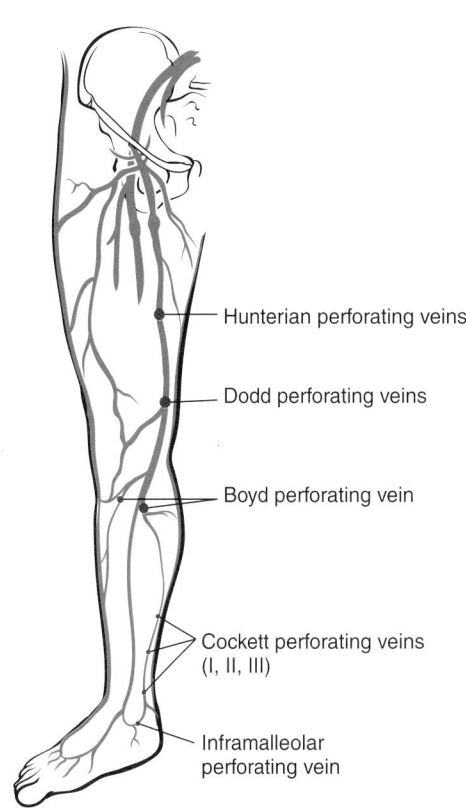

Fig. 90-4

Location of the most important perforating veins associated with the greater saphenous system are shown. Note that the Cockett and inframalleolar perforating veins are actually separate from the greater saphenous system. The Boyd perforating vein is constantly present, but it may drain the saphenous vein or its tributaries. Perforating veins in the distal third of the thigh are referred to as Dodd perforators, whereas those in the middle third of the thigh are referred to as Hunterian perforators.

TABLE 90-2

Vessel Classification

Type	Vessel Classification	Characteristics	Color
I	Telangiectasias ("spider veins")	0.1-1 mm	Red
Ia	Telangiectatic matting	<0.2 mm, very fine; can occur after injection or surgery	Red
II	Venulectasia	1-2 mm	Violaceous
III	Reticular veins	2-4 mm	Blue
IV	Nonsaphenous varicose (2° incompetent perforators)	3-8 mm	Blue
V	Saphenous varicosities	7-8 mm	Blue

Adapted from Sadick NS: *Manual of sclerotherapy,* Philadelphia, 2000, Lippincott Williams & Wilkins.

the superficial veins of the posterior thigh to the deep femoral vein.

Other connections from the superficial venous system to the deep femoral vein are the inferior gluteal vein and the veins of the medial thigh that connect through the internal pudendal system to the deep pelvic veins. It is this latter system that often results in vulvar varicosities seen frequently in pregnancy. Al-

though it is not necessary to remember all of the proper names of these perforators, it is important for the clinician to have knowledge of their location so that sclerotherapy can be carried out in a logical and effective manner.

In general, unwanted veins are referred to as *telangiectasias, reticular varicosities,* and *varicose veins* (Table 90-2).

PHYSIOLOGY

Primary Varicose Veins

The veins of the lower limb carry blood against the force of gravity back to the heart. This is accomplished by two principal means. When the muscles of the calf contract, they compress the soleal sinuses and the deep veins encased in fascia and muscle, achieving a pressure of up to 300 cm of water. Because the veins of the lower limb have valves that allow blood to flow only in a proximal direction, the column of blood is forced into the valveless veins of the abdomen.

If a person is standing still, the pressure of the veins on the dorsum of the foot will equal the distance from the foot to the right heart. This results in an average pressure of approximately of 70 to 80 cm of water. As evidenced by the pressure relationship mentioned previously, the pressure exerted by the contraction of the calf muscles is sufficient to overcome the effects of gravity and propel blood in a proximal direction. The flow of venous blood from the calf back to the heart may be considered the systolic phase. During this phase, blood is prevented from going into the superficial system by the valves of the perforating veins that close. During the relaxation phase, when the pressure in the calf compartment is diminished, blood can flow from the superficial veins through the perforators into the deep system. Therefore the superficial venous system may be likened to the atrium of the heart, and the deep veins of the calf may be likened to the ventricle.

This physiologic system breaks down when the walls of the veins dilate, causing the valves to become incompetent. The manner in which veins become incompetent is somewhat controversial. It was felt that the problem started with the valve itself. The incompetent valve allows blood to flow in a reverse direction as gravity pulls it down toward the foot. The resulting increase in venous pressure causes the veins to dilate and sequentially creates incompetence in the more distal valves. Although this still may occur, especially in patients who have had phlebitis that can destroy the structure of the valve, it now seems likely that the cause is dilation of the vein itself in patients who develop primary varicose veins.

The most proximal valve of the superficial system is at the saphenofemoral junction (SFJ). It normally allows blood to flow from the greater saphenous into the common femoral vein. When it becomes incompetent because of dilation of the saphenous, blood will flow from the common femoral into the greater saphenous, causing the vein to dilate further. This can affect a more distal valve, causing it to become incompetent; thus a cycle is begun that eventually causes dilation of the entire saphenous system.

Another mechanism for the development of varicose veins is incompetence of the valves of the perforating veins. When the calf muscles contract and greatly increase the pressure within the calf compartment, blood is prevented from flowing through the perforating vein into the superficial system by closure of its valve. If that valve is not working properly, blood will flow from the deep veins into the superficial system. The leakage of blood from the deep system into the superficial diminishes the flow of blood up the limb and back to the heart, and it greatly increases the pressure in the leg. The increase of the venous pressure, termed *venous hypertension,* is the cause of many of the sequelae seen in chronic venous insufficiency, such as edema, stasis dermatitis, pigmentation from hemosiderin, and ultimately the development of lipodermatosclerosis and venous ulceration.

Secondary Varicose Veins

Secondary varicose veins can occur as a result of the superficial or deep venous thrombosis (DVT) with resultant injury to the valves of the veins or from an arteriovenous fistula with resulting high venous pressure.

INDICATIONS

- Small bulging varicose veins up to 0.6 cm in diameter (some phlebologists treat larger veins).
- Venulectasia.
- Telangiectasia (commonly called "spider veins").
- Pain, itching, burning, tiredness, and heaviness in the lower limb (previously mentioned indications, regardless of size, may cause these symptoms).
- Cosmesis in the absence of other symptoms.
- Venous stasis ulcer.
- Venous stasis pigmentation.
- Recurrent bleeding of a vessel of any size.
- Injecting facial telangiectasias has been done and reported. It is efficacious. However, venous sinus thrombosis (in the brain) has occurred. Radiofrequency ablation or various laser/light methodologies are often as helpful without the associated risks.

CONTRAINDICATIONS

- Saphenofemoral junction (SFJ) or saphenopopliteal junction (SPJ) reflux. (Reflux from deep system into superficial creates high venous pressure, making it difficult to obliterate vein.)
- Veins larger than 0.6 cm in diameter. (If vein has large diameter, it is difficult to obtain coaptation of intimal surfaces for permanent obliteration; it is more likely that thrombus will develop within lumen of vein and recanalize over time. Some practitioners do inject these

large vessels, but recurrence and complications are more common and phlebectomy might be a wiser choice of treatment.)

- Arterial insufficiency (ankle-to-brachial ratio less than 0.7 or other signs of inadequate flow).
- Diabetes with diabetic neuropathy.
- Acute superficial or deep thrombophlebitis.
- Massive obesity.
- Anticoagulation.
- Obstruction of the deep venous system.
- Severe systemic disease (especially collagen-vascular disease, malignancy, or severe cardiac problems).
- Pregnancy.
- Lack of mobility, such as seen in stroke, arthritis, or other musculoskeletal disorders.
- Unwillingness to comply with a program of compression.
- Acute febrile illness.

Note: The clinician should use caution in patients with asthma or numerous allergies (unless hypertonic saline is used) to avoid potential hypersensitivity. Age is not a contraindication if the patient is active and has reasonably good skin turgor.

EQUIPMENT

- Camera for pictures *(optional).*
- Examination table. (A power table is helpful but not mandatory.)
- Patient stand. (The examination can be performed more optimally if the patient's feet are 24 inches off the floor. Generally this requires a made-to-order stand that includes a strong railing. The stand can be used for both examination and treatment.)
- Good lighting. (A gooseneck lamp is sufficient; however, some therapists use a more intense light source, such as a head lamp.)
- Magnification loupes (3×).
- Syringes (3.0 and 1.0 ml); ½-inch, 30-gauge needle.
- Handheld Doppler probe.
- Sclerosing solution:

Sodium tetradecyl sulfate (preferred by the author) in dilutions of 0.2%, 0.5%, 1.0%, and (rarely) 3.0%.

Hypertonic saline in a dilution of 18.7% is also commonly used (and preferred by the coauthor). It can be prepared by injecting 2 ml of 2% lidocaine into a 30-ml, multiple-dose vial of 23.4% saline (0.5 ml of this solution is injected per site). It is sterile and can be left diluted for up to 12 weeks.

Polidocanol is another common sclerosant but is not approved by the Food and Drug Administration (FDA).

Note: The assistant should have five to ten 1-ml syringes drawn up for use, depending on the sclerosant and the quantity

of veins to be injected. Each agent has benefits and risks. Hypertonic saline is effective and there are no allergic reactions; however, it is painful and the risk of extravasation necrosis of the skin is significant (Box 90-1). Polidocanol (0.05% to 3%) is a weak sclerosant but works well on small veins. Allergic reactions are possible but rare, and it is not FDA approved (in Phase III trials). It is, however, frequently used in the United States even now (Box 90-2 and Table 90-3). Sodium tetradecyl sulfate is medium in potency and relatively painless, but it must be injected carefully to avoid skin necrosis. Allergy and anaphylaxis can occur, although, again, this is rare. (See Table 90-1.)

- Cotton balls with isopropyl alcohol or benzalkonium chloride (Zephiran).

BOX 90-1

Hypertonic Saline Description

True allergic reactions are nonexistent, but side effects are more common. The degree of endothelial damage is directly proportional to the concentration used. Dilution with heparin or anesthetics can decrease effectiveness, depending on amounts. It destroys *all* cells: endothelium and red blood cells (RBCs). Significant extravasation can produce cutaneous necrosis. Hemolysis of RBCs can cause cutaneous hemosiderin staining.

BOX 90-2

Polidocanol Description

Polidocanol was originally developed as a topical anesthetic under trade name Sch 600.
There are three groups of local anesthetics:
  Esters: procaine, benzocaine, tetracaine
  Amides: lidocaine, prilocaine, mepivacaine, procainamide, dibucaine
  Urethane: polidocanol
It is generally classified as a weak detergent solution.
It should be diluted with distilled sterile water.
Patients should be warned about an Antabuse-alcohol reaction.
Elimination half-life is 4 hours with 90% elimination within 12 hours.
It does not cross the blood-brain barriers.
It is painless in injection and difficult to produce cutaneous necrosis.

TABLE 90-3

Maximum Daily Doses of Polidocanol

Concentration	Dose (ml) According to Body Weight of Patient				
	50 kg	60 kg	70 kg	80 kg	90 kg
0.5%	20	24	28	32	36
1.0%	10	12	14	16	18
2.0%	5	6	7	8	9
3.0%	3.3	4	4.6	5.3	6

Patient Questionnaire/Evaluation: Vein Injection (Sclerotherapy)

Date _____ Name _____   Birthdate _____ Age _____
Sex _____ Height _____ Weight _____
Referred by: _____

1. How many years have you noticed this problem? ____
2. Have you ever been previously treated for this problem?
                                            Yes ____ No ____
   By whom and when? _____
   _____

   With what method?
                Injection   _____
                Electrocautery   _____
                Laser   _____
                Surgery   _____

3. When did the problem with your veins occur?
                Age   _____
                Before pregnancy   _____
                After pregnancy   _____
                After trauma
                  or Premarin therapy _____
                Other   _____

4. Is there a family history of varicose or spider veins?
                Mother   _____
                Father   _____
                Sister   _____
                Brother   _____
                Children   _____
                Aunts   _____
                Uncles   _____

5. Do you have a history of:
                Smoking   _____
                Blood clots   _____
                Lupus   _____
                Bleeding disorders   _____
                Easy bruisability   _____
                Dark spots after
                  skin injury or surgery _____
                Easy scarring   _____

6. Are you developing new veins?   _____
7. Are your present veins getting bigger?   _____
8. After prolonged standing or sitting do your leges ache?   _____
9. Do your legs or veins ache before menses?   _____
10. Does walking or exercise relieve or aggravate the pain? (circle)
11. Describe any symptoms you have from your veins: _____
    _____
12. Are you required to be on your feet for long periods?   _____
13. Do you jog, run, jump rope, or do aerobics? (circle)
      How often per week?   _____
14. Are you pregnant or planning a pregnancy soon?   _____
15. Did you read and understand the patient education
    materials given to you?   _____
16. Do you understand the risks and benefits as well as
    possible complications to vein injection?   _____
17. Are you prepared to wear hose on a regular basis
    as described?   _____
18. Is your problem cosmetic or medical?   _____

PMH: MI: _____
      ALL: _____
      MEDS: _____
      FH: _____

Fig. 90-5
Patient questionnaire for sclerotherapy. (Modified from Mitchel P. Goldman, MD, Dermatology Associates of San Diego County, Inc., 9850 Genesee, Suite 480, La Jolla, CA 90237.)   *Continued*

- Tape (1 inch wide). (Some patients require paper tape.)
- Compression hose. Some clinicians stock them in the office. Patients can also be given a prescription to purchase them at a medical supply store (with proper measurement noted on the prescription) or be measured at certain retailers. Panty hose, full-length stockings, thigh-high stockings, or calf-high stockings are selected based on the areas being injected. Rubber gloves are helpful to apply the stocking or stockings.
- Elastic wraps (4 to 6 inches wide) (e.g., Ace bandages).
- Nonsterile gloves.

Note: Additional instruments that may be helpful but not necessary include a photoplethysmograph, light reflection rheograph, and a duplex scanner.

PREPROCEDURE PATIENT PREPARATION

It is best if the patient receives patient education materials before the office visit. (See the patient education handouts titled "Sclerotherapy Billing Procedures" and "Sclerotherapy (Vein Injection)" on pages 1840 and 1842, respectively, in Appendix G.) An initial visit is scheduled for 30 minutes. The patient is evaluated, venous testing is done, the legs are measured for hose, and counseling is completed. Future visits of 15 to 30 minutes are scheduled for the injections at 2- to 4-week intervals. It is best not to inject the same area any sooner than 3 to 4 weeks. Average patients will require three 30-minute injection visits.

Patient Questionnaire/Evaluation: Vein Injection (Sclerotherapy)

VARICOSITIES: R   L

          Vulvar   ____ ____
          Groin   ____ ____
          Thigh   ____ ____
          Below knee   ____ ____

PULSES: R   L

          Femoral   ____ ____
          Popliteal   ____ ____
          Dorsalis pedis ____ ____
          Post tibial   ____ ____

PRESENCE OF: R   L

          Edema   ____ ____
          Stasis pig   ____ ____
          Cellulitis   ____ ____
          Active ulcer   ____ ____
          Healed ulcer   ____ ____
          Venules   ____ ____
          Tenderness   ____ ____

                                                                    R   L

                                              PPG   ____ ____
                                              PRG   ____ ____
                                              Doppler ____ ____

IMPRESSION: _____

_____

_____

PLAN: Discussed:

        • Method
        • Cost
        • Complications
            hyperpigmentation
            blistering
            recurrence
            pain
            phlebitis
            matting
        • Stockings
        • Number of anticipated visits

        Measurements

        Ankle _____
        Calf _____
        Thigh _____
        Length _____
        Shoe size _____
        Type:
            Panty
            Thigh high
            Knee high
            20/30 or 30/40

cc: _____   _____ _____
                                 Physician Signature   Date

Fig. 90-5, cont'd

A careful history and physical examination must be performed (Fig. 90-5), and those problems that might affect treatment with sclerotherapy (e.g., anticoagulation, history of phlebitis, vein surgery, arterial disease, bleeding problems, diabetes, history of severe allergic reactions) should be sought.

Physical examination must include a careful evaluation of the pedal pulses. If they are not readily felt, it is necessary to obtain an ankle-to-brachial ratio. The only equipment needed for this is a blood pressure cuff, stethoscope, and handheld Doppler probe.

It is essential to look for the presence of saphenofemoral or saphenopopliteal reflux, also known as axial vein reflux. Its presence is a contraindication to sclerotherapy, and many insurance companies will not cover sclerotherapy if it is present. This determination can be accomplished with a careful handheld Doppler examination. The patient must be standing. The tip of the Doppler probe is held at the SFJ or SPJ while the calf muscle is firmly and sharply compressed. This creates a sound when the blood is propelled forward. As the muscle is released, there should be no retrograde flow (only silence). If it is heard, it means there is reflux at these junctions and surgical treatment is probably necessary (although some clinicians advocate duplex scan–guided sclerotherapy). Newer techniques would also include saphenous vein ablation with a radiofrequency or laser catheter.

Patients are often screened with *photoplethysmography* (PPG) and *light reflection rheography* (LRR). These are means of measuring the venous refilling time of the lower limb using a transducer to shine a certain wavelength of light into the skin about 10 cm proximal to the medial malleolus. Hemoglobin specifically absorbs this

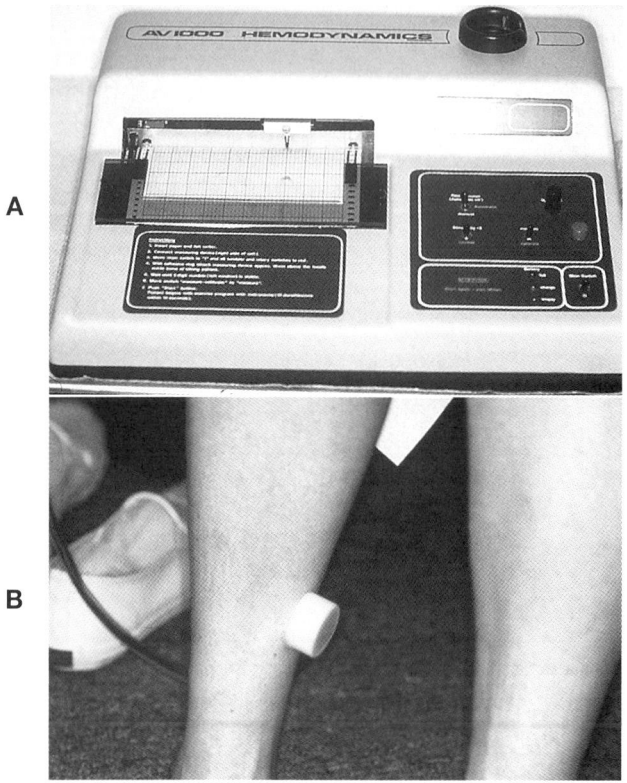

Fig. 90-6
A, Photoplethysmography (PPG) machine. **B,** PPG machine attached to a patient.

wavelength. With the patient seated, he or she dorsiflexes the foot 8 or 10 times. This compresses and empties the normal dermal venous plexus. The light that is not absorbed by hemoglobin is reflected back to the transducer and is measured. This reflection back is greater when the veins are empty (less hemoglobin to absorb the light) and decreases when the veins are full, because the vessels filled with blood (hemoglobin) absorb more light. The instrument then records how long it takes for the blood of the dermal plexus to return to baseline. A refilling time of less than 25 to 30 seconds indicates that the venous plexus is filling partially in a retrograde fashion and demonstrates incompetence of the venous system. If the test is abnormal, a tourniquet should be applied just above and then below the knee. The test is repeated; if it is normalized, it suggests that the problem is just in the superficial system (Figs. 90-6 to 90-8) and that sclerotherapy can proceed. If the filling time does not normalize with above- and below-knee tourniquets, it suggests deep venous insufficiency and further evaluation (i.e., duplex ultrasound) may be indicated.

PPG findings have been found to correlate well with venograms for the determination of DVT. In this instance, outflow of blood is blocked and the tracing is thereby flat.

A duplex scan performed when the patient is standing allows an estimate of the location of venous reflux and its magnitude. The clinician can also look for DVT, venous obstruction, and incompetent perforators. Few offices can afford this type of sophisticated equipment. However, if the clinician desires to perform duplex scan–guided sclerotherapy, obviously it is necessary. This equipment is also quite helpful if the clinician contemplates performing surgical ablation of varicosities.

Photographs of the lower limbs may be necessary. Some insurance companies require them. More importantly, photographs provide baseline information to which the patient's limbs can be compared as treatment progresses. Many phlebologists will first draw the veins in on diagrams.

The technique of sclerotherapy must be carefully explained to the patient, including possible complications and what will happen over the course of treatment. The patient must be cautioned not to expect perfection. A well-educated patient is more cooperative and satisfied.

TECHNIQUE

1. Before injecting the patient, obtain a signed consent. (See the sample patient consent form titled "Sclerotherapy" on page 1846 of Appendix G.)
2. Wipe the area to be injected with Zephiran or alcohol. This not only cleanses the area but also improves visualization of the vessels. Use a small syringe (1 or 3 ml). Stretch the skin surrounding the vessel with the nondominant hand. It is helpful to bend up the tip of the 30-gauge needle about 20 to 30 degrees to cannulate these tiny veins (Fig. 90-9).

   Direct cannulation of the vein is absolutely essential. Extraluminal injections may lead to skin necrosis. For the treatment of veins 2.0 mm in diameter or less, 0.2% sodium tetradecyl sulfate is used. Although some therapists suggest a concentration of 0.1%, it is not necessary to decrease the concentration (Table 90-4). Aspiration of blood from the small vessels cannot be accomplished. If a small wheal forms at the time of injection, the needle is not in the lumen and injection must be stopped. If the needle is properly inserted, the vessel should blanch. Once the blanching stops, withdraw and go to the next vessel. More is *not* better unless new vessels continue to blanch. The injection is carried out with extremely gentle pressure, and only 0.1 to 0.3 ml is used. Too much pressure can rupture the vein and lead to unnecessary inflammation.

   For injection of veins 3 to 5 mm, 0.5% sodium

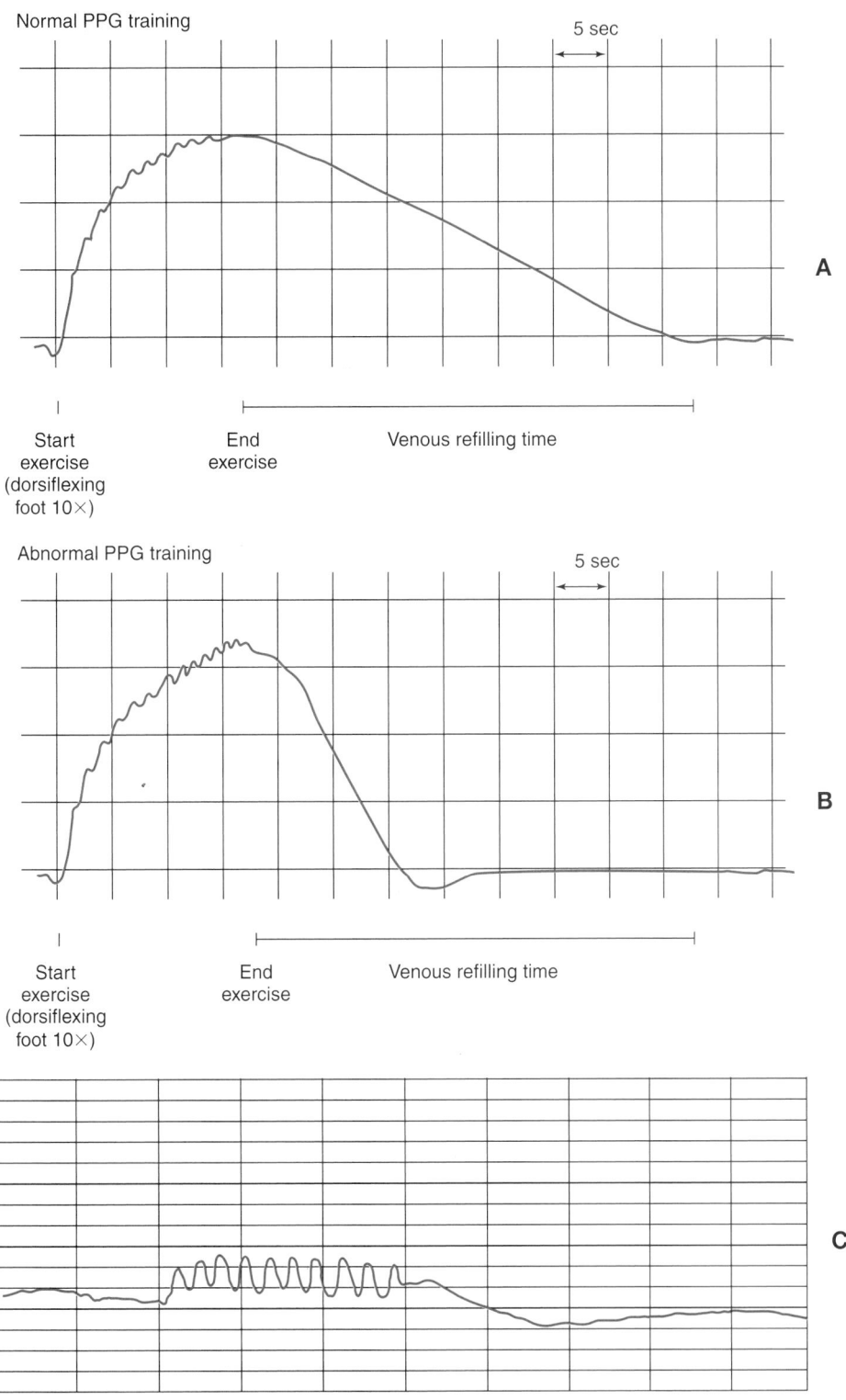

Fig. 90-7

Tracings of photoplethysmography readings. **A,** Normal. After dorsiflexing the foot 10 times, the blood has been "squeezed out" of the ankle, so less light is absorbed and more is reflected back. This gives a higher reading. As the veins refill with blood, more light is absorbed so less is reflected back. Thus a lower amplitude is recorded. A refill time over 25 seconds is normal. **B,** Abnormal. Rapid refill indicating venous insufficiency. Refill time is only 15 to 17 seconds. (Without tourniquets, this could be deep or superficial; if tourniquets are in place, this is most likely indicative of deep venous insufficiency.) **C,** Abnormal. No indication of emptying, suggesting deep venous obstruction or marked insufficiency ("picket fence" pattern).

tetradecyl sulfate is used in a quantity of 0.5 ml to a maximum of 1.0 ml. Because a stronger solution is being used, it is more likely that subcutaneous injection may lead to a slough. Therefore aspiration of blood into the hub of the needle is recommended.

For veins 5 to 6 mm in diameter, 1.0% sodium tetradecyl sulfate is used with a volume of 0.5 to a maximum of 1.0 ml (Table 90-4). Aspiration before injection is essential.

All of the previously mentioned procedures can be performed with the patient supine. Spider veins will remain visible, but at times it may be difficult to cannulate large veins in a supine patient because the veins are not dilated and collapse when the patient

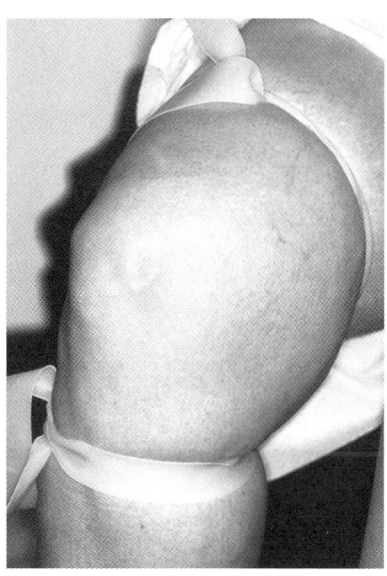

Fig. 90-8
Placement of tourniquets above and below the knee when the photoplethysmogram is abnormal. If the tracing normalizes, it indicates superficial venous incompetence. If it remains abnormal with rapid refilling, deep venous insufficiency is suggested.

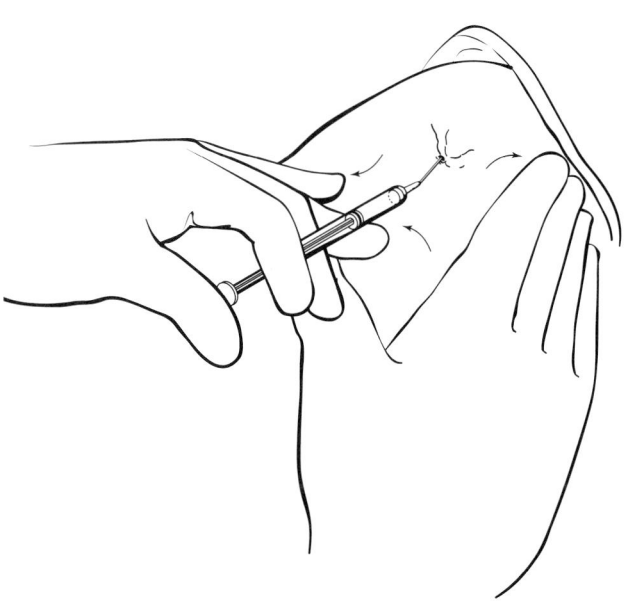

Fig. 90-9
Proper injection technique. The nondominant hand stretches the skin around the vessels. The needle bevel is up and the needle itself is bent 30 degrees upward. (Redrawn from Sadick NS: *Manual of sclerotherapy,* Philadelphia, 2000, Lippincott, Williams & Wilkins.)

TABLE 90-4

Rapid Guide for Selection of Sclerosing Solution by Vessel Type*

Vessel	Solution/Concentration	Volume (per Injection Site)
Telangiectatic matting (after previous treatment)	**Hypertonic saline, 11.7%** **Sodium tetradecyl sulfate, 0.1%** Polidocanol, 0.25% (Go slow with low injection pressures)	0.1-0.2 ml
Telangiectasia (up to 1 mm)	**Hypertonic saline, 11.7%†** **Sodium tetradecyl sulfate, 0.1%-0.2%** Polidocanol, 0.25%	0.1-0.3 ml
Venulectasia (1-2 mm)	**Hypertonic saline, 11.7%-23.4%†** **Sodium tetradecyl sulfate, 0.1%-0.25%** Polidocanol, 0.5%-0.75%	0.2-0.5 ml
Reticular veins (2-4 mm, subcutaneous blue veins)	**Hypertonic saline, 18.7%-23.4%†** **Sodium tetradecyl sulfate, 0.33%-0.5%** Polidocanol, 0.75%-1.5%	0.5 ml (may increase to 1 ml if filling of reticular vein is observed)
Nonsaphenous varicose veins (3-8 mm)	**Hypertonic saline, 18.7%-23.4%** **Sodium tetradecyl sulfate, 0.5%-1.0%** Polidocanol, 1.0%-3.0%	0.5 ml (may increase to 1 ml per injection site in large-capacity vein)
Saphenous varicose trunks (usually >5 mm)	**Hypertonic saline, 18.7%-23.4%** **Sodium tetradecyl sulfate, 1.0%-3.0%** Polidocanol, 3.0%-5.0%	0.5 ml (low-volume injection critical at high concentrations)

*Solutions in bold approved by the U.S. Food and Drug Administration.
†Many use standard 18.7% for all these indications.

lies down. In this case the patient should be asked to stand and the vein cannulated with a no. 27 butterfly that is taped in place. The patient can then be placed in a supine position and the vein injected as previously described. Alternatively, the veins are marked with a skin-marking pen in the standing position and can be injected when the patient lies down.

A compression dressing consisting of a folded piece of gauze is placed over each site and covered with a piece of Dermicel or similar tape. Paper tape is necessary for some patients to avoid allergic responses. A cotton ball and tape is used by many phlebologists and works well. The limb is then compressed either by elastic wraps or compression hose as discussed in the following section.

Note: It is often quicker and easier to just wrap Coban or Co-Flex around the entire leg followed by the compression hose. This keeps the blood off the hose and makes it easier to get the hose on the leg. It comes in 4-inch by 9-yard rolls.

A complete note should be dictated (or a form used) for at least the first injection visit (Fig. 90-10). After this, flow sheets save time (Fig. 90-11).

Sclerotherapy Treatment Note

Name: _____   Birthdate: _____
Referring physician: _____   Date: _____
Chief Complaint: Sclerotherapy injection

S: The patient has thought over what we have discussed on the last visit and has read over multiple patient education materials supplied. He/she has elected to go ahead and have the sclerotherapy performed today. We explained again the nature of the complications: hyperpigmentation, matting, recurrence, slight ulceration, phlebitis, and blebs. He/she understands these and has elected to go ahead and have the injections done. There were no further questions and subsequently we proceeded.

O: Venous sclerotherapy

Areas: _____
Sclerosant: _____
Amount: _____ ml
Number of complexes injected: _____
Complications: None or _____

Procedure note: The patient was once again examined in the supine position. The complexes of veins that were to be injected were noted. These areas were all wiped with Zephiran. Individual 1-ml syringes were used with 30-gauge needles. Each syringe was used no more than 3 to 4 times and no more than 0.5 ml of the solution was injected per vein site. In the majority of cases the vein was cannulated but in a few areas there was minimal extravasation of the sclerosant. After injection, a rolled 4 × 4 was immediately placed over the area and secured with paper tape. Upon completion of injection of the various veins, the Sigvaris/MediUSA/Jobst pantyhose/thigh high/above the knee support stockings, which were measured for the patient, were used to hold the pressure dressings in place. They were of the 20/30 gradient type. The patient tolerated this well and was discharged home.

Changes to routine: _____

Impression:
1. _____
2. _____

P: The patient will wear the stockings for at least ___ days and ___ nights without removing them. Cool baths can then soak off the tape making it easier to remove the pressure dressings. He/she is to wear the support hose for at least 4 weeks during the day but may remove them at night. After injection, he/she is to walk at least 30 minutes. Hot baths are to be avoided for at least 2 weeks. It is best to wear some type of support hose for the rest of his/her life since venous disease is an ongoing problem and the source of the problem is not resolved by the injections. It may be necessary to come back every 1-2 years to have "touch-ups" on new or recurrent veins. There may be some pigmentation from the veins. The patient should call should there be any significant problems. Follow-up in _____ weeks for a recheck and for any possible further injections.

Other: _____
cc: _____   _____   _____
                                                                    Physician Signature   Date

---

Fig. 90-10
Sample form of a sclerotherapy treatment note. (Courtesy The National Procedures Institute, Midland, Mich.)

Follow-up Sclerotherapy

Patient :_____   DOB: _____   Date: _____
Initial evaluation: _____   Referring physician: _____
PPG: _____   Sclerosant:

Working diagnosis: Support hose/Ace wrap/other:

Date	Subjective/Examination	Treatment	Impression	Plan

Fig. 90-11
Sample flow sheet for follow-up sclerotherapy appointments.
(Courtesy The National Procedures Institute, Midland, Mich.)

PEARLS

Injection sclerotherapy using hypertonic saline solution or sodium tetradecyl is a safe, relatively painless method of ablating small varicose veins, reticular venules, and spider telangiectasia, with a minimum of complications. The attending physician will have better results and happier patients if several important concepts are remembered:

1. Although spider veins may be symptomatic, most patients seek treatment because they are unhappy with the appearance of their legs. The clinician should be cautious and conservative so that a blem-ish worse than what the patient already has is not created.
2. Sclerotherapy should be viewed as a semicosmetic procedure, and the patient's high expectations must be carefully considered.
3. Careful preinjection discussion of risks must occur with patients so that they are fully aware of the protracted and tedious nature of sclerotherapy, as well as the potential complications.
4. The effect of gravity and incompetent venous valves must always be remembered. Varicose veins and spider veins tend to recur. The wearing of compression hose in the immediate postinjection period is

mandatory. Compression hose worn on a long-term basis will significantly reduce recurrence.

5. Meticulous technique is essential in sclerotherapy.
   a. The clinician must be sure the needle is in the vein.
   b. The solution should be injected slowly.
   c. A maximum of 0.5 ml of solution should be used per injection, and large bolus injections should be avoided.
   d. The clinician should watch the needle tip and stop injecting if there is extravasation.
6. The larger vessels should be injected first.
7. The clinician should begin injections proximally and work on down the leg. If injections are started distally, the proximal vessels often go into spasm and it is very difficult to inject them.
8. Telangiectasias will be visible when the patient lies down, but varicosities may disappear. It helps to mark them with a marking pen while the patient is standing.
9. The clinician should not attempt to withdraw blood before injecting telangiectasias; however, it is essential to withdraw blood before injecting larger vessels to be sure the needle is in the lumen.
10. If a wheal is seen, the clinician should stop injecting immediately. The magnification loops help identify this early in the procedure. If recognized early and the injection is stopped, the small blebs that occur generally do not lead to any sloughing. Older texts recommended diluting the area with saline for extravasation, but it is not needed with these small amounts.

Note: With careful and precise technique, the majority of small telangiectatic (i.e., spider) veins can be eliminated. Patient satisfaction with the procedure is high.

COMPRESSION

The amount and duration of compression used with sclerotherapy remains somewhat controversial. Initially Irish sclerotherapists who were treating large, bulging varicose veins used 6 weeks of continuous compression, a regimen quite difficult for the patient. Later studies suggested that 3 weeks of compression for large veins is adequate. Whether this should be used for 24 hours a day or only while the patient is standing is still an unsettled issue.

When injecting spider veins, elastic compression bandages (4 inches wide) can be used for the first 24 hours. The patient then removes the elastic bandage and the underlying dressings and wears lightweight, measured compression panty hose (15 mm of Hg-gradient hose). Many therapists use 20 to 30 mm of Hg-gradient hose or even 30 to 40 mm of Hg-gradient hose. The patient is asked to wear the hose during the course of treatment, whenever out of bed. If the patient has sclerotherapy appointments every 2 to 3 weeks, for example, and requires three visits, the patient will wear the stockings for 9 or 10 weeks. After the last treatment, the clinician can suggest that the patient wear the stockings while out of bed for at least 10 more days (preferably for 3 weeks). A recent review confirmed that wearing support hose continuously for 3 days, then while ambulatory for 3 more weeks, markedly reduced complications and recurrence.

When larger veins are injected, 30- to 40-mm Hg-compression hose are recommended. The type of stocking depends upon the areas being injected. If the thighs and both lower limbs are involved, panty hose are best. Otherwise a full-length stocking, thigh-high stocking, or calf-high stocking can be used if it compresses the areas that were injected. The physician can prescribe the stocking at the time of the patient's initial visit, and the patient can then bring it to the first therapeutic session. Many of the stocking companies are quite good in supplying physician's offices with stockings and providing prompt, next-day delivery service. Ancillary personnel can learn to measure the patient for ready-made stockings or for custom hose. The patient would then receive the hose from the physician's office.

It is recommended that patients wear lightweight compression panty hose as much as possible on an indefinite basis to diminish the recurrence of varicose veins or the development of new ones; however, many patients are resistant to such a regimen. Compression stockings are also used in the management of patients with postthrombotic syndrome, healed venous ulcers, lymphedema, and other problems. Although patients can purchase cheaper over-the-counter hose, they generally provide only compression and not a gradient of more to less pressure as the hose goes up the leg.

COMPLICATIONS

- *Bruising.* Patients must understand that they will look worse before they look better. It may take 4 to 8 weeks before the postsclerotherapy changes have resolved.
- *Hemosiderin staining (hyperpigmentation).* This occurs transiently in almost every case. It is considered a complication when it lasts for more than several weeks. In about 5% to 10% of patients, it can take up to 1 year to diminish. The discoloration follows the outline of the previously injected vein and can also be seen after stripping or phlebectomy. The larger the vein, the more likely it is to occur—especially if compression hose are not worn long enough. Unfortunately, in spite of trying many bleaching creams, little can be done to hasten

resolution. If clots are evident, their removal lessens the duration of pigmentation. Prevention (with the use of compression hose) is the key.

- *Matting (angioneogenesis).* This is the development of tiny vessels at or near the site of previous injection and occurs in 3% to 10% of patients. It may result from an injection under too high a pressure (causing rupture of the vessel) or because the volume of the sclerosing solution was too large or the solution was too strong. Matting probably develops as part of the inflammatory response that occurs as the result of these errors in technique. However, even with excellent technique, matting may occur. It may disappear in a few months. If it does not, the clinician should make a very careful search for a reticular vein leading into the area and try to obliterate it. Sometimes the matting itself can be injected or treated with light therapy, such as Photo-Derm or laser. If reinjection is done, the clinician should use low concentrations of sclerosants and inject slowly.

- *Skin slough with ulceration.* Generally this is related to extravasation of the solution. It may occur because of improper placement of the needle, rupture of the vein, having only part of the needle in the lumen, or injection of an arteriole. A tiny arteriole may also connect to a vein. In these cases, closure of the arteriole can cause a skin infarct. Ulcerations can even occur with a perfectly performed injection when the solution erodes through the wall of the vein into unhealthy skin. The ulceration often takes 4 to 8 weeks to resolve.

- *Arterial injection.* This is a dreaded complication. It will result in a large slough and even limb loss if a large artery it is injected. It is more likely to occur around the ankle, especially in the area of the posterior tibial artery.

- *Syncope.* This is more common if injections are done with the patient standing. At times standing is necessary when inserting butterfly needles and then having the patient assume a recumbent position for the injection of large veins.

- *Allergic reaction.* This will not occur with hypertonic saline, and it occurs extremely rarely with sodium tetradecyl sulfate (approximately 0.3%). When it does occur, it is usually a mild response, although anaphylaxis has been reported. Necessary equipment to treat this problem, such as an Ambu-bag, airways, epinephrine for injection, steroid for injection, and an injectable anticonvulsant should be on hand (see Chapter 203, Anaphylaxis). Pretreatment of allergic patients with 50 mg of Benadryl will obviate this problem.

- *Superficial thrombophlebitis.* Injection of sclerosant creates a chemical thrombophlebitis that is controlled and affects only the treated area. However, at times the solution can travel proximally or distally and create an area of thrombus within the veins. The area overlying this often becomes red and tender. In most cases careful technique using only a small amount of solution (0.5 to 1 ml) will prevent this outcome. It is more likely to occur when injecting larger veins. When it does occur, the patient must be reassured that nothing serious has happened. Treatment consists of compression and an antiinflammatory drug (e.g., ibuprofen).

- *Thrombus formation.* Clots can form in small veins or especially in the larger ones. They can be aspirated with a needle or incised and drained. Usually for the larger ones, a small amount of lidocaine is injected, then a no. 11 blade used to open the skin over the area. Pressure will expel the clot. No suture is needed. Thrombi are more common when larger veins are injected and if compression is not optimal postinjection. If a clot has been present more than 4 weeks, it often organizes and then is difficult to remove.

- *Postinjection itching and pain.* Patients often complain of a transient itching after injection; some phlebologists apply steroid cream immediately after injection, but this is not necessary. The site of injections may become painful. Over-the-counter pain medication, including nonsteroidal antiinflammatory drugs (NSAIDs), is adequate to control this and does not interfere with the effectiveness of treatment. Pain during the injection is minimal and well tolerated.

- *DVT and pulmonary emboli.* Fortunately this is a rare complication. It is most likely to occur if too much solution is used and it gets into the deep system. Patients who have one of the many kinds of thrombophilia are more likely to have this problem, as are patients with previous histories of DVT. Birth control pills and estrogen may slightly increase the tendency toward this complication, but it is rare and their use does not contraindicate sclerotherapy. DVT may be reduced or eliminated by having the patient walk for 20 to 30 minutes after injection of large veins to avoid pooling in the deep venous system.

POSTPROCEDURE PATIENT EDUCATION

Patients are asked to walk immediately after a session of sclerotherapy. Some therapists recommend 30 minutes, but even 5 or 10 minutes seems to be enough. Walking diffuses the solution that may have gone into the deep system and, more importantly, increases circulating fibrinolysins. (See the sample patient education handout titled "Sclerotherapy: Postprocedure Instructions" on page 1841 of Appendix G.)

The same area should not be injected again for 3 to 4 weeks. The patient can return at weekly intervals for treatment of alternate sites until treatment is complete.

Patients should be able to resume normal activities, including high-impact aerobics and jogging, 24 hours after injections for spider veins; however, some therapists would further restrict patients for 1 week. No good prospective studies indicate the effect of robust activity on sclerotherapy.

CONCLUSION

Sclerotherapy, when practiced properly, is a highly effective means of treating medium and small varicose veins and telangiectasias. Many therapists treat even large varicosities in this manner. Laser and other forms of light therapy are not as efficient and effective in most instances. At best they are useful for treating veins 3 mm in diameter and smaller. Equipment and methods may improve the results of light therapy, but sclerotherapy remains the gold standard for treating such veins.

Careful workup and management of patients with special attention to proper technique should provide good to excellent results in more than 90% of patients.

SUPPLIERS

Support hose
Sigvaris
P.O. Box 570
Branford, CT 06405
Phone: 1-800-322-7744
Website: www.sigvaris.com

BSN-Jobst Institute, Inc.
Rutherford College
100 Beiersdorf Drive
P.O. Box 390
Rutherford College, NC 28671
Phone: 1-828-879-5100
Website: www.jobst.com

MediUSA
6481 Franz Warner Parkway
Whitsett, NC 27377
Phone: 1-800-633-6334
Website: www.mediusa.com

Headlamp and ocular loupes
Welch Allyn
4341 State Street Road
P.O. Box 220
Skaneateles Falls, NY 13153-0220
Phone: 1-800-535-6663
Website: www.welchallyn.com

Luxtec
99 Hartwell Street
West Boylston, MA 01583
Phone: 1-800-325-8966
Website: www.luxtec.com

Syringes and needles
Air-Tite Products Company
565 Central Drive
Virginia Beach, VA 23455
Phone: 1-800-231-7762
Website: www.air-tite.com

Hypertonic saline/Sotradecol
Delasco
608 13th Avenue
Council Bluffs, IA 51501-6401
Phone: 1-800-831-6273
Website: www.delasco.com

Venous noninvasive diagnostic equipment (e.g., PPG, Doppler) and assistance with all sclerotherapy supplies
Sam Wagner
P.O. Box 431
202 Dodd Street
Middlebourne, WV 26149
Phone: 1-304-758-2370

Note: This is a superb resource.

Polidocanol
Pharmacy Specialists (Sam Pratt, RPh)
650 Maitland Avenue
Altemonte Springs, FL 32701
Phone: 1-800-224-7711

Patient education materials
MJD Patient Communications
4641 Montgomery Avenue, Suite 350
Bethesda, MD 20814
Phone: 1-301-657-8010
Website: www.mjdpc.com

Contemporary Health Communications
16714 Benton Taylor Drive
Chesterfield, MO 63005
Phone: 1-800-234-1742
Website: www.patient-info.com

American Academy of Dermatology Association
930 North Meacham Road
P.O. Box 4014
Schaumburg, IL 60168-4014
Phone: 1-847-330-0230
Website: www.aadassociation.org

CPT/BILLING CODES

Injections for telangiectasia, even if symptomatic, are rarely covered by insurance. Coverage for varicosities is quite variable. It is often necessary to document conservative therapy (e.g., use of compression hose) that has failed. Frequently, preapproval and photographs will be required.

Most sclerotherapists do not deal with insurance companies and ask the patient to pay at the time of service. Some will charge by the number of injections and others by the amount of solution used; still others will inject for a certain time period (15 to 30 minutes). There are no routine standards.

36468	Injection; multiple telangiectasias, leg
36469	Injection; multiple telangiectasias, face (see caution in the "Indications" section)
36470	Injection of single varicose vein
36471	Injection of multiple varicose veins, same leg
−50	Modifier for bilateral procedure
10160	Aspiration, hematoma
10140	I&D hematoma
93965	Impedance plethysmography
93970	Duplex scan

ICD-9-CM DIAGNOSTIC CODES

448.1	Spider vein/telangiectasia
448.9	Capillary vein
454.1	Varicosity with inflammation
454.1	Stasis dermatitis
454.2	Varicosity with ulceration
454.9	Varicose vein, leg
457.1	Lymphedema
459.1	Postphlebitic syndrome
459.81	Chronic venous insufficiency
709.0	Dyschromia of skin (hyperpigmentation)
729.5	Pain in leg
729.81	Swelling in leg
782.0	Burning, hyperesthesia
782.3	Edema
924.5	Hematoma, lower extremity

ADDITIONAL RESOURCES

• See the sample patient education handouts titled "Sclerotherapy Billing Procedures," "Sclerotherapy: Postprocedure Instructions," and "Sclerotherapy (Vein Injection)" on pages 1840, 1841, and 1842, respectively, of Appendix G.

• See the sample patient consent form titled "Sclerotherapy" on page 1846 of Appendix G.

BIBLIOGRAPHY

Bergan JJ, Kistner RL, editors: *Atlas of venous surgery,* Philadelphia, 1992, WB Saunders.

Conrad P, Malouf GM, Stacey MC: The Australian polidocanol (aethoxysklerol) study. Results at 2 years, *Dermatol Surg* 21:334, 1995.

Goldman MP, Bergan JJ: *Sclerotherapy: treatment of varicose and telangiectatic leg veins,* ed 3, St Louis, 2001, Mosby.

Note: This is the "Bible" and a must for anyone performing sclerotherapy!

Goldman MP, Bergan JJ, editors: *Ambulatory treatment of venous disease,* St Louis, 1996, Mosby.

Goldman MP, Beaudoing D, Marley W, et al: Compression in the treatment of leg telangiectasia: a preliminary report, *J Dermatol Surg Oncol* 16:4, 1990.

Goldman MP, Sadick NS, Weiss RA: Cutaneous necrosis, telangiectatic matting, and hyperpigmentation following sclerotherapy. Etiology, prevention, and treatment, *Dermatol Surg* 21:19, 1995.

Goldman MP, Weiss RA, Bergan JJ, editors: *Varicose veins and telangiectasias,* St Louis, 1999, Quality Medical Publishing.

Goldman MP, Weiss RA, Brody HJ, et al: Treatment of facial telangiectasia with sclerotherapy, laser surgery, and/or electrodesiccation: a review, *J Dermatol Surg Oncol* 19:899, 1993.

Green D: Sclerotherapy for varicose and telangiectatic veins, *Am Fam Physician* 46:827, 1992.

Isaacs MN: Symptomatology of vein disease, *Dermatol Surg* 21:321, 1995.

Kanter AH: The effect of sclerotherapy on restless legs syndrome, *Dermatol Surg* 21:328, 1995.

Olivencia JA: Varicose veins: not just a cosmetic problem, *Patient Care* 15:140, 1996.

Pfeifer JR, Hawtof GD: Injection sclerotherapy and CO_2 laser sclerotherapy in the ablation of cutaneous spider veins of the lower extremity, *Phlebology* 4:231, 1989.

Sadick NS: *Manual of sclerotherapy,* Philadelphia, 2000, Lippincott, Williams & Wilkins.

Note: This source is superb, concise, thorough, and practical.

Tibbs DJ, Sabiston DC, Davies MG, et al, editors: *Varicose veins: venous disorders and lymphatic problems in the lower limb,* New York, 1997, Oxford University Press.

Tretbar LL: Injection sclerotherapy for spider telangiectasias: a 20-year experience with sodium tetradecyl sulfate, *J Dermatol Surg Oncol* 15:223, 1989.

Weiss RA, Dover JS: Leg vein management: sclerotherapy, ambulatory phlebectomy, and laser surgery. In Kaminer MS, Dover JS, Arndt KA, editors: *Atlas of cosmetic surgery,* Philadelphia, 2002, WB Saunders.

Weiss RA, Sadide NS, Goldman MP, et al: Controlled comparative study of duration of compression and its effect on clinical outcome, *Dermatol Surg* 25:105, 1999.

CHAPTER 91

Radiofrequency Sclerotherapy: New Technique for Varicose Vein Treatment

Gary L. Snyder

Sclerotherapy is the act of introducing an agent—be it physical, chemical or mechanical—into a vessel to produce destruction of the endothelium and subendothelium (see Chapter 90, Sclerotherapy). The primary objective of any sclerotherapy procedure or modality is to destroy the intima (endothelium) and part of the media while keeping the outer adventitia intact. Destruction of the intima must be carried out in a manner where activation of the intrinsic pathway of coagulation discourages formation of thrombi and the extrinsic pathway is avoided. Activation of the extrinsic pathway would lead to thrombus formation, which in turn can be a major source of recanalization and recurrence. Given this rationale, any treatment or modality that causes clot or thrombus, by its very nature, goes against primary objective of sclerotherapy.

Radiofrequency sclerotherapy (RS) is the process of using high-frequency radiowaves to vaporize the thinly layered endothelium and the innermost portions of the muscular media of large veins (see Chapter 31, Radiofrequency Surgery). (The technique described here is not applicable to telangiectasias and small reticular veins.) Once this physical phenomenon has been achieved, the injured vessel must be compressed to maintain apposition of the vessel walls until wound healing gains sufficient tensile strength to maintain sclerosis. Numerous animal models have shown that the lag phase of wound healing encompasses a typical 3- to 7-day period where little or no gain in tensile strength is noted. Further, maximal tensile strength is achieved between 7 and 21 days in most animal models; therefore compression must be applied for at least 7 days, if not longer.

The instruments for RS are a high-radiofrequency generator system and a coated protective needle. The Ellman Surgitron FFPF (Fig. 91-1) emits a 3.8-MHz–frequency radiowave, which is ideal for intravascular vaporization. Radiofrequency waves with a frequency below 3.8 MHz generate more heat than vaporization and are not well suited for RS; likewise, solid core electrodes have a high current density and emanate

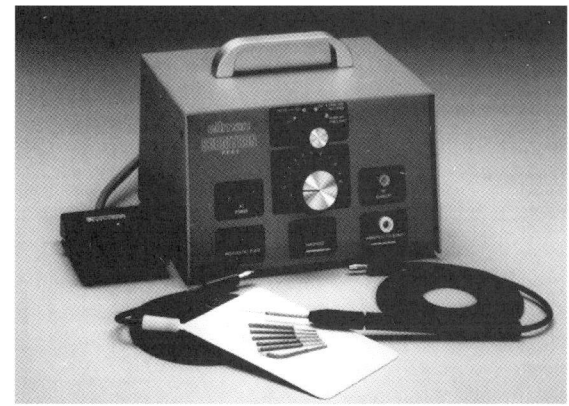

Fig. 91-1
Ellman Surgitron FFPF radiosurgery unit. (Courtesy Ellman International, Hewlett, NY.)

significant heat, which can burn surrounding tissues and cause rupture of the vessel. A specially coated metal hub hypodermic needle has been developed. It allows vaporization without the unwanted thermal effects and aids in visualization of correct intravascular placement of the needle electrode. All of the instrumentation and the needles and materials are approved by the Food and Drug Administration (FDA). The FDA does not approve procedures.

INDICATIONS

- Linear reticular and collateral varicose veins: Highly branched reticulars have too many sources of supply and lend themselves better to injection procedures.
- Truncal and non-truncal varicose veins after control of perforators and valvular insufficiency.
- An alternative to more invasive ambulatory phlebectomy, ligation and division procedures, and venous stripping. Morbidity and mortality are greatly reduced and the complete eradication of physiologic and ana-

tomic abnormalities can be overcome without scarring and debilitation.

CONTRAINDICATIONS

- Previous history of deep venous thrombosis (DVT)
- Previous history of pulmonary embolism (PE)
- Previous history of any embolism
- Current anticoagulation therapy
- Immunologically compromised states
- Deep venous incompetency
- Postphlebitic limbs
- Nonambulatory or orthopedically comprised patients
- Peripheral vascular insufficiency (relative)

EQUIPMENT

- Ellman Surgitron FFPF or other radiofrequency generator producing 3.5- to 4.0-MHz frequency (Fig. 91-1).
- Coated Scleroneedles or other coated electrodes of appropriate length and thickness. Common sizes are 30 gauge, ½-inch; 27 gauge, 1 to 1¼ inch; 25 gauge, 1 to 1½ inch; and 23 gauge, 1 inch.
- Ellman Luer-Lok adapter.
- Alcohol wipes.
- Small emesis basin or container to catch the backflow from venipuncture.
- Nonsterile gloves.
- Gauze 2 × 2–inch or greater or dental cotton rolls.
- Gradient compression hose (class II or class I).
- Xylocaine plain (0.5% to 1%), single dose vials (0.5 to 1 ml at each treatment site).
- 1-inch pillow foam (can be purchased at any hobby or sewing store in varying densities).
- Antibiotic ointment of choice.
- Nonsticking, nonabsorbent dressing (Adaptic, Xeroform, or Telfa).

PREPROCEDURE PATIENT PREPARATION

The patient should be well rested, calm, and in a warm environment to allow maximum dilation of the vein or veins to be cannulated. Treatment should not be undertaken at the initial visit. The initial visit should consist of clinical evaluation and dispensation of educational materials, including a fact sheet, explaining the most frequently asked questions (see the sample patient education handout titled "Radiofrequency Sclerotherapy" on page 1847 of Appendix G). A thorough assessment of the superficial and perforator systems should be carried out.

This may include clinical evaluations such as evaluation for perforator or saphenofemoral reflux using a handheld continuous wave Doppler. Evaluation of reflux with the handheld Doppler is essential to understanding the etiology of varicose veins. (See Chapter 85, Noninvasive Venous and Arterial Studies of the Lower Extremities, and Chapter 90, Sclerotherapy.)

An appropriate consent form should be signed (see the sample patient consent form titled "Radiofrequency Treatment of Varicose Veins" on page 1849 of Appendix G) indicating, at a minimum, patient understanding of "alternative treatments" and the ramifications of "no treatment." In addition, the patient must understand and consent to the possibility of permanent skin marks from the thermal effects of the procedure and the possibility of recurrence, without promise of cure or resolution of the problem. A signed copy of the consent and fact sheet should be retained in the medical record. Clinical before-and-after photographs help document the course and results of treatment. The office staff should document what instructions were presented and that the patient was provided additional explanation where appropriate. The patient is normally seen several days to 1 week after treatment; he or she very rarely has a medical reason to be seen in the interim.

TECHNIQUE

Appropriate sedation may be used; however, the author prefers an alert and mobile patient without sedation.

1. Have the patient stand or position the limb in a position that allows full distension of the superficial venous system.
2. Insert the metal-hubbed Scleroneedle, beginning bevel up, and rotate to bevel down with minimal advancement (Figs. 91-2 and 91-3) at a point of reflux or an incompetent valve. The gauge and length of the Scleroneedle will depend on the size of the vein, the degree of tortuosity, and the practitioner's preference. Large gauge needles are stiffer and more easily seen with Duplex-guided procedures. Longer needles will penetrate straight (less tortuous) veins further. Aspiration is generally not necessary, since a flashback will be immediate upon venipuncture of a distended vein.
3. Advance the needle carefully, taking care not to penetrate the posterior wall. Keeping the bevel down (flush with the posterior wall) is key to eliminating penetration or tearing of the wall.
4. Have the patient lie down, either prone or supine, to allow freedom of access to the needle. Elevate the limb, if necessary, to fully exsanguinate the vein.

Note: Do not attempt the procedure with a distended vein. Ulcers and severe skin burns may result from an increased need for power or time of application of energy.

5. Anesthetize the *perivascular* tissue with 0.5 to 1 ml of local anesthesia. Ballooning the tissue will make postprocedure evaluation difficult.
6. With the Luer-Lok adapter already attached to the handpiece, connect the metal-hubbed needle that was inserted. Hold and stabilize the needle intravascularly (Fig. 91-4) while the Luer-Lok adapter is twisted securely in place. The cord at the other end of the handpiece is plugged into the unit ("handpiece port").
7. Place the antenna from the radiofrequency unit near the treatment site. The antenna *does not* have to contact skin.
8. Set the power and waveform settings.
    Power (does not control frequency): 1 to 1¼
    Waveform: cut/filter (not *hemostasis,* as labeled for telangiectasias)
    The intent is to vaporize the intima, not coagulate it.
9. Activate the unit for 0.5- to 1-second intervals. Place a gloved finger over the treatment (needle tip) site. If

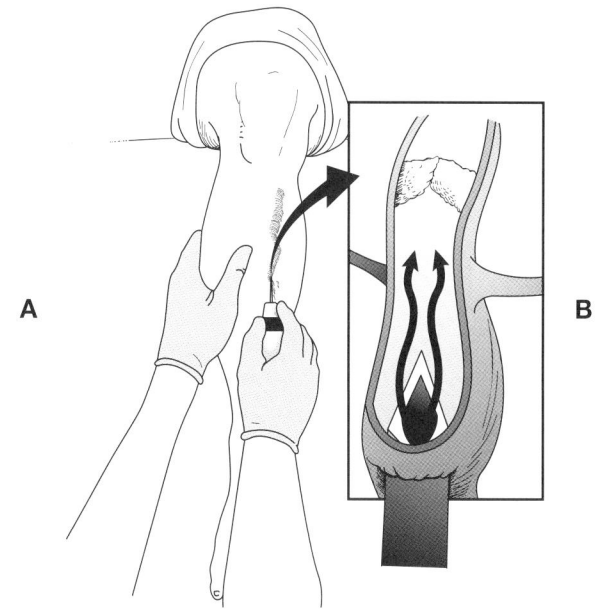

Fig. 91-2
Needle insertion. **A,** Stabilize the leg in a dependent position. **B,** Enlargement of the venous insertion site showing the bevel of the needle facing up as it is inserted. Once in the vein, it is rotated 180 degrees so the bevel is down.

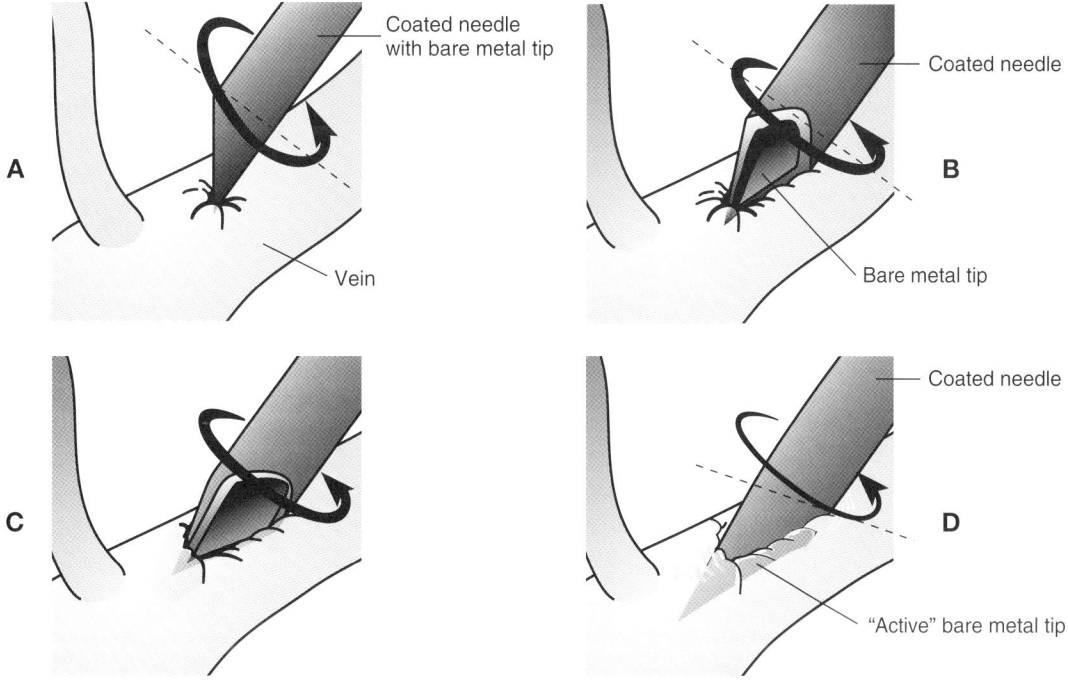

Fig. 91-3
Close-up of needle insertion. **A,** Starting bevel up. **B,** Needle rotation without advancement. **C,** Continued rotation without advancement. **D,** Complete 180-degree rotation without advancement.

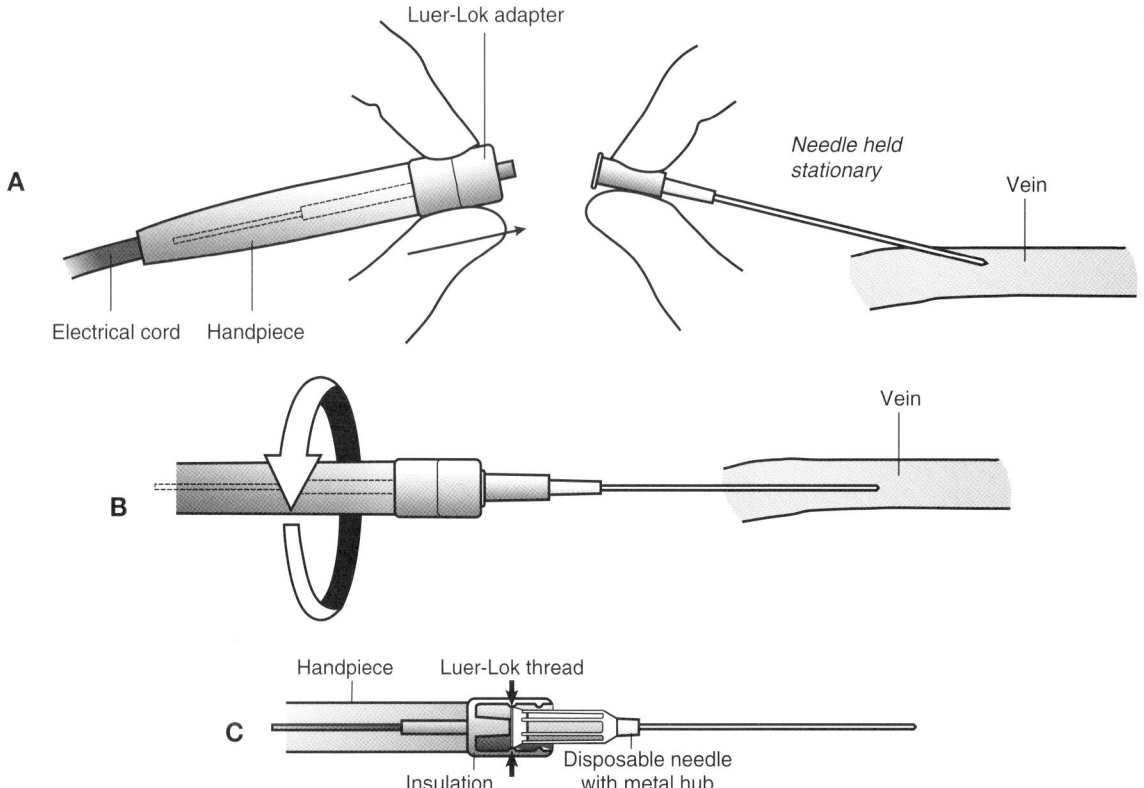

Fig. 91-4
A, The needle is held stationary to keep it in the vein while the hub adapter (connected to the handpiece and power source) is connected. **B,** The Luer-Lok is twisted onto the hub of the needle. **C,** Luer-Lok adapter shown attached to the Scleroneedle.

the tissue feels warm, use longer rest periods of 1 to 4 seconds to allow cooling. Listen for a sound (snap, crackle, or pop ["Rice Krispie effect"]) that indicates interaction of residual blood and the radiowaves. As the unit is activated, move the bare needle tip side to side horizontally to contact as much vein wall as possible. The tip can be withdrawn slowly enough to allow vaporization of additional length of vein. *Take care to keep the bare tip intravascular;* do not allow it to become intracutaneous.

10. *Stop immediately if any of the following occur:*
    - Skin starts to contract around the needle
    - Withdrawal is difficult because of tissue sticking to the needle
    - The skin feels warm at the tip of the needle treatment site
    - The tip is contacting the skin
    - A hematoma or ecchymotic area forms near the treatment site. This indicates disruption of the vessel. The area should be allowed to heal completely (up to 2 months) before retreating.
    - The skin surrounding the entry site turns white or develops a bleb or raised contour.

11. Withdraw the needle completely and observe for bleeding from the puncture. If bleeding occurs, "channel" back into the vessel and retreat as above.

12. Place pressure over the treated area for 30 to 60 seconds and then place the limb in dependency just long enough to observe for distention. If it occurs, reelevate and retreat. If no distension occurs, reelevate and proceed to compression application. Vessel spasm can give a false impression of success, and inadequate sealing of the vessel may be evident after 24 to 48 hours when the physiologic spasm releases. Indentation of the previously distended vein is the most reliable and successful indicator of appropriate sclerosis (Fig. 91-5).

13. Follow these guidelines for dressings and compression:
    - Apply an antibiotic *ointment* of choice.
    - Apply a nonsticking, nonabsorbent dressing of choice
    - Cover the treated area with foam or gauze (to increase convexity into the concave area created by the collapsed vein and allow the hose to exert greater pressure).

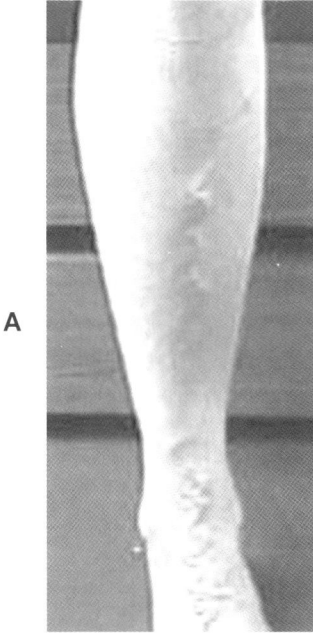

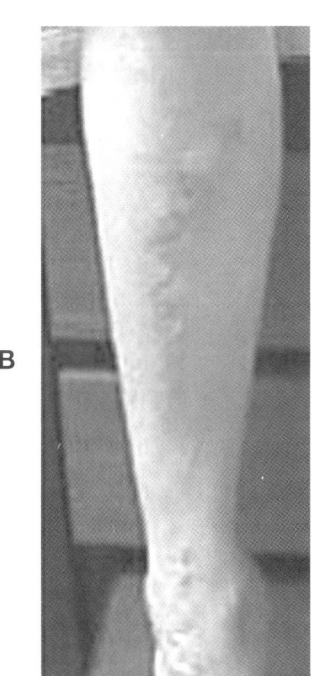

Fig. 91-5
A, Distended vessels. **B,** Indentation of vessel following procedure.

Note: DO NOT tape the foam or gauze, since even nonallergenic tape holds moisture when used with compression hose. This often causes skin reactions.

14. Follow these general guidelines:
   • The number of vessels or treatment sites will vary with the clinical condition.
   • The goal is to localize the most cephalad point(s) of reflux (usually the point where the vein(s) is/are first visible). If more than one vein is present

at a given level, it would be prudent to treat all veins at a given horizontal level.
   • After treatment at a given level, the results should be analyzed by placing the extremity into dependency and assessing return or absence of venous distention.
   • Typically, a 6- to 9-inch collapse of the proximal segment would be expected. Although there is no contraindication to treating additional distal vein segments, the author prefers to wait 5 to 7 days and bring the patient back for additional treatments. This will help minimize failure of the proximal treatment site.
   • Points of perforator reflux will guide the spacing of venipuncture. Each major point of reflux needs separate treatment.
   • Average appointment times will vary with the varicose vein presentation. Typically 15 to 30 minutes will be necessary for the experienced physician or an additional 15 minutes should be allowed for the uninitiated.
   • If multiple points are treated, pressure should be applied and maintained over the treated sites. This can be cotton or other suitable stiff material held in place with tape. The tape *must be removed* before stocking application.
   • Apply gradient compression hose over the dressings and bolsters (foam/gauze). Class II (30 to 40 mm Hg gradient) is preferred, but Class I (20 to 30 mm Hg) can be used. Since all certified gradient compression hose are manufactured with essentially the same materials and computer-controlled machines, price and personal preference will determine the brand to be used.
   • The hose should be worn for the first 48 hours continuously (thigh high types will allow the patient to go to the bathroom without removing them). The hose should then be worn with the pads in place for the next 5 days during the daytime hours when the leg is bearing weight.

COMPLICATIONS

The following are the most prominent complications.
1. Overtreatment or undertreatment represented by the following:
   a. *Thermal injury to the skin and subcutaneous structures and the vein wall* (overtreatment). Thermal injury is markedly lessened as the clinician gains skill and improves his technique through experience. The learning curve after adequate instruction is between 10 and 20 patients. Unwanted thermal effects cannot be eliminated completely, and each patient must understand that an

area of minimal discoloration may permanently exist despite successful elimination of one or more varicose veins. Each patient's skin will have different characteristics that may be predisposed to unwanted and unintended permanent skin discolorations. With experience the thermal complications can be 5% or less.

   b. *Inadequate vaporization* either at an area other than a perforator or incompetent valve or in an area where tortuosity precludes adequate vaporization of the intima and media *leads to a recurrence (undertreatment)*.

2. The second most common complication of recurrence or partial recurrence often relates to incomplete understanding of the predisposing significant factors of the development of a varicose vein. Duplex examination, with and without color, is a significant advancement in gaining the anatomic and physiologic information that is essential to proper treatment principles. Advancements in pneumoplethysmography and photoplethysmography likewise provide invaluable information. The contemporary practice of sclerotherapy is rapidly mandating the vascular evaluation to be the basis of treatment.

3. Other theoretical and infrequently experienced complications include the following:
   - Infection/cellulitis
   - Thrombosis/embolization
   - Skin ulcerations
   - Injury to the deep venous system

All of these practical and potential complications are minimized with appropriate attention to detail both during and after the procedure.

INTERPRETATION OF RESULTS/ FINDINGS AND CONSIDERATIONS

The results of radiofrequency sclerotherapy can be classified as successful (complete elimination of an unwanted vein), partially successful (incomplete elimination of an unwanted vein) or unsuccessful (recurrence or persistence of an unwanted vein after the procedure).

The *successful result* is obvious to the physician and the patient. Preprocedure videos, photographs, or leg diagrams depicting the area of treatment are helpful in documenting success. It is not unusual for a patient to focus on some minor obscure remnant of the treatment procedure and feel it is of the same significance as the preprocedure findings.

A *partially successful result* is generally accepted when the patient has been properly prepared mentally. The usual course of action would be additional treatment, which is generally acceptable.

The *unsuccessful result* may or may not be troublesome, depending on the preprocedure preparation. Since radiofrequency sclerotherapy is often performed for cosmetic reasons and occasionally physiologic abnormalities, patients expect perfection. This is particularly true when cash payments are involved.

Patients must understand from the inception, treatment of venous disease is symptomatic rather than etiological. Ambulatory phlebectomy and stripping procedures often result in immediate eradication of a visible venous structure but can be accompanied by scarring and a protracted course of healing or rehabilitation. Radiofrequency sclerotherapy can eliminate the scarring but may not be as definitive for total eradication as the vessel remains in situ. Patients must understand the risks and anticipated outcomes of all procedures to fully comprehend the anticipated course and progression of treatment.

Accurate diagnosis of the vascular abnormality gives the clinician the best chance of successful treatment. Radiofrequency sclerotherapy is most successful when directly applied at a point of incompetency either within a perforator or at the site of a valvular leak. Often this finding can only be understood with the aid of color duplex ultrasonography. A clinician can be skilled with a continuous wave handheld Doppler; however, a handheld Doppler cannot offer the benefit of direct visualization nor can sophisticated physiologic parameters be assessed as thoroughly as with duplex examination. A clinician does not have to have in-house duplex capability, since many mobile laboratories exist. Many vascular technologists are not trained to effectively map and assess the superficial and perforator systems, and their expertise is limited to ruling out DVT and cerebral assessments. The clinician may need to evaluate the results of a duplex examination himself to appreciate the significance of the findings.

The major impediment to successful radiofrequency sclerotherapy is the lack of understanding and appreciation of the effects of major superficial points of incompetency. The saphenofemoral junction (SFJ) is the most common responsible entity for failure of any sclerotherapy treatment. Volumes exist on the significance of SFJ incompetence. The practical significance can be summed up in terms of round figures. Roughly 60% of all patients with presenting signs of varicose, reticular, or telangiectatic leg veins will exhibit reflux at the saphenofemoral junction, as assessed with retrograde flow on dependency or with Valsalva's maneuver.

Of that 60% just mentioned, roughly 50% of varicose or linear reticular veins will respond to appropriate radiofrequency sclerotherapy. Based on the foregoing, approximately 70% of the patients with varicose or reticular deformity respond to appropriate radiofrequency sclerotherapy. The 30% that fail either injection or radiofrequency sclerotherapy in the presence of SFJ incompetency will need some form of intervention to correct or eliminate the SFJ incompetency prior to successful additional sclerotherapy.

ANATOMICAL, TREATMENT, AND SURGICAL CONTROVERSIES

What should be done for the 30% in question? The remaining available treatments are high ligation and/or division of the greater saphenous vein at the junction with the femoral vein (crossectomy), ligation and stripping, or endovenous obliteration of the greater saphenous vein with either laser or radiofrequency energy. Many phlebologists and surgeons also advocate simultaneous crossectomy (complete ligation of the normal four to six branches and any variants) during ligation. Stripping, when used, should be groin to knee, not groin to ankle. These procedures, when used, may not alter the course of the varicose or reticular process. In fact, the 5-year outcome of stripping procedures is no better than lesser-invasive procedures, such as ligation and division, followed by appropriate and adequate radiofrequency or injection sclerotherapy and differing kinds or ambulatory phlebectomy (see Chapter 78, Ambulatory Phlebectomy).

The newer radiofrequency and laser endovenous procedures are likely to have the same consequences as ligation and stripping if appropriate follow-up sclerotherapy and ambulatory phlebectomy are not performed. The major advance in phlebology is the ability of appropriately trained practitioners to perform endovenous procedures, sclerotherapy and ambulatory phlebectomy. This eliminates hospitalization, general anesthesia, and prolonged recuperation, which offers much more cosmetically acceptable outcomes.

When stripping is performed, it should be limited rationally from groin to just below the knee. Unfortunately, the routine procedure is groin to ankle. Anatomically, the major consistent perforators above the knee are the Hunterian and Dodds' perforators. Below the knee, Boyd's perforator attaches to the greater saphenous vein, and the vein then gives rise to the posterior arch vein, which communicates with the remaining four major perforators (namely, Sherman's and Cockett I, II, and III). Anatomically, there is no logical reason for stripping below Boyd's unless significant perforation and reflux can be demonstrated by duplex examination and/or venography with communication with the anteriorly positioned lower leg greater saphenous vein. Remember that the posterior positioned posterior arch vein receives the normal perforators below Boyd's.

GRADIENT COMPRESSION HOSE

The single most important method to prevent recurrence of varicosities is the use of true, gradient pressure support hose. (T.E.D. hose [Kendall] and other similarly designed uniform pressure hose do not qualify as gradient compression hose.) All patients must be cautioned to observe the compression rules. The physician should pay special attention to posttreatment checks to ensure that compression is being used properly. The author's compression regimen is immediate application of foam bolsters and the gradient support hose. Class II, 30 to 40 mm Hg, hose are preferred, and Class I, 20 to 30 mm Hg, hose are the minimum requirements.

Numerous manufacturers make sheer, cosmetically acceptable, gradient compression hose. All manufacturing is essentially the same with regard to the physiologic benefit derived. The real issue becomes cost. Brand name is no longer an indicator of better or lesser value.

The normal venous pressure at the ankle, with normal muscle pumps, is 15 to 20 mm Hg. Any patient with varicose or reticular venous disease must be suspect for abnormally high pressures until proven otherwise. Class III or IV gradient compression hose are extremely difficult to put on and remove; therefore many clinicians choose Class II (and even these are difficult).

One important aspect of hose containing spandex is the issue of contact allergy. Most manufacturers are using Lycra, nylon, and other materials to avoid this. Heavier medical grade stockings continue to use spandex. The physician must be cognizant of this potential problem; however, this should not be the reason to avoid use of compression. There is no rational basis in physiologic or anatomic principles to refrain from using compression support hose with any type of sclerotherapy treatment. Failure to use adequate compression is the single most frequent cause of failure of radiofrequency sclerotherapy.

POSTPROCEDURE PATIENT EDUCATION

A postoperative instruction sheet should be given and a signed copy retained in the chart. (See the sample patient education handout titled "Postsclerotherapy Treatment Instructions: Injection and Radiofrequency Sclerotherapy" on page 1848 of Appendix G.)

CONCLUSION

Radiofrequency sclerotherapy is a noninvasive, medical procedure designed to provide endovascular sclerosis, without scarring and without long periods of debilitation or recovery. The equipment and basic instrumentation is inexpensive and readily available. This is a largely operator-dependent procedure; however, the skills to complete this procedure successfully are within the reach of all physicians. Anyone wanting to practice this technique must devote the time not only to learn the technique but also to understand the vascular assessment and phlebology concepts necessary to comprehend the anatomic and physiologic basis of large vein malformation. The end result of successful treatment is spectacular. The technique provides a lower risk of significant complications, and can be delivered in the office setting on a fee-for-service basis. This makes the technique very attractive to physicians and patients alike.

SUPPLIERS

Ellman Surgitron FFPF
Ellman International, Inc.
1135 Railroad Avenue
Hewlett, NY 11557-2316
Phone: 1-800-835-5355
Website: www.ellman.com/medical

Scleroneedle
RF Scleroneedles, Ltd.
7209 South Mount Holy Cross
Littleton, CO 80127-3202
Phone: 1-800-916-7587

Training materials
Physicians Learning Unlimited Seminars (The Course Seminars)
7209 South Mount Holy Cross
Littleton, CO 80127-3202
Phone: 1-800-916-7587

Gradient compression support hose manufacturers
See the "Suppliers" section in Chapter 90, Sclerotherapy.

CPT/BILLING CODE

37799   Unlisted vascular procedure

ICD-9-CM DIAGNOSTIC CODES

454.1   Varicose veins with inflammation (stasis dermatitis, infection)
454.2   With ulcer
459.81   Chronic venous insufficiency (This should be the primary diagnosis.)
782.2   Edema, legs

ADDITIONAL RESOURCES

- See the sample patient education handouts titled "Radiofrequency Sclerotherapy" on page 1847 and "Postsclerotherapy Treatment Instructions: Injection and Radiofrequency Sclerotherapy" on page 1848 of Appendix G.
- See the sample patient consent form titled "Radiofrequency Treatment of Varicose Veins" on page 1849 of Appendix G.

WEBSITES

www.veinsaway.com (Vein Institute @ Vail, Inc.)
www.vnus.com (Endovascular Closure)

CHAPTER 92

Exercise (Stress) Testing

Grant C. Fowler
Michael Altman

Twelve million Americans have known coronary artery disease (CAD). Unfortunately, over half of individuals with CAD first discover their diagnosis *after a bad outcome,* namely a myocardial infarction (MI) or sudden cardiac death. Approximately one of every three deaths (half a million deaths a year) in the United States is caused by CAD; it is the leading cause of death in both genders. Exercise testing is not only a safe and cost-effective method for diagnosing CAD, but it is also helpful for managing CAD, including determining the prognosis. Its safety has been defined as a risk of less than 1 event per 10,000 studies if patients are selected properly. Although much money, time, and effort have been spent designing and applying new tests with greater sensitivity for diagnosing CAD, when diagnosing *significant* CAD—left main disease or multivessel disease with resultant left main equivalent (LV dysfunction)—the sensitivity of exercise testing exceeds 90% (perhaps 95%). Supporting this, one recent study (Mattera) comparing accuracy of thallium for diagnosing CAD found no benefit over exercise testing if the resting electrocardiogram (ECG) was normal. With medical management of CAD more successful than ever, primary care clinicians' skills in diagnosing and managing CAD have become more important. Performing exercise testing is one method of maximizing these skills. In fact, with the excellent prognosis data currently available that utilizes many of the parameters monitored during exercise testing, primary care clinicians can now manage certain aspects of CAD as well as their expert cardiologist colleagues.

In addition to managing those with symptoms or known CAD, primary care clinicians can use exercise testing to screen certain asymptomatic individuals. Such screening may be especially helpful for diabetics, firemen, or older individuals about to embark on a vigorous exercise program. With estimates that 12% of U.S. deaths are a result of the lack of exercise, any method to motivate patients to exercise should be beneficial. Exercise testing can be used to not only reassure individuals of the safety of exercise, but also to customize their exercise prescriptions. After almost every exercise test, the patient should receive clearance to exercise and an exercise prescription based on their true maximal heart rate (MHR), their true exercise (aerobic) capacity, and the test results. We now know that almost every patient benefits from an exercise program, even cardiac transplant patients. In fact, of all the options available, exercise may be the single best method for improving endothelial function.

Benefits of performing exercise testing in the office include having test results immediately available, improving communication and referral patterns to cardiologists, and improving ECG reading skills by primary care clinicians. Clinicians performing exercise testing also naturally improve their understanding of CAD pathophysiology as well as exercise physiology. With immediately available results, patient satisfaction is usually improved and liability for the clinician from failure to diagnose should be decreased. With nomograms now available, when there is a positive study, the patient can immediately be counseled from an outcomes or prognosis perspective. Such data will allow a patient to make a truly informed decision before undergoing a major procedure, such as coronary artery bypass surgery. With personalized data, the patient can compare his or her known risks of foregoing surgery against available known risks of surgery, thereby reserving surgery for those who choose to accept the risks.

For primary care clinicians covering emergency departments or urgent care centers, management of patients with an acute chest pain syndrome is greatly facilitated when exercise testing is available. For many patients, after myocardial damage has been excluded by serial blood tests, resolution of the symptoms, and stabilized ECG findings, an exercise test may be useful for triage. National guidelines with algorithms are available, and they have been demonstrated to be both safe and useful.

PHYSIOLOGY OF EXERCISE TESTING

Exercise increases *total* oxygen consumption, and therefore it increases oxygen demand. The amount of increase is dependent on which muscles are used (e.g., larger muscles, such as the legs, require more oxygen than smaller muscles) and the intensity of exercise. In response to increased exercise and oxygen demand, the body increases ventilation, cardiac output, and oxygen extraction by tissues. Unless there is moderate to severe lung disease (e.g., chronic obstructive pulmonary disease [COPD]) or a process severely limiting oxygen transport or extraction (e.g., severe anemia), cardiac output is usually the factor limiting an individual's maximal exercise capacity. In turn, the limiting factor for cardiac output in those with CAD is usually coronary blood flow. Maximal exercise capacity can therefore be limited by coronary blood flow. In fact, maximal exercise capacity is usually quantified by measuring or estimating an individual's maximal oxygen uptake ($Vo_{2\,max}$). In other words, exercise with large muscles can be used to measure or estimate $Vo_{2\,max}$ and to evaluate limitations in coronary blood flow.

Cardiac output can be calculated by multiplying the stroke volume by the heart rate; therefore increases in either the stroke volume or the heart rate will increase the cardiac output. Increasing the stroke volume is generally a more efficient method of increasing cardiac output (i.e., requires less oxygen). However, unless the patient is taking a β-blocker, the usual initial physiologic response to increased demand for cardiac output is to increase the heart rate. (In part, this is why β-blockers work for treating angina; they block the increase in heart rate when there is a need for increased cardiac output, thereby forcing an increase in stroke volume and minimizing the increased myocardial oxygen demand.)

In normal patients there is a linear relationship between *myocardial* oxygen demand and heart rate. In other words, the faster the heart is beating, the more oxygen it requires. Since the heart rate continues to increase as exercise intensity increases to a maximum (i.e., maximal heart rate [MHR] at maximal exertion), then so does the myocardial oxygen demand. MHR can be crudely *estimated* based on age (i.e., 220 − age ≅ MHR) or by using graphs before the procedure; however, *true* MHR is best determined with a true maximal exercise test. MHR is the heart rate noted when the patient is at maximal effort (voluntarily fatigued), and this number should be recorded and given to the patient at the end of each study when the clinician is customizing an exercise prescription.

There is also a linear relationship between myocardial oxygen demand and systolic blood pressure (SBP). In other words, the higher the heart rate and/or the higher the SBP, the harder the heart is working (and consequently the higher the myocardial oxygen demand). Therefore one method of quantifying the *myocardial* oxygen demand is to multiply the SBP by the heart rate. The product obtained is the double product or the *rate-pressure product (RPP)*. At any given moment the RPP is an estimate of total myocardial oxygen demand, and as long as the demand has not exceeded the supply, it is also a measure of total myocardial oxygen uptake or consumption. In other words, the higher the RPP, the more oxygen the heart is demanding; if supply is matching demand, the higher the capacity the heart has to deliver and use oxygen.

As the myocardium demands more oxygen, two options exist for supplying it. Either the coronary arterial *flow* increases or the *extraction* of oxygen from the flow it is already receiving increases. As it turns out, increased myocardial oxygen demand during exercise is met primarily through increases in coronary artery flow rather than through increased oxygen extraction. This is because myocardial tissue is very efficient at extracting almost all of the available oxygen from the coronary arterial flow, even in the resting state. Therefore coronary arterial *flow* is usually the limiting factor for cardiac oxygenation. This is especially true in patients with obstructive CAD.

In the patient with significant coronary artery blockage, with increasing exercise a threshold is eventually reached at which the heart's demand for oxygen exceeds the supply. At this threshold the heart becomes ischemic, first at the subendocardial layer. With subendocardial ischemia, the patient usually demonstrates ECG changes in the form of ST-segment depression. Usually and eventually this is followed by chest discomfort (i.e., angina). Because in most cases the ischemia is due to a fixed lesion, patients will develop these ECG changes at the same threshold or RPP every time. If symptoms occur, they also occur at the same RPP and follow the same pattern every time. In other words, angina caused by a fixed lesion does not radiate only into the left arm one day and into the right arm another day. If ST-segment depression occurs and angina is not experienced, silent ischemia is diagnosed.

Large muscles, such as leg muscles, rapidly increase the oxygen demand with increased exertion (e.g., using a treadmill or bicycle). $Vo_{2\,max}$ is the greatest amount (i.e., volume) of oxygen that a person can extract from inspired air while performing dynamic exercise. It is usually demonstrated when the patient is in the anaerobic range. Measuring $Vo_{2\,max}$ is a method of quantifying maximal exercise capacity, and $Vo_{2\,max}$ varies with body weight, heredity, gender, and exercise habits. It often decreases progressively with age, but this may be purely because of inadequate exercise habits. Regular aerobic exercise may maintain a constant $Vo_{2\,max}$ for a person for life. There is a nearly linear relationship between $Vo_{2\,max}$ and the maximum cardiac output; therefore the $Vo_{2\,max}$ is a measure of the functional capacity of the cardiovascular system. It can be measured directly with inspired/expired gas analysis or more easily estimated from a maximal exercise test. As mentioned previously, in those with CAD, $Vo_{2\,max}$ may be limited by coronary blood flow. With prognosis data discussed later in this chapter, $Vo_{2\,max}$ is a very important estimate or measurement for predicting outcomes from a cardiovascular perspective.

Basal oxygen consumption, or 1 metabolic equivalent (1 MET), defines the amount of oxygen an average individual consumes sitting at rest, which is approximately 3.5 ml/kg/minute (1 MET = 3.5 ml/kg/minute). $Vo_{2\,max}$ is often quantified as a multiple of the basal oxygen consumption (in METs). For instance, walking 2 miles per hour (mph) on level ground is approximately equal to 2 METs. Walking 4 mph on level ground is approximately 4 METs. Moderately active young males usually have a $Vo_{2\,max}$ of at least 42 ml/kg/min, or 12 METs. This means they are able to consume 12 times the amount of oxygen that they consume at rest. Obviously METs can also be used as a conversion factor between types of exercise. Charts are available (Fig. 92-1) to estimate exercise capacity or maximal METs by cross-referencing MET levels with different daily activities. This estimate may then be used to predict performance before placing a patient on a treadmill. Maximal exercise testing remains one of the more accurate methods of evaluating maximal METs. An individual's maximal METs, whether determined on a bicycle or a treadmill, has significant management and prognosis implications if they have CAD. Even if the test is positive for CAD, achieving certain MET thresholds can be very reassuring for prognosis.

During a maximal exercise test, a perceived exertion scale (PES) may be helpful for monitoring the patient. The PES is similar to a pain scale; however, the patient quantifies effort instead of pain during testing. Originally invented with a scale from 5 to 20, 20 was the subjective maximum that an individual could work and 5 was described as minimal or no work at all. It has now been modified to a range of from 1 to 10 (Box 92-1). Although it is a subjective measure, in most patients the PES is very reproducible; in other words, if they were asked to repeat the exercise test in 2 weeks, at the same workload and duration for both tests, they would report the same PES. As a result, in most patients the PES target for their routine exercise program can be given to the patient as part of their exercise prescription. This replaces their need to check the pulse during exercise, and anything that simplifies an exercise prescription will hopefully

VETERANS' ADMINISTRATION SPECIFIC ACTIVITY QUESTIONNAIRE

Instructions to patient: Draw a line below the activities done routinely with minimal or no symptoms, such as shortness of breath, chest discomfort, and fatigue.

1 MET: Eating, getting dressed, working at desk

2 METs: Taking a shower

3 METs: Walking slowly on a flat surface for one or two blocks
Doing a moderate amount of work around the house, such as vacuuming, sweeping the floors, or carrying groceries

4 METs: Doing light yard work (e.g., raking leaves, weeding, light carpentry, or painting)

5 METs: Walking briskly (4 mph), dancing

6 METs: Playing nine holes of golf carrying own clubs, performing heavy carpentry or mowing lawn with a push mower

7 METs: Playing tennis (singles), carrying 60 lb

8 METs: Moving heavy furniture
Jogging slowly, climbing stairs quickly, carrying 20 lb upstairs

9 METs: Bicycling at a moderate pace, sawing wood, jumping rope (slowly)

10 METs: Swimming briskly, bicycling up a hill, walking briskly uphill, jogging 6 mph

11 METs: Skiing cross-country
Playing basketball (full court)

12 METs: Running briskly and continuously (level ground, 8-minute miles)

13 METs: Rowing, backpacking, any competitive activity, including those that involve intermittent sprinting, running competitively

Fig. 92-1
Veterans' Administration specific activity questionnaire.

BOX 92-1

Perceived Exertion Scale

0	Nothing at all
0.5	Very, very weak
1	Very weak
2	Weak
3	Moderate
4	Somewhat strong
5	Strong
6	
7	Very strong
8	
9	
10	Very, very strong

increase the chance of compliance. In addition, if the clinician always checks the PES during an exercise test, they may discover those individuals who cannot be relied upon to use their PES as a measure of effort. Certain patients have a poor perception of their level of exertion, and even at maximal effort they will describe their PES as a 1 or 2. Those patients must be taught how to check the heart rate during exercise as part of their exercise prescription.

A positive test result occurs when "global" subendocardial ischemia causes *ST-segment depression* on the ECG tracing. Because this is a global phenomenon, it will usually be seen in more than one lead; if suspected it should be confirmed in an area of the ECG tracing where the baseline is relatively flat. True ischemia will cause ST-segment depression for at least three beats in a row, and the ischemia (ST changes) usually persists or worsens during the recovery period. ST-segment depression occurs because ischemia impairs the sodium/potassium adenosine triphosphatase (Na^+/K^+ ATPase) pump at the cellular level. Such an ST-segment change can also be noted in patients taking digitalis, whose site of action is the Na^+/K^+ ATPase pump. When the pump is affected, there is a resultant change in the Na^+/K^+ intracellular gradient, and a subsequent small shift in polarity. This shift in polarity is what is noted on the electrical ECG tracings as ST-segment depression.

With exercise-induced ischemia, ST-segment depression becomes a "global" phenomenon, meaning it involves the entire subendocardium. When one area of the subendocardium becomes ischemic, it reduces its workload or shuts down before becoming permanently damaged. As a result, the remaining and surrounding subendocardium must work harder. This area subsequently becomes ischemic, and a domino effect occurs, cascading around the entire subendocardium. Consequently, ST-segment depression is usually seen in multiple leads. In fact, this is such a global phenomenon that the coronary vessels involved cannot be predicted by which of the leads are demonstrating ST-segment depression.

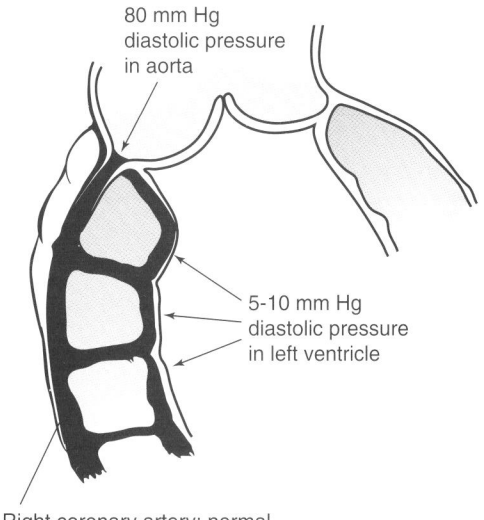

80 mm Hg diastolic pressure in aorta

5-10 mm Hg diastolic pressure in left ventricle

Right coronary artery: normal

Fig. 92-2

Normal myocardial perfusion. Note perfusion gradient is from 80 mm Hg to 5 to 10 mm Hg. (Redrawn from Ellestad MH: *Stress testing: principles and practice,* ed 4, Philadelphia, 1996, FA Davis.)

If the entire wall of the myocardium (full-thickness) becomes ischemic, such as from severe CAD, *ST-segment elevation* may be noted. It may appear very similar to that seen with a transmural infarct or a ventricular aneurysm. In this situation, the exercise test should be stopped. If either transmural ischemia is occurring or an infarct has occurred, the potential for an arrhythmia is very high. However, transmural ischemia is rare. In almost all positive exercise tests, *ST-segment depression* is what is noted, the same as with a subendocardial infarct. The subendocardial layer is usually the first to become ischemic because it is the "watershed" area of the heart, or the farthest from the arteries that are located in the epicardium (Figs. 92-2 and 92-3).

Certain other conditions may also make it difficult to perfuse the subendocardial layer, even in the absence of CAD. Normally the subendocardial layer is perfused during diastole and relies on perfusing "downhill" from 80 to 90 mm Hg of diastolic pressure (DBP) to an area where there is only 5 to 10 mm Hg pressure (i.e., end-diastolic pressure [EDP]). Thus the pressure gradient, or the difference between "uphill" DBP and "downhill" EDP, is 80 or 90 minus 5 or 10, which is a 75 to 85 mm Hg difference (DBP – EDP = 75 to 85). If hypertension is poorly controlled, EDP may be elevated, reaching as high as 30 to 40 mm Hg, with a resultant drop in this pressure gradient (DBP – EDP = 40 to 60). In other words, there is much less "pressure" for blood to flow "downhill." Anything causing diastolic dysfunction, such as profound hypothyroidism, can also result in a decreased pressure gradient. A thickened

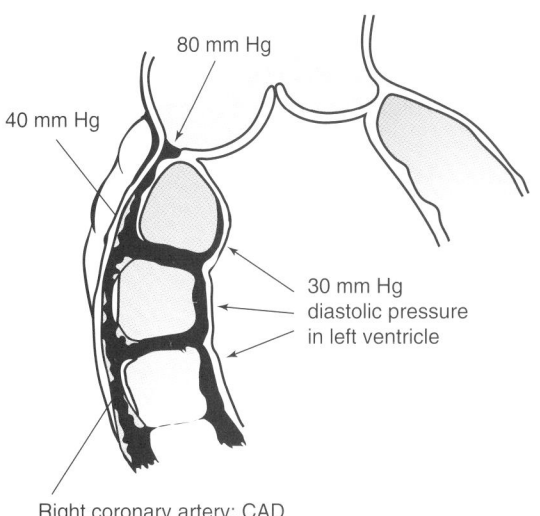

80 mm Hg

40 mm Hg

30 mm Hg
diastolic pressure
in left ventricle

Right coronary artery: CAD

Fig. 92-3
Myocardial perfusion in coronary artery disease (CAD). Note perfusion
gradient is only from 40 mm Hg to 30 mm Hg. (Redrawn from Ellestad
MH: *Stress testing: principles and practice,* ed 4, Philadelphia, 1996,
FA Davis.)

myocardial wall, as seen in left ventricular hypertrophy,
can make it physically difficult to perfuse through the
wall, thereby causing subendocardial ischemia and
ST-segment depression, even without CAD. In addition
to physical causes, other situations possibly resulting in
false positives include hypokalemia or other electrolyte
imbalances. Inadequate potassium prevents the Na^+/K^+
ATPase pump from functioning correctly, resulting in
ST-segment changes. As mentioned previously, digitalis
may also result in ST-segment depression, even at
physiologic doses.

Normal Clinical Responses to Exercise Testing

1. A gradual increase in pulse to MHR (220 −
   age ≅ MHR).

Note: If a heart rate of 120 cannot be achieved and the patient
is not on a β-blocker, the diagnosis of chronotropic incompetence is made, possibly indicating severe CAD or early sick
sinus syndrome.

2. Return of the heart rate to resting values within the
   first few minutes after exercise. The rate of return of
   the heart rate to its resting value is partly dependent
   on conditioning. In addition, recent evidence defines
   an *abnormal heart rate recovery* as a heart rate not
   decreasing by at least 12 beats per minute (bpm) in
   the first minute of recovery. An abnormal heart rate
   recovery can also be used for determining prognosis.
3. A gradual rise in SBP. Systolic pressure is usually
   the highest at maximal workload. A drop in SBP,

especially if it drops below resting SBP, may indicate
severe CAD.
4. A return of SBP to its resting value by approximately
   6 minutes after exercise.
5. Minimal change or a decrease in diastolic blood
   pressure (DBP) during exercise. During exercise
   the legs produce lactic acid, one of the most
   potent vasodilators known to man. As a result, a
   significant amount of blood volume flows into the
   legs. Because of vasodilation and its effects on
   Korotkoff sounds, diastolic pressure by auscultation
   can decrease all the way to zero in normal
   individuals.

Note: An increase in diastolic pressure of more than 10 mm Hg
is designated a *hypertensive response to exercise* (see the
"Interpretation" section).

6. Most patients perceive an increase by 1 to 3 points on
   the PES per stage of exercise. Few ever admit to
   reaching a full 10 points on the scale. Many patients'
   PES increases rapidly from 7 to 9 when they are near
   maximal effort.

INDICATIONS

Comprehensive, national guidelines are available regarding the appropriate use of exercise testing, including
special cases and situations (e.g., diabetics, patients in
the emergency department, firemen). The most common
and appropriate indications for primary care clinicians
include diagnosing CAD (especially helpful when evaluating atypical chest pain and screening asymptomatic
patients at significant risk), managing CAD, and to
provide data for an exercise prescription while determining exercise capacity and safety. In certain cases, several
of these indications end up being evaluated during the
same procedure. An example would be a patient who
has an intermediate pretest likelihood and is found to
have CAD on the treadmill. Since the diagnosis has
now been made, if it is considered safe to continue the
procedure, prognosis may also be determined by continuing the procedure. Exercise capacity (i.e., aerobic capacity) would also be determined if the patient were
allowed to complete a maximal exercise test. In this
manner, the diagnosis, prognosis, and exercise capacity
could all be determined with the same study, thereby
enhancing management.

A. General Indications

There are three general indications for cardiac testing:
1. Diagnosing CAD
   a. Patients with an intermediate (20% to 70%) pretest
      probability of CAD, based on gender, age, and

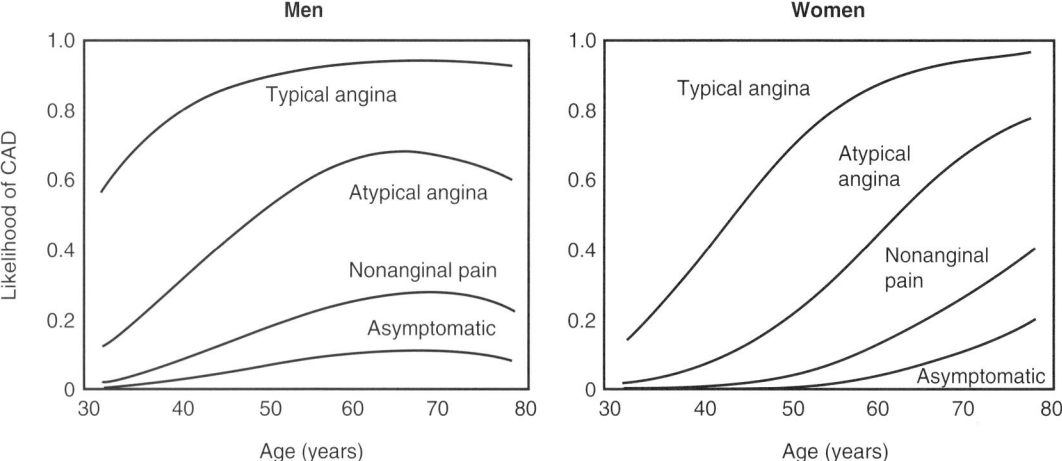

Fig. 92-4

Pretest likelihood of coronary artery disease (CAD). (Redrawn from Diamond GA, Forrester JS: *N Engl J Med* 300:1350, 1979.)

TABLE 92-1

Pretest Likelihood of Coronary Artery Disease Based on Symptoms

Age	Asymptomatic	Nonanginal Chest Pain	Atypical Angina	Typical Angina
Women				
35	0.3	1	4	26
45	1	3	13	55
55	3	8	32	79
65	8	19	54	91
Men				
35	2	5	22	70
45	6	14	46	87
55	10	22	59	92
65	12	28	67	94

Adapted from Diamond GA, Forrester JS: Analysis of probability as an aid in the clinical diagnosis of coronary artery disease. In Fowler GC, Evans CH, Altman MA: *Prim Care* 24(2):375, 1997.

TABLE 92-2

Absolute Risk of Total* Coronary Artery Disease (CAD) and Hard† CAD (see Table 92-3)

Risk Points	Women*	Women†	Men*	Men†
0	2%	1%	2%	2%
1	2%	1%	3%	2%
2	3%	2%	4%	3%
3	3%	2%	5%	4%
4	4%	2%	7%	5%
5	4%	2%	8%	6%
6	5%	2%	10%	7%
7	6%	3%	13%	9%
8	7%	3%	16%	13%
9	8%	3%	20%	16%
10	10%	4%	25%	20%
11	11%	7%	31%	25%
12	13%	8%	37%	30%
13	15%	11%	45%	35%
14	18%	13%	>53%	>45%
15	20%	15%		
16	24%	18%		
>17	>27%	>20%		

"Total CAD" equates to all forms of clinical coronary disease, whereas "hard CAD" includes clinical evidence of myocardial infarction and coronary death. CAD risks are approximated from the Framingham data.
*10-year absolute risk of total CAD based on Framingham data.
†10-year absolute risk of hard CAD based on Framingham data.

symptoms (see the "Determination of Pretest Likelihood" section, Fig. 92-4, and Table 92-1).

  b. Asymptomatic patients with multiple risk factors (Tables 92-2 and 92-3) or an abnormal coronary calcium score from electron beam CT scan (EBCT).

Note: For diagnosing CAD, determining pretest likelihood is important. This is explained for patients with symptoms by examples in Section F, Determination of Pretest Likelihood.

Although Tables 92-1 through 92-3, as well as other tables, are available for "guesstimates" of pretest likelihood in the asymptomatic population with risk factors, applying these tables often becomes very complex. As a result, many clinicians simply use good clinical judgment to determine which patients should be screened. This judgment must be weighed against the risk of a false positive in an asymptomatic individual. These particular tables are listed despite the fact that they were originally designed to determine who should receive lipid-lowering medical therapy. It is now recommended that lipid-lowering therapy be targeted to high-risk individuals. These same risk assessments should be adaptable to

TABLE 92-3

Table to Be Used for Calculating Risk Points for Table 92-2

Risk Factor	Risk Points	
	Men	Women
Age (yr)		
<34	−1	−9
35-39	0	−4
40-44	1	0
45-49	2	3
50-54	3	6
55-59	4	7
60-64	5	8
65-69	6	8
70-74	7	8
Total Cholesterol (mg/dl)		
<160	−3	−2
169-199	0	0
200-239	1	1
240-279	2	2
>280	3	3
High-Density Lipoprotein Cholesterol (HDL-C) (mg/dl)		
<35	2	5
35-44	1	2
45-49	0	1
50-59	0	0
>60	−2	−3
Systolic Blood Pressure (mm Hg)		
<120	0	−3
120-129	0	0
130-139	1	1
140-159	2	2
>160	3	3
Diabetes		
No	0	0
Yes	2	4
Smoker		
No	0	0
Yes	2	2

Adding up the points
  Age:
  Cholesterol:
  HDL-C:
  Blood pressure:
  Diabetes:
  Smoker:

Total points:

predict CAD for exercise testing. Therefore these tables serve a dual purpose in this chapter (in addition to assisting with the calculation of pretest likelihood, they can also be used to determine which asymptomatic individuals at high risk of CAD should also be receiving lipid-lowering therapy).

2. Managing CAD*:
  a. Patients with known, or a high probability of CAD, for initial assessment or for a change in symptoms
  b. After MI or revascularization, for prognostic assessment, activity prescription, evaluation of medical therapy, or cardiac rehabilitation
  c. Demonstrating proof of ischemia before revascularization
3. Determining exercise prescription data, exercise capacity, and safety
  a. Evaluation of exercise-related symptoms, including possible exercise-induced arrhythmias* (also see Chapter 84, Ambulatory Electrocardiography: Holter and Event Monitoring)
  b. Graded treadmill exercise testing is one of the best methods for determining an individual's maximum heart rate (MHR). The exception is the elite athlete, where a sport-specific exercise test should be used.
  c. MHR must be known to calculate a training heart rate range, which can be used as a guideline for aerobic training.
  d. An exercise test can also be used to estimate an individual's $Vo_{2\,max}$, which is helpful in determining a current level of fitness or conditioning.

B. Specific ACC/AHA Indications

The American College of Cardiology (ACC) and the American Heart Association (AHA) have produced guidelines for exercise testing, which have subsequently been endorsed by the American College of Sports Medicine. For the sake of completeness of this chapter and for further stratification, most of the guidelines for routine adults will be listed. Guidelines for special cases (e.g., valvular heart disease, children, exercise testing with expired ventilatory gas analysis) may be found in the ACC/AHA reference or on the AHA web page, under "Science and Professional, Scientific Publications, Scientific Statements" (www.americanheart.org). The ACC/AHA guidelines use the following classification system for indications: *Class I:* Conditions for which there is evidence or general agreement that a given procedure or treatment is useful and effective.

---

*Patients with left ventricular dysfunction, history of recent (within 7 to 10 days) acute coronary syndrome, severe valvular (aortic) stenosis, or complex or life-threatening arrhythmias are considered a higher-risk group. Exercise testing for them should be performed in the hospital by a clinician with significant experience treating patients with CAD or with consultation by a cardiologist.

Class II: Conditions for which there is conflicting evidence, a divergence of opinion, or both, about the usefulness and efficacy of a procedure or treatment.

Class IIa: Weight of evidence or opinion is in favor of usefulness and efficacy.

Class IIb: Usefulness and efficacy is less well established by evidence and opinion.

Class III: Conditions for which there is evidence or general agreement that the procedure or treatment is not useful or effective and, in some cases, may be harmful.

1. Exercise Testing in Diagnosis of Obstructive Coronary Artery Disease

Class I: Adult patients (including those with complete right bundle branch block [RBBB] or less than 1 mm of resting ST-segment depression) with an intermediate pretest probability of CAD based on gender, age, and symptoms (see "Determination of Pretest Likelihood" section, Fig. 92-4, and Table 92-1).

Class IIa: Patients with vasospastic angina.

Class IIb: Patients with a high pretest probability of CAD by age, symptoms, and gender; patients with a low pretest probability of CAD by age, symptoms, and gender; patients with less than 1 mm of baseline ST-segment depression and taking digoxin; patients with electrocardiographic criteria for left ventricular hypertrophy (LVH) and less than 1 mm of baseline ST-segment depression.

Class III: Patients with the following baseline ECG abnormalities: preexcitation syndrome (i.e., Wolff-Parkinson-White [WPW] syndrome), electronically paced ventricular rhythm, greater than 1 mm of resting ST-segment depression, complete left bundle branch block (LBBB); patients with a documented MI or prior coronary angiography demonstrating significant disease and who have an established diagnosis of CAD. (Note that for diagnostic purposes, exercise testing may not be useful. However, overall risk for individuals can be determined from obtaining $Vo_{2\,max}$ [see following sections 2, 3, and 5] if it is deemed safe to test.)

2. Risk Assessment and Prognosis in Patients with Symptoms or a History of Coronary Artery Disease

Class I: Patients undergoing initial evaluation with suspected or known CAD; patients with suspected or known CAD previously evaluated but now with a significant change in clinical status (specific exceptions noted in Class IIb).

Class IIb: Patients with the following ECG abnormalities: preexcitation (i.e., WPW syndrome), electronically paced ventricular rhythm, greater than 1 mm of resting ST-segment depression, complete LBBB; patients with

a stable clinical course who undergo periodic monitoring to guide treatment.

Class III: Patients with severe comorbidity likely to limit life expectancy or candidacy for revascularization.

3. Exercise Testing After Myocardial Infarction

Class I: Before discharge for prognostic assessment, activity prescription, or evaluation of medical therapy (submaximal at about 4 to 7 days); early after discharge for prognostic assessment, activity prescription, evaluation of medical therapy, and cardiac rehabilitation if the predischarge exercise test was not done (do a symptom limited ET at about 14 to 21 days); late after discharge for prognostic assessment, activity prescription, evaluation of medical therapy, and cardiac rehabilitation if the early exercise test was submaximal (do a symptom limited ET at about 3 to 6 weeks).

Class IIa: After discharge for activity counseling or exercise training as part of cardiac rehabilitation in patients who have undergone coronary revascularization.

Class IIb: Before discharge in patients who have undergone cardiac catheterization to identify ischemia in the distribution of a coronary lesion of borderline severity; patients with preexcitation syndrome (i.e., WPW syndrome), electronically paced ventricular rhythm, greater than 1 mm of resting ST-segment depression, complete LBBB, digoxin therapy, LVH.

Class III: Patients with severe comorbidity likely to limit life expectancy or candidacy for revascularization.

4. Asymptomatic Patients Without Known Coronary Artery Disease

Class I: None.

Class IIb: Evaluation of patients with multiple risk factors; evaluation of asymptomatic men older than 45 years of age and women older than 55 years of age planning to start vigorous exercise (especially if sedentary), involved in occupations in which impairment might impact public safety, or at high risk for CAD because of other diseases (e.g., chronic renal failure).

Class III: Routine screening of asymptomatic men or women.

Note: The Class IIb indication evokes considerable controversy because of the increased risk of false positive results. However, with good clinical judgment and/or the tables provided (e.g., Tables 92-1 through 92-3), the clinician may determine that the patient has a pretest likelihood as high as 15% to 20%, making the patient a reasonable candidate for exercise testing.

5. Exercise Testing Before and After Revascularization

Class I: Demonstration of proof of ischemia before revascularization; evaluation of patients with recurrent symptoms suggesting ischemia after revascularization.

Class IIa: After discharge for activity counseling or exercise training as part of cardiac rehabilitation in patients who have undergone coronary revascularization.

Class IIb: Detection of restenosis in selected, high-risk asymptomatic patients within the first 12 months after angioplasty; periodic monitoring of selected, high-risk asymptomatic patients for restenosis, graft occlusion, or disease progression.

Class III: Localization of ischemia for determining site of intervention; routine, periodic monitoring of asymptomatic patients after percutaneous transluminal coronary angioplasty (PTCA) or coronary artery bypass grafting without specific indications.

6. Investigation of Heart Rhythm Disorders

Class I: Identification of appropriate settings in patients with rate-adaptive pacemakers.

Class IIa: Evaluation of patients with known or suspected exercise-induced arrhythmias; evaluation of medical, surgical, or ablative therapy in patients with exercise-induced arrhythmias (including atrial fibrillation).

Class IIb: Investigation of isolated ventricular ectopic beats in middle-aged patients without other evidence of CAD.

Class III: Investigation of isolated ectopic beats in young patients.

C. Indications for Diabetics

Because of a disproportionate burden of CAD in diabetic patients, the American Diabetes Association has developed five indications for cardiac testing in diabetic patients:

1. Typical or atypical cardiac symptoms
2. Resting ECG suggestive of ischemia or infarction
3. Peripheral or carotid occlusive arterial disease
4. Two or more of the following risk factors in addition to diabetes:
   a. Total cholesterol ≥240 mg/dl, LDL cholesterol ≥160 mg/dl, or high-density lipoprotein (HDL) cholesterol <35 mg/dl
   b. Blood pressure (BP) >140/90 mm Hg
   c. Smoking
   d. Family history of premature CAD
   e. Microalbuminuria
5. Sedentary lifestyle and plan to begin a vigorous exercise program with one of the following criteria:
   a. Age 35 and over
   b. Type 2 diabetes of >10 years' duration
   c. Type 1 diabetes of >15 years' duration
   d. Presence of any additional risk factor for CAD
   e. Presence of microvascular disease (e.g., retinopathy or nephropathy, including microalbuminuria

f. Peripheral vascular disease or autonomic neuropathy

D. Indications in the Emergency Department

Patient has or had chest pain and fulfills the following requirements:

1. Two sets of negative cardiac enzymes from each of two different types of assays (troponin, myoglobin, or creatinine kinase MB) at 4-hour intervals.
2. Preexercise 12-lead ECG shows no significant changes when compared with original ECG at the time of presentation to the emergency department.
3. Absence of baseline (resting) ECG abnormalities that would preclude accurate assessment of the exercise ECG.
4. From admission to the time that results are available from the second set of cardiac enzymes, the patient has become asymptomatic, has had lessening of chest pain symptoms, or has had persistent atypical symptoms.
5. Absence of ischemic chest pain at the time of exercise testing.

E. Indications for Firemen (from National Fire Protection Association [NFPA] in 2000)

1. At age 40, periodic treadmill testing should be performed. The frequency should increase with age, but at a minimum, the test should be done every 2 years.
2. At age 35, periodic treadmill testing should be performed for individuals with one or more coronary risk factors (premature family history [less than age 55], hypertension, diabetes mellitus, cigarette smoking, and hypercholesterolemia [total cholesterol >240 or HDL <35]).

F. Determination of Pretest Likelihood

If the goal of the exercise test is to exclude CAD, determining pretest likelihood will help in the decision of whether exercise testing is the indicated and proper procedure. For diagnostic purposes, exercise testing is most valuable for patients with an intermediate (20% to 70%) pretest likelihood. Simple graphs and tables are available that require only three variables to estimate pretest likelihood in symptomatic individuals (Fig. 92-4 and Table 92-1). With a pretest likelihood in the 20% to 70% range, an abnormal or positive test provides strong justification for additional studies, including invasive studies. A negative study may provide justification for merely close observation with frequent follow-up visits.

The value of using this range (20% to 70%) is further demonstrated with graphs of posttest likelihood of CAD

(Fig. 92-5). From these graphs, the clinician should be able to see that the most information is obtained from patients with an intermediate pretest likelihood. In other words, for Fig. 92-5 the vertical gap between what would be a positive test and what would be a negative test is the largest for patients in the intermediate pretest range. In this group, positive studies are most clearly delineated from negative studies. Therefore the most information is obtained. In this range, a positive test significantly increases the likelihood of CAD, especially if greater than 2 mm ST-segment depression, whereas a negative test can be very reassuring. Using an example, a patient with a pretest likelihood of 40% with 2 mm or more of ST-segment depression now has more than an 85% likelihood of CAD. Such a posttest likelihood would justify an invasive procedure. Whereas in this same patient, less than 1 mm of ST-segment depression (a negative test) lowers their risk of CAD to less than 20%. Close follow-up of this patient may be adequate.

For patients with low (less than 20%) pretest likelihoods, although there may be other benefits of performing exercise testing, positive studies are more likely to be bothersome false positives that lead to unnecessary patient anxiety and further expensive diagnostic testing. On the other hand, a negative test in the high pretest likelihood group (more than 70%) may not be sufficient to exclude CAD. For the young or very active individual with a high pretest likelihood, coronary angiography is diagnostic and might be a more appropriate study. Again, to use examples, a patient with a pretest likelihood of 90% that has a positive study (greater than 2 mm ST-segment depression) has approximately a 96% posttest likelihood (using Fig. 92-5). There is only a 6% gain in probability, which is

very little information. If the study is negative, the patient still has a 75% likelihood of CAD. For diagnostic purposes, this probability certainly does not rule out CAD, so exercise testing has been of little value.

It should be noted that even in patients where little diagnostic information is gained with exercise testing, performing testing may be helpful for other reasons, such as for managing CAD. ACC/AHA guidelines call for "objective evidence of myocardial ischemia while on medical therapy" before angioplasty. Exercise testing is one objective method of demonstrating ischemia.

Pretest likelihood can be estimated by a description of the chest pain and the patient's gender and age. *Typical angina* is described (Diamond and Forrester) as substernal, exertional, and relieved by rest or nitroglycerine. Chest discomfort with two of these three characteristics is *atypical angina*. Chest discomfort with only one of these characteristics is considered *nonanginal chest pain*. Using these three descriptions, pretest likelihood tables and their corresponding graphs (Table 92-1 and Fig. 92-4) can be readily applied to determine pretest likelihood.

In the asymptomatic group, tables are also available to estimate absolute risk of coronary events over the next 10 years (Table 92-2) based on risk points (Table 92-3). Combining these data with clinical gestalt, clinicians can estimate which asymptomatic patients with risk factors would possibly reach the 20% pretest likelihood and benefit from exercise testing. These tables are based on Framingham data, and it should be kept in mind that additional risk should be added for *severe* abnormalities in each of the risk categories, such as severe hypertension, heavy smoking, and severe hypercholesterolemia. It should also be kept in mind

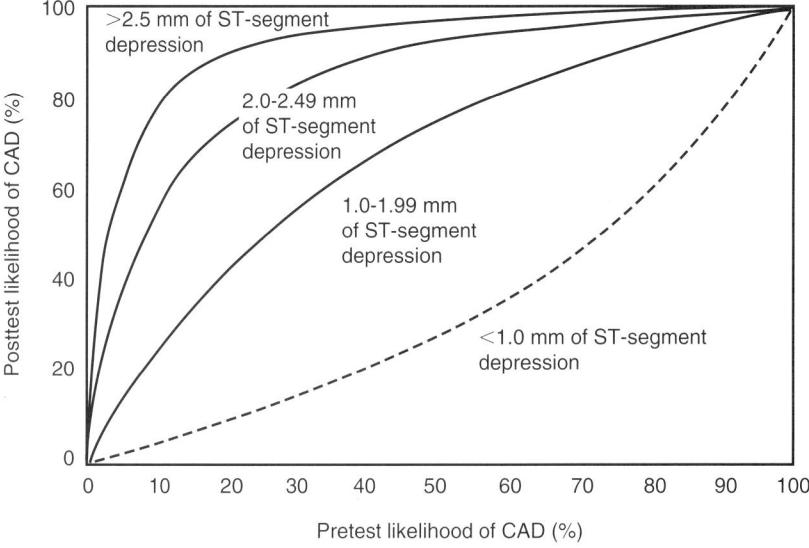

Fig. 92-5
Posttest likelihood with positive (>1 mm ST-segment depression) and negative (<1 mm ST-segment depression). (Redrawn from Epstein SE, *Am J Cardiol* 46:491, 1980.)

that approximately one third of individuals who developed CAD in Framingham had none of the usual risk factors, so generous estimates should be made when assessing risk. As newer risk factors (homocystine, ferritin, high-sensitivity C-reactive protein [cardio CRP], fibrinogen, lipoprotein (a) [LP(a)], etc.) are studied, for individuals having these risk factors the clinician may again have to use clinical judgment or gestalt when estimating an individual's pretest likelihood.

CONTRAINDICATIONS

- Very recent acute MI (generally less than 6 days) or other acute cardiac event
- Angina pectoris at rest or unstable angina
- Severe symptomatic left ventricular dysfunction
- Potentially life-threatening or uncontrolled ventricular arrhythmia or an atrial arrhythmia that compromises cardiac function
- Third-degree atrioventricular block or second-degree Mobitz Type II block without pacemaker
- Acute pericarditis, myocarditis, or endocarditis
- Severe aortic stenosis
- Suspected dissecting aneurysm
- Severe arterial hypertension (resting >200 mm Hg systolic or >115 mm Hg diastolic)
- Acute pulmonary edema, embolus, or infarction
- Acute thrombophlebitis, deep vein thrombosis, or intracardiac thrombi
- Acute or serious general illness or infection
- Neuromuscular, musculoskeletal, or arthritic condition that precludes exercise
- Uncontrolled metabolic disease, such as diabetes, thyrotoxicosis, or myxedema
- Medication intoxication from drugs such as digoxin, sedatives, or psychotropic agents
- Patient inability or lack of desire or motivation to perform the test, including severe emotional distress
- Nonavailability of advanced cardiac life support (ACLS) equipment or of an individual certified to perform ACLS

Note: Some of these contraindications are relative. In selected cases, a skilled cardiologist may perform testing for patients with these diagnoses (generally in a referral center). All are contraindications to testing in the office.

Contraindications in the Emergency Department

1. New or evolving abnormalities on the resting ECG.
2. Abnormal cardiac enzymes.
3. Inability to perform exercise.
4. Worsening or persistent ischemic chest pain symptoms from admission to the time of exercise testing.

5. Clinical risk profiling indicates coronary angiography is likely.
6. Any routine contraindications from the previous section.

Relative Contraindications to Exercise Testing

There are certain conditions that produce a study that is difficult to interpret or that will have results that add very little clinical information. Most relative contraindications fall into this category.

- Ventricular aneurysm
- Chronic infectious disease (e.g., mononucleosis, hepatitis, advanced HIV)
- Fixed-rate pacemaker (rarely used)
- Advanced or complicated pregnancy
- Frequent or complex ventricular ectopy or uncontrolled atrial arrhythmia
- Moderate hypertension (>105 mm Hg diastolic)

EQUIPMENT

- A treadmill with adjustable speed and grade—this is by far the most common equipment used for exercise testing (Fig. 92-6). Advantages include the ability to test most patients under the actual physiologic conditions of exercise. The most common types of exercise performed by patients in the United States are walking and running. In addition, a variation in patient motivation during the treadmill test is less common than with the bicycle method. Disadvantages include the fact that the treadmill may be difficult to use for patients with lower-extremity or lower-back problems or for patients who are very obese. The equipment is

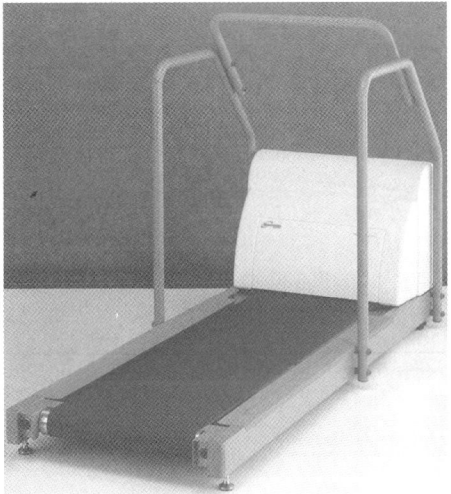

Fig. 92-6
Treadmill. (Courtesy Burdick, Inc. Deerfield, Wisc.)

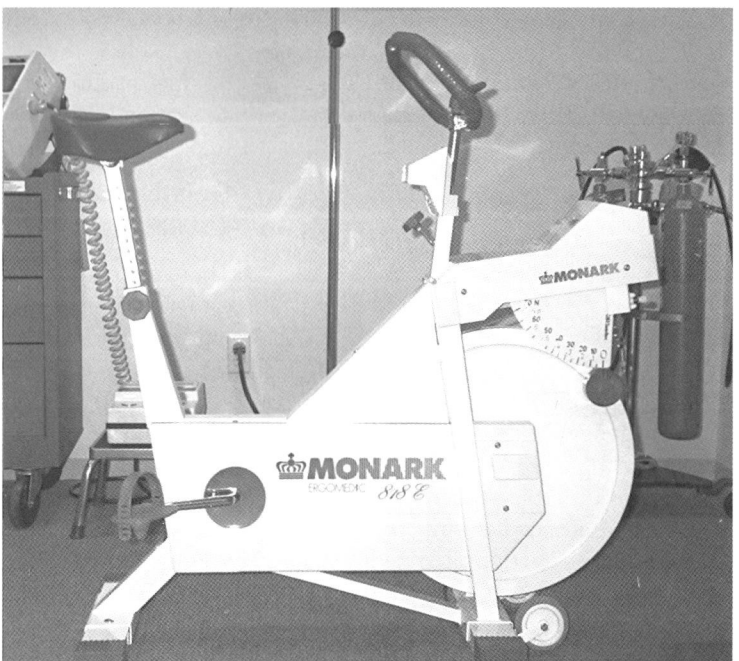

Fig. 92-7
Bicycle ergometer.

also more expensive, causes more motion artifact, and is noisier than a bicycle ergometer.

Note: If a treadmill is chosen, it should have a warm-up speed of about 0.5 to 1.5 mph, with testing speeds ranging from 2.0 mph up to 12 mph. For elite athletes, the speed may need to reach 15 mph. The slope or grades possible should range from 0% (flat) to 20%. If testing elite athletes, the grade may need to reach 25%.

- Bicycle ergometers—Bicycle ergometers use adjustable resistance and pedal frequency to exert the patient (Fig. 92-7). Advantages with the bicycle ergometer include the fact that the test can be terminated instantly. Many patients feel more secure sitting on the bicycle. If they have arthritis preventing them from walking on a treadmill, often patients can tolerate a bicycle. This method is also associated with less artifact, and BP measurements are easier to obtain. Bicycles are less expensive and quieter. Unfortunately, in the United States leg fatigue is common because most patients do not bike. In fact, as a result of leg fatigue the procedure often fails to determine $Vo_{2\,max}$. Bicycle ergometry is also dependent on motivation throughout its duration. As a result, in the United States if the patient can tolerate the treadmill, most clinicians prefer to use it.
- Arm ergometer—The arm ergometer (Fig. 92-8) enables patients with severe orthopedic problems to be tested. However, muscle fatigue often occurs before the maximum heart rate is achieved.
- ECG—A continuous monitor (Fig. 92-9) is needed (a three-channel model with continuous tracing and a screen-freeze option is desirable) as well as a

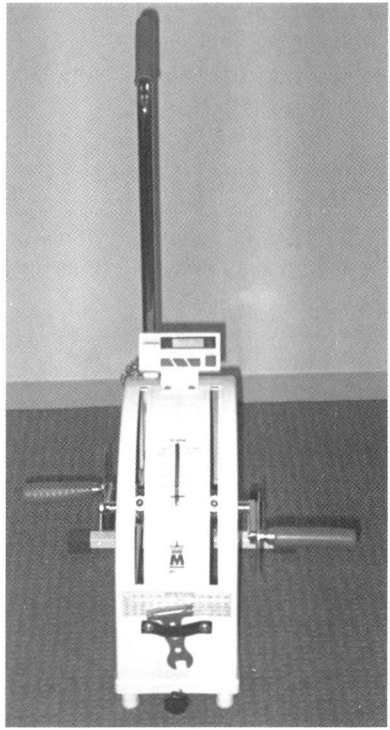

Fig. 92-8
Arm ergometer.

twelve-lead ECG recorder. With modern equipment, the recorder also runs the treadmill. Recent developments for primary care offices (e.g., wider wheelbase) allow the recorder to be wheeled from room to room for routine ECGs. Interpretive packages for 12-lead ECGs are also very convenient. Most equipment is

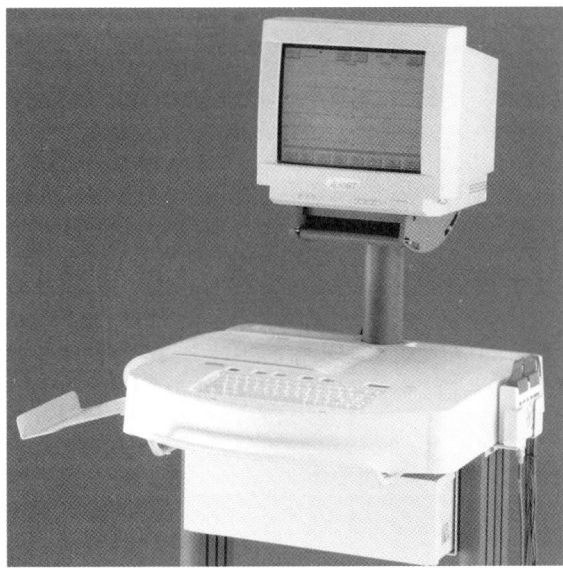

Fig. 92-9
ECG monitor. (Courtesy Burdick, Inc. Deerfield, Wisc.)

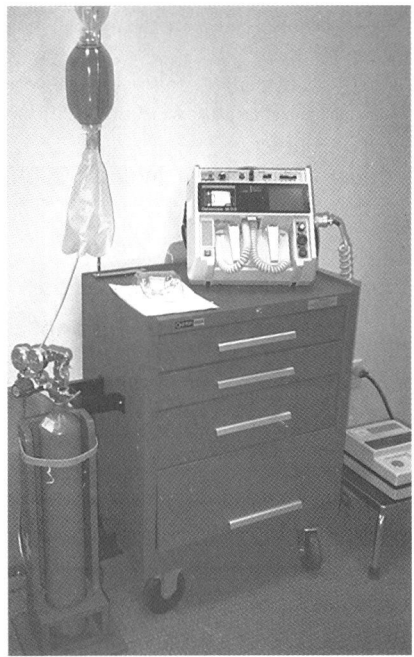

Fig. 92-10
Emergency equipment (see text for details).

now digital, allowing data to be filtered to provide a smooth baseline. However, it is important to avoid overfiltering the data and, in so doing, filtering out ST-segment depression.

- Electrodes, cables, and belt—A disposable or washable belt is preferred because patients usually sweat.
- Sphygmomanometer, including various cuff sizes—A gauge manometer is adequate because the most important readings are those relative to resting pressures (not the absolute pressures).
- Stethoscope.
- Razor, rubbing alcohol.
- Electrodes—Most clinicians now use disposable electrodes.
- Electrode cream—If not using disposable electrodes.
- Emergency equipment—This equipment (Fig. 92-10) includes a monitor/defibrillator; oxygen; airways, intubation, and suction equipment; and an emergency drug kit containing intravenous (IV) fluids and tubing (available drugs should be able to support ACLS protocols).

Note: It is also helpful to have a trained technician (Fig. 92-11) assisting. Technician certification for exercise testing is available through the American College of Sports Medicine. In many centers the technician prepares the patient; monitors the ECG and the patient's response to exercise, the heart rate, and the BP; and prepares the results for interpretation. For low-risk patients, they may actually perform the entire study without a physician being present. Otherwise, the clinician should examine the patient before, during, and after the procedure, confirm which protocol to use, and terminate the study. The clinician should also monitor the ECG tracing when the technician is taking BP readings, and the clinician should interpret the final results.

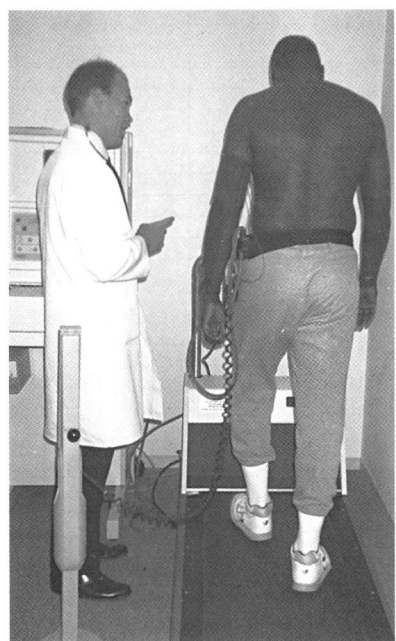

Fig. 92-11
Trained technician monitoring patient.

Written Procedure Protocols

- Informed consent procedure (see the sample patient consent form titled "Cardiac Exercise Testing" on page 1851 of Appendix G)
- Medical history, physical examination, handwritten report form (Fig. 92-12)

- Criteria for stopping exercise test (see the "Technique" section)
- Emergency response plan (should be designed for every office and kept on file in event of a complication from exercise testing)
- Quality assurance plan, including calibration and testing of equipment

Note: All emergency equipment should be checked daily, and medications should be checked weekly to monthly, depending on their use. The exercise-testing equipment should be inspected and calibrated periodically, based on manufacturer recommendations. ACLS certification cards should be kept on file along with the information and protocols listed above.

Cardiac Exercise Testing

Patient's name ________________
Medications: ________________
Reason for study: ______________

Time (min)

Date ____________
Protocol ___________
Age _____ Wt _____

Heart rate (beats per minute): 200, 190, 180, 170, 160, 150, 140, 130, 120, 110, 100, 90, 80, 70, 60

Blood pressure —

Speed															
Grade	%	%	%	%	%	%	%	%	%	%	%	%	%	%	%
Min	1	2	3	4	5	6	7	8	9	10	11	12	13	14	15
RPE															
Functional class (AHA) if Bruce protocol	IV	III			II		I								

	100%	85%
PMHR		

True MHR ____________
METS ___ Double prod ___

Reason for stopping ________________________________
Angina began ________________ Angina subsided ________________ Arrhythmias ________________
Interpretation: negative positive incomplete (<85% MHR) test
Heart rate recovery: normal abnormal
Comments: ________________________________
____
Symptoms: ________________________________
Repeat study in ________ mo/yr
Exercise prescription given? Y N

Clinician ____________________

Fig. 92-12
Exercise test results form. *METS,* Metabolic equivalents; *PMHR,* predicted maximum heart rate (220 – age). (Modified from Evans CH, Karunaratne HB: *Am Fam Physician* 45:121, 1992.)

PREPROCEDURE PATIENT PREPARATION

Before arrival:

- The clinician should instruct the patient to minimize alcohol, over-the-counter medications, and caffeine consumption the day before and the day of the procedure. He or she should encourage the patient to get a good night's sleep the night before the procedure. Patients should not eat for 2 hours before the test. It might be advisable for the most recent meal to be a small and predominately liquid meal. To minimize the risk of patient fatigue, many clinicians prefer performing exercise testing in the morning. They then instruct the patient to avoid breakfast or to have only a liquid breakfast that day.
- The procedure should be rescheduled, if possible, if the patient has a cold or other viral illness or is not feeling well in general.
- If the indication for the test is to screen for disease or to make the diagnosis (instead of for management of CAD), the clinician should instruct the patient to avoid taking β-blockers the day of the test.

Note: Digoxin can cause artifact even at therapeutic doses. If possible, digoxin should not be taken for 2 weeks before a test, the amount of time necessary for its elimination. However, a negative study in a patient taking digitalis is a good study. Estrogen has a very similar effect and can be managed the same way in postmenopausal women. β-Blockers can suppress the heart rate and prevent determination of the MHR. Patients who discontinue β-blockers should watch closely for "rebound" symptoms and, if they develop, should restart their β-blockers. Because ACE inhibitors have little or no effect on performance of a stress test, frequently they may be used as a substitute for other antihypertensives. If necessary, they can be taken on the day of the test and usually work within an hour. Clonidine may be used in the same manner.

- If the indication for the test is to determine pharmacologic efficacy in patients with CAD, obviously β-blockers should be taken the day of the study.
- The clinician should instruct the patient to bring shoes and clothing that are comfortable for walking and possibly for jogging.
- To minimize patient worry and stress (which often cause an elevated resting SBP), the clinician should explain that the risk of death for patients being tested using a treadmill is very small (1 per 10,000 patients). Because exercise testing in an office setting is an elective procedure, patients should never be exposed to excess risk (i.e., patients should be chosen very carefully to ensure that the actual risk of death is much less than even 1:10,000).

After arrival:

- The clinician should again explain the reasons for the test and answer any questions.
- The procedure should be explained again to the patient (e.g., how frequently the workload will be increased, how BP measurements will be taken, how the PES works).
- The patient should be assured of close monitoring and reassured that although the procedure stresses the heart, it is a relatively safe procedure (less than 1:10,000 mortality rate).
- The patient should know what symptoms to report during the test.
- The clinician should explain to the patient how to terminate the procedure should he or she have severe symptoms or an emergency arise.
- Signed, written informed consent should be obtained (see sample titled "Cardiac Exercise Testing" on page 1851 of Appendix G).

TECHNIQUE

1. Review the patient's interval medical history and examine the patient. Based on the history and re-examination, make sure no contraindication has developed since the last time the patient was seen.
2. Select the mode of exercise testing (e.g., treadmill, bicycle ergometer, arm ergometer), based on the individual's ability to exercise.
3. Select the protocol. There are many excellent protocols in use; therefore the choice is often dependent on the patient's predicted exercise capacity and on clinician preference. The Veterans' Administration (VA) Specific Activity Questionnaire (Fig. 92-1) may be very helpful for predicting exercise capacity and helping decide between an aggressive protocol and a modified protocol. Choose a protocol that starts at a low level of exertion (2 to 3 METs).
   a. A protocol with stage durations of at least 3 minutes (2 minutes for bicycle ergometer) allows more physiologic adaptation to the workload of each stage.
   b. Workload increases that are no greater than 1 to 3 METs per stage also allow more physiologic adaptation.
   c. Choose a protocol (Fig. 92-13) that will allow completion of the study in less than 15 minutes (even more preferable is 10 minutes or less). Tests lasting more than 15 minutes may produce fatigue and overheating, which may independently affect results.

The Bruce protocol (Table 92-4) is the most frequently used protocol, and it has been the most extensively studied and validated. It is especially useful in active patients and takes less time than other protocols because it rapidly increases workload. It does have its disadvantages: By the fourth or fifth stage, the patient must run, which increases artifact. In addition,

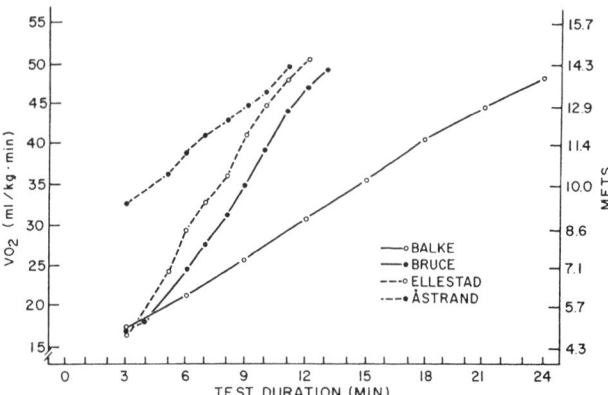

Fig. 92-13
Oxygen uptake measured according to time of exercise on four different protocols. (From Pollock MI: *Am Heart J* 92:39, 1976.)

TABLE 92-4
Standard Bruce Protocol

Stage*	Speed (mph)	Grade (%)	Metabolic Equivalents (METS)	Oxygen Consumption (ml/kg/min)
I	1.7	10	4	13
II	2.5	12	6.6	25
III	3.4	14	10	34
IV	4.2	16	14.2	46
V	5.0	18	17.2	58
VI	5.5	20	20.5	70

From Fowler GC, Evans CH, Altman MA: Exercise testing, *Prim Care* 24(2):375, 1997.
*Each stage lasts 3 minutes.

the patient often experiences difficulty in accommodating to increases in both slope and speed at the same time. Elderly patients usually have decreased proprioception in their toes and some degree of impairment of vision, making it especially difficult for them to adjust to changes in both slope and speed at the same time. In general, most "modified" protocols, such as the modified Bruce or modified Balke protocol, have a reduced progression of workload and are better tolerated by elderly or debilitated patients. Modified protocols usually maintain the same speed and only vary the elevation. Gradual but continuously increasing workload protocols (e.g., ramp) are being studied in several large centers and show promise toward becoming the preferred protocol. Table 92-5 indicates various protocols, and Fig. 92-13 graphically compares METs per minute and Vo$_{2\,max}$ as measured for four protocols.

Again, to assist in choosing between the Bruce protocol and a less aggressive protocol, such as the Modified Bruce protocol, the VA questionnaire may be helpful (Fig. 92-1). If a patient can readily achieve greater than 5 METs, they should be able to tolerate the Bruce protocol. The number of METs the patient will achieve is about the same as the number of minutes an individual can complete on the Bruce protocol. The VA questionnaire is also helpful when setting up the ramp protocol, which must be customized for each patient based on their estimated exercise capacity in METs.

The ability to directly measure expired gases (e.g., oxygen, carbon dioxide) and total ventilation during an exercise test is helpful in certain situations. With additional equipment, the clinician can do four things: (1) actually measure the maximal aerobic capacity, (2) determine the anaerobic threshold (i.e., the point during exercise when marked lactic acid production begins), (3) give a more accurate exercise prescription, and (4) decide if impaired exercise capacity is being caused by a pulmonary condition as opposed to the more common cardiac causes. The equipment needed for gas analysis during an exercise test is becoming smaller and more affordable. Adding gas analysis equipment broadens the indications for exercise testing and increases the reimbursement (see the "Suppliers" section). To avoid large capital equipment costs, there are service companies that will bring portable equipment to your office for this procedure and split the fees.

4. Obtain the resting BP.
5. Prepare the patient for the ECG machine to be used in the test (Fig. 92-9).
   a. Locate sites on the chest for electrodes, which are the same locations as for the office ECG (see Chapter 86, Office Electrocardiograms), except that the arm electrodes are placed in the infraclavicular fossae (midclavicle) and the leg electrodes are placed on the lower abdomen just above the beltline (Fig. 92-14).
   b. Cleanse the skin at these sites with alcohol preps and let them dry thoroughly.
   c. Shave any hair from the electrode sites. The cornified outer layer of skin should be removed with gentle dermabrasion. Fine sandpaper or other abrasives are usually provided in the preparation kit for this purpose.
   d. Apply electrodes to these sites.
   e. Attach lead wires from the *octopus* to the appropriate electrodes. (An ECG octopus is the set of leads usually provided by the equipment manufacturer to accompany the ECG machine.)
   f. Stabilize the exercise ECG octopus with a belt around the patient's waist. The octopus can be bundled and affixed to the patient with extra expansion loops to allow variation in distance from the ECG machine and to minimize motion artifact. Fortunately, most equipment is now digital and can use filters to minimize motion artifact.
   g. If desired, for female patients, a gown or

TABLE 92-5
Various Exercise Protocols

Treadmill Protocols

AHA Functional Class	Clinical Status	O₂ Cost (ml/kg/min)	METs	Bicycle Ergometer (1 W ≈ 6.1 kpm/min) For 70 kg body weight kpm/min	Bruce 3-Min Stages mph	Bruce %gr	USAFSAM mph	USAFSAM %gr	"Slow" USAFSAM mph	"Slow" USAFSAM %gr	McHenry mph	McHenry %gr	Stanford % Grade at 3 mph	Stanford % Grade at 2 mph	ACIP mph	ACIP %gr	CHF mph	CHF %gr	METs
Normal and I — Healthy, Dependent on Age, Activity / Sedentary Healthy		56.0	16		5.5	20													16
		52.5	15		5.0	18													15
		49.0	14	1500											3.4	24.0			14
		45.5	13	1350	4.2	16	3.3	25			3.3	21			3.1	24.0			13
		42.0	12	1200			3.3	20			3.3	18	22.5		3.0	21.0			12
		38.5	11	1050	3.4	14	3.3	15	2	25	3.3	15	20		3.4	24.0	3.4	14.0	11
		35.0	10	900					2	20	3.3	12	17.5		3.1	24.0	3.0	15.0	10
		31.5	9	750			3.3	10			3.3	9	15		3.0	21.0	3.0	12.5	9
		28.0	8	600					2	15	3.3	6	12.5	17.5	3.0	17.5	3.0	10.0	8
		24.5	7		2.5	12	3.3	5	2	10			10	14.0	3.0	14.0	3.0	7.5	7
		21.0	6								2.0	3	7.5	10.5	3.0	10.5	2.0	10.5	6
II — Limited		17.5	5	450	1.7	10	3.3	0	2	5			5	7.0	3.0	7.0	2.0	7.0	5
III		14.0	4	300	1.7	5	2.0	0	2	0			2.5	3.5	3.0	3.0	2.0	3.5	4
III		10.5	3	150	1.7	0					2.0	3	0		2.5	2.0	2.0	3.5	3
IV — Symptomatic		7.0	2												2.0	0.0	1.5	0.0	2
IV		3.5	1														1.0	0.0	1

Balke-Ware: % Grade at 3.3 mph, 1-Min Stages: 26, 25, 24, 23, 22, 21, 20, 19, 18, 17, 16, 15, 14, 13, 12, 11, 10, 9, 8, 7, 6, 5, 4, 3, 2, 1

From Froelicher VF: *Exercise and the heart: clinical concepts,* ed 3, St Louis, 1993, Mosby.

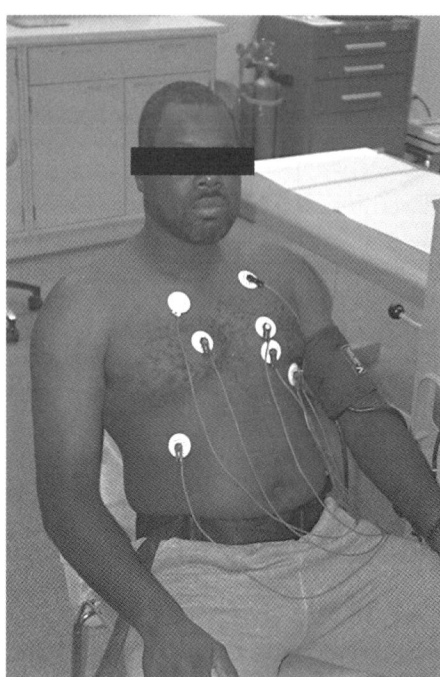

Fig. 92-14
Patient with electrodes attached.

loose-fitting shirt can be worn over the lead wires. Jog bras work well, but underwire bras should be avoided.

6. Obtain the supine, resting ECG. Because a recent MI is a contraindication to exercise testing, if there is even the remote chance of there having been a recent MI or an interval MI since the last clinician visit, a routine ECG must be repeated. For maximal diagnostic sensitivity, this supine routine ECG should be obtained with the leads in the standard limb positions to allow you to compare with any prior standard ECGs. If this ECG reveals no changes, the limb leads can then be moved back to the exercise positions to obtain the baseline supine preexercise ECG.

Note: In an occasional patient, hyperventilation alone will produce ST-segment depression. Because patients naturally hyperventilate during exercise, if there is ST-segment depression during the procedure, it may be difficult to determine whether hyperventilation caused it or if there is true ischemia. However, hyperventilation artifact is rare enough that most authorities now recommend hyperventilating only those patients with a positive test (after recovering them) to determine if hyperventilation caused the ST-segment deviation. This technique of hyperventilating only those patients with a positive result, after the procedure, saves not only time but also expense, including the expense of ECG paper. This method is especially effective in the office setting where fewer positives typically occur.

Treadmill Exercise Testing

7. Have the patient stand and obtain an ECG. If it is digital, the equipment will take 15 to 20 seconds to acquire the standing ECG. The equipment uses an average of 15 to 20 seconds of ECG tracings to measure the "signal average" against for later comparison.

Note: Occasionally, ST-segment depression occurs with standing. Therefore the isoelectric standard to measure against for ST-segment depression during exercise is the standing ECG before the test.

8. Begin the exercise test using the preselected protocol. Try to discourage the patient from gripping the handrail during the study because this will falsely elevate the maximal exercise capacity. It may also increase ECG artifact and falsely elevate BP. Time may be saved if staff demonstrates the procedure and allows the patient to practice before the clinician arrives. Staff should show the patient how to rest two fingers or the wrists on the handrail while walking near the front of the treadmill and looking straight ahead. (If the patient looks down, they will often get dizzy.)

9. Monitor and record the patient's symptoms, overall condition, pulse rate, and ECG at all times. *Instruct the patient to give adequate warning before they want to stop the test.* With the exception of submaximal testing, encourage the patient to go as far and as long as possible.

10. Record a 12-lead ECG at the end of each stage, at any time when an abnormality is noted on the monitor, immediately on stopping, and every minute for 8 minutes postexercise during recovery.

Note: Real data are obtained only from a hard copy of the 12-lead ECG. The monitor merely provides ongoing information, estimates or ST-segment changes, and allows the clinician to monitor for arrhythmias. If there is any question regarding ST-segment changes, print a hard copy for measurement and interpretation.

11. During each stage, at the start of the final minute, ask the patient if there is any chest discomfort, what point he or she has reached on the PES, and whether he or she wants to continue into the next stage. Also record the BP and heart rate near the end of each stage or at the time of any problems.

Note: For most patients, their perceived exertion (Box 92-1) is reproducible at a given level of exercise and correlates fairly well with their heart rate. Ask patients to indicate on a scale of 0 to 10 how hard they feel they are working with each stage. On the average, most patients feel they increase by 2 to 3 on the exertion scale with each stage in the early part of the study. PES usually increases more rapidly, from 7 to 9, near the end of the study. Rarely will anyone declare a

10. Individuals with good exertion perception may not have to measure their pulse as frequently while following their exercise prescription. They can simply be instructed to exercise to the level of perceived exertion that matched their appropriate heart rate for the aerobic range (60% to 80% MHR). Patients who highly underestimate their effort must be taught to measure their pulse before receiving an exercise prescription.

12. After completion of the exercise test, if it has been done for diagnostic purposes and the study has been negative, immediately ask the patient to lie down. Although this may not be comfortable for certain patients, especially if they are overweight or having slight difficulty breathing, it minimizes false positives during the recovery. Record the heart rate at 1 minute.

13. The patient should be monitored for at least 8 minutes in recovery or until symptoms or ECG abnormalities are gone.

Bicycle Ergometer Exercise Testing

7. After completing Steps 1 through 6 for treadmill exercise testing, have the patient sit on the bicycle and obtain a sitting ECG.

8. Begin the exercise test using the preselected protocol. The usual protocol starts at 25 W of resistance and increases by 25 W every 2 minutes.

9. Monitor the patient's symptoms, overall condition, pulse rate, and ECG at all times. Instruct the patient to give adequate warning before stopping the test. With the exception of submaximal testing, encourage the patient to go as far and as long as possible.

10. Record a 12-lead ECG at the end of each stage, at any time when an abnormality is noted on the monitor, immediately on stopping, and every minute for 8 minutes postexercise during recovery.

11. During each stage, at the start of the final minute, ask the patient if there is any chest discomfort, what point he or she has reached on the PES, and whether he or she wants to continue into the next stage. Also record the BP and heart rate near the end of each stage or at the time of any problems.

12. After completion of the exercise test (if it has been done for diagnostic purposes and the study has been negative), immediately ask the patient to lie down. Although this may not be comfortable for certain patients, especially if they are overweight or having slight difficulty breathing, it minimizes false positives during the recovery. Record the heart rate at 1 minute.

13. The patient should be monitored for at least 8 minutes in recovery or until symptoms or ECG abnormalities are gone.

For Both Treadmill and Bicycle Ergometer Testing, the Following Steps Are Also Necessary:

1. If the study is positive or being performed for CAD management purposes, keep the patient exercising for 3 to 4 minutes during recovery at a very low workload to prevent venous pooling and to minimize the risk of an arrhythmia. The patient may then either sit or lie down for the remainder of recovery.

2. Monitor the BP, HR, any symptoms, and the ECG tracing during recovery. Observe the patient in recovery until symptoms or ECG changes have resolved completely (or for at least 8 minutes if symptoms or ECG changes resolve earlier).

Note: For positive studies—even for those profoundly positive—very rarely are medications necessary. Simply stopping the exertion and having the patient sit up to improve oxygenation should be adequate. If there is strong suspicion that a plaque has been destabilized, aspirin, if not contraindicated, is the best choice for a medication. In the absence of contraindications, oxygen may also be considered. Sublingual nitroglycerin is risky in a vasodilated patient because it may drop the BP. Sublingual calcium channel blockers are contraindicated.

Test Termination Criteria

A good rule of thumb for stopping the study is *after* the necessary information is obtained and *before* there is a complication. In the young or fit individual, when they reach their maximal predicted heart rate (220 − age), it may be prudent to explain that all the necessary information has been obtained; however, the patient may continue to exercise for as long as he or she desires. (Allowing the patient to make this choice is also indirectly obtaining informed consent.)

Note: In the past, authorities denoted two possible definitions of a maximal stress exercise test (MSET): (1) achieving a target heart rate of greater than 85% of the predicted MHR for that patient's age (i.e., roughly 85% of 220 − age) or (2) exercise to the point of symptoms. Most authorities now encourage patients to exercise to the point of symptoms (usually generalized or voluntary fatigue).

Predicted MHR (220 − age) is not patient specific and is frequently a bad prediction. The only contraindications for going to the point of symptoms are for debilitated or elderly patients or if a submaximal test is indicated. Maximal effort is usually indicated by maximal perceived exertion and the inability to continue at that workload.

Benefits to using the point of symptoms as the endpoint include the ability to measure true exercise capacity and the patient's true MHR. It also gives the clinician knowledge about a patient's cardiac response at a level of exercise beyond what the patient is likely to reproduce independently. This is certainly reassuring to the clinician when giving an exercise prescription (i.e., it should be safe for the patient to exercise at a lower level of exertion). Disadvantages include discomfort for the patient, especially if they are significantly deconditioned.

How does the clinician know if the patient gave their maximal effort? Following the PES is often helpful. Also, an RPP greater than 25,000 indicates to the clinician that the patient has given a good effort. Many other physiologic parameters have also been studied in an attempt to predict maximal effort (e.g., heart rate, respiratory rate, BP response), and none have been found to be predictive. However, if the patient is aware that it is important for them to give maximal effort to exclude heart disease, they are usually motivated.

1. Absolute indications to terminate a study include the following:

- SBP drops below resting value, especially after the first minute or two of the study (most dangerous if it reflects LV dysfunction; in that situation there is a high risk of life-threatening arrhythmias).
- Worsening anginal chest pain (severe enough that the patient desires to stop); it is not prudent for the patient to exercise beyond the point of where they obtain their "usual" amount of chest discomfort. In other words, there is no reason for the patient to demonstrate his or her worst chest pain while performing the study.
- Central nervous system (CNS) symptoms (e.g., dizziness, disorientation).
- Signs of poor perfusion (e.g., cyanosis, pallor) or severe ventricular dysfunction (e.g., dyspnea).
- Serious arrhythmias (e.g., three PVCs in a row [i.e., ventricular tachycardia] is an indication to terminate the test), increasingly frequent PVCs associated with ischemia (chest pain or ST changes), or atrial arrhythmia with cardiovascular compromise.
- Technical problems with equipment, ECG monitor, or SBP monitoring.
- Marked ECG changes (>3 mm of horizontal or downsloping ST-segment depression, or 1 mm of ST-segment elevation).
- When maximal effort has been attained.
- Patient wants to stop the test (especially elderly patients, where there may be little warning of a complication about to happen).

2. Relative indications to terminate a study:

- Worrisome ST or QRS changes (e.g., excessive junctional depression, marked axis shift).

- Significant fatigue, shortness of breath, wheezing, leg cramps, or intermittent claudication.
- Worrisome appearance (especially important in the elderly, where stability can deteriorate very rapidly; poor perfusion may be indicated solely by a loss of color in an elderly patient) .
- Elevated BP (SBP >250 mm Hg, DBP >115 mm Hg).
- Less serious dysrhythmia, including supraventricular tachycardia.
- Development of a bundle branch block pattern that cannot be distinguished from ventricular tachycardia.

INTERPRETATION

I. Normal ECG Responses to Exercise

- P-wave amplitude increases.
- T-wave amplitude often increases.
- RR and PR intervals decrease in length.
- Below a heart rate of 150, the R-wave amplitude is unchanged or increased; above 150 or near maximal exercise, the R wave in a healthy heart usually decreases in amplitude, and the overall QRS amplitude also usually decreases (the so-called Brody effect).
- J-point (i.e., the junction between the S wave and ST-segment) is depressed in the lateral (possibly all) leads especially at maximum exercise and gradually returns to normal during recovery. The PQ junction is also usually depressed (Fig. 92-15).
- ST-segment slope is usually upsloping; however, from the J-point, the tracing rapidly returns to baseline. In other words, at 0.04 to 0.06 second after the J-point, the final position of the ST-segment is at the baseline level.

II. ST-Segment Analysis

- A positive test is determined by ECG criteria. However, the test should not be labeled simply as normal, positive, or abnormal, but rather the specific responses to exercise should be identified and documented.
- Age and risk factors for heart disease should be taken into account when interpreting results.
- Many conditions and circumstances can cause a false-positive or a false-negative test (Box 92-2).
- The lateral leads (e.g., V_4, V_5, V_6) are the most important leads to monitor for ischemia. Their electrodes are located directly over the left ventricle and are the most likely to show ischemic ST-segment changes. Although it is always recommended to use three leads, studies have found that lead V_5 is the most sensitive lead if a single lead were to be used.

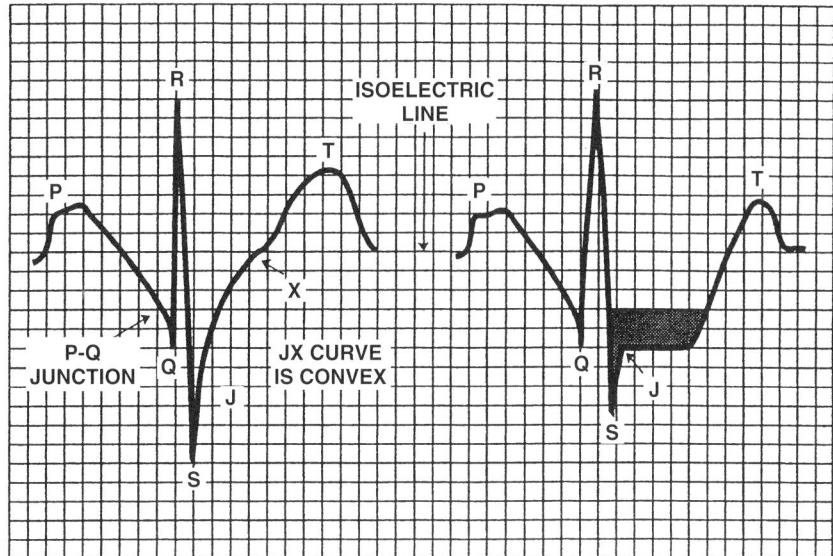

Fig. 92-15

Left, Normal exercise ECG complex. Note that the P-Q junction is deflected below the resting isoelectric line. This point is considered to be the baseline for determining ST-segment deviations. *Right,* A horizontal ST-segment depression of 2.0 mm as measured from the PQ junction. (From Ellestad MH: *Stress testing: principles and practice,* ed 4, Philadelphia, 1996, FA Davis.)

Note: The actual data are the hard copy printouts of the monitored leads and 12-lead recordings. It is recommended that these be interpreted separately, in a quiet room, scanning the entire printout, before giving the patient the results and recording them.

1. An exercise test is considered positive when 1 mm of ST-segment depression occurs in at least three beats in a row, in more than one lead, and in an area of the tracing where the baseline is relatively flat. If it is truly positive, ST-segment depression usually occurs in almost all of the leads; in most cases it will continue more than 1 minute into recovery. In fact, the ST-segment depression may worsen in recovery.

2. ST-segment deviation (depression or elevation) should be measured down or up from the level of the PQ junction. A line drawn horizontally from the PQ junction denotes the isoelectric line (Fig. 92-15).

3. ST-segment deviation (depression or elevation) should be measured at the J-point (i.e., ST zero, also known as the beginning of the ST-segment or end of the QRS complex).

4. One expert (Froelicher) only considers the study positive if the slope for 80 msec after the J-point is horizontal or downsloping. Other experts also consider a slow upsloping ST-segment pattern as positive (Fig. 92-16). They will consider a slow upsloping pattern positive if the tracing fails to reach within 1.5 mm of the baseline level of the PQ junction at 80 msec after the J-point. It should be understood that although a slow upsloping pattern may be positive, it is much more likely to be a false positive; however, accepting this pattern as a possible positive result slightly increases the sensitivity of the test for CAD. Slightly increasing the sensitivity should be weighed against the fact that such a positive usually indicates insignificant CAD. A slow upsloping pattern is more likely to be a true positive if it persists beyond 1 minute into recovery and is seen in not only the inferior leads (i.e., II, III, AVF), but also in other leads.

5. Although occasionally ST-segment elevation (i.e., transmural ischemia) can indicate the vessel involved, ST-segment depression does not localize ischemia. It cannot detect which blood vessel is involved. Subendocardial ischemia is a "global" phenomenon (i.e., for significant CAD, ST-segment changes will be seen in most leads).

6. If ST-segment elevation occurs over or adjacent to diagnostic Q waves, it may be caused by a ventricular aneurysm or a wall motion abnormality. If it occurs in a patient with a normal resting ECG or without a history of previous infarction, it indicates transmural ischemia and the test should be stopped. Transmural ischemia is extremely arrhythmogenic.

7. If downsloping or flat-pattern ST-segment depression occurs, and it is less than 1 mm or only in recovery, it may be indicative of early disease. Management options include ordering a perfusion study or a stress echo, or repeating the exercise test in 6 months.

BOX 92-2

Causes of False-Positive and False-Negative Tests

Causes of False-Positive Tests

Preexisting abnormal resting ECG (e.g., ST-segment abnormalities and bundle-branch block, especially left bundle branch block)

Cardiac hypertrophy

Female gender (Under Interpretation, see section titled "III. ST-Segment Analysis in Special Situations, B. ST Analysis in Women")

Wolff-Parkinson-White syndrome and other preexcitation variants

Short PR interval

Anemia

Hypertension (poorly controlled)

Hyperventilation

Drugs (e.g., digitalis, estrogen)

Nonfasting state

Cardiomyopathy

Hypokalemia and other electrolyte abnormalities

Hypoxemia

Vasoregulatory abnormalities

Excessive rate-pressure product (>45,000)

Sudden intense exercise

Mitral valve prolapse syndrome and valvular heart disease

Congenital heart disease

Pericardial disorders

Ventricular pacemaker

Pectus excavatum

Inadequate recording equipment, incorrect criteria, improper interpretation, or improper lead system or placement

Technical or observer error

Atrial repolarization (usually seen in inferior leads only, and short PR interval occurs on resting ECG)

Tricyclic antidepressants

Causes of False-Negative Tests

Right bundle branch block

Failure to reach an adequate exercise workload

Insufficient number of leads to detect ECG changes

Failure to use other information (e.g., systolic blood pressure drop, symptoms, dysrhythmia, heart rate response) in test interpretation

Single vessel disease

Excessive digital filtration on tracing

Tricyclic antidepressants

Technical or observer error

Medications (long-acting nitrates, β-blockers, and calcium-channel blockers have antianginal effects; they may "prolong the positive" or prolong the time of the study before the test becomes positive)

ECG Indicators of Significant or Extensive Coronary Artery Disease (Three-Vessel with LV Dysfunction or Left Main CAD)

- Markedly positive ST-segment response in multiple leads (>2.5 mm downsloping or horizontal ST-segment depression)
- Early positive ST-segment response (stage 1 of Bruce protocol or at ≤4 to 5 METS)
- Unable to complete stage 2 of Bruce protocol (especially if unable to complete stage 1)

TABLE 92-6

Recommended Criteria to Declare a Study Positive When There Are Baseline ECG Abnormalities

Abnormal Resting ST-T Configuration	Exercise or Postexercise ST Configuration	ST Depression and Point of Measurement
Flat or sagging ST and T	Horizontal	1.0 mm more depressed than at rest
	Upsloping	1.5 mm more depressed than at rest at 80 msec from J-point
	Downsloping	1.0 mm more depressed than at rest
Inverted T	Horizontal	1.5 mm at 60 msec from J-point
	Upsloping	1.5 mm at 80 msec from J-point
	Downsloping	1.5 mm at 20 msec from J-point

Note that these current criteria are slightly different depending on the configuration of the resting ST-segment and T-wave.

From Ellestad MH: Horizontal and downsloping ST segments. In *Stress testing: principles and practice,* ed 4, Philadelphia, 1996, FA Davis.

- Exercise-induced ST-segment elevation (unless it is certain that this is not from transmural ischemia)
- Worrisome ventricular arrhythmias (especially if associated with ST-segment depression or at a heart rate <130)
- Fall in exercise SBP (>10 mm Hg below baseline), especially when associated with angina or significant ST-segment changes
- Prolonged positive ST-segment response (>6 minutes of recovery)

III. ST-Segment Analysis in Special Situations

A. Baseline Abnormalities

When the ST-segments are abnormal on the resting ECG, new criteria are used to declare a test positive (Table 92-6).

B. ST Analysis in Women (Pratt)

False positives are less common in women over 50 years of age.

1. True positives are associated with four factors:
   a. Absence of mitral valve prolapse
   b. An exercise duration of less than 5 minutes
   c. The ability to reach the target heart rate
   d. The time it takes for the ST-segment to normalize is ≥6 minutes

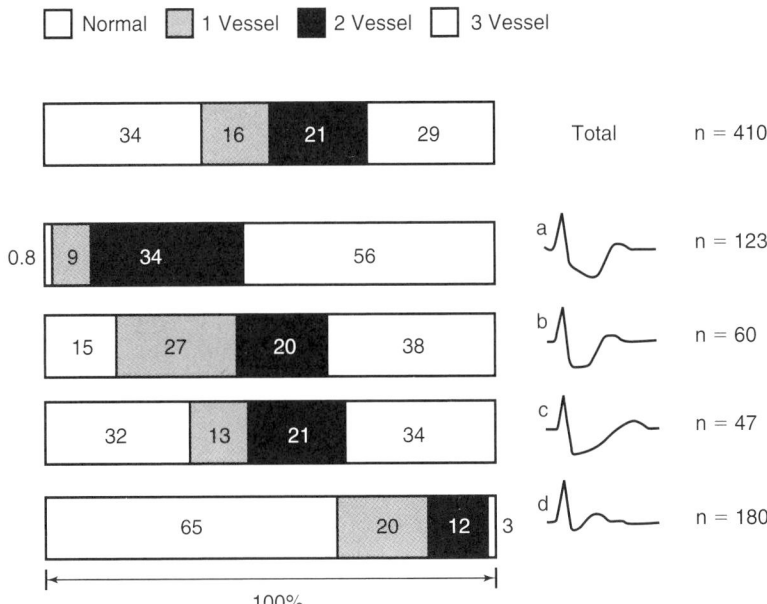

□ Normal ▨ 1 Vessel ■ 2 Vessel □ 3 Vessel

| | | | | | |
| Total | n = 410 |

Fig. 92-16
Three patterns of ST-segment depression. While downsloping pattern, *a,* usually represented 3-vessel disease (56%) and flat pattern, *b,* occasionally represented 3-vessel disease (38%), slow-uploading pattern, *c,* had 3-vessel disease in 34% and at least 1-vessel disease in 68%. Rapid-upsloping pattern, *d,* has been accepted as the normal physiologic pattern. (Redrawn from Goldschlager N, Selzer A, Cohn K: *Ann Intern Med* 85:277, 1976.)

2. False positives are associated with two factors:
   a. The ability to exercise to stage 3 of the Bruce protocol
   b. Rapid (<4 minutes) normalization of the ST-segment shift after cessation of exercise

C. Scenarios with decreased sensitivity and false positives and negatives

- If left bundle branch block (LBBB) or WPW syndrome is present, ST-segment depression does not necessarily indicate ischemia.
- If right bundle branch block (RBBB) is present, the ST-segments can only be analyzed in V_4, V_5, or V_6; the sensitivity of the test may be decreased.

Note: Recent data indicate that the presence of complete RBBB on the resting ECG is associated with a 50% greater risk of death, a rate similar to that of LBBB. The mechanism underlying the relationship is unclear.

- If ST depression occurs only in inferior leads II, III, or AVF (or any combination of the three) and not in the lateral leads, it is usually a false positive result caused by atrial repolarization. When reviewing, these patients frequently have a short PR interval on the resting ECG. (The atrial repolarization wave, which is negative, "pulls down" the ST-segment when superimposed.) Frequently, the ST-segment depression will return to normal in less than 1 minute of recovery in the false-positive cases.
- If coronary artery bypass surgery has been performed, sensitivity of the test may be decreased.

- If anterior or lateral Q waves or both are present (after MI), the sensitivity of the test may be decreased.
- See Box 92-2 for a complete listing of causes of false-positive and false-negative tests.

IV. Arrhythmias

- Prognosis in supraventricular and ventricular arrhythmias appears to be more related to underlying or coexisting conditions. Patients who are symptomatic should be referred.
- If the arrhythmia is associated with signs or symptoms of ischemia, in most cases management should be directed at treating the ischemia to minimize the arrhythmia.
- Premature ventricular contractions are common. They are only ominous in patients with LV dysfunction, severe ischemia, valvular heart disease, a cardiomyopathy, or a history of sudden cardiac death.
- Three unifocal PVCs in a row are defined as ventricular tachycardia and are an indication to terminate the test. Interestingly, asymptomatic, nonsustained ventricular tachycardia in an individual with a normal ejection fraction is not associated with increased cardiovascular mortality. However, a Holter monitor, echocardiogram, or both may be indicated.
- Young (i.e., less than 40 years of age) but otherwise healthy individuals with no CAD risk factors may have frequent PVCs at rest that resolve with exercise. If the exercise test is negative, further evaluation is usually not necessary. PVCs that go away with exercise in this population are almost always benign.

V. Exercise Capacity

The ability to achieve 15 METs indicates an excellent prognosis, even in those with known three-vessel CAD. The ability to achieve 10 METs indicates that medical management is reasonable. An inability to achieve 5 METs indicates a poor prognosis, especially if the test is positive.

- $Vo_{2\,max}$ can be estimated from various exercise protocols using standard formulas, tables, or graphs.
- Tables 92-7 and 92-8 show $Vo_{2\,max}$ estimated for individuals according to the length of time they are able to exercise on a treadmill with a Bruce protocol.
- Using estimated $Vo_{2\,max}$, an individual's approximate level of aerobic conditioning can be determined using age- and sex-matched tables. Table 92-9 and Fig. 92-17 also estimate the exercise capacity based on the number of METs a patient can achieve.

VI. Other Parameters Followed

- *Heart rate.* Failure to obtain a heart rate of 120 bpm is chronotropic incompetence with a resultant poor prognosis (approximately 15% per year will experience a coronary event); it may also indicate early sick sinus syndrome.
- *Heart rate recovery.* Failure of the heart rate to decrease 12 bpm in the first minute of recovery is an abnormal heart rate recovery. This indicates a fourfold increased risk of mortality over the next 5 years.
- *BP.* If the SBP drops below resting, it either predicts a poor prognosis or severe CAD. In one study, men with a maximal exercise systolic blood pressure <140 mm Hg had a 15-fold increase in the annual rate of sudden death when compared to those whose pressures exceeded 200 mm Hg.

A DBP increase of more than 10 mm Hg or an SBP greater than 240 mm Hg is a *hypertensive response to exercise.* In otherwise healthy individuals, with a hypertensive response to exercise, there is a slight risk of developing hypertension over the next few years. However, exercise testing should not be used to screen for hypertension because ambulatory BP monitoring is much more effective. In individuals with known hypertension or with other risk factors for

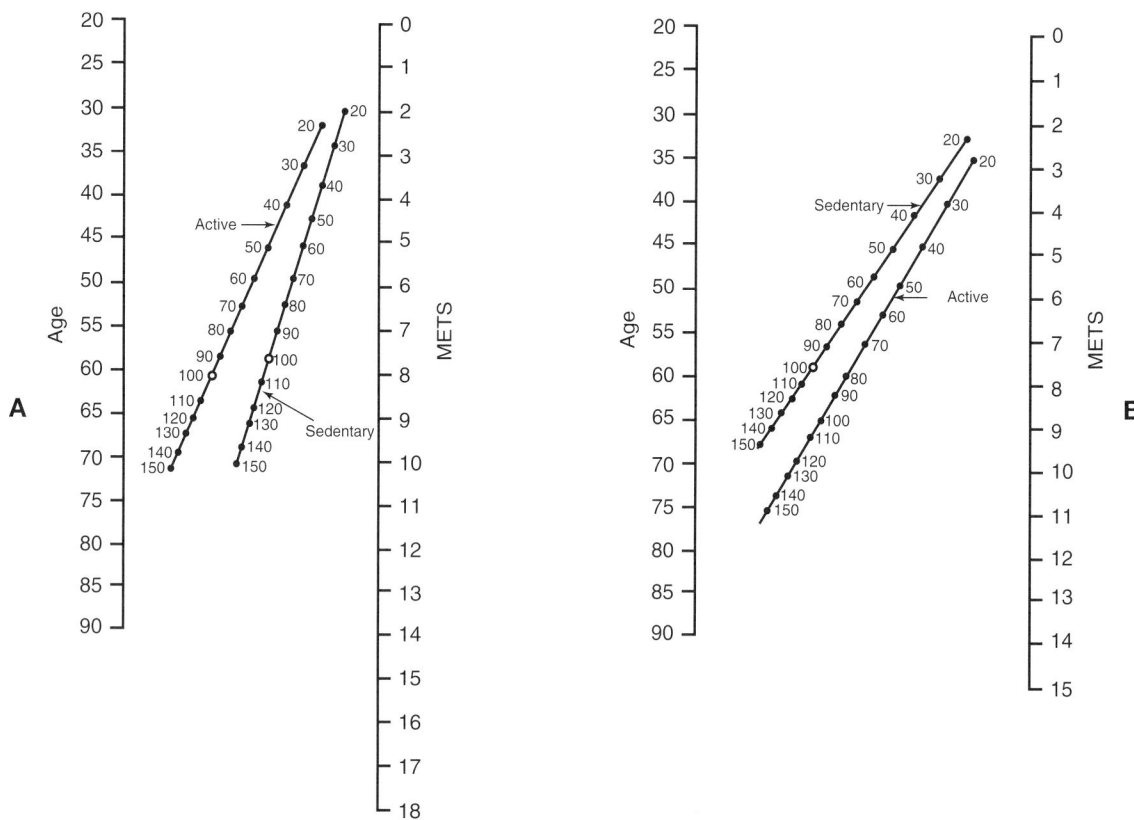

Fig. 92-17
Nomograms of percent normal exercise capacity. **A,** Percent of normal in healthy men. **B,** Percent of normal in referred men. (Redrawn from Kenney WL, editor: *ACSM's guidelines for exercise testing and prescription,* ed 5, Baltimore, 1995, Williams & Wilkins.)

TABLE 92-7
Maximal Oxygen Uptake ($Vo_{2\ max}$) from Bruce Protocol Using Treadmill Time, Female
$2.95 \times (min) + 3.74 = ml/kg/min$

TM	Vo_2	TM	Vo_2	TM	Vo_2
3.0	12.59	7.1	24.68	11.2	36.78
3.1	12.88	7.2	24.98	11.3	37.07
3.2	13.18	7.3	25.27	11.4	37.37
3.3	13.47	7.4	25.57	11.5	37.66
3.4	13.77	7.5	25.86	11.6	37.96
3.5	14.06	7.6	26.16	11.7	38.25
3.6	14.36	7.7	26.45	11.8	38.55
3.7	14.65	7.8	26.75	11.9	38.84
3.8	14.95	7.9	27.04	12.0	39.14
3.9	15.24	8.0	27.34	12.1	39.43
4.0	15.54	8.1	27.63	12.2	39.73
4.1	15.83	8.2	27.93	12.3	40.02
4.2	16.13	8.3	28.22	12.4	40.32
4.3	16.42	8.4	28.52	12.5	40.61
4.4	16.72	8.5	28.81	12.6	40.91
4.5	17.01	8.6	29.11	12.7	41.20
4.6	17.31	8.7	29.40	12.8	41.50
4.7	17.60	8.8	29.70	12.9	41.79
4.8	17.90	8.9	29.99	13.0	42.09
4.9	18.19	9.0	30.29	13.1	42.38
5.0	18.49	9.1	30.58	13.2	42.68
5.1	18.78	9.2	30.88	13.3	42.97
5.2	19.08	9.3	31.17	13.4	43.27
5.3	19.37	9.4	31.47	13.5	43.56
5.4	19.67	9.5	31.76	13.6	43.86
5.5	19.96	9.6	32.06	13.7	44.15
5.6	20.26	9.7	32.35	13.8	44.45
5.7	20.55	9.8	32.65	13.9	44.74
5.8	20.85	9.9	32.94	14.0	45.04
5.9	21.14	10.0	33.24	14.1	45.34
6.0	21.44	10.1	33.53	14.2	45.63
6.1	21.73	10.2	33.83	14.3	45.93
6.2	22.03	10.3	34.12	14.4	46.22
6.3	22.32	10.4	34.42	14.5	46.52
6.4	22.62	10.5	34.71	14.6	46.81
6.5	22.91	10.6	35.01	14.7	47.11
6.6	23.21	10.7	35.30	14.8	47.40
6.7	23.50	10.8	35.60	14.9	47.70
6.8	23.80	10.9	35.89	15.0	47.99
6.9	24.09	11.0	36.19	15.1	48.29
7.0	24.39	11.1	36.48	15.2	48.58

From Health Services Center, Kimberly-Clark Corporation, Neenah, Wisc.
Note: 1 MET = 3.5 ml/kg/min.

TABLE 92-8
Maximal Oxygen Uptake ($Vo_{2\ max}$) from Bruce Protocol Using Treadmill Time, Male
$2.94 \times (min) + 7.65 = ml/kg/min$

TM	Vo_2	TM	Vo_2	TM	Vo_2
3.0	16.47	7.4	29.40	11.8	42.34
3.1	16.76	7.5	29.70	11.9	42.63
3.2	17.06	7.6	29.99	12.0	42.93
3.3	17.35	7.7	30.28	12.1	43.22
3.4	17.64	7.8	30.58	12.2	43.51
3.5	17.94	7.9	30.87	12.3	43.81
3.6	18.18	8.0	31.17	12.4	44.10
3.7	18.52	8.1	31.46	12.5	44.40
3.8	18.82	8.2	31.75	12.6	44.69
3.9	19.11	8.3	32.05	12.7	44.98
4.0	19.41	8.4	32.34	12.8	45.28
4.1	19.70	8.5	32.64	12.9	45.57
4.2	19.99	8.6	32.93	13.0	45.87
4.3	20.29	8.7	33.22	13.1	46.16
4.4	20.58	8.8	33.52	13.2	46.45
4.5	20.88	8.9	33.81	13.3	46.75
4.6	21.17	9.0	34.11	13.4	47.04
4.7	21.46	9.1	34.40	13.5	47.34
4.8	21.76	9.2	34.69	13.6	47.63
4.9	22.05	9.3	34.99	13.7	47.92
5.0	22.35	9.4	35.28	13.8	48.22
5.1	22.64	9.5	35.58	13.9	48.51
5.2	22.93	9.6	35.87	14.0	48.81
5.3	23.23	9.7	36.16	14.1	49.10
5.4	23.52	9.8	36.46	14.2	49.40
5.5	23.82	9.9	36.75	14.3	49.69
5.6	24.11	10.0	37.05	14.4	49.98
5.7	24.40	10.1	37.34	14.5	50.28
5.8	24.70	10.2	37.63	14.6	50.57
5.9	24.99	10.3	37.93	14.7	50.87
6.0	25.29	10.4	38.22	14.8	51.16
6.1	25.58	10.5	38.52	14.9	51.46
6.2	25.87	10.6	38.81	15.0	51.75
6.3	26.17	10.7	39.10	15.1	52.05
6.4	26.46	10.8	39.40	15.2	52.34
6.5	26.76	10.9	39.69	15.3	52.63
6.6	27.05	11.0	39.99	15.4	52.93
6.7	27.34	11.1	40.28	15.5	53.22
6.8	27.64	11.2	40.57	15.6	53.52
6.9	27.93	11.3	40.87	15.7	53.81
7.0	28.23	11.4	41.16	15.8	54.10
7.1	28.52	11.5	41.46	15.9	54.40
7.2	28.81	11.6	41.75	16.0	54.69
7.3	29.11	11.7	42.04	16.1	54.98

From Health Services Center, Kimberly-Clark Corporation, Neenah, Wisc.
Note: 1 MET = 3.5 ml/kg/min.

TABLE 92-9

Cardiorespiratory Fitness Classification*
Maximal oxygen uptake (ml/kg/min)

Age (years)	Low	Fair	Average	Good	High
Women					
20-29	<24	24-30	31-37	38-48	49+
30-39	<20	20-27	28-33	34-44	45+
40-49	<17	17-23	24-30	31-41	42+
50-59	<15	15-20	21-27	28-37	38+
60-69	<13	13-17	18-23	24-34	35+
Men					
20-29	<25	25-33	34-42	43-52	53+
30-39	<23	23-30	31-38	39-48	49+
40-49	<20	20-26	27-35	36-44	45+
50-59	<18	18-24	25-33	34-42	43+
60-69	<16	16-22	23-30	31-40	41+

From American Heart Association: *Exercise testing and training of apparently healthy individuals: a handbook for physicians,* Dallas, 1972, American Heart Association.
*Data from Preventive Medicine Center, Palo Alto, Calif., and from a survey of published sources.

CAD, a hypertensive response to exercise is considered abnormal and may indicate poorly treated hypertension or evidence of CAD.

- *BP and heart rate in diabetics.* Diabetes can cause an elevated resting heart rate; BP and heart rate responses are frequently blunted in diabetics.
- *Symptoms.* Substernal chest pain in males being tested on a treadmill, even without ECG changes, is 90% predictive of CAD.
- *Lack of symptoms.* Painless ST-segment depression (i.e., silent ischemia) is common in diabetics.

DETERMINING PROGNOSIS

Normal ECG Response (Negative Test or Prognosis Is Excellent)

- Absence of any change in the ST-segment at maximal or near MHR
- Junctional or J-point depression with rapidly rising ST-segment slope
- Development of isolated T-wave inversion without ST-segment displacement
- Ventricular ectopic beats occurring infrequently, especially those occurring at heart rates exceeding 130 bpm and not associated with any evidence of ischemia
- Appearance of poorly controlled atrial arrhythmias without cardiovascular compromise
- Development of RBBB with exercise

Uninterpretable or Incomplete Exercise Test Results

- Failure to attain at least 85% of the age-predicted MHR, with absence of ischemic changes in a well-motivated patient. (β-blockers are a common cause of this.)

Note: In the geriatric or sedentary population, it is safe to exercise to a heart rate of 100, regardless of age, without testing. In those anticipated to have very poor exercise capacity, if they are not in urgent need of a cardiovascular intervention, it may be reasonable to help them increase their exercise capacity before undergoing an exercise test. This may be achieved with a walking program for several weeks or even months, four or five times a week, with a target heart rate of 100. In this manner it may be possible to avoid some uninterpretable or incomplete tests.

In addition, for uninterpretable tests through mildly positive tests, additional studies may be desirable as opposed to following serial exercise testing. This should be determined on an individual basis, frequently with cardiology consultation. In most of these instances, a radionuclide study or echocardiogram combined with the exercise test may provide additional information and increased sensitivity and accuracy. For patients suspected to be low risk and unable to complete the study because of deconditioning, it may be safe to start the patient on a low-risk exercise program and repeat the study in 6 months.

Positive and Abnormal Studies

To obtain prognosis data for abnormalities of heart rate or blood pressure, see "VI. Other Parameters Followed" in the prior section. Otherwise prognosis is poor for patients unable to achieve 5 METs or for patients demonstrating a positive study at less than 5 METs. For those patients in whom an intervention is appropriate or if the clinician is unsure of the diagnosis, prognosis, or management, a cardiologist should be consulted.

For those patients with a positive study and able to achieve 5 METs, a heart rate of 120, and an RPP of more than 25,000, a nomogram is available for determining prognosis, counseling, and follow-up. As opposed to other similar nomograms available, women (although not many) were included in the studies resulting in the nomogram in Fig. 92-18. This nomogram can be used when counseling women.

Most large coronary artery bypass surgery centers have known or published complication rates. The AHA's website (www.americanheart.org) also has excellent data for predicting complications from coronary artery bypass surgery. Using the nomogram (Fig. 92-18), patients can evaluate their annual risk of a cardiovascular event with medical management versus a surgical intervention. These are very powerful tools for what is usually a very important decision for patients to make.

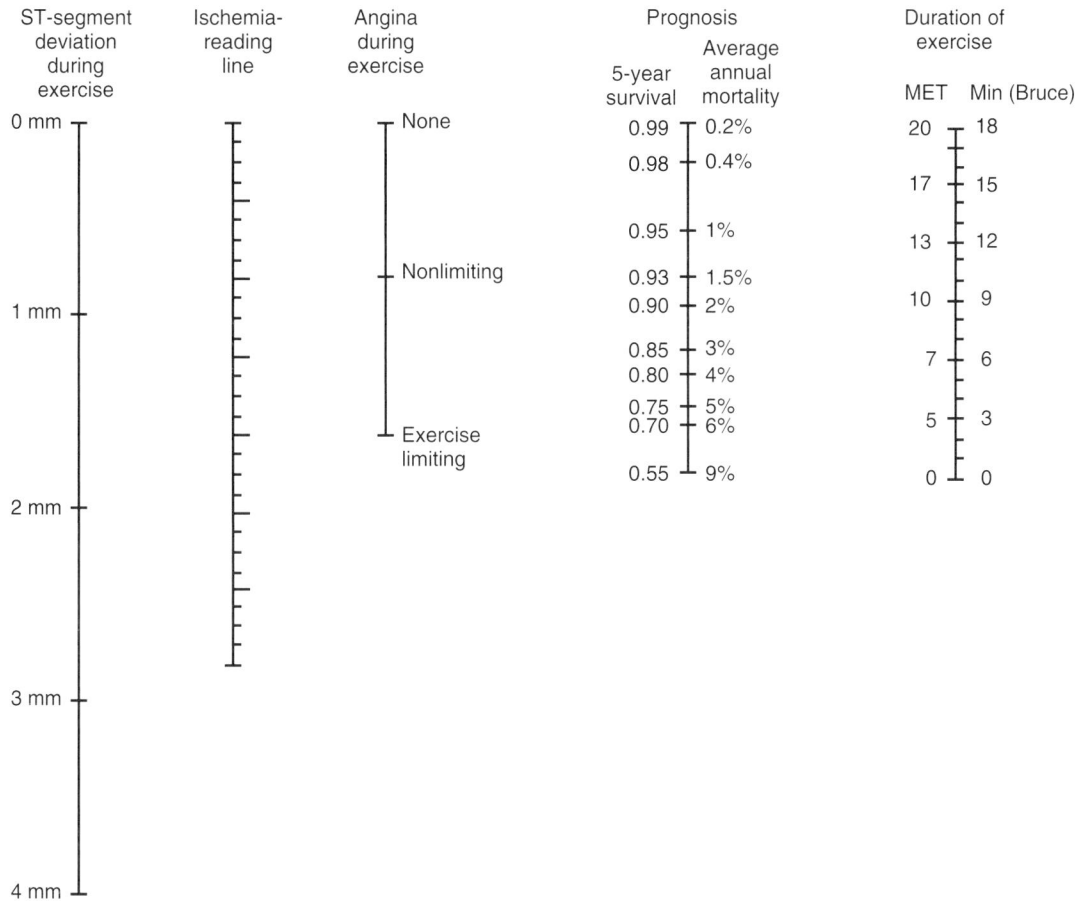

Fig. 92-18
Nomogram for Duke University Prognostic Score. (Redrawn from Mark DB, Shaw L, Harrell FE, et al: *N Engl J Med* 325:850, 1991.)

Based on several studies, for patients with CAD and able to achieve 10 METs, which is basically the level of exertion necessary to complete approximately 9 minutes of a Bruce protocol, medical management is prudent. It is also very unlikely that these patients have significant disease if they achieve a RPP of 25,000 or greater.

One study revealed that for those individuals with known three-vessel CAD and yet able to complete 15 minutes of a Bruce protocol there was a 5-year survival rate of 100%.

Negative Studies

It is important to inform patients that there is no noninvasive study that can completely exclude CAD. Thus, even after a negative study, if they experience a change in the nature or severity of their symptoms, they should discuss them with the clinician.

On the other hand, patients can be reassured that if they achieve an HR of 160 (regardless of age) and achieve 13 METS (basically equivalent to completing 12

minutes on the Bruce protocol), even with ECG evidence of ischemia, they have a very good 4- to 5-year prognosis. They basically have less than a 1% per year risk of a cardiac event for that time span. The same is true if they achieve an RPP over 35,000; they are extremely unlikely to have significant CAD. Even for positive studies, periodic evaluation with a retest in 6 to 12 months may be the most aggressive management needed.

If patients are unable to achieve these endpoints, it may indicate either inadequate effort by the patient or the presence of CAD. For a strong clinical suspicion of disease, additional testing, imaging, or angiography should be considered.

COMPLICATIONS

- Hypotension
- Congestive heart failure exacerbation
- Severe cardiac arrhythmia
- Cardiac arrest

- Acute MI
- Acute CNS event, such as syncope or stroke
- Death

Note: The overall safety of exercise testing has been confirmed with multiple studies. For patients being tested on a treadmill, the mortality rate is approximately 1 in 10,000. The hospital admission rate related to arrhythmia, prolonged chest pain, or MI is approximately 4 in 10,000. However, it should be noted that these numbers include patients with known CAD, perhaps even taking antiarrhythmics. A much smaller risk can be maintained if patients are selected carefully, which is what must be done for office testing.

POSTPROCEDURE PATIENT EDUCATION

Patients should be informed that exercise testing, just like any other noninvasive study for diagnosing CAD, is not 100% accurate. Individuals with a change in symptoms or symptoms of chest discomfort, palpitations, or any other symptoms that could be caused by CAD, should be evaluated by their clinician regardless of the result of the exercise test.

In patients with CAD or a high probability of CAD, counseling should be directed at modifying risk factors. Exercise prescriptions should be given and discussed.

Giving an Aerobic Exercise Prescription

- Exercise capacity or endurance is increased by performing regular (i.e., three episodes per week) aerobic exercise. A fourth day further increases endurance, but after the fourth day per week, the improvement reaches a plateau. While additional episodes of exercise per week may not increase exercise capacity, they may assist with weight loss.
- Aerobic exercise can be performed 3 days in a row to maintain fitness; however, the risk of an injury increases without adequate rest between exercise episodes. It is therefore recommended that individuals exercise, at an aerobic level, every other day. Participating in a less intense walking program on intervening days may also assist with weight loss.
- Aerobic exercise involves raising the heart rate to a specified point (60% to 80% of MHR) and maintaining that level of exercise for 15 to 45 minutes per session. Three 10-minute episodes in the same day accomplish the same effect.
- After testing, a safe aerobic training range is at a heart rate of 60% to 80% of MHR. This range is called the *target heart rate*. A PES of 5 to 7 can also be used in most patients (see step 11 under Technique).
- Patients should avoid dehydration and weather extremes and should warm up and cool down after each episode.

- A repeat exercise test can evaluate the improvement after implementation of an aerobic exercise program. After introduction of an exercise program, it takes approximately 12 weeks of regular exercise to achieve a new level of exercise capacity.
- To avoid boredom, it is recommended that an exercise prescription include more than one kind of aerobic exercise (e.g., swimming, biking, race walking, jogging, aerobic dance).
- An exercise prescription should include a target heart range or level of PES, duration of exercise sessions, frequency of sessions, and types of exercises that can be used to achieve the goals of cardiovascular conditioning (aerobic). The AHA recommends that a prescription include a minimum of three sessions of exercise per week for 30 minutes per session. For new exercise prescriptions, the rate of progression needs to be explained.
- Competitive athletes want to use their training program to raise their anaerobic threshold (i.e., level of exercise at which they can no longer oxygenate all tissues). Anaerobic thresholds are now best measured with expired gas analysis exercise testing.

SUPPLIERS

Note: Most manufacturers in the following list also sell defibrillators. Purchasing these as part of a package is often cost-effective.

Mortara
7865 N. 86th Street
Milwaukee, WI 53224
Phone: 1-800-231-7437
Website: www.mortara.com

Quinton Instrument Co.
3303 Monte Villa Parkway
Bothell, WA 98021
Phone: 1-888-784-6866
Website: www.quinton.com

Space Labs Burdick
500 Burdick Parkway
Deerfield, WI 53531
Phone: 1-800-777-1777
Website: www.burdick.com

Welch Allyn Schiller
4341 State Street Road
P.O. Box 220
Skaneateles Falls, NY
Phone: 1-800-535-6663
Website: www.welchallyn.com

Expired Gas Analysis or Cardiopulmonary Exercise Testing

Medical Graphics
350 Oak Grove Parkway
St. Paul, MN 55127
Phone: 1-800-950-5597
Website: www.medgraph.com

Emergency/ACLS Medication Kits

Banyan International Corp.
P.O. Box 1779
Abilene, TX 79604-1779
Phone: 1-800-782-8548
Website: www.statkit.com

ADDITIONAL RESOURCES

• See the sample patient consent form titled "Cardiac Exercise Testing" on page 1851 of Appendix G.

CPT/BILLING CODES

93000 Electrocardiogram, routine ECG with at least 12 leads; with interpretation and report
93005 Tracing only, without interpretation and report
93010 Interpretation and report only
93015 Cardiovascular stress testing using maximal or submaximal treadmill or bicycle exercise, continuous ECG monitoring, and/or pharmacologic stress; with physician supervision, with interpretation and report
93016 Physician supervision only, without interpretation and report
93017 Tracing only, without interpretation and report
93018 Interpretation and report only

ICD-9-CM DIAGNOSTIC CODES

412   Old MI (healed or no symptoms)
413.9   Other and unspecified angina pectoris
414.01 Coronary atherosclerosis, of native coronary artery
414.02 Coronary atherosclerosis, of autologous vein bypass graft
414.04 Coronary atherosclerosis, of artery bypass graft
414.05 Coronary atherosclerosis, of unspecified type of bypass graft
414.8   Chronic coronary insufficiency
427.69 Ventricular premature beats, contractions, or systoles

485.1   Palpitation
486.51 Precordial pain

BIBLIOGRAPHY

ACC/AHA clinical competence statement on stress testing: a report of the American College of Cardiology/American Heart Association/American College of Physicians—American Society of Internal Medicine Task Force on Clinical Competence, *Circulation* 102:1726, 2000. Available at circ.ahajournals.org/content/vol102/issue14. Accessed June 13, 2002.

ACC/AHA guidelines for exercise testing: executive summary: a report of the American College of Cardiology/American Heart Association Task Force on Practice Guidelines (Committee on Exercise Testing), *Circulation* 96:345, 1997. Available at circ.ahajournals.org/cgi/content/full/96/1/345. Accessed June 13, 2002.

AHA Scientific Statement: Exercise standards for testing and training: a statement for healthcare professionals from the American Heart Association, *Circulation* 104:1694, 2001.

Consensus development conference on the diagnosis of coronary heart disease in people with diabetes, *Diabetes Care* 21(9):1551, 1998.

Diabetes mellitus and exercise, *Diabetes Care* 22(suppl 1):S49, 1999.

Evans CH: Exercise testing, *Prim Care Clin Off Pract* 28(1), 2001.

Evans CH, Karunaratne HB: Exercise stress testing for the family physician, I & II, *Am Fam Physician* 45:121, 1992.

Fowler GC, Evans CH, Altman MA: Exercise testing, *Prim Care* 24(2):375, 1997.

Froelicher VF: *Exercise and the heart*, ed 3, St Louis, 1993, Mosby.

Froelicher VF, Quaglietti S: *Handbook of exercise testing*, Boston, 1996, Little, Brown.

Mattera JA, Arain SA, Sinusas AJ, et al: Exercise testing with myocardial perfusion imaging in patients with normal baseline electrocardiograms: cost savings with a stepwise diagnostic strategy, *J Nucl Cardiol* 5(5):498, 1998.

Nishime EO, Cole CR, Blackstone EH, et al: Heart rate recovery and treadmill exercise score as predictors of mortality in patients referred for exercise ECG, *JAMA* 284(11):1392, 2000.

Pratt CM, Francis MJ, Divine GW, Young JB: Exercise testing in women with chest pain: are there additional exercise characteristics that predict true positive test results? *Chest* 95(1):139, 1989.

Stein RA, Chaitman BR, Balady GJ, et al: Safety and utility of exercise testing in emergency room chest pain centers: an advisory from the Committee on Exercise, Rehabilitation and Prevention, Council on Clinical Cardiology, American Heart Association, *Circulation* 102:1463, 2000.

Vivekananthan K, Lavie CJ, Milani RV: Stress testing, *Atlas Office Proc* 3(3):377, 2000.

CHAPTER 93

Swan-Ganz (Pulmonary Artery) Catheterization

Len Scarpinato

The use of the balloon-flotation, flow-directed pulmonary artery (PA) thermodilution (Swan-Ganz) catheter perhaps best symbolizes modern care of the critically ill patient. Yet, in the more than 40 years since its introduction, no large, randomized, double-blind sham-controlled study has ever shown that the PA catheter reduces morbidity or mortality. As a result, when recent observational studies indicated increased morbidity and mortality, most clinicians were quite surprised. It also resulted in several intense reviews of the literature. There was even consideration of a moratorium on PA catheters in both the United States and Europe. Increased costs related to the use of PA catheters has also been under scrutiny.

Reviewing the literature, one will find only a few very small studies (Boyd et al, 1993; Shoemaker et al, 1988) demonstrating improved outcomes with the use of a PA catheter in high-risk surgical patients. Likewise, only sporadic, small studies (Mimoz et al, 1994) on critically ill ICU patients have demonstrated an advantage for patients using a Swan-Ganz catheter. Despite minimal evidence supporting a benefit and some evidence indicating otherwise, the U.S. Food and Drug Administration did not call for a ban following their review. Instead, they called for improved collaborative educational programs. They recommended that these be focused on when to use, how to insert, and how to maintain PA catheters, as well as how to obtain and interpret the data from PA catheters. PA catheters should only be used for solid indications and in centers where adequately trained support staff are available.

There has also been a call for additional studies; however, the money to support large randomized trials would probably be better spent on developing newer, less invasive technologies than on studying what has become a mainstay for most ICUs.

Despite the fact that the PA catheter has occasionally been maligned in the literature and abused in practice, there are particular times during the care of critically ill patients that the use of a PA catheter is unquestioned. Although urine output, blood pressure, central venous pressure (CVP), and the physical examination are all very useful parameters for monitoring critically ill patients, in certain situations there is no substitute for the PA catheter.

This chapter was written for the primary care clinician preparing to insert a PA catheter, and thus it deals only with those applications that are not controversial. Almost all PA catheters are capable of measuring cardiac output; therefore, primary care clinicians using PA catheters should be capable of obtaining this result. However, there are also "special function PA catheters," such as those that can monitor continuous cardiac output or continuous mixed venous oxygen saturation (S_vO_2) (oximetric Swan). Additional specialized catheters provide a port or built-in electrode for pacing, provide four lumens, or provide right ventricular function data. These catheters are beyond the scope of this chapter.

Although many clinicians are proficient with similar procedures and may have crossover skills, beginners should first observe PA catheter placement several times. Attempts to place the first few catheters should be supervised by a trained, skilled, and experienced clinician. After the clinician gains mastery of the skill of insertion, further study and use of the catheter should increase his or her skills, interest, knowledge, and abilities in the maintenance of a PA catheter as well as with obtaining data. Attending courses devoted to the technology will further enhance proficiency, especially for the subtle applications.

INDICATIONS

Diagnostic Indications

- Evaluation of valvular lesions
- Evaluation of chronic congestive heart failure (CHF)
- Evaluation of left ventricular function
- Suspected right ventricular dysfunction or infarction
- Suspected pulmonary arterial hypertension
- Suspected pulmonary embolism
- Oxygen transport assessment

Note: Contrary to the beliefs of many housestaff members, hypotension alone is not an indication for PA catheter placement; however, hypotension with no response to an adequate fluid bolus may be an indication. This exemplifies the primary use of the PA catheter: to obtain more data for making decisions when the patient's parameters are mixed or confusing.

Differential Diagnostic Indications

- Pulmonary edema (cardiogenic versus noncardiogenic)
- Shock (cardiogenic versus noncardiogenic)
- Low cardiac output syndrome
- Ventricular septal defect versus pericardial tamponade versus acute mitral regurgitation (especially if more than one of these is present)
- Electromechanical dissociation

Monitoring Indications

- Titration of drug or other intervention in a highly unstable patient (e.g., vasodilators, inotropes, and pacemakers)
- CHF or cardiac ischemia
- Hemodynamically unstable patient unresponsive to conventional therapy
- Myocardial infarction
- Postinfarction angina
- Cardiac tamponade
- Cor pulmonale or chronic obstructive pulmonary disease (COPD) in a patient with both cardiac and pulmonary disorders
- Right-sided heart failure resulting from severe obstructive lung disease, adult respiratory distress syndrome (ARDS), or pulmonary embolism
- Sepsis
- Optimization of conditions for a high-risk, perioperative patient
- Fluid management in certain complex situations (e.g., shock, postoperative state, ARDS, acute renal failure)

Therapeutic Indications

- Pacing
- Aspiration of air emboli during seated neurosurgery

CONTRAINDICATIONS

Contraindications are the same as those for central venous catheterization (see Chapter 81, Central Venous Catheter Insertion), plus the following relative contraindications:
- Prosthetic right heart valve
- Cardiac-paced patient (temporary, internal, or permanent)*
- Severe hypotension

- Known pulmonary hypertension
- Highly unstable arrhythmias (especially ventricular)
- Highly unstable respiratory status
- Lack of nursing staff trained in use of PA catheters
- Lack of a compatible pressure-monitoring apparatus

Note: If the underlying relative contraindication can be altered, catheterization may be worth the risk.

EQUIPMENT

- Central venous access (see Chapter 81, Central Venous Catheter Insertion)
- Radiopaque PA catheter (7 French for adults, 5 French for pediatric use; see Fig. 93-1) with syringe for balloon inflation.

Note: Standard thermodilation catheters are triple lumen catheters: distal lumen at tip for measuring pulmonary artery pressure (PAP), pulmonary artery occlusion pressures, and for blood sampling; proximal lumen for injecting a thermal bolus 30 cm proximal to tip; third lumen for inflating the balloon. Most contain a wire that runs the entire length of the catheter and terminates in a thermistor bead, approximately 4 cm from the catheter tip. (Heparin-coated catheters have been produced to decrease the risk of thrombosis, and chlorhexidine- and silver sulfadiazine–impregnated catheters may decrease the risk of infection. These may become more popular as more data become available.)

- Pressure transducer and monitor
- High-pressure tubing, connectors, and two three-way stopcocks (Fig. 93-2)
- Heparinized saline flush system
- Sterile gowns, drapes, gloves, masks, and goggles
- Guidewire
- Suture
- Fully stocked code cart and defibrillator nearby

PREPROCEDURE PATIENT PREPARATION

Because PA catheterization is usually an emergency procedure, written informed consent cannot always be obtained. However, explain the indications, risks, benefits, and any possible alternatives to the patient and the family, if possible. The implied consent should then

---

*Left bundle branch block (LBBB) was previously a contraindication because of the high occurrence rate of natural or induced right bundle branch block (RBBB) during passage of a PA catheter. This could cause complete heart block (i.e., RBBB + LBBB = complete heart block). A chronic indwelling catheter may also increase the risk of RBBB. Evidence suggests that the risk of complete bundle branch block is low; however, it may be prudent to use fluoroscopy when placing a PA catheter in a patient with an LBBB. A transvenous or transcutaneous pacer or a PA catheter with pacing capabilities should be available.

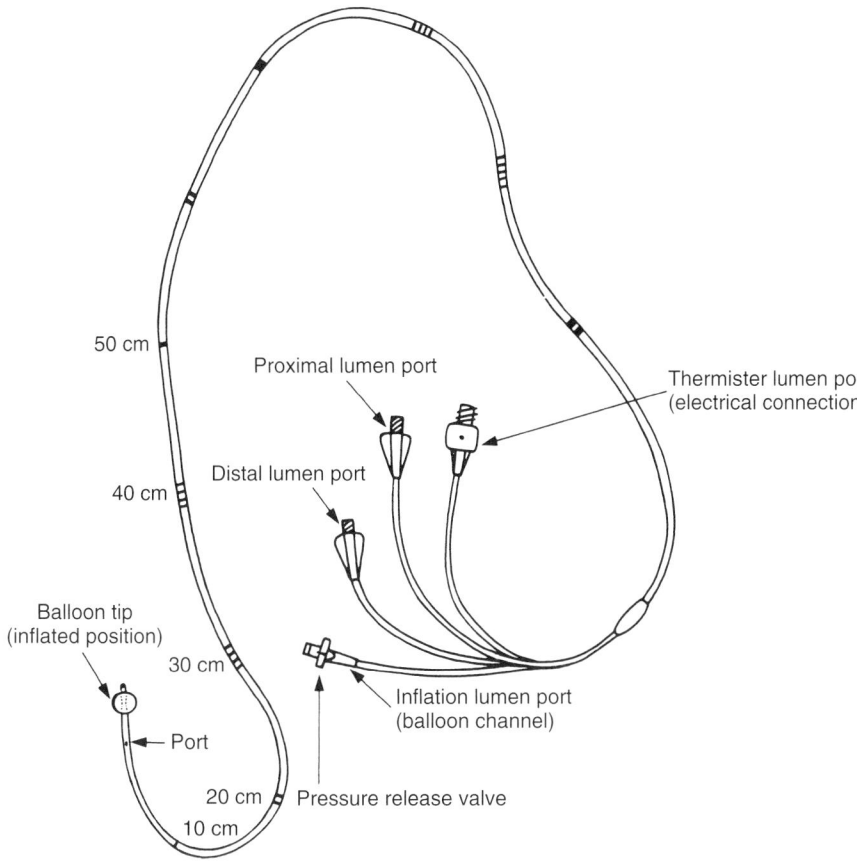

50 cm

Proximal lumen port

Thermister lumen port
(electrical connection)

Fig. 93-1
Balloon-tipped thermodilution catheter.

Distal lumen port

40 cm

Balloon tip
(inflated position)

30 cm

Port

Inflation lumen port
(balloon channel)

20 cm

Pressure release valve

10 cm

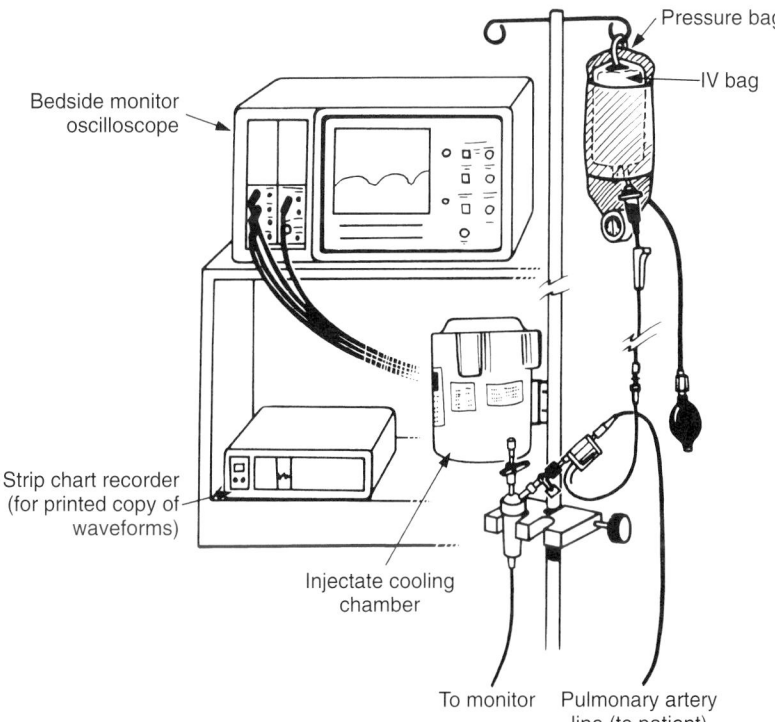

Pressure bag

IV bag

Bedside monitor
oscilloscope

Fig. 93-2
Pulmonary artery catheter set-up.

Strip chart recorder
(for printed copy of
waveforms)

Injectate cooling
chamber

To monitor   Pulmonary artery
line (to patient)

be documented. If time allows, the patient should sign for informed consent. Venous access may be established by the procedure outlined in Chapter 81, Central Venous Catheter Insertion. As delineated in Chapter 94, Temporary Pacing, catheterization of the right internal jugular vein provides the most direct access to the right atrium and ventricle, but its use may restrict patient mobility. The broad curve of the left subclavian vein may make it more difficult to traverse than the right. The most common central access used for PA catheterization is the right subclavian, which is the approach used in this chapter.

A venous cutdown into a median basilic vein in the right antecubital fossa is another option for access. To minimize the risk of pulmonary hemorrhage, this site may actually be the preferred site for patients who have undergone intravenous thrombolysis. This site also avoids the risk of pneumothorax. However, this approach usually takes more time and results in the patient having to restrict their arm motion, both during and after the procedure. If using this site, the clinician must also be familiar and comfortable with the process because it changes the technique of insertion. This site is also further from the central circulation; therefore all of the distances noted as landmarks in this chapter (i.e., when pressure waveforms should change) must be adjusted.

TECHNIQUE

Before Insertion and General Guidelines

- If the patient is on a ventilator, the ventilatory settings and alarms should be checked. The endotracheal tube should be secured and suctioned.
- Before the heart undergoes invasive monitoring or an area of the heart is traversed for any reason, record a baseline ECG.
- Since this procedure may induce arrhythmias, an additional, separate intravenous access site should be available.
- To prevent the loss of a guidewire in a patient, *never* let go of the guidewire during catheter manipulation.
- Observe strict sterile technique. Scrub after donning hair cover, goggles or eye protection, mask, and gown; wear sterile gloves and maintain sterile technique throughout the procedure. Drape as large of an area as possible, including the majority of the patient and the bed. Follow universal blood and body fluid precautions.

Conversion to a Sheath or an Introducer

If the venous catheter in place is not large enough to accept the PA catheter, it must be converted. Use an

8 French sheath for a 7 French PA catheter, or a 6 French sheath for a 5 French catheter.

1. Insert a guidewire of sufficient length through the existing venous access line.
2. Leaving the guidewire in place, remove the catheter over the guidewire.
3. Advance the dilator from the kit over the guidewire to enlarge the lumen.
4. Leaving the guidewire in place, remove the dilator.
5. Place the obturator in the sheath and pass them over the guidewire and into the patient's central circulation.
6. Remove the guidewire and the obturator, and cap the sheath with the special cap that allows for PA catheter placement.

Insertion of the Pulmonary Artery Catheter

1. Have an assistant set up, check, calibrate, and zero the electrical equipment. He or she should also level the transducer.
2. Remove the PA catheter from its sterile packaging. If used, thread the protective shield over the distal end of the catheter (distal to the clinician or the end that will remain inserted). Make sure that the docking mechanism is facing the correct direction. It should be able to be connected to the sheath that was inserted earlier. Flush the catheter by injecting sterile heparinized saline into the two open ports of the catheter. Make sure that both ports are patent. Saline is used because it conducts pressure gradations better than air.
3. Next, test the balloon before insertion. Attach the smaller syringe to the balloon port and fill the balloon with air. Usually a built-in safety mechanism prevents overdistention of the balloon. Place the balloon under sterile water or saline to check for bubbles, which indicates a leak. A leaking catheter should be replaced. If possible, test the thermistor by connecting the catheter connector cable to the cardiac output computer. It should read "ambient temperature"; if an indicator for thermistor continuity exists, it should be positive. Deflate the balloon.
4. Hand the proximal end of the catheter to the assistant. Three-way stopcocks should be attached to both the right atrial (proximal) and PA (distal) lumens. Have the assistant connect the catheter to the pressure tubing after internally flushing it with sterile saline.
5. Mark the patient's lateral mid-chest with an indelible ink spot so that the equipment can be lined up horizontally; this spot is considered the zero point. Record this height and the height of the bed mattress from the floor. The strict recording of heights is necessary, because a change in height of 1 inch

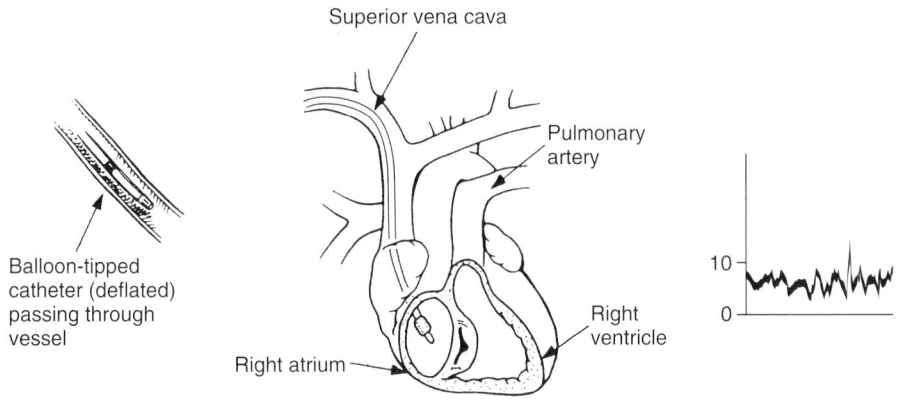

Fig. 93-3
Balloon-tipped catheter passing through vessel to the 10- to 15-cm mark. If passed through internal jugular or subclavian vein, it enters right atrium at 15- to 20-cm mark. Note pressure.

corresponds to a 1.8 mm Hg change in monitored pressure.

Note: Passage of the catheter through the PA can take as little as 10 to 20 seconds. However, there are no prizes for the most rapid passage, and more than likely, it will take longer than 20 seconds, especially with abnormal blood flow. Abnormal blood flow may be caused by valve abnormalities (tricuspid or pulmonic, stenosis or insufficiency), cardiac dysfunction, and pulmonic disease with increased right ventricular pressure. If the catheter is not passed in a short length of time, it may soften (as it is supposed to do when exposed to body heat) and become more difficult to advance. Therefore the catheter should usually be passed from the right atrium to the wedge position in 20 to 30 seconds.

6. ECG monitoring should be continuous throughout the procedure. Pass the deflated balloon-tipped catheter through the sheath to the 10- or 15-cm mark; it is marked in 10-cm increments.

7. Watch the waveform monitor for a characteristic central venous tracing or a right atrial tracing. The normal range of pressure for the right atrium should be from 0 to 10 mm Hg, and the monitor should show respiratory variation. Record these pressures (Fig. 93-3). Three positive deflections can be seen if the scale is enlarged enough on the monitor: the a, c, and v waves.

8. Verify that the appropriate scale was picked on the monitor. If the patient is asked to cough, there should be an abrupt increase in the pressure tracing correlating with the abrupt increase in intrathoracic pressure.

9. Using the syringe provided with the kit, inflate the balloon with air to the recommended full volume as indicated on the package or the syringe (0.8 to 1.5 ml of air). To avoid vessel damage, never advance

the catheter beyond this point without an inflated balloon, unless using fluoroscopy.

Note: The author uses 1.5 ml of carbon dioxide for patients with intracardiac shunts to prevent left-sided air emboli.

The provided syringe is designed to prevent the entry of undesired air. As long as it is not overdistended, the balloon will typically provide a buffer around the distal hard tip of the catheter. Avoid overfilling the balloon! It can burst with dire consequences, especially if already inserted or if bursting goes unrecognized. Never force air into a PA catheter (Fig. 93-4).

10. Pass the catheter to the 30- or 40-cm mark in a quick but not too rapid fashion. While passing the catheter, watch the pressure monitor for the characteristic right ventricular tracing. This tracing looks like a large square root sign without a dicrotic notch. A dramatic rise in the systolic pressure should occur during this manipulation, but there should be no change in the diastolic pressure (Fig. 93-5, *A*). Record the right ventricular pressures. Also watch the ECG tracing for any ectopy at this stage.

11. Once in the right ventricle, without delay, pass the catheter rapidly to the 40- to 50-cm mark, into the PA. The PA gives a peculiarly shaped tracing, like a triangle with a dicrotic notch on the downhill distal side of the triangle (Fig. 93-5, *B*). Record the pressures. Normal PA pressures are 15 to 25 mm Hg systolic, 8 to 16 mm Hg diastolic, with a mean of 10 to 20 mm Hg. Diastolic pressures are higher in the PA than in the right ventricle.

12. Once in the PA, continue passing the catheter at a much slower pace, watching for the characteristic

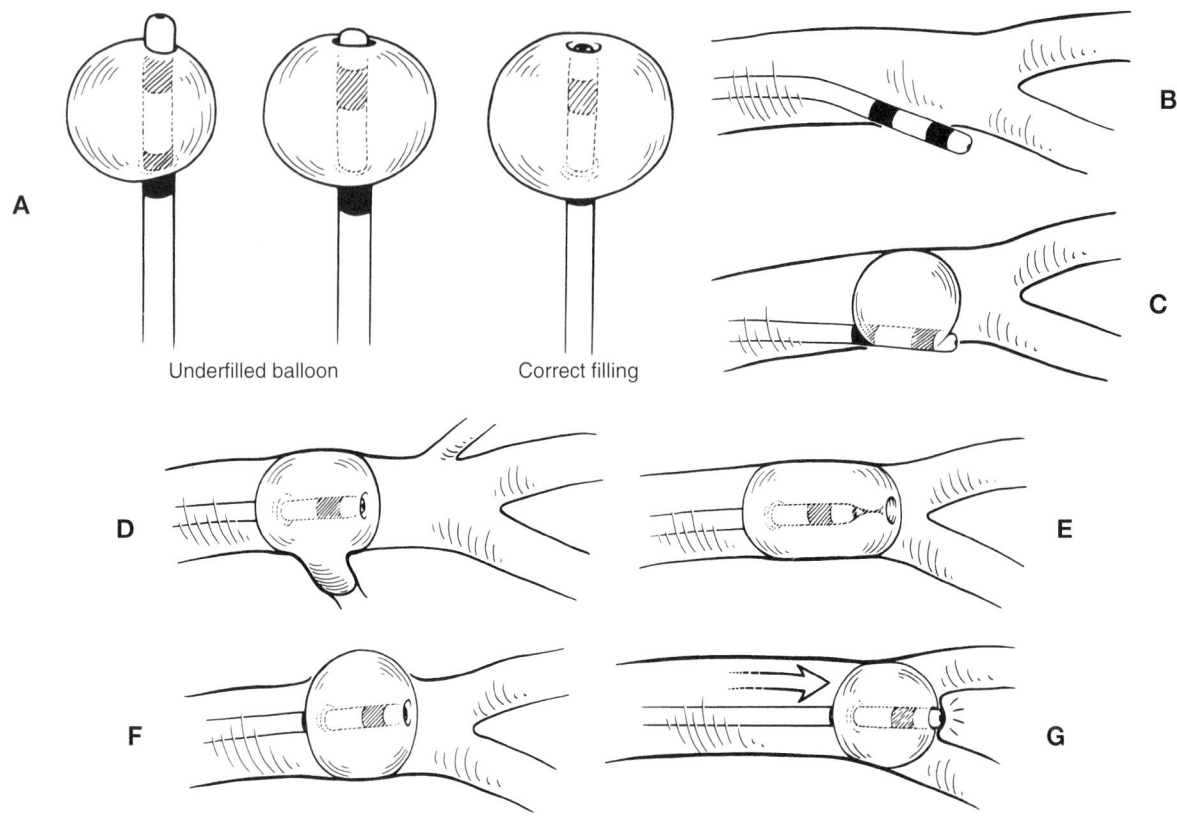

Fig. 93-4
Correct filling of the balloon and possible complications. **A,** Underfilled and correct filling. **B,** Tip perforates wall of vessel when balloon is not inflated. **C,** Eccentric balloon (inaccurate wedge) and risk of wall rupture. **D,** Overfilled balloon inadvertently distending down side of vessel. **E,** Inaccurate and overdistention of balloon can cause catheter tip occlusion. **F,** Over wedge (see the "Troubleshooting" section). **G,** Underinflated catheter with protruding tip.

pulmonary capillary wedge pressure (PCWP) tracing at about the 50-cm mark on the catheter (Fig. 93-5, *C*). With PCWP tracings, the characteristic PA pattern is lost, and the mean pressure decreases. This is the somewhat magical place where the vessel has become occluded and the catheter starts reading the "back pressure" from the other side of the heart. The catheter no longer reads PA pressures; rather, it reads pressure reflected back from the left atrium through the capillaries. If the mitral valve is not obstructed and is open during ventricular diastole, when finally wedged the PCWP approximates the left ventricular diastolic pressure (Fig. 93-5, *D*). In the absence of elevated end-expiratory pressures or obstruction of the pulmonary veins, PCWP approximates left atrial mean pressure to within 2 mm Hg. If desired, using the Starling pressure-volume relationships, left ventricular end diastolic volume can even be estimated.

13. Once the balloon is wedged, allow it to passively deflate, and watch for the phasic PA tracing. Do not aspirate to deflate the balloon; active deflation may cause rupture.

14. Inflate the balloon again and allow it to deflate to observe the two different tracings. If the syringe and balloon were designed to hold 1.5 ml, this should be the amount required to wedge the catheter safely. If any less accomplishes it, the catheter's location is too distal; withdraw it until 1.5 ml wedges it. If 1.5 ml does not wedge the balloon, pass the catheter further. Although the PCWP is called an occlusion pressure, the inflated balloon actually floats distally and *then* occludes the vessel. The vessel is not occluded from inflation at a fixed location.

15. Extend the catheter protective shield, if used, and attach it to the sheath with the docking mechanism.

16. Secure the entire assembly with suture and adequate tape. Apply a sterile dressing.

17. Order a chest x-ray (portable anteroposterior and a cross-table lateral) and auscultate the patient's chest bilaterally to exclude a pneumothorax.

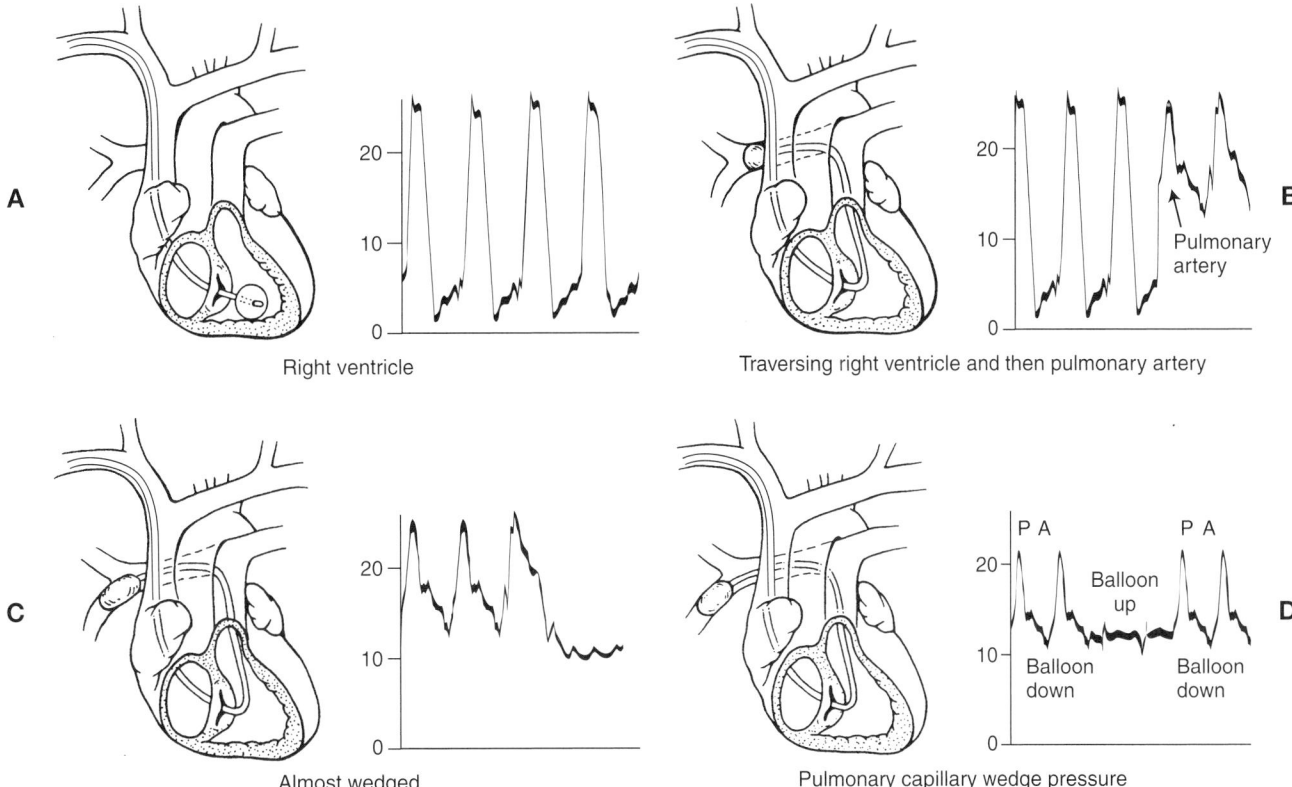

Fig. 93-5
Tracings recorded through the catheter as it traverses the ventricle and artery and is wedged, **A,** the right ventricle, **B,** the pulmonary artery, **C** almost wedged, and finally, **D,** the wedged position.

18. Begin infusion of necessary fluids and/or medications.

19. If the patient was moved, ask the assistant to rezero the equipment.

20. Document the procedure in the chart, including the tracings, and record end expiratory values. Additional documented values should include the PA pressure, the PCWP, and the cardiac output (performed by the assistant and not detailed here).

Confirmation of Proper Placement

1. Obstruction is excluded by the ability to flush the catheter before inflating the balloon.

2. When the balloon is inflated, the typical PA tracing disappears. It reappears promptly after the balloon deflates.

3. PCWP is lower than or equal to pulmonary artery diastolic pressure.

4. Oxygen levels or oxygen saturation of blood drawn from the occlusive position is greater than or equal to that of systemic arterial blood.

TROUBLESHOOTING

If salvos of premature ventricular contractions occur during catheter advancement, deflate the balloon and withdraw the catheter into the right atrium. It may be coiled in the right ventricle. If further attempts to pass it are unsuccessful, administer an intravenous bolus of lidocaine (75 to 100 mg) and attempt passage under fluoroscopy.

If a PA or PCWP tracing cannot be obtained, keep the balloon deflated, pull the catheter back to 12 cm, and try inserting again. Consider inserting the catheter using a clockwise twisting action. If this fails, try counterclockwise reinsertion. Having the patient take some deep breaths may also help pass the catheter.

Some clinicians recommend injecting cold, sterile saline solution to enhance passage; this may stiffen the catheter, which may have softened because of the warmth of the body. Occasionally, a guidewire and fluoroscopy are necessary to advance the catheter. Repositioning the patient may help.

In patients with a very low ejection fraction, an inotrope may have to be administered to facilitate passage. Difficulty may also occur in patients with tricuspid regurgitation or pulmonary hypertension. Again, having the patient take deep breaths may facilitate passage in all of these situations.

For a normal-sized adult, from the subclavian or internal jugular site, insertion beyond 50 cm (or 15 cm after entering the right ventricle) predisposes the catheter to coiling, which can lead to knotting.

When a catheter's location is too distal in the vessel, a tracing called an overwedge may be seen. This is likely to occur when the balloon is not filled with enough air. After allowing the balloon to deflate, withdraw the catheter and attempt to wedge it again, this time with the balloon fully inflated to its correct volume (Fig. 93-4). Persistent underinflation of the balloon when wedging can damage the pulmonary vessels or the endocardium, and may cause arrhythmias, especially if the catheter tip is exposed (Fig. 93-4, *A* and *G*). There are several mechanisms that are proposed to even cause rupture of the PA, an unlikely but possible consequence related to either overinflation or underinflation of the balloon (Fig. 93-4, *B, C, F,* and *G*).

When air is present in the catheter, damping can occur, which has an effect that is opposite to that of overwedging. It characteristically appears like a regular tracing, but the variations are damped. Air bubbles should be removed from the connecting tubes by aspirating and flushing the catheter. If blood cannot be aspirated, yet the catheter flushes easily, suspect a ball-valve thrombus at the catheter tip. Inject 5000 U of heparin into the lumen; allow 15 to 30 minutes for it to take effect. Initiate a continuous drip of heparin (not to exceed 20,000 U for 24 hours). If still unsuccessful, withdraw the catheter gradually 5 cm at a time, watching for waveforms.

Lesions obstructing the mitral valve, such as mitral stenosis, can interfere with the accuracy of the PCWP as an estimate of left ventricular diastolic pressure. Respirations can also cause significant variations in the pressure readings for the PA catheter. Make calibrated strip-chart recordings for all measurements derived from the catheter and then measure again at end expiration (Fig. 93-6). PCWPs may not reflect left atrial pressures for patients on a ventilator and requiring positive end-expiratory pressure (PEEP).

COMPLICATIONS

- Same possible complications as for central venous catheterization (see Chapter 81, Central Venous Catheter Insertion), *plus* the following

During Pulmonary Artery Catheter Placement

- Pulmonary infarction: can result from leaving the balloon inflated too long.

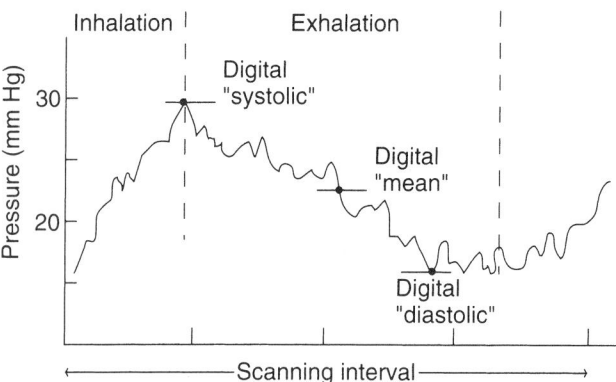

Fig. 93-6
Respiratory variation of the pulmonary artery catheter tracing. (From Wiedemann HP, Matthay MA, Matthay RA: *Chest* 85:537, 1984.)

- Atrial and ventricular ectopy or conduction changes: advancement into the PA may decrease ectopy. However, withdrawal of the catheter may be necessary. If ectopy or an unstable rhythm persists, medical treatment or electrical conversion may be necessary.
- Knotting of the catheter, inside or outside of the heart (more likely with smaller-bore catheters [e.g., 5 French]) and injury to intracardiac structures: with insertion, partially inflating the balloon while in the subclavian vein or superior vena cavae may minimize the risk of knotting. On the contrary, to avoid injury to either the pulmonic valve or tricuspid valve, do not withdraw the catheter with the balloon inflated. Also, if resistance is noted with attempted withdrawal, obtain a chest x-ray to exclude the possibility of knotting or entanglement in the heart. The catheter may become looped around the papillary muscle of the tricuspid valve so that removal is impossible.
- Malposition: can cause many problems including vessel wall puncture and possible insertion into various organs, such as the trachea, the subclavian artery, or even the endotracheal tube.
- Cardiac perforation and tamponade.

With Continued Presence of the Pulmonary Artery Catheter in the Central Circulation

- Pulmonary infarction: leaving the balloon inflated too long or downstream displacement of the deflated balloon can block an artery and cause infarction. Infarction can also result from thrombosis.
- Pulmonary hemorrhage: more common in presence of PA hypertension, possibly associated with the higher pressures forcing the tip through the vessel wall. Cautiously obtain PCWP in patients with pulmonary hypertension. Hemorrhage can also result from pulmonary infarction.

- Mural (or elsewhere) thrombus formation: thrombosis may develop anywhere throughout the course of the catheter. It can occlude any of the veins through which the catheter has passed (or elsewhere).
- Balloon rupture or catheter fracture: if balloon rupture is suspected, aspirate into the syringe the same gas volume as used for inflation, disconnect the syringe, and leave the stopcock open to vent the balloon. Remove the catheter immediately to prevent latex fragments from embolizing.
- Endocarditis: aseptic vegetations are found in approximately 30% of autopsied patients who have had a PA catheter. Both aseptic and septic vegetations may be more common in burn patients.
- Sepsis: frequent manipulations of the catheter, as well as leaving the catheter in place more than 3 days, increases the risk of positive blood cultures. After 24 to 48 hours, if the catheter has become partially withdrawn, advancing the catheter may introduce bacteria from the skin insertion site or the catheter itself. No data show that aseptic protective sleeves prevent this from happening.
- Hemoptysis: can be caused by flushing the catheter when it is in the wedged position.
- Embolism (air or thrombotic)
- Pulmonary artery rupture
- Pseudoaneurysm
- Inaccurate diagnosis because of malfunctioning or malpositioned catheter

POSTPROCEDURE CATHETER CARE

- Flush the catheter with heparinized saline every 30 minutes.
- Inflate the balloon only when measuring the PCWP. To avoid pulmonary infarction, only leave it inflated for a *maximum* of 60 seconds. To exclude the possibility of catheter obstruction before inflation, flush the catheter each time before inflating the balloon. If the catheter is occluded, there is no point in inflating the balloon.
- For obstruction, attempt to reposition the catheter. If a thrombus is suspected, see the previous page and use the same technique as used for clearing a ball-valve thrombus.
- Adjust the position of the catheter as necessary. Otherwise, the catheter may soften and migrate to a more distal site, predisposing to distal or branch-vessel occlusion. If the PAP tracing shows a loss in phasicity and begins to resemble the PCWP tracing (without balloon inflation), withdraw the catheter until the typical phasic PA tracing reappears. Always deflate when withdrawing to avoid damage to intracardiac structures.

- Remove, inspect, and replace the sterile dressing daily.
- Obtain daily chest radiographs to check for catheter migration and to exclude pulmonary infarction.

SUPPLIERS

Arrow International
2400 Bernville Road
Reading, PA 19605
Phone: 1-800-233-3187
Website: www.arrowintl.com

Edwards Lifesciences Corp (formerly a division of Baxter)
One Edwards Way
Irvine, CA 92614
Phone: 1-800-424-3278
Website: www.edwards.com

Weslee Medical, Inc.
1187 Wilmette Avenue, PMB 149
Wilmette, IL 60091-2719
Phone: 1-877-624-6681
Website: www.wesleemedical.com

CPT/BILLING CODE

93503   Insertion and placement of flow-directed catheter (e.g., Swan-Ganz) for monitoring purposes

ICD-9-CM DIAGNOSTIC CODES

401.0   Accelerated or malignant hypertension
410.11   Myocardial infarction, initial episode, anterior wall (can include damage such as ruptured myocardium)
410.91   Myocardial infarction, acute, unspecified, initial episode (can include damage such as ruptured myocardium)
411.1   Angina, unstable
415.0   Cor pulmonale, acute
415.11   Pulmonary embolism or infarct, postoperative
415.19   Pulmonary embolism or infarct, unspecified
416.0   Pulmonary hypertension, chronic primary
416.8   Pulmonary hypertension, chronic secondary
423.9   Pericardial effusion, tamponade heart, or unspecified disease of pericardium
424.0   Mitral valve disorder
424.1   Aortic valve disorder
424.2   Tricuspid valve disorder

424.3	Pulmonic valve disorder
427.1	Paroxysmal ventricular tachycardia
427.5	Cardiac or cardiorespiratory arrest
428.0	Right heart failure, secondary to left
428.0	Heart failure, congestive
428.1	Pulmonary edema (left heart failure)
518.5	Pulmonary insufficiency after trauma and surgery
785.50	Shock, unspecified
785.51	Shock, cardiogenic
785.59	Shock, other (hypovolemic, septic)

ADDITIONAL RESOURCES

• See the sample patient education handout titled "Pulmonary Artery Catheterization" on page 1852 of Appendix G.

BIBLIOGRAPHY

American Heart Association: *Textbook of advanced cardiac life support,* Dallas, 1997, AHA.

Bernard GR, Sopko G, Cerra F, et al: Pulmonary artery catheterization and clinical outcomes: National Heart, Lung, and Blood Institute and Food and Drug Administration Workshop Report Consensus Statement, *JAMA* 283(19): 2568, 2000.

Boyd O, Grounds RM, Bennett ED: A randomised clinical trial of the effect of deliberate perioperative increase of oxygen delivery on mortality in high-risk surgical patients, *JAMA* 270:2699, 1993.

Connors AF Jr, Speroff T, Dawson NV, et al: The effectiveness of right heart catheterization in the initial care of critically ill patients: SUPPORT Investigators, *JAMA* 276:889, 1996.

Hall JB: Use of the pulmonary artery catheter in critically ill patients: was invention the mother of necessity? *JAMA* 283(19):2577, 2000.

Mimoz O, Rauss A, Rekik N, et al: Pulmonary artery catheterization in critically ill patients: a prospective analysis of outcome changes associated with catheter-prompted changes in therapy, *Crit Care Med* 22:573, 1994.

Mueller HS, Chatterjee K, Davis KB, et al: ACC expert consensus document: present use of bedside right heart catheterization in patients with cardiac disease, American College of Cardiology, *J Am Coll Cardiol* 32(3):840, 1998.

Shoemaker WC, Appel PL, Kram HB, et al: Prospective trial of supranormal values of survivors as therapeutic goals in high-risk surgical patients, *Chest* 94:1176, 1988.

WEBSITES

www.asahq.org (American Society of Anesthesiologists: Practice guidelines for pulmonary artery catheterization: a report by the American Society of Anesthesiologists Task Force on Pulmonary Artery Catheterization)

www.manbit.com (Manbit Technologies: PA catheter insertion simulators are available, and the online text describes the procedure.)

www.acc.org (American College of Cardiology: Policy guidelines for cardiac catheterization, pulmonary artery catheterization, and the consensus statement on right heart catheterization)

CHAPTER 94

Temporary Pacing

Len Scarpinato

In rural or underserved healthcare settings, or if first on the scene, primary care clinicians may need to perform temporary cardiac pacing. Various options are available, with the primary purpose being to maintain circulatory stability until either the situation resolves or a permanent pacemaker can be installed. This chapter deals primarily with the intravenous route of emergency ventricular pacing. External (transcutaneous) pacing is also covered briefly. Transesophageal pacing, usually limited to atrial pacing, and transmyocardial transthoracic pacing are beyond the scope of this chapter.

The basic uses for temporary cardiac pacing are as a standby should complete heart block occur and as a way to increase heart rate during periods of symptomatic bradycardia. In addition, overdrive pacing may be used to terminate arrhythmias (e.g., sustained supraventricular or ventricular tachycardia) and atrioventricular sequential pacing used to prevent arrhythmias; however, these are generally performed by cardiologists. "Medicinal" pacing is also available and may be beneficial when used in accordance with advanced cardiac life support (ACLS) guidelines (atropine, isoproterenol, etc.). Overall, the indications for temporary pacing can be divided into therapeutic, prophylactic, and diagnostic categories. For the purposes of this chapter, only therapeutic and prophylactic pacing are covered. It should be noted that national recommendations (American College of Physicians, American College of Cardiology, American Heart Association) have been made for both obtaining and maintaining competence with temporary transvenous pacing.

EXTERNAL (TRANSCUTANEOUS) PACING

Most defibrillators are now capable of performing external transcutaneous pacing. Modern transcutaneous pacing represents a major improvement over the units first developed in the 1950s. Those units frequently inflicted severe chest and back muscle stimulation and discomfort, and they often left burns on the skin. At least one suicide was recorded of a pacer-dependent patient who removed the leads from one of the older units to "end the

pain." In the 1960s, transcutaneous pacing was largely replaced with the newly available transvenous pacing.

Subsequent discoveries have rejuvenated transcutaneous pacing, especially since the 1980s. Researchers have found that increasing the pulse duration from 2 to 20 milliseconds (ms) not only increases the safety of transcutaneous pacing (reducing the risk of ventricular fibrillation), but also reduces the required current. Reduced current means less pain and fewer burns. The development of electrodes with a larger surface area has also decreased the pain and risk of tissue burn. Use of larger electrodes allows for a reduction in the current density, or the amount of current penetrating per square unit of skin. These developments will likely lead to more frequent use of transcutaneous pacing, especially on a standby basis, and a decrease in the overall use of transvenous pacing.

One of the shortfalls of external pacing, even with today's somewhat sophisticated equipment, is the difficulty of achieving capture in about one fifth of patients. Reasons for difficult or ineffective external pacing include: increased intrathoracic air (such as barrel chests or chronic obstructive pulmonary disease), a large pericardial effusion or tamponade, recent thoracic surgery, the size of the patient, and the placement of electrodes. Increased output for capture may be required in these individuals. Another shortfall: It is rare for patients not to complain of some pectoral muscle stimulation. Although most patients rate the discomfort as mild or moderate and easily tolerable, approximately one third of patients rate the pain as severe or intolerable. Therefore, analgesics, narcotics, and/or sedatives should be considered when using the external pacer, especially if the required mean current for capture is 50 milliamperes (mA) or more (a common threshold).

Since the high voltages required for external pacing produce significant muscle twitching, conventional ECG monitors and recorders are useless. To provide decent tracings despite the large pacer spikes and their aftermath, routine ECG monitors must be equipped with an *output adapter*. Fortunately, most external pacer units come equipped with a monitor capable of filtering the spikes. Without an adequate ECG monitor, treatable ventricular fibrillation could be masked by the large pacing spikes with disastrous results. This is one of the grave risks of transcutaneous pacing.

INDICATIONS

- Short-term pacing until transvenous pacing can be initiated or underlying conditions requiring pacing are corrected (e.g., drug overdose or hyperkalemia)
- When medical therapy is not immediately available, or when significant bradyarrhythmias have not responded to medical (e.g., atropine) therapy
- As a standby in conscious patients with hemodynamically stable bradycardia
- As a standby in conscious patients with new Type II second-degree or third-degree heart block in the setting of ischemia or infarction (a preliminary trial of pacing should be performed to ensure that capture is achievable and that the pacing is tolerated by the patient)
- In children with primary bradycardia from congenital defects or following open-heart surgery
- To be considered when fluoroscopy (the preferred technique) is not available for transvenous pacer insertion.

CONTRAINDICATIONS

- Bradycardia in patient with significant hypothermia; as the core temperature drops, the ventricles are more prone to fibrillation that is resistant to defibrillation. In addition, bradycardia may be physiologic in these individuals.
- Bradycardia in children: usually due to hypoxia or hypoventilation, the best intervention is to provide an adequate airway as opposed to pacing (exceptions as mentioned in the "Indications" section above).
- Overdrive pacing: contraindicated in tachyarrhythmias with rates greater than 180 beats per minute (bpm) because that is the maximal rate of most external pacers
- Relative contraindication: bradyasystolic arrest of more than 20 minutes duration because of the well-documented poor resuscitation rates.
- Patient is unable to cooperate.
- Lack of therapeutic benefit because of advanced disease or terminal illness.

EQUIPMENT

- Two 8-cm electrodes.
- Razor or scissors to remove body hair from the area of electrode placement.

- Pacing unit. The best units allow either fixed-rate or demand mode. Most allow a range from 30 to 180 bpm, with current output from 0 to 200 mA. Pulse durations vary from 20 to 40 ms and are not adjustable by the operator. Some pacers shut off when an electrode falls off the chest to protect healthcare providers.
- ECG capable of monitoring during transcutaneous pacing. If not purchased as part of the pacing system, *an output adapter to a separate ECG monitor* is required to "blank" or neutralize the large electrical spikes from the pacer.

TECHNIQUE

1. After clipping or shaving body hair in the area, attach the exposed adhesive surfaces of two large electrode patches to the anterior and posterior chest walls (Fig. 94-1).
2. If time allows, prepare the patient with analgesia such as a narcotic and/or sedation with a benzodiazepine.
3. Turn on the power generator unit. Set the heart rate (e.g., 80 bpm) to demand pacing. Set the current output and sensing thresholds at levels similar to those used for internal pacing; however, remember that larger outputs are necessary. Keep in mind that for demand pacing, external units often do not have sensing thresholds. The final current output setting is usually 1.25 times the initial capture threshold. Pa-

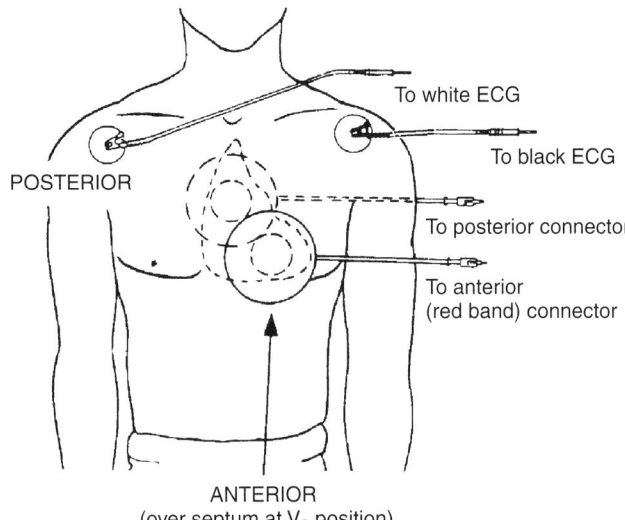

Fig. 94-1
External (transcutaneous) pacing. The anterior electrode is placed to the left of the sternum over the point of maximal impulse. The posterior electrode is placed to the left of the spinal column on the back, directly behind the anterior electrode. (From Dahlberg ST, Benotti JR: Temporary cardiac pacing. In Rippe JM, et al, editors: *Intensive care medicine,* ed 2, Boston, 1991, Little, Brown.)

tients with conditions that cause difficult or ineffective pacing may require higher outputs for capture. At these higher outputs, the resultant muscle twitches may be so serene as to preclude external pacer use.

4. Apply the electrical stimulation to the electrodes. For conscious patients, slowly increase the output (mA) from the minimal setting until capture is achieved. Electrical capture is usually indicated by a widening of the QRS complex and especially by a broad T wave. For asystolic patients, begin at full output (mA) and decrease if capture is achieved.

5. After successful pacing, prophylactic intravenous access (central venous [CV] catheter) through the right internal jugular vein may be helpful in case an internal pacer is needed urgently. Since external pacers have up to a 20% failure rate, having central venous access available minimizes the risk of having to obtain it during a "code" situation.

6. Monitor continuously for capture and potential complications (treatable ventricular fibrillation, burns, etc.). The only sure sign of electrical capture is the presence of a consistent ST segment and T wave after each pacer spike. Palpation of the carotid to confirm a pulse is not helpful because the muscle stimulation and contractions produced by the pacer simulate a carotid pulse.

Note: The increased use of external pacers has surely reduced the number of prophylactic internal pacers placed. However, in nontransient situations, external pacing is always a temporary measure until an internal (probably transvenous, as described below) pacer can be placed.

COMPLICATIONS

- Failure to recognize the presence of underlying treatable ventricular fibrillation
- Failure to recognize that the pacer is not capturing (e.g., prolonged use is often associated with leads becoming dislodged; occasionally prolonged pacing is associated with a change in pacing threshold, requiring increased pacing current)
- Third-degree burns have been reported in children, even when large electrodes were used. The risk of a burn increases if the electrodes are placed improperly or if prolonged pacing is necessary.

INTERNAL (TRANSVENOUS) PACING

INDICATIONS

Therapeutic Indications

- Symptomatic, hemodynamically compromising or life-threatening bradyarrhythmias, including sick sinus syn-

drome (systolic blood pressure <80 mm Hg, change in mental status, angina, pulmonary edema)
- Bradycardia with ventricular escape rhythms, unresponsive to pharmacologic therapy
- Asystole and bradyasystole; not routinely recommended because of poor prognosis, unless performed as early as possible after arrest (e.g., within 20 minutes)

Note: For tachyarrhythmias of less than 150 bpm, neither immediate cardioversion nor an immediate pacer is necessary.

Prophylactic Indications, in Setting of Acute Myocardial Infarction

- Symptomatic sinus node dysfunction
- Second-degree heart block (Mobitz type II)*
- Third-degree heart block*
- Newly acquired right bundle branch block (RBBB), left bundle branch block (LBBB), or alternating bundle branch block or bifascicular block

CONTRAINDICATIONS

Contraindications include those listed in Chapter 81, Central Venous Catheter Insertion, and those listed previously for external pacing. Other contraindications include the following:
- Presence of a prosthetic tricuspid valve
- Depending on access site, planned neck or clavicle surgical procedures
- Distortion of local anatomy or landmarks; for insertion from subclavian, moderate to severe chest wall deformities that distort local anatomy
- Suspected injury to the superior vena cava (e.g., superior vena cava syndrome; in that situation, insertion from below the diaphragm is preferable)
- Bleeding diathesis or anticoagulation therapy (unless emergent pacing is required, antecubital venous cutdown access is preferred)
- Concurrent thrombolysis
- Full-thickness burn, cellulitis, or other infection over the anticipated insertion site
- Pneumothorax or hemothorax on the contralateral side
- Inability to tolerate pneumothorax on ipsilateral side

---

*In patients with an inferior myocardial infarction, relatively asymptomatic second- or third-degree heart block can occur. Pacing in such patients should be reserved for symptoms or the presence of a deteriorating bradycardia. If not paced, patients should be monitored closely with a pacer nearby and on standby. It should have been tested for capture and patient tolerance.

RELATIVE CONTRAINDICATIONS

- Suspected prior injury to the vein intended for insertion.
- Vasculitis that predisposes to sclerosis or thrombosis of the veins.
- Previous long-term catheterization, injection of hyperosmotic or irritant solution, or recently discontinued catheter in the same vein.
- Contraindications specific to *internal jugular vein* access include significant carotid artery disease, distorted cervical anatomy, and recent, unsuccessful contralateral cannulation (to prevent bilateral neck hematomas, which could compromise the patient's airway).
- Subclavian insertion during CPR. (If CPR can be halted briefly, this may be beneficial; jugular access can usually be obtained without stopping CPR. Otherwise peripheral access may be preferable.)
- Children. (Rarely needed; better intervention is to treat the cause [e.g., hypoxia]. If pacing is needed, the internal jugular vein is the best access.)
- Patients receiving ventilatory support with high end–expiratory pressures (e.g., PEEP). If possible, ventilation should be interrupted briefly while attempting to cannulate the vein for access.)
- Patients with morbid obesity, marked cachexia, or severe hypovolemia may be better served by using common femoral or peripheral vein access.
- Severe hypovolemia.

EQUIPMENT

- Bipolar transvenous pacing catheters (Fig. 94-2), 4 to 6 French, may be soft and pliable and made from extruded plastic or firm, relatively nonpliable and made from woven Dacron. Some practitioners prefer soft, flexible, semifloating catheters; however, these are more difficult to maneuver and less stable once positioned. Flow-directed, flexible, balloon-tipped pacing catheters are also available. They are similar to balloon-tipped pulmonary artery catheters, but without an open lumen (Fig. 94-2). Stiffer catheters are usually easier to maneuver than balloon-tipped catheters; however, balloon-tipped catheters are easier to insert without fluoroscopy. There is also always the option of using a balloon-tipped, pacer-equipped pulmonary artery catheter (Swan-Ganz).
- Unipolar electrode catheters are available; however, unipolar catheters must rely on a second, external electrode to be placed on the skin. This electrode is very susceptible to any external electrical interference; therefore bipolar catheters are preferred.
- A flexible J-shaped catheter is available specifically for temporary atrial pacing.
- Pacer pulse generator (Fig. 94-3) with a new battery.
- Extension cable to connect pacer to catheter.
- ECG monitoring capability during insertion. (Availability of fluoroscopy is ideal.)
- Venous insertion site.

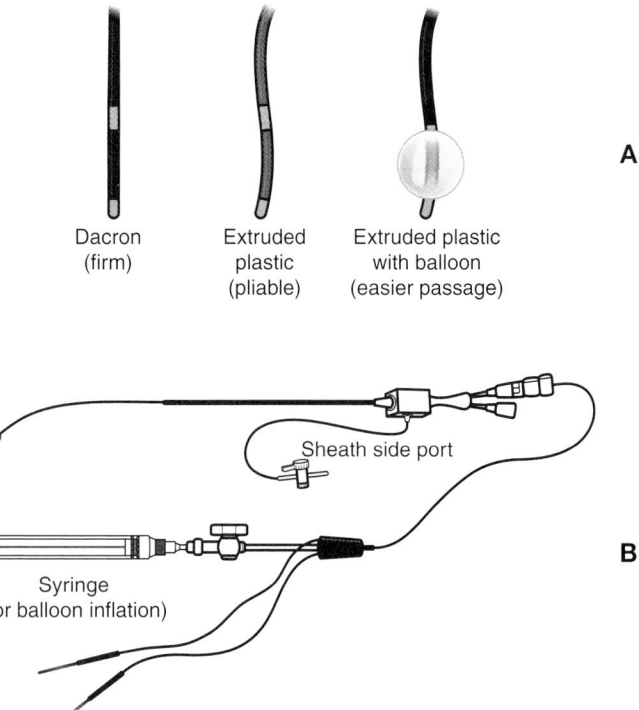

A, Distal tips of transvenous pacers. **B,** Transvenous balloon-tipped temporary pacer.

Dacron (firm)

Extruded plastic (pliable)

Extruded plastic with balloon (easier passage)

Sheath side port

Syringe (for balloon inflation)

Fig. 94-3
A, Distal tips of transvenous pacers. **B,** Transvenous balloon-tipped temporary pacer.

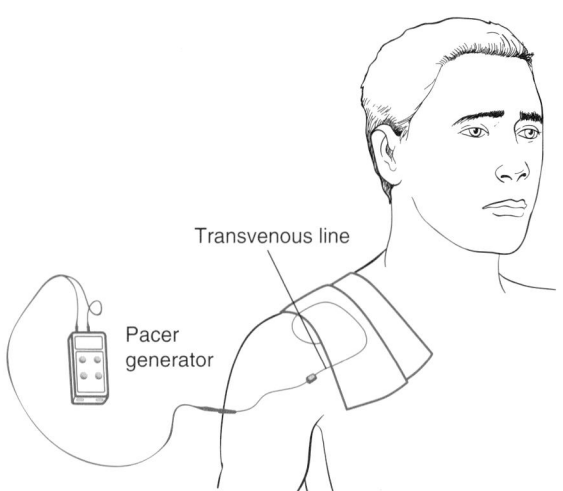

Transvenous line

Pacer generator

Fig. 94-2
Transvenous line and pacer in place.

PREPROCEDURE PATIENT PREPARATION

See Chapter 81, Central Venous Catheter Insertion.

If possible, obtain written informed consent. In many cases, pacing is an emergency procedure and written informed consent cannot be obtained. However, after the patient is stabilized, the situation, risks, and benefits should be explained to the patient and family. Implied consent should be documented. Always outline the complications of either performing or withholding the procedure.

TECHNIQUE

All steps should be performed using aseptic technique and following universal blood and body fluid precautions. Venous access is established by the procedure outlined in Chapter 81, Central Venous Catheter Insertion. Inspect the leads on the pacing catheter for any breaks or manufacturing defects.

Access Route

The most direct route for internal pacemaker insertion is through a CV catheter in the right internal jugular. The right subclavian vein can be used, especially for relatively long-term use, but this route of insertion may be more difficult because of the turns the electrode has to negotiate (Fig. 94-4). The final options include the right common femoral vein or a large peripheral vein.

Catheter Conversion

If necessary, insert a larger catheter into the established venous access site.
1. Place a guidewire down the CV access line.
2. Remove the catheter.
3. Use an obturator over the wire to enlarge the lumen.
4. Pass an introducer with catheter assembly over the guidewire.
5. Remove the introducer.
6. Check for venous return.

Pacer Placement

Fluoroscopy Technique

By far, the best method of temporary pacer placement involves fluoroscopic guidance of the semifloating or balloon-tipped bipolar pacing leads. Many intensive care units and some emergency rooms have beds that will accommodate C-arms for fluoroscopy. If C-arms cannot be accommodated, and if time and clinical conditions

permit, the patient might also be moved to the radiology suite.
1. Pass the catheter to the 10- to 12-cm mark (10-cm segments are marked on the catheter).
2. If the balloon is used, blow it up and advance the catheter; it should move easily into the right atrium (RA).
3. Pass the tip across the tricuspid valve and advance it to the apex of the right ventricle (RV). Ask the patient to take deep breaths or to cough; this will facilitate passage across the valve. Under fluoroscopy, once the radiopaque tip is at the apex, the last 2 to 3 cm of the lead should show minimal or no longitudinal motion if an attempt is made to advance the catheter farther. The remainder of the catheter may have horizontal and longitudinal motion (Fig. 94-5), but not the tip. If a balloon is used, deflate it as soon as it passes across the tricuspid valve and washes to the ventricular wall.

If the catheter tip curls up against the atrial wall,

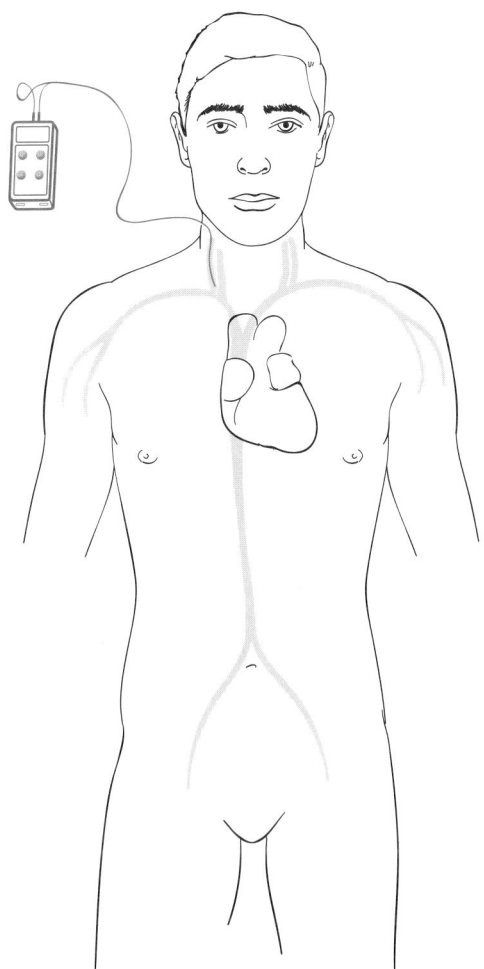

Fig. 94-4
Temporary pacer in right internal jugular vein.

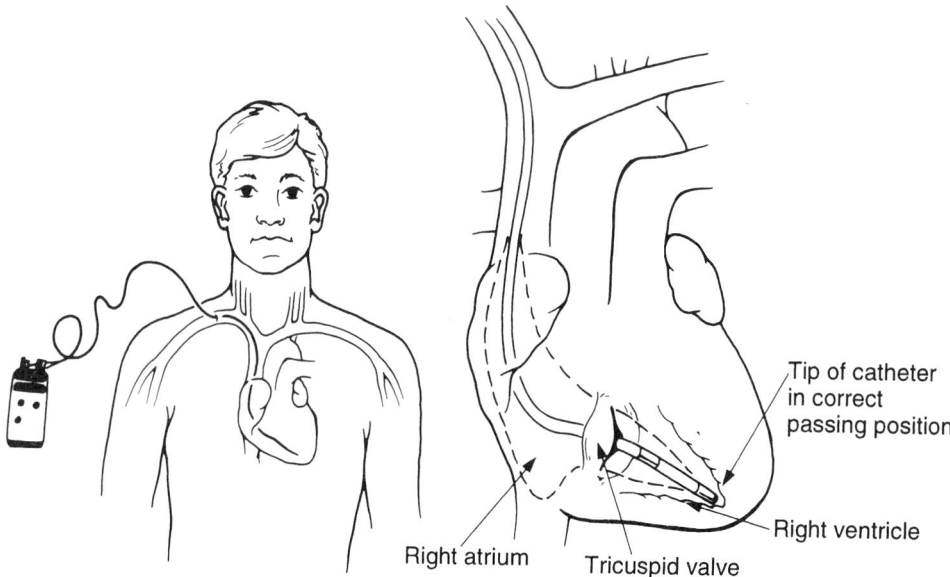

Fig. 94-5
Correct positioning of pacer catheter. When the tip reaches the apex, it quits moving under fluoroscopy.

advance it 1 to 2 cm to create a loop. Next, rotate it clockwise and watch it straighten as it enters the plane of the tricuspid valve.

4. The best final position for the catheter tip is at the apex. Electrodes remaining in the pulmonary outflow tract or along the free wall are less stable and more likely to perforate.
5. If a balloon is used, it must be deflated before withdrawal for repositioning.
6. Coiling the proximal electrode catheter around the insertion site and firmly taping it to the skin prevents inadvertent dislodgement of the distal electrode. Using the extension cable, connect the pacer electrodes to the pacer unit.

Nonfluoroscopy Technique

Initially, the patient is connected to the limb leads of an ECG. A flexible, semiflotation or balloon-tipped catheter can be advanced and positioned much like the pulmonary artery catheter (see Chapter 93, Swan-Ganz Catheterization), except that the distal negative electrode catheter is attached to an ECG machine (usually the V_1 lead, a unipolar lead). The change in the recorded QRS complex allows the practitioner to approximate the tip location (Fig. 94-6). Follow the same passage route: into the RA, across the tricuspid valve, and to the apex of the RV. While the lead is in the atrium, the P wave appears quite large; as it passes the tricuspid valve, the QRS amplitude increases. Once the catheter is correctly placed, a large, elevated ST segment should be seen. If the catheter does not advance across the tricuspid valve,

rotate it clockwise while advancing it 1 cm to flip the tip across the valve.

Emergency Technique

Unfortunately, situations frequently arise requiring placement of a temporary pacer under emergent or extreme conditions, such as during a code with the patient lying in a hospital bed. The catheter may be inserted blindly to about 12 cm, attached to the pacemaker, and turned on. Set the rate higher than the patient's highest heart rate, the amperage (ventricular output current) at the highest setting, and the mode at asynchronous (sensitivity off). A surface or conventional ECG or rhythm strip should be running while the catheter is being passed. Multiple attempts at passage may be necessary. Capture is noted by an obviously paced rhythm seen on the surface ECG. Unfortunately, even experienced clinicians occasionally fail despite multiple attempts, underscoring the benefits of fluoroscopic guidance.

Parameter Settings

Determine the parameters, and record each when it is set. Once the pacer guidewire is in place, the pacer's positive terminal should be attached to the positive lead and negative to negative, much like a car battery.

1. *Rate:* If the patient shows no intrinsic heart rate, set the pacing rate at 70 to 80 bpm to simulate the normal beating heart. If the patient is bradycardic, the same range can be used to raise the blood pressure and

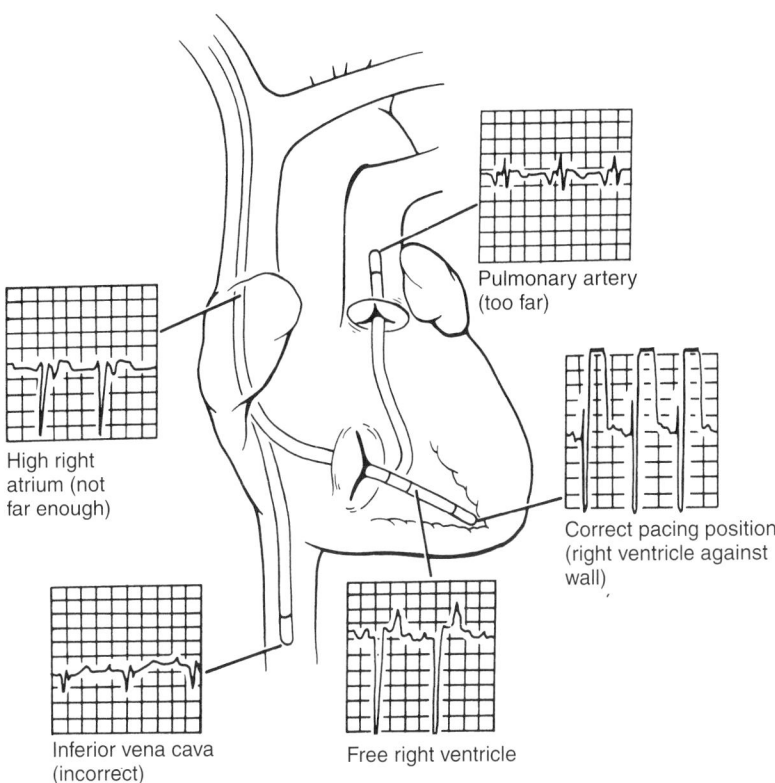

Fig. 94-6
Pattern of recorded electrocardiogram from intracardiac pacemaker electrodes at various locations in the venous circulation.

High right atrium (not far enough)

Pulmonary artery (too far)

Correct pacing position (right ventricle against wall)

Inferior vena cava (incorrect)

Free right ventricle

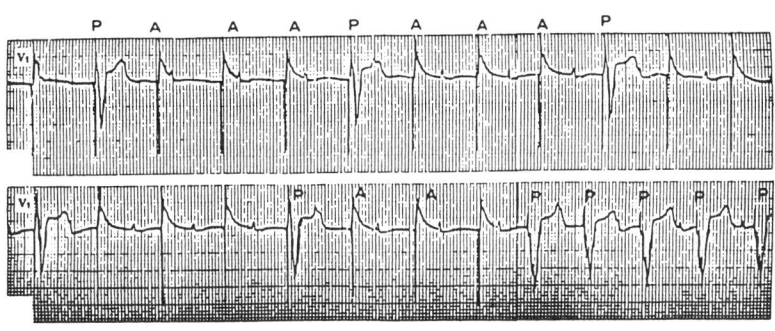

Fig. 94-7
Pacing with intermittent capture. *P,* Indicates paced beats. *A,* Indicates pacer artifact without capture. (From Dahlberg ST, Benotti JR: Temporary cardiac pacing. In Rippe JM, et al, editors: *Intensive care medicine,* ed 2, Boston, 1991, Little, Brown.)

heart rate. Record the rate chosen after setting the machine.

2. *Ventricular output:* The ventricular output is the current generated by the pacer, adjustable from 0.1 to 20 mA. Most situations discussed in this chapter require the maximum output at initiation of pacing, with gradual reduction afterward. After reaching the level of output necessary to capture the ventricle, large spikes followed by bundle branch block (BBB) pattern complexes (wide QRS complexes, ST-segment depression, and T-wave inversion depending on the lead) are seen. The bundle branch pattern occurs because the complex originates in the ventricle. A pulse should also be palpable and should generate a blood pressure. The ventricular output setting can then be reduced gradually, and capture should occur at less than 2 mA. If less than 0.5 mA, the catheter may

have become deeply embedded in the ventricular wall. Be aware that withdrawal may cause perforation. If spikes are seen but no capture occurs, catheter manipulation is indicated. If spikes and BBB pattern are seen with no pulse, the possibility of pulseless electrical activity (electromechanical dissociation [EMD]) must be considered. With EMD the proper ACLS management protocol should be followed.

3. *Stimulation or pacing threshold:* To determine the actual stimulation or pacing threshold, set the rate at 10 to 15 beats per minute above the patient's intrinsic rate (not below 60 beats per minute). Next set the sensitivity between 1.5 and 3 millivolts (mV), and use a ventricular output of about 5 mA. With the pacer turned on, the ECG should show capture (Fig. 94-7). Decrease the milliamperes until the capture of the heart is lost and the patient's heart reverts to its

intrinsic rhythm. The amperage of the ventricular output current at the time that capture is lost is the *stimulation* or *pacing threshold*. Optimally, this should be less than 2 mA, which indicates that the electrode is in adequate contact with the endocardium. In actual use, the output is maintained well above this setting (usually about twice the milliamperes, and some clinicians suggest three to five times this threshold level). If levels of 5 to 6 mA or greater are required (which is common in fibrosis, but is usually a result of poor electrode positioning), attempt to reposition the electrode.

Demand Pacing

If the patient's intrinsic rhythm is inadequate, a sensing threshold must be determined with the sensitivity knob. Occasionally a sensing threshold cannot be determined when the patient has a very slow rhythm.

Sensitivity is the control on the pacer that detects the amplitude of the patient's intrinsic R wave. The most sensitive setting is 1 mV, corresponding to full clockwise rotation of the knob. In the least sensitive setting, called *asynchronous pacing,* the pacer does not care if there is a rhythm, and functions oblivious to the intrinsic rate. The asynchronous setting should be avoided when there is an intrinsic rhythm because the additional electric spikes generated by the pacer can cause an arrhythmia.

To determine sensing threshold, first set the rate about 10 bpm below the patient's intrinsic rate. Gradually adjust the sensitivity control toward the highest sensitivity or entirely clockwise (to detect even the lowest amplitude waves), which is known as the *full demand* setting. Pacer pulses should no longer be seen because all deflections are sensed and interpreted as QRS complexes. Every intrinsic or artifactual QRS complex should generate a flash of the sense indicator on the pacer. At this level the pacer senses almost all electrical activity, and its firing is thus prevented. In fact, T waves, occasionally P waves (if the catheter is close to the atrium), chest muscle contractions, or even artifact may prevent the pacer from firing. This is called the *oversensing point.* This full demand setting is obviously too high for the pacer to function. The sensitivity control should then be turned counterclockwise, changing or decreasing the sensitivity toward higher numbers until ECG pacer spikes are seen that correspond to the patient's intrinsic rhythm, regardless of their capture. This level is the *sensing threshold* of the pacer. The pace indicator light (if the machine has one) should also flash. For *demand pacing* the sensing should be set at a level halfway between the oversensing point and the sensing threshold. This level should be recorded.

Keep in mind that pacers can fail to sense when the sensitivity setting on the pacer is too low, when the lead is malpositioned, or when the intrinsic signal is of poor quality. Once pacing is performing effectively, the length of wire that has been inserted transvenously should be recorded. Secure the electrode catheter to the skin with two sutures at two sites.

Confirmation of Lead Placement

1. A cross-table lateral and anteroposterior chest radiograph should be ordered. Pneumothorax should be ruled out. The tip of the catheter should be at the distal RV, in the apex, with no loops, kinks, or doublings. On the lateral view, the pacer should be to the left of the spine and slightly inferior and anterior, retrosternally.
2. A 12-lead ECG should demonstrate the expected LBBB pattern because of the origination of electrical current in the RV (Fig. 94-8).
3. The pacer pulse generator should be secured to the bed, not the patient, for at least 24 hours. It should be covered to prevent inadvertent trauma to the controls.

While a temporary pacer is in place, a hardwire or telemetry rhythm strip should be recorded frequently and monitored. Patients should be restricted to bed rest for at least 24 hours. Aseptic technique must be maintained when the catheter is handled, and appropriate skin care should be ordered. Sterile dressing changes should follow the intensive care unit's CV line protocol. Unnecessary catheter manipulations should be avoided. Pacemaker function should be checked daily with a 12-lead ECG. A change in the morphology of the paced QRS on the 12-lead may be the first sign of electrode displacement. Daily physical examination for friction rubs (a clue to perforation) or clicking noises (muscle stimulation) must be documented. Pacing threshold should also be determined daily and documented.

Troubleshooting: Failure to Pace

Failure to pace can occur from a variety of reasons, including—but not limited to—a faulty battery, dislodged or malpositioned leads, a loose connection, a damaged or fractured wire, electronic interference, or a faulty pacer. Some cardiac conditions cause very high pacing thresholds or preclude intrinsic pacing: myocardial fibrosis or ischemia, drug toxicity from cardiac agents, myocardial perforation, ventricular refractoriness from a low-grade, unsensed, intrinsic QRS complex.

If the pacer fails to work after it had been functioning previously, several questions should be considered: Has the catheter dislodged? Are the wires loose or disconnected? Are the pacemaker settings correct? Has the battery failed? Is there electrical interference? Has the ventricle been perforated as a result of synchronous diaphragmatic or intracostal muscle contractions?

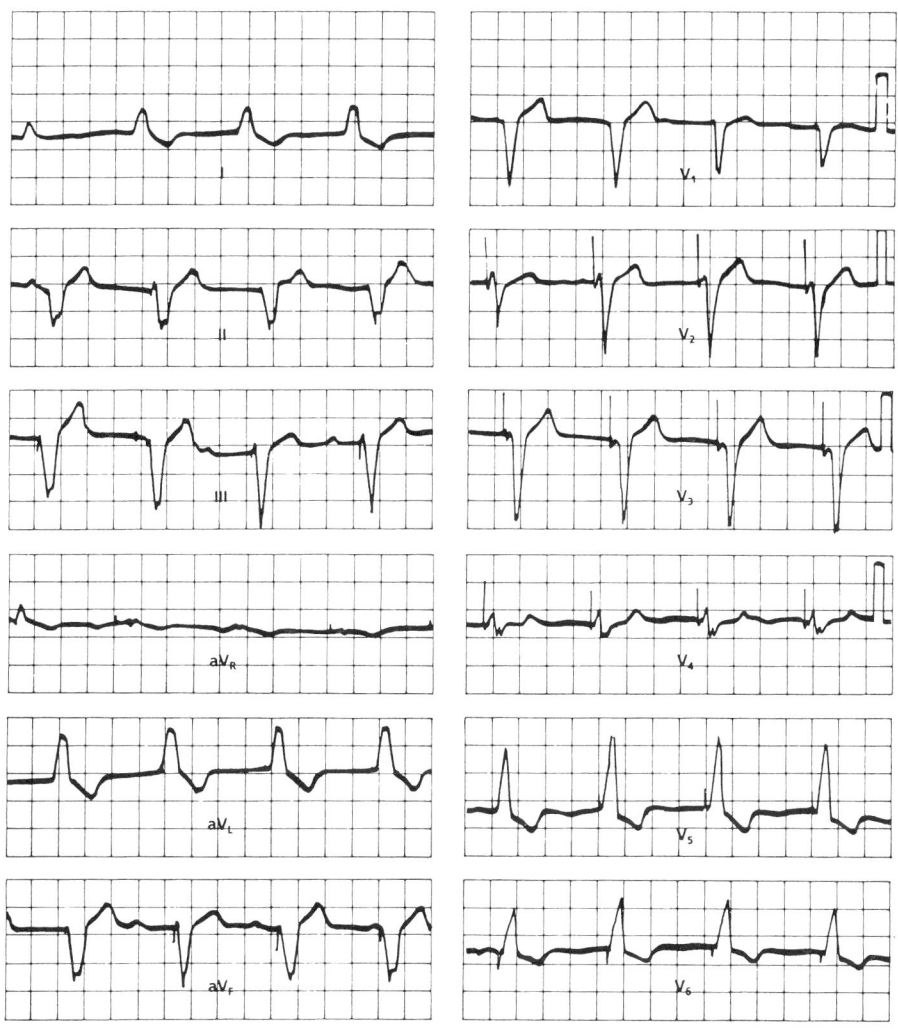

Fig. 94-8
Finished product: 12-lead ECG with pacer in place. (From Morelli RL, Goldschlager N: *J Crit Ill* 2[3]:71, 1987.)

In an emergency situation, consider increasing the stimulation or pacing threshold to regain capture. Occasionally the area in the heart near the electrode has become fibrotic, requiring a higher stimulation. Also, the catheter tip could have become partially dislodged. If the problem is oversensing, that threshold should be reset.

If all else fails, another emergency maneuver is to switch the polarity of the pacer lead connections. Occasionally this technique will regain pacing, although it has not been well documented in the medical literature.

COMPLICATIONS

(Complications include same as those for CV line insertion; see Chapter 81, Central Venous Catheter Insertion.)

Most complications are infrequent and usually minor. Life-threatening complications are rare. Complications are seen more frequently as a result of placing a pacer in an emergency situation, especially with critically ill patients and when the operator is inexperienced.

- Pacing system dysfunction (18% to 43% of cases), including failure to capture or sense the R wave properly. System malfunctions are usually due to problems with connections and lead placement or inappropriate setup of the device.
- Loss of pacing (failure of pacer, lead dislodgement, fracture of pacer wire).
- Pericardial friction rub, endocardial structural damage, myocardial damage, or infarction.
- Arrhythmia.
- Interventricular septum or right ventricular perforation, with or without cardiac tamponade.
- Infection, including bacteremia.
- Arterial or venous injury, including phlebitis and thrombosis (incidence is higher than expected).
- Diaphragmatic stimulation; chest wall stimulation.
- Pulmonary embolism.
- Air embolism.
- Electrical hazards. (Any extraneous currents, even microcurrents, can cause ventricular fibrillation if applied to a pacemaker catheter.)

POSTPROCEDURE PATIENT EDUCATION

See the "Postprocedure Patient Education" section of Chapter 81, Central Venous Catheter Insertion. Also, if a patient will need a permanent pacemaker, see the "Websites" section for patient education.

SUPPLIERS

See suppliers of pulmonary artery (Swan-Ganz) catheters, also:

Biosense Webster
3333 Diamond Canyon Road
Diamond Bar, CA 91765
Phone: 1-800-729-9010
Website: www.biosensewebster.com

Medtronic
710 Medtronic Parkway NE
Minneapolis, MN 55432-5604
Phone: 1-763-514-4000
Website: www.medtronic.com

St. Jude Medical
One Lillehei Plaza
St Paul, MN 55117-9913
Phone: 1-800-328-9634
Website: www.sjm.com

CPT/BILLING CODES

33210	Insertion or replacement of temporary transvenous single chamber cardiac electrode
36489	Placement of central venous catheter, over age 2
92953	Temporary transcutaneous pacing

ICD-9-CM DIAGNOSTIC CODES

410.11	Myocardial infarction, initial episode, anterior wall can include damage such as ruptured myocardium
410.91	Myocardial infarction, acute, unspecified location, initial episode can include damage such as ruptured myocardium
426.0	Atrioventricular block, complete or third-degree heart block
426.2	Left bundle branch hemiblock
426.3	Left bundle branch block, complete
426.4	Right bundle branch block
426.12	Mobitz Type II block
427.89	Sinoatrial node dysfunction
427.89	Sinus bradycardia, persistent, severe
427.89	Sick sinus syndrome
427.5	Cardiac arrest
427.5	Asystole

ADDITIONAL RESOURCES

- See the sample patient education handout titled "Temporary Pacing" on page 1853 of Appendix G.

BIBLIOGRAPHY

American Heart Association: *Textbook of advanced cardiac life support*, Dallas, 1997, American Heart Association.

Dahlberg ST, Mooradd MG: Temporary cardiac pacing. In Irwin RS, Cerra FB, Rippe JM, editors: *Irwin and Rippe's intensive care medicine*, ed 4, Philadelphia, 1999, Lippincott-Raven.

Davis WR: Temporary cardiac pacemakers. In Civetta JM, Taylor RW, Kirby RR, editors: *Critical care*, ed 3, Philadelphia, 1997, Lippincott-Raven.

Francis GC (writing for the Task Force): Clinical competence in insertion of a temporary transvenous ventricular pacemaker: a statement for physicians from the ACP/ACC/AHA Task Force on Clinical Privileges in Cardiology, *Circulation* 89:1913, 1994. Also located at http://216.185.112.5/presenter.jhtml?identifier=1189. (Accessed July 1, 2003.)

Jafri SM, Kruse JA: Temporary transvenous cardiac pacing, *Crit Care Clin* 8(4):713, 1992.

James DM: Temporary pacing techniques: external and transvenous. In James DM, editor: *Field guide to urgent and ambulatory care procedures*, Philadelphia, 2001, Lippincott Williams & Wilkins.

Morelli RL, Goldschlager N: Temporary transvenous pacing, *J Crit Ill* 2(3):71, 1987; 2(4):73, 1987.

WEBSITES

For diagnosis and management of third degree heart block: www.emedicine.com/EMERG/topic235.htm

For information regarding pacemakers, temporary and permanent: www.americanheart.org

For comparison of available permanent pacemakers: www.hrt.org/pacerData/pdp000421r02.html

For patient information from the manufacturers regarding permanent pacemakers: www.guidant.com (Guidant); www.medtronic.com (Medtronic); www.biotronik.com (Biotronic; available in German, English, Italian, and French); www.sjm.com (St. Jude Medical)

CHAPTER 95

Thoracentesis

Terry S. Ruhl

The pleural "space" is a potential space between the visceral pleura, which is adherent to the lung, and the parietal pleura, which is adherent to the chest wall. Normally, it contains only a thin film of lubricating fluid. When this space becomes filled with air or extra fluid, the work of breathing increases. Many diseases produce a pleural effusion, and sampling this fluid may help determine the diagnosis. Other patients may gain relief of symptoms by removal of air or fluid by thoracentesis.

INDICATIONS

- Any pleural effusion of unknown etiology (effusions with an easily explained cause, such as congestive heart failure, may be observed for response to therapy)
- Large symptomatic effusion
- Spontaneous pneumothorax (a minimally symptomatic spontaneous pneumothorax of less than 20% may be observed)

CONTRAINDICATIONS

- Patient refuses the procedure
- When chest tube placement is more appropriate

CONDITIONS ASSOCIATED WITH INCREASED RISK

- Coagulopathy or patient undergoing anticoagulant therapy
- Inability of patient to cooperate
- Very small effusions (less than 10 mm thick on a lateral decubitus film)
- Removal of large amounts of fluid (more than 1 L)
- Local skin compromise (cellulitis, burn, pyoderma, herpes zoster, etc.)
- Unstable medical condition

- Patient's receiving positive pressure ventilation
- Ruptured diaphragm
- Pleural adhesions (resulting from previous tuberculosis infection, hemopneumothorax, or empyema)

EQUIPMENT

Commercial thoracentesis trays are available. If a commercial tray is used, the manufacturer's instructions *must* be reviewed because equipment varies. Alternatively, the following equipment can be assembled:

Preparation

- Sterile tray
- Sterile 4 × 4–inch gauze pads
- Povidone-iodine solution
- Sterile gloves
- Mask
- Fenestrated drape or sterile towels
- Oxygen by nasal cannula

Anesthesia

- 10-ml Luer-Lok syringe
- 25-gauge or smaller needle
- 1½- to 2-inch, 22-gauge needle
- 10-ml lidocaine 1% with epinephrine

Insertion

- 50-ml Luer-Lok syringe
- 2-inch, 18-gauge needle (for air)
- 2-inch, 15-gauge needle (for fluid) or 16-gauge Angiocath (use of an Angiocath can decrease risk of pneumothorax, but kinks can increase the "dry tap" rate)
- 3-way stopcock
- 2 curved clamps
- Specimen tubes: 1 red top, 1 lavender top, culture tubes (aerobic and anaerobic), 10- to 50-ml red top for cytology, possibly 1 green top

Optional

- Sterile plastic tubing
- 1-inch, 15-gauge needle
- 500- or 1000-ml vacuum bottles

Dressing

- Sterile gauze pads
- Adhesive tape

PREPROCEDURE PATIENT PREPARATION

Explain the procedure and its risks to the patient. Provide a patient education handout detailing the procedure. (See the sample patient education handout titled "Thoracentesis" on page 1854 of Appendix G.) Obtain informed consent. (See the sample patient consent form titled "Thoracentesis" on page 1855 of Appendix G.)

TECHNIQUE

Insertion Site and Patient Position

1. Position the patient comfortably (Fig. 95-1). For *fluid removal,* have the patient sit and lean forward with arms supported on a table. For *air removal,* the patient should be lying supine, with the head of the bed elevated at a 30- to 45-degree angle.
2. Confirm the location and extent of fluid or air by percussion, auscultation, and study of posteroanterior, lateral, and lateral decubitus (fluid-affected side down) chest radiographs.
   Note: If available, ultrasound may be very helpful for completing this step. See Chapter 209, Emergency Department and Office Ultrasound.
3. Select the needle insertion site. For *fluid removal,* use an area one or two interspaces below the fluid level and 5 to 10 cm lateral to the spine. Do not insert below the eighth intercostal space. For *high-risk patients* or for *small effusions,* consider the use of ultrasound to guide the insertion. Perform the thoracentesis at the time of the ultrasound or in exactly the same location as fluid was shown on ultrasound, with the patient in the same position. For *air removal,* use the second or third intercostal space, in the midclavicular line or more laterally.
4. Mark the insertion site with a marker or by applying pressure from the hub of a needle.

Preparation and Anesthesia

1. Prepare the skin with povidone-iodine. Use sterile technique and universal blood and body fluid precautions. Wear a mask, and drape with sterile towels.
2. Raise a skin wheal using lidocaine with epinephrine, using a 25-gauge or smaller needle attached to a 10-ml syringe.
3. To infiltrate with the anesthetic, change to a 1½-inch 22-gauge needle. Angle the needle slightly downward, and insert it through the skin wheal so that the needle tip touches the superior border of a rib, aspirating and injecting as you advance. "Walk" the needle over the superior margin of the rib and deeper into the interspace, anesthetizing the intercostal muscle layers (Fig. 95-2, *A*).

   Note: Do not remove the needle before performing Step 4.

4. Confirm the presence of fluid or air with the small anesthesia needle; continue advancing the needle, while aspirating and injecting, until the parietal pleura has been penetrated. (A pop may be felt, or fluid or air will be aspirated.) Warn the patient that there may be a twinge of pain as you go through the pleura. Place a clamp on the needle at skin level to mark the depth (Fig. 95-2, *B*). Withdraw the needle. If no fluid is obtained, try the next higher intercostal space. If air is unexpectedly obtained, try a lower intercostal space. Do not insert the needle

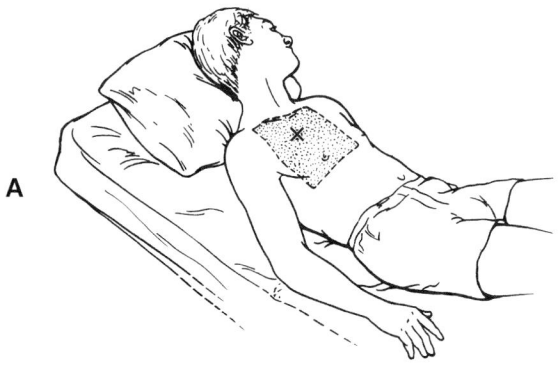

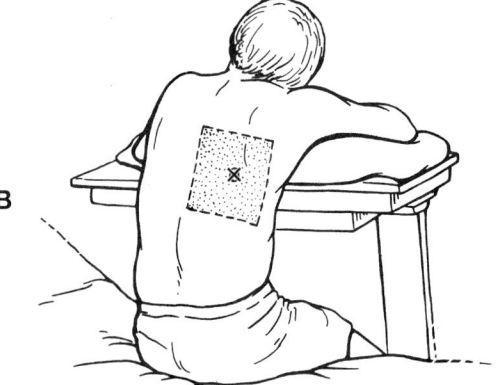

Fig. 95-1
Position for air removal **(A)** and fluid removal **(B)**.

immediately below the rib, since this is where the vessels lie.

Needle-Only Insertion Technique

1. Prepare the equipment. Attach a 15-gauge needle (for fluid) or an 18-gauge needle (for air) to a 50-ml syringe with a 3-way stopcock. Mark the previously measured depth on this needle with a clamp. Test the equipment to be sure you are well acquainted with the use of the stopcock. Open the stopcock to the syringe.

2. Insert the thoracentesis needle in the same tract as the anesthesia needle, and advance it to the level of the clamp. (Again, "walk" over the rib, not under it, to avoid vessels and nerves). Aspirate to confirm place-

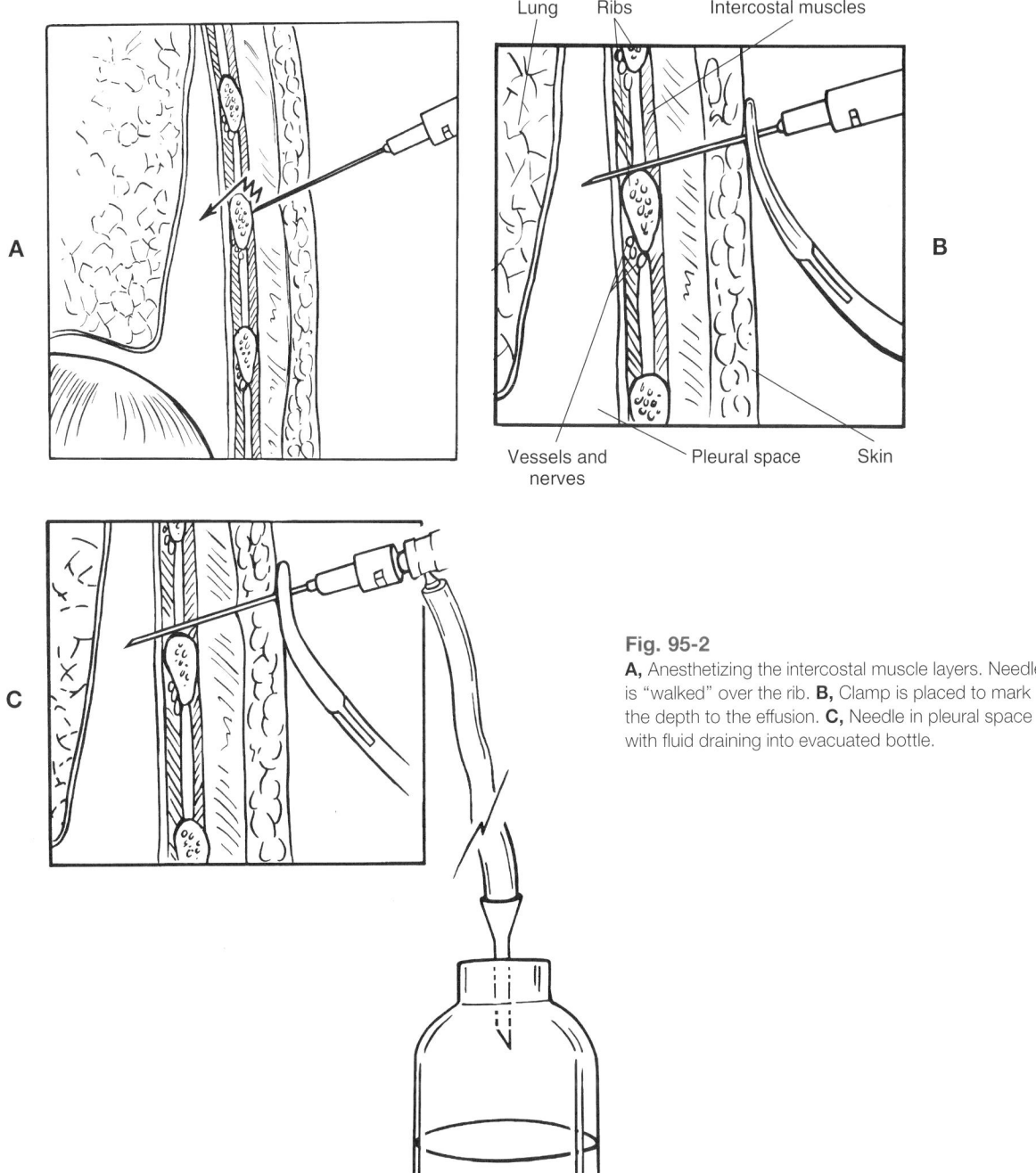

Fig. 95-2
A, Anesthetizing the intercostal muscle layers. Needle is "walked" over the rib. **B,** Clamp is placed to mark the depth to the effusion. **C,** Needle in pleural space with fluid draining into evacuated bottle.

ment. Keep the clamp attached to prevent penetrating too deeply.

Catheter-Over-Needle Insertion Technique

(Use a commercially prepared thoracentesis needle. Read the manufacturer's instructions carefully.)

1. Prepare the equipment. Familiarize yourself with the stopcock. Visualize the measured insertion depth on the needle.
2. Insert the thoracentesis needle in the same tract as the anesthesia needle, aspirating on the syringe until fluid is obtained.
3. Making sure the stopcock is off to the side port, completely withdraw the needle, leaving the catheter in the pleural space.

Catheter-Through-Needle Insertion Technique

(Use a commercially prepared thoracentesis needle. Read the manufacturer's instructions carefully.)

1. Prepare the equipment. Place the syringe and stopcock on the Y sidearm. Advance and then retract the catheter to break the seal. Mark the measured depth on this needle with a clamp.
2. Insert the thoracentesis needle in the same tract as the anesthesia needle, and advance it to the level of the clamp. Aspirate to confirm placement. Keep the clamp attached to prevent penetrating too deeply.
3. Insert the catheter. While holding the hub, advance the Y sidearm until it engages the hub. Remove the split tube. Withdraw the needle, leaving the catheter in the pleural space.

Completing the Procedure

1. *For stopcock and open container:* Pull the fluid into the syringe. Turn the stopcock off to the needle, being careful not to open the needle to the environment. Push the fluid out of the syringe into the containers. Alternate aspiration into the syringe with deposition of the syringe contents into the container by rotating the stopcock.

    For stopcock and evacuated container: Attach one end of the tube to the stopcock and the other end to a second 15-gauge needle. Place the needle in an evacuated container, and open the stopcock to the thoracentesis needle (Fig. 95-2, *C*).
2. After withdrawal of necessary fluid, remove the needle while the patient is exhaling.
3. Dress the site with a sterile dry dressing.
4. Send the fluid for study (see the following section for details). In most cases, a volume of 100 ml is sufficient for diagnostic tests.
5. Check end expiratory chest radiograph for pneumo-

thorax, especially if the patient is short of breath or has chest pain.

COMPLICATIONS

- Pneumothorax may result if air is introduced through the needle or catheter, or if the visceral pleura is punctured. Between 5% and 20% of procedures produce a pneumothorax, which requires treatment with a chest tube about 20% of the time. Pneumothorax incidence may be reduced with ultrasound-guided thoracentesis. Insert the needle only as far as needed to obtain fluid. Be comfortable with the equipment, especially the stopcock, before insertion. Smaller needles, short bevels, and removal of less fluid may also decrease the risk of pneumothorax.
- Hemothorax may result from laceration of intercostal vessels or internal mammary vessels. To reduce the risk of hemothorax, insert the needle just above the rib, avoiding the neurovascular bundle that runs below each rib. Never puncture medial to the midclavicular line.
- The spleen, liver, or diaphragm may be lacerated. To avoid lacerations to these organs, do not allow the needle to penetrate lower than the eighth intercostal space posteriorly. Mark the intended depth of penetration each time with a clamp.
- Hypoxia is very common and is caused by ventilation-perfusion mismatch in the newly expanded lung. To prevent hypoxia, you may administer oxygen for several hours after the procedure and evaluate oxygenation with pulse oximetry or by obtaining arterial blood gases.
- Reexpansion pulmonary edema can be minimized by removing no more than 1 L of fluid at a time (although many experts advocate draining the effusion dry). Remove fluid slowly and stop if the patient develops a cough, dyspnea, or chest pain.
- A catheter fragment may be left in the pleural space. To avoid this possibility, *never* withdraw the catheter through the needle. Use the needle guard, when provided.
- Failure to obtain fluid can occur. For better success, pay close attention to landmarks obtained by auscultation, percussion, and x-ray examination. Consider ultrasound guidance.
- Infection can occur. To minimize this possibility, use sterile technique and avoid inserting through infected skin.
- Hypovolemia can occur. To reduce the incidence of hypovolemia, remove less than 1 L of fluid at a time.
- Pain is associated with thoracentesis. Use adequate local anesthesia.
- Hypoproteinemia is a possibility. To reduce this problem, avoid repeated thoracenteses.

PLEURAL FLUID ANALYSIS

Many tests can be performed on, and much money wasted on, pleural fluid. Specific tests depend on the clinical situation, and many times the fluid does not yield a definitive answer. If the lactate dehydrogenase (LDH) levels in the fluid and the pleural fluid/serum ratios for LDH and protein are all normal, the fluid is a transudate and studies are unlikely to give useful information. Most transudates are from congestive heart failure, with the rest associated with hypoalbuminemia, ascites, hydronephrosis, pulmonary embolism, peritoneal dialysis, or atelectasis. One diagnostic approach is to send some of the fluid for protein, pH, and LDH measurement, while storing the remaining fluid for the other tests if the fluid proves to be an exudate. Low pH can indicate a complicated parapneumonic effusion, which may require chest tube drainage. See Table 95-1 for potentially useful tests and their significance, and see the bibliography for references on pleural fluid analysis.

TABLE 95-1

Potentially Useful Tests in the Evaluation of Pleural Effusions

Test	Abnormal Values	Frequently Associated Condition
Protein (PF/S)	>0.5	Exudate
LDH (PF/S)	>0.6	Exudate
LDH (IU)	>200	Exudate
Red blood cells (per mm³)	100,000	Malignancy, trauma, pulmonary embolism
White blood cells (per mm³)	10,000	Pyogenic infection
Neutrophils (%)	>50	Acute pleuritis
Lymphocytes (%)	>90	Tuberculosis, malignancy, sarcoidosis, fungal infection
Eosinophilia (%)	>10	Asbestos effusion, pneumothorax, resolving infection
Mesothelial cells	Absent	Tuberculosis
Glucose (mg/dl)	<60	Empyema, tuberculosis, malignancy, rheumatoid arthritis
pH	<7.20	Complicated parapneumonic process, empyema, esophageal rupture, tuberculosis, malignancy, rheumatoid arthritis
Amylase (PF/S)	>1	Pancreatitis
Bacteria	Positive	Infection
Cytology	Positive	Malignancy

Adapted from Kinasewitz GT: Pleural fluid dynamics and effusions. In Fishman AP, editor: *Pulmonary diseases and disorders,* vol 1, New York, 1998, McGraw-Hill.
IU, Concentration in international units; *LDH,* lactate dehydrogenase; *PF/S,* pleural fluid/serum ratio.

SUPPLIERS

Thoracentesis trays
Allegiance Healthcare Corp.
1430 Waukegan Drive
McGaw Park, IL 60085-6787
Phone: 1-800-964-5227
Website: www.allegiance.net

CPT/BILLING CODE

32000*   Thoracentesis, puncture of pleural cavity for aspiration, initial or subsequent

ICD-9-CM DIAGNOSTIC CODES

Effusion
511.9   Pleural
511.1   Bacterial
197.2   Malignant
012.0   Tuberculous
Pneumothorax 512.8
512.1   Iatrogenic
512.8   Spontaneous
512.0   Tension
860.0   Traumatic

ADDITIONAL RESOURCES

- See the sample patient education handout titled "Thoracentesis" on page 1854 of Appendix G.
- See the sample patient consent form titled "Thoracentesis" on page 1855 of Appendix G.

BIBLIOGRAPHY

American College of Physicians: Diagnostic thoracentesis and pleural biopsy in pleural effusions, *Ann Intern Med* 103:799, 1985.

American Thoracic Society: Guidelines for thoracentesis and needle biopsy of the pleura, *Am Rev Respir Dis* 140:257, 1989.

Barrter T, Akers SM, Pratter MR: The evaluation of pleural effusion, *Chest* 106:1209, 1994.

Ferrer JS, Munoz XG, Orriols RM, et al: Evolution of idiopathic pleural effusion: a prospective, long-term follow-up study, *Chest* 109:1508, 1996.

Fishman AP, editor: *Pulmonary diseases and disorders,* vol 1, New York, 1998, McGraw-Hill.

Queshi N, Momin ZA, Brandstetter RD: Thoracentesis in clinical practice, *Heart Lung* 23:376, 1994.

*Health Care Financing Administration (HCFA) allows additional payment for a tray for this procedure when performed in a physician's office. Charge appropriately using code "99070—surgical tray."

CHAPTER 96

Venous Cutdown

Pauline M. Aham-Neze
Grant C. Fowler

Venous cutdown has been widely used for venous access in trauma patients since Kirkman first described using the saphenous vein in 1945. When percutaneous venous access is not available, venous cutdown (i.e., venesection) is the procedure of choice for administering large volumes of fluids, including blood products. Very large bore lines can be used, allowing even more rapid infusion of fluids than through central lines. However, it should be noted that venous cutdown provides only temporary access. Even under optimal conditions using excellent technique, phlebitis is common within 3 days. Therefore if adequate staff is available, attempts should also be made to obtain large-bore percutaneous antecubital venous access while venesection is being performed elsewhere. Central venous access should be obtained if there is need for prolonged infusions or for infusion of hypertonic fluids.

INDICATIONS

- Lack of percutaneously accessible vein (e.g., obesity, unusually small or fragile veins as found in some adults and most infants, or venous sclerosis from aging, intravenous [IV] drug abuse, or previous multiple venipunctures)
- When subclavian catheterization is needed but is impractical or undesirable (e.g., in children)
- Hypotensive patient in whom major injury is suspected
- Patient with suspected large volume depletion
- Patient requiring emergency venous access or a large IV line and antecubital or other vein cannot be visualized, palpated, or cannulated percutaneously

Note: Opinion ranges widely about the best location for venous cutdown. The three most common locations, each with inherent advantages and disadvantages, are (1) the distal saphenous vein at the ankle, (2) the proximal saphenous vein at the groin, and (3) the basilic vein in the antecubital fossa. These veins are utilized here to minimize the risk of complications. Other peripheral locations are possible; however, before attempting to recall the complete anatomy of the venous system in an urgent situation, obtaining central access may be prudent.

CONTRAINDICATIONS

- Less invasive alternatives exist (i.e., routine venous catheterization)
- Inability to perform in a timely manner (when there is urgent need)
- Evidence of severe venous obstructive disease, previous thrombosis, previous prolonged hypertonic fluid infusion, or vein stripping (clinician should consider different site)
- Hypertonic fluids are to be infused for a prolonged period
- Local infection (clinician should consider different site)
- Local arterial supply inadequate (to hasten postprocedure healing of the venesection incision and to minimize complications, clinician should consider different site)

EQUIPMENT

- Tourniquet
- Antiseptic skin preparation, such as isopropyl alcohol or povidone-iodine
- Sterile gloves and drapes
- Gauze sponges (4 × 4)
- Lidocaine (1%) *without* epinephrine
- A 3-ml syringe with 25-gauge, ⅝-inch (1.6-cm) needle for anesthetic
- A 5- or 10-ml syringe for aspiration of blood after cannulation
- Silk ligatures (4-0)
- Nonabsorbable skin suture (4-0)
- Fine forceps, one set with and one set without teeth

- Tissue dissection and suture scissors
- Curved hemostats and a mosquito hemostat
- No. 15 or no. 11 scalpel blade with handle
- Needle holder
- IV fluids and setup
- Antibiotic ointment
- Adhesive tape
- Sterile cannula (anything from a 2-, 3-, or 4-French Silastic catheter to a section of IV connector tubing can be used, based on the size of the vein to be cannulated)
- Goggles
- Venous cutdown kit or tray (available in most hospitals and from commercial sources; clinician should check with central supply office of local hospital for availability of trays or vendors)

PATIENT PREPARATION AND OVERVIEW

1. If the patient is alert, explain the need for IV access and the procedure. Obtain informed consent.
2. In the basilic or distal saphenous cutdown, have an assistant apply a tourniquet proximal to the incision site and control it. This will enable the clinician to more easily visualize and palpate the vein. A tourniquet applied high on the thigh may help with locating the proximal saphenous vein. To minimize bleeding, tourniquets should be released at the time of venipuncture. Observe universal blood and body fluid precautions.
3. Cleanse the area around the vein and incision site thoroughly with either 70% isopropyl alcohol or povidone-iodine.
4. To provide ample working space, extend a wide sterile field 8 to 10 cm proximally and distally and apply sterile drapes.
5. For conscious patients, administer a local anesthetic to the area of incision using the smaller syringe.
6. Regardless of which cutdown site is chosen, incisions can all be made horizontally (i.e., laterally), which is also transversely. When subcutaneous fat protrudes through the incision, use blunt dissection and spread the tissue longitudinally along the axis of the vein. All of these veins are in superficial fat layers; therefore with a basilic or proximal saphenous cutdown, if the incision exposes muscle fascia, it is too deep.
7. The vein should appear pulseless and thin walled, and it should blanch with the application of distal traction. If a vein is not readily identified, have an assistant tighten the tourniquet, which may make it more apparent or palpable.
8. With all cutdowns, the vein should be dissected free and isolated for 2 to 4 cm along its axis.

CUTDOWN

Distal Saphenous Vein (Fig. 96-1)

Advantages

- Most consistent vein of the lower extremity, especially in its location anterior to the medial malleolus.
- No valves at this level of the vein because of minimal volume and pressure.
- Does not disrupt other resuscitative measures, such as obtaining blood gases at the femoral artery or chest compressions during cardiopulmonary resuscitation (CPR).
- Provides IV access on both sides of the diaphragm if additional central access is obtained.
- Requires minimal training and involves minimal risk of complications compared with obtaining central access. Only the minor saphenous nerve is near the incision.

Disadvantages

- Phlebitis is more common in veins of the lower extremity.
- Infection is more common in the presence of phlebitis.
- Poor route for administration of cardiac drugs during CPR.
- Hypertonic solutions should not be used.
- The saphenous vein cannot be used if it has been used for a previous surgical procedure (e.g., for coronary artery bypass grafting, previous cutdown).

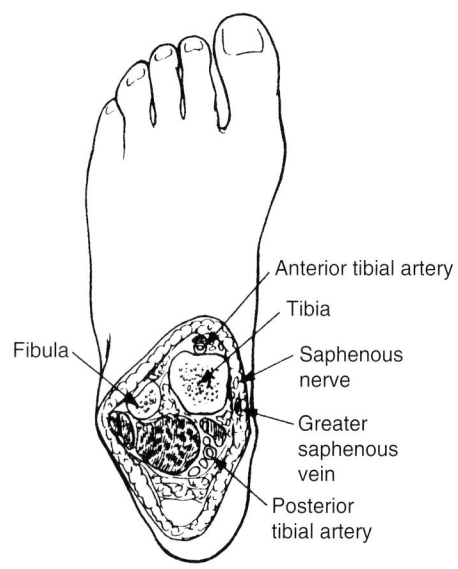

Fig. 96-1
The greater saphenous vein may be isolated easily and safely at the ankle. Only the minor saphenous nerve lies nearby.

- Older patients may have thrombosis or vein narrowing.
- Cannot be used in the presence of pelvic fracture or major knee trauma because of ileofemoral venous interruption.

Technique

1. As mentioned previously, a tourniquet should be applied (in this case, to the distal one third of the leg). Palpate the distal saphenous vein just anterior to the medial malleolus (Fig. 96-2).
2. Just above (1.5 to 2 cm) the medial malleolus, make a 2-cm transverse incision (only through skin) going from anterior to posterior tibia.
3. Using a curved closed hemostat pointing downward, scrape across/around the tibia in the line of the incision, from anterior to posterior, and pick up the tissue contained within the incision. In other words, allow the tissue to slide over the back of the hemostat.
4. While holding this tissue, turn the hemostat around (Fig. 96-3) so that its tip is directed upward; open the hemostat widely. This will improve visualization when separating the vein from the saphenous nerve and other fibrous tissue. These structures are readily identified against the silver background of the hemostat (Fig. 96-3).
5. Proceed to cannulation as described below.

Proximal or Greater Saphenous Vein at the Groin

Advantages

- Provides IV access on both sides of the diaphragm if additional central access is obtained.

- Requires minimal training and involves minimal risk of complications compared with obtaining central access.
- Large veins are easier to cannulate than distal veins; larger cannulas can be used, enabling larger volumes of infusion for patients with profound hypovolemia.

Disadvantages

- Phlebitis is more common in veins of the lower extremity.
- Infection is more common in the presence of phlebitis.
- Poor route for administration of cardiac drugs during CPR.
- Hypertonic solutions must be avoided.
- If dissection is too deep, there is a possibility of damage to nearby structures.
- Cannot be used in the presence of pelvic fracture because of ileofemoral venous interruption.

Technique

1. With the patient supine, start a horizontal (i.e., lateral) incision (skin only) at the point where the scrotal fold (or labial fold) meets the medial thigh and extend it laterally. A tourniquet applied high on the thigh (above the incision) may be helpful.
2. Imagine a vertical (i.e., longitudinal) line drawn straight downward from the most lateral aspect of the pubic tubercle (or the outer portion of the mons) (Fig. 96-4). The proximal saphenous vein is located most frequently at the point where this line crosses the incision.
3. The saphenous vein is located in the superficial fat layer. If muscle fascia is visible, the incision is too deep. The femoral artery and vein are located deeper than the superficial fat layer.
4. Proceed to cannulation as described below.

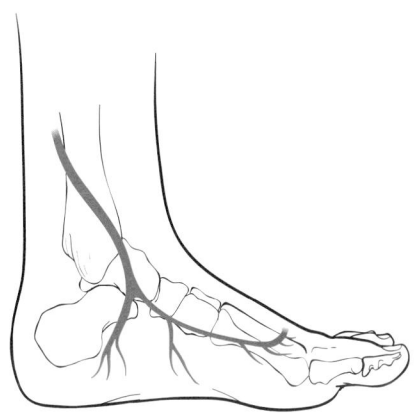

Fig. 96-2
Anatomic relationships of the saphenous vein.

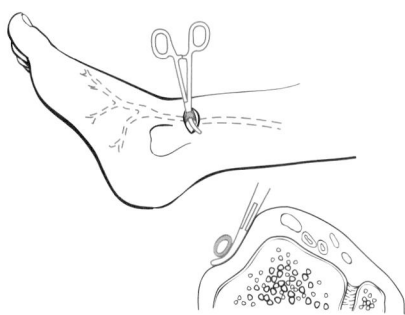

Fig. 96-3
Curved mosquito clamp is inserted into the anterior angle of the skin incision. It is then advanced under the saphenous vein and swept posteriorly. Then the clamp is turned over and lifted upward with the vein.

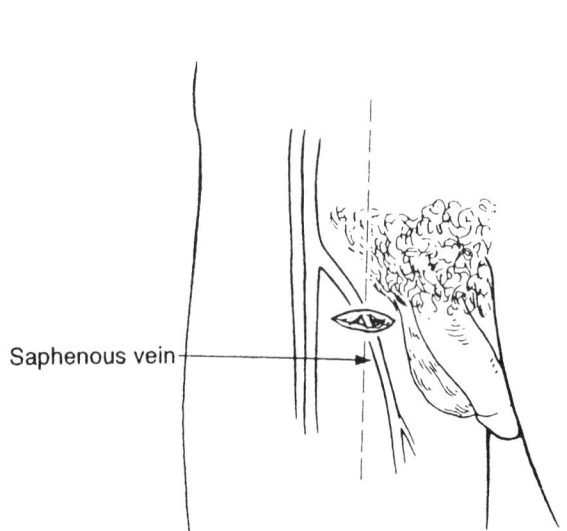

Fig. 96-4
Cutdown location for greater saphenous vein at the groin.

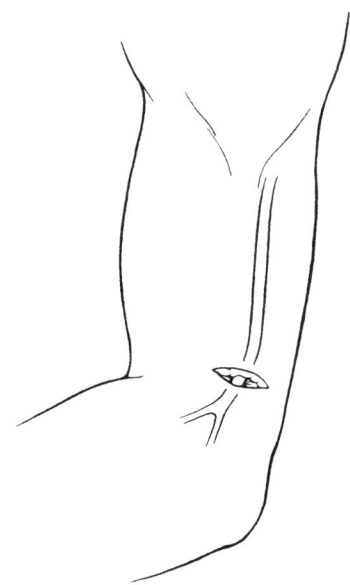

Fig. 96-5
Incision is made between the biceps and triceps for basilic vein cutdown (right arm).

Basilic Vein

Advantages

- Located closer to the heart than the saphenous vein, it affords a superior route of drug administration during CPR (although not as effective as central access).
- Less risk of infection than the saphenous vein.
- Requires minimal training and involves minimal risk of complications compared with obtaining central access.

Disadvantages

- In CPR situations, ongoing attempts at percutaneous cannulation or chest compression can make this a difficult site.
- Compared with the proximal saphenous vein, the smaller diameter of the basilic vein may limit the volume of infusions. However, the cannulas used in both of these locations are frequently the same size.
- If dissection is too deep, it is possible to damage nearby structures.

Technique

1. Take the distance between the olecranon and the acromion and divide it into thirds; the basilic vein will be located in the middle of the distal third. Apply a tourniquet proximal to this location, and palpate the vein where it lies in the groove between the triceps and the biceps muscles. On the medial arm, the vein follows a course slightly anterior and superficial to the brachial artery.
2. Make a horizontal, superficial incision from the biceps across this groove to the triceps (Fig. 96-5).
3. Locate the basilic vein by dissecting the superficial fat

layer. If muscle fascia or brachial artery is seen, the dissection is too deep.
4. Proceed to cannulation as described below.

CANNULATION

Technique

1. Pass a 4-0 silk suture under the vein as distal as possible; use this as a retractor to bring the vein into the incision.
2. Free 2 to 4 cm of the vein by spreading the scissors longitudinally along the length of the vein and dissecting aside any loose adipose or adventitial tissue. Pass another 4-0 silk suture under the proximal vein.
3. If the distal vein is to be sacrificed, the distal ligature should be tied and left long to help control and manipulate the vein. Clamp the ends of the ligature with a hemostat and use its weight to maintain tension on the ligature.
4. Place traction on the proximal ligature to minimize later bleeding; it should not be tied at this point. Select a site near the distal ligature for venotomy.
5. Loosen the tourniquet.
6. If the vein is large enough, it can be directly catheterized. Otherwise, using a scalpel or fine scissors in a distal-to-proximal direction, incise one third of the vein diameter at a 45-degree angle (Fig. 96-6, *A*). Next, expand the diameter of the lumen with the mosquito hemostat while maintaining proximal traction on the ligature (Fig. 96-6, *B*).

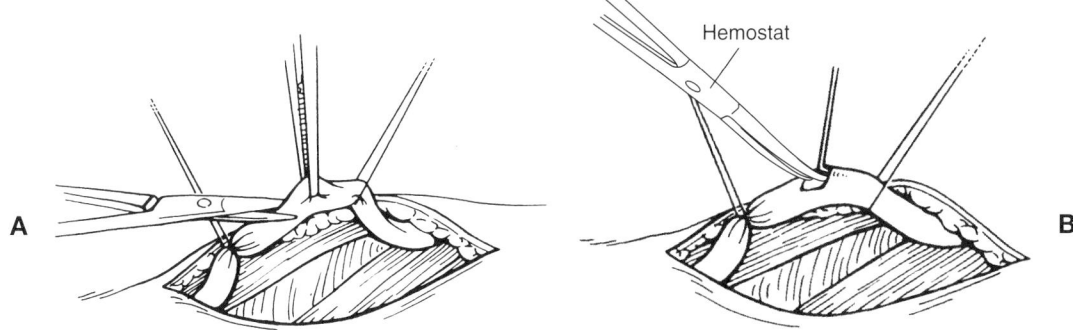

Fig. 96-6
A, Angled wedge cut is made in the anterior wall of the vein. Traction should be maintained on the vein with proximal and distal ligatures. If sacrificed, the distal vein ligature can be tied. **B,** The vein is dilated with a hemostat.

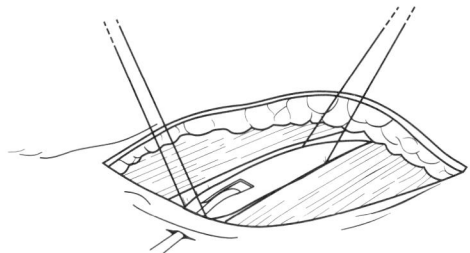

Fig. 96-7
Catheter is threaded through a separate skin stab wound and then into the vein.

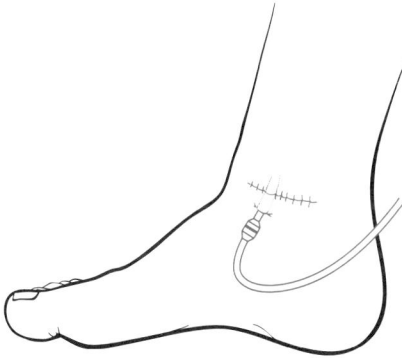

Fig. 96-8
Incision closed to minimize infection and catheter sutured in place.

7. Once the skin has been entered through a separate stab wound, introduce the cannula through the vein incision following the 45-degree angle of the incision (Fig. 96-7). Threading the catheter into the vein is usually the most difficult portion of the procedure and requires patience and foresight. Relax slightly on the proximal ligature. If the catheter cannot be threaded, the posterior wall of the vein may have been punctured, a valve may have been encountered, or a false lumen may have been created. A catheter that is too large is another possible source of difficulty. If cannulation has not succeeded after multiple attempts, repeated dilation of the vein with the mosquito hemostat followed by enlargement of the vein incision, as a last effort, may be considered.

Note: In greater saphenous vein cannulations, take caution to not cannulate beyond the saphenous vein. Further cannulation could block the lumen of the femoral vein, which would block all venous return from that lower extremity.

8. Using the larger syringe, aspirate air from the cannula by withdrawing blood. Blood may not be obtained with aspiration if the patient is in vascular collapse or if there is a valve in the vein just proximal to the cannula tip. In that case, advance the tip and attempt aspiration again. If successful, tie the proximal ligature around the vein wall and the cannula. Cut both ligatures and close the wound with skin suture (Fig. 96-8) to minimize risk of infection.

9. Completely remove the tourniquet and observe the incision for leakage of fluid or blood.

10. Secure the catheter to the skin with an additional stitch, and apply antibiotic ointment and a dressing. Risk of infection is minimized if the cutdown is removed within 48 hours of placement (Fig. 96-9).

11. If the cannula must be left in place for more than 48 hours, the IV tubing should be changed daily.

COMPLICATIONS

- Local hematoma and infection
- Phlebitis
- Embolism
- Bacteremia and sepsis
- Injury to nearby structures during cutdown

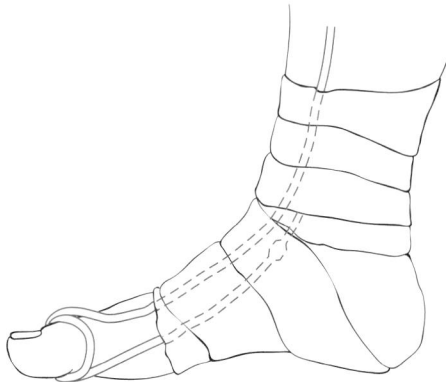

Fig. 96-9
Dressing to prevent decannulation.

CPT/BILLING CODES

36410   Venipuncture, child over age 3 years or adult, necessitating physician's skill, for diagnostic or therapeutic purposes. Not to be used for routine venipuncture.
36415   Routine venipuncture or finger, heel, or ear stick for collection of specimen(s)
36425   Venipuncture, cutdown; aged 1 year or older

ICD-9-CM DIAGNOSTIC CODES

427.5   Cardiopulmonary arrest
785.59   Hypovolemic shock (NEC)

958.4   Hemorrhage shock or shock syndrome due to trauma
772.9   Hemorrhage, unspecified in newborn (NOS)
799.1   Respiratory arrest
785.50   Shock (without trauma), unspecified
785.59   Shock, endotoxic
995.0   Shock, anaphylactic
276.5   Volume depletion, dehydration
459.89   Venofibrosis
459.0   Hemorrhage, unspecified

ADDITIONAL RESOURCES

• See the sample patient education handout titled "Venous Cutdown" on page 1856 of Appendix G.
• See the sample patient consent form titled "Venous Cutdown" on page 1857 of Appendix G.

BIBLIOGRAPHY

Johnson JD, Page JC: The distal saphenous vein cutdown procedure, *J Am Podiatr Med Assoc* 81:8, 1991.
Kirkham J: Infusion into the internal saphenous vein at the ankle, *Lancet* 2:815, 1945.
Klofas ED: A quicker saphenous vein cutdown and a better way to teach it, *J Trauma* 43:6, 1997.

PART SIX

Gastrointestinal System Procedures

CHAPTER 97

Abdominal Paracentesis

Kenneth Hu
Brett White

Paracentesis remains an important clinical technique for primary care clinicians. With the advent of new radiologic techniques, including CT scan and ultrasound, diagnosis of intraabdominal pathology has become less invasive. Nevertheless, paracentesis is the diagnostic test of choice in patients who have new onset ascites, in patients with a suspected malignant ascites, and to rule out infection in those with preexisting ascites.

Abdominal anatomy must be considered during the abdominal paracentesis procedure. Recall that large volumes of ascitic fluid tend to float the air-filled bowel toward the midline when in the supine position, where it is more easily perforated during paracentesis. In addition, the cecum is relatively fixed and less mobile than the sigmoid colon; thus bowel perforations are more frequent in the right lower quadrant than in the left. Although entering the peritoneal cavity with a paracentesis needle does present certain risks, the procedure, when performed carefully and with proper technique, can safely provide useful diagnostic and therapeutic results.

Once ascitic fluid is obtained, the fluid should be inspected and then sent to the laboratory for Gram's stain, culture, albumin content, and cell count. Additional studies may include lactate dehydrogenase, amylase, acid-fast bacilli, glucose, or total protein as clinically indicated (Table 97-1). Cytologic analysis by a pathologist should be considered when a malignancy is suspected. In immunocompromised patients the culture and testing of opportunistic infections is indicated.

INDICATIONS

Diagnostic Indications

- New onset ascites
- To rule out infection

Therapeutic Indications

- Relief of tense ascites (causing gastrointestinal or cardiorespiratory symptoms)

CONTRAINDICATIONS

Absolute Contraindications

- Acute abdomen requiring immediate surgery

Relative Contraindications

- Severe bowel distension
- Previous abdominal surgery
- Pregnancy (ultrasound guidance is preferred after the first trimester)
- Distended bladder that cannot be emptied with a Foley catheter
- Obvious infection at the intended site of needle insertion (cellulitis or abscess)
- Coagulopathy
- Thrombocytopenia

EQUIPMENT

Commercially prepared kit or the following equipment:
- Skin cleansing solution (povidone-iodine)
- Sterile gloves and mask
- Sterile marking pen (if area has not been marked indelibly before skin preparation)
- Sterile drapes
- 1% or 2% lidocaine with or without epinephrine
- 10-ml syringe for anesthetic
- 20-ml syringe for diagnostic tap
- 50-ml syringe, if using stopcock technique
- 18-gauge, 1½- to 3-inch needle (alternatively, an 18- or 20-gauge, 1½- to 3-inch Angiocath needle or spinal needle may be substituted)

- 25- or 27-gauge, 1½-inch needle for skin anesthesia
- Sterile IV tubing
- 1-L vacuum bottles, a sufficient number for draining more than 1 L of fluid if ascites volume is large
- Three-way stopcock (for use with 50-ml syringe) *(optional)*

PREPROCEDURE PATIENT PREPARATION

- Explain the procedure and its risks and benefits to the patient (see the "Complications" section).
- Obtain verbal or written informed consent.

TABLE 97-1
Ascitic Fluid Analysis

Lab Value	Exudate	Transudate
Specific gravity	>1.016	<1.016
Protein (g/dl)	>3.0	<3.0
Protein (fluid:serum)	>0.5	<0.5
LDH (U/L)	>200	<200
LDH (fluid:serum)	>0.6	<0.6

Causes of transudate: Cirrhosis, nephrotic syndrome, congestive heart failure, pseudomyxoma peritonei, inferior vena cava obstruction, Budd-Chiari syndrome, hypoalbuminemia.
Causes of exudate: Spontaneous bacterial peritonitis (SBP), malignancy, tuberculosis (TB), pancreatitis, chylous ascites, bilious or chemical causes (e.g., in the case of abdominal trauma resulting in bile duct rupture or pancreatic enzyme release).
Normal ascitic fluid cell count = <250 WBC
  • Increased WBC count seen in SBP, TB, malignancy, pancreatitis
  Cell counts often >500
  • Increased RBC count can also be seen in malignancy, TB, endometriosis, mesenteric thrombosis, pancreatitis, abdominal trauma, and perforated viscus.

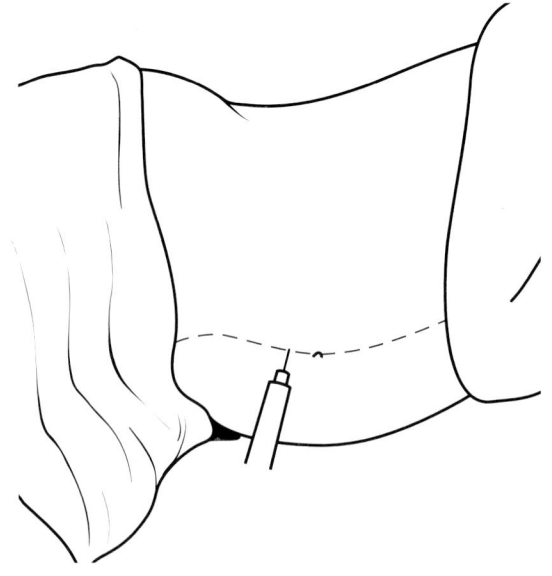

Fig. 97-1
View of patient in lateral decubitus position, demonstrating insertion of the paracentesis needle in the midline 2 to 3 cm below the umbilicus.

- Take plain and upright x-ray films of the abdomen before performing the procedure. (Air is introduced during the procedure and may confound a diagnosis of perforated viscus.)
- Examine the abdomen, delineate areas of shifting dullness, and find landmarks. Mark if necessary.
- Check for bowel distension.
- Place patient in the supine position if the lateral approach is taken (patient may be tilted slightly to the side of collection for improved fluid positioning) or in the lateral decubitus position if the infraumbilical approach is used (see the illustrations and the "Technique" section).
- Use a Foley catheter and nasogastric tube, if necessary, to decompress the bladder or stomach.
- Use wrist restraints in patients with altered mental status to prevent the patient from contaminating the sterile field or causing injury.

TECHNIQUE

1. Prepare the abdominal skin at the puncture site with povidone-iodine solution.
2. Apply sterile drapes to outline the area to be tapped. Place the patient in the left lateral decubitus position. The site to enter is in the midline about one third the distance from the umbilicus to the symphysis (usually 2 to 3 cm below the umbilicus [Fig. 97-1]). Alternatively, with the patient supine, a point about one third the distance from the umbilicus to the anterior iliac crest can be used, with the left side preferred (Fig. 97-2).
3. Infiltrate the skin and subcutaneous tissues with lidocaine (with epinephrine, if possible).
4. Direct the needle perpendicular to the skin and infiltrate the peritoneum with anesthetic (resistance will be felt as the needle perforates the peritoneum).
5. Direct the 18-gauge needle perpendicular to the skin at the preferred site. A 20- or 22-gauge needle may be preferred for diagnostic taps to minimize subsequent leakage of ascitic fluid. (An alternative method of entry is the "Z-tract" technique [Fig. 97-3]. The needle is inserted through the skin and moved 1 to 2 cm from the original site before proceeding though the deep tissue structures into the peritoneum. The theoretical advantage of this technique is the "self sealing" of the tract created by the needle, thus minimizing leaking of peritoneal fluid once the needle is removed.) With either method it is important to avoid continuous suction during entry. Suction may attract bowel loops, occlude flow, and create the appearance of an unsuccessful tap. Worse yet, continuous suction may increase the likelihood of bowel perforation. Insert the needle until fluid returns in the syringe. Apply the suction intermit-

tently as the needle is inserted to determine if fluid is present.

6. After entry into the peritoneal cavity, fluid may be withdrawn and collected for analysis. If a therapeutic paracentesis to remove excess fluid is indicated, the needle may be attached to sterile tubing and connected to vacuum bottles. The needle may need to be repositioned to allow for continuous flow. Alternatively, the patient may need to be repositioned slightly. There are numerous anecdotal reports of hypotension caused by large-volume fluid removal (greater than 5 L), although this phenomenon is poorly studied. Some physicians may give colloid replacement as prophylaxis; however, there is no evidence that this practice should be adopted universally.

7. After the fluid is removed, gently remove the needle or catheter and apply pressure to the wound; have the first 100 ml of fluid analyzed. If the wound is still leaking fluid after 5 minutes of direct pressure, suture the puncture site using a mattress suture, and apply a pressure dressing.

COMPLICATIONS

The following complications are rare but have occurred:
- Bladder perforation
- Small and large bowel perforation
- Stomach perforation
- Lacerations of major vessels (mesenteric, iliac, aorta)
- Abdominal wall hematomas
- Infection (local or intraperitoneal)
- Persistent ascitic fluid leak

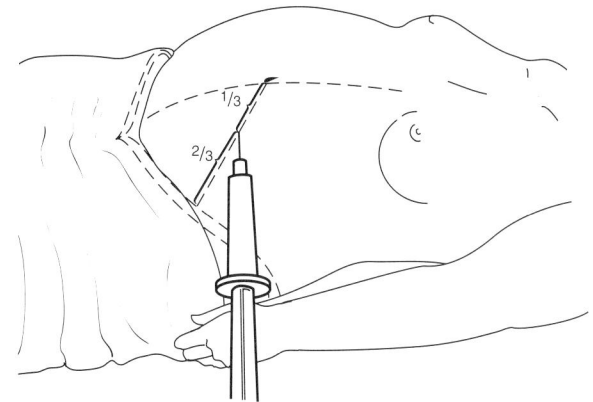

Fig. 97-2
View of abdominal wall, demonstrating insertion of paracentesis needle one third of the distance between the umbilicus and anterior iliac spine. Patient is supine.

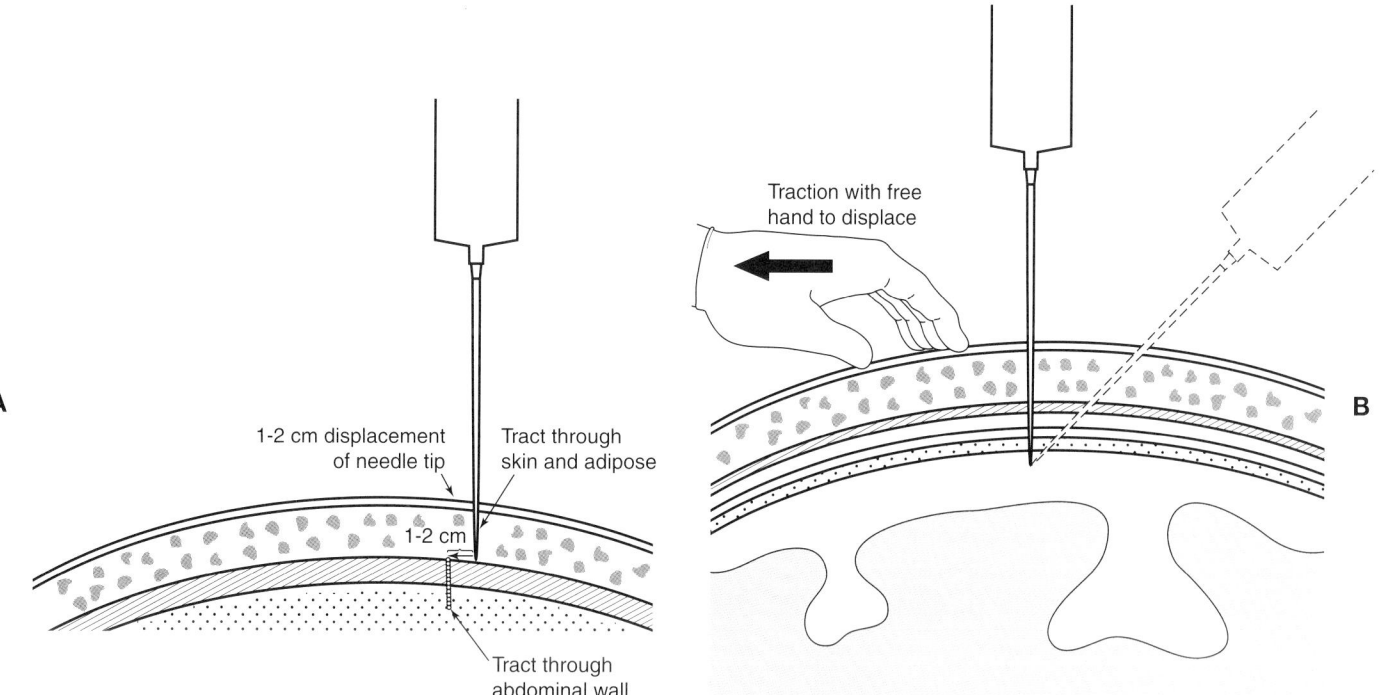

Fig. 97-3
Methods to limit leakage of ascites after a tap. **A,** Transverse view through the abdominal wall demonstrating the "Z-tract" technique. **B,** Skin on the abdominal wall is retracted a few centimeters caudad by the non-needle-bearing hand *(arrow)*. When fluid is first obtained, skin retraction can be released and the needle will lean rostrally *(broken lines)*. When the procedure is finished, the needle is withdrawn and the abdominal wall layers will facilitate closure of the needle tract.

POSTPROCEDURE PATIENT EDUCATION

Educate the patient about bleeding, pain, infection, hypotension from reaccumulation of fluid, and other complications.

SUPPLIER

Abdominal paracentesis kit
Arrow International
2400 Bernville Road
Reading, PA 19605
Phone: 1-800-233-3187
Website: www.arrowintl.com/products/critcare.html

CPT/BILLING CODES

49080*   Peritoneocentesis, abdominal paracentesis, or peritoneal lavage; initial
49081   Peritoneocentesis, abdominal paracentesis, or peritoneal lavage; subsequent

*Health Care Financing Administration (HCFA) allows additional payment for a tray for this procedure when performed in a physician's office. Charge appropriately using code "99070—surgical tray."

When either procedure is performed at an initial visit (for a new patient) and it is the major service performed, the procedure code 99025 may be used instead of the usual initial visit, as an additional service.

ICD-9-CM DIAGNOSTIC CODES

789.5   Ascites
197.6   Ascites, malignant
428.0   Ascites, cardiac
457.8   Ascites, chylous
014.0   Ascites, tuberculous
567.2   Subacute bacterial peritonitis, etc.

BIBLIOGRAPHY

Feldman M, Scharschmidt BF, Sleisenger MH: *Sleisenger & Fordtran's gastrointestinal and liver disease,* ed 6, Philadelphia, 1998, WB Saunders.

Keating KP, Yeston NS: Diagnostic peritoneal lavage: indications, results, complications, *Res Staff Phys* 37(11):31, 1991.

Roberts JR, Hedges JR: *Clinical procedures in emergency medicine,* ed 3, Philadelphia, 1998, WB Saunders.

Rosen PR: *Emergency medicine: concepts and clinical practice,* ed 4, St Louis, 1998, Mosby.

CHAPTER 98

Anal Fissure/Lateral Sphincterotomy

James A. Surrell

Anal fissure is defined as a painful linear ulcer (tear) of the distal anal canal, located just inside the anal opening (Fig. 98-1). The history of a patient with anal fissure is so characteristic that the diagnosis can usually be made accurately, based on the history alone. Patients complain of moderate-to-severe pain during and after bowel movements and have a variable amount of bleeding. Rarely, the patient with an anal fissure complains of severe and constant pain. This is usually seen only with an acute anal fissure with significant anal spasm.

The history must include whether the fissure is acute or chronic. *Chronic fissure* can arbitrarily be defined as one that has been present with signs and symptoms of pain and/or bleeding for more than 3 months. Unless the symptoms are extremely disabling, all fissures should be given a trial of conservative management, as discussed

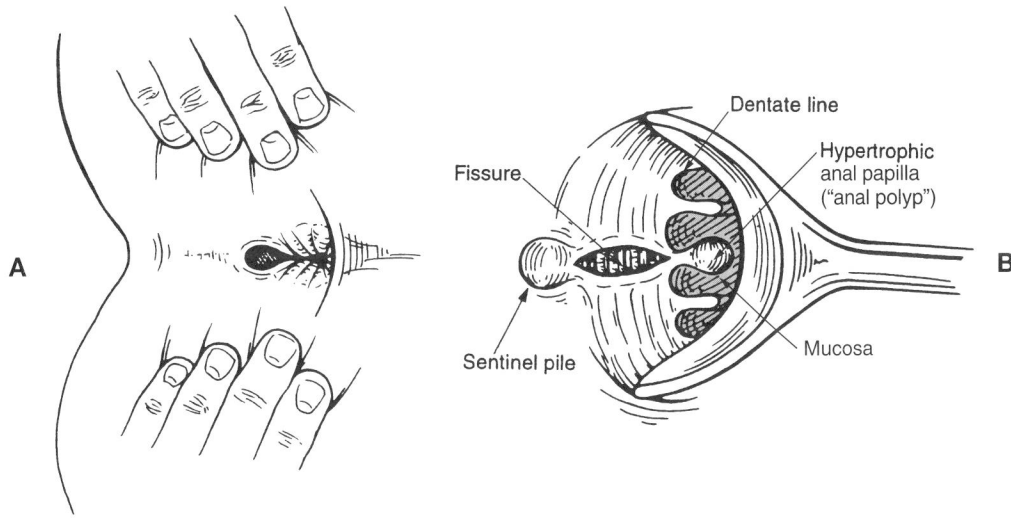

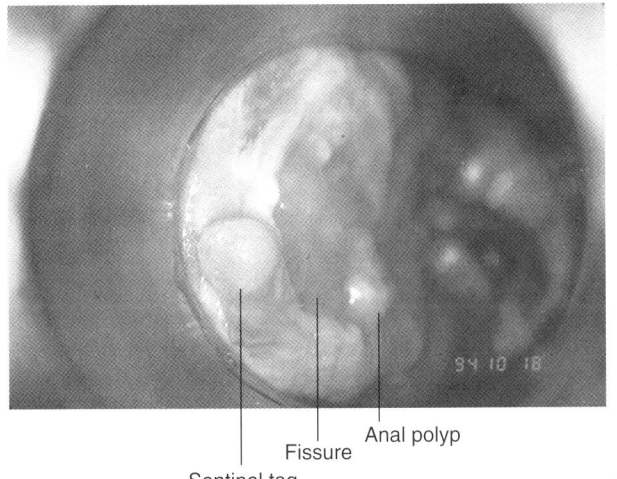

Fig. 98-1
Anal fissures. Patient is in the left lateral decubitus position. **A,** External examination. Gentle eversion of the buttocks reveals a posterior midline anal fissure. **B,** Anoscopic examination. Chronic posterior anal fissure with a distal "sentinel tag" and a proximal hypertrophic anal papilla at the level of the dentate line. **C,** Chronic anal fissure seen through an anoscope, with sentinel tag and proximal anal "polyp," which is really granulation tissue.

later. If conservative management fails, lateral internal sphincterotomy is the procedure of choice for treatment of an anal fissure.

Once the history suggests an anal fissure, the diagnosis can usually be made easily upon visual examination of the external anus and with gentle digital examination. The left lateral decubitus position is recommended for patients undergoing anorectal examination. With gentle eversion of the anoderm, one can usually directly visualize the fissure. Touching the fissure with a cotton-tipped applicator confirms the diagnosis if this reproduces the painful symptoms experienced with bowel movements. If necessary, a digital examination with good lubrication will confirm not only pain, but marked increased sphincter tone. Finally, the anoscopic examination provides more direct visualization. In classic cases, the insertion of the anoscope may be so painful that it has to be deferred. Eventually it will need to be performed at a later time to identify other possible diseases.

INDICATIONS

If the patient has symptoms of moderate-to-severe pain and/or bleeding during and after bowel movements, he or she probably has an anal fissure. If these symptoms are severe, disabling, and constant, surgical intervention should be considered sooner rather than later.

However, for most fissures, a 1- to 3-month trial of conservative management is indicated. This includes a high-fiber diet of at least 30 g of dietary fiber per day, 6 to 8 glasses of water per day, and 3 to 6 g of commercially available fiber supplements per day. If the fissure pain is severe, consider prescribing 5% lidocaine ointment to be applied to the fissure 30 minutes before and again after bowel movements. Commercially available nonprescription ointments and creams are minimally effective in the treatment of anal fissures. They may, however, be used to lubricate the anal canal for bowel movements. Steroid preparations may or may not be helpful, but they are not intended for long-term use.

Specifically advise patients not to use any ointment or cream with a rectal tube-tipped applicator or any suppositories because these products and devices tend to worsen the symptoms of an anal fissure. Advise patients to apply a small amount of any recommended ointment or cream directly to the fissure with a finger because an anal fissure is always located just inside the anal verge. The application of silver nitrate to or the use of electrocautery on the fissure site is *not* recommended and may even exacerbate the symptoms. Anal dilators should *not* be used because of the unpredictable disruption of the anal sphincters and the potential for causing incontinence.

For persistent fissures, a trial of 0.2% to 0.5% nitro-glycerin ointment may be tried. It is recommended that a small amount of this ointment (about the size of a pencil eraser) be applied directly to the fissure two to three times a day. It must be rubbed in and not just applied superficially. Patients must be cautioned that if they experience a headache, they are using too much nitroglycerin ointment. Usually, using a lesser amount will eliminate the headaches. As of this date, the 0.2% to 0.5% nitroglycerin ointment is not yet commercially available (it comes as 2%), but it can be made up by any reputable local pharmacist from a physician's prescription. The prescription usually reads as follows: "Ṛ: 0.2% nitroglycerin ointment, DISP: 60 g, SIG: apply small amount to anal fissure, as directed, three to four times a day for 6 to 8 weeks for anal fissure pain." (Be sure to clarify 0.2%, not 2.0%.) Most studies use white soft paraffin to dilute it or lidocaine or Anusol ointment. If headache does occur, aspirin should be taken an hour beforehand.

Some practitioners now question the efficacy of nitroglycerin and have switched to using nifedipine gel 0.2%. (Mix ten 20-mg capsules in 100 g of Surgilube or K-Y Jelly.) The mixture is rubbed in two to three times a day.

Both medications purportedly relax the anal sphincter to reduce spasm and pain and to induce healing (a "chemical sphincterotomy").

Lateral internal sphincterotomy is indicated if conservative management has been recommended, the patient has complied for approximately 1 month, and the symptoms of pain or bleeding are still present during and after bowel movements, and there is no improvement.

CONTRAINDICATIONS

Anal fissures occur most commonly in the posterior midline. Approximately 90% of fissures are in this location, and 10% are located in the anterior midline. If the clinician sees an anal fissure in any location other than the anterior or posterior midline, a thorough gastrointestinal workup is necessary to rule out the presence of inflammatory bowel disease or other very rare causes such as tuberculosis, syphilis, occult abscesses, leukemic infiltrates, carcinomas, herpes, or AIDS.

If it is present, inflammatory bowel disease with an atypical fissure is most commonly Crohn's disease. Another physical examination feature that should raise the suspicion of perianal Crohn's disease is the presence of fleshy edematous skin tags (see Chapter 110, Removal of Perianal Skin Tags [External Hemorrhoidal Skin Tags]). If the examiner suspects inflammatory bowel disease, upper gastrointestinal with small-bowel x-ray films are necessary, as well as colonoscopy, or barium enema x-ray combined with flexible sigmoidoscopy.

Another contraindication to lateral internal sphincterotomy is preexisting anal incontinence, although the coexistence of an anal fissure and incontinence is uncommon.

EQUIPMENT

The only special equipment required for lateral internal sphincterotomy are an assortment of various-sized ano-scopes and a surgical electrocautery unit. The Hill-Ferguson anal retractor is available in sizes small, medium, and large. Any modern electrosurgery device with a cutting and coagulation setting should suffice.

PREPROCEDURE PATIENT PREPARATION

Inform the patient that lateral internal sphincterotomy is a procedure to divide only the fibers of the involuntary internal sphincter to allow the anal canal to relax during bowel movements. Inform the patient of an approximate 5% recurrence rate and a 3% to 5% infection rate. Patients should expect mild-to-moderate postprocedure pain, which usually is well controlled with oral analgesics. Generally no more than a day or two is required for recovery, and postoperative pain is minimal compared with the preoperative discomfort from the fissure. There will be minimal bleeding and spotting for up to 6 weeks after the procedure. With proper technique combined with a thorough understanding of the anal sphincter anatomy, alteration of anal continence is uncommon.

As always, before any surgical procedure, patients should be made aware of nonoperative treatment options as discussed above. If the fissure is not resolved with either conservative or surgical treatment, the patient generally persists with symptoms intermittently. Fibrosis of the internal anal sphincter can lead to anal stenosis. Development of a subcutaneous fistula originating through the base of a long-standing anal fissure is not uncommon.

TECHNIQUE

Note: I prefer to use intravenous sedation and local anesthesia. This is an outpatient procedure, generally performed in the operating room. Only a clinician who is thoroughly familiar with the technique and with anorectal anatomy should perform this procedure.

1. Place the patient on the operating table in the left lateral decubitus position, with the buttocks just off the edge of the table and the knees flexed. It is essential that the clinician be able to clearly identify the intersphincteric groove between the internal and external sphincters so that only the fibers of the internal sphincter are divided; this is done to preserve anal continence for both flatus and feces.

2. Use the electrocautery unit to make a superficial 1-cm radial incision just distal and perpendicular to the palpable intersphincteric groove in the left lateral quadrant of the anal area (Fig. 98-2, *A*).

3. Grasp the skin edge, and clearly identify the inter-sphincteric groove using the dissecting scissors. The darker-red external sphincter should not be damaged. The lighter-colored internal sphincter is bluntly elevated with forceps. It normally extends 1 to 1.5 cm into the canal (Fig. 98-2, *B* and *C*).

4. Divide the full thickness of the internal sphincter from its distal margin up to the level of the dentate line, which is visible in the anal canal (Fig. 98-2, *D*). Because the internal sphincter is immediately subjacent to the internal hemorrhoidal vessels, significant bleeding may be encountered if these hemorrhoidal vessels are divided. If proper hemostasis cannot be obtained by using pressure or electrocautery, figure-of-eight suture ligation of these vessels may be necessary for persistent bleeding (rare).

5. Leave the primary incision site open and allow it to close secondarily. If there is a prominent sentinel skin tag distal to the fissure site or a prominent hypertrophic anal papilla proximal to the fissure site, you may excise the tag or papilla with the electrocautery unit at the time of the sphincterotomy procedure. Generally, no specific operative treatment is performed at the fissure site itself. The average operative time is 15 minutes or less.

POSTPROCEDURE PATIENT EDUCATION

Following lateral internal sphincterotomy, give the patient a prescription for nonconstipating pain medication (ibuprofen). Advise the patient to continue to follow a high-fiber diet of at least 30 g of dietary fiber per day and to use psyllium-based powder fiber supplements once or twice a day. Instruct the patient to expect some discomfort, slight bleeding, and discharge from the operative site because the wound is generally left open. Bedrest is not recommended, inasmuch as the pain from the sphincterotomy is often minimal and may even be less than that of a severe fissure.

COMPLICATIONS

Approximately 5% of patients have nonhealing fissures following sphincterotomy and may need repeat sphincterotomy. Various studies have shown a postoperative infection rate of approximately 3% to 5%, and a smaller percentage of these patients will go on to develop an associated anal fistula. The most morbid long-term com-

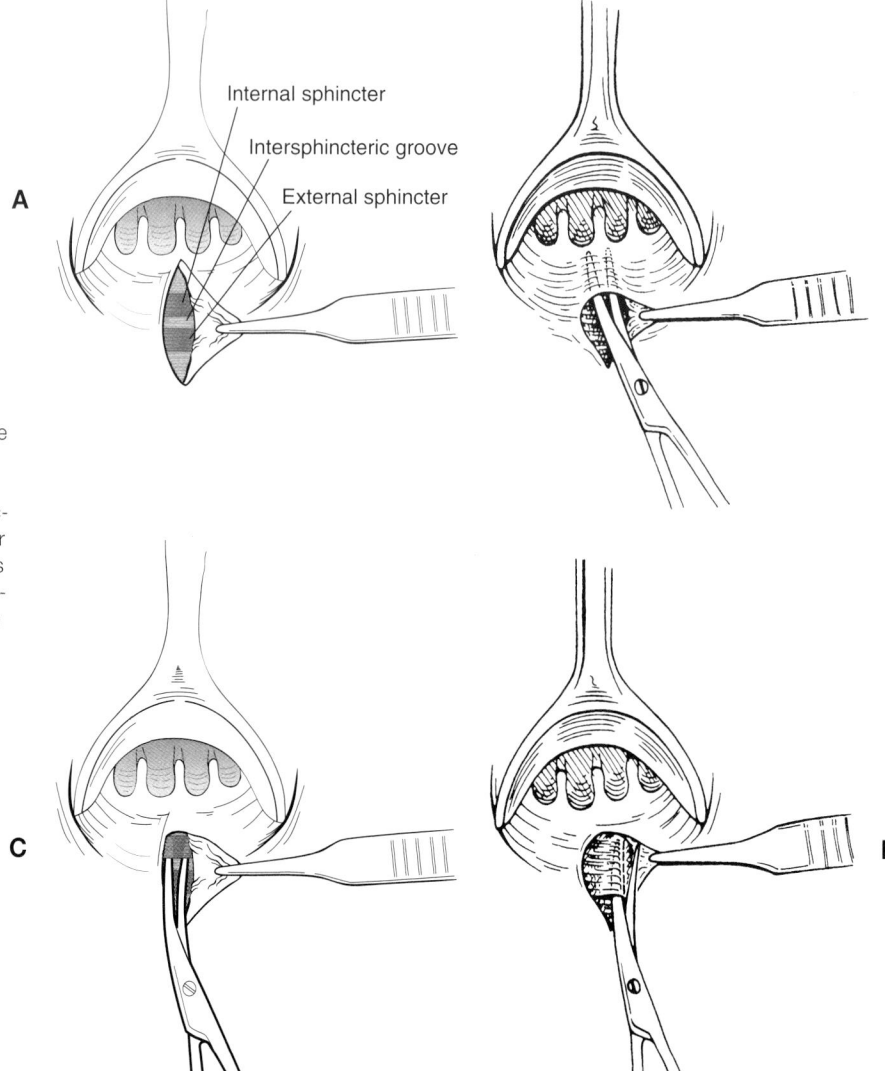

Fig. 98-2
Lateral internal anal sphincterotomy using the open technique. The patient is placed in the lateral or the prone (jackknife) position. **A,** A radial incision is made across the intersphincteric groove. A narrow Hill-Ferguson retractor is in place. **B** and **C,** The internal sphincter is separated from the anoderm by blunt dissection. **D,** The internal sphincter is divided. The wound may be closed or left open.

plication is the development of anal incontinence, either for flatus or feces. Postoperative anal incontinence can result from technical operative error during the procedure, whereby muscle fibers other than those of the internal sphincter muscle are divided. Another factor that can contribute to postoperative anal incontinence is unrecognized preexisting anal incontinence.

SUPPLIERS

Anal retractors
Anoscope product codes are SU180, SU181, and SU182.
V. Mueller
Allegiance Healthcare Corp
1430 Waukegan Road
McGaw Park, IL 60085-6787
Phone: 1-800-323-9088 or 1-800-964-5227
Website: www.allegiance.net

Davol Surgical Electrocautery Unit
Davol, Inc.
100 Sockanossett Crossroad,
P.O. Box 8500
Cranston, RI 02920
Phone: 1-401-463-7000
Website: www.davol.com

Also see Chapter 31, Radiofrequency Surgery.

CPT/BILLING CODE

46080   Anal sphincterotomy

ICD-9-CM DIAGNOSTIC CODE

565.0   Anal fissure

ADDITIONAL RESOURCES

- See the sample patient education handout titled "Fine Anal Fissures and Pruritis Ani ('Itchy Anal Area')" on page 1858 of Appendix G.

BIBLIOGRAPHY

Altomare DF, Rinaldi M, Milito G, et al: Glyceryl trinitrate for chronic anal fissure—healing or headache? Results of a multicenter, randomized, placebo-controlled, double-blind trial, *Dis Colon Rectum* 43(2):174, 2000.

Antropoli C, Perrotti P, Rubino M, et al: Nifedipine for local use in conservative treatment of anal fissures: preliminary results of a multicenter study, *Dis Colon Rectum* 42(8): 1011, 1999.

Carapeti EA, Kamm MA, Evans BK, Phillips RK: Topical diltiazem and bethanechol decrease anal sphincter pressure without side effects, *Gut* 45(5):719, 1999.

Corman ML: *Colon and rectal surgery,* Philadelphia, 1998, JB Lippincott.

Gordon P, Nivatvongs S: *Principles and practice of surgery for the colon, rectum, and anus,* St Louis, 1992, Quality Medical Publishing.

Gorfine SR: Topical nitroglycerin therapy for anal fissures and ulcers, *N Engl J Med* 333(17):1156, 1995.

Jost WH, Schimrigk K: Therapy of anal fissure using botulinum toxin, *Dis Colon Rectum* 37(12):1321, 1994.

Loder PB, Kamm MA, Nicholls RJ, Phillips RK: "Reversible chemical sphincterotomy" by local application of glyceryl trinitrate, *Br J Surg* 81(9):1386, 1994.

Lund JN, Scholefield JH: A randomised, prospective, double-blind, placebo-controlled trial of glyceryl trinitrate ointment in treatment of anal fissure, *Lancet* 349:11, 1997.

Mazier W, Levien D, Luchtefeld M, Senagore A: *Surgery of the colon, rectum, and anus,* Philadelphia, 1995, WB Saunders.

Pernikoff BJ, Eisenstat TE, Rubin RJ, et al: Reappraisal of partial lateral internal sphincterotomy, *Dis Colon Rectum* 37(12): 1291, 1994.

Richard CS, Gregoire R, Plewes EA, et al: Internal sphincterotomy is superior to topical nitroglycerin in the treatment of chronic anal fissure: results of a randomized, controlled trial by the Canadian Colorectal Surgical Trials Group, *Dis Colon Rectum* 43(8):1048, 2000.

Schouten WR, Briel SW, Auwerda JJA, de Graaf EJR: Ischemic nature of anal fissures, *Br J Surg* 83:63, 1996.

Sharp RF: Patient selection and treatment modalities for chronic anal fissure, *Am J Surg* 171:512, 1996.

CHAPTER 99

Clinical Anorectal Anatomy and Digital Examination

James A. Surrell

A practical knowledge of anorectal anatomy is necessary for the proper evaluation and treatment of patients with anorectal complaints, such as hemorrhoids and anal fissures. A basic anorectal examination includes visual inspection of the perianal tissues and digital palpation of the anorectal area. Depending on patient complaints, anoscopy and sigmoidoscopy may also be necessary. This chapter describes the practical and the clinically important features of anorectal anatomy. See Chapter 100, Anoscopy, for the actual anoscopic examination.

BASIC ANATOMY

Fig. 99-1 is a diagram of the anatomy of the anal canal and lower rectum.
- *Rectum:* The distal 10 to 12 cm of the colon.
- *Anus:* The outlet of the gastrointestinal tract, consisting of the lower 6 to 8 cm of the bowel.
- *Anal verge:* Most distal extent of the anal canal just at the opening.
- *Dentate or pectinate line:* The squamocolumnar junction located 2 to 3 cm proximal to the anal verge where

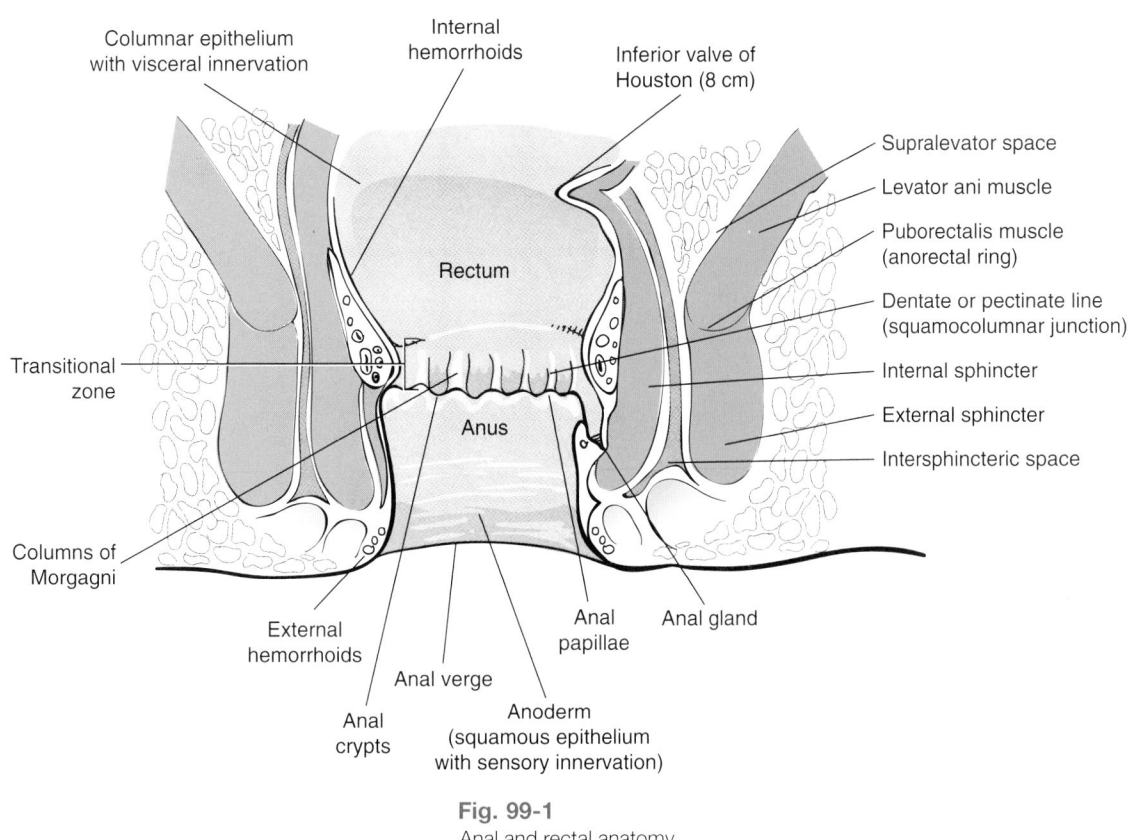

Fig. 99-1
Anal and rectal anatomy.

there is an abrupt change from squamous, sensory anoderm to columnar or mucosal epithelium. There are no sensory nerve fibers above the dentate line—only visceral type.

- *Transitional zone:* Comprised of mixed columnar and squamous epithelium; where the anal canal merges with the rectum.
- *Internal sphincter:* The innermost circular muscle.
- *External sphincter:* Located outside of the internal sphincter. Note that the external sphincter is external to the internal sphincter not only from a medial to lateral aspect, but also from a cephalad to caudad aspect at the anal verge.
- *Puborectalis muscle (anorectal ring):* Located about 1 to 2 cm above the dentate line. The distal rectum and anal canal are surrounded by two sleeves of circular muscles. This palpable anorectal ring represents the puborectalis muscle, which encircles the very distal rectum from its anterior point of attachment at the pubis.
- *"Valves of Houston":* These are not really "valves" but just folds of mucosa. There are generally three located at approximately 8, 11, and 13 cm (inferior, middle, and superior, respectively.)
- *Anal papillae:* The mucosal tips of the anal glands at the dentate line. (They can become hypertrophied and elongated and be confused with a polyp.)
- *Anal crypt:* A small pocket along the dentate line. Usually the site of cryptitis, which can lead to a fistula.
- *Anal glands:* Located at dentate line. They secrete mucus to lubricate canal and can become infected or plugged (cryptitis).
- *Columns of Morgagni:* Folds of tissue above the anal crypts/dentate line.
- *Internal hemorrhoids:* Located at and just proximal to the dentate line.

- *External hemorrhoids:* Located distal to the dentate line at the anal verge.
- *Arteriovenous vessels:* Located above, below, or at the dentate line, or both above and below the dentate line.

PATIENT POSITION

A complete anorectal examination can be accomplished with the patient on the examining table in the left lateral decubitus position (Fig. 99-2). The patient's knees are flexed and drawn toward the chest, and the buttocks are drawn toward the examiner to a point just slightly off the table. The patient's head and shoulders should remain well toward the middle of the examination table so that the patient is confident that he or she will not fall. This position also directs the axis of the anal canal and rectum directly toward the examiner. Alternatively, the rectum may be examined with the patient in the pelvic position after a genital examination or in a flexed position while bending 90 degrees over an examination table.

EXTERNAL ANAL EXAMINATION

After appropriately advising the patient, visually inspect the external anus. Look for any sign of perianal inflammation that may suggest pruritus ani or other dermatologic conditions. Gently separate the buttocks; this will generally evert the anoderm to a sufficient degree so that a posterior or anterior anal fissure may be directly visualized.

If there is a *sentinel skin tag* present in either the posterior midline or the anterior midline, be diligent in evaluation for a fissure, especially if the history is consistent with anal fissure (see Chapter 98, Anal Fissure/

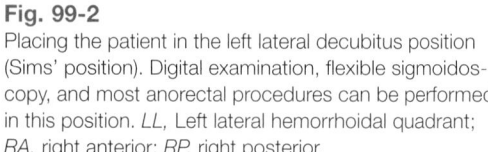
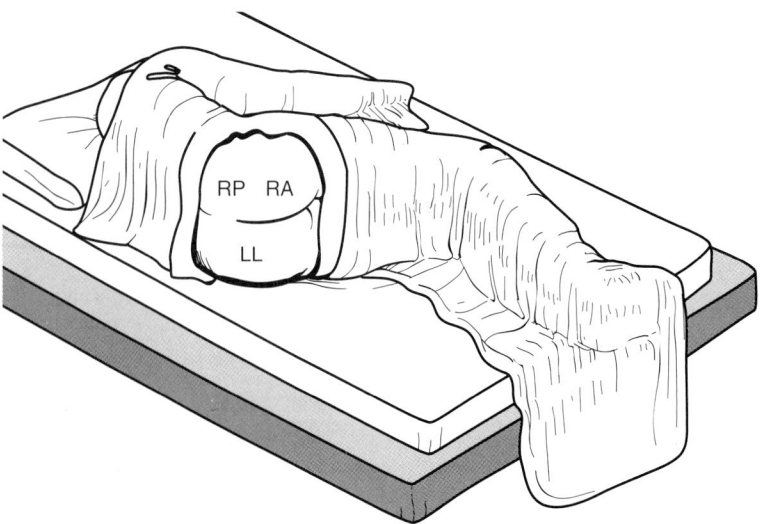

Fig. 99-2
Placing the patient in the left lateral decubitus position (Sims' position). Digital examination, flexible sigmoidoscopy, and most anorectal procedures can be performed in this position. *LL,* Left lateral hemorrhoidal quadrant; *RA,* right anterior; *RP,* right posterior.

Lateral Sphincterotomy). If present, anal skin tags, perianal abscess, or thrombosed external hemorrhoids should be readily visible at this time. Internal and external hemorrhoids are classically located in the right anterior, right posterior, and left lateral quadrants.

Internal hemorrhoids are located at and just proximal to the dentate line; *external hemorrhoids* are located distal to the dentate line at the anal verge. Hemorrhoids are collections of arteries and veins that, if not enlarged, represent normal anatomy and are not considered varicosities (see Chapter 108, Office Treatment of Hemorrhoids).

It is recommended that clinical anorectal findings be described in terms of right anterior, right posterior, or left lateral locations to provide consistency, regardless of the position of the patient.

DIGITAL ANORECTAL EXAMINATION

Inform the patient that the anus will be touched with a lubricated, gloved examining finger. Apply gentle pressure to the anal verge to allow the examining finger to enter the anal canal. If an anal fissure is present, you may feel palpable induration, most commonly in the posterior midline and less commonly in the anterior midline. Increased tone will also be noted.

In males, assess the prostate gland with your gloved examining finger in the anal canal.

To assess continence and anal sphincter function, flex your index finger slightly posteriorly and ask the patient to "squeeze down" as if to try to stop a bowel movement. If the patient has normal anatomic sphincter function, you will feel the tightening of the distal extent of the external sphincter at the base of your examining finger. The puborectalis muscle of the anorectal ring will also contract, pulling the tip of the examining finger from posterior to anterior. You should then be able to sweep the examining finger around the circumference of the distal rectum at the level of the anorectal ring and note the point of fixation of the puborectalis muscle at the symphysis pubis. Advise the patient to relax as the examination continues.

Generally, internal hemorrhoids and the dentate line are not palpable to the gloved examining finger. However, a large hypertrophic anal papilla present at the level of the dentate line may be palpable. If necessary, obtain a small sample of stool on the tip of the gloved examining finger for occult blood testing.

The procedure for anoscopic examination can be found in Chapter 100, Anoscopy.

ANAL CONTINENCE

The external sphincter and puborectalis muscle of the anorectal ring are the two muscles generally thought to afford *voluntary* anal continence. The external sphincter extends from the anal verge to the anorectal ring. The anorectal ring consists primarily of the puborectalis muscle, which encircles the very distal rectum. From a practical standpoint, it is generally accepted that either an intact functional external sphincter or an anorectal ring can provide near-perfect anal continence. The internal sphincter plays little role in maintaining voluntary anal continence. This is important when counseling patients during consideration of surgical treatment of anal fissures (see Chapter 98, Anal Fissure/Lateral Sphincterotomy).

SUMMARY

A practical understanding of the anatomy of the anal canal is essential to conducting an adequate anorectal examination. Lesions commonly seen may include pruritus ani or perianal dermatitis, anal fissures, fistulas, thrombosed external hemorrhoids, prolapsing bleeding internal hemorrhoids, hypertrophic anal papilla, perianal abscess, pilonidal disease, condyloma, polyps, cancer, and others. When anal continence is an issue, the physician must be able to evaluate the function of the external sphincter and of the puborectalis muscle of the anorectal ring on digital anorectal examination. With appropriate patient preparation and technique, the anorectal examination should not be an uncomfortable or painful experience. See Chapter 100, Anoscopy, for a description of the anoscopic examination.

BIBLIOGRAPHY

Corman ML: *Colon and rectal surgery,* Philadelphia, 1998, JB Lippincott.

Gordon P, Nivatvongs S: *Principles and practice of surgery for the colon, rectum, and anus,* St Louis, 1992, Quality Medical Publishing.

Mazier W, Levien D, Luchtefeld M, Senagore A: *Surgery of the colon, rectum, and anus,* Philadelphia, 1995, WB Saunders.

Pfenninger JL, Zainea G: Common anorectal conditions: Part I: Symptoms and complaints, *Am Fam Physician* 63(12): 2391, 2001.

Pfenninger JL, Zainea G: Common anorectal conditions: Part II: Lesions, *Am Fam Physician* 64(1):77, 2001.

CHAPTER 100

Anoscopy*

John L. Pfenninger

Anoscopy is a common procedure in both ambulatory and emergency medical care. It is used primarily to evaluate the patient with perianal and anal complaints. It is also generally performed just before or after withdrawing the colonoscope or flexible sigmoidoscope. Chapter 99, Clinical Anorectal Anatomy and Digital Examination, includes a review of clinical anatomy.

INDICATIONS

- Initial evaluation of rectal bleeding
- Anal or perianal pain
- Perianal itching (pruritus ani)
- Anal discharge
- Prolapse of the rectum
- External or internal hemorrhoids
- Fissures in ano
- Fistulae in ano
- Painful digital rectal examination
- Perianal condyloma
- Palpable masses on digital examination
- In association with sigmoidoscopy and colonoscopy (screening or diagnostic)
- Evaluation of intraanal trauma
- Follow-up of inflammatory bowel
- Retrieval of foreign body
- Evaluation of sexual abuse
- Fecal impaction
- Anal polyps, cancer

CONTRAINDICATIONS

- Unwilling patient
- Severe debilitation

---

*Dr. Jay Varma wrote this chapter in the previous edition.

- Acute myocardial infarction or similar cardiovascular condition
- Acute abdomen *(relative contraindication)*
- Marked anal canal stenosis

EQUIPMENT

- Anoscope
- Light source
- Gloves
- Lubricant
- Large-tipped cotton swabs
- Biopsy forceps, if needed
- Monsel's solution

The anoscope is a small cylindrical tool made of disposable plastic or reusable metal (Figs. 100-1 and 100-2). The size varies from 7 to 10 cm in length. They may or may not have handles. Distal diameter is approximately 2.5 cm.

Some anoscopes are readily attachable to battery light sources, whereas others require an external light source (e.g., a goose-neck lamp or headlight).

The Ive's slotted anoscope provides an unobstructed view of the walls of the anal canal (Fig. 100-2). This instrument is extremely useful not only for evaluation but also when treating various conditions. The advantage of the slotted instrument is that the mucosa is not compressed; thus small lesions and hemorrhoids may be more easily visible and treated. The diameter is also larger than most other anoscopes, and instruments are more easily manipulated within the lumen. Rather than looking out the end of the tube, the mucosal wall can be visualized in a more direct fashion.

PREPROCEDURE PATIENT PREPARATION

Patients dread inspection of the anal canal. They perceive this examination as unpleasant and uncomfortable

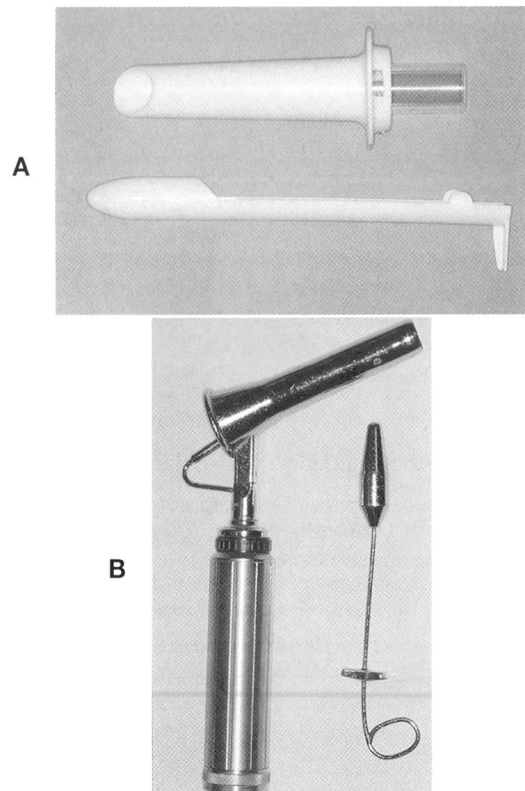

Fig. 100-1
Various types of anoscopes. **A,** Disposable plastic anoscope requiring external light source. **B,** Reusable type for use with battery-powered light source. Inserting trochars have been removed. The Ive's slotted anoscope provides the best visualization and most operative space for any interventional procedures.

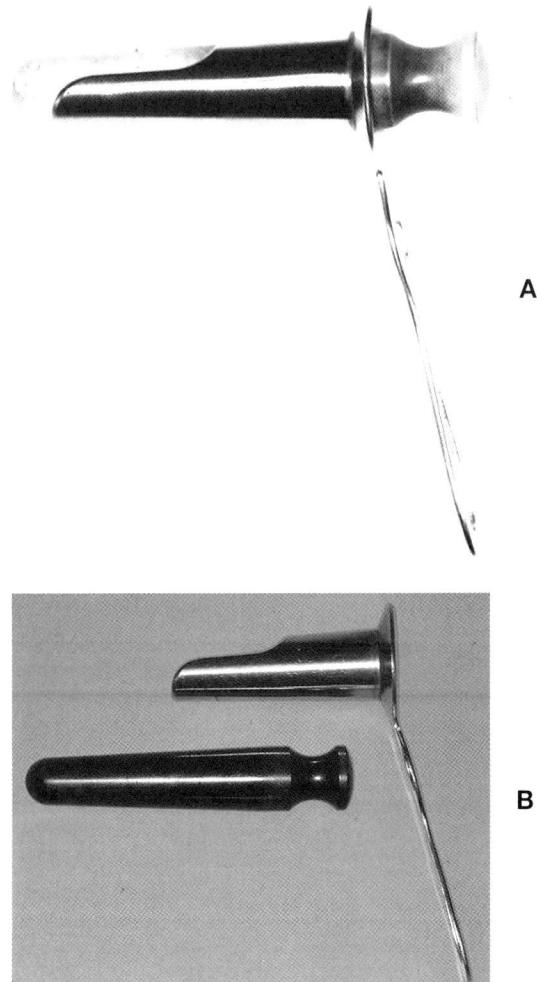

Fig. 100-2
Ive's slotted anoscope, **A,** with obturator in place and, **B,** obturator removed.

short of painful. Their concerns of embarrassment are overwhelming. This alone mandates that the patient be prepared mentally for what is involved. The patient must be cooperative and relaxed. Frank admission that the procedure will be unpleasant and uncomfortable, but not painful, is helpful. Explain the reasons necessitating the examination and the implications of not performing it. Reassure the patient that there are no significant complications resulting from anoscopy alone. However, if a biopsy sample is obtained or a lesion is removed, there may be some bleeding. If the biopsy is from below the dentate line, it will also be painful and an anesthetic will be needed.

If the reason for the exam is to evaluate anal pain (e.g., possible fissure), patients can be extremely tender and apprehensive. In addition, the anal sphincter contracts, making the examination difficult. Application of topical anesthetics, such as 5% xylocaine, 30 minutes before the examination can markedly reduce discomfort (see Chapter 11, Topical Anesthesia).

TECHNIQUE

An assistant is helpful. Both physician and assistant must wear gloves on both hands. An enema is generally not needed but may be helpful. Consider eye protection.

1. Place the patient in the left lateral position and drape. This position is most comfortable for the patient and is adequate in 95% or more situations. At times, placing the patient in stirrups or in the head-down position may be needed.

2. Have the assistant separate the glutei laterally, allowing full visibility of the perianal area. Alternatively, have the patient pull up on the right glutens. Check for any obvious lesions and possible fistulous tracks.

3. Inspect the tissue closely. Ask the patient to bear down, and observe for hemorrhoid or polyp prolapse.

```
┌─────────────────────────────────────────────────────────────────────────┐
│                              ANOSCOPY                                     │
│                                                                           │
│   Patient name _____  B.D. _____  Sex _____ │
│   Patient ID # _____                         │
│   Procedure _____  Date _____ │
│   Chief complaint: _____       │
│   Subjective: _____       │
│   Past medical history: _____       │
│   _____       │
│   _____       │
│   Medications: _____       │
│   _____       │
│   _____       │
│   Family history: _____       │
│   _____       │
│   _____       │
│                                                                           │
│   FINDINGS              Normal              Abnormal                      │
│                                                                           │
│   Perianal Skin                                                           │
│   Prostate                                                                │
│   Sphincter tone                                                          │
│   Anal canal                                                              │
│   Mucosa                                                                  │
│   Tears                                                                   │
│   Vasculature                                                             │
│   Tumor/polyps                                                            │
│   Bleeding                                                                │
│   Hemorrhoids                                                             │
│   Imp          _____         │
│                _____         │
│                _____         │
│   Follow-up date _____                                    │
│   Physician _____  Date _____  │
└─────────────────────────────────────────────────────────────────────────┘
```

Fig. 100-3
Procedure form for anoscopy.

4. Perform a careful circumferential digital examination with an index finger that has been lubricated with K-Y Jelly or 2% lidocaine jelly. Note the sphincter tone. (See Chapter 99, Clinical Anorectal Anatomy and Digital Examination.)

5. In male patients, palpate the prostate for size and masses.

6. Lubricate the anoscope well with K-Y Jelly with the obturator in place.

7. Gently insert the anoscope into the anal aperture, gradually overcoming the resistance of the sphincters. Gently advance the instrument in the direction of the umbilicus until the full length of the anoscope is inserted (subject to patient acceptance and tolerance). The procedure is better tolerated and accomplished by asking the patient to gently take a few deep breaths at the beginning of the procedure and to bear down just slightly.

8. After inserting the full length of the instrument, remove the obturator so that the mucosa of the anal canal can be visualized. Fecal material is often encountered and can be removed with a large swab. Note the gross appearance of the mucous membrane, the pectinate line, and the vasculature, as well as the presence of blood, mucus, pus, hemorrhoidal tissue, etc.

9. Gradually withdraw the instrument, observing the anal canal as the anoscope is extracted. Rotate the long cylinder anoscopes to the right and left to ensure that the entire canal has been visualized. The Ive's slotted instrument must be inserted four times so that each quadrant can be examined. Allowing it to remain in place for a minute or two allows any hemorrhoids that are present to engorge with blood and be more readily visible. Do not rotate this instrument, since it causes discomfort.

10. If a biopsy specimen is to be obtained, a variety of long-handled biopsy instruments can be used. The instruments used for cervical biopsy work well. The clinician can also use the biopsy forceps—normally used for flexible sigmoidoscopy. In this case it is applied with direct visualization of the areas. Expect some bleeding, but it is usually readily controlled with Monsel's or silver nitrate and natural pressure

when the scope is removed. Stay superficial; only 3 or 4 mm of tissue is necessary.
11. Complete the procedure form (Fig. 100-3).

COMPLICATIONS

Anoscopy, when performed gently, has few complications. Likely or possible complications include discomfort, tearing of the perianal skin or mucosa, and abrasion or tearing of hemorrhoidal tissue. There may be bleeding after biopsy, but infection almost never occurs.

POSTPROCEDURE PATIENT EDUCATION

Thoroughly explain the findings to the patient, and use pictures and drawings in the explanation. Discuss the etiology, treatment, and course of resolution of each finding as thoroughly as possible.

CPT/BILLING CODES

46600	Anoscopy, diagnostic
46604	Anoscopy with dilation
46606	Anoscopy with biopsy, single or multiple
46608	Anoscopy with removal of foreign body
46610	Anoscopy with polypectomy, hot or bipolar forceps
46611	Anoscopy with polypectomy, snare technique
46614	Anoscopy with control of bleeding
46615	Anoscopy with ablation of tumor(s), polyp(s), or other lesion(s)
46900	Destruction, lesions (e.g., condy), chem
46910	Destruction, lesions, electrodesiccation
46916	Destruction, lesions, cryocautery
46917	Destruction, lesions, laser
46922	Destruction, lesions, excision

See also the CPT billing codes for Chapter 108, Office Treatment of Hemorrhoids.

ICD-9-CM DIAGNOSTIC CODES

154.1	Cancer, rectum
154.2	Cancer, anus
211.4	Benign neoplasm, colon
455.0	Int. hemorrhoids
455.1	Int. hem, thrombosed
455.2	Int. hem, bleeding
455.3	Ext. hemorrhoid
455.9	Hemorrhoidal skin tags
555.1	Crohn's disease: colon
556.9	Ulcerative colitis
558.1	Radiation colitis
558.9	Colitis, nonspecific
564.0	Constipation
564.1	Irritable colon
565.0	Anal fissure
565.1	Fistula
566.0	Perirectal abscess
566.0	Perianal abscess
566.0	Ischiorectal abscess
566.0	Intersphincteric abscess
569.0	Anal polyp
569.3	Anal hemorrhage
569.42	Anal pain
698.0	Pruritus ani
787.6	Stool incontinence
787.99	Tenesmus
937.0	Foreign body, anus

		Malignant				
	Primary	Secondary	Ca in situ	Benign	Uncertain behavior	Unspecified
Anus	173.5	198.2	232.5	216.5	238.2	239.2
Gluteal region	173.5	198.2	232.5	216.5	238.2	239.2
Perianal	173.5	198.2	232.5	216.5	238.2	239.2

CHAPTER 101

Colonoscopy

John Bartels Pope

Colonoscopy is a procedure that allows for visual inspection of the entire large bowel from the distal rectum to the cecum. The procedure is generally well accepted by patients and, in the proper hands, is a safe and effective means of examining the large bowel. A well-trained endoscopist can generally perform a total colonoscopy in 30 to 45 minutes in greater than 90% of attempted procedures.

Colonoscopy has a greater sensitivity and specificity for the detection of colonic polyps and colorectal cancers (CRC) than air contrast barium enema. Colonoscopy is the procedure of choice in the workup of most cases of lower gastrointestinal bleeding. Another significant advantage of colonoscopy over radiologic evaluation of the large intestine is the ability to perform additional diagnostic and therapeutic measures, such as biopsy, polypectomy, and control of bleeding. Although traditionally performed in the hospital, colonoscopy can also be performed in freestanding offices or in ambulatory endoscopy centers.

It is widely accepted that the vast majority of colon cancers arise from adenomatous (neoplastic) polyps. It has been shown that the removal of adenomatous polyps by colonoscopic polypectomy can reduce the incidence of colorectal cancer by 76% to 90%. Colonoscopy then provides an opportunity to greatly influence the incidence of colorectal cancer by allowing the removal of polyps throughout the entire colon.

INDICATIONS

Diagnostic Indications

- Total colon evaluation after the finding of adenomatous polyps, especially high-risk polyps (i.e., those larger than 1 cm, small polyps with advanced histopathology, or multiple small adenomatous polyps) during flexible sigmoidoscopy
- Evaluation of abnormal or equivocal barium enema
- Evaluation of overt or occult colonic or rectal bleeding

- Evaluation of iron deficiency anemia of undetermined cause
- Surveillance of neoplastic disease after removal of polyps or cancer
- Screening for neoplastic disease in patients with family history of colorectal cancer or adenomatous (neoplastic) polyps before age 60; screening should begin at 40 years of age or 10 years before the age of discovery in relative
- Screening and surveillance for neoplastic disease in hereditary cancer syndromes:
  - Familial adenomatous polyposis syndrome (FAP) (should begin flexible sigmoidoscopy or colonoscopy at puberty). Thousands of polyps occur.
  - Hereditary nonpolyposis colon cancer syndrome (HNPCC) (should begin colonoscopy at age 21). HNPCC is defined as CRC in three or more family members, two of whom are first-degree relatives of the third, with at least two generations involved and at least one person diagnosed with CRC at less than 50 years of age. Use of the term "nonpolyposis" is a misnomer. Polyps do indeed occur in HNPNCC; it is just not to the extent seen with FAP.
- Evaluation and surveillance of inflammatory bowel disease (after 8 years in pancolitis and after 12 years in left-sided colitis)
- Evaluation of chronic diarrhea of undetermined cause
- Intraoperative evaluation of polypectomy site, bleeding lesions, or anastomotic leaks
- Endosonography for local staging (primary tumor, regional nodes, and metastasis [TNM]) of colorectal cancer
- Screening in average-risk population (controversial)
- Evaluation of significant weight loss
- Evaluation of abdominal pain

Note: Colonoscopy is often of little benefit in determining the causes of chronic lower abdominal pain, changes in bowel movements without rectal bleeding, weight loss, and anorexia.

Therapeutic Indications

- Biopsy of suspected lesion
- Polypectomy
- Therapy of bleeding lesions
- Removal of foreign body
- Reduction of sigmoid volvulus
- Decompression of pseudo-obstruction of colon
- Dilation of colonic strictures
- Laser therapy of lesions

CONTRAINDICATIONS

- Acute abdomen
- Suspected peritonitis
- Significant pelvic or abdominal adhesions
- Acute diverticulitis with systemic symptoms
- Acute exacerbation of inflammatory bowel disease
- Suspected bowel perforation
- Unstable cardiopulmonary status
- Recent myocardial infarction or pulmonary embolism
- Blood coagulation abnormalities
- Recent (within 1 week) bowel surgery
- Hyperplastic polyps on flexible sigmoidoscopy with no other indication
- Poorly prepped patient if electrocautery is to be used
- Uncooperative patient
- Metastatic adenocarcinoma of unknown primary site in the absence of colonic symptoms when it will not influence management

Note: Again, colonoscopy is often of little benefit in determining the causes of chronic lower abdominal pain, changes in bowel movements without rectal bleeding, weight loss, and anorexia.

EQUIPMENT

Basic equipment necessary to perform colonoscopy includes the following:
- Fiberoptic colonoscope
- Light source (i.e., halogen or xenon)
- Suction apparatus
- Biopsy forceps
- Snares
- Electrocautery unit
- Conscious-sedation setup

Additional instruments that may also be useful include injection needle catheter, heater probe or multipolar cautery, polyp retrieval baskets, and three-prong grasping forceps. Lubricating jelly, gauze pads, saline, sterile water, protective gowns, and eyewear are also recommended.

The colonoscope is similar to that described for flexible sigmoidoscopy, only longer. The outside diameter of the tube varies from 10 to 13 mm, and the length of the shaft varies from 105 to 185 cm. The scopes have an eyepiece with focusing controls; control wheels to deflect the tip through a range of positions, including deflection over 180 degrees; a biopsy port; suction and air and water control knobs; and locking levers to fix control wheels in a particular position (see Chapter 104, Flexible Sigmoidoscopy).

Most colonoscopies are now performed with video endoscopes. Videoscopes are fiberoptic devices; however, they use a charged coupled device (CCD) to convert light energy into electronic signals that can be converted by a computer processor into images. Videoscopes provide recording capability of entire procedures, and they also allow transmission of images to remote sites. Videoscopes also provide for a more comfortable posture for the endoscopist during the procedure. Videoendoscopy setups are significantly more expensive than conventional setups.

Cleaning and disinfecting the instrument and equipment is very important to prevent iatrogenic infections. Strict adherence to appropriate cleaning protocols virtually eliminates these risks. The American Society of Gastrointestinal Endoscopy (ASGE) provides practice guidelines for infection control during gastrointestinal endoscopy. Company representatives also provide excellent guidelines and videotapes demonstrating the process.

PREPROCEDURE PATIENT PREPARATION

Informed consent is a necessary component of colonoscopy. (See the sample patient consent form titled "Colonoscopy, Biopsy, and Polypectomy" on page 1863 of Appendix G.) Consent should be obtained by the physician and should include discussion of the nature of the procedure (how it is performed), expected benefits of the procedure, risks of the procedure (including sedation, procedure complications, and possibility of missed lesions), and alternatives to the procedure. The consent process may be facilitated with the use of procedure videotapes or written materials available from various organizations (e.g., American Society of Gastrointestinal Endoscopy, Society of American Gastrointestinal Endoscopic Surgeons). See the sample patient education handouts titled "Colonoscopy" and "Colonoscopy Preparation" on pages 1860 and 1862, respectively, of Appendix G.

A focused history should be obtained before the procedure to ensure that an appropriate indication exists for the procedure and to identify factors that may influence safe and effective performance of the procedure and subsequent management of the patient. Pertinent history should include present illness, past medical and surgical history (hysterectomy or abdominal surgeries may increase intubation difficulty), current medications, allergies, and tobacco and alcohol use. The patient should also be asked about any previous complications from anesthesia, as well as any history of coagulation abnormalities or chronic use of narcotics or tranquilizers (which may influence the ability to properly sedate) (Fig. 101-1). (See the sample patient education handout titled "Anesthesia for Colonoscopy" on page 1859 of Appendix G.)

Physical examination should include (as a minimum) assessment of vital signs and sensorium, and heart, lung, and abdominal examination.

Laboratory testing is not routinely performed before colonoscopy; however, in specific circumstances testing may be warranted (e.g., severe anemia with anticipation of polypectomy, known fluid and electrolyte abnormality).

A clean bowel is essential for colonoscopy. Three of the most common and effective preparations for cleansing the bowel include the following:

1. Polyethylene glycol (PEG) solution (4 L) taken orally (COLYTE, GOLYTELY) over a 1- to 3-hour period
2. Magnesium citrate solution (10 oz) taken with four bisacodyl tablets (5 mg)
3. Fleet Phospho-Soda (1.5 oz) added to 4 oz of water, followed by three 8 fl oz portions of clear liquids (process repeated 3 hours before procedure)

One of the previously mentioned bowel preparations should be administered starting at 4 pm the day before colonoscopy. After the preparation the patient can only have clear liquids until midnight, then NPO. One or two tap water enemas administered 1 or 2 hours before the procedure may also be helpful. In some instances it is necessary to place the patient on a liquid diet for 1 to 2 days before the procedure to achieve adequate bowel preparation.

It is important for the clinician to individualize the preparation for each patient and to take time to explain the reasons for the bowel-cleansing preparation. Patients undergoing drug therapy with certain medications (e.g., insulin, sulfonylureas, ferrous sulfate) may require special adjustments. If patients are chronically dependent on laxatives, it is advisable to continue those medicines in addition to the particular cleansing preparation chosen for that patient. Optimal examination may be better accomplished if the patient has received an electrolytic purgative solution; however, many physicians claim "less is best." Electrolytic purgative solutions may be more palatable when taken chilled or mixed with a sugar-free drink mix (red-colored mixes should be avoided). A new colon-cleansing preparation, sodium phosphate monobasic monohydrate and sodium phosphate dibasic anhy-

drous (Visicol), is available for patients unable to tolerate the taste of PEG solutions. Forty tablets are taken orally over a 2-day period in concert with copious quantities of water. Caution should be used when administering this prep to patients with renal insufficiency, ascites, or congestive heart failure.

Bowel cleansing is essential, not only to provide an unobstructed view, but also to eliminate all methane gas, which can literally explode should cautery by used during polypectomy or to stop bleeding.

ANTIBIOTIC PROPHYLAXIS

The Standards of Training and Practice Committee of the ASGE has developed practice guidelines for the use of antibiotic prophylaxis in gastrointestinal endoscopy. Antibiotic prophylaxis should be considered only for high-risk groups, as listed in Table 101-1, and only in those endoscopic procedures with increased risk of transient bacteremia, which *does not* include colonoscopy with or without biopsy or polypectomy. Although data recommending routine prophylaxis for patients at "high risk" for infective endocarditis are insufficient, the decision about antibiotic prophylaxis must be made by the individual physician and must take into account the circumstances presented by the individual patient. If there is any doubt about prophylaxis, the clinician should seek appropriate cardiology consultation. There are several antibiotic prophylaxis regimens for endoscopic procedures (Table 101-2). Further information can also be found in Chapter 204, Antibiotic Prophylaxis.

ANTICOAGULATION

The Standards of Training and Practice Committee of the ASGE has developed practice guidelines for the use of colonoscopy in conjunction with anticoagulated patients. Management is determined by establishing risk of bleeding versus risk of thromboembolic events. Colonoscopy with polypectomy is considered a high-risk procedure for bleeding. Conditions considered high risk for thromboembolic events are chronic atrial fibrillation with associated valvular heart disease, mechanical valve in the mitral position, and mechanical valve and prior thromboembolic event. High-risk procedures (i.e., colonoscopy with polypectomy) performed in high-risk conditions should be managed by discontinuing warfarin 3 to 5 days before the procedure. Consider heparin while international normalized ratio is below therapeutic level. Low-risk conditions require only discontinuation of warfarin 3 to 5 days before the procedure without use of heparin. The ASGE no longer considers recent aspirin or NSAID use a contraindication to colonoscopy with

Colonoscopy, Biopsy, and Polypectomy

Name: _____ DOB _____ Age _____
Telephone (H) _____ (W) _____
Your referring doctor: _____
Primary care doctor: _____ Want a copy sent to him/her?   Y   N
Blood pressure: _____ Received, read, and understood handouts?   Y   N

SYMPTOMS/HISTORY:
Reason for consult: _____
787.99 Change in stools
285.9 Anemia, NOS
578.9 Blood
783.2 Weight loss
455.6 Hemorrhoids, NOS
780.9 Chills
Frequency _____ daily _____ weekly
Pain: 780.9 Abdomen   Where? _____
           569.42 Rectum
                  w/BM

564.0   Constipation
780.6   Fevers
578.1   Black stools
562.11 Diverticulitis/diverticulosis
787.91 Diarrhea
211.3   Polyps
V10.05 Personal Hx colon Ca
V16.0   Family Hx Colon Ca
           Who? _____
           Age _____

Hemoccults: Date _____ Neg   Pos   Not done
Previous sigmoid: Date _____ Who? _____ OR findings: _____
Findings: _____
_____

Previous barium enema: Date _____ Findings _____
Previous abdominal surgery: _____
Hysterectomy (for women)   Y   N

PMH:
Bleeding problems   Coronary artery disease
Artificial joints   Heart murmur needing prophylaxis
Artificial heart valve   COPD
Asthma   Smoker _____ PPD × _____ years
Other medical problems: 1. _____   2. _____
                         3. _____   4. _____
Medications _____
Allergies _____

OBJECTIVE:
General:
Neck:
Lungs:
Cor:
Abd:

IMPRESSION: _____
_____
_____

COUNSELING:
Indications
Sedation
Bowel prep   Mag Citrate-Dulcolax-Fleets or GoLYTELY
Alternatives   Not performing examination/flex sig and ACBE
Risks   Bleeding
               Perforation
               Infection
               Need for hospitalization
               Sedation related
Expected results
Monitoring: BP Pulse Oxygen concentration

RECOMMENDATIONS:
1. Mag Citrate-Dulcolax-Fleets bowel prep or GoLYTELY bowel prep
2. Driver when receiving sedation
3. Sedation type   IV _____ oral _____
4. _____
5. _____

_____   _____
Physician   Date

Fig. 101-1
Sample patient counseling form for colonoscopy, biopsy, and polypectomy.

TABLE 101-1

Risk of Infection from Colonoscopy

Condition	Risk
Cardiac Conditions*	
History of endocarditis	High
Surgically constructed systemic pulmonary shunts or conduits	High
Prostheses	
Prosthetic cardiac valves, including bioprosthetic and homograft valves	High
Vascular graft material:	
First year	High
After first year	Low
Orthopedic prosthesis	Low
Central nervous system ventricular shunts	Low
Penile prosthesis	Low
Intraocular lens	Low
Pacemaker	Low
Local tissue augmentation material	Low

*The American Heart Association does not generally recommend preendoscopy prophylaxis for most congenital cardiac malformations, rheumatic and other acquired valvular dysfunction (even after valvular surgery), hypertrophic cardiomyopathy, or mitral valve prolapse with valvular regurgitation.

TABLE 101-2

Antibiotic Prophylaxis Regimens

Drug	Preprocedure Dose	Postprocedure Dose
Ampicillin	2 g IV or IM	
Gentamicin	1.5 mg/kg (up to 60 mg) IV (over 1 hr) or IM	
Amoxicillin		1.5 g PO 8 hr later
Vancomycin*	1 g IV over 1 hr	Repeat initial doses 8 hr later
Gentamicin	1.5 mg/kg (up to 80 mg)	
Amoxicillin†	3 g PO	1.5 g PO 6 hr later

Also see Chapter 204, Antibiotic Prophylaxis.
*For penicillin allergy.
†For low-risk groups.

polypectomy in the absence of a preexisting bleeding disorder.

An alternative is to use "bridge anticoagulation" with low-molecular-weight heparin. See Pearl no. 52 of Appendix I.

SEDATION

Most colonoscopic examinations are performed while the patient is under conscious sedation (see Chapter 2, Conscious Sedation [Sedation and Analgesia]). Sedation may allow for a more thorough examination of the colon because of increased patient comfort and decreased anxiety. Appropriate equipment must be available to monitor blood pressure, pulse, and respiration. A pulse oximeter is now commonly used to monitor oxygen saturation as well. During colonoscopy, it is mandatory to have an assistant available to monitor the patient. Intravenous (IV) access should be established and maintained during the entire procedure in patients receiving IV sedation. However, some physicians who use a colonoscope have reported the ability to reach the cecum in 25% to 30% of nonsedated patients during routine flexible sigmoidoscopy screens.

Benzodiazepines are the drugs most commonly used for sedation: midazolam (Versed) 2 to 5 mg or diazepam (Valium) 5 to 10 mg. Meperidine 25 to 50 mg is often used in conjunction with benzodiazepines to achieve optimal sedation. These medications should be administered slowly through the IV route. Dangerous side effects can be reversed with flumazenil (Romazicon) or naloxone (Narcan), although properly titrating these medications will minimize the need for these drugs. Endoscopists should be thoroughly familiar with the pharmacology of all these drugs. Further discussion is found in Chapter 102, Esophagogastroduodenoscopy, and Chapter 2, Conscious Sedation [Sedation and Analgesia].

A crash cart should be immediately available in case of cardiopulmonary arrest. See Chapter 203, Anaphylaxis, and the discussion regarding Banyan kits.

TECHNIQUE

Colonoscopy

The procedure for colonoscopy is as follows (also see Chapter 104, Flexible Sigmoidoscopy):

1. Place the patient on the examining table in the left lateral decubitus position.
2. Check all of the equipment for proper functioning.
3. After appropriately sedating the patient, perform a digital anorectal examination with a well-lubricated, gloved examining finger. Lubricate the shaft of the colonoscope and gently insert its tip into the anal canal. The lumen of the bowel should be directly visualized at all times during the colonoscopy procedure.
4. Insufflate air into the rectum until the lumen becomes readily apparent. The three "valves" of Houston (i.e., prominent mucosal folds) are often seen as consistent landmarks. The plexus of blood vessels is usually very apparent in the rectal mucosa (Fig. 101-2). The scope can generally be advanced without difficulty as far as the rectosigmoid junction at 15 to 18 cm.
5. Enter the sigmoid colon by passing the scope through the rectosigmoid angle. The sigmoid colon is the most common site of difficulty in passage of the instrument. There may be fixation of the bowel

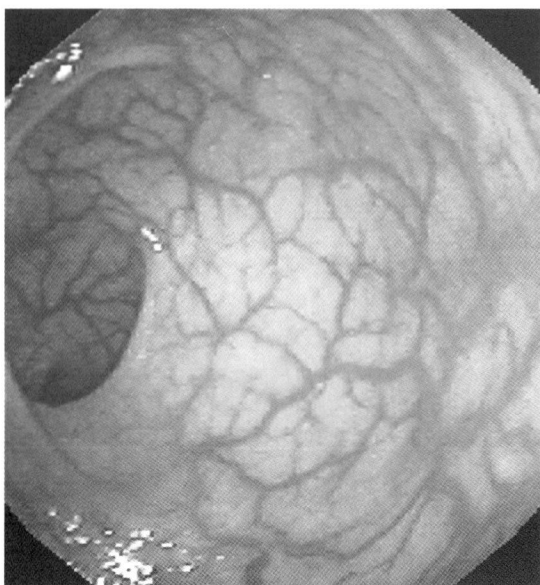

Fig. 101-2
Endoscopic view of hemorrhoidal plexus of blood vessels in normal rectum mucosa.

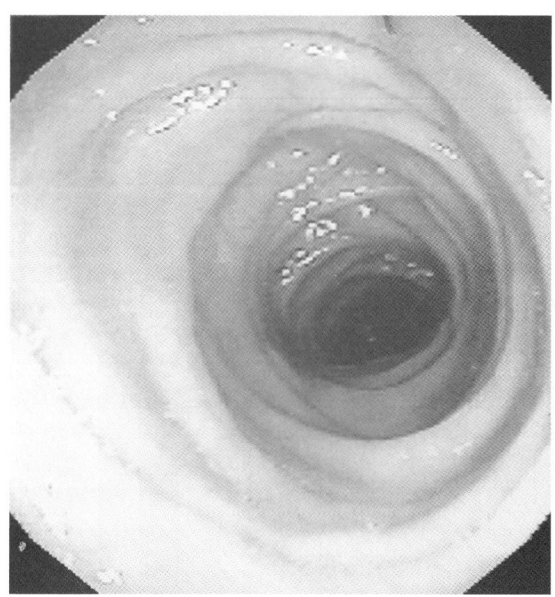

Fig. 101-3
Endoscopic view of descending colon.

from diverticular disease or adhesions from prior surgery, including a hysterectomy. The sigmoid colon is the most common site of perforation during colonoscopy. Successful passage through the sigmoid colon may require a series of maneuvers including torquing to the right and withdrawing the scope to reduce loops, applying abdominal pressure, repositioning the patient (even into a supine position), or deflating the lumen of excess air. An essential but difficult lesson to learn is that when passage of the scope is impeded, torque to the right and *withdraw* the scope to straighten out the bowel.

6. The descending colon can be recognized by a relatively straight passage through the circular-shaped bowel (Fig. 101-3) to the splenic flexure. Transversing the angle of the splenic flexure may resemble transversing the rectosigmoid junction. The transverse colon can be recognized by its characteristic triangular appearance (Fig. 101-4), and it generally has a fairly straight configuration. The hepatic flexure is often recognizable by the "liver shadow" (Fig. 101-5), which appears as a bluish-brown area where the liver is in direct contact with the bowel wall. The hepatic flexure is seen as another angle to traverse with the scope. The ascending colon may also appear triangular.

7. Advance the scope into the cecum by pulling back, keeping the tip of the scope in the center of the lumen, and applying full suction. The cecal landmarks, which may or may not be prominent, include the ileocecal valve (Fig. 101-6) and the appendiceal orifice (Fig. 101-7). Convergence of the terminal

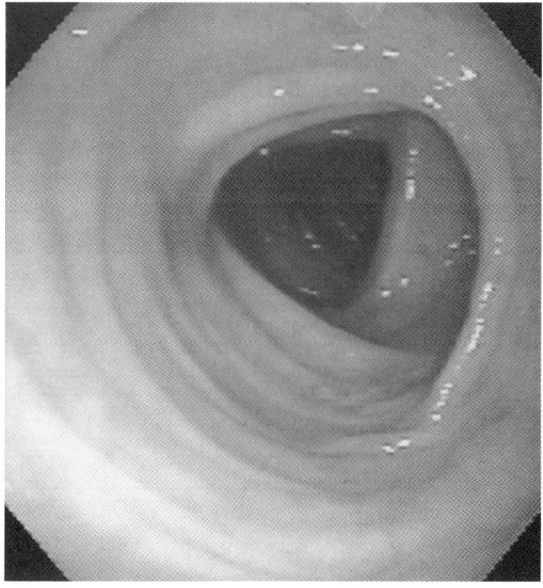

Fig. 101-4
Endoscopic view of transverse colon.

portion of the taenia coli in the cecum forms a characteristic appearance known as the "crow's foot" (Fig. 101-6). Other methods to ascertain if the cecum has been reached are to check for ballottement externally above the right inguinal canal or for transillumination in the right lower quadrant (less consistent findings).

8. Intubate the terminal ileum by advancing the tip just beyond the ileocecal valve and then deflecting the tip toward the valve as the scope is carefully withdrawn. As the tip of the scope meets the valve

3

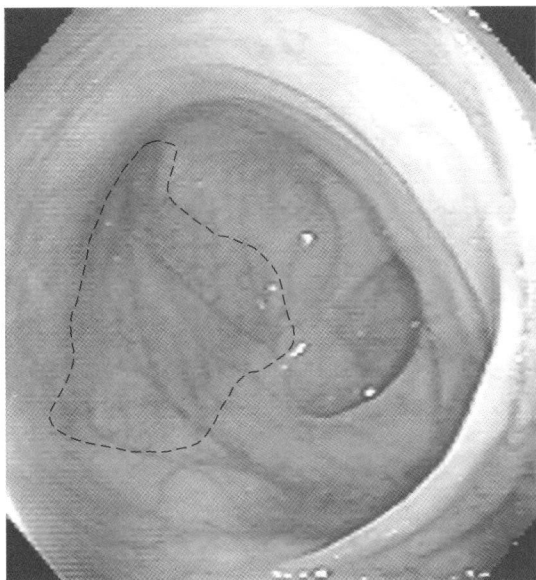

Fig. 101-5
Endoscopic view of hepatic flexure. The characteristic liver shadow is outlined here by the dashed line.

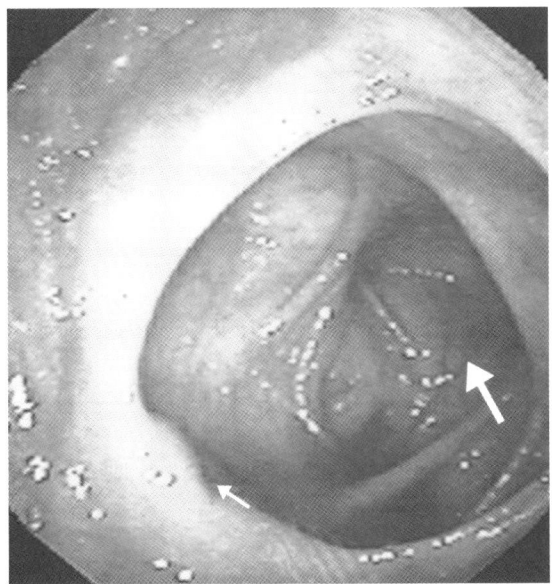

Fig. 101-6
Endoscopic view of ileocecal valve *(small white arrow)* and "crow's foot" *(large white arrow)* in cecum.

opening, torque the scope gently to allow the tip to advance briefly into the terminal ileum.

9. Carefully inspect the colon wall as the scope is withdrawn. Use a circular motion of the tip to inspect behind every mucosal fold. Lavage with water any areas of the bowel with inadequate preparation and carefully reinspect. Obtain any necessary biopsy specimens and remove polyps during this portion of the procedure.

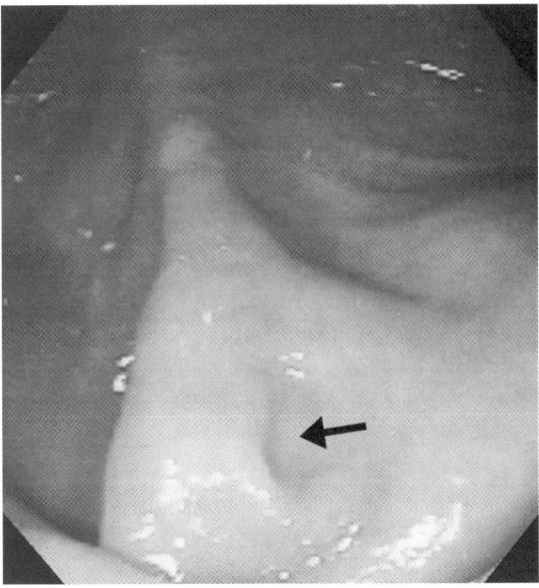

Fig. 101-7
Endoscopic view of appendiceal orifice *(arrow)*.

10. Inspect the distal rectum and anorectal junction before completely withdrawing the scope. As the tip of the scope passes the dentate line, reinsert the scope approximately 5 to 10 cm while simultaneously rotating both control wheels counterclockwise to completely deflect the tip back upon itself (retroflexion or turn around maneuver). Torque the shaft to inspect all around the anorectal junction. Alternatively, use an anoscope (Ive's slotted anoscope recommended) to complete the examination of this area.

General principles for safe and efficient intubation of the colon to the cecum include the following:
- Minimize air insufflation.
- Keep the instrument straight.
- Avoid loop formation (pull back frequently).
- Avoid advancing the scope blindly (i.e., slide-by technique) when at all possible.
- Do not oversedate the patient more than is necessary.

Polypectomy

Polyps may be sessile (i.e. broad-based polyps) or pedunculated (i.e., with a stalk) (Figs. 101-8 and 101-9). Pedunculated polyps are much more easily removed with the electrocautery snare, and the risk of perforation and bleeding is less than with a sessile polyp. The patient experiences no pain with polypectomy.

The procedure for polypectomy is as follows:
1. Position the scope so that the polyp can be visualized approximately 2 to 3 cm beyond the tip of the colonoscope. Positioning the polyp at the 5 o'clock

position where the port for the electrocautery snare exits can be helpful for biopsy and polypectomy.

2. Under direct vision at all times, pass the electrocautery snare through the colonoscope port. Position the tip of the sheath of the snare near the polyp, advance the wire loop, and open it, always under direct vision. Manipulate the snare and maneuver the tip of the colonoscope to place the snare around the polyp. Slowly secure the wire loop around the pedicle or polyp base. Maneuver the colonoscope to draw the polyp and snare away from the bowel wall to avoid excess burn injury and possible perforation.

3. Apply the electrocautery current (coagulation only) until a white eschar forms around the polyp stalk. Use the least amount of current necessary to achieve the eschar in 2 to 3 seconds (amount varies with each electrocautery unit). Tighten the snare as coagulation continues until the stalk is transected. (Thorough bowel prep is mandatory because residual gas in the colon could cause an explosion with the use of electrocautery.)

4. Retrieve the excised polyp using suction or forceps. At times this may require removal and reinsertion of the entire colonoscope. Unretrieved polyps may occasionally need to be retrieved later by straining stools after further bowel preparation solutions and cathartics are given. Large polyps may require multiple snare-resection excisions. Tissue desiccation without prior biopsy should be avoided because it is very important to have pathologic diagnosis of all colonic lesions.

5. Cancerous polyps do not need further resections if the tumor is well differentiated, if there is no lymphatic or vascular invasion, and if there is at least 2 mm between the tumor and the line of resection. With an obvious advanced colon cancer that is friable or ulcerated, biopsies will usually provide sufficient tissue for diagnosis. However, because only tiny samples can be obtained, the cancer may occasionally be missed and the specimens only reveal benign adenomatous tissue. If a strong clinical suspicion of cancer exists, the lesion should be reexamined and rebiopsied.

After colonoscopy, monitor the patient (i.e., clinical assessment, blood pressure, pulse, oxygen saturation) for at least 30 minutes and until a return to baseline cognitive function has occurred. Explain the results of the procedure to the patient, including the treatment plan

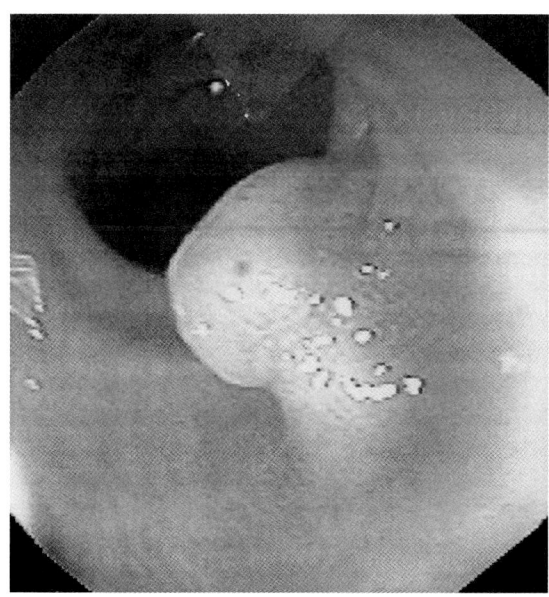

Fig. 101-8
Endoscopic view of sessile polyp.

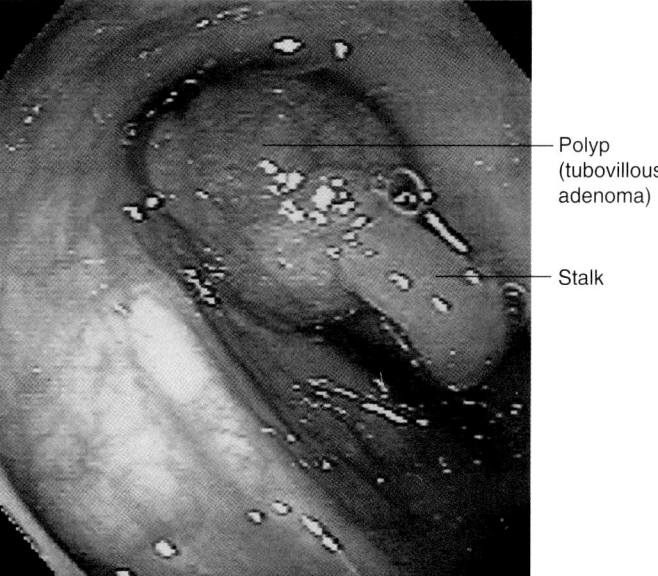

Polyp
(tubovillous
adenoma)

Stalk

Fig. 101-9
Endoscopic view of pedunculated polyp.

and follow-up appointments. Patients may resume a normal diet upon discharge even when polypectomy has been performed. Clearly explain precautions concerning possible delayed bleeding or unrecognized perforation when clinically indicated.

A well-documented procedure note is essential. It can be dictated (Fig. 101-10) or detailed in a routine form (Fig. 101-11).

COMPLICATIONS

Complications occur infrequently with diagnostic colonoscopy and only slightly more frequently with therapeutic colonoscopy. Major complications include the following:

- Cardiopulmonary over 60% related to sedation and medications used

---

Procedure: Colonoscopy
Equipment: Olympus Colonoscope
Pre-op diagnosis: History of previous colon polyps
Post-op diagnosis: Diminutive polyp
Endoscopist:
Assistant:

HPI:
Patient is a 71-year-old African-American male who was seen by Dr. Smith on 6-26-2001 and scheduled for screening colonoscopy. The patient was asymptomatic at the time. The patient had a history of colonic polyps dating back to 1996. The patient was found on that colonoscopy to have a colonic polyp reported as an adenoma by pathology report. Patient was recommended at that time to have a repeat colonoscopy in one year. The patient denied any history of colon cancer. Patient had no iron-deficiency anemia. Patient received one gallon of GoLYTELY yesterday, and the patient was NPO for the procedure today.

Informed consent was obtained from the patient after a full discussion of the risks, benefits and alternatives to the procedure. Patient was also advised of the risk of missed lesions with this procedure. He expressed an understanding of these issues and desired to continue with the colonoscopy. All questions were answered.

Medications: Conscious sedation was obtained with 50 mg of Demerol IV push with Versed 1 mg IV push. Conscious sedation was maintained throughout the procedure.

After conscious sedation was obtained, the patient was placed in the left lateral position. Digital rectal examination was performed, which showed normal sphincter tone, no masses, no external hemorrhoids. Prostate gland was not enlarged. After rectal examination was performed, the regular colonoscope was introduced via the anus and advanced inside the colon into the cecum. The procedure was difficult as a result of redundancies of the colon. External compressions of the abdomen and multiple changes in the position of the patient were required throughout the procedure in order to advance into the cecum. The bowel preparation was adequate. The extent of the exam was to the cecum. The cecum was identified by the ileal-cecal valve and appendiceal orifice was clearly visualized. After reaching the cecum, the scope was slowly withdrawn with careful inspection of all aspects of the colon in a circular fashion. Retroflexion was performed inside the rectum before completely straightening the scope, and the scope was subsequently removed from the patient. Patient was transported to recovery area and monitored for 30 minutes until return to baseline state was observed.

Complications: None

Findings: There was a diminutive polyp approximately 3 mm in size in the ascending colon that was removed with cold-force biopsy forceps. The colonic mucosa was otherwise normal. Neither diverticula nor internal hemorrhoids were seen.

Impression: Diminutive polyp

Recommendation: Given the small size of this polyp and patient's previous history, I would recommend that the patient repeat colonoscopy in 5-10 years. Other methods of colon cancer screening would not be necessary over this 10-year period (i.e., no need for checking fecal occult blood test). Patient will return to the primary care doctor for follow-up, and I have ordered Metamucil, 1 Tbsp mixed with a glass of water once a day for constipation. This can be increased to twice a day if needed.

Fig. 101-10
Sample procedure note for colonoscopy.

Procedure Note
Date:
Patient Name:
Identification Number:
Procedure:
Equipment:

Pre-op diagnosis:

Post-op diagnosis:

Endoscopist:

Assistant:

HPI:

Informed consent:

Medications:

Procedure:

Complications:

Findings:

Impression:

Recommendations:

Signature

Fig. 101-11
Sample procedure form for colonoscopy.

— Vasovagal reactions (i.e., hypotension, brady-cardia)
— Arrhythmias (including ventricular tachycardia and fibrillation)
— Myocardial infarction
• Colon perforation
• Postpolypectomy bleeding
• Postpolypectomy syndrome

• Missed lesions
• Painful experience for patient

Other rare complications include the following:
• Preparation complications
— Aspiration
— Dehydration
— Hyperphosphatemia, hyponatremia

— Mallory-Weiss tears
— Toxic megacolon
- Infections without perforation
  — Bacteremia
  — Endocarditis
  — Joint infection
  — Scope transmission of infectious agent
- Sigmoid or cecal volvulus
- Splenic rupture
- Pancreatitis
- Diverticulitis
- Incarcerated snare or colonoscope

Perforation of the colon occurs at a rate of up to 0.8% (approximately) for diagnostic colonoscopy and 0.3% to 3% for therapeutic colonoscopy. Perforations can occur for a number of reasons but occur most commonly from excessive force of insertion of the endoscope tip or with the side of the scope during slide-by, loop formation, loop reduction, or advancement despite presence of fixating lesions. Other causes of perforation include rupture of diverticulum, rupture of stricture site, transmural injury with electrocautery current with subsequent perforation, or polypectomy- and biopsy-induced perforations. Perforations may also rarely occur from pneumatic rupture of the proximal colon.

Perforations are more common with patients who are oversedated or who are under general anesthesia. It is uncommon for the scope to actually penetrate the bowel, but this type of perforation is usually noticed immediately. More frequently the perforation is small and occurs away from the scope tip. It may go unrecognized until the patient later experiences abdominal pain, fever, and distention. A radiographic film of the abdomen or chest will show pneumoperitoneum. In the majority of perforations, immediate surgery is indicated. With fecal soiling a diverting colostomy is needed; however, in the absence of obvious contamination, primary closure may be sufficient. Perforation can occur even in experienced hands and does not per se imply negligence on the part of the endoscopist.

Bleeding from postcolonoscopy and postpolypectomy occurs in approximately 1 in 1000 procedures. Bleeding may occur immediately or up to 4 weeks postprocedure. Most cases of bleeding resolve spontaneously, but some may require repeat colonoscopy with attempts to coagulate the area (i.e., epinephrine injection followed by multipolar cautery or heater probe) or laparotomy. Avoiding aspirin prophylaxis for 10 days postpolypectomy may decrease late bleeding risk.

Postpolypectomy syndrome is caused by a transmural thermal injury (i.e., burn) resulting in full-thickness bowel necrosis, which may lead to serosal inflammation. Postpolypectomy syndrome may be accompanied by fever, leukocytosis, and localized and rebound tenderness over the polypectomy site without evidence of intraperitoneal air. A conservative approach generally leads to a good outcome.

Missed neoplastic lesions have been shown to occur even with "expert" endoscopists. In one study, colonoscopy detected 95% of all lesions present. Of the 5% missed, half were not appreciated because of inability to pass the scope far enough; however, in the other half, lesions were passed without being seen.

LEARNING COLONOSCOPY

For a basic overview of colonoscopy principles and technique, the reader is directed to Raskin and Nord's *Colonoscopy: Principles and Techniques.* Additional information on endoscopic technique is found in Coller's article, *Technique of Flexible Fiberoptic Sigmoidoscopy,* and in Chapter 9 of Shinya, *Colonoscopy: Diagnosis and Treatment of Colonic Diseases,* which contains excellent diagrams, photographs, tips, and techniques. The endoscopic anatomy of the various landmark locations of the colon and rectum is well described and illustrated in Chapter 8 of Shinya's text. Silverstein and Tytgat's *Atlas of Gastrointestinal Endoscopy* contains excellent photographs of colorectal pathology. For an in-depth review of colonoscopic polypectomy, see Chapter 15 in Shinya's textbook, Chapter 44 in Bauer's textbook, Chapter 3 in Gordon's textbook, and Chapter 5 in Corman's textbook, *Colon and Rectal Surgery.*

Before attempting to perform colonoscopy, it is useful to become proficient and skilled in flexible fiberoptic sigmoidoscopy. The instrument controls and techniques used for flexible sigmoidoscopy are identical to those used to perform colonoscopy. Formal courses are available to teach colonoscopy concepts, skills, and techniques through the American Academy of Family Practice (AAFP) (Phone: 1-800-274-2237) and the National Procedures Institute (Phone: 1-800-462-2492).

One method often used for obtaining colonoscopy skills in the postresidency environment is to form a teaching relationship with a proficient endoscopist willing to act as a preceptor until adequate proficiency is obtained. Performance of colonoscopy can be mastered without fellowship training. Studies show that high-quality care and complication rates essentially identical to fellowship-trained gastroenterologists can be attained (Hopper, Kyler, Rodney, 1996), and that physician assistants may also become qualified to perform colonoscopy (Lieberman and Ghormley, 1992). The AAFP has published a position paper on family physicians performing colonoscopy. It can be found on the organization's website (www.AAFP.org/policy/issues/c-colonoscopyposition.html) and includes guide-

BOX 101-1

Overview of Colonoscopy Privileges

From American Academy of Family Physicians Position Paper

- "It is the position of the American Academy of Family Physicians (AAFP) that clinical privileges should be based on the individual physician's documented training and/or experience, demonstrated abilities and current competence, and not on the physician's specialty."
- More than 1440 family physicians across the United States perform colonoscopy in the hospital setting.
- In the 1998 AAFP Practice Profile Survey, 1163 family physicians reported performing colonoscopy in their offices.
- Twenty-six percent of family practice residencies provide training in colonoscopy.
- "Skills for performing colonoscopy are most often acquired during three years of family practice residency training. Another possible route to acquire colonoscopy skills is through preceptorship with a physician who already has such training and privileges. Established experience in flexible sigmoidoscopy examination is helpful in developing colonoscopy skills."
- "The American Society for Gastrointestinal Endoscopy (ASGE) recommends that physicians perform a minimum of 100 diagnostic colonoscopies and 20 snare polypectomies as a threshold for determining clinical competence. However, this recommendation was based on expert opinion, not scientific data."
- ". . . the AAFP strongly believes that all medical staff members should realize that there is overlap between specialties, and that no one department has exclusive rights to privileges."
- "A legal opinion on privileges for endoscopy submitted to the AAFP in 1993 stated the following:
  A. Hospitals and peer review participants risk liability under state law if they base credentialing decisions solely on whether or not a physician has obtained specialty certification.
  B. The Council on Ethical and Judicial Affairs of the AMA has issued the opinion that competitive factors must be disregarded in making decisions about credentials and privileges.
  C. There is no evidence that only board-certified gastroenterologists are qualified to perform endoscopic procedures.
  D. Hospitals violate the Medicare Conditions for Participation if they base credentialing decisions solely on specialty board certification.
  E. Hospitals and peer review participants risk loss of federal and state immunity from liability by basing credentialing decisions solely on whether or not a physician has obtained specialty certification."

From American Medical Association Clinical Privileges

- Regarding clinical privileges, the 1993 AMA Policy Compendium states, "The accordance and delineation of privileges should be determined on an individual basis, commensurate with an applicant's education, training and experience, and demonstrated current competence." It also states that "in implementing these criteria, each facility should formulate and apply reasonable nondiscriminatory standards for the evaluation of an applicant's credentials, free of anticompetitive intent or purpose."

From American Society of Gastrointestinal Endoscopy

- Competency is the minimum level of skill, knowledge, and/or expertise, attained through training and experience, required to perform a procedure safely and proficiently."
- "Departments often develop criteria for recommending privileges and, not surprisingly, these suggested criteria may vary significantly depending on the particular departmental discipline and whether the department represents mainly generalists or specialists."
- "Highly motivated family physicians or internists can acquire a level of training adequate to perform endoscopic examinations of high quality."

Information from the articles, Worthington DV: Colonoscopy: procedure skills, AAFP Position Paper, Amer Fam Phys 1:1177, 2000; American Medical Association: Clinical Privileges. In AMA Policy Compendium, Chicago, 1993, American Medical Association; and American Society of Gastrointestinal Endoscopy (ASGE): President's Message, October, 1999.

lines for establishing and maintaining proficiency and suggestions for obtaining privileges in colonoscopy.

Videotapes on endoscopy technique can be ordered from the ASGE's website (www.asge.org).

OBTAINING HOSPITAL PRIVILEGES

Most hospitals have credentialing standards regarding colonoscopy privileges. Hospitals vary widely in those standards but generally will require a minimum number of procedures and possible proctoring of applicants until competency is established. In general, credentialing becomes more restrictive where a high number of specialists perform colonoscopy in the hospital. It is advisable to carefully document all endoscopy experience and related experience and

provide a plan for continued medical education and quality assurance when applying for colonoscopy privileges.

See the AAFP Position Paper for further information. For articles that may assist in obtaining colonoscopy privileges, see the bibliography (Worthington DV, 2000; AMA, 1993; ASGE, 1999) (Box 101-1).

SUPPLIERS

Extensive marketing and technical information about colonoscopy equipment is readily available. When selecting a supplier, the clinician should consider local availability for education, equipment service, and technical support. It may be desirable to ask for local references from suppliers.

New equipment

Olympus Corp.
Medical Instrument Division
8370 Dow Circle
Strongsville, OH 44136
Phone: 1-800-627-6264
Website: www.olympusamerica.coma

Pentax Corp.
30 Ramland Road
Orangeburg, NY 10962
Phone: 1-800-431-5880
Website: www.pentaxmedical.com

Fujinon Corp.
10 High Point Drive
Wayne, NJ 07470
Phone: 973-633-5600
Website: www.fujinon.com

Used or refurbished equipment

Allegiance Equipment Management Services
1430 Waukegan Road
McGaw Park, IL 60085-6787
Phone: 1-800-726-7312
Website: www.allegiance.net

America's Endoscopy Corporation
24865 Five Mile Road, Suite 2
Redford, MI 48239
Phone: 1-800-845-8863

B-Met Endoscopic, Inc.
72 South Wyoming Avenue
Edwardsville, PA 18704
Phone: 1-877-498-2638

Corthel, Inc.
1202 Technology Drive
Aberdeen, MD 21001
Phone: 1-410-297-6512
Website: www.corthelinc.com

DunnAmics, Inc.
3502 Fairview Way
West Linn, OR 97068
Phone: 1-800-690-8824
Website: www.dunnamics.com

Endoscopy Support Services, Inc.
2 Fallsview Lane
Brewster, NY 10509
Phone: 1-845-277-1700
Website: www.endoscopy.com

Factory Authorized Medical Scope Repair, Inc.
2859 West McNab Road
Pompano Beach, FL 33069
Phone: 1-954-984-1844
Website: www.famsr.com

Fujinon, Inc.
10 High Point Drive
Wayne, NJ 07470
Phone: 1-973-633-5600
Website: www.fujinon.com

GE Medical Systems, Clinical Services
5020 Campbell Boulevard
Baltimore, MD 21236
Phone: 1-410-931-4411
Website: www.gemedicalsystems.com

Instrument Specialists, Inc.
32390 IH-10 West
Boeme, TX 78006
Phone: 1-800-537-1945
Website: 1-800-537-1945

Integrated Medical Systems, Inc.
1823 27th Avenue South
Birmingham, AL 35209
Phone: 1-800-783-9251
Website: www.imsservices.com

Karl Storz Endoscopy – America
600 Corporate Pointe
Culver City, CA 90230
Phone: 1-310-338-8100
Website: www.karlstorz.com

Matlock Endoscopic
2969 Armory Drive, Suite 400
Nashville, TN 37204
Phone: 1-800-394-9822
Website: www.matlockendo.com

Medical Optics
559 Sawgrass Corporate Parkway
Sunrise, FL 33325
Phone: 1-800-286-9542
Website: www.medicaloptics.com

Mobile Instrument Service
333 Water Avenue
Bellefontaine, OH 43311
Phone: 1-800-722-3675
Website: www.mobileinstrument.com

Nuell, Inc.
P.O. Box 55
Warsaw, IN 46581-0055
Phone: 1-800-829-7694
Website: www.nuell.com

Richard Wolf Medical Instruments
353 Corporate Woods Parkway
Vernon Hills, IL 60061-3110
Phone: 1-800-323-9653
Website: www.richardwolf.com

The Scope Exchange
4210 Tudor Lane
Greensboro, NC 27410
Phone: 1-888-299-3977
Website: www.scopex.com

SOS Medical
740 East Arrow Highway
Covina, CA 91722
Phone: 1-888-592-5550
Website: www.sos-medical.com

Spectrum Surgical Instruments
4575 Hudson Drive
Stow, OH 44224
Phone: 1-800-444-5644
Website: www.spectrumsurgical.com

Surgical Optics LLC
1900 Wyatt Drive, Suite 7
Santa Clara, CA 95054
Phone: 1-888-884-6887
Website: www.surgical-optics.com

Surgical Repair Technologies
930 Blue Gentian Road, Suite 1400
Eagan, MN 55121
Phone: 1-800-495-0297
Website: www.sohniks.com

United Endoscopy
10405 San Sevaine Way, Suite B
Mira Lorma, CA 91752-1150
Phone: 1-800-899-4847
Website: www.endoscope.com

Universal Endoscopic Services
6861 SW 196th Avenue, Suite 402
Pembroke Pines, FL 33332
Phone: 1-800-266-1464
Website: www.ues1.com

U.S. Medical Inc
4601 DTC Boulevard, 7th Floor
Denver, CO 80237
Phone: 1-800-607-7455

Used Medical Equipment and Devices Medline
278 S. Lincoln Street
Minster, OH 45865
Phone: 1-888-355-9692
Website: www.1-medical-equipment.com

Medical Replacement Parts LLC
6302 Manatee Avenue West, Suite F1
Bradenton, FL 34209
Phone: 1-800-363-6726
Website: www.endoscopepartsplus.com

CPT/BILLING CODES

45378 *	Colonoscopy beyond splenic flexure
45379 *	Colonoscopy with foreign body removal
45380 *	Colonoscopy with biopsy (single or multiple)
45382 *	Colonoscopy with control of bleeding (any method)
45383 *	Colonoscopy with ablation of tumor
45384 *	Colonoscopy with removal of lesion by hot forceps or bipolar cautery
45385 *	Colonoscopy with removal of lesion by snare technique
G0105	Screening colonoscopy in patients at high risk for CRC, if 23 months since last screening colonoscopy or barium enema (Medicare)

If colonoscopy is abnormal, the applicable CPT and ICD-9-CM codes (not G-codes) should be used. Conscious sedation is considered part of the colonoscopy and is not billed separately unless performed by a different provider.

In July 2001, Medicare began reimbursing for screening colonoscopy in patients 50 years old or older at average risk for CRC.

ICD-9-CM DIAGNOSTIC CODES

153.0	Ca, colon-hepatic flexure
153.1	Ca, colon-transverse
153.2	Ca, colon-descending
153.3	Ca, colon-sigmoid

*Health Care Financing Administration (HCFA) allows additional payment for a tray for this procedure when performed in a physician's office. Charge appropriately using code "99070—surgical tray."

153.4   Ca, colon-cecum
153.6   Ca, colon-ascending
154.1   Ca, rectum
211.3   Benign neoplasm, colon
211.4   Benign neoplasm, rectum-anus
455.0   Internal hemorrhoids
455.3   External hemorrhoids
555.1   Crohn's disease, colon
556.9   Ulcerative colitis
558.9   Colitis, nonspecific
562.1   Diverticulosis
562.12   Diverticulosis with hemorrhage
564.0   Unspecified constipation
564.5   Chronic diarrhea
569.84   Angiodysplasia
578.9   GI hemorrhage
787.6   Stool incontinence
789.0   Abdominal pain
793.4   Radiographic abnormality, GI tract
V76.51   Screening, cancer, colon (to be used with G-codes; see above)

ADDITIONAL RESOURCES

• See the sample patient education handouts titled "Anesthesia for Colonoscopy," "Colonoscopy," and "Colonoscopy Preparation" on pages 1859, 1860, and 1862, respectively, of Appendix G.

• See the sample patient consent forms titled "Colonoscopy, Biopsy, and Polypectomy" on page 1863 of Appendix G.

BIBLIOGRAPHY

Ackermann RJ: Performance of gastrointestinal tract endoscopy by primary care physicians: lessons from the US Medicare database, *Arch Fam Med* 6(1):52, 1997.

American Medical Association: *Clinical privileges*. In AMA policy compendium, Chicago, 1993, AMA.

American Society of Gastrointestinal Endoscopy (ASGE): *President's message*, October 1999.

American Society for Gastrointestinal Endoscopy (ASGE): *Standards of Training and Practice Committee: Antibiotic prophylaxis in endoscopy*, Pub No 1028, Manchester, Mass, 1995, ASGE.

American Society for Gastrointestinal Endoscopy (ASGE): *Standards of Training and Practice Committee: Guideline on the management of anticoagulation and antiplatelet therapy for endoscopic procedures*, Pub No 1029, Manchester, Mass, 1997, ASGE.

Atkin WS, Whynes DK: Improving the cost-effectiveness of colorectal cancer screening, *J Natl Cancer Inst* 92(7):513, 2000.

Bauer JJ: Colorectal surgery illustrated: a focused approach, St Louis, 1993, Mosby.

Bond JH et al: Polyp guideline: diagnosis, treatment, and surveillance for patients with colorectal polyps: Practice Parameters Committee of the American College of Gastroenterology, *Am J Gastroenterol* 95(11):3053, 2000.

Carr KW, Worthington JM, Rodney WM, et al: Advancing from flexible sigmoidoscopy to colonoscopy in rural family practice, *Tenn Med* 91(1):21, 1998.

Coller JA: Technique of flexible fiberoptic sigmoidoscopy, *Surg Clin North Am* 60(2):465, 1980.

Corman ML: *Colon and rectal surgery*, ed 4, Philadelphia, 1988, Lippincott, Williams & Wilkins.

Frazier AL, Colditz GA, Fuchs CS, Kuntz KM: Cost-effectiveness of screening for colorectal cancer in the general population, *JAMA* 284:1954, 2000.

Gordon PH, Nivatrongs S: *Principles and practice of surgery for the colon, rectum, and anus*, ed 2, St Louis, 1998, Quality Medical Publishing.

Harper MB, Pope JB, Mayeaux EJ: Colonoscopy experience at a family practice residency: a comparison to gastroenterology and general surgery services, *Fam Med* 29:575, 1997.

Hopper W, Kyker K, Rodney WM: Colonoscopy by a family physician: a 9-year experience of 1048 procedures, *J Fam Pract* 43(6):561, 1996.

Leard LE, Savides TJ, Ganiats TG: Patient preferences for colorectal cancer screening, *J Fam Pract* 45:211, 1997.

Lieberman DA, Ghormley JM: Physician assistants in gastroenterology: should they perform endoscopy? *Am J Gastroenterol* 87:940, 1992.

Lieberman DA, Weiss DG: One-time screening for colorectal cancer with combined fecal occult-blood testing and examination of the distal colon, *N Engl J Med* 345(8): 555, 2001.

Pierzchajlo RP, Ackermann RJ, Vogel RL: Colonoscopy performed by a family physician: a case series of 751 procedures, *J Fam Pract* 44(5):473, 1997.

Raskin JB, Nord HJ: *Colonoscopy: principles and techniques*, New York, 1995, IGAKU-SHOIN.

Reed DN, Collins JD, Wyatt WJ, et al: Can general surgeons perform colonoscopy safely? *Am J Surg* 163:257, 1992.

Rex DK, Johnson DA, Lieberman DA, et al: Colorectal cancer prevention 2000: screening recommendations of the American College of Gastroenterology, *Am J Gastroenterol* 95(4): 868, 2000.

Roetzheim RG, Pal N, Gonzalez EC, et al: The effects of physician supply on the early detection of colorectal cancer, *J Fam Pract* 48:850, 1999.

Shinya H: *Colonoscopy: diagnosis and treatment of colonic diseases*, New York, 1982, IGAKU-SHOIN.

Silverstein FE, Tytgat G: *Atlas of gastrointestinal endoscopy*, ed 3, London, 1997, Mosby.

Smith RA, von Eschenbach AC, Wender R, et al: American Cancer Society guidelines for the early detection of cancer: update of early detection guidelines for prostate, colorectal, and endometrial cancers. Also: update 2001—testing for early lung cancer detection, *CA Cancer J Clin* 51(1):38, 2001.

Volkers N: How can physicians define and improve procedural competency? *Ann Intern Med* 125(12):I39, 1996.

Worthington DV: Colonoscopy: procedural skills AAFP Position Paper, *Am Fam Physician* 1:1177, 2000.

For additional pertinent references, also see Chapter 2, Conscious Sedation (Sedation and Analgesia), and Chapter 104, Flexible Sigmoidoscopy.

WEBSITES

www.asge.org (American Society of Gastrointestinal Endoscopy)

www.gastro.org (American Gastroenterological Association)

www.sages.org (Society of American Gastrointestinal Endoscopic Surgeons)

www.acg.gi.org (American College of Gastroenterology)

www.gastroatlas.com (Feldman's GastroAtlas Online)

www.mindspring.com/~dmmmd/atlas_1.html (The Atlas of Gastrointestinal Endoscopy)

AAFP.org/policy/issues/c-colonoscopyposition.html (Information concerning hospital privileges and credentialing process)

CHAPTER 102

Esophagogastroduodenoscopy

Edward G. Zurad
John L. Pfenninger

The use of fiberoptic esophagogastroduodenoscopy (EGD), or gastroscopy, has revealed a myriad of diseases of the upper gastrointestinal tract to the practicing physician during the last 25 years. Refinements in equipment, technology, and ongoing developments in pharmacology have allowed this valuable tool to be used by primary care physicians, surgeons, and medical subspecialists. Advancements have allowed any interested physician to evaluate and treat patients with both simple and complex problems of the esophagus, stomach, and the duodenum.

The procedure is relatively quick and can be completed within 10 to 20 minutes. It can be performed in various settings, including the hospital, the office, and the outpatient endoscopic suite. One study (Rodney et al, 1990) indicated that when primary physicians performed EGD, it was associated with enhanced management and improved diagnostic accuracy in 89% of cases. Primary care physicians now perform flexible sigmoidoscopy, EGD, and colonoscopy on an increasingly frequent basis in their offices.

Both the fiberoptic and video gastroscopes are similar to the flexible sigmoidoscope, with which many primary care physicians have become familiar. It can be moved in multiple directions. It has channels for air insufflation, air aspiration, biopsy, and water installation. This technology, like flexible sigmoidoscopy, is increasingly being incorporated into primary care in both urban and rural areas.

INDICATIONS

In many instances, it is a symptom that results in the performance of EGD. These symptoms could include the following:
- Dyspepsia
- Dysphagia
- Odynophagia
- Early satiety
- Recurrent regurgitation
- Epigastric pain
- Sensation of food sticking
- Meal-related heartburn
- Severe indigestion
- Chronic nausea and vomiting
- Substernal or paraxiphoid pain
- Severe weight loss
- Noncardiac chest pain

Because over-the-counter (OTC) histamine-2 (H_2) antagonist therapy is available today, many patients report to their primary care physician only after failing a self-directed trial of H_2 antagonists. In addition, many patients have tried antacids or other agents for their upper gastrointestinal symptomatology that have failed, which results in their seeking further evaluation of the upper GI tract. EGD provides a precise evaluation to obtain a direct endoscopic assessment of the esophagus, stomach, and duodenum and to retrieve tissue for pathologic analysis.

Signs

Patients display many signs that stimulate the clinician's desire for further evaluation with EGD. Some of these signs include the following:
- Abdominal mass
- Hematemesis
- Unexplained anemia
- Gross or occult gastrointestinal bleeding
- Radiographic abnormality of the upper GI tract
- Weight loss

Preexisting Conditions

Many patients report to the primary care physician with a preexisting condition that requires further evaluation or surveillance with direct EGD. These conditions include the following:
- Cancer surveillance in high-risk patients (e.g., those with Barrett's esophagitis, Ménétrier's disease, gastric polyposis, pernicious anemia)

- Esophageal stricture
- Gastric retention
- Acute or chronic duodenitis
- Acute or chronic esophagitis
- Acute or chronic gastritis
- Symptomatic hiatal hernia
- Gastric ulcer monitoring
- Duodenal peptic ulcer disease
- Pyloroduodenal stenosis
- Esophageal or gastric varices
- Angiodysplasia in other area of the GI tract

CONTRAINDICATIONS

There are relatively few contraindications to the performance of EGD. The diameter of the currently used fiberoptic endoscopes used for EGD are similar to the diameter of the nasogastric (NG) tubes that are inserted on a daily basis in most hospitals. The safety of the procedure is readily acknowledged. Most primary care physicians inserted NG tubes during their medical school education and residency training. This experience should help clinicians feel more confident about the insertion of an EGD scope.

Contraindications include the following:

- History of bleeding disorder (e.g., platelet dysfunction, hemophilia)
- History of profusely bleeding esophageal varices
- Cardiopulmonary instability from any cause
- Recent myocardial infarction
- Suspected perforated viscus
- Uncooperative patient
- Absence of informed consent

EQUIPMENT

- Video gastroscope (insertion tube diameter of 7.0 to 9.5 mm, channel diameter of 2.8 mm, field of view of 120 degrees, working length of approximately 120 cm, angulation up to 210 degrees, downward angulation of 90 degrees, right and left angulation of 100 degrees, and the proper standard accessories) or a flexible fiberoptic scope as endoscope
- Light source (halogen light source versus xenon)
- Camera source
- Color video printer
- Video monitor
- Video recorder
- Biopsy forceps/brush
- Endoscopy table
- IV stand and IV sets
- Mouth guard

- Stool with wheels for the endoscopist (if he or she sits during the performance of the procedure)
- Sphygmomanometer versus continuous blood pressure monitor
- Stethoscope
- Electrocardiogram (ECG) machine or continuous cardiac monitor
- Oxygen saturation monitor (pulse oximeter) (consider Welch Allyn system that performs all necessary monitoring functions)
- Dextrose 5% and 0.45% sodium chloride solution (1 L)
- Suction equipment and tubing
- Specimen jars with formalin solution
- Syringes and needles
- K-Y Jelly scope lubricant
- Protective gloves (remember latex sensitivity in certain patients)
- Rapid urease test (CLO test) materials
- Anesthetic, sedative, and narcotic medications (see Chapter 2, Conscious Sedation [Sedation and Analgesia])
- Oxygen and delivery mask or nasal cannula
- "Crash cart" supplies (see Chapter 203, Anaphylaxis) (consider Banyan kit—a readily available "package" for the office [i.e., a "crash cart in a suitcase"])
- Toothpicks to remove tissue from biopsy forceps
- Dictation capabilities or computer for completion of the record
- Sink supplies for cleaning the scope

Cleaning Supplies

- Plastic containers for the endoscope tube
- Surgical scrub solution and water
- Enzyme solution
- 70% isopropyl alcohol
- Glutaraldehyde soaking solution
- Brushes and various channel insertion devices provided by manufacturer for internal channel cleaning

PREPROCEDURE PATIENT PREPARATION

As with any procedure, EGD needs to be explained to the patient in detail. The possible risks and complications also need to be detailed. It is wise to include a patient education handout and instructions for the patient to follow before the procedure (see the "Additional Resources" section toward the end of this chapter). The patient should also be given a copy of these to take home to share with a spouse or other family members. Informed consent must be obtained before performance of EGD (see the sample patient consent form titled

---

Staff Gastroscopy Instructions Guidelines

1. Be sure the patient has a copy of the patient teaching guides and that he or she understands and has read the instructions.
2. Advise the patient that the purpose of the study is to insert a tube through the mouth into the stomach and into the beginning of the small intestine in order to inspect the upper GI tract. We will be looking for inflammation, ulcers, growths, bleeding points, a hiatal hernia, and abnormal growths.
3. The following medications will probably be used: a "Caine" topical anesthetic, Demerol, and Valium or Versed. Be sure to inquire about sensitivity or allergy to any of the medications just mentioned.
    These medications act to depress the central nervous system. The patient's current medications, particularly tranquilizers, sedatives, sleeping pills, and muscle relaxants, must be reviewed, and their effects when taken with preprocedure medication must be considered.
4. Possible serious side effects are extremely unlikely, but they include bleeding, perforation of the GI tract, tearing of the vocal cords (voice box), aspiration of stomach contents into the lungs, tearing of the mucosa, or even death from a severe reaction (e.g., to medications).
5. All patients will have gagging, but very few (if any) will experience any discomfort with gagging if they take the full prep. Patients who take the full prep will be groggy, sleeping, or lethargic for a variable period after the procedure. They must not drive or do anything "delicate" for at least 4 hours following the procedure if they received a prep. If grogginess persists, they should wait until they are fully alert. We recommend waiting 8 hours, if possible. If patients have a medical condition that affects medication metabolism, the wait will most likely be longer.
6. The procedure can be performed in a highly motivated patient without any preparation, but the gagging is uncomfortable and tends to persist throughout the procedure. It does, however, decrease after the scope is partially inserted. A topical anesthetic spray will greatly decrease gagging in the patient who chooses to not have IV sedation.
7. Query the patient about prophylactic antibiotics and any heart valve disease and artificial joints or heart valves, and get the details about any recommendations previously given the patient. Be sure to advise the physician if the patient's understanding may be different from what is planned.

EGD Checklist
Be sure to be aware of the following:
Recent use of: ASA   Persantine   Motrin   Advil   NSAIDs   Coumadin
Preexisting disease: Asthma   Heart disease   COPD   Phlebitis   Prosthetic valves or joints

If plans to deal with any of the above medications or preexisting diseases are not recorded in the chart, please discuss with the physician how we should handle the situation.

Notes: _____

Fig. 102-1
Sample form of instruction guidelines for gastroscopy staff. (From The Medical Procedures Center, Midland, Mich.)

"Esophagogastroduodenoscopy [EGD]" on page 1869 of Appendix G). A preprocedure video that the patient and spouse or family member can view will reduce anxiety. This video, which can be obtained from various pharmaceutical companies free of charge, will also introduce the subject of conscious sedation and review contraindications to the procedure; it may even reduce the amount of conscious sedation agents required.

Figs. 102-1 to 102-6 show other helpful forms for office use.

ANTIBIOTIC PROPHYLAXIS

According to the latest American Heart Association guidelines, antibiotic prophylaxis for endoscopy with or without gastrointestinal biopsy is not recommended (see Chapter 204, Antibiotic Prophylaxis).

SEDATION AND MONITORING
(See Chapter 2, Conscious Sedation)

EGD has traditionally been performed in a hospital laboratory specializing in gastrointestinal disorders, known as a GI suite. It has also commonly been performed in an emergency room setting, an outpatient surgery facility, or a hospital operating room specially equipped for endoscopic procedures. Facility fee costs exceed physician reimbursement several fold. Many physicians have completed the procedure in their offices simply using a topical anesthetic spray.

Modern small-diameter scopes allow for a comfortable examination with little trauma to the cricopharyngeal region. As stated previously, the diameter of the scope is approximately that of an NG tube inserted daily by hospital nursing staffs.

The current move to office endoscopy has begun because of its many benefits, including safety and cost

COUNSELING FOR EGD (Upper Endoscopy)

Name: _____ DOB _____ Age _____

Telephone   (H) _____   (W) _____

Your referring doctor: _____

Primary care doctor: _____   Want a copy sent to him/her?

Blood pressure _____   Received, read, and understood handouts?

SYMPTOMS/HISTORY: Reason for consult: _____

Nausea	Previous gastric ulcer	Food getting stuck
Vomiting	Duodenal ulcer	Black, tarry stools
Heartburn	Esophagitis	Anemia
Need for antacids/H_2 blockers	Bloating	Belching
Early satiety	Pain with swallowing	Atypical chest pain
Positive *H. pylori* test	Difficulty swallowing	
Family Hx of stomach Ca	Who? _____	

PAST MEDICAL HISTORY:

Ulcer treatment	Other medical problems	Current Medications
Ex-smoker–quit _____	(1) _____	(1) _____
Aspirin use	(2) _____	(2) _____
NSAID use	(3) _____	(3) _____
Bleeding problems	(4) _____	(4) _____
Pulmonary disease	(5) _____	(5) _____
Heart disease		
Allergies _____		

OBJECTIVE:

General

Mouth   Dentures or partials   Teeth: chips

Neck: ability to hyperextend

Lungs

Heart

Abdomen

IMPRESSION:

(1) Good candidate for EGD

(2)

(3)

(4)

COUNSELING:

Bleeding	Sore throat
Aspiration	Infection
Perforation	Medication reaction

Sedation options:

Halcion/Stadol vs. IV sedation (Demerol/Versed) or topical only

Driver if sedated

PLAN:

(1) Halcion 0.25 mg 2 tablets PO 1 hr PRN with sip of water   or IV sedation   or topical

(2) NPO after midnight

(3) Driver if sedation

(4) Scheduled for EGD

(5)

(6)

_____ Date _____

Physician's signature

Fig. 102-2

Sample form for EGD counseling. (From The Medical Procedures Center, Midland, Mich.)

Guidelines for Monitoring the Patient Receiving Conscious Sedation for Gastrointestinal Endoscopy: a Summation

1. Monitoring is one aspect of endoscopy unit policy. It should be part of the overall quality assurance program for the endoscopy unit.
2. A well-trained gastrointestinal assistant, working closely with the endoscopist, is the most important part of the monitoring process.
3. The use of extracorporeal equipment to monitor patients may be a useful adjunct to patient surveillance, but it is never a substitute for conscientious clinical assessment.
4. Although changes in blood pressure, pulse, cardiac rhythm, and oxygen saturation do occur during endoscopy, no controlled studies address the question of whether noninvasive monitoring with extracorporeal equipment decreases complications.
5. The amount of monitoring should be proportional to the perceived risk of the patient undergoing the procedure. It may vary from one procedure to the next.
6. The minimal clinical monitoring for all sedated patients should include the determination of heart rate, blood pressure, and respiratory rate before sedation, during the procedure, immediately after the procedure, and when the patient is released from the endoscopy area.
7. The proper role for pulse oximetry and continuous electrocardiographic monitoring during endoscopic procedures is controversial and unsettled.
8. Given the cost of the equipment and the manpower to use it, the best decision as to whether such monitoring should be used would be based on data showing an effect on clinical outcome. Such data do not exist.
9. However, in those situations in which the individualized need of the patient indicates that measurement of cardiac rhythm or oxygen saturation will complement the clinical assessment, the use of EKG monitoring or pulse oximetry may be beneficial.

Fig. 102-3
Sample form of monitoring instructions for gastroscopy staff. (From Fleisher D: *Gastrointest Endosc* 35:262, 1989.)

EGD NURSING CHECKLIST

Patient _____ Date _____ Age _____

Notify the physician if an unexpected, unusual, or negative answer is obtained.

Have the patient change into a gown.
Orient the patient to the room and the equipment.
Confirm the patient read the handouts and took oral medication at home.
Consent signed.
NPO since _____
Someone is present to drive the patient home.
Current meds _____
Drug allergies _____
Recent use of anticoagulants _____
Preexisting and/or existing disease: None   Lung Disease   Other
Biopsy forceps, specimen cups, and slides ready.
Gloves, lubricant, and 4 × 4s available.
Resuscitation equipment available and ready, including oxygen.
Scope leakage tested.
Suction and water bottles prepared and connected.
If needed: IV 500 ml D5W /D5½ NS /NS started in LUE/RUE with # _____ Intracath/butterfly
    by _____ at _____ AM/PM.
Assist with obtaining and processing biopsies.
Secure the safety of the patient after the procedure.
Print record of vital signs and disconnect monitoring equipment.
Vital signs record attached.
Clean the equipment.
Disconnect IV fluids if used.
Prepare the patient for the physician conference.
Escort patient out with instruction sheets.

	Time
Patient in room	
Sedation started	
Procedure started (scope inserted)	
Procedure ended	
Patient discharged	

Medications	Dosage	Time

Fig. 102-4
Sample form of EGD nursing checklist. (From The Medical Procedures Center, Midland, Mich.)

EGD PROCEDURE

Name: _____ BD: _____ Date: _____

The patient gave informed consent for the procedure. Intravenous access was obtained in the R/L upper extremity. Topical anesthesia was used in the pharynx. The patient was placed in the left lateral position, and the neck flexed to the chest. The bite block was placed gently, and the scope lubricated and passed through the bite block over the tongue. The hypopharynx was visualized, the vocal cords visualized, and the scope passed through the cricopharyngeus. The scope was passed into the distal esophagus with the GE junction seen and diaphragmatic indentation noted by the sniff test. The scope was advanced into the stomach and the gastric lake suctioned. The scope was passed through the pylorus and maneuvered into the descending duodenum. The duodenum and duodenal bulb were visualized and the scope brought back into the stomach. A biopsy for CLO testing was obtained. The scope was retroflexed to view the cardia. The scope was pulled into the esophagus and the esophagus closely examined. The scope was withdrawn, and the patient tolerated the procedure well. Monitoring showed normal cardiac/oxygen status. The patient was informed of the procedure results. Pulse oximetry monitoring was used throughout the procedure to evaluate the patient for hypoxemia. A printed report is attached. Changes to above procedure: None or _____

_____

Anesthesia: Versed _____ mg IV   Monitoring: Oximetry
                   Demerol _____ mg IV   Cardiac monitoring
                   Topical Cetacaine spray   Blood pressure
                   Xylocaine 2% liquid

Complications: _____
Areas not well visualized: _____

Abnormalities noted:

Bleeding	Erythema	Friability	Erosion	Polyp	Tumor
Ulcer, gastric	Ulcer, duo	Barrett's	Diverticula	Gastric bile	Varices
Dilation	Hiatal hernia	Carcinoma	Stenosis	Scarring	Angiodysplasia

Biopsies performed: _____
Diagnoses:

535.00	Gastritis, acute	531.00	Gastric ulcer, acute w/hemo
530.81	Esophageal reflux	535.60	Duodenitis
532.00	Duodenal ulcer,	553.3	Hiatal hernia acute with hemorrhage
530.1	Esophagitis, reflux	Other	

Plan: _____   Stop smoking   Low fat diet
        _____   Avoid NSAIDs   Elevate head of bed 4-6 in
                                     Avoid chocolate/mints Do not eat 2 hours before bedtime
                                     Avoid offending foods

cc: _____   Physician: _____

Fig. 102-5
Sample form for the EGD procedure. (From The Medical Procedures Center, Midland, Mich.)

---

effectiveness. The American Academy of Family Physicians and the Joint Commission for Accreditation of Hospitals and Organizations do not recommend continuous ECG monitoring or continuous pulse oximetry for low-risk patients. More extensive monitoring becomes necessary when the following conditions exist:

- Procedures that last longer than 30 minutes
- Large bore scopes
- High-risk patient
- Situations where more than "light" sedation is used

In these scenarios more extensive clinical monitoring, including continuous ECG monitoring and pulse oximetry, is wise. All patients should have clinical monitoring of skin color, degree of sedation, loss of reflexes, blood pressure, pulse, and respiratory rate in a well-lighted room.

Table 102-1 provides a summary of the agents usually used for sedation in the United States. Sufficient anesthesia or sedation can often be accomplished without intravenous (IV) drug administration, using new approaches that are called *non-IV conscious sedation*. These have been detailed in several articles, including work sponsored by the National Procedures Institute. In such a situation a patient can be given diazepam 10 mg orally 1 hour before the procedure, or lorazepam 1 to 2 mg sublingually, 30 to 60 minutes before the procedure. Halcion 0.5 mg PO, can also be used. Table 102-1 reviews the medications used in conscious sedation.

An optional intramuscular dose of ketorolac (Toradol) 60 mg may be given 30 to 60 minutes before the procedure. Butorphanol tartrate (Stadol), 1 to 2 sprays

---

ROLE OF THE ASSISTANT

The well-trained and motivated assistant makes the EGD examination a pleasant task for the physician. It is not necessary for the attendant to attend a special course, but it is necessary to spend time learning each step of the procedure. Representatives from the endoscope manufacturer will assist in training assistants in the cleaning and care of the scopes. It is important to have assistants trained in CPR.

Before the patient arrives for the procedure, the assistant must do the following:
1. Prepare the room.
2. Have the IV set up, medications, endoscope, and the resuscitation equipment ready (but not opened).
3. Prepare the paperwork.

When the patient arrives, the assistant must do the following:
1. Bring the patient to the procedure room.
2. Orient the patient to the room and the equipment.
3. Make sure consent forms are signed, and that the patient has read and understands the instructions.
4. Verify that the patient is properly prepared (NPO, has a qualified adult to accompany the patient home). Check patient allergies. Review and record current patient medications.
5. Review the EGD procedure with the patient.
6. Record baseline vital signs.
7. Place EKG monitor pads and initiate oximetry and cardiac monitoring.
8. Initiate IV fluids at KVO if IV sedation used.
9. Give the patient topical anesthesia within 3 to 5 minutes of starting the procedure.

During the procedure, the assistant must do the following:
1. Record vital signs every 15 minutes during the procedure.
2. Assist the endoscopist with the scope, if needed.
3. Watch the monitoring equipment, and notify the physician of changes in patient status.
4. Assist with obtaining multiple biopsies and brushings.
5. Receive and process biopsy specimens and paperwork.

After the procedure, the assistant must do the following:
1. Monitor the patient's vital signs for 15 minutes.
2. Secure the safety of the patient, raise the gurney rails, etc.
3. Complete the paperwork associated with the procedure.
4. Remove monitoring equipment from the patient.
5. Clean the equipment.
6. Discontinue the IV fluids, if used.
7. Clean the room for the next procedure.
8. Prepare the patient for the physician conference.
9. Give the patient the instruction sheets.
10. Inform the person accompanying the patient of signs to observe.

Fig. 102-6
Sample form detailing the role of the assistant. (From The Medical Procedures Center, Midland, Mich.)

(intranasally), generally provides both sedation and analgesia sufficient to carry out EGD.

Benzocaine and lidocaine spray is often used in the context of EGD. It can sometimes cause significant coughing and gagging, which may then increase the patient's anxiety during the procedure.

An alternative choice for topical anesthesia includes the "Popsicle stick" method. In this scenario, Xylocaine jelly (2%) is squeezed on a tongue blade that is covered with the patient's favorite food flavoring, and this is placed into the back of the patient's throat. The patient sucks on the tongue blade while vital signs are completed, and the patient is prepared for the procedure. A tongue blade can be pressed into the posterior oral pharynx to ascertain that appropriate topical anesthesia has been obtained before insertion of the endoscope. Lack of a gag reflex ensures the desired effect.

An angiocath is usually placed when IV medications are to be used during the performance of EGD. This is connected to an IV line with IV fluids that are usually composed of D_5 (5% dextrose and one half normal saline) and normal saline. It is essential that resuscitation equipment and reversal drugs are readily available throughout the course of the procedure.

The inclusion of a benzodiazepine antagonist (Romazicon) and a narcotic antagonist (Narcan) provides a safety net for the conscious sedation segment of the procedure. If Narcan shortages occur, nalmefene (Revex) injection can be substituted to reverse opioid depression. If IV sedation is used, the endpoint to be titrated is when the patient has slurred speech while still able to be aroused.

Diazepam and other benzodiazepines can rarely cause paradoxical excitement. If this occurs, different medication (i.e., pure narcotics) should be used to complete the EGD. If significant excitation occurs, it may

TABLE 102-1

Drugs Used for Esophagogastroduodenoscopy

Medication	Dose
Narcotics	
Meperidine (Demerol) IV	10-75 mg (0.5-1 mg/kg)
Fentanyl (Sublimaze) IV	1-2 mg
Butorphanol tartrate (Stadol Nasal Spray)	1-2 mg (1-2 sprays in nostril)
Benzodiazepines	
Diazepam (Valium) IV	1-10 mg
Midazolam (Versed) IV	2-5 mg (0.035-0.1 mg/kg)
Lorazepam (Ativan) SL (onset in 10 min)	1-2 mg
Triazolam (Halcion) PO	0.5 mg
Anticholinergic	
Glycopyrrolate (Robinul)	0.002 mg (0.01 ml/kg) IM 1 hour before procedure or 0.1 mg (0.5 ml) repeated every 2-3 minutes as needed
Miscellaneous	
Simethicone (Mylicon) drops	0.6 ml (30-40 mg) in 30 ml of water PO (can also be flushed through the gastroscope with 5 ml of water)
Ketorolac (Toradol)	60 mg IM; 15 mg IV
Topical Local Anesthetics	
Lidocaine 2% viscous solution gargle	
Benzocaine 20% (Hurricaine) spray	
Benzocaine 14% and tetracaine 2% (Cetacaine)	
Antagonists	
Naloxone (Narcan) IV	0.2-0.8 mg
Flumazenil (Romazicon) IV	0.2-1 mg (start with 0.2 mg; repeat every 60 sec to a maximum of 1 mg or until reversal of benzodiazepine effect has been achieved)
Nalmefene hydrogen chloride (Revex)	1-2 ml IV

These are the drugs most commonly used. The endoscopist should become familiar with each category and fully understand the common actions, side effects, and doses of these agents. Many physicians do not use an anticholinergic, and it is contraindicated in gastric atony, dysmotility, gastric retention, or tachycardia.

BOX 102-1

High-Risk Groups

Older than 70 years old
Younger than 12 years old
Agitated, uncooperative patient
Uncontrolled coronary artery disease
Significant valvular heart disease
Prosthetic cardiac valves
Significant chronic obstructive pulmonary disease
Cardiopulmonary instability of any type
Recent cerebrovascular accident
Significant bleeding disorder or coagulopathy
Current active bleeding
Barium administration within a few hours of the procedure

tions can be handled and normal aggressive monitoring procedures can be carried out.

Many endoscopists now routinely use oxygen delivered through nasal cannula, 2 L per minute, to prevent any likelihood of hypoxemia that can occur during EGD, resulting from the mechanical nature of the tube in the upper airway region. This allows for continuous source of oxygen delivery. The patient can be stimulated to inhale by simply advising him or her to take a deep breath. If oxygen is not used in a continuous fashion during the performance of the procedure, oxygen must be available in the event that hypoxemia is encountered.

TECHNIQUE

It is essential to ensure that aspirin and platelet-inhibiting nonsteroidal antiinflammatory drugs (NSAIDs) have been discontinued at least 7 days before the procedure. The patient must take nothing by mouth after midnight on the day before the examination (or at least 8 hours must have elapsed since eating).

The assistant should initiate the IV angiocath and connect it to the IV line. If pulse oximetry and continuous ECG monitoring is to be used, these connections can be initiated at this time. Blood pressure monitoring, pulse, and respiration monitoring can also be started at this time and recorded.

1. Examine the oral cavity while the patient is in a sitting position. Any dentures or foreign objects should be removed.
2. Have the patient swallow 40 mg of simethicone in 30 ml of tap water before the initiation of the procedure. This tends to reduce reflective bubbles in the stomach that present considerable impediment to visibility during the procedure. Alternatively, simethicone can be used only if needed during the procedure (0.6 ml of simethicone liquid can be injected down the gastroscope followed by 5 ml of water).

be wise to cancel the procedure and have the patient return at another time.

It is rarely necessary to supplement the initial doses of sedative or to exceed the dose range outlined in Table 102-1, as noted previously.

It is important to select patients wisely for office-based EGD. This is a critical step. In individuals who are in the high-risk group (Box 102-1), the clinician should consider performing EGD in a facility where complica-

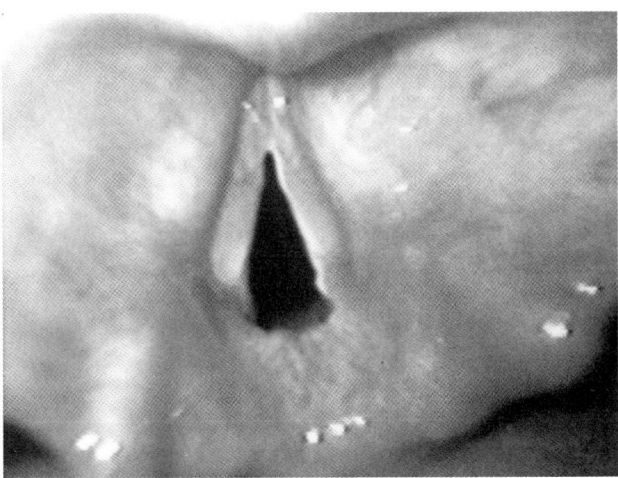

Fig. 102-7
Open vocal cord.

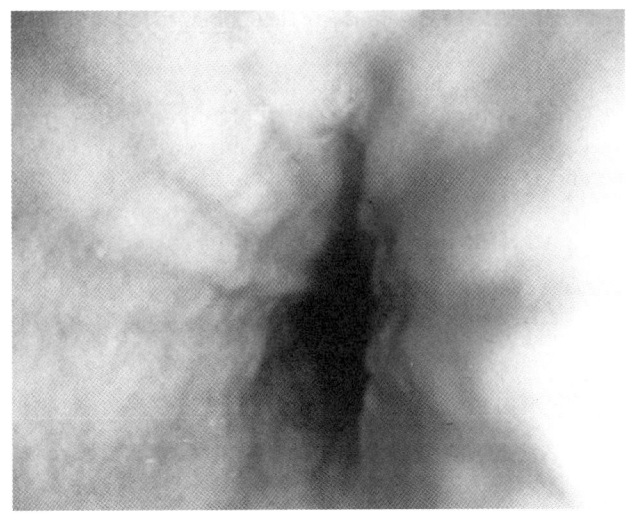

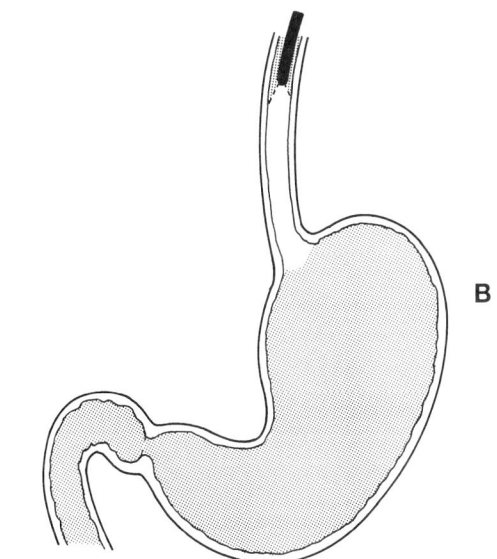

Fig. 102-8
A, Proximal esophagus. **B,** Unshaded area is seen by lighted scope.

3. The topical anesthesia should be completed at this point, as noted previously.
4. After good topical anesthesia is ensured, the patient should be placed in the left lateral decubitus position.
5. Lubricate the distal 10 cm of the scope with K-Y Jelly.
6. Insert the mouth guard into the patient's mouth; the teeth should grip this guard. The guard not only protects the patient's teeth, tongue, and oral mucosa but it also prevents the patient from damaging the scope. Introduce the scope through the mouth guard and direct it across the superior aspect of the tongue into the posterior oral pharynx.

   In the edentulous patient, the mouth guard can be placed over the scope and the scope can then be introduced through a channel created by placing the left second and third fingers of the examiner's hand over the back of the tongue.

   Guide the scope across the back of the tongue into the cricopharyngeal region. This is usually the first point of resistance encountered (approximately 17 cm from the incisor teeth and at the level of the vocal cords) (Fig. 102-7). Under direct vision, or blindly, ask the patient to swallow repeatedly while applying gentle pressure. The scope will easily pass through the cricopharyngeus region without difficulty and can then be advanced down through the esophagus (Fig. 102-8).
7. *Never* use force as the scope passes the cricopharyngeus region. The patient's normal swallowing mechanism will assist in advancing the endoscope.
8. Once the tip of the endoscope has entered the esophagus, insufflate a small puff of air to dilate the esophagus to easily visualize the mucosa throughout the cylindric esophagus. Additional air will need to be insufflated after the scope reaches the stomach and duodenum.

Note: Identify the channel in front of the scope before attempting to pass the scope to prevent injury to the patient. The lumen should always be seen.

   The endoscope should be advanced quickly but gently through the esophagus. The first landmark typically seen as the bronchioaortic constriction (Fig. 102-9).
9. As the scope is advanced, the GE junction is typically found at approximately 40 cm from the incisor teeth. It is essential to evaluate the esophagus and GE junction at the "first pass," because the mucosa may become irritated by the passage of the scope. This can distort the appearance of the GE junction

(Fig. 102-10). There is a typical mucosal color demarcation that occurs at the GE junction, with the esophageal lining being pale pink and the gastric mucosa represented by a darker pink or orange hue.

10. At this time, ask the patient to sniff through his or her nose (i.e., the "sniff test"). As the patient sniffs, the crura of the diaphragm extrinsically compress the GE junction at the esophageal hiatus. If the Z line is visualized above the level of the extrinsic compression seen from the crura of the diaphragm, then the patient is suffering from a hiatal hernia. Repeat the sniff test when viewing the Z line from below, while the scope is in the stomach in a retroflexed position.

Note: Use air, water, suction, and "miniwithdrawals" as needed to pass the scope and to fully evaluate all surfaces of the mucosa.

11. After passing through the GE junction, the endoscope is inserted into the stomach. After the scope reaches the stomach, the gastric lake, which is a collection of fluids in the dependent portion of the stomach, will typically impair visibility (Fig. 102-11). Air should be insufflated sufficiently to spread the mucosal walls apart so that this fluid can be aspirated. Many clinicians aspirate the gastric fluid and test the pH of the fluid to record the acidity of the gastric lake. After the fluid is removed and the lumen again is clearly visualized, the scope can rapidly be advanced following the rugae along the lesser curvature to the angular notch.

The scope is subsequently passed below the angularis, then into the antrum up to the pylorus (Figs. 102-12 and 102-13).

Note: The scope should be adjusted so that the small black arrow is at the top of the field and so it corresponds with the incisura. This provides proper orientation with the patient in the left lateral position.

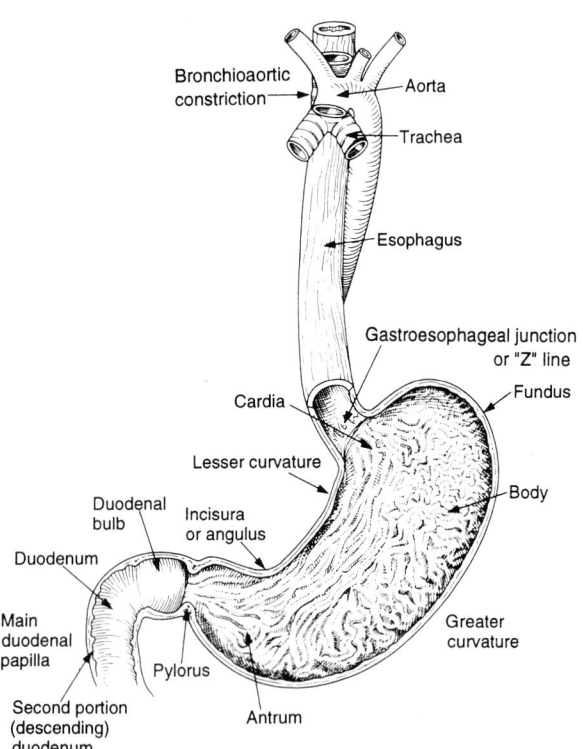

Fig. 102-9
Relevant anatomy for gastroscopy. The *cardia* is that portion of the stomach immediately surrounding the esophageal opening. The *gastroesophageal junction* is also known as the GE junction, the Z line, ora serrata, or gastric rosette. The upper end or dome of the stomach is the *fundus.* The upturn of the "J" of the stomach is separated from its vertical portion by the *angular* notch (also known as the angulus, angularis, or incisura). The *antrum* lies to the right of the angulus and ends at the *pylorus,* or greatly thickened muscular wall. The *duodenum* lies beyond the pylorus. The *lesser curvature* is the upper right border of the stomach, whereas the *greater curvature* is the left inferior margin.

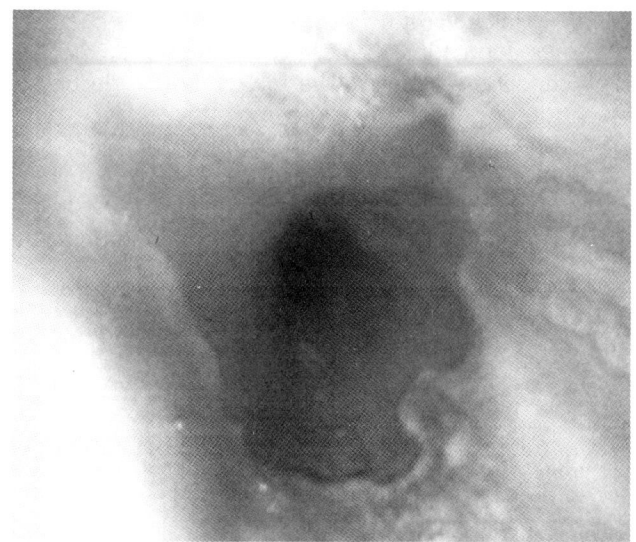

A

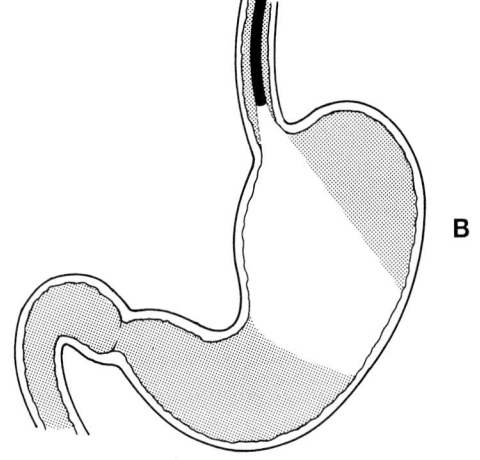

B

Fig. 102-10
A, Distal esophagus Z line. **B,** Unshaded area is seen by lighted scope.

12. Guide the endoscope through the relaxed pyloric sphincter into the duodenal bulb (Fig. 102-14). Do not attempt to pass the scope through a tightly closed pylorus. The repetitive trauma of attempting to do this will simply cause greater pylorospasm and prevent good evaluation of the duodenum. When the scope is passed through the pylorus into the duodenal bulb, it is common to encounter a *whiteout* or a *redout*. This is because the scope typically tends to rapidly advance to the junction of the first and second portions of the duodenum. At this point it is wise to withdraw the scope very slowly to reestablish the lumen and complete the duodenal exam. Biopsies are rarely needed in this area.

13. The second portion of the duodenum becomes retroperitoneal. Thus it is wise to turn the scope to the right and pass the scope downward so that it can enter the second portion of the duodenum (Fig. 102-13). The second portion of the duodenum is recognizable because of the vertical, cylindric nature of the viscera in this region. In addition, the Kerckring's folds will readily appear. Vater's ampulla can be seen along the medial aspect of the second portion of the duodenum 20% to 30% of the time. It is not essential to evaluate this area for the completion of an EGD.

14. The scope can be advanced occasionally into the third portion of the duodenum or the horizontal portion of the duodenum.

Note: At this point of the procedure, the insertion portion of the procedure is complete and it is time to withdraw the scope.

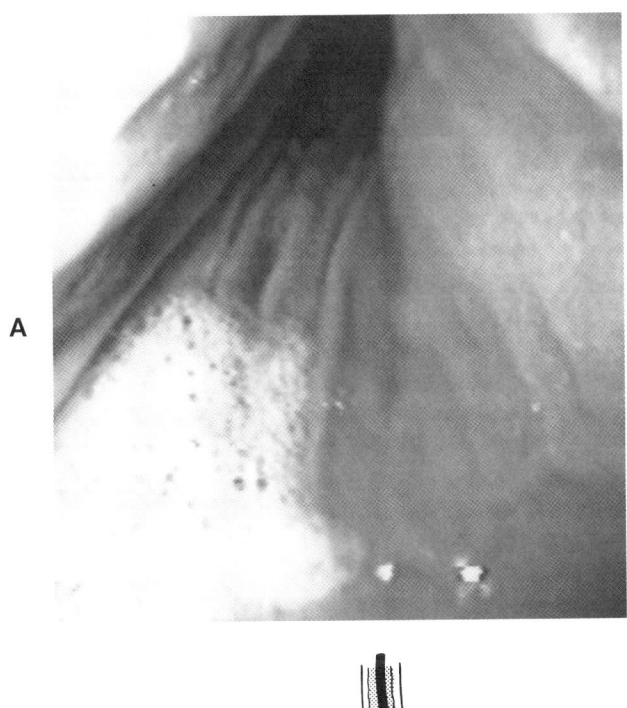

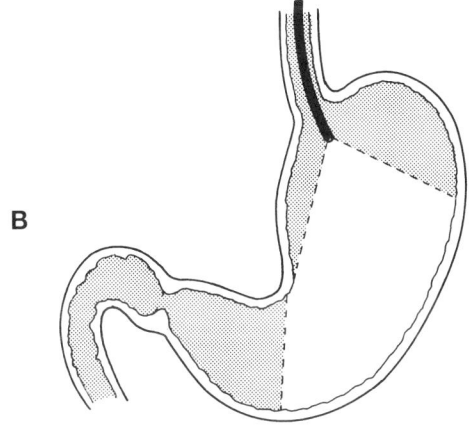

Fig. 102-11
A, Gastric lake and rugae at the 8 o'clock position. **B,** Unshaded area is seen by lighted scope.

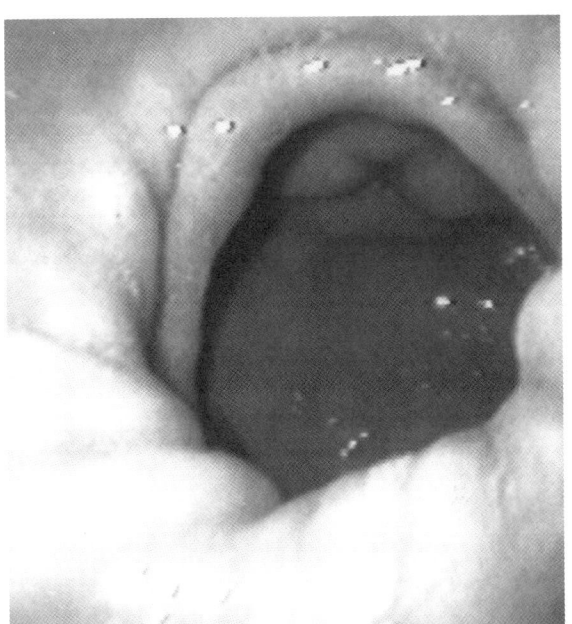

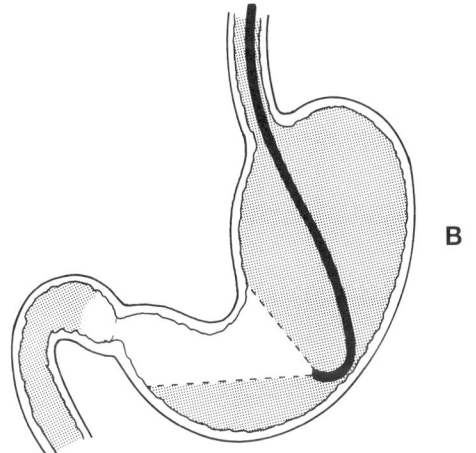

Fig. 102-12
A, Angularis at the 12 o'clock position. Closed pylorus. Prepylorus at the 6 o'clock position. **B,** Unshaded area is seen by lighted scope.

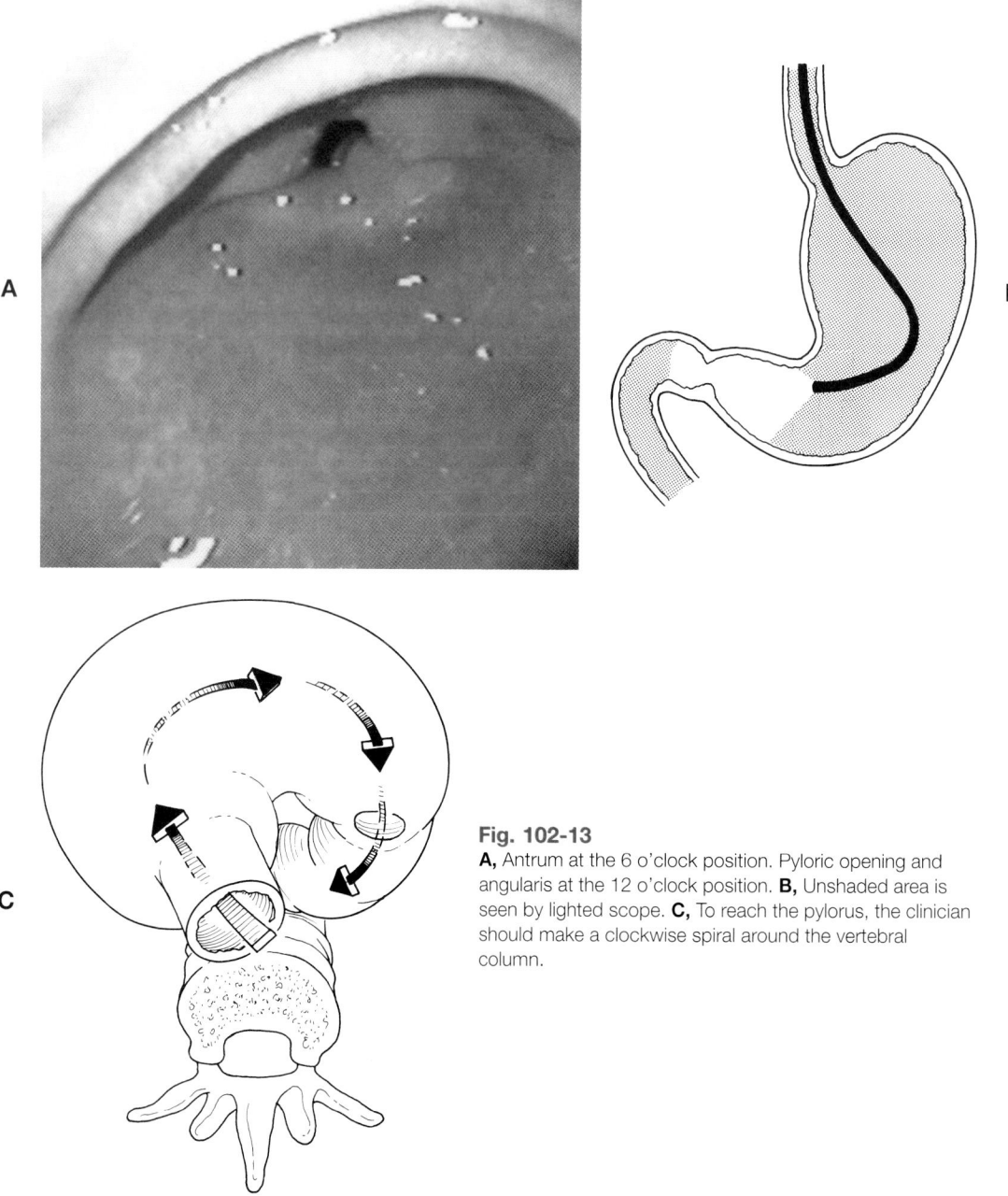

A

B

C

Fig. 102-13
A, Antrum at the 6 o'clock position. Pyloric opening and angularis at the 12 o'clock position. **B,** Unshaded area is seen by lighted scope. **C,** To reach the pylorus, the clinician should make a clockwise spiral around the vertebral column.

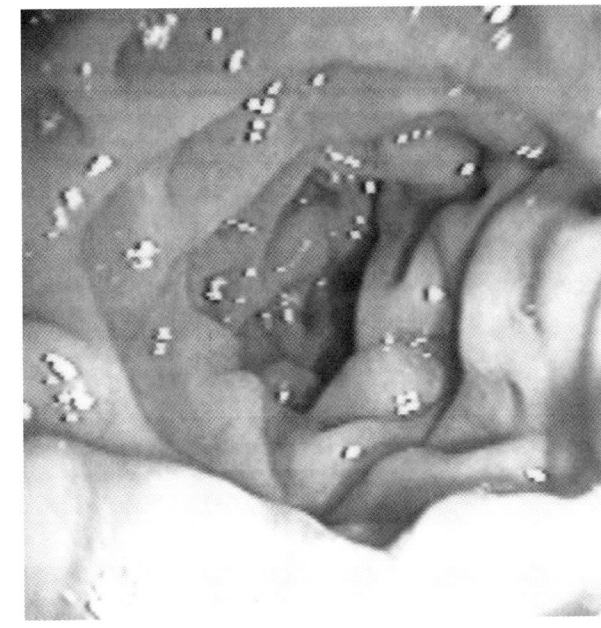

A

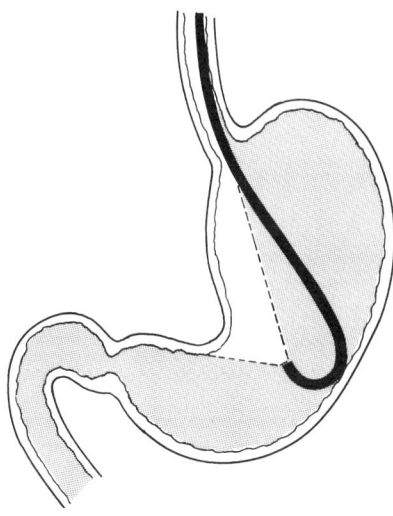

Fig. 102-15
A 180-degree angulation retroflexes the tip to see the lesser curve.

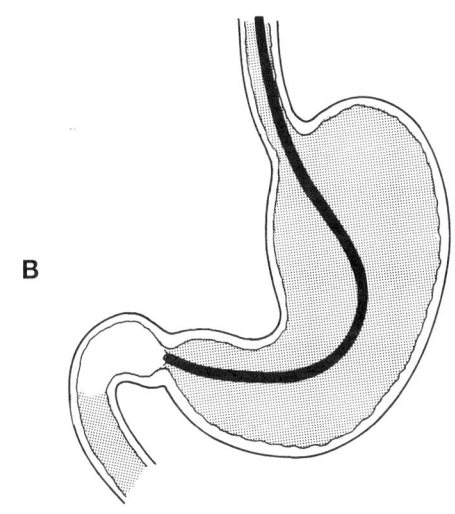

B

Fig. 102-14
A, Duodenum. **B,** Unshaded area is seen by lighted scope.

15. Withdraw the endoscope slowly with the attempt to evaluate the entire 360-degree circumferential portion of the mucosal surface. The second and sometimes the third portions of the duodenum can be evaluated readily.

16. The duodenal bulb is difficult to assess because, as it is being withdrawn, the scope typically tends to rapidly retract through the pyloric junction, back into the stomach. It is therefore necessary to reinsert it through the pylorus so that the duodenal bulb mucosa can be closely examined to rule out pathology.

17. Once back into the stomach, it is helpful to deflect the scope tip up and down as the control head is rotated right and left to ensure that the entire gastric

mucosal surface has been evaluated. If not done previously, retroflex the scope so that it is looking at itself and observe the GE junction. Examine the cardia (Figs. 102-15 and 102-16).

18. Straighten the scope tip deflections before removing the scope through the GE junction. One way to do this is to align the letters on the large inner wheel and the small outer wheel before withdrawing the instrument. If the scope is withdrawn with the tip retroflexed, it could result in mucosal damage of the GE junction or an esophageal tear.

19. The scope is withdrawn through the GE junction slowly. Again, close evaluation of the GE junction is completed. Complete a sniff test at this region one final time.

20. As the procedure is being carried out, photographs can be taken on a continuing basis, both during the initial insertion and during withdrawal.

21. Biopsies during EGD are completed as the scope is withdrawn to prevent significant downstream bleeding that can impair visibility of the mucosal surface (see the "Biopsy" section).

22. It is important to record the appearance of the vocal cords before the scope is withdrawn. The documentation of an attempt to view the vocal cords is an important component of EGD before the removal of the scope, even if they cannot be seen because of coughing or gagging.

23. The assistant should complete the monitoring process of the patient after the scope is withdrawn. The mouth guard should also be removed, and the physician may want to reexamine the patient before discharge from the facility. A 30-minute observation period after the procedure is typical if only minimal sedation is used (Box 102-2).

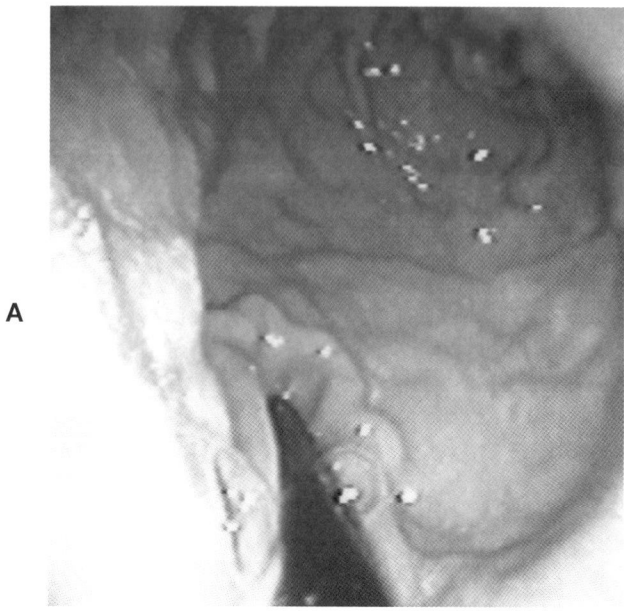

A

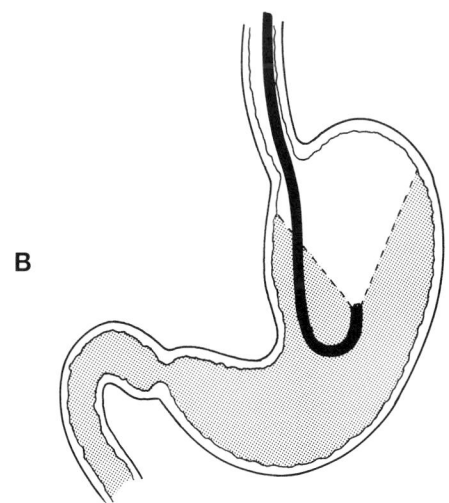

B

Fig. 102-16

A, Turnaround maneuver (i.e., retroflexing) showing the endoscope emerging from a snug EG junction at the 6 o'clock position and the cardia at the 12 o'clock position. **B,** Unshaded area is seen by lighted scope.

24. Discuss the findings with the patient (and the person who has accompanied the patient to the office) before discharge. If the patient has received significant administration of benzodiazepines, such as Versed, he or she may be amnestic or forgetful of any information provided. Photographic records of the findings, along with graphic demonstration or written comments, are extremely helpful in reviewing the results of the procedure with the patient and his or her family. Complete and review all monitoring forms.

25. The gastrointestinal assistant should document the condition in which the patient was discharged.

BOX 102-2

Intravenous Sedative Administration Recovery Nursing Documentation Parameters

Note level of consciousness on arrival.
Note response and anxiety level.
Note patency of airway, spontaneous respiratory effort.
Note status of IV access site (redness or edema).
Note breathing effort and fall of chest wall.
Note vital signs every 5 minutes.
Place the cardiac monitor.
Place the pulse oximeter.
Note body temperature.
Administer oxygen at 2 L through a nasal cannula.
Raise head of the bed 30 to 45 degrees.
Note skin turgor.
Note quality of speech (clearness and ease of speech).
Note presence or absence of nausea, gagging, spasmodic coughing, and ability to swallow.
Note presence or absence of abdominal distention or tenderness.
Note quality of bowel sounds.
Note expulsion of gas.
Note abdominal cramping.
On admission, perform an assessment of the patient's medial conditions
Note any untoward symptoms as they occur.
Note the patient's condition after 15 minutes.
Note discharge status.
Record vital signs every 5 minutes and post monitor strips, with a simple explanation, every 15 minutes or when there is an unusual occurrence.
Report any unusual responses immediately to the physician.

26. It is helpful to call the patient at home at the end of the day (before the office closes) to document that the patient is not experiencing any untoward effects after the completion of EGD.

UNSEDATED TRANSNASAL ESOPHAGOGASTRODUODENOSCOPY

With the advent of newly developed ultra-slim diameter endoscopes (5.1- to 6-mm insertion tube), the age of unsedated transnasal EGD (T-EGD) has literally "just arrived." Unsedated EGD obviously eliminates the danger of medication-related complications from sedative drugs. More than half of the morbidity and mortality attributed to EGD are due to cardiopulmonary complications from sedation effects.

Significant cost reduction is associated with the absence of fees for sedation and monitoring equipment. This alone has become a significant motivational factor to encourage office-based T-EGD.

Previously, either the patient or the physician may have opted for an empiric therapeutic trial of medications for a myriad of upper gastrointestinal complaints rather than having an EGD. Such choices may have been based on patient anxiety and physician concerns about the procedure. Such a delay in diagnosis will no longer be necessary, since T-EGD can be completed in the office, eliminating the need for nursing time and anesthesia personnel. Also preoperative, concurrent, and postoperative monitoring with a pulse oximeter are no longer issues.

Other hidden costs can also be eliminated. Such costs include the drain on the economy's workforce associated with the current need for family members or friends taking time off to assist and transport patients for EGD. Patient convenience is enhanced, since endoscopies can be performed during office hours. No lengthy recovery period or check-in or discharge time is required. Patients can return to work almost immediately following T-EGD. Physicians can perform more endoscopies in less time after they are trained and familiar with the insudated technique.

A remaining hurdle is the fact that most patients experiencing EGD have come to expect that they will sleep through their procedure and awaken with little or no awareness of what was done. Patient apprehension can be a major obstacle. This can be overcome with good patient education (such as videos of actual procedures), which will increase acceptability and tolerance. Patients can actually watch their anatomy on the screen and actively communicate (talk during the procedure), providing feedback to the physician. Immediate demonstration and explanation of the pathology is possible with a conscious patient who is viewing the procedure as it occurs.

BIOPSY

Biopsy samples are taken when visible changes are seen in the stomach or esophagus. Routine, blind biopsy specimens of the esophagus, stomach, or duodenum are not indicated. The clinician should perform a biopsy on any gastroesophageal abnormality unless it is vascular in appearance (i.e., pulsating or bluish in color). Any intended areas of biopsy should be approached with a closed biopsy forceps to assess the vascularity and/or induration of the subject area. The clinician should ensure that the intended biopsy site can be successfully reached with the scope in its current position. Biopsy of duodenal ulcers is rarely necessary because the risk of cancer is extremely small in this region.

During biopsy, the forceps are advanced through the end of the scope by the examiner, and the assistant is in charge of the operating controls. The closed forceps are directed at the area to be biopsied. When the area is reached, the assistant is advised to open the forceps and the forceps are passed directly into the biopsy area. The examiner asks the assistant to close the forceps. A gentle tug is given, and the biopsy forceps are pulled through the opening of the scope by the examiner. A tenting of the mucosa can be seen with the removal of the tissue. The assistant then retrieves the tissue by opening the

biopsy forceps over a container with formalin. A toothpick is placed into the teeth of the open biopsy forceps, dislodging the tissue material into the formalin container.

For gastric ulcers, the clinician should biopsy all four quadrants at the edges. If diffuse intestinal metaplasia is present, multiple biopsies are indicated. Because the biopsies are small, there is generally minimal bleeding. In most cases bleeding from esophageal biopsies stops within 4 to 5 minutes.

It is not necessary to continuously monitor a biopsy site during the performance of the procedure. Commonly, the examiner can complete the examination by looking at other areas of the upper GI tract and then return to reevaluate a biopsy site before the completion of the procedure. If bleeding does occur and is profuse, it must be controlled and noted on the operative report before withdrawing the scope. In most cases the acidic milieu of the stomach coagulates bleeding sites. Occasionally the distal esophagus will bleed more persistently after the completion of a biopsy; therefore many examiners perform brush "biopsies" in this region rather than the surgical biopsy.

Gastric biopsies are also commonly done to obtain tissue samples for CLO tests or for histologic analysis for *Helicobacter pylori*. *H. pylori*–associated gastritis often cannot be diagnosed by endoscopic appearance alone. When assessing a patient with chronic dyspepsia, the clinician should remember that normal-appearing gastric mucosa may exhibit marked histologic gastritis.

When performing the CLO test, the examiner should warm the slide to room temperature before the endoscopy. The absence of bismuth preparations and a 4-week abstinence from antibiotics should be documented before the performance of the procedure.

When performing *H. pylori* biopsies, the clinician should obtain tissue samples from the *normal-appearing* portions of the gastric antrum. The normal-appearing area of the mucosa is chosen because *H. pylori* may be scarce in areas where the epithelium is eroded or where the mucous layer is denuded.

Many physicians read and interpret the results of a CLO test themselves (a simple color change). However, the tissue can be sent to a pathologist. Some physicians collect two specimens: one for a CLO test and one for histologic analysis (the histologic analysis specimen is sent only if the CLO test is negative, and if there is a strong suspicion of *H. pylori*). A single biopsy has a sensitivity of approximately 95%, whereas two biopsies approach 100% sensitivity. *H. pylori* has a patchy distribution.

COMPLICATIONS

The complication rate of endoscopy performed by primary care physicians from eight clinical sites was

0.0014 (1 in 717). All cases were collected sequentially from the beginning of each physician's experience. The complication rate in subspecialty populations is 0.0013 (1.3 in 1000). Therefore complications from EGD are extremely rare. Sixty percent of the morbidity and mortality associated with EGD is due to cardiopulmonary complications that arise directly from the conscious sedation used in the procedure. True complications might include the following:

- Perforation
- Bleeding secondary to trauma or biopsy
- Infection
- Cardiopulmonary complications from conscious sedation
- Inadequate interpretation

TRAINING

Most physicians who are performing primary care endoscopy have received training either in a residency situation or in short courses. Both of these training situations provide excellent introduction to the technique of EGD, the use of conscious sedation, and the interpretation of common pathology seen with the endoscope.

It is essential for the clinician to obtain preceptor training from a skilled endoscopist who can assist with the proper insertion technique and the proper interpretation of anatomic findings during the performance of EGD.

There is no common agreement concerning how many procedures a clinician who is already competent at other endoscopic procedures (e.g., flexible sigmoidoscopy) should perform before performing EGD without supervision. Many skilled primary care endoscopists believe that approximately 5 to 15 examinations under the supervision of a competent endoscopist should be completed before performing the procedure alone. This is significantly less than a specialist who will be doing more advanced therapeutic care rather than diagnostic evaluation.

OBTAINING HOSPITAL PRIVILEGES

Hospital privileges remain a strongly contested area; the debate over who should receive these privileges is primarily motivated by subspecialty concerns. There are absolutely no study-supported data in the literature denoting a minimal number of procedures that should be supervised before obtaining hospital privileges. Although many numbers are reported by subspecialty organizations as a

proposed minimum, these numbers are subject to debate and are not in any way a demonstration of individual competency. Thus it is essential to have a skilled endoscopist precept an individual to ascertain adequate eye-hand coordination and good visual-spatial skills. For more information, the clinician should review the American Academy of Family Physicians' position paper on endoscopy (Worthington DV, 2000) and the American Medical Association's clinical privileges (AMA, 1993) (see Box 101-1).

SUPPLIERS

Banyan kit ("crash cart" in a suitcase)
Banyan International Corporation
2118 E. Interstate 20
P.O. Box 1779
Abilene, TX 79604-1779
Phone: 1-800-351-4530
Website: www.statkit.com

Welch Allyn vital signs monitor
Welch Allyn
4341 State Street Road, Box 220
Skaneateles Fall, NY 13153-0220
Phone: 1-800-769-4014, Ext. 4502
Website: www.welchallyn.com

Gastroscopes
Olympus
2 Corporate Ct. Drive
Melville, NY 11747
Phone: 1-631-844-5534
Website: www.olympus.com

Pentax
30 Ramland Road
Orangeburg, NY 10962-0822
Phone: 1-845-365-0700, Ext. 3072
Website: www.pentax.com

Fujinon
10 High Point Drive
Wayne, NJ 07470
Phone: 1-800-872-0196, Ext. 320
Website: www.fujinon.com

Patient education materials
American Society for Gastrointestinal Endoscopy
13 Elm St.
Manchester, MA 01944
Phone: 1-508-526-8330
Website: www.asge.org

CPT/BILLING CODES

36000	Introduction of needle or intracatheter, vein
43200*	Esophagoscopy with or without brush
43202	Esophagoscopy with biopsy, single or multiple
43215	Esophagoscopy foreign body removal
43234	Simple upper endoscopy
43235*	EGD with or without brushings
43239*	EGD with biopsies
43247*	EGD with foreign body removal
90780	IV therapy 1 hour
90781	IV therapy each additional hour
90784	IV injection
94761	Oximetry
99070	Surgical tray/IV tubing/supplies

ICD-9-CM DIAGNOSTIC CODES

150.3	Ca, esophagus, upper third
150.4	Ca, esophagus, middle third
150.5	Ca, esophagus, lower third
151.1	Ca, stomach, pylorus
151.2	Ca, stomach, antrum
151.3	Ca, stomach, fundus
151.4	Ca, stomach, body
152.0	Ca, duodenum
211.0	Benign lesion, esophagus
211.1	Benign lesion, stomach
211.2	Benign lesion, duodenum
464.0	Acute laryngitis/tracheitis
476.1	Chronic laryngitis
530.10	Esophagitis, unspecified
530.11	Esophagitis, reflux
530.12	Acute esophagitis
530.2	Esophageal ulcer
530.3	Esophageal stricture
530.6	Esophageal diverticulum
530.7	Mallory-Weiss tear
530.81	Esophageal reflux
530.82	Esophageal hemorrhage
530.83	Esophageal leukoplakia
531.0	Gastric ulcer, acute with hemorrhage (hem)
531.40	Gastric ulcer, chronic with hem
531.70	Gastric ulcer, chronic
532.71	Gastric ulcer, chronic with obstruction
532.0	Duodenal ulcer, acute with hem
532.40	Duodenal ulcer, chronic with hem
532.70	Duodenal ulcer, chronic
532.71	Duodenal ulcer, chronic with obstruction

535.00	Acute gastritis
535.01	Acute gastritis with hem
535.10	Atrophic gastritis
535.60	Duodenitis
536.2	Persistent vomiting
536.8	Dyspepsia
537.1	Gastric diverticulum
553.3	Hiatal hernia
578.0	Hematemesis
784.49	Hoarseness
786.09	Wheezing
786.50	Chest pain
787.01	Nausea and vomiting
787.1	Heartburn (i.e., pyrosis)
787.2	Dysphagia
787.3	Belching
789.0	Abdominal pain
793.4	X-ray abnormality, GI tract
V16.0	Family history, GI tract Ca (not primary diagnosis)
V18.5	Family history, GI disorders (not primary diagnosis)

ADDITIONAL RESOURCES

- See the sample patient education handouts found in Appendix G: "Anesthesia for Upper Endoscopy" on page 1864; "Esophagogastroduodenoscopy (EGD)" on page 1865; "Esophagogastroduodenoscopy (EGD) Preparation" on page 1867; and "Esophagogastroduodenoscopy (EGD): Postprocedure Instructions" on page 1868.
- See the sample patient consent form titled "Esophagogastroduodenoscopy [EGD]" on page 1869.

BIBLIOGRAPHY

American College of Physicians, Health and Public Policy Committee: Clinical competence in diagnostic endoscopy, *Ann Int Med* 107:937, 1987.

American Society for Gastrointestinal Endoscopy: *Appropriate use of gastrointestinal endoscopy*, Manchester, Mass, 1992, ASGE.

American Society of Gastrointestinal Endoscopy: Sedation and monitoring of patients undergoing gastrointestinal endoscopic procedures, *Gastrointest Endosc* 42(6):626, 1995.

Bell GD, Jones JG: Routine use of pulse oximetry and supplemental oxygen during endoscopic procedures under conscious sedation: British beef or common sense, *Endoscopy* 28:718, 1996.

Blackstone MD: *Endoscopic interpretation: normal and pathologic appearances of the gastrointestinal tract*, New York, 1984, Raven Press.

*Health Care Financing Administration (HCFA) allows additional payment for a tray for this procedure when performed in a physician's office. Charge appropriately using code "99070—surgical tray."

Bremang JA: Neuroleptanalgesia in ambulatory (nasal) endoscopies, *Am J Otol* 20(6):435, 1993.

Carrougher JG, Kadakia S, Shaffer RT, Barrilleaux C: Venous complications of midazolam versus diazepam, *Gastrointest Endosc* 39:396, 1993.

Coleman WH: Gastroscopy: a primary diagnostic procedure, *Prim Care* 15(1):1, 1988.

Council on Scientific Affairs, American Medical Association: The use of pulse oximetry during conscious sedation, *JAMA* 270(12):1463, 1993.

Craig A, Hanlon J, Dent J, Schoeman M: A comparison of transnasal and transoral endoscopy with small-diameter endoscopes in unsedated patients, *Gastrointest Endosc* 49(3 Pt 1):292, 1999.

Crump WJ, Phelps TK: Teaching lower gastrointestinal endoscopy: a comparison of family medicine and internal medicine residencies, *J Am Board Fam Pract* 4(1):1, 1991.

Dajani AS, Taubert KA, Wilson W, et al: Prevention of bacterial endocarditis: recommendations by the American Heart Association, *JAMA* 277:1794, 1997; *Circulation* 96:358, 1997.

Diab FH, King PD, Barthel JS, Marshall JB: Efficacy and safety of combined meperidine and midazolam for EGD sedation compared with midazolam alone, *Am J Gastroenterol* 91(6):1120, 1996.

Dies DF, Clarkston WK, Schratz CL: Intravenous ketorolac tromethamine versus meperidine for adjunctive sedation in upper gastrointestinal endoscopy: a pilot study, *Gastrointest Endosc* 43:6, 1996.

Dumortier J, Ponchon T, Scoazec JY, et al: Prospective evaluation of transnasal esophagogastroduodenoscopy: feasibility and study on performance and tolerance, *Gastrointest Endosc* 49(3 Pt 1):285, 1999.

Gorelick AB, Inadomi JM, Barnett JL: Unsedated small-caliber esophagogastroduodenoscopy (EGD): less expensive and less time-consuming than conventional EGD, *J Clin Gastroenterol* 33(3):210, 2001.

Hacker JF III, Chobanian SJ, Johnson DA, et al: Patient preference in upper gastrointestinal studies: roentgenography versus endoscopy, *South Med J* 80(4):1091, 1987.

Hocutt JE Jr, Rodney WM, Zurad EG, et al: Esophagogastroduodenoscopy for the family physician, *Am Fam Physician* 49(1):109, 1994.

Kankaria A, Lewis JH, Ginsberg G et al: Flumazenil reversal of psychomotor impairment due to midazolam as a premedication to conscious sedation for upper endoscopy, *Gastrointest Endosc* 44:416, 1996.

Keefe EB: Determinants of safe endoscopy, *Gastrointest Endosc* 40(3):379, 1994.

Larimore WL, Weber TJ: Coding and reimbursement for gastrointestinal endoscopic procedures in primary care, *J Fam Pract* 39:153, 1994.

Lazzaroni M, Bianchi Porro G: Preparation, premedication and surveillance, *Endoscopy* 30:53, 1998.

Lewis BS, Wayne JD: Upper gastrointestinal endoscopy: state of the art, *Hosp Med* 79, 1991.

Liacouras CA, Mascarenhas M, Poon C, Wenner WJ: Placebo-controlled trial assessing the use of oral midazolam as a premedication to conscious sedation for pediatric endoscopy, *Gastrointest Endosc* 47:455, 1998.

Lieberman DA, Ghormley JM: Physician assistants in gastroenterology: should they perform endoscopy? *Am J Gastroenterol* 7:940, 1992.

Mai HD, Sanowski RA, Waring JP: Improved patient care using ASGE guidelines on quality assurance, *Gastrointest Endosc* 37:597, 1991.

McCloy R: Asleep on the job: sedation and monitoring during endoscopy, *Scand J Gastroenterol Suppl* 27:97, 1992.

Morrissey JF, Reichelderfer M: Gastrointestinal endoscopy (1), *N Engl J Med* 325(16):1142, 1990.

Overholt BF, Chobanian SJ, editors: *Office endoscopy,* Baltimore, 1990, Williams & Wilkins.

Reed DN Jr, Collins JD, Wyatt WJ, et al: Can general surgeons perform colonoscopy safely? *Am J Surg* 163(2):257, 1992.

Rodney WM, Hocutt JE Jr, Coleman WH, et al: Esophagogastroduodenoscopy by family physicians: a national multisite study of 717 procedures, *J Am Board Fam Pract* 3:73, 1990.

Rodney WM, Weber JR, Swedberg JA, et al: Esophagogastroduodenoscopy by family physicians—phase II: a national multisite study 2500 procedures, *Fam Pract Res J* 13(2):121, 1993.

Sanders LD et al: Comparison of diazepam with midazolam as IV sedation for outpatient gastroscopy, *Br J Anaesth* 63:726, 1989.

Shaker R: A wake-up call? Unsedated versus conventional esophagogastroduodenoscopy, *Gastroenterology* 117(6):1492, 1999.

Smucny J: Evaluation of the patient with dyspepsia, *J Fam Pract* 50:538, 2001.

Sorbi D, Gostout CJ, Henry J, Lindor KD: Unsedated small-caliber esophagogastroduodenoscopy (EGD) versus conventional EGD: a comparative study, *Gastroenterology* 117(6):1301, 1999.

Tan CC, Freeman JG: Throat spray for upper gastrointestinal endoscopy is quite acceptable to patients, *Endoscopy* 28:277, 1996.

Thomas JM, Bredfeldt R, Easterling G, Massie M: Esophagogastroduodenoscopy training in family practice residency program, *Fam Med* 29(8):572, 1997.

Tremain SC, Orientale E, Rodney WM: Cleaning, disinfection, and sterilization of gastrointestinal endoscopes: approaches in the office, *J Fam Pract* 32(3):300, 1991.

Volkers N: How can physicians define and improve procedural competency? *Ann Intern Med* 125(12):I39, 1996.

Wayne JD et al: *Techniques in therapeutic endoscopy,* Philadelphia, 1987, WB Saunders.

Wilkins T, Brewster A, Lammers J: Comparison of thin versus standard esophagogastroduodenoscopy, *J Fam Pract* 51(7):625, 2002.

Zaman A, Hapke R, Sahagun G, Katon RM: Unsedated peroral endoscopy with a video ultrathin endoscope: patient acceptance, tolerance, and diagnostic accuracy, *Am J Gastroenterol* 93(8):1260, 1998.

Zuber TJ: A pilot project in office-based diagnostic esophagogastroduodenoscopy comparing two nonintravenous methods of sedation and anesthesia, *Arch Fam Med* 4(7):601, 1995.

Zuber TJ, Jones JG: Physician payment reforms and family physicians (letter), *JAMA* 267:2034, 1992.

Zuber TJ, Pfenninger JL: Interspeciality wars over endoscopy, *J Fam Pract* 37(1):21, 1993.

CHAPTER 103

Management of Fecal Impaction

George G. Zainea

Fecal impaction is a common condition that typically occurs in the bedridden or nursing home patient. Individuals who suffered a cerebral vascular accident are at particular risk. Fecal impaction is the most common gastrointestinal disorder occurring in patients with a spinal cord injury. Medications such as narcotics predispose to this problem. It is also a common complication of anorectal procedures as a result of reflex spasm of the anal sphincter.

DIAGNOSIS

Fecal impaction should be suspected when a patient has unexplained constipation or diarrhea. Diarrhea occurs as liquid stool passes around the hard fecal bolus. Rectal distention from the fecaloma causes reflex relaxation of the internal anal sphincter. The patient may have acute or chronic large bowel obstruction, both clinically and by x-ray examination. The chronic obstruction will increase mucosal water and electrolyte secretion, leading to frequent, loose, watery stools that pass around the bolus. The spinal cord patient may demonstrate autonomic hyperreflexia with pain, fever, tachycardia, and abdominal distention.

Digital rectal examination reveals impacted feces palpated in the rectum. It is important to assess for size and consistency of the bolus as well as for the presence of blood. In the normal situation, the rectal ampulla remains empty. A fecal bolus does not pass beyond the rectosigmoid junction until the act of defecation commences. Complications of fecal impaction can include acute or chronic bowel obstruction, mucosal ulceration, and hemorrhage.

After disimpaction, particularly in the recurrent setting, it is important to rule out an anatomic cause of obstruction. This may require proctosigmoidoscopy. Impaction may be associated with an anal or rectal stricture. The practitioner must assess for the presence of a tumor. Lastly, a deep mucosal ulcer may cause bleeding or infection as a result of fecal impaction.

TECHNIQUE

An attempt at medical therapy in an otherwise ambulatory patient is a reasonable first step. Careful administration of one or two Fleet enemas into the bolus to soften and hydrate the stool should be followed in 1 hour by the administration of a mineral oil enema to assist in passage of the softened stool.

Manual disimpaction is required in most patients. This is best performed after a circumanal block of the anal musculature with local anesthetic. A four-quadrant field block allows for complete muscle relaxation and a painless disimpaction.

Use 0.5% lidocaine drawn up in a 10-ml syringe. A 22-gauge, 1½ inch–long needle is used. Insert the needle all the way to the hub in three directions in the right, left, anterior, and posterior positions 1 cm away from the anal verge (Fig. 103-1). "Fan it out" in three directions at each of the injection sites, depositing a total of 2 to 3 ml of local anesthetic in each of the four sites as the needle is slowly withdrawn. The left decubitus position with hips

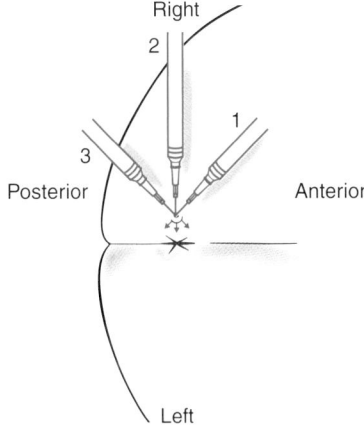

Fig. 103-1
Technique of circumanal block with local anesthetic. Patient is in the left lateral decubitus position. Repeat the injection as shown, 1 cm from the anal verge in all four quadrants (right, left, posterior, and anterior).

and knees flexed to the chest is the most comfortable for the patient. A large, rigid proctoscope may be necessary to soften and break up stool residing higher in the rectum. After passing the rigid scope up to the fecal bolus, phosphate enema solution is passed through the scope to soften the stool. A long rigid aspirator is then passed through the scope to break up the softened stool and allow for evacuation. This process is repeated as many times as necessary to empty the bowel of stool.

Disimpaction may be facilitated by intravenous or intramuscular administration of a narcotic and/or anxiolytic. Early posthemorrhoidectomy impaction may be managed best in the operating room under general or regional anesthesia.

After disimpaction, it is prudent to institute a bowel program that includes laxatives, stool softeners, or enemas along with a regular time to evacuation to prevent reimpaction.

CPT/BILLING CODES

45915   Removal of fecal impaction or foreign body under anesthesia
45300   Rigid proctosigmoidoscopy
45999   Procedure rectum (unspecified)

ICD-9-CM DIAGNOSTIC CODE

560.39   Fecal impaction

BIBLIOGRAPHY

Wexner SD, Bartolo DC: *Constipation: etiology, evaluation, and management,* Oxford, 1995, Butterworth-Heinemann.

CHAPTER 104

Flexible Sigmoidoscopy

John L. Pfenninger

The sigmoidoscope has become an essential component in the primary care physician's office to detect and prevent colorectal cancer (CRC). To decrease morbidity and mortality, the clinician must not only detect this cancer earlier, but also identify and remove precursor polyps. Approximately 150,000 cases of CRC occur each year, with 50,000 deaths. In nonsmokers of both sexes, it is the second-highest major cancer killer. Appropriate screening and removing of all precursor polyps could reduce CRC approximately 85% to 90%. The instrument, although intended initially for screening, has also evolved into a valuable tool in evaluating symptomatic patients.

During the writing of the first edition of this textbook, the debate was still focused on whether or not routine colorectal cancer screening should be performed. The current debate is not "if," but "how." An extensive review of the literature (Frazier, 2000) concluded that the best and most cost-effective method for CRC screening in patients not at risk was flexible sigmoidoscopy every 5 years, along with hemoccult testing every year, beginning at age 50. Although many now promote colonoscopy every 10 years as the "gold standard," the data are simply not there to support it—yet. "More" is not better of and by itself. A patient education handout is available (see the sample titled "Flexible Sigmoidoscopy" on page 1871 of Appendix G) to inform patients of the controversy between colonoscopy and flexible sigmoidoscopy with hemoccult cards. This will enable a more thorough informed consent.*

Studies have concluded that patients will undergo whatever test their physician recommends. Unfortunately, less than 40% of the general population over 50 has been screened following current guidelines. Not recommending routine colon cancer screening following one of the acceptable methods is now a medical-legal issue. Since 1995, all organized groups have recommended CRC screening. *It is time for physicians to implement and encourage proper screening.*

*See the editor's note at the end of this chapter.

INDICATIONS

- Screening

  The American Society of Gastroenterology (ASGE), the American Cancer Society (ACS), the American College of Physicians (ACP), the National Cancer Institute (NCI), the American College of Obstetricians and Gynecologists (ACOG), the American Academy of Family Physicians (AAFP), and the prestigious United States Preventive Services Task Force (USPSTF) all recommend routine screening of not-at-risk patients 50 years of age and older for colon polyps and colon cancer. The Michigan Cancer Consortium provides an excellent protocol based on risk status (Table 104-1) that summarizes data available through January 1, 2001 and incorporates the ACS guidelines. Note that no one is considered at "low risk" for screening purposes.

  (The consortium's recommendations for follow-up of abnormal screening tests and evaluation of rectal bleeding are also listed in Tables 104-2 and 104-3, respectively, since they are concise and practical.)

- Surveillance after previous polypectomy
- Surveillance for effectiveness of treatment for ulcerative colitis/Crohn's disease
- Abdominal pain
- Rectal bleeding (bright red or occult); see Tables 104-2 and 104-3
- Constipation or diarrhea
- Persistent change in usual bowel habits
- Unexplained weight loss, fever, or anemia
- Suspected inflammatory bowel disease or antibiotic-associated colitis
- Anorectal symptoms (Note, however, that hemorrhoids alone are not an absolute indication for flexible sigmoidoscopy or ACBE and must be put into the context of the entire patient history and examination. Medicare no longer reimburses for an endoscopy procedure with the sole diagnosis of "hemorrhoids.")
- Evaluation of radiographic abnormality or to confirm a radiologic finding with biopsy results.

TABLE 104-1

Colorectal Cancer Screening Recommendations (Michigan Cancer Consortium)

Average Risk			
Risk Category	Recommendation*	Age to Begin	Interval
All people ages 50 and over not in the categories below	Either: 1. Fecal occult blood testing plus flexible sigmoidoscopy or 2. Total colon examination (TCE)†	Age 50 Age 50	1. Fecal occult blood testing (FOBT) every year, and flexible sigmoidoscopy every 5 yr 2. Colonoscopy every 10 yr or double-contrast barium enema (DCBE) every 5-10 yr

Moderate Risk			
Risk Category	Recommendation	Age to Begin	Interval
People with single, small (<1 cm) adenomatous polyps	Colonoscopy	At time of initial polyp diagnosis	Colonoscopy *within* 3 yr after initial polyp removal; if normal, as per average risk recommendations (above)
People with one large (≥1 cm) adenomatous polyp *or* multiple adenomatous polyps of any size	Colonoscopy	At time of initial polyp diagnosis	Colonoscopy *within* 3 yr after initial polyp removal; if normal, colonoscopy every 5 yr
Personal history of curative-intent resection of colorectal cancer	Colonoscopy	Within 1 yr after resection	If normal, colonoscopy in 3 yr; if still normal, colonoscopy every 5 yr
Colorectal cancer or adenomatous polyp in first degree relative before age 60	Colonoscopy	Age 40 (or 10 yr before the youngest case in the family, whichever is earlier)	Every 5 yr
Colorectal cancer or adenomatous polyps in two *or* more first-degree relatives of *any* age	Colonoscopy	Age 40 (or 10 yr before the youngest case in the family, whichever is earlier)	Every 5 yr
Colorectal cancer in any other relatives (not included above)	As per average risk recommendation (above); may consider beginning screening before age 50.		

High Risk			
Risk Category	Recommendation	Age to Begin	Interval
Family history of familial adenomatous polyposis syndrome (FAPS)	Early surveillance with endoscopy, counseling to consider genetic testing, and referral to a specialty center	Puberty	If familial polyposis is confirmed, consider colectomy; otherwise, endoscopy every 1-2 yr
Family history of hereditary non-polyposis colon cancer (HNPCC) syndrome	Colonoscopy and counseling to consider genetic testing	Age 21	Every 2 yr until age 40, then every year
Inflammatory bowel disease‡	Colonoscopies with biopsies for dysplasia	8 yr after the start of colitis	Every 1-2 yr

The above recommendations are based on the best available evidence as of December 14, 2000.
Adapted from the Michigan Cancer Consortium Recommendations for Colorectal Cancer Screening, March 21, 2001, with permission from the Michigan Cancer Consortium.
*Digital rectal examination should be performed at the same time as sigmoidoscopy or colonoscopy.
†TCE includes either colonoscopy or DCBE. The choice of procedure should depend on the medical status of the patient and the relative quality of the medical examinations available in a specific community.
‡The available scientific evidence is much stronger for ulcerative colitis than it is for other forms of inflammatory bowel disease such as Crohn's disease.

Also see Box 104-2 (after the bibliography) for the just published 2002 U.S. Preventive Services Task Force recommendations.

Because of redundant loops of sigmoid colon and because the insertion tube that is used for barium enema can obscure a lesion, flexible sigmoidoscopy (or at the minimum, an anoscopy) is generally needed along with most air contrast barium enemas (ACBEs). ACBE is indicated in addition to flexible sigmoidoscopy if the entire bowel must be visualized. Individual circumstances dictate whether a flexible sigmoidoscopy alone or in conjunction with an ACBE is needed.

TABLE 104-2

Follow-up of Abnormal Screening Results (Michigan Cancer Consortium)

Abnormal Screening Test Result	Recommended Procedure	Future Screening Protocol
Fecal occult blood test (If only one of three cards tests positive, this is considered a positive test.)	Colonoscopy	Reassess risk status based on results of colonic examination and follow appropriate future screening protocol.
Flexible sigmoidoscopy	If biopsy done: If hyperplastic polyp: colonoscopy not necessary If adenoma: colonoscopy *or* If no biopsy done: colonoscopy	Reassess risk status based on results of biopsy and follow appropriate protocol.
Double contrast barium enema	Colonoscopy	Reassess risk status based on results of biopsy and follow appropriate protocol.
Colonoscopy	Biopsy or polypectomy	Reassess risk status based on results of biopsy and follow appropriate protocol.

Adapted from the Michigan Cancer Consortium Recommendations for Colorectal Cancer Screening, March 21, 2001, with permission from the Michigan Cancer Consortium.

TABLE 104-3

Diagnostic Evaluation of Rectal Bleeding (Michigan Cancer Consortium)

Symptom Report by Patient	Recommended Procedure	Future Screening Protocol
Bright red rectal bleeding, on tissue, in bowl, or on stool	Age 50 and up: Colonoscopy or flexible sigmoidoscopy with double contrast barium edema Age 40-50: If obvious anorectal disease, and no risk factors: flexible sigmoidoscopy. Otherwise: colonoscopy or flexible sigmoidoscopy with double contrast barium enema If obvious anal source and below age 40: treat symptomatically. If recurrent or persistent symptoms then flexible sigmoidoscopy. Further testing if clinically indicated.	Reassess risk status based on results of colonic exam and follow appropriate future screening protocol.
Burgundy-colored blood marbled into the stool	Colonoscopy	Reassess risk status on results of colonic examination and follow appropriate future screening protocol.

Adapted from the Michigan Cancer Consortium Recommendations for Colorectal Cancer Screening, March 21, 2001, with permission from the Michigan Cancer Consortium.

ABSOLUTE CONTRAINDICATIONS

- Acute abdomen
  - Suspected perforation
  - Peritonitis or intraabdominal sepsis
  - Diverticulitis
  - Bowel infarct
  - Fulminant colitis
- Severe cardiopulmonary disease
- Inadequate bowel preparation
- Lack of subacute bacterial endocarditis (SBE) antibiotic prophylaxis when indicated (see Chapter 204, Antibiotic Prophylaxis for Bacterial Endocarditis, and below)
- Uncooperative patient
- Marked bleeding disorder

RELATIVE CONTRAINDICATIONS

The following conditions require additional caution before performing flexible sigmoidoscopy:

- Pregnancy.
- Recent abdominal surgery.

- Distorted pelvic anatomy.
- History of pelvic irradiation.
- Recent barium enema (if still passing barium).
- When colonoscopy is indicated (such as in high-risk patients with inflammatory bowel disease who should receive a colonoscopy 8 years after the diagnosis was first made and every 5 years thereafter, for follow-up of colon cancer, and for patients with familial polyposis syndromes). An ACBE may also be indicated.

The following basic equipment is necessary to carry out routine fiberoptic sigmoidoscopy:

- 60- to 70-cm-long submersible scope consisting of the body with controls (Fig. 104-1) and the shaft of the scope with tip and apertures (Figs. 104-2 and 104-3; see Fig. 104-6)
- Light source (Fig. 104-4)
- Suction apparatus (Fig. 104-5)

EQUIPMENT

The flexible sigmoidoscope is available as the self-contained fiberoptic scope or the video endoscope. Although the fiberoptic scope is the traditional, most common version, the video sigmoidoscope is state of the art, using computer chip and video technology. The image from the tip of the scope is transmitted to a video monitor. This equipment facilitates videotape recording, sound narration, and other patient information storage.

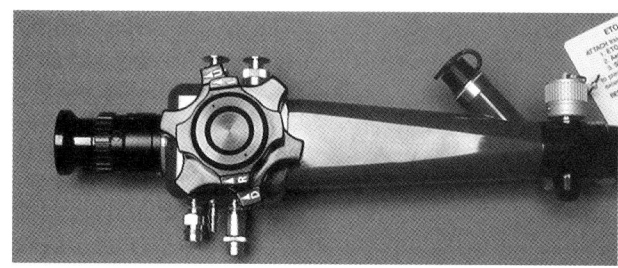

Fig. 104-1
Control head and body of the fiberoptic sigmoidoscope.

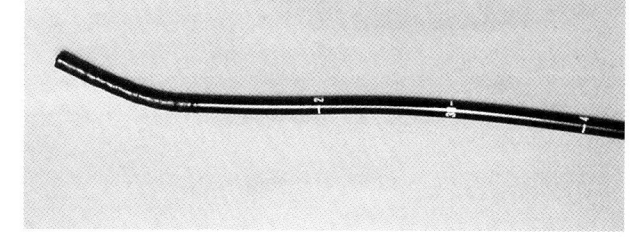

A

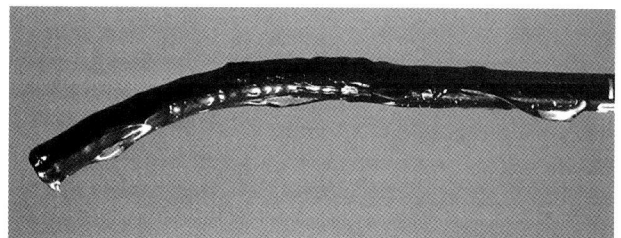

B

Fig. 104-2
A, Tip of the sigmoidoscope. **B,** Tip lubricated with K-Y Jelly.

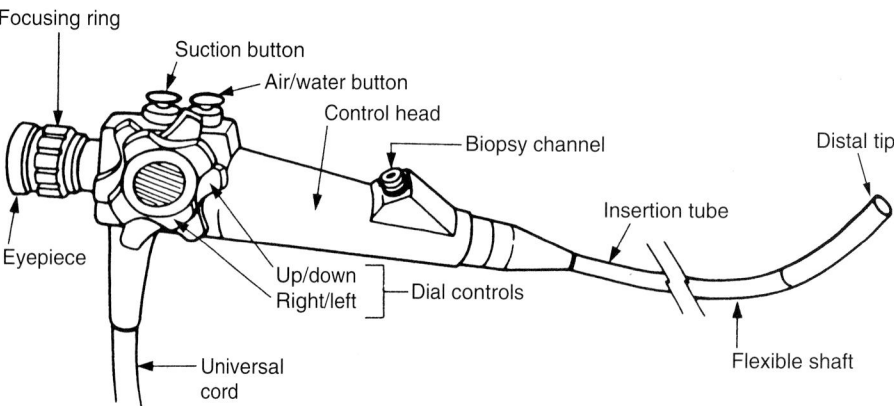

Fig. 104-3
Schematic diagram of a fiberoptic sigmoidoscope.

- Biopsy forceps (Fig. 104-6)
- K-Y Jelly
- 4 × 4–inch gauze pads
- Nonsterile gloves
- Shielded glasses (should be considered)

- Anoscope (Ive's slotted anoscope preferred) (see Fig. 100-2)
- Basin of soapy water (immediately upon completion of the procedure, suction water through the scope then place the scope in the basin)

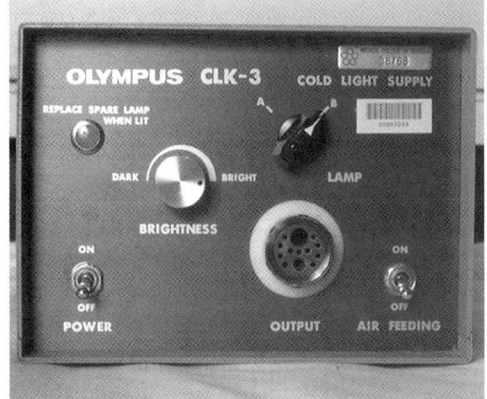

Fig. 104-4
Light source with air supply.

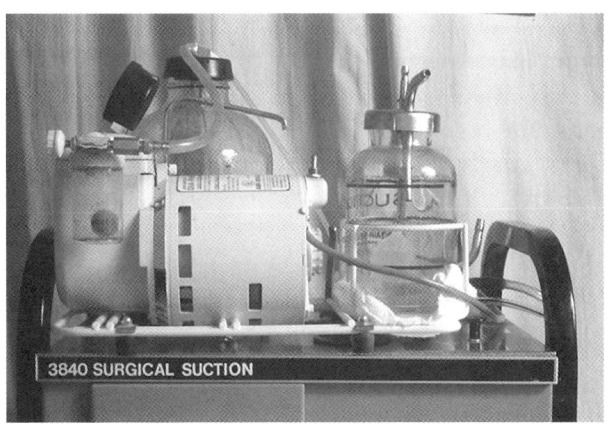

Fig. 104-5
Suction apparatus.

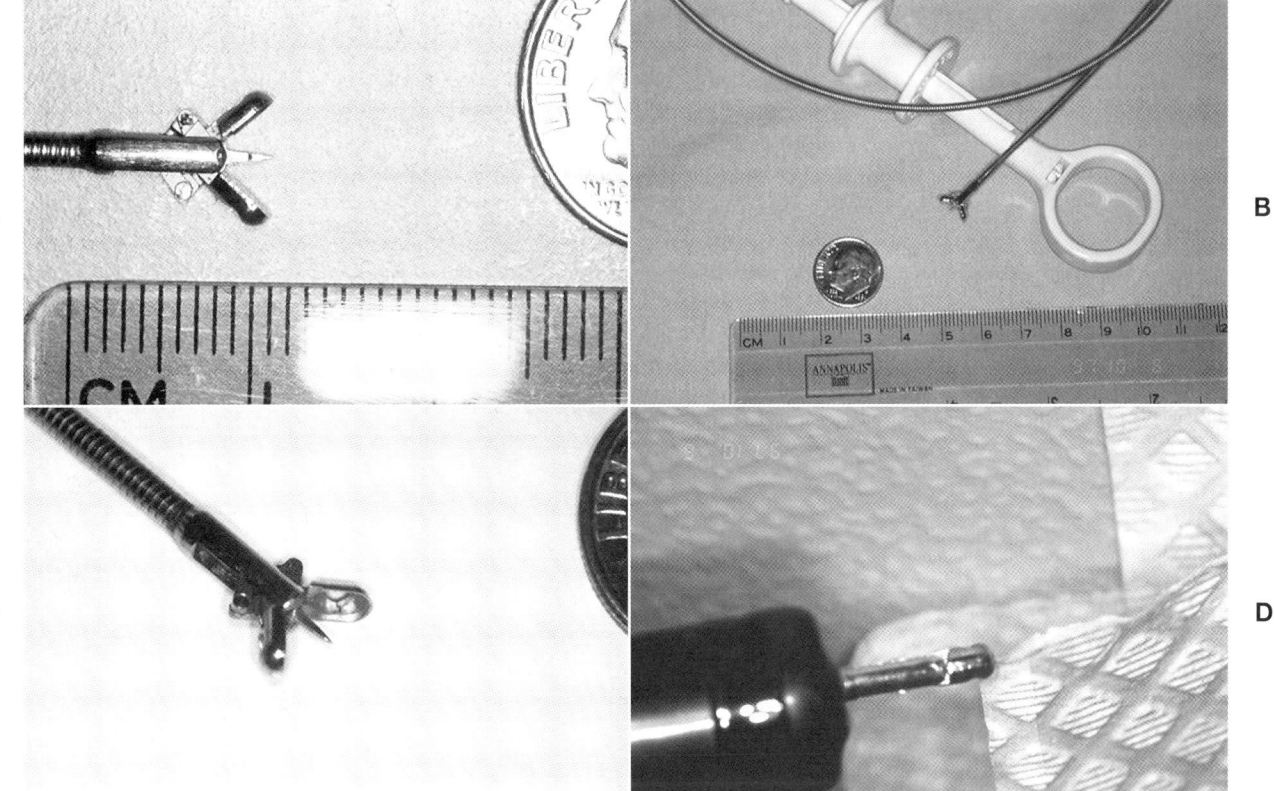

Fig. 104-6
Biopsy forceps. **A,** Relative size of forceps. **B,** Control handle. **C,** Stabilizing needle. **D,** Biopsy forceps protruding from end of scope, closed on a piece of paper. (Courtesy The National Procedures Institute, Midland, Mich.)

- Formalin jars
- Disinfecting cleanser
- Nursing assistant
- Video unit and monitor (for videoscopes only)

PREPROCEDURE PATIENT PREPARATION

Flexible sigmoidoscopy in most patients is an easy procedure performed in less than 15 minutes. However, for some patients the very thought of a tube in the rectum provokes anxiety, apprehension, and reluctance. This makes it necessary for the physician to reassure the patient and allay apprehension and anxiety with a thorough explanation. Use simple words with the aid of charts and figures. Explain the procedure to be performed, why and how it will be done, and the possible complications. The components of this patient-education process include the following:

1. Bowel cleansing instructions (usually two Fleet enemas) (see the sample patient education handout titled "Bowel Preparation for Sigmoidoscopy" on page 1870 of Appendix G)
2. The equipment used
3. Anatomy of the colon
4. The procedure
5. The discomfort experienced during the procedure ("crampy distention" especially at the second curve around 40 cm and with insufflation of air)
6. The complications that are remotely likely (e.g., perforation, bleeding)
7. Possible diseases likely to be detected
8. Biopsy technique, if needed
9. Whether photography or videotape will be used
10. Management of any findings
11. The need to continue all prescribed medications

See the patient education handout and patient consent forms, both titled "Flexible Sigmoidoscopy," in Appendix G for further clarification.

It is highly advisable to have the patient sign the informed consent form for this procedure after reading the patient information materials. (See the sample patient consent form on page 1874 of Appendix G.)

Flexible sigmoidoscopy is well tolerated by the vast majority of patients. Mild analgesia or sedation, whether given orally or intramuscularly, is rarely needed. Oral diazepam and/or ibuprofen can be used as needed in the individual situation.

Patient Bowel Preparation

Simple enemas (Fleet) administered until clear fluid is passed is the only requirement. This usually entails two enemas (occasionally three) 30 to 60 minutes before the procedure. Patients are allowed to take their medications and eat normally. If the patient tends to be constipated, a laxative should be given the day before the procedure.

In one study (Sharma and Chockalingham, 1997), two Fleet enemas given on arrival to the endoscopy suite were compared with one bottle of magnesium citrate and two Ducolax tablets the evening before the procedure. Both patients and endoscopists preferred the oral method. Another study (Manoucheri et al, 1999) showed no difference in results comparing four bowel prep regimens.

Antibiotic Prophylaxis (see Chapter 204, Antibiotic Prophylaxis; Tables 204-1 and 204-2)

Antibiotic prophylaxis is not recommended for lower endoscopy procedures with or without the performance of biopsies (see Chapter 204, Antibiotic Prophylaxis for Bacterial Endocarditis). However, the physician may choose to administer prophylactic antibiotics to high-risk patients with prosthetic heart valves, a history of endocarditis, complex cyanotic congenital heart disease, or surgically constructed systemic-pulmonary shunts or conduits; or to moderate-risk patients, which include most other congenital cardiac malformations, acquired valvular dysfunction (e.g. rheumatic heart disease), hypertrophic cardiomyopathy, or mitral valve prolapse with regurgitation and/or thickened leaflets. Prophylactic antibiotics would include parenteral ampicillin (or vancomycin) and gentamicin in most cases as noted in Table 104-4.

TECHNIQUE

The procedure of flexible sigmoidoscopy has developed its own vocabulary and terminology. Box 104-1 summarizes this "language" that must be understood before learning the procedure.

1. If sedation is to be used, record the patient's temperature, pulse, respiration, blood pressure, heart/lungs auscultation, and abdominal examination.
2. Position the patient in the *left lateral Sims' position* (see Fig. 99-2).
3. The endoscopist and assistant should wear nonsterile gloves on both hands. Double glove the right hand. (Remove the extra glove after the tip has been lubricated, the rectal examination performed, and the scope initially inserted.) Place the body and shaft of the scope alongside the patient. *Lubricate the distal 3 to 4 cm of the shaft tip with K-Y Jelly* (avoid the lens). Notice where the dials are positioned when the shaft is completely straight.

TABLE 104-4

Drug Regimens for Antibiotics for Subacute Bacterial Endocarditis Prophylaxis in Adults

Situation	Agents*	Regiment†
High-risk patients	Ampicillin plus Gentamicin	Adults: ampicillin 2 g intramuscularly (IM) or intravenously (IV) plus gentamicin 1.5 mg/kg (not to exceed 120 mg) within 30 min of starting the procedure; 6 hr later, ampicillin 1 g IM/IV or amoxicillin 1 g orally
High-risk patients allergic to ampicillin/amoxicillin	Vancomycin plus Gentamicin	Adults: vancomycin 1 g IV over 1-2 hr plus gentamicin 1.5 mg/kg IV/IM (not to exceed 120 mg); complete injection/infusion within 30 min of starting the procedure
Moderate-risk patients	Amoxicillin or Ampicillin	Adults: amoxicillin 2 g orally 1 hr before procedure, or ampicillin 2 g IM/IV within 30 min of starting the procedure
Moderate-risk patients allergic to ampicillin/amoxicillin	Vancomycin	Adults: vancomycin 1 g IV over 1-2 hr; complete infusion within 30 min of starting the procedure

From Dajani AS, Taubert KA, Wilson W, et al: *JAMA* 277:1794, 1997.
*Total children's dose should not exceed adult dose.
†No second dose of vancomycin or gentamicin is recommended.

BOX 104-1

Flexible Fiberoptic Sigmoidoscopy Terminology

Tip
Distal end of the shaft of the sigmoidoscope (Fig. 104-2).

Dials
Tip control knobs. Large inner dial moves the tip up and down. Small outer dial moves the tip left and right (Fig. 104-3). The clinician should note the neutral position for future reference when in the bowel.

Biopsy Channel
The slot through which the biopsy forceps and also the brush wire are passed through the body and shaft of the scope (Figs. 104-1, 104-3, and 104-6, *D*).

Suction Control Button (nearest the operator)
When pressed all the way down, this button allows the suction to operate continuously.

Air Insufflation/Lens Cleaner (water) Button (furthest from the operator)
This button has a small opening that can be occluded to allow air to pass into the colon continuously (Fig. 104-3). Pressing the button completely down will squirt water across the lens of the tip and will clear away debris. It must be pressed repeatedly like a squirt gun to eject the water.

Suction, Air, and Water Connection Ports
The location of tubes connecting on the bottom of the handpiece that go to suction, air, and water sources.

Slide-by
A technique of passing the flexible sigmoidoscope where the advancing tip of the scope is advanced proximally into the colon without the complete visualization of the lumen. As the scope advances, the practitioner sees the vascular mucosa "slide by." This maneuver is often unavoidable but should be used very sparingly, and the scope should be advanced only 5 to 10 cm. If the lumen is not fully visualized or if pressure, resistance, or pain is encountered, the clinician should pull back and look again for the lumen.

Pullback
Withdrawing the shaft of the scope to diminish or eliminate whiteout, redout, stretching, or looping.

One-on-one
As the scope is advanced into the rectum, there is an equal advance of the scope into the segment of colon (versus just stretching the colon without true advancement).

Redout
The tip of the scope lies flat against the mucosal surface, resulting in a red appearance through the lens.

Whiteout
The mucosal surface is stretched by the tip of the scope pressing against the mucosal surface. The vessels are thus blanched, giving a white appearance.

Tip Deflection
The tip can be directed in four directions by rotating the dials: up ("north"), down ("south"), left ("west"), and right ("east"). The deflection should always be moderate and gentle. Alternatively, the head of the scope itself can be rotated right and left to turn the tip to the right or left after being flexed up or down.

Dithering
A to-and-fro advance and withdrawal process performed with an amplitude of 5 to 6 cm and repeated every 2 to 4 seconds, coupled with a clockwise torque on the shaft on the pullback motion and a counterclockwise torque on the inward motion. This maneuver helps straighten the sigmoid colon, allowing it to compress like an accordion over the scope (Fig. 104-11).

Jiggling
A to-and-fro, 5 to 6 cm inward and outward motion of the shaft performed every 2 to 4 seconds. It helps in the visualization of a segment of colon, and can often aid scope advancement (Fig. 104-12).

Alpha Maneuver
Used only after much practice by the experienced endoscopist to assist in shortening or pleating the segments of the colon. (See Fig. 104-13 as well as text for explanation.)

Torquing
Twisting the distal shaft of the scope by rotating the head either clockwise or counterclockwise.

Retroflexion
Maximally flexing the tip of the scope, enabling it to look back upon itself. This is often used to evaluate the rectum.

4. Separate the gluteal folds laterally with the hands to expose the anal area and the anal aperture for inspection. *Perform a digital rectal examination* with K-Y Jelly or lidocaine ointment to ensure there is no obstruction or stool in the anal canal. Examine the prostate (in males) carefully. A painful examination should alert the endoscopist to a fissure, proctitis, or colitis. The examination is uncomfortable, but should not be painful if it is done gently. The digital examination helps to relax the sphincter and lubricates the anal canal. (See Chapter 99, Clinical Anorectal Anatomy and Digital Examination.)

5. Now hold the body of the scope in your left hand (Fig. 104-7). *Hold the tip of the scope shaft in the right hand, and, with the index finger alongside and stabilizing the tip, gently insert it.* Hold the tip at an oblique angle pointing posteriorly, and stretch the sphincter as the tip is slipped into the anal canal. The shaft tip can be blindly inserted 10 to 20 cm. Stop when resistance is felt. Remove the second glove on the right hand.

6. With the distal 10 cm or more of the scope in the anal canal, *switch on the light source, air, and suction, and view* at the eyepiece or on the video screen.

7. Keep holding the body of the scope in your left hand so that your thumb controls the large dial and your index finger controls the suction, irrigation, and air valves. *Hold the shaft and advance it* with your right hand, which is also available to control the small dial. *Alternatively, an assistant may advance the scope,* and you may use your right hand to manipulate the dials. The assistant must be cautioned never to advance the scope against resistance and to advance the scope only when told to do so. This latter method is often easier and makes the procedure go much more smoothly and quickly. *There is no "glory" in doing everything alone if the patient experiences more and prolonged discomfort.*

8. *Insufflation-Advance Technique. Air is needed* to maintain patency of the lumen and to obtain a clear view adjacent to the tip and a few centimeters beyond. The air button (and water button) are the same. Just covering the button introduces air, whereas rapidly pushing it down all the way ejects a small amount of water to clean the lens. (The water button must be pushed repeatedly to eject water—"just like a squirt gun"—while air continues to flow as long as the button is occluded.) This button is the one closest to the patient. *(Remember: the button closest to the patient puts things in, the button closest to the endoscopist "sucks" things out.)* A sufficient amount of air must be used to expand the bowel, but too much air may cause cramping or, in extreme cases, even perforation. Use patient comfort as a guide. With a clear view ahead, gently advance the shaft forward. The scope is generally advanced up to 15 to 18 cm without difficulty. There are three "valves" that are encountered in the rectum: the valves of Houston (Fig. 104-8). These are semilunar in shape, are not really "valves," and are located 6, 9, and 12 cm from the anal verge. Negotiating advancement into the rectosigmoid can be hampered by these folds, and the tip needs to be deflected away from the fold and toward the lumen to avoid redout or whiteout. The clinician can get "lost" in the vast arena of the rectal vault and have difficulty in locating the rectosigmoid orifice. This is more likely if too much air is insufflated, which causes the ampulla to expand upward.

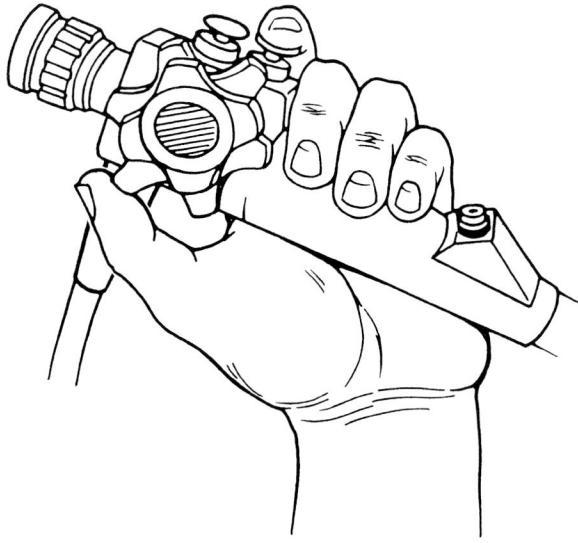

Fig. 104-7
Control head of the sigmoidoscope should be held in the left hand so that the thumb rests on the up/down control dial and the index finger can regulate the suction and air/water buttons.

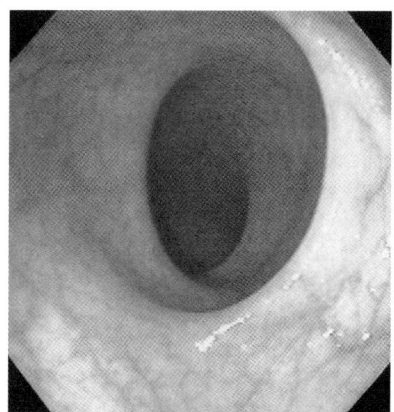

Fig. 104-8
Semilunar valves of Houston. (From Wilcox CM: *Atlas of clinical gastrointestinal endoscopy,* Philadelphia, 1995, WB Saunders.)

There is always a question of how much air to use. The answer: enough! Generally, as long as the patient is not sedated, he or she will tell if too much pressure is being generated. Some clinicians are too timid and will never see the lumen if "enough" air is not used.

At this stage, you do not need to attempt to visualize the entire circumference of the bowel. Rather, the primary goal is to insert the scope as far as possible. It is critical that the complete circumference of the bowel be closely inspected, lest a lesion be missed. This is generally performed during withdrawal of the scope.

It is ideal if the scope is only passed when the lumen is seen, but, practically speaking, *the slide-by method is used fairly commonly* and is safe as long as the scope passes easily and the patient (unsedated) is not feeling excessive pain (see Box 104-1).

9. *Advancing the scope into the sigmoid and descending colon may require using different maneuvers* in the presence of redundancy, adhesions, angulation, and loops. At times, especially in young persons, the scope can be advanced all the way up to the transverse colon without any difficulty. In older patients, especially those who have had abdominal or pelvic surgery, the presence of adhesions may make further advancement difficult. The rectosigmoid junction is at 15 to 18 cm (Fig. 104-9). Advancement may be hampered here by the angulation of the bowel toward the left into the left iliac fossa. The length of the sigmoid itself varies from 20 to 45 cm. Certain maneuvers—individually or in combination—can then be attempted in order to advance the scope into the descending colon and into the proximal parts of the splenic flexure.

Advancement by hook, rotation, and pullback. When the scope will not advance, deflect the tip of the shaft 30 to 90 degrees behind a mucosal fold (Fig. 104-10, *A-D*), and withdraw the shaft 5 to 10 cm, pulling the segment of the colon downward, twisting the head of the scope to the right, and creating a pleating and straightening-out effect. Repeat this maneuver several times as needed to achieve the desired goal of compressing the bowel over the shaft of the scope, much like an accordion. It should be done very gently with minimal (if any) resistance. *When you cannot go forward, flex the tip down, torque to the right, and withdraw. It is a difficult concept to master, but to go forward you must pull back as noted.*

Dithering-torque maneuver (Fig. 104-11). The dithering-torque maneuver is a to-and-fro advance-and-withdrawal process performed with an amplitude of 5 to 6 cm every 2 to 4 seconds. It is coupled with a clockwise torque of the shaft of about 45 to 60 degrees on the pullback motion and a counterclockwise torque on the inward motion. This process "accordionizes" the colon onto the shaft of the scope, thereby shortening the colon and enabling a larger length of the colon to be traversed and examined. Gentle tip deflection of 30 degrees with the torque motion is recommended. The clockwise torque tends to loop the sigmoid, whereas the counterclockwise torque tends to straighten it. This

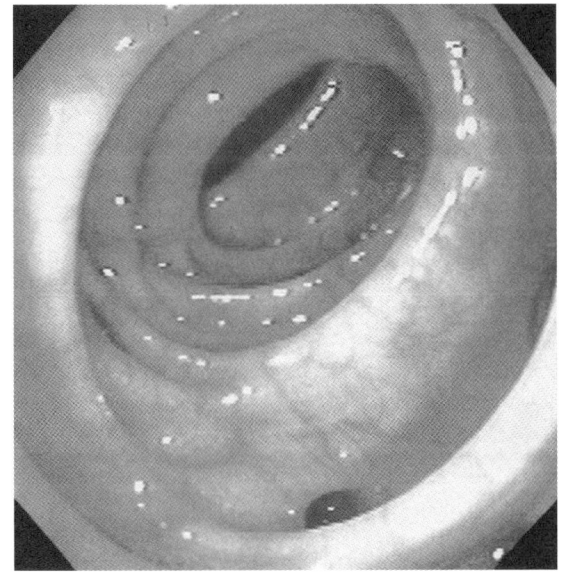

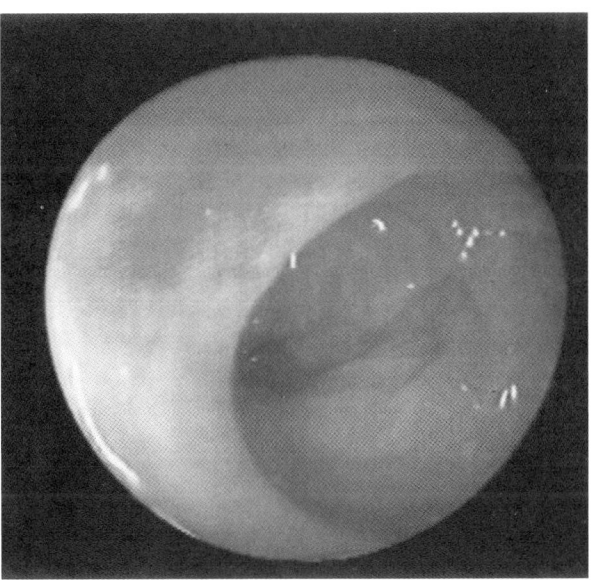

Fig. 104-9
Rectosigmoid junction. **A,** Sigmoid colon. **B,** Sigmoid colon beyond valves of Houston. (**A,** From Wilcox CM: *Atlas of clinical gastrointestinal endoscopy,* Philadelphia, 1995, WB Saunders.)

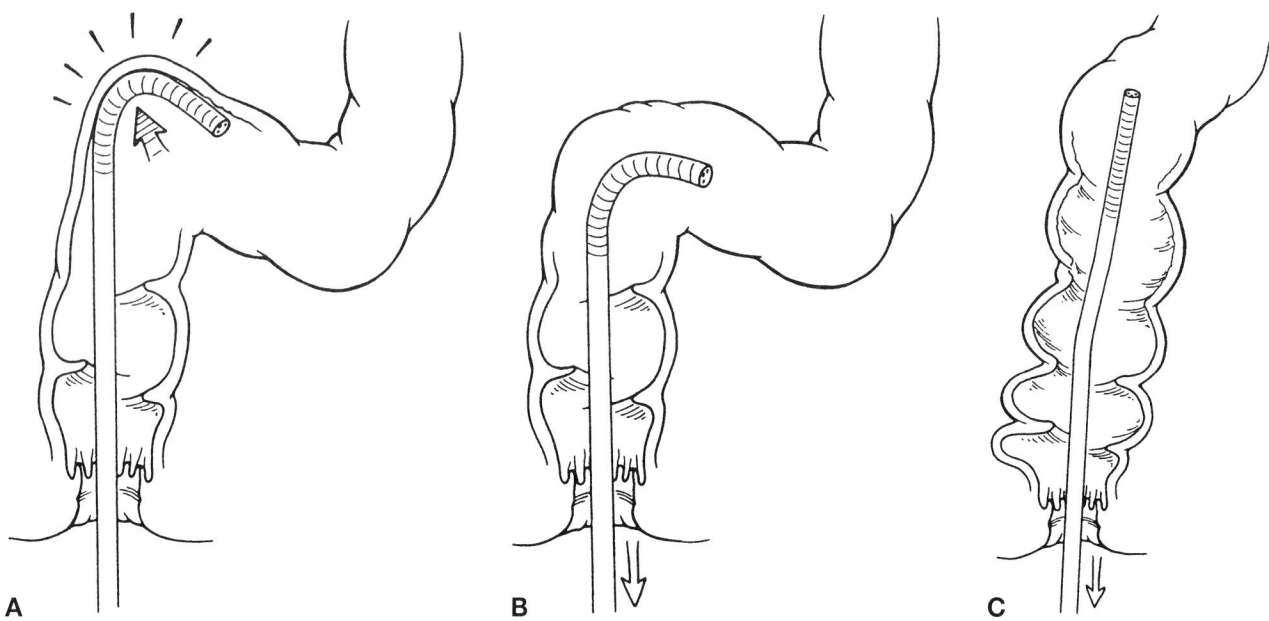

Fig. 104-10
Method of advancement at the rectosigmoid junction. Various maneuvers are needed. **A,** The scope is entering into the anus, but the view from the end of the sigmoidoscope is not changing. There is no "one-on-one" advancement; rather, the segment of colon is merely being stretched, often causing pain. **B,** Try the simple hook and pullback technique initially. **C,** Pulling back on the scope causes an accordion effect and straightens the curve.

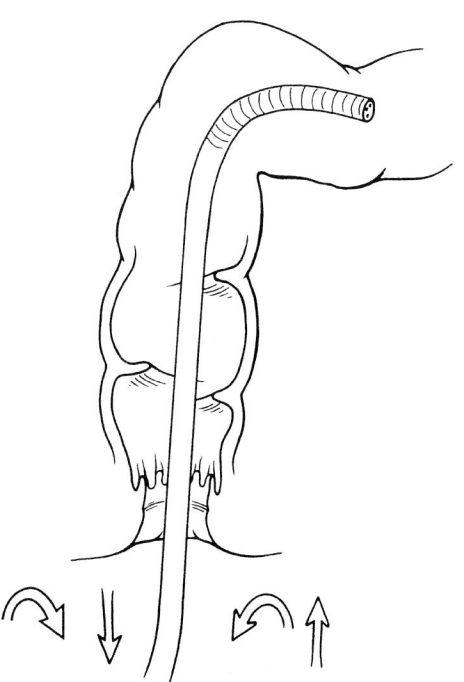

Fig. 104-11
Dithering maneuver. Rotate counterclockwise when withdrawing and clockwise when inserting. See text for details.

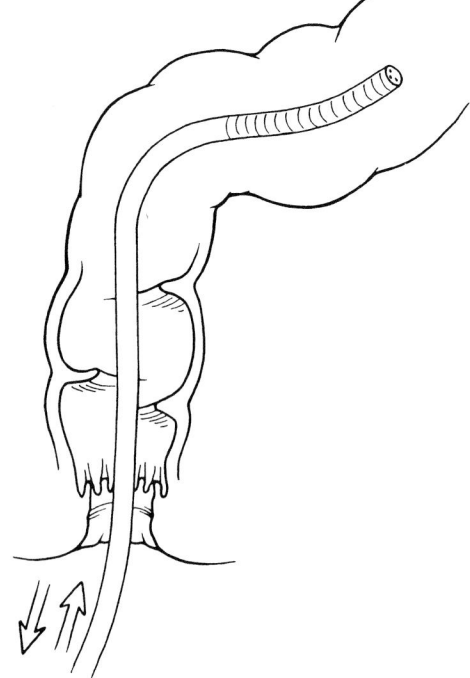

Fig. 104-12
Jiggle maneuver. See text for details.

is an effective maneuver in shortening the sigmoid, and it is of greatest use in a redundant sigmoid colon. Excessive tip deflection can become a hindrance to further advancement; therefore it should be kept to the minimum to maintain visualization of the lumen. If the tip needs greater deflection, it should be straightened soon after the lumen is located.

Jiggling is merely an in-and-out motion deflecting the tip slightly, trying to get the scope to advance. In performing flexible sigmoidoscopy, it is best to keep the scope moving in some manner to maximize the opportunity of seeing the lumen (Fig. 104-12).

Alpha maneuver (for experienced endoscopist). Advance the scope into the sigmoid. At about 25 to 30 cm deflect the tip to visualize the lumen anteriorly, and then torque the shaft counterclockwise about 145 to 180 degrees (Fig. 104-13, *A*). This swings the proximal part of the sigmoid over the distal part, so that the sigmoid colon forms a loop over itself (Fig. 104-13, *B* and *C*). Here, minimally deflect the tip to locate the lumen and then straighten it as much as possible. Further advancement of the scope will lead it into the descending colon. If resistance is encountered, rotate the shaft clockwise

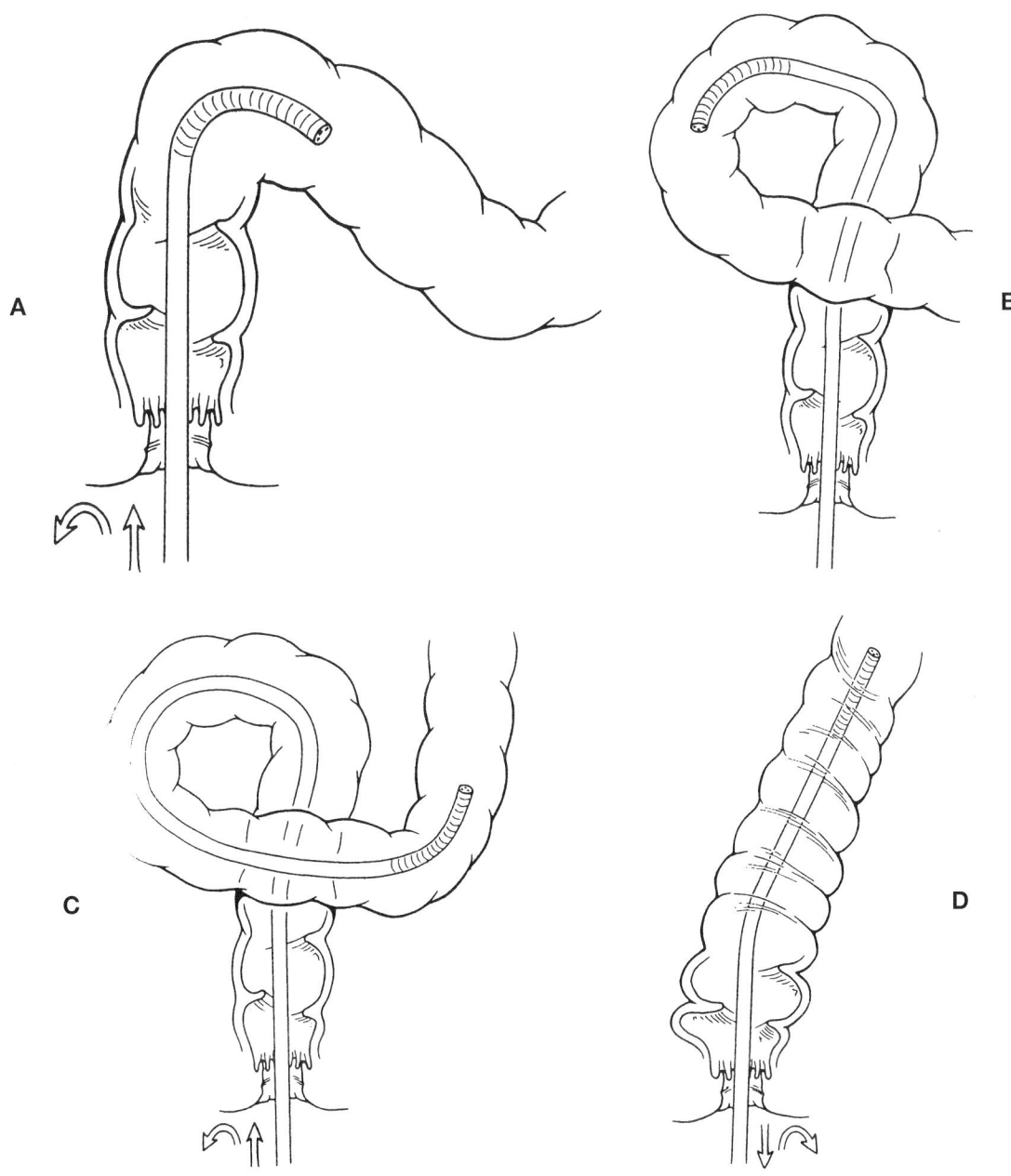

Fig. 104-13
A-D, Alpha maneuver. See text for details.

and withdraw to "accordionize," or shorten, the sigmoid (Fig. 104-13, *D*). The shaft can then be advanced into the descending colon, to the splenic flexure. The alpha maneuver is rarely needed but may be necessary in the redundant bowel. It should be used only by the experienced endoscopist.

10. Opinions vary as to whether or not *changing patient position* will improve visualization or aid in advancement of the scope. Many will roll patients onto their backs. Try it if other maneuvers do not work.

11. Once past the "second curve," the scope is generally advanced with minimal manipulation into the descending colon by jiggling, hooking, and pulling back; just simply maintaining mild inward pressure on the shaft generally suffices.

    The area of the splenic flexure can often be recognized by the bluish hue superiorly, which represents the transmitted vascularity of the spleen sitting on the colon exteriorly. The colon takes a turn anteriorly and to the patient's right at this point, and the triangular folds of the transverse colon can be identified easily (Fig. 104-14).

12. *Withdrawal of the scope is easy.* With the combination of tip deflection and torquing in both directions, gradually withdraw the shaft, visually inspecting the entire circumference of the intubated colon. Pay careful attention to all areas of the mucosal surface, particularly behind mucosal folds. Make note of diverticula and any masses. (See the "Biopsy" section.) If any segment is not seen completely, advance and withdraw again. Continue withdrawing until the rectum is reached.

13. The *anal canal must be inspected* thoroughly in one of two ways: by using an anoscope or by completely deflecting the sigmoidoscope tip to look back on itself. Either procedure is performed after completing the examination of the more proximal bowel. The sigmoidoscope can simply be withdrawn completely and the anal canal examined with the anoscope. Alternatively, after the first semilunar valve is passed, the tip of the sigmoidoscope can be retroflexed (i.e., deflected to its maximum), and the shaft withdrawn gradually. Essentially, you will be looking back up the shaft of the scope and will see the scope in the view piece or on the monitor. At about 4 to 5 cm, inspect the inner aspect of the anal canal and papillae to detect masses and hemorrhoids (although these are much better appreciated with an Ive's slotted anoscope). After a 360-degree visual inspection of the entire anal orifice, straighten the tip and withdraw it very slowly. Grasp the tip of the scope as it slips out of the anus so that it does not drop on the table, damaging its delicate construction.

14. *Reinsert the scope 5 to 6 cm and remove all the air.* Use a to-and-fro motion, rotation, and intermittent suction to prevent the mucosa from being drawn into the suction port, thus occluding it (see following Step 15). After the patient indicates that the air is gone, remove the scope and immediately draw soapy water through the suction port. Also, occlude the air port to "blow out" any accumulated debris. These last two steps will enhance cleaning and preserve proper functioning of the scope. Lay the submersible scope into the basin with soapy water.

15. *Removing fluid and air.* Only mucousy, watery fluid should be suctioned out through the scope. The channels are extremely small and are easily plugged. When suctioning (button closest to the endoscopist), push the button all the way down, intermittently, while pulling the scope back and forth a few centimeters. Constant suctioning at one position will suck mucosa into the scope, causing what appears to be a polyp ("suction polyp"). Moving the scope and varying the suction will eliminate unnecessary biopsy procedures and confusing findings. Do the same when removing air.

BIOPSY

There are many opinions about when and if biopsies should be obtained during flexible sigmoidoscopy. Some points of view with countering arguments include the following:

1. Primary care physicians should not perform a biopsy on any lesion. (*Counter:* The biopsy technique is simple and virtually without complication when only the nonelectrical biopsy forceps are used. It only samples 2 to 3 mm of the mucosa, and unless the tissue is ulcerated or inside a diverticulum, perforation is almost impossible.)

2. It is useless to obtain a biopsy sample, since the colonoscopist will need to remove the polyp anyway. (*Counter:* If the biopsy result shows a hyperplastic polyp, there is no need for colonoscopy. Documentation of an abnormality aids in categorizing the patient's risk status and reinforces the physician's rationale for the patient to have the often-resisted colonoscopy performed. It also confirms the diagnosis for the colonoscopist and mandates that the lesion be found. Even if very small "diminutive" polyps have been found but are adenomatous on histological examination, they carry the same significance as larger adenomatous ones.)

3. Do not perform a biopsy on small polyps (less than 5 mm). (*Counter:* It is precisely these lesions that are difficult to diagnose accurately with an endoscope, so they require biopsy to determine if they are adenomatous and thus require full colonoscopy.)

4. Performing a biopsy may increase malpractice in-

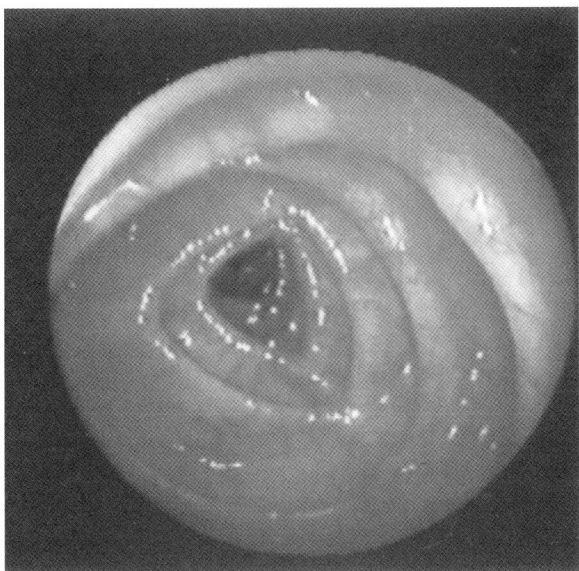

Fig. 104-14
Transverse colon with triangular folds.

surance. (*Counter:* Not doing it may miss a crucial diagnosis. Generally, premiums are not increased for this very-low-risk diagnostic procedure.)

Editors' note: It is our practice to perform a biopsy on essentially all nonvascular lesions. No complications have been encountered. If it doesn't look like the mucosa on the inside of your mouth, if it is not pulsating, if you are not inside of a diverticulum, and if you do not know what it is, perform a biopsy!

Some caveats regarding biopsy:
1. A vascular lesion (especially if pulsating!) may best be left for later biopsy under more controlled situations.
2. Do not perform electrosurgical removal of a polyp except in a fully prepped bowel (bowel gases in the colon can explode).
3. After the procedure, ensure and document that all bleeding has stopped.
4. Document the location from which each polyp was removed, and place each polyp in a separate specimen container.

The biopsy technique is straightforward. The closed forceps are passed down the biopsy channel by the endoscopist. Once they have emerged from the distal tip of the scope, the assistant opens the jaws of the forceps. The operator advances the cable firmly and fixes the forceps on the desired area using the central needle point. The assistant closes the jaws and the endoscopist sharply withdraws the forceps. The biopsy sample is placed in formalin and the site observed for bleeding. Occasionally a second or even a third biopsy sample of the lesion may be indicated (Fig. 104-5).

FINDINGS

- Polyps (iatrogenic "suction polyps," hyperplastic, and adenomatous [tubular, tubular-villous, and villous adenomas])
- Cancer
- Inflammation (inflammatory bowel [Crohn's and ulcerative colitis], antibiotic-associated colitis)
- Diverticuli
- Melanosis coli
- Arteriovenous malformations
- Foreign bodies

DOCUMENTATION

It is important that all findings be noted and documented. A comment should be made on each of the following: scope used, distance inserted, quality of preparation, patient tolerance, vascular and mucosal patterns, size of any polyps identified and depth where they were found, ease of biopsy and control of any bleeding, final impression, and follow-up recommendations (Fig. 104-15).

SIGNIFICANCE OF VARIOUS POLYPS

It is beyond the scope of this chapter to discuss the significance of various polyps. All adenomatous (neoplastic) polyps (tubular, tubulovillous, and villous lesions) have a malignant potential. Recent articles document the reduction of colorectal cancer if all neoplastic polyps are removed. The significance of hyperplastic polyps is still somewhat being debated. Most experts would suggest that their presence has little prognostic significance. Colonoscopy is not recommended for hyperplastic polyps, whereas it is essential with neoplastic polyps.

COMPLICATIONS

- Bowel perforation (extremely rare)
- Bleeding (more likely if a biopsy sample was obtained, but still very uncommon)
- Abdominal distention and pain
- Infection (Although very rare, subacute bacterial endocarditis and transmission of microorganisms between patients may occur.)
- Vasovagal symptoms
- Missed disease

Complications from flexible sigmoidoscopy are very rare. Their incidence is higher in patients with previous bowel or pelvic surgery, or irradiation. These patients

Flexible Sigmoidoscopy

Name: _____ Birthdate: _____ Phone: (H) _____

Age: _____ (W) _____

Your usual doctor: _____   Send a copy of report to him/her?   Y N

Blood pressure: _____   Received and understood handouts?   Y N

SYMPTOMS/HISTORY

Frequency _____   Pain: Abdomen   Rectum   w/BM

Consistency: Loose   Formed   Hard   Anemia _____

Change in stools _____   Weight loss: _____

Diarrhea _____   Fever _____

Constipation _____   Polyps _____

Blood _____   Hemorrhoids _____

Black stools _____   F. H. _____

TESTS:

Hemoccult: Date _____

   positive/negative   not done

Previous sigmoidoscopy/colonoscopy: Date _____

   Findings _____

Previous barium enema: Date _____

   Findings _____

PMH
Bleeding problems?   Yes   No
Artificial joints?   Yes   No
Artificial heart valve?   Yes   No
Heart murmur needing prophylaxis?   Yes   No

Allergies _____

Other medical problems? _____

Medications? _____

Health maintenance? _____

PROCEDURE   **Scope: OSF-3**
Abdominal exam: Megaly Y N   Mass Y N   Tenderness Y N

Preparation: Adequate/Inadequate   Fleets give in office Y N

Rectal: _____

Depth: _____

Reason for stopping: Limits of scope or _____

Tolerance: _____

Complications: none or _____

Findings: _____

Biopsy: _____ cm _____ cm _____ cm   Bleeding controlled   Y N

Proctoscopy: _____

IMPRESSION: _____

RECOMMENDATIONS: _____

Daily aspirins, vitamins, diet, estrogen

Repeat exam _____

cc: _____   _____   _____

               Physician's signature   Date

Fig. 104-15
Sample procedure form for flexible sigmoidoscopy. (From The Medical Procedures Center, P.C., Midland, Mich.)

have more adhesions, which tether the bowel to a fixed position, predisposing it to perforation. If the scope is advanced blindly, without seeing the lumen, the risk of perforation also increases. However, at times it is necessary and safe as long as no resistance is felt and the patient is not overly uncomfortable.

Care must be taken in the presence of diverticulosis. The mouth of the diverticulum can be interpreted as the bowel lumen, and if the scope is inserted, perforation can occur.

CLEANING AND DISINFECTION OF SCOPES

The various instrument representatives will detail the exact cleaning mechanism for each brand of scope. Tremain (1991) presents an excellent review, and reading of this article is strongly encouraged. Jackson and Ball (1997) also summarize the essential steps in disinfecting scopes. It is essential that the clinician's staff pay meticulous attention to cleaning directions for the scope. The orifices are very small, and a small amount of debris can prevent optimal functioning.

POSTPROCEDURE PATIENT EDUCATION

After completion of the procedure, explain the following:
- The findings
- Where the biopsy samples have been taken from and the necessity for pathological evaluation
- Further management or referral, and future surveillance plans
- The implications of the presence of cancer or polyps for the patient's siblings and children
- The necessity of reporting any excessive bleeding or abdominal pain
- Primary prevention methods including the use of an NSAID drug, not smoking, and a high-bulk, low-fat diet with at least five helpings of fruits and vegetables a day. A multivitamin a day, estrogen use, and statins have also been shown to reduce the incidence of CRC.

SUPPLIERS

Sigmoidoscopes
Fujinon, Inc.
10 High Point Drive
Wayne, NJ 07470-7434
Phone: 1-973-633-5600
Website: www.fujinon.com

Olympus America, Inc.
2 Corporate Center Drive
Melville, NY 11747
Phone: 1-800-645-8160
Website: www.olympus.com

Pentax Medical
30 Ramland Rd.
Orangeburg, NY 10962-2699
Phone: 1-800-431-5580
Website: www.pentaxmedical.com

(Also see the "Used or Refurbished Equipment" list in the "Suppliers" section of Chapter 101, Colonoscopy.)

CPT/BILLING CODES

45330	Sigmoidoscopy, flexible fiberoptic; diagnostic
45331	Sigmoidoscopy with biopsy and/or collection of specimen by brushing or washing
45332	Sigmoidoscopy with removal of foreign body
45333	Sigmoidoscopy with removal of polypoid lesion(s)
45334	Sigmoidoscopy with control of hemorrhage (e.g., electrocoagulation)
45336	Sigmoidoscopy with ablation of tumor or mucosal lesion
46600	Anoscopy; diagnostic (separate procedure)

Medicare will pay for *screening* flexible sigmoidoscopy after 47 months have passed since the flex sigmoidoscopy or barium enema. The code GO104 should be used. If a biopsy is taken, the code 45331, not the "G" code, should be used.

ICD-9-CM DIAGNOSTIC CODES

153.2	Ca, colon–descending (L)
153.3	Ca, colon–sigmoid
154.1	Ca, rectum
154.2	Ca, anus
211.3	Benign neoplasm, colon
211.4	Benign neoplasm, rect/anus
455.0	Internal hemorrhoids
455.2	Internal hemorrhoids, bleeding
555.1	Crohn's disease–colon
556.9	Ulcerative colitis
558.1	Radiation colitis
558.9	Colitis, nonspecific
562.1	Diverticulosis
562.12	Diverticulosis with hem
562.13	Diverticulitis with hem

564.00	Unspecified constipation
564.1	Irritable colon
565.0	Anal fissure
566.0	Perirectal abscess
569.0	Anal polyp
569.3	Anal hemorrhage
569.42	Anal pain
569.82	Ulcer, colon
569.84	Angiodysplasia, colon
578.1	Melena
578.9	GI hemorrhage, hematochezia
783.21	Weight loss
787.4	Hyperperistalsis
787.6	Stool incontinence
787.99	Tenesmus
789.0	Abdominal pain
793.4	X-ray abnormality, GI tract
V10.05	Personal Hx colon Ca (not primary Dx)
V16.0	Family Hx colon Ca (not primary Dx)
V16.0	Family Hx GI tract Ca (not primary Dx)
V18.5	Family Hx GI disorders (not primary Dx)

Medicare covered codes include:
Hx adenomatous polyps (V6700, V12.72), malignant and benign GI tract neoplasm (150.0-154.8, 159.0, 159.8, 211.0-211.4), and ca-in-situ (230.1-230.7, 235.2, 235.5, 239.0); infectious GI diseases and colitis (555.0-556.9, 558.2-558.9), ischemic lesions (557.0-557.1), other diseases (560.0-566, 568.0-569.9, 619.1, 759.6, V12.70); hematochezia, melena, change in bowel habits, abdominal pain, abdominal or pelvic mass, occult blood, anemia, abnormal x-ray exam, personal history of GI cancer.

ADDITIONAL RESOURCES

- See the sample patient education handouts titled "Bowel Preparation for Sigmoidoscopy" on page 1870, and "Flexible Sigmoidoscopy" on page 1871 of Appendix G.
- See the sample patient consent form titled "Flexible Sigmoidoscopy" on page 1874 of Appendix G.

BIBLIOGRAPHY

Bazzoli F, Fossi S, Sottili S, et al: The risk of adenomatous polyps in asymptomatic first-degree relatives of persons with colon cancer, *Gastroenterology* 109:783, 1995.

Bond JH, Levin B: Screening and surveillance for colorectal cancers, *Am J Manag Care* 4:431, 1998.

Brill JR, Baumgardner DJ: Establishing proficiency in flexible sigmoidoscopy in a family practice residency program, *Fam Med* 29(8):580, 1997.

Byers T, Levin B, Rothenberger D, et al: American Cancer Society guidelines for screening and surveillance for early detection of colorectal polyps and cancer: Update 1997, *CA Cancer J Clin* 47:154, 1997.

Cohen LB: A new illustrated, "how to" guide to flexible sigmoidoscopy, *Prim Care Cancer* Nov:13, 1989.

Dajani AS, Taubert KA, Wilson W, et al: Prevention of bacterial endocarditis: recommendations by the American Heart Association, *JAMA* 277:1794, 1997.

DeCosse JJ, Tsioulias GJ, Jacobson JS: Colorectal cancer: detection, treatment, and rehabilitation, *CA Cancer Clin J* 44:27, 1994.

Elwood JM, Ali G, Schlup MM: Flexible sigmoidoscopy or colonoscopy for colorectal screening: a randomized trial of performance and acceptability, *Cancer Detect Prev* 19(4):337, 1995.

Endoscope Repair Directory, *Outpatient Surgery* 2(9):65, 2001.

Esber EJ, Yang P: Retroflexion of the sigmoidoscope for the detection of rectal cancer, *Am Fam Physician* 51:1709, 1995.

Frazier AL, Colditz CA, Fuchs CS, et al: Cost-effectiveness of screening for endorectal cancer in the general population, *JAMA* 284:1954, 2000.

Holman JR, Marshall RC, Jordan B, Vogelman L: Technical competency in flexible sigmoidoscopy, *J Am Board Fam Pract* 14:424, 2001.

Holt WS: Factors affecting compliance with screening sigmoidoscopy, *J Fam Practice* 32:585, 1991.

Jackson FW, Ball MD: Correction of deficiencies in flexible fiberoptic sigmoidoscope cleaning and disinfection techniques in family practice and internal medicine offices, *Arch Fam Med* 6:578, 1997.

Johnson BA: Flexible sigmoidoscopy: screening for colorectal cancer, *Am Fam Physician* 59(2):313, 1999.

Leard LE, Savides TJ, Gamiats TG: Patient preferences for colorectal cancer screening, *J Fam Pract* 45:211, 1997.

Levin TR, Palitz A, Grossman S, et al: Predicting advanced proximal colonic neoplasia with screening sigmoidoscopy, *JAMA* 281:1611, 1999.

Levine R, Tenner S, Fromm H: Prevention and early detection of colorectal cancer, *Am Fam Physician* 45:663, 1992.

Lieberman DA, Weiss DG: One-time screening for colorectal cancer with combined fecal occult-blood testing and examination of the distal colon, *N Engl J Med* 345:555, 2001.

Loeve F, Brown RB, van Ballezooijen M, et al: Endoscopic colorectal cancer screening: a cost-saving analysis, *J Natl Cancer Inst* 92(7):557, 2000.

Mandel JS, Church TR, Ederer F, Bond JH: Colorect cancer mortality: effectiveness of biennial screening for fecal occult blood, *J Natl Cancer Inst* 91:434, 1999.

Manoucheri M, Nakamura DY, Lukman RL: Bowel preparation for flexible sigmoidoscopy: which method yields the best results? *J Fam Pract* 48(4):272, 1999.

Mills LR: Colon polyps, *J Fam Physician* 35:194, 1992.

Pfenninger JL, Zainea GG: Common anorectal conditions: Part I. Symptoms and complaints, *Am Fam Physician* 63:2391, 2001.

Pfenninger JL, Zainea GG: Common anorectal conditions: Part II. Lesions. *Am Fam Physician* 64:77, 2001.

Pfenninger JL: Flexible sigmoidoscopy. In Pfenninger JL, Fowler GC (eds): *Procedures for primary care physicians,* St Louis, 1994, Mosby.

Pignone M, Rich M, Tentsch SM, et al: Screening for colorectal cancer in adults at average risk: a summary of the evidence for the U.S. Preventive Services Task Force, *Ann Intern Med* 137:132, 2002.

Provenzale D, Garrett JW, Condon SE, Sandler RS: Risk for colon adenomas in patients with rectosigmoid hyperplastic polyps, *Ann Int Med* 113:760, 1990.

Read TE, Read JD, Butterly LF: Importance of adenomas 5 mm or less in diameter that are detected by sigmoidoscopy, *N Engl J Med* 336:8, 1997.

Read TE, Kodner IJ: Colorectal cancer: risk factors and recommendations for early detection, *Am Fam Physician* 59(11):3083, 1999.

Report of the U.S. Preventive Services Task Force: *Guide to clinical preventive services* (ed 2), Baltimore, 1996, Williams & Wilkins.

Rodney WM: Flexible sigmoidoscopy: the unkept promise of cancer prevention, *Am Fam Physician* 59(2):270, 1999.

Roetzheim RG, Pal N, Gonzalez EC, et al: The effects of physician supply on the early detection of colorectal cancer, *J Fam Pract* 48:850, 1999.

Groveman HD, Sanowski RA, Klauber MR: Training primary care physicians in flexible sigmoidoscopy performance: evaluation of 17,167 procedures (abstract), *West J Med* 148(2):221, 1988.

Selby JV, Friedman GD, Quesenberry CP Jr, Weiss NS: A case control study of screening sigmoidoscopy and mortality from colorectal cancer, *N Engl J Med* 326:653, 1992.

Sharma V, Chockalingham S: Randomized, controlled comparison of two forms of preparation for screening flexible sigmoidoscopy, *Am J Gastroenterol* 92:809, 1997.

Smith RA, von Eschenbach A, Wender R: American Cancer Society guidelines for the early detection of cancer: Update of early detection guidelines for prostate, colorectal, and endometrial cancers, *CA Cancer J Clin* 51(1):44, 2001.

Tremain SC, Orientale E, Rodney WM: Cleaning, disinfection, and sterilization of gastrointestinal endoscopes: approaches in the office, *J Fam Pract* 32:300, 1991.

Trilling JS, Robbins A, Meltzer D, Steinbardt S: Hemorrhoids: associated pathologic conditions in a family practice population, *J Am Board Fam Pract* 4:389, 1991.

U.S. Preventive Services Task Force: Screening for colorectal cancer: recommendations and rationale, *Am Fam Physician* 66(12):2287, 2002.

Winawer SJ, Zauber AG, Gerdes H, et al: Risk of colorectal cancer in the families of patients with adenomatous polyps: National Polyp Study Workgroup, *N Engl J Med* 334:82, 1996.

Zuber TZ: Flexible sigmoidoscopy, *Am Fam Physician* 63:1375, 2001.

WEBSITES

www.gastro.org (American Gastroenterological Association [AGA])

www.fascrs.org (American Society of Colon and Rectal Surgeons)

www.ca-journal.org (CA: A Cancer Journal for Clinicians [American Cancer Association])

BOX 104-2

New United States Preventive Services Task Force Recommendations

Editor's note: As this chapter goes to press, the **latest 2003 updates from the U.S. Preventive Services Task Force (USPSTF) on colon cancer screening** were published (see 2002 reference in the bibliography). A summary is as follows:

- The USPSTF *strongly recommends* that clinicians screen men and women 50 years of age or older for colorectal cancer.
- *Good evidence* that periodic *fecal occult blood test (FOBT) reduces mortality* from colorectal cancer and *fair evidence that sigmoidoscopy* alone or in combination with FOBT reduces mortality. The USPSTF *did not find direct evidence that screening colonoscopy is effective in reducing colorectal cancer mortality.*
- *Double contrast barium enema* offers an alternative of whole bowel examination, but is less sensitive than colonoscopy, and there is no direct evidence that it is effective in reducing mortality rates.
- Insufficient evidence that newer screening technologies (e.g., computer tomographic colography) are effective in improving health outcomes.
- Insufficient data to determine *which strategy is best* in terms of the balance of benefits and potential harms or cost-effectiveness. Studies reviewed by the USPSTF indicate that CRC screening is likely to be cost-effective (less than $30,000 per additional year of life gained), regardless of the strategy chosen.
- It is unclear whether increased accuracy of colonoscopy compared with alternative screening methods offsets the procedure's additional complications, inconvenience, and cost.
- The *choice of specific screening strategy should be based on patient preferences,* medical contraindications, patient adherence, and available resources for testing and follow-up. Clinicians should talk to patients about the benefits and potential harms associated with each option before selecting a screening strategy.
- A 10-year interval has been recommended for colonoscopy on the basis of evidence regarding the natural history of adenomatous polyps. Shorter intervals (5 years) have been recommended for sigmoidoscopy and double contrast barium enema because of their lower sensitivity, but there is *no direct evidence with which to determine the optimal interval for tests other than FOBT.*

- *In persons at higher risk* (for example, those with first-degree relatives who receive the diagnosis of CRC before 60 years of age), initiating screening at an earlier age is reasonable.
- Expert guidelines exist for high-risk patients. Early screening with colonoscopy may be appropriate. Genetic counseling or testing may be indicated for patients with genetic syndromes.
- The appropriate *age at which CRC screening should be discontinued is not known.* Discontinuing screening is therefore reasonable in patients whose age or comorbid conditions limit life expectancy.
- *Proven methods of FOBT screening use guaiac-based test cards prepared at home by patients from three consecutive stool samples* that are forwarded to the clinician. Whether patients need to restrict their *diet* and avoid certain *medications* is not established. *Rehydration* of the specimens before testing increase the sensitivity of FOBT but substantially increases the number of false positive tests. Neither *digital rectal examination* nor the testing of single stool specimen obtained during rectal exam is recommended as an adequate screening strategy for colorectal cancer.
- *FOBT should precede sigmoidoscopy* because a positive test result is an indication for colonoscopy, obviating the need for sigmoidoscopy.
- Colonoscopy is the most sensitive and specific test for detecting cancer in large polyps but associated with higher risk than other screening tests for colorectal cancer. *It is not certain whether potential added benefits of colonoscopy relative to screening alternatives are large enough to justify the added risk and inconvenience for all patients.*
- The complete recommendations and rationale statement on this topic, which includes a brief review of the supporting evidence, is available through the USPSTF website *(www.preventiveservices.ahrq.gov)* through the National Guideline Clearinghouse *(www.guideline.gov)* and in print through the AHRQ Publications Clearinghouse (Phone: 1-800-358-9295; e-mail: ahrqpubs@ahrq.gov).

Colon Cancer Screening Options Vary

(A WORD FROM DR. PFENNINGER)*

How quickly things change. People no longer need to be informed about the importance of colon cancer screening. Instead, they ask for colonoscopy rather than flexible sigmoidoscopy for screening. Since Katie Couric had her colonoscopy live on TV, everyone wants "the thing that Katie Couric got."

For women who do not smoke, breast cancer is the number one cancer killer. For non-smoking men, it is prostate cancer. However, the number two cancer killer for both men and women is colon cancer. What is unique about the disease is that it can be easily detected at an early stage and prevented.

Colon cancer starts in polyps. It takes approximately 10 years to go from nothing through the polyp stage into a cancer. Even when cancer does form, if found early before it is symptomatic, it is generally curable. As of 1996, virtually every major organization has recommended that everyone be screened for colon cancer. For those not at risk, this begins at 50 years of age and every five years thereafter. For those who are at risk, such as those with inflammatory bowel disease or those with a family history of colon cancer or polyps before the age of 60, it begins earlier. Patients over 65 are also more likely to have a cancer higher up. Scientists agree that for those in whom colon cancer is suspected, that the entire bowel must be examined with colonoscopy. The debate arises however in those who are not at risk. What is the best method of screening?

The flexible sigmoidoscopic exam involves using a fiberoptic tube about the size of your little finger to look into the lower 60 to 70 cm (2 feet) of the large bowel. The colonoscopic exam visualizes 160 cm of the lower bowel, or a little over 4 feet.

At first glance, it would seem that certainly the longer procedure would be more advantageous. However, no studies have been done that document doing the longer exam is truly cost effective in those patients not at risk.

One medical journal stated that doing just a sigmoidoscopy is like doing a mammogram of only one breast. However, using that argument, one could say that all of us should have a MRI or CT scan of the entire body every year, beginning at 50. One cannot jump to conclusions. In this case, more may not be better. The objective data are not in yet.

Although the advantage of the colonoscopy is that it examines the entire bowel, there are disadvantages. Whereas flexible sigmoidoscopy only requires two enemas 1 hour before the procedure, colonoscopy patients must have a full 1- to 2-day purge of the bowel. Most people find this quite displeasing. Many patients say that they'll "never go through that again." Thus, if they avoid future exams because of the preparation, it may actually increase their likelihood of developing cancer.

Although some physicians do carry out colonoscopy in the office, the majority of exams are done in the hospital. This increases the cost by 250 to 300 percent. In contrast, flexible sigmoidoscopies are usually performed in a physician's office. Doing a colonoscopy in a GI lab generally costs 500% to 600% more than the screening sigmoidoscopy in the office. Although complications are rare for colonoscopy, the patient is heavily sedated and there are complications from this. Also, perforation of the bowel is more common than with sigmoidoscopy. This would lead to hospitalization and further surgery. Because of the sedation, the patients will also lose an entire day of work. This too is a major cost to society for just a "screening procedure."

A few would argue that if a colonoscopy is done for screening, it need only be repeated once every 10 years instead of screening with the sigmoidoscopy every 5 years. However, I have seen colon cancers develop at 6, 7, and 8 years after that area of the bowel was screened. In the long run, I am not sure that the 10-year recommendation will stand up to scrutiny.

Approximately 1 in 11 patients will have either polyps or cancer found on the screening flexible sigmoidoscopy and will then need colonoscopy to check the entire bowel. The colonoscopy will detect 95% to 98% of all lesions in the bowel. Those missed are generally quite small. A study carrying out colonoscopy immediately after a flexible sigmoidoscopy found that 5% of patients will have lesions that were not found with the flexible sigmoidoscopy. Another way of looking at it, if sigmoidoscopy is done alone, it will pick up approximately 75% of all lesions present. When combined with stool cards that check for blood every year, approximately 90% of significant lesions will be identified.

All things considered, this is an excellent position to be in when arguing about the best method of screening, instead of trying to convince patients to obtain screening. Screening does definitely save lives. If colonoscopy was cheaper, it had less complications, it was usually carried out in an office setting, there were a significant number of adequately trained physicians to perform all the colonoscopies needed, and the preparation were easier and did not require the amount of time it does, perhaps colonoscopy could be recommended as a "routine" method. However, for that patient not at risk, flexible sigmoidoscopy and hemoccult cards may still present the best option. Research studies are pending.

Doctor's note: An article from the Journal of American Medical Association (October 18, 2000) compared 22 strategies for screening for colorectal cancer in persons at average risk. The most cost-effective strategy for the reduction of colorectal cancer mortality in white men was doing the stool cards for blood every year and a sigmoidoscopy every 5 years from 50 to 85 years of age. This resulted in a 60% reduction in cancer and an 80% reduction in cancer deaths. Some recommend only one colonoscopy at 55. This led to a 27% reduction in cancer and a 31% reduction in deaths. Others recommend a routine screening colonoscopy every 10 years. This led to a 58% reduction in cancer and a 64% reduction in mortality.

CHAPTER 105

Gastric Lavage

John Harlan Haynes III
Andrew Thomas Haynes

Gastric lavage may be the most effective means available for rapid gastric evacuation. Therapeutic evacuation of undesirable stomach contents using a large-bore tube has been medically advocated for the past 200 years. Flushing the stomach with isotonic solutions using manual or suction-assisted emptying is quite effective for treating ingestion of toxic substances or upper gastrointestinal hemorrhage. Given proper patient selection, the procedure may be performed with minimal risk.

An alternative to lavage is induced emesis. After a known toxic ingestion, immediate administration of syrup of ipecac (15 ml for children, 30 ml for adults) will usually induce vomiting and gastric evacuation. Ipecac should be *avoided* in patients who are semiconscious or obtunded or who may be prone to seizures (to avoid aspiration). Induced emesis is also *contraindicated* after ingestion of caustic or alkali substances. It should not be used for petroleum distillates, such as viscous oils, that are not absorbed well in the gastrointestinal tract. Viscous substances carry a high risk if aspirated, especially oils (e.g., mineral, seal, or signal oil used in some furniture polishes), and oils will often pass through the gastrointestinal tract undisturbed, anyway. Emesis *should* be induced for ingestion of petroleum distillates carrying more toxic substances such as insecticides, heavy metals, aniline, or nitrobenzene, as well as for hydrocarbons that carry a risk of central nervous system toxicity if they are absorbed. In addition, induction of emesis is indicated after ingestion of chemicals or drugs that are likely to rapidly produce coma or seizures (e.g., sedative-hypnotics, cyanide, tricyclic antidepressants, camphor, strychnine). Also, because of a high risk of aspiration and jaw dystonia, attempts should be made to induce emesis for ingestion of phenothiazines or other antiemetics.

Pulmonary aspiration and chemical pneumonitis can be a devastating complication of both induced emesis and gastric lavage. In one study, the incidence of pneumonitis was found to be 56% with lavage and 28% with induced emesis. Risks versus benefits must be considered when performing either induced emesis or gastric lavage.

Lavage can be performed with either an open or a closed system. Open systems are generally more time-consuming and potentially messy, but they are also less expensive. Open systems use either an active (syringe and flush) or a passive (gravity siphon) process.

A passive lavage process simply uses gravity to drain the stomach contents. Once the intragastric tube is in place, it is used as a siphon. An active lavage process uses a syringe to generate pressure as well as to aspirate and irrigate the stomach. A large syringe is used to inject and remove the fluid from the stomach through the gastric tube. This syringe must be disconnected from the tube to be filled and emptied after each lavage cycle. Alternatively, two tubes may be inserted, one in each nostril. One tube is used as the input port and the other as the output port.

Closed systems are also available prepackaged in commercial kits, self contained, and easy to use. They generally provide more protection to the healthcare provider. Closed systems usually apply active lavage processes. A well-tested closed and active system, EASI-LAV, uses a double-barrel syringe with automatic two-way valves. The syringe remains attached to the gastric tube. Its stroke volume of 125 ml allows for rapid fluid movement and the creation of fluid turbulence, resulting in fast, easy removal of toxic substances or clots.

INDICATIONS

- Poisoning by recent ingestion of a toxic substance in which attempts to induce emesis are unsuccessful or contraindicated

Note: The Regional Poison Control Center can be of great help in determining whether gastric emptying by catheter lavage is indicated.

- Upper gastrointestinal hemorrhage
- Poisoning associated with obtunded or comatose patients
- Poisoning associated with rapid onset of seizures, predicted central nervous system toxicity, or respira-

tory depression in drug overdoses (e.g., sedative-hypnotics, tricyclic antidepressants, cyanide, strychnine, camphor)
- Poisoning with resultant large pill fragments
- Severe hyperthermia (cold gastric lavage)

CONTRAINDICATIONS

- Lack of mechanical airway protection in an obtunded patient
- Caustic ingestions (acids, alkalis)
- Ingestion of hydrocarbons, especially those not absorbed (contraindicated in obtunded patient without endotracheal intubation)

EQUIPMENT

- 3 L of normal saline at body temperature
- Activated charcoal (1 g/kg) for poisonings
- Tape
- Eye protection, mask, gloves, and gown
- Suction tube with vacuum generator
- Endotracheal tube for obtunded patients, especially if they ingested by hydrocarbons
- 2% viscous lidocaine gel, or benzocaine; phenylephrine decongestant nasal spray for nasal insertion

Open System

- Large-diameter gastric tube with extra holes cut near the tip (A 32- to 50-French orogastric tube is recommended for adults; a 16- to 32-French orogastric tube is recommended for children. If the practitioner prefers a nasogastric tube, an 18 French or smaller tube should be used.)
- 50-ml tube syringe
- Y connector and clamp, with or without suction apparatus, and tubing

Closed System

- The EASI-LAV kit is an example of a closed system. It includes a fluid bag and tubing, a waste bag and tubing, a double-barrel syringe mechanism, a gastric tube, and a sample cup.

PREPROCEDURE PATIENT PREPARATION

Insertion of a nasogastric or orogastric tube can be very distressing for the conscious patient. Although gastric lavage is typically performed as an urgent or emergent procedure and most hospitals do not require written informed consent, the risks, benefits, indications, and any possible alternatives should be explained to the patient or his or her family. The patient should be prepared for any discomfort he or she might experience. (See the "Preprocedure Patient Preparation" section in Chapter 107, Nasogastric Tube, Nasoenteric Tube, and Salem Sump Insertion, for additional information for patient preparation.)

Airway protection with a cuffed endotracheal tube is very important for a patient whose level of consciousness is depressed or whose airway-protective reflexes are diminished. (The absence of blinking after touching the eyelashes is strong evidence of inability to protect the airway from vomitus.) The patient should be positioned in the left lateral recumbent position with the head lowered approximately 10 degrees. This decreases the risk of aspiration should vomiting occur.

TECHNIQUE

1. Premeasure and mark the length of the tube needed by estimating the distance from the nose, around the ear, and down to the midepigastrum. To prepare the tube, larger holes may be cut in the end of the tube to accommodate larger pill or charcoal fragments.
2. In most cases, nasal intubation for gastric lavage offers no advantage over orogastric intubation, and it may cause injury to the mucosa and turbinates and severe hemorrhage. If the tube is to be inserted nasally, spray both nostrils with the decongestant nasal spray. Lidocaine gel may be placed into the tube syringe and slowly instilled into one nostril. Ask the patient to "sniff and swallow," if he or she is able to do this. Use an 18 French tube or smaller. (See the procedure for nasogastric tube insertion in Chapter 107, Nasogastric Tube, Nasoenteric Tube, and Salem Sump Insertion.)
3. For orogastric tube insertion, if the patient is alert spray the posterior pharynx with topical benzocaine or Cetacaine spray. Position the patient's head so that it is flexed as far forward as possible, and insert your gloved index and middle finger over the base of the patient's tongue. Guide the lubricated orogastric tube over the dorsum of your fingers as the patient swallows (Fig. 105-1). If the patient gags, advance the tube immediately after gagging. Advance the tube to the previously measured distance marked on the tube.
4. Confirm intragastric tube placement initially by auscultating the stomach while introducing air with the syringe. Verify the final placement by aspirating and confirming gastric contents. This may be sent for toxicologic analysis. Secure the tube with tape.

Open System Procedure (Fig. 105-2)

5. Introduce the normal saline at a rate of 1 to 2 ml/kg per cycle from an IV bag or large syringe attached to the tube with a Y connector in the proximal circuit.

6. During saline infusion, clamp the efferent drainage arm. After instilling approximately 150 to 200 ml (50 to 100 ml in children), clamp the afferent reservoir arm. Then open the drainage arm to allow "passive" gravity to siphon and evacuate the stomach contents. Intermittent suction may be applied to facilitate gastric emptying. Manual agitation of the stomach by gentle massage of the upper abdominal wall will enhance recovery of gastric contents.

7. With active systems, use a syringe and/or vacuum suction equipment, instead of gravity, to irrigate and evacuate the gastric contents.

8. Continue gastric irrigation until at least 3 L of lavage have been utilized and the return is clear on visual inspection.

9. After gastric lavage has been completed, in cases of toxic ingestion, a slurry of activated charcoal should be used. It may be administered cleanly by adding 1 g/kg of the powder through an opened upper corner of a partially full, hanging IV bag. Infuse this mixture through the nasogastric circuit with the efferent arm clamped. Additional saline lavages should be performed until the slurry is cleared of charcoal.

10. When the procedure is completed, clamp or pinch the gastric tube during removal to prevent contaminating the lung with charcoal or gastric contents. If repeated doses of charcoal are deemed necessary, the large tube may be replaced with a standard, smaller nasogastric tube. In the obtunded, intubated patient, leave the endotracheal tube in place for at least 15 minutes after gastric tube removal to prevent aspiration. Confirm adequate spontaneous respirations and oxygenation by pulse oximetry before removing the endotracheal tube.

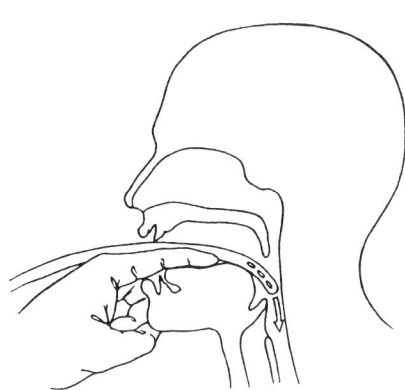

Fig. 105-1
Orogastric tube insertion.

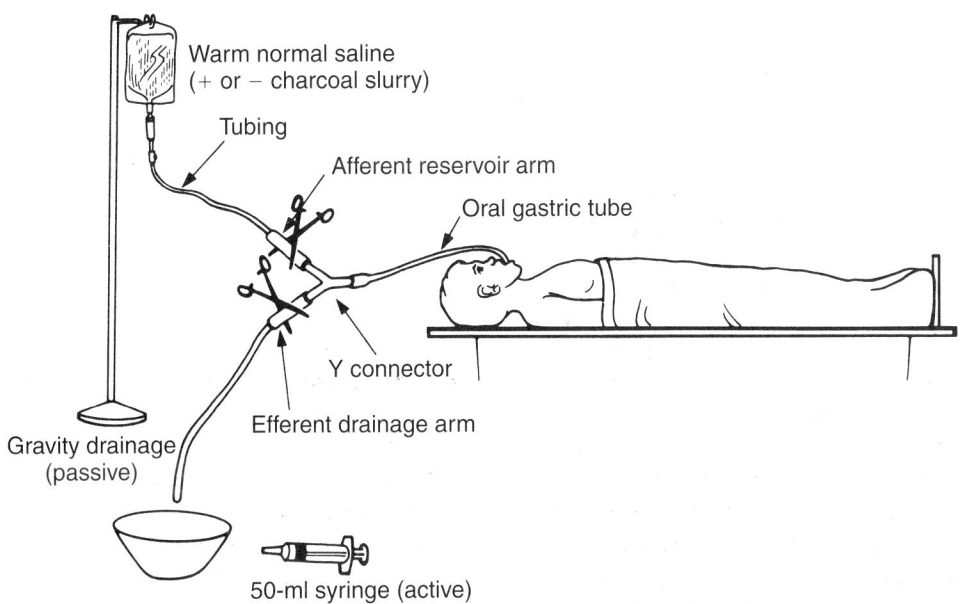

Fig. 105-2
Open gastric lavage system assembly with components.

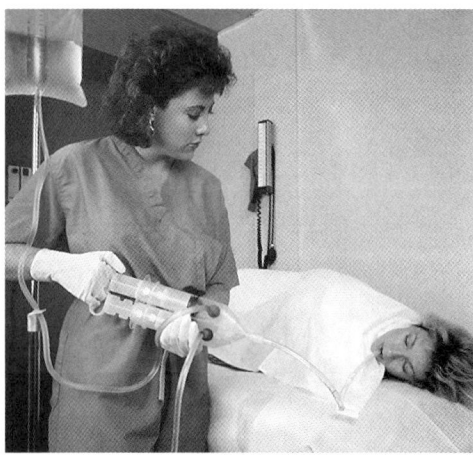

Fig. 105-3
Performing gastric lavage with the closed double-barrel syringe system. (From Haynes JH: *Fam Pract Recert* 14(10):45, 1992. Courtesy Ballard Medical Products.)

Closed System Procedure (e.g., EASI-LAV; Fig. 105-3)

5. Hang a waste bag from the bed. Close the sampling port clamp and cap. Close the fluid bag clamp, and fill the fluid bag with normal saline solution. You can rest the fluid bag on the countertop when sealing it. Finally, hang the fluid bag from an IV pole.

6. Next, evaluate the already inserted orogastric tube. Bending or kinking of the gastric tube may cause malfunction of the system. Ensure airway protection.

7. Advance both syringe plungers to the fully forward position. Attach the syringe to the gastric lavage tube and pinch the retaining collar in place.

8. Ensure proper tube placement, initially, by locking the red output plunger in the fully forward position and pumping the blue input plunger alone while listening for air bubbles in the stomach. Verify correct placement finally by aspirating gastric fluid and confirming that it is indeed gastric fluid.

9. Next, attach the blue tubing connection from the fluid bag to the blue input port on the syringe. Attach the red tubing connection from the waste bag to the red output port on the syringe. Ensure that both syringe plungers are in the fully forward position. Always leave the blue input plunger forward when not in use or fluid will flow into the patient's stomach. Open the clamp on the fluid bag.

10. To empty the stomach, first confirm that the clamp on the waste bag line is opened. Next, pump the red output plunger alone until resistance is encountered or no return is obtained. To avoid mucosal injury, never pull the red plunger against stiff resistance.

Alkali
Ethanol and other alcohols
Ethylene glycol
Fluoride
Iron
Lithium
Mineral acids
Potassium

11. Lock the red output plunger in the forward position by pushing the plunger completely forward and rotating it clockwise 90 degrees. Prime the system by pumping the blue input plunger three times to partially fill the stomach.

12. Unlock the red output plunger by rotating it 90 degrees counterclockwise. Perform the lavage as follows (Fig. 105-3):
    a. Grasp both plunger handles, pull back, and then push forward. This will wash out and empty the stomach.
    b. Perform this lavage three times.
    c. With the blue input plunger fully forward, pump the red output plunger three times (or less, if resistance is met).
    d. Repeat Steps 11 and 12a, 12b, and 12c until the gastric return fluid is clear.

13. To administer charcoal (Box 105-1 lists drugs and toxins poorly absorbed by activated charcoal), the following procedure is effective:
    a. Lock the red output plunger in the forward position by pushing it completely forward and rotating it clockwise 90 degrees.
    b. Pour charcoal into the fluid bag and reseal the bag.
    c. Lavage fluid (50 to 75 ml) may be added to make slurry and to speed administration.
    d. Pump the blue input plunger until all of the charcoal is in the stomach. Repeat Step 12 above to remove charcoal.

COMPLICATIONS

- Mucosal injury or perforation of the upper gastrointestinal tract
- Fluid and electrolyte disturbances (more common when water is used instead of saline)
- Hypothermia (prevented by using warmed saline)
- Pulmonary aspiration (over 50% in some studies)
- Hypoxemia
- Laryngospasm
- Cardiac dysrhythmias

• Same as for a nasogastric tube (See Chapter 107, Nasogastric Tube, Nasoenteric Tube, and Salem Sump Insertion.)

SUPPLIERS

Closed System

Easi-Lav
Kimberly-Clark/Ballard Medical Products
12050 Lone Peak Parkway
Draper, UT 84020
Phone: 1-800-528-5591
Website: www.kchealthcare.com

TUM-E-VAC
Ethox Corp.
251 Seneca Street
Buffalo, NY 14204
Phone: 1-800-521-1022
Website: www.ethoxcorp.com

Open System

Argyle Edlich gastric lavage tray
The Kendall Company
15 Hampshire Street
Mansfield, MA 02048
Phone: 1-800-962-9888
Website: www.kendallhq.com

CPT/BILLING CODE

91105   Gastric intubation, and aspiration or lavage, for treatment (e.g., for ingested poisons)

ADDITIONAL RESOURCES

• See the sample patient education handout titled "Gastric Lavage" on page 1875 of Appendix G.

BIBLIOGRAPHY

Haynes JH: Gastric lavage for serious poisonings, *Fam Pract Recert* 14(10):45, 1992.
Reisdorff EJ, Roberts MR, and Wiegenstien JG: *Pediatric emergency medicine,* Philadelphia, 1993, WB Saunders.
Rosen P: *Emergency medicine: concepts and clinical practice,* ed 5, St Louis, 2001, Mosby.
Rumack BH: Hydrocarbon management. In Rumack BH (ed): *Poisindex,* Englewood, Colo, 1975, Micromedix.
Tandberg D, Troutman WG: Gastric lavage in the poisoned patient. In Roberts JR and Hedges JR (eds): *Clinical procedures in emergency medicine,* ed 3, Philadelphia, 1998, WB Saunders.
Tintinalli JE, Kelen GD (eds): *Emergency medicine: a comprehensive study guide,* New York, 2000, McGraw-Hill.

CHAPTER 106

Inguinal Hernia Reduction

George G. Zainea

The indirect inguinal hernia is the most common type of groin hernia. It occurs lateral to the inferior epigastric vessels. The hernia sac passes through the internal inguinal ring. It is associated with patency of the processus vaginalis. This hernia is typically seen in children and young adults (Figs. 106-1 and 106-2).

The direct inguinal hernia occurs medial to the inferior epigastric vessels. It protrudes through the posterior inguinal floor. It is more commonly seen in adults (Figs. 106-1 and 106-3). The risk of incarceration is less than that of indirect inguinal hernia. Femoral hernias, usually found in adult women, are seen far less commonly. The protrusion occurs beneath the inguinal ligament just medial to the femoral vessels in the upper thigh. The risk of incarceration and strangulation is high with this type of hernia (Figs. 106-1 and 106-2).

DIAGNOSIS

Diagnosis involves palpation with the patient both supine and standing. An incarcerated groin hernia manifests as a nonreducible painful groin bulge. Associated intestinal obstruction may also be present.

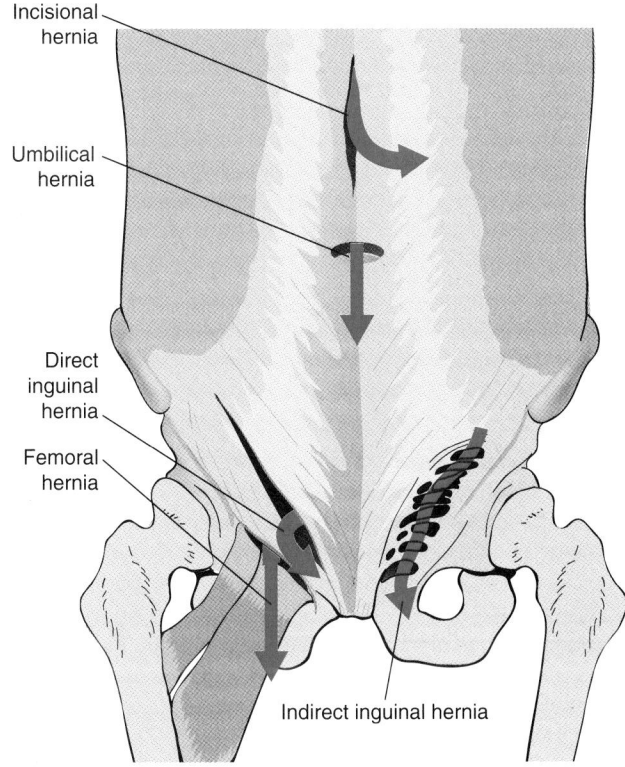

Fig. 106-1
Hernia locations in the abdominal wall. (Modified from *The hernia surgery book,* San Bruno, CA, 1998, The StayWell Company.)

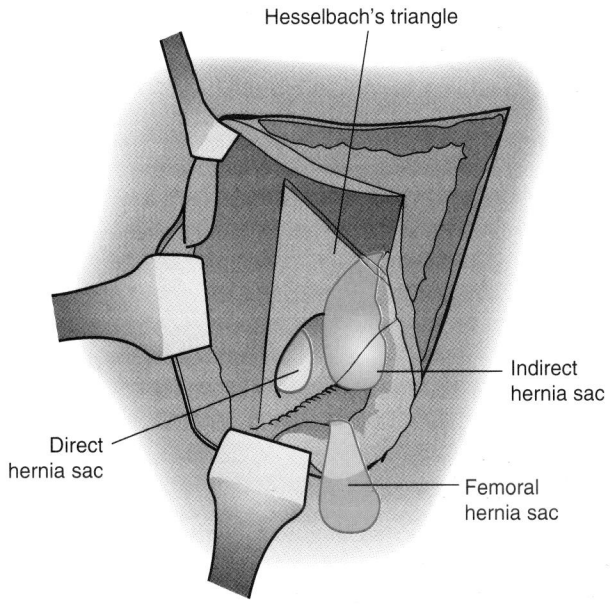

Fig. 106-2
Operative view of inguinal and femoral hernias.

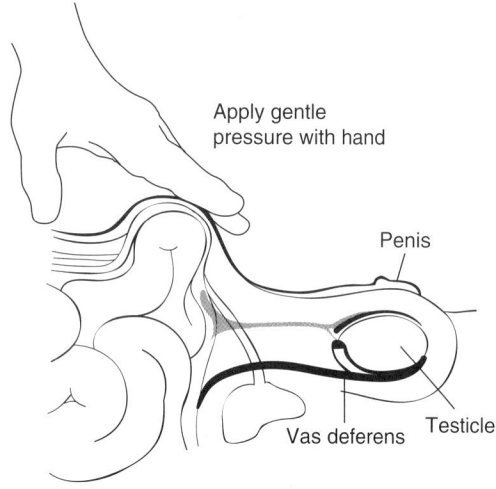

Fig. 106-3
Application of gentle pressure to reduce inguinal hernias. (Modified from *The hernia surgery book,* San Bruno, CA, 1998, The StayWell Company.)

A Valsalva maneuver allows the appreciation of a palpable impulse in a true hernia. Auscultation may reveal bowel sounds. Transillumination can be performed to assist with diagnosis.

DIFFERENTIAL DIAGNOSIS

The history and physical examination usually allows the physician to exclude other disorders that may mimic an incarcerated groin hernia, such as: an *inflamed lymph node,* which is usually evident by history and on palpation; a *dilated varicose vein,* which may appear as a bulge in the inguinal region; and a *hydrocele* of the spermatic cord, which is typically not tender, does transilluminate, and rarely is associated with an acute presentation. Other disorders to consider include *testicular torsion,* which manifests as extreme scrotal pain and swelling. With torsion, pain may be intensified with scrotal elevation, and swelling is usually confined to beneath the pubic tubercle. Finally, an *undescended testicle* may appear as an isolated groin bulge. This should be suspected if the gonad is not present in the scrotal sac.

TECHNIQUE

By definition, a hernia that is nonreducible is incarcerated. Incarceration usually involves either the bowel or the omentum. The practitioner may see intestinal obstruction with bowel incarceration; however, the most feared complication of incarceration is strangulation. With strangulation, the blood supply to the intestine is compromised, and ischemic necrosis and gangrene may result.

The decision to reduce incarcerated hernias requires clinical judgment. If strangulation is suspected, the situation is best dealt with immediately in the operating room. Patients with strangulation typically appear ill. They may be febrile. The bulge is extremely tender, and overlying skin erythema may be present.

If strangulation is not suspected, then the clinician may attempt closed reduction as follows.

1. Place the patient in the supine Trendelenburg position. This allows gravity to assist with hernia reduction.
2. Administer a narcotic for analgesia and intravenous diazepam for muscle relaxation. After sedation, allow for passive reduction of the hernia over a 30- to 40-minute period.
3. If the attempt at passive reduction is not successful, proceed with an attempt at active reduction. Place one hand over the neck of the hernia sac to guide its contents into the peritoneal cavity. Use the other hand to provide gentle and steady distal-to-proximal compression over the hernia (Fig. 106-3).

Using these techniques, the clinician should be able to reduce one third to one half of incarcerated groin hernias. Patients with irreducible groin hernias or incarcerated femoral hernias (which are seldom reducible) should be referred to a surgeon immediately.

Infants and children who successfully undergo closed reduction of inguinal hernias should be admitted to the hospital for surgical repair. An adult patient with suspected compromised bowel in the reduced hernia should be admitted to the hospital for observation. Adults who undergo successful closed reduction and return home should soon thereafter undergo elective hernia repair. A truss should be used only to prevent recurrent protrusion up to the date of surgery.

BIBLIOGRAPHY

Kauffman HM, O'Brien DP: Selective reduction of incarcerated inguinal hernia, *Am J Surg* 119:660, 1970.

Leape LL, Holder TM: Pediatric surgery. In Sabiston DC, editor: *Davis-Christopher textbook of surgery,* Philadelphia, 1981, WB Saunders.

Shandling B: Hernias. In Behrman RE, Vaughn VC, editors: *Nelson textbook of pediatrics,* ed 13, Philadelphia, 1987, WB Saunders.

Ziegler MM: Lumps and bumps. In Schwartz MW et al, editors: *Principles and practice of clinical pediatrics,* St Louis, 1990, Mosby.

CHAPTER 107

Nasogastric Tube, Nasoenteric Tube, and Salem Sump Insertion

Ramiro Sanchez

First mentioned in the medical literature in 1760, the nasogastric (Ng) tube was initially used for gastric feeding. In the early 1800s it was also used for gastric lavage in cases of poisoning. One current design, by Dr. Levin, became available in 1921. Within a few years, his invention became popular for preventing intraoperative and postoperative gastric distention. In the 1960s, improved technology allowed the manufacture of a double-lumen tube. In recent years, special soft tubes have also become available for prolonged nasoenteric feeding.

An Ng tube can be used for either diagnostic or therapeutic purposes. The Levin tube is a firm, straight, nonradiopaque and single-lumen tube used predominantly for diagnostic aspiration or to instill materials into the stomach. In contrast, the Salem sump Ng is a radiopaque, double-lumen tube. The second lumen, or vent lumen, is smaller than the main suction lumen and runs alongside the larger lumen. It provides continuous air flow when suction is applied to the main lumen. The blue "pigtail" is an extension of this vent lumen.

To further compare the Salem sump with the Levin tube, the suction lumen of a Salem tube is smaller than that of a Levin tube. A Salem tube also has graduated markings to determine the length that has been inserted. Both tubes have multiple openings at the distal end (Fig. 107-1). Even though the Levin tube is still manufactured and available, hospitals predominantly stock the Salem sump tube because it can be used for most applications.

Other specialized Ng tubes are also manufactured. While the Salem sump or the Levin tube can be used for short-term feeding, most facilities now have softer, longer, and smaller-diameter tubes designed for this purpose. These usually have a mercury- or tungsten-weighted tip to facilitate passage (Fig. 107-2). They may also have a stiffening wire or stylet available. Another

specialized Ng tube has a balloon near the tip to facilitate passage beyond the stomach (Miller-Abbott, Cantor). Tubes with a larger, esophageal balloon can be used to tamponade varices (Sengstaken-Blakemore). Larger gastric tubes are also available for gastric lavage (Ewald).

Clinicians should understand the mechanics of Ng suction before deciding which type of tube to use. Suction strength is inversely proportional to flow; therefore the lower the flow rate through the suction lumen, the higher the suction strength. In addition, a suction force of more than 25 mm Hg causes tissue capillary fragility and may damage the gastric mucosa. Also, when the suction is turned on, if there is no air to flow through the suction lumen, gastric mucosa may be pulled into the lumen instead. Besides obstructing the lumen, this can also damage the mucosa. Based on these mechanics, one advantage of the double-lumen Salem sump tube over the Levin tube is that it allows constant airflow through the secondary lumen, keeping the necessary suction in the main lumen at a minimum. By requiring less suction, the lumen is also less likely to become occluded with tissue. Salem sump tubes reduce the suction in the main tube to a maximum of 20 mm Hg, or certainly below 25 mm Hg, thereby avoiding capillary tissue damage.

If a Levin tube is used, it should be attached to an intermittent suction pump (Gomco is the most common). Intermittent pumps work in cycles and increase the suction in stages. However, although the initial setting may be only 20 mm Hg, final stages can reach 120 mm Hg. As a result, the suction reaching the patient's tissue at the drainage openings of a Levin tube can be unsafe, even with an intermittent pump. This lack of control over how much suction reaches the gastric mucosa is the biggest disadvantage of a Levin tube. For short-term use, however, or for simply instilling medications, Levin tubes are certainly adequate.

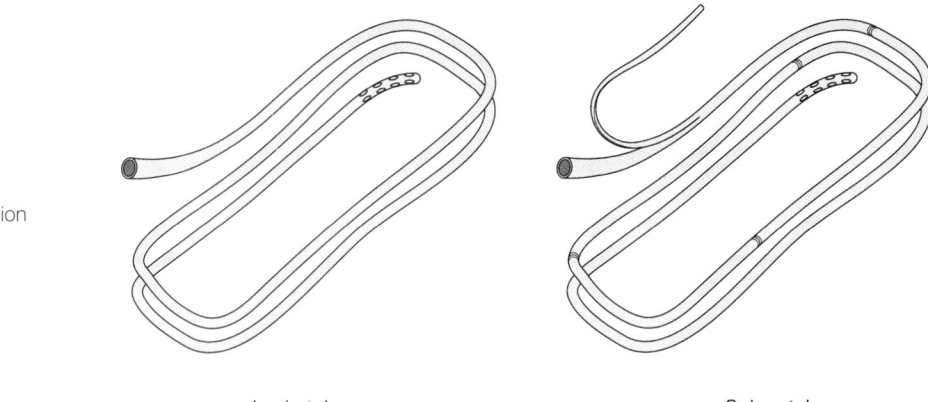

Fig. 107-1
Firm, straight (Levin) tube and sump suction (Salem) tube.

Levin tube   Salem tube

Fig. 107-2
Feeding tube with weighted, radiopaque tip.

INDICATIONS

Therapeutic Indications

- Drainage of gastric contents. Examples include small bowel obstruction, gastric outlet obstruction, paralytic ileus, upper gastrointestinal (GI) bleeding, refractory vomiting, severe pancreatitis (with obstruction or ileus), gastric lavage (especially for drug overdose or for upper GI bleeding when clots might not fit through the tube without dilution), prevention of aspiration, and decompression of stomach before diagnostic peritoneal lavage (DPL).
- Instillation of feedings or medications for patients unable to take by mouth. Examples include antacids, nutritional supplements, and activated charcoal for drug overdoses. (See Chapter 105, Gastric Lavage.)

Diagnostic Indications

- Sampling gastric contents. Examples include hematochezia (exclusion of a GI bleed proximal to the ligament of Treitz) or when a mycobacterial infection is suspected (obtaining a morning gastric aspiration may increase the chance of a positive test).
- Instillation of diagnostic agents. Examples include radiopaque contrast media for delineation of a transdiaphragmatic hernia, or for a small bowel radiologic procedure.

In the diagnosis of suspected upper GI bleeding, Lutz (1979) instilled 200 ml of saline solution in the stomach in adults (10 ml/kg in children) and then aspirated. He defined an aspirate as "positive for blood" if he obtained a grossly bloody aspirate of 10 ml or more. The withdrawal of 30 ml of pinkish fluid with at least a fourth of the volume filled with flecks of blood was also considered positive. In addition, obtaining 30 ml of dark fluid strongly positive for occult blood (i.e., positive guaiac card) should also be considered positive. These rigorous definitions are the only ones studied prospectively.

Unfortunately, there are several problems with using these definitions. A false positive may occur if epistaxis was caused by insertion of the Ng tube. This is a frequent occurrence, especially in children. Also, the low pH in the gastric aspirate can cause equivocal results when using the standard guaiac slide tests. This can be neutralized by adding buffers such as sodium hydroxide (NaOH) to the aspirate; however, this is cumbersome. Fortunately, there is a commercially available product, Gastroccult, which is not only more sensitive, but also provides information about the fluid's pH.

Regarding overall sensitivity, using endoscopy as the gold standard, up to 16 percent of patients with negative aspirates will have documented upper GI bleeding. This may be due to the intermittent nature of the bleeding. In addition, the findings of a pink aspirate with no flecks of blood may be called negative; however, a pink aspirate with no flecks of blood may be merely the result of having washed away previously clotted blood.

CONTRAINDICATIONS

- Facial fractures or basilar skull fractures with suspected cribriform plate injuries (may result in intracranial intubation)
- Esophageal obstruction, strictures, or a history of alkali ingestion (increase the possibility of esophageal perforation)
- Comatose patients without protected airways (increase the risk of aspiration)
- Penetrating neck wounds in the awake trauma victim (gagging might stimulate increased bleeding from the wound)

TABLE 107-1

Enteral Alimentation Tubes

Trade Name	Material	Circumference (French)	Length (in/cm)	Feeding	Duration of Use
Keofed	Silicone	5, 7.3, 9.6	43/107.5	Gastric or intestinal	Up to 6 weeks
Dobbhoff	Polyurethane	8	43/107.5	Gastric or intestinal	Up to 6 weeks
Duo-Tube	Silicone	5, 6, 8	40/100	Gastric or intestinal	Up to 6 weeks
Entriflex	Polyurethane	8	36, 43/90, 107.5	Gastric or intestinal	Up to 6 weeks

- Choanal atresia
- Recent oropharyngeal, nasal, or gastric surgery
- Zenker's diverticulum
- Percutaneous endoscopic gastrostomy (PEG) tube indicated
- Tube feeding in patients with advanced dementia (relative contraindication, since there is little evidence that the outcome will be improved)

Note: Esophageal varices are not a contraindication to Ng intubation. Also, extreme care should be taken in trauma patients whose cervical spines have not been cleared radiologically. Oral placement may be indicated if there is bilateral nasal obstruction, head or facial trauma, presence of nasal packing, or undue risk of precipitating hemorrhage (e.g., coagulopathies or hereditary hemorrhagic telangiectasia).

EQUIPMENT

- Gloves, mask, goggles, and impervious gown.
- Towel or surgical Chux for covering patient's clothing.
- Paper tissues.
- Emesis basin.
- Ng tube (For adults, use a 16 or 18 French Salem sump tube with antireflux valve. Use 10 French for children.) For feeding tubes (5 to 12 French) see Table 107-1. While larger tubes (12 French) are less comfortable and should be used for shorter time periods, they are less likely to become occluded than smaller tubes (5 to 8 French).
- Tincture of benzoin
- Hypoallergenic tape (e.g., Hy-Tape)
- Stethoscope
- Large (60 ml) syringe with catheter tip (Toomey)
- Suction equipment
- Cup of water with drinking straw
- Water soluble lubricant gel (Surgilube) or 2% lidocaine gel (Xylocaine Jelly)
- Topical anesthetic spray such as benzocaine (Hurricaine) or tetracaine hydrochloride (Cetacaine)
- Laryngoscope for difficult insertions
- Phenylephrine hydrochloride (Neo-Synephrine, Afrin) *(optional)*.
- Soft nasal trumpet airway *(optional)*.

PREPROCEDURE PATIENT PREPARATION

Although the insertion of an Ng tube is a common, fairly simple procedure, serious complications can occur. The risk for complications can be minimized by taking a few precautions: obtaining the full cooperation of the patient, informing the patient carefully at each step of the process, using anesthesia for the nasal and retropharyngeal mucosa, premeasuring the length of the Ng tube needed for insertion, using a gentle technique for insertion of the tube, and carefully confirming that the tube is in the proper position before instilling any liquid.

Insertion of an Ng tube is one of the most distressful procedures for patients. Although most hospitals do not require written informed consent, the risks, benefits, indications, and any possible alternatives should be explained to patients. In addition, patients should be prepared for the discomfort they will experience. The unpleasant nature of the procedure should not be minimized. Patients should be aware that their full cooperation is needed to facilitate passage of the tube down the correct path. The risks of additional complications should be explained if the insertion must be performed forcefully.

If a topical anesthetic is going to be used, patients should be informed that it should minimize the discomfort. However, they should be aware that even with the anesthetic, their eyes may water or tear, and they may experience an intense tickling sensation, and/or an urge to sneeze. After the tube has been placed, they will usually adapt to it very soon and no longer notice it. During insertion, they may experience a slight gagging sensation. Swallowing rapidly will minimize this response. At some point during the procedure, they will probably be asked to assist insertion by swallowing. To help them swallow, give them a glass of water and a straw.

TECHNIQUE

Observe universal blood and body fluid precautions during the procedure. Wear gloves, goggles, a face mask, and an impervious gown. Place unconscious patients in the left lateral position with their head turned to the downward side to prevent aspiration. Extreme care should be taken when placing a tube in unconscious patients, because their cough reflex may not be intact (they may not cough with tracheal intubation). They also cannot be asked to talk and demonstrate that there has not been a tracheal intubation.

The technique for the conscious and cooperative patient is discussed in this chapter.

1. Elevate the head of the bed into a high Fowler (sitting) position. Rest the back of the patient's head on a pillow or directly on the bed for support. The patient's clothing needs to be protected with a towel or surgical Chux. An emesis basin should be available on the patient's lap.

2. Various conditions may cause asymmetric nostril openings (e.g., septal deviation, nasal polyps, septal spurs), so examine both nostrils to determine which is the largest and most open (usually the right nostril). You can also watch the patient inhaling through his or her nose to determine which nostril is more open.

3. Topical anesthesia usually increases the patient's comfort, and application of a nasal decongestant such as phenylephrine hydrochloride (Neo-Synephrine, Afrin) may minimize damage to the nasal mucosa. Although this procedure is usually brief, application of the decongestant before the anesthesia usually results in the anesthesia lasting longer. Topical cocaine solution can be used for its combined anesthetic and vasoconstrictive properties. Another option for topical anesthesia is to inject 5 ml of 2% lidocaine gel (Xylocaine Jelly) into the nostril before insertion. The pharynx can then be sprayed with a topical anesthetic spray such as benzocaine (Hurricane) or tetracaine hydrochloride (Cetacaine) to minimize the gag reflex. If possible, allow time for the anesthetics and decongestants to take effect before inserting the tube.

4. A different option is to lubricate a soft nasal airway with 2% lidocaine gel and allow the patient to insert the lubricated airway into his or her nares. The Ng tube can then be inserted through the soft airway. As the patient swallows the gel, it will anesthetize the pharynx. A soft airway will not only minimize patient discomfort, but it can also decrease the risk of severe epistaxis, intracranial intubation, and kinking of the Ng tube into the mouth.

Note: In emergencies, patients do well with adequate lubrication alone. There may not be time for anesthesia.

5. A large-bore Ng tube (16 or 18 French) Salem sump tube (with antireflux valve, if available) should be used for adults. Select the largest tube possible for the patient's nostril size. The Levin tube should be selected in the same manner. The Salem sump tube

has marks at 18, 22, 26, and 30 inches from the distal end. Measure the tube to fit the patient by holding the Ng tube above the patient, with the distal end near the xiphoid process and the proximal end extended to the nose. Loop the midportion over the patient's ear lobe. Note the tube marks based on these measurements or mark the tube with a piece of tape to avoid inserting the tube too far.

6. Lubricate the tip of the tube with anesthetic jelly or a water-soluble lubricant. Curl the tube by rolling 18 to 20 inches of the distal tube clockwise onto the first three fingers of your nondominant hand.

7. Introduce the lubricated tube tip into the nostril, pointing straight to the back of the base of the head (Fig. 107-3). Feed the tube slowly with the dominant hand into the nostril using continuous movement while unrolling the curled tube with the nondominant hand. The patient can sniff to assist the insertion. Never force a tube against resistance; however, spinning or twisting the tube slightly may overcome resistance.

8. When the tip of the tube reaches the retropharynx, a slight increase in resistance will be noted. Have the patient flex his or her head slightly forward to narrow the pharyngeal airway. Continue to advance the tube, and when the resistance decreases again, ask the patient to swallow (Fig. 107-4). Continue to push the tube with the same motion while asking the patient to continue swallowing. If the patient starts coughing or becomes distressed, the tube has probably entered the trachea. The tube should be withdrawn a few inches, but not entirely, twisted slightly,

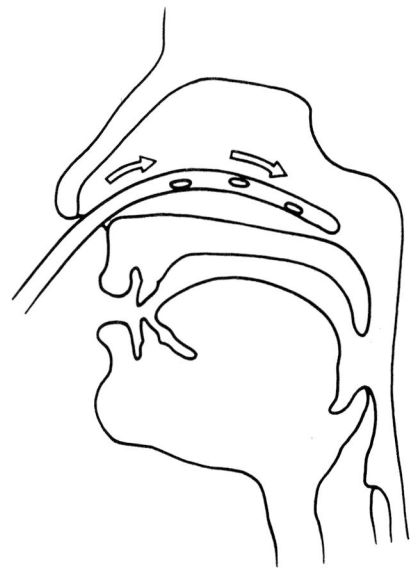

Fig. 107-3
Nasogastric tube insertion.

and the process started again. Ask the patient to start swallowing again.

Note: Occasionally, it is difficult for a patient to swallow on command. If a cup of water with a straw is available, the patient can often swallow some water while the tube is being advanced.

9. If the patient is not coughing, continue to push the tube until the desired mark is reached. In adults, this is usually around the 18-inch mark—the first mark—on a Salem sump tube. The gastroesophageal junction is usually about 16 inches from the nose. If the stomach is full, an immediate return of fluid may occur. Use the emesis basin to collect this. If there is no return of fluid, open the patient's mouth to confirm that the tube is not curled in the mouth or pharynx.

10a. Extra steps to facilitate placement of a nasoenteric feeding tube:
    i. Having placed the tube into the stomach, leave some extra tubing or slack to facilitate passage of the tip into the duodenum.
    ii. Place the patient in a right-side-down decubitus position.
    iii. A 60-ml syringe (Toomey) can be used to inject 400 ml of air to distend the stomach. This may allow a feeding tube coiled in the fundus of the stomach to uncoil and pass more freely into the duodenum.
    iv. In refractory cases, metoclopramide (Reglan) 10 mg may be given intravenously to increase gastric motility.

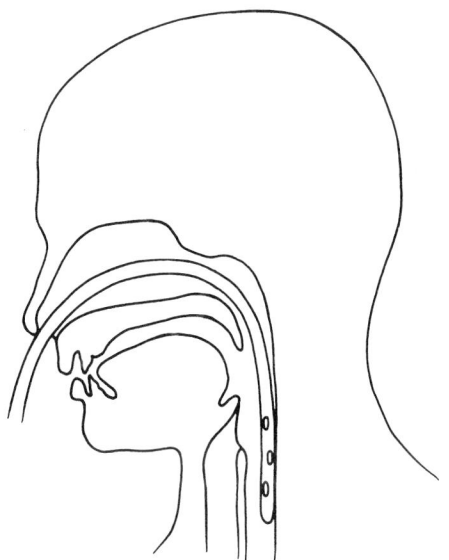

Fig. 107-4
Have the patient flex his or her head. Next, gently advance the tube while asking the patient to swallow.

10b. Extra steps to facilitate any tube placement:
    i. If the tube persistently kinks or coils into the mouth, cooling the tube in ice chips or a refrigerator may stiffen it to prevent coiling.
    ii. Placement may be facilitated manually through the oropharynx with three fingers, if necessary.
    iii. In difficult cases, a laryngoscope may be helpful for guiding or confirming proper placement.
    iv. Fluoroscopic or endoscopic assistance may be necessary.

11. Once the tube is passed, confirm the location of the tip as soon as possible. Ask the patient to speak following placement. If he or she is unable to speak, the tube is in the trachea and should be withdrawn. Be aware that cases have been reported in which the patient could talk despite tracheal placement of a small-bore feeding tube.

12. There are two previous, traditional methods for confirming proper Ng placement: (a) by confirming absence of rhythmic airflow, and (b) by auscultation. As it turns out (see Note below), both of these techniques have been found to be inadequate. Fortunately, placement can also be confirmed (c) by aspiration to check for gastric contents, and (d) radiographically.
    a. Rhythmic airflow. With this method, the clinician listens for rhythmic airflow at the distal end of the Ng tube. If breath sounds are heard, the tube has been placed incorrectly into the respiratory tract. An adaptation of this technique is to place the distal end of the Ng tube into a glass of water. If the tube has been placed incorrectly into a bronchus or the trachea, bubbles will appear.
    b. Auscultation. Using a large irrigation syringe, such as a 60-ml syringe with a catheter-tip (Toomey), rapidly inject 40 to 60 ml of air into the tube while auscultating in the epigastric area. According to this method, proper Ng placement is confirmed when a rush of air is heard in the stomach. The patient may also belch as a result of the air being injected into the esophagus.

Note: In 1994, Barbara Rakel reviewed these traditional techniques for assessing Ng tube placement and found that they were unreliable. Cases have been reported of bubbles being formed despite gastric placement of the Ng and not being formed despite the tube being located in the left lower lobe of the lung. With x-ray films used as the gold standard, a high number of tubes (almost 50%) thought to be in the stomach following auscultation were found to be in the esophagus, duodenum, or jejunum. She also found studies and case reports in which tubes were found in the respiratory tract despite auscultation having been performed. This is especially true for smaller-bore feeding tubes. In addition, Rakel reported four pneumothoraces caused by the insufflation used with the auscultation method of confirming placement.

    c. Aspiration. Aspiration through the Ng tube with a syringe is an acceptable method of confirming placement. If gastric juices are aspirated, correct placement has been demonstrated. Testing the pH of the aspirate will further verify placement. Rakel reviewed several studies regarding the significance of the pH value of the aspirate. She found that gastric fluid should have a pH of from 0 to 4. If the patient is on antiacids or H_2 inhibitors, the pH is between 0 and 6 approximately 70% to 80% of the time. Fluid aspirated from the duodenum averaged a pH of 6.5. Fluid aspirated from tracheobronchial secretions ranged from 6.74 to 8.79 pH. In other words, suspect that it is fluid from the respiratory tract when the pH is greater than 6.

    d. Radiographs. The gold standard to confirm placement of radiopaque tubes is the radiograph. Confirmation in this manner *must* be done on all small-bore Ng or nasoenteric tubes used for feeding purposes *prior to feeding*. The distal tips of these tubes should be allowed to migrate to the duodenum before enteral feeding is initiated.

13. After confirmation of proper Ng tube placement, the tube must be secured. One method is to tape it to the patient's nose (Fig. 107-5). First, apply tincture of benzoin to the dorsum of the nose. Using 1-inch-wide hypoallergenic tape, obtain a 5-inch piece of tape. Make a 3-inch cut length-wise in the middle, thereby forming two narrow strips of tape at one end of the 5-inch piece. Apply the uncut part of the tape to the patient's nose. The two narrow strips of tape should then be applied in a spiral down and around the Ng tube, going away from the patient's nose. They should be applied one strip at a time. Attempt to tape the tube so that it will rest in the middle of the nostril. This minimizes direct contact of the tube with the skin of the nose to hopefully avoid pressure necrosis.

14. Next, secure the Ng tube to the patient's gown. Place a slipknot over the tube with a rubber band, and then pin it to the patient's gown. This should minimize the risk of the Ng tube being tugged out of position. The Salem sump tube vent, or blue pigtail, must remain above the patient's waistline at all times to prevent gravity from siphoning fluid. Inadvertent siphoning of gastric contents could block the sump vent. When suction is discontinued during ambulation, the pigtail should be attached to the connector of the main lumen to close the system. This maneuver should help avoid the spillage of gastric fluids.

COMPLICATIONS

The most common complication is patient discomfort. The traumatic insertion of an Ng tube can cause epistaxis, but this is often avoided by using careful technique. Epistaxis can be massive and require packing, or it can even compromise the airway. If the tube is forced against resistance, a cribriform plate fracture can occur.

Gagging can occur and induce vomiting with aspiration of gastric contents. This can cause an aspiration pneumonitis or pneumonia, which are frequent causes of morbidity/mortality. In one study of 108 cases, 11.6% of surgical patients and 12.5% of nonsurgical patients developed aspiration pneumonitis, directly related to Ng tubes. Overall mortality rates reached 30% in the study. Patients with an altered mental status from severe trauma or another cause should have their airway secured with an endotracheal tube before attempting to place an Ng tube. This may prevent bronchoaspiration.

A common complication is intubation of the trachea. This should be recognized rapidly in the conscious patient when it causes them to cough, choke, or develop respiratory distress and/or an inability to talk. The vocal cords may also be traumatized. In a patient with decreased consciousness, tracheal intubation can go undetected, creating multiple complications such as atelectasis, pulmonary edema, pneumonia, or lung abscess.

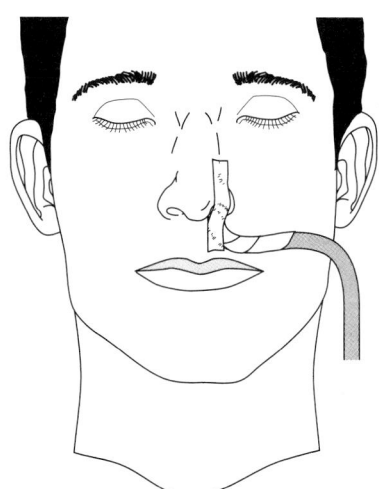

Fig. 107-5
Secure the tube with a 5-inch long piece of 1-inch wide hypoallergenic tape, partially cut lengthwise. Apply to the dorsum of the nose and spiral the cut portions down the Ng away from the nose.

The penetration of an Ng tube into the pleural space is a rare but reported complication. A case of perforation of the cervical esophagus has also been reported. This event was heralded by the production of subcutaneous emphysema of the neck and chest. Otherwise, perforation of the esophagus may occur when the esophagus has been damaged (e.g., chemical burns) or if strictures are present. Bleeding from esophageal varices is not usually caused by Ng intubation.

With long-term use, sinusitis, erosion of nasal tissue, or even a tracheoesophageal fistula can occur. Tracheoesophageal fistulas are usually associated with simultaneous use of an endotracheal tube. Sinusitis can cause a fever of unknown origin in ICU patients.

Individuals with facial or maxillofacial trauma have a significantly increased risk of inadvertent intracranial intubation. This can obviously cause severe and catastrophic complications. The risk of this complication can be reduced by initially introducing a nasotracheal tube or a soft rubber nasal airway. A smaller-diameter Ng tube can then be passed through it. This technique decreases the danger of penetrating the cranium, reduces the discomfort during insertion, decreases epistaxis, and decreases the frequency of the Ng tube kinking into the mouth.

SUPPLIERS

Latex-free, zinc oxide tape

Hy-Tape International
P.O. Box 540
Patterson, NY 12563-0540
Phone: 1-800-248-0101
Website: www.hytape.com

Salem sump and feeding tubes

The Kendall Company
15 Hampshire Street
Mansfield, MA 02048
Phone: 1-800-962-9888
Website: www.kendallhq.com

Cook Incorporated
P.O. Box 489
Bloomington, IN 47402-0489
Phone: 1-800-457-4500
Website: www.cookincorporated.com

Feeding tubes

Corpak MedSystems/VIASYS Healthcare
100 Chaddick Drive
Wheeling, IL 60090
Phone: 1-800-323-6305
Website: www.corpakmedsystems.com

Topical anesthetic

Cetacaine
Cetylite Industries, Inc.
9051 River Road
Pennsauken, NJ 08110
Phone: 1-800-257-7740
Website: www.cetylite.com

Xylocaine
AstraZeneca L.P.
725 Chesterbrook Boulevard
Wayne, PA 19087
Phone: 1-610-695-1000
Website: www.astrazeneca.com

Guaiac cards

Gastroccult (formerly from Smith-Kline Diagnostics)
Beckman Coulter, Inc.
4300 N. Harbor Boulevard
P.O. Box 3100
Fullerton, CA 92834-3100
Phone: 1-800-877-6242
Website: www.beckmancoulter.com

60-ml syringe with catheter tip (Toomey)

Becton, Dickinson and Co.
1 Becton Drive
Franklin Lakes, NJ 07417
Phone: 1-201-847-6800
Website: www.bd.com

CPT/BILLING CODES

43752	Nasogastric or orogastric tube placement, necessitating physician's skill
89130	Gastric intubation and aspiration, diagnostic, each specimen, for chemical analysis or cytopathology
91105	Gastric intubation, and aspiration or lavage, for treatment (e.g., for ingested poisons)

ICD-9-CM DIAGNOSTIC CODES

014.82	Tuberculosis, gastrocolic, labs pending
261	Calorie deficiency, severe
263.9	Malnutrition, calorie
536.2	Vomiting, persistent, nonpregnant
537.0	Gastric outlet obstruction
560.1	Ileus, paralytic
561.81	Small intestine obstruction, due to adhesions
577.0	Pancreatitis, NOS or acute
577.1	Pancreatitis, chronic
578.0	Hematemesis

578.1   Hematochezia
578.9   Gastrointestinal bleeding, unspecified
787.03   Vomiting, NOS
787.01   Vomiting, NOS with nausea
977.9   Poisoning, unspecified drug or medicinal substances

REFERENCES

Chen YS, Wang SM: A modified method to insert a nasogastric tube without kinking in the nasal cavity, *Am J Emerg Med* 10(6):614, 1992.

Fisman DN, Ward ME: Intrapleural placement of a nasogastric tube: an unusual complication of nasotracheal intubation, *Can J Anaesth* 43(12):1252, 1996.

Katz MI, Faibel M: Inadvertent intracranial placement of a nasogastric tube, *AJR Am J Roentgenol* 163(1):222, 1994.

LeFrock JL, Clark TS, Davies B, Klainer AS: Aspiration pneumonia: a ten year review, *Am Surg* 5(5):305, 1979.

Lutz GD, Bynum TE, Hendrix TR: Gastric aspiration in localization of gastrointestinal hemorrhage, *JAMA* 241:576, 1979.

Rakel BA, Titler M, Goode C, et al: Nasogastric and nasointestinal feeding tube placement: an integrative review of research, *AACN Clin Issues Crit Care Nurs* 5(2):194; quiz 218, 1994.

Wrenn K: The lowly nasogastric tube: still appropriate after all these years (at times), *Am J Emerg Med* 11:84, 1993.

WEBSITES

www.merck.com/pubs/mmanual/section3/chapter19/19a.htm (article: "Diagnostic and Therapeutic Gastrointestinal Procedures")

CHAPTER 108

Office Treatment of Hemorrhoids

George G. Zainea
John L. Pfenninger

Hemorrhoidal disease occurs in approximately 50% to 80% of the U.S. population. Although this disease is rarely fatal, it accounts for a great deal of human pain and suffering. Internal hemorrhoids are the most common cause of lower gastrointestinal (GI) bleeding. Nonetheless, it is imperative that the clinician confirm that bleeding is indeed originating from hemorrhoidal disease and not from a more proximal lesion. Occasionally, bleeding can be severe and is associated with anemia.

Most hemorrhoidal symptoms can be managed with medical therapies that include suppositories, topical agents, and fiber supplementation. Patients who fail medical therapies are appropriate candidates for in-office treatments of hemorrhoids. Only the minority of individuals requires definitive treatment for severe symptomatic hemorrhoids with a surgical hemorrhoidectomy. A hemorrhoidectomy requires general or regional anesthesia and is associated with significant discomfort and loss of time from work or usual activities after surgery.

Rubber-band ligation is a time-tested and proven method for treating internal hemorrhoids. However, other approaches have been developed. Newer modalities include infrared photocoagulation (IRC). Sclerotherapy is also occasionally used. These therapies can be used selectively or in combination depending on the extent and severity of internal disease. Lasers have also been used for the treatment of internal disease (see Chapter 27, Laser Therapy). The treatment for external hemorrhoid disease has been unchanged for decades.

Two metaanalyses have been reported on the treatment of internal hemorrhoids. One concludes that band ligation is best, whereas the other supports IRC. In both instances, hemorrhoid symptoms resolved in 80% to 90% of properly selected cases.

The physician must know the anorectal anatomy (see Chapter 99, Clinical Anorectal Anatomy and Digital Examination) and must be able to perform a thorough anoscopic examination (see Chapter 100, Anoscopy) to appropriately assess and treat hemorrhoids.

After completion of any of these procedures, a medi-

cal program to regulate bowel habits should be implemented to prevent recurrence, which is as important as the surgical intervention itself.

Note: Two previous methods of treating internal hemorrhoids (bipolar electrocoagulation [BICAP] and low amperage direct current [Ultroid]) are no longer available since manufacturers discontinued production of the units. If information is needed, see the first edition of this text or the article by Pfenninger and Surrell, 1995.

CLASSIFICATIONS/SYMPTOMS

Hemorrhoids are enlarged arteriovenous vessels and are classified according to their origin from above or below the dentate (pectinate) line. Those developing from above the dentate line are internal hemorrhoids; those from below are external hemorrhoids. It should be clear that classification is dependent on *origin,* not on the location of the most distal portion of the hemorrhoid (Fig. 108-1).

Hemorrhoids above the dentate line—*internal hemorrhoids*—are covered by mucosa and do not have somatic sensory innervation. Thus internal hemorrhoids are well suited for treatment in the office setting without anesthesia, since they lack pain fibers. Those below the dentate line—*external hemorrhoids*—are covered by skin (anoderm) and are extremely sensitive. Treatment of external hemorrhoids requires some form of anesthesia. *Mixed hemorrhoids* refers to those vessels that originate right at the dentate line or the presence of both internal and external hemorrhoids.

The anal canal can be divided into eight segments, and are as noted with the patient lying in the left lateral decubitus position (Fig. 108-2, *A*). Internal hemorrhoids usually occur in three major positions based on the vascular architecture of the anal canal: the right anterior, right posterior, and left lateral positions (Fig. 108-2, *B*).

Internal hemorrhoids are also characterized by their

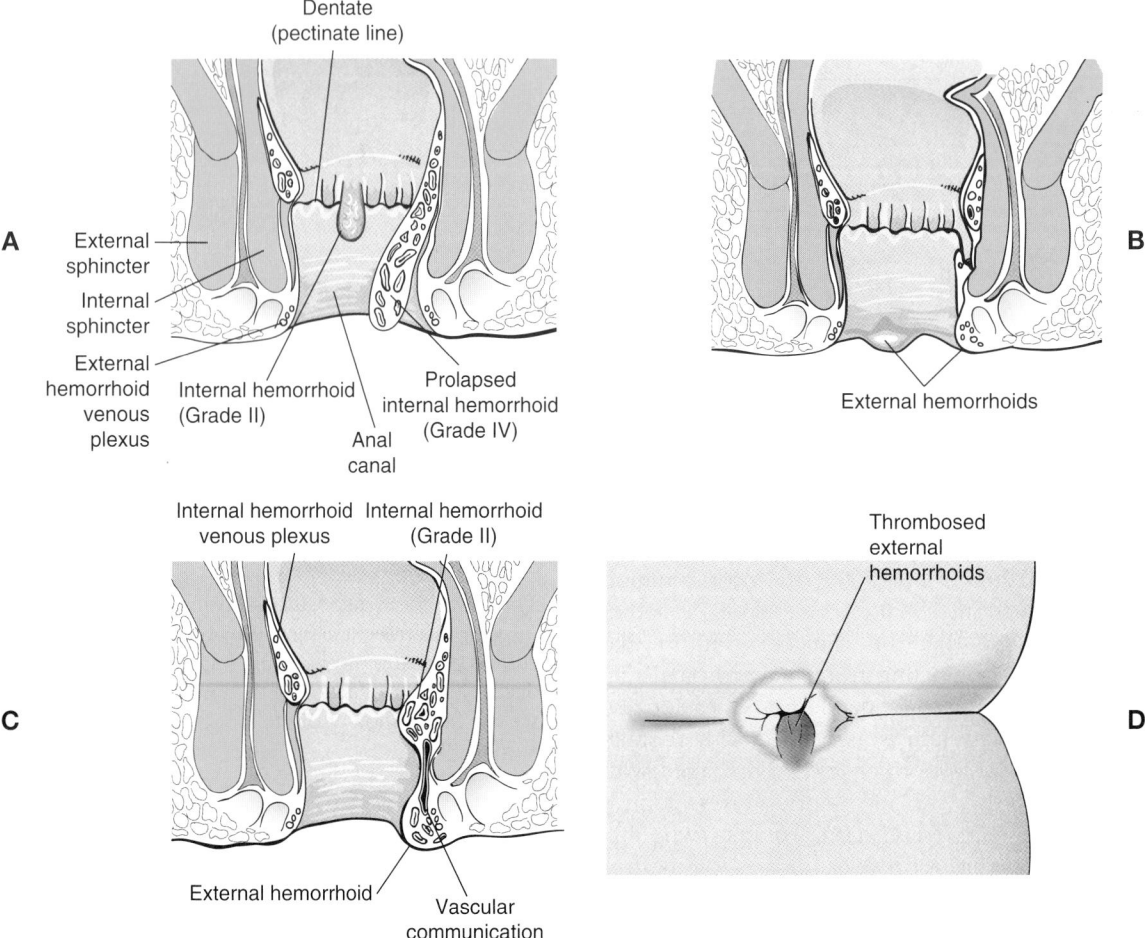

Fig. 108-1
Various types of hemorrhoids. **A,** Internal hemorrhoid. Note that although an internal hemorrhoid may be visible "externally" (Grade IV), it is classified by its origin, which, as shown here, is above the dentate line. **B,** External hemorrhoid. **C,** Mixed hemorrhoid disease (both internal and external hemorrhoids with a vascular communication). **D,** Thrombosed external hemorrhoid. (Redrawn from Pfenninger JL, Surrell J: *Am Fam Physician* 52:821, 1995.)

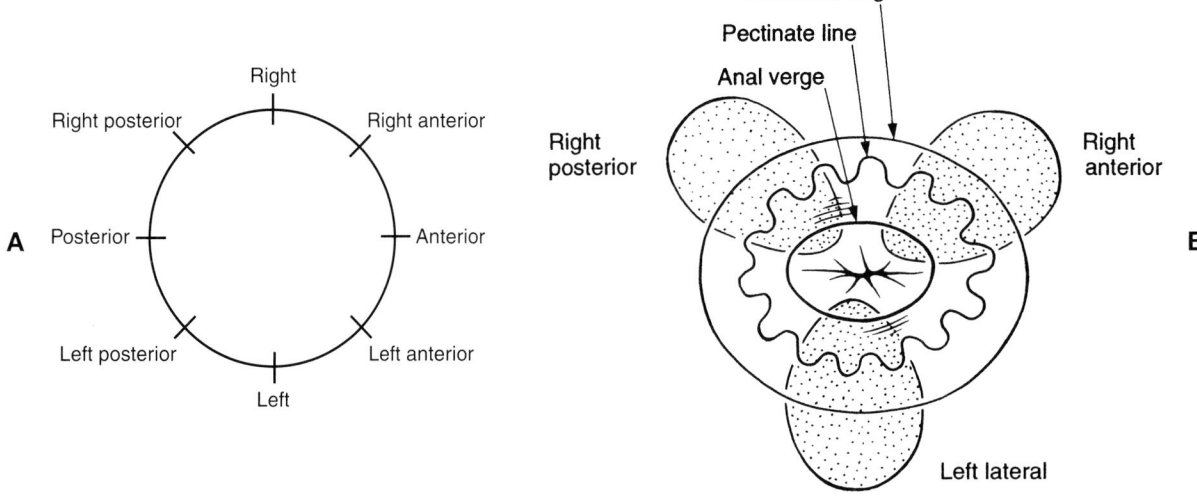

Fig. 108-2
A, Representation of eight segments in the rectum as seen through a slotted (Ives) anoscope, with the patient in the left lateral decubitus position. **B,** Usual three primary hemorrhoidal groups.

size from Grade I to IV, as noted in Table 108-1 and Fig. 108-3. Symptoms of internal hemorrhoids include painless bleeding, prolapse, aching after defecation, and discharge. The key step in diagnosis and classification of internal hemorrhoids is anoscopic examination (see Chapter 100, Anoscopy). External hemorrhoids can form clots that are painful. Patients then present with a "painful lump."

Approximately 25% of internal hemorrhoid symptoms do not respond adequately to medical treatment and require further therapy. Most thrombosed external hemorrhoids require evacuation to provide symptomatic relief.

TABLE 108-1

Classification of Internal Hemorrhoids

Grade	Description
I	Small, do not prolapse
II	Medium, prolapse and return spontaneously
III	Large, prolapse but reduce manually
IV	Largest, prolapse, not reducible

INDICATIONS

Bleeding or other symptomatology from internal hemorrhoids that has failed medical management (bulk agents, suppositories, topical preparations, and sitz baths).

Note: The mere presence of hemorrhoids alone, without symptoms, is not necessarily an indication for treatment.

CONTRAINDICATIONS

- Bleeding diathesis
- Pregnancy or immediate postpartum period (less than 8 weeks)
- Inflammatory bowel disease
- Anorectal fissures
- Active anorectal infections
- AIDS or other immunodeficiency states
- Portal hypertension
- Rectal wall mucosal prolapse
- Anorectal tumors

Recommendations for cardiac prophylaxis are not specific (see Chapter 204, Antibiotic Prophylaxis). Al-

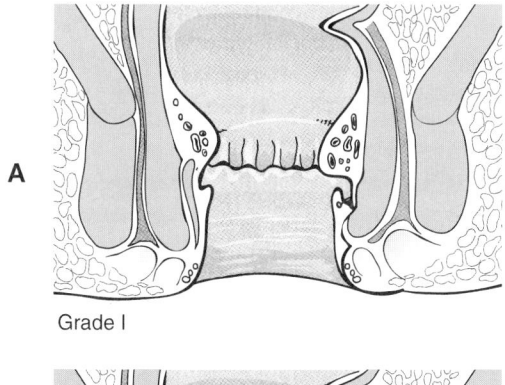
Grade I

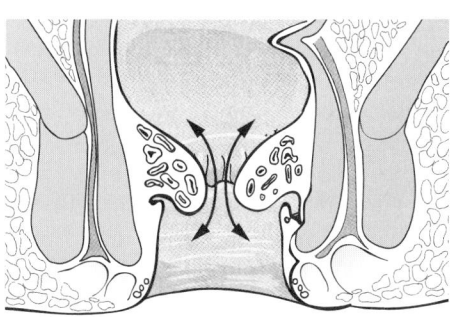
Grade II

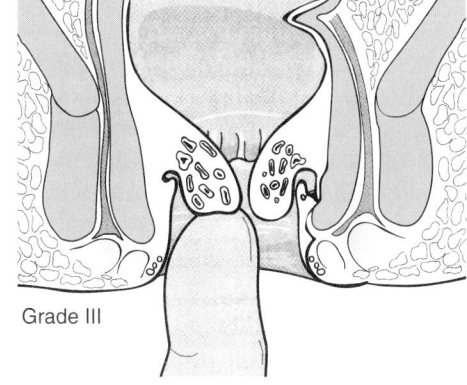
Grade III

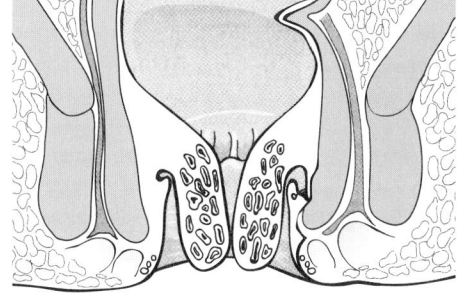
Grade IV

Fig. 108-3
Grading of *internal* hemorrhoids. **A,** Grade I hemorrhoids are present and identifiable. **B,** Grade II hemorrhoids prolapse with a bowel movement but return spontaneously. **C,** Grade III hemorrhoids prolapse and can be replaced manually. **D,** Grade IV hemorrhoids remain prolapsed in spite of all efforts at reduction and are often associated with varying amounts of mucosal prolapse. (From Pfenninger JL, Surrell J: *Am Fam Physician* 52:821, 1995.)

though it is recommended for high-risk patients with procedures that involve intestinal mucosa, it is not recommended for endoscopy with biopsy. Those at high risk for subacute bacterial endocarditis (SBE) (previous history of SBE, artificial valves, history of rheumatic fever, or very-high-risk murmurs) should be treated with caution. The duration of antibiotic treatment necessary is unknown, and antibiotic therapy may be impractical, since the treated areas may remain irritated and open for 2 to 3 weeks after each treatment.

PREPROCEDURE PATIENT PREPARATION

1. Give the patient one or two Fleet enemas before the procedure. Although not absolutely necessary, it is aesthetically helpful.
2. Ask the patient to avoid aspirin for 1 week before treatment.
3. Provide a patient education handout to ensure informed consent (see the sample patient education handout titled "Hemorrhoids" on page 1876 of Appendix G).
4. A complete history and pertinent physical examination are essential. Record these on the sample encounter forms (Figs. 108-4 and 108-5) that summarize the information.
5. The patient may be examined and treated in the left lateral decubitus, which is generally more comfortable, or the prone jack-knife position when exposure is difficult. No sedation is necessary for a patient having only anoscopy and hemorrhoid treatment. The patient may take four ibuprofen 200-mg tablets 1 to 2 hours before the office visit. Before performing anoscopy, perform an external visual and a digital anorectal examination. Ask the patient to perform a Valsalva maneuver (bearing down) to rule out full-thickness rectal prolapse. (Occasionally, examination with the patient sitting on the commode is necessary to assess for this.)

Note: Only internal hemorrhoids are treated by these methods (IRC, banding, sclerotherapy). Treatment of external hemorrhoids requires excision and is associated with pain; thus local anesthetics are needed.

TREATMENT

Rubber-band ligation (Barron or McGivney ligation), infrared coagulation (IRC), and sclerotherapy for internal hemorrhoids, and the treatment of thrombosed external hemorrhoids are discussed below. A summary of techniques and their indications is found in Table 108-2. The treatment of perianal skin tags is dealt with separately in Chapter 110, Removal of Perianal Skin Tags (External Hemorrhoidal Skin Tags). Because of the discharge and poor patient acceptance, cryotherapy is not covered in this discussion.

RUBBER-BAND LIGATION

Rubber-band ligation involves placing a rubber band around the base of an internal hemorrhoid. The ensnared tissue undergoes necrosis and sloughs. Rubber-band ligation is used for treatment of second- or third-degree bleeding or prolapsing internal hemorrhoids.

Equipment

- Slotted Ives anoscope (see Fig. 100-2)
- McGivney ligator with bands (or an acceptable alternative device) (Fig. 108-6)

Editor's note: It just came to my attention that a new disposable hemorrhoid ligator has been released on the market: the O'Regan Hemorrhoid Banding Kit (Fig. 108-7). I have not had a chance to use it yet, but it looks intriguing as does the anoscope (see "Suppliers" section).

- Alligator forceps (similar to long-handled Allis clamp)
- External light source
- Large ob-gyn cotton swabs

Technique (Figs. 108-8 and 108-9)

1. Load the ligating drum with two bands. A small amount of soapy water on the cone will facilitate this.
2. Insert the anoscope, and visualize the hemorrhoid to be ligated. Treat the largest hemorrhoid group, or the obviously bleeding source, first. Have an assistant stabilize the anoscope.
3. With one hand, draw the hemorrhoidal tissue into the ligating drum with an alligator forceps. If the patient experiences pain, grasp the hemorrhoidal tissue more proximally. Pull just hemorrhoidal tissue into the ligator; avoid excessive mucosa.
4. With the other hand, grasp the handle of the ligator and push forward slightly. Squeeze the handle. The outer drum slides over the inner drum, displacing the rubber bands around the hemorrhoid.
5. Reposition or withdraw the anoscope. Patient tolerance is highest if only one hemorrhoid group is treated per visit. However, some physicians treat more than one segment per visit. Avoid circumferential ligation, since it may increase pain, and the tension on the mucosa may lead to nonhealing fissures.

Text continued on p. 847

INITIAL ENCOUNTER FORM
HEMORRHOIDS

NAME _____ DOB _____ Age _____ M/F _____ Date _____

SUBJECTIVE:
Original onset: _____ Present trouble started: _____

SYMPTOMS/HISTORY:

Anal itching	Bleeding	Weight loss
Pain	TP/with BMs/dripping	Fevers
with BM	Change in BMs	Chills
between BMs	frequency/consistency	Sweats
rectum	Fecal incontinence	Colon polyps
abdomen	Protrusion	

PRIOR TREATMENT:
Medical: _____
Surgical: _____

Previous exams:
   anoscopy   Date _____ Who_____ Findings_____
   sigmoidoscopy   Date _____ Who_____ Findings_____
   barium enema   Date _____ Who_____ Findings_____

Other: _____
Has patient read over and understood handouts? Y   N

PMH:
  MI: _____
  Meds: _____
  Allergies : _____
  Other: _____

FH:
  Colon polyps?
  Cancers: Colon   Breast   Uterine

HEALTH MAINTENANCE:

Pap	exercise stress test	dt
mammo	colon ca screen	pneumorax
bone density	PSA	flu
	chol	

Please turn page

Fig. 108-4
Sample of initial encounter form for hemorrhoids.

Continued

OBJECTIVE:
Abdomen:
External:
    Visual
        redundant tissue
        external hemorrhoidal disease
        prolapse
        fissure
        fistula
        infection
        other
Digital:
    Masses:
    Tenderness:
    Prostate:
Anoscopic:
    Fissure
    Fistula
    Hemorrhoids

RP   RA

LL
Patient in LL decubitus

IMPRESSION:

PLAN:

Patient education: -Diet
                    -Hygiene
                    -Control of symptoms
                    -Technique of destruction
                    -Risks
                    -Benefits
                    -Complications

Treatment: IRC   Banding

    Surgical:

    Other:

    Referral to _____

Flex sig indicated?

    Scheduled? _____   Where? _____

Follow-up:

_____   _____
Physician Signature   Date

cc: _____

Fig. 108-4, cont'd
Sample of initial encounter form for hemorrhoids. Used with permission of The Medical Procedures Center, P.C., Midland, Mich.

HEMORRHOID TREATMENT SUMMARY

Patient _____ Birthdate _____ Date _____

Initial evaluation date _____ Referring physician _____

Colonoscopy, flexible sigmoidoscopy, barium enema _____   Date _____

Results _____

	Grade	Segments	Settings	Comments/Date/Signature
◯				
◯				
◯				
◯				
◯				
◯				

Fig. 108-5
Summary of treatment/follow-up visit sheet. (Courtesy William Everts, DO, Zephyr Cove, Nev.)

TABLE 108-2

Comparison of Therapeutic Modalities for Treatment of Internal Hemorrhoids

Method	Grade of Internal Hemorrhoid				Ease of Performing Method	Complications
	I	II	III	IV		
Infrared coagulator	+++	+++	±	−	+++	Rare
Rubber band	±	+++	+++	−	++	Some
Sclerotherapy	++	+++	±	−	+	Common

Scale: −, Not recommended (does not work); +++, easiest (best suited).

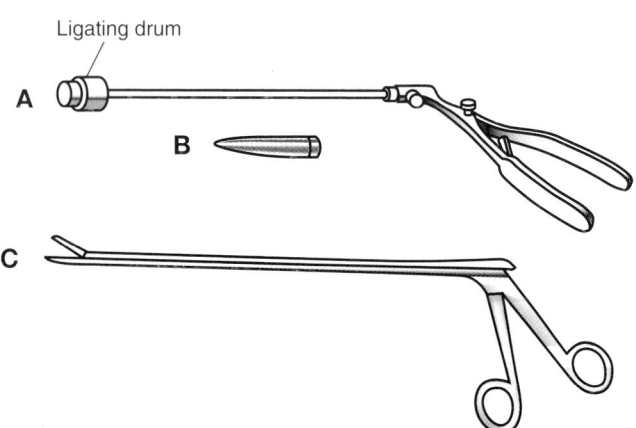

Fig. 108-6
McGivney ligator. **A,** Ligator. **B,** Cone to load bands. **C,** Forceps to grasp hemorrhoid.

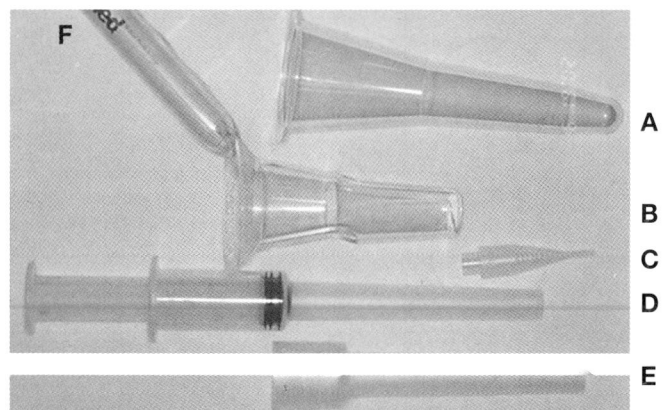

Fig. 108-7
O'Regan disposable banding unit. **A,** Trocar for insertion of anoscope. **B,** Anoscope. **C,** Loading cone for bands. **D,** Syringe for suction to pull up hemorrhoid. **E,** Sleeve that fits over syringe apparatus that pushes bands off onto hemorrhoids. **F,** Penlight inserted into anoscope handle for light.

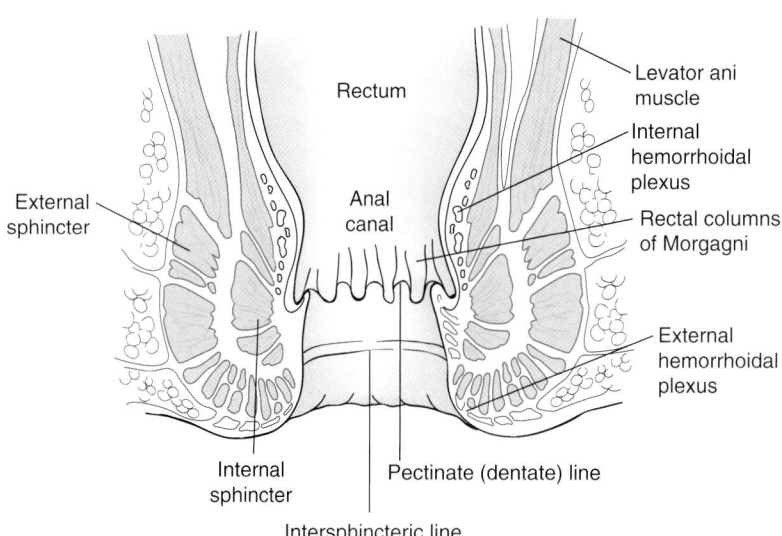

Fig. 108-8
Anatomy of the anal region. Also see Chapter 99, Clinical Anorectal Anatomy and Digital Examination. Note the location of origin of internal and external hemorrhoids.

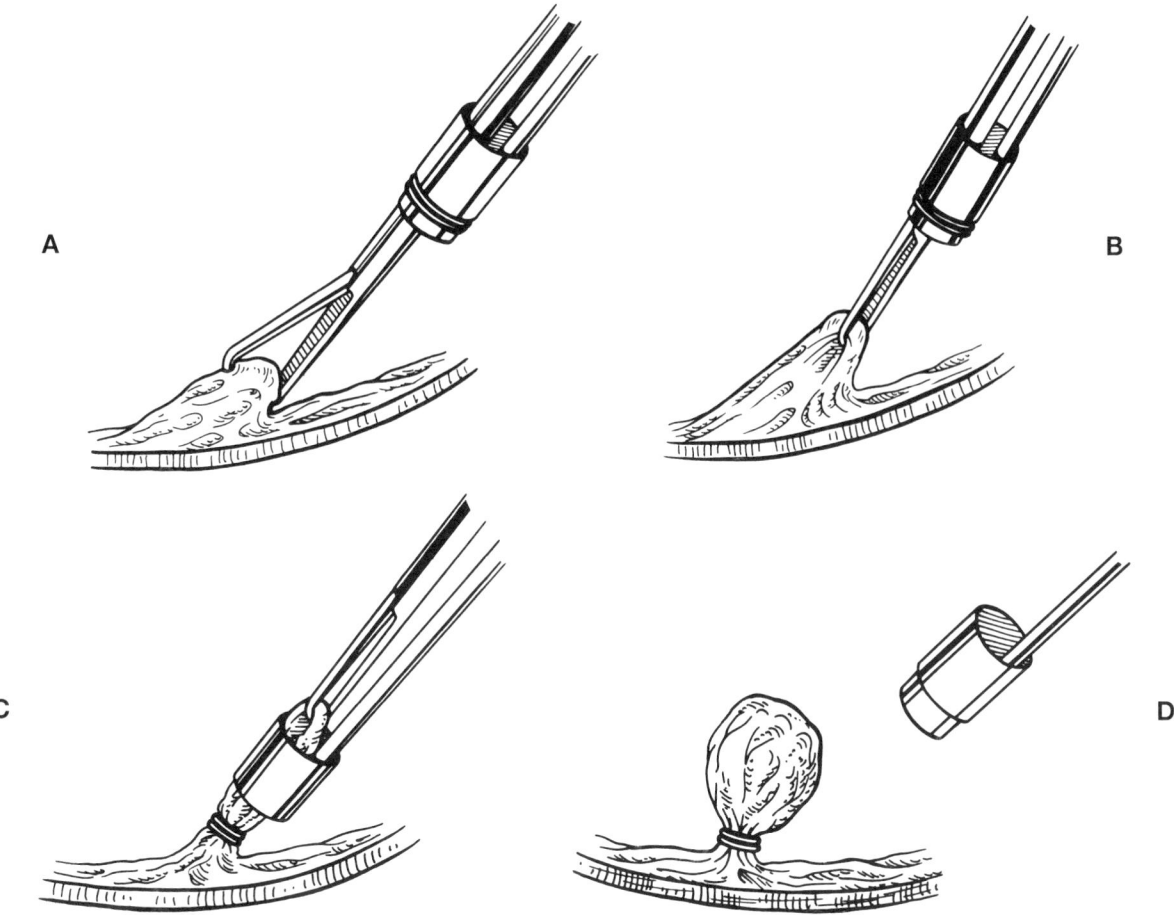

Fig. 108-9
Rubber-band ligation. The hemorrhoid is, **A,** grasped and, **B,** firmly tethered. **C,** The tissue is drawn into the drum, and, **D,** two rubber bands are released. If the patient tolerates the grasping of the hemorrhoid with forceps, ligation can be performed with minimal or no discomfort.

Complications

- Spotting can be expected for 8 to 10 days, then bleeding usually occurs 1 to 2 weeks after the procedure, when the hemorrhoidal tissue sloughs. Bleeding can be significant but rarely requires active intervention.
- Patients may experience a dull ache for 2 days after the procedure. If severe pain is experienced during the procedure, the band will need to be removed with a scissors. It was applied too far distal.
- Thrombosis of external hemorrhoids occurs rarely. Treat symptomatically or with excision.
- Sepsis with pelvic cellulitis (perineal sepsis) is a serious complication, but it rarely occurs. Patients complain of fever, increasing perineal pain, swelling, inability to urinate, or dysuria. Treatment requires hospitalization, broad-spectrum antibiotic administration, and debridement.

Advantages

- The instrument itself is inexpensive, and there are no disposable tips to replace.
- Higher grades of hemorrhoids can be treated.
- The procedure is quick.
- The procedure is easy to learn.

Disadvantages

- The procedure is somewhat more uncomfortable than other techniques, and significant complications have been reported (e.g., perineal sepsis).
- Two people are needed to perform the procedure (the operator and the assistant, who holds the anoscope).

Postprocedure Patient Education

- Inform the patient that mild aching discomfort may be experienced over the next 2 days (see the patient education handout titled "After Hemorrhoid Treatment" on page 1879 of Appendix G).

- Ask the patient to report any excessive bleeding, fever, dysuria, inability to urinate (a sign of perineal sepsis), or increasing pain.
- Ask the patient to follow up in 4 to 6 weeks for reexamination and further banding, as needed.

INFRARED COAGULATION

Equipment

- Infrared coagulator (Redfield) (Fig. 108-10)
- Slotted Ive's anoscope (Redfield) (see Fig. 100-2)
- External light source
- Large ob-gyn cotton swabs

Note: The new units are not submersible for cleaning. Instead, they use a disposable sheath that is changed for each visit. It is imperative not to immerse the newer units (in contrast to the older units) in sterilizing solutions.

Technique

Infrared light is applied to the *base* of the internal hemorrhoid, forming a white coagulum that ulcerates and then forms a scar. The diameter of burn correlates with the size of the probe tip, which is usually 6 mm. The depth of penetration correlates with the time of the pulse, which is generally 1.5 to 2.0 seconds. Infrared coagulation is used for first- and second-degree and smaller third-degree internal hemorrhoids. It can be used for larger hemorrhoids, but treatment may need to be repeated in 4 to 6 weeks. It is a painless procedure, and although more than one hemorrhoid group is sometimes treated, most clinicians begin by treating only one complex to determine patient tolerance. Treatment of more than one complex of hemorrhoids at a time may increase posttreatment discomfort and the other complications, especially bleeding. A teaching video describing this technique is available from Redfield Corp.

1. With the patient in the left lateral decubitus position, insert the Ives slotted anoscope and identify the hemorrhoid to be treated. Insert a 6-mm probe.
2. Press the probe tip firmly onto or preferably immediately just above the hemorrhoid. Only light pressure is needed.
3. Pull the trigger. The unit has an incorporated time switch that limits exposure. The typical setting is 1.5 seconds. Generally, three to five separate applications are made for each hemorrhoid group. One group is treated per visit at 4- to 6-week intervals. For the first treatment, select the hemorrhoid that is bleeding or that is the largest. Larger hemorrhoids

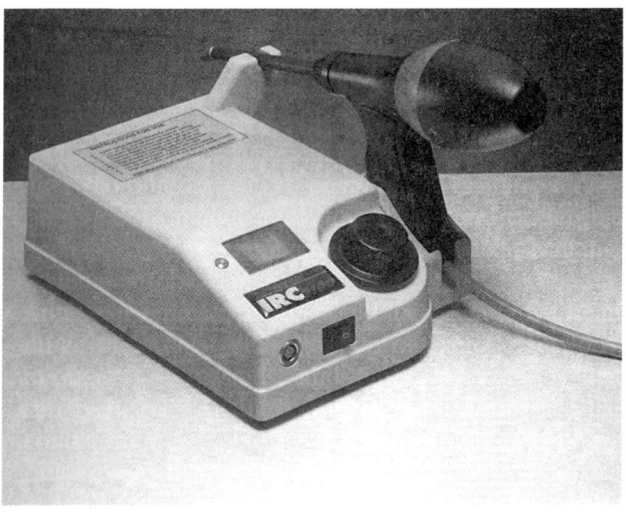

Fig. 108-10
Infrared coagulator unit, base, and handpiece. (Courtesy Redfield Corp, Rochelle Park, NJ.)

may require more than one treatment session or a longer exposure (2 seconds).

Caution: Do not overlap treatment sites. Overlapping increases the depth of burn. Place the probe adjacent to a previous site in a linear fashion or in a diamond shape, but do not overlap if possible (Fig. 108-11).

4. Realign the anoscope and apply treatment to another hemorrhoidal group if more than one group is to be treated.
5. Wipe off the tip with saline-soaked gauze between applications. This allows the tip to cool and cleans the end. If a loud "pop" is heard, there is debris or mucus between the tip and the mucosa. No damage is done, but the sudden noise can be frightening to the patient (and the clinician).
6. Remove the anoscope. No special aftercare is needed.

Complications

- Patients may experience a mild, dull, aching pain lasting up to 2 days after treatments.
- Minor bleeding may be encountered for up to 2 weeks after the procedure. More bleeding can be expected at 10 to 14 days when the eschar sloughs. This can usually be managed conservatively but very rarely will require topical astringents or maybe even a suture.
- Rarely, patients experience a thrombosed external hemorrhoid in the area after treatment.
- Rarely, slow-healing ulcers can be encountered.

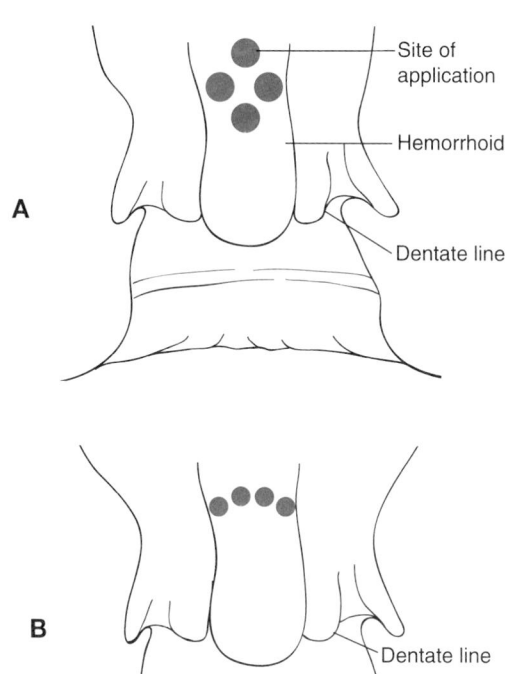

Fig. 108-11
Treatment of internal hemorrhoids using infrared coagulation. **A,** Diamond shape. **B,** Linear method. Each circle indicates a single application for 1.5 to 2 sec. Up to six applications per visit may be needed per hemorrhoid segment.

Advantages

- It is an essentially painless procedure.
- There have been no reported cases of perineal sepsis.
- The procedure is quick, simple to learn, and cost effective.
- The procedure is well tolerated by patients.
- No costs for disposable probes, but new units require disposable vinyl sheaths.
- It can be used in patients with pacemakers.
- The unit can also be used to remove tattoos, reduce nasal turbinates, stop bleeding from biopsy and hair donor sites, and treat verruca and condyloma.
- The unit is well made and requires little maintenance.

Disadvantages

- The procedure is not very effective for advanced third-degree hemorrhoidal disease and works poorly for fourth-degree hemorrhoidal disease.
- The unit costs more than the materials for band ligation.

Postprocedure Patient Education

- Ask the patient to follow up in 4 to 6 weeks to treat residual disease or another group. In the elderly or compromised patients (e.g., diabetics), it is best to wait longer.
- Ask the patient to report any severe symptoms of pain, fever, or inability to urinate (see the patient education handout titled "After Hemorrhoid Treatment" on page 1879 of Appendix G).

SCLEROTHERAPY

Sclerotherapy is used for treatment of first- or second-degree internal bleeding hemorrhoids. Injection of 1 to 2 ml of sclerosant into the internal hemorrhoid causes sclerosis and fixation of the submucosa to the underlying muscularis. This technique is relatively quick. All three major hemorrhoidal groups can be treated at one sitting. Unfortunately it has not been as effective as other modalities and has been associated with impotence, the reason for which is unknown.

Equipment

- Ive's slotted anoscope
- 5-ml syringe
- 25-gauge spinal needle
- Sclerosant (sodium morrhuate, sodium tetradecyl sulfate, or phenol in almond oil)

Technique (Fig. 108-12)

1. Insert the anoscope and visualize the hemorrhoid group to be injected.
2. Insert the spinal needle into or immediately above the hemorrhoid group. Withdraw the plunger of the syringe and aspirate for blood to ensure that the sclerosant will not be injected directly into a vein.
3. Inject 1 to 2 ml of sclerosant. A wheal should be noted during injection. Take care to inject well *above* the level of the dentate line.
4. Document the location of the injection and the amount of sclerosant used.
5. Reposition the anoscope to visualize the next hemorrhoid group to be treated.

Complications

- The procedure is painful if the sclerosant is injected below the level of the dentate line.
- Thrombosis of internal or external hemorrhoids may occur, causing pain. Thrombosis is managed with topical creams, analgesics, and sitz baths.

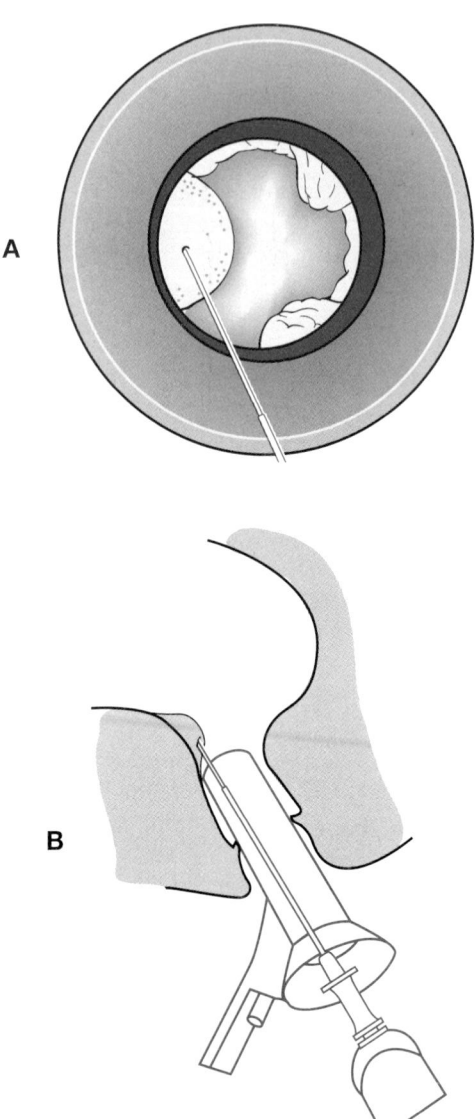

Fig. 108-12
A, Sclerotherapy as viewed through the anoscope. If a wheal is not produced, the injection is too deep and the needle should be withdrawn. An injection that is too superficial will produce necrosis of the lining of the anal canal. **B,** Injection technique.

- Bleeding is usually the result of injection into the mucosa rather than the submucosa. Necrosis and ulceration with bleeding occur 2 to 3 weeks after injection. Healing usually occurs in 3 to 6 weeks.
- Abscess occurs very rarely.
- Anaphylaxis from sclerosant is rare.
- Impotence has been reported, but the etiology is uncertain.

Advantages

- The procedure is effective.
- The equipment cost is minimal.

- It can be used concomitantly with banding or other therapies.

Disadvantages

- The procedure is associated with more significant complications.
- The technique is harder to master.

Postprocedure Patient Education

- Inform the patient that mild rectal discomfort may occur after treatment, and tell the patient to report any severe symptoms (see the sample patient education handout titled "After Hemorrhoid Treatment" on page 1879 of Appendix G).
- Instruct the patient to return to the office in 4 weeks for repeat examination and further treatments if necessary.

THROMBOSED EXTERNAL HEMORRHOIDS

External hemorrhoids occur below the dentate (pectinate) line. Patients with thrombosed external hemorrhoids have a painful, tender, swollen, bluish lump at the anal orifice. If the patient is seen within 48 hours of the onset of symptoms, the thrombosed hemorrhoid should be incised or excised. After 48 hours, symptoms have usually improved and symptomatic care is recommended. However, *if the patient is still experiencing significant pain,* the hemorrhoid can be surgically relieved even after 48 hours.

There are three basic surgical approaches: (1) excise an ellipse over the clotted hemorrhoid and evacuate the clot, (2) excise the hemorrhoid completely, and (3) simple incision over the clot with expression of the contents.

Equipment

- No. 11 blade and tissue scissors
- Mosquito hemostats
- Fine tissue forceps
- Lidocaine (2%) with epinephrine; 27-gauge, 1½-inch needle, and 3-ml syringe
- Antiseptic solution
- 4-0 or 5-0 absorbable suture (if closure is desired)

Technique (Fig. 108-13)

1. Cleanse the perianal area with antiseptic solution.
2. Infiltrate the base of the thrombosed external hemorrhoid with lidocaine with epinephrine (2 to 5 ml).

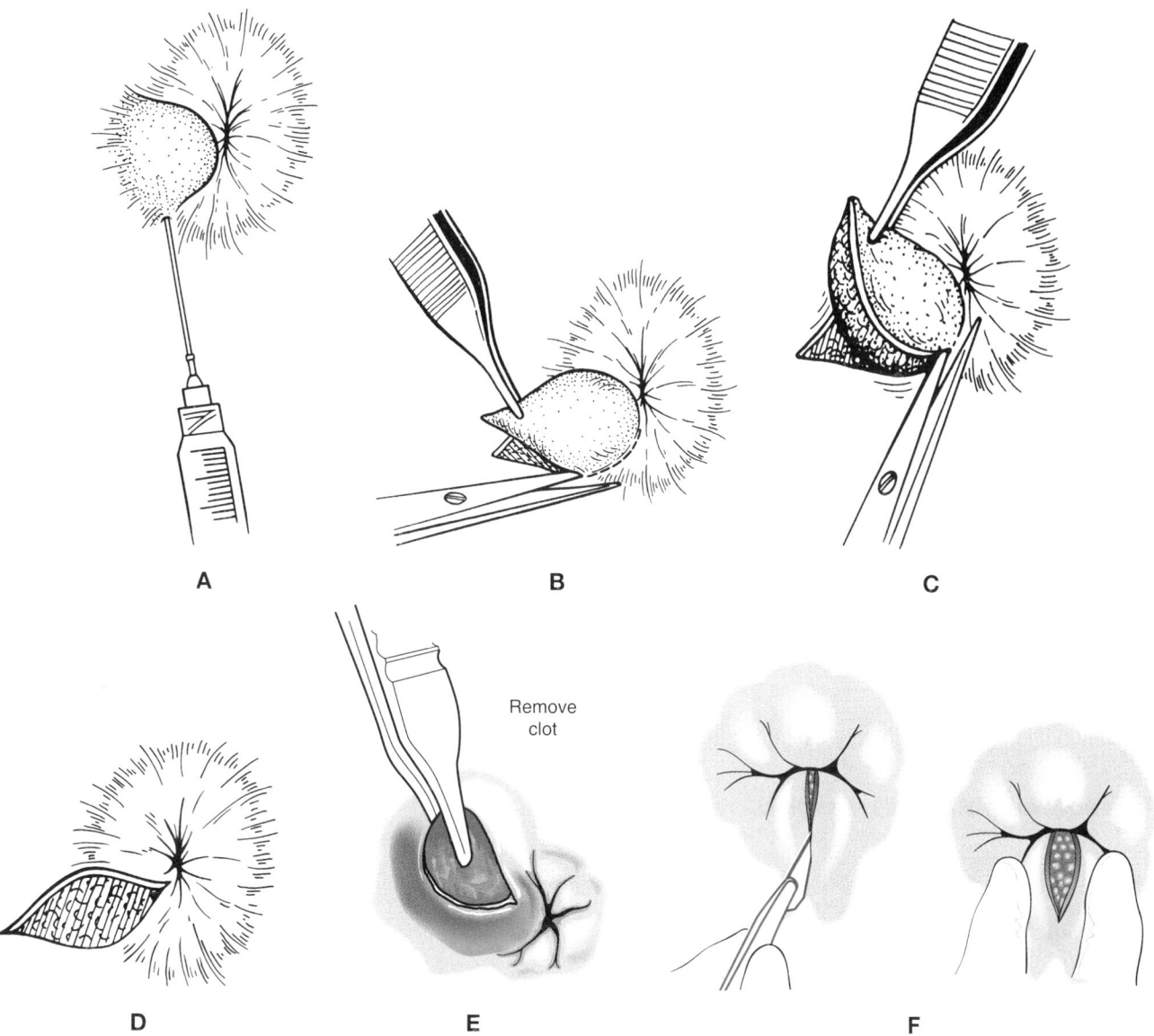

Fig. 108-13

Excision of a thrombosed hemorrhoid. **A,** The area is infiltrated with 2% lidocaine with epinephrine. **B** and **C,** The thrombosed hemorrhoid is excised along with a small wedge of skin. **D,** Skin edges are sufficiently separated to permit adequate drainage, thereby preventing clot reaccumulation. They can also be closed with fine absorbable suture. **E,** Instead of removing the entire hemorrhoid, a small elliptical incision is made over the hemorrhoid and the clot is expressed. No suture closure is needed. **F,** A simple incision and drainage with expression of all clots can also be performed. Multiple clots are often present and should be removed. After the initial clot is removed, spread the incision to expose the base of the hemorrhoid to remove other thrombi. The disadvantage of this approach is that the incision can seal over, allowing the clot to reaccumulate.

3. Excise the hemorrhoid as an ellipse, or perform an elliptical excision over the hemorrhoid and remove the skin. Be sure to evacuate all clots.
4. Control any bleeding with cautery or silver nitrate sticks.
5. The wound may be left open to heal by secondary intention without adverse sequela. The skin edges may also be approximated with interrupted fine absorbable suture (unless silver nitrate was used).
6. Alternatively, after anesthetization, the base of the clotted hemorrhoid can be clamped with a hemostat. The tissue over the hemostat is excised. With the hemostat still in place, a suture is placed proximal to

the tip. If interrupted sutures are used, leave the ends long and use them for traction to pull down the upper portion of the incision. If a running stitch is used, the long end can be used in the same manner. Then remove the hemostat and complete closure. This ensures that the entire excisional site has been sutured closed.

7. Some physicians *simply incise* over the thrombus and evacuate the clot. If this is done, it is imperative that *all* clots be removed. After the incision is made, express the clot, and then explore the cavity with hemostats to break down any septa. Another incision inside the cavity may be necessary. Frequently more than one clot will be evacuated. Re-express the area to be sure all clots have been removed. This technique is quicker, but warn the patient that there is a higher likelihood of reaccumulation with this approach.

Complications

- Bleeding
- Pain
- Recurrence
- Chronic fissure
- Infection

Postprocedure Patient Education

See the sample patient education handout titled "After Hemorrhoid Treatment" on page 1879 of Appendix G.

- Recommend that the patient take sitz baths two to three times per day for 1 week.
- Oral analgesics, topical anesthetic cream (e.g., xylocaine ointment 5%), and stool softeners are helpful.
- A follow-up examination should be scheduled for 4 weeks.
- Emphasize that the patient avoid prolonged sitting on the toilet to prevent recurrent thrombosis.
- Explain to the patient that a high-bulk, high-fluid diet is essential.

SUPPLIERS

Infrared Coagulator (IRC)

Ive's slotted anoscope
Redfield Corp.
210 Summit Avenue
Montvale, NJ 07645
Phone: 1-800-678-4472
Website: www.IRC2100.com

Band ligator
Most medical supply stores or Redfield Corp.

Sclerosing agents
See Table 90-1.

O'Regan Hemorrhoid Banding Kit
Medsurge Medical, Inc.
210-828 Harbourside Drive
North Vancouver, BC V7P 3R9
Phone: 1-888-287-1958
Website: www.medsurgemedical.com

CPT/BILLING CODES

46600	Anoscopy
46221	Hemorrhoidectomy, by simple ligature (e.g., rubber band)
46220	Excision, single anal tag
46230	Excision of external hemorrhoid tags and/or multiple papillae
46320	Enucleation or excision of external thrombosed hemorrhoid
46083	I & D thrombosed external hemorrhoid
46500	Injection of sclerosing solution, hemorrhoids
46934	Destruction of hemorrhoids, any method; internal (e.g., IRC)
46935	Destruction of hemorrhoids, any method; external
46936	Destruction of hemorrhoids, any method; internal and external

Note: This last code is not appropriate when only IRC, band ligation, or sclerotherapy techniques are used for treatment of internal hemorrhoids.

ICD-9-CM DIAGNOSTIC CODES

455.9	Hemorrhoid tag
455.0	Internal hemorrhoids
455.1	Internal hemorrhoids, thrombosed
455.2	Internal hemorrhoids, bleeding
455.3	External hemorrhoids
455.4	External hemorrhoids, thrombosed

ADDITIONAL RESOURCES

- See the sample patient education handouts titled "Hemorrhoids" and "After Hemorrhoid Treatment" on pages 1876 and 1879, respectively, of Appendix G.

BIBLIOGRAPHY

Bleday R, Pena JP, Rothenberger DA, et al: Symptomatic hemorrhoids: current incidence and complications of operative therapy, *Dis Colon Rectum* 35:477, 1992.

Bullock N: Impotence after sclerotherapy of haemorrhoids: case report, *BMJ* 314:419, 1997.

Corman ML: *Colon and rectal surgery,* Philadelphia, 1984, JB Lippincott.

Dennison AR, Whiston RJ, Rooney S, Morris DL: The management of hemorrhoids, *Am J Gastroenterol* 84:475, 1989.

Devine R, Ory S: Treatment of hemorrhoids in pregnancy, *JFP* 17:65, 1992.

Fazio VW: *Current therapy in colon and rectal surgery,* Philadelphia, 1990, BC Decker.

Goligher JC: *Surgery of the anus, rectum and colon,* ed 5, London, 1984, Bailliere-Tindall.

Johanson JF, Rimm A: Optimal nonsurgical treatment of hemorrhoids: a comparative analysis of infrared coagulation, rubber band ligation, and injection sclerotherapy. *Am J Gastroenterol* 87:1600, 1992.

Leibach J, Cerda J: Hemorrhoids: modern treatment methods, *Hosp Med* August:53, 1991.

MacRae HM, McLeod RS: Comparison of hemorrhoidal treatment modalities: a meta-analysis, *Dis Colon Rectum* 38:687, 1995.

Pfenninger JL: Modern treatments for internal haemorrhoids, *BMJ* 314:1211, 1997.

Pfenninger JL, Surrell J: Nonsurgical treatment options for internal hemorrhoids, *Am Fam Physician* 52:821, 1995.

Pfenninger JL, Zainea GG: Common anorectal conditions: Part I: symptoms and complaints, *Am Fam Physician* 63:2391, 2001.

Pfenninger JL, Zainea GG: Common anorectal conditions: Part II: lesions, *Am Fam Physician* 64:77, 2001.

Russell TR, Donahue JH: Hemorrhoidal banding: a warning, *Dis Colon Rectum* 28:291, 1985.

Schrock TR: Examination of the anorectum, rigid sigmoidoscopy, flexible sigmoidoscopy, and diseases of the anorectum. In Sleisenger MH, Fordtram JC, editors: *Gastrointestinal disease,* ed 4, Philadelphia, 1989, WB Saunders.

Schussman LC, Lutz LJ: Outpatient management of hemorrhoids, *Prim Care* 13(3):527, 1986.

Smith LE: Hemorrhoidectomy with lasers and other contemporary modalities, *Surg Clin North Am* 3:665, 1992.

Standards Task Force of American Society of Colon and Rectal Surgeons: Practice parameters for the treatment of hemorrhoids, *Dis Colon Rectum* 36:1118, 1993.

Templeton JL, Spence RA, Kennedy TL, et al: Comparison of infrared coagulation and rubber band ligation for first and second degree haemorrhoids: a randomised prospective clinical trial, *Br Med J* 286:1387, 1983.

Walker AJ, Leicester RJ, Nicholls RJ, Mann CV: A prospective study of infrared coagulation, injection and rubber band ligation in the treatment of haemorrhoids, *Int J Colorectal Dis* 5:113, 1990.

Zinberg SS, Stern DH, Furman DS, Wittles JM: A personal experience in comparing three non-operative techniques for treating internal hemorrhoids, *Am J Gastroenterol* 84:488, 1989.

CHAPTER 109

Perianal Abscess Incision and Drainage

James A. Surrell

A perianal abscess is clearly one of the most painful anal conditions seen in the outpatient setting. The pain of a perianal abscess is severe, disabling, and progressive, and the only relief these patients obtain is with spontaneous rupture of the abscess or when they seek medical attention for incision and drainage (I & D). The most common etiology of perianal abscess is thought to be an infection originating at the dentate line in the anal crypts (see Chapter 99, Clinical Anorectal Anatomy and Digital Examination). The infection then usually migrates through the path of least resistance to the perianal tissues, where there is a closed-space environment ideal for proliferation of this mixed bacterial infection.

The four locations where abscesses can occur and their relative incidence are shown in Fig. 109-1. The most common site (60%) of a perianal abscess is in the *perianal* tissues immediately adjacent to the anal verge. If the abscess is located 2 to 3 cm away from the anal verge, then it is most likely in the *ischiorectal* location

(25%) just outside the anal sphincters. A perianal abscess can occur in the intersphincteric plane, between the internal and external sphincters. (An abscess in this location may not be externally visible or palpable in the perianal tissues.) The pain of a perianal abscess is present with an *intersphincteric* abscess, but the diagnosis will be confirmed only on digital anorectal examination, where the fluctuant mass is easily palpable. The least common location for a perianal abscess is the *supralevator* location, and this truly is a peri*rectal* abscess as opposed to a peri*anal* abscess. Most clinicians would agree that if a supralevator abscess is diagnosed, they must look for an intraabdominal or pelvic source. A supralevator abscess may be associated with appendicitis, diverticulitis, pelvic inflammatory disease, or other pelvic or abdominal disease.

Patients with a perianal abscess may develop an associated fever and often have a marked leukocytosis, depending on the severity of the infection. Once the

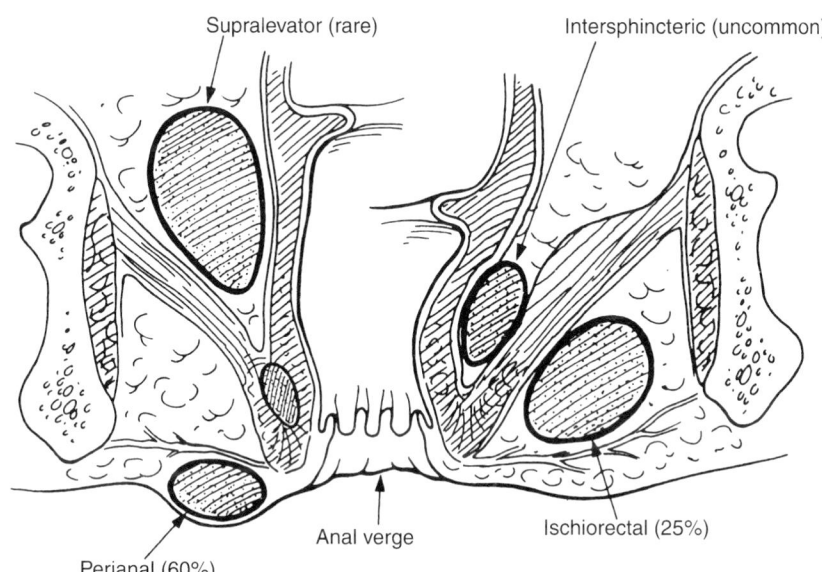

Fig. 109-1
Various anatomic locations of anorectal abscesses.

Supralevator (rare) Intersphincteric (uncommon)

Anal verge

Ischiorectal (25%)

Perianal (60%)

diagnosis of perianal abscess is made, it is essential to proceed with adequate I & D treatment without delay. This is especially important in any patient who may be immunocompromised, is on steroids, or who has diabetes or any other debilitating comorbidity. The treatment of choice for perianal abscess is clearly I & D—*not* antibiotic therapy. If adequate I & D of a perianal abscess is not performed, patients can rapidly develop severe infectious problems such as *necrotizing fasciitis,* which can become life threatening, or *perineal sepsis,* which is a medical emergency identified with the classic triad of pain, fever, and inability to void.

INDICATIONS

Nearly every perianal abscess should be incised and drained. The only reason not to perform this procedure would be if spontaneous drainage of the abscess has occurred and if, in the judgment of the examining clinician, adequate drainage has resulted. These abscess cavities can have multiple loculations and, if spontaneous drainage has occurred, the abscess cavity must still be explored with a digital examination or hemostats to break down any loculated areas within the abscess.

CONTRAINDICATIONS

Patients with underlying hematologic diseases may have perianal abscesses. The associated hematologic disease may include leukemia, granulocytopenia, and lymphoma. The infecting organisms seen with this type of perianal abscess may be quite different from those seen with an otherwise uncomplicated perianal abscess. In those patients with an associated hematologic disorder and a perianal abscess—for example, with leukemia under poor control—conservative treatment with antibiotics combined with local radiotherapy may be advised. Other clinicians recommend aggressive surgical management of perianal abscess in patients with hematologic disorders, but clearly this is never to be attempted in the outpatient setting.

EQUIPMENT

A minor surgical instrument setup includes the following:
- Local anesthesia (2% xylocaine with epinephrine).
- 25- to 30-gauge, 1½-inch needle with 5-ml syringe.
- Hemostats.
- No. 11 blade.
- 4 × 4–inch gauzes or iodoform gauze.

- Penrose drain.
- Suction may be needed if the abscess is large.
- Surgical electrocautery unit is often helpful to achieve hemostasis at the I & D site of the infected and hyperemic tissue.
- Ive's slotted anoscope or various-sized Hill-Ferguson anal retractors to facilitate visualization (available from most medical supply companies).

PREPROCEDURE PATIENT PREPARATION

Advise the patient that, in all likelihood, rather dramatic pain relief will follow the procedure. Further advise the patient that, unless adequate I & D is accomplished, further tissue damage may result. Clearly, the most effective way to afford adequate pain relief is to drain the abscess. Recurrence, bleeding, and pain are all possible. Further workup may also be necessary to rule out other disease processes, such as inflammatory bowel, once the infection is controlled.

TECHNIQUE

Patients with a perianal abscess have a clear need for prompt pain relief. Local anesthesia may be used in an attempt to anesthetize the skin at the intended I & D site, but this is often only marginally effective. The infected perianal tissues usually do not respond well to local anesthetic agents because of the highly acid environment. Either spinal or general anesthesia for this outpatient procedure may be required, depending on the specific patient circumstances. Before I & D of the abscess cavity, it is appropriate, if not essential, to perform anoscopy to look for an internal opening of a fistula tract feeding the abscess cavity. The advantage of doing the anoscopy before I & D of the abscess is that, with gentle pressure on the abscess cavity, the physician may see pus expressed from an internal opening at the level of the dentate line. This then clearly establishes the diagnosis of an associated anal fistula. Textbooks of colon and rectal surgery vary widely on the incidence of associated fistula with perianal abscess, but most experts would agree that it is at least in the range of 50%.

1. Anesthetize the area using 2% xylocaine with epinephrine and a 27- or 30-gauge needle.
2. Make an incision over the fluctuant area near the anal canal in a plane radial to the circumference of the anal canal. The advantage of this type of incision is that it can be extended easily to perform anal fistulotomy if a fistula is present and if fistulotomy is indicated. Another option is to remove an ellipse of tissue such

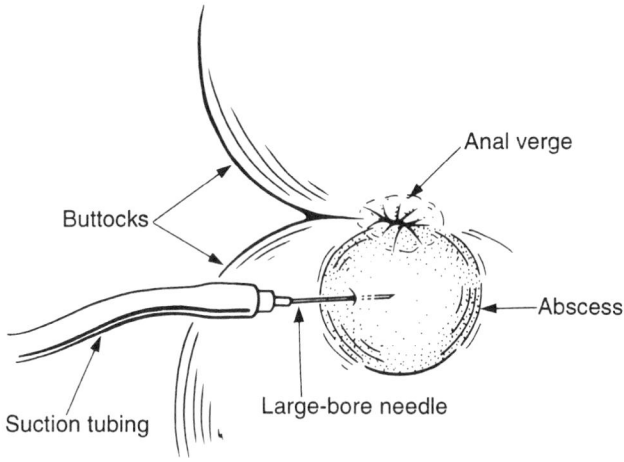

Fig. 109-2
Needle (16 gauge or larger) and suction aspiration of a perianal abscess.

that you can easily place a gloved examining finger into the abscess cavity (if it is that large) to break down any loculations and to place drains. At this time, express all of the purulence.

3. Irrigate the abscess cavity, and, if deemed necessary, place a Penrose drain loosely into the abscess cavity and suture it at the skin edge level. A Penrose drain will not adhere to surrounding tissue, which makes its subsequent removal generally painless. (Alternatively, pack small wounds with ¼- or ½-inch iodoform gauze.)

4. Remove the Penrose drain within 24 to 48 hours. With a small perianal abscess, in the office setting, the iodoform gauze is removed in 10 to 14 days. Earlier removal may lead to recurrence of the abscess.

5. In selected patients with a well-defined fluctuant perianal abscess, drainage can be accomplished without anesthesia by placing a large-bore, 16-gauge needle (attached to suction) into the abscess (Fig. 109-2). This can be an effective *temporizing* measure to afford dramatic and prompt pain relief if definitive surgical treatment is not readily available. The disadvantage of this needle suction technique is that evaluation for an associated anal fistula becomes more difficult.

6. Antibiotics are generally not required postoperatively. Consider them in immunocompromised patients or if there is extensive cellulitis or sepsis.

COMPLICATIONS

The most common complication after I & D of a perianal abscess is recurrence. The most common cause of recurrence of a perianal abscess is an unrecognized, and therefore untreated, associated fistula. The patient with a recurrent perianal abscess must be thoroughly evaluated for the presence of an associated anal fistula. Another cause of recurrent perianal abscess includes the presence of inflammatory bowel disease, most commonly Crohn's disease. Bleeding, excessive pain, and fasciitis are rare complications.

POSTPROCEDURE PATIENT EDUCATION

After an adequate drainage procedure of a perianal abscess, advise the patient to take sitz baths for 10 to 15 minutes two to four times a day. Spend some time with the patient and his or her family to reinforce the fact that the infected wound must heal from the inside out. Most patients understand that they must keep the wound from closing with either sitz baths or showering. Explain that daily wound irrigations may be needed to prevent the skin edges from closing prematurely before the abscess cavity has resolved. This will help to avoid a secondary infection and a recurrent abscess. These instructions usually serve as adequate motivation to follow the recommended postprocedure care.

CPT/BILLING CODES

10060	Incision and drainage of one abscess
10061	Incision and drainage of multiple abscesses or complex (placement of drain)
10180	Incision and drainage of complex-postoperative infection
45005	Incision and drainage submucosal rectal abscess
46040	Incision and drainage of perirectal abscess
46050	Incision and drainage of superficial perianal abscess

ICD-9-CM DIAGNOSTIC CODES

566	Perirectal abscess
566	Perianal abscess
566	Ischiorectal abscess
566	Intersphincteric abscess

BIBLIOGRAPHY

Corman ML: *Colon and rectal surgery*, Philadelphia, 1998, JB Lippincott.

Gordon P, Nivatvongs S: *Principles and practice of surgery for the colon, rectum, and anus,* St Louis, 1992, Quality Medical Publishing.

Mazier W, Levien D, Luchtefeld M, Senagore A: *Surgery of the colon, rectum, and anus,* Philadelphia, 1995, WB Saunders.

Pfenninger JL, Zainea G: Common anorectal conditions. Part I: symptoms and complaints, *Am Fam Physician* 63:2391, 2001.

Pfenninger JL, Zainea G: Common anorectal conditions. Part II: lesions, *Am Fam Physician* 64:77, 2001.

CHAPTER 110

Removal of Perianal Skin Tags (External Hemorrhoidal Skin Tags)

James A. Surrell

Perianal skin tags represent a stretching and enlargement of the normal perianal skin (Fig. 110-1). As such, they are not true external hemorrhoids. Perianal skin tags are believed to occur as a result of the stretching of the perianal skin as a result of a previously thrombosed external hemorrhoid. Perianal skin tags are not painful; patients most often seek treatment for them when they begin to interfere with anal hygiene. It is important to note that perianal skin tags do not cause pain, bleeding, or itching. If these symptoms are present, then another source must be sought as the cause of these symptoms.

INDICATIONS

- Large perianal skin tags interfering with anal hygiene
- Perianal skin tags that annoy the patient or are symptomatic (e.g., pruritus)

Generally, a conservative approach to the management of perianal skin tags is recommended, since the vast majority of these benign lesions are asymptomatic. If the patient is bothered by pruritus, try local measures

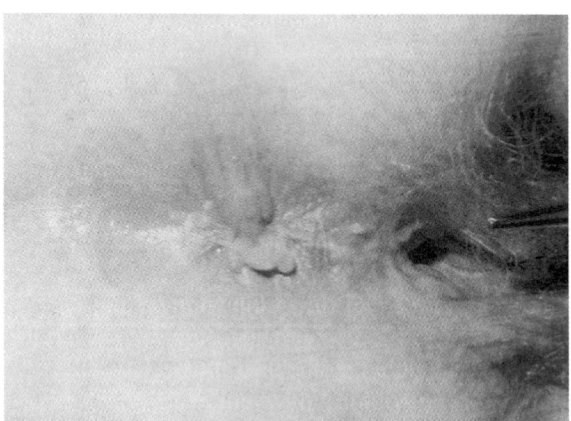

Fig. 110-1
Perianal skin tags.

first (see the sample patient education handout titled "Anal Fissures and Pruritus Ani ['Itchy Anal Area']" on page 1858 of Appendix G).

CONTRAINDICATIONS

- If the patient with perianal skin tags complains of pain, bleeding, or itching, then another source for these symptoms must be sought. Skin tag excision will *not* relieve these symptoms. Even when the patient complains of pruritus "from the tag," be sure he or she is following proper hygiene practices noted in the aforementioned patient education handout, since the tag itself may not be the cause of symptoms.
- If the perianal skin tags have a fleshy edematous appearance (Fig. 110-2), a diagnosis of anal Crohn's disease must be strongly considered. Nearly all patients with anal Crohn's disease will develop fleshy edematous skin tags and will have associated signs and symptoms of pain, discharge, bleeding, and atypical anal fissures (see Chapter 98, Anal Fissure/Lateral Sphincterotomy). Excision of perianal skin tags in Crohn's disease may lead to significant morbidity because of the creation of an indolent, nonhealing wound.

EQUIPMENT

- 2% xylocaine with epinephrine
- 25- to 30-gauge needle

Since the perianal skin tags are external to the anal canal, no anal retractor is needed. Any standard surgical forceps are adequate to grasp the skin tag, which is generally removed with electrocautery. The electrocautery unit should have both coagulation and cutting capability. (See Chapter 31, Radiofrequency Surgery, and Chapter 150, Loop Electrosurgical Excision Procedure (LEEP) for Treating Cervical Intraepithelial Neoplasia, for listings of suppliers of various modern electrosurgery

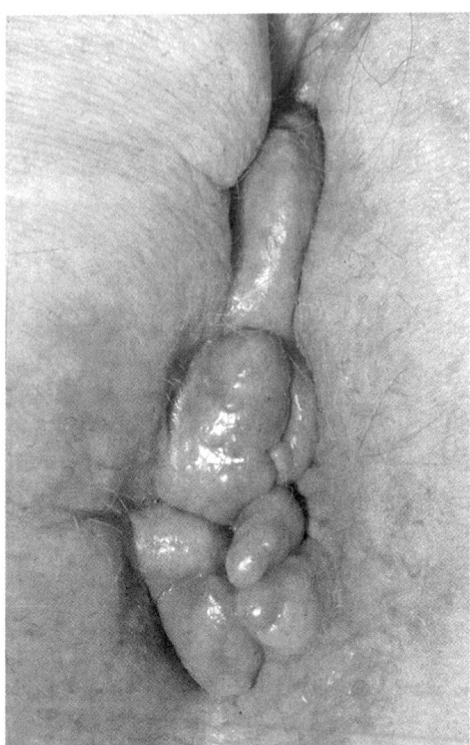

Fig. 110-2
Crohn's disease: edematous skin tags. (From Thomson J: Disorders of the anus and anal canal. In Misiewicz JJ et al, editors: *Slide atlas of gastroenterology,* London, 1986, Gower Medical Publishing.)

units.) Alternatively, the lesion can be excised with sharp tissue scissors or a knife blade, but this will increase the likelihood of bleeding.

PREPROCEDURE PATIENT PREPARATION

Most patients should be discouraged from having their perianal skin tags excised. Perianal skin tags per se generally cause no significant symptoms. Question the patient in-depth as to his or her reasons for wanting the skin tags excised. The most common indication is interference with anal hygiene resulting from the presence of one or more large perianal tags. Advise the patient that there will be some mild to moderate "burning" postoperative pain at the site of the excision. Postoperative bleeding is generally negligible, and infection is rare because the cauterized operative site is generally left open. The chances for infection increase if the site is sutured (Vicryl, chromic).

TECHNIQUE

1. Place the patient in the left lateral decubitus position on the procedure table.

2. Infiltrate the base of the skin tag with approximately 1 ml of local anesthetic (e.g., 2% lidocaine with epinephrine). To minimize discomfort, inject the anesthetic solution (at room temperature) very slowly at the base of the skin tag with a 25- or 30-gauge ½-inch hypodermic needle. When performed properly, this injection technique affords minimal discomfort to the patient. Do not use too much volume because this will distort the area to be excised and may leave an excessively large wound. Alternatively, do a field block around the lesion to maintain undisturbed anatomy near the tag.

3. After approximately 1 minute, grasp the skin tag with a 4 × 4–inch gauze pad between the thumb and index finger and compress it to reduce the edema caused from the infiltration of the local anesthetic. This also restores the skin tag to its "normal" anatomy so the site of excision can be identified properly.

4. Grasp the skin tag with forceps (which will confirm that appropriate anesthesia has been induced), and hold perpendicular to its base on the perianal skin. Care must be taken not to put any undue tension on the skin tag, since this will also serve to "tent up" and broaden the base of the skin tag and create an excision site that is much larger than needed.

5. Excise the skin tag, using the electrocautery unit in the cutting or blend mode. The site of excision should be approximately 3 mm above the normal perianal tissues because there will be electrocautery tissue destruction below the site of excision. If the skin tag is held taut and/or excised right at the level of the perianal skin, the resulting wound defect and patient discomfort will be greater than needed.

6. Cauterize any residual small bleeding sites. No more than three perianal skin tags are recommended to be excised during any one procedure.

7. Leave the site of excision open, since suture closure of this site will contribute to an increase in postoperative pain and a greater likelihood of perianal abscess.

8. Apply antibiotic ointment to soothe the area and prevent it from drying on clothing.

COMPLICATIONS

- A perianal abscess can develop at the site of excision of a skin tag, although this is uncommon and occurs less than 5% of the time. If an abscess does occur, appropriate incision and drainage will be necessary.
- If the skin tag excision site is very close to the anal verge, a chronic fissure may develop, although this is uncommon. Should a fissure develop and persist, then lateral internal sphincterotomy would be recommended.

- Perianal cellulitis can occur. Should this be diagnosed, appropriate antibiotic therapy should be instituted.
- Bleeding or hematoma may occur.

Excision of skin tags should not alter anal continence because of the lack of involvement of this procedure with the anal sphincters.

POSTPROCEDURE PATIENT EDUCATION

Wash the area gently three to four times a day and after defecation with mild soap and water. Xylocaine ointment 5% or an antibiotic ointment may be used to decrease discomfort. Prescribe a nonconstipating pain medication (e.g., ibuprofen). Further advise the patient to follow a high-fiber diet with commercial fiber supplements and four to six glasses of water per day. Time off from work is usually minimal and would range from 0 to 3 days, depending on the extent of excision. Total healing time may take up to 6 weeks for complete new skin coverage. Perianal discomfort will generally be present for 1 week or less.

CPT/BILLING CODE

46230   Excision of perianal skin tag

ICD-9-CM DIAGNOSTIC CODE

4559   Hemorrhoidal tag

BIBLIOGRAPHY

Corman ML: *Colon and rectal surgery*, Philadelphia, 1998, JB Lippincott.

Gordon P, Nivatvongs S: *Principles and practice of surgery for the colon, rectum, and anus*, St Louis, 1992, Quality Medical Publishing.

Mazier W, Levien D, Luchtefeld M, Senagore A: *Surgery of the colon, rectum, and anus*, Philadelphia, 1995, WB Saunders.

Pfenninger JL, Zainea GC: Common anorectal conditions. Part I: symptoms and complaints, *Am Fam Physician* 63:2391, 2001.

Pfenninger JL, Zainea GC: Common anorectal conditions. Part II: lesions, *Am Fam Physician* 64:77, 2001.

Pilonidal Cyst and Abscess: Current Management

James A. Surrell

A pilonidal cyst and/or abscess is located in the gluteal crease, usually within 5 to 10 cm of the anal verge. This lesion was originally described in the mid-1800s, and there has been considerable debate in the literature over whether it is an acquired or a congenital lesion. Most experts now believe that this is an acquired lesion resulting from penetration of the skin at this level from shafts of hair. A pilonidal sinus frequently contains multiple hairs that are microscopically noted to be tapered at both ends like shed hairs. The existence of hair follicles in the wall of the pilonidal sinus tract has never been demonstrated conclusively. Pilonidal sinus and abscess is a disease of the younger population, and 75% of cases are seen in males. Most patients develop symptoms of pilonidal disease between the ages of 20 and 25 years. A typical patient develops an abscess or recurrent infection and drainage at the base of the spine. The disease is characterized by a recurrence of the infection with the development of multiple sinus tracts in this location.

Examination of the patient with suspected pilonidal disease generally reveals an area of inflammation in the midline of the gluteal crease, with one or more sinus openings (Fig. 111-1). The openings may be slightly off the midline. Careful inspection of this site may reveal loose hairs projecting from the sinus openings. If the pilonidal sinus has an associated abscess, the patient will complain of pain and the examiner may note swelling and erythema at this site. Spontaneous and ongoing drainage is the common indicator, however, and if an abscess is present it is usually small. As a general guideline, if the patient gives a history of recurrent infection at the base of the spine, this in itself is almost diagnostic of a pilonidal sinus. Some difficulty in diagnosis may occur if the pilonidal sinus is located in the more caudad position closer to the anal canal. This raises the possibility of an anal fistula as the cause of the

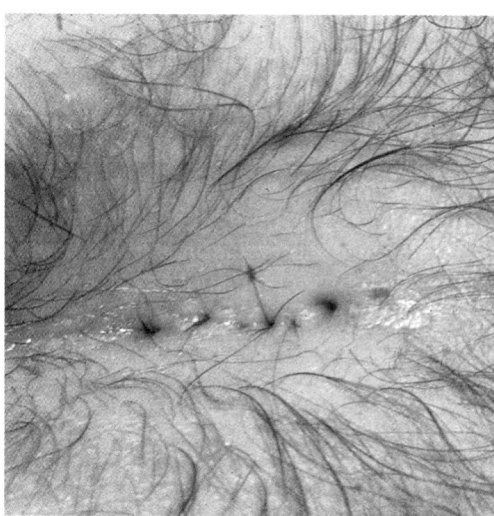

Fig. 111-1
Multiple (six) pilonidal sinus openings in the natal cleft. (From Thomson J: Disorders of the anus and anal canal. In Misiewicz JJ et al, editors: *Slide atlas of gastroenterology,* London, 1986, Gower Medical Publishing.)

infection. If, however, hairs are found in the lesion, this offers convincing confirmatory evidence that the physician is dealing with a pilonidal sinus.

INDICATIONS

Surgical treatment should be performed for the following:
- Acute abscess formation in the superior gluteal crease area (simple incision and drainage [I & D])
- Patients with a history of recurrent infections and drainage at the base of the spine (excision of the area). (Antibiotic therapy should only be considered as tem-

porizing and palliative, since recurrence will be the rule until adequate I & D excision is accomplished.)

CONTRAINDICATIONS FOR SURGICAL TREATMENT OF PILONIDAL CYST AND ABSCESS

- Patient with a paucity of symptoms, such as only minimal drainage with little or no discomfort or inflammation occurring perhaps only once or twice per year
- Marked bleeding dyscrasia

EQUIPMENT

- Local anesthesia.
- No special equipment is needed to perform a simple incision and drainage; a no. 11 blade is adequate.
- Only a minor surgical setup is required for excision plus a derm curette.

PREPROCEDURE PATIENT PREPARATION

The procedure of choice is I & D; for recurrent abscesses or persistent draining, excision of the involved area is needed. The wound is left open to heal by secondary intention. With this technique the patient needs to be informed of a prolonged healing time. The wounds are not at all disabling, and they can be expected to close in 8 to 12 weeks. Other options for treatment of pilonidal disease must be reviewed to include excision and primary closure, as well as skin flap and other plastic procedures for more extensive and complex pilonidal disease.

TECHNIQUE

A simple I & D may be all that is needed for a small abscess or first-time presentation. For recurrent disease, perform an elliptical incision at the site of the pilonidal disease to include the obvious sinus tract(s) (Fig. 111-2). The lateral and deep margins should extend to noninfected tissue that appears healthy. This procedure can be performed under local anesthesia (with intravenous sedation) or under general anesthesia in the operating room. Because of the proximity of the infected site, spinal anesthesia is *not* recommended. Thoroughly inspect the wound during the procedure, and curette all chronically infected granulation tissue so that the remaining wound defect is lined with healthy-appearing tissue with no obvious remaining sinus tracts. If the resultant

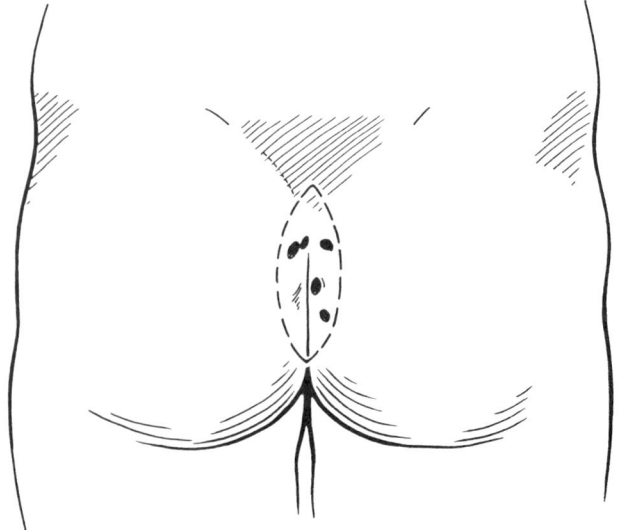

Fig. 111-2
Area of elliptical excision for pilonidal sinus.

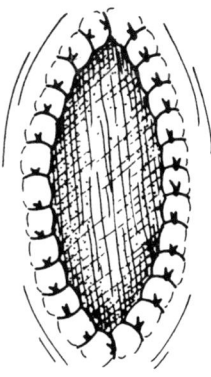

Fig. 111-3
Marsupialization after excision of pilonidal sinus, closed with interrupted absorbable sutures.

wound defect is not too deep, depending on the extent of the disease and the body habitus of the patient, consider marsupialization of the wound by tacking the skin edges to the base of the wound with an absorbable running simple suture (Fig. 111-3). This tends to prevent premature secondary wound closure. Total procedure time is generally 30 minutes or less.

COMPLICATIONS

Clearly, the most common complication of surgery for pilonidal disease is recurrence. The results of reported pilonidal disease surgery are variable, but most physicians report that the open technique has less of a recurrence rate than the closed technique. The obvious disadvantage to the open technique is the prolonged healing time, but these wounds generally do not afford significant morbidity to the patient during this longer healing process. Bleeding, excessive pain, and infection are rare.

POSTPROCEDURE PATIENT EDUCATION

If the procedure is performed with the pilonidal disease excised and the wound left open, instruct the patient on proper wound management. An open wound should be cleansed several times daily with soap and water, either by showering or other irrigation.

During the early stages of wound healing, the wound is packed with moistened gauze sponges and changed twice daily. During the early phases of the postprocedure recovery, examine the patient on a weekly basis to assess adequate progress. At this time, if hair regrowth is occurring, wound edges may be shaved. Every attempt to prevent loose hairs from entering the healing wound should be made. Instruct the patient on the concept of the wound's healing from the inside out so that premature skin bridging does not occur before the entire cavity is obliterated. Typical time off from work is approximately 1 week.

CPT/BILLING CODES

10080	Incision and drainage of pilonidal cyst, simple
10081	Incision and drainage of pilonidal cyst, complicated
11770	Excision of pilonidal cyst or sinus, simple
11771	Excision of pilonidal cyst or sinus, extensive
11772	Excision of pilonidal cyst or sinus, complicated

ICD-9-CM DIAGNOSTIC CODES

685.0	Pilonidal cyst with abscess
685.1	Pilonidal cyst, without mention of abscess

BIBLIOGRAPHY

Corman ML: *Colon and rectal surgery,* Philadelphia, 1998, JB Lippincott.

Gordon P, Nivatvongs S: *Principles and practice of surgery for the colon, rectum, and anus,* St Louis, 1992, Quality Medical Publishing.

Mazier W, Levien D, Luchtefeld M, Senagore A: *Surgery of the colon, rectum, and anus,* Philadelphia, 1995, WB Saunders.

CHAPTER 112

Peritoneal Lavage, Diagnostic

Brett White
Kenneth Hu

Diagnostic peritoneal lavage (DPL) is a procedure that consists of two components. The first part involves the attempt to aspirate any free blood that may be present in the peritoneal cavity. If this initial portion of the procedure reveals hemoperitoneum, the test is considered positive and the remainder of the procedure is aborted. Hemoperitoneum in this circumstance is highly predictive of intraperitoneal injury and warrants a laparotomy.

If no free blood is obtained during the initial aspiration, the second portion of the procedure is conducted. This next step involves the introduction of normal saline into the peritoneal cavity. The instilled fluid is subsequently drained from the peritoneal cavity and analyzed for a number of laboratory tests, which may ultimately point toward the nature of the intraabdominal pathology.

Newer radiologic techniques, in particular CT scan and ultrasound, have supplanted DPL as procedures of choice for stable patients with blunt abdominal trauma in the diagnosis of intraabdominal injury that may necessitate surgical intervention. DPL continues to be the diagnostic test of choice in many centers, however, particularly in cases of penetrating abdominal injuries. It is also used in patients with blunt abdominal trauma who are hemodynamically unstable and cannot be transported safely from the emergency department to radiology.

INDICATIONS

- Following penetrating injuries (such as a stab wound or gunshot wound) to the abdomen, flank, back, or lower chest in order to assess intraperitoneal hemorrhage or organ injury
- Following blunt abdominal trauma in a patient that is either hemodynamically unstable or has an altered mental status in order to assess intraperitoneal hemorrhage or organ injury.

CONTRAINDICATIONS

Absolute Contraindications

- Acute abdomen requiring immediate surgery

Relative Contraindications

- Previous abdominal surgery
- Coagulopathy
- Pregnancy
- Obesity

EQUIPMENT

Commercially prepared kit or the following equipment:
- Skin-cleansing solution (povidone-iodine).
- Sterile gloves and mask.
- Sterile marking pen (if area has not been marked indelibly before skin prep).
- Sterile drapes.
- 1% or 2% lidocaine with or without epinephrine.
- Scalpel, no. 11 blade.
- 9 to 18 French peritoneal catheter.
- 10-ml syringe for anesthetic.
- 20-ml syringe for diagnostic tap.
- 50-ml syringe, if using stopcock technique.
- 18-gauge, 1½- to 3-inch needle. Alternatively, an 18- or 20-gauge 1½- to 3-inch spinal needle may be substituted.
- 25- or 27-gauge, 1½-inch needle.
- Instruments for retractions such as hemostats or Army-Navy retractors.
- Needle holder.
- Nylon skin suture (4-0 or 5-0) on cutting needle.
- Absorbable sutures (2-0 Vicryl) for peritoneum and fascia, if peritoneum is to be opened.
- Sterile IV tubing.
- Three-way stopcock (for use with 50-ml syringe) *(optional)*.

PREPROCEDURE PATIENT PREPARATION

• Explain the procedure and its risks and benefits to the patient if possible (see the "Complications" section).
• Obtain verbal or written informed consent if possible.
• Place patient in the supine position.
• Use a Foley catheter and nasogastric tube for decompression of the bladder or stomach, respectively, if necessary.
• If necessary, use wrist restraints, especially for patients with altered mental status, to prevent contamination of the sterile field or injury from needle stick.

Editor's Note: Reviewing Chapter 97, Abdominal Paracentesis, may also be helpful.

TECHNIQUE

The procedural setup and fluid removal are identical for the open and closed techniques.
1. Decompress the stomach and bladder. (See Chapter 107, Nasogastric Tube and Salem Sump Insertion, and Chapter 113, Bladder Catheterization.)
2. Prepare the abdominal skin at the puncture site with povidone-iodine solution, and apply sterile drapes

as appropriate. The ideal site is immediately inferior to the umbilicus (Fig. 112-1). The supraumbilical approach may be used in pregnant patients or those patients with pelvic fractures.
3. Infiltrate the skin and subcutaneous tissues with lidocaine with epinephrine

Open Technique

4a. Using the no. 11 blade scalpel, create a 4- to 6-cm vertical skin incision.
4b. By blunt dissection, proceed down to rectus fascia. Open the rectus fascia by scalpel and proceed down to the peritoneum by sharp and blunt dissection.
4c. The peritoneum is visualized and opened. The catheter can then be inserted into the peritoneal space by direct visualization (Fig. 112-2). Proceed to step 5.

Closed Technique

4a. Insert an 18-gauge needle through the skin and directly into the peritoneal space.
4b. The guidewire may be introduced through the 18-gauge needle. Remove the needle.
4c. Slide the peritoneal catheter over the wire, using gentle twisting motions. With the closed technique, it may be necessary to make a small skin nick at the entry site with the scalpel to allow passage of the lavage catheter.
4d. Remove the wire after the catheter is in the peritoneum.

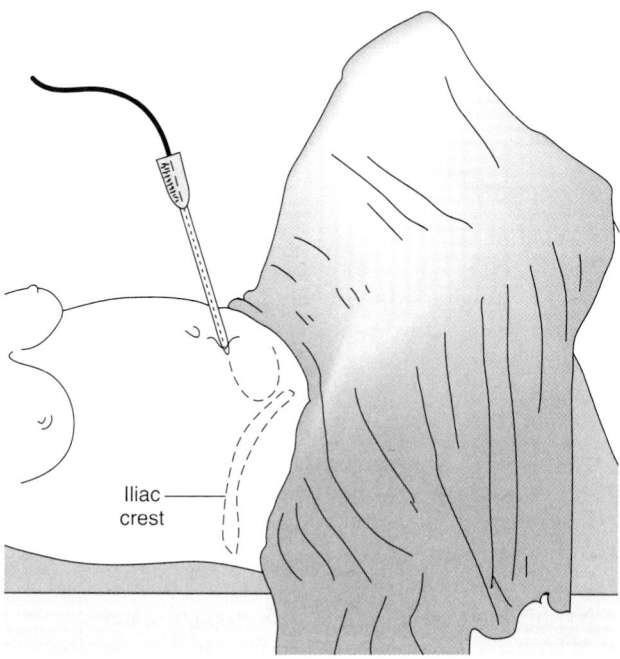

Fig. 112-1
Insertion of the needle into the peritoneal cavity in the midline, immediately inferior to the umbilicus.

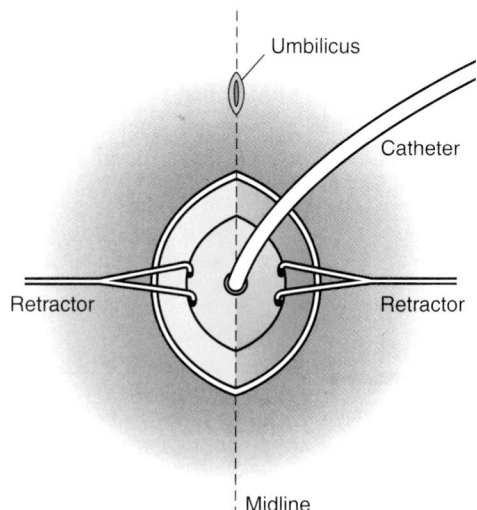

Fig. 112-2
Open technique, view from above. Superficial layers have been opened and are retracted away from the field of view. Catheter is inserted through the opened peritoneum directly into the peritoneal space.

5. Attach the syringe to the catheter and attempt to withdraw fluid. If more than 10 ml of blood is obtained, the patient should be prepared for emergent laparotomy immediately. If the tap is dry, proceed to lavage.

6. Connect the intravenous tubing and infuse lactated Ringer's solution or normal saline. The amount infused is 1 L for adults and 15 ml/kg for children.

7. The infused fluid is removed by placing the IV bag on the floor and allowing the fluid to return by gravity. Alternatively, the IV tubing may be connected to a 1-L vacuum jar.

8. The aspiration of greater than 10 ml of gross blood is considered a positive finding. Findings of more than 100,000 red blood cells (RBCs) per cubic millimeter are also considered positive. Findings of 20,000 to 100,000 RBCs should be considered equivocal. In these patients an observation period of 12 to 24 hours should be considered. Two situations provide exceptions to these general rules: (1) stab wounds to the low chest where diaphragmatic injury is suspected, and (2) gun shot wounds. The threshold for a positive RBC count should be 5000 RBC/mm^3 in these situations. Always be mindful of the hemodynamic stability of the patient when interpreting these results.

9. After the fluid is removed, gently remove the catheter and apply pressure to the wound. When the open technique is used, close the peritoneum and rectus fascia with absorbable suture. The skin is then closed with nylon suture. If the closed technique was used, placement of a pressure dressing alone may suffice, although a single suture may be necessary if the wound continues to leak.

COMPLICATIONS

- Bladder perforation
- Small and large bowel perforation
- Stomach perforation
- Lacerations of major vessels (mesenteric, iliac, aorta)
- Abdominal wall hematomas
- Abdominal wall dehiscence
- Infection (local, intraperitoneal, or systemic)
- False positive (vessel laceration during procedure) and false negative (poor catheter placement or loss of fluid into the thoracic cavity) results

POSTPROCEDURE PATIENT EDUCATION

Educate the patient about the potential for bleeding, pain, infection, and other complications.

SUPPLIER

Peritoneal lavage kit
Arrow International
2400 Bernville Road
Reading, PA 19605
Phone: 1-800-233-3187
Website: www.arrowintl.com/products/critcare.html

CPT/BILLING CODES:

49080   Peritoneocentesis, abdominal paracentesis, or peritoneal lavage; initial
49081   Peritoneocentesis, abdominal paracentesis, or peritoneal lavage; subsequent

ICD-9-CM DIAGNOSTIC CODES

568.81   Hemoperitoneum
868.00   Injury, abdomen or abdominal viscera, internal
868.03   Injury, internal peritoneum

BIBLIOGRAPHY

Roberts JR, Hedges JR: *Clinical procedures in emergency medicine*, ed 3, Philadelphia, 1998, WB Saunders.

Rosen PR: *Emergency medicine: concepts and clinical practice*, ed 4, St Louis, 1998, Mosby.

Schwartz GR, editor: *Principles and practice of emergency medicine*, ed 3, Philadelphia, 1992, Lea & Febiger.

Tintinalli JE, Kelen GD, Stapczynski JS, *Emergency medicine, a comprehensive study guide*, New York, 2000, McGraw-Hill.

PART SEVEN

Urinary System Procedures

CHAPTER 113

Bladder Catheterization

Robert E. James
James R. Palleschi

Urethral catheterization may be performed for diagnostic or therapeutic indications. Familiarity with the anatomy of the urethra and with the catheters that are available will increase the ease and success of bladder catheterization.

In the male patient with a normal lower urinary tract, there are two points of potential obstruction when passing a urethral catheter: The first is at the point of acute upward angulation between the bulbous and the membranous urethra. The second is at the bladder neck, where a bladder neck stenosis or an enlarged median lobe of the prostate gland may be present (Fig. 113-1).

In the female patient, the angle between the urethra and the bladder neck increases with age. Consequently, in the older patient, the urethra is normally directed toward the sacrum, whereas in the younger patient it is angled toward the umbilicus. Keeping these urethral angles in mind will improve the physician's technique, thereby reducing the patient's discomfort and facilitating the passage of a urethral catheter. Catheter size is measured in French units. As the number increases, the size increases (i.e., a 16-French catheter is larger than a 12-French). One "French unit" is approximately 0.33 mm.

INDICATIONS

Short-Term Catheterization

- Acute urinary retention
- Collection of uncontaminated urine specimen for analysis, culture, and sensitivity
- Diagnostic studies of the lower urinary tract (voiding cystourethrogram and urodynamics)
- Monitoring of urinary output
- Measurement of residual urine volume
- Surgery on structures adjacent to urinary tract
- Urinary tract surgery

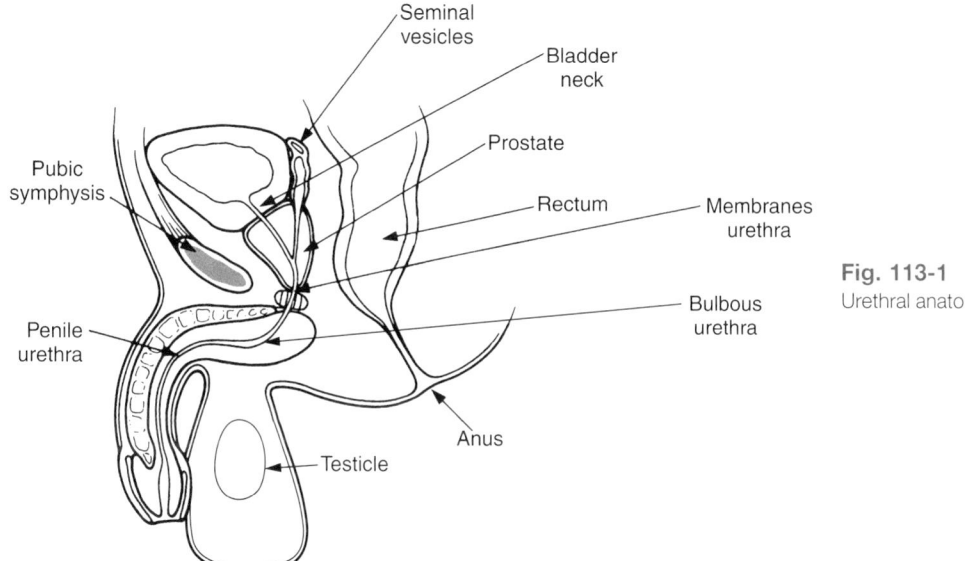

Fig. 113-1
Urethral anatomy of the male.

Long-Term Catheterization

- Chronic urinary retention
- Neurogenic bladder and retention in patient with inability to intermittent self-catheterize
- Incontinence with complicating skin breakdown
- Comfort measure for terminally ill or severely disabled patient with incontinence

CONTRAINDICATIONS

- Known urinary tract obstruction, such as urethral stricture
- Recent reconstructive surgery of the urethra or bladder neck
- A combative or uncooperative patient
- Known or suspected urethral disruption resulting from pelvic trauma
- Acute infection of the prostate and/or urethra

EQUIPMENT

- Urethral catheters:
  - *Foley catheter:* The Foley catheter is a straight urethral catheter with a single port that is used to inflate the retaining balloon (Fig. 113-2). A 16- to 18-French Foley catheter may be used for adults who require either a temporary or chronic indwelling catheter.
  - *Coudé catheter:* This catheter is similar to a Foley catheter with one exception: The terminal 2 inches are curved upward (Fig. 113-3). This is used in adult males for whom a Foley catheter cannot be inserted because of an enlarged median lobe of the prostate

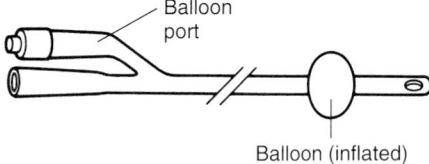

Fig. 113-2
Foley catheter with balloon inflated.

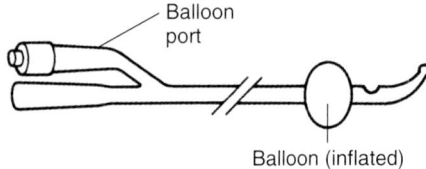

Fig. 113-3
Coudé catheter with balloon inflated.

gland or an elevated bladder neck. Some physicians advocate using a coudé catheter in all men more than 50 years of age. A 16- to 18-French catheter is normally used.

Note: Silastic catheters are available for latex-sensitive patients. Catheters impregnated with various substances such as antibiotics are of little value and are expensive.

- Lubricant: Either a water-soluble lubricant (K-Y Jelly) or a lubricant with a local anesthetic (2% lidocaine jelly) may be employed. When available, the latter is preferred; 10 ml is sufficient for female patients and 10 to 20 ml for male patients.
- Sterile towels and gloves
- Antiseptic solution
- Closed urinary drainage system

PREPROCEDURE PATIENT PREPARATION

The specific indications for catheterization and the technique should be reviewed with the patient. Catheter care should be discussed with the patient if it is to remain in place. (See the sample patient education handout titled "Urinary Catheter Care" on page 1880 of Appendix G.)

TECHNIQUE

1. The *female patient* is placed in the lithotomy or the supine position with the legs abducted. The *male patient* is placed in the supine position; the legs may be either abducted slightly or straight.
2. Cleanse the urethral meatus and surrounding area with antiseptic solution, and isolate the genitalia with sterile drapes or towels. Maintain sterile technique throughout.
3. Insert the 2% lidocaine jelly into the urethra with a syringe and leave it in place for approximately 5 to 10 minutes (longer is better to maximize effect). Some manufacturers place the anesthetic jelly in a syringe with a smooth conical end that can be inserted into the urethra. Otherwise, draw the anesthetic jelly into a 10-ml syringe. Place the end of the syringe *(without a needle)* gently inside the urethral meatus and inject the lidocaine jelly into the urethra. The *male patient* should be asked to compress the midurethra between his index finger and thumb to prevent the jelly from leaving the urethra.
4. For an adult patient, select a 16- or 18-French catheter. A Foley catheter is used for *female* patients. Following the anticipated course of the urethra, pass the catheter 3 inches into the bladder. Once urine is obtained, the balloon may be inflated with 5 ml of normal saline or

water. Then gently pull the catheter outward until the balloon is resting against the bladder neck.

For *male patients less than 50 years of age,* a Foley catheter may be used. Pass the catheter into the bladder the full length until the junction of the Foley catheter and inflation port for the balloon is all that is visible (Fig. 113-4).

Caution: If this is not done, the balloon may be inflated within the urethra. The balloon is normally inflated with 5 ml of normal saline or water. If the balloon does not inflate easily, or if the patient experiences discomfort in the perineum or penis as the balloon is being inflated, you should suspect that the balloon is located within the urethra. In such a case, the balloon should be deflated, and the catheter reinserted.

Once the balloon has been inflated, pull it gently down against the bladder neck.

For *male patients more than 50 years of age,* select a coudé catheter. The curve at the tip of the catheter should be directed at the 12 o'clock position. This will permit the catheter to glide over an enlarged median lobe of the prostate gland or an elevated bladder neck. If the catheter does not pass easily, it should be removed and the procedure should be repeated. Occasionally, the tip of the catheter will rotate as it is being inserted. If this occurs, the catheter will not pass through the prostatic urethra into the bladder. If you

cannot pass a 16-French Foley or coudé catheter into the male urethra, there is usually a urethral stricture, bladder neck stenosis, or very large median lobe of the prostate gland. *After resection of the prostatic urethra,* the tip of the catheter may hang up at the widened outlet of the prostatic urethra. In such a case, you may consider using a 12-French Foley or coudé catheter. Directing the catheter tip into the prostatic urethra with a gloved finger in the rectum while passing the catheter with the opposite hand also can be attempted. If the smaller catheter does not pass, a urology consultation is advised.

5. In most instances the catheter needs to be secured to the leg with tape or other means to prevent trauma to the urethra.

Difficult Catheterizations

Women

Postmenopausal women with a narrow introitus or women with a recessed or a high-riding urethra may be very difficult to catheterize because the urethral meatus cannot be clearly visualized. In either case, the following technique is usually successful. After preparing the patient as described, identify the urethral meatus with the tip of one of your index fingers. Then, slide a 16-French catheter along the index finger and into the urethra. If this cannot be accomplished, the patient may have a stenotic meatus. Using the same technique, use a 12-French Foley or coudé catheter. If this is unsuccessful, a urology consult is advised.

Men

In men with a severe phimosis, the prepuce cannot be retracted enough to see the urethral meatus. If the os of the prepuce is large enough to pass a catheter, you may be successful using the following technique. Fix the glans penis in its normal position with the meatus at the 6 o'clock position. Using a coudé catheter, rotate the catheter until the tip is pointing down in the 6 o'clock position. The tip of the catheter will be directed through the os of the prepuce in this position. Once the catheter has entered the urethra, it may be rotated until the tip is pointed up in the 12 o'clock position. The catheter then may be advanced into the bladder. If the os of the prepuce will not permit the passage of a catheter, a dorsal slit of the prepuce may be performed (see Chapter 121, Dorsal Slit for Phimosis), and the catheter inserted. Otherwise, a suprapubic catheter may be inserted (see Chapter 115, Suprapubic Catheter Insertion/Change).

COMPLICATIONS

- Urinary tract infection (see Box 113-1 for prevention guidelines)

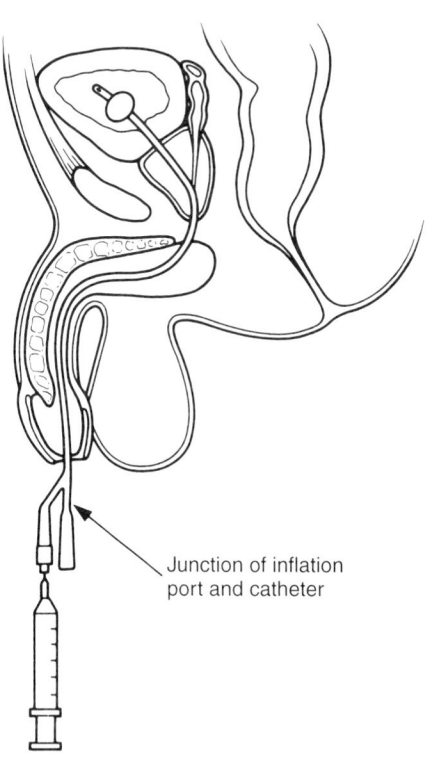

Fig. 113-4
In the male, the Foley catheter is passed into the bladder until the junction of the catheter and inflation port for the balloon is met.

Junction of inflation port and catheter

BOX 113-1

Centers for Disease Control and Prevention Guidelines for
Prevention of Catheter-Associated Urinary Tract Infection

Category I: Strongly Recommended

Catheterize only when necessary.
Educate personnel in correct techniques of catheter insertion
    and care.
Emphasize handwashing.
Insert catheter using aseptic technique and sterile equipment.
Secure catheter properly.
Maintain closed sterile drainage.
Obtain urine specimens aseptically.
Maintain unobstructed urine flow.

Category II: Moderately Recommended

Periodically reeducate personnel in catheter care.
Use smallest suitable catheter bore.
Avoid irrigation unless needed to prevent or relieve obstruction.
Refrain from daily meatal care.
Do not change catheter at arbitrary intervals.

From Cravens DD, Zweig S: *Am Fam Phys* 61(2):369, 2000. Information from
http://aepo-xdv-www.epo.cdc.gov/wonder/prevguid/p0000416/p0000416.asp
(accessed June 20, 2002).

- Transient hematuria
- Creation of a false passage resulting from the use of a small catheter, excessive force, or the presence of a urethral stricture
- Urethral stricture
- Obstruction of flow

CPT/BILLING CODES

53670	Simple catheterization
53675	Complicated catheterization

ICD-9-CM DIAGNOSTIC CODES

788.20	Urinary retention or stasis, NEC
788.30	Urinary incontinence
625.6	Stress urinary incontinence, female
788.32	Stress urinary incontinence, male
596.54	Neurogenic bladder, without cauda equina syndrome
344.61	Neurogenic bladder, with cauda equina syndrome
596.0	Bladder neck obstruction, acquired
753.6	Bladder neck obstruction, congenital
598.9	Urethral stricture, (anterior), (posterior), (organic)
598.1	Urethral stricture, caused by trauma
602.8	Prostatic stricture
600.0	Prostatism

ADDITIONAL RESOURCES

- See the sample patient education handout titled "Urinary Catheter Care" on page 1880 of Appendix G.

BIBLIOGRAPHY

Cancio LC, Sabanegh ES, Thompson IM: Managing the Foley catheter, *Am Fam Physician* 48(5):829, 1993.

Cravens DD, Zweig S: Urinary catheter management, *Am Fam Physician* 61(2):369, 2000.

Hopkins TB: Urethral catheterization. In Vander Salem TJ, editor: *Atlas of bedside procedures,* Boston, 1979, Little, Brown & Co.

Kunin CM, Chin QF, Chambers S: Indwelling urinary catheters in the elderly, *Am J Med* 82:405, 1987.

Moore KN, Kelm M, Sinclair O, Cadrain G: Bacteriuria in intermittent catheterization users: the effect of sterile versus clean reused catheters, *Rehabil Nurs* 18(3):306, 1993.

Pomfret IJ: Catheters: design, selection and management, *Br J Nurs* 5(4):245, 1996.

Thuroff JW: Retrograde instrumentation of the urinary tract. In Tanagho EA, Macanich JW, editors: *General urology,* East Norwalk, Conn, 1988, Lange Medical Publications.

Warren JW: Catheter-associated urinary tract infections, *Infect Dis Clin North Am* 11:609, 1997.

Wong ES: Guideline for prevention of catheter-associated urinary tract infections, Feb 1981. Available at http://aepo-xdv-www.epo.cdc.gov/wonder/prevguid/p0000416/p0000416.asp (accessed June 20, 2002).

CHAPTER 114

Diagnostic Cystourethroscopy

Andrew C. Steele

Neeraj Kohli

The construction of the cystoscope has progressed from the original tube-and-candle, first described in the early 1800s, to the flexible fiberoptic cystoscope available today. The discussion in this chapter is confined to the use of the rigid endoscope. This instrument's ease of use in the female patient, superior visualization, and similarity to the familiar hysteroscope all make it preferable to the flexible cystoscope for many providers. The technique of cystourethroscopy greatly enhances the provider's ability to diagnose and treat a variety of genitourinary tract conditions. Diagnostic cystourethroscopy can be performed routinely and comfortably in the office.

Editor's note: It might be helpful to also review Chapter 113, Bladder Catheterization, along with this chapter.

INDICATIONS

- Urinary incontinence
  - Intrinsic sphincter deficiency, confirms the diagnosis and allows treatment with periurethral bulking agents
  - Obstructive or irritative voiding symptoms (urgency, frequency, urge incontinence) unresponsive to conservative measures
  - Suspected diverticulum, fistula, or ectopic ureter
- Known or suspected urogynecologic malignancy
  - Gross or microscopic hematuria
  - Staging for bladder, cervical, or endometrial cancer
- Recurrent urinary tract infections
- Pelvic pain symptoms
  - Dyspareunia
    - Suspected interstitial cystitis or urethritis
    - Endometriosis of the bladder
- Traumatic injury to the lower genital tract
- Intraoperative assessment of the bladder or urethra
  - Exclusion of inadvertent intraluminal suture placement or bladder trauma following incontinence correction procedures

- Assessment of coaptation of the urethra following suburethral sling procedures
- Evaluation of ureteral patency with intravenous indigo carmine dye

CONTRAINDICATIONS

Cystourethroscopy is generally safe and well tolerated. Acute cystitis or pyelonephritis should be treated before cystourethroscopy is performed, since sepsis has been reported following cystoscopy in an infected patient.

EQUIPMENT

- Cystoscope (Fig. 114-1)
  - Sterile rigid telescopes with 0- and 70-degree lenses.
  - Sterile sheath of 17- to 22-French diameter with inflow and outflow ports.

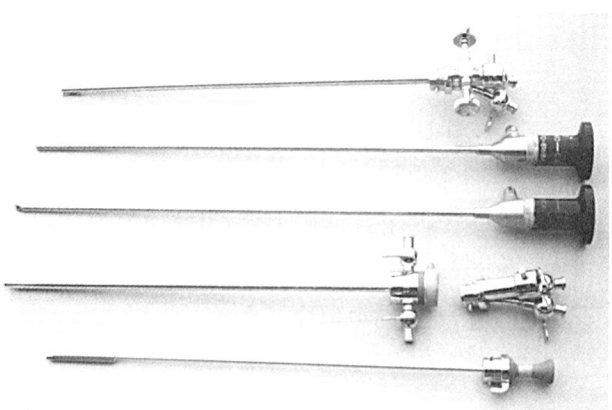

Fig. 114-1
Cystoscope components, including (from top to bottom) operative sheath, telescopes (2), sheath and bridge, and obturator.

— Sterile scope-to-sheath bridge. This bridge may have one or two operative ports that admit the passage of biopsy instruments or urethral catheters.

— A light source and fiberoptic cable compatible with the telescope.

- Irrigation tubing
- Distension medium in 500-ml to 3-L bags. Saline or Ringers' lactate may be used if electrocautery is not anticipated. If electrocautery is anticipated, then a nonconductive medium such as mannitol, sorbitol, or glycine should be used.
- Cotton balls moistened with an antiseptic solution (Betadine)
- Sterile gloves
- Sterile cotton-tip applicators
- 1% to 2% xylocaine gel
- Blue towel for tray top
- Basin to capture irrigation runoff
- Video equipment *(optional),* including camera, high-resolution monitor, videocassette recorder, and printer

PREPROCEDURE PATIENT PREPARATION

Consent to perform cystourethroscopy should be obtained before the procedure. The patient should be informed of the possibility of discomfort during and after the procedure, as well as the potential for postprocedure urinary tract infection. Patients with valvular disease (e.g., mitral valve prolapse) require antibiotic prophylaxis before the procedure (see Chapter 204, Antibiotic Prophylaxis).

TECHNIQUE

Preparation

1. After the patient has emptied the bladder, *cleanse the urethral meatus* with an antiseptic solution.
2. Generously *lubricate the cotton-tipped applicator* with 2% xylocaine gel, and insert it into the urethral meatus to the level of the bladder neck. Observe the angle of the urethra as an aid to inserting the cystoscope.

Note: Use sterile technique and wear sterile gloves from this point throughout the procedure.

3. Prepare the cystourethroscope as follows:
   a. *Assemble the cystourethroscope* by attaching the 0-degree telescope to the bridge and sheath (Fig. 114-2).

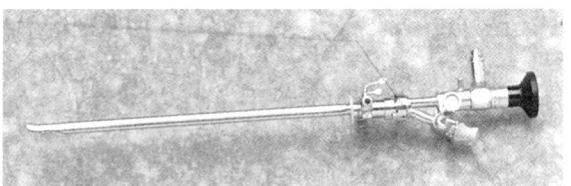
Fig. 114-2
Assembled cystoscope with telescope, bridge, and sheath.

   b. *Attach the light cable* to the cystourethroscope and the light source. Turn on the light source before insertion to ensure proper illumination.
   c. *Attach the infusion tubing* to the infusion port on the sheath, and attach this in turn to the appropriate instillation medium hung on a nearby IV pole. The tubing is then flushed.
4. *Lubricate the distal portion of the cystoscope* sheath with 2% xylocaine gel. Remove the applicator. After ensuring that all ports are in the closed position, *start the flow of the infusion medium* by opening the stop-cock of the inflow port. The operator should have sole control of the fluid infusion through this port.

Urethroscopy

5. *Insert the lighted and assembled cystoscope* into the urethral meatus, following the line of the urethra. Initial insertion may be achieved using fluid as the obturator. Fluid is infused during inspection to a maximum of 350 to 500 ml or until the patient is uncomfortable. If resistance is encountered, the scope should not be forced; rather, the angle of insertion of the cystoscope should be reassessed. Continued difficulty in inserting the cystourethroscope may be an indication for urethral dilation before proceeding. Dilation can be performed serially using urethral dilators beginning with 14 French and dilating up to 32 French. Alternatively, a smaller size sheath can be used.
6. *Advance the cystoscope* under direct visualization into the bladder lumen. Then withdraw it slowly until the internal urethral meatus is visualized. While slowly withdrawing the cystourethroscope, examine the entire length of the urethral mucosa for pathology (Fig. 114-3). Gentle palpation of the anterior vaginal wall during withdrawal may help to identify a urethral diverticulum, which tends to occur on the posterior aspect of the urethra.

Cystoscopy

7. *Remove the cystoscope* and discontinue the infusion flow. *Replace the 0-degree telescope with an angled*

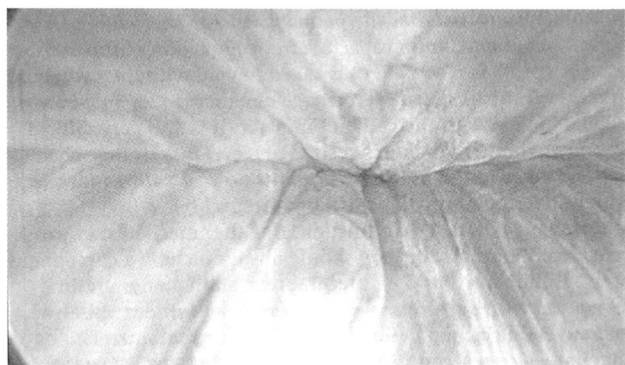

Fig. 114-3
View of normal urethral mucosa.

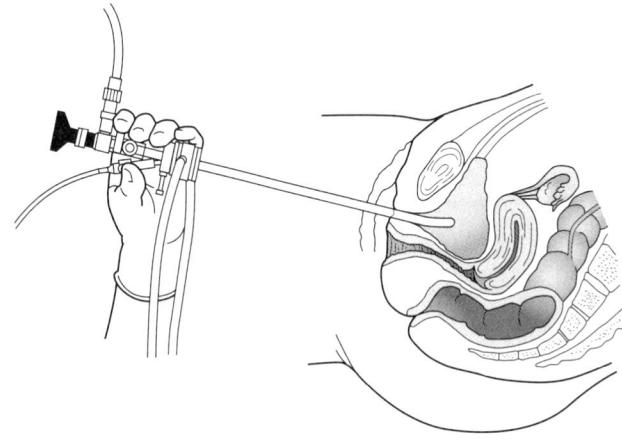

Fig. 114-4
Technique of cystoscopy using angled telescopic lens.

lens (30- or 70-degree) telescope and reinsert the reassembled cystoscope as described above. For adequate cystoscopy the bladder should be filled to approximately 250 ml or greater. If the patient notes discomfort from overdistension of the bladder, open the outflow port on the sheath and drain an appropriate amount of fluid from the bladder.

8. *Perform a systematic examination of the bladder lumen,* and identify a small air bubble, which is usually present at the bladder dome. With this as a landmark, examine the anterior and lateral sidewalls in a stepwise fashion. To visualize the entire bladder dome, rotate the angled lens about the long axis of the telescope while keeping the camera in a fixed orientation (Fig. 114-4). Lateral torque, with the urethral meatus as the fulcrum, can cause pain and should be avoided. Intraluminal pathology, including the presence of tumor, endometriosis, trabeculations, stones, chronic cystitis, and hemorrhage, should be noted (Fig. 114-5). Intraluminal sutures inadvertently placed at the time of a previous urethropexy are generally identified on the lateral sidewalls at the 2 and 10 o'clock positions.

9. *Visualize the trigone,* located posteriorly just proximal to the internal urethral meatus at the 6 o'clock position. Any abnormalities should be noted. Rotating the scope 20 to 30 degrees to each side will allow visualization of the *ureteral orifices.* If one orifice is visualized, identification of the *interureteric ridge* will lead to the contralateral orifice. (In patients with large cystoceles, reduction of the prolapse may be necessary in order to see the orifices.) If possible, *identify ureteral peristalsis with efflux of urine.*

10. For patients with pelvic pain or interstitial cystitis, bladder distention with at least 600 to 1000 ml may be therapeutic but usually requires general anesthesia because of poor tolerance in the office as a result of severe pain.

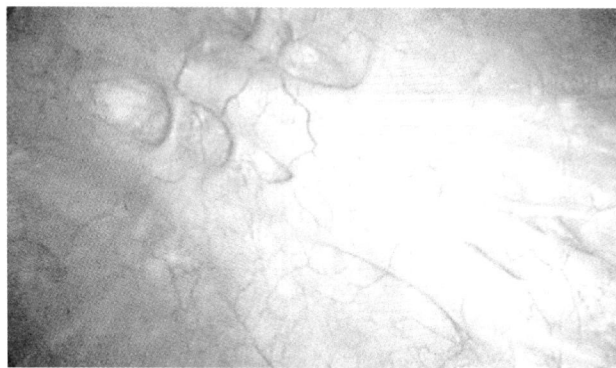

Fig. 114-5
Cystoscopic evaluation of bladder lumen demonstrating coarse trabeculations (ridges).

11. After completing the procedure, *turn off the infusion of distension medium and drain the patient's bladder* with the ancillary port on the cystoscope sheath. Samples of this drainage can be sent for cytologic analysis if desired. Remove the cystoscope and turn off the light source to prevent accidental injury from the hot light.

12. Disassemble the cystoscopic telescopes, bridge, and sheaths and clean them by immersion in glutaraldehyde solution (Cidex) for 20 minutes before reuse.

BLADDER BIOPSY

Bladder biopsy is useful for evaluation and histologic confirmation of suspicious lesions including malignancy and interstitial cystitis. Although it can be performed in the office, bladder biopsy usually requires a larger sheath to accommodate the biopsy forceps, is associated with patient discomfort, and occasionally requires electrocautery to control bleeding. Given these considerations, it is recommended that cystoscopic biopsies be performed in the ambulatory surgical suite.

COMPLICATIONS

- Bacteriuria
- Sepsis
- Urethral or bladder neck trauma
- Bleeding
- Pain

Complications following cystourethroscopy are rare. The reported rates of bacteriuria following this procedure are 2% to 7%. Rare cases of systemic sepsis associated with performance of cystoscopy in the presence of untreated infection have been reported. Although the use of prophylactic antibiotics is controversial, it is reasonable to prescribe one to two doses of an antibiotic such as Macrodantin or trimethoprim/sulfamethoxazole after the procedure. Rarely, trauma to the urethra and bladder neck can result from instrumentation.

INTERPRETATION OF RESULTS

A complete review of abnormal findings at the time of cystoscopy is beyond the scope of this chapter. However, the physician who routinely performs cystoscopy should be familiar with the normal appearance of the bladder and urethra. Abnormal anatomic findings should correlate with the patient's symptoms. In patients with overactive bladder symptoms (urgency, frequency, nocturia, enuresis, or urge incontinence), the urethra should be inspected for diverticulum and the bladder inspected for trabeculations, infectious changes, and foreign bodies.

For the evaluation of incontinence, cystoscopy is useful in the evaluation of intrinsic sphincter deficiency (the internal urethral meatus is open at rest) and vesicovaginal and urethrovaginal fistulas. In patients with genitourinary pain syndromes, the urethra may appear atrophic and the bladder may reveal petechial hemorrhages or Hunner's ulcers consistent with interstitial cystitis. Bladder distention, which is often therapeutic, can be accomplished at the time of cystoscopy with instillation of 600 to 1000 ml of solution.

Cystoscopy is useful for evaluation of lower urinary tract injury. Cystoscopy may reveal a bladder laceration or penetration of the bladder by sutures placed during surgery. To assess ureteral integrity and patency, patients can be given 5 ml intravenous indigo carmine at the time of cystoscopy. Both ureteral orifices should be noted to eject dye 5 to 10 minutes after intravenous injection. In some cases dye spillage may be delayed up to 15 minutes.

POSTPROCEDURE PATIENT EDUCATION

Each patient should be provided with instructions concerning expected postprocedure symptoms. A preprinted informational handout may be useful for this purpose. Specific information should include the following:

1. Patients should take antibiotic prophylaxis, if prescribed. They should be instructed to follow up immediately if dysuria, pyuria, or fever greater than 100.4° F develops within 72 hours of the procedure.
2. A small amount of transient hematuria within the first few hours after cystoscopy is normal. If it persists or is excessive, the patient should be instructed to follow up immediately.
3. The patient may have some discomfort following the procedure. A short course of the bladder analgesic, phenazopyridine, may be used to alleviate this. If the discomfort persists, the patient should be instructed to follow up for evaluation.

CONCLUSION

Cystourethroscopy is an easy and safe procedure that can be performed in the office setting or the operating room to allow the clinician to visualize the lower urinary tract. It can be useful in the diagnosis of various conditions ranging from urinary incontinence to pain syndromes. Before routinely performing cystoscopy, physicians should familiarize themselves with the equipment and feel comfortable recognizing abnormal pathology on visualization of the urethra or bladder. The results of the cystourethroscopy, in conjunction with the patient's history and physical examination, can provide diagnostic information needed to implement an effective treatment plan.

SUPPLIERS

ACMI Corporation
300 Stillwater Avenue
Stamford, CT 06902-3695
Phone: 1-888-524-7266
Website: www.circoncorp.com

Karl Storz Endoscopy-America, Inc.
600 Corporate Pointe
Culver City, CA 90230-7600
Phone: 1-800-421-0837
Website: www.karlstorz.com

Olympus America, Inc.
2 Corporate Center Drive
Melville, NY 11747
Phone: 1-800-645-8160
Website: www.olympusamerica.com

CPT/BILLING CODES

52000	Cystourethroscopy (separate procedure)
52005	Cystourethroscopy, with ureteral catheterization
52204	Cystourethroscopy, with biopsy
52260	Cystourethroscopy, with dilation of bladder for interstitial cystitis; general or conduction anesthesia
52281	Cystourethroscopy, with calibration and/or dilation of urethral stricture or stenosis
52285	Cystourethroscopy for treatment of the female urethral syndrome with any or all of the following: urethral meatotomy, urethral dilation, internal urethrotomy, lysis of urethrovaginal septal fibrosis, lateral incisions of the bladder neck, and fulguration of polyp(s) of urethra, bladder neck, and/or trigone

ICD-9-CM DIAGNOSTIC CODES

788.1	Dysuria
788.21	Incomplete bladder emptying
788.31	Incontinence: urge
788.37	Incontinence: continuous leakage
788.41	Urinary frequency
569.0	Bladder neck obstruction
595.1	Cystitis: interstitial
599.2	Diverticulum: urethral
596.2	Fistula: bladder
597.31	Urethral syndrome
599.7	Hematuria
788.30	Incontinence: unspecified
788.33	Incontinence: mixed
625.6	Incontinence: stress
788.2	Urinary retention
592.1	Calculus: ureteral
595.2	Cystitis: chronic
867.0	Injury: bladder/urethra
599.1	Fistula: urethral

BIBLIOGRAPHY

Albala D: *Color atlas of endourology,* Philadelphia, 1999, Lippincott, Williams & Wilkins.
Bavetta S, Olsha O, Fenely J: Spreading sepsis by cystoscopy, *Postgrad Med J* 66:734, 1990.
Clark KR, Higgs MJ: Urinary infection following out-patient flexible cystoscopy, *Br J Urol* 66:503, 1990.
Harris RL, Cundiff GW, Theofrastous JP, et al: The value of intraoperative cystoscopy in urogynecologic and reconstructive pelvic surgery, *Am J Obstet Gynecol* 177:1367, 1997.
Howard RS, Golin AL: Long-term follow-up of asymptomatic microhematuria, *J Urol* 145:335, 1991.
Nickel JC, Wilson J, Morales A, et al: Value of urologic investigation in a targeted group women with recurrent urinary tract infections, *Can J Surg* 34:591, 1991.
Rosenzweig BA: Endoscopic evaluation of the lower urinary tract. In Walters MD, Karram MM (eds): *Clinical urogynecology,* St Louis, 1993, Mosby.

WEBSITES

www.healthy.net/library/articles/ahcpr/incont.htm (Patient information on incontinence from the Agency for Health Care Policy and Research Guidelines)
www.niddk.nih.gov (Information on a wide range of topics on urologic conditions from the National Institutes for Health)
www.circoncorp.com (Official website for a leading supplier of endoscopic equipment; this site also has a number of instructional videos available on performing endoscopy)
www.karlstorz.com (Another major supplier of endoscopy equipment)

CHAPTER 115

Suprapubic Catheter Insertion/Change

Robert E. James
James R. Palleschi

Suprapubic catheters are normally used to provide short-term urinary drainage. If the patient's age or comorbid conditions preclude corrective surgery, the temporary catheter may be left in place or, with the aid of an exchange wire and appropriate dilators, may be replaced with a permanent suprapubic catheter.

INDICATIONS

- Impassable urethral stricture, bladder neck contracture or obstruction
- Inability to pass a urethral catheter over an elevated bladder neck or an enlarged median lobe of the prostate gland
- Urethral trauma
- Recent urethral or bladder neck reconstructive surgery
- Inability to tolerate a urethral catheter and unwilling or unable to perform intermittent self-catheterization
- Bladder drainage required in the presence of a significant urethral or prostate infection
- Severe phimosis precluding the insertion of a urethral catheter

CONTRAINDICATIONS

- Uncooperative patient
- Bleeding disorder or the use of systemic anticoagulants
- Cellulitis over the insertion site

EQUIPMENT

- Local anesthetic: 10-ml lidocaine 1% to 2%
- 10-ml syringe; 1½-inch, 22-gauge spinal needle
- Antiseptic skin preparation
- Sterile towels
- Mask and sterile gloves
- Mounted scalpel blade (no. 11 or no. 15)
- Suture scissors, needle holder, and 2-0 silk suture
- Closed urinary drainage system
- Suprapubic catheter set

Note: There are many manufacturers of suprapubic catheters and insertion kits, including the following: Bonnano catheter (Becton-Dickinson Corp.), Stamey percutaneous suprapubic catheter set (Cook Urological), the Simplastic suprapubic catheter (Franklin Medical), and the Lawrence SupraFoley suprapubic catheter introducer (Rusch Inc.).

The principal components of each set, except for the SupraFoley suprapubic catheter introducer, are a metal obturator and the suprapubic catheter. The metal obturator is placed down through the suprapubic catheter and is subsequently removed when the catheter is appropriately positioned within the bladder. The end of the catheter may consist of a *Coudé, Malecot tip, Robinson*, or *Foley bulb*. All of these are equally effective in retaining the catheter within the bladder (Fig. 115-1).

PREPROCEDURE PATIENT PREPARATION

Explain to the patient that mild to moderate suprapubic discomfort may be experienced for a few hours to days after this procedure. As long as the catheter is in place, intermittent hematuria and irritating voiding symptoms may be present. Review catheter care, including the use of a leg bag and overnight drainage bag. Tell the patient to contact the physician if increasing pain, excessive bleeding, temperature greater than 101° F, or a nonfunctioning catheter is noticed. Informed consent should be obtained.

TECHNIQUE

1. Place the patient in the supine position. If the bladder is not palpable, the procedure should be delayed until the bladder can be easily identified, or

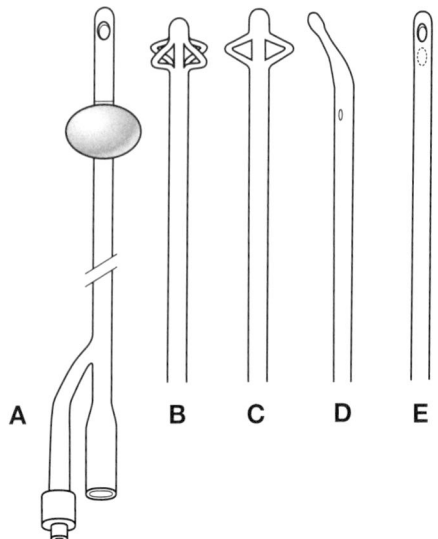

Fig. 115-1
Commonly used catheters. **A,** Foley-type balloon catheter. **B,** Malecot self-containing, four-wing urethral catheter. **C,** Malecot self-retaining, two-wing catheter. **D,** Coudé hollow, olive-tip catheter. **E,** Robinson urethral catheter. (From Walsh PC, Retik AB, Vaughn ED Jr, Wein AJ: *Campbell's urology,* ed 7, Philadelphia, 1998, WB Saunders.)

the insertion should be completed with ultrasound guidance.

Note: If the patient has a bladder or pelvic anatomic abnormality from previous surgery, cancer, or trauma, the procedure should be completed with the aid of ultrasound guidance.

2. Maintain sterile technique. Prepare the suprapubic skin with an antiseptic solution, and drape with sterile towels. Inject the local anesthetic into the skin overlying the abdominal wall and dome of the bladder.

3. Make a 1-cm horizontal skin incision 5 cm above the symphysis pubis in the midline (in both adult and pediatric patients). At this point, some physicians prefer to pass a 22-gauge spinal needle into the bladder. This will verify the bladder location before the suprapubic catheter is inserted. If the bladder is distended, this procedure is not necessary.

4. Once the skin incision has been made, place the metal obturator into the lumen of the suprapubic catheter, with the sharp oblique end of the obturator extending beyond the tip of the catheter (Fig. 115-2). Advance the obturator and catheter together through the skin incision at a 60-degree caudal angle toward the bladder neck (approximately the mid-perineal area) (Fig. 115-3). With momentary pressure, advance the catheter through the rectus sheath and muscle and into the dome of the bladder. This requires inserting it a total of approximately 5 cm below the skin in adults.

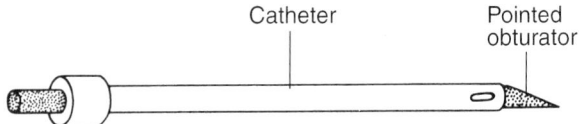

Fig. 115-2
Suprapubic catheter with obturator in place.

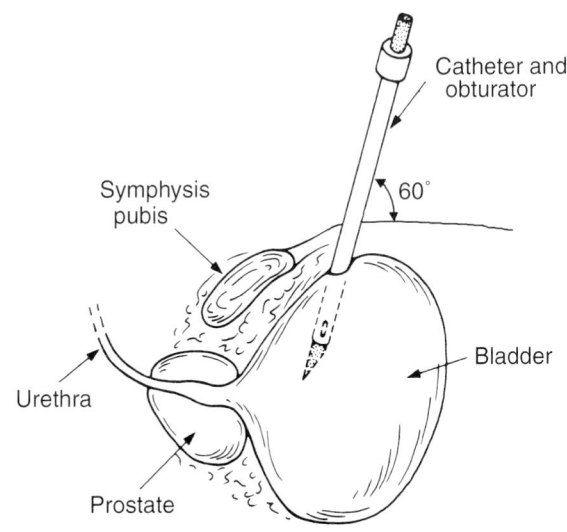

Fig. 115-3
Insertion and advancement of the catheter and obturator.

5. Advance the catheter and obturator an additional 5 cm in adults to assure appropriate positioning. Remove the obturator; urine will be seen passing from the suprapubic catheter. After the obturator is removed, the wings of the Malecot type of catheter (Stamey suprapubic catheter) will expand, or the pigtail tip of the Bonnano catheter will coil inside the bladder to prevent it from falling out.

6. If the catheter has a balloon tip, once it has been appropriately positioned within the bladder, inflate the balloon with sterile saline.

   The SupraFoley suprapubic catheter introducer consists of a plastic sheath, through which a sharp, plastic obturator is inserted. Make a 1-cm incision just above the symphysis, over the dome of the distended bladder. Advance the obturator through the anterior rectus sheath, into the bladder. Then remove the obturator and advance a Foley catheter down through the plastic sheath into the bladder. The balloon is filled with 5 to 10 ml of water or saline. A tab is located on the top edge of the plastic sheath; pull down and remove it. This removes a strip of the sheath, allowing the removal of the sheath; leave the catheter in place in the bladder.

7. Pull back the catheter until the balloon, coil, or wings are resting against the dome of the bladder.

8. Secure the catheter in place with a silk suture.
9. Using sterile saline, irrigate the catheter to ensure appropriate drainage and position.
10. Connect a drainage bag to the catheter.

COMPLICATIONS

- Perivesicle bleeding
- Gross hematuria
- Failure to drain
- Infection
- Intestinal perforation (more likely when the bladder is not distended, when the normal anatomy is distorted by previous surgery or trauma, or when the obturator and catheter are not introduced at the correct angle; normally, a small perforation usually will seal spontaneously without consequence)

SUPRAPUBIC CATHETER REPLACEMENT

If the catheter has been in place for several weeks and a mature tract is established, the existing catheter may be removed and replaced with a similar catheter. To replace a percutaneous suprapubic catheter, fill the bladder with sterile saline or water, and remove the catheter. The sterile water or saline will begin to pass through the suprapubic catheter site and, consequently, the catheter needs to be replaced promptly. Place an obturator in the new catheter, and advance it down the tract until the sterile water or saline begins to exit through or around the catheter. Usually a local anesthetic is not required.

If the catheter needs to be replaced before the tract is mature, the bladder should be filled with sterile saline or water before removing the catheter. If the catheter is obstructed, it should be removed and another catheter inserted once a distended bladder can be palpated. At that time, a new catheter may be inserted in the same tract, employing the technique described previously. Ultrasound guidance should be used if the bladder cannot be positively identified or palpated.

With a Malecot or winged-tip catheter, frequently the wings are soft enough that they will retract as the catheter is removed. If there is difficulty removing the catheter, insert the obturator in the catheter to straighten the wings before removing the catheter. The tension in the pigtail is maintained by a silk suture that runs through the catheter and exits near its end. There it is tied around a small post. When the suture is cut or released, the pigtail will uncurl and can be removed.

If an open suprapubic cystotomy has been performed, a mature tract between the skin and the bladder usually is formed within 4 to 6 weeks. If the catheter must be replaced, select a similar-sized catheter. Normally, a catheter guide or obturator is not required. The new catheter should be introduced into the bladder immediately after removing the original one. After inflating the balloon with 5 to 10 ml of sterile saline, irrigate the bladder to ensure that the catheter is draining properly. Usually, a suprapubic catheter is replaced every 6 to 8 weeks, or whenever it is not draining properly.

SUPPLIERS

Bonnano catheter kit
Becton-Dickinson Corp.
1 Becton Drive
Franklin Lakes, NJ 07417
Phone: 1-201-847-6800
Website: www.bd.com

Stamey percutaneous suprapubic catheter kit
Cook Urological
1100 West Morgan Street
P.O. Box 227
Spencer, IN 47460
Phone: 1-800-457-4448
Website: www.cookurological.com

Simplastic suprapubic catheter
Franklin Medical
1320 Airport Road
Montrose, CO 81401
Phone: 1-800-255-1196
Website: www.franklinmedical.com

Lawrence Supra Foley suprapubic catheter introducer
Rusch Inc.
2450 Meadowbrook Parkway
Duluth, GA 30096
Phone: 1-770-623-0816
Website: www.ruschinc.com

CPT/BILLING CODES

51010   Insertion of a percutaneous suprapubic catheter
51705   Changing a suprapubic catheter, simple

ICD-9-CM DIAGNOSTIC CODES

596.0   Bladder neck contracture/obstruction
597.8   Urethritis, unspecified
599.6   Urinary obstruction, stricture
601.0   Acute prostatitis with urinary obstruction

602.8   Prostatic stricture
605.0   Phimosis, severe
867.0   Urethral injury, with no open wound
867.1   Urethral injury, with open wound

BIBLIOGRAPHY

Carter BH: Instrumentation and endoscopy. In Walsh PC, editor: *Campbell's urology,* vol 1, Philadelphia, 1998, WB Saunders.

Hagen IK: Instrumental examination of the urinary tract. In Smith DR, editor: *General urology,* East Norwalk, Conn, 1984, Lange Medical Publications.

Hopkins TB: Percutaneous suprapubic cystostomy. In Vander Salem TJ, editor: *Atlas of bedside procedures,* Boston, 1979, Little, Brown.

Landrigan RR, Hopkins SC: Suprapubic urinary diversion by percutaneous insertion of a council tip catheter, *Urology* 27(2):168, 1986.

CHAPTER 116

Suprapubic Taps or Aspirations

Robert E. James
James R. Palleschi

Suprapubic aspiration is a valuable diagnostic procedure, and, occasionally, it may even be a valuable therapeutic tool. In most cases, suprapubic aspiration can be performed safely at the bedside or in the physician's office. (For insertion of suprapubic catheters, see Chapter 115, Suprapubic Catheter Insertion/Change.)

INDICATIONS

- Collection of a urine specimen for analysis, culture, and sensitivity using sterile technique
- Temporary relief of acute urinary retention

CONTRAINDICATIONS

- Blood dyscrasia, coagulation disorder, or anticoagulant therapy
- An uncooperative patient
- Infection or cellulitis of the suprapubic area

EQUIPMENT

- Local anesthetic: 10 ml lidocaine, 1%
- Needles:
  For anesthetic: 1½-inch, 25- to 30-gauge needle
  Localization needle: 4-inch, 22-gauge spinal needle
  Aspiration needle: In most cases, the localization needle will be sufficiently large to obtain an adequate urine specimen. If not, an 18- or 20-gauge intravenous needle may be used.
- 10-ml syringe
- Microscope slide for direct examination, methylene blue, and Gram's stain
- Sterile urine culture collection container

PREPROCEDURE PATIENT PREPARATION

Review the purpose of the procedure and the technique with the patient and family. The patient may experience pain in the suprapubic area or mild hematuria for 24 to 48 hours after this procedure. Obtain informed consent.

TECHNIQUE

1. Place the patient in the supine position on the examination table. Examine the suprapubic area by palpation and percussion to identify the distended bladder. If the distended bladder cannot be identified positively, the procedure should be delayed until the bladder can be identified, or the procedure may be performed with ultrasound guidance.
2. Cleanse the suprapubic area with an antiseptic solution, and drape in a sterile fashion. Maintain the sterile technique.
3. In the midline, anesthetize the skin approximately 2 inches above the symphysis pubis (in both the adult and the pediatric patient). Next, inject sequentially down to the fascia and bladder, aspirating each time before injection. In the adult, usually 10 ml is required to anesthetize the skin, abdominal wall, and abdominal bladder. In a child, the same can be accomplished with 3 to 5 ml of anesthetic. Infants may only require 1 to 2 ml.
4. Direct the 22-gauge spinal needle with the obturator in place (Fig. 116-1) through the anesthetized skin at a 60-degree caudal angle directed toward the bladder neck. If the bladder is distended, the needle will enter the abdominal bladder after it has been advanced approximately 2 inches in the adult.
5. Remove the obturator and connect a sterile syringe

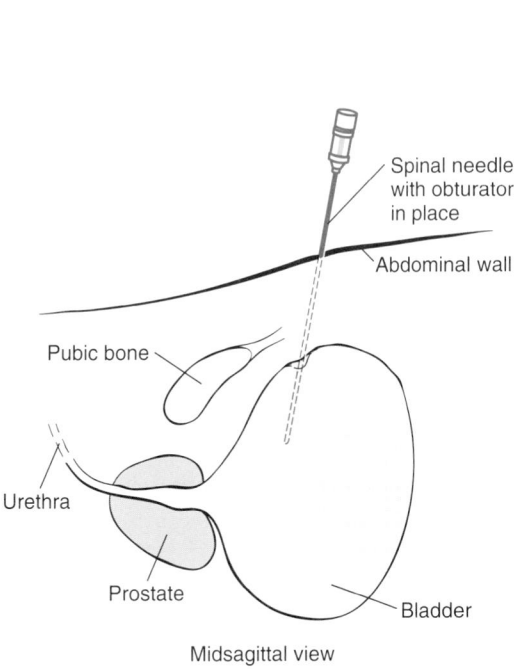

Fig. 116-1
Insertion of the spinal needle with the obturator in place.

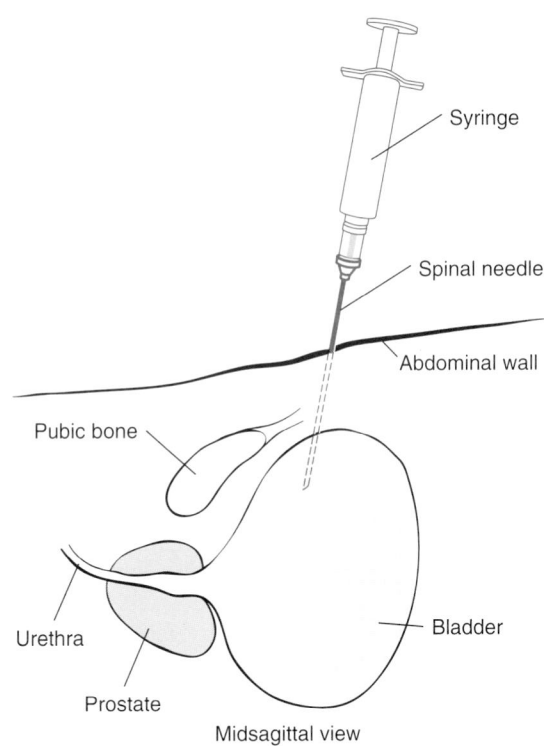

Fig. 116-2
Connection of the syringe to aspirate urine from the bladder.

(Fig. 116-2) to aspirate urine from the bladder. If urine is not obtained, slowly advance the needle, applying continuous suction on the syringe. If the specimen cannot be obtained after advancing the needle an additional 2 inches, terminate the procedure and start once again as outlined above. If you are unsuccessful a second time, the procedure should be delayed until the bladder is further distended, or the procedure should be performed with ultrasound guidance. If continued difficulties are encountered, a urology consultation should be obtained.

COMPLICATIONS

- Transient hematuria
- Perivesical hematoma
- Intestinal perforation (If this occurs with a 22-gauge needle, it should seal spontaneously and should not be a problem.)

POSTPROCEDURE PATIENT EDUCATION

The patient should notify the physician in case of persistent (lasting longer than 2 days) or increasing blood in the urine, increasing abdominal pain, difficulty urinating, or a temperature above 101° F.

CPT/BILLING CODE

51000   Suprapubic bladder aspiration

ICD-9-CM DIAGNOSTIC CODES

780.6   Fever
788.20   Urinary retention or stasis NEC
599.0   Urosepsis

BIBLIOGRAPHY

Hagen IK: Instrumental examination of the urinary tract. In Smith DR, editor: *General urology,* East Norwalk, Conn., 1984, Lange Medical Publications.

Hopkins TB: Percutaneous suprapubic cystotomy. In Vander Salem TJ, editor: *Atlas of bedside procedures,* Boston, 1979, Little, Brown & Co.

CHAPTER 117

Bedside Urodynamic Studies

Neeraj Kohli
Judy Wynne Neff

The diagnosis and management of urinary incontinence and voiding dysfunction in females is often challenging. Urinary incontinence has many etiologies, but it is most often the result of urethral incompetence *(genuine stress incontinence)*, detrusor instability *(urge incontinence)*, a combination of both *(mixed incontinence)*, or poor bladder emptying *(overflow incontinence)*. Urodynamic testing, specifically the cystometrogram, is used to demonstrate and differentiate among these conditions. Establishing the correct diagnosis during the initial workup is critical for developing an effective management plan. Although the patient history and physical examination may provide preliminary data regarding the underlying cause of incontinence, urodynamic testing provides objective assessment of lower urinary tract dysfunction while increasing the sensitivity and specificity of the diagnostic workup.

Urodynamics is the study of hydrodynamics and muscle activity to define the functional status of the lower urinary tract. Cystometry and uroflowmetry are the mainstays of urodynamic testing. Cystometry assesses the filling-storage phase by measuring the pressure-volume relationship of the bladder as it distends and contracts. It helps diagnose abnormalities of detrusor activity, sensation, capacity, and compliance. In contrast, uroflowmetry evaluates the voiding phase by measuring the urine volume voided over time. This allows detection of anatomic (obstructive) or physiologic (functional) voiding abnormalities.

Studies have shown that bedside (simple) urodynamic testing has a sensitivity of *up to 75%* in the evaluation of urinary incontinence. They are easy to perform and cost-effective in the office setting. Often they can be performed by office personnel. Correlation of these test results with patient history and physical examination can often determine the cause of urinary incontinence during the initial workup. Most conservative management protocols can be initiated on the results of these simple tests alone, without the need for complicated multichannel urodynamic studies.

However, in certain patients, greater sensitivity or specificity or more precise measurements may be needed. Examples include males; diabetics; individuals with neurologic disorders; and patients before surgery for incontinence, especially if they are at high surgical risk. Additional examples include following pelvic radiation or surgery or for patients with incontinence and a confusing diagnosis or mixed etiology. Incontinence following failed surgery for incontinence or failing routine treatment or where the treatment progress needs to be monitored quantitatively may need more precise measurements. For all of these situations, complex uroflowmetry or complex cystometry are indicated (see Chapter 118, Urodynamic Testing [Multichannel]).

INDICATIONS

- Urinary incontinence
- Overactive bladder symptoms (urgency, frequency, nocturia, enuresis)
- Urinary retention or incomplete bladder emptying
- Pelvic pain
- Painful voiding syndromes

CONTRAINDICATIONS

- Active cystitis
- Gross hematuria
- Intolerance of urethral catheterization
- Uncooperative patient
- Multichannel urodynamic testing indicated (see Chapter 118, Urodynamic Testing [Multichannel])

Patients with active cystitis or gross hematuria should be evaluated and treated before urodynamic testing. Patients unable to tolerate urethral catheterization in the office or who are uncooperative are not candidates for bedside urodynamic testing.

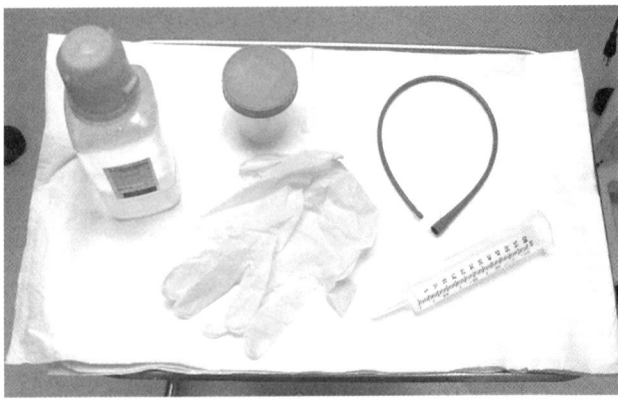

Fig. 117-1
Equipment used for urodynamic testing.

EQUIPMENT (Fig. 117-1)

- Nonsterile gloves
- Stopwatch
- Graduated voiding container
- Iodine swabs
- Water-based lubricating gel (nonanesthetic)
- 14-French red rubber urinary catheter
- Sterile urine specimen container
- Urinalysis chemstrips
- 50-ml catheter tip syringe with bulb or plunger removed
- 500-ml of room temperature sterile saline or sterile water
- Sterile cotton-tipped swab with anesthetic gel

PREPROCEDURE PATIENT PREPARATION

All patients should be counseled regarding the indications, techniques, alternatives, and complications associated with urethral catheterization and bedside urodynamics. Clear communication and instructions allow the patient to be comfortable during testing and thereby improve the results obtained. Patients should be instructed to come to the office with a full bladder to maximize information obtained from initial uroflowmetry. Each step of the procedure should be explained to the patient before proceeding.

TECHNIQUE

Simple Uroflowmetry

1. The patient's bladder should be very full. If not, provide fluids and time to fill the bladder. Since urine flow parameters are dependent on volume voided, the patient needs to be able to void at least 200 ml for the test to be reliable.

2. In a relaxed, private setting, tell the patient to void into a graduated container placed over the commode. The total time to void is recorded with the stopwatch, and total volume voided is measured.

Simple Cystometry

3. After the patient has voided, clean the external urethral meatus with iodine swabs and insert the lubricated tip of the urinary catheter into the bladder lumen. Drain the residual urine into the sterile specimen container and record the postvoid residual volume. After completion of the cystometry and cough stress test, perform a urinalysis on this specimen to rule out urinary tract infection. In patients with a positive urinalysis, send the specimen for urine culture.

4. With the urinary catheter in place, attach the 50-ml syringe (with bulb or plunger removed) to the proximal end of the urinary catheter and hold it approximately 15 cm above the pubic symphysis. Fill the bladder by pouring the sterile saline or sterile water through the open top syringe in increments of 50 ml (Fig. 117-2). Take care to keep the tip of the catheter within the bladder lumen and to prevent withdrawing it into the urethra.

5. During filling, ask the patient to report when she feels the first sensation of fullness, the first urge to void, as well as when she has reached her maximum bladder capacity. Record the total volume infused for each of these sensations.

6. Observe the water level in the syringe during filling; it should fall steadily. A sudden rise in the water level with or without associated urgency or incontinence may indicate an uninhibited detrusor contraction or detrusor instability (Fig. 117-3). Other causes of a "water hiccup" may be artifact, including Valsalva's maneuver or cough by the patient or the catheter tip slipping into the proximal urethra.

Cough/Valsalva Stress Test

7. After the bladder is filled to maximum capacity, remove the catheter and examine the patient in the supine dorsolithotomy position. The patient is asked to cough or perform a Valsalva maneuver, and the external urethral meatus is observed for signs of urine leakage. Abrupt urine leakage with a cough suggests *stress urinary incontinence* whereas prolonged leakage following cessation of the cough indicates cough induced *detrusor instability*. If urinary leakage is observed in the vagina from the

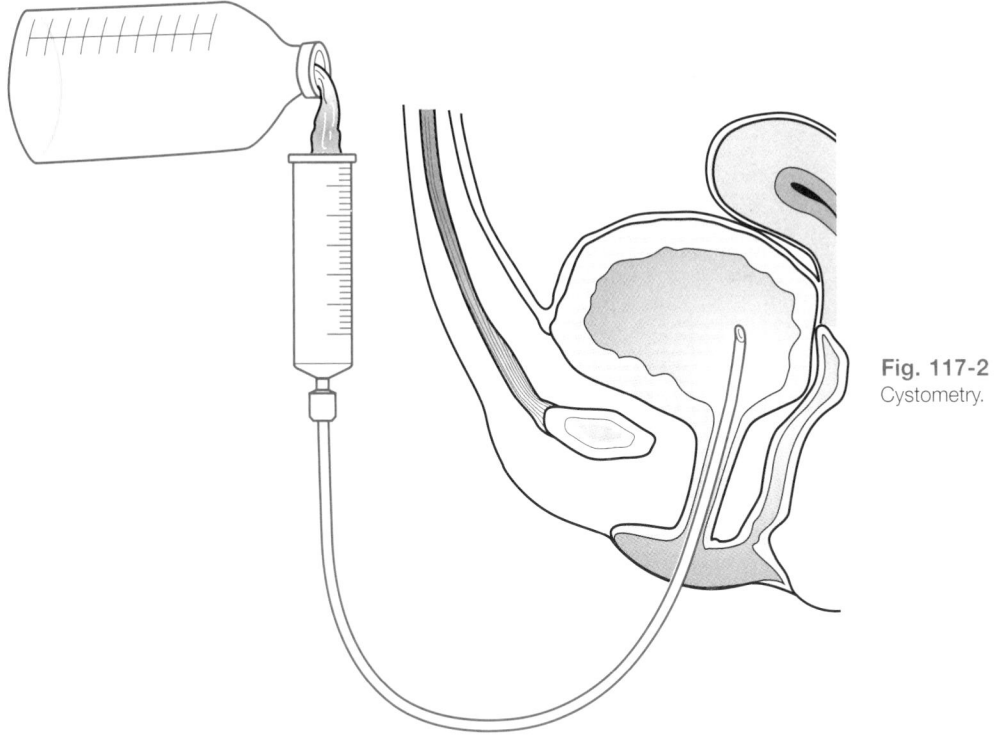

Fig. 117-2
Cystometry.

anterior vaginal wall, a *vesicovaginal fistula* should be considered.

8. Repeat the test with the patient standing.

Cotton Swab Test (Q-Tip Test)

9. After the supine and standing cough stress test, place the patient in the supine dorsolithotomy position and reexamine her. Insert a cotton-tipped swab with anesthetic gel into the urethra until resistance is overcome; this indicates its position at the bladder neck. Record the swab resting angle relative to the horizontal plane. Ask the patient to cough or perform a Valsalva maneuver again, and measure the maximum angle of deflection. The difference between this value and the resting angle is the *angle of change.* An angle of change of greater than 30 degrees indicates *urethral hypermobility* (Fig. 117-4).

Measurement of Post-Void Residual

10. Next, instruct the patient to void into the graduated container. Measure the amount voided (total void).

11. Determine a second postvoid residual by subtracting the measured total void from the maximum bladder capacity noted on filling cystometry.

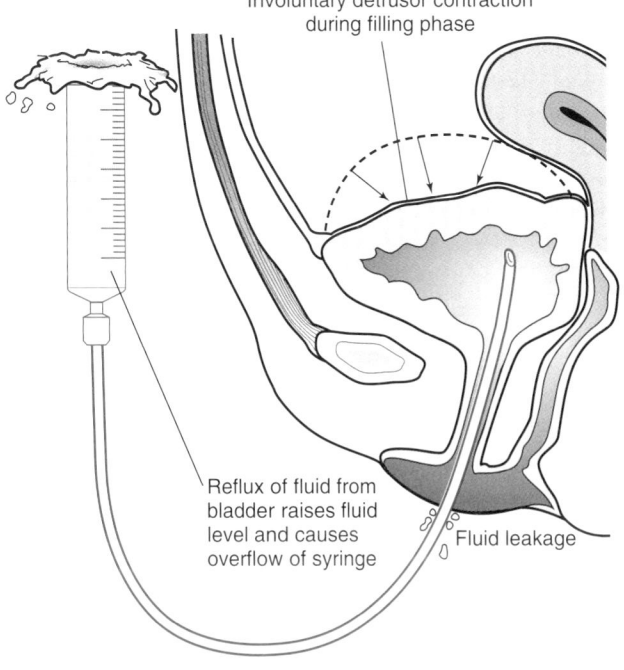

Involuntary detrusor contraction during filling phase

Reflux of fluid from bladder raises fluid level and causes overflow of syringe

Fluid leakage

Fig. 117-3
Involuntary detrusor contraction.

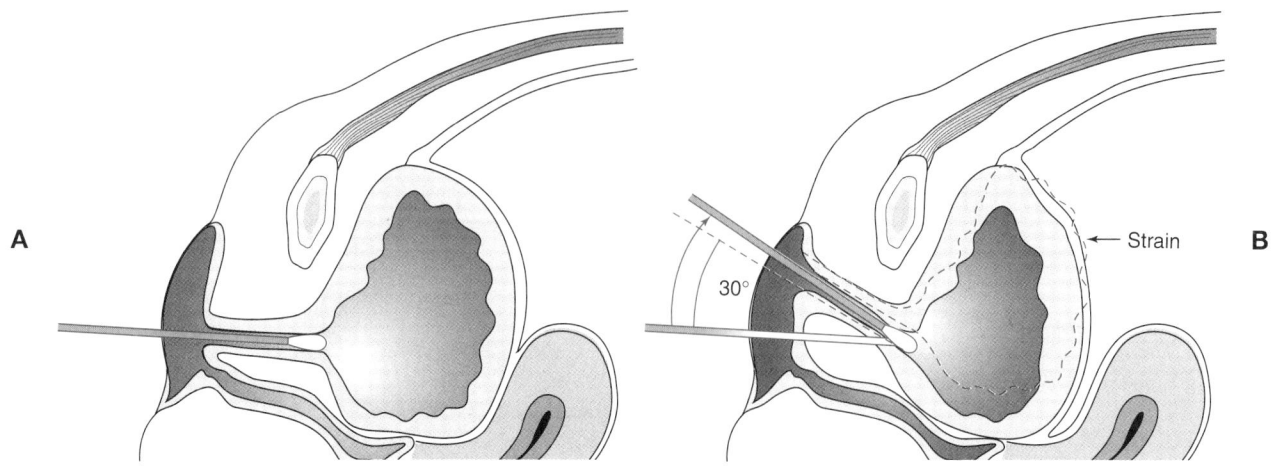

Fig. 117-4
Cotton swab test for ureterovesical junction mobility. **A,** Cotton swab at rest. **B,** Cotton swab with strain (Valsalva).

COMPLICATIONS

- Urinary tract infection (rare)
- Transient gross hematuria
- Urethral discomfort, transient
- Pelvic pain, transient

Bedside urodynamics are associated with few complications. In rare cases, patients may develop a urinary tract infection following the procedure. These patients should be treated accordingly, and routine prophylactic antibiotics following the procedure is not usually indicated.

Transient gross hematuria may be noted after the procedure, especially after a difficult catheterization in a postmenopausal woman with urethral atrophy. This usually resolves spontaneously within 48 hours. Some patients may complain of urethral discomfort or pelvic pain after testing. These symptoms are usually self limited, but these patients may benefit from a short course of phenazopyridine (Pyridium). Cystoscopy-urethroscopy should be considered in patients with hematuria or lower urinary tract pain that persists beyond 48 to 72 hours.

INTERPRETATIONS OF RESULTS

Uroflowmetry with measurement of a post-void residual assesses bladder emptying and evaluates for overflow incontinence. Most experts consider a uroflowmetry study to be normal if the patient *voids at least 200 ml in the course of 15 to 20 seconds.* Prolonged voiding times may indicate an obstructed voiding pattern resulting from increased outlet resistance *(urethral obstruction)* or poor propulsive force *(detrusor dysfunction).* Normal values for a post-void residual are not universally established, but various experts have defined *a normal postvoid residual measurement as less than 100 ml and less than 20% of the total void.*

Cystometry evaluates bladder function, including sensation, compliance, and detrusor activity during filling. Most patients experience a *first sensation of filling at 100 to 150 ml, first urge to void at 200 to 350 ml,* and *maximum bladder capacity at 400 to 550 ml. Urge incontinence* should be considered in patients with reduced bladder capacity, with or without a spontaneous detrusor contraction and coexisting overactive bladder symptoms. Patients with increased bladder capacity should be evaluated for a *neurogenic bladder. Urge incontinence from detrusor instability* is documented when an involuntary contraction results in an overflow of the filling syringe (Fig. 117-3).

A positive cough stress test indicates *genuine stress incontinence* (GSI). In patients with GSI and a positive Q-Tip test, *urethral hypermobility* is suspected. In patients with GSI and a fixed urethra on Q-Tip test *intrinsic sphincter deficiency* is the presumed diagnosis. These patients require complex multichannel urodynamics for further evaluation (see Chapter 118, Urodynamic Testing [Multichannel]).

POSTPROCEDURE PATIENT EDUCATION

The results of the testing and various management options should be discussed in detail with the patient. Patients should be instructed to call the clinician's office for pain or hematuria lasting longer than 48 hours and for symptoms of a urinary tract infection. Patients with persistent incontinence despite conservative therapy are candidates for complex urodynamics.

CPT/BILLING CODES

51725   Simple cystometrogram
51736   Simple (nonelectronic) uroflowmetry
81000   Urinalysis (Chemstrip)

ICD-9-CM DIAGNOSTIC CODES

788.3   Urinary incontinence—unspecified
788.31   Incontinence—urge
788.33   Incontinence—mixed
625.6   Incontinence—stress
788.21   Incomplete bladder emptying
788.41   Urinary frequency
788.36   Nocturnal enuresis
625.9   Pelvic pain
619.0   Vesicovaginal fistula
595.0   UTI

BIBLIOGRAPHY

Fantl JA, et al: *Urinary incontinence in adults: acute and chronic management,* Clinical Practice Guideline, No 2, 1996 update, Rockville, Md, US Department of Health and Human Services. Public Health Services, Agency for Health Care Policy and Research 2:5, 1996.

Kohli N, Karram MM: Urodynamic evaluation for female urinary incontinence, *Clin Obstet Gynecol* 4(1): 672, 1998.

Wall LL, Norton PA, Delancey JO: Practical urodynamics. In *Practical urogynecology,* Baltimore, 1993, Williams & Wilkins.

WEBSITES

www.healthy.net/asp/templates/article.asp?PageType=Article&ID=409 (Patient information on incontinence from the Agency for Health Care Policy and Research)

www.niddk.nih.gov (Information on a wide range of topics on urologic conditions from the National Institutes for Health)

CHAPTER 118

Urodynamic Testing (Multichannel)

Neeraj Kohli
Briana Walton

Urinary incontinence is a common problem among a growing population: the elderly. Given the broad range of etiologic factors that can cause both acute and chronic incontinence (Box 118-1), accurate diagnosis is the cornerstone for formulating an effective treatment plan. In addition to a careful history and physical exam, urodynamic testing—the study of hydrodynamics and muscle activity to define the functional status of the lower urinary tract—can quantify abnormalities to facilitate arriving at an accurate diagnosis. Urodynamic testing is also useful for objective assessment of patient improvement after a prescribed treatment protocol.

Bedside urodynamics as described in Chapter 117, Bedside Urodynamic Studies for Urinary Incontinence, provides objective qualitative data regarding the etiology of urinary incontinence, overactive bladder symptoms, and voiding dysfunction and can be performed easily by primary care providers in the office setting. These screening tests are useful before attempting conservative treatment after an initial visit in the uncomplicated patient. However, some patients require a more precise, quantitative analysis of lower urinary tract function as it pertains to their presenting symptoms of

BOX 118-1
Differential Diagnosis of Urinary Incontinence

Genitourinary
Genuine stress incontinence
Detrusor instability (idiopathic)
Detrusor hyperreflexia (neurologic)
Mixed incontinence
Overflow incontinence
Fistula (vesical, ureteral, urethral)
Congenital abnormalities (ectopic ureter)

Nongenitourinary
Functional
Neurologic
Cognitive
Environmental
Pharmacological
Metabolic

incontinence, pain, or voiding dysfunction. Multichannel urodynamics (MCUD) provides specific quantitative information about detrusor and urethral function during filling, storage, and emptying of urine.

MCUD involves the simultaneous measurement of pressure from multiple sites during bladder filling and emptying and allows precise measurement of intravesical, intraurethral, and intraabdominal pressure (Fig. 118-1). MCUD refers to a set of tests used to evaluate the bladder and urethra. *Complex uroflowmetry* is the measurement of urine volume voided over time, allowing detection of anatomic (obstructive) or physiologic (functional) voiding abnormalities. *Complex cystometry,* a filling test of the bladder, measures the pressure-volume relationship of the bladder as it distends and contracts, determining abnormalities of detrusor activity, sensation, capacity, and compliance consistent with urge incontinence or detrusor instability. *Urethral pressure profilometry* evaluates the urethral continence mechanism as a possible cause of stress urinary incontinence (SUI). Finally, *pressure-flow studies* allow determination and quantification of a patient's voiding mechanism and help establish the etiology of voiding dysfunction.

The basic goal of multichannel urodynamics is to obtain the simultaneous measurement of pressure from multiple sites (multichannel) during bladder filling to allow precise measurement of detrusor and urethral sphincter function. Bladder (P_{ves}) and urethral (P_{ura}) pressure are measured directly with a single intravesical catheter that contains two microtransducers, one located in the bladder and other in the urethra. A separate, single microtransducer catheter is placed either in the rectum or the vagina and indirectly measures simultaneous intraabdominal pressure (P_{abd}). Detrusor pressure (P_{det}) and urethral closure pressure (P_{ucp}) are derived from electronic subtraction of one measured pressure from a second measured pressure. Detrusor pressure is derived by subtracting intraabdominal pressure from intravesical pressure ($P_{det} = P_{ves} - P_{abd}$), whereas urethral closure pressure is the difference between urethral pressure and bladder pressure ($P_{ucp} = P_{ura} - P_{ves}$) (Fig. 118-2).

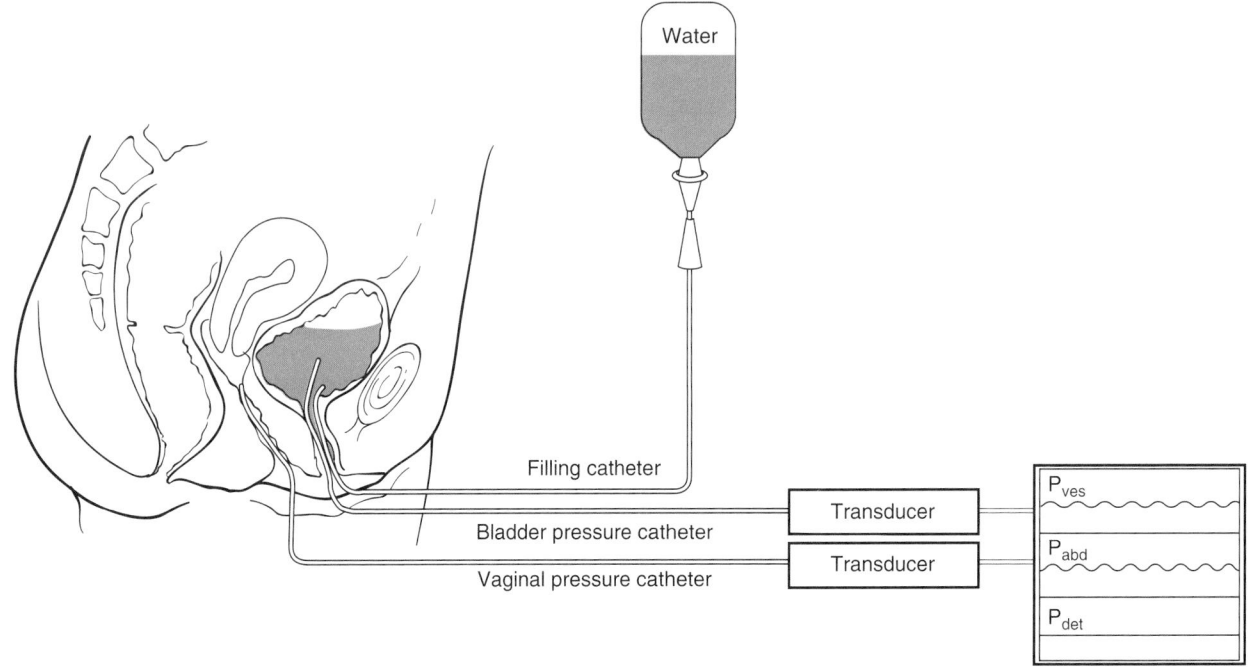

Fig. 118-1
Multichannel urodynamics (MCUD) with measurement of vesical and abdominal pressure using separate catheters. P_{abd}, Intraabdominal pressure; P_{det}, detrusor pressure; P_{ves}, bladder pressure.

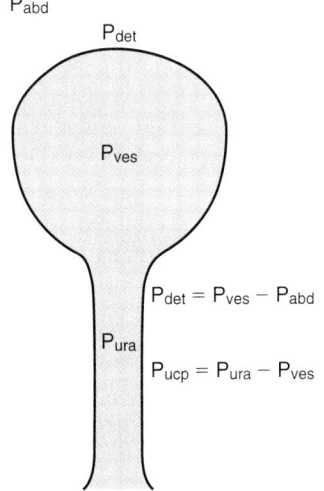

Fig. 118-2
Mathematical formulas deriving detrusor pressure and urethral closure pressure from multichannel urodynamics measurements. P_{abd}, Intra-abdominal pressure; P_{det}, detrusor pressure; P_{ucp}, urethral closure pressure; P_{ura}, urethral pressure; P_{ves}, bladder pressure.

DEFINITIONS

1. Valsalva leak point pressure (VLPP): the pressure required to open the urethra.
2. Urethral pressure profile (UPP): the pressure along the functional length of the urethra. The maximal urethral closure pressure (MUCP) is recorded as maximal pressure minus the baseline urethral pressure (P_{ves}). It reflects the highest pressure the sphincter has at rest in order to keep it closed.
3. Intravesical pressure (P_{ves}): the pressure within the bladder.
4. Abdominal pressure (P_{abd}): the pressure surrounding the bladder. It is approximated by the pressure within the vagina or the rectum.
5. Detrusor pressure (P_{det}): the component of the intravesical pressure that is created from the force in the bladder wall alone. It is estimated by subtracting abdominal pressure from intravesical pressure. The simultaneous measurement of both abdominal and intravesical pressure is required to obtain this measurement.
6. Urethral pressure (P_{ura}): the pressure within the urethra, which reflects both the urethral closure pressure and the vesical pressure.
7. Functional bladder capacity: the amount of urine the bladder can hold under natural conditions.
8. Cystometric capacity: a subjective measure of the total volume of fluid the patient can tolerate comfortably during bladder filling.

INDICATIONS

Many cases of uncomplicated incontinence can be initially diagnosed and treated by using bedside urodynamic studies (see Chapter 117, Bedside Urodynamic

Studies.) Should bedside urodynamic studies reveal ambiguous results or the subsequent treatment fail, MCUD studies are recommended. Other indications for MCUD include the following:

History

- Mixed incontinence
- Unclear etiology of incontinence
- Continuous leakage
- Coexisting neurologic disorders or diabetes

After Bedside Urodynamic Studies

- Simple cystometry that is inconclusive
- Mixed incontinence results

Stress Incontinence

- Before surgical correction
- Potential stress incontinence with significant pelvic prolapse
- Recurrent incontinence after previous surgery for SUI

Therapeutic Failures

- Urge incontinence
- Frequency, urgency, and pain syndrome
- Nocturnal enuresis

Miscellaneous

- Lower urinary tract dysfunction after pelvic radiation
- Lower urinary tract dysfunction after radical pelvic surgery

CONTRAINDICATIONS

- Untreated cystitis
- Unevaluated and untreated gross hematuria
- Uncooperative patient
- Inability to tolerate urinary catheterization

There are few contraindications to MCUD. Patients with active cystitis or gross hematuria should be evaluated and treated prior to urodynamic testing. Patients who are unable to tolerate urethral catheterization or are uncooperative in the office setting should not be considered candidates for multichannel urodynamic testing.

EQUIPMENT

- Nonsterile gloves
- Commode with graduated voiding container
- Adjustable urodynamics chair (recommended)
- Urodynamics unit (includes cystometer and uroflowmeter) with printer
- Microtip or dual-lumen measuring catheters
- IV pole with 1-L bag of room-temperature infusion solution (sterile water, saline, or lactated Ringer's solution)
- Iodine swabs
- Water-based lubricating gel (nonanesthetic)
- Red rubber urinary catheter
- Sterile urine specimen container
- Urinalysis chemstrips
- Roll of tape (to secure the measuring catheters in place)
- Large cotton-tipped applicators or vaginal speculum (to reduce uterine prolapse)

PREPROCEDURE PATIENT PREPARATION

All patients should be counseled regarding the indications, techniques, and complications associated with urethral catheterization (see the sample patient education handout titled "Urodynamic Testing" on page 1881 of Appendix G). Clear communication and instructions allow the patient to be comfortable during testing and thereby improve the results obtained. Patients should be instructed to come to the office with a full bladder so as to maximize information obtained from initial uroflowmetry. Each step of the procedure should be carefully explained to the patient before proceeding with it. Drug allergies should be noted prior to prescribing prophylactic antibiotics or phenazopyridine.

TECHNIQUE

Complex Uroflowmetry

1. The patient is asked to come to the office with a full bladder, since urine flow parameters are dependent on volume voided (the patient should void at least 200 ml for the test to provide reliable data).
2. In a relaxed, private setting, the patient is instructed to void into a graduated container placed over the commode (Fig. 118-3). Uroflowmetry measurements, including time and flow rate, are recorded with the urodynamic unit set to "uroflowmetry."

Complex Cystometry

3. After the patient has voided, place her in the sitting position and cleanse the external urethral meatus

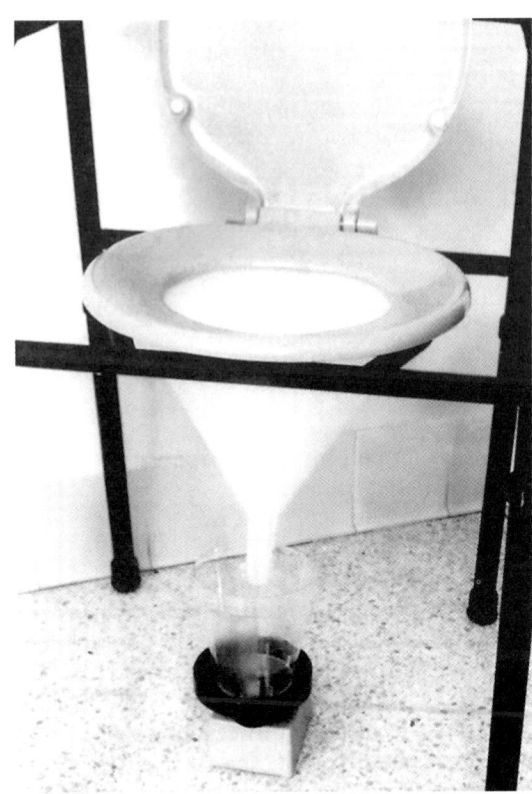

Fig. 118-3
Typical complex uroflowmetry setup with commode and uroflow instrument.

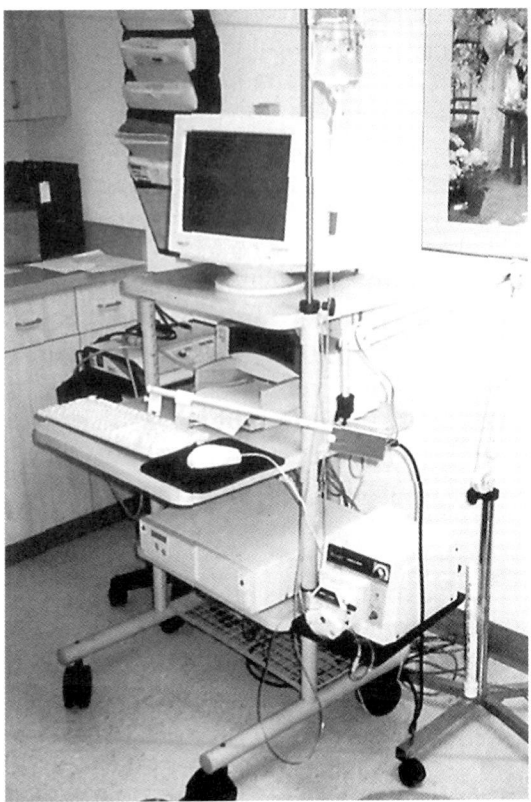

Fig. 118-4
Complex cystometry setup with fluid, water pump, multichannel transducers, and recording device (computer).

with iodine swabs. Insert the lubricated tip of the red rubber catheter into the bladder lumen. The residual urine is drained into the sterile specimen container, and the postvoid residual volume is recorded. Dipstick urinalysis is routinely performed. In patients with a positive test for leukocytes, MCUD should be postponed until after treatment of the urinary tract infection. Urine culture may be sent on the catheterized specimen.

4. Turn on the urodynamic unit and printer, and attach the pressure catheters to the appropriate channels. Connect the bladder catheter infusion port to the IV tubing of the infusion solution, which is attached to a water pump to regulate flow (Fig. 118-4).

5. Calibrate the urodynamic unit with the catheters in water, and set all channels to zero. Introduce the bladder catheter into the bladder through the external urethral meatus with the microtransducer at the 3 o'clock position. Take care to place the proximal transducer near the midurethra. Then place the abdominal catheter into the vagina, or into the rectum if the patient has pelvic prolapse beyond the hymenal ring. The catheters are secured to the patient's inner thigh with tape. In patients with significant prolapse, to reduce artifact, we recom-

mend performing the cystometry with the prolapse reduced using a large cotton-tipped applicator.

6. Activate the cystometrogram recording device, and ask the patient to cough to confirm correct placement. A cough should produce a pressure spike on the tracing. The bladder is then filled with water at a medium fill rate, which is defined as 10 to 100 ml per minute.

7. Record bladder volumes corresponding to first sensation, normal desire, strong desire, urgency, and maximum bladder capacity. This is most easily accomplished by correlating bladder sensations with normal experiences (Table 118-1). Instruct the patient to periodically cough (cough stress test), and inspect the external urethral meatus for sudden urine loss. Determine the minimum volume at which leakage occurs (when leakage is first noted).

8. Continue bladder filling until bladder pressure shows a progressive rise above baseline (reduced compliance) or maximum bladder capacity.

Urethral Pressure Profile

9. After completion of the cystometry, a UPP is performed by recording the pressure while pulling

TABLE 118-1

Correlation of Interval Bladder Sensations to Normal Experiences

	Sensation	Normal	Life Circumstance
First	Awareness of bladder filling	100-200	While watching TV, aware that urine is in the bladder
Second	Normal desire to void	200-300	Sensation that she would usually and normally empty her bladder
Third	Strong desire to void	300-400	She would attempt to hold urine during good TV program
Fourth	Urgent desire to void		She would go straight to the bathroom at a department store during a sale
Fifth	Maximum capacity	400-600	She would consider pulling the car of the road to urinate in the woods

the transducer from the internal to the external urethral meatus at a constant speed. It can be pulled by hand or with a mechanical pulling device. Multiple measurements can be performed by re-inserting and withdrawing the pressure catheter. The MUCP is calculated by subtracting the baseline urethral pressure from the maximum (Fig. 118-5).

Pressure-Flow Studies

10. If a pressure-flow study is required to evaluate voiding dysfunction, the catheters are left in place and the patient is instructed to void into the commode. Intravesical, intraabdominal, and intraurethral pressures are measured, and, using subtraction analysis, the mechanism of voiding is determined.

COMPLICATIONS

- Bladder infection
- Gross hematuria

Like bedside urodynamics, MCUD is associated with few complications. In rare cases, patients may develop a urinary tract infection after the procedure. Routine prophylactic antibiotics as well as phenazopyridine, a bladder analgesic, are recommended after the procedure. Transient gross hematuria may also be noted after the procedure, especially after difficult catheterization in a postmenopausal woman with urethral atrophy. This usually resolves spontaneously within 48 hours. Cystoscopy-urethroscopy should be considered in patients with persistent hematuria or lower urinary tract pain beyond 48 to 72 hours.

INTERPRETATION OF RESULTS

Uroflowmetry with measurement of a postvoid residual assesses bladder emptying and evaluates for overflow incontinence. Most experts consider a uroflowmetry study to be normal if the patient voids at least 200 ml during the course of 15 to 20 seconds (Fig. 118-6). Prolonged voiding times may indicate an obstructed voiding pattern resulting from increased outlet resistance (urethral obstruction) or poor propulsive force (detrusor dysfunction). Normal values for a postvoid residual are not universally established, but previous investigators have advocated a normal postvoid residual measurement to be less than 100 ml and less than 20% of the total void.

Cystometry will document abnormalities of bladder sensation and compliance (Box 118-2). With normal bladder capacities, the detrusor pressure should remain stable (less than 15 cm H_2O change) throughout filling. A gradual rise and decline of the detrusor pressure indicates detrusor instability, which may or may not be associated with observable urge incontinence episodes. Sudden urine loss associated with periodic coughing or Valsalva's maneuvers during filling cystometry are diagnostic of SUI (Fig. 118-7).

Urethral pressure profiles provide static evaluation of the urethral sphincter mechanism. MUCP values less than 20 cm H_2O are consistent with intrinsic sphincter deficiency, values between 20 and 30 cm H_2O are borderline, and values greater than 30 cm H_2O are considered normal (Fig. 118-8).

POSTPROCEDURE PATIENT EDUCATION

After MCUD testing, results should be reviewed in detail with the patient. The diagnosis should be confirmed on the basis of careful review of the urodynamic tracing, and management options should be discussed. Patients with voiding dysfunction may benefit from urethral dilation, smooth muscle relaxants, or intermittent self-catheterization. For patients who demonstrate detrusor instability or reduced bladder capacity with coexisting overactive bladder symptoms, nonsurgical treatment modalities, including anticholinergic medications, bladder retraining, dietary modification, and neuromodulation, should be initiated. Patients with SUI should be offered both surgical and nonsurgical treatment modalities (see Chapter 154, Pessaries), depending on the severity of their incontinence, the anticipated outcomes, and surgical risk factors.

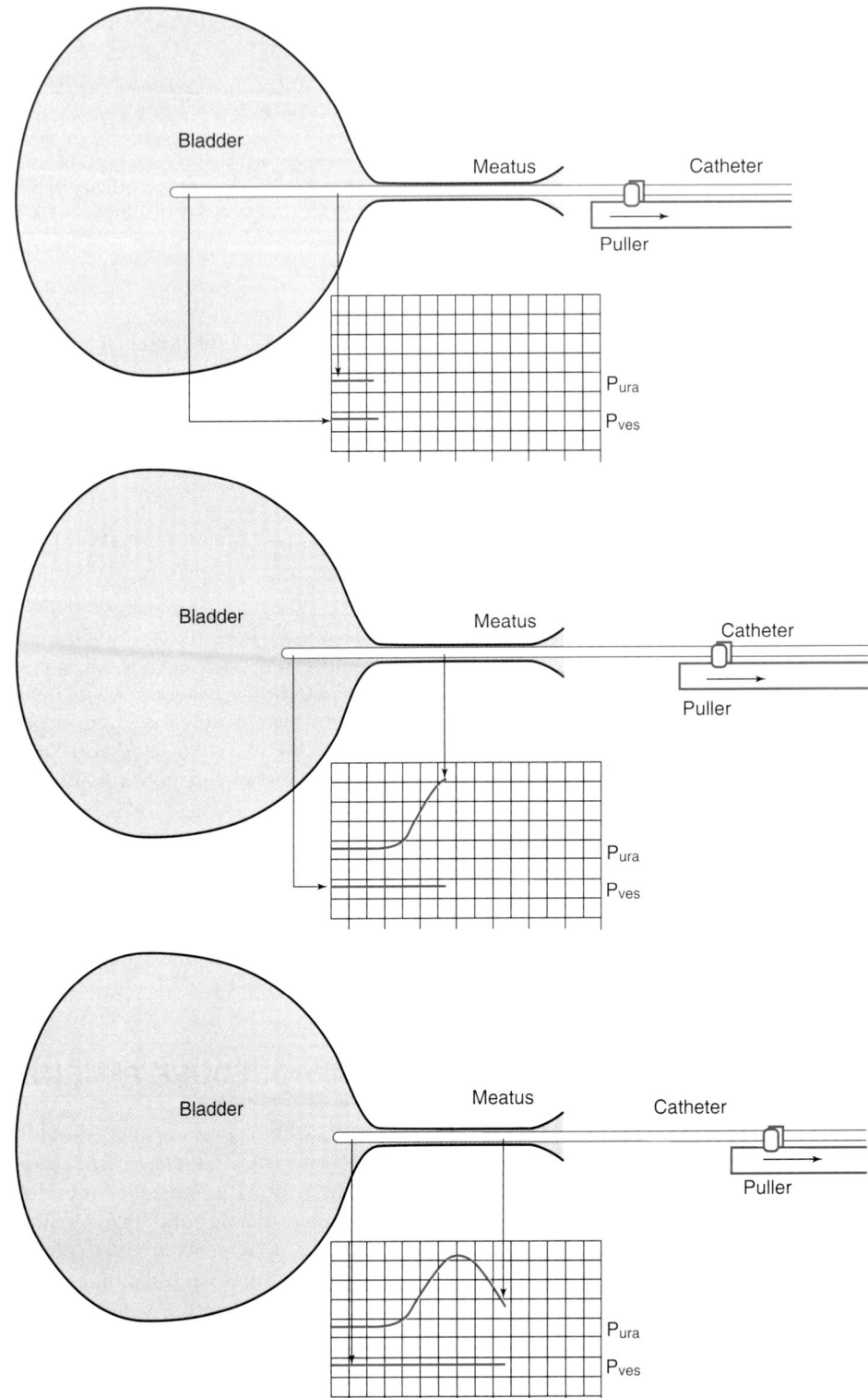

Fig. 118-5
Sample urethral pressure profile created during retraction of the urethral catheter. P_{ura}, Urethral pressure; P_{ves}, bladder pressure.

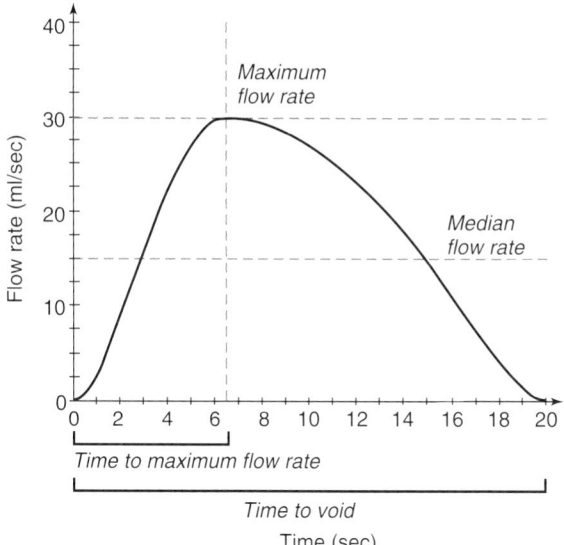

Fig. 118-6
Normal uroflow tracing in women without obstruction.

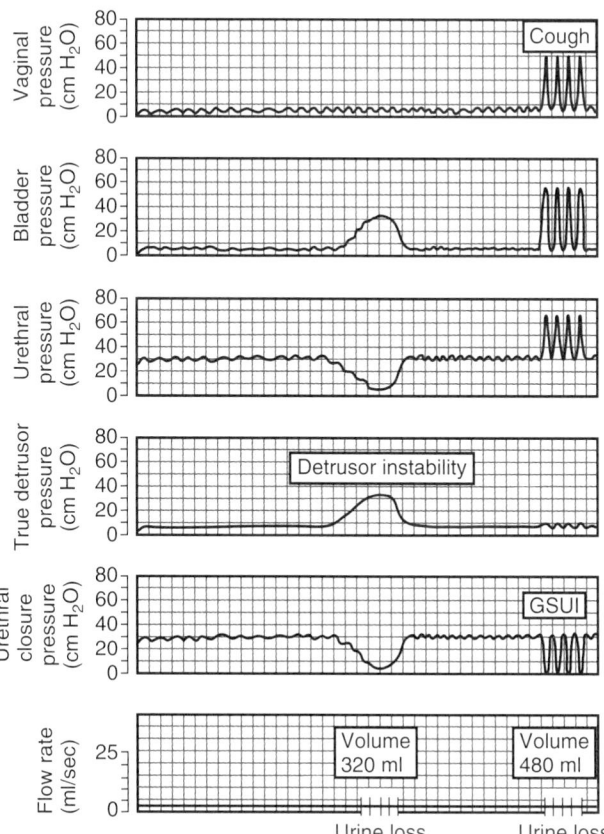

Fig. 118-7
Typical complex cystogram tracing in woman with mixed incontinence: detrusor instability (at 320 ml) and genuine stress incontinence (at 480 ml). *GSUI,* Genuine stress urinary incontinence.

BOX 118-2
Diagnosis and Conditions of Bladder Capacity

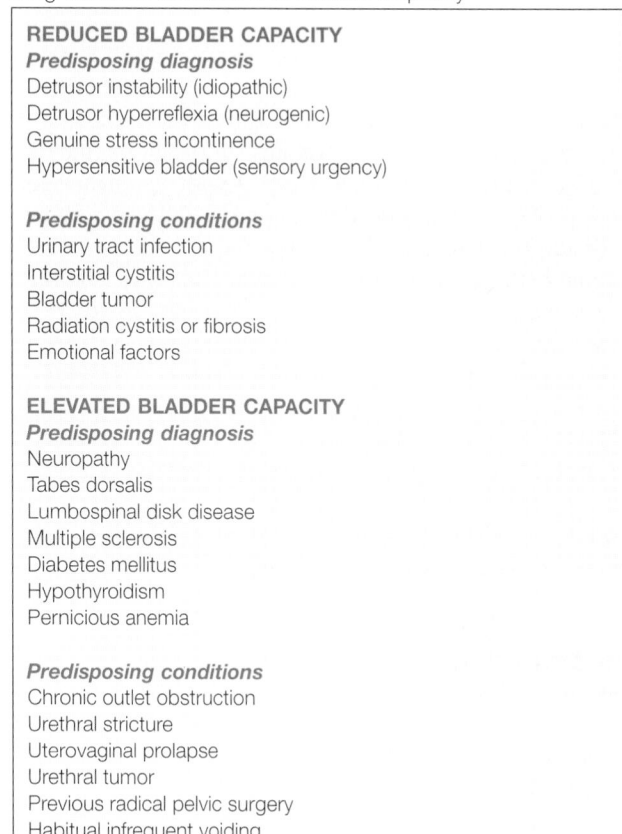

REDUCED BLADDER CAPACITY
Predisposing diagnosis
Detrusor instability (idiopathic)
Detrusor hyperreflexia (neurogenic)
Genuine stress incontinence
Hypersensitive bladder (sensory urgency)

Predisposing conditions
Urinary tract infection
Interstitial cystitis
Bladder tumor
Radiation cystitis or fibrosis
Emotional factors

ELEVATED BLADDER CAPACITY
Predisposing diagnosis
Neuropathy
Tabes dorsalis
Lumbospinal disk disease
Multiple sclerosis
Diabetes mellitus
Hypothyroidism
Pernicious anemia

Predisposing conditions
Chronic outlet obstruction
Urethral stricture
Uterovaginal prolapse
Urethral tumor
Previous radical pelvic surgery
Habitual infrequent voiding

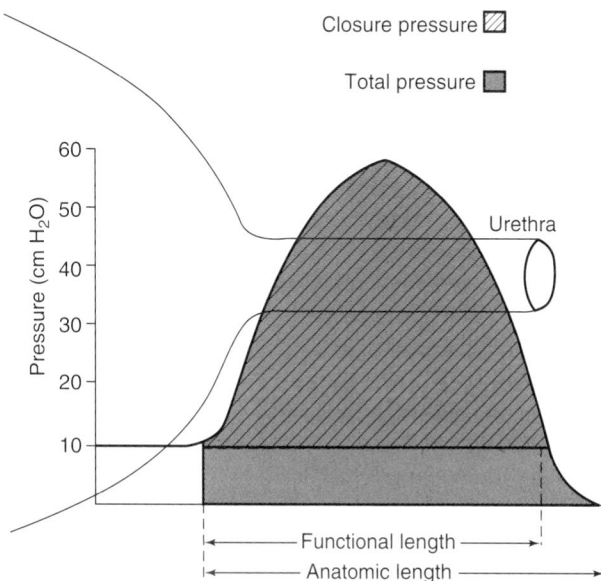

Fig. 118-8
Normal urethral pressure profile curve, also demonstrating relationship of functional to anatomic length.

CONCLUSION

Multichannel urodynamic testing and its role in the clinical management of patients with complex urogynecologic pathology are still controversial. The primary goal of such an evaluation should be to reproduce and quantify the patient's symptoms. Indications include refractory urinary incontinence, SUI with significant pelvic prolapse, voiding dysfunction, and inconclusive bedside urodynamic studies. For those who frequently manage these conditions, the availability of complex urodynamic testing equipment is recommended. It allows quantitative evaluation and more precise determination of the underlying disease processes. In addition, for patients who are currently undergoing treatment, it allows quantitative measurement of improvement or deterioration from their baseline states. However, given the complexity of the lower urinary tract, results of multichannel urodynamics should always be correlated with the physical examination and clinical history.

SUPPLIERS

MedAmicus, Inc.
15301 Highway 55 West
Plymouth, MN 55447
Phone: 1-800-559-2613
Website: www.medamicus.com

Laborie Medical Technologies
310 Hurricane Lane #2
Williston, VT 05495
Phone: 1-802-878-1110
Website: www.laborie.com

Medtronic Functional Diagnostics
3850 Victoria Street North, MS V215,
Shoreview, MN 55126-2978
Phone: 1-612-514-1700
Website: www.medtronic.com

Life-Tech, Inc.
4235 Greenbriar Drive
Stafford, TX 77477-3995
Phone: 1-281-491-6600
Website: www.life-tech.com

CPT/BILLING CODES

51726	Complex cystometrogram (e.g., calibrated electronic equipment)
51741	Complex uroflowmetry (e.g., calibrated electronic equipment)
51772	UPP studies, any technique
51784	Electromyography studies of anal or urethral sphincter, other than needle, any technique
51795	Voiding pressure studies, bladder voiding pressure, any technique
51797	Voiding pressure studies, intraabdominal voiding pressure (rectal, gastric, intraperitoneal)

When multiple procedures are performed in the same session, either modifier -51 or code 09951 is used. All procedure codes above imply that procedures were performed by or under the direct supervision of a physician and include supplies.

ICD-9-CM DIAGNOSTIC CODES

625.9	Pelvic pain
788.21	Incomplete bladder emptying
788.31	Incontinence—urge
788.37	Incontinence—continuous leakage
788.41	Urinary frequency
788.36	Nocturnal enuresis
788.35	Incontinence w/postvoid dribbling
596.55	Detrusor sphincter dyssynergia
596.52	Low bladder compliance
596.5	Bladder dysfunction
788.30	Incontinence—unspecified
788.33	Incontinence—mixed
625.6	Incontinence—stress
788.2	Urinary retention
788.43	Nocturia
599.82	ISD
596.59	Detrusor instability
788.36	Nocturnal enuresis

ADDITIONAL RESOURCES

- See the sample patient education handout titled "Urodynamic Testing" on page 1881 of Appendix G.

BIBLIOGRAPHY

Fantl JA et al: *Urinary incontinence in adults: acute and chronic management. Clinical Practice Guideline, no 2, 1996 update,* Rockville, Md, 1996, US Department of Health and Human Services. Public Health Service, Agency for Health Care Policy and Research 2:5.

Karram MM: Urodynamics: voiding studies. In Walters MD, Karram MM, editors: *Clinical urogynecology,* St Louis, 1993, Mosby.

Kohli N, Karram MM: Urodynamic evaluation for female urinary incontinence, *Clin Obstet Gynecol* 4(1):672, 1998.

Wall LL, Norton PA, Delancey JO: Practical urodynamics. In *Practical urogynecology*, Baltimore, 1993, Williams & Wilkins.

WEBSITES

www.healthy.net/library/articles/ahcpr/incont.htm (patient information on incontinence from the Agency for Health Care Policy and Research Guidelines)

www.laborie.com (leading manufacturer of urodynamic equipment)

www.medamicus.com (maker of small portable urodynamic systems)

www.sghurol.demon.co.uk/urod/ (comprehensive review of various urodynamic tests)

PART EIGHT

Male Reproductive System

CHAPTER 119

Adult Circumcision*

John R. Holman
Donald E. DeWitt

Adult circumcision is a procedure about which little is written, even in the urological literature. It is often performed for reasons that are not purely medical, yet it also has clearly defined medical indications. Some patients have their own nonmedical reasons.

General anesthesia may be necessary, but usually local anesthesia is sufficient in the outpatient setting, including the properly equipped office. Informed consent should be obtained after a thorough discussion with the patient (and partner, if appropriate), during which the indications, procedure, postprocedure care, and potential complications are explained. (See the sample patient education handout titled "Adult Circumcision" on page 1883 of Appendix G and the sample patient consent form titled "Circumcision/Dorsal Penile Nerve Block" on page 1884 of Appendix G.) This is required for all patients, and it must always be documented. This serves as a record of the authenticity of the complaint of the patient, and it is important because individual physicians may vary in their judgments of the need for surgery. The physician must make sure that the patient's reasons for requesting circumcision are medically sound and that his expectations of the results are realistic.

INDICATIONS

- Phimosis (tightness of the foreskin so that it cannot be drawn back from over the glans); possibly related to complaints of pain with erections and intercourse
- Paraphimosis (retraction of a narrow, inflamed foreskin that cannot be replaced)
- Penile hygiene; recurrent balanitis (inflammation of the glans penis)
- Posthitis (inflammation of the prepuce) not relieved by medical treatment

---

This chapter was originally submitted in the previous edition by the late Dr. DeWitt. Dr. Holman has updated and revised it for this edition. The opinions contained herein are those of the authors and should not be construed as official or as reflecting the views of the Department of the Navy or the Department of Defense.

- Preputial neoplasms
- Excessive foreskin redundancy
- Frenular tears
- Patient or spouse preference after informed discussion.

Patients may also have social, religious, or personal reasons for requesting a circumcision. Exploration of these reasons ensures a thorough understanding of the risks and benefits as well as alternatives to the procedure.

CONTRAINDICATIONS

- Active inflammation in the genital area
- Infection in the genital area
- Psychiatric disorder or history (relative contraindication; these patients must be screened carefully)
- Bleeding dyscrasias (evaluate appropriately)
- History of penile surgery, significant trauma, or unusual-appearing or ambiguous genitalia (consider a referral to a specialist)

EQUIPMENT

- 10-ml syringe with a 1- to 1½-inch, 27-gauge needle and a ½-inch, 30-gauge needle
- Prep bowl with a dozen 4 × 4–inch gauze sponges
- Iodine solution or other antiseptic for scrub
- Ring forceps
- Pack of sterile 4 × 4–inch gauze bandages
- 1 fenestrated drape
- 6-inch segment of half-inch Penrose drain
- 6 straight mosquito forceps
- 1 large straight forceps
- 1 curved Mayo scissors
- 1 medium-size straight Metzenbaum scissors
- 1 suture scissors
- 5-inch needle holder
- 1 Brown-Adson thumb forceps
- 4-0 or 5-0 absorbable suture (Vicryl, Dexon, etc.)
- Petrolatum gauze

- 1-inch Kling bandage
- 1 malleable 4- to 6-inch silver probe *(optional)*
- Needle-tip electrocautery unit
- Sterile marking pen

PREPROCEDURE PATIENT PREPARATION

The patient should be properly counseled and evaluated before the surgery. A patient education handout is provided, and a consent form is signed. (See the sample patient consent form titled "Circumcision/Dorsal Penile Nerve Block" on page 1884 of Appendix G.) If the patient is anxious, a preprocedural dose of an oral, sublingual, intramuscular, or intravenous anxiolytic (such as diazepam) may be administered. If this is used, someone must drive the patient home after the procedure.

The patient should be supine and comfortable. Shav-

ing and clipping of hair should be avoided to minimize the infectious complications. Surgically prep the entire genitalia, scrotum, and pubic area with an appropriate antiseptic solution. Use a fenestrated drape.

Anesthesia

Ring Block

1. Using a 10-ml syringe filled with 1% lidocaine *without* epinephrine and a 1-inch, 27-gauge needle, inject 0.5 to 1 ml subcutaneously over the superficial dorsal vein so that the wheal is raised at the junction of the penis and the pubis (Fig. 119-1, *A*).
2. Without withdrawing the needle, angle it toward both sides of the dorsal vein and inject additional lidocaine.
3. Extend the needle subcutaneously downward to the deep fascia of the penis—an area of firm resistance—and continue injecting circumferentially, staying close

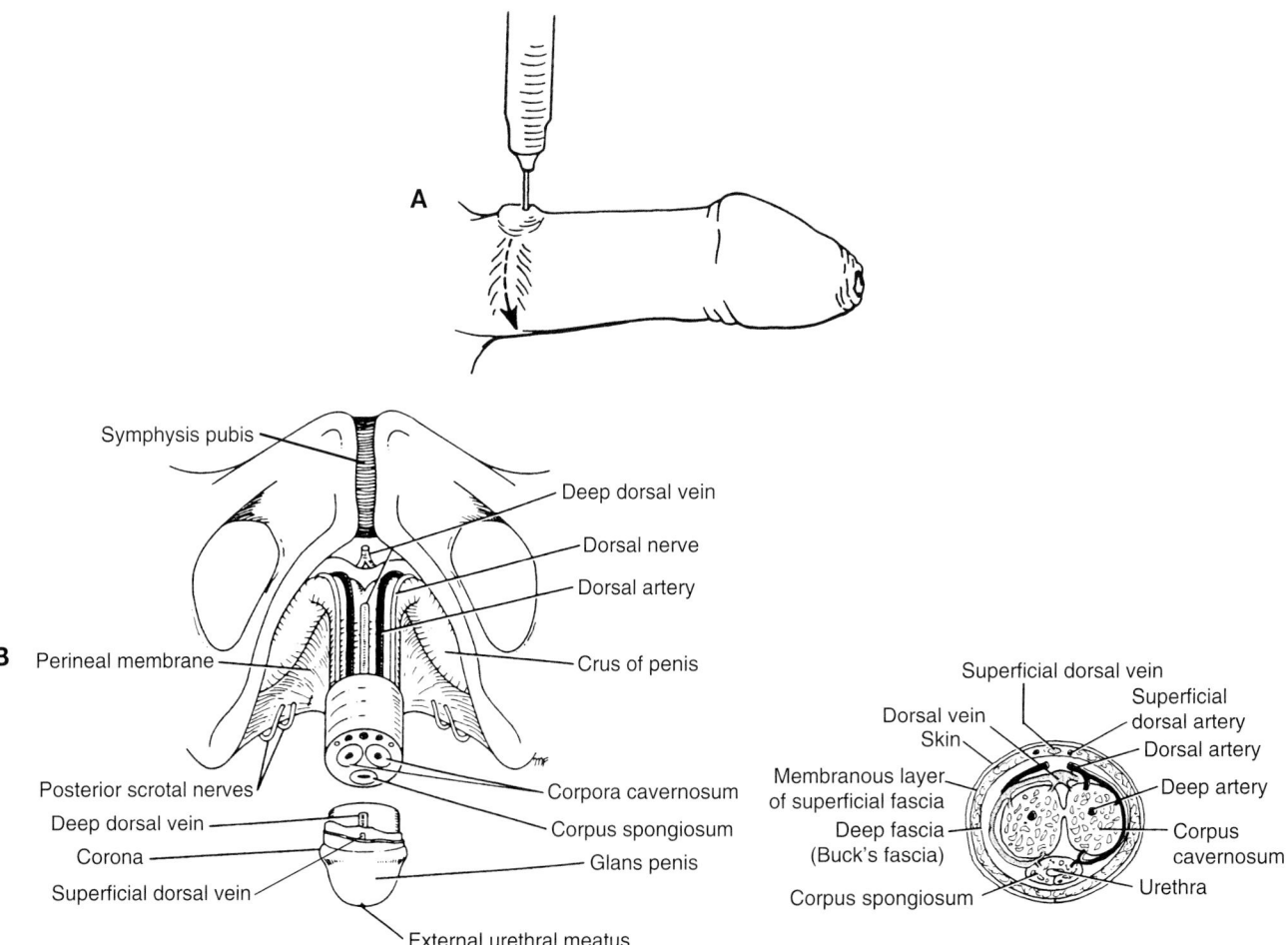

Fig. 119-1
A, Site of initial injection over dorsal vein. **B,** Cross-section view of the penis. (**B** from Snell RS, Smith MS: *Clinical anatomy for emergency medicine,* St Louis, 1993, Mosby.)

to the deep fascia of the penis. The penile skin is loose; therefore complete circumferential deployment of the anesthetic agent can be accomplished, and the ventral surface can be reached from both sides. This is called a *ring block*. Inject approximately 4 ml in this manner on each side. Do not penetrate the fascia.

4. Wait a few minutes, and then inject 1 ml of the local anesthetic subcutaneously into the frenulum using a ½-inch, 30-gauge needle (Fig. 119-2).

5. Wait several more minutes and then test the depth of local anesthesia by cautiously grasping the edge of the foreskin with a mosquito hemostat. Should more anesthesia be required, use a Penrose drain as a tourniquet around the midportion of the penis. Tie the tourniquet tightly or hold the Penrose drain with a clamp to obstruct venous return. Inject an additional 2 ml lidocaine into both corpora cavernosa just distal to the tourniquet (Fig. 119-3).

6. After approximately 5 minutes, retest for anesthesia; if anesthesia is adequate, remove the tourniquet.

Dorsal Penile Nerve Block

As an alternative or in addition to the ring block, the surgeon may perform a *dorsal penile nerve block*. The dorsal penile nerve is blocked by injecting local anesthetic solution deep to Buck's fascia, where the nerves emerge from under the pubic bone.

1. The patient is placed in the supine position.

2. After preparation of the skin, two injection sites are identified over the inferior edge of the pubic bone at approximately the 10 and 2 o'clock positions relative to the base of the penis.

3. A 27-gauge (1½-inch) needle is inserted directed ventrally until the pubic bone is contacted.

4. The needle is "walked" caudad off the pubis and through Buck's fascia.

5. After aspiration, 5 ml of local anesthetic is injected at each site. A mixture of equal volumes of 0.5% bupivacaine (Marcaine) and 1% or 2% lidocaine without epinephrine provides rapid onset of anesthesia and suitable duration for circumcision.

DORSAL SLIT TECHNIQUE

The dorsal slit technique is preferred if the patient has phimosis or paraphimosis. An assistant is of considerable help in carrying out this procedure.

1. Using small straight hemostats, grasp the distal foreskin at the 11, 1, 5, and 7 o'clock positions, and gently pull the foreskin over the glans (Fig. 119-4).

2. Use a malleable silver probe or the hemostats on the undersurface of the dorsal foreskin to determine a point 1 cm distal to the corona.

3. Place a large straight hemostat at the 12 o'clock position, close it firmly, and compress and crush the foreskin to the point that you previously determined with the silver probe.

4. After 5 or more minutes (time it by the clock), remove the forceps and use a straight Metzenbaum scissors to incise through the *center* of this crushed area (Fig. 119-5). Crushing the tissue reduces the bleeding from this incision.

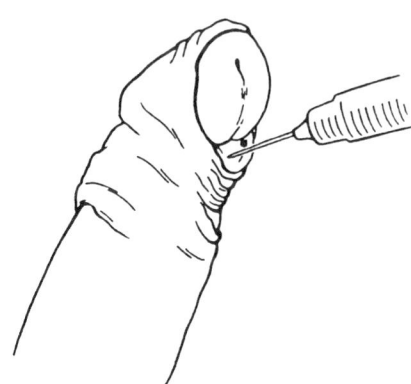

Fig. 119-2
Additional anesthetic injected into the frenulum.

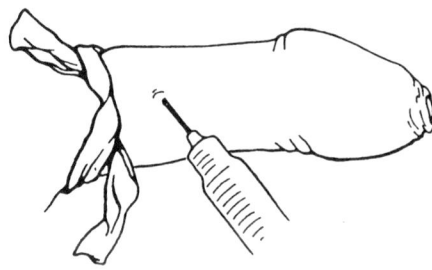

Fig. 119-3
Injection of anesthetic into corpora cavernosa with tourniquet applied.

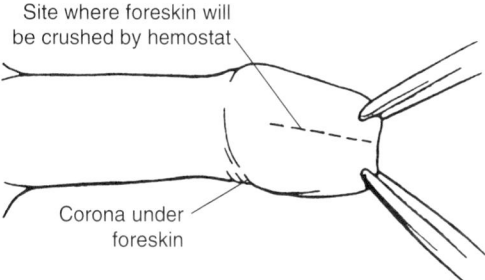

Site where foreskin will be crushed by hemostat

Corona under foreskin

Fig. 119-4
Straight hemostats (4) applied at the dorsal and ventral aspects of the tip of foreskin at the 11, 1, 5, and 7 o'clock positions.

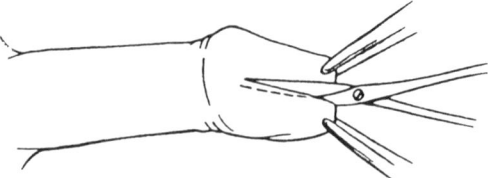

Fig. 119-5
Cutting through crushed tissue.

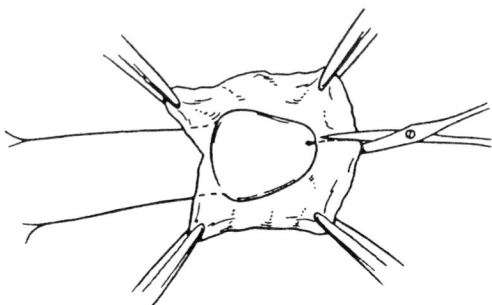

Fig. 119-6
Ventral slit to base of frenulum. It can be crushed as for the dorsal incision.

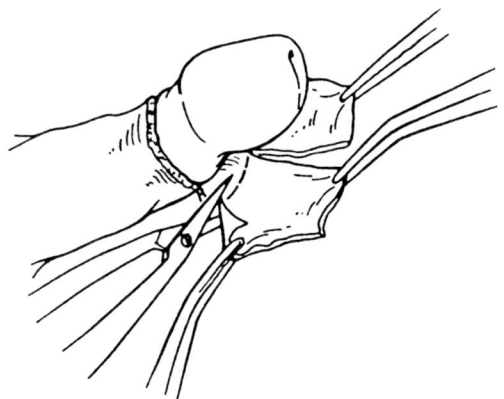

Fig. 119-7
Excision of foreskin.

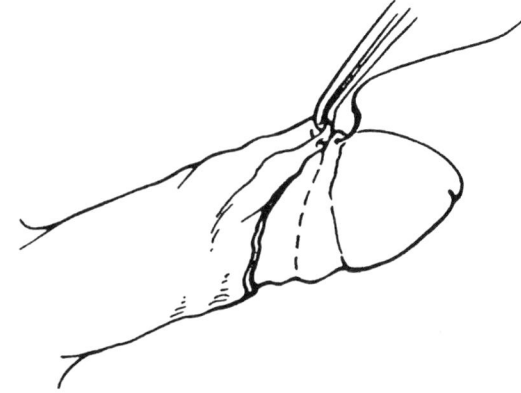

Fig. 119-8
Suturing of the skin to the shaft mucosa just proximal to the corona.

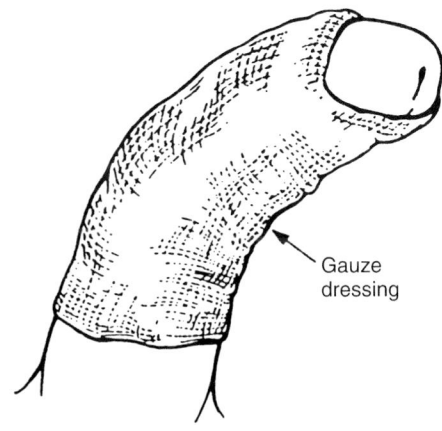

Fig. 119-9
Suture covered with gauze dressing.

5. Repeat this procedure of clamping at the 6-o'clock position and make an incision *up to the base of the frenulum* (Fig. 119-6).

6. After the dorsal and ventral areas are clamped, but before they are incised, mark a line where the circumferential excision of the foreskin is to occur. Use a marking pen to connect the dorsal point with the inferior point on each side.

7. Using a curved Mayo scissors, carefully excise these two lateral tissue flaps, maintaining a 1-cm margin from the corona, except at the frenulum where the foreskin is tapered only 2 to 3 mm (Fig. 119-7). Fulgurate all bleeders or tie with a 5-0 plain catgut.

8. If the large dorsal vein is cut, ligate with absorbable sutures.

9. After complete hemostasis, sew the outer layer of skin just proximal to the glans to the underlying mucosal layer (1 cm skin remnant of prepuce) with multiple 4-0 or 5-0 absorbable sutures (Fig. 119-8). If performing the procedure alone, leave some sutures long dorsally. These can be used (and cut off later) for retraction to stabilize the penis when suturing ventrally. Use hemostats to fix the long suture to the drape.

10. Place two layers of petrolatum gauze dressing over the suture line around the entire circumference and overlay with a light layer of Kerlix or Kling (Fig. 119-9).

SLEEVE TECHNIQUE

The sleeve technique uses two circumferential incisions. One is made on the internal aspect of the foreskin distally, near the coronal sulcus. The other is made on

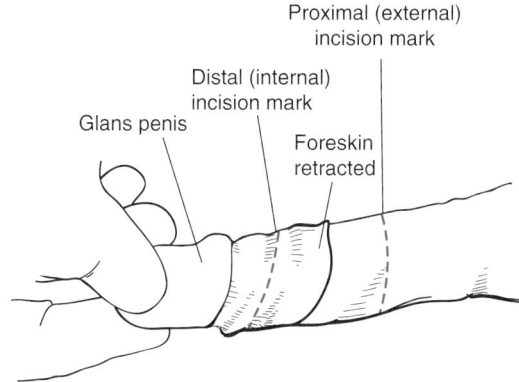

Fig. 119-10
External and internal preputial skin incision sites are marked. (Redrawn from Holman JR, Stuessi KA: *Am Fam Physician* 59[6]:1514, 1999.)

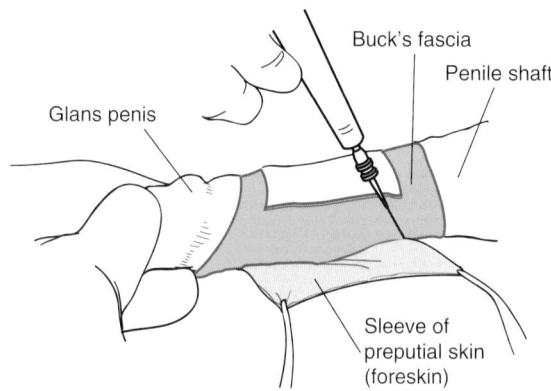

Fig. 119-12
Sleeve excised with electrocautery, tissue scissors, or scalpel. (Redrawn from Holman JR, Stuessi KA: *Am Fam Physician* 59[6]:1514, 1999.)

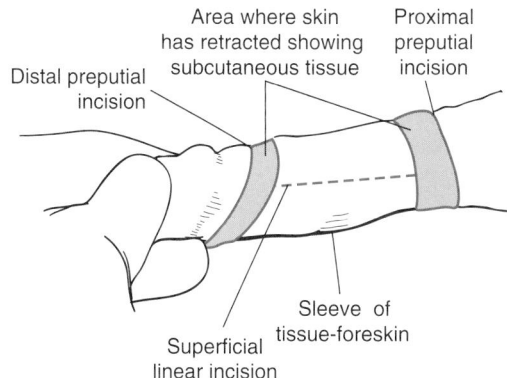

Fig. 119-11
After incisions are made, a "sleeve" of preputial skin remains. The shaded (pink) areas show where the skin has retracted, showing subcutaneous tissue. (Redrawn from Holman JR, Stuessi KA: *Am Fam Physician* 59[6]:1514, 1999.)

the external part of the foreskin proximally and defines an amount of prepuce removed. A "sleeve" of tissue between the two incisions will be excised.

1. The external preputial incision is outlined with a marking pen at the level of the corona.
2. After retracting the foreskin, the internal preputial incision is marked with the pen approximately 1 cm proximal to the coronal sulcus. It is important to apply gentle downward pressure on the prepubic fat pad at the base of the penis while making the initial outlines to remove the correct amount of skin (Fig. 119-10).
3. The external proximal circumferential preputial incision is made with the scalpel and carried to Buck's fascia.
4. After retracting the foreskin, a second circumferential incision is made in the inner prepuce at the previous mark. The internal incision is carried straight across the frenulum ventrally (Fig. 119-11).

5. A sleeve of tissue now exists between the two incisions. This sleeve is the foreskin. Hemostats are placed dorsally for traction.
6. After making a superficial linear incision on the "sleeve" with the electrocautery tool, subcutaneous attachments are separated between Buck's fascia and the prepuce. The sleeve is excised with electrocautery (Fig. 119-12).
7. The frenulum is reapproximated initially with the "U" stitch.
8. Four quadrant sutures are located on the dorsum and both sides, and the remaining interrupted sutures are placed at 4- to 7-mm intervals (Fig. 119-8).
9. A sterile dressing of petroleum gauze can be applied (Fig. 119-9).

COMPLICATIONS

- Bleeding
- Hematoma
- Infection
- Pain with erection (prevented by leaving an adequate "cup" [1 cm margin] of coronal skin [see Step 7 under the "Dorsal Slit Technique" section])
- Stricture and scarring (rare)
- Dehiscence resulting from nocturnal erections

POSTPROCEDURE PATIENT EDUCATION

- Prescribe 5 days' worth of adequate analgesics appropriate for the patient's pain tolerance. A combination product containing codeine (such as Tylenol #3), a nonsteroidal antiinflammatory drug, or a similar product is sufficient.

- Instruct the patient to soak in a tub of warm water 24 to 36 hours later and to remove all of the dressing at that time.
- Give the patient instructions on how to replace the petroleum gauze and Kling gauze, which should be done every day until the patient returns to the office for the follow-up visit in 1 week.
- Tell the patient to call if there is any undue pain, active bleeding, or signs of infection (e.g., streaks of redness, fever, purulent drainage).
- Instruct the patient to avoid sexual arousal and sexual intercourse for about 4 weeks.
- One ampule of amyl nitrate (crush and inhale one to six times as needed; may be repeated once after 5 minutes) can be used as abortive therapy for erections during the 1-week recovery period.

CPT/BILLING CODE

54161 Circumcision, surgical excision other than clamp device, or dorsal slit, other than newborn

ICD-9-CM DIAGNOSTIC CODES

605 Phimosis
605 Paraphimosis
607.1 Balanitis
607.9 Penile pain
302.70 Psychosexual dysfunction

ADDITIONAL RESOURCES

- See the sample patient education handout titled "Adult Circumcision" on page 1883 of Appendix G.
- See the sample patient consent form titled "Circumcision/Dorsal Penile Nerve Block" on page 1884 of Appendix G .

BIBLIOGRAPHY

Fakjian N, Hunter S, Cole GW, Miller J: An argument for circumcision: prevention of balanitis in the adult, *Arch Dermatol* 126(8):1046, 1990.

Holman JR, Stuessi KA: Adult circumcision, *Am Fam Physician* 50:1514, 1999.

Pienkos EJ: Circumcision at the 121st Evacuation Hospital: report of a questionnaire with cross-cultural observations, *Mil Med* 154:169, 1989.

Pories WJ, Thomas FT: *Office surgery for family physicians*, Stoneham, Mass, 1985, Butterworth.

Szmuk P, Ezri T, Ben Hur H, et al: Regional anaesthesia for circumcision in adults: a comparative study, *Can J Anaesth* 41:1181, 1994.

Wakefield SE, Elewa AA: Adult circumcision under local anaesthetic, *Br J Urol* 75:96, 1995.

CHAPTER 120

Androscopy

John L. Pfenninger

Androscopy is an office procedure used to identify condyloma. It examines the male genitalia under magnification after acetic acid has been applied. Another term for this procedure is "penoscopy."

Recent literature documents the close association of the human papillomavirus (HPV) with cervical dysplasia and cervical cancer. Whether the virus alone leads to cancer is unknown. It is likely, however, that HPV is the necessary cause (if not the single sufficient cause) for cervical cancer. Human papillomavirus is very contagious, and it is most readily spread through sexual contact; it may be transmitted in yet unknown ways in a minority of cases. Condoms provide little protection from HPV.

The clinical significance of condyloma and HPV in men is uncertain, but men act as carriers and may transmit the disease to sexual partners. Although rare, HPV can cause penile carcinoma. Anal-receptive homosexuals have 50 times the rate of anal carcinoma. An increased rate of anal carcinoma in anal-receptive females can also be anticipated, but there is no literature to document this.

There are over 100 types of HPV. Eight to ten of these characteristically infect the genital areas. Condyloma acuminata, the visible lesions that we commonly see, are caused by noncarcinogenic strains, such as types 6 and 11. The subclinical types, identified only by examination under magnification after acetic acid staining, are more likely to cause neoplastic changes; frequently these are types 16 and 18.

There is no evidence that treatment of male partners of women who have dysplasia lessens the likelihood of persistence or recurrence in the female. Wearing a condom has little benefit, since the infection is a regional disease. In men, it is present on the penis, scrotum, perineum, and perianal areas. What is visible is only a focal manifestation of a diffuse involvement. In women, it is present on the cervix, the vagina, the vulva, and the perineal and perianal areas.

Some clinicians question the value of carrying out an androscopic examination. Identification and treatment of condyloma is not the only reason to perform androscopy. Patient education is perhaps the most valuable aspect of this procedure. The male must be informed of the significance of his disease and the necessity of maintaining a single-partner committed relationship. It is no longer a matter of moral or religious persuasion, but rather a good health practice to be monogamous (as is exercising, not smoking, eating low-fat foods, and so forth). Men spread the disease even when visible lesions are not apparent. Only through education can they change their habits.

Men who have HPV affect their partners in several ways. Not only do they spread the virus by skin-to-skin contact, but HPV has been shown to be present in the semen and in the sperm cell itself. Men who smoke have nicotine and by-products in the ejaculate as well as on their hands (important during manual stimulation). Those who are subject to passive smoking have lower folate levels—a known risk factor for cervical cancer.

The common factors for penile carcinoma include lack of hygiene, sex outside of marriage, smoking, and HPV. Differentiating mild, moderate, and severe dysplasia of the penis (penile intraepithelial neoplasia [PIN]) is nearly impossible without obtaining biopsy samples. Anorectal cancer frequently contains the human papillomavirus, and some now recommend obtaining a Pap smear of the pectinate line (or dentate line) on a regular basis to detect anal dysplasias in high-risk individuals.

INDICATIONS

- Visible condyloma on the penis, scrotum, or anus. (Staining and examination with magnification will identify smaller lesions that are easier to treat. It also confirms that the entire lesion has been removed when surgical or ablative therapies are used. Early and complete treatment may reduce the recurrence of the disease.)
- Partner with recurrent or persistent condyloma acuminata or cervical dysplasia. (There is some evidence

that if the male presents a high viral load, the immune system response of the partner may be overwhelmed by the virus. High viral load exists if the male has visible acuminate lesions or a diffuse acetowhite staining of the penis.)

- Psychological reassurance.
- Chronic perineal or perianal irritation.
- Recurrent condyloma.
- Medical-legal examinations in child abuse cases.
- History of other sexually transmitted diseases.
- Necessity for patient education. (Performing the procedure is better received by the patient than "just talking." A biopsy-proven diagnosis speaks a thousand words of reinforcement.)

EQUIPMENT

- Spray bottle with 5% acetic acid (white vinegar)
- Colposcope (or a high-quality handheld magnifying lens)
- High-quality fine-tissue scissors (e.g., 5-inch curved Metzenbaum)
- Pickups
- Formalin jars
- Monsel's solution
- 1- to 5-ml lidocaine 1% or 2% without epinephrine
- 30-gauge needle
- 1- to 5-ml syringe (depending on size and number of lesions)
- Radiofrequency unit with smoke evacuator, 85% trichloroacetic acid, or an infrared coagulator (IRC) if condylomata are to be treated. (See Chapter 157, Treatment of Noncervical Condyloma Acuminata.)

PREPROCEDURE PATIENT PREPARATION

It is always best if the patient is well informed about the nature of the disease prior to the procedure. Provide the patient with a teaching guide (see the sample patient education handout titled "Androscopy" on page 1885 of Appendix G). Encourage the patient to watch a 30-minute videotape (available from Creative Health Communications) that discusses the implications of HPV infection in men and women prior to the visit. Viewing the videotape will help the patient focus on questions that he or his partner may have, and it will allow the practitioner to avoid repetitious explanations of the same counseling information. No preoperative medication is needed for the procedure, and the patient can be reassured that there will be minimal discomfort, even if biopsies are obtained.

TECHNIQUE

1. After the patient is placed in the examination room, the nurse instructs the patient to spray the entire genital and anal area with 5% acetic acid (white vinegar) and allow to soak for 5 minutes.
2. Obtain a detailed sexual history (Fig. 120-1).
3. Place the patient on an examination table with stirrups, and position as a female is positioned for a Pap smear. Conduct a visual inspection and note any lesions.
4. Spray the entire genital and perineal area again. Allow the solution to run freely over the perineum and anus.
5. Inspect the entire anogenital area under magnification, including the meatus of the penis. Generally a colposcope is used on low power (3× to 5×). Move the penis and scrotum forward and back to bring them into focus (unlike colposcopy, where the cervix is stationary and the scope is adjusted into focus). There is no study comparing good handheld magnification with colposcopic evaluation.
6. Grossly apparent warts that were previously seen will turn white with the acetic acid. Previously unseen, small, "flat," or subclinical lesions will also now be identifiable on the penis, scrotum, perineum, or rectum. They will show up as white areas known as acetowhite changes.
7. Biopsy any atypical lesions with an unusual vascular pattern (mosaicism or punctation; see Chapter 139, Colposcopic Examination) or pigmentation. The pigmentation in worrisome lesions will look different from that of a freckle or nevus; it will be a nondiscrete, brownish discoloration. If no atypical lesions are seen, biopsy one or two of the acuminate lesions or the acetowhite areas to document the presence of HPV and that there is no dysplasia. It is very convincing to have the pathology report confirm your clinical diagnosis, which reinforces the findings to the patient.
8. A penile biopsy specimen is easily obtained by using sharp tissue scissors. (A punch biopsy is not needed—you are not sampling the cavernosa!) If only one or two small lesions are to be sampled, simply tent up the skin by pinching it at its base (Fig. 120-2). Looking through the colposcope, obtain a 3- to 4-mm sample with the sharp tissue scissors or remove the entire lesion. No anesthetic is required, and this method is often less painful than the injection. Only a very superficial sampling is needed. If the lesions are larger, or more than two samples are to be obtained, it is best to anesthetize with 1% to 2% lidocaine without epinephrine. Using a 30-gauge needle minimizes any discomfort.

Androscopy Encounter Form

Patient to Fill Out:

Date _____ Referring Physician
Name _____ DOB _____ Age ____
Phone _____
Reason for Examination _____
History:

Age _____	History of genital warts	Y N
Smoker Y N	Treated	Y N Method _____ When ____
Age at first intercourse _____	Visible warts now	Y N
No. of sexual partners	Partners with warts	Y N
(total in lifetime) _____	Previous partners	
History of sexual abuse Y N	w/abnormal Pap	Y N

Other history of venereal disease (circle):   Gonorrhea   Syphilis   AIDS   Herpes

Do you desire testing for any of the above diseases?   Y   N

Physician Section:
Procedure: _____
PMH: _____
Illnesses: _____
Medications: _____
Allergies: _____
Health maintenance: _____
Family history: _____

    Gross Inspection:

    5% acetic acid   penis
    and examination   urethra
    with colposcope: scrotum
                                groin
                                perineum
                                rectum

Biopsy:_____
Impression:_____
Treatment: _____

Plan: Discourage smoking
            Counseling regarding safer sex, cause for cancer, reporting penis lesions, partner evaluation
            Instruction sheets on androscopy?   Efudex?   Videotapes?
            Consider other VD Testing
            Follow-up in _____ weeks

                                    _____ Date _____
                                              Physician's signature

Fig. 120-1
Patient encounter form. Used with permission of the Medical Procedures Center, P.C., Midland, Mich.

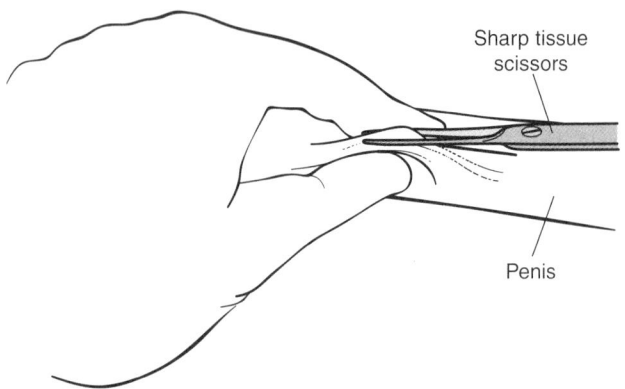

Fig. 120-2
Tenting up the penile skin to obtain a biopsy.

9. If lesions are numerous, diffuse, or large, they may need to be removed with radiofrequency surgery, 85% trichloroacetic acid, cryosurgery, 5-fluorouracil (Efudex), the IRC, or excisional (shave) therapy. A dorsal penile nerve block may facilitate this removal (see Chapter 157, Treatment of Noncervical Condyloma Acuminata).
10. Monsel's solution may be needed as an astringent to limit postoperative bleeding.
11. If only flat asymptomatic acetowhite changes appear on the penis, anus, or scrotum, treatment is unnecessary, although the biopsies will confirm HPV.
12. Unless the patient has had an extensive area of warts treated, he can return to full activity with no modification of his daily routine.

POSTPROCEDURE CARE

See the sample patient education handout titled "Genital Condyloma (Wart) Removal" on page 1887 of Appendix G.

Topical 5% lidocaine (Xylocaine) ointment (a prescription) not only soothes the area but prevents treated sites from adhering to the undergarments. A nonsteroidal inflammatory drug is recommended to reduce pain and swelling.

No definite recommendations can be made regarding treatment of dysplastic lesions on the penis, since studies of long-term follow-up have not been conducted. Between 5% and 10% of the lesions biopsied will come back with a report of mild or moderate bowenoid dysplastic change. Rarely, a severe dysplasia will be found. (Unlike dysplastic cervical lesions in females, it is difficult to predict the degree of dysplastic change observed during the examination, even with magnifica-

tion, in the male.) In such situations, the patient should return for reexamination to confirm that the entire dysplastic lesion(s) was removed. The patient should report any unusual growths or ulcerations at once, and he should discuss his HPV history with his physician during future examinations. Sexual partners should be examined and should obtain regular Pap smears. Smoking is strongly discouraged. Supplemental vitamins with folic acid may reduce recurrences.

COMPLICATIONS

There are essentially no complications. There may be minimal depigmentation, scarring or bleeding. The penile skin is very thin, and the biopsy should be kept very superficial. Condyloma acuminata can be confused with other lesions, such as condyloma lata, molluscum contagiosum (commonly seen), keratoses, bowenoid dysplasia, nevi, hemorrhoidal tags, and other nondescript papular lesions. Care must be taken that men do not become psychological cripples because of HPV, but at the same time know that each new sexual partner is at risk of contracting the wart virus and should receive annual Pap smears for the rest of her life.

CPT/BILLING CODES

There presently is no CPT code for androscopy. Use 55899, unlisted procedure, male genital system (documentation suggested). Insurance companies still rarely pay. Consider charging for a more extended visit (if new patient) and for treatment of warts or penile biopsy only.

54100 Biopsy, penis, cutaneous
54050 Simple destruction of penile lesions: chemical
54055 Simple destruction of penile lesions: electrosurgical
54056 Simple destruction of penile lesions: cryocautery
54057 Simple destruction of penile lesions: laser
54060 Simple destruction of penile lesions: excision
54065 Destruction of penile lesions, extensive, any method
54105 Biopsy of penis, deep

ICD-9-CM DIAGNOSTIC CODES

07811 Condyloma
607.9 Penile pain

Skin Lesions	Penis	Scrotum	Anus
Primary malignancy	187.4	187.7	173.5
Metastatic	198.82	198.82	198.2
Cancer-in-situ	233.5	233.6	232.5
Benign	222.1	222.4	216.5
Uncertain	236.6	236.6	238.2
Unspecified	239.5	239.5	239.2

ADDITIONAL RESOURCES

• See the sample patient education handouts titled "Androscopy" on page 1885 and "Genital Condyloma (Wart) Removal" on page 1887 of Appendix G.

BIBLIOGRAPHY

Barrasso R, DeBrux J, Croissant O: High prevalence of papilloma virus: associated penile intraepithelial neoplasia in sexual partners of women with cervical intraepithelial neoplasia, *N Engl J Med* 317:916, 1987.

Bosch FG, Castelisague X, Munoz N, et al: Male sexual behavior and human papilloma DNA, *J Natl Cancer Inst* 88:1060, 1996.

Brinton LA, Li JY, Rong SD, et al: Risk factors of penile cancer: results from a case-control study in China, *Int J Cancer* 47:504, 1991.

Burmer GC, True LD, Krieger JN: Squamous cell carcinoma of the scrotum associated with human papillomavirus, *J Urol* 149:374, 1993.

Daling JR, Weiss NS: Are barrier methods protective against cervical cancer? *Epidemiology* 1:261, 1990.

Demeter LM, Stoler MH, Bonnez W, et al: Penile intraepithelial neoplasia: clinical presentation and an analysis of the physical state of human papilloma DNA, *J Infect Dis* 168:38, 1993.

Epperson WJ: Androscopy for anogenital HPV, *J Fam Pract* 332:143, 1991.

Epperson WJ: Preventing cervical cancer by treating genital warts in men: why male sex partners need androscopy, *Postgrad Med* 88:229, 1990.

Frisch M, Fenger C, Vanden Brule AJ, et al: Variants of squamous cell carcinoma: cancer of the anal canal and perianal skin and their relation to human papillomavirus, *Cancer Res* 59:753, 1999.

Goldie SJ, Kuntz KM, Weinstein MC: The clinical effectiveness and cost effectiveness of screening for anal squamous intraepithelial lesions in homosexual and bisexual HIV-positive men, *JAMA* 281:1822, 1999.

Koutsky L: Epidemiology of genital human papillomavirus infections, *Am J Med* 102:3, 1997.

Krebs HB: Management of human papilloma virus: associated genital lesions in men, *Obstet Gynecol* 73:312, 1989.

Krebs HB, Helmkamp F: Does the treatment of genital condylomata in men decrease the treatment failure rate of cervical dysplasia in the female sexual partner? *Obstet Gynecol* 76:660, 1990.

Krogh G: Clinical relevance and evaluation of genito-anal papillomavirus infections in the male, *Semin Dermatol* 11:229, 1992.

Lai YM, Yang FP, Pao CC: Human papillomavirus deoxyribonucleic acid and ribonucleic acid in seminal plasma and sperm cells, *Fertil Steril* 65:1026, 1996.

Malek RS, Goellner JR, Smith T, et al: Human papillomavirus infection and intraepithelial-in-situ, and invasive carcinoma of the penis, *Urology* 42:159, 1993.

Noel JC, Vancenbossche M, Peny MO: Verrucous carcinoma of the penis: importance of human papilloma typing for diagnosis and therapeutic decisions, *Eur Urol* 22:83, 1992.

Palefsky JM: Anal cancer and its precursors: an HIV-related disease, *Hosp Physician* 29:35, 1993.

Palefsky JM, Holly EA, Gonzales J, et al: Detection of human papillomavirus DNA in anal intraepithelial neoplasia and anal cancer, *Cancer Res* 51:1014, 1991.

Patton D, Rodney WM: Androscopy of unproven benefit, *J Fam Pract* 332:135, 1991.

Pfenninger JL: Androscopy: technique for examining men for condyloma, *J Fam Pract* 29(3):286, 1989.

Pfenninger JL: Letter to the editor, *J Fam Pract* 33(6):566, 1991.

Pfenninger JL: Androscopy: examination of the male partner. In Apgar BS, Brotzman GL, Spitzer M, editors: *Colposcopy: principles and practice: an integrated text and atlas,* Philadelphia, 2002, WB Saunders.

Poblet E, Alfaro L, Ferdander-Segoviano P, et al: Human papillomavirus associated with penile squamous cell carcinoma in HIV-positive patients, *Am J Surg Pathol* 23:1119, 1999.

Rando RF: Human papilloma virus: implications for clinical medicine, *Ann Intern Med* 108:628, 1988.

Richart R: Men and HPV, *Prim Care Cancer* Aug:5, 1995.

Rosenberg SK: Sexually transmitted papilloma viral infections: IV: The white scrotum, *J Urol* 33(6):462, 1989.

Tokudome S: Semen of smokers and cervical cancer risk (letter), *J Natl Cancer Inst* 89:96, 1997.

Von Krogh G: Clinical relevance and evaluation of genitoanal papilloma virus infection in the male, *Semin Dermatol* 11(3):229, 1992.

Weiner JS, Liu ET, Waither PJ: Oncogenic human papillomavirus type 16 in association with squamous cell cancer of the male urethra, *Cancer Res* 52:5018, 1992.

Whidden P: Cigarette smoking and cervical cancer (letter), *Int J Epidemiol* 23:1099, 1994.

Wikström A, Hedblad MA, Johasson B, et al: The acetic acid test in evaluation of subclinical genital infection: a competence study on penoscopy, histopathology, virology and scanning electron microscopy findings, *Genitourin Med* 68:90, 1992.

Xi LF, Critchlow CW, Wheeler CM, et al: Risk of anal carcinoma-in-situ in relation to human papillomavirus type 16 variants, *Cancer Res* 58:3839, 1998.

Zabbo A, Stein BS: Penile intraepithelial neoplasia in patients examined for exposure to human papillomavirus, *J Urol* 41(1):24, 1993.

Dorsal Slit for Phimosis

Scott A. Cota

A continued debate exists of medical versus surgical management of phimosis. Some recommend topical steroids or topical nonsteroidals, whereas others advocate surgical correction. Although the exact definition of phimosis is still controversial, this condition has been recognized since ancient times. Phimosis can be physiologic, congenital, or acquired as a result of inflammation or infection. Rickwood (1980) described phimosis as a stricture of the preputial orifice caused by lichen sclerosus et atrophicus, also known as balanitis xerotica obliterans. American literature describes phimosis as scar formation of the foreskin because of any injury or inflammatory condition and the inability to retract the foreskin over the glans penis. Poor hygiene, diabetes, and zipper injuries are conditions that may increase the risk of phimosis. Acute phimosis may occur with infection or as a complication from various treatments for verruca, which can cause inflammation (85% trichloroacetic acid, electrocoagulation, etc.). Phimosis may lead to urinary retention or infection as well as paraphimosis (nonreducible retracted foreskin), which may require urgent or emergent intervention. The surgical options for phimosis include dorsal slit, ventral slit, lateral preputioplasty, lateral preputioplasty procedure, and circumcision. Dorsal slit is a simple procedure involving a single cut along the dorsal foreskin that allows rapid access to the urethral meatus and glans penis.

INDICATIONS

- To gain emergency access to the urethral meatus for bladder catheterization in the presence of phimosis
- To prevent recurrent balanitis with abscess formation
- Adjunct treatment before circumcision or after phimotic ring incision for paraphimosis

CONTRAINDICATIONS

- Active infection of the genitalia
- Anatomic abnormalities of the external genitalia (refer to urologist)

EQUIPMENT

- 10-ml syringe with 1¼-inch, 27-gauge needle
- 1% Lidocaine without epinephrine
- Three small straight hemostats
- Straight iris or small Metzenbaum scissors
- Suture scissors
- Absorbable suture (4-0) on small reversed cutting needle
- Needle driver
- Fenestrated drape
- Iodine solution or other antiseptic scrub
- Prep bowl with 4 × 4–inch gauze sponges
- Adson forceps

PREPROCEDURE PATIENT PREPARATION

Provide appropriate information to the patient about the procedure while obtaining informed consent. Risks include pain, bleeding, infection, damage to the glans, poor cosmetic result, and hematoma formation. Benefits include resolution of phimosis, prevention of paraphimosis, increased ease of hygiene, decreased risk of urinary retention, and decreased pain with intercourse.

Place the patient in a comfortable supine position on an examination table in a well-lit room. Using sterile technique, surgically prep the genital area with an antiseptic solution. Place the penis through a fenestrated drape and onto the surgical field.

Anesthesia

1. Dorsal penile nerve block or modified "ring block" is used to obtain anesthesia after prepping and draping the penis.
2. Dorsal penile nerve block anesthetizes the right and left dorsal nerves where they branch from the pudendal nerve from under the pubic bone.
3. The lateral and ventral portions of the penile shaft are innervated by branches arcading from the dorsal

midline, radiating toward the ventral surface. The axons innervating the glans are in a constant dorsal, midline location along most of the penile shaft.

4. A 27-gauge, 1¼-inch needle is inserted at the base of the penis just under the pubic bone and into Buck's fascia at the 2 o'clock and 10 o'clock position (Fig. 121-1).

5. After aspirating inject 3 to 5 ml of lidocaine into the base of the penis at the 2 o'clock and 10 o'clock positions deep to Buck's fascia at the inferior edge of the pubic bone.

6. Wait 5 minutes and test for the adequacy of anesthesia by grasping the dorsal foreskin with a hemostat.

7. A modified ring block can be used if anesthesia is incomplete. This is performed by interconnecting the two positions across the dorsal midline at the base of the penis in a subcutaneous fashion (Fig. 121-2).

TECHNIQUE

1. After achieving local anesthesia, the operator grasps the distal dorsal foreskin in the 2 o'clock and 10 o'clock positions with two of the small straight hemostats (Fig. 121-3). Use the instruments to apply countertraction when performing the procedure.

2. Identify the corona of the glans, which determines the proximal extent of the dorsal slit.

3. Gently retract the foreskin and attempt to identify the urethral meatus.

4. The closed third straight hemostat is horizontally introduced into the opening of the foreskin between the inner layer of the foreskin and the glans penis. Advance it proximally to the coronal sulcus. Avoid entering the urethral meatus.

5. Tent up the foreskin and spread open the hemostat. Withdraw the instrument and twist to the right and left to break up adhesions around the circumference of the glans (Fig. 121-4).

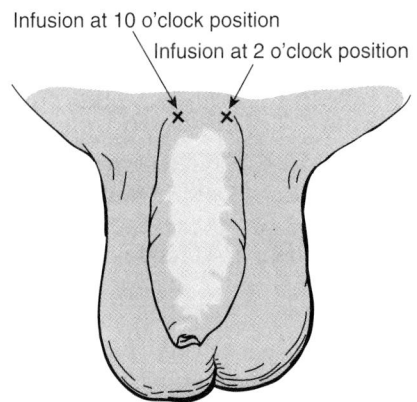

Infusion at 10 o'clock position
Infusion at 2 o'clock position

Fig. 121-1
Dorsal nerve block.

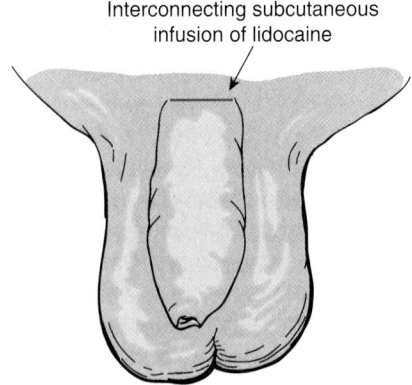

Interconnecting subcutaneous infusion of lidocaine

Fig. 121-2
Ring block.

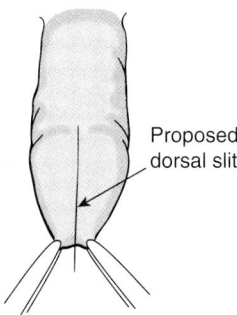

Proposed dorsal slit

Fig. 121-3
Grasp foreskin at the 2 o'clock and 10 o'clock positions. Attempt to identify urethral meatus.

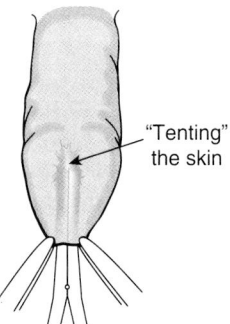

"Tenting" the skin

Fig. 121-4
Adhesiolysis. Separate the foreskin from the glans by spreading while withdrawing the hemostat.

6. When lysis of adhesions is complete, the hemostat is withdrawn, opened, and reinserted with one jaw of the hemostat in the plane between the glans and the inner layer of the foreskin while the other is placed on the outer skin. This should be at the 12 o'clock position with the instrument in a longitudinal position. Advance the instrument to the level of the coronal sulcus and clamp tightly. This crushes the interposed anesthetized foreskin. Leave in place for 5 minutes (Fig. 121-5).

7. Remove the hemostat and cut the foreskin longitudinally with iris or Metzenbaum scissors along the entire distance of the serrated, crushed foreskin.

8. If crush hemostasis is inadequate and there is bleeding after cutting the dorsal slit, absorbable sutures should be used to allow adequate hemostasis. This is performed by placing two running 4-0 Vicryl or Dexon sutures beginning at the apex of the dorsal slit and running distally to reapproximate the two layers of each side of the incision of the foreskin (Fig. 121-6).

9. Placement of sterile petroleum jelly or antibiotic ointment on the wound edges prevents the dressing from adhering to the wound.

COMPLICATIONS

- *Bleeding:* Late bleeding can be controlled with direct pressure, Monsel's solution, Gelfoam, or the placement of hemostatic ligatures.
- *Injury to the urethral meatus or glans:* Avoid blind introduction of hemostat and scissors when performing the procedure to prevent injury to the urethral meatus or glands.
- *Infection:* Antibiotics can be used to control infection commonly due to skin pathogens such as *Streptococcus* or *Staphylococcus*.
- *Pain:* Hyperesthesia with intercourse may occur.
- *Anesthesia complications:* May include hematoma formation at the site of injection.
- *Poor cosmetic result.* Elective circumcision may be recommended if the patient is not satisfied with the cosmetic "dog-ear" appearance of the foreskin.

POSTPROCEDURE PATIENT EDUCATION

1. After successful dorsal slit for phimosis, the prepuce is easily retracted to access the urethral meatus and cleanse the glans penis.
2. Once retracted, the foreskin should be reduced on completion of catherterization or cleansing to avoid iatrogenic paraphimosis.
3. Between 3 and 5 days of analgesics should be prescribed for postprocedure pain.
4. The patient should wear loose briefs and gently cleanse the wound for 5 to 7 days with soap and water three to four times a day.
5. The patient should avoid intercourse or masturbation for 4 to 6 weeks to prevent disruption of the wound.
6. The patient should be instructed to return for postprocedure wound check in 1 to 2 weeks and to return immediately if excessive bleeding occurs.
7. Instruct the patient on signs of infection that should not be confused with fibrinous exudate (a straw-colored exudate), which is part of normal healing.

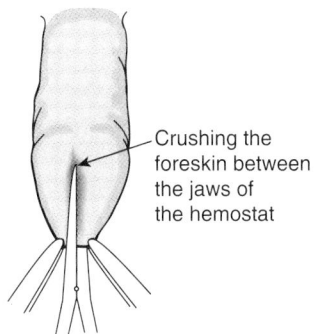

Fig. 121-5
Crush hemostasis. Place the clamp longitudinally in the 12 o'clock position for 5 minutes.

Crushing the foreskin between the jaws of the hemostat

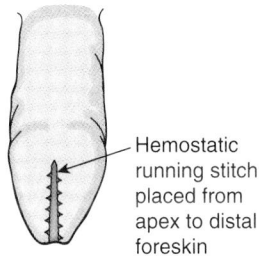

Hemostatic running stitch placed from apex to distal foreskin

Fig. 121-6
Placement of sutures to control bleeding.

CONCLUSION

Dorsal slit is an effective procedure that permits easy retraction of the foreskin, without the need for circumcision. It can be performed in the office setting or emergency room for complications related to phimosis.

CPT/BILLING CODE

54160   Dorsal slit for phimosis

ICD-9-CM DIAGNOSTIC CODES

605   Phimosis
605   Paraphimosis

ADDITIONAL RESOURCES

- See the sample patient education handout titled "Dorsal Slit for Phimosis" on page 1888 of Appendix G.
- See the sample patient consent form titled "Dorsal Slit for Phimosis" on page 1890 of Appendix G.

BIBLIOGRAPHY

Chu CC: Topical steroid treatment of phimosis in boys, *J Urol* 162(3Pt1):861, 1999.

Hodges FM: Phimosis in antiquity, *World J Urol* 17(3):133, 1999.

Holman J, Steussi K: Adult circumcision, *Am Fam Physician* 59(6):1514, 1999.

Rickwood AMK, Hemalatha V, Batcup G, Spitz L: Phimosis in boys, *Br J Urol* 52:144, 1980.

Roberts JR, Hedges JR: *Roberts and Hedges: clinical procedures in emergency medicine,* ed 3, Philadelphia, 1998, WB Saunders.

Szmuk P, Ezri T, Ben Hur H, et al: Regional anaesthesia for circumcision in adults: a comparative study, *Can J Anaesth* 41(12):1181, 1994.

Van Howe RS: Cost-effective treatment of phimosis, *Pediatrics* 102(4):E43, 1998.

Yang CC, Bradley WE: Neuroanatomy of the penile portion of the human dorsal nerve of the penis, *Br J Urol* 82(1):109, 1998.

CHAPTER 122

Prostate Biopsy

Robert S. Tan
Grant C. Fowler

Primary care clinicians often perform prostatic specific antigen (PSA) screening in their offices, and abnormally elevated PSAs are not rare. An elevated PSA could indicate inflammation or infection of the prostate or carcinoma. Although some clinicians consider it controversial, the blood test known as a "free PSA" (Table 122-1) may help further differentiate between inflammation, infection, or cancer. An elevated PSA velocity, which is an increase of more than 0.75 ng/ml per year, may also indicate cancer. After further evaluation or treatment, a prostate biopsy may be warranted.

Similar to finding an abnormal PSA, routine rectal examination by a primary care clinician may reveal an abnormality in the consistency of the prostate. For individuals at risk of prostate cancer, or for males over 50, biopsy may be warranted. Biopsy may even be warranted with a normal PSA. If transrectal ultrasound of the prostate and seminal vesicles (TRUSP-SV) is available and a rapid diagnosis is desired, patients with easily palpable, discrete lesions, those with abnormal findings on TRUSP-SV, or those with abnormal PSAs may be excellent candidates for biopsy in the office. If TRUSP-SV is not available, prostate biopsy may be performed on palpable lesions. However, it must be understood that a negative biopsy in such a situation does not exclude carcinoma. See Fig. 122-1 for a sample algorithm.

As primary care clinicians continue to perform wellness examinations and to check PSAs, and as babyboomers age, the number of patients who will need a prostate biopsy will increase. The overall rate of prostate cancer is about 15%; about 1 in 8 males will eventually be diagnosed with prostate cancer. Diagnosis rates are higher in individuals with abnormal PSA levels, with results varying from 26% to 33%.

Approximately 97% of all prostate cancers are adenocarcinoma, the remainder being neuroendocrine tumors, sarcoma, carcinoid, melanoma, or metastatic cancer. Early detection of prostate cancer may lead to improved survival in the treated group. In some countries, the geriatrician or primary care clinician may perform the prostate biopsy. Early confirmation of diagnosis by the primary care clinician or geriatrician can be helpful for the individual and the family. Unfortunately with today's technology, it is not always easy to predict who will have a problem from the prostate cancer. Often it lies dormant. However, blood tests are someday expected to detect the overall 15% to 20% of prostate cancers that are very aggressive so that treatment can be focused on these. The other 80% to 85% would be left alone. When this blood test is available, primary care clinicians will be able to stratify their referrals after confirming the cancer by biopsy.

Considering the fact that prostate biopsies in the United States are not performed by many primary care clinicians, not all patients with elevated PSAs are candidates for biopsy by primary care clinicians. In certain cases, referral to the urologist is always prudent, such as in individuals with an elevated PSA but no evidence of prostatitis, no palpable lesion, and no abnormality on TRUSP-SV. However, even this scenario is discussed in the "Technique" section ("sextant" biopsy). TRUSP-SV is often not available to primary care clinicians; therefore this may be another reason for referral for biopsy.

The introduction of TRUSP-SV (see Chapter 124, Prostate and Seminal Vesicle Ultrasonography) has im-

TABLE 122-1

Association of Percent-Free Prostate Specific Antigen (PSA)*
with Prostate Cancer

Percent Free PSA	Probability of Cancer
Up to 10%	56%
10%-15%	28%
15%-20%	20%
20%-25%	16%
Greater than 25%	8%

From Catalona WJ, Partin AW, Slawin KM, et al: *JAMA* 279:1542, 1998.
*The "free" PSA is a measure of unbound PSA. Whereas the majority of PSA from benign prostatic hyperplasia is unbound or "free," much of the PSA from cancer is bound. In this table, free PSA was studied in men aged 50 and older with a total PSA between 4 and 10 ng/ml and a negative digital rectal examination.

proved the accuracy of prostate tissue sampling. The sole reliance on digital rectal examination (DRE) to guide biopsy may depend on the experience of the clinician. As stated above, although a DRE-guided biopsy may indeed confirm cancer, a negative study without TRUSP-SV cannot exclude cancer in all regions of the gland. Fortunately, by evaluating the whole gland, TRUSP-SV improves the ability of the clinician to exclude cancer. Equally fortunate, especially for underserved areas, technicians or sonographers will now bring TRUSP-SV equipment to your office. Overreading services by a radiologist for TRUSP-SV are also available over the Internet (see the "Suppliers" section).

Note: TRUSP-SV should not be used to screen the general population. If a hypoechoic area is seen on TRUSP-SV (and they are common), it probably should be biopsied, regardless of PSA. Therefore some experts warn against performing TRUSP-SV unless a biopsy is indicated and will probably be performed. It is more helpful for guiding the biopsy than for excluding the diagnosis.

INDICATIONS

- A situation clinically suspicious of prostate cancer (Fig. 122-1) (elevated PSA, PSA velocity; low percentage of free PSA; or a DRE revealing abnormal consistency or a

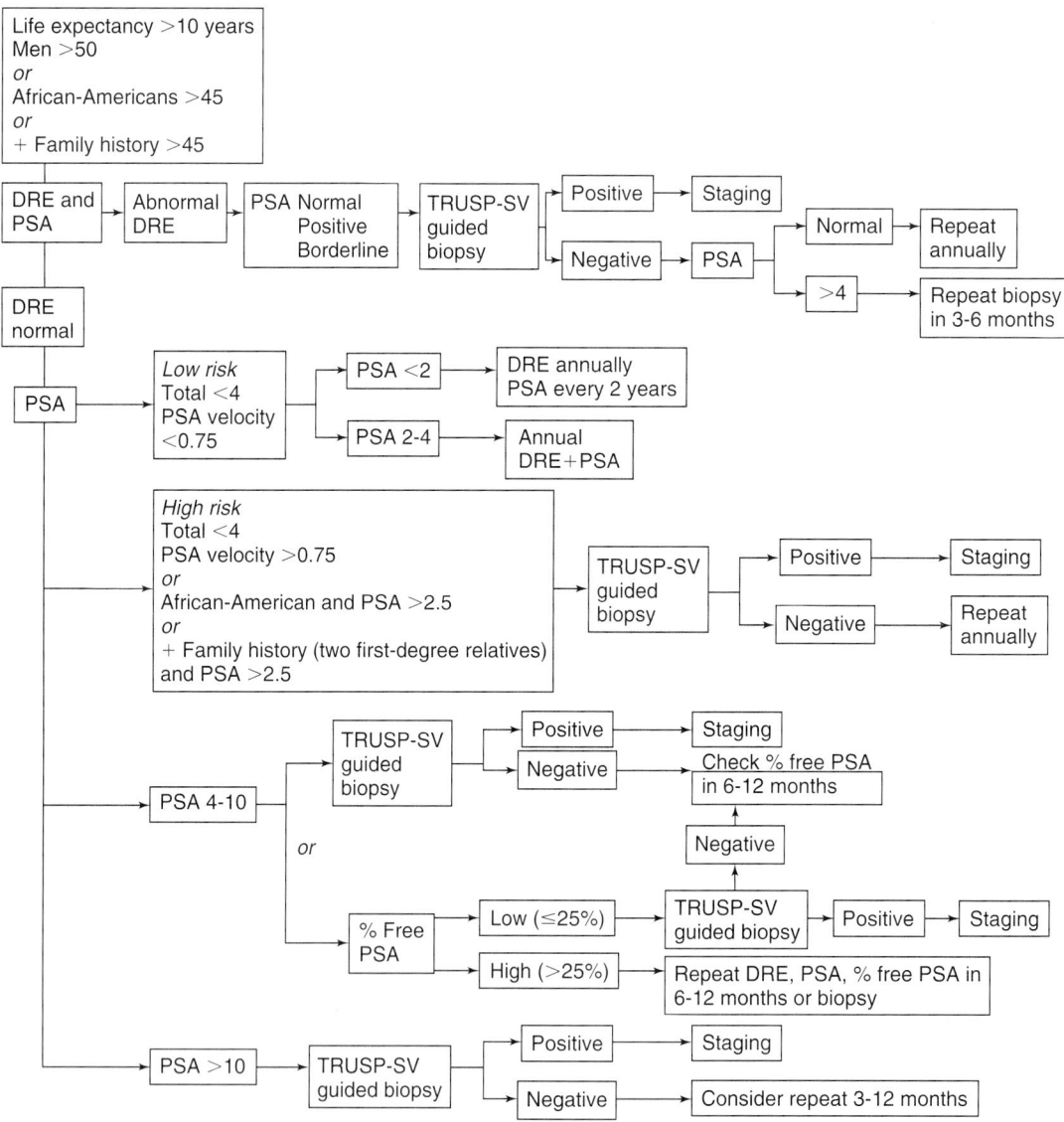

Fig. 122-1
Sample algorithm for men who desire early cancer detection after discussion of pros and cons with their clinician. *DRE*, Digital rectal examination; *PSA*, prostatic specific antigen; *TRUSP-SV,* transrectal ultrasound of the prostate and seminal vesicles. (Redrawn from Braunwald E, Fauci AS, Kasper DL, et al: *Harrison's principles of internal medicine,* ed 15, New York, 2001, McGraw-Hill.)

change in consistency of the prostate). Approximately one in three patients with elevated PSA have cancer.

CONTRAINDICATIONS

- Local infection (proctocolitis)
- Prostatitis
- Operator not familar with the procedure, TRUSP-SV, or the anatomy
- Coagulopathy or anticoagulated patient (heparin, lovenox, clopidogrel, etc.)
- Life expectancy less than 10 years *(relative contraindication)*

Note: The functionality and comorbid status of the patient should be taken into account and discussed with the patient and family before a biopsy is performed. In a patient with a shortened life span from anticipated comorbid medical conditions, a prostate biopsy may not be indicated to improve prognosis. In that situation, the patient's outcome may not be affected significantly, even with treatment of the cancer. However, biopsy might be indicated for other management purposes. Such a biopsy certainly could be performed by a primary care clinician or geriatrician (e.g., in a demented patient with an elevated PSA, knowing that the patient has metastatic prostate cancer might help the family decide about hospice care.) Alternatively, a bone scan might confirm metastatic prostate cancer (PSA higher than 10 ng/ml). These options should be discussed and biopsy performed only if having a tissue diagnosis would be important to the hospice, the clinician, or the family.

PREPROCEDURE CONSIDERATIONS AND PATIENT PREPARATION

1. Urinalysis should be performed to rule out infection. If present, it should be treated with a course of antibiotics. Prostatic excretions should be evaluated, and a postprostatic massage (see Chapter 123, Prostate Massage) urinalysis should be evaluated. If positive, these should be sent for culture.

Note: Prostatitis should be excluded in patients with an elevated PSA (PSA higher than 4 but below 50 ng/ml). One study of males over the age of 50 with elevated PSAs (mean 11.5 ng/ml) reported a reduction by 18% in the number of patients requiring biopsy when prostatitis was aggressively ruled out. In that study, 41% of patients tested positive for infection by either expressed prostatic secretions or a postprostatic massage urinalysis. These patients were treated with a 4-week course of antibiotics (trimethoprim-sulfamethoxazole or a quinolone if sulfa allergic). Two to four weeks after antibiotic therapy, 20% had normal PSA levels. Of those that did not respond to antibiotics, cancer was found by biopsy in 29%. Of those men without a positive postprostatic massage urinalysis or expressed prostatic secretions positive for infection, 50% had cancer.

2. Blood work, including complete blood count (CBC) with platelets, partial thromboplastin time (PTT), and international normalized ratio (INR), should be performed before the procedure to ensure that there are no bleeding problems. The patient should refrain from nonsteroidal antiinflammatory drugs and aspirin for 2 weeks, if possible, before the procedure. At a minimum the patient should refrain for 72 hours.
3. Analgesics and antianxiety medications can be given before the procedure. Extra-strength acetaminophen (Tylenol, two tablets) and a sedative such as lorazepam (Ativan) 1 mg or diazepam (Valium) 5 mg is recommended an hour before biopsy. Another option is rofecoxib (Vioxx) 50 mg an hour before the procedure. (COX-2 inhibitors have no platelet effect and therefore minimal bleeding effect.) All three of these classes of medications can be given together.
4. A cleansing enema is given the night before the procedure.
5. A quinolone antibiotic is given prophylactically the day of the procedure (e.g., ciprofloxacin 500 mg bid or gatifloxacin 400 mg qd) and for 3 days after the procedure.
6. Preprocedural education for the patient should include a discussion of diagnostic sampling errors, pain, and possible rare complications. The patient should also be aware that, even if the biopsy results are positive, the cancer may not always be aggressive. Treatment should be individualized based on the functional status of the patient, especially for the elderly.
7. A signed consent form should be obtained and the patient given a patient education handout.

EQUIPMENT

- Nonsterile gloves, eye protection, and gown
- Bard Biopty cut instrument and needle
- Transrectal ultrasound unit with needle guide, sterile sheath, and sterile lubricant gel
- Sterile tray, drapes, and gloves

TECHNIQUE

1. Place the patient in the left lateral decubitus position with knees flexed to his chest (Fig. 122-2). Follow universal blood and body fluid precautions.
2. Perform a rectal examination with nonsterile gloves, and palpate the prostate for areas of abnormal or different consistency. Next, change to sterile gloves.
3. Under sterile conditions, attach the external needle guide to the sterile, sheathed, ultrasound probe

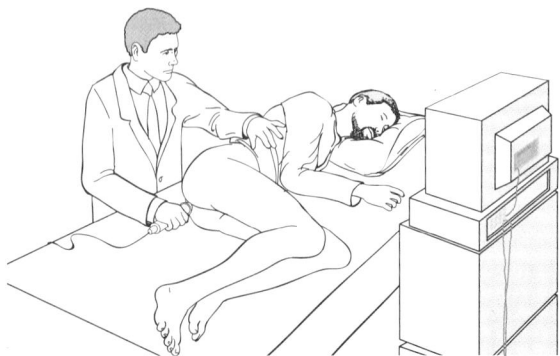

Fig. 122-2
Positioning of patient.

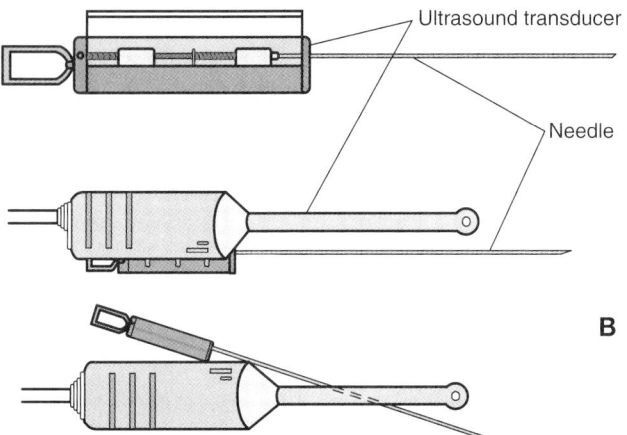

Fig. 122-3
Needle can be introduced through, **A,** an internal or, **B,** external puncture guide. (Redrawn from Brackman J, Denis LJ: Prostate ultrasound and needle biopsy. In Graham Jr SD, ed: *Glenn's urologic surgery,* ed 5, Philadelphia, 1998, Lippincott-Raven.)

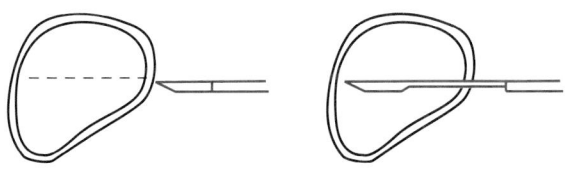

Fig. 122-4
Tru-cut biopsy of prostate.

(Fig. 122-3). A sterile condom or glove can be used as a sheath. Some probes may have a balloon that can be filled with water to produce a clearer ultrasound image. Sterile gel is placed on the tip of the probe, and the ultrasound probe, along with the external needle guide, is then inserted into the rectum.

4. Evaluate the prostate for abnormalities with the ultrasound. Abnormalities include the presence of hypoechoic (can be cancerous) or hyperechoic (occasionally cancerous) lesions, asymmetries, or discontinuities of the echo at the prostate boundary. Hypoechoic areas are more commonly fibrous or muscular structures in the prostate; however, they are also suspicious for cancer, especially in the peripheral zone (10% to 20% are cancer). They should be the focus of the ultrasound study as well as the biopsy. Hyperechoic areas are usually indicative of periprostatic fat, yet they can also be cancer (see Chapter 124, Prostate and Seminal Vesicle Ultrasonography). The overall prostate volume should be noted.

5. An 18-gauge Tru-Cut type needle is introduced into the mechanical actuating device (e.g., Biopty). This device is placed into the external needle guide.

6. Locate the target in the prostate by moving the probe in the rectum in the different planes. Two or three directed tissue samples should be taken from the suspicious lesion or area (Fig. 122-4). To avoid any surprises, the patient should be warned just before the biopsy is performed.

7. In patients with an indurated prostatic nodule on palpation, but no abnormality on the TRUSP-SV, geographic biopsies may be indicated in addition to biopsies of the nodule. The site of the biopsy should be noted and biopsies repeated on the opposite, normal side. The Biopty device should then be removed from the external needle guide, and if the palpable area has not been biopsied, the biopsy should be repeated manually at the site of palpable induration.

8. In patients with an elevated PSA, yet no palpable abnormality or TRUSP-SV abnormality, a "sextant biopsy" may be indicated. Three biopsies are taken on each side: one at the apex, one at the base, and one in between. This method of biopsy is certainly more invasive and can be more painful for the patient; however, it is an acceptable technique to exclude prostate cancer. Certain centers, such as M.D. Anderson Hospital, are now even taking 10 core samples each time, and this may become the standard.

COMPLICATIONS

- Rectal bleeding
- Hematuria
- Hemospermia
- Fever and chills, prostatitis
- Hematoma
- Failure to diagnose prostate cancer

POSTPROCEDURE PATIENT EDUCATION

Patients should be aware that, even with a negative biopsy, they may have microscopic cancer in a small area of the prostate. If the biopsy was for an abnormal PSA and it remains abnormal, a repeat biopsy may be necessary at a later date. These facts should be explained to the patient again during a follow-up appointment.

The use of prophylactic antibiotics may decrease the incidence of infections. Patients should call the primary care clinician's office for significant rectal bleeding (any bleeding more than just spotting on the toilet paper), for severe hematuria (resulting in passage of clots), for a temperature above 100° F, for inability to void, or for any other change in clinical status.

SUPPLIERS

Bard Biopty cut instruments and needle

Bard Peripheral Technologies
13183 Harland Drive NE
Covington, GA 30014
Phone: 1-770-385-2300
Website: www.bard.com

Note: In the past, Tru-Cut needles were commonly used; however, spring-driven biopsy guns such as the Biopty make it much easier to obtain prostate tissue and are currently the favored instrument. Biopty has also been compared against fine needle aspiration and the studies showed better results as well as higher patient satisfaction with Biopty.

Transrectal ultrasound unit with needle guide

See Chapter 209, Emergency Department and Office Ultrasound, for a list of manufacturers. Most of those manufacturers make TRUSP-SV units with needle guides.

Radiology overreading services

Overread Corp.
3037 Hopyard Road, Suite I
Pleasanton, CA 94588
Phone: 1-888-426-6331
Website: www.overread.com

CPT/BILLING CODE

55700   Biopsy, prostate needle or punch, single or multiple, any approach

ICD-9-CM DIAGNOSTIC CODES

185	Prostate cancer
600	Prostate nodule
600.2	Prostatic hyperplasia, benign
600.9	Prostatism
601.9	Prostatitis
601.0	Prostatitis, acute
601.1	Prostatitis, chronic
790.93	PSA elevated

BIBLIOGRAPHY

Braeckman J, Denis LJ: Prostatic ultrasound and needle biopsy. In Graham SD Jr, editor: *Glenn's urologic surgery,* ed 5, Philadelphia, 1998, Lippincott-Raven.

Catalona WJ, Partin AW, Slawin KM, et al: Use of the percentage of free prostate-specific antigen to enhance differentiation of prostate cancer from benign prostatic disease: a prospective multicenter clinical trial, *JAMA* 279:1542, 1998.

Cooner WH, Mosley BR, Rutherford CL, et al: Prostate cancer detection in a clinical urological practice by ultrasound, digital rectal examination and prostate specific antigen, *J Urol* 143:1146, 1990.

Renfer LG, Kiesling VJ Jr, Kelley J, et al: Digitally-directed transrectal biopsy using Biopty gun versus transrectal needle aspiration: comparison of diagnostic yield and comfort, *Urology* 38(2):108, 1991.

Vallencien G, Prapotnich D, Veillon B, et al: Systematic prostatic biopsies in 100 men with no suspicion of prostate cancer on digital rectal examination, *J Urol* 146:1308, 1991.

WEBSITE

www.nccn.org (National Comprehensive Cancer Network; guidelines are available)

CHAPTER 123

Prostate Massage

Robert E. James
James R. Palleschi

Prostate massage has been used therapeutically and diagnostically in the management of recurrent or chronic prostatitis and prostatodynia. At this time, its primary benefit is in establishing the diagnosis of chronic prostatitis.

INDICATIONS

- Diagnosis of chronic or subacute prostatitis
- In the management of prostatitis and prostatodynia *(infrequent)*

CONTRAINDICATIONS

- Acute prostatitis
- Prostatic abscess
- Significant difficulty voiding

EQUIPMENT

- Examination glove and water-soluble lubricant
- Microscope
- Sterile culture container

PREPROCEDURE PATIENT PREPARATION

Tell the patient that he may have an urge to urinate and may feel rectal pressure for 15 to 60 minutes after prostatic massage. Tell the patient to contact the physician or the nearest emergency room if he experiences chills, myalgia, rigors, or temperature above 101° F.

TECHNIQUE

1. Place the patient in a comfortable position for the prostate examination. A variety of positions may be used: the knee-chest position, left lateral decubitus position, or bent over the examination table. (With this position, the patient should place his elbows on the examination table and spread his heels apart. The patient is thus immobilized, which facilitates the prostate examination and the subsequent massage.) In addition, the patient may assist you in collecting the expressed prostatic fluid by holding the microscope slide below the urethral meatus of the glans penis.

2. Apply a generous amount of lubricant to the anus and to your gloved index finger. The examination will be more comfortable for the patient if he performs a mild Valsalva's maneuver as the finger passes through and into the anal opening. In patients with a high-riding prostate, a Valsalva's maneuver may bring the gland down to the examining finger.

3. For the prostate massage, press the pad of your index finger into the substance of the prostate. Start on the superior and lateral aspect of the prostate and move your index finger toward the midline or median sulcus. Gradually work from the base or superior aspect of the prostate gland down to the inferior portion or apex (Fig. 123-1). This motion is carried out several times bilaterally. Lastly, massage the median furrow, or midaspect, of the prostate gland, from the base to the apex. The prostatic secretions are massaged toward the prostatic urethra. These secretions then pass through the distal urethra and can be collected for microscopic examination and culture and sensitivity if desired. Normally, you need to repeat the prostatic massage for a period of 30 to 90 seconds before any secretions are obtained. The quantity collected may vary from a few drops to 2 to

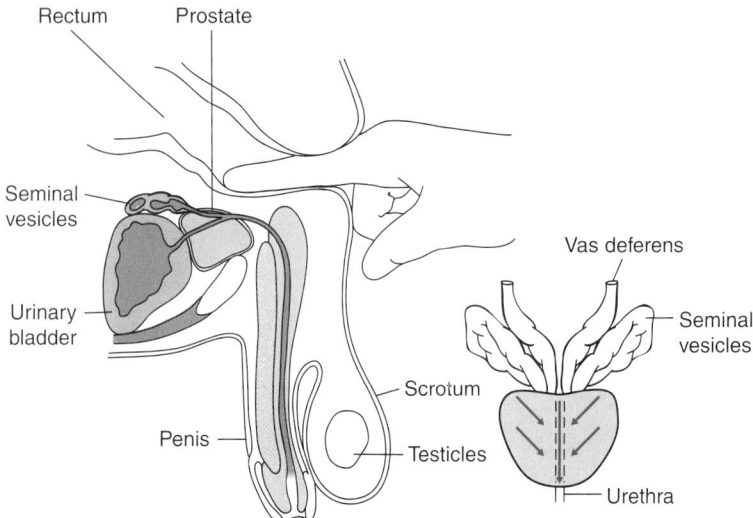

Fig. 123-1
Technique of prostatic massage. The glandular substance is compressed from its lateral edges to the urethra, which lies in the center. (Drawing at right shows direction of pressure.) The seminal vesicles are then stripped from above downward.

3 ml. Some patients will not discharge any secretions (despite correct performance of the prostate massage as described) or may have discomfort sufficient to abort the procedure. Clinically, more than 15 white blood cells per high-power field suggest an infectious process.

COMPLICATIONS

• Rarely, bacteremia or urosepsis may occur after a prostate massage. This can be avoided by not performing prostate massage on a patient suspected of having acute prostatitis or a prostate abscess.
• Occasionally, a patient with significant prostatism resulting from prostatic hypertrophy may develop sufficient prostate edema after a massage, leading to temporary difficulty urinating or urinary retention.
• Hematuria and hematospermia occur infrequently after a prostate massage.

CPT/BILLING CODE

87205   Prostatic smear
There is no CPT code for prostate massage.

ICD-9-CM DIAGNOSTIC CODES

600.0   Prostatitis, hypertrophic
600.9   Prostatitis
601.0   Prostatitis, acute
601.1   Prostatitis, subacute
601.1   Prostatitis, chronic
601.3   Prostatocystitis
601.2   Abscess of prostate (note: avoid prostate massage)
601.9   Prostatitis (congestive)
602.9   Unspecified disorder of prostate, prostatodynia
602.1   Congestion or hemorrhage of prostate

BIBLIOGRAPHY

Tanagho EA: Physical examinations of genitourinary tract. In Tanagho EA, Macaninch JW, editors: *General urology,* Norwalk, Conn, 1988, Lange Medical Publications.

CHAPTER 124

Prostate and Seminal Vesicle Ultrasonography

Philip J. Aliotta

Transrectal ultrasound of the prostate and seminal vesicles (TRUSP-SV) is an essential tool in the assessment of these organs. Useful for defining anatomy, evaluating blood flow, and diagnosing and treating benign and malignant diseases of these glands, it is now the standard in most urologists' practices.

Although TRUSP-SV has proved helpful in the investigation of the infertile couple, more importantly, the introduction of TRUSP-SV has improved the accuracy of prostate tissue sampling (see Chapter 122, Prostate Biopsy). Even though a digital rectal examination (DRE)–guided biopsy may indeed confirm cancer, a negative study without TRUSP-SV cannot definitively exclude cancer. TRUSP-SV improves the ability of the clinician to exclude cancer in all regions of the gland.

One important recent development for TRUSP-SV, especially for underserved areas: technicians or sonographers are now making services available on-site for primary care clinicians. Overreading services for TRUSP-SV by a radiologist are now also available over the Internet (see the "Suppliers" section). This may revolutionize the management of suspected prostate cancer. However, an understanding of anatomy is necessary before scanning. The prostate can be described by its general anatomy, zonal anatomy, tissue anatomy, or ultrasound anatomy.

GENERAL ANATOMY (Fig. 124-1)

Prostate

The prostate is a chestnut-shaped gland surrounded by a pseudocapsule of dense fibrous tissue and smooth muscle that connects with the muscular layers of the prostatic urethra. The pseudocapsule cannot be separated from the gland itself. It has an anterior, posterior, and lateral surface. The prostate base is contiguous with the bladder superiorly. The apex of the prostate is contiguous with the striated urethral sphincter. Lateral to the prostate is the pubococcygeal portion of the levator

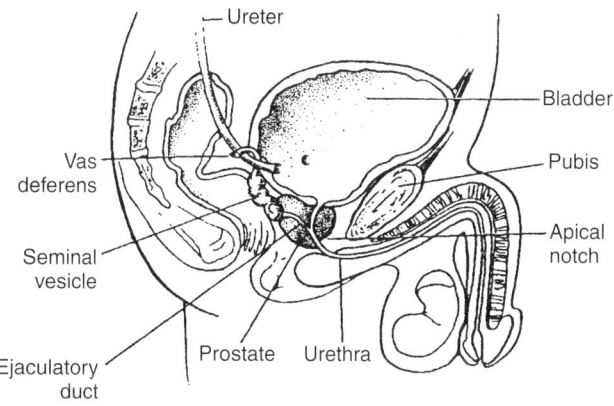

Fig. 124-1
General anatomy of prostate and seminal vesicles. (From Brooks JD: Anatomy of the lower urinary tract and male genitalia. In Walsh PC, Retik AB, Vaughn ED Jr, Wein AJ, editors: *Campbell's urology,* ed 7, Philadelphia, 1998, WB Saunders.)

ani and endopelvic fascia. Denonvilliers' fascia, which separates the prostate from the rectum, is posterior to the prostate.

Vas Deferens and Seminal Vesicles

Arising from the tail of the epididymis, the vas deferens consists of a tortuous proximal portion and a dilated terminal portion called the ampulla. The ampulla is capable of storing sperm and lies posterior to the bladder. Superior to and bordering the base of the bladder, posteriorly, are the seminal vesicles. They also lie adjacent to the ampullae of the vasa deferentia and the distal ureters.

ZONAL ANATOMY

Traditionally, the prostate was divided into five major lobes (anterior, middle, posterior, and two lateral lobes) and two minor lobes (trigonal and subcervical lobes).

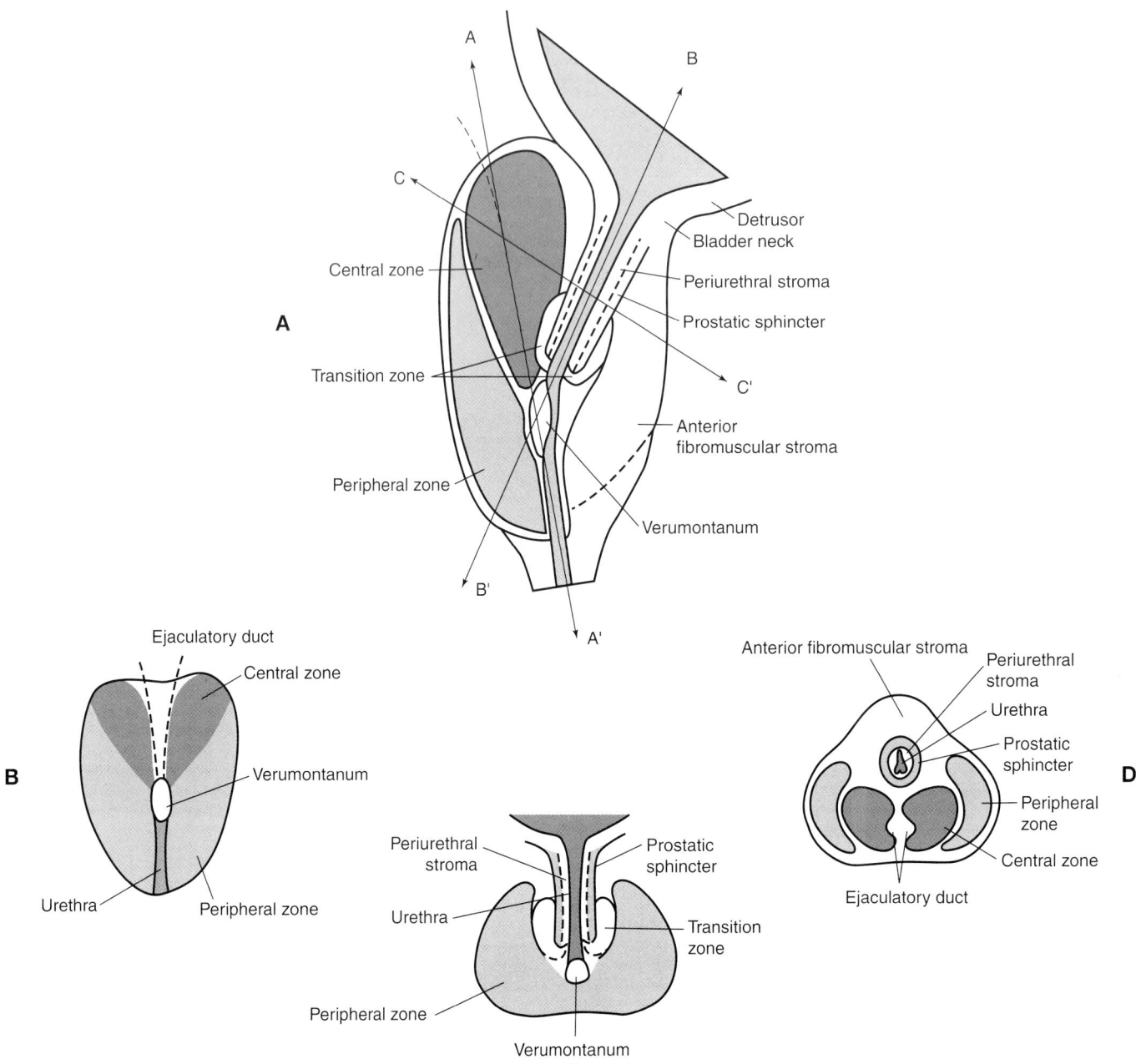

Fig. 124-2
A, Midsagittal plane. **B,** Coronal section (through the plane A-A' in **A**). **C,** Oblique coronal section (through the plane B-B' in **A**). **D,** Transverse section (through the plane C-C' in **A**). (**A,** Redrawn from McNeal JE: *Urology* 17[suppl]:11, 1981. **B-D,** Redrawn from Muldoon LD, Resnick MI: Normal anatomy of the prostate. In Resnick MI: *Prostatic ultrasonography,* Philadelphia, 1990, BC Decker.)

McNeal derived a three-dimensional model of the prostate, as illustrated in Fig. 124-2.

TISSUE ANATOMY

The normal prostate consists of a combination of *glandular tissue* and *fibromuscular structures*.

Glandular Tissue

Glandular tissue accounts for roughly 66% of the prostate. There are four identified glandular zones, each with a distinct ductal system draining into a specific part of the urethra. These first three zones share similar histologic and embryologic origin. The fourth zone is the central zone (CZ) and differs histologically from the rest of the gland. It is derived from the Wolffian duct.

1. *Peripheral zone (PZ) (less than 75% of the glandular tissue).* The largest area of glandular tissue comprising the lateral and most of the posterior aspect of the prostate except at the base is in the PZ. The PZ ducts drain into the distal urethral segment. The majority (greater than 65%) of prostate cancers occur in the PZ.
2. *Transition zone (TZ) (5% or more of the glandular tissue).* Between 5% and 10% of the glandular tissue is in the TZ. The TZ comprises two small lobules on either side of the proximal urethral segment just lateral to the periprostatic sphincter. The TZ is the site of origin of most of the symptomatic benign prostatic hyperplasia (BPH) and approximately 20% of carcinomas.
3. *Periurethral glands (PUG) (1% or more of the glandular tissue).* These glands are embedded in the smooth muscle wall of the urethra entirely within the preprostatic sphincter. Involved in the BPH process, these glands can give rise to an enlarged middle lobe.
4. *Central zone (CZ) (less than 25% of the glandular tissue).* The CZ is cone shaped and surrounds the ejaculatory ducts. The major distinction between the CZ and the PZ is that the CZ is relatively resistant to the development of cancer. Only 10% of cancers occur in the CZ. Interestingly, BPH does not occur within the CZ.

Fibromuscular Structures

Fibromuscular structures make up 33% of the prostate. There are four fibromuscular structures:
1. Anterior fibromuscular stroma (AFS)
   - A continuation of the detrusor muscle
   - Covers the anterior and anterolateral aspects of the glandular tissue from base to apex
2. Preprostatic sphincter (PPS)
   - Smooth muscle fibers of the lower ureters and superficial trigone
   - Intimately related to the TZ
   - Prevents pooling of urine in the proximal segment of the urethra
   - Prevents retrograde ejaculation
3. Postprostatic sphincter (POPS)
   - The proximal extension of the striated external urethral sphincter muscle covering the anterior and lateral aspects of the distal urethra
   - Contributes to continence
4. Longitudinal smooth muscle (LSM)
   - Part of the urethra.

The key to understanding prostate tissue anatomy is to understand the anatomy of the prostatic urethra, which is approximately 3 cm long. It should be used as a primary reference point. Proximally, the prostatic urethra takes a sharp 35-degree anterior angulation with its posterior wall. The point of angulation divides the urethra into its proximal and distal urethral segments. The proximal urethral segment is related to two tiny glandular regions, the TZ and PUG, and to the preprostatic sphincter. The verumontanum lies solely in the distal segment. In addition, the distal urethral segment is related to the function of ejaculation. The ejaculatory ducts and the excretory ducts (PZ and CZ) empty into the distal urethral segment.

ULTRASOUND ANATOMY

(For definitions of *hyperechoic, isoechoic,* and *hypoechoic,* see the "Interpretation" section.)

With ultrasound, the anatomy is divided into two general areas that are immediately obvious to the examiner:
1. The outer area, or *outer gland,* is close to the rectum and generally described as isoechoic.
2. The inner area, or *inner gland,* is more hypoechoic in appearance.

Composition of the Inner and Outer Glands

Inner Gland
- Anterior fibromuscular stroma
- Preprostatic sphincter
- Periurethral glands
- Longitudinal smooth muscle
- Postprostatic sphincter

Outer Gland
- Transition zone
- Central zone
- Peripheral zone

BASIC ULTRASOUND PHYSICS

Ultrasound imaging is based on the "pulse echo" principle, whereby a short burst of ultrasound is emitted from a transducer and directed into the tissue. Echoes are produced as a result of the interaction of sound with tissue, and some of these echoes travel back to the transducer. By timing the period elapsed between the emission of the pulse and the reception of the echo, the distance between the transducer and the echo-producing structure can be calculated and an image formed. (See Chapter 209, Emergency Department and Office Ultrasound.)

Sound consists of longitudinal vibrations that propagate through a medium such as water or soft tissue. It consists of the repetitive (or periodic) production of such compressions, which travel in regular succession. The number of compressions produced each second is the *frequency* (measured in Hertz [Hz]), and the distance between successive compressions, which depends on the speed at which the sound travels in the medium, is the *wavelength* (measured in millimeters). Tissues that are very elastic, dense, or compressible tend to transmit sound waves through them. Inelastic, less dense, or noncompressible tissues tend to reflect the sound waves.

Gain adjustment refers to the amount of amplification applied to a returning echo signal. *Contrast and brightness* adjustments can also be made to provide a homogeneous midrange echo pattern of the normal peripheral zone.

Sound Frequency

The characteristics of sound transmission are as follows:
- The lower the frequency, the longer the wavelength.
- The higher the frequency, the shorter the wavelength.
- The lower the frequency of sound, the greater the ability to penetrate tissue, but the poorer the quality (resolution) of the ultrasound picture obtained.
- The higher the sound frequency, the poorer the tissue penetration by sound, but the better the quality of the picture.

There is an ideal frequency for imaging the prostate, which is about 7 MHz. A 10-MHz probe shows only the part of the prostate closest to the rectum, whereas a 3-MHz probe, with its lower frequency, delivers higher penetration but poorer quality imaging (Fig. 124-3).

INDICATIONS

- Evaluation of a palpable prostatic nodule or induration
- Suspicion of prostatic abscess

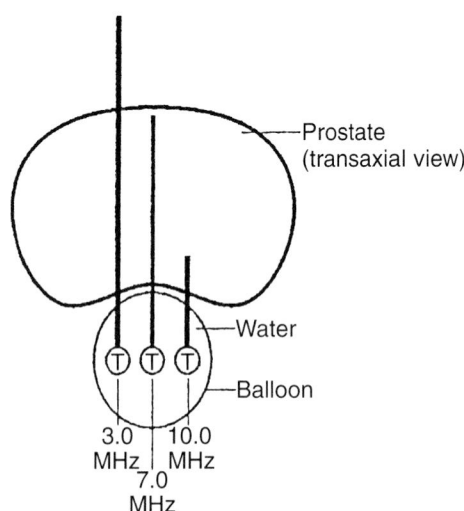

Fig. 124-3
Ideal frequency for imaging the prostate is about 7 MHz. (From Cooner WH: Physical principles of prostate ultrasonography. In Stamey TA, editor: *Monographs in urology,* Montverde, Fla, 1990, Medical Directions Publishing.)

- Azoospermia
- Brachytherapy
- Abnormal prostate specific antigen (PSA) (Fig. 122-1 shows an algorithm combining PSA, free PSA, PSA velocity, and TRUSP-SV):
  - Elevated PSA (greater than 4.0 ng/ml)
  - Low free PSA II (less than 25%) in individual with PSA in the range of 4 to 10 ng/ml
  - Elevated PSA velocity (greater than 0.75 ng/ml rise in PSA per year)
  - Elevated PSA density (greater than 0.15 ng/ml)
- Prostatitis
  - Acute
  - Chronic
  - Chronic pelvic pain syndrome
  - Prostatitis with an elevated PSA
- Prostate volume study
- Prostate cancer staging
- Detection of posttreatment prostate cancer recurrence
- Prostatic intraepithelial neoplasia (PIN) on prior biopsy
- Adenosis on prior biopsy

Note: In the patient with cancer, when attempting to determine the extent of local disease, TRUSP-SV is generally restricted to determining whether the tumor has invaded the seminal vesicles or not.

CONTRAINDICATIONS

- Bleeding disorders
- Anticoagulant therapy
- Significant rectal disease:
  - Obstructing lesions
  - Fissures
  - Thrombosed hemorrhoids
  - Proctitis
- Untreated bacterial urinary tract infection
  - Cystitis
  - Prostatitis

Note: If a hypoechoic area is seen on transrectal ultrasonography (TRUSP-SV), it probably should be biopsied, regardless of PSA. Therefore some experts warn against performing TRUS unless a biopsy is indicated. It should probably not be used for screening. The primary role of ultrasound is to ensure accurate sampling of any lesions and of the entire gland during biopsy.

PREPROCEDURE PATIENT PREPARATION

1. Serum PSA on record
2. Documented DRE
3. Informed consent
4. Fleet enema 1 to 2 hours before the procedure

5. Fluoroquinolone therapy:
   a. The author prefers a 3-day regimen using a quinolone the day before, the day of, and, if a biopsy is performed, the day after.
   b. For patients undergoing repeat TRUSP-SV and biopsy (for persistent abnormalities in PSA despite negative biopsies and normal DRE), use a 5-day protocol of quinolone therapy, extending the quinolone for 3 days after the biopsy. Also, add metronidazole 500 mg twice a day by mouth for 3 days after the biopsy.
6. Patient vital signs before procedure
7. Patient positioning options:
   a. Knee-chest
   b. Lithotomy
   c. Left-lateral decubitus with knees flexed 90 degrees

EQUIPMENT

Types of Prostate Ultrasound

- Transabdominal
- Transperineal
- Endourethral
- Transrectal (with and without color flow Doppler enhancement)

Types of Transducer Design

- Radial array (with cephalocaudad or right-to-left oscillation)
- Linear array (piezoelectric crystals are placed in a line, and each crystal fires and receives echoes in sequential order)

Recent advancements in ultrasound technology have resulted in the following:
- The development of biplanar probe transducers
- The development of a single probe to image the gland in both the transverse and sagittal planes
- A single probe that can have:
  - Two perpendicularly positioned transducers,
  - A single transducer that can rotate, or an
  - End-fire transducer that can provide a transverse and sagittal view by rotating the probe 90 degrees.

TECHNIQUE

General Principles

- The performance of prostate ultrasonography requires the examiner to know which aspects of the procedure are operator dependent so that the best possible study can be obtained. No mandatory technical standards exist for performance of prostatic ultrasound.

The examination sequence remains a matter of personal preference. Practitioners should develop a technique that is reproducible and with which they are comfortable.
- Prostate ultrasonography and examination should be carried out in at least two planes:
  a. Transaxial-transverse (across the long axis). Images from this orientation offer several advantages in the assessment of the prostate:
     i. Increased information about the lateral margins
     ii. Assessment of capsular integrity
     iii. Accurate volume assessment
  b. Longitudinal-sagittal (parallel to the body axis or long axis). Images from this orientation provide more information about the apex and base of the prostate and facilitate biopsy.

Procedure

1. Perform a DRE before insertion of the probe. This serves many purposes:
   a. Dilates the anal sphincter, reducing the discomfort from probe insertion.
   b. Assesses the gland for size, shape, and areas of irregularity or suspicion. This enables the sonographer to associate what he or she feels with what is being viewed during the study.
   c. Rules out a rectal obstructive process of either benign or malignant etiology.
2. Position the patient. Various positions will work, but the left lateral decubitus position is comfortable for the patient and will reduce bowel gas interference.
3. Have the patient perform a slight Valsalva's maneuver during probe insertion to relax the sphincter and to further facilitate probe insertion.
4. After insertion, while scanning in the transaxial mode, advance the probe to the level of the seminal vesicles. Making parallel images (cuts), scan from superior to inferior. Examination of the seminal vesicles should focus on the following:
   a. Symmetry
   b. Size
   c. Echo pattern
   d. Mass
   e. Cystic changes
   Because the seminal vesicles do not always lie symmetrically in the body, it is occasionally difficult to comment on their symmetry on a cut-by-cut basis. Often they must be studied and their images interpreted as they appear in their entirety (Fig. 124-4). If prostate cancer is present, it is important to determine whether there has been local invasion to the seminal vesicles.
5. From the seminal vesicles, the probe is withdrawn to the level of the base of the prostate and imaging includes all areas from the base to the apex. Evaluate

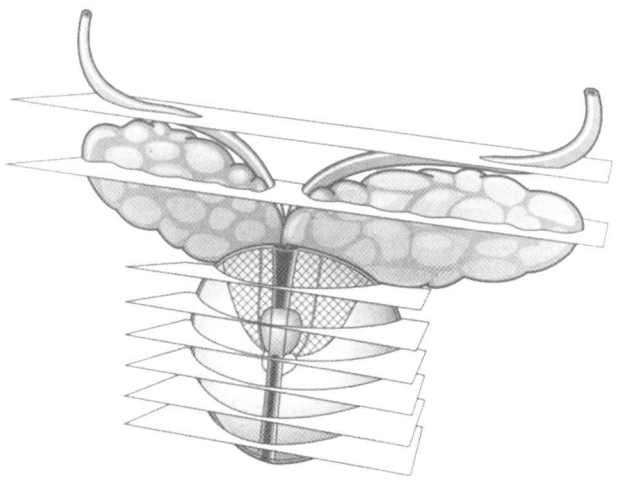

Fig. 124-4
Ultrasonographic examination of the seminal vesicles and prostate using parallel images from superior to inferior. (From Rifkin MD: *Ultrasound of the prostate: imaging in the diagnosis and therapy of prostatic disease,* ed 2, Philadelphia, 1997, Lippincott-Raven.)

the prostate for symmetry, its lateral margins, and the integrity of the capsule. Assess the inner and outer gland for irregularities. The periprostatic "environment" is also assessed at this time.

Normal peripheral zone echogenicity represents the *baseline* or is *isoechoic*. Any lesion that is less echogenic is labeled *hypoechoic;* anything giving rise to more echoes is *hyperechoic.*

6. Prostate biopsy

Outer gland lesion: The needle is placed just in front of the lesion before penetration of the capsule.

Inner gland lesion: The biopsy needle must first penetrate the capsule and outer gland.

7. Volume determination should be performed. Various software applications or technical features of individual ultrasound machines enable the examiner to estimate prostate volume.

Special case: Ultrasound and biopsy of a man without a rectum: this requires transperineal ultrasound in conjunction with magnetic resonance imaging (MRI). The MRI defines the areas of suspicion as a region of low signal intensity on T2-weighted sequences. Transperineal ultrasound helps localize the area of the prostate but seldom demonstrates the specific lesion.

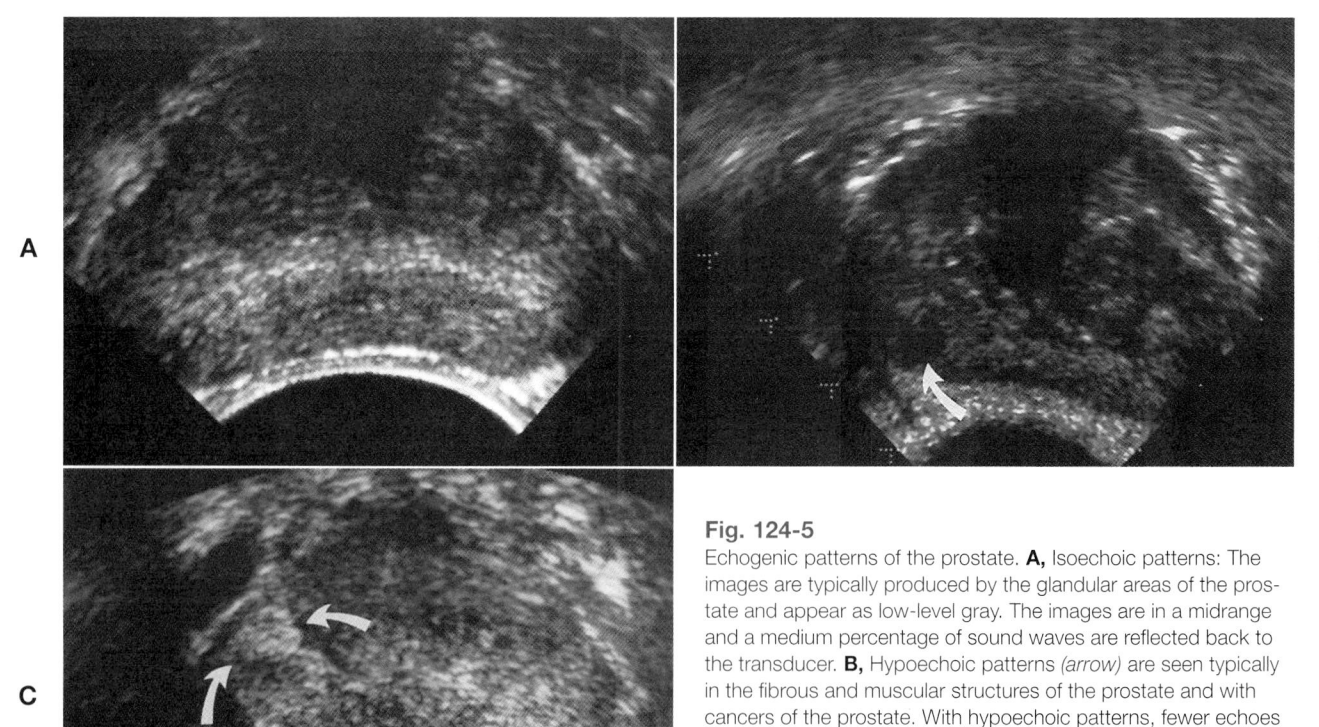

Fig. 124-5
Echogenic patterns of the prostate. **A,** Isoechoic patterns: The images are typically produced by the glandular areas of the prostate and appear as low-level gray. The images are in a midrange and a medium percentage of sound waves are reflected back to the transducer. **B,** Hypoechoic patterns *(arrow)* are seen typically in the fibrous and muscular structures of the prostate and with cancers of the prostate. With hypoechoic patterns, fewer echoes are reflected back and more actually pass through the tissues, making them appear darker. **C,** Hyperechoic patterns *(arrows)* result when more sound waves are reflected back to the transducer, producing images that are light gray to white. The periprostatic fat is hyperechoic, as are some cancers. (From Rifkin MD: *Ultrasound of the prostate: imaging in the diagnosis and therapy of prostatic disease,* ed 2, Philadelphia, 1997, Lippincott-Raven.)

INTERPRETATION AND EVALUATION OF THE PROSTATE

Interpretation

From the prostate, three types of echogenic pattern are described: isoechoic (Fig. 124-5, *A*), hypoechoic (Fig. 124-5, *B*), and hyperechoic (Fig. 124-5, *C*). Unfortunately, no single finding on ultrasound permits universal distinction between cancer and benign conditions. However, most cancers are hypoechoic. Cancers less than 5 to 7 mm, those that are well differentiated, and those located in the TZ are difficult to distinguish from normal prostate.

Evaluation

1. General appearance
2. Inner gland status
3. Outer gland status
4. Anterior prostate status
5. Any focal intraprostatic abnormalities
6. Status of the internal architecture
   a. Normal
   b. Disrupted
7. Integrity of capsule
8. Urethral position
9. Focal lesion(s)
   a. Number
   b. Location
   c. Echogenic pattern: hypoechogenic, isoechogenic, hyperechogenic, mixed, anechoic
   d. Margin of the focus: well defined, poorly defined
   e. Calculi
   f. Cysts
10. Ejaculatory duct status
    a. Normal
    b. Dilated
    c. Infiltrated
11. Neurovascular bundles present?
12. Lymph nodes visible?
13. Seminal vesicles
    a. Overall, symmetric or asymmetric
    b. Size
    c. Shape
    d. Echo pattern
    e. Cystic changes
    f. Solid mass effect
14. Rectal wall integrity

COMPLICATIONS

- Rectal bleeding from the following:
  - Hemorrhoidal vessels
  - Rectal wall laceration
  - Arterial-venous malformation
- Hematuria
- Hematospermia
- Urinary retention
- Urosepsis
- Bacteremia
- Needle tract seeding of cancer
- Vasovagal response with or without seizure

POSTPROCEDURE PATIENT EDUCATION

Postprocedure vital signs should be performed and fluids offered or provided (e.g., sport drink or fruit juice). The findings and any instructions should be reviewed with the patient. A follow-up appointment should be made. The patient should call the facility for difficulty urinating, rectal bleeding, high fever, or further questions.

SUPPLIERS

Transrectal Ultrasound Units with Needle Guides
Available from most ultrasound manufacturers (see Chapter 209, Emergency Department and Office Ultrasound, for a list of manufacturers).

Radiology Overreading Services
Overread Corp.
3037 Hopyard Road, Suite I
Pleasanton, CA 94588
Phone: 1-888-426-6331
Website: www.overread.com

Probes and Scans
See Figs. 124-6 to 124-11.

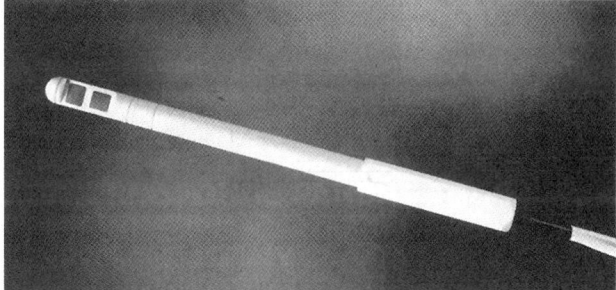

Fig. 124-6
Biplane probe. (From Rifkin MD: *Ultrasound of the prostate: imaging in the diagnosis and therapy of prostatic disease,* ed 2, Philadelphia, 1997, Lippincott-Raven.)

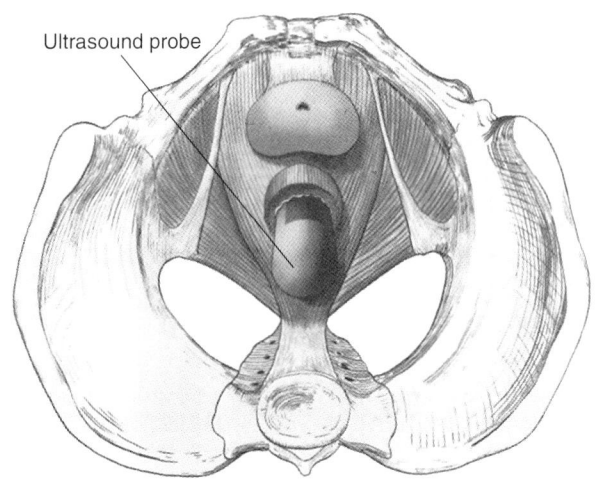

Fig. 124-7
Endorectal scan. (From Rifkin MD: *Ultrasound of the prostate: imaging in the diagnosis and therapy of prostatic disease,* ed 2, Philadelphia, 1997, Lippincott-Raven.)

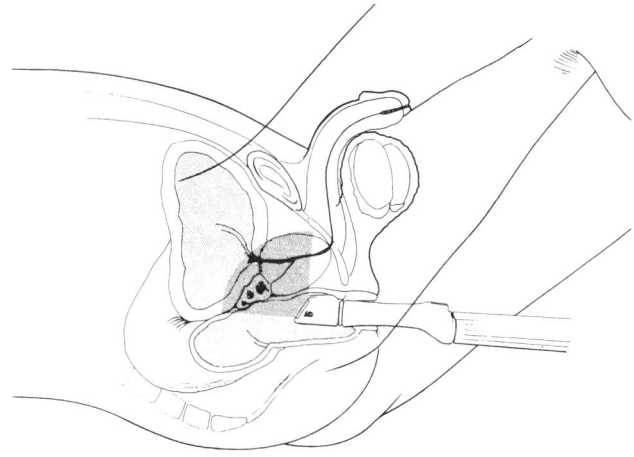

Fig. 124-9
Oblique end-fire scanning. (From Rifkin MD: *Ultrasound of the prostate: imaging in the diagnosis and therapy of prostatic disease,* ed 2, Philadelphia, 1997, Lippincott-Raven.)

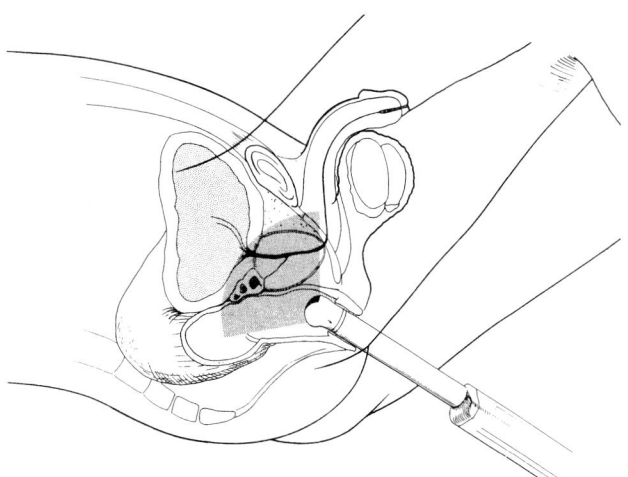

Fig. 124-8
Oblique end-fire endorectal probe. (Modified from Rifkin MD: *Ultrasound of the prostate: imaging in the diagnosis and therapy of prostatic disease,* ed 2, Philadelphia, 1997, Lippincott-Raven.)

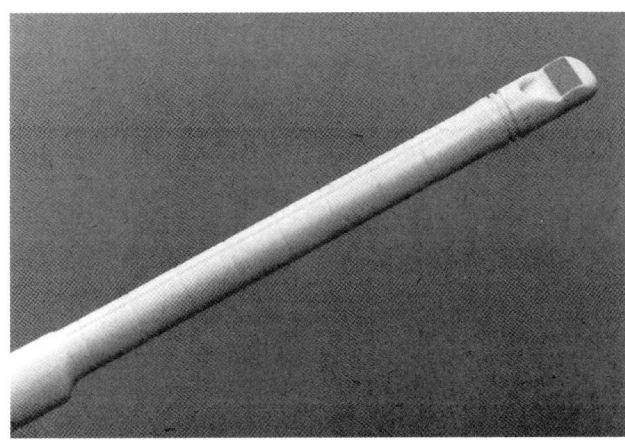

Fig. 124-10
Side-fire probe. (From Rifkin MD: *Ultrasound of the prostate: imaging in the diagnosis and therapy of prostatic disease,* ed 2, Philadelphia, 1997, Lippincott-Raven.)

CPT/BILLING CODES

76942	Ultrasonic guidance for needle biopsy, radiologic supervision, and interpretation
76872	Echocardiography, transrectal
55700	Prostate biopsy; needle or punch, single or multiple, any approach

ICD-9-CM DIAGNOSTIC CODES

600	Prostate nodule
185	Prostate cancer
601.0	Prostatitis, acute
601.1	Prostatitis, chronic
608.83	Hemospermia
236.5	Neoplasm of uncertain origin

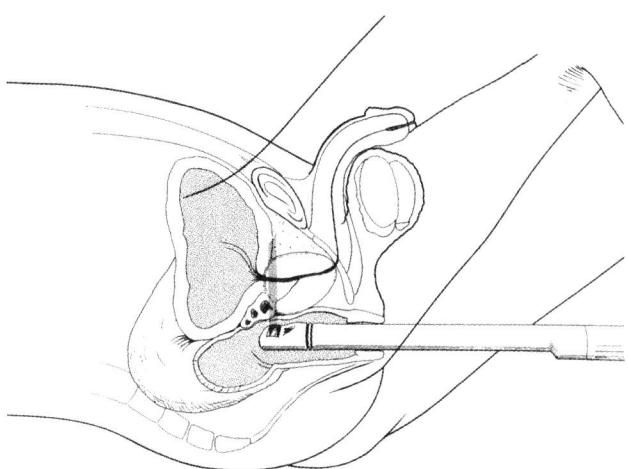

Fig. 124-11
Side-fire scanning. (From Rifkin MD: *Ultrasound of the prostate: imaging in the diagnosis and therapy of prostatic disease,* ed 2, Philadelphia, 1997, Lippincott-Raven.)

ADDITIONAL RESOURCES

- See the sample patient education handout titled "Prostate Ultrasound and Biopsy" on page 1891 of Appendix G.
- See the sample patient consent form titled "Transrectal Ultrasound of the Prostate With or Without Biopsy" on page 1892 of Appendix G.

BIBLIOGRAPHY

Brawer MK: Techniques of examination in prostatic ultrasonography. In Resnick MI, editor, *Prostatic ultrasonography,* Philadelphia, 1990, BC Decker.

Brawer MK, Chetner MP: Ultrasonography of the prostate and biopsy. In Walsh PC, Retik AB, Vaughan ED Jr, Wein AJ, editors: *Campbell's urology,* ed 7, Philadelphia, 1998, WB Saunders.

Brooks JD: Anatomy of the lower urinary tract and male genitalia. In Walsh PC, Retik AB, Vaughan ED Jr, Wein AJ, editors: *Campbell's urology,* ed 7, Philadelphia, 1998, WB Saunders.

Cooner WH: Physical principles of prostate ultrasonography, *Monogr Urol* 11(2):18, 1990.

Kaye KW: Ultrasound of the normal prostate, *Contemp Urol* 3(7):64, 1991.

McNeal JE: The prostate gland: morphology and pathology, *Monogr Urol* 9(3):36, 1988.

Muldoon LD, Resnick MI: Normal anatomy of the prostate. In Resnick MI, editor, *Prostatic ultrasonography,* Philadelphia, 1990, BC Decker.

Rifkin MD: *Ultrasound of the prostate: imaging in the diagnosis and therapy of prostatic disease,* ed 2, Philadelphia, 1997, Lippincott-Raven. (This book is a must-read for the individual serious about prostate ultrasonography.)

CHAPTER 125

Self-Injection Therapy for the Treatment of Erectile Dysfunction

Robert E. James
James R. Palleschi

Significant advances have been made in the diagnosis and treatment of erectile dysfunction. Although the introduction of oral drugs has decreased the need and the use of injection therapy, it is still indicated in some patients. The self-injection of vasoactive agents into the corpora cavernosa now enables many patients to resume satisfactory sexual activities without surgery. The last two medications approved by the Food and Drug Administration (FDA) for the treatment of impotence are alprostadil (Caverject [powder for injection], Edex [powder for injection], and MUSE [urethral suppository]) and oral sildenafil citrate (Viagra). Alprostadil is prostaglandin E_1 (PGE_1). In the near future, two additional oral medications for the treatment of impotence will be reviewed by the FDA: tadalafil and vardenafil.

Sildenafil citrate (Viagra) is most effective in patients with mild-to-moderate impotence. This would include men who are able to obtain a good erection but cannot maintain it and those men who have an erection that is at least a 5 out of 10 in rigidity, where 10 is defined as the best erection they can remember.

The transurethral form of alprostadil (MUSE) was approved by the FDA in 1996 for the treatment of impotence. It is most effective in men who have difficulty maintaining an erection, and in those who have a partial erection, or 5 out of 10 in rigidity.

Despite the advances in the treatment of erectile dysfunction, vacuum erection devices remain an attractive option or adjunct. These devices are attractive to patients who have failed oral therapy and decline or fail intraurethral or intracavernosal alprostadil. Patients using intracavernosal therapy who want to have intercourse more than three times a week usually meet their goal by using vacuum erection devices. (See Chapter 128, Vacuum Devices for Erectile Dysfunction.)

In the treatment of moderate to severe erectile dysfunction, intracavernosal therapy with vasoactive agents still has a very important role.

In July of 1995 the FDA approved *injectable alprostadil (PGE_1)* for the treatment of organic erectile dysfunction. The American Urological Association's guidelines for the treatment of erectile dysfunction recommend alprostadil as the drug of choice, and it is the only intracavernosal vasoactive agent approved by the FDA.

There is also *papaverine hydrochloride,* a nonspecific smooth muscle relaxant. In addition to alprostadil, which is a vasodilator and a smooth muscle relaxant, papaverine hydrochloride may be used with *phentolamine mesylate,* a smooth muscle relaxant that enhances the effect of papaverine. For several years these agents have been used extensively for impotence, although this remains an unlabeled indication.

These vasoactive agents induce an erection by increasing arterial blood flow, relaxing the sinusoidal spaces within the cavernosal tissue, and increasing venous resistance. An excellent erection that lasts for 30 to 90 minutes usually occurs in patients with mild to moderate arterial insufficiency, mild to moderate venous incompetence, psychogenic impotence, neurogenic impotence, and medication-induced impotence.

INDICATIONS

- Impotence resulting from arterial insufficiency
- Impotence resulting from mild to moderate venous incompetence
- Psychogenic impotence (Patients with performance anxiety may be treated with counseling, oral agents, short-term intracavernosal agents, or a combination of these.)
- Neurogenic impotence
- Medication-induced impotence, when drug therapy cannot be altered or terminated
- Diagnostic erection
- Intolerance to or ineffective oral drugs

CONTRAINDICATIONS

- Blood dyscrasia, coagulation disorder, or anticoagulation drug therapy
- Unstable cardiovascular disease
- Impaired manual dexterity or vision
- Presence of a prosthetic penile device
- Valvular heart disease
- Intolerance to the test dose of the vasoactive agent
- Patients taking monoamine oxidase (MAO) inhibitors
- Patients with a propensity toward secondary forms of priapism, such as individuals with sickle cell disease or trait, leukemia, and multiple myeloma

Although many urologists use intracavernosal pharmacotherapy for the treatment of erectile dysfunction in men with Peyronie's disease who have mild-to-moderate penile curvature, this is listed on the alprostadil (Caverject) insert as an exclusion at this time. If a physician elects to use this treatment in men with Peyronie's disease, a special informed consent is advised.

EQUIPMENT

- 1- to 3-ml syringes with ½-inch, 27- and 30-gauge needles
- Alcohol swabs
- Vasoactive agents

Papaverine HCl 30 mg/ml is available in 10-ml multidose vials.

Papaverine and phentolamine solution: Inject 5 mg (or 10 mg) of phentolamine (Regitine) into a 100-ml vial of papaverine 30 mg/ml. The (approximate) concentrations will be papaverine 30 mg/ml and phentolamine 0.5 or 1.0 mg/ml.

PGE₁ (alprostadil) is also available in 1-ml ampules from Upjohn as Prostin VR Pediatric 500 μg/ml. For the desired concentration, inject 0.2 ml of this preparation into each of five 10-ml vials of bacteriostatic normal saline for injection. Each vial will contain PGE_1 10 μg/ml.

Alprostadil: Both Caverject and Edex come in a prepackaged, single use kit, containing the diluent, alprostadil, needles, syringe, and alcohol swabs.

Open vials or compounded solutions should be refrigerated to maintain sterility and effectiveness. A 30-day expiration date is recommended; however, sufficient effectiveness has been reported for up to 3 months.

Antidote for priapism: α-Adrenergic agents will cause vasoconstriction and thus will usually result in prompt detumescence should priapism occur. Some of the available agents include *ephedrine sulfate, epinephrine,* and *phenylephrine hydrochloride* (Neo-Synephrine).

(See the "Treatment of the Persistent Erection [Priapism]" section for dilutions and use.)

PREPROCEDURE PATIENT PREPARATION

Discuss the self-injection program, alternatives, and potential complications with the patient and, when possible, his partner. Patients using this program may experience bruising at the injection site and local or systemic infection (less than 0.05% incidence). Chronic fibrosis at the injection site may occur with repeated injections, and this may result in pain or penile curvature. Papaverine may elevate the results of liver function tests. Consequently, patients should obtain pretreatment liver function tests, and should be retested every 3 months while using papaverine. If the liver function test values begin to rise, the medication should be discontinued. If the initial liver function tests are elevated, use PGE_1 instead of papaverine. Approximately 20% of patients using PGE_1 may experience an ache in the penis that may last for several hours and that may recur with each injection. *Priapism,* an erection lasting longer than 4 hours, may occur in up to 10% of patients receiving any of the vasoactive agents, but it reportedly occurs less frequently with PGE_1. Systemic side effects, such as dizziness and orthostatic hypotension, occur in 2% of patients receiving these vasoactive agents and are believed to be secondary to penile venous incompetence.

Instruct the patient to contact the physician if he experiences a significant erection that persists for more than 4 hours. This will need to be treated promptly to prevent intracorporeal fibrosis and failure to respond to future therapy.

TECHNIQUE

1. Complete the patient's history and physical examination to provide a preliminary diagnosis.
2. Select the agent and the dose. If psychogenic or neurogenic impotence is suspected, use a smaller dose of the vasoactive agent. In patients with psychogenic impotence, one fourth of the maximum dose should be used; and in patients with neurogenic impotence, no more than one sixth of the maximum dose should be used initially. The maximum dose of *papaverine* is 60 mg, and that of PGE_1 is 20 μg. To reduce the risk of priapism and to prevent other untoward reactions, even when vascular disease is suspected as the cause of impotence, the initial dose should not exceed 30 mg of papaverine or 10 μg of PGE_1. If a satisfactory erection does not occur, the

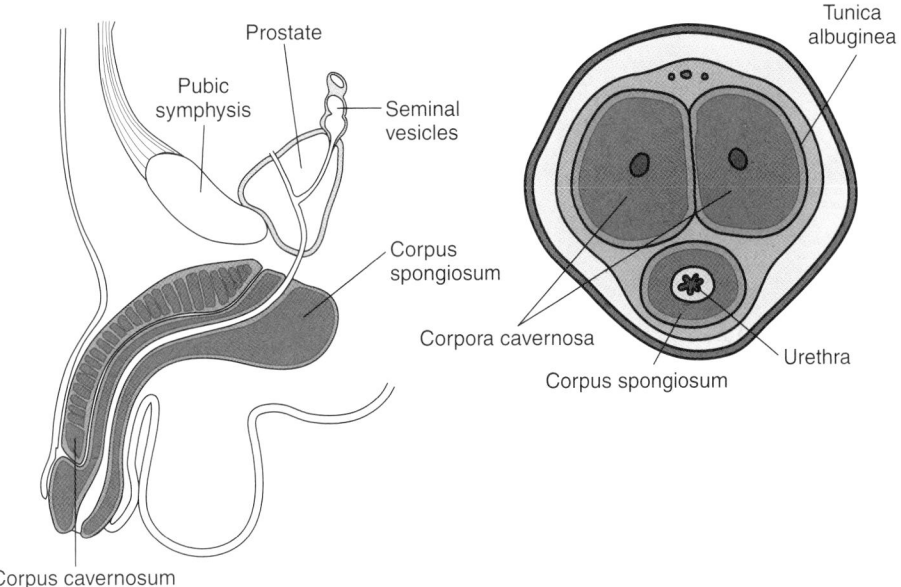

Fig. 125-1
Side view of penis and scrotum *(left)* and cross-sectional view of penis *(right)*.

dose may be appropriately increased at the time of the next office appointment. Although the usual dose of *alprostadil* is between 10 and 20 µg, urologists have used as up to 40 µg in some cases. In patients with psychogenic or neurogenic impotence, you should begin with 2 to 5 µg, and gradually increase the dose as needed. Otherwise, the usual starting dose is 10 µg.

3. Once the desired dose of the vasoactive agent has been selected, extend the patient's penis and prepare the lateral surface with an alcohol swab. Locate the neurovascular bundle at the 12 o'clock position and the urethra at the 6 o'clock position (Figs. 125-1 and 125-2). Select as the injection site an area between these two structures (1 to 5 on the patient's left, 7 to 11 on the patient's right) in which there are no superficial veins. The injection site may be anywhere between the base of the penis and just proximal to the glans penis. It is strongly recommended that only Caverject or Edex be used. With the patient standing, gently direct the penis to the left or the right, to expose its lateral surface. Introduce a 27- or 30-gauge needle perpendicular to the skin and tunica albuginea and into the corpora cavernosum. Normally, the needle is advanced 0.5 inch. Inject the vasoactive agent rapidly as a bolus into the corpus cavernosum. The medication will enter the opposite corpus cavernosum through cross-circulation. If resistance is met as the medication is injected, withdraw the needle slowly as you continue to inject. The resistance normally occurs because the needle is against the opposite wall of the corpus cavernosum.

To prevent injection of the medication into the subcutaneous space, *advance the needle the entire ½ inch and then withdraw slowly.*

4. Once the injection is completed, have the patient apply pressure to the injection site for 2 minutes.

5. Evaluate the condition of the patient periodically during the first 15 minutes following the injection. The patient's comfort, presence of side effects, and the quality of the erection should be evaluated at 15-minute intervals for 30 to 60 minutes. To evaluate the quality of the erection the patient will experience with sexual stimulation, you may ask the patient to apply manual stimulation. The patient may be discharged from the office within 30 to 60 minutes after the injection, provided he is comfortable and not experiencing any side effects. Instruct the patient to contact you if priapism occurs. Once the appropriate dose has been determined and the patient is skilled and comfortable with self-injection therapy, he may perform it independently, but *no more than three times per week.* Priapism rarely occurs after the appropriate dose has been determined, unless the patient independently increases the dose.

Treatment of the Persistent Erection (Priapism)

If the patient does not have significant hypertension or unstable cardiac or cerebrovascular disease, an intracavernosal α-adrenergic agonist is safe and very effective in the treatment of priapism. Priapism is defined as an erection that lasts over 4 hours. Before injecting the

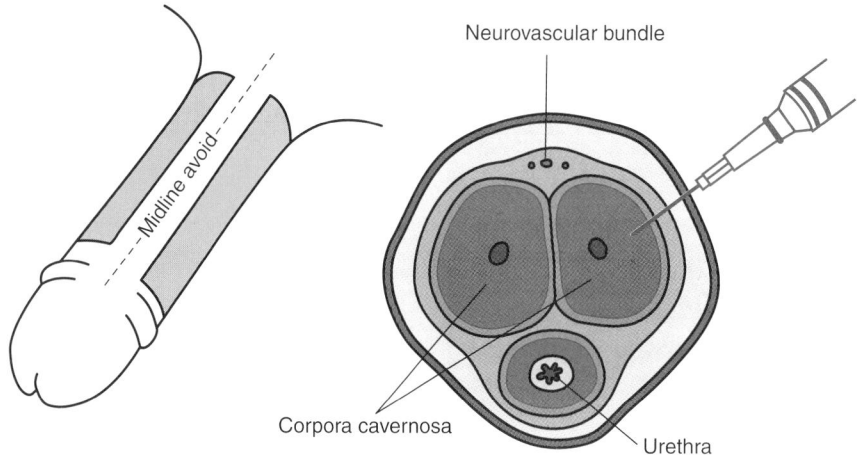

Fig. 125-2
Intracavernous injection site. The clinician grasps the glans and pulls firmly outward to tense penis without rotating.

antidote, you should attempt to treat the priapism by first irrigating blood from the corpora cavernosum with saline. Inject the skin over the aspiration site (shaft of the penis) with 0.5 to 1 ml of local anesthetic (1% to 2% lidocaine). If ineffective, the patient may benefit from a penile block with 1% to 2% xylocaine and intravenous morphine sulfate. Then irrigate using aseptic technique with a 30-ml syringe and a 16- to 18-gauge needle. Insert the needle ½ inch into the midlateral corporal body and irrigate with saline. If the priapism does not resolve with irrigating with 250 to 500 ml of saline, proceed with injection of β-adrenergic agonists.

The following agents may be considered for the treatment of priapism if aspiration and irrigation of blood is unsuccessful:

- *Ephedrine sulfate:* A vial contains 50 mg (25 mg/ml). Initially inject 10 to 25 mg into the corpus cavernosum. If detumescence does not begin within 15 to 30 minutes, the dose may be repeated. A maximum of 50 mg may be given. Ephedrine is the drug of choice because of its efficacy, simplicity, and safety. If ineffective, a urology consult is advised.
- *Epinephrine:* Inject 1 ml of diluted epinephrine (10 to 20 μg/ml) slowly into the corpus cavernosum every 5 to 10 minutes. This may be repeated twice, and if satisfactory detumescence does not occur, a urology consultation should be obtained. (To prepare the proper dilution, use epinephrine 1:10,000 solution. For 10 μg/ml, dilute 0.1 ml of epinephrine with 0.9 ml of normal saline. For 20 μg/ml, dilute 0.2 ml of epinephrine with 0.8 ml of normal saline.)
- *Phenylephrine hydrochloride* (Neo-Synephrine) 1%: Inject 1 ml slowly into the corpus cavernosum every 5 to 10 minutes. If satisfactory detumes-

cence does not occur after the second dose, a urology consultation should be obtained. (To prepare the proper dilution, use phenylephrine hydrochloride 0.1 ml diluted with 0.9 ml of normal saline for 100 μg/ml. Use phenylephrine hydrochloride 0.2 ml diluted with 0.8 ml of normal saline for 200 μg/ml.)

These medications should be given individually and never in combination. Monitor the blood pressure and pulse closely in all patients. Cardiac arrhythmias and significant hypertension may occur. If these measures are ineffective, obtain a urology consultation. Surgical intervention may be required at this time.

Complications

- Priapism (an erection that lasts over 4 hours)
- Infection
- Subcutaneous ecchymosis or hematoma
- Fibrosis to the corpora cavernosum with repeated injections
- Curvature of the penis occurring after repeated injections
- Painful erections
- Dizziness or postural hypotension
- Myocardial infarction, stroke, or both in patients with unstable cardiac or cerebrovascular disease
- Elevated liver function tests (papaverine)

POSTPROCEDURE PATIENT EDUCATION

As many as 50% of men using self-injection therapy will discontinue this treatment within 1 year. This may be for many reasons, including: lack of a suitable partner; fear of needles; inadequate response to therapy; fear of complications; lack of sexual spontaneity; and the desire for alternate therapy, including a permanent solution, such as a penile prosthesis. Consequently the patient should be seen periodically and should be asked about his sexual activity and satisfaction with self-injection therapy.

CPT/BILLING CODE

54235   Injection of corporus cavernosum
54250   Nocturnal tumescence and/or rigidity test

J-CODES

J2440   Papaverine HCl up to 60 mg
J0170   Epinephrine, adrenalin up to 1 ml
J2370   Phenylephrine HCl up to 1 ml
J0270   Alprostadil injection 1.25 μg
J0275   Alprostadil urethral suppository

ICD-9-CM DIAGNOSTIC CODES

302.72   Impotence (sexual, psychogenic)
607.84   Impotence, organic origin NEC

ADDITIONAL RESOURCES

• See the sample patient education handout titled "Self-Injection Therapy for Impotence" on page 1893 of Appendix G.

BIBLIOGRAPHY

Armstrong DK, Convery A, Dinsmore WW: Intracavernosal papaverine and phentolamine for the medical management of erectile dysfunction in a genitourinary clinic, *Int J STD AIDS* 4:214, 1993.

Barada JH, McKimmy RM: Vasoactive pharmacotherapy. In Bennett AH, ed: *Impotence*, Philadelphia, 1994, WB Saunders.

Bennett AH, Carpenter AJ, Barada JH: An improved vasoactive drug combination for a pharmacological erection program, *J Urol* 146:1564, 1991.

Bernard F, Lue TF: The roles of the urologist in patient auto-injection therapy for erectile dysfunction, *Contemp Urol J* 4:21, 1990.

Broderick GA, Lue TF: Treatment of priapism. In Rafer J, editor: *Common problems in infertility and impotence*, St Louis, 1990, Yearbook Medical Publishers.

Bucher A, Mrstik C, Stogermayer F: Therapeutic effect of PGE$_1$ in the treatment of erectile dysfunction, *Aktuel Urol* 21:17, 1990.

Burnett AL et al: Long-term follow-up of patients receiving injection therapy for erectile dysfunction, *Urology* 49:932, 1997.

Corporal Pharmacotherapy for Erectile Dysfunction and Priapism: 1966 monographs in urology, vol 2.

Padma-Nathan H: Erectile dysfunction, *Patient Care* 17(suppl 4):2, 1998.

Floth A, Schramek P: Intracavernous injection of prostaglandin E$_1$ in combination with papaverine: enhanced effectiveness in comparison with papaverine plus phentolamine and prostaglandin E$_1$ alone, *J Urol* 145(1):56, 1991.

Gerber GS, Levine LA: Pharmacological erection program using prostaglandin E$_1$, *J Urol* 146:786, 1991.

Kerfoot WW, Carson CC: Pharmacologically induced erections among geriatric men, *J Urol* 146:1022, 1991.

Kulmala RV, Tamelia TL: Effects of priapism lasting 24 hours or longer caused by intracavernosal injection of vasoactive drugs, *Int J Impot Res* 7(2):131, 1995.

Lee M, Cannon B, Sharifi R: Chart for preparation of dilutions of alpha-adrenergic agonists for intracavernous use in treatment of priapism, *J Urol* 153(4):1182, 1995.

Lewis R: Review of intraurethral suppositories and iontophoresis therapy for erectile dysfunction, *Int J Impot Res* 12(suppl 4):586, 2000.

Lue TF: Priapism after transurethral alprostadil, *J Urol* 15(5):1231, 1999.

Lui S M-C, Lin J S-N: Treatment of impotence: comparison between the efficacy and safety of intracavernous injection of papaverine plus phentolamine (regitine) and prostaglandin E$_1$, *Int J Impotence Res* 1:147, 1990.

Peterson A, Wessells H: Improving prospects for patients with priapism, *Contemp Urol* 14(2):30, 2002.

Sur RL, Kane CJ: Sildenafil citrate-associated priapism, *Urology* 55(6):950, 2000.

Virag R, Shoukry K, Floresco J, et al: Intracavernous self-injection of vasoactive drugs in the treatment of impotence: 8-year experience with 615 cases, *J Urol* 145:287, 1991.

Zorgniotti AW: Pharmacologic erection therapy. In Rafer J, editor: *Common problems in infertility and impotence*, St Louis, 1990, Yearbook Medical Publishers.

WEBSITES

www.caverject.com
www.socsi.com
www.viagra.com

CHAPTER 126

Sperm Banking

James A. Daitch
Anthony J. Thomas, Jr.

The most common malignancies affecting men between 20 and 35 years of age are testicular cancer, Hodgkin's disease, lymphoma, and leukemia. Improved chemotherapeutic and radiation treatment modalities have significantly increased cancer survival in this age group. These treatments, however, can drastically reduce or eliminate a patient's fertility. Persistent azoospermia occurs in approximately 20% to 40% of men treated for testicular cancer, and in 70% of men after combination chemotherapy with mechlorethamine, vincristine, procarbazine, prednisone (or MOPP) for Hodgkin's disease. Presently, there are no methods to predict which men will remain profoundly oligospermic or azoospermic after treatment and which will regain normal spermatogenesis. Patients undergoing radiation therapy, even if administered supradiaphragmatically and with a gonadal shield, may still receive testicular radiation doses high enough to impair fertility. Consequently, therapeutic sperm banking, or cryopreservation, has become an important part of the management of men with malignancies, who may desire to have children in the future.

Successful pregnancy after sperm cryopreservation was first reported in 1953. Follow-up, large-scale studies have demonstrated the safety and efficacy of sperm freezing. There has been no increase in fetal abnormalities reported with the use of cryopreserved sperm when compared with fresh sperm.

Cryopreservation with subsequent thawing does decrease sperm motility by 25% to 50% and may induce structural damage to some of the sperm. Improved cryopreservation methods as well as newer assisted reproductive techniques (ARTs), such as in vitro fertilization (IVF) with intracytoplasmic sperm injection (ICSI), have dramatically improved pregnancy rates using even a few, thawed, cryopreserved sperm. Pregnancy rates may approach 30% per attempt.

INDICATIONS

Sperm cryopreservation should be discussed as a routine part of the therapeutic management of adolescents or adult men with malignancies who may desire to preserve their ability to reproduce. This includes men who will undergo surgery, chemotherapy, or radiation therapy. Many men with malignancies have impaired semen quality even before treatment. If the quality of sperm obtained is poor, simple insemination may not be appropriate. More sophisticated techniques (IVF, ICSI) may be necessary to establish a pregnancy. Discussions with the patient and his family should also address the fate of the cryopreserved sperm if the patient does not survive the disease or if he becomes unable to make decisions for himself.

CONTRAINDICATIONS

Cryopreservation of sperm is not contraindicated in any patient as long as he does not have a disease communicable through his semen. Patients with extremely poor semen quality have the potential to initiate pregnancies using new ARTs. Future developments in cryobiology and ARTs may enable even the most severely impaired stored semen samples to be used effectively when thawed.

Cryopreservation should be performed before the onset of chemotherapy or radiation therapy. After these therapies have been initiated, chromosomal abnormalities in the sperm of these men may increase.

PREPROCEDURE PATIENT PREPARATION

The patient should abstain from ejaculation for 48 hours before collection. If this will significantly delay cancer treatment, abstinence lengths as short as 24 hours can still be used effectively. Patients are asked to complete semen cryopreservation forms (consent forms, the fate of the cryopreserved sperm if the patient does not survive the disease or becomes unable to make decisions for himself, fee schedule), and a blood sample is required to test for sexually transmitted diseases (cytomegalovirus, hepatitis virus, human immunodeficiency virus, human T-cell leukemia virus, and rapid plasma reagin). The patient is provided a sterile collection cup and asked to collect a semen sample by masturbation (at the laboratory where the sperm will be preserved). After collection, abstinence time, collection method, entirety of the collected specimen, and the time of collection are recorded. The specimen and the vials to be used for cryopreservation are then labeled with the patient's name and identification number, and a semen identification form is signed by the patient after he confirms the labeling accuracy. A Polaroid picture of the patient can be taken to provide future positive identification.

Typically, three to six semen samples are collected and cryopreserved. The cost of cryopreservation for three specimens ranges from approximately $700 to $900. Most sperm banks also assess annual storage fees that can range from $40 to $130 for each frozen ejaculate.

CONCLUSION

Sperm cryopreservation is a safe and effective way to help preserve fertility in men before treatment for malignancies or before elective sterilization. Cryopreservation may be the only way to ensure effective reproductive capability after therapy. Physicians should discuss sperm cryopreservation with all young men who are about to begin cancer treatment, since even very poor quality sperm can be preserved for future use with ART.

CPT/BILLING CODE

89259   Sperm cryopreservation

ICD-9-CM DIAGNOSTIC CODES

v26.8   Cryopreservation (procreative management)
606.0   Azoospermia
606.1   Oligospermia

186.9   Testis tumor
208.90   Leukemia
202.80   Lymphoma
201.9   Hodgkin's disease

BIBLIOGRAPHY

Agarwal A, Sidhu RK, Shekarriz M, Thomas AJ Jr: Optimum abstinence time for cryopreservation of semen in cancer patients, *J Urol* 154:86, 1995.

Berthelsen JG, Skakkebaek NE: Gonadal function in men with testis cancer, *Fertil Steril* 39:68, 1983.

Cohen J, Garrisi GJ, Congedo-Ferrara TA, et al: Cryopreservation of single human spermatozoa, *Hum Reprod* 12:994, 1997.

Hallak J, Hendin BN, Thomas AJ Jr, Agarwal A: Investigation of fertilizing capacity of cryopreserved spermatozoa from patients with cancer, *J Urol* 159:1217, 1998.

Khalifa E, Oehninger S, Acosta AA, et al: Successful fertilization and pregnancy outcome in in-vitro fertilization using cryopreserved/thawed spermatozoa from patients with malignant diseases, *Hum Reprod* 7:105, 1992.

Meistrich ML: Potential genetic risks of using semen collected during chemotherapy, *Hum Reprod* 8:8, 1993.

Petersen PM, Giwercman A, Skakkebaek NE, Rorth M: Gonadal function in men with testicular cancer, *Semin Oncol* 25:224, 1998.

Petersen PM, Skakkebaek NE, Rorth M, Giwercman A: Semen quality and reproductive hormones before and after orchiectomy in men with testicular cancer, *J Urol* 161:822, 1999.

Rousseaux S, Sele B, Cozzi J, Chevret E: Immediate rearrangements of human sperm chromosomes following in-vivo radiation, *Hum Reprod* 8:903, 1993.

Witt MA: Sperm banking. In Lipshultz LI, Howards SS: *Infertility in the male*, ed 3, St Louis, 1997, Mosby.

WEBSITES

www.asrm.org (American Society for Reproductive Medicine)
www.resolve.org (RESOLVE: The National Infertility Association)

CHAPTER 127

Implantable Hormone Pellets for Testosterone Deficiency in Adult Men

John Harlan Haynes III

Testosterone is responsible for normal growth and development of male sex organs and maintenance of secondary sex characteristics. As the primary androgenic hormone, its production and secretion are the end product of hormonal and biochemical interactions. Gonadotropin releasing hormone (GnRH) is secreted by the hypothalamus and controls the pituitary secretion of luteinizing hormone (LH) and follicle-stimulating hormone (FSH). LH regulates production of testosterone by the testes, and FSH stimulates spermatogenesis. Testosterone can be converted in the body to either dihydrotestosterone (DHT) by 5-alpha reductase or into estradiol by aromatase. DHT preferentially binds to androgen receptors and becomes the more active form involved in hair growth and sebum production. Estradiol may be important in maintaining libido and bone mass but may contribute to truncal obesity and feminine characteristics.

Testosterone deficiency is common, occurring in 1 in 200 men. The prevalence increases with age as testosterone levels decrease and sex hormone–binding globulin levels increase (causing a further decrease in free or bioavailable testosterone). More than 50% of men over the age of 55 may suffer from low testosterone, increasingly referred to as *andropause*. Treatment should be considered in all men with testosterone deficiency as long as contraindications do not exist. Abnormally low testosterone levels are associated not only with sexual dysfunction, but also with other comorbid conditions such as lipid disorders, cardiovascular disease, insulin insensitivity, osteoporosis, and cognitive and mood changes. Testosterone deficiency may be a cause of sarcopenia, a condition of aging senescence characterized by muscular weakness and atrophy.

In general, there are two basic types of testosterone deficiency:

- *Primary*, or hypergonadotropic, hypogonadism results from primary testicular failure. In this situation, testosterone levels will be low and levels of pituitary gonadotropins (LH and/or FSH) will likely be high-normal or elevated.

- *Secondary*, or hypogonadotropic, hypogonadism is the result of inadequate secretion of pituitary gonadotropins. In addition to a low testosterone level, LH and/or FSH levels will be low or low-normal.

Hypogonadism is defined as a free testosterone level that is below the lower limit of normal for young adult control subjects. Previously, age-related decreases in free testosterone were once accepted as "normal." Currently, they are not considered normal. No agreement exists on the exact normal level of testosterone as men age or the serum testosterone level at which a man loses his sexual function.

The definition of *relative hypogonadism* is also uncertain. Many men have perfectly normal sexual function even if their testosterone levels decline into the age-adjusted lower normal range. Patients with low-normal to subnormal range testosterone levels warrant a clinical trial of testosterone. The threshold of response to and dosage of testosterone varies with age. If LH is increased and the testosterone level is low, the patient will have decompensated primary testicular failure. Testosterone replacement therapy is then essential.

An effect of testosterone on endothelial function in men is supported by a recent study that reported on the effects of intravascular administration of physiologic doses of testosterone on coronary blood flow in men with coronary artery disease. The results showed an increase in coronary vasodilation and blood flow in the testosterone test subjects.

HEALTH IMPLICATIONS OF TESTOSTERONE DEFICIENCY

Testosterone deficiency can result in the following:
- Anemia
- Decreases in or loss of libido and erectile function
- Absence or regression of secondary sexual characteristics
- Oligospermia or azoospermia

BOX 127-1

Testosterone Deficiency Screening

The "low testosterone syndrome" often seen in healthy older men is thought to play a role in a number of clinical problems occurring in the growing elderly male population. A checklist has been developed to help heighten awareness of the presence of testosterone deficiency in the older male. Physicians may find the following questions helpful in screening their older patients.

Screening Questions

1. Do you have a decrease in libido (sex drive)?
2. Do you have a lack of energy?
3. Do you have a decrease in strength or endurance?
4. Have you lost height?
5. Have you noticed a decreased "enjoyment of life"?
6. Are you sad or grumpy?
7. Are your erections less strong?
8. Have you noted a recent deterioration in your ability to play sports?
9. Are you falling to sleep after dinner?
10. Has there been a recent deterioration in your work performance?

- Decrease in energy, increased fatigue
- Depressed mood
- Increase in fat mass
- Progressive decrease in lean body mass and in muscle strength
- Decrease in bone density and increased risk of osteopenia/osteoporosis

Men with testicular failure may suffer from sexual dysfunction, as well as osteoporosis, muscle weakness, depression, and lassitude, which is the clinical spectrum of hypogonadism. The sexual dysfunction, especially decreased libido and decreased erectile capacity, often reverses with testosterone replacement therapy. The variability of response in some patients may be related to comorbid medical illnesses, vascular dysfunction at the penile level, or psychological factors (Box 127-1).

MEN AT INCREASED RISK FOR TESTOSTERONE DEFICIENCY

- Decreased secondary sexual characteristics
- Erectile dysfunction or reduced libido
- An unexplained decrease in energy and/or muscle weakness
- Unexplained osteopenia or osteoporosis
- Testicular atrophy
- HIV/AIDS with weight loss
- Long-term systemic glucocorticoids
- Chronic alcoholics or substance abusers
- Chronic systemic diseases (chronic renal failure, chronic inflammatory diseases, etc.)
- Recent-onset gynecomastia
- Morbid obesity

- Family history of endocrine failure
- Hypothyroidism

DIAGNOSIS OF TESTOSTERONE DEFICIENCY

In symptomatic men, follow these guidelines:

- Measure total testosterone (Total T) by blood measurement taken between 7 and 10 AM.
- If Total T is less than 200 ng/dl, therapy is indicated after ruling out treatable endocrine causes (see below).
- If Total T is less than 200 ng/ml or between 200 and 400 ng/ml, repeat the test and measure LH, FSH, and prolactin levels.
- If repeat Total T is still low and LH and/or FSH is normal or elevated, consider initiating therapy.
- If repeat Total T is still low and LH is low, or prolactin is elevated, obtain an MRI of the sellar and pituitary region and consider a referal to an endocrinologist for further evaluation.
- A Total T above 400 ng/ml is considered normal and clinical judgment should guide the next steps. Treatment of levels between 200 and 400 mg/ml with other values being normal is a clinical judgment.

CONTRAINDICATIONS

- Known or suspected prostate cancer or breast cancer
- Severe benign prostatic hypertrophy (BPH) related bladder outlet obstruction
- Treatment for improved athletic performance, body building, or short stature

PATIENTS IN WHOM TREATMENT REQUIRES CAREFUL MONITORING

- Untreated sleep apnea
- Prostate problems and uncorrected obstructive symptoms caused by BPH
- Edema, fluid retention
- Gynecomastia
- Polycythemia or exacerbated erythropoiesis

Note: It is important to closely monitor those patients with a family history (i.e., presence in a first-degree relative) of prostate cancer.

TREATMENT

Testosterone should be administered only to men who are testosterone deficient, as evidenced by distinctly

BOX 127-2
Insurance Criteria for Reimbursement of Testosterone Pellets

Aetna, U.S. Healthcare, BlueCross/Blue Shield, and Medicare cover FDA-approved implantable testosterone pellets (Testopel Pellets) subject to the following patient selection criteria only:

- As *second-line testosterone replacement therapy* in males with congenital or acquired endogenous androgen absence or deficiency associated with primary or secondary hypogonadism when neither transdermal nor intramuscular testosterone replacement therapy is effective or appropriate.
- Primary hypogonadism includes conditions such as testicular failure as a result of cryptorchidism, bilateral torsion, orchitis, or vanishing testis syndrome and inborn errors in testosterone biosynthesis or bilateral orchiectomy.
- Secondary hypogonadism (hypogonadotropic hypogonadism) conditions include gonadotropin-releasing hormone deficiency or pituitary-hypothalamic injury as a result of surgery, tumors, trauma, or radiation and are the most common form of hypogonadism seen in older adults.

subnormal serum testosterone levels (less than 400 ng/dl or subnormal based on specific assay used).

The principal goals of testosterone therapy are to alleviate symptoms and to reduce health risks by restoring the serum testosterone concentration to the normal range.

There are currently four acceptable modes of drug delivery:

Note: Oral androgens (methyltestosterone, fluoxymesterone) are associated with significant risk of hepatotoxicity and are therefore not recommended.

Transdermal testosterone (Testoderm, Androderm): Transdermal therapeutic systems are replaced every 24 hours. Serum levels of testosterone peak 2 to 8 hours after application of a patch.

Testosterone gel (Androgel 1%) 2.5 to 5 mg: Applied daily to skin, "T gel" replacement improves sexual function and mood, increases lean muscle mass and strength, and decreases fat mass in hypogonadal men with less skin irritation and discontinuation as compared with the transdermal patch. These positive results occur within 30 days. Because of the amount of skin to which the gel is applied, the serum concentrations are more even and higher over 24 hours than is the patch.

Injectable testosterone esters: The principal esters available in North America are testosterone enanthate and testosterone cypionate. Injections of testosterone enanthate or testosterone cypionate may be given at intervals ranging from 7 to 14 days. Dosing typically is 100 mg IM per week or 200 mg IM per 2 weeks. A weekly injection of 100 mg causes less variation outside of the normal range.

Implantable hormone pellets: The implantable pellets are perhaps the most convenient, dependable, and best tolerated method of testosterone delivery. Subcutane-

ous pellets are used as a second-line therapy when other methods have failed or have not been tolerated. Placed subcutaneously in the buttocks through a special trocar device, 450 mg usually provides sustained adequate blood levels (e.g., 400 to 600 ng/dl) for 4 to 6 months (Box 127-2).

MONITORING PATIENTS ON TESTOSTERONE REPLACEMENT

- Clinical symptoms and signs of testosterone deficiency
- Frequency and duration of erections
- Acne and breast size and tenderness
- Possible skin irritation with transdermal therapy
- Serum testosterone levels
- Lipid profiles
- Sleep apnea

Transdermal testosterone delivery systems: Serum testosterone should be drawn 8 to 12 hours after application or per patch label instructions. Skin irritation at the site of the patch is common.

Injectable and/or implantable testosterone: Monitor nadir testosterone levels at 3 months, before the next injection or implantation. Levels that exceed 800 ng/dl or are less than 200 ng/dl require adjustment of the dose or frequency.

Digital rectal examination (DRE) and prostate specific antigen (PSA): DRE should be performed and a PSA level checked in all men before initiating treatment, again at 3 months, and then annually in men more than 40 years of age. An abnormal DRE, a confirmed increase in PSA more than 2 ng/ml, or a total PSA more than 4.0 ng/ml requires evaluation by a urologist.

Hematocrit: Level should be checked at baseline, then periodically thereafter. A hematocrit more than 52% warrants evaluation for hypoxia and sleep apnea and/or a reduction in the dose of testosterone therapy. Testosterone is known to stimulate erythropoiesis.

Liver function, cholesterol, and HDL-cholesterol: Levels should be checked periodically. Testosterone lowers total cholesterol, LDL, and HDL.

Breast examination: Regular breast examinations are recommended.

Bone mineral density: Measurement of bone mineral density of the lumbar spine and/or the femoral necks at 1 year may be considered in hypogonadal men with osteopenia, especially those younger than 80 years old.

EQUIPMENT

- Resusable Bardini implanter kit (includes the trocar and stylet plunger)

- 5-cm trocar pellet implanter (3.2-mm bore diameter)
- Forceps
- Stainless steel tray
- Sterile gloves
- 1% Lidocaine with epinephrine 2 to 3 ml
- 3-mm syringe; 27-g, 1½-inch needle
- No. 11 scalpel blade
- 75-mg testosterone pellets (usually six) having a diameter of approximately 3.2 mm
- Lidoderm 5% patch placed 15 minutes before the procedure at site of insertion *(optional)*

Note: The implanter kit *must be sterilized before use* and should be sterilized by steam in an autoclave at 121° C, for a minimum of 15 minutes. The standard procedures for sterilizing surgical instruments should be followed.

PREPROCEDURE PATIENT PREPARATION

All potential risks, benefits, and alternatives to testosterone replacement therapy should be discussed, specifically the potential complications regarding trocar insertion subcutaneously (including infection and bleeding). The patient should understand that once the pellets are inserted, they are not able to be removed. They slowly dissolve and the effects will last for at least 3 months.

TECHNIQUE

Implantation Area

The 75-mg pellets are fat soluble and so are implanted subcutaneously. In most men, an area on either lateral buttock between the gluteus maximus and the tensor fascia latae muscle may be chosen so that implantation is made below the skin and above the muscle and fascia, just inferior to the iliac spine, directed posteriorly and inferiorly.

Preparation

1. Place patient in the prone position.
2. Cleanse the skin over the lateral buttocks with Betadine antiseptic (Fig. 127-1, *A*).
3. Create a skin wheal using lidocaine 1% with epinephrine (Fig. 127-1, *B*).
4. Inject 2 to 3 ml of 1% lidocaine with epinephrine along the track of the trocar insertion.

Implantation

1. Place as many pellets (usually six) as are indicated clinically in the sterile tray.
2. Make a small puncture with a no. 11 scalpel blade.
3. Insert the Bardani implanter with stylet (solid rod with pointed end) in place; direct it subcutaneously the full depth (about 5 cm) (Fig. 127-2, *A*).

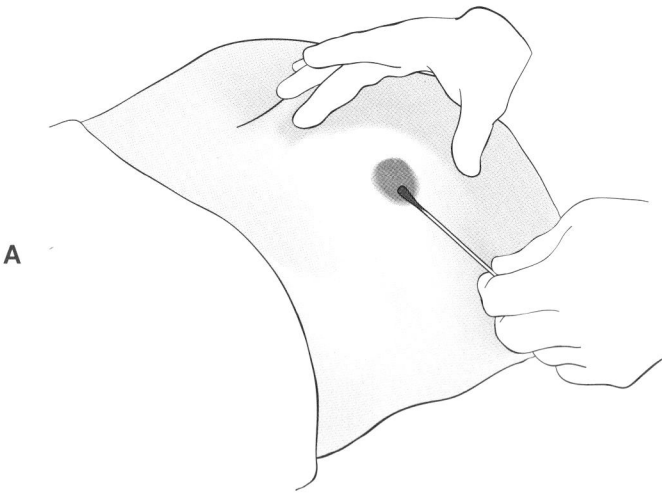

A

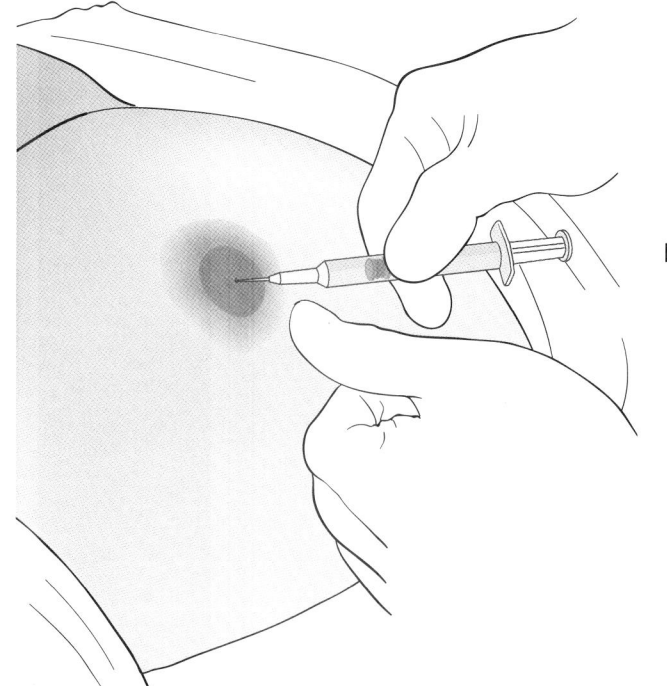

B

Fig. 127-1
Preparation for implantation of testosterone pellets. **A,** Cleanse skin with an accepted antiseptic preparation. **B,** Create skin wheal using lidocaine 1% with epinephrine. (Redrawn from Bartor Pharmacal, Rye, NY.)

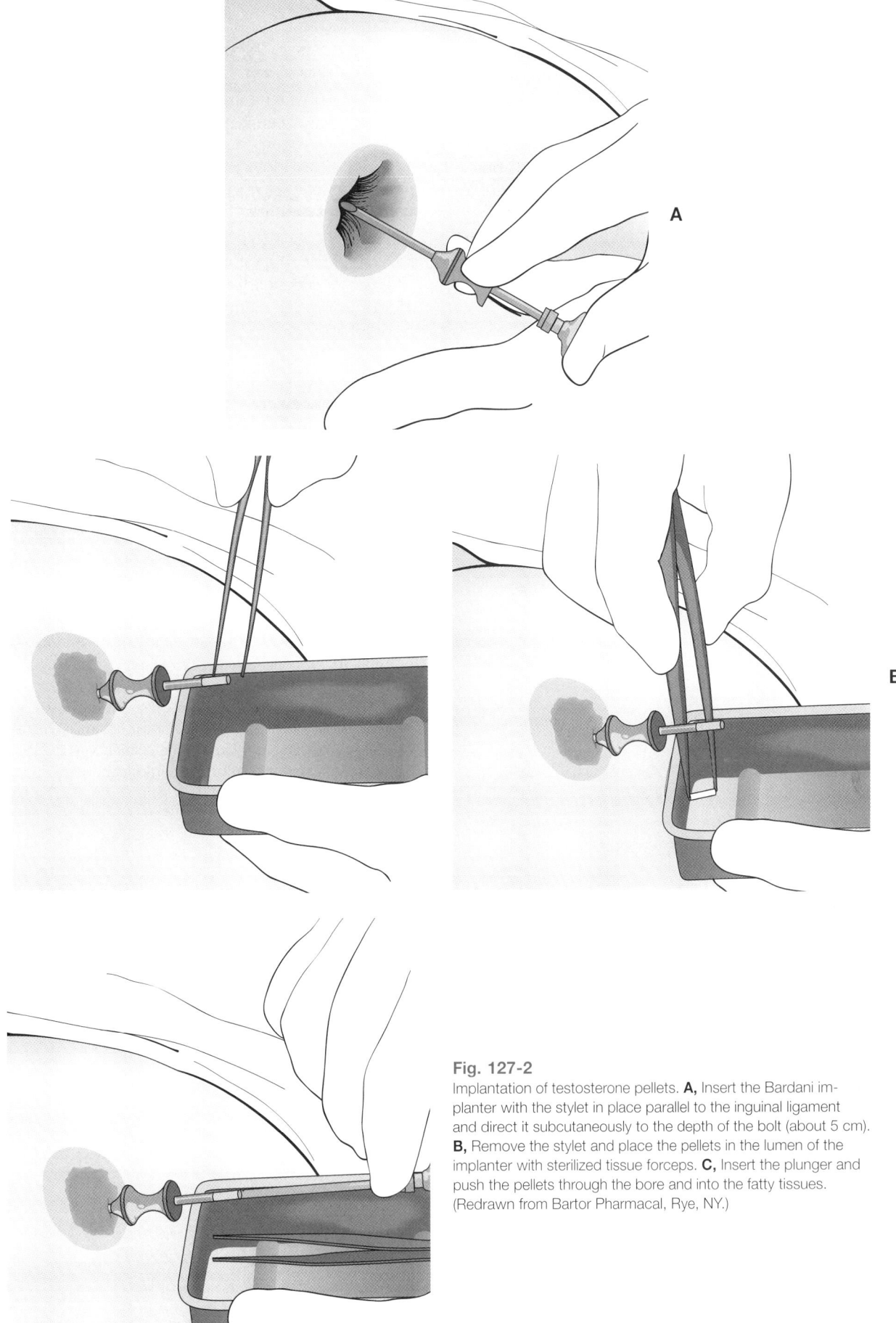

Fig. 127-2

Implantation of testosterone pellets. **A,** Insert the Bardani implanter with the stylet in place parallel to the inguinal ligament and direct it subcutaneously to the depth of the bolt (about 5 cm). **B,** Remove the stylet and place the pellets in the lumen of the implanter with sterilized tissue forceps. **C,** Insert the plunger and push the pellets through the bore and into the fatty tissues. (Redrawn from Bartor Pharmacal, Rye, NY.)

4. When the stylet is removed, place the pellets in the hollow tube of the implanter with the sterilized tissue forceps. The sterilized tray should be held beneath the implanter as the pellets are inserted in case one is inadvertently dropped (Fig. 127-2, *B*). A pellet that falls into the sterilized tray may be replaced, but a pellet that becomes contaminated must be discarded because it cannot be resterilized.
5. The plunger (solid tube with blunt end) is then inserted and the pellets are pushed through the bore and eased into the fatty tissues (Fig. 127-2, *C*).
6. Remove the implanter with a twisting motion.
7. Give the patient a dry dressing to apply with pressure for a few minutes.
8. Clean and close the puncture site with Steri-strips, and cover with an adhesive bandage.

The pellets are slowly absorbed, and there is no need to ever remove them. The procedure may be repeated on the opposite buttock in 3 to 6 months, depending on the adequacy of serum testosterone. Have the patient return in 3 months to check for efficacy and tolerability.

COMPLICATIONS

- Hematoma, bleeding
- Infection
- Pain at insertion site
- Increased fluid retention
- Gynecomastia
- Worsening sleep apnea
- Increased hematocrit
- Worsening prostate symptoms
- Testicular atrophy
- Mood swings

POSTPROCEDURE PATIENT EDUCATION

For the first 24 hours, the patient should keep a dry pressure bandage on the insertion site and limit strenuous activity. Watch for any complications as noted previously.

SUPPLIER

Bartor Pharmacal Co.
70 High Street
Rye, NY 10580
Phone: 1-914-967-4219

CPT/BILLING CODE

11980   Subcutaneous implantation of testosterone pellets

ICD-9-CM DIAGNOSTIC CODES

253.4   Pituitary hypogonadism
257.2   Male hypogonadism, testicular, primary or secondary
353.4   Hypogonadotrophic hypogonadism

BIBLIOGRAPHY

Cunningham GR, Snyder PJ, Swerdloff RS, Tenover JS: *Testosterone replacement therapy in men: emerging clinical issues.* Newsletter from the Endocrine Society's 82nd Annual Meeting, June 24, 2000, Toronto, Ontario, Canada.

Guay AT, Nankin HR: AACE clinical practice guidelines for the evaluation and treatment of male sexual dysfunction (developed by the American Association of Clinical Endocrinologists and the American College of Endocrinology), 1980. Available at www.aace.com/clin/guidelines/sexdysguid.pdf (accessed June 21, 2002).

Nezhat C, Karpas AE, Greenblatt RB, Mahesh VB: Estradiol implants for conception control, *Am J Obstet Gynecol* Dec 15;138(8):1151, 1980.

Petak SM, Baskin HJ, Bergman DA, et al: AACE Clinical Practice Guidelines for the Evaluation and Treatment of Hypogonadism in Adult Male Patients (developed by the American Association of Clinical Endocrinologists and the American College of Endocrinology), 1980. Available at www.aace.com/clin/guidelines/hypogonadism.pdf (accessed June 21, 2002).

Replacing testosterone in men, *Drugs Therapeutics Bull* 37(1): 3, 1999.

Rosano GM, DeZiegier D, Pagnotta P, et al: Plasma testosterone levels in males with coronary disease, *Eur Heart J* 19S(abstr):141, 1998.

Tenover JL: Testosterone and the aging male, *J Androl* 18:103, 1997.

Thom MH, Studd JW: Hormone implantation, *Br Med J* 280:848, 1980.

Wang C, Swerdloff RS, Iranmeanesh A, et al: Transdermal testosterone gel improves sexual function, mood, muscle strength, and body composition parameters in hypogonadal men, *J Clin Endo Met* 85(8):2839, 2000.

Webb CM, McNeill JG, Collins P: Testosterone increases coronary blood flow in men with coronary heart disease, *J Am Coll Cardiol* 131(S2A):405, 1998.

CHAPTER 128

Vacuum Devices for Erectile Dysfunction

Chad J. Smith

Erectile dysfunction is a common medical problem occurring in nearly 30 million American males. Vacuum devices to promote erection are safe and have overall clinical success rates of approximately 90%. They are useful in nearly all men with erectile dysfunction, except those with severe cavernous fibrosis. Therapy depends on the ability to transfer blood into the corpus cavernosa (see Fig. 125-1), which is limited by fibrosis.

A number of devices are available for use. The majority have three common components: a vacuum chamber or cylinder, a vacuum pump that creates a negative pressure within the chamber, and an elastic constriction band.

The device creates a nonphysiologic erection by trapping blood in both the intracorporeal and extracorporeal compartments of the penile shaft by means of the negative pressure vacuum. The constrictor band is then placed above the chamber, over the proximal shaft, constricting blood flow into and out of the penis and maintaining an erection for sexual intercourse. Erection is maintained distal to the constricting band. Most manufacturers recommend that the vacuum-induced erection be maintained for less than 30 minutes because penile distension, edema, and cyanosis may ensue with prolonged use.

INDICATIONS

- Erectile dysfunction resulting from vascular disorders
- Erectile dysfunction resulting from neurologic disorders
- Erectile dysfunction resulting from psychogenic disorders
- Erectile dysfunction resulting from hormonal disorders
- Erectile dysfunction as a result of medications, when the medication cannot be altered or terminated

CONTRAINDICATIONS

- Blood dyscrasias, coagulation disorders, or anticoagulation drug therapy
- Impaired manual dexterity to operate the device

EQUIPMENT

- Vacuum erection device, including chamber, vacuum pump, and constriction bands. Battery-operated suction devices may be preferable in patients with impaired manual dexterity or after debilitating neurologic events such as stroke or quadriplegia. Constriction bands come in a variety of sizes to fit the penile shaft. (See Fig. 128-1.)
- Lubricant as needed.

PREPROCEDURE PATIENT PREPARATION

Discuss use of the suction device, alternatives, relative benefits, and potential complications with the patient and, when possible, his partner. The patient should be aware that a vacuum-induced erection, unlike a physiologic erection, causes rigidity distal to the constrictor band and may allow the penis to pivot at its base and requires positioning for vaginal penetration. Although it is generally well tolerated, patients using this device may experience painful ejaculation, penile pain, ecchymoses, hematomas, petechiae, and decreased penile temperature or numbness distal to the constriction band. Painful ejaculation has been reported in 10% to 15% of men because the constriction band at the base of the penis causes distension of the proximal urethra during ejaculation. The semen then drains out the penile meatus once the constriction band is removed. Hematomas have been reported in 9.8% and local skin injury in 2.2% of long-term

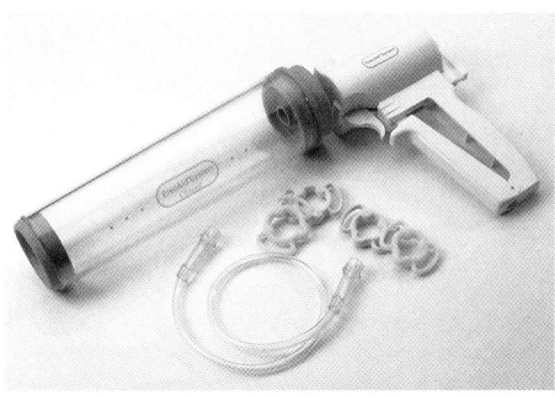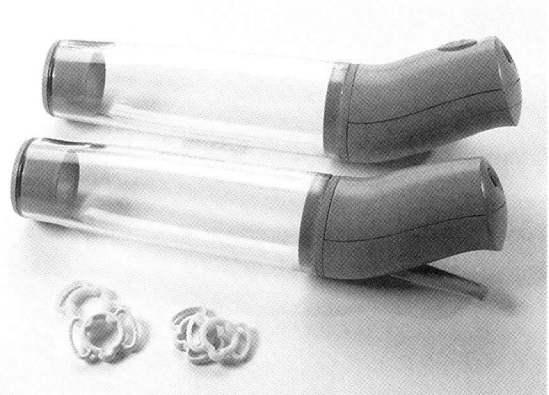

Fig. 128-1
Typical vacuum devices for erectile dysfunction. (Courtesy TIMM Medical Technologies, Eden Prairie, Minn.)

users. These various complications can be reduced or eliminated by increased experience with the device and by emphasizing the need to remove the constriction band after 30 minutes. Most manufacturers provide instructional materials, videos, and customer service availability by phone to assist with appropriate use of their equipment.

TECHNIQUE

1. Complete the patient's history and physical to establish a diagnosis of erectile dysfunction.
2. Select a desired device for use.
3. Apply the open end of the vacuum chamber over the penis. A seal should be made with the skin at the base of the penis, usually with the help of lubricant jelly.
4. Activate the vacuum pump to create negative pressure within the chamber, thereby drawing blood into the penis and producing an erection-like state. Most devices have release valves in the chamber that prevent formation of excessive pressure.
5. Once adequate tumescence is achieved, slide the constrictor band at the base of the chamber onto the penile shaft. This effectively traps blood within the penis to maintain the erection. The chamber and pump may now be removed. Constrictor bands are available in a variety of sizes.
6. After intercourse, remove the band from the penile shaft. The vacuum-induced erection will subside.
7. Inspect the penis for evidence of injury.
8. After use, submerge all parts of the suction devices in soapy water for cleaning except the vacuum pump.

COMPLICATIONS

- Decrease in penile temperature or numbness distal to the constriction band
- Local skin injury
- Painful ejaculation
- Penile pain
- Subcutaneous ecchymoses, petechiae, or hematoma
- With prolonged use greater than 30 minutes, progressive penile distension, edema, and cyanosis may occur.

SUPPLIERS

ErecAid
TIMM Medical Technologies
6585 City West Parkway
Eden Prairie, MN 55344
Phone: 1-800-438-8592
Website: www.timmmedical.com

Vacuum Erection Device (VED)
Mission Pharmacal Co.
10999 IH-10 West Suite 1000
San Antonio, TX 78230
Phone: 1-800-531-3333
Website: www.missionpharmacal.com

CPT/BILLING CODE

55899   Unlisted procedure, male genital system (documentation suggested)

ICD-9-CM DIAGNOSTIC CODES

607.84   Impotence of organic origin
302.72   Impotence, nonorganic or unspecified

ADDITIONAL RESOURCES

- See the sample patient education handout for "Vacuum Devices for Erectile Dysfunction" on page 1896 of Appendix G.
- See the sample patient consent form for "Vacuum Devices for Erectile Dysfunction" on page 1897 in Appendix G.

BIBLIOGRAPHY

Derouet H, Caspari D, Rohde V, et al: Treatment of erectile dysfunction with external vacuum devices, *Androlgia* 31(Suppl 1):89, 1999.

Lewis RW, Witherington R: External vacuum therapy for erectile dysfunction: use and results, *World J Urol* 15(1):78, 1997.

NIH Consensus Development Panel on Impotence: Impotence, *JAMA* 270:83, 1993.

CHAPTER 129

Vasectomy

George C. Denniston
John L. Pfenninger

Vasectomy is a safe, inexpensive, permanent form of contraception. Unlike tubal ligation for women, vasectomy is usually performed in an office setting, is less expensive, and is associated with fewer and less severe complications. No mortality from vasectomy has been reported, whereas approximately 10 women die annually from complications of tubal ligation in the United States. Although both procedures have low failure rates, failure of vasectomy can be detected easily when men bring in their postprocedural semen specimens.

In the chain of events that leads to choosing vasectomy, the key person is usually not the surgeon. Rather it is the person who helps the man make the decision to have a vasectomy; this is often the primary care physician. Therefore it is important those who wish to help men come to a decision about vasectomy to be well informed about the procedure (see the sample patient education handout titled "Vasectomy [Permanent Male Sterilization]" on page 1898 of Appendix G).

A vasectomy can be performed in many ways. The Association for Voluntary Surgical Contraception (AVSC) is promoting the "no-scalpel" method. Whether it is "better" than the traditional methods is still debated, but it certainly is quicker and lends itself to a significant psychologic advantage. The no-scalpel approach is a *method of entry*—what is done to the vas deferens inside is variable and a matter of preference. "Laser vasectomy" does not exist (unless one uses the laser to cut into the scrotum or to seal the vas edges). It has no practical advantages and may even be detrimental to a quick procedure.

INDICATIONS

- Vasectomy is appropriate for a man who does not wish to have children—or to have any more children—but who wishes to continue having sexual intercourse.

CONTRAINDICATIONS

- Local infection
- Coagulation disorders
- Inability to palpate and elevate both vasa
- Marked stress from a recent event, such as divorce or financial setback *(relative)*
- Lack of adequate informed consent
- Potential for hysterectomy in wife
- Inappropriate reasons for wanting vasectomy (e.g., improving a troubled marriage, curing sexual problems)
- Frail, insecure masculine image and overconcern about ability to function sexually after the surgery *(relative)*

PREPROCEDURE PATIENT PREPARATION

Fully informed consent can be obtained and confirmed by providing the patient with a vasectomy fact sheet (see the sample patient education handout titled "Vasectomy [Permanent Male Sterilization]" on page 1898 of Appendix G), and having the patient answer several true-or-false questions in writing (Fig. 129-1). Questions answered incorrectly should be discussed, and the patient should correct the answer and initial it. The patient should sign the filled-out questionnaire and the formal consent form (see the sample patient consent form titled "Request for Vasectomy" on page 1904 of Appendix G). This is an improvement over other methods of obtaining informed consent for vasectomy, because it ensures adequate knowledge by the patient and offers better legal protection to the physician. It is wise to include the wife or partner, if any, in the consent process; however, a man has a right to vasectomy even in the absence of spousal consent.

The standard "consent form" has been changed here to a "request for vasectomy." Men are not consenting to

---

Vasectomy Questionnaire

After you have read the vasectomy fact sheet, please answer the following questions. It is simply to confirm that you understand the procedure. If you answer some of the questions incorrectly, the counselor or the doctor will discuss them with you.

Please circle the correct answer. Correct answers to these questions confirm that you understand the basic facts about vasectomy.

1. Vasectomy keeps the sperm from getting out.	False	True
2. Most vasectomies are performed using local anesthetic.	False	True
3. After vasectomy men are still fertile for some time.	False	True
4. After vasectomy the amount of fluid ejaculated is about the same as before the procedure.	False	True
5. A complication can occasionally occur after a vasectomy.	False	True
6. Vasectomy is very different than castration.	False	True
7. Vasectomy should be considered permanent.	False	True

Patient signature: _____ Date_____

Fig. 129-1
Sample patient questionnaire for vasectomy. Note: The correct answer to all questions is True.

---

vasectomy, they are requesting that it be done. This puts more of the decision-making responsibility on the patient. Standard policy has always been to operate on any man who is fully informed and is certain that he wants a vasectomy. It should be made clear that it is his decision. It also makes it more difficult for the patient to say later, "You should never have permitted me to have a vasectomy." If the patient is young and without children, the physician must be sure of the patient's decision; however, these are not absolute grounds to deny the vasectomy. The doctor still retains responsibility to help the patient make a decision that will not cause regret in the patient in the future.

The vasectomy questionnaire (Fig. 129-1), and the patient education handouts and consent forms in Appendix G, help achieve fully informed consent. The preprocedure counseling visit can be documented using the encounter form in Fig. 129-2, which reviews the patient's pertinent history, physical and counseling points, and documents the follow-up semen specimen checks. Fig. 129-3 is a checklist of the counseling material reviewed with the patient. The original sheet is for the patient. It is a good summary of all points that should be covered and a reminder for the patient of what to do just before and after the surgery. A copy is

placed in the chart. (For a more detailed description of the preprocedural counseling visit, see Pfenninger [1984b].)

The clinician should note the questions, "How well do you tolerate pain" and "Do you have a tendency to faint?" on the encounter form (Fig. 129-2). If the patient tolerates pain well, only ibuprofen (not Valium) is needed. If the patient selects "OK" on the form as an indication of pain tolerance, the clinician should give Valium 10 mg PO and the ibuprofen. If the patient tolerates pain poorly or has a tendency to faint, the clinician should give Valium, ibuprofen, and atropine. Atropine 0.5 mg is given IM on arrival to the office before surgery. This effectively blocks any vasovagal response (nausea, fainting, seizure-like activity, etc.). This optimizes the "vasectomy" experience for both the patient and physician.

Many now recognize the educational value of patient education videotapes. The patient can review the material several times privately at home. A vasectomy counseling videotape is available from Creative Health Communications or The National Procedures Institute (see the "Suppliers" section).

Federal agencies require that a specific consent form be signed. These are usually available from local health

Vasectomy Encounter Form
To be filled out by patient:

Date: _____
Referring physician: _____

Patient's name: _____
Age: _____ DOB: _____
Education level: _____
Occupation: _____
Marriage: 1st, 2nd, 3rd
     years: _____

Phone: (H) _____ (W) _____
Wife or partner's name: _____
Age: _____
Education level: _____
Occupation: _____
Marriage: 1st, 2nd, 3rd
     years: _____

What is the quality of your marriage/relationship? _____
Any marital problems? _____
How is sexual functioning? _____
Any sexual problems? _____
Children's ages and sexes: _____
Religion: _____
Do you have religious conflict with vasectomy?   Yes   No
Current contraceptive: _____
Are you or your wife experiencing any problems with this form of contraception?   Yes   No
Have you considered a tubal ligation?   Yes   No
Have you considered other temporary methods?   Yes   No
Why do you want a vasectomy? _____
How long have you been thinking about limiting the size of your family? _____
Patient's health?   Good   Poor
Partner's health?   Good   Poor
Is there any genetic disease in the family?   Yes   No
If "Yes," please explain: _____
Do you have any particular concerns about undergoing a vasectomy? If so, describe them:
_____
How well do you tolerate pain?   Well   OK   Poorly
Do you have a tendency to faint?   Yes   No

Have you had, or do you have any of the following?
1. Epididymitis?   Yes   No   6. Bleeding tendencies?   Yes   No
2. Lumps in the testicles?   Yes   No   7. Any major illness?   Yes   No
3. Hernia or hernia surgery?   Yes   No   8. Psychological counseling? Yes   No
4. Trauma in the groin?   Yes   No
5. VD, prostatitis, urine infection? Yes   No

Do you take aspirin?   Yes   No
Do you take regular medications?   Yes   No
If "Yes," please list these medications: _____
Do you have any allergies to certain medications?   Yes   No
If "Yes," please list these medications: _____
Have you read and understood the handouts explaining vasectomy?   Yes   No
Have you viewed and understood the videotape, if provided?   Yes   No
(If you have not seen it, please come 30 minutes early for the counseling visit to see it)
Any questions regarding videotape or handouts?   Yes   No

Fig. 129-2
Sample vasectomy encounter form. (Courtesy Medical Procedures Center, P.C., Midland, Mich.)
Continued

departments or the state Medicaid agency. Forms must be filled out meticulously, since any excuse the agency can use to deny payment will be used! Note that consents are only valid from more than 30 days after the counseling session (when it must be signed by the patient) until 180 days after it is signed.

EQUIPMENT

- Scalpel handle with a no. 15 blade or the no-scalpel dissecting vas forceps (Fig. 129-4, *A*)
- Vas clamps for isolating vas (Fig. 129-4, *B* and *C*). Dr. Li's (AMI) traditional no-scalpel vas clamp and

Physical examination
(To be filled out by physician):

Hernia?	Yes	No
Testicles?	Normal	Abnormal _____
Vas-palpable bilaterally?	Yes	No
Urethral discharge?	Yes	No

Scrotal contents?   Variocele   R   L
                     Spermatocele   R   L
Skin: Normal   Abnormal _____

Impression: _____
_____

Plan: Valium 10 mg   ibuprofen 800 mg   atropine 0.5 sub q   Dt
       Vas scheduled?   Yes   No
       Diagram given to patient and explained?*   Yes   No
Other: _____

_____   _____
        Physician signature   Date
cc: _____

Postoperative Information

Date surgery performed: _____
Complications during surgery: None or _____
          Technique: NSV   Open-ended

	Result	Date	Initials	Patient Notified
Semen check no. 1:	_____	_____	_____	_____
Semen check no. 2:	_____	_____	_____	_____

It is OK to give the results to: _____

It is OK to leave message on answering machine: Yes   No

Problems (see dictated note)   Date
I. _____   _____
II. _____   _____

Fig. 129-2, cont'd
(Courtesy Medical Procedures Center, P.C., Midland, Mich.) Asterisk refers to diagram and summary sheet found in Fig. 129-3.

Dr. Wilson's adaptation (Zinnanti) are most commonly used.

Dr. Soonawala of Bombay, India, developed the Soonawala vasectomy forceps. If these are not available, they can easily be made by filing off both sides of a baby Allis forceps until only three teeth are left: one tooth on one side, and two teeth on the other (i.e., 1×2 teeth). As an alternative the clinician can use sharp or blunted towel clips.

- Cautery unit, either an electrocautery unit and handpiece, with a fine-needle electrode (unit should be set at the lowest level that quickly cauterizes small "bleeders") or battery unit.

A battery-powered cautery is now available with sterile sheaths and disposable tips from Advanced Meditech International (AMI) (Fig. 129-5). Based on Schmidt's findings, a battery-powered cautery unit may be the instrument of choice for optimal sealing of the vas ends compared with an electrosurgical unit.

- Three hemostats (small)
- Adson tissue forceps (1×2 teeth)
- Tissue scissors
- Method to seal vas sheath; either needle holder with a 4-0 chromic catgut suture on an atraumatic needle or a medium hemoclip applicator with clips
- A 10-ml syringe ($1\frac{1}{2}$-inch, 27-gauge or smaller bore needle)
- Lidocaine (1%) without epinephrine (10 ml)
- Sterile sodium bicarbonate solution for less pain during anesthetic infiltration

Patient Education Worksheet

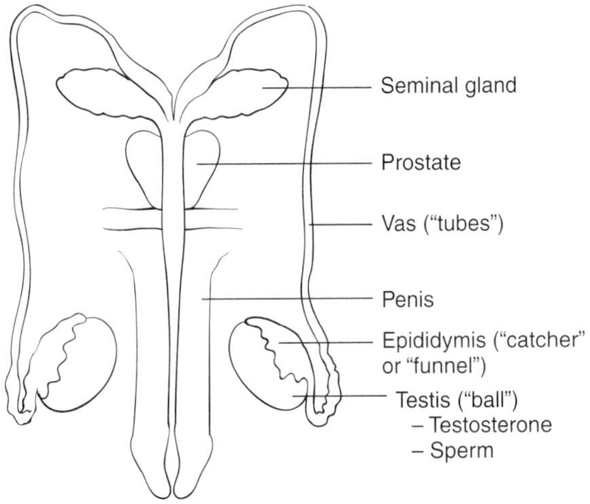

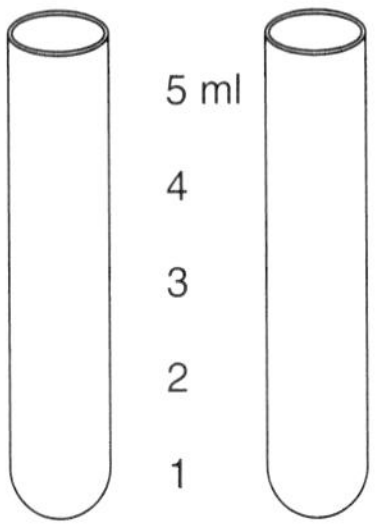

1. Anatomy

2. Procedure
- Lidocaine numbing
- Clamp around vas
- Insert forceps or make incision
- Remove 1/4 inch
- Cauterize
- Tissue wall separating ends
- No suture closure

3. Complications
- Pain
- Bleeding
- Infection
- Granuloma
- Long-term complications
- Failure

Seminal gland

Prostate

Vas ("tubes")

Penis

Epididymis ("catcher" or "funnel")

Testis ("ball")
- Testosterone
- Sperm

5 ml

4

3

2

1

4. Preparation (day of surgery)
- No aspirin for 10 days
- Clip scrotal hair with scissors, 1 to 2 hours before surgery
- Shower after clip
- Take four (4) 200-mg ibuprofen (Advil, Nuprin, Motrin) and Valium if needed 1 hour before surgery
- If any type of sedative used, someone else needs to drive patient to and from the office
- Sign permit if not already done
- Jock strap (supporter-type strap, not one that holds a cup)

5. After surgery
- Day of surgery: Home, feet up, ice, jock; three (3) 200-mg ibuprofen four times per day
- Day 2: Walk, shower, wear jock; three (3) 200-mg ibuprofen four times per day
- Day 3: Whatever is comfortable, but not vigorous activity
- Day 4: Return to work

6. Sex
- Week 1: One time at end of week
- Week 2: Two times
- Thereafter as desired (use contraception until two semen checks are negative)

7. Follow-up specimens
- After 6 weeks (or 15 ejaculations) and after 3 months (sample no more than 2 hours old)
- Call the office and be sure the doctor is in
- No need for appointment, just drop off specimen (but be sure doctor available)
- Label container with patient name

8. Costs
- Counseling
- Procedure
- Semen checks
- Follow-up problems for 1 year

Patient's signature: _____ Date _____
Physician's signature: _____ Date _____

Fig. 129-3

Sample vasectomy patient education worksheet. (Courtesy Medical Procedures Center, P.C., Midland, Mich.)

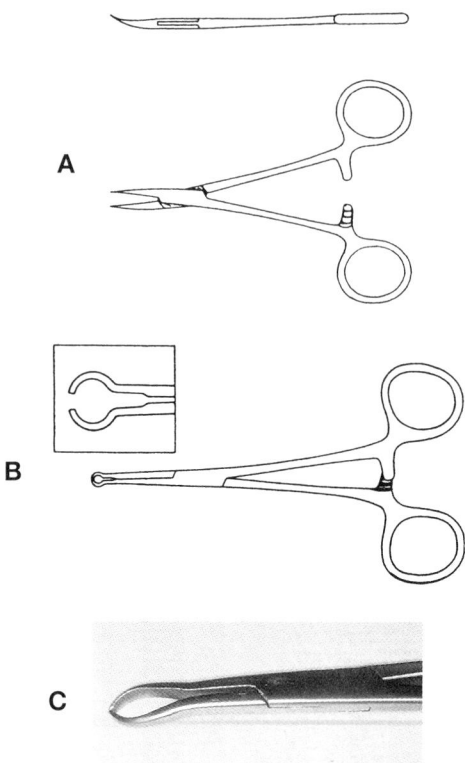

Fig. 129-4
No-scalpel vasectomy instruments. **A,** The dissecting forceps. **B,** Percutaneous vas clamp. **C,** Wilson vas clamp (Zinnanti). (**A-B,** From Li SQ, Goldstein M, Zhu J, Huber D: *J Urol* 145:341, 1991.)

Note: Just before injection of the anesthetic, the clinician should draw up 1 ml of sodium bicarbonate and then 10 ml of the lidocaine.

- Large pack of 4 × 4–inch gauze
- Povidone-iodine or Hibiclens preparation
- Fenestrated sterile drape and nonfenestrated drape
- Sterile gloves and mask
- Single sterile glove (into which the cautery device is placed)
- Pair of nonsterile gloves for iodine prep
- Specimen jar

TECHNIQUE

A vasectomy can be performed in many ways. Some clinicians use one incision in the midline, whereas others recommend two separate incisions. The no-scalpel technique from China is only a method of entering the scrotum and isolating the vas. Once this is accomplished, any number of occlusion techniques may be used. Some surgeons merely incise the vas and cauterize both ends. Others resect 1 to 2 cm of vas and cauterize both ends or they cauterize just the

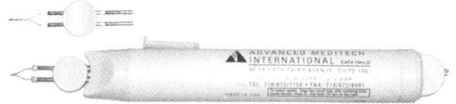

Fig. 129-5
Battery-operated cautery with disposable tip (AMI).

prostatic end. Ligation of the vas has been generally replaced by cautery of the ends (or end) and interposing a layer of fascia between the two ends. The fascia can be closed over with chromic suture or with hemoclips. The latter are quicker and avoid the bleeding seen occasionally when placing a suture. (For an excellent discussion of various techniques, see Lipshultz [1980].)

The open-ended technique is described here, using cautery only on the **prostatic** end of the cut vas and chromic catgut suture to close the fascia over that end. It differs from other techniques in that the testicular end of the vas is indeed left open. The open-ended technique was first recommended and used more than 50 years ago. Errey and Edwards (1986) recently documented its merits. It minimizes the problem of back pressure on the testicle and the associated long-term pain in the occasional patient (i.e., congestive epididymitis). Symptomatic sperm granulomas may be reduced. The incidence of vasectomy failure is probably not increased **if the cauterized end is properly covered with surrounding fascia.** This step, interposing the fascia, is critical if only the distal (i.e., prostatic) end is cauterized. Numerous authors have reported increased failure rates using the open-ended technique, since fascial interposition is somewhat difficult for those less experienced. It is for this reason that most surgeons still routinely cauterize both the prostatic and testicular resected ends in addition to using the fascial sheath. Finally, with the open-ended technique, dilation of the proximal vas (i.e., testicular end) does not occur, making surgical reanastomosis at a later date, if desired, easier. (See Denniston and Kuehl [1994].) Some vasectomists use this technique only for men less than 30 years old because they may be more likely to request reversal, and cauterize both ends in those over 30.

The technique is as follows:

1. Have the patient lie down undressed but draped from the waist down. Clip any remaining excess scrotal hair that has not already been removed.
2. After cleaning the site with an alcohol wipe, anesthetize the skin in the midline. Use 0.5 to 1 ml of lidocaine to infiltrate subcutaneously along the median raphe. The small volume will help prevent anesthetic distortion over the site of entry.

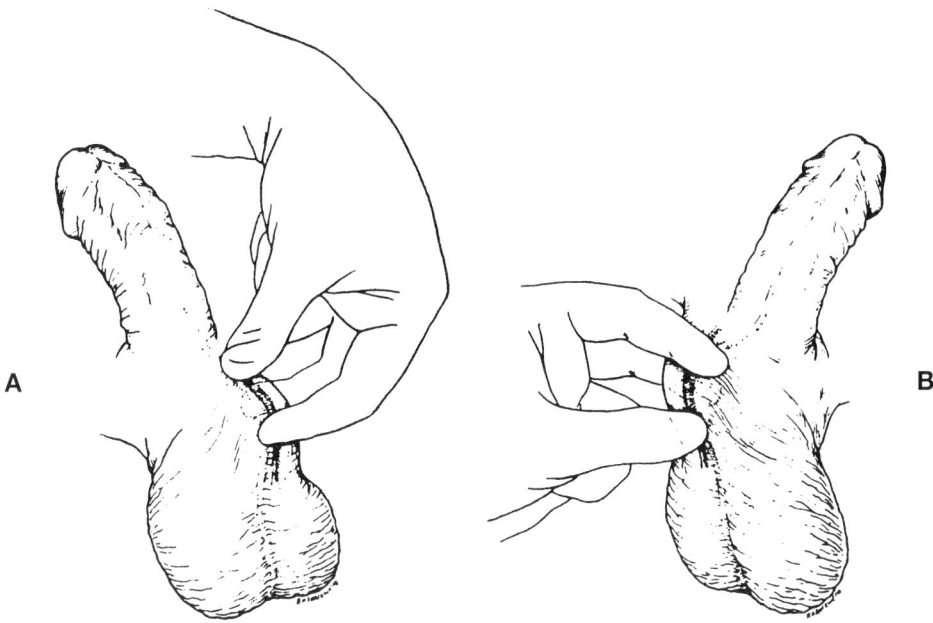

Fig. 129-6
Three-point fixation of the vas beneath the skin. **A,** Left side. **B,** Right side. Proper immobilization of the vas is a crucial factor in ease of performing a vasectomy. For single entry, the clinician should isolate the vas beneath the midline raphe. (From Li SQ, Goldstein M, Zhu J, Huber D: *J Urol* 145:341, 1991.)

3. Isolate the left vas between the fingers high in the scrotum and bring it to the surface. The vas has the diameter and consistency of a ballpoint pen refill. Roll it gently upwards until it is immediately beneath the skin. Use three-point fixation to secure the vas. Using the middle finger of the left hand (if right-handed), press up from beneath the scrotum. On top of the scrotum, hold the vas between the thumb and index finger (Fig. 129-6, *A*). Although the vas can be resected close to the epididymis (even in the convoluted portion), it is desirable to do the surgery as distal (i.e., as close to the groin) as possible. A longer testicular remnant of the vas may reduce long-term postoperative discomfort and also enhance the chances for reanastomosis, if desired. Therefore secure the vas "as high up" as possible.
4. Anesthetize the vas (Fig. 129-7). Enter the skin from the anesthetized midline and inject 3 to 5 ml around the vas high on the left in several areas. Let the vas fall back, then grasp the right vas (Fig. 129-6, *B*). Redirect the needle from the midline to the right vas and inject another 3 to 5 ml. The anesthetic will block the nerves in both proximal and distal directions.
5. Now perform the surgical scrub and draping. This gives the anesthetic time to work. Nonsterile gloves are used with *warm* disinfectant scrub. Warm solutions will help relax the scrotum, which allows easier palpation of the vas. Prep well down onto the perineum, since the hands will often be in this area when grasping for the vas. Cover the area with sterile surgical drapes. A fenestrated drape usually goes over the scrotum while a nonfenestrated drape is placed over the thighs.
6. Use one of the types of vas clamps suggested to anchor the vas in the midline (Fig. 129-8, *A, B*).

Editor's note: The more experienced vasectomist will generally make one midline entry and resect each vas through the same site. For those less experienced, it is easier to make two entries (over each isolated vas). In this case additional lidocaine will be needed to anesthetize the skin over the entry sites.

7. Using the vas dissecting forceps with the tips spread apart, pierce the skin going down to the vas with one of the tips (Fig. 129-8, *C*). The step replaces making the incision that was done in the past with a scalpel.
8. Close the dissecting forceps and enter the previously made opening with the forceps closed (Fig. 129-8, *D*). Again, go deep enough to penetrate the perivas fascia.
9. Spread the dissecting forceps several times to reveal

the vas. It is usually more white; if the vas itself is entered, it will tear, revealing muscle fibers. You only want to separate the perivas fascia off the vas and widen the skin wound to about 6 to 8 mm (Fig. 129-8, *E*).

10. Now insert only one jaw of the dissecting forceps into the vas and, rotating clockwise, deliver the vas through the skin (Fig. 129-8, *F[1]*). If the fascia has been penetrated up to the vas, and there are no perivas adhesions from previous infections, trauma, or surgery, this step goes easily. However, many times the vas does not slide out easily. Alternatively, use the dissecting forceps or hemostats to pull and tease the fascia away from the vas, clearing about a 1-cm section (Fig. 129-8, *F[2]*). Release the vas clamp (Fig. 129-8, *G*).

11. Grasp the vas through the incision with the vas clamp (Fig. 129-8, *H*). Place the clamp **through** the vas itself. Strip away any remaining adherent fascia. Use a hemostat or preferably the sharp vas-dissecting forceps to create a small loop of vas. Using a twisting motion, push it through the tissue under the loop of vas and apply downward pressure to "strip" the tissue off the vas (Fig. 129-8, *I*).

12. Apply hemostats to the **fascial** tissue only at each end of the isolated vas as a safety measure (Fig. 129-8, *J[1]*).

13. Incise the vas, but not completely through. If a piece of vas is going to be removed, make two partial incisions 1 to 1½ cm apart (Fig. 129-8, *J[2]*). The specimens may be sent for pathologic examination; however, once the physician is able to identify the vas in vivo with certainty, this is no longer necessary.

Editor's note: Instead of sending the segments for histologic examination, some clinicians give the 1 cm vas segments in formalin (some put each side in a separate bottle) to their patients and instruct them to keep the segments in a medicine cabinet, away from children, until they have two negative semen checks. They can then dispose of the segments. Considering that 500,000 vasectomies are performed each year in the United States, that each pathology specimen costs between $150 and $200 to process, and that some physicians put each side in separate bottles, clinicians can save the healthcare system $75 million to $150 million per year by not sending in the specimens! If the patient keeps the specimens, and if the vas should fail (which is rare), the patient can then take the tissue to the lab to confirm they were resected, if desired.

14. Cauterize the prostatic end only (open-ended technique) or both ends of the vas by inserting the cautery tip 5 to 10 mm into the lumen, activating the cautery unit and then withdrawing the tip (Fig. 129-8, *K*). The objective is to create a graduated burn, minimal at the upper portion and maximal at the cut tip so that fibroblasts can close the vas somewhere in between. If too much burning is done, the entire tip may slough.

15. With the hemostats still in place, complete the transection through the entire vas. At this point, if a section of vas is removed, it is placed in formalin (Fig. 129-8, *L*).

16. With 4-0 chromic, create a "purse-string closure" and draw the fascia over the *prostatic* end of the vas, being careful to prevent the open *testicular* end from falling back into the sheath (Fig. 129-8, *M*).

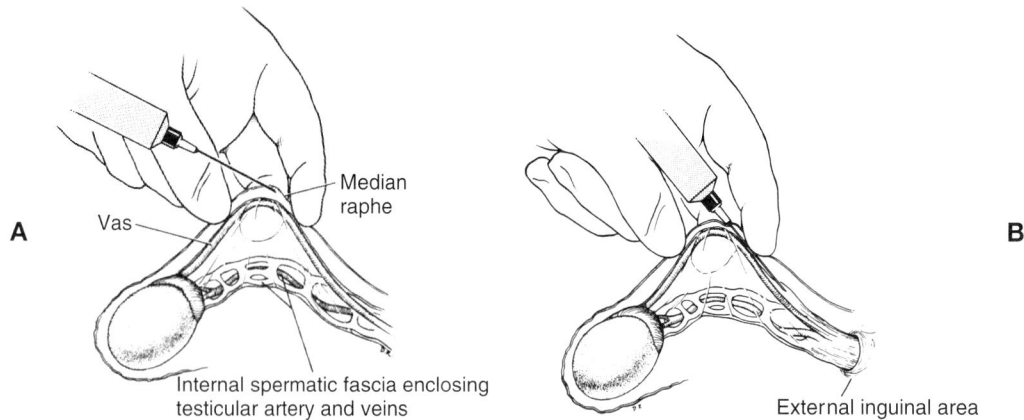

Fig. 129-7

Technique of perivas nerve block. **A,** To anesthetize the skin, a wheal with anesthetic is placed into the median raphe (superficially) from midscrotum up to the base of the penis. **B,** To anesthetize the vas, the 1½-inch needle is inserted in the midline and tracks along the vas toward the inguinal area. The vas has been pulled to the midline. Anesthetic is injected around the vas at the base of the scrotum. This is now repeated with the other vas. (From Li SQ, Goldstein M, Zhu J, Huber D: *J Urol* 145:341, 1991.)

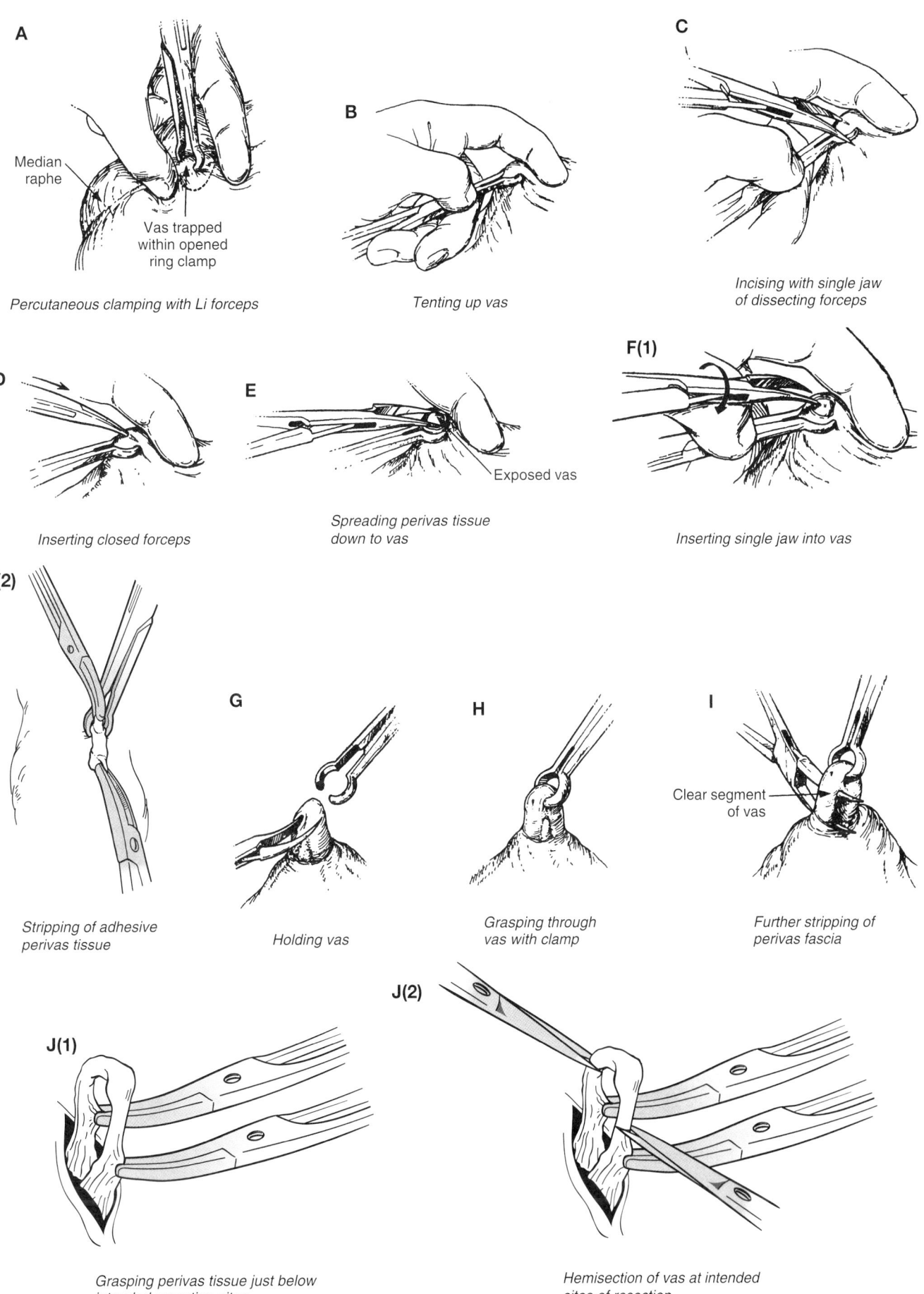

A

Median raphe

Vas trapped within opened ring clamp

Percutaneous clamping with Li forceps

B

Tenting up vas

C

Incising with single jaw of dissecting forceps

D

Inserting closed forceps

E

Exposed vas

Spreading perivas tissue down to vas

F(1)

Inserting single jaw into vas

F(2)

Stripping of adhesive perivas tissue

G

Holding vas

H

Grasping through vas with clamp

I

Clear segment of vas

Further stripping of perivas fascia

J(1)

Grasping perivas tissue just below intended resection sites

J(2)

Hemisection of vas at intended sites of resection

Fig. 129-8

Sequence of the vasectomy procedure showing several alternatives. See text for details.

Continued

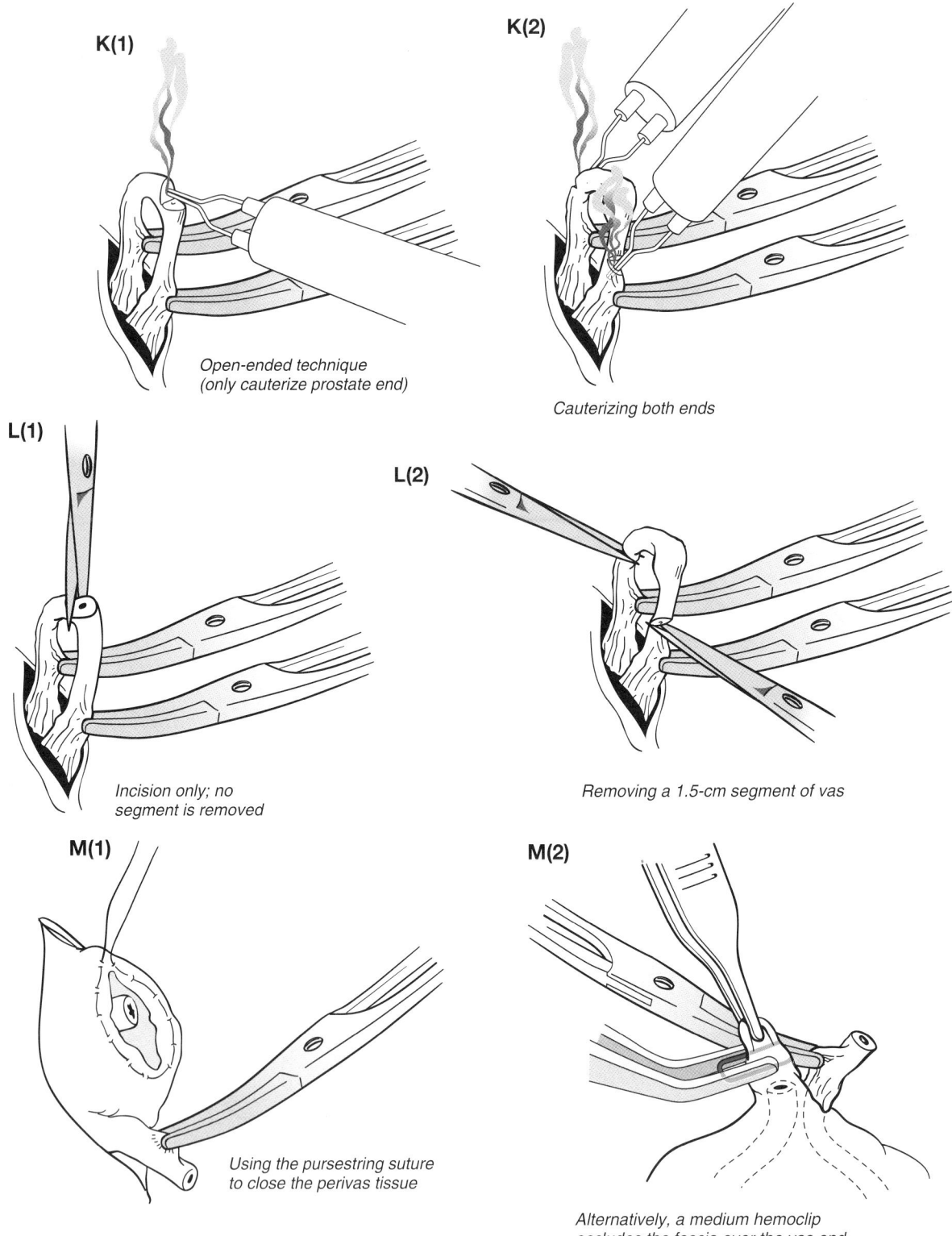

K(1)

*Open-ended technique
(only cauterize prostate end)*

K(2)

Cauterizing both ends

L(1)

*Incision only; no
segment is removed*

L(2)

Removing a 1.5-cm segment of vas

M(1)

*Using the pursestring suture
to close the perivas tissue*

M(2)

*Alternatively, a medium hemoclip
occludes the fascia over the vas end*

Fig. 129-8, cont'd

Release the hemostat only from the prostatic end at this point. (Some close over the testicular end.)

Note: The suture is placed only on the fascia, not on the vas itself. Rarely is the vas itself ligated. If not tight enough, the suture serves no purpose. If it is too tight, the end necroses, often leaving an open tip.

Alternatively a medium hemoclip is applied (only on the fascia). This is quicker and may cause less bleeding (Fig. 129-8, *M[2]*).

17. After hemostasis is ensured, drop the vas back into the scrotum. If bleeding is identified at any time during the procedure, use cautery to control it. Alternatively, the bleeding can be sutured or included under the vas clip.
18. Now identify the right vas. (If a second incision is made, provide additional anesthesia on the skin.) Isolate the right vas. Confirm that it is the right vas by tugging gently to move the right testicle. The procedure that was carried out on the left side is now carried out on the right.
19. A single 4-0 chromic catgut or Vicryl suture may be needed to close the skin, although generally the small openings (incisions) can be left open.
20. Antibiotic ointment is often placed on the wound, then covered with several 4 × 4–inch gauze pads to provide a compression dressing. This may be held in place with an athletic supporter or tight underwear.
21. Give the patient appropriate instructions for care, provide two containers for semen samples, and caution the patient to use alternative birth control until the semen checks are negative.
22. Discharge the patient after the instructions on postprocedure care and follow-up are understood. (See the sample patient education handout titled "Now That You Have Had Your Vasectomy" on page 1902 of Appendix G.)
23. Document the procedure with the appropriate operative report (Fig. 129-9).

Note: As with most invasive surgeries, it is advisable to call the patient in 1 to 3 days for follow-up. The call will be appreciated and will allow the clinician to answer any questions the patient may have.

CAUTERY INSTRUMENT STERILITY

It is difficult to maintain sterility of any reusable cautery instrument. The method shown in Figure 129-10 can be used for an electric unit with handpiece or a battery unit. Alternatively, disposable sterile sheaths can be obtained from AMI.

COMPLICATIONS

- *Swelling and discomfort* are prevented routinely by using an ice pack and mild analgesic (acetaminophen or ibuprofen). The pack is usually placed over the supporter but may need to be applied directly to the skin if bleeding is suspected.
- *Ecchymosis* makes the scrotum look bad but is harmless. Careful cautery of any bleeding, especially on the skin margins of the incision, usually prevents it.
- *Hematoma,* a major concern, may be prevented through good hemostasis. If it occurs, it may take 6 to 8 weeks to resolve. The scrotum can be as large as a grapefruit. Expectant waiting is generally advised. Surgical intervention can lead to trauma to neurovascular structures because they are hard to identify in the clots. Not evacuating the clot can also lead to calcification changes. Prevention by limiting activity the day of and the day after surgery is essential.
- *Infection* is always a risk, but is prevented by careful sterile technique. Prophylactic antibiotics are generally not indicated. The examination postoperatively is difficult because the patient is always somewhat tender. Suspect an infection if the postoperative course is generally good and improving, but in 3 to 14 days the patient experiences an increase in pain. Fever is rare. A urinalysis is usually normal. Clinicians can empirically begin a nonsteroidal antiinflammatory drug (NSAID) for pain and an antibiotic (for 10 to 14 days) if infection is suspected. Treatment with Augmentin, doxycycline, trimethoprim sulfa, or a cephalosporin is indicated.
- *Sperm granuloma* is only a problem if symptomatic; the risk of symptomatic sperm granuloma is surprisingly not increased if the open-ended technique is used.
- *Vasectomy failure* is a rare occurrence—about 1 in 1200 (slightly more if open-ended technique is used). The clinician should stress to the patient the importance of returning for semen specimen testing.
- There are some *uncommon complications.* For example, neuroma is characterized by exquisite sensitivity at the vasectomy site and can be definitively treated by a single injection of procaine. Congestive epididymitis may occur weeks to months after the procedure and is associated with the occlusion of the testicular end of the vas. It may cause chronic testicular pain in vasectomized patients. Leaving the testicular end of the vas open should prevent this complication.
- In large, long-term studies of vasectomized men, no increase in incidence of *chronic disease* has been found, including, among other diseases studied, hypertension, diabetes, autoimmune diseases, cardiovascular diseases, and prostate cancer.

No-Scalpel Vasectomy Operative Report

Patient name: _____ Date: _____

The patient has been previously counseled and given informed consent. The patient had all questions answered before the start of the procedure. The patient understands alternate contraceptive choices and that vasectomy is considered a permanent change. The patient was laid supine, the anterior scrotum was wiped with alcohol, and the penis was lifted cephalad. The skin of the anterior scrotum over the median raphe was anesthetized using 1 ml of a 1:1 mixture of 2% xylocaine with epinephrine and 1% xylocaine without epinephrine. The 25-gauge, 1^{1}/4-inch needle was then inserted alongside the left vas in the upper scrotum, and an external spermatic sheath block was accomplished. The needle was withdrawn. The right vas was brought to the midline. The needle was inserted and an external spermatic sheath block performed on the left. A total of __ ml of Xylocaine was administered. The patient tolerated the anesthetic administration well.

The scrotum was prepped with Betadine solution, and sterile drapes were placed. The left vas was swung to the midline using three-finger technique and grasped just below the anesthetized skin using the ring clamp. The skin above the vas was punctured using the vas dissecting forceps. The skin was spread, and the vas forceps was used to lift the vas through the small skin puncture site. The loop of vas was regrasped with the vas clamp. The fascial tissues were dissected off the vas. The vas was then hemitransected on both sides of the elevated loop of vas. The proximal and distal cut ends of the vas were cauterized using the battery cautery unit. The distal vas (prostatic end) was then fully transected. The distal cut vas was placed below the fascial tissues. The fascia was sealed over the distal vas using a medium metal hemoclip. The clip was placed up to but not over the proximal (testicular) vas. The end of the proximal vas protruded above the hemoclip. The proximal end was cut free from the upper loop, and the ^{1}/4-inch piece of vas was placed in formalin. Good hemostasis was noted. The structures were then returned to the scrotum. The right side was swung to the midline using the three-finger technique. The vas was grasped through the previous skin incision using the vas clamp. The patient reported tugging in the right groin, confirming grasp of the right vas. The vas was delivered through the skin, and the same procedure as performed on the left side was performed on the right.

After completion of the procedure, the scrotum was washed off with saline solution. Good hemostasis was noted at the skin site. Gauze was placed over the incision, and a supporter was placed. The patient was given extensive postoperative instructions. The patient will watch for signs of infection (e.g., pus, redness, swelling). The patient will rest, use acetaminophen and ibuprofen for discomfort, and apply ice to the scrotum as needed. The patient will refrain from heavy lifting or straining for a week. The patient will attempt sexual activity in 1 week and is aware that the first ejaculation may contain a drop of blood or produce a sharp pain. It was emphasized to continue contraception until two sperm evaluations were noted to be clear. The patient will return for sperm checks in approximately 6 and 12 weeks. The patient was informed to return if other problems develop. The patient will keep the two vas specimens in formalin in a safe location until the sperm checks are cleared (then the patient can dispose of them). The patient was referred to the patient instruction sheets.

Premedication: 800 mg ibuprofen   Valium 10 mg   atropine 0.5 mg   Dt
Assistant: _____
Present in room: Wife   Partner   Friend
Driver: _____
Tolerance: Good   Poor
Estimated blood loss: _____ ml
Changes to procedure: None or _____
Complications: None or _____

Impression: Uncomplicated vasectomy using no-scalpel technique
Other instructions: _____

cc: _____ Physician:_____

Fig. 129-9
Sample form of a no-scalpel vasectomy operative report. In this case, the open-ended technique was not used. (Courtesy Medical Procedures Center, P.C., Midland, Mich.)

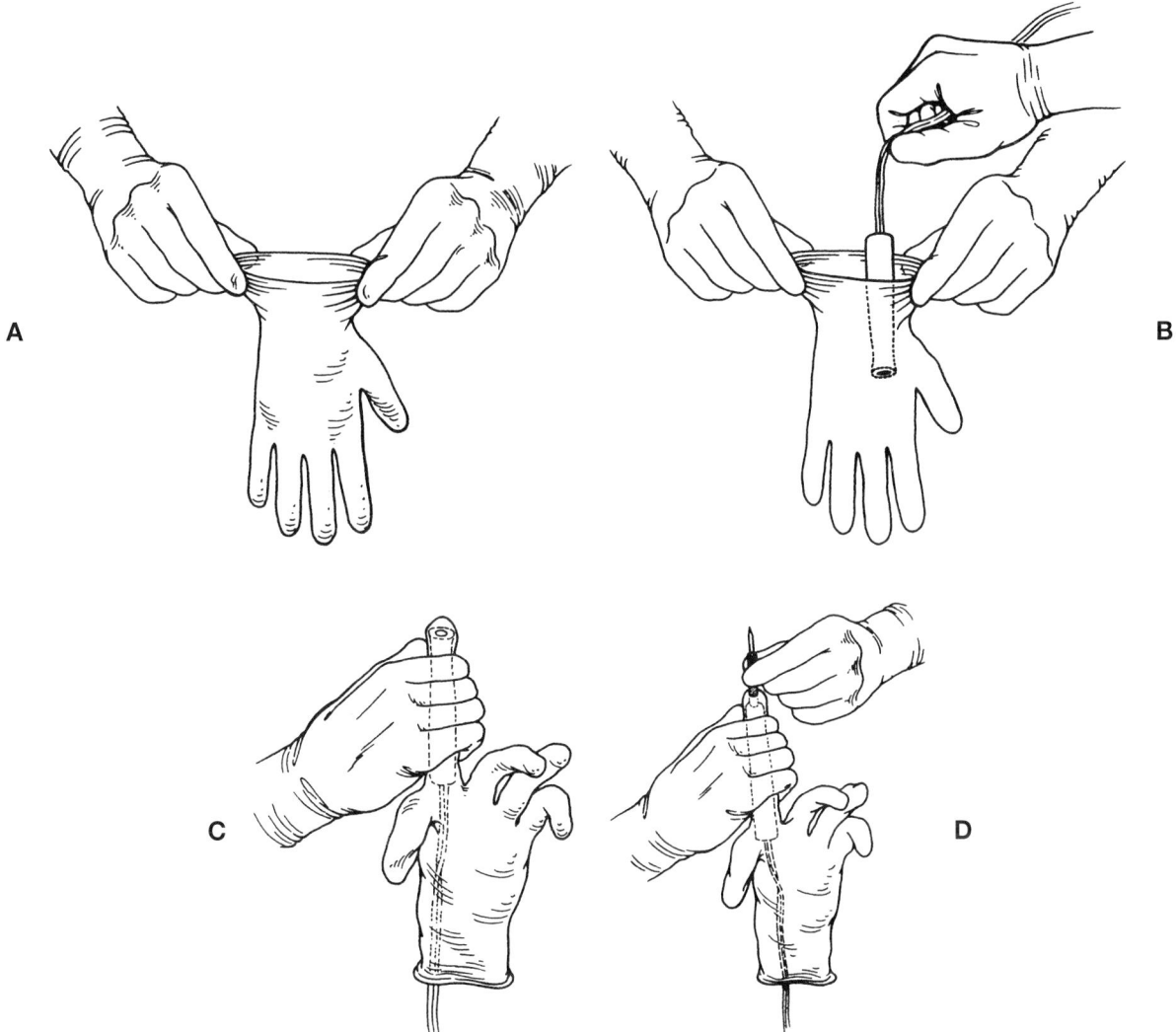

Fig. 129-10
Maintaining a sterile cautery instrument. **A,** Gloved physician holds the sterile glove. **B,** Assistant holds the cautery unit without the tip by the wire and carefully drops into finger of glove. **C,** Gloved physician grasps the cautery handle inside the glove finger. **D,** Sterile tip is punctured through rubber glove. The unit can now be handled in a sterile fashion; the clinician is careful not to contaminate the surgical field with the wire. (If it is a battery unit without wire, the unit can be activated so that the tip will burn through the glove to be exposed for use.)

- Studies show patients are 98% to 99% satisfied with the vasectomy decision. However, some *regret* having the procedure, either because of the complications discussed previously or later desire for children.
- *Pregnancy* can occur either because contraception was not used until the sperm were cleared or because of failure (i.e., spontaneous recanalization). Two studies also document rare pregnancy (DNA proven) in men who have negative checks both after vasectomy and again after the pregnancy! Apparently a

sperm can slip through in some cases of apparent successful vasectomy.

REVERSAL

Many patients request vasectomy reversal because a new partner wishes to have children. With fully informed consent, the true regret rates are extremely low, and patient and partner satisfaction with the procedure are extremely high. (Rosenfeld showed it is the only contraceptive method with which 100% of women are satisfied. With tubal ligation, the method with next highest acceptance rate, only 78% of women are satisfied.) Reversal can be accomplished using either a macroscopic or microscopic approach and results in pregnancy approximately 80% of the time. Intracytoplasmic sperm injection (ICSI) can be used but is much more costly. The use of previously frozen sperm is least expensive.

POSTPROCEDURE PATIENT CARE

No routine postprocedure examination is necessary. For the physician who is just beginning to perform vasectomy procedures, it may be advisable to see the patients in 1 to 2 weeks to gain an appreciation for the normal postprocedure changes.

It is customary to obtain two postprocedure semen checks: the first after 6 weeks or 15 ejaculations (whichever is later) and the second in 3 months. Sperm can persist in the ejaculate for many weeks. This method will detect essentially all failures. If recanalization occurs, it generally takes place in the early postprocedure period. Some define a positive specimen as any visualized sperm under high power (unspun specimen). Others claim that only live sperm are significant. It may be prudent to document at least one *completely* sperm-free sample. If the specimen is obtained too soon after vasectomy, sperm (live or dead) may be seen in the ejaculate even though the procedure was successful.

Edwards (1993) reported that testing can be done 4 weeks after vasectomy, regardless of the number of postvasectomy ejaculations. As long as the examination was done within 12 hours of collection, the specimen was read as negative if no motile sperm were seen. Repeat tests were recommended only if motile sperm were seen. This study has not become the accepted standard.

If a true surgical failure is suspected based on semen analysis, it may be advisable to have the patient produce a specimen in the office before proceeding with repeat vasectomy.

POSTOPERATIVE SEMEN ANALYSIS

The clinician places a drop or two of unspun fresh ejaculate onto a slide (no staining is necessary). The sample is covered with coverslip and examined under 40× magnification for the presence of live or dead sperm (higher power with oil immersion is not necessary). Fig. 129-11 shows the appearance of sperm in a *failed* vasectomy (no sperm should be seen). Semen checks are included as part of the procedure code.

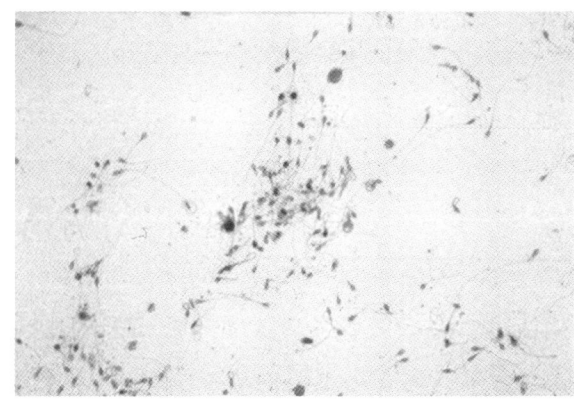

Fig. 129-11
Postoperative semen check. The appearance of sperm in the ejaculate of a failed vasectomy. (Courtesy Nicholas Hruby, MD, Saginaw, Mich.)

SUPPLIERS

Videotapes for patient education
The National Procedures Institute (NPI)
4909 Hedgewood Drive
Midland, MI 48640
Phone: 1-800-462-2492
Website: www.npinstitute.com

EngenderHealth (formerly Association for Voluntary Surgical Contraception)
440 Ninth Avenue
New York, NY 10001
Phone: 1-212-561-8000
Website: www.engenderhealth.org

Written patient education handouts
EngenderHealth (see previous listing)

Procter & Gamble Pharmaceuticals
1 or 2, Procter & Gamble Plaza
Cincinnati, OH 45201
Phone: 1-513-983-1100
Website: www.pgpharma.com

Advanced Meditech International (AMI)
86-38 53rd Avenue, Suite 100
Flushing, NY 11373
Phone: 1-800-635-2452
Website: www.ameditech.com

American Urological Association
1120 North Charles Street
Baltimore, MD 21201
Phone: 1-800-908-9414
Website: www.auanet.com

Krames Communications
1100 Grundy Lane
San Bruno, CA 94066
Phone: 1-800-333-3032
www.krames.com

Other patient information

EngenderHealth online patient information Website: www.engenderhealth.org

EngenderHealth vasectomy information line
Phone: 1-888-VASEC-4-U

Vasectomy and vasectomy reversal online information
Website: www.vasectomy.medical.com

Advanced Meditech International (AMI) (see previous listing)

Technique videotapes for physicians

Advanced Meditech International (AMI) (see previous listing)

EngenderHealth (see previous listing)

Health Sciences Center for Educational
     Resources
University of Washington
T-252 Health Sciences Bldg, Box 357161
Seattle, WA 98195-7161
Phone: 1-206-685-1158
Website: www.hscer.washington.edu/hscer

The National Procedures Institute (NPI) (see previous listing)

Dr. Charles Wilson
The Vasectomy Clinic
5402 47th Avenue NE
Seattle, WA 98105
Phone: 1-206-525-4090
Website: www.thevasectomyclinic.org

American Academy of Family Physicians
11400 Tomahawk Creek Parkway
Leawood, KS 66211-2672
Phone: 1-800-274-2237
Website: www.aafp.org

No-scalpel vasectomy brochure

Advanced Meditech International (AMI) (see previous listing)

No-scalpel Instrument Suppliers

Advanced Meditech International (AMI) (see previous listing)

CooperSurgical (Wilson clamp and dissecting forceps)
95 Corporate Drive
Trumbull, CT 06611
Phone: 1-800-243-2974
Website: www.coopersurgical.com

Hemoclips and clip applicators

Ethicon, Inc.
P.O. Box 151
Somerville, NJ 08876-0151
Phone: 1-800-438-4426
Website: www.ethiconinc.com

Weck Closure Systems
2917 Weck Drive
P.O. Box 12600
Research Triangle Park, NC 27709
Phone: 1-800-234-9325
Website: www.weckclosure.com

Battery-operated cautery

Advanced Meditech International (AMI) (see previous listing)

Ellman
1135 Railroad Avenue
Hewlett, NY 11557
Phone: 1-800-835-5355
Website: www.ellman.com

Note: Most medical suppliers also carry battery-operated cautery equipment.

Teaching models

Advanced Meditech International (AMI) (see previous listing)
The National Procedures Institute (NPI) (see previous listing)
Dr. Charles Wilson (see previous listing)

ADDITIONAL RESOURCES

- See the sample patient education handouts titled "Vasectomy (Permanent Male Sterilization)" and "Now That You Have Had Your Vasectomy" on pages 1898 and 1902, respectively, of Appendix G.
- See the sample patient consent form titled "Request for Vasectomy" on page 1904 of Appendix G.

BIBLIOGRAPHY

Alderman PM: Complications in a series of 1224 vasectomies, *J Fam Pract* 33:576, 1991.

Benger JR: Persistent spermatozoa after vasectomy: a survey of British urologists, *Br J Urol* 76:376, 1995.

Cox B, Sneyd MJ, Paul C, et al: Vasectomy and risk of prostate cancer, *JAMA* 287:3110, 2002.

Davis JE: Male sterilization, *Curr Opin Obstet Gynecol* 4:522, 1992.

Denniston GC: The effect of vasectomy on childless men, *J Reprod Med* 21(3):151, 1978.

Denniston GC: Vasectomy by electrocautery: outcomes in a series of 2,500 patients, *J Fam Pract* 21(1):35, 1985.

Denniston GC, Kuehl L: Open-ended vasectomy: approaching the ideal technique, *J Am Board Fam Pract* 7:285, 1994.

DerSimonian R, Clemens J, Spirtas R, Perlman J: Vasectomy and prostate cancer risk: methodological review of the evidence, *J Clin Epidemiol* 46(2):163, 1993.

Edwards IS: Early testing after vasectomy, based on the absence of motile sperm, *Fertil Steril* 59(2):431, 1993.

Errey BB, Edwards IS: Open-ended vasectomy: an assessment, *Fertil Steril* 45:843, 1986.

Giovannucci E et al: A long-term study of mortality in men who have undergone vasectomy, *N Engl J Med* 326(1):1392, 1992.

Giovannucci E, Ascherio A, Rimm EB, et al: A prospective cohort study of vasectomy and prostate cancer in US men, *JAMA* 269:873, 1993.

Greenberg MJ: Vasectomy technique, *Am Fam Physician* 39(1):131, 1989.

Guess HA: Is vasectomy a risk factor for prostate cancer? *Eur J Cancer* 29A(7):1055, 1993.

Haws JM, Feigin J: Vasectomy counseling, *Am Fam Physician* 52(5):1395, 1995.

Haws JM, Morgan GT, Pollack AF et al: Clinical aspects of vasectomies performed in the US in 1995, *J Urol* 52:685, 1998.

Healy B: From the National Institutes of Health, *JAMA* 269:2620, 1993.

Hendry WF: Vasectomy and vasectomy reversal, *Br J Urol* 73:337, 1994.

Howards SS, Peterson HB: Vasectomy and prostate cancer—chance bias, or a casual relationship, *JAMA* 269:913, 1993.

John EM, Whittemore AS, Wu AH, et al: Vasectomy and prostate cancer: results from a multicentric case-control study, *J Natl Cancer Inst* 87:662, 1995.

Kendrick JS, Gonzales B, Huber DH, et al: Complications of vasectomy in the United States, *J Fam Pract* 25:245, 1987.

Li PS, Li SQ, Schlegel PN, Goldstein M: External spermatic sheath injection for vasal nerve block, *Urology* 39(2):173, 1992.

Li SQ, Goldstein M, Zhu J, Huber D: The no-scalpel vasectomy, *J Urol* 145:341, 1991.

Lipshultz LI, Benson GS: Vasectomy 1980, *Urol Clin North Am* 7:89, 1980.

McDonald S: Is vasectomy harmful to health? *Br J Gen Pract* 47:381-386, 1997.

McKay W, Morris R, Mushlin P: Sodium bicarbonate attenuates pain on skin infiltration with lidocaine, with or without epinephrine, *Anesth Analg* 66:572, 1987.

O'Brien TS, Cranston D, Ashwin P, et al: Temporary reappearance of sperm 12 months after vasectomy clearance, *Br J Urol* 76:371, 1995.

Pfenninger JL: Complications of vasectomy, *Am Fam Physician* 30(5):111, 1984a.

Pfenninger JL: Preparation for vasectomy, *Am Fam Physician* 30(4):177, 1984b.

Raspa RF: Complications of vasectomy, *Am Fam Physician* 48(7):1264, 1993.

Reynolds RD: Vas deferens occlusion during no-scalpel vasectomy, *J Fam Pract* 39:577, 1994.

Rosenfeld JA, Zahorik PM, Saint W, Murphy G: Women's satisfaction with birth control, *J Fam Pract* 36(2):169, 1993.

Schmidt SS: Prevention of failure in vasectomy, *J Urol* 109:296, 1973.

Schmidt SS: Vasectomy: principles and comments, *J Fam Pract* 33:571, 1991.

Schmidt SS: The vas after vasectomy: comparison of cauterization methods, *J Urol* 40(5):468, 1992.

Stockton MD, Davis LE, Bolton KM: No-scalpel vasectomy: a technique for family physicians, *Am Fam Physician* 46(4):1153, 1992.

Vasectomy: Procedures for your practice, *Patient Care* 24:116, 1991.

WEBSITE

www.vasectomymedical.com (An excellent Internet resource on vasectomy and vasectomy reversal, that includes physician directories for providers. This popular site walks the prospective patient through the decision-making process, explaining in simple, understandable language all that should be considered.)

PART NINE

Gynecology and Female Reproductive System Procedures

CHAPTER 130

First-Trimester Abortion and Emergency Oral Contraceptives

Steven H. Eisinger

Abortion became legal in every state in the United States as a result of the *Roe v Wade* Supreme Court decision in 1973. The decision was based on a person's constitutional right to privacy; thus abortion of a pregnancy during the first trimester is a private issue to be settled between the woman and her doctor. More than 1.2 million elective abortions are now performed in the United States annually. Over half of these are 8 weeks or less in gestational age, and 88% are in the first trimester. A patchwork of state laws now exists that regulates abortion, ranging from highly restrictive to highly liberal. Recent trends have placed increasing legal constraints on abortion, although these are being challenged in the courts. *It is imperative for any physician performing abortion to have an accurate working knowledge of any state and local restrictions governing abortion.*

Abortion differs from other medical procedures because it can generate strong feelings not just among patients and family, but among the practitioners as well. Before providing abortion services, the thoughtful physician should examine the emotional, ethical, and societal aspects of abortion. He or she must consider the effect of abortion on his or her practice, office staff, and community. Security must be considered. The decision to perform abortions is complicated; however, those physicians who decide to offer the procedure may take satisfaction in knowing that they are providing service to their patients.

The suction curettage technique explained in this chapter can be used for *a missed or incomplete abortion* (see Chapter 144, Dilation and Curettage). Although the suction curettage technique is detailed in this chapter, two other techniques warrant discussion: manual vacuum aspiration and medical abortion. In addition, a brief discussion of emergency oral contraception is included.

EMERGENCY ORAL CONTRACEPTION

Primary contraception is always best. Emergency contraception may be needed at times when an unwanted pregnancy is a possibility.

Emergency oral contraception is treatment intended for women who have had unprotected intercourse but who wish to avoid pregnancy. This includes women who have used no contraception during intercourse, whose method of contraception has failed (such as a broken condom), or who have been victims of sexual assault. Appropriate candidates must be at risk for pregnancy (i.e., cycling regularly with presumed ovulatory cycles and neither pregnant, premenarchal, postmenopausal, nor otherwise already using other effective contraception). Women at midmenstrual cycle are at greatest risk, but risk exists at any time in the cycle. This method is also called *postcoital contraception* and *"the morning-after pill."*

High doses of sex steroids administered within 72 hours of exposure are known to prevent pregnancy. The mechanism is unclear but probably involves interference with implantation of a fertilized ovum. Some regard this as a form of abortion, but others feel that abortion occurs only after implantation. The medications do not interrupt an ongoing pregnancy.

Two regimens are commercially available by prescription for emergency contraception: Preven (Gynetics) and Plan B (Women's Capital). Preven uses the Yuzpe or combination pill method, developed many years ago, which consists of tablets containing ethinyl estradiol 50 μg and levonorgestrel 0.25 mg. Two pills must be taken as soon as possible after the exposure but within 72 hours. Two additional pills are taken 12 hours later. Plan B consists of tablets containing 0.75 mg of levonorgestrel. One pill is taken as soon as possible after exposure (again within 72 hours) and the second pill is taken 12 hours later.

TABLE 130-1

Commercially Available Emergency Oral Contraceptives and Their Equivalents from Regular Oral Contraceptive Brands*

Name	Formulation	Dosage
Dedicated Progestin-Only Product		
Plan B	0.75 mg levonorgestrel	One pill immediately; one pill in 12 hours
Equivalent dose from oral contraceptive brand		
Ovrette	0.075 mg norgestrel	20 pills immediately; 20 pills in 12 hours
Dedicated Combination Estrogen/Progestin Product		
Preven	50 µg ethinyl estradiol	Two pills immediately; two pills in 12 hours
	0.25 mg levonorgestrel	
Equivalent dose from oral contraceptive brand		
Ovral	50 µg ethinyl estradiol	Two pills immediately; two pills in 12 hours
	0.50 mg norgestrel	
Ovral-28	(White tablets)	
Ogestrel	50 µg ethinyl estradiol	Two pills immediately; two pills in 12 hours
	0.50 mg norgestrel	
Lo/Ovral	30 µg ethinyl estradiol	Four pills immediately; four pills in 12 hours
	0.30 mg norgestrel	
Lo/Ovral-28	(White tablets)	
Low-Ogestrel	30 µg ethinyl estradiol	Four pills immediately; four pills in 12 hours
	0.30 mg norgestrel	
Nordette	(Light orange tablets)	Four pills immediately; four pills in 12 hours
	30 µg ethinyl estradiol	
	0.15 mg levonorgestrel	
Levlen	30 µg ethinyl estradiol	Four pills immediately; four pills in 12 hours
	0.15 mg levonorgestrel	
Levora	30 µg ethinyl estradiol	Four pills immediately; four pills in 12 hours
	0.15 mg levonorgestrel	
Triphasil	(Yellow tablets)	Four pills immediately; four pills in 12 hours
	30 µg ethinyl estradiol	
	0.125 mg levonorgestrel	
Tri-Levlen	(Yellow tablets)	Four pills immediately; four pills in 12 hours
	30 µg ethinyl estradiol	
	0.125 mg levonorgestrel	
Trivora	(Pink tablets)	Four pills immediately; four pills in 12 hours
	30 µg ethinyl estradiol	
	0.125 mg levonorgestrel	
Alesse	20 µg ethinyl estradiol	Five pills immediately; five pills in 12 hours
	0.1 mg levonorgestrel	
Alesse-28	(Pink tablets)	
Levlite	(Pink tablets)	Five pills immediately; five pills in 12 hours
	20 µg ethinyl estradiol	
	0.1 mg levonorgestrel	

*All regimens must begin within 72 hours of the unprotected intercourse.

The components of the products just described are hormones commonly found in certain oral contraceptives, including a number of generic preparations. Therefore it is possible to put together comparable doses by taking the right number of pills from appropriate oral contraceptive packs. Note that the sole estrogen represented in these preparations is ethinyl estradiol, but that two progestins are represented: norgestrel and levonorgestrel. Since levonorgestrel is the active isomer of norgestrel, twice as much norgestrel is required for the same therapeutic effect. Table 130-1 provides the equivalent dosages.

The *prescribing regimen* is the same for all the options: the first dose is taken immediately, and the second dose is taken 12 hours later. Evidence shows that early administration enhances efficacy. The greatest efficacy occurs when the regimen starts within 24 hours of exposure, but the treatment may be initiated up to 72 hours after exposure. With the Yuzpe method (Preven and all its equivalents), which contains estrogen, nausea and vomiting is a common problem. Therefore a prophylactic antiemetic is recommended before the hormones are administrated. Breast tenderness may also occur. Side effects are less with the progestin-only method (Plan B and its equivalent).

Medical contraindications to oral contraceptives, such as severe hypertension and history of thromboembolism, are listed in product information for Preven but have not been shown to be significant with the short dosage schedule. The progestin-only method (Plan B or its equivalent) has no known medical contraindications. The World Health Organization has stated that the only contraindication to emergency contraception is an ongoing pregnancy. No teratogenic effects have been identified.

Efficacy of both methods is good, but in a head-to-head randomized, blinded study the progestin-only method (Plan B) had an efficacy of 85%, whereas the Yuzpe method (Preven) had an efficacy of 57%. This is a significant difference. Menses may be early, on time, or delayed after treatment. If the delay is 21 days or more from the date of treatment, a pregnancy test should be performed.

The cost of emergency contraception varies from $23 to $36 retail. Availability has been sporadic in the past. Some pharmacies, including a large discount chain, have refused to stock the medications.

Access appears to be the major issue for emergency contraception. Both doctors and patients are often unaware of the possibility of the treatment. Education is a major component in getting this valuable treatment to the patients who need it. Critical delays in treatment may occur when doctors require an office visit before prescribing or the patient has to search for a pharmacy that carries the prescription. For these reasons, the American College of Obstetricians and Gynecologists has advocated the practice of discussing emergency contraception with all patients who are sexually active and at risk for a contraceptive failure. They may even be given a prescription to be held in reserve in case of an exposure. Prescribing over the telephone appears to be safe. Other alternatives under discussion designed to increase access include distribution by pharmacists and over-the-counter availability. A national telephone hotline (not associated with the manufacturers) has been established to provide the names and numbers of local clinics that provide emergency contraceptive services: 1-888-not-2-late (668-2528).

Another approach to emergency contraception is the placement of an intrauterine device (IUD). The IUD is probably effective up to a week after exposure. See Chapter 148 for a full discussion of IUD insertion.

MANUAL VACUUM ASPIRATION

Manual vacuum aspiration is a technique of early abortion undergoing a resurgence in recent years. It is based on a handheld and operated nonelectrical syringe to provide the vacuum to evacuate the uterus. Small double-portal flexible cannulae are available for early abortions.

There are two principal advantages to this system. First, it is highly portable, inexpensive, and inconspicuous, and it can provide a means for a practitioner to offer early abortions without having a large investment in equipment. This is ideal for practitioners who perform only an occasional procedure, or who need the capability only for the occasional complication of a medical abortion. It is also suitable for third world applications.

The second advantage is that the system is quiet. Although there is still some suction sound, there is no machine noise. Patients have related that the noise of the machine can be a disquieting part of the experience. Less disruption of the tissue is another attribute described with this technique. Frequently a tiny gestational sac can be identified intact upon performing the *float test,* thus confirming that the abortion is complete. (See the "Suction Abortion" section, step 12.)

The key component of manual vacuum aspiration is the preparation and use of the syringe (see Fig. 130-1, *A*). The 60-ml syringe has an auto-vacuum feature, which is activated by closing the valve or pushing the buttons forward. Then the plunger can be drawn back using a moderate amount of force to create the vacuum, until the arms of the plunger spring outward over the end of the syringe barrel (Fig. 130-1, *B*). This preserves the vacuum until the valve is opened. The syringe may then be attached to a cannula placed into the uterus, and the vacuum activated by pushing the buttons backward. The procedure then proceeds much as it does with machine vacuum (Fig. 130-2).

MEDICAL ABORTION

Medical abortion has come into use in the past few years. Hopefully, medical abortion will be easy and safe enough for any physician to offer it through the physician's office, thus making abortion more private and more available than it is at present.

Two basic forms of medical abortion are presently available—mifepristone and methotrexate—and each is followed by a prostaglandin.

Mifepristone Medical Abortion

Mifepristone, formerly known as RU-486, is an antiprogesterone developed in France in 1980. It has undergone extensive clinical trials in France, China, Sweden, and many other countries. Although initially kept out of the United States for political reasons,

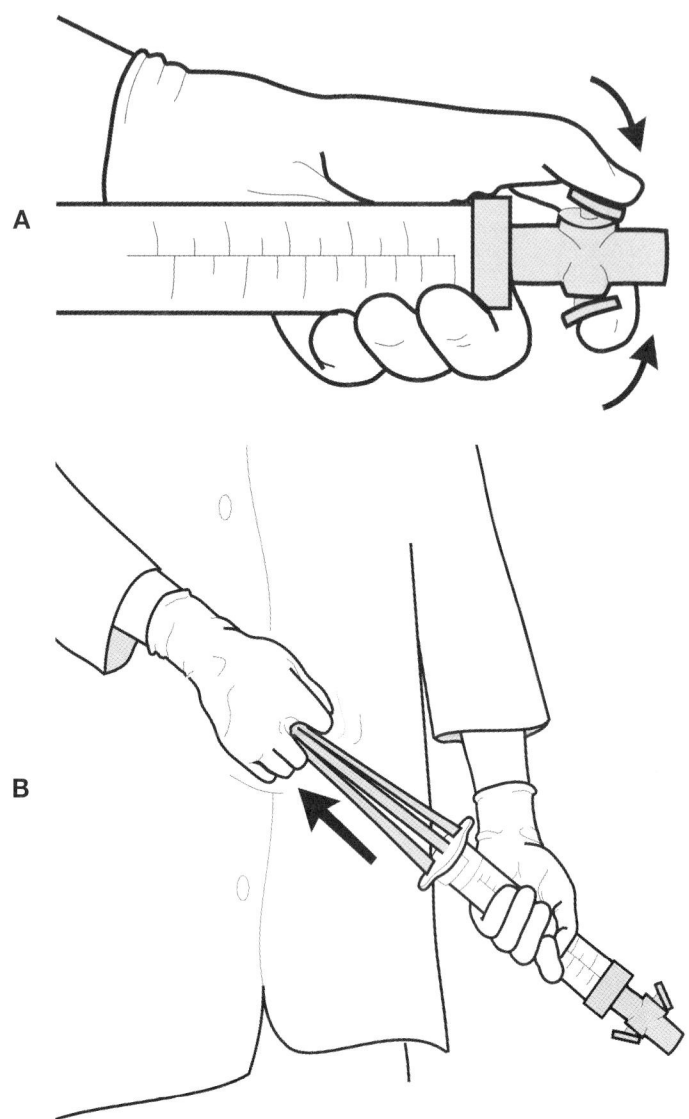

Fig. 130-1
Auto-vacuum feature of IPAS double-valve syringe. **A,** Valve is closed by pushing the buttons down and forward until they lock in place. **B,** Vacuum is created when plunger is drawn back until its arms snap outward and over the end of the syringe barrel. (From Winkler J, Blumenthal P, Greenslade F: Early abortion services: new choices for providers and women. *Advances in abortion care,* IPAS, Carrboro, NC, 5[2]:1996.)

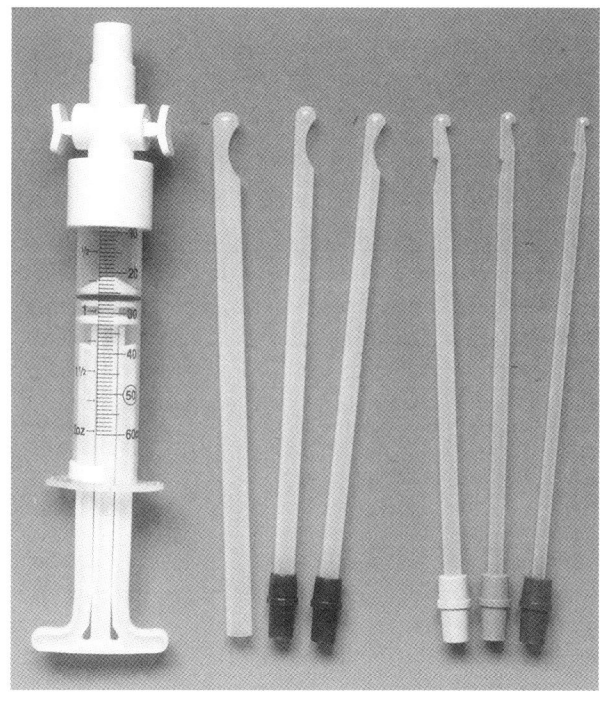

Fig. 130-2
IPAS manual vacuum instruments. (From Winkler J, Blumenthal P, Greenslade F: Early abortion services: new choices for providers and women. *Advances in abortion care,* IPAS, Carrboro, NC, 5[2]:1996.)

Medical *contraindications* to mifepristone are rare, but they include adrenal failure, severe asthma, porphyria, and long-term glucocorticoid therapy. An IUD in utero is also a contraindication. Great caution should be used in treating patients with coagulopathies or who are anticoagulated or in patients who are severely anemic. Side effects of mifepristone are usually minor when compared with the side effects of misoprostol during medical abortion (see below).

Mifepristone has proved to be remarkably safe and effective, and it provides women with a real alternative to surgical abortion.

Misoprostol is an important adjunct to medical abortion. Misoprostol is a prostaglandin E_1 analog available in tablet form for oral administration, marketed under the brand name Cytotec. It is indicated for the prevention and treatment of ulcers, is inexpensive, and comes in 100- and 200-µg tablets. Misoprostol is a powerful uterotonic. Given orally or vaginally, it causes strong uterine cramping and greatly enhances the success rates and rapidity of medical abortion. Studies have shown higher efficacy and lower side effects when it is administered vaginally. Typical prostaglandin side effects that occur with misoprostol are nausea, vomiting, chills, and fever. Misoprostol is believed to be a teratogen when administered in early pregnancy if abortion should fail to occur. Pregnancy is the sole

mifepristone was available for abortion research. After many years of delay and debate, it was approved by the Food and Drug Administration (FDA) for use as an abortifacient in September of 2000. It is distributed in the United States by Danco Laboratories under the brand name Mifeprex. Mifepristone is not available by prescription through standard pharmacies; it is distributed directly to clinics and physician offices, which in turn dispense it directly to patients. The current cost of mifepristone from the distributor is about $90 per 200-mg tablet.

contraindication listed in the FDA-approved literature for misoprostol. Other prostaglandins have been used for medical abortion, but none have the combination of safety, efficacy, and low cost of misoprostol.

Two basic protocols exist for the use of mifepristone and misoprostol: the *Standard Protocol* and the *Evidence-based Protocol,* also referred to as *Acceptable Alternatives to the FDA Regimen*. The Standard Protocol, described by the product literature and reflecting FDA-imposed restrictions, is very conservative and cautious. The Evidence-based Protocol is more flexible. Both protocols are described here, with the similarities and differences pointed out.

Patient Selection

Medical abortion is suitable for early pregnancies only. The FDA-approved *Standard Protocol* limits gestational age to 49 days or less from the last menstrual period. The *Evidence-based Protocol* permits abortion up to 63 days. *Transvaginal ultrasound dating is essential* in both protocols, to establish accurate dates and to rule out ectopic pregnancy. Medical abortion is quite different from surgical abortion, and patients should be counseled carefully in order to make a free and informed choice between the two procedures. Patients must understand what to expect and be screened for their ability to cope, since the method includes several hours of cramping and bleeding. With the Evidence-based Protocol patients can be treated at home. Table 130-2 compares the medical and surgical abortion methods.

Protocols

The *Standard Protocol* calls for the oral administration of 600 mg of mifepristone (three 200-mg tablets), followed by oral misoprostol 400 μg 48 hours later. The physician is obligated to give the misoprostol to the patient in the office or clinic and to observe the patient for 4 hours, during which approximately half of patients will abort. Several studies have verified that lower doses of mifepristone are equally effective. The *Evidence-based Protocol* calls for 200 mg of mifepristone (one 200-mg tablet) given orally, followed by 800 μg of misoprostol administered vaginally 24 to 72 hours later. Several studies have allowed patients to insert the vaginal misoprostol tablets at home. The Standard Protocol calls for follow-up within 14 days; the Evidence-based Protocol calls for follow-up much sooner—within 4 to 7 days. Both protocols call for the ready availability of surgical backup should a suction dilation and curettage (D & C) become necessary. Table 130-3 compares the two regimens.

Efficacy

All protocols have a high rate of success in many studies. The Standard Protocol has success rates between 90%

TABLE 130-2

Comparison of Medical and Surgical Abortion

Medical Abortion	Surgical Abortion
Suitable for early pregnancy only	Suitable for early and later pregnancy
Oral medications only	Surgical procedure
Higher level of patient involvement	Lower level of patient involvement
Abortion may take place in the office or clinic (Standard Protocol) or at home (Evidence-based Protocol)	Occurs in office, clinic, or hospital
Takes two or three visits over several days; sometimes longer	Takes one to two visits, the actual procedure is brief
High success rate, but significant chance of failure	Very high success rate
Requires very careful patient follow-up	Requires follow-up, but less important
Oral pain medication over several hours	Local and/or IV sedation or general anesthesia
Treats missed abortion	Treats missed abortion
Does not treat ectopic pregnancy (mifepristone)	Does not treat ectopic pregnancy, but may provide diagnosis
Resembles miscarriage	Surgical procedure
May be more private	Requires office or clinic visits during surgical hours; may be less private

TABLE 130-3

Comparison of Standard Food and Drug Administration Regimen and the Evidence-Based Regimen

	Standard Regimen	Evidence-Based Regimen
Maximum gestational age	Up to 49 days (ultrasound confirmed)	Up to 63 days (ultrasound confirmed)
Mifepristone dose	600 mg (three tablets)	200 mg (one tablet)
Misoprostol dose	400 μg orally (two tablets)	800 μg vaginally (four tablets)
Misoprostol timing	48 hours after mifepristone	24 to 72 hours after mifepristone
Misoprostol location	MD office or clinic	Home
Follow-up office visit	Day 14	Day 4 to 8
Minimum number of office visits	3	2
Cost	Higher	Lower

and 98%, with success defined as complete abortion without the need of surgical intervention. Comparable success rates—between 96% and 99%—are attributed to the Evidence-based Protocol.

Complications

The major complications of medical abortion with mifepristone and misoprostol are continuation of the pregnancy, retained products, and heavy bleeding resulting from incomplete abortion. Continuation of pregnancy is related to gestational age. In the gestational age-group of 54 to 63 days, ongoing pregnancy rates vary between 5% and 9%, but they are substantially lower at lower gestational ages (down to less than 1% for gestational age of less than 42 days). Cramping and bleeding are expected when the medical method is used, but bleeding heavy enough to require emergency care (or heavy enough to require transfusion) is generally less than 1%. In the Population Council American Trial, 4 patients out of more than 2000 required a transfusion. In other large studies, no patients have required transfusion. The treatment of both of these major complications is the same: a suction D & C. Endometritis following medical abortion is very rare, although one patient in Canada is known to have died from sepsis after a mifepristone medical abortion.

Teratogenicity of mifepristone is unknown. Patients should be counseled carefully, however, that a significant risk of congenital defects occurs with an ongoing pregnancy after use of misoprostol in the first trimester. Therefore a surgical abortion is recommended in the event of a medical failure. Sensitization to Rh factor is very low, *but anti-D immune globulin is indicated in Rh-negative patients.*

Mifepristone is not recommended until a gestational sac is visible by transvaginal ultrasound. Mifepristone is apparently not effective in treating an ectopic pregnancy. Because the tissue is so scant and is usually discarded when the patient aborts at home, there is no possibility of diagnosing an ectopic pregnancy by showing the absence of products of conception on pathologic examination.

Psychological Reactions

Most patients seem highly accepting of medical abortion; many find it more "natural" or more resembling a miscarriage than surgical abortion. In the home setting, under the Evidence-based Protocol, patients can be supported by loved ones in private. Patients attending doctors' offices or clinics for medical abortion are less likely to be subjected to harassment than patients undergoing surgical abortion. On the other hand, some patients want the experience to be finished as quickly as possible, and some do not tolerate the several hours of cramping and bleeding that accompany most medical abortions. Some women prefer not to see the aborted products of conception, which can happen with medical abortion. All in all, women usually react well to the procedure, and it provides a real choice in safe abortion methods.

Methotrexate Medical Abortion

Methotrexate followed by misoprostol is also an effective means of accomplishing medical abortion.

Methotrexate is a folic acid antagonist that has been available since the 1950s. It interferes with trophoblastic development and thus interrupts an early first trimester pregnancy. The medication is widely available in the injectable and oral form, and it is inexpensive. Methotrexate is usually viewed as an antineoplastic drug and is used for gestational trophoblastic disease, blood dyscrasias, and other cancers. However, it is also used in nonneoplastic conditions such as rheumatoid arthritis, Crohn's disease, and psoriasis.

Patient selection is similar to medical abortion with mifepristone. Most protocols limit gestational age to 49 to 56 days. Accurate dating is essential. The dosage of methotrexate is 50 mg/m^2, given intramuscularly. Most American women fall between 1.5 and 2.0 m^2, so the usual dosage is between 75 and 100 mg of methotrexate. The square meter value of an individual patient is most often calculated by a nomogram using height and weight, available in most pharmacies. A formula can also be used:

$$m^2 = \text{square root ([height in inches} \times \text{weight in pounds]/3131)}$$

Fifty mg given orally is also effective.

Misoprostol 800 μg vaginally is given at some time interval later, usually 3 to 7 days. Close follow-up is mandatory by performing transvaginal ultrasounds or serial βHCG determinations, because methotrexate is much slower than mifepristone. Abortion occurs in 75% of women within the first week, but the remaining 25% may take up to 28 days to abort. The dose may be repeated in a week if necessary.

Efficacy is 82% to 96%, which approaches the efficacy of mifepristone, but it takes much longer. The primary complications of the method are the same as with mifepristone: heavy bleeding, retained pregnancy, and ongoing pregnancy. The treatment for these conditions is also the same: suction D & C.

Methotrexate has potential side effects such as hepatic and hematologic toxicity, which are fortunately rare in the one-time moderate dosage used in this protocol. It is also a teratogen when it fails to interrupt the pregnancy.

Overall, methotrexate seems clearly inferior to mifepristone in most respects. Three exceptions exist. Methotrexate costs much less than mifepristone, particularly when mifepristone is given in the full standard dose. In addition, two uncommon clinical dilemmas favor the use of methotrexate: the situation where a patient cannot take oral medication, and the situation in which the location of a pregnancy (intrauterine versus ectopic) cannot be determined with certainty. Methotrexate has become a standard of care in the treatment of early unruptured ectopic pregnancy, whereas mifepristone is believed to be ineffective for ectopic pregnancy. Therefore, when a gestational sac cannot be located by ultrasound, or signs and symptoms suggest the possibility of ectopic pregnancy, methotrexate may be a better choice than mifepristone.

COUNSELING

A full discussion of counseling is beyond the scope of this chapter, but several techniques and principles can be outlined. Six areas of importance may be described.

1. *Explore the patient's feelings.* This may be done through asking nonjudgmental and open-ended questions as well as active listening. The clinician should empathize and help the patient reflect on her own feelings. Ambivalence should be acknowledged and discussed.
2. *Explore options.* The patient has three options: terminating the pregnancy, carrying it and keeping the baby, or adopting it out. The risks, advantages, and disadvantages of each may be explored, in the context of the woman's particular life situation. If she chooses abortion, then certain options are available, such as medical abortion or surgical abortion.
3. *Making decisions.* Strategies for decision-making and the need for any additional counseling may be explored. The patient should be encouraged to seek advice from others whom she trusts: partner, parents, siblings, friends, teachers, or spiritual counselors. A timetable for decision-making must be established based on the gestational age.
4. *Screening for special problems.* Extreme anxiety or ambivalence, drug or alcohol use, or medical or psychological problems may require special and individualized measures.
5. *Informed consent.* The risks of the procedure must be reviewed and any questions answered. The patient's ability to give informed consent must be reviewed with regard to her age, mental status, and any possibility of coercion. A support person may be able to be present during any procedure.
6. *Postprocedure issues.* These include the need for any additional counseling, contraception, follow-up visits, and reporting any complications.

INDICATIONS

Very few strictly medical indications exist for elective first-trimester abortion. Evaluation of these patients is highly individualized and probably would involve the input of consultants. Rarely, a woman may have a life-threatening illness such as a cancer for which treatment cannot begin until the pregnancy is terminated. Occasionally, a patient may have a progressive life-threatening illness that so limits her life expectancy that childbearing and child rearing may be unwise or impossible. Abortion is generally considered acceptable for pregnancies resulting from rape or incest, or those in which a major birth defect exists. Exposure to a teratogenic drug may also be a consideration. Most abortions are requested for nonmedical reasons, such as psychological, economic, educational, or personal relationship factors.

CONTRAINDICATIONS

Medical contraindications are quite rare. Active pelvic infection is one such contraindication as is any serious medical condition that might complicate surgery. In such cases the patient's condition should be stabilized before abortion. The procedure is probably best performed in the hospital by consultants.

SURGICAL ABORTION
EQUIPMENT

- An instrument for dilating the cervix: Pratt, Hegar, or Denniston cervical dilators; or laminaria (inserted 6 to 12 hours before the procedure) (see Chapter 137, Cervical Stenosis and Cervical Dilation)
- Large Graves' speculum
- Povidone-iodine or other antiseptic solution
- Ring forceps
- Cotton balls
- 4 × 4–inch gauze pads
- Single-toothed cervical tenaculum
- Uterine sound
- 10 ml of anesthetic (1% lidocaine or 2% chloroprocaine) with 22-gauge spinal needle, or 22-gauge needle on 3-inch needle extender
- Suction curettes in a variety of sizes (from 6 to 12 mm)
- Suction machine with tubing, or manual vacuum aspiration syringe (Figs. 130-1 and 130-2)
- Formalin jar
- Roberts, Stone, or small ring forceps to explore uterine cavity
- IV solutions, tubing, and oxytocics (for treatment of excessive bleeding)

PREPROCEDURE PATIENT PREPARATION

1. Perform a standard, accurate pregnancy test. It should be positive, and this should be documented. A home pregnancy test is technically adequate but may not have been performed correctly. Transvaginal ultrasound demonstrating an intrauterine pregnancy is also acceptable proof of pregnancy.
2. Consider performing a hematocrit or hemoglobin determination.

3. Determine the blood type, including Rh factor (*mandatory*). Rh-negative women who have been pregnant less than 13 weeks should receive the 50 μg dose of D immunoglobulin (MICRhoGAM 50 μg); Otherwise, Rh sensitization occurs in 1% or more of untreated patients.

4. Optional testing—depending on patient risk factors, the nature of the practice, and financial considerations—includes urinalysis, Pap smear, gonorrhea and chlamydia screening, and blood tests for syphilis and HIV antibodies.

5. Gestational age *must* be determined. This can usually be accomplished by correlating weeks from the last normal menstrual period with a pelvic examination to size the uterus. Of course, abnormal bleeding in pregnancy, contraception use, menstrual irregularities, poor recall of dates, denial, and even the possibility of falsification may hinder a physician in calculating an accurate gestational age from historical data.

   Sizing the uterus by examination requires practice and may be complicated when a patient is obese, is uncooperative, has uterine or ovarian tumors, or has a retroverted uterus. As a rough guideline, up to the sixth week of pregnancy, the uterus is the size of a golf ball or plum in nulliparous women and slightly larger in parous women. By 8 to 9 weeks the uterus is the size of a tennis ball or small orange but is softer and often asymmetrically enlarged. By 10 weeks the uterus is the size of a medium orange. By 12 weeks the uterus is as large as a grapefruit and becomes palpable suprapubically in thin or normal weight women. A retroverted uterus will pop forward out of the pelvis between 12 and 13 weeks. By 15 or 16 weeks the uterus is the size of a cantaloupe. The uterine isthmus becomes softened (Hegar's sign) in early pregnancy, occasionally to the point where the globular uterine corpus feels like a separate pelvic mass.

6. When there is any doubt at all of the gestational age, perform a transvaginal ultrasound examination. Ultrasound examination is highly accurate in dating a pregnancy and may be accepted as accurate, regardless of historical data or results of the physical examination. Transvaginal ultrasound also sheds light on several important complications of pregnancy such as first-trimester fetal demise, ectopic pregnancy, and gestational trophoblastic disease or molar pregnancy.

7. Perform a standard brief history and physical examination.

8. Premedication is optional. Ibuprofen 600 to 800 mg orally or diazepam 5 mg or 10 mg orally an hour before the procedure may be given.

9. Establishment of an IV line is optional. An IV line may be useful for sedatives and oxytocics but is generally not necessary. However, oxytocin, methylergonovine (Methergine), and other injectable drugs must be readily available should an unexpected hemorrhage occur.

10. Conscious sedation may be offered. A simple and effective regimen is midazolam (Versed) given intravenously at the rate of 1 mg per minute up to 5 mg. The patient should be monitored for respiratory depression with a pulse oximeter and frequent vital signs, and a crash cart should be available (see Chapter 2, Conscious Sedation [Sedation and Analgesia]).

11. Atropine 0.4 mg may be given intravenously or subcutaneously in patients with a history of a vagal reaction to prior cervical manipulations (bradycardia, loss of consciousness, diaphoresis, etc.).

12. Prophylactic antibiotics are becoming the standard of care. The practice remains controversial and regimens differ, but doxycycline (200 mg given preoperatively) or metronidazole (1 g orally preoperatively), then 500 mg every 6 hours for three doses postoperatively, are two acceptable regimens. Special consideration must be given to women with active infections, cardiac defects, prostheses, and other high-risk conditions (see Chapter 204, Antibiotic Prophylaxis).

TECHNIQUE (SUCTION CURETTAGE)

Laminaria Insertion

The patient should be seen the day before the planned abortion for insertion of the laminaria. If only minor dilation is required, a morning insertion for an afternoon procedure will suffice. *Laminaria digitata* is a seaweed stem, 2 to 3 mm wide and several centimeters long, resembling a brown twig with a string attached to one end. It is hygroscopic and in a moist environment will swell to five times its original size within 12 hours. (See Fig. 137-2.) Laminaria dilation of the cervix is a common adjunct to abortions, especially for pregnancies 8 weeks and beyond. It accomplishes dilation safely and gently, minimizes trauma to the cervix, and causes less pain than surgical dilation. Insertion of the laminaria is usually an easy and brief procedure, but it requires an extra visit, since one visit is required for the laminaria insertion and another for the definitive procedure (Fig. 130-3).

Laminaria insertion is not always necessary. Very early abortions (up to 7 weeks) can usually be performed with a small Karman cannula (No. 5 or 6) without dilation of any kind. Alternatively, the operator

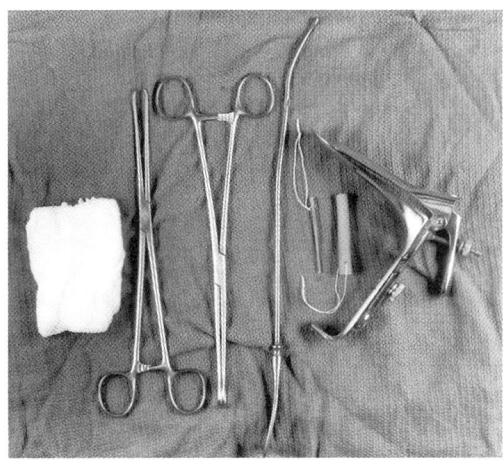

Fig. 130-3
Laminaria setup. *Left to right,* Gauze pads, single tooth tenaculum, ring forceps, small dilator, two sizes of laminaria, and Graves' speculum.

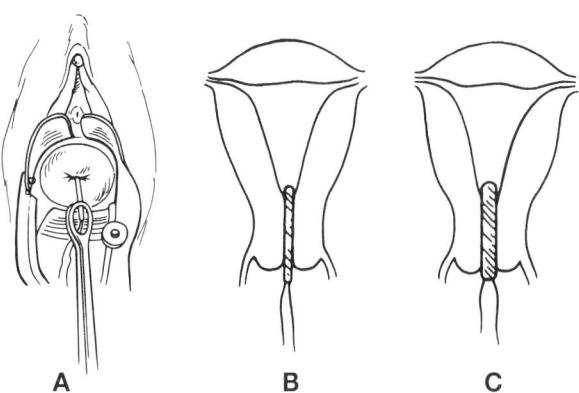

Fig. 130-4
A, Insertion of the laminaria; **B,** immediately after insertion; **C,** 12 to 24 hours after insertion.

may choose to dilate the cervix surgically with tapered dilators (Pratt or Denniston). This procedure has the advantage of not requiring an additional visit, but the disadvantages of more patient discomfort and a greater risk of damaging the cervix. Most physicians do not use a laminaria for the vast majority of early abortions because of the extra visit required.

1. Size the uterus and detect its position with bimanual examination, place the speculum to expose the cervix, and then cleanse the cervix with an antiseptic.
2. Grasp the cervix on the anterior lip with a single-toothed tenaculum. Two to four ml of 1% lidocaine may be instilled submucosally at the 12 o'clock position, so the tenaculum will not be felt. Next, delicately pass a uterine sound through the cervical os. The purpose of sounding is not to determine the depth of the uterus, but rather to determine the axis of the cervical canal and to accomplish slight dilation. Insert the uterine sound just past the internal os and then remove it.
3. The laminaria may then be inserted with little difficulty. Grasp the laminaria lightly with a ring forceps, oriented vertically. Insert the laminaria into the cervix, allowing it to pivot in the ring forceps so that the tip "finds" the cervical canal. Push the laminaria all the way into the cervix (Fig. 130-4). It is particularly important to maintain traction on the tenaculum if the uterus is markedly flexed forward or backward, in order to straighten out its axis.
4. Remove the tenaculum and place a sponge against the laminaria to help hold it in position. Usually several 4 × 4 gauze pads are used.

A confident and experienced operator may skip the tenaculum and sounding steps and simply slide the laminaria directly into the cervix. Direct insertion is easy if the patient is parous and if the uterus is neither severely retroflexed nor anteflexed.

When the gestational age is more than 11 weeks, a second laminaria—placed alongside the first laminaria in the exact same fashion—will permit use of a large suction curette and expedite the procedure.

In most patients the laminaria is left in overnight. In some patients it may cause significant cramping, which can be controlled with nonprescription pain medication like ibuprofen 800 mg.

Although the laminaria is inexpensive and has proved itself effective, a synthetic osmotic dilator is available that accomplishes the same goal (Lamicel).

Dilation with Surgical Dilators

For early abortions, up to 8 weeks in nulliparas and 9 weeks in parous women, surgical dilation is satisfactory and eliminates the extra visit for laminaria.

After paracervical block is administered (see Chapter 174, Paracervical Block), the cervix is sounded with a uterine sound, not to determine depth but to determine the axis of the canal. Then progressively larger dilators are introduced. These are held with a delicate pencil grip, and applied with just enough force to pass. Traction on the tenaculum on the cervix is essential at all times while instrumenting the uterus to straighten out the cervico-uterine canal. A slight pop or giving sensation will be felt as the dilator passes through the internal os. Each dilator may be left in place for a moment before going to the next one. Dilation is complete when the size of dilator matches the intended size of curette. Most patients experience some cramping during dilation.

Dilation with Misoprostol

Another method of dilating the cervix has emerged in recent years: administration of misoprostol. Misoprostol is known to cause softening and dilation of the cervix and cramping of the uterus. Although studies are few, they show that 400 μg of misoprostol, given vaginally 3 to 4 hours before the procedure, works well, especially for surgical abortions at an early gestational age. Oral administration works less well, and higher doses given vaginally have no greater effect and cause more side effects. Patients commonly experience cramping and bleeding before the actual surgical procedure with the preoperative administration of vaginal misoprostol.

Paracervical Block

Paracervical block (see Chapter 174, Paracervical Block) is a simple, safe, and effective means of providing local anesthesia for abortion in the office setting (see Fig. 130-5). Remove the laminaria and sponge if previously placed, cleanse the cervix and vagina with an antiseptic, and grasp the anterior lip of the cervix with a single-toothed or atraumatic tenaculum.

An alternative to the standard paracervical block is the *cervical block,* as described by Eugene Glick, MD. This technique creates a field block around the cervix at the level of the internal os.

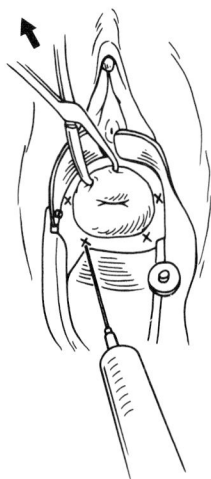

Fig. 130-5
Paracervical block technique. *X* shows locations where submucosal injections can be made. Ten ml of local anesthetic (1% lidocaine or 2% chloroprocaine) with a 22-gauge needle is injected into four sites at the 3, 5, 7, and 9 o'clock positions. (Some clinicians prefer to inject in the 4 and 8 o'clock positions only.) Ideally the injection should be given submucosally, near the junction of the cervix and vagina. The injection should be superficial enough to raise a bleb or wheal under the mucosa. Since the area is vascular, care must be taken not to inject the anesthetic directly into a vessel. The tenaculum may be used to elevate the cervix and hold it to either side for better exposure of the injection sites.

The technique uses ½% lidocaine 22.5 ml, with one unit of Vasopressin and 2.5 ml of 8.4% sodium bicarbonate added, to total 25 ml. This mixture is then injected as follows: 1 to 2 ml at the 12 o'clock position superficially on the cervix; then 2 ml at the 10 and 2 o'clock positions superficially; then 1 ml at the 3, 4, 5, 7, 8, and 9 o'clock positions. Then deeper injections are given, about 4 cm into the outer third of the myometrium about at the level of the internal os. These injections are angled up into the uterus from near the cervicovaginal junction at the 3, 5, 7, and 9 o'clock positions. About 2 ml should be injected at each site, and the anesthetic should be "tracked" to avoid a large bolus at any single location. Many variations of this technique exist.

Suction Abortion

Note: Suction abortion can also be used for a missed or incomplete spontaneous abortion.

After administering the paracervical block, the operator may perform the actual abortion.

1. Sound gently with a uterine sound, primarily to determine the direction of the canal rather than its depth. Traction on the tenaculum is necessary at all times while instrumenting the uterus (Fig. 130-6).
2. Cervical dilators may be used to assess the adequacy of cervical dilation (Fig. 130-7). Even when the laminaria is used, further dilation may occasionally be useful.
3. Select a suction curette (Fig. 130-8). As a general rule, the size of the curette in millimeters should correspond to the gestational age in weeks. Place

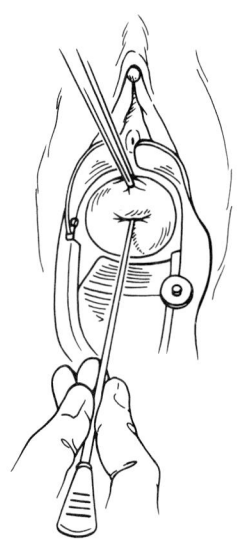

Fig. 130-6
Sounding the uterus.

the curette into the uterus as far as it will easily go, until it meets resistance (Fig. 130-9).

4. Attach the curette to the suction machine by means of the tubing. Turn on the machine. Close any valves on the curette to create intrauterine suction. A suction pressure of 60 to 65 cm Hg or greater is required to accomplish the procedure. If suction is inadequate, there is probably a leak in the system that should be identified and corrected (Fig. 130-10).

5. Using the rotating metal handle on the tubing, rotate the suction curette vigorously in place—first one way, then the other—several times. Gentle in-and-out piston motions may accompany the rotation.

6. Watch the tissue that appears in the curette and tubing. The products of conception have a characteristic appearance. First, clear fluid is noted, followed by tan "fluffy" material, which are the remnants of the placenta and decidua usually mixed with blood. Fetal parts cannot usually be identified until the pregnancy borders on the second trimester. The appearance of abnormal tissue (such as omental fat or bowel) in the curette is a sign of *perforation*. Absence of tissue is also important to note.

7. After several rotations in each direction, remove the curette while the suction is still on. Reinsert it into the uterus with the suction off. (The suction is controlled with the slide control on the metal handle. It is not necessary to turn the machine on and off.) Turn the suction back on, rotate, and remove it again, repeating this until no further tissue is seen in the curette. As the uterus is evacuated, it tends to clamp down, bringing additional tissue into the range of the curette portal. Patients will experience more discomfort at this point, and the operator will feel more resistance to rotating the curette.

8. With a medium-sharp uterine curette, curette and feel all quadrants of the uterine cavity. A clean uterus will have a firm, slightly gritty or rough feel. Additional tissue adherent to the uterine walls feels spongy or slippery. Alternatively, a Roberts, Stone, or small ring forceps may be used to grasp within the uterine cavity for any additional tissue (Fig. 130-11).

9. Pass the suction curette once more to remove any debris or blood from the sharp curettage (if performed).

10. A follow-up transvaginal ultrasound may be performed immediately after the procedure. This is to demonstrate that the gestational sac and products of conception have been removed from the uterus. This examination is particularly appropriate for very early abortions.

11. The procedure is now completed. Remove all instruments and observe the patient for 10 to 15 minutes for bleeding or any unusual reaction. If more sedation or general anesthetic was used, follow the usual guidelines. The patient is then free to leave, with appropriate follow-up information (see the sample patient education handout titled "Instructions After Termination of Pregnancy" on page 1905 of Appendix G).

12. Examine all tissue using the "*float test,*" and/or send all tissue for pathological examination. The "float test" is to identify products of conception grossly, at the time of the procedure. It is particularly important in very early abortions, procedures in which scant tissue is obtained, and patients who are at risk for ectopic pregnancy. The tissue obtained should be washed free of blood with saline or tap water. Fragments of tissue can then be suspended in

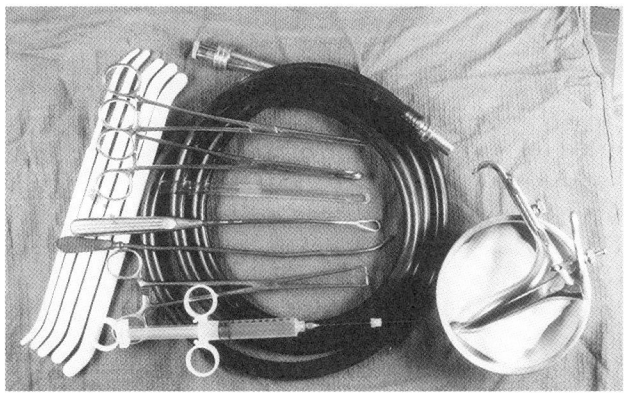

Fig. 130-7
Suction abortion set up includes cervical dilators, suction tubing, polyp and ring forceps, suction curette, blunt uterine sound, tenaculum, syringe, and speculum.

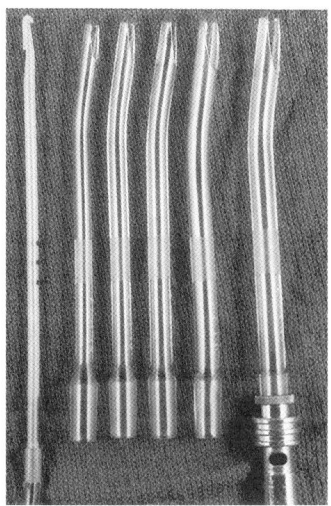

Fig. 130-8
Suction curettes.

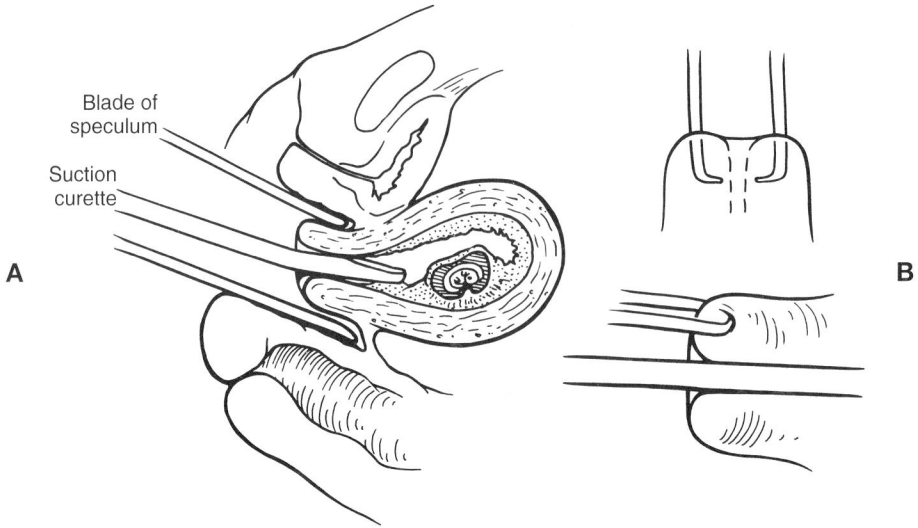

Fig. 130-9
A, Initial placement of the suction curette into the uterus. Advance until there is resistance. **B,** The tenaculum is used to stabilize the cervix.

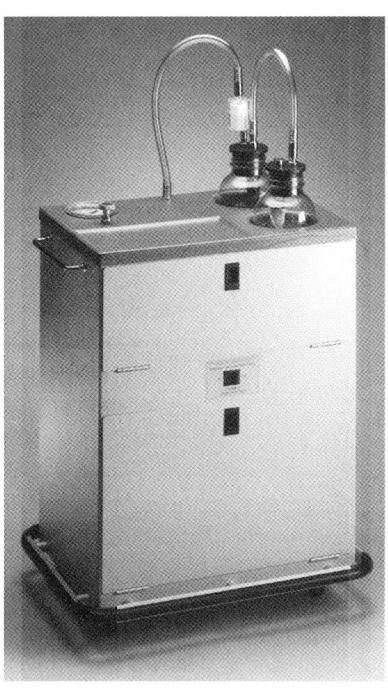

Fig. 130-10
Berkeley Synevac vacuum curettage machine.

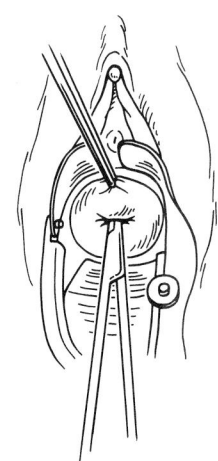

Fig. 130-11
Exploration of the uterus with Stone forceps.

placenta and membranes can be distinguished easily from decidua and clot.

COMPLICATIONS

The overall complication rate of first-trimester abortion is low (probably less than 5%) and certainly lower than that of delivery. However, complications can and do occur, including those resulting in major disability or even death. Careful attention to technique and constant vigilance for complications are mandatory.

any clear fluid—saline, tap water, and formalin all work—and carefully inspected. Placental tissue has a characteristic "fronding" or finely arborized appearance caused by the villi. Backlighting and low-power magnification such as a colposcope or a magnifying glass is helpful. With a little practice,

Complications of abortion fall into four categories: laminaria complications, paracervical block complications, suction curettage complications, and obstetric and gynecologic complications.

Laminaria Complications

If the laminaria perforates the cervix and creates a false passage, the abortion cannot be accomplished. Proper placement is essential. If the laminaria is left in over 24 hours, infection may result.

The laminaria may fall out, migrate up into the uterus, or fragment. If the laminaria falls out before dilation is effected, mechanical dilation or replacement of the laminaria must be carried out. If migration or fragmentation (a piece breaks off and remains intrauterine) is suspected, a careful search of the uterine cavity must be carried out to remove it.

Occasionally, the internal os will be stenotic and dilate with more difficulty. The laminaria may assume an hourglass configuration, which makes it difficult to remove because the area that is intrauterine is difficult to pull back through the narrowed, stenotic area. This may also lead to fragmentation.

Some patients may experience a vasovagal reaction, which consists of bradycardia, diaphoresis, nausea, and (rarely) convulsions. Atropine may be administered for treatment and prevention (0.4 mg IV or SC); the patient's legs should be elevated and her head lowered. If the patient admits to having a low pain threshold or tendency to faint easily, give the atropine prophylactically 15 to 30 minutes before the procedure of inserting and again with removal.

Occasionally, a patient will change her mind after the laminaria has been placed. The laminaria can be removed at any time, and in most cases, the pregnancy will continue unaffected. However, the patient must be warned of the risk of miscarriage.

Paracervical Block Complications

- Some bleeding usually results.
- Intravascular injection is common, despite efforts to prevent it. Patients experience dysphoria, tinnitus, an unusual taste in the mouth, and visual disturbances. These sensations are transient.
- More severe reactions, such as convulsions or allergic reactions are rare.
- Anesthetic effect may not be total, but it is usually adequate to carry out the procedure.

Suction Curettage Complications

- The most feared complication is uterine *perforation.* Perforation is identified by increased pain, hemor-

rhage, or signs of an acute condition in the abdomen. Fat or bowel tissue observed in the suction apparatus is diagnostic, as is passing a blunt instrument up through the perforation. Culdocentesis may help in diagnosing internal bleeding (see Chapter 142, Culdocentesis [Colpocentesis]). Treatment must be individualized and depends on whether the abortion is complete or not and whether there is the likelihood of intraabdominal injury. Minimum treatment includes admission for close observation and antibiotics. If the risk of hemorrhage or visceral injury is great, laparoscopy or laparotomy may be necessary. If perforation occurs before the uterus is emptied, the procedure may be finished under direct laparoscopic observation.

- *Hemorrhage* that occurs during the procedure suggests laceration or perforation, or, more commonly, uterine atony with incomplete evacuation of the uterus. Coagulopathy is also a possibility.
- *Lacerations* of the cervix can sometimes occur on the exocervix because of a tenaculum tearing out. These are usually quite superficial. Tamponade may be required, and suturing is rarely needed. Puncture sites on the cervix can also bleed briskly and respond to tamponade or packing the vagina for a few minutes.
- *Atony* can occur when the pregnancy is greater than 10 or 11 weeks. Oxytocics, such as methylergonovine (Methergine) 0.2 mg IM, may be helpful; some clinicians give them routinely when terminating pregnancies of 11 weeks and beyond. Some physicians will also routinely run an oxytocin infusion during the procedure. Carboprost tromethamine injection (Hemabate, Pharmacia-Upjohn Pharmaceuticals) given intramuscularly or directly into the cervix is indicated if atony is severe.
- *Retained products* may be present along with atony. The procedure must be repeated if retained products are suspected. If bleeding is severe, repeating the procedure may require deeper anesthesia to ensure complete evacuation of all tissue. Excessive bleeding in the days or weeks after the abortion suggests incomplete abortion. Carefully repeating the procedure is the best course.
- *Postabortal infection,* often called *endometritis,* is relatively common but usually is not severe. Symptoms of endometritis include uterine tenderness, lower abdominal pain, fever, and elevated white blood cell count. Oral antibiotics may be prescribed; however, repeat suction curettage may be required. Rarely, a patient will have severe sepsis or septic shock and require aggressive treatment, including hospital admission, IV antibiotics, fluids, and even hysterectomy.
- *Late sequelae,* such as *infertility, premature labor,* and *incompetent cervix,* have been studied extensively. Most modern studies, especially since laminaria

dilation became common, have been very reassuring that serious obstetric and gynecologic consequences are rare.

- About 10% of women will have lasting emotional sequelae, or *postabortal depression*. The majority of these women will have been emotionally unstable or highly ambivalent before the procedure. Counseling is recommended.

Obstetric and Gynecologic Complications

- *Ectopic pregnancy* may be unsuspected when a patient requests an early abortion. Pathologic examination or a float test of the tissue obtained from such a procedure would show only decidua and not the actual products of conception. Additional studies, such as ultrasound and serial quantitative βHCG determinations, are indicated. Obviously, prompt action is required when ectopic pregnancy is suspected.
- *Miscarriage.* About 15% of pregnancies end in miscarriage or spontaneous abortion, also known as *first trimester fetal demise.* Symptoms include bleeding, cramping, and passage of tissue. Modern means of diagnosing miscarriage in the first trimester include transvaginal ultrasound and serial quantitative βHCG determinations. Patients who are already bleeding may request an abortion. If miscarriage is suspected, going ahead with the procedure makes sense medically, since eventually the patient may require suction completion in the emergency room setting in any event. It is of some importance to the patient's future reproductive capacity to know if the present pregnancy is viable or a miscarriage, since miscarriage may be recurrent.
- *Scant tissue.* Occasionally, tissue obtained during an abortion is very scant. This may indicate that the patient has already spontaneously aborted, that she has an ectopic pregnancy, that she was not pregnant, or that the procedure failed to interrupt the pregnancy. Ultrasound examination and repeat HCG determinations may be necessary, and clinical follow-up is essential. With a failed abortion, the procedure may be attempted again at a later date.
- *Myomata or fibroids.* These muscular tumors of the myometrium complicate abortion in two ways. First, they may disguise the gestational age of a pregnancy by greatly enlarging the uterus. In this case, ultrasound is necessary to reveal the true age. Second, depending on their location, myomata may prevent or limit access to the uterine cavity. Performing the procedure under anesthesia and ultrasound guidance may be the only recourse. Medical abortion has been successful in cases in which surgical abortion is impossible because of myomata.

- *Ovarian tumors* may also inhibit the accuracy of an examination. Again, ultrasound will clarify the issue. Usually the abortion can be performed under ultrasound guidance, and the ovarian tumor dealt with appropriately at a later time.
- *Duplication anomalies of the female genital tract* result from the failure of the uterus to fuse completely during embryonic development; these anomalies range from arcuate uterus, to total duplication of the internal genitalia, including a double-barreled vagina. The critical point in abortion is determining on which side the pregnancy is and gaining access to it. Rarely, a pregnancy in a hemiuterine horn is inaccessible to surgical evacuation. In such cases medical means of abortion are usually successful.

POSTPROCEDURE PATIENT EDUCATION

Methylergonovine 0.2 mg administered orally every 6 hours for six to ten doses may assist in contracting the uterus and prevent bleeding. An alternative, not approved for the purpose by the FDA, is misoprostol (Cytotec), which has powerful uterotonic activity. Doxycycline 100 mg orally twice a day for 7 days is advised by some clinicians.

No sexual activity is advisable for 2 weeks. Also see the sample patient education handout titled "Instructions After Termination of Pregnancy" on page 1905 of Appendix G.

SUPPLIERS

All special equipment, including suction machines, hosing curettes, dilators, laminaria, and ancillary instruments
Berkeley Medevices, Inc.
1330 South 51st Street
Richmond, CA 94804
Phone: 1-510-526-4046

Most instruments are available from general medical suppliers or the following:
CooperSurgical
95 Corporate Drive
Trumbull, CT 06611
Phone: 1-800-243-2974
Website: www.coopersurgical.com

Miltex, Inc.
700 Hicksville Road
Bethpage, NY 11714
Phone: 1-800-645-8000
Website: www.miltex.com

Mifeprex
Danco Laboratories
P.O. Box 4816
New York, NY 10185
Phone: 1-877-432-7596
Website: www.dancolaboratories.com

CPT/BILLING CODE

581.20	Dilation and curettage, diagnostic and/or therapeutic (nonobstetrical)
592.00	Insertion of cervical dilator (e.g., laminaria, prostaglandin)
598.12	Treatment of incomplete abortion, any semester, completed surgically
598.20	Treatment of missed abortion, completed surgically, first trimester
598.21	Treatment of missed abortion, completed surgically, second trimester
598.30	Treatment of septic abortion, completed surgically
598.40	Induced abortion, by dilation and curettage
598.41	Induced abortion, by dilation and curettage and evacuation
598.55	Induced abortion, by one or more vaginal suppositories (e.g., prostaglandin) with or without cervical dilation (e.g., laminaria), including hospital admission and visits
598.71	Removal of cerclage suture under anesthesia (other than local)

ICD-9-CM DIAGNOSTIC CODES

622.4	Cervical stenosis
632	Abortion, missed
634.91	Abortion, spontaneous, incomplete
634.92	Abortion, spontaneous, complete
635.90	Abortion, elective
637.90	Abortion, inevitable
637.91	Abortion, incomplete
637.92	Abortion, complete
640.00	Abortion, threatened, unspecified
646.30	Abortion, habitual or recurrent

ADDITIONAL RESOURCES

- See the sample patient education handout titled "Instructions After Termination of Pregnancy" on page 1905 of Appendix G.

- See the sample patient consent form titled "Termination of Pregnancy" on page 1906 of Appendix G.

BIBLIOGRAPHY

American College of Obstetricians and Gynecologists: *Emergency oral contraception,* ACOG Practice Bull No 25, Washington, DC, March 2001, ACOG.

American College of Obstetricians and Gynecologists: *Medical management of abortion,* ACOG Practice Bull No 26, Washington, DC, April 2001, ACOG.

American College of Obstetricians and Gynecologists: *Mifepristone for medical pregnancy termination,* ACOG Committee Opinion No. 245, Washington, DC, Dec 2000, ACOG.

American College of Obstetricians and Gynecologists: *Prevention of D isoimmunization,* ACOG Tech Bull No 147, Washington, DC, Oct 1990, ACOG.

Blumenthal PD, Remsburg RE: A time and cost analysis of the management of incomplete abortion with manual vacuum aspiration, *Int J Gynaecol Obstet* 45:261, 1994.

Christin-Maitre S, Bouchard P, and Spitz I: Medical termination of pregnancy, *N Engl J Med* 342(13):946, 2000.

Creinen MD, Edwards J: *Early abortion: surgical and medical options, current problems in obstetrics, gynecology, and fertility,* January/February 20(1), 1997.

Glick, E: *Surgical abortion,* West End Women's Medical Group, Reno, Nev., 1998.

Grimes D, Raymond E, Jones B: Emergency contraception over-the-counter: the medical and legal imperatives, *Obstet Gynecol* 98(1):151, 2001.

Macisaac L, Grossman D, Balistreri E, Darney P: A randomized controlled trial of laminaria, oral misoprostol, and vaginal misoprostol before abortion. *Obstet Gynecol* 93(5):766, 1999.

National Abortion Federation: *Clinical Policy Guidelines,* Washington, DC, 1998, National Abortion Federation.

National Abortion Federation Medical Education Series—Early Options: *A provider's guide to medical abortion (training and resource binder),* Washington, DC, 2001, NAF.

Pastuszak AL, Schüller L, Speck-Martins CE, et al: Use of misoprostol during pregnancy and Möbius syndrome in infants, *N Engl J Med* 338(26):1881, 1998.

Policar MJ, Pollack AE: *Clinical training curriculum in abortion practice,* Washington, DC, 1995, National Abortion Federation.

Pymar HC, Creinin MD: Offering mifepristone as an abortion option, *Contemp Ob Gyn* Feb:113, 2001.

Randomised controlled trial of levonorgestrel versus the Yuzpe regimen of combined oral contraceptives for emergency contraception. Task Force on Postovulatory Methods of Fertility Regulation, *Lancet* 352:428, 1998.

Schaff EA, Eisinger SH, Franks P, Kim SS: Combined methotrexate and misoprostol for early induced abortion, *Arch Fam Med* 4:774, 1995.

Schaff EA, Eisinger SH, Stadalius LS, et al: Low-dose mifepristone 200 mg and vaginal misoprostol for abortion, *Contraception* 59:1, 1999.

Singh K, Fong YF, Prasad RN, Dong F: Randomized trial to determine optimal dose of vaginal misoprostol for preabortion cervical priming, *Obstet Gynecol* 92(5):795, 1999.

Spitz IM, Bardin CW, Benton L, Robbins A: Early pregnancy termination with mifepristone and misoprostol in the United States, *N Engl J Med* 338(18):1241, 1998.

Stewart FH, Wells ES, Flinn SK, Weitz TA: Early medical abortion: issues for practice, San Francisco, Calif., 2001, UCSF Center for Reproductive Health Research & Policy.

Turk P: Abortion. In Lichtman R, Papera S, editors: *Well-woman care,* Norwalk, Conn., 1991, Appleton & Lange.

Walsh N: Woman dies of sepsis in abortion pill study, *Ob Gyn News* Oct 15:4, 2001.

Winkler J, Blumenthal P, Greenslade F: Early abortion services: new choices for providers and women, IPAS, *Adv Abort Care* 5(2):1, 1996.

WEBSITE

www.ipas.org/pdf/adv52eng.pdf

CHAPTER 131

Barrier Contraceptives: Cervical Caps, Condoms, and Diaphragms*

Edward J. Mayeaux, Jr.
Barbara S. Apgar

CERVICAL CAPS

The cervical cap is a barrier contraceptive method that is applied to the cervix like a "suction cup." It is much less commonly used than other barrier methods, and physician training in this method is sometimes difficult to obtain. The Food and Drug Administration (FDA) approved the Prentif Cavity Rim Cervical Cap in May 1988. It is the only type of cervical cap available in the United States. The cervical cap's efficacy is similar to that of the diaphragm. If it is used properly, pregnancy will occur in only 6.5% of cervical cap users at the end of 1 year. The pregnancy rate rises to about 12% after 2 years. Because some women do not use the device regularly or properly, the overall pregnancy rate among cervical cap users is about 18% at 2 years.

Early studies suggested that cervical cap use was associated with development of cervical dysplasia. Although subsequent studies have not found cervical dysplasia to be increased, careful monitoring of cervical cytology in cervical cap users is appropriate.

INDICATIONS

• Prevention of pregnancy

CONTRAINDICATIONS

• Inability of patient to be properly fitted
• Inability of patient to understand instructions for use

---

*Barry D. Weiss, MD, wrote the text on cervical cap and condoms in the first edition of *Procedures for Primary Care Physicians*. Dr. Mayeaux has reviewed and updated that material for this edition. Dr. Apgar has updated the section on diaphragms.

• Inability of patient to insert and remove device correctly
• History of toxic shock syndrome
• Known or suspected uterine or cervical malignancy, including unresolved abnormal Pap smear test result
• Congenital or other anatomic abnormalities of the cervix (e.g., polyps) that would preclude proper fitting
• Current vaginal or cervical infection
• Use during menses
• Use during postpartum or postabortal period

ADVANTAGES

• Can be used when medical indications or patient intolerance preclude use of hormone-based contraception (e.g., birth control pills)
• Better tolerated in diaphragm users who experience recurrent urinary tract infection
• May be worn longer than a diaphragm and requires less spermicide
• Not affected by weight gain or weight loss
• May be used in women with pelvic relaxation who cannot retain a diaphragm

EQUIPMENT

A cervical cap fitting set that includes one of each of the four sizes of cervical caps is needed. The sizes are based on the internal diameter of the rim: 22, 25, 28, and 31 mm (Fig. 131-1). Fitting sets are available from the manufacturer. The manufacturer also provides an excellent information packet, monograph, and videotape to instruct the clinician on use and fitting of the cervical cap. After fitting is completed, the cervical cap is dispensed directly by the physician to the patient.

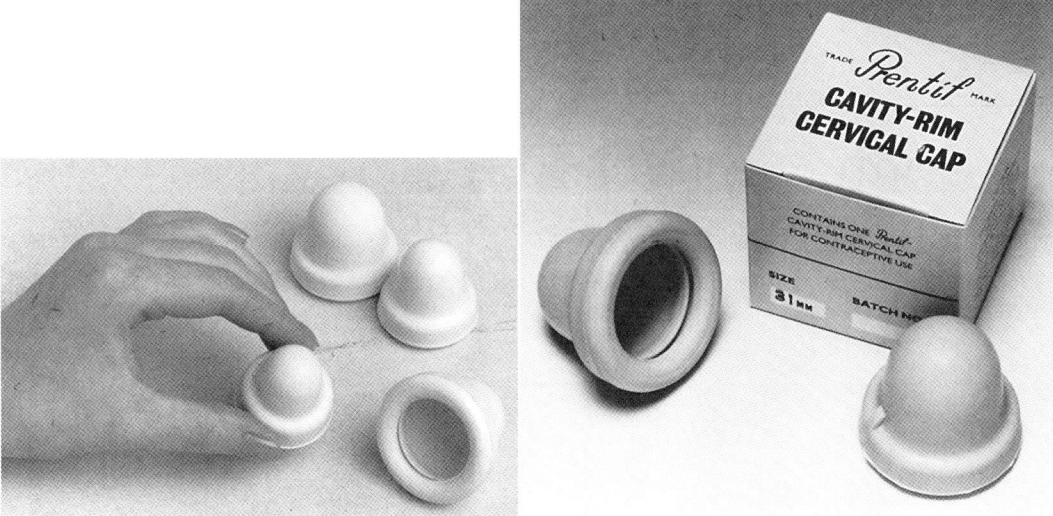

Fig. 131-1
Prentif cavity-rim cervical cap. (Courtesy Cervical Cap Ltd, Los Gatos, Calif.)

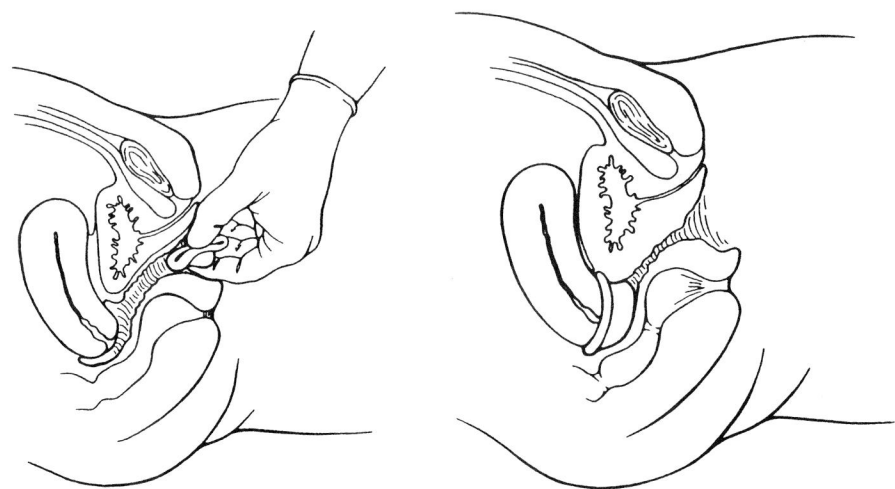

Fig. 131-2
Properly fitted cervical cap.

TECHNIQUE

Before fitting the cervical cap, the clinician should perform a pelvic examination and obtain a Pap smear to exclude cervical or vaginal infection. (Cultures should be obtained as indicated.) A patient should not be fitted for a cervical cap during pregnancy or until 6 weeks postpartum.

1. Lubricate the cap rim, compress the sides together, and insert it into the vagina. The cavity of the cap should fit over the cervix (Fig. 131-2).
2. Try each size of cervical cap until the correct one is identified. The correct size is the smallest that fits satisfactorily. The majority of women (80% to 90%) will be fitted with a 22-mm or 25-mm cap.
   a. Ideally the cap should cover the entire cervix.
   b. The cap should adhere firmly to the cervix by its own self-generated suction.
   c. The dome of the cap should be closely applied to the cervix. If there is good suction, squeezing the tip of the rubber wall between the fingers will cause a dent that is maintained for 30 seconds.

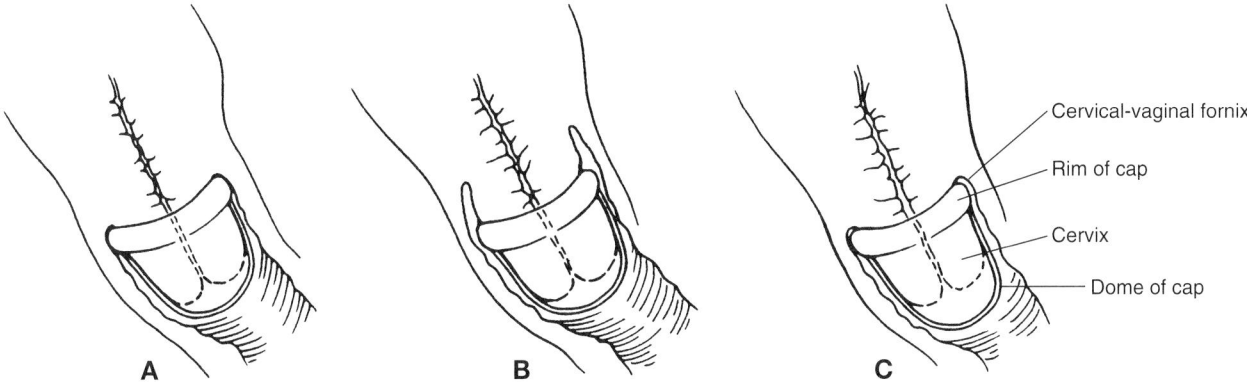

Fig. 131-3
Properly and improperly fitted cervical caps. **A,** The properly fitted cap is closely applied to the cervix, and the rim of the cap fills the cervicovaginal fornix. **B,** The cap is too small. Although the dome of the cap is closely applied to the cervix, the rim does not reach into the fornix, leaving the base of the cervix exposed. **C,** The cap is too large. Although the dome covers the cervix and the rim extends into the fornix, the cap is not closely applied to the cervix and may be easily dislodged.

d. The rim of the cap should tuck evenly into the cervicovaginal fornix around the entire circumference.

e. No gaps should exist between the rim of the cap and the cervix itself.

f. No parts of the cervix should be exposed or palpable below the rim of the cap.

g. The cap should not be easily dislodged. Light tugging on the dome should not affect it (Fig. 131-3).

3. The correct technique for removing the cap involves pushing the rim away from the cervix to break the suction, then pulling the cap out of the vagina. Do not pull on the dome of the cap. A cap that fits too tightly will be difficult to remove. (The patient can apply the cap up to 40 hours prior to intercourse. It should remain in place for at least 8 hours after intercourse, but removed within 48 hours after the last episode. The cap may remain in place a total of 72 hours before removal.)

4. After the correct size has been determined and the techniques have been demonstrated, the patient should satisfactorily perform insertion and removal.

5. Up to 20% of women cannot be fitted properly with the four currently available sizes. These women are not candidates for the cervical cap.

6. The manufacturer recommends cleaning fitting caps by soaking them in 70% alcohol for 20 minutes, followed by air drying.

COMPLICATIONS

• Dislodgement during intercourse can lead to contraception failure.

• Dislodgement is the most frequent reason that women discontinue using the cervical cap.

• Vaginal odor or discharge occurs in 5% to 27% of cervical cap users.

• Lacerations and abrasions of the vagina and cervix can occur if the cap is left in place too long.

• The cervical cap causes vaginal discomfort in less than 3% of users.

• Toxic shock syndrome is a possible complication.

• The cervical cap has a higher failure rate than diaphragms in the first year postpartum.

When using these contraceptive methods, the possibility of system failure or patient noncompliance must be anticipated. Many patients could benefit from discussion of emergency contraception when a barrier method is selected (and periodically thereafter). A prescription for emergency contraception should be considered. (See Chapter 130, First-Trimester Abortion and Emergency Oral Contraceptives.)

POSTPROCEDURE PATIENT EDUCATION

See the sample patient education handout titled "Cervical Cap: Use for Contraception" on page 1908 of Appendix G.

• The FDA-approved labeling states that a Pap smear should be performed after 3 months of cervical cap use. If the test is abnormal, cap use must be discontinued and cytologic abnormality should be evaluated and treated. If the 3-month Pap smear is normal, annual screening cytology exams should be performed.

• When the patient returns for the annual refitting, the cap should be worn into the office so that proper application and fit can be assessed.

CONDOMS (MALE AND FEMALE)

The *male condom* is a contraceptive device that covers the penis and acts as a barrier to sperm. It is applied by unrolling it onto the erect penis while leaving a space at the end to contain the ejaculate. The FDA approved the *female condom* (Reality Female Condom) in 1993. It consists of a lubricated polyurethane sheath with one sealed end and flexible rings on each end. It does not need to be fitted since there is only one size and no prescription is required. One end is inserted into the vagina like a vaginal diaphragm, and the other end rests on the outside against the vulva. When used in combination with a spermicide, pregnancy rates range from 2 to 10 pregnancies per 100 users per year. Condoms also serve as a barrier to sexually transmissible infectious organisms. However, male condoms do not protect the user or the partner from transmission of the human papillomavirus. Most modern condoms are latex based, but animal product and polyurethane-based prophylactics are readily available without a prescription and are relatively inexpensive for episodic use. The clinician should discuss appropriate use with patients, because condoms are frequently used incorrectly and patients are often reticent about asking questions. (See the sample patient education handout titled "How to Use Condoms for Contraception and Disease Prevention" on page 1909 of Appendix G.)

INDICATIONS

- For prevention of pregnancy
- For prevention of the spread of sexually transmitted disease (STD) (often used for this purpose regardless of other contraception used)

CONTRAINDICATIONS

- Allergy or hypersensitivity to latex rubber or spermicides (for latex condoms)

COMPLICATIONS

- Condom rupture during intercourse can lead to contraception failure. If rupture occurs, intravaginal spermicidal contraceptive jelly or foam should be used immediately. Emergency contraception should be considered. (See Chapter 130, First-Trimester Abortion and Emergency Oral Contraceptives.)
- Local or systemic hypersensitivity because of latex rubber allergy can occur.
- Condom efficacy can be adversely affected by

BOX 131-1

Common Oil-Based Preparations that Adversely Affect Condom Efficacy

Medications
Butoconazole (Femstat)
Conjugated estrogens (Premarin)
Estradiol (Estrace)
Miconazole (Monistat)
Tioconazole (Vagistat-1)

Lubricants
Baby oil
Butter
Cocoa butter
Cold cream
Mineral oil
Hand lotion
Petroleum jelly
Shortening
Suntan oil
Vegetable oil

oil-based preparations and lubricants, so they should not be used. (See Box 131-1 and the sample patient education handout titled "How to Use Condoms for Contraception and Disease Prevention" on page 1909 of Appendix G.)

DIAPHRAGMS

The diaphragm is a barrier contraceptive device that mechanically blocks sperm from entering the cervical opening (Fig. 131-4). It acts with spermicidal jelly to produce a theoretical contraceptive effectiveness rate of 98%, but it has an actual rate of 80% to 93% for new users and 97% for long-term users. In one study only 45% of users were satisfied with use of the diaphragm for contraception (compared with 57% of birth control pill users).

INDICATIONS

- Personal desire for barrier contraception without hormonal influence
- Intolerance to hormonal contraceptive agents
- Desire for STD protection even though using another contraceptive method

CONTRAINDICATIONS

- Vaginal stenosis or significant pelvic abnormalities
- Allergy to spermicidal jelly
- Recurrent urinary tract infections associated with diaphragm use

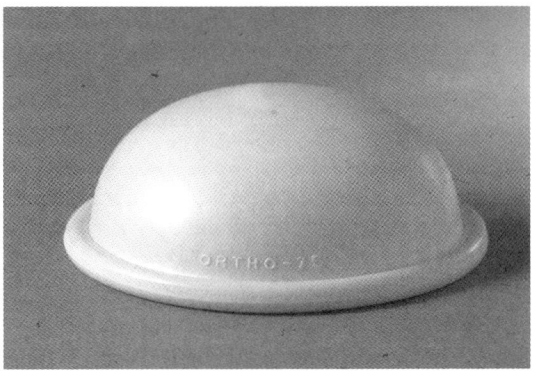

Fig. 131-4
Vaginal diaphragm. (Courtesy of Ortho-McNeil Pharmaceutical, Inc., Raritan, NJ.)

- Allergy to rubber or latex
- Aversion to touching the genital area
- Fitting sooner than 6 weeks postpartum or before the uterus has involuted
- Uterine prolapse
- Large cystocele or rectocele

EQUIPMENT

Diaphragms (sizes 65 to 90) come in three types:

1. *Arching spring:* Molded one-piece spring and dome with firm rim that forms an arc when rim is compressed in center. It needs no introducer and is recommended for women with decreased pelvic support, cystocele or rectocele, retroverted uterus, or for those who find a firmer rim easier to insert. This is the most popular type in the United States.
2. *Coil spring:* Molded one-piece spring and dome with a softer, more flexible rim than arching spring. It may be used with an introducer and is recommended for women with good vaginal support; with no cystocele, rectocele, or pelvic floor relaxation; and with a cervix in midplane or anterior position.
3. *Flat spring:* Molded one-piece spring and dome with a softer and more flexible rim than arching spring or coil spring. It has flat plane flexibility, may be used with an introducer, and is recommended for smaller women with a narrow or shallow pelvic shelf. It is excellent for nulliparous women or athletic women with strong pelvic musculature.

    Other equipment includes the following:
- Spermicidal jelly (nonoxynol-9 recommended)
- Set of fitting rings (measured in millimeters and ordered by size in 5-mm increments) or diaphragms can be obtained from Ortho Pharmaceutical Company,

usually at no cost to practitioner (preferable to fit with rings that have domes rather than rings only so patient can feel what real diaphragm will be like)
- Diaphragm introducer *(optional)*

PREPROCEDURE PATIENT PREPARATION

The clinician should explain the fitting procedure and diaphragm use to the patient. (See the patient education handout titled "How to Insert and Use a Diaphragm" on page 1911 of Appendix G.) The manufacturer will supply educational handouts for patients at no charge. The patient must understand how to use the diaphragm properly and the potential failure rate.

The clinician should explain that the fitting rings are cleaned by soaking them in a disinfectant between uses.

TECHNIQUE

1. Place the patient in the lithotomy (i.e., pelvic) position.
2. Measure for the correct size of diaphragm: Hold the index and middle fingers together and straight and insert both into the vagina. With the middle finger touching the posterior fornix, raise the hand to bring the surface of the index finger in contact with the pubic arch. Use the thumb to mark the point directly under the pubic bone and withdraw the fingers from the vagina, holding the thumb in position (Fig. 131-5, *A*).
3. To determine the diaphragm size, place one end of the diaphragm rim on the tip of the middle finger with the opposite side of the rim lying just in front of the thumb tip. This is the approximate diameter of the diaphragm needed (common sizes are 75 to 80 mm; Fig. 131-5, *B*).
4. A water-soluble lubricant placed on the fitting rings or diaphragms will aid insertion and make the fitting procedure more comfortable for the patient. Prepare to insert a fitting diaphragm or a ring of the approximate size into the vagina by folding the diaphragm in half: Press the middle of the opposite sides together between the thumb and fingers of one hand (Fig. 131-6). Hold the vulva open with the other hand. Gently slide the folded diaphragm into the vagina and aim toward the posterior fornix (Fig. 131-7). If the placement is correct, the cervix should be palpable through the dome of the diaphragm (Fig. 131-8, *A*) and the proximal rim should fit behind the pubic arch without undue pressure (Fig. 131-8, *B*).
5. When correct fit is determined, remove the diaphragm from the vagina by inserting the index finger

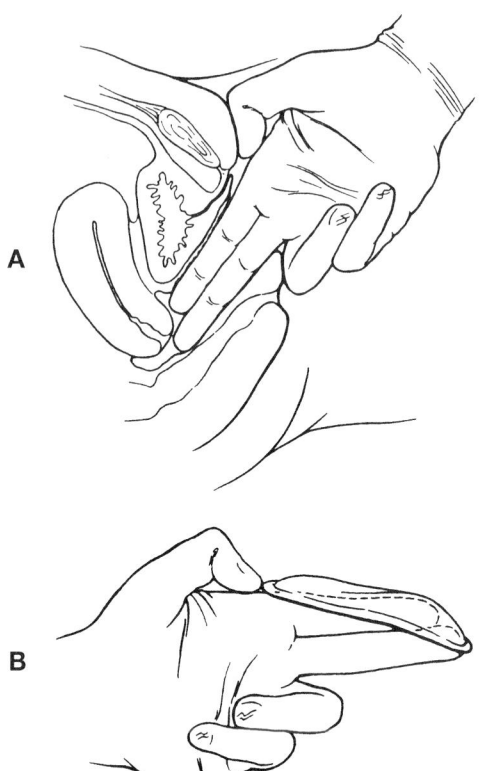

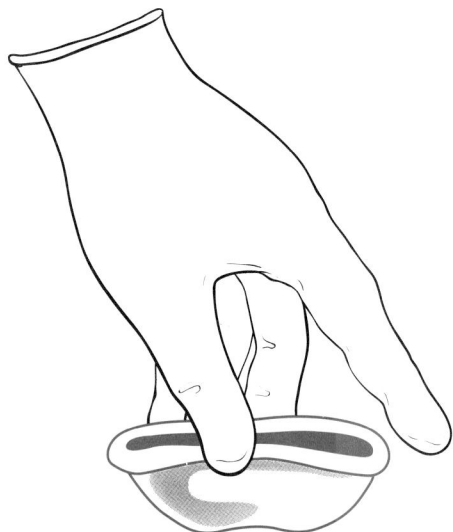

Fig. 131-5
A-B, Clinical examination to measure for appropriate diaphragm size (see text for details).

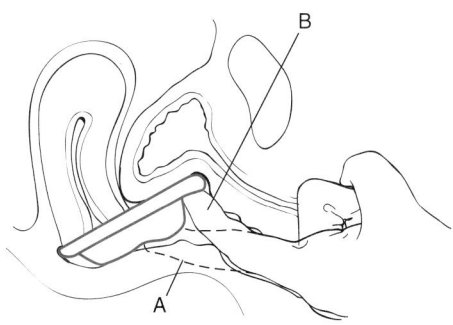

Fig. 131-6
Diaphragm is folded for insertion.

into the vagina under the symphysis pubis and hooking it under the proximal rim. Gently pull the diaphragm down and out (Fig. 131-9). The diaphragm may be slippery from the lubricant, so it should be grasped tightly to avoid inadvertent slippage.

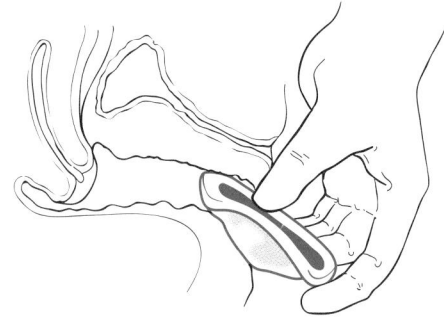

Fig. 131-7
Inserting the diaphragm.

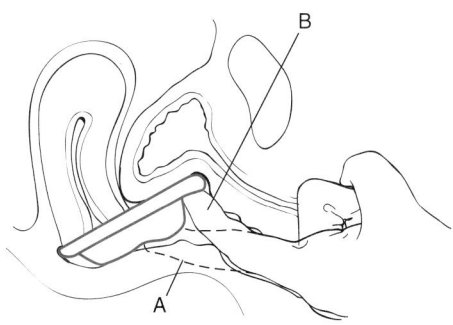

Fig. 131-8
Proper positioning of the diaphragm. *A,* Cervix is palpable behind the diaphragm. *B,* Rim fits snuggly but without discomfort behind the symphysis pubis.

COMPLICATIONS

- If a diaphragm is too small, it may not completely cover the cervix. A diaphragm that is too small may merely push the cervix proximally but not actually cover it. If a diaphragm is too large, it may be uncomfortable and not provide a tight seal. A diaphragm that is too large may slip out the vagina and be too loose to maintain a correct fit.
- Toxic shock syndrome has been reported in women who have worn diaphragms continuously for more than 24 hours.
- The pregnancy rate is increased if spermicide is not used with the diaphragm.
- A change in weight (i.e., a gain or loss of 10 lb), pregnancy, or pelvic surgery may alter the fit of the diaphragm.
- Pressure ulcerations can occur. These are caused by excessive pressure of the diaphragm against the lateral vaginal walls because of improper fit.
- Increased rates of urinary tract infections have been reported in longstanding diaphragm users, but barrier methods may also decrease the risk of cervical dysplasia.

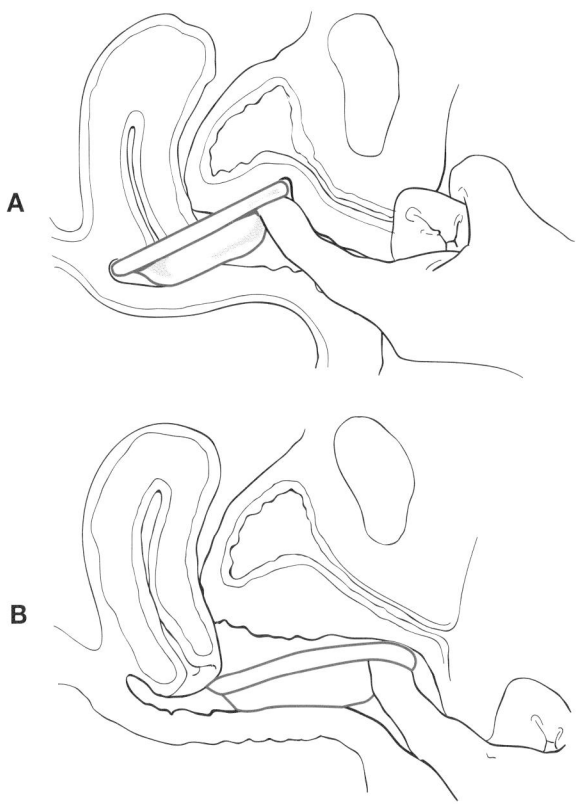

Fig. 131-9
Removal of the diaphragm. **A,** Finger is hooked under the rim. **B,** Diaphragm is pulled out through the introitus.

- Pregnancy may occur if the diaphragm is removed immediately after coitus or improperly fitted.

POSTPROCEDURE PATIENT EDUCATION

See the sample patient education handout titled "How to Insert and Use a Diaphragm" on page 1911 of Appendix G.

- The patient should be shown (and should practice) how to insert and remove the diaphragm and how to apply spermicidal jelly to the rim and the dome (Fig. 131-10). Nonoxynol-9, the spermicidal jelly that is recommended, supplies both contraceptive and STD protection. It should be applied to the concave surface of the dome and the rim of the diaphragm so that the uterus is sealed off mechanically and chemically. The patient should place approximately 1 tbsp of jelly in the dome and apply a thin layer around the rim.
- The patient should be instructed to make sure that the diaphragm rim is firmly in place proximally behind the pubic bone and below and behind the cervix. In addition, the patient should feel for the cervix through the dome of the diaphragm to ensure correct placement.

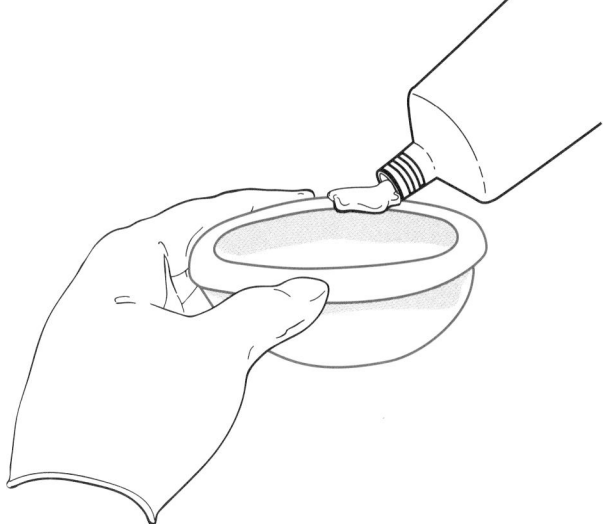

Fig. 131-10
Proper application of spermicidal jelly to diaphragm and dome.

- The patient should be told not to douche or remove the diaphragm for 6 hours after intercourse and to leave the diaphragm in place and insert additional spermicidal jelly into the vagina should additional coitus occur during this time.
- The patient should be asked to walk around the examination room with the diaphragm in place to ensure a comfortable fit.
- The prescription for the diaphragm should include: the manufacturer's name (if desired), the type, and the size. A refill should be given in event that a new diaphragm is needed when the practitioner is unavailable.

Note: The sponge is currently awaiting FDA approval. See www.contraceptivesponges.com for more information.

SUPPLIERS

Cervical caps
Cervical Cap Ltd
430 Monterey Ave, Suite 1B
Los Gatos, CA 95030
Phone: 1-408-395-2100
Website: www.cervcap.com

Diaphragms
Ortho-McNeil Pharmaceutical Company
1000 Route 202 South
Raritan, NJ 08869-0602
Phone: 1-800-682-6532
Website: www.ortho-mcneil.com

Vaginal condoms

Reality Female Condom
Female Health Company
515 North State Street, Suite 2225
Chicago, IL 60610
Phone: 1-312-595-9123
Website: www.femalehealth.com

CPT/BILLING CODE

57170   Diaphragm or cervical cap fitting with instructions

ICD-9-CM DIAGNOSTIC CODES

Cervical Caps

V2509   Family planning advice
V2502   Initiation of other contraceptive measures

Condoms

V2509   Family planning advice
V259   Unspecified contraceptive management

Diaphragms

V2502   Initiation of contraception (diaphragm)
V2509   Family planning advice
V259   Unspecified contraception

ADDITIONAL RESOURCES

• See the sample patient education handouts titled "Cervical Cap: Use for Contraception" on page 1908, "How To Use Condoms for Contraception and Disease Prevention" on page 1909, and "How to Insert and Use a Diaphragm" on page 1911 of Appendix G.

BIBLIOGRAPHY

Can you rely on condoms? *Consum Rep* 54(3):135, 1989.

Craig S, Hepburn S: The effectiveness of barrier methods of contraception with and without spermicide, *Contraception* 26:347, 1982.

Davis KR, Weller SC: The effectiveness of condoms in reducing heterosexual transmission of HIV, *Fam Plann Perspect* 31(6):272, 1999.

Faundes A, Elias C, Coggins C: Spermicides and barrier contraception, *Curr Opin Obstet Gynecol* 6(6):552, 1994.

Fihn SD, Latham RH, Roberts P, et al: Association between diaphragm use and urinary tract infection, *JAMA* 254(2):240, 1985.

Fortney JA: Contraception for American women 40 and over, *Fam Plann Perspect* 19(1):32, 1987.

Gillespie L: The diaphragm: an accomplice in recurrent urinary tract infections, *Urology* 24(1):25, 1984.

Hatcher RA, Stewart F, Trussel J, et al: *Contraceptive technology,* ed 15, New York, 1992, Iverting.

Heaton CJ, Smith MA: The diaphragm, *Am Fam Physician* 39(5):231, 1989.

Jackson M, Berger GS, Keith LG: *Vaginal contraception,* Boston, 1981, GK Hall.

Jaffe R: Toxic shock syndrome associated with diaphragm use, *N Engl J Med* 305:1585, 1981.

Procedures for your practice: fitting a cervical cap, *Pat Care* 25:140, 1991.

Richwald GA, Greenland S, Gerber MM, et al: Effectiveness of the cavity-rim cervical cap: results of a large clinical study, *Obstet Gynecol* 74:143, 1989.

Rosenfelt JA et al: Women's satisfaction with birth control, *J Fam Psychol* 36(2):169, 1993.

Speroff L, Darney P: *A clinical guide for contraception,* ed 2, Baltimore, 1996, Williams & Wilkins.

Tagg PI: The diaphragm: barrier contraception has a new social role, *Nurse Pract* 20(12):39, 1995.

Vessey M, Lawless M, Yeates D: Efficacy of different contraceptive methods, *Lancet* 1:841, 1982.

Vinson RP, Epperly TD: Counseling patients on proper use of condoms, *Am Fam Physician* 43:2081, 1991.

Weiss BD, Bassford T, Davis T: The cervical cap, *Am Fam Physician* 43:517, 1991.

Widaholm MV: Vaginal lesion: etiology—a malfitting diaphragm? *J Nurse Midwifery* 24:39, 1979.

CHAPTER 132

Bartholin's Cyst/Abscess: Word Catheter Insertion, Marsupialization

Barbara S. Apgar

Michael L. Tuggy

Simple incision and drainage (I&D) of a Bartholin duct cyst or gland abscess may give immediate and dramatic results, but the recurrence rate after such a procedure is unacceptably high. The Bartholin's glands are located at the vaginal opening at the crease between the hymen and labia minora (at approximately the 5 and 7 o'clock positions). Total excision of the gland and duct is rarely required. Total excision is not an office procedure and can be associated with increased morbidity. It is preferable to create an epithelialized tract from the vulvar vestibule to the cyst, which allows for continued functioning of the Bartholin's gland, proper drainage, and minimal recurrence. Use of a Word catheter creates a fistulous tract that preserves the gland and allows for adequate drainage. Recurrence using this technique is between 2% and 15%. The Word catheter has a short latex stem with an inflatable bulb at the distal end (Fig. 132-1) and can be used if either an abscess or a cyst is present. Marsupialization is reserved for treatment of Bartholin duct cysts.

INDICATIONS

* Treatment of symptomatic Bartholin's gland duct cyst (painful, growing)
* Treatment of Bartholin's gland abscess

CONTRAINDICATIONS

Any condition that would preclude normal I&D of a vulvar cyst or abscess would preclude use of the Word catheter. Small asymptomatic glands do not need to be drained.

EQUIPMENT

* Word catheter (Rusch and Milex)
* 3-ml syringe (for catheter inflation)
* 22-gauge, 1-inch needle (for catheter inflation)
* 1% to 2% lidocaine for anesthesia
* 30-gauge, 1½-inch needle (for anesthesia)
* 3-ml syringe (for anesthesia)
* No. 11 blade
* Pickups with teeth
* Small hemostats (2)
* 4 × 4–inch gauze pads
* Normal saline for irrigation
* Antiseptic solution (povidone-iodine if not allergic)

PREPROCEDURE PATIENT PREPARATION

The clinician should explain the procedure to the patient and obtain informed consent. A nonnarcotic oral analgesic may be administered before the procedure, if desired.

TECHNIQUE

1. Place the patient in the dorsal lithotomy position.
2. Prepare the vestibule with the antiseptic solution. It is preferable to enter the cyst or abscess from the vaginal side of the introitus unless it requires a much deeper incision. Inject lidocaine just inside the introitus. If the incision is to be made external to the introitus where the abscess is "pointing," plan to insert the catheter approximately in the area of the original duct orifice, immediately adjacent to the hymenal ring.

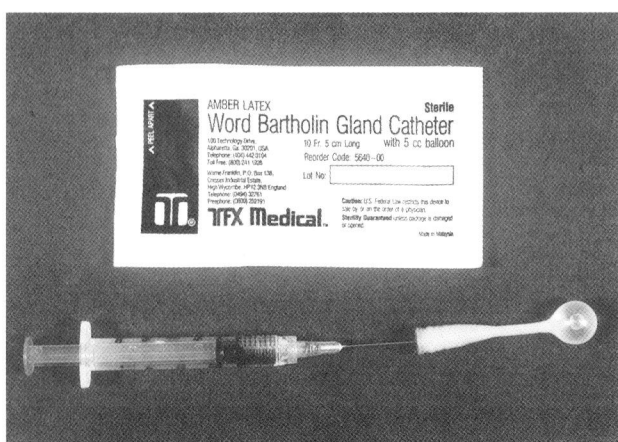

Fig. 132-1
Word catheter.

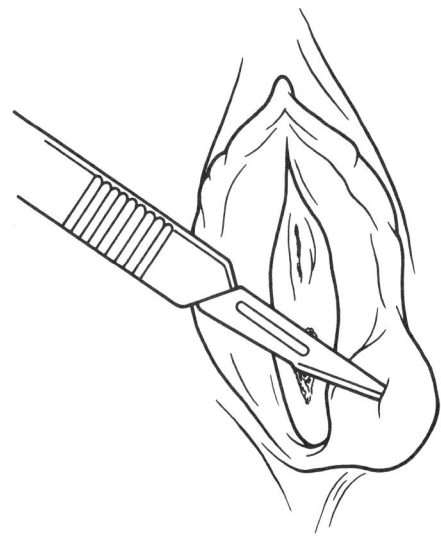

Fig. 132-2
Incision should be just large enough to admit the uninflated Word catheter.

3. Lance or incise the cyst or abscess with a no. 11 scalpel blade. It is essential that the stab wound penetrate the cyst or abscess wall, which will be evidenced by the free flow of pus or mucus. Culture contents if indicated. Although the majority of simple cysts are sterile, abscesses are typically polymicrobial with many others containing *Neisseria gonorrhoeae*. Culturing generally will not change initial management. The stab wound must be just large enough for the catheter to be inserted, usually 3 to 4 mm (Fig. 132-2).

It may be difficult to insert the catheter into the cyst after the incision is made, the contents are extruded, and the cyst/abscess has collapsed. If the catheter is inserted, it may be in a false tract and not in the cyst/abscess itself. Therefore, to preserve the tract, dissect *carefully* through the skin until the cyst/abscess wall is visualized. The cyst wall is grasped tightly with one hemostat while avoiding rupture. The other hemostat is placed gently about 5 mm from the first hemostat. This enables stabilization of the cyst wall while the incision is made. The cyst is incised in the area between the two hemostats. The hemostats continue to hold the cyst wall while the cyst cavity is gently evacuated with pressure and irrigated with 25 to 50 ml of normal saline. Alternatively, to ensure proper placement of the catheter within the cavity, insert pickups with teeth as the incision is made. One arm of the pickup slides down the side of the blade into the lumen while the other gently grasps externally. This stabilizes the tissue while the Word catheter is inserted, prevents the creation of false tracts outside the cavity, and ensures proper placement. This latter technique can also be used should the cyst/abscess be inadvertently incised while attempting the first approach described previously.

4. Insert a small hemostat into the stab wound and break away any loculations, being careful to maintain integrity of the cyst wall.

5. Insert the sterile catheter into the incision first, and then inflate the bulb by injecting 2 to 3 ml of saline through the sealed-stopper end. Use just that quantity of saline necessary to ensure that the catheter will not fall out with normal activity (usually 2.5 to 3 ml) (Fig. 132-3). Do *not* use air to inflate the catheter. A *common problem* occurs when the clinician injects the fluid into the balloon, releases the syringe plunger, and checks the tightness of the balloon in the cavity by tugging on it. Although it may seem secure then, the increased pressure in the balloon will push the saline back up into the syringe; the balloon then deflates to a smaller size and the catheter inadvertently falls out before it is time to be removed. To prevent this, *maintain pressure on the syringe plunger while checking the bulb placement*.

6. If the incision was made inside the hymen, tuck the catheter stem into the vagina, where it will rest perpendicular to the perineum. With the catheter in the vagina, the patient has freedom of movement and activity without the added awareness of protrusion of the catheter stem, which can occur if an external incision site is used. Most patients tolerate the catheter without discomfort if excessive amounts of saline are not introduced into the catheter bulb.

Bartholin's Cyst Marsupialization (Fig. 132-4)

1. Place the patient in the dorsal lithotomy position. Local anesthetic with 2% xylocaine with epinephrine,

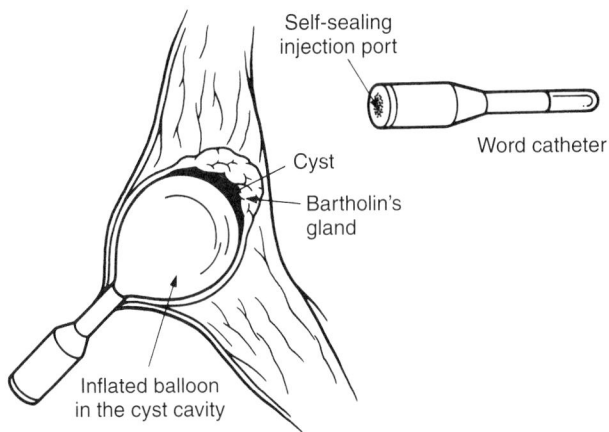

Self-sealing
injection port

Word catheter

Cyst

Bartholin's
gland

Inflated balloon
in the cyst cavity

Fig. 132-3
Balloon is inflated within the cavity of the cyst so that it will not fall out
through the stab wound.

a pudendal block with 2% xylocaine without epinephrine, or a spinal block can be used for anesthesia (rarely necessary)

2. Clean the perineum with providone-iodine solution (if not allergic).

3. Inspect the external genitalia to determine the extent of the duct cyst. Retract the labium laterally to identify the incision site internal to the hymeneal ring. Make the incision longitudinal with respect to the vagina. Generally an elliptical incision 1 or 2 cm in width at the center is needed to allow for removal of a substantial portion of the Bartholin cyst wall. Avoid excising any portion of the external skin (versus mucosa).

4. Usually during this excision of the ellipse, the cyst contents and the cyst wall will collapse. Therefore the mucosa over the cyst should be excised first and the cyst wall grasped with two small hemostats before the segment is removed. Explore the cyst with small hemostats and remove any loculated portions of the cyst.

5. Thoroughly irrigate the cyst cavity with normal saline.

6. When suturing the Bartholin cyst wall, approximate the cut edge of the cyst wall to the adjacent edge of the vaginal mucosa. This allows for more rapid transformation of the Bartholin cyst wall into a normal mucosa lining that will blend into the vaginal mucosa. Use 4-0 Vicryl and place interrupted sutures around the ellipse.

7. After placing an anchoring stitch with long tags to grasp and stabilize the tissue, pass the stitches from the inside through just the Bartholin cyst wall. Bring the needle to the surface and between the cyst wall and submucosal layer. Now insert the needle under the vaginal epithelium and pull it to the surface of the vaginal wall. This effectively imbricates the two layers

(cyst wall and vaginal mucosa) over the submucosal tissue, which allows them to heal together.

8. After the entire ellipse has been sutured open, irrigate the wound and inspect it for bleeding. There should be at least a gap of 1 cm across the open marsupialization. Normally no dressing is needed; only a pad is needed to allow for collection of blood or drainage from the wound.

9. Instruct the patient to perform sitz baths daily for 3 or 4 days and to return for follow-up in about a week. At that time, the ellipse will be probed for patency. Use of prophylactic antibiotics are unnecessary in the majority of cases and the need should be assessed individually. The degree of induration within the local tissue, or other risk factors such as pregnancy or diabetes where the possibility of infection can lead to more significant complications and is more likely, should be ascertained. Sutures will absorb on their own.

COMPLICATIONS

- Continuous pain after insertion of the Word catheter may occur. The bulb may be too large for the cyst cavity, which may be corrected by withdrawing some of the fluid, thus reducing the size of the bulb.

- With an abscessed Bartholin's gland, there may be cellulitis around the vulvar opening of the duct. Insertion of the catheter may not correct the cellulitis, and antibiotics may need to be administered for 48 to 72 hours after insertion of the catheter. If gonorrhea is cultured, appropriate actions need to be taken.

- If the needle used to introduce the saline into the catheter punctures the stem, the catheter will gradually deflate and fall out before epithelialization is complete.

- If the stab wound is too large, the catheter will fall out. It may be necessary to suture the stab wound around the catheter to keep it in place. If it falls out in less than 4 weeks, the likelihood of recurrence is high. Because of only partial formation of a new tract, placement of another Word catheter is indicated but it may not be possible because of constriction of the opening.

- Excessive bleeding is rare. Recurrence is always a possibility. Scarring is usually minimal.

POSTPROCEDURE PATIENT EDUCATION

Word Catheter

- Tell the patient to expect a discharge, since the catheter will allow for drainage of the cyst or abscess.

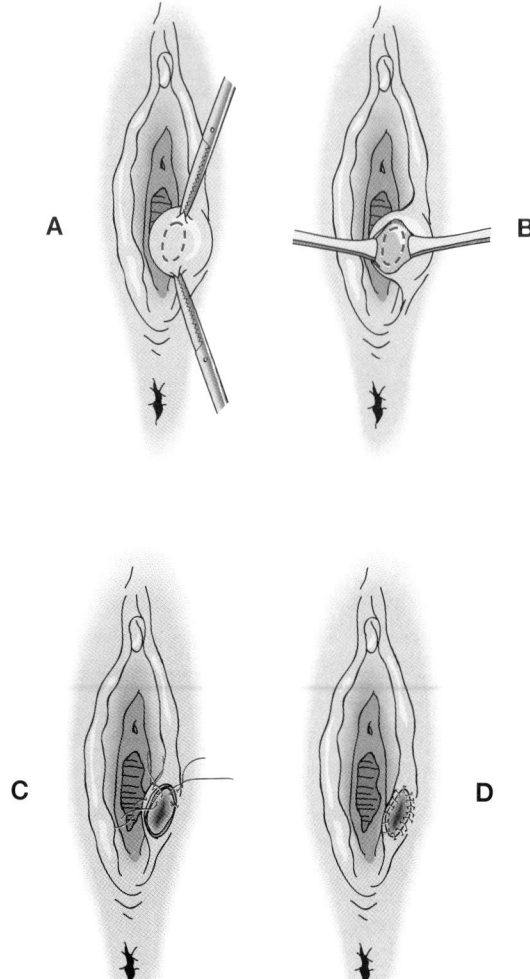

Fig. 132-4
Bartholin's cyst marsupialization. **A,** Use local anesthesia and excise an ellipse in the mucosa proximal to the hymenal ring. **B,** Identify cyst wall and grasp with hemostats. Then excise ellipse in cyst. Evacuate all contents. **C,** Suture the cyst lining to the mucosa incision margin. Place an "anchoring" stitch and leave long tags for traction. **D,** Completed marsupialization using interrupted absorbable sutures.

- The Word catheter is left in place for 4 to 6 weeks until epithelization of the new tract is complete.
- Advise the patient that sexual activity may be resumed after 2 weeks, but it may increase the risk of expulsion of the catheter. If this happens, another catheter may need to be inserted. If possible, it is best to defer sexual activity until the catheter is removed.
- Encourage daily showers or tub baths.
- Schedule a return visit in 4 to 6 weeks. At that time, the catheter is removed by inserting a needle into the catheter sealed-stopper end and drawing out the saline. The catheter is then withdrawn from the incision.

Marsupialization

- Daily sitz baths are encouraged for 3 to 5 days.
- Avoid sexual activity until after the first post-op check at one week.

SUPPLIERS

Word Bartholin's gland catheter
Milex Products, Inc.
4311 North Normandy
Chicago, IL 60634
Phone: 1-800-621-1278
Website: www.milexproducts.com

Rusch, Inc.
2450 Meadowbrook Parkway
Duluth, GA 30096
Phone: 1-770-623-0816
Website: www.ruschinc.com

CPT/BILLING CODES

56405	I&D of vulvar or perineal abscess
56420	I&D of Bartholin's gland cyst/abscess
56440	Marsupialization of Bartholin's gland cyst
56740	Excision of Bartholin's gland or cyst

ICD-9-CM DIAGNOSTIC CODES

616.2	Bartholin's cyst
616.3	abscess
616.4	Other vulvar abscess

BIBLIOGRAPHY

Cohen SD, et al: Management of the Bartholin's abscess, *Am J Gynecol Health* 4(3):42, 1990.

Goldberg JE: Simplified treatment for disease of Bartholin's gland, *Obstet Gynecol* 35:109, 1970.

Heah J: Methods of treatment for cysts and abscesses of Bartholin's gland, *Br J Obstet Gynecol* 95:321, 1988.

Hill DA, Lense JJ: Office management of Bartholin gland cysts and abscesses, *Am Fam Physician* 57(7):1611, 1998.

Lashgari M, Curry S: Preferred methods of treating Bartholin's duct cyst, *Contemp Obstet Gynecol* 40:38, 1995.

Oliphant MM, Anderson GV: Management of Bartholin's duct cysts and abscesses, *Obstet Gynecol* 16:476, 1960.

Word B: New instrument for office treatment of cyst and abscess of Bartholin's gland, *JAMA* 190:777, 1964.

CHAPTER 133

Breast Biopsy

Helen A. Pass

An excisional breast biopsy is a technically straightforward outpatient procedure readily performed under local anesthesia. With appropriate training and experience, primary care physicians can become qualified to perform most simple breast biopsies. The challenge is to correctly identify which lesions are amenable to biopsy and which require referral to a breast (general) surgeon. The goals in the management of a patient with a breast mass should be to obtain the diagnosis in the most expedient manner, to achieve good cosmesis, and to preserve all therapeutic options if the mass is unexpectedly found to be malignant at biopsy.

The only definitive method for ensuring that a mass is benign is to remove the tissue for pathologic examination. The missed or delayed diagnosis of a breast mass that ultimately proved to be cancerous is currently the most litigious aspect of medical practice. Failure to be impressed with physical examination findings was cited as the most common reason for the delay in diagnosis of breast cancer. Benign masses are usually smooth, well circumscribed (round), and freely mobile, and many cancers (e.g., colloid, medullary, and expansive intraductal) may mimic this presentation. Similarly, even though the incidence of breast cancer rises dramatically after age 65, 63% to 80% of lawsuits resulted from the missed diagnosis of cancer in women below age 50. In addition, whereas the presence of a significant positive family history increases the suspicion that a palpable abnormality may prove to be malignant, two thirds of all women with the diagnosis of breast cancer have no identifiable risk factor. Nevertheless, it is important to remind our patients and ourselves that not all breast masses are cancerous.

The role of mammography in women with a breast mass is twofold. First, it can offer clues as to the degree of suspicion that the mass may be malignant. Worrisome mammographic features include the findings of a spiculated lesion, a mass associated with pleomorphic microcalcifications, or dermal edema and retraction. Secondly, it allows assessment of the remainder of the breast parenchyma both in the involved and contralateral breasts. Before proceeding with excisional biopsy, a baseline mammogram must be obtained to rule out the presence of an occult synchronous lesion that may alter the surgical approach. Moreover, if the mass is highly suspicious, *referral to a surgeon* may be indicated to facilitate management of a presumed breast cancer.

Note: Failure of mammography or ultrasound to visualize a discrete palpable abnormality should *not* be construed as evidence of the benignity of the lesion. Up to 10% of breast cancers are radiographically occult. Thus a lesion should be removed if it meets the criteria for biopsy based on the clinical breast examination, regardless of the breast-imaging characteristics. Likewise, if a woman identifies an area of change in her breasts, the complaint should be taken seriously.

In addition to highly suspicious lesions, *referral to a general surgeon* should be considered for an additional small subset of patients. Masses in prepubertal or pubescent females (prepubertal gynecomastia) could represent the forming breast buds and must not be biopsied unless highly suspicious, since lifelong cosmetic deformity may result. Masses greater than 4 cm are best approached by core biopsy provided that if the lesion proves to be malignant, consideration should be given to neoadjuvant chemotherapy; if the lesion is benign, special surgical techniques will be necessary to minimize the cosmetic deformity associated with subsequent removal. Finally, lesions requiring preoperative mammographic localization with wire placement should not be performed by primary care practitioners unless they have received specific training in this technique.

Consideration should be given to performing fine needle aspiration (FNA) prior to excisional biopsy (see Chapter 210, Fine Needle Aspiration Cytology and Biopsy). FNA is both diagnostic and therapeutic for simple cysts, thereby avoiding unnecessary anxiety and surgery. If the mass is solid, a specimen for cytologic examination can be obtained, and breast cancer can be diagnosed prior to excisional biopsy. The false negative rate of FNA is 0.4% to 35%, and the false-positive rate is less than 1%. Thus concordance among the clinical breast examination, the breast imaging, and the FNA must be established, especially if the decision is made not to proceed to biopsy.

INDICATIONS

- The presence of a palpable, dominant abnormality in a male or female patient
- A cystic lesion if:
  — The FNA contained bloody fluid
  — A palpable abnormality remains after FNA
  — The cyst recurred after two FNAs
- After an FNA that was equivocal, nondiagnostic, or not concordant with the clinical breast examination or breast imaging
- Unresolved patient anxiety and a desire for removal of the mass
- Physician anxiety or uncertainty about the true nature of the lesion

CONTRAINDICATIONS

- Mass that is highly suspicious for breast cancer (refer to breast or general surgeon) (relative)
- Mass greater than 4 cm (consider diagnosis by core biopsy or referral to surgeon) (relative)
- Mass in a prepubertal or pubescent female (consider referral) (relative)
- Lesion requiring preoperative mammographic localization (i.e., it is nonpalpable) (consider referral) (relative)
- Allergy to local anesthetics
- Uncorrected bleeding disorder

EQUIPMENT

- Surgical marking pen
- Betadine or other antiseptic skin preparation solution
- Fenestrated drape
- Local anesthetic (the addition of 1 ml of 8.5% sodium bicarbonate solution to each 10 ml of 1% lidocaine without epinephrine creates a buffered solution with a more neutral pH, allowing less discomfort during infiltration, and a more rapid onset of action)
- Sterile 4 × 4–inch gauze
- Scalpel with no. 10 and no. 15 blades
- Two curved hemostats
- Needle driver
- Adson pickups
- DeBakey pickups (optional)
- Metzenbaum tissue scissors
- Allis clamp

- Small self-retaining retaining retractor (e.g., mastoid retractor, or small Wheatlander retractor) (optional)
- Electrocautery unit
- 3-0 or 4-0 Vicryl suture
- 4-0 or 5-0 Monocryl or PDS suture
- Steri-Strips
- Jobst postoperative brassiere (optional)

PREPROCEDURE PATIENT PREPARATION

All women over 35 years of age should have a preprocedure mammogram. Provide calm reassurance to the patient, since the discovery of a breast mass and the knowledge that biopsy is necessary is a highly stressful event for the patient. Provide detailed explanations of the procedure supplemented by written educational material.

TECHNIQUE

Determining the optimal placement of the incision for an excisional breast biopsy is a balance between achieving the most desirable cosmetic result and preserving further surgical options should the lesion prove to be cancerous. Use of preoperative FNA can minimize the number of breast masses unexpectedly found to be malignant. Generally, incisions placed along Langer's lines—the natural lines of skin tension and creasing—produce the best cosmetic result. However, a radial incision may be preferable in the most medial part of the breast (much easier to reexcise if a mastectomy is subsequently required) or in the lower half of the breast if the mass is larger, or subsequent removal of skin will be required (e.g., with reexcision lumpectomy) (Fig. 133-1). A better cosmetic result is achieved in the lower half of the breast by narrowing the breast when removing breast volume through a radial incision than by shortening the distance between the areolar complex and inframammary fold with a curvilinear incision. In a young woman in whom the mass is likely benign, consideration may be given to placing the incision in a circumareolar location.

Benign lesions may either be enucleated or removed with a small rim of normal tissue. Care should be taken to ensure that the mass is not morcellated. The specimen should be oriented for pathologic examination in case it is found to be malignant and reexcision is necessary.

After removing the breast mass, most surgeons no longer reapproximate the remaining deep breast parenchyma ("dead space"). Meticulous hemostasis must be achieved to avoid hematoma formation. Drains should not be used. Closure of the superficial fascia provides good restoration of the breast contours and, furthermore,

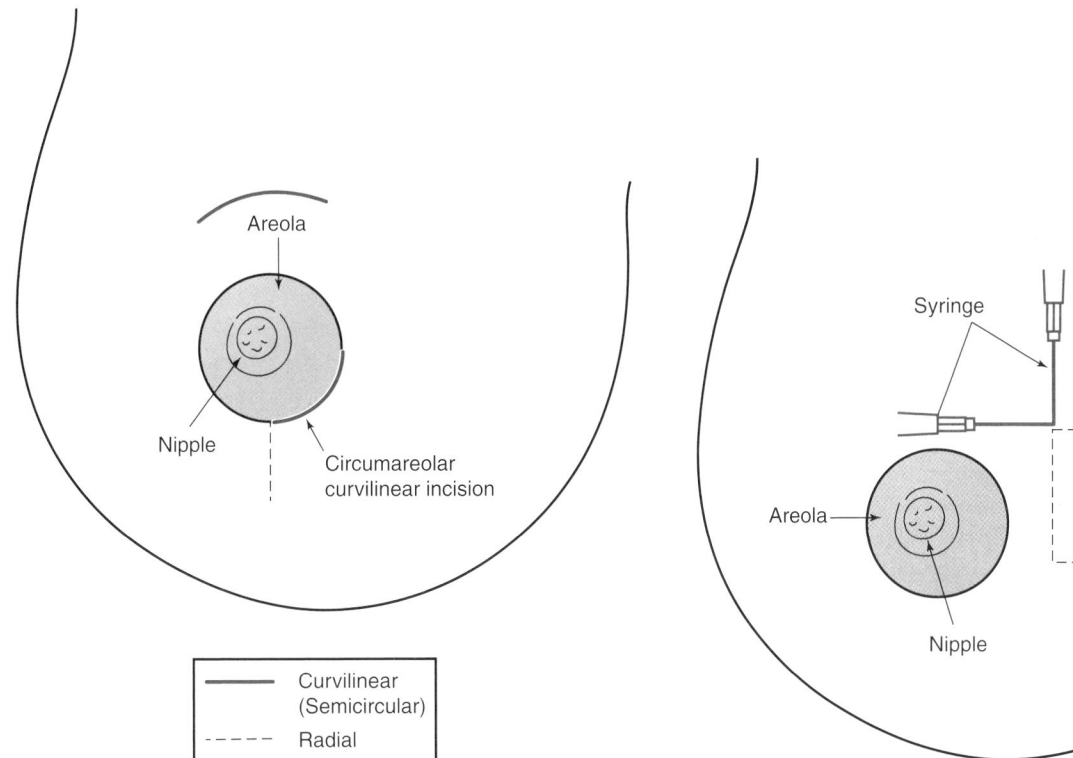

Fig. 133-1
Proper planning of incisions limits postoperative scarring. See text for details.

Fig. 133-2
Field block local anesthesia technique to preserve the ability to palpate the lesion in the center of the field. Infiltration of excessive amounts of local anesthetic directly over the mass makes palpation of the abnormality difficult.

eliminates the breast distortion with poorer cosmesis and greater mammographic distortion that occurs when the "dead space" is reapproximated.

1. Obtain written informed consent.
2. Using sterile technique, cleanse and drape the breast.
3. Using a surgical marking pen, outline the incision and the borders of the mass.
4. Give local anesthesia (1% lidocaine without epinephrine mixed 10:1 with 8.5% sodium bicarbonate). Infiltrate the incision with the local anesthetic to create a dermal wheal. Use the anesthetized wheal for all subsequent needle inserts, and infiltrate circumferentially around the lesion to be removed. Excess local anesthetic directly overlying the mass may obscure the nodule, hindering identification. (Alternatively, do a field block by injecting circumferentially around the lesion but not over the lesion itself. This allows easier palpation of the mass in the center of the field without the distortion created by the volume of anesthetic.) (Fig. 133-2)
5. Incise the skin with a no. 15 blade, making sure to hold the blade at right angles to the skin edges to avoid beveling the incision. Carry the incision vertically to the subcutaneous layer.
6. Use tissue scissors to dissect the subcutaneous tissue from the mass.
7. Cauterize bleeders with the electrocautery.
8. Circumferentially excise the specimen using the tissue scissors, a no. 10 blade, or the electrocautery unit. Exercise care to avoid harming the skin edges. An Allis clamp may be used on the mass to provide countertraction, facilitating removal of the mass. Provide more local anesthesia in the deeper layers as needed.
9. Orient the specimen for pathologic evaluation using marking sutures (this can facilitate localization of inadequate margins should the lesion be found to be an incompletely excised malignancy).
10. Submit all specimens for pathologic evaluation. Use of frozen section analysis is optional, since hormone receptor analysis is now routinely performed on paraffin-embedded tissue in case of malignancy.
11. Obtain meticulous hemostasis with electrocautery.
12. Reapproximate the subdermal tissue with buried interrupted Vicryl sutures. To prevent deformity, do not reapproximate the deep tissues, and do not

incorporate excessively large amounts of tissue, since this may lead to dimpling.

13. Close the skin with a running subcuticular suture of 4-0 or 5-0 Monocryl or PDS.

14. Wash off remaining skin preparation solution, then apply Steri-Strips and a sterile bandage (for larger biopsies, a pressure dressing or Jobst brassiere may be applied).

15. Provide adequate oral analgesia, emergency phone numbers, and written postoperative instructions.

16. The patient may remove the dressing in 24 to 48 hours and resume showering. Submersion of the incision (e.g., swimming) and vigorous exercise should be avoided for 1 week.

17. The sutures will dissolve and should not require removal.

COMPLICATIONS

- Hematoma (may mimic recurrence of the mass)
- Infection (cellulitis or abscess formation)
- Scarring or skin distortion
- Pain (generally minimal)
- Fluid collection (may require aspiration if symptomatic)
- Failure to identify the correct mass or incomplete removal of the lesion
- Need for subsequent surgery (if the mass is malignant, incompletely excised, or a complication occurs)

INTERPRETATION OF RESULTS AND CONSIDERATIONS

- The closure of the incision is all the patient sees; your surgical skill will be judged by the scar left on her breast. Plan the incision carefully, and use plastic surgical technique for skin closure.
- It is imperative to communicate the pathology results in a timely manner and to refer to specialists if necessary. It is imperative to communicate the results from pathology and arrange for any specialist referrals in a timely fashion.
- Avoid biopsying large or complicated lesions; refer instead.
- Management of breast complaints is very litigious. Adequately document the workup. Obtain informed consent. Diligently follow up all biopsy results, and recognize when referral is appropriate.

POSTPROCEDURE PATIENT EDUCATION

Give the patient written instructions regarding removal of the dressing, resumption of showering, and follow-up appointment. The patient should report excessive pain, drainage from the wound, redness, fever, or abnormal swelling. A follow-up appointment will ensure the lesion has been removed, although induration may be palpable for several weeks. See the sample patient education handout titled "Breast Biopsy" on page 1913 of Appendix G.

CONCLUSION

Accurate interpretation of the clinical breast examination can be difficult. Any persistent palpable abnormality or asymmetric finding must be evaluated with physical examination, breast radiologic imaging, tissue diagnosis, and possibly ultrasound. All findings must be concordant, and, if not, workup must proceed even if the mammogram is normal. With sufficient training and experience, most primary care practitioners can perform excisional breast biopsies in the office setting expeditiously and with a good cosmetic outcome. Complex or highly suspicious masses may prompt referral to a breast specialist.

SUPPLIERS

Jobst Postoperative Brassiere
Fredericks–Jobst Institute Inc.
P.O. Box 653
Toledo, OH 43697-0653

CPT/BILLING CODES

88170	Fine needle aspirate (FNA) with or without preparation of smears
19100	Biopsy of breast, needle (FNA)
19101	Biopsy of breast, incisional*
19120	Excision of cysts or breast lesions*
19125	Excision of breast lesion radiographically guided*
19126	Excision radiographically guided, each additional lesion*

ICD-9-CM DIAGNOSTIC CODES

174.9	Malignant neoplasm of breast (female), unspecified
217	Benign neoplasm of the breast
611.72	Lump or mass in the breast

*Health Care Financing Administration (HCFA) allows additional payment for a tray for this procedure when performed in a physician office. Charge appropriately using code "99020—surgical tray."

793.8   Abnormal radiologic and other examination of breast (mammographic lesion, microcalcifications)

ADDITIONAL RESOURCES

- See the sample patient education handout titled "Breast Biopsy" on page 1913 of Appendix G.
- See the sample patient consent form titled "Breast Biopsy" on page 1916 of Appendix G.

BIBLIOGRAPHY

Cady B, Steele GD, Morrow M, et al: Evaluation of common breast problems: guidance for primary care providers, *CA Cancer J Clin* 48:49, 1998.

Coury C: Evaluation of a breast complaint: is it cancer? *Am Fam Physician* 49:445, 1994.

Donegan WL: Evaluation of a palpable breast mass, *N Engl J Med* 327:937, 1992.

Gamble WG: Breast surgery. In Benjamin RB, editor: *Atlas of outpatient and office surgery*, Philadelphia, 1994, Lea & Febiger.

Layfield LJ, Glasgow BJ, Cramer H: Fine-needle aspiration in the management of breast masses, *Pathol Annu* 24:23, 1989.

Physician Insurers Association of America: *Breast cancer study*, Lawrenceville, NJ, 1990, PIAA.

CHAPTER 134

Cervical Cerclage

Charles E. Werner, Jr.

Cerclage is a procedure designed to manage cervical incompetence, which is usually defined as a painless dilation of the cervix with expulsion of the products of conception in the second or early third trimesters. The first procedure to attempt to treat this condition, the Shirodkar cerclage, was introduced in the early 1950s. Since that time, several other cerclage techniques have been described. Some are performed transabdominally in a nonpregnant state, such as the Lash procedure. The more common vaginal approaches include the previously mentioned Shirodkar and the much more common McDonald, because of its technical ease and relative lack of complications. It can be placed prophylactically in the nonemergent setting as well as in the emergent situation when the diagnosis of incompetent cervix has been made but the pregnancy is yet to be lost irretrievably.

This chapter deals only with the McDonald cerclage in the nonemergent setting (i.e., as a prophylactic procedure). Before performing a cerclage procedure, the clinician must have sufficient technical training, the ability to arrive at a diagnosis, and the capability of handling consequent complications.

Further compounding the decision to place a cerclage is the relative paucity of well-designed randomized prospective studies serving to demonstrate its use. Most of the available data come from retrospective case-controlled reporting in which the patient serves as her own control. If the clinician clearly believes that cervical cerclage has an important role to play in preventing a disastrous reproductive outcome, it would be unethical to design a study that would deny treatment. This, obviously, creates a difficult dilemma.

INDICATIONS

- A classic history of cervical incompetence: a painless dilation of the cervix with expulsion of the products of conception in the second or early third trimester. A careful history is required to delineate this condition from preterm labor. Old records should be obtained and studied.

- Extensive surgical trauma to the cervix, either from cone biopsy, loop electrosurgical excision procedure, or obstetric laceration
- Abnormally foreshortened cervix (exactly what constitutes abnormal is somewhat in dispute, but usually between 2.5 and 2.8 cm)
- Wedging of the amniotic membranes into the cervical canal on transvaginal or transabdominal ultrasound
- Diethylstilbestrol exposure
- Some uterine anomalies

CONTRAINDICATIONS

- Nonviable pregnancy
- Known or suspected abnormal pregnancy
- Undiagnosed vaginal bleeding
- Ruptured membranes
- Acute cervical or intrauterine infection

TECHNIQUE

A cerclage can be placed as soon as an intrauterine pregnancy is confirmed, but it is most commonly accomplished between the fourteenth and eighteenth week of the pregnancy. This allows most pregnancies that will be spontaneously lost to do so and therefore avoids placing a cerclage in a hopeless situation. It is usually not placed if the fetus has reached a gestational age at which viability can be anticipated.

1. Obtain informed consent (see the sample patient consent form titled "McDonald Cerclage" on page 1917 of Appendix G).
2. Document intrauterine viability. (This should be confirmed afterwards as well.)
3. The patient is brought to the operating room where a suitable anesthesia, usually either a general or regional, is provided. Local anesthesia or paracervical anesthesia is avoided because of concern for alteration in uterine blood flow.
4. Place the patient in the dorsolithotomy position; prep and drape her in a sterile fashion.

5. Drain the bladder (a Foley catheter is not necessary).
6. Perform a pelvic examination.
7. Place a weighted speculum in the posterior vagina.
8. Use a ring forceps to manipulate the cervix while an assistant handles a right angle or Deaver retractor to retract the vagina, thus providing adequate exposure.
9. A nonabsorbable large diameter suture (e.g., no. 5 Mersilene or Ethibond [not to be confused with "5-0," which is much smaller]) with a large needle is used. Grasp the anterior lip of the cervix and displace it inferiorly. Place the stitch in the mid portion of the cervix equidistant from the ectocervix and the vaginal reflection. If right handed, enter the cervix at the 12 o'clock position and, proceeding in a counter-clockwise manner (clockwise if left handed), pass the stitch to the 9 o'clock position where it is again removed from the cervix, immediately looped back into the cervix, and then passed out again at the 6 o'clock position. Attempt to pass the suture through the mid position of the cervical stroma without entering the endocervical canal. (Sutures that are placed too shallowly [e.g., too close to the epithelium] will tear out when drawn tight.) Reinsert the suture at the 6 o'clock position, then withdraw it at the 3 o'clock position, reinsert it, and then withdraw it again at a point very close to the starting position (Fig. 134-1, *A*).
10. Cinch down the suture like a purse string—without drawing too tightly—and tie it.
11. Some surgeons prefer to place a second cerclage somewhat lower, perhaps 5 to 10 mm below the first, if cervical length allows (Fig. 134-1, *B*). (Care must be taken not to rupture membranes or inadvertently enter the bladder by attempting to aggressively place a stitch too cephalad.)
12. After adequate recovery, the patient can usually be discharged the same day; however, if there is concern about possible complications, she can be admitted for observation. Tocolytics or hormonal therapies are of no benefit. It is extremely important that the postoperative note, which should also be placed in the obstetric record, indicates the type of suture used, the type of cerclage performed (McDonald), and the location and number of knots placed in the cervix. A diagram is very helpful.

COMPLICATIONS

Complications can be devastating and usually lead to the very situation cerclage was designed to avoid.
• Pregnancy loss either from rupture of membranes or chorioamnionitis.
• Scarring of the cervix, which may cause significant cervical and potential uterine injury during labor.

• Quite commonly a bothersome vaginal discharge results from the foreign body reaction of the non-absorbable suture in the cervix. This is usually well tolerated but is best explained thoroughly prior to placement.

REMOVAL

The cerclage is left in place until the 37th week of the pregnancy, at which time it can usually be removed

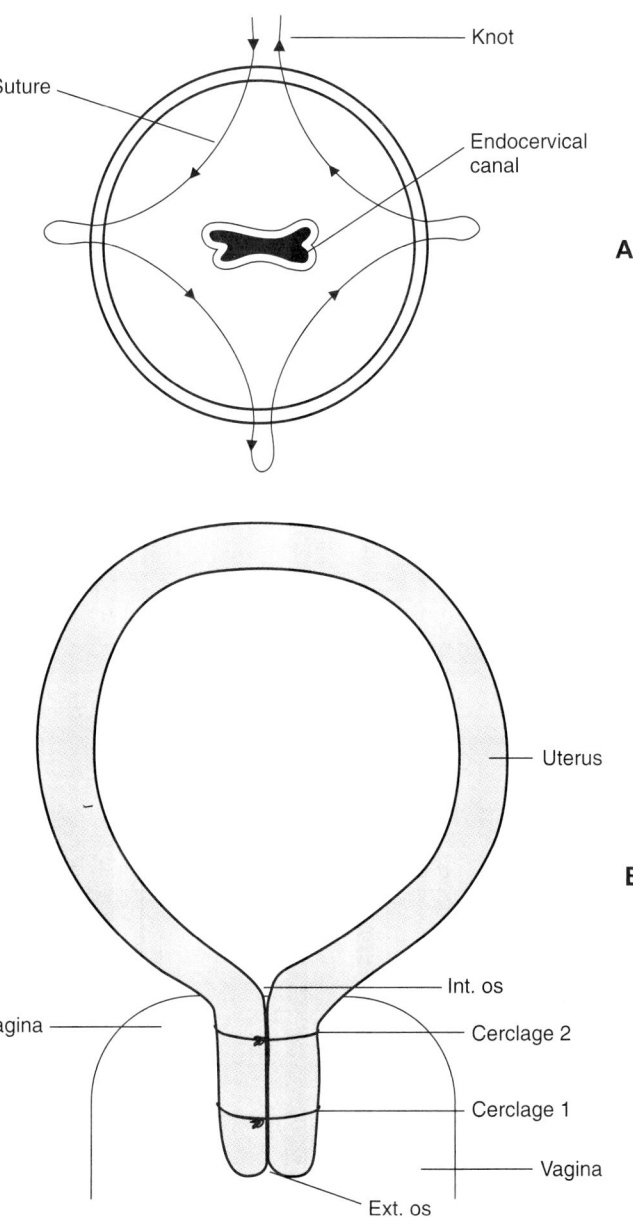

Fig. 134-1
Cervical cerclage. **A,** Cross section of cervix showing four bites in the cervix. **B,** Second cerclage is sometimes placed 5 to 10 mm below the first cerclage. Suture would be within cervical stroma.

easily in the office. The patient is placed in the usual examination position with the speculum placed. The knot is then grasped with the pickups (such as a Russian), the knot is elevated, and the Metzenbaum's scissors are used to cut the cerclage stitch, which is then easily removed. If, however, difficulty arises when attempting to remove the stitch, the clinician should not hesitate to proceed to the operating room. If preterm labor is encountered later in the pregnancy and tocolysis is not successful, the cerclage should be removed at that time to avoid damage to the cervix.

POSTPROCEDURE PATIENT EDUCATION

Controversy exists regarding the optimal postoperative recommendations. It is not unreasonable to ask the patient to refrain from vaginal intercourse and to limit her physical activity. This recommendation can vary from several weeks to the duration of the pregnancy. The vast majority of patients who have experienced such a devastating event as a pregnancy loss are more than willing to bear the burden of these short-term restrictions. However, there is little evidence to support these recommendations, and they may be modified to fit the individual situation.

CONCLUSION

Cervical cerclage is a procedure that holds out the hope that a patient may have a successful pregnancy. It is extremely important to perform a careful history and examination, to be as confident in the diagnosis as possible, and to use scrupulous technique to arrive at a good outcome.

CPT/BILLING CODES

59320	Cerclage
59871	Removal of cerclage suture under anesthesia (other than local)

ICD-9-CM DIAGNOSTIC CODES

6225	Incompetent cervix
65453	Incompetent cervix in pregnancy (affecting fetus or newborn, 761.0)

ADDITIONAL RESOURCES

- See the sample patient consent form titled "McDonald Cerclage" on page 1917 of Appendix G.

BIBLIOGRAPHY

Abdelhak YE, Aronov R, Roque H, Young BK: Management of cervical cerclage at term: remove the suture in labor? *J Perinat Med* 28:453, 2000.

Abdelhak YE, Sheen JJ, Kuczynski E, Bianco A: Comparison of delayed absorbable suture v nonabsorbable suture for treatment of incompetent cervix, *J Perinat Med* 27:250, 1999.

ACOG criteria set: cervical cerclage, Int J Gynaecol Obstet 56:211, 1997.

ACOG criteria set: cervical cerclage, Int J Gynaecol Obstet 56:298, 1997.

Althuisius SM, Dekker GA, Hummel P, et al: Final results of the Cervical Incompetence Prevention Randomized Cerclage Trial (CIPRACT): therapeutic cerclage with bed rest versus bed rest alone, *Am J Obstet Gynecol* 185(5):1106, 2001.

Althuisius SM, Dekker GA, van Geijn HP, et al: Cervical incompetence randomized cerclage trial (CIPRACT): study design and preliminary results, *Am J Obstet Gynecol* 183(4):823, 2000.

American College of Obstetricians and Gynecologists: Preterm labor, *ACOG Tech Bull* June 206:710, 1995.

Cunningham FG, MacDonald PC, Gant NF, et al (eds): *Williams obstetrics,* ed 20, Stamford, Conn., 1995, Appleton & Lange, pp 588-590.

Funai EF, Paidas MJ, Rebarber A, et al: Change in cervical length after prophylactic cerclage, *Obstet Gynecol* 94:117, 1999.

Gabbe SG, Niebyl JR, Simpson JL (eds): *Obstetrics: normal and problem pregnancies,* ed 4, New York, 2001, Churchill Livingstone, pp 790-792.

Guzman ER, Forster JK, Vintzileos AM, et al: Pregnancy outcomes in women treated with elective versus ultrasound-indicated cervical cerclage, *Ultrasound Obstet Gynecol* 12:323, 1998.

Hassan SS, Romero R, Berry SM, et al: Patients with an ultrasonographic cervical length ≤15 mm have nearly a 50% risk of early spontaneous preterm delivery, *Am J Obstet Gynecol* 182:1458, 2000.

Hassan SS, Romero R, Maymon E, et al: Does cervical cerclage prevent preterm delivery in patients with a short cervix? *Am J Obstet Gynecol* 184(7):1325, 2001.

Heath VC, Souka AP, Erasmus I, et al: Cervical length at 23 weeks of gestation: the value of Shirodkar suture for the short cervix, *Ultrasound Obstet Gynecol* 12:318, 1998.

Kelly S, Pollock M, Maas B, et al: Early transvaginal ultrasonography versus early cerclage in women with an unclear history of incompetent cervix. *Am J Obstet Gynecol* 184(6):1097, 2001.

Lazar P, Gueguen S, Dreyfus J, et al: Multicentred controlled trial of cervical cerclage in women at moderate risk of preterm delivery, *Br J Obstet Gynaecol* 91:731, 1984.

Macdonald R, Smith P, Vyas S: Cervical incompetence: the use of transvaginal sonography to provide an objective diagnosis, *Ultrasound Obstet Gynecol* 18:211, 2001.

McElrath TF, Norwitz ER, Lieberman ES, Heffner LJ: Management of cervical cerclage and preterm premature rupture of the membranes: should the stitch be removed? *Am J Obstet Gynecol* 183:840, 2000.

Novy MJ, Gupta A, Wothe DD, et al: Cervical cerclage in the second trimester of pregnancy: a historical cohort study, *Am J Obstet Gynecol* 184(7):1447, 2001.

OB/GYN Clinical alert: Is prophylactic cerclage in patients with a history suggestive of incompetent cervix better than waiting for ultrasound signs of cervical shortening? *Am Health Consultants* 17(9):65, 2001.

O'Connell MP, Lindow SW: Reversal of asymptomatic cervical length shortening with cervical cerclage: a preliminary study, *Hum Reprod* 16:172, 2001.

O'Connor S, Kuller JA, McMahon MJ: Management of cervical cerclage after preterm premature rupture of membranes, *Obstet Gynecol Surv* 54:391, 1999.

Rust OA, Atlas RO, Reed J, et al: Revisiting the short cervix detected by transvaginal ultrasound in the second trimester: why cerclage therapy may not help, *Am J Obstet Gynecol* 185(5):1098, 2001.

Te Linde RW, Rock JA, and Thompson JD (eds): *Te Linde's operative gynecology*, ed 8, Philadelphia, 1997, Lippincott-Raven.

Rush RW, Isaacs S, McPherson K, et al: A randomized controlled trial of cervical cerclage in women at high risk of spontaneous preterm delivery, *Br J Obstet Gynaecol* 91:724, 1984.

Rust OA, Atlas RO, Jones KJ, et al: A randomized trial of cerclage versus no cerclage among patients with ultrasonographically detected second-trimester preterm dilatation of the internal os, *Am J Obstet Gynecol* 183(4):830, 2000.

Surico N, Ribaldone R, Arnulfo A, Baj G: Uterine malformations and pregnancy losses: is cervical cerclage effective? *Clin Exper Obstet Gynecol* 27:147, 2000.

Treadwell MC, Bronsteen RA, Bottoms SF. Prognostic factors and complications rates for cervical cerclage: a review of 482 cases, *Am J Obstet Gynecol* 165(3):555, 1991.

Yang JH, Kuhlman K, Daly S, Berghella V: Prediction of preterm birth by second trimester cervical sonography in twin pregnancies, *Ultrasound Obstet Gynecol* 15:288, 2000.

CHAPTER 135

Cervical Conization

Lydia A. Watson

In most cases, proper evaluation of abnormal Pap smears and cervical lesions include colposcopy, multiple-punch biopsy sampling, and endocervical curettage. However, conization of the cervix plays an important role in both the diagnosis and the management of abnormalities of the cervix. Cold-knife conization (CKC) is considered the gold standard by which all other outpatient techniques are critiqued. "Cold knife" refers to a surgical blade versus the old "hot-wire" cone, or the newer loop procedure.

Conization of the cervix consists of the removal of a cone-shaped wedge of tissue from the cervix uteri. To be considered an adequate specimen, the tissue removed must include the entire transformation zone with the squamocolumnar junction and the entire lesion surrounded by uninvolved margins. The large loop electrical excision procedure is described in Chapter 150, Loop Electrosurgical Excision Procedure (LEEP) for Treating Cervical Intraepithelial Neoplasia. A review of Chapter 139, Colposcopic Examination, and Chapter 141, Cryotherapy of the Cervix, is also recommended.

INDICATIONS

A conization may be indicated for diagnosis and/or treatment. Usually any conization method can be used interchangeably, although using a knife blade causes less tissue artifact (pathological distortion) than other methods and may allow a better histologic examination.

Indications for Diagnosis

- Inadequate colposcopic evaluation of the cervix:
  — The lesion is not seen on colposcopic examination, but Pap smear is significantly abnormal
  — Incomplete visualization of a lesion that extends into the endocervical canal on colposcopic examination
  — Inadequate visualization of entire transformation zone, including the squamocolumnar junction (e.g., goes into the os where it cannot be evaluated)

- Positive endocervical curettings (i.e., dysplasia or cancer)
- If there are inconsistencies between cytologic findings, histologic diagnoses, and colposcopic impression (i.e., a Pap smear that is at least two stages worse than colposcopic biopsy)
- If invasive cancer has not been ruled out satisfactorily by colposcopic evaluation.

Indications for Therapy

- If a cytology or biopsy specimen suggests micro invasive carcinoma of the cervix (clinician must rule out frank invasion to define the proper treatment; in this case, procedure may also be therapeutic)
- For high-grade dysplasia (i.e., moderate or severe dysplasia by biopsy) greater than 2 cm or more than two quadrants (some would argue all high-grade lesions require conization)
- When cervical cryotherapy is contraindicated (Chapter 141, Cryotherapy of the Cervix)
  — Lesion too large for cryotip
  — Markedly irregular surface of cervix with crevices that cryo will not reach
  — Glandular involvement on biopsy (relative)
  — Lesion extends more than 5 mm into the os
- For unreliable patients (e.g., patients unlikely to be compliant with follow-up after cryotherapy and during attempts to monitor lesser cervical intraepithelial neoplasia lesions without treatment)
- To correct, cervical stenosis (although the os is more likely to be opened using a shallow LEEP excision than a CKC)

CONTRAINDICATIONS

- Pregnancy (relative contraindication)

Note: Pregnancy is not an absolute contraindication to conization; however, only a well-trained obstetrician/gynecologist or surgeon capable of managing complications should perform the procedure on a pregnant patient (see the "Complications" section).

- Known frank invasive carcinoma of the cervix or endocervix ("Carcinoma in situ" is not a cancer, but rather a severe dysplasia. With microinvasive cancer, a conization procedure must be performed to rule out frank invasion.)
- Patient with contraindications for general or regional anesthesia
- Unstable medical conditions (rarely is conization an emergency)
- Unstable bleeding disorders
- Inflammatory cervicitis (causes increased bleeding)
- Heavy menses at time of surgery (relative; just makes more difficult)

PREPROCEDURE PATIENT PREPARATION

- The procedure and complications should be explained to the patient, and written informed consent should be obtained. (See the patient education handout titled "Cold-Knife Conization of the Cervix [Cone Biopsy]" on page 1918 and the sample patient consent form titled "Cervical Conization" on page 1920 of Appendix G.)
- The need for general, local, or regional anesthesia should be explained.
- All options for treatment and evaluation should be explained.

EQUIPMENT

- Povidone-iodine
- Colposcope with green filter
- Acetic acid and full-strength Lugol's solution
- Vasopressin 20 U in 20 ml of normal saline for infiltration of the cervix
- Long scalpel handle with no. 11 blade
- Long, fine-tooth forceps
- Kevorkian endocervical curette
- Electrocautery unit
- 0-Chromic or 0-Vicryl suture (or Surgicel, Gelfoam, or Avitene) for hemostasis; long needle holders
- Large Graves' speculum
- Uterine sound

TECHNIQUE

1. *Special considerations:* Most lesions are found on the ectocervix in premenopausal women, so the cone should have a broad base and the top should have a wide angle (Fig. 135-1, *A*). In postmenopausal women, the specimen will be long and narrow, with an acute angle at the cone top. The squamocolumnar

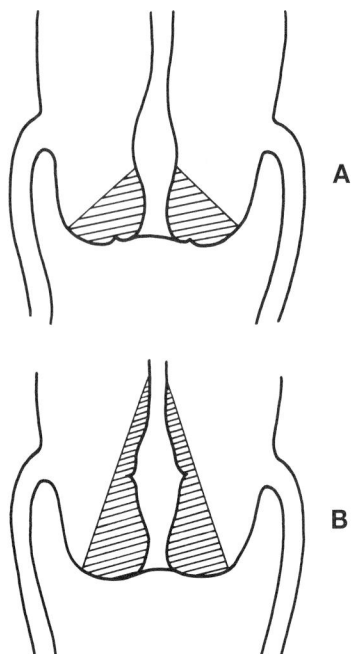

Fig. 135-1
Variation in size and shape of cervical tissue removed during conization. **A,** For large ectocervical lesion. **B,** For canal lesions.

junction in these patients has generally moved inside the endocervical canal, and lesions are more likely to be endocervical. The transformation zone in older women is generally quite small (Fig. 135-1, *B*).

2. Administer general, local (intrastromal), or regional anesthesia to the patient, and obtain adequate exposure of the cervix.

3. Apply full-strength Lugol's solution to the cervix to aid in determining the width of the cone base. All areas that do not stain will be removed. Alternatively, perform colposcopy using acetic acid and the green filter to demarcate the lesion and the transformation zone.

4. Obtain hemostasis by circumferentially infiltrating the cervical stroma with a solution of 20U of Vasopressin diluted in 20 ml of normal saline (Fig. 135-2).

Note: Hemostatic retention sutures are no longer routinely used.

5. Gently sound the uterine canal to determine position and size of the uterus.

6. Incise the cervix in a circular fashion, making the incision outside of the Lugol's-negative or aceto-white area. Begin at the 6 o'clock position. This will prevent the blood that runs down from obscuring the incision line (Fig. 135-3, *A*). Angle the blade centrally to the width and depth desired.

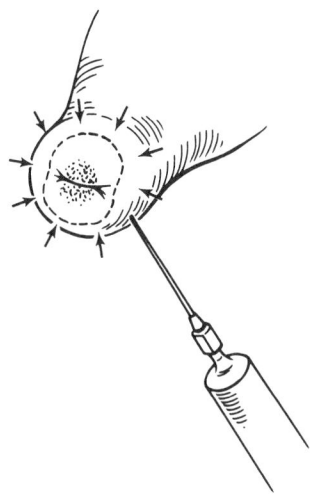

Fig. 135-2
Intracervical injection.

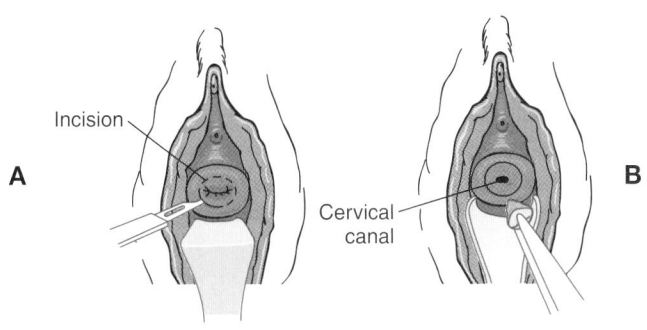

A

Incision

Cervical
canal

B

Fig. 135-3
A-B, Conization technique (see text for details).

7. Use a fine-toothed forceps to elevate the cone away from the underlying bed. Avoid damaging the cervical epithelium (Fig. 135-3, *B*).
8. Mark the 12 o'clock position of the specimen for the pathologist with a single suture placed into the cervical stroma.
9. Curette the remainder of the endocervical canal (ECC) with a small curette to rule out disease above the upper margins of the cone.
10. Perform a dilation and curettage, *if indicated*, at this time.
11. Obtain hemostasis with superficial electrocoagulation by using a ball electrode or individual suture ligatures to control bleeding. The cone site may also be packed with an absorbable gelatin sponge (e.g., Gelfoam) or similar hemostatic material. Most apply Monsel's solution to the base of the excision after coagulation.
12. Place the cone specimen in fixative to send for pathologic interpretation.

COMPLICATIONS

Complications for the nonpregnant patient include the following (overall complication rate 10%):
- Pain and cramping generally minimal.
- Immediate or delayed hemorrhage. (Eschar sloughs in 7 to 10 days. Delayed hemorrhage can occur at this time; some spotting is to be expected for 10 to 14 days.) If bleeding is excessive at the time of surgery, inject 1 ml of 2% xylocaine with epinephrine into each bleeding spot. This will generally slow bleeding enough to allow electrocoagulation. Alternatively, and rarely, a "figure of 8" stitch may need to be placed over the bleeding vessel.
- Cervical stenosis (less than 3 mm) that prevents menses or obtaining a good endocervical Pap smear.
- Uterine perforation.
- Pelvic cellulitis (very rare) or cervicitis.
- Damage to the bladder or rectum. (This is usually seen in cases of significant vaginal atrophy with shallow vaginal fornices.)
- Cervical incompetence.
- Infertility caused by loss of mucus-producing endocervical glands.
- Anesthetic complications.
- Positive margins or positive ECC. (If ectocervical margins show only dysplasia, the patient should be followed closely but a repeat cone is not indicated. Usually the lesion will resolve during the inflammatory healing process. A repeat cone may be indicated in older patients who are at a high risk and do not desire pregnancy, those who have had pelvic irradiation, or both the margins and ECC are positive. If the ECC above the excisional site is positive with a high-grade lesion, repeat conization should be considered.)
- Missing the lesion (rare).

In addition to the complications mentioned for the nonpregnant patient, complications for the pregnant patient include the following:
- Fetal loss rate of 10% (secondary to rupture of the membranes, premature labor, and excessive hemorrhaging)
- Postoperative hemorrhage rate of 30%

POSTPROCEDURE PATIENT EDUCATION

- A follow-up appointment should be scheduled for 4 to 6 weeks.
- The patient should be instructed to avoid intercourse, douching, and tampon use until follow-up examination confirms healing.
- The patient should be asked to notify the clinician of

elevated temperature, excessive vaginal bleeding, or purulent discharge.
- The first follow-up Pap smear should be scheduled in 3 to 4 months if all margins are clear.

CPT/BILLING CODES

57520	Conization, with or without fulguration, cold knife or laser
57522	Conization, loop electrode
57505	Endocervical curettage
99070	Surgical tray

ICD-9-CM DIAGNOSTIC CODES

180.9	Cervical neoplasm, malignant (excludes carcinoma in situ)
078.11	Condyloma
219.0	Benign neoplasm, cervix
233.1	Carcinoma in situ, cervix
622.0	Cervical erosion or ulcer
622.1	Cervical atypia
622.1	Cervical dysplasia (mild, moderate, severe)
622.2	Cervical leukoplakia
622.4	Cervical stenosis
622.7	Cervical polyp

ADDITIONAL RESOURCES

- See the sample patient education handout titled "Cold-Knife Conization of the Cervix (Cone Biopsy)" on page 1918 of Appendix G.

- See the sample patient consent form titled "Cervical Conization" on page 1920 of Appendix G.

BIBLIOGRAPHY

American College of Obstetricians and Gynecologists: Cervical cytology: evaluation and management of abnormalities, *Tech Bull* 183, August 1993.

Disaia P, Creasman W, editors: *Clinical gynecologic oncology,* ed 5, St Louis, 1997, Mosby.

Narducci F, Occelli B, Boman F, et al: Positive margins after conization and risk of persistent lesion, *Gynecol Oncol* 76(3):311, 2000.

Parsons L, Ulfelder H: *An atlas of pelvic operations,* Philadelphia, 1968, WB Saunders.

Pfenninger JL: Good things still come in old packages: cryosurgery vs LEEP. Loop electrosurgical excision procedure, *J Am Board Fam Pract* 12(5):416, 1999.

Ryan KJ, Berkowitz R, Barbieu RL, editors: *Kistner's gynecology principles & practice,* Chicago, 1990, YearBook Medical Publishers.

Schaefer G, Graber A, editors: *Complications in obstetrics and gynecologic surgery,* New York, 1981, Harper & Row.

Thompson D, Rock JA, editors: *Te Linde's operative gynecology,* ed 7, Philadelphia, 1992, JB Lippincott.

Turner RJ, Cohen RA, Volt RL, et al: Analysis of tissue margins of cone biopsy specimens obtained with "cold knife," CO_2 and Nd:YAG lasers and a radiofrequency surgical unit, *J Reprod Med* 37:607, 1992.

Wheeless CR, editor: *Atlas of pelvic surgery,* ed 2, Philadelphia, 1988, Lea & Febiger.

White CD, Cooper WL, Williams RR: Cervical intraepithelial neoplasia extending to the margins of resection in conization of the cervix, *J Reprod Med* 36(9):635, 1991.

CHAPTER 136

Cervical Polyps

Edward J. Mayeaux

Cervical polyps are pedunculated tumors that usually arise from the endocervical canal mucosa (endocervical polyps) or, rarely, that originate from the ectocervical epithelium (ectocervical polyps). They are often single but may be multiple, and they are usually bright red and have a rather fragile, spongy structure. Polyps can also originate from the endometrium (endometrial polyp), then appear in the cervical os (Figs. 136-1 to 136-4).

Vascular congestion and edema are frequently present. There may be ulceration at the tip of the polyp. Many endocervical polyps show extensive squamous metaplasia, which may mimic dysplasia. Squamous cell dysplasia and cancer (also sarcomas) may originate in such a polyp, but they are rare. If a polyp is discovered, the polyp should be removed and sent for pathologic study.

EPIDEMIOLOGY

Cervical polyps are common and are found in approximately 4% of all gynecologic patients. They are most commonly seen in perimenopausal and multigravid women between ages 30 and 50. Cervical polyps are usually endocervical and are almost always benign. The cause of most polyps is unknown, but they may result from inflammation, trauma, or pregnancy. Postmenopausal women with cervical polyps have higher incidence of coexisting endometrial polyps, and hormone replacement does not affect this association. Patients on Tamoxifen therapy have a very high association of cervical polyps with endometrial polyps and may need evaluation with a dilation and curettage (D & C). Malignant degeneration of polyps is rare.

SYMPTOMS/PHYSICAL FINDINGS

Polyps may vary in size from extremely small (a few millimeters) to large (larger than 4 cm). Polyps are most commonly asymptomatic and are usually found during the annual gynecologic pelvic examination. The pedicle can become so elongated that the polyp may protrude from the vaginal orifice. Large polyps can cause some cervical dilatation. There may be a vaginal discharge associated with cervical polyps if the polyp becomes infected.

Ulceration of the tip and vascular congestion often lead to postcoital or dysfunctional uterine bleeding. Larger polyps may bleed periodically, producing intermenstrual spotting and postcoital bleeding. Straining efforts, as in defecation, also may cause slight bleeding. Symptoms may be exactly the same as in the early stages of cervical cancer.

The differential diagnosis of cervical polyps is shown in Box 136-1. Since an association exists between cervical polyps and endometrial polyps, some authors consider performing a D & C with all cervical polyp removals. However, most physicians simply perform a polypectomy in the office if the patient is otherwise asymptomatic.

INDICATIONS

Removal of the polyp(s) is usually indicated, since it may cause irritation and bleeding. It is also necessary to rule out a neoplastic process. Be sure to identify the location of the base of the polyp to exclude the possibility of an endometrial polyp. Endometrial polyps may have more extensive blood supplies and require more extensive postremoval workup.

CONTRAINDICATIONS

- Uncooperative patient
- Bleeding dyscrasia

EQUIPMENT

- Vaginal speculum
- Nonsterile gloves

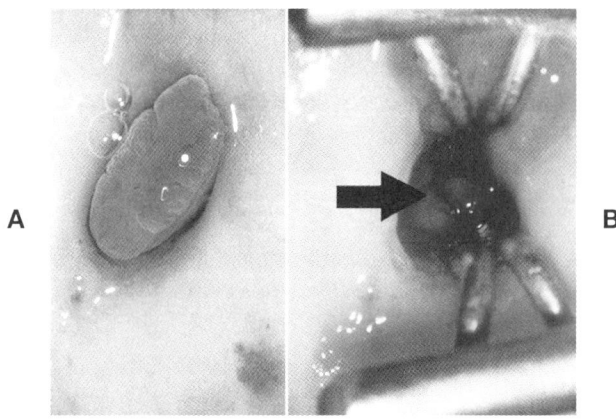

Fig. 136-1
A, Endocervical polyp. **B,** Identifying the base of the polyp *(arrow)* with an endocervical speculum. (Courtesy Duane Townsend, MD.)

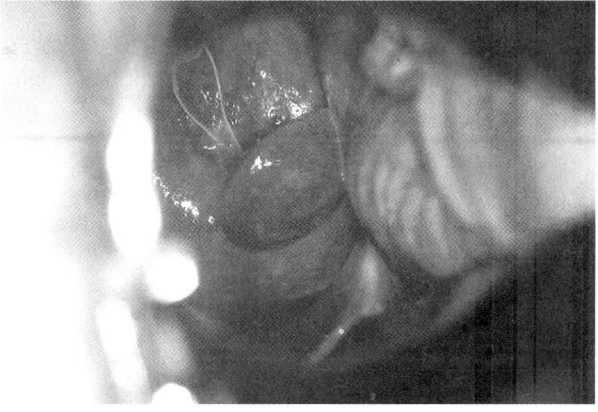

Fig. 136-2
Ectocervical polyp. Stalk is attached to the ectocervix. Note the IUD strings. (Courtesy The National Procedures Institute, Midland, Mich.)

- Topical anesthesia (lidocaine jelly or benzocaine solution) may be used but is not usually needed
- Ring forceps or cervical biopsy forceps
- Kogan's endocervical speculum *(optional)*
- Pathology container
- Silver nitrate sticks
- Colposcope *(optional)*
- Endocervical (Kevorkian) curette

TECHNIQUE

1. Insert the speculum and obtain a Pap smear if not recently done.
2. Identify the base of the polyp to exclude the possibility of an endometrial polyp. This can usually be accompanied with gentle manipulation of the cervix and the cervical os with a cotton-tipped applicator or ring forceps. If the pedicle extends deeper than can be

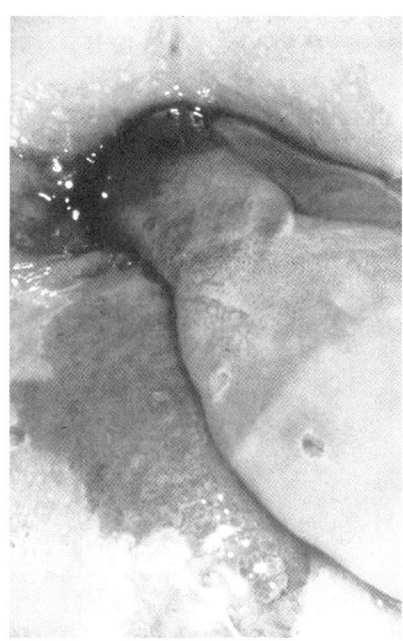

Fig. 136-3
Dysplastic endometrial polyp. Stalk originates in endometrial cavity. (Courtesy of Duane Townsend, MD.)

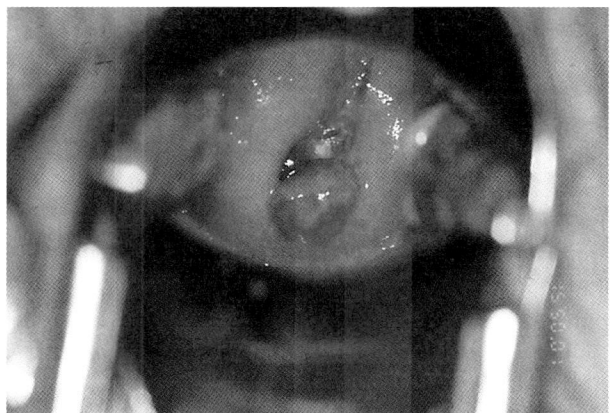

Fig. 136-4
Apparent cervical polyp, which is really a large nabothian cyst. (Courtesy The National Procedures Institute, Midland, Mich.)

BOX 136-1
Differential Diagnosis of Cervical Lesions

Cervical polyp
Condyloma
Endometrial polyp
Prolapsed myoma
Retained products of conception
Squamous papilloma
Sarcoma
Cervical malignancy

easily visualized, a Kogan's endocervical speculum or colposcopic magnification are often helpful.

3. Once it is determined that the polyp is cervical in origin, it may be gently grasped with ring forceps and twisted until it falls off. This may cause slight discomfort. Another common method of removal is to use the cervical biopsy forceps, which is placed at the attachment of the stalk and clipped off. The base of the polyp is then scraped with an endocervical (Kevorkian) curette. Alternatively, a small polyp may just be scraped off in its entirety with a sharp curette. Magnification with the use of a colposcope greatly aids in removal.

4. Bleeding is usually self limited but can be controlled with pressure, silver nitrate, Monsel's solution, or cautery. Silver nitrate is more caustic and is most frequently used because it not only stops the bleeding, but also destroys any residual remnant of the polyp.

5. If multiple polyps are present, it is best to curette the canal thoroughly. It may also be prudent to perform a D & C, especially if the patient is postmenopausal or has had irregular bleeding or is on Tamoxifen therapy.

6. Submit the polyps for pathologic examination.

Editor's note: My preferred method is to examine the polyp with a colposcope, identify the base, then remove it with cervical biopsy forceps. The base of the stalk is then curetted vigorously, followed by curettement of the entire canal. This material is sent in a separate container to pathology. The base is then cauterized with silver nitrate. Recurrence is rare.

COMPLICATIONS

- Bleeding or spotting
- Pain
- Recurrence

ALTERNATIVE PROCEDURES

Since most polyps are benign, they are often just observed on routine examinations. However, there is no sure way of knowing the true nature unless they are removed and examined histologically. Polyps may also be removed by curettage during D & C or with hysteroscopic wire or snare removal. During pregnancy, the cervix is highly vascularized. If the polyps are stable and appear benign, they should just be observed during the pregnancy and removed only if they are causing bleeding. Polyps can also be excised by electrocautery and loop electrosurgical excision procedure. In the case of large polyps, an outpatient surgical suite should be considered. Endometrial polyps are often best removed during a hysteroscopic examination. They should be suspected when a stalk is still visible inside the os after removal of the polyp itself.

POSTPROCEDURE PATIENT EDUCATION

Instruct the patient to avoid sexual intercourse, douching, and tampon usage for a week. If active bleeding occurs, the patient should be seen immediately. Reevaluate the patient in 6 to 8 weeks.

After that, the cervix should be checked at the patient's routine gynecologic visits. Since polyps are almost always benign, usually no further treatment is needed.

CPT/BILLING CODES

There is no separate CPT code for cervical polyp removal.

57500	Cervix uteri biopsy
57505	Endocervical curettage
58100	Endometrial sampling (biopsy) with or without endocervical sampling (biopsy), without cervical dilation, any method.

ICD-9-CM DIAGNOSTIC CODES

622.7	Polyp of cervix
621.0	Endometrial polyp
219.0	Benign neoplasm of the cervix
078.11	Condyloma acuminatum

BIBLIOGRAPHY

Abramovici H, Bornstein J, Pascal B: Ambulatory removal of cervical polyps under colposcopy, *Int J Gynaecol Obstet* 22(1):47, 1984.

Coeman D, Van Belle Y, Vanderick G, et al: Hysteroscopic findings in patients with a cervical polyp, *Am J Obstet Gynecol* 169(6):1563, 1993.

David A, Mettler L, Semm K: The cervical polyp: a new diagnostic and therapeutic approach with CO_2 hysteroscopy, *Am J Obstet Gynecol* 130(6):662, 1978.

Golan A, Ber A, Wolman I, David MP: Cervical polyp: evaluation of current treatment, *Gynecol Obstet Invest* 37(1):56, 1994.

Goudas VT, Session DR: Hysteroscopic cervical polypectomy with a polyp snare, *J Am Assoc Gynecol Laparosc* 6(2):195, 1999.

Neri A, Kaplan B, Rabinerson D, et al: Cervical polyp in the menopause and the need for fractional dilatation and curettage, *Eur J Obstet Gynecol Reprod Biol* 62(1):53, 1995.

CHAPTER 137

Cervical Stenosis and Cervical Dilation

Kathleen T. Dor
John L. Pfenninger

Cervical stenosis is a stricture of the cervix that most commonly occurs at the internal os. Cervical stenosis can be either congenital or, more commonly, acquired. Acquired causes include postoperative scarring (from cone biopsy, cautery, or cryotherapy of the cervix), cancer (endometrial or endocervical), radiation complications, infections, or atrophy. In acquired cases the external os is most frequently affected (Fig. 137-1).

Narrowing of the cervical canal can impede menstrual flow, causing intrauterine pressure at the time of menses. Premenopausal women with cervical stenosis can have pelvic pain, dysmenorrhea, amenorrhea, infertility, or abnormal bleeding. In some cases retrograde menstrual flow may occur, causing endometriosis. Women may have a soft, slightly tender midpelvic mass as a result of hematometra. Postmenopausal women may have pyometra, which is highly suspicious for endometrial carcinoma. Postmenopausal women with pyometra usually do not require antibiotics.

Cervical stenosis is diagnosed by the inability to pass a 2-mm dilator into the uterus. Ultrasonography can assess canal diameter while evaluating the patient for hematometra and a pyometra, but this is much more expensive. Some physicians differentiate an anatomic stenosis (less than 2-mm canal) with a functional stenosis (the canal may be larger than 2 mm, but the patient is still symptomatic).

CERVICAL DILATION

Treatment of cervical stenosis consists of dilation by using either progressive metal or "plastic" dilators or osmotic tents. Laminaria tents are made from the stems of seaweed, usually *Laminaria japonica,* that is dried and made into sticks. Synthetic self-expanding cervical dilators (Dilateria, Lamicel) that resemble laminaria tents can also be used. Once the tents are placed into the endocervical canal, they rehydrate and expand, thereby allowing dilation of the cervical canal (Figs. 137-2 and 137-3). Laminaria tents should not be used if pyometra is present or infection is suspected. The os and canal must be patent enough to admit the tents, which are available in different diameters. Some mechanical dilation may be

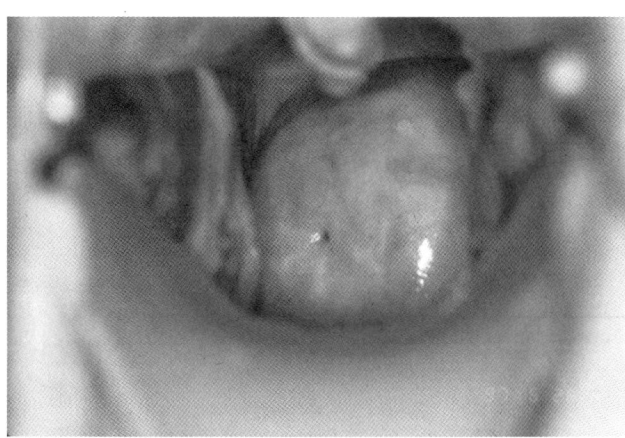

Fig. 137-1
External os stenosis after loop electrosurgical excision procedure.

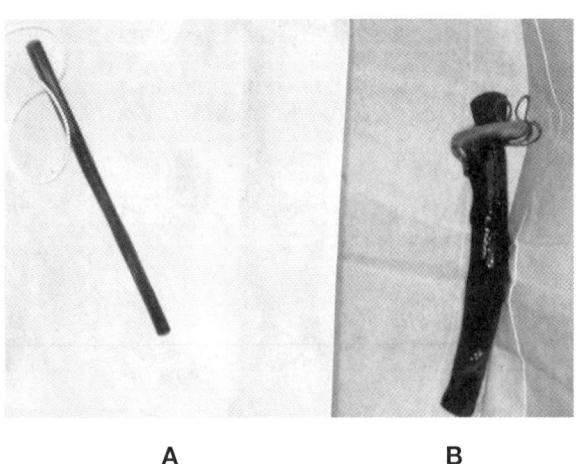

A   B

Fig. 137-2
A, Laminaria before insertion. **B,** Swollen laminaria after removal.

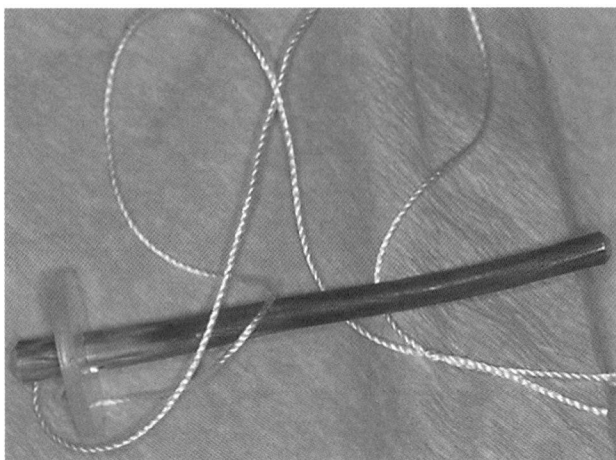

Fig. 137-3
Close-up of laminaria in Fig. 137-2, *A*.

necessary first to allow their placement. Other options for the treatment of external os stenosis are the use of the carbon dioxide laser or a small radiofrequency loop excision. The latter two methods can remove a stricture that is readily visible externally.

The majority of dilations can be performed in the office. For those extremely anxious patients or those in whom pain cannot be controlled easily, the procedure may need to be performed in the operating room.

INDICATIONS

- Symptomatic stenosis (e.g., dysmenorrhea)
- Inability to obtain adequate pap smears
- For IUD insertion
- To perform an indicated endocervical curettage or dilation and curettage (D & C)
- To perform medical abortion
- If needed for hysterosalpingogram
- Before hysteroscopy
- Before endometrial ablation techniques
- To perform an endometrial biopsy

CONTRAINDICATIONS

- Pregnancy
- Pelvic inflammatory disease; vaginal or cervical infections (treat before dilation)
- Laminaria tents not for use in the case of pyometra

EQUIPMENT

- Table that allows the patient to be placed in the lithotomy position

- Needle extender or long spinal needle to provide local anesthesia, if needed (see Chapter 151, Loop Electrosurgical Excision Procedure [LEEP] for Treating Cervical Intraepithelial Neoplasia)
- 5 ml 2% xylocaine with epinephrine
- Adequate light source
- Large vaginal speculum
- Nonsterile gloves; use sterile gloves if a D & C is to be performed
- Ring forceps
- Uterine sound (malleable, formed to the position of the uterus)
- Metal cervical dilators (1 to 6 mm) and/or osmotic tent (various sizes) (see Fig. 144-1)
- OS Finder or os locator *(optional)*
- Cervical single-toothed tenaculum
- Paracervical block kit with 10 ml 1% lidocaine in a 10-ml syringe with a 6-inch, 20-gauge needle; may be helpful if dilation of more than 4 to 6 mm is done (see Chapter 174, Paracervical Block)
- 4 × 4–inch gauze; Betadine solution

PREPROCEDURE PATIENT PREPARATION

- Obtain consent from the patient. (See the sample patient consent form titled "Cervical Stenosis and Cervical Dilation" on page 1921 of Appendix G.)
- Generally 800 mg of ibuprofen 1 hour before the procedure is all that is required. Occasionally, Diazepam 10 mg by mouth is helpful.
- If further sedation is to be given, the patient should not eat or drink 6 hours before the procedure (see Chapter 2, Conscious Sedation). This may be necessary if curettage is to be performed. Consider anesthesia with 2 mg IV midazolam and 50 mg meperidine with 25 mg promethazine IM. In this case, the patient should also be monitored with pulse oximetry.

TECHNIQUE

1. Place the patient in a lithotomy position.
2. Perform a pelvic examination to evaluate the uterine size and position.
3. Prepare the cervix and vagina with Betadine (or diluted chlorhexidine if the patient is allergic to Betadine).
4. Try to cannulate the cervical canal with a small silver probe, the 2-mm dilator, or the OS Finder or os locator. If the patient becomes uncomfortable, provide anesthetic. Administer 5 ml of a local anesthetic *submucosally* at the 12, 3, 6, and 9 o'clock positions on the cervix (see Chapter 151, Loop Electrosurgical Excision Procedure for Treating CIN), or use a

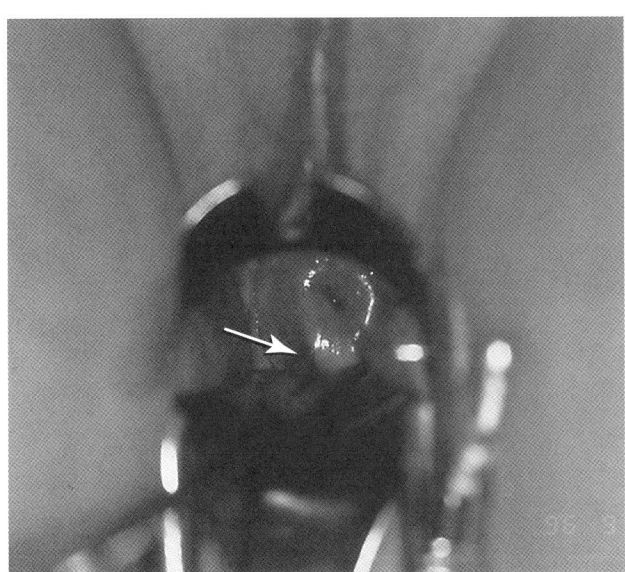

Fig. 137-4
Single-toothed tenaculum placed posteriorly *(arrow)* on the cervix.

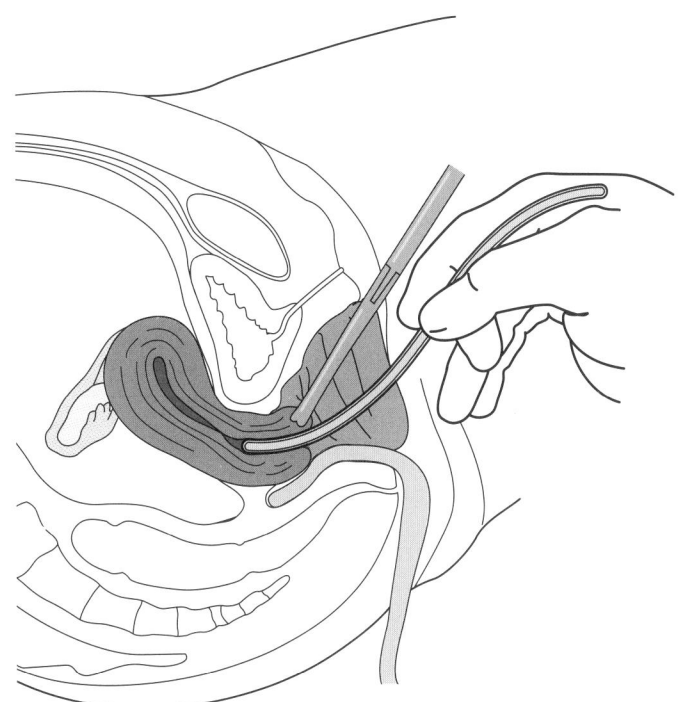

Fig. 137-5
Cervical dilation using a Hegar dilator. During the procedure, the fourth and fifth fingers rest against the perineal area in order to prevent uncontrolled movements of the dilator, which can lead to uterine perforation. A weighted speculum is in the posterior vagina. The tenaculum is applied to the anterior lip of the cervix. (Adapted from Cunningham FG et al, editors: *Williams obstetrics,* ed 20, Stamford, Conn, 1997, Appleton & Lange.)

paracervical block with 5 ml lidocaine at the 4 and 8 o'clock positions (see Chapter 174, Paracervical Block). Aspirate for blood before injecting to ensure that the needle is not in a blood vessel. The use of a local injection (not a paracervical technique) really makes this procedure easier on the patient and easier for the physician to accomplish good pain control.

5. If the cervix is too mobile, place a tenaculum at the 12 o'clock or 6 o'clock position and use it to apply traction on the cervix while dilating it (Fig. 137-4). Use progressively larger dilators.

6. Once the external os is entered, the most difficult part of the procedure is passing through the internal os. If the sound-dilator does not pass readily, apply the tenaculum if not already done. The OS Finder or os locator generally enters the lumen without creating a false passage. It often takes firm, steady pressure on metal dilators to penetrate the internal os. (This step causes significant anxiety in the physician!) As the tenaculum is pulled outward, the dilator is pushed forward until a "give" is felt. Insert the dilator just through the internal os and gradually insert the larger dilators until the uterine sound can be admitted.

7. Bend the uterine sound to conform to the shape of the uterus (anteverted, midline, or retroverted), insert, and determine the size of the uterine cavity. Up to 10 cm is normal. The sound should pass easily before resistance is felt. Unless the clinician examination suggests an enlarged uterus, this should be no more than 10 cm (possibly 12 cm). If the sound goes beyond this, suspect perforation and stop all further attempts.

8. Dilation to 4 to 6 mm is sufficient for most procedures and usually readily accomplished in the office. If a curettage or surgical abortion is to be performed, dilate the cervix to 11 mm, if possible, using progressively larger Hegar dilators. These patients probably require more aggressive sedation. When inserting the dilator, rest your fourth and fifth fingers on the perineum and buttocks to prevent uncontrolled movements of the dilator (Fig. 137-5).

9. Perform the procedure indicated.

10. If endometrial or endocervical carcinoma is being ruled out, curette the endocervix with a Kevorkian curette, using firm motions from the internal os to the external os around the entire endocervix (360 degrees twice). Collect the tissue on a Telfa pad or on a 2 × 2–inch piece of lens paper (see Chapter 139, Colposcopic Examination). To collect uterine fragments from an endometrial curette, place a Telfa pad in the posterior vagina and use the sharp curette to scrape the walls of the uterus. Both Telfa pads should be submitted in separate jars of formalin and

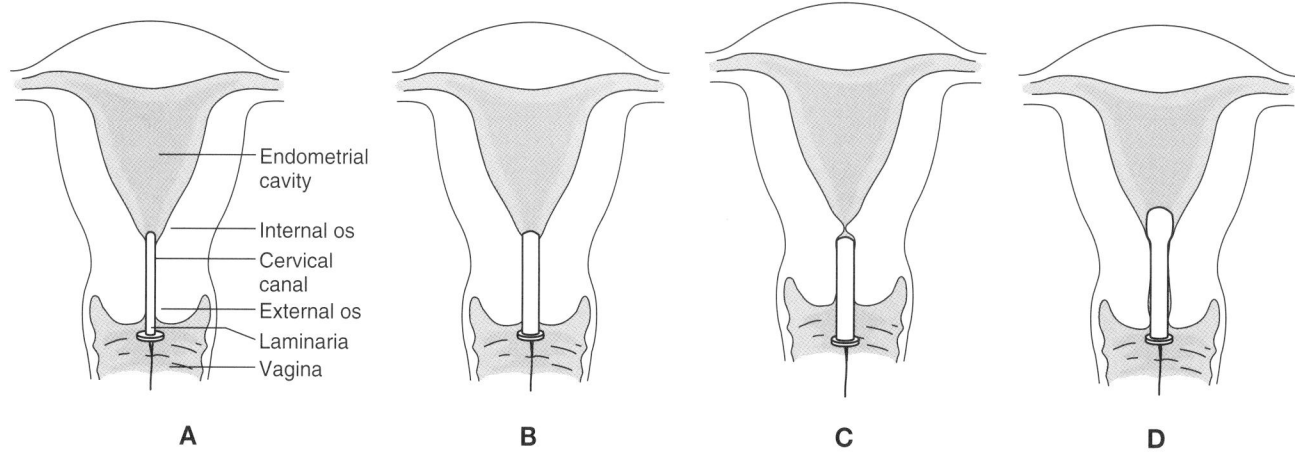

Fig. 137-6

Insertion of a laminaria tent. **A,** The laminaria tent immediately after placement. Note that the upper end is just through the internal os. It is difficult to determine this "optimal" position, and it is not possible to obtain it with internal os stenosis. **B,** The laminaria tent 24 hours later. **C,** The laminaria tent not placed far enough to dilate the internal os. **D,** The laminaria tent inserted too far, making it difficult to remove. (Adapted from Cunningham FG et al, editors: *Williams obstetrics,* ed 20, Stamford, Conn, 1997, Appleton & Lange.)

sent to pathology. (See Chapter 144, Dilation and Curettage, and Chapter 146, Endometrial Biopsy.)

LAMINARIA TENT PLACEMENT

1. In order for laminaria tents to be used, the external os must be patent. Subsequently, they are used either for internal os stenosis or for a gradual dilation of the canal for larger procedures. They come in various sizes, and more than one may be inserted for greater dilation.
2. Prepare the patient and cervix as described above.
3. Sound the endocervix. Do not go much beyond the internal os.
4. Grasp the cervix with the tenaculum if necessary and use it to apply traction on the cervix (Fig. 137-4).
5. Hold the string end of the laminaria with ring forceps and insert it into the os, ensuring that the laminaria tent does not extend into the uterine cavity. Use the largest laminaria tent that will fit into the os. Sometimes, however, this may be quite small. If unable to insert the laminaria tent, you may have to dilate the os further before its insertion (Figs. 137-6 and 137-7).
6. Laminaria are quite long and usually protrude out of the cervix for several centimeters.
7. Cover the cervix with inserted laminaria with a sterile 4 × 4–inch gauze that has been dipped into *dilute*

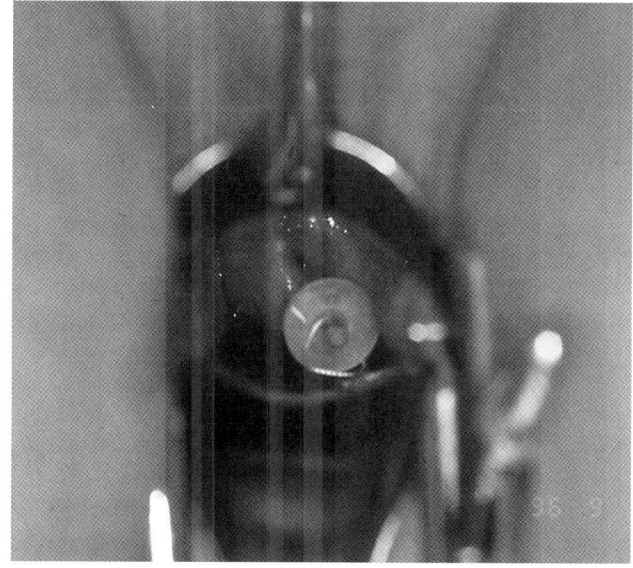

Fig. 137-7

Laminaria tent has been inserted. It is difficult to appreciate that the tent actually protrudes 2 cm outside the cervix.

Betadine solution, and tuck the edges in the fornices. Then place several dry 4 × 4–inch gauzes over the first one to hold the laminaria tent in place (Fig. 137-8).
8. Remove the speculum while holding the gauze in place with the ring forceps.
9. To prevent infection, the laminaria tent should be removed within 24 hours by grasping it with a ring

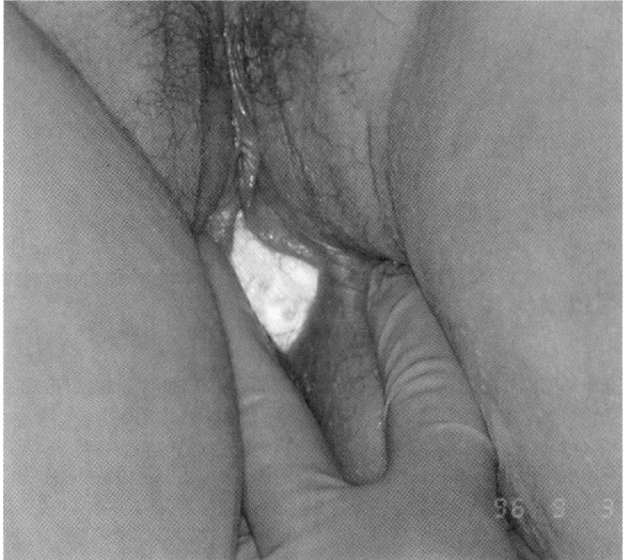

Fig. 137-8
Laminaria held in place with 4 × 4–inch gauze inserted in the vagina. Patients tolerate this surprisingly well.

forceps, rotating it 360 degrees, and pulling it out. Lesser procedures may only require 8 to 12 hours. Often the laminaria is inserted at the end of the day and removed the next morning; alternatively, the patient is the first one seen during the morning, with the laminaria removed when she is seen again as the last patient of the day. It may be necessary to replace the initial smaller laminaria with a larger one if the dilation is not adequate on removal.

10. Dilation can cause significant cramping, and ibuprofen 600 mg every 6 hours is advised.

COMPLICATIONS

- Pain
- Hemorrhage
- Infection (especially if the laminaria tent is left in over 24 hours)
- Perforated uterus
- Anaphylaxis from the laminaria tent (rare)
- Inability to dilate the os
- Synthetic tents, which can break or separate on removal, making it difficult to retrieve all of it

Many physicians are fearful of a perforation, but it is generally uneventful unless it is not recognized and the dilator is advanced too far or unless other procedures are attempted outside the uterine cavity. If suspected, no further instrumentation should be done. Explain to the patient what is suspected. After 30 minutes of observation she can go home if vital signs are stable and there is no pain. She should report any fever, pain, or excessive bleeding. A follow-up visit or phone call within 24 hours is advisable. Repeat attempts at cannulation or dilation can be done after 6 to 8 weeks.

POSTPROCEDURE PATIENT EDUCATION (also see Chapter 144, Dilation and Curettage)

- If a laminaria tent is placed, the patient should be instructed to return within 24 hours for removal of the laminaria tent. Between 8 and 12 hours is generally adequate.
- The patient should not engage in sexual intercourse while the laminaria is in place. If curettage is performed, sexual intercourse should be avoided for 2 weeks.
- If dilation was performed for cervical stenosis, the patient should be instructed to return in 4 to 6 weeks for repeat examination and possible repeat dilation.
- The patient should return or call for fever, abdominal or pelvic pain, purulent vaginal discharge, or bleeding.
- In postmenopausal women not on estrogen replacement, or those with low estrogen states (e.g., Depo-Provera or Norplant users), estrogen cream helps maintain patency of the os. This is especially important if dilation was done for postsurgical (conization) scarring complications.

CONCLUSION

Cervical dilation may need to be repeated several times on a monthly basis if performed for cervical stenosis. Pregnancy and vaginal delivery may actually lead to a more lasting cure. As long as the patient is menstruating and is asymptomatic, and a Pap smear can be obtained, then physician intervention is not needed.

SUPPLIERS

Laminaria, mechanical dilators
McKesson HBOC Inc.
12555 West Jefferson Blvd., Suite 101
Los Angeles, CA 90066
Phone: 1-800-523-9626

Laminaria and lamicel, all mechanical dilators, os locator, canal finder
MedGyn
328 N. Eisenhower Lane
Lombard, IL 60148
Phone: 1-800-451-9667
Website: www.medgyn.com

Mechanical dilators and os locators

Cooper Surgical
15 Forest Parkway
Shelton, CT 06484
Phone: 1-800-645-3760
Website: www.coopersurgical.com

CPT/BILLING CODES

57800	Dilatation of cervical canal, instrumental
59200	Cervical dilation, laminaria
58120	Dilation and curettage, diagnostic and/or therapeutic (nonobstetrical)
57505	Endocervical curettage

ICD-9-CM DIAGNOSTIC CODE

622.4	Cervical stenosis

ADDITIONAL RESOURCES

• See the sample patient education handout titled "Cervical Stenosis and Cervical Dilation" on page 1921 of Appendix G.

• See the sample patient consent form titled "Cervical Stenosis and Cervical Dilation" on page 1923 of Appendix G.

BIBLIOGRAPHY

Clarke-Pearson DL, Dawood MY, editors: *Green's gynecology: essentials of clinical practice,* ed 4, Boston, 1990, Little, Brown.

Cunningham FG et al, editors: *Williams obstetrics,* ed 20, Stamford, Conn, 1997, Appleton & Lange.

DeCherney AH, Pernoll ML, editors: *Current obstetric and gynecologic diagnosis and treatment,* ed 8, Norwalk, Conn, 1994, Appleton & Lange.

Mishell DR, Stenchever MA, Droegemueller W, Herbst AL, editors: *Comprehensive gynecology,* ed 3, St Louis, 1997, Mosby.

Ryan KJ, Berkowitz RS, Barbieri RL, Dunaif A, editors: *Kistner's gynecology & women's health,* ed 7, St Louis, 1999, Mosby.

CHAPTER 138

Cervicography

Richard C. Cherkis

The cervicography system is a universally unified, organized, quality-controlled screening procedure for the detection of cervical cancer and precancerous conditions. It combines colposcopic principles with a noninvasive photographic technique that permits quality-controlled expert evaluation of normal and abnormal cervical findings, and it provides permanent and objective documentation of these findings on a 35-mm slide. The concept of cervicography is similar to that of cytology.

The cervicography system lends itself to use in any women's cancer–screening setting, including the private office, the hospital, the family planning clinic, and the mass screening drive. It can be used in conjunction with the Pap smear; it is significantly more sensitive than the Pap smear; it has a high negative predictive value; and, when combined with the Pap smear, it is one of the best methods of screening for cervical cancer.

A cerviscope cervical camera (Fig. 138-1) is used to take photographs of the cervix. The cerviscope stan-dardizes color, depth of field, lighting, and focal length; thus it provides images that enable uniformity in evaluation. The handheld cerviscope is focused on the cervix by moving the instrument back and forth (Fig. 138-2). When the cervix is in focus, a picture is taken. The film is sent to National Testing Laboratories, where it is developed into photographic slides (cervigrams). These are projected onto a screen that is at least 6 feet wide, allowing the evaluator to view an image of the cervix with a magnification and resolution comparable to that of colposcopy (Fig. 138-3). Only certified evaluators—gynecologists specializing in colposcopy who have passed stringent written and oral examinations given by the National Testing Laboratories—are used to interpret the films.

Cervicography findings are divided into four categories: negative, atypical, positive, and technically defective (Fig. 138-4). A print of the cervigram with the expert evaluation is returned to the clinician and can be entered into the patient's record. It also provides an excellent medium for patient education.

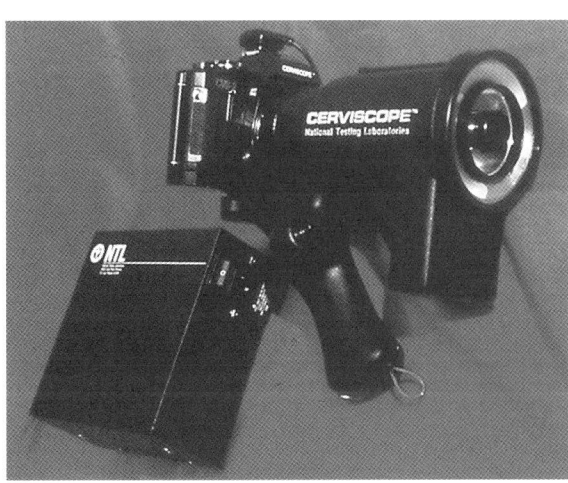

Fig. 138-1
Cerviscope.

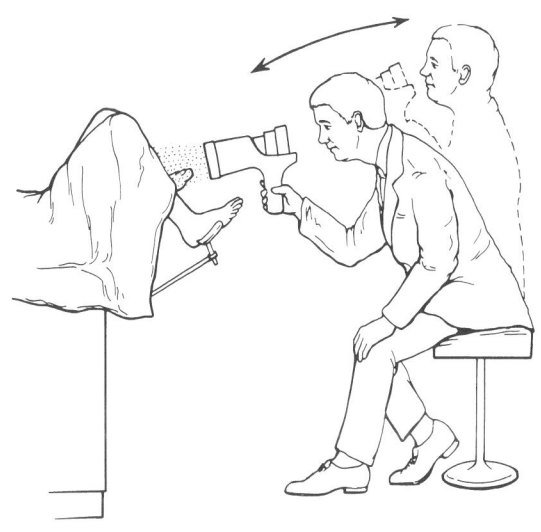

Fig. 138-2
Focusing of the cerviscope.

The cerviscope, the evaluation method, and the terminology used in the evaluation process are standardized worldwide by National Testing Laboratories. Quality control is strictly maintained in every aspect of the cervicography system.

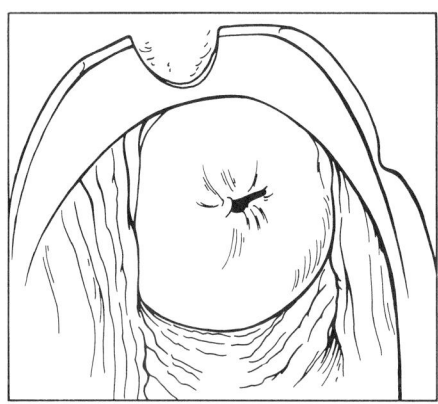

Fig. 138-3
Cervigram is obtained by focusing through the vaginal speculum.

RATIONALE FOR CERVICOGRAPHY SCREENING

- The Pap smear has a significant false-negative rate.
- The specificity of the Pap smear is unclear.
- Colposcopic screening is not always practical because of the time, equipment, and expertise necessary.
- Cervicography identifies high- and low-risk patients for development of cervical neoplasia.
- Cervicography adds an important quality-control dimension to screening.
- A print of the cervigram is invaluable in minimizing patients' health concerns and sexual apprehensions when an abnormality exists.

INDICATIONS

- Routine screening in conjunction with the Pap smear
- Documentation of ectocervical findings
- Documentation of cervical findings before ablative procedures
- Evaluation of the patient with an atypical Pap smear
- Evaluation of low-grade abnormalities
- Evaluation of the patient with suspicious or positive Pap smears where colposcopy is not available

---

CERVIGRAM REPORT

NEGATIVE: Repeat the cervigram picture and Pap smear on a routine basis.
1. _____ Components of the transformation zone are visible.
2. _____ Components of the transformation zone are not visible.

ATYPICAL: A cervigram picture and Pap smear are recommended in _____ 6 months or _____ 12 months.
1. _____ A lesion of doubtful significance is visible inside the transformation zone.
2. _____ A lesion of doubtful significance is visible outside the transformation zone.

POSITIVE: Colposcopy is recommended.
0. _____ Probable normal variant appearance warrants colposcopy to exclude significant disease
1. _____ Compatible with a low-grade lesion: _____ A _____ B
2. _____ Compatible with a high-grade lesion
3. _____ Compatible with cancer

Morphology:
_____ Acetowhite epithelium   _____ Erosion or ulceration
_____ Punctation   _____ Discoloration
_____ Mosaic   _____ Irregular surface contour
_____ Atypical vessels

TECHNICALLY DEFECTIVE: Please retake cervigram picture.
1. _____ View of cervix obscured by:
        ___ mucus ___ blood ___ position of cervix ___ other: _____
2. _____ Insufficient acetic acid reaction when reaction is anticipated
3. _____ Other problems: ___ Out of focus ___ Overexposed ___ Underexposed

Fig. 138-4
Elements of the cervigram report.

CONTRAINDICATIONS

Although cervigrams can be obtained in any situation, they will have little value (or are more likely to miss) cervical dysplasia if there is significant bleeding or marked inflammation. The cervix must also have estrogen stimulation for the acetic acid to stain abnormalities. Thus estrogen replacement may at least temporarily be needed after menopause, with progesterone-only contraception, and after delivery if breastfeeding.

EQUIPMENT

- Cerviscope, power supply, and patient log sheet
- Speculum
- 5% acetic acid
- Large cotton swabs

TECHNIQUE

1. Insert the speculum for adequate visualization of cervix. Obtain a Pap smear if necessary.
2. Apply the 5% acetic acid. This step requires 15 seconds of swabbing or dabbing.
3. View the cervix with a cerviscope camera (Fig. 138-2). Do *not* take a cervigram now. (There would be a 50% false-negative rate.) In this step, look for obstructions of the view: mucus, blood, prolapse of vaginal walls, retroverted or anteverted cervix, and pubic hair across the opening of the speculum. This step is critical because it also allows time for the first application of acetic acid to take effect.
4. Apply a second application of 5% acetic acid. This step requires 15 seconds of swabbing or dabbing.
5. View the cervix with the cerviscope and eliminate any obstructions described in Step 3. Look for acetic acid pooling that obstructs the view of the posterior lip of the cervix. If present, remove any excess with a swab.
6. Take two pictures (cervigrams) of the cervix now. This should be done within 30 seconds of the second application of acetic acid. If one or both of the cervigrams is not taken within the 30 seconds, reapply the acetic acid before taking another cervigram(s).
7. Record the required patient information on the patient log sheet.
8. Send the film to National Testing Laboratories (NTL).

SUPPLIERS

The clinician who decides to use cervicography can obtain instructional videotapes and appropriate information from the following:

National Testing Laboratories
400 Biltmore Drive, Suite 407
Fenton, MO 63026
Phone: 1-800-842-7135
Website: www.ntlworldwide.com

National Testing Laboratories schedules a full day in-service to explain the various aspects of the system, to train the appropriate office personnel, and to ascertain that the individuals taking the cervigrams are doing the procedure properly. National Testing Laboratories furnishes the film (as well as the film developing and processing), evaluations, appropriate forms, mailers, and patient educational pamphlets.

NTL offers three choices for setting up the Cervicography system, based on the individual practitioner's needs and capabilities:

1. The Cerviscope equipment can be purchased and used apart from NTL. The clinician would then be responsible for purchasing and developing the film, evaluating the slides, maintaining the computer system, and billing the patient. The cost of all necessary equipment and initial supply of film is $3500.
2. The equipment can be purchased, but NTL will provide all supplies and film, develop the film, evaluate the slides, and maintain the computer system. The cost is the same as in Option 1, but the office is charged $25 per patient for NTL's services.
3. NTL places the equipment on consignment in the office and provides the services described in Option 2. In addition, NTL bills the patients $45 for the service, although this can be negotiated if the patient is unable to afford this price.

Cost

National Testing Laboratories' current fee to the healthcare provider for cervicography screening in the United States ($25) is comparable to the cost of a Pap smear. The patient cost from the healthcare provider is approximately $40 to $50. Cervicography costs may be covered by insurance. The cost of a cerviscope and related equipment is approximately $3500.

CPT/BILLING CODE

58999   Miscellaneous gynecologic procedure, Cervicography system

BIBLIOGRAPHY

August N: Cervicography for evaluating the "atypical" Papanicolaou smear, *J Reprod Med* 36:89, 1991.

Campion MJ, Reid R: Screening for gynecological cancer, *Obstet Gynecol Clin North Am* 17:695, 1990.

Eskridge C, Begneaud W, Landwehr C: Cervicography combined with repeat Papanicolaou test as triage for low-grade cytologic abnormalities, *Obstet Gynecol* 92:351, 1998.

Ferris D, Payne P: Cervicography: adjunctive cervical cancer screening by primary care clinicians, *J Fam Pract* 37:158, 1993.

Greenberg MD, Campion MJ, Rutlege LH: Cervicography as an adjunct to cytologic screening. In Wright VC, editor: *Obstetrics and gynecology clinics in North America,* vol 20, Philadelphia, 1993, WB Saunders.

Stafl A: Cervicography: a new method for cervical cancer detection, *Am J Obstet Gynecol* 139:815, 1981.

Stafl A: Cervicography in cervical cancer detection, *Postgrad Obstet Gynecol* 10(3):1, 1990.

Tawa K, Forsythe A, Cove JK, et al: A comparison of the Papanicolaou smear and cervigram: sensitivity, specificity, and cost analysis, *Obstet Gynecol* 71:229, 1988.

CHAPTER 139

Colposcopic Examination

Gary R. Newkirk

Colposcopy is nothing more than the observation of a cervix under magnification after it has been stained with acetic acid in order to identify the most abnormal areas for biopsy, so that the patient can be triaged to appropriate care.

Addressing the widespread human papillomavirus (HPV) and genital epithelial dysplasia epidemic requires mastery of colposcopy, cervical biopsy, and endocervical curettage (ECC). The most frequent indications for these procedures include evaluation of an abnormal Pap smear (see Chapter 152, Pap Smear and Related Techniques for Cervical Cancer Screening), visible cervical abnormalities, or evidence of clinical HPV infection. Current evidence suggests that the majority of cases of cervical dysplasia can be managed entirely in the outpatient setting. Successful colposcopy requires *strict compliance with established protocol* and the support of the pathologist, urologist, and gynecologist. Mechanisms for excellent documentation and rigorous follow-up are mandatory. Physicians who assimilate colposcopy skills into their practices will benefit from responding to a major public health problem and will enhance their patients' access to care.

The colposcope is essentially a stereoscopic (3× to 40×), portable operating microscope with a focal distance appropriate to examine the genitalia and cervix. The colposcopic examination serves to (1) identify normal landmarks, (2) identify abnormal areas in relation to these landmarks, (3) facilitate directed biopsy of abnormal areas for histologic diagnosis, and (4) rule out invasive cancer. Based on the findings, patients are triaged for observation, for outpatient procedures (e.g., cryotherapy, loop electrical excision procedure [LEEP]), inpatient intervention (e.g., cervical conization, whether laser or conventional), or definitive therapy for invasive carcinoma.

Colposcopic-directed biopsy provides histologic clarification of abnormal Pap smears; this is mandatory before definitive therapy. Premalignant and malignant cervical conditions produce colposcopically identifiable epithelial changes that are often characteristic and generally occur within the transformation zone, which can be examined carefully during the colposcopic examination. Ultimately, the pathologist is the one who provides the histologic diagnoses for abnormalities identified during the colposcopic examination. Therefore the major challenge for the colposcopist is to distinguish the normal from the abnormal and to sample the most abnormal appearing changes for histologic confirmation. The ECC is performed as part of the routine colposcopic examination (in nonpregnant patients) to confirm the absence of occult disease within the endocervical canal.

Colposcopy itself, without the benefit of histologic confirmation, is not considered a diagnostic tool. Even though colposcopically defined visual abnormalities correlate with cervical dysplasia or frank carcinoma, the ultimate diagnosis rests on the traditional histologic interpretation of submitted samples and not with the visual pattern recognition. Accordingly, diagnostic accuracy requires that the colposcopist perform *liberal* biopsy of the abnormal cervix.

In the past decade, major changes in our understanding of the epidemiology and science of cervical carcinoma have yielded efforts to develop a unified terminology to be used throughout the international scientific community. The International Federation of Cervical Pathology and Colposcopy (IFCPC) approved a basic colposcopic terminology at its Seventh World Congress in Rome in May 1990 (Box 139-1). These terms should be used to describe findings during the colposcopic examination.

COLPOSCOPIC FINDINGS

The prudent colposcopist must be completely familiar with the normal findings and the visual abnormalities that correlate with dysplasia and malignancy (Fig. 139-1; also see Fig. 152-1).

Normal Colposcopic Findings

Original Squamous Epithelium. This is a featureless, smooth, pink epithelium. There are no features suggest-

I. Normal colposcopic findings
   A. Original squamous epithelium
   B. Columnar epithelium
   C. Normal transformation zone
   D. Squamocolumnar junction
   E. Squamous metaplasia
II. Abnormal colposcopic findings
   A. Within the transformation zone
      1. Acetowhite epithelium (areas of white after application of acetic acid-vinegar)†
         (a) Flat
         (b) Micropapillary or microconvoluted
      2. Punctation (red dots)
      3. Mosaicism (linear, tilelike patterns)
      4. Leukoplakia (white change *before* application of vinegar)
      5. Iodine-negative epithelium (tissue that is *not* deeply stained by iodine [full-strength Lugol's solution])†
      6. Atypical vessels
   B. Outside the transformation zone (ectocervix, vagina)
      1. Acetowhite epithelium
         (a) Flat
         (b) Micropapillary or microconvoluted
      2. Punctation
      3. Mosaicism
      4. Leukoplakia
      5. Iodine-negative epithelium
      6. Atypical vessels
III. Colposcopically suspect invasive carcinoma
IV. Unsatisfactory colposcopy
   A. Squamocolumnar junction not visible
   B. Severe inflammation or severe atrophy
   C. Cervix not visible
   D. Entire lesion not seen (i.e., goes into canal)
   E. Most advanced lesion not biopsied (i.e., in canal)
V. Miscellaneous findings
   A. Nonacetowhite micropapillary surface (micropapillomatosis vaginalis)
   B. Exophytic condyloma
   C. Inflammation
   D. Atrophy
   E. Ulcer
   F. Other (polyp, hemorrhage, cysts, etc.)

Adapted from Stafl A, Wilbanks GD: *Obstet Gynecol* 77(2):313, 1991.
*See text for definitions.
†For the effects of acetic acid and iodine to be appreciated, the cervical and vaginal tissues **must** have estrogen stimulation.

ing columnar epithelium, such as gland openings or nabothian cysts. The epithelium was "always" squamous and was not transformed from columnar to squamous after birth.

Columnar Epithelium. This is a single layer of mucus-producing, tall epithelium that extends between the endometrium and the cervical squamous epithelium. Columnar epithelium appears irregular, with stromal papillae and clefts. With acetic acid application and magnification, columnar epithelium has a grapelike or "sea-anemone" appearance. It turns mildly acetowhite. Columnar epithelium is found in the endocervix, sur-

rounding the cervical os, and is generally visible on the ectocervix in the reproductive age group.

Transformation Zone (TZ). This is the geographic area between the original squamous epithelium and the columnar epithelium that is occupied by metaplastic epithelium in varying degrees of maturity. There is no way to define where the *original* transformation begins. The *active transformation zone* contains gland openings, nabothian cysts, and, typically, islands of columnar epithelium surrounded by metaplastic squamous epithelium. It is the area of most active metaplasia. The *active* transformation zone then extends from the squamocolumnar junction (SCJ) (see below) to the outermost visible gland. For all practical purposes, when the term "transformation zone" is used, it is generally referring to the "active" TZ, since that is where disease processes occur.

Squamous Metaplasia. Columnar epithelium on the ectocervix is transformed over time into mature squamous epithelium by undergoing squamous metaplasia. Squamous metaplasia typically occupies the TZ to varying degrees. At the SCJ, it appears as a "ghost white" film when acetic acid is applied.

Squamocolumnar Junction. Generally, this is a clinically visible line seen on the ectocervix or within the distal canal (e.g., postcryotherapy or postmenopausal age group) that demarcates endocervical tissue from squamous tissue or from squamous metaplastic tissue. Conceptually, the SCJ is comparable to the vermilion border around the mouth and the dentate or pectinate line in the rectum where the mucosa meets squamous epithelium.

Abnormal Colposcopic Findings

Atypical Transformation Zone. This is a TZ with findings suggesting cervical dysplasia or neoplasia

1. *Acetowhite.* Epithelium that transiently whitens following the application of acetic acid. Areas of acetowhite correlate with higher nuclear density. The white staining fades within minutes.
2. *Punctation.* A stippled appearance of capillaries viewed end-on; often found within acetowhite areas, where they appear as fine-to-coarse red dots.
3. *Mosaicism.* An abnormal change made up of small red blood vessels appearing in linear form, suggesting a confluence of tile or chicken-wire patterns. This is best viewed after staining with acetic acid under magnification.
4. *Leukoplakia (hyperkeratosis).* Typically an elevated, white plaque seen *before* the application of acetic acid. There is generally no change, or the area

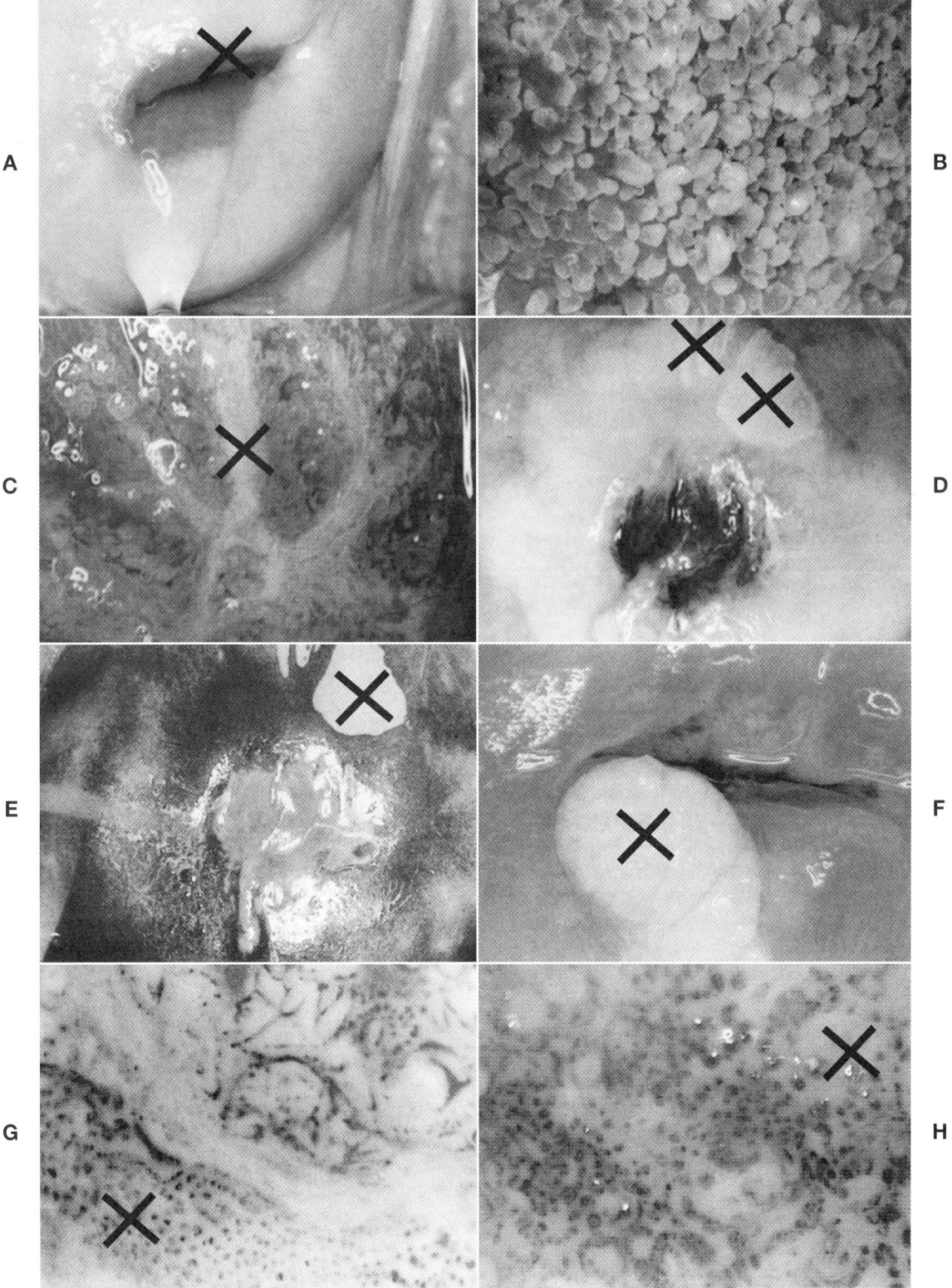

Fig. 139-1
Colposcopic findings. *Normal:* **A,** Squamocolumnar junction; **B,** Endocervical tissue (high magnification); **C,** Squamous metaplasia overlying endocervical tissue. *Abnormal:* **D,** Acetowhite areas from the 12 to 2 o'clock positions; **E,** Lugol's solution highlighting acetowhite area in **D** (nonstaining with Lugol's); **F,** Leukoplakia, abnormal white lesion before acetic acid; **G,** Punctation in lower left corner; **H,** Coarse punctation. *Continued*

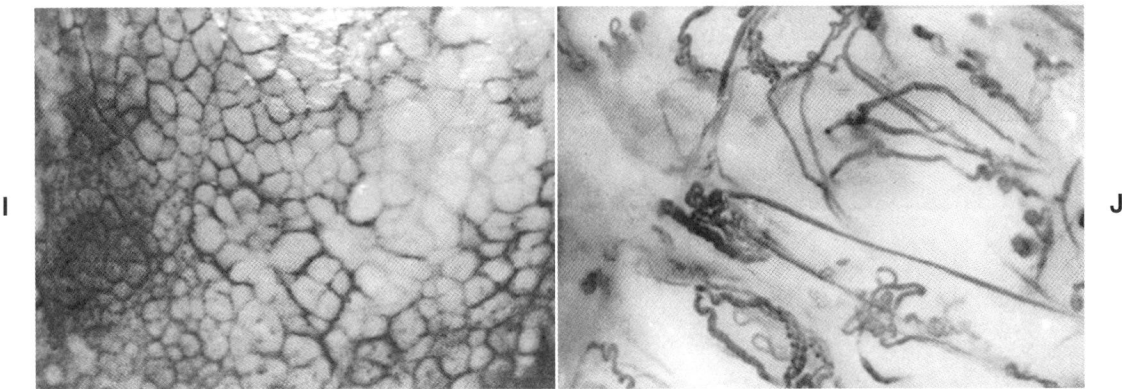

Fig. 139-1, cont'd
I, Mosaicism; **J,** Abnormal blood vessels. The *X* identifies findings noted. (From Cartier R, Cartier I: *Practical colposcopy,* Paris, 1993, Cartier Laboratoire.)

becomes more densely white, after application of acetic acid.

5. *Abnormal blood vessels.* Atypical, irregular true vessels with abrupt courses and patterns; often appear as commas, corkscrews, or spaghetti shapes. No definite pattern is recognized as there is with punctation or mosaicism.

Suspect Invasive Cancer. This is a complex pattern consisting of roughened, irregular cervical epithelium, typically with abundant abnormal vessel patterns and dense acetowhite change with a slightly yellowish hue. It may also appear as ulcerated, friable, necrotic tissue. There may be a bulk effect or tumorlike appearance.

Unsatisfactory Colposcopy

The entire SCJ or the limits of all lesions cannot be completely visualized. Proper examination can also be hampered if an active inflammatory process is present, if the patient is not estrogen primed (e.g., postmenopausal without replacement therapy, on progesterone-only types of contraception, lactation) or if heavy menses is present.

Other Colposcopic Findings

- Vaginocervicitis
- Traumatic erosion
- Atrophic epithelium
- Endocervical polyps
- Changes from diethylstilbestrol (DES)
- Abnormal pigmentation
- Nabothian cysts
- Vaginal, vulvar, perineal, perianal lesions

Guidelines regarding visual colposcopic findings help ensure sampling of the most advanced sites of cervical dysplasia. *The classic hallmark of cervical dysplasia in-cludes the change that dysplastic epithelium undergoes following the application of 3% to 5% acetic acid (vinegar) or Lugol's (concentrated iodine) solution.* Following the application of acetic acid, *dysplastic epithelium* typically turns whiter than the surrounding normal epithelium *(acetowhite epithelium).* More advanced dysplasia typically appears denser white, thicker, and more sharply bordered; areas have straight edges, few or no satellite lesions, and become more rough or thickened as the severity of dysplasia advances. There may begin to be a "yellowish" hue. Changes in the vasculature pattern also correlate with cervical dysplasia. These abnormal patterns, which often occur within an acetowhite or leukoplakia patch, include *punctation, mosaicism,* and frankly *abnormal vessel variations.* The more coarse the punctation or mosaicism, the more severe the dysplasia. Frankly abnormal vessel patterns imply severe dysplasia or potential invasive carcinoma. Following the application of Lugol's solution, there is an immediate blackening (staining) of normal epithelium (iodine uptake is high in normal cells that are rich in cytologic glycogen); abnormal dysplastic tissue, which has cells that contain much less intracellular glycogen, are *not* stained by iodine (*Lugol's negative epithelium*) and remain a white or faint yellow.

Squamous metaplasia, a normal finding, may appear slightly acetowhite and may take up Lugol's iodine incompletely; therefore this tissue can cause some degree of confusion for the novice colposcopist. Squamous metaplasia is the physiologically normal tissue where the columnar epithelium is being transformed into mature squamous epithelium. This occurs in the TZ—the same site where dysplasia generally occurs. Squamous metaplasia is especially prominent with certain conditions such as active cervicitis and where healing and reparative activities occur such as after treatment. *Questionable areas always warrant biopsy.* If squamous metaplasia without dysplasia is reported on biopsy, when the Pap smear was abnormal, the prudent colposcopist must look elsewhere to explain the finding of dysplasia on the Pap smear. A report of squamous metaplasia among other biopsies revealing dysplasia reflects the difficulty encountered by the colposcopist in evaluating this normal variant of acetowhite change. (Indeed, not all appendixes removed for an acute abdomen are the source of the pain either!) The only other common areas that normally turn slightly white with acetic acid are the *endocervical (columnar) cells,* which are located within the cervical canal and extend a variable distance onto the exocervix. Endocervical tissue can generally be differentiated from abnormal areas by colposcopic examination because of its grapelike appearance on high-power magnification. Biopsy is still warranted if there is any confusion.

This chapter focuses on the evaluation of the abnormal Pap smear as it typically relates to cervical disease. *The complete examination also includes the colposcopic examination of the remainder of the genital system in women.* The colposcope can also be used to examine male genitalia (see Chapter 120, Androscopy). Ultimately, the patient's cytologic, colposcopic, and histologic data are used in concert to direct appropriate management. A well-managed colposcopy program provides effective treatment for all patients with identified abnormalities of the cervix and genital tract.

Many colposcopists keep their scopes immediately available to augment the routine Pap and pelvic examination. Although complete formal colposcopic examination and biopsy can be performed when visual abnormalities are identified, many clinicians prefer to reschedule patients for full colposcopic examination at a later date. This allows more time for patient education and thorough evaluation.

INDICATIONS

- Pap smear consistent with dysplasia or cancer.
- Pap smear with unexplained or persistent *squamous* atypia.
- Pap smear with atypical *glandular* cells (*always* perform colposcopy)
- Worrisome history despite Pap smear findings (e.g., postcoital bleeding)
- An atypical Pap smear in which the patient tests positive for high-risk HPV.
- Pap smear with evidence of HPV infection (koilocytosis).
- Suspicious visible lesion or palpable lesion of the cervix.
- Abnormal vaginal bleeding, especially if postcoital, regardless of Pap smear status.
- History of intrauterine DES exposure.
- Evaluation or follow-up of previously treated or high-risk patients.
- The colposcope can be used for other reasons such as removal of a cervical polyp or to find a lost IUD string,

to evaluate rape patients, etc., but in these instances, a full colposcopic examination protocol may not be indicated.

STRONG CONSIDERATIONS FOR COLPOSCOPY

- Patient with visible genital condylomata or sexual partner with evidence of condylomata
- History of genital warts or sexual partner with history of genital warts
- Unexplained vaginal discharge, vulvodynia, cystitis
- Multiple sexual partners
- Early age of first coitus
- History of or current sexually transmitted disease
- Intravenous drug abuse
- Positive findings of HPV-DNA on cervical screening (see Chapter 145, Human Papillomavirus DNA Sampling)
- Patients with HIV infection (Pap smear is less reliable)

CONTRAINDICATIONS

Most contraindications relate to temporary or treatable conditions that alter the timing of the colposcopic examination rather than absolutely preventing it from occurring. The adequate colposcopic examination requires excellent visualization with a compliant and cooperative patient.

- Active, inflammatory cervicitis.
- Uncooperative patient.
- Postmenopausal patient who is not estrogen primed (intravaginal or oral estrogens for 2 to 4 weeks, respectively).
- Some patients on progesterone-only contraception or lactating mothers may also need estrogen to gain the effect of acetic acid and iodine.
- Heavy menses (may prevent adequate examination).

Note: Pregnancy is not a contraindication to colposcopy and biopsy, although a slightly different protocol is used and more bleeding can be expected from biopsies.

EQUIPMENT

The equipment and supplies used during routine colposcopy should be within reach in the colposcopy examination room (Figs. 139-2 to 139-5). Monsel's (ferric subsulfate) solution should be thoroughly shaken in its original bottle and then allowed to evaporate until it is the consistency of a thick, yellowish-brown paste; this renders it a potent astringent to control biopsy-induced bleeding.

Fig. 139-2
Colposcope and colposcopist (the author) in position for examination and biopsy.

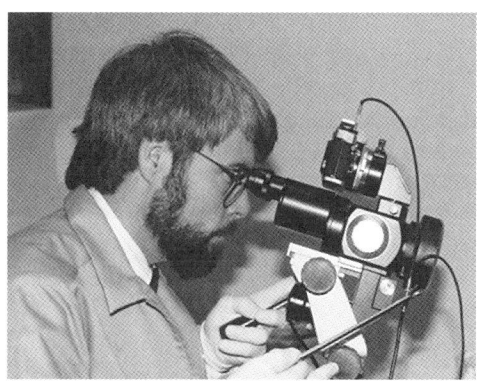

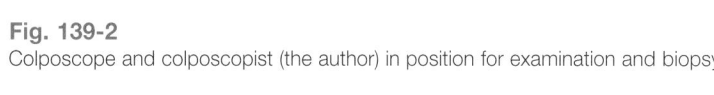

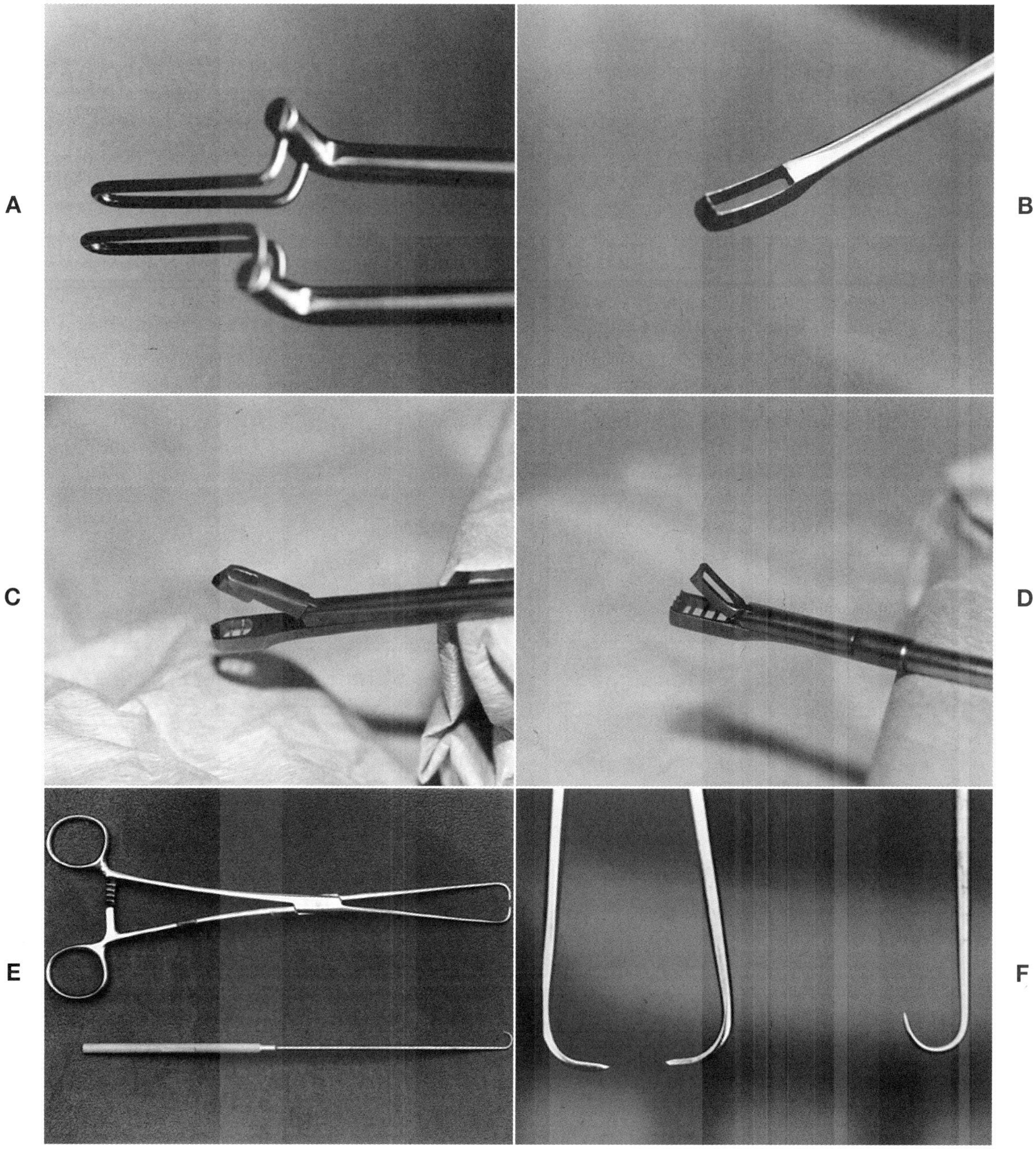

Fig. 139-3
Key instruments required for the colposcopic examination with biopsy. **A,** Kogan endocervical speculum; **B,** Kevorkian endocervical curette without basket; **C,** Tischler cervical biopsy forceps; **D,** Kevorkian biopsy forceps; **E,** cervical tenaculum and hook; **F,** close-up of tenaculum and hook.

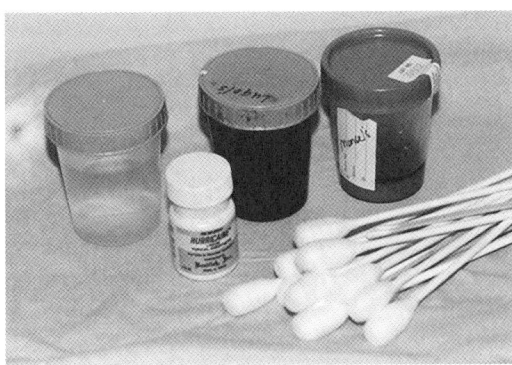

Fig. 139-4
Typical colposcopy materials on a Mayo stand, which is holding plastic cups (sputum cups) of acetic acid, Lugol's and Monsel's solution, specimen bottles, and cotton-tipped swabs.

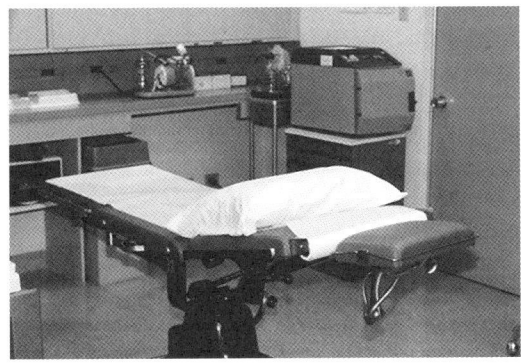

Fig. 139-5
Typical power table, which facilitates patient positioning during colposcopic examination.

- Colposcope: variable fixed power or zoom lens (3× to 7× low power to 15× to 40× high power)
- Biopsy forceps* (e.g., Tischler, baby Tischler, mini Townsend, Kevorkian)
- Endocervical curette* (Kevorkian, no basket)
- Endocervical speculum† (Kogan, both narrow and wide types)
- Ring forceps*
- Tenaculum† (rarely used)
- Cervical hook† (rarely used)
- Pap smear materials†
- Vaginal speculums (e.g., metal Graves' or disposable plastic speculum) in various sizes and lengths (use largest tolerated), or a clear, lighted, plastic speculum setup (e.g., Welch-Allyn) for selected cases

---

*Included in "colpo pack." These must be sterilized before procedures. "No touch" technique is used on the ends of instruments touching the patient. Reusable instruments are sterilized, but colposcopy is not a "sterile" procedure per se.

†Available in colposcopy room but not used at every procedure.

‡Hospital pharmacy.

§Grocery store or mix to make 3% to 5% acetic acid.

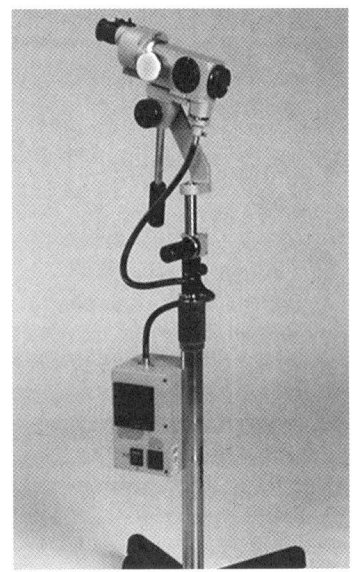

Fig. 139-6
Wallach TriStar colposcope on rolling pedestal stand.

- Full-strength Lugol's iodine solution (30 ml) (not always necessary after experience is gained but must be readily available)†,‡
- Monsel's solution (ferric subsulfate), 1 ml‡
- Acetic acid solution 3% to 5% (white vinegar; 4 to 6 oz or 120 to 180 ml)§
- Cotton- or rayon-tipped swabs (8 to 10)
- Junior scopettes/OB-GYN applicators (6 to 10)
- 4 × 4–inch gauze
- Urine or sputum cups for vinegar
- Vaginal side wall retractor (see Chapter 150, Loop Electrosurgical Excision Procedure [LEEP] for Treating Cervical Intraepithelial Neoplasia)‡
- Underpads ("chuck pads") (17 × 24 inch)
- Cotton balls (15 to 20)
- Power-assisted patient examination table that can be raised or lowered (Minimum height should be no more than 24 inches from floor, or older and disabled patients will have a difficult time getting on to it.)

Optional items include: a preprocedural dose of an oral nonsteroidal antiinflammatory agent, aromatic ammonium capsules ("smelling salts") for vasovagal responses, and a camera-video attachment.

Some clinicians now use a cytobrush to obtain the endocervical assessment instead of performing a formal ECC.

Colposcopes come in a variety of "shapes and sizes" (Fig. 139-2) but are basically the same. The stands may be like joysticks, may be on rollers, or may project out on an arm (Fig. 139-6). There is a dial for changing magnification and another for fine focusing. The eyepieces also focus independently. A simple mechanism is usually available for inserting a green filter into the visual field,

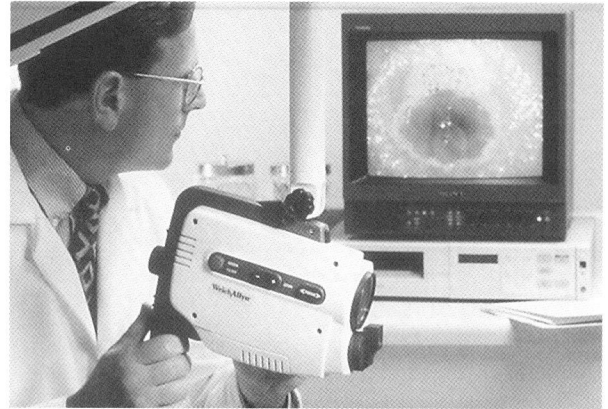

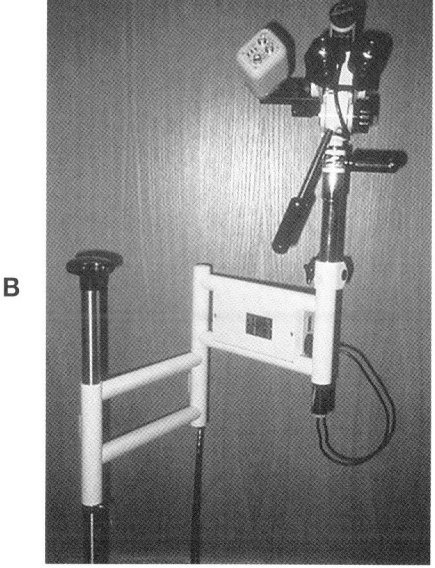

Fig. 139-7

A, Welch Allyn video colposcope. **B,** Leisegang colposcope with swing arm tripod and video camera attached.

which makes identifying abnormalities easier. The unit is turned on to the highest light intensity and then used basically as a "set of binoculars," but with a short focal distance to observe cervical tissues.

Some scopes have video options rather than binocular vision options (i.e., Welch Allyn) (Fig. 139-7, *A*). Most other scopes can be adapted for video use (Fig. 139-7, *B*). In teaching situations some type of video mode or teaching-head adapter is mandatory. It is not necessary (and is rarely performed) to videotape colposcopic examinations for medical-legal purposes.

PREPROCEDURE
PATIENT PREPARATION

- Discuss the indications for colposcopy with the patient. The patient should acknowledge the importance of long-term follow-up. The patient should advise the physician's clinic of change of address or telephone number.

- Instruct the patient to continue contraceptive practices before and after the colposcopic examination until treatment or management decisions have been made. There is no evidence that any type of contraception or estrogen replacement therapy affects cervical dysplasia.

- Explain to the patient that a pregnancy test will be performed on the day of the procedure if pregnancy is a possibility, but the test with or without biopsies will have no effect on a pregnancy.

- Instruct the patient to consume a regular diet on the day of the procedure and not to skip a meal before the procedure. This lessens the possibility of a vasovagal episode.

- Warn against taking aspirin, or medications containing aspirin, for 7 days before the procedure. Aspirin consumption within the past week does not ordinarily contraindicate colposcopy with biopsy, but you should be aware of the potential for more bleeding. Normally, nonsteroidal antiinflammatory drugs, such as ibuprofen, do not significantly prolong bleeding; therefore they may be taken before the procedure for pain control.

- Review the medical history with particular attention to in-utero exposure to DES; drug allergies; asthma; diabetes mellitus; history of vagal sensitivity (frequent fainting); bleeding disorder; recent symptoms of cervicitis or pelvic inflammatory disease; symptoms suggesting pregnancy; symptomatology suggestive of an endometrial disorder that may require endometrial sampling; and history of prior cervical treatment, including conization, laser therapy, or cryotherapy (Figs. 139-8 and 139-9).

- Explain that the procedure will take about 20 to 30 minutes. Most clinics ask patients to arrive at least 15 minutes early to allow for appropriate education, a pregnancy test, and questions.

- If pictures will be taken, inform the patient, and establish consent before the actual procedure (see the sample patient consent form titled "Clinical Photography and/or Videotaping" on page 1928 of Appendix G).

- Review the risks before the procedure: pain, infection, bleeding, discharge, and missing disease (all very rare).

- Explain that colposcopy with biopsy ordinarily renders a diagnosis and is not a therapeutic procedure per se. Definitive therapy will be determined by correlation of historical, colposcopic, cytologic, and histologic data.

- Discuss treatment options. Ordinarily, cervical cryotherapy, if indicated, is performed after the cervix has had time to heal from the biopsy and pathology reports are available. This typically can be performed as early as 2 weeks after colposcopy or after the next menstrual cycle.

Colposcopy

PATIENT INSTRUCTIONS: Please complete questions down to "Procedure."

Date_____ Age_____ Birthdate _____
Name_____ Referring physician _____
Phone (home)_____ (work)_____ Reason for colposcopy _____

HISTORY

Previous abnormal paps?	Y N	Age of first Pap___ How often_____
History of previous cryocautery (freezing)?	Y N	Number of pregnancies___ Children___
History of previous cervical surgery?	Y N	Date of last menstrual period_____
Personal history of cancer?	Y N	Type of contraception_____
Family history of cancer?	Y N	Number of sexual partners (lifetime)___
History of venereal diseases (circle)		Age at first sexual intercourse_____
• gonorrhea • AIDS • herpes • syphilis		Do you smoke? Y N
Do you desire testing for any of these diseases?	Y N	Partner(s) with warts? Y N
History of genital warts?	Y N	History of sexual abuse? Y N
Visible warts now?	Y N	Other PMH:
Previously treated?	Y N	Meds:_____
If so, how?_____		Allergies:_____
		Other:_____

PROCEDURE (Doctor will fill out)

Observation without staining:_____

Pap repeated?	Y N	LK= Leukoplakia
SCJ seen?	Y N	WE= White epithelium
Endo spec needed?	Y N	PN= Punctation
ECC done?	Y N	MO= Mosaicism
Entire lesion seen?	Y N	ATZ= Abnormal transformation zone
		AV= Abnormal vessels
Vaginal vault:		BE= Bulk effect
		AG= Atypical glands
Urethra:		X= Biopsy sites

Labia:

Perineum:

Rectum:

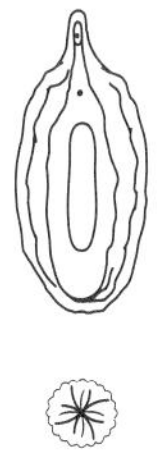

IMPRESSION: Adequate colposcopy? Y   N

_____

RECOMMENDATIONS:			**PLAN:**
Cryocautery	Y N	Tip:_____	Discourage smoking
Referral to specialist	Y N		Partner needs information
LEEP	Y N		Need at least annual Paps for rest of life
Other:			no matter what others say
			Handout on cryocautery/LEEP/Andro/HPV
			vitamins/smoking

cc: _____   _____
                                                        Physician's Signature

Fig. 139-8
Sample patient form for colposcopy. (Courtesy The National Procedures Institute, Midland, Mich.)

Follow-up Colposcopy Visits

Name_____   Referred by_____

Initial colposcopy date:_____   Findings: Cervix _____

                                                     ECC   _____

                                                     Other _____

Laser

Cryo

Treatment date: _____   TCA

Efudex

LETZ: Ecto _____ Endo _____ ECC _____

Problem: _____

Partner evaluated?   Y   N   Viewed tapes: Self?   Y   N

                                                  Partner? Y   N

Smoker?   Y   N

Diet: _____

Vitamins?   Y   N

Date	History Findings/Treatments	Pap/Bx's: Done	Pap/Bx's: Results	Plan	Copy Sent

Physician

Fig. 139-9

Sample patient form for colposcopy follow-up. All data are summarized in one place. Additional sheets would omit upper portion. (Courtesy The National Procedures Institute, Midland, Mich.)

- If applicable, inform the patient that she may likely receive a separate bill for the interpretation of the pathology samples obtained during the biopsy procedure.
- Subacute bacterial endocarditis (SBE) prophylaxis is not necessary.

Many physicians mail patient education information to their patients before their colposcopy examination (see the sample patient education handout titled "Colposcopy" on page 1924 of Appendix G). This decreases patient anxiety and improves understanding of the disease process. Videotapes are available to further enhance patient education and informed consent (Creative Health Communications; see the "Suppliers" section). Commercial brochures are also available from the American College of Obstetricians and Gynecologists as well as Krames Communications.

TECHNIQUE

Figs. 139-8 and 139-9 provide a summary protocol for the colposcopic examination and highlight the key patient management issues. Clinicians are also advised to either dictate or write their findings in the medical record to supplement the colposcopic examination form. See Box 81-1 for the suggested terminology to be used to describe findings.

With practice and skill, the colposcopic examination with appropriate tissue sampling can be assimilated effectively into the contemporary clinician's practice. In addition to the necessary technical skills, the successful colposcopy program requires close attention to data interpretation and careful patient follow-up. The patient who has an abnormal Pap smear and who ultimately has biopsy-confirmed cervical dysplasia remains at an increased lifetime risk for recurrence or reexpressions of genital malignancy.

1. *Prepare the colposcopy room.* Make sure the room is warm. Some patients benefit from quiet background music. Have all necessary solutions and equipment readily at hand. Make sure the appropriate culture media, KOH, and wet prep materials are in the room. Keep all sizes of speculums in your colposcopy room.
2. *Prepare the patient.* Mail information before the procedure. Answer her questions. Use a pelvic model or diagrams when you explain the procedure. Review medical history. Are there significant medical conditions such as diabetes or bleeding disorders? Is there a recent history of symptoms suggesting pregnancy, vaginosis, or pelvic inflammatory disease? What are her drug allergies? Is she sensitive to iodine? Ibuprofen 800 mg may be offered 30 minutes before the procedure.

3. *Obtain informed consent.* Before the office visit, allow the patient to review a written description of the procedure, its risks, and complications (see the sample patient education handout titled "Colposcopy" on page 1920 of Appendix G). Address questions and concerns. Obtain informed consent, which may include a signed permit.
4. *Obtain a pregnancy test as necessary.* An ECC is contraindicated in pregnancy. Occult pregnancy at the time of colposcopy is common.
5. *Warm and insert the speculum.* Colposcopy requires the widest speculum the patient can comfortably tolerate. The examination requires greater cervical and vaginal exposure than a screening Pap smear. Because of the relative duration of the colposcopic examination, the vaginal walls may migrate inward, which makes visualization more difficult. (A carefully inserted, wide, large Graves' speculum is far more comfortable in the long run than constant prodding and manipulating of the vagina to move the vagina out of the field of view if an inappropriately narrow speculum is used.) If necessary, use a vaginal side wall retractor. A thin layer of water-soluble vaginal lubricant can be applied on the speculum. This thin coating significantly facilitates the insertion of the speculum, will rarely interfere with Pap smear testing (if necessary), and does not interfere with biopsy interpretation. Use both thumbscrew dimensions of the speculum to gain maximum exposure. Ideally, the colposcopic examination is facilitated by having the cervix facing anteriorly and virtually "suspended" between the blades of the speculum.
6. *Grossly examine the cervix and vaginal fornices.* Does the cervix appear inflamed or infected? An active cervicitis confuses colposcopic detail. Characterize the vaginal and cervical discharge. Once the Pap smear has been obtained, it is permissible to gently blot (not rub) excess secretions away to view the cervix more clearly. Use magnification to quickly scan the cervix to identify landmarks, such as the TZ with its SCJ. Are there areas of gross vessel atypia? It is important to scan the cervix for gross leukoplakia before applying acetic acid. Although acetic acid greatly enhances the elucidation of diseased areas, its mild vasoconstricting properties can render significant vessel detail less obvious.
7. *Obtain specimens for cultures, KOH and wet preparations, HPV-DNA probe, and Pap smear, as necessary.* Even a correctly performed Pap smear irritates the cervix, may cause bleeding, and may change fine colposcopic detail. The Pap smear may need to be repeated because the original Pap smear was performed at a different lab; because more than 3 months have elapsed since the last Pap smear; because the patient is pregnant (Pap smears are less

reliable during pregnancy and colposcopy is more difficult; it is important to maximize clinical assessment); and because of the need to allay any concern or confusion regarding the adequacy or interpretation of the original Pap smear results.

8. *Perform a bimanual examination if one has not been done recently.* (If a Pap smear is desired, do it before the bimanual examination.) Is the uterus enlarged or tender? What position is the cervix? Can the cervix be moved? How long is the vagina? Are there palpated abnormalities of the introitus, vagina, fornices, or cervix? Examine the vulva for obvious condylomata.

9. *Apply 5% acetic acid.* One method is to use 4 × 4–inch gauze rolled up tightly and held longitudinally in a ring forceps. This saturates the cervix with vinegar quickly and without trauma. Cotton balls or large swabs also work well. Use large swabs or junior scopettes to repeat the application. Refer to acetic acid as "vinegar" or simply as "douche solution" when discussing it with the patient. Warn her of brief stinging and coldness. Repeat application every 5 minutes, because the acetowhite effect is only temporary.

10. *Perform the colposcopic examination.* Start with low power (typically 5×). Scan the entire cervix with bright white light. Use a vinegar-soaked, cotton-tipped swab to help manipulate the cervix and TZ into view. It is almost never necessary to use the tenaculum to move the cervix. The cervical hook can be used; however, it is rarely needed. The Kogan endocervical speculum greatly aids the examination of the distal endocervical canal. It should be used when either the entire SCJ or the entire lesion cannot be seen because it (or they) is up inside the endocervical canal. Use this instrument gingerly to prevent bleeding and pain. Use higher magnification to carefully document abnormal findings. The entire TZ, including the SCJ, must be seen and evaluated. Abnormalities will turn white (acetowhite).

11. *Use the green filter to enhance vascular detail.* All abnormal areas demand biopsy. Lugol's solution aids with the identification of abnormal (dysplastic) areas but is rarely used (it is unnecessary and messy). Both dysplasia and reparative (metaplastic) tissue will incompletely stain with concentrated iodine because of low levels of cellular glycogen (as compared with the staining of healthy, mature squamous epithelium). The sharply outlined borders afforded by Lugol's can be dramatic, and this can help clarify biopsy sites. Iodine staining does not interfere with histology. However, Lugol's may obscure the underlying vascular pattern. Lugol's solution should be used when further clarification of potential biopsy sites is necessary or when no lesion is seen with acetic acid. Applying Lugol's solution will also help delineate the SCJ for the beginning colposcopist (endocervical cells do not stain with Lugol's) and is used for performing cervical loop electrosurgery procedures (LEEP, large loop excision of the transformation zone) because its effects last longer than those of acetic acid.

12. *Mentally map the cervix.* The main goal of colposcopy is to identify areas for biopsy. The colposcopist must be able to differentiate normal tissues from abnormal. Acetowhite areas that are unifocal; that have sharp, flat, straight borders; that stain white quickly; and those that appear thick or raised are likely to be more abnormal histologically. The presence of coarse punctation or mosaic patterns, or of frankly abnormal vessels, is associated with a more severe degree of dysplasia. Ultimately, however, the histopathologist is the one who makes the diagnosis from biopsy samples. Be prepared to draw a careful record of what is observed and where biopsy samples were taken. The colposcopic impression of severity of disease must be recorded to compare and correlate later findings. Coppleson and associates (1986) have proposed scoring indexes to help discern colposcopically identifiable lesions. Many physicians find these helpful when beginning colposcopy (Reid, 1993).

13. *Is the colposcopic examination satisfactory?* The entire TZ, including all the SCJ, must be visualized. The borders of all lesions must be seen in their entirety (lesions should not disappear into the canal, for example). Patients who are uncooperative or who have a severely flexed uterus with inadequate visualization are potential "real world" causes of inadequate colposcopy. An inadequate colposcopic examination coupled with cytologic evidence of dysplasia may necessitate a cervical cone biopsy sample for evaluation. In summary, the *adequate* colposcopic examination requires the following: (1) visualizing the entire TZ including the SCJ, (2) identifying the area of abnormality producing the abnormal Pap smear, (3) confirming that the limits of all abnormal areas are clearly seen, (4) obtaining a biopsy sample of all abnormal areas, and (5) verifying no colposcopic evidence of malignancy. *The patient is a candidate for ablative therapy* if (1) the aforementioned conditions are met *and* no lesion extends more than 5 mm into the canal, (2) the ECC is negative, (2) there is no colposcopic evidence of malignancy, (3) any high-grade lesion is only focal in size, and (4) there is correlation between Pap, colposcopic impression, and histology.

14. *Perform the ECC.* Some colposcopists elect to omit the ECC in instances where a clear source of cervical dysplasia is identified on the ectocervix, the SCJ is clearly seen, and the canal appears colposcopically clear of dysplasia. Others consider replacing the ECC

with careful cytobrush sampling of the canal at the time of the colposcopic examination. Nonetheless, most colposcopists still perform the ECC as a necessary component of the colposcopic examination, and that is the preferred method of the author, especially if ablative therapy such as cervical cryotherapy is performed later (see Chapter 141, Cryotherapy of the Cervix). Generally, local anesthesia is not necessary.

Use a Kevorkian curette without basket. Insert gently until the internal cervical os is reached, about 1.5 to 2 cm within the canal. This can be manifested by a slight puckering of the cervix with further advancement. In multiparous women the internal os is not well defined; the curette should not be advanced farther than 2 cm. Scrape the entire lining of the canal *(360 degrees) twice*. The procedure may be done with or without colposcopic observation. The American Society for Colposcopy and Cervical-Pathology recommends using the colposcope to avoid inadvertently sampling lesions near the os. The curetted sample appears as a coagulum of mucus, blood, and small gray or tan tissue fragments. The scope can then be used to examine tissue and to further tease the loosened sample from the canal. Sometimes a cytobrush will retrieve the remnants of the ECC sample, which may persistently remain stuck in the canal. Submit the ECC in a separate bottle on a piece of paper towel, lens paper, or Telfa. Ordinarily, it is not necessary to place a sample pad in the posterior vaginal fornix as it is with formal dilation and curettage (D & C). Do *not* perform an ECC on pregnant patients or patients with evidence of active cervicitis or PID. All other patients must have a documented negative ECC prior to ablative therapy. Some physicians prefer to perform the ECC after the cervical biopsy samples are obtained because (1) bleeding caused by the ECC can obscure lesions on the lower lip (but a cervical biopsy can bleed and "wash away" or dilute the curettage sample) and (2) the ECC, which takes only 30 seconds, is still the most uncomfortable part of the procedure. If performed first, however, the patient can be assured early that "the worst is over."

15. *Obtain cervical biopsy samples.* Sample the posterior (lower) areas first to prevent blood from dripping over future biopsy sites. The cervix can be manipulated with a cotton-tipped swab, a junior scopette, or a hook to provide an adequate angle for obtaining the biopsy sample. A 3-mm–thick sample is all that is necessary. It is *not* necessary to include normal-appearing tissue with biopsy samples (that is, to include the margins of lesions in the sample). Beginning colposcopists can enhance their skills by placing samples from different biopsy

sites in separate bottles and subsequently correlating them with colposcopic impression. After sufficient experience colposcopists can place all biopsy samples together. The cervix will be treated based on the most severe lesion as well as the size of the lesion. Putting different biopsies in separate containers only increases cost, but it does not change therapy. For learning experience, an unusual or atypical-appearing lesion may be placed in a separate container to provide better feedback. If bleeding is profuse from a particular site and more samples are needed, hold a cotton-tipped swab to the area and proceed with obtaining the next sample. (To control persistent bleeding, see the "Complications" section.) Do not apply Monsel's solution until all samples are obtained. Monsel's solution in a biopsy specimen can ruin good histology. As noted above, some physicians prefer to obtain the cervical biopsy samples before the ECC.

16. *Apply Monsel's solution to bleeding areas after all biopsies have been obtained.* To be most effective, the Monsel's should be as thick as toothpaste. This consistency can be achieved by allowing the Monsel's solution to evaporate down to a pasty consistency. Swab out the excess Monsel's and bloody debris in the posterior vault, which appears as a black mass of coagulum that may alarm the patient and irritate the vulva. Observe the cervix until all evident bleeding ceases.

17. *Remove the speculum and examine the vagina.* Reapply acetic acid to the vaginal sidewalls. Gently retract the speculum with a back-and-forth twisting motion to the right and left and observe through the colposcope as the vaginal wall collapses around the receding blades. Are abnormal vaginal areas apparent? Be sure to colposcopically examine vaginal areas that were abnormal when palpated during the bimanual examination. Biopsies of the vagina can be obtained with the same biopsy forceps but are placed in separate containers.

18. *Examine the vulva and anus.* Vulvar examination may be performed at this time. Acetic acid application will yield an acetowhite effect in most sites with condylomata. It is mandatory to do a careful vulvar colposcopic examination with acetic acid in women at high risk for vulvar dysplasia (those with HPV infection and smokers), including those with unexplained vulvar itching, smokers over age 40, those with abnormal-appearing areas of vulvar tissue, and especially those with vulvar symptoms.

The easiest way to examine the vulva is to begin superiorly. Use two hands to separate the vulva and slowly raise the power table with the foot pedal. Examine carefully from clitoris to anus. *The finding of perianal condylomata warrants anoscopy.* The Ive's slotted anoscope is ideal (see Chapter 100,

Anoscopy). If condylomata are grossly visible, it may be best to resolve the lesions first before inserting the scope and risking spread internally. Acetic acid can be used in the anal canal but is rarely necessary. Small anal canal condylomata can usually be palpated. For the technique of biopsying the vulva, see Chapter 161, Vulvar Biopsy.

19. *Allow the patient to recover.* Have the patient rest supine for at least several minutes, then sit up slowly and rest again.

20. *Document your findings.* Carefully draw a picture of lesions and biopsy sites. Photos of the cervix do not replace accurately drawn diagrams of the colposcopic cervical findings. These should be included regardless of whether the colposcopic examination is considered adequate.

    Chart whether the colposcopic impression supports outpatient cervical cryotherapy and which cryotip should be used (size and shape). This is not a decision based solely on colposcopic appearance. Only histologic reporting and correlation of cytologic, colposcopic, and histologic data together can define the appropriate therapeutic intervention. Factors such as lesion location, grade of severity, number, and size also dictate treatment options. For instance, large lesions (over 25 mm in diameter, more than 15 mm from the os, or involving more than two cervical quadrants), even if they are only mildly dysplastic, are treated more appropriately with loop excision or laser therapy as opposed to a small focal severe dysplasia, which may respond to ambulatory cryotherapy very well. (See Chapter 150, Loop Electrosurgical Excision Procedure [LEEP] for Treating Cervical Intraepithelial Neoplasia, and Chapter 141, Cryotherapy of the Cervix.)

21. *Discuss the findings, and give postprocedure instructions.* After the patient has recovered and is dressed, review your impressions but withhold the specific diagnosis until the histology report has returned and review of all the clinical data have been examined. Provide careful postprocedure instructions (see the sample patient education handout titled "After Colposcopy and Biopsy Information" on page 1927 of Appendix G). Advise abstaining from intercourse for 24 hours and using tampons for 5 days. Instruct the patient to return if she experiences unusual vaginal odor, discharge, pelvic pain, or fever. Make a specific agreement as to how the results of the biopsy are to be reported. Unless a problem arises, the patient does not need a follow-up pelvic examination. Discussing the results of the biopsy sampling and subsequent treatment options on the telephone may be an appropriate follow-up mechanism for some patients; however, most will appreciate a visit to the physician for this important interaction.

HISTOLOGY, CYTOLOGY INTERPRETATION OF DATA

If at all possible, the same pathologist (or at least the same group of pathologists) should interpret both the cytology and histology results for a given patient. The clinician should be concerned if significant discrepancy is found between the Papanicolaou cytology and the biopsy histology. In general, a report that a greater degree of abnormality was found on the biopsy compared with the Pap smear (e.g., Pap = CIN 2; biopsy = CIN 3) is common and acceptable. The clinician should be concerned, however, if biopsy-generated histology reports are significantly less advanced than Papanicolaou cytology (two or greater grades of severity less). For instance, a cytology smear indicating carcinoma in situ, with biopsy samples of only mild dysplasia, might indicate that the worst area was missed on evaluation, and that the patient may have in situ or invasive carcinoma in another site. A good rule of thumb is not to freeze or ablate any cervix until the discrepancy between histology and cytology has been explained adequately and sufficiently. Repeating colposcopy and biopsy sampling to reconcile the difference is forgivable, even in the hands of the most experienced clinicians. Freezing invasive cancer is never acceptable.

A negative ECC sample will show strips or fragments of orderly, benign columnar epithelium with mucus and blood. Lack of identifiable endocervical tissue constitutes an inadequate ECC sample. An inadequate ECC sample is not uncommon, and in the overwhelming majority of patients it simply means that the ECC must be repeated before definitive therapy. If the ECC sample indicates dysplasia, it is a positive ECC and an indication for cone biopsy procedure (see Chapter 135, Cervical Conization and Chapter 150, Loop Electrosurgical Excision Procedure [LEEP] for Treating Cervical Intraepithelial Neoplasia). Current protocol does not support freezing the canal with a long narrow probe to treat endocervical dysplasia. Some "positive" ECCs result from contamination with dysplastic lesions at the verge of the os. *Nonetheless, do not assume this!* The beginning colposcopist must remain comfortable referring patients with equivocal or problematic colposcopic, cytologic, and histologic correlation. Know your limitations!

POSTPROCEDURE PATIENT EDUCATION

See the sample patient education handout titled "After Colposcopy and Biopsy Information" on page 1923 of Appendix G.

• Agree on a time to discuss and interpret biopsy findings by phone or follow-up visit.

- Explain that mild vaginal discharge may occur following a cervical biopsy procedure, especially if Monsel's solution was used to control bleeding. This discharge is often grainy and black, which is the result of Monsel's mixing with mucus and blood. This discharge may last approximately 24 hours.
- Advise the patient that she may have spotting for at least 48 hours. Although there may be some spotting, it is safe to resume intercourse after 24 hours.
- Instruct the patient to report passage of clots, onset of fresh profuse bleeding, foul vaginal odor, fever, or pelvic pain. Women with these complaints following a cervical biopsy procedure require evaluation.
- Encourage the patient to continue contraception.
- Patients rarely require vaginal creams (e.g., triple sulfa) after a cervical biopsy has been obtained. Nonetheless, some women may have vaginitis caused by organisms such as yeast, bacteria, or *Trichomonas,* and therapy aimed at these pathogens may be helpful. Women who feel comfortable douching may use a nightly (or morning) dilute povidone-iodine solution as desired.
- *Emphasize the importance of returning for definitive therapy.* Reemphasize the relationship of cervical dysplasia with sexually transmissible disease, poor diet, smoking, and nonmonogamous sexual practices. Be sure the patient understands the lifelong risks of HPV infection.

COMPLICATIONS

- Most *postcervical biopsy* or *ECC bleeding is minimal* and handled completely with Monsel's solution. Rarely, the patient experiences a fresh, bloody discharge. Often, a simple reapplication of Monsel's solution is all that is necessary. Very rarely, a simple cervical stitch of 4-0 absorbable suture across a particularly deep biopsy site may be required. Avoid obtaining a cervical biopsy sample immediately before the menses; subsequent bleeding may be confused with menstrual flow, and the uterus may potentially be more prone to infection. Some clinicians will saturate the end of a vaginal tampon with Monsel's solution and insert this to provide pressure and astringent action for persistent cervical oozing. The tampon can then be removed several hours later by the patient. At times, it may be necessary to cauterize the biopsy site. An effective way to control fairly brisk bleeding is to inject 1 to 2 ml of 2% lidocaine with epinephrine into the bleeding site. This will either stop or reduce the bleeding enough to effectively apply Monsel's solution or cauterize the site. Use a needle extender (see Chapter 150, Loop Electrosurgical Excision Procedure [LEEP] for Treating Cervical Intraepithelial Neoplasia) or a spinal needle to reach the cervix.
- A *foul cervical discharge, fever,* or *pelvic pain* may

indicate postprocedure infection. Infection is extremely rare but typically occurs on the third or fourth day after the biopsy sample has been taken. A cervical biopsy sampling should be avoided if there is clinical evidence of invasive cervicitis.
- Despite correct technique, there is the potential risk that the most advanced *cervical disease may be missed* by the colposcopist at the time of the biopsy sampling or potentially by the histologist at the time of tissue analysis. Careful, timely transport of all samples to a reputable lab is important. Some pathologists prefer all cervical biopsy samples to be placed in the same container, whereas others prefer separate containers for each, but the ECC sample should remain separate. (Each bottle costs between $150 and $200 for processing.) The colposcopist is well advised to be liberal in obtaining biopsies of all abnormal-appearing areas of the cervix for histologic interpretation. Widespread four-quadrant cervical disease challenges the colposcopist to sample areas most likely to contain cervical carcinoma. Lack of correlation between the Papanicolaou cytology and subsequent histology can suggest situations when potentially the worst area has not been sampled. The main goal of colposcopy is to rule out invasive cervical cancer and to select patients who are candidates for outpatient treatment. When the colposcopist cannot safely accomplish this goal, cervical conization—rarely, but importantly—is the only way of accomplishing this task. "Blind biopsies" where random samples are obtained are generally discouraged.
- Some women will experience *vaginal discharge* after a cervical biopsy sample is obtained. This will typically last 1 or 2 days and should diminish with time.
- Cervical biopsy sampling typically causes *brief pain and discomfort.* Ordinarily, this pain is well tolerated by most women. Careful explanation of the procedure, a warm room, and a caring, careful manner all minimize the discomfort. Studies have shown preoperative oral nonsteroidal antiinflammatory drugs decrease discomfort associated with the procedure. Application of topical anesthetics actually increases the pain experience!
- Rarely, *vasovagal reactions* occur with the procedure but are much more likely to occur with cervical cryotherapy.

SUPPLIERS

Physician teaching slides and tapes
Bio-Vision, Inc.
350 Fifth Avenue, Suite 3304
New York, NY 10118
Phone: 1-800-665-VIRUS (8478)
Website: www.bio-v.com

National society for promotion of quality education and patient care for cervical/vaginal disease
American Society for Colposcopy and Cervical Pathology (ASCCP)
20 West Washington Street, Suite 1
Hagerstown, MD 21740
Phone: 1-800-787-7227
Website: www.asccp.org

Colposcopy training courses
American Academy of Family Physicians
11400 Tomahawk Creek Parkway
Leawood, KS 66211-2672
Phone: 1-913-906-6000
Website: www.aasp.org

American Society for Colposcopy and Cervical Pathology (ASCCP)
20 West Washington Street, Suite 1
Hagerstown, MD 21740
Phone: 1-800-787-7227
Website: www.asccp.org

The National Procedures Institute, Inc.
4909 Hedgewood Drive
Midland, MI 48640
Phone: 1-800-462-2492
Website: www.npinstitute.com

Patient education videotapes
Creative Health Communications
4675 South Portsmouth Road
Bridgeport, MI 48722
Phone: 1-800-462-2492

Patient education brochures and support groups
American Social Health Association
P.O. Box 13827
Research Triangle Park, NC 27709
Phone: 1-919-361-8400
Website: www.ashastd.org

American College of Obstetricians and Gynecologists
409 12th St., S.W., PO Box 96920
Washington, D.C. 20090-6920
Phone: 1-800-762-2264
Website: www.acog.org

Krames Communications
1100 Grundy Lane
San Bruno, CA 94066
Phone: 1-800-333-3032
Website: www.krames.com

Colposcope and instrument manufacturers
Accuscope/Vineland Medical Products, Inc.
P.O. Box 575
1471 E. Chestnut Avenue
Vineland, NJ 08360-0575
Phone: 1-609-692-5140

CooperSurgical, Inc.
95 Corporate Drive
Trumbull, CT 06611
Phone: 1-203-601-5200

Gyne-Tech Instrument Co.
1115 Chestnut Street
Burbank, CA 91506
Phone: 1-323-849-1512

Jedmed Instruments Co.
5416 Jedmed Court
St Louis, MO 63129
Phone: 1-314-845-3770
Website: www.jedmed.com

MedGyn
328 N. Eisenhower Lane
P.O. Box 1491
Lombard, IL 60148
Phone: 1-800-451-9667
Website: www.medgyn.com

Olympus
2 Corporate Center Drive
Melville, NY 11747
Phone: 1-800-848-9024
Website: www.olympus.com

Wallach Surgical
235 Edison Road
Orange, CT 06477
Phone: 1-800-243-2463
Website: www.wallachsurgical.com

Welch Allyn, Inc.
4341 State Street Road, Box 220
Skaneatles Falls, NY 13153-0220
Phone: 1-800-535-6663
Website: www.welchallyn.com

DS Vasconelles
19260 NE 22nd Road
North Miami Beach, FL 33179
Phone: 1-800-933-0009
Website: www.dfv.com.br

Zeiss
One Zeiss Drive
Thornwood, NY 10594
Phone: 1-800-442-4020
Website: www.zeiss.com

Other colposcopy equipment/supplies (also see Chapter 150, Loop Electrosurgical Excision Procedure [LEEP] for Treating Cervical Intraepithelial Neoplasia, and Chapter 141, Cryotherapy of the Cervix)

Medscand (Cytobrush)
CooperSurgical
95 Corporate Drive
Trumbull, CT 06611
Phone: 1-800-645-3760
Website: www.medscand.se

Milex (Amino Cerv Creme; pap supplies)
4311 N. Normandy
Chicago, IL 60634
Phone: 1-800-621-1278
Website: www.milexproducts.com

National Testing Lab (cerviscopes, cervicography)
400 Biltmore Drive, Suite 407
Fenton, MO 63026
Phone: 1-800-325-9737
Website: www.ntlworldwide.com

Roche Biomedical Labs (Viral Typing)
1447 York Court
Burlington, NC 27215
Phone: 1-800-334-5161

Trylon Corporation (speculoscopy)
970 West 190th Street, Suite 850
Torrance, CA 90502
Phone: 1-800-486-8979
Website: www.tryloncorp.com

Wallach Surgical (Papette, Pap smear samplers)
(See contact information above.)

Welch Allyn, Inc.
(See contact information above.)

CPT/BILLING CODES

56605	Biopsy of vulva
56606	Biopsy of each additional
56820*	Colposcopy of the vulva
56821*	Colposcopy of the vulva; with biopsy(s)

*Revised for 2003.

57100	Biopsy of vaginal mucosa
57420*	Colposcopy of the entire vagina, with cervix if present
57421	Colposcopy of the entire vagina, with cervix if present; with biopsy(s)
57452*	Colposcopy of the cervix including upper/adjacent vagina
57454*	Colposcopy of the cervix including upper/adjacent vagina with biopsy(s) of the cervix and endocervical curettage
57455*	Colposcopy of the cervix including upper/adjacent vagina with biopsy(s) of the cervix
57456*	Colposcopy of the cervix including upper/adjacent vagina; with endocervical curettage
57460	Colposcopy of the cervix including upper/adjacent vagina with loop electrode biopsy(s) of the cervix (do not report 57456 in addition to 57461)
57461*	Colposcopy of the cervix including upper/adjacent vagina; with loop electrode conization of the cervix
57500*	Biopsy of cervix only, single or multiple (also use this code for removal of a cervical polyp since there is no other specific code)
57505	Endocervical curettage (not done as part of a D & C)
57510	Electrocautery of cervix
57511	Cryosurgery of cervix
57513	Laser ablation of cervix
57520	Conization cervix
57522	Conization, LEEP technique

ICD-9-CM DIAGNOSTIC CODES

180.09	Cervical neoplasm, malignant (excludes Ca in situ)
078.11	Condyloma acuminatum
219.0	Benign neoplasm, cervix
233.1	Ca in situ, cervix
616.0	Cervicitis
616.10	Vaginitis
622.0	Cervical ectropion
622.0	Cervical erosion/ulcer
622.1	Cervical atypia
622.1	Dysplasia, cervix
622.2	Cervical leukoplakia
622.4	Cervical stenosis
622.7	Cervical polyp
622.8	Cervical atrophy
622.8	Nabothian cyst
623.0	Dysplasia, vagina
623.1	Vaginal leukoplakia
623.5	Vaginal leukorrhea

623.7   Vaginal polyp
623.8   Vaginal bleeding
623.8   Vaginal cyst
624.0   Vulvar dystrophy
624.1   Vulvar atrophy
624.6   Vulvar or labial polyp
795.0   Nonspecific abnormal Pap (many insurance companies will not pay for colposcopy with this nonspecific code)

ADDITIONAL RESOURCES

• See the sample patient education handouts titled "Colposcopy" and "After Colposcopy and Biopsy Information" on pages 1924 and 1927, respectively, of Appendix G.
• See the sample patient education handout titled "Clinical Photography and/or Videotaping" on page 1928 of Appendix G.

BIBLIOGRAPHY

Apgar BS, Brotzman GL, Spitzer M: *Colposcopy principles and practice: an integrated textbook and atlas,* Philadelphia, 2002, WB Saunders.

Brotzman GL, Apgar BS: Assessing colposcopic skills: the instructor's handbook, *Fam Med* 30(5):350, 1998.

Burke L, Antonioli DA, Ducatman BS: *Colposcopy: text and atlas,* East Norwalk, Conn, 1991, Appleton & Lange.

Clifton P, Shaughnessy AF, Andrews S: Ineffectiveness of topical benzocaine spray during colposcopy, *J Fam Pract* 46:242, 1998.

Coppleson M, Pixley E, Reid B: The tissue basis of colposcopic appearances. In *Colposcopy: a scientific and practical approach to the cervix, vagina, and vulva in health and disease,* ed 3, Springfield, Ill, 1986, Charles C Thomas.

Cox T: ASCCP Practice Guidelines: Management of glandular abnormalities in the cervical smear, *J Lower Genital Tract Dis* 1(1):41, 1997.

Curry SL, Pfenninger JL, Sarma S: Colposcopy: when? why? how? *Patient Care* 15:167, 1994.

Dunn TS et al: Comparing endocervical curettage and endocervical brush at colposcopy, *J Low Genital Tract Dis* 4:76, 2000.

Ferris DG, Willner WA, Ho JJ: Colposcopes: a critical review, *J Fam Pract* 34(1):25, 1992.

Gibson CA, Trask CE, House P: Endocervical sampling: a comparison of endocervical brush, endocervical curette, and combined brush with curette techniques, *J Low Genital Tract Dis* 5(1):1, 2001.

Goldie SJ, Weinstein MC, Kuntz KM, Freedberg KA: The costs, clinical benefits, and cost-effectiveness of screening for cervical cancer in HIV-infected women, *Ann Intern Med* 130(2):97, 1999.

Gordon PR, Weiss BD: Family physician colposcopy practices, *J Am Board Fam Pract* 5:27, 1992.

Guerra B, De Simone P, Gabrielli S, et al: Combined cytology and colposcopy to screen for cervical cancer in pregnancy, *J Reprod Med* 43(8):647, 1998.

Harper D, Roach MS: Cervical intraepithelial neoplasia in pregnancy, *J Fam Pract* 42:79, 1995.

Hatch KD: *Handbook of colposcopy,* Boston, 1989, Little, Brown.

Hatch KD: Colposcopy of vaginal and vulvar human papillomavirus and adjacent sites, *Obstet Gynecol Clin North Am* 20(1):203, 1993.

Khanna N, Phillips MD: Adherence to care plan in women with abnormal Papanicolaou smears: a review of barriers and interventions, *J Am Board Fam Pract* 14:123, 2001.

Kim JJ, Wright TC, Goldie SJ: Cost-effectiveness of alternative triage strategies for atypical squamous cells of undetermined significance, *JAMA* 287(18):2382, 2002.

Kim TJ, Kim HS, Park CT, et al: Clinical evaluation of follow-up methods and results of atypical glandular cells of undetermined significance (AGUS) detected on cervicovaginal Pap smears, *Gynecol Oncol* 73(2):292, 1999.

Krumholz BA: Colposcopy in pregnancy: directed brush cytology compared with cervical biopsy, *Obstet Gynecol* 94(6):1054, 1999.

Li J, Rousseau MC, Franco EL, Ferenczy A: Is colposcopy warranted in women with external anogenital warts? *J Low Genital Tract* 7(1):22, 2003.

Lonky NM, Sadeghi M, Tsadik GW, Petitti D: The clinical significance of the poor correlation of cervical dysplasia and cervical malignancy with referral cytologic results, *Am J Obstet Gynecol* 181(3):560, 1999.

Mandelblatt JS, Lawrence WF, Womack SM, et al: Benefits and costs of using HPV testing to screen for cervical cancer, *JAMA* 287(18):2372, 2002.

Manetta A, Keefe K, Lin F, et al: Atypical glandular cells of undetermined significance in cervical cytologic findings, *Am J Obstet Gynecol* 180(4):883, 1999.

Massad LS, Meyer PM: Predicting compliance with follow-up recommendations after colposcopy among indigent urban women, *Obstet Gynecol* 94(3):371, 1999.

McKee MD, Lurio J, Marantz P, et al: Barriers to follow-up of abnormal Papanicolaou smears in an urban community health center, *Arch Fam Med* 8(2):129, 1999.

Melnikow J, Nuovo J, Willan AR, et al: Natural history of cervical squamous intraepithelial lesions: a meta-analysis, *Obstet Gynecol* 92(4 Pt 2):727, 1998.

Mitchell MF, Schottenfeld D, Tortolero-Luna G, et al: Colposcopy for the diagnosis of squamous intraepithelial lesions: a meta-analysis, *Obstet Gynecol* 91(4):626, 1998.

Moniak CW, Kutzner S, Adam E, et al: Endocervical curettage in evaluating abnormal cervical cytology, *J Reprod Med* 45:285, 2000.

Newkirk GR: Teaching colposcopy and androscopy in family practice residencies, *J Fam Pract* 31(2):171, 1990.

Pfenninger JL: Colposcopy in a family practice residency: the first 200 cases, *J Fam Pract* 34(67):67, 1992.

Pfenninger JL: Colposcopy, LEEP, and other procedures: the role for family physician, *Fam Med* 28(7):505, 1996.

Pretorius RG, Belinson JL, Zhang W: The colposcopic impression, *J Reprod Med* 46:724, 2001.

Reid R: Biology and colposcopic features of human papillomavirus—associated cervical disease, *Obstet Gynecol Clin North Am* 20(1):123, 1993.

Rodney WM, Felmar E, Morrison J, et al: Colposcopy and cervical cryotherapy: Feasible additions to the primary care physician's office practice, *Postgrad Med* 81(8):79, 1987.

Solomon D, Davey D, Kurman R, et al: The 2001 Bethesda System: terminology for reporting results of cervical cytology, *JAMA* 287(16):2114, 2002.

Shaw E, Sellors J, Kaczorowski J: Prospective evaluation of colposcopic features in predicting cervical intraepithelial neoplasia: degree of acetowhite change most important, *J Low Genital Tract* 7(1):6, 2003.

Stafl A, Wilbanks GD: An international terminology of colposcopy: report of the nomenclature committee of the International Federation of Cervical Pathology and Colposcopy, *Obstet Gynceol* 77(2):313, 1991.

Stewart DE, Lickrish GM, Sierra S, Parkin H: The effect of educational brochures on knowledge and emotional distress in women with abnormal Papanicolaou smears, *Obstet Gynecol* 81:280, 1993.

Stoler MH: New Bethesda terminology and evidence-based management guidelines for cervical cytology findings, *JAMA* 287(16):2140, 2002.

Stoler MH, Schiffman M: Interobserver reproducibility of cervical cytologic and histologic interpretations-realistic estimates from the ASCUS-CSIL Triage Study, *JAMA* 285:1500, 2001.

Wright TC Jr, Cox JT, Massad LS, et al: 2001 Consensus Guidelines for the management of women with cervical cytological abnormalities, *JAMA* 287(16):2120, 2002.

Wright VC, editor: Contemporary colposcopy. In *Obstetrics and gynecology clinics of North America,* vol 20, Philadelphia, 1993, WB Saunders.

Zahm DM, Nindl I, Greinke C, et al: Colposcopic appearance of cervical intraepithelial neoplasia is age dependent, *Am J Obstet Gynecol* 179(5):1298, 1998.

CHAPTER 140

Contraceptive Implants (Norplant): Insertion and Removal*

Ronald D. Reynolds

The Norplant System (levonorgestrel implants), the first sustained-release subdermal contraceptive delivery system, provides highly effective contraception for 5 to 7 years. This progestin-only contraceptive differs from the progestin-only "mini pill" in that it maintains a constant blood level of levonorgestrel.

The Norplant System was first marketed by Wyeth Laboratories in the United States in 1991. It was developed by the Population Council (which manufactures the implants in Finland) and has been in use elsewhere in the world since 1986. The system consists of six thin, flexible implants of soft silastic tubing sealed at each end with silicone. The implants are 3.4 cm long and 2.4 mm in diameter, and each contains 36 mg of dry, crystalline levonorgestrel. Placement involves a counseling visit, followed by a brief office procedure in which the implants are inserted in a fanlike pattern just beneath the skin of the distal medial upper arm.

Norplant has three possible mechanisms of action: (1) It suppresses ovulation in the majority of cycles by maintaining a consistently low level of progestin, (2) it creates an inhospitable uterine environment for ovum implantation, and (3) it prevents sperm penetration by increasing the viscosity of cervical mucus. Studies of women who continue using Norplant beyond the FDA-approved 5-year period show that if body weight is 150 pounds or less, there is continued contraceptive efficacy out to 7 years.

One significant concern about long-term contraceptives is whether women will continue to have their routine Pap smears. Clinicians should stress the necessity of annual Pap smears to patients using long-term contraceptive methods—even though they do not need a new prescription.

A few years after its release in the United States, Norplant became the focus of a large number of class action lawsuits alleging problems with counseling, side effects, and removal difficulties. Wyeth feels that these are baseless and is vigorously defending them in court. They have promised to defend any practitioners that become involved in these suits. Physicians should not be afraid to use this highly effective contraceptive option.

A further setback occurred in August 2000 when Wyeth embargoed a lot of Norplant because of worry over warehouse stability testing. As of September 2002, the lot in question has been shown to be problem free, but Wyeth has decided to stop marketing Norplant altogether in the United States. Norplant remains available in the rest of the world.

The litigation and embargo has held up the release of an already FDA-approved new version of Norplant (called Norplant 2 in the rest of the world), consisting of two solid levonorgestrel-impregnated rods that work for 3 to 5 years. Yet another implantable progestin *single* rod system called Implanon is also in clinical trials.

INDICATIONS

Norplant should be considered for women who:
- Desire long-term reversible contraception
- Are considering sterilization but are not ready to make the final decision
- Have difficulty remembering to take birth control pills daily
- Cannot tolerate other forms of contraception, such as birth control pills and coitus-dependent techniques (e.g., condoms, diaphragm)

---

*Editor's note: The Norplant System is no longer being offered to patients in the United States; however, this chapter is included here for completeness for physicians who may be following patients who now have Norplant implants inserted and for physicians in countries where it is still used.

- Cannot tolerate estrogen administration
- Have contraindications to IUD use (nulliparous, history of ectopic pregnancy or pelvic inflammatory disease, nonmonogamous relationship)

CONTRAINDICATIONS

- Possible pregnancy
- Active thrombophlebitis or thromboembolic disease
- Undiagnosed abnormal vaginal bleeding
- Acute liver disease
- Benign or malignant liver tumors
- Known or suspected carcinoma of the breast
- Unwillingness to accept metrorrhagia for at least 6 to 18 months or amenorrhea
- Excessive concern over the minimal scar that will occur at the site of placement and removal
- Lack of informed consent

EQUIPMENT

Insertion supplies

The Norplant System contains the following items in a *non-sterile tray, with each item in a sterile wrap:*
- Set of six Norplant implants
- Norplant insertion trocar
- Disposable no. 11 scalpel blade
- 6-ml syringe
- Two needles (18 and 22 gauge)
- Skin closure tapes
- Three packages of two 4 × 4–inch gauze sponges
- 3-inch roller gauze bandage
- Three surgical drapes (one is fenestrated)
- Forceps
- Patient booklets (one is informational; the other is a menstrual cycle diary)
- FDA patient insert, with tear-off consent attached

The inserting physician must provide:
- 6 ml of 1% or 2% lidocaine with or without epinephrine
- Sterile gloves
- Povidone-iodine (Betadine) solution
- Sterile water to wash off antiseptic when done
- Tape for the roller bandage

Optional, but highly recommended, supplies include the following:
- 1¼-inch, 27-gauge needle for infiltration of anesthetic
- Bicarbonate solution to neutralize the lidocaine
- "Bulldog" paper clamp to hold implants in package during opening
- Fan-shaped template (available from Wyeth)
- Skin marker

Removal Supplies

A minor skin surgery tray (as might be used for a skin biopsy) is used for removal. At a minimum, instruments include the following:
- No. 11 scalpel blade
- Straight and curved delicate hemostats (e.g., Miltex 7-8 and 7-10)
- Adson forceps

Depending on the removal procedure chosen, the following may also be needed:
- Norgrasp ring-tipped forceps (greatly simplifies procedure)
- No-scalpel vasectomy dissecting forceps

Disposable supplies include the following:
- Skin marker
- Local anesthetic supplies as for insertion
- Povidone-iodine (Betadine) solution
- Sterile gloves
- Sterile fenestrated drape
- 4 × 4–inch gauze sponges
- Skin closure tapes
- Sterile water to wash off antiseptic when done
- 3-inch roller gauze bandage
- Tape for the roller bandage

PREPROCEDURE PATIENT PREPARATION

To ensure that the patient is not pregnant, Norplant is generally placed during menses. Although the patient can be counseled and have Norplant inserted the same day, this entails an arduously long visit and might not give the patient time to fully consider her decision after becoming fully informed about risks and benefits. Consequently, the patient usually has separate counseling and placement visits.

When the patient schedules her counseling visit, she should receive an educational handout (see the sample patient education handout titled "Norplant System" on page 1929 of Appendix G) and a copy of the FDA patient insert from the manufacturer. Ask her to review these before the office visit and to come in early for the counseling visit to review an educational videotape (provided by Wyeth). Before the counseling visit, have the patient complete her portion of the encounter form (Fig. 140-1)

During the counseling visit, patients need to be informed of other choices for contraception such as the pill, patch, vaginal ring, IUD, depomedroxyprogesterone injections (Depo-Provera) and barrier methods, as well as permanent surgical contraception. The fact that Norplant offers no protection from sexually transmitted diseases must be emphasized. The clinician should review the effectiveness of Norplant and tell the patient

Patient Encounter Form
Norplant System

Patient to fill out:

Name _____   Date _____

Birth date _____ Age _____   Family doctor _____

Number of pregnancies _____   Last menstrual period _____

Miscarriages or abortions _____

Current contraceptive method _____

What contraception have you tried? _____

How long is your usual period? _____ days

Last Pap smear   date _____ result _____

Last physical/pelvic examination   date _____

When would you like to get pregnant again? _____

Have you ever had the following?

A pregnancy in your tubes?	Y	N	Any liver tumors?	Y	N
Infection in your tubes?	Y	N	A personal or family		
Any venereal disease?	Y	N	history of breast cancer?	Y	N
Genital warts?	Y	N	Any problems with		
An IUD?	Y	N	diabetes?	Y	N
Blood clots in your legs			Any problems with		
or a stroke?	Y	N	high cholesterol?	Y	N
Any type of liver disease?	Y	N	Any swelling in your legs?	Y	N
Any unusual vaginal bleeding?	Y	N	A low blood count?	Y	N

Did you read and understand the handouts we gave you?   Y   N

Did you see the Norplant videotape?   Y   N

For the doctor:

Model used to show insertion technique   Y   N

Effectiveness reviewed   Y   N

Advantages:

¥ Cost (includes counseling, insertion, follow-up)

¥ Lack of estrogen

¥ Good for 5 years

¥ Nothing to remember

¥ Reversible

Disadvantages/complications:

¥ Irregular bleeding/lack of periods

¥ Headache, nausea, weight gain, nervousness

¥ Insertion

¥ Removal

¥ Cysts

¥ Failure

¥ Costs

Contraindications: none or _____

Manual reviewed?   Y   N

Impression: _____

Plan: _____

Physician s signature _____ date _____

cc: _____

Fig. 140-1

Sample patient encounter form for the Norplant System. (Modified from Wyeth Pharmaceuticals Division of Wyeth, St. David's, Penn.)

that, although this method is not absolutely foolproof, it is one of the best contraceptive devices available, with a failure rate of less than 1%.

The clinician should discuss the advantages of Norplant, including the absence of estrogen, the long duration of effectiveness, reversibility, and the fact that nothing needs to be remembered daily as with birth control pills. Although the initial cost is high, Norplant costs less than birth control pills for the same duration. Overall, after 1 year, 81% of all patients continue to use Norplant. The implants do not interfere with activity in any way. Norplant is effective within 24 hours of insertion if inserted within 7 days after the onset of a menstrual period. For women weighing 150 lb or less, Norplant can provide continued contraception for 7 years (although FDA approval is for only up to 5 years).

The clinician should review the side effects and disadvantages of the Norplant system. Many of these are progestin-related, and a statement to the effect that "Norplant makes your body think it's pregnant" helps to explain them. Discussion should include the following:

Irregular bleeding. Almost all women can expect to experience an alteration of menstrual pattern during the first year. The menstrual cycle usually becomes more regular or the patient becomes amenorrheic within 6 to 18 months.

Headache, nausea, dizziness, fluid retention. Pregnancy-like effects.

Mood changes. Particularly irritability and depression.

Weight gain. Rare, but quite profound in some cases.

Acne and hair loss. Levonorgestrel has androgenic properties to which some women are sensitive.

Ovarian cysts. Can cause some discomfort but generally resolve on their own. Rarely clinically apparent.

Pregnancy. Rare, but possible. Patients need to obtain a pregnancy test if they miss their period once periods normalize or if pregnancy symptoms develop. Should pregnancy occur, the implants must be removed immediately, although there are no studies showing adverse effects on the fetus.

Thromboembolic phenomena. Low incidence; however, women who will be subjected to prolonged immobilization because of surgery or other illnesses should consider having the implants removed before surgery or receive thrombophlebitis prophylaxis.

Although cost is an advantage, it is also a disadvantage because the patient must pay the entire price initially. Premature removal of the implants resulting from side effects is also a disadvantage. The patient should be reassured that there is currently no known relationship between this method and any type of genital cancer or silicone problem. However, abnormal bleeding caused by the Norplant itself could mask bleeding from cervical or endometrial cancers.

If there are no contraindications and the patient indicates that she would like to use Norplant, the clinician should show her some sample implants and the site of insertion in the distal medial aspect of the nondominant upper arm. The clinician should briefly review how the implants are inserted and removed and tell the patient of the *surgical* effects and possible complications of insertion, including the following:

• Pain at the time of insertion, and afterwards (minimal)
• Bleeding
• Bruising
• Infection
• Damage to deep structures including blood vessels and nerves
• Skin damage if the implant is placed too superficially
• Reaction to the anesthetic
• Two small scars (one for insertion, one for removal)

Informed consent is a medicolegal necessity for any procedure, but especially for Norplant. The clinician should always document that the patient has read over both the patient education handout (see the sample patient education handout titled "Norplant System" on page 1929 of Appendix G) and the FDA patient package insert, and that the risks, benefits, possible complications, and alternatives have been discussed. The patient insert contained in each Norplant system has a detailed checklist for the patient to initial and sign as well as for the implanting physician to sign. It is highly recommended that this form be used in addition to the usual consent form.

If the patient has not had a Pap smear and pelvic examination within the past 6 months, these should be performed at this time. The patient's Pap smear should be normal before insertion of Norplant.

If she still desires placement after this full informed consent process, an appointment should be scheduled on a day that falls within 7 days after the start of her next menstrual period.

TECHNIQUE

Insertion

Wyeth standardizes the method of insertion, shown in the copy of the package insert (Fig. 140-2). Some important additional details follow:

1. The Norplant system's white tray is *not* sterile and cannot be used during the insertion process. Sterile fields (patient's arm, and side-table for instruments) must be created with the drapes provided in the kit. Sterile technique must be rigorously followed because a foreign body is being implanted.

2. Use of a fan-shaped template and skin marker before skin prep helps to ensure accurate place-

INSERTION PROCEDURE

Insertion should be performed within seven days from the onset of menses. However, NORPLANT SYSTEM capsules may be inserted at any time during the cycle provided pregnancy has been excluded and a nonhormonal contraceptive method is used for at least 7 days following insertion. It is recommended that a complete history and physical examination, including a gynecologic examination, be performed before the insertion of NORPLANT SYSTEM capsules. Determine if the subject has any allergies to the antiseptic or anesthetic to be used or contraindications to progestin-only contraception. If none are found, the capsules are inserted using the procedure outlined below.

One NORPLANT SYSTEM set consists of six capsules in a sterile pouch. The insertion is performed under aseptic conditions using a trocar to place the capsules under the skin.

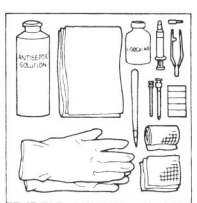

Figure 1: The following equipment is recommended for the insertion:
— an examining table for the patient to lie on.
— sterile surgical drapes, sterile gloves (free of talc), antiseptic solution.
— local anesthetic, needles, and syringe.
— #11 scalpel, #10 trocar, forceps.
— skin closure, sterile gauze, and compresses.
The plastic cover and tray are NOT STERILE.

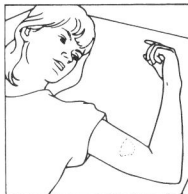

Figure 2: Have the patient lie on her back on the examination table with her left arm (if the patient is left-handed, the right arm) flexed at the elbow and externally rotated so that her hand is lying by her head. The capsules will be inserted subdermally through a small 2-mm incision and positioned in a fanlike manner with the fan opening towards the shoulder.

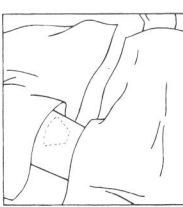

Figure 3: Prep the patient's upper arm with antiseptic solution; cover the arm above and below the insertion area with a sterile cloth. The optimal insertion area is in the inside of the upper arm about 8 to 10 cm above the elbow crease.

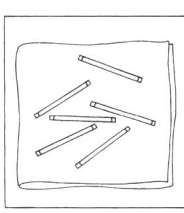

Figure 4: Open the sterile NORPLANT SYSTEM package carefully by pulling apart the sheets of the pouch, allowing the capsules to fall onto a sterile drape. Count the six capsules.

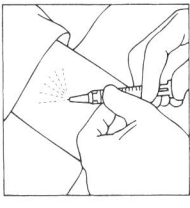

Figure 5: After determining the absence of known allergies to the anesthetic agent or related drugs, fill a 5-mL syringe with the local anesthetic. Since blood loss is minimal with this procedure, use of epinephrine-containing anesthetics is not considered necessary. Anesthetize the insertion area by first inserting the needle under the skin and injecting a small amount of anesthetic. Then anesthetize six areas about 4 to 4.5 cm long, to mimic the fanlike position of the implanted capsules.

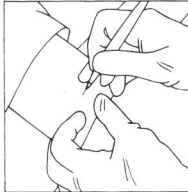

Figure 6: Use the scalpel to make a small incision (about 2 mm) just through the dermis of the skin. Alternatively, the trocar may be inserted directly through the skin without making an incision with the scalpel. The bevel of the trocar should always face up during the insertion.

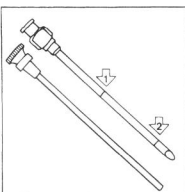

Figure 7: The trocar has two marks on it. The first mark is closer to the hub and indicates how far the trocar should be introduced under the skin before the loading of each capsule. The second mark is close to the tip and indicates how much of the trocar should remain under the skin following the insertion of each implant.

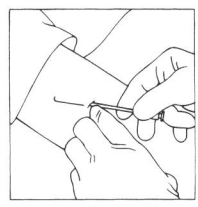

Figure 8: Insert the tip of the trocar through the incision beneath the skin at a shallow angle. Once the trocar is inserted, it should be oriented with the bevel up toward the skin to keep the capsules in a superficial plane. It is important to keep the trocar subdermal by tenting the skin with the trocar, as failure to do so may result in deep placement of the capsules and could make removal more difficult. Advance the trocar gently under the skin to the first mark near the hub of the trocar. The tip of the trocar is now at a distance of about 4 to 4.5 cm from the incision.
Do not force the trocar, and if resistance is felt, try another direction.

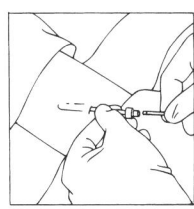

Figure 9: When the trocar has been inserted the appropriate distance, remove the obturator and load the first capsule into the trocar using the thumb and forefinger.

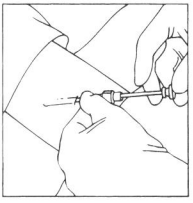

Figure 10: Gently advance the capsule with the obturator towards the tip of the trocar until you feel resistance. Never force the obturator.

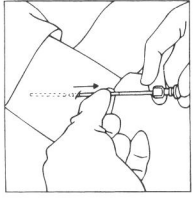

Figure 11: Hold the obturator steady, and bring the trocar back until it touches the handle of the obturator.

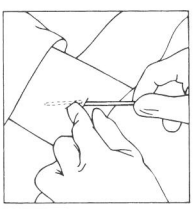

Figure 12: The capsule should have been released under the skin when the mark close to the tip of the trocar is visible in the incision. Release of the capsule can be checked by palpation. It is important to keep the obturator steady and not to push the capsule into the tissue.

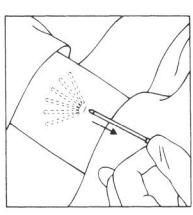

Figure 13: Do not remove the trocar from the incision until all capsules have been inserted. The trocar is withdrawn only to the mark close to its tip. Each succeeding capsule is always inserted next to the previous one, to form a fanlike shape. Fix the position of the previous capsule with the forefinger and middle finger of the free hand, and advance the trocar along the tips of the fingers. This will ensure a suitable distance of about 15 degrees between capsules and keep the trocar from puncturing any of the previously inserted capsules.
Leave a distance of about 5 mm between the incision and the tips of the capsules. This will help avoid spontaneous expulsions. The correct position of the capsules can be ensured by feeling them with the fingers after the insertion has been completed.

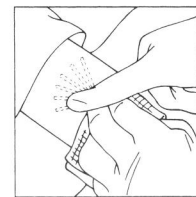

Figure 14: After placement of the sixth capsule, a sterile gauze may be used to apply pressure briefly to the insertion site to ensure hemostasis. Palpate the distal ends of the capsules to make sure that all six have been properly placed.

Fig. 140-2
Norplant System insertion technique, from the package insert. (Courtesy Wyeth Pharmaceuticals Division of Wyeth, St. David's, Penn.)
Continued

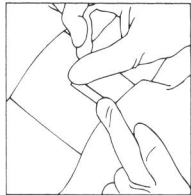

Figure 15: Press the edges of the incision together, and close the incision with a skin closure. Suturing the incision should not be necessary.

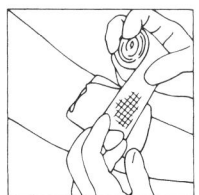

Figure 16: Cover the insertion area with a dry compress, and wrap gauze around the arm to ensure hemostasis.

Observe the patient for a few minutes for signs of syncope or bleeding from the incision before she is discharged.

Advise the patient to keep the insertion area dry and avoid heavy lifting for 2 to 3 days. The gauze may be removed after 1 day, and the butterfly bandage as soon as the incision has healed, i.e., normally in 3 days.

HINTS
Insertion
— Counselling of the patient on the benefits and side effects of the method prior to insertion will greatly increase patient satisfaction.
— Correct subdermal placement of the capsules will facilitate removal.
— Before insertion, apply the anesthetic just beneath the skin so as to raise the dermis above the underlying tissue.
— Never force the trocar.
— To ensure subdermal placement, the trocar with bevel up should be supported by the index finger and should visibly raise the skin at all times during insertion.
— To avoid damaging the previous implanted capsule, stabilize the capsule with your forefinger and middle finger and advance the trocar alongside the finger tips at an angle of 15 degrees.
— After insertion, make a drawing for the patient's file showing the location of the 6 capsules and describe any variations in placement. This will greatly aid removal.

Fig. 140-2, cont'd
(Courtesy Wyeth Pharmaceuticals Division of Wyeth, St. David's, Penn.)

ment. If the patient is very thin, rotate the fan posteriorly toward the triceps to prevent the upper tip of the rightmost (in a left arm placement) implant from causing pain by impinging on the biceps.

3. To prevent the assistant from flinging the implants into the air while opening the long implant bag, place a Bulldog paper clamp halfway up the implants on the outside of the bag (Fig. 140-3). The implants have a tendency to stick to the wrap. When the bag is opened, the upper half of the implants are exposed to grasp but cannot be ejected without releasing the clamp.

4. There is controversy over the use of lidocaine *with* epinephrine. This was reported to cause cutaneous ulcerations in one three-patient case report, but there are other possible explanations for these cases. Many physicians use lidocaine with epinephrine without problems and find that it safely minimizes postoperative bruising.

5. When making the skin incision, do not push the no. 11 blade in deep enough to complete the incision in one motion. To do so could bring the tip close to the brachial artery as well as the ulnar and median nerves. Instead, use a shallow sawing motion to lengthen the incision after skin entry.

6. Correct subdermal placement of the implants will facilitate easy removal. To ensure this the obturator must be inside the trocar and the bevel must be up as the trocar is advanced. The skin should be visibly tented up at all times during trocar advancement. *Stay superficial* (subdermal) even though this typically requires slightly more force to insert than deeper subcutaneous insertion.

7. Do not push on the obturator to release the implant into the skin; this will create a corkscrew implant that is difficult to remove. The trocar creates a tract in the tissue for the implant. The obturator pushes the implant down just until it is at the end of the trocar. The obturator then simply holds the implant

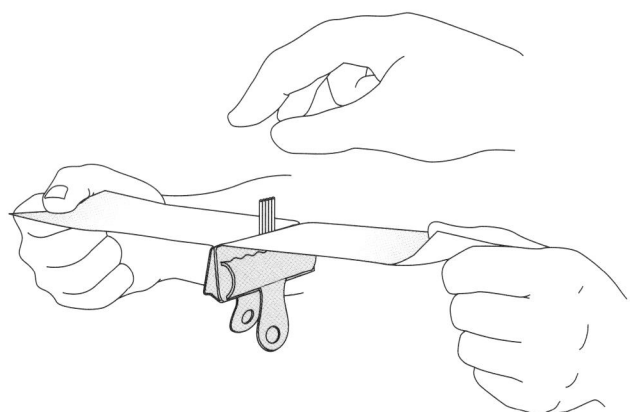

Fig. 140-3
Use of a Bulldog paper clamp to hold the implants in their sterile bag during opening.

in place while the trocar is pulled back, depositing it into the tissue.

8. There are two circular ringed grooves on the trocar. These indicate how far to insert and withdraw the trocar. As the trocar is withdrawn to the mark near the tip, the implant should be felt falling from the tip. If this does not happen, the trocar must be actively disengaged from the implant by withdrawing slightly, then depressing the trocar tip, and sliding the tip over towards the next intended tract. To ensure that the implant can disengage easily, the trocar must be held with the bevel up. The secret to this is to keep the "10" stamped into the trocar hub always facing upward.

9. Do not remove the trocar from the incision between insertions or the implants will end up in different tissue planes and will be difficult to remove.

10. Place your index finger over each newly inserted implant to prevent the trocar (with obturator in place) from catching on it as you readvance the trocar (Fig. 140-2, *12*). If the trocar catches an

implant, it could damage it or force its distal end back up the arm, creating a U-shaped implant that will be difficult to remove.

11. *Before inserting the implants, always count with the patient to be sure that there are indeed six implants present. After insertion, palpate to again identify all six* subdermal implants. If implants are dropped or the patient expels an implant, they can be returned to Wyeth for a free replacement.

12. Use a sterile water–soaked gauze to *remove antiseptic from the arm after the procedure.* The skin closure tape will stick better, and the patient will not have to endure a week of cracked brown skin at the site.

Complications of Insertion

Most patients have a large but minimally painful ecchymotic area around the site of insertion, which can be expected to resolve within approximately 2 weeks. Applying ice to the area immediately after insertion and using epinephrine in the anesthetic may minimize this.

Infection around the area of insertion is very uncommon (0.7%). However, if infection does occur, a trial of a first-generation cephalosporin such as cefadroxil may be attempted. If not successful, or if there is abscess formation, the implants should be removed and the area allowed to heal. Whether all implants need to be removed or not is the decision of the physician. Whenever less than six implants are in place, the woman must use another method of contraception.

Expulsion of an implant can occur. This is more common if the placement is too shallow or if infection occurs at the time of insertion. If any part of an implant is exposed through the skin, it *must* be removed. A new sterile implant must be placed, since less than six implants do not provide adequate contraception.

Removal

Removal can be more difficult and often takes more time than insertion. Within a few weeks of placement the implants become surrounded with a fibrous envelope. This must be opened to deliver the implant, so being able to grasp the implant is only part of the challenge.

Wyeth initially recommended only the Population Council method shown in Fig. 140-4. This uses a curved and straight hemostat to grasp the implants for removal. In experienced hands, this often takes about 20 minutes.

Since removals can be difficult at times, a number of innovative methods have been developed. The "Modified U" technique and the Pop Out method are detailed later, along with some comments on how to deal with difficult removals.

Regardless of the method chosen, all implants should be palpated and marked on the skin before removal. The patient's arm needs to be in the same position as when they were placed, and she should verify this arm placement before removal. A few moments of preplanning can save significant operative time. If U-shaped or corkscrewed implants are found, the incision may need to be moved or a second incision planned. If one or more implants are not palpable, the patient can be referred to a practitioner with experience in removing difficult implants.

Anesthesia and Skin Prep

All removal methods require infiltration anesthesia. For the most bloodless view possible, 1% lidocaine with epinephrine is used. Buffering of the lidocaine and injecting through a 27-gauge needle minimize pain for the patient. Infiltration only needs to be performed in areas that will be manipulated during the removal, not along the entire length of the implant. If anesthetic volume is restricted to no more than 3 ml and the implants have each been marked, infiltration on top of the implants (where the nerve endings are) is acceptable. Otherwise, infiltration should be performed underneath the implants. Use of too much anesthetic can obscure palpation of the rods.

The skin is prepped with Betadine *after* anesthesia, and a sterile fenestrated drape is applied. This allows time for good anesthesia onset.

Population Council Method

Fig. 140-4 shows step-by-step instructions for the Population Council method. Dissection with a hemostat around the tips of the implants frees up the area to ease removal. Use of fine-tipped, extra delicate, mosquito hemostats (e.g., Miltex 7-8 [straight] and 7-10 [curved]) makes dissection much easier.

Frequently, the implant tip cannot be pushed down into the newly made incision, so it must be grasped by palpation through the incision with the upfacing tips of the curved hemostat. Traction is then applied. Unfortunately, the skin is often grasped along with the implant, making the implant difficult to withdraw.

Only the tip of the implant has a thicker section of material that is durable enough to be grasped with a hemostat. Incision of the fibrous envelope that surrounds the implant can be done readily at the tip with a no. 11 blade. However, along the implant's shaft, great care must be exercised to not tear or break the implant.

"Modified U" Technique

The "Modified U" technique is the author's method of choice for removal. It has three advantages: a positive grasp on the implant, the ability to go after a line (the implant's shaft) rather than a point in space (the tip), and ease of removal even during difficult procedures. Removal times are 5 to 10 minutes in experienced hands. A number of studies have shown that it is easier to learn and quicker to perform than the Population Council

REMOVAL PROCEDURE

Described below is a removal procedure which was developed and used during the clinical trials for the NORPLANT SYSTEM. As with many surgical procedures, variations of the technique have appeared and some have been published. No one particular procedure routinely appears to have any advantage over another.

It is recommended that removals be prescheduled so that preparations for carrying out the procedure can be facilitated.

Removal of the capsules should be performed very gently and will usually take more time than insertion. Capsules are sometimes nicked, cut, or broken during removal. The incidence of overall removal difficulties, including damage to capsules, has been 13.2 percent. Less than half of these removal difficulties have caused inconvenience to the patient. If the removal of some of the capsules proves difficult, have the patient return for another visit. The remaining capsule(s) will be easier to remove after the area is healed. It may be appropriate to seek consultation or provide referral for patients in whom initial attempts at capsule removal prove difficult. If contraception is still desired, a barrier method should be advised until all capsules are removed. The position of the patient and the asepsis are the same as for insertion.

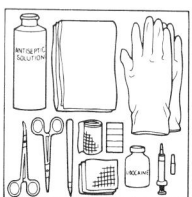

Figure 17: The following equipment is needed for the removal:
— an examining table for the patient to lie on.
— sterile surgical drapes, sterile gloves (free of talc), antiseptic solution.
— local anesthetic, needles, and syringe.
— #11 scalpel, forceps (straight and curved mosquito).
— skin closure, sterile gauze, and compresses.

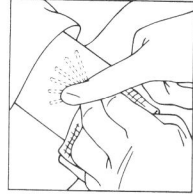

Figure 18: Palpate the capsules to make sure that all six capsules have been located, marking their position with a sterile marker. If all six capsules cannot be palpated, they may be localized via ultrasound (7 MHz), X ray, or compression mammography.

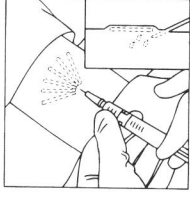

Figure 19: Once all six capsules are located, apply a small amount of local anesthetic *under* the capsule ends nearest the original incision site. This will serve to raise the ends of the capsules. Anesthetic injected over the capsules will obscure them and make removal more difficult. Additional small amounts of the anesthetic can be used for the removal of each of the capsules, if required.

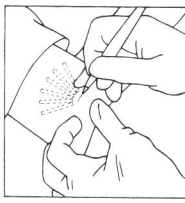

Figure 20: Make a 4-mm incision with the scalpel close to the ends of the capsules. Do not make a large incision.

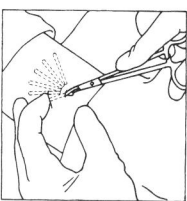

Figure 21: Push each capsule gently towards the incision with the fingers. When the tip is visible or near to the incision, grasp it with a mosquito forceps.

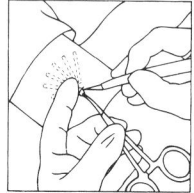

Figure 22: Use the scalpel, forceps, or gauze to very gently open the tissue sheath that has formed around the capsule.

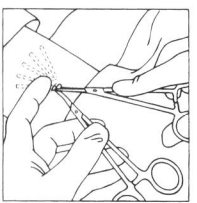

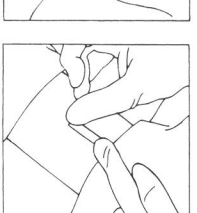

Figures 23 and 24: Remove the capsule from the incision with the second forceps.

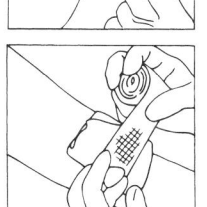

Figures 25 and 26: After the procedure is completed, the incision is closed and bandaged as with insertion. The upper arm should be kept dry for a few days. Following removal, fertility rates return to levels comparable to those seen in the general population of women using no method of contraception, and a pregnancy may occur at any time. If the patient wishes to continue using the method, a new set of NORPLANT SYSTEM capsules can be inserted through the same incision in the same or opposite direction.

HINTS
Removal
— Alternate removal techniques have been developed.
— The removal of the implanted capsules will usually take a little more time than the insertion.
— Before initiating removal, all capsules should be located by palpation. If all six capsules cannot be palpated, they may be localized via ultrasound (7 MHz), X ray, or compression mammography.
— Before removal, apply the anesthetic *under* the capsule ends nearest the original incision site.
— If the removal of some of the capsules proves difficult, interrupt the procedure and have the patient return for another visit. The remaining capsule(s) will be easier to remove after the area is healed.
— It may be appropriate to seek consultation or provide referral for patients in whom initial attempts at capsule removal prove difficult.

Fig. 140-4

Norplant System Population Council removal technique, from the package insert. (Courtesy Wyeth Pharmaceuticals Division of Wyeth, St. David's, Penn.)

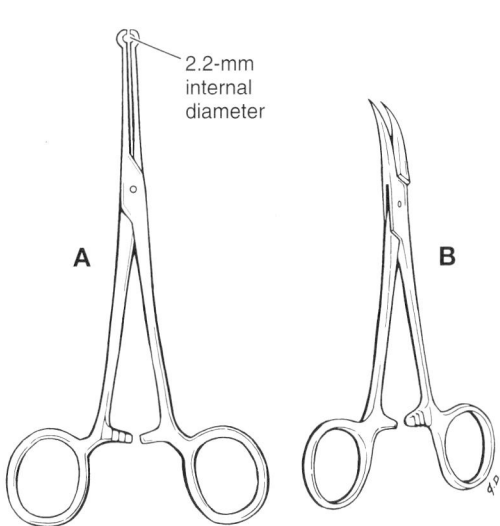

Fig. 140-5
A, Norgrasp forceps and, **B,** no-scalpel vasectomy dissecting forceps used for the "Modified U" technique. (Courtesy Jef Dirig, Cleveland, Okla.; originally appeared in Reynolds RD: *J Fam Pract* 40:173, 1995.)

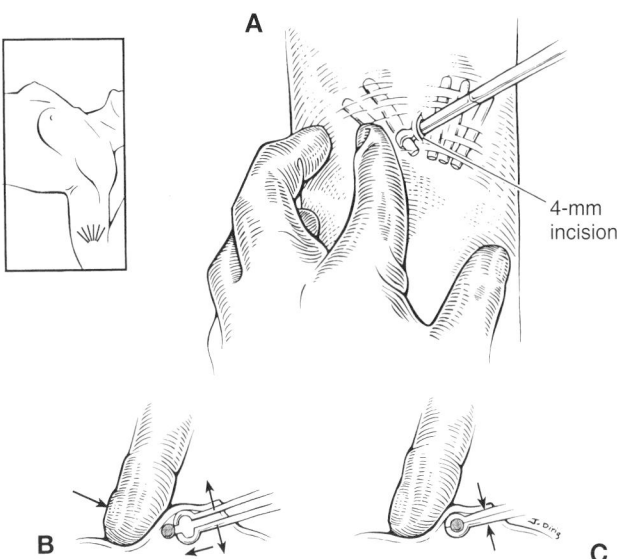

Fig. 140-6
A-C, Grasping the implant by palpation using Norgrasp forceps. See text for details. (Courtesy Jef Dirig, Cleveland, Okla.; originally appeared in Reynolds RD: *J Fam Pract* 40:173, 1995.)

method. Two specialized instruments are used for the "Modified U" technique: (1) Norgrasp forceps and (2) no-scalpel vasectomy dissecting (NSV) forceps (Fig. 140-5).

Use a skin-marking pen to mark the location of a 4-mm incision parallel to the implants, between implants 3 and 4. Place the distal end of the *mark* about 5 mm proximal to the distal end of the *implant tips*. Make a 4-mm-long shallow stab incision at the premarked location with a no. 11 scalpel blade. Use the fine-tipped curved delicate hemostat to bluntly dissect a 4- to 5-mm-wide tissue plane both superficial and deep to the shafts of all the implants through the incision.

Using Norgrasp forceps, grasp each implant somewhere along its shaft (Fig. 140-6, *A*, shows removal from the left upper arm). If an implant can be seen directly in the incision, it is simply grasped in the ring tip under direct vision. This can often be done with implants 3 and 4.

To grasp implants that can only be palpated, place your nondominant index finger along the axis of, and just lateral to, the closest palpable implant. Close—but do not lock—the Norgrasp forceps and insert the tip through the incision. Advance the closed ring tip until it touches the implant. As the forceps is opened, use your palpating finger to push the implant into the grasp of the ring tip (Fig. 140-6, *B*). Close and lock the forceps around the implant (Fig. 140-6, *C*).

After the implant is firmly grasped, apply traction to bring it to the incision. When the ring is visible in the incision, direct the handles of the Norgrasp forceps toward the patient's shoulder. If the grasp is within 4 to

5 mm of the tip, the tip itself may deliver out of the incision (Fig. 140-7). More often, a few millimeters of the implant's shaft is exposed in the inferior end of the incision.

The tissue envelope that surrounds the implant must be opened before the implant is free to be removed. NSV dissecting forceps are used both for this task and to deliver the implant. If the *tip* has delivered out, use the left blade of the dissecting forceps to sharply puncture the surrounding tissue envelope at the center of the implant's tip (Fig. 140-8, *A*). The depth of this puncture is about 1 to 2 mm, through the tissue envelope and into the thick end of the implant. After withdrawing the left blade, close but do not lock the blades and insert them in the hole just made (Fig. 140-8, *B*). Stretch open the envelope by opening the blades, exposing the bare end of the implant (Fig. 140-8, *C*). Rotate the dissector clockwise around its long axis until its blades curve upwards. Push the envelope back along the shaft of the implant with the blades (Fig. 140-8, *D*), and then grasp the implant itself (Fig. 140-8, *E*). Unlock the Norgrasp forceps, which frees the implant for removal, and pull it out.

More commonly, the *shaft* of the implant will be exposed in the incision. Use a 4 × 4–inch gauze pad to wipe toward yourself along the incision, further exposing the implant in its tissue envelope. In this situation, the closed blade tips of the dissecting forceps work well to tear the tissue envelope open along the axis of the implant (Fig. 140-9, *A*). The exposed bare implant has a characteristic shiny surface unlike the tissue envelope. If it is unclear

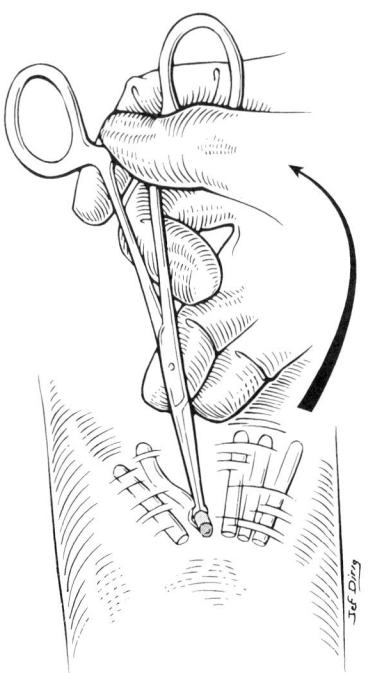

Fig. 140-7
Rotation of Norgrasp forceps toward the shoulder to expose the implant. (Courtesy Jef Dirig, Cleveland, Okla.; originally appeared in Reynolds RD: *J Fam Pract* 40:173, 1995.)

whether the envelope is open, rub the closed dissecting forceps tips on top of what appears to be the bare implant. If a tissue layer is still present, it will move with the tips. The implant surface itself will not move.

The envelope opening needs to be enlarged to allow the implant to be lifted out. Hold the closed dissecting forceps with the blade's curve facing downwards and your index finger on the hinge for better control. Place the blade tips in the plane between the implant and left side of the opening in the tissue envelope. When the forceps blades are opened along the axis of the implant, the tissue envelope opening will be enlarged (Fig. 140-9, *B*). Stretch the length of the opening to twice the width of the implant.

Skewer and deliver the implant through the opening in the tissue envelope. Hold the dissecting forceps with the blade's curve facing downwards and open them. Firmly skewer the implant with the right blade in the center of the envelope opening (Fig. 140-9, *C*). The blade tip punctures the front wall of the implant and enters its cavity by 2 to 3 mm. Rotate the forceps 180 degrees clockwise along its axis by supinating the hand to palm up (Fig. 140-9, *D*) to hang a small loop of the implant on the now upwards-facing forceps blade tip (Fig. 140-9, *E*).

Close the forceps to gently hold the implant. To avoid cutting through the Silastic material, do not lock the instrument. Be careful not to apply too much lifting force at this point. The implant will not lift very far since it is still constrained by the Norgrasp ring. Release the

Fig. 140-8
A-E, Use of the no-scalpel dissecting forceps to deliver an implant if the tip pops out. See text for details. (Courtesy Jef Dirig, Cleveland, Okla.; originally appeared in Reynolds RD: *J Fam Pract* 40:173, 1995.)

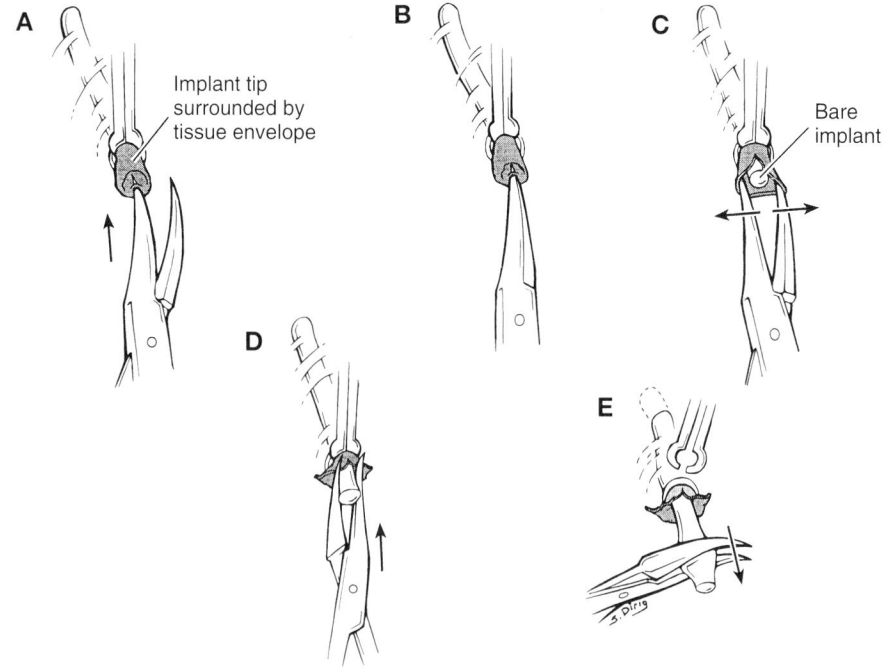

Norgrasp forceps to allow delivery of the implant as a U-shaped loop (Fig. 140-9, *F*).

The remainder of the implants are removed in the same manner. They usually come out in a 3-2-1-4-5-6 order. After removing the antiseptic, close the wound with a skin closure tape and apply a sterile bandage. This bandage is left in place for 24 hours, and the skin closure tape is allowed to fall off on its own. The wound should be kept dry for 24 hours.

Pop-Out Method

The pop-out method is an "instrument-free" technique that works well for very superficial, well-placed, easily palpable implants. Removal times are in the 15- to 20-minute range in experienced hands.

Make the 4-mm incision very close to the implant's lower tips. Apply digital pressure with your non-dominant hand to the proximal end of an implant, pushing it down to the incision (Fig. 140-10, *A*). Manipulate the skin to guide the lower tip into the incision. When the tip becomes visible, use the no. 11 scalpel blade to open the tissue envelope surrounding the tip (Fig. 140-10, *B*). Continued digital pressure on the far end pushes the implant out to where it can be grasped in the fingers or with forceps and removed (Fig. 140-10, *C*). Closure of the wound and postoperative instructions are the same as the other removal techniques.

Tips for Difficult Removals

Norplant removal is essentially six separate procedures in one. It is not unusual for one or more implants to be difficult to remove. Experienced clinicians often use a combination of the above methods during the same procedure. For all techniques, further dissection around a difficult implant can often help, especially if the implant is attached to the underside of the skin.

- If an implant is deeply placed, it can be lifted up to the skin surface with the proximal blades of the Norgrasp ring. When the ring is withdrawn, the implant will drop. It can be guided by the palpating finger into the ring for removal (Fig. 140-11).
- If the implants seem excessively deep, a needle can be placed perpendicularly underneath the midshaft of the implants to prop them up toward the skin and stabilize them.
- If a poorly placed implant is found on initial palpation, the "Modified U" technique is best suited for the removal because a single incision can usually be placed in a nontraditional location and still allow removal of all the implants.
- If one implant cannot be palpated at the start, and the clinician feels confident in his or her removal skills, it is reasonable to proceed with removal. Often, the "hidden" implant is next to or under another, and it becomes apparent during the procedure.

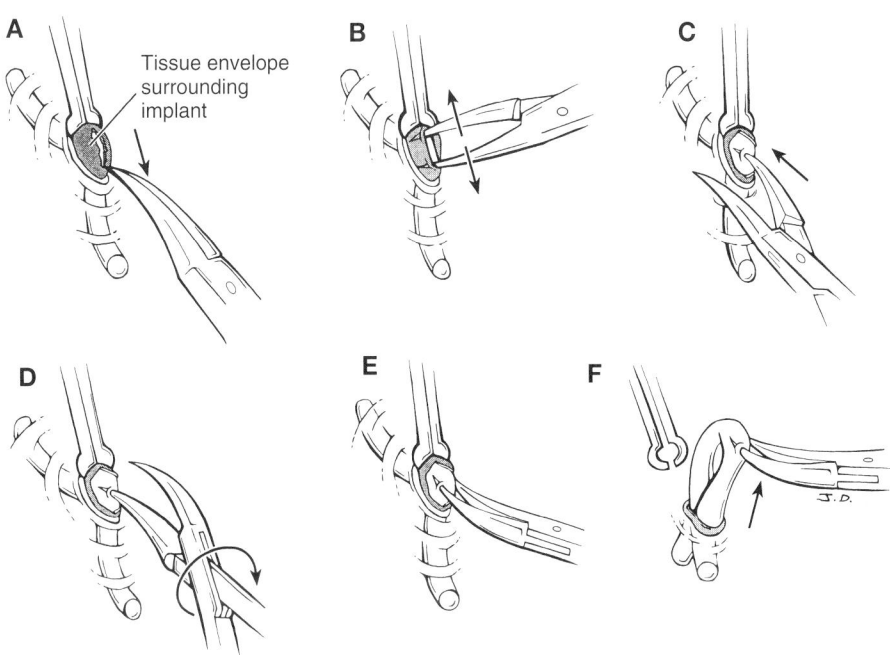

Fig. 140-9
A-F, Use of the no-scalpel dissecting forceps to deliver an implant if the shaft is grasped. See text for details. (Courtesy Jef Dirig, Cleveland, Okla.; originally appeared in Reynolds RD: *J Fam Pract* 40:173, 1995.)

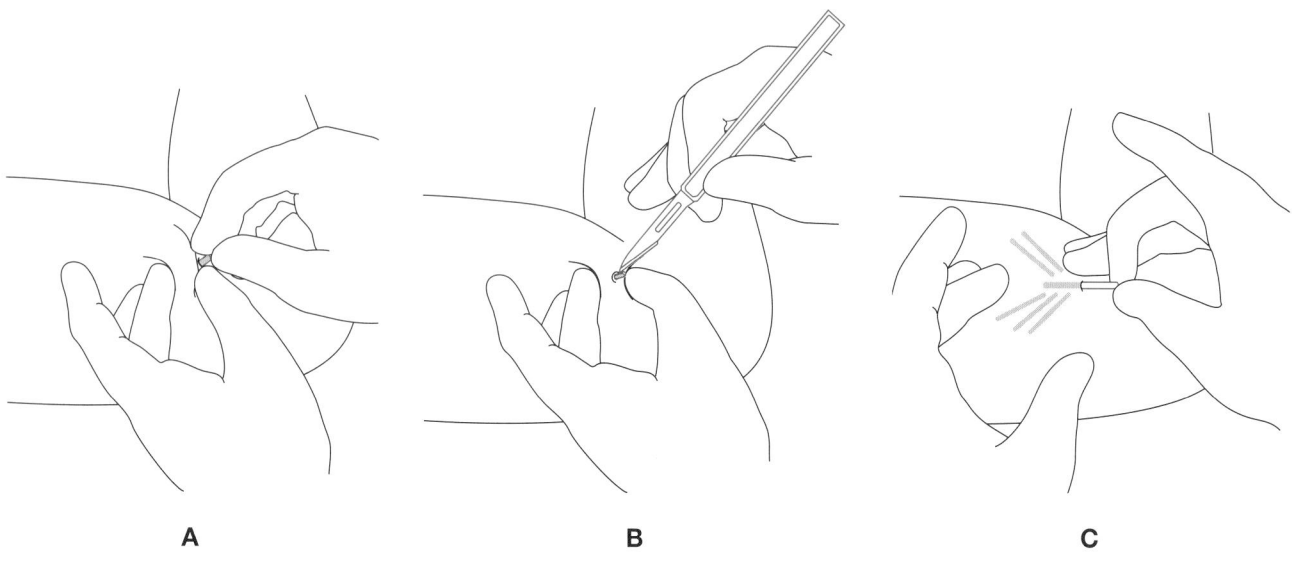

A **B** **C**

Fig. 140-10
A-C, Pop-out method of Norplant removal. See text for details.

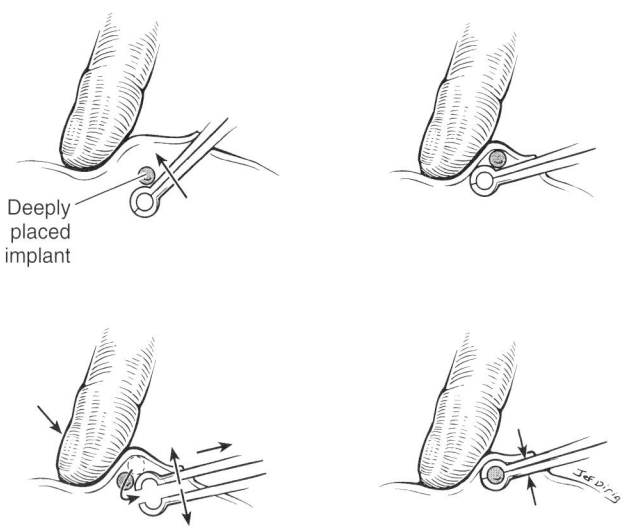

Deeply
placed
implant

Fig. 140-11
Norgrasp forceps used to lift and deliver a deeply placed implant.
(Courtesy Jef Dirig, Cleveland, Okla.; originally appeared in Reynolds
RD: *J Fam Pract* 40:173, 1995.)

- If the sixth implant cannot be located after some effort during the procedure, the clinician should *stop* and use an imaging study to find it. Excessive dissection can very rarely traumatize the brachial artery, or the ulnar or median nerves, with devastating consequences.

- Compression mammography techniques and ultrasound work best for finding a lost implant. Implants do not show up well on plain films. The "mammogram" film needs to be taken in the same arm position in which the implants were placed, but with the patient standing. A BB taped over the insertion incision provides a landmark. The disadvantages of "mammography" are lack of depth information and interference of the localization by the humerus.

- Ultrasound with a 7-MHz linear array transducer and a standoff pad will show the implant in cross section as a ring with posterior acoustic shadowing, and axially as two parallel lines. Lower frequencies do not focus well close to the skin surface. The ultrasonographer should relax pressure on the transducer once the implants are found to provide an accurate depth. A permanent surgical marker can localize the implant on the skin to ease removal.

- A deep implant, once localized and the depth determined, can often be removed by making a 4-mm incision with a no. 11 blade over the midshaft, dissecting to the implant with a delicate straight hemostat, and grasping it for removal with Norgrasp forceps.

- Ultrasound during a difficult removal may not be helpful because of gas within the tissues. The area should heal for a week or so before getting the preoperative localization study.

- Wyeth maintains a Norplant System Consultants Network (1-800-922-0877) of experienced clinicians who can assist with difficult removals. This same number can be used to request instruction and patient education materials as well as to answer any questions about Norplant.

Complications of Removal

- Most patients have little to no pain after removal.
- As with any minor skin procedure, infection can occur. This can be managed with a first-generation cephalosporin.
- Bleeding is rare but some bruising (although less than with insertion) generally occurs.
- The worrisome (but extremely rare) complications of removal are damage to deep structures such as the brachial artery, cephalic vein, and median and ulnar nerves. If these develop, immediate consultation with a vascular surgeon or neurosurgeon is indicated.

Reinsertion

Reinsertion can be carried out at the same location, usually on the same visit. The "Modified U" removal technique is especially well suited for this, since the incision for removal becomes the insertion site about 1.5 cm up the arm from the original set. For sterility's sake, it is wise to redrape and reglove between removal and reinsertion. There is no need to use the opposite arm or to place the implants in the opposite direction during reinsertion. The patient should be prepared for 6 to 18 months of irregular bleeding again, since levonorgestrel levels will be higher from the new implants.

CONCLUSION

Norplant is a highly effective progestational contraceptive that is well suited for the woman who desires 5 to 7 years of reversible contraception but has difficulty with remembering daily medication or does not like coitus-dependent methods. It offers no STD protection. Attention to detail in the insertion procedure eases removal difficulties. A number of removal techniques are available to suit almost any situation.

SUPPLIERS

Norplant System professional assistance, including patient educational supplies, training, and free Norgrasp forceps

Wyeth Laboratories
Philadelphia, PA
Phone: 1-800-922-0877

Norgrasp forceps and no-scalpel vasectomy dissecting forceps

Advanced Meditech International
86-20 53rd Avenue, Suite A
Flushing, NY 11373
Phone: 1-800-635-2452
Website: www.ameditech.com

Extra delicate 5-inch Halsted mosquito hemostats (straight is 7-8, curved is 7-10)

Miltex Instrument Co., Inc.
700 Hicksville Road
Bethpage, NY 11714
Phone: 1-800-645-8000

Bulldog paper clamp

Any local office supply store

CPT/BILLING CODES

11975   Insertion, implantable contraceptive capsules
11976   Removal, implantable contraceptive capsules
11977   Removal with reinsertion, implantable contraceptive capsules

Many states have their own "X" codes for Medicaid Norplant billing. These codes divide the charges into separate kit and professional parts, and they sometimes distinguish between procedure locations, giving a facility charge to hospitals and proportionally reducing the professional charge at this location.

ICD-9-CM DIAGNOSTIC CODES

V25.02   Contraception, counseling of specific agent NEC
V25.5   Contraception, insertion of subdermal implantable
V25.43   Contraception, surveillance of subdermal implantable
V45.52   Contraception, device in situ subdermal

ADDITIONAL RESOURCES

- See the sample patient education handout titled "Norplant System" on page 1929 of Appendix G.

BIBLIOGRAPHY

Burns EA, Driscoll CE: Norplant insertion and removal, *Patient Care* March 15:69, 1995.

Darney PD, Klaise CM, Walker DM: The "Pop-out" method of Norplant removal, *Adv Contracept* 8:188, 1992.

Flattum-Riemers J: Norplant: a new contraceptive, *Am Fam Physician* 44:103, 1991.

Gu S, Sivin I, Du M, et al: Effectiveness of Norplant implants through seven years: a large-scale study in China, *Contraception* 52:99, 1995.

Nelson AL, Sinow RN: Real-time ultrasonographically guided removal of nonpalpable and intramuscular Norplant capsules, *Am J Obstet Gynecol* 178:1185, 1998.

Praptohardjo U, Wibowo S: The "U" technique: a new method for Norplant implants removal, *Contraception* 48:526, 1993.

Reynolds RD: The "Modified U" technique: a refined method of Norplant removal, *J Fam Pract* 40:173, 1995.

Wyeth-Ayerst Laboratories: Norplant System Video Library for the Health Care Professional, Philadelphia, 1995.

Zuber TJ, DeWitt DE, Patton DD: Skin damage associated with the Norplant contraceptive, *J Fam Pract* 34:613, 1992.

CHAPTER 141

Cryotherapy of the Cervix

Madeline R. Lewis
John L. Pfenninger

Cryotherapy is the treatment of choice for select cervical intraepithelial lesions. This procedure is easy to learn, well tolerated by the patient, and has a success rate of 85% to 94%. It requires a refrigerant gas under pressure, such as nitrous oxide, and a hollow applicator probe. The cryoprobe allows rapid freezing of cervical tissue, causing a controlled destruction of the transformation zone and the epithelial lesion. Cellular destruction is greatest when a rapid freeze, slow thaw, and refreeze method is used. This procedure has few complications, can be performed quickly, is low in cost, and preserves cervical tissue.

Cryotherapy treats cervical dysplasia by destroying the lesion and the transformation zone. Cell death occurs as a result of ice crystal penetration into the intracellular space. The depth of destruction is directly proportional to the lateral spread of the freeze, which is measured by the size of the ice ball that forms around the tip of the cryoprobe. An ice ball of 5 to 7 mm will result in adequate cellular destruction, since severe dysplasia (CIN III) can extend to a depth of about 3 to 5 mm into the glands within the transformation zone. The frequency and depth of gland involvement seems to be directly proportional to the grade of the squamous intraepithelial lesion. However, the overall success of cryotherapy is related more to the size of the lesion than the grade of the lesion. Low-grade and small high-grade lesions may be adequately treated with cryotherapy. The lesion should be less than 3 cm in diameter (some recommend less than 2 cm), involve no more than two quadrants of the cervix, and extend less than or up to 5 mm into the endocervical canal. Large high-grade lesions, microinvasive, or invasive lesions need more aggressive treatment such as loop electrosurgical excision procedure (LEEP), conization, or even hysterectomy.

Treatment failures do occur with cryotherapy as with any other treatment modality. "Cure rates" have been in the 95% range for CIN I and CIN II which is consistent with other modalities. For CIN II, it drops to 89% overall but this has been correlated more to lesion size and depth, not to severity of disease. High-grade lesions are often larger in size and extend deeper down into the glands making them more difficult to treat.

INDICATIONS

Cryotherapy may be used for treatment of squamous dysplasia that was confirmed with a biopsy after a complete and adequate colposcopic examination. *It is essential* that the Pap smear results, the appearance of the cervix upon colposcopic examination, and the histologic report from the biopsy do not vary more than one degree of severity. That is, colposcopic impression and histologic findings can only be one degree less than the Pap smear. If there is "lack of correlation," this must be resolved or a conization of the cervix is indicated because it presumed the most advanced lesion has not been identified. It is common for histology to be worse than the Pap smear. The patient would then be treated based on biopsy findings. Cryotherapy may be used to treat low-grade squamous intraepithelial lesions (LSIL) and small, focal high-grade intraepithelial lesions (HGSIL) which includes carcinoma-in-situ. Large high-grade lesions will usually have deeper gland involvement, and these patients will need to have an excisional treatment, such as LEEP or conization.

Selection criteria include the following:
- Complete colposcopic examination done, with good correlation between Pap smear results, visual examination, and histologic biopsy report. (see above)
- Entire squamocolumnar junction (SCJ) and the entire lesion must be visible. ("adequate colposcopy")
- Lesions should be less than 3 cm in diameter (some recommend no more than 2 cm) and involve no more than two quadrants of the cervix.
- The probe tip must be able to cover the entire lesion and the entire transformation zone.
- The lesion does not extend more than 5 mm into the endocervical canal.

- The endocervical canal sampling is negative for dysplasia.
- The cervix should be relatively flat without large crevices.
- There should be no significant glandular involvement on biopsy.
- The patient must be reliable.

Cryotherapy also may be useful to treat patients with *chronic cervicitis* that is culture negative, unresponsive to antibiotic therapy, and has negative colposcopy and biopsy findings. External genital HPV lesions may be treated with cryotherapy, although a different freezing technique is used (see Chapter 15, Cryosurgery, and Chapter 157, Treatment of Noncervical Condyloma Acuminata).

CONTRAINDICATIONS

- Patients with colposcopic or histologic findings more than one degree less than the Pap smear. These patients need to have a complete reevaluation before any treatment (see discussion above).
- Positive endocervical curettage (ECC) (i.e., dysplasia or cancer).
- Lesion is so large that the cryoprobe will not cover it completely.
- Lesion extends into the endocervical canal more than 5 mm.
- Large high-grade lesions or carcinoma-in-situ lesions; LEEP is the treatment of choice for most of these lesions and will result in a better cure rate than cryotherapy.
- Invasive lesions (including microinvasion); these will need more aggressive treatment, such as a conization, hysterectomy, radiation, etc.
- Cryotherapy is not appropriate for any invasive lesion. The practitioner must be sure to differentiate too between "carcinoma-in-situ" and "microinvasive cancer." Although select patients with carcinoma-in-situ that meet the criteria can be treated with cryotherapy, *no one with microinvasive lesions can be treated this way.* Patients with microinvasive disease need a conization procedure to determine the true extent of the disease.
- Patient is within 1 week of menses or is having heavy menstrual flow; the resulting canal edema from cryotherapy could obstruct the normal menstrual outflow.
- Pregnancy. Although there would probably be no adverse effect, it would be best to wait until after delivery if possible.
- Acute cervicitis; in these patients it is best to treat the acute infection before cryotherapy.
- Immunosuppressed patients *(relative).*

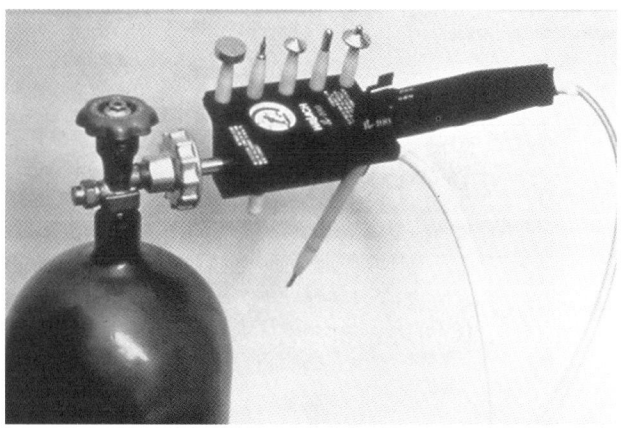

Fig. 141-1
Nitrous oxide tank with the yoke adapter for the cryogun. Several cryotips attached. (Courtesy Wallach Surgical Devices, Milford, Conn.)

- Cryoglobulinemia.
- Women exposed to DES in-utero; they are at greater risk for cervical stenosis.
- Markedly irregular cervix where the indentations are deep and the cryo probe just won't reach the areas.
- Significant glandular involvement on ECC or biopsy.
- Noncompliant patient (best to do definitive excisional procedure

Editor's note: Many would suggest that all CIN III lesions (which includes carcinoma-in-situ) be treated with conization procedures. However, the data strongly supports the efficacy of properly performed cryotherapy for small lesions that meet the criteria listed above. Cryotherapy is much more cost effective with potentially fewer and less significant complications.

EQUIPMENT

- Nitrous oxide 20-lb tank with a pressure gauge and gas cut-off valve (Figs. 141-1 and 141-2)
- Flexible tubing from tank to probe
- Probe gun
- Probe tips: 19- and 25-mm diameter tips, slightly coned and flat; do not use any tips with nipples that are more than 5 mm in length (Fig. 141-3)
- Water-soluble lubricant, such as K-Y Jelly
- Vaginal speculum
- Vaginal wall retractors or glove to place over the speculum (to prevent injury to vaginal sidewalls in patients with redundant vaginal walls) (See the "Technique" section of Chapter 152, Pap Smear and Related Techniques for Cervical Cancer Screening, for instructions on how to retract sidewalls with a "homemade" vaginal stint.)
- "O" ring supply; these are round rubber washers that attach at the base of the probe tip. They may

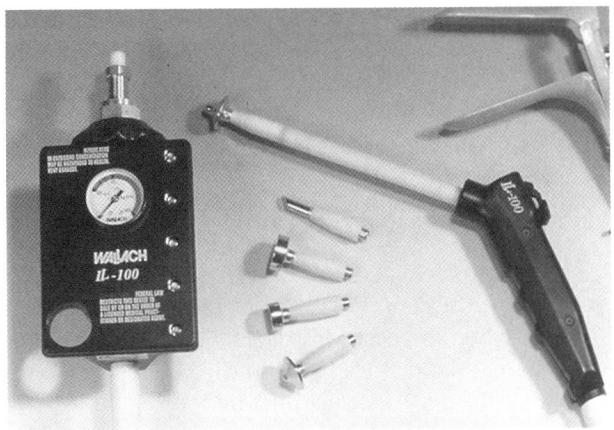

Fig. 141-2
Closeups of yoke adapter with pressure gauge and cryogun. (Courtesy Wallach Surgical Devices, Milford, Conn.)

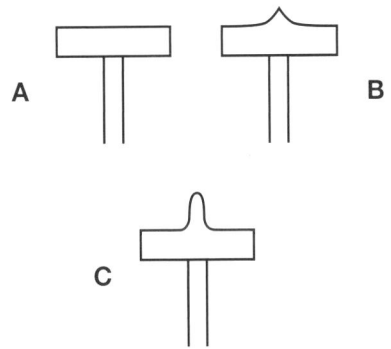

Fig. 141-3
Tips used for nitrous oxide cryotherapy of the cervix. Probe tips with 19 and 25 mm diameters are generally used. Acceptable tips are, **A,** flat and, **B,** slightly conical. **C,** Example of older cryotherapy tip with long endocervical nipple. These tips should not be used if the nipple is longer than 5 mm.

crack over time, which could result in leakage of the refrigerant at the joint between the probe and the tip. They are easily replaced by simply removing the old one and putting on the new one (a matter of seconds).

PREPROCEDURE PATIENT PREPARATION

• Provide the patient with a patient education handout (see the sample patient education handout titled "Cryotherapy of the Cervix" on page 1931 of Appendix G).
• Discuss the risks, benefits, and possible complications of cryotherapy.

• Before the procedure, review the indications with the patient.
• Obtain written informed consent.
• Update the menstrual history and do a pelvic examination if one has not been done within the previous few months. Be sure the patient is not pregnant, or postpone the procedure until you are sure. If there is any doubt, a pregnancy test should be performed.
• Confirm the biopsy report and note any area where disease is concentrated to ensure that the cryoprobe readily covers the area.
• Have the office staff premedicate the patient on her arrival to the office (if appropriate) with ibuprofen 800 mg or another nonsteroidal antiinflammatory drug (NSAID) to reduce the cramping that accompanies the procedure if not already taken. For maximum effectiveness, the NSAID should be taken approximately 30 to 60 minutes before the procedure. This has been shown to markedly reduce discomfort and cramping.

TECHNIQUE

Prepare Equipment

1. Be sure the tank has adequate pressure; for most tanks the needle on the pressure gauge will be in the "green zone."
2. Be sure the "O" ring (the small rubber washer) at the base of the probe tip is intact.
3. Select the proper size and shape of probe tip. If the 19-mm tip covers the entire lesion and all of the transformation zone, it can be used. If all areas aren't covered, use the larger 25-mm tip. If the lesion and SCJ are well out on the ectocervix, use a flat tip. If they approach the os or are slightly (less than 5 mm) into the os, use the conical tip. Avoid tips with long extensions because these may cause cervical stenosis.
4. Select the proper size vaginal speculum; the entire cervix and transformation zone must be well visualized, so consider using the largest speculum the patient can tolerate.

Prepare the Patient

1. Place the patient in a comfortable dorsal lithotomy position.
2. Even if NSAIDs have been used, some consider using a paracervical or mucosal block. (See Chapter 174, Paracervical Block, and Chapter 150, Loop Electrosurgical Excision Procedure [LEEP] for Treating Cervical Intraepithelial Neoplasia, for information on these procedures.) Both have been shown to reduce the discomfort associated with cryotherapy.

Editor's note: The "pain" associated with cryotherapy is more of a crampy discomfort. Although in general, only NSAIDs have been used, the mucosal block seems reasonable and is easy to accomplish using a needle extender. It too however has some discomfort. The paracervical block is more difficult to administer, takes significant time, and is associated with its own complications. Most do not use it.

3. Insert speculum. If necessary, use a speculum cover or vaginal wall retractors to prevent vaginal sidewall injury in those with redundant sidewalls.

Perform Cryotherapy

1. Apply water-soluble lubricant (such as K-Y Jelly) to the cryoprobe tip.
2. Turn on the gas valve (pressure gauge in the "green zone").
3. Apply the probe firmly to the cervix and begin freezing by pulling the trigger or pushing the freeze button. The tip will adhere in about 3 to 5 seconds (Fig. 141-4). After the tip adheres, pull back slightly. There is a tendency to push in on the probe. This stretches the uterosacral ligaments and causes discomfort. Pulling back slightly will also cause the vagina to "billow out" reducing the likelihood of the probe sticking to the sidewalls.
4. Watch the probe tip carefully to monitor the rim of ice. A 5- to 7-mm ice ball is required for cellular destruction. This generally takes at least 3 minutes. A timed freeze is no longer recommended, since the size of the tip used, the amount of cervical vascularity and fibrous tissue, and the pressure in the nitrous tank all alter the amount of time required to effect the 5- to 7-mm ice ball. Some "over freezing" is not going to cause a problem (Fig. 141-5).
5. When the ice ball around the probe tip reaches 5 to 7 mm, defrost by pushing the defrost button (on most machines) or releasing the freeze button. The probe tip will detach in about 15 seconds. Do not try

to pull the probe off until it has thawed because that may result in laceration of cervical tissue. (The "active" defrost requires that the gas be left on—*do not* turn off the gas from the tank. A "passive" defrost will take at least 5 minutes just for the probe to release from the tissues.) If the probe does not easily release, check to be sure no one has turned off the gas. Switch back and forth between freeze and defrost. Sometimes the valve can stick.

6. Allow for a complete thaw of the cervix, which is seen when the cervix resumes a normal pink color. This may take 8 to 10 minutes. The patient often feels "flushed" during this period. Refreeze; the second freeze may take less time. Again, a 5- to 7-mm ice ball is required. A rapid freeze, slow defrost, and rapid refreeze have been shown to be the most efficacious method of treatment. The double freeze is also recommended by the American College of Obstetricians and Gynecologists.
7. Thaw as above.
8. Remove speculum and turn off tank.
9. Have the patient sit up slowly to avoid any vasovagal symptoms, such as lightheadedness or flushing. This has occurred up to 10 minutes after completing the procedure.
10. Give the patient follow-up information; she will have a profuse watery or blood-tinged discharge for 2 to 4 weeks. The next Pap smear should be scheduled for 4 months after this procedure (see the sample patient education handout titled "After Cryotherapy of the Cervix" on page 1933 of Appendix G).
11. Consider prescribing Amino-Cerv Vaginal Creme to help reduce the discharge; patient should use one applicator full in the vagina at bedtime for 2 weeks. Ask the patient to bring the tube into the office and insert the first applicator prior to removing the speculum.

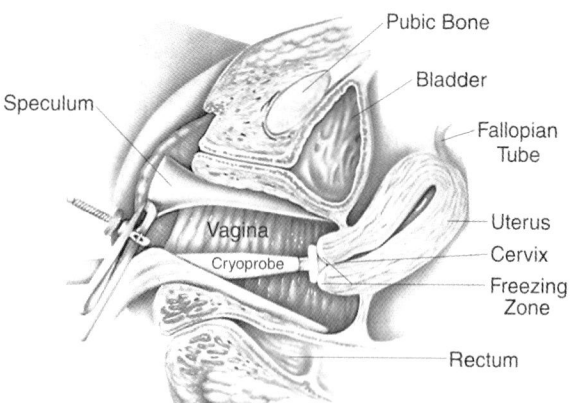

Fig. 141-4
Proper application of the cryotip to the cervix.

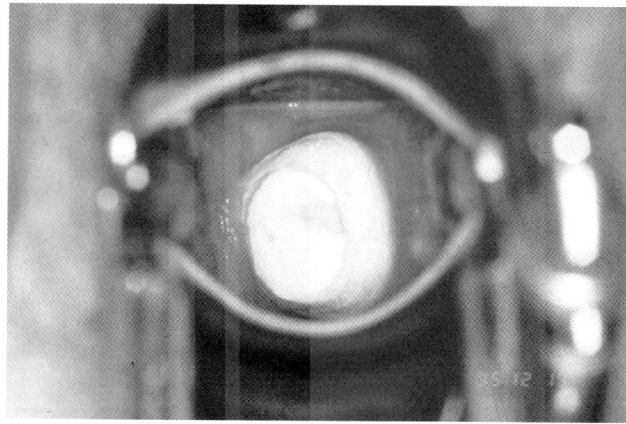

Fig. 141-5
Appearance of the cervix immediately after cryotherapy. (Courtesy The National Procedures Institute, Midland, Mich.)

COMPLICATIONS

- Vaginal mucosal injury is possible; avoid this by being certain that the cryoprobe does not touch the vaginal sidewalls. Use a speculum cover or vaginal wall retractors if necessary. If small areas are frozen, there are generally no significant adverse outcomes.
- The patient may experience vasovagal symptoms after the procedure; avoid this by having the patient sit up slowly and rest a while before standing.
- Pain and cramping may occur during cryotherapy; medicate patients with a NSAID about 30 to 40 minutes before the procedure. In an especially anxious patient, consider a paracercival or mucosal block. Avoid aggressive pulling on the cryoprobe during freezing because this may cause more intense cramping.
- The profuse watery discharge that follows cryotherapy is the most unpleasant consequence. It will last at least 2 weeks but begins in a day or two. The Amino-Cerv Vaginal Creme may help some and can be refilled for a total use of four weeks. Do not confuse this discharge with a cervicitis.
- A cervicitis is possible after therapy. If the discharge is not improving after 2 weeks, consider metronidazole (Flagyl) by mouth.
- A pelvic inflammatory disease is extremely rare. Consider it only if there is extreme pelvic tenderness and fever.
- Should the patient surprisingly start her period within 4 to 5 days of cryotherapy, she may retain menses causing severe discomfort. The cervix can be probed with a cotton-tipped applicator which will usually release the blood.
- A very rare complication is cervical stenosis; using the proper probe tip should prevent this. Avoid any tip with projections greater than 5 mm. (The study by Steinstra and associates [1992] found no stenosis, and they were able to identify the SCJ 100% of the time in a follow-up visit.)
- Asymmetric freeze of the cervix. If a cervix is very irregular in shape, consider freezing in segments, starting with the small, slightly nippled tip, then using the flat tip to cover the remaining areas.
- Treatment failure. Close follow-up is essential.

POSTPROCEDURE PATIENT CARE

1. Amino-Cerv Vaginal Creme: see above. A peri-pad is needed for a few weeks.
2. Normal bathing is acceptable. Showers work best.
3. Tampons are best avoided. They can irritate the friable cervix and cause bleeding.
4. Sex is best avoided for 2 to 3 weeks. It too may irritate the cervix and the discharge can make for an unpleasant experience (see the sample patient education handout titled "After Cryotherapy of the Cervix" on page 1933 of Appendix G).
5. A follow-up Pap smear should be performed 4 months after cryotherapy, which allows adequate repair time of the cervical tissues. If that Pap smear is normal, the Pap smear should be repeated 8 and 12 months after treatment. If all three of these postcryotherapy Pap smears are normal, annual Pap examinations are resumed (Some will do the first pap at 4 months then two more at 6 month intervals. Statistically it is important to perform three Pap smears to rule out recurrence). Most recurrences are within the first year after cryotherapy. If any of the postcryotherapy Pap examinations are abnormal, a complete reevaluation should be done, including colposcopy, biopsy, and endocervical sampling. For high-grade lesions, repeat colposcopy may be performed when performing the Pap at 8 months. The cervix will have an altered appearance after cryotherapy (Figs. 141-6 to 141-9). It takes 4 to 8 months to return to a totally normal appearance.

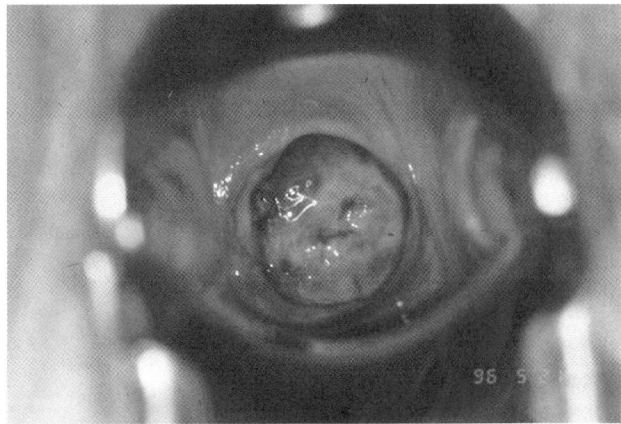

Fig. 141-6
Appearance of the cervix with large eschar 10 days after cryotherapy. (Courtesy The National Procedures Institute, Midland, Mich.)

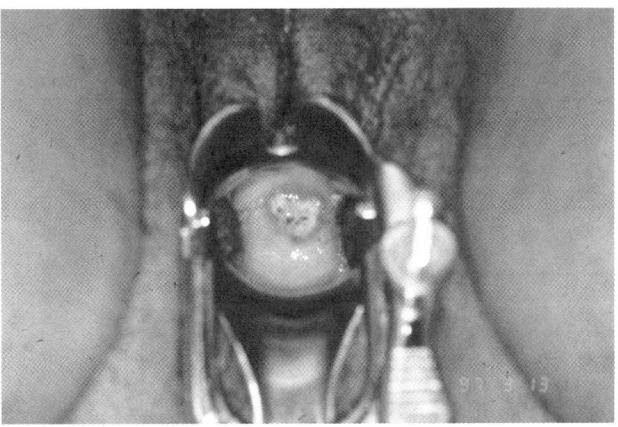

Fig. 141-7
Cervix 6 weeks after cryotherapy. (Courtesy Duane Townsend, MD.)

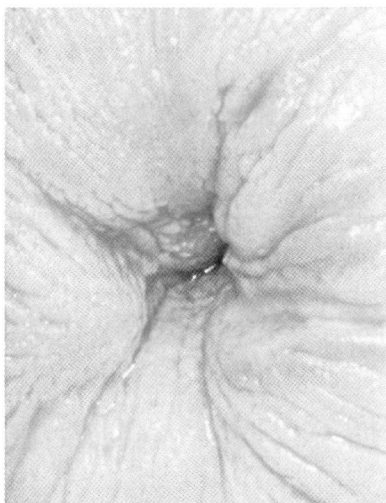

Fig. 141-8
Cervix 8 to 10 weeks after cryotherapy. Note radial striations. (Courtesy Duane Townsend, MD.)

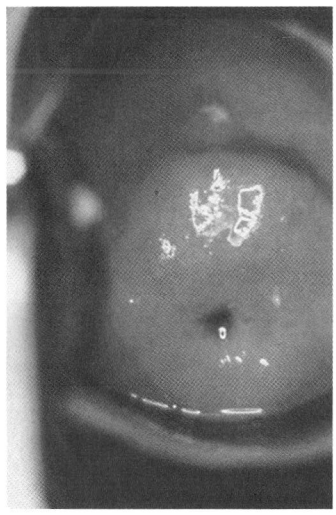

Fig. 141-9
Cervix 8 months after cryotherapy. Note the smooth ectocervix and lack of ectocervical transformation zone. The squamocolumnar junction is located right at the os. (Courtesy Duane Townsend, MD.)

SUPPLIERS

CooperSurgical, Inc. (Frigitronics, Leisegang)
95 Corporate Drive
Trumbull, CT 06611
Phone: 1-800-645-3760
Website: www.coopersurgical.com

Wallach Surgical Devices, Inc.
235 Edison Road
Orange, CT 06477
Phone: 1-203-799-2000
www.wallachsurgical.com

Welch Allyn Medical Products
4341 State Street Road
P.O. Box 220
Skaneateles Falls, NY 13153-0220
Phone: 1-800-535-6663
Website: www.welchallyn.com

CPT/BILLING CODE

57511   Cryocautery of cervix, initial or repeat

ICD-9-CM DIAGNOSTIC CODES

078.1   Condyloma acuminatum
622.1   Cervical dysplasia
233.1   CIN III/carcinoma-in-situ
616.0   Chronic cervicitis
Neoplasm, cervix, SCJ (os, canal)
219.0   Benign
236.0   Uncertain
233.1   CIS
180.8   Malignancy

ADDITIONAL RESOURCES

• See the sample patient education handouts titled "Cryotherapy of the Cervix" and "After Cryotherapy of the Cervix" on pages 1931 and 1933, respectively, of Appendix G.

BIBLIOGRAPHY

Brown KS: In from the cold: cryotherapy gets a second look, *J Natl Cancer Inst* 90:351, 1998.

Burke L: Evolution of therapeutic approaches to cervical intra-epithelial neoplasia, *J Lower Genital Tract Dis* 1:267, 1997.

Ferris DG: Cryotherapy of the cervix, *J Lower Genital Tract Dis* 2:98, 1998.

Ferris DG, Ho JJ: Cryosurgical equipment: A critical review, *J Fam Pract* 35:185-193, 1992.

Harper DM: Paracervical block diminishes cramping associated with cryosurgery, *J Fam Pract* 44:71, 1997.

Harper DM: Cervical mucosal block effectively reduces the pain and cramping from cryosurgery, *J Fam Pract* 47:285, 1998.

Harper DM: Pain and cramping associated with cryotherapy, *J Fam Pract* 39:551, 1994.

Harper DM, Mayeaux EJ, Daraleman TP, et al: Healing experiences after cervical cryosurgery, *J Fam Pract* 39:551, 1994.

Kurman RJ, Heusur DE, Herbst AL: Interim guidelines for management of abnormal cervical cytology, *JAMA* 271(23):1866, 1994.

Mayeaux EJ, Spigener SD, German JA: Cryotherapy of the uterine cervix, *J Fam Pract* 47:99, 1998.

Mitchell MF, Tortolero-Luna G, Cook E, et al: A randomized clinical trial of cryotherapy, laser vaporization, and loop electrosurgical excision for treatment of squamous intraepithelial lesions of the cervix, *Obstet Gynecol* 92:737, 1998.

Noller KL: Cryotherapy, laser vaporization, and loop electrosurgical excision for treatment of squamous intraepithelial lesions of the cervix, *Comment OB/GYN Clin Alert* 61, Dec 1998.

Noller KL: Colposcopy: The evolution of a technique, *Colposcopist* 26(4):2, 1994.

Persad VL, Pierotic MA, Guijon FB: Management of cervical neoplasia: a 13-year experience with cryotherapy and laser, *J Lower Gen Tract Dis* 5(4):199, 2001.

Pfenninger JL: Good things still come in old packages: cryosurgery vs LEEP, *J Am Board Fam Pract* 12(5):416, 1999.

Richart RM, Townsend DE, Crisp W, et al: An analysis of "long term" follow-up results in patients with CIN treated by cryotherapy, *AM J Obstet Gynecol* 137:823, 1980.

Steinstra KA, Brewer BE, Franklin LA: A comparison of flat and shallow conical tips for cervical cryotherapy, *J Fam Pract* 35:185, 1992.

Culdocentesis (Colpocentesis)

Steven H. Eisinger

Culdocentesis is a procedure performed in female patients to detect and sample free intraperitoneal fluid. With this procedure, critical diagnostic information can be obtained for a variety of important gynecologic conditions, such as ectopic pregnancy and pelvic inflammatory disease. The implications of the results are usually clear-cut but must always be considered in the context of the patient's total clinical picture.

INDICATIONS

Broadly speaking, any suspicion of free fluid within the peritoneal cavity of women may be an indication for culdocentesis.

Ectopic Pregnancy

The classic and most widely applied indication for culdocentesis is a suspected leaking or ruptured tubal ectopic pregnancy. Approximately 1 in 100 pregnancies is ectopic.

In a typical tubal ectopic pregnancy, intraperitoneal hemorrhage will eventually occur. Hemoperitoneum will cause pelvic peritonitis, which is manifested by rebound tenderness in the lower abdomen without guarding and by tenderness on pelvic examination. Surprisingly, the signs of hemoperitoneum may be subtle or absent, even in the presence of relatively large amounts of blood. Eventually, more generalized peritonitis will occur, causing abdominal pain and distension, ileus, shoulder pain, and a "doughy" feel to the abdomen. The cul-de-sac may bulge into the vagina on speculum examination. When these signs of hemoperitoneum are combined with the classic signs of ectopic pregnancy—positive pregnancy test, amenorrhea followed by vaginal bleeding—emergency culdocentesis may be indicated.

Although other more sophisticated methods exist to diagnose a ruptured or leaking ectopic pregnancy (such as ultrasound, β-human chorionic gonadotropin determi-nations, and laparoscopy), in the emergency room setting, culdocentesis remains the fastest, easiest, and surest way to confirm the diagnosis. Indeed, a culdocentesis showing blood, along with a positive pregnancy test, is associated with ectopic pregnancy more than 99% of the time.

Acute Salpingitis

The second major indication for culdocentesis is acute salpingitis, also known as pelvic inflammatory disease (PID). Clinical signs and symptoms of acute salpingitis vary and are sometimes difficult to interpret. Classically, a woman has progressive aching lower abdominal pain, often beginning during or after her menstrual period. On examination she will have fever, rebound tenderness, and exquisite tenderness on motion of the cervix or palpation of the adnexa, which may be enlarged. Again, pelvic peritonitis is the key finding, indicating irritating fluid (in this case, pus) free in the lower abdomen. Accurate diagnosis is important; however, false-negative and false-positive diagnoses of acute salpingitis are quite frequent. The fastest means of establishing the diagnosis is by obtaining pus through culdocentesis. Many authorities now advocate that culdocentesis be considered in all cases of suspected acute salpingitis when laparoscopic diagnosis is not feasible.

Other Indications

A ruptured cyst may cause pain. Culdocentesis demonstrates the cyst fluid free in the abdomen. Occasionally, a ruptured cyst will create a hemoperitoneum as dramatic and dangerous as that associated with a ruptured ectopic pregnancy.

Ascitic fluid may be obtained through culdocentesis either for diagnostic purposes—such as obtaining fluid for cytologic analysis to assess for ovarian cancer—or for relief of the symptoms of excessive ascites. In this regard the procedure is similar to paracentesis.

CONTRAINDICATIONS

- A cul-de-sac mass is a contraindication for culdocentesis, because such a mass could be a benign or malignant neoplasm, an endometrioma, an abscess, or an unruptured ectopic pregnancy whose rupture would be harmful.
- If the uterus is in fixed retroversion, the cul-de-sac will be obliterated and culdocentesis will be impossible.

EQUIPMENT

The equipment required for culdocentesis is simple and should be available in any well-equipped office or emergency room (Fig. 142-1).
- Speculum
- Single-tooth tenaculum or Allis forceps
- 10- or 20-ml syringe
- 20-gauge spinal needle or a 3-inch needle extender
- 1½-inch, 20-gauge needle
- Sterile swabs or sponges
- Ring forceps
- Antiseptic solution
- Three-finger control syringe (allows the clinician to aspirate with one hand)

The instruments should be sterile. Universal blood precautions should be followed, although technically face masks, drapes, and so forth are not necessary.

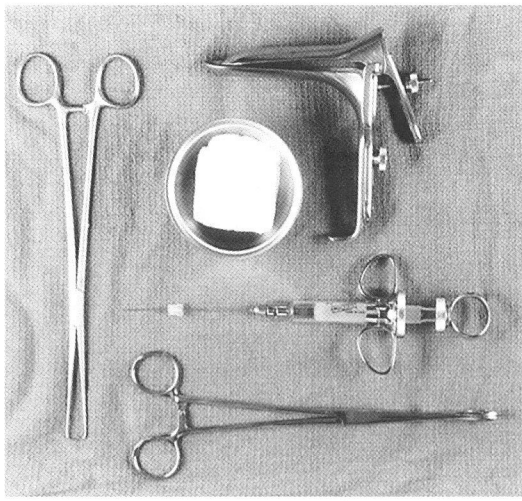

Fig. 142-1
Equipment required to perform culdocentesis: single-tooth tenaculum, sponges, ring forceps, Betadine, and a Graves' speculum. A three-finger control syringe with 20-gauge spinal needle is helpful, but a 10-ml syringe with spinal needle may suffice. A needle extender (3 to 5 inches) will also facilitate the procedure, making it easier to reach the posterior cul-de-sac.

TECHNIQUE

1. *Perform a standard pelvic examination* before culdocentesis. During the speculum examination, vaginal cultures may be obtained or other tests performed. A bulging of the cul-de-sac into the posterior fornix of the vagina is a finding suggestive of the presence of intraperitoneal fluid.
2. During the bimanual examination, *determine the size, position, and mobility of the uterus.* If the uterus is fixed in retroversion, culdocentesis should not be performed. On the other hand, a mobile retroverted uterus may be manipulated and moved out of the way by lifting or pulling on the cervix with a tenaculum. An anterior uterus presents no problem. The cul-de-sac must be determined to be free of masses. A fixed mass in the cul-de-sac contraindicates culdocentesis.
3. *Position the patient.* Allow the patient to walk or sit up for a short time before the procedure. Fluid will then collect in the cul-de-sac. To prevent a syncopal episode, obtain orthostatic vital signs before raising the patient to an upright position.

   The correct position for culdocentesis is the lithotomy position, with the head and shoulders *raised* slightly. The procedure may be performed in the office or emergency room setting on a regular examination table with stirrups.
4. *Place the speculum.* A medium Graves' speculum is suitable for most patients. Open it as wide as the patient can tolerate. This will expose the posterior vaginal fornix and stretch the mucosa taut, making the procedure easier.
5. *Cleanse the vagina* with a suitable antiseptic solution.
6. *Grasp the cervix with a tenaculum* or Allis forceps (Fig. 142-2). The tenaculum may be placed vertically or horizontally on the anterior or posterior lip of the cervix, as the clinician desires. Grasping the cervix with a tenaculum causes discomfort for most women; therefore a small amount of local anesthetic may be injected prior at the tenaculum site.
7. *Choose the puncture site.* Manipulate the cervix gently with the tenaculum by pulling either in and out or up and down. This maneuver will identify the line of reflection where the mucosa sweeps off the cervix and crosses or covers the cul-de-sac. Insert the needle about 1 cm below this reflection, in the midline (Fig. 142-3). If the puncture site is too high, the needle will hit the cervix. If the needle is placed too low, it may enter the rectum or tunnel beneath the posterior peritoneum of the cul-de-sac.
8. *Administer anesthesia,* if desired. Culdocentesis is generally perceived by women as quite painful. Some clinicians recommend injecting a small amount

of local anesthetic into the puncture site; others have used anesthetic gel on the mucosa. The patient may be reassured that although the pain is sharp, it is bearable and will only last for a few seconds. Judiciously selected intravenous narcotics or seda-

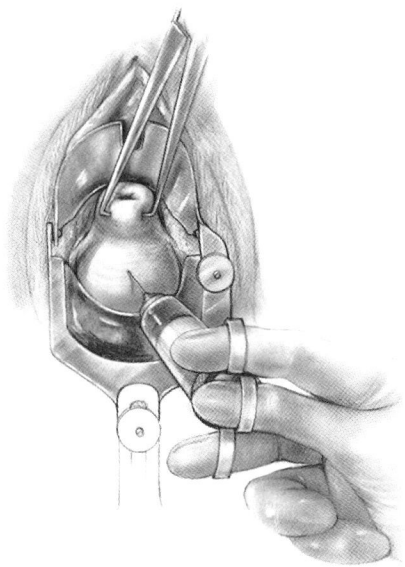

Fig. 142-2
Operator's view of culdocentesis. Note the widely opened speculum, the tenaculum grasping the lower lip of the cervix and elevating it in the vagina, and the bulging posterior vaginal fornix. The puncture site is about 1 cm below the deflection of the mucosa from the cervix onto the posterior fornix. The needle is held approximately horizontally to seek the pool of fluid and to avoid puncturing the rectum. (From Eisinger SH: *J Fam Pract* 13:95, 1981.)

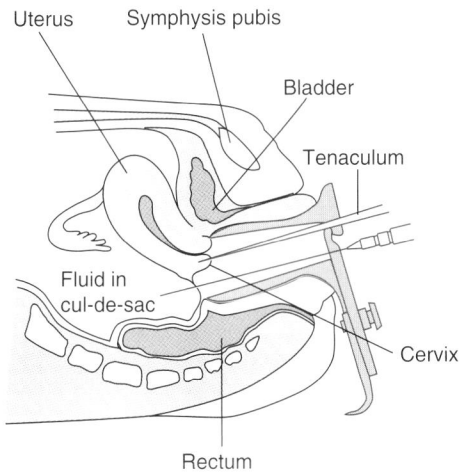

Fig. 142-3
Midline sagittal view of pelvis during culdocentesis showing anatomic relationships and position of instruments. Note the depth of the needle puncture and the proximity of the tip to adjacent structures. (Redrawn from Eisinger SH: *J Fam Pract* 13:95, 1981.)

tives, such as 50 mg of meperidine (Demerol) or 3 to 5 mg of midazolam (Versed), can be helpful.

9. *Make the puncture.* Elevate the cervix in the vagina to stretch the mucosa, and retract it outward to pull the uterus out of retroversion. Between 2 and 3 ml of air may be placed in the syringe prior to puncture, although this step should be omitted if infection is suspected. The needle should be approximately horizontal. Perform the puncture itself with a bold, smooth movement, inserting the needle 3 to 4 cm through mucosa.

10. *Inject the air in the syringe.* If there is resistance to air injection, the needle tip is in a solid organ, such as the uterus, and should be repositioned; usually, the air passes freely. Sometimes the air may be heard bubbling through free fluid.

11. *Pull back on the syringe plunger,* strongly aspirating while withdrawing the needle slowly. Stop when fluid returns in the syringe. The syringe should be filled and the needle withdrawn. If no fluid is obtained, a second or even third attempt may be made at a slightly different location or angle. A spray of bloody, frothy fluid is often seen just as the needle emerges from the mucosa. This is blood from the venus plexus of the vaginal mucosa and should not be interpreted as a bloody tap.

12. *Terminate the procedure when fluid is obtained,* or when three taps fail to yield any fluid. Remove all instruments from the vagina and allow the patient to rest. Bleeding from the puncture and tenaculum sites is usually slight.

13. *Examine the fluid from the cul-de-sac.* Observe blood from the cul-de-sac for several minutes for clotting that would indicate a traumatic tap. Blood-tinged or frankly bloody fluid should be spun for a hematocrit. Turbid or clear fluid should be examined microscopically by means of Gram's stain, and cultures—both aerobic and anaerobic—should be obtained.

COMPLICATIONS

Culdocentesis is generally quite free of complications. Both small and large bowel may occasionally be pierced, but ill effects have not been described. A serious potential complication is in puncturing or rupturing various pathologic pelvic structures listed in the "Contraindications" section.

Intrapelvic hemorrhage as a result of the procedure is very rare, since the great vessels of the pelvis lie away from the midline and should not be approached by the needle tip. The most significant hazard of the procedure is a deceptive result, providing unwarranted reassurance or leading to unnecessary treatment.

INTERPRETING RESULTS

Blood obtained from the cul-de-sac should be tested in two ways: for clotting ability and hematocrit. Pooled blood within the peritoneal cavity is usually defibrinated and will not clot. However, in exceptional cases, bleeding is so brisk that the blood does not have time to become defibrinated.

Fluid may appear quite bloody even when the hematocrit is low. As a rough rule, a hematocrit below 15% indicates either a minor amount of bleeding or a bloody tap. Frank blood is an indication for immediate surgery, either laparoscopy or laparotomy. Blood-tinged fluid can usually be managed more conservatively. Medical therapy for ectopic pregnancy with methotrexate may be chosen.

Pus or turbid fluid should always be Gram stained and microscopically examined; white blood cells and bacteria are often identified. Cultures of specimens obtained from the cul-de-sac are the best means of assessing the bacteriology of a pelvic infection without performing surgery. However, cultures obtained from culdocentesis fluid do not always accurately reflect the bacteriology of the infection. Pus, particularly watery pus, indicates that acute salpingitis is the problem in most cases, and treatment should be medical. Appendicitis can also produce an exudate with white blood cells.

Clear fluid is commonly obtained in three situations: it may be the contents of a ruptured ovarian cyst; it may be ascites; or, in small amounts, it may be normal. In general, aspirated clear fluid is reassuring, and no active management is required. Dark brown, chocolate-like material is old blood. A ruptured endometrioma is the most likely cause.

Somewhat less than half the time, no fluid at all can be obtained, even with repeated efforts. This phenomenon should be referred to as a dry tap, not a negative tap. *No diagnostic assumptions should be made on the basis of a dry tap.* The needle simply may not have found the pool of fluid. When a dry tap occurs, physicians must resort to ultrasound or laparoscopy, or they must rely wholly on their clinical acumen, to make the correct diagnosis.

CPT/BILLING CODE

57020   Colpocentesis

ICD-9-CM DIAGNOSTIC CODES

633.9   Ectopic pregnancy ruptured
381.51   Salpingitis (acute)

BIBLIOGRAPHY

Eisinger SH: Procedures in family practice: culdocentesis, *J Fam Pract* 13:1, 1981.

Hager WD, Eschenbach DA, Spence MR, Sweet RL: Criteria for diagnosis and grading of salpingitis, *Obstet Gynecol* 61(1): 113, 1983.

Mishell DR, Jr, Stenchaver MA, Herbst AL, Droegemueller W: *Comprehensive gynecology,* ed 3, St Louis, 1997, Mosby.

Romero R, Copel JA, Kadar N, et al: Value of culdocentesis in the diagnosis of ectopic pregnancy, *Obstet Gynecol* 65(4): 519, 1985.

Vermesh M, Graczykowski JW, Sauer MV: Reevaluation of the role of culdocentesis in the management of ectopic pregnancy, *Am J Obstet Gynecol* 162:411, 1990.

CHAPTER 143

Diagnostic Hysteroscopy

Lydia A. Watson
Barbara S. Apgar

The hysteroscope has recently emerged as one of the most valuable tools for viewing the endocervical canal and uterine cavity. Hysteroscopy is now being taught routinely as the method of choice for diagnosing, sampling, and treating intrauterine pathology. The hysteroscopist has three goals: (1) to transform the uterine cleft into a cavity by the use of distending agents, (2) to illuminate the uterine cavity by a light source and light transmission, and (3) to transmit the image by an optical system. Hysteroscopes are designed to apply optical physics to a small dark space (the endometrial cavity) through a narrow aperture (the cervical canal). With the smaller-diameter scopes, diagnostic hysteroscopy can be performed in the office setting without the need for cervical dilation or local anesthesia. Controlled-rate carbon dioxide insufflators as well as Hyskon delivered by a Cook OB/GYN handheld pump allow safe distension of the uterine cavity with minimal side effects. Saline and Ringer's lactate can also be used as distending media; however, larger volumes may be required for adequate visualization, making these less than ideal for routine office use.

Hysteroscopy is best performed in the proliferative phase of the cycle when the endometrium is the thinnest.

INDICATIONS

- Suspicion of endometrial polyps or submucous uterine myomas
- Evaluation of persistent abnormal uterine bleeding in a premenopausal or postmenopausal patient when an endometrial biopsy is inconclusive
- Localization of lost intrauterine devices
- Diagnosis of uterine or cervical carcinomas
- Infertility evaluations (with hysterosalpingography), including recurrent miscarriage
- Evaluation of postpartum bleeding
- Evaluation prior to endometrial ablation
- In future, possibly for the insertion of a tubal occlusion device for contraception

CONTRAINDICATIONS

- Acute pelvic infections
- Acute uterine bleeding (relative contraindication)
- Pregnancy
- Recent uterine perforation
- Known uterine or cervical carcinoma

EQUIPMENT

- For office use, a flexible or rigid (0- or 30-degree viewing angle) panoramic hysteroscope, 3.6 to 5 mm in diameter (see the "Suppliers" section) (Figs. 143-1 and 143-2). The *flexible hysteroscope* has ultrathin glass fibers. The scope is rotated by a movement of the hand; the distal end has a maximum up-and-down deflection of approximately 100 to 120 degrees (Fig. 143-3). Deflection of the distal tip is accomplished by the thumb, which moves the deflection control lever on the handle of the scope. The distal tip can be maneuvered around lesions so that structures obscured by masses (such as polyps) can be visualized. The *rigid hysteroscope* consists of a telescope with a 0- or 30-degree viewing angle and a sheath measuring 3 to 5 mm in diameter. The telescope consists of an eyepiece, a barrel, and a terminal lens. The sheath that fits over the telescope has a port for carbon dioxide insufflation. The 0-degree scope provides a straight-on view, whereas the 30-degree scope provides a view that is 30 degrees off the horizontal. The 0-degree scope approximates normal vision, whereas the 30-degree scope allows dexterous examination of the cornual area.
- Carbon dioxide insufflator (constant flow/variable pressure).

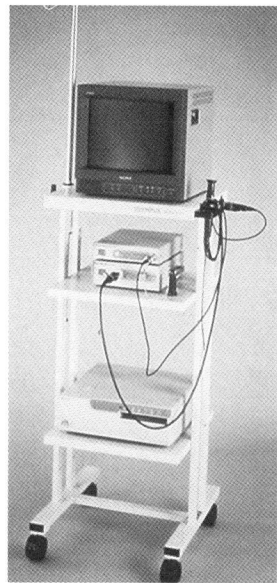

Fig. 143-1
Video hysteroscopy setup. (Courtesy Olympus Corp., Melville, NY)

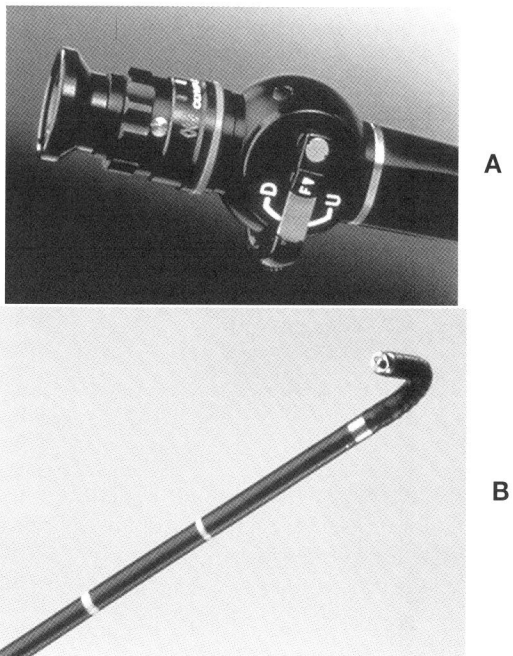

A

B

Fig. 143-3
A, Hysteroscope head. **B,** Mobile tip at the end of the hysteroscope.
(Courtesy Olympus Corp., Melville, NY)

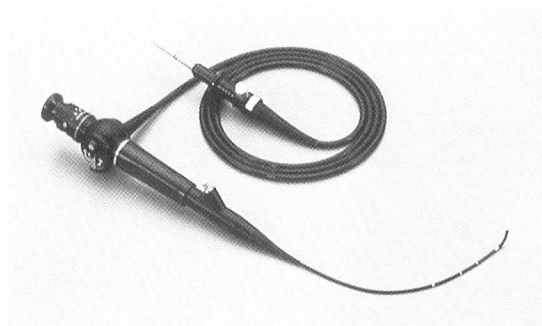

Fig. 143-2
Olympus hysteroscope. (Courtesy Olympus Corp., Melville, NY)

- Xenon lamp light source (xenon provides best illumination).
- Vaginal speculum (unhinged on one side).
- Antiseptic solution.
- Lidocaine 1% *without* epinephrine *(optional)*
- 10-ml syringe, 4-inch needle extender, 27-gauge needles *(optional)*
- Tenaculum.
- Uterine sound.
- Endocervical curette.
- Standard accessory instruments (used through a 3-mm operating channel sheath):
  –7 French grasping forceps
  –Biopsy forceps
  –Scissors

PREPROCEDURE PATIENT PREPARATION

The clinician should explain the procedure to the patient and obtain informed consent (see the sample patient consent form titled "Diagnostic Hysteroscopy" on page 1934 of Appendix G). Full resuscitative equipment must be available. A pregnancy test should be considered for patients of reproductive age who are not using reliable birth control. Cervical or uterine cultures should be obtained for patients at high risk for pelvic infection before hysteroscopy is performed.

Nonsteroidal inflammatory drugs (NSAIDS) administered 30 minutes before the procedure can significantly diminish the discomfort of the procedure. Alternatively, an intrastromal cervical injection of 1% lidocaine (10 to 15 ml) can be administered. Patients requiring subacute bacterial endocarditis prophylaxis should be prescribed appropriate antibiotics. (See Chapter 204, Antibiotic Prophylaxis.)

TECHNIQUE

1. Place the patient in the dorsal lithotomy position. Perform a bimanual pelvic examination to determine uterine position and size.
2. Place a sterile vaginal speculum (unhinged on one side), and cleanse the cervix with antiseptic solution.

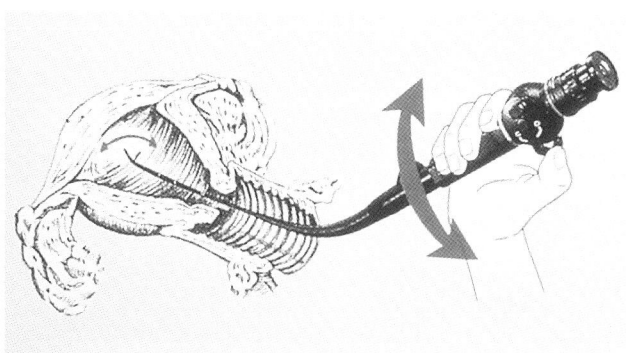

Fig. 143-4
Hysteroscopic examination of the uterine cavity.

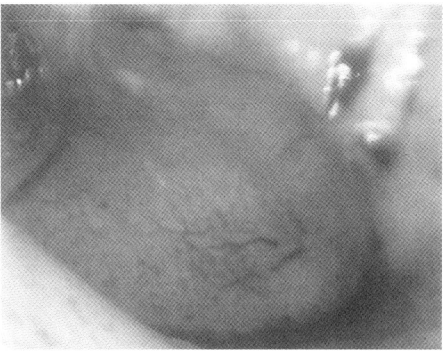

Fig. 143-6
Endometrial polyp.

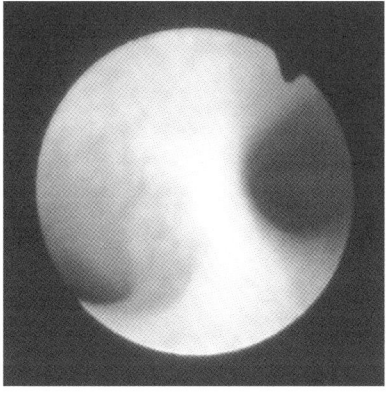

Fig. 143-5
Typical view inside the uterus showing the fundus with bilateral tubal ostia.

3. Grasp the anterior cervix with a tenaculum. Perform endocervical curettage if indicated. Sound the uterus to determine the depth and direction of the central axis.

4. Engage the hysteroscope at the external os, and begin carbon dioxide insufflation through the instillation port on the scope at an initial rate of 30 ml/min. As the hysteroscope traverses the endocervical canal, the carbon dioxide will create a visual space ahead of the scope. Advance the scope only if the view is clear. The internal os is seen as a narrow constriction at the upper portion of the endocervical canal. Increase the carbon dioxide insufflation rate to 40 to 60 ml/min, when the isthmus of the uterus is entered. The spacious cavity above the isthmus is the corpus, and it should be examined systematically (Fig. 143-4). The central point of müllerian duct fusion projects down from the fundus. The cornua are located on both sides of this fused tissue. Tubal ostia are seen at the uppermost portion of the fundal cornua bilaterally. The endometrial lining appears pink-white and smooth (Fig. 143-5). Endometrial glands open into the cavity through white-ringed elevations. A biopsy

of the suspicious areas should be performed, and then stalked endometrial polyps may be removed with grasping forceps (Fig. 143-6).

5. Diagnostic hysteroscopy takes an average of 5 to 10 minutes to perform. The carbon dioxide insufflation must be critically controlled during the procedure. If the gas is instilled too quickly, obstructive bubbles of carbon dioxide will form.

6. After the uterus is inspected, withdraw the hysteroscope.

7. Perform endometrial sampling if indicated.

8. Clean the scope with a disinfectant solution.

9. Dictate the procedure in standard operative note form, recording all abnormal findings in detail.

COMPLICATIONS

- Uterine perforation can occur if the hysteroscope is forcibly advanced without a panoramic, unobstructed view.
- Infection is rare if strict protocols are followed in screening for pelvic infections in high-risk patients.
- Complications related to carbon dioxide insufflation are rare with use of a constant-flow insufflator. Acidosis and hypercarbia are rare events.
- Patients can experience shoulder pain after carbon dioxide insufflation.

POSTPROCEDURE PATIENT EDUCATION

- The patient should be placed in the Trendelenburg position if she experiences shoulder pain as a result of the carbon dioxide instillation.
- Analgesics should be administered to control mild uterine cramping.
- If infection develops after the procedure, therapy with broad-spectrum antibiotics effective against anaerobes should be initiated.

- The patient is allowed to go home after the procedure and resumes normal activities the following day.

CPT/BILLING CODES

58558   Hysteroscopy, surgical; with sampling (biopsy) of endometrium and/or polypectomy; with or without D & C
58562   Hysteroscopy, surgical; with removal of impacted foreign body
58555   Hysteroscopy, diagnostic (separate procedure)
58559   Hysteroscopy, with lysis of adhesions
58560   Hysteroscopy, with division or resection of intrauterine septum
58561   Hysteroscopy, with removal of leiomyomata
58563   Hysteroscopy, with endometrial ablation (e.g., endometrial resection, electrosurgical ablation, thermal ablation) (Also see Chapter 158, Endometrial Ablation.)

ICD-9-CM DIAGNOSTIC CODES

1820   Cancer, uterus
2180   Submucous leiomyoma, uterus
2181   Intramural leiomyoma
2191   Benign neoplasm, uterus
2332   Ca in situ, uterus
6210   Uterine polyp
6212   Enlarged uterus
6213   Endometrial hyperphasia
6215   Intrauterine synechiae
6238   Vaginal bleeding
6253   Dysmenorrhea
6259   Pelvic pain
6271   Postmenopausal bleeding
V1042   Personal history, ca uterus

SUPPLIERS

Olympus America Inc.
2 Corporate Center Drive
Melville, NY 11747
Phone: 1-800-645-8160
Website: www.olympusamerica.com

CooperSurgical
95 Corporate Drive
Trumbull, CT 06611
Phone: 1-800-645-3760
Website: www.coopersurgical.com

ACMI (Circon).
136 Turnpike Road
Southborough, MA 01772-2104
Phone: 1-888-524-7266
Website: www.circoncorp.com

ADDITIONAL RESOURCES

- See the sample patient consent form titled "Diagnostic Hysteroscopy" on page 1934 of Appendix G.

BIBLIOGRAPHY

American College of Obstetricians and Gynecologists: *Hysteroscopy*, Tech Bull No 191, Washington DC, April 1994, ACOG.

Apgar B, DeWitt D: Diagnostic hysteroscopy, *Am Fam Physician* 46(5):19S, 1992.

Frey DL: Should you be doing hysteroscopy? *Fam Pract Management* 63, April 1994.

Gimbleson RJ, Rappold HO: A comparative study between panoramic hysteroscopy with directed biopsies and dilatation and curettage, *Am J Obstet Gynecol* 158(3):489, 1988.

Heury LA: A buyer's guide to hysteroscopes, *Fam Pract Management* 68, April 1994.

Julian TM: Hysteroscopic complications, *J Low Genital Tract Dis* 6(1):39, 2002.

March CM: Hysteroscopy, *J Reprod Med* 37(4):293, 1992.

Mencaglia L, Perino A, Hamou J: Hysteroscopy in premenopausal and postmenopausal women with abnormal uterine bleeding, *J Reprod Med* 32(8):577, 1987.

Obermair A, Geramou M, Gucer F, et al: Does hysteroscopy facilitate tumor cell dissemination? *Cancer* 88:139, 2000.

Rock A, Thompson JD: *Te Linde's operative gynecology*, ed 8, Philadelphia, Lippincott-Raven, 1997.

Shapiro BS: Instrumentation in hysteroscopy, *Obstet Gynecol Clin North Am* 15(1):13, 1988.

Taylor PJ: Hysteroscopy: where have we been, where are we going? *J Reprod Med* 38(10):757, 1993.

Valle RF: Hysteroscopy in the evaluation of female infertility, *Am J Obstet Gynecol* 137(4):425, 1980.

Wheeler JM, DeCherney AH: Office hysteroscopy, *Obstet Gynecol Clin North Am* 15(1):29, 1988.

CHAPTER 144

Dilation and Curettage

Verneeta L. Williams
Sheila Thomas

The dilation and curettage (D & C) is a valuable diagnostic and therapeutic tool in the management of abnormal uterine bleeding (AUB) and pregnancy-related disorders. Endometrial biopsy techniques have replaced D & C in most diagnostic situations, and hysteroscopy (see Chapter 143, Diagnostic Hysteroscopy) is now often performed in place of the "blind" D & C when initial diagnostic and therapeutic interventions fail. When the operator is experienced and the proper ancillary personnel are available, the office D & C proves to be a very cost-effective and safe procedure for the patient. Alternatively it can be performed in outpatient day surgery centers and in inpatient hospital settings. In many instances of abnormal bleeding, diagnosis is facilitated if the sampling is done just before an anticipated period (e.g., anovulatory bleeding). Unless the procedure is pregnancy related, the clinician should ensure that the patient is not pregnant and should know the status of the Pap smear before the surgery. In addition to this chapter, it would be helpful for the clinician to review Chapter 146, Endometrial Biopsy.

INDICATIONS

Screening Indications

- As a prehysterectomy measure in postmenopausal women to exclude the possibility of endometrial or endocervical cancer
- As a part of postmenopausal vaginal surgery without hysterectomy

Note: In general, a D & C will not be performed for screening purposes. When "screening" is selected in high-risk cases, an endometrial biopsy or ultrasound technique is generally selected.

On reaching menopause all women should be informed about the risks and symptoms of endometrial cancer and strongly encouraged to report any unexpected bleeding or spotting to their physicians. Smith and associates (2001) found no evidence, however, to support the screening of asymptomatic women and some evidence against screening for women at risk (Chapter 146, Endometrial Biopsy).

Diagnostic Indications

- To determine the cause of abnormal premenopausal bleeding that has not been corrected by medical management
- To determine the cause of abnormal premenopausal bleeding that occurs in women over 40 years of age with inadequate endometrial biopsies
- To determine the cause of postmenopausal bleeding when endometrial aspiration is nondiagnostic
- To rule out cancer and adenomatous hyperplasia with atypia when complex hyperplasia (adenomatous hyperplasia) is found on endometrial biopsy
- When the endometrial lining (stripe) measures more than 5 mm on ultrasound
- To determine the cause of significant uterine bleeding that is too excessive for an endometrial biopsy
- When a reliable pelvic examination is required but cannot be obtained to evaluate the internal organs prior to endometrial biopsy and thus anesthesia would be helpful
- For a debilitating medical condition or apprehensive patient when endometrial biopsy cannot be obtained
- When cervical stenosis cannot be resolved and prevents an office procedure
- When pregnancy-related causes are suspected for AUB
- When atypical glandular cells are reliably found and confirmed on Pap smear, but no cause is found in less invasive workup

Therapeutic Indications

- For removal of a suspected endometrial polyp
- For removal of retained products of conception associated with postpartum infection or hemorrhaging

- For removal of retained products after an incomplete abortion
- For therapy of excessive hemorrhaging
- For use in combination with hysteroscopy

Note: Performing a D & C to resolve hormonally related AUB has not been found to be effective.

Other:
- Elective termination of pregnancy (Chapter 130, First-Trimester Abortion and Emergency Oral Contraceptives)

CONTRAINDICATIONS

- The presence of an active pelvic infection
- Signs of a systemic coagulopathy (i.e., diffuse intravascular coagulation [DIC]) or unknown anticoagulation status
- Existence of comorbid medical conditions that

are unstable (e.g., renal failure, active cardiac compromise)
- Uncertainty concerning the viability of an intrauterine pregnancy
- Patient's preference to defer procedure in anticipation of a spontaneous resolution of a miscarriage
- Prior history of uterine procedures and the development of Asherman's syndrome (i.e., endometrial synechiae)

Note: A D & C should be performed in the office only with a cooperative patient with no other significant health risk factors and the availability of adequate resuscitation equipment.

EQUIPMENT (Fig. 144-1)

- Sterile gowns *(optional)*.
- Sterile gloves.
- Sterile drapes.
- Sterile sponge gauze.

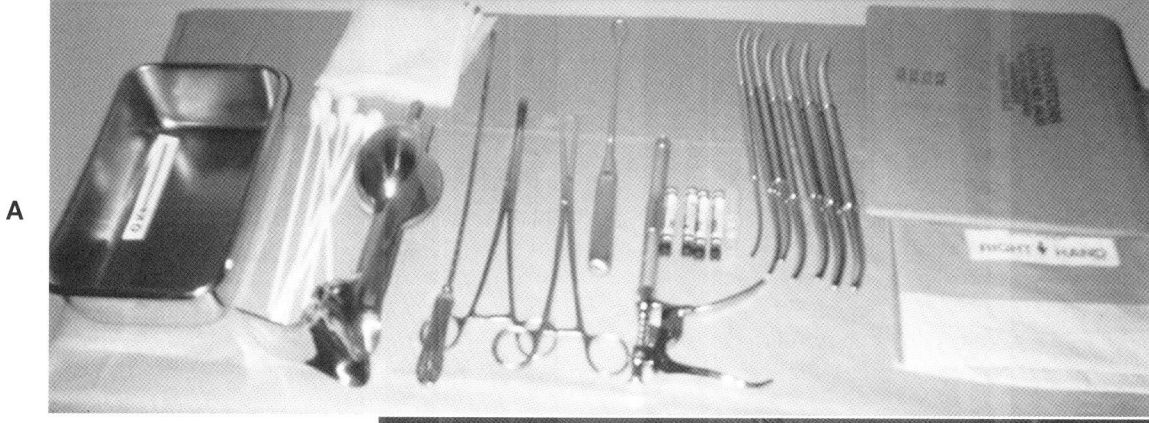

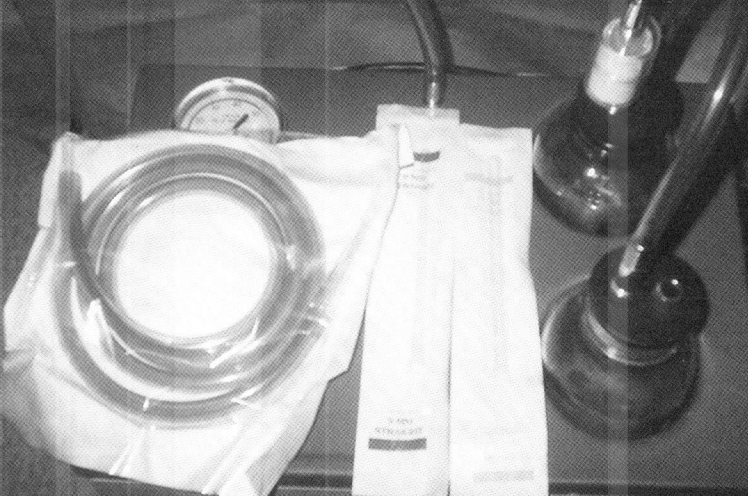

Fig. 144-1
A, Equipment used for dilation and curettage (D & C) *(left to right):* sterile basin, 4 × 4 sterile sponge gauze, large OB-GYN applicators, weighted speculum, uterine sound, ring forceps, single-tooth tenaculum, curette, dental gun, 1.8 ml of 2% lidocaine with epinephrine, uterine dilators, leggings, and sterile covering. **B,** Suction device and tubing.

- Formalin bottles.
- Lens paper or Telfa pads for endocervical curettage and uterine curettage tissue.
- Antiseptic cleansing solution.
- Sterile bowl.
- Suction hosing and suction apparatus with pump (for some situations).
- Ring forceps.
- Uterine sound.
- Graves' or weighted (Auvard) speculum.
- Polyp (Stone) forceps.
- Cervical dilators.
- Kevorkian endocervical curette for endocervical curettage.
- Curved and straight suction catheters (size 8 to 12 mm) when applicable.
- Sharp uterine curette.
- IV needle, catheter, and tubing.
- IV fluids *(optional)*.
- IV antibiotics *(optional)*.
- A 20-gauge spinal needle and syringe, dental anesthetizing gun, or needle extender when local anesthesia (submucosal block) will be used.
- Lidocaine 5 ml (2%) with epinephrine for submucosal block or 10 ml 2% lidocaine without epinephrine for paracervical block or equivalent.

Note: Review Chapter 150, Loop Electrosurgical Excision Procedure (LEEP) for Treating Cervical Intraepithelial Neoplasia, for information regarding local anesthetic use (it is not needed if general anesthesia is given).

- Tenaculum.
- Ultrasound *(optional)*.
- Pulse oximeter if IV sedation is given.

PREPROCEDURE PATIENT PREPARATION

Each patient should be comfortable with the decision to perform a D & C. All questions regarding the procedure, alternatives, and risks should be explained carefully so that the patient can make an informed consent (see the sample patient consent form titled "Dilation and Curettage (D & C) Request" on page 1938 of Appendix G). If performed in the office with sedation, appropriate knowledge and equipment must be available for possible complications and resuscitation. The physician will need a nurse available throughout the entire procedure to aid with preparing the patient for the procedure, injecting IV medications, handling equipment, and for the postoperative and recovery periods. The patient's vital signs must be stable for the clinician to perform an office D & C. If bleeding has been prolonged or heavy, a hemoglobin or hematocrit should be obtained. The ability to obtain IV access is also important should the need arise to correct hemodynamic instability.

Anesthesia and Analgesia

In the outpatient setting, anesthetic and analgesic choice is somewhat limited. For D & C procedures performed in the hospital, the choice of sedation is much more variable. No matter which drug regimen is selected, it is important that persons and equipment used for resuscitation be available should anaphylaxis, bleeding, or oversedation occur.

When making anesthetic and analgesic choices for D & C, the clinician should consider the following:

- A paracervical block is useful before placement of a tenaculum onto the cervix and before cervical dilation, unless a general anesthetic is used.
- The clinician should use 10 ml of 1% or 2% lidocaine without epinephrine, injected at the 3 to 4 o'clock and 8 to 9 o'clock positions (being careful not to inject intravascularly) (see Chapter 174, Paracervical Block).
- Many times a submucosal cervical local block is sufficient (see Chapter 150, Loop Electrosurgical Excision Procedure [LEEP] for Treating Cervical Intraepithelial Neoplasia).
- The clinician should consider giving nonsteroidal antiinflammatory drugs (NSAIDs) 1 hour before the procedure for office procedures to reduce cramping and decrease uterine bleeding. Diazepam (Valium) 10 mg PO 1 hour before the procedure combined with a maximum dose NSAID and local lidocaine are often sufficient to accomplish a D & C.
- IV medication can be used for more sedation (Chapter 2, Conscious Sedation [Sedation and Analgesia]).
- Meperidine (Demerol) should be given in 25- to 50-mg doses. Onset of action is immediate, and it can cause nausea. Therefore it should be administered with 12.5 to 25 mg of Phenergan.
- Diazepam (Valium) (1- to 5-mg doses) or Midazolam (Versed) (1- to 5-mg doses) can be used to augment the effect of Demerol.

Note: Demerol can be reversed with Naloxone (Narcan), whereas flumazenil (Romazicon) reverses the effects of Valium and Versed.

TECHNIQUE

1. A hematocrit and hemoglobin, Rh, blood type, and screen should be considered if the patient's problem is pregnancy related. Platelet count, prothrombin time (PT), partial thromboplastin time (PTT), and fibrin split products (FSP) may be indicated in some

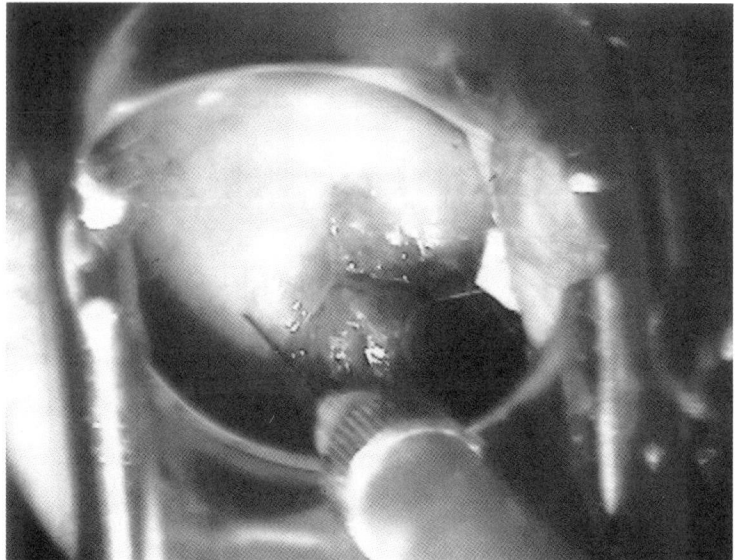

Fig. 144-2
Dental gun used for submucosal block.

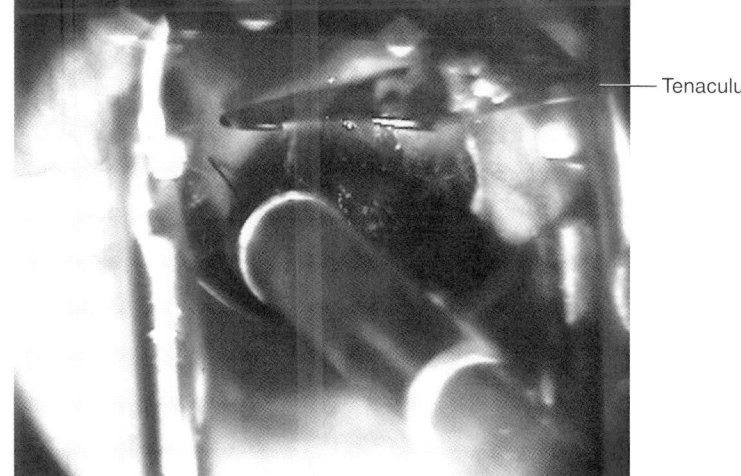

Tenaculum

Fig. 144-3
Dental gun used for a paracervical block at fornix. The single-tooth tenaculum has been placed on the anterior tip of the cervix.

situations. If uncertain of pregnancy status, obtain a pregnancy test.

2. Start an IV and administer fluids. Sedate the patient if needed.

3. Prophylactic antibiotics are not indicated in routine D & Cs.

4. Place the patient in the dorsal lithotomy position.

5. Determine the position of the uterine fundus by performing a bimanual examination or under ultrasound guidance if skilled in its use.

6. Expose the cervix using a Graves' or Auvard's speculum, and cleanse the vagina, cervix, and posterior fornix with an antiseptic solution (e.g., Betadine, cyproheptadine).

7. Put on a sterile gown and gloves.

8. Place sterile drapes around the perineum.

9. Empty the bladder (if full) with an in-and-out catheter.

10. Perform a paracervical block (see Chapter 174, Paracervical Block) or submucosal block (Fig. 144-2). This can be omitted if the patient has general anesthesia.

11. Grasp the cervix at the 12 o'clock position and elevate it using a tenaculum (Fig. 144-3).

12. Perform an endocervical curettage unless the problem is pregnancy related or if one has been performed during a recent evaluation (Chapter 139, Colposcopic Examination). This is called a "frac-

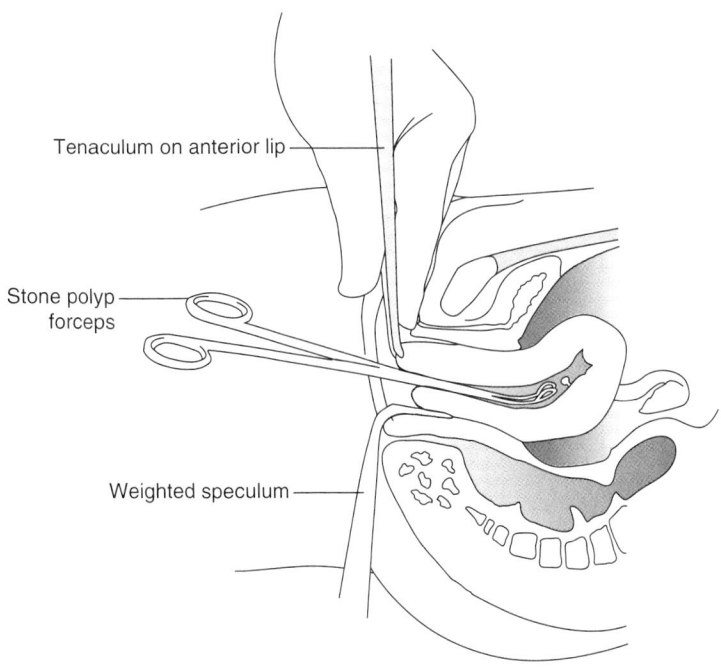

Fig. 144-4
Stone polyp forceps used to remove polyp from uterine cavity. (Redrawn from Junnila RD: Dilation and curettage. In Benjamin RB: *Atlas of outpatient and office surgery,* ed 2, Philadelphia, 1994, Lea & Febiger.)

tional curettage" because the endocervical canal is being evaluated separately from the uterine cavity.

13. Use short, firm, in-and-out strokes from the internal os to the external os, curetting in a full 360-degree circle, twice.

14. Place the collected tissue on a Telfa pad or lens paper, and send this specimen in a separate container to the pathology laboratory.

15. Insert a uterine sound into the os to determine the axis of the cervix and uterine cavity, as well as the depth of the uterus. Greater than 10 cm is abnormal in a premenopausal woman. Most postmenopausal uteri sound less than 8 cm. (For information regarding steps to take when either external or internal os stenosis is encountered, see Chapter 137, Cervical Stenosis and Cervical Dilation.)

16. Dilate the os to 8 to 12 mm using dilators.

17. If using the suction methods, insert the largest suction curette that can easily pass through the os and attach the other end to the suction hosing.

18. Make sure the suction hosing has a tissue trap.

19. Place the curette in the center of the uterus, turn on the suction machine, and close the suction valve on the handle of the curette. To achieve adequate suction, 60 cm or greater of mercury is needed. Use a rotary, slightly in-and-out motion, until an increased resistance to rotation is achieved.

20. Remove the curette slowly with the suction on without touching the vaginal sidewalls. Curette the entire endometrial lining using a "to-and-fro" motion. Do not pull the curette past the internal os. Remove curette with suction off.

21. Place a Telfa pad or large sheet of lens paper into the posterior vaginal vault.

22. Insert a sharp curette and lightly scrape all sides of the uterine cavity. Collect the material on the Telfa pad or lens paper and send in separate lab container.

23. Search the cavity for polyps by systematically opening and closing the Stone polyp forceps while moving across the dome, anterior, and posterior walls of the uterus (Fig. 144-4). Remove any tissue grasped with the forceps with gentle pressure or twisting.

24. Reinsert the curette and suction out any remaining tissue *(optional)*.

Optional Methods

- The entire procedure can be performed under ultrasound guidance (Fig. 144-5).
- Luminaria can be placed in the os the night before the procedure for dilation of the cervix (Chapter 137, Cervical Stenosis and Cervical Dilation).
- A sharp curette alone can be used instead of a suction curette to remove endometrial tissue.

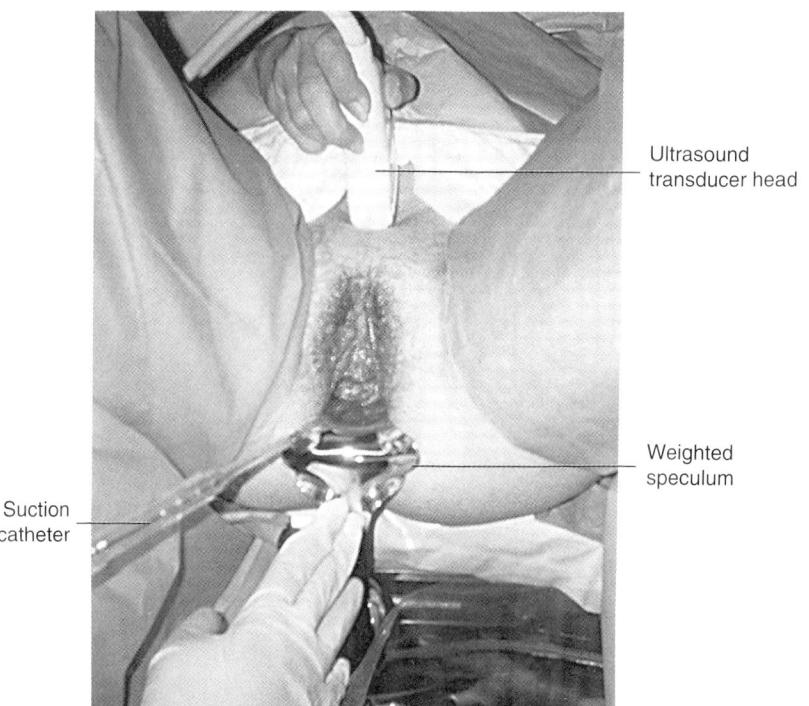

Fig. 144-5
Weighted speculum and suction equipment used in dilation and curettage (D & C). Ultrasound is used to guide the physician during the procedure.

- A curved suction curette is used if the uterus is anteflexed or retroflexed. A straight suction curette is used if the uterus is in midposition.

COMPLICATIONS

- *Hemorrhage:* This is very rare unless the problem is pregnancy related (occurs in less than 1%). Most women will have some spotting for a few weeks afterwards.
- *Infection:* This is extremely rare; treatable with a broad-spectrum antibiotic covering anaerobes.
- *Perforated uterus:* This is more likely to occur in the presence of uterine infection; with a stenotic cervical os, especially in elderly postmenopausal women; in cases in which a sharp (as opposed to vacuum) curette is used; and in patients who are less than 8 weeks' postpartum.
  — With lateral perforation, injury to uterine artery is possible.
  — Anterior-posterior perforation is usually not serious if a small curette is used.
  — Perforation with a blunt object (usually the sound) is generally uncomplicated.
  — Perforation with a sharp object is more significant.
  In most cases, treatment for perforation is simple observation. Perforation should be suspected if the uterine sound or curette passes beyond 9 to 10 cm in the postmenopausal or beyond 12 cm in menstruating women (unless the uterus actually palpates this large). If perforation occurs, the procedure should be terminated. Before discharging the patient, the clinician should look for unstable vital signs and significant pelvic pain or bleeding. Some physicians provide antibiotic coverage, although this is not generally done. The patient should report any fever, pelvic pain, or discharge. The risk of perforation is reduced if the D & C is carried out under ultrasound guidance.
- *Asherman's intrauterine adhesions* may cause secondary amenorrhea, infertility, recurrent abortion, or other menstrual irregularities. Postoperative adhesions are more common when the D & C is performed on the puerperal uterus.
- *Disease may be missed*—in most vigorous D & Cs, studies show only 50% to 60% of the endometrial cavity is actually curetted. The patient and physician must understand that if symptoms persist, a further or repeat diagnostic test may be needed.

POSTPROCEDURE PATIENT EDUCATION

Immediately After the Procedure

- Subsequent to completing the D & C, observe the vital signs for any indication of deleterious effects (i.e., lowered blood pressure or elevation in pulse rate).

- If continued vaginal bleeding is evident after the procedure, give 10 to 20 U of IV oxytocin (Pitocin) in a liter of lactated Ringer's (LR) solution, and methylergonovine maleate (Methergine) 0.2 mg IM. This is especially helpful in pregnancy-related procedures.
- If bleeding does not stop, the clinician should inspect for lacerations and use ultrasonography to visualize intrauterine contents to rule out an incomplete evacuation.
- If a significant decrease in blood volume has occurred, it may be necessary to replenish body fluids intravenously using normal saline or LR solution.
- Provide RhoGAM if patient's blood type is Rh negative and procedure is pregnancy related.

Before Discharge

- The patient should be alert and ambulatory and should have stable vital signs before discharge.
- Instruct the patient to insert nothing in vagina for 2 weeks. This includes sexual activity.
- The patient is to call the office if bleeding is greater than one sanitary napkin per hour or if there is fever, purulent discharge, or unrelieved abdominal pain.
- Consider NSAIDs for pain.
- If the patient is at risk for vaginal infection, consider Doxycycline 100 mg bid for 7 to 10 days.
- Ergonovine 0.2 mg every 4 hours for 1 to 2 days can be given to decrease bleeding in pregnant patients.

After discharge, consider a postoperative check in 1 to 2 weeks to discuss pathological tissue findings and assess the patient's well-being.

Pathological Findings on Dilation and Curettage

Normal Findings
- Proliferative endometrium
- Secretory endometrium
- Atrophic endometrium
- Products of conception

Abnormal Findings
- Endometrial polyp
- Chronic endometritis
- Cystic (simple) hyperplasia
- Adenomatous (complex) hyperplasia
- Adenomatous hyperplasia with atypia
- Adenocarcinoma in-situ
- Endometrial carcinoma (i.e., adenocarcinoma)
- Hydatidiform mole (i.e., trophoblastic disease)
- Variations of cervical dysplasia (from endocervical curettage)

CPT/BILLING CODES

58120	D & C (diagnostic or therapeutic but nonobstetric)
59160	D & C (postpartum)
78630	Transvaginal ultrasound
76700	Transabdominal ultrasound
00946	Paracervical block
36415	Venipuncture
36000	Starting an IV
57505	Endocervical curettage*

ADDITIONAL RESOURCES

- See the sample patient education handout titled "Dilation and Curettage (D & C)" on page 1936 of Appendix G.
- See the sample patient consent form titled "Dilation and Curettage (D & C)" on page 1938 of Appendix G.

BIBLIOGRAPHY

American Academy of Family Practice: *Advanced life support in obstetrics* (course material), Leawood, Kan, 1996, AAFP.

Canavan TP, Doshin R: Endometrial cancer, *Am Fam Physician* 59(11):3069, 1999.

Carcinoma of the endometrium, Tech Rep 162, Washington, DC, Dec 1991, American College of Obstetricians and Gynecologists.

Feldman S, Berkavitz RS, Tostesan AN: Cost-effectiveness of strategies to evaluate postmenopausal bleeding, *Obstet Gynecol* 81:968, 1993.

Grimes DA: Diagnostic dilation and curettage, *Obstet Gynecol* 142:1, 1982.

Hacker N, Moore JG: *Essentials of obstetrics and gynecology,* ed 3, Philadelphia, 1998, WB Saunders.

Johnson BE, Johnson CA, Murray JL, Apgar BS: *Women's health care handbook,* Philadelphia, 1996, Hanley & Belfus.

Junnila RD: Dilation and curettage. In Benjamin RB: *Atlas of outpatient and office surgery,* ed 2, Philadelphia, 1994, Lea & Febiger.

Oriel KA, Schrager S: Abnormal uterine bleeding, *Am Fam Physician* 60:1371, 1999.

Smith RA, von Eschen Bach AC, Wender R, et al: American Cancer Society guidelines for the early detection of cancer, *CA Cancer J Clin* 51:38, 2001.

---

*The endocervical curettage is now "bundled" with a D & C and cannot be charged separately (unless it is not performed as part of D & C).

Human Papillomavirus DNA Typing

The Papanicolaou (Pap) smear has been the principal screening device for cervical cancer since the 1940s, dramatically decreasing the incidence and mortality of this disease. Because of the limitations of traditional Pap smear–based screening, new technologies may serve as worthwhile adjuncts for earlier and more directed diagnosis and serve to decrease health care costs. In spite of new technologies, it is important to note that only about *half* of the women in the United States with cervical cancer *have been screened*. Efforts to enhance screening numbers by any method hold the most promise for reducing the incidence and mortality of this disease.

The current Bethesda system has increased the use of colposcopic triage programs. An equivocal or "atypical squamous cells of undetermined significance (ASCUS)" classification presents a medical dilemma. Of the 2 to 3 million U.S. women diagnosed with ASCUS each year, 75% do not have cervical disease. Although only 5% to 10% of these women harbor serious cervical disease, more than one third of high-grade lesions in screening populations were identified from ASCUS Pap test results. Human papillomavirus (HPV) DNA typing is being studied to help define triage pathways to better identify those women whose disease may progress.

There is overwhelming evidence that human papillomavirus (HPV) is the primary agent in the development of cervical cancer and its precursor, cervical intraepithelial neoplasia (CIN). HPV is the most common sexually transmitted virus. Clinical manifestation is dependent on the epithelial location, HPV type, host-immune status, viral titers, and age.

There are more than 40 genotypes of genital HPV. Subtypes are further categorized as "low risk" (types 6, 11, 42, 43, 44) and "high/intermediate risk" (types 16, 18, 31, 33, 35, 39, 45, 51, 52, 56, 58, 59, 68). Specific HPV types have also been associated with other lesions (Table 145-1).

Studies have shown the following:

- High-risk HPV DNA is found in virtually all (99.7%) cervical carcinomas and precursor lesions worldwide. HPV 16 is the subtype most commonly isolated in cervical cancer specimens.

TABLE 145-1

Human Papillomavirus (HPV) Types Associated with Various Lesions

Lesion	HPV Type
Common warts	2
Planar	4
Butcher's	7
Flat	3
Plantar	1
Epidermodysplasia verruciformis	3, 5, 8, 9, 10, 12, 14, 15, 17, 19, 26, 27
Respiratory	11, 16, 30, and others
Genital	
Low risk	6, 11, 42, 43, 44
High risk	16, 18, 31, 33, 35, 39, 45, 51, 52, 56, 58, 59, 68

- The higher the grade of the neoplasia, the greater the association with HPV.
- HPV detection in Pap smear–negative women is predictive of an increased risk of subsequent detection of CIN.
- The risk of progression may be correlated with viral type.

Despite HPV's causative role in cervical neoplasia, most women with HPV will have spontaneous regression of the infection and never develop cervical cancer. Delineating those women more likely to progress to neoplasia by having persistent, high-risk infection would aid in risk stratification and surveillance/treatment strategies. The use of HPV DNA typing is hoped to be a useful adjunct to the standard Pap test, which would aid in decreasing the time and costs associated with repeat Pap smears, colposcopy, biopsy, and treatment.

Two large studies in the United States have provided strong evidence that testing for HPV DNA high-risk subtypes is a useful tool for managing women with equivocal results. These studies have demonstrated that HPV DNA testing with or without repeat cytology, detects over 90% of high-grade squamous intraepithelial lesions (HSIL) in ASCUS patients and reduces unnecessary colposcopies and treatment by 38% to 60%.

The Kaiser Permanente Study showed that in women with an ASCUS diagnosis, HPV testing identified 89.2% of women with underlying high-grade disease with a specificity of 64%. Repeat Pap testing had a sensitivity of 76% and a specificity of 64%. In women under age 30, the sensitivity and negative predictive values were 100%.

The ASCUS/LSIL (Atypical Squamous Cells of Undetermined Significance/Low-Grade Squamous Intraepithelial Lesions) Triage Study (ALTS), which is still in progress, concluded that HPV DNA testing for cancer-associated HPV subtypes was a viable option for management of ASCUS. The sensitivity to detect CIN 3 or greater lesions by testing for cancer-associated HPV was 96.3% in women with ASCUS, exceeding the 85% sensitivity of a single repeat cytologic specimen using a triage threshold of ASCUS or above on Pap smear. The predictive value of a negative HPV DNA test was 98.9%. Earlier results concluded that the use of HPV DNA typing in LSIL was *not recommended* because of the high percent of women with LSIL who were positive for HPV DNA (at least 75%).

The use of HPV DNA typing after an ASCUS Pap result can lead to improved outcomes by earlier treatment, anxiety relief, and reduction of unnecessary medical tests and interventions for women without cervical disease.

A 2001 editorial in *CA: a Cancer Journal for Clinicians* (Rubin, 2001) concluded that "HPV typing is being investigated as a means of triaging patients with minor abnormalities or Pap smear, but at this point, such testing seems to be of limited use." However, the recommendations published in the April 2002 *JAMA* article suggest using DNA typing to triage ASCUS, evaluating treatment "cure," and screening women over 30 years old. As of May 2002, the Food and Drug Administration (FDA) had not yet approved HPV DNA cytologic typing for primary screening.

In addition to cytologic specimens, DNA typing can also be performed on tissue samples.

INDICATIONS

- To screen patients with ASCUS Pap smear results to determine the need for colposcopy
- To provide quality control for cytologic and histologic diagnosis in laboratories
- To determine HPV types in cases of suspected sexual abuse
- To correlate HPV types in victims and perpetrators of sexual abuse
- Research applications

The HPV test is not intended to be used as a screening device in the general population. Future applications may include HPV DNA typing in immunocompromised women. It is not approved by the FDA for use in males.

However, tissue samples can be used to determine HPV types in cases of suspected sexual abuse to correlate HPV types in the victim and the perpetrator.

CONTRAINDICATIONS

Manufacturers do not recommend use of the conical brush in pregnancy, although several studies have documented its safety.

EQUIPMENT

Many tests can be used to document HPV disease including polymerase chain reaction, Southern blot, in situ, and hybrid capture. These tests can detect HPV even before there are visible microscopic cell changes. The detection rate varies with laboratory accuracy, essay variability, physiologic changes, and age. Comparison of multiple clinically useful testing methods revealed that a second generation hybrid capture method (hybrid capture 2 [HC2]) yielded the optimal test results for evaluating HPV.

Currently the only FDA-approved, commercially available test for HPV DNA typing is the Hybrid Capture HPV DNA Assay manufactured by Digene. All national reference laboratories use this assay.

Cervical specimens can be tested with the Digene HPV test as follows:
- Digene cervical sampler kit with conical brush and transport tube and medium.
- While obtaining a Pap smear, specimens are collected using the broom type collection device or brush and "swished" in Cytyc PreservCyt solution for ThinPrep determinations.
- Cervical biopsies collected in Digene specimen transport medium.

Tissue biopsies (cervical, penile, anal, etc.) can also be placed in formalin for in situ hybridization in paraffin-embodied tissue. A pathologist can help determine which test is available, the costs, and which assay should be done.

TECHNIQUE

Collection of Cervical Sample with Brush

1. Remove excess mucus from the cervical os and surrounding ectocervix using a cotton or Dacron swab. Discard the swab.
2. The specimen is collected with a cervical conical brush using Digene's Specimen Collection Kit by inserting the brush 1 to 1.5 cm into the os of the cervix until the largest outer bristles of the brush touch the ectocervix. The Digene brush is different

than the standard Pap smear brush. It is softer and has a conical shape (2 mm distally and 7 mm up the shaft end near the clinician).

3. Do not insert the brush completely into the cervical canal.
4. Rotate the brush three full turns in a counterclockwise direction.
5. Insert the brush to the bottom of transport tube and snap off shaft at score line and cap securely.

Specimens in Cytyc PreservCyt Solution

1. Cervical plastic broom or cytobrush specimens collected and rinsed thoroughly in Cytyc PreservCyt solution for use in making ThinPrep Pap test slides can be used. Using a brush to collect the sample instead of the plastic "broom" almost doubles the pickup of abnormal cells. Whether this has any beneficial effect for HPV typing is unknown.
2. The ThinPrep test slide should be prepared by the laboratory. There must be at least 4 ml of solution remaining for the Digene HPV test, or lack of sufficient material could lead to false negatives. The HPV testing sample should be collected after the Pap smear sample has been taken if both are done in the same visit. A second sample for the Digene HPV test is not necessary if the Cytyc ThinPrep Pap test is performed, unless the laboratory prefers two samples for ease in processing. If the sample is collected during colposcopy, the HPV sample should be collected before use of acetic acid or any other type of solution.

Direct Cervical Biopsies

Direct cervical biopsies collected in Digene specimen transport medium can be used and must be 2 to 5 mm in cross section. The sample needs to be frozen immediately at $-20°$ C.

As noted previously, samples can be placed directly into formalin for in situ hybridization in paraffin-embodied tissue. Your pathologist can help determine which test is available to you and the costs involved.

COMPLICATIONS

No complications have been reported.

TEST INTERPRETATION

The Digene HPV test can differentiate between two groups: low-risk (HPV types 6, 11, 42, 43, 44) and high/intermediate-risk (types 16, 18, 31, 33, 35, 39, 45, 51, 52, 56, 58, 59, 68) but does not determine the specific HPV type present.

The presence of high or intermediate risk HPV in women with ASCUS Pap results indicates a higher risk for cervical disease and should engender subsequent stronger consideration of colposcopy and possible treatment. Studies currently taking place may generate algorithms that could be used to help make a determination.

Specific HPV types can be determined in select cases but are not usually clinically relevant and markedly increase cost.

SUPPLIERS

Digene Corp.
1201 Clopper Road
Gaithersburg, MD 20878
Phone: 1-800-344-3631
Website: www.digene.com

CPT/BILLING CODE

87621   HPV amplified probe technology × 2 (two test results per patient specimen: include low-risk and high-risk)

Note: This is the code for *interpretation* of the test. There is no code for the practitioner to use for collection of the specimen.

BIBLIOGRAPHY

Atypical Squamous Cells of Undetermined Significance/Low-Grade Squamous Intraepithelial Lesions Triage Study: Human papillomavirus testing for triage of women with cytologic evidence of low-grade squamous intraepithelial lesions: baseline data from a randomized trial, *J Natl Cancer Inst* 92(5):397, 2000.

Cohn DE, Herzog TJ: New innovations in cervical cancer screening, *Clin Obstet Gynecol* 44(3):538, 2001.

Cox JT, Lorincz AT, Schiffman MH, et al: Human papillomavirus testing by hybrid capture appears to be useful in triaging women with a cytologic diagnosis of atypical squamous cells of undetermined significance, *Am J Obstet Gynecol* 172:946, 1995.

Ferenczy A: The Bethesda system (TBS): advantages and pitfalls. In Franco E, Monsonego J, editors: *New developments in cervical cancer screening and prevention,* Malden, Mass, 1997, Blackwell Science.

Janicek MF, Averette HE: Cervical cancer: prevention, diagnosis, and therapeutics, *CA Cancer J Clin* 51(2):92, 2001.

Manos MM, Kinney WK, Hurley LB, et al: Identifying women with cervical neoplasia: using human papilloma DNA testing for equivocal Papanicolaou results, *JAMA* 281(17):1605, 1999.

National Institutes of Health: *Cervical cancer: consensus development conference statement,* vol 14, no 1, Bethesda, Md, April 1996, NIH.

Peyton CL, Schiffman M, Lorincz AT, et al: Comparison of PCR– and hybrid capture–based human papillomavirus detection systems using multiple cervical specimen collection strategies, *J Clin Microbiol* 36(11):3248, 1998.

Rubin SC: Cervical cancer: successes and failures, *CA Cancer J Clin* 51(2):89, 2001.

Shen L, Rushing L, McLachlin CM, et al: Prevalence and histologic significance of cervical human papillomavirus DNA detected in women at low and high risk for cervical neoplasia, *Obstet Gynecol* 86:499, 1995.

Solomon D, Schiffman M, Tarone B: Comparison of three management strategies for patients with atypical squamous cells of undetermined significance: baseline results from a randomized trial, *J Natl Cancer Inst* 93(4):293, 2001.

Sulik SM, Kroeger K, Schultz JK, et al: Are fluid-based cytologies superior to the conventional Papanicolaou test? A systematic review, *J Fam Pract* 50(12):1040, 2001.

CHAPTER 146

Endometrial Biopsy

Barbara S. Apgar
John L. Pfenninger

Endometrial biopsy (EB) is a safe and cost-effective diagnostic method of evaluating the endometrium for causes of abnormal uterine bleeding and infertility, and to rule out the presence of precursor changes or invasive adenocarcinoma of the endometrium.

It is the preferred *first* procedure for evaluating abnormal uterine bleeding and has virtually replaced the dilation and curettage (D & C). The *ACOG Technical Bulletin* (1991) concludes that the accuracy of office endometrial biopsy under optimal conditions approaches that of D & C (the false negative rate of endometrial biopsy is 5% to 15% whereas for D & C it is 2% to 6%). Some advocate using endometrial thickness as determined by transvaginal ultrasonography as an alternative, but exact safe cutoff measurements vary among authors and vary by patient race. (Also see Chapter 144, Dilation and Curettage, and Chapter 209, Emergency Department and Office Ultrasound.)

INDICATIONS

- To determine the cause of abnormal uterine bleeding (pre and post menopausal) secondary to ovulation/anovulation disorders, hormonal therapy, and malignancy/hyperplasia
- To evaluate infertility (short luteal phase, ovulation/anovulation)
- To evaluate endometrial cells on a Papanicolaou smear in a woman over the age of 40 years.
- For the evaluation of atypical glandular cells (AGC) in a woman over the age of 40 years or in a younger woman if abnormal bleeding is present or if other causes cannot be identified.
- To evaluate abnormal endometrial thickness on transvaginal ultrasound (generally felt to be 5 mm or more).
- Lower thresholds for diagnostic intervention is appropriate for women with abnormal uterine bleeding who are at higher risk of endometrial cancer (obesity, hypertension, family history, infertility, diabetes, chronic anovulation, other cancers, chronic unopposed estro-

gen therapy if uterus present, late menopause [over 55 years old], nulliparity, tamoxifen therapy)
- Follow-up to previous diagnosis of endometrial hyperplasia or atypia
- To evaluate an enlarged uterus (in conjunction with ultrasound examination)
- To reassure women who are not satisfied by discussions of likely benign nature of vaginal bleeding
- As screening for women with hereditary non-polyposis colon cancer syndrome (HNPCC). The latest American Cancer Society Guidelines (2001, 2003) suggest that this is the only true *screening* indication for EB. HNPCC is defined as three relatives with histologically verified colorectal cancer, with one a first-degree relative of the other two. At least two successive generations must be affected and at least one case must be diagnosed before the age of 50. Women should be screened if they are known carriers of the autosomal dominant gene or in the absence of genetic testing, if there is a strong suspicion of its presence. Annual screening should begin at age 35 due to the high risk of endometrial cancer. (The American Cancer Society does note that this recommendation is made on the basis of expert opinion and that strong scientific evidence is not yet available to substantiate their recommendation.)

CONTRAINDICATIONS

- Pelvic inflammatory disease/cervicitis
- Pregnancy

PREPROCEDURE PATIENT PREPARATION

1. Explain the procedure to the patient and obtain informed consent. (See the sample patient education handout titled "Endometrial Biopsy" on page 1939 of Appendix G and the sample patient consent form

titled "Endometrial Biopsy" on page 1940 of Appendix G.) Obtain the appropriate clinical history and clinical records (Fig. 146-1).

2. Offer the patient a nonnarcotic oral analgesic 1 hour before the procedure (e.g., ibuprofen 600 to 800 mg). A sedative such as oral diazepam (Valium) 10 mg may be administered an hour before the procedure in extremely anxious patients.

3. Antibiotic prophylaxis is not indicated.

4. Endometrial biopsy should be performed on Day 22 or 23, counting from the first day of the last menstrual period in reproductive age women. By that time, evidence of secretory glands (indicating that ovulation has occurred) should be present. Avoid doing a biopsy during the menstrual period because stromal breakdown can simulate malignancy resulting from fragmentation of cells and hemorrhage. Endometrial biopsy can be performed anytime in postmenopausal women, but avoid bleeding episodes if possible in order to optimize sample size.

EQUIPMENT

Various instruments are used to obtain endometrial tissue (Fig. 146-2 through 146-6). The more popular ones are described here for comparison. Small cervical dilators are helpful for stenotic cervices (see Chapter 137, Cervical Stenosis and Cervical Dilation) and should be readily available when performing these procedures.

Flexible Plastic Endometrial Aspirator (Disposable)

• Vaginal speculum (preferably large Graves')
• Antiseptic solution (povidone-iodine) if not allergic and cotton balls
• Ring forceps
• Endometrial aspirator (various manufacturers); some aspirators are calibrated in centimeters
• Single-toothed tenaculum, (may or may not be necessary)
• Uterine sound (may or may not be necessary)
• Scissors
• Sample bottle with buffered formalin and labels for patient identification
• Endocervical curette without basket (e.g., Kevorkian) or some method of adequately sampling the endocervical canal

Stainless-Steel Curette (reusable)

• Vaginal speculum (preferably large Graves')
• Antiseptic solution (povidone-iodine) if not allergic and cotton balls

• Ring forceps
• Novak or Randall curette
• Single-toothed tenaculum
• Uterine sound
• 20-ml syringe
• Sample bottle with buffered formalin and labels for patient identification
• Endocervical curette without basket (or some method of sampling the endocervical canal)

Tis-u-Trap Endometrial Curette and Vabra Aspirator (Disposable)

• Vaginal speculum (preferably large Graves')
• Antiseptic solution (povidone-iodine) if not allergic and cotton balls
• Ring forceps
• Tis-u-Trap sampler device (Fig. 146-3, *A*) or Vabra Aspirator—requires external suction pump
• Single-toothed tenaculum
• Uterine sound
• Sample bottle with buffered formalin and labels for patient identification
• Endocervical curette without basket

Brush Sampler

• Tao brush (Fig. 146-5). Some suggest using the Tao brush after the endometrial biopsy to reduce false negatives. Studies now report using it as a "stand-alone" method for endometrial sampling.
• Antiseptic solution (povidone-iodine) if not allergic and cotton balls.
• Ring forceps.
• Vaginal speculum (preferably large Graves').
• Uterine sound.
• CytoRich Red solution.
• Endocervical curette without basket (or some method of sampling the endocervical canal).

TECHNIQUE

Place the woman in stirrups and perform a Pap smear first if it is indicated. Perform a bimanual examination to determine the position of the uterus. Insert the large Graves' speculum in the usual fashion and wipe the cervix clear of any blood, mucous or debris. Use the ring forceps and cotton balls to swab the cervix and vaginal cuff with antiseptic solution.

When using an endometrial biopsy to rule out neoplasm, an endocervical curettage (ECC) generally precedes endometrial sampling (just as with a D & C). Introduce a Kevorkian endocervical curette without a basket or similar disposable curette through the external os and into the endocervical canal. Curette the entire endocervical canal 360 degrees twice, scraping from the internal os to the external os (see Chapter 139, Colposcopic Examination). A gritty sensation should be appreciated and the patient generally feels some cramping. Collect the tissue obtained onto 2 × 2–inch squares of lens paper then place in formalin. The endometrial biopsy itself should follow the ECC.

The plastic endometrial aspirators are self-contained instruments that require no external suction pump and are currently the most commonly used instrument for

---

Endometrial Biopsy Encounter Form

Date: _____

Name _____ Date of Birth _____ Age _____

Regular Doctor _____

Referring Doctor _____

Symptoms _____

_____

Age of first period _____ Pregnancies _____ Deliveries _____ Miscarriages/Abortions _____

Last menstrual period _____ Weight _____ Smoker _____ Packs/day _____

Periods regular in past?   Y   N   How often? _____

    No. of days? _____ Flow? _____

Last Pap smear

Date _____ Performed where _____ Result _____

Any Pap smears abnormal in past?   Y   N

Any history of genital warts in self or partner?   Y   N

Previous uterine or cervical procedures? _____

Ever take birth control pills?   Y   N

Ever take hormones?   Y   N

Ever use IUD/coil?   Y   N

Ever have infection or pregnancy in tubes?   Y   N

Ever have a tubal ligation?   Y   N   Age _____

Risk Factors:

    Obesity   Excessive hair growth   Hypothyroidism

    Breast, ovarian, colon ca   Alcohol abuse   Unopposed estrogen

    Tamoxifen   Liver disease   Family hx breast, colon or ovarian ca

    Anovulation/infertility   Diabetes   HNPCC

PMH:

    Meds: _____

    Allergies: _____

    Illnesses: _____

    Surgeries: _____

    Health Maintenance: _____

FH: _____

Preparation: Handouts read and understood?   Y   N

    Complications explained (perforation, bleeding, pain, missing lesion, infection)   Y   N

Fig. 146-1

Sample of endometrial biopsy encounter form. (Used with permission from The National Procedures Institute, Midland, Mich.)

Examination:

Abdomen

Pap performed?   Y   N

Bimanual: Uterus

Position: Ant   Mid   Post

Size: Normal or _____

Tenderness: Y   N

Ovaries

Palpable: Y   N   Size _____

Tenderness: Y   N

Speculum: Cervix

Procedure: Prep with _____

Tenaculum   Y   N

ECC done?   Y   N

Sounding _____ cm

Instrument used _____

Number of insertions _____

Amount of tissue _____

Bleeding _____

Complications: None or _____

Impression: _____

_____

_____

Plan: _____

_____   _____

Physician's signature   Date

cc: _____

Fig. 146-1, cont'd
For legend see previous page.

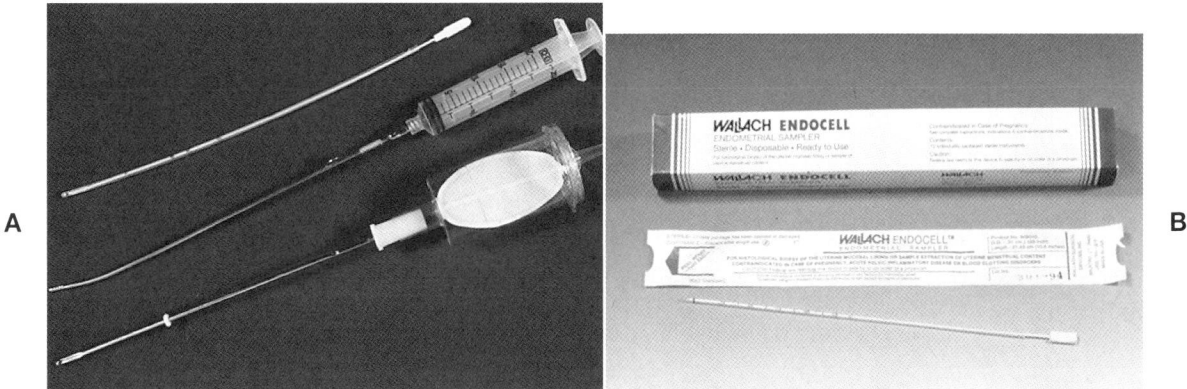

Fig. 146-2
A, Three common instruments used to obtain an endometrial sample. *Upper,* Plastic disposable aspirator; *middle,* the Novak curette; *lower,* the Tis-u-Trap. **B,** Wallach biopsy unit.

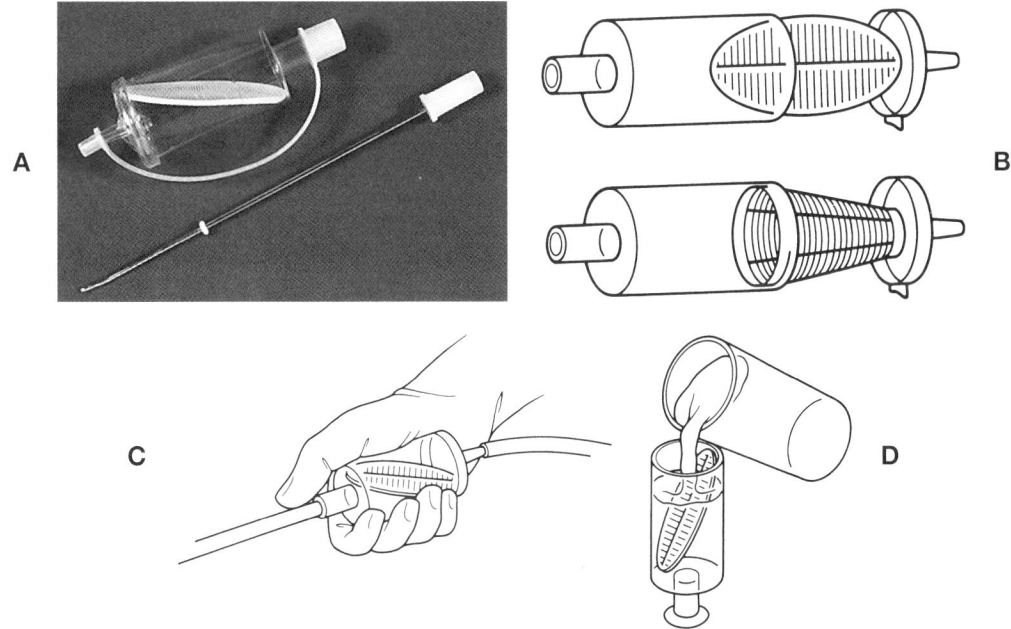

Fig. 146-3
A, Tis-u-Trap sampler device. **B,** The plastic grid onto which the tissue will rest. **C,** Initiate suction by covering the suction hole on the curette. **D,** Remove the curette from the tissue trap and cap the opening. Pour formalin into the container to cover the plastic grid, then seal with cover.

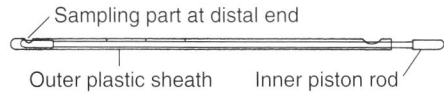

Fig. 146-4
Typical plastic, flexible, disposable endometrial suction aspirator.

obtaining an EB. The stiffer-tipped aspirators may be more successful in obtaining a sample in the presence of a stenotic os. More flexible types may be "stiffened" by placing them in a freezer for 10 to 15 minutes. The aspirator consists of an outer plastic sheath with a circular opening in the distal end. An internal plastic rod functions as a piston that creates negative pressure within the instrument sheath when it is retracted. These units are inexpensive, require little office setup, and are associated with diagnostic accuracy at least equal to that of D & C (except for the diagnosis of endometrial polyps) (Fig. 146-4).

If the aspirators are calibrated, they can be used to sound the depth of the uterus (6.5 to 10 cm is normal). Without calibration or if they cannot be inserted even

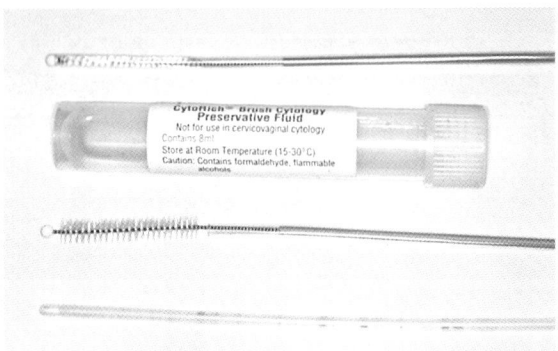

Fig. 146-5
Top, Tao brush and plastic cover over bristles. *Middle upper,* Liquid medium for Tao brush sample. *Middle lower,* Tao brush. *Lower,* Plastic aspirator for size comparison.

with methods noted above, then a metal uterine sound should be used.

In addition to the typical aspirators, there is also a disposable setup that allows more suction by attaching a locking syringe on the end of the plastic aspirator (Milex). This may be helpful when there is significant bleeding or one expects to find a generous amount of tissue (Fig. 146-6).

The Novak curette, the Tis-u-Trap endometrial curette, and the Vabra aspirator may be used to obtain a microcurettage of the endometrium. The latter two instruments obtain suction by using an external electric pump. The Novak curette or Randall curette is attached to a syringe.

The Tao brush is the newest method of obtaining an endometrial sample and is described below.

With all endometrial biopsy techniques, cleanse the cervix with antiseptic solution, and insert the sterile sampling device through the cervical os without touching the vulva or vaginal walls. Do not touch or contaminate the part of the sampler that is placed into the uterus. Sterile gloves and speculum are not necessary if a "no touch" technique is used. An endocervical curette is used to perform an endocervical curettage before the endometrial biopsy specimen is obtained (see Chapter 139, Colposcopic Examination). The endocervical and endometrial samples are placed in separate formalin containers.

Plastic Endometrial Aspirators (most common method)

1. Perform a bimanual examination to determine the position of the uterus.
2. Insert a vaginal speculum, and visualize the cervix.
3. Cleanse the cervix with antiseptic solution.
4. Perform the endocervical curettage if a neoplastic process is suspected.

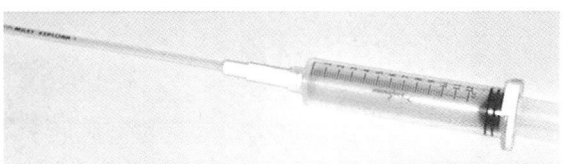

Fig. 146-6
Milex endometrial suction curette with locking syringe attached.

5. If the aspirator is not calibrated, then a uterine sound should be used to record the depth of the endometrial cavity.
6. Introduce the aspirator (with the piston fully inserted to the distal tip of the sheath) through the external os and endocervical canal, into the uterine cavity, and up to the fundus. A tenaculum may be placed on the cervix to stabilize it as the aspirator is inserted (Fig. 146-7, *A*).
7. Document the depth of the endometrial cavity if this has not already been done. If the aspirator cannot be inserted even after the tenaculum has been applied for stabilization, it may be necessary to use a metal uterine sound or dilators first. (See Chapter 137, Cervical Stenosis and Cervical Dilation.)
8. With the aspirator fully inserted, stabilize the sheath with one hand, so it will not be removed during the procedure. Draw the piston completely back in one continuous motion with the other hand to create negative pressure within the lumen of the sheath (Fig. 146-7, *B*).
9. Rotate the sheath between the thumb and index finger, while moving it in and out between the fundus and the internal os until adequate sample is obtained. These combined actions cause the aspirator opening to go through a helical arc against the walls of the uterus. The negative pressure within the sheath draws the endometrial tissue into the aspirator opening, where it is sheared away and carried into the sheath lumen. Do not remove the aspirator outside the cervix or suction will be lost. Fill the sheath lumen with as much tissue as possible (Fig. 146-7, *C*).
10. Withdraw the entire device from the uterus. Do not push the piston back in the sheath before withdrawal or the sample will be lost.
11. Cut off the distal tip of the aspirator (Fig. 146-7, *D*) with the scissors, and expel the sample into the formalin by advancing the piston into the sheath (Fig. 146-7, *E*).

Note: Although the manufacturers do not recommend it, I [JLP] do not cut off the tip but rather just gently express the contents into formalin. If the aspirator does not become contaminated, I will reinsert the unit to obtain more tissue if I feel it may be beneficial.

12. Remove the speculum from the vagina.

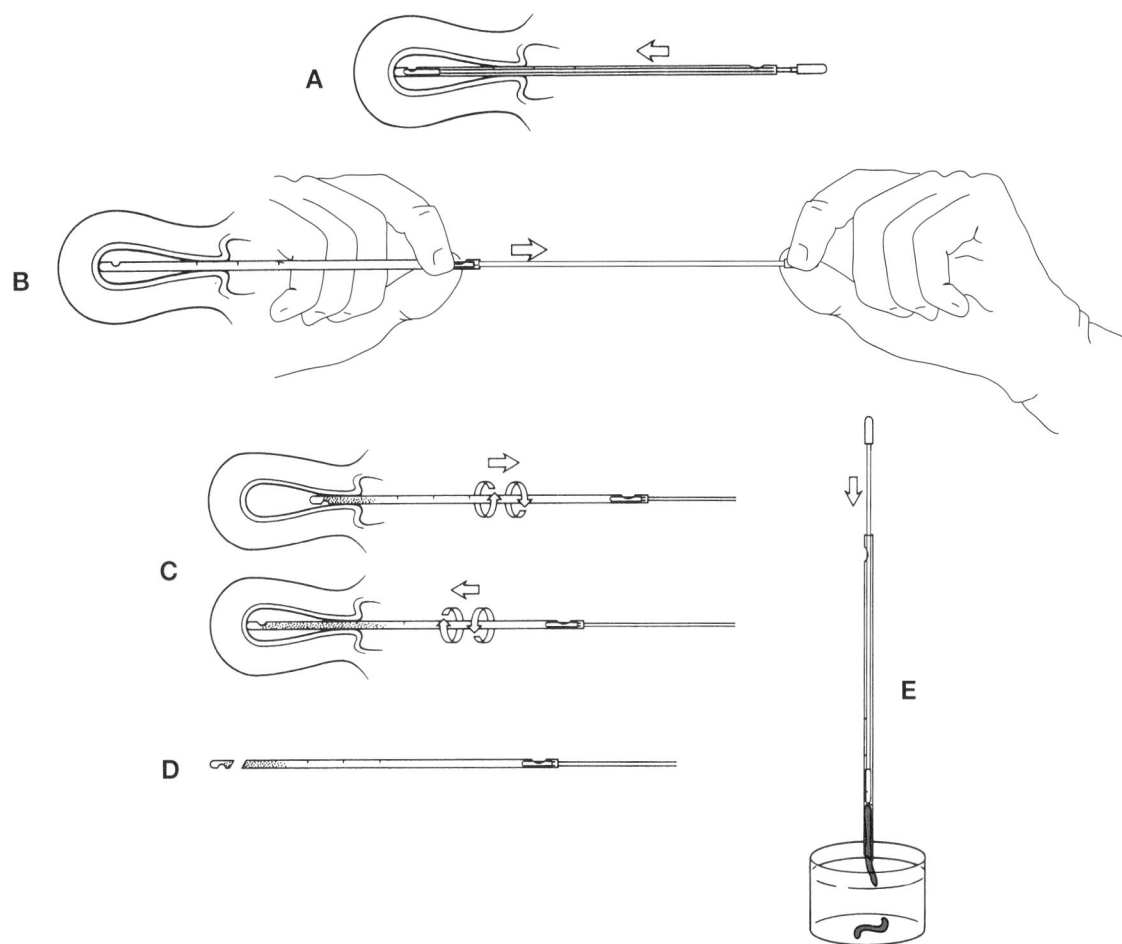

Fig. 146-7
A, With the piston fully advanced within the sheath, insert the aspirator through the cervical canal into the uterine cavity. **B,** While holding the outer sheath, pull the piston back completely creating maximum negative pressure within sheath. **C,** Simultaneously roll the sheath between your fingers while pushing the sheath laterally and back and forth from the fundus to internal os at least three or four times (more is better) to obtain the sample. **D,** Remove the aspirator from the uterus and cut off the distal tip just proximal to the curette opening. **E,** Advance the piston rod to expel the sample into the formalin.

Novak or Randall Curette

1. Perform a bimanual examination to determine the position of the uterus.
2. Insert a vaginal speculum, and visualize the cervix.
3. Cleanse the cervix with antiseptic solution.
4. Perform the ECC if the procedure is being done to rule out a neoplastic process (see above).
5. Apply a tenaculum to the anterior or posterior lip depending on the position of the uterus. Grasp the cervix with the tenaculum in the horizontal position. Avoid grasping the cervix when the tips are vertically oriented at the 3 or 9 o'clock position, thereby decreasing the diameter of the external os. Use of local anesthesia (2 ml 2% xylocaine) at the site of the tenaculum tips may help to decrease discomfort that would be experienced.

6. Apply gentle traction on the tenaculum and insert a uterine sound to the top of the fundus, and measure the length of the endometrial cavity. If stenosis is present, see Chapter 137, Cervical Stenosis and Cervical Dilation.
7. Apply gentle traction with the tenaculum as the curette is inserted into the endometrial cavity up to the fundus.
8. Attach a 20-ml syringe to the curette hub. Create suction by pulling the syringe plunger back to the 10- to 15-ml mark.
9. Perform four to six single-strip curettages, by applying pressure against the side walls of the uterus, and sampling from the fundus to the lower uterine segment. One sample from each quadrant is advised.
10. Withdraw the curette from the uterus and express

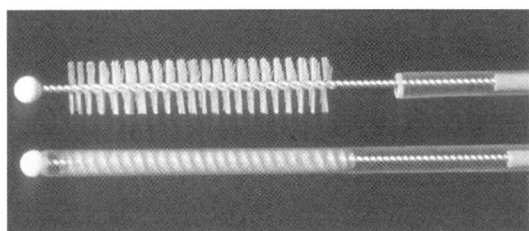

Fig. 146-8
Tao brush for obtaining an endometrial sample. *Top,* The brush. *Bottom,* The brush with a plastic cover around it for insertion.

the sample into the formalin sample bottle by pushing the plunger of the syringe toward the curette. Label the formalin bottle.

11. Remove the speculum from the vagina.

Tao Brush Method

The Tao Brush may be used alone, or, either before or after the plastic aspirators are used (Fig. 146-8).

1. Perform a bimanual examination to determine the position of the uterus.
2. Insert a vaginal speculum, and visualize the cervix.
3. Cleanse the cervix with antiseptic solution.
4. Perform the ECC if the procedure is being done to rule out a neoplastic process (see above). Grasp the cervix if necessary.
5. Sound the uterus (up to 10 cm is normal). If stenosis is present, see Chapter 137, Cervical Stenosis and Cervical Dilation.
6. Insert the Tao brush protected by the plastic outer sheath until it reaches the fundus.
7. Withdraw the outer sheath to expose the plastic bristles and rotate 360 degrees 10 times against the uterine walls (Fig. 146-9).
8. Cover the brush with the outer sheath and then remove entire apparatus.
9. Place the brush into supplied fixative and pull the sheath back and forth 10 times to dislodge the endometrial tissue. The "kit" supplied with the Tao brush includes CytoRich Red, which hemolyzes the blood. The pathologist then prepares a "thin-layer" sample (liquid-based cytology).

Tis-u-Trap or Vabra Aspirator

1. Perform a bimanual examination to determine the position of the uterus.
2. Insert a vaginal speculum, and visualize the cervix.
3. Cleanse the cervix with antiseptic solution.
4. Perform the ECC if the procedure is being done to rule out a neoplastic process (see above).
5. Apply a tenaculum to the anterior or posterior lip of the cervix.

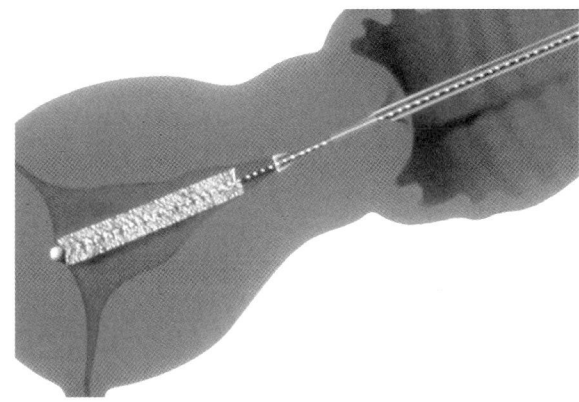

Fig. 146-9
Tao brush inserted into endometrial cavity with cover removed. (Courtesy of Cook ObGyn, Spencer, Ind.)

6. Insert a uterine sound to the fundus, and measure the depth of the endometrial cavity (up to 10 cm is normal). If stenosis is present, see Chapter 137, Cervical Stenosis and Cervical Dilation.
7. Attach the device to the external suction pump, and activate the pump to 55 cm H_2O.
8. Insert the curette through the os and into the uterine cavity and up into the fundus. The depth is determined by the previous uterine sounding. Now initiate the suction by covering the suction hole.
9. Perform a curettage of the entire endometrium. The tissue will travel through the curette and into the trap, where it will collect on the grid.
10. When sufficient tissue is in the trap, discontinue the suction and remove the curette from the uterus.
11. Turn off the suction pump and remove the curette from the trap.
12. Add formalin to the trap, ensuring that all the tissue is exposed to the solution. Cap and label the trap, preparing it for transport to pathology (Fig. 146-3).
13. Remove the speculum from the vagina.

COMPLICATIONS

- *Bacteremia, septicemia,* and *endocarditis* have been reported after endometrial biopsy, although they are very rare.
- Reports indicate a 0.1% to 1.3% risk for *uterine perforation* with use of rigid devices while sounding, or with dilation for stenosis. Patients in whom perforation is suspected should be observed closely for bleeding complications and infection, but no other intervention is indicated unless symptoms develop. They may be sent home if there are no symptoms and vital signs are stable after 30 minutes of observation. Caution should be taken regarding signs of infection and bleeding. Repeat biopsy can be attempted in 6 to 8 weeks.

- Excessive *uterine bleeding* may occur after endometrial biopsy, especially in patients with undiagnosed coagulation disorders or perforation.
- *Missing the lesion* on biopsy is always a possibility and could be considered a complication. There is a 5% to 15% false negative rate for endometrial biopsy.
- Up to 10% of patients have been reported to have some degree of *vasovagal reaction* after the procedure.
- *Pain* is generally minimal, and if present after 24 hours, the patient should report it. There will generally be significant cramping at the time of the ECC but this should be short-lived.

POSTPROCEDURE PATIENT EDUCATION

- Ask the patient to remain supine for 10 minutes after the endometrial biopsy has been taken. Assess for vasovagal reaction.
- Painful uterine cramps (if present) usually subside rapidly or are relieved by nonsteroidal antiinflammatory agents.
- If heavy bleeding is not observed and the vasovagal reaction (if it has occurred) has resolved, the patient may be discharged from the clinic.
- The patient may resume sexual relations after bleeding has stopped.
- Instruct the patient to report any fever, cramping after 48 hours, or bleeding that is heavier than a normal menses.
- No follow-up visit is necessary, but if patient's bleeding symptoms persist, she may need further evaluation with a repeat endometrial biopsy, a D & C, hysteroscopy, or a pelvic ultrasound.

INTERPRETATION OF THE ENDOMETRIAL BIOPSY SAMPLE
(Box 146-1)

1. Interpretation of the biopsy sample is determined by the status of the functionalis layer (upper two thirds of the endometrium). Minimum changes occur in the basalis layer.
2. Atrophic, denuded, or scarred endometrium may not yield sufficient sample for diagnosis. Inadequate samples may be obtained immediately after menses, in the presence of a hypoestrogenic state, if prolonged bleeding has occurred, or intrauterine adhesions or synechiae are present. Menopausal status has more effect on the quality or adequacy of the sample than does the type of instrument used.
3. Types of hyperplasia range from simple hyperplasia to invasive carcinoma:

BOX 146-1
Findings on Endometrial Biopsy Sampling

Insufficient Tissue
Follow-up depends on clinical situation; may need to repeat or use other diagnostic techniques

Normal
Proliferative endometrium
Secretory endometrium
Atrophic endometrium

Pregnancy Related
Retained products of conception
Decidua (consider an ectopic or missed abortion)

Infectious Etiology
Endometritis, treat as indicated

Abnormal
Rarely, endometrial polyp
Simple (cystic) hyperplasia
- Progression to risk for cancer extremely small. Little need for follow-up unless symptoms present
Complex (adenomatous) hyperplasia
- Low but some risk for progression to cancer
- Treat with progestational agents and follow-up with tissue sampling in 6 months
Atypical hyperplasia
- Significant risk for progression to cancer
- Consider hysterectomy because of significant risk of progression to invasion and need for long-term follow-up to detect progression. If child bearing not complete, treat with progestational agents and follow with frequent biopsies. Referral and consultation should be strongly considered.
Adenocarcinoma
- Referral indicated for appropriate workup and treatment

Note: If the ECC is positive for dysplasia, a conization is indicated. If symptoms persist, in spite of treatment, regardless of biopsy results, further evaluation is indicated.

a. *Simple hyperplasia* (back-to-back crowding of endometrial glands is absent; glands are evenly distributed throughout stroma, and hypertrophy is absent). Also known as *cystic hyperplasia*. There is no clinical significance to this finding.
b. *Complex hyperplasia* (endometrial glands are hypertrophied and stroma is obliterated by glands). Also known as *adenomatous hyperplasia*. This is a low-grade precancerous change and needs proper treatment, assessment, and follow-up.
c. *Atypical hyperplasia* (cytologic atypia of glands). Atypical hyperplasia has a significant risk of developing into adenocarcinoma. It may be difficult for the pathologist to differentiate atypical hyperplasia from well-differentiated adenocarcinoma. There is the potential for overdiagnosis and inappropriate treatment if histologic diagnosis is inaccurate (Box 146-1).
4. Histology determines therapy. The degree of endo-

metrial hyperplasia and the presence of other conditions cannot be determined by the amount of bleeding, when bleeding occurs in the menstrual cycle, the gross appearance of the endometrial biopsy sample, or the volume of tissue obtained at the time of biopsy. The histopathology must be determined. Transvaginal endometrial thickness measurement does not reduce the need for histologic determination in symptomatic women.

SUPPLIERS

Plastic Endometrial Aspirator

Pipelle
CooperSurgical
15 Forest Parkway
Shelton, CT 06484
Phone: 1-800-243-2974
Website: www.coopersurgical.com

Pipet Curet
Milex Products
4311 N. Normandy
Chicago, IL 60634
Phone: 1-800-621-1278

Endocell Endometrial Sampler
Wallach Surgical
235 Edison Road
Orange, CT 06477
Phone: 1-203-799-2000
Website: www.wallachsurgical.com

Other Samplers

Tao Brush
Cook OBGyn
1100 West Morgan Street
P.O. Box 227
Spencer, IN 47460
Phone: 1-812-829-4891
Website: www.CookOBGyn.com

Tis-u-Trap Sampler Device, endometrial suction curette
Milex Products
(Same contact information as above)

Vabra Aspirator
Berkeley Medevices
1330 South 51st. Street,
Richmond, CA 94804-4628
Phone: 1-800-227-2388
Website: www.berkeleymedevices.com

Stainless-Steel Novak or Randall Endometrial Curettes, and Endocervical Curettes
Most medical supply companies will have these curettes.

(For ECC units, also see Chapter 139, Colposcopic Examination)

CPT/BILLING CODES

58100,	Endometrial biopsy, any method (including Tao brush) without dilation, with or without endocervical curettage
57800	Cervical dilation (instrument)
59200	Cervical dilation (laminaria)

ICD-9-CM DIAGNOSTIC CODES

182.0	Ca uterus
219.1	Benign neoplasm, uterus
233.2	Ca in situ, uterus
621.0	Uterine polyp
621.2	Enlarged uterus
621.3	Endometrial hyperplasia
625.9	Pelvic pain
626.5	Functional vaginal bleeding
626.8	Dysfunctional uterine bleeding
626.9	Abnormal uterine bleeding
627.0	Premenopausal menorrhagia
627.1	Postmenopausal bleeding
622.1	Atypical glandular cells
V07.4	Postmenopausal HRT
10.42	Personal Ca uterus

ADDITIONAL RESOURCES

- See the sample patient education handout titled "Endometrial Biopsy" on page 1939 of Appendix G. See the sample patient consent form titled "Endometrial Biopsy" on page 1940 of Appendix G.

BIBLIOGRAPHY

Apgar BS, Newkirk GR: Endometrial biopsy in primary care office procedures, Primary Care Clincs of North America 24(2):303, 1997.

American College of Obstetricians and Gynecologists: ACOG Committee Opinion, *Tamoxifen and endometrial cancer,* no. 169, Feb 1996, ACOG.

Baugham DM: Office endometrial aspiration biopsy, *Fam Pract Recert* 15(5):45, 1993.

Carcinoma of the endometrium, *ACOG Tech Bull* 162:1, 1991.

Canavan TP, Doshi NR: Endometrial cancer, *Am Fam Physician* 59:3069, 1999.

Check JH et al: Clinical evaluation of the Pipelle endometrial suction curette for timed endometrial biopsies, *J Reprod Med* 34(3):218, 1989.

Del Priore G, Williams R, Harbatkin CB, et al: Endometrial brush biopsy for the diagnosis of endometrial cancer, *J Reprod Med* 46:439, 2001.

Dunn TS, Stamm CA, Delorit M, Goldberg G: Clinical pathway for evaluating women with abnormal uterine bleeding, *J Reprod Med* 46(9):831, 2001.

Farquhar CM, Lethaby MA, Sowter M, Verry J, Baranyai J. An evaluation of risk factors for endometrial hyperplasia in premenopausal women with abnormal uterine bleeding. *Am J Obstet Gynecol* 1999; 181:525-9.

Franehi M, Ghezzi F, Donadello N, et al. Endometrial thickness in tamoxifen-treated patients: An independent predictor of endometrial disease. *Obstet Gynecol* 1999; 93:1004-8.

Grimes DA: Diagnostic dilation and curettage: a reappraisal, *Am J Obstet Gynecol* 142(1):1, 1982.

Guido RS, Kanbour-Shakor A, Rulin MC, Christopherson WA: Pipelle endometrial sampling: sensitivity in the detection of endometrial cancer, *J Reprod Med* 40:553, 1995.

Her-Juing H, Casto BD, Elsheilch TM: Endometrial brush biopsy: an accurate outpatient method of detecting endometrial malignancy, *J Reprod Med* 48:41, 2003.

Jaber R: Detection of and screening for endometrial cancer, *J Fam Pract* 26(1):67, 1988.

Kaunitz AM, Masciello A, Ostrowski M, Rovira EZ: Comparison of endometrial biopsy with the endometrial Pipelle and Vabra aspirator, *J Reprod Med* 33(5):427, 1988.

Koonings PP, Grimes DA: Endometrial sampling techniques for the office, *Am Fam Physician* 40(4):207, 1989.

Koonings PP, Moyer DL, Grimes DA: A randomized clinical trial comparing Pipelle and Tis-u-Trap for endometrial biopsy, *Obstet Gynecol* 75(2):293, 1990.

Kurman RJ, Kaminshi PF, Norris HJ: The behavior of endometrial hyperplasia: a long-term study of "untreated" hyperplasia in 170 patients, *Cancer* 56:403, 1985.

Larson DM, Bronste SK: Histopathologic adequacy of office endometrial biopsies taken with the Z-Sampler and Novak curette in premenopausal and postmenopausal women, *J Reprod Med* 39(4):300, 1994.

Larson DM, Johnson KK, Broste SK, et al: Comparison of D&C and office endometrial biopsy in predicting final histopathologic grade in endometrial cancer, *Obstet Gynecol* 86:38, 1995.

Oriel KA, Schrager S: Abnormal uterine bleeding, *Am Fam Physician* 60:1371, 1999.

Perkins RL, Hernandez E, Berenberg JL: Septicemia in a postmenopausal woman after endometrial biopsy, *Am J Gynecol Health* 4(2):20, 1990.

Runowicz C, Saslow D, Smith RA, et al: 2001 ACS guidelines for the cancer-related check-up: an update for endometrial cancer, *CA Cancer J Clin* 51(1):59, 2001.

Schneider L: Causes of abnormal vaginal bleeding in a family practice center, *J Fam Pract* 16(2):281, 1983.

Silver MM, Miles P, Rosa C: Comparison of Novak and Pipelle endometrial biopsy instruments, *Obstet Gynecol* 78:828, 1991.

Smith RA, Cokkinides V, Eyre HJ: American Cancer Society Guidelines for the Early Detection of Cancer, 2003, *CA Cancer J Clin* 53:27, 2003.

Smith RA, von Eschenbach AC, Wender R, et al: American Cancer Society guidelines for the early detection of cancer: update of early detection guidelines for prostate, colorectal, and endometrial cancers, *CA Cancer J Clin* 51:38, 2001.

Stovall TG, Photopulos GJ, Poston WM: Pipelle endometrial sampling in patients with known endometrial carcinoma, *Obstet Gynecol* 77:954, 1991.

Tabor A, Watt HC, Wald NJ. Endometrial thickness as a test for endometrial cancer in women with postmenopausal vaginal bleeding. *Obstet Gynecol* 2002; 99:663-670.

Wu HH, Harshbarger KE, Berner HW, Elsheika FM: Endometrial brush biopsy (Tao brush), *Am J Clin Pathol* 114:412, 2000.

Young GCH, Wan LS: Endometrial biopsy using the Tao brush method, *J Reprod Med* 45:109, 2000.

CHAPTER 147

Hysterosalpingography/ Sonohysterosalpingography

Steven Fettinger

Hysterosalpingography (HSG) is a radiologic examination of the female genital tract. It allows for the evaluation of the cervical canal, endometrial cavity, tubal lumen, and the periadnexal area. The basic infertility work-up includes an HSG, although some physicians feel that it has been superseded by laparoscopy with hysteroscopy. However, it remains an integral part of many other diagnostic work-ups. HSG is a relatively easy procedure, requires no anesthesia, and has a low complication risk. Its use as a *therapeutic* procedure for enhancing fertility is promoted by some clinicians. The addition of selective cannulation of the cornual ostia has eliminated many false positives and opened new therapeutic options. This possibility, however, requires special training and currently limits its use to an infertility specialist or an interventional radiologist. The radiation exposure is usually minimal, in the 50 to 500 mrem ranges.

Sonohysterosalpingography (SHSG) is a newer technique of visualization of the reproductive tract using ultrasound and the injection of ultrasonic contrast media. The ease of this procedure and the availability of ultrasound in the office have been responsible for its rapid growth. The discomfort involved is less, but the complications and contraindications are similar. The anatomy is imaged using a vaginal probe ultrasound and catheter-injected normal saline (or ultrasonic contrast media). The procedure itself is simple, but the expertise and experience needed for interpretation are beyond the average practitioner. The limitations of accuracy in visualizing the fallópian tubes are made up for by the ability to identify endometrial pathology. Evaluation of the endometrial stripe thickness in the work-up of abnormal uterine bleeding has been enhanced greatly by using SHSG in combination. Some clinicians rely solely on the thickness of the endometrial stripe to rule out endometrial cancer. However, ethnic variations exist and cancer has been found frequently in Japanese women with stripes only 3 to 4 mm thick. The American College of Obstetricians and Gynecologists' (ACOG) technical bulletin advises that if an endometrial biopsy and endocervical curettage are negative, no further work-up is needed unless bleeding persists or there are other indications to suspect cancer. Hormone replacement and tamoxifen also affect uterine lining thickness.

INDICATIONS

- Infertility (uterine)
  - Endometrial adhesions (Asherman's syndrome)
  - Polyps
  - Pedunculated leiomyomata
  - Uterine anomalies
  - Diethylstilbestrol (DES): T-shaped uterus
- Infertility (tubal)
  - Assessment of tubal patency
  - Salpingitis isthmica nodosa
  - Periadnexal adhesive disease
  - Tubal cannulation procedures
- Habitual abortions
  - Asherman's syndrome
  - Uterine anomaly
  - DES changes
  - Leiomyomata
- Cervical incompetency (controversial indication)
- Preoperative and postoperative evaluation
  - Tubal reanastomosis/reimplantation, tuboplasty
  - Uterine septal resection, metroplasty
  - Myomectomy
- Localization of lost intrauterine contraceptive device (IUD); ultrasound alone is the procedure of choice
- Abnormal uterine bleeding (SHSG)
- Confirmation of tubal occlusion after Essure contraceptive coil insertion

CONTRAINDICATIONS

- Allergy to contrast medium
- Recent history of or active salpingitis
- Pregnancy

- Recent dilation and curettage
- Untreated sexually transmitted disease (STD)

GENERAL EQUIPMENT

- Cannulas

Many types of HSG cannulation devices are available. The choice of catheters used may depend on procedure indication and physician preference. Three general types are in common use, with multiple modifications (the flexible balloon cannulas are also used for SHSG):
1. *Olive-tipped cannulas.* A small cannula traverses the cervical canal, and an olive- or cone-shaped seat is held against the inner cervix to seal it.
2. *Suction cannulas.* A small cannula is held in place and sealed by a suction cup on the ectocervix.
3. *Balloon cannulas.* One or two balloons are used to fix and seal the cervix. A primary intrauterine balloon is pulled down against the internal cervical os by a second balloon, a spring-loaded platform, or manual traction. The balloon catheters (including pediatric Foley catheters) obscure the lower uterine anatomy; however, the balloon can be deflated after the procedure, and additional contrast dye can be injected to evaluate this area.

Special selective cannulation catheterization systems (Cook Balloon Cervical Catheter) are available from most vendors (see the "Suppliers" section). These catheters are used to selectively cannulate and evaluate a fallopian tube in special circumstances (e.g., unilateral or bilateral nonvisualization, salpingitis isthmica nodosa, or prior ectopic pregnancy). They may also be used therapeutically in some patients to open a blockage in the proximal tubes.
- Contrast medium

Most centers currently use water-soluble dye. There has been continued controversy regarding the use of water-soluble versus oil-based media (Table 147-1). The question of ionic or nonionic water-soluble dye depends on the preference of the radiologist. The majority of centers are using the cheaper ionic dyes, except in patients with a history of an iodine allergy.

SPECIFIC EQUIPMENT

- Prep tray, including 4 × 4–inch gauze pads, ring forceps, povidone-iodine solution, medicine cups, lubricating jelly, and a plastic speculum
- Cannula (Fig. 147-1)
  - Jaco, or Kuhn (nondisposable)
  - Hysterocath (Cook)
  - HUI (CooperSurgical)
  - HUI Mini-Flex (CooperSurgical)

- ZUMI 2.0/4.0/4.5 (BEI/Zinnanti)
- H/S Elliptosphere Catheter Set (Ackrad)
- Pediatric Foley catheter
- Contrast medium
  - HSG Contrast
    - Water soluble: Salpix (Ortho Pharmaceutical), Sinografin (Squibb),
    - Conray 60 (Mallinckrodt Pharmaceutical)
    - Oil based (Lipoidal or Ethiodol)
    - Nonionic water soluble: Hypaque-60 (Winthrop-Breon Pharmaceutical)
  - SHSG Contrast
    - Normal saline
    - Echovist (Schering-Berlin Pharmaceutical)
    - Albunex (Mallinckrodt Pharmaceutical)
- Vaginal speculum
  - One-armed Graves' (removable after placement of cannula)
  - Plastic nonradiopaque (disposable)
- Tenaculum (if needed to fixate cervix for cannula placement)
- Syringe, 10 or 20 ml

TABLE 147-1

Selection of Contrast Medium

Medium	Advantages	Disadvantages
Water soluble	Rapidly absorbed Less need for delayed films Improved visualization of details Extravasation tolerated	No enhancement of fertility
Oil based	Possible fertility enhancement	Delayed films may be needed Granuloma formation possible Embolism if extravasation occurs

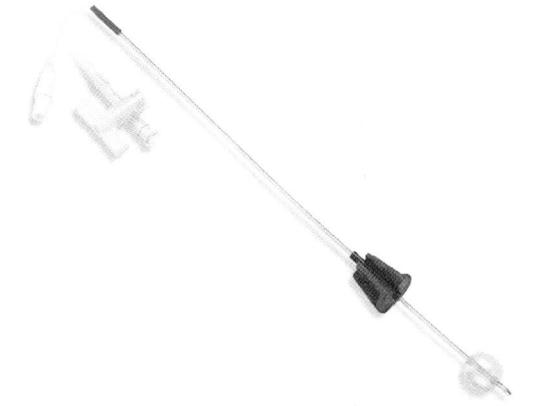

Fig. 147-1

Example of uterine catheter for injection of dye for hysterosalpingography. (Courtesy CooperSurgical, Trumbull, Conn.)

PREPROCEDURE EVALUATION

- HSG should be performed in the preovulatory phase of the menstrual cycle to avoid exposing an embryo to radiation and to decrease the risk of infection (infection rates are higher if the procedure is performed during the secretory phase). HSG during the preovulatory phase will avoid the possibility of dislodging a preimplantation conception, and thereby prevent an ectopic pregnancy.
- Patients with a history of salpingitis require negative cultures for sexually transmitted disease, and a nontender preprocedure pelvic examination.
- Patients with a history of pelvic inflammatory disease or prior tuboplasty should be treated with prophylactic antibiotics. One option shown to be effective is doxycycline 200 mg the morning of the procedure and 100 mg twice a day for 5 days following the procedure. Antibiotic prophylaxis is controversial for patients without a history of pelvic inflammatory disease or prior tuboplasty. Many physicians now use prophylaxis with all patients undergoing HSG, despite the lack of evidence of its usefulness in low-risk patients.
- Preoperative medications may include a nonsteroidal antiinflammatory agent, such as ibuprofen 600 mg, given 1 to 2 hours preoperatively to decrease pain and cramping. Diazepam 10 to 20 mg 1 to 2 hours preoperatively may be given for extreme apprehension.

PREPROCEDURE PATIENT PREPARATION

- Discuss the procedure, the typical findings, alternatives to, risks of, and possible complications of the procedure with the patient; obtain informed consent.
- Explain to the patient that mild discomfort will be experienced during the procedure, and that spotting for up to a few days after the procedure is expected.
- Educate the patient about the warning signs of complications (e.g., increasing pain, heavy bleeding, and fever).

TECHNIQUE (Fig. 147-2)

Hysterosalpingography

1. Check all equipment to ensure that the setup is complete and in proper working condition.
2. Draw up the contrast material and preload the cannula (bubbles may obscure intrauterine disease).
3. Position the patient on a high-resolution image-intensifier fluoroscopy table in the dorsal lithotomy position. An adequate light should be available.
4. Perform a bimanual pelvic examination to assess the degree of flexion or retroflexion of the uterus and to exclude pelvic tenderness (the latter is a contraindication to HSG if there is suspected inflammation).
5. Insert the vaginal speculum.
6. Cleanse the cervix and upper vagina with povidone-iodine.
7. If indicated by the cannula choice, grasp the anterior lip of the cervix with the tenaculum (slowly, to minimize pain).
8. Insert the cannula and seat it as indicated by the specific cannula:
   Inflate the upper balloon, then the lower balloon (Cook).
   Inflate the upper balloon and set the spring platform (CooperSurgical).
   Inflate the balloon and pull down (pediatric Foley and Zinnanti).
   Insert the cannula and set spring to tenaculum (Jaco).
   Insert the cannula and seat suction cup onto the cervix, then apply suction to the cup (Cook).
9. Remove the speculum (nonradiopaque plastic speculum may be left in place).
10. Place the patient in the recumbent position for fluoroscopy.
11. Inject the contrast slowly. Between 1 and 3 ml may be sufficient to show intrauterine detail; greater volumes may obscure small polyps or adhesions. The injection should be viewed concurrently, and a single spot film taken. Upward or downward movement of the tenaculum will often change the degree of flexion to obtain a better view.
12. Continue to inject dye until the tubes start to fill. A spot film at this point may show tubal detail that will be obscured after dye spills.
13. Continue to inject dye until intraabdominal spill of dye is seen bilaterally. A spot film at this point will sometimes show peritubal detail. A delayed film may be needed to confirm location of dye in peritubal adhesions.
14. Rolling the patient from side to side during the procedure sometimes helps the clinician to visualize lesions.
15. If visualization of one tube cannot be accomplished initially, try relaxing the tubal spasm by relieving the pressure on the syringe and waiting 1 to 2 minutes.

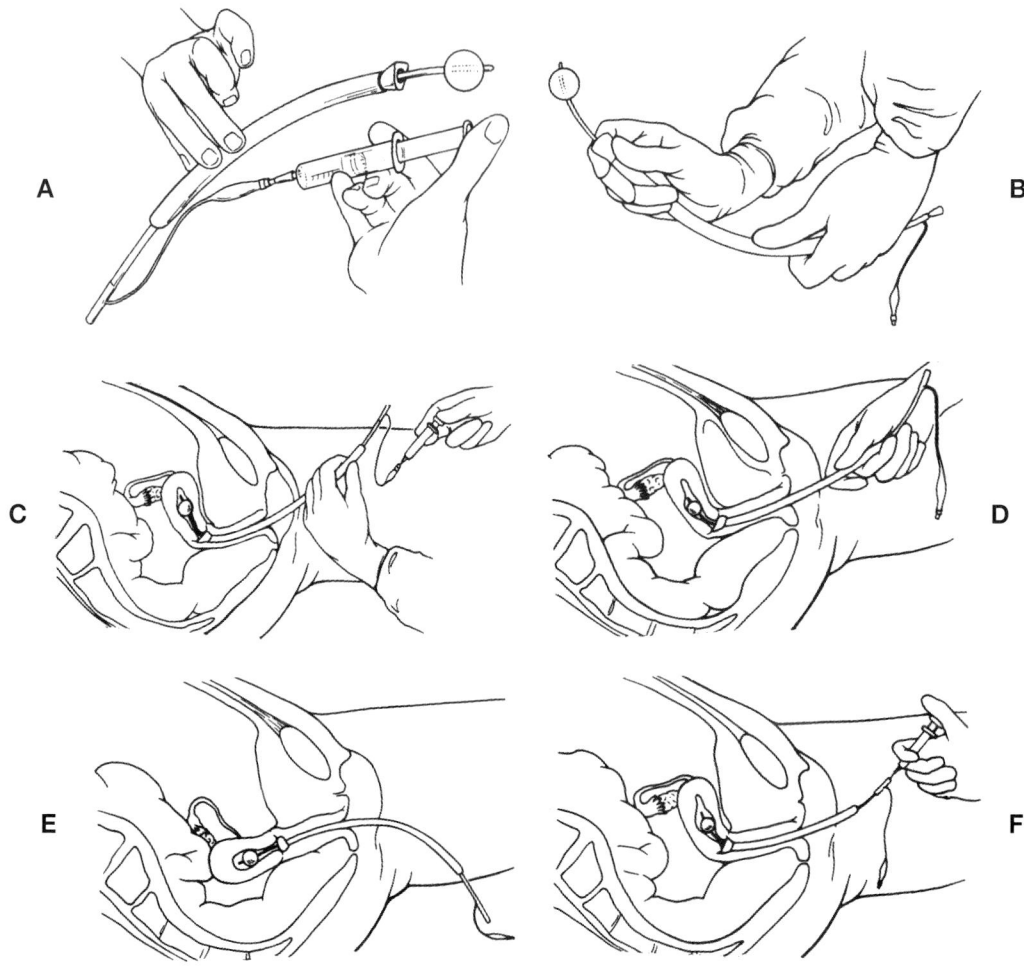

Fig. 147-2
Technique of using ZUMI 4.5 (Zinnanti) for HSG. **A,** Testing catheter cuff balloon. **B,** Adjusting catheter for uterine depth. **C,** Placement of catheter and inflation of cuff. **D,** Gentle downward traction to test placement and to seal against cervix. **E,** Placement for posteriorly flexed uteri. **F,** Injection of contrast media. For more detail, refer to the product package instructions.

16. Remove the instruments.
17. Observe the patient for 30 minutes for allergic reactions and heavy bleeding.
18. Selective cannulation of the ostia is briefly done as follows:
    a. Preassemble coaxial catheter portions to be used or add portions as indicated, for the given patient (Fig. 147-3, *A*).
    b. Place the cervical access catheter (CAC) as above (catheter type must match the system used) (Fig. 147-3, *B*).
    c. Introduce the uterine ostial access catheter (UOAC) through the CAC under radiologic guidance until the tip reaches the tubal ostia (this may be aided by the injection of a small amount of a contrast) (Fig. 147-3, *C*).
    d. Pass the uterine cornual access catheter (UCAC)

through the UOAC until the ostia is reached (Fig. 147-3, *D*).
    e. Advance the guidewire into the tube for a short distance, advance the UCAC over the wire, and then repeat the process until the UCAC is well within the tubal lumen.
    f. While holding the UCAC in place, remove the wire.
    g. Confirm placement by injecting contrast into UCAC.

Sonohysterosalpingography

1. Using the infusion port of the catheter, fill the catheter with sonomedia, purging all air.
2. Position the patient in the lithotomy position and insert a speculum.

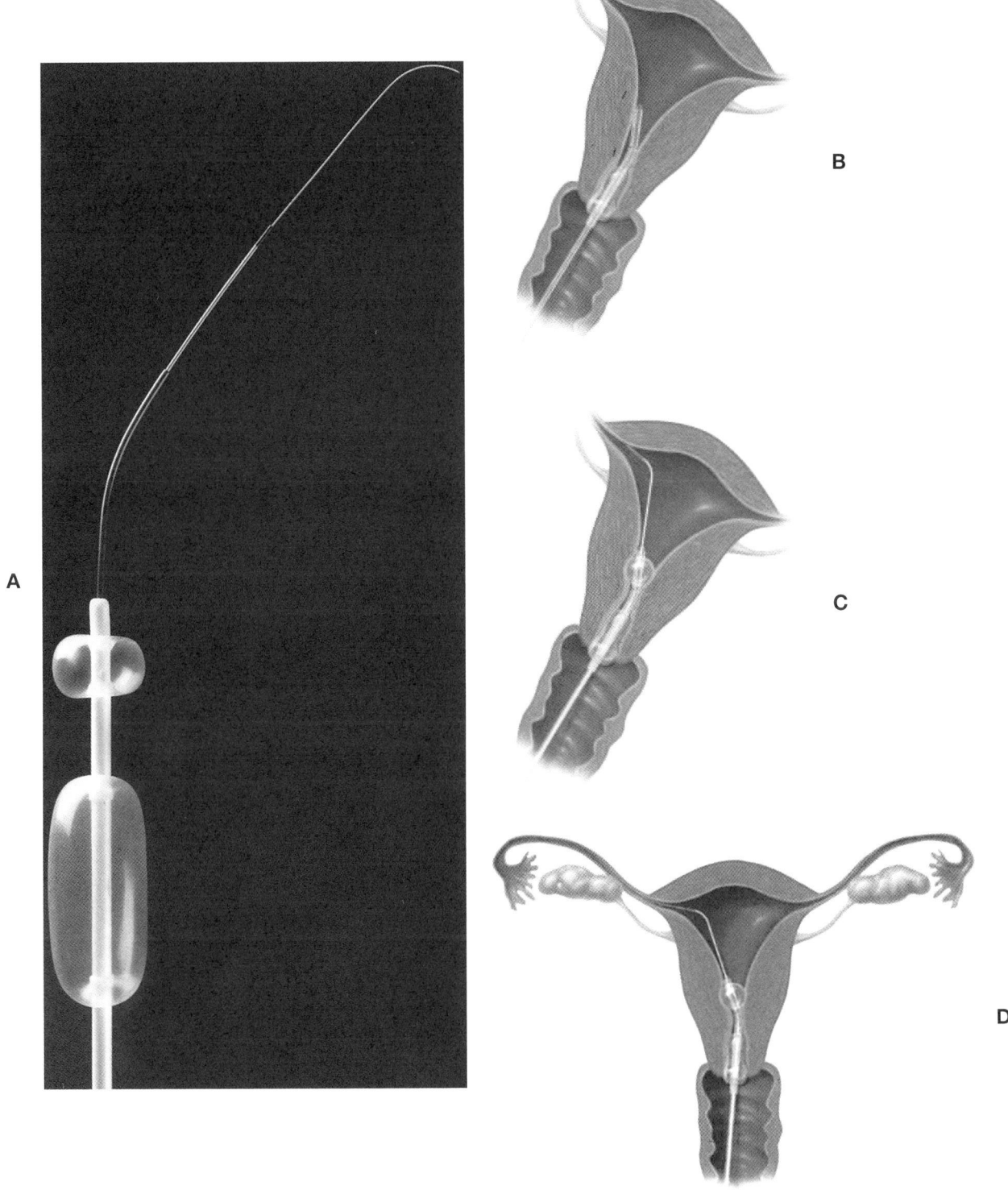

Fig. 147-3
Selective cannulization of the ostia. **A,** Preassembled Cook balloon cervical cannula (BCC), the selective salpingography catheter (SSC), and the inner catheter with wire guide (IC). **B,** BCC in uterus. **C,** SSC passes through BCC. **D,** IC through SSC. (Courtesy Cook Ob/Gyn, Spencer, Ind.)

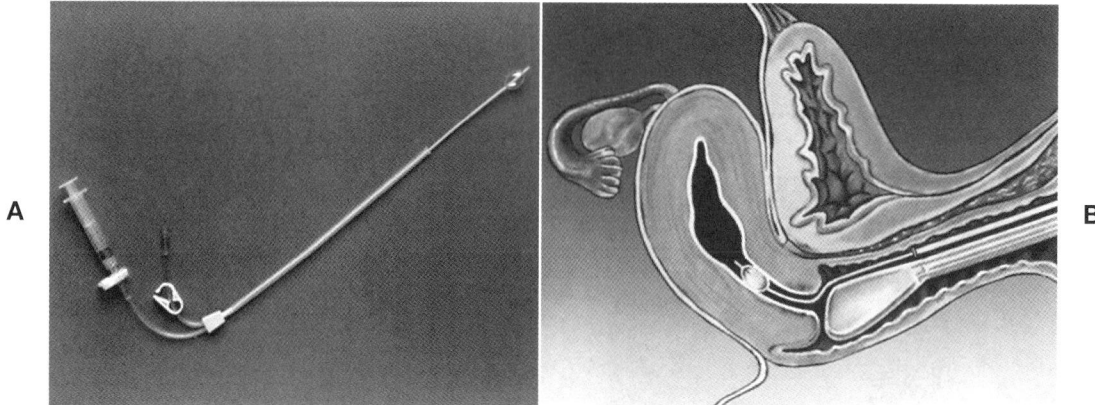

Fig. 147-4
Sonohysterosalpingography. **A,** H/S Elliptosphere catheter set. **B,** Catheter placed in cervical canal. (Courtesy Ackard Laboratories, Inc., Cranford, NJ.)

3. Prep the vagina and cervix with povidone-iodine prep or equal.
4. Insert the SHSG catheter of choice and inflate the balloon (Fig. 147-4).
5. Remove the speculum and insert the transvaginal ultrasound transducer into position.
6. While imaging the uterus, slowly inject 10 to 20 ml of contrast.
7. The uterine distention allows evaluation of the cavity for polyps or other pathology.
8. Continued injection (especially if Albunex is used) fills the tubes for study; if spillage into the abdomen occurs, patency is verified.

COMPLICATIONS

• Infection rates may be as high as 3%. Antibiotic prophylaxis is indicated in select patients (as mentioned previously) to decrease this risk.
• Tenaculum site bleeding is rare but may require suturing.
• Extravasation of dye into the intravascular space warrants discontinuation, especially if an oil-based dye is used (there is a risk of oil pulmonary embolus).
• Granuloma formation after oil-based dye is a rare late complication.
• Uterine perforation should prompt discontinuation.
• Rupture of a hydrosalpinx.

INTERPRETATION

Interpretation is beyond the scope of this chapter, but a few points may be helpful.

• The normal HSG should show: (1) a smooth triangular endometrial cavity, (2) a narrow smooth isthmic tube, (3) a progressively enlarging, increasingly convoluted ampullary tube with internal mucosal folds, and (4) spillage into the peritoneal cavity with dispersion between bowel loops.
• The correlation of HSG and laparoscopy may be as poor as 25% false-positive and false-negative (the use of selective cannulation may decrease this). Therefore absolute statements regarding tubal patency should not be made.
• Uterine anomalies are classified according to Buttram and Gibbons, but may also require laparoscopy to fully define the abnormality.
• The association of renal with uterine developmental anomalies may be as high as 20%; therefore renal evaluation may be indicated.
• As noted previously, regardless of study results, HSG can be "therapeutic" and assist pregnancy success for unknown reasons.

SUPPLIERS

Ackrad Laboratories, Inc.
70 Jackson Drive
Cranford, NJ 07016
Phone: 1-800-684-4252
Website: www.ackrad.com

Cook Ob/Gyn
1100 West Morgan Street
P.O. Box 271
Spencer, IN 47460
Phone: 1-800-541-5591
Website: www.cookobgyn.com

CooperSurgical
95 Corporate Drive
Trumbull, CT 06611
Phone: 1-203-601-5200
Website: www.coopersurgical.com

CPT/BILLING CODE

58340   Hysterosalpingography
74740   Hysterosalpingography, radiologic supervision and interpretation
58345   Transcervical introduction of fallopian tube catheter for diagnosis and/or treatment
74742   Transcervical introduction of fallopian tube catheter for diagnosis and/or treatment, radiologic supervision and interpretation
99070   Supplies and materials
76830   Transvaginal ultrasound combined with SHSG
76831   Transvaginal ultrasound combined with SHSG, radiologic supervision and interpretation

ICD-9-CM DIAGNOSTIC CODES

218.XX*   Uterine leiomyoma
628.XX*   Infertility, female (628.2 of tubal origin)
622.5   Incompetence of cervix
629.9   Unspecified disorder of female genital organs (habitual aborter without current pregnancy)
V26.2   Investigation and testing (fallopian insufflation)

*See ICD-9 code book for more specific codes.

BIBLIOGRAPHY

American College of Obstetricians and Gynecologists: Compendium of selected publications, ACOG Educational and Practice Bulletins No 125, 212, 215, 237, Washington, DC, Dec 2000, ACOG.

Buttram VC Jr, Gibbons WE: Mullerian anomalies: a proposed classification, *Fertil Steril* 32:40, 1979.

Fleischer A, Javitt MC, Jeffrey RB: *Clinical gynecologic imaging,* Philadelphia, 1996, Lippincott Williams & Wilkins.

Garcia CR: *Current therapy of infertility,* ed 3, Toronto, 1988, BC Decker.

Kempers RD, Cohen J, Haney AF, Younger JB: *Fertility and reproductive medicine,* New York, 1998, Elsevier Science.

Mishell DR Jr: *Infertility, contraception & reproductive endocrinology,* ed 3, Montvale, NJ, 1991, Medical Economics Company.

Oriel K, Schrager S: Abnormal uterine bleeding, *Am Fam Physician* 60(5):1371, 1999.

Rock JA, Murphy AA, Jones HW: *Female reproductive surgery,* Baltimore, 1992, Williams & Wilkins.

Sciarra JJ: *Gynecology and obstetrics,* vol 26, Philadelphia, 2002, Lippincott Williams & Wilkins.

Smith-Bindman R, Kerlikowske K, Feldstein VA, et al: Endovaginal ultrasound to exclude endometrial cancer and other endometrial abnormalities, *JAMA* 280(17):1510, 1998.

Speroff L, Glass RH, Kase NG: *Clinical gynecologic endocrinology and infertility,* ed 6, Baltimore, 1989, Lippincott Williams & Wilkins.

Stovall DW: The role of hysterosalpingography in the evaluation of fertility, *Am Fam Physician* 55(2):621, 1997.

Taymor ML: *Infertility,* New York, 1990, Plenum Publishing.

Tsuda H, Kawabata M, Kawabata K, et al: Differences between Occidental and Oriental postmenopausal women in cutoff level of endometrial thickness for endometrial cancer screening by vaginal scan, *Am J Obstet* 172(5):1494, 1995.

Watson A, Vanderkerckhove P, Lilford R, et al: A meta-analysis of the therapeutic role of oil soluble contrast media at hysterosalpingography: a surprising result? *Fertil Steril* 61:470, 1994.

CHAPTER 148

Intrauterine Device Insertion

Ashley K. Christiani

John L. Pfenninger

The intrauterine device (IUD) has been available as a birth control method for over 25 years. Although the precise mechanism of action remains elusive, it is thought that the IUD works to prevent pregnancy in several ways. The primary action appears to be by interfering with sperm migration through thickening of the cervical mucus. When the IUD is in place, few sperm ever reach the oviducts. High copper concentrations may also mitigate sperm penetration and fertilization of the ovum. A mild "foreign-body" inflammatory reaction within the uterine lining also occurs, thus interfering with implantation should any fertilization occur. For the progesterone systems, ovulation may be inhibited.

Although the IUD fell out of favor for many years after a reported increase in the incidence of pelvic inflammatory disease (PID) and the highly publicized Dalkon Shield lawsuits, contemporary IUDs (considered much safer than their predecessors) are now gaining in popularity. The risk of PID is elevated only for the first month after insertion of the IUD.

Some features that make the IUD an attractive form of birth control for many women are its high efficacy rate (less than 1% risk of pregnancy), its ease of use once inserted, and its relative lack of systemic effects (Tables 148-1 and 148-2). Two IUDs are currently available in the United States: (1) the ParaGard T380A, a copper IUD containing no hormones that may be left in place for 10 years, and (2) the Mirena Levonorgestrel Intrauterine System (LNG IUS), a progesterone-secreting device effective for 5 years.

Clinicians have often avoided the use of IUDs, particularly in nulliparous women, for fear of litigation. However, studies now show little risk of infection with the device, no increased risk of infertility in the absence of chlamydia, and numerous advantages to the IUD as a long-term reversible contraceptive. In addition to other benefits, IUDs have been shown to decrease the risk of uterine cancer by as much as 49%.

Although the IUD has not been shown to increase risk of cervical dysplasia, women using this form of contraception may be less likely to present for routine gynecological examinations and should be specifically instructed to continue regularly scheduled pelvic examinations and PAP smears.

INDICATIONS

- The *ideal* candidate for an IUD is a parous woman in a stable, mutually monogamous relationship, with no history of PID, ectopic pregnancy, or any condition that would predispose to ectopic pregnancy (Box 148-1). The patient should be willing to check for the presence of IUD threads on a monthly basis.
- The IUD is especially appropriate for women who have difficulty remembering to take oral contraceptives or are intolerant to them, who wish to maintain fertility, and who want to avoid systemic hormones.
- Women over 35 who are smokers and have an increased risk of thromboembolic events are *ideal* candidates.

  Although not an indication listed by the company, the LNG IUS may be a preferred method in women with hypermenorrhea or dysmenorrhea. Even though spotting or bleeding may increase for a few months, menstrual bleeding and cramping decrease significantly within 3 to 6 months. Approximately 20% of women will experience absence of bleeding because of the localized progestin effect.

  Another possible off-label use for the LNG IUS is for treating postmenopausal women on estrogen replacement who are intolerant to oral progestins. The progesterone component in this case ensures endometrial lining suppression and decreases the risk of endometrial hyperplasia and uterine cancer.

CONTRAINDICATIONS

- Pregnancy or suspicion of pregnancy (except in the setting of emergency contraception).
- After unprotected intercourse for emergency contra-

ception (see Chapter 130, First-Trimester Abortion and Emergency Oral Contraceptives).

- History of ectopic pregnancy or any condition that would predispose to ectopic pregnancy.
- Congenital or acquired uterine cavity malformations, including large fibroids or abnormally large or small uterine cavity (smaller than 6 cm or greater than 9 cm).
- Acute sexually transmitted disease (STD).
- Current or prior history of PID.
- Untreated acute cervicitis, vaginitis, bacterial vaginosis, genital actinomycosis, or other uncontrolled genital-tract infections.
- Postpartum endometritis or infected abortion within the past 3 months.
- Less than 8 weeks postpartum or after second-trimester abortion until uterine involution has occurred (slight increased risk of perforation persists in lactating women).
- Known or suspected uterine or cervical neoplasia.
- Unresolved abnormal Pap smear.
- Genital bleeding of unknown cause.
- Multiple current sexual partners or a partner who is not monogamous.
- Acute liver disease (benign or chronic, including Wilson's disease).

- Immunodeficiency states including, but not limited to, leukemia, uncontrolled diabetes, acquired immunodeficiency syndrome (AIDS), intravenous drug use, or chronic systemic steroid use *(relative)*.

Some studies suggest it is safe to use IUDs in patients with well-controlled human immunodeficiency virus (HIV), but caution is advised.

- History of a previously inserted IUD that has not been removed.
- Allergy to copper (for ParaGard); hypersensitivity to any component of the IUD including levonorgestrel, silicone, or polyethylene; or any past history of IUD intolerance.
- Known or suspected carcinoma of the breast (for LNG IUS).
- Artificial heart valves.
- Wilson's Disease (for ParaGard).

TABLE 148-1
Rate of Continuation of Contraceptive Method at 1 Year

Method	Continuing Method After 1 Year (%)
Mirena intrauterine device (IUD)	81%
ParaGard Cooper IUD	79%
Oral contraceptive pill	71%
Depo-Provera	70%
Condom	61%
Diaphragm	56%
Spermicide	40%

From Trussell J: Contraceptive efficacy. In Hatcher RA, Trussell J, Stewart F, et al (eds): *Contraceptive technology,* ed 17 (rev), New York, 1998, Irvington Publishers.

BOX 148-1
Characteristics of Candidates for Intrauterine Device (IUD) Use

Desire for a reversible, long-term, cost-effective birth control method that allows spontaneity (first choice for these patients)
Failure of a previous birth control method because of forgetfulness
Multiparity
Not ready for tubal ligation
Breast-feeding mother (Mirena not advisable)
Low risk for sexually transmitted diseases
After delivery or abortion
Childbearing complete, but patient objects to sterilization
Contraindications to hormonal contraception (excluding progesterone-releasing IUDs)
Previous uncomplicated use of IUD

From Canavan, Timothy P: *Am Fam Physician* 58:2077, 1998.

TABLE 148-2
Annual Failure Rates for Birth Control Methods

Method	"Typical Use" Failure	"Ideal Use" Failure
Sterilization		
Male sterilization	0.15%	0.1%
Female sterilization	0.5%	0.5%
Hormonal Methods		
Implant (Norplant*)	0.05%	0.05%
Hormone shot (Depo-Provera)	0.3%	0.3%
Combined pill (Estrogen/Progestin)	5%	0.1%
Minipill (Progestin only)	5%	0.5%
Intrauterine Devices		
Copper T	0.8%	0.6%
LNG 20	0.1%	0.1%
Barrier Methods		
Male latex condom†	14%	3%
Diaphragm*	20%	6%
Vaginal sponge (no previous births)‡	20%	9%
Vaginal sponge (previous births) ‡	40%	20%
Cervical cap (no previous births)*	20%	9%
Cervical cap (previous births)*	40%	20%
Female condom	21%	5%
Spermicide (Gel, Foam, Suppository, Film)	**26%**	**6%**
Natural Methods		
Withdrawal	19%	4%
Natural family planning (e.g., calendar, temperature, cervical mucus)	25%	1%-9%
No Method	85%	85%

Data adapted from Trussell J: Contraceptive efficacy. In Hatcher RA, Trussell J, Stewart, F et al (eds): *Contraceptive technology,* ed 17, New York, 1998, Irvington Publishers.
*Used with spermicide.
†Used without spermicide.
‡Contains spermicide.

- Uninformed patient without full consent.
- Nulliparity. Although the manufacturers list nulliparity as a contraindication to an IUD, many authorities state that any nulliparous woman who feels confident she can avoid sexually transmitted infections should be considered a possible candidate for an IUD. These women should be warned of the risk of PID and of the slightly elevated risk of IUD expulsion.
- Desire for short-term contraceptive use (may be more cost-effective to use any other method).

EQUIPMENT

- The desired prepackaged IUD (ParaGard, LNG IUS) (Fig. 148-1)
- Speculum
- Sterile basin with cotton balls moistened with a water-based antiseptic, such as iodine (Betadine) or chlorhexidine gluconate
- Ring forceps
- Cervical tenaculum
- Uterine sound
- Nonsterile gloves (for bimanual examination before insertion procedure)
- Sterile gloves (for IUD insertion phase)
- Sterile towel to cover tray
- Long suture scissors (to cut IUD threads after insertion)

Optional Equipment

- Nonsteroidal antiinflammatory drug (NSAID), to be taken before procedure (e.g., 800 mg ibuprofen)
- Cervical dilators (see Chapter 137, Cervical Stenosis and Cervical Dilation)
- Lidocaine 2% without epinephrine and equipment for paracervical block or submucosal block (10-ml syringe, needle extender with a 22-gauge long needle, Monsel's solution, and cotton-tipped swaps) (see Chapter 174, Paracervical Block and Chapter 150, Loop Electrosurgical Excision Procedure [LEEP] for

Treating Cervical Intraepithelial Neoplasia, for the submucosal injection technique)
- Heating pad (low to medium setting) for patient's abdomen (may decrease pain, nausea, and cramping some women experience with cervical manipulation)

Clinicians should not use a heating pad in women who have had recent abdominal surgery, any abdominal rash, a wound, an injury, or who have sensory neurologic impairment.

PREPROCEDURE PATIENT PREPARATION

A separate office visit for patient counseling, consent, and preparation should be scheduled before the IUD insertion visit. At this visit the patient has the opportunity to review the material, consider her contraceptive options, ask questions, and plan for the procedure. Similarly, the clinician has the opportunity to assess potential risks and benefits of IUD insertion, provide counseling, and perform the screening evaluation.

Patient Counseling and Consent

Federal guidelines require that patients be given an IUD patient information brochure as part of the consent process before IUD insertion. Brochures are provided through the manufacturers of ParaGard and the Mirena LNG IUS (see the "Suppliers" section). These brochures are excellent resources and can serve as consent documents when the patient reviews the checklists and signs the forms.

The clinician should confirm that the patient understands her risks, benefits, and alternatives to IUD placement and the common side effects experienced with this form of contraception. The clinician should also advise of the cramping and discomfort associated with IUD insertion as well as removal and the potential for transient nausea, dizziness, or faintness during and immediately after the procedure. It is common to have mild spotting and cramping for a few days after the procedure, but if these symptoms are severe or the discomfort is not alleviated with over-the-counter analgesics, the patient will need medical evaluation. Patients must be willing to check for the presence of IUD threads after the first menstrual period and each month thereafter. If the threads cannot be found or seem to be migrating upward, the patient must notify her physician. Although patients may expect reliable birth control immediately after IUD insertion,* it is advisable to

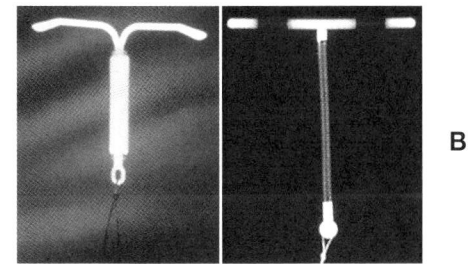

Fig. 148-1
Various intrauterine devices. A, Mirena LNG IUS. **B,** ParaGard T380A. (**A,** Courtesy Berlex Laboratories, Wayne, NJ. **B,** Courtesy Ortho-McNeil Pharmaceutical, Inc., Raritan, NJ)

*The American College of Obstetricians and Gynecologists (ACOG) has suggested the use of a second method of birth control during the first month following IUD insertion.

observe 1 to 2 weeks of pelvic rest after the procedure to minimize the risk of infection and other complications. The importance of a mutually monogamous relationship should be emphasized with the explanation that any new partners will significantly increase the risk of pelvic inflammatory disease while the IUD is in place.

Screening Evaluation

Prior to IUD insertion, a Pap smear (within 6 months) and pelvic examination along with any appropriate STD screening should be performed and the results documented as negative. The pelvic examination should include assessment of uterine size and position, examination for signs of cervicitis or vaginitis, and evaluation of the general morphology of the cervix and os, including signs of cervical stenosis.

Pretreatment

Patients should consider taking ibuprofen or other NSAID 45 to 60 minutes before IUD insertion to minimize cramping and discomfort during the procedure. Routine antibiotic prophylaxis for bacterial endocarditis is no longer recommended. However, given the increased risk of PID in the first 3 weeks following IUD insertion, some clinicians prefer to administer doxycycline 200 mg 1 hour before the procedure or erythromycin 500 mg orally 1 hour before and 6 hours after IUD insertion, since prophylaxis is for PID.

TECHNIQUE

The IUD insertion technique described here provides general guidelines for the procedure. For further details, the clinician should refer to the physician insert provided by each manufacturer within the respective packaging.

Initial Steps

1. Ensure that the patient understands the method and alternatives to IUD placement and that the consent form has been signed. Confirm that the patient is still a candidate for the IUD (i.e., is in a stable, monogamous relationship and has not developed any contraindications as listed previously). Confirm a negative Pap smear result.
2. Confirm a negative pregnancy test if patient is not menstruating or there is any question of status.
3. Reassess the need for a NSAID, antibiotic prophy-

laxis (not routinely recommended), heating pad (low to medium heat) for the patient's abdomen, or other special accommodations.
4. Perform a speculum examination and bimanual pelvic examination to establish the size, position, consistency, and mobility of the uterus and to screen for the presence of any signs or symptoms of acute vaginal infection.
5. Change to sterile gloves and observe sterile technique from this point on in the procedure.
6. Prepare a sterile field containing the supplies discussed previously. Request an assistant, if desired.
7. With the patient in the lithotomy position, insert another warm sterile speculum into the vagina. The cervix should be well-visualized and the os centered in the midline.
8. Using the ring forceps, cleanse the cervix with the antiseptic-soaked cotton balls.
9. Perform a paracervical block (see Chapter 174, Paracervical Block) if desired, although it is rarely if ever needed.
10. Clamp a single-tooth tenaculum to the anterior lip of the cervix. It may be helpful to ask the patient to cough as you apply the device or to inject 1 to 2 ml of 2% lidocaine into the tenaculum site before placement. Apply gentle downward traction on the tenaculum to correct for any angulation and to stabilize the cervix.
11. Gently and slowly sound the uterus. Careful technique will decrease the patient's discomfort and the risk of perforation, laceration, and other complications. The uterine depth should be between 6.5 and 8.5 cm. Do not place an IUD if the depth is outside the normal range (there is an increased risk of complications in this setting). If the sound cannot be inserted because of stenosis, dilate the cervix (see Chapter 137, Cervical Stenosis and Cervical Dilation).
12. Prepare the IUD for insertion. Fig. 148-2 is a graphic depiction of the Mirena IUS system. The inserter tube refers to the hollow cylinder in which the IUD or IUS fits.

    It may be possible to load the IUD into the inserter while it is still in the original packaging. This is referred to as the "no-touch technique" and is described in the packaging information of IUDs that provide this loading option (see Fig. 148-3). Alternatively, sterile gloves are used to "load" the unit by folding the arms down and inserting them in the inserter tube. The inserter "rod" for the Paragard refers to the solid trocar that fits inside of the inserter tube.
13. Insert the chosen IUD, as noted below and in Fig. 148-4 (ParaGard) and Fig. 148-5 (LNG IUS).

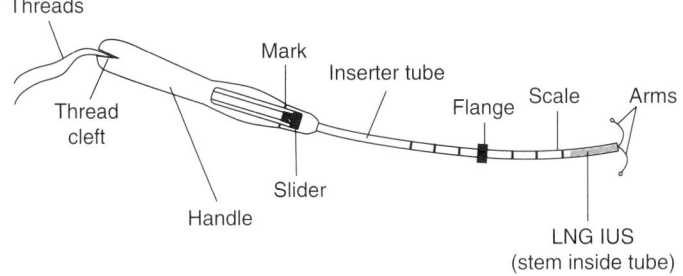

Fig. 148-2
Mirena Levonorgestrel Intrauterine System (LNG IUS) and inserter.
(Redrawn from Berlex Laboratories, Wayne, NJ.)

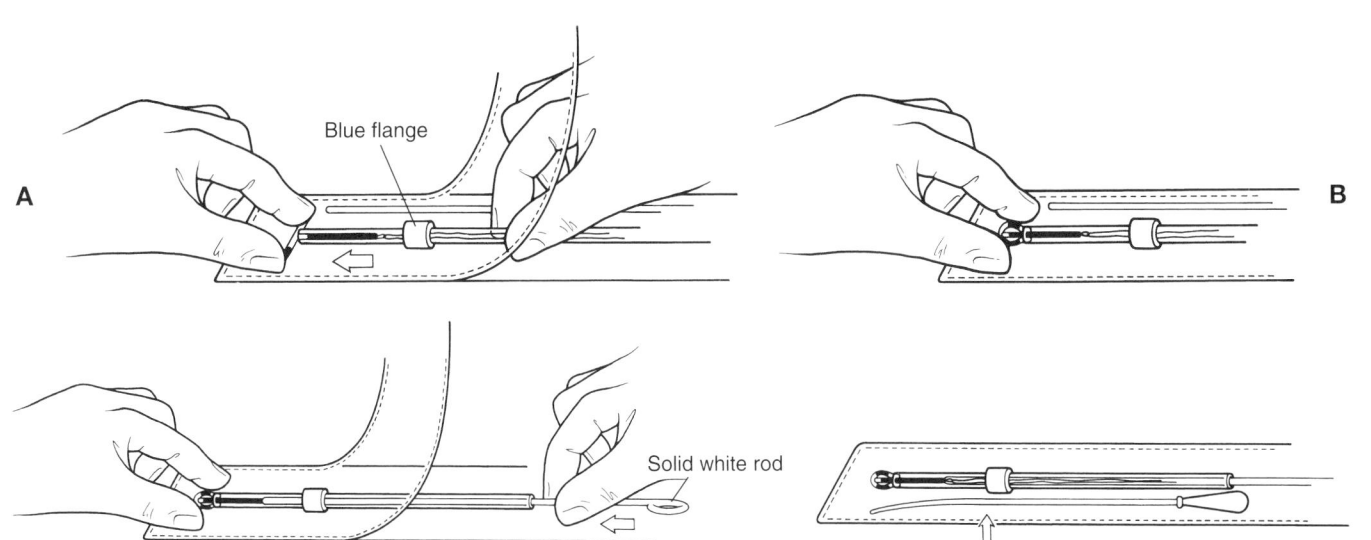

Fig. 148-3
Loading the ParaGard intrauterine device (IUD) using the "no-touch" technique just before insertion. A, After the bimanual examination and antiseptic solution preparation and after the uterus has been sounded, the IUD is inserted into the hollow inserter tube. **B,** The arms are bent down and inserted just far enough to retain them in the tube. **C,** The solid white inserter rod is placed into the hollow insertion tube from the other end so that it just touches the bottom of the vertical arm of the IUD. **D,** The blue flange is set so that the distance from the tip of the IUD to the flange is the same distance as the depth of the uterus (as determined by the uterine sound). (Redrawn from Pfenninger JL: *Fam Pract Res J* 14[2]:131, 1992.)

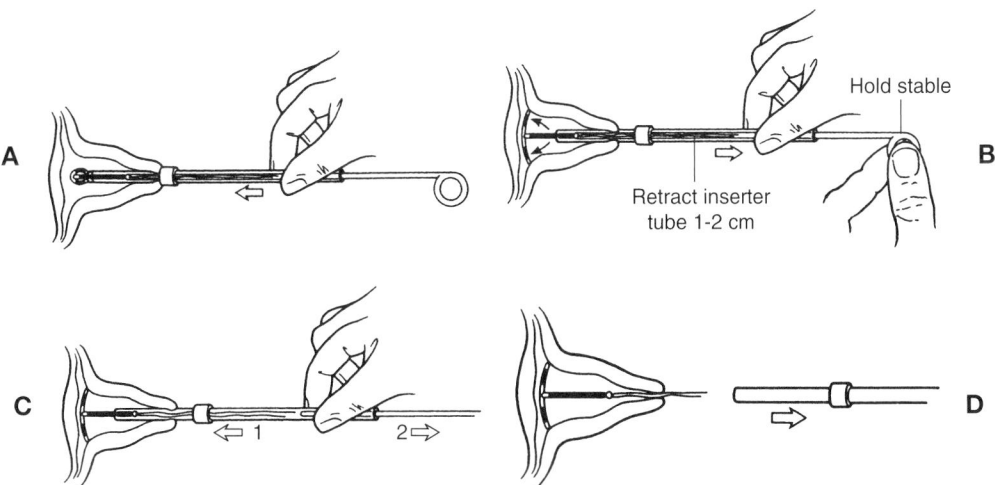

Fig. 148-4
Inserting the ParaGard intrauterine device (IUD). A, The single-tooth tenaculum is applied to stabilize the cervix and the IUD-inserter unit is placed into the cervical canal up to the flange. **B,** While an assistant holds the tenaculum, the clinician holds the solid white rod stable in the dominant hand, and withdraws the insertion tube approximately 2 cm. **C,** *1,* The inserting tube (with rod still in place) is gently advanced to ensure high placement of IUD; *2,* the solid inserting rod is withdrawn while holding the tube steady. **D,** The insertion tube is withdrawn and the threads are cut, ensuring adequate length. (Redrawn from Pfenninger JL: *Fam Pract Res J* 14[2]:131, 1992.)

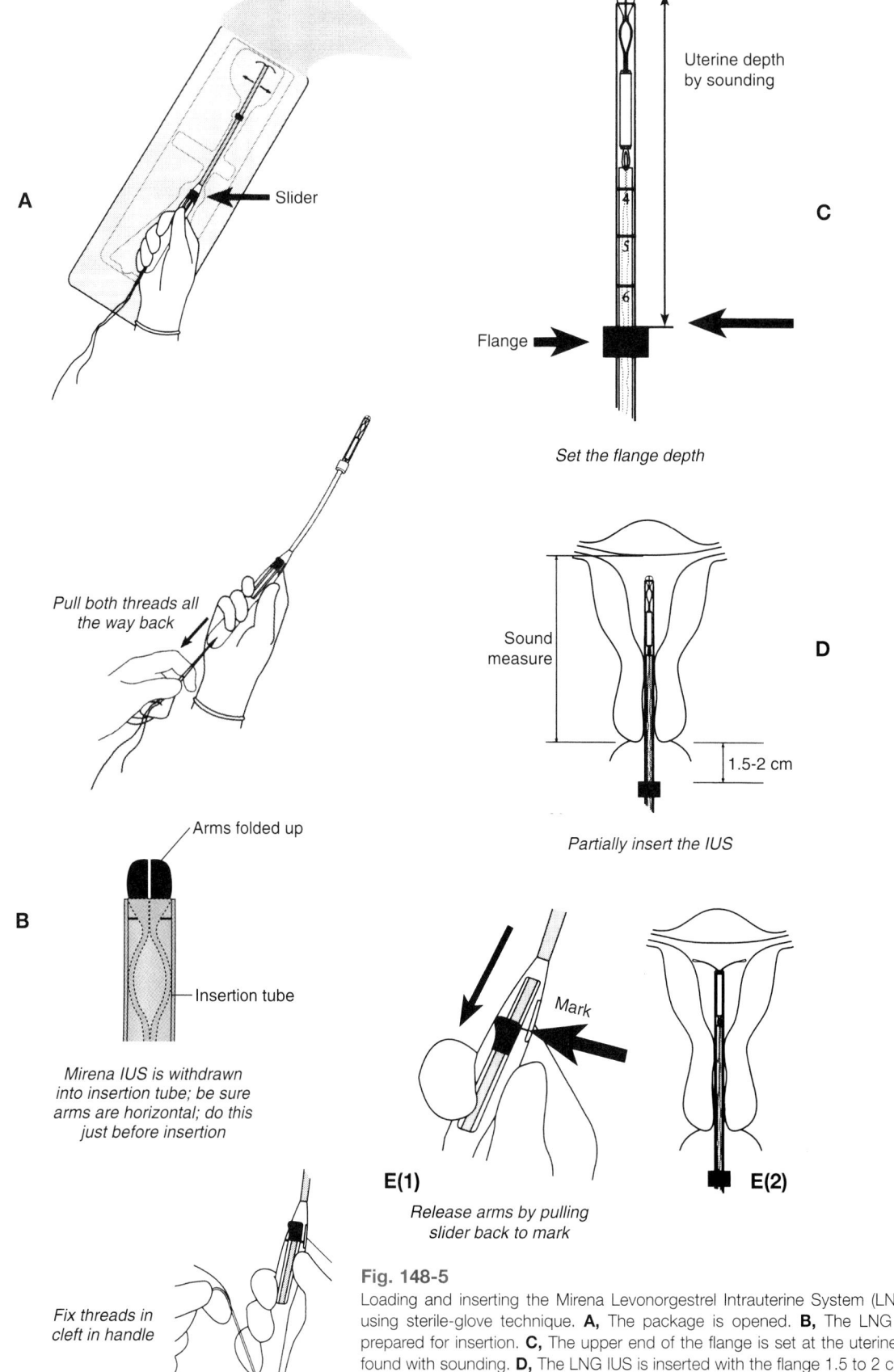

A — Slider

Uterine depth by sounding

C

Flange

Set the flange depth

Pull both threads all the way back

Sound measure

D

1.5-2 cm

Partially insert the IUS

Arms folded up

B

Insertion tube

Mirena IUS is withdrawn into insertion tube; be sure arms are horizontal; do this just before insertion

Mark

E(1)

E(2)

Release arms by pulling slider back to mark

Fix threads in cleft in handle

Fig. 148-5
Loading and inserting the Mirena Levonorgestrel Intrauterine System (LNG IUS) using sterile-glove technique. **A,** The package is opened. **B,** The LNG IUS is prepared for insertion. **C,** The upper end of the flange is set at the uterine depth found with sounding. **D,** The LNG IUS is inserted with the flange 1.5 to 2 cm from the ectocervix. **E,** The arms are released by pulling the slider back to the mark.

Continued

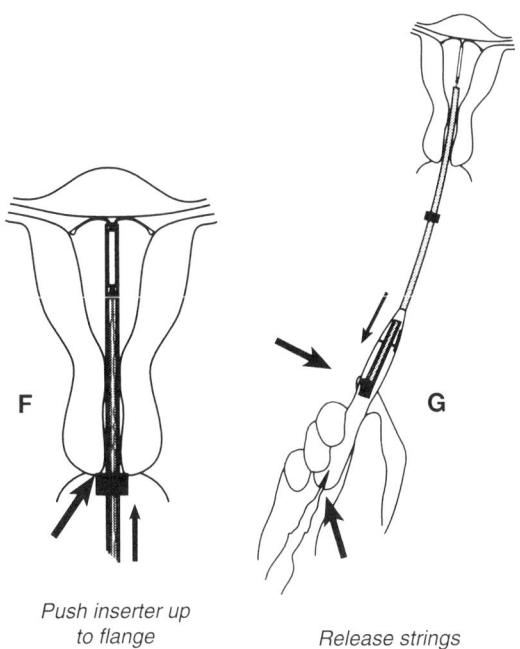

Push inserter up
to flange

Release strings

Fig. 148-5, cont'd
F, For fundal positioning, the clinician holds the slider in position at the mark and pushes the inserter gently inward until the flange touches the cervix. The LNG IUS should now be in the fundal position. **G,** Finally, the LNG IUS is released by pulling the slider all the way back, which releases the strings. The insertion tube is then removed. Cut the strings to leave 2 to 3 cm visible outside the cervix. (Courtesy Association of Reproductive Health Professionals, Ithaca, NY, copyright 2000, used by permission. **B** *(center),* Redrawn from Association of Reproductive Health Professionals, Ithaca, NY.)

ParaGard Insertion

After following the initial steps above, insert the ParaGard IUD as follows:

1. Make certain that the horizontal arms of the IUD are parallel to the horizontal orientation of the blue flange to ensure proper placement within the uterus. The blue flange is held horizontal on insertion.
2. Grasp the single-tooth tenaculum to stabilize the cervix. Insert the IUD inserter unit into the cervical canal up to the flange (Fig. 148-4, *A*). Have an assistant hold the tenaculum. With the solid white rod in your dominant hand, use the other hand to withdraw the clear plastic inserter tube toward you approximately 2 cm as the white rod is held in place (Fig. 148-4, *B*) This maneuver will allow the IUD to "fall" into place. Pushing in on the solid rod could cause a perforation. A small "pop" can often be felt as the IUD unfolds.
3. Now gently and slowly push the hollow tube inserter toward the fundus until resistance is felt to allow "high placement" of the IUD (Fig. 148-4, *C[1]*). Fundal placement of the IUD decreases the risk of expulsion, accidental pregnancy, and other complications. Withdraw the solid rod only (Fig. 148-4, *C[2]*). *Do not*

withdraw the tube before removing the rod first. The strings are inside the tube and compressed against the tube by the rod. Pulling both out at the same time could immediately pull out the IUD.
4. Withdraw the insertion tube (Fig. 148-4, *D*).
5. Complete the procedure as noted below.

LNG IUS Insertion

After following the initial steps above, insert the LNG IUS (Mirena) as follows:

1. After opening the sterile package, release the threads, making sure the slider is in furthest position from you. Use the sterile packaging to rotate the arms of the system to be horizontal when the lettering on the handle is facing upward (Fig. 148-5, *A*).
2. Prepare the LNG IUS for insertion. Pull on both threads to draw the LNG IUS into the insertion tube. The arms will fold upward, whereas the Paragard arms fold down. The knobs at the ends of the arms close the open end of the inserter. Fix the threads tightly in the cleft at the near end of the inserter shaft (Fig. 148-5, *B*).
3. Set the upper end of the flange at the uterine depth measured previously (Fig. 148-5, *C*).
4. Holding the slider with the forefinger or thumb firmly in the furthermost position, advance the inserter into the cervical canal until the flange is about *1.5 to 2 cm from the cervix.* This gives sufficient space for the arms to open in the uterus (Fig. 148-5, *D*).
5. While holding the inserter steady, release the arms of the LNG IUS by pulling the slider back until it reaches the mark (i.e., raised horizontal line) (Fig. 148-5, *E*).
6. Holding the slider in position, push the inserter gently inward until the flange now touches the cervix. The LNG IUS should now be in the fundal position (Fig. 148-5, *F*).
7. Holding the inserter steady, release the LNG IUS by pulling the slider all the way back. The threads will be released automatically (Fig. 148-5, *G*). Remove the inserter carefully from the uterus.
8. Complete the procedure as noted below.

Completion of Procedure

1. After the inserter is removed from the uterus, cut the IUD threads to a length of 2 to 5 cm beyond the os (Fig. 148-6). It is better to leave the threads too long than too short because they can be shortened on subsequent visits (if necessary) and short threads may be irritating or painful for a male partner.
2. Remove the tenaculum and observe the site for bleeding. If bleeding is seen, apply pressure or Monsel's solution to achieve hemostasis.
3. Remove the speculum.
4. Provide postprocedure counseling to the patient and

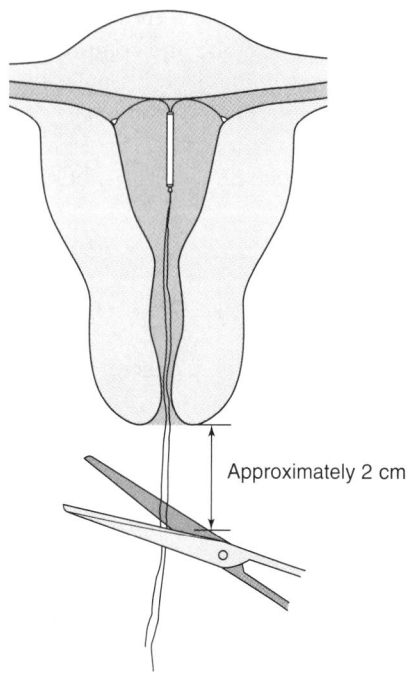

Fig. 148-6
Threads are cut (leaving about 2 to 3 cm visible outside the cervix). (Redrawn from Berlex Laboratories, Wayne, NJ.)

arrange a follow-up appointment for an IUD and symptom check after the first postinsertion menses.
5. Complete the encounter form (Fig. 148-7) or dictate a complete note.

COMPLICATIONS

In general, IUD placement is a relatively safe procedure with significantly less morbidity and mortality than pregnancy and delivery. The IUD itself is generally well tolerated, as demonstrated by the 1-year continuation rate for this birth control method in comparison to other methods.

Nonetheless, it is important to counsel the patient on the risk of complications and common side effects of the IUD. These include, but are not limited to the following:

Contraception Failure

Although rare (less than 1%), pregnancy is possible even with the IUD in place. Should this occur, the IUD should be removed as soon as the possible. Although there is a risk of inducing an abortion with removal of an IUD, if it is left in place, premature labor, sepsis, and spontaneous abortion are possible. It is also important to rule out ectopic pregnancy immediately, because nearly 50% of pregnancies achieved with the IUD in place will be in a location outside the uterus. Patients with IUDs do not have a higher ectopic pregnancy rate—it is actually lower. However, if a woman does become pregnant with an IUD in place, it is more likely to be ectopic.

Pelvic Inflammatory Disease

The risk of PID is only elevated the first 20 days after IUD insertion or in the setting of exposure to a new sexual partner. If the clinician suspects PID, the IUD should be removed immediately and broad-spectrum antibiotics should be initiated.

Perforation

Perforation of the uterus or cervix is extremely rare (less than 0.1%). It generally occurs at the time of uterine sounding or occasionally with insertion. The clinician should avoid IUD placement in a woman if her uterus has not fully involuted after pregnancy or abortion to minimize the risk of perforation. (The IUD should only be inserted 8 to 10 weeks after delivery.) Good visualization and stabilization of the cervix during sounding and IUD insertion are important. Perforation should be suspected if the sound enters the uterine cavity more than 12 cm while uterine palpation indicates a normal size. The perforation itself is usually painless and often occurs in the setting of forceful pressure through a tight cervical os. Should perforation be suspected, the clinician should pull out the IUD (if already inserted) and observe the patient for 30 minutes. If stable, the patient can be discharged and told to report any signs of infection, abdominal pain, rapid pulse, or shortness of breath. Generally there is an uncomplicated resolution, and insertion can be attempted again in 6 to 8 weeks (no prophylactic antibiotics are indicated). Unstable patients may require immediate surgical consultation.

Spontaneous Expulsion

Although uncommon, most IUD expulsions occur within the first 6 months after insertion. The patient may not realize that the IUD has spontaneously passed through the cervical os. For this reason the patient must check for the IUD thread each month after menstruation.

Occasionally the IUD will become lodged in the cervical os, which may cause cramping and discomfort. In this case the IUD should be removed and a new one may be placed if desired.

If an IUD is spontaneously passed or it is removed because of a complication, it may be returned to the company for a free replacement. Similarly, if the device

---

IUD ENCOUNTER FORM

Patient to fill out:

Name _____ Date _____

Birthdate _____ Age _____

Number of pregnancies _____ Miscarriages or abortions _____

Current contraceptive method _____

Have you had:

A pregnancy in your tubes?	Y N	
Infection in your tubes?	Y N	
Any venereal disease?	Y N	
An IUD before?	Y N	
Leukemia, AIDS, heart murmur?	Y N	
Rhematic fever, diabetes?	Y N	
Are you on steroids?	Y N	

Are you allergic to copper?   Y N

How long is your usual period? _____ days

Have you ever had a low blood count?   Y N

Number of lifetime sexual partners? _____

Current number of sexual partners? _____

Last Pap smear: Date _____ Result _____

Did you read and understand the company handout?   Y N

For the Doctor:

Company handout explained   Y N

Impression _____

Plan _____

PMH: PMI: _____

       All: _____

       Meds: _____

       Surgeries: _____

Procedure/(Insertion):   **Date** _____

LMP _____

Pap: Y N   Type of IUD: Paragard T380A

Bimanual: uterus: adnexa: Mirena IUS

Prep with Tenaculum   Y N

Sound   cm.

Insertion:

Patient Tolerance:

Complications:

Reinforce: bleeding, pregnancy, infection, pain, expulsion

Remove on: _____

Given new company handout?   Y N

Given card?   Y N

Follow-up: _____

_____

Physician Signature

cc: _____

Fig. 148-7

Sample intrauterine device encounter form. (From The Medical Procedures Center, Midland, Mich.)

becomes contaminated during the insertion process and cannot be used, it may be returned to the manufacturer for a full refund.

Embedded or Lost Intrauterine Device String

If the strings are not visible in the os, the clinician should first rule out pregnancy. On occasion the IUD may become embedded into the uterine lining, complicating removal. If the IUD cannot be removed either because the strings are not visible or because it is too difficult to do so, an IUD remover may be needed. If still unsuccessful, it may be necessary to have an imaging study to confirm an intrauterine location. Although IUDs are radiopaque, a flat plate of the pelvis and abdomen is only two dimensional (2-D) and cannot confirm an intrauterine location. Ultrasound provides a three-dimensional (3-D) location and is preferred. Hysteroscopy may be needed to locate the IUD for removal (see Chapter 149, Intrauterine Device Removal).

Actinomyces

Actinomyces is an anaerobic, gram-positive bacteria. It is more frequently found in IUD users and is generally asymptomatic. It is usually detected on a routine Pap smear. Controversy exists as to proper treatment. Some would treat with ampicillin or tetracycline and remove the IUD only if the condition persists or if symptomatic. Others would always remove the IUD and treat. Rarely does the bacteria cause a systemic problem in healthy individuals. If a present or past infection is known, it is best not to insert the IUD. Actinomyces is less likely in copper-containing IUDs.

Uterine Bleeding and Cramping

IUDs may cause abdominal or low-back pain and cramping, as well as irregular uterine bleeding, particularly in the first 3 months of use. Some women will have heavier bleeding and increased dysmenorrhea with the IUD, particularly when using the ParaGard. Conversely, approximately 20% of women using the Mirena LNG IUS will cease having periods after 3 to 6 months. Menstruation returns rapidly once the device is removed.

Ovarian Cysts

Ovarian cysts may develop in patients using the Mirena LNG IUS because of hormonal stimulation. Enlarged follicles are seen in about 12% of LNG IUS users. Most of the cysts are asymptomatic and self-limiting, but on occasion they may cause pelvic pain or dyspareunia.

Breast Cancer

Women who use hormone-containing IUDs, such as LNG IUS, may have a minimal increase in breast cancer risk.

Hormonal Side Effects and Use During Lactation

Hormone-containing IUDs, such as the LNG IUS, may have side effects such as mood changes, acne, headache, breast tenderness, dysmenorrhea, nervousness, vaginitis, hypertension, or nausea. Weight gain is generally not a problem. Other forms of contraception may be preferable for lactating women.

Pap Smears/Cervical Dysplasia

Although no known association has been shown between cervical dysplasia and use of the IUD, it is essential that the Pap smear be normal before insertion. Should the patient develop an abnormal Pap smear, the IUD may complicate the process of cervical and endocervical canal sampling and procedures such as the loop electrosurgical excision procedure or conization. Because patients using IUDs do not require annual renewal of their contraception, they are at greater risk of neglecting their annual Pap smears. When treating these patients, the clinician should emphasize that they must return for their annual Pap smear and pelvic examinations.

Wilson's Disease

The copper containing IUDs may precipitate symptoms in Wilson's disease.

Medical Diathermy

Medical diathermy is contraindicated in women with copper-containing IUDs.

POSTPROCEDURE PATIENT EDUCATION

Give the patient a copy of the IUD handout provided by the manufacturer. Reiterate the major concerns and keep the following in mind:
- The patient must check for the presence of IUD threads after each menstruation. If she cannot feel them or they are much longer than they were previously, the physician should be contacted immediately.
- The patient should be clear on the signs and symptoms of IUD expulsion (most importantly, cramping).
- The patient should be instructed to report any of the

following: excessive pain, malodorous discharge, excessive bleeding (other than spotting for a few months), pain with intercourse, prolonged amenorrhea, unexplained fever, prolonged pelvic discomfort, any type of genital lesions, abnormal vaginal discharge, signs of STD, signs of pregnancy, or any other concerns.

- The patient should be counseled that the IUD will not prevent infection from HIV, herpes, HPV, Chlamydia, gonorrhea, or any other STD.

CONCLUSION

Recent research indicates that the IUD should receive strong consideration as a long-term contraceptive method in patients who have a monogamous relationship and who do not have a history of PID or ectopic pregnancy. IUDs have high efficacy (less than 1% failure rate), require little maintenance, provide long-term yet reversible contraception, and are cheaper than birth control pills over a 5-year period. The LNG IUS offers the additional benefit of decreased vaginal bleeding and may provide use in hormone replacement to protect against uterine malignancy and hyperplasia. Because the IUDs primary function is to prevent conception (as opposed to preventing implantation), it has become a more acceptable birth control method for both patients and physicians.

SUPPLIERS

ParaGard T380A
Ortho-McNeil Pharmaceutical
P.O. Box 300
Raritan, NJ 08869-0602
Phone: 1-800-682-6532
Website: www.paragardiud.com

Mirena
Berlex Laboratories
300 Fairfield Road
Wayne, NJ 07470-7358
Phone: 1-973-694-4100
Website: www.berlex.com

Note: Most companies will provide videotapes and training models for their devices.

CPT/BILLING CODES

58300   Insertion of intrauterine device (IUD), not including device

58301   Removal of IUD

J7300   Charge for cost of copper IUD (ParaGard T380A)

J3490   Unclassified drug (Mirena)

Note: The Mirena reimbursement support line can be reached at 1-866-647-3646.

ICD-9-CM DIAGNOSTIC CODES

V 25.1   Encounter of contraceptive management; insertion of intrauterine contraceptive device

V 2542   Intrauterine contraceptive device; checking, reinsertion, or removal of intrauterine device

BIBLIOGRAPHY

Alvarez F, Brache V, Fernandez E, et al: New insights on the mode of action of intrauterine contraceptive devices in women, *Fertil Steril* 49:768, 1988.

American College of Obstetricians and Gynecologists: The intrauterine device, *ACOG Tech Bull* 164:1, 1992.

Berlex Laboratories: Mirena package insert, November 2000.

Canavan TP: Appropriate use of the intrauterine device, *Am Fam Physician* 58:2077, 1998.

Connell EB: The intrauterine device. Reassessing its role as a contraceptive option, *Female Patient* 21:40, 1996.

Farley TM, Rosenberg MJ, Rowe PJ, et al: Intrauterine devices and pelvic inflammatory disease: an international perspective, *Lancet* 339:785, 1992.

Fortney JA, Feldblum PJ, Raymond EG: Intrauterine devices: the best long-term contraceptive method? *J Reprod Med* 44:269, 1999.

Gilbert DN, Moellering RC Jr, Sande MA: The Sanford guide to antimicrobial therapy, ed 32, Hyde Park, VT, 2002, Antimicrobial Therapy.

Guines DA, Hubacher D: IUDs: time for renaissance, *Am Fam Physician* 58(9):1963, 1998.

Hatcher RA (ed): *Contraceptive technology*, ed 17, New York, 1998, Ardent Media.

Pfenninger JL: IUD insertion. In Pfenninger JL, editor: *Procedures for primary care physicians*, St Louis, 1994, Mosby.

Hubacher D, Lara-Ricalde R, Taylor DJ, et al: Use of copper intrauterine devices and the risk of tubal infertility among nulliparous women, *N Engl J Med* 345:561, 2001.

Kronmal R, Whiney C, Rumford S: The intrauterine device and pelvic inflammatory disease: the women's health study reanalyzed, *J Clin Epidemiol* 44:109, 1991.

Ortho Pharmaceutical Corp: ParaGard package insert, July 1995.

Ortiz ME, Croxattott B, Bardin CW: Mechanism of action of intrauterine devices, *Obstet Gynecol Surv* 51(12 suppl):542, 1996.

Prior IUD use not associated with infertility among nulliparous women, *Contraceptive Report* 12:6, 2001.

Skegg DCG: Safety and efficacy of fertility-regulating methods: a decade of research, *Bull World Health Organ* 77:713, 1999.

Speroff L: Levonorgestrel and copper IUDs are excellent contraceptive devices, *Ob Gyn Clin Alert* 10(12):89, 1994.

Speroff L: The IUD and PID, *Ob Gyn Clin Alert* 9:9, 1992.

Spinmato JA: Mechanism of action of intrauterine contraceptive devices and its relation to informed consent, *Am J Obstet Gynecol* 176:503, 1997.

Thomsen RJ, Rayl DL: Dr. Lippes and his Loop: four decades in perspective, *J Reprod Med* 44:833, 1999.

Walsh T, Grimes D, Frezieres R, et al: Randomized controlled trial of prophylactic antibiotics before insertion of intrauterine devices, *Lancet* 351:1005, 1998.

CHAPTER 149

Intrauterine Device Removal

John L. Pfenninger

Generally, intrauterine device (IUD) removal is a simple and uncomplicated procedure that takes only a few minutes. The rare case in which the IUD string is not visible ("lost" IUD) presents a more challenging situation.

INDICATIONS

- Desire for pregnancy
- Postmenopause
- Pregnancy confirmed
- Suspicion of infection
- Inability to identify strings in the cervical os
- Before loop electrosurgical excision procedure conization
- Patient intolerance: pain, bleeding, other
- Manufacturer recommendations:
    Paragard T380   10 years
    Mirena   5 years
- Anticipated new sexual partner (?)

CONTRAINDICATIONS

There are no contraindications.

REMOVAL WITH IDENTIFIABLE STRINGS

The usual IUD removal is straightforward, and there is no need for sterile technique although nonsterile gloves are worn. Insert the speculum, and visualize the IUD strings. Using ring forceps, grasp the strings and pull toward the introitus in a firm and deliberate motion until the IUD is delivered. The patient will likely experience momentary discomfort, which may be prevented somewhat by premedicating with 800 mg of ibuprofen. Remove the speculum and send the patient home. Some minor spotting may be expected for a few days. There is no need to culture the IUD unless infection is suspected.

WHEN THE INTRAUTERINE DEVICE STRINGS ARE NOT VISIBLE

If the speculum is inserted and IUD strings cannot be visualized after a diligent search, one of several approaches may be used. *First,* try using a cytobrush or similar instrument and insert it (the brush portion) the full depth into the cervical canal (2 cm). After insertion, rotate and extract the brush in a repeated, continuous motion. In one study, 24 of 27 lost strings were retrieved in this maneuver when other methods had failed.

If this fails, try a *second* method. Insert a long-handled, hemostat-like instrument (such as a uterine packing forceps) into the os, with the instrument opened as much as the os will allow. Close the jaws in hopes that the strings are grasped. If the strings are indeed grasped, resistance will be felt when the instrument is removed. Carry out this maneuver four or five times in an attempt to grasp the strings. If unsuccessful, or if the os is too small, other methods will be needed to find the strings.

A *third* approach uses an endocervical speculum along with a colposcope to identify the strings. Frequently, the end of the string is just within the os. Once visualized, it is much more easily grasped with forceps and removed.

Should these techniques fail, proceed with a more invasive technique. (See Chapter 137, Cervical Stenosis and Cervical Dilation, for the instrumentation to be used.) Perform a bimanual examination to identify the position of the uterus. Prepare the area with an antiseptic solution. Grasp the anterior lip with a single-toothed cervical tenaculum and apply slight traction to straighten the uterus. A uterine sound may be used to dilate the internal os. Alternatively, one of the varieties of IUD removers can be used to enter the intrauterine cavity (Fig. 149-1). Using the larger-sized instruments will prevent or minimize the potential for perforation of the uterus. The double IUD extractor and flexible IUD hook are commonly used. The double IUD extractor resembles a crochet hook that "hooks" the IUD (Fig. 149-2). Use a twist-and-pull motion to "catch" the IUD. Frequent, repeated passes are often needed. The

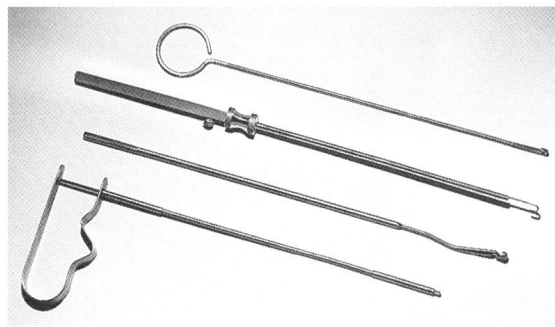

Fig. 149-1
Intrauterine device (IUD) removal instruments. From top to bottom: simple IUD hook, universal IUD hook, double IUD extractor, and flexible IUD hook.

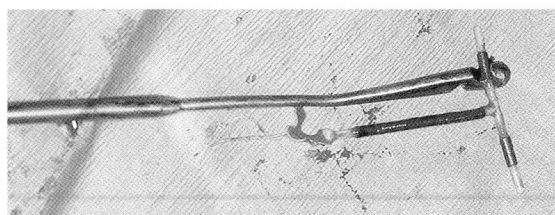

Fig. 149-2
Double intrauterine device (IUD) extractor after retrieving a "lost" IUD (ParaGard T380).

flexible IUD hook is actually a forceps. Insert the stem into the uterus and compress the handle to open the jaws. When the handle is released, the jaws grasp the IUD as they close. Then withdraw the unit. With either instrument, if the string or the IUD is grasped, resistance will be felt.

If the IUD has been in place for a significant length of time, it may have become embedded in the endometrium, and significant force will be required to remove it. If the force seems to be extreme or there is any question whether the IUD is still in place, it may be best to defer removal. Although a flat plate x-ray of the abdomen will identify whether the IUD is present (IUDs are radiopaque), the x-ray film will not indicate whether the IUD *is intrauterine.* A pelvic ultrasound examination, on the other hand, will confirm whether it is present *and* whether it is intrauterine. If the IUD has moved to an extrauterine position, surgery will be required.

If an intrauterine IUD is confirmed by ultrasound, the patient must return for a visit when further, more aggressive attempts can be made to remove it. If all else fails, the patient may require a dilation and curettage procedure, with the IUD removed under anesthesia or

with the aid of a hysteroscope. No prophylactic antibiotics are needed.

COMPLICATIONS

Other than slight discomfort, there are usually no complications from the routine IUD removal. If other instrumentation is required because of lost strings, rare complications include perforation, infection, and bleeding.

SUPPLIERS

The various IUD removal instruments should be available from most medical supply firms. Those shown in Fig. 149-1 are from the following:

CooperSurgical, Inc.
95 Corporate Drive
Trumbull, CT 06611
Phone: 1-800-645-3760
Website: www.coopersurgical.com

CPT/BILLING CODES

58300	IUD insertion
58301	IUD removal

ICD-9-CM DIAGNOSTIC CODES

Contraceptive device

996.32	Complications (lost IUD)
996.76	Causing menorrhagia
V25.1	Insertion
V25.42	Reinsertion
V25.42	Removal
V25.42	Maintenance/surveillance/checking IUD

BIBLIOGRAPHY

Ben-Rafael Z, Bider D: A new procedure for removal of a "lost" intrauterine device, *Obstet Gynecol* 87:785, 1996.
Bounds W, Hutt S, Kubba A, et al: Randomized comparative study in 217 women of three disposable plastic IUCD thread retrievers, *Br J Obstet Gynaecol* 99:915, 1992.

Loop Electrosurgical Excision Procedure (LEEP) for Treating Cervical Intraepithelial Neoplasia

Thomas C. Wright, Jr.
Ralph M. Richart

A variety of techniques can be used to treat cervical intraepithelial neoplasia (CIN). The appropriateness of a particular technique to treat a particular lesion depends on a number of factors, including lesion size, location, and extension into the endocervical canal. Many clinicians now use an electrosurgical excisional procedure that uses thin-wire loop electrodes to excise CIN lesions and atypical transformation zones (TZs) in their entirety. This procedure is known as the *loop electrosurgical excision procedure (LEEP)*. Another term that refers to this procedure is *LLETZ* (large loop excision of the TZ). It is also simply called the *loop procedure*. Many clinicians subdivide LEEP into two procedures: (1) routine LEEP, which is used for excision for lesions confined to the exocervix (or visible portion of the cervix), and (2) LEEP conization, which is used when lesions extend into the endocervical canal. LEEP has a number of advantages over other treatment modalities for CIN, including the following:

- It produces little if any pain.
- It is easy to learn and perform.
- It involves inexpensive equipment.
- It enables the entire lesion to be assessed histologically to rule out an invasive cervical cancer.
- It allows many patients to be diagnosed and treated in a single office visit.
- It results in an excellent pathologic specimen with minimal loss of blood and minimal thermal artifact.
- It enables cervical conization to be performed in the office at significantly reduced cost (referred to as LEEP conizations).
- Complications are few and long-term studies confirm its safety.

INDICATIONS

Routine LEEP

- Biopsy-confirmed CIN of any grade and a satisfactory colposcopic examination.
- LEEP is preferred over ablative therapies such as cryotherapy in the following conditions:
  - High-grade lesion is greater than 2 cm or two quadrants
  - Lesion is not covered by cryoprobe
  - Ectocervix is irregular
  - Whenever "screen and treat" (e.g., colposcopic evaluation and treatment) at a single visit is advantageous
  - Patients have recurrent CIN after previous therapy (e.g., cone biopsy, LEEP, cryotherapy)

LEEP Conization

- Unsatisfactory colposcopy in women with biopsy-confirmed CIN of any grade (e.g., cannot see entire lesion, SCJ, or TZ).
- HSIL referral cytology and unsatisfactory colposcopy.
- HSIL referral cytology with satisfactory colposcopy and either no CIN or only CIN I identified ("lack of correlation principle").
- Positive endocervical sampling (e.g., neoplasia of any grade present)
- Microinvasive lesions on cervical biopsy

CONTRAINDICATIONS

- Bleeding diathesis
- Severe cervicitis

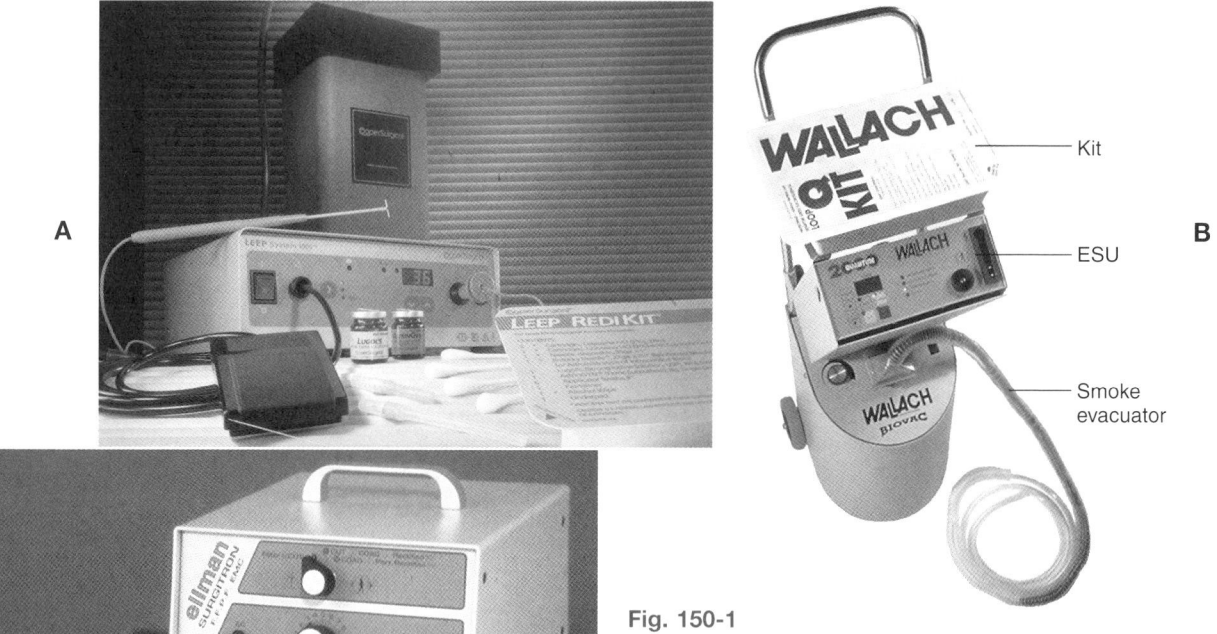

Fig. 150-1
Electrosurgical units used for LEEP procedures. **A,** CooperSurgical electrosurgical (LEEP) unit with handpiece, loop electrodes, and foot switch. **B,** Wallach Q2000 electrosurgery unit, with smoke evacuator beneath the unit and a kit with all the supplies for the procedure on top. This smoke evacuator automatically turns on when the unit is activated and turns off 20 seconds after it is deactivated. **C,** Ellman radiofrequency unit. (**A,** Courtesy CooperSurgical, Trumbull, Conn. **B,** Courtesy Wallach Surgical Devices, Orange, Conn. **C,** Courtesy Ellman International, Hewlett, NY.)

- Patient exposed in utero to diethylstilbestrol
- Pregnancy
- Less than 12 weeks after delivery
- Clinically apparent invasive carcinoma of the cervix
- Equivocal cervical abnormalities
- Heavy menses
- A preexisting short cervix (relative contraindication—clinician should consider referral)
- Special precaution is needed in patients with pacemakers (relative contraindication)
- Lack of expertise to control potential severe cervical bleeding

Note: It is imperative that the LEEP procedure not just be used to excise the TZ indiscriminately in women with atypical Pap smears. The procedure should be reserved to treat CIN lesions, not just atypical Pap smears. Cryotherapy is less expensive, has fewer complications, and has equal outcomes in properly selected patients (while at the same time removing less tissue) (see Chapter 15, Cryotherapy). Cold-knife conization is preferred when conization is being performed for a glandular abnormality.

EQUIPMENT

- Electrosurgical generator or unit (ESU) (Fig. 150-1) with the following features:

—Minimum output capability of 50 watts in both cutting and coagulation modes
—Rapid-start features
—Patient-grounding pad monitor (beneficial if the patient is under anesthesia)
—Isolated circuitry

Editor's note: Although the Ellman Surgitron does not meet some of these qualifications, it has been used extensively for the LEEP procedure.

- Loop electrodes of the appropriate size and a ball electrode for fulguration (Fig. 150-2) (These can be either of the disposable or of the reusable variety.)

   It is recommended that clinicians use only the shallow loop electrodes (i.e., either 0.8 or 1.0 cm deep) for routine LEEP. Larger electrodes can be used with large cervices or when lesions extend into the endocervical canal (e.g., LEEP conization). A variation is the Fischer electrode, which provides a true "cone" specimen.
- Electrode handle and a patient return electrode (grounding pad or antenna)
- Nonconductive speculum (either coated with a nonconductive material or made of plastic) capable of being used in conjunction with a smoke evacuator
- Smoke evacuator equipped with an adequate viral and odor filter

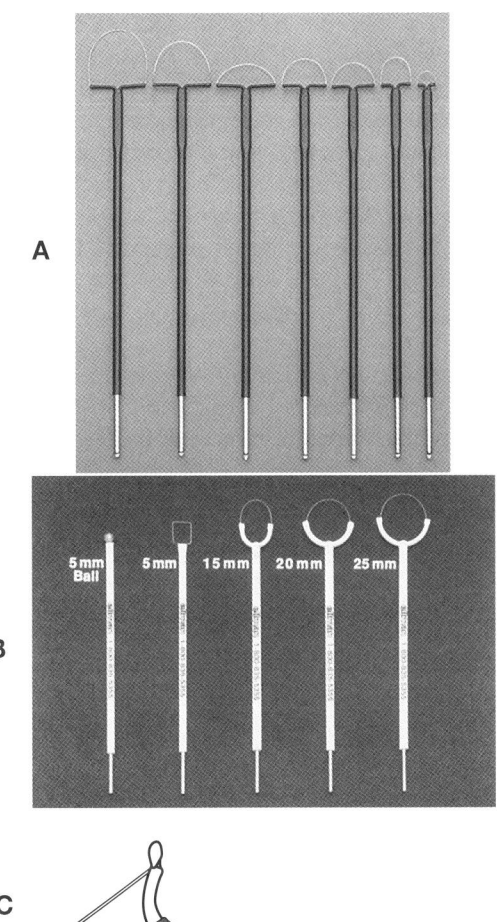

Fig. 150-2
Wire loop electrodes for loop electrosurgical excision procedure (LEEP). **A,** Loop electrodes come in a variety of sizes and shapes. **B,** The Ellman electrodes. **C,** The Fischer electrode, which removes more of a conical piece.

- Colposcope capable of low magnification (4× to 7.5×)
- Nonsterile gloves
- Acetic acid (5%)
- Full-strength aqueous Lugol's solution
- Cotton balls and large OB-GYN applicators
- Ring forceps
- Syringe (5 ml) with 4-inch needle extender and 1½-inch, 25-gauge needle as well as 5 ml of 2% lidocaine with epinephrine), or dental type of syringe equipped with a 25- to 27-gauge needle at least 1½ inches long with two 1.8-ml ampules of 2% lidocaine with 1:100,000 epinephrine (Fig. 150-3)
- Vaginal sidewall retractor
- Kevorkian endocervical curette
- Monsel's paste, which is made by allowing Monsel's solution to evaporate until it forms a thick yellow paste
- Containers of histology fixative (usually 10% formalin)
- A 12-inch needle holder and 2-0 Vicryl suture material together with a vaginal pack in the event that large-vessel bleeding occurs

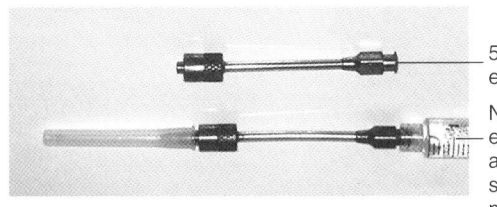

5-inch needle extender   **A**

Needle extender attached to syringe and needle   **B**

Fig. 150-3
A, Needle extender (5 inch). **B,** Needle extender placed on the end of a 5-ml syringe with 25-gauge, 1½-inch needle attached.

- A power examination table with adjustable height (recommended)

PREPROCEDURE PATIENT PREPARATION

- Provide a patient education handout (see the sample patient education handout titled "Loop Electrosurgical Excision Procedure [LEEP]" on page 1941 of Appendix G).
- Instruct the patient to take 600 to 800 mg of ibuprofen or a preferred nonsteriodal antiinflammatory 1 to 2 hours before the procedure.
- Obtain informed consent.

TECHNIQUE

The procedure is best performed immediately after menses so that any vaginal bleeding is not confused with menses.

1. Have the patient undress from the waist down and lie on the gynecologic examination table. It is important that the patient not move, cough, or change position once the excision is started. Thus a cooperative patient is essential.
2. Attach the patient return electrode grounding pad to the patient's thigh and connect the grounding pad to the ESU (or place the "antenna plate" under the hip).
3. Insert a nonconductive speculum with the smoke evacuator attachment into the vagina and connect it to the smoke evacuator. It is important that the speculum be large enough to allow complete, unobstructed visualization of the cervix. If the vaginal sidewalls remain in the way, use a vaginal sidewall retractor (Fig. 150-4).
4. Apply the acetic acid solution, examine the cervix colposcopically, and identify all lesions and the TZ.
5. Apply full-strength Lugol's solution to the cervix (this lasts longer than acetic acid). Use cotton balls or a large OB-GYN applicator.
6. Inject approximately 0.5 to 1.5 ml of 2% lidocaine with epinephrine 1:100,000 intracervically (submu-

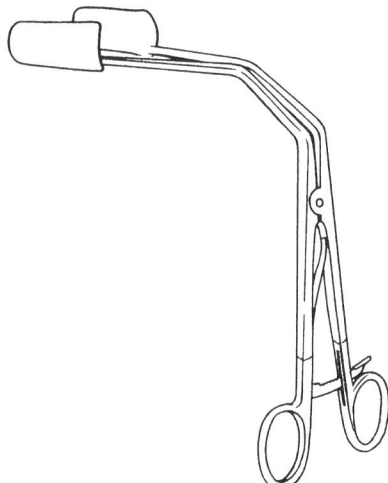

Fig. 150-4
Vaginal sidewall retractor.

cosally) at each of the 12, 3, 6 and 9 o'clock positions (to a total of 2 to 6 ml). Take care to inject the cervix superficially, only 3 to 5 mm deep. Additional injections may be needed at intervals between those noted previously, depending on the size of the cervix.

7. Although loops of many different sizes are available from various manufacturers, a round loop 2 cm wide by 0.8 cm deep (R2008) is most frequently used for CIN lesions confined to the portio. For a small, nulliparous cervix, use a 1.5 × 0.7–cm loop (R1507). For LEEP conizations when lesions extend into the endocervical canal, a 1 × 1–cm loop electrode can be used to excise the endocervical canal itself. This can be combined with the ectocervical loop to perform a "cowboy hat" type of procedure (See Fig. 150-7, *C*).

The power required will depend on the ESU used and the diameter of the loop. In general, a 2.0 × 0.8 cm loop will require between 35 and 45 watts of power, whereas a 1 × 1–cm loop will require only 20 to 30 watts of power. For LEEP, the use of a blended (cut and coag) current provides the best combination of minimal tissue artifact and minimal amounts of bleeding. Many use a pure cutting setting, which provides even less burn artifact for the pathologist while still controlling bleeding. It allows for the use of less power so less tissue is damaged.

Three different types of cervical LEEP excisions can be performed, depending on the size and location of the CIN lesion. For practical purposes, we further subdivide these into two groups: LEEP for lesions confined to the exocervix, and LEEP conization for lesions extending into the endocervix.

For *small lesions confined to the ectocervix,* the clinician should perform the following:

a. Select a loop electrode 1.5 to 2.0 cm wide and 0.8 cm deep.
b. Place the loop several millimeters lateral to the edge of the CIN lesion and make a test pass over the lesion to ensure that the path is clear.
c. Hold the loop just above the surface, activate the loop, and then push it perpendicularly, gradually, into the tissue to a depth of about 4 mm.
d. While pushing the loop deeper into the cervical stroma to the full depth of 8 mm, draw it laterally and through the endocervical canal. Pull it to the other side several millimeters past a lesion or several millimeters beyond the TZ, whichever is more lateral, before removing it (Fig. 150-5).

Note: In most instances the entire CIN lesion and the TZ can be removed in a single pass. This produces a donut-shaped specimen with the endocervical canal in the center.

For larger lesions confined to the ectocervix, the clinician should perform the following:

a. In some instances, CIN lesions may be too extensive to be removed in a single pass. In this event, remove the central portion of the lesion using a 2-cm-wide loop electrode, as previously described.
b. Then, excise the remaining CIN and TZ with additional, more superficial passes using the same loop electrode. Alternatively, the remaining tissue can be ablated using electrocoagulation and a ball electrode (Fig. 150-6).

For CIN extending into the endocervical canal, LEEP conizations are performed and lesions are removed in a two-step procedure that uses a 2-cm-wide exocervical electrode in conjunction with a 1 × 1–cm loop or square endocervical electrode to produce a cowboy hat type of excision. For this procedure, one of two methods can be used.

The first method involves excising the endocervical portion of the lesion, first using the 1 × 1–cm endocervical electrode. Once the endocervical portion of the lesion is excised, the exocervical portion is excised using a standard 2.0 × 0.8 cm loop electrode (Fig. 150-7, *A*).

In the second method, the large ectocervical portion is excised first, followed by the smaller endocervical portion (Fig. 150-7, *B*). Care should be taken not to excise the endocervical canal too deeply. Both approaches leave a cowboy hat shape excision on the cervix (Fig. 150-7, *C*). The endocervical and exocervical excisional specimens should be submitted for pathologic assessment in separate containers.

Occasionally the electrode "stalls" midway through the excision and will not cut. This occurs

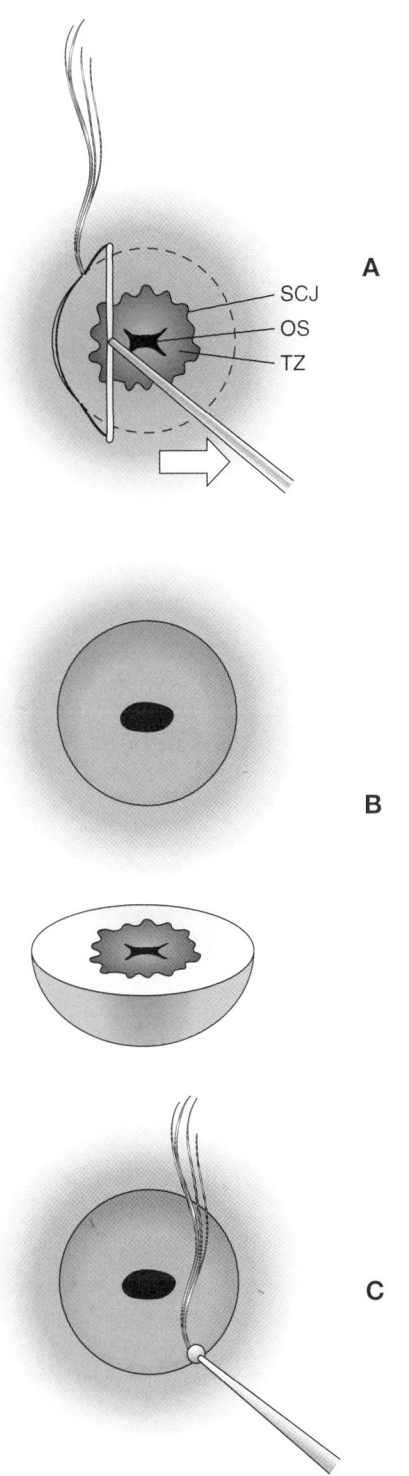

Fig. 150-5
Standard loop electrosurgical excision procedure (LEEP) for cervical intraepithelial lesions that can be removed in a single pass. After painting the cervix with Lugol's solution and injecting lidocaine, the clinician uses an ectocervical loop (2 cm wide and 0.8 cm deep) to resect the entire lesion (**A** and **B**). Then the crater base is coagulated using a 5-mm ball electrode followed by the application of Monsel's paste **(C)**.

when there is significant bleeding, the movement is too rapid, the ground is not attached properly, the cutting power is too low, or the reusable electrode is not clean (i.e., carbon buildup). If stalling occurs, it is best to remove the electrode and approach from the opposite side.

Some pathologists prefer that after the specimen is excised, it be removed from the cervix using forceps, opened along one side, and placed in a plastic holder to allow it to fix in formalin in the proper orientation. Other pathologists prefer the specimen be tagged at a certain location. Clinicians should check with the particular pathologist to determine preferences. Generally "tagging" the tissue to provide location provides little practical information.

The average cervix is 3 to 4 cm long. Removing 1 to 1.5 cm generally has minimal adverse consequences. It is only after numerous cervical procedures that one begins to see significant long-term complications.

8. Inspect the cervix and endocervical canal to ensure that all nonstained (with Lugol's) and all acetowhite epithelium has been excised. (More acetic acid may need to be applied with a Q-Tip to the canal.) If WE remains, another excision should be carried out (until no WE is remaining). Care should be taken not to interpret thermal cautery effect in the endocervical canal as residual neoplasia.

9. Perform an ECC above the excisional base. This helps confirm there was no dysplasia above the excision.

10. Fulgurate any bleeding points at the base of the excision using a ball electrode with the "coagulation" setting on the ESU. For 5-mm ball electrodes, power settings of 40 to 55 watts are usually required to obtain adequate arcing between the electrode and the tissue. (Excessive bleeding is more frequent in patients with severe cervicitis and in those less than 12 weeks after delivery.) Frequently the entire base of the excision is lightly coagulated. Perform the coagulation up to the endocervical canal, but take care not to insert the electrode into the canal. Excessive coagulation is not warranted and may be detrimental to optimal healing.

11. Apply Monsel's paste to the entire area. Fig. 150-8 shows the typical cervix upon completion of the procedure *(A)* and 6 weeks after the procedure *(B)*.

COMPLICATIONS

- Significant *intraoperative bleeding* is an uncommon but potentially serious complication. It sometimes occurs when the electrode is inserted too deeply into

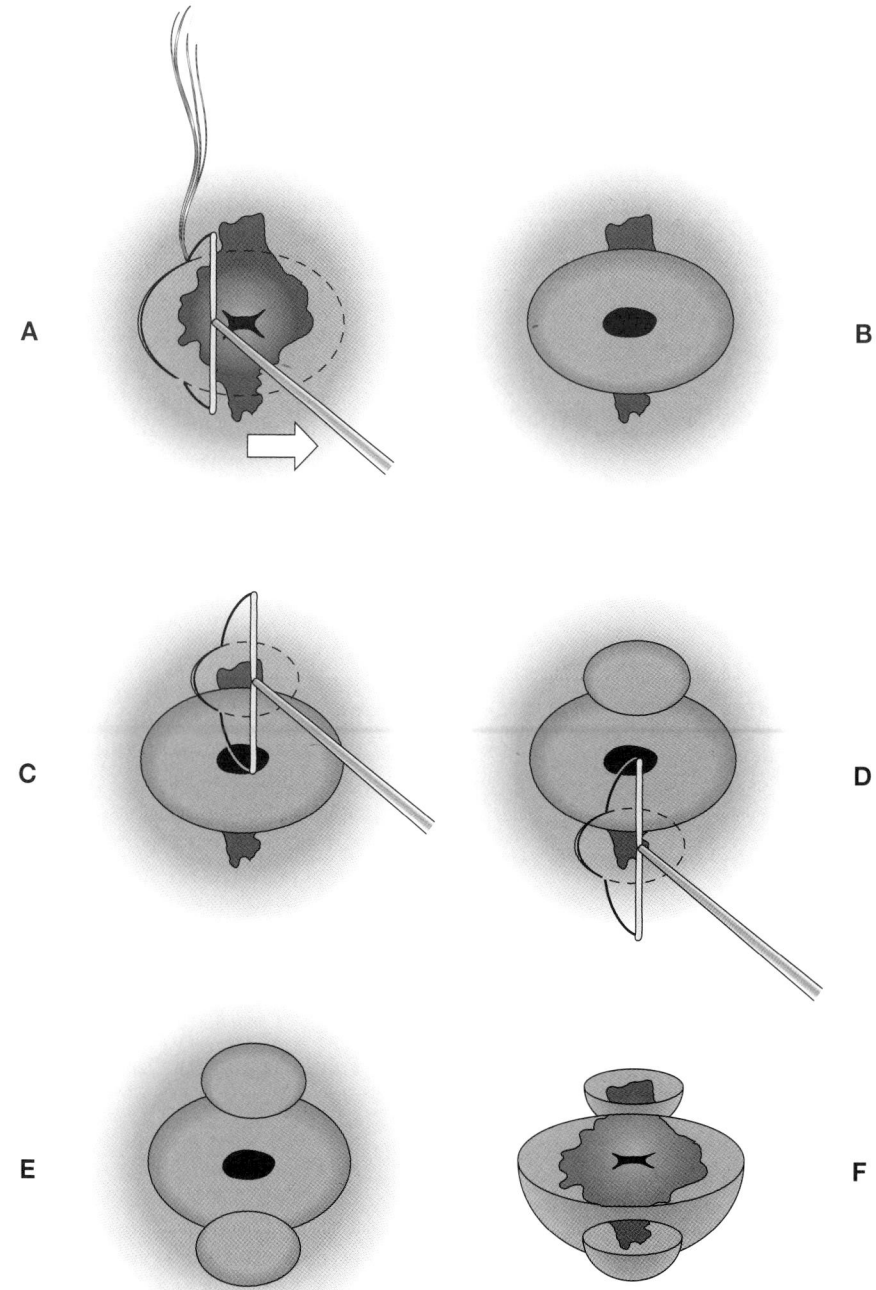

Fig. 150-6
For lesions too large to be removed in a single pass, the clinician uses a 2 × 0.8 cm loop electrode to resect the central portion of the lesion (**A** and **B**). Then, the remaining tissue is resected with additional passes using the same electrode (**C-E**). Tissue specimens (**F**) are placed in formalin.

the tissue at the 3 and 9 o'clock positions (where the cervical branches of the uterine artery are located) or when the patient has severe cervicitis. The most effective way to control bleeding is to first apply pressure directly to the bleeding site using a large cotton-tipped applicator. Once the bleeding has slowed, the ball electrode is then placed in direct contact with the bleeding site and tissue is "desic-cated" using coagulation current. If it is not controlled with pressure, the clinician should inject 1 to 2 ml 2% Xylocaine with epinephrine into the bleeding site. With the bleeding slowed or stopped, the ball electrode can then be effective.

For rare cases of persistent bleeding a "figure of eight" hemostatic stitch can be placed or the vagina and cervix should be packed tightly with 4 × 4 gauze

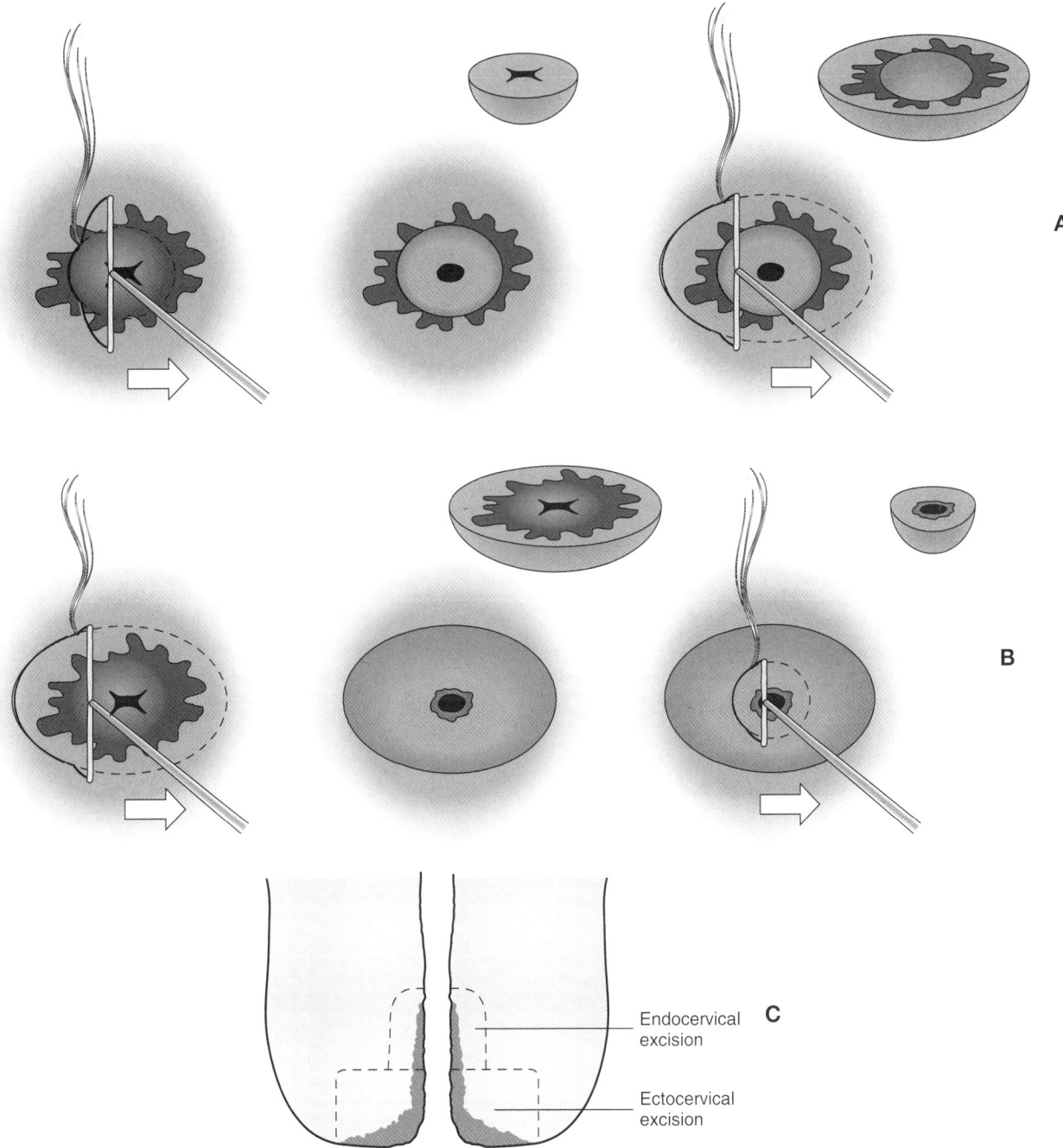

Fig. 150-7
Two methods for obtaining an endocervical sample with the loop electrosurgical excision procedure: **A,** The clinician resects the endocervical portion of the lesion using a 1 × 1–cm loop. Then a 2.0 × 0.8–cm loop is used to resect additional cervical intraepithelial neoplasia extending on to the portio. **B,** In some cases it may be necessary to excise the ectocervical portion first. Excising to a depth greater than 1.5 cm into the canal increases the chances of significant bleeding. **C,** Longitudinal section showing the "cowboy hat" procedure.

and the patient should be transported to the emergency room.

• *Postoperative bleeding* occurs in less than 5% of patients. These patients experience a modest amount of bleeding 4 to 10 days after LEEP. It can usually be managed by electrofulguration or by packing the crater base with Monsel's paste. Minimal spotting is to be expected up to 14 days after the procedure and after initial intercourse.

• Posttreatment *cervical stenosis* is an uncommon complication (less than 1%) and occurs predominately in postmenopausal women and those lacking estrogen

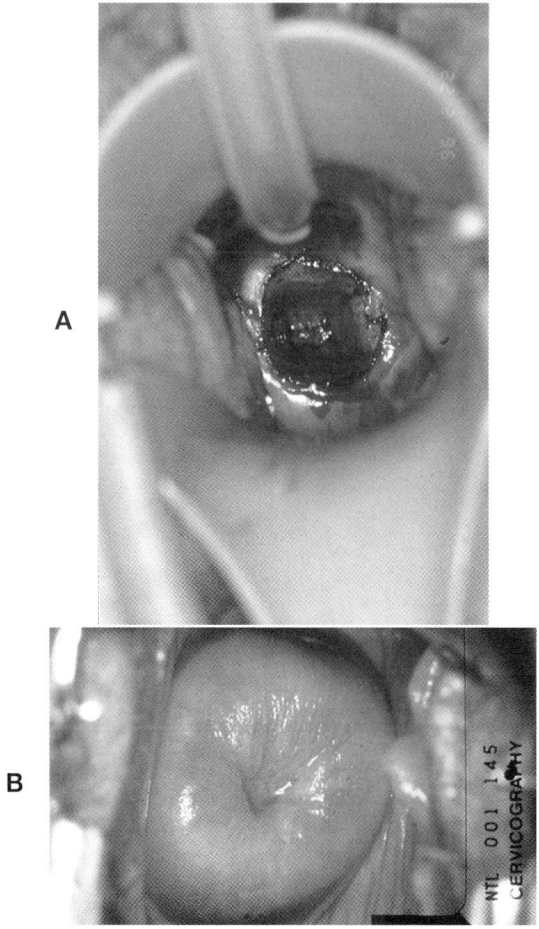

Fig. 150-8
A, Appearance of the cervix as seen through a nonconductive speculum immediately after the loop electrosurgical excision procedure (LEEP). **B,** Appearance of cervix 6 weeks after LEEP. Note the absence of an ectocervical transformation zone. (**A,** Courtesy The National Procedures Institute, Midland, Mich; **B,** courtesy National Testing Laboratories, St Louis, Mo.)

(postmenopausal; Norplant and Depro-Provera users; lactating women). For postmenopausal patients, or if a hypoestrogen state is suspected, the clinician should consider replacement estrogen for 2 to 3 weeks after the procedure (one applicator of Premarin in the vagina every night).

- Using a coated, nonconductive speculum prevents *electric shock,* which is caused by touching the speculum with the electrode during the procedure. An "electric shock" sensation can make the patient jump, causing significant injury.
- *Inadvertent burns or lacerations* to the lateral vaginal wall or other sites can occur but are rare. The clinician should instruct the patient not to move. Ureters, bowel, and bladder are only millimeters away from the vaginal sidewalls.
- *Stalling of the electrode* can occasionally occur (see previous discussion).

- *Pain and discomfort* are minimal and generally can be controlled with nonsteroidal antiinflammatory drugs (NSAIDs).
- *Infection* is rare. Metronidazole or doxycycline can be used.
- *Recurrence or persistence of disease* occurs in 5% to 10% of cases.
- *Cervical incompetence* is unlikely, unless numerous procedures have been performed on the cervix. Infertility is not generally a concern unless stenosis occurs or the majority of the endocervical canal has been removed, reducing the number of mucus-producing glands. The clinician should avoid overuse of the procedure when it is not indicated.
- Positive margin. If the ectocervical or endocervical excisional margins are "positive" on histology or if the ECC is positive for neoplasia, the patient is at higher risk for recurrence. However, even in these situations, less than one third of lesions will persist. The cautery and inflammatory response appears to resolve most of these. In these cases it is prudent to perform colposcopy with endocervical curettage and repeat cytology approximately 3 to 4 months after the initial LEEP. In some instances, especially high-risk and postmenopausal patients, consideration should be given to performing a diagnostic conization procedure (e.g., either a cold-knife or LEEP conization) once the cervix has healed.

POSTPROCEDURE PATIENT EDUCATION

See the sample patient education handout titled "Loop Electrosurgical Excision Procedure (LEEP)" on page 1941 of Appendix G.
- The clinician should instruct the patient to avoid vaginal intercourse, douching, use of tampons, and heavy exercise (especially weight lifting) for 3 weeks.
- If significant bleeding persists for more than 2 weeks (if the volume is comparable to that of a normal period or greater), if the patient begins passing large blood clots, if the vaginal discharge becomes foul smelling, or if there is significant pelvic pain (especially if it is associated with a fever), the patient should call the physician or return to the clinic.

POSTPROCEDURE PATIENT CARE

Patients are seen 4 to 6 weeks after the procedure for a review of the pathology report and for a brief postoperative check. This helps reassure the patients and decreases their anxiety about how well they have healed. It also provides an opportunity to reinforce prevention methods, such as not smoking. It is important to check for cervical stenosis. The os is easier to dilate early rather than waiting for a more mature scar (see Chapter 137, Cervical Stenosis and Cervical Dilation).

The clinician should then reevaluate the patient using either a program of repeat cytology at 6 and 12 months, a single HPV DNA test for high-risk types of HPV at 12 months, or a combination of cytology and colposcopy at 6 and 12 months. If a program of repeat cytology is used for follow-up, patients with a cytologic result of atypical squamous cells or greater should be referred for colposcopy. If HPV DNA testing at 12 months is used, patients with high-risk types of HPV identified should be referred for colposcopy.

SUPPLIERS

Equipment
Aspen Labs
952 S. Zephr Court
Lakewood, CO 80226
Phone: 1-303-699-9854

CooperSurgical
95 Corporate Drive
Trumbull, CT 06611
Phone: 1-203-601-5200
Website: www.coopersurgical.com

Ellman International Inc
1135 Railroad Avenue
Hewlett, NY 11557
Phone: 1-800-835-5355
Website: www.ellman.com

ERBE USA, Inc.
2225 Northwest Parkway
Marietta, GA 30067
Phone: 1-770-955-4400

Leisegang Medical
95 Corporate Drive
Trumbull, CT 06611
Phone: 1-203-601-5200
Website: www.leisegang.com

MedGyn Products, Inc.
328 N. Eisenhower Lane
Lombard, IL 60148
Phone: 1-800-451-9667
Website: www.medgyn.com

Premier Medical Products
1710 Romano Drive, Box 4500
Plymouth Meeting, PA 19462
Phone: 1-888-773-6872
Website: www.premusa.com

Utah Medical Products, Inc.
7043 South 300 West
Midvale, UT 84047-1048
Phone: 1-800-533-4984
Website: www.utahmed.com

Valleylab, Inc.
5920 Longbow Drive
Boulder, CO 80301-3299
Phone: 1-800-255-8522

Wallach Surgical Devices, Inc.
235 Edison Road
Orange, CT 06477
Phone: 1-800-243-2463

WelchAllyn
4341 State Street Road
P.O. Box 220
Skaneateles Falls, NY 13153-0220
Phone: 1-800-535-6663
Website: www.welchallyn.com

Booklet on patient education
Krames Communications
1100 Grundy Lane
San Bruno, CA 94066-3030
Phone: 1-800-333-3032
Website: www.krames.com

CPT/BILLING CODES

57460	Colposcopy with loop electrosurgical excision or excisions of the cervix (LEEP)
57500	Cervical biopsy
57520	Cervical conization, with or without fulguration
57522	Cervical conization using loop technique
57505	Endocervical curettage
99070	Supplies and materials for kits and electrodes (a surgical tray charge is generally allowed for an office LEEP)

ICD-9-CM DIAGNOSTIC CODES

180.9	Cervical cancer
622.1	CIN I and II (mild to moderate dysplasia)
233.1	CIN III (severe dysplasia, ca-in-situ)

ADDITIONAL RESOURCES

• See the sample patient education handout titled "Loop Electrosurgical Excision Procedure (LEEP)" on page 1941 of Appendix G.

BIBLIOGRAPHY

ACOG committee opinion. Role of loop electrosurgical excision procedure in the evaluation of abnormal Pap test results. Number 195, November 1997. Committee on Gynecologic Practice. American College of Obstetricians and Gynecologists, *Int J Gynaecol Obstet* 61:203, 1998.

Apgar B, Wright T, Pfenninger J: Loop electrosurgical excision procedure for CIN, *Am Fam Physician* 46:505, 1992.

Bigrigg A, Haffenden DK, Sheehan AL, et al: Efficacy and safety of large-loop excision of the transformation zone, *Lancet* 343:32, 1994.

Bigrigg MA, Codling BW, Pearson P, et al: Pregnancy after cervical loop diathermy, *Lancet* 337:119, 1991.

Dobbs SP, Asmussen T, Nunns D, et al: Does histological incomplete excision of cervical intraepithelial neoplasia following large loop excision of transformation zone increase recurrence rates? A six year cytological follow up, *Br J Obst Gynecol* 107:1298, 2000.

Duggan BD, Felix JC, Muderspach LI, et al: Cold-knife conization versus conization by the loop electrosurgical excision procedure: a randomized, prospective study, *Am J Obstet Gynecol* 180:276, 1999.

Eilers GM, Swanson T, Kitowski J, Smith M: Is LEEP a feasible addition to the family physician's office? *Fam Pract Res J* 14(1):87, 1994.

Felix JC, Muderspach LI, Duggan BD, et al: The significance of positive margins in loop electrosurgical cone biopsies, *Obstet Gynecol* 84:996, 1994.

Ferenczy A, Choukroun D, Arseneau J: Loop electrosurgical excision procedure for squamous intraepithelial lesions of the cervix: advantages and potential pitfalls, *Obstet Gynecol* 87:332, 1996.

Ferenczy A, Choukroun D, Falcone T, et al: The effect of cervical loop electrosurgical excision procedure on subsequent pregnancy outcome: North-American experience, *Am J Obstet Gynecol* 172:1246, 1995.

Ferris DG, Hainer BL, Pfenninger JL, et al: "See and treat" electrosurgical loop excision of the cervical transformation zone, *J Fam Pract* 42:253, 1996.

Ferris DG, Hainer BL, Pfenninger JL, et al: Electrosurgical loop excision of the cervical transformation zone: the experience of family physicians, *J Fam Pract* 41:337, 1995.

Flannelly G, Langhan H, Jandial L, et al: A study of treatment failures following large loop excision of the transformation zone for the treatment of cervical intraepithelial neoplasia, *Br J Obstet Gynecol* 104:718, 1997.

Gonzalez DI, Jr., Zahn CM, Retzloff MG, et al: Recurrence of dysplasia after loop electrosurgical excision procedures with long-term follow-up, *Am J Obstet Gynecol* 184:315, 2001.

Haffenden DK, Bigrigg A, Codling BW, et al: Pregnancy following large loop excision of the transformation zone, *Br J Obstet Gynaecol* 100:1059, 1993.

Hallam NF, West J, Harper C, et al: Large loop excision of the transformation zone (LLETZ) as an alternative to both local ablative and cone biopsy treatment: a series of 1000 patients, *J Gynecol Surg* 9:77, 1993.

Harper DM, Walstatter BS, Lofton BJ: Anesthetic blocks for loop electrosurgical excision procedure, *J Fam Pract* 39:249, 1994.

Irvin WP, Jr., Andersen WA, Taylor PT, Jr., et al: "See-and-treat" loop electrosurgical excision. Has the time come for a reassessment? *J Reprod Med* 47:569, 2002.

McLucas B, McGill J: Pure cutting for loop excision of squamous intraepithelial lesions, *J Reprod Med* 39:373, 1994.

Mitchell MF, Tortolero-Luna G, Cook E, et al: A randomized clinical trial of cryotherapy, laser vaporization, and loop electrosurgical excision for treatment of squamous intraepithelial lesions of the cervix, *Obstet Gynecol* 92:737, 1998.

Murdoch JB, Morgan PR, Lopes A, et al: Histological incomplete excision of CIN after large loop excision of the transformation zone (LLETZ) merits careful follow up, not retreatment, *Br J Obstet Gynaecol* 99:990, 1992.

Noller KL: Cryotherapy, laser vaporization, and loop electrosurgical excision for treatment of squamous intraepithelial lesions of the cervix, *Ob Gyn Clin Alert* Dec:61, 1998.

Paraskevaidis E, Koliopoulos G, Paschopoulos M, et al: Effects of ball cauterization following loop excision and follow-up colposcopy, *Obstet Gynecol* 97:617, 2001.

Paraskevaidis E, Lolis ED, Koliopoulos G, et al: Cervical intraepithelial neoplasia outcomes after large loop excision with clear margins, *Obstet Gynecol* 95:828, 2000.

Pfenninger JL: Colposcopy, LEEP, and other procedures: the role for family physicians, *Fam Med* 28:505, 1996.

Pfenninger JL: Good things still come in old packages: cryosurgery vs LEEP. Loop electrosurgical excision procedure, *J Am Board Fam Pract* 12:416, 1999.

Robinson WR, Webb S, Tirpack J, et al: Management of cervical intraepithelial neoplasia during pregnancy with LOOP excision, *Gynecol Oncol* 64:153, 1997.

Suh-Burgmann EJ, Whall-Strojwas D, Chang Y, et al: Risk factors for cervical stenosis after loop electrocautery excision procedure, *Obstet Gynecol* 96:657, 2000.

Wright TC, Gagnon MD, Richart RM, et al: Treatment of cervical intraepithelial neoplasia using the loop electrosurgical excision procedure, *Obstet Gynecol* 79:173, 1992.

Wright TC, Jr., Koulos J, Schnoll F, et al: Cervical intraepithelial neoplasia in women infected with the human immunodeficiency virus: outcome after loop electrosurgical excision, *Gynecol Oncol* 55:253, 1994.

Wright TC, Richart RM, Ferenczy A, et al: Comparison of specimens removed by CO_2 laser conization and loop electrosurgical excision procedures, *Obstet Gynecol* 79:147, 1992.

Wright TC, Richart RM, Ferenczy AF: *Electrosurgery for HPV-related lesions of the anogenital tract*, New City, NY, 1992, ArthurVision.

Zaitoun AM, McKee G, Coppen MJ, et al: Completeness of excision and follow up cytology in patients treated with loop excision biopsy, *J Clin Pathol* 53:191, 2000.

CHAPTER 151

Modern Methods of Natural Family Planning (NFP)

John Thomas Littell

Natural family planning (NFP) is to be viewed as an effective, natural alternative to other, more invasive and/or artificial, methods of birth control. It is also a means of enhancing a woman's understanding of her own fertility.

REASONS FOR CHOOSING NATURAL FAMILY PLANNING

Clearly not all women and couples wish to choose the chemical and mechanical methods presently available to delay pregnancy. Their decision is not based solely on economic variables, since these artificial methods are widely available and generally affordable. Rather, couples are interested in NFP for one or more of the following reasons:

- *Religious conviction:* Both Catholicism and Islam forbid artificial contraception and abortion or abortifacient methods of birth control.
- *Health reasons:* The increased risks and fears of vascular accidents and breast cancer associated with oral contraceptive use, or osteoporosis associated with long-acting depo-progestins, are not acceptable to many women. More often, women abandon the artificial methods after experiencing significant mood disturbances, weight gain, or intolerable cycle abnormalities.
- *"Natural is better":* Many women simply want to preserve their normal cycle of fertility, rather than alter or permanently limit their fertility for the sake of avoiding pregnancy. NFP allows women to maintain (or, at times, improve) their usual cycle.
- For some, *costs* of other contraceptive methods are still a disincentive.

EARLY FORMS OF NATURAL FAMILY PLANNING

The "rhythm" method, also known as the *calendar* or *Ogino-Knaus* method, was named after two physician researchers in Japan and Austria in the 1930s. This method involves calculating the fertile period by counting days from the first day of the last menses. It was the only reasonably effective method of birth control in the world (except abstinence) for three decades until the introduction of oral contraceptives in the 1960s. Couples calculate the approximate time of ovulation based on the fact that ovulation usually takes place 11 to 16 days before the next menses. This "fertile window" is derived from a review of the previous 6 to 12 cycles, taking into account the shortest and longest cycles. By subtracting 19 days from the shortest cycle and 10 days from the longest cycle, the woman can determine the first and last days, respectively, of the fertile phase. The method takes into account the possibility of 3 days of sperm life before this fertile window and a 24-hour maximal life of the ovum. Although women with regular cycles approached 99% method effectiveness with rhythm, those with irregular cycles had typical effectiveness rates of about 50%. It is rarely in use now because of the availability of more effective natural methods.

SYMPTOTHERMAL METHOD

After Vollman first published findings in 1940 correlating midcycle (periovulatory) pain with an upwards temper-

Author's note: As a family physician practicing obstetrics and as an instructor in natural family planning (NFP), I was honored to be asked to write this chapter. Yet, as the founder of Family Physicians for Life, I state at the outset my commitment to preserving and protecting all human life from the moment of conception, that is, fertilization. Hence I differ with the editor's decision to include potentially abortifacient methods of birth control and surgical abortion in this textbook. The message of NFP, however, is certainly not restricted only to "pro-life" physicians and patients.

ature shift, the symptothermal (ST) method emerged as the first natural method of family planning to rely upon the observations made by the woman with regards to her period of fertility. Temperature variations during the reproductive cycle are recorded on a chart, including the luteal phase elevation or "thermal shift" (i.e., postovulatory sustained increase from basal body temperature of about 0.4° F). These readings are combined with other periovulatory observations, including the appearance of fertile cervical mucus during the days leading up to ovulation, the opening of the cervical os and raising of cervix at ovulation, "mittelschmerz" (i.e., periovulatory pain), and midcycle breast tenderness. These multiple signs and symptoms of fertility enable the woman or couple to either avoid or achieve pregnancy. Couples may choose to emphasize one observation more than the others, using the others to "crosscheck" their primary observation (e.g., temperature shift used to "crosscheck" cervical mucus observations).

The ST method allows for several different "rules" for avoiding pregnancy. Each rule recognizes the appearance of cervical mucus at the vulva or vagina as the first sign of fertility. In determining the end of the fertile window, couples may choose to emphasize mucus observations over temperature observations (and vice-versa). The most conservative rule recognizes both observations equally. For example, postovulatory infertility commences after the third day (or more) of a thermal shift (> 0.4° F), crosschecked by 4 or more days of "drying up" of the cervical mucus—whichever comes first.

By combining the many signs of fertility on a single chart, couples using the ST method are able to practice natural family planning effectively in any situation, for example, when breast-feeding, "coming off" of artificial contraception, or having irregular cycles. For the sake of simplicity, many couples eventually choose to rely solely upon cervical mucus observations for determining their fertile period—in a manner quite similar to the ovulation method described below.

OVULATION METHOD (BILLINGS METHOD)

The ovulation method was developed by Drs. John and Lynn Billings of Melbourne, Australia. In the 1950s this method evolved from the symptothermal method after researchers confirmed that women were able to predict the time of ovulation by using cervical mucus observations alone, reflecting changing levels of estrogen being produced by the developing ovarian follicle. Cervical mucus observations are external only, with a strong emphasis on sensation (e.g., feeling slippery or dry), either while wiping with toilet paper or simply while

walking about. The "peak" of fertility is defined as the last day of slippery sensation at the vulva. The basis of the method is that sperm without receptive cervical mucus will die within hours, whereas with the presence of good cervical mucus, sperm may survive up to 5 days. After the peak day, the woman typically notices a transition to a dry or sticky sensation at the vulva, reflecting a rise in the progesterone level during the luteal phase.

To avoid pregnancy, couples are advised to avoid intercourse or any genital contact between them from the time when the cervical mucus first appears (generally, a few days after the end of menses) until 3 days after the last "slippery" day. Although known as the "ovulation" method, this method does not pinpoint the exact day of ovulation, but rather identifies a "peak" sign of fertility (i.e., last day of "slippery" mucus). Ovulation is known to occur anywhere from 3 days before "peak" through 3 days after peak, with the majority of ovulations occurring on peak or peak plus 1 day. In addition, the cervical os remains open for 3 days after "peak," with mucus within the cervical crypts allowing for continued sperm life—hence the instruction to avoid genital contact for 3 full days after the peak day if the couple wishes to avoid pregnancy. Variations of the ovulation method exist; these include the "Creighton model," which quantifies the cervical mucus observations and standardizes all observations. Stamps and charts are used by most methods, although more recently the Billings have proposed the use of universal symbols and a charting system using handheld computer systems (e.g., Palm Pilot).

EFFECTIVENESS OF NATURAL FAMILY PLANNING

The effectiveness of modern methods of NFP for avoiding pregnancy, when taught and used correctly (i.e., method effectiveness), ranges from 97% to 100% in all published studies. However, it must be emphasized that, given that these methods rely upon the ability of the couple to abstain from genital contact during periods of fertility, the "use effectiveness" rate typically approaches about 80%. The use effectiveness rate approaches the method effectiveness rate of 100% when couples have compelling reasons for avoiding pregnancy. It can be used effectively by women of all ages, including those with irregular cycles or constant vaginal discharge, those "coming off" of oral contraceptives or other artificial methods, and nursing mothers.

The ability to use modern methods of NFP relies ultimately upon the acceptance of the technique(s) by physicians and other health care providers as legitimate and effective methods of family planning, and also upon the availability of trained instructors and other resources that readily convey the needed information.

CONCLUSION

Modern methods of NFP are increasing in popularity for reasons of personal well-being and/or religious conviction. The two principle methods available in the United States—the symptothermal and ovulation methods—have demonstrated effectiveness approaching 100% in all studies when used correctly and 80% efficacy in typical use situations. In addition to avoiding or spacing out pregnancies, many women have turned to these methods to also assist them in achieving pregnancy and in attempting to manage a number of other gynecologic and reproductive health concerns. Physicians wising to learn more about NFP may contact any of the organizations listed below for further information, including physician seminars, which are regularly held by the Couple-to-Couple League and by the Pope Paul VI Institute.

RESOURCES

Symptothermal method

The Couple to Couple League International
P.O. Box 111184
Cincinnati, OH 45211-1184
Phone: 1-513-471-2000
Website: www.ccli.org

Northwest Family Services, Inc.
4805 NE Glisan Street
Portland, OR 97213
Phone: 1-503-215-6377

Ovulation method

Billings Ovulation Method-USA
  (BOMA)
P.O. Box 16206
St. Paul, MN 55116
Phone: 1-800-637-6371
  or 1-651-699-8139
Website: www.boma-usa.org

Pope Paul VI Institute
6901 Mercy Road
Omaha, NE 68106-2604
Phone: 1-402-390-6600
Website: www.popepaulvi.com

Family of the Americans Foundation
P.O. Box 1170
Dunkirk, MD 20754
Phone: 1-301-627-3346

Natural Family Planning Teaching Aides and Books

Symptothermal method

Kippley J, Kippley S: *The art of natural family planning*, ed 4, Cincinnati, 1997, Couple to Couple League International.

Ovulation method

Billings E, Westmore A: *The Billings Method*, Australia 1997, Penguin Books.

Wilson MA: The ovulation method of birth regulation: the latest advances for achieving or postponing pregnancy—naturally, New York, 1980, Van Nostrand Reinhold.

Hilgers TW: *The medical applications of natural family planning*, Omaha, Neb, 1992, Pope Paul IV Institute.

All methods

Aguilar N: *No pill, no risk birth control*, New York, 1986, MacMillan.

Weschler T: *Taking charge of your fertility*, New York, 1995, Harper Perennial.

ICD-9-CM DIAGNOSTIC CODES

V25.09	Family planning advice
V29.9	Unspecified contraceptive management
599.0	Vaginal discharge
626.4	Irregular menses
259.9	Hormonal imbalance

BIBLIOGRAPHY

Febring R, Kitchen S, Shivanandan M: *An introduction to natural family planning* (booklet), Washington, DC, 1999, Diocesan Development Program for Natural Family Planning, National Conference of Catholic Bishops.

Geerling JH: Natural family planning, *Am Fam Physician* 52(6):1749, 1995.

Howard M, Stanford J: Pregnancy probabilities during use of the Creighton Model Fertility Care System, *Arch Fam Med* 8(5):391, 1999.

Indian Council of Medical Research: Field trial of Billings ovulation method of natural family planning, *Contraception* 53:69, 1996.

Ryder REJ: "Natural family planning": effective birth control supported by the Catholic Church, *BMJ* 307:723, 1993.

Stanford J, Lemaire JC, Thurman PB: Women's interest in natural family planning, *J Fam Pract* 46(1):65, 1998.

WEBSITE

www.woomb.org (World Organization of Ovulation Method – Billings)

CHAPTER 152

Pap Smear and Related Techniques for Cervical Cancer Screening

Gary R. Newkirk

Despite the controversies surrounding cervical Papanicolaou (Pap) smear testing, it remains an effective tool for cancer prevention and detection. Numerous studies have documented a statistically valid drop in the incidence and mortality rates of invasive cervical carcinomas since the introduction of the Pap smear. Unfortunately, cervical cancer screening has not eradicated this potentially preventable disease. The current cervical cancer detection system relies on a complex system of clinical and laboratory procedures that have potential for error at numerous points. Koss' (1989) landmark discussion summarizes major sources of error, including (1) problems with the initial clinical examination, (2) inappropriate smear collection technique, (3) laboratory errors in sample preparation and interpretation, (4) errors in report interpretation, (5) failure of the clinician to understand or appropriately respond to Pap smear–generated data, and (6) failure of the patient to follow the clinician's recommendations.

Compelling arguments link cervical neoplasia with human papillomavirus (HPV) infection. Epidemiologic data further document the epidemic proportions of new genital HPV infections. There appears to be escalating pressure to rely on Pap smear screening methodology, yet recent reports documenting between 20% and 50% false-negative results alarm patients and clinicians alike. Clinicians can continue to make significant contributions to cancer prevention in women by refining their method of Pap smear sampling, by enhancing their understanding of Pap smear report interpretation, and by clarifying their recommendations for patient management. This chapter focuses on a contemporary approach to Pap smear screening; it is assumed that basic pelvic examination skills have been mastered. Box 152-1 offers a brief summary of the terminology used throughout this discussion. Figure 152-1 provides a graphic representation of the changes involved with preinvasive and invasive disease of the cervix as well as a depiction of histological and cytological correlates. Figure 152-2 depicts the anatomy involved.

The Pap smear is a *screening test only;* it is *not diagnostic.* Thus, if an abnormality is seen or palpated at the time of the pelvic examination, it should be examined with a colposcope and a directed biopsy performed. The physician cannot rely on the Pap smear alone to be diagnostic for that particular lesion.

INDICATIONS

- *Screening:* All women by age 18 or with onset of sexual activity; annually thereafter. (Some clinicians will screen a subset of women with no risk factors every 3 years, providing that there are three negative yearly Pap smears and the risk factors do not change. Box 152-2 summarizes these risk factors for cervical dysplasia. As this chapter goes to press, the American Cancer Society has just released the latest Pap smear screening recommendations. See Box 152-3 for a summary. Many clinicians find this modified screening methodology impractical and clinically difficult to apply. Medicare limits screening in not-at-risk patients to every 3 years.) Lesbians also require regular Pap smears.
- *Follow-up* after borderline abnormal Pap smears (atypical squamous cells [ASC])
- *Diethylstilbestrol (DES)–exposed offspring:* At least by age 14, onset of menstruation, or initial sexual activity; every 6 to 12 months thereafter if colposcopy and biopsy are performed and tissue is found to be benign. DES-exposed offspring require colposcopic evaluation (and repeat colposcopy with biopsy as necessary). The appropriate Pap smear follow-up usually requires modified routines determined by coordinated exchange of expert opinion between the clinician, pathologist, and, quite often, a gynecologist familiar with this small subgroup of women. The vagina must also be observed closely, since it has a much higher risk for dysplasia and cancer.

BOX 152-1

Terminology and Definitions

Atypical glandular cells (AGC): In the past these were called "AGUS" (atypical glandular cells of undetermined significance), but since the incidence of pathology is so high (10% cancers and 25% high-grade lesions), the "US" has been dropped by Bethesda-2001. All need further investigation.

Atypical squamous cells (ASC): Bethesda-2001 divides these into ASC-US (atypical squamous cells of undetermined significance) and ASC-H (atypical squamous cells, cannot exclude HSIL).

Carcinoma in situ (CIS): Dysplasia involves the entire squamous epithelium but does *not* penetrate the basement membrane. Included in CIN III and HGSIL designations.

Cervical intraepithelial neoplasia (CIN): See "Dysplasia." CIN I refers to mild dysplasia, CIN II to moderate dysplasia, and CIN III to severe dysplasia, including carcinoma in situ (CIS).

Columnar epithelium: Single-layer, mucin-secreting epithelium on the surface of the endocervix. It can often be seen on the ectocervix and is proximal to the SCJ.

Dysplasia: Premalignant change in the cervical epithelium displaying proliferation of parabasal cells with disordered polarity, loss of cellular junctions, coarse nuclear chromatin clumping, abnormal nuclear cytoplasmic ratio, and high mitotic index. Reported as mild, moderate, and severe dysplasia. Usually refers to histology.

Ectocervix: Also called exocervix. The flat portion of the cervix that is readily visible. The cervical os is located centrally.

Endocervical cells: Glandular, columnar-shaped cells obtained from the endocervical (columnar) epithelium in the endocervical canal.

Endocervix: The area within the endocervical canal.

Exocervix: See "Ectocervix."

Frankly invasive squamous cell carcinoma of the cervix: Invasion greater than 3 mm (or 5 mm depending on classification used) below the basement membrane.

Koilocytotic or koilocytic: Equivalent terms include condylomatous atypia and human papillomavirus (HPV) effect; these terms describe cells that have perinuclear halos or vacuoles that vary in shape and configuration, and that show a distinct zone of clearing between the nucleus and cytoplasmic membrane. The abnormal nuclei are characterized by wrinkling, variation in size and shape, binucleate forms, and hyperchromasia. Usually indicative of HPV infection.

Microinvasive cervical cancer: Invasion 3 mm or less below the basement membrane. Some terminologies allow 5 mm of invasion and include other descriptive factors.

Squamocolumnar junction (SCJ): The line where the squamous epithelium of the ectocervix joins the mucus-secreting columnar epithelium of the endocervix.

Squamous cells: Epithelial cells on the surface of the ectocervix. These cells appear smooth and pink on the cervix.

Squamous intraepithelial lesion (SIL): Reported as either low (LGSIL, LSIL) or high grade (HGSIL, HSIL), corresponding to increasing severity of dysplasia (Bethesda terminology). Originally referred to cytology diagnosis, but now often used to describe histology as well.

Squamous metaplasia: A type of tissue present where the columnar epithelium is being replaced (transformed) by squamous epithelium. This normal tissue occurs within the cervical transformation zone, and the transformation of columnar to squamous epithelium is a totally normal process.

Transformation zone (TZ): Area of transformation or replacement of the cervical columnar epithelium by squamous epithelium through a process called metaplastic change. The *active* TZ goes from the outermost gland to the SCJ. The TZ is the principal site of origin for precancerous and invasive squamous cell carcinomas of the cervix.

Also see Chapter 139, Colposcopic Examination, and Figs. 152-1 and 152-2.

- *Any visible or palpable lesion of the cervix:* Follow precaution that the Pap smear is *not* diagnostic and further assessment is usually done with a biopsy directed by the colposcope.
- *Any abnormal vaginal bleeding or discharge.*
- *Posthysterectomy* (hysterectomy for benign disease): Every 3 years if patient's risk for cancer remains low.
- *Posthysterectomy* (hysterectomy for dysplasia, carcinoma): Annually after three or four normal Pap smears at 4- to 6-month intervals.
- *Posttreatment for cervical dysplasia, malignancy:* Every 4 months for at least three visits; every 6 months for two visits where indicated; annually thereafter.
- *Victims of rape, incest, abuse:* As part of initial workup. Repeat in 6 to 12 months.

There are numerous schemes for follow-up after treatment for cervical dysplasia and carcinoma. All involve increased frequency of Pap smear testing for a period of time. Repeat colposcopic examination is often performed with endocervical curettage or cervical biopsy, if necessary. All women with a history of cervical dysplasia remain at significant risk for disease recurrence and should undergo Pap smear testing at least annually for life.

CONTRAINDICATIONS

There are no absolute contraindications to obtaining a Pap smear. Relative contraindications include clinical circumstances in which sample collection is difficult to obtain or difficult to interpret (e.g., active vaginitis or cervicitis, pelvic inflammatory disease [PID], or menses). The clinician must weigh the benefits versus the risk of obtaining the screening Pap smear under these circumstances. For instance, if a woman presents with abnormal vaginal bleeding, a Pap smear is advised, despite the presence of blood. This contrasts with a patient who comes in for a routine Pap smear screening and has begun to menstruate. In the latter instance, the Pap smear can be deferred to a more favorable time. See the sample patient education handout titled "Pap Smear Information" on page 1943 of Appendix G, which includes advice on what women can do to optimize Pap smear results.

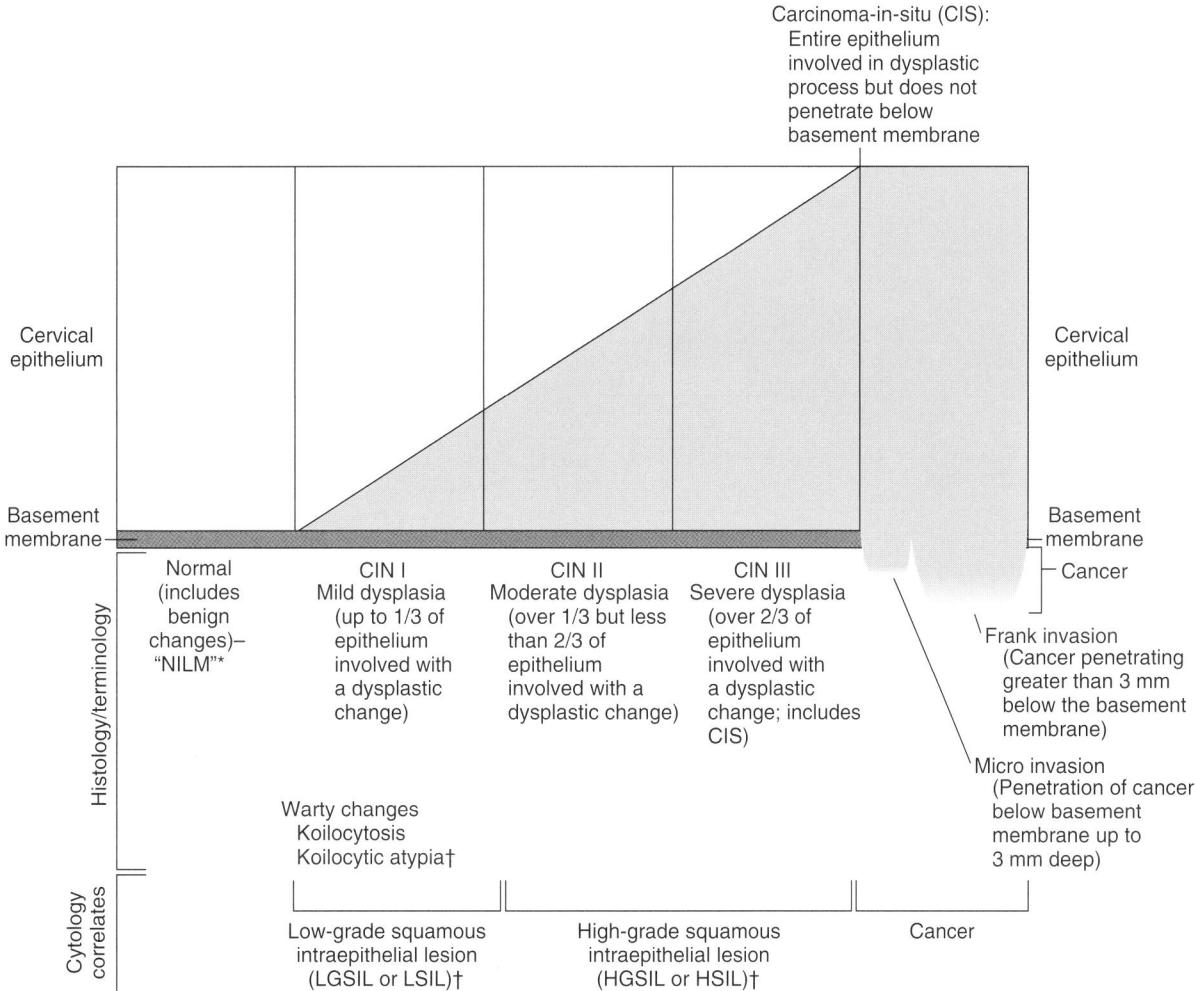

Fig. 152-1
Histologic and cytologic correlations of various terms used to describe preinvasive and invasive squamous cell disease of the cervix. Also see Box 152-1 for further description of the terms. The degree of epithelial involvement correlates with the severity of cytology as well as the total degree of involvement of the dysplastic tissue in relation to the thickness of the cervical squamous epithelium. On histology, involvement below the basement membrane supports a diagnosis of invasive cancer.

EQUIPMENT

- Examination table appropriate for placing the patient in the lithotomy position
- A warm, well-lit examination room
- Various-sized speculums: Graves' (metal), many suppliers, $14 to $20 each; Pederson (metal); plastic, disposable, 25 per box, about $1.60 each (Welch-Allyn, Inc; Durr-Fillauer Medical, Inc.

- Water-soluble lubricant (e.g., K-Y Jelly)
- Nonsterile examination gloves for the clinician
- Large swabs for gently blotting excess discharge
- Cotton swabs (numerous sources)
- Method for warming the speculum (warm water or speculum drawer warmer [light bulb])
- Wooden spatulas (Cervical Scraper No. 7, Hardwood Products Co.) or plastic spatula (Cervical Scraper [8½ inch], Milex Products) for ectocervical sample

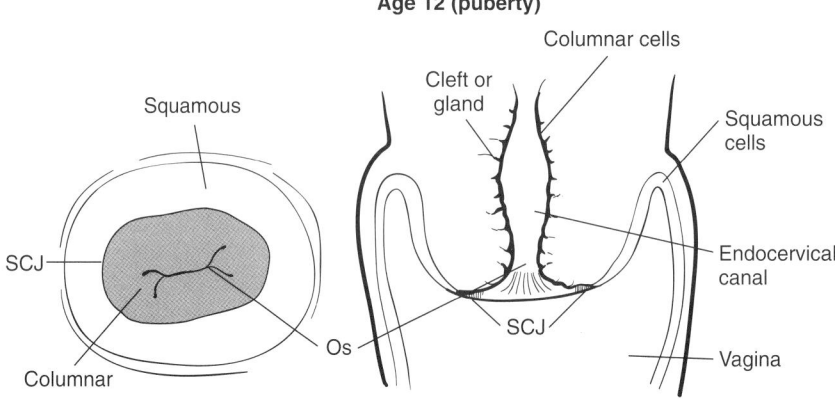

Age 12 (puberty)

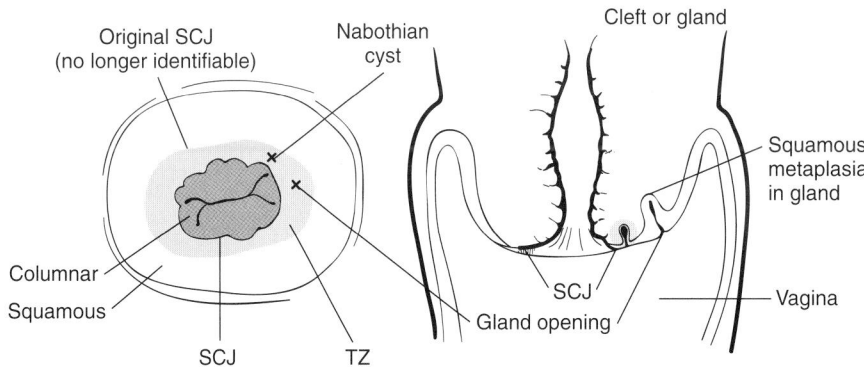

Age 21 (reproductive)

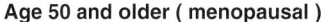

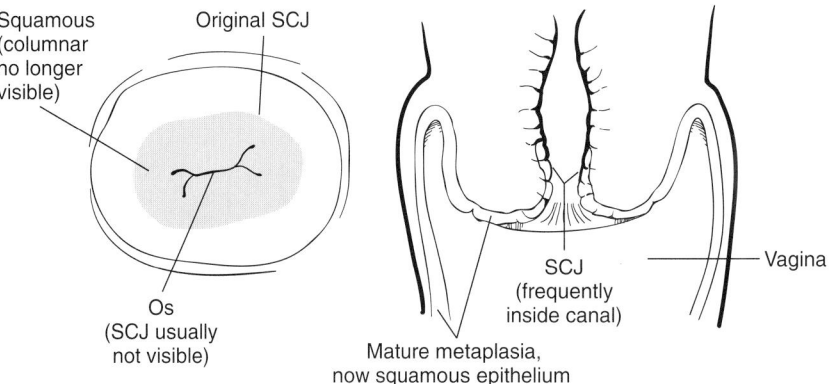

Age 50 and older (menopausal)

Fig. 152-2

Appearance of cervix in various age groups. The area most at risk in all age groups is the transformation zone *(TZ),* including the squamocolumnar junction *(SCJ).* Note how location varies with age. The SCJ and TZ are readily visible in younger women and may be quite large. The SCJ migrates inward with aging and by menopause, it is usually within the canal and is not visible. The entire TZ must be sampled to maximize efficacy of the Pap smear.

BOX 152-2

Risk Factors and Historical Characteristics Correlated with Abnormal Pap Smears

Tobacco smoking
Early age of first intercourse (under age 16)
Multiple sexual partners (more than three)
History of sexual abuse
Other sexually transmitted disease history
Illicit drug use (intravenous or oral)
History of genital or anal condyloma
History of abnormal Pap smear, cervical dysplasia, or cervical
    cancer
Sexual partner with condyloma or history of intercourse with a
    woman with cervical dysplasia or cancer
Sexual partner with more than three sexual partners
Immunocompromised patient, including HIV-positive status
History of vulvar dysplasia
Diethylstilbestrol (DES) exposure (should be extremely rare now)

- Cytobrush Plus for endocervical sample (Medscand)
- As an alternative to taking two samples, a "broom" device can be used for ectodermal and endocervical sample (Cervex-Brush, CooperSurgical, Inc; Papette, Wallach Surgical Devices)
- Microscope slides, fixative (common hairspray; consult with reference laboratory performing cytology for their preference)
- Appropriate patient identification, history forms to accompany Pap smear and other tests
- Culture or transport media and swabs as necessary for gonorrhea, chlamydia, herpes, fungal, and KOH/wet mount
- Cervical tenaculum or cervical hook *(rarely needed)*
- Ring forceps
- Lugol's solution (approximately $6/pint, local pharmacy) *(optional)*
- 5% acetic acid solution ($3/gal, white vinegar, local grocery store) *(optional)*
- Materials and solutions for liquid-based Pap smears (e.g., ThinPrep [CYTYC Corp., Boxborough, Mass.]), if desired or indicated.

SAMPLING DEVICES

Concern over the frequency and occurrence of false-negative Pap smears has led to the development of newer Pap smear sampling, preparation, and processing techniques. Despite the higher costs for these sampling devices (nominally $0.40 to $0.80 each), the increased quality of smears, the improved detection rates, and, ultimately, the fewer patients who must return for "inadequate" repeat smears more than justify this added expense. The routine use of the Cytobrush, Cervex-Brush, Papette, or similar devices is recommended (see

below for liquid-based technologies). A Pap smear consists of sampling the endocervical canal and the entire transformation zone (Figs. 152-2 to 152-4). At times, the broom device will not be wide enough to sample the entire area at risk (the TZ). Additional sampling of the area missed is then required.

The Pap smear test is considered exfoliative cytology; the transformation zone need not be dermabraded of its mucosa to obtain an adequate sample. There are enough cells from one Cytobrush and a wooden spatula sample to provide material for cytologic interpretation for five slides! Sharp, fine-edged plastic devices are advocated by some physicians; however, wood works fine for sampling of the ectocervix. A bloody Pap smear sample decreases detection rates. Fig. 152-5 illustrates several of the common sampling devices that achieve satisfactory sampling. Clinicians should not be locked into using a single method of transformation zone sampling; they should choose a technique based on patient anatomy. The days of the "one size fits everybody" Pap smear sampling device should be over.

The **ThinPrep method** (Fig. 152-4) is the latest introduction into Pap smear technology and relies on "liquid-based samples." The same principles apply regarding collection of cells. The collection device then, instead of being spread on a slide, is "swished" in a vial of liquid that is spun and processed to eliminate blood and other debris. In addition to being more sensitive and specific, another advantage of the ThinPrep technique is that the residual cytologic material left over after the Pap smear is completed can be used for HPV-DNA typing when Pap smears are equivocal (atypical). This is termed "reflex DNA typing." Those with high-risk viral types would be further evaluated with colposcopy, whereas those *without* evidence of high-risk HPV-DNA would be returned to the not-at-risk pool and annual Pap testing. Evidence supports that women with Pap smears indicating "atypical squamous cells" may benefit from this "reflex" HPV-DNA testing, wherein the residual ThinPrep material is automatically tested for HPV-DNA types. Alternatively, women would have to be called back for repeat Pap smear sampling immediately for DNA typing. If done, the testing only needs to be for the high-risk group of HPV, not for specific HPV types or for low-risk types. A Cytobrush can be used in the same way as the broom (Cervex-Brush) and may actually collect more cells than the broom! Although there are fewer false-positives and fewer false-negatives, the benefit of this methodology has still not proved cost effective, nor has it been shown to be superior in reducing morbidity and mortality. The ability for automatic DNA testing, however, would

BOX 152-3

American Cancer Society Guidelines for the Early Detection of Cervical Neoplasia and Cancer—2002

1. When to start screening
- Begin approximately 3 years after the onset of vaginal intercourse but no later than 21 years of age.
- Adolescents who may not need a Pap smear should still obtain appropriate preventive health care, including contraception and education, other screening, and treatment of sexually transmitted diseases.

2. When to discontinue screening
- Women who are age 70 and older with an intact cervix and who have had three or more documented consecutive technically satisfactory, normal/negative cervical cytology tests, and no abnormal/positive cytology tests within a 10-year period prior to age 70 may elect to cease cervical cancer screening.
- When comorbid or life-threatening illnesses are present, Pap smears are not needed.
- Screening should be continued for women over 70:
  - —If they have not been previously screened
  - —When previous Pap smear screening information is unavailable
  - —If there was in utero exposure to diethylstilbestrol (DES)
  - —For immunocompromised women (including HIV positive)
  - —For women over 70 but who have tested positive for HPV DNA

3. Screening after hysterectomy
- After a total hysterectomy with removal of the entire cervix for benign lesions, Pap smears using vaginal cytology are not indicated.
- The presence of CIN II/III is not considered a "benign lesion," so continued screening would be indicated.
- Women who have had a subtotal hysterectomy should continue cervical cancer screening.
- With history of CIN II/III, or it is not possible to document the absence of the same prior to the hysterectomy, three documented consecutive technically satisfactory normal/negative cervical cytology tests should be obtained before ceasing screening. In addition, there should have been no abnormal tests within the previous 10-year period.
- Women with DES exposure and/or history of cervical carcinoma should continue screening after hysterectomy as long as they are in reasonably good health and do not have a life-limiting chronic condition.

4. Screening interval
- Perform annually with conventional cervical cytology smears OR every 2 years using liquid-based cytology. At or after age 30, women who have had three consecutive technically satisfactory normal/negative cytology results may be screened every 2 to 3 years (unless they have a history of in utero DES exposure, are HIV positive, or are immune compromised).

5. New technologies
- The panel did not issue a statement on new technologies that are under development. These include aided visualization (i.e., speculoscopy), cervicography, computer-assisted screening devices, optical probe devices, self-collected vaginal samples for HPV DNA testing, and spectroscopy/electronic detection devices.
- Liquid-based Pap technology: as an alternative to conventional cervical cytology smears, conventional screening may be performed every 2 years using liquid-based cytology; at or after age 30, women who have had three consecutive, technically satisfactory normal/negative cytology results may be screened every 2 to 3 years (unless they have a history of in utero DES exposure, are HPV positive, or are immune compromised).
- HPV/DNA testing with cytology – **Primary** cervical cancer **screening** has **not** been approved by the FDA. Should the FDA approve HPV DNA testing for primary screening, it would be reasonable to consider it for women age 30 and over, as an alternative to cervical cytology testing alone. Cervical screening may be performed every 3 years using conventional or liquid-based cytology combined with a test for DNA for high-risk HPV types.

6. Additional recommendations
- Patients need to be educated (especially teens) that a pelvic examination does not equate with a cytology (Pap) test. They still need regular healthcare visits.
- No recommendation was made regarding pelvic and rectal examinations. They are not effective in detecting cervical cancer early enough, but there are other reasons to consider them. These should be discussed on an individual basis with the primary care physician.
- Referrals of women with low-grade lesions for colposcopy may be less necessary for adolescents given the self-limited nature of many low-grade squamous intraepithelial lesions (LSILs) in this age group. Detection and treatment of high-grade squamous intraepithelial lesions (HSILs) should be the goal of adolescent screening and referral.
- Health insurance payers should not exclude adolescents or women of any age from coverage for cervical health on the basis of false positive cytology results and/or mild abnormalities on cervical cytology.
- Health insurance coverage for new cervical screening technology is not uniform. Patients should be advised of this by their primary care provider.
- There is considerable clinical evidence with the use of the cytobrush in pregnant women with no apparent complications.
- Cervical broom instruments and other single sampling instruments are comparable to the spatula and brush.
- An endocervical swab is less sensitive than an endocervical brush and its use is discouraged. It may be considered for pregnant women.

Adapted from Saslow D, Runowicz CD, Solomon D, et al: American Cancer Society guidelines for the early detection of cervical neoplasia and cancer, *CA Cancer J Clin* 52(6):342, 2002.

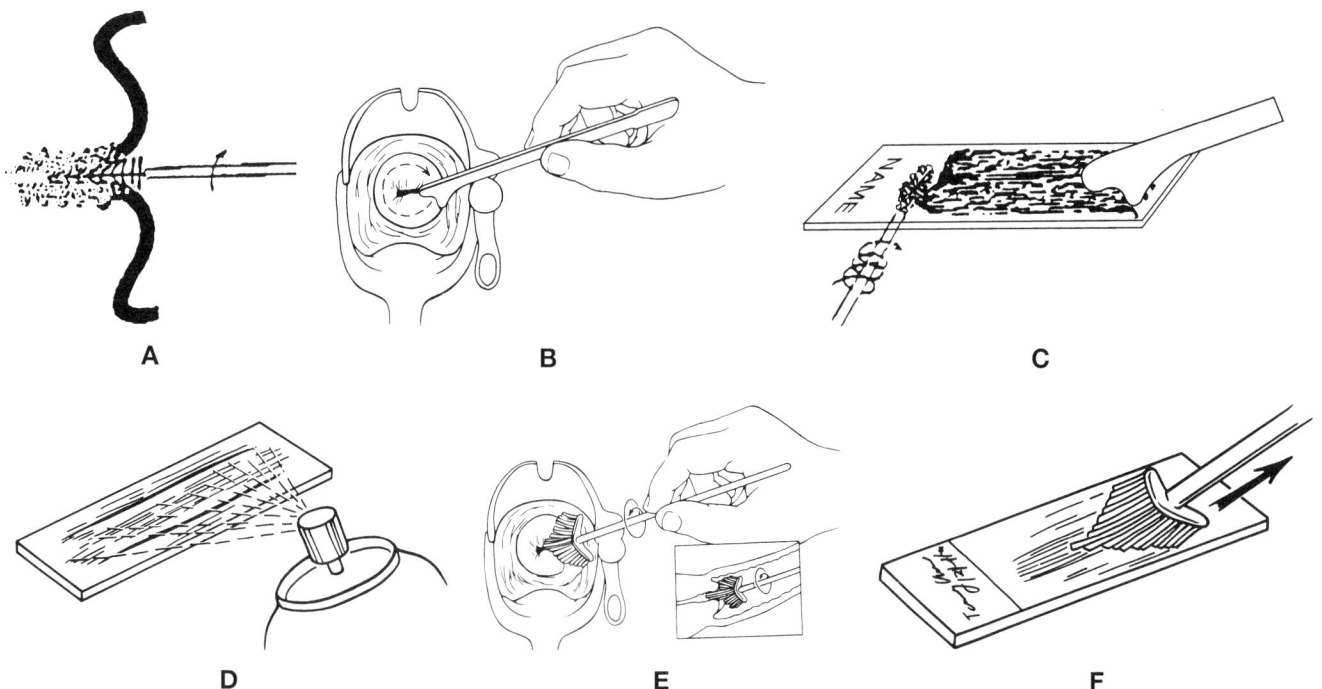

Fig. 152-3

Obtaining the Pap smear. **A,** Endocervical sample with Cytobrush; rotate 90 to 180 degrees. **B,** Ectocervical sample obtained with a wooden or plastic spatula. **C,** A single-slide technique is preferred. First, the spatula sample is spread, which is then followed by "unrolling" of the brush sample directly over the first sample. **D,** Immediate fixation of the slide with cytologic fixative. **E,** Alternatively, a single sampling device may be used (Papette, Cervex-Brush, or "broom") to obtain both ectocervical and endocervical samples at the same time. Rotate 360 degrees five times. **F,** Spreading the sample from broom device onto slide.

obviate the need for another pelvic examination and collection of cervical material. Women who are negative for HPV-DNA would not require colposcopy, whereas most others would. Some researchers feel, however, that it is premature to use automatic or "reflex" HPV-DNA screening strategies because the cost-benefit and ultimate morbidity and mortality data have yet to be produced. Many clinicians still believe that typing should currently be limited to research purposes. Until more investigation is completed and widespread consensus is reached, few would argue that a more immediate way of reducing mortality from cervical cancer is by screening more women who currently are not obtaining their Pap smears.

Editor's note: In addition to the reflex DNA testing potential and better specificity and sensitivity, a third argument is being made for liquid-based technologies. Several methods are pending FDA approval for computer-based reading of screening Pap smears. (Currently the only approval for computer systems is for overreading previously read Pap smears or for selecting cells for technicians to view.) Computers can only deal with liquid-based preparations. The time for the traditional Pap smear as we have known it may be limited.

PREPROCEDURE PATIENT PREPARATION

The patient should understand the reason for performing the Pap smear. The Pap smear is best performed during midcycle. The patient should avoid douching, vaginal medications, and intercourse for 24 hours prior to the procedure. Reschedule the examination if the patient is actively menstruating. The patient should void before unclothing for the examination. Inform the patient of the mechanisms you use to follow up on test results (Pap smear, cultures, etc.). (See the sample patient education handout titled "Pap Smear Information" on page 1943 of Appendix G.)

TECHNIQUE

1. Obtain history (especially sexual aspects of age at first intercourse, number of sexual partners, and history of sexual abuse or rape), review of systems, and answer questions. Clarify the patient's risk factors for cervical dysplasia. Review past Pap results if available.

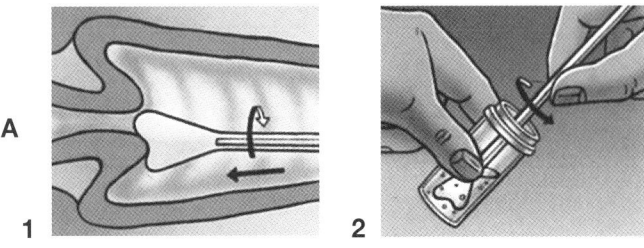

A 1   2

1, **Obtain** an adequate sampling from the ectocervix using a *plastic* spatula.
2, **Rinse** the spatula as quickly as possible into the PreservCyt Solution vial by swirling the spatula vigorously in the vial 10 times. Discard the spatula.

AND

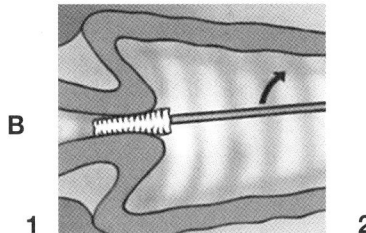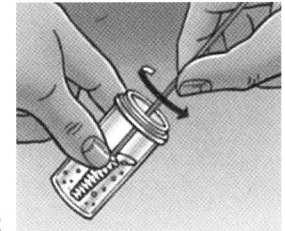

B 1   2

1, **Obtain** an adequate sampling from the endocervix using an endocervical brush device. Insert the brush into the cervix until only the bottom-most fibers are exposed. Slowly rotate ¼ or ½ turn in one direction. DO NOT OVER-ROTATE.
2, **Rinse** the brush as quickly as possible into the PreservCyt Solution by rotating the device in the solution 10 times while pushing against the PreservCyt vial wall. Swirl the brush vigorously to further release material. Discard the brush.

OR

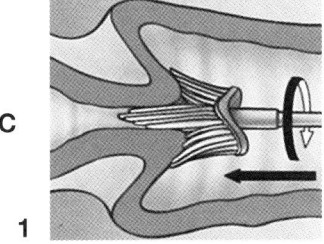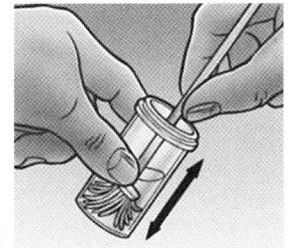

C 1   2

1, **Obtain** an adequate sampling from the cervix using a broom-like device. Insert the central bristles of the broom into the endocervical canal deep enough to allow the shorter bristles to fully contact the ectocervix. Push gently, and rotate the broom in a clockwise direction five times.
2, **Rinse** the broom as quickly as possible into the PreservCyt Solution vial by pushing the broom into the bottom of the vial 10 times, forcing the bristles apart. As a final step, swirl the broom vigorously to further release material. Discard the collection device. Be sure entire transformation zone has been sampled.

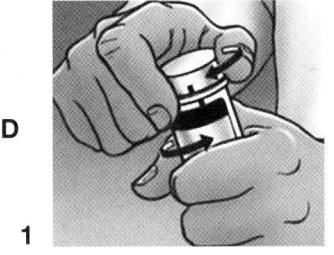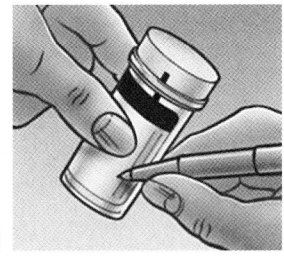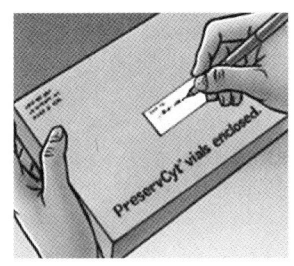

D 1   2   3

1, **Tighten** the cap so that the torque line on the cap passes the torque line on the vial.
2, **Record** the patient's name and ID number on the vial, and record the patient information and medical history on the cytology requisition form.
3, **Place** the vial and requisition in a specimen bag for transport to the laboratory.

Fig. 152-4
Liquid-based (ThinPrep) methods using, **A,** plastic spatula, **B,** endocervical brush, or, **C,** broom-like device. **D** shows final three steps for each method. (Courtesy CYTYC Corp., Boxborough, Mass.)

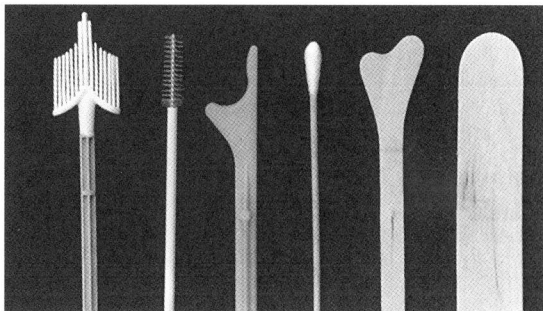

Fig. 152-5
Papanicolaou sampling devices. *Left to right:* Cervex-Brush, Cytobrush, Miltex plastic sampler, cotton swab, wooden Ayre spatula, and tongue blade. The swab and tongue blade are discouraged.

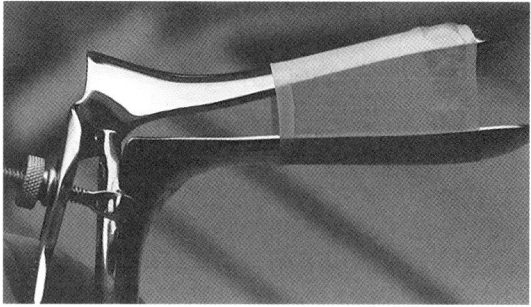

Fig. 152-6
Vaginal speculum stent. To aid in the visualization of the cervix, a single finger of a latex examination glove can be cut off and placed over the blades of a standard vaginal speculum. This is helpful if there is redundant vaginal mucosa, as seen with pregnancy, obesity, or multiparity.

2. Proceed with the general medical and breast examination, leaving the pelvic examination for last.

3. Label the frosted end of the glass slide or the vial with the patient's name and other identifying data as necessary.

4. Place the patient in the lithotomy position, and begin the examination. Wear nonsterile gloves. Inspect the vulva, and assess hair pattern, anatomy, estrogen effect, discharge, and any abnormal areas. Ask the patient if she has any concerns.

5. Place a small amount of water-soluble lubricant on the warmed speculum and insert it. Carefully advance the speculum, applying gentle pressure posteriorly. In patients whose vaginal walls prolapse and obstruct view, consider using a vaginal stent. This can be fashioned by cutting off both ends of a single finger of a latex rubber glove and placing it over the blades of the speculum (Fig. 152-6). For those who are very obese or have excessively deep vaginas, a special, long "Snowman" speculum is available from CooperSurgical, Inc.

6. Adjust the speculum to obtain adequate visualization of the cervix, and tighten the screw or lock the speculum open.

7. Determine whether the vagina or cervix appears inflamed or infected. Avoid rubbing or otherwise traumatizing the cervix.

8. Identify cervical landmarks, including the transformation zone with its squamocolumnar junction. Note the nature of the cervical mucus. Markedly excessive mucus or discharge may be gently blotted, not rubbed, from view. However, mucus may actually contain the exfoliated cells needed for the microscopic exam. So, unless truly necessary, do not remove this mucus; include it in the sample. Note any gross cervical lesions, such as erosions (ulcerations), leukoplakia (white areas), nabothian cysts, or condylomata. Examine the vaginal fornices for obvious abnormalities.

9. Obtain the Pap smear by using an endocervical sampling device (Cytobrush, Papette, or Cervex-Brush). Q-tips are not to be used. If the Cytobrush is used, first insert the Cytobrush into the canal and rotate 90 to 180 degrees. Do not rotate more than this, since it may cause bleeding, which can wash away or obscure abnormal cells. Follow this by a gentle sampling of the entire transformation zone with a spatula device, rotating it 360 degrees. If broom devices (Papette, Cervex-Brush) are used, insert and rotate 360 degrees five times. The broom will obtain both endocervical and ectocervical samples at the same time but must be rotated multiple times to collect an adequate number of cells.

Sampling the vaginal pool has little advantage during Pap smear screening unless the patient has had a hysterectomy. In this instance, be sure to sample the vaginal cuff itself. If vaginal abnormalities are seen, another Pap smear of these areas (using a spatula) may be submitted on a separate slide. Areas that appear abnormal on visualization will ultimately require colposcopy and biopsy.

10. If a one-slide smear technique is suggested by your reference lab (check with your pathologist), withhold smearing the endocervical Cytobrush sample on the slide until the spatula sample is smeared first. Follow this quickly by rolling out the Cytobrush sample (which is less subject to drying artifact) over the spatula smear and spray immediately with cytofixative. If a two-slide technique is used, each preparation is evenly applied to its appropriate slide immediately after sampling, and then the slide is sprayed or dipped in preservative within 5 seconds. The broom devices will provide only a single slide.

11. If a thin-layer technology Pap smear method is utilized, follow the instructions of the manufacturer, which usually require swishing the Pap sample

directly into a vial of transport liquid rather than smearing the sample on glass slides (CYTYC Corp.).

12. Perform the appropriate cervical cultures after cytologic sampling, if indicated. (The CDC recommends that all sexually active females under 30 be routinely screened for chlamydia and rechecked after treatment is completed.)

13. Some experienced colposcopists have recognized the benefit of routinely using acetic acid staining of the cervix following the Pap smear, especially in women who have significant risk factors for cervical dysplasia. Three to five percent acetic acid (white vinegar) applied to the cervix turns abnormalities white. Any observed cervical abnormality that cannot be readily explained by normal anatomic variants (e.g., nabothian cysts), either before or after acetic acid application, warrants colposcopic evaluation, even if the Pap smear report is normal. Some have labeled this the "naked-eye inspection of the cervix." Although significant cervical dysplasia can be detected by this technique, there is also significant risk of obligating women to unnecessary colposcopy for insignificant acetic acid changes on the cervix as seen with the naked eye.

14. Examine the vagina by slowly withdrawing the speculum, which is held slightly open, allowing the vagina to collapse over the blades. Note abnormalities.

15. Lubricate the gloved hand as necessary and proceed with the bimanual examination. Pay particular attention to palpated abnormalities of the introitus, vagina, fornices, and cervix. Palpate the areas of Skene's and Bartholin's glands. Ask your patient to bear down, and observe for uterine or pelvic floor prolapse and for leaking of urine. Having her cough facilitates assessment of pelvic support.

16. Complete the remainder of the bimanual examination, noting the size, contour, tenderness, and mobility of the uterus and adnexal structures.

17. Perform a rectal examination on women with rectal complaints who are under age 40. Perform it routinely after this age. Be sure to put on a new glove before the rectal examination to prevent the spread of HPV or other infectious agents to the anus.

18. Allow the patient to dress.

19. Make sure the Pap smear requisition form includes all pertinent data regarding your patient. Include clinical findings, patient risk factors, or your concerns as part of this "referral" (Bethesda recommendation).

COMPLICATIONS

The Pap smear is only a screening test. False-negative rates are high (20% to 50%, with an average of 25%), and significant disease can be missed or underestimated. More frequent Pap smear screening or colposcopy may be indicated, depending on patient history and risks for having or developing genital malignancy.

"GOLDEN RULES"

- Identify cervical landmarks and gross abnormalities, and sample both the endocervical canal and the entire transformation zone. Choose a transformation zone sampler that fits your patient.
- All Pap smears reported as abnormal require some form of intervention. A report of dysplasia warrants colposcopy. Many clinicians also recommend colposcopy for reports of ASC, especially in patients with numerous risk factors. At the least, repeat Pap smear is indicated in most cases, or DNA typing to determine which ASC Pap has high-risk HPV. Atypical glandular cells (AGCs) definitely need further evaluation. (See Chapter 139, Colposcopic Examination.)
- Clarify your patient's risk factors for having HPV infection and cervical dysplasia as part of the routine examination. Anyone with substantial risks requires at least annual Pap smears.
- An observed abnormality on the cervix that cannot be readily explained by normal variants (e.g., nabothian cysts) warrants colposcopic examination. A normal Pap smear report in the face of an observed abnormal cervix should not dissuade the clinician from performing colposcopy and biopsy.
- The presence of cervicovaginitis alters the *timing* for colposcopic examination, not the indication.
- Know your cytopathologist. Interpretive problems should be discussed directly with the pathologist, who can address your questions, including the option to review the cytology at issue.
- The optimal way to reduce morbidity and mortality from cervical cancer may not be new technology but rather, convincing women who have not been screened for large intervals, or at all, to have a Pap smear.

INTERPRETATION

Adequacy

The Pap smear report should indicate whether the smear was adequate. Unless the patient has had a hysterectomy, this should include cytologic evidence that the transformation zone was sampled. Ordinarily, the reporting of endocervical cells along with squamous cells implies adequate sampling. Many cytologists attribute to "squamous metaplasia" the same significance as the reporting of "endocervical cells present."

Either is considered objective evidence that the transformation zone was sampled, which implies an adequate sample. Many reports will in some way use or check the word "adequate." Bethesda-2001 further delineates adequacy (Box 152-4).

Interpretation System

Table 152-1 summarizes and compares the various Pap smear reporting systems, whereas Box 152-4 defines the latest Bethesda-2001 terminology. The "Bethesda system" named after the national consensus conference for Pap smear interpretation has provided a uniform nomenclature for Pap smear cytology interpretation and attempts to address much of the confusion regarding Pap smear terminology. In September 2001, the Bethesda consensus conference convened for the third time and provided revisions of the reporting system, with general recommendations as follows:

- The Pap smear report should use terminology that is understood by the clinician.
- The clinician should be able to discuss the Pap report with the cytopathologist if questions arise.
- All abnormal Pap smears require some form of intervention in addition to the routine yearly screening interval.
- See additional notes below regarding findings in postmenopausal women.

Follow-up Recommendations

A consensus group hosted by the American Society of Colposcopy and Cervical Pathology (ASCCP) recently convened and published guidelines for the management of abnormal cervical cytology. These recommendations used the 2001 Bethesda interpretation system and are applicable to clinical circumstances. (Also see Chapter 139, Colposcopic Examination.)

The following is a summary of recommendations for follow-up.

Pap Report
- Atypical Squamous Cells (ASC).
  a. ASC-US (atypical squamous cells of undetermined significance):
  Three follow-up approaches are possible:
  (1) Do DNA typing. If high-risk HPV present, colposcopy is indicated. If not, perform routine annual Pap smears.
  (2) Immediately refer to colposcopy, especially if risk factors are present.
  (3) Repeat the Pap smear and perform colposcopy only on those with repeated abnormal Pap smear results.
  b. ASC-H (atypical squamous cells cannot rule out high-grade dysplasia): All require colposcopy.

These patients all need colposcopy:
- Evidence of SIL of any degree (low- and high-grade SIL): All require colposcopy. This category includes any indications that HPV is present. Note that all LGSIL/mild dysplasias require colposcopy, not a repeat Pap smear or DNA typing.
- Evidence of malignant cells: colposcopy.
- Evidence of glandular atypia/atypical glandular cells (AGS): colposcopy with ECC.

Note: A report describing *glandular* or adenomatous atypia (to be differentiated from squamous atypia) warrants immediate colposcopy with endocervical curettage to rule out a high-grade lesion and cervical adenocarcinoma. Furthermore, *endometrial* carcinoma may be suggested by abnormal cytology detected by a Pap smear. In such instances, formal endometrial sampling is mandated in patients over 40 years of age. In postmenopausal women not on estrogen replacement, estrogen effect or endometrial cells on the Pap smear is not normal. Evaluate the ovaries and uterus. If the findings of AGS are definite, conization, pelvic ultrasound, and even laparoscopy may be indicated.

Pelvic Examination Findings Requiring Colposcopy
- Abnormal-appearing cervix
- Abnormal-feeling cervix or vagina
- Genital condylomata at any site

Other Indications for Colposcopy
- Positive high-risk HPV-DNA screen (DNA screens should not be routine)
- DES offspring
- Partner with genital condylomata
- History of sexual abuse or rape
- Other sexually transmissible disease (relative)

SUPPLIERS

CooperSurgical, Inc.
95 Corporate Drive
Trumbull, CT 06611
Phone: 1-800-645-3760
Website: www.coopersurgical.com

CYTYC Corp.
85 Swanson Road
Boxborough, MA 01719
Phone: 1-800-442-9892
Website: www.cytyc.com

Hardwood Products Co.
P.O. Box 149
Guilford, ME 04443
Phone: 1-800-321-2313
Website: www.hwppuritan.com

BOX 152-4

2001 Bethesda Pap Smear Reporting Terminology (abridged)

Specimen Adequacy

Satisfactory for evaluation *(note presence/absence of endocervical/ transformation zone component)*

Unsatisfactory for evaluation . . . *(specify reason)*

Specimen rejected/not processed *(specify reason)*

Specimen processed and examined, but unsatisfactory for evaluation of epithelial abnormality because of *(specify reason)*

General Categorization *(optional)*

Negative for intraepithelial lesion or malignancy (NILM)

Epithelial cell abnormality

Other

Interpretation/Result

Negative for intraepithelial lesion or malignancy

Organisms

Trichomonas vaginalis

Fungal organisms morphologically consistent with *Candida* species

Shift in flora suggestive of bacterial vaginosis

Bacteria morphologically consistent with *Actinomyces* species

Cellular changes consistent with herpes simplex virus

Other non-neoplastic findings *(optional to report; list not comprehensive)*

Reactive cellular changes associated with the following:

Inflammation (includes typical repair)

Radiation

Intrauterine contraceptive device

Glandular cells status posthysterectomy

Atrophy

Epithelial cell abnormalities

Squamous cell

Atypical squamous cells (ASC)

Of undetermined significance (ASC-US)

Cannot exclude HSIL (ASC-H)

Low-grade squamous intraepithelial lesion (LSIL)

Encompassing: human papillomavirus/mild dysplasia/ cervical intraepithelial neoplasia (CIN) I

High-grade squamous intraepithelial lesion (HSIL)

Encompassing: moderate and severe dysplasia, carcinoma in situ; CIN II and CIN III

Squamous cell carcinoma

Glandular cell

Atypical glandular cells (AGC) *(specify endocervical, endometrial, or not otherwise specified)*

Atypical glandular cells, favor neoplastic (specify endocervical or not otherwise specified)

Endocervical adenocarcinoma in situ (AIS)

Adenocarcinoma

Other (list not comprehensive)

Endometrial cells in a woman ≥40 years of age

Automated Review and Ancillary Testing *(include as appropriate)*

Educational Notes and Suggestions *(optional)*

From Wright TC Jr, Cox JT, Massad LS, et al: *JAMA* 287(16):2120, 2002.

TABLE 152-1

Classification and Approximate Comparative Nomenclature of Cervical Smears

Papanicolaou (Numerical)	National Cancer Institute Class	CIN System* (Cytodescriptive)	Bethesda-2001
Class I Normal smear; no abnormal cells	Negative	Normal	Negative for intraepithelial lesion or malignancy (NILM)
Class II Atypical cells; no neoplasia	Atypical	Reparative or atypical	Atypical squamous cells (ASC) of undetermined significance (ASC-US) or cannot exclude HSIL (ASC-H)
Class III Smear contains abnormal cells consistent with dysplasia	Suspicious	CIN I (mild dysplasia), CIN II (moderate dysplasia), CIN III (severe dysplasia) }	Low-grade SIL (HPV changes and CIN I) High-grade SIL
Class IV Smear contains abnormal cells consistent with carcinoma in situ	Positive	CIN III	High-grade SIL (CIN II, CIN III, CIS)
Class V Smear contains abnormal cells consistent with carcinoma of squamous origin*	Positive	Carcinoma*	Invasive carcinoma*

CIN, Cervical intraepithelial neoplasia; *CIS,* carcinoma in situ; *HSIL,* high-grade squamous intraepithelial lesion; *SIL,* squamous intraepithelial lesions.
*Further subcategorization of carcinoma is confirmed by histologic features demonstrated by biopsy. Microinvasion = <3 mm penetration; frankly invasive >3 mm (some argue 5 mm as depth of differentiation).

Milex Products
4311 N. Normandy
Chicago, IL 60634
Phone: 1-800-621-1278
Website: www.milexproducts.com

Wallach Surgical Devices, Inc.
235 Edison Road
Orange, CT 06477
Phone: 1-800-243-2463
Website: www.wallachsurgical.com

CPT/BILLING CODES

99201-99215	Pap smear*; use office visit codes
88150	Pap smear interpretation†
57500	Biopsy of cervix‡
57505	Endocervical curettage‡

ICD-9-CM DIAGNOSTIC CODES

622.0	Cervical ulcer
622.1	Cervical atypia
622.1	Cervical dysplasia
622.1	Cervical leukoplakia
622.7	Cervical polyp
622.8	Cervical atrophy
623.8	Abnormal vaginal bleeding
626.8	Uterine bleeding
233.1	Cervical carcinoma in situ
795.0	Abnormal Pap (some insurances will not reimburse for this code)
219.0	Neoplasm of the cervix, benign
180.9	Malignant condyloma or SIL

ADDITIONAL RESOURCES

- See the sample patient education handout titled "Pap Smear Information" on page 1943 of Appendix G.

---

*Many clinicians include the professional fee for performing the Pap smear as part of the female annual examination by upgrading to an "extended visit."

†A code used by the cytopathologist for billing. Very few clinicians (i.e., nonpathologists) interpret their patients' cytology.

‡The majority of cervical biopsies and the endocervical curettage (ECC) will be performed as part of the formal colposcopic examination. Please refer to the chapter on colposcopy for appropriate billing information.

BIBLIOGRAPHY

American American Academy of Family Physicians: *Clinical recommendations 2001: introduction to AAFP summary of policy recommendations for periodic health examination,* January 2001, order no. 962, reprint 510, p 4.

Cox JT: Evaluating the role of HPV testing for women with equivocal Papanicolaou test findings, *JAMA* 281(17):1645, 1999.

Follen M, Richards-Kortum R: Emerging technologies and cervical cancer, *J Natl Cancer Inst* 92(5):363, 2000.

Jones W: Impact of the Bethesda system, *Cancer* 76:1914, 1995.

Kaufman RH, Adam E: Is human papillomavirus testing of value in clinical practice? *Am J Obstet Gynecol* 180:1049, 1999.

Khauna N, Phillips MD: Adherence to care plan in women with abnormal Papanicolaou smears: a review of barriers and interventions, *J Am Board Fam Pract* 14:123, 2001.

Kim JJ, Wright TC, Goldie SJ: Cost-effectiveness of alternative triage strategies for atypical squamous cells of undetermined significance, *JAMA* 287(18):2382, 2002.

Koss LG: The Papanicolaou test for cervical cancer detection: a triumph and a tragedy, *JAMA* 261:737, 1989.

Lee KR, Asjfaq R, Bordsmg GG, Corkill ME, et al: Comparison of conventional Papanicolaou smears and a fluid-based, thin-layer system for cervical cancer screening, *Obstet Gynecol* 90(2):278, 1997.

Lonky NM, Sadeghi M, Tsadik GW, Petitti D: The clinical significance of the poor correlation of cervical dysplasia and cervical malignancy with referral cytologic results, *Am J Obstet Gynecol* 181(3):560, 1999.

Lundber GD: The 1988 Bethesda system for reporting cervical/vaginal cytological diagnoses, *JAMA* 262(7):931, 1989.

Mandelblatt JS, Lawrence WF, Womack SM, et al: Benefits and costs of using HPV testing to screen for cervical cancer, *JAMA* 287(18):2372, 2002.

Noller K: AGUS reports scare me, *ObGyn Clin Alert* June 1998, p. 15.

Reed BD, Ruffin MT, Gorenflo DW, Zazove P: The psychosocial impact of HPV cervical infection, *J Fam Pract* 48:110, 1999.

Saslow D, Runowicz CD, Solomon D, et al: American Cancer Society guidelines for the early detection of cervical neoplasia and cancer, *CA Cancer J Clin* 52(6):342, 2002.

Smith RA, VonEssenland AC, Wender R, Levin B, et al: American Cancer Society guidelines for the early detection of cancer: update of early detection guidelines for prostate, colorectal and endometrial cancer, *CA Cancer J Clin* 51:38, 2001.

Solomon D, Davey D, Kurman R, et al: The 2001 Bethesda System: terminology for reporting results of cervical cytology, *JAMA* 287(16):2114, 2002.

Solomon D, Schiffman M, Tarone R: Comparison of three management strategies for patients with atypical squamous cells of undetermined significance: baseline results from a randomized trial, *J Natl Cancer Inst* 93(4):293, 2001.

Stoler MH: New Bethesda terminology and evidence-based management guidelines for cervical cytology findings, *JAMA* 287(16):2140, 2002.

Stoler MH, Schiffman M: Interobserver reproducibility of cervical cytologic and histologic interpretation: realistic estimates from the ASCUS-LGSIL Triage Study, *JAMA* 285:1500, 2001.

Wright TC Jr, Cox JT, Massad LS, et al: 2001 Consensus Guidelines for the management of women with cervical cytological abnormalities, *JAMA* 287(16):2120, 2002.

Zweizig S, Noller K, Reale F: Neoplasia associated with atypical glandular cells of undetermined significance on cervical cytology, *Gynecol Oncol* 65:314, 1997.

WEBSITES

jama.ama-assn.org (Journal of the American Medical Association: Bethesda 2001 Guidelines)

www.asccp.org (American Society for Colposcopy and Cervical Pathology: Consensus guidelines for abnormal cytology)

CHAPTER 153

Permanent Female Sterilization (Tubal Ligation)

Gary R. Newkirk

In the United States, voluntary sterilization remains one of the most widely used contraceptive methods, chosen by nearly 20% of married women. Family physicians who are skilled with basic surgical technique are in an ideal position to discuss and perform permanent sterilization procedures for both men and women. Approximately 500,000 tubal ligations are performed each year in the United States. A similar number of vasectomies are carried out. No man has ever died from the vasectomy procedure itself. Between 10 and 14 women die each year (in the United States) from tubal ligation and have a potential for more serious complication. The failure rate for vasectomy is 1 in 1200, whereas tubal ligation failures occur in 1 in 250 procedures. Although vasectomy allows detection of failures, no simple technique allows the surgeon to find tubal ligation failures. Cost is also a consideration with a tubal ligation, requiring hospitalization and raising the total charges to five to six times that of an office vasectomy. When a patient asks about permanent contraception, it behooves the primary care physician to point out the benefits of vasectomy over a tubal ligation. Even the American College of Obstetricians and Gynecologists (ACOG) agrees that all things considered, a vasectomy is the procedure of choice.

Nevertheless, when vasectomy is not appropriate for whatever reason, tubal ligation remains an excellent choice for permanent surgical contraception.

Despite numerous variations, female sterilization consists of two basic steps: (1) exposing the fallopian tubes, and (2) partially resecting or occluding the tubes to prevent conception. This chapter discusses the minilaparotomy approach to permanent female sterilization, both as an interval and as a postpartum procedure.

Box 153-1 outlines basic terminology related to permanent female sterilization methodology. Minilaparotomy and laparoscopy are abdominal surgical approaches that are considered safe, quick, and readily available. Basic anatomy is outlined in Fig. 153-1.

Table 153-1 shows advantages and disadvantages of the minilaparotomy and the laparoscopic techniques. Despite the recognized advantages of laparoscopy for certain situations, minilaparotomy—because of its reliance on readily available surgical equipment, fewer technical demands, and applicability to both interval and postpartum periods—is the method of choice for many primary care physicians. Box 153-2 summarizes the more common methods for ligating the tubes.

This chapter outlines the minilaparotomy approach and the modified Pomeroy or "Parkland" method (Figs. 153-2 and 153-3) for ligation. The ideal method is still under debate; however, the modified Pomeroy or Parkland methods (with their variations) remain popular in this country. Prudent physicians should identify patients who may benefit by referral either for alternative methods that they cannot offer because of their lack of skill, training, equipment, or facility; or because of the patient's clinical condition.

INTERVAL TUBAL LIGATION

INDICATIONS

- Desire for permanent sterilization
- Medical conditions that place the patient at significant risk for irreversible morbidity or death if she should become pregnant
- Known severe inheritable genetic disease where childbearing is not desired

Absolute Contraindications

- Active peritoneal infections
- Severe chronic heart, lung, or metabolic disease (abdominal insufflation [laparoscopy] and the head-down [Trendelenburg's] position can cause acute cardiopulmonary decompensation)
- Any unstable medical condition
- Lack of informed consent
- Inability to tolerate anesthesia
- Patient unsure of desire for permanent sterilization

BOX 153-1

Female Sterilization Terminology

Laparotomy

A relatively large abdominal incision performed to optimize surgical exposure for a variety of intraabdominal surgeries.

Minilaparotomy

Sometimes referred to as minilap; involves a small abdominal incision usually less than 5 cm (2 inches).

Laparoscopy

Involves inserting an illuminated telescope-like instrument into the abdomen that allows visualization of the fallopian tubes in order to accomplish electrocoagulation or application of clips or rings. For *open* laparoscopy, a small incision is made within or just below the umbilicus to allow passage of a special cannula, around which the skin makes an airtight seal. The cannula allows for insufflation of the abdomen, passage of the laparoscope and instruments, and occlusion of the tubes. Open laparoscopy is considered safer than traditional *closed* laparoscopy, especially in women with prior pelvic or abdominal surgery or infection. With the *closed* laparoscopic procedure, the laparoscope is inserted blindly through the abdominal wall.

Postpartum Tubal Ligation

Tubal ligation performed within 72 hours of delivery.

Interval Tubal Ligation

Tubal ligation performed at times other than during the immediate postpartum period—generally 6 weeks after delivery or more.

Technical Failure

Inability to complete the planned sterilization during the operation, which results in a change of method or failure to perform the sterilization.

Colpotomy

A vaginal approach to tubal ligation through the posterior vaginal fornix.

Relative Contraindications

- Prior significant pelvic or abdominal infection; minilaparotomy or laparoscopy may be more difficult (laparotomy may be necessary.)
- Severe obesity, especially with a history of pelvic or abdominal infection
- Chronic heart disease, irregular pulse, uncontrolled hypertension, pelvic masses, uncontrolled diabetes, bleeding disorders, severe nutritional deficiencies, severe anemia, and umbilical or hiatal hernia (The risks of future pregnancies must be weighed against the risks of permanent sterilization procedures.)

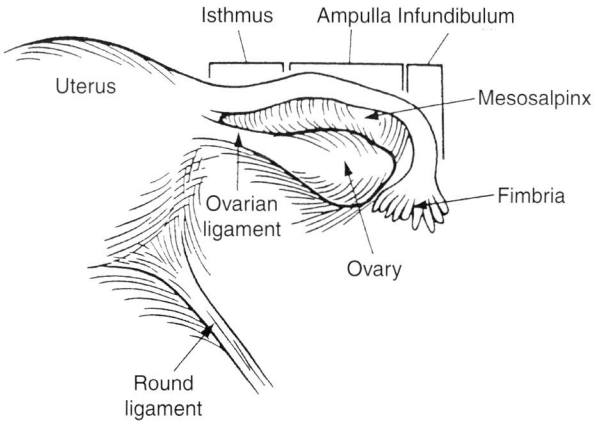

Fig. 153-1
Basic anatomy of the parauterine structures.

TABLE 153-1

Advantages and Disadvantages of Minilaparotomy and Laparoscopy

	Advantages	Disadvantages
Minilaparotomy	Easy to learn Basic surgical training and skill Inexpensive instruments Complications are usually minor Can be performed as a postpartum or interval	Takes longer than laparoscopy Difficult to perform on patients who are obese or who have pelvic scarring or adhesions Scar slightly larger More pain from the abdominal incision Higher infection rate than laparoscopy procedure
Laparoscopy	Very low complication rate Quick procedure (10-15 min) Very small incision Useful for other diagnostic and therapeutic purposes Less painful	Complications may be serious Requires abdominal insufflation, with its added risk More difficult to learn; requires specialized training for physician and staff Equipment is more expensive and requires more maintenance and repair Not recommended as a postpartum procedure

EQUIPMENT

- A laparotomy pack contains most of the instruments necessary for basic abdominal surgery and is available in most hospital outpatient or inpatient surgical suites.
- Suction catheter (Generally, suction is not used during a routine minilaparotomy tubal ligation. Suction is available on demand at most surgical suites; it is mandatory if complications such as bleeding develop.)
- Coagulation device (Most operative suites have a Bovie or similar coagulation device available. Some surgeons prefer to have this available for all cases; others use this electively, or when complications develop. Since a Bovie requires grounding, it should be set up in advance. A ground plate can be attached before the patient is draped and scrubbed.)

- Sutures, according to the following:

Anatomical site	Suture
Tubal ligation	0 Plain or chromic
Peritoneum	2-0 Chromic
Fascia	0 Dexon
Scarpa's fascia	2-0 Chromic
Skin	Metal clips, 4-0 Dexon

- 8-inch Babcock forceps to separate and retract fallopian tube (Fig. 153-4, *A*)
- Ring sponge (ring forceps holding a tightly folded gauze pad)
- Small Richardson or Army-Navy retractors for holding the incision open (Fig. 153-4, *B*)
- Adson tissue forceps with teeth for skin manipulation (Fig. 153-4, *C*)
- Metzenbaum scissors for general tissue blunt dissection and incision (Fig. 153-4, *D*)
- Kelly clamps for blunt dissection, and for grasping and

BOX 153-2

Common Tubal Ligation Methods

Minilaparotomy ("Open" Procedure)
Pomeroy technique
The most common procedure performed for both interval and post-partum tubal ligations. Absorbable catgut sutures are used to tie the base of a loop of midportion (ampullary) tube. The ligated loop of tube is then removed. As the suture absorbs, the ends pull apart and are obstructed by the healing and scarring process. From 3 to 6 cm of the tube is destroyed (Fig. 153-2).

Parkland technique
A small length of tube is separated from the mesosalpinx and ligated at each end about 2 cm apart; the free segment between the ligatures is removed (Fig. 153-3).

Irving technique
An extremely effective yet more difficult method that cannot be reversed easily. The tube is cut and the uterine end buried beneath the peritoneum within the wall of the uterus. The remaining end is buried within the mesosalpinx.

Uchida technique
A technically demanding yet extremely effective method that is becoming more popular in the United States. The tube is severed and the uterine end is buried within the mesosalpinx.

Fimbriectomy
Accomplished by complete removal of the fimbriated end of the tube. The procedure appears to have a higher pregnancy failure rate, and reversal is unlikely.

Laparoscopy Clips
Under laparoscopic guidance, clips are applied to occlude the tubal lumen. Hulka (spring-loaded) and Filshie clips (titanium and silicone rubber) are commonly used. Clips destroy less than 1 cm of tissue, and reversals are considered much easier.

Electrocoagulation
A bipolar probe is passed through a small segment of tube to cauterize and obstruct the lumen.

Tubal ring
A small Silastic ring is stretched and placed over a loop of fallopian tube and then released. The tube is blocked by compression. Usually a 2- to 3-cm segment of the tube is involved. Reversal is more successful than with electrocauterization, Irving, or Uchida techniques.

Vaginal Approaches
Ligation, clips, electrocoagulation rings
Two varieties have been used. *Colpotomy* involves a surgical incision in the posterior vaginal fornix through which the tube is delivered and occluded by ligation, clips, or rings. In *culdoscopy,* a culdoscope is passed through a smaller colpotomy incision to allow identification of the tubes and application of the electroprobe, clips, or rings. Both of these less popular methods share higher complication and failure rates. They are not postpartum methods.

Transcervical approaches
Still considered experimental procedures, these methods of blocking the tubes from a transcervical-intrauterine approach continue to evoke interest. One method is to use Silastic "plugs" placed under hysteroscopic guidance. Various techniques are under development to provide a reversible sterilization by "pulling the plugs" when a pregnancy is desired.

In the fall of 2002, the Food and Drug Administration approved a new method whereby a small stainless steel inner coil and superelastic outer coil (4 cm × 0.8 mm, after release 4 cm × 1.5 - 2 mm) is inserted hysteroscopically into the fallopian tubes for permanent sterilization. It is called Essure. See the "Suppliers" section for more information.

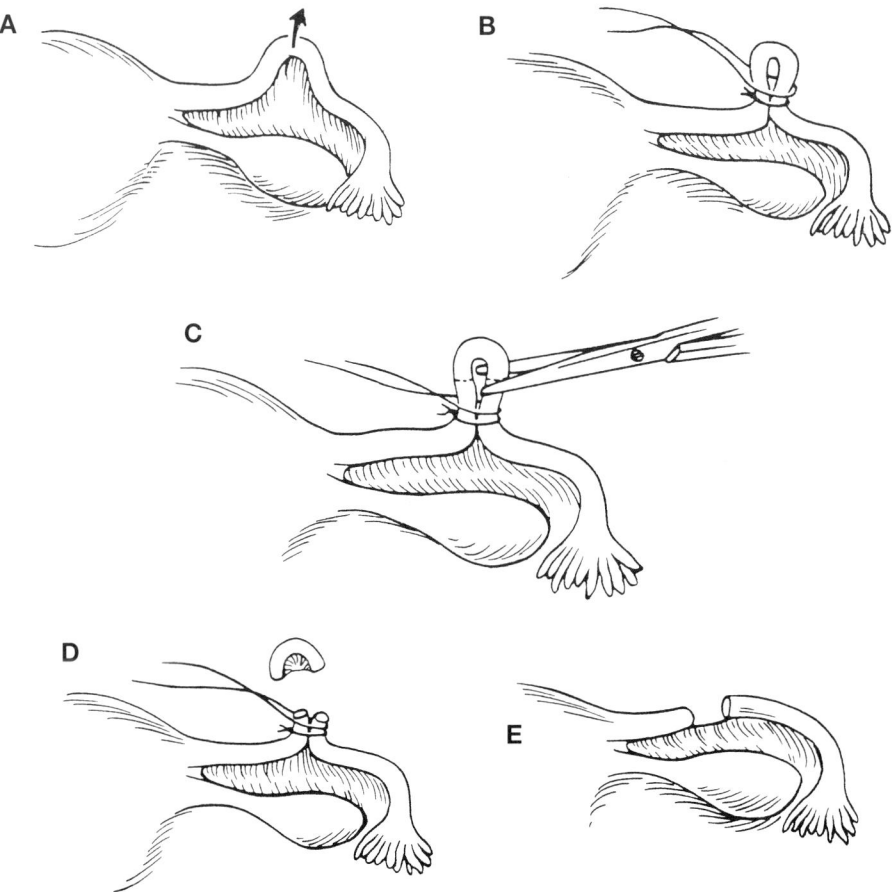

Fig. 153-2
Modified Pomeroy technique. **A,** Lift loop. **B,** Double ligation 0 or 2-0 plain gut suture, no crushing. **C,** Each limb of tubal loop is cut separately. **D,** Loop is cut off. **E,** Later results.

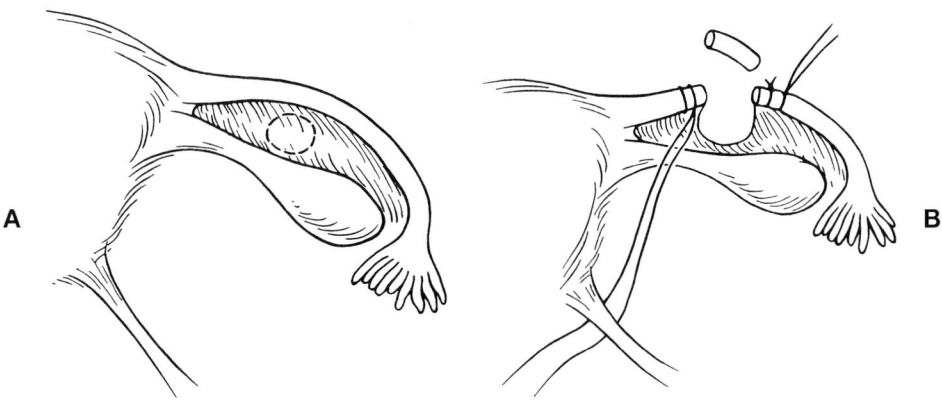

Fig. 153-3
Parkland method of tubal ligation. **A,** A relatively bloodless area of the mesosalpinx is identified within the isthmic portion of the tube. **B,** A segment of tube is isolated and removed after double ligation with chromic suture.

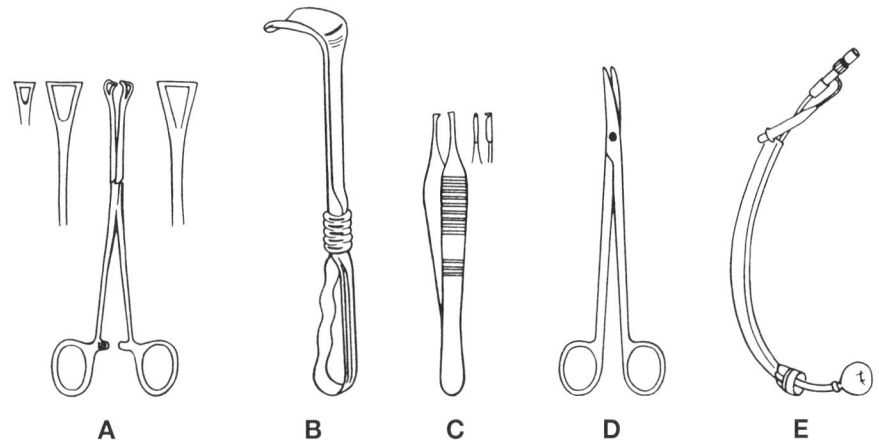

Fig. 153-4
Instruments for tubal ligation. **A,** Babcock forceps; **B,** small Richardson retractor; **C,** Adson tissue forceps; **D,** Metzenbaum scissors; **E,** uterine manipulator. (Also see Chapter 147, Hysterosalpingography/ Sonohysterosalpingography.)

tagging suture, bleeders, or tissue planes (fascia, peritoneum)
- Uterine manipulators for use with the cervical tenaculum or the newer uterine manipulators (Fig. 153-4, *E*) (CooperSurgical)
- 5-ml, 0.5% bupivacaine (Marcaine) *(optional)*

PREPROCEDURE PATIENT PREPARATION

Preprocedure Visits

Preprocedure evaluation and counseling for women who want permanent sterilization warrants focused attention. A special visit should be scheduled to discuss contraceptive options, risks, technique, and follow-up demands of sterilization surgery. (See the sample patient education handout titled "Permanent Female Sterilization [Tubal Ligation]" on page 1946 of Appendix G.) In addition, many insurance companies require preauthorization, which should be obtained at this visit. The counseling session should not be hurried or tacked on to the end of a visit for an acute illness. Written materials should be given to the patient at this time. Federal payment programs require that counseling precede surgery by at least 30 days and not more than 180 days. Special forms need to be signed and the patient must be at least 21 years of age. If the patient is involved in a monogamous relationship, it is wise to have the partner present during the consultation to address his concerns. His written consent is not mandatory, but if he disagrees with his partner's decision, his reasons should be explored. It is also important to address the issues and benefits of vasectomy (refer to the opening paragraph of this chapter).

A preprocedure examination, which requires a reasonable amount of time, should occur within 10 days (some hospitals require less than 5 days) of anticipated surgery. Review the patient's complete medical history, paying particular attention to prior pelvic or abdominal surgery and to infection. Are there drug allergies or drug intolerances? Is there a history of heart disease, diabetes, bleeding disorder, endometriosis, or dysfunctional uterine bleeding? Is other concomitant surgery necessary (e.g., dilation and curettage [D & C], breast biopsy, or procedure for urinary incontinence)? Is the Pap smear normal? Discuss the method of anesthesia that is to be used. Carefully review anticipated postprocedure morbidities (e.g., pain, the necessity of limited lifting). Remain mindful of the risk factors for regret. Review current contraceptive methods. Is pregnancy a possibility at the time of surgery? If the patient smokes, can she quit before surgery?

Preprocedure examination should be thorough. Focus on the heart, lung, breast, and abdominal examinations. During the pelvic examination, assess for the presence of vulvar, vaginal, or cervical disease. Obtain specimens for culture (e.g., gonorrhea, chlamydia) as necessary. Assess the degree of uterine prolapse and urinary incontinence; have the patient bear down and cough. Perform a bimanual examination to assess uterine size, shape, and tenderness. Palpate the ovaries for enlargement. Pay particular attention to uterine mobility. Can the uterus be brought out of the pelvis easily, or is it frozen in a particular direction? Estimate the degree of abdominal wall obesity. Show the patient the location and size of the anticipated abdominal incision and eventual scarring.

Perform laboratory tests as necessary. Typically, hospitals require hemoglobin levels and a urinalysis as the minimum prerequisites for general anesthesia. Perform a pregnancy test if there is any question of pregnancy. If there is clinical evidence of cervicitis or pelvic inflammation, obtain specimens for culture, and treat the condition accordingly. In this case, schedule the surgery only when treatment and clinical response have been adequate. Some hospitals require a copy of the patient's normal, recent Pap smear on the chart.

Many same-day and outpatient surgery services offer preanesthesia counseling. The patient can meet with the anesthesia clinician to discuss anesthesia, risks, time to arrive at the hospital, how long to fast before surgery, and other issues. This counseling should be used whenever available; for many hospitals, it is a requirement.

Call the hospital surgery personnel with any special requests for the anticipated surgery. Will a D & C be performed? (If so, it should be done *after* minilaparotomy.) Is a uterine manipulator necessary and what type?

General Information

- Minilaparotomy is the safest sterilization method in the postpartum period, with a complication rate approaching that of interval sterilization, which is usually less than 3%. Laparoscopy is not as safe during the immediate postpartum period as at other times.

- Average rates for tubal sterilization failures are 1 in 250 at 1 year.

- Postpartum and postabortion sterilization appears to be somewhat less effective than interval sterilization.

- Of the women who have tubal sterilization, 1% to 2% seek reversal; however, sterility is not easily reversed. Only 30% to 70% of these women are candidates for reversal surgery, and pregnancy occurs in about 50% of those who do undergo it. Reversal is most successful if less than 3 cm of the tubes was originally damaged or removed. The most "reversible" techniques include those that do not involve electrocautery and those in which the smallest segment is removed from within the isthmic portion of the tube. Women with the following risk factors for regret should not necessarily be denied surgery; however, the prudent physician should counsel these patients before performing sterilization.

  —Marital disharmony at the time of sterilization. (Remarriage is the reason 90% of women request reversal.)

  —Age less than 30 years at the time of sterilization. (Some clinicians debate whether this is a significant risk factor.)

  —Religious, socioeconomic, and educational background shows much less correlation with regret. Low parity or number of live children is also less well correlated.

  —Regret may be slightly more prevalent after postpartum sterilization procedures; however, as a risk factor, this is less well defined.

  —Regret is more likely when sterilization is chosen because of financial difficulties, health, or emotional problems.

TECHNIQUE

Check in with the preoperative holding area. Is the patient's chart complete and informed consent form available and signed? Are the laboratory values within normal range? Does your patient have any questions? Is the family in the waiting room?

Tell the operating room scrub or float nurse what equipment and sutures you will need. Clarify the position that the patient will be placed in for the surgery (e.g., lithotomy, frog-legged, or standard supine position). Request a specific cleansing agent for patients who are allergic to iodine.

1. Cleanse the vulva and vagina. A vaginal prep is necessary if the bladder is to be catheterized or a uterine manipulator is to be applied.

2. Drain the bladder. Perform a quick, gentle, straight catheterization to decompress a distended bladder from the operative field. Catheterization of the bladder is not universally performed. This is particularly true for patients under local anesthesia who can void sufficiently just before anesthesia. However, when the surgeon is new to this technique or when delay is anticipated in completing the abdominal entry (obesity, prior pelvic surgery, or infection), bladder injury is more likely. Draining the bladder helps reduce this risk. "Fluid bolusing" at the time of general anesthesia induction is common, and the bladder can fill quickly.

3. Apply the uterine manipulator (for interval minilaparotomy). Traditional devices include acorn or Hulka devices. Newer adaptations, such as Cooper-Surgical's uterine manipulator (Fig. 153-4, *E*), are easy to apply and are rarely traumatic. Many clinicians use manipulators routinely; others reserve them for anticipated problems with adequate exposure (abdominal obesity, prior pelvic surgery or infection, or retroversion or flexion of the uterus). Less-experienced surgeons will find them helpful. The patient must be in either the lithotomy or the frog-leg position, and general anesthesia is required.

4. Sterile gloves may be used without formal gowning for insertion of the uterine manipulator or for straight catheterization of the urinary bladder. In fact, it is advisable for the surgeon not to perform these procedures with the same formal gowning and gloving worn for the minilaparotomy, because

contamination is likely when the patient is in the lithotomy position.

5. Prepare and scrub the abdomen. Minilaparotomy should not be performed through pubic hair. Depending on patient pubic hair distribution, shaving a small strip of pubic hair over the operative site may be necessary.

6. Perform the procedure after thorough surgical scrub and gowning. Wipe any powder from the latex gloves with sterile, saline-soaked sponges.

7. Apply surgical drapes as for abdominal surgery.

8. Palpate three fingerbreadths above the symphysis pubis (Fig. 153-5). With one hand on the abdomen above the symphysis, move the uterine manipulator. Often the uterus can be felt with the abdominal hand, which offers reassurance that the incision will provide ready access to the uterus and adnexa.

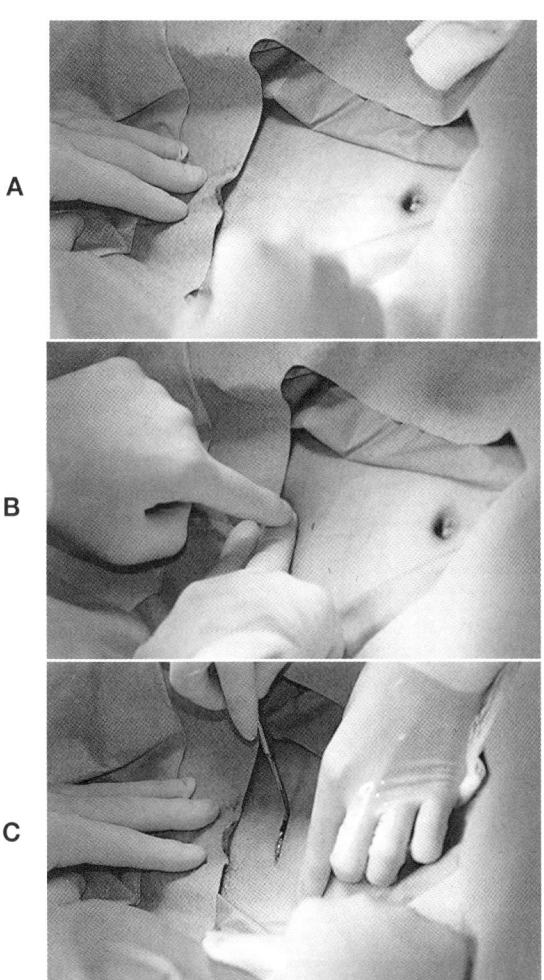

Fig. 153-5
Locating the site of the abdominal incision. **A,** The top of the upper border of the escutcheon has been shaved. **B,** The area 2 to 3 fingerbreadths above the symphysis pubis is identified. **C,** A 5-cm transverse incision is made.

Using the skin scalpel with a no. 10 blade, make a transverse incision. There is no need to arc this incision. Often the linea nigra, the faint line demarcating the midline, can be visualized. The incision should be no more than 5 cm long, and often a smaller incision will suffice.

9. Switch to the deep knife (new no. 10 blade) and progress through Scarpa's fascia (within the fat) until the rectus sheath is encountered. Often, once Scarpa's fascia is divided, the sub-Scarpa's fat can be brushed away with a sponge, using a wiping motion. Bleeders can be cauterized using the electrocoagulator. Do not tunnel the incision, especially in the obese abdomen; this can be prevented by ensuring that the subcutaneous fat has been divided all the way to both edges of the skin incision. The subcutaneous fat presents an excellent opportunity to test the power on the Bovie before entering the abdomen. The Bovie device should never be used for the first time on intraabdominal tissue, in case the power is set dangerously high.

10. Once the rectus fascia is identified by its dense, white fibrous appearance, make a small transverse incision on each side of the linea alba. Using a Metzenbaum scissors, carefully extend the fascial incision to the lateral margin of the skin incision and across the midline. Place two Kelly clamps on the incised lower fascial edge and gently retract and elevate the fascia. Gently place the index finger (preferably) or the blunt end of the scalpel along the midline under the incised fascial edge, and gently roll toward the lateral margins, freeing the sheath from the underlying rectus muscle. In the midline, the pyramidalis remains adherent; use the Metzenbaum scissors to carefully cut along the inferior linea alba, freeing the muscle and making more room. Apply Kelly clamps to the upper segment of the anterior rectus sheath, and free the underlying muscles in a similar fashion. You do not need to roll the index finger under the rectus sheath any further than the skin incision. Perforating vessels arise more laterally and can be ruptured. Carefully use cautery to control bleeding.

11. Using blunt dissection with the index finger or the blunt end of the knife, separate the rectus muscles from the transversalis fascia and peritoneum in the midline. A gentle rolling action of the index finger (or the blunt end of the scalpel) under each lateral band of rectus muscles ensures adequate room.

12. Using two Kelly clamps or pickups, opposing each other, lift the transversalis and peritoneum, thereby tenting these layers away from underlying abdominal structures. Using either the scalpel or Metzenbaum scissors, make a small buttonhole incision between the two clamps. This incision should be

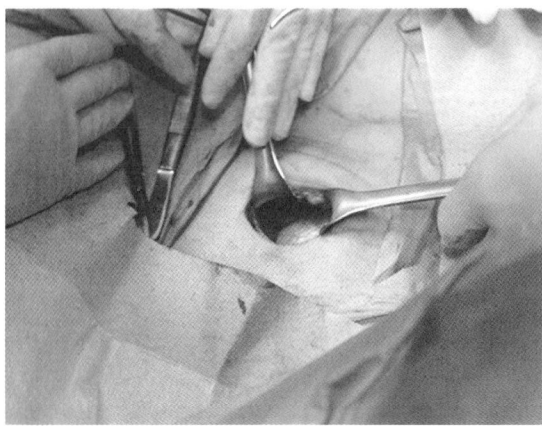

Fig. 153-6
Small Richardson retractors used in pairs and gently lifted upward offer excellent exposure.

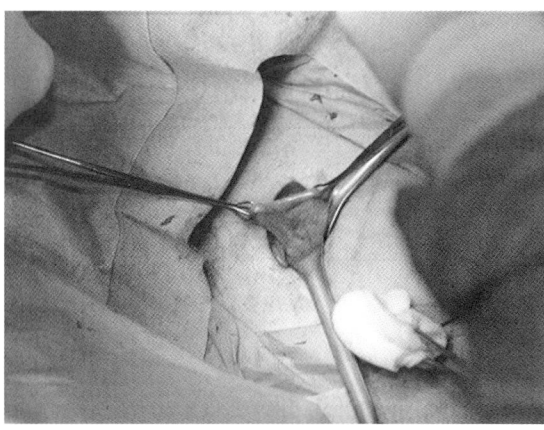

Fig. 153-7
Using Babcock forceps, gently bring the tube through the incision and identify a portion of the mesosalpinx relatively devoid of vessels.

well above the symphysis pubis, favoring the cephalad (toward the umbilicus) portion of the wound to avoid the bladder. At this point, use a Kelly clamp to enter the small incision, and with a combination of blunt dissection and retraction of tissues, enter the abdomen. The key maneuver is to maintain this elevation of the incision edges to expose abdominal viscera. The obese abdomen may contain a significant amount of fat below the peritoneum, which requires special care when dissecting. It may be difficult to distinguish this tissue from omentum or mesenteric fat that may be adherent in the lower pelvis, especially in women with a history of abdominal surgery or infection. The peritoneal incision may be extended either transversely (preferred) or vertically.

13. Place the small Richardson retractors, and with gently opposed and elevating retraction, lift the abdominal wall and inspect the abdominal cavity (Fig. 153-6). If the small intestine obscures the view, place the patient in the reverse Trendelenburg position (head down) to allow the bowel to gravitate cephalad out of view. Use a gauze pad rolled tightly on a ring clamp to brush the bowel and adnexal structures aside if they are obstructing the view. Using Babcock forceps, identify the adnexal structures. Once the fallopian tube is identified, use two Babcock forceps to gently retract the tube until the ovary and fimbriated end are clearly identified. Apply slight traction on the Babcock to deliver the tube through the incision for the ligation procedure (Fig. 153-7). A tube can be avulsed at the uterus with subsequent bleeding, so be careful to avoid forceful retraction. Use the uterine manipulator to help with visualization and exposure.

14. Carefully elevate the fallopian tube and identify a relatively avascular area of the mesosalpinx. Using a Kelly to gently penetrate or the Bovie on "coag" (*not "cutting"*) to avoid making too large of a hole, make a small hole through the mesosalpinx (Fig. 153-8). Then clamp the tube with a Kelly, placing one jaw through this hole and the other across the tube. Place another Kelly clamp 2 cm distal to the first one, isolating a segment of tube. Using a 2-0 chromic suture on a needle, place a stick tie on the uterine side of the tube proximal to the Kelly clamp and encircle the tube. Tag this tie (Kelly is placed on the suture to maintain control). Most surgeons place a second tie on the same side and cut (Fig. 153-9). Place a similar tie on the fimbriated side of the tube. Remove the Kelly clamps. Incise through each of the two crush marks made by the Kelly clamps and remove the segment of the tube (Fig. 153-10). Lightly cauterize the exposed mesosalpinx if bleeding is observed. Cut the tags and repeat this procedure on the other tube. Current evidence supports the use of preemptive analgesia using infiltration of the incised skin and uterine tubes at cut ends with 0.5% bupivacaine. Postoperative pain, nausea, vomiting, and cramping were significantly lessened by this practice.

15. Perform a sponge count and, if it is correct, close the abdomen.

16. Identify and hold the edges of the peritoneum with Kelly clamps or pickups (Fig. 153-10, *A*). Use a running 3-0 chromic suture to reapproximate the cut edges. Identify and tag the fascial sheath edges with Kelly clamps. Close this sheath with a running 0 Dexon suture (Fig. 153-10, *B*). Palpate the closure to make sure there are no buttonhole defects in the

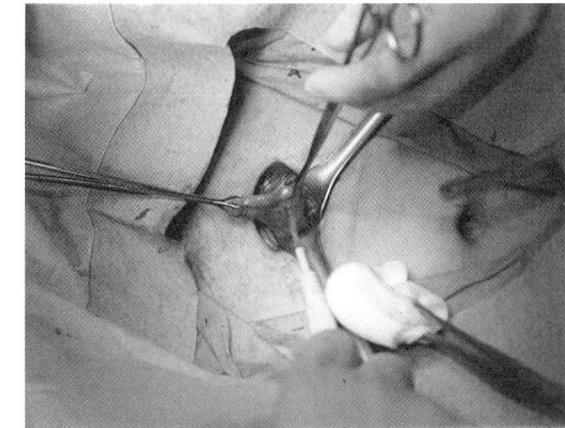

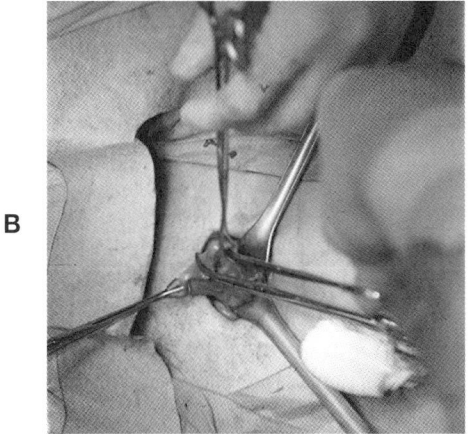

Fig. 153-8
Using the Bovie on "coagulation," make a 2- to 3-cm incision in the mesosalpinx **(A)** through which two Kelly clamps can be passed to isolate a segment of tube **(B).**

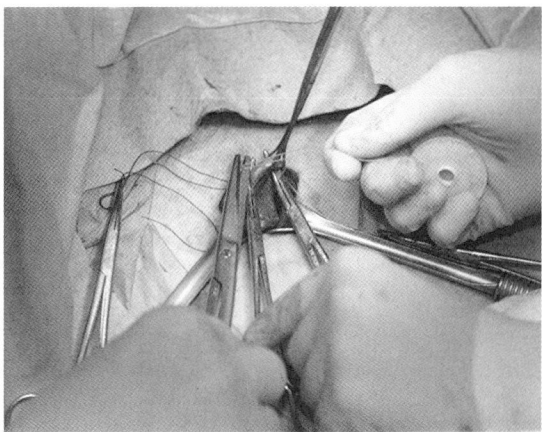

Fig. 153-9
Tie chromic sutures on each side of the tube next to the Kelly clamps on the portion of the tube that will remain.

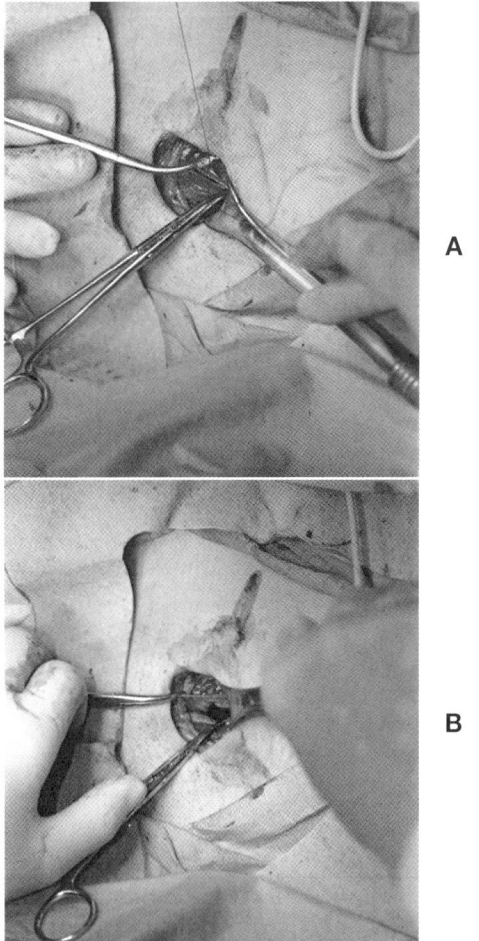

Fig. 153-10
A, For closure, identify the peritoneum and retract it with Kelly clamps.
B, Suture the peritoneum with a running 3-0 chromic suture.

fascial repair that could later manifest as incisional hernias. If there is more than 1 cm of subcutaneous fat, close Scarpa's fascia with interrupted 2-0 chromic sutures. The skin may be closed with staples or by running a subcuticular stitch of 3-0 chromic suture on a Keith needle.

17. Cleanse the surgical site with normal saline and apply a gauze dressing.

18. Take the patient to the recovery room. She may be discharged when she is awake, is tolerating oral liquids, and is ambulatory. Send the tubal segments for routine pathologic examination; place them in separate bottles marked "right" and "left." Write a brief operative note in the chart. State any complications, blood loss, and other findings. Dictate a complete operative report immediately after surgery. The patient should be seen in the office within 7 to 14 days or at any time a complication develops. Review the tubal histology report.

POSTPROCEDURE PATIENT EDUCATION

Give the patient postprocedure instructions and inform the family of any follow-up instructions. (See the patient education handout titled "After Tubal Ligation" on page 1948 of Appendix G.)

POSTPARTUM TUBAL LIGATION

Postpartum tubal ligation (PTL) has many similarities with interval tubal ligation, but there are also major differences. Despite the convenience, cost savings, and ultimate desires of the patient, PTL remains an elective surgery. Numerous contraindications include maternal fever, pregnancy-related hypertension, uncontrolled diabetes mellitus, and excessive blood loss. Concerns regarding the viability and health of the newborn must be considered as well. Women who must postpone their postpartum sterilization should be reassured that interval tubal ligation as early as 6 weeks after delivery is also an excellent method of sterilization surgery. PTL can readily be performed during cesarean section; however, never assume that PTL remains the patient's desire if the cesarean section was performed because of concern over the condition of the fetus. (See the patient education handout titled "Postpartum Tubal Ligation" on page 1949 of Appendix G.)

TECHNIQUE

Review the technique described earlier for interval tubal ligation.

1. PTL can often be performed with the same block (epidural, caudal) that was used during labor. If this is not desirable or possible, there are many advantages to allowing the patient to rest and recover from labor and to schedule the PTL procedure for the next morning. A repeat hemoglobin determination will be much more meaningful after equilibration of fluid, especially if there is concern over blood loss during delivery. This delay also allows more time to observe the condition of the newborn.

2. The bladder should be drained either by having the patient void immediately before surgery or by straight catheterization (preferred method). Prepare the abdomen in the immediate umbilical area. Surgical scrub and draping are required.

3. Make a curved infraumbilical incision in the abdomen with the skin knife (no. 11 blade) (Fig. 153-11). Gentle inferior retraction on the abdominal skin at the time of this incision ensures that the scar will be close to or within the umbilical crater.

4. Carry the incision deeper with the deep knife (no. 10 blade). Once the skin and subcutaneous fat have been divided, enter the abdomen by favoring the

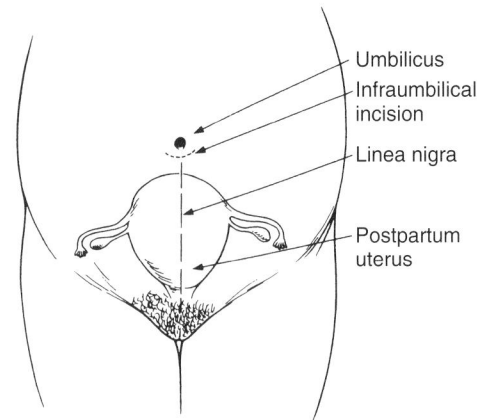

Fig. 153-11
Postpartum tubal ligation by minilaparotomy requires a small transverse infraumbilical incision.

inferior portion of the wound. (Dissecting through the substance of the umbilicus can be frustrating because tissue planes are not well defined.) Blunt dissection with Kelly clamps, which can probe and spread, is the preferred method for exploring and defining the portal of entry into the abdominal cavity. Some surgeons prefer to grasp each lateral side of the incision with towel clamps and elevate the entire incision away from underlying structures, such as the bowel and the uterus, when entering the peritoneum. Once the abdominal cavity is identified, the incision through the fascia and peritoneum can be extended, but it rarely needs to be longer than 4 to 5 cm.

5. Push the uterus gently to one side to rotate the adnexal structures into view. Use Babcock clamps to identify the fallopian tube, which in the postpartum period is typically swollen and engorged compared with the nonpregnant state. Follow each tube until the fimbriated ends and ovaries are identified. Extremely gentle traction is warranted because vessels within the mesosalpinx can be huge and easily damaged by traction. Tears in these vessels can cause profound bleeding.

6. Once the tube has been identified clearly, perform a tubal ligation as described previously for the interval sterilization technique. If the mesosalpinx is extremely fragile, many clinicians prefer the more traditional modified Pomeroy technique. The loop, tie, and cut features of the Pomeroy render a quick hemostatic procedure that can minimize the traction injuries or raw cut edges of the mesosalpinx produced by other procedures. Remember that if the tube cannot be delivered through the incision for a tubal ligation procedure, clips may be applied to the correctly identified fallopian tube.

7. Close the abdomen in a layered fashion as previously described. With periumbilical incisions, it is some-

times difficult to clearly redefine the peritoneal edges for closure. However, closure of the fascia is crucial and time should be spent clearly identifying the edges of this layer for definitive suturing.

8. The patient should be seen within 2 weeks of PTL. At this time, the histology report should be reviewed.

COMPLICATIONS

Major Complications

- Major factors related to the development of complications include clinician inexperience, patient obesity, prior pelvic or abdominal surgery, and other medical problems such as diabetes mellitus, heart disease, asthma, bronchitis, and emphysema.
- Major complications occur in less than 2% of all procedures and may require prolonged hospitalization (0.3% requiring 3 or more nights in the hospital) or laparotomy (0.02% to 1.2% in large studies) to resolve complications.
- Delayed complications requiring readmission to the hospital occur after less than 1% of procedures.
- Minilaparotomy and laparoscopy have similar complication rates.
- Female sterilization causes very few deaths (10 to 15 deaths per 500,000 procedures per year in the United States), and most are related to anesthetic complications (overdose or drug reaction), infection, and hemorrhage.
- Mortality rates from sterilization are far lower than with childbirth.
- Rare complications of tubal litigations include pregnancy (intrauterine and ectopic) and luteal phase pregnancy.

Minor Complications

- Minilaparotomy appears to have a higher rate of minor complications (12% versus 7%) and a longer average operating time when compared with laparoscopy. Minilaparotomy convalescence appears to be slightly longer and more painful. High complication rates have been reported when laparoscopy is performed by inexperienced physicians.
- Minor minilaparotomy complications include wound infections, slight blood loss, uterine perforation by uterine manipulation instruments, and bladder injury. Most minor injury complications are immediately recognized and managed intraoperatively.
- Laparoscopy complications include those of minilaparotomy, as well as unique problems related to insertion of the instrument and gas insufflation of the abdomen. These include gas embolism, subcutaneous emphysema, or cardiac arrest. Vessel or organ

laceration may occur. Open laparoscopy may make some of these complications less likely.

- Pain occurs after both minilaparotomy and laparoscopy. Chest and shoulder pain is common after laparoscopy; this is caused by trapped gas under the diaphragm after insufflation of the abdomen. Most postprocedure and recovery pain can be managed with oral drug therapy, and narcotics are rarely necessary after the third postprocedural day.
- There is no compelling evidence that female sterilization causes long-term complications. Menstrual cycles do not significantly change as a result of sterilization; but abnormalities may persist if they existed before surgery. Among women who do experience menstrual changes, about half observe improvements and half experience irregular cycles or increased bleeding.
- Sterilized women do not appear to have different rates of pelvic inflammatory disease, cervicitis, hysterectomy, or D & C. Ovarian cancer may be diminished.
- Sterilized women are no more likely to experience severe psychiatric problems than unsterilized women.

SUPPLIERS

Essure
Conceptus, Inc.
1021 Howard Avenue
San Carlos, CA 94070
Phone: 1-650-628-4900
For training information: 1-877-377-8732
Website: www.essure.com

CPT/BILLING CODES

58600	Interval tubal ligation
58605	Postpartum tubal ligation
58982	Laparoscopic tubal ligation

ICD-9-CM DIAGNOSTIC CODES

V2509	General counseling and family planning advice
V252	Sterilization; admission for interruption of fallopian tubes or vas deferens

ADDITIONAL RESOURCES

- See the sample patient education handouts titled "Permanent Female Sterilization (Tubal Ligation)" on page 1946, "After Tubal Ligation" on page 1948, and "Postpartum Tubal Ligation" on page 1949 of Appendix G.

BIBLIOGRAPHY

American College of Obstetricians and Gynecologists: *Sterilization*, Tech Bull 113, Feb 1988, ACOG, Washington, DC.

Chi IC, Potts M, Wilkens L: Rare events associated with tubal sterilizations: an international experience, *Obstet Gynecol Surv* 41(1):7, 1986.

Green LR, Laros RK: Postpartum sterilization, *Clin Obstet Gynecol* 23(2):647, 1980.

Hillis SD, March Banks PA, Tylor LR, Peterson HB: Poststerilization regret: findings from the United States Collaborative Review of Sterilization, *Obstet Gynecol* 93(6):889, 1999.

Mattingly RF: Surgical conditions of the fallopian tube. In Linde TE, editor: *Operative gynecology*, ed 5, Philadelphia, 1982, JB Lippincott.

McGonigle KF, Huggins GR: Tubal sterilization: epidemiology of regret, *Contemp Obstet Gynecol* 35(10):15, 1990.

Peterson HB, Xia Z, Hughes JM, et al: The risk of pregnancy after tubal sterilization: findings from the U.S. Collaborative Review of Sterilization, *Am J Obstet Gynecol* 174(4):1161, 1168, 1996.

Peterson HB, Xia Z, Hughes JM, et al: The risk of ectopic pregnancy after tubal sterilization: U.S. Collaborative Review of Sterilization Working Group, *N Engl J Med* 336(11):762, 1997.

Rulin MC, Davidson AR, Philliber SG, et al: Long-term effect of tubal sterilization on menstrual indices and pelvic pain, *Obstet Gynecol* 82(1):118, 1993.

Visalyaputra S, Lertakyamanee J, Pethpaisit N, et al: Intraperitoneal lidocaine decreases intraoperative pain during postpartum tubal ligation, *Anesth Analg* 88(5):1077, 1999.

Wittels B, Faure EA, Chavez R, et al: Effective analgesia after bilateral tubal ligation, *Anesth Analg* 87(3):619, 1998.

CHAPTER 154

Pessaries

Penny Jenkins
Francie Bernier
Timothy J. Downs*

Historically, pessaries have been used to correct pelvic floor deformities and dysfunctions, and symptoms associated with genital prolapse, uterine retrodisplacement, and cervical incompetence in women. In addition to hanging women by their heels, physicians as early as Hippocrates reported the use of half a pomegranate in the vagina for women with prolapse! In 1860, Hugh Lenox Hodge, Professor of Gynecology at the University of Pennsylvania, designed a pessary using Goodyear's newly patented vulcanized rubber. Since that time, technological advances in composition and a wide variety of sizes and shapes now make fitting pessaries an art (Fig. 154-1).

INDICATIONS

- Stress urinary incontinence (including athletic stress urinary incontinence)
- Uterine prolapse
- Vaginal vault prolapse
- Uterine retrodisplacement
- Pelvic relaxation
- Cystocele
- Enterocele
- Rectocele
- Cervical incompetence†
- Poor surgical candidates with significant symptoms while awaiting surgery
- Prophylactic postoperatively
- Preoperative diagnostic aid

---

*The authors thank Ms. Ruth Cogan of Milex Corp. for her review of this chapter.

†The pessary has been advocated for patients at risk for preterm labor and those diagnosed with cervical incompetence. Until the results of randomized controlled studies now in progress are known for pessary use with an incompetent cervix and women at risk for preterm delivery, cervical cerclage and bed rest should remain standard of care. (See Chapter 134, Cervical Cerclage.)

Indications for pessary use include reduction of pelvic organ prolapse and relief of symptoms associated with prolapse, such as stress urinary incontinence. Preoperative use of pessaries as a diagnostic tool for any of the above indications can be helpful to estimate the amount of normal function that may be restored after surgery. A pessary can also help determine if the patient will develop incontinence if a prolapse is surgically corrected. A short-term use may be to simply postpone surgery. Although surgery generally produces a more permanent cure, a pessary may be the treatment of choice for women who are poor surgical candidates, who want to postpone surgery indefinitely, or who prefer a nonsurgical treatment option. Pessaries may also be used postoperatively in women at risk for recurrent prolapse.

CONTRAINDICATIONS

- Vaginal ulceration
- Active vaginitis
- Any pelvic infections or lacerations
- Severe atrophic changes
- Endometriosis has been suggested as possible contraindication to pessary use
- Noncompliant patient
- Impaired mental capacity
- Lack of manual dexterity

There are few absolute contraindications to pessary use; however, certain patients may require more careful monitoring. Active vaginitis including atrophic changes and vaginal ulcerations should be treated and resolved before pessary use. Although ulcerations are generally considered a contraindication, when they are a direct result of an exteriorized prolapse, a pessary may prevent further injury and promote healing. Severe atrophic changes are a contraindication to immediate pessary use; however, once the vagina is reestrogenized, the

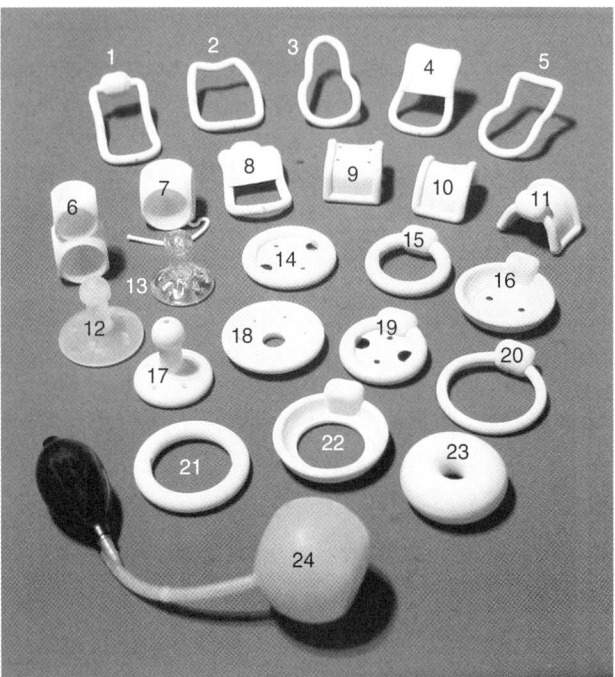

Fig. 154-1

Various type of pessaries. *1,* Hodge with knob; *2,* Risser; *3,* Smith; *4,* Hodge with support; *5,* Hodge; *6,* Tandem Cube; *7,* Cube; *8,* Hodge with support and knob; *9,* Regula; *10,* Gehrung; *11,* Gehrung with knob; *12,* Gellhorn 95% rigid (silicone); *13,* Gellhorn rigid (acrylic silicone); *14,* ring with support; *15,* ring with knob; *16,* incontinence dish with support; *17,* Gellhorn flexible; *18,* Shaatz; *19,* ring with knob and support; *20,* incontinence ring; *21,* ring; *22,* incontinence dish; *23,* donut; *24,* Inflatoball. (Courtesy Milex Production, Inc., Chicago, Ill.)

woman may begin using the device. The woman using a pessary must be mentally and physically capable of using the device as recommended and able to return for appropriate follow-up.

FITTING PESSARIES

Fitting kits are available from the two largest manufacturers of pessaries in the United States. Milex has kits for the Ring pessary and Gellhorn pessary, and Mentor Corporation has a kit with the Ring pessary and a conversion chart for converting the size of the ring pessary to other types it manufactures. Conversions of pessary sizes remain difficult, however. The totally different shape of each pessary and whether the pessary fits in front of the cervix (e.g., the Gellhorn, Donut, or Cube), behind the cervix (e.g., the lever pessaries), or over the cervix (e.g., the Gehrung) precludes simple conversions. The manufacturer should be contacted for product information and obtaining pessary fitting kits.

A properly fitted pessary should be comfortable for the patient; should remain in place despite walking, standing or provocative maneuvers; and should not interfere with bladder and bowel function. Although the goal of treatment for stress incontinence is to make the patient completely dry, the patient may view even a small improvement positively.

Pessary manufacturers typically recommend voiding before the fitting session. The literature does not provide a clear rationale for this recommendation. There are two reasons why the patient should not void before the fitting session. First, there are a number of pessaries now available for the treatment of stress incontinence, and correct sizing is partially determined by whether the woman continues to lose urine with a pessary in place. Many women do not lose urine when the bladder has been emptied recently. Second, a pessary that is too large can obstruct the urethra, so the patient must void before leaving the office to ensure proper fit. Some patients cannot void twice within the scheduled appointment time. It is important that the incontinence pessaries with a knob be fitted *before* the patient empties her bladder.

In certain cases, it may be more advantageous not to teach the patient insertion and removal at the initial pessary fitting appointment. It will not only save time; it will allow the patient to wear the device for a short time to determine effectiveness and proper sizing before purchasing the device. On the other hand, the Cube and Inflatoball pessary *must* be removed nightly and cleaned, so removal and insertion must be taught to the patient at the fitting visit. Many women are skeptical about wearing a pessary and may be more motivated once they experience improvement in their symptomatology.

Once the goal of treatment is determined, the vagina should be inspected for estrogen status, erythema, erosions, and ulcerations. A Pap smear should be obtained if indicated. *Determining pessary size is similar to fitting a contraceptive diaphragm* (see Chapter 131, Barrier Contraceptives: Cervical Cap, Condom, and Diaphragm). The fingers are spread apart to measure width. A rough estimate of length is determined by measuring the distance from the posterior fornix or vaginal apex to the symphysis pubis. The second and third finger are placed in the vagina with the third finger in the posterior fornix, and the depth of insertion is marked on the proximal second finger. The distance between the tip of the third finger and the mark on the second finger approximates vaginal depth (see Fig. 131-8). This is also a good opportunity to evaluate pelvic floor strength and teach the patient how to do Kegel exercises.

The patient should be examined in the standing position after initial placement and reexamined after performing provocative maneuvers and voiding. Provocative maneuvers include standing, sitting, walking, squatting and Valsalva's maneuver. Then the patient should try to void. If difficulty is experienced while trying to void or if discomfort is noted during these maneuvers, the next smaller size of pessary should be tried. If the pessary has shifted position after the above maneuvers, a larger size *or* different pessary should be tried.

PESSARY SELECTION

Pessaries are available in a wide range of sizes and shapes, each with a specific indication and function. Selection depends on anatomy, symptomatology, and the overall goal of treatment. Identifying the best choice is often a trial-and-error process; clinicians should not be discouraged if the first selection is not successful. *The most commonly prescribed pessaries are the Ring, the Gellhorn and the Donut.* For the novice starting to fit pessaries for the first time, obtaining fitting kits and samples of the most commonly used pessaries may decrease the difficulty of pessary fitting.

Nontoxic and nonallergenic silicone has replaced the red rubber material of previous pessaries. Silicone has greater longevity, does not absorb odors, and can be sterilized by most methods.

Pessaries are made with several modifications of the same theme. For example, the Ring pessary has a version "with support," which has a silicone web across the central opening. This "supports" the bladder, effectively reducing a mild to moderate cystocele. The "Ring with Knob" has a bulbous portion that is placed retropubically to restore the urethral-vesical (U-V) angle and increase urethral closing pressure. The addition of the "Knob" is for stress urinary incontinence from a hypermobile U-V angle. Some devices have both modifications.

PESSARY TYPES BY INDICATION

- *Stress incontinence:* Ring with Knob, Hodge, Hodge with Knob, Smith, Risser, Incontinence Ring, Incontinence Dish, Mar-Land, Gehrung with Knob (Fig. 154-2)
- *Preoperative evaluation for Burch Procedure for stress incontinence:* Hodge, Risser, and Hodge with Support
- *Uterine retrodisplacement:* Smith, Risser, and Hodge
- *Uterine prolapse, first or second degree:* Smith, Risser, Hodge, Ring, Ring with support, Shaatz, Legula (A pessary can be used to be sure that correction of uterine prolapse does not take a "kink" out of the urethra, leading to urine leakage.)
- *Uterine or vaginal vault prolapse, third or fourth degree:* Donut, Inflatoball, Cube, and Tandem Cube (The Gellhorn is not as well suited for severe vaginal

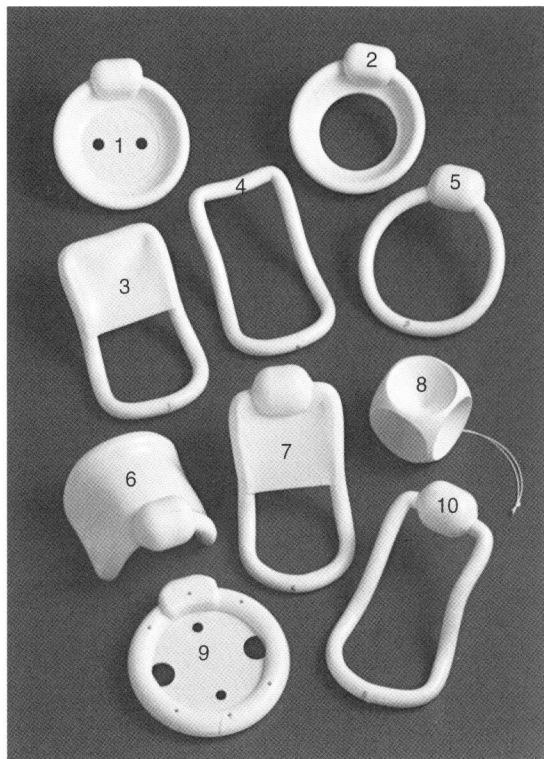

Fig. 154-2
Stress urinary incontinence pessaries (made with silicone). *1,* Incontinence dish with support; *2,* incontinence dish; *3,* Hodge with support; *4,* Hodge; *5,* Incontinence ring; *6,* Gehrung with knob; *7,* Hodge with support and knob; *8,* Cube; *9,* Ring with support and knob; *10,* Hodge with knob. (Courtesy Milex Production, Inc., Chicago, Ill.)

wall prolapse, because walls have been known to prolapse and encompass the pessary. It is adequate for uterine prolapse.)
- *Stress incontinence with cystocele, first or second degree:* Hodge with Support, Hodge with Knob with Support, Mar-Land with Support, Incontinence Dish with Support, Gehrung with Knob, and Ring with Support (with or without Knob).
- *Stress incontinence with uterine prolapse, first or second degree:* Hodge with Knob, Hodge with Knob with Support, Hodge, Hodge with Support, Incontinence Ring, Incontinence Dish, Incontinence Dish with Support, Mar-Land, Mar-Land with Support, Ring, Ring with Knob, Ring with Support and Knob
- *Cystocele:* Gehrung, Gehrung with Knob, Ring with Support, Gellhorn, Donut, Inflatoball, Cube, and Tandem Cube
- *Enterocele:* Gellhorn, Gehrung, Donut, Inflatoball, Cube, Tandem Cube
- *Rectocele:* Gellhorn, Gehrung, Donut, Inflatoball, Cube, Tandem Cube
- *Incompetent cervix:* Hodge (discuss with obstetrical consultant)

USE OF SPECIFIC PESSARIES

Ring Pessary/Ring Pessary with Support/ Ring Pessary with Support with Knob

Since the Ring is one of the easiest pessaries to insert and remove, it may be one of the first devices to try in cases of *prolapse without accompanying stress incontinence,* or with a knob when mild *prolapse is accompanied by stress incontinence* (Fig. 154-2, 5).

Indications
- *First- or second-degree uterine or vault prolapse.*
- Ring with Support may also be used *with a first- or second-degree cystocele.* The Ring with Support with Knob is used for *first- or second-degree prolapse accompanied by stress incontinence.* Both are available in sizes 0 to 10, although approximately 85% of patients are fit with sizes 3 through 6. (Ring pessaries are also available in sizes 10 through 13 through special order.)

Insertion
The device is hinged and will fold in only one direction. Compress the sides, creating a half-moon effect. Insert with the posterior end directed down toward the rectum. Once the device is fully intravaginal, rotate a quarter turn, placing the hinge transverse in the vagina to decrease the chance of expulsion, and open.

Removal
Insert the index finger in the notch and rotate the hinge anteriorly; fold end; pull down and out.

Other Pessaries to Try
Gellhorn, Donut, Gehrung, Shaatz, Oval Ring, or Inflatoball

Gellhorn

The Gellhorn (Fig. 154-1) will stay in when most other devices will be expelled and is *ideal for third-degree or greater prolapse.* Although this device looks intimidating, it is surprisingly comfortable. The stem functions to stabilize the device in the vagina and facilitates removal. A shorter stem is available by special order. Available in diameter sizes of 1½- through 3½-inch in increments of quarter inches (85% are fit with sizes 2¼ through 3 inches).

Indications
- *Third-degree uterine or vault prolapse*
- *Complete procidentia*
- *Any degree of cystocele, enterocele, or rectocele* (not the first choice in cases of mild prolapse)

Insertion
Position the disc portion parallel to the introitus, angling it such that the device avoids contact with the urethra. Apply strong pressure posteriorly and advance the device until it is fully intravaginal, then rotate with an upward motion until only the stem is palpable in the vagina.

Removal
Pull the knob down until it meets resistance, rotate parallel to the introitus while pulling down and out (use a "barber pole" action). It may also be removed by pulling the knob down toward the rectum until it meets resistance, then pulling the knob caudally. It may be necessary to insert the index finger of the opposite hand between the device and the posterior vaginal wall to break the suction.

Other Pessaries to Try
Donut, Inflatoball, or Gehrung

Donut

The most commonly recognized pessary, the space-occupying donut is very useful in patients with *excessive redundant tissue* (Fig. 154-1). It is available in diameters of 2 through 3¾ inches in increments of quarter inches (85% of patients will be fit with sizes 2¼ through 3 inches).

Indications
- *Third-degree uterine or vault prolapse*
- *Complete procidentia*
- *Any degree of cystocele, enterocele, or rectocele* (not the first choice in cases of mild prolapse)

Insertion
Turn the device parallel to the introitus, exert pressure posteriorly, and advance until it is fully intravaginal. Then rotate with an upward motion until the device is transverse.

Removal
Hook the index finger in the center hole, pull down while rotating the device parallel to the introitus, and remove while exerting pressure posteriorly.

Other Pessaries to Try
Gellhorn, Inflatoball, or Gehrung

Lever Pessaries (Hodge, Smith, Risser)

Originally designed for uterine retrodisplacement, the Lever pessaries now offer greater versatility. The

Smith and Risser are modifications of the Hodge. The Smith (Fig. 154-1) is rounded at both ends and is designed for the patient with a well-defined pubic notch and narrow introitus. The Hodge (Fig. 154-1 and Fig. 154-2, *4*), a modification of the Smith, is squared on one end and is designed for patients with a shallow pubic notch. This device is also designed to decrease pressure on the urethra. A further modification, the Risser (Fig. 154-1), has a wider heel, which provides a larger weight-bearing zone. All three pessaries are manually shapeable which allows the provider to bend the device to conform to the needs of the patient. For those patients who require more retropubic support, this can be accomplished by bending the anterior part of the device. The Lever is available in sizes 0 to 9 (85% of patients will use sizes 2 to 5).

Indications

- *Stress incontinence associated with urethral hypermobility*
- *First- or second-degree uterine prolapse*
- *Uterine retrodisplacement*

The Hodge and Risser may also be used as a test for effectiveness of the Burch procedure for stress incontinence.

Insertion

Compress the sides and insert the rounded end into the vagina, direct the heel into the vault or posterior fornix, and position the anterior portion retropubic. The device should fit snugly, should not rotate, and should remain retropubic.

Removal

Hook the device with the index finger to fold it, and pull the device down and out. It may be necessary to grasp the device between two fingers or with the index finger and thumb.

Other Pessaries to Try

Hodge with a knob, Incontinence Ring, Incontinence Dish, or Mar-Land

Hodge with Support

The Hodge with Support is exactly like the Hodge, only with a silicone platform (Figs. 154-1 and 154-2, *3*). This device is also manually shapeable and available in sizes 0 to 9 (the most common sizes are 2 to 5).

Indications

- *Stress incontinence associated with urethral hypermobility coupled with a first- or second-degree cystocele,*

first- or second-degree uterine prolapse, and uterine retrodisplacement.
- May be used as a test for effectiveness of the Burch procedure.

Insertion and Removal

Same as for the Hodge.

Other Pessaries to Try

Hodge with a Knob with Support, Mar-Land with Support, Incontinence Dish, or Gehrung with a Knob

Hodge with a Knob, with and without Support

An adaptation of the Hodge and the Incontinence Ring, the Hodge with a Knob *restores continence* by stabilizing the bladder base and increasing urethral closure pressure and functional urethral length (Fig. 154-1 and Fig. 154-2, *7*). This device is manually shapeable and available in sizes 0 to 9 (the most common sizes are 2 to 5).

Indications

- *Stress incontinence*
- *Stress incontinence associated with first- or second-degree uterine prolapse*
- *Uterine retrodisplacement*

In addition, the device is available with support for a first- or second-degree cystocele.

Insertion and Removal

Same as for the Hodge.

Other Pessaries to Try

Hodge, Hodge with Support, Incontinence Ring, Incontinence Dish, Incontinence Dish with Support, Mar-Land, or Mar-Land with Support

Incontinence Ring

The incontinence ring *restores continence* by supporting the bladder base and increasing urethral closure pressure and functional urethral length (Figs. 154-1 and 154-2, *5*). It is available in sizes 0 to 10 (sizes 11, 12, and 13 are by special order), and 85% of patients use sizes 2 to 7.

Indications

- *Urinary stress incontinence*

Insertion

Compress the sides like a contraceptive diaphragm, insert the heel into the vault or posterior fornix, and center the ball in the retropubic space.

Removal

Hook the index finger posterior or lateral to the ball, and pull down and out.

Other Pessaries to Try

Hodge, Smith, Risser, Mar-Land, or Incontinence Dish

Incontinence Dish, with and without Support

The incontinence dish (Figs. 154-1 and 154-2) is an adaptation of the incontinence ring. By stabilizing the bladder base, increasing urethral closure pressure, and lengthening the functional urethral, *continence* is restored. *It also offers support to an accompanying mild prolapse.* Incontinence dishes are available in diameter sizes of 55 through 85 mm in increments of 5 mm (85% of patients will use sizes 60 to 75 mm).

Indications

- Stress incontinence coupled with a first- or second-degree cystocele or first- or second-degree uterine prolapse.

Insertion

Compress the sides and turn the device parallel to the introitus. Rotate the device once it is intravaginal so that the heel is posterior to the cervix and the knob is retropubic.

Removal

Hook the device with the index finger, and pull down and out. Alternatively, insert your index finger between the device and the symphysis, grasp between the finger and thumb, and pull down and out.

Other Pessaries to Try

Hodge with Support, Hodge with a Knob with Support, or Mar-Land with Support

Mar-Land, with and without Support*

An adaptation of the Ring pessary, the Mar-Land has a round Silastic base with a half-moon support that fits retropubic (Fig. 154-3). Application of gentle pressure to the urethra *restores continence.* The device is available in sizes 2 to 8 (the most common sizes are 2 to 5).

Indications

- *Stress incontinence*
- *First- or second-degree uterine or vault prolapse*

Insertion

Compress the sides and turn the device parallel to the introitus. Rotate the device once it is intravaginal so

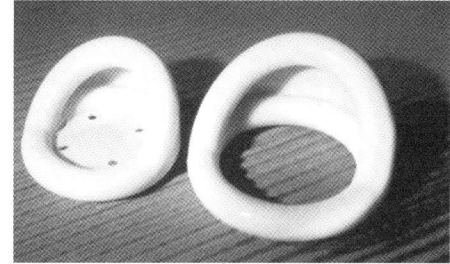

Fig. 154-3
Mar-Land pessaries, with *(left)* and without *(right)* support. (Courtesy Mentor Corporation, Santa Barbara, Calif.)

that the heel is in the vault or posterior fornix and the arch is positioned retropubic. It may also be inserted by folding the pessary in half so that the back ring collapses the supportive sling. The folded pessary should now be in a crescent shape. Insert by directing the crescent shape downward, and advance it until the device is fully intravaginal with the supportive sling retropubic.

Removal

Hook the device with the index finger, and rotate parallel while pulling down and out.

Other Pessaries to Try

Hodge, Hodge with Support, Hodge with a Knob, Hodge with a Knob with Support, Incontinence Ring, Incontinence Ring with Support, or the Incontinence Dish

Gehrung, with or without a Knob*

The Gehrung is manually shapeable, which allows the provider to bend and shape it to conform to the needs of the patient (Figs. 154-1 and 154-2, 6). Support is derived from the lateral remnants of the levator sling. The device is available in sizes 0 through 9 (the most common sizes are 2 through 5).

Indications

- *Cystocele*
- *Rectocele*
- *Uterine prolapse*
- *Cystocele coupled with stress urinary incontinence*

Insertion

Compress the sides of the device and turn it parallel to the introitus. Insert the left heel, advance until the device is fully intravaginal, and rotate the anterior arch forward such that the cystocele rests on the bridge. The heels of the pessary should rest on vaginal floor.

---

*Available from Mentor Corp.

*Available from Milex.

Removal

Push the anterior arch posteriorly toward the rectum; grasp the lateral heel and fold to remove.

Other Pessaries to Try

Hodge, Hodge with Support, Incontinence Ring, Incontinence Dish, or Incontinence Dish with Support

Shaatz*

The Shaatz device has a round silicone base with a slightly concave surface (Fig. 154-1). This pessary is available in diameters of 1½ through 3½ inches in quarter-inch increments (the most common sizes are 2¼ through 3 inches).

Indications

- *First- or second-degree uterine or vault prolapse*
- *Cystocele, enterocele, or rectocele*

Insertion

Compress the sides and turn the device parallel to the introitus advancing until it is fully intravaginal, then rotate with an upward motion until the device is transverse with the concave surface facing up. The cervix rests behind the disc.

Removal

Hook the index finger in the center hole, bringing the device to the introitus. Then rotate parallel and pull the device down and out.

Other Pessaries to Try

Gellhorn, Gehrung, Inflatoball, Ring with Support, Oval Ring with Support, or Donut

Inflatoball (Latex Rubber)

Manual dexterity is a requirement for use of the Inflatoball (Fig. 154-1). It is available in sizes small through extra-large. Medium and large are the two most common sizes.

Indications

- *Third-degree uterine or vault prolapse*
- *Complete procidentia*
- *Any degree of cystocele, enterocele, or rectocele* (not the first choice in cases of mild prolapse)

Insertion

Compress all of the air out of the ball before inserting and attach the inflator bulb to the open end of the stem. Position high in the vagina and inflate to the desired pressure.

Removal

Deflate and remove nightly. The latex rubber will absorb secretions and odors, and the pessary should be left out overnight if possible. Do not pull on the stem to remove.

Other Pessaries to Try

Gellhorn, Gehrung, or Donut

Cube and Tandem Cube*

The Cube is available with holes (special order).

Extreme caution must be exercised with use of this pessary (Figs. 154-1 and 154-2, *8*). The patient must be mentally and physically competent to properly insert and remove the device and comply with follow-up recommendations. Support is achieved from the negative pressure created by the suction action of the six concave surfaces on the vaginal mucosa. Atrophic changes increase the risk of ulceration and erosion, thus a well-estrogenized vagina is essential. The cube is available in sizes 0 through 7 (the most common sizes are 2 through 5). The Tandem Cube is a double cube design with the larger cube inserted first and placed against the uterine cervix. The larger cube is 2 sizes bigger than the small one. Sizes range from 2/0 to 7/5, and the most common sizes are 4/2 to 7/5. There are no holes in the device for drainage.

Indications

- *Third-degree uterine or vaginal vault prolapse*
- *Complete procidentia*
- *Any degree of cystocele, enterocele, or rectocele* (not the first choice in cases of mild prolapse)

The Cube should be tried first. If the Cube fails, then try the Tandem Cube. Young women who experience *stress urinary incontinence when exercising vigorously* (e.g., tennis, aerobics, or jogging) may benefit from this pessary ("athletic support pessary").

Insertion

Compress and insert high in the vagina.

Removal

Removal must be performed nightly. Break the suction by slipping two to three fingers between the vaginal wall and the pessary, then pinch the device between the thumb and index finger, and pull down and out. Do *not* try to remove without breaking the suction or you could damage vaginal mucosa. *Do not pull on the string to remove.* This pessary should be removed, cleaned daily, and left out overnight as often as possible. Regular use of vaginal estrogen cream is recommended in the postmenopausal patient not on replacement hormones.

*Available from Milex.

*Available from Milex.

Other Pessaries to Try

Gellhorn, Inflatoball, Donut, or Gehrung

COMPLICATIONS

- Vaginitis
- Vaginal erosion or ulceration
- Discomfort
- Obstructed defecation and/or urination
- Impaction of the pessary

It is normal for the patient to experience an increase in vaginal discharge. However, odor, itching, change in color, or bleeding should be reported to the provider. Many healthcare providers overlook the importance of estrogen in maintaining the acid pH balance necessary to prevent vaginitis. The vagina should be reestrogenized by using vaginal estrogen cream, 1 g every other night for 1 month, then two to three times per week thereafter. Alternating a pH-adjusted vaginal gel (e.g., Trimo San gel, half applicator, two or three times per week) with the estrogen cream is beneficial as well. In addition to atrophic changes, ulcerations may be associated with a device that is too large or not removed on a regular basis. Discomfort is usually associated with anterior displacement during Valsalva's maneuver or a device that is too large. The patient should wash and push the pessary further in the vagina. If that does not alleviate the discomfort, a smaller size should be tried. Obstruction of defecation should be promptly reported to the provider. Removal of the pessary should resolve the problem, and delay in removal may lead to obstipation. Obstruction of urination should be uncommon if voiding was performed in the office with the device in place. A smaller pessary should resolve the problem. Impaction of the device is rare and typically associated with "forgotten pessaries." A reminder system such as a tickler file will help to alleviate this problem and ensure appropriate follow-up.

PESSARY CARE

Patients should remove the pessary and wash it with warm, soapy water. Soap with deodorants, perfumes, or detergents should not be used. Autoclaving is the recommended method of sterilization for pessaries from the fitting sets between fittings.

FOLLOW-UP CARE

Although much has been written about pessaries, there is no consensus in the literature regarding frequency of removal and follow-up. Ideally, the pessary should be removed nightly, and cleaned and replaced the next morning. Realistically, women are reluctant to comply with such frequency. In many cases, pessaries have been left in the vagina for months at a time without complication. (The Cube and Tandem Cube must be removed nightly because there are no holes for drainage.) The final decision is left to the healthcare provider and should be based on several factors: the patient's mental and physical capacity to insert and remove the device, and her willingness to do so on a regular basis; the health of the vaginal mucosa; the potential for complications; how well the device fits; and the patient's ability to comply with follow-up visits.

In general, the patient should be seen 1 week after the initial fitting, and then 1 month, 3 months, and finally every 6 months thereafter. Patients unable to care for the device themselves should be seen at least every 2 to 3 months. At each visit the patient should be questioned about bowel and bladder function, symptoms associated with vaginitis, vaginal bleeding, and problems with insertion and removal. The vaginal mucosa should be inspected for erythema, ulceration, laceration, and estrogen status. The device may be cleaned and reinserted if there are no complications. The pessary is a foreign body in the vagina. Inspections of the vaginal vault at 3-month intervals seems prudent and warranted.

TIPS

The following are anecdotal helpful hints and not manufacturers' recommendations.

- *Diaphragms:* Do not overlook the usefulness of a simple diaphragm for mild degrees of prolapse or incontinence.
- *Dental tape:* One of the most frequent complaints by women is that they cannot reach the device. A long piece of dental tape placed, for example, on the stem of the Gellhorn or through a hole in the Shaatz may facilitate removal. The tape should be wrapped around the device several times, since it may slice through the silicone.
- *Stay relaxed for device removal:* The patient should keep the pelvic floor muscles relaxed and even give a gentle Valsalva to assist with removal.
- *Estrogen:* Regular use of vaginal estrogen cream should be strongly encouraged. The Estring may also be used with several of the pessaries.
- *Double pessaries:* A small Donut coupled with a Gellhorn pessary may be useful for patients with excessive redundant tissue. The stem of the Gellhorn does not fit through the hole in the Donut (Fig. 154-4).

- *Kegel exercises:* Ongoing performance of Kegel exercises cannot be stressed enough. Useful patient devices include *Kegel Kones* (a set of six weighted devices, which get progressively smaller and heavier). The *Kegel Exersizer* is an intravaginal device that measures intravaginal pressure. The cone-shaped device has an approximately 2-foot flexible hose to transmit the pressure to a gauge to give the patient positive feedback with a proper perineal (Kegel) contraction. Some physical therapy departments have assisted patients with proper technique for Kegel exercises by using this type of device.
- *A woman with very little or no vaginal muscle tonicity and/or marked vaginal wall prolapse* may have difficulty even retaining a Donut or a Gellhorn pessary. In such cases the Cube pessary is indicated. The six concavities of this pessary cling to the vaginal walls, preventing the walls, uterus, bladder, and/or rectum from expelling the pessary. The reason this pessary should be removed nightly is that the Cube fills the entire vaginal cavity so there is no drainage of vaginal-cervical secretions. By adding holes to the Cube, which can be done on request, the suction is lost (bulk is the only thing left). The other, equally important, reason for daily removal of this pessary is that the negative pressure (suction) builds up, making it much more difficult to break the suction and remove the Cube.
- *Sexual activity:* Another factor influencing pessary selection is whether the patient is still sexually active. Since few women are able to insert or remove a Donut or Gellhorn pessary, these pessaries should not be inserted in a woman who wants to remain sexually active.
- *Pessaries and x-rays:* Some pessaries contain wire coils; these pessaries must be removed before an x-ray or MRI. The face page of each pessary instructional brochure indicates whether the pessary contains metal. An instructional brochure is enclosed with each pessary shipped.

CONCLUSION

Although surgical repair remains the treatment of choice for many urogynecologic dysfunctions, pessaries are a viable option for a variety of situations. Their rise in popularity is due in part to the versatility associated with the numerous sizes and shapes now available and in part to the "aging" of the U.S. population.

SUPPLIERS

Kegel Kones, Kegel Exersizer, and related pessary products
Milex Products, Inc.
4311 N. Normandy
Chicago, IL 60634
Phone: 1-800-621-1278
Website:www.milexproducts.com

Mentor Corporation
201 Mentor Drive
Santa Barbara, CA 93111
Phone: 1-805-879-6000
Website: www.mentorcorp.com

Note: UroMed Corporation, holder of the patent on the Introl pessary, is no longer manufacturing this device and no longer stocks the item.

Estring
Pharmacia Corp.
100 Route 206 North
Peapack, NJ 07977
Phone: 1-888-768-5501
Website: www.pharmacia.com

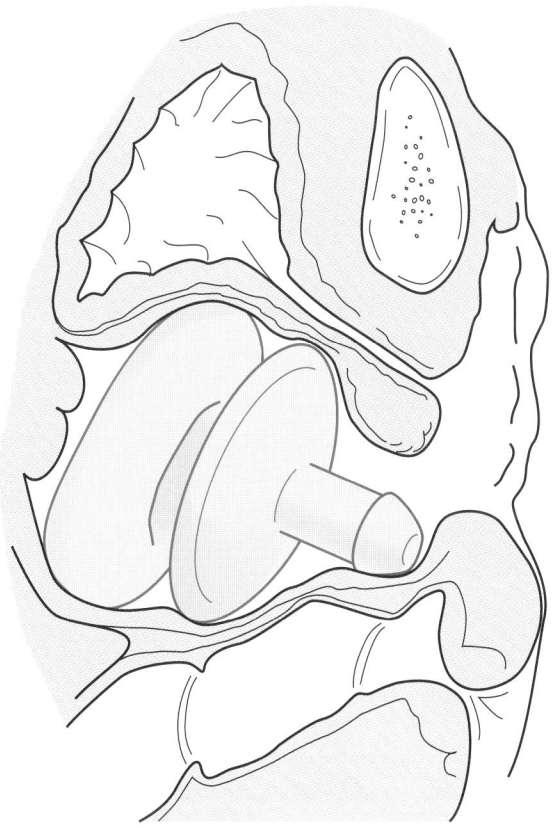

Fig. 154-4
Double pessaries in place. The Donut pessary is inserted first, and the Gellhorn pessary (stem out) is inserted second. (Redrawn from Myers DL, Lasala CA, Murphy JA: Instruments and methods: Double pessary used in grade 4 uterine and vaginal prolapse, *Obstet Gynecol* 91[6]:1019, June 1998.)

CPT/BILLING CODES

The pessary cost is now billed to the local Medicare carrier. A doctor no longer needs a medical supplier number, and routine insurance forms will provide reimbursement.

57160   Pessary fitting and insertion. An E/M code 99211-99215 can be billed in addition depending on documented examination and decision-making complexity. (Only the E/M Code is to be used when the patient comes in for removal and cleaning and reinsertion.)

A4561   Rubber pessaries or intravaginal devices (average reimbursement: $21)

A4562   Nonrubber pessaries or intravaginal devices (average reimbursement: $44.25 to $53.11, depending on the particular region in the country)

The alternative for Part B providers is to write a prescription for the device, have the patient fill the prescription at a local pharmacy, and return with the pessary for insertion. Place of service is the home of the patient. Milex pessaries are not available at pharmacies.

ICD-9-CM DIAGNOSTIC CODES

618.0   Vaginal wall prolapse (w/o uterine prolapse)
618.0   Rectocele, female (w/o uterine prolapse)
618.0   Cystocele, female (w/o prolapse)
618.1   Uterine prolapse (w/o vaginal wall prolapse)
618.2   Uterovaginal prolapse
618.4   Rectocele, female (w/ uterine prolapse)
618.4   Cystocele, female (w/ prolapse)
618.5   Posthysterectomy vault prolapse
618.6   Enterocele, vaginal
618.8   Pelvic relaxation
621.6   Retroflexed uterus, symptomatic
625.6   Incontinence, stress
654.5   Cervical incompetence in pregnancy

ADDITIONAL RESOURCES

- See the sample patient education handout titled "Patient Education for Your Pessary" on page 1950 of Appendix G.

BIBLIOGRAPHY

Bernier F, Harris L: Treating stress incontinence with the bladder neck support prosthesis, *Urol Nur* 16:1, 1995.

Bernier F, Jenkins P: The role of vaginal estrogen in the treatment of urogenital dysfunction in postmenopausal women, *Urol Nur* 17:3, 1997.

Bhatia N, Bergman A: Pessary test in women with urinary incontinence, *Obstet Gynecol* 65:2, 1985.

Davila GW: Vaginal prolapse: management with nonsurgical techniques, *Postgrad Med* 99:4, 1996.

Deger R, Menzin A, Mikuta J: The vaginal pessary: past and present, *Post Grad Obstet Gynecol* 13:18, 1993.

Myers DL, LaSala CA, Murphy JA: Instruments and methods: double pessary use in grade 4 uterine and vaginal prolapse, *Am Coll Obstet Gynecol* 91:6, 1998.

Newcomer J: Pessaries for the treatment of incompetent cervix and premature delivery, *Obstet Gynecol Surv* 55(7):443, 2000.

Sulak R, Kuehl T, Shull B: Vaginal pessaries and their use in pelvic relaxation, *J Reprod Med* 38:12, 1993.

Sultana C: Pessaries for pelvic organ prolapse, *Female patient* 28:59, 2003.

Viera AJ, Larkins-Pettigrew M: Practical use of the pessary, *Am Fam Physician* 61:2719, 2000.

Wu V, Farrell S, Baskett T, Flowerdew G: A simplified protocol for pessary management, *Obstet Gynecol* 90:6, 1997.

Zeitlin MP, Lebherz TB: Pessaries in the geriatric patient, *J Am Geriatr Soc* 40:6, 1992.

CHAPTER 155

Postcoital Examination Test (Sims-Huhner Test)

Barbara S. Apgar

The postcoital test (PCT) is an evaluation of the survival and motility of sperm in the cervical mucus. The test is performed just before ovulation, usually between days 12 and 14 of the normal menstrual cycle. In infertility investigations the incidence of sperm or mucous abnormalities ranges from 20% to 30%. Whether cervical factors are the cause of infertility remains controversial. The PCT does not reliably test for defective cervical function. Results vary because of lack of standardization of the PCT. The PCT should be viewed as a means of detecting if sperm are present in the ejaculate and cervical mucus, rather than as a diagnostic test. The PCT should not be used as a substitute for a semen analysis.

INDICATIONS

- Investigation of the sperm and cervical mucous interaction
- Monitoring the cervical mucus during the first ovulatory cycle of treatment with clomiphene citrate

CONTRAINDICATIONS

- Any condition that would preclude unprotected sexual intercourse followed by examination and sampling of the cervix

EQUIPMENT

- Vaginal speculum
- Vaginal swabs
- Tuberculin syringe with cap
- Microscope
- Glass slides and coverslips
- Plastic endometrial aspirator (see Chapter 146, Endometrial Biopsy) *(optional)*

PREPROCEDURE PATIENT PREPARATION

- Explain the proper timing of intercourse (just before ovulation) to the couple. The PCT should be performed as near as possible to ovulation, when the cervical mucus is the most estrogenic. The test is usually performed on days 12 to 14 of an ideal 28-day cycle. Basal body temperature (BBT) charts will help in determining this diagnostic interval.
- Instruct the couple to abstain from intercourse for 2 days before the test but to have intercourse 6 to 10 hours before the office visit. Before performing the PCT, determine that the BBT is in accord with the proper timing of the menstrual cycle for the performance of the test. An ovulation kit may also be used to determine the correct testing interval.
- Explain that vaginal lubricants, medications, and douches should not be used near the time of intercourse or up to the time of the office visit.
- Instruct the patient to come to the office 6 to 10 hours after intercourse.

TECHNIQUE

1. Place the patient in the lithotomy position. Insert a vaginal speculum and visualize the cervix. Gently wipe the cervix with a vaginal swab.
2. Insert a tuberculin syringe (without the needle) into the endocervical canal and retract the plunger to draw the mucus into the syringe. An endometrial aspirator (which is longer) may also be used to obtain the mucus. If the volume of the specimen is inadequate (usually 2 ml), the procedure may be repeated until a sufficient sample is obtained. Place the syringe cap over the hub once the sample is obtained so that the mucus will be stored in an airtight container until it is ready for processing.
3. Note the amount and clarity of the mucus.

4. Record the degree of stretchability (i.e., spinnbarkeit) of the mucus. A ring forceps or Kelly clamp may be used to grasp the mucus at the cervical os. The stretch of the mucus may be measured as the forceps is removed from the vagina. The mucus can also be placed between the index finger and thumb. The stretch of the mucus is determined as the fingers are drawn apart. A mucous stretch greater than 10 cm is indicative of a high estrogenic state conducive for ovulation. A spinnbarkeit of less than 3 cm indicates a low likelihood that sperm could penetrate through the mucus and an unfavorable situation for ovulation.

5. Place a drop of the mucus from the syringe on a glass slide, and immediately place a coverslip over the sample.

6. Examine the cervical mucus under low power for the presence of sperm and other components, such as trichomonads, leukocytes, squamous cells, or *Candida*. Make a note of the number of sperm. Examine the specimen under high power. The number of sperm in at least five different fields should be averaged. Record an average number or range of numbers of sperm present. Note whether the sperm are mobile, whether they have normal or abnormal morphology, and, if possible, whether they exhibit forward progression. For a normal study, if specimens are examined 6 to 10 hours after intercourse, *there should be an average of at least 10 actively motile sperm per high-power field*. Actively moving sperm are facilitated by the presence of optimal cervical mucus. A decrease in the quality of the cervical mucus and an increase in viscosity and cellularity caused by rising progesterone levels after ovulation impair sperm survival.

The presence of ferning, increased elasticity, and decreased viscosity of the cervical mucus is an indirect indication of estrogen production and ovulation.

Interpretation of Results of the Postcoital Test

All abnormal PCTs should be repeated. The primary cause of a negative or abnormal PCT is failure to accurately time the test. PCTs are usually abnormal in anovulaory cycles. If the initial PCT yields poor results, a second test should be performed 1 to 3 hours after intercourse.

COMPLICATIONS

- The validity of the PCT has been questioned because of varying standards for normal results and because there are numerous techniques for obtaining and interpreting the samples.

- Falsely abnormal results can result from poor timing of the menstrual cycle, poor mucus quality because of infection, faulty coital positions not favoring vaginal sperm retention, and low semen volume or low numbers of sperm. Although a normal PCT is encouraging, an inadequate test does not necessarily preclude fertilization.

POSTPROCEDURE PATIENT EDUCATION

If the test is inconclusive or abnormal, the clinician should ask the patient to return the next month for a repeat examination, or the test strategy should be abandoned and the infertility workup should proceed.

CPT/BILLING CODE

89300　　Semen analysis; presence or motility (or both) of sperm, including Huhner test

ICD-9-CM DIAGNOSTIC CODE

628.9　　Infertility, female
628.4　　　with dysmenorrhea
628.4　　　due to cervical origin
606.9　　Infertility, male
606.0　　　due to azoospermia
606.1　　　oligospermia

BIBLIOGRAPHY

Griffith CS, Grimes DA: The validity of the postcoital test, *Am J Obstet Gynecol* 162(3):615, 1990.

Harrison RF: The diagnostic and therapeutic potential of the postcoital test, *Fertil Steril* 36:71, 1981.

Jones HW, Toner JP: The infertile couple, *N Engl J Med* 329(23):1710, 1993.

Moghissi K: Postcoital test: physiologic basis, technique and interpretation, *Fertil Steril* 27:117, 1976.

Moghissi KS: Cervical factors in infertility, *Contemp Ob Gyn* 38:19, 1993.

Muasher SJ: Infertility. In Rosenwaks Z, Benjamin F, Stone ML, editors: *Gynecology principles and practice*, New York, 1987, Macmillan.

Shane JM: Evaluation and treatment of infertility, *Ciba Found Symposia* 45(2):1, 1993.

Wentz AC: The cervical factor: evaluation and therapy. In Wentz AC, editor: *Gynecologic endocrinology and infertility for the house officer*, Baltimore, 1988, Williams & Wilkins.

CHAPTER 156

Speculoscopy

A Visual Adjunct for Cervical Cancer Screening as part of the PapSure Procedure

Neal M. Lonky

Visual inspection is an essential component of any screening examination of the female lower genital tract. Complete visualization of the cervix during the speculum examination has been traditionally accomplished with standard projected incandescent, fluorescent, or fiberoptic illumination. During the standard Pap smear procedure, after adequate visualization, global cytologic sampling of the exocervix and endocervical canal with sampling devices (cervical spatula and endocervical brush) is performed. Clinicians have increasingly relied on the results of the Pap smear (microscopic evaluation of exfoliative and surface cervical cytology) as the "gold standard" for cervical screening during the past 50 years. Although the implementation of the Pap smear in the United States and other developed countries around the world has led to a reduction of incident cases and deaths associated with cervical cancer since its introduction, that trend has leveled and may have increased over the last 10 to 15 years.

A large proportion of new cases, advanced stage cases, and deaths related to squamous cell carcinoma and adenocarcinoma of the cervix arise in women who do not avail themselves of cancer screening (unscreened or under-screened) because of financial or cultural barriers, or by choice. An appreciable false-negative rate of the standard cervical screening examination also contributes to missed opportunities to discover and treat patients at an earlier stage. The sensitivity of a single Pap smear may be under 50% for the detection of cervical cancer or cancer precursors, and there is a time delay between its performance and the final report. In addition, close to half of all invasive cancers arise in women who received negative standard cervical cancer screening Pap smear results performed within 3 years of their diagnosis. Thus there is a need for more sensitive primary care screening tests that are cost effective and provide timely information to the clinician regarding a patient's risk of harboring cervical neoplasia. This can lead to immediate counseling and triage to a more definitive procedure (colposcopy and cervical biopsy) to establish a diagnosis. The biopsy result may guide treatment and ultimately prevent the morbidity and mortality related to cervical cancer.

The U.S. Food and Drug Administration (FDA) has approved the use of speculoscopy, which is an enhanced method of visualization. After a prewash of the vaginal and cervical tissues with acetic acid, the cervix is viewed with low-power portable magnification (ideally 5× power) and a unique chemiluminescent light source (Speculite). Abnormal areas turn white (acetowhite change). The combination of the Pap smear and speculoscopy is commercially available as PapSure (Torrance, Calif). The FDA has confirmed that screening with PapSure is at least twice as sensitive as using the Pap smear alone for the detection of cervical pathology.

Speculoscopy was developed in the late 1980s to increase the ability of the clinician to identify women with neoplastic lesion(s) of the cervix during the vaginal speculum examination. Not all acetowhite lesions viewed under conventional light represent pathology. However, acetowhite lesions detected during speculoscopy correlate highly (over 90%) with lesions identified during colposcopy (a more expensive diagnostic examination performed after obtaining abnormal findings on cytologic screening). When colposcopic biopsy and histology are used as the basis for comparison, cervical lesions detected with speculoscopy are twice as likely to represent neoplasia (as opposed to metaplasia or inflammation) when compared with naked eye observation after staining. Studies document that this is due to the unique electromagnetic spectral frequency and energy level of the blue-white chemiluminescent light source. Intraepithelial neoplasms appear sharply marginated in contrast to surrounding normal epithelium that take on a bluish hue. This enhancement could not be replicated with blue-filtered, projected traditional illumination.

The cost of speculoscopy is only a small fraction of the charge for a colposcopy. Low cost combined with higher sensitivity make speculoscopy a more ideal screening method. When speculoscopy is used in screening, the clinician can expect an overcall (false positive) rate—the number of false positives divided by the number of women screened—of 4% to 6% (lesions seen and biopsied without histologic evidence of cancer, intraepithelial neoplasia, or human papillomavirus infection [HPV]). Speculoscopy increases the detection of low-grade cervical lesions twofold to threefold and high-grade or cancerous lesions by as much as 40% when compared with the Pap smear alone. Much like colposcopy, speculoscopy cannot aid the clinician in detecting lesions deep in the endocervical canal. Their detection requires the endocervical brush (cell sampling) portion of the PapSure procedure.

The majority of screening errors associated with the traditional Pap smear are due to inadequate cytologic sampling. Lesions (1) may be missed with the sampling device, (2) may be covered by barriers such as keratin, (3) may be deeply embedded in the epithelium, or (4) may never be shed sufficiently to be collected on the sampling device. This occurs in by a subset of patients ("nonshedders") whose cell-to-cell adherence is increased and whose lesions cannot be detected through examination of exfoliative cytology. Adjunctive techniques that rely on cell processing (thin layer preparations), biological testing (e.g., DNA hybridization or probes), or specialized reading of slides (computerized analysis that may use neural networks) cannot address the problem when cells from cervical lesions are not captured for analysis. Research has demonstrated numerous cases in which biopsy-proven intraepithelial lesions and cancers are visualized by the clinician in "real time" with speculoscopy that failed detection with the Pap smear. This improvement in sensitivity provides the opportunity to immediately inform, educate, and manage the patient.

Speculoscopy should not be considered a "stand-alone" screening test in the United States. It should be used as an adjunct to the Pap smear. The combination of visual screening and cervical cytology provides improved sensitivity in identifying women with true mucosal abnormalities or when compared to screening using the Pap smear alone. The combined results of PapSure allow more women with cervical lesions to be identified. They may then be referred for colposcopy, or at least followed more closely.

INDICATIONS

- Any woman coming in for their interval gynecologic screening examination.
- To screen women at high-risk for cervical neoplasia. High-risk status includes, but is not limited to: women with prior cervical neoplasia (treated or untreated); women who are underserved and cannot avail

themselves of regular checkups; women who are unreliable to return for follow-up care because of social or economic barriers; daughters of women who took diethylstilbestrol (DES daughters); women who suffer from immunodeficiency, including the human immunodeficiency syndrome (HIV or AIDS); and women with a history of HPV or other STD infection.

CONTRAINDICATIONS

- In the United States, speculoscopy results should not be used without Pap smear results.
- Speculoscopy is contraindicated in patients in whom a Pap smear is contraindicated. This includes women who have douched or used intravaginal medications within 2 to 3 days of the screening visit.
- Speculoscopy should not be performed in patients in whom acetic acid (5% solution) wash is contraindicated.
- Menses or significant bleeding.
- Vaginal or cervical infection.

Precautions

- The manufacturer warns that, although speculoscopy alone is highly sensitive in detecting neoplastic lesions, only the *combination* of the two tests (Pap plus speculoscopy) provides the most sensitive approach in identifying women with cervical abnormalities.
- Although speculoscopy enhances the examiner's ability to discern acetowhite lesions, it is not intended to grade such lesions or direct biopsies.
- The examiner is reminded to refer any woman with an abnormal Pap smear for colposcopy, even in the presence of a negative speculoscopy result.

EQUIPMENT

The manufacturer provides the following:
- A small, self-contained, plastic capsule (Speculite) that holds the chemiluminescent activator and fluorescent chemicals (similar to the chemiluminescent wands that children use at Halloween, only significantly smaller [3 cm × 1 cm]).
- A disposable, double-sided, adhesive strip for attachment of the Speculite to the upper dilator blade of any speculum or examination tool.
- A small (10 cm × 3 cm), handheld, monocular, low-power (5× to 6×) telescope to provide magnification during the inspection phase of the speculoscopy examination. (A 5× commercially available set of binocular loupes is also acceptable.)
- A clinical data sheet for the medical record and triage chart (Fig. 156-1).

SPECULOSCOPY REPORT

PF#

PATIENT NAME: _____

DATE: _____ AGE: _____ LMP: _____

PREVIOUS PAP SMEAR RESULT: _____ DATE: _____

PATIENT TREATMENT HISTORY: (Cryotherapy, Laser, LEEP)

TYPE: _____ DATE: _____

THE FOLLOWING IS TO BE COMPLETED BY THE EXAMINER

RISK ASSESSMENT: (Circle One)

1. Patient age at first intercourse?   <15   15-20   21-30   >30

2. Patient lifetime number of partners?   1-4   5-10   >10

3. Patient family history of cervical cancer?   YES   NO

4. Does the patient smoke?   YES   NO

5. Patient history of STD?   YES   NO

SPECULOSCOPY EXAM RESULT: (Check One)   ☐ **NEGATIVE**   ☐ **POSITIVE**

DIAGRAM SPECULOSCOPY RESULTS HERE ➤

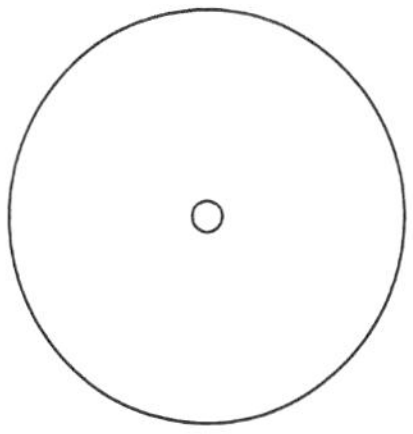

_____ Clinician

MANAGEMENT PLAN: Routine _____   Follow-up In_____ Months Refer to Colposcopy _____

RECORD TODAY'S PAP SMEAR RESULTS HERE: _____

COMMENTS: _____

_____

_____

_____

_____

PapSure™   (FILE IN PATIENT CHART)

Fig. 156-1
Sample speculoscopy report form. (Courtesy of PapSure, Torrance, Calif.)

• A patient educational brochure that describes the rationale behind speculoscopy. It also answers the commonly asked questions about the procedure and the significance of the results.

Other supplies needed include the following:
• A vaginal speculum.
• A 5% acetic acid solution (vinegar).
• Pap smear supplies.

PREPROCEDURE PATIENT PREPARATION

The patient should not be screened if she is actively bleeding or suspects she is suffering from a vaginal infection. She should refrain from douching or using intravaginal medication at least 3 days before the examination. Sexual intercourse should be avoided for 1 to 2 days before the test. A brochure that explains the rationale underlying the use of aided visual testing, the improved sensitivity, and the reduced specificity associated with combining speculoscopy

with cytologic screening is helpful. The brochure also describes the procedural steps in detail, the possible stinging associated with the application of dilute acetic acid, the possible bleeding associated with obtaining an exocervical and endocervical cytologic specimens with a spatula and brush device, the time required to perform the test, and the costs associated with testing. The patient should have time to review it before the examination. The manufacturer provides a modified consent form to document the patient's informed discussion regarding PapSure (see the sample patient consent form titled "PapSure" on page 1949 of Appendix G).

TECHNIQUE

A. Prepare and Activate the Speculite Light Source

1. Remove the Speculite from the foil packet.
2. Firmly bend the Speculite capsule until you feel a "snap" (Fig. 156-2, *A*).

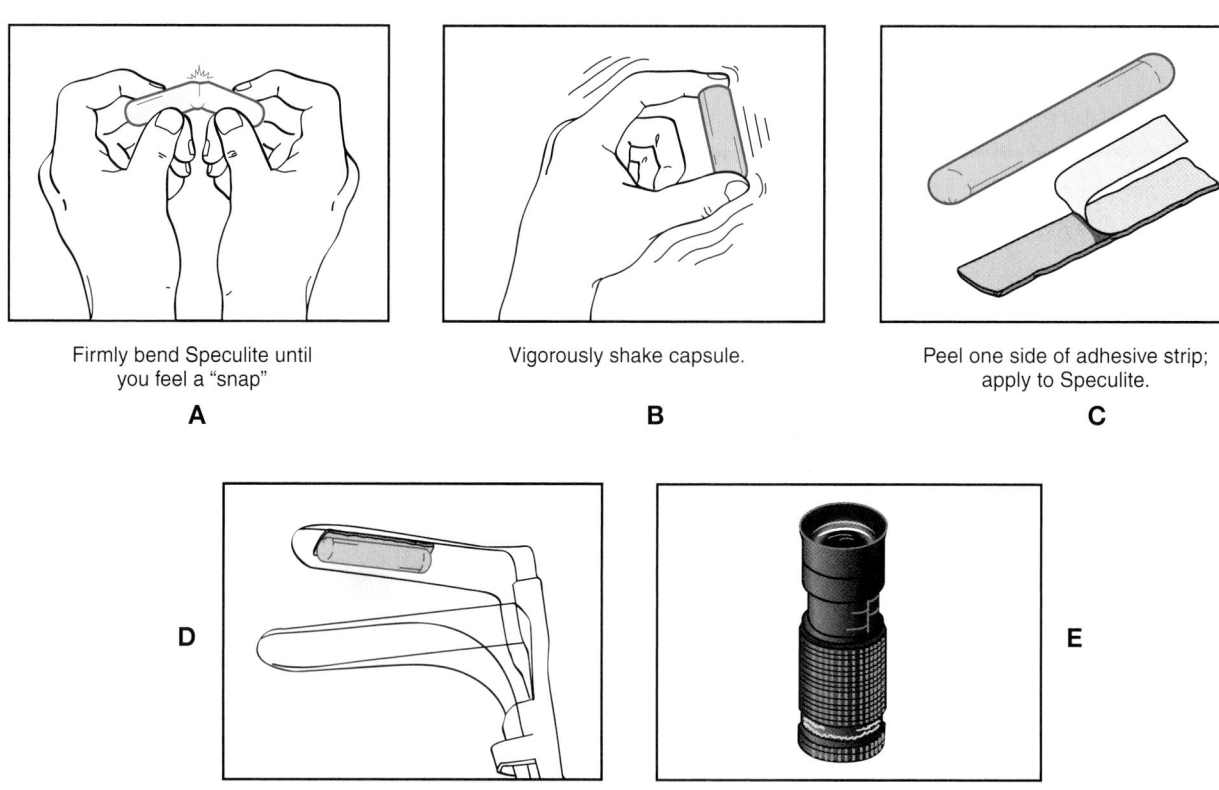

Firmly bend Speculite until
you feel a "snap"

A

Vigorously shake capsule.

B

Peel one side of adhesive strip;
apply to Speculite.

C

D   Speculite applied to
the speculum

E   The telescope "optic"
provided by manufacturer

Fig. 156-2
A, Firmly bend the Speculite until you feel a "snap." **B,** Vigorously shake the capsule. **C,** Peel one side of adhesive strip and apply it to the Speculite. **D,** Speculite applied to the speculum. **E,** Telescope "optic." (**D** and **E,** Redrawn from Trylon Corporation, Torrance, Calif.)

3. Vigorously shake the capsule, distributing the chemicals that produce a "blue-white" light (Fig. 156-2, *B*).
4. Peel off the protective layer from one side of the two-sided adhesive strip and apply to the illuminated Speculite (Fig. 156-2, *C*).
5. Remove the remaining protective layer from the adhesive strip.
6. Attach the light to the inner, upper blade of the speculum (metal or plastic). The brightest illumination produced by the Speculite light source is during the first 5 minutes after the capsule has been activated.

B. Perform the Routine Pap Smear

1. With the patient in the lithotomy position, insert the illuminated speculum, into the vaginal vault.
2. Additional projected incandescent light can be used during this part of the examination.
3. Visually examine the vaginal and cervical mucosa before obtaining the Pap smear and before performing speculoscopy.
4. Perform the routine Pap smear, using the method you prefer. Obtain both an endocervical and exocervical sample at the transformation zone. Be sure to apply fixative to the slide immediately after obtaining the routine Pap smear. If indicated, perform a cervical culture at this time. (See Chapter 152, Pap Smear and Related Techniques for Cervical Cancer Screening.)

C. Perform the Speculoscopy Examination

1. After completing the routine Pap smear, liberally apply 5% acetic acid (common table vinegar) to the vaginal and cervical mucosal surfaces, using a large ob-gyn cotton-tipped applicator, a 4 × 4–inch gauze square, or a cotton ball held with ring forceps.
2. Dim or turn off the room lights. This is a critical step to allow for adequate visualization of the cervix and any lesions. This is analogous to viewing the glow of a white substance under ultraviolet light.
3. With the low-power magnifying optic (5×), prefocused to 16 to 18 inches from the cervix, perform the visual speculoscopy examination. Wait at least 60 seconds after the acetic acid wash before this visualization step.
4. Inspect the mucosa for the presence or absence of white areas. If an aceto-whitened area is present, the speculoscopy result is *positive*. The aceto-whitened areas should have at least one sharply demarcated border between the whitened area and the darker blue or purple normal adjacent cervical tissue. The lesions are not graded with respect to their morpho-

logic appearance or associated vascular patterns. The speculoscopy is either *positive* (+) or *negative* (–). If no distinct aceto-whitened area is seen, the examination is *negative*. If a faint white area is seen with amorphous borders (not sharply demarcated), the examination is *negative*.

5. Possible additional steps include the following:
   a. You may reapply the 5% acetic acid to the cervix to help distinguish acetowhite lesions from mucus.
   b. On occasion, light from the Speculite may reflect from the cervix, causing a slight glare. To distinguish between a reflection and an aceto-whitened area, move the speculum slightly, or press on the cervix with a cotton-tipped applicator to change the contour of the cervix. True lesions remain fixed whereas the shape and location of the glare vary with any movement or compression. This may help differentiate light reflection from a true acetowhite lesion.

D. Document the Results of PapSure and Complete the Pelvic Examination

1. Restore the normal room lighting.
2. Remove the speculum from the patient's vagina.
3. Remove the adhesive strip and the Speculite from the speculum (if it is not a disposable speculum), and discard the strip and Speculite. If the speculum is disposable, discard everything.
4. Complete the pelvic examination.
5. Document speculoscopy findings on the speculoscopy report form (Fig. 156-1).

SUGGESTED CLINICAL MANAGEMENT USING PAPSURE

By combining the routine Pap smear with speculoscopy, a triage plan that uses the results of *two tests* must be considered. A consensus panel led by Dr. Groesbeck P. Parham (Division of Gynelogic Oncology) from the University of Arkansas suggested the following options for clinician's managing patients who are screened with PapSure (Table 156-1).

DEFINITIONS

Positive Pap smear: Bethesda System classification of low-grade squamous intraepithelial neoplasia or worse.

ASC (atypical squamous cells) Pap smear: Bethesda System classification of atypical squamous cells of uncertain significance (ASC-US).

TABLE 156-1

Suggested Clinical Management Using PapSure

Pap Smear Result	Speculoscopy Result	Clinical Management
Positive	Positive	Colposcopy
Positive	Negative	Colposcopy
Negative	Positive	Follow or colposcopy*
Negative	Negative	Routine screening†
ASC	Positive	Colposcopy
ASC	Negative	Follow or colposcopy*

ASC, Atypical squamous cells.

*Patients with concomitant risk factors for cervical disease that include but are not exclusive to: history of cervical neoplasia, prior treatment for cervical neoplasia, smoking history, exposure in utero to diethylstilbestrol, a patient who is unreliable to follow up with the clinician, an underserved patient (rarely or never presents for health services), history of human papillomavirus or human immunodeficiency virus infection, and an immunocompromised patient should receive immediate referral for colposcopy. Those without risk factors should undergo repeat PapSure at approximately 6 months.

†Data from peer review journal publications representing more than 10,000 women examined with PapSure show the negative predictive value of PapSure is 99%. The decision to lengthen cervical cancer screening intervals in low-risk patients may be justified more strongly by using the results of these two tests.

Negative Pap smear: Benign-appearing cytology; adequate specimen.

Positive speculoscopy: The presence of at least one well-demarcated, easily visible acetowhite lesion in which at least one well-defined linear margin can be seen adjacent to the blue or purple normal cervical epithelium.

Negative speculoscopy: Homogeneous blue-purple appearance of the cervical epithelium, which may be interspersed with glossy white reflection of the light source onto the moist cervical epithelium.

Alternatively, faint acetowhite lesions without well demarcated borders are to be considered negative.

Speculoscopy and cytologic sampling can be performed in women who are "status-post hysterectomy," and the presence of vaginal intraepithelial neoplasia or cancer can be determined. The algorithm in Table 156-1 can be used to triage patients with cellular (Pap smear) abnormalities or visible acetowhite lesions.

COMPLICATIONS

- To date, there have been no adverse events associated with the use of chemiluminescence and acetic acid wash during the speculoscopy examination.
- If the capsule that contains the chemiluminescent chemicals should leak during activation or during the examination, there is no potential for injury to epithelial surfaces, but clothing may be stained.

- The possibility that speculoscopy will reveal lesions that lead to colposcopy and biopsy as well as result in normal (no pathology) on biopsy represent false positive tests (both speculoscopy and colposcopy). Prior studies estimated this to occur in 4% to 6% of women screened, which is the lowest rate of all the visual screening modalities.
- The potential for false-negative speculoscopy exists in patients with lesions too small to visualize under low-power magnification or lesions inside the endocervical canal (where no visual test of any magnification strength can reach).

POSTPROCEDURE PATIENT EDUCATION

Although the results of the Pap smear traditionally take days to weeks to return to the clinician, the result of the speculoscopy examination is immediate. This affords the opportunity for immediate counseling and education. The patient should already be familiar with the rationale behind visual testing by reviewing the patient education handout (see the sample titled "PapSure" on page 1947 of Appendix G) before the examination. Patients who are unlikely to return for follow-up should be actively managed into a colposcopy triage plan if their PapSure result is positive by virtue of a visual lesion. This can be stressed at the point of service during the screening visit. Patients with negative speculoscopy screening should be advised that the final result will require the results of cervical cytology, and a phone number or address where the patient can be reach to plan any follow-up visits should be secured before the patient leaves the office. If this poses a problem, immediate colposcopy can be arranged for patients with positive tests.

Patient Consent Form

Speculoscopy is cleared by the FDA for use along with the Pap smear during routine screening for cervical abnormalities. Therefore a patient consent form is required for financial more than for medical reasons (see the sample patient consent form titled "PapSure" on page 1949 of Appendix G).

CONCLUSION

The single-test sensitivity of the Pap smear in detecting cervical neoplasia is less than 50% when colposcopy and biopsy are used as the "gold standard." This should not be confused with laboratory error, which averages 5% to 10% in most laboratories (a Pap smear is reported, then overread by a second expert). Women who exit from the primary cervical screening examination with persistent undiscovered neoplastic lesions (false-negative screening) represent the cohort of "screened" women who are still at risk for progression and death from cervical cancer. By adding the speculoscopy procedure (PapSure: blue-white chemiluminescent light, low-power magnification, and the acetic acid prewash) to the routine Pap smear, the detection of cervical cancer and precancer lesion(s) increases twofold to threefold. The negative predictive value of a negative PapSure examination approaches 99% and allows women to be assigned to a lower-risk status. This may provide additional information to support lengthening screening intervals for low-risk women. Prior data suggest that the routine use of PapSure may lead to an overcall (positive test in women without neoplastic lesions) of 4% to 6% of the population screened.

The probability that unscreened or underscreened women (who are traditionally less likely to follow up) will harbor neoplastic lesions is much higher than the well-screened population, and attention should be paid to screening tests that improve sensitivity and allow for meaningful patient education before the patient leaves the examination setting. The results of speculoscopy are immediate and interpreted by the clinician, as opposed to the delay associated with Pap smears. Because the average cost of speculoscopy is less than one tenth that of colposcopy, it is more affordable in an adjunctive screening role and is ideally suited for primary healthcare providers.

SUPPLIER

PapSure
Trylon Corp.
970 West 190th Street, Suite 850
Torrance, CA 90502
Phone: 1-800-486-8979
Website: www.papsure.com

BILLING AND CODING

CPT/Billing Codes

Note: A specific CPT code has not been established at this time for speculoscopy.

New and Established Patients

Evaluation and management (E & M) codes should be upgraded when PapSure is used as follows:
• Upgrade code (to the next level) for history, physical, and medical decision making.

• When maximum code is used (99215 or 99205), use the Misc. GYN code (58999) and/or the supply code (99070). (To cover cost of speculoscopy supplies, charge cost plus 15%.)

Preventive Medicine (E&M) Age Specific Codes

Add the following:
   Modifier –21 or –22 *or* use code 09922
   or use miscellaneous GYN code 58999 in addition to preventive health code and/or supply code: 99070 (to cover cost of speculoscopy supplies, charge cost +15%)

Capitated and Cash-Paying Patients

Cash: Many offices currently are charging $20 to $25

ICD-9-CM DIAGNOSTIC CODES

622.1	Cervical dysplasia or atypia
233.1	Cervical carcinoma in situ
219.0	Benign neoplasm cervix
6160	Cervicitis
7950	Abnormal Pap

(*Note:* Some insurance will not pay for colposcopy with only this nonspecific code)

6230	Vaginal dysplasia
180.9	Cervical cancer
1840	Vaginal cancer

ADDITIONAL RESOURCES

• See the sample patient education handout titled "PapSure" on page 1947 of Appendix G.
• See the sample patient consent form titled "PapSure" on page 1949 of Appendix G.

BIBLIOGRAPHY

Fahey M, Irwig L, Macaskill P: Meta-analysis of Pap test accuracy, *Am J Epidemiol* 141:680, 1995.
Landis SH, Taylor M, Bolden S, Wingo PA: Cancer statistics for 1998, *CA Cancer J Clin* 48:6, 1998.
Lonky N, Edwards G: Comparison of chemiluminescent light versus incandescent light in the visualization of acetowhite epithelium, *Am J Gynecol Health* VI:11, 1992.
Lonky N, Mann W, Massad L, et al: Ability of visual tests to predict underlying cervical neoplasia, *J Reprod Med* 40:530, 1995.
Mann W, Lonky N, Massad S, et al: Papanicolaou smear screening augmented by magnified chemiluminescent exam, *Int J Gynecol Obstet* 43:289, 1993.
Phillips TJ: Current approaches to venous ulcers and compression, *Am Soc Dermatol Surg* 27:611, 2001.

Taylor LA, Sorensen SV, Ray NF, et al: Cost-effectiveness of the conventional Papanicolaou test with a new adjunct to cytological screening for squamous cell carcinoma of the uterine cervix and its precursors, *Arch Fam Med* 9(8):713, 2000.

Wertlake P, Francus K, Newkirk G, et al: Effectiveness of the Papanicolaou smear and speculoscopy as compared with the Papanicolaou smear alone: a community-based clinical trial, *Obstet Gynecol* 90:421, 1997.

WEBSITES RELATED TO THE PROCEDURE

medicalreporter.health.org/tmr0596/lonky.html (Patient information about Pap smears and cervical cancer prevention)

www.medscape.com/Medscape/womens.health/1996/v01.n10/w155.korn/w155.korn.html (Innovations in screening for cervical neoplasia)

www.papsure.com

Treatment of Noncervical Condyloma Acuminata

Edward J. Mayeaux, Jr.

With the increasing prevalence of human papillomavirus (HPV) infections, effective treatment is of major concern to practicing physicians. HPV infection may be found as acuminate lesions or as acetowhite epithelium (epithelium that turns white after application of acetic acid). Careful inspection and, if possible, colposcopy of the genital area is of great value for locating areas to be treated. HPV is a multicentric disease. Coexisting external and internal lesions or multiple lesions involving the entire lower genital system of both men and women may be present. *Because of the risk of neoplastic transformation, biopsy should be performed if anything is atypical or suspicious about the lesion.* Pigmentation is particularly worrisome. Biopsy should be performed before treatment is initiated. If biopsy is performed after treatment, it is important to communicate to the pathologist the type and amount of preceding treatment. *Any lesion that does not resolve after two treatments of any type should be biopsied.*

The clinician must decide which treatment modality is best, based on clinical skill, extent of disease, and overall chance of success. Because there is no specific "cure" for the HPV virus itself, the goal of treating HPV infections is the elimination of obvious or troublesome lesions (the disease caused by the virus). Since eradication of the virus is probably impossible, the treatment of asymptomatic intraurethral, intravaginal, or cervical condylomata (without dysplasia) exposes the patient to treatment risk without obvious benefit. The patient may harbor HPV-DNA for life; therefore patient education is important to prevent unreasonable expectations. Treating male sexual partners with HPV infection has not appeared to change the posttreatment failure rate in women with cervical dysplasia. These findings should not deter the clinician from appropriately counseling, examining, and treating HPV-infected men. See Chapter 120, Androscopy. All methods of treating HPV have significant failure and recurrence rates. Common modalities for treatment are noted in Table 157-1.

INDICATIONS

- Visible, acuminate condylomata
- Symptomatic condylomata

CONTRAINDICATIONS

- Any known adverse reactions to the selected treatment modality.
- Any lesion that is possibly cancerous. (These lesions should be biopsied before treatment.)

PREPROCEDURE PATIENT PREPARATION

Explain the procedure to the patient, along with the risks and benefits of the procedure. If an investigational drug is to be used, such as 5-fluorouracil (5-FU) (Efudex), the non–FDA approved nature of the therapy should be explained and informed consent should be obtained.

CRYOSURGERY

See Chapter 15, Cryosurgery, and Chapter 141, Cryotherapy of the Cervix.

Equipment

Cryosurgery may be carried out with a variety of cryosurgical methods:
- Cryogun with nitrous oxide tank and small dermal tips
- Liquid nitrogen and cotton-tipped applicators
- Liquid nitrogen pressurized sprayer (Brymill Cryogun, Wallach Ultrafreezer)
- Verruca-Freeze, Ellman MEDI-FRIG

TABLE 157-1

Therapies Currently Available for the Treatment of Genital Warts*

Treatment Modality	Average No. of Treatments	Success Rate†	Recurrence <6 months	Average Length of Study Follow-Up	Total Cost to Patient‡
Ablative Therapy					
CO₂ laser	1.3	89%	8%	13.9 months	$174.50
Cryotherapy	1.9	83%	28%	2.7 months	$156.50
Electrocautery	1.4	93%	24%	3 months	$181.00
Infrared coagulator	1.5	80%	20%	6 months	$178.00
Chemical–Ablative Therapy					
Topical 5-fluorouracil	6.6	71%	13%	10.9 months	$165.00
85% Trichloroacetic acid	4	81%	36%	2 months	$237.50
Podophyllin	4.2	65%	39%	6 months	$237.00
Podophyllotoxin (Condylox)	10.5 (pt applied)	61%	34%	3.2 months	$180.00
Chemical–Immune Enhancer Therapy					
Imiquimod (Aldara)	30 (pt applied)	56%	— §	7 months	$233.00
Interferon (local injection)	11	52%	25%	7.8 months	$805.00
Excisional Therapy					
Blade/scissors	1.1	93%	24%	8.3 months	$161.50
Radiofrequency (loop)	1	90%	— §	8 months	$155.00

*Based on author's best estimate as compiled from available English-language literature. Very small studies, study results that fell 2 standard deviations beyond the means, and very poorly designed studies were excluded.
†Defined as clearance of all condyloma at end of therapy or healing from therapy.
‡Based on hypothetical patients without other medical problems and local prices. Cost based on all of the following that apply: $75.00 for initial visit, $50.00 for any second follow-up, and $35.00 for each additional follow-up; $30.00 for anesthetic or therapeutic injections; $55.00 for the pharmacy cost of Condylox; $40.00 for SFU; $7.50 for TCA; and $108.00 for Imiquimod. One posttreatment follow-up is assumed. Local prices usually vary.
§No data or not recorded.

Techniques

General Techniques for All Methods

1. No anesthetic is required for cryotherapy, although if there are large or multiple lesions, patients may prefer it.
2. Place the patient in the lithotomy position and examine the vulva, perineum, and rectum (or scrotum and penis). If the lesions cover a large area, it may be prudent to treat sections at separate visits to prevent excessive posttreatment discomfort. Treatment should be directed at the acuminate warts rather than at subclinical condylomata that cannot be seen with the naked eye. Staining with dilute acetic acid may make smaller acuminate lesions more prominent.

Nitrous Oxide, Method

1. Select the proper size of cryotip based on the size of the lesion. The tip should cover small lesions; larger lesions may be frozen in sections or clusters.
2. Moisten the lesion with water-soluble gel before positioning the probe to improve tip-to-tissue adhesion. With the cryotip at ambient temperature, place the tip on an individual lesion. Activate the cryogun to initiate the flow of gas within the probe, which begins the freezing process. Apply gentle traction on the lesion to lift the skin away from underlying tissue as soon as ice appears on the tissue (this is

especially important on the penile shaft). This traction isolates the lesion from the surrounding tissue, minimizes discomfort, and ensures cold transfer. Clumped lesions may be frozen in clusters but will require longer freezing times. Clusters also require the freeze-thaw-refreeze technique to produce the necessary cryonecrosis. (The tissue is frozen until it appears solid white, then thawed until it turns pink again, and then frozen a second time.) Stop freezing as soon as the ice extends just 2 to 3 mm beyond each lesion's border. All lesions are frozen. Some practitioners prefer a second application after the initial thaw in all cases.

3. Explain to the patient that a tingling or burning sensation is normal, especially with thawing.

Gases (Verruca-Freeze and MediFrig), Liquid Nitrogen (Cotton-Tipped Applicator and Spray)

1. Standard or large cotton-tipped applicators may be used to apply liquid nitrogen. Standard applicators (Q-Tips) work better if wisps of cotton are pulled from a cotton ball and twirled to add bulk to the end of the applicator. Pour liquid nitrogen into a Styrofoam cup. Dip the cotton-tipped applicator into the liquid nitrogen and apply immediately to the lesion. Reapply until the lesion turns white. Avoid freezing more than 2 to 3 mm beyond the

border of the lesion. Thaw time should take at least 1 minute.

2. With the Thermos-type container (Brymill Mini-Freezer and Wallach Ultrafreezer), spray a jet of liquid nitrogen on the lesions. Select an orifice large enough to have the site of the spray cover the lesion, but do not overspray. (This is a quick and economical use of liquid nitrogen.) Apply the liquid nitrogen until the lesion turns white. Avoid freezing more than 2 to 3 mm beyond the lesion. Thaw time should take at least 1 minute. A spray guard is available to protect surrounding skin. Alternatively, the physician can use an ear speculum to place around the lesion and limit excessive overspray.

3. Verruca-Freeze and MEDIFRIG work similar to liquid nitrogen and an ear speculum is placed over the wart. Compressed gas in a can is sprayed into it. A speculum should be selected that just covers the lesion. The compressed gas liquefies with spraying, and rapid evaporation results in freezing of the lesion. Use of this agent obviates the need for maintaining large amounts of liquid nitrogen. The speculum must be positioned so that it is perpendicular to the lesion; in this way it acts like a funnel. This position requirement may be impractical on the genitalia. Once the material is sprayed into the speculum, it is held in place until the bubbling stops. Care must be taken that the liquid does not leak out from under the speculum and freeze normal tissue. One application may suffice on small lesions. If the lesions are large, a second application may be necessary after thawing. There are also cotton-tipped applicator-like attachments that allow this device to be used in a manner similar to step 1.

Postprocedure Patient Education

- Usually no postprocedure medication is needed. Topical anesthetic ointments may be used to minimize discomfort. Sitz baths may aid resolution when large areas are treated. Silver sulfadiazine (Silvadene) ointment or other antibiotic ointments may not only be soothing but may also reduce the possibility of superficial infection. They also help keep the denuded tissue from sticking to underclothing. Moist environments also promote healing with less scarring. No dressing is required, but some patients may request a sanitary napkin. Ice packs are helpful.

- Lesions that are cryonecrosed progress from erythema to edema and then turn black. They may also blister up. The blister may be left intact or removed. The lesions disappear within a few days, and healing should be complete in 7 to 8 days.

- The patient should be advised to report any signs of infection or excessive discomfort.

- Treated areas should be washed with mild soap and water several times each day. Postcryotherapy management is similar to a second-degree burn.

Complications

- If the area treated at one visit is too large, extensive necrosis and pain may occur. It is prudent to treat large areas over multiple visits. Infection may occur at the treatment site if the area is not kept clean by normal hygienic measures.
- Recurrence or persistence of lesions is common.
- Cryotherapy is probably the safest therapy for treating HPV lesions during pregnancy.
- Cryoguns are associated with a higher risk of perforation and fistula formation inside the vagina when compared with the cotton-tipped applicator method.

Suppliers

See Chapter 15, Cryosurgery.

CHEMICAL CAUTERY

Equipment

- Bichloracetic acid (BCA), 85% trichloroacetic acid (TCA), podophyllin, or 0.5% podofilox (Condylox)
- Cotton-tipped applicators or toothpicks

Technique

1. For BCA, TCA, or podophyllin, identify the lesions to be treated. For small lesions, use the wooden end of the cotton-tipped applicator or a toothpick to apply the solution directly on the lesion. Avoid getting the solution on normal skin. However, the wart virus can be identified 3 mm beyond the obvious lesion. Also, do not apply Vaseline or other ointment around the lesions; besides being time consuming, it often gets on the lesion itself and protects exactly what is meant to be treated. For larger lesions, use the cotton-tipped end of the applicator to apply the solution, again being careful to avoid getting the solution on normal skin. Continue in the same manner until all the lesions are treated. The patient may experience intense pain, which will subside in about 5 minutes. In 1 to 2 days the skin will slough. Patients may need retreatment every 2 weeks until the lesions resolve.

Note: Use of podophyllin in pregnant patients and on occluded mucous membranes is contraindicated.

2. Patients may apply topical 0.5% podofilox solution or gel themselves at home. Podofilox is a pure standardized compound of the active ingredient in podophyl-

lin. Podofilox is indicated for topical treatment of external genital warts, but it is not indicated for the treatment of mucous membrane (urethra, rectum, vagina) condyloma. Podofilox is applied to the warts with a cotton-tipped applicator supplied with the medication. Treatment should be limited to an area less than 10 cm², and no more than 0.5 ml of the solution should be used each day. The solution is applied in the morning and evening for 3 consecutive days; then a 4-day waiting period is observed, during which the solution is not applied. This 1-week treatment cycle may be repeated six times or until there is no visible wart tissue. Remember the "2-3-4-6 Rule": twice a day for 3 days, off for 4 days, used for 6 weeks. Later, the entire treatment can be repeated. There are no established guidelines for use in pregnant women, young children, and nursing mothers.

Complications

- Treatment with too much solution can lead to excessive tissue damage and prolonged healing.
- Persistence and recurrence is not uncommon.
- Systemic reactions with extensive exposure to podophyllin may include nausea, vomiting, fever, confusion, coma, renal failure, ileus, and leukopenia. Local reactions include erosions, ulcerations, scarring, balanitis, and phimosis.
- Seizures have occurred with application of podophyllin to mucous membranes.

Postprocedure Patient Education

- For lesions that are cauterized chemically, the healing process is usually less than 1 week but may take longer.
- Patient education sheets are supplied by the manufacturer of podofilox.

INTERFERON THERAPY

Indications

- Recalcitrant condyloma unresponsive to other modalities

Contraindications

- Pregnancy

Equipment

- Recombinant interferon alfa-2b
- 27- to 30-gauge needle and a 1-ml syringe

Technique

1. The manufacturer recommends that only five warts be treated at one time, making this treatment time consuming and expensive.
2. The standard dose is 1 million U of interferon (0.1 ml) three times a week for 3 weeks (total of nine injections).
3. Use a 25- to 30-gauge needle to inject the interferon directly into the center of the wart's base (intralesional).
4. Maximum response should occur within 4 to 6 weeks. If there is no clinical response after 16 weeks, a second 3-week course should be completed.

Complications

- Flulike symptoms such as myalgias, fatigue, headache, chills, and fever may occur.
- May cause menstrual problems in adolescents.
- Treatment beyond 3 weeks may cause reversible leukopenia and liver enzyme elevations.

Postprocedure Patient Education

- The patient may take an analgesic if flulike symptoms develop.

ELECTROSURGERY OR LASER THERAPY

Treatment of warts with electrosurgery can be ablative or excisional. Lesions that are small or few in number can be cauterized easily with a ball or needle electrode. Modern electrosurgery uses radiofrequency technology and a loop electrode (see below). Place the electrosurgical unit on coagulation (or hemostasis) with just enough power to "cook" the wart. Wipe away the debris. If viable tissue remains, touch the wart again with the electrode. Condylomata are epidermal, and there is little need or desire to go deep. With "just enough" current there will be little scarring. An alternative approach would be laser ablation, but it is expensive. It is more commonly used when there are extensive condyloma on the vulva or when the vagina and/or cervix also need treatment. (See Chapter 27, Laser Therapy.)

SURGICAL REMOVAL

Condyloma can be excised surgically with sharp iris scissors or a knife blade after appropriate anesthesia. However, the penile and vulvar skin is thin; it is easy to resect too deeply, which may result in scarring. Warty lesions also tend to be vascular and bleed easily. Although this can be controlled with Monsel's solution, it is often easier to use radiofrequency (loop) excisional surgery, especially for bigger lesions (see below as well as Chapter 31, Radiofrequency Surgery). For small pedunculated growths, scissor excision may be ideal.

LOOP ELECTROSURGICAL EXCISION

Also see Chapter 31, Radiofrequency Surgery.

Equipment

- Square or round loop electrodes (Use loop size consistent with the size of the warts. Use dermatology electrodes with shorter shafts rather than the longer ones used to carry out the loop electrosurgical excision procedure [LEEP] procedure. The shorter shafts allow better control of depth, and the operator's hand can be stabilized against surrounding tissue.)
- Electrosurgical generator (ESU)
- Colposcope or 3× to 5× magnification lens
- Grounding pad or antenna
- Smoke evacuator
- 2% lidocaine with or without epinephrine (Epinephrine should not be used on the penis.)
- Syringe with 30-gauge needle
- Ball electrodes (5 mm)
- Macroneedle electrodes
- Silvadene or other antibiotic cream
- Virus-filtering (submicron) mask and nonsterile gloves
- 4 × 4–inch sterile gauze pads
- Acetic acid
- Monsel's solution
- Formalin bottles

Suppliers

See list of companies for radiofrequency units in Chapter 31, Radiofrequency Surgery, and Chapter 150, Loop Electrosurgical Excision Procedure (LEEP) for Treating Cervical Intraepithelial Neoplasia.

Preprocedure Patient Preparation

Explain the procedure to the patient, and obtain informed consent. The major risks are pain, bleeding, infection, recurrence, and scarring.

Technique

1. Apply 5% acetic acid (or vinegar) to the warts. Keep the tissue moist by repeated acetic acid application.
2. Turn on the ESU power supply. Check the manufacturer's guidelines for proper power settings (usually around 15 to 20 watts).
3. Place the grounding pad on the thigh or buttocks.
4. With a 27- to 30-gauge needle, inject 2% lidocaine under the base of the wart to make a wheal that extends beyond the margin of the wart.
5. Activate the smoke evacuator and place the hose close to the excisional site.
6. Select the cutting (preferred) or blend mode on the ESU.
7. Using a method of magnification allows more precise removal and assurance that small lesions are not missed. The loop should not excise deeper than 1 mm to the dermal-epidermal junction (looks like chamois cloth). Often it is best just to "debulk" the wart on the first pass. Then make fine, superficial "feathering" strokes to remove the remaining tissue. Significant bleeding may be a signal that the excision is too deep or, paradoxically, that there is residual wart tissue. To control the depth of excision, place the fifth finger of the hand holding the pencil wand with the electrode on the index finger of the opposite hand that is used to expose the lesion. The loop will travel between the spread index finger and thumb of the nondominant hand. Hold the pencil wand close to where the electrode inserts into the wand. Use caution, because the loops cut very quickly.
8. After the loop electrode has been used to excise the wart, the ball electrode or macroneedle may be used to coagulate any bleeders or residual tissue, although this is rarely necessary.
9. Remove the coagulated remnants with cotton-tip applicators or gauze sponges soaked with acetic acid (5%).
10. Upon completion, inspect the excised area with the colposcope to ensure that the entire wart has been excised and that no coagulated remnants are left at the base of the excised lesion. Also be sure no small lesions have been missed.
11. Apply an antibiotic ointment to the excision area, and use gauze pads to cover the excision site.

Note: Many patients prefer this modality over chemical cautery methods because healing is often more rapid and less painful.

Complications

- Hypopigmentation may rarely occur at the excision site. Keloids may form on skin that has a tendency for keloid formation.
- Postprocedure bleeding and wound infections are extremely rare.
- According to Ferenczy (1990), treatment failure at 8 months (average two treatments) is 19%.

- If the procedure is performed correctly, scarring is minimal and comparable with that of laser excision.

Postprocedure Patient Education

- Provide the patient with the sample patient education handout titled "Genital Condyloma (Wart) Removal" on page 1887 of Appendix G. Instruct the patient that postprocedure discomfort may last for up to 2 weeks. However, initial discomfort should resolve in 24 to 48 hours. When large areas have been treated during the initial recovery period, sitz baths may be taken two to three times a day. At a minimum, the area should be washed three to four times per day, followed by application of an antibiotic ointment or other ointment. This is continued for 5 to 7 days until reepithelialization has taken place. Ice packs may also be used initially. For those patients who have perianal removals, stool softeners (docusate sodium) are important throughout the entire recovery period.
- If acute discomfort persists beyond 48 hours, instruct the patient to contact the physician. Rarely, a mixture of equal parts of 20% benzocaine (Hurricaine) ointment and silver sulfadiazine may be used. Lidocaine ointment 5% provides excellent relief and also keeps the tissues moist. NSAIDs are also beneficial.
- Instruct the patient to return to the office in 4 to 6 weeks, and to call if fever, chills, or purulent discharge develop.

INFRARED COAGULATION

Infrared coagulation (IRC) can be used to ablate warts on the external genitals as well as mucous membranes. The advantages are that it is quick, and depth of destruction is readily controlled by the automatic timer. (See Chapter 108, Office Treatment of Hemorrhoids.) Destruction occurs when infrared light travels down the light guide and concentrates on the lesion. There is no electrical current involved.

Technique

1. Anesthetize lesions.
2. Set timer on 1 to 1.25 seconds for the average lesion. If the lesion is quite thick, the unit can be set up to 3 seconds. The depth of penetration will be roughly 1 mm/sec applied.
3. Apply the Teflon-coated tip to the lesion using slight pressure.
4. Pull the trigger and hold it in place until it automatically turns off. The light will not harm the eyes,

although it is bright and uncomfortable if directly viewed.
5. Wiping the tip and allowing the tip to cool for a few seconds between applications is recommended.
6. If the lesion was large, reapplication is carried out with slight overlapping.
7. Wipe away the ablated tissue with moistened gauze and determine if depth is adequate.
8. Treat the next lesion.
9. Postoperative treatment is the same as noted for other ablative treatments with electrocautery and acids.
10. Reexamine and retreat if necessary in 3 to 4 weeks. Expect slight denuding of the epithelium and mild ulceration as seen with topical acid treatments. There is generally little residual scarring.

IMIQUIMOD CREAM (ALDARA)

Imiquimod (Aldara) cream is a unique approach to HPV treatment. It acts as an immune stimulator by inducing multiple subtypes of interferon-alpha (INF-α). This causes induction of several cytokines, including tumor necrosis factor and interleukins. These in turn activate natural killer cells, T-cells, polymorphonuclear neutrophil leukocytes, and macrophages, thus increasing antitumor activity. The drug has almost no systemic side effects. Use of this drug in children has not been evaluated. It can be used after other treatments to reduce recurrences.

Indications

- Can be used on all external HPV-infected sites.
- It is a pregnancy class B drug.

Technique

The cream comes in small packets (box of 12) and is applied to the lesions three times a week for up to 16 weeks. The cream may be applied to the affected area, not strictly to the lesion itself. For best results, it must be rubbed in well, not just lightly applied to the involved areas.

Complications

- Side effects can include erythema, erosion, itching, skin flaking, and edema. Therapy may be temporarily halted if symptoms become problematic.
- Not for use on occluded mucous membranes or on the uterine cervix.
- Not recommended for use with condoms or diaphragms because of possible latex damage.
- Persistence or recurrence of infections.

5-FLUOROURACIL (5-FU)

Treatment with 5-FU should be considered only for extensive intractable condyloma resistant to other modalities or for the treatment of vaginal intraepithelial neoplasia (VAIN). The Food and Drug Administration has not approved labeling of 5-FU for treatment of condylomata, and the patient should be advised that this is technically an investigational use. Because of the reported teratogenic potential, 5-FU should be used with extreme caution—if at all—in nonsterile women of reproductive age. If used, a signed consent form should be obtained with the patient indicating she will not become pregnant. Although commonly used historically, 5-FU use has fallen into disfavor for HPV treatment because of complications of vaginal scarring and the development of other more acceptable methods.

Indications

- Extensive vulvar, perianal, penile, or vaginal condyloma
- Vaginal intraepithelial neoplasia (VAIN)
- Vulvar intraepithelial neoplasia (VIN)
- Urethral meatus lesions

Caution: Patients with blond or red hair, or with very light complexions, may be more sensitive to 5-FU. Also use cautiously in patients with known skin sensitivities such as atopic dermatitis. Mucosal areas are much more sensitive than keratinized skin.

Contraindications

- Pregnancy
- Lack of birth control method (relative contraindication)

Equipment

- 5% 5-FU (Efudex, Fluoroplex) cream
- Vaginal applicator marked with dosage lines

Preprocedure Patient Preparation

- Obtain informed consent before initiating treatment.
- Advise the patient of alternative methods of treatment. Frequently when 5-FU is being considered, laser or LEEP therapy is also an option.
- The patient should know that the inflammatory response is delayed by 3 to 4 days. The patient may believe the medication is not working and apply it more frequently, leading to complications.
- Use of 5-FU should be limited to clinicians experienced with managing side effects, which are similar to those experienced when treating the face for actinic changes (e.g., chemical burns). See the sample patient teaching guide titled "Efudex Protocol" on page 1954 of Appendix G.

Technique

1. For the vagina, instruct the patient to use 1.5 g of 5-FU per week for 10 weeks. A standard Ortho vaginal applicator will hold 10 ml of cream (5 g of 5-FU). Patients should then use only one third of an applicator of cream for each treatment. The 5-FU should be inserted intravaginally and/or applied directly to any external lesions at bedtime (for perianal, etc.).
2. Instruct the patient to apply zinc oxide to the vulva or scrotum (where treatment is not necessary) to protect it in the event that the 5-FU should leak out onto the vulva or the sacs come into contact with perineal or perianal application. This is not necessary if external condyloma exist in this area, but the scrotum is extremely sensitive to this drug and should be protected at all times.
3. The patient may insert a small tampon into the vagina to keep the 5-FU within the introitus.
4. If there is no inflammatory response after 3 weeks, the patient may increase the frequency of application to every 5 days.

Complications

- Pain.
- Bleeding.
- Persistence of disease.
- Persistent vaginal ulcers may develop in patients who are extremely sensitive to the 5-FU or in patients who overuse the medication. For some patients, the vaginal ulcers may fail to heal with time, and they may have persistent vaginal discharge and bleeding (rare). Patients who fail to heal may require surgical excision of the ulcer and primary closure of the defect.
- Vaginal stenosis (rare).
- If 5-FU is to be used after cryotherapy of the cervix, wait at least 4 weeks before initiating 5-FU therapy to avoid cervical stenosis.

Postprocedure Patient Education

Instruct the patient to contact the physician if severe inflammation or any hypersensitivity reaction occurs. Intravaginal estrogens or steroid creams may be used to decrease the inflammatory reaction. See the sample patient education handout titled "Genital Condyloma (Wart) Removal" on page 1887 on Appendix G.

PERIANAL AND INTRAANAL LESIONS

Treatment of perianal and intraanal lesions is similar to treatment for vaginal condylomata. Additional guidelines are as follows:

• Podofilox and imiquimod should not be used on mucous membranes (i.e., inside the anus). TCA, excisional therapy, electrocautery, and the infrared coagulation may be used intraanally.
• Anoscopy should be performed on all patients with perianal lesions to rule out more proximal lesions. This is often done after resolution of the external lesions to avoid possible trauma and potential spread of the virus proximally.
• The risk of rectal carcinoma is increased 50 times in receptive homosexual men, and HPV appears to be involved in the process. Some suggest Pap smears of the dentate line of the anus to detect early dysplastic lesions just as with the cervix.

CONDYLOMA IN PREGNANCY

Condyloma may grow rapidly in size and multiply quickly especially during the second trimester immune suppression. After delivery, they may and often do resolve spontaneously. Women who have warts in the perineum with subsequent tears or episiotomies have a higher risk of dehiscence of the wound. Most physicians recommend treatment of perineal condyloma during the third trimester. Safe modalities include cryotherapy, 85% TCA, electrocautery, laser therapy, IRC, and radiofrequency (loop) or sharp tissue scissor excision. Although cryotherapy may be used, there is often more swelling and discomfort.

It appears that HPV is in the amniotic fluid of infected mothers, so there is no indication for C-section unless the lesions are so large that they inhibit normal delivery.

GENERAL CONSIDERATIONS FOR ALL METHODS

• HPV is associated with cervical cancer, and women must be followed closely with Pap smears and/or colposcopy.
• The patient and partner must not smoke. Even passive smokers have been found to have lower folate levels—a known risk for HPV. Reducing smoking does lead to reduction in cervical dysplasia, whereas continuing to smoke encourages progression.
• The patient should consume a diet with at least five helpings of fruits and vegetables.
• A multivitamin with 400 µg of folic acid is recommended to enhance the immune system.
• Patients must be informed that they can spread the disease at any time and that monogamy is most prudent.
• Condoms are not needed with current partners, since they already have the virus; once infected, the patient will always have the virus. Although condoms protect from other STDs, the FDA is considering requiring all condom manufacturers to state that they do not protect the patient from HPV, since it is all around the area including the vulva, scrotum, and perineum, which are not protected by the condom. See Box 157-1 for a summary of treatment options for various locations.

BOX 157-1

Methods of Preferred Treatment for Various Locations of Condylomata

External Genital/Perianal Condylomata
Cryotherapy
Podofilox, podophyllin
Imiquimod
85% TCA
Electrocautery
Electro/radiofrequency excision
Laser

Cervical Warts
Must rule out dysplasia before treatment (perform colposcopy), then the following:
    Cryotherapy
    85% TCA
    Electrocautery
    Excision with radiofrequency or multiple biopsies

Vaginal
Cryotherapy
85% TCA
Electrocautery
5-FU (extensive disease)
Laser

Urerthral Meatus
Cryotherapy
Electrocautery
85% TCA
Excision
5-FU (small amount on a Q-Tip bid × 7 days)

Anal
Cryotherapy
85% TCA
Surgical
Electrocautery

Oral
Cryotherapy
Electrocautery
Excision

Pregnancy
Cryotherapy
Electrocautery/excision
85% TCA

5-FU, 5-Fluorouracil; *TCA,* trichloroacetic acid.

CPT/BILLING CODES

11900 Injection, intralesional; up to and including seven lesions *(interferon)*

11901 Injection intralesional; more than seven lesions

46900 Destruction of lesion(s); *anus* (e.g., condyloma), simple; chemical

46910 Destruction of lesion(s); *anus* electrodesiccation, simple

46916 Destruction of lesion(s); *anus* cryosurgery, simple

46922 Destruction of lesion(s); *anus* surgical excision, simple

46924 Destruction of lesion(s); *anus, extensive; any method*

Note: Use this code if removal takes more than 15 minutes or if there are more than 15 large lesions.

54050 Destruction of lesion(s); *penis* (e.g., condyloma), simple; chemical

54055 Destruction of lesion(s); *penis* electrodesiccation, simple

54056 Destruction of lesion(s); *penis* cryosurgery, simple

54060 Destruction of lesion(s); *penis* surgical excision, simple

54065 Destruction of lesion(s); *penis, extensive, any method* (see guidelines above for 46924)

54100 Biopsy, cutaneous, *penis*

56501 Destruction of lesion(s); *vulva*, simple; any method

56515 Destruction of lesion(s); *vulva, extensive, any method* (see guidelines above for 46924)

56605 Biopsy, *vulva* introitus

57061 Destruction of lesion(s); *vagina*, simple; any method

57065 Destruction of lesion(s); *vagina*, extensive; any method (see guidelines above for 46924)

57100 Biopsy, *vagina*

ICD-9-CM DIAGNOSTIC CODE

07811 Condyloma, any site

ADDITIONAL RESOURCES

- See the sample patient education handouts titled "Efudex Protocol" and "Genital Condyloma (Wart) Removal" on pages 1954 and 1887, respectively, of Appendix G.

BIBLIOGRAPHY

Baker DA, Douglas JM Jr, Buntin DM, et al: Topical podofilox for the treatment of condylomata acuminata in women, *Obstet Gynecol* 76(4):656, 1990.

Bekassy Z, Westrom L: Infrared coagulation in the treatment of condyloma acuminata in the female genital tract, *Sex Trans Dis* 14:209, 1987.

Bergman A, Bhatia NN, Broen EM: Cryotherapy for the treatment of genital condylomata during pregnancy, *J Reprod Med* 29:432, 1984.

Brown DR, Fife KR: Human papillomavirus infections of the genital tract, *Med Clin North Am* 74:1455, 1990.

Chamberlain MJ, Reynolds AL, Yeoman YB: Toxic effects of podophyllum application in pregnancy, *Br Med J* 3:391, 1972.

Edwards L, Ferenczy A, Eron L, et al: Self-administered topical 5% Imiquimod cream for external anogenital warts, *Arch Dermatol* 134:25, 1998.

Eron LJ, Judson F, Tucker S, et al: Interferon therapy for condyloma acuminata, *N Engl J Med* 315(17):1059, 1986.

Felmar E et al: Primary care office procedures: treatment of genital lesions via cryocautery, *Prim Care Cancer* 6:1, 1988.

Ferenczy A et al: *Loop electrosurgical excision procedure (LEEP) syllabus,* Shelton, Conn, 1991, Cooper Surgical.

Ferenczy A: Diagnosis and treatment of anogenital warts in the male patient, *Prim Care* 10:11, 1990.

Fletcher JL: Perinatal transmission of human papillomavirus, *Am Fam Physician* 43:143, 1991.

Friedman-Kien AE, Eron LJ, Conant M, et al: Natural interferon alfa for treatment of condyloma acuminata, *JAMA* 259(4):533, 1988.

Frisch M, Fenger C, van den Brule AJ, et al: Variants of squamous cell carcinoma of the anal canal and perianal skin and their relation to human papillomaviruses, *Cancer Res* 59(3):753, 1999.

Greenberg MD, Rutledge LH, Reid R, et al: A double-blind, randomized trial of 0.5% podofilox and placebo for the treatment of genital warts in women, *Obstet Gynecol* 77:735, 1991.

Human papillomavirus infection, *MMWR* 42:83, 1993.

Kling AR: Genital warts: therapy, *Semin Dermatol* 11:247, 1992.

Krebs HB: Treatment of vaginal condylomata acuminata by weekly topical application of 5-fluorouracil, *Obstet Gynecol* 70(1):68, 1987.

Krebs HB: Treatment of vaginal intraepithelial neoplasia with laser and topical 5-fluorouracil, *Obstet Gynecol* 73(4):657, 1989.

Krebs HB, Helmkamp BF: Chronic ulcerations following topical therapy with 5-fluorouracil for vaginal human papillomavirus-associated lesions, *Obstet Gynecol* 78(2):205, 1991.

Krebs HB, Helmkamp BF: Treatment failure of genital condylomata in women: role of the male sexual partner, *Obstet Gynecol* 165:337, 1991.

Ling MR: Therapy of genital human papillomavirus infections. Part I: Indications for and justification of therapy, *Int J Dermatol* 31(10):682, 1992.

Ling MR: Therapy of genital human papillomavirus infections. Part II: Methods of treatment, *Int J Dermatol* 31(11): 769, 1992.

Maw RD: Treatment of anogenital warts, *Dermatol Clin* 16: 829, 1998.

Miller DM, Brodell RT: Human papillomavirus infection: treatment options for warts, *Am Fam Physician* 53(1):135, 148, 1996.

Patsner B: A patient applied topical solution for genital warts, *Contemp Obstet Gynecol* 12:27, 1991.

Pfenninger JL: The male role in cervical cancer. In Apgar BS, Brotzman GL, Spitzer M: *Colposcopy: principles and practice: an integrated text and atlas,* St Louis, 2002, Mosby.

Richart R et al: Ways of using LEEP for external lesions, *Contemp Obstet Gynecol* 5:138, 1992.

Slattery ML, Robison LM, Schuman KL, et al: Cigarette smoking and exposure to passive smoke are risk factors for cervical cancer, *JAMA* 261(11):1593, 1989.

Szarewski A, Jarvis MJ, Sasieni P, et al: Effect of smoking cessation on cervical lesion size, *Lancet* 347(9006):941, 1996.

Tyring SK et al: Alpha interferon in the management of genital warts, *Female Patient* 18:33, 1993.

Vance JC, Bart BJ, Hansen RC, et al: Intralesional recombinant alfa-2 interferon for the treatment of the patient with condyloma acuminatum or verruca plantaris, *Arch Dermatol* 122:272, 1986.

Welander CE, Homesley HD, Smiles KA, Peets EA: Intralesional interferon alfa-2b for the treatment of genital warts, *Am J Obstet Gynecol* 162(2):348, 1990.

CHAPTER 158

Endometrial Ablation (Roller Ball, Cryoablation, Thermal Balloon)

Duane E. Townsend

For over a century, physicians have attempted a variety of methods to control abnormal uterine bleeding as an alternative to hysterectomy. It is estimated that nearly 50% of women will have significant, heavy menstrual bleeding during their lifetime, particularly during the fifth and sixth decades of life. In the late 1880s there was a report of a physician placing a uterine sound into the endometrial cavity of patients and attaching the sound to a series of batteries. It was noted that women who did not have uterine fibroids had significant improvement in their heavy bleeding. However, because of the lack of suitable equipment and delivery systems, interest in endometrial ablation for the treatment of abnormal bleeding was essentially nonexistent. The technique dilation and curettage (D & C) was introduced and became the gold standard for the treatment of abnormal bleeding, even though this procedure continues to be ineffective in controlling abnormal uterine bleeding. During the last four decades, different methods of hormone manipulation have been used with limited success.

Modern methods of achieving endometrial coagulation by heat had their beginning when Goldrath successfully used the Nd:YAG laser in the early 1980s. His technique was quickly followed by other methods in which a urologic resectoscope was used to remove the endometrial lining. Resection was soon followed by roller ball endometrial ablation, in which the lining is not removed but is destroyed by cauterization. For the past decade the use of the Nd:YAG laser, uterine resection, and roller ball ablation have been the primary methods used to control abnormal bleeding when hysterectomy was not desired and hormones were ineffective.

Unfortunately, the majority of women are unaware of endometrial ablation, and their physicians do not offer the procedure. Many physicians prefer to perform a hysterectomy, often for financial reasons (i.e., "hysterectomy pays better and is more definitive").

This chapter focuses on the most commonly used method of endometrial ablation: roller ball ablation. Cryosurgical endometrial ablation, which is the safest, most versatile method and the easiest to master, is also discussed. The thermal balloon, which was approved by the Food and Drug Administration (FDA) several years ago, is also reviewed in detail.

INDICATIONS

The indications for performing endometrial ablation focus on the woman who complains of heavy uterine bleeding, has completed her family, and wishes to avoid hysterectomy. Invariably, conservative means, such as hormone manipulation and D & C, have failed to control the bleeding. Endometrial ablation is effective in controlling postmenopausal bleeding resulting from benign disease (e.g., polyps, submucous myomas) or hormone replacement therapy. The desire to avoid hysterectomy in a patient with significant medical problems is also an indication.

CONTRAINDICATIONS

- Pregnancy
- Active or subacute pelvic infection
- Complex endometrial hyperplasia (i.e., adenomatous hyperplasia with atypia)
- An enlarged uterus (i.e., uterine cavity sounds to 12 cm or greater)
- Myomatous uterus in excess of 14 weeks' gestational size
- Total cervical stenosis
- Previous endometrial ablation

• Unusual anatomical variations that might prevent an ablation (e.g., markedly retroflexed uterus or some type of uterine anomaly)

ADVANTAGES

• Minimal anesthesia (cryoablation)
• Short operating time
• Performed in outpatient facility (roller ball and thermal balloon ablation) or office (cryoablation)
• Few complications
• Rapid postoperative recovery and return to normal activity
• Highly effective in controlling bleeding (95% success rate)
• Highly effective in controlling or eliminating associated symptoms (e.g., premenstrual syndrome, dysmenorrhea, moodiness)
• Easily mastered (cryoablation)

EQUIPMENT

The equipment required for roller ball endometrial ablation includes the following:
• A standard urologic resectoscope and associated equipment
• A video system
• An electrocautery system
• Laminaria

CRITERIA FOR PROCEDURE

1. The patient should document periods of abnormal bleeding by a menstrual calendar.
2. The patient should have had a normal Pap smear within the previous 12 months.
3. An endometrial biopsy should not show any type of endometrial atypia.
4. Uterine sounding should be done to determine cavity size, and it should be less than 12 cm.
5. If the uterus is abnormal on palpation or if any adnexal pathologic condition is present, ultrasound is required before roller ball ablation.
6. If cryoablation, thermal balloon ablation, or other type of endometrial destructive techniques is to be performed, prior ultrasound is mandatory to determine the presence or absence of submucous fibroids or endometrial polyps.
7. The patient does not want additional pregnancies and has been informed of her inability to become pregnant after ablation.

8. Although there are few age limits, most patients are over 35.

PREPROCEDURE PATIENT PREPARATION

Once the patient has been evaluated for roller ball ablation and desires to proceed, she should receive a single injection of a gonadotropin-releasing hormone (Gn-RH) agonist, 3 to 5 weeks before surgery. This is important so that the uterine lining is as thin as possible for the surgery. Most patients will bleed about 2 weeks after the injection. The agonist may be given anytime during the menstrual cycle. Other medications that have been used with limited success include Danocrine, birth control pills, and progestins.

Should endometrial roller ball ablation be performed without endometrial preparation, it requires that endometrial resection occur first, followed then by roller ball ablation.

A Laminaria tent is strongly recommended for insertion into the cervical canal and through the internal os, 24 hours before the planned procedure. This will soften the cervix and facilitate the cervical dilation. The patient is given a prescription for pain medication (e.g., hydrocodone bitartrate) and antibiotics (e.g., doxycycline hyclate) at the time of the Laminaria insertion. Antibiotics should be continued for 3 days after surgery.

CONSENT FOR SURGERY

No special consent form is needed in addition to that used by the center in which surgery is being performed. To be approved for ablation, many insurance companies and health management organizations (HMOs) require that the patient receive a variety of other treatments before ablation is performed. When counseling a patient for ablation, the complications listed in the text should be discussed with the patient and carefully noted in the physician's progress notes.

TECHNIQUE

Operative hysteroscopic procedures (Figs. 158-1 and 158-2) are performed in a surgical center or outpatient facility. General anesthesia is recommended to attain adequate uterine relaxation. Local blocks (e.g., paracervical) and conduction anesthesia (e.g., spinal or epidural) have been used, but these do not give the same degree of uterine relaxation that general anesthesia does.

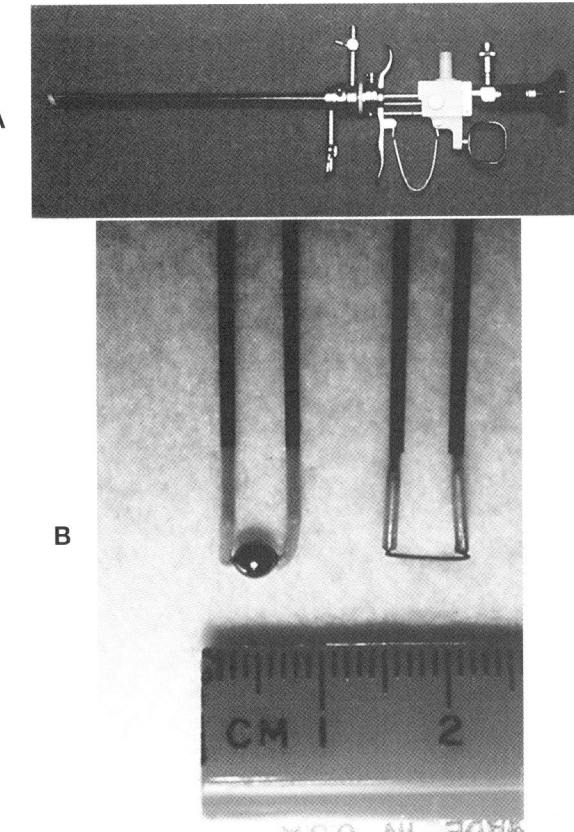

Fig. 158-1
A, Standard resectoscope used for roller ball endometrial ablation.
B, Roller ball electrodes *(left)* and loop electrodes *(right)*.

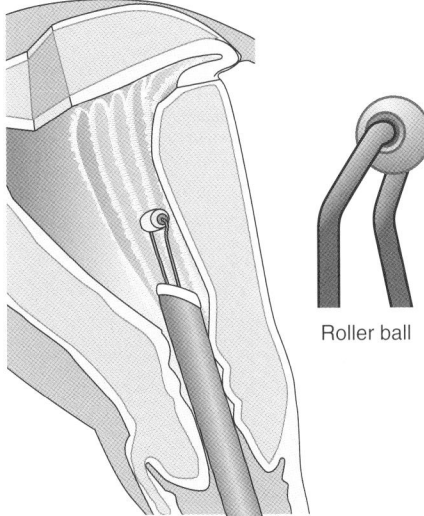

Fig. 158-2
Artist's conception of roller ball electrodes cauterizing endometrial cavity.

1. After administering anesthetic, position the patient and drape in the standard fashion for a D & C. Expose the cervix and grasp the anterior lip with a single-toothed tenaculum, and perform a paracervical block (see Chapter 174, Paracervical Block). Then dilate the internal os to a 12 mm size with Hegar dilators.

2. Once the cervix has been dilated, set up all the necessary equipment for performing the procedure, such as video systems, electrocautery units, and resectoscope. The camera is attached to the eyepiece, irrigating fluid tubing is attached to the resectoscope, and the electrocautery cord and light source are attached to the appropriate posts.

3. Since a large amount of irrigating fluid may be used during the course of surgery, try to collect all of the fluid that is used during the procedure. A collecting drape made from a Mayo Stand Cover in which the closed end has been removed is placed beneath the buttocks to serve as a funnel. The other end is placed into a large collecting bucket. A 15-L plastic water cooler bucket is ideal. Cut off the small neck and shoulders of the water cooler bucket. Pour in 1000 ml of water and make a mark. Continue pouring and marking until 15 lines have been made. The average water cooler bucket will hold about 16,000 to 17,000 ml of fluid. This system is reproducible, inexpensive, and accurate.

4. After all systems have been properly attached and determined to be operable, place the resectoscope into the uterine cavity and remove it several times as irrigating fluid flows through the resectoscope. This process should clear the cavity. The irrigating fluids the author has used include Sorbitol, Glycine, and Resectisol. No single fluid has an advantage over the others.

5. Once the cavity is cleared of clots, note the anatomic landmarks showing that the resectoscope is in the endometrial cavity (e.g., both tubal ostia and the internal os of the cervix). If any polyps or fibroids are present in the cavity, remove them with the loop electrode. Once the cavity has been cleared, attach the roller ball electrode. (See Chapter 143, Diagnostic Hysteroscopy.)

6. Set the cautery unit at 110 W coagulation. Place the resectoscope into the endometrial cavity. With the roller ball electrode slightly extended and the cautery activated, gently touch the top of the endometrial cavity with the roller ball electrode for 1 second. Continue this maneuver across the entire top of the fundus between the tubal ostia, using overlapping touch applications. After cauterizing a line between the ostia, withdraw the resectoscope and the roller ball to a point 1.5 cm below the internal os. The internal os is the narrowing that is present immediately proximal to the endometrial cavity. Create a burn ring at this point. The area of the uterine lining

that needs to be coagulated has now been delineated. The endometrial cavity is destroyed by placing the electrode at the horizontal burn line between the ostia and then slowly withdrawing the electrode to the burn ring. Carry out this method of cauterization using overlapping passes until the entire cavity is destroyed. Perform a second pass, making certain that the tubal ostia are treated. During surgery, note the fluid balance. Have the circulating nurse check the output every time 3000 ml is infused and announce this. If the irrigating fluid intake and output show a discrepancy, it must be accounted for. If the fluid balance reveals a 1000-ml deficit, the operation is terminated to avoid hyponatremia. Hyponatremia has never been reported with a normal-sized uterus.

7. At the conclusion of the operation, remove the tenaculum and cauterize the tenaculum sites on the cervix with the ball electrode to minimize bleeding at the tenaculum site. Remove the drapes and place a pad on the perineum. Return the patient to the recovery room. Surgical personnel are responsible for cleaning the scope after the procedure is completed.

Although this technique has been criticized as being too difficult, the author has taught over 1000 physicians, including primary care physicians, to perform the technique. Unfortunately, it may take the average physician up to 25 cases before he or she can expect to become proficient with operative hysteroscopy. This slow learning curve has been the primary impediment in popularizing this technique.

COMPLICATIONS

- Uterine perforation may occur during the insertion of the Laminaria.
- Cervical laceration may occur during dilation (occurs primarily when a Laminaria is not used).
- Uterine perforation may occur during cervical dilation. This is minimized with the use of the Laminaria.
- Infection may occur (seldom occurs if antibiotics are used).
- Bleeding may occur during ablation. This has never occurred with roller ball ablation but may occur during resection of polyps, fibroids, and endometrial tissue.
- Postoperative hemorrhage may occur, usually when patients are too active in the first few weeks after ablation. Patients should rest for a few weeks following the procedure.
- Perforation with roller ball electrodes may occur, which usually happens because improper technique was used. A perforation requires immediate laparoscopy to determine if the bowel has been injured and if the perforation site is bleeding.

- Absorption of too much fluid during surgery (i.e., dilutional hyponatremia). This has not been observed in patients with a uterus of normal size, but it can occur if the patient has a large cavity. It may also occur during resection of fibroids.
- Pain as a result of postablation tubal syndrome. The pain, which feels similar to menstrual cramps, is severe and located lateral to the uterus. It is usually cyclic and associated with light uterine bleeding.

INTERPRETATION, RESULTS, FINDINGS, AND CONSIDERATION

The success of endometrial ablation is not determined until 1 year after the procedure. Over 95% of the patients report significant diminution of their bleeding, with 85% having amenorrhea, or minimal spotting. Success of ablation is directly dependent upon the training and skill of the surgeon. Some patients may begin to experience light bleeding 2 to 3 years after surgery, but it is rarely excessive.

POSTPROCEDURE PATIENT EDUCATION

Patients are advised to resume normal activities 2 to 3 weeks after the procedure. They can expect a watery discharge, which may be brownish or tinged with blood. Some patients have spotting and light bleeding for up to 2 months after the operation. If the patient engages in vigorous exercise, she may have severe bleeding, which may be controlled by bed rest for 24 to 36 hours. Infection has not been observed in those patients who take antibiotics.

Lethargy has been noted rarely in patients and seems to be related to anesthesia.

CRYOABLATION

Drogmueller was the first to report that freezing the uterine cavity was practical and safe. His intent was to achieve sterility by freezing the uterine ostia. Because cryosurgery is rarely associated with scarring, he was unable to sterilize the patients. However, he did note significant reduction of menstrual flow in the treated individuals. He then reported on the successful use of cryosurgery in controlling abnormal uterine bleeding. However, the equipment he used was large and cumbersome, and as a consequence, interest in cryoablation did not attract much attention until recently. A new, compact cryosurgical unit has been developed, which uses recirculating refrigerants (Figs. 158-3 and 158-4). Also, special lightweight probes accompany the unit. The cryosurgical system includes a mobile console that contains the compressor and refrigerants. A flexible delivery line that is about 5 feet long carries the gases to a permanent cryoprobe. A disposable cryoprobe is mounted over the permanent probe, and it is the disposable probe tip that comes in contact with the endometrium.

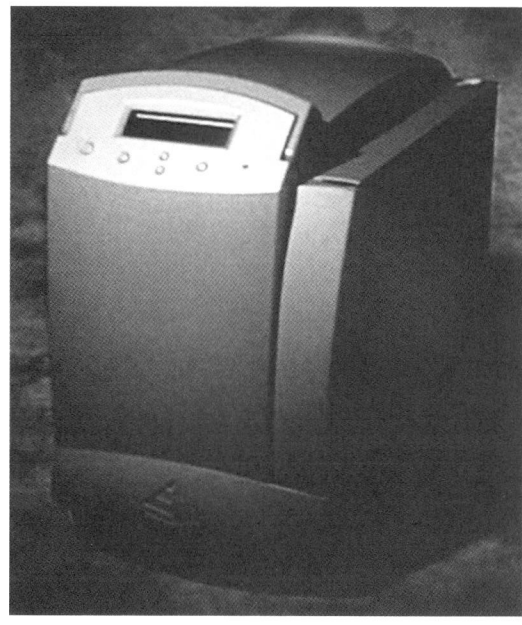

Fig. 158-3
Cryosurgical unit for performing endometrial cryoablation.

A recently completed study directed by the FDA demonstrated the safety and effectiveness of the cryoablation system in controlling abnormal uterine bleeding. Cryoablation was found to be as effective as roller ball ablation, but it is much easier to learn and causes no significant side effects to the patient. It is safer than roller ball ablation because it does not require distension of the uterus or the use of large amounts of fluid that are necessary with operative hysteroscopy. Moreover, cryoablation requires little anesthesia and can be performed in a physician's office.

The workup and preparation of a patient for a cryoablation procedure are similar to that for roller ball ablation, except that all patients must have an ultrasound performed to determine whether she has endometrial polyps or myomas. If submucous fibroids or polyps are found within the uterine cavity, the tissue should be sampled to rule out a premalignant or malignant process. This is accomplished by hysteroscopy and D & C, either in the office or an outpatient facility. If the submucous myomas are greater than 3 cm in diameter or extend over halfway into the uterine cavity, the patient is not a good candidate for cryoablation. The resectoscope should be used to remove the myomas before ablation. Pretreatment with a Gn-RH agonist is not necessary. Cryoablation is best performed in the early proliferative phase of the menstrual cycle (i.e. days 3 through 8). The urinary bladder should contain at least 300 ml of fluid since

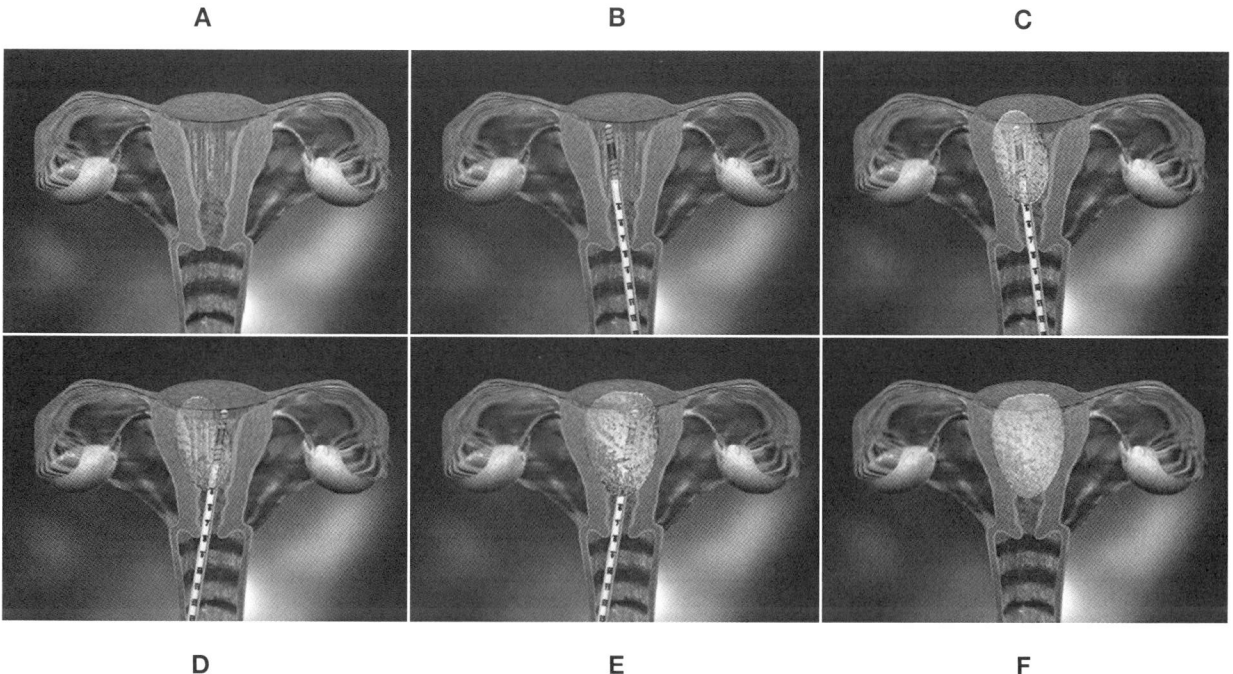

Fig. 158-4
Stages of cryoablation. **A,** Uterus before freezing. **B,** Cryoprobe in right cornua. **C,** End of first freeze.
D, Cryoprobe in left cornua. **E,** End of second freeze. **F,** Cryozone after cryoprobe removed.

abdominal pelvic ultrasound is used to both direct the insertion of the cryoprobe and monitor the treatment. (See Chapter 209, Emergency Department and Office Ultrasound, and Chapter 173, Obstetric Ultrasound.) The procedure can be performed either in the physician's office or outpatient facility, since little anesthesia or analgesia is required.

TECHNIQUE

1. Whether cryoablation is performed in a physician's office or outpatient facility, the methodology is identical. The patient should not eat or drink anything 6 hours before the treatment. After arrival in the treatment facility, she may be given light sedation (e.g., 10 mg of Valium or titrate 2 to 5 mg of Versed). She is taken to the treatment or operating room and placed on the treatment table in low stirrups. The legs should not be elevated more than 10 degrees above the horizontal. This position is important for visualizing the ultrasound that is used to monitor the treatment session.

2. Prep the perineum and vagina for surgery, and drape the perineum in a sterile fashion. Perform a pelvic ultrasound to ascertain the volume of fluid in the urinary bladder. The bladder should be at least three to four times as large as the uterus. Add sterile saline as necessary through a Robinson or Foley catheter.

3. Carefully place a large, open-sided, or weighted speculum into the vagina to expose the uterine cervix. Inject the anterior cervical lip with 1 to 2 ml of local anesthetic.

4. Use a single-toothed tenaculum to grasp the anterior cervical lip in order to stabilize the uterus, and carry out a paracervical block (see Chapter 174, Paracervical Block).

5. Sound the uterus in the midline and in each cornu. The internal os does not usually require dilation, since the outside diameter of the cryoprobe is only 5 mm.

6. Place the cryoprobe into the uterine cavity and direct it into one of the cornua under ultrasound monitoring. Then inject 5 ml of sterile saline into the uterine cavity through the injection port located on the underside of the cryoprobe. Apply gentle traction to the tenaculum as the cryoprobe is positioned in the cornual area.

7. Depress the freeze button, commencing the circulation of the refrigerants and the freezing process. Monitor the progress of the cryozone by ultrasound. The cryozone appears as a hyperechoic (dark) area on the sonogram, because the cryozone is frozen water. The initial treatment session continues until the edge of the cryozone is at least halfway through the uterine wall (about 5 to 6 minutes).

8. Depress the heat button and warm the probe tip until it can be removed from the uterine cavity (about 60 to 90 seconds). Then direct the cryoprobe into the unfrozen cornua. Once the position of the probe in the untreated cornua is confirmed by sonogram, inject 5 ml of sterile saline, apply gentle traction to the tenaculum, and depress the freeze button. The developing cryozone is once again observed on the sonogram.

9. Stop treatment once the second cryozone has extended as least halfway through the myometrium and has coalesced with the first cryozone (about 5 to 6 minutes). This will appear as one large cryozone on the sonogram. Depress the heat cycle button to heat the probe tip, and remove the probe from the uterus.

10. Hand the probe to the assistant, who removes the disposable probe and cleans the permanent inner probe. Then place the permanent cryoprobe into the probe housing within the console.

11. The urinary bladder is emptied, and the patient is transferred to a gurney and taken to recovery. She should be ready for discharge in about 1 hour. She should be sent home with a prescription for ibuprofen and doxycycline hyclate, 50 mg # 10. The amount of pain is usually minimal after the procedure. The patient should be instructed to take the antibiotics until they are gone, one twice a day.

RESULTS, INTERPRETATION AND CONSIDERATIONS

At 1 year after the procedure, over 95% of patient are extremely pleased with the results of treatment. Many women who have menometrorrhagia also experience mood swings, premenstrual syndrome, and dysmenorrhea. After undergoing cryoablation, over 95% of the patients noted that their symptoms had disappeared, and 96% of the patients treated in the FDA study would recommend cryoablation to a friend.

COMPLICATIONS AND PATIENT POSTPROCEDURE EDUCATION

In patients who participated in the FDA study and in over 1000 patients treated with cryoablation, no significant side effects or complications were noted. In contrast to cryosurgery of the uterine cervix, which is invariably followed by a profuse watery discharge for up to 4 weeks,, there is no or very little discharge after cryoablation. The patient's postsurgical course is benign.

she may return to normal activities immediately but should be asked to refrain from vigorous exercise or sexual relations for about 1 week after the procedure.

THERMAL BALLOON ABLATION

The thermal balloon ablation technique (Figs. 158-5 and 158-6) received FDA approval several years ago. The preoperative workup and preparation is similar to that for cryoablation, except that a Gn-RH agonist is once again not needed before thermal balloon ablation. A D & C is performed before balloon ablation. The balloon is inserted into the uterine cavity, and warm fluid (i.e., 87° C) is circulated for 8 minutes. The total time for treatment is about 20 to 25 minutes. The technique is performed under either anesthesia or paracervical block and heavy sedation. Preliminary results indicate that most patients have bleeding after the treatment, but it is less than the amount of bleeding they had before the treatment.

Initially, thermal balloon ablation was met with much enthusiasm, because it was proposed as a technique that could be performed with little anesthesia or analgesia in a physician's office. As more experience was gained with the balloon ablation, the degree of pain associated with this technique and its high failure rate has dampened this enthusiasm. Use of thermal balloon ablation is limited to women who have a uterus of normal size. Moreover, because of the pain associated with treatment, patients require heavy sedation and often some degree of anesthesia. Many women continue to complain of significant pain in the first 24 to 36 hours after treatment.

Other Methods

In addition to roller ball ablation, cryoablation, and thermal balloon ablation, two additional techniques have recently received FDA approval for endometrial ablation. The first technique is called *hydrothermablation,* which requires significant cervical dilation and hysteroscopy. This procedure is performed under heavy sedation or anesthesia. The uterine cervix must be dilated to at least 8 to 9 mm. A hysteroscope is placed into the uterine cavity, and very hot saline is circulated throughout the cavity. Slightly enlarged uteri and even those with submucous myomas may be treated. Lupron should be given to the patient before treatment to get the necessary 2 to 4 mm penetration into the myometrium to reduce the menstrual flow. The circulating hot saline "cooks" the surface of the endometrium and extends about 2 to 4 mm into the tissue. Total treatment time is about 30 minutes. Short term results after hydrothermablation are no better than with roller ball ablation or cryoablation. Because significant dilation is required and considerable pain is associated with the hot saline, heavy sedation or anesthesia is required. Many woman experience moderate to severe pain during the first 24 hours after treatment.

The second and most recent technique to receive FDA approval uses bipolar cautery delivered though an expandable mesh (Novacept, Inc.) that is inserted into the uterine cavity. Once the mesh has been properly positioned, which takes up to 30 minutes, the actual treatment time is 2 minutes. Results with this method are identical to those previously discussed. This treatment is restricted to women who have a uterus of normal size that does not contain polyps or myomas.

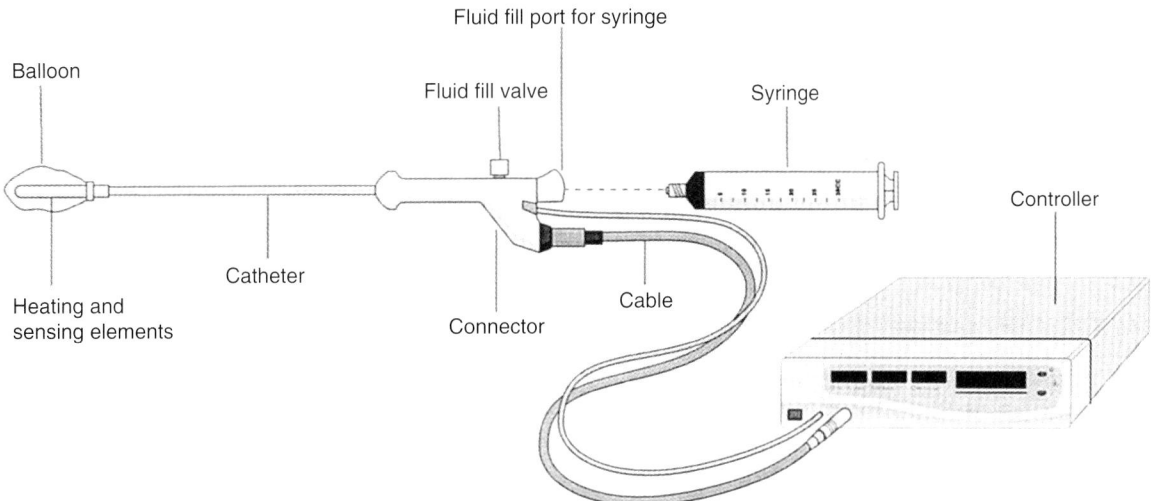

Fig. 158-5
Complete Thermachoice system for performing thermal balloon ablation.

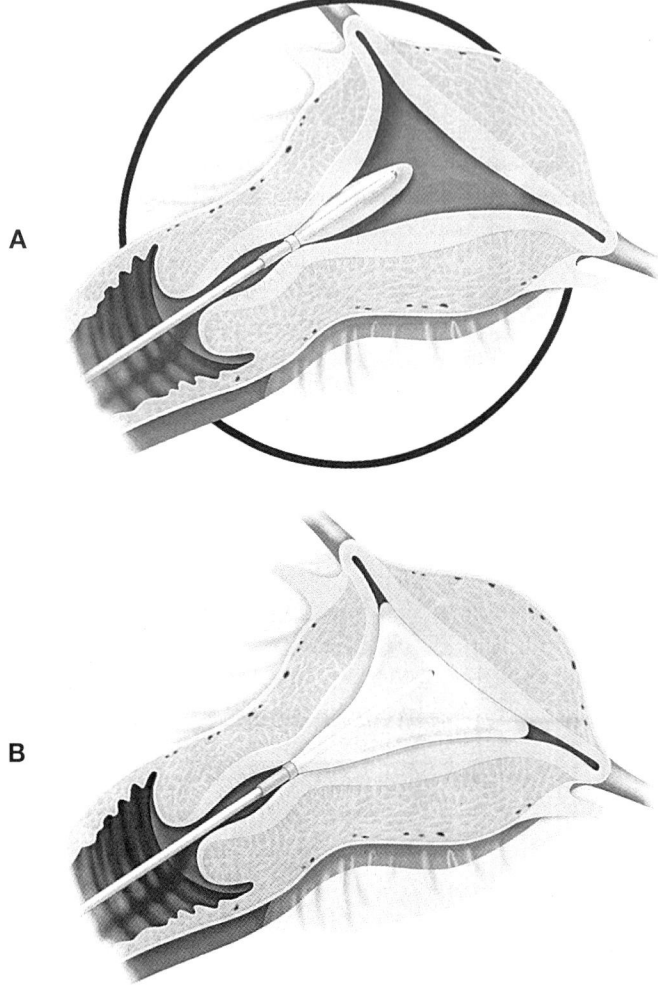

Fig. 158-6
A, Thermal balloon within uterine cavity before filling balloon fluid.
B, Thermal balloon distended with 87° C fluid for 8 minutes.

CONCLUSION

Endometrial ablation has become an important tool in the control of abnormal uterine bleeding in women who no longer wish to have children. It is ideally suited for patients in the fifth and sixth decades of life. There are many ablation methods from which to choose. Operative hysteroscopy with roller ball ablation represents the "gold standard." It has a fairly long learning curve but is the most versatile. It must be performed in a surgical center or outpatient facility. The remaining techniques discussed in this chapter are all autoablative and are controlled by time, except cryosurgery. Cryoablation is probably the safest of all methods and can be used in uteri that are large or contain submucous myomas or polyps. Because of the natural analgesic properties of cold, patients usually experience little pain. When cryoablation is coupled with ultrasound, it is the only

method whereby one can see in real time the depth of destruction of the uterine wall.

SUPPLIERS

Roller ball endometrial ablation
The equipment required for roller ball endometrial ablation includes a standard urologic resectoscope, a video system, and an electrocautery system. The following companies manufacture these systems:

Karl Storz Endoscopy-America, Inc.
600 Corporate Pointe
Culver City, CA 90230-7600
Phone: 1-800-421-0837
Website: www.karlstorz.com

Olympus America Inc.
Endoscope Division
2 Corporate Center Drive
Melville, NY 11747
Phone: 1-800-848-9024
Website: www.olympusamerica.com

ACMI Circon
300 Stillwater Avenue
Stamford, CT 06902-3695
Phone: 1-203-357-8300
Website: www.circoncorp.com

Richard Wolfe Medical Instruments Corp.
353 Corporate Woods Parkway
Vernon Hills, IL 60061
Phone: 1-847-913-1113
Website: www.richard-wolf.com

CooperSurgical
95 Corporate Drive
Trumbull, CT 06611
Phone: 1-800-645-3760
Website: www.coopersurgical.com

Cryoablation
Cryogen, Inc.
11065 Sorrento Valley Ct.
San Diego, CA 92121
Phone: 1-888-634-0444
Website: www.cryogen-inc.com

Thermal balloon
Gynecare, Inc. (Division of Ethicon, Inc.)
P.O. Box 151
Somerville, NJ 08876-0151
Phone: 1-800-255-2500
Website: www.gynecare.com

Hydrothermablation
Bei Medical Systems Company, Inc.
100 Hollister Road
Teterboro, NJ 07608
Phone: 1-210-727-4900
Website: www.beimedical.com

Bipolar cautery equipment/mesh
Novacept, Inc.
1047 Elwell Court
Palo Alto, CA 94303
Phone: 1-650-428-0300
Website: www.novacept.com

Brochures
Each company listed in this chapter has its own brochure for physicians and patients. The websites should be reviewed for examples.

CPT/BILLING CODES

58555	Hysteroscopy, diagnostic (separate procedure)
58558	Hysteroscopy, surgical with sampling, with or without D & C
58561	Hysteroscopy with removal of leiomyomata
58563	Hysteroscopy with endometrial ablation (any method)
59200	Laminaria insertion

ICD-9-CM DIAGNOSTIC CODES

626.8	Dysfunctional uterine bleeding
626.2	Menometrorrhagia

BIBLIOGRAPHY

Bieber EJ, Loffer FD: *The gynecologic resectoscope*, Cambridge, Mass, 1995, Blackwell Science.

Bongers MY et al: *A prospective, double-blind, randomized, and controlled trial of two second-generation ablation devices, NovaSure GEA and Thermachoice.* Paper presented at the 30th Meeting of the AAGL, San Francisco, November 16-19, 2001.

Decherney AM, Polan ML: Hysteroscopic management of intrauterine lesions and intractable uterine bleeding, *Obstet Gynecol* 61:392, 1983.

Drogmueller W et al: Cryosurgery of the uterus, *Am J Obstet Gynecol* 110:27, 1972.

Drogmueller W, Greer BE, Makowski EL: Preliminary observations of cryoablation of the endometrium, *Am J Obstet Gynecol* 107(6):958, 1970.

Goldrath MH, Fuller TA, Segal S: Laser photovaporization of endometrium for the treatment of menorrhagia, *Am J Obstet Gynecol* 140:14, 1981.

Goldrath MH, Barrionuevo M, Husain M: Endometrial ablation by hysteroscopic instillation of hot saline solution, *J Am Assoc Gynecol Laparosc* 4:235, 1997.

Hepard M et al: *Uterine cryoablation therapy in women with menorrhagia.* Paper presented at the 30th meeting of the AAGL, San Francisco, November 16-19, 2001.

Hidlebaugh DA: Relative costs of gynecologic endoscopy vs traditional surgery for treatment of abnormal uterine bleeding, *Am J Manag Care* Sep 25:7 Spec No:SP31, 2001.

Loffer FD: Complications of hysteroscopy—their cause, prevention and correction, *J Am Assoc Gynecol Laparosc* 3:11, 1995.

Serden SD, Brooks PG: Treatment of abnormal uterine bleeding with the gynecologic resectoscope, *J Reprod Med* 36:676, 1991.

Townsend DE, Fields G, McCausland A, Kauffman K: Diagnostic and operative hysteroscopy in the management of persistent post menopausal bleeding, *Obstet Gynecol* 82:419, 1993.

Townsend DE, McCausland V, McCausland A, et al: Post-ablation-tubal sterilization syndrome, *Obstet Gynecol* 82:422, 1993.

Townsend DE, Richart RM, Paskowitz RA, Woolfork RE: "Rollerball" coagulation of the endometrium, *Obstet Gynecol* 76:310, 1990.

CHAPTER 159

Management of the Adult Victim of Sexual Assault

Olasunkanmi W. Adeyinka

Current statistics indicate that a sexual assault occurs every 4 seconds in this country. One in every four women will be sexually assaulted in her lifetime. But it is not only women; almost 10% of assault victims are male. Sexual assault is the fastest growing, most frequently committed, and most underreported violent crime in the United States.

Sexual assault is underreported for many reasons, including societal misconceptions about the victims of sexual assault, feelings invoked by such an assault, and the burden of reporting an assault. Misconceptions persist, despite enhanced public education, that individuals who are assaulted may have encouraged the act by their behavior, dress, lack of resistance, or previous promiscuity. Complex law enforcement and healthcare systems are often perceived as being impersonal and nonsupportive. An estimated 75% of victims know their perpetrators, possibly enhancing feelings of embarrassment, guilt, and fear of retribution. These feelings and misconceptions combined with inadequate support systems often prevent victims from reporting a sexual assault.

The purpose of the medical evaluation after sexual assault is to assess the patient for physical injuries or possible disease, to document injuries and to collect the necessary evidence. The remainder of the encounter should be used to treat any injuries, to prevent pregnancy and disease, and to find the proper support services for the victim. The examination and treatment should be done as soon as possible after the assault, especially the collection of evidence. While an evaluation within 48 hours is preferred, victims are encouraged to see a clinician even if more than 72 hours have elapsed (this still allows a clinician to treat and prevent many problems).

Collaboration between hospitals, community services and local law enforcement agencies for the establishment of protocols is very helpful and such protocols will ease victims' pain and suffering. Primary care clinicians can be instrumental in assuring that this collaboration takes place. Such collaboration is effective at not only streamlining the evaluation process but also for easing the burden of reporting. Some institutions offer 24-hour availability of specially trained and experienced volunteers, such as a nurse on every shift. These volunteers can provide the victim continuous support during the cumbersome process of answering questions and the examination. They can also act as a witness for the chain of evidence. A supportive volunteer system can offer such simple things as a change of clothing (victims often need to leave their clothing as evidence), which are hugely appreciated by victims.

INDICATIONS

- Sexual assault

Note: Sexual assault is any form of nonconsenting sexual activity. It encompasses all unwanted sexual acts from fondling to forcible penetration.

EQUIPMENT

- Camera and film
- Wood's light
- Sexual assault kit: most emergency departments have a standard kit that contains a protocol for care and all the necessary specimen containers. These should be in compliance with and fulfill state laws for sexual assault (Table 159-1). In general, kits should contain the following:
  a. Information for the victim
  b. Consent form for the examination
  c. Instructions, checklist, and chain of custody form
  d. History and physical examination forms
  e. Diagrams for use in documentation of injuries (Fig. 159-1; see also www.forensicdocumentation.com)

TABLE 159-1

Sexual Assault Kit Equipment*

Contents	Purpose
Two urine containers	Urine for microscopic urinalysis, pregnancy test, and drug screen
Fingernail clippers, file, and envelope	Fingernail clippings and scrapings
Forceps, scissors, two envelopes	Pubic hair trimming in one envelope, head hair trimming in other envelope
Plastic comb, large paper towel, two envelopes	Pubic hair combing in one envelope, head hair combing in other envelope
Vaginal speculum, aspiration pipette, red-topped test tube and stopper	Aspiration of vaginal contents
Four cotton-tipped swabs and a test tube or envelope, one slide	Vaginal (or penile) swabbing, and smear (same for rectal swabbing and smear if indicated)
Saline, 10 ml; two aspiration pipettes and bulbs; two test tubes, two slides	Vaginal washing (and rectal if indicated using second pipette and test tube)
Cervical scraper, brush, slides, Pap smear fixative	Pap smear
Thayer-Martin plates and chlamydia cultures *and/or* sample tubes for gonorrhea/chlamydia enzymatic probes	Gonorrhea and chlamydia evaluation (positive cultures are the gold standard for court, but probes have greater sensitivity)
Four cotton-tipped swabs and a test tube or envelope, one slide	Oral swabs and smear
Two cotton-tipped swabs and a test tube or envelope	Saliva collection for secretor status
Three red-topped test tubes and stoppers, tourniquet, nonalcohol swab to prepare skin, syringe and needle	Blood samples
Labeled paper bags	Collection of clothing and dried body fluids
Necessary and helpful forms:	Information, consent, and documentation
• patient education handout	
• consent form	
• history and physical examination form	
• diagrams for documentation of injuries	
• chain of custody form	
• any necessary instructions	
• check list	

*Contents should be refrigerated after collection.

f. Specimen containers, equipment, and labels
• Colposcope *(optional)*

PREPROCEDURE PATIENT PREPARATION

If a patient calls before presenting to the emergency department, first make sure that the patient is safe. If not, encourage the patient to call the police. Next, encourage the patient to not take a bath or remove the clothing worn during the assault. If possible, they should postpone urinating, defecating, brushing their teeth, or drinking anything until samples are collected. Also, ask them to bring a change of clothing. Patients should sign for informed consent before starting the evaluation (see the sample patient consent form titled "General Patient Consent Form/Forensic Evaluation" on page 1959 of Appendix G).

Explain the process of the evaluation to the patient. Let them know that you will explain every step of the examination before performing it. Even if she or he may not want to report the assault, a very thorough examination is necessary in case they later change their mind. Continue to reassure the patient that they are safe and that someone else will always be in the room to comfort them during the evaluation.

TECHNIQUE

1. Open the sexual assault kit. Once the kit is opened, the chain of evidence must be maintained and evidence must not be left unattended. Signatures of those in attendance must be documented on the form for any and all evidence collected. (See Fig. 160-8 for a sample chain of evidence form.) The kit should be labeled as a biohazard. After the patient has signed the consent form, proceed with taking the history.

History

2. The history should be taken in a quiet room, with a witness present, after the patient has been assured that she or he is safe. Be cautious about the terms used in stating patient complaints. Avoid

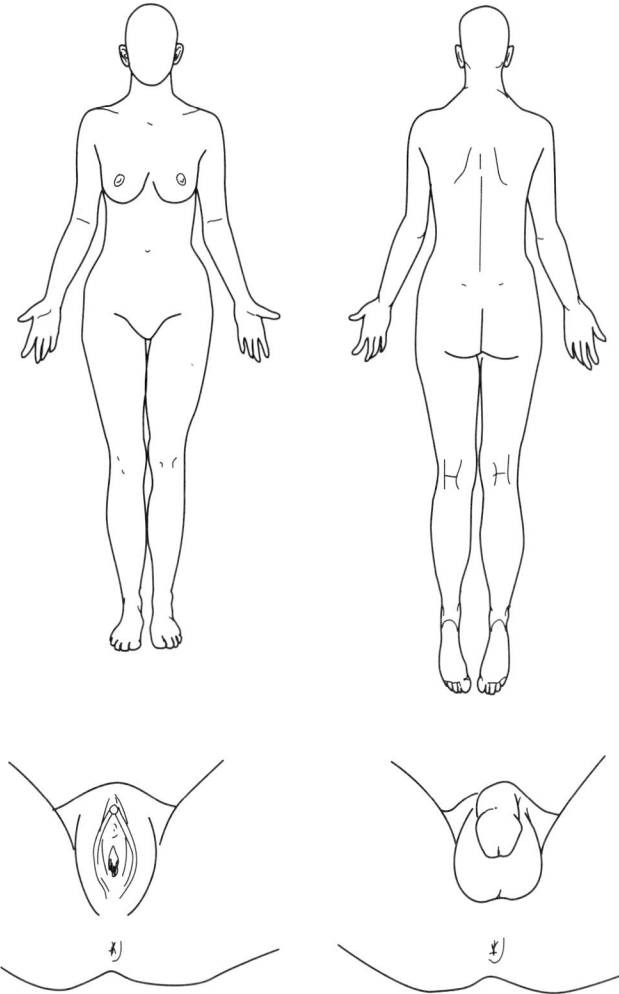

Fig. 159-1
Traumagram. Mark and label locations where there is evidence of trauma. (From Botasch AS, Braen GR, Gilchrist VJ: Acute care for sexual assault victims, *Patient Care* 28[13]:112, 1994. Copyright of Marcia Hartsock, Artist.)

use of the word "rape" because this is a legal term. Instead, state the patient complaint as being a "sexual assault." Also, try to avoid the terms "why didn't you. . ." or "you shouldn't have. . ." or "Did you do anything to lead them on?" In fact, try to avoid the words "why" and "alleged" altogether; "why" implies blame and "alleged" implies disbelief.

Questions should be directed to the victim in a nonjudgmental way, and the patient should be allowed to talk about the assault at a comfortable pace, using her or his own words. It is important to observe nonverbal communication that may indicate a need for further questioning. Supportive terms worth using include "I'm glad you're alive," "You did what you needed to survive," "I'm sorry

this happened to you," and "It was not your fault." Allow the victim to express her or his feelings. To build rapport, it may be worth obtaining the medical and sexual history before obtaining the assault history.

Note: If you have a long-term relationship with the patient, the patient may prefer to be examined in your office. However, in many jurisdictions, legally admissible evidence of a sexual assault cannot be collected without using the kit and other resources that are often available only in the emergency department. It is important for practitioners to know the assault and rape laws in their state so that they can comply with any legal requirements.

A. Medical and Sexual History (Gynecologic History for Women)

- Medical disease, if present, should be documented.
- Last voluntary sexual encounter up to one week prior to the assault and the race of that individual should be documented. If the encounter is less than 48 hours ago, blood and fluid samples may be requested from that individual at a later date.
- The victim's alcohol and drug intake should be documented.
- For women, the date of the victim's last menstrual period, their contraceptive use, pregnancy history, use of tampons, and any previous episode of gynecologic infection or pelvic surgery should be documented.

B. Assault History

An accurate but brief description of the assault is crucial for proper collection and analysis of the physical evidence. This includes documenting the following:

- Age and identifying information for victim, and assailant(s), if available
- Date, time, and location of the alleged assault
- Details of sexual contact, such as actual or attempted oral, rectal, or vaginal penetration of the victim. Attempt to determine whether there was an ejaculation, digital penetration or penetration with foreign objects. It should be documented whether a tampon was present, or if a lubricant, contraceptive foam, a spermicide, or a condom was used. If any of these are unknown, that should be documented.
- Type of physical restraints used, if any, and whether there were any threats, weapons, drugs, or alcohol involved. Was the assailant injured during the assault?
- Activities of the victim after the assault, such as changing clothes, wiping, washing, bathing, douching, dental hygiene, urination, vomiting, smoking, eating, drinking, or defecation.

Physical Examination

3. Having a trained, experienced volunteer in the room in addition to the nurse may help distract the victim from her or his emotional and physical pain during the examination. The physical examination and collection of evidence are performed congruently. Carefully examine the entire body and photograph and/or make drawings of the injured areas (Fig. 159-1). The clinician should search for bruises, abrasions, or lacerations about the head, neck, back, buttocks, or extremities. A victim who was choked may have petechiae on the face and conjunctiva. Physical trauma may be greater in sexually assaulted men, perhaps because only those who have been more seriously injured are likely to report the crime.

4. Examine the oral cavity. Broken teeth, a torn frenulum of the tongue or lip, or pharyngeal trauma may indicate that the mouth was forced open. Using two swabs simultaneously, swab the oral cavity and along the teeth for evidence of semen. Do not moisten the swabs prior to sample collection.

   Repeat with two additional swabs. Prepare one smear on the slide by gently smearing the swabs over the surface. Allow the swabs and smear to air dry. Place swabs in envelope or test tube provided.

5. The victim's clothing should be collected and placed in a paper bag that is sealed and signed. Allow any wet clothing to air dry before packaging. If additional bags are needed, use only new paper (grocery-type) bags.

   It may be helpful to photograph the patient before she or he disrobes. Semen may appear as flaking, crusty stains on clothing and it will fluoresce under a Wood's light. Have the patient disrobe while standing on paper from the examination table. Each item of clothing should be placed in a separate paper bag. Do not use plastic bags for clothing collection because they promote bacterial growth on blood or semen. Use gloves when touching the victim's clothes to avoid contaminating the evidence with your DNA or blood type from sweat.

6. For women, a pelvic examination should be performed to complete the physical examination. Lesions around the vulva or rectum may be present because of trauma from a hand, penis, or other foreign body. Superficial or extensive lacerations of the hymen and vagina, injury of the urethra, and, occasionally, rupture of the vaginal wall may be present. Swab and preserve any semen for later DNA analysis. A Wood's light can be used to examine the perineum or inner thigh for semen. Semen fluoresces more brightly than feces, urine, or pus.

   a. Lubricate the speculum with water. Standard lubricants may adversely affect the results of the acid phosphatase test and alter sperm motility. Examine the vaginal wall and cervix for abrasions, ecchymoses, and lacerations. A colposcope may be helpful to document any microtrauma to the cervix or vagina. It can also be used to take photographs. The cervix should be swabbed and cultures and probes sent for gonorrhea and chlamydia. Four swabs should be utilized and a smear prepared in a manner similar to the oral swabs. They should be allowed to air dry before sealing.

   b. A Pap smear should be performed. Intact spermatozoa may be seen several days later on a Pap smear.

   c. Any fluid from the posterior fornix should be aspirated and examined under the microscope. A sample of the aspirated fluid should be saved for DNA testing, as well as for testing for acid phosphatase, and blood group antigens.

   d. If no secretions are visible, a small amount of saline (about 5 ml) may be used to lavage the cervix and posterior fornix. Aspirate this fluid and save while using some to prepare slides. Examine the slides under the microscope for spermatozoa. Lavaging with normal saline may enhance motility of spermatozoa for up to 2 hours. Motile sperm from the vagina imply intercourse within the past 6 hours (rarely within the past 12 hours) and their presence should be documented. Immotile sperm imply intercourse within the past 12 to 18 hours (in rare cases, up to 24 hours). In addition to examining for spermatozoa with a wet smear, the slide should be examined for trichomonas, bacterial vaginosis, or the presence of any candida species.

7. The victim's pubic hair should be combed to detect foreign bodies, as well as for perpetrator pubic hair samples. If found, approximately 15 to 20 perpetrator hairs should be collected as part of the evidence. In a separate container, 15 to 20 of the victim's trimmed pubic hairs should be saved. This process should be repeated for head hair, using separate specimen containers.

8. Bimanual and rectal examinations should be performed. Anal assault is more common in men. Look for erythema, edema, bleeding, mucosal tears, fissures, a hematoma, or sphincter laxity or spasm. The digital rectal examination is usually sufficient if nothing suspicious is palpated and bleeding is absent or insignificant.

9. Anoscopy or proctoscopy are difficult for the patient, but may be required if you suspect a tear. The rectal area should be swabbed for chlamydia. If anal intercourse is known to have occurred, four anal swabs should be utilized and a smear prepared

in a manner similar to the oral swabs. Anal swabs can be moistened with sterile normal saline before using, if necessary. They should be allowed to air dry before sealing. (Penile swabs and smears can be performed in the same manner by swabbing the outside of the penile shaft.)

Next, wash the rectal vault with 5 to 10 ml of normal saline introduced through the anus with the hub of a syringe. Allow the saline to stand for 5 to 10 minutes, then aspirate and preserve as evidence. These samples can be examined for motile sperm, immotile sperm, and acid phosphatase. Fecal contamination precludes their use for blood group antigen analysis.

Note: Pelvic, rectal and proctoscopic examinations should be done gently and with careful explanation because the victim may not only experience severe discomfort because of the local trauma but they may also experience flashbacks.

Laboratory Tests

10. Obtain fingernail clippings and scrapings. These may harbor bits of the assailant's blood, skin, or hair. Photographs of bite marks may also be used to match dental records.
11. Saliva samples should be taken. The victim should not be allowed to smoke or eat for 30 minutes prior to taking a sample. If there is trauma to the mouth, this procedure should be delayed until the wound is healed. The swabs should be allowed to air dry before sealing. They should not be removed from the victim's mouth by anyone other then the victim or the examiner.
12. Guided by the history of the assault, the victim's symptoms, and any local protocol, determine which laboratory tests are appropriate. Recommended laboratory tests in all cases of sexual assault include the following:
- A Venereal Disease Research Laboratory (VDRL) test for syphilis or rapid plasma reagin (RPR) test should be obtained at the initial visit and repeated in 4 to 6 weeks
- Hepatitis B serology should be checked (hepatitis B surface antigen and antibody and the hepatitis B core antibody).
- Serology for HIV should be obtained at the initial visit and repeated at 3, 6, and 12 months after exposure, following proper patient counseling.
- The patient's blood type should be determined from blood or saliva swabs.
- For women, a urine or serum beta–human chorionic gonadotropin (HCG) pregnancy test at the initial examination is needed to rule out existing pregnancy.

Treatment

13. Treatment of major or life-threatening injuries should occur before initiating the evaluation. After the patient is stable, treatment of other physical injuries should be dependent on the type sustained.
14. Sexually transmitted disease prevention:
    a. Gonorrhea and chlamydia prophylaxis. The current recommendation for the treatment of gonorrhea and chlamydia trachomatis is 400 mg of cefixime orally or 250 mg of ceftriaxone intramuscularly (or 2 g of spectinomycin for those allergic to cephalosporins) followed by 100 mg of doxycycline twice daily for 7 days or 500 mg of tetracycline four times per day for 7 days or 1 g of azithromycin. Doxycycline should not be prescribed for pregnant patients.

       This regimen will probably treat incubating syphilis. Although the overall risk of acquiring a sexually transmitted disease from a single sexual encounter is only 5% to 10%, the above treatment should be prescribed for all victims of sexual assault.
    b. Hepatitis B prophylaxis. If the patient has not been immunized, hepatitis B virus vaccine should be given at the initial visit, then repeated at 1 and 6 months. Hepatitis B immunoglobulin (HBIG) 0.06 ml IM should be offered if the assailant is thought to be in a high risk group for hepatitis B and the victim has experienced vaginal or anal bleeding from the assault. The same dose can be repeated in 1 month if the victim's serology is negative.
    c. HIV prophylaxis. HIV prophylaxis is not universally recommended. However, it should be understood that if the assailant cannot be apprehended and tested (most cases), the victim's infection status may not be known for 6 to 12 months. Treatment should be tailored to the patient's needs after counseling for medication costs and potential toxicity.
15. For women, if the pregnancy test is negative, pregnancy prevention should be offered. Recommended treatment is Ovral tablets (50 mg of ethinyl estradiol), two tablets initially, followed by two tablets in 12 hours. Another option is conjugated estrogen (Premarin) 50 mg/d IV for 2 days or 30 mg/d PO for 5 days. These treatments are 97% effective for prevention of pregnancy if used within 72 hours of intercourse.

Note: Since up to half of all victims do not report for their follow-up visit, it is very important to perform adequate prophylaxis on patients during the initial visit.

Follow-up

16. The patient should have a follow-up visit with a clinician within 72 hours to again document bruising and to evaluate the results of cultures if prophylactic antibiotics were not given. HIV testing should be repeated at 3, 6, and 12 months and a test for syphilis repeated after a month. Follow-up counseling referrals should be made at the first visit. An additional follow-up visit should be made at 1 to 2 weeks to monitor patient progress (and to evaluate for pregnancy in women) as a result of the assault. If the patient did not receive prophylaxis for infection, cultures should be taken. For pregnant women, options can be discussed.

POSTPROCEDURE PATIENT EDUCATION

Sexual assault is associated with major emotional and psychologic sequelae. Most women go through the three stages of rape trauma syndrome: (1) trauma (e.g. fear of being alone, fear of men, sexual problems, depression); (2) denial (not wanting to talk about it); and (3) resolution (dealing with fears and feelings, regaining a sense of control over life). During the first two stages, patients may experience flashbacks, numbness or constriction of feeling, or hypervigilance. Mood swings, irritability, and anger are common and may indicate signs of healing. Insomnia, tension headaches, anorexia, fatigue, nausea, abdominal pain, and genitourinary symptoms are not uncommon. The last stage may take years to reach. The patient should be aware that should the case go to court, it may be necessary to gather additional evidence at a later time. Adequate follow-up and a counseling referral are an essential component of management. Men go through similar stages and need similar counseling.

Patients should receive a written outline of what was performed with the initial evaluation and what treatments were provided. They should also be given a written list of specific instructions and follow-up appointments. It should be written because most assault victims will not remember the evaluation and treatment they received, much less the instructions they were given following the treatment. Many communities have sexual assault centers that will provide advocates and support personnel for the victims during medical visits and for follow-up appointments. It is very important for the patient to connect with the assault center. If they don't connect, after obtaining the victim's permission, a trained counselor should be consulted. The most important contributing factor to the patient's recovery is contact with a trained advocate or counselor within the first 72 hours of a sexual assault.

The Rape, Assault and Incest National Network (RAINN; phone: 1-800-656-HOPE; website: www.rainn. org) can assist with finding local agencies and counselors trained to assist sexual assault victims.

SUPPLIERS

Sexual Assault Evidence Collection Kit

Gieserlab Equipment and Supply
P.O. Box 659
Chestertown, MD 21620
Phone: 1-888-778-7829
Website: www.gieserlab.com

MedTech International
P.O. Box 162992
Altamonte Springs, FL 32716-2992
Phone: 1-800-447-0014
Website: www.1ivenue.com/medtechinternational/item 123593.ctlg

Sirchie Fingerprint Laboratories, Inc. (standardized kit available that fulfills laws for many Western states)
100 Hunter Place
Youngsville, NC 27596
Phone: 1-800-356-7311
Website: www.sirchie.com

CPT/BILLING CODE

Use E/M codes for established or new patients for the noncolposcopic portion of the examination.

57452   Colposcopy

In some states, the law enforcement agency is required to pay for the evidence collection examination in the case of a reported sexual assault. The patient should sign a consent form to allow the law enforcement agency to be billed.

ICD-9-CM DIAGNOSTIC CODES

V71.5	Rape, alleged, observation or examination, victim or culprit
V71.8	Observation for other specified conditions
V71.81	Abuse and neglect
V72.3	Gynecologic examination, Papanicolaou smear as part of general gynecologic examination, pelvic examination (annual) (periodic)
878.4	Open wound, vulva, without mention of complication
878.5	Open, wound, vulva, complicated

878.6   Open wound, vagina, without mention of complication
878.7   Open wound, vagina, complicated
995.83   Adult sexual abuse

ADDITIONAL RESOURCES

- See the sample patient education handout titled "Sexual Assault" on page 1957 of Appendix G.
- See the sample patient consent form titled "General Patient Consent Form/Forensic Evaluation" on page 1959 of Appendix G.

BIBLIOGRAPHY

Adolescent victims of sexual assault, ACOG Technical Bulletin 252, Washington, DC, October 1998, American College of Obstetricians and Gynecologists.

Anderson A: "Don't scream, Miss Annie. Don't scream," *Am Fam Physician* 59(1):213, 1999.

Dunn S: Lavage fluid in sexual assault examination, *CMAJ* 138(5):400, 1988.

Holmes MM, Resnick HS, Frampton D: Follow-up of sexual assault victims, *Am J Obstet Gynecol* 179(2):336, 1998.

Lenahan LC, Ernst A, Johnson B: Colposcopy in evaluation of the adult sexual assault victim, *Am J Emerg Med* 16(2):183, 1998.

Petter LM, Whitehill DL: Management of female sexual assault, *Am Fam Physician* 58(4):920,929, 1998.

Young WW, Bracken AC, Goddard MA, Matheson S: Sexual assault: review of a national model protocol for forensic and medical evaluation, *Obstet Gynecol* 80(5):878, 1992.

WEBSITE

www.forensicdocumentation.com

CHAPTER 160

Management of Young Female as Possible Victim of Sexual Abuse

David B. Bosscher

Sexual abuse is so common that primary care clinicians should consider it as a possibility even during routine office visits. Although child abuse experts are available in many communities, the generalist clinician is often critical for the first line of evaluation. Unfortunately, family turmoil, anger, or resentment toward a current or ex-spouse or significant other is frequently associated with complaints of sexual abuse, making assessment more difficult.

In young females, common initial complaints include itching, redness, burning, irritation, discharge, or bleeding at the vagina. The abuse may be disclosed initially or discovered later. Occasionally, the abuse will be discovered when a parent wants a child examined following their use of sexually explicit language or their demonstration of a sexual act on their doll. Often the complaints are nonspecific and the parent(s) simply hopes that some test can prove or disprove sexual abuse. Since children are exposed often to sexually explicit media, the examiner must carefully sift through such allegations. Unfortunately, the majority of children are seen long after the incident may have occurred. However, if the alleged incident was less than 72 hours ago, immediate examination is mandatory, using a carefully structured protocol (e.g., a rape kit; see Chapter 159, Management of the Adult Victim of Sexual Assault).

Note: Clinicians may be uncomfortable performing a gynecologic examination on a young child. For known abuse or those cases indicating abuse, clinicians must balance the need to obtain evidence in a timely, thorough, and efficient manner against appearing uncomfortably hurried or unconcerned. However, for very low probability or negative cases (see Table 160-2), the examination might be used to educate the child and the parents about perineal hygiene. In that situation, the clinician can model for parents appropriate ways to discuss anatomy and gynecologic issues with children. Perhaps the examination can be used to prevent future health problems and provide a powerful, lasting influence on a child's future gynecologic care and reproductive health. In certain very low probability situations, it may be critical to take an unhurried approach and to attempt to make the examination a positive experience to avoid traumatizing or embarrassing the child.

Note that sexual abuse is also common in young males (12% to 25% of girls versus 8% to 10% of boys by age 18). Although this chapter focuses on females, it is not meant to deny the possibility of abuse in males. If it is suspected in a young male, many of the same principles apply.

INDICATIONS

- Suspicion of sexual abuse after initial questioning or preliminary physical examination
- Referral from teacher, parent, or other responsible person alleging sexual abuse

Note: The Federal Bureau of Investigation has identified sexual assault as the most rapidly increasing violent crime in America. Retrospective studies of adult women indicate that more than half of all cases of sexual victimization occur before age 18, and 32% of all rapes occur among girls between the ages of 11 and 17.

CONTRAINDICATIONS

- Lack of needed instruments or supplies to carry out the examination
- Lack of forms to preserve the chain of evidence
- Lack of a witness for the examination to preserve the chain of evidence
- Lack of consent to examine or treat a minor if a parent or guardian is not present

EQUIPMENT

- Either a handheld lens with an adequate examination light or a colposcope to examine details. If neither is available, an otoscope may be helpful. One major benefit of a colposcope is that it allows the clinician to use both hands for the examination. If a handheld lens or an otoscope is used, an assistant will be needed.

- Camera.
- A rape kit should be available in case it is necessary to document rape. If alleged sexual contact was within the past 72 hours, consider using the rape kit to collect evidence in an organized manner. (See Chapter 159, Vaginal Examination of the Female for Rape.)

Equipment on a Mayo Stand

- Room-temperature culture media for gonorrhea (modified Thayer-Martin-Jembec).
- Chlamydia and herpes culture media.
- Materials for wet prep and KOH prep.
- Cotton swabs, calcium alginate swabs (Calgiswab) or equivalent.
- Viscous lidocaine may be helpful, applied to the introitus, if any instruments are used.

Note: Although chlamydia cultures, and possibly gonorrhea cultures, are more expensive than slide tests or DNA probes and usually take longer for results, the gold standard for testimony in court regarding *all* sexually transmitted diseases is a positive culture (if the organism can be cultured). A DNA probe kit may also be used, and may still be positive in partially treated cases; however, there is a slight false-positive rate with all DNA probes, making them almost useless in court.

PREPROCEDURE PATIENT PREPARATION

Explain the entire procedure to the caregiver and the child at a language level that both will understand. The child needs to know that she will be asked a lot of questions and that some may seem "silly." Explain that after the questions, the child will be examined.

It is often helpful to allow a young girl to maintain her sense of control over the process. After establishing rapport with the child, assure her that she will be allowed to be as active a participant as possible. If possible, she should know that she will be asked for permission before proceeding with any part of the examination.

Issues of privacy and confidentiality are important when examining older children. Although most young girls will prefer to have a parent, usually the mother, in the room at all times, in some cases it will be helpful to later spend time alone with the child. When alone with an examiner, a child may disclose abuse or other concerns. Letting her and the parent(s) know ahead of time (before the examination) that the clinician will be spending time alone with her may increase her comfort. Allowing that time alone may give her a greater sense of control and a feeling of responsibility for her own health.

Parents should be reassured that the child's hymen will not be altered in any way by the examination. Anatomic diagrams may be helpful for demonstration.

TECHNIQUE

Taking the History

1. One goal of the history is to establish or enhance rapport with the child; therefore it is helpful to talk to children at eye level. Most abusers and clinicians are physically larger than children; minimizing that discrepancy is usually appreciated. Therefore sit at or below eye level throughout the history. (If at all possible, try to minimize the time standing above the child, even during the examination!)

2. Be sure to take notes while obtaining the history. It is often complicated. Obtain the names of persons potentially involved. It is important to note if there is a previous history of sexual abuse, especially if this may alter examination findings. While building rapport, ask about the current family structure, recent life changes, and which activities she enjoys. It is also good to ask about school and her friends.

3. Document the descriptions of any potential sexual abuse in the child's own words. When the meaning of a word is not clear, ask clarifying questions. Document the meaning of the word in her terms. For example, if the child mentions sex, ask her what that means. Because of depictions on television, children often think that sex means just being naked and in bed with another person.

4. Do not be any more leading in questioning than is absolutely necessary. Begin with very general questions and go to more specific ones if the child does not offer sufficient information. For example, ask "Has anyone touched you in a way that made you feel funny or bad?" before asking "Has anyone touched your bottom?" Leading questions can not only misdirect the child and subsequently the examiner, but they can also be neutralized by a defense attorney.

5. Do not allow the caregiver(s) to adopt a coaching role. Such a role may impugn the clinician's testimony as well as the child's.

6. Do not attempt to gather the complete history a second time if it has already been done by another professional (the Protective Service worker, the social worker, etc.). Obtain only enough history to determine which parts of the physical examination and what laboratory tests are important to perform.

7. Small children are challenged by the concepts of numbers and time. They often cannot tell how many times something occurred; however, they can often specify in general terms: "a lot," "once in a while," or "one time." Likewise, regarding time, small children

do not understand the difference between "3 months ago" and "8 months ago." However, they can usually recall what happened today or yesterday.

Preparing for the Vaginal Examination

1. A medical assistant or nurse can be very helpful if they will use a toy or book or stuffed animal to distract the child during the examination.
2. Again, explain the examination to the caregiver and the child at a language level they will comprehend. This is an important step toward reinforcing the child's sense of control over the examination. Begin by describing familiar portions of the examination ("I'm going to listen to your heart and then feel your tummy"). Then, simply state that you are going to examine her genitalia ("Then I'm going to look at your bottom").
3. Explain to the child that the most important part of the examination is when the examiner merely "looks" around and that it is important for her to communicate with the examiner during the examination. Reassure the child that the examination will not hurt, and that if instruments are used, they are specially designed for little girls.
4. Perform the physical examination except for the vaginal-rectal portion. The examination should proceed from the least to the most intrusive while gaining the confidence of the child with each step.
5. Before performing the vaginal examination, it is helpful to recall normal anatomy (Fig. 160-1). The vagina is 4 to 5 cm long with thin, red epithelium in premenarchal girls. In perimenarchal girls, the hymen and vaginal mucosa are thickened. The vagina is approximately 8 cm long, and normal leukorrhea may be present.

Performing the Vaginal Examination

1. Talk constantly ("verbal anesthesia"). A calm, quiet, confident voice can be hypnotic. Use of a relaxed and unhurried approach may decrease the child's anxiety. Having the parent sit close by or hold the child's hand may also provide comfort. If the child is provided a hand mirror, it may provide distraction for her, promote education, and allow her to participate more actively in the process.
2. Tell the child that it is acceptable to undress because they are in a clinician's office.
3. Frog-leg examination
   a. Begin with the frog-leg examination. The child is supine with knees apart and feet touching in the midline (Fig. 160-2). Alternatively, the mother may assist with the frog-leg position (Fig. 160-3). Older children may be placed in adjustable stirrups (Fig. 160-4).
   b. Inspect the vulva and areas lateral to it. Use the colposcope, a hand lens with adequate lighting, or an otoscope to better visualize the introitus.
   c. Gently open the labia by applying lateral traction, just lateral to the vulva at the level of the posterior introitus. Do not force the labia open; they will usually open with persistent gentle traction or the child may assist by holding her labia apart. Sometimes, traction with just two index fingers is all that is needed to open the labia.
   d. Examine carefully the entire circumference of the introitus and hymen. Normal hymenal variants

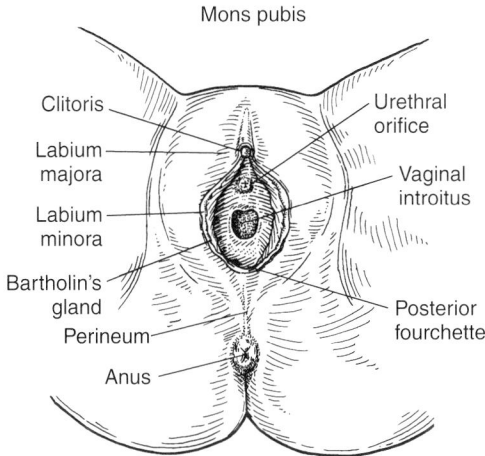

Fig. 160-1
Anatomy of genitalia in prepubertal girl. (From Dieckmann RA, Fiser DH, Selbst SM: *Illustrated textbook of pediatric emergency and critical care procedures,* St Louis, 1997, Mosby.)

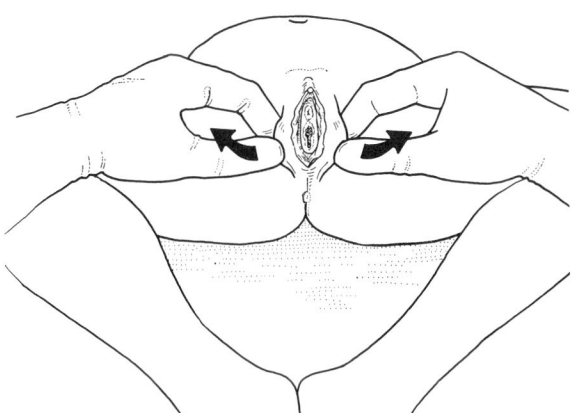

Fig. 160-2
Frog-leg position. Note gentle traction on posterior labia to enhance visualization. (From Dieckmann RA, Fiser DH, Selbst SM: *Illustrated textbook of pediatric emergency and critical care procedures,* St Louis, 1997, Mosby.)

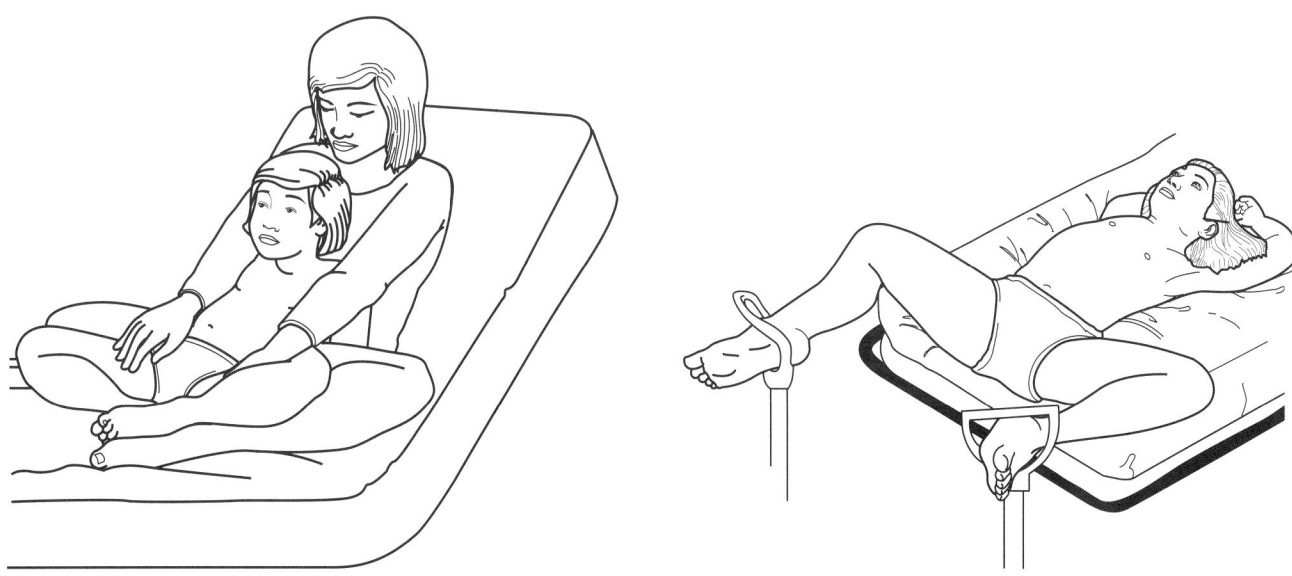

Fig. 160-3
Frog-leg position with mother's assistance. (Redrawn from Khan JA, Emans SJ: Gynecologic management of rape in adolescent girls, *Patient Care* 33[6]:71, 1999.)

Fig. 160-4
Lithotomy position with use of stirrups. (Redrawn from Khan JA, Emans SJ: Gynecologic management of rape in adolescent girls, *Patient Care* 33[6]:71, 1999.)

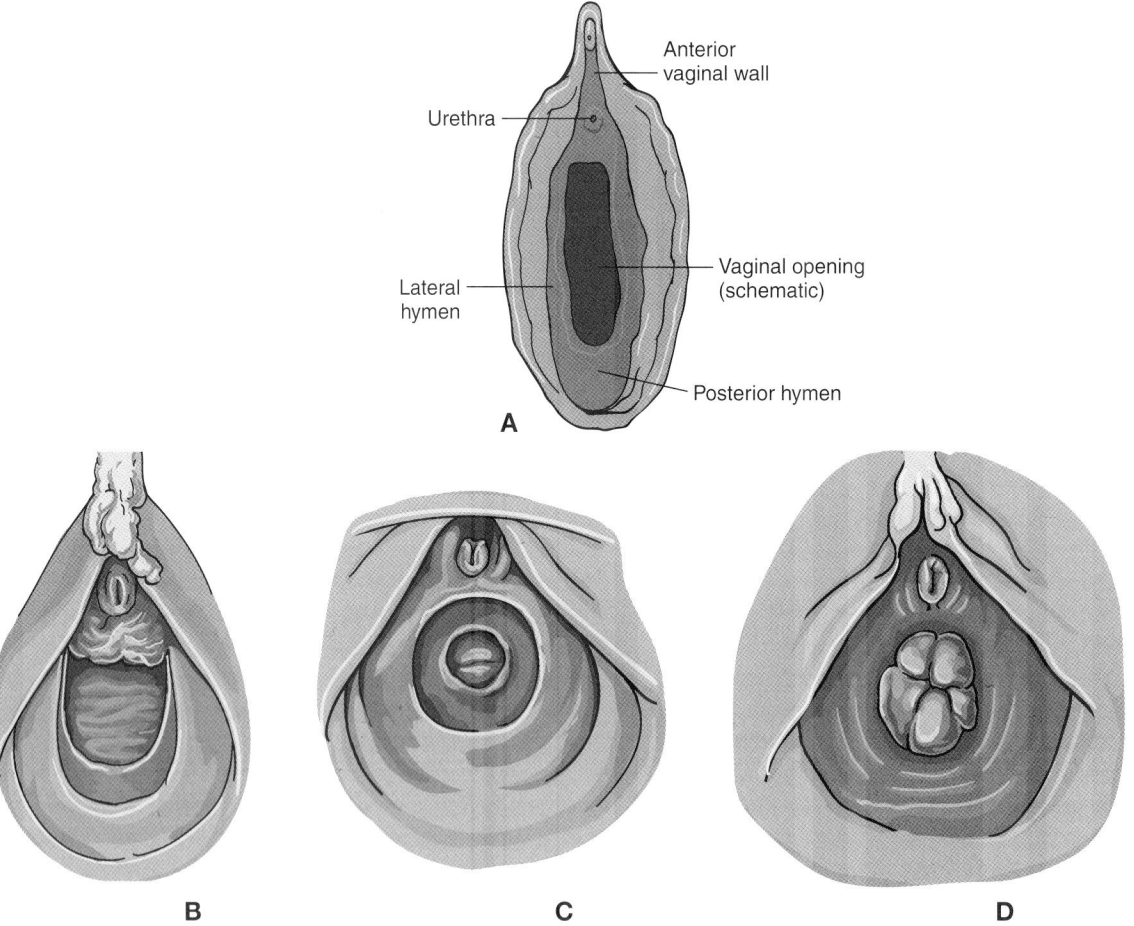

Fig. 160-5
Variants of normal hymen. **A,** Normal hymen. **B,** Posterior rim or crescentic hymen. **C,** Circumferential or annular hymen. **D,** Fimbriated or redundant hymen. (**B-D,** Redrawn from Khan JA, Emans SJ: Gynecologic management of rape in adolescent girls, *Patient Care* 33[6]:71, 1999.)

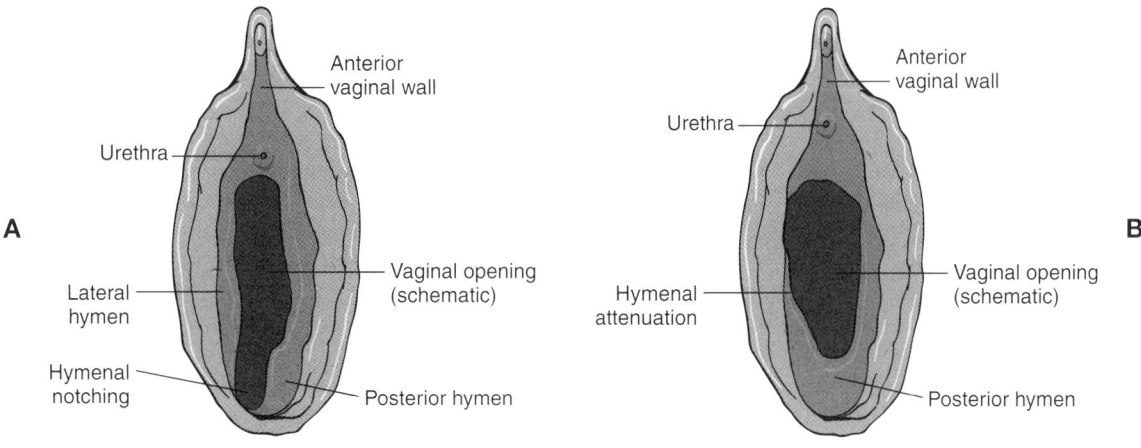

Fig. 160-6
A, Hymenal notching. **B,** Hymenal attenuation.

are illustrated (Fig. 160-5). Look carefully for asymmetry, for notching in the posterior hymen, or for attenuation (thinning) (Fig. 160-6) of the hymen around its lateral edges. These findings are usually caused by sexual abuse, and rarely by accidental trauma. The significance of the diameter of the hymenal orifice is controversial; a large orifice may be consistent with a history of abuse, but it is not an absolute criterion. If the hymen cannot be fully visualized, ask the child to cough or take a deep breath. Pull the labia gently forward and down or laterally. A colposcope is helpful at this stage. A hand lens or an otoscope can also be used if an assistant can help with the examination.

e. Acute trauma from sexual abuse is evidenced by the presence of hematomas, abrasions, lacerations, hymenal transections, and/or vulvar erythema. These conditions usually resolve within 10 to 14 days.

f. No cultures should be taken at this time. Wait until after the knee-chest examination.

4. Knee-chest examination (for children older than 2 years)

a. Surprisingly, most young children readily adopt this position. It is particularly helpful if the vagina and cervix need to be visualized. Buttocks should be higher than the back, with legs apart. It is important that the knees be approximately 25 cm (12 inches) apart. The child can rest her head to one side on her folded arms (Fig. 160-7).

b. Gentle traction laterally will often open up the labia. Ask the patient to take 10 slow deep breaths, since this will also relax the perineal structures.

c. Use the colposcope (otoscope or hand lens with an assistant) to look at the posterior hymen,

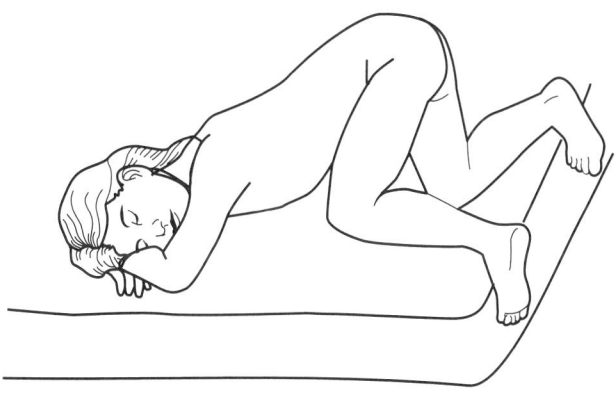

Fig. 160-7
Knee-chest position. (Redrawn from Khan JA, Emans SJ: Gynecologic management of rape in adolescent girls, *Patient Care* 33[6]:71, 1999.)

which is the preferred position for detecting small but significant abnormalities of the hymen. Again, look for asymmetries, notching, or attenuation. Take photographs if abnormalities are seen.

d. The lower vagina will be visualized in this position, and the upper vagina and cervix in 80% to 90% of prepubertal girls. Also, examine the rectum in this position.

5. Resume the frog-leg position to collect cultures. Perform the following *only* if a vaginal discharge or pain is noted, if there is genital itching or odor or urinary symptoms, or if there are genital ulcers or lesions. Consider cultures if the prevalence of STDs in the community is high, if a sibling or another child or adult in the household has an STD, or a known assailant has an STD or is at high risk.

a. Culture (not DNA probe) for chlamydia. Collect the specimen as deeply in the posterior vagina as you can. Use a cotton or calcium alginate swab. If possible, it should be moistened with nonbacteriostatic saline to minimize the discomfort. Before inserting, allow the child to feel a similar swab on her skin. Avoid touching the hymen when obtaining the culture. It may also be helpful to ask the child to cough in order to distract her and open the hymen.

Alternatively, a male urethral swab may be used to gently scrape the vaginal wall.

b. Alternatively, a vaginal wash and aspiration can be obtained. Using a small feeding tube attached to a small syringe, insert the tube into the vagina and inject and aspirate 0.5 to 1 ml of sterile saline. A soft plastic or glass eyedropper with 4 to 5 cm of IV plastic tubing attached can also be used in the same manner. A catheter-in-a-catheter technique is another option. Insert the needle of an IV butterfly into the distal end of a no. 12 bladder catheter. Attach a 1-ml tuberculin syringe to the hub of the butterfly tubing. Insert the catheter into the vagina, and inject and aspirate the saline.

Chain of Evidence Form

* PLEASE COMPLETE CAREFULLY—THIS FORM IS REQUIRED FOR LEGAL PURPOSES

1. Use this LOG to document specimen transfer so that "chain of evidence" can be preserved.
2. Each time the specimen changes hands, the new carrier-technologist must place his or her initials on the form in the appropriate location and must mark the date and time.
3. When the final laboratory report is prepared, staple securely to the LOG before sending the report to the ordering clinician.
4. Please use separate forms if specimens of different types are submitted (e.g., blood specimen and GC culture) or if specimens are sent to different labs.
5. If you perform the laboratory test in your office, have each staff member who handles the specimen initial the form. Anyone in attendance during the history and examination should sign as a witness at the bottom of the form.
6. If you have questions, call the ordering clinician.

Patient's name: _____   Date: _____

Laboratory test(s) ordered (circle):   RPR   Urine culture   Culture for GC/Chlamydia   HIV

Other: _____

Patient's medical record number: _____   Date of birth: _____

Ordering clinician: _____

Each person handling the specimen should *PLACE INITIALS in the first column, then mark the TIME and DATE.*

1. SPECIMEN COLLECTED by _____   1. DATE _____ TIME _____
2. DELIVERED TO LAB by _____   2. DATE _____ TIME _____
3. RECEIVED IN LAB by _____   3. DATE _____ TIME _____
4. PROCESSED by _____   4. DATE _____ TIME _____
5. PROCESSED by _____   5. DATE _____ TIME _____
6. FINAL REPORT PREPARED by _____   6. DATE _____ TIME _____

WITNESSES TO EXAMINATION:

1. _____   1. DATE _____ TIME _____
2. _____   2. DATE _____ TIME _____
3. _____   3. DATE _____ TIME _____
4. _____   4. DATE _____ TIME _____
5. _____   5. DATE _____ TIME _____
6. _____   6. DATE _____ TIME _____

Fig. 160-8
Chain of evidence form.

c. For gonorrhea (GC), use a cotton or calcium alginate swab to obtain slides of the following: throat, deep in the posterior vagina, and rectum. Place them on a single plate partitioned into thirds.

Note: If any area is actually positive, you will need to reculture each area separately to confirm the location. A false-positive chlamydia or GC culture is very rare so it should be investigated.

d. Obtain a herpes culture if there is any lesion resembling herpes.
e. Cultures for other organisms can be obtained by placing the calcium alginate swab into a transport Culturette II (contains medium) or by sending the aspirated fluid to the lab for direct plating.
f. Obtain a wet prep or KOH prep if indicated.
g. Note and document the presence of any condyloma.

6. In addition to the above studies, obtain a urine culture, syphilis serology, and HIV testing on all patients because of the paucity of findings with these diseases.

Note: Foreign bodies are often found as the cause of a discharge. Removal may be possible with a cotton-tipped applicator or by lavaging the vagina with saline or warm water. Viscous lidocaine may be useful for anesthesia at the introitus.

7. Send all cultures to the lab, using *chain of evidence* form and precautions (Fig. 160-8).
8. After the examination, congratulate the child for her cooperation. Discuss the results and the diagnosis and management plan with the child and her parent(s) after she is dressed. Since the results of the examination are often inconclusive, help the parent(s) to understand that a careful and complete investigation includes Protective Services and/or law enforcement officials.
9. Implications of positive laboratory findings are set out in Table 160-1. Table 160-2 contains guidelines for making reporting decisions.

Uncooperative Patients

The uncooperative patient calls for artistry on the part of the examiner. Often (but not always), proceeding through the examination slowly will result in a satisfactory examination. Leaving the room and returning when she is ready often allows a child to regain control.

TABLE 160-1

Implications of Commonly Encountered Sexually Transmitted Diseases (STDs) in Prepubertal Children

STD Confirmed	Sexual Abuse	Suggested Action
Gonorrhea	Certain	Report
Syphilis	Certain	Report
Chlamydia	Probable	Report
Condyloma	Probable	Report
Trichomonas	Probable	Report
Herpes 1 (on genitals)	Possible	Report
Herpes 2	Probable	Report
Bacterial vaginosis	Uncertain	Medical follow-up
Candida albicans	Unlikely	Medical follow-up

Adapted from American Academy of Pediatrics Committee on Child Abuse and Neglect: *Pediatrics* 87:254, 1991.

TABLE 160-2

Guidelines for Making the Decision to Report Sexual Abuse of Children

History	Physical Examination	Laboratory Abnormality	Level of Concern About Sexual Abuse	Action
None	Normal	None	None	None
Behavioral changes	Normal	None	Low	+/– report, follow closely
None	Nonspecific	None	Low	+/– report, follow closely
Nonspecific history by child or history by parent only	Nonspecific	None	Possible	+/– report, follow closely
None	Specific findings	None	Probable	Report
Child's clear statement	Specific findings	None	Probable	Report
None	Normal, nonspecific, or specific findings	Positive culture for GC, chlamydia, +RPR, *Trichomonas,* presence of sperm	Definite	Report
Behavioral changes	Nonspecific changes	Other sexually transmitted diseases	Probable	Report

Adapted from American Academy of Pediatrics Committee on Child Abuse and Neglect: *Pediatrics* 87:254, 1991.
RPR, Rapid plasma reagin test.

Nasally administered Versed, a short-acting benzodiazepine (dosage: 0.2 to 0.4 mg/kg of the injectable solution) can enhance cooperativeness. When administered by this route (use a TB syringe without a needle), the drug will be effective within 15 minutes. Side effects are rare. Versed syrup is available as another option. The child must be observed by a knowledgeable parent or by your staff for about 1 to 2 hours after the drug is given. This technique, considered Class 1 conscious sedation under most hospitals' sedation protocols, requires no intensive monitoring. (See Chapter 7, Pediatric Sedation.)

CPT/BILLING CODES

Use E/M codes for the noncolposcopic portion of the examination.

57452   Colposcopy

ICD-9-CM DIAGNOSTIC CODES

V71.5   Rape, alleged, observation or examination, victim or culprit
878.4   Open wound, vulva, without mention of complication
878.5   Vulva, complicated
878.6   Open wound, vagina, without mention of complication
878.7   Vagina, complicated
995.53   Child sexual abuse

BIBLIOGRAPHY

American Academy of Pediatrics Committee on Child Abuse and Neglect: Guidelines for the evaluation of sexual abuse of children, *Pediatrics* 103(1):186, 1999.

American College of Obstetricians and Gynecologists: *Adolescent victims of sexual assault,* ACOG Tech Bull 252, Washington, DC, October 1998.

Holmes MM: Clinical management of rape in adolescent girls, *Patient Care* 3(7):42, 1999.

Khan JA, Emans SJ: Gynecologic examination of the prepubertal girl, *Patient Care* 33(6):71, 1999.

O'Connell BJ: Evaluation of the sexually abused child, including the role of colposcopy, *J Lower Gen Tract Dis* 5(2):87, 2001.

Sexually Transmitted Diseases Treatment guidelines—2002, *MMWR* 51(RR06):1, 2002.

Wissow L: *Child advocacy for the clinician,* Baltimore, 1990, Williams and Wilkins.

ADDITIONAL RESOURCES

• See the sample patient education handout titled "Sexual Abuse" on page 1960 of Appendix G.

CHAPTER 161

Vulvar Biopsy

Gregory L. Brotzman

Evaluation of the vulva is an important component of a routine gynecologic examination. Fig. 161-1 shows basic vulvar anatomy as well as the orientation of lines of skin tension. Skin tension lines are important in considering excisional or punch biopsies of the vulva. With the index finger and thumb of the nondominant hand, the skin should be stretched in the opposite direction of (perpendicular to) the tension lines, so that the excision margins form an ellipse after release. This allows an easier closure if sutures are used. Although most lesions found at vulvar examination are benign, such as skin tags or simple nevi, biopsy is occasionally needed to obtain a clearer understanding of the lesion present. This is especially true in older women and in those who smoke, since they have a significantly increased risk of developing vulvar intraepithelial neoplasia (VIN) or cancer.

Depth of biopsy is an important consideration. Disease of the non–hair-bearing areas of the vulva (labia minora, forchette, interior aspect of the labia majora) is usually only 1 to 2 mm in depth. In contrast, hair-bearing areas (outer aspect labia majora) may have disease that follows the hair shaft and is several millimeters in depth. Deep biopsies are not necessary for non–hair-bearing vulvar skin areas, but biopsies should go down full depth to adipose tissue where hair is present. An elevated lesion can be shaved off (see Chapter 33, Skin Biopsy) if it is certain not to be a melanoma (seborrheic keratosis, condyloma, nevus, etc.).

Examination of the vulva is aided by the use of a colposcope (low-power setting, 5×) or a magnifying glass after staining with 3% to 5% acetic acid (vinegar). Staining helps delineate dysplastic tissue and warty changes by turning it white (acetowhite epithelium).

In addition to this chapter, see Chapter 157, Treatment of Noncervical Condyloma Acuminata, Chapter 33, Skin Biopsy, and Chapters 22 to 26 on excision of lesions and follow-up repair.

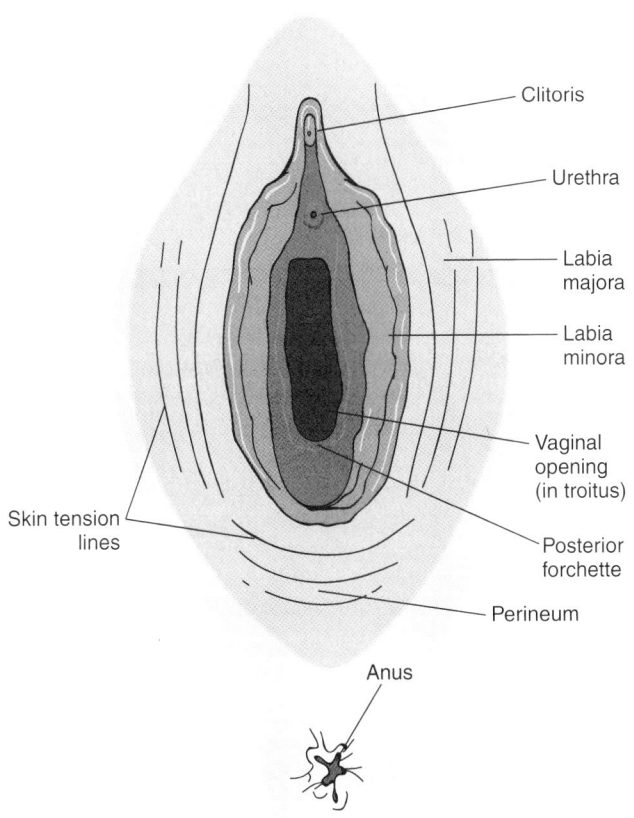

Fig. 161-1
Vulvar anatomy. The vertical and horizontal lines demonstrate the lines of skin tension. When a biopsy is being performed, stretch the skin in the direction opposite to the skin tension lines, so that after the biopsy is done, the skin will form an ellipse when relaxed, making it easier to close if sutures are needed.

INDICATIONS

- Pigmented lesions
- Vulvar ulceration of uncertain etiology
- White epithelium (skin that turns white after the application of 5% acetic acid)
- Leukoplakia (white skin before the application of acetic acid)
- Presumed condylomata that do not readily respond to

conventional therapy (if not resolved or significantly improving after two treatment attempts of any kind)
• Any skin abnormality that needs definitive diagnosis

CONTRAINDICATIONS

• Allergy to local anesthetic
• Bleeding diathesis (relative)
• Recent (<3 weeks) chemical destruction attempts. These may result in false-positive histologic findings. It is best to wait until healing has occurred after any treatment before attempting a biopsy of such lesions.

EQUIPMENT

• 3-mm Keyes punch biopsy (4 and 5 mm also accepted but may require suturing, whereas 3 mm does not) (Fig. 161-2, *A*) or sharp tissue scissors, or a no. 15 blade for elevated or non–hair-bearing areas
• No. 15 scalpel blade for excision
• 1% lidocaine (Xylocaine) with or without epinephrine (can mix 1:10 with sodium bicarbonate solution to decrease discomfort)
• 30-gauge, ½-inch needles
• 1- to 5-ml syringe
• Nonsterile gloves
• Formalin containers
• Iris scissors (Fig. 161-2, *B*)
• Pickups (Fig. 161-2, *C*)

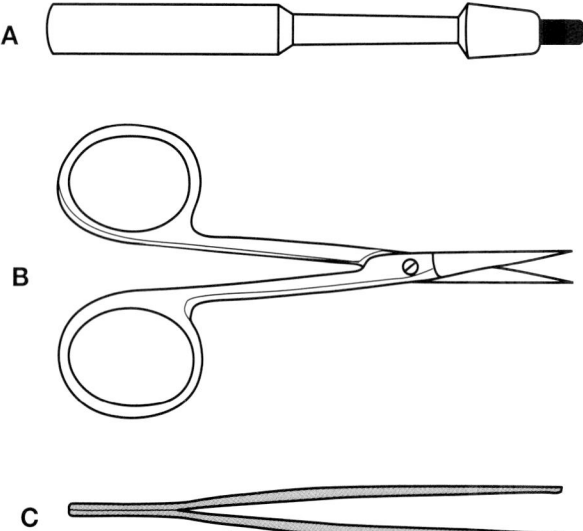

Fig. 161-2
A, Keyes punch biopsy. **B,** Iris scissors. **C,** Tissue forceps.

• Povidone-iodine or alcohol swabs
• Monsel's solution (thickened ferric subsulfate solution)
• Small cotton-tipped applicators
• Antibiotic ointment

PREPROCEDURE PATIENT PREPARATION

If there are no contraindications, have the patient use 600 mg of ibuprofen 1 hour before the procedure to help with postprocedure discomfort.

TECHNIQUE

There are three ways to perform a biopsy of the vulva:
• Punch biopsy (with a Keyes punch)
• Excisional biopsy (using a no. 15 scalpel blade)
• Shave excision (using tissue scissors or a blade)

Deciding which type of biopsy technique to use depends on the size and location of the lesion (see above). A large lesion would likely require punch biopsies to sample it, or it may be possible to excise it in its entirety with an excisional biopsy technique. Frequently, small lesions can be excised completely with punch biopsy. Most punch biopsies do not require suturing, whereas excisional biopsies do.

General Technique

1. Draw up 1 to 5 ml Xylocaine with or without epinephrine, mixed with a 10:1 ratio of Xylocaine to bicarbonate solution, 1 mEq/ml.
2. Identify the lesion (Fig. 161-3, *A*).
3. Prep the skin with a povidone-iodine swab or alcohol.
4. Inject around and under lesion with local anesthetic to raise the lesion (Fig. 161-3, *B*).
5. Test skin with needle to be sure anesthesia is adequate (should be immediately effective).
6. Stretch the skin in direction opposite of skin tension lines in the vulvar area (i.e., stretch horizontally for a labial biopsy and stretch vertically for a perineal biopsy).

Technique for a Keyes Punch

1. Place punch over lesion perpendicular to the surface and slowly twist with minimal pressure on the punch instrument (let the cutting occur with the instrument) (Fig. 161-3, *C*).
2. Continue until you feel a "give" and the punch is loose from the surrounding tissues.

3. Gently grasp the edge of the lesion or the subcutaneous portion of the biopsy with the tissue forceps and lift up (avoid grasping the central portion of the lesion, as this may cause crush artifact to the specimen).
4. Snip the base of the specimen with iris scissors, and remove the biopsy sample (if multiple biopsies of the same lesion are obtained, each lesion should be in its own container) (Fig. 161-3, *D*).
5. Apply a small amount of Monsel's solution or aluminum chloride solution to the biopsy crater, using a small cotton-tipped applicator.
6. More resistant bleeding may be treated with a small piece of Gelfoam or an absorbable suture.
7. Wipe away any excess hemostatic agent or blood with saline-moistened gauze.

Note: After either the punch biopsy or the excisional biopsy, apply a small amount of antibacterial ointment to the biopsy site.

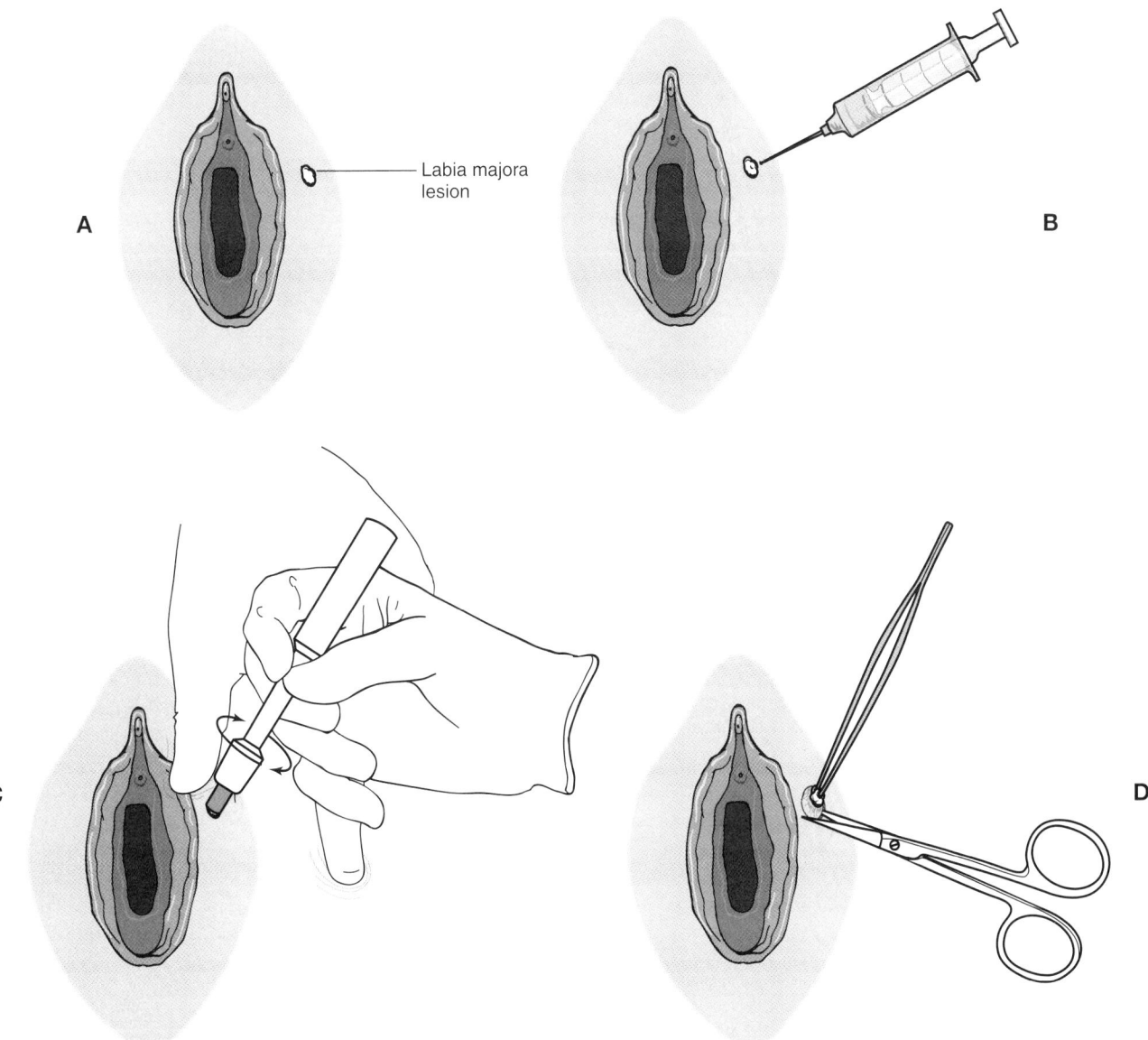

Fig. 161-3
Example of punch biopsy. **A,** Lesion of left labia majora. **B,** Lesion anesthetized. **C,** Biopsy performed with a Keyes punch. **D,** If Keyes punch used, once the skin is free from surrounding tissues, snip base with iris scissors.

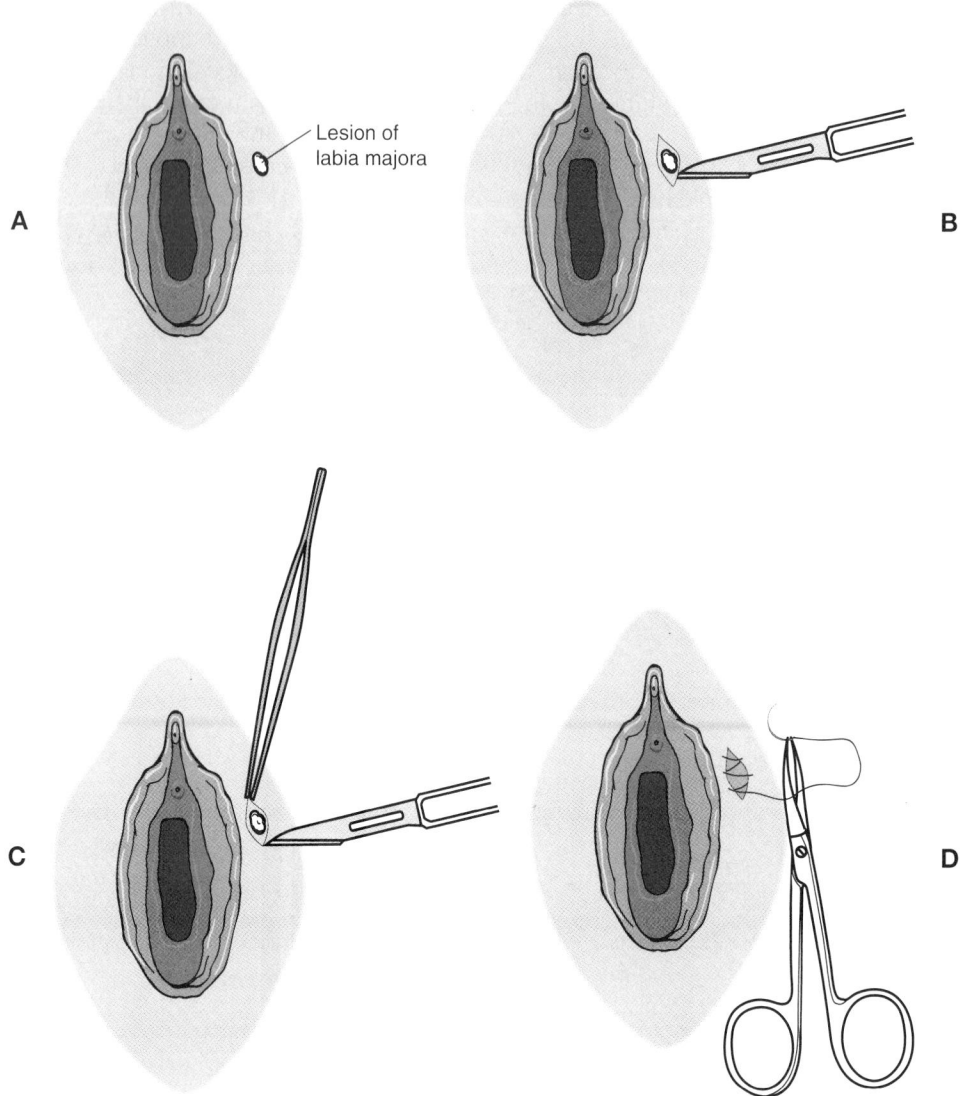

Fig. 161-4

Example of excisional biopsy. **A,** Lesion of labia majora. **B,** After anesthesia, elliptical incision made along skin tension lines. **C,** Scalpel used to free base from apex toward center of excised area. **D,** Skin closed with subcuticular running absorbable suture.

Technique for an Excisional Biopsy

Fig. 161-4 illustrates an excisional biopsy. See Chapters 22 to 26 for further details on performing an excisional biopsy with repair.

- Pain
- Scar
- Recurrence
- Not sampling the most advanced part of the lesion

COMPLICATIONS

The following complications are extremely rare:
- Infection
- Bleeding, hematoma, ecchymosis
- Hypopigmentation

POSTPROCEDURE PATIENT EDUCATION

Instruct the patient to perform the following after the procedure:
- Wash the area twice a day with soap and water.
- Apply antibiotic ointment after each cleansing.

- Use acetaminophen or ibuprofen for discomfort (Note: First determine any contraindications on the use of these medications in the patient).
- Take sitz baths as needed for discomfort if extensive removals are performed.
- Use ice packs as needed.
- For more recalcitrant pain, use over-the-counter benzocaine gel (toothache-type pain reliever) as needed.
- Call for persistent pain, redness, or swelling.
- Avoid intercourse until discomfort is gone (usually 3 to 5 days).
- Arrange a follow-up appointment or phone call to discuss biopsy results.

CONCLUSION

Vulvar biopsy is a straightforward, easy-to-perform office skill that allows the practitioner to differentiate benign from neoplastic lesions, often being curative when the entire lesion is encompassed by the biopsy.

CPT/BILLING CODES

56605	Biopsy of vulva or perineum (one lesion)
56606	Biopsy of each additional vulvar or perineal lesion

For complete excisional removals, also see excision codes.

ICD-9-CM DIAGNOSTIC CODES

624.9	Unspecified noninflammatory disorder of vulva and perineum
078.11	Condyloma acuminatum
701.9	Skin tag
221.2	Benign vulvar neoplasm
624.8	Vulvar dysplasia
233.3	VIN 3
616.10	Vulvitis

ADDITIONAL RESOURCES

- See the sample patient education handout titled "Vulvar Biopsy" on page 1961 of Appendix G.
- See the sample patient consent form titled "Vulvar Biopsy" on page 1962 of Appendix G.

BIBLIOGRAPHY

Apgar B: Vulvar/vaginal pathology. In *Basic colposcopy for the family physician,* AAFP, 1992.

Apgar BS, Brotzman GL, Spitzer M: *Colposcopy: principles and practice: an integrated textbook and atlas,* Philadelphia, 2002, WB Saunders.

Clarke-Pearson DL, Dawood MY, editors: *Green's gynecology: essentials of clinical practice,* ed 4, Boston, 1990, Little, Brown.

DiSaia P, Creasman W, editors: *Clinical gynecologic oncology,* ed 5, St Louis, 1997, Mosby.

Kurman R, editor: *Blaustein's pathology of the female genital tract,* ed 4, New York, 1994, Springer-Verlag.

Scott J, DiSaia P, Hammond C, Spellacy W, editors: *Danforth's obstetrics & gynecology,* ed 6, Philadelphia, 1990, JB Lippincott.

Wheeler C Jr, editor: *Atlas of pelvic surgery,* ed 2, Philadelphia, 1988, Lea & Febiger.

CHAPTER 162

Wet Smear and KOH Preparation

Barbara S. Apgar

GYNECOLOGY AND FEMALE REPRODUCTIVE WET SMEAR AND KOH PREPARATION

The wet smear is an important tool in the office evaluation of vaginitis and estrogen status. It should be performed on patients with vaginal symptoms, even if the diagnosis seems obvious. The wet smear is an accessory tool to the clinical history, the inspection of the vulvar and vaginal mucosa and the cervix, and the determination of the pH of the vaginal secretions.

INDICATIONS

- Vaginal discharge
- Vulvar or vaginal pain
- Abnormal vaginal secretions

CONTRAINDICATIONS (RELATIVE)

- Recent douching
- Intravaginal medications
- Menses

EQUIPMENT

- Vaginal speculum
- Small cotton-tipped applicators
- Small test tubes
- Normal saline
- 10% potassium hydroxide (KOH) solution
- Glass slides and coverslips
- Microscope
- pH test tape

PREPROCEDURE PATIENT PREPARATION

- Explain the procedure to the patient. Written consent is not required.
- Instruct the patient to avoid vaginal medication, douches, and coitus for 24 hours before the procedure.

TECHNIQUE

1. Place the patient in the lithotomy position and insert vaginal speculum.
2. Rub a cotton-tipped applicator along the lateral vaginal walls and the lateral fornices to collect the specimen. Avoid collecting only the secretions in the fornices. Put the cotton-tipped applicator in a small test tube (3 to 4 inches long) that contains approximately 1 ml of normal saline. Leave the applicator in the test tube until the wet smear is prepared in the laboratory. Remove the speculum from the vagina.
3. Take the test tube to the laboratory to prepare the wet smear. Remove the cotton-tipped applicator from the test tube, place a drop on the left side of the glass slide, and immediately place a coverslip over the drop. Place another drop from the cotton-tipped applicator on the right side of the slide. Add a drop of 10% KOH solution to the drop and immediately place a coverslip over it. Two separate slides may also be prepared.
4. Examine the saline and KOH-prepared samples under low (10×) and high (40×) power of the microscope. Examine the saline preparation for the presence of *Lactobacillus* species (normal vaginal flora) (Fig. 162-1), leukocytes (more than 5 to 10 cells per high power field [HPF] may indicate infection), parabasal cells (may indicate low estrogenic state),

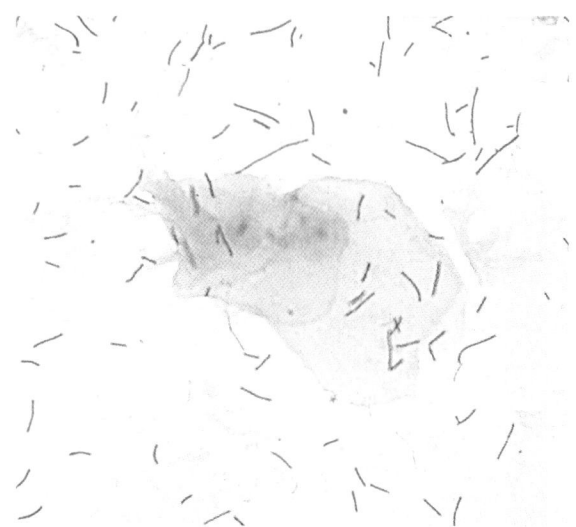

Fig. 162-1
Lactobacillus species. (From Morse SA, Moreland A, Holmes K: Atlas of sexually transmitted diseases and AIDS, ed 2, London, 1996, Gower Medical Publishing.)

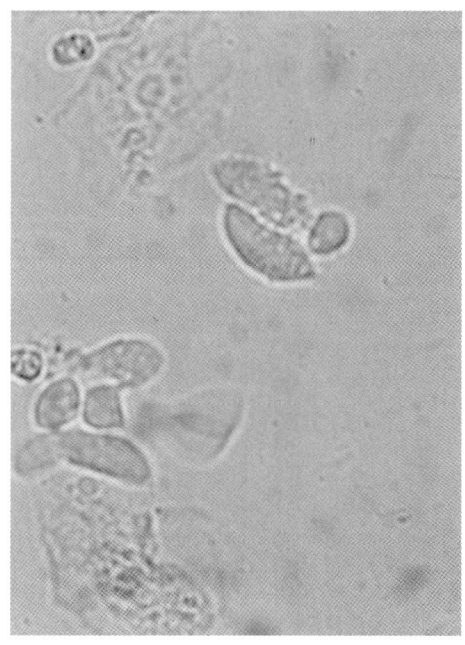

Fig. 162-2
Microscopic examination of a wet mount reveals multiple motile trichomonads. (From Zitelli BJ, Davis HW: *Atlas of pediatric physical diagnosis,* ed 4, St Louis, 2002, Mosby.)

trichomonads (trichomoniasis vaginalis) (Fig. 162-2), and clue cells (bacterial vaginosis) (Fig. 162-3). A clue cell is a large epithelial cell with indistinct borders and adherent multiple coccobacilli organisms clinging to it. At least five different microscopic fields should be surveyed to observe an adequate number of representative fields. Scan the KOH-prepared sample for the presence of hyphae or buds (candidiasis). The absence of hyphae but presence of budding spores suggests infection with a non-albicans type of *Candida,* such as *C. glabrata* (Fig. 162-4). If the number of leukocytes exceeds the number of squamous cells, an inflammatory process should be suspected.

Note: Lactobacilli are large, long bacillary rods. Their absence or decrease, coupled with an abundance of clue cells and a vaginal pH greater than 4.7, may be consistent with the clinical findings observed in bacterial vaginosis.

5. pH test tape may be used to screen for the specific type of vaginitis. A piece of the pH test tape may be directly applied to the vaginal wall, or the tape can be applied to the vaginal secretions adhering to the speculum when it is removed from the vagina. Compare the color of the test tape that has been in contact with the secretions to the color guide on the tape dispenser. The range of values will be determined by the color of the tape.

Normal flora—pH ≤4.5
Candidiasis—pH 4 to 5
Bacterial vaginosis—pH ≥4.7
Trichomonas—pH >6

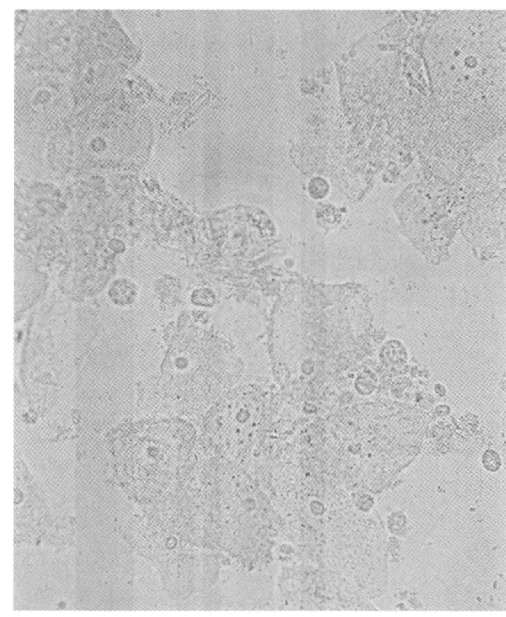

Fig. 162-3
"Clue cells" on wet mount consist of vaginal epithelial cells covered with adherent refractile bacteria. (From Zitelli BJ, Davis HW: *Atlas of pediatric physical diagnosis,* ed 4, St Louis, 2002, Mosby.)

The combination of pH reading and the microscopic impression help make an accurate diagnosis. However, the results may be invalid if blood, semen, or douche solution is present.

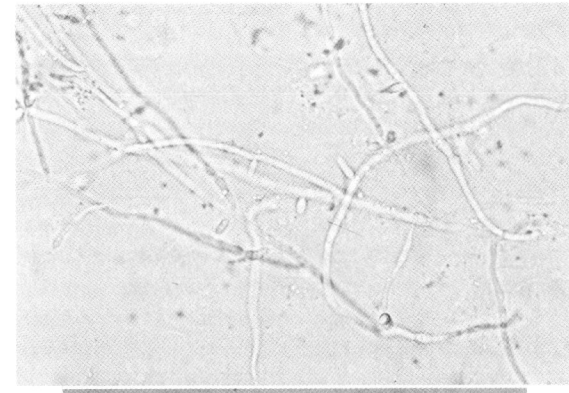

A

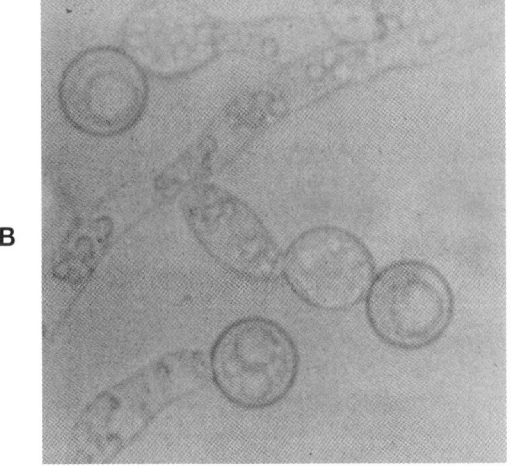

B

Fig. 162-4
A, Yeast hyphae and, **B,** budding yeast. (From Zitelli BJ, Davis HW: *Atlas of pediatric physical diagnosis,* ed 4, St Louis, 2002, Mosby.)

6. At the time that the vaginitis evaluation is performed, specimens from the cervix may be obtained to ascertain the presence of chlamydial and gonorrheal infections. The proper sampling devices and proper preparation are important and depend on the type of test the laboratory uses. If a cotton-tipped swab is used for sample collection, the cervix does not need to be wiped clean before the procedure. Insert the applicator directly into the cervical canal until the cotton tip is completely inside the os. Gently twirl the tip several times in the os. Withdraw the applicator and place it in the proper container. Your laboratory should provide specific directions for obtaining the sample and transporting it to the laboratory.

POSTPROCEDURE PATIENT EDUCATION

Instruct the patient about medication, if needed, and the need for follow-up appointments.

CPT/BILLING CODES

58999	Wet smear and KOH preparation
87220	Tissue examination by KOH slide from skin, hair, or nails

ICD-9-CM DIAGNOSTIC CODES

616.10	Vaginal infection (vaginitis)
112.1	Yeast (candidiasis)
131.01	Trichomonas
616.10	Bacterial vaginosis
627.3	Atrophic vaginitis
623.5	Vaginal discharge
625.9	Vulvar pain
625.9	Vaginal pain

BIBLIOGRAPHY

Berthholf ME, Stafford MJ: An office laboratory panel to assess vaginal problems, *Am Fam Physician* 32(3):113, 1985.

Carr PL, Felsenstein D, Friedman RH: Evaluation and management of vaginitis, *J Gen Int Med* 13(5):335, 1998.

Centers for Disease Control: 1998 sexually transmitted diseases guideline, *MMWR* 47(RR-1):70, 1998.

Eschenbach DA, Hillier SL: Advances in diagnostic testing for vaginitis and cervicitis, *J Reprod Med* 34(8):555, 1989.

Landers DV: Vaginitis/cervicitis: diagnosis and treatment options in a limited resource environment, *Womens Health Issues* 6(6):342, 1996.

Majeroni BA: Bacterial vaginosis: an update, *Am Fam Phys* 57(6):1285, 1998.

Pandit L, Ouslnader JG: Postmenopausal vaginal atrophy and atrophic vaginitis, *Am J Med Sci* 314(4):228, 1997.

Priestly CJ, Jones BM, Dhar J, Goodwin L: What is normal vaginal flora? *Genitourinary Med* 73(1):23, 1997.

Shesser R: Common vaginal infections: a concise work-up guide, *Female Pat* 15:53, 1990.

Sobel JD: Vaginitis, *N Engl J Med* 337:1896, 1997.

PART TEN

Obstetrics

CHAPTER 163

Amniocentesis

Clark B. Smith

Amniocentesis is very helpful for evaluating an inaccessible in utero patient. Although genetic studies were first performed on amniotic fluid in the 1950s, before 1970 the primary indication for amniocentesis was the Rh-immunized patient. Since that time, the indications have expanded to include evaluation of fetal lung maturity, fetal genetics, rupture or infection of the amniotic membranes or fluid, and other factors related to fetal health. In some centers caring for high-risk patients, amniocentesis is a routine procedure in approximately 15% of pregnancies. However, the overall frequency of amniocentesis has decreased every year since 1989—down to 2.4% of pregnancies (2000). It is important to remember that complications from amniocentesis can be serious—some can even be lethal.

INDICATIONS

Prenatal Diagnosis (First and Second Trimester)

1. *Chromosomal studies.* Amniotic fluid contains fetal and amniotic cells. The fetal cells include desquamated squamous cells and cells from the gastrointestinal tract, respiratory tract, and urinary system. Although it requires 2 to 3 weeks for results, culture of these cells allows accurate fetal chromosome analysis for chromosomal, sex-linked, and metabolic disorders. For chromosomal analysis, amniocentesis is usually performed at 15 to 17 weeks; when there are sufficient numbers of desquamated fetal cells to allow successful culture. Although amniocentesis can be performed in the late first trimester (i.e., 10 to 14 weeks' gestation), chorionic villus sampling (CVS) is usually performed because the risk of fetal loss is less and there is an increased risk of talipes equinovarus with amniocentesis. Indications for early amniocentesis include the following:
   a. Advanced maternal age (i.e., 34 years of age or older)
   b. Parent who is a carrier of a genetic disease that can be diagnosed by amniocentesis
   c. Mother who is a carrier of an X-linked disorder
   d. History of a child with a chromosomal disorder, neural tube defect, inherited biochemical disorder, or multiple anomalies
   e. Mother with a history of three or more spontaneous abortions

Note: Some experts recommend that mothers be referred to specialized medical centers for first trimester or early second-trimester amniocentesis and genetic studies. Less fluid is available at this stage, and there may be less risk of complications with more operator experience. This is particularly important if the procedure must be performed *through* the placenta. A cell culture is also very fragile, and proper transport and assurance against loss or mix-up are essential. It may be best to perform the study at the institution where the cells will be cultured.

2. *Abnormal triple screen.* Serum α-fetoprotein, unconjugated estriol, and β-HCG levels together are known as a *triple screen.* Careful sonographic fetal evaluation in patients with abnormal triple-screen results may diagnose (or exclude) an open neural tube defect or Down syndrome. Occasionally, amniocentesis may be required for clarification.
3. *Evaluation for amnionitis.* In a patient with ruptured membranes and clinical signs of amnionitis, Gram's stain and culture of amniotic fluid may be performed before initiation of treatment (i.e., antibiotics and prompt delivery of the infant).

Evaluating Fetal Health (Late Second or Third Trimester)

1. Bilirubin levels, measured spectrophotometrically as $\Delta OD450$, remain the standard for following the Rh or other blood group isoimmunized (not including ABO incompatibility) pregnancy. There is an excellent correlation between this measurement, gestational age, and intensity of hemolytic disease.

Following American College of Obstetricians and Gynecologists (ACOG) guidelines, amniocentesis is performed at 24 to 26 weeks and repeated at 1- to 3-week intervals, depending on the severity of disease. Some centers prefer cordocentesis (under ultrasound guidance) because of the low risk of fetal loss and the ability to determine fetal blood type. However, this procedure is highly specialized and has not been shown to produce better outcomes.

2. If the color of the fluid indicates meconium passage by the fetus, this may be an indicator of some degree of fetal distress. Clear fluid, although reassuring, does not completely exclude fetal distress.

3. Amniography may be useful in assessing the fetal gastrointestinal tract, particularly when an anomaly (e.g., tracheoesophageal fistula, duodenal atresia) is suspected. Normal amniography may also be indirect reassurance of fetal well-being.

Evaluating Fetal Maturity (Third Trimester)

The most common reason for performing amniocentesis is to assess fetal lung maturity. Lecithin (L), sphingomyelin (S), and phosphatidylglycerol (PG) are phospholipids in the newborn lung that act as surfactants and lower the surface tension in the alveoli. Using amniocentesis to determine the L/S ratio, the presence of PG, or both may minimize the risk of delivering an infant that will develop respiratory distress syndrome (RDS). Kits are commercially available to help determine these measurements, or variations on them, and are therefore useful for predicting fetal lung maturity.

1. PG by itself can be used as an indicator of fetal lung maturity. Fortunately, blood, meconium, or vaginal secretions (as contaminants) in the amniotic fluid do not affect PG. PG does not appear until 35 weeks of gestation; although not an absolute guarantee that respiratory distress will not occur, the presence of PG provides considerable reassurance against it. Also important, the absence of PG is not necessarily a strong predictor of respiratory distress after delivery. Although commercially available kits can be used to document PG presence rapidly and with considerable accuracy, it still usually takes several hours to obtain the results. That is why L/S studies are usually more convenient and still considered the "gold standard" for fetal lung maturity.

2. At about 34 weeks' gestation, the concentration of L relative to S begins to rise, and both can be measured directly. It has been frequently reported that the risk of RDS is very slight when the L/S ratio is greater than 2, and there is an increased risk of RDS when the ratio is below 2. It should be noted that with some complications of pregnancy, such as maternal diabetes, RDS may occur despite a mature L/S ratio. As a result, some clinicians require the presence of PG before an elective delivery of a diabetic mother. In addition, the presence of blood has been reported to both increase and decrease the ratio, and the presence of meconium can produce falsely mature results.

3. The "shake test" is a rapid screening test for L/S ratio in which varying dilutions of amniotic fluid are shaken with ethanol. Ethanol is a nonfoaming, competitive surfactant that eliminates the contributions of protein, bile salts, and salts of free fatty acids to the formation of a stable foam. At an ethanol concentration of 47.5%, stable bubbles that foam after shaking are due entirely to lecithin in the amniotic fluid. Positive tests, a complete ring of bubbles at the meniscus with a 1:2 dilution of amniotic fluid, are rarely associated with RDS. The shake test is moderately good, but not excellent, at predicting RDS, and it should therefore be regarded as a screening procedure.

To perform the shake test, the clinician should mix 1 ml of amniotic fluid with 1 ml of 95% ethanol. This vial should be compared with a second vial of 1 ml of amniotic fluid mixed with 0.5 ml of 95% ethanol and 0.5 ml of normal saline. After 30 seconds of vigorous shaking, a ring of bubbles in the second vial indicates an L/S ratio of 2 or greater. Bubbles in the 1:1 mix, but not in the second vial, indicate that the fetus is in a bordering stage of development but not yet mature.

4. The foam stability index (FSI) is a commercially available variation of the shake test. The kit has test wells built into it containing predispensed amounts of ethanol. Amniotic fluid (0.5 ml) is added to each well and shaken. A "control" demonstrates an example of the stable foam end point. The FSI is read as the highest reading corresponding to a well in which a ring of stable foam persists. This test appears to be a reliable predictor of fetal lung maturity if the FSI is 47 or higher; however, this test is unreliable if the amniotic fluid is contaminated with blood.

5. Although results are not available as rapidly as with the shake test, the fetal lung maturity (FLM) assay usually provides results faster than a PG assay. The FLM assesses overall surfactant activity, using a 2-ml sample of amniotic fluid. An FLM result greater than 55 indicates maturity, from 40 to 50 indicates borderline maturity, and less than 39 indicates immaturity.

6. Lamellar counts on the amniotic fluid are also quite reliable if they show fetal lung maturity. They are quick, inexpensive, and readily available anywhere that platelet counts are done. Clinicians experienced with lamellar counts often use them as a quick screen to decide who needs the full L/S or PG evaluation.

Therapeutic Interventions

1. Relief of hydramnios, although this is temporary because the fluid rapidly reaccumulates
2. Intrauterine transfusion for Rh-hemolytic disease

CONTRAINDICATIONS

- Infected lesions of the abdominal wall where amniocentesis must be performed
- Patient refusal
- When the results of tests will not change the clinical course (e.g., patient would refuse termination regardless of laboratory data)
- Maternal coagulopathy *(relative contraindication)*
- Placental abruption *(relative contraindication)*
- Problems not diagnosable by evaluation of the amniotic fluid (e.g., teratogen exposure, radiation exposure, drug use early in pregnancy, history of genetic disorders not diagnosable by amniocentesis) *(relative contraindication)*

EQUIPMENT

- Real-time diagnostic ultrasound unit
- Commercial amniocentesis tray or sterile tray containing at least three plain sterile specimen tubes (5 to 10 ml each) with caps; standard-length 20- or 22-gauge spinal needle (no larger than 20 gauge should be used); 20-ml syringe; 5-ml syringe; 1½-inch, 22- or 23-gauge needle; sterile 4 × 4 gauze pads; sterile Band-Aids; and sterile towels for drapes
- Skin antiseptic (e.g., povidone-iodine, chlorhexidine gluconate)
- Local anesthetic solution (e.g., 1% or 2% lidocaine [*without* epinephrine])
- Fetal heart rate monitor
- Sterile gloves

Note: To obtain disposable amniocentesis trays, the clinician should check with a local surgical supplier.

PREPROCEDURE PATIENT PREPARATION

The clinician should discuss the procedure with the patient (and the patient's partner, if available) beforehand. Both people should be informed of the risks and told the benefits of having an amniocentesis. In addition, the clinician should describe alternative modes of evaluation or treatment (if any) and obtain signed informed consent. (See the sample patient consent form titled "Amniocentesis" on page 1964 of Appendix G.)

TECHNIQUE

1. Have the patient lie on the examining table or bed with the head elevated 20 to 30 degrees. Alternatively, perform the procedure with the patient in the slight (15 degrees) left lateral decubitus position. Monitor the fetal heart rate for 5 minutes to establish a baseline.
2. Locate a pocket of fluid with real-time ultrasound (Fig. 163-1, *A-E*). Try to find a pocket that the needle will be able to reach without going through the placenta or near the fetal face. The best locations (associated with low risk of cord puncture) are usually in the area of the fetal extremities. Sometimes it is necessary to elevate the fetal head from the pelvis to insert the needle below the head (however, very low amniocentesis is associated with increased risk of rupture of membranes or spontaneous abortion). Use the ultrasound *electronic* calipers to measure the depth from the skin that the needle must penetrate to enter the pocket. Note the desired longitudinal angle for the needle. If not perpendicular to the abdomen, note the lateral angle of the probe used to locate the pocket. The needle should be directed at the same lateral angle. Mark the location of the puncture site on the skin using pressure from a needle hub.
3. Prepare the abdomen with antiseptic solution.
4. Wearing sterile gloves, raise a skin wheal with the anesthetic at the puncture site, then continue to anesthetize along the course of the needle track to the parietal peritoneum and serosal surface of the uterus (requires 4 to 5 ml of anesthetic solution). Remove the needle.
5. With the stylet in place and with concurrent real-time ultrasound guidance (transducer in sterile plastic bag, glove, or cover), insert the 20- or 22-gauge spinal needle along the selected track (at the correct angles) to the previously measured depth (Fig. 163-1, *E*). Remove the stylet.

Note: The clinician should feel a little "pop" as the needle moves through the fascia. When it penetrates the amniotic membrane, there is sudden free movement.

In most cases the amniotic fluid will flow through the needle. If not, rotate the needle (this may move the tip away from membranes, fetal parts, etc.). If there is no flow of fluid, attach the empty 5-ml anesthetic syringe to the needle hub and apply gentle suction. If there is still no fluid, replace the stylet and advance the needle another 0.5 to 1.0 cm or until resistance is felt. Again, remove the stylet. If there is no fluid, reattach the small syringe and withdraw the needle slowly with gentle suction, rotating it as it is withdrawn.

6. Once the fluid pocket is located, withdraw 2 or 3 ml of fluid in the small syringe and then discard it. This

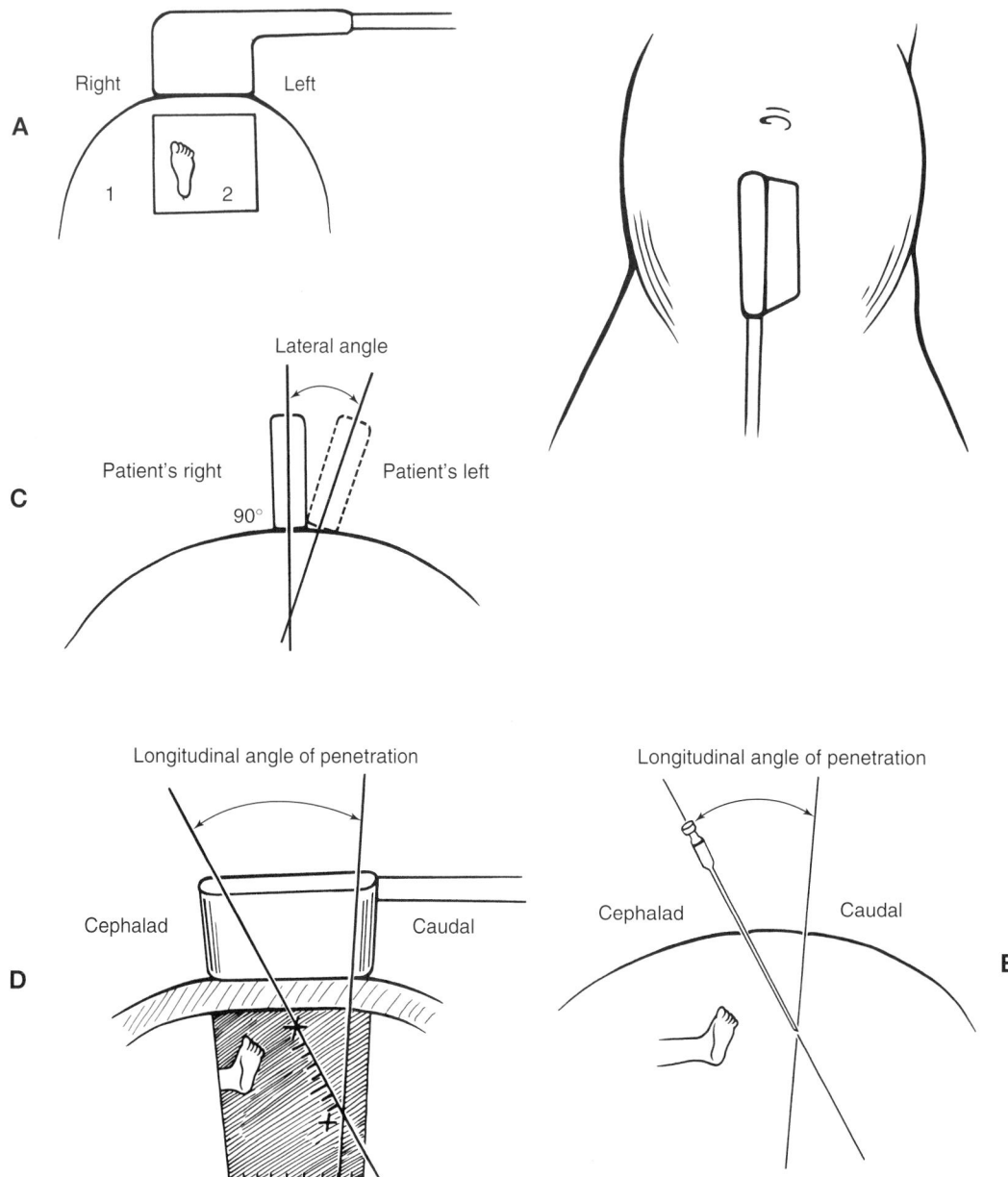

Fig. 163-1

A, Locating a pocket of fluid with a transverse view. An area near the fetal extremities is usually associated with the lowest risk: *1*, maternal abdomen/pelvis, *2*, intrauterine amniotic fluid and fetal foot. **B,** The clinician should turn the probe to a longitudinal position to assess the other dimensions of the fluid pocket. If possible, the probe should be kept perpendicular to the anterior abdominal wall by moving it laterally to position it over the best pocket. **C,** Transverse view of the probe turned longitudinally. Note that the probe is held perpendicular to the abdomen. If not, note the lateral angle. **D,** Longitudinal view. Note measurements with calipers; the needle direction is also determined. **E,** Longitudinal view. Needle is inserted to previously measured depth at the proper angle.

minimizes the amount of blood in the remaining fluid sample (blood can affect laboratory results). Next, withdraw 15 to 25 ml of fluid (or the volume needed for the tests planned). Remove the needle, clean the excess antiseptic from the abdominal wall, and cover the puncture wound with a Band-Aid. If the patient is unsensitized Rh-negative, administer 300 mg of Rh-immune globulin.

7. If grossly bloody amniotic fluid is encountered in the specimen, it is important to determine whether it is

maternal or fetal blood. If the blood is fetal, use the Kleihauer-Betke technique to estimate the volume in the specimen. In addition, monitor the fetal heart rate closely for 1 to 2 hours for the development of tachycardia. If the volume of fetal blood loss is significant for the fetal age and the fetus is judged mature enough to survive extrauterine life, fetal tachycardia is an indication for intervention and delivery.

8. If no amniotic fluid is obtained, repeat the ultrasound examination and again localize the fluid pocket, its angle, and its distance from the skin; prepare the skin with antiseptic and repeat the tap (again under continuous ultrasound guidance).

Note: It is recommended that no more than two attempts be made because repeated attempts increase the risk of significant fetal injury or induction of labor. It is also important not to use a needle larger than 20 gauge because the incidence of complications rises with needle gauge.

9. Following a normal successful amniocentesis, monitor the fetal heart rate and the mother's response for 20 to 30 minutes, after which time the patient may leave.

COMPLICATIONS

A wide variety of complications have been reported, including injuries or even fetal death. However, serious complications are uncommon and the procedure is considered relatively safe in experienced hands. Complications from amniocentesis include the following:

- Pain, bruising, or infection at the puncture site
- Uterine contractions, occasionally progressing to labor but usually self-limited
- Occasional (1% to 2% risk) spontaneous abortion after late first trimester or midtrimester amniocentesis
- Premature rupture of membranes
- Placental separation or abruption
- Fetal injury, such as skin scars, dimpling, eye injury, genital injury (risk increases with oligohydramnios)
- Cord or placental blood vessel injury with resultant fetal hemorrhage
- Rh-factor isoimmunization
- Uterine or amniotic fluid infection
- Fluid leak with resultant oligohydramnios *(rare)*

POSTPROCEDURE PATIENT EDUCATION

Printed instructions help patients remember what they are told. The clinician should give the patient an instruction sheet to use after amniocentesis. (See the sample patient education handout titled "Following Amniocentesis" on page 1963 of Appendix G.)

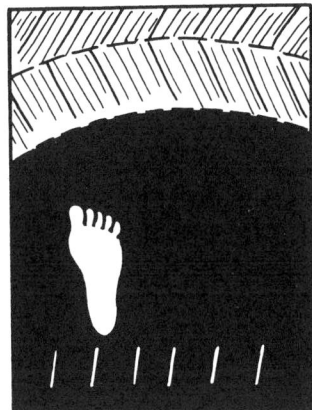

Fig. 163-2
Example of a good image to be photographed for documenting the site chosen for amniocentesis. Note the large pocket of fluid near an extremity and the absence of the cord.

The patient was placed in low semi-Fowler's position and the fetal heart tones were monitored for 5 minutes. Real-time ultrasound was used to locate a collection of amniotic fluid in the area of the fetal extremities at a depth of 5 cm. No loops of cord were noted. The overlying skin was marked, prepped with povidone-iodine solution, and draped with sterile towels. After local anesthesia with 1% lidocaine, a 20-gauge spinal needle was inserted into the fluid pocket under continuous ultrasound guidance. A total of 15 ml of clear (or "meconium stained," "slightly blood tinged," "grossly bloody") amniotic fluid was removed without (with) difficulty. A sterile dressing was applied to the puncture site, and the fetal heart tones were monitored for another 20 minutes. These remained normal; the patient felt well and was discharged with warnings and instructions for follow-up.

Fig. 163-3
Example of an amniocentesis procedure note.

CPT/BILLING CODES

The clinician should include a picture of the amniotic fluid pocket from the ultrasound examination (when possible) (Fig. 163-2) and a procedure note (Fig. 163-3) in the documentation.

59000   Amniocentesis, any method
76946   Ultrasonic guidance for amniocentesis, radiologic supervision and interpretation

ICD-9-CM DIAGNOSTIC CODES

These are illustrative codes for conditions commonly associated with amniocentesis. A fifth digit (represented by the * symbol) is used in codes 640 to 648 and 651 to 659. Following are the fifth digits used and the episodes of care they represent:

0   Unspecified
1   Delivered, with or without mention of antepartum condition
2   Delivered, with mention of postpartum complication
3   Antepartum condition or complication
4   Postpartum condition or complication

655.2*   Hereditary disease in family, possibly affecting fetus
655.1*   Chromosomal abnormality in fetus
659.6*   Advanced maternal age, primiparous or multiparous
656.1*   Rh isoimmunization
657.0*   Polyhydramnios
658.4*   Chorioamnionitis
658.1*   Premature rupture of membranes
644.0*   Threatened premature labor (after 22 weeks)
646.3*   Habitual aborter
655.8*   Other known or suspected fetal abnormality, not elsewhere classified
645.2*   Prolonged pregnancy
654.2*   Previous cesarean delivery, NOS
642.5*   Severe preeclampsia
656.3*   Fetal distress

ADDITIONAL RESOURCES

- See the sample patient education handout titled "Following Amniocentesis" on page 1963 of Appendix G.
- See the sample patient consent form titled "Amniocentesis" on page 1964 of Appendix G.

BIBLIOGRAPHY

Jauniaux E, Rodeck C: Use, risks and complications of amniocentesis and chorionic villus sampling for prenatal diagnosis in early pregnancy, *Early Pregnancy* 1(4):245, 1995.

Liley AW: Liquor amni analysis in management of the pregnancy complicated by rhesus sensitization, *Am J Obstet Gynecol* 82:1359, 1961.

Queenan JT: Amniocentesis. In Queenan JT: *Management of high-risk pregnancy,* ed 3, Ann Arbor, 1994, Blackwell Scientific Publications.

Reece EA: Early and midtrimester genetic amniocentesis: safety and outcomes, *Obstet Gynecol Clin North Am* 24(1):71, 1997.

Silver RK, Russell TL, Kambich MP, et al: Midtrimester amniocentesis: influence of operator caseload on sampling efficiency, *J Reprod Med* 43(3):191, 1998.

Simpson JL, Elias S: Prenatal diagnosis of genetic disorders. In Creasy RK, Resnick R: *Maternal-fetal medicine,* ed 3, Philadelphia, 1994, WB Saunders.

Yankowitz J, Weiner CP: Modern management of Rhesus disease, *Curr Opin Obstet Gynecol* 8(2):139, 1996.

Cesarean Section

Rebecca H. Gladu

Cesarean section is the operative delivery of a baby to decrease perinatal morbidity and mortality. Currently in the United States, cesarean section is performed at an average of 22.6% of all deliveries. There is nationwide emphasis on reducing this rate to a more reasonable 12% to 15%; for many years before 1960, the rate was 3% to 5%.

Nationally, about 1.5% of urban and 12.2% of rural family physicians have cesarean section privileges in their hospitals. This represents approximately 600 urban and 2600 rural family physicians. These family physicians are found in a wide variety of practice settings, ranging from urban teaching institutions to isolated rural practices. Many family practice obstetrics fellowships exist for training family physicians to perform cesarean sections.

This chapter discusses one standard technique for performing an uncomplicated low cervical transverse cesarean section. It is not intended to discuss all of the possible techniques or medical situations in which a cesarean section may be necessary.

INDICATIONS

Maternal Indications

- Repeat section when mother declines to have a trial of labor
- Repeat section when a trial of labor is not indicated
- Antepartum hemorrhage
- Pelvic, vaginal, or vulvar tumors
- Cervical cancer

- Severe hypertension or severe preeclampsia
- Contracted pelvis (cephalopelvic disproportion [CPD])
- Labor intolerance resulting from medical disease
- Uterine rupture
- Maternal thrombocytopenia
- Active maternal herpes simplex genital infection
- Condyloma too large to allow vaginal delivery

Fetal Indications

- Transverse lie
- Transverse arrest
- Brow presentation
- Failed trial of forceps
- Arrest of the active stage
- Fetal distress
- Fetal anomalies
- Breech in a primigravida patient
- Cord prolapse
- Very low birthweight infant (less than 1500 g)
- Multiple gestation (e.g., three to five fetuses)
- Perimortem
- Macrosomia

CONTRAINDICATIONS

Patient refusal of operation with clear consequences explained and accepted by the mother. Since cesarean section is considered a lifesaving procedure in many instances, there are no other contraindications. Of course, a cesarean section cannot be performed if there are inadequate facilities, inadequate availability of anesthesia, or a lack of blood availability.

EQUIPMENT

Standard operating room cesarean section package to include the following:

Quantity Needed	Instrument
2	Babcock clamps (if tubal ligation planned)
6	Allis clamps
4	Pennington clamps (8 inch)
2	Tissue forceps (toothed) (6 and 8 inch)
2	Dressing forceps (smooth) (6 and 8 inch)
2	Russian forceps (6 and 8 inch)
4	Sponge forceps
2	Adson forceps with teeth
2	No. 20 blade (skin)
1	No. 10 blade (deep)
6	Curved hemostats (5½ inch)
6	Curved Kelly clamps
2	Needle holder
4	Kocher or Ochsner clamps (7½ inch)
2	Army-Navy retractor
1	DeLee, Fritsch, or Rochard universal retractor
3	Richardson retractor (small, medium and large)
1	Bandage scissors (7¼ inch)
1	Metzenbaum scissors (7 inch)
1	Curved Mayo scissors (6½ inch)
1	Suture scissors
1	Straight Mayo scissors (6½ inch)
1	Poole suction tip
1	Yankauer tonsil suction tip
4	Packages of suture (two packages each of 0-chromic and 1-0 Vicryl)
20	Lap sponges
1	Surgical stapler
1	Bovie cautery device
1	Cervical dilators

PREPROCEDURE PATIENT PREPARATION

A consent form should be explained and signed, and the patient's questions should be answered. A standard hospital consent form can be used emphasizing the following risks to the patient undergoing cesarean section:

- Risk of anesthesia
- Injury to the bladder and ureters
- Injury to the bowel
- Possible hysterectomy
- Possible hemorrhage requiring transfusion

BOX 164-1

Typical Preoperative Orders for Cesarean Section

Lab: H/H, urinalysis
Type and hold 2 units PRBCs
Foley to gravity
Anesthesia pre-op for epidural, spinal or general anesthesia.
NPO
Bicitra (Sodium citrate) 30 ml po
IV D5RL at 125 ml/hr

- Potential for infection
- Rare chance of injury to the fetus
- Risk of rupture of the uterus with future labors

A consent for use of blood products in the event of hemorrhage should also be obtained.

Box 164-1 shows typical preoperative orders for a cesarean section.

TECHNIQUE

1. Tilt the operating table to the left when regional anesthesia is used. (This displaces the uterus to the left, which permits better venous return and fetal oxygenation.)
2. After anesthesia is induced by regional (epidural), spinal, or general anesthetic, test for anesthesia of the abdominal skin with the Allis clamp.
3. When anesthesia is certain, perform a Pfannenstiel skin incision by incising the abdominal skin to a width of approximately 13 to 15 cm, two finger-breadths above the symphysis pubis, using a no. 20 blade (Fig. 164-1). Maintain hemostasis from dermal bleeding with Bovie cautery.
4. Carry the incision down through the subcutaneous fat to the fascia with the no. 10 knife blade. Incise the fascia horizontally in the midline about 2 cm with the scalpel. Lift the fascia and extend the cut edges laterally and superiorly in a curvilinear fashion with the curved Mayo scissors.
5. Grasp the superior edge of the fascia with two Ochsner clamps to elevate the fascia off of the underlying muscle, bluntly dissecting the fascia and the heavier fibers of the linea alba away from the muscle with fingers (Fig. 164-2). This may be more difficult in a repeat case because of adhesion scar formation. In such cases, use the Mayo scissors to cut the adhesions. Then use the Mayos again to cut through the midline fibers of the linea alba. Be careful not to cut the muscle tissue or to cut a "buttonhole" through the fascia. Repeat this dissection on the inferior edge of the fascia, bluntly and sharply dissecting the fascia away from the muscular tissue.

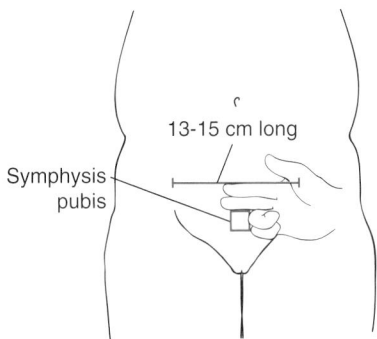

Fig. 164-1
Pfannenstiel skin incision. The horizontal incision is carried out two fingerbreadths above the symphysis pubis.

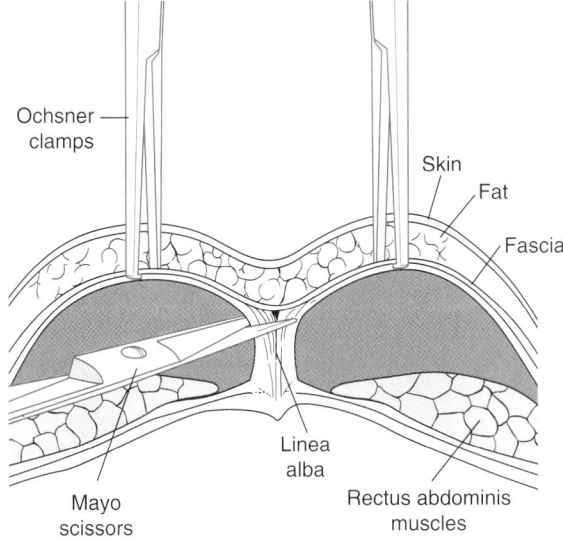

Fig. 164-2
Dissection of the linea alba.

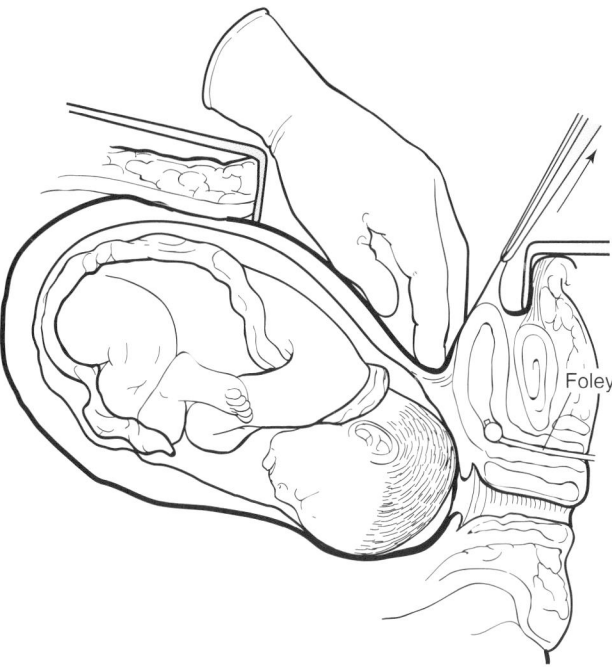

Fig. 164-3
Dissection of the bladder away from the uterus.

6. Bluntly separate the rectus muscle in the midline in a vertical fashion to expose the peritoneum. Grasp the peritoneum superiorly with two hemostats, tent it away from the underlying viscera, and incise with the no. 20 blade. Extend this incision vertically superiorly and inferiorly bluntly, being careful not to extend to the bladder inferiorly.

7. Place the DeLee bladder blade to retract and identify the bladder.

8. Develop the bladder flap. Pick up the peritoneum over the lower uterine segment with tissue forceps and incise it laterally to make a flap approximately 12 cm long (Figs. 164-3 and 164-4). Dissect the peritoneum off of the uterus with a sponge on a ring forceps or bluntly with the fingers. Reapply the DeLee bladder blade to include the inferior bladder flap just created.

9. Determine the position of the lateral uterine vessels. Next, incise the lower uterine segment over the fetal head, which is known as "scoring the uterus." Announce this so that the anesthesiologist and nursery attendant can prepare for imminent delivery. It is best to use a no. 20 blade and a 2- to 3-cm incision, proceeding millimeter by millimeter in depth to avoid injuring the presenting fetal part below (Fig. 164-5).

10. Extend the uterine incision (protecting the fetal parts with two fingers inside the opening, just under the muscle) by cutting with bandage scissors in a superior and lateral direction through the lower uterine segment for a total incision of approximately 10 to 11 cm (Fig. 164-6). Be careful to avoid the uterine arteries.

11. Rupture the membranes with the Allis clamp.

12. Deliver the fetal head by inserting a cupped hand over the head and occiput, keeping the wrist straight. Gently lift upward without flexing the wrist, bringing the head out of the incision along with your hand (Fig. 164-7). It may be necessary for the assistant to exert gentle fundal pressure after the occiput has cleared the incision.

Note: If the head is flexed tightly or stuck from excessive pushing before the procedure, as is common in arrest of descent cases or true CPD, have an assistant push the head inward and upward from below (Fig. 164-8). Occasionally it may be necessary to inject 0.25 mg terbutaline SC or IV to relax the uterus in order to move the baby upward far enough

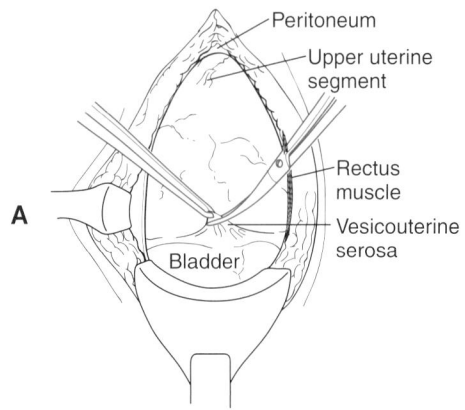

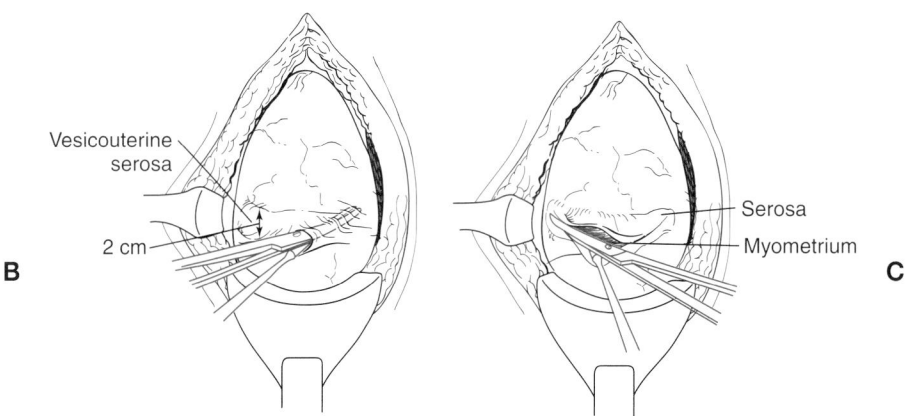

Fig. 164-4
Development of the bladder flap. **A,** Tenting of the peritoneum. **B,** Undermining the peritoneum. **C,** Incising the peritoneum. (Redrawn from Cunningham FG, MacDonald P, Gant NF, et al, editors: *Williams obstetrics,* ed 19, Norwalk, Conn, 1993, Appleton & Lange.)

to allow for delivery. Note that this could increase blood loss from uterine atony.

13. Suction the fetal mouth and nose, deliver the anterior shoulder, the posterior shoulder, then the rest of the infant as in a vaginal delivery. Clamp and cut the cord and hand the infant to the nurse in attendance. Obtain cord blood if necessary, and then manually extract the placenta bluntly with the fingers (Fig. 164-9). Remove the last adherent membranes with the aid of ring forceps.

14. Give one dose of perioperative antibiotics after the cord is clamped. This has proved to reduce postoperative wound infection by 50%. A broad-spectrum cephalosporin, such as cefoxitin 1 g IV, can be used to prevent wound infection. In penicillin-allergic patients, use clindamycin 600 mg IV in one dose.

15. Exteriorize the uterus. To control blood loss, place two Pennington clamps at the edges of the incision

where bleeding is most vigorous. Wrap the uterine fundus in a clean moist lap sponge as you massage the uterus; gently clean the inner endometrium with moist lap sponges so that it is free of any clots, membranes, and debris. Should the cervix be closed, dilate it with cervical dilators at this point.

16a. Now close the hysterotomy incision with a running locked stitch of 0-chromic catgut (Fig. 164-10). Should bleeding or oozing continue after a one-layer closure, imbricate with another layer of 0-chromic catgut. Do not include the endometrial layer in the closure of the myometrium. Should an extension of the incision occur (typically inferiorly toward the cervix), repair the extension first, and then repair the hysterotomy incision. Occasionally, one small area of the hysterotomy incision may bleed and can be repaired with a "figure of 8" stitch for hemostasis.

16b. Optional: Close the bladder flap with 2-0 chromic. Most sources do not recommend closing the

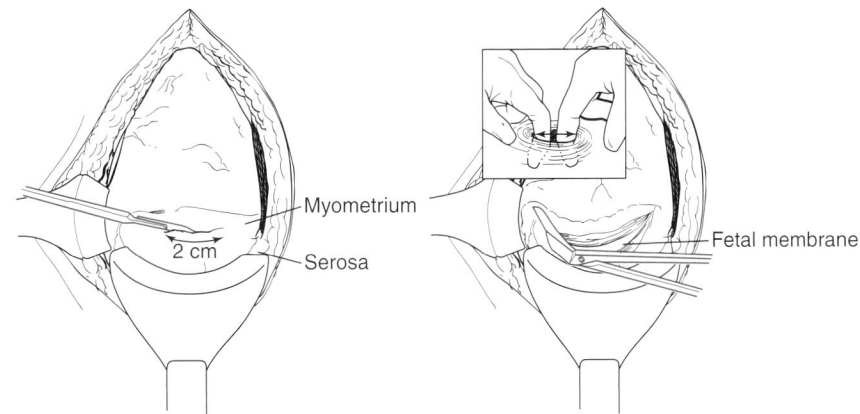

Fig. 164-5
Low cervical transverse incision. The uterine incision is developed in a curvilinear fashion. (Redrawn from Cunningham FG, MacDonald P, Gant NF, et al, editors: *Williams obstetrics,* ed 19, Norwalk, Conn, 1993, Appleton & Lange.)

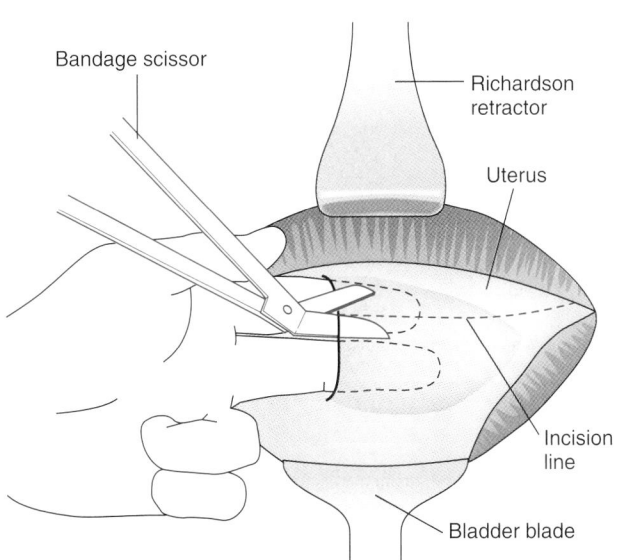

Fig. 164-6
Protecting the fetal head from the bandage scissors when incising the uterus. Two fingers are placed under the incision to protect the infant from the bandage scissors.

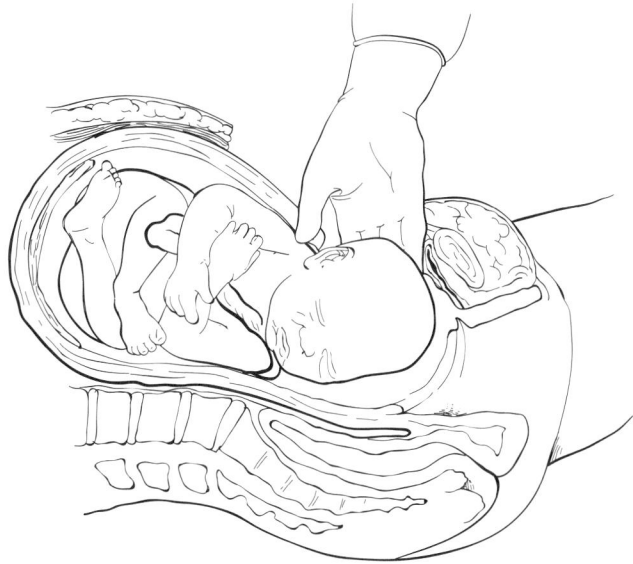

Fig. 164-7
Lifting the fetal head out of the uterus. Keep the wrist straight to avoid using the uterus as a fulcrum.

peritoneum. It will reapproximate on its own without suturing.

17. Inspect the uterus, tubes, and ovaries. If a bilateral tubal ligation is desired, this is the time to do it.

18. Return the uterus to the abdominal cavity.

19a. Irrigate the abdominal cavity of clots and debris using warm saline and a tonsil suction tip. Palpate the right and left colic gutters for abnormal structures, and inspect the appendix and gallbladder.

19b. Optional: Close the parietal peritoneum using a 2-0 chromic suture. However, it will reapproximate on its own.

20. Close the two-layered fascia in a running stitch with 1-0 Vicryl or any other strong monofilament suture. Make sure that the sutures are placed equally across the incision and no more than 1 cm apart.

21a. Irrigate the subcutaneous fat and stop any bleeding with Bovie cautery.

21b. Optional: Close the subcutaneous dead space. This is only necessary for patients with a very large pannus in which it is difficult to reapproximate the skin without this step. Remember that every suture placed is a nidus for possible infection, so keep the amount of suturing to the required steps only. If suturing is required for closure, use interrupted

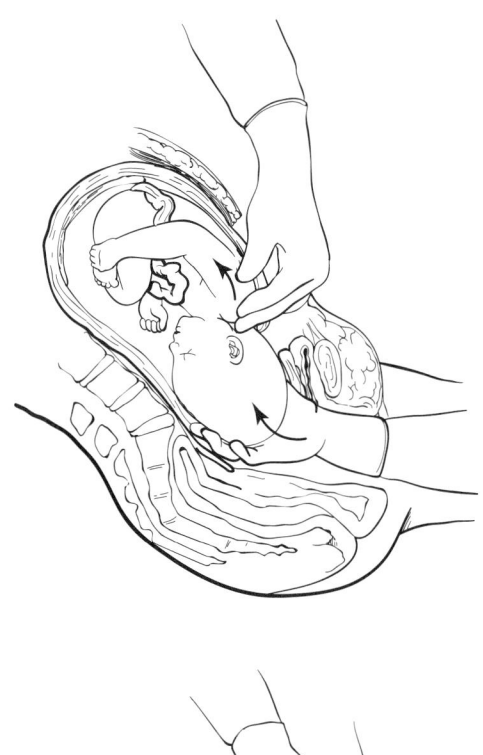

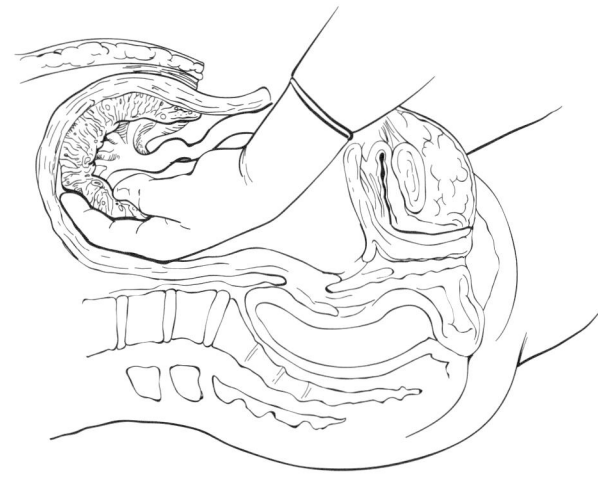

Fig. 164-9
Manual extraction of the placenta.

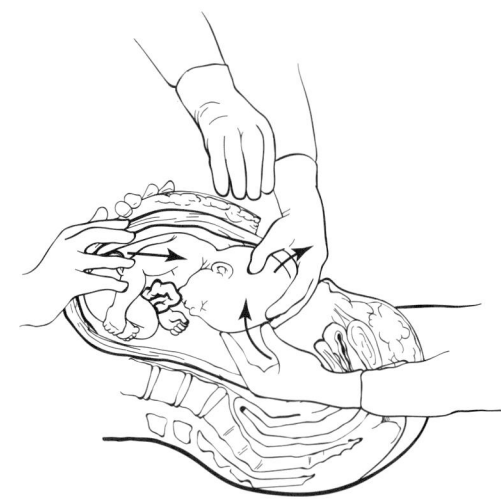

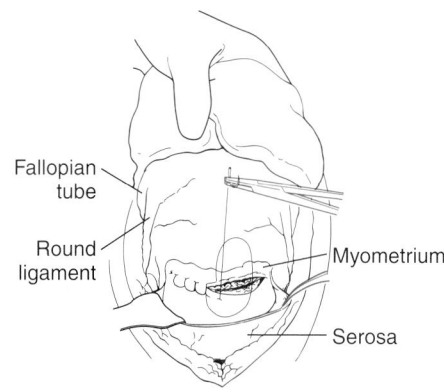

Fig. 164-10
Uterine closure with a running locked stitch of 2-0 chromic catgut suture. (Redrawn from Cunningham FG, MacDonald P, Gant NF, et al, editors: *Williams obstetrics,* ed 19, Norwalk, Conn, 1993, Appleton & Lange.)

Fig. 164-8
Technique to extract an impacted fetal head. An assistant exerts gentle upward force on the head from the vagina as the operator exerts steady upward pressure on the shoulders. (Redrawn from Plauch WC, Morrison JC, O'Sullivan MJ: *Surgical obstetrics,* Philadelphia, 1992, WB Saunders.)

sutures with absorbable suture material, such as 3-0 chromic gut.

22. Close the skin. Most surgeons prefer the skin stapler, which does an excellent job when staples are placed 1 cm apart. However, a plastic skin closure with deep buried sutures and a final subcuticular stitch is certainly acceptable if time permits.

Choice of Uterine Incision

Three types of uterine incisions are used for cesarean sections: low cervical transverse, low vertical, and classical (Table 164-1).

1. Low cervical transverse incision (Kerr incision): The uterus is incised transversely in the thin lower uterine segment 2 cm above the detached bladder. The incision is extended on either side so that it is large enough to allow delivery of the baby, depending on the baby's size. The incision should not be so large as to encounter the uterine arteries laterally.

2. Low vertical incision (Krönig incision): A midline vertical incision made in the lower uterine segment, with care taken not to extend the incision inferiorly to the cervix. It may be extended superiorly into the body of the uterus if more room is needed to deliver the baby.

3. Classical incision: A vertical midline incision made into the body of the uterus above the lower uterine segment, extending into the uterine fundus of sufficient length to allow delivery of the baby.

TABLE 164-1

Types of Uterine Incisions

	Advantages	Disadvantages
Low cervical transverse	Lower uterine segment is thin and less vascular Incision heals well, less risk of subsequent dehiscence Most popular, >90% of all cesarean births	Risk of lateral extension into the uterine vessels
Low vertical	Useful if lower uterine segment is thick or has fibroids For transverse lie with back down For fetal anomalies such as hydrocephalus	Need for greater separation of the bladder from lower uterine segment Need for repeat cesarean section if upper segment entered
Classical incision	Suitable for emergent cases, easiest and fastest access to the infant Better exposure Ability to develop a larger opening for delivery	Increased blood loss Difficult repair (3 layer) Increased risk of rupture in subsequent pregnancies Adhesion formation between incision and abdominal organs Eight times greater risk of dehiscence than transverse incision

Example of an Operative Note

Fig. 164-11 shows an example of an ordinary, uncomplicated case. Any complications should be added and noted in the dictation.

COMPLICATIONS

- Anesthesia
- Injury to the bladder and ureter
- Injury to the bowel
- Uterine hemorrhage
- Infection: endometritis, urinary tract infection, respiratory infection, atelectasis, wound infection, septic pelvic thrombophlebitis
- Pulmonary embolism
- Risk of rupture in future deliveries
- Injury to the child

POSTOPERATIVE ORDERS

Box 164-2 shows typical postoperative orders for cesarean section.

POSTPROCEDURE PATIENT EDUCATION

First 24 Hours

The patient should be told what to expect, such as pain control issues (e.g., patient-controlled analgesia [PCA] pump versus IV narcotic analgesia). She will experience some uterine cramping and receive fundal massage by

BOX 164-2

Typical Postoperative Orders for Cesarean Section

1. Admit to the Family Practice Service.
2. Admit to recovery room, then to floor as follows.
3. Monitor vital signs every 15 minutes until stable, then every 30 minutes until anesthesia wears off, then every 4 hours on the floor.
4. Instruct nothing by mouth.
5. Give IV D5 Half NS at 125 ml/hr with 20 U of oxytocin to the first liter only.
6. Obtain hematocrit on first postoperative day.
7. Insert Foley to gravity.
8. Perform incentive spirometry if patient is a smoker.
9. Call doctor for the following:
   - Fever over 100.4° F
   - Pulse over 110
   - Increasing uterine tenderness
   - Foul-smelling lochia
   - Excessive vaginal bleeding
10. Provide pain medication: PCA pump if available, otherwise Demerol 50 to 75 mg with Phenergan 25 mg IM every 3 to 4 hours as needed.
11. Provide RhoGAM if indicated.

the nurses. Her Foley catheter remains in place. She may have the baby with her as early as possible to start breastfeeding and bonding. Most patients stay in the hospital 3 to 5 days after a cesarean section.

First Postoperative Day

The patient should ambulate to prevent atelectasis and pneumonia. If bowel sounds are present, diet should be advanced to clear liquids and then to full liquids as tolerated. If she is ambulating well, the Foley catheter can be removed and she can walk to the bathroom. The

Operative Report

Procedure: Primary low cervical transverse Pfannenstiel cesarean section

Indication:

Anesthesia:

Surgeon:

Surgical assistant:

Findings (gender, weight, Apgar scores):

Estimated blood loss:

Complications:

Specimens to pathology:

Operative Procedure in Detail:

The patient was taken to the operating room and placed in the supine position. The abdomen was prepped and draped in the sterile fashion for an abdominal procedure, and anesthesia was satisfactorily induced. A Pfannenstiel incision was carried out with the skin knife two fingerbreadths above the symphysis pubis and taken through the subcutaneous tissue with the deep knife. The rectus sheath was incised transversely in the midline, undermined bilaterally with the Mayo scissors, and incised. The superior edge of the fascia was grasped with the Ochsner clamps on both sides of the midline, and the rectus muscles were bluntly dissected from the fascia. The linea alba was taken down sharply. A similar procedure was carried out inferiorly. The rectus and pyramidalis muscles were sharply and bluntly divided in the midline. The parietal peritoneum was identified and grasped in the midline with two hemostats, tented, and entered sharply with the Metzenbaum scissors. The incision was extended longitudinally, transilluminating the bladder to define the lower limits of the dissection. The DeLee bladder retractor was placed, and the lateral colic gutters were grasped in the midline with Russian forceps and entered with Metzenbaum scissors. After bilateral undermining, the incision was extended in a curvilinear fashion and the bladder flap created using blunt dissection. The bladder blade was repositioned to further retract the bladder.

The lower uterine segment was entered transversely in the midline using the knife and extended laterally in a curvilinear fashion using the bandage scissors, with two fingers protecting the presenting fetal part. The infant was encountered in the vertex position and was delivered atraumatically. The nose and mouth were suctioned with the bulb syringe; the cord was clamped and cut, and the infant was handed to the attendant. Cord blood was obtained and the placenta was manually extracted with ring forceps, gently dissecting the final adherent membranes.

The uterine fundus was exteriorized through the abdominal incision and wrapped in a moist lap. The uterine cavity was swabbed with a moist lap and was inspected to ensure removal of all membranes and placental fragments. The hysterotomy incision was then closed with a running locked stitch of 1-0 chromic catgut in a single layer. Hemostasis was excellent. The retrouterine space was inspected, irrigated, and suctioned to remove all blood, clots, and amniotic fluid.

The fundus was then replaced in the peritoneal cavity and the hysterotomy incision reinspected for hemostasis, which was good. The vesicouterine peritoneum was reapproximated using a continuous stitch of 2-0 chromic. Laps were removed from the colic gutters, which were individually inspected, irrigated, and suctioned until clean.

The subfascial space was inspected for hemostasis. The fascia was then closed with a running simple stitch of 1-0 Vicryl. The skin was closed with staples and the incision dressed with a Telfa pad and a pressure dressing. The patient was transferred in good condition by stretcher with the Foley draining clear urine.

Fig. 164-11
Example of operative form for typical cesarean section.

IV should be changed to a heparin lock. Oral narcotic analgesia can replace a PCA pump, IV, or IM narcotics. She should note some flatus, and urination should increase from postpartum diuresis.

Second Postoperative Day

The criteria for going home include a bowel movement, ability to tolerate a regular diet, lack of fever, and full ambulation on oral pain medication only. Many patients can be discharged 36 hours after a cesarean section. *If the skin is closed,* staples can be removed and replaced with Steri-Strips. If not, this can be done at postoperative Day 5 on an outpatient basis.

Discharge Instructions

- No driving for 10 days.
- Refrain from intercourse for 4 weeks.
- Care of the surgical incision is relatively simple. Water can wash over the wound as long as there is no direct impact of water onto the wound. Keeping the wound clean and dry is important for adequate healing. This includes avoiding coverage by skin folds, which can lead to excessive moisture and infection.
- Notify the physician's office for the following problems: pus seeping out of the wound, fever, painful urination, difficulty breathing, shortness of breath, or increasing pain.
- Follow up in the clinic for a wound check in 1 week.
- Limit activity to walking for the first week, back to full activity by 6 weeks.

CONCLUSION

This chapter is limited to the performance of the uncomplicated cesarean section. For a more exhaustive review of how to handle complications or more complex surgical deliveries, review the Yasin et al (1992) reference listed in the bibliography.

CPT/BILLING CODES

59510   Routine obstetric care including antepartum care, cesarean delivery, and postpartum care

59514   Cesarean delivery only
59515   Cesarean delivery including postpartum care
59618   Routine obstetric care including antepartum care, cesarean delivery, and postpartum care, following attempted vaginal delivery after previous cesarean delivery
59620   Cesarean delivery only, following attempted vaginal delivery after previous cesarean delivery
59622   Cesarean delivery only, following attempted vaginal delivery after cesarean delivery, including postpartum care

BIBLIOGRAPHY

Abuhamad A, O'Sullivan MJ: Operative techniques for cesarean section. In Plauche WC, Morrison JC, Sullivan MJ, editors: *Surgical obstetrics,* Philadelphia, 1992, WB Saunders.

American Academy of Family Physicians: *Facts about family practice,* Kansas City, 1993, AAFP.

Damos J, et al: Intrapartum procedures, Section G. Cesarean Section. In Ratcliffe S, Sakornbut E, Byrd J, editors: *Handbook of pregnancy and perinatal care in family practice,* Philadelphia, 1996, Hanley & Belfus.

Hankins GDV, Gilstrap L, Clark SL, editors: *Operative obstetrics,* East Norfolk, Conn, 1995, Appleton & Lange.

Kahn NB Jr, Schmittling G: Obstetric privileges for family physicians: a national study, *J Am Board Fam Pract* 8(2):120, 1995.

Kirschner CG, et al: *CPT 98: Physicians' current procedural terminology,* Chicago, 1997, American Medical Association.

Raimer KA, O'Sullivan MJ: Cesarean section: history, incidence, and indications. In Plauche WC, Morrison JC, O'Sullivan MJ, editors: *Surgical obstetrics,* Philadelphia, 1992, WB Saunders.

Yasin SY, Walton DL, O'Sullivan MJ: Problems encountered during cesarean delivery. In Plauche WC, Morrison JC, O'Sullivan MJ, editors: *Surgical obstetrics,* Philadelphia, 1992, WB Saunders.

CHAPTER 165

Cervical Ripening/Vaginal Prostaglandins

Scott T. Henderson

When the induction of labor is warranted, traditional methods (oxytocin administration and amniotomy) are not always successful. Possible hindrances include the fact that 10% of women requiring induction have an "unripe" cervix. Clinicians continue to search not only for the best method of preinduction cervical ripening, but also for a dependable method for induction of labor. Among available options, mechanical cervical dilators (24 French Foley and osmotic dilators such as Laminaria) facilitate ripening by stimulating the natural release of prostaglandins. However, these can be uncomfortable and probably should be reserved for use when all other methods have failed or for a fetal demise. Membrane stripping has been studied, but the range of results is large, from low patient satisfaction and low efficacy to excellent in both measures. Artificial prostaglandins are probably now the most frequently used method. Dinoprostone (prostaglandin E_2 [PGE_2]) can be used intravaginally or intracervically. Intravaginal misoprostol (Cytotec), a synthetic PGE_1 approved to treat gastric mucosa, is the most recent addition to the prostaglandins used for cervical ripening and labor induction.

Compared with the dinoprostone insert, misoprostol (25 to 50 μg) inserted vaginally is slightly more effective clinically and much more cost effective. Misoprostol (25 μg every 3 hr) has also been compared with dinoprostone gel (0.5 mg every 6 hr) and found to have a higher rate of successful inductions, a shorter time to delivery, and a significantly lower need for oxytocin augmentation. Oral misoprostol has also been used for labor induction, but reports indicate mixed results. At this time, there is insufficient evidence to determine optimal dosing and to verify safety for oral misoprostol.

Editor's note: It has been our experience that repeated low doses (25 mg) of intravaginal misoprostol are very safe and cost-effective and often eliminate the need for oxytocin.

One large advantage of both the dinoprostone insert and the vaginal misoprostol over the dinoprostone gel is that they can be inserted without putting the patient in stirrups. Their application can be performed with a simple bimanual examination. Another difference between the dinoprostone preparations and misoprostol is that, in certain centers, otherwise stable patients can be sent home when dinoprostone (either gel or insert) is used. After monitoring for 30 minutes to 2 hours, if there is no increase in uterine activity and the fetal heart rate does not change, patients can be transferred. On the contrary, when vaginal misoprostol is used—because of a higher incidence of uterine hypertonicity—the patient should be monitored continuously. Most centers require that the patient remain in the hospital for monitoring. Also, while misoprostol remains an excellent choice for the usual postdates pregnancy, due to the higher incidence of hypertonicity, it should be used with caution if there is even soft evidence of fetal or placental compromise (e.g., oligohydramnios or intrauterine growth retardation).

A hospital protocol for cervical ripening and labor induction should be written and followed. The protocol should indicate whether the patient needs to remain hospitalized if there is no uterine activity. If a commercially prepared insert or gel or misoprostol is not available and a compounded gel is used, the protocol should also allow the pharmacy to compound the gel.

A cervical scoring system—the Bishop's system (Table 165-1)—has been developed for assessing multiparous women at the time of induction. The maximum Bishop score is 13; when the score exceeds 8, the likelihood of a successful vaginal delivery with oxytocin induction approaches that of spontaneous labor. Otherwise, the duration of pregnancy before spontaneous labor and the success of an induction is inversely correlated with the score. A low Bishop score (especially if under 6) correlates with a prolonged labor or failed induction. A modified Bishop score with a maximum of 10 has also been studied in a study to quantify results: For a score of 9 or more, there is basically a 100% chance of successful oxytocin induction; for a score from 5 to 8, there is a 5% risk of failure; and for a score of 4 or less, there is a 20% risk of failure.

TABLE 165-1

Bishop Score

Assessment Score	Dilation (cm)	Effacement (%)	Fetal Station*	Consistency	Position
0	0	Up to 30	−3	Firm	Posterior
1	1-2	40-50	−2	Medium	Mid
2	3-4	60-80	−1, 0	Soft	Anterior
3	5-6	90-100	+1, +2, +3		

Add the score for each of the clinical assessments. If the total score is greater than 8, the success of induction approaches that of spontaneous labor.
*−3 = engaged, +3 = on the perineum.

INDICATIONS FOR CERVICAL RIPENING

- Induction or delivery indicated and Bishop's score less than 4/13. Consider if Bishop score is less than 8/13.

Induction or delivery may be indicated in the following situations:

- Postdate pregnancy
- Chronic hypertension or other maternal medical problem (diabetes, renal disease, severe chronic pulmonary disease)
- Pregnancy-induced hypertension
- Chorioamnionitis
- Suspected fetal jeopardy (intrauterine growth retardation or isoimmunization)
- Fetal demise
- Logistical factors (e.g., risk of rapid labor in a patient living a long distance from hospital, psychosocial indications)
- Premature rupture of membranes (PROM) (i.e., no labor within 4 hours after membranes have ruptured)

Management options include expectant management, prostaglandins, and oxytocin. So far, studies show no differences in cesarean section rates between these options. One study found that the use of prostaglandins had a decreased risk of chorioamnionitis, neonatal infection, and neonatal admission to NICU when compared with expectant management. It was also preferred by patients when compared with expectant management.

Another study by the same group (Hannah et al.) found that the use of oxytocin had the same trend toward benefits and decreased risks when compared with prostaglandins (decreased risk of chorioamnionitis, neonatal infection, neonatal admission to NICU, and patient preference); however, the results were not statistically significant. In theory, the increased risk of infection with use of prostaglandins for PROM is due to the fact that prostaglandins must be inserted vaginally. Increased numbers of vaginal examinations with PROM are associated with an increased risk of infection. Therefore dinoprostone should be used with caution in patients with ruptured membranes. However, despite the need to be inserted vaginally, misoprostol has been found by at least three studies to be an excellent alternative to oxytocin in women with premature rupture of membranes near term.

CONTRAINDICATIONS

- Nonreassuring fetal heart tracing or definite evidence of fetal distress.
- Hypertonic, tachysystolic, or other hyperactive uterine patterns (see the "Complications" section for definition).
- If oxytocic drugs are contraindicated or prolonged, contractions of the uterus may be detrimental to fetal safety or uterine integrity.
- Unexplained vaginal bleeding.
- Known hypersensitivity to prostaglandins.
- Multiparity with six or more previous term pregnancies.
- High probability of cephalopelvic disproportion (CPD).
- Breech position.
- Previous cesarean delivery or major uterine surgery.
- Vaginal delivery is not indicated.

EQUIPMENT

- PGE$_2$ gel (compounded Prostin gel or Prepidil) or vaginal insert (Cervidil or misoprostol tablet 25 μg). Prostin is also available as a 20-μg suppository that can be compounded into a gel (see compounding instructions below), but most hospitals now have commercial Prepidil gel available. Since Misoprostol is only available commercially in a 100-μg dosage, certain references strongly recommend that the pharmacist cut the tablet into quarters to ensure correct dose.
- Applicator (if gel is used). The Prepidil kit (Upjohn) 0.5 mg PGE$_2$ (2.5 ml) in syringe supplied with two shielded catheters (10- and 20-mm tip) or an infant endotracheal tube (3-mm inner diameter) with proximal end removed (a normal intravenous catheter without needle works if gel is thin enough).
- Sterile gloves.

- Terbutaline 0.25 mg. (Two doses should be available.)
- Fetal heart tone and uterine tocographic monitors.
- Heparin lock *(optional).*

Editor's note: The price range on the prostaglandin preparations is quite extraordinary. One hospital charged the following: Prostin 20 µg suppository: $770; Prepidil: $273; and Cervidil: $423. The charge for Cytotec is $2 for a 100-µg tablet!

Compounding Equipment and Instructions

- Dinoprostone 20 mg suppository
- Sterile lubricating gel (K-Y Jelly) (80 ml)
- Methylene blue 1% solution
- 10-ml plastic syringes

The following compounding technique should be performed aseptically:

1. Slice the suppository into several pieces and place a drop of methylene blue solution onto each slice.
2. Mix until a smooth, uniform-color paste is formed.
3. Slowly add the lubricating gel to the paste, making a smooth, uniform-color gel without large suppository pieces visible.
4. Store the desired dose of gel in 10-ml syringes (1 mg/4 ml).
5. Replace the cap of the syringe and store in a freezer for up to 90 days.

PREPROCEDURE PATIENT PREPARATION

The indications for cervical ripening or the use of vaginal prostaglandins should be discussed with the patient. Alternatives (if any) as well as potential benefits should be discussed. Only dinoprostone has been approved by the Food and Drug Administration (FDA) for this indication. Review the possible complications with the patient (and family, if present). Be familiar with the package insert information.

Misoprostol is *not* approved by the FDA for this use. Patients should be informed of the off-label use and possible complications of any prostaglandin as listed below. It may be helpful to remind the patient that clinicians frequently use medications off label (e.g., most of the common medications used to halt preterm labor are off label).

TECHNIQUE

Dinoprostone Gel

1. Thaw the PGE$_2$ gel for 1 to 2 hours before the procedure. (Do not force the warming with a water bath or microwave.)

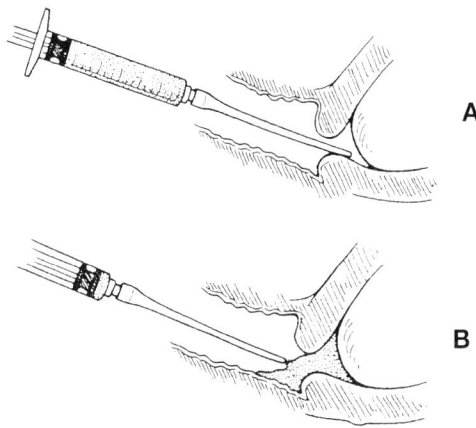

Fig. 165-1
Application of PGE$_2$ gel, **A,** intracervically or, **B,** intravaginally.

2. Apply an external fetal monitor. Obtain a nonstress test (NST) and assess for regular uterine contractions. If the NST is nonreactive or a normal uterine contraction pattern is noted, do not proceed with insertion.
3. Obtain intravenous access *(optional).*
4. Connect the modified infant endotracheal tube or the appropriate shielded catheter (20 mm in length if no cervical effacement is present or 10 mm if greater than 50% effacement) to the filled syringe.
5. To properly administer the gel, the patient should be in a dorsal position with the cervix visualized, using a speculum.
6a. *If a compounded gel is used,* attach the filled syringe to the tube. An additional air-filled syringe will be needed to express all the gel into the vagina or cervix.
6b. *If a commercial gel preparation is used,* use a gentle expulsion technique under sterile conditions. The gel is easily extruded from the syringe. Use the contents of one syringe for one patient only. After injection, do *not* attempt to administer the small amount of gel remaining in the catheter. The syringe, catheter, and any unused package contents should be discarded after use.
7. Insert the endotracheal tube or catheter into the vagina and express a total of 4 ml (1 mg) of compounded PGE$_2$ gel onto the exocervix and into the posterior vaginal fornix. The endotracheal tube or catheter acts as a guide. Alternatively, the tube may be placed approximately 2 cm into the cervical canal; take care not to pass beyond the internal cervical os. This is similar to how Prepidil should be administered. Instill 0.5 mg of PGE$_2$ gel into the cervical canal (Fig. 165-1). (The commercially available gel is packaged as a single 2.5-ml [0.5-mg] unit dose.) If the tube becomes disconnected, spread the remaining contents of the syringe onto the cervix

with your fingers. If the compounded gel was used, either fill the syringe with air after emptying or attach a second air-filled syringe and push any remaining PGE_2 through the tube to make sure all of the PGE_2 is inserted.

8. The patient should remain supine for at least 15 to 30 minutes to minimize leakage from the cervical canal. Maintain external fetal monitoring for 2 hours after the installation. Monitoring may be discontinued after 2 hours if there is no uterine activity.

9. Reevaluate the cervix after 6 hours. If there is minimal change, the procedure may be repeated with a second dose. If needed, a third dose may be administered after 6 more hours.

10. The package insert recommends an interval of 6 to 12 hours between the use of dinoprostone gel and oxytocin. However, some clinicians will initiate oxytocin in 4 hours if there is no uterine hyperactivity. The maximum recommended cumulative dose for a 24-hour period is 1.5 mg of dinoprostone (6 ml of compounded preparation or 7.5 ml of Prepidil). Some clinicians use up to double this amount.

Dinoprostone Insert

1. Apply an external fetal monitor. Obtain an NST and assess for regular uterine contractions. If the NST is nonreactive or a normal uterine contraction pattern is noted, do not proceed with insertion.

2. Obtain intravenous access *(optional)*.

3. On bimanual examination, place the insert transversely in the posterior fornix of the vagina (Fig. 165-2). A minimal amount of water-soluble lubricant can be used to assist with insertion.

4. The patient should remain supine for at least 2 hours after insertion but thereafter may be ambulatory. Maintain external fetal monitoring for 2 hours after

the installation. Monitoring may be discontinued after 2 hours if there is no uterine activity.

5. The insert should be removed upon onset of labor or 12 hours after insertion. Reevaluate the cervix after 12 hours.

6. The insert should be removed at least 30 minutes before oxytocin administration, if uterine hyperstimulation is encountered, or before amniotomy.

Misoprostol

1. Apply an external fetal monitor. Obtain an NST and assess for regular uterine contractions. If the NST is nonreactive or a normal uterine contraction pattern is noted, do not proceed with insertion.

2. Obtain intravenous access *(optional)*.

3. On bimanual examination, insert 25 μg of misoprostol (one quarter of 100-μg tablet) into the posterior vaginal fornix. Certain protocols recommend continuous uterine and fetal monitoring after insertion.

4. Reevaluate the cervix after 4 hours. If there is minimal change, the procedure may be repeated with a second dose.

5. Misoprostol should be held if two or more contractions occur in 10 minutes, a Bishop score of 8/13 has been achieved, active labor begins, or the fetal heart rate is nonreassuring. Oxytocin should not be administered sooner than 2 hours after the last dose of misoprostol.

6. Misoprostol is not recommended for use in this manner for more than 24 hours.

Editor's note: For all three techniques, keep terbutaline 0.25 mg for subcutaneous injection at the patient's bedside in case of hyperstimulation. Remember that once applied (except for Cervidil, which can be removed by using its retrieval system), prostaglandins cannot be removed or reduced like oxytocin; therefore, if at all possible, hyperstimulation should be avoided. Start low and go slow! For practical purposes, all

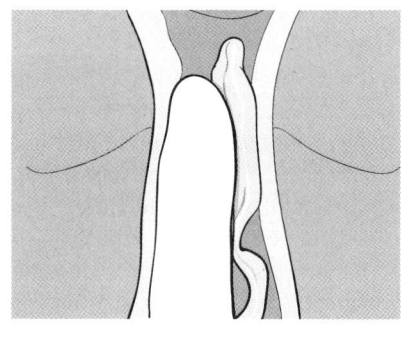
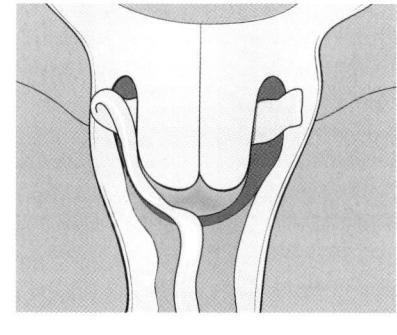
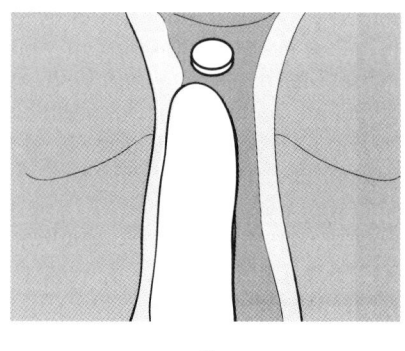

A   B   C

Fig. 165-2
Application of PGE_2 insert (**A-B**) or misoprostol intravaginally (**C**). (**A-B,** Redrawn from Cervidil insert, Forest Pharmaceuticals, Inc., St Louis, MO.)

of these techniques can be performed in the evening and overnight, with planned oxytocin administration and/or amniotomy the following morning.

COMPLICATIONS

- Vomiting, fever, diarrhea (0.5% to 8%)
- Uterine hyperstimulation (0.5% to 5%): defined as five or more contractions in 10 minutes or contractions lasting longer than 2 minutes
- Fetal heart rate abnormalities (Treatment: the patient should be positioned on her left side and administered an IV fluid bolus. Oxygen should be applied with a mask. If necessary and not contraindicated, 0.25 mg of terbutaline should be injected subcutaneously or intravenously; this injection may be repeated once.)

CPT/BILLING CODE

59200   Insertion of cervical dilator (e.g., laminaria, prostaglandin), separate procedure

ICD-9-CM DIAGNOSTIC CODES

The fifth digit (X) is required for Codes 640-648 and 651-659 to denote the following:

0	Unspecified
1	Delivered, with or without mention of antepartum condition
2	Delivered, with mention of postpartum complication
3	Antepartum condition or complication
4	Postpartum condition or complication

645.0X	Postterm pregnancy or pregnancy which has advanced beyond 42 weeks of gestation
642.0X	Hypertension
	benign essential hypertension complicating pregnancy
	chronic NOS
	essential
	preexisting
642.4X	Mild or unspecified preeclampsia

642.5X	Severe preeclampsia
642.6X	Eclampsia
642.7X	Preeclampsia or eclampsia superimposed on preexisting hypertension
648.0X	Diabetes mellitus
648.8X	gestational
646.2X	Unspecified renal disease, without mention of hypertension
658.1X	PROM (membranes ruptured <24 hours before onset of labor)
658.2X	Delayed delivery after spontaneous or unspecified rupture of membranes (ruptured >24 hours before onset)
658.4X	Chorioamnionitis
656.5X	Intrauterine growth retardation
656.1X	Rh isoimmunization
656.4X	Fetal demise

BIBLIOGRAPHY

American College of Obstetricians and Gynecologists: *Induction of labor*, ACOG Practice Bulletin no 10, Washington, 1999, ACOG.

Apgar BS: Current trends in cervical ripening and labor induction, *Am Fam Physician* 60(2):418, 1999.

Cochrane Abstracts. Available at www.cochrane.org (accessed June 30, 2002).

Hannah ME, Ohlsson A, Farine D, et al: Induction of labor compared with expectant management for prelabor rupture of the membranes at term, *N Engl J Med* 334(16):1005, 1996.

Harman JH, Kim A: Current trends in cervical ripening and labor induction, *Am Fam Physician* 60(2):477, 1999.

Hofmeyr GJ, Gulmezoglu AM: Vaginal misoprostol for cervical ripening and labour induction in late pregnancy (Cochrane Review), *The Cochrane Library* 3:1999, Oxford: Update Software.

Kierse MJNC: Prostaglandins in preinduction cervical ripening: meta-analysis of worldwide clinical experience, *J Reprod Med* 38:89, 1993.

Lydon-Rochelle M, Holt VL, Basterling TR, Martin DP: Risk of uterine rupture during labor among women with a prior cesarean delivery, *N Engl J Med* 345(1):3, July 5, 2001.

Sanchez-Ramos L, Peterson DE, Delke I, et al: Labor induction with prostaglandin E_1 misoprostol compared with dinoprostone vaginal insert: a randomized trial, *Obstet Gynecol* 91:401, 1998.

Wing DA: Labor induction with misoprostol, *Am J Obstet Gynecol* 181(2):339, 1999.

CHAPTER 166

Fetal-Movement Counting, Nonstress Test, and Contraction Stress Test

Stephen Ratcliffe

FETAL-MOVEMENT COUNTING

Both human and animal studies indicate that a fetus in trouble (hypoxic) will reduce its oxygen requirements by reducing its activity. In addition, maternal perception of fetal movement appears to be an accurate reflection of fetal activity. As a result, fetal-movement counting (FMC) is a potentially useful tool for monitoring the fetus during the third trimester of pregnancy. In fact, FMC is now a common practice in high-risk pregnancies and studies continue to evaluate its use in low-risk pregnancies. The primary purpose of FMC is to identify pregnancies needing an intervention to prevent fetal demise or stillbirth.

Several studies have evaluated the outcomes of pregnancies in which patients complained of decreased fetal movement (Ahn et al, 1987; Whitty et al, 1991). Approximately 5% of those patients required immediate delivery for either a maternal or a fetal indication. Another 6.8% had abnormal fetal tracings requiring additional follow-up. These outcomes suggest that decreased fetal movement in late pregnancy requires further antenatal testing. Since decreased fetal movement may be the earliest sign of placental insufficiency, evaluation should be performed in a timely fashion. However, the literature has conflicting results on whether other parameters need to be followed as well. One recent study (Harrington et al, 1998) concluded that decreased fetal movement as an isolated finding was not associated with adverse outcomes.

Although approximately 50% of stillbirths occur in normal pregnancies, FMC has not assumed a routine role in all pregnancies. This is for a number of reasons. Previous studies used different protocols and therefore had varying results. Several protocols required women to perform FMC for up to an hour, three times a day. These regimens resulted in poor patient compliance. The largest of these studies (n = 68,000), which used FMC on all women during the third trimester, found no benefit to screening all pregnancies (Grant et al, 1989). A more recent prospective, nonrandomized study demon-strated a reduced perinatal mortality rate. This study used routine FMC with the count-to-ten method described in this chapter.

INDICATIONS

The clinician needs to decide for which of the following scenarios to use fetal movement counting (FMC):

1. All pregnancies as a routine practice:
   The scientific evidence does not support daily FMC in all pregnancies. However, the available evidence *does* support women being on the alert for overall decreased fetal movement. It seems prudent for a patient who senses decreased fetal activity to have been instructed, beforehand, either to report to labor and delivery or to self-administer some type of FMC.
2. High-risk pregnancies (e.g., hypertension, diabetes or other high-risk conditions):
   Randomized controlled trials have not been performed in these settings. However, it is a common practice to recommend FMC as a secondary method of fetal surveillance in all high-risk pregnancies.

Editor's note: At present, antenatal testing (e.g., nonstress test, contraction stress test, biophysical profile) has been so effective that the likelihood of fetal death in high-risk, tested populations is lower than in low-risk, untested populations. This paradox will force us to consider other methods of fetal monitoring as well as to possibly perform antenatal testing in all pregnancies. In the meantime, questions about patient acceptability of FMC, the burden of further testing precipitated by nonreassuring FMCs, and the risks of unwarranted early interventions need to be answered.

CONTRAINDICATIONS

- Impaired mental status or significant linguistic or cultural barrier—any barrier preventing adequate communication or the proper use of FMC could cause screening errors or failures.

- Mother unable to sense fetal movements—there are cases where the clinician can actually *see* the baby moving (e.g., during a routine visit, while measuring the fundal height, or otherwise observing the anterior abdomen), and yet the patient cannot sense the movement. In that situation the patient will not be able to perform FMC.

TECHNIQUE

1. The patient should be instructed in the count-to-ten method of FMC (see the sample patient education handout titled "Fetal-Movement Counting" on page 1966 of Appendix G). The count-to-ten method, described by Moore, has been studied and compared to the Sadovsky method (three 30- to 60-minute counts at preset times each day) and the Rayburn method (FMC for 60 minutes, once a day). The count-to-ten method is the clear favorite of patients. Instruct the patient to time how long it takes to count 10 fetal movements (swishes, rolls, kicks, etc.). The test is completed and considered to be "reassuring" when 10 movements are counted in less than 2 hours. Tests are usually performed in the evening and, as it turns out, are often completed within 20 minutes.
2. The patient is instructed to report to labor and delivery or to notify her clinician if 10 movements are not recorded within a 2-hour period. Such a result is a "nonreassuring" screening test.

Editor's note: Although the evidence does not support daily FMC in every pregnancy, it is unlikely to be harmful if it is used several times a week in most pregnancies starting at 34 weeks.

COMPLICATIONS

- False-positive results: unfortunately, in order to identify those fetuses that are experiencing true distress, FMC produces a large number of false-positive results. A nonreassuring FMC may be complicated by a false-positive follow-up antenatal test. These abnormal results may even culminate in the decision to induce labor, thereby exposing the mother and child to the risks of induction (e.g., fetal distress, cesarean section). The risk of these complications is a large part of the controversy surrounding the use of FMC with every pregnancy.

INTERPRETATION OF RESULTS

A reassuring test is described above. Patients arriving at labor and delivery with a complaint of decreased fetal movement should undergo antenatal testing (e.g., a nonstress test and an amniotic fluid index [AFI]; or a biophysical profile [BPP]). If any of these tests are abnormal, a contraction stress test should be considered (or a delivery if mature). If the nonstress test and AFI or the BPP are found to be normal, no further testing is generally indicated unless additional factors warrant surveillance (Ahn et al, 1987).

NONSTRESS TEST

The nonstress test (NST) was introduced in the United States in the early 1970s. Despite a paucity of randomized controlled trial evidence to support its use, the NST has become a mainstay of antenatal testing. In fact, the NST is the most commonly used first-line antenatal test for high-risk fetuses (e.g., prolonged pregnancy, growth restricted fetus, underlying maternal medical condition(s), decreased fetal movement, other events or diagnoses occurring during pregnancy). An NST involves the use of fetal monitoring to document fetal heart rate accelerations that occur in conjunction with fetal movements. In a "reassuring" or "reactive" NST, there are at least two accelerations of greater than 15 beats/min that last for 15 seconds in a 20-minute period.

Extensive clinical observations have repeatedly shown a strong correlation between absent or less frequent fetal heart rate accelerations and progressive fetal hypoxia. On the contrary, the presence of fetal heart rate accelerations associated with fetal movement (a reactive NST) is a reassuring indicator of good fetal health. Although this is not a complex procedure, the clinician must be adept at the proper interpretation of the NST, taking into consideration the reason the test was ordered, gestational age, and whether there are any congenital anomalies or maternal medical condition(s). The clinician should also know whether the patient has taken any medications (e.g., narcotics or barbiturates) that might affect the reactivity of the fetal tracing.

INDICATIONS

The NST is used to monitor the fetal health status of high-risk pregnancies as early as 34 weeks' gestation. Some of these high-risk conditions include the following:

- Suspected or confirmed intrauterine growth restriction (IUGR) or growth retardation

- Maternal or gestational diabetes
- Essential hypertension or preeclampsia
- Postdates or prolonged pregnancy
- Decreased fetal movement
- Maternal trauma
- Other maternal or fetal condition posing risk to fetus (renal disease, multiple gestation, substance abuse, prior fetal demise, etc.)

Some investigators have used the NST as early as 28 to 34 weeks' gestational age. However, different criteria have to be used to define a reactive or reassuring tracing because the premature fetus will have less pronounced heart rate accelerations than the more mature fetus.

CONTRAINDICATIONS

There are no specific contraindications to performing an NST other than a gestational age less than 28 to 34 weeks.
- Gestational age less than 34 weeks (relative contraindication, modified criteria can be used for interpretation)

EQUIPMENT (See the "Suppliers" section)

- Fetal heart rate and uterine pressure monitor (Fig. 166-1)
- Blood pressure cuff
- Fetal stimulation device (vibro-acoustic stimulator, such as an artificial larynx)
- Ultrasonic gel for monitor
- Bed or comfortable reclining chair

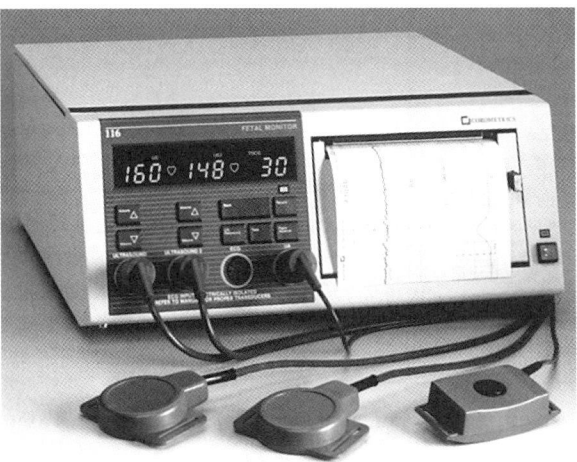

Fig. 166-1
Intrapartum fetal and uterine monitor. (Courtesy GE Medical Systems Information Technologies, Inc.)

PREPROCEDURE PATIENT PREPARATION

Before the NST is performed, the patient should be given a handout outlining the procedure and the steps to follow (see the sample patient education handout titled "Nonstress Test" on page 1967 of Appendix G). Many testing centers use standardized protocols in an attempt to minimize environmental variables. These protocols encourage the patient to eat about 2 hours before the NST, to not smoke or take sedative drugs before the test, and to remain sedentary during the hour before testing.

TECHNIQUE

1. Place the patient in a semi-recumbent (semi-Fowler's) position, tilted slightly to her left or with slight left lateral hip displacement. She can also be seated in a reclining chair at a 30- to 45-degree angle.
2. Apply external uterine and fetal monitors (tocodynamometer and Doppler) to record any uterine contractions and the fetal heart rate. Record the patient's blood pressure before the test to make sure she does not have supine hypotension, which could cause a falsely abnormal test. Check the blood pressure every 10 to 15 minutes during the test.
3. Ask the patient to report or record any fetal movements.
4. Monitor the patient for a 30-minute baseline period. Two additional 30-minute monitoring periods should be considered if the tracing is nonreactive. A fetal tracing is considered reactive if there are two or more accelerations of more than 15 beats/min lasting for at least 15 seconds. These accelerations should occur within a 20-minute interval.
5. If there is insufficient fetal movement in the first or second 30-minute observation period, some studies support the use of a vibro-acoustic stimulator (e.g., an artificial larynx) to induce fetal movement. The presence of reactivity to these induced movements has been shown to correlate well with reactivity to spontaneous fetal movements during an NST (Marden et al, 1997). In other words, using the stimulator does not seem to affect the sensitivity of the test.

COMPLICATIONS

- False-positive results: the NST itself poses no known risks to the mother or fetus. However, the improper interpretation of the test may lead to premature or unnecessary interventions that could lead to iatrogenic morbidity or mortality. Unfortunately, false-positive tests are common, partly dependent upon the reason the test was ordered.

INTERPRETATIONS OF RESULTS

In a low-risk pregnancy, nonreactivity usually indicates the infant is sleeping. The clinician should extend the observation period for as long as 90 minutes total to decrease the likelihood of a false-positive test. At least one study has shown that a reactive NST remains predictive of a good outcome regardless of the length of time (up to 100 minutes) needed to demonstrate reactivity. Alternatively, the clinician may choose to use a vibro-acoustic stimulation device as described above to induce fetal movements. Again, make sure the patient did not get hypotensive from being in the semi-recumbent position. This can cause a falsely abnormal test.

The clinician must take into account the risk status of the patient and the indication for ordering an NST when interpreting a nonreactive NST and before proceeding with further interventions. The positive predictive value of an abnormal NST ranges from 15% for evaluating a postdates pregnancy to 69% for evaluating IUGR. Hence false-positive tests are common. The low-risk patient at 41 weeks' gestation who has a nonreactive NST most likely has a healthy fetus, and the clinician must undertake further steps to confirm this without subjecting the patient and fetus to unnecessary iatrogenic interventions. However, persistent absence of reactivity in the absence of an obvious etiology (maternal medications, prematurity, or congenital anomalies) is associated with fetal compromise in most cases.

Of the few infants who do not do well after a normal NST, most succumb to an unpredictable, untoward event such as a cord accident, an abruption, a congenital anomaly, or preterm labor. Otherwise, reactive NSTs that have no other abnormalities on the tracing (e.g., variable decelerations) have a very low false-negative rate (3 in 1000). However, to improve on even this risk, studies indicate that performing NSTs twice a week may produce better outcomes. This is especially true for high-risk pregnancies. The other protocol that many centers have adopted utilizes an NST combined with an AFI (see Chapter 173, Obstetric Ultrasound) also known as the *modified biophysical profile*. When used to assess the at-risk pregnancy, this combination of tests reduces the false-negative rate by more than two thirds to less than 1 in 1000 (Miller et al, 1996). This false-negative rate is comparable to that of either the BPP or a contraction stress test.

Options available to the clinician for evaluating a persistently nonreactive NST include proceeding with a contraction stress test, obtaining a BPP, or proceeding with induction when the infant is mature and favorable conditions exist. A sample flowchart for the management of NST results, as used in a private family practice clinic in Colorado, is shown in Fig. 166-2. In settings that do not routinely obtain an AFI, the occurrence of repetitive variable decelerations in an otherwise reactive NST should prompt a measurement of the AFI (Jaschevatzky et al, 1998). This subgroup of fetuses is at increased risk of cord compromise during labor.

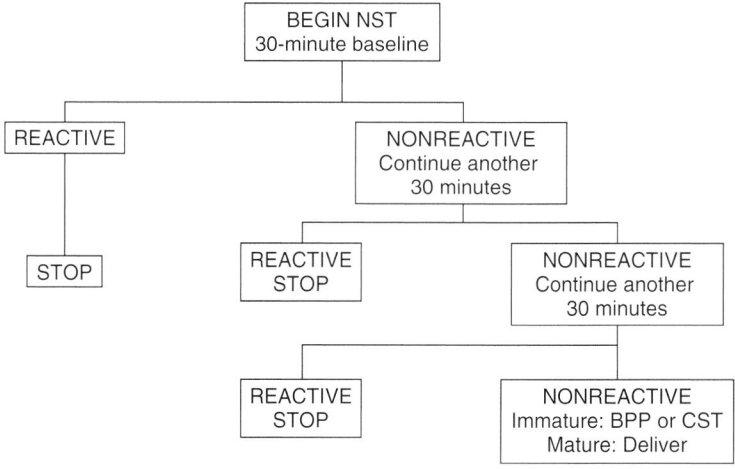

Fig. 166-2
Sample flowchart for management of the nonstress test. *BPP,* Biophysical profile; *CST,* contraction stress test. (Courtesy Kent Petrie, MD.)

POSTPROCEDURE PATIENT EDUCATION

It is essential that patients receive a detailed explanation of the results of the NST and the specific signs and symptoms (e.g., decreased fetal movement, vaginal bleeding, leakage of fluid) for which they should watch. Patients should receive explicit instructions regarding follow-up appointments and when to go to labor and delivery.

CONTRACTION STRESS TEST

The contraction stress test (CST) was one of the first antepartum fetal tests. It is designed to identify fetuses at risk from either uteroplacental insufficiency or cord compression. A CST is usually a secondary antenatal test used when an NST, AFI, or BPP does not provide the reassurance needed to continue an expectant course of pregnancy management. The basis of the test is to determine whether uterine contractions cause late decelerations in the fetal heart tracing.

Normally, when the uterus contracts, there is a brief decrease in the oxygen supply to the placenta. With an adequate placenta and cord, there is an adequate oxygen reserve so that the fetus is not affected. With placental or cord insufficiency, the fetal oxygen reserves are diminished. As a result, a brief hypoxic episode from a uterine contraction can cause a vagus-mediated bradycardia that in turn produces a late deceleration. (Hypoxia can also directly affect the myocardium causing a late deceleration.) Therefore, if a CST results in a late deceleration, it usually indicates inadequate fetal and placental oxygen reserve.

Research in the mid 1960s found that late decelerations correlated with stillbirths and low Apgar scores. In 1972, Ray and Freeman began systematic trials of CSTs in the United States. They called this test the *oxytocin challenge test* because it relied on an infusion of synthetic oxytocin (Pitocin). Contemporary clinicians often use spontaneous contractions or those induced by breast stimulation in place of oxytocin administration. Not only has this simplified the procedure, but it has also resulted in the procedure being called the *contraction stress test*.

The CST, NST, and BPP (see Chapter 173, Obstetric Ultrasound) are used to screen for fetal compromise or to evaluate a pregnancy when fetal compromise is suspected. The CST is a more sensitive test of fetal well-being than the NST; however, the CST is a more expensive test and requires more staff and clinician time to perform. As a result, it is generally used to follow up abnormal or suspicious NSTs or BPPs.

INDICATIONS

- Suspected fetal compromise in a high-risk pregnancy (e.g., IUGR, pregnancy-induced hypertension, or postdates pregnancy)
- Evaluation of a suspicious NST or BPP

Note: Combining an NST with an assessment of amniotic fluid volume (i.e., modified BPP) produces an evaluation with equal the sensitivity of a BPP. The sensitivity also approaches that of the CST; therefore the modified BPP appears to be emerging as the screening test of choice.

CONTRAINDICATIONS

- If labor is contraindicated, CST is contraindicated (e.g., advanced cases of premature labor when considerable dilation and effacement have already occurred, incompetent cervix with nonmature fetus, placenta previa, classical cesarean scar).
- Breech or other fetal indication for cesarean *(relative contraindication)*.

EQUIPMENT (See "Suppliers" Section)

- Fetal heart rate and uterine pressure monitors (Fig. 166-1)
- Ultrasonic gel for monitors
- Blood pressure cuff
- Intravenous setup
- Terbutaline
- Bed or comfortable reclining chair

Note: CSTs are usually performed in a hospital or nearby setting.

PREPROCEDURE PATIENT PREPARATION

Give the patient a teaching guide explaining the CST (see the sample patient education handout titled "Contraction Stress Test" on page 1965 of Appendix G) and answer any questions she may have.

TECHNIQUE

1. Place the patient in a semi-recumbent (semi-Fowler's) position, tilted slightly to her left, or with slight left lateral hip displacement. She can also be sitting in a reclining chair at a 30- to 45-degree angle. Attach fetal and uterine monitors.

2. Take a baseline blood pressure to ensure that supine hypotension, which could cause a false-positive CST, does not exist. Repeat every 10 to 15 minutes during the test.

3. Record a baseline fetal heart rate/contraction tracing for 20 to 30 minutes to assess for reactivity and to determine whether there are spontaneous uterine contractions. Subcutaneous terbutaline, which relaxes uterine muscle in the event of serious uterine hyperstimulation and hypertonic contractions, should be readily available. If there are adequate spontaneous contractions (three or more per 10 minutes, lasting greater than 45 seconds), monitor the fetal heart rate during these contractions and complete the study.

4. If there are not enough adequate spontaneous contractions, obtain a baseline NST. Next, ask the patient to stimulate one nipple by massaging it for about 2 minutes. She can then stop the stimulation for 2 minutes before repeating the process on the other side. If intermittent stimulation does not achieve the desired uterine contractions, bilateral stimulation should be performed for about 10 minutes.

5. Once an adequate contraction pattern is achieved, the breast stimulation should be stopped. Uterine hyperstimulation patterns occur in 3% to 4% of CSTs using breast stimulation. Provide continuous fetal and uterine monitoring.

Note: The nipple-stimulation CST is being used more frequently because it bypasses the need for placing an intravenous line. If successful, it also reduces the testing time.

6. If nipple stimulation does not produce an adequate contraction pattern, oxytocin can be administered. Initiate the intravenous infusion of oxytocin at 0.5 to 1.0 mU/min. This rate may be increased every 15 minutes by increments of 0.5 to 1.0 mU/min until regular uterine contractions are achieved. An adequate CST has been achieved when there are three contractions lasting greater than 45 seconds within a 10-minute period. If oxytocin is used, the majority of patients will achieve this contraction pattern by the time they reach an infusion level of 4 to 8 mU/min. Uterine hyperstimulation (more than five contractions per 10 minutes or contractions lasting 90 seconds or more) occurs during oxytocin challenge testing in about 1% of patients and generally responds to stopping the oxytocin infusion. If the contractions do not decrease rapidly after stopping the oxytocin, subcutaneous terbutaline, 0.25 to 0.5 mg, should be administered.

COMPLICATIONS

- Uterine hyperstimulation: often provides a false-positive CST that may lead to improper management if not correctly identified.
- Fetal distress requiring an emergency intervention is a rare complication of uterine hyperstimulation. Uterine hyperstimulation almost always resolves if the oxytocin infusion or breast stimulation is stopped. If this is not sufficient, subcutaneous terbutaline may be used as described above.

INTERPRETATIONS OF RESULTS

"Negative" test results are reassuring; "positive" or "suspicious" results are cause for concern. A CST is positive if more than 50% of the contractions are accompanied by late decelerations in the absence of uterine hyperstimulation. The reactivity of the fetal tracing (see "Nonstress Test" section) is an important factor to weigh when evaluating a positive CST. A *reactive,* positive CST is associated with a high incidence of false positives, whereas a *nonreactive,* positive CST has a much higher predictive value for identifying a compromised fetus (Fig. 166-3).

A suspicious or equivocal CST is one in which less than 50% of the contractions result in late decelerations. The result is also labeled equivocal if the decelerations occur during hyperstimulation because it cannot be determined whether the CST is negative or positive.

A negative CST is one in which no late decelerations occur when the contraction frequency is at least three per 10 minutes. In addition, no significant variable decelerations should occur. A negative CST that is *nonreactive* is uncommon. This test result deserves further scrutiny to determine if the cause is a medication (e.g., narcotics or phenobarbital), a fetal central nervous system defect, subtle fetal distress, or a premature infant.

A positive or suspicious CST should be given careful consideration. Maternal factors that affect placental function such as dehydration or hypotension should be addressed. If improvement in the fetal heart rate tracing cannot be attained, and if fetal pulmonary maturity has been confirmed, labor is often induced.

POSTPROCEDURE EDUCATION

A CST must be interpreted in the context of the patient's overall clinical condition. Because CSTs are

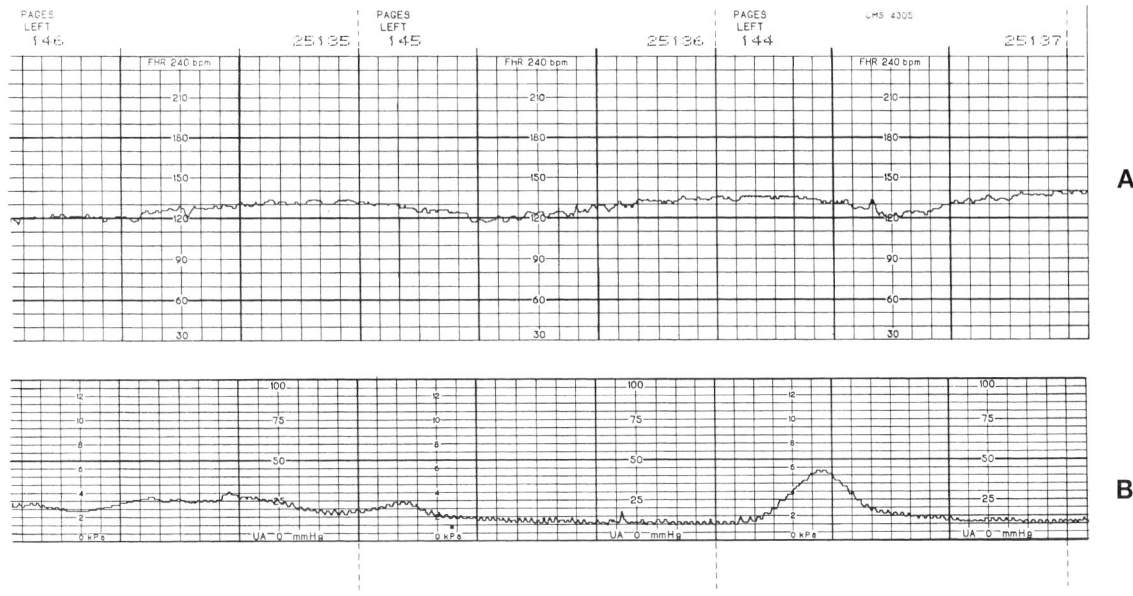

Fig. 166-3
Nonreactive positive contraction stress test. **A,** Fetal heart rate. **B,** Uterine contractions.

generally reserved for high-risk patients, clear post-procedure instructions for these patients are essential. Even patients with negative CSTs require explicit instructions for follow-up antenatal testing, clinician visits and any signs and symptoms for which they should be watching. The fetal deaths that have been reported after negative CSTs are often attributed to congenital malformations, placental abruption, and poor glucose control in women with diabetes; counseling for patients at risk should be appropriate.

SUPPLIERS

Hewlett-Packard/Agilent (now owned by Philips Medical)
Philips Medical Systems
3000 Minute Man Road
Andover, MA 01810
Phone: 1-800-225-0230
Website: www.medical.Philips.com *or* shop.medical.philips.com

Corometrics (now owned by GE Medical Systems)
General Electric Medical Systems, Inc
P.O. Box 414
Milwaukee, WI 53201
Phone: 1-800-433-5566
Website: www.gemedicalsystems.com

CPT/BILLING CODES

59020	Fetal contraction stress test
59025	Fetal nonstress test

If the patient has a diagnosis in addition to normal pregnancy, counseling for FMC (fetal movement counting) is coded with an E/M code:

99203	Physician typically spends 30 minutes face-to-face with a new patient and/or family
99214	Physician typically spends 25 minutes face-to-face with an established patient and/or family

If there is no additional diagnosis (normal pregnancy), preventive medicine codes should be used:

99401	Preventive medicine counseling and/or risk factor reduction intervention(s) provided to an individual (separate procedure); approximately 15 minutes
99402	approximately 30 minutes

ICD-9-CM DIAGNOSTIC CODES

V22.0	Supervision of normal first pregnancy
V22.1	Supervision of other normal pregnancy
642.03	Benign, essential hypertension complicating pregnancy, antepartum
642.43	Mild or unspecified preeclampsia, antepartum
642.53	Severe preeclampsia, antepartum

642.63	Eclampsia, antepartum
642.73	Preeclampsia or eclampsia superimposed on preexisting hypertension, antepartum
645.03	Prolonged pregnancy, advanced beyond 42 weeks of gestation, antepartum
645.13	Postterm pregnancy, over 40 completed to 42 completed weeks, antepartum
646.33	Habitual aborter, antepartum
648.03	Diabetes mellitus, preexisting, antepartum
648.83	Diabetes mellitus, gestational, antepartum
648.93	Maternal trauma complicating pregnancy, antepartum
646.23	Unspecified renal disease, without mention of hypertension, antepartum
656.53	Intrauterine growth restriction or retardation, antepartum
656.43	Fetal demise, antepartum

ADDITIONAL RESOURCES

- See the sample patient education handouts titled "Contraction Stress Test," "Fetal-Movement Counting," and "Nonstress Test" on pages 1965, 1966, and 1967, respectively, of Appendix G.
- See the sample patient consent forms titled "Contraction Stress Test," "Fetal-Movement Counting," and "Nonstress Test" on pages 1968, 1969, and 1970, respectively, of Appendix G.

BIBLIOGRAPHY

Fetal-movement counting

Ahn MO, Phelan JP, Smith CV, et al: Antepartum fetal surveillance in the patient with decreased fetal movement, *Am J Obstet Gynecol* 157:860, 1987.

Grant A, Elbourne D, Valentin L, Alexander S: Routine formal fetal-movement counting and risk of antepartum late death in normally formed singletons, *Lancet* 2(8659):345, 1989.

Harrington K, Thompson O, Jordan L, et al: Obstetric outcome in women who present with a reduction in fetal movements in the third trimester of pregnancy, *J Perinat Med* 26:77, 1998.

Moore TR, Piacquadio K: A prospective evaluation of fetal-movement screening to reduce the incidence of antepartum fetal death, *Am J Obstet Gynecol* 160:1075, 1989.

Smith CV, Davis SA, Rayburn WF: Patients' acceptance of monitoring fetal movement: a randomized comparison of charting techniques, *J Reproduc Med* 37:144, 1992.

Whitty JE, Garfinkel DA, Divon MY: Maternal perception of decreased fetal movement as an indication for antepartum testing in a low-risk population, *Am J Obstet Gynecol* 165:1084, 1991.

Nonstress test

Jaschevatzky OE, Marom D, Ostrovsky P, et al: Significance of sporadic decelerations during antepartum testing in term pregnancies, *Am J Perinatol* 15:291, 1998.

Marden D, McDuffie RE, Allen R, et al: A randomized controlled trial of a new fetal acoustic stimulation test for fetal well-being, *Am J Obstet Gynecol* 176:1386, 1997.

Miller DA, Rabella YA, Paul R: The modified biophysical profile: antepartum testing in the 1990s, *Am J Obstet Gynecol* 174:812, 1996.

Nageotte MP, Towers CV, Asrat T, Freeman RK: Perinatal outcome with the modified biophysical profile, *Am J Obstet Gynecol* 170:1672, 1994.

Rayburn WF: Monitoring fetal body movement, *Clin Obstet Gynecol* 30:899, 1987.

Sandovsky E, Polishuk WZ. Fetal movements in utero, *Obstet Gynecol* 50:49, 1997.

Tan KH, Smyth R: Fetal vibroacoustic stimulation for facilitation of tests of fetal wellbeing, *Cochrane Database Syst Rev* 1:CD002963, 2001.

Contraction stress test

Berkus MD, Langer O: Intrapartum fetal surveillance: a reappraisal, *Pediatr Ann* 25:200, 1996.

Hanley ML, Vintzileos AM: Antepartum and intrapartum surveillance of fetal well-being. In Reece EA, Hobbins JC, editors: *Medicine of the fetus and mother,* ed 2, Philadelphia, 1999 Lippincott-Raven.

Hoskins IA, Frieden FJ, Young BK: Variable decelerations in reactive nonstress tests with decreased amniotic fluid index predict fetal compromise, *Am J Obstet Gynecol* 165:1094, 1991.

Lagrew DC: The contraction stress test, *Clin Obstet Gynecol* 38:11, 1995.

Pircon RA, Freeman RK: The contraction stress test, *Obstet Gynecol Clin North Am* 17:129, 1990.

CHAPTER 167

Episiotomy

Donald N. Marquardt

Episiotomy is the second most commonly performed surgical procedure in the United States, surpassed only by circumcision. Episiotomy is used to facilitate the second stage of labor in approximately 60% of all deliveries (and up to 90% of primiparous deliveries) in the United States. However, nurse-midwives and physicians in Europe perform the surgery much less frequently (approximately one eighth the frequency), which is consistent with their view that delivery is a natural process that does not necessarily benefit from intervention. The European view is slowly being supported by the scientific evidence and increasingly being adopted in the United States.

In a comprehensive review in 1983, Thacker and Banta concluded that "the widespread use of episiotomy did not withstand scientific scrutiny . . . [and] the risks of episiotomy had been widely ignored." Since that time, additional exhaustive reviews have indicated that, despite a slightly increased risk for labial and anterior vaginal lacerations, *avoidance* of episiotomy leads to *less* overall perineal trauma. Other studies have concluded that avoiding episiotomies minimizes the risk of fourth-degree lacerations. Six studies that compared a restrictive policy of episiotomy with a policy of its routine use were reviewed for the Cochrane database. Although "severe trauma" occurred with similar frequency with both policies, there was less posterior vaginal or perineal trauma with a restrictive policy and less overall need for suturing. Episiotomy therefore falls into the category of "Forms of Care Likely to be Ineffective or Harmful" (ineffectiveness or harm demonstrated by clear evidence) in the Cochrane database.

It seems reasonable to conclude that episiotomy should not be performed routinely. In fact, avoiding episiotomy may improve quality of life in several areas as determined by a study at McGill University (Klein et al, 1991). However, for certain situations and indications, episiotomy may be unavoidable or extremely useful.

An episiotomy is performed to enlarge the vaginal outlet to facilitate delivery. In a midline or median episiotomy, the incision is made in a direct line posteriorly from the vagina toward the anus, and down to—but not including—the external anal sphincter. Alternatively, in a mediolateral episiotomy, the incision is directed 45 degrees laterally from the midline at the base of the introitus. The latter is associated with more bleeding, a more difficult surgical repair, faulty healing, and a higher risk of postoperative pain, including dyspareunia. The only usual benefit to mediolateral episiotomy is a decreased risk of extension to a third or fourth degree tear. As a result, it is performed much less frequently in the United States. This chapter is limited to the median episiotomy, although a modified version is also discussed. Readers interested in the classic mediolateral episiotomy are referred to a technical review by Varner (1986).

INDICATIONS

Any situation that prolongs the second stage of labor and thereby significantly endangers the life of the mother, the integrity of her perineum, or the brain of the fetus could warrant episiotomy. The fact that episiotomy is a surgical procedure with attendant risks and potentially fatal complications should be weighed against the decision to speed the second stage of labor by a few minutes.

Current obstetric literature suggests that episiotomy may be indicated when vaginal delivery is anticipated and one of the following maternal or fetal indications exists:

Maternal Indications

- Significant cardiac disease (e.g., mitral stenosis)
- Prolonged second-stage labor (greater than 2 hours for primiparous or 1 hour for multiparous or with regional anesthesia greater than 3 hours for primiparous or 2 hours for multiparous)

Note: The evidence is changing regarding these time guidelines and there is disagreement as to whether this is still an indication.

- Risk of significant perineal trauma (e.g., large infant, use of forceps or vacuum)

Fetal Indications

- Significant fetal distress in second stage
- Prematurity
- Breech presentation
- Shoulder dystocia

As mentioned earlier, several previous indications (e.g., prevention of pelvic relaxation and decreased incidence of perineal morbidity) are not supported by clinical trials. Current indications may change as further evidence replaces speculation. Clinical trials are necessary to demonstrate whether less invasive maneuvers (e.g., perineal massage, changes in maternal position, breathing, or pushing) are helpful in alleviating second-stage complications or in reducing trauma for a premature infant or breech delivery. Readers are encouraged to remain up to date with the literature.

CONTRAINDICATIONS

- Patient refusal
- Severe scarring or malformation of perineum (e.g., from inflammatory bowel disease or lymphogranuloma venereum) *(relative contraindication)*
- Extensive or large condyloma that may lead to frank hemorrhage if incised *(relative contraindication)*

EQUIPMENT

Episiotomy is usually performed with blunt-tipped surgical scissors (a scalpel may also be used). Equipment for repair includes the following:
- Needle holder
- Nontraumatic forceps
- Allis clamps
- Ring forceps
- Vaginal retractor(s)
- 4 × 4–inch gauze pads
- 3-0 and 4-0 glycolic polymer sutures (preferred over chromic, which is associated with more discomfort during healing) on a large, curved needle
- Cutting needle, or a tapered point needle (decision based on clinician's preference)

If effective regional (e.g., epidural, pudendal) anesthesia is not in place, a 10-ml syringe with a 1½-inch, 27-gauge needle should be available to locally infiltrate the anesthetic of preference (usually 1% lidocaine *without* epinephrine).

PREPROCEDURE PATIENT PREPARATION

Discuss an episiotomy with the patient (and partner) during prenatal care, *before* an emergent moment of need when neither the clinician nor the patient is in an optimal situation for exchange of information. Ideally, the patient's desires are part of a written birth plan (see Chapter 178, Vaginal Delivery). Discuss the potential risks and possible benefits to allow the patient to make an informed decision concerning liberal or restricted use of episiotomy at the time of delivery. Also discuss the specific circumstances in which episiotomy may be medically necessary.

TECHNIQUE

In the second stage of labor, as the fetal cranium begins to distend the maternal perineum, effort should be directed toward assisting with the natural thinning of the perineum and dilation of the introitus. These efforts include placing tension on the perineum and gently stretching it, from inside the introitus, with the index and middle fingers. Labeling posterior as the 6 o'clock direction, rotate these fingers, under gentle tension, from about the 4 o'clock to the 8 o'clock positions. Gentle exterior massage with the thumb and/or other hand at the same time, in this same location, may also help with thinning of the perineum.

The decision for episiotomy is usually made after the fetal cranium (not just the caput) distends the introitus. Waiting until a minimum of 3 to 4 cm of the fetal scalp diameter is visible and delivery is imminent will prevent excessive blood loss. Until that time, massaging the perineum, as described above, may not only minimize bleeding, but may also provide some anesthesia by placing pressure on the local nerve endings. As the head further distends the introitus, an episiotomy is needed if it appears that the head will not be deliverable without an episiotomy or that there will be so much tension on the perineum that it will tear. An episiotomy may also be necessary for one of the other indications.

1. In preparation for cutting, the index and middle fingers of the nondominant hand are inserted between the fetal scalp (or presenting part) and the maternal perineum, directed toward the maternal anus (toward the 6 o'clock position). The thumb should be placed on the exterior perineum. The thumb and fingers serve two functions: to protect the fetus and to palpate the anal sphincter as a reminder of its location for the clinician. The thumb defines the bottom of the episiotomy (Fig. 167-1).

2. Check for anesthesia by gently scratching or pinching the perineum with tissue forceps or the Allis clamp. If anesthesia is not already adequate, administer additional local anesthetic if not otherwise contraindicated. Anesthetize the midline of both the perineum (for a median episiotomy) and the floor of the vagina. The middle and index fingers should be in place between the fetus and the perineum/

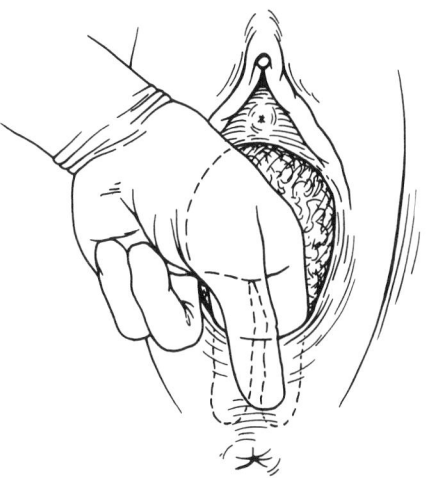

Fig. 167-1
Palpating and attempting to stretch and thin the perineum before episiotomy.

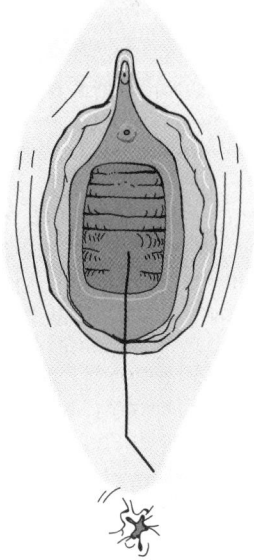

Fig. 167-3
"Hockey stick" extension of midline episiotomy.

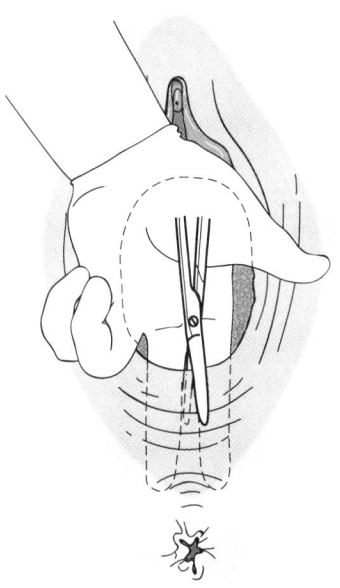

Fig. 167-2
Performing the midline episiotomy.

floor of the vagina to avoid fetal injection with anesthetic.

3. Insert one blade of the scissors to cut parallel to and between the fingers. Again, take care to protect the fetal-presenting part. After the incision has passed the fetus, avoid cutting the external sphincter of the anus (Fig. 167-2) by keeping pressure posteriorly with the fingers. Under direct visualization, extend the incision up the vaginal mucosa an additional 2 to 4 cm,

through the hymenal ring, to release tension and prevent tearing. Delivery should proceed expeditiously to minimize blood loss.

Note: In the patient with a very short perineum, consider performing a variant of the median episiotomy: the "hockey stick" episiotomy. After the usual median incision has reached the rectal sphincter, veer off of the midline, laterally, for 1 or 2 cm (Fig 167-3). In this manner, the perineal incision is L-shaped or the shape of a hockey stick. At delivery, if the incision extends by tearing, it should naturally follow the L-shape, avoiding the rectal sphincter.

Repair

1. Most clinicians prefer to repair the episiotomy after the third stage of labor. This avoids disturbing the episiotomy repair with the delivery of the placenta. Also, if the placenta separates in the middle of the repair, bleeding may make visualization difficult. As with any surgical repair, accurate assessment of the extent of injury (both by palpation and by direct visualization) is crucial. Carefully and closely inspect for "extensions" or tears beyond the episiotomy. This examination may reveal damage (complete or partial) to the anal sphincter (third-degree laceration) or rectal mucosa (fourth-degree laceration).

2. A rectal examination should be performed after every delivery. After donning an additional sterile exam-

ination glove and lubricating a finger with antiseptic solution, palpate the distal 6 cm of the rectal mucosa. Determine whether the sphincter has sufficient "bulk" remaining (i.e., produces the sensation of a small doughnut being palpated). In the absence of this sensation, evaluate closely for a third-degree extension.

3. Next, exclude occult damage to the rectal mucosa, even in the absence of injury to the sphincter or anus. Such a tear or "buttonhole," usually located superior to the sphincter, could later produce a rectovaginal fistula if left unrepaired. Remove the additional examination glove after the rectal examination, before repairing the episiotomy, to prevent contamination. Carefully examine the remainder of the lower urogenital tract for lacerations not contiguous with the episiotomy. Repair those that need it.

Repair of Third- and Fourth-Degree Extensions (Tears)

1. If the rectal mucosa is no longer intact (fourth-degree laceration), it must be repaired to prevent fistula formation. One method involves reapproxi-mating the submucosa with interrupted subcuticular stitches. Use 4-0 polyglycolic suture, stitched 3 to 5 mm apart, which will invert the mucosa into the lumen. Sutures should begin at the apex of the laceration and proceed distally (Fig. 167-4, *A*).

Note: If the apex of the laceration is not visible, an interrupted suture can be placed distally and used to apply gentle traction toward the surgeon, bringing the apex of the wound into view. The distal interrupted suture can be removed or tied later. (This technique can be applied to *any* vaginal, or even a cervical laceration, when there is difficulty visualizing the apex.)

2. Following reapproximation of the mucosa, a second layer of interrupted stitches may be made laterally (horizontally if the patient is in the standard lithotomy delivery position) over the submucosal stitches. This should give the wound additional strength and decrease the chance of fistula formation between rectum and vagina.

3. After the rectal mucosa and submucosal tissues are repaired, any damage to the sphincter (third-degree laceration) must be identified and repaired (Fig. 167-4, *B,C*) before closure of the episiotomy or

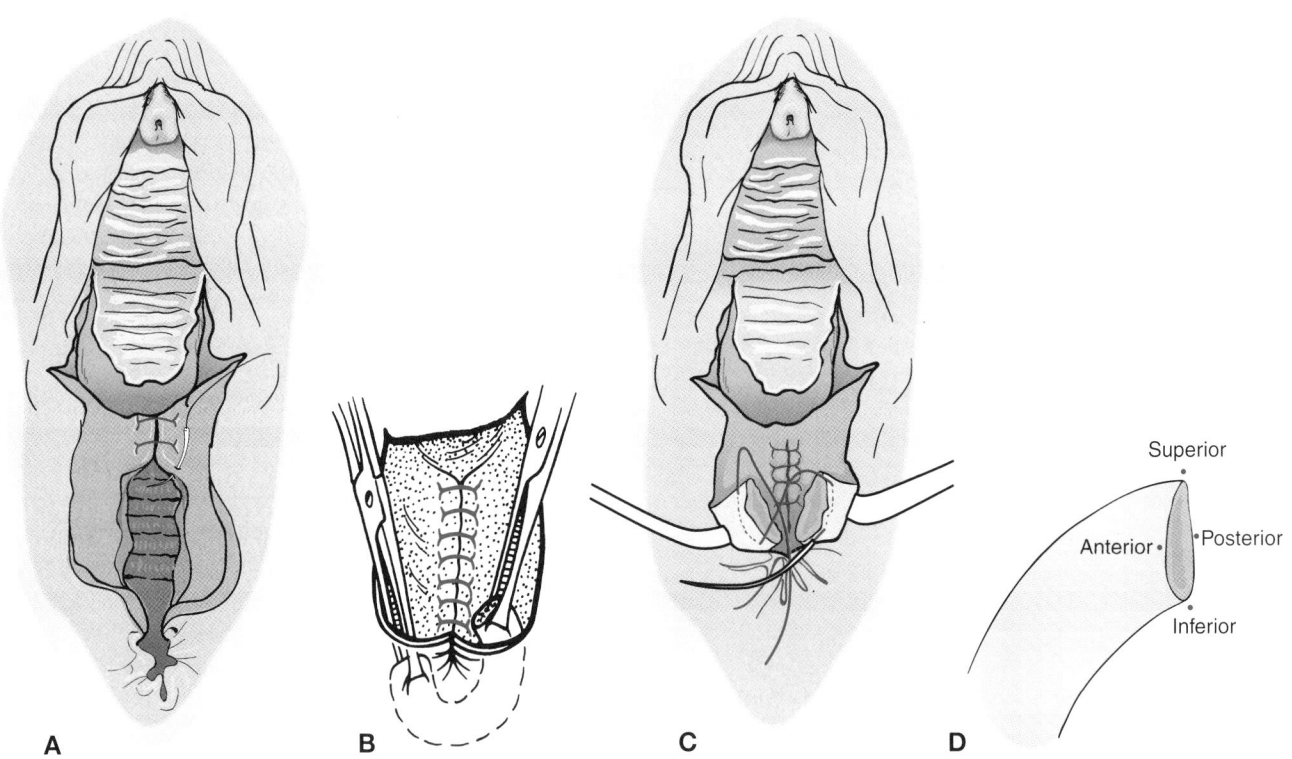

A   **B**   **C**   **D**

Fig. 167-4
Repair of fourth-degree extension of a midline episiotomy. **A,** The rectal mucosa is repaired using interrupted submucosal stitches. **B,** The sphincter is retrieved with Allis forceps. **C,** The ends are reapproximated with figure-eight sutures through the muscle sheath. **D,** Four locations are stitched in order from posterior to superior or inferior and then anterior. When the sphincter has been repaired, the remainder of the wound is closed as a median episiotomy.

vaginal mucosa. Since suturing the sphincter muscle alone will not provide sufficient strength to hold until healing is complete, the fibrous sphincter sheath (fascia) must also be reapproximated. It is identified as a tenacious white sheath, often retracted further laterally than the muscle edges. Search for the sheath on the posterior, inferior, superior, and anterior planes of the muscle. Often, lateral probing with the Allis clamp will be necessary. When the opposing ends of the sphincter sheath are located, grasp each with the Allis and reapproximate. To provide adequate strength for successful repair, a figure-eight suture (Fig. 167-4, *C*) should be placed in four locations (Fig. 167-4, *D*): the posterior, inferior, superior, and anterior planes of the rectal sheath. Upon completion, a repeat rectal examination should confirm adequate sphincter reapproximation and adequate "bulk"/support.

Repair of the Episiotomy

1. Once any injury to the rectal mucosa and the anal sphincter have been well repaired, carefully examine the wound. Use the 3-0 polyglycolic suture to place a stitch above the apex on the vaginal incision. Tie here, and then run it down to the introitus and reapproximate the hymenal ring (Fig. 167-5). Either locked or unlocked sutures may be used. If locked sutures are used, take care to avoid too much tension, possibly causing tissue necrosis. Current evidence from the literature supports a running nonlocked stitch on the vaginal mucosa (to decrease tissue ischemia and necrosis). Deep placement of the perineal subcuticular stitches (only leaving the perineal wound gaping 2 to 3 mm) also significantly decreases itching during healing with no loss of cosmesis or function. It is also critical that these stitches provide hemostasis, close all dead space, and not enter the rectum. One way to accomplish all of this is to take wide bites laterally on each side, and then to bring the needle out at the base of the incision, ensuring that it does not go deep into the rectum. The bulbocavernosus should be approximated carefully at the base of the introitus with a crown stitch, before the perineum is repaired.

2. Reexamine the wound. If the deep perineal tissues are not yet reapproximated, close with an additional layer (Fig. 167-6). For a "hockey stick" extension, run the stitch to the perineal apex. Deep interrupted sutures (Fig. 167-7) can also be used to reapproximate the deep perineal tissue.

3. Repair is completed with a continuous subcuticular stitch up the perineum (Fig. 167-8). Interrupted transcutaneous sutures were associated with more pain in the immediate postpartum period when compared with continuous subcuticular sutures (Kettle, 2002).

4. Once repair is complete, perform a final rectovaginal examination. Verify again that the rectal mucosa is intact. This examination should also ensure that the rectum has not been violated or obstructed by suture, and that no gauze sponges or instruments remain in either the rectum or the vagina. If either of the first two conditions is not met, immediate correction (by removal of the existing repair and repeating the procedure with care) is imperative to minimize the risk of infection and fistula formation.

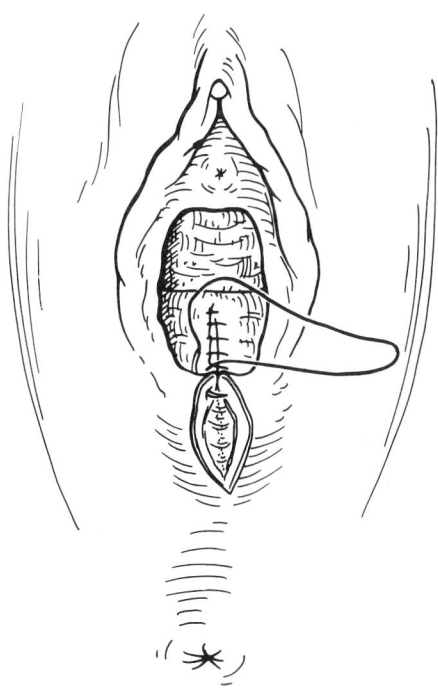

Fig. 167-5
Closure of the vaginal mucosa. The first stitch is placed *above* the apex of the wound and tied. This stitch is then continued as a running or locked stitch down to the introitus. The hymenal ring has been reapproximated and the needle is then taken to the depth of the bulbocavernosus.

COMPLICATIONS

- Blood volume loss is reported to be approximately 300 ml from an uncomplicated median episiotomy, but easily may be more if there is an unexpected delay in delivery or repair. Observe the patient carefully and treat proactively, especially if other conditions threaten to compromise the patient's blood volume (e.g.,

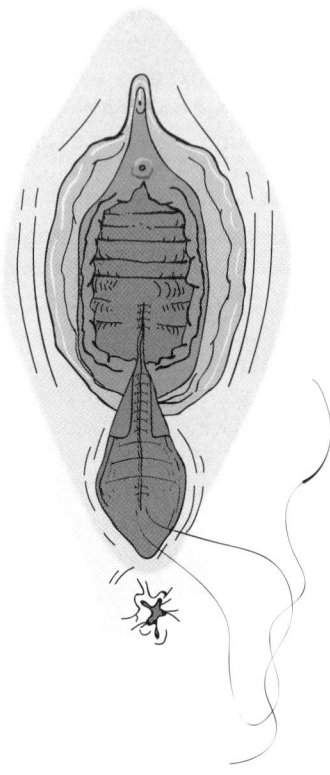

Fig. 167-6
Repair of the vaginal mucosa has been completed with locked stitches. The hymenal ring and bulbocavernosus has been reapproximated and a deep running layer of perineal sutures have been placed, using the same suture. Finishing the perineal closure would entail running the subcuticular stitches back to the introitus.

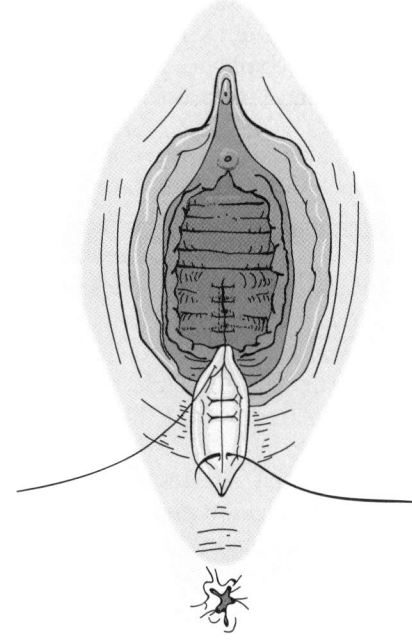

Fig. 167-7
Alternative method of closing the deep perineal space, using another piece of suture and deep interrupted stitches. The perineal skin is closed with a subcuticular stitch using the remaining suture from the vaginal repair.

intravascular hypovolemia resulting from other blood loss or preeclampsia).

- Hematoma formation is unusual but not rare. Acute swelling and pain, frequently severe, must alert the clinician to a possible hematoma. The patient must be reexamined in a timely manner, and if a hematoma is present, it must be opened immediately. The bleeding must then be arrested, and the space either closed or drained to prevent recurrence.
- Infection is probably the most serious threat to episiotomy recovery. A range of wound infections is possible, from a minor superficial exudative wound infection, to a life-threatening septic hematoma, to fatal necrotizing fasciitis. Maternal fever and unusual pain or swelling in the perineum must be evaluated thoroughly to rule out serious infection.
- Rectovaginal and urogenital fistulae (vesicovaginal, vesicocervicovaginal, urethrovaginal, and ureterovaginal) may occur from either direct trauma (hence the importance of careful examination of the entire lower genital tract) or from infection or necrosis associated with suturing. Incontinence of either feces or urine starting 10 or more days after delivery

should alert the clinician to the possibility of these complications.
- Pelvic relaxation and poor perineal tone, once thought to be minimized by performing an episiotomy, may actually be exacerbated by the procedure. While not life threatening, they may lead to a lifetime of misery and disability for the unfortunate woman.
- Local pain or wound breakdown and dyspareunia are usually self-limited complications. Bartholin's duct cysts, inclusion cysts, and endometriosis at the wound site are rarely encountered but may require surgical repair.
- In addition to maternal complications, episiotomies place a nearby patient in jeopardy: the fetus. Fetal complications may range from injecting the scalp with anesthetic, producing lidocaine toxicity, to minimal abrasions, to rare but significant lacerations on the presenting part (e.g., eyelid lacerations and even castration of a male breech infant).

POSTPROCEDURE PATIENT EDUCATION

After delivery, patients with sutures are less comfortable than patients without sutures, and women with episiotomies may experience more pain than women

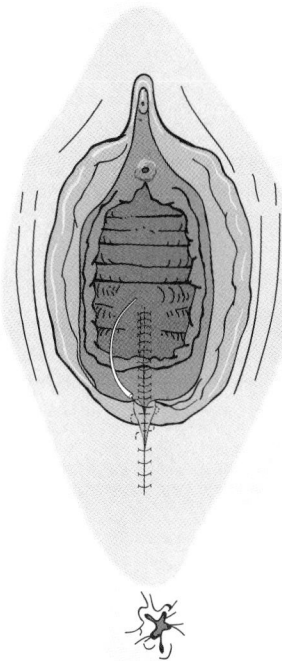

Fig. 167-8
Running subcuticular stitch is used to close the skin of the perineum.

with minor lacerations. Many women will desire analgesia, and nonsteroidal antiinflammatory drugs (e.g., ibuprofen) are increasingly used instead of acetaminophen with codeine. Codeine can be constipating, and this is a great inconvenience for women after a third- or fourth-degree repair. Warm sitz baths and heat lamps aid in comfort and healing, but recently, the application of ice packs to the perineum to reduce swelling and postpartum pain has gained credibility.

Potential complications must be discussed with the patient so that she is aware of the signs and symptoms for which she must immediately contact the clinician.

CPT/BILLING CODES

59400   Routine obstetric care, including antepartum care, vaginal delivery (with or without episiotomy, and/or forceps) and postpartum care

59409   Vaginal delivery only (with or without episiotomy and/or forceps)

59300   Episiotomy or vaginal repair by other than the attending physician

ICD-9-CM DIAGNOSTIC CODES

650   Normal delivery

The fifth digit (X) is required for Codes 660-669 to denote the following:
0   Unspecified
1   Delivered, with or without mention of antepartum condition
2   Delivered, with mention of postpartum complication
3   Antepartum condition or complication
4   Postpartum condition or complication

Codes related to deliveries with forceps or vacuum:
662.2X   Prolonged second stage of labor
659.7X   Abnormality in fetal heart rate or rhythm

Codes related to episiotomy and episiotomy repair, and for repair of low vaginal lacerations:
664.0X   First-degree perineal laceration
664.1X   Second-degree perineal laceration
664.2X   Third-degree perineal laceration
664.3X   Fourth-degree perineal laceration
664.4X   Unspecified perineal laceration

BIBLIOGRAPHY

Carroli G, Belizan J: Episiotomy for vaginal birth, *Cochrane Database Syst Rev* 2:CD000081, 2000.

Fleming N: Can the suturing method make a difference in postpartum perineal pain? *J Nurse Midwifery* 35(1):19, 1990.

Kettle C, Johanson RB: Continuous versus interrupted sutures for perineal repair, *Cochrane Database Syst Rev* 2:CD000947, 2000.

Klein M et al: The McGill/University de Montreal multicentre episiotomy trial. Proceedings of the nineteenth annual meeting of the North American Primary Care Research Group, 1991 Quebec City.

Renfrew MJ, Hannah W, Albers L, Floyd E: Practices that minimize trauma to the genital tract in childbirth: a systematic review of the literature, *Birth* 25: 143,1998.

Thacker SB, Banta HD: Benefits and risks of episiotomy: an interpretive review of the English Language Literature, 1860-1980, *Obstet Gynecol Surv* 38:322, 1983.

Varner MW: Episiotomy: techniques and indications, *Clin Obstet Gynecol* 29:309, 1986.

WEBSITES

www.cochrane.org (Cochrane abstracts)

CHAPTER 168

External Cephalic Version

Andrew S. Coco

In about 4% of term pregnancies, the fetus is in the breech position. Because the risk of complications with vaginal breech delivery is generally considered high, almost 90% of these fetuses are delivered by cesarean section without a trial of labor. Practiced since the time of Aristotle, external cephalic version (ECV) is a procedure that externally rotates the fetus from a breech presentation to a vertex presentation. Trials of ECV conducted over the past 15 to 20 years demonstrate an extremely strong safety record and a success rate of about 65%. As a result of these studies, ECV has made a resurgence in the past 20 years. In addition to being safe and effective, the manual skills to perform ECV are easily acquired. Despite these favorable features, ECV is still underutilized. In fact, breech presentation is the third most frequent indication for cesarean section (after labor dystocia and repeat cesarean), and it accounts for 12% of the cesarean sections in the United States. Routine use of ECV could substantially reduce the rate of cesarean section, especially since it can be performed in basically any setting that has an ultrasound machine and an experienced sonographer. Clinicians must also be equipped and prepared for cesarean section if the need for an immediate delivery arises.

INDICATIONS

- Low-risk gestation at 37 weeks or more, by good dating criteria.
- The type of breech (e.g., frank, complete, footling) is not a factor in determining suitability. Women with a fetus in transverse lie are also candidates, as are those who are attempting vaginal birth after cesarean (VBAC).

Note: To perform ECV, it is preferable that the diagnosis of breech be made before the patient is in active labor! The further the breech is engaged in the pelvis, the more difficult the ECV; therefore the clinician should screen for breech, at least with Leopold's maneuvers, in every pregnancy near term.

CONTRAINDICATIONS

- Multiple pregnancy
- Evidence of uteroplacental insufficiency
- Significant third-trimester bleeding
- Suspected intrauterine growth restriction
- Amniotic fluid abnormalities
- Uterine malformation
- Placenta previa
- Maternal cardiac disease
- Pregnancy-induced hypertension
- Uncontrolled hypertension
- Nonreassuring fetal monitoring pattern
- Major fetal anomaly

EQUIPMENT

- Intravenous catheter with heparin lock
- Blood-drawing equipment for a complete blood count (CBC) and blood type and screen
- Syringe with 0.25 mg of terbutaline (Brethine)
- Fetal heart rate monitor
- Examination table with Trendelenburg's position
- Ultrasound machine
- Ultrasonic gel
- Towels
- Sterile gloves and lubricant (if vaginal exam is required)
- Syringe of Rh_0 (D) immune globulin (RhoGAM) for Rh-negative patients

PREPROCEDURE PATIENT PREPARATION

Generally the patient is examined and counseled at one visit (see the sample patient education handout titled "External Cephalic Version [ECV]" on page 1971 of Appendix G) and returns for ECV at another visit. This allows time for both the patient and her partner to make an informed decision about ECV. At the ECV visit, the patient should bring a signed consent form (see the sample patient consent form titled "External Cephalic Version [ECV]" on page 1972 of Appendix G). The procedure should be scheduled as close to (but not before) 37 weeks' gestational age to maximize the chances of success while avoiding a preterm birth. The patient should be instructed not to eat a heavy meal during the 3 hours before ECV. The clinician should also reassure the patient that ECV causes only minimal discomfort.

TECHNIQUE

1. Perform an ultrasound examination to confirm a singleton in breech presentation, determine the amniotic fluid index, note the placental location, and rule out uterine malformations or congenital anomalies. The patient should empty her bladder after the ultrasound examination.
2. Perform a nonstress test to confirm a reassuring fetal heart rate tracing.
3. Draw blood for a CBC, type and screen. Establish IV access.
4. Administer a tocolytic agent, such as terbutaline (Brethine), subcutaneously about 15 minutes before the procedure. (This is optional because studies show conflicting efficacy. However, some type of relaxation technique should be used. One study in the literature demonstrates efficacy of hypnosis for spontaneous version. See Chapter 212, Medical Hypnosis.)

5. Place the patient in slight Trendelenburg's position to facilitate disengagement and mobility of the breech. Liberally coat the abdomen with ultrasonic gel to decrease friction and lessen the chances of an overly vigorous manipulation.
6. One or two persons may perform ECV. Determine the degree of pelvic engagement of the breech and perform gentle disengagement, if possible. Sometimes this requires a second operator to attempt vaginal disengagement. Successful disengagement is usually the key factor in achieving success.

Note: The breech (i.e., buttocks) is what is actually manipulated during the maneuver. The head is merely guided gently toward the pelvis while the breech is actively moved cephalad.

7. Attempt either the classic forward roll or the back flip. Most clinicians tend to try the forward roll first (Fig. 168-1). However, some base their preference on whether the baby is mostly on one side of the uterus (e.g., fetal head and spine are on the same side of the maternal midline) or not. A forward roll is chosen if the fetal head and spine are on different sides of the maternal midline, and a back flip (Fig. 168-2) is chosen if they are on the same side. Emphasis should be on gentle persuasion of the fetus, as opposed to forceful movements.
8. In most cases, if it is going to occur at all, success is attained quite easily. If the first attempt is unsuccessful, a second attempt is made in the opposite direction. After two failed attempts, if another attempt is to be made, it should be rescheduled.

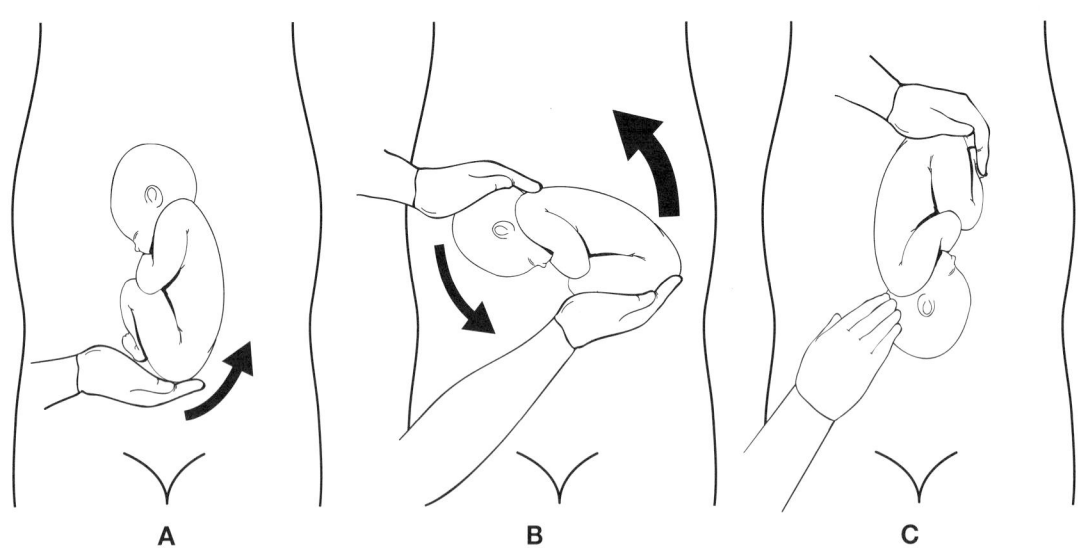

A B C

Fig. 168-1
External cephalic version using the classic forward roll. **A,** The breech is mobilized. A second person is sometimes needed to vaginally disengage the baby. **B** and **C,** At the same time, the breech is gently pushed upward while the head is directed into the pelvis.

9. It is important to monitor the fetal heart rate with the ultrasound probe for fetal bradycardia, immediately after all attempts. If fetal bradycardia is noted after a successful version, return the infant to its previous breech presentation in hopes of reducing umbilical cord compression. Ultrasound imaging is also used after all attempts to confirm success or failure.

10. Regardless of success or failure, perform a nonstress test after the procedure to exclude fetal heart rate abnormalities.

11. Administer Rh_0 (D) immune globulin (RhoGAM) after the procedure to all Rh-negative patients because of a 4.1% risk of fetomaternal blood exchange.

12. If an attempt is unsuccessful and no evidence of fetal compromise is found, it is safe and cost-effective to repeat ECV several days to 1 week later.

Note: ECV is easier to perform with multiparous mothers and when there is plenty of amniotic fluid. ECV may be worth considering, even in early labor, in multiparous women while en route to cesarean. It should never be performed under anesthesia unless the clinician is very experienced or is preparing for cesarean section. The technique should never be so forceful as to cause so much discomfort that anesthesia is necessary.

COMPLICATIONS

In general, ECV is very safe. When a protocol is used that includes fetal heart rate monitoring, ultrasonography, and ready access to operative delivery, the complication rate has ranged from about 1% to 2% since 1979. Most important, the literature provides overwhelmingly reassuring evidence against the risk of fetal death. Since 1980, only two fetal deaths have been reported with ECV. Both occurred when ECV was performed without the use of fetal heart rate monitoring or ultrasonography in preterm infants in Zimbabwe. In other words, there are no reports of fetal death when a protocol has been used similar to that outlined in this chapter.

- The risk of spontaneous reversion to a breech presentation after successful version is about 7%.
- Occasionally, the procedure needs to be discontinued because of excessive maternal discomfort.
- There is a small risk of premature rupture of membranes or active labor within several days after the procedure. If the ECV was unsuccessful, either of these events could lead to a cesarean section for breech presentation, depending on patient and provider interest in an attempt at vaginal breech delivery.
- Transient, benign changes in fetal heart rate tracings are common (up to 39% in one study). There is a small risk of more worrisome changes, such as severe variable decelerations, late decelerations, or persistent bradycardia. These changes could signify placental abruption or umbilical cord entanglement and therefore necessitate an urgent cesarean section.

POSTPROCEDURE PATIENT EDUCATION

- Clinicians should teach women how to check for reversion to breech, and women should do so daily.

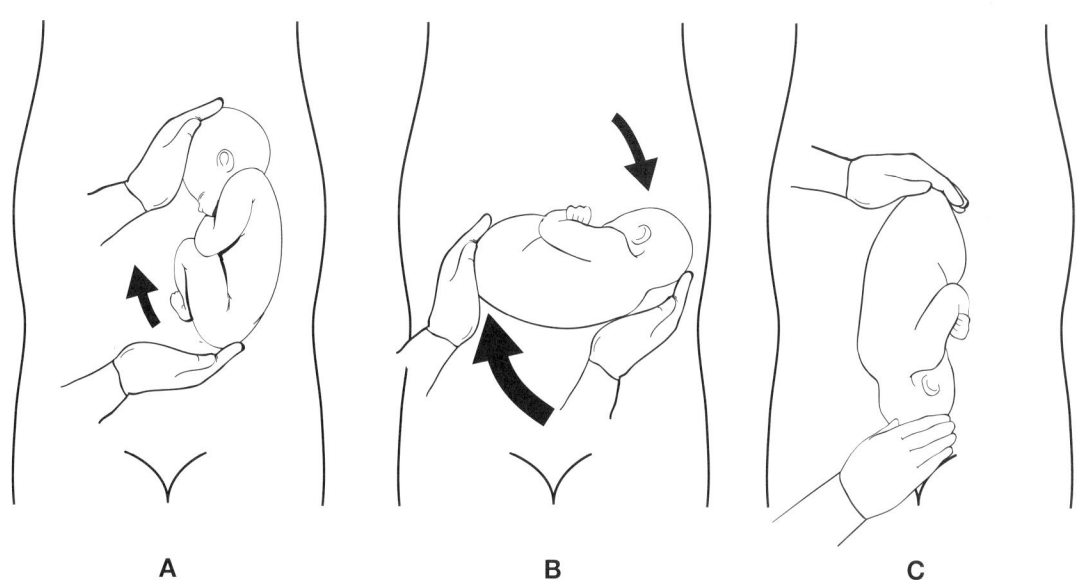

Fig. 168-2

External cephalic version using the back flip. **A,** As with the forward roll, the breech is mobilized, possibly using a second person to vaginally disengage the baby. **B** and **C,** At the same time, the breech is gently pushed upward while the head is directed into the pelvis.

- The clinician should go over the postprocedure information on the sample patient education handout (see page 1971 of Appendix G), reemphasizing the major concerns.
- Women who have undergone a successful ECV should check their abdomen daily for reversion to breech. If the fetus has reverted, they should call or return to the clinic. One study has shown that training women to make regular self-assessments of the presenting part after successful ECV could improve the ultimate rate of vaginal delivery through the use of prompt, repeat ECV when reversion is detected before labor.
- Patients should call for any signs of premature rupture of membranes or labor. They should be instructed about the symptoms of both.
- Follow-up visits, plans for a repeat attempt at ECV (in the event of an unsuccessful attempt), a possible trial of vaginal breech delivery, or a cesarean section when labor ensues are important to discuss with the patient.

SUPPLIERS

For a list of ultrasound suppliers, see Chapter 173, Obstetric Ultrasound.

CPT/BILLING CODE

59412   External cephalic version (ECV)

ICD-9-CM DIAGNOSTIC CODES

625.2   Breech presentation without version
625.3   Transverse or oblique fetal presentation

ADDITIONAL RESOURCES

- See the sample patient education handout titled "External Cephalic Version (ECV)" on page 1971 of Appendix G.

- See the sample patient consent form titled "External Cephalic Version (ECV)" on page 1972 of Appendix G.

BIBLIOGRAPHY

American College of Obstetricians and Gynecologists: *ACOG practice bulletin no. 13,* Washington, DC, 2000, The College.

Bergstrom S: External cephalic version and daily post-versional maternal self-assessment: a prospective study, *Gynecol Obstet Invest* 33:15, 1992.

Coco AS, Silverman SD: External cephalic version, *Am Fam Physician* 58(3):731, 1998.

Hannah ME, Hannah WJ, Hewson SA, et al: Planned caesarean section versus planned vaginal birth for breech presentation at term: a randomised multicentre trial: Term Breech Trial Collaborative Group, *Lancet* 356(9239):1375, 2000.

Hofmeyr GJ: External cephalic version facilitation for breech presentation at term (Cochrane Review), *Cochrane Database Syst Rev* 4:CD000184, 2001.

Lau TK, Lo KW, Rogers M: Pregnancy outcomes after successful external cephalic version for breech presentation at term, *Am J Obstet Gynecol* 176:218, 1997.

Phelan JP, Stine LE, Mueller E, et al: Observations of fetal heart rate characteristics related to external cephalic version and tocolysis, *Am J Obstet Gynecol* 149:658, 1984.

Rosen DJ, Illeck JS, Greenspoon JS: Repeated external cephalic version at term, *Am J Obstet Gynecol* 167:508, 1992.

Zhang J, Bowes WA Jr, Fortney JA: Efficacy of external cephalic version: a review, *Obstet Gynecol* 82:306, 1993.

WEBSITES

www.cochrane.org (for updates on most obstetrical issues)
www.obfocus.com/resources/breech.htm (information on breech deliveries)
familydoctor.org/handouts/310.html ("Breech Babies: What Can I Do if My Baby is Breech?")

CHAPTER 169

Fetal Scalp Electrode Application

Timothy J. Downs

Intrapartum fetal heart rate monitoring has been an important part of maternal fetal care for decades. Invasiveness ranges from intermittent auscultation with a fetoscope, to external electronic cardiac Doppler monitoring, to internal electronic monitoring with fetal scalp electrodes. Controversy persists on how frequent or invasive fetal monitoring should be for any particular patient because labor and delivery is a dynamic process, no single indicator predicts fetal asphyxia, and monitoring has its price. Using continuous external monitoring limits maternal movement and has been shown to increase dysfunctional labor and cesarean rates. Internal monitoring has the same limitations in maternal movement and increases the risk of injury or infection for both mother and infant. On the contrary, inadequate fetal monitoring increases the risk of asphyxia to the fetus.

The use of internal monitoring with a scalp electrode should be limited to situations with concern for or evidence of fetal distress that cannot be appropriately monitored by external means. Improvements in the electronics used to externally monitor fetal heart rate have decreased the need for internal monitoring. The newer-generation monitors can now even convey beat-to-beat variability with minimal loss of signal. Unfortunately, with fewer applications of the internal electrodes, training opportunities have been less common. However, internal monitoring will continue to be needed in specific situations, as will the ability to know how and when to safely apply fetal scalp electrodes. Discussion of the subtleties of the abnormal fetal heart rate tracing is beyond the scope of this chapter. The practitioner of maternal and fetal care is referred to a number of good references. The evaluation of the entire clinical picture, including stage of labor, concurrent medical problems, current medications, and availability of operative delivery and obstetric consultation should be considered when making management decisions.

Note: In randomized clinical trials comparing intermittent auscultation with routine use of continuous electronic fetal monitoring (EFM), EFM is associated with an increase in cesarean and operative vaginal delivery.

FETAL SCALP ELECTRODE APPLICATION

INDICATIONS

A reassuring pattern found in a normal-risk pregnancy can be monitored safely by intermittent auscultation. Continuous monitoring is indicated if a nonreassuring pattern is found.

- Laboring patient with inability to demonstrate reassuring fetal heart rate patterns with external monitoring.
- High-risk pregnancies (e.g., maternal hypertension, diabetes, drug abuse, previous fetal demise) generally require continuous monitoring. This can be either external or, if needed, internal monitoring. A baseline 20-minute external tracing upon admission to the labor suite is commonly recommended.
- Nonreassuring fetal heart rate patterns, including the following possibilities:
  — Persistent fetal bradycardia (fetal heart rate [FHR] at or below 120 beats per minute [bpm])
  — Persistent fetal tachycardia (FHR at or greater than 160 bpm)
  — Decreased beat-to-beat variability by external monitoring
  — Lack of FHR accelerations during early contraction
  — Lack of FHR accelerations with scalp stimulation
  — Persistent late decelerations
  — Deep variable decelerations
  — Poor or intermittent external monitor tracing caused by fetal movement or maternal body habitus
  — Inability to differentiate between early benign decelerations (from head compressions) and late decelerations possibly indicating fetal distress
- Inadequate staffing to provide intermittent auscultation

PREREQUISITES

- Vertex presentation
- Cervical dilation of 2 to 3 cm
- Ruptured membranes

- Head well engaged in maternal pelvis (to decrease risk of prolapsed cord when applying electrode)

The clinician should determine the fetal presentation, station, and position by vaginal examination. When in doubt, ultrasound examination in the labor or delivery suite can be invaluable and may detect a condition that requires a different intervention (e.g., footling breech in a primipara requiring cesarean). The amniotic sac can prevent application of the scalp electrode and should be ruptured. The clinicians should note the color of the amniotic fluid; clear fluid can be reassuring. Meconium-stained fluid indicates that fetal distress may have occurred at some time during the pregnancy, and continuous monitoring is indicated during labor.

CONTRAINDICATIONS

- Persistent fetal distress requiring emergency cesarean in which delay would be detrimental to the fetus
- Presentation other than vertex presentation
- Application of electrode to fontanel
- Uncooperative patient
- Refusal of mother
- Untreated group B streptococcus infection
- Imminent delivery (relative)
- Placenta previa or vasa previa
- Inadequate cervical dilation to allow introduction and accurate placement of scalp electrode over one of the skull plates (to avoid the fontanels)

There are situations, such as placental abruption, in which any delay in emergency cesarean delivery can be critical. The clinician should not delay the operative delivery to place a scalp electrode. Fetal injuries have occurred if the presentation is not vertex. These include eyelid or ocular injury, as well as scrotal, labial, and buttock lacerations. Meningitis, cerebrospinal fluid (CSF) leak, or both are possibilities if the electrode is applied to a fontanel. In one study, when group B streptococcal (GBS) sepsis occurred in the early neonatal period, application of a scalp electrode increased the rate of CSF-positive cultures and mortality in the neonatal period by eightfold compared with no scalp electrode. Therefore treatment of known GBS infection is recommended. For unknown GBS status, obtaining a vaginal culture for GBS would be prudent if a fetal scalp electrode is used. A case could be made for presumptive treatment of GBS if a scalp electrode is used and the status is unknown, but data is lacking regarding the risks and benefits of this action.

EQUIPMENT

- Scalp electrodes
- Intrapartum monitor

- Sterile gloves
- Connecting wires
- Surgical lubricant or Betadyne solution

Note: Suction scalp electrodes have been designed that attach to the surface of the fetal scalp, but these have a significantly higher failure-to-attach rate.

TECHNIQUE

The clinician should perform the following when applying a fetal scalp electrode:

1. Read the package insert accompanying the scalp electrode.
2. Confirm that the presenting part is the vertex, and ensure that the cervix is appropriately dilated.
3. Rupture the membranes if they are still intact.
4. Apply, or have staff apply, the connecting cord to the maternal thigh closest to the monitor and connect it to the monitor.
5. Aseptically handle the scalp electrode.
6. Free the tail wire to allow for free clockwise rotation of the electrode in the applicator (i.e., stiffening) tube.
7. Place the tip of applicator tube between the pads of the index and long fingers of the hand used for vaginal examination.
8. Place the examining fingers in the vagina and inside the cervix (up against the vertex of the fetus).

Note: The fontanels must be avoided.

9. For safety, wait for the next contraction (when the vertex will be well engaged and will not become disengaged). During the contraction, turn the outer handle of the scalp electrode clockwise until the screwlike tip stops (usually about two turns). Fundal pressure by an assistant can prevent the vertex from floating out of the pelvis, away from the scalp electrode, and will further decrease the risk of prolapsing the umbilical cord.
10. Gently retract the electrode handle and ensure that the scalp electrode tip does not pull free.
11. Palpate around the scalp electrode to ensure that it is not applied to the maternal cervix.
12. Release the wire ends for the handle, and carefully remove both the applicator tube and the handle from the vagina. Allow the electrode wires to slide through the applicator tube until they emerge from the patient end of the tube.
13. Connect the red and green wires to the monitor

connector and ensure that the monitor is switched from Doppler reading to ECG reading.

14. Check the ECG tracing.

15. Watch for signs of possible fetal distress, such as persistent tachycardia, loss of beat-to-beat variability, late decelerations, or persistent bradycardia.

16. Consider insertion of an internal pressure monitor (see Chapter 172, Intrauterine Pressure Catheter Insertion). If variable decelerations are noted, the internal pressure monitor can also be used for amnioinfusion, which often resolves the compression on the umbilical cord and variable decelerations (see Chapter 177, Transcervical Amnioinfusion).

17. If a severe deceleration occurs immediately after application of the scalp electrode, reexamine the cervix immediately and check for a prolapsed umbilical cord. If present, disengage the presenting part by pushing the vertex cephalad with the examining fingers to relieve pressure on the cord and restore umbilical blood flow while preparations are made for immediate cesarean birth.

REMOVAL OF FETAL SCALP ELECTRODE

INDICATIONS

- Imminent delivery
- Need to replace electrode because of loss of tracing
- Inadvertent application of the electrode to maternal tissue
- Application of vacuum-assisted device
- Cesarean delivery

CONTRAINDICATIONS

- Concern for fetal distress and inability to externally monitor before delivery

TECHNIQUE

1. The electrode should be removed when delivery is imminent (but before the head is delivered).

2. Remove the electrode by grasping the two wires, pulling the ends apart, and untwisting the wires. This spins the electrode tip in the counter-clockwise direction and unscrews it from the scalp.

3. In case of a precipitous delivery, cut the wire leads close to the perineum to prevent them from catching and pulling on the fetal scalp. The wires can then be removed after delivery of the infant.

COMPLICATIONS

- Randomized, clinical trials indicate an increase in cesarean and operative vaginal deliveries when continuous electronic fetal monitoring is used routinely.
- Fetal scalp abscess
- Increased CSF seeding and mortality rate in untreated early (first 7 days) neonatal group B streptococcal sepsis
- Cephalohematoma (especially if vacuum-assisted birth is performed)
- Subcutaneous emphysema of scalp with vacuum-assisted birth
- CSF leak
- Trauma to structures other than scalp when electrode is misplaced or presentation is not vertex (e.g., eyelid or ocular injury with face presentation; scrotal, labial, and buttock lacerations with breech presentation)
- Umbilical cord prolapse resulting from dislodging the vertex when applying force in the cephalic direction (while applying the electrode)
- Inaccurate monitoring of second twin because of scalp electrode placement on first twin, especially if first twin is deceased (rare)
- Infectious exposure (from sharps injury) to clinician applying electrode

CONCLUSION

Application of a fetal scalp electrode can be very helpful when monitoring a high-risk labor. In situations where concern for fetal distress cannot be dismissed by external monitoring, the use of a fetal scalp electrode justifies its increased risks. Precautions must be taken to apply the scalp electrode to the scalp over the skull plates only. Depending on the experience of the operator, forceps delivery should be considered over vacuum-assisted delivery after scalp electrode placement.

SUPPLIERS

Scalp electrodes and fetal monitoring equipment are always provided by the hospitals in which they are used. Becoming familiar with locally available equipment is recommended.

CPT/BILLING CODES

There is no separate code for application of fetal scalp electrode.

59050	Fetal monitoring during labor by consulting physician (not attending physician) with written report; supervision and interpretation
59051	Fetal monitoring during labor by consulting physician (not attending physician) with written report; interpretation only
59400	Routine obstetric care including antepartum care, vaginal delivery with or without episiotomy, forceps, or both) and postpartum care
59409	Vaginal delivery only (with or without episiotomy, forceps, or both)
59410	Vaginal delivery including postpartum care (excluding antepartum care)
59610-14	Successful vaginal birth after previous cesarean (VBAC)

ICD-9-CM DIAGNOSTIC CODES

656.3X	Fetal distress, affecting management of pregnancy or delivery
663.0	Umbilical cord prolapse
762.2	Placental insufficiency, affecting fetus or newborn
767.1	Cephalohematoma, because of birth injury
792.3	Meconium-stained amniotic fluid

BIBLIOGRAPHY

Achiron R, Zakut H: Misinterpretation of fetal heart rate monitoring in case of intrauterine death, *Clin Exp Obstet Gynecol* 11(4):126, 1984.

Birenbaum E, Robinson G, Mashiach S, Brish M: Skull subcutaneous emphysema: a rare complication of vacuum extraction and scalp electrode, *Eur J Obstet Gynecol Reprod Biol* 22(4):257, 1986.

Feder HM, MacLean WC, Moxon R: Scalp abscess secondary to fetal scalp electrode, *J Pediatr* 89(5):808, 1976.

Fehrmann H: Misdiagnosis of fetal heart rate during a twin labour. Case report, *Br J Obstet Gynaecol* 87(12):1174, 1980.

Freedman RM, Baltimore R: Fatal Streptococcus viridans septicemia and meningitis: relationship to fetal scalp electrode monitoring, *J Perinatol* 10(3):272, 1990.

Freud E, Orvieto R, Merlob P: Neonatal labioperineal tear from fetal scalp electrode insertion: a case report, *J Reprod Med* 38(8):647, 1993.

Gill P, Sobeck J, Jarjoura D, et al: Mortality from early neonatal group B streptococcal sepsis: influence of obstetric factors, *J Matern Fetal Med* 6(1):35, 1997.

Lauer AK, Rimmer SO: Eyelid laceration in a neonate by fetal monitoring spiral electrode, *Am J Ophthalmol* 125(5):715, 1998.

McGregor JA, McFarren T: Neonatal cranial osteomyelitis: a complication of fetal monitoring, *Obstet Gynecol* 73(3):490.

Rhoton-Vlasak A, Duff P: Glove perforations and blood contact associated with manipulation of the fetal scalp electrode, *Obstet Gynecol* 81(2):224, 1993.

Thacker SB, Stroup DF: Continuous electronic heart rate monitoring for fetal assessment during labor, *Cochrane Database System Rev* 2:CD000063, 2000.

CHAPTER 170

Forceps- and Vacuum-Assisted Deliveries

Carol Osborn

INSTRUMENT-ASSISTED DELIVERY

Knowledge and experience with instrument-assisted (forceps or vacuum) delivery is important for all obstetrics (OB) providers managing the second stage of labor, particularly in an emergency such as severe fetal or maternal compromise. In unexpected situations the knowledgeable use of an assisted delivery may be lifesaving and help reduce morbidity. Assisted deliveries are also a safe alternative to an operative delivery, as long as criteria and indications are followed. Currently as many as 15% of all vaginal deliveries are assisted deliveries. The safe use of these procedures depends on understanding and clinically establishing the station and position of the vertex.

Because of difficulties in estimating engagement and in defining different stations, the American College of Obstetrics and Gynecology (ACOG) defined and reclassified instrumented deliveries. The intention of this reclassification is to improve the safety of assisted deliveries and is as follows:

Outlet Forceps or Vacuum

- Fetal skull has reached the pelvic floor.
- Fetal scalp is visible between contractions.
- Sagittal suture is in an anteroposterior diameter (i.e., OA, ROA, LOA, OP, ROP, or LOP) that is less than 45 degrees from the midline.

Low Forceps or Vacuum

- Leading edge of the vertex is at +2 or greater station.
- Fetal head at this station fills the hollow of the sacrum.
- Head is not on the pelvic floor.
- Rotations are less than 45 degrees.

Midforceps or Vacuum

- Head is engaged.
- Vertex is higher than +2 station.
- Advisable only in emergency situations.

With the classification change, the term *high forceps* has been eliminated. High forceps describes application of the forceps before engagement of the vertex. This procedure has no place in modern obstetrics because of unacceptably high morbidity rates. Midinstrumentation is reserved for providers who are experienced with this application. If an OB provider is uncomfortable with the evaluation or application of forceps, a cesarean section is likely a safer route of delivery.

Before any forceps or vacuum application proceeds, the position and station of the vertex presentation must be determined. First, fetal engagement is verified. By definition, engagement indicates the biparietal diameter has passed the plane of the inlet. Clinically the fetal skull is at or below the ischial spines (i.e., 0 station). Checking the amount of space between the fetal head and the symphysis gives an additional measurement of station (Fig. 170-1).

Two things that complicate the clinician's ability to ensure complete engagement and assess descent are: (1) molding, which leads to overestimation of descent or station, and (2) asynclitism or occipitoposterior presentation, which also leads to overestimation of station. To avoid this miscalculation, the clinician should always confirm that the fetal head fills the sacral hollow. The sacral hollow should not admit the fingers of the examining hand when the vertex fills the sacral hollow.

Position can be difficult to determine, especially if the head has marked caput. The following method helps determine position:
- Anterior fontanelle is shaped like a cross or plus (+) and is usually larger than the posterior fontanelles.
- Posterior fontanelle is shaped like a Y.
- When in doubt, the clinician should find the fetal ears to determine position.

If the position and descent meet criteria for an outlet or low instrumentation, then the provider needs to consider whether to use forceps or a vacuum to assist the delivery. The pros and cons of forceps versus vacuum extraction are described in Box 170-1.

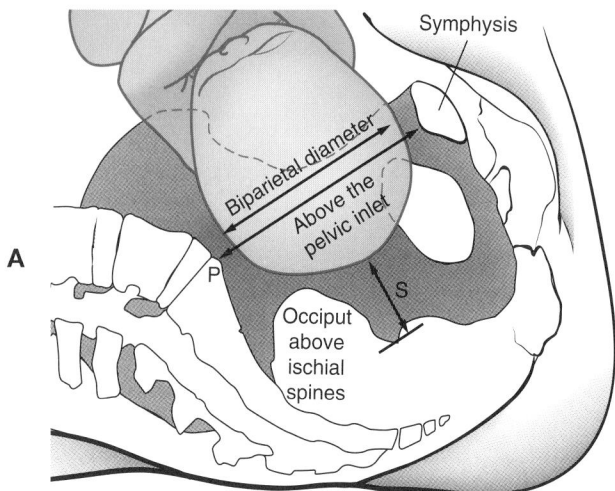
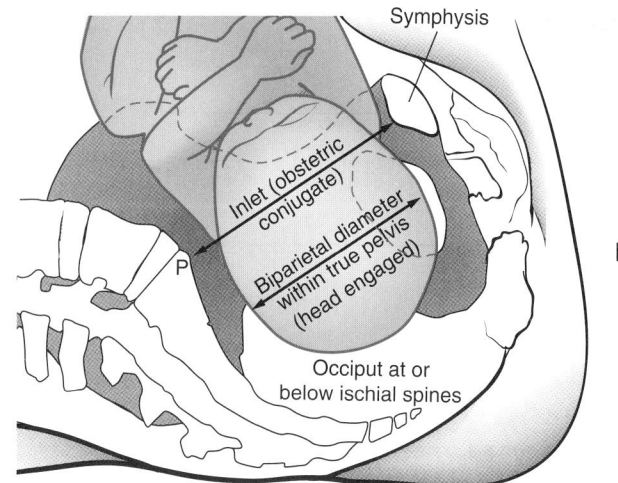

Fig. 170-1

A, When the lowermost portion of the fetal head is above the ischial spines, the biparietal diameter of the head is not likely to have passed through the pelvic inlet and therefore is not engaged. **B,** When the lowermost portion of the fetal head is at or below the ischial spines, it is usually engaged. Exceptions occur when there is considerable molding, caput formation, or both. *P,* Sacral promontory; *S,* ischial spine. (Modified from Cunningham FG, MacDonald P, Gant N, et al, editors: *William's obstetrics,* ed 19, East Norwalk, Conn, 1993, Appleton & Lange.)

BOX 170-1

Forceps versus Vacuum Extraction

Forceps
Pros
Effects a more rapid delivery (e.g., for fetal distress)
Useful in breech (for the aftercoming head) and face presentations
Useful for rotations if experienced

Cons
Requires significant experience
Increased risk of intracranial hemorrhage
Requires more maternal anesthesia
Associated with more cervical, vaginal, and perineal lacerations

Vacuum
Pros
Easy to apply
Teaches the clinician to follow the pelvic curve
Allows autorotation from occiput posterior and occiput transverse positions
Less force to the head
Requires less anesthesia
Results in fewer vaginal and cervical lacerations
Fewer perineal lacerations
Use if not completely sure of head position

Cons
Difficult to maintain vacuum if head is molded or the infant has a full head of hair
Pull only with contractions, which increases the time to successful delivery
Associated with intracranial hemorrhage at a greater rate than spontaneous deliveries
Only useful in vertex presentations
Increased incidence of cephalohematomas

TABLE 170-1

Limits of the Duration of the Second Stage of Labor Before Intervention

Parity	Without Regional Anesthetic	With Regional Anesthetic
Nullipara	2 hr	3 hr
Multipara	1 hr	2 hr

INDICATIONS

Maternal Indications for Instrument Delivery

- *Maternal exhaustion.* This is associated with prolonged second-stage pushing. Maternal exhaustion is especially common in the nulliparous labor. The lack of a trained labor companion during the second stage is associated with a longer labor and increased use of instrumentation.
- *Prolonged second stage.* The average second stage for primiparous patients is 50 minutes and 20 minutes for multiparous patients. Regional anesthesia prolongs the second stage by inhibiting the maternal urge to push (Table 170-1).
- *Medical conditions for which the strain of the second stage of labor would be deleterious.* Examples include cardiac valvular disease, respiratory disease (e.g., active asthma), toxemia, and chronic hypertension.

Maternal and Fetal Indications for Instrument Delivery

- Relative cephalopelvic disproportion.
- Malposition (OP or OT).
- Malpresentation (face or breech); use forceps only. For breech deliveries, forceps are often needed for the aftercoming head once the body has been delivered.
- Hemorrhage.

Fetal Indications for Instrument Delivery

- Nonreassuring fetal heart tracing
- Rapid deterioration of the tracing or any condition that makes it unsafe for the fetus
- Premature placental separation

CONDITIONS REQUIRED FOR INSTRUMENTATION

- Vertex presentation (As noted previously, instrumentation may also be required to deliver the head in breech presentation as well. However, vertex presentation is required for the usual suction and outlet or low forceps applications.)
- Complete cervical dilatation
- Ruptured membranes
- No known severe cephalopelvic disproportion
- If unsuccessful, willingness to abandon procedure and proceed to cesarean section

EQUIPMENT

Include all equipment listed for normal vaginal delivery in Chapter 178, Vaginal Delivery. Simpson or Tucker-McLean forceps are the most commonly used forceps with vertex presentation of term infants. Modern vacuum extractors (e.g., Mityvac, Columbia, Kiwi) use a soft Silastic cup. If a Silastic extractor is chosen, a separate vacuum pump operated by hand or foot is necessary. Both forceps and vacuum equipment should be readily available on all labor decks (Fig. 170-2).

FORCEPS DELIVERY
CONTRAINDICATIONS

- Fetal head not engaged
- Position of the head not determined
- Incomplete dilatation
- History of a failed forceps delivery with a macrosomic fetus

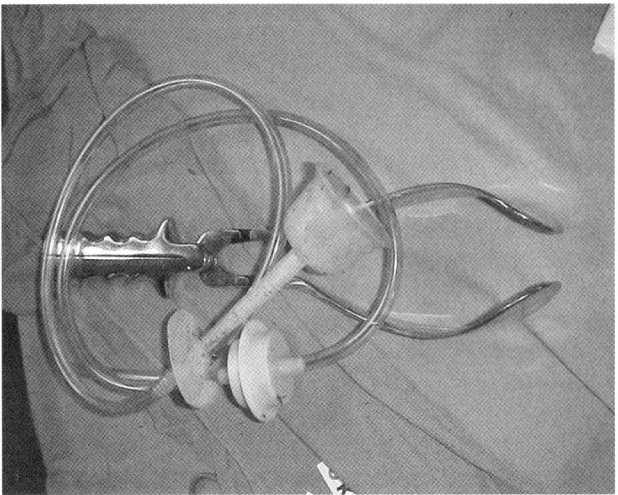
Fig. 170-2
Mityvac extractor and Tucker-McLean forceps.

TECHNIQUE

The forceps are interlocking parts with a right and a left side that correspond to the side of the maternal pelvis in which they lie when applied. Each side has a handle, shank, and blade. The Simpson forceps is most commonly used for low and outlet deliveries.

Initially developed by Dr. J. Bachman, the acronym *ABCDEFGHIJ* has become part of the Advance Life Support in Obstetrics (ALSO) curriculum; it is useful when training for forceps- and vacuum-assisted deliveries. Except for *F, G,* and *H,* the acronym is essentially the same for both procedures:

A: Is the *Anesthesia* adequate? Consider a local or pudendal block or both. *Ask* for help.
B: Is the *Bladder* empty? Straight catheterize if needed.
C: Is the *Cervix* completely dilated?
D: *Determine* the position of the fetal head. Consider shoulder *Dystocia* (i.e., why is there a delay?).
  - Anterior fontanelle is larger and forms a cross.
  - Posterior fontanelle is smaller and forms a Y.
  - Find the ear, feeling which way it bends.
  - The descent should be to a +2 station, with the vertex filling the sacrum.
E: Is the *Equipment* ready (e.g., suction, cord clamp, instrument table)?
F: Are the *Forceps* ready for application?
  1. Articulate the forceps to ensure a proper fit.
  2. Disarticulate the handles and take the left handle in the left hand (holding it like a pencil with concave cephalic curve toward the vulva and the shank perpendicular to the floor).

3. Begin to ease the forceps along the left side of the fetal head (OA); use the right hand to protect the maternal sidewalls and guide the blade into position. (The right thumb is placed on the heel of the blade and gently inserted.)

4. Right forceps handle is then held in the right hand.

5. Insertion is along the right side of the fetal head, with the left hand protecting the maternal right pelvis and guiding the blade into place.

6. If correctly applied, the handle should fit together and lock.

7. Check the application **P**osition **F**or **S**afety (**P**osterior fontanelle, **F**enestration, **S**agittal suture).
   - **P**osterior fontanelle is midway between the shanks and 1 cm above the plane of the shanks.
   - **F**enestrations of the forceps should admit no more than one fingertip.
   - **S**agittal suture should be midline and midway between the shanks.

G: Use *Gentle* traction (i.e., Pajot's maneuver) (Fig. 170-3).

1. The pelvic curve from the inlet through the outlet is described as a J-shaped curve.

2. Initially, one hand pulls the forceps handles in the same direction that the handles extend (an approximately horizontal vector, outward and away from the mother).

3. The other hand is placed on the shaft close to the perineum and pushes in a downward vector.

4. The summation of these two vectors creates an outward-and-downward force.

5. As the crown of the head moves from under the symphysis, the traction should begin upward.

H: The *Handle* is elevated to follow the J-shaped pelvic curve (Fig. 170-3, *B*).

 I: Evaluate for the need of an episiotomy *Incision*. A lack of distension of the perineum will dictate the need.

J: The forceps are removed when the *Jaw* is reachable.

COMPLICATIONS

- Vaginal or cervical lacerations or both
- Postpartum hemorrhage from the previously mentioned lacerations
- Fetal birth trauma (e.g., fractured clavicle, cephalohematoma, lacerations, abrasions, facial nerve palsy, intracranial hemorrhage)

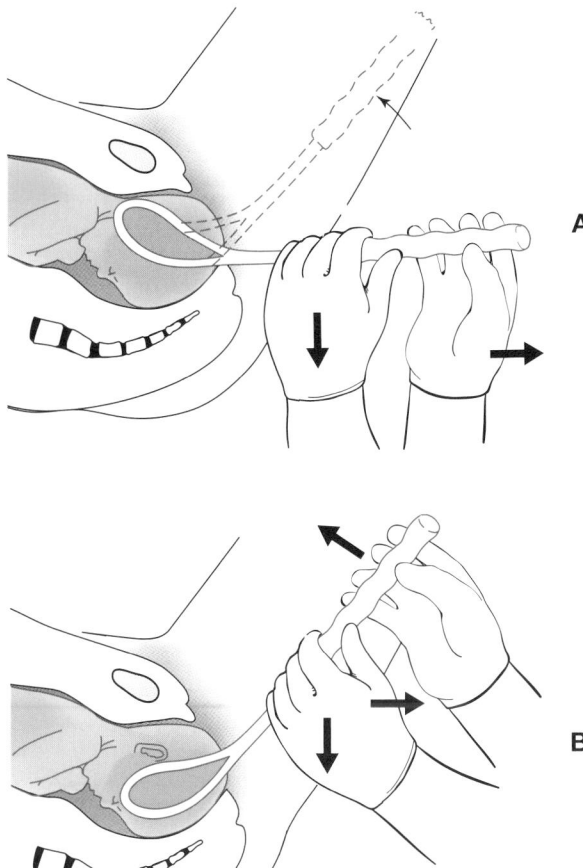

Fig. 170-3
Occiput anterior delivery by outlet forceps (Simpson). The direction of gentle traction for delivery of the head is indicated. Initially, the forceps are horizontal *(a)* and gradually rotated forward *(b)*. Forces are as noted.

VACUUM DELIVERY
CONTRAINDICATIONS

- Prematurity (not recommended before 37 weeks' gestation because of increased risk of intracranial hemorrhage)
- Malpresentation (e.g., breech, face, brow, transverse lie)
- Incomplete cervical dilatation (only exceptions are the urgent delivery of a second twin or a severely abnormal tracing without immediately available cesarean section)
- Head not engaged
- Cephalopelvic disproportion (patient with a history of failed instrumented delivery or a macrosomic fetus at a high station [concern for shoulder dystocia])

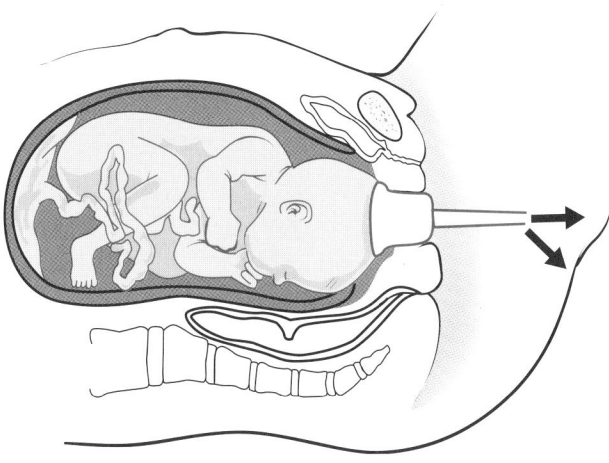

Fig. 170-4
Correct position of the vacuum cup and the correct direction of traction before the vertex clears the symphysis pubis. (Modified from Epperly T, Breitinger R: Vacuum extraction, *Am Fam Physician* 38:205 1988.)

- Delivery requiring excessive traction
- Prior scalp sampling

TECHNIQUE

A: Is the *Anesthesia* adequate? *Ask* for help.
B: Is the *Bladder* empty?
C: Is the *Cervix* completely dilated?
D: *Determine* the position of the fetal head. Consider shoulder *Dystocia* (i.e., why is there a delay?).
  - Anterior fontanelle is larger and forms a cross.
  - Posterior fontanelle is smaller and forms a Y.
  - Find the ear, feeling which way it bends.
  - Descent should be to a +2 station, with the vertex filling the sacrum.
E: *Equipment* and *Extractor* ready (suction, cord clamp, instrument table, etc.)?
F: Insert and apply the cup over the posterior *Fontanelle*.
  - Wipe vertex clean of blood and fluid.
  - Spread the labia.
  - Compress and insert the cup.
  - Place the cup over the posterior fontanelles.
  - Sweep the finger around the cup to check for trapped maternal tissue.
  - Calibrate the vacuum dials, noting that yellow (10 mmHg) is the resting suction and that red (50 mmHg) is the suction pressure required for traction during contractions.
G: Use *Gentle* traction (Fig. 170-4).
  1. Apply traction at right angles to the plane of the cup.

2. Do not rock or torque the vacuum. Only use gentle, steady traction.
3. As the fetal head moves around the symphysis and extends, the vacuum handle will rise from a horizontal to a nearly vertical position.
4. If the cup detaches, consider the following problems: inadequate vacuum suction, trapped maternal tissue, a fetal scalp electrode in the way, incorrect application of the extractor (not over the flexion point), or bending or rotation of the shaft.
H: *Halt* traction when the contraction is over.
  1. Reduce the vacuum to 10 mm Hg between contractions.
  2. Repeat the gentle-traction cycle with the next contraction.
  3. *Halt* the procedure if the cup disengages more than 3 times, if no progress is noted after three consecutive pulls, or if a delivery does not occur after 20 minutes of intermittent traction.
  4. Use caution when attempting a forceps delivery after a failed vacuum extraction (only if the vertex is right on the perineum). A cesarean section may be a better choice (intracranial hemorrhage is most common after a failed vacuum followed by a forceps delivery).
I: Make an *Incision* for episiotomy, if necessary. A midline episiotomy may be associated with increased risk of third- and fourth-degree perineal lacerations.
J: Remove the vacuum cup when the *Jaw* is delivered.
  A suction application can also be used to rotate the head from an OP to an OA position before delivery (Fig. 170-5).

COMPLICATIONS

- Subgaleal hematoma
- Shoulder dystocia
- Neonatal scalp emphysema
- Cephalohematomas
- Hyperbilirubinemia
- Fetal cervical trauma
- Perineal tears

The Food and Drug Administration (FDA) published a public advisory in 1998 concerning complications resulting from vacuum deliveries. The FDA found a fivefold increase in death and serious injury after vacuum deliveries. Although part of this increase may be due to the increased use of this procedure, the blame may also lie in failing to follow established protocols. The most concerning complication is a life-threatening subgaleal hematoma.

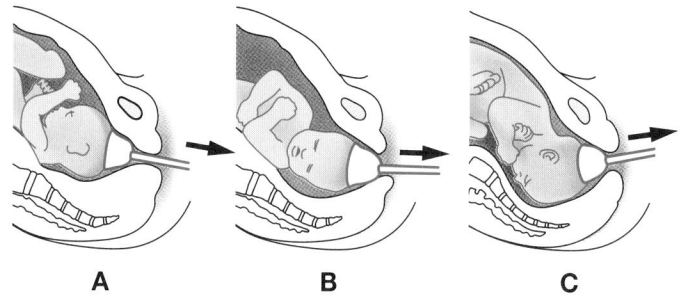

Fig. 170-5
Illustration showing, **A,** OP application, **B,** rotation, and **C,** delivery using vacuum extractor. (Modified from Lowdermilk DL, Perry SE, Bobak IM: *Maternity and women's health care,* ed 7, St Louis, 2000, Mosby.)

RECOMMENDED OUTLINE FOR OPERATIVE NOTE AFTER INSTRUMENT-ASSISTED DELIVERY

- Preoperative diagnosis (note indication for the assistance, such as maternal exhaustion)
- Postoperative diagnosis (note preoperative diagnosis and result of the procedure [e.g., vaginal delivery, term infant, weight, Apgar score, cord pH])
- Operation (note outlet forceps or vacuum extraction)
- Instrument (e.g., Simpson forceps)
- First stage (note length, interventions, or complication)
- Second stage (same information as in first stage, including type of fetal monitoring)
- Third stage (type of placenta delivery, description of placenta)
- Repairs
- Bladder
- Estimated blood loss
- Anesthesia

POSTPROCEDURE PATIENT EDUCATION

Instrumented deliveries increase the level of maternal concern for the infant. The provider should discuss the need for the instrument delivery and maternal perceptions regarding the delivery on the first postpartum day.

After the procedure, the patient should be advised to monitor the following and report any changes to the practitioner:
- Bleeding
- Fevers
- Dysuria and urinary retention
- Pelvic pain (could indicate hematoma)

CPT/BILLING CODES

59400	Global vaginal delivery (antepartum, vaginal delivery with or without episiotomy and with or without forceps or suction)
59409	Vaginal delivery *only*
59409	including postpartum care
59610	VBAC (global)
59899	Induction

ICD-9-CM DIAGNOSTIC CODE

669.51	Forceps or vacuum delivery

BIBLIOGRAPHY

American College of Obstetricians and Gynecologists: *Operative vaginal delivery ACOG practice bulletin no. 17,* Washington, DC, June 2000, The College.
Bachman J: Forceps delivery (letter), *J Fam Pract* 29(4):360, 1989.
Damos J: *ALSO curriculum,* Leawood, Kans, 2000, American Academy of Family Practitioners.
Ratcliffe S, Byrd J, Sakornbut E: *Pregnancy and perinatal care in family practice,* Philadelphia, 1996, Hanley & Belfus.
Warenski JC: Managing difficult labor: avoiding common pitfalls, *Clin Obstet Gynecol* 40:525, 1997.

CHAPTER 171

Intrathecal Analgesia

Thomas E. Howard

Intrathecal analgesia uses the subarachnoid (dural) space for the injection of analgesic narcotics. This space is filled with cerebrospinal fluid (CSF) and is the same space used for a spinal block. For intrathecal analgesia, injected opioids diffuse through the CSF and coat the visceral pain receptors in the dorsal horn of the spinal cord (T10-L1). Although it does not provide complete pain relief, this technique provides considerably more pain relief than the parenteral route. In addition, pain relief is more rapid than with epidural anesthesia. In contrast to spinal or epidural anesthesia, local anesthetics are not injected. This allows for profound analgesia (not anesthesia) without clinically significant motor or autonomic blockade.

This procedure is not technically difficult to perform and has no reported adverse effects on either the infant or the progress of labor. Clinicians comfortable with performing lumbar puncture can easily learn this procedure and perform it without an anesthesiologist. It is useful in many clinical settings, especially where epidural anesthesia is not readily available, or when complete anesthesia is not necessary (Box 171-1).

Intrathecal analgesia is ideally suited for patients in the first stage of labor. The pain in this stage is primarily due to uterine contractions and dilation. Pain in the second stage of labor is due to both uterine contractions and fetal descent through the birth canal. Since fetal descent also stimulates the pudendal nerve (S2-S4), intrathecal analgesia is less effective; however, it does continue to help with the discomfort from uterine contractions. The real overall benefit for intrathecal analgesia is the improved ability of the laboring mother to tolerate the contractions, thereby resulting in a more rested mother for the second stage of labor. This in turn should enhance the overall birthing experience.

Because the duration of intrathecal analgesia is limited, it should be used when the expected remaining duration of the first stage of labor is less than 6 hours. Although the procedure can be repeated later in labor, each additional dural puncture increases the risk of post–dural puncture headache (PDPH). If a cesarean section becomes necessary, general, spinal, or epidural anesthesia may also be used following intrathecal analgesia.

INDICATIONS

- Active first stage of labor
- Epidural anesthesia not available (many rural and community hospitals), not needed, or not desired

CONTRAINDICATIONS

- Patient refusal
- Allergy to selected narcotics
- Spinal abnormalities, such as marked scoliosis, making the procedure technically difficult
- Active systemic infection, such as maternal bacteremia
- Cutaneous lesion of the lower back, such as cellulitis or dermatitis
- Known coagulopathy or patient anticoagulated (heparin or its analogues warfarin, or clopidogrel [Plavix])

BOX 171-1

Advantages and Disadvantages of Intrathecal Narcotics in Labor

Advantages
Prolonged, superior analgesia compared with IV administration
No effect on expulsive forces in labor
Rapid onset of analgesia
Technique similar to lumbar puncture
Low incidence of serious side effects
Cost advantages compared with epidural anesthesia

Disadvantages
Analgesia is usually inadequate for second stage of labor
No anesthesia for instrumented delivery or episiotomy
Does not provide surgical anesthesia
Risk of respiratory depression
High incidence of mild side effects
May require a repeat injection, which increases the risk of post–dural puncture headache

EQUIPMENT

- Spinal anesthesia kit, which includes: sterile prep materials, local anesthetic, a 25-gauge or smaller spinal anesthesia needle, and an 18- or 19-gauge introducer
- Syringe with filter tip needle for drawing up narcotic for injection
- Narcotics for injection (Table 171-1)
- Ephedrine
- Naltrexone 25 mg tablet
- Naloxone ampules (0.4 mg)
- Continuous fetal monitor (internal or external)
- Sterile gloves
- Personnel to monitor for side effects, including monitoring blood pressure
- Pulse oximeter

PREPROCEDURE PATIENT PREPARATION

Ideally the patient should be informed of the available analgesia and anesthesia options during the prenatal period to aid in giving informed consent. (See the sample patient consent form titled "Intrathecal Analgesia" on page 1974 of Appendix G.) Preferably, desired analgesia or anesthesia should be determined as part of a written birthing plan. Staff providing prenatal education should be knowledgeable of this technique and offer information to their clients. An education handout can be given to them to read before the onset of labor. (See the sample patient education handout titled "Intrathecal Narcotic Analgesia" on page 1973 of Appendix G.)

During labor, the clinician should review the benefits and risks with the patient and obtain informed consent. Ideally, since the pain of labor might impair the mother's understanding of this information, the counseling should be done in the presence of the mother's labor coach.

TECHNIQUE

1. Ensure continuous fetal monitor is in place and check for contraindications to intrathecal analgesia.
2. Obtain informed consent.
3. Establish IV access and, if possible, give a 500-ml bolus to help prevent the rare side effect of maternal hypotension (give this bolus very slowly for women with pregnancy-induced hypertension).
4. Place the patient in the desired position for dural puncture (sitting or lying on left side) and locate the L3-4 or L4-5 interspace.
5. Perform sterile preparation and draping. Administer the local skin anesthetic as you would for a lumbar puncture.
6. Insert the introducer needle through the anesthetized skin and into the supraspinous ligament. It is especially important to use an introducer in larger patients because the spinal needle is otherwise difficult to direct. Spinal anesthetic needles used for this procedure are less rigid than those needles most clinicians use for lumbar puncture.
7. Insert a narrow gauge, bullet-type or pencil-point anesthetic needle (25 to 27 gauge) through the introducer into the intrathecal space. You will detect a distinct pop or snap when passing through the ligamentum flavum. Whereas minimal or no fluid returns when passing through the epidural space, CSF returns when the intrathecal space has been entered (just as with a lumbar puncture). Remove the trocar from the anesthesia needle and confirm that CSF is flowing into the hub of the needle.
8. Draw up selected narcotics into a syringe with a filter-tip needle (filter prevents drawing up tiny glass particles). Selection of narcotics depends on the duration of action and desired effect (Table 171-1). A commonly used combination is Fentanyl 25 mcg with preservative-free morphine 0.25 mg. This allows for the rapid onset of action of the lipid soluble Fentanyl and a longer duration of analgesia from morphine. These may be drawn up and mixed in the same syringe.
9. Place the syringe with the narcotic onto the spinal needle. Aspirate slightly before injecting over 5 to 10 seconds. Aspiration and injection should be performed between contractions.
10. Remove the spinal needle and syringe as a unit and place the patient on her left side for uterine displacement. Monitor her pulse and blood pressure every 5 minutes for 15 minutes; if stable, she can then

TABLE 171-1

Duration and Onset of Action for Intrathecal Narcotics

Medication	Dosage	Onset of Action (min)	Duration of Action (hr)
Fentanyl	10-30 mcg (usual dose 25 mcg)	5	1.5-3.5
Sufentanil	5-10 mcg	5	1-3
Meperidine	10-20 mg	5-10	2-4
Morphine (preservative free*)	0.1-1.0 mg† (usual dose 0.25 mg)	15-60	2-6

*Astramorph and Duramorph are commercially available, preservative-free morphine preparations. It is important to use preservative-free medications to avoid the complication of arachnoiditis from the preservative.
†Morphine at doses of 0.5-1.0 mg can have a duration of action of up to 12 hours but with a higher rate of side effects; it is therefore not recommended.

move to a more comfortable position. Maternal hypotension (rare) occurs soon after the medication is given if it is going to happen. If this occurs, it should be treated with another fluid bolus and with ephedrine 5 to 10 mg IV push. This ephedrine dose can be repeated every 5 minutes as necessary.

11. Vital signs (respiratory rate, heart rate, and blood pressure) are then monitored every 30 minutes for the duration of labor. Increased monitoring should be maintained after delivery until the analgesic is metabolized. Nursing staff should assess for sedation and arousability (Table 171-2).

If moderate or somnolent sedation is noted by nursing staff, the clinician should be notified and the patient's oxygen saturation (SaO_2) should be checked. Use naloxone for treatment of respiratory depression at doses of 0.2 to 0.4 mg IV. This can be repeated every 3 minutes until the respiratory depression or sedation is reversed. Administer oxygen if the SaO_2 is diminished. Naloxone can also be given by a continuous IV infusion at 0.4 mg/hr if necessary. While the exact mechanism is unknown, respiratory depression may be caused by ascending spread of the analgesic agent. In theory, if the narcotic spreads too far cephalad, it can suppress the respiratory centers in the fourth ventricle of the brain. The incidence of respiratory depression peaks at between 4 and 9 hours, but it has been noted as late as 12 hours after administration of intrathecal narcotics. The time of highest risk for the mother is after delivery when her respiratory drive may be decreased. Unfortunately, this is also a time when mothers are monitored less frequently, while resting. Some protocols call for postpartum continuous pulse oximetry or frequent hands-on measurements of vital signs and mental status.

12. Oral naltrexone 12.5 to 25 mg is given within 30 minutes after the delivery. This is a long-acting narcotic antagonist that reduces the side effects of the intrathecal narcotics, including the risk of respiratory depression, and is generally free of side effects at these dosages.

13. If pain relief diminishes before delivery, there are four options:
   a. Intrathecal narcotic injection can be repeated, especially if the patient is still in the first stage of labor.
   b. A supplemental parenteral narcotic injection can be given. However, it is important to give this at half the usual dose to avoid the side effect of respiratory depression.
   c. Epidural anesthesia can be administered.
   d. Some anesthesiologists perform a combination intrathecal/epidural. An epidural catheter is placed at the time of the intrathecal injection and can be used later if operative delivery is necessary, or if added pain relief is desired.

TABLE 171-2

Sedation Scale to Monitor for Respiratory Depression from Intrathecal Narcotics

Sedation Level	Assessment
None	Awake and alert
Minimal	Drowsy or sleeping but easily aroused
Moderate	Drowsy or sleeping but not easily arousable
Somnolent	Drowsy or sleeping and cannot be fully aroused

COMPLICATIONS

Although serious complications with intrathecal narcotics analgesia are rare, the incidence of less severe side effects is high (Table 171-3). Pruritus, although seldom severe, is quite common. Approximately one-third of patients request treatment for pruritus. It responds best to naloxone at the doses listed, especially if it is associated

TABLE 171-3

Side Effects and Their Management for Intrathecal Analgesia in Labor

Side Effects	Incidence	Treatment
Pruritus (usually mild)	≥50%	May not be related to histamine release, but can try diphenhydramine (Benadryl) 20-50 mg orally, IM, or IV every 6 hr prn or naloxone (Narcan) 0.2-0.4 mg IV.
Nausea and vomiting	30%-50%	Metoclopramide (Reglan) 10 mg orally or IV every 6 hr or promethazine (Phenergan) 25 mg IM every 6 hr.
Urinary retention	4%-20%	In-and-out catheterization prn.
Postdural puncture headaches	1%-6%	Usually no treatment is necessary. Blood patch if not resolved with conservative management (rest, fluids, analgesics, caffeine).
Maternal hypotension	Up to 15%	Generally transient. If systolic blood pressure <90 or any fetal distress, use IV fluid bolus, uterine displacement, and/or ephedrine (5-10 mg IV push). Repeat every 5 min as necessary.
Respiratory depression	0.2%-0.4%	Naloxone (Narcan) 0.2-0.4 mg IV. Consider oxygen with decreased SaO_2.

with respiratory depression. However, the analgesic effect may be affected by naloxone. Nalbuphine (Nubain) is an opioid agonist-antagonist that can be used for pruritus alone. Another option is diphenhydramine (Benadryl). Nausea and vomiting are treated symptomatically.

With this procedure, there have been no adverse effects on APGAR scores, and no bad fetal outcomes reported. Rarely (less than 10%), fetal heart rate decelerations are seen and these are generally transient. Fetal heart rate monitoring is recommended according to institutional protocols.

There is no effect on the normal course of labor at the suggested dosages. Higher doses of morphine (up to 2 mg) may more frequently require oxytocin augmentation.

CPT/BILLING CODE

62274   Injection of diagnostic or therapeutic anesthetic or antispasmodic substance (including narcotics); subarachnoid or subdural, single

ICD-9-CM DIAGNOSTIC CODE

650   Normal delivery

ADDITIONAL RESOURCES

- See the sample patient education handout titled "Intrathecal Narcotic Analgesia" on page 1973 of Appendix G.
- See the sample patient consent form titled "Intrathecal Analgesia" on page 1974 of Appendix G.

BIBLIOGRAPHY

Herpolsheimer A, Schretenthaler J: The use of intrapartum intrathecal narcotic analgesia in a community-based hospital, *Obstet Gynecol* 84:931, 1994.

Rust LA, Waring RW, Hall GL, Nelson EI: Intrathecal narcotics for obstetric analgesia in the community hospital, *Am J Obstet Gynecol* 170:1643, 1994.

Stephens MB, Ford RE: Intrathecal narcotics for labor analgesia, *Am Fam Physician* 56(2):463, 1997.

Wildman KM, Mohl VK, Cassel JH, et al: Intrathecal analgesia for labor, *J Fam Pract* 44:535, 1997.

Zapp J, Thorne T: Comfortable labor with intrathecal narcotics, *Mil Med* 160:217, 1995.

CHAPTER 172

Intrauterine Pressure Catheter Insertion

Christian Raigosa

To monitor uterine pressure during labor has been a quest of clinicians since the mid-nineteenth century. Early investigators developed intrauterine balloons to measure pressure changes in both the pregnant and the nonpregnant uterus. As knowledge of uterine physiology increased, methods of recognizing dysfunctional labor patterns and assessing adequacy of contractions rose to the forefront of the field of obstetrics. External tocometers were introduced as early as 1930, using pressure transducers placed on the abdominal wall. Modern external tocometers are only a slight variation from these earlier prototypes. Although the information obtained from external monitors is still useful today, there is often a poor correlation between the information obtained from an internal versus an external monitor. Maternal body habitus, position, and movement often affect the external measurement method. To assess adequacy of contractions, the intrauterine method remains the gold standard.

The intrauterine pressure catheter (IUPC) allows for the determination of true uterine pressure, as well as contraction frequency, and is relatively unaffected by the maternal factors previously listed. Now mostly solid, the first IUPCs were a hollow tube filled with sterile saline solution (hence the name *catheter*) and were connected at the bedside to a pressure transducer. Some of these catheters are still in use today. In fact, in parts of the world where electricity is not available, internal uterine *manometers* are used and their measurements correlate fairly well with those of IUPCs. In addition to measuring pressure, IUPCs have a hollow tube (channel or port) that can be used for amnioinfusion or amniotic fluid sampling, if desired. (See Chapter 177, Transcervical Amnioinfusion.)

The ideal candidate for IUPC insertion is a patient in the second stage of labor. Because of the risks associated with insertion, not all laboring patients warrant catheterization. When the adequacy of contractions is questioned, IUPC insertion may be needed to determine if the patient has a dysfunctional labor curve. Data from the IUPC can be used to calculate Montevideo units (i.e., mean active contraction pressure multiplied by the number of contractions in 10 minutes). Uterine contraction strength is generally considered adequate when it falls between 180 and 200 Montevideo units. If there are inadequate contractions, the clinician may choose to initiate oxytocin therapy to augment labor and potentially shorten its duration (and improve the likelihood that the patient will deliver vaginally). If oxytocin is already in use, the dose may be adjusted to attain adequate uterine contractions as determined by the Montevideo units. If the contractions are adequate and the labor is not progressing, the decision may be made to perform a cesarean section.

In women with a scarred uterus undergoing a trial of labor, the IUPC may increase safety by monitoring for any sudden variations in pressure. These variations could signify a life-threatening obstetric complication such as a uterine rupture. The IUPC can also be used for amnioinfusion to dilute meconium or to manage severe variable decelerations. Cord compression is believed to be the cause for severe variable decelerations, and infusing a fluid bolus into the amniotic sac often cushions the cord and abolishes the abnormal fetal heart rate pattern. Amnioinfusion entails the instillation of sterile fluids (most commonly normal saline) into the amniotic cavity as an initial bolus followed by a continuous infusion. By simultaneously monitoring fetal heart rate activity, the clinician can then determine the efficacy of such an intervention.

Lastly, the IUPC is useful for withdrawing amniotic fluid in a sterile fashion for the purpose of evaluating possible amnionitis or meconium staining.

INDICATIONS

- Dysfunctional labor curve with concern for adequacy of contractions
- Failure to progress or suspected arrest of labor
- Vaginal birth after cesarean delivery with concern for uterine rupture
- Amnioinfusion
- Amniotic fluid sampling for culture or meconium evaluation

It is estimated that less than 5% of patients in labor have indications for internal pressure monitoring. External monitoring should be used for patients with uncomplicated labor and no anticipated problems. Internal monitoring is indicated when the labor is not progressing and external monitoring cannot determine whether there are adequate labor forces.

CONTRAINDICATIONS

- Unruptured fetal membranes
- Inadequately dilated cervix
- Placenta previa
- Uterine bleeding (undetermined cause)
- Acute fetal distress
- Labor not indicated (e.g., preterm, breech)

EQUIPMENT

- Intrauterine pressure catheter
- Reusable cable that connects catheter to fetal monitor
- Sterile gloves
- Fetal monitor with adequate supply of tracing paper
- Amniotomy hook (if indicated)
- IV tubing, pole, and fluid (if amnioinfusion desired)

PREPROCEDURE PATIENT PREPARATION

Before insertion of an IUPC, the provider should review the patient's medical record to ensure that there are no contraindications to its insertion. Once this is verified, the clinician should counsel the patient regarding the need for an IUPC in a manner consistent with providing informed consent. An explanation should be offered about why an amnioinfusion is needed or how information regarding the uterine contractions, strength, and pattern will help make clinical decisions. Such decisions may affect labor augmentation, hopefully shortening the labor without unduly increasing the risk of uterine rupture or fetal distress. Ultrasound may also be performed before the procedure to determine placental location and to plan the direction of catheter insertion in order to avoid the placenta.

After a thorough discussion, the patient should be placed in a dorsal lithotomy position. A cervical examination should be performed to assess the degree of cervical dilation and the status of the membranes. If intact, and an IUPC is indicated, the fetal membranes should then be ruptured.

TECHNIQUE

1. Obtain assistance from a qualified nurse or assistant to allow for sterile handling of the IUPC.
2. Ensure that all necessary supplies are present. Prepare a sterile field on the delivery bed or table.
3. Turn on the fetal monitor. Connect the interface cable to the fetal monitor. (The cable is not sterilized between patients but is cleansed with alcohol. It should not go into the sterile field.) Switch the fetal monitor from the external tocometer setting, if used, to the IUPC setting.
4. Open the IUPC package. Using sterile gloves, remove the IUPC and plastic catheter guide from its package. Note the 45-cm depth mark on the IUPC. Hand off the correct end of the IUPC to be connected to the interface cable.
5. Establish a "0" baseline for the monitor as described by the manufacturer.
6. Flush the amnioport with infusion solution, if amnioinfusion is desired.
7. Perform a second cervical examination to ensure that the amniotic membranes are ruptured and that the cervix is adequately dilated. Position the tips of the examining fingers (index and middle) away from the side of the uterus that the placenta is located, if known.
8. While the examining fingers are still in the cervical os and the pads of the fingers are touching the presenting fetal part, use the opposite hand to insert the IUPC and the plastic catheter guide. Insert them along the palmar aspect of the examining hand, through the vagina, and into the cervical os. The IUPC should remain inside the catheter guide until the next step. The tip of the catheter guide should be advanced until it is placed between the examining fingers (index and middle) and the presenting fetal part.
9. While holding the end of the catheter guide in place between the examining fingers, use the opposite hand to advance the IUPC through the catheter guide past the presenting part and into the amniotic sac. Minimal, if any, resistance should be noted. Stop advancing the IUPC when the 45-cm mark is at the introitus or if resistance is noted. This mark usually corresponds with the proper fundal positioning of the IUPC tip.
10. Once the IUPC tip is in the proper position, hold the IUPC in place with the examining fingers at the cervical os. Use the opposite hand to retract the catheter guide out of the vaginal tract; remove it from the IUPC. Next, snap the catheter guides in place on the IUPC near the connection with the interface cable. Secure the external components of the IUPC to the patient's thigh. Some slack should be left between the introitus and the belt securing

the IUPC to the patient's thigh. This should prevent inadvertent removal of the IUPC with patient repositioning or if the patient moves around a lot. It should also ensure continued proper positioning of the catheter tip.

11. Confirm that the connections between the IUPC and the reusable monitor cable and from the monitor cable to the monitor are both secure.

12. Demonstrate proper functioning of the IUPC. Have the patient cough or perform the Valsalva maneuver and note the proper changes. Palpable changes in the uterine tone should correlate with an increase in intrauterine pressure on the uterine monitor strip.

13. Finally, document IUPC insertion in the medical record. See Chapter 177, Transcervical Amnioinfusion, if needed.

Note: The advancement of the IUPC should proceed smoothly, without resistance. If resistance is felt during catheter advancement, change the direction of the catheter tip until insertion proceeds easily. Never force the catheter against resistance, because such force increases the risk of complication. Always try to insert the IUPC directed away from the placental site.

Intrauterine Pressure Catheter Removal

Removal of the IUPC is relatively simple and is usually performed just before delivery. Wait until the last uterine contraction has ceased and gently apply traction to the external end of the IUPC cable until the catheter is outside the uterus. If any resistance is encountered while removing the IUPC, stop and redirect the catheter until it can be removed with minimal resistance.

COMPLICATIONS

- Uterine rupture.
- Placental trauma and abruption.
- Hemorrhage.
- Fetal trauma.
- Chorioamnionitis: risk of chorioamnionitis increases with the duration of labor, the number of vaginal examinations, and intrauterine instrumentation.

SUPPLIERS

Intran Plus IUP-400
Utah Medical Products, Inc. (United States)
7043 South 300 West
Midvale, UT 84047-1048
Phone: 1-800-548-8667
or

Utah Medical Products, Inc. (Europe)
Garrycastle Industrial Estate
Athlone, County Westmeath, Republic of Ireland
Phone: 353-902-73932
Website: www.utahmed.com

Softrans IUPC
Kendall LTP
The Ludlow Company LP
Two Ludlow Park Drive
Chicopee, MA 01022
Phone: 1-800-962-9888
Website: www.kendall-ltp.com

CPT/BILLING CODES

There are no current CPT codes for IUPC insertion. However, labor that is postterm, induced, augmented, or otherwise complicated (blood pressure problems, arrest of labor, fetal distress, etc.) is not included in a routine delivery. It should be coded with hospital evaluation and management codes.

59610   Routine obstetric care including antepartum care, vaginal delivery (with or without episiotomy, and/or forceps) and postpartum care, after previous cesarean delivery.
59618   Routine obstetric care including antepartum care, cesarean delivery, and postpartum care, following attempted vaginal delivery after previous cesarean delivery.
99356   Prolonged physician service in the inpatient setting, requiring direct (face-to-face) patient contact beyond the usual service (e.g., maternity fetal monitoring for high-risk delivery or other physiological monitoring); first hour
99357   Each additional 30 minutes
99358   Prolonged evaluation and managed service before and/or after direct (face-to-face) patient care (e.g., review of extensive records and tests, communication with other professionals and/or patient/family); not face-to-face care; first hour
99359   Each additional 30 minutes

ICD-9-CM DIAGNOSTIC CODES

658. 0   Oligohydramnios
658.4   Infection of amniotic cavity
661   Abnormality of forces of labor
662   Long labor

665.1   Rupture of uterus during labor
792.3   Nonspecific abnormal findings in fluid surrounding fetus

BIBLIOGRAPHY

Cunningham FG: *Williams obstetrics,* ed 20, Stamford, Conn, 1997, Appleton & Lange.

Gibb DMF: Measurement of uterine activity of labour—clinical aspects, *Br J Obstetr Gynaecol* 100(9):28, 1993.

Handwerker SM, Selick AM: Placental abruption after insertion of catheter tip intrauterine pressure transducers: a report of four cases, *J Reprod Med* 40(12):845, 1995.

Scott JR, editor: *Danforth's obstetrics and gynecology,* ed 7, Philadelphia, 1994, Lippincott-Raven.

Smith RP: A brief history of intrauterine pressure measurement, *Acta Obstet Gynecol Scand Suppl* 129:5, 1984.

Strong TH Jr, Ahn MO, Lipscomb KR, et al: Intrauterine manometry: reapplication of an old concept, *Int J Gynaecol Obstet* 34(4):315, 1991.

Trudinger BJ: Fetal hazards of the intrauterine pressure catheter: five case reports, *Br J Obstetr Gynaecol* 85(8):567, 1978.

WEBSITE

www.aafp.org/practice/ob/coding3.html (Coding for intrapartum care: using other evaluation and management services in maternity care)

CHAPTER 173

Obstetric Ultrasound

Richard E. A. Brunader

Ultrasound is defined as the range of sound waves with frequencies greater than 20,000 Hz, which are undetectable by the human ear. Most ultrasound scanners use frequencies of 1 to 10 MHz; 3.5 to 5 MHz is the most commonly used frequency range for obstetric examinations. According to natality data, ultrasound is being used more commonly in the United States. In 2000, 67% of mothers who had live births underwent ultrasound during pregnancy, compared with 48% in 1989.

To evaluate the use of ultrasound as a routine screening procedure during pregnancy, the National Institutes of Health sponsored a landmark Consensus Development Conference in 1984. The consensus was that routine screening was not justified and that ultrasound should be used only for specific indications. (Those indications have remained somewhat constant and are similar to those listed in the "Indications" section.) This consensus was further supported by evidence from the RADIUS study, published in 1993 (Ewigman et al), although there continues to be controversy regarding this study. The current position of the American College of Obstetrics and Gynecology (ACOG) also continues to support this consensus.

However, this is not a worldwide consensus. The Royal College of Obstetricians and Gynecologists and the European Committee for Ultrasound Radiation Safety endorse routine prenatal ultrasound examinations. Ultrasound is routinely used in several European countries, including Sweden and Germany. The Canadian Task Force on Preventive Health Care finds fair evidence for routine ultrasound screening in the second trimester, even in women without clinical indications. Many U.S. insurers, including managed care organizations, now also reimburse for routine obstetrical ultrasound screening.

Editor's note: Routine first trimester scanning in a high-risk population to confirm gestational age is very helpful when later managing intrauterine growth retardation (IUGR) or postdates pregnancies. It may also improve maternal bonding.

Obstetric ultrasound can be performed either transabdominally (TAUS) or transvaginally (TVUS). Transvaginal scanning is performed predominately in the first trimester and it usually facilitates visualization of fetal structures 1 week earlier than transabdominal scanning.

Ultrasound can be very successful when attempting to detect anomalies in high-risk patients, but it is very technician- or clinician-dependent. It is important for the clinician performing the examination to have adequate training and equipment and a willingness to seek appropriate consultation for complicated cases.

Obstetric ultrasound studies are classified in two different ways: for billing purposes and radiologically. For billing purposes, the scan is either a *complete* study (survey) or a *limited* scan (a single organ or to answer a clinical question [e.g., "Is there fetal heart activity," or "Is there a placenta previa?"]). A limited study is typically performed in clinical emergencies or as a follow-up to a complete study. Radiologically, scans are defined as either *basic* (survey) or *targeted*. A targeted evaluation is done to identify, characterize, or exclude fetal anomalies. Targeted evaluations are usually performed by individuals with considerable experience in scanning fetal anomalies.

Adequate documentation for every ultrasound study is essential. This should include a permanent written report, complete with the ultrasound images incorporating measurement parameters and anatomical findings. Fig. 173-1 is an example of an ultrasound report form. Suggested documentation for first, second/third, and intrapartum scans are noted below, adapted from American Institute of Ultrasound in Medicine (AIUM) guidelines. Only basic obstetric ultrasound studies are discussed here and they should include the elements described below:

First Trimester Basic Ultrasonography Documentation

1. Document the location of the gestational sac. If visible, the embryo should be identified and the crown-rump length (CRL) measured and recorded.
2. Report the presence or absence of fetal life (e.g., cardiac or somatic activity).

OBSTETRIC ULTRASOUND

PATIENT IDENTIFICATION:

Name_____

Age_____ DOB_____

PMD_____

LMP_____EDC_____

Age	Gravidity	Term	Preterm	Abortion	Living

Parameter	Measurement	Gestational age	Indices	
GEST SAC			CI	
CRL			HC/AC	
BPD			FL/AC	
OFD			FL/BPD	
HC			AC/BPD	
AC			distal femoral epiph?	
FL			proximal tibial epiph?	
OTHER			proximal humeral epiph?	
Estimated fetal age			Other	
Estimated fetal weight	EFW	Percentile		

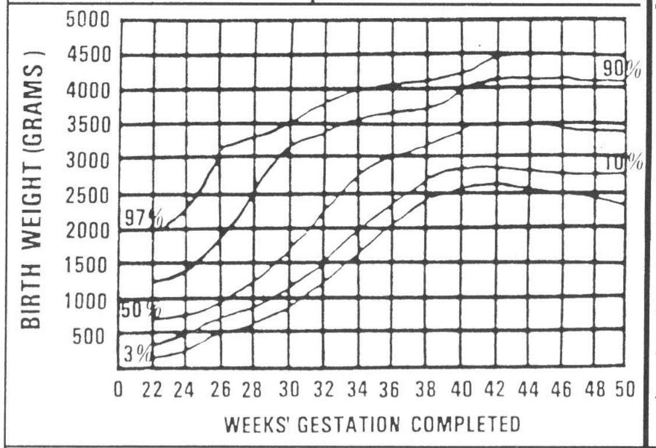

Reason for examination

Requested by

Estimated gestational age at examination

Number of fetuses / Presentation

Placental location / Placental grade

AFI =

- ❑ Septum cavum pellucidum
- ❑ Cisterna magna
- ❑ Lateral ventricle
- ❑ Extremities
- ❑ 4 Chamber heart
- ❑ Stomach
- ❑ Fetal kidneys
- ❑ Fetal bladder
- ❑ Normal abd. wall
- ❑ Normal spine
- ❑ 3-Vessel cord
- ❑ Normal diaphragm

Biophysical profile score =

Movement _____
Breathing _____
Tone _____
Fluid _____
NST _____

TOTAL _____

IMPRESSIONS/RECOMMENDATIONS:

Uterus _____

Adnexa _____

_____

_____

_____

_____

_____

_____

PREPARED BY:

(Signature and Title)

DATE OF EXAMINATION:

[Graph: BIRTH WEIGHT (GRAMS) vs WEEKS' GESTATION COMPLETED, showing percentile curves 90%, 10%, 97%, 50%, 3%; y-axis 500–5000, x-axis 0, 22 24 26 28 30 32 34 36 38 40 42 44 46 48 50]

Fig. 173-1
Sample obstetric ultrasound report form.

3. Document fetal number (This portion of the study deserves special attention. It is very easy to overlook a second or third gestational sac in first trimester scans and it is the most common time that one is overlooked).

4. Perform an evaluation of the uterus (including the cervix), adnexal structures, and the cul-de-sac.

Note: The most accurate assessment of gestational age with transabdominal scanning is by CRL at age 9 to 11 weeks. It depends on the population being scanned, but liberalizing the number of scans performed during this time may decrease the number of postdate pregnancies to be managed. In other words, if many women are unsure of their dates, routine ultrasound may provide more accurate gestational ages and expected dates of confinement (EDCs). Therefore, the overall number of women thinking that they are 42 weeks, when they are actually less than 42 weeks, may decrease. Liberalizing the number of early scans to establish dates in a high-risk population may also improve the management of IUGR.

Second and Third Trimester Basic Ultrasonography Documentation

1. Document fetal life, number, presentation, and activity.

2. Report a quantitative and qualitative estimate of the amount of amniotic fluid (increased, decreased, normal; AFI or deepest vertical pocket).

3. Record the placental location and determine its relationship to the internal cervical os.

4. Assess gestational age using a combination of biparietal diameter (or head circumference) and femur length.

5. Assess fetal growth with the abdominal circumference measurements. If previous studies have been performed, give an estimate of the appropriateness of the interval growth. Fetal weight should be estimated in late second and all third trimester scans.

6. Perform an evaluation of the uterus, cervix, and adnexal structures.

7. The study should include, but not necessarily be limited to, the following fetal anatomy: cerebral ventricles, posterior fossa, heart, spine, stomach, diaphragm, kidneys, urinary bladder, umbilical cord insertion site, extremities, and intactness of the anterior abdominal wall.

Intrapartum Basic Ultrasonography Documentation

1. Document fetal life, number, and presentation.

2. Report an estimate of the amount of amniotic fluid.

3. Record the placental location and determine its relationship to the internal cervical os.

INDICATIONS

- Estimation of gestational age
- Evaluation of fetal growth
- Vaginal bleeding of undetermined etiology
- Determination of fetal presentation/presenting part
- Suspected multiple gestation
- Adjunct to amniocentesis
- Significant uterine size/dates discrepancy
- Pelvic mass
- Suspected hydatidiform mole
- Adjunct to cervical cerclage placement
- Suspected ectopic pregnancy
- Adjunct to special procedure
    —In-vitro fertilization
    —Embryo transfer
    —Chorionic villous sampling
- Suspected fetal death (see Chapter 209, Emergency Department and Office Ultrasound)
- Suspected uterine abnormality
- Intrauterine contraceptive device localization (see Chapter 209, Emergency Department and Office Ultrasound)
- Ovarian follicle development surveillance for infertility
- Biophysical profile (BPP)
- Observation of intrapartum events
    —Management of second twin
    —Manual removal of placenta
- Suspected polyhydramnios or oligohydramnios
- Suspected placental abruption
- Adjunct to external version
- Estimation of fetal weight and/or presentation and/or cervical dilation in premature rupture of membranes and/or preterm labor
- Abnormal serum alpha-fetoprotein values*
- Follow-up observation of identified anomaly*
- Follow-up evaluation of placental location for identified placenta previa
- History of previous infant with congenital anomaly*
- Serial evaluation of fetal growth in multiple gestation
- Evaluation of fetal condition in late registrants for prenatal care

CONTRAINDICATIONS

- Maternal refusal

---

*Usually a targeted examination performed by individuals experienced in this area.

EQUIPMENT

- Real-time ultrasound machine with either a 3-MHz or higher transducer for transabdominal scans or a 5-MHz or higher transducer for transvaginal scans. Among state-of-the-art machines, differences between different manufacturers are primarily subjective. (See the "Suppliers" section.)
- Ultrasonic gel
- Towels to remove gel when study completed
- Sheaths or probe covers for transvaginal scanning
- Appropriate forms for documentation

PREPROCEDURE PATIENT PREPARATION

If the pregnancy is greater than 20 weeks, it is not necessary to have a full bladder for transabdominal scanning. The patient's bladder should be empty or only slightly full for transvaginal scanning.

Issues to be discussed with patients who undergo obstetric ultrasound include the following:
- Safety
- Purpose of the examination
- Detection of birth defects
- Accuracy of measurements
  —Dating
  —Estimated fetal weight

After many years, no study of safety has ever indicated more than a theoretical risk to the fetus from routine ultrasound scanning (see the "Complications" section). AIUM is a not-for-profit national professional organization that continues to monitor ultrasound safety. They have never noted any safety problems (for mother or child) with ultrasound.

In the office setting, when asked why they think an ultrasound is being performed, patients commonly state "to make sure the baby is okay." If applicable, it may be important to explain that the ultrasound is being performed to answer a particular clinical question, not for general screening. They should be aware, especially if a limited study is being performed, that no ultrasound study can ensure a perfect baby. Patients also frequently request an ultrasound to determine the sex of the infant. They should be informed that national guidelines (NIH or otherwise) do not list this as an indication for ultrasound. After providing this information, it is the clinician's choice as to whether to attempt to determine the sex of the infant.

A handout for the patient to review before scanning can be quite helpful. (See the sample patient education handout titled "Obstetric Ultrasound" on page 1975 of Appendix G.) After scanning, giving the patient a picture of the fetal hand profile, the facial profile, or even the genitalia should enhance bonding with minimal legal hazard.

TECHNIQUE

1. Follow a routine when scanning an apparently normal pregnancy. However, even with a normal pregnancy you should have a low threshold for varying from the routine. For example, if you see an excellent sonographic view of something that will later need to be documented (e.g., placenta), freeze it and record an image. You may not get another chance. If an abnormality is noted, document it but do not forget to complete the routine scan.

2. First, briefly sweep the entire uterus to check for fetal viability and gross pathology as well as to determine the direction in which the fetus is lying. For first trimester scans, it is important to methodically sweep the entire uterus to exclude multiple gestations. After gross pathology is excluded, it may enhance bonding to allow the patient and family to watch the images during scanning.

3. Next, evaluate the lower uterine segment before the bladder fills and distorts the cervical length or its relationship to the placenta.

4. To maintain orientation, evaluate the long axis and transverse views of the spine if the fetus is in a convenient position. After getting oriented to the fetal spine, you will be three-dimensionally oriented to how the baby is lying (e.g., on all fours). Transverse views of various organs will then be easier to locate and will make more sense.

5. Evaluate the fetus in transverse views from head to pelvis. In particular, transverse views of the brain, chest, heart, abdomen, stomach, kidneys, and bladder should be obtained. The cord insertion site should be imaged. Record appropriate images for documentation.

6. Longitudinal views of the diaphragm, stomach, kidneys, and bladder should also be visualized. Take appropriate documentation photos.

7. Next evaluate the extremities. The clinician should visualize all four extremities. Record an image of a femur for measurements.

8. A final sweep should be made through the entire fetus and an informal BPP performed for late trimester pregnancies.

9. Finally, the placental site and amniotic fluid volume should be evaluated. If the placenta has not already been visualized during the previous scanning, it is usually located posteriorly. If there has been difficulty imaging the fetus, the amount of amniotic fluid is probably reduced.

10. While scanning, the necessary measurements listed in the next section should be obtained. Techniques and formulas for obtaining specific measurements are also discussed in the following sections. Use the appropriate sections when attempting to answer particular clinical questions or for certain situations as needed.

Measurements

The biparietal diameter, abdominal circumference, and femur length are measured as the basis of most obstetric ultrasound evaluations. Early in pregnancy, crown-rump length and gestational sac measurements are also important. Certain early developmental landmarks, if noted, may also provide worthwhile information for estimating gestational age (Table 173-1).

1. Crown-rump length (CRL)
   a. Formula:

   Gestational age (weeks) = (CRL [mm] + 65)/10

   b. The CRL is the longest length of the fetus, excluding the fetal limbs and the yolk sac. One should average crown-rump measurements from three satisfactory images.

   Note: Determining CRL is the most accurate method of establishing gestational age.

   c. Transabdominally, CRL is most accurate between 9 and 11 weeks. Even more accurate is CRL by transvaginal scanning between 7 and 9 weeks. The greatest problem with measuring CRL transabdominally earlier than 9 weeks is that the fetus is very small and the borders may be unclear. As a result, it may be very difficult to obtain the maximum longitudinal diameter (CRL) of the fetus. After 11 or 12 weeks, the fetus flexes and extends so much that it may be difficult to obtain the true maximal diameter (Fig. 173-2).

2. Gestational sac (GS) diameter
   a. Formula:

   Gestational age (weeks) = (Avg GS [mm] + 25.43)/7.02

TABLE 173-1

Developmental Landmarks by Abdominal Ultrasound*

Landmark	Fetal Age (from LMP)
Visualization of gestational sac	5-6 weeks
Embryonic pole	6-7 weeks
Fetal heart motion	7-8 weeks
Fetal movement	8-9 weeks
Biparietal diameter measurable	12-13 weeks

*Many of these may be visualized up to a week earlier with transvaginal scanning.

b. The GS measurement is not the best value to use for estimating gestational age, and it should be used only if other dating parameters are *not* available.

c. The GS consists of a hypoechogenic area, which corresponds to the chorionic vesicle, and an echogenic rim or ring, which corresponds to the trophoblast. The GS of a normal pregnancy also may be characterized by a *double echogenic ring.* The inner ring is the decidua capsularis plus the chorion laeve. The outer ring is the decidua vera. At the implantation site, the hyperechoic rim is thicker, and it comprises the decidua basalis and chorion frondosum (Fig. 173-3).

d. The presence of a normal in utero GS, complete with contents (Fig. 173-4), usually confirms an intrauterine pregnancy and indirectly excludes ectopic gestation. In some cases, however, it may be difficult to differentiate between the gestational sac seen with an early intrauterine pregnancy and the *pseudogestational sac* sometimes seen with an ectopic pregnancy (see the "First Trimester Scanning" section and Chapter 209, Emergency Department and Office Ultrasound).

Note: This method of exclusion of ectopic pregnancy may not be helpful for patients taking ovulation-induction medications for fertility (see the "First Trimester Scanning" section).

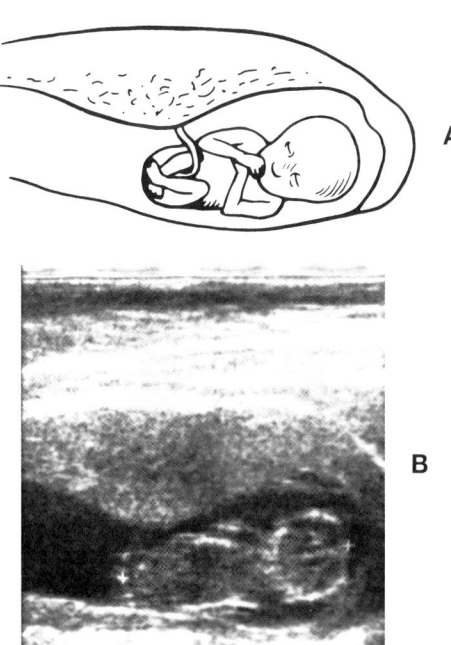

Fig. 173-2
Measurement of the crown-rump length. **A,** Fetus at 12 to 13 weeks. **B,** Ultrasound scan showing the longest length of a 12-week fetus. Measurement should be made from the top of the crown (head) to the bottom of the rump.

First Trimester

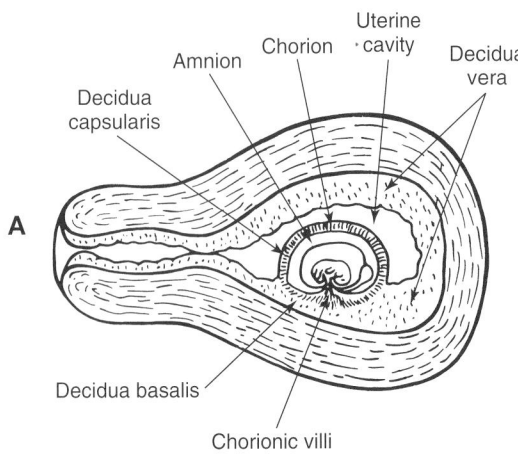

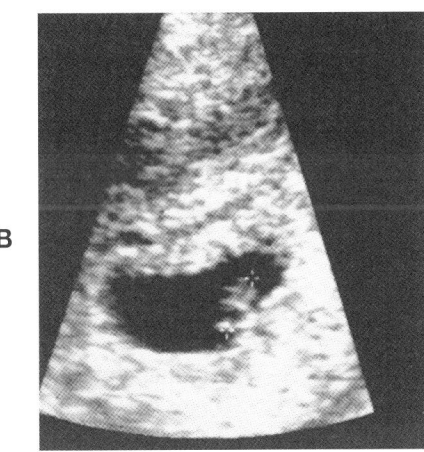

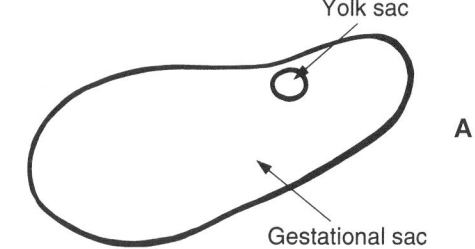

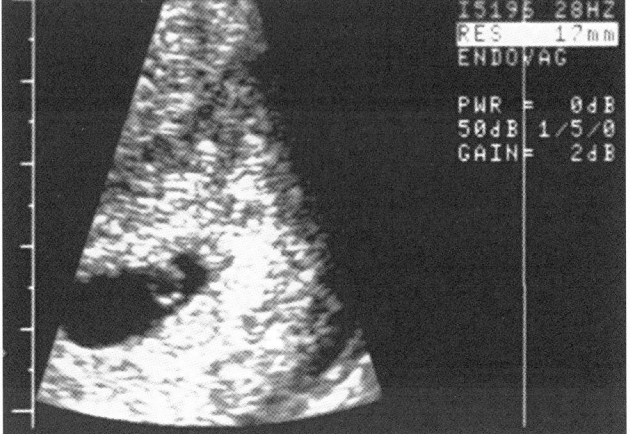

Fig. 173-4

Gestational sac with yolk sac on transvaginal ultrasound. **A,** Yolk sac is generally first seen at about 5 weeks' gestation by transvaginal scanning and at 6 to 7 weeks' gestation by transabdominal scanning. Its presence confirms an intrauterine gestation, but does not rule out a rare concomitant ectopic pregnancy (see text). **B,** Ultrasound scan of gestational sac with yolk sac demonstrated.

Fig. 173-3

Illustration accompanying a transvaginal photograph detailing an early gestation. **A,** The decidua capsularis and the decidua vera form the double echogenic ring. **B,** The ultrasound scan contains a fetal pole with 7-mm crown-rump length, which corresponds to a 6-week gestation. Pregnancies earlier than 5 weeks by transvaginal scanning and earlier than 6 weeks by transabdominal scanning generally do not show a fetal pole. Usually, only a hypoechogenic area corresponding to the chorionic vesicle is seen at this age.

Note: The BPD is one of the only outer-to-inner diameter measurements used in all of sonography. Inner diameter is used because the posterior calvarium causes a lot of artifact and tends to distort outer-to-outer diameter measurements (Fig. 173-5).

b. The most commonly accepted reference plane for BPD is a cross-section parallel to the canthomeatal line and slightly above it. This cross-sectional plane cuts through the falx cerebri, the thalamus, the cavum septum pellucidum, and the medial cerebral artery. The head shape should be oval at this plane.

4. Head circumference (HC)
   a. Formula:

   HC = 1.57 (BPD + occipital-frontal diameter [OFD]).

   Note: Some clinicians use HC = 1.57 (BPD + 0.3 cm + OFD) because of the manner in which BPD is measured.

   b. The OFD is measured in the same plane as the BPD. The OFD diameter measurement should be made from the skull's outer-to-outer aspect.

e. The sac is measured inside the hyperechoic rim, including only the anechoic (dark or fluid-filled) space. If the sac is round, only one dimension is needed; if ovoid, three measurements are taken and an average diameter calculated (Avg GS).

3. Biparietal diameter (BPD)
   a. The BPD is measured ideally when the fetus is lying in an occiput transverse position. In this position, BPD is the distance measured between the outer table of the proximal fetal skull and the inner table of the contralateral side of the skull.

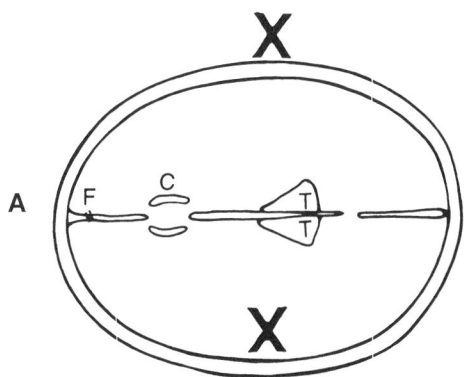

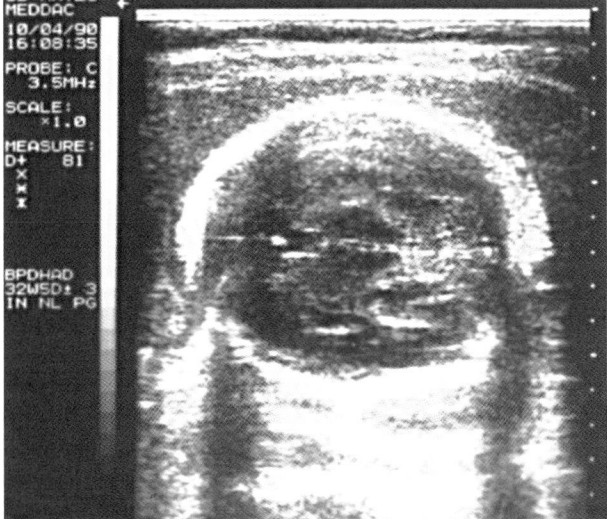

Fig. 173-5
A, Biparietal diameter (BPD) is measured from outer to inner aspects of the skull. *C,* Cavum septum pellucidum; *F,* falx cerebri; *T,* thalami. **B,** Ultrasound scan of the fetal cranium at the proper level for a BPD, the level of the cavum septum pellucidum and thalamus. Note artifact behind posterior skull table.

5. Cephalic index (CI)
   a. Formula:

$$CI = BPD/OFD$$

   b. Prenatal molding of the fetal skull is common and may result in an inaccurate determination of the BPD. The cephalic index (the ratio of the BPD to the OFD) can be used to screen for cranial shape abnormalities. The CI is a constant throughout pregnancy. The normal value is 78.3% ± 8% (±2 standard deviations [SD]). Values below this normal range indicate a dolichocephalic head (an ellipse with a BPD that is shorter than expected or "too flat"). Values above this normal range indicate a brachycephalic head (an ellipse with a BPD that is wider than expected or "too round").
   c. If the CI is significantly above or below the normal range, the BPD may not be a reliable estimation of

gestational age. Instead, the HC should be used for estimating gestational age.

6. Abdominal circumference (AC)
   a. Formula:

$$AC = 1.57 (D_1 + D_2)$$

   b. Two diameters (D_1 and D_2), the anteroposterior abdominal diameter and the transverse abdominal diameter, are taken at the level of the junction of the umbilical vein and the left portal vein. This junction appears as an echolucent structure shaped like a hockey stick. These diameters should be at right angles to each other, and the plane in which they are taken should be at a right angle to the fetal spine. These measurements should also be outer-to-outer diameter measurements.
   c. For estimating gestational age, the AC is only useful when there is no clinically apparent maternal or fetal condition that would modify liver growth. The AC is most useful for establishing gestational age in midgestation and late pregnancies (Fig. 173-6).
7. Femur length (FL)
   a. The central diaphysis of the shaft of the femur should be measured. This is not necessarily the largest or longest measurement that can be obtained. The longest measurement may include the femoral neck, which, if included, would overestimate the true value (Fig. 173-7).

Fetal Body Ratios

1. *Cephalic index (CI).* (See previous discussion.)
2. *Head circumference/abdominal circumference (HC/AC).* This ratio has a positive predictive value of 62% for detecting asymmetric IUGR and a negative predictive value of 98%. The HC/AC is normally about 1.2 at 20 weeks and drops linearly to about 1 at 36 to 38 weeks' gestation. From that time, it remains about 1 or below until delivery. Screening for an HC/AC greater than 1 after 36 weeks detects 85% of IUGRs. This method fails to detect symmetric IUGR.
3. *Femur length/abdominal circumference (FL/AC).* The FL/AC ratio will not detect symmetric IUGR, but it is sensitive for asymmetric IUGR. This ratio has the further advantage of having normal-range values that do not change with time after 20 weeks. The normal value for this ratio expressed as a percentage is 22% ± 2% (±2 SD). A value greater than 24% indicates IUGR. A value less than 20.5% is suggestive of macrosomia. However, even though the negative predictive value is 92% to 93%, the positive predictive value is only 18% to 20%.

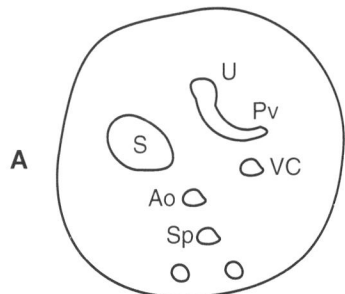

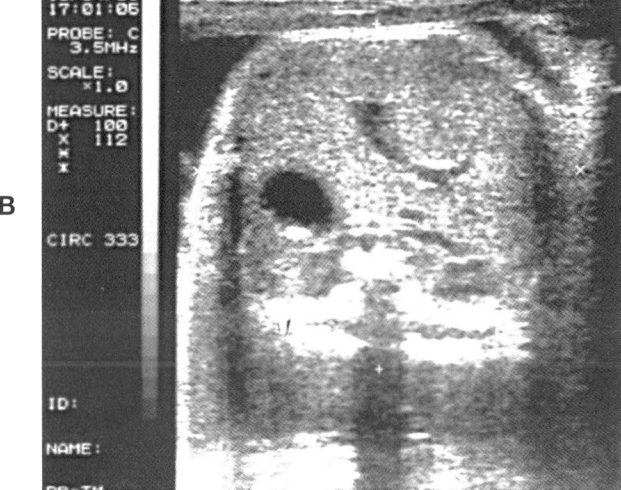

Fig. 173-6

Abdominal circumference. **A,** This third trimester cross-section of the fetal abdomen shows the junction of the umbilical vein and left portal vein. The stomach is seen on the left side of the fetus. *Ao,* Aorta; *VC,* vena cava; *Pv,* portal vein; *S,* stomach; *Sp,* spine; *U,* umbilical vein. **B,** Ultrasound scan of abdominal cross-section.

4. *Femur length/biparietal diameter (FL/BPD).* After 22 weeks' gestational age, the FL/BPD ratio is almost constant, with a normal range of 79% ± 8% (±2 SD) from 22 to 40 weeks. The predictive values of this ratio are similar to those for FL/AC. The FL/BPD has three important uses: (1) evaluation of the ultrasound examination for measurement error, (2) detection of diseases of the fetal head and limbs, and (3) classification of IUGR.

Ultrasonographic Dating

1. Because of biologic variability, traditional clinical methods can only estimate gestational age with 90% certainty to within 2 weeks. This is the limit when even the best clinical methods are applied (using last menstrual period, date when uterus reaches umbilicus, first heard fetal heart tones, fundal height, and quickening). In part, this is because 25% to 45% of women are unable to provide an accurate menstrual history. For this and other reasons, the EDC derived from the last menstrual period differs by more than 2

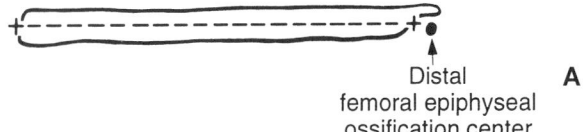

Distal femoral epiphyseal ossification center

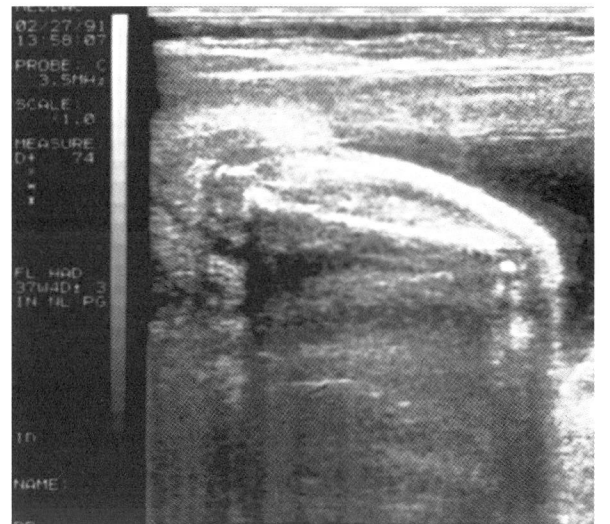

Fig. 173-7

A, Third trimester femur is measured along the central shaft of the diaphysis. **B,** Ultrasound scan demonstrating the echogenic distal femoral epiphyseal ossification center on the right, which indicates a gestational age of 33 weeks or more.

TABLE 173-2

Outline of Ultrasonographic Dating of Pregnancy

Weeks of Gestation	Recommended Dating Measurement	Accuracy
3-5	None	
5-6	GS	± 1 week
6-12	CRL	± 3-5 days
12-20	1. BPD	± 1 week
	2. FL	± 1 week
20-30	1. BPD	± 2 weeks
	2. FL	± 2 weeks
	3. AC	± 3 weeks
30-40	1. BPD	± 3 weeks
	2. FL	± 3 weeks
	3. AC	± 3.5 weeks

AC, Abdominal circumference; *BPD,* biparietal diameter; *CRL,* crown-rump length; *FL,* femur length; *GS,* gestational sac.

weeks from the actual date of birth in nearly one quarter of pregnancies. Ultrasound dating early in pregnancy can be helpful for correcting the EDC.

2. Ultrasound-determined size of certain body parts correlates with gestational age. In general, growth is quite uniform in the first 20 weeks of gestation. Thereafter the progressive increase in variability makes estimation of gestational age difficult and less accurate (Table 173-2).

Indicated Dating Parameters Based on Gestational Age

1. From 7-10 wk: use an average of GS and CRL
2. From 11-14 wk: use an average of CRL, BPD, and FL
3. From 15-28 wk: use an average of BPD, HC, FL, and AC
4. After 28 wk: use an average of BPD (with CI), HC, FL, and AC

AC, Abdominal circumference; *BPD,* biparietal diameter; *CI,* cephalic index; *CRL,* crown-rump length; *FL,* femur length; *GS,* gestational sac; *HC,* head circumference.

3. When reporting ultrasound estimates of age, it is very important to understand and report the associated uncertainties. The uncertainty or variability is usually expressed as plus or minus two standard deviations (± 2 SD), which should be applicable to 95% of fetuses in a normal population. Reporting a single age estimate for a given fetal measurement gives a false impression about the accuracy of the method. Thus the variability of the estimate (in SD) should be given as well.

4. Pregnancy dating often uses an average of estimates of age from several methods; see Box 173-1 for suggestions as to which parameters to use with each stage of pregnancy. Any of the measurements may be technically incorrect. However, it is unlikely that several measurements will be incorrect in the same direction. Therefore, when averages are used, measurement errors tend to be self-canceling and a more accurate overall estimate of gestational age is made.

5. When using the multiple parameter dating approach, or an averaged estimate of age, it is critical to avoid using any measurements that might have been affected by a pathologic process in the fetus (e.g., hydrocephaly, microcephaly, macrosomia, IUGR, or fetal dwarfism). After 22 weeks' gestational age, potential errors can be minimized by making certain that the fetal body ratios are within normal limits (see the "Fetal Body Ratios" section). If the CI indicates a normally shaped head, the FL/BPD ratio can be calculated. If the FL/BPD ratio is below 70%, the FL should be eliminated; if the ratio is above 86%, the fetal head measurements should be discarded. If the FL/BPD ratio is normal, the FL/AC ratio can be calculated. If the FL/AC ratio is less than 20%, the AC should not be used because of possible macrosomia; if the ratio is above 24%, the AC should not be used because of possible IUGR.

6. The presence of certain fetal epiphyseal ossification centers may be helpful when estimating gestational age for pregnancies beyond 30 weeks. This is especially useful at this stage of pregnancy because we know dating by other ultrasound parameters has limited reliability (Table 173-2). A visible distal femoral epiphysis (Fig. 173-7) indicates a menstrual age of at least 33 weeks, a visible proximal tibial epiphysis indicates a menstrual age of at least 35 weeks, and a visible proximal humeral epiphysis indicates a gestational age of at least 38 weeks.

Placental Imaging

1. Maturational changes of the placenta occur in its three basic anatomic areas (the amniochorionic plate, the placental body, and the basal layer) and form the basis for the following grading system of placental maturity (Fig. 173-8):

   Grade 0: Placenta has a chorionic plate that is very smooth. The placental substance is homogenous and without calcifications.

   Grade I: There is some undulation and some indentations in the chorionic plate. There are also scattered echogenic areas, which represent calcifications within the placental substance.

   Grade II: The chorionic plate has more indentations, but they do not reach the basal plate. The grade II placenta is characterized by a straight line of echoes with calcifications present along the axis of the basal plate. These echoes are high-amplitude, bright, white, and linear or comma-shaped.

   Grade III: The chorionic plate indentations reach the basal plate. There is complete compartmentalization of the placenta with extensive echogenic areas representing calcifications. They may cast shadows.

   Note: In a third trimester scan, if the placenta has not been located by the time the other parameters have been obtained, it is usually located posteriorly, having been obscured by infant body parts.

2. Grade 0 is most common in the first trimester; grade I appears after 14 weeks' gestation and is most common until around 34 weeks. Grade II may appear after 26 weeks' gestation and is most common at around 36 weeks. Grade III most commonly appears after 35 weeks' gestation. Even with a grade III placenta, there is a 4% chance of fetal pulmonary immaturity.

3. A grade II placenta before 26 weeks or a grade III placenta before 35 weeks is abnormal.

4. IUGR, oligohydramnios, and hypertension are associated with accelerated placental maturation. Diabetes mellitus and Rh sensitization are associated with delayed maturation. Preeclampsia and pregnancy-induced hypertension do not affect placental maturation.

5. The principal purposes of the ultrasound examination for bleeding in the second and third trimesters are to delineate the placental implantation site, to exclude placenta previa, and to attempt to determine whether there has been an abruption.

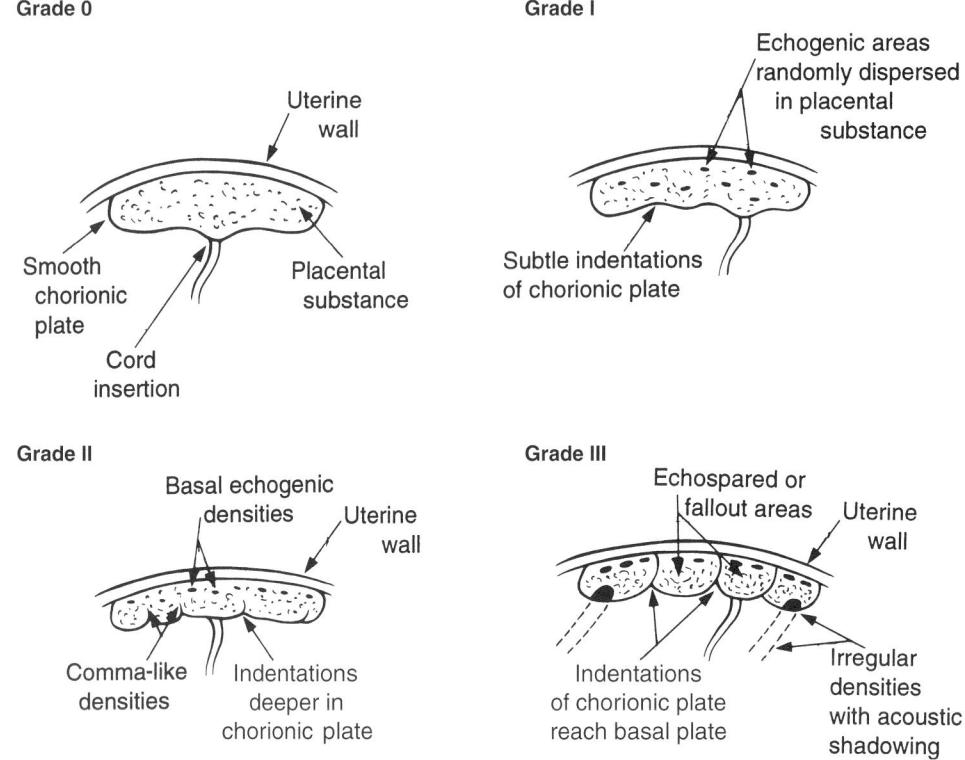

Fig. 173-8
Four grades of placental maturity. (Redrawn from Grannum P, Berkowitz R, and Hobbins J: *Am J Obstet Gynecol* 133:915, 1979.)

Note: In the proper scenario, unless a large abruptio placenta is clearly confirmed on ultrasound, the possibility should be managed clinically (as if there is an abruptio placenta). With ultrasound, there is a risk of false negatives; most abruptio placenta are small and easy to miss. There is also the risk of false positives; venous lakes can appear very similar to an abruptio placenta.

Amniotic Fluid Volume

1. Estimation and documentation of amniotic fluid volume (AFV) is the standard of care during routine ultrasound examinations. Although there is no precise method of determining amniotic fluid volume, there are several indirect methods of estimation.
   a. *Subjective assessment:* Although simple and rapid, if used alone a subjective assessment (e.g., increased, decreased, or normal fluid volume) requires a highly trained sonographer. Since the result lacks a numerical value, it is difficult to follow trends; therefore most centers prefer an amniotic fluid index (AFI) over subjective assessment for estimating AFV. Even if a maximal vertical pocket or AFI will be measured, clinicians should practice making a subjective assessment and record it.
   b. *Maximum vertical pocket:* This technique involves measuring the single deepest vertical pocket of amniotic fluid, not including segments of the umbilical cord. *Oligohydramnios* is defined as the absence of a pocket of fluid at least 2 cm in depth, and *polyhydramnios* is diagnosed when any pocket exceeds 8 cm. This technique is most helpful for quantitating fluid with a multiple gestation pregnancy or in the assessment of polyhydramnios.
   c. *Amniotic fluid index (AFI):* This is the quantitative approach to estimating the AFV used by most centers. The uterus is divided into four quadrants. The ultrasound transducer is then held in a vertical and sagittal alignment (marker dot on the probe turned toward the mother's head or cephalad). With the patient supine, the transducer is held perpendicular to the plane of the floor and aligned longitudinally with the mother's spine. Starting in one quadrant, the pocket of fluid with the largest vertical dimension is identified, measured, and recorded. Care must be taken not to include segments of the umbilical cord in the measurement. Coiled cord can fill the space and appear to be fluid. This procedure is repeated in each quadrant and the values

summed. If the sum (AFI) is less than 8 cm, perform the four-quadrant evaluation 3 times and average the values.

2. Polyhydramnios
   a. In nondiabetic women, polyhydramnios is defined as an AFI of 24 cm or more.
   b. The most likely etiology is idiopathic (34.6%), followed by diabetes mellitus (24.6%), congenital anomalies (20.1%), erythroblastosis fetalis (11.5%), and multiple gestation (9.2%).
   c. Once identified, a patient with an AFI of 24 cm or more should have a detailed or targeted ultrasound examination to rule out fetal anomalies.
   d. Abnormal fetal lie, operative delivery, and abruptia all occur more frequently during labor in patients with polyhydramnios.

3. Oligohydramnios
   a. Significant oligohydramnios is defined as an AFI of less than 5 cm.
   b. Excluding patients with premature rupture of membranes, approximately 83% of patients with oligohydramnios will have fetal intrauterine growth retardation; however, only 16% of patients with IUGR fetuses will have oligohydramnios.
   c. Fetal weight should be estimated whenever oligohydramnios is present.
   d. Premature rupture of membranes can cause severe oligohydramnios or anhydramnios.
   e. Fetal causes of oligohydramnios are usually related to urinary tract anomalies.
   f. Fetal heart rate abnormalities, depressed Apgar scores, and passage of meconium all occur more frequently during labor in patients with oligohydramnios.
   g. In most cases, oligohydramnios in a term infant is an indication for delivery.

Fetal Assessment (Biophysical Profile)

1. A combination of biophysical variables (the BPP) was first introduced by Manning in 1980. The most important aspect in the sensitivity of this test is that it combines both acute and chronic markers of the fetal and placental condition. Documenting the acute markers (fetal heart rate reactivity [FR], fetal movement [FM], fetal breathing movement [FBM], and fetal tone [FT]) is very similar to performing an in-utero neurologic examination of the infant. It can demonstrate acute oxygenation of the various parts of the neurologic system. Documenting the chronic marker (AFI) is similar to obtaining a "hemoglobin A1C" of fetal oxygenation. It demonstrates how well the fetus has been oxygenated over the last few days, weeks, or maybe even a month.

2. A normal BPP is indirect evidence that each of the portions of the central nervous system that control particular activities are functioning and, therefore, oxygenated. When all of the various portions of the central nervous system are active, it indicates that overall the fetus is well oxygenated at that time. The absence of a given BPP activity, however, is difficult to interpret because it may reflect either pathologic depression or normal periodicity.

3. In chronic sustained fetal hypoxia, a protective redistribution of fetal cardiac output may occur, with blood being directed away from nonvital fetal organs (kidneys or lung) toward vital fetal organs (heart, brain, and adrenals). This leads to decreased urine production, oligohydramnios, and a low AFI. A low AFI may be the earliest marker of placental insufficiency.

4. A fetal BPP score of 8 or more is reassuring of fetal well-being; however, a BPP score of less than 8 is nonreassuring, and repeated testing or delivery is indicated. The presence of oligohydramnios constitutes an abnormal biophysical assessment regardless of the overall score (Table 173-3).

Fetal Size

1. Many formulas and tables are available for prediction of fetal weight. These formulas are based on a variety of combinations of BPD, HC, AC, and FL. The predictive accuracy of these formulas ranges from ±14.8% to ± 20.2% (±2 SD). Formulas are often compared against a commonly used table (Shepard et al, 1997).

2. On clinical examination, a discordance between size and dates should arouse suspicion of specific disorders, depending on gestational age. In early pregnancy, suspect multiple gestation, a hydatidiform mole, incorrect menstrual history, and genetic or developmental defects. Later in pregnancy, fetal malposition, IUGR, fetal dysmaturity, genetic or developmental defects, multiple gestation, fetal macrosomia, and abnormal amniotic fluid volume are causes to consider. Many of these possibilities can be further evaluated with ultrasound.

a. Intrauterine Growth Retardation

1. Clinical signs of IUGR include poor increase in either fundal height (>4 cm difference from expected fundal height) or maternal weight gain (<100 to 200 g [3.5 to 7 oz] per week in third trimester) or both. However, diagnosis of IUGR by clinical means is possible in only approximately 33% of pregnancies.

2. By comparison, a diagnosis of IUGR by ultrasound is much more accurate than a clinical diagnosis, especially if dating is accurate (e.g., from transabdominal ultrasound at 9 to 11 weeks). However, even with ultrasound, sensitivities and specificities are

variable, so ultrasound information should be correlated with clinical data. This combination of information will significantly improve a clinician's ability to diagnose IUGR.

3. Important ultrasound parameters for evaluating potential IUGR.

   a. Oligohydramnios

      i. For the general population the sensitivity of oligohydramnios in the diagnosis of IUGR is approximately 16%.

      ii. For high-risk populations, the predictive value and sensitivity of oligohydramnios is enhanced (sensitivity can exceed 85%). If oligohydramnios is present and there is no evidence of premature rupture of membranes or congenital anomalies, IUGR is the likely cause. The combination of oligohydramnios and IUGR portends a less favorable outcome, and early delivery should be considered. Generally, if the pregnancy is at 36 weeks or more, the high risk of intrauterine loss may mandate delivery.

   b. Biparietal diameter (BPD). BPD alone is not a very helpful parameter when diagnosing IUGR. With symmetric IUGR, both head and body measurements fall off the growth curve together and result in an erroneous estimate of gestational age. Even with asymmetric IUGR, the BPD remains normal until late in the course.

   c. Head circumference (HC). The HC is a more shape-independent measurement of fetal head size than the BPD. In cases of cranial shape abnormalities, its inclusion in the growth profile will significantly decrease the high number of false-positives seen when BPD is used. However, because IUGR may not selectively affect brain and head growth, or is "relatively head-sparing," HC alone is also not a very useful measurement. The HC is most useful when it is used with another measurement as a ratio.

   d. Femur length (FL). The FL can also be misleading when trying to diagnose IUGR. In asymmetric IUGR, FL usually parallels the gestational age as calculated from the last normal menstrual period. Therefore, for asymmetric IUGR, FL may not be helpful. In symmetric IUGR, all measurements will be small and result in an erroneously early gestational age estimate, so again FL is not helpful. Similar to HC, FL is most useful for prediction of IUGR when it is used in a ratio.

   e. Abdominal circumference (AC). The AC is useful for assessing fetal nutritional status. The AC involves measurement of the liver, which is smaller in chronic hypoxia. With inadequate oxygen or nutrition, the liver cannot produce substrate (glycogen); thus the AC is the best single predictor of IUGR.

   f. Calculation of fetal body ratios (see the "Fetal Body Ratios" section).

   g. Placental grade. When fetal growth pattern and estimated weight suggest a small fetus, the finding of a prematurely grade III (before 35 weeks) placenta is further evidence of IUGR.

   h. Use of fetal epiphyseal ossification centers (see the "Ultrasonographic Dating" section).

TABLE 173-3

Fetal Biophysical Profile Scoring According to Manning and Colleagues

Variable	Score 2	Score 0
Fetal breathing movement (FBM)	The presence of at least 30 sec of sustained FBM in 30 min of observation	<30 sec of FBM in 30 min
Fetal movement (FM)	Three or more gross body movements in 30 min of observation; simultaneous limb and trunk movements are counted as a single movement	Two or fewer gross body movements in 30 min of observation
Fetal tone (FT)	At least one episode of motion of a limb from a position of flexion to extension and a rapid return to flexion	Fetus in a position of semi- or full-limb extension with no return to flexion with movement; absence of fetal movement is counted as absent tone
Fetal reactivity (FR)*	The presence of two or more fetal heart rate accelerations of at least 15 bpm and lasting at least 15 sec and associated with FM in 40 min	No acceleration or less than two accelerations of the fetal heart rate in 40 min of observation
Qual AFV†	A pocket of amniotic fluid that measures at least 1 cm in two perpendicular planes	Largest pocket of amniotic fluid measures <1 cm in two perpendicular planes
Maximal score	10	—
Minimal score	—	0

From Manning FA, Platt LD, Sipos L: *Am J Obstet Gynecol* 136(6):787, 1980.
AFV, Amniotic fluid volume; *FBM,* fetal breathing movement; *FM,* fetal movement; *FT,* fetal tone.
*Modern centers perform a nonstress test.
†Modern centers usually determine an amniotic fluid index.

4. Suspect IUGR by ultrasound if the following occur:
   a. AC falls in the lower 15th percentile. (Sensitivity of ultrasound is >95% if AC <2.5th percentile.)
   b. Weight falls in the lower 15th percentile.
   c. HC/AC ≥0.95 (HC/AC >1.0 after 36 weeks detects 85% of IUGR).
   d. FL/AC ≥23.5%.
5. In the absence of an accurate gestational age, the assessment of risk for IUGR predominantly relies on fetal disproportionality and asymmetry. This may lead to the diagnosis of asymmetric IUGR. However, to diagnose symmetric IUGR, unless dates are very accurate, serial ultrasounds must be performed to assess fetal growth. Some experts recommend serial scans at 2- or 3-week intervals to identify IUGR in the absence of reliable dating. Therefore, for those at risk, liberalizing the use of early ultrasound for establishing gestational age may be the best way to diagnose symmetric IUGR.
6. Newer techniques to identify IUGR are being evaluated, including Doppler ultrasonography of the umbilical artery and M-mode echocardiography of the fetal heart.

b. Macrosomia

1. Fetal macrosomia is defined in absolute terms as a fetal weight of greater than 4000 g, regardless of gestational age. However, macrosomia is also considered when a fetal weight falls in the upper 90th percentile for any gestational age at any point during the pregnancy.
2. Symmetric macrosomia occurs when the excessive fetal weight is the result of proportionate growth of all fetal parameters. For example, the weight, length, and head size may all be above the 90th percentile for age. Symmetric macrosomia is usually the result of a prolonged gestation or genetics (i.e., large parents). The HC/AC and the FL/AC ratios are usually within the normal range for age.
3. Asymmetric macrosomia generally occurs in patients with class A to C diabetes mellitus. Although the values of HC and FL are higher than average, they usually fall below the 90th percentile for age. The excessive weight results from profound increases in soft tissue mass that are reflected by an AC and an estimated fetal weight above the 90th percentile. The HC/AC and the FL/AC ratios usually fall below the 10th percentile for age.

Note: Sonographic diagnosis of macrosomia does *not* predict prognosis for vaginal delivery. In fact, for suspected macrosomia, the accuracy of estimated fetal weight by ultrasound is no better than that obtained with clinical palpation (Leopold's maneuvers). As a result, ACOG guidelines (November 2000) state that suspected macrosomia is not a contraindication to attempted vaginal birth. However, they do state that prophylactic cesarean delivery may be considered with estimated fetal weights of more than 5000 g in women without diabetes and more than 4500 g in diabetic women.

Preterm Labor

1. Preterm labor is defined as onset of labor before a gestational age of 37 weeks. Preterm labor affects 10% of pregnancies, and it accounts for 75% of perinatal morbidity and mortality.
2. Ultrasound parameters that are important when evaluating the patient in preterm labor include the following:
   a. Fetal number. Multiple gestations have an increased risk of preterm labor.
   b. Estimated fetal weight. Preterm labor is associated with IUGR.
   c. Amniotic fluid index. Preterm labor is associated with both oligohydramnios and polyhydramnios.
   d. BPP score. A low BPP may contraindicate tocolysis.
   e. Other possible contraindications to tocolysis:
      i. Fetal malformations.
      ii. Evidence of concealed placental abruption.
   f. Ultrasonic cervical evaluation:
      i. Cervical shortening (present if the distance from internal os to the leading edge of the portio vaginalis is less than 3 cm).
      ii. Dilation of the endocervical canal (present if the maximal diameter of the endocervical canal exceeds 1 cm).
      iii. Bulging of the fetal membranes into the endocervical canal (conical rather than rounded shape of the isthmic region).
      iv. Thinning of the lower uterine segment (anterior wall thickness less than 0.6 cm).

Postdates Pregnancy

1. Expected date of confinement is defined as 40 weeks (280 days) from the first day of the last normal menstrual period, or 266 days after ovulation, providing cycles are regular and occur at 28-day intervals. Normal term ranges from 38 to 42 weeks.
2. A postdates pregnancy is one with a duration that has exceeded 42 weeks (294 days) from the last normal menstrual period, assuming a 28-day cycle.
3. One study showed that the incidence of post-dates pregnancy was overestimated by 7.5% when gestational age was determined using just the menstrual history; but it fell to 2.6% when using early ultrasound examination, and to 1.1% when both menstrual and early ultrasound measurements were used.
4. Complications detectable by ultrasound include the following:
   a. Physiologic oligohydramnios (detectable by AFV determination).

b. Macrosomia (detectable by calculation of estimated fetal weight).

c. Dysmaturity resulting from chronic uteroplacental insufficiency (detectable by evidence of asymmetric IUGR).

d. Congenital anomalies (detectable by anatomic survey).

e. Patient that should not be induced (e.g., a preterm delivery could be prevented by having good estimates of gestational age).

5. The contraction stress test is still regarded as the most reliable method of antenatal surveillance for the postdates pregnancy. However, it has basically been replaced by BPP used on a weekly basis. The results of studies comparing the use of twice weekly nonstress tests and an AFI with both of these are acceptable. All are characterized by minimal morbidity and mortality but unfortunately high intervention and cesarean section rates. The benefits of obtaining twice weekly nonstress tests (NSTs) and an AFI over the other techniques include the fact that a sonographer or physician is not required to perform an NST/AFI. Specially trained personnel (nursing) are certainly capable of performing these two evaluations.

First Trimester Scanning (See Chapter 209, Emergency Department and Office Ultrasound, for a detailed description)

1. The most common causes of bleeding in the first trimester:
   a. Unknown causes.
   b. Embryonic resorption/ blighted ovum.
   c. Threatened, missed, incomplete, or complete abortion.
   d. Ectopic pregnancy.
   e. Abortion of one member of a multiple gestation.
   f. Hydatidiform mole.

2. When evaluating for ectopic pregnancy by transabdominal scanning, an extrauterine gestational sac is seen in less than 10% of cases (rates are higher with transvaginal scanning). Ultrasound is more helpful for excluding ectopic pregnancy by demonstrating an intrauterine gestation. When an intrauterine gestation is clearly demonstrated, the likelihood of simultaneous extrauterine and intrauterine gestations (i.e., a combination pregnancy) is only one in every 7000 to 8000 cases* or one in 30,000 low-risk pregnancies.

   An ectopic pregnancy becomes almost certain with transvaginal scanning if (a) there is no intrauterine pregnancy, (b) the patient has no vaginal bleeding, and (c) the quantitative HCG is more than 2000 international units.

3. The sonographic appearance of a gestational sac can be simulated by the exfoliation of hyperplastic endometrium associated with an ectopic pregnancy. This sonographic finding, known as a *pseudogestational sac,* can appear very similar to a gestational sac. A pseudogestational sac occurs in 10% to 20% of ectopic pregnancies. Thus the unequivocal diagnosis of an intrauterine pregnancy should not be made until the gestation sac contains two concentric rims, a fetal pole, and a yolk sac, or fetal heart activity can be identified within the sac.

4. In a normal pregnancy, the mean serum human chorionic gonadotropin (HCG) doubling time is 1.98 days. If serial HCG titers show a plateau or fall, an abnormal (ectopic) or nonviable pregnancy is deemed likely.

5. There are many reasons variations can exist between institutions when measuring HCG. Purity differences among test kits (different manufacturers) can contribute to variations in measurement. Variations can even exist in the same laboratory in different runs, or occasionally in the same run. With this much variation, even using a given standard, it is important to be aware which test kit is being employed when correlating the sonographic findings with the quantitative HCG levels.

6. Optimally, each institution should correlate its ultrasound equipment and sonographers' skill with quantitative HCG levels obtained from its own reference laboratory. When this is accomplished, externally published quantitative HCG reference levels and expected ultrasound findings should be used only as rough guidelines. Current published quantitative HCG levels and ultrasound correlations are outlined in Table 173-4.

7. If a gestational sac is absent at an HCG value above the institution's threshold, ectopic pregnancy, recent spontaneous abortion, and early hydatidiform degeneration should be considered. Suspicion of an ectopic pregnancy should be even higher if there is significant fluid in the cul de sac.

8. Ultrasonic examination can be very helpful for evaluating whether tissue is remaining after a spontaneous abortion, for diagnosing the vanishing twin syndrome (abortion of one member of a multiple gestation), and for establishing fetal viability in threatened abortion. It is the procedure of choice for evaluation of gestational trophoblastic disease.

9. With ultrasonic examination alone, a normal gestational sac can often be distinguished from an abnormal sac doomed to miscarriage, even before

---

*The rate of combination pregnancies in women on ovulation-inducing drug therapy (clomiphene or human chorionic gonadotropin) has been reported as high as 1:100.

TABLE 173-4

Possible Outcomes Based on Ultrasound Quantitative Human Chorionic Gonadotropin (HCG) Combinations

HCG Level (mIU/ml)*	Presence/Absence of Gestational Sac (GS) on Transabdominal Ultrasound (TAUS)	Significance
>1800	+ GS	Intrauterine pregnancy; if fetal pole or yolk sac is identified, no further ultrasound is required. Ectopic pregnancy is basically ruled out. (<1:7000 risk unless patient taking fertility ovulation induction medications [see text].)
<1800	+ GS	Failed intrauterine pregnancy or absorbed pregnancy (Mde); ectopic pregnancy with pseudogestational sac; or very rarely, an early pregnancy that may continue.
>1800	– GS	Suspect ectopic pregnancy.
<1800	– GS	Indeterminate. May be result of an early intrauterine pregnancy, ectopic or failed pregnancy. Follow HCG titer every 2 to 4 days; for normal pregnancies, HCG should double. However, normal HCG trends occur in 15% of ectopic pregnancies. Thus, as soon as the level crosses the threshold for the practitioner's facility, repeat the ultrasound examination.

*Actual values will vary from institution to institution based on particular assay used, quality of TAUS machine, and the skill of the ultrasonographer.

the embryo is visible. The size and appearance of the gestational sac should be evaluated according to major and minor criteria for normalcy. A gestational sac of abnormal size or appearance correlates highly with an abnormal outcome.

a. Major criteria for a normal-appearing gestational sac:
   i. A sac of 25 mm or more in diameter must reveal an embryo within it.
   ii. The sac must be round in shape.
b. Minor criteria for a normal appearing gestational sac:
   i. The gestational sac is located in the fundus of the uterus.
   ii. A thick, echogenic decidual ring surrounds the gestational sac.
   iii. There is evidence of the double ring sign.
10. When a gestational sac with a mean diameter greater than 25 mm lacks an embryo or when the gestational sac is grossly distorted, abnormal pregnancy is almost certain. Using these criteria, 76% of abnormal pregnancies and 93% of normal pregnancies will be correctly classified by only one ultrasound scan. Failure to meet any single major criterion or all three minor criteria will identify 53% of abnormal pregnancies but will be 100% specific in predicting spontaneous abortion.
11. Once embryonic cardiac motion is seen on ultrasound, the likelihood of spontaneous abortion is very low (less than 16% for pregnancies less than 8 weeks; less than 2% to 4% after 12 weeks).

COMPLICATIONS

Although there are theoretical risks of ultrasound damaging human fetuses, no proven harm has been documented to any human fetus or mother. The only other possible complications from an obstetric ultrasound are failure to diagnose an anomaly or condition, an inaccurate estimate of gestational age or weight, inappropriate reassurance of a perfect infant, or inaccurate determination of the sex of the infant. Because fetal anomalies can remain undetected even by the best sonographer with the best equipment, the patient should never be unequivocally assured that the fetus is "fine." However, the patient can be reassured with answers to certain specific questions provided by the scan.

POSTPROCEDURE PATIENT EDUCATION

If follow-up scans or other management will be needed, the patient must know when and where to go for them.

SUPPLIERS

Acuson (owned by Siemens)
1220 Charleston Road
P.O. Box 7393
Mountain View, CA 94039-7393
Phone: 1-800-422-8766
Website: www.acuson.com

Advanced Technology Laboratories (ATL) (owned by Phillips)
22100 Bothell Everett Highway
P.O. Box 3003
Bothell, WA 98041-3003
Phone: 1-800-526-4963
Website: www.atl.com

Agilent Technology (formerly Hewlett-Packard)
3000 Minuteman Road
Andover, MA 01810
Phone: 1-800-934-7372
Website: www.agilent.com

Aloka
10 Fairfield Boulevard
Wallingford, CT 06492
Phone: 1-203-269-5088
Website: www.aloka.com

Biosound Esaote, Inc.
8000 Castleway Drive
Indianapolis, IN 46250
Phone: 1-800-428-4374
Website: www.biosound.com

General Electric Medical Systems
P.O. Box 414
Milwaukee, WI 53201
Phone: 1-800-558-5102
Website: www.gemedicalsystems.com

Hitachi Medical Corp.
660 White Plains Road
Tarrytown, NY 10591-5107
Phone: 1-800-852-2080
Website: www.hitachiultrasound.com

Medison USA
6616 Owens Drive
Pleasanton, CA 94588
Phone: 1-800-829-7666
Website: www.medisonusa.com

Phillips Medical Systems of North America, Inc. (also owners of ATL)
20 Center Point Drive, Suite 110
La Palma, CA 90623
Phone: 1-800-843-7572
Website: www.medical.philips.com

Pie Medical
8000 Castleway Drive
Indianapolis, IN 46250-1943
Phone: 1-800-927-0708
Website: www.piemedicalusa.com

Siemens Medical Solutions, Inc. (also owners of Acuson)
22010 SE 51st Street
Issaquah, WA 98029
Phone: 1-800-367-3569
Website: www.siemansmedical.com

Toshiba America Medical Systems
2441 Michelle Drive
Tustin, CA 92780
Phone: 1-800-421-1968
Website: www.medical.toshiba.com

CPT/BILLING CODES

76801	Ultrasound, pregnant uterus, real time with image documentation, fetal and maternal evaluation, first trimester (<14 weeks 0 days), transabdominal approach; single or first gestation
76802	Each additional gestation (use in conjunction with 76801)
76805	Ultrasound, pregnant uterus, real time with image documentation, fetal and maternal evaluation, after first trimester
76810	Each additional gestation (use in conjunction with 76805)
76815	Limited (fetal heart beat, placental location, fetal position, and/or qualitative amniotic fluid volume)
76816	Follow-up or repeat
76818	Fetal biophysical profile; with non-stress testing
76819	Fetal biophysical profile; without non-stress testing

ICD-9-CM DIAGNOSTIC CODES

623.8	Vaginal bleeding
630	Hydatidiform mole
632	Missed abortion
633.9	Ectopic pregnancy
634.91	Abortion or miscarriage, incomplete, without complications
634.92	Abortion or miscarriage, complete, without complications
640.03	Threatened abortion, antepartum
641.03	Placenta previa without hemorrhage, antepartum
641.13	Placenta previa with hemorrhage, antepartum
641.21	Placental abruption, delivered
641.23	Placental abruption, antepartum
644.20	Preterm labor
644.21	Preterm labor, delivered
645.13	Postterm pregnancy (40 to 42 weeks), antepartum
645.23	Prolonged pregnancy (>42 weeks), antepartum

ADDITIONAL RESOURCES

- See the sample patient education handout titled "Obstetric Ultrasound" on page 1975 of Appendix G.
- See the sample patient consent form titled "Obstetric Ultrasound" on page 1977 of Appendix G.

BIBLIOGRAPHY

American College of Obstetricians and Gynecologists: *Routine ultrasound in low-risk pregnancy,* ACOG Practice Patterns No 5, Washington, DC, August 5, 1997, ACOG.

American College of Obstetricians and Gynecologists: *Fetal macrosomia,* ACOG Practice Bulletin No 22, Washington, DC, November 2000, ACOG.

Brunader R: Accuracy of prenatal sonography performed by family practice residents, *Fam Med* 28(6):407, 1996.

Callen PW, editor: *Ultrasonography in obstetrics and gynecology,* ed 3, Philadelphia, 1994, WB Saunders.

Ewigman BG, Crane JP, Frignoletto FD, et al: Effect of prenatal ultrasound screening on perinatal outcome, *N Engl J Med* 329:821, 1993.

Keith R, Frisch L: Fetal biometry: a comparison of family physicians and radiologists, *Fam Med* 33(2):111, 2001.

Manning FA, Platt LD, Sipos L: Antepartum fetal evaluation: development of a fetal biophysical profile, *Am J Obstet Gynecol* 136(6):787, 1980.

Routine prenatal ultrasound screening. In Canadian Task Force on Preventive Health Care: *Canadian guide to clinical preventive health care,* Ottawa, 1994, Health Canada (rev 1998).

Sabbagha RE, editor: *Diagnostic ultrasound applied to obstetrics and gynecology,* ed 3, Philadelphia, 1994, JB Lippincott.

Sanders RC, Miner NS, editors: *Clinical sonography: a practical guide,* ed 3, Philadelphia, 1998, Lippincott-Raven.

Screening ultrasonography in pregnancy. In: *Guide to clinical preventive services,* ed 2, Baltimore, 1996, Williams & Wilkins.

Seeds JW: The routine or screening obstetrical ultrasound examination, *Clin Obstet Gynecol* 39:814, 1996.

Shepard MJ, Richards VA, Berkowitz RL, et al: An evaluation of two equations for predicting fetal weight by ultrasound, *Am J Obstet Gynecol* 156:80, 1987.

Smith CB, Sakornbut EL, Dickinson LC, Bullock GL: Quantification of training in obstetrical ultrasound: a study of family practice residents, *J Clin Ultrasound* 19(8):479, 1991.

Timor-Tritsch IE, Rottem S, editors: *Transvaginal sonography,* ed 3, New York, 1997, Elsevier.

Vandenbosche RC, Kirchner JT: Intrauterine growth retardation, *Am Fam Physician* 58(6):1384, 1998.

CHAPTER 174

Paracervical Block

Scott T. Henderson

A paracervical block anesthetizes Frankenhäuser's ganglion, which contains the visceral sensory nerve fibers from the uterus, cervix, and upper vagina. By injecting local anesthetic submucosally into the fornix (cervicovaginal junction) of the vagina, effective anesthesia during the first stage of labor (cervical dilation) can be attained. This procedure may provide great comfort to mothers in early labor, especially primiparous women who spend the most time in early labor. Although a paracervical block should enhance the experience, the pudendal nerves are not blocked. Therefore additional anesthesia may be required for delivery. It should also be noted that these anesthetics are relatively short acting, so the procedure may need to be repeated during labor. A paracervical block can also be used for anesthesia for other procedures involving the cervix (e.g., conization, dilation and curettage).

INDICATIONS

- First stage of labor
- Cervical conization or ablation procedures
- Dilation and curettage

Note: Paracervical block may be especially useful for women giving birth in hospitals where other obstetric anesthesia services are not available. However, a submucosal block may be more effective for cervical procedures (e.g., IVD, cryotherapy; see Chapter 150, Loop Electrosurgical Excision Procedure [LEEP] for Treating Cervical Intraepithelial Neoplasia).

CONTRAINDICATIONS

- Uteroplacental insufficiency
- Preexisting fetal distress
- Allergy to anesthetic agent
- Presence of local infection
- Known coagulopathy or anticoagulated patient (e.g., heparin or its analogues, warfarin, clopidogrel [Plavix]) *(relative contraindication)*

EQUIPMENT

- 10-ml syringe (with finger rings if available [see Fig. 175-1]; otherwise a plain syringe can be used)
- Iowa trumpet with a 6-inch, 20-gauge needle (a must during labor) (see Fig. 175-1) or a 3-inch needle extender on the end of a syringe with a 1½-inch, 22-gauge needle
- Lidocaine* 1% (or chloroprocaine 1.5% or mepivacaine 1%)
- Sterile gloves
- Antibacterial solution and sterile gauze pads
- Sterile speculum for nonpregnant cervix
- Fetal heart monitor (if patient is pregnant)

PREPROCEDURE PATIENT PREPARATION

Obtain informed consent, and outline the possible complications, risks, benefits, and alternatives for anesthesia. (See the sample patient consent form titled "Paracervical Block" and the sample patient education handout titled "Paracervical Block" on pages 1979 and 1978, respectively, of Appendix G.)

TECHNIQUE

1. Place the patient in the lithotomy position.
2. In the gravid patient, assess the cervix and proceed if dilation is 5 to 9 cm. If the cervix is dilated greater than 7 or 8 cm, proceed with caution to preclude injecting the fetal scalp.

---

*Volumes and doses are for 1% lidocaine (10 mg/ml) *without* epinephrine. Toxicity may occur with doses greater than 1 mg/kg (70 mg or 7 ml in a 70-kg patient), with rapid absorption, or with intravascular administration. Maximum dosage should not exceed 4.5 mg/kg or a maximum of 30 ml of a 1% solution (300 mg), and maximum dose should not be repeated in less than 2 hours.

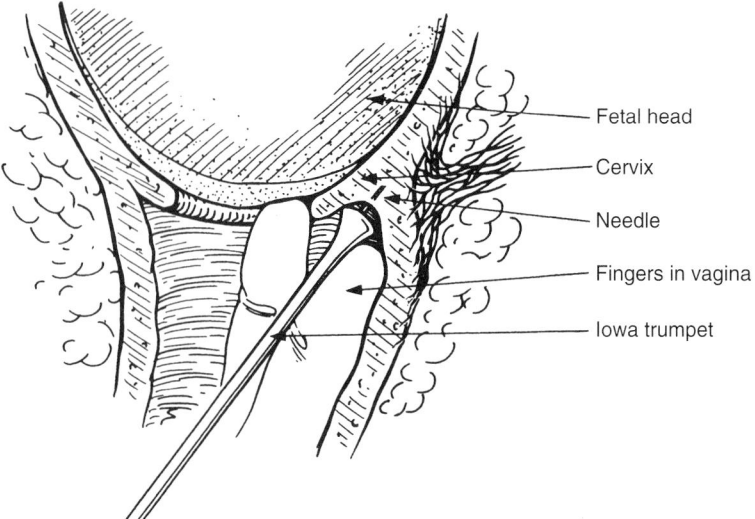

Fig. 174-1
Technique of administering a paracervical block during labor using an Iowa trumpet.

3. Prepare the perineal area with an antibacterial solution.
4. Using your sterile-gloved lubricated index and middle fingers as a guide, lay the trumpet against them and insert it into the vagina. (For a nonpregnant cervix, paracervical block is usually performed under direct visualization, using the sterile speculum.)
5. Place the 20-gauge needle within the trumpet (or 1½-inch needle on an extender) through the mucosa at the *cervicovaginal junction* at the 3 o'clock position. Take care not to insert the needle deeper than 0.5 cm into the tissue (Fig. 174-1).

Note: The positions of the paracervical nerves actually "migrate" superiorly during progressive dilation. In the nonpregnant cervix and in early labor, the nerves are located at the 4 and 8 o'clock positions, respectively (Fig. 174-2). As dilation progresses, they are found more in the 3 and 9 o'clock areas. Proper location of injection is important to gain maximum effect.

6. After aspirating for blood, inject 5 to 10 ml of 1% lidocaine. (Alternatively, 2 to 3 ml may be placed in two or three locations around the probable location of the nerve.)
7. For pregnancy, monitor the fetal heart rate for approximately 5 minutes. If no bradycardia is apparent, repeat the procedure on the contralateral side. Then monitor the fetal heart rate for 20 to 30 minutes, along with maternal blood pressure and pulse. (For non-pregnant patients, simply repeat the procedure on the contralateral side).

Note: It may be necessary to repeat the entire procedure, depending on the duration of activity of the anesthetic agent. A good response is generally maintained for 45 to 75 minutes.

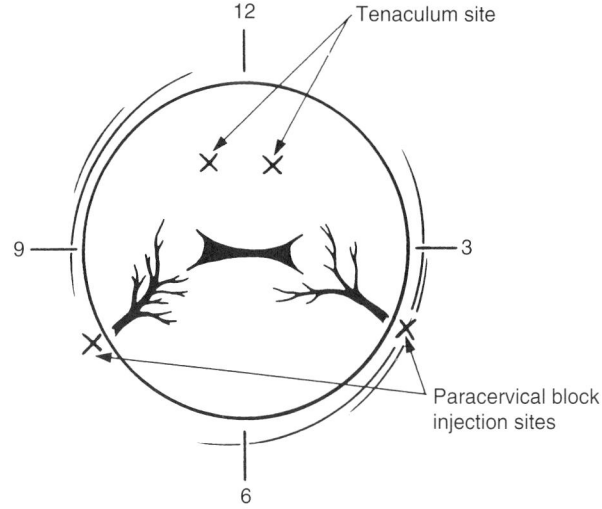

Fig. 174-2
Paracervical block location and where to place the tenaculum in nonpregnant cervix.

However, the effect may only last 30 minutes, or as long as 90 minutes. If lidocaine is used, use no more than 30 ml of a 1% solution and do not repeat in less than 2 hours.

COMPLICATIONS

- Intrafetal injection.
- Idiosyncratic fetal bradycardia. This may occur in 10% to 70% of blocks. However, there is generally no adverse outcome unless the child is delivered during the bradycardia. The most common adverse outcome is the anxiety that patients and clinicians often

experience for the 3 to 6 minutes it takes for this condition to resolve. Despite the fact that this bradycardia is not associated with adverse outcomes, it is the reason many providers choose not to use paracervical blocks. Based on studies of pregnant ewes, the bradycardia may result from drug-induced uterine artery vasoconstriction and myometrial hypertonus; therefore, paracervical block is contraindicated in situations of potential fetal compromise.

- Inhibition of labor if given too early in the first stage of labor.
- Subgluteal or retropsoal hematoma or infection.
- Neuropathy resulting from hematoma formation.
- Intravascular injection.

CPT/BILLING CODE

64435   Paracervical block

ICD-9-CM DIAGNOSTIC CODE

650   Normal delivery

ADDITIONAL RESOURCES

- See the sample patient education handout titled "Paracervical Block" on page 1978 of Appendix G.
- See the sample patient consent form titled "Paracervical Block" on page 1979 of Appendix G.

BIBLIOGRAPHY

Cunningham FG, McDonald PC, Gant NF, et al: *Williams obstetrics,* ed 21, Stamford, Conn, 2001, McGraw-Hill.

Day T: Community use of paracervical block in labor, *J Fam Pract* 26:545, 1989.

Eberle RL, Norris MC: Labour analgesia: a risk-benefit analysis, *Drug Saf* 14(4):239, 1996.

Goins JR: Experience with mepivacaine paracervical block in obstetric private practice, *Am J Obstet Gynecol* 167:342, 1992.

Levy BT, Bergus GR, Hartz A, et al: Is paracervical block safe and effective? A prospective study of its association with neonatal umbilical artery pH values, *J Fam Pract* 48(10):778, 1999.

Shnider SM, Levinson G: *Anesthesia for obstetrics,* ed 3, Baltimore, 1993, Williams & Wilkins.

CHAPTER 175

Pudendal Anesthesia

Donald N. Marquardt

The pudendal nerve supplies both sensory and motor innervation to the perineum. It is composed of parts of the second, third, and fourth sacral nerves, and has three branches. In a female, these branches supply the following structures:

1. The dorsal nerve of the clitoris, which innervates the clitoris and its erectile tissues
2. The perineal nerve, which innervates the muscles of the perineum and the skin of the labia minora, labia majora, and vestibule
3. The inferior hemorrhoidal nerve, which innervates the external sphincter of the anus and perianal skin (responsible for the anal "wink" reflex)

Pudendal anesthesia attempts to block the nerve as it enters the lesser sciatic foramen, usually inferior and medial to the insertion of the sacrospinous ligament on the ischial spine. The pudendal vessels lie lateral to the nerve at this location, so care must be taken to avoid intravascular injection. Although total block of the pudendal nerve should abolish pain and sensation over this entire area, the nerve or its branches may take aberrant pathways and be missed by the block. The transvaginal approach to blockade seems more reliable than a transperineal approach; however, even a transvaginal approach is totally effective, bilaterally, in only about half of patients.

INDICATIONS

- Obstetrical anesthesia for spontaneous vaginal delivery, episiotomy and episiotomy repair, repair of low vaginal lacerations, and low (outlet) forceps or vacuum
- When epidural is incomplete or inadequate
- For minor surgery of the lower vagina and perineum

Note: Because the upper vagina, cervix, and uterus receive separate innervation from the lower thoracic nerves, pudendal anesthesia alone is not sufficient for midforceps application or for high vaginal, cervical, or uterine manipulation or repair. Again, pudendal anesthesia is less than 100% reliable, even in the best of hands. The patient must be checked bilaterally for loss of the anal "wink" reflex (demonstrates adequate anesthesia) before proceeding with whatever procedure is requiring anesthesia

CONTRAINDICATIONS

- Patient refusal
- Allergy to local anesthetic agents
- Current infection in the ischiorectal space or neighboring structures, including the vagina and perineum

Relative Contraindications

- Coagulopathy or anticoagulant therapy (e.g., warfarin, heparin or its analogues, clopidogrel [Plavix]).
- A successful pudendal block will impair some reflexive maternal pushing. This may prolong the second stage of labor in women who are ineffective at pushing.

EQUIPMENT

- 10-ml syringe with finger ring, filled with anesthetic (usually lidocaine without epinephrine*; alternative anesthetics include 10 ml per side or 20 ml total of either 3% 2-chloroprocaine [low toxicity], 1% mepivacaine, or 0.5% bupivicaine [longer duration].)
- Iowa trumpet (Fig. 175-1) or similar guide to facilitate placement of the needle
- Needle, usually 6-inch, 20- or 22- gauge (The operator should check, before the procedure, that the needle is longer than the guiding device and equipped with a "stop" to prevent penetration of tissue deeper than 10 to 15 mm.)

---

*Volumes and doses are for 1% lidocaine *without* epinephrine, 10 mg/ml. Toxicity may occur above 1 mg/kg (70 mg or 7 ml in a 70-kg patient) with rapid absorption or intravascular administration. Maximum dosage should not exceed 4.5 mg/kg or a maximum of 30 ml of 1% solution (300 mg), and maximum dose should not be repeated in less than 2 hours. See step 5 in the following section for usual doses.

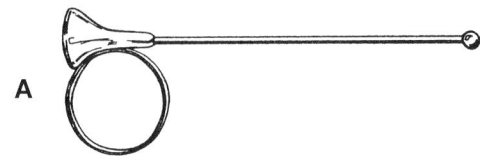

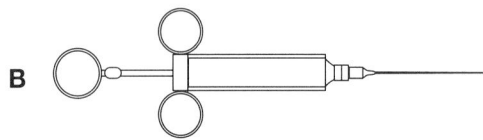

Fig. 175-1
A, Iowa trumpet. **B,** Syringe with finger rings.

- Resuscitation equipment and medications to support the patient if an adverse reaction to an anesthetic is encountered (see the "Complications" section)
- Sterile gloves

PREPROCEDURE PATIENT PREPARATION

Explain the potential risks (see the "Contraindications" and "Complications" sections) and the potential benefits to the patient so she may make an informed decision. This discussion should include alternatives and occur before the moment of greatest anesthetic need, when neither the patient nor the clinician can communicate optimally. Ideally, desired anesthesia should be indicated as part of a birth plan written well before the pregnancy is at term.

TECHNIQUE

Appropriate monitoring of the patient (and, in obstetric cases, the fetus) is mandatory, with IV access secure. Since a fairly large volume of anesthetic agent is given, there must be provision for speedy resuscitation should toxicity or an adverse reaction occur. See the following "Complications" section, or Chapter 5, Local and Topical Anesthetic Complications, for symptoms of adverse reactions.

1. Timing is important for pudendal anesthesia. Approximately 5 to 10 minutes must be allowed for the anesthetic to infiltrate the nerve and cause its effect. However, for obstetric indications, the anesthetic should be administered neither so early that it blocks effective reflex pushing, nor so late that it wears off before delivery. In nulliparous women, it is usually administered after the cervix has completely dilated and the head has descended to a +2 to +3 station. In multiparous women, the pudendal may be adminis-

tered earlier when rapid delivery is expected, but never before the cervix has dilated to 5 cm because it may slow or arrest labor. Anesthesia may last for 20 to 60 minutes, depending on the agent used.

2. Prepare and drape the patient in the dorsal lithotomy position; usually no vaginal prep is used. In obstetric procedures, (a) the length of time the patient is flat should be minimized and (b) *the fetus must be carefully monitored* throughout the procedure and after anesthesia.

3. Grasp the Iowa trumpet or needle guide with your sterile-gloved, nondominant hand. The wrist should be pronated, with the thumb through the ring and the shaft between the index and middle fingers. Adequately lubricate the index and middle fingers and use them to protect the vaginal mucosa (and, in obstetric cases, the fetal head). Insert the fingers into the vagina and direct the tip of the guide to the patient's ipsilateral ischial spine (i.e., the left hand of the right-handed operator is used to direct the guide to the patient's left ischial spine). Maintain the guide at an angle nearly parallel to the patient's back (Fig. 175-2).

4. Carefully define the anatomy to increase the likelihood of a successful procedure. Attempt to delineate the ischial spine. On its inferior surface, the sacrospinous ligament is attached. Next, attempt to palpate the pudendal artery laterally. Locating these landmarks helps prevent injection of the anesthetic directly into the vessels. It also helps to define the location of the nerve, which is medial to the vessels. If the anatomy is particularly difficult to define, injection just below the ischial spine should be sufficient (but only after aspirating to be certain the needle is not in a vessel).

Note: For those inexperienced at identifying the ischial spine, the bony prominence of the nose at the inner canthus of the eye provides a reasonable facsimile of the small and somewhat sharp ischial spine. Attempt to palpate your own eye before putting on gloves, to provide a sense of what it will be like to locate the ischial spine.

5. With your dominant hand, grasp the syringe and direct the needle through the guide to a point on the vaginal mucosa just beneath the tip of the ischial spine.

Note: Aspirate for blood with the syringe before injecting anesthetic each time the needle placement is changed. If blood is aspirated, intravascular injection is likely; withdraw the needle and redirect medially, away from the vessels.

Raise a mucosal wheal with 1 ml lidocaine. Through this wheal, inject the desired sites. Usually two to three sites are injected on each side: (1) posterior to the tip of the ischial spine, (2) inferior or medial to the tip of the spine, and (3) through (and into) the sacrospinous ligament.

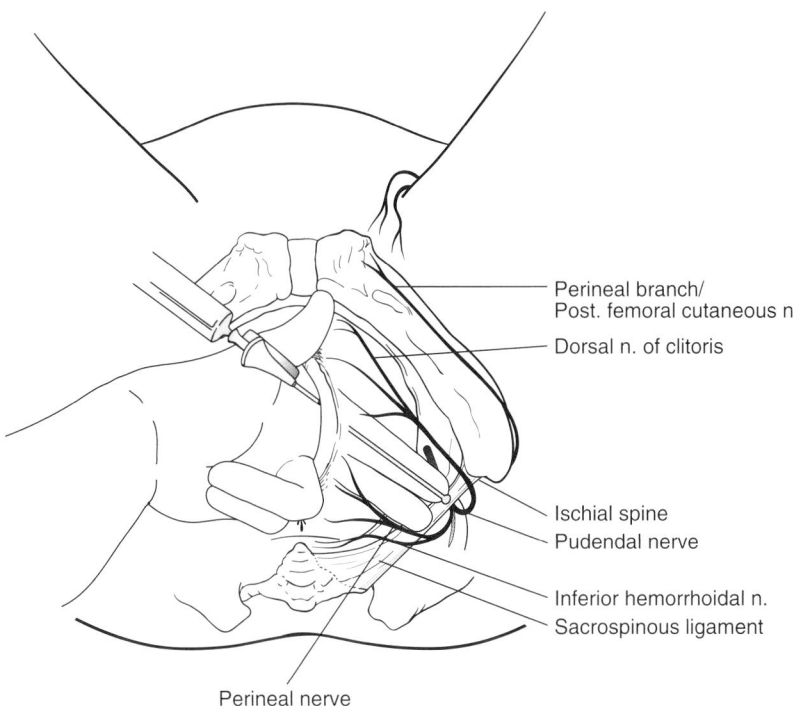

Perineal branch/
Post. femoral cutaneous n.

Dorsal n. of clitoris

Ischial spine
Pudendal nerve

Inferior hemorrhoidal n.
Sacrospinous ligament

Perineal nerve

Fig. 175-2
Practitioner's left hand is directing guide and
needle toward the patient's left pudendal nerve.

Inject each site with 2 to 4 ml 1% lidocaine, with a maximum of 10 ml per side.

Note: Each time the needle is redirected, the tip should be drawn back into the guide, the guide redirected, and then the needle advanced to the desired site.

6. Withdraw the needle, refill the syringe, and inject into the opposite side if bilateral anesthesia is desired. Most operators prefer to use the same hand for the guide; however, some say that switching hands for the opposite side is more effective. If switching hands, make sure the needle tip is withdrawn to protect yourself from a puncture wound.

7. After 5 minutes, check anesthesia on *each* side. Using an Allis forceps, gently scratch over the perineum and watch for the anal "wink" reflex. If there is no reflex to mild stimulus, confirm that the anesthesia is complete with a pinch on each side.

8. A smaller repeat dose on a side not demonstrating adequate anesthesia may be used, but care must be taken to avoid doses at which, even with slow absorption from the tissues, toxic serum levels could be reached. Local anesthesia may be used on the perineum to augment the effect, if necessary (when the pudendal block is not completely effective).

9. As discussed earlier, a pudendal block usually does not provide anesthesia for the upper vagina or cervix. This is important to remember after delivery when attempting to visualize the entire cervix and upper vagina. If manual exploration of the uterus is necessary, the addition of an IV narcotic analgesia, such as 50 mg of meperidine, may be helpful and appreciated.

COMPLICATIONS

- Systemic anesthetic toxicity, which usually results from intravascular administration or inappropriate doses, may initially cause palpitations, tinnitus, dysarthria, or drowsiness. It may progress to confusion, loss of consciousness, convulsions, hypotension, and bradycardia. Although complications are usually transient, support of the patient's oxygenation and blood pressure is essential (especially to minimize fetal complications in obstetric cases). See Chapter 5, Local and Topical Anesthetic Complications, for management of complications.

- The most frequent complication with pudendal anesthesia is failure to provide adequate anesthesia. Local or regional (e.g., saddle block or epidural) anesthesia should be offered if available.

- Hematomas and infections have been reported but are rare. Infections may be life threatening (up to 30% mortality in one series), in part because they are difficult to diagnose. Infection frequently spreads either superiorly along the psoas muscle or laterally along the obturator internus muscle. Infections must be suspected when there is severe pain in the back or hip or limitation of motion, and especially if there is increasing fever. Full evaluation and therapeutic measures are immediately indicated.

- Despite the fact that the anesthetic reaches the neonatal bloodstream after regional anesthesia, studies have failed to demonstrate neonatal neurobehavioral effects or other adverse effects.

POSTPROCEDURE PATIENT EDUCATION

There is little need for specific postanesthesia instruction. Remind the patient of the rare but possible complications so that she will report to her clinician if any symptoms develop.

CPT/BILLING CODE

64430   Introduction/injection of anesthetic agent (nerve block), diagnostic or therapeutic

ICD-9-CM DIAGNOSTIC CODES

650   Normal delivery

The fifth digit (X) is required for Codes 651-659 and 660-669 to denote the following:

0   Unspecified
1   Delivered, with or without mention of antepartum condition
2   Delivered, with mention of postpartum complication
3   Antepartum condition or complication
4   Postpartum condition or complication

Codes related to deliveries with forceps or vacuum:
662.2X   Prolonged second stage of labor
659.7X   Abnormality in fetal heart rate or rhythm

Codes related to episiotomy and episiotomy repair, and for repair of low vaginal lacerations:
664.0X   First-degree perineal laceration
664.1X   Second-degree perineal laceration
664.2X   Third-degree perineal laceration
664.3X   Fourth-degree perineal laceration
664.4X   Unspecified perineal laceration

BIBLIOGRAPHY

Bonica JJ, McDonald JS: Other regional analgesic/anesthetic techniques. In Bonica JJ, McDonald JS, editors: *Obstetric analgesia and anesthesia,* ed 2, Baltimore, 1995, Williams & Wilkins.

Huffnagle HJ, Huffnagle SL: Alternatives to conduction analgesia. In Morris NC, editor: *Obstetric anesthesia,* ed 2, Philadelphia, 1999, Lippincott, Williams & Wilkins,.

Svancarek W, Chirino O, Schaefer G Jr, Blythe JG: Retropsoas and subgluteal abscesses following paracervical and pudendal anesthesia, *JAMA* 237:892, 1977.

CHAPTER 176

Saddle Block Anesthesia

Thomas H. Corbett

With the advent of more complex techniques for producing analgesia and anesthesia, including single-dose intrathecal opiates and continuous spinal or epidural infusion, traditional saddle block (low spinal) anesthesia is used less often. However, a saddle block is occasionally the most useful technique available. An ideal "saddle block" anesthetizes the area that would touch a saddle if the patient were riding a horse. In practice, saddle block anesthesia occasionally extends beyond these borders. Saddle block anesthesia has been used for many years for both surgical procedures and obstetric deliveries. In obstetrics, saddle block anesthesia is limited to near the time of delivery because of the profound motor paralysis it produces.

Clinicians administering saddle block anesthesia must have a good understanding of not only the anatomy involved and needle insertion techniques, but also the pharmacology and physiology involved. They must be familiar and experienced with the diagnosis and management of possible complications. Saddle block anesthesia should be performed only in a hospital, surgery center, or facility where equipment and adequately trained personnel are available to manage any and all possible complications.

INDICATIONS

- For use in obstetrics when time or other circumstances do not allow the use of continuous catheter spinal or epidural anesthetic techniques (e.g., routine delivery, assisted delivery [forceps, vacuum], episiotomy or perineal repair, or other obstetric procedures).
- Genital surgery (e.g., dilation and curettage [D & C], hysteroscopy, vaginal surgery, adult circumcision, orchiectomy, or complicated vasectomy).
- Anorectal surgery (e.g., hemorrhoidectomy, fistulectomy, or rectal-anal biopsy).

CONTRAINDICATIONS

- Patient declines
- Moderate to severe hypovolemia
- Cutaneous lesions of the lower back
- Blood dyscrasias; coagulopathy; prolonged international normalized ratio (INR), prothrombin time (PT) or activated partial thromboplastin time (APTT); or severe anemia
- Anticoagulant therapy (e.g., heparin, warfarin, enoxaparin [Lovenox], clopidogrel [Plavix])
- Allergy to specific local anesthetics
- Spinal abnormalities including scoliosis and other structural abnormalities
- Active systemic infection
- Lack of proper resuscitative equipment, skills, or trained staff
- Preexisting neurologic diseases (amyotrophic lateral sclerosis, other degenerative nerve diseases, polio)
- Preoperative headache *(relative contraindication)*

EQUIPMENT

- Disposable sterile gloves.
- Equipment for the clinician to observe universal blood and body fluid precautions.
- Disposable spinal tray containing the following:
  1. Appropriate prep solutions, swabs, and sterile 4 × 4–inch gauze pads
  2. Disposable drapes
  3. Syringes
     a. 3-ml plastic Luer-Lok for local infiltration of lidocaine 1%
     b. 5-ml procedural syringe for administration of intrathecal agent
  4. Needles
     a. 3½-inch, 25-gauge spinal needle
     b. 20-gauge introducer needle

c. 19-gauge filter needle for drawing solutions into the syringes

d. 25- or 27-gauge skin wheal needle

5. Medications

a. Lidocaine 1% (available in 5-ml vial) for local infiltration

b. Hyperbaric anesthetic

i. Lidocaine 5% (preservative free) in 7.5% glucose for intrathecal administration (2-ml vial), *or*

ii. Tetracaine 1% (2-ml vial) is mixed at the time of use with an equal volume of dextrose 10% (5-ml vial) to make the solution hyperbaric, *or*

iii. Bupivicaine 0.75% in 8.25% dextrose (2-ml vial)

c. Epinephrine 1:1000 (1-ml vial). The addition of 0.2 to 0.3 mg (0.2 to 0.3 ml of 1:1000) epinephrine to tetracaine will produce vasoconstriction and prolong the duration of anesthesia by about 50%

d. Ephedrine 5% (1-ml) for use if hypotension develops (the usual dose to treat hypotension is 10 mg [0.2 ml] IV)

Note: A 1% solution equals 10 mg/ml.

- Continuous fetal monitoring equipment if used for labor and delivery.
- Patient monitoring equipment including automated blood pressure (BP) device, continuous ECG, and pulse oximeter.
- Emergency and resuscitative equipment, including suction, positive-pressure breathing device (Ambu-Bag), oxygen, and defibrillator. Having general anesthesia equipment available may be useful.
- Emergency and other drugs not included in the spinal kit:

1. Atropine
2. Diphenhydramine (Benadryl)
3. Ephedrine (not included in all commercial spinal kits)
4. Lidocaine for IV injection
5. Metoclopramide (Reglan)
6. Neo-Synephrine

ANESTHETIC AGENTS AND DOSES

For saddle block, the three commonly used local anesthetics are lidocaine, tetracaine, and bupivicaine. Lidocaine produces a more rapid onset of anesthesia than tetracaine or bupivacaine; however, it is the shortest acting of the three. Lidocaine generally produces adequate surgical analgesia for 45 to 90 minutes, whereas tetracaine and bupivicaine will last 1½ to 3 hours.

Recently, reports of neurologic sequelae have raised concerns about the use of lidocaine for intrathecal anesthesia. The risk appears to be reduced if the lidocaine solution is diluted before injection with an equal volume of spinal fluid. Tetracaine and bupivicaine are excellent alternatives to lidocaine; however, their increased duration of action requires a longer recovery period.

Note: For a rapidly progressing obstetric patient, lidocaine may be the only option that will work fast enough.

Hyperbaric solutions (solutions more dense than cerebrospinal fluid [CSF]) are used for saddle block anesthesia so that in the sitting position, the anesthetic solution travels caudally, affecting only the lower levels of the spinal cord. It is important to remember that during pregnancy, inferior vena cava compression will cause engorgement and distention of the vertebral venous system. As a result, there is a decrease in the spinal fluid capacity of the subarachnoid space; therefore, the dose requirements are generally reduced in the pregnant patient.

Near delivery, the usual dose of lidocaine for a saddle block is 25 to 50 mg of 5% lidocaine in 7.5% dextrose (0.5 to 1.0 ml). It should be mixed with equal amounts of CSF before injecting. The equivalent dose of 1% tetracaine is 4 to 6 mg (0.4 to 0.6 ml) plus an equal volume of 10% dextrose solution. For bupivicaine, 5 to 6 mg (0.66 to 0.8 ml of the 0.75% bupivicaine in 8.25% dextrose) should be used. In surgical procedures for the nonpregnant patient, the doses should be increased.

Confining the anesthetic to a saddle block distribution depends on the dosage and the time that the patient remains in the sitting position after administration of the anesthetic. Too little time in the sitting position (lying down too soon) may produce a higher level of anesthesia than desired, placing the patient at higher risk of hypotension.

Note: From an anesthetic perspective, the *level* of anesthesia refers to an anatomic level or segment of effect (e.g., up to the level of the umbilicus [T10], the lower border of the ribs [T8] or the level of the xiphoid [T6]), whereas *depth* refers to the amount of remaining sensation. With saddle block, both motor and sensation are blocked; however, the level of the sensory block is usually two segments above the motor block.

PREPROCEDURE PATIENT PREPARATION

A thorough medical history and physical examination should be performed to rule out any contraindications to saddle block anesthesia. Laboratory studies, including a coagulation profile, should be performed if indicated. The medical history should include questions about any previous history of spine trauma, neurologic disease, blood dyscrasias or coagulopathies, and whether the patient is currently taking any medications. Physical examination should include careful observation of the back to rule out anatomic deformities or other physical problems that might make performing a saddle block more difficult.

Patients should be informed of the available options for anesthesia and analgesia. A fact sheet should be given to the patient to read preoperatively or before the onset of labor. Preferably the fact sheet is given to the patient as a part of their preoperative assessment or prenatal care. Shortly before labor or surgery or during early labor, the clinician should review the options again with the patient, including the benefits and specific risks, answer any questions, and obtain signed informed consent. Desired anesthesia or analgesia should be included in the patient's birth plan. They should be informed that during labor and delivery any anesthetic procedure is optional and that there are associated risks.

TECHNIQUE

1. Patients in labor should be considered to have a full stomach and treated orally with an H_2 blocker (e.g., ranitidine [Zantac], 150 mg), metoclopramide (Reglan, 10 mg), and Bicitra (30 ml) at least 30 minutes before undergoing saddle block anesthesia.
2. Confirm that informed consent and permission forms are signed and in order.
3. Establish IV access with a 20-gauge or larger catheter and give a bolus of 500 to 1000 ml of IV fluids. The patient should be well hydrated before the procedure to minimize the risk of developing hypotension.

Note: Administer IV fluids slowly in women with pregnancy-induced hypertension.

4. For patients in labor, fetal monitoring should be used. For all patients, secure the continuous BP, ECG, and pulse oximetry monitors and record the initial values. Thereafter, monitor carefully for hypotension by cycling the BP monitor to take measurements at least every 2.5 minutes. Vital signs should be recorded on the anesthesia chart at least every 5 minutes.
5. Open the disposable spinal kit and mix the appropriate solutions. Use the filtered needle to draw up any solutions that will be administered intrathecally.
6. Place the patient in the sitting position with the back and neck flexed and the spine straight and not rotated. An assistant should stand in front of the patient during the procedure, helping the patient to maintain the proper position.
7. Locate the L2-3, L3-4, or L4-5 interspace. Perform the sterile preparations and drape the area.
8. Administer the local anesthesia (lidocaine 1%) to the interspace area by first making a skin wheal, then injecting into the deeper tissues in the same direction that the spinal needle will be advanced.
9. Insert the introducer needle into the supraspinous ligament at the proper angle to later direct the spinal needle into the subdural space.

Note: The proper angle depends on which interspace is used. At the L4-5 interspace, the proper direction for the needle tip is basically perpendicular (90 degrees) to slightly cephalad, whereas it decreases to about 70 degrees (and aimed cephalad) at the L2-3 interspace. The proper location is usually just below the inferior edge of the spinous process or slightly below that level (Fig. 176-1). For saddle block anesthesia, insertion angle and location are identical to those used for epidural anesthesia; however, the depth of insertion is unique to each procedure.

10. Insert the 3½-inch, 25-gauge spinal needle into the introducer. Next, advance the spinal needle into the intrathecal space. A "pop" is usually felt when the needle passes through the ligamentum flavum and into the space. Confirmation is obtained when spinal fluid flows from the hub of the spinal needle and continues to do so after the needle is rotated 360 degrees. Rotating the needle ensures that there is no tissue right at the tip of the needle that could later cause an obstruction and prevent injection (Fig. 176-2).

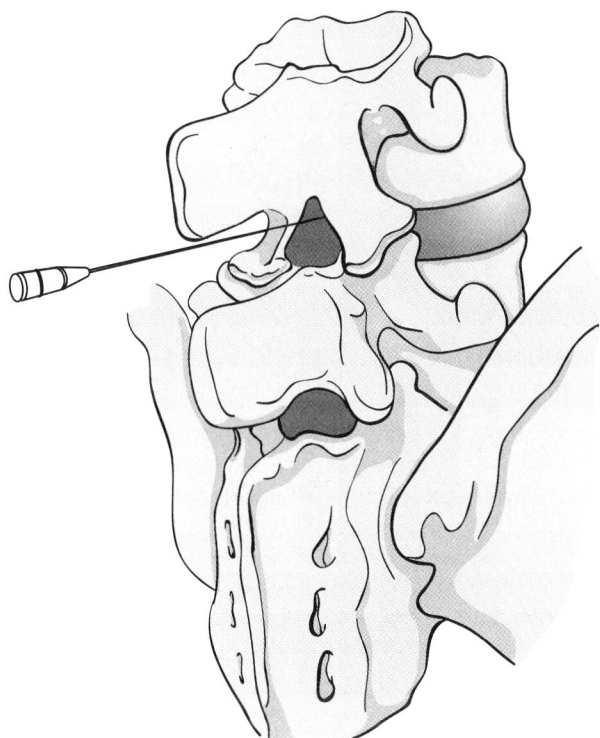

Fig. 176-1
Spinal needle introduced through the L-4 and L-5 interspace. Note that the needle is introduced just below the inferior border of the L-4 spinous process. The tip is directed at 90 degrees to the spine or slightly cephalad.

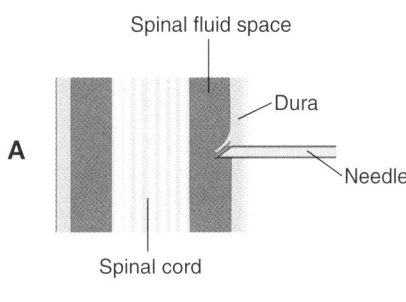

Spinal fluid space

Dura

Needle

A

Spinal cord

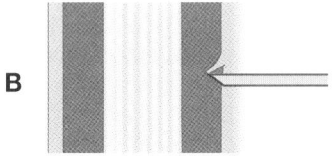

B

Fig. 176-2
A, Bevel of spinal needle occluded by a dural flap following puncture. The flap prevents free flow of spinal fluid through the spinal needle. **B,** Rotating the needle 180 degrees separates the dural flap from the bevel, allowing free flow of spinal fluid through the needle.

11. With the anesthetic solution syringe connected onto the hub of the spinal needle, a small amount of spinal fluid to confirm the placement of the needle. Next, if using lidocaine, withdraw an equal amount of CSF (0.5 to 1 ml) as the amount of lidocaine already in the syringe. Reinject the lidocaine/CSF–mixed solution through the spinal needle, slowly, over a period of 5 to 10 seconds. Tetracaine or bupivicaine should also be injected slowly. Do not aspirate or inject during a uterine contraction.

12. Remove the spinal needle, syringe, and introducer as a unit. Have the patient remain in the sitting position for 2 to 5 minutes to allow the anesthetic to "set" while it drifts downward into the spinal canal. Allowing the patient to become recumbent or lie in the lithotomy position too soon can result in a higher level of anesthesia than desired. However, if the patient becomes hypotensive, he or she should be returned to the recumbent position immediately and treatment initiated. Otherwise, at the end of the sitting period, place the patient in the lithotomy position. For pregnant women, left uterine displacement should be performed by lifting the uterus slightly and either manually pushing or pulling it toward the patient's left side. An assistant should perform this maneuver. This maneuver may be facilitated by having the patient turn slightly toward her left side. Left uterine displacement helps minimize or avoid vena caval compression syndrome (decreased venous return to the heart combined with venous congestion around the spinal cord). In a late

trimester pregnancy, this syndrome can lead to prolonged hypotension.

13. Check sensation to sharp objects (e.g., a needle) and record the level of anesthesia on the anesthesia record. Once adequate anesthesia has been established, the patient is prepared for delivery.

Note: The factors affecting the level of anesthesia include (1) the lumbar puncture site, (2) the volume of solution used, (3) the rate of injection, (4) the specific gravity of the solution used, and (5) the position of the patient.

COMPLICATIONS

Intraoperative and postoperative complications of saddle block anesthesia are essentially the same as for higher levels of spinal anesthesia.

Intraoperative Complications

- Hypotension may occur at any time, particularly during and shortly after administration of the anesthetic. It must be corrected rapidly by (1) placing the patient in a recumbent position, (2) infusing a rapid bolus of IV fluids (500 ml), (3) rapid administration of ephedrine 10 mg (IV), and (4) relieving pressure on the vena cava from the pregnant uterus by left uterine displacement.
- High spinal block with respiratory insufficiency or total spinal block with total respiratory arrest must be treated immediately with respiratory assistance and continued as needed for the duration of the block. Hypotension commonly occurs concurrently.
- Nausea and/or vomiting may occur concurrently with a drop in blood pressure and usually is relieved with correction of the hypotension by ephedrine (10 mg IV). If accompanied by bradycardia, the nausea and/or vomiting may regress after treatment with atropine (0.4 to 0.6 mg IV). Nausea and vomiting in the absence of other symptoms may be treated with metoclopramide (Reglan) (10 mg IV).
- Allergic reactions: use Benadryl 25 to 50 mg IV.
- Systemic reactions, including cardiac arrhythmia/ arrest, are rare. To treat this, routine advanced cardiac life support protocols should be followed.

Postoperative Complications

- Headache may occur, with an incidence as high as 5%. Most postspinal headaches can be treated conservatively (oral analgesics, fluids, rest), but some require more aggressive treatment, including a blood patch (see Chapter 213, Lumbar Puncture, for instructions on performing a blood patch).

- Urinary retention sometimes occurs, requiring catheterization.
- Neurologic sequellae (rare), including arachnoiditis, meningitis, palsies, and paralysis.

SUPPLIERS

Disposable trays, infusion pumps, needles, etc.
B. Braun Medical Inc.
824 12th Avenue
Bethlehem, PA 18018
Phone: 1-800-854-6851
Website: www.bbraunusa.com

Baxter Healthcare Corporation
Anesthesia & Critical Care
Pharmaceuticals
95 Spring Street
New Providence, NJ 07974
Phone: 1-908-286-7000
Website: www.Baxter.com

Becton, Dickinson and Co.
1 Becton Drive
Franklin Lakes, NJ 07417
Phone: 1-888-237-2762
Website: www.bd.com

Rusch Inc.
2450 Meadowbrook Parkway
Duluth, GA 30096
Phone: 1-770-623-0816
Website: www.ruschinc.com

Sims Portex Inc.
10 Bowman Drive
Keene, NH 03431
Phone: 1-800-258-5361
Website: www.portexusa.com

Epidural and saddle block needles
The Kendall Company
15 Hampshire Street
Mansfield, MA 02048
Phone: 1-800-962-9888
Website: www.kendallhq.com

CPT/BILLING CODES

62273   Injection, lumbar epidural, of blood or clot patch
62274   Injection of diagnostic or therapeutic anesthetic or antispasmodic substance (including narcotics); subarachnoid or subdural, single

ICD-9-CM DIAGNOSTIC CODES

(For other than pregnancy codes, see the appropriate procedure chapter for ICD-9-CM codes.)
650   Normal delivery
V22.2   Pregnant state, NOS

The fifth digit (X) is required for codes 640-648, 651-659, and 660-669 to denote the current episode of care.
0   Unspecified
1   Delivered, with or without mention of antepartum condition
2   Delivered, with mention of postpartum complication
3   Antepartum condition or complication
4   Postpartum condition or complication

652.2x   Breech presentation
653.5x   Unusually large fetus causing disproportion
660.4x   Shoulder dystocia
644.2x   Premature labor with delivery (<37 weeks)

Codes Related to Deliveries with Forceps or Vacuum
662.2x   Prolonged second stage of labor
659.7x   Abnormality in fetal heart rate or rhythm or fetal distress

Codes Related to Episiotomy and Episiotomy Repair and Codes for Repair of Low Vaginal Lacerations
664.0x   First-degree perineal laceration
664.1x   Second-degree perineal laceration
664.2x   Third-degree perineal laceration
664.3x   Fourth-degree perineal laceration
664.4x   Unspecified perineal laceration

ADDITIONAL RESOURCES

- See the sample patient education handout titled "Saddle Block Anesthesia" on page 1980 of Appendix G.

BIBLIOGRAPHY

Gerancher JC: Cauda equina syndrome following a single spinal administration of 5% hyperbaric lidocaine through a 25-gauge Whitacre needle, *Anesthesiology* 87(3):687, 1977.
Johnson ME: Potential neurotoxicity of spinal anesthesia with lidocaine, *Mayo Clin Proc* 75(9):921, 2000.

CHAPTER 177

Transcervical Amnioinfusion

David Glenn Weismiller

Amnioinfusion is an inexpensive, minimally invasive and proven therapeutic measure used since 1983 to restore or replace amniotic fluid during labor. It is performed by infusing normal saline or lactated Ringer's transcervically through a catheter, and there are two common applications: (1) to assist with the management of severe variable fetal heart rate decelerations and (2) to dilute thick meconium fluid. Overall, the procedure appears to pose little risk while offering considerable benefit in properly selected patients.

In theory, artificially increasing the amniotic fluid volume should protect the umbilical cord from compression, thus reducing the number and severity of variable decelerations. If decelerations become severe and persistent, it is possible for the fetus to become distressed and even require emergency operative delivery. A recent metaanalysis of nine randomized trials provides supportive evidence for amnioinfusion in this situation. Another summary of 12 published randomized trials suggests that using amnioinfusion for babies at risk of cord compression (e.g., repetitive variable decelerations, especially in the presence of oligohydramnios or amniotomy) decreases not only the occurrence of variable decelerations but also the number of cesarean sections. Yet another reference actually quantifies the reduction in variable decelerations and cesarean sections by nearly one half. Interestingly, amnioinfusion is also associated with a reduction in postpartum endometritis for women at risk.

Previous randomized controlled trials had suggested that the *prophylactic* use of amnioinfusion for oligohydramnios might reduce the incidence of fetal distress and cesarean intervention. However, recent comparison studies found no advantage to prophylactic amnioinfusion as opposed to using amnioinfusion only when fetal heart rate decelerations occur.

Diluting thick meconium fluid may also reduce the risk of meconium aspiration syndrome. Meconium passage occurs in three distinct situations: (1) as a physiologic maturational event, (2) as a response to acute hypoxic events, and (3) as a response to chronic intrauterine hypoxia. It has long been known that the risk of meconium aspiration is high in patients with thick meconium, particularly if associated with an episode of fetal hypoxia. In contrast, thin meconium is not associated with an increased perinatal mortality rate or incidence of meconium aspiration syndrome. Therefore, diluting meconium in the already potentially compromised fetus is postulated to have a positive effect on neonatal outcome.

A recent summary of 10 published randomized trials indicates that the use of amnioinfusion for moderate to thick meconium is associated with (1) a reduction in heavy meconium staining of the liquor, (2) a reduction in variable fetal heart rate decelerations, and (3) a trend toward reduced caesarean section rates. No perinatal deaths were reported. Where facilities for perinatal surveillance were limited, amnioinfusion was associated with a reduction in meconium aspiration syndrome, neonatal hypoxic ischemic encephalopathy, and need for neonatal ventilation or intensive care unit admission. Although most of the studies involved small numbers of participants (i.e., firm conclusions cannot be reached), there was a trend toward reduced overall perinatal mortality.

Different protocols for amnioinfusion are used, but they all appear to be safe, easy to perform, and are associated with few complications. Future academic attention should be directed not toward finding the perfect protocol but rather toward publicizing the effectiveness of amnioinfusion.

INDICATIONS

- Repeated severe variable fetal heart rate decelerations not responsive to conventional therapy (e.g., left-sided labor, intravenous hydration, oxygen therapy, etc.)
- Thick or particulate meconium staining of the amniotic fluid

Editor's note: Obviously amnioinfusion might be a consideration during labor in *many* pregnancies because variable decelerations are very common. In reality, experienced clinicians use amnioinfusion in certain selected situations. An example is the multiparous pregnancy that has only an hour or so remaining before the second stage of labor, yet the fetal strip shows very deep, severe variables that last a long time (perhaps as long as the contraction). We have all nervously watched such a labor knowing that these deep variables may exhaust the fetus. It is nice to have amnioinfusion available as a possible preventive measure. A similar situation may be seen with oligohydramnios, or even borderline oligohydramnios. Often these infants endure a stormy labor with deep variables early in labor. Amnioinfusion may be an option in these situations.

One study at our institution (University of Texas Medical School at Houston) indicated that amnioinfusion for thick meconium reduced the number of infants with meconium below the cords. Although this was not convincing enough evidence for all of our obstetricians to use amnioinfusion for thick meconium, the information was beneficial to most of our primary care clinicians.

CONTRAINDICATIONS

- Amnionitis
- Polyhydramnios
- Uterine hypertonus
- Multiple gestation
- Known fetal anomaly
- Known uterine anomaly
- Severe fetal distress
- Nonvertex presentation
- Fetal scalp pH <7.20
- Placental abruption or placenta previa (known or suspected)
- Patient refusal or uncooperative patient

EQUIPMENT

- Intrauterine pressure catheter
- Normal saline or lactated Ringer's at room temperature
- Fetal monitor
- Intravenous tubing
- Intravenous pump
- Fetal scalp electrode*
- Sterile gloves (for insertion)
- Vaginal lubricant (for insertion)
- Fluid warmer (if the fluid is to be infused at a rate of more than 15 ml/min)

---

*Recommended, not required.

PREPROCEDURE PATIENT PREPARATION

Before performing the procedure, discuss it with the patient (and family, if present). Inform her of the risks and explain why amnioinfusion should be beneficial. (For severe repetitive variable decelerations, amnioinfusion decreases the number of variable decelerations and cesarean sections and possibly the risk of postpartum endometritis. Diluting thick meconium fluid may reduce the risk of meconium aspiration syndrome.) Describe alternative modes of intervention (if applicable) and obtain informed consent. Answer any questions that the patient (or family) may have.

TECHNIQUE

1. Perform a sterile vaginal examination to confirm cephalic presentation, determine the degree of dilation, and exclude a cord prolapse.
2. Place a fetal scalp electrode (recommended, not required) or ensure adequate fetal monitoring.
3. Insert an intrauterine pressure catheter, and document the resting tone. The resting tone should be less than 15 mm Hg.
4. Link normal saline (or lactated Ringer's) at room temperature to the intravenous tubing. Prime the tubing, as it would be done for intravenous use.
5. Attach the tubing to the infusion port of the intrauterine pressure catheter (Fig. 177-1).
6a. For patients with repetitive severe variable decelerations:
    a. Start the infusion with an initial bolus of 250 ml of fluid over 20 to 30 minutes.
    b. Next, adjust the rate of infusion according to the severity of decelerations. The usual infusion rate is 10 to 20 ml/min up to a total of 600 ml infused, or until resolution of the variable decelerations, if that occurs first.
    c. With resolution, continue the infusion for an additional 250 ml beyond the volume at which the decelerations resolved.
    d. Terminate the infusion if 800 to 1000 ml of saline does not resolve the decelerations. However, if decelerations do not resolve completely, yet there is an increase in frequency and severity when the fluid is discontinued, it may be prudent to resume the infusion.
6b. In patients with thick meconium-stained fluid:
    a. Start with a bolus of 250 to 500 ml of fluid over 30 minutes.
    b. Follow the bolus by a constant infusion of 1 to 3 ml/min.

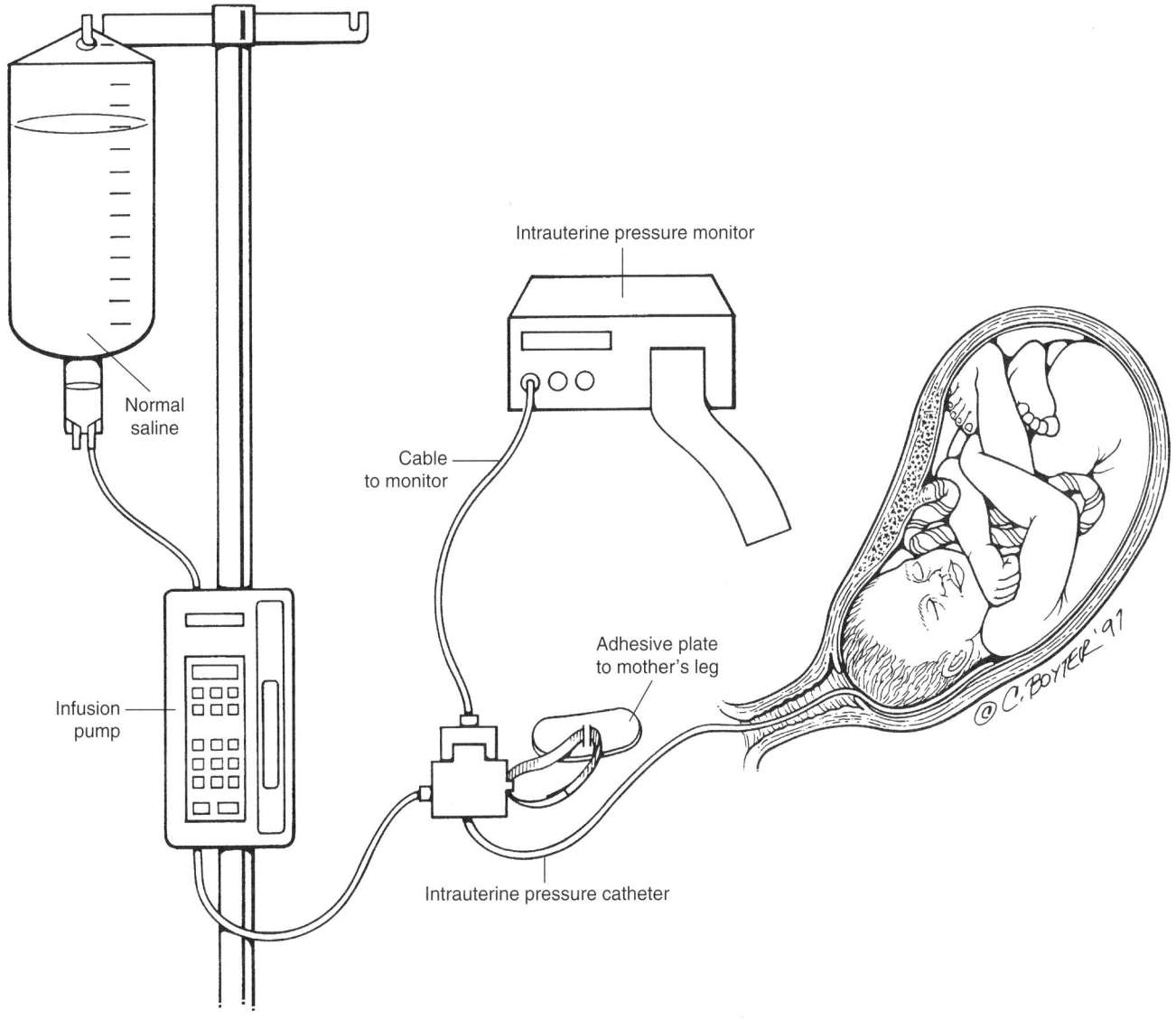

Fig. 177-1
Procedure for amnioinfusion. (From Weismiller DG: *Am Fam Phys* 157[3]:509, 1998 [artist: Charles Boyer].)

7. Warm the fluid to body temperature if it is administered at a rate of greater than 15 ml/min.
8. Monitor fetal heart rate and resting uterine tone continuously during the intervention; monitor intrauterine pressure via the same intrauterine pressure catheter, a second one, or a double-lumen catheter.
9. Discontinue the infusion if uterine tone becomes persistently elevated or if the flow of fluid from the vagina stops. Allow the uterine pressure to equilibrate over 5 minutes, and reassess the resting uterine tone. Discontinue the infusion if the new resting tone is 15 mm Hg above the baseline resting tone or 30 mm Hg maximum.
10. After the initial bolus, it is extremely important to verify that fluid is flowing from the vagina and that volume overload is not occurring.

COMPLICATIONS

There are occasional amnioinfusion failures. The possible causes for failure include inadequate infusion volume or rate, rapid progression to second stage of labor, or cord complications; however, the cause of the majority of failures is unknown (Fig. 177-1).

In one study, all teaching hospitals were surveyed to determine how, when, and with what results amnioinfusion is being performed in the United States. It was found that neither the method employed nor the number of infusions performed appeared to significantly increase the risk for complications. The fact that the mean number of amnioinfusions performed per year is similar between centers that did and centers that did not report complications suggests that complications are generally infrequent or, perhaps, that the risk of complication decreases as clinician experience increases. (It also might indicate a reporting problem!)

- Isolated cases of umbilical cord prolapse have been reported, but they are well within the usual occurrence rate of prolapse in pregnancies with vertex presentation, even when amnoinfusion is not used.
- Uterine tone may increase, and hypertonus has been reported; thus monitoring intrauterine pressure, the total volume infused, and the continuous flow of fluid from the vagina is important.
- Prolonged fetal bradycardia has been reported following rapid administration (50 ml/min) of unwarmed fluid.
- Prophylactic amnioinfusion (although not recommended) was associated with increased intrapartum fever.
- Other reported rare complications:
  — Uterine scar disruption (one reported case)
  — Iatrogenic polyhydramnios and elevated intrauterine pressure resulting in fetal bradycardia (one reported case)
  — Amniotic fluid embolism (five reported cases, all associated with previously reported risk factors for amniotic fluid embolism)
- Rare complications associated with placement of an intrauterine pressure monitor (IUPC):
  — Uterine perforation
  — Umbilical cord trauma
  — Placental abruption
- Prolonged use of an IUPC is associated with an increased risk of perinatal infection.

Note: Most trials reviewed have been too small to address the possibility of rare but serious adverse maternal effects of amnioinfusion.

CPT/BILLING CODE

59899   Unlisted procedure, maternity care and delivery

ICD-9-CM DIAGNOSTIC CODES

792.3   Nonspecific abnormal findings in fluid surrounding fetus
656.3   Fetal distress

ADDITIONAL RESOURCES

- See the sample patient education handout titled "Transcervical Amnioinfusion" on page 1981 of Appendix G.
- See the sample patient consent form titled "Transcervical Amnioinfusion" on page 1983 of Appendix G.

BIBLIOGRAPHY

Hofmeyr GJ, Gulmezoglu AM, Nikodem VC, de Jager M: Amnioinfusion, *Eur J Obstet Gynecol Reprod Biol* 64:159, 1996.

Hofmeyr GJ: Amnioinfusion for meconium-stained liquor in labour (Cochrane Review). In *The Cochrane Library*, 3, 2002, Oxford: Update Software.

Hofmeyr GJ: Amnioinfusion for umbilical cord compression in labour (Cochrane Review). In *The Cochrane Library*, 3, 2002, Oxford: Update Software.

Hofmeyr GJ: Prophylactic versus therapeutic amnioinfusion for oligohydramnios in labour (Cochrane Review). In *The Cochrane Library*, 3, 2002, Oxford: Update Software.

Klingner MC, Kruse J: Meconium aspiration syndrome: pathophysiology and prevention, *J Am Board Fam Pract* 12(6):450, 1999.

Morrison EH: Common peripartum emergencies, *Am Fam Physician* 58(7):1593, 1998.

Schrimmer DB, Macri CJ, Paul RH: Prophylactic amnioinfusion as a treatment for oligohydramnios in laboring patients: a prospective, randomized trial, *Am J Obstet Gynecol* 165:972, 1991.

Wenstrom K, Andrews WW, Maher JE: Amnioinfusion survey: prevalence, protocols, and complications, *Obstet Gynecol* 86:572, 1995.

WEBSITES

www.cochrane.org

CHAPTER 178

Vaginal Delivery

Carol Osborn

The management of a vaginal delivery begins with the onset of labor. Labor is a complex process of coordinated uterine contractions resulting in cervical effacement and dilation, followed by descent and delivery of the newborn and placenta. This can be a rapid, precipitous process lasting only 1 to 2 hours or a long, slow process taking 1 to 2 days. Routinely the birth occurs following a 6- to 12-hour period of labor.

Over the last 30 years, labor in this country has evolved from being a period of maternal isolation to being a patient- or family-focused experience. During this same evolution, practitioners have begun to question the scientific evidence surrounding many of their routine interventions. For example, interventions such as perineal shaves and enemas, when studied, have turned out to be cultural or habitual interventions that do not produce better outcomes. Even the routine use of electronic fetal monitoring (EFM) has not been proven to produce healthier babies. Although EFM technology may seem helpful, at least eight randomized clinical trials have failed to show improvement in fetal morbidity or mortality with its use. Meanwhile, cesarean section rates have increased dramatically, largely the result of tracings falsely indicating severe fetal distress. Such interventions have certainly "medicalized" and complicated the process, but they have not necessarily improved the outcomes. Since the evidence relating to labor is slowly evolving, clinicians are encouraged to remain up to date. An excellent resource for reviewing the current evidence on labor management and its associated interventions is the Cochrane Collaboration (see the "Websites" section at the end of this chapter).

Editor's note: It has become one editor's practice to avoid *any* intervention, except perhaps a heparin lock IV, as long as labor is progressing and no more data is needed. Any intervention has its risks, and perhaps none should be performed unless indicated. An example is amniotomy: Unless there is evidence of fetal distress (e.g., where it would be useful to check for meconium) or labor has been prolonged, amniotomy may not be helpful and could cause problems (e.g., uterine tetany). What does the evidence show? Early amniotomy is associated with both benefits and risks. Benefits include a reduction in

labor duration and a possible reduction in abnormal 5-minute Apgar scores. However, at least one metaanalysis failed to find that routine early amniotomy reduced the risk of cesarean delivery; rather, there was a trend toward increased numbers of cesarean sections. This suggests that amniotomy should be reserved for women with abnormal labor progress, for nulliparas in an active management of labor protocol (AML) or for possible fetal distress. Another example: A fetal scalp clip may not need to be applied if external EFM is adequate. In fact, the evidence indicates that if there is an adequate nursing to patient ratio, results from intermittent auscultation may be superior to either internal or external EFM.

This chapter focuses on delivering the infant, the dramatic result of labor, which is often an unpredictable process for both the mother and the fetus. Understanding the process of labor maximizes the potential for appropriate management and a successful outcome. The following discussion outlines a normal labor for a vertex, singleton fetus. The technique that follows is for the same. During this process, mother and fetus should be monitored by the method of choice.

LABOR

Labor begins with the identification of true labor, whose onset is often confused with false or prodromal labor. True labor is characterized by contractions that are regular, of increasing intensity, lasting a minute each, and associated with cervical change. False labor contractions do not progress in intensity and are usually irregular, but they can produce discomfort. In addition, sedation may stop false labor but rarely halts true labor.

Labor is divided into three progressive stages: *first stage*, from onset of true labor until complete cervical dilation; *second stage*, from complete dilation to delivery of the infant; *third stage*, from delivery of the infant to delivery of the placenta. The median time of each stage is different for nulliparas than for multiparas (Table 178-1). Protraction disorders are defined by a slow rate of either dilation or of descent, after onset of active labor (e.g., low end of normal range: 1 cm/hour dilation for

TABLE 178-1

Parameters for Progression of Spontaneous Labor*

Parameter	Median
Nulliparas	
Total duration	10.1 hr
Stages	
First	9.7 hr
Second	33.0 min
Third	5.0 min
Latent phase (duration)	6.4 hr
Dilation (rate)	3.0 cm/hr
Descent (rate)	3.3 cm/hr
Multiparas	
Total duration	6.2 hr
Stages	
First	8.0 hr
Second	8.5 min
Third	5.0 min
Latent phase (duration)	4.8 hr
Dilation (rate)	5.7 cm/hr
Descent (rate)	6.6 cm/hr

Modified from Gabbe SG, editor: *Obstetrics: normal & problem pregnancies,* ed 3, New York, 1996, Churchill Livingstone.

*Protraction disorders are defined by either a slow rate of dilation or of descent after onset of active labor (e.g., low end of normal for dilation and descent: 1 cm/hr dilation for nulliparas, 1.2 cm/hr for multiparas; 1 cm/hr descent for nulliparas, 2 cm/hr for multiparas). Progression at a rate below these numbers may warrant an intervention such as oxytocin augmentation.

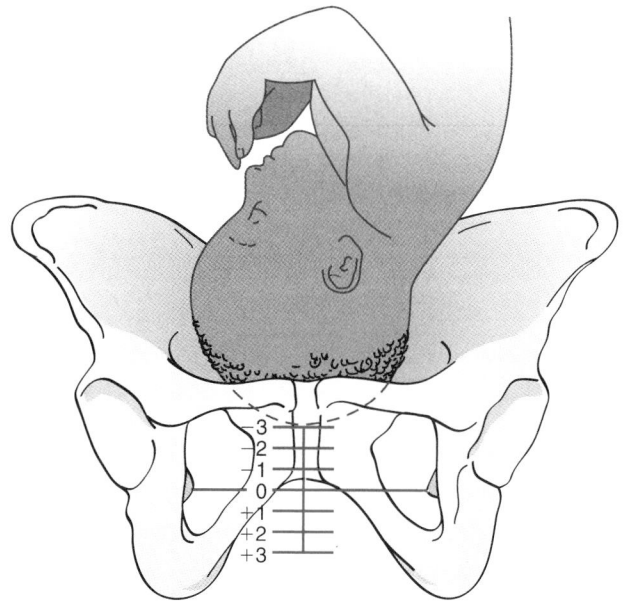

Fig. 178-1

Descent of fetal head into the pelvis. Zero station is diagnosed when the fetal vertex has reached the level of the ischial spines. (Redrawn from Niswander K: *Obstetrics: essentials of clinical practice,* ed 2, Boston, 1981, Little, Brown.)

nulliparas, 1.2 cm/hour for multiparas; 1 cm/hour descent for nulliparas, 2 cm/hour for multiparas). Progression at a rate below those defined numbers may warrant an intervention such as oxytocin augmentation.

Editors' note: Most women in the United States have heard a horror story of "pain" and a prolonged "labor" associated with a delivery. It is one editor's opinion that clinicians could do no harm by avoiding or minimizing the use of such terms. These terms have negative connotations, or at the least they invoke fear and anxiety, especially among nulliparas. One simple change is to use the word contraction instead of "pain." This would be more in keeping with pregnancy and delivery being a healthy process as opposed to being a condition and a remedy. If women hear the word "labor," it could clearly be considered hard work as opposed to being an anticipated and desired set of strong contractions. If she hopes for the strong contractions needed to produce the long-awaited and desired delivery of a new life, it may not seem like pure "labor." (See Chapter 212, Medical Hypnosis, for more information to enhance deliveries.)

As the cervix dilates, the fetus descends through the birth canal. Using the force of each contraction, the fetal head negotiates incrementally through the angles of the maternal pelvis, following a standard pattern of movements known as the cardinal movements of labor:

1. Engagement
   - Defined by descent of the biparietal diameter of the fetus to a level below the maternal pelvic inlet.
   - Often occurs before the onset of labor, especially in nulliparas.
   - Is verified clinically when the lowest portion of the occiput (not caput) is palpated at or below the maternal ischial spines (0 station).
   - In almost every case, it indicates the maternal bony pelvis is sufficient to allow full descent of the head. In turn, this confirms that the pelvis is adequate to allow delivery of the infant.
   - Verification may be difficult if the fetal head is molded or in an occiput posterior presentation.

2. Descent (Fig. 178-1)
   - Slow and intermittent process.
   - Most rapid at the end of the first stage and during the second stage of labor.
   - Measured by station (level of presenting part). Quantified by how many centimeters the presenting part is above or below the ischial spines (e.g., −2 station is 2 cm above the ischial spines, +2 station is 2 cm below the ischial spines).

3. Flexion
   - The force of contractions pushes the head into a flexed position (Fig. 178-2, *A*). It remains in this position until the head has descended to the level of the vulva.
   - This position aids with descent by minimizing the diameter of the presenting part.
   - Normally, the posterior fontanel is in the center of the dilating cervix.

A   **B**   **C**

D   **E**

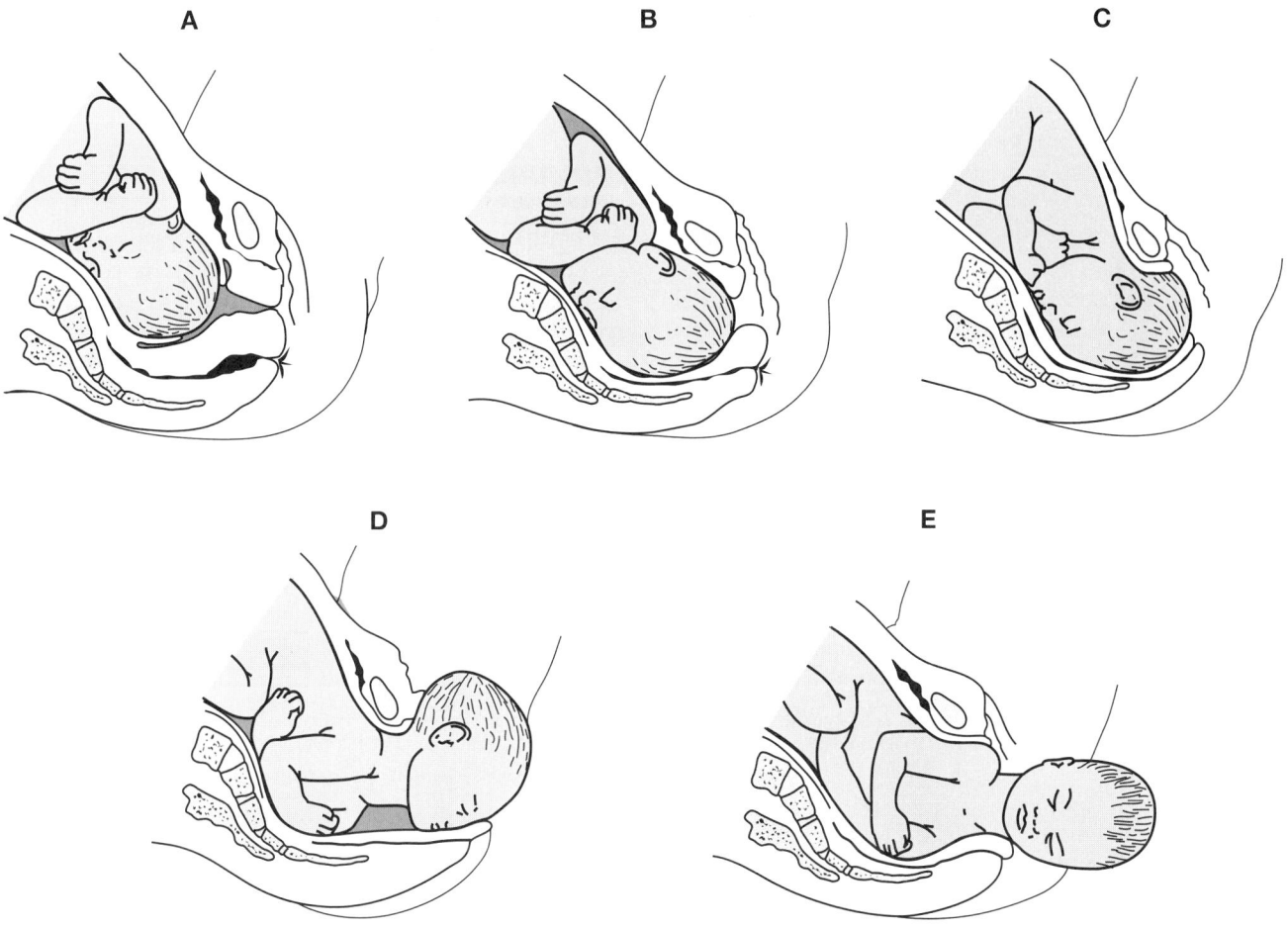

Fig. 178-2
A, Engagement of flexed head. **B,** Left occipitoanterior (LOA) position. **C,** Anterior rotation of head to occipitoanterior (OA) position. **D,** Extension of head. **E,** External rotation of head. (Redrawn from Pernoll M: *Benson and Pernoll's handbook of obstetrics and gynecology,* ed 9, New York, 2001, McGraw-Hill.)

4. Internal rotation
• Takes place during descent and is a passive fetal motion.
• After engagement, the head rotates transversely but must eventually rotate anteriorly (Fig. 178-2, *B*) (or posteriorly) to pass the maternal ischial spines and reach the perineum.
• The final position of the vertex is usually left occipitoanterior (LOA), occiput anterior (OA) (Fig. 178-2, *C*), or right occipitoanterior (ROA); however, it is occasionally (5% to 10%) occiput posterior (OP).
5. Extension
• The force of contractions from above meets the force of resistance from the pelvic muscles below and interacts to use the pubic symphysis as a fulcrum. This combination of forces and a fulcrum pushes the head around the pubic bone (Fig. 178-2, *D*).
• The head becomes extended with delivery as a result of these forces.

• Extension occurs fairly rapidly and is observed clinically when the perineum distends.
6. External rotation and restitution
• After delivery, the head rotates back to a transverse position and the shoulders rotate into an antero-posterior (AP) position, before they are delivered (Fig. 178-2, *E*).

Although dilation and descent may occur rapidly, the path is often full of stops and starts, which may lead to a misinterpretation of the progress and a desire to intervene. There are three common pitfalls of labor management that can increase the risk of the patient having an operative delivery (If practiced commonly they can also increase a hospital's operative delivery rate): (1) failing to differentiate true from false labor (leading to premature interventions), (2) being impatient during the management of a slowly progressing nullipara, and (3) attempting to induce an unfavorable cervix.

In an attempt to reduce prolonged labor in nulliparas, the AML protocol was created and studied at the National Maternity Hospital in Dublin, Ireland. It was successful in not only decreasing the average length of labor but it also decreased the overall cesarean section rate to 7%. The AML protocol for nulliparas has six underlying tenets:

1. Extensive prenatal education
2. A specific definition of labor
   a. Painful contractions and presence of bloody show (blood-stained mucus), or
   b. Painful contractions and complete cervical effacement, regardless of dilation, presence of bloody show (blood-stained mucus)
3. Early amniotomy (1 hour after admission)
4. Close assessment of labor progress (recheck 1 hour after artificial rupture of membranes [AROM]; if cervix has dilated less than 1 cm, start oxytocin)
5. High-dose oxytocin (start with 6 mU/min and increase every 15 minutes)
6. Continuous support by an experienced (parous) laywoman or doula. Emotional support early in labor may be more critical than support given to a woman after she is admitted to the hospital and may have already chosen an epidural.

Randomized controlled trials of AML in the United States have shown that while AML may shorten the duration of labor, it does not necessarily reduce the numbers of operative deliveries. Some researchers have shown a reduction in cesarean deliveries, but none as dramatic as in the Irish studies. As it turns out, having clinicians continuously review cesarean delivery cases in the hospitals for these studies may have had more of an impact on the rates than the AML protocol.

INDICATIONS

- Vertex presentation, active labor, vulva distended, and deliverable baby
- Fetal distress in a deliverable baby

CONTRAINDICATIONS

- Cord prolapse
- Placenta previa or vasa previa
- Abnormal fetal lie (e.g., footling breech, transverse lie, persistent brow presentation)
- Prior classical cesarean section
- Active herpes simplex infection
- Pelvic deformities
- Congenital deformities (hydrocephalus)
- Invasive cervical carcinoma

Note: New American College of Obstetricians and Gynecologists (ACOG) guidelines recommend against delivering breech babies vaginally.

EQUIPMENT

Although equipment setups vary, depending on the hospital or the staff, the following list is considered standard for a *birthing room*. In addition to what is listed below, deliveries in an *operating room* require a full gown, a mask, and foot and head covers.

- Oxygen with flowmeter (one setup for mother and another for infant)
- Delivery bed (should be able to break down into a modified lithotomy position, if needed)
- Setup for infant (infant warmer, oxygen with bag and mask, suction with DeLee, infant laryngoscope, intubation equipment, umbilical catheter, medications, and monitoring equipment for resuscitation [see Chapter 182, Neonatal Resuscitation])
- Sterile equipment tray or table containing the following (see also Fig. 178-3):
  — 10-ml tube for cord blood
  — Scissors (blunt or sharp-ended, for cutting the cord)
  — Bulb syringe
  — One plastic cord clamp (may use artery forceps for the other)
  — Two curved artery forceps
  — Two ring forceps clamps
  — Drapes and towels
  — Placenta basin
  — Gown and sterile gloves (gown is optional)

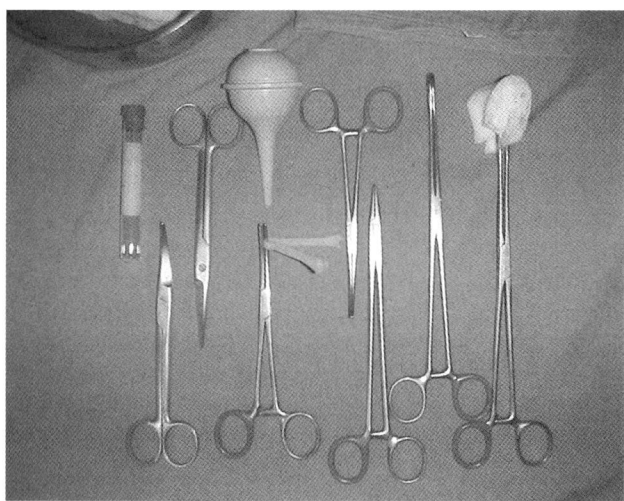

Fig. 178-3
Instruments for vaginal delivery. *Left to right:* Cord blood tube, two scissors (blunt and sharp edge), bulb syringe, cord clamp, two curved artery forceps, needle holder, two ring forceps.

- Optional equipment for sterile tray or table (also see Chapter 167, Episiotomy):
  — Second pair of scissors (blunt-ended for episiotomy)
  — Needle holder nontraumatic forceps, Allis clamps
  — 10-ml syringe
  — 22-gauge, 1½-inch needle (for local anesthesia)
  — 1% lidocaine, without epinephrine
  — Two 3-0 absorbable sutures with tapered needles
  — Gauze pads (4 × 4)
  — Sterile speculum
  — Betadine or surgical soap for prep and betadine solution
- Emergency kit (for precipitous deliveries):
  — Sterile gloves (large size)
  — Two sterile towels
  — One pair of blunt-ended scissors
  — One plastic cord clamp
  — Two curved artery forceps
  — Gauze pads (4 × 4)
  — Bulb syringe
  — Placenta basin

PREPROCEDURE PATIENT PREPARATION

Amazingly, there has been a recent increase in the rate of cesarean sections in certain parts of the country. A certain expert has even called for a 50% cesarean rate! The controversy seems to revolve around three issues: (1) whether women should have the choice of cesarean, with or without an indication, (2) whether reducing the rate of cesarean deliveries below a certain threshold will actually increase the number of poor outcomes, and (3) recent vaginal birth after cesarean (VBAC) safety data.

1. *Choice:* Advocates on behalf of childbearing women have been asking for "freedom of choice" in many areas for years. With modern anesthesia being safe, why should a cesarean be different than any other elective surgery? One answer is that no other form of intraabdominal or pelvic surgery is performed without a medical indication. Without trivializing the patient, the clinician must explore the reasons why they might want such surgery. A common misperception is that the risks of perineal injury, pelvic floor and rectal sphincter damage, sexual dysfunction, or damage to the baby outweighs the risks of major surgery.
2. *Risk of reducing rate of cesareans:* This has been explored from many angles, and after an exhaustive review of the evidence, recent national guidelines call for a further reduction in the cesarean section rate. By 2010, the guidelines call

for a rate for primary cesarean sections of 15.5% (down from 17.8% in 1997). They call for a rate for repeat cesarean sections of 63% (down from 71% in 1997).

3. *VBAC safety:* Although (ACOG) has modified their position on VBAC, the risk of complications from a spontaneous VBAC remains less than that for a cesarean section. The risks of augmentation depend on many things, including the availability of the clinician, the length of time required to perform an immediate operative delivery, and many other aspects of facility support.

It is likely that these debates will continue and that the cesarean rate will continue to increase. Therefore advocates of vaginal delivery need to stay up to date with the statistics, remain involved in their community, and be prepared to educate patients and communities regarding these issues. They may even have to get involved in preventing their hospital from requiring informed consent for every vaginal birth (as opposed to for operative deliveries), which some hospitals are doing. (See the sample patient consent form titled "Vaginal Delivery" on page 1986 of Appendix G.)

In addition to being prepared to discuss the pros of vaginal delivery over a cesarean, the clinician can help the patient develop a birth plan. This will often enhance her birthing experience. Such a plan usually gives her a sense of control over the situation, a sense of security with the process and it may decrease her anxiety. In addition, it is always best to have discussed preferences and procedures before the patient is anesthetized, uncomfortable, or stressed (Fig. 178-4).

Completing a birth plan also helps the clinician assess the patient's preparedness for a baby. Certain aspects of anticipatory guidance should be discussed.

TECHNIQUE

Typically, as the cervix begins to fully dilate, the intensity of the contractions increases and the patient starts to feel the urge to push. Even if the patient has regional anesthesia, she will feel pressure as the fetus begins to descend more rapidly. When the cervix is completely dilated, the second stage of labor has begun.

Note: Following the onset of active labor, if no change in dilation occurs in 2 hours despite adequate contractions, oxytocin stimulation or augmentation is indicated. If the adequacy of contractions is uncertain, an intrauterine pressure monitor can be placed (see Chapter 172, Intrauterine Pressure Catheter Insertion). If contractions are deemed adequate for 2 hours, some will consider performing a cesarean delivery. Recent guidelines suggest that up to 4 hours of oxytocin augmentation with arrest of active labor is also safe and effective.

Anticipatory Guidance and Patient Preferences for Birthing Plan (checklist completed by clinician)

Patient name: _____

Date: _____ Clinician: _____

Answers to the following will help determine the patient's individual preferences and amount of preparation during prenatal care, labor, and postpartum care:

Is prenatal birth education (Lamaze) planned? ☐ Yes ☐ No

   Who will attend Lamaze? _____

If no rupture of membranes has occurred (ROM), is an enema desired? ☐ Yes ☐ No

Pubic hair prep? ☐ No prep ☐ Mini prep ☐ Full prep

Diet preferences: ☐ Clear liquids ☐ Ice chips ☐ Nothing

IV access preferences: ☐ Hep-Lock ☐ None ☐ IV with lactated Ringer's at 100 ml/hr

Fetal assessment (low-risk patient):

   ☐ Continuous electronic fetal monitoring for 20 minutes (baseline strip); then, if baseline is reassuring, periodic auscultation every 30 minutes in first stage, then every 15 minutes in second stage (auscultation done during contraction and for 30 seconds following).

   ☐ Continuous electronic fetal monitoring.

   ☐ Scalp clip okay.

Preferences for maximizing comfort during labor (anesthesia?): _____ Position _____

Father to be present during labor? ☐ Yes ☐ No

Female support person (doula) to be present? ☐ Yes ☐ No

Patient attitude toward episiotomy? _____ (desired) _____ (only if necessary)

Infant feeding preferences? ☐ Breast-feeding ☐ Bottle feeding

For male infant, is circumcision desired? ☐ Yes ☐ No

Preferred clinician for baby: _____

Rooming-in with baby? ☐ Yes ☐ No

Postpartum contraception preference: _____

Baby's name? _____

Hospital preregistration? ☐ Yes ☐ No

Mother has visited labor and delivery? ☐ Yes ☐ No

Encouraged intrapartum ambulation, frequent position changes? ☐ Yes ☐ No

Practiced positions for emergencies (e.g., knee chest, rolling onto hands/knees)? ☐ Yes ☐ No

If the clinician provides anticipatory guidance, it may not only improve the outcomes, but it may also give mother a greater sense of security. The results of this questionnaire should be dictated or copied, signed by the patient, and a copy given to the patient. She should bring it to labor and delivery when admitted.

Fig. 178-4
Anticipatory guidance and patient preferences for birthing plan.

After the second stage of labor has begun, the length of time until delivery varies (Table 178-1). Two or three explosive pushes may be enough to deliver a multipara, whereas a nullipara with regional anesthesia may take 3 hours. If labor stalls during this stage, consider oxytocin stimulation. To prevent maternal exhaustion, if the infant is stable, alternating periods of rest and pushing is recommended. In fact, recent publications indicate that for women with epidural anesthesia, it may be beneficial to have the mother refrain from actively pushing until the vertex is at the introitus.

Note: It is imperative for the mother to reach full dilation before allowing her to push, especially for nulliparas. Pushing against a portion of undilated cervix may result in a cervical tear, soft tissue dystocia, or an exhausted mother. Soft tissue dystocia can sometimes be confirmed by examination (e.g., a previously 100% effaced and dilated cervix has become thickened and regressed to only 8 cm dilation). In other situations, the swelling and edema of soft tissues will be located around the cervix. If the fetus is stable, management options include allowing the mother to rest and to not push for as long as possible if contractions are adequate. Oxytocin augmentation may also be helpful. Even sedation may be helpful until the soft tissue dystocia resolves.

One of the most common reasons for a prolonged second stage of labor is persistent OP position. On average, the OP position will prolong labor by 1 hour in multiparas and 2 hours in nulliparas. Consider the possibility of OP position if labor is predominantly felt in the back. A persistent anterior cervical lip or an easily palpable anterior fontanel may also be associated with the OP position. To confirm the OP position by examination, the infant's skull sutures should be followed until the posterior fontanel can be palpated. If an ear is palpable, the direction that the ear is facing will also help determine which direction the baby is facing.

Preparation for delivery should begin at the onset of the second stage for the multipara and as the vertex reaches the pelvic floor in the nullipara.

Preparation

1. Put on sterile gloves and consider a gown. Remember to observe universal blood and body fluid precautions.
2. Prepare the delivery tray.
3. Turn on the warmer for the bassinette and notify the nursery staff for meconium-staining or fetal distress. Make sure that all necessary equipment is available for a neonatal resuscitation (see Chapter 182, Neonatal Resuscitation).
4. Verify that all needed equipment is on the sterile tray or table and within reaching distance. Empty the mother's bladder (usually requires using a catheter with aseptic technique if she has an epidural).
5. Make an attempt to rotate a persistent OP vertex to an OA position (see the note in the following section).
6. Wash the perineal area with a surgical soap *(optional).*

Position of the Woman

Allow the patient to find a comfortable position for pushing and resting. The rationale for each position is noted below as well as possible inconveniences or complications for each position.
1. Modified dorsal

- Semisitting position with knee flexed and legs widely separated; the mother can grip below her knees for leverage when pushing
- Good position for multipara deliveries
2. Squatting, kneeling
- More physiologic for pushing
- Less discomfort with pushing
- Fewer perineal tears
- Increased incidence of hemorrhage
3. Lithotomy
- Better access for the provider, so this position is often used for instrumentation
- Difficult position for pushing
- Increased risk for maternal aspiration
4. Left lateral
- Left side with knees flexed and separated
- Offers better clinician access for head control
- Need an assistant to hold upper leg

Note: To rotate the fetus from the OP position, any maternal position that causes her to curl forward from the hips is felt to be helpful. Various positions and activities can be tried, such as squatting or ambulating, or placing mother on her hands and knees, on her side, or with her back arched. The theory is that with most of these positions, the infant will become uncomfortable and be encouraged to turn itself. If the various positions fail to cause rotation, manual rotation can be attempted. Place the mother in the lithotomy, lateral Sims', or hands and knees position. With a hand in the posterior pelvis behind the occiput, attempt to rotate and flex the head with a contraction, while the mother is pushing. If the fetus is straight OP, the clinician's dominant hand should be used. If the fetus is partially rotated, use whichever hand is easiest to rotate it in the direction of the shortest distance to OA.

Anesthesia Options (if Desired)

- Regional anesthesia. (See Chapter 3, Epidural Anesthesia and Analgesia, and Chapter 176, Saddle Block Anesthesia. Also see Chapter 171, Intrathecal Analgesia, for the first stage of labor and for part of the second stage.)
- Pericervical block, for first stage of labor to decrease the discomfort with contractions (see Chapter 174, Paracervical Block).
- Pudendal block, for perineal pain (see Chapter 175, Pudendal Anesthesia).
- Local infiltration of lidocaine if episiotomy is considered (see Chapter 167, Episiotomy).

Delivery

1. Observe the perineum for distention due to the fetal head. The time to consider an episiotomy is when the introital opening is at least 3 to 4 cm in diameter. Compare the head size with the elasticity of the perineum, as well as with the amount of room in the pel-

vis. Will the perineum stretch around the head, and how much tension will there be in case it tears?

2. If an episiotomy is to be performed, the best time to perform it is when the opening is 5 to 6 cm (see Chapter 167, Episiotomy). This procedure is clearly optional. It is usually only performed if it is unsafe for the mother to push (cardiac disease or prolonged second stage), for significant fetal distress (to expedite delivery), before reducing a shoulder dystocia, if an infant is premature or breech, or to make room if there is risk of perineal trauma (e.g., large infant or use of forceps or vacuum).

3. Next, the clinician should support the perineum during contractions, using either hand. As the head advances, make sure to control its progress. Maintain flexion of the head with pressure applied through a towel placed on the perineum. The head should be delivered slowly, in a controlled manner, as it edges forward with each contraction. Between contractions the head will gradually extend. Recall that as the head extends, it will increase in diameter. Therefore, do not allow the head to extend too rapidly or the chin may tear the perineum. In other words, palpate the chin (through the towel over the perineum), and prevent it from "popping" (suddenly extending) and tearing the perineum.

4. If a rapid delivery is necessary (e.g., fetal distress) or assistance is needed (e.g., inadequate pushing because of regional anesthesia or maternal exhaustion), a modified Ritgen maneuver can be used. The Ritgen maneuver merely assists or exacerbates the extension of the fetal head. To perform it, while palpating the infant's chin (through the towel on the perineum), pull outward on the chin and then press it upward to extend the head. Again, this effort should be weighed against the possibility of the chin "popping" through the perineum and tearing it. In most cases, the chin can be controlled and extended enough for delivery without "popping" the perineum.

5. For an OP delivery, the head is usually delivered more readily by applying flexion, not extension. The tension on the perineum can be very high, resulting in a third- or fourth-degree laceration. Again, assisting and controlling the amount of flexion with a hand, through the towel on the perineum, may minimize the risk of lacerations.

6. As the head is slowly delivered, reach around the neck to reduce any nuchal cords (occurs in 20% of deliveries). Wipe the mucus off the infant's nose and mouth while suctioning both orifices with a bulb syringe. The head has now externally rotated to allow the shoulders to assume an AP position.

7. Delivery of the shoulders should be performed with slow and deliberate motions and without exerting excessive traction. Gently depress the head toward

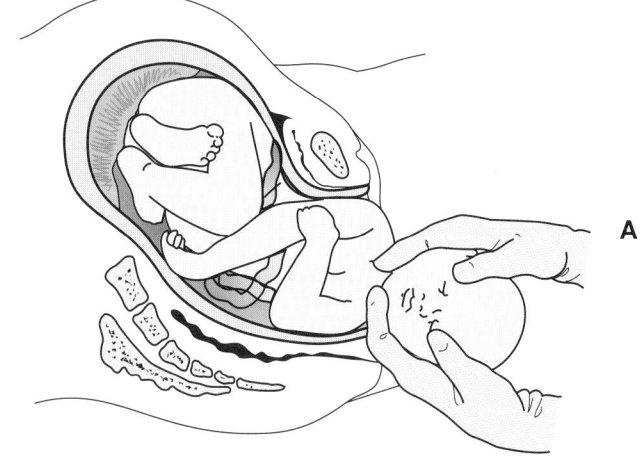

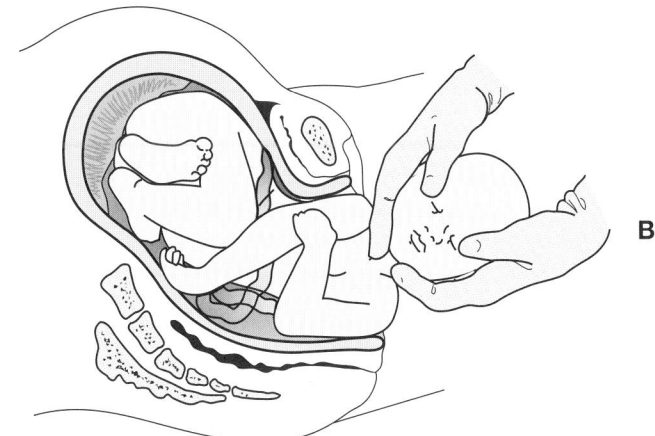

Fig. 178-5
A, Gentle downward traction to bring about descent of anterior shoulder. **B,** With delivery of the anterior shoulder completed, applying gentle upward traction delivers the posterior shoulder. (Redrawn from Ratcliffe S, Baxley EG, Byrd J, Sakornbut E: *Family practice obstetrics,* ed 2, Philadelphia, 2001, Hanley and Belfus.)

the maternal coccyx (Fig. 178-5, *A*), and when the anterior shoulder has passed the symphysis, lift the fetal head upward (Fig. 178-5, *B*). This allows for delivery of the posterior shoulder. It is important to protect the perineum again with one hand through a sterile towel. As the posterior shoulder is delivered, it should also be prevented from "popping" through the perineum and tearing a third- or fourth-degree laceration. If shoulder dystocia is a concern, attempt to deliver the head and shoulders in one continuous motion. This may prevent the anterior shoulder from lodging or becoming impacted against the symphysis.

Editor's note: Although management of shoulder dystocia is beyond the scope of this chapter (see "Useful

Continuing Education" section), one or two of the maneuvers used in that situation, known as the Rubin II or Woods' screw maneuvers, can be used for all large babies (or small pelvises), even in the absence of dystocia. It is the editor's opinion that by using such maneuvers with all large babies, it may minimize the number of tears and the amount of local trauma. Having practiced these maneuvers during routine deliveries may also be beneficial when a shoulder dystocia finally occurs. To perform the Rubin II maneuver, enter the vagina with your hand and apply two fingers to the back of the anterior shoulder of the infant. Apply pressure to rotate it toward the front of the infant and in effect "shrug" the baby's shoulders (adduct them). This will decrease their AP diameter. At the same time, the clinician's other hand can be applied to the infant's posterior shoulder from the front of the infant. Applying pressure here will abduct this shoulder, and rotate it toward the back of the infant. With both maneuvers applied at the same time, the infant's shoulders turning together approximates the turning of a threaded screw (Woods' screw).

8. Next, grasp the baby around the neck and place a finger in the infant's axilla to maintain lateral flexion of the trunk. The trunk is easily delivered with gentle, continuous traction. Support the trunk with the hand not supporting the neck.

   Many clinicians feel that the infant should be held just below the level of the introitus to be suctioned. The cord should then be clamped. In vitro data support that this is the proper level and time for optimal placental-fetal transfusion. However, no outcome studies support this assertion. In an attempt to increase bonding, some clinicians place the newborn on the mother's chest while clamping the cord.

9. Clamp the cord about 3 to 4 cm from the umbilicus with a plastic cord clamp and a curved artery clamp. Cut the cord and, as clinically indicated, pass the infant to the mother, nurse, or nursery personnel. Finally, collect 7 to 10 ml of cord blood while verifying that the cord has two arteries and a vein. Fetal anomalies are associated with cords having less than three vessels.

10. While waiting to deliver the placenta, place one hand (on a sterile drape) over the fundus and palpate it. Use the other hand to apply firm traction on the cord. Controlled cord traction may not only facilitate placental removal; it may also decrease the risk of postpartum hemorrhage. Avoid overaggressive traction, however, which may detach the placenta from the cord and cause hemorrhage. Monitor the uterus for atony and uterine inversion (see "Complications" section) by continuous palpation.

   Note that the active management of the third stage of labor calls for oxytocin to be given at the time of delivery of the anterior shoulder. The cord is then clamped and cut immediately. Next apply,

continuous, controlled traction to the cord until delivery of the placenta. Oxytocin, methylergonovine (Methergine), or prostaglandins are later used as indicated to contract the uterus. These maneuvers have been shown to reduce postpartum hemorrhage by two thirds, yet to not increase the need for manual placental removal. They have also not been shown to endanger an undiagnosed twin.

As opposed to active management, expectant management of the third stage of labor allows the placenta to deliver spontaneously, aided by gravity or nipple stimulation. When studied, active management has been found to be superior to expectant management in terms of blood loss, postpartum hemorrhage, and other serious complications. However, active management has been associated with an increased risk of unpleasant side effects (e.g., nausea and vomiting), and hypertension, especially if methylergonovine is used.

11. As the uterus becomes rounded, the cord will usually lengthen and a gush of vaginal blood indicates placental separation. Usually the placenta separates within 5 minutes of the delivery but it can take as long as 30 minutes. Once the separation occurs, have the mother bear down gently. This is normally enough pressure to expel the placenta. If not, milk the placenta out of the birth canal. This is done by placing one hand on the fundus and using it to exert a slight to moderate amount of pressure. This should propel the placenta into the vagina (Fig. 178-6). After the placenta has passed through the introitus, gently remove any remaining or attached membranes with a ring forceps. This prevents tearing the membranes and decreases the chance of any being left behind.

   If the placenta has not delivered within 30 minutes, it may be trapped by a contracted cervical ring. This diagnosis is likely if the uterus has already contracted, the gush of vaginal blood occurred, and the cord lengthened. The Brandt maneuver will often deliver the placenta: apply firm pressure suprapubically to hold the uterus in place, apply firm traction on the umbilical cord, and attempt to deliver the placenta.

Manual Delivery of the Placenta

Manual removal of the placenta is indicated (3% of vaginal deliveries) if the placenta does not deliver within 30 minutes or if significant bleeding occurs and the uterus does not contract. For failure of the uterus to contract, the injection of oxytocin (Pitocin) (2 ml/20 IU in 20 ml of normal saline) into the placental side of the clamped cord may be helpful. It will occasionally result in contraction of the uterus and delivery of the placenta.

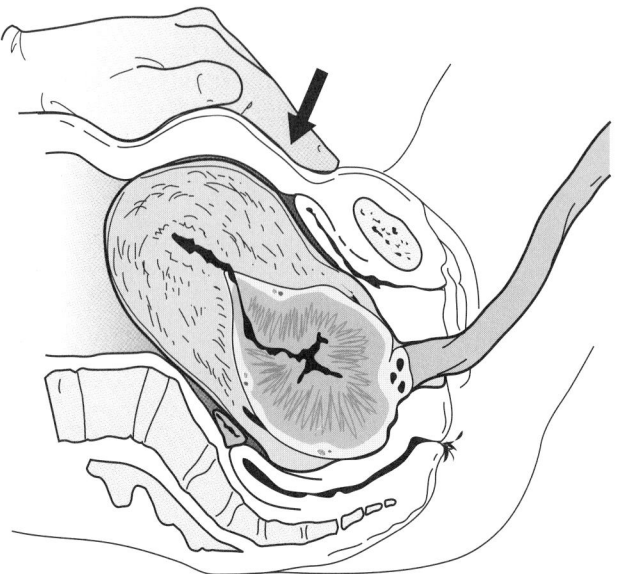

Fig. 178-6

Expression of placenta. Note that the hand is *not* trying to push the fundus of the uterus through the birth canal! As the placenta leaves the uterus and enters the vagina, the uterus is elevated (fundus pushed upward and posteriorly) by the hand on the abdomen *(arrow)* while the cord is held in position. The mother can aid in the delivery of the placenta by bearing down. As the placenta reaches the perineum, the cord is lifted, which in turn lifts the placenta out of the vagina. Adherent membranes are eased away from thin attachments to prevent their being torn off and retained in the birth canal. (Redrawn from Cunningham FG, Gant NF, Leveno KJ, et al, editors: *Williams' obstetrics,* ed 18, East Norwalk, Conn, 1989, Appleton & Lange.)

For manual removal, change gloves and enter the vagina with your dominant hand, palpating for lacerations. Next, find the cervix and enter the uterus. With two or three fingers, and then the whole hand if necessary, find the plane between the placenta and the uterine wall. Gently follow this plane and use your hand to separate the placenta from the uterine wall. After complete separation, hold onto the placenta with the dominant hand, and slowly withdraw the hand with the placenta. If the cleavage plane cannot be separated or parts of the plane cannot be developed completely, prepare for surgical removal of the placenta.

After the third stage, always examine the placenta while it is in the basin or on the table for completeness. If incomplete, reenter the vagina and uterus manually to perform this same maneuver to retrieve any fragments. Covering the sterile glove on the inserted hand with one 4 × 4 gauze pad may give additional traction when sweeping the uterus. Such sweeps may also be useful in patients after VBAC, for those bleeding excessively or for premature deliveries.

If it has not already been given, intravenous oxytocin should be given and gentle uterine massage performed to prevent atony. Currently, in the United States, it is the clinician's choice as to whether to give oxytocin with the delivery of the shoulders or after the placenta is expelled. Usually this is given IV (20 to 40 units in 1 L of isotonic solution over 8 hours). If atony and bleeding persist, methylergonovine can be given (2 mg IM [normotensive patients only]) or 15-methyl prostaglandin (250 µg IM). After the uterus is firm, begin any necessary repair.

COMPLICATIONS

Maternal Complications

- Hemorrhage (4% with postpartum greater than 500 ml in 24 hours) and risk of hemodynamic instability
- Maternal tissue damage: uterine rupture, cervical or vaginal lacerations, perineal injury or rectal tears
- Uterine inversion followed by massive hemorrhage (1 in 2000 deliveries)

Endometritis

- Retained placenta; placental fragments or membranes

Editor's note: There has never been a proven association between uterine inversion and excessive cord traction. However, uterine inversion is associated with fundal placentas, uterine atony, and congenital weakness of the uterus. Management begins with calling for assistance, including general anesthesia, and immediately attempting to replace the uterus. If possible, it should be replaced without removing the placenta. If the uterus is not replaceable immediately, there is an 85% to 90% success rate of replacing the uterus with tocolysis. (Oxytocin should be discontinued and the uterus relaxed with intravenous beta-mimetic medications or magnesium sulfate [preferred]). The remaining 15% to 20% of patients will require general anesthesia for the abdominal relaxation needed for uterine replacement. After replacement, oxytocin should be restarted and the postpartum hemorrhage managed just like any other. (Preparation should be made for intravenous resuscitation with large bore intravenous catheters, etc.)

Fetal Complications

- Intracranial hemorrhage
- Brachial plexus damage
- Fractures of the humerus or clavicle
- Asphyxia and associated problems
- Neonatal sepsis

Editor's note: The likelihood of a malpractice lawsuit appears to be related to the number of deliveries a clinician performs, rather than their specialty. In the past, statistics indicated that clinicians were sued about once every 3125 deliveries. In other words, a primary care clinician could perform 300 deliveries a year for 10 years, on the average, before being involved in a lawsuit. This is a large number of deliveries for most primary care clinicians!

POSTPROCEDURE PATIENT EDUCATION (POSTPARTUM INSTRUCTIONS)

Upon discharge from the hospital, patients should be given specific instructions about their medications and other postpartum care. Any and all questions should be answered. Whether patients are breast-feeding or not, new mothers will require instructions for breast care. They should also be instructed about sitz baths, peri-pads, and other perineal care. Inform them about when to call the clinician. Pelvic rest should be maintained for at least a month. The follow-up appointment for a Pap smear should be 6 weeks after the delivery.

SUPPLIERS

Although prenatal care is beyond the scope of this chapter, good prenatal patient education and documentation enhances this procedure as well as lowers the malpractice risk.

Information on MOM (Management of Maternity)—a prenatal care, clinician and patient education program—and free samples of the MOM Care Chart Documentation Form
American Academy of Family Physicians
11400 Tomahawk Creek Parkway
Leawood, KS 66211-2672
Phone: 1-800-274-2237, Ext. 4148
Website: www.aafp.org/momcare/index.html

Prenatal care record and patient education system
(Note: This system has been used nationally for over 20 years, with only seven malpractice claims filed despite more than 700,000 deliveries)
Advanced Medical Systems, Inc.
440 E. Cheyenne Mountain Boulevard, #26
Colorado Springs, CO 80906
Phone: 1-800-876-7145
Website: www.amsintl.com

CPT/BILLING CODES

00946	Anesthesia (paracervical block or pudendal block) for vaginal procedures; vaginal delivery
59400	Global vaginal (routine obstetric care, including antepartum care, vaginal delivery [with or without episiotomy, and/or forceps] and postpartum care)
59409	Vaginal delivery *only*
59510	Global cesarean section (routine obstetric care, including antepartum care, cesarean delivery, and postpartum care)
59514	Cesarean section *only*
59610	Global VBAC delivery *only* (routine obstetric care including antepartum care, vaginal delivery [with or without episiotomy and/or forceps] and postpartum care after previous cesarean delivery)
59899	Induction

Labor that is postterm, induced, augmented, or otherwise complicated (blood pressure problems, arrest of labor, fetal distress, etc.) is not included in a routine delivery. It should be coded with hospital evaluation and management codes.

99356	Prolonged physician service in the inpatient setting, requiring direct (face-to-face) patient contact beyond the usual service (e.g., maternity fetal monitoring for high risk delivery or other physiologic monitoring); first hour
99357	Each additional 30 minutes

And, if prolonged care, but not face-to-face care:

99358	Prolonged evaluation and management service before and/or after direct (face-to-face) patient care (e.g., review of extensive records and tests, communication with other professionals and/or patient/family); first hour

Note: A good reference for coding is provided by the American Academy of Family Physicians (AAFP) at www.aafp.org/practice/ob.

ICD-9-CM DIAGNOSTIC CODES

645	Postdates pregnancy
650	Normal delivery
654.21	Previous cesarean section
656.31	Fetal distress
658	Oligohydramnios
659.21	Pyrexia in labor
663.01	Prolapse of cord
664.1	Perineal laceration—degree 4
666.1	Postpartum hemorrhage
667.1	Retained placenta/membranes
792.3	Meconium staining

USEFUL CONTINUING EDUCATION

Other than performing supervised deliveries or completing an obstetrics rotation or fellowship, there is no better resource for practicing the skills for a delivery than the AAFP's Advanced Life Support in Obstetrics (ALSO) course. This course provides practice for both the cognitive and the manual skills for simple or complicated deliveries. Excellent, lifelike pelvis and infant mannequins allow the learner to practice in a calm environment, even using assisted delivery equipment. Courses are taught throughout the United States as well as internationally. More information can be found at www.aafp.org/also.

ADDITIONAL RESOURCES

- See the sample patient education handout titled "Care Following a Vaginal Delivery" on page 1984 of Appendix G.
- See the sample patient consent form titled "Vaginal Delivery" on page 1986 of Appendix G.

BIBLIOGRAPHY

American Academy of Family Physicians: *Advanced Life Support in Obstetrics (ALSO) provider course syllabus,* ed 4, Kansas City, 2000, AAFP.

Beischer NA, Mackay EV, Colditz P: *Obstetrics and the newborn,* ed 3, London, 1996, WB Saunders.

Evans AT, Niswander KR: *Manual of obstetrics,* ed 6, Philadelphia, 2000, Lippincott, Williams & Wilkins.

Fraser WD, Turcot L, Krauss I, Brisson-Carrol G : Amniotomy for shortening spontaneous labour, *Cochrane Database Syst Rev* (2):CD000015, 2000.

Gabbe SG, Niebyl JR, Simpson JL: *Obstetrics: normal and problem pregnancies,* ed 3, New York, 1996, Churchill Livingston.

Niswander KR, Evans AT: *Manual of obstetrics,* ed 5, Philadelphia, 1996, Little, Brown.

Pitkin RM, Scott JR: Active management of labor: the American experience, *Clin Obstet Gynecol* 40(3):510, 1997.

Prendiville WJ, Elbourne D, McDonald S: Active versus expectant management in the third stage of labour, *Cochrane Database Syst Rev* (2):CD000007, 2000.

Ratcliffe SD, Byrd JE, Sakornbut EI: *Pregnancy and perinatal care in family practice,* Philadelphia, 1996, Hanley & Belfus.

WEBSITES

www.aafp.org/momcare/index.html (AAFP's Management of Maternity program)

www.aafp.org/practice/ob (AAFP: Coding for intrapartum care and other obstetrical services)

www.cochrane.org (The Cochrane Collaboration database: reviews are available online; the abstracts can be browsed and searched for free.)

PART ELEVEN

Pediatrics

CHAPTER 179

DeLee Suctioning

David B. Bosscher

Suctioning, using a DeLee suction device, is a means by which the upper airways of the neonate can be cleared and the stomach emptied of meconium-stained secretions. Meconium is present in the amniotic fluid in 9% to 20% of deliveries. Initially it was felt that DeLee suctioning of the oropharynx and stomach carried out before delivery of the neonate's chest would prevent meconium aspiration syndrome (MAS). It is now known that some infants aspirate before delivery and therefore no intrapartum intervention can prevent all meconium aspiration. DeLee suctioning after delivery of the anterior shoulder and before delivery of the chest (before the neonate's first breath) prevents further meconium aspiration with the first breath and still remains a cornerstone in the resuscitation of infants at risk for meconium aspiration. Further intervention, such as endotracheal intubation and suctioning of the trachea, may be indicated for premature infants or those with respiratory distress.

INDICATIONS

- To minimize meconium aspiration in the neonate when meconium-stained amniotic fluid is present
- To help relieve respiratory distress in the newborn when the stomach is full or when regurgitated stomach contents partially occlude the airway
- To assist in the diagnosis of choanal atresia
- To help exclude certain types of tracheoesophageal fistulae

CONTRAINDICATIONS

- A neonate with choanal atresia should not receive DeLee suctioning via the nasal route.
- Thick particulate meconium cannot be adequately suctioned with a DeLee suction device alone. In the newborn infant with depressed or absent respirations, heart rate less than 100 beats per minute (bpm), or poor muscle tone, DeLee suctioning

immediately after the neonate's head and anterior shoulder are delivered should be followed with more definitive suctioning of the trachea below the vocal cords with an endotracheal tube after completion of the delivery.

EQUIPMENT

- A DeLee suction device or similar suction device, 8 to 10 French (Fig. 179-1)
- A bulb syringe to clear the mouth and nasal openings
- Gloves, facial coverings, and other necessary items for universal blood and body fluid precautions (Many hospitals now use mechanical or wall suction for the DeLee to maintain these precautions.)

TECHNIQUE

1. Prepare the equipment. Be certain that the rolled-up latex covering the suction end of the DeLee suction device is functioning. Place this end into your suction source. Make certain the suction is functioning. Human suctioning is not recommended.
2. Quickly clear the mouth and nose of the neonate with a bulb syringe.
3. Gently insert the mouth end of the suction device into the mouth of the neonate. Attempt to keep the catheter sterile.
4. Slowly advance the catheter into the oropharynx, then direct it down into the esophagus (hypopharynx) with your finger.
5. Continue to advance the catheter until approximately 5 cm of its length remains outside the infant's mouth. The distal end is now in the infant's stomach.
6. Using a vacuum source that does not exceed 100 mm Hg, apply vacuum to the suction end of the DeLee device. Occlude the thumb opening on the vacuum device. After vacuum application for a few seconds, slowly withdraw the catheter while maintaining

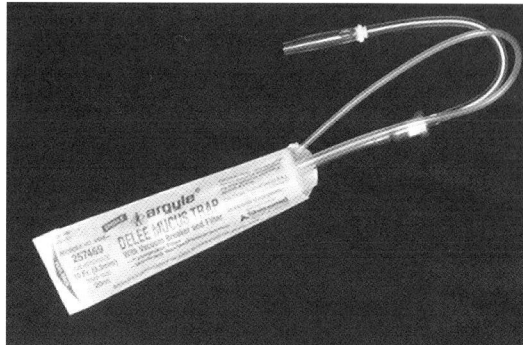

Fig. 179-1
DeLee suction device.

vacuum. If time allows, use the same technique to suction the infant's nose also.

7. After delivery of the infant, check for any respiratory distress. Treat minor degrees of distress with proper positioning and oxygen administration if necessary (see Chapter 182, Neonatal Resuscitation).

8. As part of documenting the care of the newborn in the postdelivery period, always mention that DeLee suctioning was performed. Document any complications.

COMPLICATIONS

- Stimulation of the neonatal oropharynx with any suction device during the first few minutes after delivery can evoke a vagal response and induce apnea or bradycardia and resultant fetal distress.
- Vigorous DeLee suctioning could cause trauma to the upper airways, the esophagus, and the stomach.
- In a neonate with a tracheoesophageal fistula, the DeLee suction device could enter the airway below the larynx, causing respiratory distress.
- Older DeLee suction devices, and even some of the newer ones that use human suction, allow aspirated neonatal stomach contents to enter the mouth of the person applying suction. This method has the potential for spreading infectious diseases. Do not use your mouth to apply suction. Newer models use mechanical or wall suction and are safer for the clinician; however, they are more cumbersome and difficult to use in a sterile field.

INDICATIONS FOR FURTHER RESUSCITATION EFFORTS

Prevention of meconium aspiration syndrome (MAS) and sequelae is the goal of resuscitative efforts. Some

have suggested that the airways of all infants with meconium-stained amniotic fluid be intubated and suctioned. Metaanalysis of four randomized controlled trials of endotracheal intubation at birth in vigorous term infants with meconium-stained fluid failed to reveal benefit of intubation over expectant observation when evaluating both morbidity and mortality as end points. Expectant management after suctioning of the upper airway and stomach before delivery of the chest is recommended for vigorous term infants until further research is available. For other infants with cardio-respiratory distress, neonatal resuscitation efforts are indicated (see Chapter 182, Neonatal Resuscitation).

CPT/BILLING CODE

99440   Newborn resuscitation; care of the high-risk newborn at delivery, including, for example, inhalation therapy, aspiration

ICD-9-CM DIAGNOSTIC CODES

792.3   Meconium in amniotic fluid
656.8   Meconium noted during delivery

BIBLIOGRAPHY

American Heart Association: *Guidelines for neonatal resuscitation,* Dallas, 1993, AHA.

American Heart Association and American Academy of Pediatrics: *Textbook of neonatal resuscitation,* Dallas, 1993, AHA/AAP.

Falciglia HS et al: Does DeLee suction at the perineum prevent meconium aspiration syndrome? *Am J Obstet Gynecol* 167:1243, 1992.

Halliday HL: Endotracheal intubation at birth for preventing morbidity and mortality in vigorous, meconium-stained infants at term, Abstract, *Cochran Database Syst Rev* CD 000500: 2000.

Houlihan CM, Knuppel RA: Meconium-stained amniotic fluid: current controversies, *J Reprod Med* 39:888, 1994.

Katz VL, Bowes WA: Meconium aspiration syndrome: reflections of a murky subject, *Am J Obstet Gynecol* 166:171, 1992.

Niermeyer S et al: International Guidelines for Neonatal Resuscitation: an excerpt from the Guidelines 2000 for Cardiopulmonary Resuscitation and Emergency Cardiovascular Care: International Consensus on Science. Contributors and reviewers for the Neonatal Resuscitation Guidelines, *Pediatrics* 106(3):E29, 2000.

Peng TC, Gutcher GR, Van Dorsten JP: A selective aggressive approach to the neonate exposed to meconium-stained amniotic fluid, *Am J Obstet Gynecol* 175:296, 1996.

CHAPTER 180

Dorsal Penile and Subcutaneous Ring Block for Newborn Circumcision

Grant C. Fowler
Ronald D. Reynolds

Most of the controversy about whether or not infants should receive analgesia or anesthesia for circumcision has ended. Previously, the controversy weighed whether the incompletely developed neonatal nervous system was capable of experiencing pain against the risk of anesthesia. Many clinicians chose not to use circumcision anesthesia, due in part to this controversy, as well as due to their lack of training or experience in the techniques available, the additional steps (and time) required to perform the procedure, and the time required for the anesthesia to take effect. However, with proper planning, the number of steps and the time required are minimal. In addition, studies have documented the safety of anesthesia as well as the improved outcomes in neonates. In fact, the American Academy of Pediatrics now recommends routine use of analgesia for circumcision.

Common analgesic and anesthetic techniques for circumcision include dorsal penile nerve block (DPNB), subcutaneous ring block, precircumcision oral analgesics, and topical anesthesia (see Chapter 11, Topical Anesthesia). Several studies have reported that the subcutaneous ring block is the most effective. This chapter discusses DPNB, an alternative technique of DPNB using a single injection, and subcutaneous ring block. All three techniques appear to be more effective than oral or topical anesthesia, and no major complications have been reported with any of these methods. Studies have found that anesthetized infants show less crying, tachycardia, and irritability, and exhibit fewer behavior changes for the 24 hours following circumcision. They also have less variability in oxygen saturation and blood pressure during the procedure, and lower serum cortisol levels after the procedure.

INDICATIONS

• Parental desire. Should be considered in any healthy newborn undergoing circumcision

CONTRAINDICATIONS

• Known hypersensitivity to anesthetic
• A known bleeding disorder *(relative contraindication)*

Other contraindications are the same as for circumcision:
• Hypospadias, epispadias, or megaurethra*
• Unusual appearing genitalia*
• Inability to determine the phenotype of the child* (ambiguous genitalia)
• Age less than 12 hours (physiologic adaptation requires 12 to 24 hours)
• Severe illness
• Prematurity (until the child is ready for discharge from hospital)

EQUIPMENT

• 1% lidocaine without epinephrine.
• 1-ml syringe with 27-gauge needle (some tuberculin syringes come with this combination). If the needle is removable, using a 30-gauge needle to administer the anesthetic may minimize bleeding and discomfort.
• Alcohol wipe.
• Infant restrainer (papoose board or Circumstraint) if assistant not available to hold infant.

---

*Urologist should be consulted.

PREPROCEDURE PATIENT PREPARATION

Discuss the risks, benefits, and alternatives with the parents, and obtain informed consent. Most clinicians combine this consent with the circumcision consent form.

TECHNIQUE

Before the procedure, note the anatomy as shown in Fig. 180-1. Consider giving the infant a few swallows of glucose water or a sugar-coated pacifier to minimize distress. In a warm room, have an assistant hold the infant or place the infant's legs in restraints. Fold back the diaper to expose the penis.

Note: As the clinician becomes more comfortable performing DPNB or ring block, time may be saved by performing the procedure *before* the infant is prepped. This allows time for the anesthetic to take effect while other preparations are being made.

DORSAL PENILE NERVE BLOCK (TWO TECHNIQUES)

Standard Technique

1. Using an index finger, palpate the lateral side of the penis to determine the depth of the root of the penis, which is usually about 0.75 to 1 cm beneath the skin surface. Often it is about the size, shape, and consistency of a large blueberry just under the symphysis pubis.

2. Prepare the skin at the base of the penis with an alcohol pad. Using aseptic technique and stabilizing the penis by gentle, slightly downward or ventral traction, insert the needle at the 1 o'clock position (the dorsal or cephalad direction being the 12 o'clock position, and the ventral direction being the 6 o'clock position) in a posteromedial direction (Fig. 180-2). Insert to a depth of 0.3 to 0.5 cm. This depth corresponds to 0.5 to 0.7 cm distal to the penile root, or slightly proximal to where the dorsal nerves branch (Fig. 180-3). The tip of the needle should be freely movable, indicating that it is in loose connective tissue. This prevents injection into the corpus cavernosum. Taking care not to inject into a blood vessel (check by aspirating), inject 0.4 ml of lidocaine. Repeat the injection at the 11 o'clock position. Do not exceed a total of 0.8 ml of lidocaine.

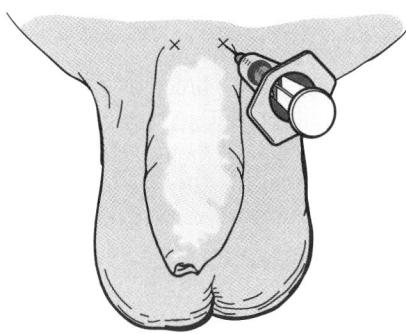

Fig. 180-2
Injection sites and direction of needle for administering dorsal penile nerve block.

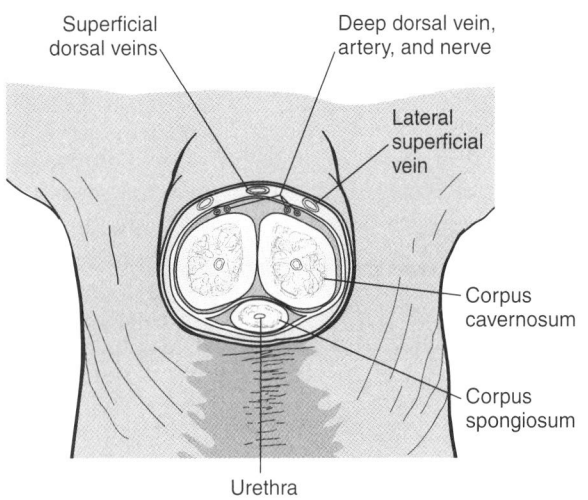

Fig. 180-1
Anatomy of the penile root (cross section).

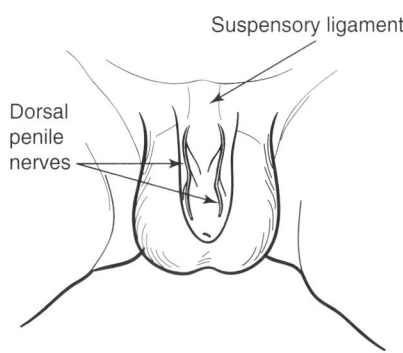

Fig. 180-3
Location of dorsal penile nerves. Note branching begins after emerging from the suspensory ligament of the penis.

3. In the infant whose penile root is not palpable because it is embedded in pubic fat, the anesthetic can be injected at the same locations, depth, and direction: about 0.3 to 0.5 cm inferolateral to the penile-suprapubic skin junction (Fig. 180-4).

Alternative Technique Using Single Injection Site

1. Instead of making two skin punctures (at the 11 and 1 o'clock positions), insert the needle at the 12 o'clock position and angle the needle toward the 11 and 1 o'clock positions. The 12 o'clock position is where the dorsal skin of the penis reflects onto the abdomen (penile-suprapubic skin junction). Insert the needle here and angle toward the 1 o'clock

position to a depth of about 0.5 cm. The tip of the needle should be freely movable, indicating that it is in loose connective tissue. This prevents injection into the corpus cavernosum. Taking care not to inject into a blood vessel (check by aspirating), inject 0.4 ml of lidocaine.

2. Withdraw the needle until the tip is just below the skin surface and then advance to place the injection directed at the 11 o'clock position (Fig. 180-5). Do not exceed a total of 0.8 ml of lidocaine.

Note: DPNB has also been demonstrated to be effective in adults. Obviously, larger doses of lidocaine are used in adults.

SUBCUTANEOUS RING BLOCK

1. Prepare the skin both at the base of the penis as well as around the penis, with an alcohol pad. Using aseptic technique and stabilizing the penis by gentle, slightly downward or ventral traction, insert the needle into the lateral side of the penis at the base (Fig. 180-6). Staying superficial to Buck's fascia, place a subcutaneous bleb of lidocaine. Then advance the needle circumferentially around the base of the penis while injecting. A couple of punctures may be necessary to accomplish this.

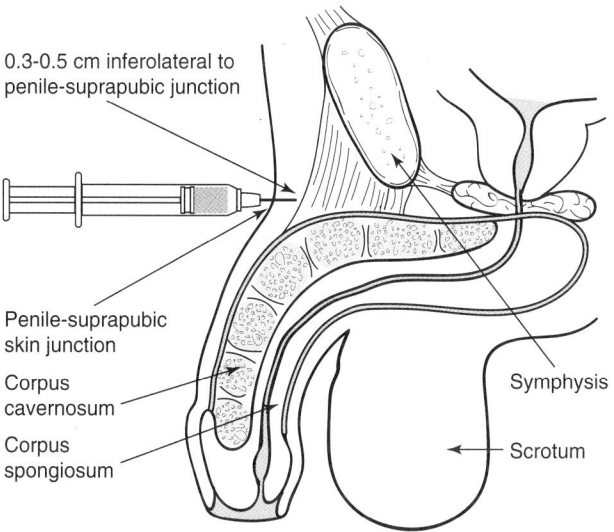

Fig. 180-4
Sagittal view through the perineum showing anesthetic injection in a posteromedial direction at a depth of 0.3 to 0.5 mm.

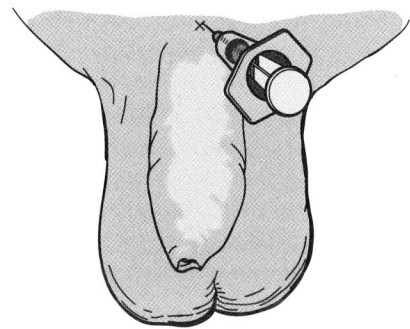

Fig. 180-5
Dorsal penile nerve block using a single injection site at the 12 o'clock position.

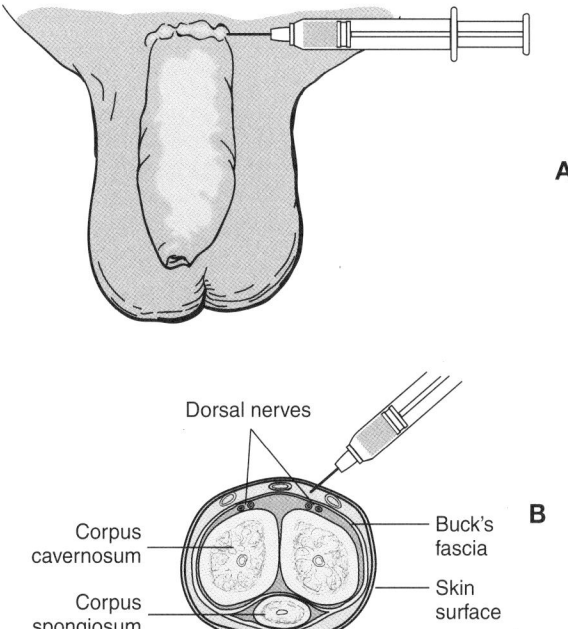

Fig. 180-6
Subcutaneous ring block. **A,** Needle is inserted at base of penis, and a subcutaneous bleb of lidocaine is placed. A 360-degree ring of anesthesia is completed around the penis. **B,** Cross-section of penis at base showing paired dorsal nerves deep to Buck's fascia.

2. After completing a 180-degree half circle, the same procedure is followed on the opposite side of the penis. A maximum of 1 ml of lidocaine should be used to complete the 360-degree circumferential ring. Intravascular injection can be avoided by frequently aspirating with the syringe while injecting the subcutaneous ring.

Notes Regarding Optimal Effects

- One study in adults has found that using slower injection rates (i.e., longer injection times, such as 100 to 150 seconds) caused less pain than shorter injection times (40 to 80 seconds). A 30-gauge needle provides slower injection rates as well as overall increased patient comfort. It also causes less bleeding.
- Another study comparing plain and buffered lidocaine in newborns failed to demonstrate a difference in oxygen saturations, crying, heart rate, or any other measure of distress.
- Although some anesthesia will take effect in as little as 2 to 3 minutes, ideally 3 to 5 minutes should be allowed for the full effect of the anesthesia before performing circumcision. Conveniently, this is about the amount of time it takes to prep and drape the infant and appropriately arrange the instruments.
- Avoid injecting air, which can cause pain.

COMPLICATIONS

- Inadequate anesthesia
- Localized edema, bleeding, or hematoma at the injection site
- Local skin infection or necrosis
- Allergic reaction to lidocaine
- Systemic reaction to intravascular lidocaine
- Penile necrosis (This is theoretical, since it has not been reported. Only lidocaine *without* epinephrine should be used, since epinephrine can cause vasospasm of the penile arteries.)

SUPPLIERS

Circumstraint
Olympus Medical Corp.
5900 1st Avenue South
Seattle, WA 98108
Phone: 1-800-426-0353
Website: www.olymed.com

CPT/BILLING CODE

64450-47   Nerve block, diagnostic or therapeutic, other peripheral nerve, anesthesia by surgeon (A few insurers will pay for this as a separate procedure from the circumcision.)

BIBLIOGRAPHY

American Academy of Pediatrics: Committee statements: report of the task force on circumcision, *Pediatrics* 103(3):686, 1999.

Lander J, Brady-Fryer B, Metcalfe JB, et al: Comparison of ring block, dorsal penile nerve block, and topical anesthesia for neonatal circumcision: a randomized controlled trial, *JAMA* 278(24):2157, 1997.

Lenhart JG, Lenhart NM, Reid A, et al: Local anesthesia for circumcision: which technique is most effective? *J Am Board Fam Pract* 10(1):13, 1997.

Mattson SR: Routine anesthesia for circumcision, *Postgrad Med* 106(1):107, 1999.

Serour F, Mandelburg A, Mori J: Slow injection of local anesthetic will decrease pain during dorsal penile nerve block, *Acta Anaesthesiol Scand* 42:926, 1998.

CHAPTER 181

Intraosseous Venous Access

Rafael F. Cruz

One of the most frustrating and difficult challenges faced by clinicians is the establishment of vascular access in the critically ill pediatric patient. Establishment of peripheral IV access is notoriously difficult in the small pediatric patient who is in shock or cardiac arrest. For children less than 5 years of age, thin bones and a vascular marrow make intraosseous venous access (IOVA) an excellent alternative. With IOVA, the marrow cavity (Fig. 181-1) functions as a rigid "vein" or conduit for fluid that does not collapse with hypovolemia or even shock.

Intraosseous venous access was originally described in the 1920s. However, with the introduction of plastic catheters and improved peripheral IV access skills, the need and interest for IOVA diminished. In the 1980s IOVA saw a resurgence in use as a rapid method for vascular access in pediatric shock emergencies. It has now been studied and proven to be a safe, reliable, and rapid temporary method for vascular access, especially when compared with percutaneous IV access. In addition, almost any intravenous medication can be administered by IOVA, often without changing the dosage or concentration (Box 181-1). With IOVA, there is immediate absorption of the medication or fluids into the systemic circulation, and drug concentrations remain elevated longer than with IV administration.

The disadvantages of IOVA include the temporary nature of the procedure, since it should not be used for more than 24 to 48 hours. Although the infusion rates may be limited, they can also reach more than 24 ml/min with a 20-gauge needle and a pressure infusor bag (blood pressure cuff inflated to 300 mm Hg around the IV fluid bag). The rate-limiting factor is usually the size of the marrow cavity. Unfortunately IOVA is especially limited in children over 5 years of age because, beyond this age, the red bone marrow has mostly been replaced by the less vascular yellow marrow.

One retrospective study of pediatric cardiopulmonary arrest patients revealed that, although the time to obtain peripheral IV was occasionally minimal, the average time was a disappointing 7.9 minutes ± 4.2 minutes. The overall peripheral IV success rate was only 17%. Of all techniques used, the success rate was highest with IOVA (83%), next most successful was surgical cutdown (81%), and central venous line placement (CVP) (77%) came in third. The average time required to establish vascular access was 4.7 minutes for IOVA, followed by 8.4 minutes for CVP, in turn followed by 12.7 minutes for venous cutdown.

In the pediatric cardiopulmonary arrest situation, it is reasonable to use IOVA as the initial approach for vascular access because of the high success rate and the rapidity of the procedure. In fact, all providers of emergency care should be familiar with IOVA, since in certain situations it may be the only available means of obtaining vascular access. To learn the procedure or to maintain skills for IOVA, clinicians can practice on raw chicken drumsticks, swine ribs, or piglet tibias.

INDICATIONS

- Any emergency condition that requires immediate vascular access (with critically ill patients who are hemodynamically unstable but still perfusing, it is customary to make two to three attempts at peripheral venous access before relying on the IOVA route)
- Shock (e.g., infection, bleeding, burns, severe dehydration)

Note: When a large volume of IV replacement fluid is needed very rapidly, bilateral IOVA may be necessary as well as the use of a pressure infusor bag or a large syringe.

- Cardiopulmonary arrest
- Prolonged status epilepticus (life threatening)
- Inability to secure endotracheal intubation for medication administration
- Need for administration of IV fluids or medications that cannot be given through an endotracheal tube (e.g., blood, sodium bicarbonate, dextrose)
- Inability to obtain peripheral vascular access due to obesity or edema of the patient's extremities

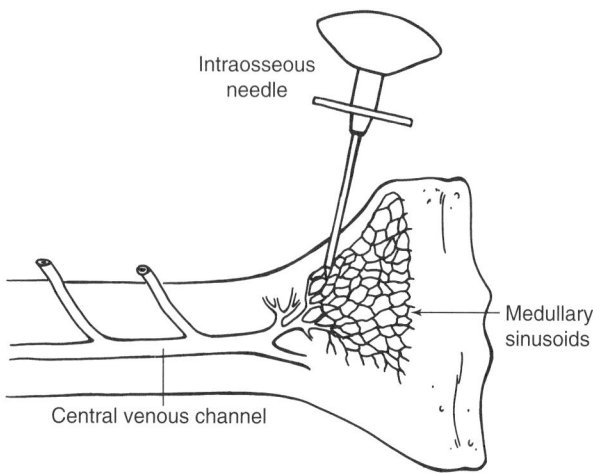

Fig. 181-1
Intramedullary venous system. With intraosseous venous access, the marrow cavity functions as a "vein" that will not collapse.

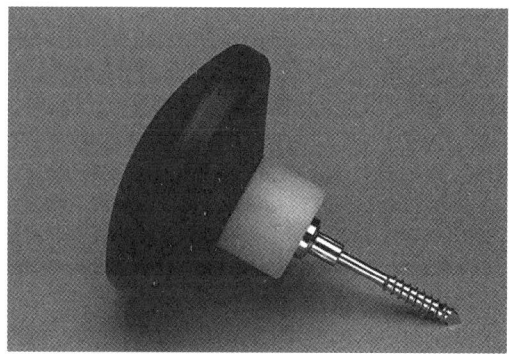

Fig. 181-2
Intraosseous infusion needle. (Courtesy Cook Critical Care, Bloomington, Ind.)

BOX 181-1
Products Acceptable for Intraosseous Infusion

Drugs	Solutions
Antibiotics	Calcium gluconate
Atropine sulfate	Colloids
Dexamethasone	Contrast media
Diazepam	Dextrose (D-glucose)
Digoxin	Plasma
Dobutamine	Ringer's lactate
Dopamine	Sodium bicarbonate
Epinephrine	Sodium chloride
Heparin	Whole blood
Insulin	Packed red blood cells
Lidocaine	Parenteral nutrition
Morphine sulfate	
Phenytoin	
Succinylcholine	

CONTRAINDICATIONS

Contraindications to IOVA are few and are all relative, especially since this is a very temporary, and occasionally a life-saving, procedure. However, the risks and benefits of the procedure should be considered.

- Ipsilateral fracture of an extremity (increases the risk of subcutaneous extravasation, so the other lower extremity should be used).
- Unsuccessful attempt in ipsilateral lower extremity (the other lower extremity should be used).
- Skin compromise at the selected site (e.g., burn or infection).
- Osteogenesis imperfecta (increased risk of fracture).
- Osteoporosis (increased risk of fracture).

- Sepsis or bacteremia (potential risk of bacterial seeding of marrow space).

EQUIPMENT

- Disposable intraosseous needle, 16 to 20 gauge (Fig. 181-2)
- Sterile latex gloves
- Goggles
- Sterile drapes
- Antiseptic solution (povidone-iodine, Hibiclens, or alcohol)
- Local anesthetic (1% lidocaine)
- Two 5-ml syringes and 25-gauge needles for local anesthetic administration
- Two 10-ml syringes for aspirating medullary contents and flushing with normal saline
- 2 × 2–inch gauze pads
- 4 × 4–inch gauze pads
- Tape
- IV solution, tubing, and pressure infusor bag (can use a blood pressure cuff)
- Extremity or torso restraints for the uncooperative patient
- Plastic or Styrofoam cup

PREPROCEDURE PATIENT PREPARATION

In most cases, IOVA is performed emergently. When time allows, the indications should be documented and explained to the parents. If performed electively, the

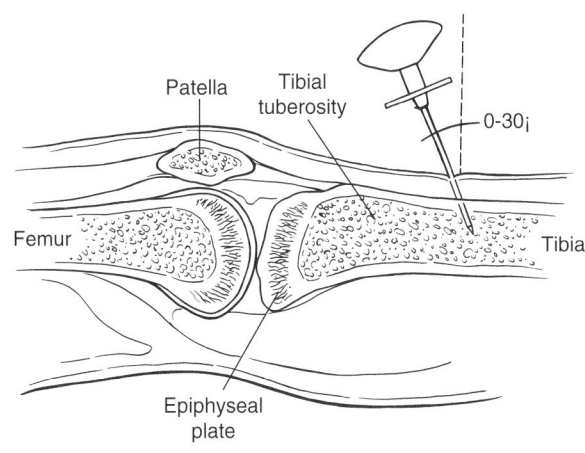

Fig. 181-3
Proximal tibial needle insertion.

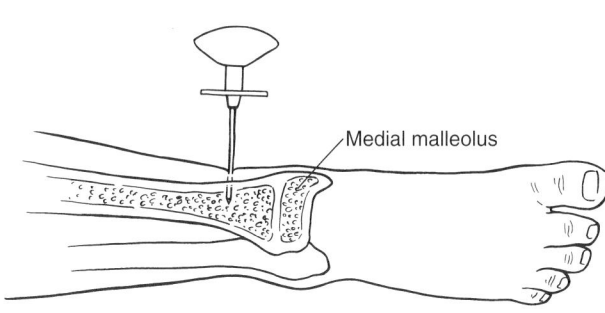

Fig. 181-4
Distal tibial needle insertion.

indications, alternatives, benefits, and risks should be explained to the parents. Signed informed consent should be obtained.

CHOICE OF LOCATION

The proximal tibia (Fig. 181-3) is the preferred site of infusion for children under 5 years of age. In CPR situations, this location is advantageous because it is located away from the area where CPR is taking place. In addition, the proximally located tibial tuberosity is a broad flat surface close to the skin where there are few intervening muscles, nerves, and blood vessels; therefore bony landmarks are easily recognized. After the age of 5, thickening of the cortex makes it very difficult to penetrate the proximal tibia.

The distal tibia (Fig. 181-4) and distal femur (Fig. 181-5) are alternative sites for IOVA. Whereas the distal tibia is a good second choice because the bone and tissues are thin, the distal femur is covered with muscles and fat, often making palpation of bony landmarks difficult. The distal femur should probably be reserved for those cases in which the proximal and distal tibia cannot be used. The sternum and ilium are seldom used because the width of the marrow space is inadequate in children under 3 years of age, and insertion may be technically difficult and dangerous. The sternal site carries a substantial risk of mediastinal puncture.

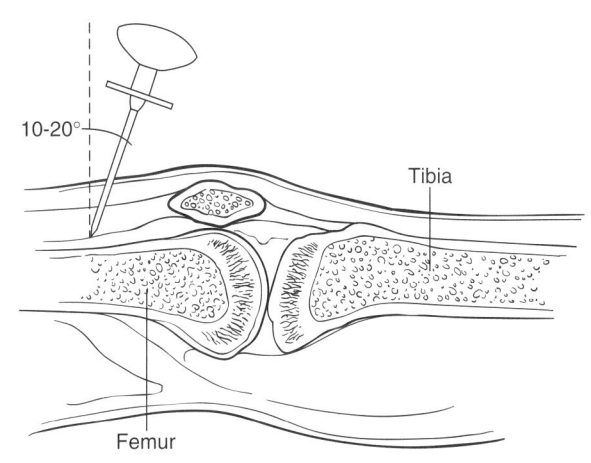

Fig. 181-5
Distal femoral needle insertion.

TECHNIQUE

1. With the infant restrained, place a small sandbag beneath the extremity. An assistant may be useful to help restrain the infant.
2. Prepare the skin with antiseptic solution and drape the area. Follow universal blood and body fluid precautions.
3. Administer local anesthetic down to the periosteum (this is optional; it may not be necessary for patients with an altered mental status).
4. To avoid through-and-through bony penetration, hold your index finger approximately 1 cm from the needle tip and avoid pushing past this mark.

5. Perform the procedure according to the selected insertion site:
   a. Proximal tibia
      (1) Palpate the tibial tuberosity with your finger. Select a site below the tibial tuberosity on the flat surface of the proximal, anteromedial tibia.
      (2) Grasp the medial aspect of the tibia with the thumb or fingers of your nondominant hand to secure it.
      (3) Using your dominant hand, insert the IOVA needle with a boring or screwing motion at up to a 30-degree angle from the vertical (Fig. 181-3). It should be pointed caudally, in the direction of the long axis of the bone, away from the epiphysis.
   b. Distal tibia
      (1) Insert the IOVA needle into the distal medial tibia at the broad flat area proximal to the medial malleolus and posterior to the saphenous vein. It should be inserted at an angle perpendicular to the skin (Fig. 181-4).
   c. Distal femur
      (1) Insert the needle 2 to 3 cm above the epicondyles in the anterior midline.
      (2) Direct the needle cephalad at an angle of 10 to 20 degrees from the vertical (Fig. 181-5).
6. Placement in the marrow space is confirmed by the following:
   a. There is a decrease in resistance (or "it gives") as the needle passes through the cortex into the softer medulla. The skin-to-cortex distance is rarely more than 1 cm in infants and children.
   b. The needle should stand upright without support when the stylet is removed.
   c. Marrow should be easily aspirated into a syringe.
   d. Fluids should infuse easily without extravasation.
7. Radiographs can be used to confirm needle position if time and the clinical situation permits (optional).
8. Flush the needle with saline solution (heparin is optional).
9. A sterile 2 × 2–inch gauze pad cut to fit around the needle should be taped down as a dressing. Next, place a cup (Styrofoam or plastic, with the bottom removed) over the IOVA site and firmly secure it with tape (Fig. 181-6).

   Note: This cup will offer additional protection for the IOVA in the case of inadvertent extremity movement.

10. Attach the pressure bag infusor to the IV bag and tape the IV tubing in place.
11. Restrain the limb with soft restraints to avoid inadvertent movement.

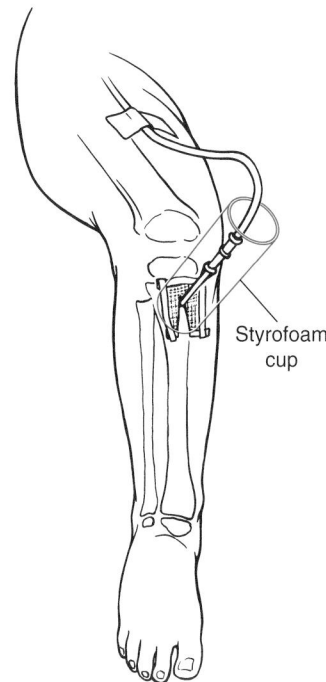

Fig. 181-6
Completed intraosseous venous access with cup protector.

12. Observe the infusion site for evidence of extravasation. Establish peripheral IV access within 24 to 48 hours after IOVA placement, then remove the IOVA.

For Removal

1. Rotate the needle slightly to loosen its seal. Withdraw the needle with a firm, quick motion.
2. Place a sterile pressure pad over the puncture site; apply firm pressure for 5 minutes to prevent hematoma formation. Next, apply a sterile dressing to the extremity. Do not constrict the extremity with the dressing.

POSTPROCEDURE PATIENT CARE AND EDUCATION

Following IOVA removal, the dressing must be changed daily. Dressings may be discontinued after 48 hours. The patient, his or her family, and the nursing staff should be taught to monitor for signs of infection or other possible complications.

COMPLICATIONS

• The most common complication is unsuccessful placement. This occurs in up to 20% of patients and is often due to the technical difficulty of the procedure. Technical failure can result from a lack of familiarity with the landmarks, improper technique, inadequate size of the marrow cavity, or the amount of red versus yellow marrow present.

- Clotting of marrow in the needle or displacement of the needle may lead to loss of vascular access.
- Subcutaneous, or occasionally subperiosteal, infiltration of fluid or leakage from the puncture site is common. This is especially common with use of pressure infusor bags or long-term use of intraosseous infusion. Extravasated crystalloid is usually not a problem, but solutions containing sodium bicarbonate (or other potentially cytotoxic agents) should be stopped or slowed to minimize extravasation. Muscle or tendon compartment syndromes from excessive fluid extravasation are a possibility.
- Slow infusion rates may be due to a small, fibrotic marrow cavity. Initially, flow rates may be slow because of plugging of the needle by marrow contents. Flushing the needle with 5 to 10 ml of saline often clears the needle.
- No lasting effects have been noted in bone, growth plate, or marrow elements after IOVA. The needle is directed away from the growth plate to avoid inadvertent injury to this structure. After successful placement, a small defect is created in the cortex that is visible as a small radiolucent area on radiographs. It should resolve in 30 to 40 days. In one case report, tibial fractures were seen after unsuccessful IOVA attempts, but these are very rare.
- Localized cellulitis or a subcutaneous abscess may be observed in less than 1% of cases. Osteomyelitis in most studies is at an incidence of less than 1%. Infections were usually associated with prolonged catheter placement, placement in bacteremic patients, or use of hypertonic infusions.
- Hematomas are most likely caused by local trauma from needle insertion.
- Pain is possible with insertion and when intramedullary pressure is increased during infusion. It is generally not a problem with slow infusions or in the unconscious patient. Slowing the infusion rate in the conscious patient may relieve symptoms.
- A theoretical complication is creation of a bone embolus when a needle without a stylet is used. No documented cases of a bone embolism have been reported. A fat embolism has been reported from tibial infusion in adults but not in children, probably because the marrow in children is relatively fat free.
- Bone marrow elements (immature blood cells, including blasts) have been observed in venous blood sampled proximal to IOVA infusion sites. Before more invasive diagnostic measures are undertaken, a repeat complete blood count with differential should be performed, preferably from the more permanent replacement IV site on another extremity.
- With sternal puncture, death has occurred from mediastinitis, hydrothorax, or injury to the heart or great vessels. This is avoidable if the tibia or femur is used rather than the sternum.
- Through-and-through placement of the needle can occur. Advancement of the needle through the opposite side of the bone can be prevented by placing your index finger approximately 1 cm from the needle tip. Your finger will prevent pushing too deep. (Some intraosseous needles have a preset depth indicator on the shaft.)

SUPPLIER

Cook Critical Care
P.O. Box 489
Bloomington, IN 47402
Phone: 1-800-457-4500
Website: www.cookcriticalcare.com

CPT/BILLING CODE

36680   Placement of needle for intraosseous infusion

ICD-9-CM DIAGNOSTIC CODES

427.5   Cardiorespiratory arrest
785.59   Hypovolemic shock (NEC)
958.4   Hemorrhagic shock or shock syndrome due to trauma
772.9   Hemorrhage, unspecified in newborn (NOS)
799.1   Respiratory arrest
785.50   Shock (without trauma), unspecified
785.59   Shock, endotoxic
995.0   Shock, anaphylactic
276.5   Volume depletion, dehydration
345.11   Status epilepticus

ADDITIONAL RESOURCES

- See the sample patient education handout titled "Intraosseous Venous Access (IOVA)" on page 1987 of Appendix G.
- See the sample patient consent form titled "Intraosseous Venous Access (IOVA)" on page 1988 of Appendix G.

BIBLIOGRAPHY

American College of Surgeons: *Advanced Trauma Life Support for doctors,* Chicago, 1997, ATLS.

Chameides L, editor: *Textbook of pediatric advanced life support,* Dallas, 1998, American Heart Association.

Driggers DA, Johnson R, Steiner JF, et al: Emergency resuscitation in children: the role of intraosseous infusion, *Postgrad Med* 89(4):129, 1991.

Glaeser PW, Losek JD, Nelson DB, et al: Pediatric intraosseous infusions: impact on vascular access time, *Am J Emerg Med* 6:330, 1988.

Hedges R: *Clinical procedures in emergency medicine,* Philadelphia, 1998, WB Saunders.

Schwartz GR: *Principles and practice of emergency medicine,* Philadelphia, 1986, WB Saunders.

CHAPTER 182

Neonatal Resuscitation*

Eric M. Hughes

The first few moments of a newborn's life can be the most critical. If needed, effective emergency care during this transition can prevent lifelong consequences. Proper resuscitation requires essential equipment and knowledge of necessary protocols before delivery.

INDICATIONS

Neonate with the following:
• Inadequate or ineffective respirations
• Inadequate heart rate
• Central cyanosis
• Other evidence of cardiorespiratory distress

EQUIPMENT

• Suction equipment, including a bulb syringe, mechanical suction device, suction catheters (6, 8, 10 French), pediatric feeding tube (8 French), and meconium aspirator (DeLee)
• Oxygen source with flow meter, infant resuscitation bag (≤750 ml) with appropriately sized facemasks, laryngoscope with no. 0 and no. 1 straight blades, and sterile newborn endotracheal tubes (2.5, 3.0, 3.5, and 4.0 mm)
• Drugs, including epinephrine 1:10,000 (0.1 mg/ml), naloxone (0.04 mg/ml), normal saline for injection, and sodium bicarbonate 4.2% (0.5 mEq/ml)
• Miscellaneous items, including a radiant warmer, pediatric stethoscope, needles (25, 21, and 18 gauge), syringes (1, 3, 10, 20 ml), adhesive tape (½-inch width), and umbilical catheter (3.5 or 5 French)

TECHNIQUE

As with all medical procedures, universal precautions against exposure to blood and other body fluids should

be followed. Initial measures, including proper positioning, drying, suctioning, and stimulation, should be provided to all newborns. Fig. 182-1 is a flow diagram of the protocol for neonatal resuscitation explained below.

Positioning, Suction, and Stimulation

1. Prevent heat loss by placing the infant under a radiant heat source, then quickly drying him or her and removing wet linen. (Recovery from acidosis is delayed by hypothermia.)
2. Open the airway by positioning the infant on the back with the neck slightly extended. Extreme hyperextension or flexion of the infant's neck may diminish airflow.
3. Clear the airway by suctioning the mouth, then the nose, with a bulb syringe or mechanical device (suction catheter). If mechanical suction is used, pressure should not exceed 100 mm Hg. Deep suctioning of the oropharynx may produce a vagal response and cause bradycardia and apnea. Infants with meconium-stained amniotic fluid (whether light or heavy) should have the mouth, pharynx, and nose suctioned as soon as the head is delivered and before the body is delivered (see Chapter 179, Delee Suctioning). Direct tracheal suctioning should only be carried out if the newborn has absent or depressed respirations, a heart rate below 100 bpm, or poor muscle tone. A meconium aspirator is very helpful in performing this procedure (Fig. 182-2). This unique piece of equipment is used only for neonates. One end of the device is for a neonatal endotracheal tube, the other end for suction, and the top hole is for the operator's thumb.
4. Promote respiratory activity by providing tactile stimulation (slap the sole of the foot or gently rub the back).

Initial Assessment

1. Assess the infant's respiratory status, heart rate, and color.

*Marvin DeWar wrote this chapter in the previous edition.

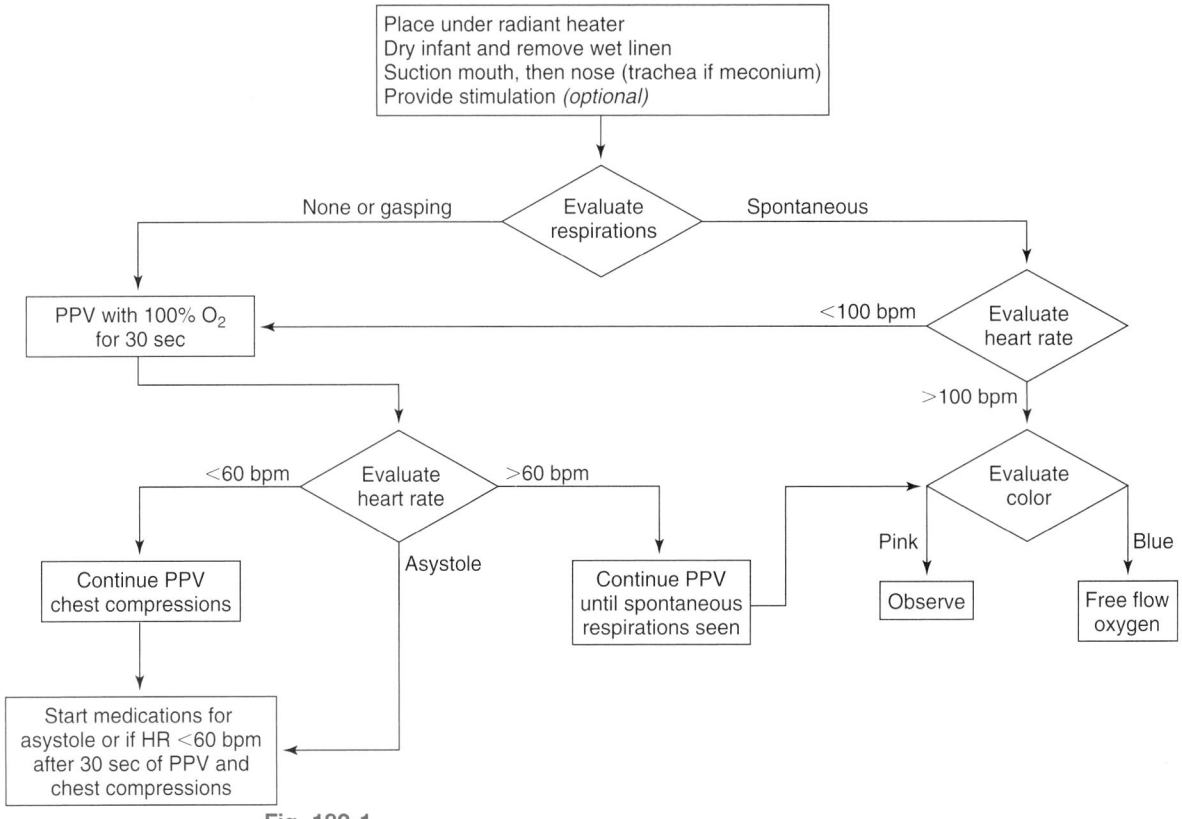

Fig. 182-1
Resuscitation flowchart. *HR,* Heart rate; *PPV,* positive pressure ventilation.

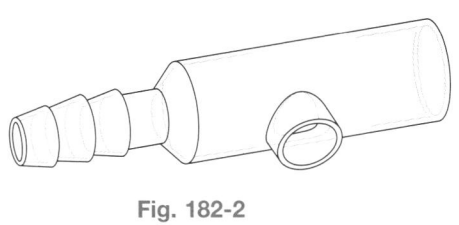

Fig. 182-2
Meconium aspirator.

2. Infants with adequate respiratory and cardiac function (good ventilation and heart rate greater than 100 bpm), and with no evidence of central cyanosis, can be merely observed.
3. Infants with depressed respiratory function (shallow, slow, or absent respirations), an abnormal heart rate, or central cyanosis should undergo further resuscitation.

General Guidelines of Resuscitation

As with all resuscitations, the order of importance is **A**irway, **B**reathing, and **C**irculation. The three cardinal indicators in neonatal resuscitation are **R**espirations, **H**eart **R**ate, and **C**olor. In general the initial assessment should take no more than 30 seconds; should the need for further resuscitation occur, reassessment of interven-

tions should occur every 30 seconds. APGAR scores should be kept at appropriate intervals. Special circumstances may arise which may be treated more adequately with procedures used in general pediatric resuscitation (e.g., chest tube for pneumothorax).

Ventilation

1. Ventilatory insufficiency produces the majority of respiratory and circulatory abnormalities in the newborn period. *Rapid* institution of ventilatory support in newborns with abnormalities of respiratory function or heart rate, or central cyanosis, maximizes the chances of a successful outcome.
2. Positive pressure ventilation (PPV) with 100% oxygen is indicated for infants with inadequate respiratory effort or a heart rate less than 100 bpm. Free-flow oxygen administration may be adequate for the infant with central cyanosis if respiratory function is adequate and the heart rate is over 100 bpm. (The cause for cyanosis should be sought.) If central cyanosis persists despite oxygen administration, PPV should be applied.
3. PPV is usually accomplished with a bag and mask, using either a self-inflating bag or an anesthesia bag. Appropriately sized facemasks with cushioned rims

TABLE 182-1

Endotracheal Tube Selection

Infant Weight (g)	Gestation Age (wk)	Endotracheal Tube Size (mm)
<1000	<26	2.5
1000-2000	26-34	3.0
2000-3000	34-40	3.5
>3000	>40	3.5-4.0

should be used. A pressure gauge or pop-off valve should be used to ensure adequate ventilatory pressures.

4. Ventilate the infant at a rate of 40 to 60 breaths per minute with a tidal volume of 6 to 8 ml/kg. Adequate ventilation is verified clinically by observing bilateral symmetrical chest expansion and the presence of bilateral breath sounds. Inadequate ventilation may indicate an inadequate facemask seal, a blocked airway, or inadequate ventilation pressure. After initial ventilations, pressures of less than 30 to 40 cm H$_2$O should be adequate.

5. Perform an endotracheal intubation when prolonged PPV is required, when a bag and mask ventilation is ineffective, or when diaphragmatic hernia is suspected. Select an endotracheal tube of appropriate size (Table 182-1), and insert it under direct visualization using the laryngoscope. The tip should rest above the tracheal bifurcation. Appropriate endotracheal tube location is verified clinically by the presence of bilaterally symmetrical breath sounds and is confirmed with a chest x-ray film.

6. Oral airways are rarely required during neonatal resuscitation but are indicated for bilateral choanal atresia, Pierre Robin syndrome, and when necessary for adequate ventilation.

7. Use of a laryngeal mask airway (LMA) (Fig. 182-3) can be an acceptable alternative when bag-mask ventilation and endotracheal intubation has failed. (The LMA is a substitute in certain cases for traditional endotracheal intubation.) The LMA should only be used by properly trained personnel and is not considered a routine substitute for endotracheal intubation.

8. Gastric catheter placement (8 French) is indicated in prolonged resuscitation efforts to prevent stomach distension, a frequent problem in newborns who are being ventilated by mask.

Chest Compressions

1. Administer chest compressions if the infant's heart rate is below 60 bpm after adequate positive pressure ventilation (PPV) for 30 seconds. Chest compressions can be accomplished with the thumbs placed on the sternum, and the hands encircling the chest (preferred method), or with the tips of the middle and

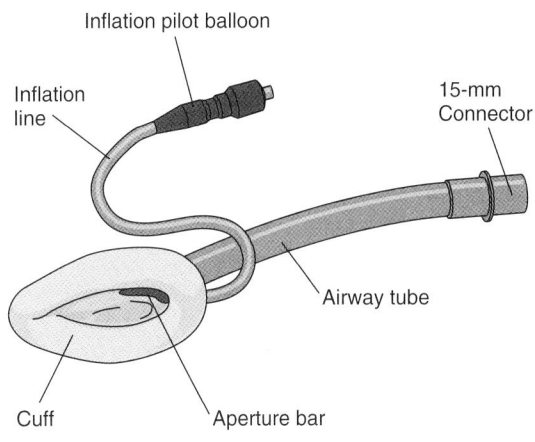

Fig. 182-3
Laryngeal mask airway.

index fingers (Fig. 182-4). Chest compressions should be applied to the lower third of the sternum. The sternum should be depressed one third to half of the anterior-posterior dimension of the chest or one third the depth of the chest, rather than an exact depth of compression. The compression depth must be adequate to produce a palpable pulse.

2. Chest compressions should be administered at a ratio of 3:1 with PPV, at a rate of 90 compressions and 30 ventilations every minute. Reassess the pulse every 30 seconds. The umbilical cord stump is a convenient location to palpate the pulse.

3. Continue chest compressions until the spontaneous heart rate is 60 bpm or higher (Fig. 182-1).

Medications (Table 182-2)

Administer medication for asystole or when the heart rate remains less than 60 bpm after adequate PPV and chest compressions for a minimum of 30 seconds. Medication may be administered through the umbilical vein with a 3.5 or 5 French umbilical catheter placed just below the skin level. (See Chapter 186, Umbilical Vessel Catheterization.) Alternative access can be obtained through a peripheral vein, or, in the event that no other access is available, by intraosseous access (see Chapter 181, Intraosseous Venous Access). Intraosseous access can be very difficult to obtain in premature infants. Alternative routes of administration (endotracheal [ET], intramuscular [IM], or subcutaneous [SQ]) are available for some medications.

Termination of Resuscitation

Discontinuation of resuscitative efforts may be appropriate if resuscitation of an infant with cardiorespiratory arrest does not produce spontaneous circulation within

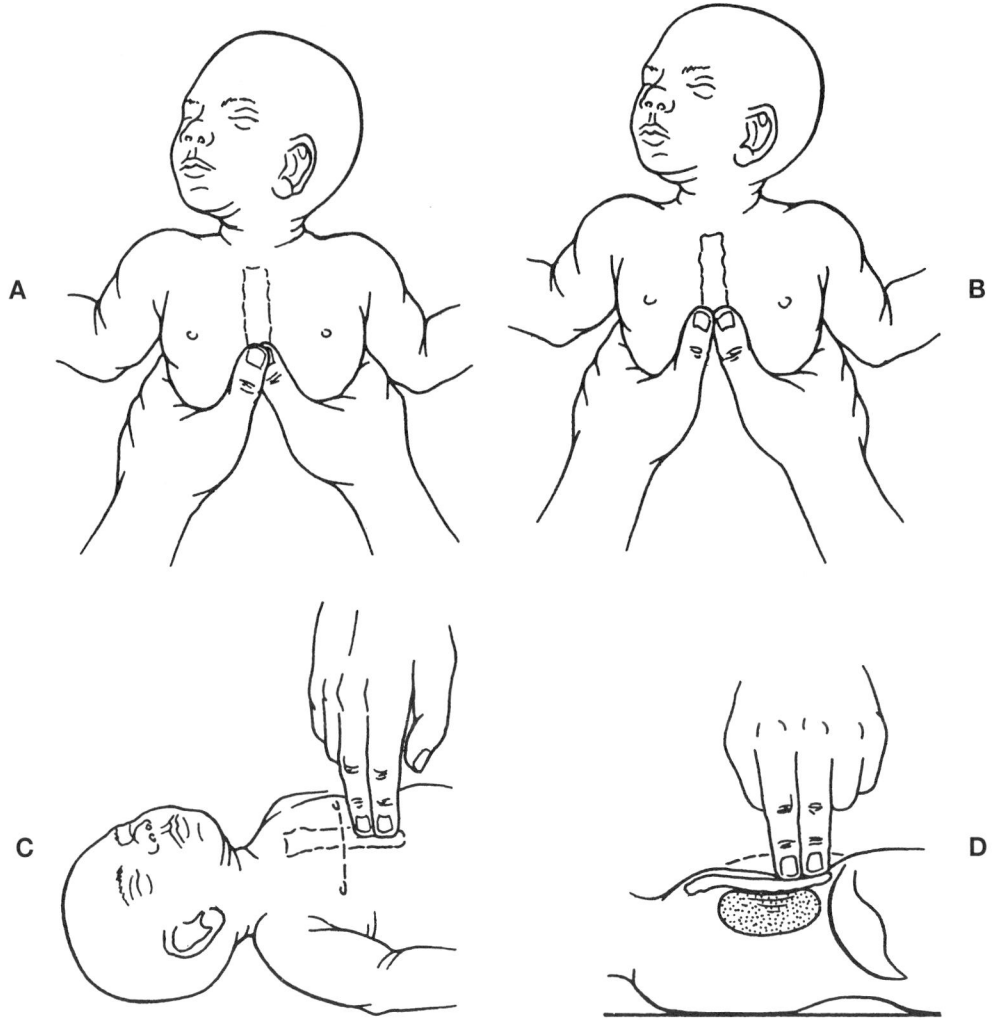

Fig. 182-4
Chest compression. Two-thumb technique with, **A,** thumb over thumb and, **B,** side by side. **C,** Two-finger technique. **D,** Chest compression depth is one third to one half of the anterior-posterior diameter of the chest or one third of the depth of the chest.

TABLE 182-2

Medications Used for Neonatal Resuscitation

Medication	Indication	Dose	Route of Administration
Epinephrine	Asystole or HR <60 despite adequate PPV and chest compressions for 30 sec	0.1-0.3 ml/kg of a 1:10,000 solution or 0.01-0.03 mg/kg	IV or ET, can repeat every 3-5 min
Volume expander (crystalloid or blood)	Evidence of acute blood loss with signs of hypovolemia, or failure to respond to resuscitation or signs of shock	10 ml/kg	IV over 5-10 min
Sodium bicarbonate	Prolonged arrest unresponsive to other therapy or for documented metabolic acidosis	1-2 mEq/kg	IV over at least 2 min
Naloxone	History of maternal narcotic administration within 4 hr of delivery and respiratory depression	0.1 mg/kg	ET, IV preferred, IM, SQ acceptable

ET, Endotracheal; *HR,* heart rate; *IM,* intramuscular; *IV,* intravenous; *PPV,* positive pressure ventilation; *SQ,* subcutaneous.

15 minutes. Resuscitation of newly born infants after 10 minutes of asystole is also very unlikely to result in survival or survival without severe disability. Those involved in neonatal resuscitation should pursue local discussions to formulate guidelines consistent with local resources and outcome data.

POSTPROCEDURE PATIENT MANAGEMENT AND EDUCATION

* Maintain careful monitoring in an appropriately staffed intensive care unit.
* Continue evaluation with serial arterial blood gases, frequent determination of fluid and electrolyte status, chest x-ray films, and other modalities as indicated by clinical findings.
* Completely document the resuscitation effort in the medical record.
* Discuss situation with parents.

COMPLICATIONS

Suction

* Vagal response (bradycardia or apnea)
* Hypoxia

Ventilation

* Pneumothorax
* Hypoxia resulting from inadequate ventilation
* Complications from intubation (see Chapter 83, Tracheal [Endotracheal and Nasotracheal] Intubation)

CPT/BILLING CODES

99440   Newborn resuscitation: provision of positive pressure ventilation and/or chest compressions in the presence of acute inadequate ventilation and/or cardiac output

99431   History and examination of the normal newborn infant, initiation of diagnostic and treatment programs and preparation of hospital records

99436   Attendance at delivery (when requested by delivering physician) and initial stabilization of newborn
(99436 may be reported in addition to 99431)
(99436 may not be reported in addition to 99440)

ICD-9-CM DIAGNOSTIC CODES

427.5   Asystole (heart)
768.5   Asphyxia, newborn, severe
768.6   Asphyxia, newborn, mild/moderate
769   Respiratory distress syndrome, newborn, idiopathic
768.4   Respiratory distress, fetus or newborn
770.8   Cyanosis, newborn
763.83   Bradycardia, newborn
770.8   Bradypnea
779.8   Arrest, fetus or newborn
770.1   Meconium aspiration

BIBLIOGRAPHY

An advisory statement from the Pediatric Working Group of the International Liaison Committee on Resuscitation, *Circulation* 99:1927, 1999.
American Academy of Pediatrics: *Neonatal resuscitation,* ed 4, Washington, DC, 2000, AAP.
Niermeyer S, Kattwinkel J, Van Reempts P, et al: International Guidelines for Neonatal Resuscitation: An excerpt from the Guidelines 2000 for Cardiopulmonary Resuscitation and Emergency Cardiovascular Care: International Consensus on Science, *Pediatrics* 106:E29, 2000.

Newborn Circumcision

Ronald D. Reynolds
Grant C. Fowler

Newborn circumcision is the most commonly performed surgical procedure in the United States. Controversy exists as to the need for the procedure. Studies have shown a lower incidence of urinary tract infection and some sexually transmitted diseases in circumcised males. There also may be a slightly decreased risk of HIV infection in circumcised males. Circumcision clearly prevents penile cancer. However, these problems (penile cancer, HIV, STDs, and UTIs) are rare even in uncircumcised males.

In developed countries that do not circumcise boys, there is not a high incidence of foreskin problems later in life. Behavioral factors appear to be far more important than circumcision status in the acquisition of HIV infection and sexually transmitted diseases. Therefore, the decision to circumcise is not currently based on scientific evidence. Rather, this decision is generally made based on cultural, familial, or ethnic precedence.

Clinicians performing circumcision are encouraged to remain current with guidelines and the scientific evidence. Recent evidence suggests that sexual partners of uncircumcised males may be at higher risk of abnormal Pap smears and cervical cancer. This is probably due to human papillomavirus (HPV). Research results need to be more clearly defined in this area, however, before guidelines are changed, because abnormal Pap smears are common. The most recent American Academy of Pediatrics (AAP) circumcision position reads as follows:

Existing scientific evidence demonstrates potential medical benefits of newborn male circumcision; however, these data are not sufficient to recommend routine neonatal circumcision. In circumstances in which there are potential benefits and risks, yet the procedure is not essential to the child's current well-being, parents of all male infants should be given accurate and unbiased information and be provided the opportunity to discuss this decision. If a decision for circumcision is made, procedural analgesia should be provided.

Of note, this is the first time that the AAP has recommended procedural analgesia for circumcision. Common methods of analgesia administration include dorsal penile nerve block or subcutaneous ring block (see Chapter 180, Dorsal Penile and Subcutaneous Ring Block for Newborn Circumcision), precircumcision oral analgesics, and topical anesthesia such as EMLA cream (see Chapter 11, Topical Anesthesia). Although studies have shown EMLA cream to be effective, blocks appear to be more effective. Studies have shown that infants anesthetized with a block cry less, are less likely to have tachycardia, are less irritable, and have fewer behavior changes during the 24 hours after the procedure. They also have less variability in oxygen saturation and blood pressure during, and lower serum cortisol levels after, the procedure.

Three techniques of newborn circumcision are common in the United States: Mogen, Gomco, and Plastibell. Most clinicians continue to use the technique they were taught in their training. Both Gomco and Plastibell require a dorsal slit, considerable manipulation to prepare the foreskin for excision, and result in removal of a cylindrical sleeve of tissue. Both techniques carry the risk of removing too much tissue from the ventral side. In addition, Plastibell leaves behind a foreign body that may contribute to infection. One study comparing Gomco to Plastibell indicated that there was not only a higher rate of infection with Plastibell, but also a slightly higher rate of bleeding.

Most clinicians who learn to use the Mogen clamp tend to prefer this technique because it is quicker and simpler, and it follows the angle of the corona for an excellent cosmetic result. Contrary to popular belief, the Mogen clamp is not a guillotine. It is simply a crushing device with a narrow slot that, when used appropriately, does not allow entry of the glans into the slot.

Note: Occasionally, meatal stenosis occurs in the first few years of life. Although rare, it may be the most common late complication of circumcision and is probably a result of meatitis or a meatal ulcer. Following circumcision, the glans and meatus are no longer protected by the foreskin, and diaper irritation may cause an inflammatory membrane to form. If the meatus is less than 2 mm in length or less than 25% to 30% of the diameter of the glans, meatotomy can be performed in the office (see the "Technique" section). Parents should be instructed to watch for the development of meatal stenosis.

INDICATION

* Parental desire

CONTRAINDICATIONS

* Hypospadias, epispadias, or megaurethra*
* Unusual appearing genitalia*
* Inability to determine the phenotype of the child* (ambiguous genitalia)
* Age younger than 12 hours (physiologic adaptation requires 12 to 24 hours)
* Severe illness
* Prematurity (until the child is ready for discharge from the hospital)
* Gomco is relatively contraindicated for an abnormally short penile shaft (less than 1 cm); see the "Gomco Technique" section*

If there is a family history of bleeding problems, appropriate laboratory studies should be performed before the procedure. If the mother is thrombocytopenic, the infant's platelet count should be checked.

One relative contraindication to circumcision is age greater than 6 to 8 weeks. By this age, maternal clotting factors have been metabolized, possibly predisposing the infant to increased blood loss. The foreskin may also develop significant edema after defining the plane between the glans and the foreskin, making it difficult to use the Gomco clamp.

PREPROCEDURE PATIENT PREPARATION

Discuss the risks and benefits of the procedure with the parents. Informed consent is obtained, and a patient teaching guide is given to the parents. (See the sample patient education handout titled "Newborn Circumcision" on page 1989 of Appendix G.) The AAP has two brochures that may be used: (1) *Circumcision: Pros and Cons* and (2) *Newborns: Care of the Uncircumcised Penis.* (See the "Suppliers" section.)

Because of the risk of regurgitation, infants being circumcised should be at least 1 hour postprandial.

*Consult a urologist.

Confirm that the infant has had at least one void since birth.

EQUIPMENT

Equipment Common to All Techniques, Including Meatotomy

* Infant restraint board (Circumstraint), leg straps, and padding if chair or assistant not available to hold infant
* Glucose water or sugar-coated pacifier
* Analgesic and anesthetic supplies
* Sterile gloves
* Betadine swabsticks
* Sterile drape with 1-inch fenestration
* Sterile 2 × 2–inch gauze pads
* Three straight mosquito hemostats
* White petrolatum (Vaseline) gauze, ½ inch wide
* Disposable diaper
* Adequate light source
* One 5- to 6-inch flexible blunt probe *(optional)*
* Skin marking pen *(optional)*

Equipment for Mogen Technique

* Mogen clamp, neonatal size (2.5-mm slot)

Note: The larger adult size is dangerous to use on a newborn because the glans can become trapped in the larger slot. The clinician should confirm that the neonatal size does not open more than 2.5 mm.

* No. 10 blade scalpel

Equipment for Gomco Technique

* Straight scissors with one blunt tip
* Gomco circumcision clamps (1.1-, 1.3-, and 1.45-cm sizes)

Note: The most commonly used size is 1.3 cm. The 1.1-cm size is usually for a very small infant, whereas the 1.45-cm clamp usually fits a large infant. Even larger sizes are available for children and adults.

* No. 10 blade scalpel
* Sterile safety pin *(optional)*
* Adson forceps *(optional)*

Equipment for Plastibell Technique

* Straight scissors with one blunt tip
* Plastibell device (1.1-, 1.2-, 1.3-, and 1.4-cm sizes)

Note: Similar to Gomco, 1.3 cm is the most commonly used Plastibell size.

* Iris scissors

Equipment for Bleeding Complications of All Three Techniques

- Topical epinephrine
- Gelfoam or Surgicel
- 5-0 absorbable suture (chromic or catgut) on a taper needle
- Needle holder and suture scissors

MOGEN TECHNIQUE

1. Position the infant appropriately in a warm room. An infant may experience discomfort when you extend his legs on a circumcision-restraint board. As a result, special circumcision chairs have been developed for exposure of the penis without extension of the legs. If such a chair is not available, an assistant can hold the infant on a pillow with the knees flexed and legs abducted for adequate exposure. If an assistant is not available, a Circumstraint can be used. Leave the baby's arms free to minimize distress. Offer him a swallow or two of glucose water or a sugar-coated pacifier to calm him.

2. Consider using a skin marker to mark the coronal edge. Inspect the penis for abnormalities and for the location of the meatus on the glans. For epispadias or hypospadias, terminate the procedure.

3. If penile anatomy is normal, anesthetize the penis (preferably with a dorsal penile nerve block or subcutaneous ring block [see Chapter 180, Dorsal Penile and Subcutaneous Ring Block for Newborn Circumcision]).

4. Using Betadine swabsticks, prepare the entire penis and a 1-inch area surrounding the penis. Wear sterile gloves when placing the fenestrated drape.

5. Grasp the very edge of the foreskin with hemostats at the 2 and 10 o'clock positions, taking care not to grasp the glans. (When describing the penis, use the dorsal midline as the 12 o'clock position. To identify the true dorsal midline, identify the frenulum and consider the foreskin 180 degrees opposite it to be the 12 o'clock position. This orientation technique can even be used if the penile shaft is rotated.)

6. Place gentle traction on the foreskin by holding the two hemostats side by side in your nondominant hand. Gently insert the third hemostat, closed and from below the grasping hemostats, at the 12 o'clock position between the foreskin and the glans. Advance to the depth of the coronal sulcus (Fig. 183-1). To ensure that the meatus is not entered, keep the foreskin tented up as this hemostat is advanced. Open this hemostat and sweep it clockwise and counterclockwise to free the foreskin off the glans. Usually this takes a number of open-close cycles starting at different places around the corona. Do not free the area from the 5 to 7 o'clock positions (the frenulum) because it contains an arteriole. Do not dissect beyond the depth of the coronal sulcus. As an alternative to opening and closing a hemostat, a blunt probe may be used to free the foreskin off of the glans.

7. Tent the foreskin away from the glans by gently lifting the grasping hemostats. Ensure that no part of the glans is in the way. Advance the lower blade of a third hemostat between the glans and foreskin at the 12 o'clock position to a position no less than 5 mm distal to the coronal sulcus (Fig. 183-2). Do not apply traction to the grasping hemostats as this dorsal hemostat is applied or you will remove too much foreskin. Close and lock the hemostat in place.

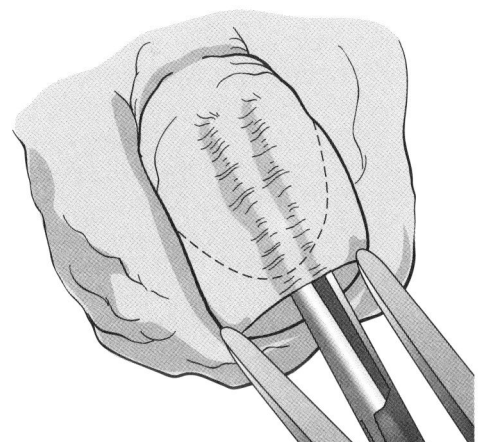

Fig. 183-1
Insert the third hemostat between the foreskin and the glans, tenting the foreskin as it is advanced. Here the surgeon is just beginning to open the hemostat to free the foreskin off the glans.

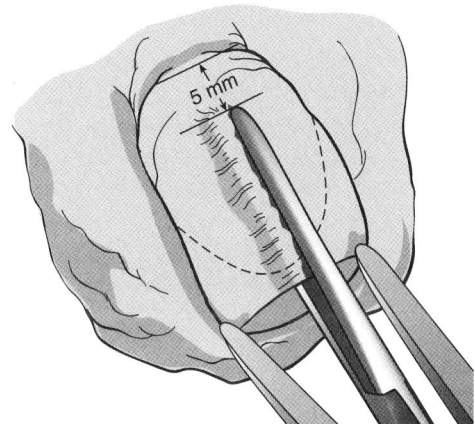

Fig. 183-2
Place a dorsal hemostat with its tip 5 mm from the corona.

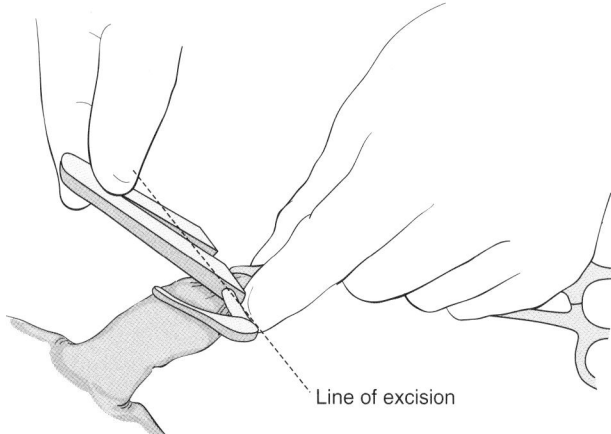

Line of excision

Fig. 183-3
Pinch the foreskin to push the glans back while advancing the Mogen clamp vertically along the angle of the corona.

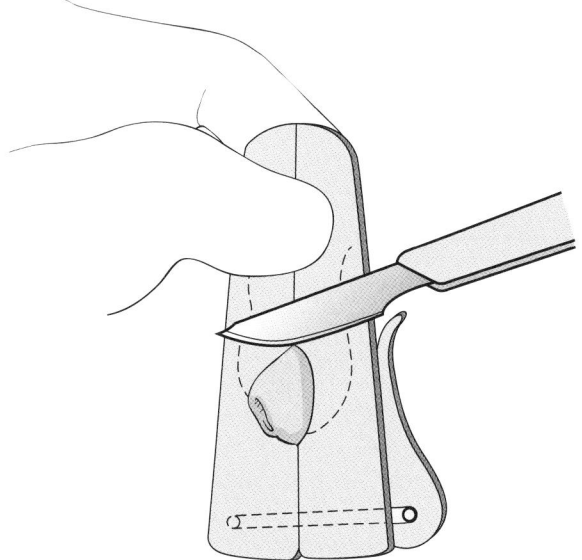

Fig. 183-4
Excise the foreskin.

8. Remove the two foreskin edge grasping hemostats.
9. Using the thumb and index finger of your nondominant hand, pinch the free foreskin underneath the dorsal hemostat while curling your other fingers of the same hand around the handles of the hemostat. This pushes the glans back out of the way of the Mogen clamp. Release any traction on the hemostat and foreskin because traction on the frenulum can rotate the glans and bring the meatus into the path of the Mogen clamp. Maintain the pinch while the Mogen clamp is placed.
10. Inspect the Mogen clamp to be sure it is a neonatal size, then open it fully. Hold it so that the open end of the slot is down and the flat surface faces you. With your dominant hand, advance the Mogen slot across the foreskin, starting immediately behind the tip of the dorsal hemostat (Fig. 183-3). Angle the Mogen's advancement to remove more foreskin dorsally than ventrally, following along the angle of the corona (dorsum of the glans). Slide the clamp across the foreskin as far as it will go easily. At this point, use of the skin markings can assure that an adequate, but not excess, amount of foreskin is removed.
11. Before locking the Mogen clamp, drop the foreskin pinch and attempt to move the glans beneath the slot. You should be able to move the glans freely for a few millimeters up-and-down and side-to-side. If the glans is not free, *do not* lock the Mogen clamp.
12. Lock the Mogen clamp by moving the bar across the slot and closing the cam lever fully.
13. Use the scalpel to cut the foreskin off flush with the flat surface of the Mogen clamp (Fig. 183-4). Discard the foreskin in a biohazard waste container.
14. Unlock and remove the Mogen clamp.

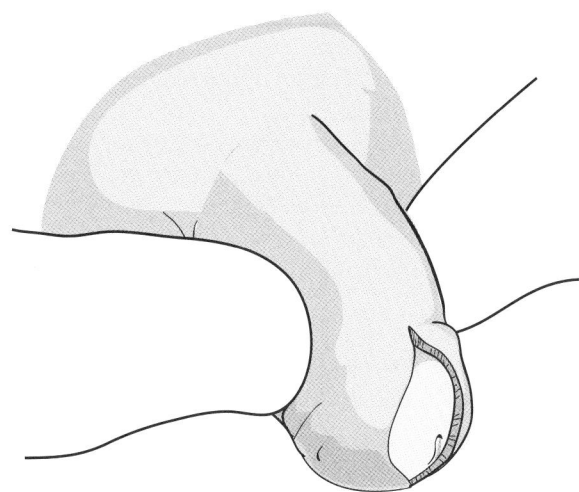

Fig. 183-5
Liberate the glans with thumb pressure.

15. Gently separate the crushed edges of the foreskin to liberate the glans. Grasp the penile shaft skin at the 3 and 9 o'clock positions to pull the crush line apart (Fig. 183-5). Be sure to separate fully to avoid the possibility of causing a paraphimosis. It is not unusual to have a few remaining attachments between the glans and the mucosal surface of the remaining foreskin next to the corona. The easiest way to divide these is to use the tip of a closed and locked hemostat to follow the coronal sulcus. Do not be too vigorous or try to free the frenular area or you will cause bleeding.
16. Check for hemostasis. To control any bleeding, apply pressure or topical epinephrine to the specific

source. In rare cases of persistent bleeding, Gelfoam or Surgicel can be applied with pressure to hasten clotting. Rarely will bleeding require suturing. In the event that it does, use an absorbable suture at the site of the bleeding, which is usually an arteriole. Do not use silver nitrate for hemostasis because it can leave a permanent stain in the tissue. Persistent bleeding after circumcision is a common presenting sign for a factor-deficient bleeding disorder hemophilia. If bleeding persists following the described measures, obtain clotting studies and consider a hematology consultation.

17. Wrap white petrolatum gauze around the site, and reapply the diaper.
18. Administer an oral dose of acetaminophen (10 to 15 mg/kg).
19. Document the procedure and time in the chart. To ensure continued hemostasis, do not discharge the infant for about an hour after the procedure.

GOMCO TECHNIQUE

1. Choose an appropriate sized Gomco clamp, which is 1.3 cm for most newborns. (The bell diameter should be slightly larger than the glans' diameter. The bell should cover the glans completely, but just barely.) Carefully inspect the clamp. If the clamp was packaged disassembled, reassemble it in the sterile field. Since there is more than one manufacturer for Gomco clamps, make sure the reassembled clamp parts fit together properly. Reassembled parts may be from different manufacturers. Make sure the bell is the correct size for the clamp and that there are no defects. Lightly tighten the clamp with the bell in place. Make sure that no light can be seen around the bell where it meets at the base plate. This ensures a complete circumferential crush for optimal hemostasis. Next, verify that the top surface of the base plate is flat. Last, there should be at least 2 mm between the back of the lever arm and the base plate beneath the nut before tightening. This also ensures adequate clamping.
2. As in steps 1 through 6 of the "Mogen Technique" section, position the infant (restrain if necessary), inspect his penis for abnormalities, consider marking the coronal edge, administer analgesia or anesthesia, apply antiseptic and drapes, and free the foreskin from the glans. Use of a Gomco clamp is relatively contraindicated in infants with unusually short penile shafts. If the shaft appears short, use your index and middle finger to expose the entire shaft by pushing the skin down at (around) the base of the penis. For a shaft shorter than 1 cm when measured in this manner, obtain consultation before

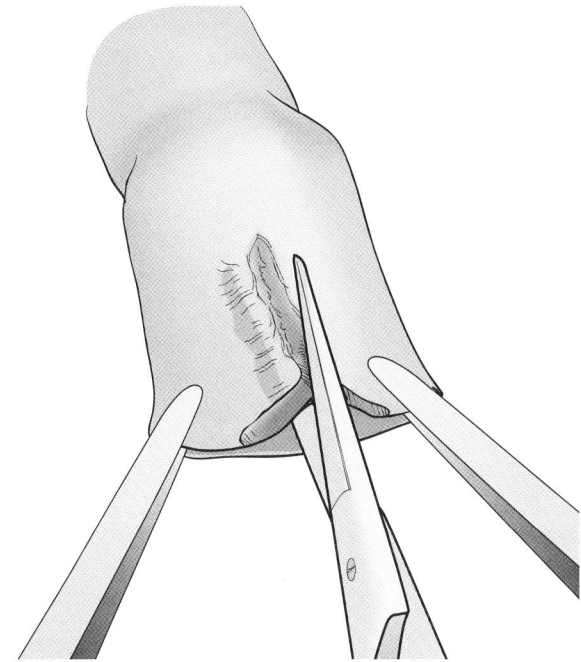

Fig. 183-6
Incise the dorsal slit.

using a Gomco clamp; a Mogen clamp is usually preferred in this situation.

3. As in step 7 of the "Mogen Technique" section, place a crushing dorsal hemostat at the 12 o'clock position, but only apply it to the distal third or half of the length of the foreskin (the total length of the foreskin extends from the foreskin edge to the coronal sulcus). This hemostat is not applied more proximal than 1 cm from the coronal sulcus. Make sure that the crushing hemostat contains both the mucosal and skin layers of the foreskin.
4. The hemostat can be removed immediately after crushing. Removal reveals a crushed area of foreskin that has been devitalized and therefore will not bleed when cut. Tent the foreskin with the edge hemostats. Make sure the edge hemostats hold both mucosal and skin foreskin layers. Using scissors with their blunt blade down, cut a dorsal slit through the center of the crush line (Fig. 183-6). Be careful to cut only in the crush line; do not extend laterally or past the apex of the crush line. Venturing beyond or outside the crush line results in unnecessary bleeding.
5. Retract the foreskin back from around the glans. If, at this point, you cannot fully retract the foreskin, recrush a bit further dorsally, and extend the dorsal slit. Lyse any remaining adherence between the foreskin and glans with the closed tips of a locked hemostat or the blunt probe. You should be able to fully reveal the sulcus behind the corona. Do not

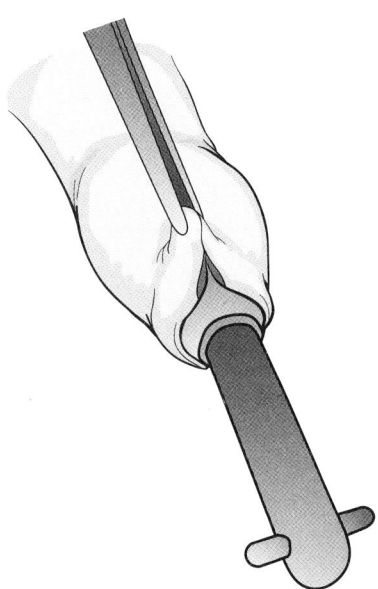

Fig. 183-7
Reapproximate the dorsal slit around the Gomco bell.

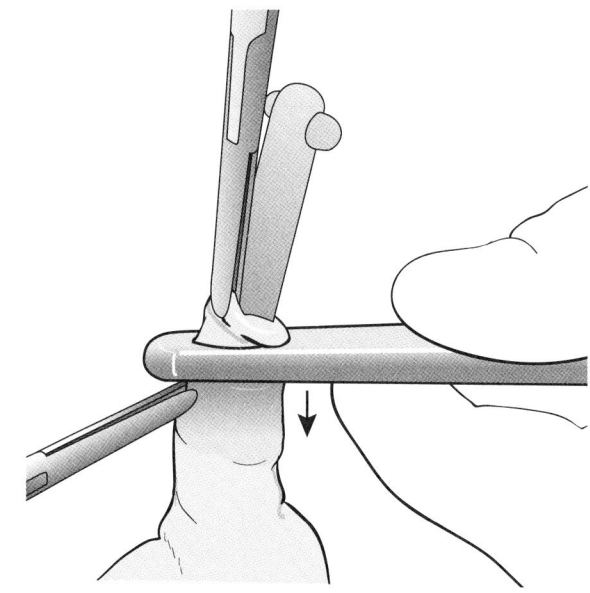

Fig. 183-8
Bring the bell's stem and foreskin through the ring by exchanging hemostats.

dissect at all between the 5 and 7 o'clock positions to avoid the frenulum and its arteriole.

Note: If the clinician notices hypospadias or epispadias after the dorsal slit has been made, terminate the procedure. After termination, if there is bleeding from the dorsal slit, whipstitch the edges or close the dorsal slit using fine chromic suture. Repair of penile congenital anomalies may require foreskin tissue; do not remove any, if possible.

6. Place the bell of an appropriate sized Gomco clamp over the glans.
7. Use the still-attached edge hemostats to reapproximate the foreskin around the bell while applying gentle downward pressure on the bell's stem. Make sure that both mucosal and skin layers of the foreskin are reapproximated. The bell should occupy the space between the glans and the foreskin and sit against the coronal edge.
8. When the Gomco bell is appropriately placed, grasp both sides of the dorsal slit, near the middle of the incision, in the tips of a third hemostat. This reapproximates the foreskin around the stem (Fig. 183-7). The approach with the hemostat is from above at a low angle, with handles up near the infant's umbilicus. This will ease the next step. (Some clinicians use a safety pin to hold the dorsal slit edges together in this step, but this unnecessarily increases the risk of a puncture injury to the clinician.)
9. Remove the two foreskin edge hemostats.
10. Place the end of the stem through the hole in the Gomco baseplate as far as it will go without dislodging the foreskin.

11. Reaching through the baseplate hole with a hemostat, regrasp across the foreskin's dorsal slit just above the tips of the lower hemostat (Fig. 183-8). Remove the lower hemostat. Pull the stem fully up through the baseplate hole. (If using a safety pin, pull the entire pin along with the bell through the baseplate hole. The safety pin will need to be turned parallel to the stem of the bell to pull it through the hole. The safety pin can then remain in place throughout the remainder of the procedure.)
12. Assemble the Gomco clamp by grasping the wings of the bell's stem in the rocker arm's end, placing the rocker arm in its fulcrum slot, and loosely placing the nut on its screw.
13. Make sure that the foreskin has been drawn through the hole in the Gomco clamp evenly from all sides. The apex of the dorsal slit must be above the baseplate. Using a hemostat or forcep, pull on the mucosal edge of the dorsal slit to be sure that the mucosal apex of the dorsal slit is also above the baseplate. When you are sure that the foreskin is evenly pulled through the Gomco clamp and the apex of the dorsal slit is visible above the baseplate, firmly tighten the clamp. Remove the hemostat.
14. On the top side of the baseplate, the scalpel can be used to immediately excise the foreskin. It should be excised circumferentially and completely at the junction of the baseplate and the bell (Fig. 183-9). The top side of the baseplate is on the same side as the stem of the bell. Make sure that all skin and mucosal layers are removed. Any remaining tissue above the clamp will become necrotic and a

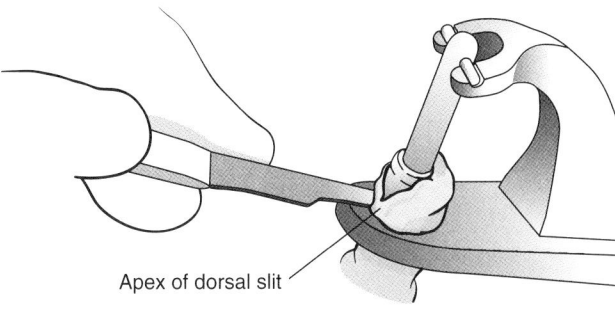

Fig. 183-9
Excise the foreskin. The apex of the dorsal slit should be visible above the baseplate.

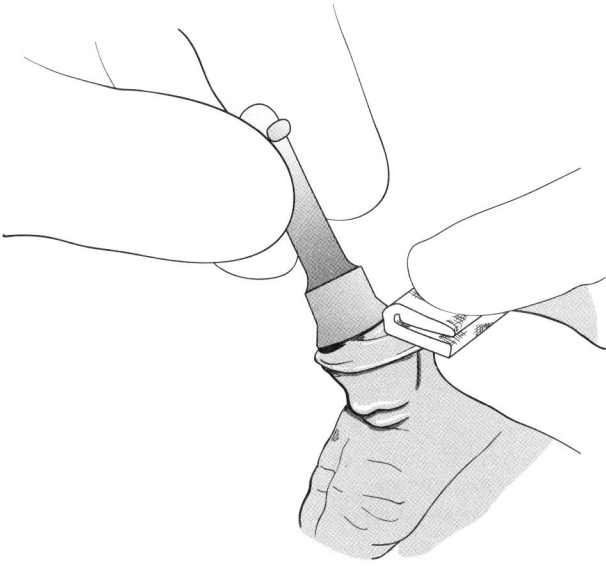

Fig. 183-10
Tease the adherent tissue off the bell edge with gauze.

possible source of infection. Cut the excised ring of foreskin away from the stem with scissors and discard it in a biohazard waste container.

15. Loosen and disassemble the Gomco clamp.
16. To remove the adherent foreskin edge from the bell, gently tease it away using a piece of gauze (Fig. 183-10).
17. Follow steps 16 through 19 of the "Mogen Technique" section to check hemostasis, dress the wound, and document the procedure.

Note: A rare complication of using a Gomco clamp that is too large, or from pulling too much foreskin through the baseplate hole, is degloving of the penile shaft skin. In this situation, after the clamp and bell are removed, the shaft skin will retract too far and expose the underlying tissue proximal to the coronal

sulcus. Attempts to control bleeding in the usual manner often fail. A primary closure with four absorbable (5-0 chromic) sutures should be made. Sutures are placed circumferentially to reposition the retracted shaft skin to a point just proximal to the corona. Care must be taken in the ventral area to avoid the urethra. Some clinicians catheterize the infant with a 5-French feeding tube before performing the repair. Otherwise, no special aftercare is needed.

PLASTIBELL TECHNIQUE

1. Choose an appropriate sized Plastibell, which is 1.3 cm for most normal newborns. (The Plastibell should fit like an appropriate-sized Gomco bell.) Drop the device into the sterile field.
2. As in steps 1 through 6 of the "Mogen Technique" section, position the infant (restrain if necessary), consider marking the foreskin at the coronal edge, inspect the penis for abnormalities, administer a dorsal penile nerve or subcutaneous ring block, apply antiseptic, drape, and free the foreskin from the glans.
3. As in steps 4 and 5 of the "Gomco Technique" section, place a dorsal crushing clamp and remove it, cut a dorsal slit, and retract and fully free the foreskin. Leave the two foreskin edge hemostats in place.
4. Place the Plastibell string loosely around the base of the penis and put two twists in the string to start a surgeon's knot.
5. Place the Plastibell over the glans (Fig. 183-11) with its "wishbone" vertical. The edge of the Plastibell should just touch the coronal edge. Exchange the Plastibell for an appropriate size if this is not the case. It is particularly dangerous to use too large a Plastibell because the glans can push through its center and cause a paraphimosis, with resultant necrosis of the glans. If the size is correct, pull the foreskin over the device by manipulating the grasping hemostats.
6. When the Plastibell is appropriately placed, with the handles of a third hemostat, grasp both sides of the dorsal slit with the hemostat tips at about the middle of the incision. This will reapproximate the foreskin around the device and hold it in place (Fig. 183-12).
7. Ensure that the string groove of the Plastibell is below the apex of the dorsal slit and at the appropriate place on the foreskin. Adjust the grasping hemostat if necessary. When you are sure that everything looks fine, remove the foreskin edge hemostats.
8. Place the string over the groove in the Plastibell, and tighten the string just until it remains in place (Fig. 183-13).
9. Check the placement of the string and bell again,

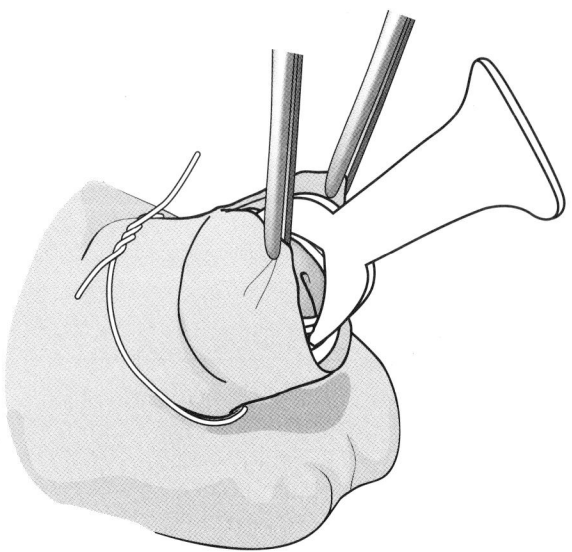

Fig. 183-11
Place the Plastibell on the glans and check for proper size.

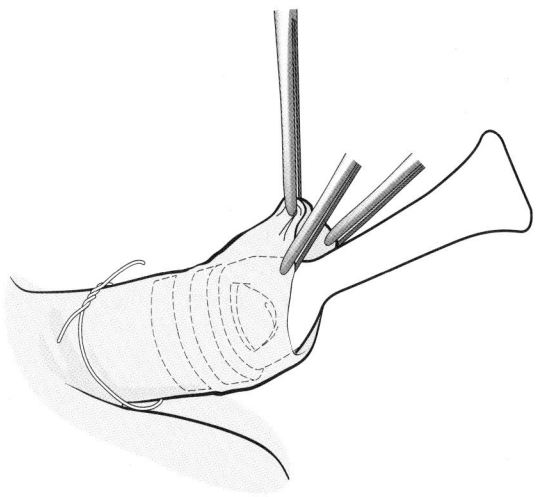

Fig. 183-12
Reapproximate the foreskin around the Plastibell and hold it in place with a hemostat.

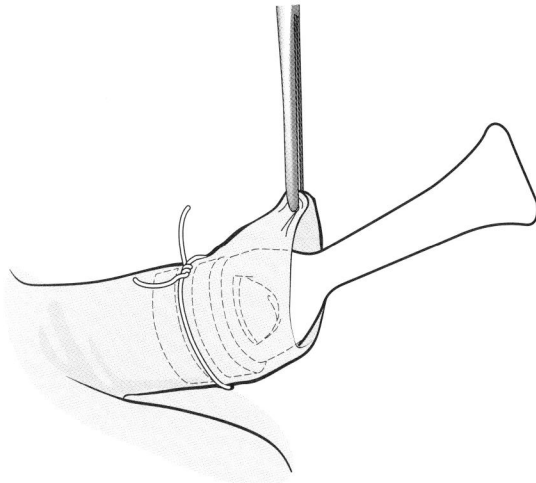

Fig. 183-13
Start of a surgeon's knot in the groove of the Plastibell.

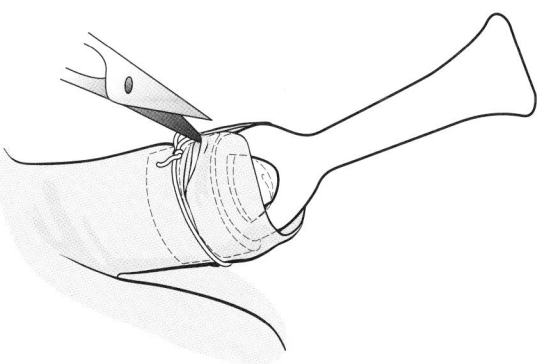

Fig. 183-14
Trim the excess foreskin with iris scissors.

making sure that the apex of the foreskin incision is distal to the string. Be sure that you are not removing too much foreskin, and that the Plastibell can move freely on the glans.

10. Tighten the string as much as possible and hold at this tension for a few seconds. Complete the surgeon's knot in the string and trim the excess string to ¼ inch in length.

11. Remove the hemostat that has been approximating the dorsal slit.

12. Using iris scissors, cut the foreskin away to within 3 mm of the string. Be careful not to cut the string (Fig. 183-14). Discard the foreskin in a biohazard waste container.

13. Holding the body of the Plastibell between the index finger and thumb of one hand, bend the wishbone with the other hand until it snaps at its junction with the bell (Fig. 183-15).

14. Verify again that the Plastibell can move up and down on the glans and that the meatus is not occluded.

15. As in steps 16 through 19 of the "Mogen Technique" section, check for bleeding, cover with petrolatum gauze, reapply the diaper, and record the procedure in the chart.

MEATOTOMY

1. For a meatus of less than 2 mm in length or less than 25% to 30% of the diameter of the glans, meatotomy is indicated. Local anesthesia (EMLA cream) or a block (dorsal penile nerve or subcutaneous ring) can be used to minimize discomfort. Lidocaine without epinephrine can also be injected in the perimeatal area. Wrapping the penis with gauze soaked in plain

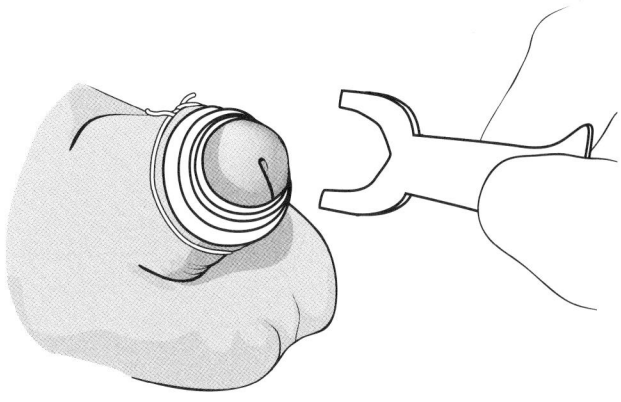

Fig. 183-15
Snap the Plastibell at the junction of the ring and the wishbone.

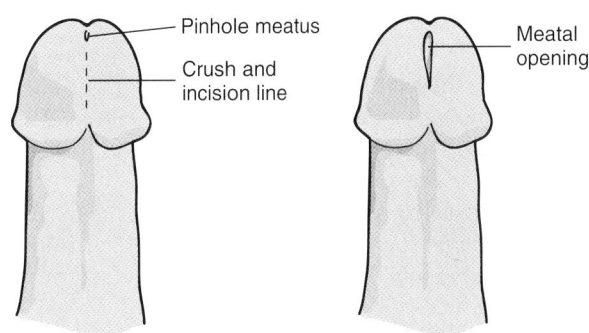

Fig. 183-16
A, Meatal stenosis and location of crush line. **B,** Meatus following meatotomy.

2% lidocaine for a few minutes before the anesthetic injection and using a 30-gauge needle may decrease some of the discomfort of the injection.

2. Apply Betadine to the penis and place a fenestrated drape.

3. Place the upper tip of a straight mosquito hemostat inside the meatus at the 6 o'clock position. The tip should be several millimeters inside the meatus, with the opposite tip no further than the frenulum. Close the hemostat to obtain a crush line of hemostasis between the inferior side of the meatus and the frenulum (Fig. 183-16). Frequently the majority of the crush line will be located on the thin, sometimes translucent, inflammatory membrane that has caused the meatal obstruction.

4. Using fine iris scissors, cut through the center of the crush line. Be careful to cut only in the crush line. If you extend laterally or past the crush line, bleeding and discomfort will occur.

5. A closed hemostat can then be inserted into the urethra to blindly palpate for distal urethral webs. If webs are noted, urologic referral is indicated.

6. Parents are instructed to insert a small dilator into the meatus daily for 2 weeks to prevent recurrence of the stenosis. Use either a small eyedropper or the tip of a tube of ophthalmic ointment as the dilator. White petrolatum ointment can be used as a lubricant.

POSTPROCEDURE PARENT EDUCATION

Mogen and Gomco Techniques

Parents should report any bleeding or signs of infection. It is normal to have a red, angry looking glans, often with a yellowish crust that may last for a week. Acetaminophen (10 to 15 mg/kg every 6 hours) is given for any apparent pain or irritability. Rarely is any analgesic needed beyond 24 hours. The patient

education handout includes postprocedure instructions for parents. (See the sample handout titled "Newborn Circumcision" on page 1989 of Appendix G.)

Parents are instructed to remove the white petrolatum gauze when it becomes soiled. Following Mogen and Gomco, they are told to retract the penile shaft skin back from the corona and to apply white petrolatum to the area at each diaper change. After the Plastibell falls off, this same procedure is followed. This should continue for a week to prevent adhesions from forming. To prevent the glans from sticking to the diaper, parents should apply a smear of white petrolatum to the front of the diaper for the first week. They can wash the penis with soap and water the day after surgery.

Plastibell Technique

In addition to following all of the same basic instructions as patients who undergo circumcision using the Mogen or Gomco clamp, parents need to know what to expect with a Plastibell. They should know that the foreskin remaining beyond the string will turn black and necrotic and fall off along with the Plastibell within 1 week. Each Plastibell device comes with a postoperative education card that is given to the parents.

All Techniques

Parents are instructed to watch for meatal stenosis. Meatal stenosis appears as a pinhole urethra causing a narrow or angulated urinary stream. This can be associated with enuresis or incontinence. Meatotomy in the office is a simple procedure and will usually correct the problem.

COMPLICATIONS

• Bleeding
• Infection (most common with Plastibell because of the

retained tissue and the foreign body nature of the device)
- Trauma to the glans or urethra
- Poor cosmetic result due to remaining adherence of mucosa to glans, removal of too much or too little foreskin, or uneven removal of foreskin
- Paraphimosis from inadequate opening of the Mogen crush line after the procedure is completed or from the use of too big a Plastibell. A Plastibell may be removed with an orthopedic bone-cutting forceps.
- Degloving of penile shaft skin (Gomco only, see the "Gomco Technique" section)
- Meatal stenosis: rare, but a possible late complication

SUPPLIERS

Circumstraint
Olympic Medical Corp.
5900 First Avenue South
Seattle, WA 98108
Phone: 1-800-426-0353
Website: www.olymed.com

Gomco circumcision clamps (1.1-, 1.3-, and 1.45-cm sizes)
Gomco Division
Allied Healthcare Products, Inc.
1720 Sublette Avenue
St. Louis, MO 63110
Phone: 1-800-444-3940
Website: www.alliedhpi.com

Mogen clamp
Mogen Instrument Co.
437 Crown Street
Brooklyn, NY 11225
Phone: 1-718-604-8833

Plastibell device (1.1-, 1.2-, 1.3-, and 1.4-cm sizes)
Plastibell
Hollister Inc.
2000 Hollister Drive
Libertyville, IL 60048
Phone: 1-800-323-4060
Website: www.hollister.com

Brochures
American Academy of Pediatrics
Division of Publications
141 Northwest Point Boulevard
Elk Grove Village, IL 60007-1098
Phone: 1-800-433-9016
Website: www.aap.org

CPT/BILLING CODES

54150   Circumcision, using clamp or other device; newborn
53025   Meatotomy, infant

ICD-9-CM DIAGNOSTIC CODES

V50.2   Circumcision, routine
599.6   Urinary obstruction, unspecified
597.89 Meatitis, urethral

ADDITIONAL RESOURCES

- See the sample patient education handout titled "Newborn Circumcision" on page 1989 of Appendix G.

BIBLIOGRAPHY

American Academy of Pediatrics: Policy statements: report of the task force on circumcision, *Pediatrics* 103:686, 1999. Available at www.aap.org/policy/re9850.html. (Accessed October 29, 2002.)

Castellsague X, Bosch FX, Munoz N, et al: Male circumcision, penile human papillomavirus infection, and cervical cancer in female partners, *N Engl J Med* 346(15):1105, 2002.

Haouari N, Wood C, Griffiths G, Levene M: The analgesic effect of sucrose in full term infants: a randomized controlled trial, *BMJ* 310:1498, 1995.

Kunz HV: Circumcision and meatotomy, *Prim Care* 13(3):513, 1986.

Laumann EO, Masi CM, Zuckerman EW: Circumcision in the United States: prevalence, prophylactic effects, and sexual practice, *JAMA* 227:1052, 1997.

Peleg D, Steiner A: The Gomco circumcision: common problems and solutions, *Am Fam Physician* 58:891, 1998.

Reynolds RD: Use of the Mogen clamp for neonatal circumcision, *Am Fam Physician* 54:177, 1996.

Spach DH, Stapleton AE, Staum WE: Lack of circumcision increases the risk of urinary tract infection in young men, *JAMA* 267:679, 1992.

WEBSITES

www.fda.gov/cdrh/safety/circumcision.pdf ("Potential for Injury from Circumcision Clamps")

CHAPTER 184

Pediatric Arterial Puncture and Venous Minicutdown

Rebecca H. Gladu*

ARTERIAL PUNCTURE

Arterial blood may be needed for blood gas analysis or for routine laboratory analysis. In the infant or child, the radial artery is the most appropriate and most common site selected for arterial puncture. The brachial, posterior tibial, and dorsalis pedis arteries are optional sites, but each has its own risk of complications. Because of the risk of thrombosis, the femoral artery should not be used for arterial puncture in the infant or child.

INDICATIONS

- To obtain arterial blood from the pediatric patient in respiratory distress or for other studies that require arterial blood
- To guide the management of the pediatric patient receiving ventilatory support or undergoing intensive respiratory therapy
- To obtain blood for routine laboratory analysis when venous blood cannot be obtained

Note: The last indication is controversial. The benefit must outweigh the higher risk of obtaining an arterial sample.

CONTRAINDICATIONS

- Infection, burns, or local skin damage at the site of the intended puncture

EQUIPMENT

- Tuberculin syringe
- 25-gauge butterfly scalp vein needle or standard 25- or 26-gauge needle
- Alcohol swabs

- Heparin
- Container of crushed ice for sample transport
- Sterile 4 × 4–inch gauze pads
- Sterile gloves
- Goggles or eye protection
- Lidocaine 1%, without epinephrine *(optional)*
- An arm or leg board *(optional)*

TECHNIQUE

1. Always perform an Allen's test to confirm adequate collateral circulation (Chapter 79, Arterial Puncture and Percutaneous Arterial Line Placement).
2. Draw heparin into a tuberculin syringe, eject the heparin, and attach a 25-gauge butterfly needle (preferred for infants and neonates) or a 25- or 26-gauge needle.
3. Immobilize the upper extremity by taping it to an arm board or by having an assistant manually stabilize it.
4. Identify the radial artery by dorsiflexing the wrist and palpating over the distal volar radius. Grasp the wrist with the nondominant hand, and cleanse the site of intended puncture with an alcohol swab (as an option, infiltrate with 1% lidocaine without epinephrine).
5. Universal blood and body fluid precautions should be followed. Insert the needle at the point of maximum pulsation at a 30- to 45-degree angle (Fig. 184-1). Continuous suction should be applied with the plunger of the syringe because, in a child, arterial blood will not flash into the syringe as in the adult patient. If using the butterfly needle, have an assistant maintain gentle suction while the needle is advanced.
6. If resistance is encountered, it is most likely that the needle has made contact with underlying bone (radius). At this point, withdraw the needle very slowly while maintaining suction on the plunger until there is blood return. If there is no blood return and the tip of the needle has been withdrawn to a point just beneath

*Dr. Gregg K. Phillips wrote this chapter in the first edition.

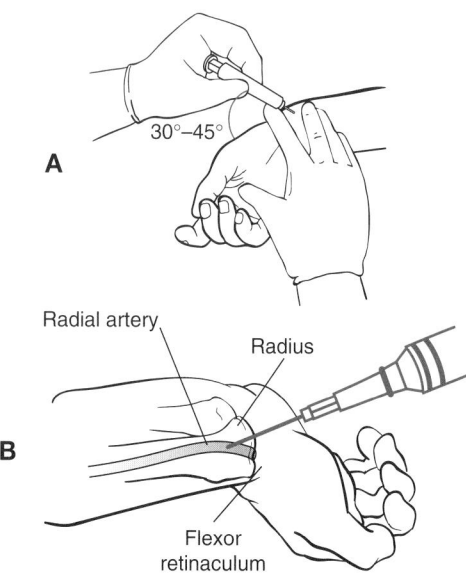

Fig. 184-1
Pediatric arterial puncture. **A,** Anatomic location of the radial artery with immobilization of the wrist in hyperextension. **B,** The artery is entered with the bevel up and the needle at 30 to 45 degrees from horizontal.

the skin, readvance the needle toward the point of maximal pulsation before withdrawing it from the skin. Several attempts can be made in this manner causing minimal trauma to the infant before choosing another site.

7. When arterial blood is encountered, withdraw 0.3 to 0.5 ml into the syringe before removing the needle. Leave the butterfly needle in place (with its extension tubing) if more blood is needed for other analyses. This will facilitate changing the syringe. For blood gas analysis, place the syringe on ice and immediately transport to the laboratory.

8. After removing the needle, always maintain manual compression at the arterial puncture site for a minimum of 5 minutes to prevent the formation of a hematoma.

COMPLICATIONS

- Bleeding and hematoma formation
- Formation of an intraarterial thrombus
- Nerve injury
- Infection

Note: Because the radial artery is not in close proximity to a nerve or vein, its puncture usually results in fewer complications than puncture of the brachial, posterior tibial, or dorsalis pedis arteries. Repeated puncture at the same site increases the chance of complications but may not be avoidable.

VENOUS MINICUTDOWN

Obtaining percutaneous venous access in infants or in hypovolemic children can be a challenge. Venous cutdown can be used to gain vascular access after a failed percutaneous attempt or simultaneously while trying to place a percutaneous venous line. If the situation is emergent and a percutaneous line cannot be placed in a matter of minutes, venous cutdown can often be performed rapidly. An additional alternative is placement of an intraosseous line, which may in fact be technically less difficult and quicker (Chapter 181, Intraosseous Venous Access). Chapter 96, Venous Cutdown, offers technical advice on the overall mechanics of venous cutdown. This chapter offers an abbreviated and clinically easier method for pediatric patients in emergency situations: the minicutdown. Standard venous cutdown takes 5 to 15 minutes, even in the hands of a skilled clinician. Minicutdown is less complicated and can usually be performed in less than 5 minutes. The saphenous vein is the most common site for cutdown in the pediatric patient.

INDICATIONS

- In an emergency situation, inability to obtain needed percutaneous venous access in a matter of minutes or inability to maintain a peripheral IV

CONTRAINDICATIONS

- Infection or trauma at the site of the intended cutdown

EQUIPMENT

- Mounted no. 15 scalpel
- Mosquito hemostats
- Antiseptic solution
- 4-0 silk suture
- Skin retractors
- Sterile 4 × 4–inch gauze pads
- Sterile gloves
- Goggles or eye protection
- Leg board *(optional)*

TECHNIQUE

1. Immobilize the lower extremity by securing it to a board or by having an assistant manually hold the patient.

2. The saphenous vein is a consistent anatomic structure and is located a finger breadth anterior to and a finger breadth superior to the medial malleolus at the ankle.

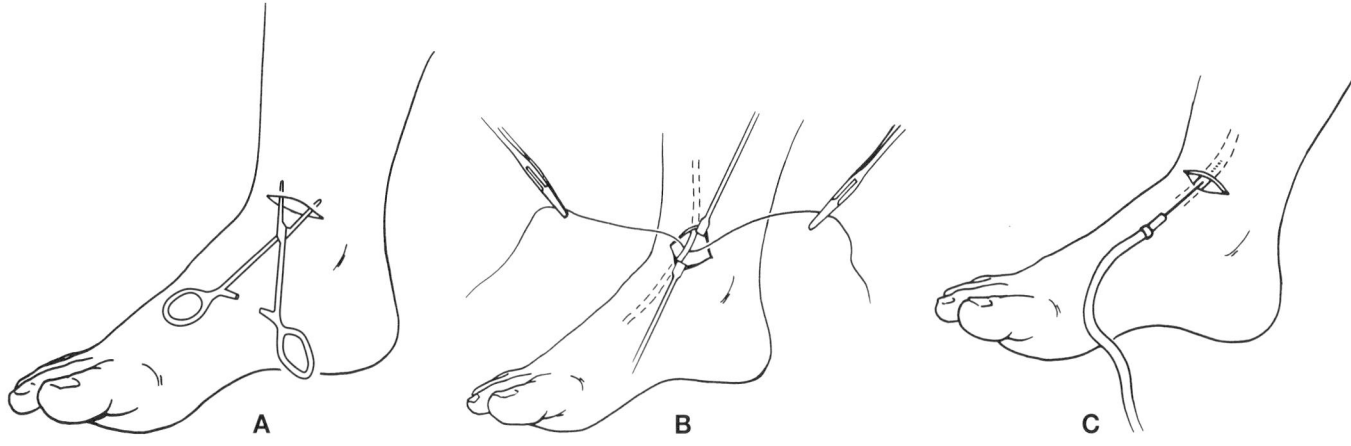

Fig. 184-2
Venous minicutdown. **A,** Blunt dissection after making a transverse incision. **B,** Localization of the vein.
C, Cannulating the vein.

Cleanse this area with an antiseptic solution. Follow universal blood and body fluid precautions. Make a 1-cm transverse incision through the dermis, exposing the underlying subcutaneous tissue.

3. Exposure of the vein is accomplished with skin retractors and blunt dissection with a mosquito hemostat, staying parallel to the course of the vein (Fig. 184-2, *A*). When the saphenous vein is identified, pass a 4-0 silk suture beneath the vessel and clamp both ends of the suture with a hemostat (Fig. 184-2, *B*).

4. Using upward traction on the vein with the suture to stabilize it, cannulate the vessel with an intravenous catheter under direct visualization (Fig. 184-2, *C*). Advance the catheter in the usual fashion, then attach intravenous tubing and begin infusing fluid. As with percutaneous line placement, steady fluid flow is indicative of successful cannulation. With the minicutdown technique, the vein is not ligated after cannulation. Although the catheter is not as secure with this technique, because the vein can be directly visualized, cannulation can be performed very rapidly when time is crucial. Since the minicutdown technique does not destroy the vein, standard cutdown can still be performed when the clinical situation becomes less emergent.

COMPLICATIONS

- Wound infection
- Local hematoma
- Phlebitis
- Damage to adjacent structures from incision and dissection

Note: Because this is only a temporary procedure, the risk of these complications is minimal.

CPT/BILLING CODES

36420	Venipuncture, cutdown; under age 1
36425	Venipuncture, cutdown; age 1 or over
36600	Arterial puncture, withdrawal of blood for diagnosis

Pediatric Arterial Puncture

276.4	Acid-base mixed disorder
276.2	Acidosis
276.2	Acidosis, lactic
276.3	Alkalosis
493.01	Asthma, extrinsic, with status asthmaticus
493.90	Asthma, unspecified, with status asthmaticus
986	Carbon monoxide, toxic effect
427.5	Cardiac or cardiorespiratory arrest
780.01	Coma
250.1	Diabetic ketoacidosis
493.9	Dyspnea, asthma
428.1	Dyspnea, cardiac
786.09	Hypercapnia
799.0	Hypoxia
770.1	Meconium aspiration syndrome
428.1	Pulmonary edema (left heart failure)
518.5	Pulmonary insufficiency following trauma and surgery
799.1	Respiratory arrest
518.82	Respiratory distress: acute
786.09	Respiratory distress: NOS or respiratory insufficiency
769	Respiratory distress syndrome of newborn
518.81	Respiratory failure, NOS
518.83	Respiratory failure, chronic
518.84	Respiratory failure, acute and chronic
785.50	Shock

785.51   Shock, cardiogenic
770.6   Transient tachypnea of newborn

Venous Minicutdown

785.59   Hypovolemic shock, NEC
958.4   Hemorrhagic shock due to trauma
459.0   Hemorrhage, unspecified
772.9   Hemorrhage, in newborn, NOS
458.0   Orthostatic hypotension
459.89   Venofibrosis

BIBLIOGRAPHY

John Hopkins Hospital: *Harriet Lane handbook,* ed 15, St Louis, 2000, Mosby.

Kofas E: A quicker saphenous vein cutdown and a better way to teach it, *J Trauma* 43(6):985, 1997.

Roberts JR: *Clinical procedure in emergency medicine,* Philadelphia, 1998, WB Saunders.

Simon RR: *Emergency procedures and techniques,* Baltimore, 1987, Williams & Wilkins.

Stovroff M: Intravenous access in infants and children, *Pediatr Clin North Am* 45(6):1390, 1998.

Sweeny MN: Vascular access in trauma, options, risks, benefits, and complications, *Anesth Clin North Am* 17(1): 104, 1999.

CHAPTER 185

Suprapubic Bladder Aspiration

Carlos A. Moreno

Suprapubic bladder aspiration is a method of obtaining a sterile urine specimen in a young infant when other methods are unsatisfactory. This procedure is most successful in an infant less than 2 years of age because the bladder is an abdominal organ. After 2 years, as the child grows, the bladder moves into the pelvis, increasing both the difficulty of the procedure and the risk of complications. (See Chapter 209, Emergency Department and Office Ultrasound, for a method of confirming a full bladder and determining where to direct the needle.)

INDICATIONS

- To obtain sterile urine for culture in an infant or child under the age of 2 (e.g., suspected urinary tract infection or sepsis)
- To decompress the urinary bladder when there is urethral obstruction (after decompression, a referral should be made to pediatric urology)

CONTRAINDICATIONS

- Bleeding abnormality or coagulopathy
- Infection or loss of integrity of skin or fascia at the site of needle insertion (e.g., burn, cellulitis, etc.)
- Anatomic genitourinary tract anomalies
- Bowel distention (ileus, obstruction, etc.)
- Scars from previous lower abdominal surgery that might cause adhesions

Note: With ultrasonic directed aspiration, the last three contraindications may be overcome. (See Chapter 209, Emergency Department and Office Ultrasound.)

EQUIPMENT

- Povidone-iodine solution
- 70% isopropyl alcohol
- Sterile 4 × 4–inch gauze pads

- Sterile gloves
- 3-ml sterile syringe with 1 or 1½-inch, 22- or 23-gauge needle
- Sterile urine specimen container
- Adhesive bandage

TECHNIQUE

1. Before bladder aspiration, the infant's diaper should be dry and urination should not have occurred within the previous hour. This should ensure a full bladder. An alternative is to perform a quick ultrasound to confirm a full bladder.
2. Hold the infant in the supine, frog-leg position. Observe universal blood and body fluid precautions.
3. Urination can be prevented by gently pinching the penis or by applying anterior rectal pressure in a female infant.
4. Cleanse the lower abdomen with povidone-iodine and then remove the iodine with 70% alcohol.
5. With the needle attached to a 3-ml sterile syringe, direct it into the midline of the abdomen at a point 1 cm above the symphysis pubis. Hold the needle perpendicular to the abdomen or direct it slightly caudal (Fig. 185-1).
6. Aspirate gently with the syringe while advancing the needle. To avoid puncturing the posterior bladder wall or retroperitoneal structures, do not advance the needle after urine begins to enter the syringe. If the bladder if full, urine is usually obtained before the needle is inserted to its full depth.
7. If no urine is obtained, withdraw the needle without removing from the skin and attempt bladder puncture again, angling 20 degrees more caudal. If three attempts are unsuccessful, the bladder is considered empty. The procedure can be repeated in an hour if the patient is stable. Some urine should have accumulated in an hour.

Note: An alternative is to catheterize the infant, especially when they are too unstable to wait an hour. If ultrasound is

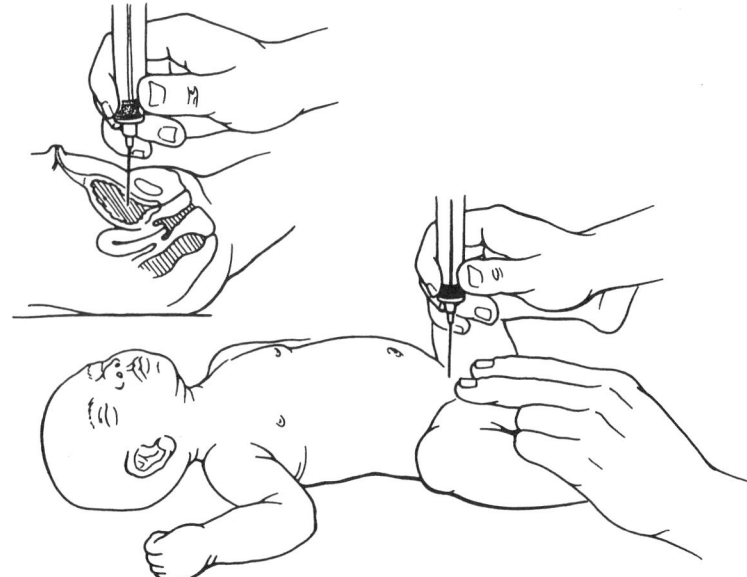

Fig. 185-1
Proper technique of suprapubic bladder aspiration.

available, it can be helpful in the unstable patient to confirm the presence of urine before subjecting them to catheterization and risk of iatrogenic urinary tract infection (UTI).

8. After withdrawing the needle, apply pressure to the puncture site and cover it with a sterile dressing. Next, apply mild pressure to the dressing for a minute. After a minute, if there is adequate hemostasis and no urine is draining from the puncture site, pressure can be discontinued.
9. Transfer the aspirated urine to a sterile container and transport to the laboratory for analysis, culture, and sensitivity.

COMPLICATIONS

- Microscopic hematuria (typically transient, resolving without specific treatment)
- Iatrogenic UTI (risk is minimized by the use of sterile technique)
- Perforation of the bowel (rare and may be managed by close observation and, if necessary, antibiotic administration)
- Retroperitoneal hematoma or damage to retroperitoneal structures (very rare)
- Infection of the abdominal wall

CPT/BILLING CODE

51000   Aspiration of bladder by needle

ICD-9-CM DIAGNOSTIC CODES

771.8	Newborn; other infection specific to the perinatal period;
771.8	Neonatal urinary tract infection
771.8	Septicemia (sepsis) of the newborn
788.20	Urinary retention, unspecified
788.21	Incomplete bladder emptying
595.0	Acute cystitis

BIBLIOGRAPHY

Greene MG, editor: *Harriet Lane handbook,* St Louis, 2000, Mosby.

Finberg, L, editor: *Saunders manual of pediatric practice,* St Louis, 1998, WB Saunders.

Hoekelman RA, editor: *Primary pediatric care,* ed 4, St Louis, 2001, Mosby.

CHAPTER 186

Umbilical Vessel Catheterization

Susan E. Murphey

Since the vessels are directly visualized, umbilical vessel catheterization is a convenient method for obtaining central vascular access. Catheterizing the umbilical artery provides direct access to the aorta, whereas catheterizing the umbilical vein provides direct access to the inferior vena cava (Fig. 186-1). Primary care clinicians may need to perform umbilical vessel catheterization in the delivery room for a newborn resuscitation or occasionally in the emergency department for a newborn or infant in distress. In addition, they may need to perform it in the nursery or neonatal intensive care unit (NICU) for an infant requiring continuous monitoring or frequent infusions of medications or fluids. In fact, both vessels are frequently catheterized in the NICU for premature infants requiring prolonged vascular access or monitoring.

Compared with the vein, the umbilical artery is a more durable vessel with higher velocity blood flow; therefore there is a slightly lower risk of complications when catheterized. Inserting an umbilical artery catheter (UAC) or an umbilical vein catheter (UVC) is easier if performed in the first 30 to 60 minutes of the infant's life. However, a UAC may be inserted up to the seventh day of life and a UVC at up to 2 weeks of age. Despite the fact that the vessels are easily accessible, placing a UAC can be a time-consuming procedure. If a UAC is not obtainable, a UVC is an alternative for infusion. It is also an option if peripheral intravenous access is difficult to obtain. After the first day of life, there are little data supporting benefit of a UAC over a UVC for infusion, although an attempt should always be made to obtain peripheral venous access before either of these is inserted.

INDICATIONS

Umbilical Artery Catheterization

- Newborn resuscitation requiring: monitoring for cardiorespiratory distress (i.e., needed arterial pressure monitoring, frequent arterial sampling)

- Newborn or infant in an NICU requiring:
  - —Mechanical ventilation for respiratory distress (i.e., needs frequent arterial sampling)
  - —Oxygen hood and greater than 40% oxygen (FIO_2 0.4) requirement with an abnormal chest x-ray (i.e., needs frequent arterial sampling)
  - —Exchange transfusion that can be performed through a UAC (e.g., newborn weighing less than 1800 g)

Umbilical Vein Catheterization

- Newborn resuscitation requiring:
  - —Administration of drugs, blood, blood expanders, or fluids
  - —Monitoring for cardiorespiratory distress (central venous pressure [CVP] monitoring)
- Newborn or infant in an NICU requiring:
  - —Greater than 12.5% dextrose to maintain blood glucose while taking nothing by mouth (NPO)
  - —Pressor drips, total parenteral nutrition (TPN) solution, or hypertonic medications (e.g., newborn weighing less than 1000 g or who is critically ill)
  - —Exchange transfusion that can be performed through a UVC (e.g., newborn weighing less than 1800 g)

Note: By convention, a newborn is defined as an infant less than 1 month old.

CONTRAINDICATIONS

- None, during the first hours of life if the newborn has normal anatomy and no local skin infections.
- Vascular insufficiency of a lower extremity is a contraindication for UAC.
- Local infection (e.g., omphalitis, impetigo), or abdominal distention (possibly caused by intestinal hypoperfusion or necrotizing enterocolitis) are contraindications that can develop after the first few hours of life.

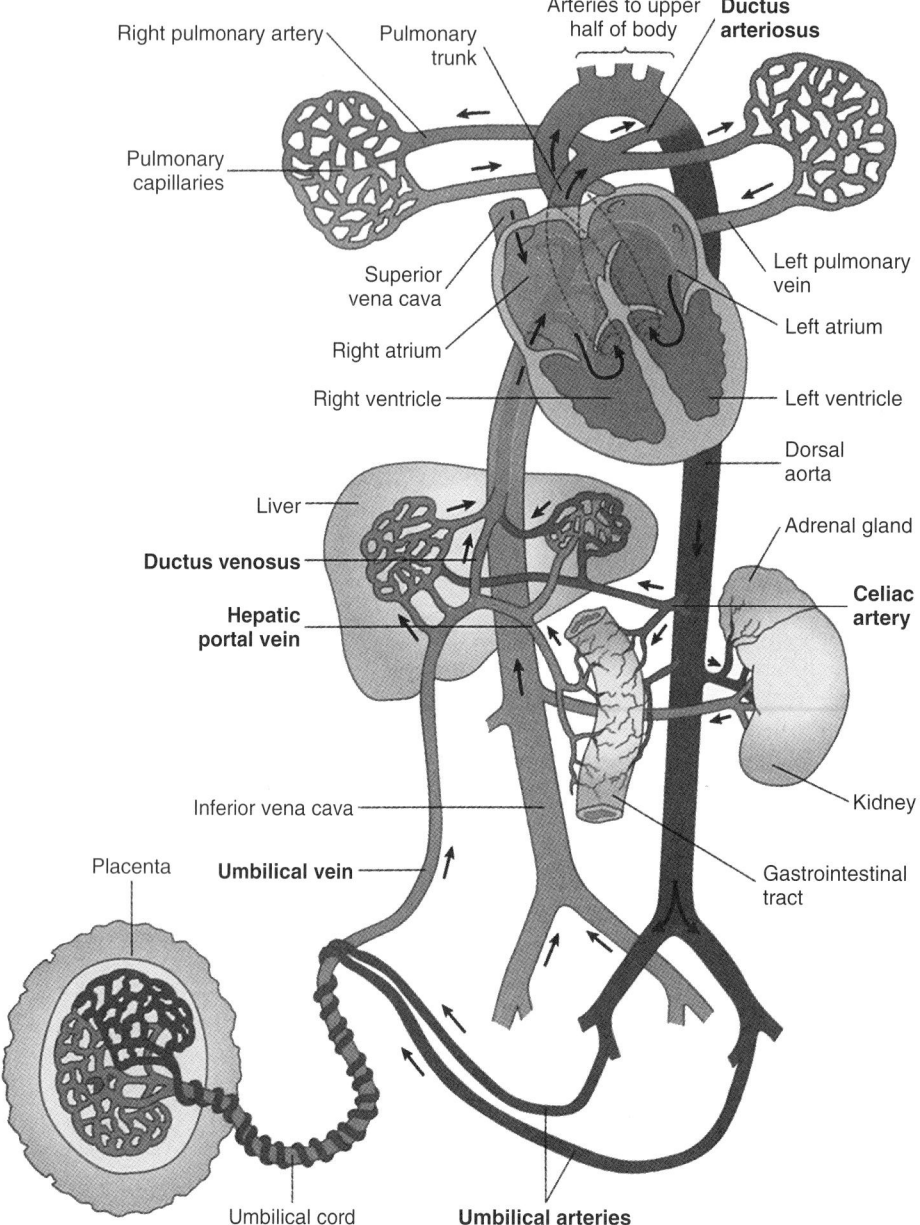

Fig. 186-1
Fetal circulation at term. (Modified from Carlson B: *Human embryology and developmental biology,* ed 2, St Louis, 1999, Mosby.)

EQUIPMENT

- Sterile measuring tape
- 3.5 to 5.0 French umbilical catheter for UAC; up to 8 French umbilical catheter for UVC
- Surgical cap and mask; sterile gown and gloves
- Eye protection for clinician
- Povidone-iodine or antiseptic scrub solution
- Three-way stopcock (sterile); locking connectors
- Heparin for flush (1 to 2 units heparin/ml of 0.25 normal saline [NS])
- Sterile instrument tray with small hemostats, forceps (iris curved), scissors, needle holder, mounted no. 11 scalpel blade and drapes
- Antibiotic ointment
- 4-0 or 5-0 silk suture with a small needle or a catheter stabilizer
- Sterile umbilical tape
- Infant radiant warmer, means of restraint, cardiac and oxygen saturation monitors, supplemental oxygen
- D_5W, $D_{10}W$, or NS infusion setup (use heparin 1 unit/ml, unless medications are to be administered that

are incompatible with heparin) with fluid chamber, 0.22-µg filter and infusion pump
- Adhesive tape

A rule of thumb for selecting umbilical artery catheter size is to use a 5 French for infants weighing more than 2000 g and a 3.5 to 4 French for infants weighing less. Because the lumen of the vein is larger, a 5 to 8 French catheter can be used for UVC in term infants (more than 1800 g), especially infants requiring exchange transfusion. The catheter may be composed of any FDA-approved material; double lumen catheters are also now available.

PREPROCEDURE PATIENT PREPARATION

The newborn needing umbilical catheterization will typically demonstrate signs and symptoms of cardiorespiratory distress shortly, if not immediately, after birth. If performed as an emergency procedure, implied consent and the indications should be documented in the chart. Explain the need for the procedure to the parent(s) when there is time. For less urgent insertions, obtain informed consent from the parent(s) after discussing the alternatives, risks, and potential benefits of the procedure.

When the infant arrives at the nursery, if umbilical catheterization is probable, the umbilical stump should be left at least 4 cm long. The two thick-walled arteries and the single vein should be easily identifiable. Place the infant under an infant warmer and restrain, if possible. The cardiac rate should be monitored, and adequate oxygenation should be provided throughout the procedure.

TECHNIQUE

1. Set up the tubing, fluids, fluid chamber, 0.22-µg filter, and infusion pump. Flush and fill the tubing with heparin flush to remove air from the system.
2. Prepare the entire abdomen from xiphoid to pubis with sterile povidone-iodine or antiseptic scrub solution. Scrub the umbilical stump and apply sterile drapes. Observe universal blood and body fluid precautions when performing the procedure.
3. Calculate the insertion length of the catheter for proper placement.
   a. UAC. There are two commonly used, standard insertion depths for UAC. One results in "high" placement of the catheter tip, which is above the diaphragm at the level of the thoracic aorta (spinal level T6 to T9). This site places the tip between the ductus arteriosus and the origin of the celiac axis. The second site results in "low" placement of the catheter tip (spinal level L3 to L5), which is below the diaphragm. This site places the tip between the inferior mesenteric artery and the bifurcation of the aorta.

   i. For high placement: (a) measure the axial or longitudinal distance from the level of the umbilicus to the level of the shoulder or clavicle (shoulder-umbilicus length). Then use the nomogram (Fig. 186-2, *A*), or (b) calculate the length based on birthweight (BW). Length (cm) = [3 × BW (kg)] + 9.

   When a nomogram or the birthweight is not available or in an urgent situation, if the shoulder-umbilicus length is greater than 13 cm, simply add 1 cm to the shoulder-umbilicus length. This results in a reasonable estimate for the catheter insertion depth. When the shoulder-umbilicus length is less than 13 cm, insert the catheter 2 cm further than the shoulder-umbilicus length.

   ii. For low placement: (a) use the nomogram (Fig. 186-2, *A*) with the shoulder-umbilicus length, or (b) calculate the length based on birthweight. Length (cm) = BW (kg) + 7.

   If a nomogram or the birthweight is not available or in an urgent situation, insert the catheter until blood is first encountered and then advance it 1 additional centimeter.

   Note: One meta-analysis study found that high placement UACs (compared with low placement) have fewer acute vascular complications and no increase in permanent vascular sequelae.

   b. UVC. For central venous pressure readings, place the catheter tip 0.5 to 1 cm above the diaphragm. The insertion depth can be estimated with a nomogram (Fig. 182-2, *B*) or with one of two formulas: (a) length (cm) = shoulder-umbilicus length (cm) × 0.6, or (b) length (cm) = (UAC insertion length [cm] × 0.5) + 1. If a nomogram or the BW is not available or in urgent situations, a second option is to insert the UVC gently for 4 to 5 cm until blood return is noted. *Never insert more than 5 cm without radiographically checking the placement*. If the catheter is being placed for a single-exchange transfusion, it may be inserted to just beneath the skin (3 to 5 cm), as long as good blood flow is noted and there is no leakage around the catheter.

4. Loosely tie the sterile umbilical tape around the proximal stump. It should be tight enough to control bleeding but loose enough to allow later passage of the catheter. A silk suture can be used as a purse string ligation in the same manner.

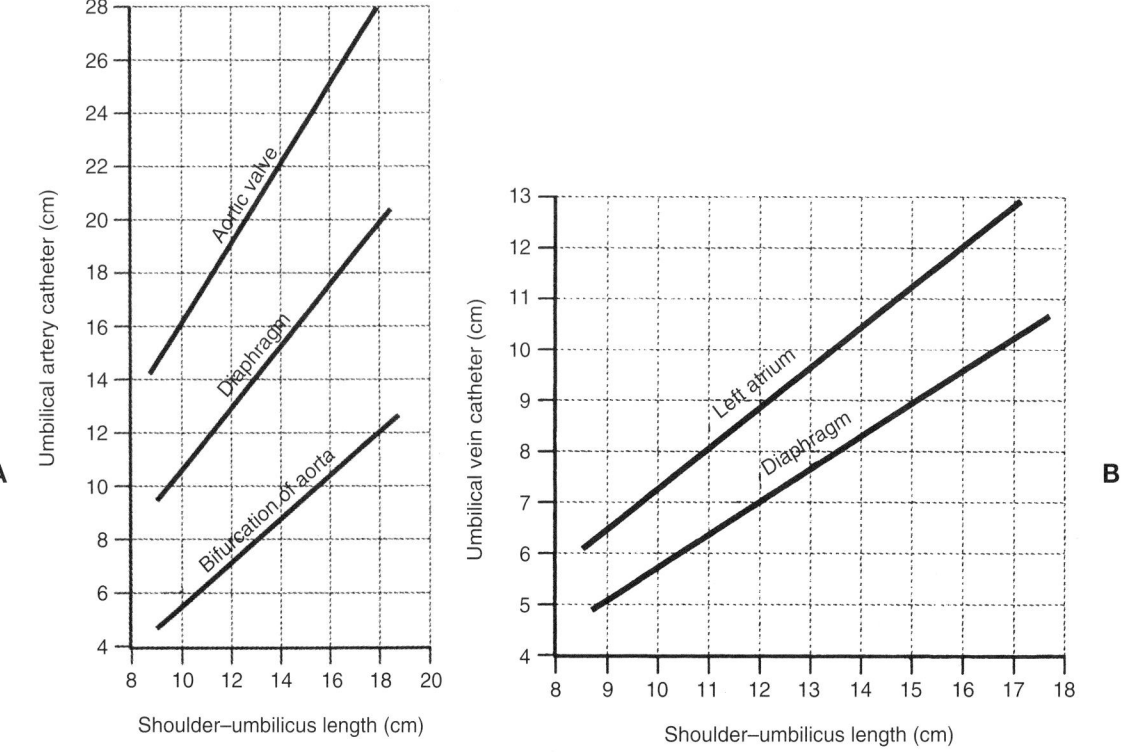

Fig. 186-2
Approximate distances for insertion, placement confirmed by x-ray after insertion. **A,** Umbilical artery catheter (avoid inserting to level of aortic valve). **B,** Umbilical vein catheter. (From Siberry G, Iannone R, editors: *The Harriet Lane handbook,* ed 15, St Louis, 2000, Mosby.)

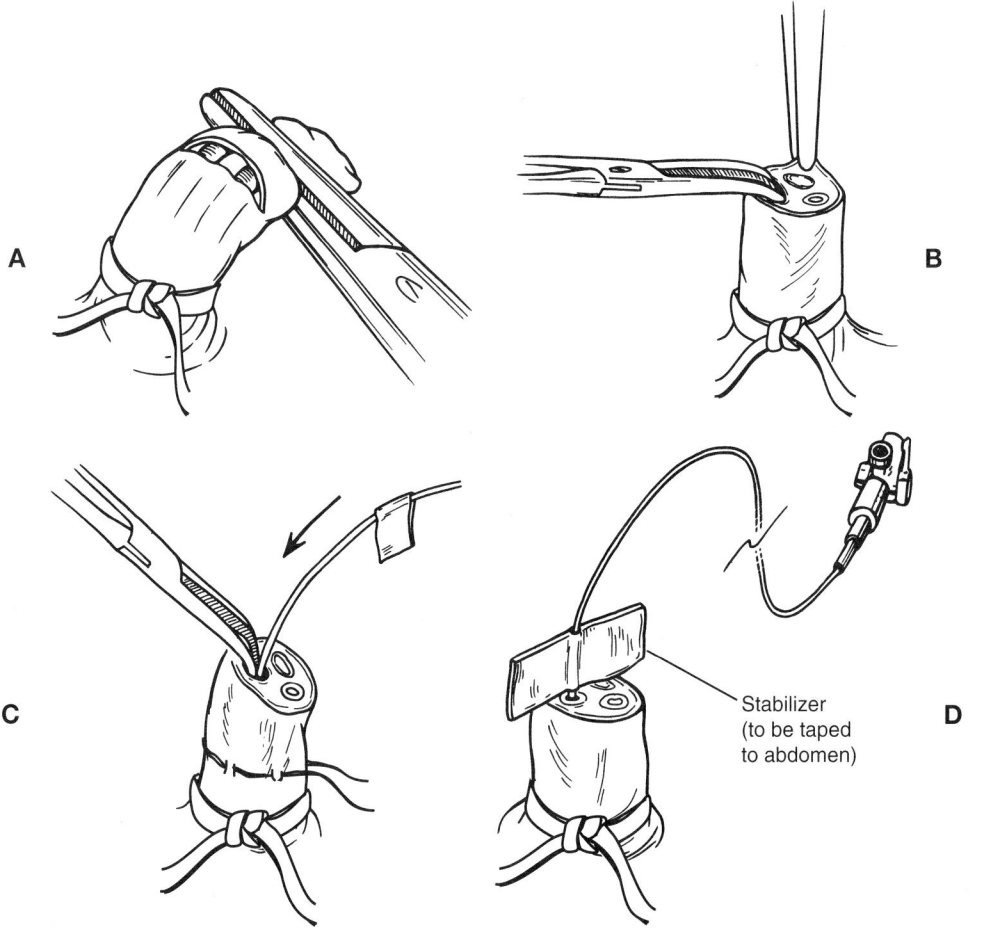

Stabilizer
(to be taped
to abdomen)

Fig. 186-3
Umbilical artery placement. See text for details.

5. With the scalpel, transect the cord approximately 1 cm above the umbilical tape (Fig. 186-3, *A*). Correctly identify the arteries and the vein. Because the vein is the single vessel and has the largest lumen, it is usually the easiest to identify. It can then be distinguished from the thicker-walled arteries that are usually lateral to the vein.

6. The cord stump should be grasped with one or two hemostats (on opposite sides of the umbilicus) and the cut edge everted. Gently dilate the desired vessel with small curved forceps (Fig. 186-3, *B*). To do so, insert one prong, then both prongs of the iris forceps, then open the forceps prongs slightly to dilate the lumen to a depth of about 1 cm. Next, grasp the catheter approximately 1 cm from the tip with your thumb and forefinger or with the forceps. Gently insert the catheter through the vessel lumen to the length previously measured (Fig. 186-3, *C*).

7a. UAC. Placing traction on the cord stump in a cephalad direction usually facilitates directing the catheter caudally. With insertion, use gentle, constant pressure to overcome any resistance. Resistance is usually encountered at a depth of about 1 to 2 cm as the vessel turns caudal. Slight resistance may again occur when the catheter enters the internal iliac artery at approximately 5 to 6 cm. At this depth, the catheter must turn cephalad. Twisting the catheter slightly may also help overcome resistance. Occasionally, resistance from vasospasm may be overcome by applying constant gentle pressure for 30 seconds, causing the spasm to subside. Another technique for relieving vasospasm is to fill the tip of the catheter with 2% lidocaine and then to flush some of it at the level where the resistance is noted. After waiting 1 to 2 minutes, attempt to advance the catheter again. Do *not* advance against significant resistance, especially at a depth of 4 to 5 cm. Resistance at this depth generally indicates a false tract has been created. Rather than continuing to advance the catheter, withdraw it and attempt to cannulate the other artery.

7b. UVC. Insert in the same manner as a UAC. At the insertion depth previously determined, CVP can be measured, hyperalimentation solutions can be administered, and medications can be infused. If an obstruction is encountered at a depth of 5 to 10 cm, the catheter has probably entered a branch of the portal vein of the liver and should be withdrawn.

8. Secure the catheter with the umbilical tape. Also use a silk suture in a purse-string fashion (Fig. 186-3, *C*), or with a stabilizer (Fig. 186-3, *D*). *Once the sterile field is taken away, the catheter may not be advanced.* For that reason, it is often more convenient to insert the catheter slightly further than is needed. (For a UAC, *never* exceed the distance to the aortic valve [Fig. 186-2].) Then it can be withdrawn slightly after an x-ray film has confirmed the location of the tip.

9. Apply sterile gauze over the antibiotic ointment, and tape the catheter to the abdomen.

10. Obtain x-ray film confirmation to ensure proper placement. Again, the ideal location of the UAC tip is either high placement at T6 to T9 (above the diaphragm and the celiac axis but below the ductus arteriosus) or low placement at L3 to L5 (above the aortic bifurcation but below the inferior mesenteric artery). If x-ray film confirmation is not possible, a UVC should be used instead of a UAC and should be inserted only 3 to 5 cm or until prompt return of blood is noted.

11. For UAC, if vasospasm occurs, causing ischemia of one buttock or leg, apply warm compresses to the contralateral limb in an attempt to trigger reflex vasodilation in the affected limb. If no improvement in limb color or pulse is observed in 15 minutes, the catheter should be withdrawn. An attempt can also be made to relieve vasospasm by repositioning the catheter. Withdraw it a short distance and/or rotate it, while observing limb color. If successful, confirm proper placement again with an x-ray film. Other options include withdrawing the line completely and catheterizing the other artery or using a smaller catheter in the same artery.

12. For catheter removal, the stopcock should be turned off. Umbilical tape should be tied loosely around the stump. The catheter should then be gradually withdrawn over 3 to 5 minutes. If there is bleeding, tighten the umbilical tape or grasp the vessel with forceps and apply pressure until it stops.

COMPLICATIONS

- Air embolization (use a three-way stopcock and flush all tubing before connecting)
- Hepatic abscess or infarction (to avoid this, confirm proper placement with an x-ray film)
- Necrotizing enterocolitis (NEC)
- Pelvic exsanguination
- Exsanguination from disconnected tubing (use locking connectors on tubing, secure the line)
- Bacteremia or sepsis (to minimize risk, remove the catheter once the infant is stabilized or within 5 days)
- Vascular perforation or malformation
- Congestive heart failure (CHF)
- Fluid around the umbilicus, if the catheter is placed too low or withdrawn too far

- Silent thrombus (difficult to diagnose without contrast studies)

UAC Complications

- Ischemia to bowel, liver or other intraabdominal organ, or lower extremity
- Systemic hypertension as a result of renovascular stenosis or thrombosis

UVC Complications

- Portal hypertension
- Pericardial perforation (if placed in the right atrium for central monitoring)
- Arrhythmias

POSTPROCEDURE PATIENT EDUCATION

Check the catheter frequently for patency and the infant for signs of infection. If signs of infection are noted, take cultures from the catheter.

As soon as the catheter is no longer needed, it should be removed. In addition, remove the catheter in the face of complications. When the catheter is no longer needed for arterial sampling or for CVP monitoring, in some NICUs it is simply pulled out enough to leave the tip in the midline. This maintains peripheral access if it is extremely critical or has been difficult to obtain. At that level, it then can be used for infusions.

CPT/BILLING CODES

36660   Catheterization, umbilical artery, for diagnosis or therapy; newborn
36510   Catheterization, umbilical vein, for diagnosis or therapy; newborn

ICD-9-CM DIAGNOSTIC CODES

779.3   Feeding problems in newborn
785.59   Hypovolemic shock, NEC
958.4   Hemorrhagic shock as a result of trauma
459.0   Hemorrhage, unspecified
772.9   In newborn, NOS
775.4   Hypocalcemia and hypomagnesemia of newborn
770.1   Meconium aspiration syndrome
775.6   Neonatal hypoglycemia
771.8   Neonatal sepsis
773.0   Newborn hemolytic disease caused by Rh isoimmunization
770.8   Other respiratory problems after birth (e.g., perinatal apnea, newborn bradycardia)
769   Respiratory distress syndrome of newborn

BIBLIOGRAPHY

Advanced Life Support Group: *Advanced paediatric life support,* ed 3, London, 2001, BMJ.

Avery GB, Fletcher MA, MacDonald MG: *Neonatology, pathophysiology, and management of the newborn,* ed 5, Philadelphia, 1999, Lippincott, Williams & Wilkins.

Barrington KJ: Umbilical artery catheters in the newborn: effects of position of the catheter tip (Cochrane Review). In *The Cochrane Library,* Oxford, 2002, Update Software.

Carlson B: *Human embryology and developmental biology,* ed 2, St Louis, 1999, Mosby.

Lipton JD, Schafermeyer RW: Umbilical vessel catheterization. In Henretig FM, King C, editors: *Textbook of pediatric emergency procedures,* Baltimore, 1997, Williams & Wilkins.

Seidel HM, Rosenstein BJ, Pathak A: *Primary care of the newborn,* ed 3, St Louis, 2001, Mosby.

Siberry GK, Iannone R: *The Harriet Lane handbook,* ed 15, St Louis, 2000, Mosby.

Spitzer AR: *Intensive care of the fetus and neonate,* St Louis, 2002, Mosby.

WEBSITE

www.cochrane.org (The Cochrane Collaboration)

PART TWELVE

Orthopedics

CHAPTER 187

Ankle and Foot Splinting, Casting, and Taping

Gregory A. Marolf

Jeffrey R. Kovan

Russell D. White

Primary care clinicians encounter a wide variety of acute and chronic foot and lower leg injuries that may benefit from immobilization. The value of immobilization as an initial means of treatment has been known for centuries. Treatment of foot and ankle injuries involves an accurate clinical evaluation and, when indicated, radiographic assessment of potential fractures, avulsions, or instability. Casting and cast splinting are commonly used in acute situations, whereas splinting and taping best control chronic instabilities and act as adjuncts in rehabilitation. Rest, ice, compression, and elevation (RICE) are often required before acute immobilization is used.

INDICATIONS

Soft Tissue Injuries

- Ankle sprains: Treatment options include a sugar tong splint or a short leg cast. Taping or braces (stirrup, or lace-up type) can be used for support as the patient returns to weight bearing.
- Plantar fasciitis: Immobilization can be achieved with a nocturnal posterior leg splint, which provides a constant stretch to the plantar fascia. Other treatments include stretching, exercises, nonsteroidal antiinflammatory drugs, corticosteroid injection, iontophoresis, off-the-shelf orthoses, or customized orthotics. (A recent study [Pfeffer, 1999] indicates stretching exercises and off-the-shelf orthoses were more effective than customized orthotics.)

Fractures

- Tibial or fibular: Stable distal tibial or fibular fractures, including malleolar fractures, can be immobilized with a short leg walking cast. Tibial fractures may need up to 10 weeks of immobilization, while fibular fractures need 3 to 4 weeks of immobilization. Stress fractures generally do not need immobilization.
- Fifth metatarsal: Immobilize avulsion fractures with a postoperative shoe, posterior splint, or short leg cast for 4 to 6 weeks, with weight bearing after 10 to 14 days. Immobilize Jones fractures with a non-weight-bearing short leg cast for 6 to 10 weeks.
- Other: Primary care clinicians may also encounter fractures of the tarsals, or 1st through 4th metatarsals. When these fractures are nondisplaced and stable, immobilization alone may be appropriate; otherwise surgical referral is necessary.

Prophylaxis Against Injuries

Ankle taping or bracing may be used as prophylaxis against injury in ankles that need additional stabilization and improved proprioception.

CONTRAINDICATIONS

- Early (premature) casting: Casting before maximal swelling has occurred can cause necrosis and possibly a compartment syndrome.
- Open wound: Never place a cast over an open wound, because of the potential for infection. If the wound is not too large, a window may be cut in the cast to monitor it.
- Unstable fractures: These need surgical repair. Splint only until definitive treatment can be provided.

BENEFITS OF DIFFERENT TYPES OF IMMOBILIZATION

The type of immobilization used may vary with the location or severity of the injury, patient preference, and the plan of treatment. The following list of benefits for each option may help when making decisions.

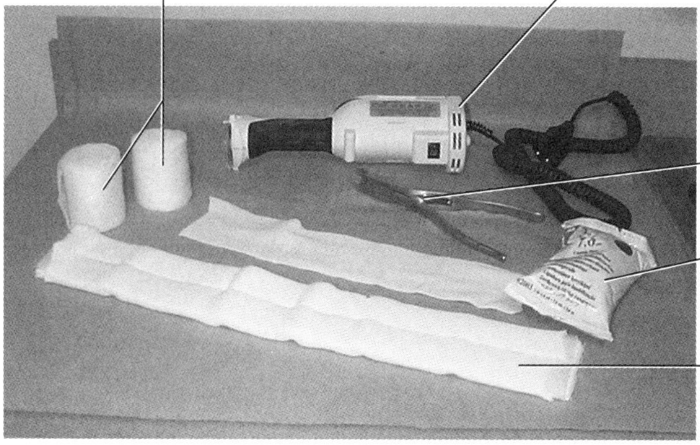

Fig. 187-1
Materials needed for casting: cotton padding, casting material, cast spreader, cast cutter, and plaster strips.

Splinting

- Stability for soft tissue injuries
- Pain relief
- Easily removable for icing, etc.
- Provides temporary support for patients needing surgery

Casting

- Marked stability
- Significant pain relief
- Immobilization for hard-to-treat soft tissue injuries as well as fractures

Taping

- Supports acutely injured ankles
- Supports chronically weak ankles or a chronically injured plantar fascia
- Enhances proprioception
- Prophylaxis against injury

EQUIPMENT

Casting (Fig. 187-1)

- Stockinette: 4-inch is appropriate for most patients, but 3-inch may be needed for smaller patients.
- Cast padding: 3- or 4-inch rolls, depending on patient size
- Cast material: 3- or 4-inch rolls, depending on patient size
- Gloves, nonsterile
- Water bucket with tepid water
- Scissors
- Foot stand *(optional)*
- Cast cutter
- Cast spreader

Splinting

- Cast padding and plaster cast material in rolls *or* premade splint material (plaster or synthetic)
- Gloves
- Water bucket with tepid water
- Scissors
- Compression wrap (Ace bandage)

Taping for Ankle

- Skin prep (benzoin)
- Lubricant *(optional)*

Note: The lubricant may be applied to the skin at sites of potential friction or irritation

- Underwrap
- 1½- or 2-inch athletic tape
- Pressure pads or mole skin

Taping for Plantar Fasciitis

Equipment is similar to that used for the McConnell method of taping for patellofemoral knee pain:
- 2-inch dressing retention sheet (skin tape, white)
- 1½-inch patellofemoral adhesive tape (high-tensile strength tape, brown; some of the original work with McConnell taping was rumored to have used duct tape!)
- Alcohol swabs
- Commercial adhesive remover

PREPROCEDURE PATIENT PREPARATION

Obtain verbal or written consent. The patient should be aware that there will be a temporary loss of flexibility following immobilization, especially in the foot. In some cases, a partial loss of flexibility can become permanent. Place the patient in a seated or supine position. Some clinicians prefer a prone position with the knee flexed 90 degrees.

TECHNIQUE

Splinting

Most clinician offices and emergency rooms have access to premade splinting materials that are fixed or inflatable (e.g., Aircast). However, inexpensive splints can be made from a plaster cast roll and cast padding:
1. Estimate the length of the splint you plan to use.
2. Unroll cast material into layers, making 11 to 13 layers.
3. In a similar fashion, unroll cast padding into layers, making 6 to 8 layers.
4. Unroll a single layer of cast padding for the outside of the splint.
5. The plaster cast material will be placed between the inner and outer layers of cast padding. The inner layers (six to eight layers) are placed between the splint and the skin, while the single outer layer of cast padding is placed on the outside of the splint. The latter is used to prevent the Ace bandage from adhering to the plaster.

Generally, when making a splint from casting materials, plaster is used. When using this type of splint, the padding will not be wet. The casting material is immersed in water separately.

Premade splints may be plaster or fiberglass. With premade materials, the padding will be wet. Premade splint material can also be simulated by rolling stockinette over the outside of the 11 to 13 layers of cast materials. Fold over the ends of the stockinette and tape them to keep the splint neat. Both the stockinette and the casting materials are then immersed in water together. Both will be wet when applying. Several layers of cast padding are then placed between the patient's skin and this splint to prevent skin breakdown.

Two types of ankle splints will be discussed: sugar tong and posterior. Application depends on the indication and degree of stabilization desired. The sugar tong splint may be used in ankle sprains, to prevent inversion or eversion.

Sugar Tong Splint
1. Measure from the fibular head (at the knee) to the calcaneus, double that measurement, and cut the splint material and padding to size.
2. Wet the splint material and remove excess water by applying gentle pressure across the width of the splint material.

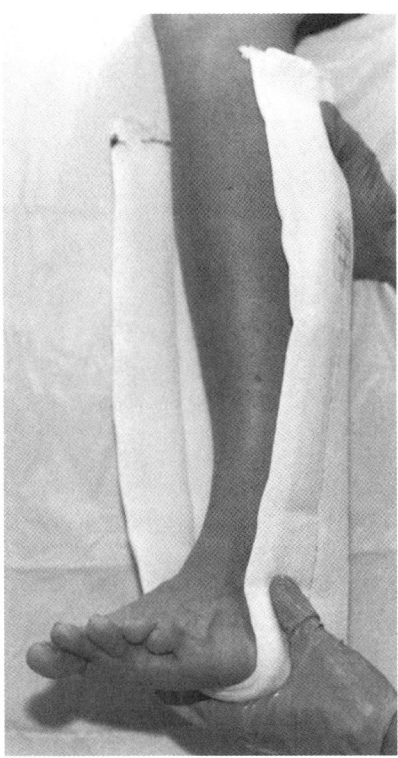

Fig. 187-2
Splint material in the shape of a U. The splint allows for swelling while providing medial and lateral support.

3. Place the padding against the patient's skin and have the patient or an assistant hold it in place.
4. Apply the splint material against the lateral aspect of the leg, starting just distal to the fibular head. Wrap the splint under the heel, and return it up the medial side of the leg to just below the knee (Fig. 187-2). (It should look like a long sugar tong, or U shaped; the anterior and posterior aspects are open.)
5. Mold the splint material to support the ankle and heel.
6. Place a layer of padding over the splint.
7. Wrap the splint material to hold it in place with an Ace bandage or a roll of cast padding (Fig. 187-3).

Posterior Splint
The posterior splint may be used with stable tibial or fibular fractures and plantar fasciitis to restrict dorsiflexion or plantar flexion of the foot and ankle complex.
1. Measure from the metatarsal heads to just distal to the popliteal fossa, and cut the splint material and padding to size.
2. Wet the splint material and remove excess water.
3. Place the padding against the patient's skin and have the patient or an assistant hold it in place.
4. Apply the splint material over the padding and against the plantar aspect of the foot and along the posterior aspect of the leg. Extend the splint from the

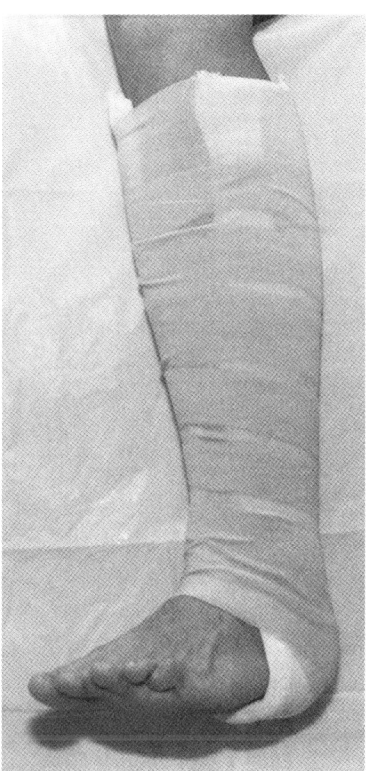

Fig. 187-3
Finished sugar tong splint held in place with a compression wrap.

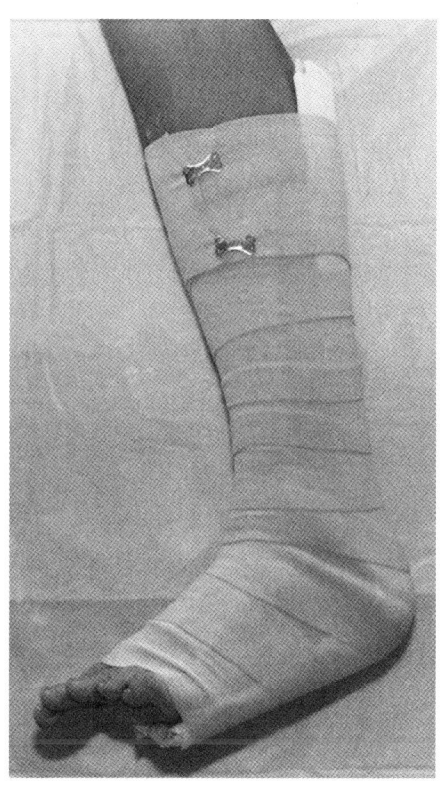

Fig. 187-5
Finished posterior splint held in place with a compression wrap.

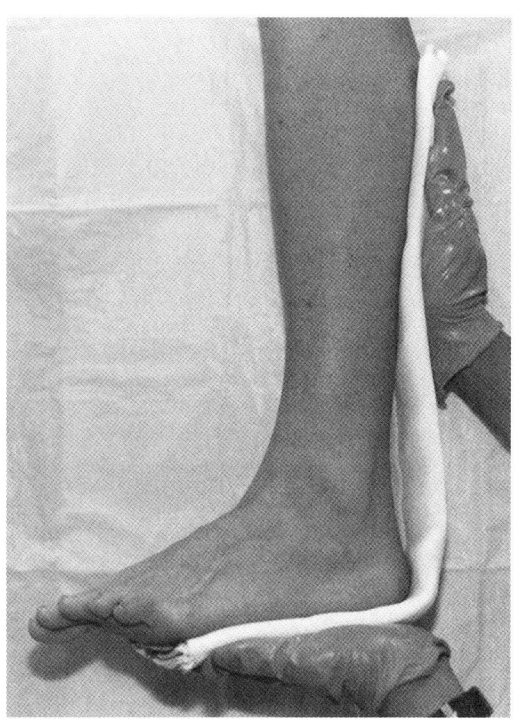

Fig. 187-4
Cast material runs along the posterior aspect of the lower leg and the plantar surface, providing immobilization for ankle dorsiflexion and plantar flexion.

metatarsal heads to just distal to the popliteal fossa (Fig. 187-4).

5. Mold the splint material to support the ankle and heel.
6. Place a layer of padding over the outside of the splint.
7. Wrap the splint material to hold it in place with an Ace bandage or a roll of cast padding (Fig. 187-5).

Casting

Short Leg Cast. May be used for stable tibial or fibular fractures, 5th metatarsal fractures, or severe ankle sprains (after acute swelling subsides).

1. Measure from the metatarsal heads to the knee and cut the stockinette to length. Be sure to allow extra stockinette to fold over the ends of the cast.
2. Slide stockinette on and smooth all wrinkles or folds. The crease that will be formed at the anterior ankle should be trimmed away (Fig. 187-6).
3. Place the ankle in neutral position (90 degrees). Failure to flex it to 90 degrees may lead to difficulty in ambulating and to Achilles tendon shortening. A foot stand may be useful to support the foot.
4. Wrap the cast padding over the stockinette, starting at the foot. The padding should overlap 50% with

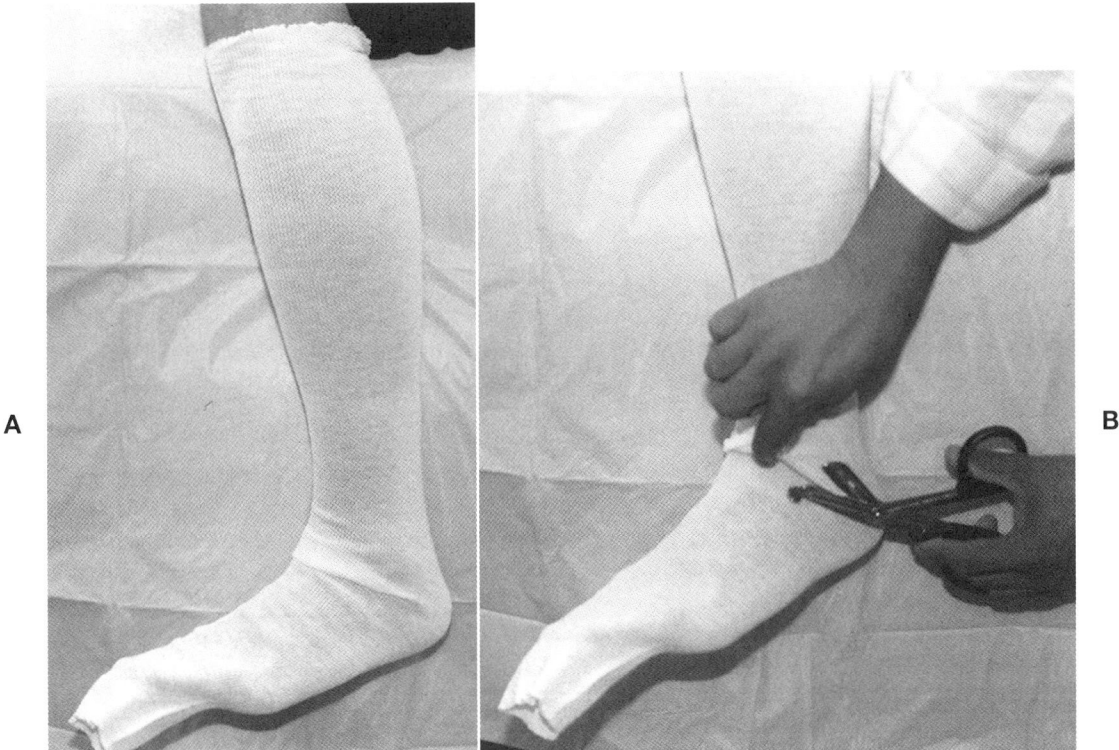

Fig. 187-6
A, Stockinette is placed on the lower leg from the knee to the toes. **B,** The transverse crease formed at the ankle should be removed.

each consecutive wrap. The padding should extend from the metatarsal heads to just distal to the fibular head. Care should be taken to provide adequate padding around the heel, the malleoli, the metatarsal heads, the proximal fibula, and the anterior tibia (Fig. 187-7).

5. Wet the cast material. Wrap the foot and ankle with the cast material in a manner similar to that already done with the cast padding. It should be wrapped over the cast padding. Maintain moderate tension, and overlap the rolls by 50% (Fig. 187-8).

6. Mold the cast to ensure neutral position of the ankle at 90 degrees.

7. Fold the stockinette over the ends of the cast to provide a smooth edge (Fig. 187-9).

8. Apply a final layer of cast material over the initial layer and the folded down edge of the stockinette at the ends (Fig. 187-10). For a walking cast, 6 to 8 layers of reinforcing strips may be placed under the heel and foot prior to the final cast layer. These are shaped like an L and go from the metatarsal heads to the midcalf to provide additional support.

9. Allow 10 minutes for the cast to set, and instruct the patient not to bear weight for at least 24 hours. Provide crutches for ambulation.

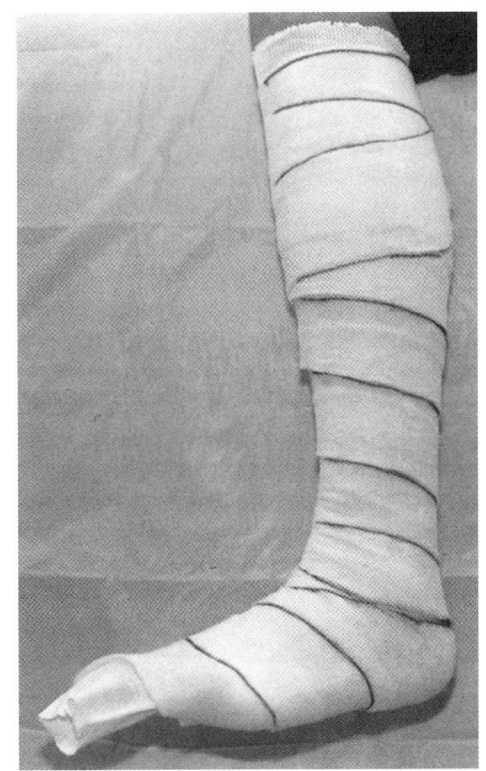

Fig. 187-7
Cast padding is applied with 50% overlap on each turn.

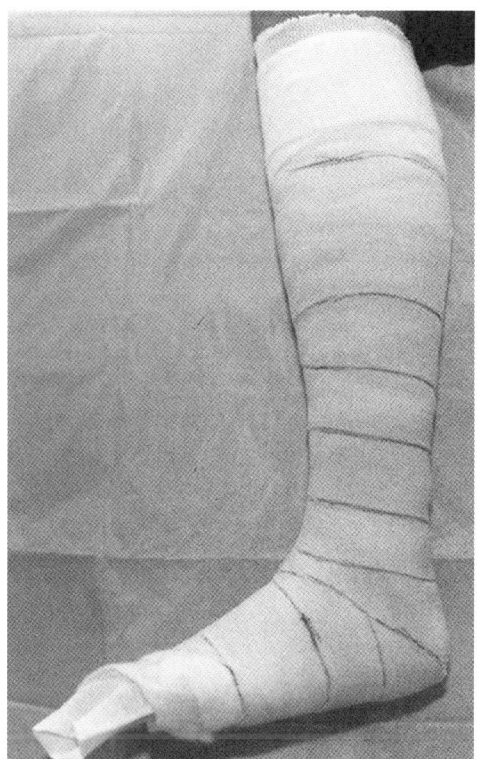

Fig. 187-8
Application of cast material with 50% overlap on each turn.

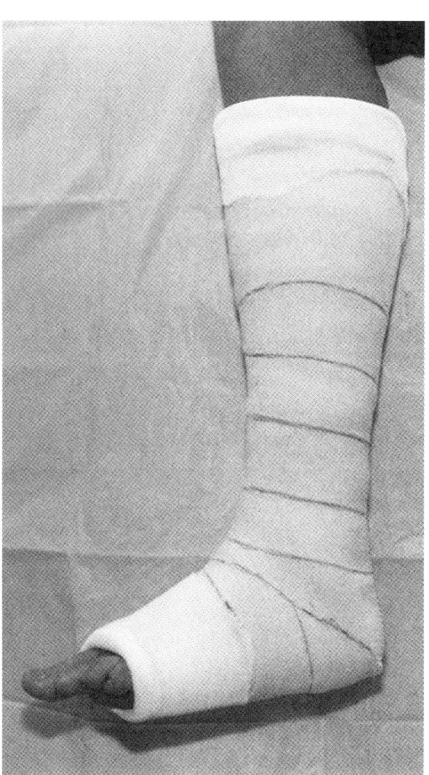

Fig. 187-9
After the first roll of cast material is placed, the stockinette is folded back over the ends.

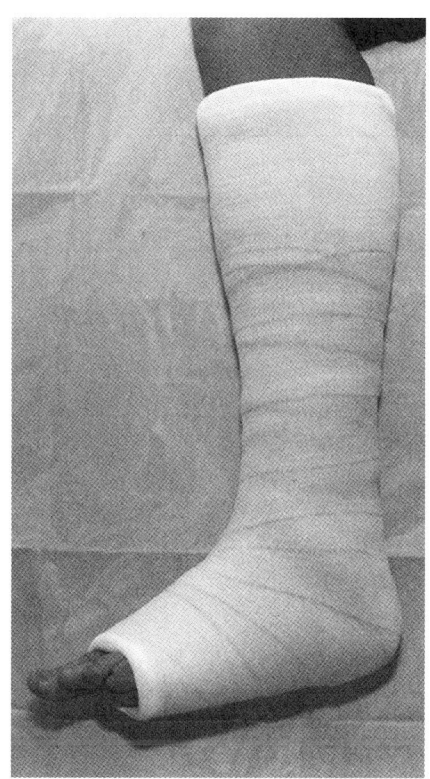

Fig. 187-10
Finished short leg cast.

10. A walking boot may be fitted to ease ambulation. Again, wait 24 hours for the cast to set before allowing weight bearing.

Note: A walking heel is unnecessary for a fiberglass cast.

Cast Removal or Bivalving

1. When splitting the cast, both the medial and lateral sides should be cut.
2. Starting at the top of the cast, make straight cuts that run posterior to the malleoli. Use a finger to stabilize the saw against the cast and to control the depth of the cut.

   Note: When using a cast saw, make plunging cuts along the length of the cut. Do not attempt to steadily drag the saw along the length of the cut, as this will cause the blade to heat up, and may burn the patient.

3. Next, make cuts along the medial and lateral sides of the foot that intersect with the initial cuts. Take care to avoid cutting over bony prominences (Fig. 187-11).
4. After the cuts are complete, a cast spreader is inserted into the cut and spread to widen the cut.
5. The cast padding and stockinette are then cut with blunt-tipped scissors.
6. The cast may then be opened and removed, or

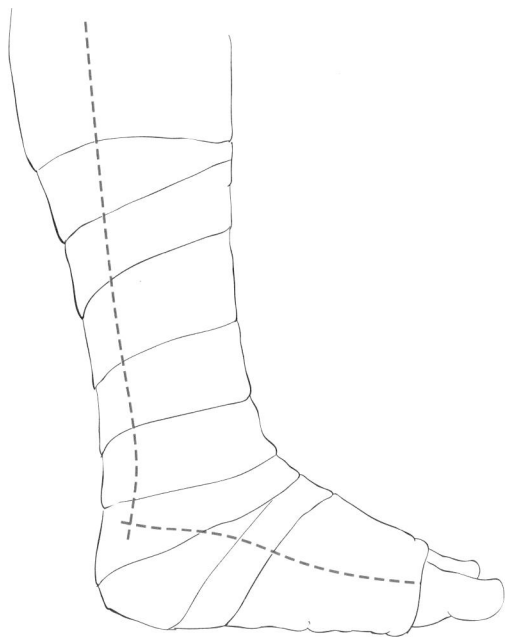

Fig. 187-11
When a cast is being removed, medial and lateral cuts are made posterior to the malleoli.

wrapped with a compression bandage to serve as a splint. Note: When wrapped with a compression bandage, the resultant splint provides almost as much support as a cast; therefore a clinician should have a low threshold for bivalving a cast to minimize complications. The same saws can be used for both plaster and fiberglass.

Bracing

Ankle bracing may be used prophylactically (to prevent injury), therapeutically, after an acute injury, or after injury to prevent reinjury. Commercial premade braces come in several styles. All styles may be used for any of these indications. Consider patient comfort and stability in choosing a brace. If the patient does not tolerate one style, consider a different one. Styles include the following:
- Lace up
- Stirrup
- Hinged

Taping

Plantar fasciitis

For this procedure, two pieces of skin tape will be applied followed by two pieces of high-tensile adhesive tape over them. The first three pieces of tape are simply applied smoothly and without wrinkles or any tension. Only the last piece of tape is applied under tension.

Skin Prep

With the patient sitting on an examination table, skin oils and other debris should be cleansed from the plantar aspect of the affected foot with alcohol. While the alcohol is allowed to dry, palpate the dorsalis pedis pulse. Document the presence or absence of the pulse.

Application

1. Place the foot in a neutral position (90 degrees), approximately the same position as if the patient were standing on it. From this position, it should be slightly inverted or "turned in" (sole of the foot facing slightly medially).
2. Apply skin tape (white tape) from the ball of the foot (Fig. 187-12, *A*) to the mid-heel (Fig. 187-12, *B*). The upper edge of the tape will extend slightly up the medial side of the foot, but it should not be higher than one third of the way up to the medial malleolus. In fact, keeping it low on the foot and simply taping around the posterior calcaneus may minimize any friction on the Achilles tendon. Smooth the wrinkles and bubbles, and there should be no tension applied to this piece of tape.
3. Locate the navicular bone. It causes the bony projection about 1 inch anterior to the medical malleolus. Apply skin tape (white tape), under no tension, from the heel (Fig. 187-12, *C*) up the medial aspect of the foot to end on top of the foot (Fig. 187-12, *D*). This tape should cover and include the navicular bone and extend past the midline of the dorsum of the foot.
4. Apply tensile tape (brown tape) of the same length in the same location and manner as the first piece of skin tape, simply covering that skin tape. Smooth any wrinkles or bubbles, but do not apply any tension.
5. Apply a second piece of tensile tape (brown tape) over the second piece of skin tape. This tape should be applied under tension, but not so much as to occlude the dorsalis pedis pulse.
6. When the patient stands, since the tape bears the weight of the plantar fascia and deloads it, he or she should be almost symptom free. For severe cases of plantar fasciitis, adding a slight degree of plantar flexion to the foot prior to taping, in addition to the slight inversion, will deload the fascia even more.
7. Since it loses strength with weight bearing, the tape should be removed and reapplied daily for 4 to 6 weeks. Outlining the outside edges of the tape with a permanent marker may be helpful for patient education purposes. This outline may help them when reapplying the tape the next day. They may want to outline it each day or use a copy of Fig. 187-12 to remind them of how to reapply the tape. When the tape is being changed, the foot should be massaged and put through range-of-motion exer-

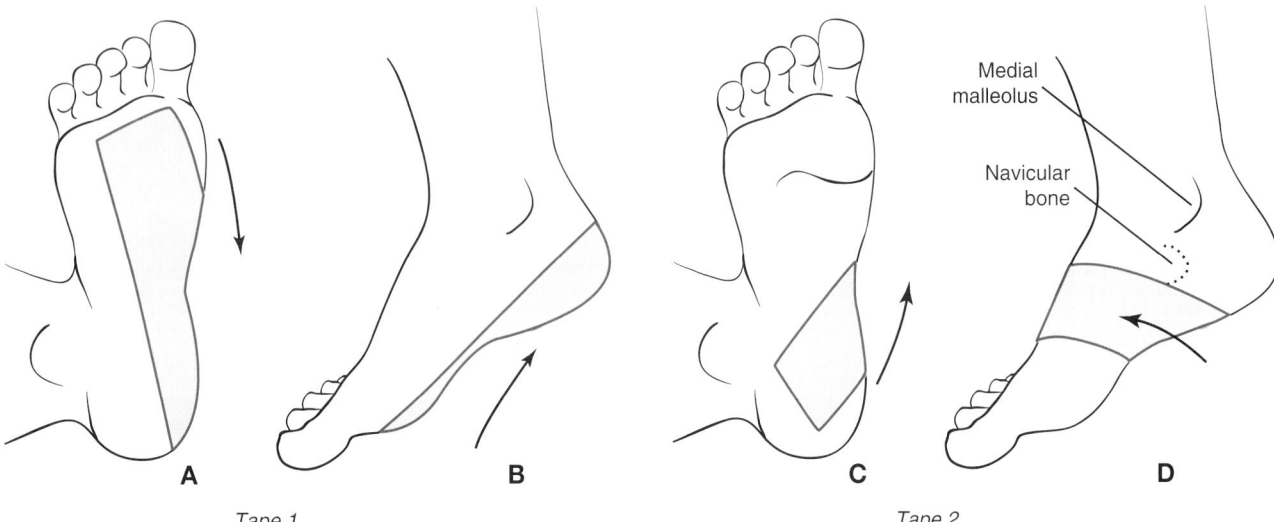

Tape 1   *Tape 2*

Fig. 187-12
Skin tape #1 (white tape) is applied from the ball of the foot **(A)** to the mid-heel **(B).** Skin tape #2 (white tape) is applied from the heel **(C)** up the medial aspect of the foot to end on top of the foot **(D).** Tensile tape pieces #1 and #2 are applied in the same locations and directions. They should be the same lengths as the skin tape.

cises. Using a commercial adhesive remover will help when cleaning off the debris from the skin tape of the day before.

8. For more severe cases, if the patient is symptomatic when bearing weight following taping, gradually more degrees of plantar flexion should be applied with each day of subsequent taping. The goal should be to bear weight with almost no symptoms for 4 to 6 weeks. This allows the fascia to heal.

9. Following resolution of symptoms and completion of the taping regimen, the foot should be rehabilitated aggressively with stretching and range-of-motion exercises.

Note: This technique was first used by Frank Ward, PT, and Dechie Bello-Rapoport, PT, MBA, at the Memorial Hermann Sports Medicine Physical Therapy Rehabilitation Center in Houston, Texas. One of their success stories included a woman who had had plantar fasciitis for 7 years!

Ankle
Skin Prep
Ankle taping provides the greatest support when applied directly against the skin. Daily application, however, will likely cause skin irritation. The use of underwrap material can prevent this. Shave the foot and ankle. Apply a coating of skin prep, usually benzoin. This will protect the skin, and provide better adhesion. Avoid the use of skin prep in patients with a history of sensitivity or allergy to these products (underwrap is recommended in these patients [Fig. 187-13, *B*]). Lubrication or padding may be applied to the skin at sites of potential friction or irritation (Fig. 187-13, *A*).

Application
There are several methods used for taping the ankle. The most commonly used is the *closed basket-weave technique,* also known as the Gibney technique, which provides strong tape support (Fig. 187-13). This extra support may be needed in either recently sprained or chronically weak ankles.

1. An anchor strip is placed around the ankle 5 to 6 inches above the malleoli (Fig. 187-13, *C*).
2. A second anchor strip is placed around the instep.
3. A stirrup strip is placed posterior to the malleoli (Fig. 187-13, *D*). For an inversion injury, hold the foot in *eversion* when applying the stirrup strips. Conversely, hold the foot in *inversion* for an eversion injury.
4. The first horizontal (Gibney) strip is placed under the malleoli, and attached to the foot anchor (Fig. 187-13, *D*).
5. A second stirrup is placed overlapping the first by 50%, followed by a second Gibney strip, also overlapping the first by 50%. A third stirrup and Gibney are then placed in similar fashion (Fig. 187-13, *E*).
6. Placement of the Gibney strips is then continued up the ankle to the anchor strip (Fig. 187-13, *F*).
7. Two or three strips are placed around the arch for added support (Fig. 187-13, *G*).
8. Last, heel locks are applied as a final support. Starting high on the instep, wrap the tape posteriorly across the Achilles tendon, downward hooking the heel, leading under the arch, and then up the opposite side and finishing at the starting point. The heel lock is completed by repeating the wrap in the opposite direction (Fig. 187-13, *H*).

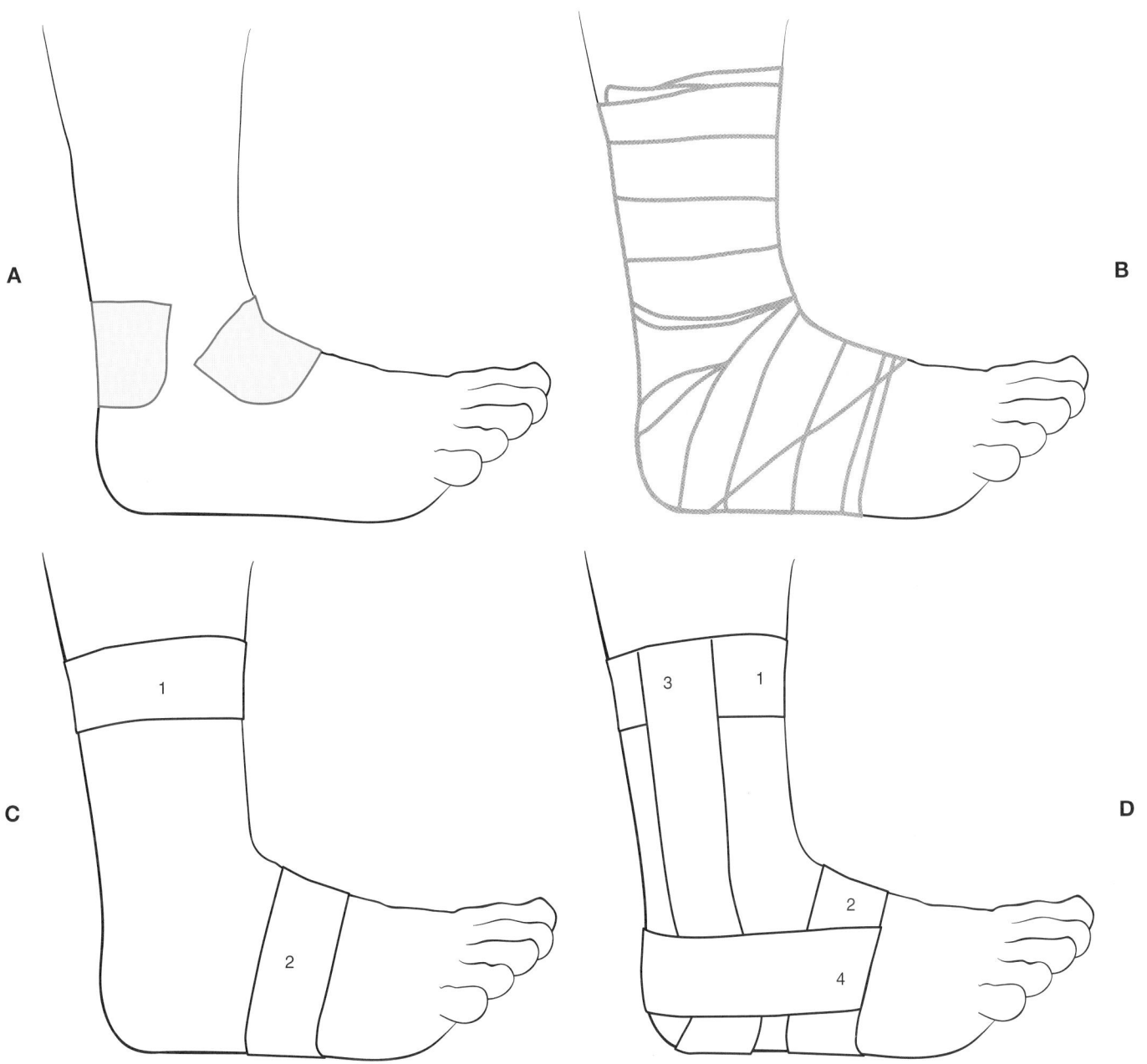

Fig. 187-13

Closed basket-weave (Gibney) technique. **A,** Application of padding at pressure points. **B,** Manner of application of thin underwrap tape. **C,** Anchor straps are placed either directly onto skin or over underwrap. **D,** Application of first stirrup and Gibney strips.

Continued

An alternative method, the *open basket-weave technique,* allows for some degree of dorsiflexion and plantar flexion. This technique accommodates swelling and may be used after acute injury. The procedure for the open basket weave is the same as for the closed basket-weave, with the notable exception of the Gibney strip placement. The Gibney strips are placed with a gap anteriorly. After the Gibney strips are placed, the gap is closed and the ends are locked by two to four strips running down the instep.

COMPLICATIONS

- *Nerve entrapment:* When casting, compression of the common peroneal nerve at the fibular head may

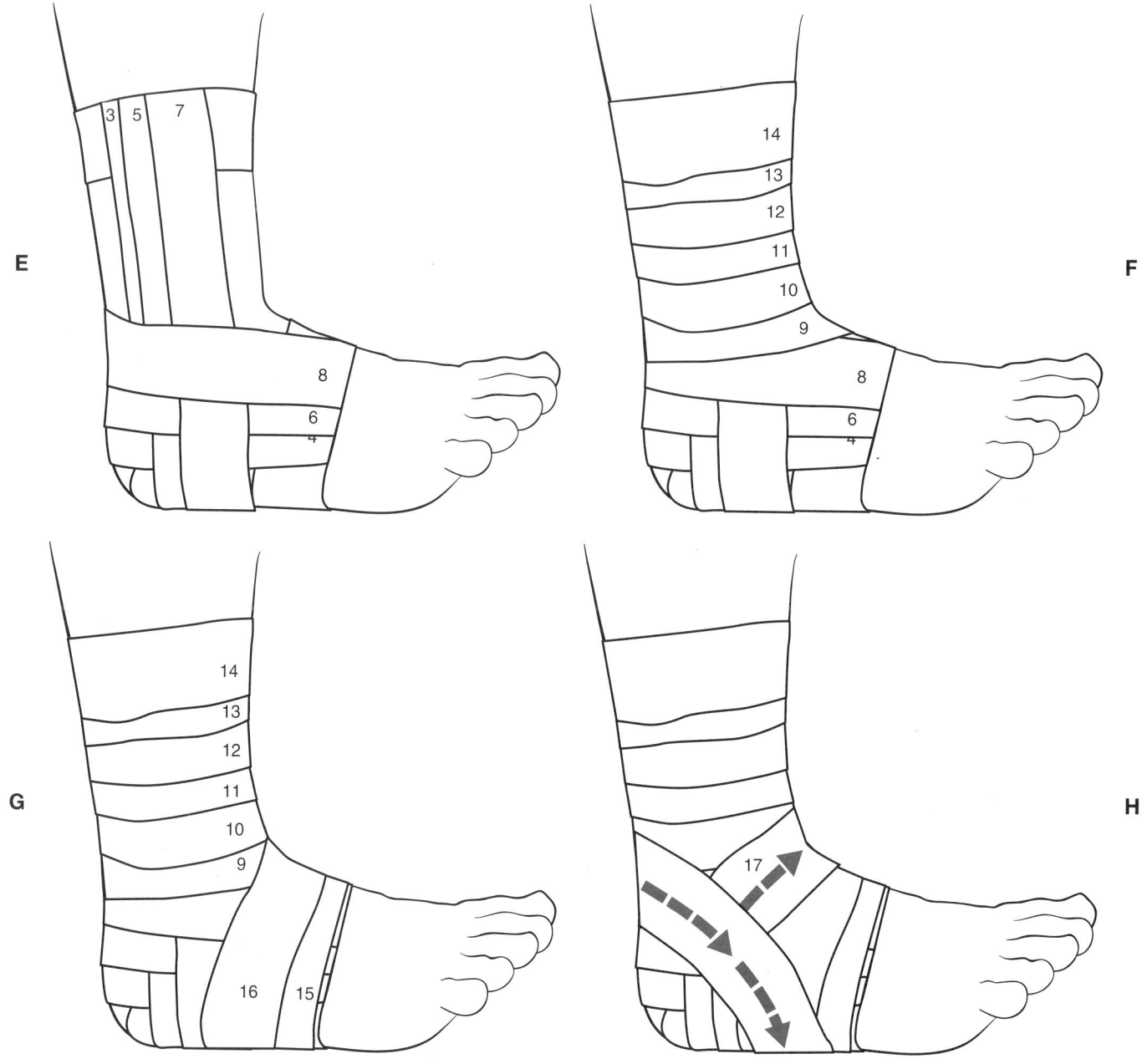

Fig. 187-13, cont'd
E, Stirrup and Gibney strips are applied in an alternating fashion. **F,** Gibney strips are continued up the ankle to the anchor strip. **G,** Application of arch strips. **H,** Heel locks are applied for additional support.

lead to foot drop. Correct placement of the proximal end of the cast is essential.

- *Compartment syndrome:* This may be caused by applying the cast before swelling has reached its maximum. If the patient notes any pain caused by the cast, the cast should be bivalved immediately to evaluate for any neurovascular compromise.

Note: One of the earliest signs of an impending compartment syndrome is pain on resisted plantar flexion

of the great toe. Have the patient dorsiflex his or her toe, and if pain radiates into the leg when the clinician attempts to plantar flex the toe, the cast should be bivalved immediately.

- *Loosening of the cast:* Application of a cast when swelling is present may lead to cast looseness when the swelling abates. A loose cast will no longer provide adequate stability and immobilization.
- *Skin necrosis:* Skin necrosis may be caused by

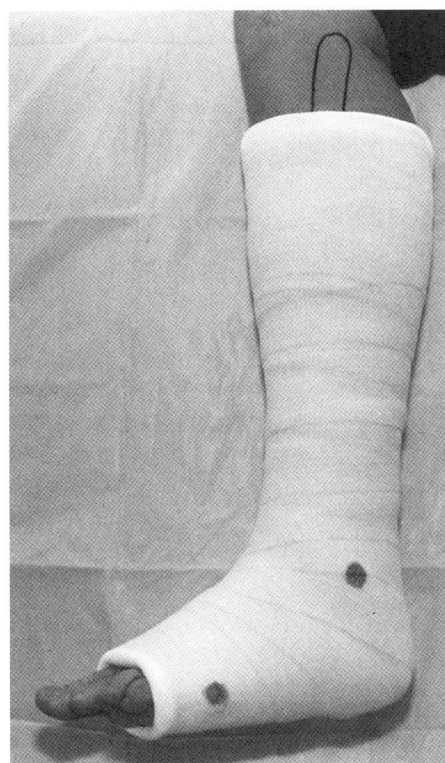

Fig. 187-14
Common locations for pressure sores are noted on the cast. Note the outline of the fibular head above the cast. This is the site of possible peroneal nerve entrapment.

pressure over bony prominences. This is best prevented by placing extra padding at potential pressure points (Fig. 187-14). If necessary, a window may be cut in the cast to remove the source of irritation. A window should not be cut, however, in areas that have acute swelling. In that case, a different form of immobilization should be employed.

• *Joint stiffness:* Patients often suffer from joint stiffness as a result of immobilization. This is best prevented by not immobilizing joints any longer than what is needed for fracture healing.

POSTPROCEDURE PATIENT EDUCATION

In an acute injury, after immobilization the patient should elevate the leg for 48 to 72 hours to prevent swelling. Ice can be used, in a sealed container, over the cast or splint to help alleviate pain. Every effort should be made to keep the cast or splint dry. Patients should remove or cover it when bathing. If the cast or splint does become wet, patients may dry it with a hair dryer set on the cool setting.

Nothing should be inserted between a cast and the skin. This may cause abrasions and undetected infections. With a cast, patients should call immediately if they notice pain, fever, tightness or irritation, numbness, or discolored or cool toes. They can be taught to test for pain on resisted plantar flexion of the great toe. For any type of immobilization, they should know to call for certain symptoms.

SUPPLIERS

Foot and Ankle

Casting and splinting materials, accessories, braces
M-Pact
1040 OCL Parkway
Eudora, KS 66025
Phone: 1-800-255-4152
Website: www.m-pactmed.com

Casting and splinting materials
Johnson & Johnson Professional, Inc.
325 Paramount Drive
Raynham, MA 02767-0350
Phone: 1-800-526-2459
Website: www.johnsonandjohnson.com

3M Health Care
3M Center, Bldg. 275-4E-01
St. Paul, MN 55144-1000
Phone: 1-800-228-3957
Website: www.3m.com

Splints and braces
Aircast, Inc.
92 River Road
Summit, NJ 07901
Phone: 1-800-526-8785
Website: www.aircast.com

DonJoy (dj) Orthopedics, Inc.
2905 Scott Street
Vista, CA 92083
Phone: 1-800-321-9549
Website: www.djortho.com

Braces

Swede-O, Inc.

611 Ash St.

P.O. Box 610 North Branch, MN 55056

Phone: 1-800-525-9339

Website: www.swedeo.com

Dressing retention sheet (skin tape)

Hypafix

Smith & Nephew, Inc.

11775 Starkey Road

P.O. Box 1970

Largo, FL 33779-1970

Phone: 1-800-876-1261

Website: www.snwmd.com

High-tensile strength adhesive tape

Leukotape-P (this brand was specifically developed for
   use with McConnell taping)

Beiersdorf, Inc.

Wilton Corporate Center

187 Danbury Road

Wilton, CT 06897

Phone: 1-203-563-5800

Website: www.beiersdorf.com

Healwell Night Splint

FLA Orthopedics

2881 Corporate Way

Miramar, FL 33025

Phone: 1-800-327-4110

Website: www.clinitex.com

Nocturnal splints

Freedom PF Night Splint II

AliMed, Inc.

297 High Street

Dedham, MA 02026

Phone: 1-800-225-2610

Website: www.alimed.com

CPT/BILLING CODES

Fracture Management

Fracture care CPT codes include initial management of
fractures, along with initial splint or cast application.
These codes include subsequent routine cast care and
removal.

Codes for closed treatment *without* manipulation
include the following:

27750	Tibial shaft fracture
27760	Medial malleolus fracture
27780	Fibular shaft fracture
27786	Lateral malleolus fracture

Codes for closed treatment *with* manipulation include
the following:

27752	Tibial shaft fracture
27762	Medial malleolus fracture
27781	Fibular shaft fracture
27788	Lateral malleolus fracture

Cast or Splint Application

The following codes can be used when not part of
comprehensive fracture management, or when used for
soft tissue injuries. If a cast needs replacement, these
codes can also be used.

29405	Application of short leg cast
29425	Walking/ambulatory type
29440	Adding walker to previously applied cast
29730	Windowing cast
29740	Wedging cast
29515	Application of short leg splint
29540	Strapping; ankle
29799	Unlisted procedure, casting or strapping
29700	Removal or bivalving of short leg cast applied by another physician

Supplies

A4565	Sling
A4570	Splint material
A4580	Plaster cast supplies
A4590	Special cast supplies (fiberglass)
99070	Miscellaneous supplies/materials

ICD-9-CM DIAGNOSTIC CODES

845.0	Ankle sprain
728.71	Plantar fasciitis
823.80	Tibial fracture
823.81	Fibular fracture
824.2	Lateral malleolus fracture
824.0	Medial malleolus fracture
825.25	Metatarsal fracture
825.20	March (stress) fracture

BIBLIOGRAPHY

Arnheim D: *Modern principles of athletic training,* St Louis, 1989, Mosby.

Crenshaw A: *Campbell's operative orthopedics,* ed 7, St Louis, 1987, Mosby.

Eiff MP, Hatch RL, Calmbach WL: *Fracture management for primary care,* Philadelphia, 1998, WB Saunders.

Kessler R: *Management of common musculoskeletal disorders,* Philadelphia, 1983, Harper & Row.

Mellion M, Walsh W, Shelton G: *The team physician's handbook,* ed 2, Philadelphia, 1997, Hanley & Belfus.

Pfeffer G, Bacchetti P, Deland J, et al: Comparison of custom and prefabricated orthoses in the initial treatment of proximal plantar fasciitis, *Foot Ankle Int,* 20(4):214, 1999.

Prentice W, Arnheim D: *Principles of athletic training,* ed 9, Madison, Wisc, 1996, Brown & Benchmark.

Richmond J, Shahady E: *Sports medicine for primary care,* Cambridge, 1996, Blackwell Science.

CHAPTER 188

Cast Immobilization

Scott W. Eathorne
Todd M. Sheperd

Cast immobilization is a technique often used for treating a variety of medical conditions that the primary care physician encounters. Although newer technologies have led to an evolution in casting materials, the general principles of this valuable technique have stood the test of time. Having a knowledge of the materials available, understanding the indications and fundamental precepts of cast immobilization, and developing the necessary manual skills can enable the primary care physician to adequately treat the patient who has an injury amenable to such therapy.

HISTORY

The use of immobilization to treat acute fractures dates back to the era of the fifth dynasty (2730-2625 BC), when splints made from bark were used to treat fractures of the forearm. Gypsum, from which plaster of Paris is derived, was initially used around the sixteenth century in parts of the Turkish Empire. The development in 1927 of the hard-coated plaster of Paris rolls that incorporated a binder allowed for improved adherence of the plaster to the cloth. Since then, various additives have been used to either accelerate (salicylic acid, zinc, or aluminum) or slow (gums or glue) the setting process.

Currently, fiberglass is the most common material used in casting. It has the advantage(s) of being stronger and lighter, and it will often create less heat during application. The cost of fiberglass continues to be more than that of plaster, but in recent years this difference has decreased significantly. In addition to newer cast material, the development of synthetic padding (Gore-Tex) has allowed the cast to survive significant water exposure without damage.

INDICATIONS

Casts are used to treat (1) a variety of stable, acute fractures, (2) reduced dislocations, (3) injuries to the soft tissues including muscle, tendon, and ligament, (4) congenital and acquired deformities (e.g., correction of talipes equinovarus, or congenital clubfoot), and (5) to stabilize and protect postoperative vascular, tendon, or nerve injuries following surgical repair. The most common diagnosis the primary care physician makes that requires cast immobilization is the stable, nondisplaced, closed fracture of a long bone. The primary care physician often treats fractures involving the radius or ulna, phalanges, metacarpals, metatarsals, or malleoli. Other conditions include some Grade III ligament sprains (e.g., ankle), Achilles tendon disruptions, and tendonitis refractory to other forms of therapy. (See Chapter 192, Fracture Care.)

CAST APPLICATION
EQUIPMENT

- Rubber gloves
- Patient drape
- Physician gown and shoe covers
- Stockinette (2-, 3-, and 4-inch widths)
- Soft cotton (e.g., Webril) or synthetic bandages (2-, 3-, 4-, and 6-inch widths)
- Felt padding
- Rubber heels (walking cast)
- Synthetic waterproof cast padding (e.g., Procel cast liner)
- Cast removal protective strip (e.g. DE-FLEX Strip)
- Casting material (Fig. 188-1)
  —Plaster (e.g., plaster of paris)
  —Synthetic (e.g., fiberglass)
- Water source (should have traps in drains if using plaster)
- Elastic (Ace) bandages
- Slings
- Scissors
- Chinese finger traps
- Leg stand

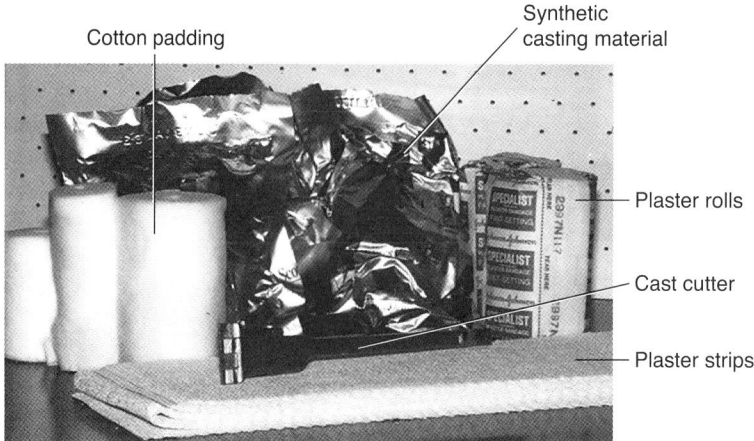

Fig. 188-1
Materials needed for casting: cotton padding, synthetic casting material or plaster rolls, cast separator, cast cutter, and plaster strips.

When water is added to the plaster, the water molecules are incorporated into the calcium sulfate hemihydrate molecules with a resultant exothermic reaction. The powdery white substance is converted into a solid, rock-hard material, with a significant amount of heat generated. A curing process then follows over the next few days, characterized by continued water evaporation; a process accelerated by low humidity, high ambient temperature, and increased air circulation.

Synthetic materials require immersion in water to activate the curing process, with generally less heat generated than with plaster. *Attention to water temperature in this process is especially important,* because water that is too warm can lead to rapid curing and significant difficulty in application.

Advantages of plaster casts over fiberglass include low cost, ease of molding, long shelf life, and low allergenicity. Synthetic cast material is more expensive, but this has narrowed in the years since fiberglass cast material was introduced. Fiberglass has also improved in its ease of application and continues to be superior in strength, durability, weight, water resistance, and drying time. Both materials are available in multiple sizes, ranging from 2 to 5 inches in width for general, circumferential cast use.

Ideally, a single room or area should be dedicated to the application of casts and splints. This room should have a plaster trap in the sink, and all materials should be easily accessible. Rubber gloves, shoe covers, gowns, and drapes should be available to protect against the inevitable exposure to casting materials. An easily cleaned examination table, stool, and leg stand can greatly facilitate the process of cast application.

COMMON CAST TYPES (see Chapter 192, Fracture Care)

Short-Arm Casts

Short-arm casts are generally indicated in the treatment of stable sprains of the wrist, as well as some stable fractures of the distal radius, carpal bones, and metacarpals. Physicians practicing cast immobilization should be aware of those fractures requiring orthopedic evaluation for possible open reduction and internal fixation. Materials required for short-arm cast applications include a 3-inch stockinette, two rolls of 3-inch cast padding (the waterproof liner replaces the need for both padding and stockinette), and two to four rolls of either 3- or 4-inch plaster bandage (or 2- or 3-inch fiberglass bandage). In general, adult males will require 4-inch plaster (3-inch fiberglass) and children will require 3-inch plaster (2-inch fiberglass). Adolescents and females may require either size depending on preference and size of extremity. The patient should be supine or seated, with the arm abducted 90 degrees and the elbow flexed 90 degrees. The wrist should be slightly extended and in a position of function (Fig. 188-2). Chinese finger traps attached to the patient and suspended from above can support the arm and assist in maintaining the position of function. The cast extends from the proximal forearm (about 1 inch distal to the flexion crease of the elbow) distally to include the palm and dorsum of the hand, completely covering the forearm. The metacarpal-phalangeal (MCP) joints are allowed complete motion, with the cast stopping just proximal to the distal palmar crease (Fig. 188-3). Short-arm casts only partially immobilize the wrist joint and allow movement of the thumb. In addition, they

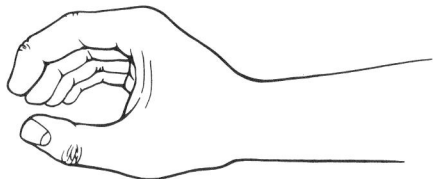

Fig. 188-2
Position of the wrist in the application of arm casts.

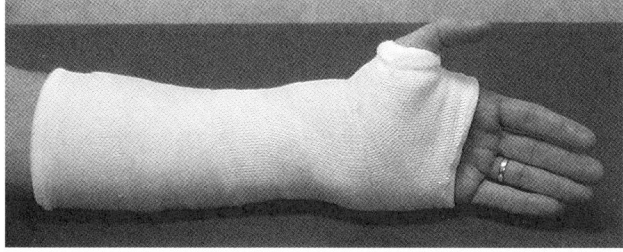

Fig. 188-3
Appearance of a completed short-arm cast. Note that the thumb and fingers are free to move.

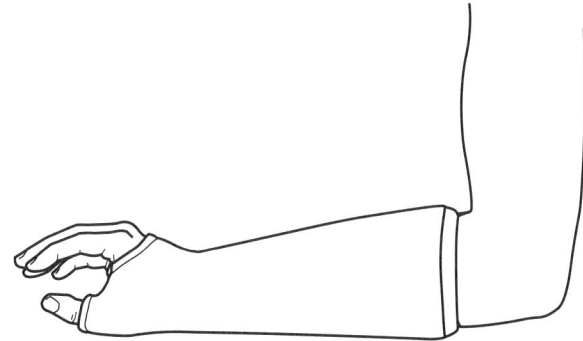

Fig. 188-4
Short-arm cast with thumb spica.

allow for supination and pronation to occur because the elbow is not included. An adaptation of the short-arm cast is the *short-arm thumb spica,* in which the thumb is included to the level of the interphalangeal (IP) joint (Fig. 188-4). This type of cast may be used for injuries to the scaphoid, trapezium, or first metacarpal, or for any injury requiring wrist and thumb immobilization.

Short-Leg Casts

Short-leg casts are generally indicated in the treatment of some stable ligamentous injuries to the ankle, and stable fractures of the ankle, calcaneus, tarsals, and metatarsals. Materials include a 4-inch stockinette and three rolls of 4-inch cast padding (or waterproof liner). With fiberglass casts, three rolls of 4-inch fiberglass bandage are generally needed. An extra reinforcing strip of heavy-duty fiberglass can also be used posteriorly along the bottom of the foot up the back of the leg. For plaster casts (used less often), materials vary widely based on personal preference, but they usually include two to three rolls of 6-inch plaster bandage and an adequate number of plaster splint strips (again for posterior and foot reinforcement), with size based on patient limb size. Application of the short-leg cast is achieved either in the sitting position with the leg hanging over the table, or prone with the knee flexed to 90 degrees to help relax the gastrocnemius muscle. The ankle is usually held at a 90-degree angle to the leg, but this may be altered depending on

the type of injury. A foot-stand or assistant can provide support to the foot. The cast extends from just below the knee joint, usually including the fibular head, distally to the base of the toes, including the metatarsal heads (Fig. 188-5). Again, the ankle joint is only partially immobilized, since the cast does not involve both the joint above and below. For *walking short-leg casts* (Fig. 188-6), a posterior reinforcing strip is placed and molded after application of the second roll of fiberglass bandage and before placing the final roll. The walker can be applied the same day or at a later time. If applied initially, patients have a tendency to walk on it before the primary cast is dry enough, leading to breakdown of the cast.

Other types of common casts and splints are shown in Fig. 188-7. Even with splints, where casting materials do not totally surround the extremity, there is generally a layer of stockinette around the entire area followed by the padding, then the casting material. This is held in place with an Ace wrap or similar material.

PREPROCEDURE PATIENT PREPARATION

After diagnosing an injury requiring cast immobilization, and before its application, the indications for casting, estimated duration of immobilization, and potential impact on activities of daily living should be discussed with the patient. Typically, discussion of common problems and potential complications from casting occur following application. Online references for patient education handouts can be found at the end of this chapter.

TECHNIQUE

Casts are generally applied to immobilize and/or protect an injured part of the body in a position that will

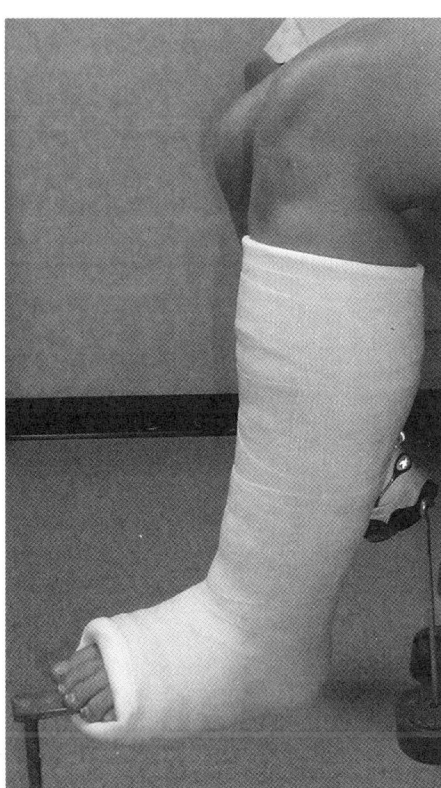

Fig. 188-5
Appearance of a completed short leg cast. The cast should hold the ankle at 90 degrees. In addition, the proximal end of the cast should far enough from the knee to eliminate the possibility of skin irritation with knee flexion.

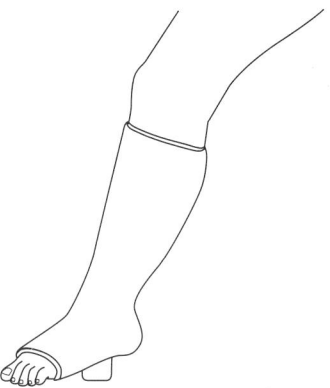

Fig. 188-6
Short-leg cast with walker.

facilitate healing. This simplistic view directs the fundamentals of cast immobilization. First, to best approach complete immobilization, *a cast must conform precisely to the anatomy of the region being immobilized*. Failure to accomplish this can lead to unacceptable movement of the injured area, leading to potential loss of reduction, malalignment of a reduced dislocation, or persistent inflammation in a refractory tendonitis. Second, *effective immobilization is achieved only by including a sufficient amount of injured area in the cast*. Ideally, this is accomplished by including the joint above and the joint below the area of injury. However, exceptions to this rule are made based on the nature of the injury. Achieving adequate immobilization requires attention to these fundamentals before application of the cast. If these goals cannot be met, the injury may best be served by another means of immobilization.

1. Before application of any casting materials, cleanse, dry, and thoroughly inspect the skin to be included in the cast for any lesions such as lacerations, abrasions, or ulcers. If present, they should be noted and, if significant, may contraindicate inclusion in the cast or may require special "window" techniques. Depending on the acuity of the injury and degree of soft-tissue swelling, immobilization using circumferential casting may be contraindicated. In this situation, the injury may require the use of a splint for immobilization until more definitive care can be given after the swelling has diminished.

2. After this assessment is completed, position the patient such that the injured area can be held most easily in the desired position throughout the application process. This often requires the use of an assistant or assistive device (e.g., leg stand or finger traps).

Note: Cast application is performed in a step-wise manner, and development of a systematic approach will help ensure consistency and minimize the potential for error.

3. The *first layer* generally applied in casting is the *stockinette*. A poorly fitting stockinette can contribute to skin breakdown, so it must be applied carefully. Use a 3-inch-wide stockinette for adult arm casts, and a 4-inch-wide for legs, with exceptions based on the extremes of limb size. The material should go well past the toes or fingertips and 4 to 5 inches above the elbow or knee (Fig. 188-8, *A*). (Cutting the stockinette too short is a common problem among those learning the procedure.) Some of this "extra" material is ultimately incorporated into the cast or, eventually, cut off.

4. Remove all transverse wrinkles; they become pressure points after cast application and can cause skin breakdown. This can be achieved by cutting the redundant material, which is usually at a joint. Fig. 188-8, *B*, shows a short-leg stockinette that has been cut and then overlayed at the anterior ankle to reduce wrinkles.

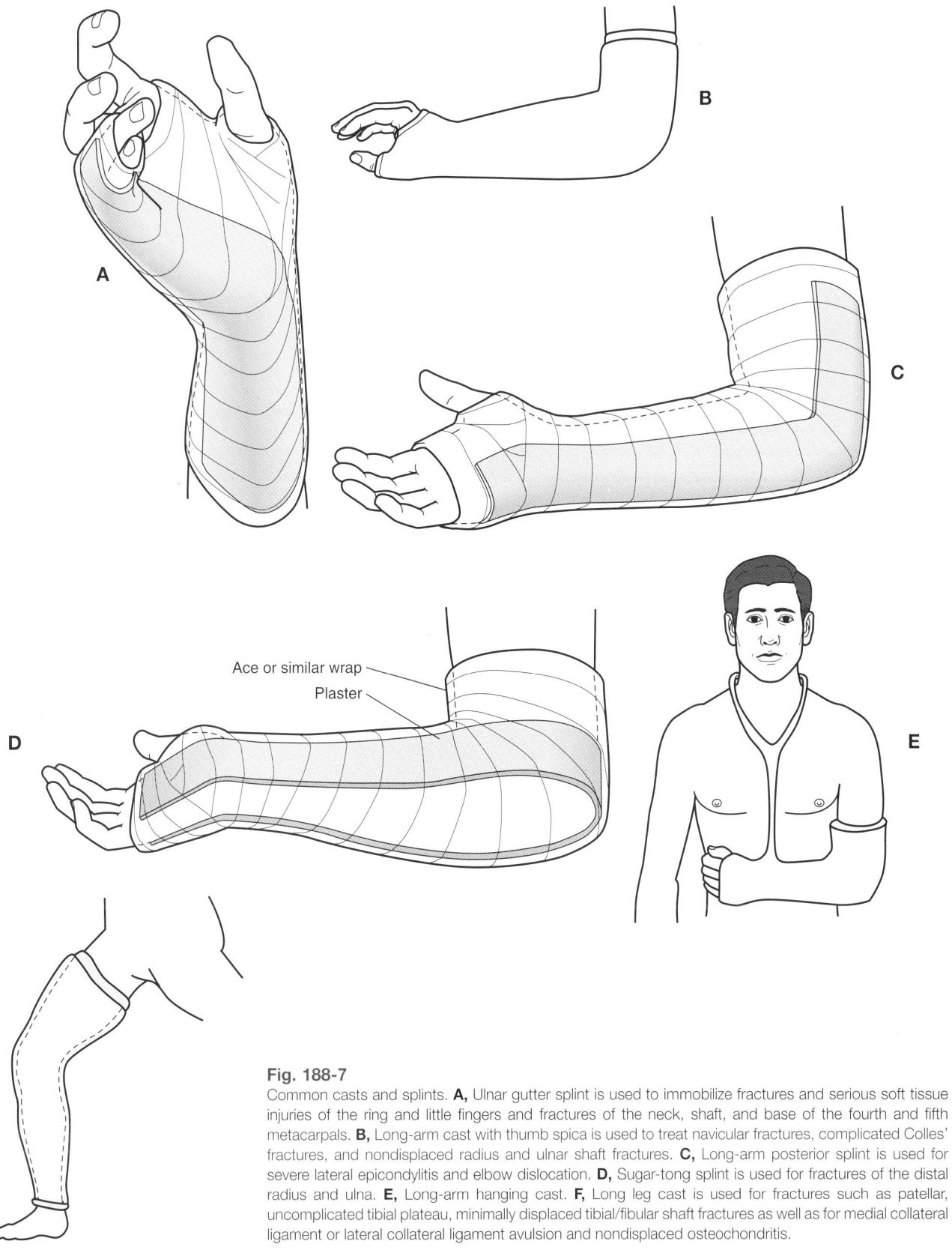

Ace or similar wrap

Plaster

Fig. 188-7
Common casts and splints. **A,** Ulnar gutter splint is used to immobilize fractures and serious soft tissue injuries of the ring and little fingers and fractures of the neck, shaft, and base of the fourth and fifth metacarpals. **B,** Long-arm cast with thumb spica is used to treat navicular fractures, complicated Colles' fractures, and nondisplaced radius and ulnar shaft fractures. **C,** Long-arm posterior splint is used for severe lateral epicondylitis and elbow dislocation. **D,** Sugar-tong splint is used for fractures of the distal radius and ulna. **E,** Long-arm hanging cast. **F,** Long leg cast is used for fractures such as patellar, uncomplicated tibial plateau, minimally displaced tibial/fibular shaft fractures as well as for medial collateral ligament or lateral collateral ligament avulsion and nondisplaced osteochondritis.

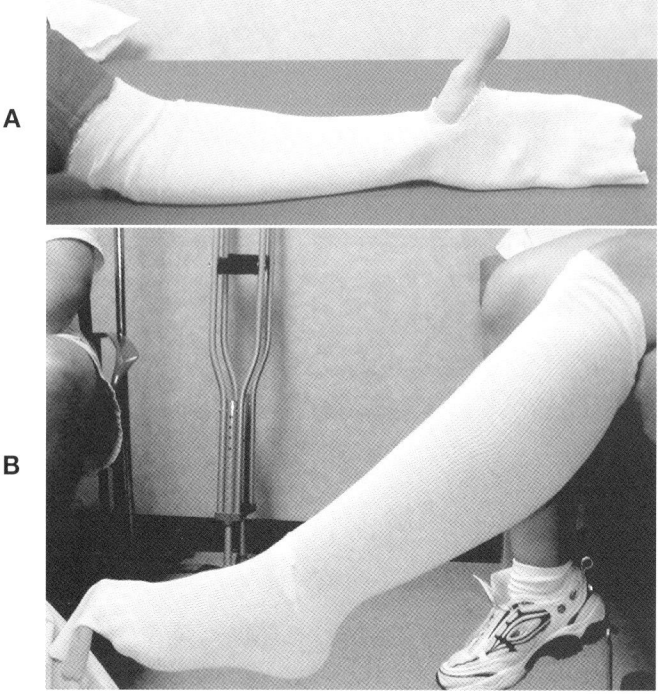

A

B

Fig. 188-8
A, Demonstration of proper stockinette application for short-arm cast. Enough excess is present to allow a cuff to be created below the final layer of casting material. **B,** Application of stockinette for a short-leg cast, demonstrating the technique to eliminate transverse wrinkle at ankle. Note the length of the stockinette for a short-leg cast.

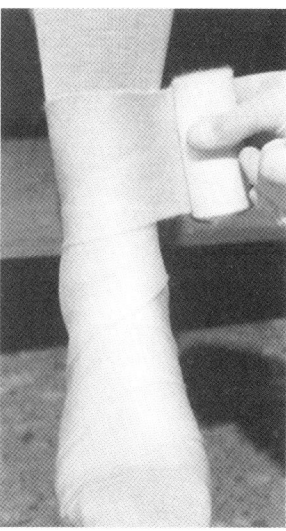

Fig. 188-9
Application of soft cast padding. Beginning at one end, cast padding is added while overlapping each turn by half. (From Mercier LR: *Practical orthopedics,* ed 5, St Louis, 2000, Mosby.)

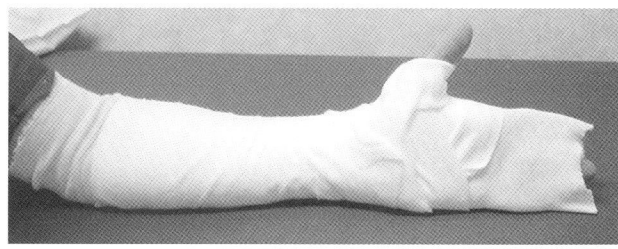

Fig. 188-10
Short-arm cast after application of cast padding and before addition of casting material.

5. After ensuring that the stockinette overlying the area to be immobilized is smooth and free of wrinkles, apply the second layer. The *second layer consists of soft cast padding material (Webril),* which comes in rolls and is applied in a circular manner. Start at one end (usually distally) and work toward the other; on the first turn around the extremity, roll the padding over itself to create an anchor. After this, each subsequent turn will overlap itself by 50% (Fig. 188-9). Two layers of cast padding can be applied, but care should be taken not to pad too much because this can lead to a loose cast. The goal with padding, as with the stockinette, is to avoid wrinkles, which may contribute to pressure points. Stretch or tear the advancing edge that is to encircle a larger portion of the extremity in order to avoid wrinkles. Keeping in mind the local anatomy, apply additional padding to bony prominences and likely areas of increased local pressure (e.g., flexion creases; fulcrum points such as the proximal anterior tibia where short-leg walking casts may rub; and common areas of nerve compression or pressure necrosis, such as over the proximal fibula). Felt pads appropriately fashioned can prevent common complications and improve comfort. Fig. 188-10 shows a short-arm cast after cast padding application and before cast material application.

6. When using the *waterproof cast liner,* it is applied in a manner identical to the application of cast padding and eliminates the need for stockinette use. By using this material, only two total layers of material are needed (cast liner and cast material). To apply, start unrolling onto the extremity from either the distal or proximal end point. Remember to keep the adhesive side of the cast liner *away* from the patient's skin. The material is applied until the opposite end of the desired endpoint is reached and is extended 4 to 5 cm beyond the desired length of the cast. The excess will allow the ends to be folded back at the margins before casting material application (Fig. 188-11, *A*). Apply additional material to bony prominences to prevent pressure-related complications. Unlike traditional cast padding, the waterproof cast liner must be cut to achieve proper sizing because it does not tear

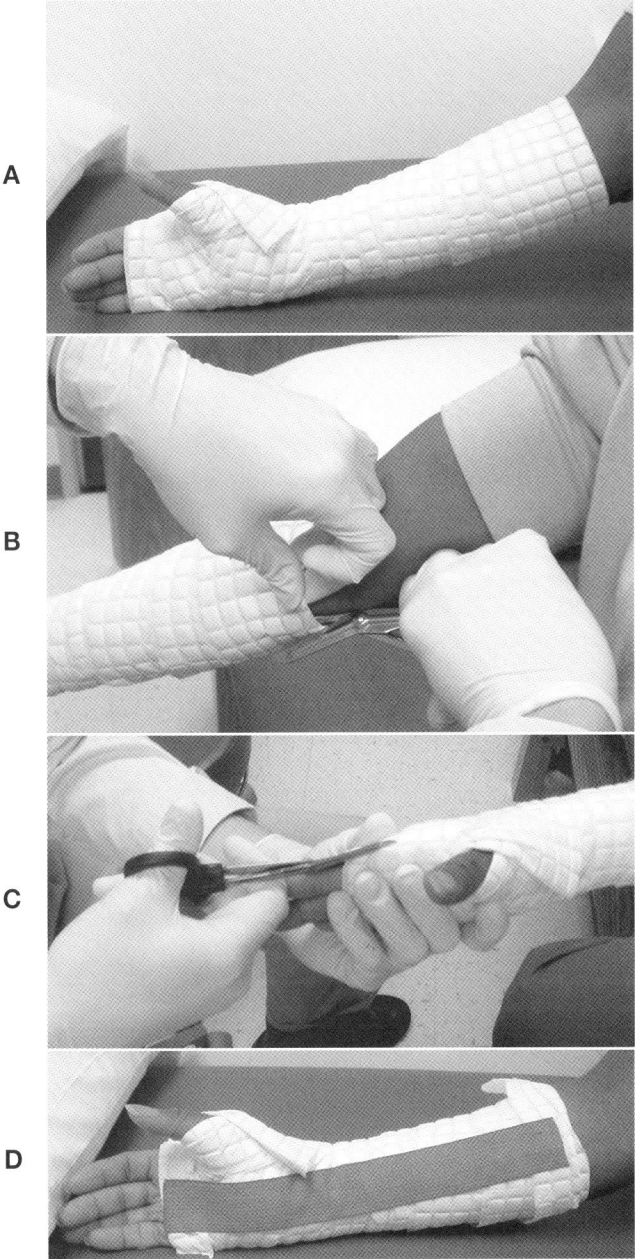

Fig. 188-11
Gore-Tex application. **A,** Gore-Tex liner applied 4 to 5 cm beyond desired cast length. **B-C,** Using scissors to cut material and allow liner to be folded. **D,** Protective strip applied before application of cast materials.

(Fig. 188-11, *B-C*). In addition, waterproof cast liner requires the use of a protective strip below the cast material (Fig. 188-11, *D*).

7. Apply the *third layer* (or second layer if cast liner was used), *which consists of the cast material itself*. The type of material used (plaster or synthetic) dictates how the next step will be completed. Although application is quite similar, a few significant differences are worth noting.

When using *plaster-impregnated rolls,* place each roll individually in water at room temperature and submerse until the bubbling stops. Cold water slows the setting process, whereas warmer water speeds it. A faster setting may be desirable when immobilizing a recently reduced dislocation. After removal from the water, gently squeeze and twist the roll to eliminate excess water and begin the application (Fig. 188-12, *A*). Placement of the plaster rolls should follow the direction of the cast padding and should be applied in a similar manner. The first turn has 100% overlap, and each additional turn overlaps approximately 50%. To avoid transverse wrinkles, plaster rolls can be tucked (folded over) at the edges when redundancy occurs and smoothed with the palm of the hand (Fig. 188-12, *B-C*). Avoid stretching and applying undue pressure with each turn. *Apply four to six layers* of plaster evenly, with extra reinforcement in areas under increased stress. Apply each roll in a consistent manner, either distal-to-proximal or proximal-to-distal, with the length of the area to be immobilized covered with each layer. Covering only a portion of the extremity and overlapping with the next roll may lead to inherent weakness and future difficulties with the cast. *Before placing the final layers, the ends of the stockinette should be folded over onto the initial layers.* Reinforcing strips or cast cushions, if used, should be added now (depending on the type of cast being applied) (Fig. 188-12, *D*).

8. Place the final layers of cast material and smooth the cast, using both hands. Make sure that it conforms to the contours of the local anatomy by using the palms to apply pressure to the cast (Fig. 188-12, *E*). If the fingers are used to conform (or mold) the cast, subtle pressure areas under the cast may be created. Position of the injured area while casting is critical. The ankle joint should be at 90 degrees and the hand and wrist in a position of function (slightly extended, relaxed). This position should be closely rechecked before hardening of the cast. See Fig. 188-2 for an example of the position of function used with short-arm casts. With certain fractures or tendon injuries, the above positions may be altered to improve tissue healing. The provider should be aware of these needs before the application of the cast.

Application of *synthetic materials* follows a similar course, with a few noteworthy exceptions. Water used to activate the curing process should be kept no warmer than room temperature to avoid rapid setting of the roll. Normally, this occurs in 2 to 3 minutes. Because of the flexibility of the synthetic bandage rolls, tucking of edges is not necessary to avoid transverse creases. However, care must still be taken

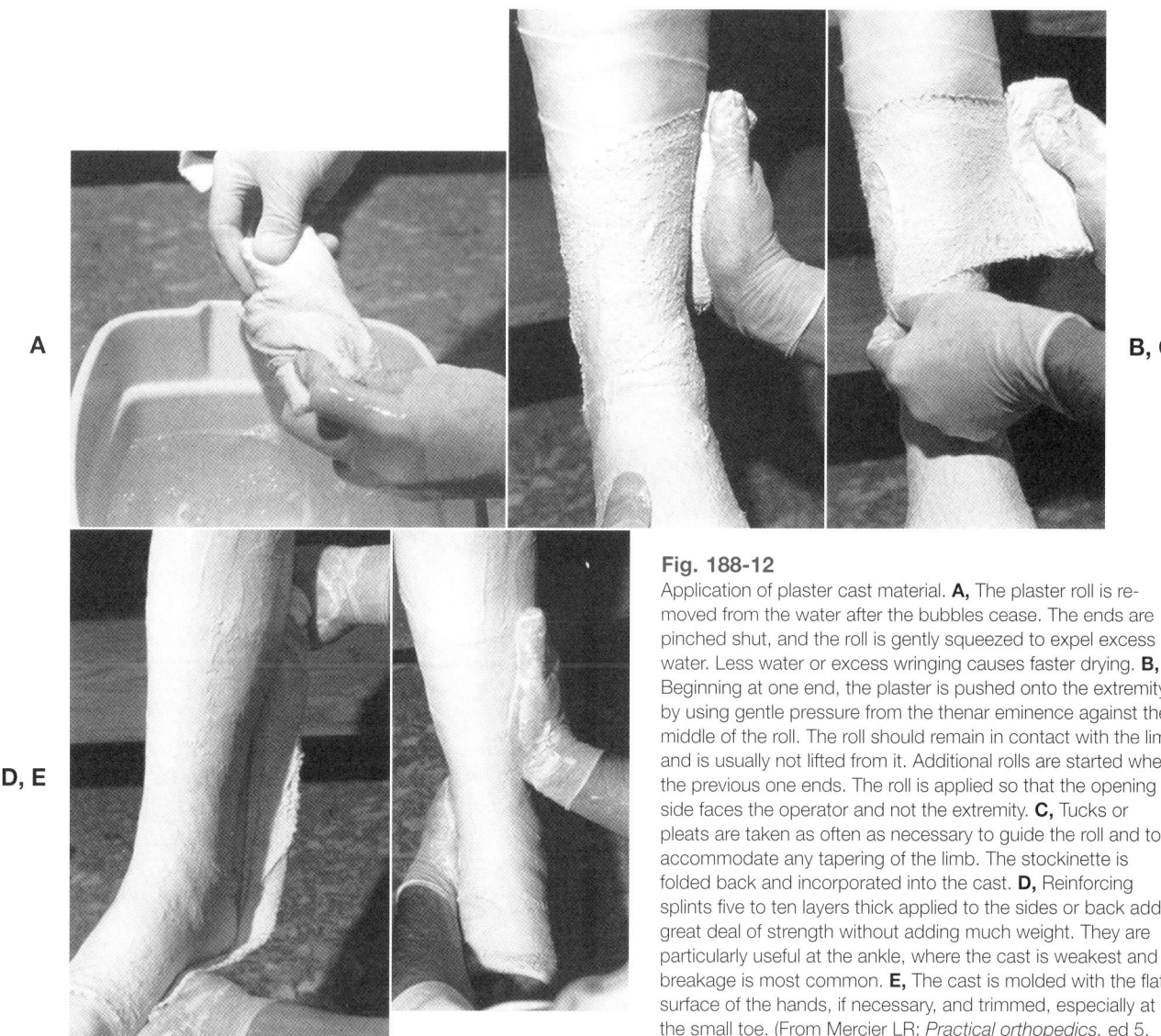

Fig. 188-12
Application of plaster cast material. **A,** The plaster roll is removed from the water after the bubbles cease. The ends are pinched shut, and the roll is gently squeezed to expel excess water. Less water or excess wringing causes faster drying. **B,** Beginning at one end, the plaster is pushed onto the extremity by using gentle pressure from the thenar eminence against the middle of the roll. The roll should remain in contact with the limb and is usually not lifted from it. Additional rolls are started where the previous one ends. The roll is applied so that the opening side faces the operator and not the extremity. **C,** Tucks or pleats are taken as often as necessary to guide the roll and to accommodate any tapering of the limb. The stockinette is folded back and incorporated into the cast. **D,** Reinforcing splints five to ten layers thick applied to the sides or back add a great deal of strength without adding much weight. They are particularly useful at the ankle, where the cast is weakest and breakage is most common. **E,** The cast is molded with the flat surface of the hands, if necessary, and trimmed, especially at the small toe. (From Mercier LR: *Practical orthopedics,* ed 5, St Louis, 2000, Mosby.)

to avoid pulling the cast material too tight. Molding should occur between each layer, with most synthetic casts requiring only two to three layers of cast material, depending on the area immobilized (Fig. 188-13, *A-C*). Strips of heavy-duty, reinforcing material are available and frequently applied (e.g., the posterior aspect of a short-leg walking cast) to increase durability (Fig. 188-13, *D*). After the final check of position, synthetic casts may require trimming of rough edges. If not performed, these edges may catch on clothing or can injure the skin and soft tissues under the cast. Trimming can be done with a file, sandpaper, cast saw, or scissors, and it is done with less difficulty when the cast is still soft (Fig. 188-13, *E*).

POSTPROCEDURE PATIENT EDUCATION

After cast application, instruct the patient in proper cast care and advise of signs and symptoms that require immediate attention. For *plaster,* avoidance of unnecessary forces to the cast, such as weight bearing, should be advised for at least the first 24 to 48 hours, as the material will still be in the curing process. *Synthetic casts* usually develop sufficient durability to bear increased forces after 12 to 24 hours. Depending on the acuity of injury, elevation for the initial 48 to 72 hours may be recommended to reduce swelling. Crutch walking is necessary for lower-extremity injuries treated with immobilization until adequate cast strength has been achieved to support weight bearing. Crutches that fit

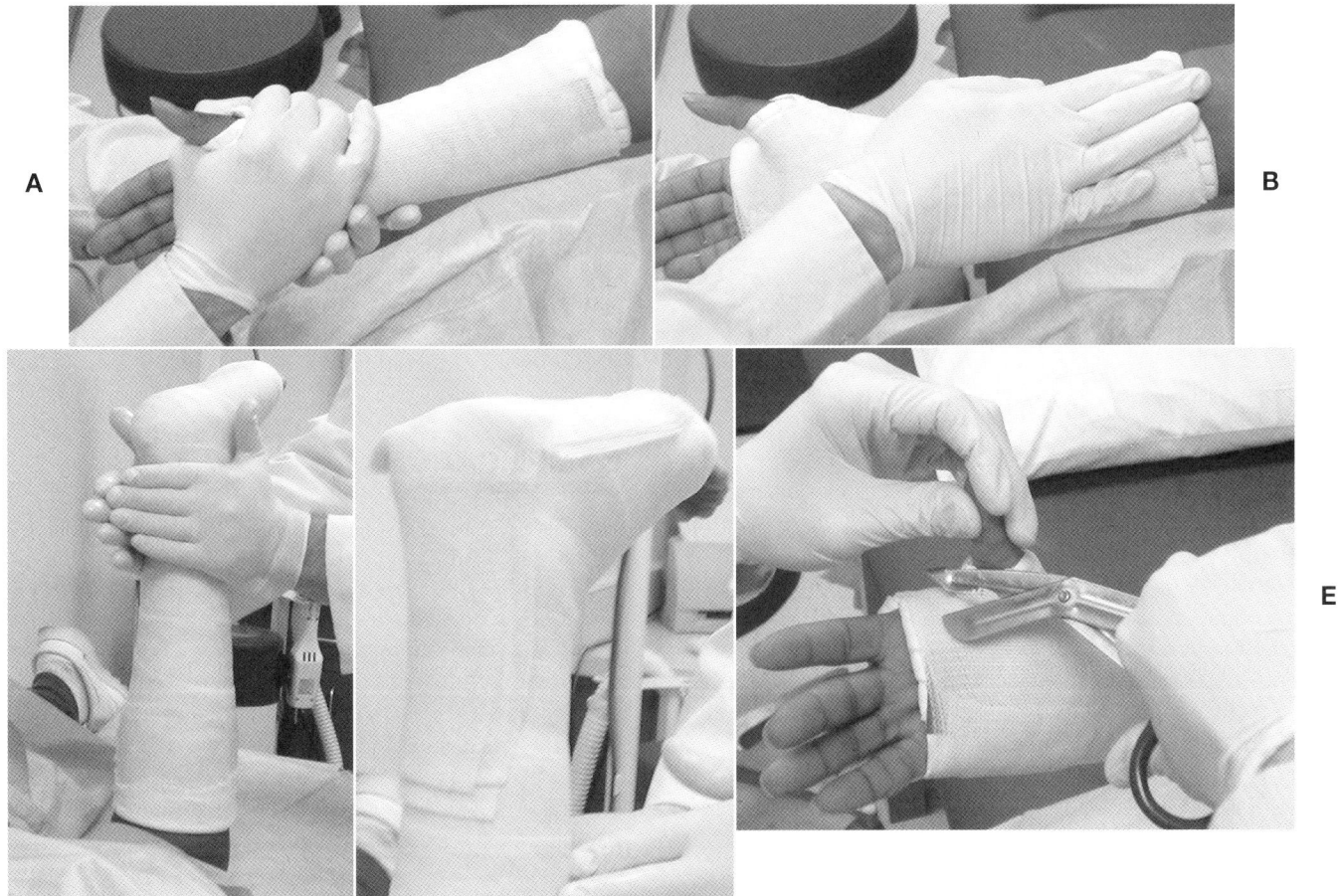

Fig. 188-13
Application of synthetic materials. **A,** Molding short-arm cast at wrist. **B,** Molding short-arm cast at forearm.
C, Molding short-leg walker at Achilles' area. **D,** Position of posterior reinforcement strip for short-leg walker. **E,** Trimming excess cast material to avoid trauma to nearby skin.

properly will be 1 to 1½ inches below the axilla when placed vertically between the arm and body. The handgrips should be adjusted to allow the patient to have slightly flexed elbows during use. It is also important to remind patients that crutches are not intended to support the weight in the axilla, since this can lead to paresthesias in the arm. The weight of the body should be supported in the hands and the unaffected lower extremity (using a three-point gait). Prior to discharging the patient, it is also helpful to observe his or her gait with the use of crutches and correct any problems that may occur.

Patients must take care to avoid getting the cast material wet and must be advised that submersion of even synthetic casts is unacceptable if routine stockinette and padding are used. If the cast should get wet, the patient may try drying it with an electric blow dryer on the cool setting, being careful not to overheat the cast material. Soaked plaster casts and synthetic casts (with

traditional stockinette and padding) that have saturated the underlying cast padding require attention by a physician and possible replacement. If not evaluated, the patient may suffer loss of immobilization, skin irritation, and maceration from moisture under the cast material. The patient *must never introduce foreign objects (e.g., coat hangers) underneath the cast for any reason.* Strategies for the patient with pruritus under the cast include using cool air from an electric blow dryer or baby powder applied under the cast.

Patients using waterproof cast liner and fiberglass cast material may allow their cast to get wet. Bathing with mild soap is permitted. In general, a synthetic cast will require 1 to 4 hours to dry after submersion. Common sense should dictate the avoidance of swimming in areas that might allow the introduction of foreign bodies beneath the cast (e.g., fish, debris).

Cast wearers should contact their physician if they develop increased *pain* in the immobilized region;

numbness, tingling or *weakness* in the affected area; *change in skin color* distal to the cast; or *persistent skin irritation.*

CAST REMOVAL

EQUIPMENT

- An electric, oscillating, cast saw
- Cast spreaders
- Bandage/trauma scissors

TECHNIQUE

Removal techniques differ based on previous experience and training. Patient counseling before starting the procedure, especially in the pediatric population, is likely to be the most effective means of minimizing fear and apprehension. Some practitioners find the solution to this potential problem in allowing ancillary staff (nurses or physician assistants) to perform this function. In either case, it is good practice to describe the technique to the patient and include descriptions of any sensations (e.g. warmth, vibration) likely to be experienced. Actually turning on the cast saw and applying it briefly to one's own skin to show that it will not cut the skin is a method sometimes used for demonstrating the relative safety of the procedure. The fear related to the noise generated by the cast saw can be reduced with the use of hearing protection. This may be especially helpful in the pediatric population. Once the patient is prepared, actual removal of the cast is fairly easy.

1. Stabilize the immobilized limb, with the patient in a comfortable position and with a drape covering any clothing likely to be exposed to cast dust. Some patients will also appreciate wearing a surgical mask to help reduce any inhaled cast dust.
2. Determine the cut line before starting and avoid potentially sensitive areas.
3. Hold the cast saw in one hand, and use the thumb and another finger (usually the index) to stabilize the saw against the cast (Fig. 188-14). This technique best allows control of the depth of cut. Constantly change the area of the blade in contact with the cast and avoid prolonged cutting in a single area to decrease the heat generated by the procedure and limit the potential for saw-induced burns. Another technique to reduce cast saw heat production is to cut in a manner similar to a sewing machine needle. With this method the depth of the cast saw is constantly changing and exposes different areas of the saw blade to cast material. Depending on casting material and type of cast, either one (univalve) or two (bivalve) cuts along the entire length of the cast will be required.
4. After full-thickness cuts have been made through the casting material, use the cast spreaders to expose the underlying padding and stockinette (Fig. 188-15), which can then be divided with bandage/trauma scissors.
5. Once all material has been divided, remove the cast and allow the patient to cleanse the skin, providing the injury has healed adequately. Postprocedure cast care is injury specific and geared toward rehabilitation of the affected limb.

COMPLICATIONS

The most well-known and feared complication is the development of a compartment syndrome (see Chapter 189, Compartment Syndrome Evaluation). The process can occur with even a simple, benign-appearing injury. If a snug circumferential cast is applied and tissue swelling continues after the initial injury, conditions are set for compromise of the microcirculation to the immobilized tissue. This may lead to ischemia of the affected area, producing muscle necrosis and further edema. If this process continues untreated and compartmental pressures reach a critical level (thought to be 30 to 60 mm Hg for 4 to 8 hours), irreversible damage to the involved tissues may ensue. Ultimately, Volkmann's ischemic contractures may occur, with loss of limb function.

Signs and symptoms of compartment syndrome include *pain* that is out of proportion to the injury or is elicited with pressure over the affected compartment or with stretching of involved muscle groups. Additional indications of impending compartment syndrome include *paresthesias* in the corresponding dermatome, the *inability to generate a forceful muscle contraction*, and *normal pulses* in the affected limb. Pulselessness and pallor are not characteristics of compartment syndrome, because pressures will never rise high enough in a compartment to completely obstruct the major blood vessels in that area. *All patients who receive a cast as part of their therapy should be counseled regarding the above signs and symptoms.* Should they occur, emphasis must be placed on the immediate need to contact the treating physician or to seek care in an emergency department. *Delayed diagnosis and treatment can lead to irreversible muscle and nerve damage.*

Initial treatment in suspected cases of compartment syndrome is relief of the pressure generated by the cast, either through bivalving or complete removal. Definitive diagnosis rests on characteristic signs, symptoms, and objective measurement of the compartmental pressure. Treatment of documented compartment syn-

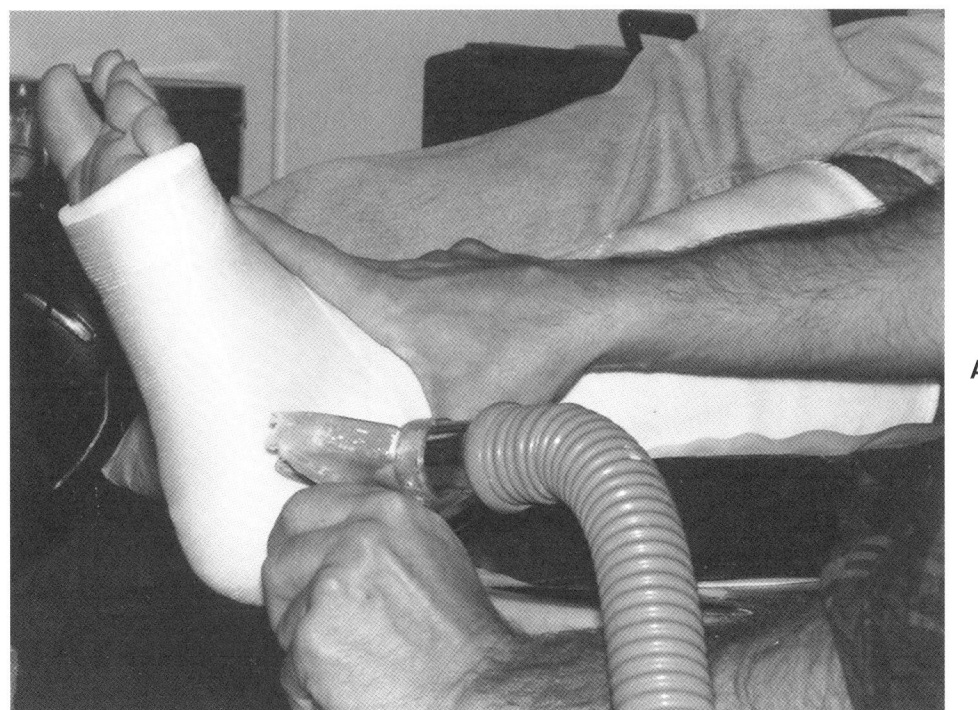

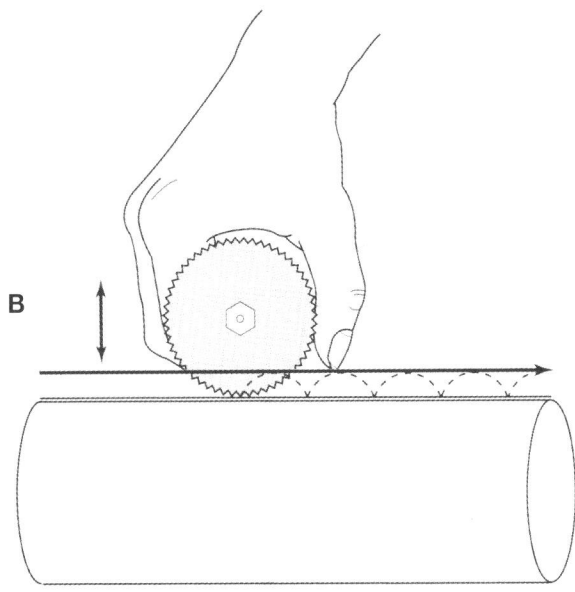

Fig. 188-14
Cast removal. **A,** Hold the cast saw in one hand, and use the thumb and another finger (usually the index) to stabilize the saw against the cast, which prevents the blade from injuring the underlying skin. **B.** Cut down through both sides of the cast. Do not saw back and forth with the blade. Cut the cast at right angles to the material. (**B** from Mercier LR: *Practical orthopedics,* ed 5, St Louis, 2000, Mosby.)

drome may require surgical intervention in the form of fasciotomy.

Various skin conditions, nerve palsy, joint stiffness, disuse osteoporosis, and *thromboembolic events* may also complicate cast therapy. Of the skin conditions, *cast dermatitis* may be the most common, usually resulting in severe, bothersome pruritus from poor ventilation to the underlying skin. Use of absorbent powders (e.g., talc or baby powder) may help limit the incidence of this condition. Two problems may result if patients introduce objects under the cast to relieve intense itching. First, the object may become trapped under the cast, producing a pressure point that can cause severe ulceration. Second, such instruments as coat hangers can easily lacerate the skin if used too aggressively, forming a nidus for infection or even requiring suture repair. *Pressure sores* may result from poorly fitting casts that are insufficiently padded over bony prominences or inadequately molded to local anatomic contours (Fig. 188-16). As mentioned, transverse wrinkles in stockinette or cast padding or ridges in the cast material can lead to pressure sores. The patient who complains of persistent skin irritation

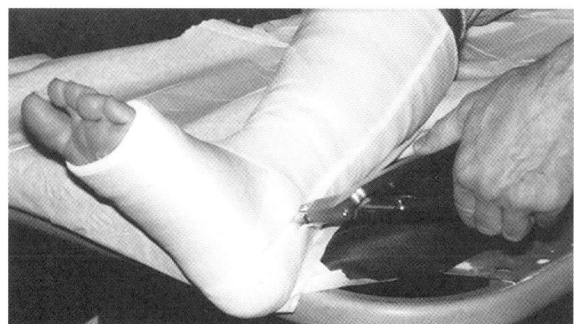

Fig. 188-15
Cast pliers separate the upper and lower portions of the cast, which has been cut on both sides.

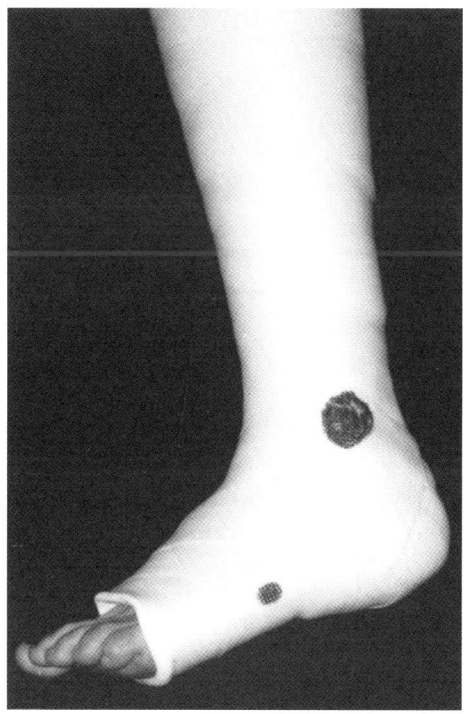

Fig. 188-16
Common location for pressure sores (noted by ink on cast).

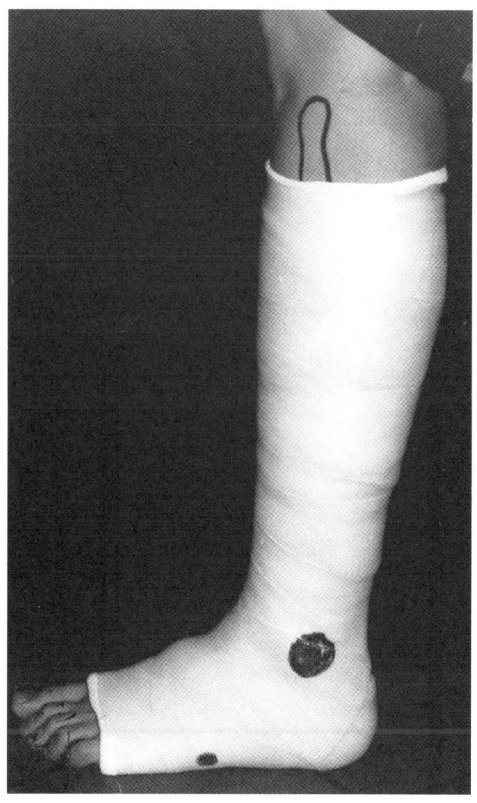

Fig. 188-17
Outline on the skin denotes the fibular head and indicates where the peroneal nerve is located. Excess pressure in this area leads to paralysis and foot drop.

characterized by burning or pain should be seen for evaluation and for possible opening of a window over the symptomatic area to facilitate direct examination. Additional skin damage may occur during cast removal as a result of heat generated by the cast saw. These burns are preventable with use of good technique, and their frequency may be reduced with the use of protective strips under the cast (e.g., DE-FLEX Strip). The use of waterproof liner under the cast material *increases* the chance of burns during cast removal (this should be discussed with patients prior to cast application), and the use of a protective strip under the cast material is highly recommended. Many providers have patients sign a

consent form prior to using waterproof liner because of increased risk of burns and because many insurance providers do not cover the additional cost of this material.

Any cast used to immobilize an anatomic region where superficial peripheral nerves lie in close proximity to underlying bone may lead to nerve *palsy*. Long-leg casts and those short-leg casts involving the head of the fibula can produce a common peroneal nerve palsy as the rigid cast compresses the nerve in its course over the fibular head (Fig. 188-17). Symptoms may include loss of sensation over the dorsolateral aspect of the involved foot, and "foot drop," or weakness in the ankle dorsiflexors. Other potential areas of involvement include the ulnar nerve as it passes through the cubital tunnel region, usually seen with long-arm casts, and the median nerve as it passes through the carpal tunnel (both short- and long-arm casts). These neurologic injuries can be complete or incomplete, reversible or irreversible, and should be recognized and treated in a timely fashion.

A nearly universal complaint following cast immobilization is *joint stiffness*, which is directly related to duration of immobilization. This fact should be discussed with the patient at the time of cast application and should be taken into consideration when determining length of treatment. Depending on the cause for initial treatment and response to therapy, the physician can initiate fairly aggressive stretching exercises after cast removal to facilitate the return of normal joint function. Use of simple range-of-motion and other exercises involving nonimmobilized joints in the affected extremity (e.g., straight-leg raising, finger or toe flexion/extension) can minimize the effects of prolonged disuse.

Thromboembolic complications, such as deep venous thrombosis or pulmonary embolism, can occur with cast use (usually of the lower extremity) and must be considered when patients have suspicious symptoms. Diagnosis is difficult because of the presence of the original injury and limitations in examination. To exclude the diagnosis of venous thrombosis may require cast removal and ancillary testing (e.g., duplex ultrasound).

CPT/BILLING CODES

Using the codes for fracture treatment includes application of casts and splints. The clinician cannot use these codes for the *initial* application. Use the cast application codes listed below when any of the following occurs:

1. Application of cast/splint is temporary and definitive treatment will be done later or by someone else (e.g., application performed in ER or office for patient comfort or to temporarily stabilize an injury).
2. The cast must be replaced.
3. The cast or splinting is performed as an initial service for treatment and no other procedure is planned (e.g., casting of a sprained ankle). Use a casting code in addition to an E/M code.

Casting and strapping codes include removal. Use removal codes only if the cast has been applied by another physician.

If not listed here, see CPT codes 29000 to 29799 in the CPT code book.

Upper Extremity Casts

29065	Shoulder to hand (long arm)
29075	Elbow to finger (short arm)
29085	Hand and lower forearm (gauntlet)
29086	Finger (e.g., for contracture)

Upper Extremity Splints

29105	Application of long-arm splint (shoulder to hand)

29125	Application of short-arm splint (forearm to hand): static
29130	Application of finger splint: static

Lower Extremity Casts

29345	Application of long-leg cast (thigh to toes)
29355	Application of long-leg cast—walker or ambulatory type
29365	Application of cylinder cast (thigh to ankle)
29405	Application of short-leg cast (below knee to toes)
29425	Application of short-leg cast—walker or ambulatory type
29435	Application of patellar tendon bearing (PTB) cast
29440	Adding walker to previously applied cast
29445	Application of rigid total contact leg cast

Lower Extremity Splints

29505	Application of long-leg splint (thigh to ankle or toes)
29515	Application of short-leg splint (calf to foot)

Lower Extremity Strapping

29530	Strapping, knee
29540	Strapping, ankle
29550	Strapping, toes
29580	Unna boot

Removal or Repair (codes for cast removals should be used only for casts applied by another physician)

29700	Removal or bivalving, gauntlet, boot, or body cast
29705	Removal or bivalving, full-arm or full-leg cast
29730	Windowing of cast
29740	Wedging of cast (except clubfoot casts)
29799	Unlisted procedure, casting or strapping

Also see Chapter 192, Fracture Care, for appropriate ICD-9 codes.

ADDITIONAL RESOURCES

• See the sample patient education handouts regarding cast care titled "Cast Care" and "Care of Casts and Splints" on pages 1991 and 1992, respectively, of Appendix G. See the sample patient education handout regarding crutch use titled "Crutch Use" on page 1995 of Appendix G.

BIBLIOGRAPHY

Anderson BC: *Office orthopedics for primary care: diagnosis and treatment,* ed 2, Philadelphia, 1999, WB Saunders.

Bucholz RW, Heckman JD: *Rockwood and Green's fractures in adults,* ed 5, Philadelphia, 2001, Lippincott, Williams & Wilkins.

Eiff MP, Hatch RL, Calmbach WL: *Fracture management for primary care,* Philadelphia, 1998, WB Saunders.

Koval KJ, Zucherman JD: *Handbook of fractures,* ed 2, Philadelphia, 2002, Lippincott, Williams & Wilkins.

Medley ES, Shirley SM, Brilliant HL: Fracture management by family physicians and guidelines for referral, *J Fam Pract* 8(4):701, 1979.

Wu K: *Techniques in surgical casting and splinting,* Philadelphia, 1987, Lea & Febiger.

Compartment Syndrome Evaluation

Robert L. Kalb

Compartment syndrome occurs when the pressure inside the fascial compartment of an extremity is higher than the pressure of the blood in the vessels going into the compartment. This leads to compromise of the circulation to the soft tissues (muscles and nerves) and causes tissue ischemia and eventual muscle necrosis. If the compartment syndrome is present for 8 hours or more, irreversible muscle damage occurs and leads to subsequent fibrosis and contracture of the flexor tendons. The flexor tendons are most involved since they are in the deepest compartments in the calf and forearm and are therefore most affected and the earliest to be involved. Surgical release using an incision through the fascial compartments is required to relieve the excessive pressure caused by bleeding and edema.

CONDITIONS ASSOCIATED WITH COMPARTMENT SYNDROME

- Soft tissue injury only (no fractured forearm, calf, hand, or foot)
- Soft tissue injury with fractured forearm, calf, hand, or foot
- Supracondylar fracture of the elbow (Volkmann's ischemia)
- Exercise-induced compartment syndrome
- Crush injury to thigh
- Prolonged tourniquet application (longer than 2 hours)
- Electrical injury
- Burns
- Gluteal compartment syndrome from trauma
- Dog or shark bites in susceptible areas

It is important to understand that compartment syndrome can occur with or without a fracture. It is most commonly present in the *calf* or the *forearm*. It can, however, occur in the hand and foot. The higher the amount of soft tissue trauma, the higher the chance of compartment syndrome. For this reason, any high-velocity injury should be treated with caution, since the energy dissipated through the soft tissue associated with the injury can cause extreme swelling. Injuries commonly associated with compartment syndrome include auto accident and pedestrian trauma, especially with bumper injuries to the calf or forearm.

CONDITIONS THAT CAN CREATE, MASK, OR WORSEN COMPARTMENT SYNDROME

- Applying heat to injury
- Spinal cord injury
- Intoxication
- Head trauma
- Changes in sensorium (alcohol, drugs, etc.)

An injury with or without fracture that is then subjected to warm water or any other form of heat energy resulting in vasodilation will have increased swelling and an increased chance of compartment syndrome.

Patients who have a severe bruise from a fall who then soak in a hot tub of water can develop compartment syndrome. It can also happen when expansion of the soft tissue envelope (skin) cannot occur because of the constriction of a cast. If any patient has pain out of proportion to objective findings, after trauma to an extremity or placement of a cast, the cast and Webril should be removed entirely and the patient examined carefully for compartment syndrome. If removal of the cast and Webril does not bring immediate and complete relief of the intense pain, evaluation for compartment syndrome with subsequent surgical treatment is indicated. Even without a cast, any feeling of tense, tight, swelling in the forearm, hand, calf, or foot should lead to suspicion of compartment syndrome.

Another presentation for compartment syndrome is that of an individual who, while intoxicated, falls and sustains an injury. Because of the intoxication, the pain is ignored. Patients who have spinal cord injury resulting from motor vehicle accidents will not have pain in the calf or forearm in spite of the swelling that may also occur as a result of the accident. For the reasons mentioned above, a fasciotomy should be carried out immediately in any such patient with a tense and swollen calf, forearm, hand, or foot.

Compartment syndrome can occur at any age but is much more common in adults than children. Be aware that the swelling following an injury sometimes will not peak until 24 to 72 hours later. For this reason compartment syndrome needs to be considered and careful physical examination carried out to detect any early signs for up to 3 days after severe injuries.

Compartment syndrome, which is referred to as "Volkmann's ischemia" in the forearm, can occur after *supracondylar fractures* that cause a large amount of swelling about the elbow.

Compartment syndrome can occur with *exercise*. This is rare, however. Athletes may report running up to 5 miles beyond the point where they experienced cramping, tenseness, and swelling in the legs. This usually resolves with cessation of the activity. If not, exercise-induced compartment syndrome, as with traumatic conditions, can be diagnosed by measuring the compartmental pressures. Compartment syndrome can also appear with symptoms of shin splints. This can be differentiated because shin splints have tenderness on the bone itself without palpable tense pressure within the compartments. Compartment syndrome can occur in both the foot and the leg in some forms of trauma. Exercise-induced compartment syndrome occurs only in the calf.

Compartment syndrome can be associated with *calcaneus fractures;* but this is rare.

Compartment syndrome can occur in the *thigh* because of a severe crushing injury or related to a *prolonged tourniquet* time (longer than 2 hours) under anesthetic. Tourniquet time less than 2 hours, however, does not produce compartment syndrome.

Compartment syndrome can be a direct result of *infection,* such as that related to scratches, cuts, or insect or snake bites in the upper or lower extremity.

Patients who have *electrical injuries,* with or without a visible skin burn, can develop a compartment syndrome. The mechanism is similar to the device available on the market to cook a hot dog. The injury, in fact, has been called the "hot dogger." As a hot dog is punctured at both ends with a metal spike, an electrical current is delivered through the hot dog. This causes intense heat, thus cooking the hot dog. The same mechanism occurs with burn injuries with an entrance and exit point for the electrical energy. The "cooked" tissue inside literally swells nearly to the point of bursting but is restrained by the surrounding tissue, and the pressure subsequently builds. The extent of injury may not be visible on the patient's initial visit but can develop during the next 1 to 3 days.

Burns from other causes, *industrial injection injuries* from various types of guns injecting fluid accidentally into the extremities, and *dog* and *shark bites* can produce compartment syndrome.

Gluteal compartment syndrome can occur related to direct trauma associated with an *automobile accident* or *fall from a height* directly onto the buttock. Immediate swelling can ensue as bleeding occurs into the muscle compartment; this is also rare. Similarly, patients who are on long-term *anticoagulation* can develop bleeding into the muscle compartments, leading to increased pressure.

DIAGNOSIS

A diagnosis of compartment syndrome made after loss of pulses and loss of capillary refill is too late for optimal treatment. The most important and earliest symptom associated with compartment syndrome is *pain.*

If pain after an injury is associated with swelling in an extremity and the pain is not relieved by medication (such as up to 1 or 2 Percocet tablets q4h), compartment syndrome should be suspected.

The earliest physical findings are (1) loss of fine-touch and (2) pain with extension of the great toe or the thumb. Compartment syndrome most commonly occurs first in the volar compartment of the forearm, where the long flexor tendon of the thumb travels, and in the calf, the location of the long flexor tendon for the great toe. By passively extending the great toe or the thumb, the muscle tendon unit in this deep compartment is stretched. If the muscle is ischemic because of early compartment syndrome, pain will be present and increased by extension of the thumb or toe. Two-point discrimination is also impaired early.

INDICATIONS TO MEASURE COMPARTMENT PRESSURES

- Excessive constriction
- Pain: earliest and most sensitive
- Pain out of proportion to objective findings
- Increasing pain not relieved by usual narcotic pain medication
- Loss of fine touch
- Loss of two-point discrimination
- Pain with extension of great toe or thumb of affected limb
- Increased discomfort when muscle trapped in fascial compartment is moved (actively or passively), especially the flexor muscles

INDICATIONS TO PERFORM FASCIOTOMY

- Compartment pressure reading over 30 mm Hg
- Suspicion of false normal pressure readings, but very high clinical suspicion of compression
- Tense compartment with clinical signs of a compartment syndrome

INDICATIONS FOR REFERRAL FOR FASCIOTOMY

- If the compartment is tense to palpation
- If there is pain out of proportion to objective findings
- If there is decreased sensation and pain with passive extension of the thumb or great toe
- To avoid missing someone who needs a fasciotomy (the same approach as with an appendicitis).
- If compartment pressures are measured at over 30 mm Hg

CONTRAINDICATIONS TO MEASUREMENT

- When compartment syndrome is clinically obvious and measurement would delay definitive treatment
- Cellulitis directly over the area to be measured
- Anticoagulation (*relative contraindication*)

EQUIPMENT

- Betadine antiseptic solution
- IV needle or catheter
- IV tubing: arterial blood pressure tubing
- Normal saline IV solution
- Pressure measurement system
- Pressure transducer
- Monitor to display pressure readings
- Local anesthetic (1% lidocaine), syringe, and needles

Emergency physicians primarily use three pressure measurement systems: the *Stryker 295 intracompartmental pressure monitor system,* which is a portable penlike compartmental pressure device made by the Stryker Company; *mercury manometer systems;* and *arterial line systems.* The Stryker 295 is much like a tonometer for measuring glaucoma (Fig. 189-1). The device uses a needle and pressure transducer and provides a reasonably accurate measurement of compartment syndrome.

Probes used to enter the compartment include the simple 18-gauge needle, 18-gauge spinal needle for deep compartments, the side-port needle, wick catheter,

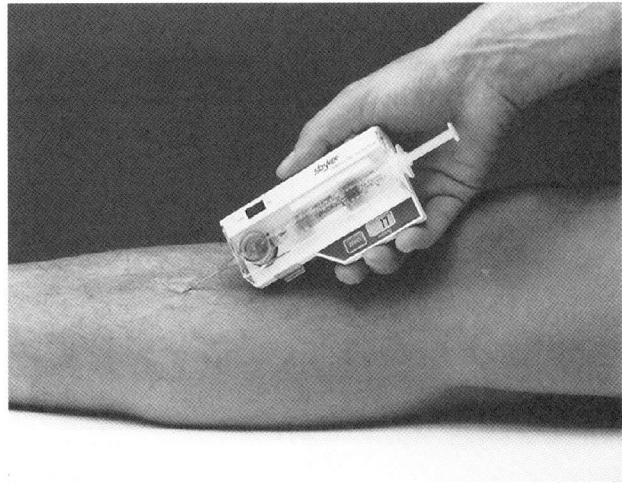

Fig. 189-1
Stryker 295 intracompartmental pressure monitor system. (Courtesy Stryker Instruments, Kalamazoo, Mich.)

slit catheter, and the solid-state transducer intracompartmental catheter. All three pressure measurement systems mentioned above can be used with the simple 18-gauge needle, 18-gauge spinal needle, and the side-port needle. The wick catheter and slit catheter are used for more prolonged in-hospital monitoring or research.

Each body "compartment" can become compromised. Various compartments are demonstrated in Figs. 189-2 to 189-13. Placement of the needle for the sites is as noted in Table 189-1.

TECHNIQUE

General

1. Obtain informed consent.
2. The compartment to be measured is at heart level, positioned so needle can enter perpendicular to compartment
3. Avoid any external pressures to area; the region tested may need to be slightly elevated off the bed by an assistant. The patient must be cooperative and not move or contract the muscle group.
4. Prep skin with Betadine.
5. A *superficial* local anesthetic can be given.
6. When the needle is pulled between measurements, flush it to be sure it has not become plugged with blood or tissue

Compartment pressures can be measured in many ways, including the wick catheter technique. The pressure measurement involves placing a needle into the compartment and injecting a small amount of normal saline to transmit pressure to a pressure transducer, similar to measuring radial artery pressure through an

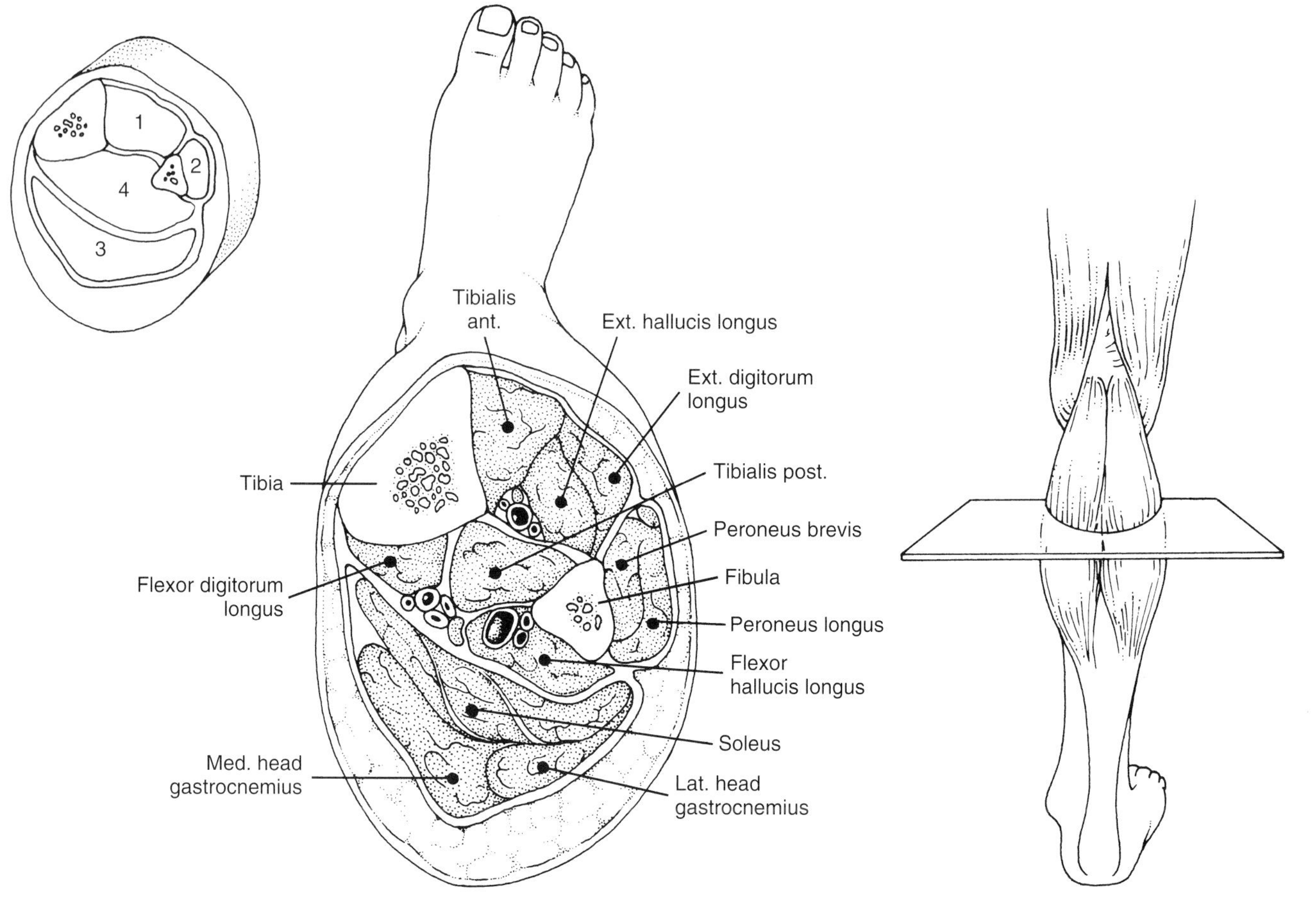

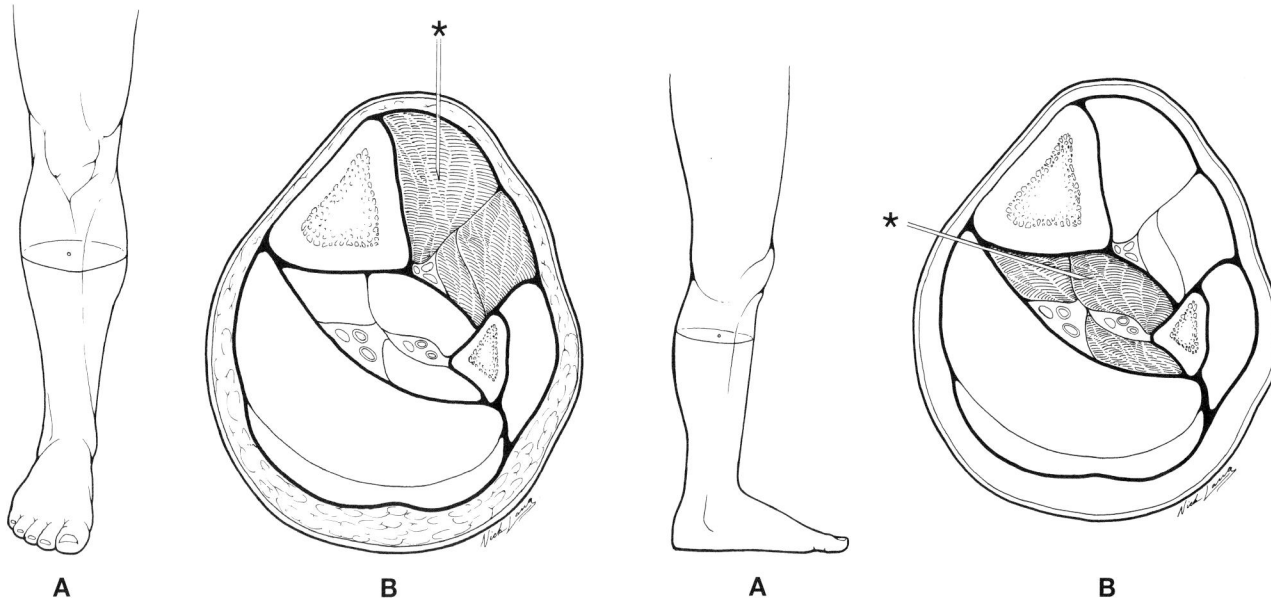

Fig. 189-2
Fascial compartments of the **lower leg** with enclosed muscle groups: *1,* anterior; *2,* lateral; *3,* superficial posterior; and *4,* deep posterior compartments. (From Stack LB: Compartment syndrome evaluation. In Roberts JR, Hedges JR: *Clinical procedures in emergency medicine,* ed 3, Philadelphia, 1998, WB Saunders.)

A

B

Fig. 189-3
Anterior compartment syndrome of the lower leg. **A,** Suggested needle entry point is indicated by the small circle. **B,** The needle should be inserted *(*)* to a depth of 1 to 3 cm. (Modified from Matsen FA, editor: *Compartmental syndromes,* New York, 1980, Grune & Stratton. In Roberts JR, Hedges JR: *Clinical procedures in emergency medicine,* ed 3, Philadelphia, 1998, WB Saunders.)

A

B

Fig. 189-4
Deep posterior compartment syndrome of the lower leg. **A,** Suggested needle entry point indicated by the small circle. **B,** The needle should be inserted *(*)* to a depth of 2 to 4 cm. (Modified from Matsen FA, editor: *Compartmental syndromes,* New York, 1980, Grune & Stratton. In Roberts JR, Hedges JR: *Clinical procedures in emergency medicine,* ed 3, Philadelphia, 1998, WB Saunders.)

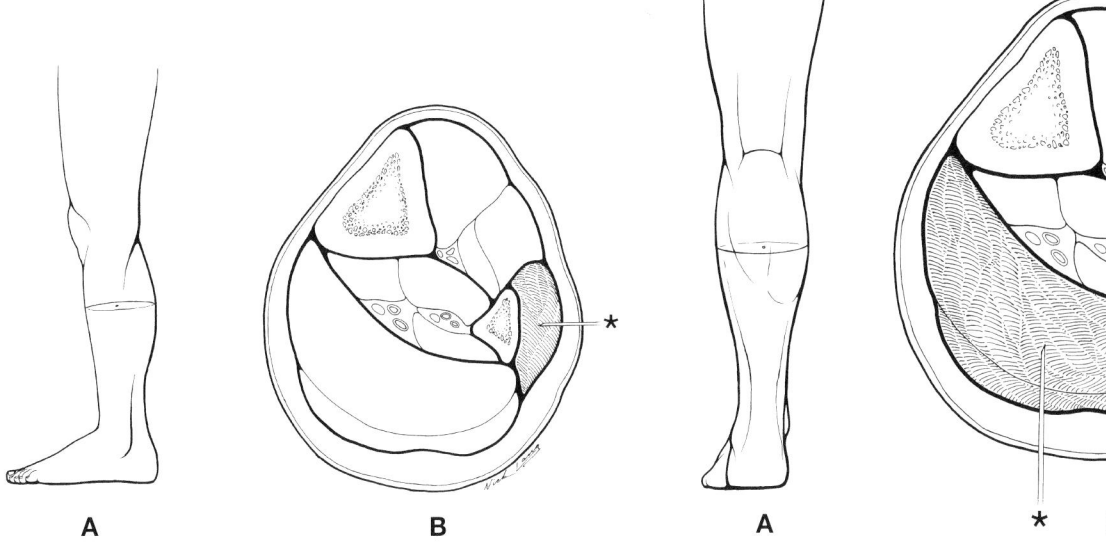

Fig. 189-5
Lateral compartment syndrome of the lower leg. **A,** Suggested needle entry point indicated by the small circle. **B,** The needle should be inserted (*) to a depth of 1 to 1.5 cm. (Modified from Matsen FA, editor: *Compartmental syndromes,* New York, 1980, Grune & Stratton. In Roberts JR, Hedges JR: *Clinical procedures in emergency medicine,* ed 3, Philadelphia, 1998, WB Saunders.)

Fig. 189-6
Superficial posterior compartment syndrome of the lower leg. **A,** Suggested needle entry point indicated by the small circle. **B,** The needle should be inserted (*) to a depth of 2 to 4 cm. (Modified from Matsen FA, editor: *Compartmental syndromes,* New York, 1980, Grune & Stratton. In Roberts JR, Hedges JR: *Clinical procedures in emergency medicine,* ed 3, Philadelphia, 1998, WB Saunders.)

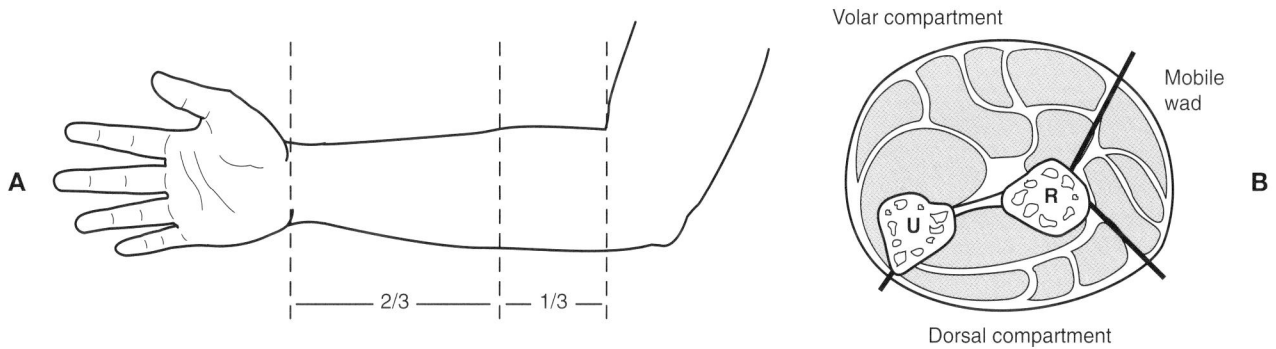

Fig. 189-7
A, Level of needle insertion of the forearm with, **B,** cross-section through the upper third of the forearm demonstrating the three forearm compartments (volar, dorsal, mobile wad). *R,* Radius; *U,* ulna. (From Green DP, editor: *Operative hand surgery,* New York, 1982, Churchill Livingstone.)

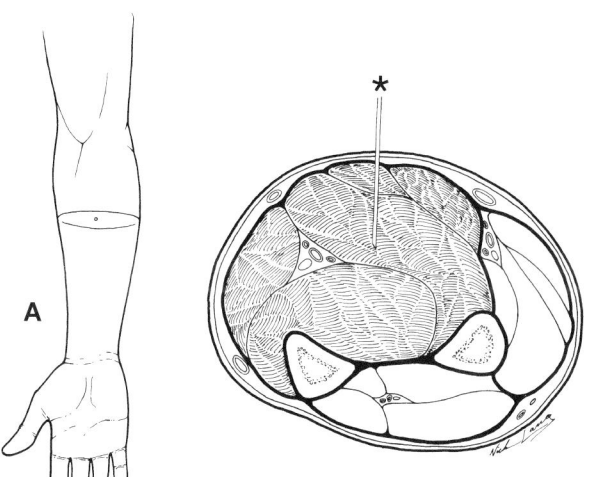

Fig. 189-8
Volar compartment syndrome of the forearm. **A,** Suggested needle entry point indicated by the small circle. **B,** The needle should be inserted (*) to a depth of 1 to 2 cm. (Modified from Matsen FA, editor: *Compartmental syndromes,* New York, 1980, Grune & Stratton. In Roberts JR, Hedges JR: *Clinical procedures in emergency medicine,* ed 3, Philadelphia, 1998, WB Saunders.)

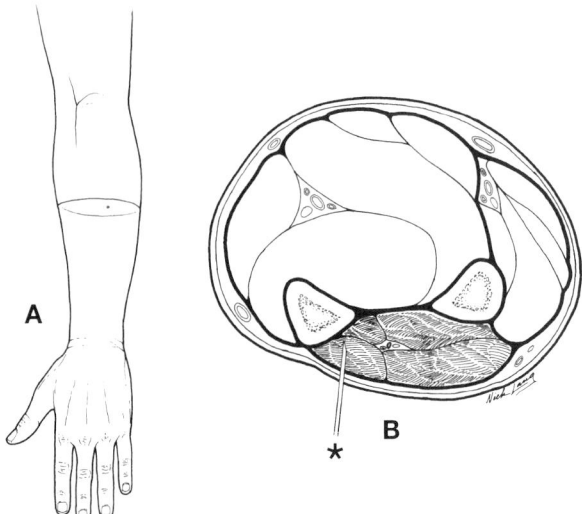

Fig. 189-9
Dorsal compartment syndrome of the forearm. **A,** Suggested needle entry point indicated by the small circle. **B,** The needle should be inserted *(*)* to a depth of 1 to 2 cm. (Modified from Matsen FA, editor: *Compartmental syndromes,* New York, 1980, Grune & Stratton. In Roberts JR, Hedges JR: *Clinical procedures in emergency medicine,* ed 3, Philadelphia, 1998, WB Saunders.)

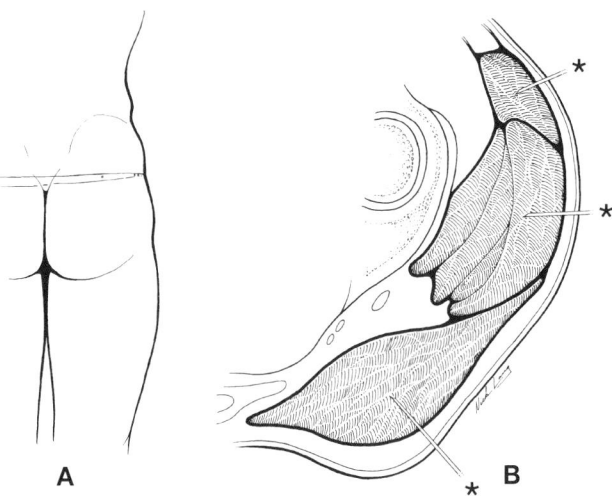

Fig. 189-11
Gluteal compartment syndrome. **A,** Suggested needle entry points are indicated by the small circles. The needle should be inserted to a depth of 4 to 8 cm depending on which compartment is being measured. **B,** Needle tips *(*)* shown entering muscle compartments. (Modified from Owen CA, Moody PR, Mubarak SJ, et al: *Clin Orthop* 132:57, 1978. In Roberts JR, Hedges JR: *Clinical procedures in emergency medicine,* ed 3, Philadelphia, 1998, WB Saunders.)

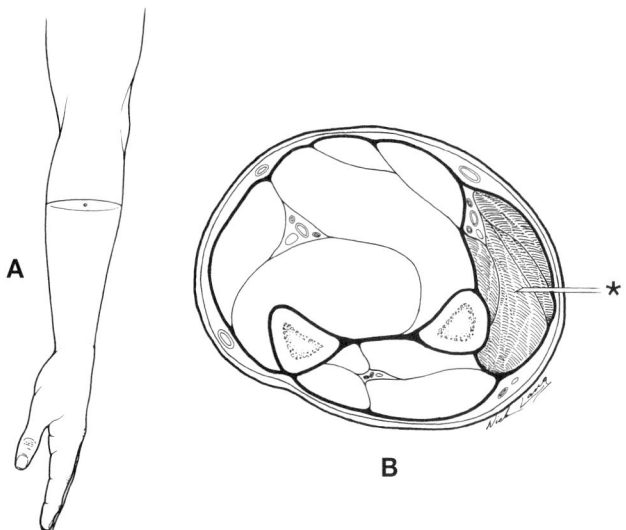

Fig. 189-10
Mobile wad compartment syndrome of the forearm. **A,** Suggested needle entry point indicated by the small circle. **B,** The needle should be inserted *(*)* to a depth of 1 to 1.5 cm. (Modified from Matsen FA, editor: *Compartmental syndromes,* New York, 1980, Grune & Stratton. In Roberts JR, Hedges JR: *Clinical procedures in emergency medicine,* ed 3, Philadelphia, 1998, WB Saunders.)

arterial line. These measurements are accurate. In the emergency room or the operating room, the *respiratory therapist can hook up an IV line and attach it to a pressure transducer.* The line is then attached to a sterile needle, which is flushed with normal saline and inserted into the muscle compartment to be tested. The pressure is transmitted. Pressure readings in all compartments *should be 30 mm Hg or below.* Any reading above that level requires immediate consultation for surgical treatment of compartment syndrome.

Do not rely only on pressure. Fasciotomy is indicated if the compartment is tense to palpation, if there is pain out of proportion to objective findings, or if there is decreased sensation and pain with passive extension of the thumb or great toe. If any of these findings are present even in the face of what appears to be normal compartment pressures, immediate referral should be carried out. Compartment pressures can give false-normal readings at times. Compartmental pressure measurements therefore are of value only when combined with the other information on physical examination and pain level.

1. Start IV line to sedate patient if needed.
2. Begin pulse oximeter to monitor conscious sedation if used.
3. Clean the site with alcohol.
4. Flush the line.
5. Zero the monitor.
6. Insert the needle.
7. Measure pressure.

Compartments of the foot

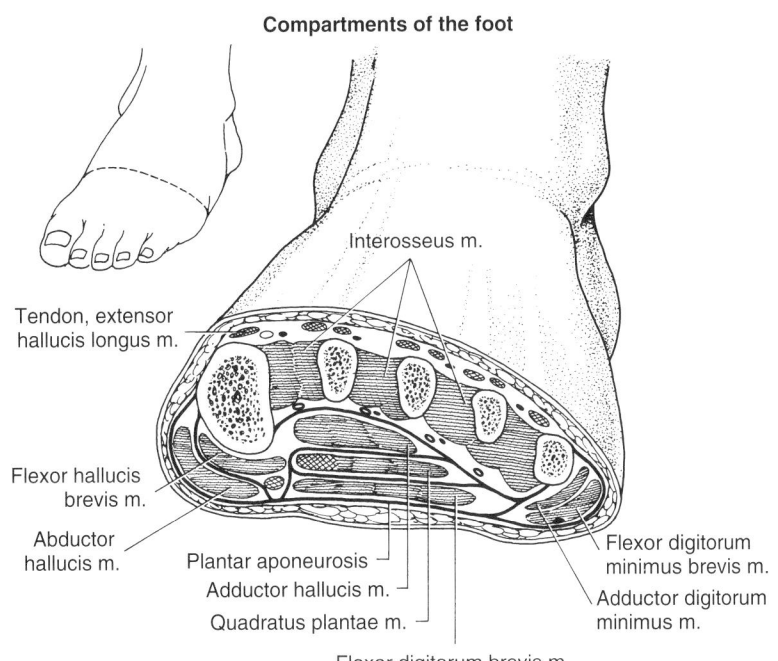

Interosseus m.

Tendon, extensor
hallucis longus m.

Flexor hallucis
brevis m.

Abductor
hallucis m.

Plantar aponeurosis

Adductor hallucis m.

Quadratus plantae m.

Flexor digitorum brevis m.

Flexor digitorum
minimus brevis m.

Adductor digitorum
minimus m.

Fig. 189-12
Compartments of the foot. (From Mubarak SJ, Hargens AR: *Compartment syndromes and Volkmann's contracture*, Philadelphia, 1981, WB Saunders.)

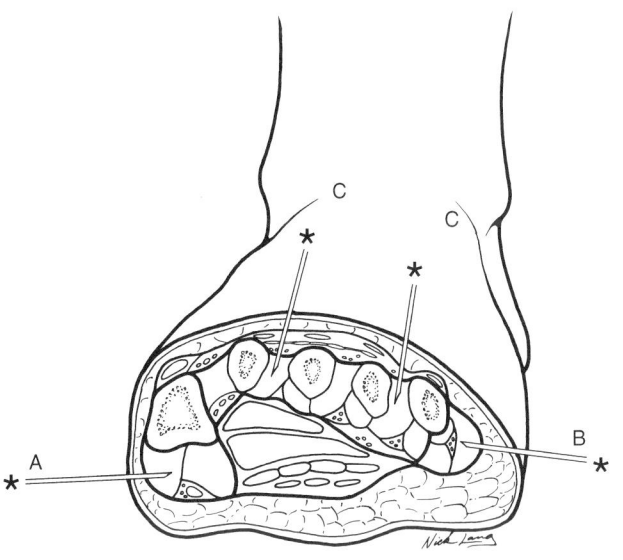

Fig. 189-13
Compartment syndromes of the foot. Suggested needle pathways (*) to measure intracompartmental pressures: *A*, Medial. *B*, Lateral. *C*, Interosseous compartments. The central compartment is located between these compartments. (Modified from Myerson M: *Bull Hosp Joint Dis* 47:251, 1987. In Roberts JR, Hedges JR: *Clinical procedures in emergency medicine*, ed 3, Philadelphia, 1998, WB Saunders.)

TABLE 189-1

Landmarks for Proper Needle Placement to Measure Compartment Pressures

Compartment	Position	Location	Insert Needle (perpendicular to skin unless otherwise stated)	Depth (cm)	Confirm Proper Position by Pressure Variation
Lower Leg					
Anterior	Supine	Junction of proximal and middle thirds of tibia anteriorly	1 cm lateral to anterior tibia (Fig. 189-3)	1-3	Compression proximal or distal Plantar flexion foot Dorsiflexion of foot
Deep posterior	Supine	Junction of proximal and middle thirds of tibia anteriorly	Just posterior to medial border of tibia. Direct at posterior border of fibula (Fig. 189-4)	2-4	Toe extension Ankle invasion
Lateral	Supine	Junction of proximal and middle thirds, posterior border of fibula	Just anterior to posterior border of fibula. Direct at fibula (Fig. 189-5)	1-1.5	Compression inferior or superior to needle Inversion of foot and ankle
Superficial posterior	Prone	Junction of proximal and middle thirds posterior leg	3-5 cm on either side of vertical line in middle of calf (Fig. 189-6)	2-4	Compression inferior or superior to needle Foot dorsiflexion
Forearm					
Volar	Forearm in supination	Junction of proximal and middle thirds of forearm	Just medial to palmaris longus. Direct needle to palpated posterior border of ulna (Fig. 189-7)	1-2	Compression proximal or distal to needle Extension of fingers or wrist
Dorsal	Forearm in supination	Junction of proximal and middle thirds of forearm, posterior aspect of ulna	1-2 cm lateral to posterior aspect of ulna (Fig. 189-9)	1-2	Compression proximal or distal to needle Flex fingers or wrist
Mobile wad	Forearm in supination	Junction of proximal and middle thirds of forearm, most lateral portion of forearm	In muscle tissue lateral to radius	1-1.5	Compression of proximal or distal to needle Ulnar deviation of wrist
Gluteal					
All three compartments	Prone	Point of maximal tenderness	Spinal needle	4-8	Compression of gluteal musculature
Foot					
Medial	Supine	Medial aspect of base of first metatarsal	Medial aspect of foot, inferior to base of first metatarsal into abductor hallucis	1-1.5	Compression of medial compartment
Central	Supine	Medial aspect of base of first metatarsal	Medial aspect foot inferior to base of first metatarsal, through abductor hallucis	3	Compression of central compartment
Lateral	Supine	Base of fifth metatarsal	Inferior to base fifth metatarsal	1-1.5	Compression of lateral compartment
Interosseous	Supine	Dorsum, bases, second and fourth metatarsal	Dorsum of second and fourth web spaces	1	Compression of interosseous compartment

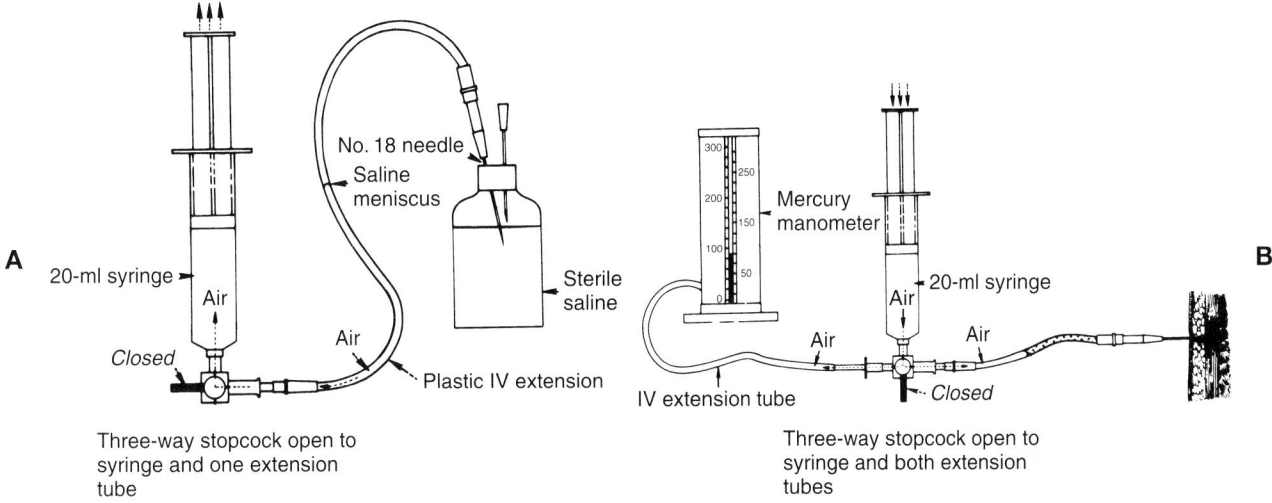

Fig. 189-14
Mercury monitor technique for compartmental pressure monitoring. **A,** Drawing up saline to partially fill tubing. **B,** Completed system set-up with needle inserted into compartment. (From Whitesides TE, Haney TC, Morimoto K, et al: *Clin Orthop* 113:43, 1975.)

8. Squeeze the involved area to see if pressure increases to confirm function.
9. Measure opposite side pressure as a control and if there is any question about proper readings on affected side.

EQUIPMENT AND TECHNIQUE FOR MERCURY MANOMETER

The following setup is readily available and least expensive but also least accurate:
* Two 18-gauge needles
* Two sets of tubing
* 20-ml syringe
* Three-way stopcock
* 50-ml vial normal saline
* Mercury manometer

1. Prepare setup (Fig. 189-14, *A*). Be sure there are no air bubbles in saline. Turn the stopcock "closed" on tubing with needle before pulling it out of the saline vial to prevent leakage.
2. Insert the needle into the desired compartment (Table 189-1).
3. Complete the hook up to the manometer (Fig. 189-14, *B*).
4. *Slowly* depress syringe plunger. This gives the mercury column time to move. Watch the column of saline. When it begins to enter tissue, the pressure in the syringe has exceeded tissue pressure. Note the reading on the manometer, which is the compartmental pressure.

5. Check a second recording by removing the needle and repeating as above.

EQUIPMENT AND TECHNIQUE FOR ARTERIAL LINE (Also see Chapter 87, Percutaneous Arterial Line Placement)

* Sterile saline
* Two three-way stopcocks
* 18-gauge needle
* 20-ml syringe
* Arterial line tubing (high pressure tubing)
* Pressure transducer and cable
* Pressure monitor
* Adjustable transducer stand

1. Connect the cable to the monitor.
2. Assemble the equipment (Fig. 189-15).
3. Fill the transducer, arterial line tubing, and needle. Close the stopcock to the arterial line tubing.
4. Open the other stopcock to air. Place the transducer at the level of the compartment.
5. Calibrate to zero and close the stopcock.
6. Open the stopcock to the "arterial line," and insert the needle into the compartment. Move the muscles of the desired compartment. Pressures should elevate. Allow the muscles to rest and measure the pressure.
7. Pull the needle and repeat for a second confirmatory measurement.

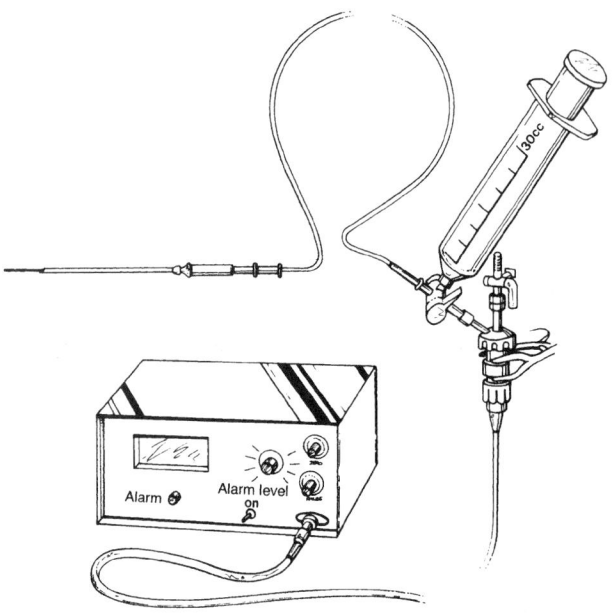

Fig. 189-15
Arterial line system for compartmental pressure measurement. (From Rorabeck CH: Compartment syndromes. In Browner BD, Jupiter JB, Levine AM, Trafton PG, editors: *Skeletal trauma: fractures, dislocations, ligamentous injuries,* vol 1, ed 2, Philadelphia, 1992, WB Saunders.)

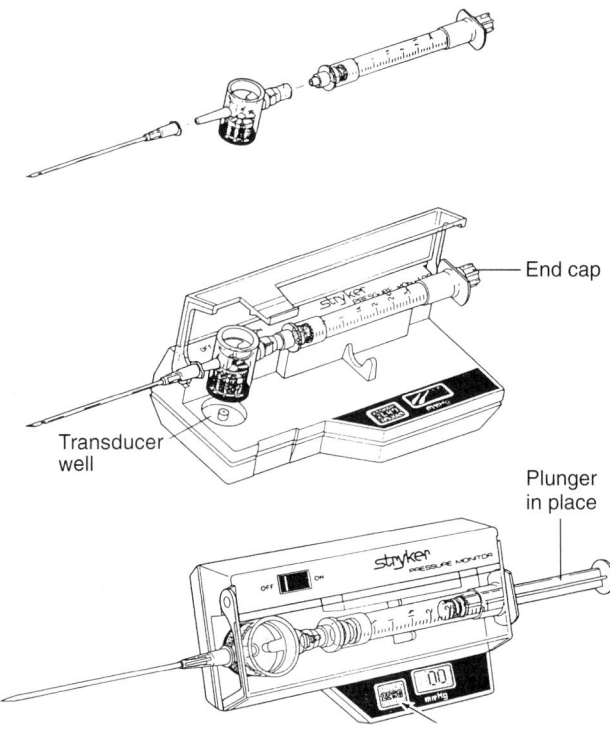

Fig. 189-16
Stryker 295 intracompartmental pressure monitor system assembly. (Courtesy Stryker Instruments, Kalamazoo, Mich.)

EQUIPMENT AND TECHNIQUE FOR THE STRYKER 295 INTRACOMPARTMENTAL PRESSURE MONITOR SYSTEM

- Prefilled syringe with saline
- Side port needle
- Diaphragm chamber
- Handheld pressure monitor
- Stryker 295 quick-pressure monitor set (disposable pouch)

1. Open the disposable 295 quick-pressure monitor setup.
2. Assemble the equipment (Fig. 189-16).
3. Open the cover of the monitor and insert the chamber into the device well with the block surface down. Be sure it is firmly in place.
4. Snap the cover closed.
5. Remove the syringe cap and insert the plunger.
6. Purge the system of air. Tilt the end of the needle up 45 degrees, and slowly fill the system with saline. *The saline must not roll back into transducer well.*
7. Turn on the unit. Readings should be between 0 and 9 mm Hg.
8. Simulate the angle of insertion and press the "zero" button. If the monitor does not read "00," there is a problem. Review the instructions supplied with the kit if necessary. A reading of "00" must be displayed or readings will be inaccurate.
9. Insert needle into the tissue.
10. Inject up to 0.3 ml of saline.
11. Read the pressure once it stabilizes.
12. Repeat readings by turning the unit off and withdrawing the needle and repeating the above steps.

COMPLICATIONS

- Bleeding
- Infection
- Increased pressure from extra fluid
- Pain
- Inaccurate, falsely reassuring readings

Each of the first three (bleeding, infection, increased volume of fluid) could exacerbate a compartment syndrome.

SUMMARY

In summary, the most important thing to understand is that compartment syndrome can cause muscle damage and lead to permanent flexion deformity.

Compartment syndrome can be avoided with early diagnosis and treatment. It is always better to err on the side of decompressing a compartment if there is any indication that decompression is required rather than delay diagnosis in anyone who needs decompression and does not receive it. No permanent harm (other than a scar) ever comes from compartment decompression even if the need for it is borderline. Permanent harm, however, will occur if the patient with borderline compartment syndrome is not treated and muscle necrosis develops. Remember that (1) permanent damage occurs after a minimum of 8 hours of compromised blood supply, and (2) pain, lack of pulse, and pallor are end-stage compartment syndrome signs. If these signs are relied on to make the diagnosis of compartment syndrome, it will be too late for optimal treatment in most cases.

SUPPLIERS

Stryker Instruments
4100 E. Milham
Kalamazoo, MI 49001
Phone: 1-800-253-3210
Website: www.inst.strykercorp.com

CPT/BILLING CODES

24999	Unlisted procedure, humerus or elbow
25999	Unlisted procedure, forearm or wrist
26989	Unlisted procedure, hand or fingers
27899	Unlisted procedure, leg or ankle

ICD-9-CM DIAGNOSTIC CODES

| 958.6 | Volkmann's ischemia |
| 958.9 | Compartment syndrome |

ADDITIONAL RESOURCES

- See the sample patient education handout titled "Trauma to Extremities and Avoidance of the Compartment Syndrome" on page 1996 of Appendix G.

BIBLIOGRAPHY

Black KP, Taylor DE: Current concepts in the treatment of common compartment syndromes in athletes, *Sports Med* 15(6):408, 1993.

d'Amato TA, Kaplan IB, Britt LD: High-voltage electrical injury: a role for mandatory exploration of deep muscle compartments, *J Natl Med Assoc* 86(7):535, 1994.

Dellaero DT, Levin LS: Compartment syndrome of the hand: etiology, diagnosis, and treatment, *Am J Orthop* 25(6):404, 1996.

Gerow G, Matthews B, Jahn W, Gerow R: Compartment syndrome and shin splints of the lower leg, *J Manipulative Physiol Ther* 16(4):245, 1993.

Griffiths D, Jones DH: Spontaneous compartment syndrome in a patient on long-term anticoagulation. *J Hand Surg (Br)* 18(1):41, 1993.

Hutchinson MR, Ireland ML: Common compartment syndromes in athletes: treatment and rehabilitation, *Sports Med* 17(3):200, 1994.

Manoli A II, Fakhouri AJ, Weber TG: Concurrent compartment syndromes of the foot and leg, *Foot Ankle* 14(6):339, 1993.

Myerson M, Manoli A: Compartment syndromes of the foot after calcaneal fractures, *Clin Orthop* 290:142, 1993.

Peters CL, Scott SM: Compartment syndrome in the forearm following fractures of the radial head or neck in children, *J Bone Joint Surg Am* 77(7):1070, 1995.

Schnall SB, Holtom PD, Silva E: Compartment syndrome associated with infection of the upper extremity, *Clin Orthop* 306:128, 1994.

Seybold EA, Busconi BD: Anterior thigh compartment syndrome following prolonged tourniquet application and lateral positioning, *Am J Orthop* 25(7):493, 1996.

Simpson NS, Jupiter JB: Delayed onset of forearm compartment syndrome: a complication of distal radius fracture in young adults, *J Orthop Trauma* 9(5):411, 1995.

Stack LB: Compartment syndrome evaluation. In Roberts JR, Hedges JR: *Clinical procedures in emergency medicine,* ed 3, Philadelphia, 1998, WB Saunders.

Vidal P, Sykes PJ, O'Shaughnessy M, Craddock K: Compartment syndrome after use of an automatic arterial pressure monitoring device, *Br J Anaesth* 71(6):902, 1993.

Diagnostic Needle Arthroscopy, Lavage (DNAL), and Biopsy of the Knee

Chantal Lemoine*

Joint lavage is a simple, low-risk and effective method of relieving pain in patients suffering from arthritis of the knee. Several studies performed over the past decade have proved lavage to be effective in osteoarthritis, a disease affecting millions of people in the United States alone, with undesirable effects in terms of morbidity and loss of productivity. The affected are increasing with the expansion of the elderly and overweight population in the United States. In addition to patient benefits of pain relief and increased walking time, arthroscopic joint lavage provides the physician the benefit of direct visualization of cartilage, synovium and ligamentous structures. This also affords a visually guided biopsy for accurate diagnosis of synovial pathology. The physician's appreciation of the pathology in the patient's knee improves from a two-dimensional, black-and-white radiograph and surface palpation to a three-dimensional visual understanding of the state of the patient's cartilage, degree of erosion, and amount of inflammation present in the synovium. This global comprehension of what is really going on inside a patient's knee can be quite surprising and totally different from what the physician has been taught to expect based on the sum of physical findings, x-ray, magnetic resonance imaging (MRI), and serologic studies. Such surprise encounters by the physician arthroscopist serve to illustrate the need for diagnosticians to use the best technology available in the 21st century in order to provide the best and most appropriate therapy for their patients suffering from arthritis of the knee.

The availability of a minimally invasive, small-diameter arthroscope with single-portal suction irrigation and side-by-side biopsy (through the same portal)

has made this procedure possible, opening up the pathology of the knee to office-based practitioners. This one-portal innovative procedure minimizes trauma to the skin and joint surfaces and reduces patient discomfort such that patients are able to tolerate the procedure with only local anesthesia and light anxiolytic premedication. They actually enjoy looking at their knee on the video monitor or sleeping through the procedure if they prefer. In the author's experience, most patients enjoy seeing what is happening. Indeed the time spent educating the patient about his or her knee pathology is invaluable in terms of ongoing comprehension of disease process and acceptance of appropriate therapeutic modalities.

The procedure, with rigorous aseptic technique, can be performed safely in the office, allowing the patient to walk in and out within 2 hours, accounting for preparation and recuperation time. Subsequent to the procedure, rest and elevation of the knee are prescribed, along with intermittent ice applications. The patient is able to resume regular activities the next day.

The procedure must be performed by a skilled arthroscopist under strictly sterile conditions, in a spacious room suited to surface disinfection to minimize the possibility of contamination. The procedure itself lasts from 45 minutes to 1 hour.

The arthroscope is used to inspect the suprapatellar fossa and the patellofemoral, medial and lateral compartments of the knee. It is also used to lavage the knee of loose bodies, cartilage fragments and "wear particles," and inflammatory factors and degradative enzymes. Synovial biopsy is performed when indicated by the degree of inflammation or other striking abnormalities of the synovium.

For the first time, visually guided synovial biopsy is available to assist the office-based practitioner in accurately diagnosing inflammatory diseases of the knee, such as rheumatoid arthritis and pseudogout in their early stages, as well as rarer conditions such as

*This is dedicated to Dr. Warren Blackburn, who taught me to fly like a bomber pilot with an arthroscope, and to Jeff Kadan, who never stopped believing in the power of fiberoptics and adapted this arthroscope to all my suggestions. Many, many thanks to both of you for opening the universe of the knee to my eyes.

pigmented villonodular synovitis. This can significantly affect treatment outcome for the patient in the early stages of an inflammatory arthritis, since neither the patient nor the physician have to wait for joint destruction to occur before initiating the newer disease modifying therapies.

INDICATIONS

Osteoarthritis

Lavage of the osteoarthritic knee is indicated for therapeutic relief from the pain of refractory osteoarthritis in patients who have failed conservative therapy with nonsteroidal antiinflammatory agents (COX-1 and COX-2 inhibitory drugs), intraarticular steroid injections, and physical therapy. In clinical trials, lavage of the knee with sterile saline or Ringer's lactate has proved to be superior to intraarticular steroid injections in both pain relief and duration of effect. Indeed, in the patient with moderate to severe osteoarthritis, joint lavage is the single most effective, minimally invasive therapeutic modality available. Combining lavage with steroid instillation at the end of the lavage has been shown to be superior to steroid injection alone, and to extend the length of symptomatic relief obtained from lavage alone. Clinical studies looking at the efficacy of lavage combined with hyaluronan are in progress.

Unexplained Knee Pain

Diagnosis of unexplained knee pain with the arthroscope is superior to MRI diagnostic capability in both sensitivity and specificity of findings. It offers the advantages of direct visualization of abnormalities, visually guided biopsy of the synovium if indicated, and therapeutic lavage when appropriate.

Removal of Loose Bodies

Calcified and noncalcified cartilaginous loose bodies can be removed easily with the arthroscope. With full suction, noncalcified loose bodies measuring up to 5 mm in diameter can be suctioned through the open cannula. Rigid, calcified loose bodies measuring more than 3.5 mm in diameter are not amenable to removal with this method.

Recurrent Knee Effusions

In patients with known osteoarthritis, recurrent knee effusions may indicate an undiagnosed coexisting inflammatory condition such as pseudogout; internal derangement caused by loose bodies, meniscal degeneration, and tears; or torn cruciate ligaments. These conditions can be assessed with a much higher degree of accuracy with the arthroscope compared with available imaging techniques, including MRI of the knee. In addition, in most patients, lavage provides an average of 6 months of relief from pain and recurrent effusion.

Crystal-Induced Arthritides

The procedure provides accurate visual and tissue diagnosis. The lavage, which reduces the crystal load, provides long-lasting benefits (6 to 12 months on average of reduced pain and effusions) in patients with persistent symptoms unresponsive to medical therapy, or in patients unable to tolerate the medications used to control crystal deposition and resultant inflammation.

Unexplained Arthritis

For patients who, despite serologic and radiologic investigation, have a diagnostic dilemma, arthroscopic evaluation can provide an early diagnosis of such conditions as rheumatoid arthritis or confirm the presence of tissue-based, crystal-induced synovitis or internal derangement. It also provides easy access to visually guided biopsy. Pigmented villonodular synovitis is a rare condition that can be diagnosed easily with visually guided synovial biopsy.

Resistant Inflammatory Arthritis

Patients with known inflammatory conditions such as rheumatoid arthritis, psoriatic arthritis, Reiter's syndrome, or crystal-induced arthritis are often well controlled with medication, with the exception of one or two persistently inflamed and symptomatic joints, most often the weight-bearing knee. In these patients, arthroscopic lavage, with instillation of steroids upon completion of the lavage, can decrease symptoms in the resistant knee joint without increasing or altering the therapeutic regimen used to control the underlying inflammatory condition to possibly toxic levels. In addition, the visual inspection and possible use of tissue biopsy can exclude a superimposed opportunistic infection in an immunocompromised host or can rule out a coexisting condition (e.g., internal derangement, loose bodies) that may respond to therapeutic lavage.

Nonsurgical Candidates

Many patients, because of severe medical conditions that preclude general or epidural anesthesia or the use of tourniquets (e.g., heart disease, severe COPD, peripheral vascular insufficiency, recurrent deep vein thromboses or pulmonary embolism, morbid obesity, or advanced age with multiple co-existing medical problems), are not surgical candidates. These patients, although the optimal approach to their knee symptoms would otherwise be surgical intervention, can still greatly benefit from the therapeutic effects of lavage. As mentioned previously, the average duration of relief is approximately 6 months, and the procedure can be repeated at 6-month intervals in order to maintain the therapeutic improvement.

Patient Alternative to Surgical Intervention

For patients who want to delay surgical arthroscopy or joint replacement surgery, this procedure provides a less invasive, palliative option while providing valuable structural information about the affected knee. This information can then be used by the surgeon to plan the appropriate type of surgery (arthroscopic reconstruction, total or partial joint replacement, etc.) that best fits the patient's needs. The patient can use this time to physically and mentally prepare for surgery (lose weight if indicated or strengthen the supporting knee musculature with physical therapy) and put in place necessary support systems for optimal recuperation from planned surgical intervention.

In all of the above situations, office-based arthroscopy of the knee with lavage and optional biopsy is designed to relieve pain, establish diagnosis, remove loose bodies and cartilage fragments, monitor the course of the disease, clarify and reassess the physician's understanding of the disease process, and thus guide further therapy.

CONTRAINDICATIONS

- Sepsis.
- Severe bleeding abnormalities (i.e., hemophilia, severe thrombocytopenia, or platelet dysfunction). Note that patients on warfarin (Coumadin) can undergo this microinvasive and nonsurgical procedure safely with the use of local epinephrine to control minor bleeding, without interruption or alteration of warfarin dosage.
- Cellulitis or other local infection at proposed site of arthroscope insertion.
- Massive obesity.
- Severe medical problems.

EQUIPMENT

- A 1.7-mm arthroscope with 30,000 pixel fiberoptic bundle and distal dual-element lens
- A 3.5-mm cannula with sharp trocar and blunt obturator

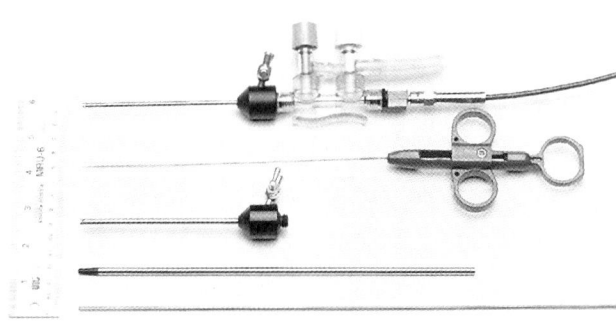

Fig. 190-1
Top row, Diagnostic cannula attached to disposable suction-irrigation handpiece with fiberoptic arthroscope locked in place. *Second row,* 1-mm biopsy instrument. *Third row,* Biopsy cannula. *Fourth row,* Dilator shaft. *Bottom row,* Cannula exchange rod. (From Troum OM: *Clin Atlas Off Proc* 5[4]:537, 2002.)

- Suction-irrigation handpiece and tubing set (that attaches to cannula) through which the arthroscope is inserted, with separate suction and irrigation channels, and exchangeable biopsy cannula (Fig. 190-1)
- High-resolution camera
- Optical coupler
- Light source
- Color video monitor
- Vacuum suction unit
- Dual 1200-ml vacuum collection canisters
- Irrigation pump with capacity for two 1000-ml hanging bags, maximum pressure 550 mm Hg with gauge indicator
- Air compressor
- Digital video-print recorder
- Video equipment cart (Fig. 190-2)
- Flexible biopsy forceps
- Adjustable arthroscopy table or chair with foot or remote controls
- Rolling stool with adjustable height for arthroscopist
- Sphygmomanometer
- Stethoscope
- Nasal oxygen setup
- Sterile normal saline or Ringer's lactate in 1-L bags for joint irrigation and lavage
- Specimen jars with formalin for biopsy specimens, and sterile specimen jars for culture specimens
- Sterile syringes and needles
- Sterile gloves, gowns, masks, shoe covers, and hair caps
- Prepackaged sterile arthroscopy kit with drapes, scalpel, etc.
- Absorbent floor pads

Disinfection Supplies

- Plastic or metal pans with covers for soaking, disinfecting, and rinsing arthroscope, cannulas, trocar, obturator, and biopsy forceps

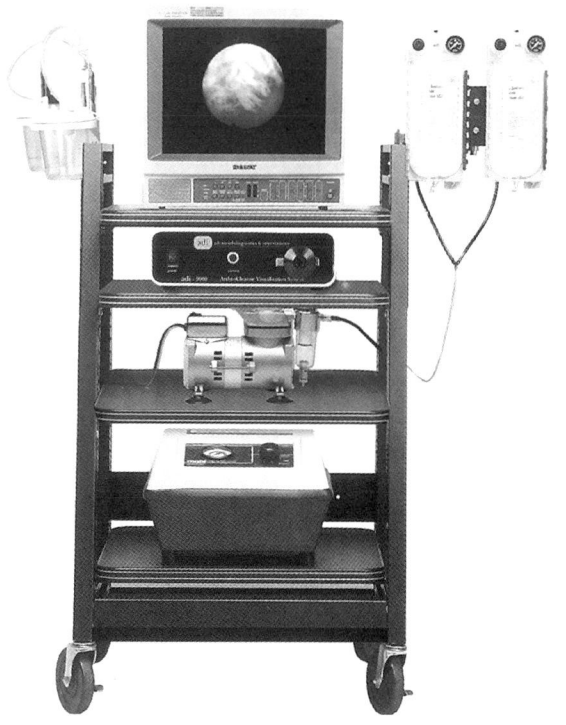

Fig. 190-2
Diagnostic needle arthroscopic lavage scope system equipment cart.
(From Troum OM: *Clin Atlas Off Proc* 5[4]:537, 2002.)

- Surgical scrub sponges, sink, and running water
- Betadine scrub solution with sterile sponges for prepping patient's leg
- Manufacturer-supplied cleaning brushes for arthroscope cannulas
- Manufacturer-specified cleaning and disinfecting solutions for instruments, arthroscope, and room surfaces (floors, counters, etc.)
- Steris Corporation Sterilization Unit *(optional)*
- Sterile water for rinsing and soaking instruments after disinfection
- Bucket, mop, and surface sponges

PREPROCEDURE PATIENT PREPARATION

At the time of the office visit when the procedure is planned and agreed on, the physician explains the procedure, its purpose, most common complications, and expectations in layman's terms. The patient should understand that this is a palliative or diagnostic procedure and not a cure; realistic expectations will greatly affect patient satisfaction. A patient education handout should be provided to the patient with encouragement to ask any questions (see the sample patient education handout on page 1997 of Appen-

dix G). When the patient arrives on the day of the procedure, a signed informed consent is obtained (see the sample patient consent form on page 1999 of Appendix G).

ANTIBIOTIC PROPHYLAXIS

Antibiotic prophylaxis is not used routinely because of the extremely low rate of infection (<0.5%) from this procedure. However, it is indicated in the immunosuppressed patient, in patients with prosthetic joints, and in patients with abnormal or artificial valves according to the guidelines of the American Heart Association.

Sedation

Upon the patient's arrival, vital signs are obtained and any abnormal values are reported to the physician and dealt with as necessary. Complete sedation is not necessary for this procedure, and only light oral anxiolytic sedation is administered with 5 to 10 mg of oral diazepam or similar anxiolytic agent. Most patients remain awake during the procedure and are able to cooperate with repositioning of their knee at the request of the arthroscopist. Some patients fall into a light sleep but are easily awakened if their cooperation is required. Intravenous access is not required because no intravenous medications are administered, and patients with serious medical problems are not candidates for this procedure.

TECHNIQUE

Room Preparation

Unless the procedure is being performed in a surgical suite, the room to be used is prepared ahead of time by removing any extraneous furniture, office supplies, papers, etc. The only items remaining should be the arthroscopy cart; the examination table or arthroscopy chair; the arthroscopist's stool and a stool for the scrub nurse; and a clean table or counter that will be draped and where the arthroscopy instruments and supplies will be set out. A smaller, nonsterile area should also be cleaned and draped with a clean, disposable drape, to display nonsterile supplies and bottles of injectables. All cabinets should be closed after removing necessary supplies, and all surfaces, including counters and floors, should be wiped down with an envirocidal solution (a surface disinfectant that kills bacteria and viruses on contact) according to supplier specifications. Once the room has been prepared, the examination room door should be closed, and only authorized personnel wearing shoe and hair covers, scrubs, and masks may enter

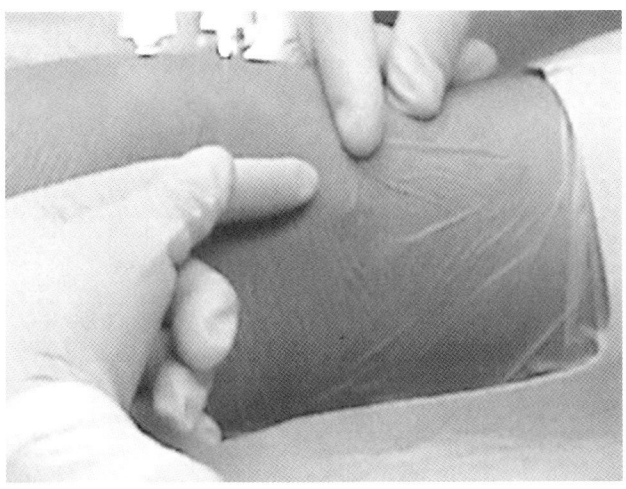

Fig. 190-3
Identification of inferolateral portal (head is to the left).

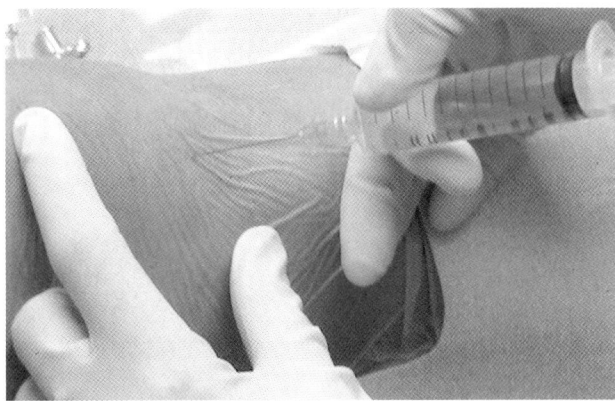

Fig. 190-4
Intradermal anesthesia is achieved by injecting 5 to 8 ml 1% lidocaine with 1:1000 epinephrine using a 25-gauge, 1½-inch needle.

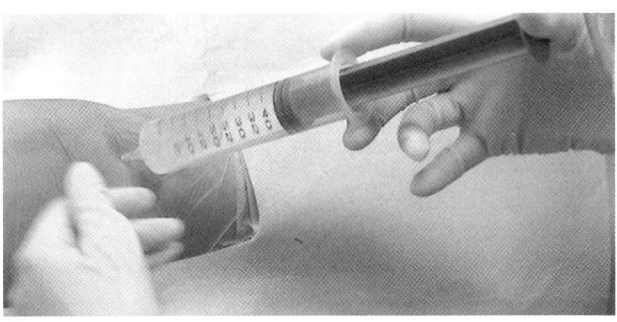

Fig. 190-5
Intraarticular anesthesia is achieved with 40-ml 0.05% bupivicaine using a 21-gauge, 1½-inch needle.

the room. Such personnel should be kept to a minimum to decrease the risk of surface or airborne contamination.

Patient Preparation

After signing the informed consent, the patient is asked to undress down to his or her underwear and is given a disposable gown, hair cover, and disposable shoe covers. (No socks or street shoes are allowed on the patient.) The patient is given 5 to 10 mg of oral diazepam for light sedation, brought to the arthroscopy room and placed on the examination table. The nurse should ask the patient which knee is being arthroscoped and should confirm this information with the arthroscopist. The proper leg is then scrubbed with Betadine scrub, using sterile sponges from midthigh down to the ankle. This is allowed to air dry, and a sterile drape is placed over the patient with a plastic window over the knee. The drape covers the patient from the shoulders down to below the toes and hangs down on each side of the table without touching the floor. The patient is instructed to keep his or her arms underneath the drape at all times.

Procedure

After scrubbing your hands and arms, don sterile gown and gloves and approach the patient. Verbally ascertain patient comfort. Inspect and palpate the patient's knee through the plastic window, and locate the inferolateral portal by following the lateral and inferior borders of the patella and palpating for the joint space at their intersection (Fig. 190-3). After locating the inferolateral portal, anesthetize this area locally with approximately 5 to 8 ml of 1% lidocaine with 1:1000 epinephrine with a 25-gauge, 1½-inch needle from the skin surface down

(but not through) the joint capsule (Fig. 190-4). Be careful to raise a skin bleb at the insertion of the needle to ensure complete surface anesthesia, and follow a straight injection path pointing the needle in the direction of the intersection of the cruciate ligaments. After full intradermal anesthesia is achieved, insert a 50-ml syringe with a 21-gauge, 1½-inch needle filled with 0.05% bupivicaine into the knee through the same needle track, penetrate the joint capsule, and insert approximately 40 ml of bupivicaine into the knee joint (Fig. 190-5). Because of the caliber of the needle, moderate effort is required to instill the bupivicaine into the joint space; however, take care not to apply extreme pressure in order to avoid instilling the bupivicaine into the tissues or intravascularly. Keep one hand pressed lightly over the suprapatellar surface of the patient's knee to feel this area expanding as the bupivicaine is instilled into the knee.

After full intradermal and intraarticular anesthesia, use a no. 11 blade scalpel to make a small incision 0.5 cm wide and 2 cm deep at the location of the inferolateral portal (Fig. 190-6). This is accomplished in

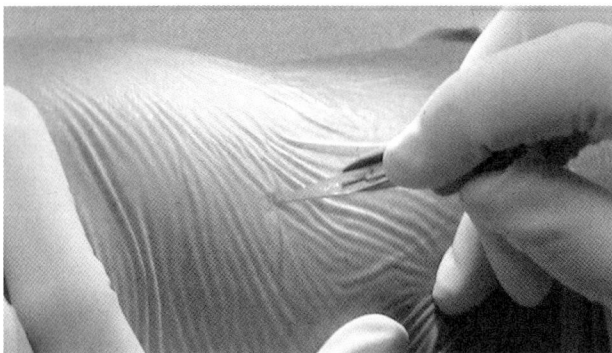

Fig. 190-6
Infereolateral portal incision 0.5 cm wide and 2 cm deep is made with a no. 11 blade scalpel.

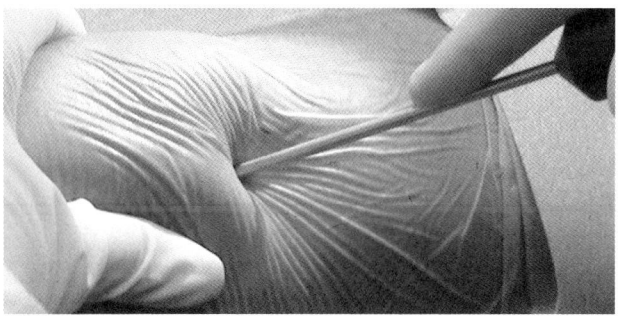

Fig. 190-7
Joint cannulation. Diagnostic cannula is inserted into knee joint. The sharp trocar is locked in place on the attached suction-irrigation handpiece.

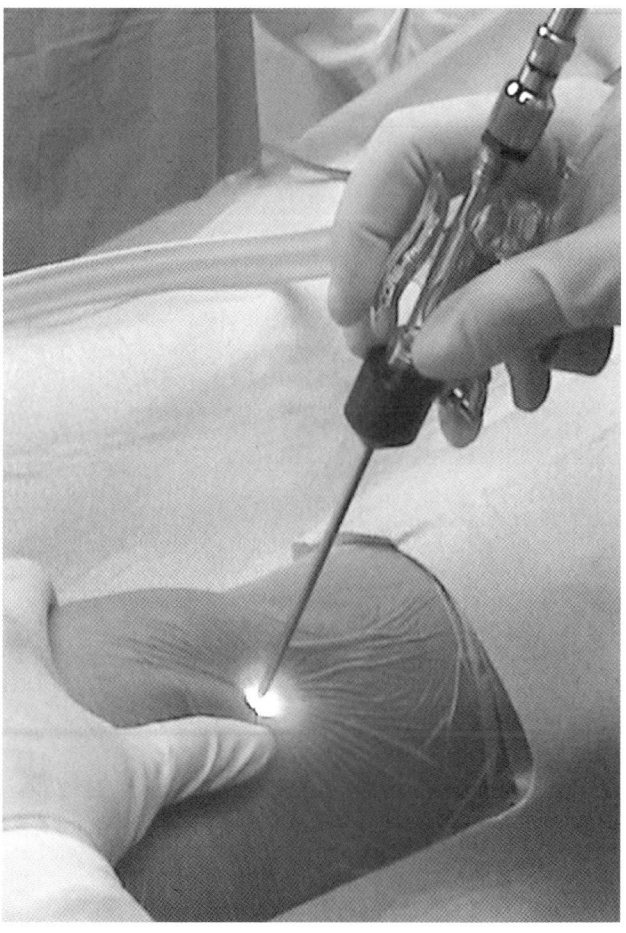

Fig. 190-8
Cannulation established. Fiberoptic arthroscope locked in place with suction-irrigation tubing set attached. Note: internal illumination viewed externally.

one smooth jabbing motion with the scalpel blade held parallel to the joint line so that the incision follows the skin folds and heals more easily with minimal scarring. Through this incision, insert the sharp trocar and cannula, attached to the handpiece and tubing, into the knee joint (Fig. 190-7). It is easiest to have the knee flexed at a 90-degree angle and to aim for the cruciate ligaments. Hold the cannula and trocar at a 45-degree angle to the lateral skin surface of the knee. Use moderate pressure to pierce through the joint capsule, but check the forward motion of the trocar and cannula in order to stop as soon as the capsule is breached to avoid injuring any internal structures with the sharp point of the trocar. Once inside the joint capsule, remove the sharp trocar and replace it with a blunt obturator. Advance the blunt trocar and cannula underneath the patella into the suprapatellar space. This is accomplished by straightening out the patient's leg in order to lift the patella away from the femur, and by angling the cannula so that it lies underneath and parallel to the undersurface of the patella. This should be achieved easily without need for any undue force. Keep one hand over the suprapatellar area and gently advance the

cannula and blunt trocar until the tip of the trocar rests against the joint surface at the superior pole of the suprapatellar space and is easily palpable though the skin without distorting the joint surface. Remove the blunt trocar and replace it with the arthroscope. Attach suction and irrigation tubing to vacuum suction and air-pressurized irrigation, respectively (Fig. 190-8). Before proceeding any further, collect an aliquot of joint fluid through one of the ports of the handpiece, and send it to the laboratory for culture and sensitivity and crystal analysis. A cell count is not reliable on this fluid because it will have been diluted by the addition of the intraarticular bupivicaine used to achieve anesthesia.

At this point a full diagnostic arthroscopy can proceed by visual examination. If there is excessive cloudiness resulting from multiple loose bodies or an inflammatory effusion, an initial lavage with 100 to 200 ml of fluid may be needed to clear the joint sufficiently to allow for adequate visualization. Throughout the procedure, fluid can be instilled into the knee by pressing down the

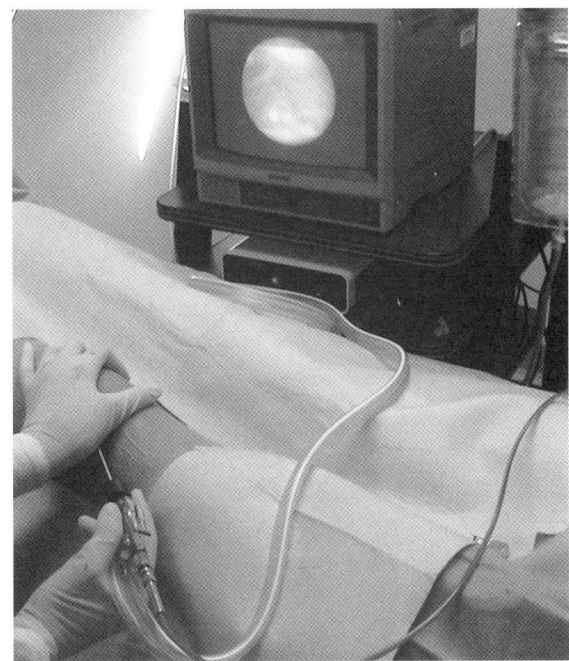

Fig. 190-9
Arthroscopist's simultaneous viewing of external knee and hand devices and internal joint space as seen on monitor.

irrigation button on the handpiece, allowing flow of pressurized sterile irrigation fluid (sterile normal saline or Ringer's lactate) into the joint. Fluid can be removed from the joint by depressing the white suction button controlling the suction channel. Pressure of fluid within the joint must be controlled and can be gauged by distention of the suprapatellar space as well as by patient tolerance for joint distention. Despite the anesthesia, the stretch receptors in the joint capsule will be activated by excessive pressure, causing some discomfort to the patient. Adequate visualization through the arthroscope necessitates distention of the knee with a moderate amount of irrigation fluid.

Begin inspection by examining the suprapatellar fossa for areas of synovial proliferation, crystal deposition, and plicae (Fig. 190-9). Withdraw the arthroscope slightly until the patella appears as a half-moon superiorly, and inspect the patellofemoral joint with attention to assessment of the articular cartilage, degree of chondromalacia, cartilage erosions, and osteophyte formation as well as possible crystal deposition. Once this has been accomplished, with the arthroscope positioned directly under the patella and the leg fully extended, guide the scope around medially into the medial gutter, following the contour of the medial femoral condyle, until the medial joint space is reached. It may be necessary to maneuver around osteophytes in order to enter the medial joint space. Once inside the medial joint space, careful attention is paid to the degree

of cartilage degeneration of both the tibial and femoral surfaces, as well as to the integrity of the meniscus. Advance the arthroscope along the joint line toward the intercondylar notch until the cruciate ligament(s) come into view. In cases in which the anterior cruciate ligament is torn, advance the arthroscope easily into the intercondylar notch; the posterior cruciate ligament is easily visualized. It is also possible to access the lateral joint space by advancing through the notch in these cases, and the arthroscope is able to sweep across the entire joint line. When the anterior cruciate ligament is intact, it is usually not possible to access the lateral joint space from a medial approach. Instead, withdraw the arthroscope from the medial joint space into the medial gutter, swing it back around the medial femoral condyle under the patella, and guide it around the lateral femoral condyle into the lateral joint space. In cases in which the joint spaces are very narrowed, have the patient bend the knee in order to open up the medial joint space and position the legs in a figure-four position (with the knee bent and the ankle crossed over the opposite leg and the hip abducted and externally rotated) in order to open up the lateral joint space. Also closely inspect the medial and lateral gutters for areas of synovial proliferation, loose bodies, and crystal deposition. If there are areas of abnormal synovial proliferation, make the decision as to whether or not to perform a biopsy on the synovium.

Before performing a biopsy on the synovium, if there are significant loose bodies and cartilage fragments, lavage the joint with the arthroscope, using tidal lavage. This is accomplished by filling the joint with irrigation fluid, then immediately suctioning the fluid to a relatively dry joint. Repeat this maneuver until there is visual clearing of loose bodies and cartilage fragments. The average joint requires about 1 L of fluid for adequate lavage, and this amount is divided into the three accessible joint compartments, starting with the suprapatellar and patellofemoral joint spaces, followed by the medial gutter and medial joint space, including the notch, and ending with the lateral gutter and lateral joint space. The author chooses this order of lavage because the highest concentration of loose bodies and cartilage fragments collect in the lateral gutter, most likely because of gravitational force. Most patients tend to allow their legs to remain externally rotated during the procedure. It thus seems logical to force the flow of fluid in a circular manner starting from the suprapatellar area, proceeding to the medial joint space, and ending with the lateral joint space and lateral gutter.

After the lavage, if biopsy is indicated, replace the suction-irrigation cannula with the biopsy cannula, which is designed with two side-by-side channels (one for the arthroscope and one for the flexible biopsy forceps). This cannula is not used for joint inspection or lavage because it has to be of larger diameter in order to accommodate the biopsy instrument, and is thus more difficult to maneuver into all the joint compartments. In order to minimize trauma to the joint capsule, change the cannula by removing the arthroscope from the handpiece and suction-irrigation cannula and replace it by a simple blunt-tipped rod introducer. When inserted fully into the handpiece and cannula, the introducer exceeds the length of the instrument by approximately 1½ inches (Fig. 190-10). Then remove the entire instrument from the joint over the rod, leaving the introducer in place and thus maintaining the path through the capsule into the joint. The removable suction-irrigation cannula is then detached from the handpiece and replaced with the biopsy cannula. Insert the biopsy cannula, now attached to the handpiece, over the rod introducer into the joint, using a twisting motion with mild pressure, in order to enlarge slightly the track into the joint. Once inside the joint, remove the introducer and replace it with the arthroscope. Synovial biopsy can then proceed under direct visualization. After visually locating the synovial area to be biopsied, insert the biopsy instrument through the biopsy channel (Fig. 190-11). As the tip of the biopsy instrument extends past the cannula, it comes into view of the arthroscope; guide it to the area of synovium to be biopsied. Open the jaws of the biopsy instrument by pulling back on the spring-loaded handle and close them around the desired piece of synovium by releasing the handle. Remove the piece of synovium (caught in the jaws of the biopsy forceps) from the joint by withdrawing the biopsy instrument from its channel. This maneuver can be repeated until adequate sampling has been obtained. Collect the biopsy specimens on a sterile gauze pad soaked with sterile saline to prevent drying out of the specimens. Later, tease them off using a sterile 21-gauge needle, and transfer them to appropriate containers for pathology (formalin containers) or culture (containers with a small amount of sterile saline without any preservatives). Forward these to the laboratory immediately for best results. If the biopsy causes visible bleeding, control this by instilling a small amount (0.5 to 1 ml lidocaine with 1:1000 epinephrine) into the joint through the medication portal of the handpiece. Also, at any point during the procedure, if there is any bleeding caused by friction of the arthroscope against friable synovium, or pain elicited by the procedure, immediately instill additional aliquots of lidocaine with 1:1000 epinephrine or 0.05% bupivicaine into the joint using this portal, which is equipped with Luer-Lok and stopcock mechanisms. After completion of the biopsy and control of any resultant bleeding by the methods described above, again lavage the joint with a small amount of irrigation fluid to clear it of any blood.

If there is significant synovial inflammation, intraarticular steroids may be injected into the joint through the medication port. This is followed by a 2-ml flush of irrigation fluid or anesthetic—usually lidocaine with

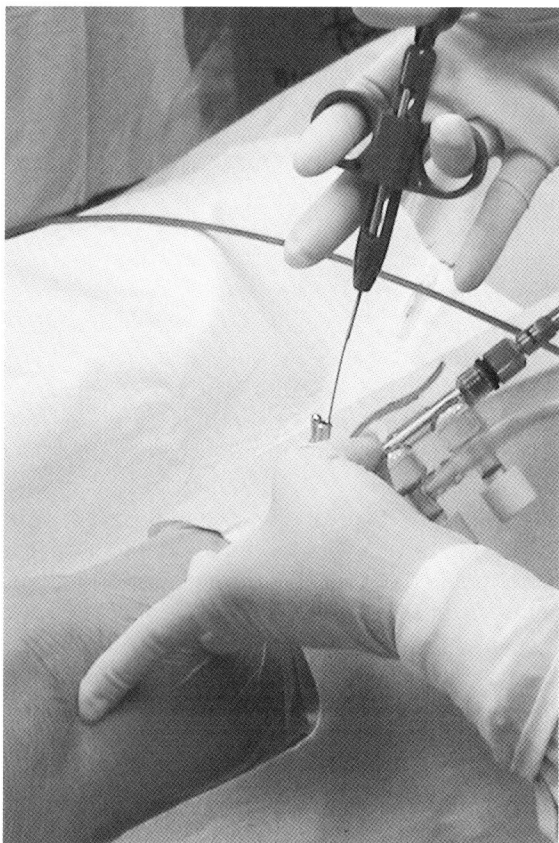

Fig. 190-11
Visually guided biopsy. With biopsy cannula and attached handpiece in place, scope is reinserted. The biopsy instrument is inserted through the working channel of the cannula.

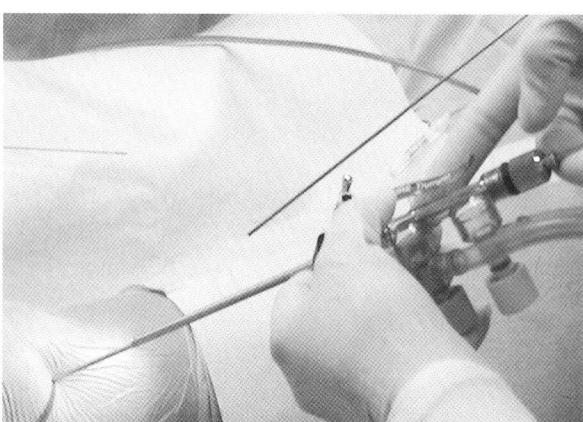

Fig. 190-10
Cannula exchange. Biopsy cannula and suction-irrigation handpiece sliding over exchange rod for easy reinsertion back into the joint.

1:1000 epinephrine—to constrict the synovial vessels and decrease systemic absorption of the steroid (Fig. 190-12). Then remove the arthroscope and cannula from the joint.

Apply a Steri-Strip to the incision site, taking care to appose the two sides of the incision, closing it before applying the Steri-Strip. Then apply a sterile dressing and light pressure bandage around the entire knee. Wash the rest of the patient's leg clean of Betadine using warm water, taking care not to touch or moisten the sterile bandage. Help the patient off the table and into an adjoining room where he or she can change back into street clothes and footwear. During this time and before the patient leaves the office, orally review postarthroscopic care and instructions with the patient and family. In addition the patient is given a copy of the same written post-arthroscopy instructions (see the sample patient education handout on page 1998 of Appendix G), which he/she is asked to sign to acknowledge receipt. A copy of this signed document is kept in the patient's permanent record.

Examine the patient before he or she leaves the office, and check the patient's knee for range of motion, pain, and bleeding through the dressing. Give the patient a potent analgesic such as codeine or hydrocodone in case of pain that may occur during the first 24 hours as well as a prescription for antibiotics if prophylaxis is indicated.

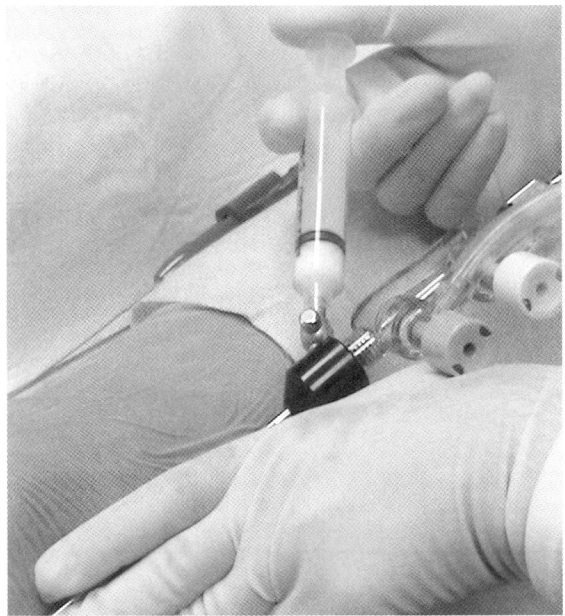

Fig. 190-12
Intraarticular injection. Identified synovial inflammation is injected with 2-ml steroid followed by 2 ml flush of saline or 1:1000 lidocaine with epinephrine.

POSTPROCEDURE PATIENT EDUCATION

The patient may resume work or normal activity the following day, but he or she should avoid excessive walking or standing. Have the patient schedule a follow-up knee check within 3 to 5 days, and instruct him or her to call immediately should any fever, bleeding, swelling, or extreme pain develop. All patients who have had this procedure are able to leave the office walking. Patients are not permitted to drive home because of the administration of the oral sedative, so advise them ahead of time to arrange for a ride from a friend or relative.

COMPLICATIONS

- *Flare of crystal-induced arthritis:* This can be prevented by instilling intraarticular steroids into the joint at the completion of the lavage.
- *Cellulitis:* Overall incidence is less than 2% and is more likely to occur in immunosuppressed patients. Use of prophylactic antibiotics in these patients significantly reduces the incidence of cellulitis around the inferolateral portal.
- *Rupture of joint capsule:* This occurs in less than 0.5% of patients and is more likely to occur in elderly patients with thinning of their joint capsules. This is easily detected by visual inspection and occurs primarily in the suprapatellar fossa. This does not affect the outcome of the procedure.
- *Septic arthritis:* This has been reported in the arthroscopic literature with a 1% to 2% incidence, which includes surgical arthroscopy; however, in over 2000 cases of office DNAL, the author has not witnessed any intraarticular infections.
- *Postoperative fall resulting in hip fracture:* One reported case in the literature
- *Synovial cysts:* Sometimes occur at the inferolateral portal and can be prevented by the use of pressure dressings during the healing of the incision track.
- *Other:* Phlebitis, vascular insufficiency, popliteal cyst rupture, reflex sympathetic dystrophy, and aseptic fistula formation have all been reported in the literature as arthroscopic complications, but they have not been seen by the author over the past 7 years and more than 2000 cases with this office procedure.

In conclusion, this DNAL, which can be safely performed in an office or other ambulatory setting, has been shown to be an effective treatment for patients suffering from the pain of osteoarthritis, with a very low rate of minor complications. In addition, it provides the practitioner with an effective tool superior to radiographs or MRI, to diagnose and treat inflammatory arthritides, and to evaluate the painful knee. It is also a nonsurgical therapeutic alternative for patients who are either not surgical candidates or are desirous of delaying surgical intervention. This procedure is currently under-used in the treatment of arthritis, but it should gain in popularity as more physicians attain the skills and the level of comfort required to perform this in the office setting.

SUPPLIERS

ADI (Advanced Diagnostics and Interventions)
216 Via Linda Vista
Redondo Beach, CA 90277
Phone: 1-310-373-6769

Steris Corp.
5960 Heisley Road
Mentor, OH 44060-1834
Phone: 1-800-989-7575
Website: www.steris.com

CPT/BILLING CODES

29870	Arthroscopy, knee, diagnostic, with or without biopsy
29874	Arthroscopic lavage for removal of loose or foreign body
99070	Bupivicaine injection (Medicare Code J0670)
99070	Normal saline irrigation, 1000 ml (Medicare Code J0670)
99070	Valium 10 mg po (Medicare Code J3360)
99070	Sterile custom tray (Medicare Code A4550)

ADDITIONAL RESOURCES

• See the sample patient education handouts titled "Diagnostic Arthroscopy and Lavage Patient Information and Instructions" on page 1997 and "After Arthroscopy and Lavage Information and Care" on page 1998 of Appendix G.

• See the sample patient consent form titled "Consent to Diagnostic or Therapeutic Procedures and Administration of Anesthesia" on page 1999 of Appendix G.

BIBLIOGRAPHY

American College of Rheumatology Subcommittee on Osteoarthritis Guidelines: Recommendations for the medical management of osteoarthritis of the hip and knee: 2000 update, *Arthritis Rheumatol* 43(9):1905, 2000.

de la Serna AR: Joint lavage is beneficial for pain reduction in the treatment of knee osteoarthritis, *J Rheumatol* 28:635, 2001.

Edelson R, Burks RT, Bloebaum RD: Short-term effects of knee washout for osteoarthritis, *Am J Sports Med* 23(3):345, 1995.

Halbrecht JL, Jackson DW: Office arthroscopy: a diagnostic alternative, *Arthroscopy* 8(3):320, 1992.

Hochberg MC, Altman RD, Brandt KD, et al: Guidelines for the medical management of osteoarthritis, *Arthritis Rheumatol* 38(11):1541, 1995.

Ike RW, Arnold WJ, Rothschild EW, et al: Tidal irrigation versus conservative medical management in patients with osteoarthritis of the knee; a prospective randomized study, *J Rheumatol* 19:772, 1992.

Koziol-Ehni LR, Cohen LM, Arnold WJ: Role of arthroscopy in the management of patients with osteoarthritis of the knee: present and future, *Resid Staff Physician* 42(9):11, 1996.

Michalska M: Knee arthroscopy in the office, *Hosp Pract (Off Ed)* 32:179, 1997.

Ravaud P, Moulinier L, Giraudeau B, et al: Effects of joint lavage and steroid injection in patients with osteoarthritis of the knee, *Arthritis Rheum* 42(3):475, 1999.

Troum OM: Office-based diagnostics: needle arthroscopic lavage. In Pfenninger JL, editor: Joint injection techniques, *Clin Atlas Off Proc* 5(4):2002.

Troum OM, Lemoine C: Conservative management of the osteoarthritic knee, *Curr Opin Orthop* 11:3, 2000.

Vad VB, Cooke PM, Weikiewicz TL, et al: *Hylan versus knee lavage and Hylan in management of knee osteoarthritis*, 67th annual meeting of American Academy of Orthopedic Surgeons, March 15-19, 2000.

Wollaston S, Brion P, Kumar A, et al: Complications of knee arthroscopy performed by rheumatologists, *J Rheumatol* 28(8):1871, 2001.

CHAPTER 191

Extensor Tendon Repair

David T. Bortel

Acute **extensor tendon** injuries are common and for the most part may be addressed surgically as an outpatient in an acute care setting with proper equipment. Extensor tendons are more superficial with a paratenon, the vascularized, filmy connective tissue that envelops the extensor tendon and allows gliding over the forearm or dorsal foot, which does not readily separate when lacerated. This makes these injuries amenable to repair with less need for significant dissection compared with flexor tendons. However, the practitioner should not ignore the complexity of the extensor mechanism. Most consider the act of extension more intricate than finger flexion. The act of extension is comprised of two separate and neurologically independent (yet interdependent) systems: the radially innervated extrinsic extensors (originating from the forearm) and the intrinsic system (originating in the hand) that is innervated by the median and ulnar nerves (Fig. 191-1).

Extensor injuries are typically classified by zones of injury (Fig. 191-2). Each zone has uniquely associated injury patterns and therefore different modes of treatment. Greater than 50% of these extensor tendon injuries will have an associated injury (e.g., fracture, dislocation/ligamentous injury, capsular damage, or flexor tendon injury). **Flexor tendon** injuries should be treated in an appropriate surgical facility with appropriate equipment and personnel trained regarding the demanding anatomic considerations.

PRINCIPLES

Penetrating trauma needs to be examined carefully for any loss of the neurovascular status and any loss of motor/tendon function. The wound should be anesthetized and explored to *visualize the potentially involved tendon* with wound extension if necessary in order to understand the personality of the specific injury pattern. When a tendon is completely transected, the cut ends can retract a considerable distance. Since a *partial tendon laceration* might appear to have full function on examination, the wound must be evaluated judiciously.

The entire tendon complex must be observed throughout the entire arc of motion at the injury location. Most practitioners feel *a repair is warranted if more than 40% cross-sectional damage has occurred.* A tendon repair must have healthy padded skin for viability, or tissue grafting will be necessary. Wounds older than 6 to 8 hours need aggressive cleansing with strong consideration toward leaving the wound open for a later staged irrigation or debridement with subsequent closure. During this interval, exposed bone, joint, and tendon tissue should be loosely covered with native tissue or a damp sterile gauze followed by a bulky dressing and an anterior-posterior splint, including fingertip through forearm. Tendon repair may be delayed up to 10 days.

A repaired tendon develops a fibroblastic bulbous connection during the first 2 weeks. Tendon collagen usually does not begin to form until the third week. At the end of the fourth week, swelling and vascularity will decrease. Once the junction becomes strong, the tendon can tolerate active gliding. Knowledge of appropriate splinting and necessary therapy is essential when caring for these injuries. Repaired tendons must be immobilized to promote healing and to prevent tendon rupture. *Joint and tendon motion is discouraged for at least the first 3 weeks because of excessive tissue reaction.* After hand extensor tendon repair, the splint typically can be placed on the dorsal surface from the forearm to the fingertips to protect and prevent active extension. The digits and wrist may be slightly flexed within the tolerances of the repair. These joints must be protected against flexion when changing dressings or splints. After this period of immobilization, depending on the particular circumstances, passive motion can then be initiated commonly under the guidance of a skilled hand therapist. Reasonable strength may be present to this repaired tendon as early as 6 weeks after the injury, again depending on the patient's reliability and health status (e.g., neurological status, tobacco use, metabolic and rheumatologic issues).

The vast majority of **flexor tendon** injuries should be treated by a surgeon skilled with these injuries in an appropriate surgical suite. Particularly, **flexor tendon**

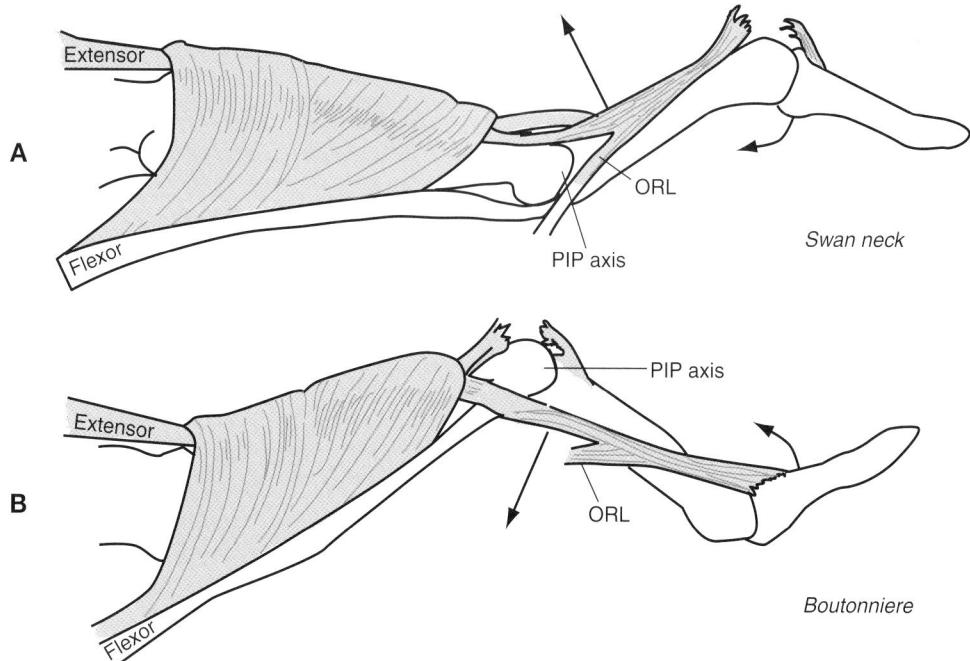

Fig. 191-1
Note the intimate working relationship of the intrinsic and extrinsic extensor mechanism. (Note that the flexor is not shown.) **A,** Mallet finger *(Zone I injury)* that has resulted in a *swan-neck deformity* because the oblique retinacular ligament (ORL), also known as the conjoined lateral bands, has subluxed dorsal to axis of rotation at the level of the PIP joint. **B,** A *Zone III injury* allows the ORL to sublux volar to the axis of rotation at the PIP joint resulting in a *Boutonniere deformity.*

injuries located in "no man's land" (between the proximal palmar crease and the proximal interphalangeal joint) are terribly challenging. Results of tendon repair are consistently better when fixed primarily (within 10 days) rather than secondarily (after 10 days or delayed). Familiarity with the chapters referenced is encouraged if managing tendon injuries (Doyle, 1999; Thompson, 1993; Wright, 1998).

EQUIPMENT

- Surgical prep (Betadine, Hibiclens); hand through elbow with particularly thorough cleansing of the contaminated tissues.
- Ruler in centimeters.
- Irrigation device for contaminated wounds: 30-ml syringe with 18-gauge angiocatheter or commercially manufactured splash shield device (see Fig. 23-1) and sterile saline.
- Appropriate anesthetic (see Chapter 4, Local Anesthesia).
- 3- to 20-ml syringe.
- 27-gauge, 1¼-inch needle (small-gauge needles are preferred to administer anesthesia).
- Additional 27-gauge, 1½-inch needles (useful to stabilize tendon end; *optional*).
- Sterile drapes; fenestrated drape applied over the lesion; appropriate larger barrier as indicated.
- 4 × 4–inch gauze sponges; cotton sterile applicators are also useful.
- Sterile pack containing: 4½-inch needle holder; curved dissecting scissors; one or more mosquito hemostats; suture scissors; Adson forceps with and without teeth; skin hooks; small self-retaining retractor (Alms, Holzheimer, or Weitlaner).
- Additional small (micro) instruments (may be helpful depending on the size of structures).
- No. 15 blade for excisions or wound lengthening with blade handle (single disposable unit also available).
- Pack of folded sterile towels for patient arm positioning and/or surgeon wrist support.
- Appropriate suture (see Chapter 25, Laceration and Incision Repair: Suture Selection, as well as following text for specifics for tendons).
- Allis forceps for removal of deeper masses *(optional)*.
- Skin-marking pen.
- Electrocautery unit.
- Specimen jar (if necessary).
- Sterile gloves.

• Operative microscope or magnifying "loops," particularly if considering neurovascular repair *(optional)*.

Suture Material Considerations

Suture preferences can be quite variable among practitioners who perform tendon repairs. Physicians experienced with tendon repairs have found nonabsorbable material to be most desirable. (Absorbable materials such as Vicryl can precipitate an undesirable inflammatory response, which might lead to excessive tendon adhesion formation. Furthermore, as absorbable suture breaks down, this commonly will occur while the tendon is very weakened at the repair site and is prone to failure.) If the tendon is of sufficient size with a transected pattern, most physicians will use one or two "core sutures" implementing a braided, nonabsorbable material such as Tycron or Ethibond (usually 4-0 is a good size for the repair, depending on the patient's tendon size). If a running or interrupted epitenon repair is performed, ideally a fine monofilament material is implemented. This commonly will range from a 5-0 to a 7-0 with nylon being a frequently used material. Other suture material can be considered, depending on the surgeon's preference and experience. Appropriate suture for the wound closure will be needed (see Chapter 25, Laceration Repair: Suture Selection).

TECHNIQUE

Radiographic evaluation to the injured area is useful to rule out any residual foreign material that might still be present within the soft tissues. Sometimes, depending on the mechanism, an unsuspected fracture might even be present. This information might influence the treatment plan. After verifying appropriate anesthesia and completion of a thorough prep and drape, the wound should be explored carefully to further delineate the injury pattern. An additional irrigation and debridement might be necessary, depending on the nature of the injured tissues and if further foreign material is discovered. Any nonviable tissue must be removed. One should have little reluctance to extend the wound proximally and distally to understand the extent of the trauma, to satisfactorily visualize the damaged tissues, and to garner access to proximal and distal segments of the involved tendon(s). Electrocautery and a tourniquet are most useful to ensure appropriate hemostasis. Since these repairs can be quite tedious, most surgeons will perform these while seated in a comfortable chair with the patient's arm positioned out to the side on an arm board. The primary surgeon will usually have his back facing the patient's head, allowing greater access to the extensor portion of the forearm and

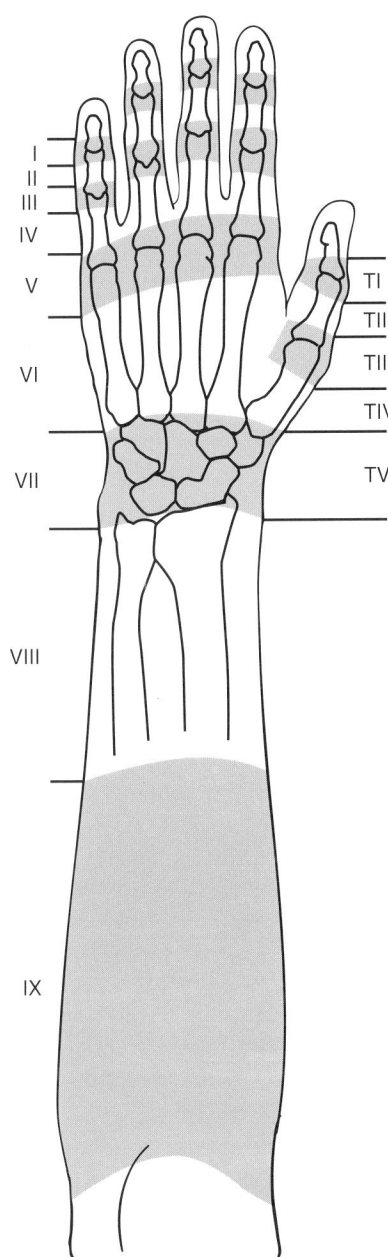

Fig. 191-2
Zones of extensor injury. The extensor mechanism can be injured from the fingertip to the proximal forearm. Corresponding zones in the thumb are referred to as "T" plus the zone number.

• Mask.
• Protective glasses with shield.
• Sterile gown.
• Arm board.
• Mayo or instrument holding stand.
• ¼-inch Penrose drain (to tag and protect critical structures).
• Appropriate finger or arm tourniquet (with routine use precautions).
• Comfortable chair.

hand. With a large sterile field including the elbow through hand and a sterile-gowned physician, contamination is less likely when positioning the patient and providing stable wrist supports for the surgeon performing these procedures.

Ragged tendon ends should be trimmed to allow a clean and direct reapproximation. It is imperative that the physician be familiar with the associated anatomy for consideration of possible neurovascular injury. If a neurovascular injury is discovered, further referral to an experienced upper extremity surgeon is warranted. If critical structures are near the repair area, the clinician should take special precaution to protect these structures. Incomplete tendon lacerations can be repaired directly or debrided if considered an insignificant portion of the tendon. Occasionally, a tendon is lacerated in an oblique fashion, which is usually amenable to a direct repair with a fine nonabsorbable material. Most surgeons recommend a direct end-to-end repair of transverse extensor tendon lacerations (rather than side-to-side). If a tendon has adequate substance, a "core" suture particularly with a braided, nonabsorbable material is implemented. Typically one or two "core" sutures are placed. The stitch ideally has a buried know (Fig. 191-3). A Kessler stitch or its modifications are commonly used. Many surgeons use an epitenon running suture with or without a "core" stitch. The epitenon repair usually is with a fine, monofilament, nonabsorbable material that is appropriate for the size of the structures being repaired (Fig. 191-4). Simple interrupted sutures commonly will fail through the tendon ends because of the fiber alignment. When the sutured tendon ends are brought together, a secured knot is present with minimal trauma to the tendon ends. During the repair, the tendon ends should be handled in an atraumatic technique with minimal tissue crushing. (Nontoothed forceps can be quite helpful.) The approximated tendon ends should not buckle or be compressed excessively. A flat end repair promotes proper healing and return of the proper gliding action to the tendon. Particular consideration to the anatomic zones are listed as follows.

BY THE ZONES

Zone I: Distal Interphalangeal (DIP) Joint

This is by definition a "mallet finger" unless the laceration is incomplete. These sometimes will progress to a "swan neck" deformity as the conjoined lateral bands sublux dorsally, resulting in proximal interphalangeal (PIP) joint hyperextension with the associated mallet deformity (flexion deformity at the DIP joint) (Fig. 191-1). Zone I injuries are commonly missed, especially when not associated with an open/laceration injury. These injuries usually occur when an athlete or manual laborer "jam" the fingertip. These frequently will lead to a poor outcome often needing a DIP fusion because the incomplete extensor mechanism at the unstable DIP joint interferes with dexterity and leads further to subsequent arthritic changes at this joint.

Zone I injuries are classified into four subtypes:

- Type I: Closed or blunt trauma with loss of tendon continuity with or without a small avulsion fracture
- Type II: Laceration proximal to the DIP joint with loss of tendon continuity
- Type III: Deep abrasion with loss of skin, subcutaneous cover, and tendon substance
- Type IV: (1) Transepiphyseal plate fracture in children, (2) hyperflexion injury with fracture of 20% to 50% of the articular surface, (3) hyperextension injury with fracture of the articular surface usually greater than 50% and with fairly early volar subluxation of the distal phalanx

A radiograph with careful detail particularly scrutinized from a lateral projection of the DIP joint should be obtained. Fractures noted (typically interarticular) should be stabilized appropriately. Commonly, the fracture will need to be pinned.

Treatment

If not open, all Zone I injuries should be splinted in extension or even hyperextension across the DIP joint (a digital block may be needed). Open lacerations can be repaired with care to avoid the vulnerable germinal nail matrix. These patients should be directed to a physician who is skilled in treating these injuries. A temporary, retrograde, buried pin in full extension is often better tolerated than external splinting.

Zone II: Middle Phalanx and Thumb Proximal Phalanx

Zone II injuries typically can be treated similarly to Zone I injuries. Many of these injuries are associated with a crush. The splint must be extended to include the PIP joint.

Zone III: Proximal Interphalangeal Joint

An injury at this location frequently will lead to a "Boutonniere" deformity (Fig. 191-1). A Zone III deformity (and the previously noted mallet finger) are the most commonly missed closed injuries of the hand. The central slip is injured and the lateral bands can migrate volar past the axis of rotation at the PIP, resulting in a PIP flexion contracture with or without hyperextension at the DIP joint. Many patients will have an associated collateral ligament or volar plate injury. If not

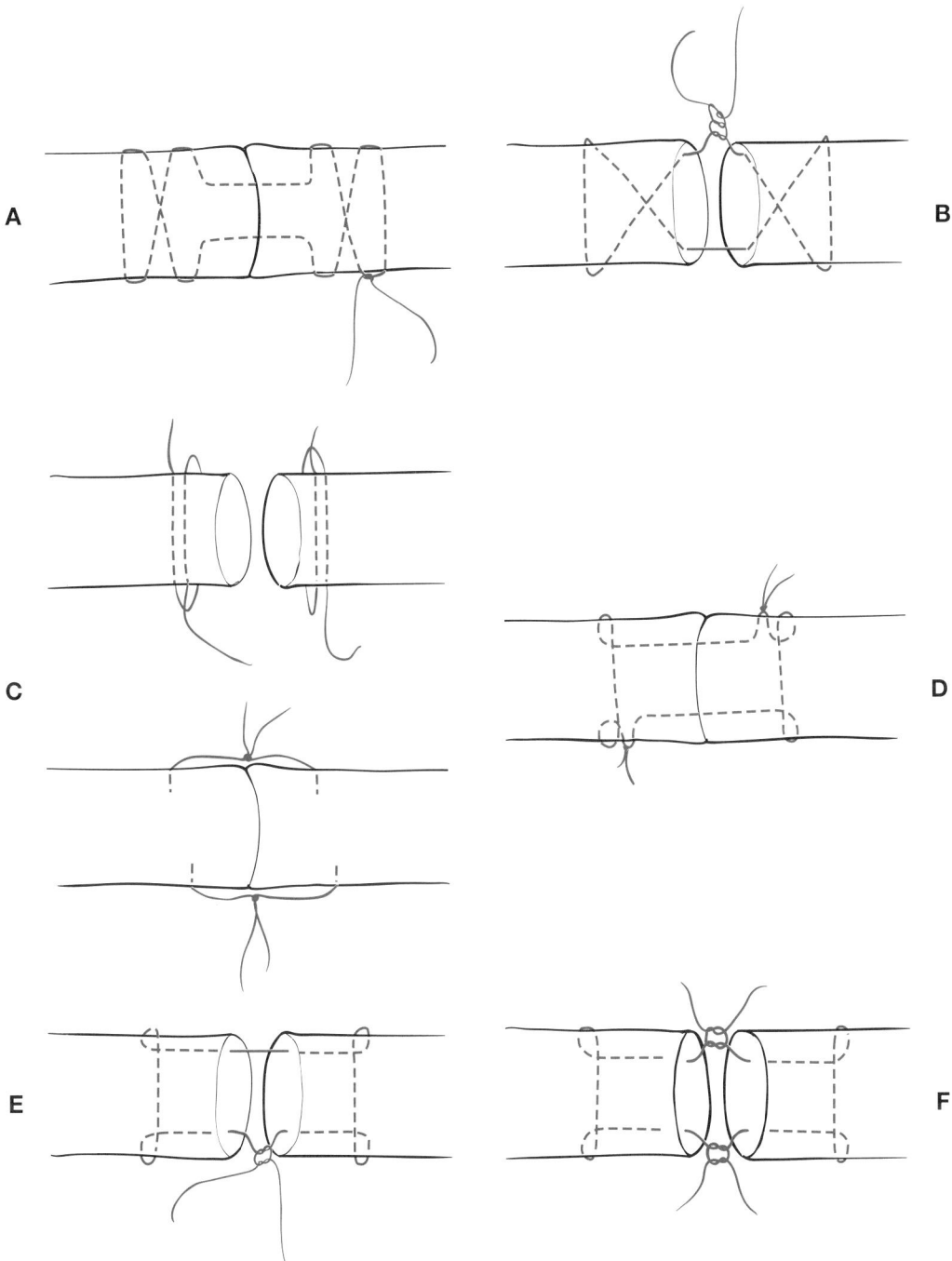

Fig. 191-3
Commonly used techniques for end-to-end tendon suture. **A,** Conventional Bunnell stitch. **B,** Crisscross stitch. **C,** Mason-Allen (Chicago) stitch. **D,** Kessler grasping stitch. **E,** Modified Kessler stitch with single buried knot. **F,** Tajima modification of Kessler stitch with double buried knots. (From Strickland JW: *J Am Acad Orthop Surg* 3:44, 1995.)

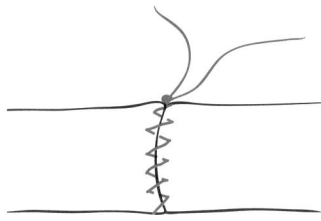

Fig. 191-4
Simple running suture used for peripheral epitenon tendon repair. A locked running suture can also be used for greater strength.

recognized and treated early, no good salvage operation can restore normal function to these injuries.

Treatment

The PIP should be splinted in extension, possibly incorporating the DIP joint in extension. The patient should be referred to a physician trained in these complex problems to have definitive care initiated within 7 to 10 days.

Zone IV: Proximal Phalanx

These are normally easy to identify. The lateral band extension expansion is rarely completely transected. A fine absorbable suture repair, followed by protected motion while the PIP joint is splinted in extension, is typically used. Consider a bite wound (see Zone V).

Zone V: Metacarpophalangeal (MP) Joint

Zone V injuries are *frequently* from a human tooth. Obtain a radiograph to rule out a fracture or foreign body. If there is *any* chance of a bite wound, it should be cleansed aggressively and *left open* with consideration of appropriate antibiotic coverage. Frequently, the MP joint capsule is penetrated. Thus these wounds should be opened, carefully explored in flexion and extension, and then normally left open. The hand should be splinted for later wound inspection and delayed tendon repair. An experienced practitioner can repair the wound primarily if it is considered *noncontaminated* and *not* associated with a bite wound.

Note: At this level, disruption of the sagittal bands of the extensor hood may occur (e.g., dislocation of the extensor tendon) acutely or spontaneously. These should be splinted and directed to a surgeon skilled with managing hand and tendon injuries.

Zone VI: Metacarpal Level

A primary repair can be pursued routinely. Buried core sutures are the typical technique used. The practitioner

must oversee a careful splinting and therapy program. Again, consider a bite wound.

Zone VII: Wrist Extensor Retinacular Area

Zone VII injuries may be repaired similarly to Zone VI injuries, realizing that the extensor retinaculum is involved and may need repair or resection. Posttraumatic adhesions are not uncommon and thus should be managed with added diligence during hand therapy.

Zone VIII: Distal Forearm

Zone VIII injuries may be treated similarly to Zone VI and VII injuries. At this level, adjacent structures can easily be injured, retracted, and difficult to appreciate. Sensory cutaneous nerves (radial branches and the antebrachial cutaneous nerve) should be protected carefully if in the field and repaired if observed to be lacerated.

Zone IX: Proximal Forearm

Zone IX injuries are frequently associated with neurovascular trauma. These injuries should be explored in an operating room by a surgeon skilled with these problems.

If the practitioner has experience with extensor tendon injuries and is comfortable with splinting and therapy programs, repairs of Zones IV through VI and maybe VIII can be addressed in an emergency room or an appropriately equipped office, if the inherent problems of each zone are understood. The remaining zones might be repaired in these settings relative to the physician's experience and available equipment. The potential complications associated with these injuries and their repairs must be followed carefully. Complications can be quite significant, including: primary failure of the repair, secondary later rupture of the tendon, stiffness, contractures with limited range of motion from resultant adhesions, residual pain, residual overlying tissue problems, infection, and problems related to other adjacent structures. The practitioner will never be faulted for leaving a wound open and splinted after an *aggressive* irrigation and debridement, especially over the MP joint. Ideally, tendon, bone, and joint tissues are kept moist within the wound with a damp sterile dressing to protect desiccation of these vulnerable structures.

Extensor tendon lacerations to the feet occur less frequently than the upper extremities because of activity patterns and protection that shoes and pants can provide. However, when these injuries do occur, they commonly are associated with additional significant trauma to other tissues including fractures. The physician must be diligent to rule out other possible injuries by considering associated anatomic structures and implementing appropriate radiographs. Isolated, lower extremity extensor tendon injuries otherwise might be managed in a similar fashion to the prior discussion regarding the correlating anatomic zones (e.g., a tendon injury at the ankle under the retinacular tissues would correlate to a Zone VII injury in the upper extremity). Foot flexor tendons should be addressed by a skilled surgeon in these areas. (It is not uncommon that an isolated flexor tendon laceration will be relatively well tolerated without repair.)

Physicians normally will give an appropriately dosed first- or second-generation cephalosporin for a clean open injury, which should provide satisfactory coverage for most gram-positive skin organisms. Consideration for gram-negative and anaerobic coverage should be entertained for contaminated wounds, especially if occurring at a farm. Cultures from contaminated wounds can be beneficial for subsequent antibiotic choices. Continued antibiotics are usually unnecessary unless there is gross contamination or a subsequent infection develops. It is safest to reevaluate these wounds and repairs at 2 to 3 days for possible early infection. Adjustment of antibiotic management might be necessary, especially when considering the patient's particular circumstances.

CPT/BILLING CODES

25270   Repair, tendon or muscle, extensor, forearm and/or wrist; *primary,* single, *each* tendon or muscle

25272   Repair, tendon or muscle, extensor, forearm and/or wrist; *secondary,* single, *each* tendon or muscle

26410   Repair, extensor tendon, dorsum of hand, single, primary or secondary; without free graft, each tendon

26418   Repair, extensor tendon, dorsum of finger, single, primary or secondary; without free graft, each tendon

26432   Closed treatment of distal extensor tendon insertion, with or without percutaneous pinning (e.g., mallet finger)

28208   Repair, tendon, extensor, foot; primary or secondary, each tendon

ICD-9-CM DIAGNOSTIC CODES

727.63   Other disorders of synovium, tendon, and bursa, rupture of tendon, nontraumatic, extensor tendons of hand and wrist

727.68   Other disorders of synovium, tendon, and bursa, rupture of tendon, nontraumatic, other tendons of foot and ankle

736.1   Other acquired deformities of limbs, mallet finger

882.2   Open wound of hand except fingers(s) alone, with tendon involvement

883.2   Open wound of fingers(s) with tendon involvement

892.2   Open wound of foot except toe(s) alone with tendon involvement

893.2   Open wound of toe(s) with tendon involvement

ADDITIONAL RESOURCES

• See the sample patient education handout titled "Repair of Extensor Tendon(s) Injury" on page 2000 of Appendix G.
• See the sample patient consent form titled "Repair of Extensor Tendon(s) Injury" on page 2001 of Appendix G.

BIBLIOGRAPHY

American Academy of Orthopaedic Surgeons: *CPT/ICD-9 cross-reference,* Rosemont, Ill, 2001, AAOS.

Dabezies EJ, Schutte JP: Fixation of metacarpal and phalangeal fratures with plates and screws, *J Hand Surg* 11:283, 1986.

Doyle JR: Extensor tendons: acute injuries. In Green DP, editor: *Operative hand surgery,* New York, 1999, Churchill-Livingstone.

Kleinert HE, Verdan C: Report of the committee on tendon injuries, *J Hand Surg* 8:794, 1983.

Newport ML, Blair WF, Steyers CM Jr: Long-term results of extensor tendon repair, *J Hand Surg* 15A:961, 1990.

Rosenthal EA: Extensor surface injuries at the proximal interphalangeal joint. In Bowers WH, editor: *The interphalangeal joints,* New York, 1987, Churchill-Livingstone.

Thompson DS, Peimer CA: Extensor tendon injuries: acute repair and late reconstruction. In Chapman MW, editor: *Operative orthopedics,* ed 2, Philadelphia, 1993, JB Lippincott.

Wright PE II: Flexor and extensor tendon injuries. In Canale ST, editor: *Campbell's operative orthopaedics,* ed 9, St Louis, 1998, Mosby.

CHAPTER 192

Fracture Care

Robert L. Kalb

Primary care clinicians are able to manage a wide range of fractures and obtain good clinical outcomes. It is important to have orthopedic rotation training, as well as supportive orthopedic backup. Primary care clinicians so equipped are able to manage more complicated fractures, including one third of fractures requiring reductions. A patient with multiple fractures or displaced, intraarticular, and epiphysial plate fractures should generally be referred to an orthopedic surgeon. Adverse outcomes can be avoided if primary care clinicians carefully select the fractures based on their level of training and use supportive backup when appropriate. This chapter covers the common guidelines for the management of fractures, which can be treated in the office by the primary care clinician.

Decisions regarding whether to manage a displaced fracture are often influenced by the state's malpractice insurance premiums. Fractures requiring reduction often require higher malpractice premiums. Those treating fractures, especially the ones that require reduction, must have a good working relationship with an orthopedic surgeon who will be willing to provide informal advice on questions of management and on specific cases. It is ideal to have a relationship with an orthopedist, who is willing to offer advice, examine the patient, and return the patient to the referring clinician for continued follow-up care.

All of the fractures discussed in this chapter can be treated in the office with local anesthesia. This chapter is intended to serve as a guide for the primary care practice. This text cannot possibly review the management of all fractures; rather, it provides a basic summary approach. Because the management of fractures differs so greatly in children than it does in adults, both patient populations are considered separately.

With all fractures, the first phase of healing involves osteoclasts going to the fracture site, causing reabsorption of the dead mineralized bone at the tip of the fractured bone. This reabsorption results in the fracture line (even in those fractures that are nondisplaced or initially only hairline cracks), appearing larger in the follow-up x-ray. As fracture healing occurs, callus forms, pain resolves, and tenderness becomes less. The radiograph will not show the fracture callus and healing until the later stage of mineralization of the callus. It is only when mineralization has occurred that the x-ray beam no longer easily penetrates the callus, which results in the image of healing observed on the x-ray film.

Box 192-1 lists types of casts, and Chapter 188, Cast Immobilization, contains more details on casts discussed in this chapter.

EQUIPMENT

- Cast material (plastic and fiberglass)
- One-step fiberglass prepadded splint material 3, 4, 5, and 6 inches
- Stockinette
- Cast padding: cotton Webril, synthetic Webril, or Gortex lining material to allow swimming in the cast
- Cast saw
- Cast spreader
- Cast scissors

TERMINOLOGY

Open fracture: A fracture that communicates through a hole in the skin, which by definition is therefore contaminated and more likely to become infected if the hole is greater than 1 cm in diameter. Open fractures should almost always be referred to an orthopedic surgeon. (The old term *compound fracture* is the same as open fracture.)

Closed fractures: All fractures, which are not openly communicating with a hole in the skin. The vast majority of fractures are closed, and the skin is not broken.

Torus fractures: A fracture in which only one of the cortices is buckled.

Greenstick fracture: A greenstick fracture is one level worse than a torus fracture. It involves an actual crack or disruption of one cortex and often a buckling of the opposite cortex. This fracture is so named because it represents a deformation of the bone, much like cracking a green twig on an apple tree in springtime. The tension side of the bent twig cracks, whereas the compression side (i.e., the concave side) buckles but does not crack.

Comminuted fracture: A fracture in which the bone is in more than two pieces. Often an additional piece, which is small and shaped like a butterfly and therefore named a *butterfly fragment,* is found at the fracture site.

Fracture dislocation: A joint dislocation associated with a fracture of the bone on one or both sides of the joint, which is dislocated.

Intraarticular fractures: Fractures that extend into the joint or articular surface. If an intraarticular fracture is displaced, the patient should be referred to an orthopedic surgeon.

Delayed union: A fracture that is not healed in twice the normal healing time is called a delayed union. For example, a radius fracture with an expected healing time of 2 months would be considered a delayed union if it had not healed in 4 months.

Nonunion: The fracture has not united with bone during a time interval of three times the normal expected healing time. For example, a distal radius fracture is expected to heal completely in 2 months. If a distal radius fracture has not healed in three times that amount or 6 months, it is considered a nonunion fracture.

Atrophic nonunion: A bone end near the fracture becomes pointed like a partially consumed pepper-mint stick or icicle without any sign of new bone formation.

Hypertrophic nonunion: The bone end forms new bone even though it is not united.

Malunion: A fracture has united with unacceptable angulation, rotation, or shortening.

FRACTURES IN ADULTS

Cervical Spine Fractures

The possibility of a cervical spine fracture being unstable and the predisposition to spinal cord complications should always be considered. The exception would be a fracture involving only the spinous process. This type of fracture is referred to as a *clayshovelers' fracture* and represents only an avulsion as a result of stress on the interspinous ligaments. These spinous process fractures require nothing more than a soft cervical collar and symptomatic management. The radiologist or orthopedist can review the x-ray studies to confirm the existence of no other associated problems.

Thoracic Spine Fractures

A thoracic spine fracture can be treated symptomatically with back support and with minimal trauma, provided the fracture is the typical compression type occurring in an older osteoporotic patient. Thoracic spine fractures after a high-velocity injury, such as a motor vehicle accident or fall from a height greater than 6 feet and all those that occur in patients under 60 years of age, should generally be referred for orthopedic surgical consultation to rule out instability, which may require surgical stabilization.

Lumbar Spine Fractures

Lumbar spine fractures are generally treated similarly to thoracic spine fractures. With a patient who has an *os calcis fracture,* always x-ray the lumbar spine, because the axial loading injury associated with an os calcis injury is often associated with a lumbar spine fractures and an ileus. Sky diving injuries commonly result in fractures of the thoracic or lumbar spine.

Pelvic Fracture

A pelvic fracture tends to occur in osteoporotic older patients after a fall. Appropriate views to assess the pelvic fracture include inlet and outlet, anteroposterior (AP) pelvis, and oblique views of the acetabulum. A radiologist or orthopedist will be able to determine from these views whether any question of acetabular involvement remains. If so, the patient should be referred if there is any associated displacement. If the fracture involves only the pubic or ischial rami, the patient can be treated with walking as tolerated or full weight-bearing walking with a walker. Although walking may be uncomfortable, explain to the patient that it is not dangerous or harmful. The pubic and ischial rami both function only as tie rods for the anterior portions of the pelvis and do not participate in weight-bearing activities. The typical older woman who falls and breaks her pelvis has a pubic or ischial ramus fracture only and does not require bed rest or surgical intervention (Fig. 192-1). Always observe for shock, and check for hematuria with a urinalysis.

If the pelvis fracture occurs in anyone under 50 years of age or in individuals involved in a motor vehicle accident, refer them to an orthopedist for evaluation and for other associated injuries, especially to the sacroiliac joint. Always palpate the sacroiliac joint to ensure that it is nontender and therefore not involved with the injury.

Intertrochanteric Femur Fractures

The *intertrochanteric femur fracture* (Fig. 192-2) is the most common type of hip fracture. It is extracapsular and involves either the greater or lesser trochanteric area of the proximal femur or hip or both. Neither this fracture nor the femoral neck fracture involves the hip joint itself; therefore both types are extraarticular fractures. The intertrochanteric fracture results from the patient tripping over a carpet, pet, or step or slipping and falling. With the intertrochanteric fracture, it is the force of the direct fall onto the intertrochanteric area that results in the fracture. This scenario is entirely different from the femoral neck stress fracture discussed below. The intertrochanteric fracture always requires hip pinning with a compression screw and bone plate device. For this reason, these patients should be referred to an orthopedic surgeon. The intertrochanteric fracture, even if nondisplaced, is at high risk for displacement even with rolling over and moving in bed. For this reason, it should not be treated without surgery.

Neck of Femur Fracture

Fracture of the femoral neck (Fig. 192-2) is the second most common type of hip fracture. It typically occurs in the older osteoporotic patient who is walking in the home and the hip suddenly gives way and the patient falls to the floor for no apparent reason. No history of tripping over a carpet, pet, or step is reported. The patient does not know the reason for the fall. The fracture through the neck of the femur is actually a stress fracture, which ultimately becomes complete, resulting in instability that causes the patient to fall. Most of these

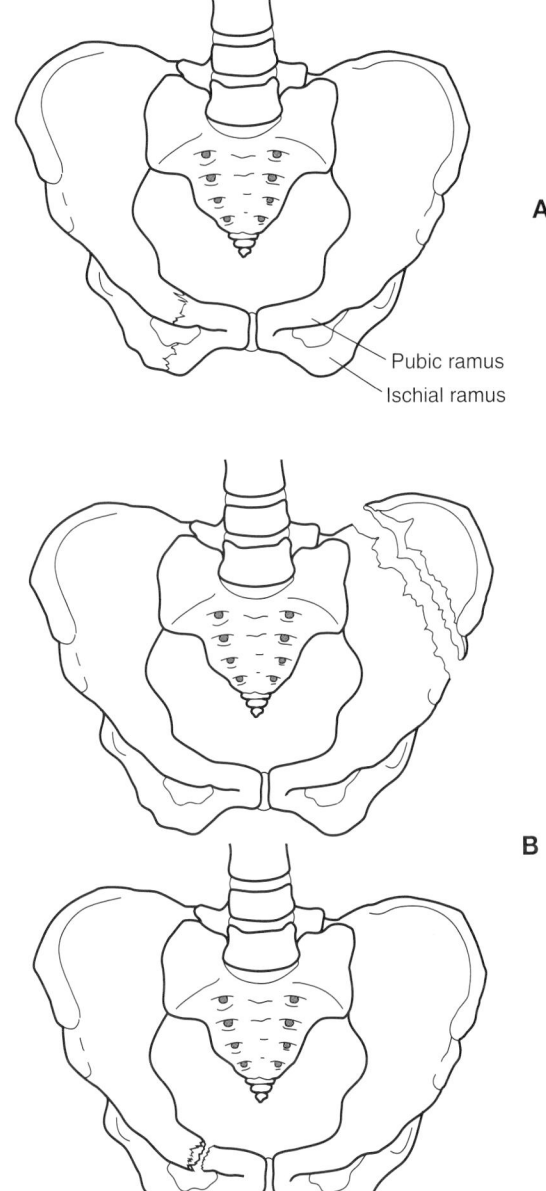

A

Pubic ramus
Ischial ramus

B

Fig. 192-1
Pelvic fractures. **A,** Stable. **B,** Tile classification of pelvic disruption. *Top,* Fractures of the pelvis not involving the ring. *Bottom,* Stable, minimally displaced fractures of the ring.

fractures are displaced and appropriately treated with a prosthetic replacement (one half of a total hip). Sometimes these fractures are nondisplaced and can be treated with pinning.

If a patient does not have a history of falling but complains of pain in the groin aggravated by walking and weight-bearing activity, rule out hip osteoarthritis with a weight-bearing radiograph. Always be certain to order a true lateral radiograph of the hip because it will often show a fracture not visible on the plain AP or "frog leg" AP view. If the hip joint is free of osteoarthritic findings, a diagnosis of *impending stress fracture* should be considered. In some patients, the fracture is not visible on the radiograph but can be observed on a magnetic resonance image (MRI). The MRI is now the standard of care evaluation technique because it is more sensitive and specific than either a bone scan or a computed tomographic (CT) scan in diagnosing femoral neck stress fractures. Patients with nondisplaced stress fractures in progress demonstrated by bone or MRI can be treated with a walker and no weight-bearing activity on the involved side. This treatment often allows the fracture to heal completely and prevents surgery.

Femoral Shaft Fractures

Femoral shaft fractures should always be referred for surgical stabilization. These fractures are at high risk for fat embolism and neurovascular problems. A distal femur fracture, which is often intraarticular (extending into the knee joint), should always be referred for surgical intervention to stabilize the fracture. This is true even if the fracture is nondisplaced.

Patella Fractures

A nondisplaced patella fracture (Fig. 192-3), whether comminuted or not, is treated with a cylinder, full weight-bearing walking cast or with a knee immobilizer, crutches, and 10% partial weight-bearing activities. A follow-up clinical examination is performed, and AP and

lateral radiographs are assessed 3 weeks after treatment. If no displacement exists and tenderness with palpation is resolved, then gentle non–weight-bearing range-of-motion exercises can be started in an arch of 0 to 45 degrees. Another x-ray film should be obtained 6 weeks after treatment. At this point, the fracture should be solidly healed and point tenderness over the patella should be resolved. Active and passive range-of-motion movements can now be initiated in therapy. During the healing phase, the patient should be encouraged to carry out quadriceps and hamstring isometrics and straight-leg raising exercises to maintain muscle function and tone.

Fibula Fractures

Fibula fractures require no immobilization or restriction of weight-bearing activities because the fibula contributes only 15% of weight bearing to the lower extremity. The fibula can be used for bone graft without a problem. *Fibula fractures, however, rarely occur alone.* Always check for associated injury around the ankle, over the medial and lateral collateral ligaments, and the tibiofibular distal joint. It is common for a severe ankle-twisting injury to result in a small fracture around the ankle and a fracture anywhere along the fibula, including the proximal fibula. Isolated fibula fractures can occur from

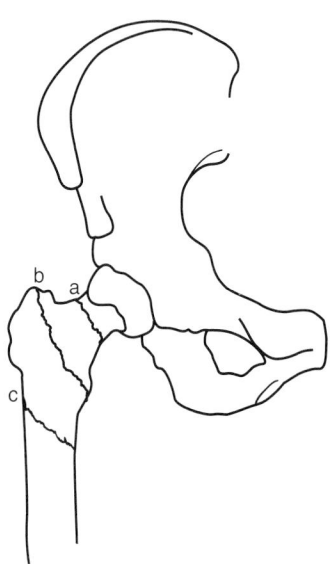

Fig. 192-2
Proximal femur fractures. *a,* Neck; *b,* intertrochanteric; *c,* subtrochanteric.

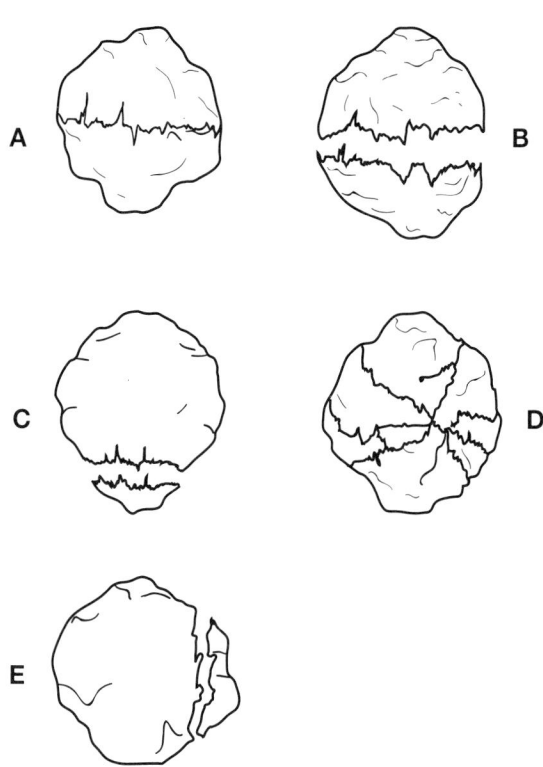

Fig. 192-3
Classification of patellar fractures. **A,** Nondisplaced transverse. **B,** Displaced transverse. **C,** Upper or lower pole. **D,** Comminuted. **E,** Vertical.

a blow directly to the side of the calf. Again, these fractures require no immobilization or restriction of weight-bearing activities and always heal uneventfully.

Always evaluate the function of the *peroneal nerve* when treating a fibula fracture by documenting the strength of active foot extension at the ankle, as well as eversion. If the peroneal nerve function is absent, document this during examination. No further treatment is required because the peroneal nerve, if injured, can only be observed to determine if and when it will recover. Surgical exploration or intervention for peroneal neuropraxia is not performed acutely.

Tibial Plateau Fracture

The clinician should be certain that a tibial plateau fracture is nondisplaced, especially if it extends into the joint surface. Tomograms are the only method to confirm no displacement. *If any displacement has* *occurred, the patient must be referred to an orthopedic* *surgeon for surgical intervention.* If the fracture is extraarticulary displaced and intrarticulary nondisplaced, it can be treated with crutches, non–weight-bearing activities for 3 months, and gentle active range-of-motion movements. These fractures need to be watched carefully with a clinical examination and radiographic recheck evaluation at 2-week intervals for the first month to be certain of no displacement, which can occur with motion of the knee joint. Again, be certain to document the strength of the peroneal nerve (see above).

Tibial Fractures

Tibial fractures (Fig. 192-4) involving the *shaft* of the tibia can be treated with a long leg cast with the knee in 30 degrees flexion and the ankle in neutral position (right angle).

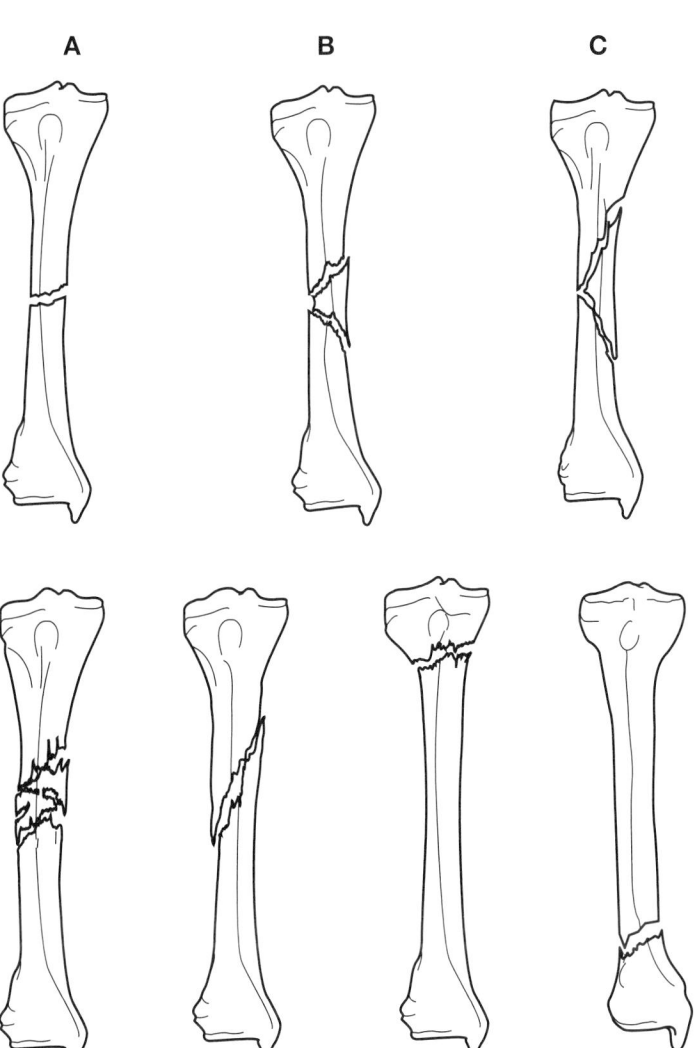

Fig. 192-4
Tibial shaft fractures. **A,** Transverse or short oblique. **B,** Small butterfly fragment. **C,** Large butterfly fragment. **D,** Segmental comminution. **E,** Spiral. **F,** Proximal one-fourth transverse or oblique. **G,** Distal one-fourth transverse or oblique. **A** is usually stable. The stability of **B** and **C** is dependent on the size of the butterfly fragment. Type **D** is usually unstable; types **E, F,** and **G** are stable but difficult to control.

If any *angulation* of the tibia shaft fracture has occurred, a *goniometer* must be used to assess the amount. Angulation up to 5 degrees in the AP radiograph and up to 10 degrees in the lateral radiograph is acceptable. Angulation over these amounts requires correction by wedging the cast.

Shortening greater than 2 cm is not acceptable and requires referral for surgical treatment. If any doubt about the amount of overlap remains, a bone length measurement radiograph can be provided by the radiologist to compare the length of one tibia with the other.

If less than 50% bone surface contact is observed in the AP or lateral views, then the patient should be referred to an orthopedic surgeon for fracture reduction.

If the fracture is satisfactory in alignment and length, then non–weight-bearing activities and a long leg cast for a period of 4 to 6 weeks is appropriate. At that point the cast is cut down to a short leg level and gentle weight-bearing movements are started for the remaining 2 additional months while in the short leg cast.

Tibia fractures are notorious for developing *compartment syndrome* (see Chapter 189, Compartment Syndrome Evaluation) when any significant soft-tissue trauma has occurred. If the tibia fracture is the result of a fall from a height greater than 6 feet or the result of a high-velocity injury such as in an automobile accident, be very cautious of compartment syndrome development. Be certain that the patient elevates the leg at home so that the calf is 2 feet higher than the heart at all times for 1 week. This elevation minimizes the chance of compartment syndrome development. Explain to the patient that the heart is the pump and that the fluid from the leg needs to drain toward the pump, which requires the fluid in the leg to be elevated higher than the pump. Seat cushions from the couch stacked three high under the calf can help achieve this elevation. The patient's chest must be flat, although pillows can be placed under the head to facilitate reading and eating. Sitting in a Laz-E-Boy recliner, however, does not provide adequate elevation because the chest is at the level of the calf.

Patients may use their crutches to go to the bathroom, placing no weight on the injured side. They should return to the bed, couch, or floor, lie down, and resume elevation of the leg as soon as possible. If there is loss of fine-touch sensation, distension and swelling of the calf, or pain is not relieved by oral pain medication, then immediate referral should be carried out in an emergency manner to rule out compartment syndrome (see Chapter 189, Compartment Syndrome Evaluation). Compartment syndrome after a tibia fracture can occur up to 10 days after the fracture. *The peak time for compartment syndrome after a tibia fracture is on the third day after the injury.*

For tibia fractures in which the fibula is not broken, very little chance exists of the tibia becoming unacceptably shortened because the fibula will splint the soft tissue at an appropriate length. *If the fibula is broken in addition to the tibia,* then a higher incidence of shortening of the tibia fracture exists as a result of unopposed muscle contraction. This is especially true in an oblique angle fracture. The oblique angle allows sliding of the fracture into a shortened position. If the fracture is transverse, then this sliding shortening cannot occur.

Ankle Fractures

Point tenderness over the lateral malleolus (distal fibula) or medial malleolus (distal tibia) distinguishes an ankle fracture from a sprain. If no point tenderness is felt over the malleoli, then an x-ray is not necessary. Point tenderness over the lateral ligaments (anterior talofibular and calcaneal fibular ligament) indicates an ankle sprain. A *first-degree ankle sprain* will have tenderness only over the anterior talofibular ligament, whereas a *second- or third-degree ankle sprain* has tenderness over the anterior talofibular ligament and the calcaneal fibular ligament, which lies more posterior.

Small fragment avulsion fractures, nondisplaced single malleolar fractures, and stable bimalleolar fractures can be treated nonoperatively.

Medial Malleolar (Distal Tibia) Fractures

If nondisplaced in the AP, lateral, and mortis views of the ankle, then treatment of medial malleolar fractures with a short leg cast is appropriate. If the fracture line is below (distal to) the level of the ankle mortis, immediate full weight-bearing activities may be allowed. If the fracture is at or above the ankle mortis, 2 weeks of non-weight-bearing movements followed by another 4 weeks with weight-bearing activities while in the cast is appropriate. (The ankle mortis is the joint space on the mortis view x-ray between the top of the talus and the bottom of the tibia.)

Medial and lateral malleolar fractures require a minimum of 6 weeks for healing. If the patient smokes, the fracture healing time can be doubled. If the medial malleolar fracture is displaced, refer the patient to an orthopedic surgeon.

Lateral Malleolar (Distal Fibula) Fractures

There are three types of *distal fibula fractures*. A *Weber A* is the first type and occurs below the level of the ankle mortis. It can be treated with an immediate weight-bearing short leg cast for 6 weeks. (Remember, the ankle mortis is the joint space on the mortis view x-ray between the top of the talus and bottom of the tibia.)

A *Weber B* is the second type of fibula fracture, which

occurs at the level of the ankle mortis. Again, if the AP, lateral, and mortis x-ray views show the fracture to be nondisplaced, it can be treated with a short leg walking cast for 6 weeks. Because this fracture is at the level of the ankle mortis, no weight-bearing activities are allowed for the first 2 weeks. This restriction prevents stress at the ankle mortis, which could cause displacement at the fracture site from weight-bearing activities.

A *Weber C* distal fibula fracture is the third type of lateral malleolus fracture. It occurs above the ankle mortis and has the greatest potential for displacement. This fracture includes a portion of the syndesmotic ligament area between the tibia and fibula distally, just above the ankle mortis. The portion of the syndesmotic ligament from the ankle mortis up to the level of the fracture is always disrupted in order for the fracture to occur at this height. This fracture is also treated in a walking cast for 6 weeks with no weight-bearing activities during the first 3 weeks.

Note: A cast boot must be prescribed for any patient wearing a short leg splint or cast or a long leg splint or cast. The cast boot protects the toes and cast and prevents material from slipping through the end of the cast up underneath the foot.

Again, medial and lateral malleolar fractures require a minimum of 6 weeks for healing. Beware of delayed union and prolonged healing time in individuals who smoke or in those who are taking antiinflammatory medications. Both *smoking and antiinflammatory medications delay fracture union.* Patients with fractures should be informed of this fact and strongly advised to discontinue smoking and antiinflammatory medication. Patients should also be informed that the incidence of *reflex sympathetic dystrophy* after any injury, including a fracture, is much higher when they smoke. The incidence of postfracture stiffness in the joint (especially at the elbow and where the fracture extends into the joint) is dramatically increased in patients who have diabetes or in those who smoke. Patients can understand this when they understand that diabetes and smoking have similar effects on the capillary blood flow.

It is now known that *reflex sympathetic dystrophy* involves, in fact, a shut down of the capillary circulation system and results in arterial blood being shunted in a bypass fashion from arterioles to venules without adequate capillary profusion. This phenomenon has been demonstrated by sampling the oxygen content of venous blood in the involved extremity compared with the uninvolved extremity. The oxygen content in the venous blood in an extremity with reflex sympathetic dystrophy is higher, which is due to the oxygen not being taken out by the tissues, as it would be if the blood were supplied normally to the capillary system.

Talus Fracture

A nondisplaced talus fracture is treated with a short leg non–weight-bearing cast for 1 month followed by an additional month of weight-bearing activities while in the cast. If displacement has occurred, the patient should be referred to an orthopedic surgeon. The patient should be aware that despite perfect reduction, healing is often complicated by avascular necrosis. The nonunion rate is 50%; and an associated high incidence of osteoarthritis exists. A talus fracture is second only to the scaphoid fracture in the wrist as the site for chronic postfracture pain and complications.

Calcaneus Fracture

Obtain axial, lateral, and oblique radiographs of the calcaneus. If any doubt remains about displacement, obtain a CT scan. A radiologist or an orthopedist can offer suggestions on when to obtain the CT scan by viewing the plain radiographs of the calcaneus. If intraarticular displacement has occurred, refer the patient for consideration for open reduction and internal fixation.

A radiograph of the thoracic and lumbar spine must be obtained because of the high incidence of associated axial fractures. This association is due to the os calcis fracture almost always being an axial-loading injury, such as falling from a ladder. These injuries have a high incidence of thoracic and lumbar spine fractures. The clinician must palpate the thoracic and lumbar spine in these patients and always check for ileus, which can occur up to 3 days after the fractures of the thoracic and lumbar spine.

If the os calcis fracture is nondisplaced, a compression soft wrap without a splint or cast is the appropriate treatment. The patient must avoid all weight-bearing activities for a minimum of 3 months and longer if the patient smokes or uses antiinflammatory medications. Plaster and fiberglass, either splint or cast, is not an appropriate treatment for an os calcis fracture. Only early gentle active range-of-motion movements are appropriate to minimize stiffness associated with these fractures. Maximal elevation is critical to minimize swelling and pain. Elevation with the patient lying down and the hip and knee flexed to 90 degrees with couch cushions under the calf is best at all times for the first week. Patients may be up on crutches to go to the bathroom; otherwise they are to be supine with the leg elevated.

If the patient is not instructed to keep the hip and knee bent 90 degrees with the elevation, then they will complain of sciatica. This complication is due to placing pillows or blankets underneath the heel, which results in the knee being straight and provides stretch on the sciatic nerve.

Midfoot Tarsal Bone (Cuneiforms, Cuboid, Navicular) Fractures

If fractures of midfoot tarsal bones are nondisplaced, apply a short leg walking cast with weight-bearing activities as tolerated after the first week. The cast should be in place for 5 weeks. If displaced, refer the patient to an orthopedic surgeon. Beware of a fracture of the *Lis-franc joint*, which is a fracture that extends into the tarsometatarsal joint at the midfoot. Always obtain AP and lateral radiographs when an injury occurs to the bridge of the foot. It is critical not to miss an unstable fracture of this area. The fracture may appear nondisplaced on the AP view; however, on the lateral view, an anterior displacement may be observed at the joint. Always check the base of the second metatarsal where there is a lock-and-key configuration to the midfoot and ensure that there is no involvement or displacement at this level. If any questions remain about an injury to the midfoot or about the radiographic views, ask an orthopedic surgeon or a radiologist to review the films in consultation. These fractures are rare because of the rigidity of the midfoot.

Metatarsal Fractures

Beware of the most common fracture, which occurs at the base of the fifth metatarsal and represents an avulsion fracture. The peroneus brevis tendon inserts into this area. With an inversion sprain mechanism to the forefoot and ankle, a small piece of bone can be pulled loose. The displacement is usually no greater than 3 mm; whether displaced or not, it is treated with a wooden sole fracture shoe with weight-bearing activities as tolerated, as well as ice and elevation for comfort. Weight-bearing movement is allowed with this injury because the fracture is stable and a cast is not required. The purpose of the wooden sole shoe is to prevent flexion at the midfoot when the patient walks, thereby preventing stress at the fracture site. The wooden sole shoe is worn for 3 weeks or longer until the patient is comfortable without it and can return to wearing a regular shoe. However, sports should be avoided for a minimum of 2 months.

A metatarsal fracture must be differentiated from a true *Jones fracture*, which is much less common and treated entirely differently. The true Jones fracture occurs in nearly the same location and extends across the entire shaft just distal to the base of the fifth metatarsal. If displaced, the patient should be referred to an orthopedic surgeon. If nondisplaced, treatment includes a short leg walking cast with non–weight-bearing activities for the first 3 weeks. This fracture is notorious for delayed union, especially in those who smoke or in patients taking antiinflammatory medication. No sport should be allowed after this injury for a minimum of 3 months.

Clinicians must beware of *compartment syndrome* in the foot. With multiple fractures of three or more metatarsals from a crushing-type injury, extreme swelling can occur in the foot, which requires decompression for compartment syndrome. This occurrence is rare, but it can develop. Elevation is critical in any crush or high-velocity injury in which soft tissue–associated damage is greater than that with a low velocity–force injury. A patient with multiple metatarsal fractures must also be treated similarly to those with a calcaneus fracture, which includes the 90-degree hip and knee flexion position and elevation with four couch cushions under the calf at all times for 1 week.

Fractures of multiple metatarsals 2, 3, 4, and 5 at the shaft level require cast treatment, as do *isolated fractures of the great toe metatarsal*. The patient should be restricted to no weight-bearing for 2 weeks, followed by a gradual return to weight-bearing as tolerated while in the cast for a total of 6 weeks. Most fractures involve the second, third, fourth, or fifth metatarsals alone and are *single* metatarsal fractures. Isolated single metatarsal fractures, including the first metatarsal and fractures of more than one of the lesser metatarsals, require cast treatment.

Toe Fractures

Rarely is surgical intervention required, even when the fractures are displaced. Displaced fractures can be managed by reduction of the fracture after a digital block anesthetic followed by manual traction and pulling the toe into a corrected position. Buddy taping the involved toe to the adjacent toe for 3 weeks stabilizes the fracture. When taping digits together (fingers or toes), place dry cotton between the toes or fingers to prevent skin maceration from moisture. Patients can change their dressing after a shower.

Fractures in the distal phalanges of the fingers or toes sometimes involve injury to the nail bed and an open fracture caused by the bone pushing up through the nail bed. In these patients, the treatment should be a digital block anesthetic followed by removal of the nail to irrigate the nail bed thoroughly at the site of the open fracture. The nail bed can be repaired with 5-0 absorbable suture, which will prevent nail deformity. Nail bed repair is more appropriate for the fingers than the toes because many individuals will accept some deformity of the nail plate in the toe but they have more cosmetic concerns when deformity occurs in the finger (see Chapter 29, Nail Bed Repair).

Clavicle Fractures

Treatment is symptomatic with figure-eight brace or sling or both or neither, depending on patient's comfort level (see Fig. 192-8). If the clavicle fracture site results in pressure and tenting of the skin, refer the patient for possible surgery. Clavicle fractures (Fig. 192-5) require a

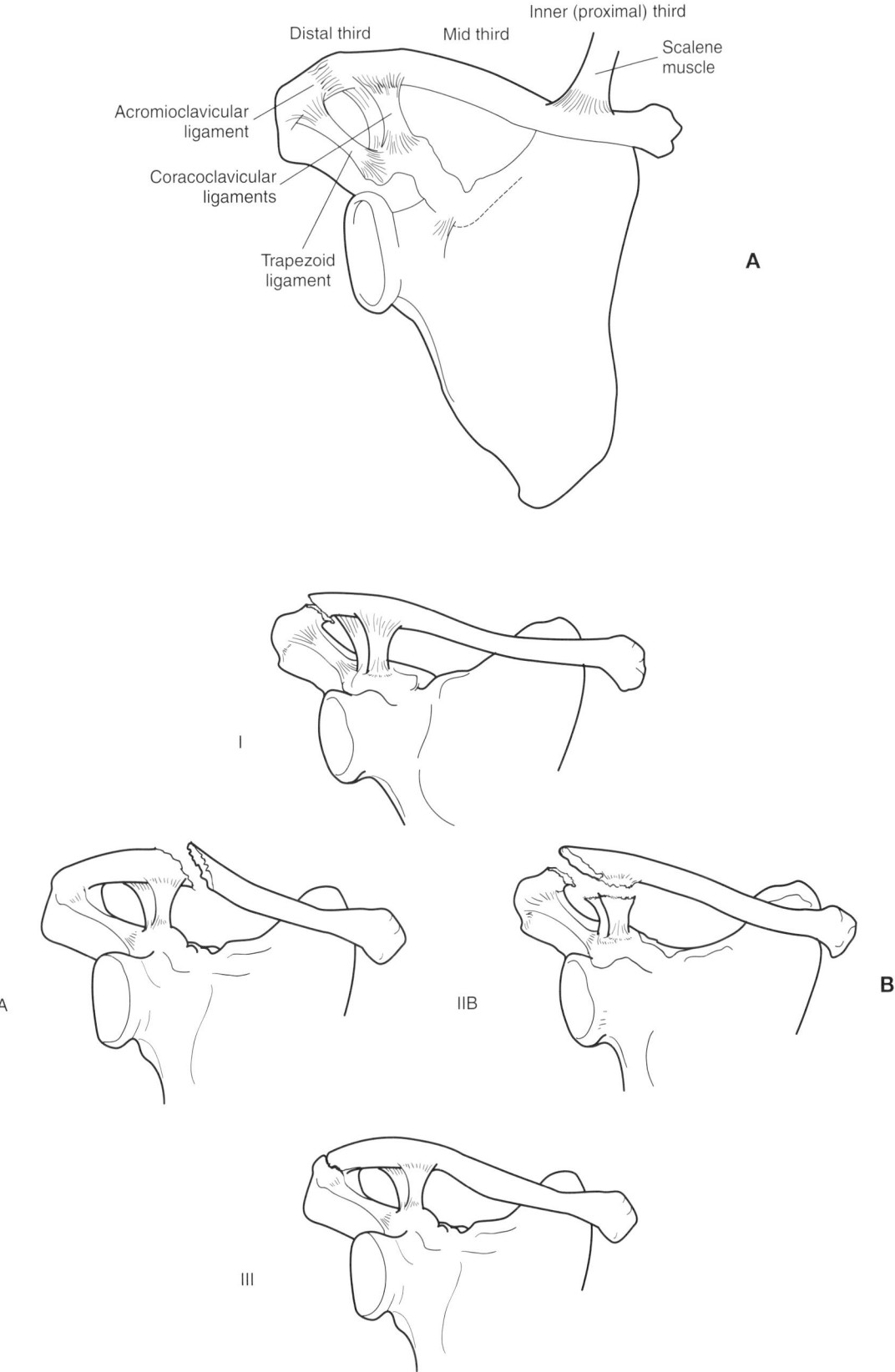

Fig. 192-5
Clavicle fracture. **A,** Fractures of the clavicle are classified by location into the distal (15%), middle (80%), and proximal third (5%). Clavicle fractures can be nondisplaced, displaced, angulated, or nonangulated. **B,** Classification of fractures of the distal third of the clavicle (Allman). Type I: minimal displacement with ligaments intact. Type IIA: proximal shaft is displaced with ligaments intact. Type IIB: Corroid ligament is ruptured but trapezoid ligament is intact. Type III: fracture of the articular surface with no disruption of the ligaments.

minimum 2 months for solid union, and contact sports should be avoided 4 months after a clavicle fracture. Remember to adjust the figure-eight splint to ensure that it is tight enough to be supportive yet loose enough to avoid tingling and numbness as a result of pressure on the brachial plexus as the splint wraps around the armpit. Instruct the patient to loosen or tighten the brace for more support, if needed, or to reduce restriction, if tingling and numbness occurs.

Always listen to the chest to ensure that no pneumothorax develops related to the clavicle fracture, especially for those fractures that occur with motor vehicle acci-dents. A chest x-ray is also appropriate. Instruct the patient to report any shortness of breath immediately.

Do not be dismayed if the 1-month follow-up x-ray shows no sign of healing. See the earlier discussion.

Scapula Fractures

The scapula is covered on all sides with muscle and therefore has excellent blood supply. For these reasons, fractures of the scapula (Fig. 192-6) heal extremely well, even when displaced. All fractures of the scapula are treated closed with a sling or shoulder immobilizer for comfort (only if needed) for 2 weeks. Range-of-motion movement of the shoulder and use of the upper extrem-ity on the side of the fracture is encouraged to minimize stiffness in the shoulder joint. In these fractures, always obtain a true AP of the glenohumeral (shoulder) joint and a true lateral scapula Y view. These views will demon-strate any intraarticular extension into the glenoid shoul-der socket. If any question remains about a fracture being intraarticular and displaced at the glenoid, then a CT scan should be assessed. If it confirms displacement, then referral to an orthopedic surgeon should be made. If no displacement is present, early range-of-motion move-ment should be used, when tolerated.

Proximal Humerus Fractures

It is a necessity to obtain true AP and scapula Y views. Fractures involving the greater tuberosity (Fig. 192-7) with displacement should be referred to an orthopedic surgeon. Most fractures in older patients are of the surgical neck. As long as 50% overlap of bone is seen on the AP and scapula Y views, treatment with a shoulder immobilizer for 2 weeks is appropriate, followed by gentle passive and active assistive range-of-motion movements of the shoulder to minimize stiffness (Fig. 192-8). The shoulder immobilizer is worn 24 hours a

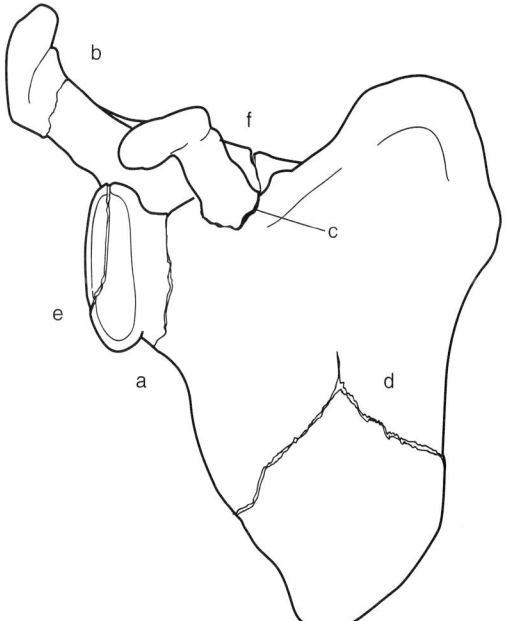

Fig. 192-6
Scapula fractures (anterior view). *a,* Neck; *b,* acromion process; *c,* coracoid process; *d,* body; *e,* glenoid rim or articular cartilage; *f,* spinous process, which is posterior and only partially seen here.

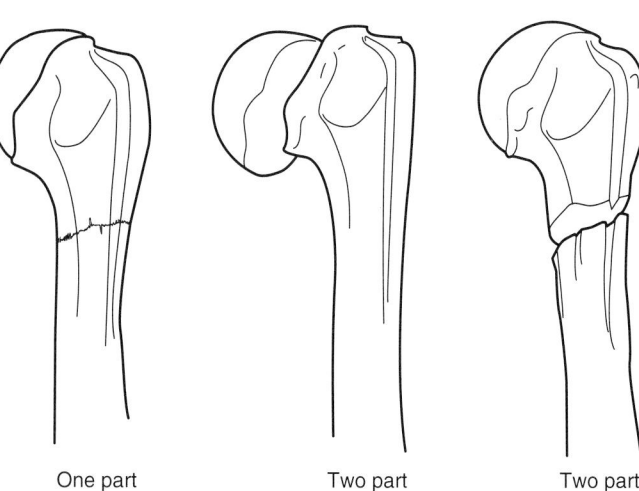

Fig. 192-7
Neer classification of proximal humerus fractures. One part or mini-mally displaced fracture occurs when no segments are displaced by more than 1.0 cm or angulated more than 45 degrees. A two-part fracture is one in which one segment is significantly displaced by more than 1.0 cm or more than 45 degrees.

One part   Two part   Two part

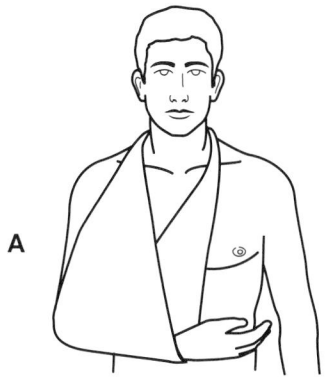

A

Simple shoulder sling used
for humerus, clavicle, and
radial head fractures.

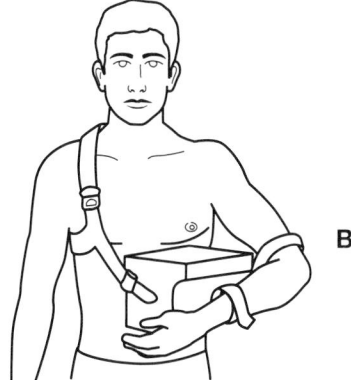

B

Abduction pillow shoulder
immobilizer used for rotator
cuff tendon tear after surgery.

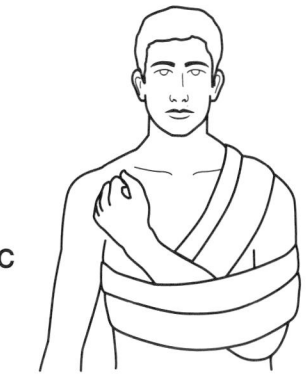

C

Sling and swathe bandage used
for severe acromioclavicular
separation and fractures of
upper humerus.

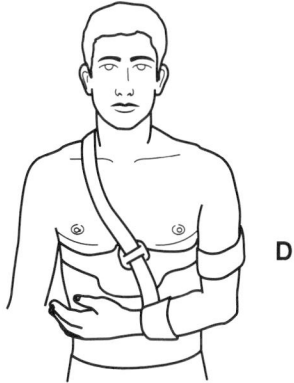

D

Shoulder immobilizer used
for humeral neck fractures.

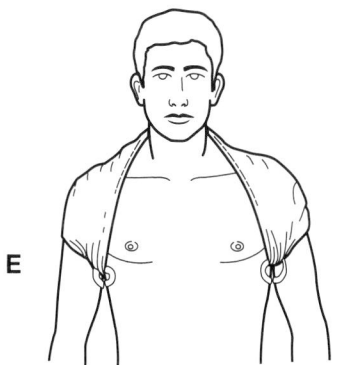

E

Figure-of-eight strap for
fractures of the clavicle.

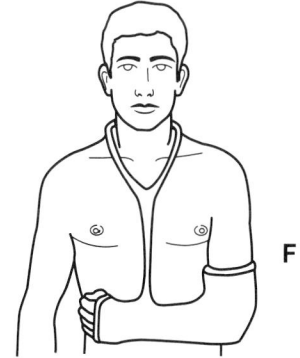

F

The hanging arm cast used
for humeral neck and humeral
shaft fractures. Provides
weight and traction to align
the fracture pieces.

Fig. 192-8
Possible methods of immobilization of the shoulder. **A,** Simple shoulder sling. Used for humerus, clavicle, and radial head fractures. **B,** Abduction pillow shoulder immobilizer used for rotator cuff tendon tear after surgery. **C,** Sling and swathe bandage used for severe acromioclavicular separation and fractures of upper humerus. **D,** Shoulder immobilizer used for humeral neck fractures. **E,** Figure-of-eight strap for fractures of the clavicle. **F,** The hanging arm cast used for humeral neck and humeral shaft fractures. It provides weight and traction to align the fracture "pieces."

day, except when performing physical therapy or an exercise program. The shoulder immobilizer prevents displacement of the fracture at night while sleeping. Remind the patient not to use the arm for heavy activity during the day. Protection of the shoulder for these fractures is appropriate for a total of 6 weeks before returning to regular activities.

In all fractures, palpation for resolution of point tenderness at the fracture site is a very reliable clinical index of solid fracture union. This finding combined with radiographic union determines when to allow patients to return to full activity without restriction. If the proximal humerus fracture involves the greater tuberosity, lesser tuberosity, surgical neck, or displacement of the structures, the patient should be referred to an orthopedic surgeon.

Humerus Shaft Fractures

Weakness in finger or wrist extension may indicate abnormal radial nerve function. If this weakness is present, it should be documented, but it does not change the treatment because radial nerve exploration is not appropriate even when the radial nerve function is absent or weak. Radial nerve function almost always returns during the 6 months after the injury.

Because of the excellent motion at the shoulder and the elbow, angulation up to 30 degrees at the humeral fracture site can be accepted. Treatment consists of a *hanging arm cast* (Fig. 192-8, *F*). The cast goes from the humerus, around the elbow flexed at 90 degrees, and down to the wrist. This position is maintained for 1 month until tenderness decreases on palpation and early fracture union is visible. At this point, the hanging arm cast and shoulder immobilizer can be removed and a *functional humerus cast brace* can be applied.

Functional humerus cast braces (Fig. 192-9) are available through local brace supply shops. These off-the-shelf braces are made from polyethylene. They wrap around the midshaft of the humerus and provide circumferential compression of the muscle belly, resulting in some hydraulic stabilization at the fracture site. The patient may then begin to move the shoulder and elbow in the brace and begin light function, including eating, brushing teeth, reading a newspaper, and using the arm. The elbow is notorious for becoming stiff with permanent limitation of motion. For this reason, any time the elbow is immobilized for treatment of a humerus fracture at the shaft or shoulder, encourage the patient to adjust the brace to allow the elbow to hang straight in full extension for 15 minutes each day to prevent loss of elbow extension.

The fracture of the shaft of the humerus is unique in the amount of angulation of the long bone that is accepted, and it is also unique in the healing rate and

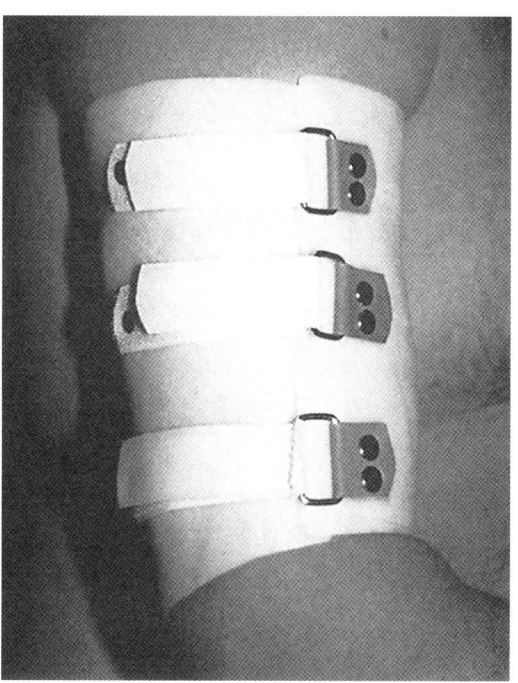

Fig. 192-9
Humeral fracture braces. (Courtesy AliMed, Inc., Dedham, Mass.)

low incidence of nonunion of a long bone fracture of the shaft. This distinction is due to the excellent blood supply surrounding the bone, which is brought there by the large amount of muscle tissue that is in contact all around the shaft of the humerus. This muscle surrounding the humerus also provides little noticeable cosmetic deformity with angulation up to 30 degrees.

If the patient's radial nerve function is initially normal but becomes impaired after the splint, a brace or shoulder immobilizer is applied and the patient is referred to an orthopedic surgeon for evaluation and treatment.

Supracondylar Humerus Fractures

Nondisplaced supracondylar fractures (Fig. 192-10) can be treated with a posterior long arm fiberglass one-step prepadded splint. The elbow should be held at 90 degrees flexion, and a shoulder immobilizer (Fig. 192-8, *D*) should be used. True AP and lateral radiographs of the distal humerus should be obtained after immobilization. These films will confirm that no displacement has occurred since the time of the immobilization. Follow-up radiographs should be reviewed 1 and 3 weeks after injury. When significant tenderness is no longer felt at the fracture site and healing is noted on the radiograph, the splint can be discontinued to allow active range-of-motion movement at 4 to 6 weeks. The patient should be instructed to avoid any passive motion at the elbow because it will predispose the elbow to

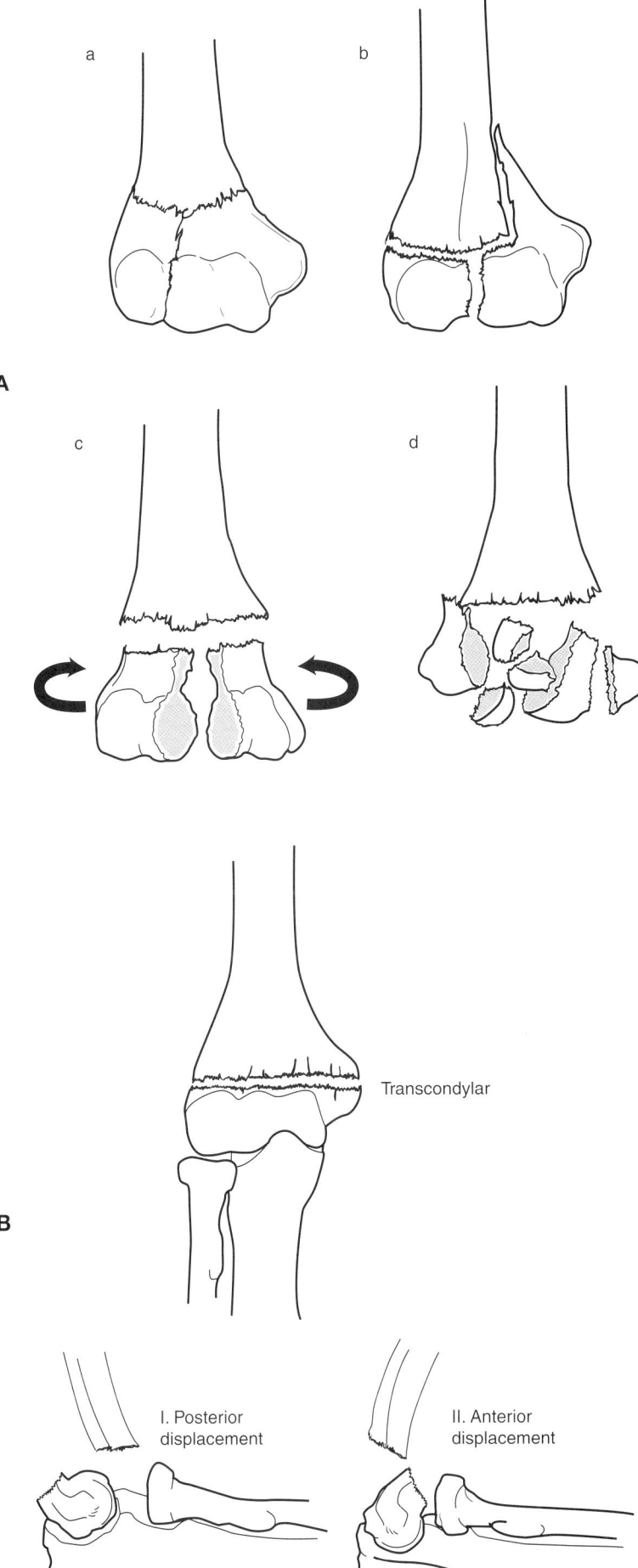

Fig. 192-10
A, Intracondylar fractures of humerus. *a,* No displacement of fragments; *b,* T-shaped fracture with the trochlear and capitellar fragments separated but not appreciably rotated in the frontal plane; *c,* T-shaped fracture with separation of the fragments and significant rotary deformity; *d,* T-shaped intercondylar fractures with severe comminution of the articular surface and wide separation of the humerus condyles.
B, Transcondylar fractures of humerus.

ectopic bone formation and permanent stiffness. The splint is used for protection for a total of 8 weeks, but it is removed for showers, bathing, and active exercise 3 weeks after injury.

Intracondylar Fractures

Intracondylar fractures are unstable and require internal fixation (see Fig. 192-10, *A*).

Fractures of the Humerus Epicondyles at the Elbow

Fractures of the humerus epicondyles (Fig. 192-11) are treated with a splint in a manner similar to the treatment of nondisplaced supracondylar fractures as previously discussed. Patients with displaced intracondylar fractures should be referred to an orthopedic surgeon.

Elbow Fractures

Elbow fractures include those intraarticular fractures of the distal humerus or proximal ulna (olecranon). If nondisplaced, treatment is similar to the treatment for a supracondylar fracture as previously discussed. If any displacement has occurred, the patient should be referred to an orthopedic surgeon (Fig. 192-12).

Radial head fractures (Fig. 192-13), which extend into the joint at the radiocapitellar area, should be referred to an orthopedic surgeon if displaced. If not displaced, then treatment is early range-of-motion movement, pronation, supination, and elbow flexion and extension. Immobilization is not required. If the patient experiences too much pain without immobilization, then a long arm fiberglass one-step splint and sling can be used but should be removed as soon as possible to minimize stiffness. With injuries to the radial head at

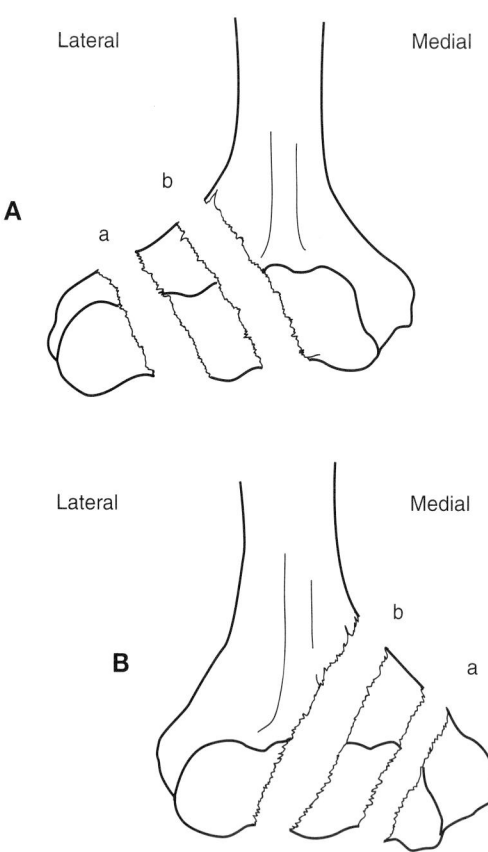

Fig. 192-11
Fractures of the humeral condyles. **A,** Lateral humeral condyle. *a,* Simple fracture of the lateral condyle with lateral wall of trochlea attached to main mass of the humerus; *b,* fracture with lateral wall of trochlea attached to fractured lateral condylar fragment. **B,** Medial lateral condyle. *a,* Simple fracture of medial condyle with lateral wall of trochlea attached to main mass of the humerus; *b,* fracture with lateral wall of trochlea attached to fractured medial condylar fragment.

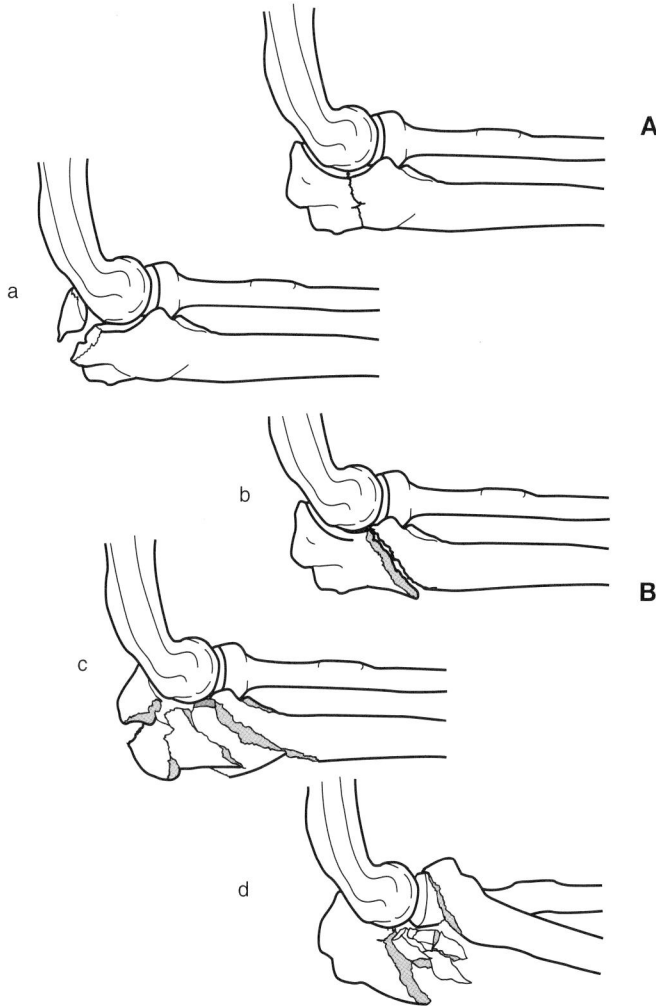

Fig. 192-12
Elbow fractures. **A,** Undisplaced. **B,** Displaced fractures. *a,* Avulsion fracture; *b,* oblique and transverse fracture; *c,* comminuted fractures; *d,* fracture dislocations.

the elbow, always check the wrist to ensure that there is no tenderness over the radius and ulna at the level of the wrist. This assessment will confirm that no associated injury to the wrist has occurred, which would result in instability. If tenderness is present also over the wrist, obtain true AP and lateral radiographs. If any displacement or dorsal subluxation of the ulna is present, with or without fracture, the patient should be referred to an orthopedic surgeon.

Mid-Forearm Fractures

Isolated fractures of the ulna shaft with no fracture of the radius can be treated with a long arm splint and sling with the elbow in 90 degrees flexion. The splint remains in place for protection for 8 weeks. The fracture of the ulna will become sticky, stable, and less painful after 3 weeks, allowing removal of the splint for gentle range-of-motion movement of the elbow, including pronation and supination of the forearm twice a day for 15 minutes to minimize stiffness.

Fracture of the radius shaft requires surgery in all cases. Even with the nondisplaced, the fractures will often become displaced. These patients should be referred to an orthopedic surgeon.

Patients with a *fracture of the radius and ulna shaft* should always be referred to an orthopedic surgeon because these fractures always require open reduction internal fixation as a result of instability.

Distal Forearm Fractures

Colles' Fracture

This is the most common wrist fracture. When it involves the distal 2 cm of the radius and is angled dorsally, it is called a *Colles' fracture* (Fig. 192-14). If nondisplaced, it can be treated in the office with a short arm cast for 6

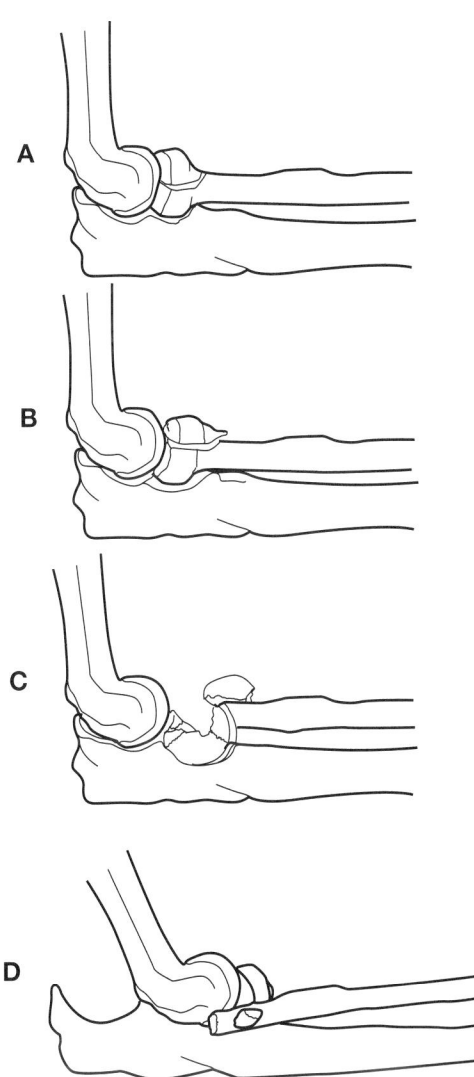

Fig. 192-13
Radial head fractures (Mason classification with Johnston modification). **A,** Nondisplaced linear or transverse fractures. **B,** Fractures with minimal displacement or comminuted fractures without displacement. **C,** Comminuted fractures with marked displacement. **D,** Radial head fractures with elbow dislocation.

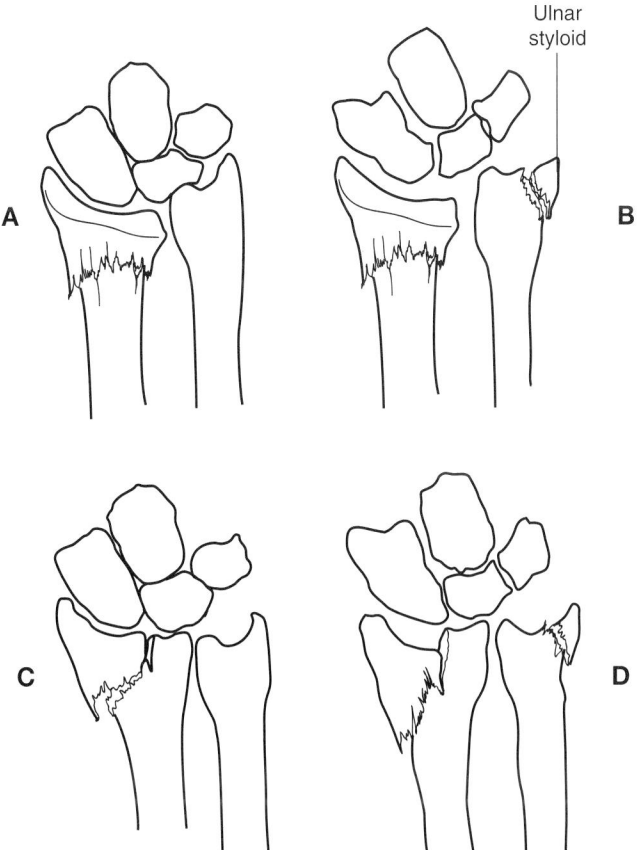

Fig. 192-14
Distal radius fractures. **A,** Colles'. **B,** Colles' commonly associated with ulnar styloid. **C,** Intraarticular fracture. **D,** Intraarticular fracture of radius with associated fracture of ulnar styloid process.

weeks. Be careful to trim the cast distally along the diagonal line of the proximal palmar crease so that full flexion of the metacarpophalangeal (MP) joints is possible to prevent stiffness. The fracture should be followed with radiographic evaluation at 1, 2, and 6 weeks after the fracture to ensure no displacement and complete healing. The fracture radiograph at 6 weeks is taken after the cast is removed so that the presence of the cast does not interfere with visualizing fracture healing. If tenderness persists at the fracture site or if evidence exists of an incomplete union, an ulnar gutter cast should be applied using 6-inch wide one-step fiberglass material over the same length of the forearm. This cast can be removed to allow gentle range-of-motion movement of the wrist to minimize stiffness, but it should be reapplied until all tenderness resolves and a solid fracture union is noted on the radiograph. This treatment is often necessary for patients who are taking antiinflammatory medication or for those who refuse to discontinue smoking.

Colles' fractures require reduction if the lateral radiographic view shows the distal radius articular surface to be facing dorsally rather than in the neutral position. The distal articular surface should face perpendicular to the long axis of the forearm with a line drawn straight through the radius lunate and capitellum. If not reducible, unstable, comminuted, or intraarticular, these fractures are best treated by an orthopedic surgeon.

On the AP view, if the radius is not equal to or longer than the length of the ulna, reduction is also required. Most all patients have a radius that is longer than the ulna; this characteristic is referred to as negative ulnar variance as seen on the AP radiograph. A few patients have the radius and ulna at the same length. If any doubt remains, a comparison AP radiograph can be assessed. If there is displacement at the fracture site, as noted by a dorsal tilt of the distal surface on the lateral view or a shortening of the radius on the AP view, reduction is required.

Reduction can be performed in the office by injecting 10 ml plain 1% Xylocaine into the fracture site hematoma. This injection should be performed slowly to prevent pain associated with distension. The surface can be sprayed with Fluro-Methane to cool the skin and decrease the discomfort associated with the injection. Always clean the skin after applying the spray with a Betadine or alcohol preparation. Lidocaine injection is then administered. Allow 10 minutes for the anesthetic block to become effective. The patient is supine during the entire procedure including the injection.

After the injection has blocked the pain, hang the patient's hand in finger traps traction with the elbow flexed 90 degrees; gradually add counterweight to the forearm with a weight hanger and orthopedic felt sling over the humerus attached to the weight hanger (Fig. 192-15). A weight of 15 to 20 lb is appropriate, and the patient should be in the suspended traction position for 15 to 20 minutes. At that point, reduction is usually achieved spontaneously by ligamentotaxis. The soft tissue attachments to the bone will pull the bone into a reduced position in response to the traction. If any visible or palpable deformity remains after 15 to 20 minutes of traction, then manual pressure can correct the deformity by pushing from dorsal to volar over the distal radius distal to the fracture site. At this point with the arm maintained in traction, a short arm, well-molded cast is applied. Take great care to mold with your thenar cone at the base of the thumb, pressing into the patient's palm to prevent a gap in the volar portion of the cast at the palm. After the cast is hard, trim it to allow full flexion at the proximal palmar crease at the MP joints.

After the cast is hard and three-point molding is applied (pushing volarly distal to the fracture site, dorsally just proximal to the fracture site, and volar against the elbow), the traction weight is removed and the cast is extended to the long arm level, which goes at least 5 inches proximal above the elbow. Be careful to pad the cast margins well proximally and distally and stop the plaster or fiberglass at least 1 inch proximally below the padding margin.

True AP and lateral postreduction radiographs are then appropriately taken. If a persisting dorsal tilt of the distal radial articular surface or a shortening of the radius

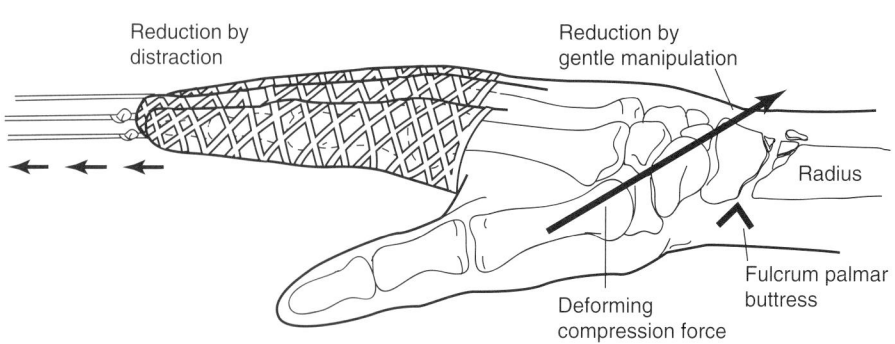

Fig. 192-15
Treatment of Colles' fracture to effect reduction.

in relation to the ulna is seen on the postreduction radiograph, then the reduction is unacceptable and referral should be made for repeat reduction under general anesthetic and the application of skeletal external frame traction.

Smith Fracture

A *Smith fracture* is similar to a Colles' fracture except that the angulation is volar. This fracture is treated in the same manner as the Colles' fracture as previously discussed. If reduction is not anatomically perfect, refer the patient to an orthopedic surgeon.

Fractures of the distal radius are often intraarticular, involving the radioulnar joint or radiocarpal joint and often involving the ulnar styloid. If any intraarticular displacement persists after reduction, the patient should be referred to an orthopedic surgeon.

Ulnar styloid fractures indicate a larger force of injury and a higher chance of loss of reduction. However, surgical treatment is never required for a displaced ulnar styloid fracture. These fractures often remain nonunited on follow-up radiographs, but this development has no clinical significance. Patients will look at the radiograph and think that they have a loose piece of bone floating. They should be reminded that this bone is attached to soft tissue and does not freely float and will not move.

After reduction, radiographs should again be obtained at 1 and 2 weeks after injury to ensure no loss of reduction. If loss of reduction is present, the patient should be referred to an orthopedic surgeon. If no loss of reduction is present, then the cast can be shortened to a short arm level cast after 2 weeks to allow elbow range-of-motion movement for the remaining 4 weeks while in the short arm cast.

Fractures of the Carpal Bones

Most often chip avulsion fractures and fractures of the carpal bones are treated with an ulnar gutter cast for comfort and protection for 4 to 6 weeks until symptoms resolve. The ulnar gutter cast can be removed for a shower.

Scaphoid (Navicular) Fractures

When there is pain in the "snuffbox," always consider a scaphoid navicular injury (Fig. 192-16). Obtain a scaphoid magnification view radiograph, and consult with a radiologist or orthopedist to confirm that the fracture is, in fact, nondisplaced. If nondisplaced, then the ideal treatment is a long arm thumb spica cast for 6 weeks, followed by shortening to a short arm thumb spica cast for the remaining 6 weeks of treatment.

A thumb spica short arm cast is appropriate for any patient who has significant tenderness only over the snuffbox (scaphoid), with follow-up radiograph and examination in 3 weeks without the cast. If at that time no tenderness is felt over the scaphoid and no fracture is visible, then there was no scaphoid fracture. Scaphoid fractures are notorious for being difficult to see acutely. For this reason, always err on the side of immobilization when a scaphoid fracture is suspected, even when not visible on the radiograph. If after 3 weeks the cast is removed and no fracture line is visible but persistent tenderness is noted over the fracture site, immobilization

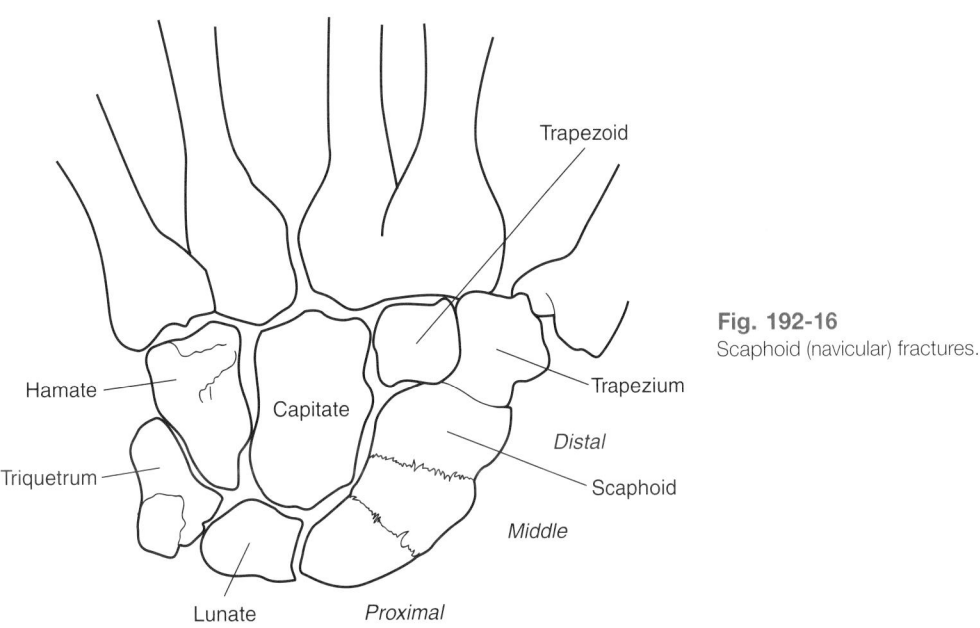

Fig. 192-16
Scaphoid (navicular) fractures.

for an additional 3 weeks would be appropriate, followed by repeat radiographs. At that point, if no fracture line is visible, then there was no scaphoid fracture and gentle range-of-motion exercises can be initiated.

For any scaphoid fracture in which displacement exists, refer the patient to an orthopedic surgeon. Avascular necrosis, delayed union, nonunion, and arthritis are common complications of scaphoid fractures, and the patient needs to be aware of these at the start.

Metacarpal Fractures

Nondisplaced metacarpal fractures, including those that are intraarticular, are treated with an ulnar or a radial gutter cast, depending on the fracture location. Fractures of the thumb metacarpal are treated with a thumb spica cast. An index finger metacarpal fracture can be treated with a radial gutter cast with a hole cut out for the thumb to allow thumb function. Fractures of the middle, ring, and small metacarpals are treated with an ulnar gutter cast. Gutter cast can be made using 6-inch wide one-step fiberglass prepadded splint material.

If the fracture is in the midportion of the shaft, angulation greater than 15 degrees is not acceptable and requires reduction and often pin fixation. Hematoma block reduction can be carried out with three-point pressure fixation in the cast, followed by postreduction radiographs. If the reduction is satisfactory, the ulnar gutter cast or radial gutter cast remains in place for 1 month, followed by cast removal for range-of-motion exercises. The metacarpal remains protected in the cast when not performing range-of-motion movements for an additional 3 weeks.

Immobilize the metacarpals with 90-degree flexion at the MP joint and full extension of the interphalangeal (IP) and distal interphalangeal (DIP) joints of the fingers. Often referred to as the "intrinsic plus," this position happens to be where the MP joint lateral ligaments and those of the DIP and PIP joints are in maximal stretch. This position prevents tightening during immobilization and secondary stiffness of the joint. The gutter cast should go from the tips of the fingers to the midforearm. Remember to place dry cotton ball padding between the fingers to prevent skin maceration from moisture accumulation.

(Immobilizing all metacarpal fractures in an MP joint flexion 90-degree position eliminates the need to worry about malrotation of the metacarpal fracture, because the flexed finger at the MP joint serves to align the metacarpal in direct rotation with the adjacent metacarpals. This alignment acts as a reference angle because their prospective fingers are also flexed 90 degrees. Also, see the comment in the "Phalangeal Fractures" section.)

Patients with *displaced intraarticular fractures* (Bennett and Rolando fractures) should be referred to an

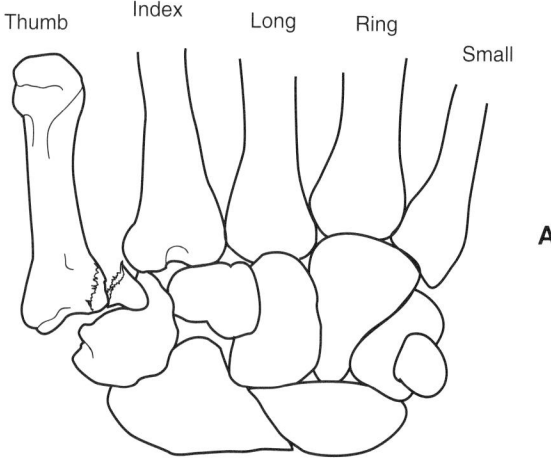

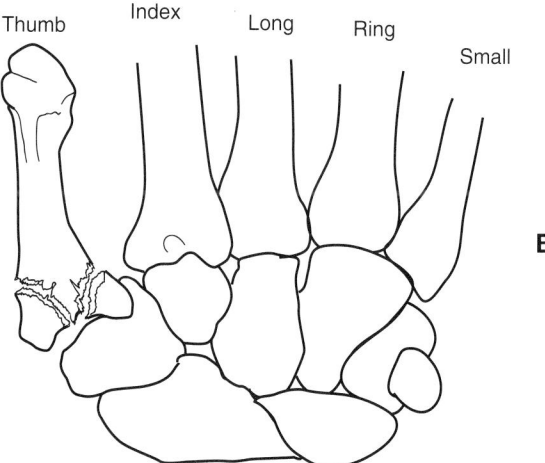

Fig. 192-17
Displaced intraarticular fractures of the proximal thumb. **A,** Bennett's fracture. **B,** Rolando's fracture.

orthopedic surgeon, especially those who have intraarticular fractures at the base of the thumb (Fig. 192-17).

Boxer fractures occur at the fifth metacarpal neck. Angulation up to 60 degrees is acceptable for this fracture. The clinician must be certain, however, not to confuse a boxer fracture (fifth metacarpal neck) with a fifth metacarpal shaft fracture, because angulation of the shaft of the fifth metacarpal greater than 15 degrees is not acceptable (Fig. 192-18).

Treatment for a boxer fracture at the metacarpal neck is immobilization for 3 weeks, followed by cast removal for early range-of-motion movement. The cast is reapplied for an additional 2 weeks to protect the fracture and complete the healing process. Hematoma block with attempted manipulation reduction is appropriate for angulation greater than 20 degrees at the metacarpal fractured neck. However, it is acceptable to allow angulation beyond this point if a reduction cannot be achieved. Explain to patients with boxer fractures that

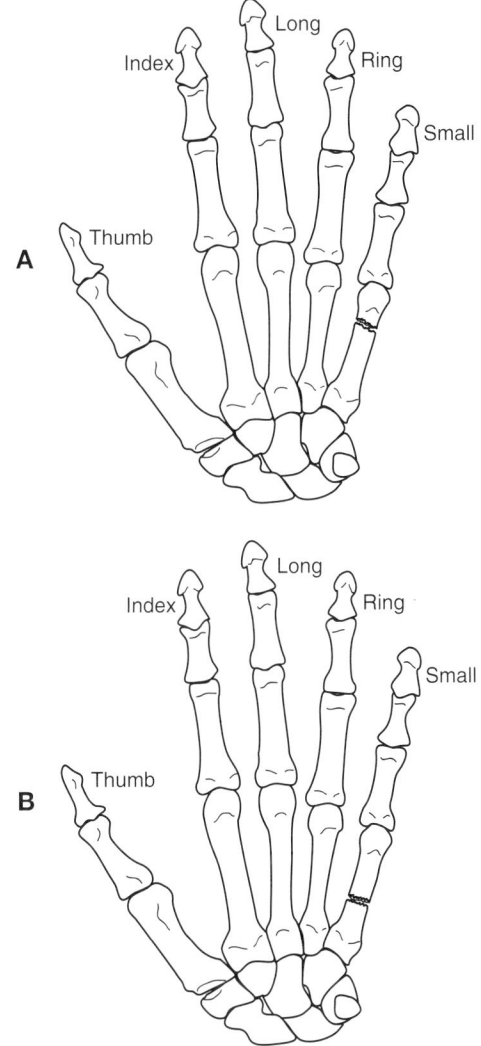

Fig. 192-18
A, Boxer's fracture. **B,** Metacarpal shaft fracture.

interosseous ligaments that run between each of the metacarpals.

Phalangeal Fractures

Phalangeal fractures can be immobilized with aluminum foam splints, buddy taping, or stack splints in the case of mallet finger involving the distal phalanx. If there is any displacement of these fractures, referral is appropriate. Volar plate avulsion fractures caused by hyperextension injuries at the PIP joint are best immobilized with a dorsal block splint holding the PIP joint in 45 degrees flexion for 3 weeks.

Always check the collateral ligaments by stress examination. Use a digital block if the examination is too painful without. If collateral ligaments are disrupted despite a negative x-ray, buddy taping is appropriate for protection for 1 month while allowing protected range-of-motion movement in the taped position.

In general, with metacarpal and phalangeal fractures, malrotation is one of the most common complications. To avoid malrotation, always hold the MP joints in 90 degrees flexion for any metacarpal fracture to ensure perfect rotational alignment. For the phalangeal fractures, always note the plane of the nail beds while looking at the fingers from the ends. Compare them with the opposite hand to ensure correct rotational alignment.

In summary, any intraarticular fracture with displacement at the joint surface should be referred to an orthopedic surgeon for reduction and fixation. Extraarticular and interarticular fractures without displacement at the joint surface can be treated without referral. If any doubt remains as to whether displacement in the joint surface is present, consult an radiologist or orthopedist.

CHILDREN'S FRACTURES

Children's bone tissue is elastic, similar to a plastic flyswatter handle. For this reason, their bones can deform and bow without actually cracking the cortex. This elastic deformation commonly occurs in the radius and ulna shaft and is referred to as a bone bow fracture. If in doubt about the normal alignment of the forearm, remember that the ulna is always straight and that a small 10- to 20-degree bow is normally present in the radius. Assessment of a comparison film can determine what is normal for the patient. When viewing comparison films, always make sure the views are taken in exactly the same projection on both forearms so that a true comparison can be made. *Comparison films* in children are beneficial because the growth plates ossify at different ages.

Comparison radiographs in children are especially important when treating any elbow injury, because

the bone will heal with abundant callus, and inform them that they will have a bump over the dorsum of the hand because the callus is subcutaneous.

When treating boxer fractures, be *cautious* of any mark on the skin over the knuckle, which could suggest an open fracture or a human bite lesion that might become infected. If either is present, begin broad-spectrum antibiotics, possibly giving the first dose intravenously (IV). The wound should be inspected again in 2 to 3 days to ensure no infection.

If an isolated *fracture involves one of the long or ring metacarpals,* it can be treated without immobilization if the patient is comfortable and wishes to use their hand out of a cast. Approximately 3 to 5 mm of shortening of the finger may occur as the metacarpal overrides itself. However, no shortening will occur beyond this point because the fractured metacarpal is being suspended between the two intact metacarpals and the associated

numerous centers of ossification exist in the elbow that develop at various ages 3 to 12 years.

Salter's classification is commonly used for children's fractures involving the growth plate (Box 192-2 and Fig. 192-19).

Upper Extremity (Pediatric)

Clavicle fractures do not require referral, reduction, or intervention unless tenting of the skin is observed with whiteness over the skin as a result of a loss of blood supply. Patients with a clavicle fracture near the acromioclavicular joint that is displaced should be referred to an orthopedic surgeon. The vast majority of fractures, however, occur in the middle third of the

clavicle and are treated with a figure-eight strap for immobilization and comfort. Remember, the figure-eight strap is only applied to increase comfort; as soon as the child is comfortable without it, the strap is no longer is required. In toddlers, a figure-eight strap is not necessary, because healing occurs so quickly. In older children, a sling may be more comfortable than a figure-eight clavicle strap. These straps and splints can be removed for bathing and then reapplied. To show patients how to put the straps back on and get the straps in the same position, instruct them to use a pen to make marks on the white straps at the level of the buckles. This "trick" will enable the patient to reapply the splint, sling, or brace in the same position with the same degree of tension as applied it in the office.

Rib fractures, similar to those in adults, do not require treatment, immobilization, or bracing. Although patients may ask for any one of these treatments, remind them that splints or rib binders for treatment of rib fractures can cause atelectasis. Always use auscultation of the chest to ensure no pneumothorax or respiratory compromise. Sometimes subcutaneous emphysema suggests lung puncture by a rib or clavicle fracture. This complication can be ruled out by palpating the skin around the area of the fracture of the clavicle or ribs to check for any crepitance.

Fractures around the shoulder usually involve only the surgical neck of the humerus. As long as there is 50%

BOX 192-2
Salter's Classification of Physical Injuries*

Salter Type I fracture is diagnosed with a normal x-ray and by point tenderness directly over the growth plate. No tenderness should be felt over the ligaments around the joint. This type of fracture is common in infants and young children. Treatment is always closed with cast immobilization.

Salter Type II involves a fracture through the growth plate and then through the metaphysis. This type of fracture is more common in older children. The prognosis for growth disturbance is very high when the fracture involves the distal femoral growth plate. Refer all patients with this type of fracture to an orthopedic surgeon if any displacement has occurred. Reduction is almost always performed with a general anesthetic to provide complete muscle relaxation. This relaxation allows the traction to decrease the force across the growth plate, which is required to set it. The less force required to set the fracture, the less recurrent injury to the growth plate itself (Fig. 192-19).

Salter Type III fracture involves the epiphysis extending into the epiphysial plate. If any displacement has occurred, the patient should be referred to an orthopedic surgeon. These fractures are most common in the distal tibia and can be associated with growth arrest. Anatomic reduction is always required, and surgery may be required.

Salter Type IV fracture extends from the joint surface through the epiphysis and on through the epiphysial plate and out through the metaphysis. These fractures are often displaced and require open surgical treatment. This fracture most commonly occurs at the lateral humeral condyle at the elbow. These injuries extend into the joint. If the fracture appears nondisplaced and any question of displacement remains, it may be beneficial for a radiologist or an orthopedist to review the film and tomograms.

Salter Type V injury is a crush injury of the epiphysial plate and is uncommon. When this fracture occurs, it is usually at the knee or ankle and associated with growth arrest. The x-ray may be normal, appearing like a Salter Type I fracture. For this reason, for any patient with tenderness over the growth plate whether it is a Salter I or Salter V fracture (and often this is difficult to determine), caution the parents that growth arrest can be a complication in children when it extends into the growth plate. Osteoarthritis can occur as a result of any fracture that extends into the joint itself, whether this occurs in an adult or a child.

*See Fig. 192-19.

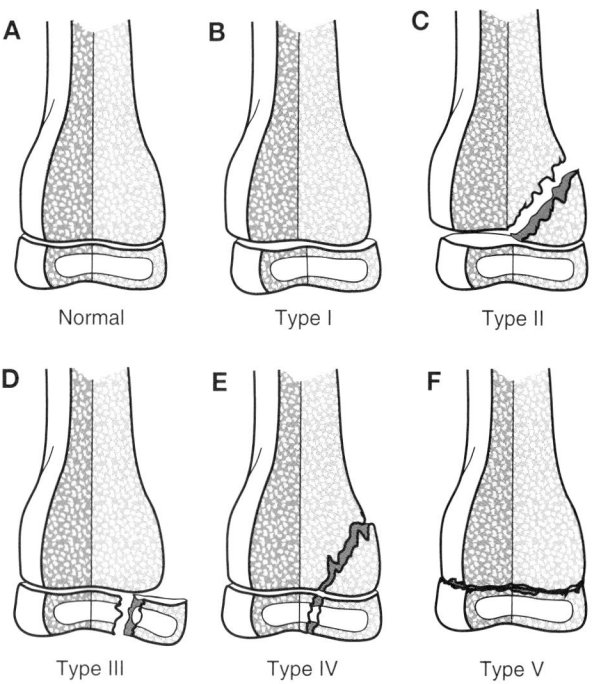

Fig. 192-19
Illustrations of Salter's classification for fractures in children (also see Box 192-2). **A,** Normal. **B,** Type I. **C,** Type II. **D,** Type III. **E,** Type IV. **F,** Type V.

bone-on-bone contact and less than 45 degrees of angulation, this fracture can be accepted without reduction. As with adults, treatment is a hanging arm cast for 3 to 4 weeks until tenderness resolves on palpation and comfort is present. Humerus shaft fractures always heal well, and angulation up to 25 degrees on AP and lateral planes can be accepted. Always check for radial nerve function.

Distal humerus supracondylar fractures can be best evaluated with comparison of true lateral radiographs. Remember that the distal humerus ordinarily has a tilt in an anterior direction. If the distal humerus is entirely straight, approximately 10 to 15 degrees of bending of the distal humerus has occurred in a posterior direction. This bending can be accepted, however, as long as it is not bent backward beyond the straight position.

A supracondylar fracture and radial head and neck fracture can be identified with a *posterior fat pad sign*. The posterior fat pad sign is the result of intraarticular bleeding in the elbow joint with any fracture that is intraarticular. The blood goes into the olecranon fossa in the distal humerus and causes the fat pad that resides there to float posteriorly; therefore it is no longer hidden in the olecranon fossa. As it floats posteriorly, it is visible as a fat pad on the true lateral radiograph of the distal humerus. In the absence of any abnormality on the radiograph, a fat pad sign indicates bleeding into the joint and leads to a diagnosis of occult fracture most likely involving the radial head or neck. This involvement can be determined by point tenderness with palpation of the radial head and neck. Fractures of the radial neck can be angulated with the acceptance of angulation up to 10 degrees. A child with any angulation beyond that point should be referred to a orthopedic surgeon for closed reduction.

Common fractures in the forearm include *torus fractures*. These are treated with a short arm cast for 1 month until all tenderness resolves. *Greenstick fractures* are one level worse than a torus fracture. These involve an actual crack or disruption of one cortex and often a buckling of the opposite cortex. These fractures are so named because they represent a deformation of the bone much like cracking a green twig on an apple tree in springtime. The tension side of the bent twig cracks, whereas the compression side (concave side) buckles and does not crack.

Any angulation greater than 10 degrees requires reduction. In any fracture of the forearm that requires reduction, a long arm cast is automatically necessary to prevent pronation and supination at the elbow. The cast is always applied with the elbow in at least 90 degrees flexion, and the sling must always hold the arm in at least 90 degrees flexion. If it does not do so or if the cast is applied in less than 90 degrees flexion, the cast will continue to slip out of the sling.

If any displacement or angulation is present, patients with *fractures of the radius or ulna shaft* should always be referred to an orthopedic surgeon for closed manipulation reduction. The fracture is treated with a long arm cast if no displacement is present. The long arm cast remains in place for a minimum of 6 weeks.

Wrist and Hand (Pediatric)

Fractures of the carpal bones are uncommon in children. With a fall on the outstretched arm, the typical fracture is of the distal radius and ulna. These fractures can be reduced by hematoma block and finger traps traction, as in the adult. This technique should be reserved for the child who is 12 years or older and very cooperative and understanding. Younger children, who are uncooperative, anxious, or otherwise frightened of injections, should have a reduction under general anesthesia. This approach will provide a more comfortable, less-frightening experience and allow maximum muscle relaxation for the least traumatic reduction affecting the growth plate.

Metacarpal and phalangeal fractures that are nondisplaced are simply treated with ulnar gutter cast or radial gutter cast immobilization. The position of immobilization and the angulation are the same as that used for treating adults. Remember, the fifth metacarpal neck can accept angulation up to 45 degrees, whereas the shaft angulation can be accepted only to 10 degrees. Phalangeal fractures including mallet fingers are treated the same for children as they are in adults.

The so-called *octave fracture* is a common fracture in children that occurs at the base of the proximal phalanx of the small finger, where it is angulated ulnarly. It is so named since playing the piano requires children to stretch their fingers into wide abduction. Reduction is required and is easily done using a finger digital block anesthetic, followed by placement of a pen in the web space between the fourth and fifth fingers. The pen acts as a fulcrum between the two fingers. The small finger is then pulled back into place with traction and radial deviation until it is perfectly straight using the pen or pencil deep in the web space as a bolster or fulcrum at the proximal phalanx at the apex of angulation at the fracture. This technique works extremely well. After this treatment, buddy taping and splint immobilization is appropriate for a minimum of 3 weeks.

Mallet fingers in children are treated with a stack splint as they are in adults. Again, a child with any displaced interarticular fracture or displaced growth plate fracture should be referred to an orthopedic surgeon for reduction.

Lower Extremity Fractures (Pediatric)

Fractures of the pelvis are uncommon except in automobile accidents or high-velocity trauma. Patients with these fractures should all be referred to an orthopedic surgeon to rule out other associated injuries to the abdomen or genitourinary and gynecologic systems.

Femur fractures are also uncommon and when present should be immediately referred to an orthopedic surgeon for further evaluation and treatment. Remember, a *slipped capital femoral epiphysis or avascular necrosis of the femoral head in children (Perthes' disease)* can present with knee pain. The knee examination and radiograph may be entirely normal. The first clue to the diagnosis is limitation of hip internal rotation on the involved side. The *Trendelenburg test* often shows weakness in the gluteus medius on the involved side. *If a child under 17 years of age complains of knee pain and the knee examination and radiographs are negative, always examine and carry out radiographs of the pelvis and hips*. AP pelvic and true lateral radiographs of the hips are appropriate studies for this purpose.

Fractures of the distal femur, which are nondisplaced and have normal radiographs, are diagnosed by point tenderness over the distal femoral epiphysis, which is located 3 cm above the joint line. Treatment involves a cylinder cast for complete immobilization, crutches, and protective partial weight-bearing activities for 1 month. During the follow-up examination, a window can be placed in the cast through which the examiner's finger can palpate for tenderness. As long as tenderness is felt at the fracture site, the cast should remain in place. The tenderness should resolve within 8 weeks or sooner, depending on the child's age.

Patella fractures are usually nondisplaced and are similarly treated with a knee immobilizer or cylinder cast. The immobilization remains in place for 1 month until all tenderness resolves.

Beware of any *intraarticular avulsion fractures along the lateral tibia plateau.* This type of fracture indicates an anterior cruciate ligament avulsion pulling loose a piece of bone. If there is any displacement associated with this, referral to an orthopedist should be carried out for surgical repair.

Proximal tibia fractures are treated the same as those of the distal femur and are diagnosed by point tenderness over the growth plate. Tibia shaft fractures can be treated in a long leg cast without reduction, provided that no angulation greater than 5 degrees is present on the AP radiograph and no greater than 10 degrees of angulation on the lateral radiograph. If angulation is present, then referral to an orthopedic surgeon should be made for closed manipulation reduction.

Fibula fractures are of no concern and will heal uneventfully without treatment. However, if any angulation is present, then referral to an orthopedic surgeon should be made for closed manipulation reduction.

Foot and Ankle Fractures (Pediatric)

Patients with any *fracture around the ankle* that is displaced should be referred to an orthopedist. Fractures that are nondisplaced can be treated with a short leg cast and non–weight-bearing movements for 2 weeks, followed by advancing to weight-bearing activities for the remaining 3 to 4 weeks while in the cast.

Fracture of the talus, navicular, and cuneiform bones can be treated with a short leg walking cast, provided there is no displacement.

Fractures of the metatarsals are treated the same in children as they are in adults. *Peroneus brevis avulsion fractures* can be treated with a wooden sole fracture shoe. Beware of the fracture of the *proximal shaft of the metatarsal,* which is different from a peroneus brevis avulsion fracture. For optimal healing, this type of fracture requires a short leg fiberglass cast and non–weight-bearing movements for 2 weeks, followed by weight-bearing activities for an additional 6 weeks.

Complications (Adult and Pediatric)

Compartment syndrome (see Chapter 189, Compartment Syndrome Evaluation)

Compartment syndrome is the most devastating complication in fracture treatment and is caused by swelling and a tight cast leading to neurovascular compromises. This syndrome most frequently occurs in the calf and forearm. Any patient who requires more than the average dose of oral pain medication for fractures of the forearm or tibia (or any other fracture, for that matter) should be immediately examined as an emergency. If the patient feels the cast is too tight or if there is excess pain beyond what would be reasonably expected, or if any swelling in the digits occurs, then the cast and padding should be immediately split. If pain relief does not occur, the entire cast should be removed and the extremity inspected for signs of tenseness of the skin. If the skin is not tense and the calf is involved, perform a Doppler study to rule out phlebitis. Treatment of the fracture and maintenance of reduction of the fracture is always a second priority to preserving the blood supply to the soft tissue and bone. If any question of compartment syndrome as a result of tenseness in the skin of the forearm and calf remains, compartmental pressure measurements must be performed and a fasciotomy preformed if pressures are elevated.

Elevation of the extremity after the injury can prevent compartment syndrome. Always instruct patients with short or long leg casts and injuries to the tibia to lie down and keep the chest flat. The head may be elevated with pillows but not the chest. The knee and hip should be bent in 90 degree flexion each, and the calf should be placed on four couch seating cushions to keep it 2 feet higher than the heart at all times for the first week.

Compartment syndrome can occur after a tibia fracture any time during the first week. The higher the velocity of the injury, the more committed the fracture, the higher the energy of the force, the more soft tissue trauma, and the higher the chance of swelling. For the upper extremity, always tell patients to carry their arm over their head in a monkeylike position for the first week. Children may go to school, but their arm should be propped up over their head or on a stack of books in front of them on their desk. At night, they should sleep with couch cushions elevating the arm. Parents should set their alarm clock for 3 am and reposition the child's arm back up on the pillows because the child will have most likely wiggled the arm off the elevated position. Be certain that patients *do not* have slings to use for a long arm cast for the first week. If they are given a sling, they will automatically carry the cast and arm down in front by their chest and it will be lower than the heart and promote swelling. The sling should not be used until after the first week.

Open Fractures

As in adult bone injuries, any patient with an *open fracture* should be referred to an orthopedist. The open fracture may be associated with only a small puncture wound in the skin, and this puncture wound may be located several inches from the fracture itself because of the forces of deformation at the time of the injury. It is also appropriate to refer all patients with fractures involving the spine or knee because fractures around the spine and knee are at high risk for growth plate arrest or neurologic injury. With any fracture around the elbow, always obtain comparison views. Because the elbow has delayed centers of ossification, if any sign of fracture is present, referral to an orthopedist or a radiologist should be carried out to review the films.

Child Abuse

Any suspicious history of child abuse should be investigated by assessing long bone radiographs of the upper and lower extremities. This long bone study should be carefully reviewed for signs of fractures in various bones in different stages of healing, which would indicate a history of numerous injuries. A corner fracture is a typical radiographic fracture pattern, which is noted at the corner of the metaphysis of the long bones.

BIBLIOGRAPHY

Herring JA: Tachdjian's *pediatric orthopedics from the Texas Scottish Rite Hospital for Children,* ed 3, Philadelphia, 2002, WB Saunders.

Korin SH, Berlet AC: *Handbook of common orthopedic fractures,* West Chester, Penn, 1989, Medical Surveillance.

Medley ES, Shirley SM, Brilliant HL: Fracture management by family physicians and guidelines for referral, *J Fam Pract* 8(4):701, 1979.

Rang M: *Children's fractures,* ed 2, Philadelphia, 1983, Lippincott.

Rockwood CA, Wilkins KE, Beaty JH, editors: *Rockwood & Green's fractures in adults,* ed 4, Philadelphia, 1996, Lippincott-Raven.

Rockwood CA, Wilkins KE, King RE, editors: *Rockwood & Wilkins' fractures in children,* New York, 2001, Lippincott.

Salter RB: *Disorders and injuries of the musculoskeletal system,* Baltimore, 1970, Williams & Wilkins. Salter RB, Harris WR: Injuries involving epiphysial plate, *J Bone Joint Surg* 45A:587, 1963.

Spinner M: Monteggia fractures in children with nerve palsies, *Clin Orthoped* 58:141, 1968.

Wilkins KE, Beaty JB, Kasser JR, editors: *Rockwood & Wilkins' fractures in children,* Philadelphia, 2001, Lippincott.

CHAPTER 193

Ganglion Treatment

David T. Bortel

The most common tumor of the hand or wrist is the ganglion, with a propensity for women. The ganglion can occur at most any location adjacent to a joint or tendon sheath. The most common site is the dorsal wrist (Fig. 193-1). The scapholunate joint is the normal site of original pathology (Fig. 193-2). Volar cysts typically originate from the scaphotrapezial or trapeziometacarpal joint (Fig. 193-3). Another site of origin is the palmar fibroosseous flexor sheath. These normally present as a hard, small, painful lesion at the proximal interphalangeal (PIP) flexion crease (Fig. 193-4). Ganglions can be located at other body sites, with the foot and ankle being the next most common location (Figs. 193-5 and 193-6). Occasionally they can even become intraosseous.

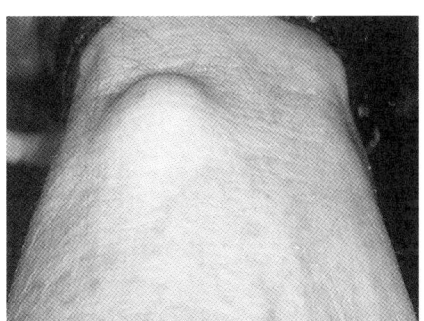

Fig. 193-1
Dorsal wrist ganglion. (Courtesy The National Procedures Institute, Midland, Mich.)

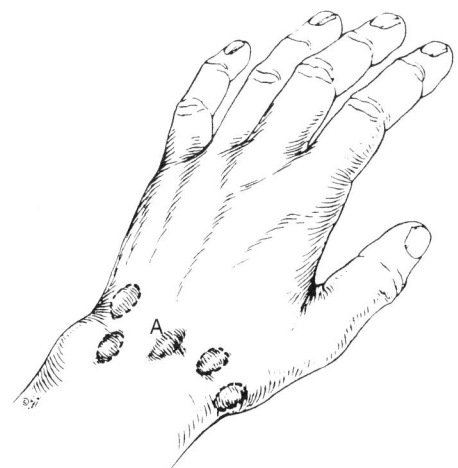

Fig. 193-2
A few of the many possible locations of dorsal wrist ganglions. The most common site, *A,* directly over the scapholunate ligament. The others are typically connected to the scapholunate ligament through an elongated pedicle. (Redrawn from Angelides AC: Ganglions of the hand and wrist. In Green DP, Hotchkiss RN, Pederson WC, editors: *Green's operative hand surgery,* New York, 1999, Churchill Livingstone.)

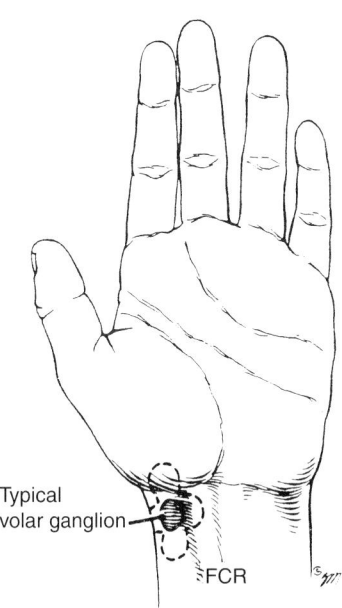

Fig. 193-3
Typical location of a volar wrist ganglion. Possible subcutaneous extensions *(dotted lines)* are often palpable. *FCR,* Flexor carpi radialis. (Redrawn from Angelides AC: Ganglions of the hand and wrist. In Green DP, Hotchkiss RN, Pederson WC, editors: *Green's operative hand surgery,* New York, 1999, Churchill Livingstone.)

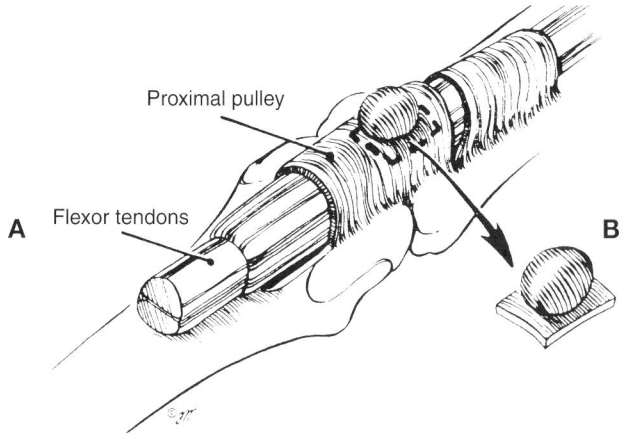

Fig. 193-4
A, Volar retinacular ganglion in situ on the proximal annular ligament (A1 pulley) of the flexor tendon sheath. **B,** Excised specimen with a surrounding margin of tendon sheath. (Redrawn from Angelides AC: Ganglions of the hand and wrist. In Green DP, Hotchkiss RN, Pederson WC, editors: *Green's operative hand surgery,* New York, 1999, Churchill Livingstone.)

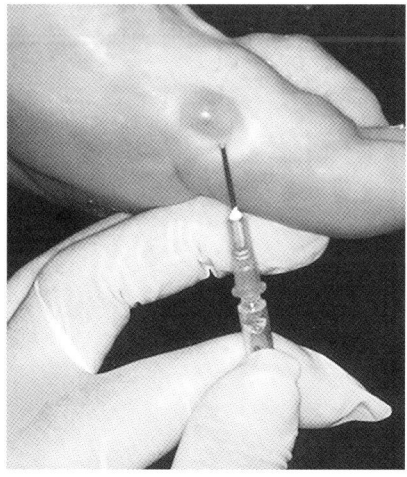

Fig. 193-5
Metatarsal phalangeal joint of toe. (Courtesy The National Procedures Institute, Midland, Mich.)

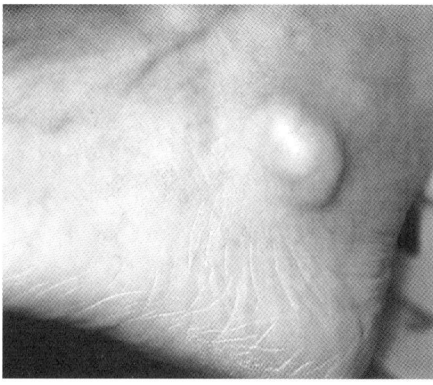

Fig. 193-6
Ganglion inferior to malleolus of ankle. (Courtesy The National Procedures Institute, Midland, Mich.)

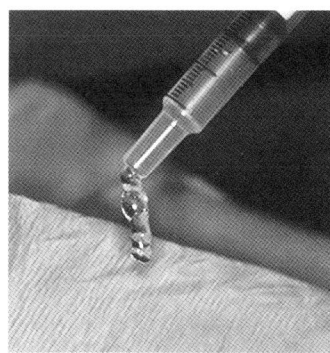

Fig. 193-7
Typical, thick, honeylike consistency of ganglion mucin. (Courtesy The National Procedures Institute, Midland, Mich.)

IDENTIFICATION AND CHARACTERISTICS

Patients usually present recognizing an obvious mass, sometimes complaining of pain and weakness. Ganglion cysts usually are easy to identify by their typical appearance. The most consistent characteristic is the typical location where they are found as noted above. The cyst is often rubbery, sometimes firm. Occasionally one may compress fluid from one septated area to another. The ganglion will transilluminate if of sufficient size. Seldom is it necessary to further investigate ganglions with additional studies. Confirmation can be verified with aspiration of the typical viscous mucoid fluid (Fig. 193-7). A differential diagnosis includes extensor tenosynovitis, lipoma, sebaceous cyst, or other hand tumors.

The ganglion cyst is a fibrous-walled, mucin-filled structure typically connected to the joint capsule or tendon sheath by a tortuous stalk. A "one-way valve" probably predicates the formation of these frequently painful, yet nonmalignant lesions. Increased use of the offending joint or tendon leads to increased production of the encapsulated mucin, thus magnifying the symptoms. The ganglion commonly is self-limiting (perhaps over several years) by rupture or resorption. These cysts are often septated and *may reflect underlying ligamentous pathology.*

Note: A close "cousin" of the ganglion cyst is the mucous (or mucinous) cyst. Both are nearly identical histologically, but the mucous cyst often involves a more ominous process. Mucous cysts arise from an arthritic distal interphalangeal (DIP) joint (i.e., the cyst is a direct drainage conduit to the DIP joint) (Fig. 193-8). Unfortunately, as these cysts enlarge with time, they commonly will erode into the germinal nail matrix, causing discomfort and nail distortion. Past treatments have included sclerosis, steroid injections, cautery with chemicals or electrically, cryotherapy, and simple incision and drainage. The thinned local subcutaneous tissue may rupture

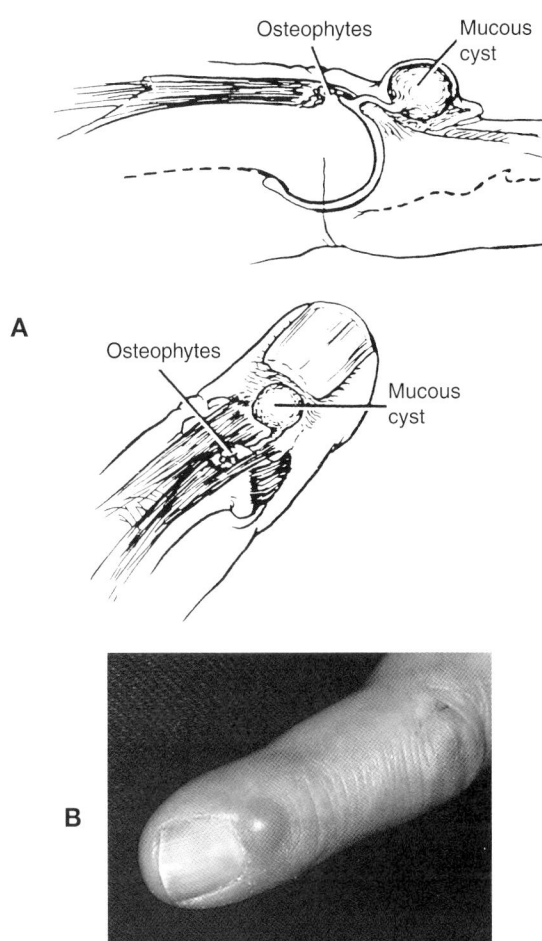

Fig. 193-8
A, Relationship between mucous cyst and marginal osteophyte of distal interphalangeal joint. Note that the cyst communicates with the joint. Marginal osteophyte produces attrition of extensor tendon expansion with motion. **B,** Distal interphalangeal joint. (**A,** Redrawn from Eaton RG, Dobranski AI, Littler JW: *J Bone Joint Surg* 55[3]:570, 1973. **B,** Courtesy The National Procedures Institute, Midland, Mich.)

spontaneously, leading to a septic joint or osteomyelitis. These lesions are particularly difficult to manage, even by skilled hand surgeons. Aspiration or injection of these mucous cysts can be attempted judiciously once the real risk of initiating an infected joint is recognized. If used, the patient needs to be aware of the signs of infection.

PREPROCEDURE
PATIENT PREPARATION

Aspiration and Injection

The patient should be informed that he or she will experience some discomfort similar to having a tooth numbed by a dentist. When the area is anesthetized, a temporary burning sensation will be felt. The Lidocaine anesthetic typically lasts for 30 to 60 minutes. While anesthetized, the involved tissue could be prone to

further unknown trauma until the anesthetic wears off. After the procedure, there will be a pressure sensation that may last for a few days. Typically a pressure dressing will be necessary for several days over the ganglion site. Any steroid placed may produce a local reaction such as a simple skin irritation or as dramatic as dermal atrophy or even significant hypopigmentation. A subsequent cutaneous slough is extraordinarily rare. Similarly, systemic manifestations are rare, since dosages and volumes are generally very small for these lesions.

Ganglion Excision

The patient should be informed of the typical anesthetic risks that are anticipated for their particular procedure technique. Furthermore, the patient should be informed of the potential risk of surgery of this nature, including infection, neurovascular injury, rarely a venous thromboembolic event (normally related to the lower extremities), or recurrence of the ganglion. If the ganglion has resulted from a capsular or ligamentous defect, additional problems such as underlying joint destabilization or stiffness may also occur.

EQUIPMENT

Please refer to specified treatment techniques. See Chapter 194, Joint and Soft Tissue Aspiration and Injection.

TREATMENT (OPTIONS)

1. *Observation*. Unless the ganglion is symptomatic (unsightly, painful, or limits motion), no treatment is necessary. Aspiration is indicated if there is uncertainty with the diagnosis.
2. *Digital pressure or rupture with a mallet, Bible, or blade*. These have all been tried historically with minimal success. Simple incision and drainage or rupturing with a needle are variants of this method.
3. *Aspiration and injection*. Aspiration with a steroid injection remains a commonly used technique. Although failure rates are high, some consider it the initial treatment of choice.
4. *Surgery*. Excision may be simple or quite complex. It is generally performed with a sterile surrounding.

TECHNIQUE OF INJECTION

Steroids

1. Using a 25-gauge needle, 1 ml or less of local lidocaine (1%) without epinephrine is deposited in a wheel fashion over the most superficial portion of

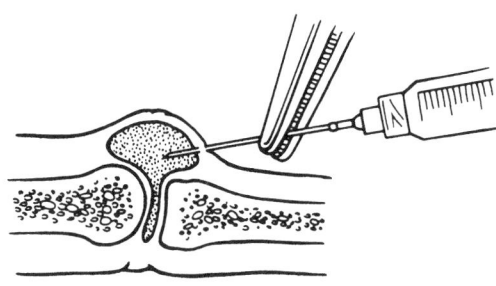

Fig. 193-9
Use an 18-gauge needle and a 1- to 3-ml syringe to enter the ganglion and aspirate its contents. The contents are often thick, and there may be only minimal return of a gel-like material. Hold the needle in position with the hemostat and remove the syringe. Attach the steroid-containing syringe and inject the contents.

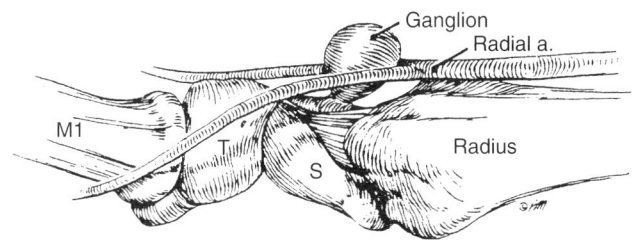

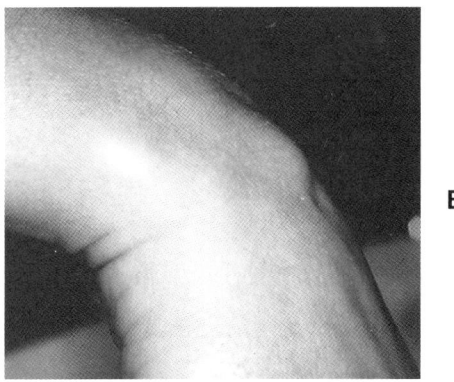

Fig. 193-10
A, Usual relationship of the ganglion to the radial artery and volar joint capsule. *M1,* First metacarpal; *S,* scaphoid; *T,* trapezium. **B,** Dorsum of wrist. (**A,** Redrawn from Angelides AC: Ganglions of the hand and wrist. In Green DP, Hotchkiss RN, Pederson WC, editors: *Green's operative hand surgery,* New York, 1999, Churchill Livingstone. **B,** Courtesy The National Procedures Institute, Midland, Mich.)

the ganglion. If the cyst is small, avoid this step since it may obscure the underlying lesion.

2. A 1- to 3-ml syringe with an 18-gauge needle is then inserted centrally into the ganglion. Assisted with digital pressure on the cyst, all the thick gelatinous fluid is aspirated (Fig. 193-9).

3. Secure this needle in place with a sterile hemostat (having verified being within the cyst) and remove the syringe with mucin.

4. Attach a prepared syringe of 50% lidocaine and 50% betamethasone or Depo-Medrol, and inject into the confines of the cyst. Variable amounts are used depending on the size of the cyst (0.1 to 1 ml). To reduce local steroid complications, consider starting with even lesser amounts of steroid.

5. Pressure is held over the needle track with a sterile gauze pad; then the area is wrapped with a small ace wrap to maintain occlusion of the cyst walls.

6. Take all precautions to maintain the tip of the aspiration needle in the cyst. *Do not* withdraw it and then attempt a second insertion to inject.

Sclerosants

1. Technique is as noted above. Instead of using steroids, substitute with 1 ml of 3% STD (sodium tetradecyl sulphate). This is the same solution used for sclerosing veins. Inject with approximately half the amount of the mucin withdrawn.

Note: This technique reportedly has an 80% resolution rate.

2. Maintain compression continuously for 2 weeks.

3. Take all precautions to maintain the tip of the aspiration needle in the cyst. *Do not* withdraw it and then attempt a second insertion to inject.

COMPLICATIONS

It is emphasized that this procedure should not be taken lightly. Consideration of medical history and location is of utmost importance. The tissue overlying the ganglion commonly is thin with a poor blood supply and can slough because of bleeding, inadequate perfusion, or immune compromise. In addition, these cysts can be intertwined with neurovascular structures (Fig. 193-10), and an intravascular or intraneural injection can have adverse results. Subcutaneous atrophy or depigmentation can occur if the steroid concentration is too high.

OPERATIVE TREATMENT

Surgical excision usually is 95% curative if the ganglion and stalk are removed with a small cuff of the adjacent joint capsule. The procedure should be approached with the same seriousness of any other hand surgery. A surgical suite with general or regional anesthesia is preferred. These operations should be performed by physicians familiar with these lesions and anatomic structures. Even with surgical excision, the cysts can recur. The small troublesome mucinous cyst on the dorsal DIP joint can actually require a fairly aggressive procedure to resolve.

CPT/BILLING CODES

10160   Puncture aspiration of abscess, hematoma, bulla, or cyst
20550   Injection tendon, ganglion, trigger point
20600   Injection, small joint or cyst
25110   Excision, lesion of tendon sheath, forearm and/or wrist
25111   Excision of ganglion, wrist (dorsal or volar); primary

ICD-9-CM DIAGNOSTIC CODE

727.41   Ganglion; joint

BIBLIOGRAPHY

Andren L, Eiken O: Arthrographic studies of wrist ganglions, *J Bone Joint Surg* 53A:299, 1971.

Angelides AC: Ganglions of the hand and wrist. In Green DP, Hotchkiss RN, Pederson WC, editors: *Green's operative hand surgery,* New York, 1999, Churchill-Livingstone.

Angelides AC, Wallace PF: The dorsal ganglion of the wrist: its pathogenesis, gross and microscopic anatomy, and surgical treatment, *J Hand Surg* 1:228, 1976.

Brown JS: *Minor surgery: a text and atlas,* ed 4, London, 2001, Oxford University Press.

Clay NR, Clement DA: The treatment of dorsal wrist ganglia by radical excision, *J Hand Surg* 13B:187, 1998.

Holm PCA, Pandey SD: Treatment of ganglia of the hand and wrist with aspiration and injection of hydrocortisone, *Hand* 5:63, 1973.

Jayson MIV, Dickson ASJ: Valvular mechanism in juxta-articular cysts, *Ann Rheum Dis* 29:415, 1970.

Kleinert HE, Kutz JE, Fishman JH, McCraw LH: Etiology and treatment of the so-called mucous cyst of the finger, *J Bone Joint Surg* 54A:1455, 1972.

Loder RT, Robinson JH, Jackson WT, Allen DJ: A surface ultrastructure study of ganglia and digital mucous cysts, *J Hand Surg* 13A:758, 1988.

Nelson CL, Sawmiller S, Phalen GS: Ganglions of the wrist and hand, *J Bone Joint Surg* 54A:1459, 1972.

Peimer CA, Thompson JS: Tumors of the hand. In Chapman MW, editor: *Operative orthopaedics,* Philadelphia, 1993, JB Lippincott.

Psaila JV, Mansel RE: The surface ultra-structure of ganglia, *J Bone Joint Surg* 60B:228, 1978.

Richman JA, Gelberman RH, Engber WD, et al: Ganglions of the wrist and digits: results of treatment by aspiration and cyst wall puncture, *J Hand Surg* 12(6):1041, 1987.

Smith DL: *Postgrad Med* 95:117, 1994.

CHAPTER 194

Joint and Soft Tissue Aspiration and Injection (Arthrocentesis)

John L. Pfenninger

Aspiration and injection of soft tissue and joints is relatively simple. Steroid injection into joints fell into disfavor for many years because the procedure was overused and abused. When appropriate guidelines are followed, complications are extremely rare. The alternative to focal treatment with injection is usually systemic nonsteroidal antiinflammatory drugs (NSAIDs), which have significant toxicity with prolonged use.

Primary care physicians should master the technique of aspiration and injection for many reasons. If the physician aspirates an inflamed joint, a diagnosis can be made immediately. If a joint is distended, pain can be relieved rapidly by aspirating the fluid. Injecting an anesthetic or steroid solution can give focal pain relief without the toxicity of the systemic medications.

The clinician should not withhold the benefits of injection therapy because there is not complete familiarity with the precise anatomy involved.

The reader may want to refer to Chapter 190, Diagnostic Needle Arthroscopic Lavage and Biopsy, and Chapter 193, Ganglion Treatment, for related information.

INDICATIONS

Diagnostic Indications

- To evaluate synovial fluid and determine whether an effusion is from an infectious, rheumatic, traumatic, or crystal-induced etiology
- To perform a therapeutic trial to differentiate between various etiologies of a condition (e.g., costochondritis from coronary artery disease, trochanteric bursitis from deep hip disease, occipital trigger points from vertebral disease)

Therapeutic Indications

- To remove exudative fluid from a septic joint
- To relieve pain in a grossly swollen joint (e.g., traumatic effusion)
- To inject lidocaine, saline, or corticosteroids for trigger points, noninfectious inflammatory arthritis, tendonitis, or neuritis

Corticosteroids have a marked effect on inflammation. There are no good data to indicate that steroid injections decrease the long-term adverse effects of chronic degenerative osteoarthritis, but there is no doubt that they result in acute symptomatic improvement.

Conditions

Box 194-1 lists the conditions that are improved with local corticosteroid therapy. Localized pain that persists more than a few weeks after a trial of NSAIDs warrants an injection with steroids. Injection can be tried primarily when the potential toxicity or intolerance to NSAIDs outweighs the risk of local corticosteroids.

Indications for Hyaluronic Acid Supplementation

Synovial fluid functions as a lubricant and a shock absorber in the joint. In osteoarthritis, it retains very little of these intrinsic physical properties. At a critical load, normal synovial fluid changes its mechanical properties from viscous lubricant to elastic shock absorber. This occurs between walking and running and is determined by the dynamic stress of both the frequency and the force of the load. This property is lost in osteoarthritis. In addition, the concentration of hyaluronan in the synovial fluid in patients with osteoarthritis is less than normal. Injected hylans and hyaluronans have properties similar to normal synovial fluid, and although they may only remain in the knee less than 2 weeks, the beneficial effects can persist up to a year (mean duration of 8.2 months). There is some evidence that they stimulate endogenous production of the synovial fluid. There is no evidence that viscosupplementation retards the progression of joint deterioration, but it shows promise of postponing for years the need for total knee replacement. The materials injected (hylans and

BOX 194-1

Conditions Improved with Local Corticosteroid Injection

Articular Conditions
Rheumatoid arthritis
Seronegative spondyloarthropathies
   Ankylosing spondylitis
   Arthritis associated with inflammatory bowel disease
   Psoriasis
   Reiter's syndrome
Crystal-induced arthritis
   Gout
   Pseudogout
Osteoarthritis
Ganglions
Coccydynia

Nonarticular Disorders
Fibrositis
   Localized (trigger points)
   Systemic
Bursitis
   Subacromial
   Olecranon
   Trochanteric
   Anserine
   Prepatellar
Periarthritis
   Adhesive capsulitis
Tenosynovitis/tendonitis
   de Quervain's disease
   Trigger finger
   Bicipital tendonitis
   Tennis elbow (lateral epicondylitis)
   Golfer's elbow (medial epicondylitis)
   Plantar fasciitis
   Rotator cuff
   Supraspinatus tendonitis
   Impingement syndrome
Neuritis
   Carpal tunnel syndrome
   Cubital tunnel
   Tarsal tunnel syndrome
Costochondritis
Tietze's syndrome
Morton's neuroma

Adapted from Pfenninger JL: *Am Fam Physician* 44:1196, 1991.

hyaluronans) are pharmacologically inert so the Food and Drug Administration (FDA) classifies them as "devices," not "drugs."
- Approved for use in knee only.
- May be used instead of, or after, intraarticular corticosteroid injections and before surgical intervention.
- Effective in all stages of osteoarthritis of the knee, although it wanes in the most advanced stages.

CONTRAINDICATIONS

- Cellulitis or broken skin over the intended entry site for the injection or aspiration

- Anticoagulant therapy that is not well controlled
- Severe primary coagulopathy
- Infected effusion of a bursa or a periarticular structure (for injection)
- More than three previous injections in a weight-bearing joint in the preceding 12-month period (relative)
- Lack of response to two or three prior injections (relative)
- Suspected bacteremia (Unless the joint itself is suspected as the source of the bacteremia, it should not be tapped. Doing so could inoculate the joint space and actually *cause* infection.)
- Unstable joints (for steroid injection)
- Inaccessible joints (For many primary care physicians, this includes the hip joint, the sarcoiliac joint, and the joints of the vertebral column.)
- Joint prostheses (If infection is suspected, consider a referral to the orthopedist who placed the prosthesis, if at all possible.)
- Pregnancy (relative)

EQUIPMENT

In the past, joint injections were frequently performed without gloves with only an alcohol wipe. In contrast, some physicians still use an extensive sterile draping procedure. Although the former is grossly inadequate, the latter is probably unnecessary unless the patient is immunosuppressed, diabetic, or at high risk of infection. Most injections are administered after an alcohol or povidone-iodine wipe. Gloves (sterile or nonsterile) should be used. When a culture is anticipated, sterile gloves are more customary. Masks are unnecessary.

Required equipment includes the following:
- Povidone-iodine wipes or alcohol wipes
- Sterile or nonsterile gloves
- Sterile drapes *(optional)*
- 22- to 27-gauge, 1½-inch needle for injections
- 18- to 21-gauge, 1½-inch needle for aspirations
- 30-gauge, ½-inch needle, if skin anesthesia is to be given (usually not needed)
- 1- to 10-ml syringe for injections (Luer-Lok is recommended.)
- 3- to 50-ml syringe for aspirations
- Single dose vials of 1% lidocaine

Note: There are two reasons to use single-dose vials. No allergic reaction has ever been reported to xylocaine (an amide), but reactions do occur to the preservative (parabens). This is still rare. Local anesthetics with an ester base (e.g., Novocaine) can cause allergic reactions. Also, many steroids will precipitate when mixed with the

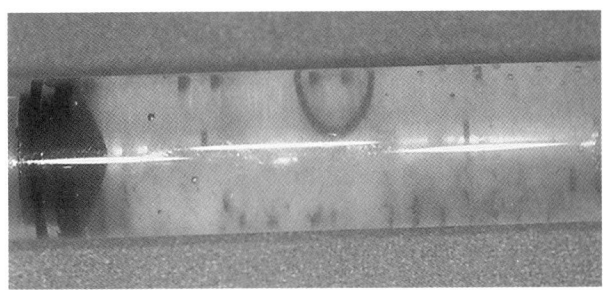

Fig. 194-1
Example of precipitation of steroid (Celestone Soluspan) when mixed with lidocaine solution from a multidose vial.

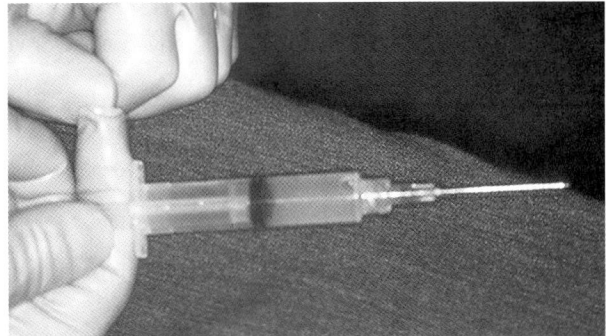

Fig. 194-2
Steroid in solution (Celestone Soluspan) when mixed with lidocaine from a single-dose vial. It is preferable to have the steroid in solution rather than in precipitated form.

TABLE 194-1
Relative Potency of Corticosteroids

Corticosteroid	Relative Antiinflammatory Potency	Approximate Equivalent Dose (mg)
Short-acting Preparations		
Cortisone	0.8	25
Hydrocortisone	1	20
Intermediate-acting Preparations		
Prednisone	3.5	5
Prednisolone tebutate (Hydeltra-TBA)	4	5
Triamcinolone (Aristocort, Aristospan, Kenalog)	5	4
Methylprednisolone acetate (Depo-Medrol)	5	4
Long-acting Preparations		
Dexamethasone (Decadron-LA)	25	0.6
Betamethasone (Celestone Soluspan)	25	0.6

Adapted from Leversee JH: *Prim Care* 13:572, 1986.

parabens preservatives. This leads to uneven distribution in the syringe as well as the injection of small crystals into the site. Theoretically, a homogenous solution would be desired and will be more efficacious, although no studies have studied the issue. Certain manufacturers do not recommend injecting precipitated steroids (Figs. 194-1 and 194-2).

- Hemostat (to be used if joint is to be aspirated then injected using different syringes but same needle)
- Tubes for culture or other laboratory studies (if aspiration is performed)
- Corticosteroid preparation (Tables 194-1 and 194-2)

Note: It is best to pick out one or two preparations and learn them well. It is not necessary to be familiar with all the drugs listed. There is no consensus in the literature as to the

"best" drug or the optimal dosages. Recommendations are given.

- Hyaluronic acid preparation (if used)
  —Sodium hyaluronate (Hyalgan, Supartz) and hylan G-F 20 (Synvisc)
  —Dosages:
    Synvisc: three injections, 1 week apart ($620)
    Hyalgan: five injections, 1 week apart ($640)
    Supartz: five injections, 1 week apart ($587)
- Band-Aid

PREPROCEDURE PATIENT PREPARATION

Inform the patient of the risks, benefits, and possible complications of injection therapy. This is especially important if steroids are used. Rarely is there ever a

TABLE 194-2

Common Corticosteroids and Recommended Dosages for Various Joint Injections

Corticosteroid	Concentration (mg/ml)	Large Joint* Dosage (mg)	Medium Joint† Dosage (mg)	Small Joint‡ Dosage (mg)	Ganglia (mg)	Tendon Sheath (mg)	Bursa (mg)
Hydrocortisone acetate	25, 50	40-100	20-40	8-20	20-40	20-50	40-90
Prednisolone tebutate (Hydeltra-TBA)	20	20-30	10-20	8-10	10-20	4-10	20
Prednisolone sodium phosphate	20	10-20	5-10	4-5	5-10	3-8	20
Triamcinolone hexacetonide (Aristospan)	5, 20	20-30	10-20	8-10	10-20	4-10	20
Triamcinolone diacetate (Aristocrat)	25, 40	20-40	10-20	8-10	10-20	4-10	20
Triamcinolone acetonide (Kenalog)	10, 40	20-40	10-20	8-10	10-20	4-10	20
Methylprednisolone acetate (Depo-Medrol)	20, 40, 80	20-40	10-40	8-10	4-20	4-10	20
Dexamethasone sodium phosphate (Decadron)	4	2-4	1-3	0.8-1	1-2	0.4-1	2-3
Dexamethasone acetate (Decadron-LA)	8	2-4	1-3	0.8-1	1-2	0.4-1	2-3
Betamethasone acetate/phosphate (Celestine Soluspan)	6	6-12	3-6	1.5-3	1-3	1.5-2	3-6

*Such as knee, shoulder, ankle.
†Such as elbow, wrist.
‡Such as metacarpophalangeal, interphalangeal, acromioclavicular, temporomandibular.

complication from the use of lidocaine alone. However, with steroids, and especially with repeated injections, there are some adverse consequences (see the "Complications" section and Table 194-3). Inform the patient that there is always a possibility for *infection* with the injection, although this is extremely rare. *Bleeding* into a joint can occur, although this generally does not happen unless the patient has a coagulopathy. The injection may actually cause more *pain* during the first 24 to 36 hours. This is called *steroid flare*. If the pain lasts for more than 72 hours, evaluate the patient for the possibility of a septic joint. Warn the patient of a possible *failure* to *obtain relief* and that a second or even a third injection may be needed. *Whether or not steroids have significant adverse effects*, and the degree of this reaction on the cartilage and bone itself when steroids are injected into the joint space, is controversial. *Allergic reactions* are very rare. *Tendon ruptures* should be avoidable if the injection is placed peritendinously instead of within the tendon itself. However, rupture is always a possibility. As a final precaution, warn the patient that a steroid placed too close to the surface of the *skin* occasionally causes *atrophy* (Fig. 194-3). This may leave the patient with *depigmentation and a slight indentation* in the skin.

For diabetics, rapidly absorbed steroids can interfere with *glucose metabolism;* therefore glucose levels need to be followed more closely in the first 24 hours.

TABLE 194-3

Adverse Effects of Local Corticosteroid Therapy

Complication	Estimated Prevalence
Postinjection flare	2%-5%
Steroid arthropathy	0.8%
Tendon rupture	<1%
Facial flushing	<1%
Skin atrophy, depigmentation	<1%
Iatrogenic infectious arthritis	0.01%
Transient paresis of injected extremity	Rare
Hypersensitivity reaction	Rare
Asymptomatic pericapsular calcification	43%
Acceleration of cartilage attrition	Unknown

From Gary RG, Gottlieb NL: *Clin Orthop* 177:253, 1983.

Pneumothorax has been reported after injection of trigger points and other conditions around the thorax. See below for the proper technique to avoid this.

TECHNIQUE

Before injection therapy, consider the differential diagnosis. If tumor or fracture is possible, radiographs should be obtained. Many times, especially with trigger-point injection (see Chapter 10, Trigger-Point

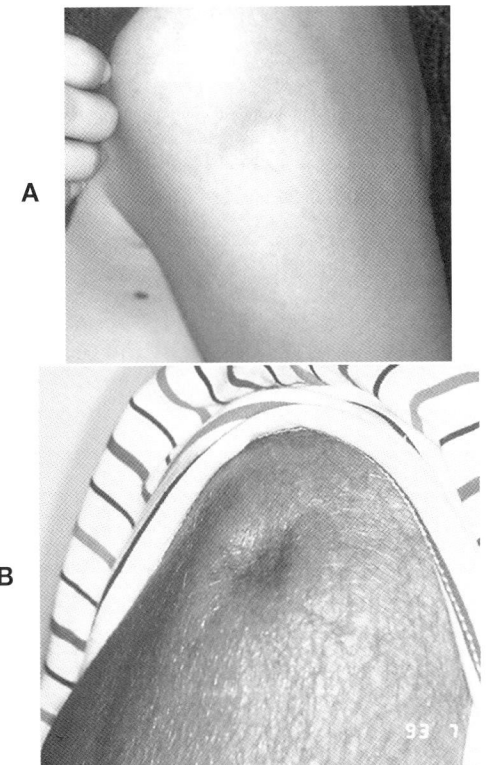

Fig. 194-3
A, This patient received a steroid injection for "allergies" approximately 6 weeks before this photo was taken. It is an example of steroid fatty atrophy. This resolved spontaneously by 6 months. **B,** An example of fat atrophy from a steroid injection received 5 years previously. This is a chronic condition that will not resolve. (Courtesy The National Procedures Institute, Midland, Mich.)

Injection), radiographs are not necessary. Other diagnoses may also be fairly straightforward and not require a prior radiograph examination. If the diagnosis is in question or if the patient is at risk for bone metastases (e.g., a history of breast or prostate cancer), it should be clarified before injection therapy.

Generally, the clinician injects a combination of lidocaine with the steroid of choice. Single-dose vials of lidocaine should be used to avoid the preservative/precipitation problems (see above and the "Complications" section). Using a rather large volume of lidocaine may be beneficial. Not only does it disburse the steroid in a less-concentrated solution, but the volume itself may have a therapeutic effect. In some instances, only a minimal amount of lidocaine can be used (e.g., ganglion cysts, trigger fingers). In other sites, larger amounts are recommended (e.g., lidocaine 5 to 10 ml in a shoulder or knee mixed with 0.5 to 1 ml of selected steroid). A good rule of thumb is to use more, not less, when it comes to lidocaine.

The recommended dosages of medications (Table 194-4) and the specific techniques for various injection sites (Figs. 194-4 to 194-26) are included in this chapter. The general approach is as follows:

1. Identify the site of entry and mark it with a thumbnail, ballpoint pen, or indelible marker.
2. Prep the area with an alcohol or povidone-iodine wipe. (Note that alcohol often removes ink and skin marker solutions.)
3. Draw up the proper amounts of steroid and anesthetic into a single syringe and mix well by tipping the syringe backwards and forward.
4. Using appropriate syringes and needles, either aspirate or inject the site as indicated. After insertion but before injection, pull back the plunger to be sure the needle is not in a blood vessel.
5. If aspiration of an effusion is to be followed by injection, there are two choices: (1) have two needle/syringe setups and enter the area twice, or (2) enter once, aspirate, grasp the needle with a hemostat (being careful not to change the position of the needle tip), remove the syringe with the aspirate, then replace it with the lidocaine/steroid syringe, and finally inject the contents.
6. If lidocaine or steroid is to be injected, it is often necessary to inject in two or three areas around the site of tenderness. This is not necessary when the joint space itself has been entered.
7. Although much has been written regarding *laboratory evaluation of joint fluid aspirates,* Schmerling and associates (1990) reported that the *white blood cell* (WBC) count and *polymorphonucleocyte percentage* (PMN) were the only helpful tests to determine the etiology of an exudate. Use lavender-topped vacutainers for these studies. It is recommended that synovial fluid be examined within 1 hour after arthrocentesis. WBC counts of mildly inflammatory fluids can decrease to "non-inflammatory range" within 5 to 6 hours. Glucose, protein, LDH, complement fixation, electrolyte, uric acid levels, rheumatoid factor, and antinuclear antibodies were of little benefit. Fluids for chemistry testing should be transported in green or red top tubes and be analyzed within 4 hours.

If the exudate is cloudy, the WBC count is elevated, or if a septic joint is strongly suspected, a *culture* is also indicated. For cultures, submit as much fluid as possible. "Swabbed samples" may not be adequate. Large-volume specimens (over 2 ml) support viability of most microorganisms for up to 24 hours at room temperature. Nevertheless, transport to the lab ASAP. *Do not refrigerate!* Large samples may be sent in the syringe used to aspirate them or in a sterile 5- or 10-ml red-topped container. For volumes less than 2 ml, consider using bottles with culture media (e.g., Port-A-Cul) inside. Lavender and green containers cannot be used.

TABLE 194-4

Needle Size and Drug Dosage for Injection Therapy

Structure	Needle Gauge (Length)	Dose of 1% Lidocaine (ml)	Dose of Methylprednisolone Acetate (mg)
Abductor tendon of thumb (de Quervain's disease)	25 (1½ inch)	3-4	10-20
Acromioclavicular joint	22-25 (1-1½ inch)	2-4	4-10
Ankle	22 (1-1½ inch)	3-5	20-40
Anserine bursa	22-25 (1½ inch)	3-5	20-40
Biceps tendon	22 (1½ inch)	5-10	10-20
Calcaneal bursa	22 (1½ inch)	5	20-40
Carpal tunnel	25 (1½ inch)	1	20-40
de Quervain's disease	25 (1½ inch)	3-4	10-20
Elbow			
Radiohumeral joint	22	3-5	20-30
Lateral or medial epicondyle ("tennis elbow," "golfer's elbow")	22-25	3-5	10-30
Olecranon bursa	22 (1-1½ inch)	2-3	10-20
Finger and toe joints (interphalangeal)	25 (1 inch)	0.5-1.0	4-10
Flexor tendon sheath (trigger finger)	25 (1 inch)	0.25-0.5	4-10
Ganglion of wrist, other	18-20 (1-1½ inch)	0.25-0.5	4-10
Hip joint	20 (2½-3 inch)	5	40-80
Knee intraarticular space	20 (1½ inch)	5	20-80
Plantar fascia	22 (1½ inch)	2-4	15-30
Prepatellar bursa	20-22 (1-1½ inch)	3	20-40
Shoulder intraarticular space	20 (1½ inch)	5-7	20-40
Shoulder rotator cuff tendon	18-20 (1½ inch)	5	20-40
Shoulder subacromial bursa	22 (1½-2 inch)	5-7	30-40
Tarsal tunnel	25 (½-1 inch)	1-2	10-20
Temporomandibular joint	25 (½-1 inch)	1-2	5-20
Trigger point	25 (1½ inch)	3-5	10-30
Trochanteric bursa	22 (1½-2 inch)	5-10	20-40
Wrist joint	22-25 (1-1½ inch)	2-4	20-40

Modified from Pfenninger JL: *Am Fam Physician* 44:1690, 1991.

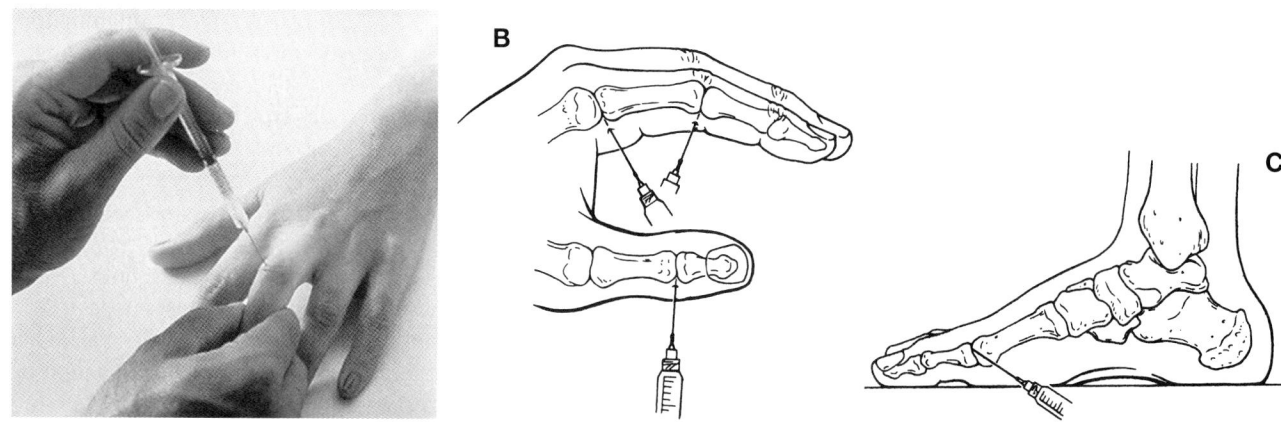

Fig. 194-4

Finger and toe joints. A, Appropriate technique for injecting a finger joint. Tendons run over the dorsum of the finger, whereas nerves and vessels run laterally. Open the joint slightly by flexing it and then inject between the ligaments and the vascular structures as noted. The needle enters at a 45-degree angle to the joint. Any of the finger **(B)** and toe **(C)** joints may be aspirated or injected in the lateral, medial, or dorsal aspect. Slightly flex the joint to open the joint space. Direct the needle to enter just medial or lateral to the extensor tendon. Avoid going too far laterally or medially where the nerve and vascular structures run. (**A,** Courtesy Pharmacia Corp.)

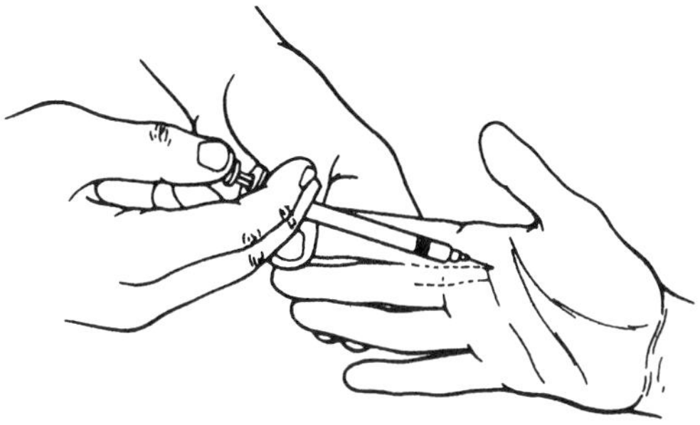

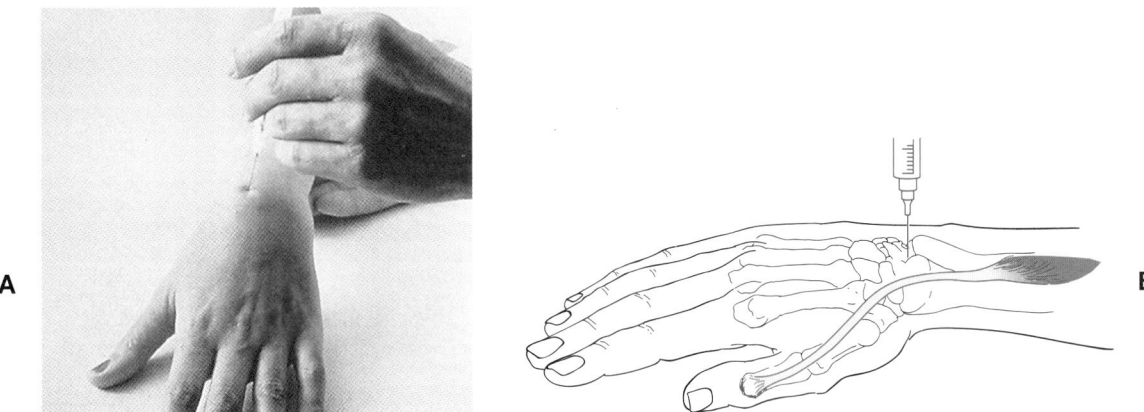

Fig. 194-5
Trigger finger. A, The anatomy of a finger showing the annular pulleys, which maintain the flexor close to the bony structures. When the tendon becomes inflamed and enlarges, it catches on the pulleys, causing a snapping with extension or a "trigger finger." **B,** Identify the flexor tendon involved. Insert the needle at the distal palmar crease. Attempt to position it peritendinously. When the needle is in position, the syringe will move with flexion of the finger.

Labels in figure A: Annular pulleys; Synovial sheath; Flexor digitorum superficialis tendon; Annular pulleys

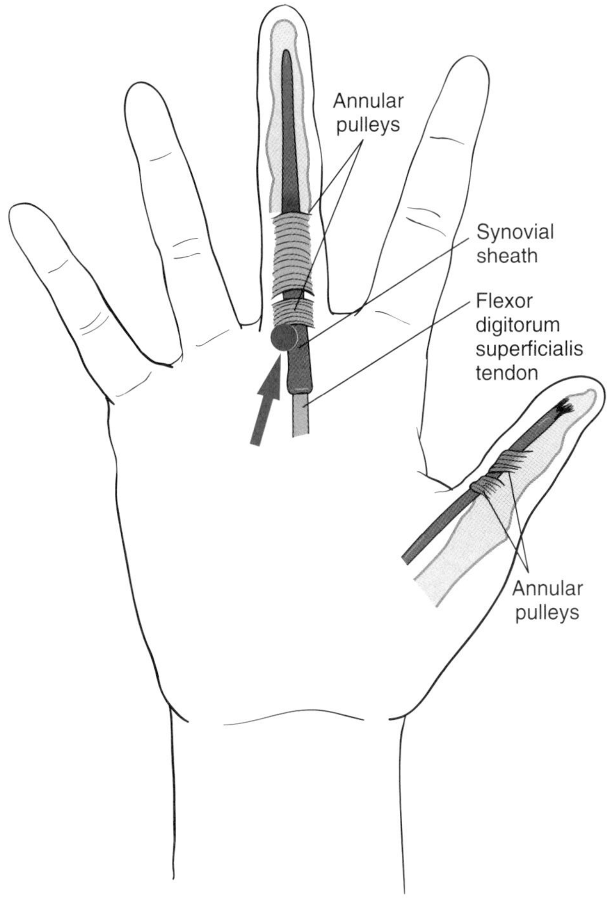

Fig. 194-6
Wrist joint. A, Injection of the wrist joint. The hand is held in slight flexion, and the needle is inserted just distal to the radius in the "snuff box." **B,** Flex the joint 20 degrees to open the joint spaces. The dorsal approach is generally used. Position the needle perpendicular to the skin surface. Enter at a site distal to the radial head and lateral to the extensor pollicis longus tendon (just ulnar to the anatomic "snuff box"). If the needle can be easily inserted to 1 or 2 cm, it is correctly positioned in the joint space. The intercarpal joints have interconnecting synovial spaces, and the contents of one correctly placed injection will disperse into the entire joint complex. (**A,** Courtesy Pharmacia Corp.)

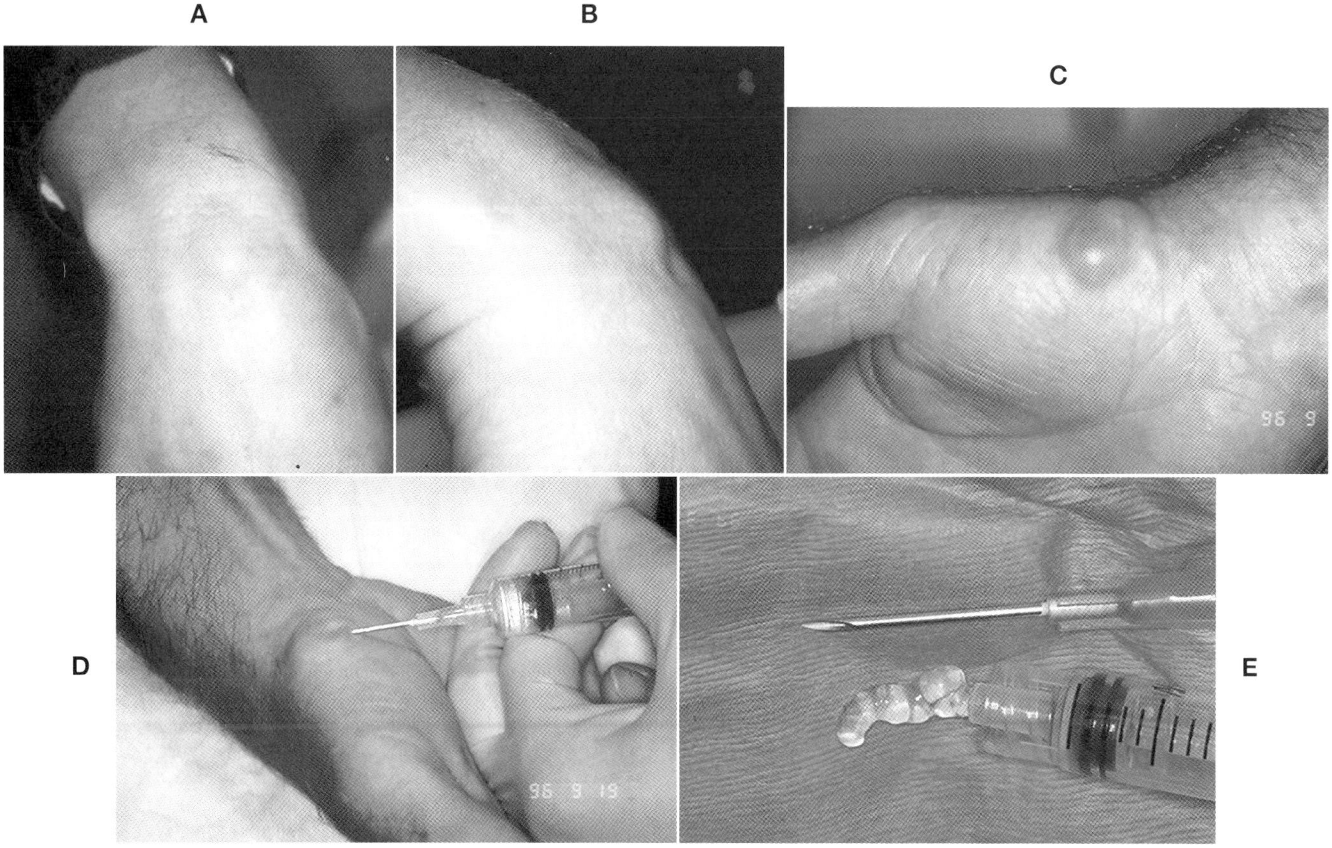

A   **B**   **C**

D   **E**

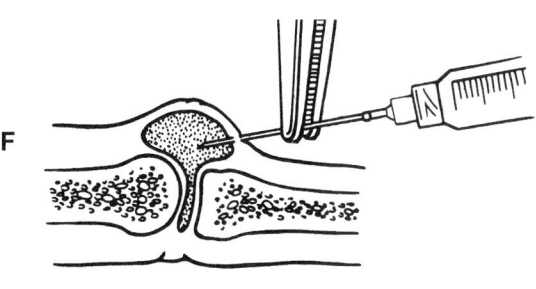

Fig. 194-7

Ganglion. A ganglion is a manifestation of joint inflammation. Typical dorsal wrist ganglion cysts as seen from the, **A,** frontal and, **B,** side views. **C,** Example of an unusual ganglion cyst on the thenar eminence. **D,** Aspiration of the cyst previously seen. **E,** Example of the thick gelatinous material removed from a ganglion cyst. A large 18-gauge needle must be used if this material is to be withdrawn. **F,** Use an 18-gauge needle with a 1- to 3-ml syringe to enter the ganglion and aspirate its contents. The contents are often thick, and there may only be minimal return of a gel-like material. Hold the needle in position with the hemostat and remove the syringe. Attach the steroid-containing syringe and inject the contents. (Some have used fibrin sealants, hypertonic saline, and other irritants for attempts to "scar down" the cyst.) (**A-E,** courtesy The National Procedures Institute, Midland, Mich.)

F

Fig. 194-8

De Quervain's disease. Maximally abduct the thumb to accentuate and identify the tendon. Insert the needle parallel to (but not into) the tendon. Inject at the areas of greatest tenderness. Postinjection splinting may still be necessary.

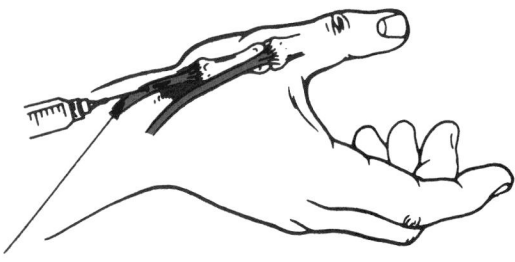

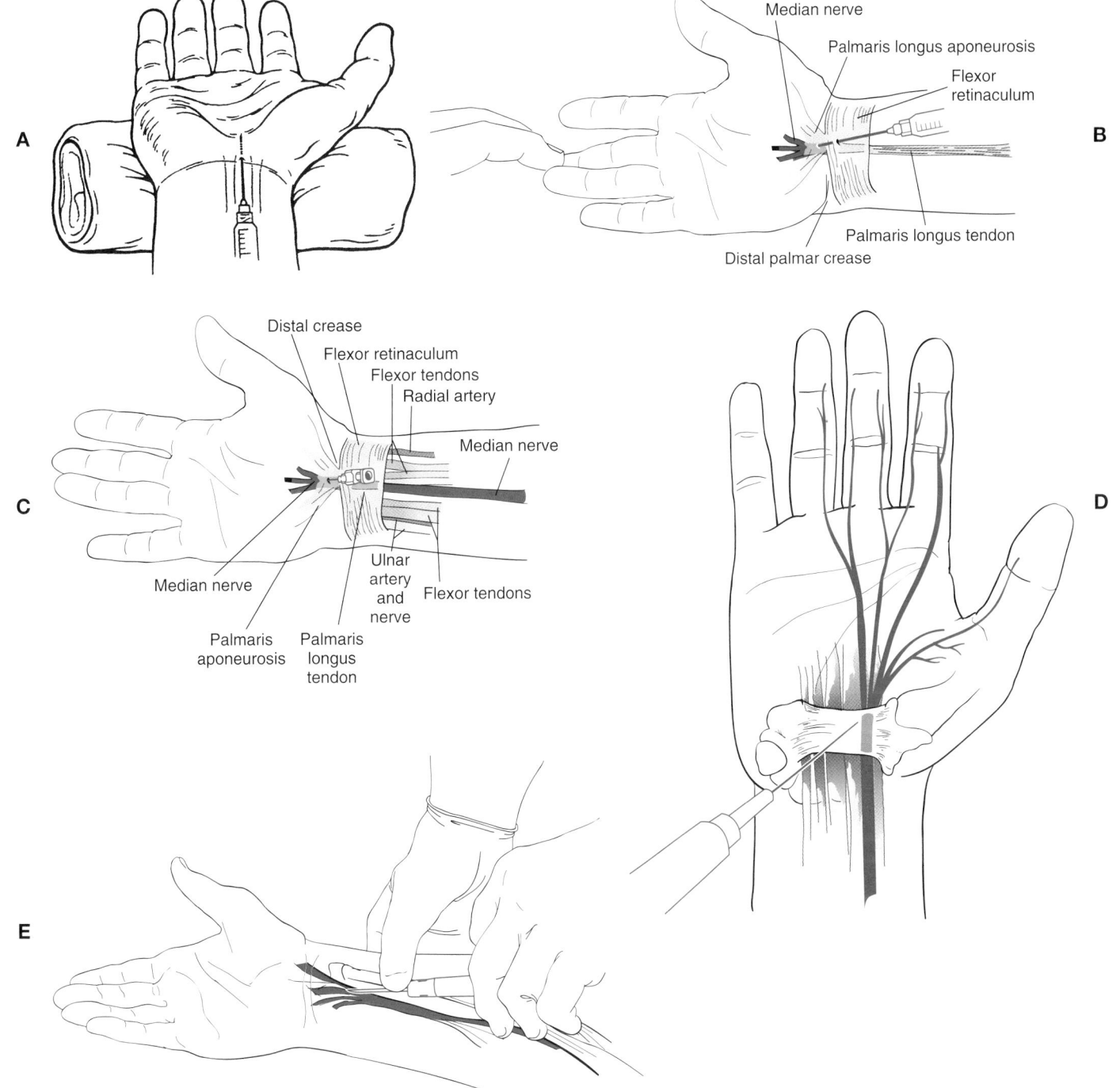

Fig. 194-9

Carpal tunnel syndrome. Four approaches to injection: **A,** *Traditional method.* Dorsiflex the wrist 30 degrees and rest it on a rolled towel. Insert the needle at the distal crease of the wrist either lateral or medial to the palmaris longus tendon. **B,** Find the tendon by having the patient flex the middle finger against resistance. Angle the needle downward at a 45-degree angle toward the tip of the middle finger. If there is any discomfort in the fingers, withdraw and reposition the needle. Advance 1 to 2 cm until there is no resistance, and then inject the medication. **C,** *Alternative method.* Insertion of the needle directly over the carpal tunnel. Use a perpendicular approach going directly through the flexor retinaculum into the median nerve space. **D,** *A third method* of injecting the carpal tunnel. The needle is inserted just radial to the pisiform bone and directed toward the carpal tunnel just beneath the transverse carpal ligament. The needle goes dorsally and distally to terminate within the carpal tunnel just to the ulnar side and dorsal to the median nerve. **E,** *A more recent approach* is to inject on the volar aspect of the forearm 4 cm proximal to the wrist crease between the palmaris longus tendon (see above) and the radial flexor tendon. The needle is inserted in a distal direction with the syringe lifted 10 to 20 degrees up from the parallel. This approach supposedly minimizes chances of trauma to the nerve. In all cases **(A-E),** the injection should be given with minimal pressure, slowly. If there is resistance or if the patient feels "pins and needles" in the fingers, stop immediately. If an intraneural injection occurs, there will be significant pain after injection and surgical decompression may be needed.

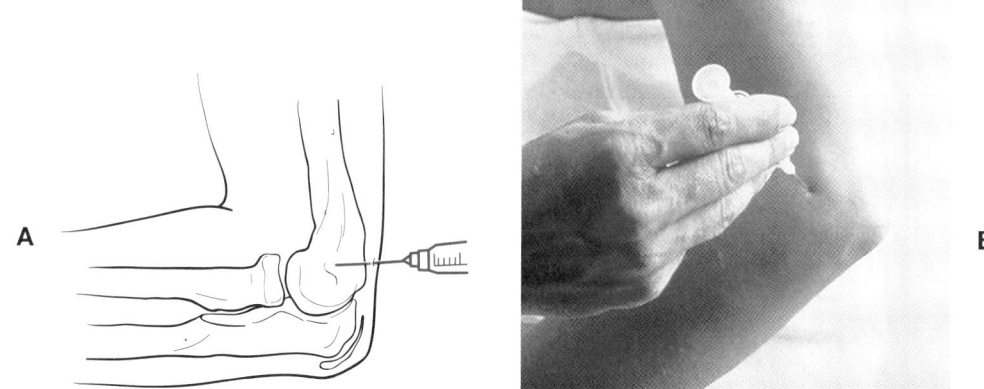

Fig. 194-10
Lateral epicondylitis (tennis elbow). A-B, Find the area of greatest tenderness over the lateral epicondyle. Insert the needle perpendicularly until bone is felt. Withdraw the needle 1 to 2 mm and inject. It may be beneficial to fan out the injections in several directions into the extensor aponeurosis and the radial collateral ligament. Massage the injection site. If distal tenderness is still present after several minutes, another injection in a fanlike pattern may be necessary. Medial epicondylitis (golfer's elbow) is treated in a similar fashion. (**B,** Courtesy Pharmacia Corp.)

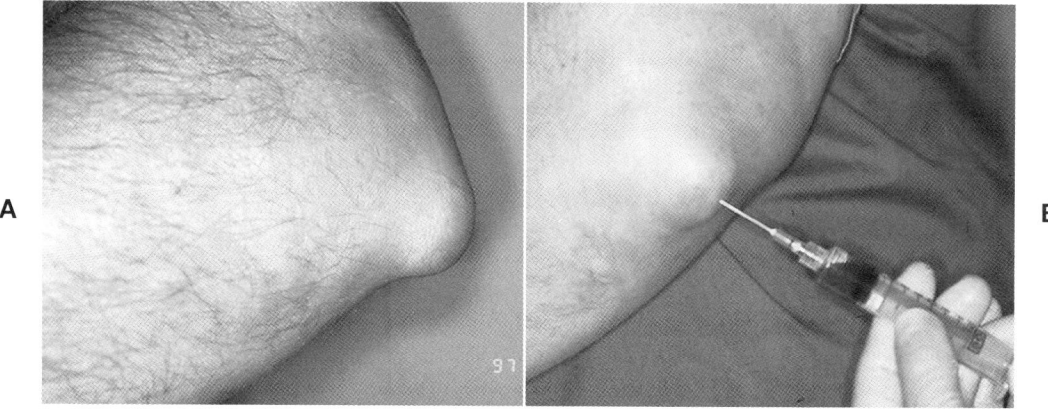

Fig. 194-11
Olecranon bursa. A, Olecranon bursitis. **B,** Aspirating the olecranon bursa. **C,** This bursa is easily identified and entered. Insert a large-bore needle directly into the bursa and aspirate until fluid is returned. Whether cloudy or not, the fluid should be submitted for culture and concurrent infection should be ruled out. Await the culture results before injecting with a steroid. It is next to impossible to tell whether the bursa is infected or not on a clinical basis. While waiting for the culture results, place the patient on nonsteroidal antiinflammatory drugs (NSAIDs) and wrap the area tightly. If infection is suspected, start an antibiotic to cover staph infection while waiting for culture results. Once infection is ruled out, steroids can be used. In a double-blind study comparing focal steroid injection into the olecranon bursa with systemic NSAIDs, the most rapid benefit and most lasting effect came from steroid injections. (**A-B,** Courtesy The National Procedures Institute, Midland, Mich.)

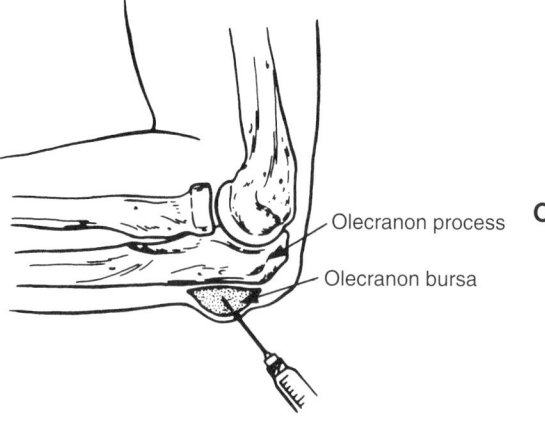

Olecranon process
Olecranon bursa

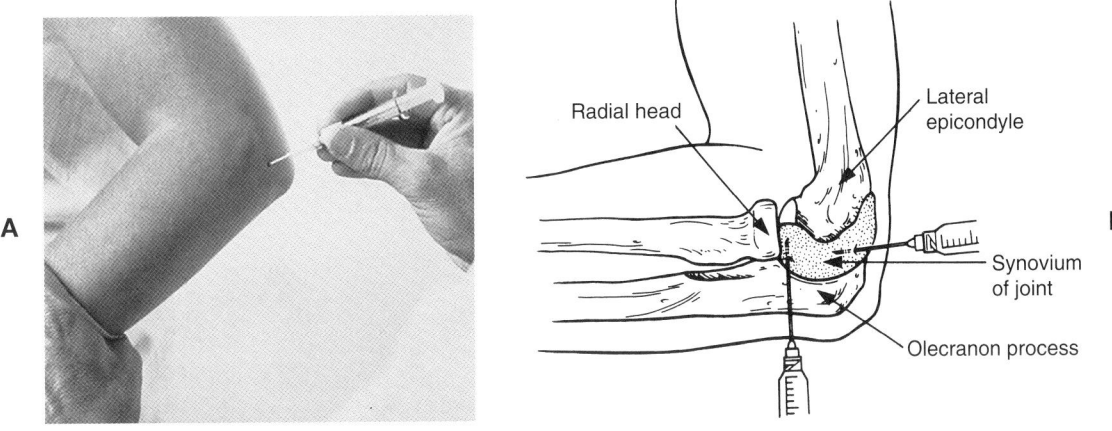

Fig. 194-12
Elbow joint. A, Injection of the elbow joint. **B,** Flex the elbow 45 degrees. Identify the lateral epicondyle. Inject into the joint space just inferior to the lateral epicondyle and superior to the olecranon process of the ulna. A slight concavity can be felt just inferior to the radial head and helps identify the proper point of insertion. (**A,** Courtesy Pharmacia Corp.)

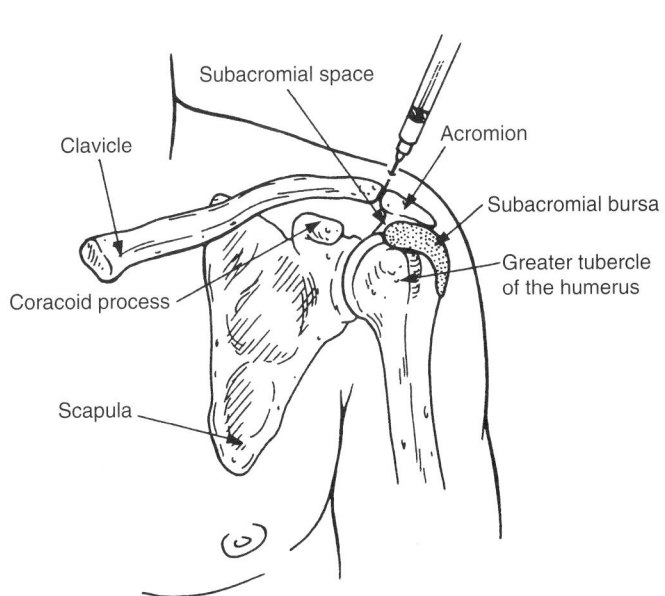

Fig. 194-13
Acromioclavicular joint. With the patient seated and arm at the side, palpate the clavicle, moving laterally until a prominence is felt. This is the acromioclavicular joint. It is about 1.5 to 2 cm inward from the lateral edge to the acromion. Insert the needle from an anterior or superior position into the joint and angle it medially, then inject.

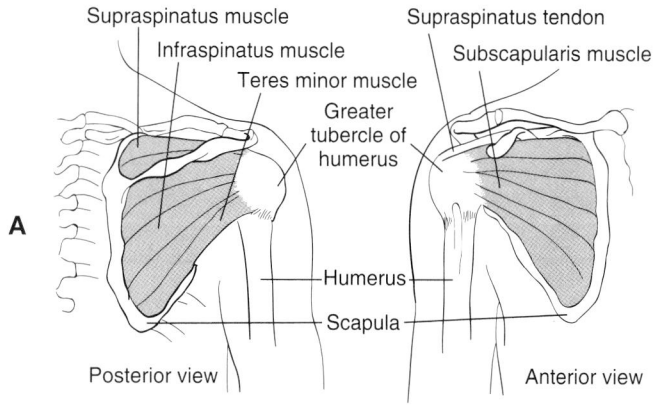

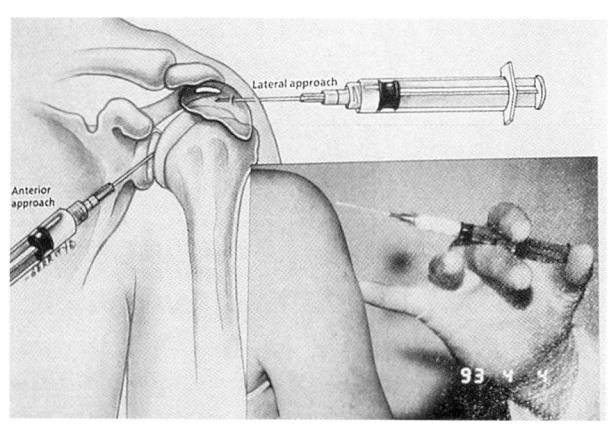

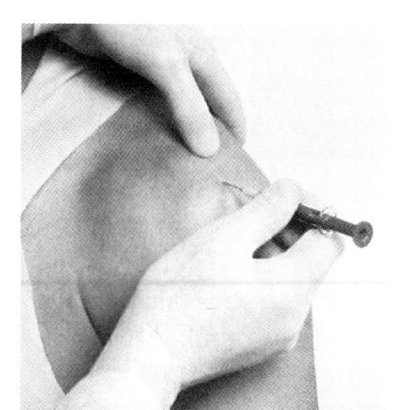

Fig. 194-14
Subacromial bursa. Most injection procedures involving the shoulder will include an injection into the subacromial bursa. Palpate the superior surface of the shoulder, progressing laterally until there is a slight drop-off. This is the lateral edge of the acromion. The now palpable soft spot above the humeral head is the location of the subacromial bursa. Direct the needle perpendicular to the surface and insert the needle through the deltoid muscle into the bursa. The needle should be free floating, since it is within a space, not a muscle or tendon. The tendon of the supraspinatus **(A),** the muscle most commonly involved in a rotator cuff syndrome, is directly medial to this bursa **(B)** and can be entered by directing the needle deeper. If the tendon is calcified as it is entered, a gritty sensation may be felt. Inject within the bursa, not within the tendon. **A,** The muscles of the rotator cuff are demonstrated. They include the supraspinatus, the infraspinatus, teres minor, and the subcapularis. **B,** Injection of the subacromial bursa and the shoulder joint itself. **C,** The technique of a subacromial bursa injection. (**B** and **C,** Courtesy Pharmacia Corp.)

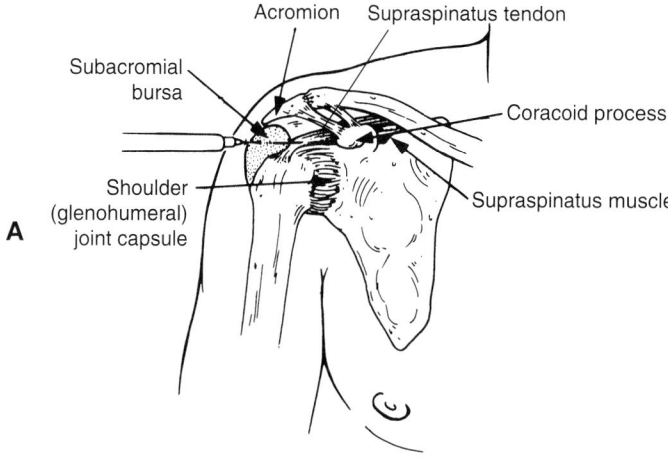

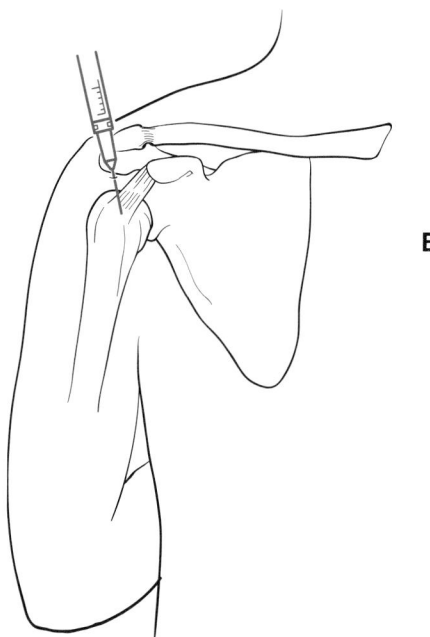

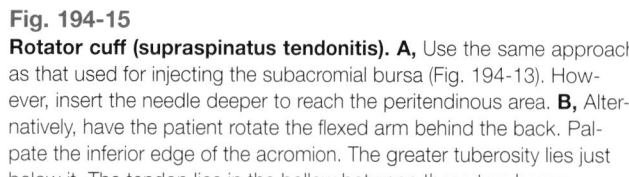

Fig. 194-15
Rotator cuff (supraspinatus tendonitis). A, Use the same approach as that used for injecting the subacromial bursa (Fig. 194-13). However, insert the needle deeper to reach the peritendinous area. **B,** Alternatively, have the patient rotate the flexed arm behind the back. Palpate the inferior edge of the acromion. The greater tuberosity lies just below it. The tendon lies in the hollow between these two bones.

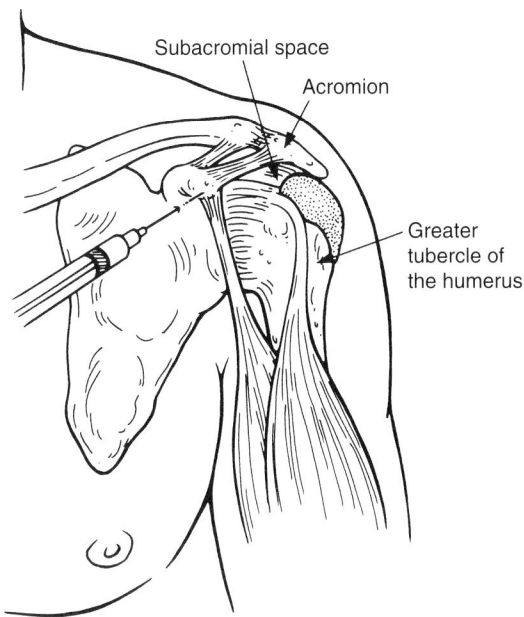

Fig. 194-16
Short head of the biceps. The short head of the biceps attaches to the coracoid process. This is the palpable bony prominence located inferior to the clavicle and medial to the humerus over the anterior portion of the shoulder. Rarely does this area have to be injected, but should a patient have pain and discomfort over the coracoid process, insert a needle directly into the point of maximal tenderness until it reaches the bone. Withdraw the needle 1 or 2 mm and inject. Only a small volume of steroid is needed along with relatively larger amounts of lidocaine. Additional steroid may be injected parallel to the tendon distally (if it is palpable).

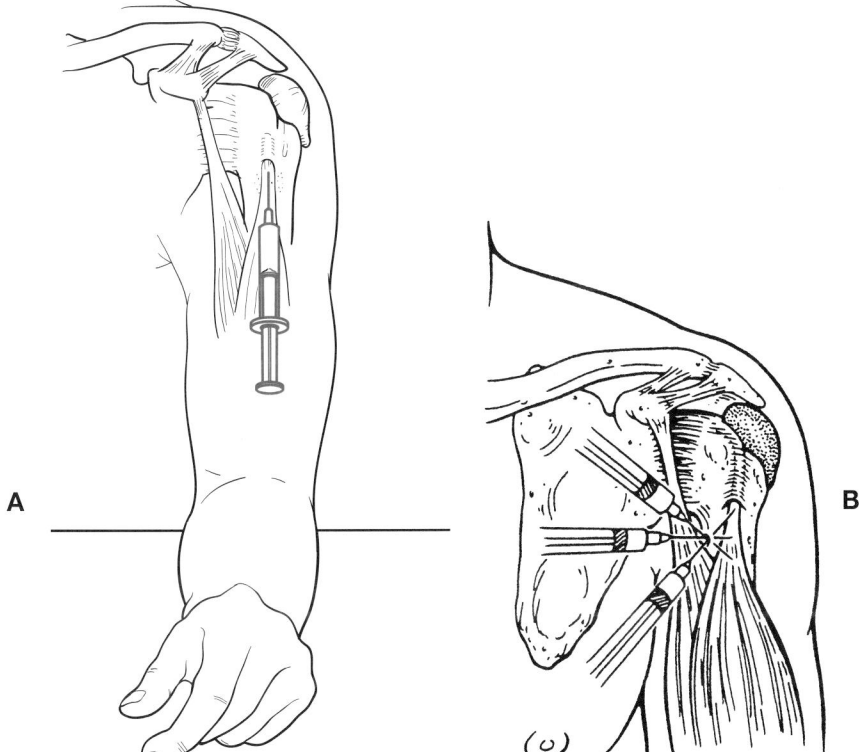

Fig. 194-17
Injection of the **long head of the biceps (bicipital tendonitis). A,** Have the patient seated with arm flexed 90 degrees. Identify the biceps tendon by placing your hand on the patient's shoulder with your fingers posteriorly and the thumb anteriorly over the proximal humerus. Rotate the patient's arm and shoulder inward and outward. The bicipital groove is palpable anteriorly and the tendon "snap" can be felt under your thumb. Identify the most tender area of the tendon (usually in the bicipital groove on the humerus). Insert the needle into this groove and attempt to make a *peritendinous* injection of steroid and lidocaine. Often, a slip of the subacromial bursa surrounds the more proximal portion of the tendon. **B,** If pain persists on palpation after the injection, further injection in a fanlike *peritendinous* pattern may be needed more distally.

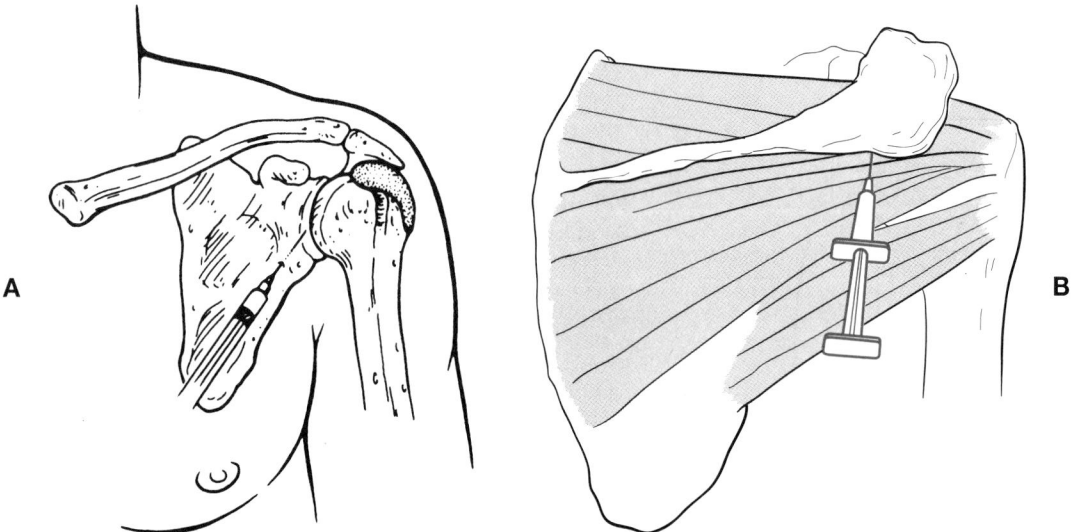

Fig. 194-18

Intraarticular shoulder joint injection. A posterior or an anterior approach can be used to inject into the space of the shoulder joint (scapulohumeral or glenohumeral joint). **A,** In the anterior approach, rotate the shoulder outward. This opens the joint space. Identify the coracoid process. Insert the needle 1 cm inferior and 1 cm lateral to the coracoid process, and direct the needle perpendicularly, or slightly laterally, into the glenohumeral joint. The properly inserted needle should not contact bone. (Also see Fig. 194-13, *B*.) **B,** With the posterior approach, the patient is again seated with the arm rotated medially across the waist. Palpate the inferior-posterior aspect of the acromion with the thumb. Place the index finger on the coracoid process. Insert the needle just below the acromion and aim towards the coracoid. Insert 2 to 3 cm deep.

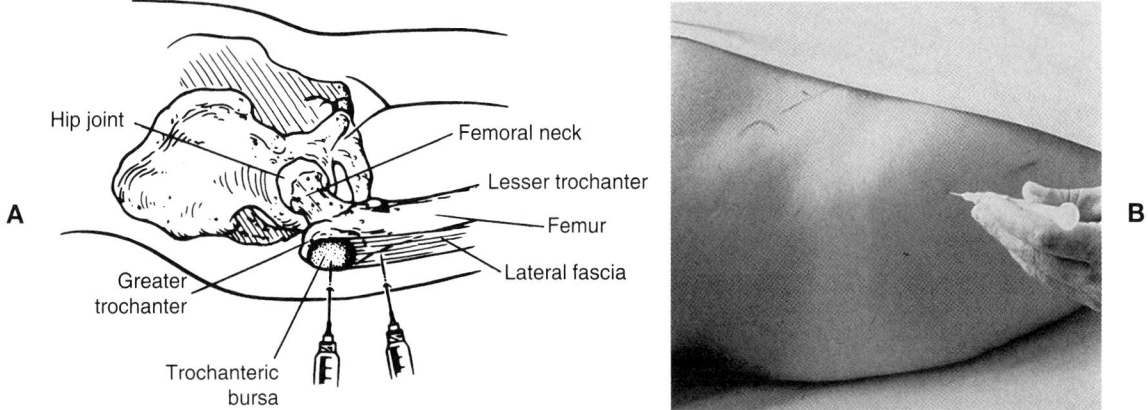

Fig. 194-19

Trochanteric bursa. A, Trochanteric bursa is located at the most superior prominent portion of the femur. Tenderness in this area generally denotes a trochanteric bursitis. Direct the needle perpendicular to the femur at the point of maximal tenderness, and insert until bone is felt. Withdraw the needle 2 to 3 mm and inject. Frequently the pain radiates more distally, as it might with lateral epicondylitis. In this case the pain radiates down the lateral portion of the femur along the fascia. If the patient is still experiencing discomfort 5 minutes after injection of the bursa and massage of the area, a more distal injection may be necessary at the areas of tenderness. **B,** Injecting for trochanteric bursitis. (**B,** Courtesy Pharmacia Corp.)

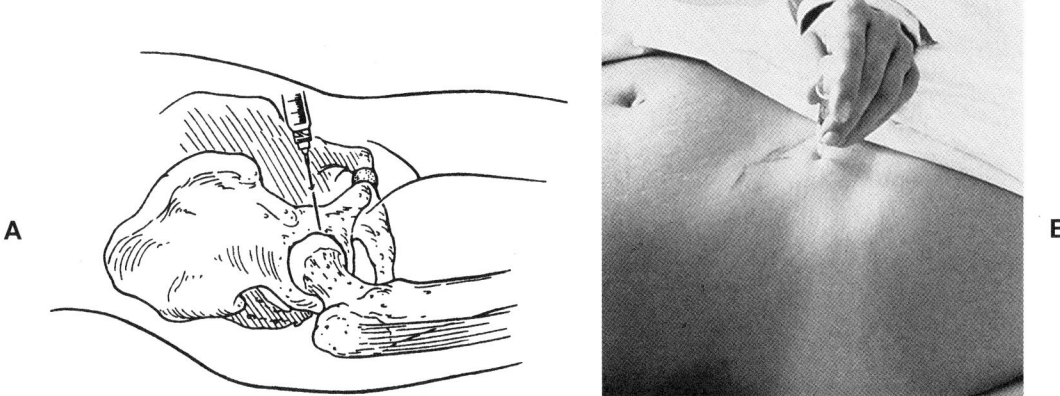

Fig. 194-20

Hip joint proper. A, Experience is necessary to inject the hip joint itself. Even experienced practitioners often use fluoroscopy. An anterior or posterior approach can be taken. However, the anterior approach is most common. Great care must be taken to avoid entering any of the blood vessels or nerves coursing through the inguinal canal area. Position the hip so that the leg is maximally extended and rotated inward. (The hip is placed in extension and internal rotation.) Use a long (2.5-inch) 20-gauge needle to enter 2 to 3 cm below the anterior superior spine of the ilium and 2 to 3 cm lateral to the femoral pulse. The needle should point posteromedially at a 60-degree angle to the skin and then should course through the capsule ligaments until it reaches bone. Withdraw the needle slightly and aspirate for fluid. Injection may then be carried out, and there should be little resistance. **B,** Injecting the hip. (**B,** Courtesy Pharmacia Corp.)

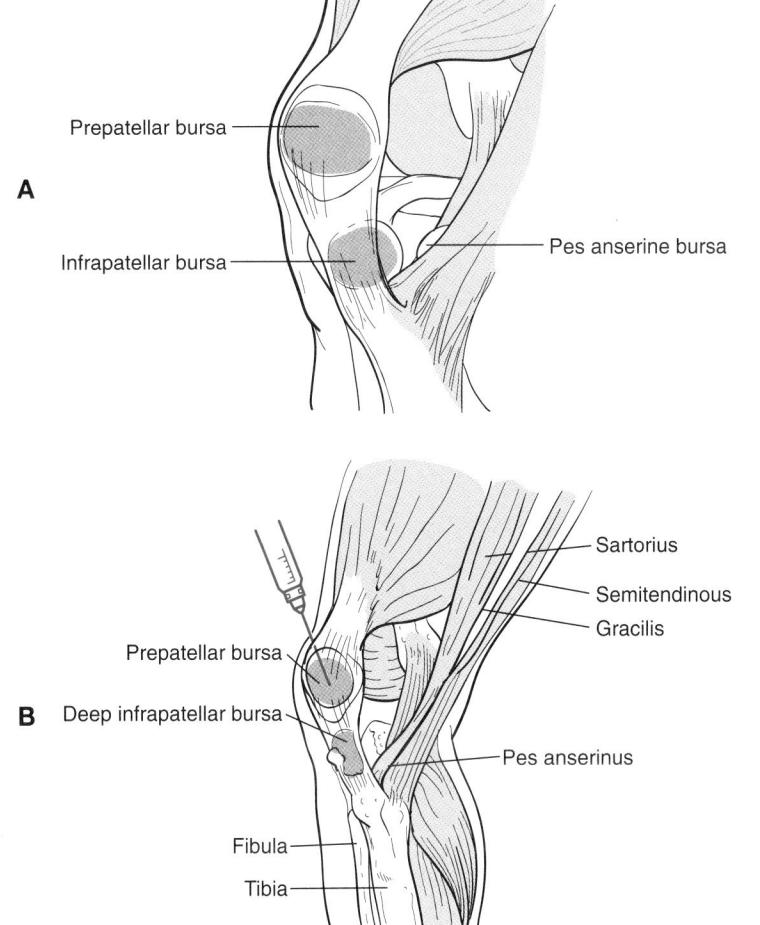

Fig. 194-21

Prepatellar bursa. A, Identify the bursa, which is located between the skin and the patella. **B,** Insert the needle just above the patella and at the lateral portion of the bursa, and direct it to the center of swelling. Aspirate fluid (for culture), switch syringes, and then inject. (Although the data are not as documented as for olecranon bursitis, the protocol for injecting this bursa can be the same.)

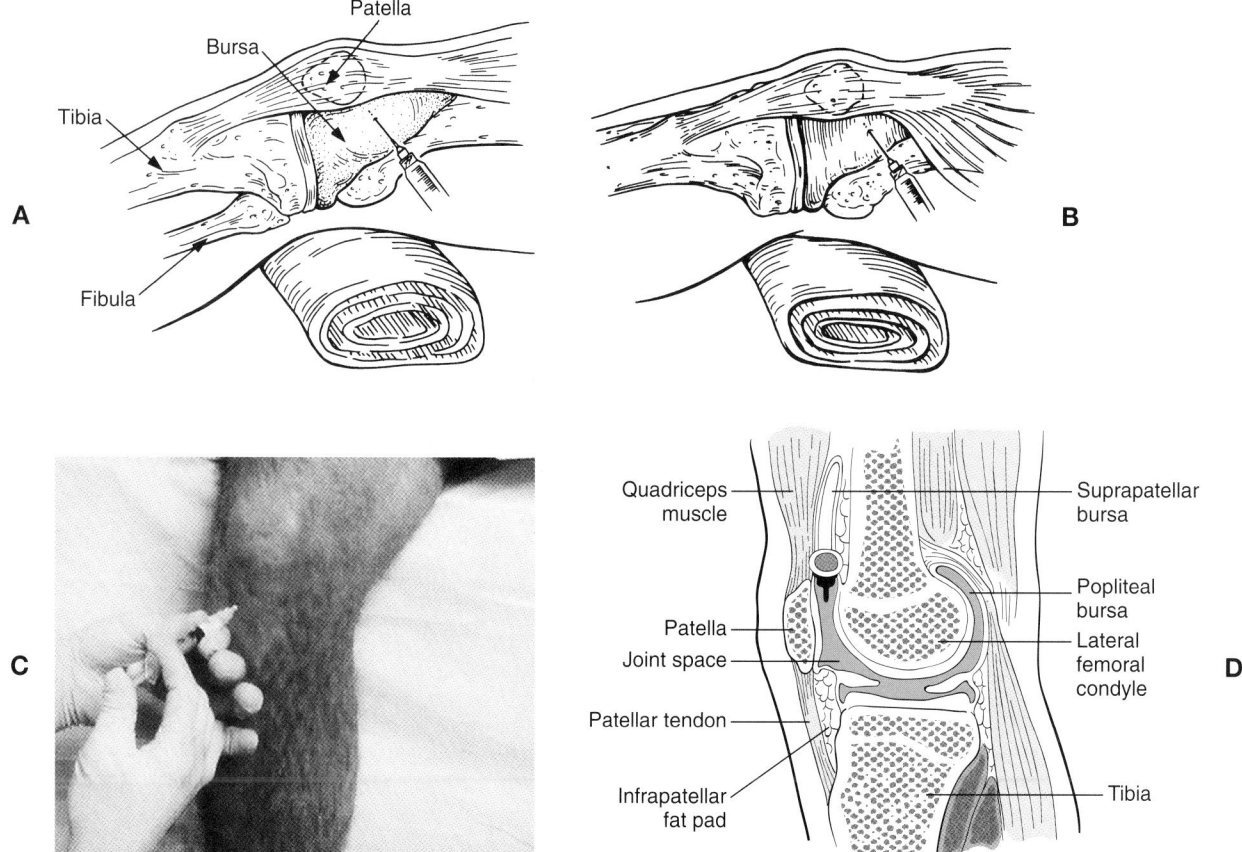

Fig. 194-22

Knee joint. The knee is one of the easiest joints to enter and one of the most common joints to aspirate and inject. Slightly flex the knee using a towel in the popliteal space with the patient lying on an examination table. Either a lateral **(A)** or medial **(B)** approach may be used. For the lateral approach, palpate the superior lateral aspect of the patella and insert the needle 1 cm superior and lateral to this point. Apply gentle pressure on the contralateral side of the knee to encourage the fluid to pool in the area of aspiration. Direct the needle under the patella at a 45-degree angle to the midjoint area. Aspirate all fluid before injection. There should be no resistance. **C,** Other approaches include entering medially or laterally directly above the joint line or with the patient seated going directly through the patellar tendon just below the patella. **D,** The knee joint space is large and is readily entered from multiple approaches.

A **Baker's cyst** is a sac of synovial fluid that has leaked out of a hole in the posterior capsule of the knee. It generally indicates significant internal knee problems, and steroid injections are only a temporary relief frowned on by many clinicians. Insert the needle 3 cm medial to the midline and 3 cm below the popliteal crease. Take care to avoid the popliteal artery, vein, and nerve.

Fig. 194-23

Anserine bursa. The anserine bursa is located on the upper medial portion of the tibia under the insertion of the sartorius, semitendinous, and gracilis tendons. This bursa frequently becomes inflamed in elderly, somewhat obese women; the symptoms are aggravated by going up and down stairs. Palpate and find the point of maximal tenderness, and insert the needle perpendicular to the tibia. When bony resistance is encountered, withdraw the needle 2 or 3 mm and inject several areas in a fanlike fashion. (Also see Fig. 194-20, *A.*)

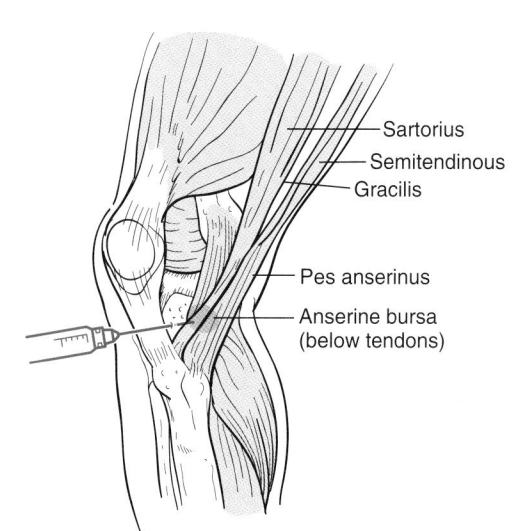

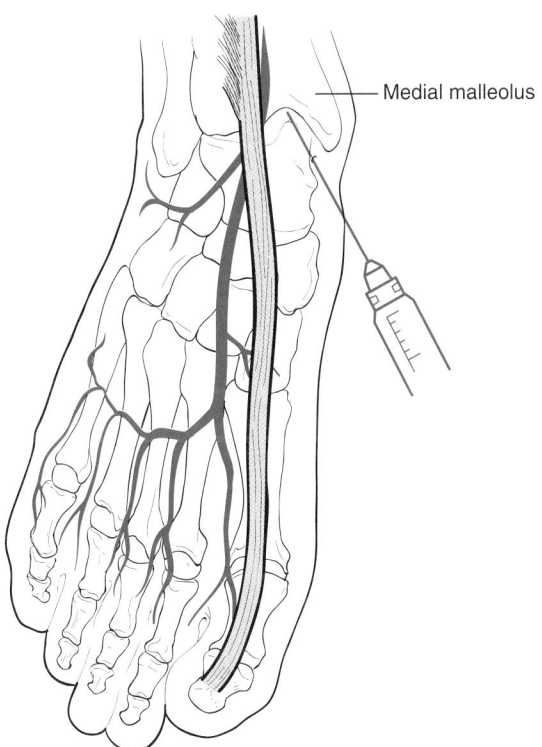

Medial malleolus

Fig. 194-24
Ankle joint. Anteromedial approach is the easiest. Have the patient maximally dorsiflex the toe, accentuating the extensor tendon. Identify the hollow between the anterior medial malleolus and the long extensor tendon. This is the spot for injection. The needle must be inserted approximately 3 cm and directed slightly lateral.

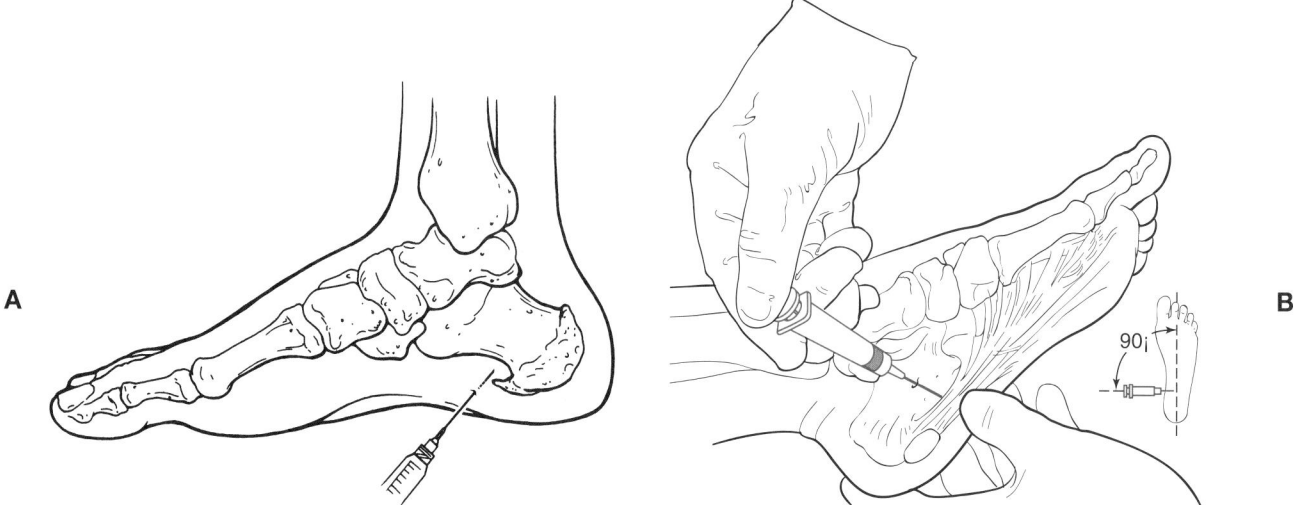

A   B

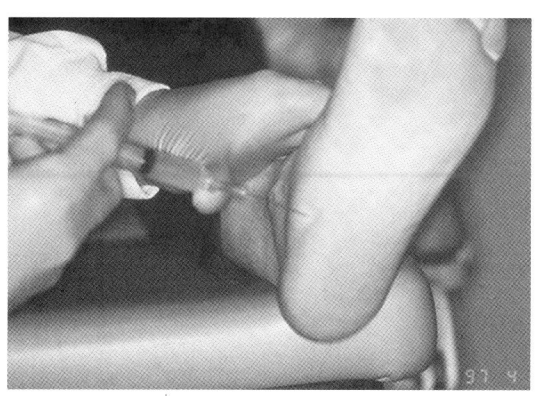

Fig. 194-25
Calcaneal spur/plantar fasciitis. A, Two approaches can be used.
Many physicians prefer to direct the needle from the lateral side of the
foot rather than from the inferior (plantar) side. The adipose tissue of the
heel is uniquely segmented to provide cushion for the foot. If the plantar approach is used and steroid leaks out through the tract, atrophy
could result and thus the patient would have heel pain while walking.
Nevertheless, many physicians approach directly from the plantar position
to inject steroid right over a calcaneal spur. Using the lateral approach,
the physician would direct the needle to enter just below the bony prominence of the calcaneus, and just anterior to the heel pad, and go to the
midline until the point of maximal tenderness is reached **(B-C).** (**C,** Courtesy The National Procedures Institute, Midland, Mich.)

C

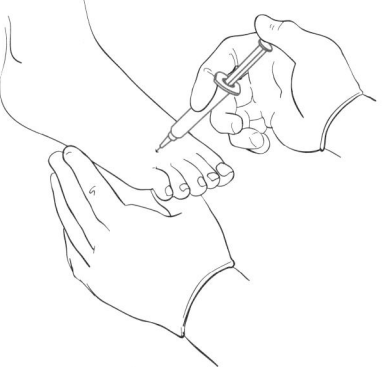

Fig. 194-26
Morton's neuroma. Approach the foot from dorsal aspect. Insert
needle 1 to 2 cm proximal to affected web space. Insert needle
perpendicularly all the way to the plantar surface. Do not penetrate skin,
but estimate depth by observing tenting of skin. Withdraw 1 cm and
inject.

If there is any suspicion of gouty arthritis, *examine the fluid for crystals under polarized light*. A *peripheral smear* may be helpful when a bloody tap is obtained after trauma. The presence of fat cells indicates a fracture. The Pfenninger articles listed in the bibliography contain many tables of other characteristics of synovial fluid for differential diagnosis, although the benefit of additional studies is unproven.

8. Technique of injection for hyaluronic acid devices:
- Must be intraarticular.
- More demanding than steroid intraarticular injections because it must be placed within the synovial space, not the surrounding soft tissue.
- Some will use fluoroscopy to be certain of intraarticular injection.
- Do not mix with xylocaine or steroids.
- Drain all effusions before injection.
- Forced injections push material into the elasticity zone and then are very difficult to administer; slow injections must be given with a 22-gauge or larger needle.
- Patient should avoid strenuous activity for 48 hours.
- Derived from chicken or rooster combs, so an allergy to eggs or feathers would dictate caution.

COMPLICATIONS (Box 194-2 and Table 194-3)

- Injection into a vein or artery
- Introduction of infection (usually *Staphylococcus*) into joint space (18 infections per 250,000 injections [0.072%])
- Trauma to articular cartilage
- Injury to nearby nerves (e.g., median nerve in carpal tunnel injection)
- Pneumothorax (when injecting thoracic trigger points)
- Subcutaneous fatty atrophy (Fig. 194-3)

- Adverse drug reaction (Table 194-3)
- Injection of steroid into a septic joint (If there is any suspicion of infection, do not instill steroids until laboratory studies have ruled it out.)
- Osteoporosis and cartilage damage (This is rare; reported cases have usually occurred after 20 to 30 injections. For joints, especially weight-bearing joints, a limit of three steroid injections per year provides a wide margin of safety.)
- Inappropriate diagnosis
- Tendon rupture (To reduce the possibility of tendon rupture, inject peritendinously instead of intratendinously. Ruptures usually occur after multiple injections and when the patient will not rest the area. Finger tendon ruptures have been reported after steroid injection. Gray and Gottlieb [1983] recommend setting a limit of five total injections per finger joint.)
- Reactions to lidocaine (True allergic reactions to lidocaine itself have not been reported. Lidocaine is an amide. Allergic reactions have been reported to the esters [e.g., "Novocaine"]; when reactions are suspected to lidocaine, it has usually been drawn up from a multidose vial. These contain parabens preservatives, which can cause a reaction. So, if suspicions of a "caine" allergy arise, single-dose vials of lidocaine should be used. Another reason to use single-dose vials is to avoid precipitation of the steroid. See earlier discussion.)
- Steroid flare (Steroid flares occur rarely but are very painful. The patient actually experiences more discomfort after the injection. It is not associated with fever, occurs within 12 to 24 hours of the injection, and resolves spontaneously within 72 hours. It may be controlled with ice and/or nonsteroidal drugs.)
- Problems with viscosupplementation injections
  —Injection site pain is more frequent.
  —Rash and itching, cramps, ankle edema, muscle pain, and tachyarrhythmia have been reported.

BOX 194-2

Possible Complications of Intraarticular or Soft Tissue Injections

Local Complications	Systemic Complications
Bleeding	Flushing of the face
Hemarthrosis	Impaired glucose tolerance
Iatrogenic infection; septic arthritis	Syncope
Skin depigmentation	Menstrual irregularity; uterine bleeding
Subcutaneous atrophy	Muscle wasting and myopathy
Pain	Osteoporosis
Postinjection flare	Psychological upset
Tendon rupture	Steroid arthropathy
Periarticular calcification	Adrenal suppression
Intraarticular calcification	Acne
Osteonecrosis	Pancreatitis
Charcot-like arthropathy	Posterior subcapsular cataracts
Fat necrosis	Avascular necrosis
Tenosynovitis	Allergic reactions and/or anaphylaxis from local or preservatives in multidose vials
Nerve damage from inadvertent injection	
Pneumothorax (thoracic trigger points)	

From McKeag D: Complication of joint aspiration/injection, *Clinics atlas of office procedures* 5(4):2002 (in press).

—A local reaction can produce a massive effusion that resembles a septic joint; 69% with pain experience relief after effusion resolves.

POSTPROCEDURE PATIENT CARE AND EDUCATION

- A Band-Aid or other dressing should be left on for 8 to 12 hours.
- It is essential that the affected area be rested. Injection therapy is not a cure itself. It is used in conjunction with other modalities. Physical therapy, NSAIDs, and hot or cold compresses may all be indicated, depending on the specific problem. If a weight-bearing joint (such as the knee) is injected, rest is indicated for a longer period than that for a wrist ganglion cyst injection.
- The patient should report immediately if he or she develops fever, chills, or any sign of infection. If the discomfort from the injection does not resolve within 72 hours, the patient should be examined to rule out a septic joint.
- The patient may bathe normally.
- A short course of an NSAID is often beneficial at the time of injection; the two modalities combined may have a markedly beneficial effect.

CPT/BILLING CODES*

20526	Injection: therapeutic (e.g. local anesthetic, corticosteroid), carpal tunnel
20550†	Injection: tendon sheath, ligament, ganglion cyst
20551	Injection: therapeutic of tendon at its origin or insertion
20552	Injection: single or multiple trigger point(s), one or two muscle group(s)
20553	Injection: single or multiple trigger point(s), three or more muscle groups
20600†	Arthrocentesis, aspiration and/or injection; small joint, bursa, or ganglion cyst (e.g., fingers, toes)
20605†	Arthrocentesis, aspiration and/or injection, intermediate joint, bursa (e.g., temporo-mandibular, acromioclavicular, wrist, elbow, ankle, olecranon bursa)
20610†	Arthrocentesis, aspiration and/or injection, major joint or bursa (e.g., shoulder, hip, knee, subacromial bursa)

*Can also charge for any injected medications using appropriate J code.
†Office visit can also be charged.

ICD-9-CM DIAGNOSTIC CODES

274.0	Gouty arthropathy
354.0	Carpal tunnel syndrome
354.2	Cubital tunnel syndrome
355.5	Tarsal tunnel syndrome
355.6	Morton's neuroma
696.0	Psoriatic arthritis
714.0	RA
715.11	DJD shoulder
715.12	DJD elbow
715.14	DJD hand
715.16	DJD knee
715.17	DJD ankle
715.17	DJD foot
719.41	Shoulder pain
723.1	Neck pain
724.5	Back pain
729.5	Arm pain
719.42	Elbow pain
719.43	Wrist pain
719.44	Hand pain
729.5	Leg pain
719.45	Knee pain
719.46	Ankle pain
719.47	Foot pain
729.5	Toe pain
719.51	Shoulder stiffness
719.56	Knee stiffness
724.3	Sciatica
724.79	Coccydynia
726.10	Bursitis, shoulder
726.10	Rotator cuff syndrome
726.11	Tendinitis shoulder
726.12	Bicipital tendinitis
726.2	Impingement syndrome
726.31	Medial epicondylitis (golfer's elbow)
726.32	Lateral epicondylitis (tennis elbow)
726.33	Olecranon bursitis
726.5	Trochanteric bursitis
726.61	Pes anserine bursitis
726.64	Patellar tendinitis
726.65	Prepatellar tendinitis
726.71	Achilles bursitis
726.73	Heel spur
727.03	Trigger finger
727.04	de Quervain's disease
727.05	Tendinitis hand/wrist
727.06	Tendinitis foot/ankle
727.3	Bursitis
727.41	Ganglion, joint
727.51	Baker's cyst
727.82	Calcific tendinitis
728.71	Plantar fasciitis
729.0	Fibrositis
729.4	Fasciitis

J CODES

Steroids

J0702   Betamethasone acetate (Celestone Soluspan)
J0810   Cortisone
J1100   Dexamethasone sodium phosphate (Decadron)
J1095   Dexamethasone acetate
J1700   Hydrocortisone acetate
J1021,   Methylprednisolone acetate
  J1040   (Depo-Medrol)
J2640   Prednisolone sodium phosphate
J1690   Prednisolone tebutate (Hydeltra-TBA)
J7506   Prednisone
J3301   Triamcinolone acetonide (Kenalog)
J3302   Triamcinolone diacetate (Aristocort)
J3303   Triamcinolone hexacetonide (Aristospan)

Hyaluronic Acid Derivatives

J7315   Sodium hyaluronate (Hyalgan)
J3490   Sodium hyaluronate (Supartz)
J7320   Hylan G-F 20 (Synvisc)

BIBLIOGRAPHY

Altman RD, Moskowitz R: Intraarticular sodium hyaluronate (Hyalgan) in the treatment of patients with osteoarthritis of the knee: a randomized clinical trial, *J Rheumatol* 25(11):2203, 1998.

Anderson B, Kaye S: Treatment of flexor tenosynovitis of the hand ("trigger finger") with corticosteroids: a prospective study of the response to local injection, *Arch Intern Med* 151:153, 1991.

Baker DG, Schumacher HR: Acute monarthritis, *N Engl J Med* 329(14):1013, 1993.

Birrer RB: Aspiration and corticosteroid injection: practical pointers for safety, *Phys Sportsmed* 20(12):57, Dec 1992.

Blair B, Rokito AS, Cuomo F, et al: Efficacy of corticosteroids for subacromial impingement syndrome, *J Bone Joint Surg* 78-A(11):1685, 1996.

Cardone DA, Tallia AF: Joint and soft tissue injection, *Am Fam Physician* 66(2):283, 2002.

Carrabba M, Paresce E, Angelini M, et al. The safety and efficacy of different dose schedules of hyaluronic acid in the treatment of painful osteoarthritis of the knee with joint effusion, *Eur J Rheumatol Inflamm* 15:25, 1995.

Dammers JW, Veering MM, Vermeulen M: Injection with methylprednisolone proximal to the carpal tunnel: randomised double blind trial, *BMJ* 321:884, 2000.

Fadale PD, Wiggins ME: Corticosteroid injections: their use and abuse, *J Am Acad Orthop Surg* 2(3):133, May 1994.

Genovese MC: Joint and soft tissue injection, *Postgrad Med* 103(2):125, 1998.

George E: Intra-articular hyaluronan treatment for osteoarthritis, *Ann Rheum Dis* 57:637, 1998.

Gray RG, Gottlieb NL: Intra-articular corticosteroids: an updated assessment, *Clin Orthop* (177):253, July-Aug 1983.

Hay EM, Paterson SM, Lewis M, et al: Pragmatic randomized controlled trial of local corticosteroid injection and naproxen for treatment of lateral epicondylitis of elbow in primary care, *BMJ* 319:964, 1999.

Jones A, Regan M, Ledingham J, et al: Importance of placement of intra-articular steroid injections, *BMJ* 307(6915):1329, Nov 20, 1993.

Kamm GL, Hagmeyer KO: Allergic-type reactions to corticosteroids, *Ann Pharmacother* 33:451, 1999.

Kotz R, Kolarz G: Intra-articular hyaluronic acid: duration of effect and results of repeated treatment cycles, *Am J Orthoped* 28:5, 1999.

Leversee JH: Aspiration of joints and soft tissue injections, *Prim Care* 13:572, 1986.

Nelson KH, Briner W, Cummins J: Corticosteroid injection therapy for overuse injuries, *Am Fam Physician* 52(6):1811, 1995.

Owens DS Jr: Aspiration and injection of joints and soft tissues. In Ruddy S, Harris ED, Sledge CB, et al, editors: *Kelley's textbook of rheumatology*, ed 6, Philadelphia, 2001, WB Saunders.

Pfenninger JL: Injections of joints and soft tissue. Part I. General guidelines, *Am Fam Physician* 44:1196, 1991.

Pfenninger JL: Injections of joints and soft tissue. Part II. Guidelines for specific joints, *Am Fam Physician* 44:1690, 1991.

Pfenninger JL editor: Joint injection techniques, *Clinics Atlas of Office Procedures* 5(4):2002.

Rifat SF, Moeller JL: Basics of joint injection, *Postgrad Med* 109(1):157, 2001.

Rifat SF, Moeller JL: Site-specific techniques of joint injection, *Postgrad Med* 109(3):123, 2001.

Rozenthal TD, Sculco TP: Intra-articular corticosteroids: an updated overview, *Am J Orthop* 29(1):18, Jan 2000.

Salzman KL, Lillegard WA, Butcher JD: Upper extremity bursitis, *Am Fam Physician* 56(7): 1797, 1997.

Saunders S, Cameron G: *Injection techniques in orthopaedic and sports medicine*, Philadelphia, 1997, WB Saunders. (*Editor's note:* This is an excellent manual.)

Schmerling RH, Delbanco TL, Tosteson ANA, et al: Synovial fluid tests: what should be ordered? *JAMA* 264(8):1009, 1990.

Scott WA: Injection techniques and use in the treatment of sports injuries, *Sports Med* 22:406, 1996.

Slotkoff AT, Clauw DJ, Nashel DJ: Effects of soft tissue corticosteroid injection on glucose control in diabetics, *Arthritis Rheum* 37:S347, 1994.

Smith DL, McAfee JH, Lucas LM, et al: Treatment of nonseptic olecranon bursitis: a controlled, blinded prospective trial, *Arch Intern Med* 149:2527, 1989.

Stefanich RJ: Intra-articular corticosteroids in treatment of osteoarthritis, *Orthop Rev* 15(2):65, 1986.

Troum OM: Office-based diagnostic needle arthroscopic lavage. In Pfenninger JL, editor: Joint injection techniques, *Clinics Atlas of Office Procedures* 5(4):2002.

Walker-Bone K, Javaid K, Arden N, et al: Medical management of osteoarthritis, *BMJ* 321:936, 2000.

Wen DY: Intra-articular hyaluronic acid injections for knee osteoarthritis, *Am Fam Physician* 62(3):565, 2000.

Wiggins ME, Fadale PD, Ehrlich MG, et al: Effects of corticosteroids on the healing of ligaments, *J Bone Joint Surg* 77-A(11):1682, 1995.

Young CC, Ruthorford DS, Neidfeldt MW: Treatment of plantar fasciitis, *Am Fam Physician* 63(3):467, 2001.

Zuckerman JD, Meislin RJ, Rothberg M: Injections for joint and soft tissue disorders; when and how to use them, *Geriatrics* 45(4):45, 1990.

CHAPTER 195

Knee Braces

Scott A. Paluska

The knee joint is the largest joint in the body, and knee trauma or overuse injuries are common. Traditionally, strength, flexibility, and technique modification have been essential components of knee rehabilitation. Improved surgical techniques have also enhanced conservative therapy for acute and chronic knee disorders over the last few decades. Recently, knee braces have been used in an attempt to prevent or limit the occurrence of knee injuries. Knee braces have gained additional recognition as adjuncts to physical therapy following a knee injury and for a variety of anterior knee pain syndromes.

Several types of knee braces are currently in common use that are manufactured by many different companies and have a wide range of styles and prices:
- *Prophylactic:* Braces designed to reduce the occurrence or severity of knee injuries during athletic endeavors
- *Functional:* Braces designed to minimize tibial rotation and translation in unstable knees
- *Patellofemoral:* Braces designed to centralize the patella in the trochlear groove and improve patellofemoral joint alignment.

Despite their popularity, appropriate indications and true benefits of knee braces have not been defined or validated by rigorous research. As a result, confusion exists regarding when or if to use knee braces for the prevention or treatment of knee injuries.

INDICATIONS

Prophylactic Knee Braces

- Medial collateral ligament (MCL) protection during valgus knee forces
- Secondary MCL injury protection after a previous MCL injury
- Athletes at high risk for MCL injuries, particularly in contact sports

Functional Knee Braces

- Mild-to-moderate anterior cruciate ligament (ACL) instability

- ACL-deficient knees treated nonsurgically
- Postoperative support following ACL reconstruction surgery
- Support for mild-to-moderate posterior cruciate ligament (PCL) or MCL instability

Patellofemoral Knee Braces

- Patellar subluxation or dislocation
- Anterior knee pain syndromes
- Patellar tendinitis
- Osgood-Schlatter disease
- Postoperative effusion control

CONTRAINDICATIONS

Prophylactic Knee Braces

- Unstable knee requiring surgical management
- Control of tibial translation or rotation in ACL-deficient knees

Functional Knee Braces

- Unstable knee requiring surgical management
- Complex knee injuries such as posterolateral corner injuries

Patellofemoral Knee Braces

- Unstable knee requiring surgical management
- Knee disorders unrelated to the patellofemoral joint

EQUIPMENT

Prophylactic Knee Braces

- Custom or off-the-shelf (prefabricated) brace with unilateral or bilateral bars
- Tape measure
- Athletic tape or hook-and-pile fasteners

- Skin razor *(optional)*
- Elastic wrap or brace cover *(optional)*

Functional Knee Braces

- Custom or off-the-shelf (prefabricated) brace
- Tape measure or specific measuring device supplied by the brace manufacturer
- Athletic tape *(optional)*
- Skin razor *(optional)*
- Elastic wrap or brace cover *(optional)*

Patellofemoral Knee Braces

- Neoprene custom or off-the-shelf (prefabricated) brace
- Tape measure
- Counterbalancing straps *(optional)*
- Patellar buttresses *(optional)*
- Inflation device for inflatable air pocket *(optional)*
- Athletic tape *(optional)*
- Skin razor *(optional)*

PREPROCEDURE
PATIENT PREPARATION

The clinician should identify the appropriate indication for using a knee brace and explain that the brace may or may not be helpful. If the patient is a minor, consent should be obtained from the parent or guardian. (See the sample patient consent form titled "Knee Braces" on page 2004 of Appendix G.) The initial fitting and brace application should be scheduled with adequate time allowed for correct sizing and an explanation of correct brace usage. See the sample patient education handout titled "Knee Braces" on page 2002 of Appendix G.

TECHNIQUE

Prophylactic Knee Braces

Prophylactic knee braces are available as custom or off-the-shelf (prefabricated) models (Fig. 195-1). Cost is greater for custom models, but both types have similar efficacy. High-level athletes may benefit from the weight distribution and fit characteristics of a custom brace. A prefabricated brace is sufficient for most patients. At-risk athletes, such as football linemen, may benefit from wearing prophylactic knee braces on both knees.

1. Obtain the longest brace that the patient can wear comfortably (at least 50 cm).
2. Select a brace with either unilateral or bilateral bars based on personal preference and cost. Bilateral bars

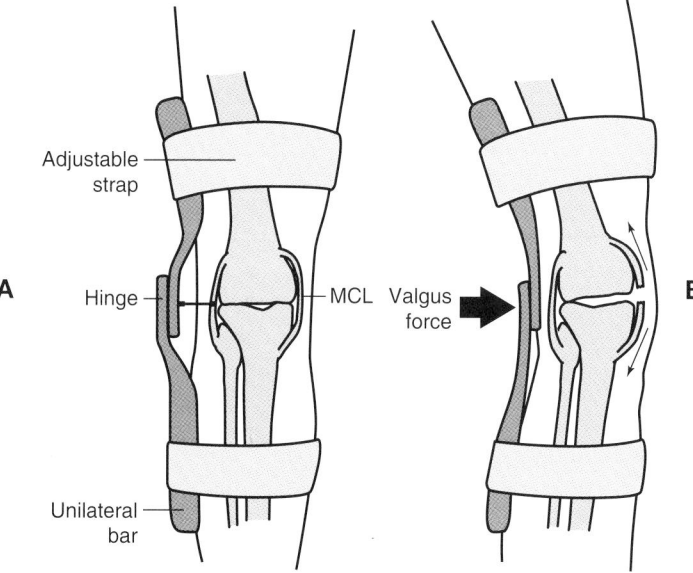

Fig. 195-1
Representative prophylactic knee brace. **A,** Unilateral hinged bar prophylactic knee brace in a neutral position. **B,** Valgus-applied force causing increased medial collateral ligament *(MCL)* tension and potential ligament rupture. Use of the brace would hopefully prevent the MCL tear seen here.

may improve a brace's ability to transfer loads placed on the free joint during impact.
3. Shave the skin under the brace, if desired, to maximize brace-to-skin contact.
4. Secure and adjust the athletic tape or brace enclosures to minimize brace movement.
5. Align the hinges with the femoral condyles to minimize knee range-of-motion attenuation. Correct hinge placement relative to the knee joint is important for brace efficacy.
6. Cover the brace with the elastic wrap or brace cover, if desired, to minimize brace deterioration or injury to others during contact activities.
7. Inspect the brace regularly for signs of deterioration or excessive wear.
8. Tighten and adjust the brace regularly during prolonged athletic activities.
9. Replace a broken or damaged brace.

Functional Knee Braces

Functional knee braces are available as custom or off-the-shelf (prefabricated) models (Fig. 195-2). They have similar designs and use either a "hinge-post-shell" or a "hinge-post-strap" design, which have differing ways of securing the brace around the user's thigh and calf. The "hinge-post-shell" braces may provide better long-term durability and enhanced soft-tissue contact. Custom braces may be more appropriate for patients

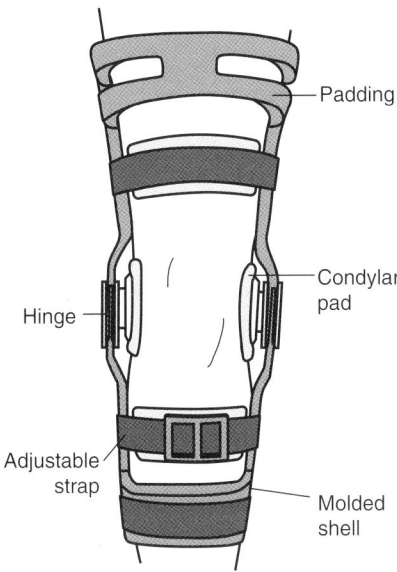

Fig. 195-2
Representative functional knee brace.

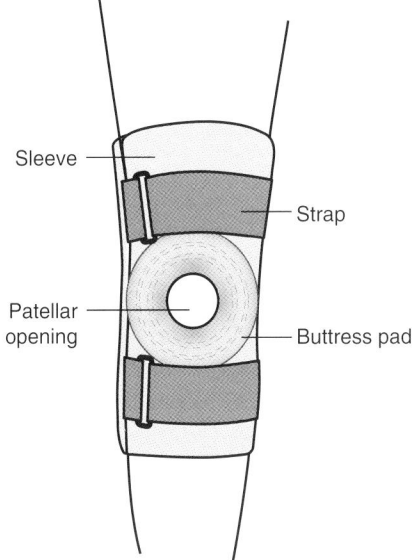

Fig. 195-3
Representative patellofemoral knee brace.

participating in high-level activities or having abnormal limb contours. Prefabricated braces are sufficient for many patients. Studies have found few significant objective differences between custom and prefabricated braces.

1. Measure the thigh circumference six inches above the mid-patella if using a prefabricated brace, and select the corresponding brace size according to the manufacturer's instructions.
2. Measure the thigh, knee, and calf dimensions with the manufacturer-specific instrument for custom braces. The submitted measurements will be used to fabricate a brace that closely meets the affected patient's leg.
3. Choose the longest length brace that the patient can comfortably wear, generally mid-thigh to mid-calf. Longer braces may be more uncomfortable, so a balanced brace length and patient comfort is important to improve compliance.
4. Set the hinge extension stop at 10 to 20 degrees of flexion to minimize potentially harmful knee hyperextension.
5. Position the condylar hinge pads in direct contact with the medial and lateral joint lines to allow the brace's flexion axis to conform to the knee joint.
6. Fasten the brace securely around the patient's leg, using the brace closures or straps.
7. Cover any exposed metal with athletic tape or use a brace cover if available.
8. Inspect the brace regularly for signs of deterioration or excessive wear.
9. Replace a broken or damaged brace.

Patellofemoral Knee Braces

Patellofemoral knee braces are available in many different styles, but most use a Neoprene sleeve, a cut-out to fit the patella, and padding around the patella (Fig. 195-3). Some braces also include adjustable straps or moveable buttresses. Most patients can use a prefabricated brace without the need for customization. No patellofemoral brace type or materials appear to be clearly superior.

1. Measure the leg circumference three inches above and three inches below the knee joint line or around the mid-patella with the leg extended and relaxed, depending on the manufacturer's instructions.
2. Obtain the corresponding brace size (XS to XXL).
3. Pull the brace onto the patient's leg and center the patellar cutout over the anterior knee.
4. Align the hinges, if present, with the femoral condyles.
5. Position the buttress, if moveable, medially to the patella for medial patellar instability (rare) or laterally for lateral instability (common).
6. Snugly secure the counterbalancing straps, if present, around the patient's thigh and calf. Moveable straps may be placed proximally to the patella for most patients, except for those with patellar tendinitis who may benefit from a distal placement.
7. Apply athletic tape to the top and bottom of the brace, if desired, to minimize brace migration while still allowing adjustment of counterbalancing straps.
8. Inspect the brace regularly for signs of deterioration or excessive wear.
9. Replace a broken or damaged brace.

COMPLICATIONS

- In general, knee braces are associated with few complications when selected and worn appropriately. Careful brace sizing may limit unwanted side effects of brace wear.
- Skin breakdown or irritation may occur from brace-to-skin contact over bony prominence.
- Athletes may note a diminished sense of speed and knee range-of-motion.
- While wearing a knee brace, a patient may harbor a false sense of security or invincibility regarding the brace's efficacy and subsequently sustain a more significant knee injury.
- Some braces may interfere with the patient's sense of knee joint proprioception.
- Brace-related contact injuries to other athletes may occur.
- Brace wear may require increased energy expenditure during vigorous activities.
- Premature muscle fatigue resulting from regional muscle ischemia and lactic acid accumulation may limit athleticism.
- Excessive preloading of the knee ligaments by the brace may potentiate the severity of a knee injury.

POSTPROCEDURE PATIENT EDUCATION

Give the patient a copy of any materials provided by the brace manufacturer. It is important to remind the patient of the following:

- Knee braces are only part of a comprehensive knee rehabilitation program. More important components of knee injury prevention and treatment include muscular strengthening, increased flexibility, and technique modification.
- He or she should report any of the following in regards to the knee brace: poor fit, mechanical dysfunction, skin breakdown or irritation, new-onset knee pain, or concerns regarding proper brace use.

CONCLUSION

Knee braces may minimize some knee injuries, but their efficacy has not been fully established by well-controlled studies. Many patients express subjective symptom improvements that exceed objective findings. Clinicians must assess the costs and potential risks of knee braces when deciding to use them for patients. In general, knee braces appear relatively safe in most athletic settings when used appropriately. A knee brace should be used only in conjunction with appropriate education, muscular rehabilitation, and activity modification.

SUPPLIERS

Prophylactic Knee Braces

McDavid Protective Knee Guard (unilateral support) or Pro Stabilizer (bilateral supports)
McDavid Sports Medical Products
10305 Argonne Drive
Woodridge, IL 60517
Phone: 1-800-237-8254
Website: www.mcdavidinc.com

DonJoy Protective Knee Guard (unilateral support) or Playmaker (bilateral supports)
dj Orthopedics
2985 Scott Street
Vista, CA 92083
Phone: 1-800-321-9549
Website: www.donjoy.com

Functional Knee Braces

Lenox Hill Precision Fit (prefabricated) or Spectra Light (custom)
Seattle Orthopedic Group, Inc.
26296 Twelve Trees Lane NW, Building One
Poulsbo, WA 98370
Phone: 1-800-248-6463
Website: www.soginc.com/SOGI

Pro 50 KS 5 ACL Brace (prefabricated)
Pro Orthopedic Devices, Inc.
2884 E. Ganley Road
Tucson, AZ 85706
Phone: 1-800-523-5611
Website: www.proorthopedic.com

Townsend Design Rebel 99 (prefabricated) or Air (custom)
Townsend Design
4615 Shepard Street
Bakersfield, CA 93313
Phone: 1-800-432-3466
Website: www.townsenddesign.com

Bledsoe Ultimate CI (prefabricated)
Bledsoe Brace Systems
2601 Pinewood Drive
Grand Prairie, TX 75051
Phone: 1-888-253-3763
Website: www.bledsoebrace.com

Donjoy Legend (prefabricated) or Defiance (custom)
dj Orthopedics
2985 Scott Street
Vista, CA 92083
Phone: 1-800-321-9549
Website: www.donjoy.com

Patellofemoral Knee Braces

Palumbo Tracker
Palumbo Orthopedics
8206 Leesburg Pike, Suite 404
Vienna, VA 22182
Phone: 1-800-292-7223
Website: www.palumbobrace.com

Ortho-Care Body Flex
Ortho-Care
11911 East 83rd Street
Raytown, MO 64138
Phone: 1-800-821-1303
Website: www.ortho-care.com

DonJoy OnTrack
dj Orthopedics
2985 Scott Street
Vista, CA 92083
Phone: 1-800-321-9549
Website: www.donjoy.com

PRProPro 180 Dr. "M-U" Universal Patella Support
Pro Orthopedic Devices, Inc.
2884 E. Ganley Road
Tucson, AZ 85706
Phone: 1-800-523-5611
Website: www.proorthopedic.com

CPT/BILLING CODE

29530   Strapping, knee

ICD-9-CM DIAGNOSTIC CODES

844.0   Sprain and strains of knee and leg
844.0   LCL strain
844.1   MCL strain
844.2   Cruciate ligament of knee
836.3   Dislocation of patella
726.64   Patellar tendinitis
726.65   Prepatellar bursitis
726.69   Knee bursitis
717.7   Chondromalacia of patella
717.83   Old disruption of ACL

ADDITIONAL RESOURCES

- See the sample patient education handout titled "Knee Braces" on page 2002 of Appendix G.
- See the sample patient consent form titled "Knee Braces" on page 2004 of Appendix G.

BIBLIOGRAPHY

Albright JP, Powell JW, Smith W, et al: Medial collateral ligament knee sprains in college football: brace wear preferences and injury risk, *Am J Sports Med* 22(1):2, 1994.

Albright JP, Powell JW, Smith W, et al: Medial collateral ligament knee sprains in college football: effectiveness of preventive braces, *Am J Sports Med* 22(1):12, 1994.

Albright JP, Saterbak A, Stokes J: Use of knee braces in sports: current recommendations, *Sports Med* 20(5):281, 1995.

Arroll B, Ellis-Pegler E, Edwards A, Sutcliffe G: Patellofemoral pain syndrome: a critical review of the clinical trials on nonoperative therapy, *Am J Sports Med* 25(2):207, 1997.

Cutbill JW, Ladly KO, Bray RC, et al: Anterior knee pain: a review, *Clin J Sport Med* 7(1):40, 1997.

Greenwald AE, Bagley AM, France EP, et al: A biomechanical and clinical evaluation of a patellofemoral knee brace, *Clin Orthop* 324:187, 1996.

Liu SH, Mirzayan R: Current review: functional knee bracing, *Clin Orthop* 317:273, 1995.

Papagelopoulos PJ, Sim FH: Patellofemoral pain syndrome: diagnosis and management, *Orthopedics* 20(2):148, 1997.

Paulos LE, France EP, Rosenberg TD, et al: The biomechanics of lateral knee bracing: Part 1: Response of the valgus restraints to loading, *Am J Sports Med* 15(5):419, 1987.

Powers CM, Shellock FG, Beering TV, et al: Effect of bracing on patellar kinematics in patients with patellofemoral joint pain, *Med Sci Sports Exerc* 31(12):1714, 1999.

Sitler M, Ryan J, Hopkinson W, et al: The efficacy of a prophylactic knee brace to reduce knee injuries in football: a prospective, randomized study at West Point, *Am J Sports Med* 18(3):310, 1990.

Wojtys EM, Huston LJ: "Custom-fit" versus "off-the-shelf" ACL functional braces, *Am J Knee Surg* 14(3):157, 2001.

Wojtys EM, Kothari SU, Huston LJ: Anterior cruciate ligament functional brace use in sports, *Am J Sports Med* 24(4):539, 1996.

CHAPTER 196

Nursemaid's Elbow: Subluxation of the Radial Head

Fred M. Hankin

James L. Telfer

Nursemaid's elbow, radial head subluxation (RHS), or "pulled elbow" is a common injury to children under 7 years old. The mechanism of injury is usually axial traction of the outstretched, pronated forearm. The child initially complains of pain and then refuses to use the arm; the concerned parents then take the child to seek medical attention. At times, however, the injury occurs unobserved by an adult.

The elbow consists of the articulation of the humerus, ulna, and radial head. The radius and ulna flex and extend against the humerus, and the radial head rotates against the ulna and capitellum (humerus) to permit forearm pronation and supination. The radial head is held in place against the proximal ulna and capitellum by the annular ligament and joint capsule. In infants and young children, sudden traction on the distal forearm is more than the annular ligament can sustain and the radial head slides distally. Presumably the annular ligament or synovial tissue becomes interposed between the radial head and capitellum, causing discomfort and preventing the radial head from spontaneous reduction.

DIAGNOSIS

Often the history suggests the diagnosis. Typical scenarios for radial head subluxation include a caregiver pulling a child out of harm's way, a reluctant child being pulled along by the hand, a child suddenly dropping to the floor while being held, or a child being swung playfully by the arms. The child expresses acute pain and refuses to move the affected extremity. The child holds the elbow in a pronated and slightly flexed position (the nursemaid's position). Examination reveals no deformity and little if any swelling around the elbow. The child resists range of motion at the elbow, including further flexion or extension as well as supination and further pronation.

Minimal tenderness is noted over the radial head, but not the supracondylar regions. Neurovascular compromise is rare with this injury. Not infrequently, a child will have no known traction injury but holds the arm against the chest, refuses to use the arm, and has only minimal tenderness over the radial head without significant deformity, swelling, or neurovascular compromise. The absence of a classic history of axial traction does not rule out the diagnosis of radial head subluxation. A small retrospective study found that a third of the 45 cases of nursemaid's elbow in the emergency department did not have a history of axial traction.

RADIOGRAPHIC STUDIES

The clinician should take standard elbow radiographs, including three views (anteroposterior, lateral, and an oblique). Comparison radiographs of the contralateral elbow are essential in the young child because incomplete ossification increases the difficulty in evaluating the immature elbow structures and alignment. Radiographs of nursemaid's elbow are usually normal or reveal longitudinal misalignment of the radial head with the capitellum.

The clinician should evaluate the radiographs for the presence of a "fat pad sign" (joint effusion), location and alignment of epiphyseal growth centers, and the longitudinal alignment of the radial head with capitellum. The fat pad sign is positive if a radiolucent stripe is visible at the posterior distal aspect of the humerus on the lateral view of the elbow and not visible on the comparison view. The periarticular fat is displaced posteriorly by an increase in intrarticular joint fluid, making it visible in the lateral view. This is a nonspecific finding. A positive fat pad sign associated with a history of trauma suggests a bloody joint effusion and intraarticular injury. In this case immediate orthopedic referral is recommended. A nursemaid's elbow can still be present despite the absence of a fat pad sign.

Misalignment of the ossification centers suggests a growth plate injury. Orthopedic referral is recommended for growth plate injury or other obvious fracture. Elbow fractures have a high complication rate.

We would never recommend manipulation of the patient, even with classic symptoms, before a radiographic study was performed, although some do.

TECHNIQUE

Supination and then flexion of the forearm has been the usual method described in modern literature, including the first edition of this text, to reduce RHS. A technique using hyperpronation and flexion has been evaluated recently, which, based on these small prospective studies, appears to be safe and at least as effective as supination and flexion. The techniques differ in the direction the forearm is rotated.

Supination and Flexion Method (Fig. 196-1)

1. The elbow is held in one of the operator's hands with either the thumb or second and third fingers exerting constant gentle pressure over the radial head in a medial direction.
2. The patient's wrist is supinated with the operator's other hand.
3. The patient's forearm is rapidly raised toward the upper arm, flexing the elbow past 90 degrees.
4. The forearm is moved so that the elbow is in 90 degrees of flexion and released.
5. The success of the manipulation is often tested by offering the child his or her favorite toy or a piece of candy on the side of the affected arm. If the child reaches with the affected arm, the manipulation was successful.
6. Repeat manipulation can be attempted after 30 minutes. Using the alternative method of hyperpronating the forearm and rapid flexion has been successful even when repeat supination and flexion has failed.

Pronation and Flexion Method (Hyperpronation) (Fig. 196-2)

1. The elbow is held with one of the operator's hands with the thumb or second and third fingers again exerting constant gentle medial pressure on the radial head.
2. The patient's wrist is hyperpronated with the operator's other hand.
3. Rapid flexion at the elbow is performed.
4. The elbow is extended to 90 degrees and released.
5. The success of manipulation is tested as noted previously.

Sometimes a snap or a satisfying clunk of the radial head may be felt, indicating reduction. The radial head is often reduced before manipulation by an x-ray technician positioning the elbow for the standard radiographic views. Sometimes, spontaneous reduction without manipulation occurs before evaluation by the physician. The caregivers generally need assurance that the child has suffered nothing serious.

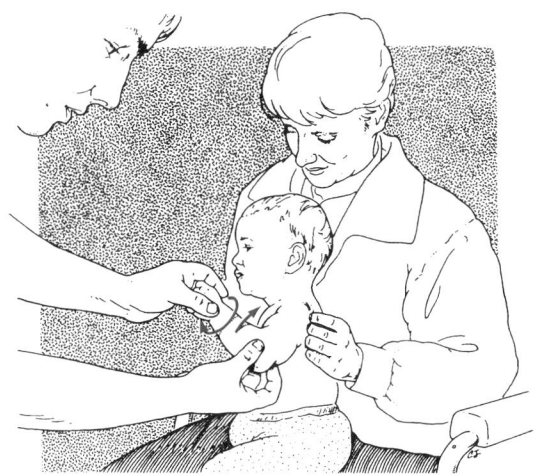

Fig. 196-1
Reduction maneuver for a subluxed radial head (nursemaid's elbow) involves gentle supination of the forearm and flexion of the elbow. The examiner's thumb can be placed over the child's elbow to help palpate the radial head during the reduction process.

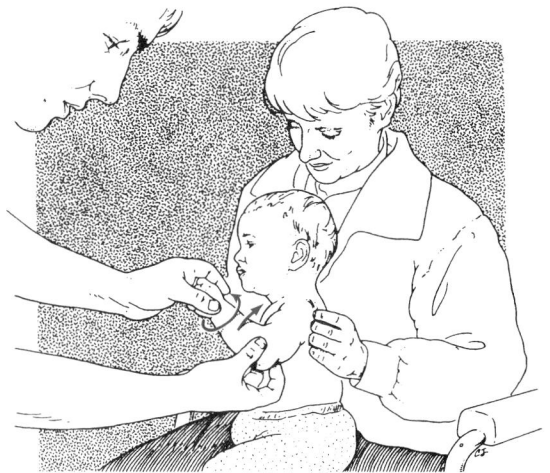

Fig. 196-2
Pronation and flexion method.

DIFFERENTIAL DIAGNOSIS

If there is concern regarding the possibility of a growth plate injury, generally the best approach is obtaining an orthopedic consultation. Rarely, an arthrogram is needed to determine the extent of injury. Sedation or general anesthesia is often required to complete the study. The radiographic contrast can help to outline articular surfaces and to give the examiner a better understanding of the nonossified anatomy.

Joint aspiration can be performed if there is concern regarding the possibility of more significant trauma or infection in the elbow (see Chapter 194, Joint and Soft Tissue Aspiration and Injection [Arthrocentesis]). Bloody fluid confirms the presence of a traumatic intracapsular injury, such as a fracture. Purulent material confirms the diagnosis of septic arthritis. Routine elbow aspiration is not recommended for a nursemaid's elbow; it is an adjunct diagnostic procedure that can be used in difficult diagnostic situations. Sedation or general anesthesia may be required. If any of the preceding diagnoses are being considered, an orthopedic surgeon should be consulted.

POSTPROCEDURE PATIENT EDUCATION

After successful reduction of a subluxed radial head, the provider should tell the child to rest the limb for several days and then reevaluate the child with follow-up clinical and possibly radiographic examination if symptoms do not totally resolve in 24 to 48 hours. A small percentage of patients will resublux the radial head within a few days of reduction, although the number and risk factors are not well defined. In a small randomized prospective study, immobilization in a flexed, supinated position with a posterior splint reduced the recurrence rate from 13% to zero (p <.05) at follow-up 2 days after manipulation. Children that remain reluctant to use their elbow in a normal fashion should be splinted. Follow-up evaluation in 2 or 3 days is recommended to determine normal joint function.

Patients with splints should not remove the splint until the short-term follow-up examination.

Generally, children will let their symptoms be their guide in regards to activity level: once they are comfortable, they will resume their activities. It may take several days for them to do so. The long-term prognosis of nursemaid's elbow is generally favorable. Occasionally the child will have several episodes of subluxation, but the incidence drops off significantly after age 7. Long-term functional or growth problems are rare after appropriate treatment of this injury. Congenital radial head dislocation is a separate entity and not related to the common pediatric problem of nursemaid's elbow.

CPT/BILLING CODES

24640   Closed treatment of radial head subluxation in child (nursemaid's elbow) with manipulation
29105   Splint, arm, long

ICD-9-CM DIAGNOSTIC CODE

755.59   Subluxation, joint, upper extremity

BIBLIOGRAPHY

Macias CG, Bothner J, Wiebe R: A comparison of supination/ flexion to hyperpronation in the reduction of radial head subluxations, *Pediatrics* 102:e10, 1998.

McDonald J, Whitelaw C, Goldsmith LJ: Radial head subluxation: comparing two methods of reduction, *Acad Emerg Med* 6:715, 1999.

Sacchetti A, Ramoska EE, Glascow C: Nonclassic history in children with radial head subluxations, *J Emerg Med* 8:151, 1990.

Taha AM: The treatment of pulled elbow: a prospective randomized study, *Arch Orthop Trauma Surg* 120:336, 2000.

CHAPTER 197

Orthotics, Corns, Calluses, and Plantar Warts

David W. Snider

ORTHOTICS

Orthotics are prescription, in-shoe devices designed to protect and improve abnormal foot function. Orthotics are custom made and, as such, may differ in the materials from which they are manufactured. Each prescription will exhibit various modifications and additions depending on the underlying diagnosis. The two most common types of orthotics are functional orthotics and accommodative orthotics. Both of these are custom made to precise casts, impressions, or scans of the patient's foot that have been made in the position in which the practitioner wishes the foot to function.

INDICATIONS

Functional Orthotics

Functional orthotics are usually rigid or semirigid thermoplastic shells with corrections or additions built in to change a foot's position or to control an abnormal foot motion. Flexible deformities of the foot are most frequently treated with this type of orthotic.

Accommodative Orthotics

Accommodative orthotics are softer and more cushioned, designed to protect painful plantar lesions or bony deformities of the foot. A number of closed-cell and open-cell foam products—as well as those made from cork, leather, rubber, and silicon—are used in the fabrication of accommodative orthotics. These designs are most frequently used with rigid foot deformities, arthritic foot changes, and diabetic conditions.

Conditions

Orthotics are extremely successful in treating a variety of common foot conditions such as plantar fasciitis, heel spur syndrome, early bunion deformities, hammer toes, painful corns and calluses, Morton's neuromas, chronic lateral ankle instability, and diabetic foot pathologies such as Charcot changes and plantar ulcerations. Arthritic patients also benefit from soft accommodative orthotic devices.

CONTRAINDICATIONS

- Usually none, although extreme care must be taken with the neuropathic diabetic foot to ensure an exact fit.
- Some difficulty exists in fitting prescription orthotics in women's and men's dress shoes, although specialty laboratories do manufacture these devices.
- When anticipating a functional rigid or semirigid orthotic, the patient's ankle dorsiflexion must be greater than 10 degrees with the knee extended.

EQUIPMENT

More than 100 prescription orthotic laboratories are accredited throughout the United States. The choice of laboratories is left to the discretion of the practitioner. Benefoot, Inc. in New York is an example of an excellent facility and can be a very helpful resource.

Impressions taken in the office can be performed with the following techniques:
- ScanCast Optical Scanner (Fig. 197-1) (Benefoot, Inc.)
- Biofoam Impression Kit (Smithers Bio-Mechanical Systems)
- Johnson & Johnson, Extra-Fast Setting casting tape (Moore Medical Corporation)

IMPRESSION TECHNIQUES

Plaster Cast Technique

Four-inch-wide Johnson & Johnson Extra Fast Setting casting splints are used usually two layers thick. The casting tape is wrapped around the foot to completely cover the heel, medial, and lateral margins; plantar aspect; and toes (Fig. 197-2). The casting tape is then smoothed to ensure full contact with the foot, and the desired positioning technique is then used. When the casting tape dries, the foot is easily released from this "slipper cast."

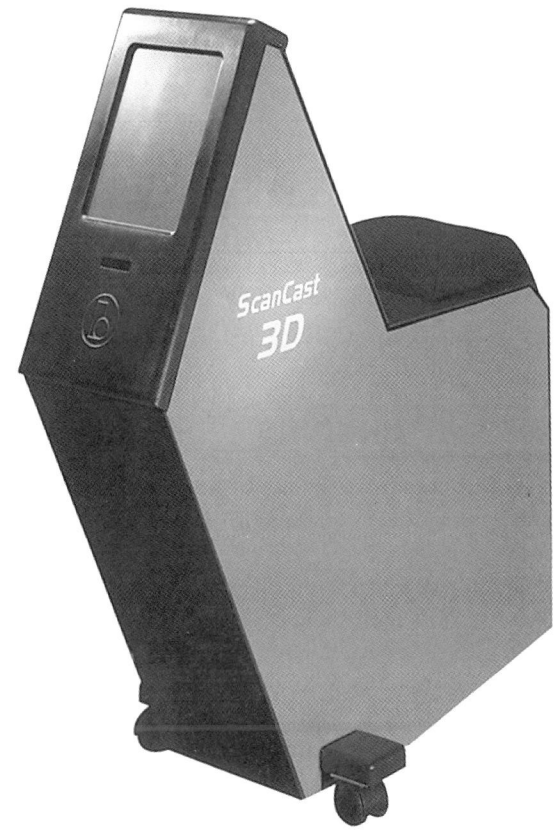

Fig. 197-1
ScanCast 3D is a portable self-contained unit. (Courtesy Benefoot, Inc.)

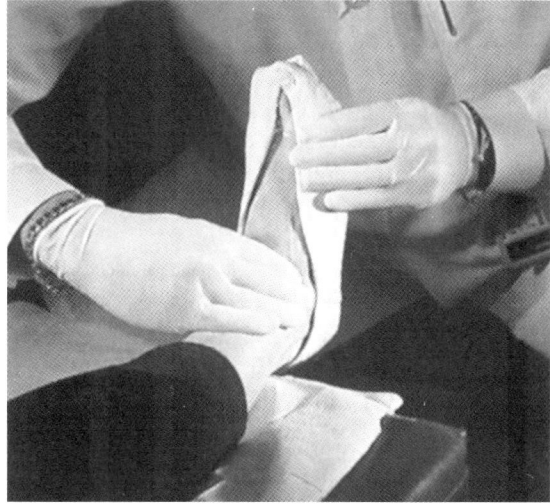

Fig. 197-2
Casting tape applied to foot. (Courtesy Benefoot, Inc.)

ScanCast Technique

With the ScanCast (Benefoot, Inc.), the foot is positioned accordingly in front of the ScanCast Screen (Figs. 197-1 and 197-3). Neutral position is confirmed and visualized. The scan function is activated. Scanning takes approxi-

mately 1 second and is then repeated for the other foot. A digital image of the plantar surface of the foot is recorded. An orthotic is developed from this scan. (A positive model of the foot is constructed and the orthotic is molded onto this model.)

Foot Position

There are four basic positions that may be used to obtain a cast of the foot for an orthotic:
1. Subtalar neutral position, non-weight bearing
2. Subtalar neutral position, partial weight bearing
3. Rectus position
4. Full weight bearing

Subtalar Neutral Position, Non-weight Bearing

This technique is used most frequently to capture the "neutral" position of the foot. The patient may be sitting, supine, or prone with the feet hanging free over the end of the examination table. The ankle is kept at right angles to the leg. This technique requires the casting tape (Fig. 197-2) or ScanCast Optical Scanner (Fig. 197-3). The foot is inverted and everted while the medial aspect of the talonavicular joint is palpated. The talonavicular joint is placed in a congruous position and stabilized. The examiner's other hand grasps dorsally and plantarly under the 4th and 5th metatarsal phalangeal joints and maximally pronates the midtarsal joint. The foot is then held in this position during scanning or until the casting tape applied to the foot dries. This procedure is then repeated for the other foot.

Indications: Useful when maximum biomechanical control of forefoot and rearfoot deformities is required (e.g., flexible flat foot deformity, tibialis posterior dysfunction, most pediatric deformities). Best indicated for flexible feet with greater than 10 degrees into ankle dorsiflexion. Most commonly used with sport orthotics.

Subtalar Neutral Position, Partial Weight Bearing

With this technique, the patient sits comfortably with the knee flexed at 90 degrees, the ankle at 90 degrees, and the center of the patella located directly over the second metatarsal phalangeal joint. The foot is either wrapped in casting tape or placed over the Biofoam Impression Kit and carefully positioned in the foam (Fig. 197-4). If casting tape is used, the patient is placed on a 2-inch-thick, plastic-wrapped foam pad until the casting tape dries. Care is taken to avoid inverting or everting the heel during the impression stage.

Indications: Most flexible foot deformities (e.g., pes cavus, pes planus, heel spurs, plantar fasciitis, bunions, painful corns, or calluses on the plantar aspect of the foot).

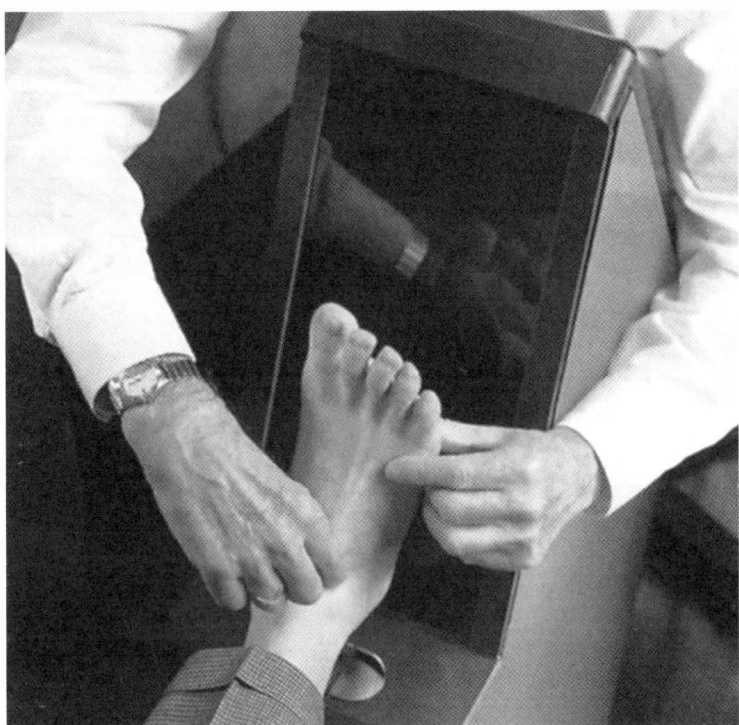

Fig. 197-3
Using the ScanCast 3D to scan the foot. (Courtesy Benefoot, Inc.)

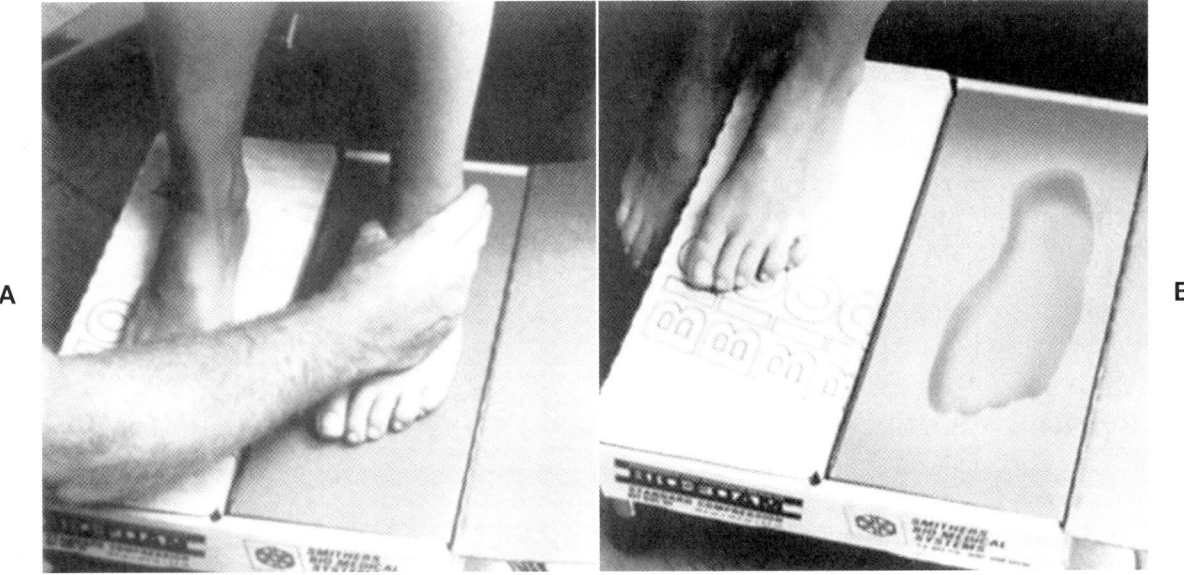

A

B

Fig. 197-4
Taking foam impressions. **A,** Ankle should not be supinated or pronated. **B,** Inspect each impression for
defects or an uneven nature of the weight-bearing surface, or abnormal plantar contour. (Courtesy Smithers
Bio-Medical Systems.)

Rectus Position

This technique is similar to the non-weight-bearing neutral position, except that the forefoot is held parallel to the plantar aspect of the rearfoot during the time plaster is drying or the foot is being scanned.

Indications: All childhood foot deformities (e.g., metatarsus adductus, pes cavus, pes planus, and calcaneal valgus).

Full Weight Bearing

The practitioner can choose the Biofoam impression or plaster. The patient is instructed to stand in a normal angle and base-of-gait.

Indications: Full-weight-bearing impressions are useful for rigid and arthritic foot deformities, where accommodative padding under pressure points will be beneficial.

COMPLICATIONS

Many adjustments can be performed in the office, usually relating to thickness, width, or position of accommodations. Shoe fitting can be difficult with some dress shoes.

POSTPROCEDURE PATIENT EDUCATION

Patients are instructed to initially wear an oxford style shoe, at least five eyelets per side, with a removable manufacturer's insole. They begin by wearing the orthotics approximately 1 hour per day to tolerance. Average break-in period is between 4 and 12 weeks. If ankle equinus is present, the patient is instructed to continue with gastroc-soleus–stretching exercises. Maximum benefit from orthotics usually takes 12 weeks.

CORNS AND CALLUSES

CORNS (HELOMAS)

Helomas are discrete localized lesions found on the toes, usually overlying bony prominences or digital deformities. They are generally painful. *Soft corns* (heloma molle) are usually interdigital lesions resulting from abnormal pressure or improper shoe fit (Fig. 197-5). Friction or structural deformities cause mechanical irritation between the toes. Soft corns are most commonly found between the fourth and fifth toes, but they can occur in any interdigital space. These lesions often become macerated and even secondarily infected. After paring, a small sinus tract can occasionally be identified. *Hard corns* (heloma durum) are usually found on the top

of the distal digit and the lateral fifth toe. These lesions result from structural deformities or bony prominences. Pressure or friction from foot gear over these prominences causes thickening of the integument. Corns have a central translucent core and can be distinguished from warts by the lack of punctate bleeding on paring. Also, skin lines pass through corns but around warts (Box 197-1).

Etiology

Corns and calluses generally occur as a result of abnormally high pressure from deformity or foot gear, shear forces, or friction from ambulation.

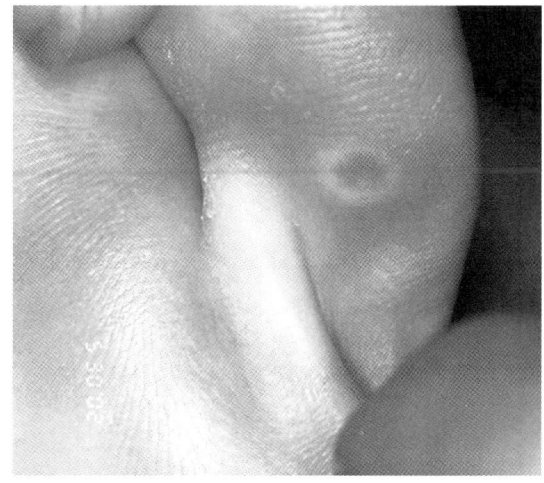

Fig. 197-5
Soft corn on lateral aspect of the toe. (Courtesy The National Procedures Institute, Midland, Mich.)

BOX 197-1
Distinguishing Features of Warts and Plantar Corns

Wart
Relatively rapid onset
May or may not be under bony prominences
Skin lines pass around lesion
Maximum pain squeezing side to side
End arteries visible as red or black dots on paring
Rapid recurrence after shaving and padding

Plantar Corn
Develops over months or years
Located under bony prominences
Skin lines pass through lesion
Maximum pain with direct pressure
No end arteries visible on paring
Slower recurrences after shaving

From Singh D, Bentley G, Trevino SG: *BMJ* 312:1403, 1996.

Clinical Appearance

Corns tend to be well circumscribed, round to oval, hyperkeratotic buildups. They are usually uniform in color and vary from whitish-gray to yellowish-gold. Subdermal hemorrhages can cause areas of discoloration that may appear dark red, brown, or black. Lesions are painful to direct and indirect pressure. When pared down, a pearl-white core is usually found over the area of greatest pressure.

Differential Diagnosis

- Verrucae
- Digital bursa
- Epidermal malignancies
- Porokeratoses

CALLUSES (TYLOMAS, PLANTAR KERATOMA)

Calluses are broad-based hyperkeratotic masses commonly found on the plantar aspect of the foot at sites of friction or high pressure. They may be quite painful when located over the metatarsal phalangeal joints. They can occur diffusely around the heel or on the margins of the toes. They do not have a "nucleus" like the corn and are more of a diffuse hyperkeratotic tissue (Figs. 197-6 and 197-7).

Intractable Plantar Keratoma

Intractable plantar keratomas (IPKs) are deep, nucleated plantar calluses found beneath a metatarsal phalangeal joint. The lesions are extremely painful with palpation and ambulation. The areas are usually circular, of smaller diameter than tylomas, and exhibit a central "clear" core upon scalpel debridement.

Treatment

Treatment should not only provide symptomatic relief, but also alleviate the underlying mechanical cause inciting the problem.

Debridement

Removing hyperkeratotic tissue from corns or calluses can be accomplished with pumice stone, scalpel, electric drill, and/or keratolytic agents such as weak salicylic acid plasters. It is easier to do this if the area has been soaked and softened. Of course, this is only a temporary cure, and the lesion will recur unless the primary cause for the excessive pressure is corrected. Shoes must be evaluated and modified if necessary. Thicker socks may also be of benefit.

Combined Approaches

Therapy for these disorders includes mechanical supportive orthotics (either functional or accommodative), nonsteroidal anti-inflammatory drugs (NSAIDs), accommodative foot gear, digital pads, and accommodations made of moleskin, cushlin (Scholl Corporation), silicone (Silipos), or Spenco (all available through Moore Medical Corp.).

Surgical Treatment

Surgical removal of bone exostosis, correction of digital deformities, or elevation of depressed metatarsals may

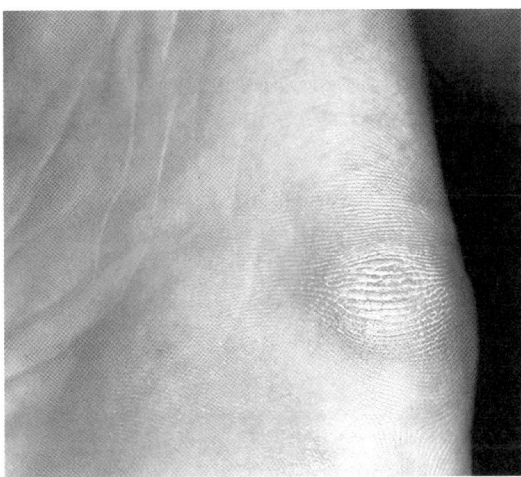

Fig. 197-6
Callus on foot. Differential is a plantar wart. (Courtesy The National Procedures Institute, Midland, Mich.)

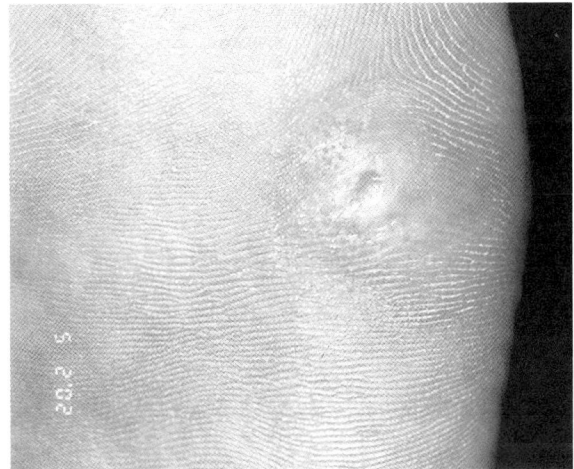

Fig. 197-7
Intractable plantar keratoma showing solid, smooth, hard central core. There are no pinpoint bleeders characteristic of a wart. (Courtesy The National Procedures Institute, Midland, Mich.)

be recommended when conservative therapies fail to provide lasting relief.

COMPLICATIONS

Secondary infections can occur with untreated corns or calluses. Ulcerations are a serious complication with diabetic neuropathy. Bursitis can occur with untreated lesions.

WARTS (VERRUCAE PLANTARIS)

Verrucae plantaris ("plantar warts") are well-circumscribed, benign, tumorigenic, dermatotrophic lesions. The diagnosis is relatively simple, judging from appearance, the production of pain upon lateral compression of the lesion, and pinpoint bleeding after debridement.

ETIOLOGY

Verrucae plantaris is caused by the human papilloma virus.

CLINICAL APPEARANCE

Verrucae are well contained within the epidermis; the dermis is relatively uninvolved. The lesion obliterates normal papillary skin lines. (This is an important diagnostic feature when treating warts. Often there is hyperkeratotic skin over the lesion. If this material is pared away after treatment and skin lines are seen, the wart is considered resolved.) The appearance typically resembles grayish or brown papules with hypertrophic capillaries creating black or brown specs within the margins of the lesion. Plantar warts can occur singularly or in multiple clusters, which are referred to as *mosaic verrucae*. Smaller lesions surrounding the large centralized clusters are referred to as *satellite lesions*.

DIFFERENTIAL DIAGNOSES

Warts are often confused with deep calluses. Pinpoint bleeding after scalpel debridement is a diagnostic hallmark of verrucae plantaris. Other differential diagnoses include porokeratosis, epidermal malignancies (amelanotic melanoma), and various epidermal inflammatory conditions.

TREATMENT OPTIONS (also see Chapter 44, Wart [Verruca] Treatment)

There are numerous treatments with a plethora of methods including injections (bleomycin, *Candida* antigen), chemical cautery with various acids, caustic chemotherapy such as 5-fluorouracil, cryotherapy, infrared coagulation, electrosurgery, immunotherapy (including Imiquimod), CO_2 pulse dye laser, and surgical excision or curettage. Even duct tape has been reported to be beneficial with an 85% cure rate!

TREATMENT TECHNIQUES

Chemocautery

Scalpel debridement of all hyperkeratotic tissue should be performed first. After debridement, the application of various acids, such as trichloracetic acid 85%, salicylic acid 60%, or pyrogallic acid 25%, should be used. Careful protection of the surrounding normal integument is paramount. The acids are usually followed by an occlusive, adhesive dressing. The patient is then instructed to keep the area dry and intact for approximately 2 to 7 days. The above procedure is repeated until normal skin lines are visualized. Treatment times vary greatly with individuals. If there is minimal improvement after a reasonable number of treatments, another form of treatment, such as cryotherapy or other options as mentioned, should be considered.

Other Techniques

Specifics of treatment using other modalities are noted in the specific chapter dealing with each technique. (See the following chapters: Chapter 27, Laser Therapy; Chapter 44, Wart [Verruca] Treatment; Chapter 108, Office Treatment of Hemorrhoids [for use of the IRC]; Chapter 13, Approach to Various Skin Lesions; Chapter 17, Cryosurgery; and Chapter 31, Radiofrequency Surgery.

COMPLICATIONS

Posttreatment pain can be controlled with ice, NSAIDs, and acetaminophen. Chemical burns can create a sterile abscessed treatment site. These rarely become infected. Painful plantar scarring should be avoided, since walking on scars can feel like stepping on a pebble.

CPT/BILLING CODES

Orthotics

A4580   Orthotic casting
L3030   Orthotics

Corns (helomas)

L3030   Prescription orthotics
11055   Debridement of corns, calluses, IPKs (intractable plantar keratosis)

Wart-verrucae plantaris

17000   Destruction (e.g., laser surgery, electrosurgery, cryosurgery, chemosurgery, surgical curettement), all benign or premalignant lesions, first lesion
17003   2 to 14 lesions (each)
17004   15 or more lesions (one set fee)

ICD-9-CM DIAGNOSTIC CODES

728.71   Plantar fasciitis
726.73   Heel spur
735.0   Bunion
735.4   Hammer toes
700   Corns (heloma molle, heloma durum)
701.1   Calluses, IPKs
355.6   Morton's neuroma
734   Pes planus, acquired
754.61   Pes planus, congenital
713.5   Charcot joint
736.73   Pes cavus
754.79   Metatarsus adductus
715.97   Osteoarthritis
078.19   Verrucae plantaris (plantar warts)

SUPPLIERS

Orthotics

Benefoot, Inc.
1507 Executive Drive
Edgewood, NY 11717
Phone: 1-800-554-3668
Website: www.benefoot.com

Smithers Bio-Medical Systems
P.O. Box 118
Kent, OH 44240
Phone: 1-800-321-8286

Moore Medical Corporation
P.O. Box 1500
New Britain, CT 06050-1500
Phone: 1-800-234-1464
Website: www.mooremedical.com

ADDITIONAL RESOURCES

- See the sample patient education handout titled "Corns and Calluses of the Feet" on page 2005 of Appendix G.

BIBLIOGRAPHY

Bedinghaus JM, Niedfeldt MW: Over-the-counter foot remedies, *Am Fam Physician* 64:791, 2001.

Birrer RB, Dellacorte MP, Grisafi PJ: *Common foot problems in primary care*, Philadelphia, 1992, Hanley & Belfus.

Dockery G: *Clinics in podiatric medicine and surgery*, Philadelphia, 1986, WB Saunders.

Ellis J: Orthoses, plantar warts, corns, and calluses. In Pfenninger JL, Fowler GC, editors: *Procedures for primary care physicians*, St Louis, 1994, Mosby.

Jahss MH, editor: *Disorders of the foot and ankle*, ed 2, Philadelphia, 1991, WB Saunders.

McGlamry ED: *Comprehensive textbook of foot and ankle surgery*, Philadelphia, 2001, Lippincott, Williams & Wilkins.

Ringold S, Mendoza JA, Tarini BA, Sox C: Is duct tape occlusion therapy as effective as cryotherapy for the treatment of the common wart? *Arch Pediatr Adolesc Med* 156(10):975, 2002.

Samit MH, Dana AS: *Cutaneous lesions of the lower extremities*, Philadelphia, 1971, Lippincott.

Singh D, Bentley G, Trevino SG: Callosities, corns, and calluses. *BMJ* 312:1403, 1996.

Yale: *Podiatric medicine*, Baltimore, 1974, Williams & Wilkins.

CHAPTER 198

Osteoporosis Screening

Susan Taylor*

Osteoporosis is a systemic disease that can affect different bones to a varying degree. Osteoporotic patients are more likely to sustain fractures, particularly of the wrist, spine, and hip. Although many factors contribute to this pathologic condition, intrinsic bone strength is one of the most important determinants of fracture risk. It is influenced by bone mineral density (BMD) and bone structure, which includes both bone size and shape and the microarchitectural characteristics of the bone. Each year more than 1.5 million fractures caused by osteoporosis occur in the United States (250,000 of these are hip fractures, which cause a 10% to 20% excess mortality rate within 1 year; 250,000 of the remaining injuries are wrist fractures; and 700,000 are spinal fractures). The lifetime incidence of osteoporotic fracture in white women is approximately 50%. BMD screening and treatment of osteoporosis could prevent many of these fractures.

Bone is in a state of dynamic equilibrium. In a normal young adult, bone resorption by osteoclasts is equal to bone formation by osteoblasts. Most people attain their level of peak bone mass between the ages of 30 and 35. In men, bone mass then normally decreases at a rate of 0.3% per year. In women this rate is normally 0.5% per year, with an accelerated rate of bone loss of 2% to 3% per year for 6 to 10 years after menopause. The risk of developing low bone mass in women is four times greater than that in men.

There are two primary types of osteoporosis. Type I occurs predominantly in women within 15 to 20 years after menopause; it affects mostly trabecular bone and results in fracture sites mainly in the distal radius and the vertebrae. Type II osteoporosis occurs in men and women over the age of 70, with a female-to-male ratio of 2:1. Cortical and trabecular bone are affected equally, and fractures occur mainly in the hip, pelvis, and humerus.

The clinical presentation of osteoporosis is usually silent, although it can present as shortened stature, kyphosis, lordosis, or fracture (usually of the vertebrae,

hip, or forearm). Osteoporosis screening does not tell a particular patient whether he or she will or will not have a fracture, just the relative risk of fracture compared with the general population. Often factors such as propensity to falling, poor vision, and medications that increase orthostatic hypotension also affect the risk of fracture for an individual. Risk factors for osteoporosis are listed in Box 198-1.

Secondary causes of osteoporosis should be suspected in any person with a bone density that is significantly lower than their age- and sex-matched counterparts. If an unknown secondary cause of osteoporosis is suspected, initial workup should include serum thyroid-stimulating hormone (TSH), serum protein electrophoresis, parathyroid hormone (PTH) and vitamin-D level, urine calcium, and AM cortisol levels. Secondary causes of osteoporosis are listed in Box 198-2.

METHODS OF MEASURING BONE MINERAL DENSITY

Standard x-ray films have very poor sensitivity, and a decrease in bone density of as much as 50% may not be detected. All currently available methods of bone density measurement are accurate in predicting risk of fractures. All of these methods also have a low effective radiation dose, less than that of a standard chest x-ray. They all appear to have a precision of 98% to 99%, except for quantitative ultrasound, which has a slightly lower precision of 92% to 98%. A summary of their characteristics is as follows:

- Dual-energy x-ray absorptiometry (DXA or DEXA) is the most widely used and thoroughly studied BMD measurement method. DXA uses two x-ray beams, one at higher energy and one at lower energy, which calculate the BMD value by measuring the absorption of each beam and subtracting the soft-tissue absorption. It can measure BMD at central or peripheral sites and has an accuracy of 90% to 99%. Axial DXA scanning uses the hip, spine, or total body. Peripheral DXA uses the forearm, finger, or heel. For an axial DXA, the patient lies on the table and the arm of the

BOX 198-1
Risk Factors for Osteoporotic Fracture

Potentially Modifiable Risk Factors
Smoking
Below normal body weight or <70 kg
Estrogen deficiency (menopause before age 45, bilateral oopho-
    rectomy, premenopausal amenorrhea for >1 year)
Lifelong low intake of calcium
Excessive alcohol or caffeine consumption or low-calcium intake
Visual impairment
Repeated falls
Inadequate physical activity
Frailty or poor overall physical condition
Lack of sunlight exposure

Nonmodifiable Risk Factors
History of fracture as an adult
Family history of fractures, especially among first-degree relatives
Caucasian, Asian
Female sex
Dementia
Elderly
Frailty or poor overall physical condition

BOX 198-2
Secondary Causes of Osteoporosis

Drugs
Alcohol
Aluminum
Anticonvulsants
Cytotoxic drugs
Steroids
Gonadotropin-releasing hormone agonists
Heparin
Lithium
Tamoxifen (premenopausal use)
Thyroxine (excessive use)
Tobacco

Diseases
Acromegaly
Adrenal atrophy and Addison's disease
Amyloidosis
Ankylosing spondylitis
Chronic obstructive pulmonary disease
Congenital porphyria
Cushing's syndrome
Endometriosis
Epidermolysis bullosa
Gastrectomy
Gonadal insufficiency
Hemochromatosis
Hemophilia
Hyperparathyroidism
Hypophosphatemia
Idiopathic scoliosis
Lymphoma
Leukemia
Malabsorption
Mastocytosis
Multiple myeloma
Multiple sclerosis
Nutritional disorders
Osteogenesis imperfecta
Parenteral nutrition
Pernicious anemia
Rheumatoid arthritis
Sarcoidosis
Severe liver disease
Thalassemia
Thyrotoxicosis
Tumor secretion of parathyroid hormone–related peptide
Type I diabetes

machine moves around the patient, who is usually clothed. For a peripheral DXA, a small, portable, easy-to-use machine takes a few minutes to scan a peripheral part of the body (Fig. 198-1).

- Single-energy x-ray absorptiometry (SXA) uses a single-energy x-ray beam for measurement while a water bath simulates a uniform soft-tissue thickness. The body site used is usually the heel, which is placed in a small, portable machine. SXA has an accuracy of 98% to 99% (Fig. 198-2).
- Quantitative ultrasound (QUS) transmits high-frequency sound waves across bone and measures broadband ultrasound attenuation (BUA) and the speed of sound (SOS) in bone, both of which are decreased in osteoporotic bone. A QUS machine is portable, provides no radiation exposure, and uses the heel, shin, wrist, radius, phalanx, or metatarsal.
- Quantitative computed tomography (QCT) uses a conventional computed tomography (CT) scanner that requires calibration and special software to measure bone mass of the spine or of the forearm (i.e., peripheral QCT) (Fig. 198-3). The peripheral machine is portable, and has an accuracy of 92% to 98%. The axial QCT uses a large CT scanner and has an accuracy of 85% to 97%. QCT is much more expensive and has significantly more radiation exposure compared with DXA.
- Peripheral BMD measurement can be used to assess fracture risk at both peripheral and central sites and performs as well as central BMD, with the exception of assessment of hip fracture risk, which is best predicted by hip BMD measurement (Siris et al, 2001).

DXA is the most widely used and has been the most extensively studied BMD measurement technology. To standardize values from different densitometers, results are reported as standard deviations (SDs) above or below the mean peak bone mass for the patient's age- and sex-matched score (i.e., Z-score) or sex-matched normal young adult reference (i.e., T-score). A difference of one SD equals a 10% to 12% difference in bone density. The T-score is the most clinically relevant value on the BMD report and can help confirm a diagnosis of osteoporosis. The World Health Organization (WHO)

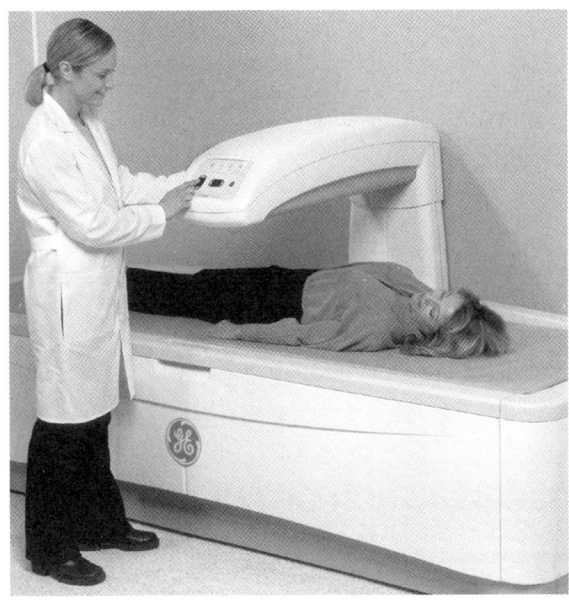

Fig. 198-1
Prodigy central (or axial) DXA scanning unit. (Courtesy GE Lunar Corp, Madison, Wisc.)

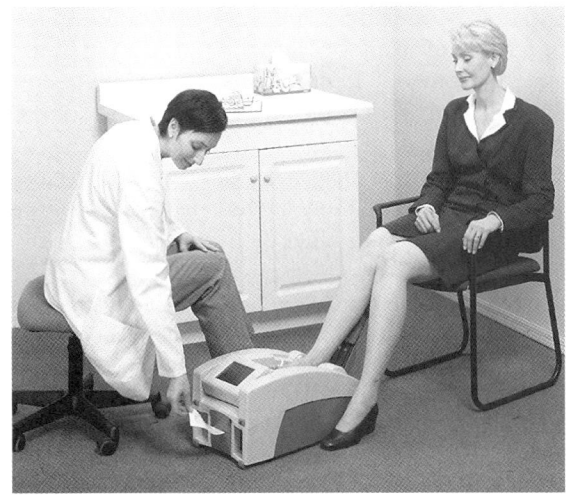

Fig. 198-2
Achilles peripheral ultrasound scanning unit. (Courtesy GE Lunar Corp, Madison, Wisc.)

defines normal bone mass as a T-score above −1, osteopenia as a T-score between −1 and −2.5, and osteoporosis as a T-score at or below −2.5. The National Osteoporosis Foundation (NOF) recommends initiating therapy to reduce fractures in women with BMD T-scores below −2 in the absence of risk factors and BMD T-scores below −1.5 in the presence of risk factors.

Note: Biochemical markers of bone turnover can also be measured, and elevated levels indicate a higher risk of hip fracture. These decrease 20% to 70% during antiresorptive treatment; however, they are not reliable in individuals for predicting bone loss or choosing treatment.

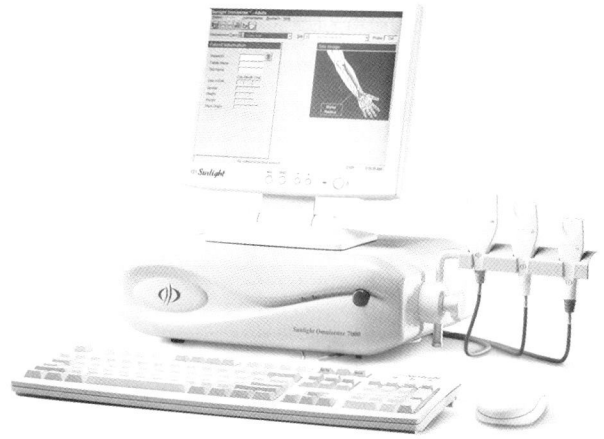

Fig. 198-3
Sunlight peripheral ultrasound unit. (Courtesy Sunlight Medical, Somerset, NJ.)

INDICATIONS

The NOF guidelines recommend BMD testing for the following:
- All women older than 65 years of age regardless of risk factors
- All postmenopausal women under 65 years of age who have at least one additional risk factor for osteoporosis other than menopause (Box 198-1)
- All postmenopausal women with fractures
- All women who are considering therapy for osteoporosis and feel that BMD test results would influence this decision
- All women who have been receiving hormone replacement therapy for a prolonged period

The U.S. Preventive Services Task Force (USPSTF) recently published its guidelines for BMD testing:
- Women 65 years of age and older should be screened routinely for osteoporosis. The USPSTF recommends that routine screening begin at 60 years of age for women with an increased risk for osteoporotic fractures.
- Recent data suggest that peripheral bone density testing (using quantitative ultrasonography) in the primary care setting can help identify postmenopausal women with a higher risk for fracture over the short term (1 year).

- A change in BMD may require a minimum of 2 years for reliable measure because the precision of testing is limited. However, longer intervals may be adequate for repeated screening to identify new cases of osteoporosis.
- No data exist that determine the appropriate age to stop screening, and there are few data on osteoporosis treatment in women older than 85.

Note: Men with hypogonadism, history of long-term steroid use, or a history of fractures are also an important population to screen. Repeat BMD testing is indicated to evaluate efficacy of treatment for osteoporosis (axial scanning only, because peripheral scanning does not accurately reflect treatment changes).

CONTRAINDICATIONS

There are no absolute contraindications to BMD testing. However, relative contraindications include the following:

- Pregnancy (although DXA scanning provides less than one tenth the radiation of a standard chest x-ray film) is a relative contraindication to DXA, but quantitative ultrasound is not contraindicated because there is no known radiation exposure.
- Patients who are not candidates for treatment of osteoporosis are not good candidates for BMD testing.
- Patients who are not interested in accepting treatment for osteoporosis, regardless of the results of BMD testing, are not good candidates for this procedure.

PREPROCEDURE PATIENT PREPARATION

In general no consent form is needed for BMD testing, although the procedure, its indications, relative contraindications, and purpose should be discussed with each patient. The patient should be informed of the safety and low level of radiation exposure and told that the procedure should take only a few minutes (see the patient education handout titled "Osteoporosis and Bone Density Screening Tests" on page 2007 in Appendix G).

TECHNIQUE

For conventional DXA-BMD testing, the patient will lie down (clothed) on an open machine and a scanning arm will be moved around the patient to obtain the measurements of the hip and spine. Peripheral DXA, SXA, and QUS machines are usually small and portable; the patient places the heel or wrist into the device for a few minutes. All methods of BMD measurement are painless and relatively fast.

COMPLICATIONS

No complications have been reported, except a very low level of radiation exposure that is less than one tenth the radiation of a conventional chest x-ray. Quantitative ultrasound has no radiation exposure.

INTERPRETATION OF BONE MINERAL DENSITY RESULTS

The results of BMD testing are standardized among the different methods listed previously. In general a patient's BMD is expressed as a relationship to two norms:

1. The T-score is the relationship to the expected BMD for "young normal" adults of the same sex. The T-score represents the number of SDs the patient's BMD is from the control. The T-score is used to define osteoporosis and osteopenia. A normal result is within 1 SD of a "young normal" adult (i.e., T-score above −1). Osteopenia is a T-score between −1 and −2.5. Osteoporosis is defined by a T-score less than −2.5 or a BMD greater than 2.5 SDs below that of a "young normal" adult.
2. The Z-score is the relationship to the expected BMD for age- and sex-matched patients; it is also expressed in terms of SDs away from the norm. T-scores decline in parallel with the steady drop in bone mass that occurs with aging; however, the Z-score should compare patients with others of their age and sex.

In more practical terms, a recent large observational study revealed that osteopenia, as measured by peripheral BMD methods, was associated with 1.73 times the risk of fracture within 1 year, and osteoporosis was associated with 2.74 times the risk of incident fracture within 1 year (Siris et al, 2001).

MONITORING

In general, monitoring of BMD while on therapy is recommended every 2 years (and, in most cases, will not be covered by Medicare if it is done more frequently). However, this procedure can be done more frequently for persons on long-term steroid therapy or if a new method of BMD monitoring is used.

Monitoring of BMD while on therapy should be done with axial measurements, because they more accurately reflect fracture risk and changes in bone density after therapy. A baseline BMD of the axial skeleton is indicated when osteoporosis is detected by peripheral scanning, because peripheral BMD scanning is a screening test (like a Pap smear). Peripheral BMD testing is an inexpensive, convenient way to pick up abnormal results in an at-risk population in need of further testing. Axial BMD testing should be used to determine and monitor treatment methods, similar to the use of colposcopy to further guide treatment of an abnormal Pap smear.

POSTPROCEDURE PATIENT EDUCATION

See the sample patient education handout titled "Osteoporosis Screening Information" on page 2006 of Appendix G.

SUPPLIERS

DXA

Hologic Inc.
35 Crosby Drive
Bedford, MA 01730
Phone: 1-781-999-7300
Website: www.hologic.com

Lunar Corporation (GE Medical Systems)
726 Heartland Trail
Madison, WI 53717-1915
Phone: 1-800-445-8627
Website: www.gemedicalsystems.com

Norland Medical Systems, Inc.
106 Corporate Park Drive, Suite 106
White Plains, NY 10604
Phone: 1-914-694-2285
Website: www.norland.com

Peripheral DXA

Lunar Corporation (contact information above)

Norland Medical Systems, Inc. (contact information above)

Osteometer MediTech, Inc.
12515 Chadron Avenue
Hawthorne, CA 90250
Phone: 1-310-978-3073
Website: www.osteometer.com

Schick Technologies, Inc
30-00 47th Avenue
Long Island City, NY 11101
Phone: 1-718-937-5765
Website: www.schicktech.com

SXA

Norland Medical Systems, Inc. (contact information above)

QUS

Hologic Inc. (contact information above)

Lunar Corporation (contact information above)

Myriad Ultrasound Systems, Ltd
Rehovot, Israel
Phone: 1-888-722-6994

Sunlight Medical, Inc
100 Davidson Avenue, Suite 108
Somerset, NJ 08873
Phone: 1-800-750-6011
Website: www.sunlightmedical.com

QCT

Computerized Imaging Reference Systems, Inc.
2428 Almeda Avenue, Suite 212
Norfolk, VA 23513
Phone: 1-800-617-1177
Website: www.cirsinc.com

Image Analysis, Inc
1380 Burkesville Street
Columbia, KY 42728
Phone: 1-800-548-4849
Website: www.image-analysis.com

Peripheral QCT

Norland Medical Systems, Inc. (contact information above)

CPT/BILLING CODES

76075	Axial DXA
76076	Peripheral (appendicular) DXA
76078	Radiographic absorptiometry (appendicular)
76977	Quantitative ultrasound (appendicular QUS)
78350	Single-photon absorptiometry (appendicular)
G0130	Single-energy x-ray absorptiometry (appendicular)
G0131	Quantitative computed tomography (axial QCT)

G0132   Peripheral quantitative computed tomography (appendicular)

ICD-9-CM DIAGNOSTIC CODES

V82.81   Screening code for osteoporosis
V49.81   Status code for postmenopausal women

ADDITIONAL RESOURCES

• See the sample patient education handouts titled "Osteoporosis Screening Information" and "Osteoporosis and Bone Density Screening Tests" on pages 2006 and 2007, respectively, of Appendix G.

BIBLIOGRAPHY

Chesnut III CH: Osteoporosis, an underdiagnosed disease, *JAMA* 286:2865, 2001.

Deblinger L: Bone mineral density testing: who, when, how, *Patient Care* 1:62, 2001.

Johnston CC, Dawson-Hughes B, Melton LJ, et al: *Physician's guide to prevention and treatment of osteoporosis,* Washington, DC, 2000, National Osteoporosis Foundation.

Kenny AM, Prestwood KM: Osteoporosis: Pathogenesis, diagnosis, and treatment in older adults, *Rheum Dis Clin North Am* 26(3):569, 2000.

Koopman WJ, editor: *Arthritis and allied conditions,* ed 13, Baltimore, 1997, Williams & Wilkins.

Levis S, Altman R: Bone densitometry: clinical considerations, *Arth Rheum* 40:577, 1998.

Miller PD, Zapalowski C, Kulak CA, Bilezikian JP: Bone densitometry: the best way to detect osteoporosis and to monitor therapy, *J Clin Endocrinol Metab* 84(6):1867, 1999.

Siris ES, Miller PD, Barrett-Connor E, et al: Identification and fracture outcomes of undiagnosed low bone mineral density is postmenopausal women: results from the National Osteoporosis Risk Assessment, *JAMA* 286:2815, 2001.

Ullom-Minnich P: Prevention of osteoporosis and fractures, *Am Fam Physician* 60:194, 1999.

U.S. Preventive Services Task Force: Screening for osteoporosis in postmenopausal women: recommendations and rationale, *Ann Intern Med* 137:526, 2002.

CHAPTER 199

Shoulder Dislocations

J. Mark Wiedemann

The shoulder is uniquely designed to permit overhead and reaching maneuvers. The proximal humerus and the scapula (glenoid portion) articulate to form the shoulder joint. The glenoid forms a shallow concave surface, which rests against the larger, convex surface of the proximal humerus. The glenoid labrum forms a soft tissue cuff around the glenoid, which increases its depth and width, thus providing a larger concavity. Surrounding capsule and ligamentous structures help hold the humerus statically against the glenoid. Superficial to this capsule, a cuff of muscles and its tendinous attachments (the rotator cuff) further stabilize (statically and dynamically) the proximal humerus against the glenoid (Fig. 199-1).

When the normal static (bone, labrum, capsule, and ligaments) and dynamic (muscles and tendons) restraints are exceeded, the shoulder can slide out of joint. This can result from chronic, repetitive, attritional injuries, which frequently cause subluxation of the shoulder. More commonly a sudden, onetime insult to the shoulder results in frank dislocation of the joint. The shoulder can dislocate in a posterior, anterior, or inferior direction, leading to multidirectional instability. *Anterior instability* occurs when a shoulder dislocates on a frequent basis in the anterior direction. *"Dead arm" syndrome* refers to the chronic shoulder subluxation syndrome that is seen in persons involved in arm-over-head activities such as baseball pitching or swimming. *Posterior dislocations* occur rarely, are often misdiagnosed, and should be considered in patients who experience a loss of external rotation, particularly after a seizure or electroshock therapy.

Most frequently the physician encounters a subcoracoid, anterior dislocation. This usually results from an abducted, extended, externally rotated upper extremity that has met with resistance, resulting in a lever arm that forces the proximal humerus anteriorly out of the glenoid socket. This discussion will be limited to anterior dislocations of the shoulder.

DIAGNOSIS

The patient will have a loss of the normal shoulder contour, although this may be hard to detect in heavyset individuals. The acromion becomes very prominent. A prominence (humeral head) may be noted in the anterior chest region. Clinically a hollow can be appreciated beneath the acromion process, due to the transposed humeral head. The arm will frequently be held in an abducted, externally rotated posture. A neurologic deficit, most frequently involving the axillary nerve (shoulder abduction and sensation over the deltoid), may be noted on careful examination. All nerves of the brachial plexus can potentially be injured, however, and a careful neurologic examination is warranted. Vascular compromise is uncommon, but proximal and distal arterial flow should be assessed.

RADIOGRAPHIC STUDIES

Radiographic studies should be conducted before attempts are made to reduce the shoulder. It is important to determine the presence or absence of fractures before the physician's manipulation. Obtain standard radiographs of the shoulder, including an anterior-posterior glenoid fossa projection. The most important projection in this series is the axillary view (Fig. 199-2). In the event of a dislocation, this view will help determine in which direction the humeral head is dislocated relative to the glenoid. Some centers prefer to use a lateral scapular or a Y-type view. Alternatively, in some obese individuals a computed tomography (CT) scan may be necessary to determine the direction of the shoulder dislocation and the presence of concomitant fractures.

EQUIPMENT

- Stretcher
- Weights

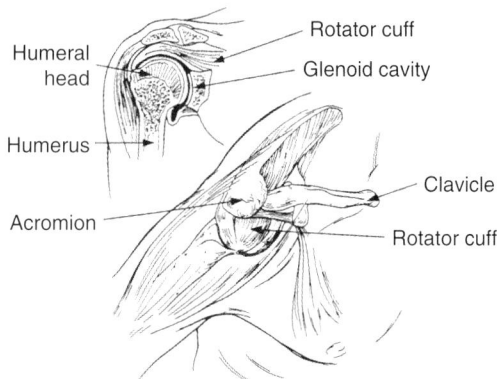

Fig. 199-1
Anatomy of the shoulder joint. The rotator cuff consists of the supraspinatus, infraspinatus, subscapularis, and teres minor. Also see Chapter 194, Joint and Soft Tissue Aspiration and Injection (Arthrocentesis).

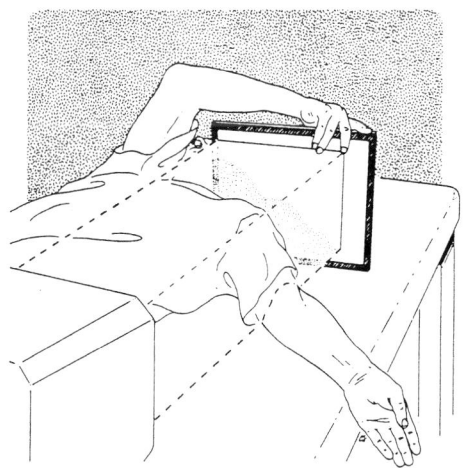

Fig. 199-2
Radiographs should include an axillary view. This projection helps document the direction (anterior versus posterior) of the shoulder dislocation and confirm position after closed reduction maneuvers.

- Analgesia
- Muscle relaxant
- Narcotics
- Benzodiazepines
- Reversal agents

TECHNIQUE

There are a number of techniques available to the physician and emergency room staff. The patient is probably best served by the Stimson technique wherein weight loading and time gently reduce the joint. Certainly, this is the least traumatic for the shoulder of the maneuvers discussed in the following section, and

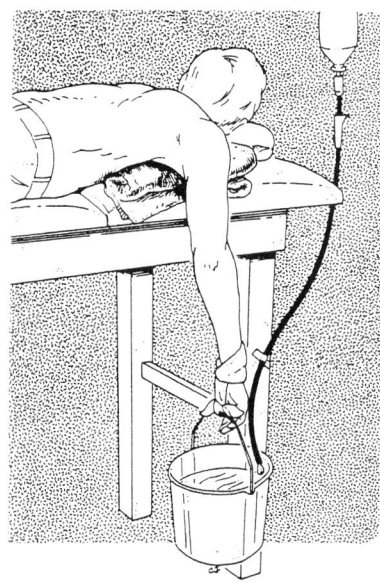

Fig. 199-3
Gentle, sustained, longitudinal traction can provide an effective means for closed reduction of an anterior dislocation. As the intravenous fluid bag slowly empties into the bucket, a gradual traction force is created.

should help minimize the chances of developing an iatrogenic fracture related to the reduction process.

Stimson Technique

1. Adequately sedate the patient. This frequently requires the use of a general anesthetic. Alternatively, under supervised conditions, good conscious sedation can frequently be achieved in the emergency room setting. If significant sedation is given in the office practice, adequate respiratory support measures and monitoring should be present.

2. The patient is placed in the prone position upon a stretcher (Fig. 199-3). After adequate levels of sedation are achieved, a rolled-up towel or blanket can be placed beneath the coracoid process and pectoralis major muscle. A weight is affixed to the wrist to provide longitudinal, sustained traction. Wrapping a gauze bandage around the wrist, rather than tape, should provide secure fixation of the weights to the limb. A bucket of water can be used if weights are not available.

3. With time and relaxation, usually the shoulder will reduce itself. Occasionally, the physician can facilitate the reduction by gently alternating internal and external rotation to the arm.

4. After the shoulder has been reduced, hold the limb in internal rotation against the abdomen and adduction (humerus against the lateral trunk) by a sling and swath device. A careful post-reduction neurovascular assessment is required.

5. Obtain appropriate postreduction radiographs to determine whether adequate reduction of the joint surfaces has been achieved. A congruous-appearing joint without significant distraction (interposed tissue) between the glenoid and the humerus should be noted. Occasionally, comparison shoulder radiographs may be required. A repeat radiographic axillary view (and sometimes a postreduction CT scan) is also required to confirm the location of the proximal humerus in the glenoid. Some recent studies question the value of postreduction imaging, but in most communities it is still the standard of care.

Scapular Manipulation

Scapular manipulation may be performed with the patient prone, sitting, or supine. When the patient is prone, traction is applied to the arm, as shown in Fig. 199-4. From 2 to 7 kg of traction is required. The patient may or may not require analgesia for this technique, since there is somewhat less manipulation (and less chance of injury) done than with most other techniques (Fig. 199-4, *A*). One hand rotates the inferior aspect of the scapula medially, and the other hand rotates the superior aspect laterally. When the patient is sitting, an assistant provides forward traction on the affected arm with countertraction against the head of the humerus. From behind the patient, the physician manipulates the scapula as described previously. There have never been complications reported from using this technique. Finally, anecdotal report has been made of successful anterior shoulder dislocation reduction using this technique in the multiply traumatized patient in the supine position. The shoulder is gently flexed upward by an assistant to a 90-degree position. The operator slides his hands under the patient's scapula and proceeds as described previously. This technique may be used when other injuries limit repositioning the patient (Fig. 199-4, *B*).

Hennipen Technique

The Hennipen technique is named after the Hennipen County Emergency Medical Center where the technique was first described. It is the technique preferred by some authors for anterior shoulder dislocations. There is less manipulation than in most other techniques, a lower probability of neurovascular or musculoskeletal damage, and little or no need for analgesia. The patient is seated upright or reclining at 45 degrees. With the physician stabilizing the patient's right elbow joint (the affected arm) with the left hand, the right hand grasps the wrist. Slowly the patient's forearm is externally rotated until there is 90 degrees of external rotation. The procedure should be stopped if the patient experiences pain or discomfort. Usually, after allowing the muscula-

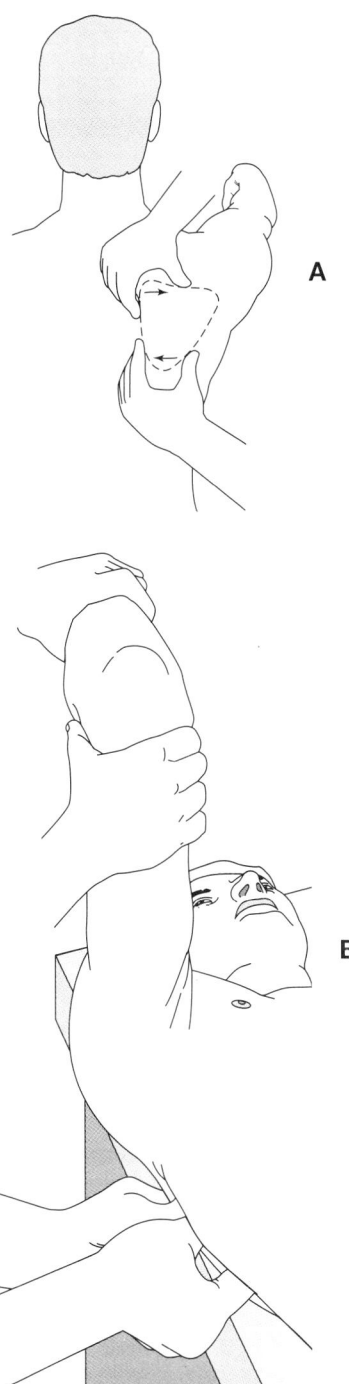

Fig. 199-4
Scapular manipulation technique. **A,** An assistant flexes the patient's arm (or it is flexed by gravity and weights, as with the Stimson technique). It must be slowly brought to a 90-degree position. The operator then rotates the inferior scapular tip medially, and superior aspect laterally (clockwise on the right shoulder and counterclockwise on the left). **B,** The same technique with the patient in a supine position. With the patient's shoulder and elbow both flexed 90 degrees, and the shoulder adducted, gentle upward pressure is maintained by an assistant while the scapula is manipulated as described.

ture to relax, the procedure can be continued without analgesia. If pain or discomfort persists, the patient may require analgesia. The reduction usually occurs by the time the forearm has reached 90 degrees of external rotation; but if it has not, the arm is slowly elevated. If reduction still does not occur, the humeral head is gently manipulated posteriorly until it reduces (Fig. 199-5).

Modified Kocher Maneuver

The modified Kocher maneuver is similar to the Hennipen technique. The patient is placed supine with the arm of the affected shoulder over the edge of the gurney. After assessing and providing for the patient's need of analgesia, the forearm, with the elbow joint held at 90 degrees and used as a pivot point, is rotated externally (abducting superiorly) over at least a 5-minute period, with gentle downward pressure on the dislocation. After the arm reaches 120 degrees of rotation, the arm is brought back to internal rotation, at which time reduction usually occurs (Fig. 199-5).

Milch-Cooper Technique

With the patient sitting or supine, the arm is moved to 10 to 20 degrees of forward flexion with slight abduction. Forward flexion with traction is continued until the patient's arm is directly overhead (Fig. 199-6). Abduction of the arm and outward traction at the shoulder are then increased until reduction occurs, which is usually signified by an audible or palpable "clunk."

Fulcrum Method

With the patient supine or sitting, a firmly rolled blanket 6 to 8 inches in diameter is placed as a fulcrum within the axilla of the affected shoulder. The distal humerus is used as lever and is adducted gently, with simultaneous posterior manipulation of the shoulder.

Boss-Holzach-Matter Method

The patient sits against the maximally raised head of a gurney and wraps his forearms around the ipsilateral

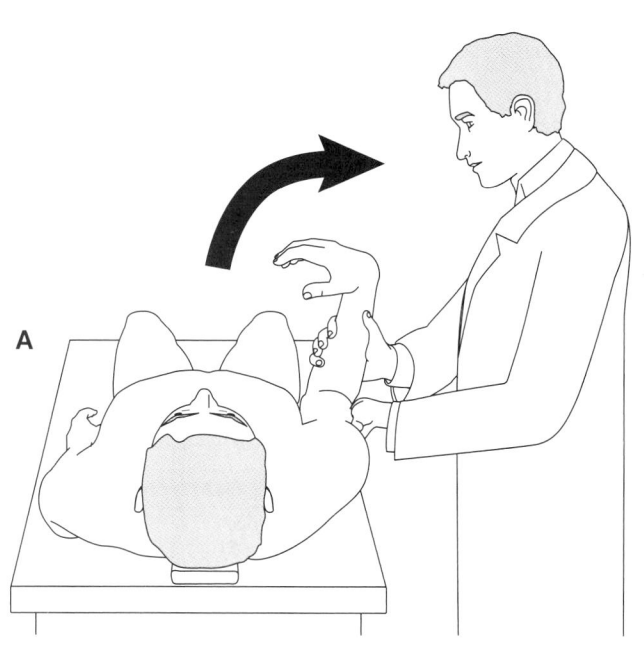

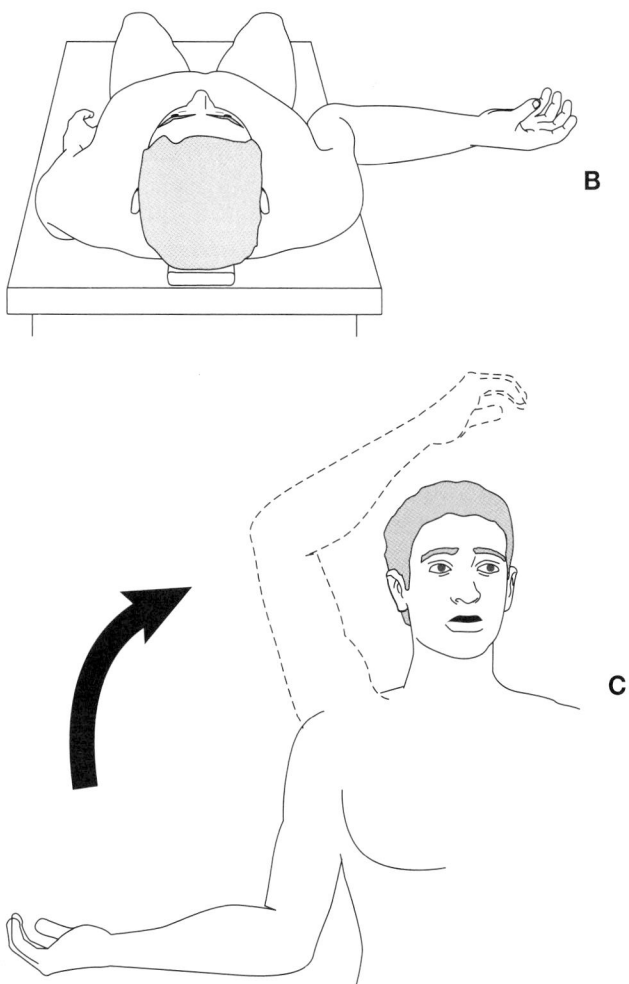

Fig. 199-5
A-B, Hennipen and modified Kocher techniques. Both techniques start as shown in **A.** The modified Kocher proceeds as shown in **B,** and then the forearm is returned to complete internal rotation with gentle shoulder joint pressure. **C,** The Hennipen technique is continued, if necessary, as shown, with elevation of the arm and manipulation of the joint posteriorly until the arm is overhead and the dislocation is reduced.

knee, flexed at 90 degrees. The head of the gurney is then lowered. The patient is asked to hyperextend his neck while leaning back and shrugging the shoulders anteriorly. This technique reportedly does not require analgesia.

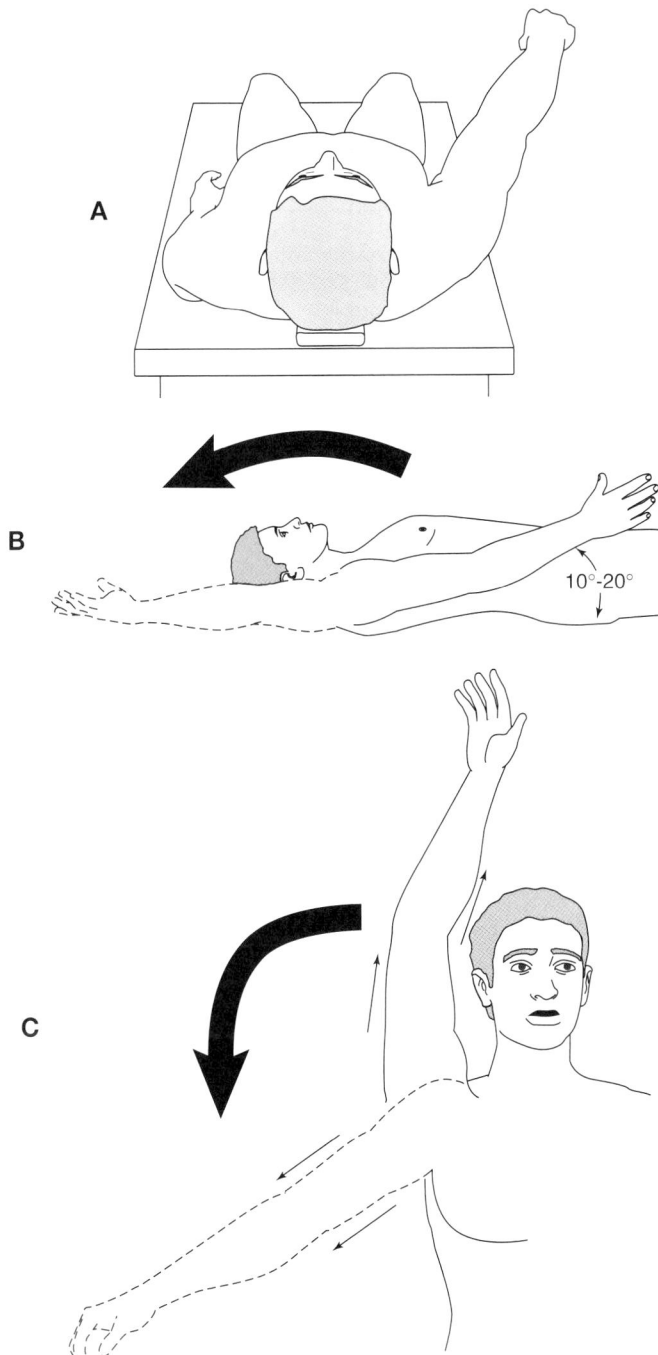

Fig. 199-6
A, Milch-Cooper technique. The arm is started at 10 to 20 degrees flexion and slight abduction. **B,** Elevation continues slowly until the arm is directly overhead. **C,** Then the arm is slowly brought through a full, lateral downward arc, maintaining constant outward traction until reduction occurs. Note that outward traction is maintained only in step C.

Hippocratic Maneuver

Because the Hippocratic maneuver is no longer recommended, it is included only for historical interest. The physician places his foot against the chest wall to provide countertraction and manipulates the arm. This technique can cause serious neurovascular trauma.

Many other techniques have been described in the literature but are not reviewed here.

COMPLICATIONS

If the shoulder dislocation proves irreducible, an orthopedic surgeon should be consulted and the use of general anesthesia should be considered. Iatrogenic fracture and neurovascular damage are ever-present risks.

One of the risks after a shoulder dislocation is redislocation. This is a very common occurrence in the young adult population. If appropriate care is not maintained and enforced, the frequency of redislocation increases. Usually immobilization for a period of 4 to 6 weeks following a successful reduction is warranted. Appropriate clinical, neurologic, and radiographic follow-up examinations should be made throughout this time to confirm maintenance of the reduction.

POSTPROCEDURE PATIENT EDUCATION

After the designated period of immobilization, assign a gentle strengthening program, with particular emphasis on the shoulder internal rotators. Unrestricted external rotation and lifting activities are usually not permitted for a period of 3 months. With recurrent dislocations, an arthrogram, CT arthrogram, or arthroscopy might be warranted to help identify an anatomic variant that might make the patient more prone to redislocation. Patients with peripheral neuropathies, syringomyelia, and psychiatric histories may be more prone to dislocating their shoulders, and these underlying conditions should be considered in patients with repeated dislocations. (See the sample patient education handout titled "Shoulder Reduction or Putting Dislocated Shoulder Back into Place" on page 2009 of Appendix G.)

CPT/BILLING CODES

23650   Closed treatment of shoulder dislocation, with manipulation, without anesthesia
23655   Closed treatment of shoulder dislocation, with manipulation, with anesthesia

ICD-9-CM DIAGNOSTIC CODES

831   Dislocation of shoulder

The following fifth-digit subclassification is for use with category 831:

    0   Shoulder, unspecified (humerus NOS)
    1   Anterior dislocation of humerus
    2   Posterior dislocation of humerus
    3   Inferior dislocation of humerus
    4   Acromioclavicular (joint) (clavicle)
    9   Other (scapula)
831.0   Closed dislocation
831.1   Open dislocation
832   Dislocation of elbow
718.1   Other derangement of joint, shoulder region
718.3   Recurrent dislocation of joint

ADDITIONAL RESOURCES

- See the sample patient education handout titled "Shoulder Reduction or Putting Dislocated Shoulder Back into Place" on page 2009 of Appendix G.

BIBLIOGRAPHY

Doyle WL, Ragar T: Use of the scapular manipulation method to reduce an anterior shoulder dislocation in the supine position, *Ann Emerg Med* 27(1):92, 1996.

Dunmire SM, Paris P: *Atlas of emergency procedures,* Philadelphia, 1994, WB Saunders.

Roberts JR, Hedges JR, editors: *Clinical procedures in emergency medicine,* ed 3, Philadelphia, 1998, WB Saunders.

Subluxations and dislocations about the glenohumeral joint. In Rockwood CA, Green DP et al: *Rockwood and Green's fractures in adults,* ed 3, Philadelphia, 1991, JB Lippincott.

Rosen P, Barkin RM, Hockberger RS, et al: *Emergency medicine: concepts and clinical practice,* ed 4, St Louis, 1998, Mosby.

WEBSITES

www.medmedia.com/06/1735.htm (Milch technique of shoulder reduction)

www.physsportsmed.com/issues/2000/11-00/joy.htm (self-reduction of anterior shoulder dislocation)

www.fpnotebook.com/ort299.htm (shoulder relocation maneuvers)

PART THIRTEEN

Osteopathic Procedures

CHAPTER 200

Manipulative Medicine

Geraldine N. Urse

References to the use of manual medicine have been found in ancient Egyptian writings. Hippocrates, father of modern medicine, used traction and leverage techniques. Manual medicine disappears from print about the time of the plague during the Middle Ages, as the barber-surgeons began to assume direct patient care and physicians distanced themselves from their patients. In the late 1800s renewed interest in manual techniques surfaced both in England and the United States. The bone-setting technique was introduced in England and had many enthusiasts, including Dr. Edward Harrison and Sir Herbert Barker. In the United States two men who would greatly influence manipulative medicine and therapy came into the forefront. Dr. Andrew Taylor Still founded the American School of Osteopathy in Kirksville, Missouri, in 1892. Dr. Still believed that structure and function were interrelated and that if the body were restored to proper alignment, it would work to heal itself. Another proponent of manual therapy was a former grocer and self-taught manipulative therapist, D.D. Palmer, who originated chiropractic medicine in 1896.

Today there are many practitioners of manual medicine, from chiropractors, physical therapists, and massage therapists to physicians. Each one of these disciplines has tenets that it holds true of its profession, but the common thread is the use of a "hands-on" approach to patient care. Today health maintenance organizations and insurance carriers demand cost-efficient management of patients. This demand, coupled with the already known and potentially serious side effects and cost of nonsteroidal antiinflammatory drugs, creates a real need for the cost-effective use of manipulative therapy. While it may not benefit all patients or be appealing to all practitioners, every medical practitioner has the basic knowledge to be trained as a proficient practitioner of manipulative medicine. Incorporation of manipulative techniques into the daily practice routine requires some commitment by the staff and the physician; however, the potential benefit for the patient is worth the effort. Potential patient benefit was revealed in a randomized controlled trial (Bove and Nilsson, 1998) conducted on the use of spinal manipulation in the treatment of episodic tension headache. The study concluded that there was a significant reduction in the amount of medications used and the number of hours per day the patient spent in pain following the use of manipulative therapy to treat the headache.

The initial component of manipulative therapy is structural examination. This examination requires that the patient be barefoot and in a gown that opens down the back. The practitioner first observes the patient's skin, looking for any changes in coloration. With the patient standing, the practitioner observes for any changes in weight-bearing posture (e.g., shifting the weight to one hip or the other); anterior, posterior, or lateral curves of the spine; and overall alignment of the body. The shoulder and hip heights are measured along with the medial malleoli for equality. Palpation is used to evaluate any areas of asymmetry. Active and passive range of motion is evaluated in flexion, extension, rotation and sidebending. All restrictions found in motion are noted, along with changes in the muscle and superficial tissue textures. These changes are referred to as *somatic dysfunctions.*

Somatic dysfunction is defined in the Yearbook and Directory of the American Osteopathic Association as "impaired or altered function of related components of the somatic (body framework) system; skeletal, arthrodial, and myofascial structures, and related vascular, lymphatic and neural elements." The diagnosis of somatic dysfunction can be a stand-alone finding or can accompany other diagnoses. Three changes are seen in the tissues of a patient with somatic dysfunction: (1) asymmetry, (2) abnormal range of motion, and (3) alteration in tissue texture. These changes can either be chronic or acute in quality.

Tissue texture changes associated with chronic dysfunctions are slightly increased tension with a ropy or stringy consistency to the muscles. The skin over a chronic dysfunction will feel dry and no edema will be present. Acute dysfunctions will have increased tissue temperature when palpated and a boggy rough consistency with a rigid, often boardlike, quality. Edema and tenderness will also be present. A quick and simple test for somatic dysfunction is to rub firmly and briskly over the area in question for a 10-second period. After completion observe for blanching (whiteness) or erythema (redness), noting the length of time it takes to return to normal. An area of acute somatic dysfunction will remain red longer than areas without dysfunction.

Comprehensive coverage of every technique and its indication is beyond the scope of this chapter. Therefore this overview encourages the practitioner to investigate the many courses offered in manipulative therapy. Some techniques use articulatory or joint mobilization, whereas others use the energy of muscles to correct the dysfunction. One method—the craniosacral technique—teaches that there is a rhythm related to respiratory function. When this rhythm is disrupted, a dysfunction results and affects the body as a whole. The goal of manipulative therapy, regardless of technique, is to return the body to its usual state of function by reducing the asymmetry, increasing the range of motion, and reversing the tissue texture changes.

INDICATIONS

- Cervical spine dysfunction
- Thoracic spine dysfunction
- Lumbar spine dysfunction
- Rib motion dysfunction
- Myofascial or soft tissue dysfunction or discomfort
- Muscle contraction headaches
- Temporal mandibular joint (TMJ) syndrome
- Many other somatic disorders

Very few conditions are not amenable to some form of manipulative therapy. Obvious surgical conditions and emergent medical problems require traditional interventions. However, when these patients are examined, there will be corresponding tender points associated with the diagnosis. For instance, the patient with an acute gall bladder will have a thoracic spine dysfunction at the T5-9 regions on the right, whereas the patient with acute myocardial infarction will demonstrate a dysfunction at the T1-5 level on the left. These are examples of viscerosomatic reflexes. A patient with acute exacerbation of asthma will have restricted rib motion in all planes as well as limited excursion of the diaphragm. These are examples of both viscerosomatic and visceroviseral reflexes. All three of these examples can be treated with manipulative techniques to help patients regain their former state of function. Multiple studies have been conducted that demonstrate patients treated with manipulative therapy have decreased use of pain medications and physical therapy modalities.

The decision to treat a patient with a manipulative technique can be made only after obtaining a careful history and performing a physical and a structural examination. The exact technique to be used depends on the proficiency of the provider. There is no substitution for adequate training.

CONTRAINDICATIONS

- Patient refusal
- Obvious surgical emergency
- Obvious medical emergencies (e.g., myocardial infarction or diabetic ketoacidosis)
- Any diagnosis that remains uncertain as to the structural integrity (e.g. fracture)

Manipulative therapy is an adaptable procedure, but certain criteria must be considered before a technique is chosen. Delay of emergency care and patient refusal are the only true contraindications.

CONDITIONS TO BE TREATED WITH CAUTION

- Osteoporosis
- Metastatic cancer to the bones
- Acute arthritis
- Bone fractures
- Spondylosis (vertebral ankylosis)
- Intense pain from acute injuries
- Pregnancy
- Anticoagulation or hemophilia
- Radicular pain resulting from herniated discs
- Posterior vertebral artery insufficiency; hyperextension of the cervical spine

Care must be exercised with the thrusting techniques in patients with known bone metastasis from carcinoma, osteoporosis, acute arthritis, fractures or spondylosis. Patients with acute injuries, such as whiplash, may be in too much pain to be treated initially; however, after a few days of conservative management, they should be easily treated. Other conditions should be approached with caution and the technique chosen with care, such as patients who are pregnant, on anticoagulation medications, or experiencing radicular pain from herniated discs. Patients can benefit from manipulative therapy after surgery as long as the technique is chosen with both the surgical procedure and the state of the patient in mind. Manipulative techniques using hyperextention should be used with caution in patients with posterior vertebral artery insufficiency.

EQUIPMENT

A flat, firmly padded table of appropriate height—although tables with adjustable heights are available—is the only equipment required. The table should allow the practitioner to work without injury to his or her back. The tabletop should be even with the fingertips of the standing practitioner. A pillow should also be available for the patient's comfort.

TECHNIQUE

Soft tissue techniques such as muscle energy, myofascial release, and counterstrain, as well as articulatory techniques including high-velocity low-amplitude (HVLA), are available to treat somatic dysfunctions (Table 200-1). The abundance of techniques precludes their full inclusion in this format. Following is an example of a muscle energy technique for the treatment of cervical somatic dysfunction. It is hoped that this information will stimulate the practitioner to seek complete and thorough knowledge of manipulative therapy.

Muscle Energy Technique for Cervical Muscle Spasm

With the patient seated comfortably on the table, an active and passive range of motion examination of the cervical spine is completed. Passive range of motion is obtained by placing a hand on the head of the patient and initiating movement in four planes: (1) flexion, (2) extension, (3) rotation, and (4) side-bending. Any decrease or restrictions to movement are noted as to plane and direction (e.g., "Decreased range of motion in flexion, rotation to the right and side-bending to the left [FR_RSB_L]"). The patient is then asked to lie supine on the table while the physician sits at the head of the table. Placing the hands on each side of the neck, the physician palpates for areas of tenderness or fullness that accompany somatic dysfunction. The physician then places the tip of the index finger over the area of dysfunction. With the other hand the physician introduces extension until motion is felt under the monitoring fingertip. This engages the first motion barrier. Side-bending is then introduced, using pressure by the monitoring finger against the restricted area. Rotation is introduced by asking the patient to turn the head toward the side of

decreased motion (in this case, to the right). The physician places a hand on the patient's cheek and requests that the patient rotate the head toward the midline while the physician isometrically resists the rotation for 3 seconds. The patient is instructed to relax and the physician simultaneously releases the counterforce. Once the patient is relaxed, the physician reintroduces motion and again engages the new motion barriers. These steps are repeated two or three times. At the end of the last engagement the patient's head is returned to neutral position and active motion reassessed for change.

COMPLICATIONS

- Muscular discomfort
- Bone fracture
- Joint dislocation
- Stroke

Adverse outcomes depend on the type of technique used. The most common side effect following all forms of manipulative therapy is muscle soreness. This is easily relieved by the use of warm packs and antiinflammatory medications. High-velocity low-amplitude (HVLA) or articulatory techniques have the potential complication of fracture or dislocation. There have been instances of strokes following manipulative therapy in patients with carotid plaques or vertebral artery disease. Correct patient selection and careful application of technique will virtually eliminate complications.

CPT-4 BILLING CODES

CPT-4 billing codes are different from ICD-9-CM codes (see below). The chiropractic codes are to be used only by chiropractors, the osteopathic manipulative codes are designed for osteopathic physicians, and the general manipulation codes are to be used by all other practitioners.

Osteopathic CPT-4 Codes

98925	1 to 2 regions
98926	3 to 4 regions
98927	5 to 6 regions
98928	7 to 8 regions
98929	9 to 10 regions

Chiropractic CPT-4 Codes

98940	Spinal levels 1 to 2
98941	Spinal levels 3 to 4
98942	Spinal level 5
98943	Extraspinal 1 to 2

TABLE 200-1
Techniques Used in Manipulative Therapy

Technique	Components
Soft tissue techniques	Muscle energy—direct and indirect
	Counterstrain
	Myofascial release
Articulatory techniques	High velocity, low amplitude
	Low velocity, high amplitude
Craniosacral technique	Myofascial release

General CPT-4 Codes

97140	One or more regions
97250	Myofascial release
97010	Hot packs

ICD-9-CM DIAGNOSTIC CODES

739.X	Somatic dysfunction (X identifies body level)
739.1	Somatic dysfunction, cervical spine
739.2	Somatic dysfunction, thoracic spine
739.3	Somatic dysfunction, lumbar spine

The ICD-9-CM code for somatic dysfunction is 739.X. The digit following the decimal point indicates what body level is being treated (e.g., 739.7 is upper extremity). The diagnostic codes are universal for all practitioners. For a complete listing please consult the ICD-9-CM code book.

AVAILABILITY OF TRAINING

There are many places available to access information regarding training in specific modalities or techniques of manipulative therapy. This list is neither exhaustive nor comprehensive.

American Academy of Osteopathy
3500 DePauw Blvd., Suite 1080
Indianapolis, IN 46268-1136
Phone: 1-317-879-1881
Website: www.academyofosteopathy.org

American Osteopathic Association
142 E. Ontario Street
Chicago Illinois 60611
Phone: 1-800-621-1773
Website: www.aoa-net.org

The Upledger Institute
11211 Prosperity Farms Road, Suite D-325
Palm Beach Gardens, FL 33410
Phone: 1-561-622-4334
Website: www.upledger.com

Sutherland Cranial Teaching Foundation
4116 Hartwood Drive
Ft. Worth, TX 76109
Phone: 1-817-926-7705

The Cranial Academy
8202 Clearvista Parkway #9D
Indianapolis, IN 46256
Website: www.cranialacademy.org

American Chiropractic Association
1701 Clarendon Boulevard
Arlington, VA 22209
Phone: 1-800-986-4636
Website: www.amerchiro.org

American Massage Therapy Association
820 Davis Street, Suite 100
Evanston, IL 60201-4444
Phone: 1-847-864-0123
Website: www.amtamassage.org

BIBLIOGRAPHY

American Osteopathic Association: *Yearbook and directory of osteopathic physicians 2000/2001,* Chicago, 2000, AOA.

Andersson GB, Lucente T, Davis AM, et al: A comparison of osteopathic spinal manipulation with standard care for patients with low back pain, *N Engl J Med* 341(19):1426, 1999.

Barker S, Kesson M, Ashmore J, et al: Professional issue: guidance for pre-manipulative testing of the cervical spine *Man Ther* 5(1):37, 2000.

Beal MC, editor: *The principles of palpatory diagnosis and manipulative technique,* Newark, Ohio, 1989, American Academy of Osteopathy.

Bove G, Nilsson N: Spinal manipulation in the treatment of episodic tension-type headache: a randomized controlled trial, *JAMA* 280:1576, 1998.

DiGiovanna EL, Schiowitz S: *An osteopathic approach to diagnosis and treatment,* Philadelphia, 1991, JB Lippincott.

Greenman PE: *Principles of manual medicine,* Baltimore, 1989, Williams & Wilkins.

Hoyt WH, Shaffer F, Bard DA, et al: Osteopathic manipulation in the treatment of muscle-contraction headache, *J Am Osteopath Assoc* 78(5):322, 1979.

Klofkorn WK: *One hundred years of osteopathic medicine,* Greenwich, Conn, 1995, Greenwich Press.

McPartland J, Miller B: Bodywork therapy systems, *Phys Med Rehabil Clin North Am* 10(3):583, 1999.

Nyiendo J, Haas M, Goodwin P: Patient characteristics, practice activities, and one-month outcomes for chronic, recurrent low-back pain treated by chiropractors and family medicine physicians: a practice-based feasibility study, *J Manipulative Physiol Ther* 23(4):239, 2000.

Stoddard Alan MB: *Manual of osteopathic technique,* London, 1980, Hutchinson.

Vickers A, Zollman C: ABC of complementary medicine: the manipulative therapies: osteopathy and chiropractic, *BMJ* 319:1176, 1999.

PART FOURTEEN

Alternative Medicine

CHAPTER 201

Acupuncture

Victor S. Sierpina

The insertion of fine needles into the body at specific points or "channels of energy flow" called meridians has been used in the treatment of human and animal disease for thousands of years. The oldest reference to this traditional oriental medical procedure dates to 2600 BC, when fine, sharpened stone or bamboo needles were reported to be used in the treatment and prevention of illness.

Contemporary use of acupuncture has become increasingly popular. It is offered not only by traditionally trained oriental medical doctors (OMDs), but also by allopathic and osteopathic physicians and clinicians alike. Patient interest and acceptance of acupuncture in this country has resulted in its investigation and recognition by such bodies as the National Institutes of Health's (NIH's) Office of Alternative Medicine. Their advisory panel recently released a consensus statement supporting the efficacy of acupuncture and acknowledging the potential benefit of acupuncture in a number of acute and chronic conditions. Furthermore, they recommended that the insurance industry consider wider coverage for this safe and effective technique. These statements have begun changing the perceptions of this ancient art of medicine from that of a curiosity or "an experimental treatment" to that of an acceptable procedure within medical science.

Although the exact mechanism of its action is not known, acupuncture is the most widely studied alternative therapy, and a wide variety of theories attempt to explain its effects. After use for many centuries, the traditional concept used by the Chinese and others to explain acupuncture is that it is a method of balancing *qi* (or *chi*), an invisible yet essential, ceaselessly flowing life energy that circulates silently and invisibly in the body. Since no scientist has ever measured or seen qi, only its effects can be observed. These effects are best demonstrated when the body is performing normally, an amalgamation of all the physiologic, immunologic, and homeostatic functions of a living organism. The blockage of the flow of qi, an inadequate or waning supply of it, or an excess amount of qi can all lead to conditions of pain, disease, and loss of homeostasis.

This quasi-mystical explanation is not always satisfying to the medical scientist's mind and theory. Thus attempts have been made over the years to derive a more robust explanation, one that is understandable in terms of western scientific tradition and terminology. The work of Pomeranz and others showed that some of the effects of acupuncture are achieved by activating the endorphin neuropeptide system and can be blocked by the opiate receptor antagonist naloxone. Others have looked into the quantum physics realm and found parallels there in nonlocal effects, standing wave theory, and other quantum principles now used by physicists. Certain hybrid models apply western medical and physiologic terminology to explain the effect of needling. These models discuss the ionic and electrical milieu of cells and tissues as well as the foreign body effect and the pattern of injury currents induced by needling. Additional theories explain acupuncture results as being due to a "neurogate blocking phenomenon," various neural or endocrinological events, effects on cytokine and prostaglandin inflammatory pathways, or an electromagnetic field realignment. Given the sheer range and diversity of these explanations, it is likely that acupuncture works through a number of mechanisms and perhaps is not yet fully explicable with our current science. However, its effects on humans and animals, its longevity as a healing art, and its resurgence in the western medical community are all inductive evidence of the value of acupuncture, whatever its mechanism of action.

Although there is considerable variability among training approaches for physicians, the annual 200-hour course offered by the University of California at Los Angeles (UCLA), called Medical Acupuncture for Physicians, is widely acknowledged as a benchmark minimum for those wanting to practice acupuncture. Classes are offered over several months and are designed to give practical knowledge without requiring too much time away from a medical practice. A number of shorter courses, such as the 2-day introductory courses offered by the National Procedure Institute (NPI) (4909 Hedgewood Dr., Midland, Mich 48640, 1-800-462-2492), provide an excellent overview and some simple treatment techniques but are not designed to provide mastery. The longer 2- to 3-year courses offered at oriental medical colleges are not usually required by states for licensure and are often impractical for the practicing clinician to complete.

Laws governing physician acupuncture are listed on the American Academy of Medical Acupuncture's website: www.medicalacupuncture.org.

Blending this ancient medical art into a medical practice can be a source of satisfaction to both professionals and their patients. It can serve as a practice builder and provide new opportunities to attract patients. With the NIH consensus panel's opinion on record, healthcare professionals have reason to anticipate better insurance coverage for acupuncture and a resulting increase in demand. In fact, some HMOs already reimburse for alternative therapies, including acupuncture.

INDICATIONS

Although acupuncture has been used to treat every imaginable human condition, to treat animals, and to prevent disease, most clinicians performing acupuncture find its greatest usefulness in the following conditions:

- Arthritis
- Asthma
- Back pain
- Carpal tunnel syndrome
- Dizziness
- Dysmenorrhea
- Gastrointestinal disorders
- Gynecological problems
- Headache
- Irritable bowel syndrome
- Mental and mood disturbances
- Musculoskeletal pain
- Neuralgia
- Sciatica
- Sinusitis
- Skin disorders
- Substance addiction
- Tendonitis
- Tennis elbow
- Upper respiratory infections
- Urological disease

CONTRAINDICATIONS

- Septic or extremely weakened patient.
- Local skin infection or loss of skin integrity (e.g., burns, cellulitis).
- Uncooperative patients or patients with delusions, hallucinations, or paranoia.

- Electroacupuncture should not be applied across the brain or heart.
- During pregnancy, a number of points are to be avoided (see acupuncture references for details), since some of these points may stimulate labor.
- The umbilicus, the nipple, points over major vessels and nerves and an infant's fontanelle are points forbidden by both classical and contemporary practitioners.
- During menses *(relative contraindication)*.
- Patient unable to lie down (relative contraindication; sitting or standing treatments should usually be avoided, especially for first treatment)

EQUIPMENT

A variety of needles are available, ranging from very fine, 34- or 36-gauge needles, to 18-gauge needles used for veterinary acupuncture. The most commonly used needles are those from 0.5 to 3.0 inches in length and in the 30- to 34-gauge size. Acupuncture needles usually have solid stainless steel shafts and a copper, silver, or wound-steel-wire handle. The longer needles are used in thicker muscle groups, such as the back, buttocks, and legs, whereas the shorter, more delicate needles are used in the hands, face, and ears.

In addition to the needles, acupuncturists both in the United States and abroad, including China, now commonly use electrostimulation units (Fig. 201-1). These are small, hand-held, battery-operated units, similar in design to transcutaneous electrical stimulation (TENS) units used for pain control. Instead of the electrode pad that is used with the TENS unit, a small alligator clip is placed onto the shaft of an acupuncture needle to deliver the electrical current.

Other materials that may be used by an acupuncturist include: imbedded ear needles; metallic or magnetic beads; the herb moxa *(Artemisia vulgaris)*, which is burned to heat the skin, needle, or acupuncture points; glass or bamboo cups used for a corollary procedure

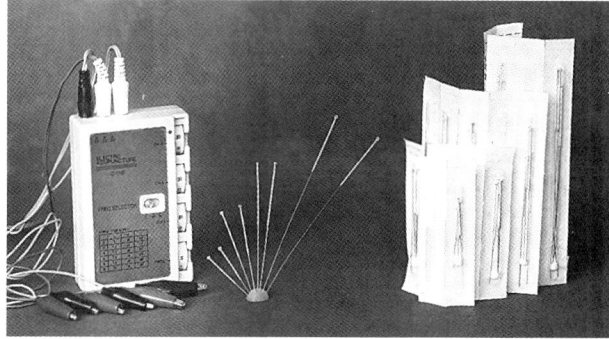

Fig. 201-1
Examples of an electroacupuncture stimulator *(left)* and acupuncture needles of various sizes *(right)*.

called *cupping;* small hammers with several needles on the tip (plum blossom or seven-star needles); and electrical point locators, probes, or stimulators.

Generally, four sizes of needles and a few electrostimulator devices are all that are necessary for most medical acupuncture applications. The cost of these supplies varies, but a reasonable, complete set of equipment will usually cost less than $1000. (See the list of suppliers at the end of the chapter.)

PREPROCEDURE
PATIENT PREPARATION

Although acupuncture is among the safest of invasive medical therapies, some precautions are needed. A thorough standard examination and diagnostic evaluation by a clinician is needed before acupuncture. Interestingly, performing them often prepares the patient for acupuncture, by giving him or her confidence in a known, established medical ritual—the routine physical. If the patient has never had acupuncture, the clinician should first show him or her the needles and stimulation devices. It is essential to assure the patient that the needles are sterile and disposed of after every treatment to allay fears of disease transmission. It is helpful to explain the risk of a needle reaction and the occasional endorphin rush, or "high," that follows some treatments.

Like any other medical treatment or procedure, it is wise to discuss the pros and cons of treatment, any conventional therapy options that may not have been tried, the likelihood of success with acupuncture, possible costs, and the expected number and length of treatments. Most conditions amenable to acupuncture will show a positive response in 4 to 10 treatments. With initial treatments, the patient may experience no response, a temporary worsening of the condition, or a gradual (or even sudden) improvement. For most chronic conditions, such as low back pain, a series of 4 to 10 treatments at $50 to $100 per treatment is often worth the investment for the patient seeking relief.

The topics just mentioned should be discussed with every patient before initiating a course of acupuncture treatments. The initial evaluation, review of records, discussion of options, and development of care plan usually occupy the entire first visit. Needle treatment is often deferred until the second visit. Generally no informed consent forms or releases are used in acupuncture therapy, although they may be useful in certain practice situations.

TECHNIQUE

Although the choice of points, their location, and the details of acupuncture therapeutics are beyond the scope of this chapter, the text below should give a general idea of how to interact with the patient, and how a treatment session is staged and integrated into a medical practice.

1. After the patient and acupuncturist agree that a trial of acupuncture is appropriate and mutually acceptable, the patient is draped or gowned. Special efforts should be made to ensure patient comfort on the treatment table, using supports such as pillows, towels, and bolsters, since the patient will be lying down for a session lasting 15 to 30 minutes or more. As noted above, sitting or standing treatments are avoided unless the patient is known to have tolerated them previously.

2. Acupuncture points are palpated on the body, extremities, ears, face, or scalp, and the needle is inserted deftly with a slight twirling motion (Figs. 201-2 to 201-4). A sufficient depth of insertion has been reached when the patient feels a slight aching sensation, indicating that the qi has been reached (de qi sensation). Needle insertion should be painless, other than the mild de qi sensation and a tiny prick the patient may feel as the needle penetrates the skin. Although some acupuncturists wipe the area of insertion with an alcohol swab, this is not necessary. However, cleansing before needling may be prudent in certain cases (e.g., patients who have an immune deficiency or diabetes or those who are concerned or worried).

3. A typical treatment may require 15 to 30 needles. After all of the needles are in place, electroacupuncture electrodes are usually attached to several but not all of the needles. The electrostimulator is turned on, and the current is gradually increased until the patient can feel a pulsing sensation. The current is then increased to the patient's maximal tolerance level, and then backed off slightly (Fig. 201-5).

4. A timer is set, and a healthcare professional should remain within hailing distance to assist the patient if needed. The patient may be given a bell to ring if assistance is needed (e.g., if a needle falls out, the patient becomes uncomfortable or for some other reason needs the presence of another person).

5. At the end of the session, a nurse or medical assistant removes the wires and clips from the needles, removes the needles and disposes of them in a sharps container, and allows the patient to dress. The clinician or acupuncturist may return to evaluate the treatment or the patient may be discharged without further attention until the next visit. Usually the clinician is seeing or managing other patients while an acupuncture session is in progress. He or she may start another or even two more acupuncture sessions while the first is occurring, or the clinician may attend to other standard medical cases.

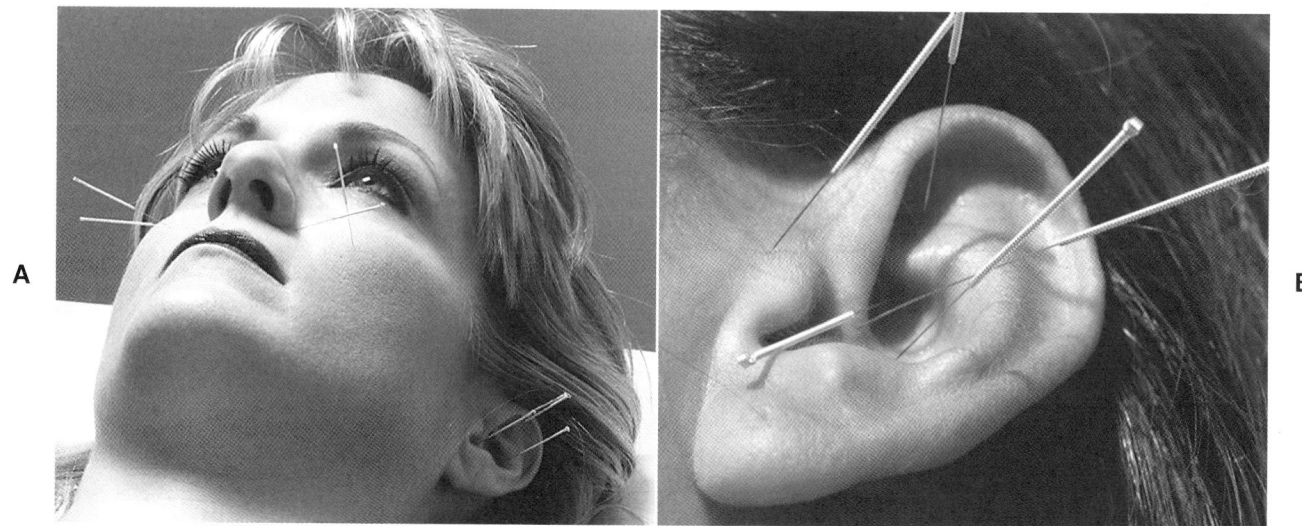

Fig. 201-2
A, Example of treatment of facial and ear points. **B,** Ear acupuncture is demonstrated.

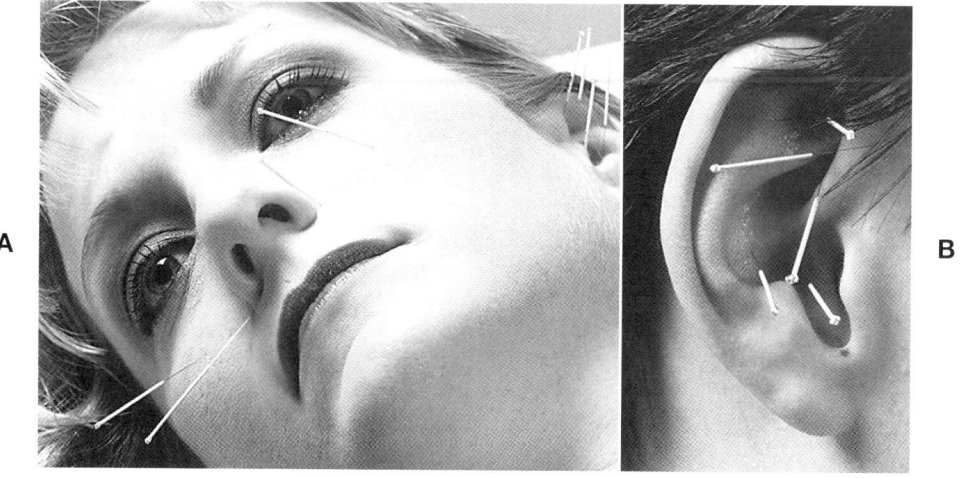

Fig. 201-3
A, Facial points used for sinus problems are demonstrated. **B,** Example of auricular points used for an addiction is shown.

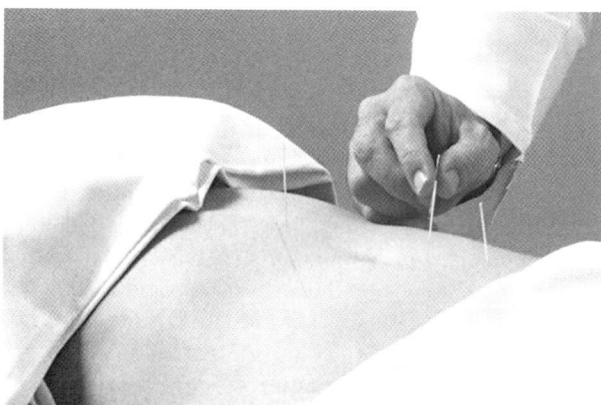

Fig. 201-4
Needle insertion in abdomen.

6. Follow-up treatments are done at intervals of up to 2 weeks. During return visits, the acupuncturist interviews, examines, and reevaluates the patient and his or her progress. Treatment and needle location may be altered based on the patient's response, or the same or similar pattern may be used. As the patient starts to improve, treatment intervals are spaced further apart. Whereas some patients obtain permanent relief from acupuncture, others may require interval "tune-up" treatments to sustain their improvement.

7. The patient's diagnosis, his or her vital signs, type of treatment, and needle application points used should be dictated into the medical record.

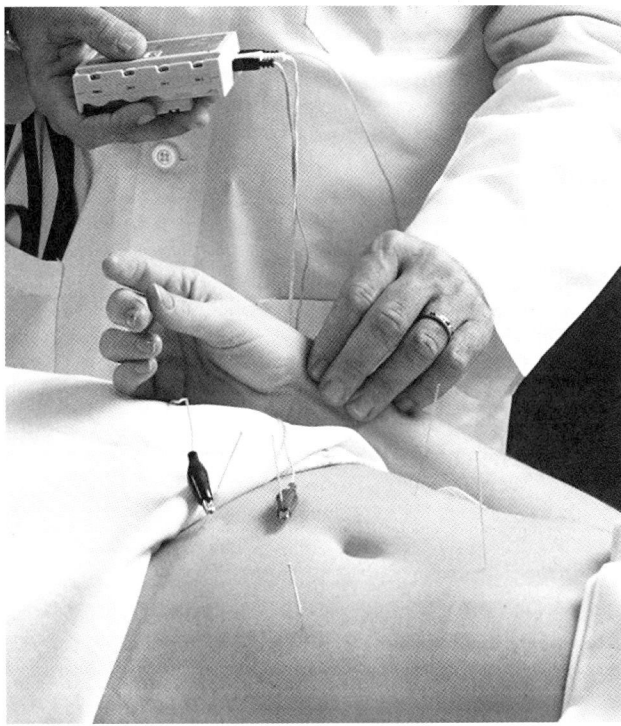

Fig. 201-5
Checking the pulse and adjusting the treatment settings.

COMPLICATIONS

Complications are rare in acupuncture, but of those reported, the most common are local pain, swelling, hematoma formation, organ puncture, pneumothorax, metal allergy, needle reaction (fainting), a posttreatment period of euphoria, local infection such as perichondritis, or even more serious infections such as endocarditis. Systemic infections, such as hepatitis and acquired immunodeficiency syndrome, have been reported as transmitted by acupuncture needle. However, poorly qualified practitioners who reused needles and did not use sterile technique were the cause of these infections.

POSTPROCEDURE PATIENT EDUCATION

Depending on the type of treatment, usually no special instructions are necessary. Band-Aids are not needed. Some patients, particularly at their first treatment, experience a euphoric spell thought to be related to endorphin release. The practitioner may instruct patients to drive carefully after a treatment or to have someone drive them home.

Some treatments are designed to increase general energy and vigor, especially in chronically weakened patients. Advice should be given to these patients to avoid heavy meals, alcoholic beverages, sexual relations,

and intense exercise for about 8 hours after the treatment. This should enhance treatment benefits.

SUPPLIERS

Acupuncture needles and other equipment
Lhasa Medical, Inc.
539 Accord Station
Accord, MA 02018-0539
Phone: 1-800-722-8775
Website: www.lhasamedical.com

OMS Medical Supplies
1950 Washington Street
Braintree, MA 02184
Phone: 1-800-323-1839
Website: www.omsmedical.com

Books and references on acupuncture
Redwing Book Company
44 Linden Street
Brookline, MA 02445
Phone: 1-800-873-3946
Website: www.redwingbooks.com

CPT/BILLING CODES

97780 Acupuncture without electroacupuncture
97781 Acupuncture with electroacupuncture

Standardized fees depend on the client population, geography, and increasingly on the rate of insurance reimbursement. However, treatments are billed in the range of $50 to $100 in most cases and locations.

ICD-9-CM DIAGNOSTIC CODES

789.00 Abdominal pain, unspecified site
303.90 Alcohol dependence syndrome, chronic, unspecified
300.0 Anxiety
714.0 Arthritis, rheumatoid, adult
715.0 Arthrosis, osteoarthrosis, site unspecified or generalized
493.0 Asthma, without mention of status asthmaticus
724.2 Back pain, low or low back syndrome
354.0 Carpal tunnel syndrome
595.1 Cystitis, chronic interstitial
311 Depressive disorder not otherwise classified
309.0 Depressive reaction, brief
309.1 Depressive reaction, prolonged
691.8 Dermatitis, atopic (eczema)

780.4	Dizziness
304.00	Drug dependence, opioid, unspecified
304.10	Drug dependence, barbiturate, unspecified
304.20	Drug dependence, cocaine, unspecified
304.40	Drug dependence, amphetamine, unspecified
625.3	Dysmenorrhea
617	Endometriosis
346.00	Headache, classical migraine, not intractable
346.10	Headache, common migraine, not intractable
346.20	Headache, cluster without intractable migraine
307.81	Headache, tension
564.1	Irritable bowel syndrome
726.32	Lateral epicondylitis
729.89	Musculoskeletal pain, limbs
729.2	Neuralgia, unspecified
625.9	Pelvic pain
696.1	Psoriasis
722.10	Sciatica, discogenic
473.9	Sinusitis, chronic
726.90	Tendonitis, site NOS
519.8	Upper respiratory infection, chronic

ADDITIONAL RESOURCES

- See the sample patient education handout titled "Acupuncture" on page 2010 of Appendix G.

BIBLIOGRAPHY

Helms J: *Acupuncture energetics,* Berkeley, Calif., 1996, Medical Acupuncture Publishers.

Helms J: An overview of medical acupuncture, *Altern Ther Health Med* 4(3):35, 1998.

Rubik B: Can Western science provide a foundation for acupuncture? *Altern Ther Health Med* 1(4):41, 1995.

Stux G, Pomeranz B: *Acupuncture: textbook and atlas,* Berlin, 1987, Springer-Verlag.

Ulett G: Scientific acupuncture: peripheral electrical stimulation for the relief of pain, part I: basics, *Pain Manag* May/June:128, 1989.

Ulett G: Scientific acupuncture: peripheral electrical stimulation for the relief of pain, part II: clinical aspects, *Pain Manag* July/August:186, 1989.

Villaire M: NIH consensus conference confirms acupuncture's efficacy, *Altern Ther Health Med* 4(1):21, 1998.

WEBSITES

www.medicalacupuncture.org (American Academy of Medical Acupuncture: a physician-oriented site)

A large number of websites can be found on the Internet by searching under the keyword *acupuncture*.

PART FIFTEEN

Miscellaneous

CHAPTER 202

Allergy Testing and Immunotherapy

Harold H. Hedges III

The primary methods of allergy skin testing are (1) single skin prick tests (SPTs) (pricking the skin at a 45-degree angle), or (2) skin puncture tests (puncturing the skin at a 90-degree angle) through each previously placed allergen, and (3) using preloaded devices with multiple allergens and applying five to eight allergens simultaneously. Multiple-test applicators have gained in popularity because of their safety, ease of use, test reproducibility, and readability. Two are available: Multi-Test II (Lincoln Diagnostics) and Quintest (Hollister Stier).

Although considered an SPT, Multi-Test II is comparable to an intradermal (ID) test using a 1:1000 dilution of antigen. Several studies have shown that a positive ID skin test (1:100 dilution) following a negative SPT has little or no clinical significance; thus it is not recommended. (See below.)

Older scratch testing methods are not as reproducible or reliable as SPT and are not recommended.

Radioallergosorbent testing (RAST) is an in vitro test performed by a reference laboratory and can be recommended. It is the test of choice for patients exhibiting dermographism, hyporeactive skin, poorly controlled asthma, eczema, or any skin condition limiting the placement of skin tests.

The identification of allergens helps direct patient avoidance measures and medical therapy; it also provides the basis for immunotherapy. As Nelson (1996) states, "Immunotherapy provides the only potentially curative treatment available because of its unique ability to change the natural history of allergic respiratory disease and Hymenoptera sensitivity. Many suggest starting immunotherapy is a reasonable option that can provide safe and cost effective management for a substantial number of patients." It has been suggested to start immunotherapy earlier in allergic disease in order to prevent (rather than just reduce) the inflammatory response, to prevent the development of asthma in children with rhinitis, and to be able to begin at lower levels of patient sensitivity. It may be the only safe modality for patients whose jobs require alertness and who cannot tolerate antihistamines (e.g., pilots, truck drivers). It is accepted that a positive SPT or RAST test does not necessarily mean clinical sensitivity, so correlation with the clinical history is essential if immunotherapy is to be successful.

INDICATIONS

Perennial or seasonal rhinitis, rhinosinusitis, rhinoconjunctivitis, rhinitis with otitis media, and anaphylaxis from Hymenoptera stings are the major symptom complexes suggesting allergy testing. Patients should be tested for tree, grass, and weed pollens; mold sensitivity; and appropriate insect or animal danders. Limited food testing may be performed. There is increased risk in testing and placing asthmatics on immunotherapy, and the risk/benefit ratio must be considered carefully. Many asthmatics have concomitant allergic rhinitis, which, when treated, aids in asthma control.

CONTRAINDICATIONS

- Any condition that compromises the patient's ability to withstand the rare anaphylactic reaction.
- Although most allergic patients can be safely tested and treated by the primary care physician, an allergist may be helpful in the evaluation and treatment of patients with anaphylactic reactions (particularly to stinging insects), reactions to anesthetics, and difficult-to-control moderate and severe persistent asthma. Great caution must be exercised.
- Immunotherapy is generally not initiated during pregnancy. Allergic patients on maintenance therapy who become pregnant may continue the desensitization process through the pregnancy.
- Patients taking β-blockers should have alternative medications prescribed before testing and immunotherapy, since β-blockers interfere with the response to epinephrine should anaphylaxis occur.

- Those with dermographism, those with chronic skin diseases that limit access to normal skin, and those (physically or psychologically) unable to communicate symptoms should be tested by RAST.
- There is no specific age limit (young or old) to check for inhaled allergens with skin testing, but generally it is not done before the age of 3. Food allergy and other adverse food reactions should be explored by limited food testing (SPT or RAST) and/or single or multiple food elimination diet.
- Patients with uncontrolled hypertension, unstable angina, or recent myocardial infarction are not candidates for immunotherapy.
- Antihistamines may blunt the response to skin testing and should be eliminated before testing. Older, short-acting antihistamines should be eliminated 48 hours before skin testing, and longer-acting antihistamines should be stopped 2 to 4 weeks before testing. Steroids may also reduce the skin response. Positive and negative controls are used to validate skin test results. The positive control (histamine) should respond with a 7- to 10-mm wheal (3+ reaction). If the response is less, it is still blunted by the antihistamine or other medication. RAST is not affected by any antihistamines, steroids, or other medication.

ALLERGY SCREENING

It is appropriate and cost effective to screen patients for allergy with a limited screen of six allergens before applying all allergens. The screen consists of a positive and negative control; house dust mite mix; cat; and the most common tree, grass, weed, and mold allergens of the geographic area. Physicians and patients reluctant to rely on only six allergens for screening may use a second panel of eight allergens consisting of dog; cockroach; feathers; silk; and secondary tree, grass, weed, and mold preparations. When all sites are negative (excluding the positive control), the probability of allergy is less than 5%. Approximately 50% of rhinitic patients tested by Multi-Test or RAST will test negative. These patients have nonallergic rhinitis. Identification of nonallergic triggers is critical for medical care. Decongestants, nasal steroids, or nasal astemizole are medications indicated for nonallergic rhinitis. Roughly 50% of patients with rhinitis have an allergic basis to their symptoms. Many patients have both allergic and nonallergic rhinitis. Screens are performed with both SPT or RAST methods. Phadiatope (Pharmacia) and the Multiple Inhalant Allergy (MIA) screen from LabCorp are two RAST screens using 10 allergens.

A history of symptoms in springtime generally correlates with positive skin tests to tree allergens. Summertime symptoms correlate with grass sensitivity, and fall symptoms correlate with weed sensitivity. In the warmer climates there is much overlap. Year-round (perennial) symptoms correlate with house dust mite, mold, or insect or animal sensitivity. Perennial symptoms with seasonal exacerbations frequently occur in the same patient.

PREPROCEDURE PATIENT PREPARATION

- Establish the history compatible with rhinitis and/or asthma.
- Explore hereditary factors, allergic and nonallergic triggers, previous and present medications, severity and duration of symptoms, secondary infections, and limitations caused by the symptoms.
- Perform a physical examination to evaluate for signs of atopic disease: rhinorrhea (especially if clear and combined with nasal congestion and pale blue swollen turbinates), allergic shiners, conjunctivitis, or evidence for reversible airway disease. Spirometry or peak expiratory flow rate is helpful to identify associated asthma. (See Chapter 89, Pulmonary Function Testing.) Poorly controlled asthmatics (FEV_1 less 70% of their *personal best effort*) should not be skin tested or receive immunotherapy until treated and stable. RAST is a safe alternative in this situation.
- Inform patients about the nature of the testing, the risk of possible reactions, the type of reactions encountered (local and systemic), and the treatment available should a reaction occur.
- Instruct patients to avoid older, short-acting antihistamines 48 hours before skin testing. Longer-acting antihistamines should be avoided 4 weeks before testing.
- Explain the frequency and duration of immunotherapy (weekly or biweekly injections for 3 to 5 years), the expected response, and the criteria for discontinuance (symptom-free control with little or no medication and no increase in symptoms with increasing intervals between injections).

EQUIPMENT

For Skin Testing

- Multiple allergen applicators and loading docks (Multi-Test II, Quintest).
- Individual applicators for the occasional testing of one or two allergens (Duotip [Lincoln Diagnostics], Morrow Brown Needle [Morrow Brown Diagnostics]).

- Alcohol sponges to clean the testing site.
- Allergen concentrates (usually 1:20 dilution; house dust mite comes only as a 1:100 dilution), usually 30 to 50 (standardized or 1:20 weight/volume [w/v] identified for the specific geographic locale by published data or suggested by providers of allergy diagnostics.
- Histamine phosphate (2.75 mg/ml) for positive control and saline for the negative control.
- Recording form (Fig. 202-1).
- Black skin-marking pen.
- Timer capable of timing at least 20 minutes.
- Millimeter ruler.
- EpiPen, Ana-Kit, or epinephrine; and albuterol.
- Resuscitation equipment in the rare event of anaphylactic reaction (the same as that for giving any injections in the office). (See Chapter 203, Anaphylaxis.)
- Disposable tuberculin syringes fitted with a 26- or 27-gauge needle for the "vial test" (see the "Intradermal Testing and the Vial Test" section).

Radioallergosorbent Testing (RAST)

- Equipment for drawing blood.
- Mailing packages or instructions provided by the RAST laboratory.

TECHNIQUE

Skin Prick Tests

SPTs are performed by placing a drop of allergen concentrate (usually 1:20 w/v) on the arm or back, then pressing a needle through the drop into the epidermis at a 45-degree angle. The tip of the needle is then lifted up, producing the pricking sensation. If performed correctly, no bleeding should occur (Fig. 202-2). The puncture test is similar, but the skin is punctured at a 90-degree angle (Fig. 202-3). Several skin testing devices are listed above. The use of Multi-Test II is described in detail here because it has been found to be safe, easily learned, reproducible, and reliable. A videotape of the procedure is available from Lincoln Diagnostics.

Skin Prick Test Multi-Test Method

Multi-Test II is a sterile, disposable, multiple-test applicator used to apply eight allergens simultaneously. Although considered an SPT, its reliability is comparable to ID techniques using a 1:1000 dilution of allergen. Laboratories that supply the allergen concentrates will help determine the most relevant allergens for the patient's geographic area based on established patterns.

The system consists of sterile disposable plastic applicators (Fig. 202-4) and the Dipwell tray (Fig. 202-5).

Loading the Dipwell Tray

1. Establish a master list of allergen panels (each containing eight allergens) to be tested and enter them on the recording form. This is the key for loading each allergen in the same test well each time. Make copies of this for recording test results and refer to it when replenishing allergens.
2. Label (number) each panel A, B, C, D, etc.
3. Allergen panels are made by adding 1 ml (enough for 100 applications) of each allergen concentrate (1:20 w/v in 50% glycerine or standardized extract) to each well numbered 1 through 8. Applicator heads are numbered 1 through 8 and correspond to the numbered wells. Each Dipwell tray accommodates three Allergen panels, each with eight testing heads (Fig. 202-5).
4. Panel A (screening panel) contains the positive control in well A1 and the negative control in well A8. A2 through A7 contain the most common tree, grass, weed, and mold allergens from a geographic area plus house dust mite mix and cat.

Note: This panel will identify over 95% of those in the allergic population. A negative (except for the positive control) screen indicates a nonallergic cause of rhinitis or asthma. No further allergy testing is indicated. This reduces the cost of total allergy testing. When the screen is positive, additional allergens of the geographic area are tested (usually 30 to 40). An additional panel can also be used to check for allergies to common foods (e.g, milk, corn, wheat, egg, soy, sugar, bakers yeast, and pork).

5. Trays are stored in the refrigerator and stack easily.

Application of Multi-Test

1. Place the Dipwell tray(s), which has been filled as noted previously, on a flat surface with the "cradle" for the "T" handle facing away from you (Fig. 202-5).
2. Remove the sterile applicator from the package (held with the blue dot at the top) by pulling the label at the blue dot. This positions the "T" handle for correct placement in the Dipwell tray.
3. Place the applicator(s) in the Dipwell tray (Fig. 202-5). The application now has the allergen on the respective tips.
4. Cleanse the skin and allow to dry.
5. Mark (number) the test sites on the skin corresponding to the placement of the applicators (A, B, C, D, etc.) with a black skin-marking pen.
6. Apply Panel A (screening panel) to the volar surface of the forearm (supported with a pillow to keep the arm flat) with the "T" handle toward the patient's

MULTI-TEST® RECORDING FORM

| Patient Name: | Age: | Sex: | Date: |

| Patient ID: | Ordered by: | Tested by: |

Initial Test ☐   Re-test ☐

BATTERY A SCREEN I   Location: Back ☐ Forearm ☐

Site	Antigen	Grade	Wheal	Flare	Comments
1	Positive Control		mm	mm	
2	Mite Mix		mm	mm	
3	Alternaria		mm	mm	
4	Cat		mm	mm	
5	Elm		mm	mm	
6	Bluegrass / June (Std.)		mm	mm	
7	Ragweed Mix		mm	mm	
8	Negative Control		mm	mm	

BATTERY B SCREEN II   Location: Back ☐ Forearm ☐

Site	Antigen	Grade	Wheal	Flare	Comments
1	Dog		mm	mm	
2	Cockroach		mm	mm	
3	Feather Mix		mm	mm	
4	Silk		mm	mm	
5	T.O.E.		mm	mm	
6	Epicoccum		mm	mm	
7	Bermuda		mm	mm	
8	English Plantain		mm	mm	

BATTERY C PANEL III (Molds)   Location: Back ☐ Forearm ☐

Site	Antigen	Grade	Wheal	Flare	Comments
1	Pullularia		mm	mm	
2	Aspergillus		mm	mm	
3	Cephalosporium		mm	mm	
4	Cladosporium		mm	mm	
5	Fusarium		mm	mm	
6	Mucor		mm	mm	
7	Penicillium		mm	mm	
8	Helminthosporium		mm	mm	

BATTERY D PANEL IV (Trees)   Location: Back ☐ Forearm ☐

Site	Antigen	Grade	Wheal	Flare	Comments
1	Alder		mm	mm	
2	Birch		mm	mm	
3	E. Cottonwood		mm	mm	
4	Hackberry		mm	mm	
5	Maple / Box Elder		mm	mm	
6	Pine		mm	mm	
7	Sweet Gum		mm	mm	
8	Sycamore		mm	mm	

SEE BACK SIDE

Fig. 202-1
Sample recording form. (Courtesy Lincoln Diagnostics, Decatur, Ill.)

Battery E PANEL V (Grass)   Location: Back ☐ Forearm ☐

Site	Antigen	Grade	Wheal	Flare	Comments
1	Oak		mm	mm	
2	Hickory / Pecan		mm	mm	
3	Mtn. Cedar		mm	mm	
4	Timothy (Std.)		mm	mm	
5	Grass Smuts		mm	mm	
6	Bermuda (Std.)		mm	mm	
7	Johnson		mm	mm	
8	Bahia		mm	mm	

Battery F PANEL VI (Weeds)   Location: Back ☐ Forearm ☐

Site	Antigen	Grade	Wheal	Flare	Comments
1	Cocklebur		mm	mm	
2	Dock		mm	mm	
3	Lambs Quarter		mm	mm	
4	Nettle		mm	mm	
5	Pigweed /Careless		mm	mm	
6	Marshelder, R.		mm	mm	
7	Russian Thistle		mm	mm	
8	W. Water Hemp		mm	mm	

Battery G FOODS   Location: Back ☐ Forearm ☐

Site	Antigen	Grade	Wheal	Flare	Comments
1	Beef		mm	mm	
2	Corn		mm	mm	
3	Egg		mm	mm	
4	Milk		mm	mm	
5	Pork		mm	mm	
6	Soybean		mm	mm	
7	Wheat		mm	mm	
8	Baker's Yeast		mm	mm	

Battery H   Location: Back ☐ Forearm ☐

Site	Antigen	Grade	Wheal	Flare	Comments
1			mm	mm	
2			mm	mm	
3			mm	mm	
4			mm	mm	
5			mm	mm	
6			mm	mm	
7			mm	mm	
8			mm	mm	

Fig. 202-1, cont'd
(Courtesy Lincoln Diagnostics, Decatur, Ill.)

head (Fig. 202-6). Apply with a rocking motion to and fro and side to side. When applied with correct pressure, a footprint of each testing head will be visible. No bleeding should occur.

7. A positive reaction to the tree, grass, weed, or mold allergen(s) is followed by testing all remaining significant allergens of the area suggested by history. Total number is variable from area to area, usually 20 to 40. These are placed on the patient's back with the patient lying face down and can be applied at this visit (Fig. 202-7). Sites must be kept flat to prevent allergens from running and contaminating other sites. Hairy sites should be avoided, since this interferes with readability. A typical positive response is shown in Fig. 202-8.

Interpretation of Results (Box 202-1)

Positive responses are noted by wheals and flares.
• The wheal is the raised area at the test site. This is

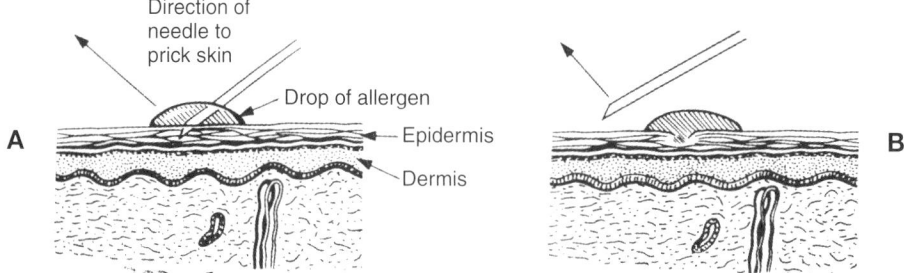

Fig. 202-2
Method for percutaneous skin prick testing. **A,** The drop of allergen is placed on the skin and a 27-gauge needle (bevel up) is placed through the allergen drop into the superficial epidermis. **B,** The needle pricks the skin at a 45-degree angle, allowing allergen to come in contact with sensitized mast cells located in the epidermis, and then is lifted up. The dermis is not violated and bleeding at the site is nonexistent or minimal.

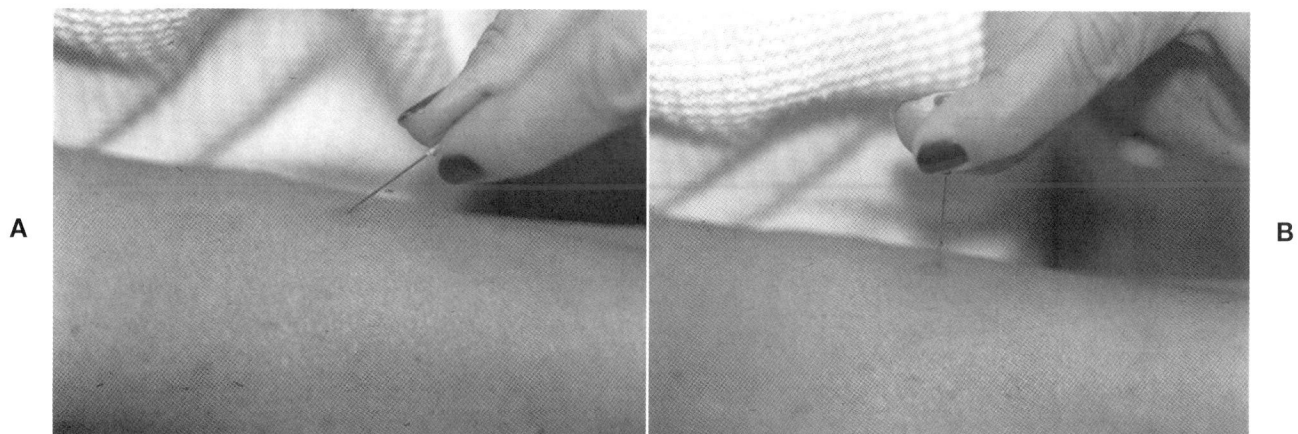

Fig. 202-3
A, Skin prick test (45-degree angle). **B,** Skin puncture test (90-degree angle). In both methods, only the epidermis is penetrated.

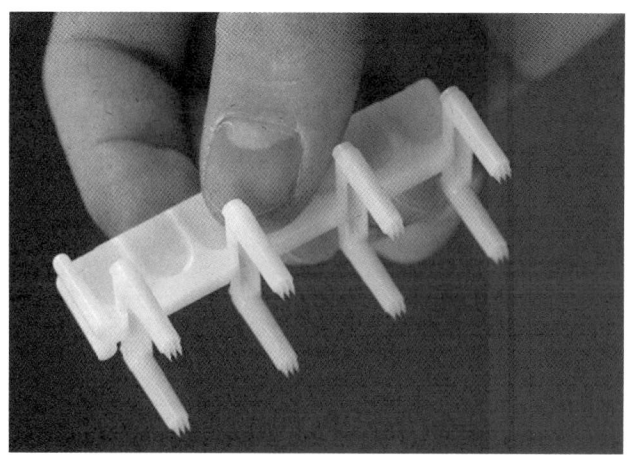

Fig. 202-4
Disposable plastic applicator for Multi-Test II.

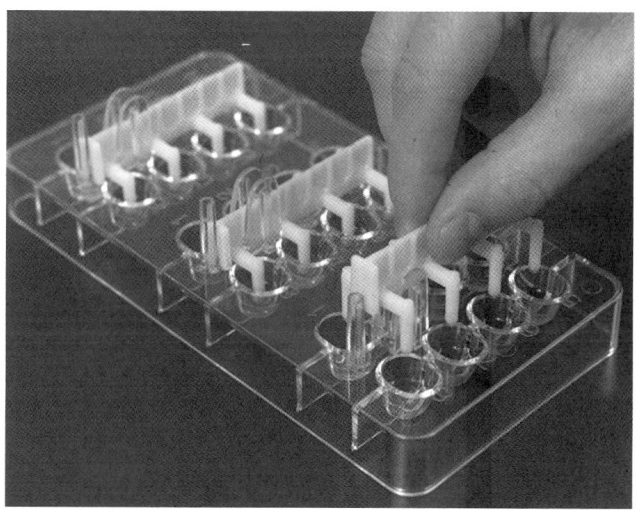

Fig. 202-5
Dipwell tray for Multi-Test II.

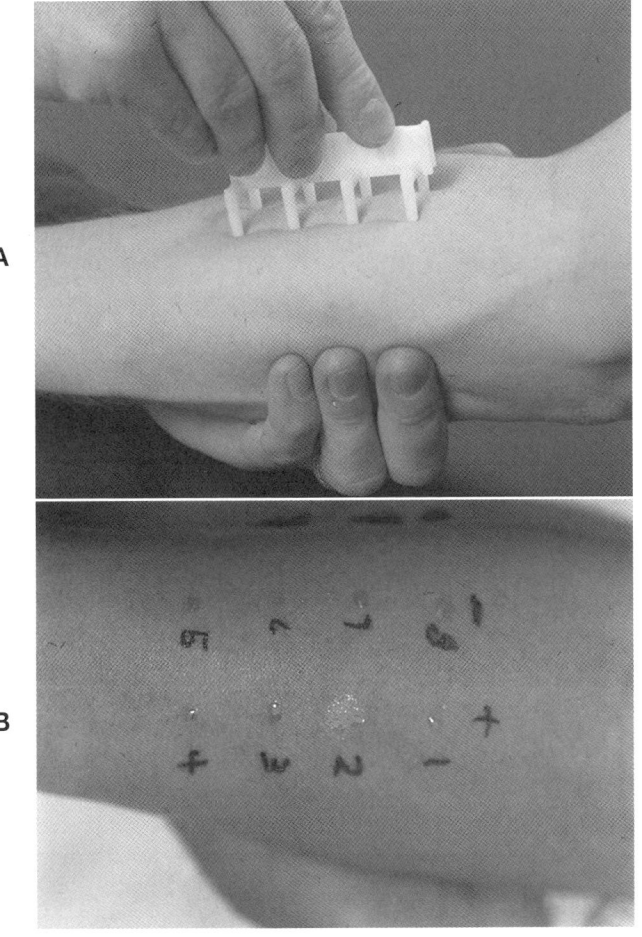

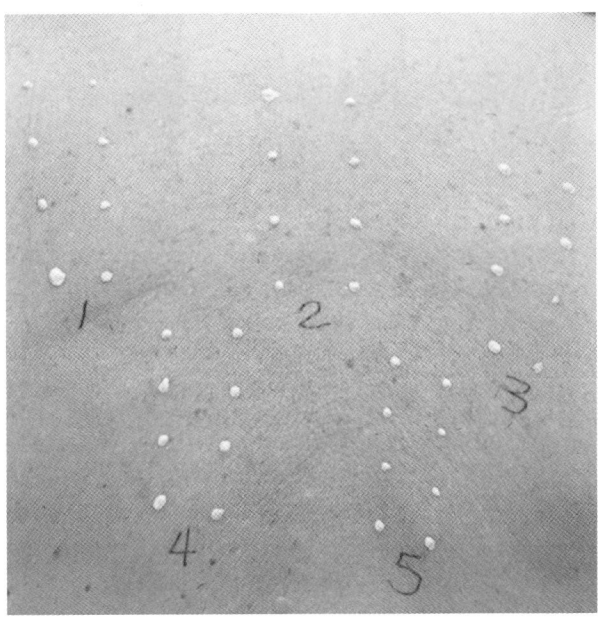

Fig. 202-6
Applicator is applied to volar surface of forearm with "T" handle toward the patient's head. **A,** Applicator with allergen is placed on the forearm with "T" handle toward patient. Skin is tightened with the opposite hand. Rocking motion to and fro and side to side ensures good allergen contact. **B,** Footprint of application of Multi-Test (Midwest screen). Positive and negative controls are at sites 1 and 8. House dust mite, *Alternaria,* cat, elm tree, bluegrass, and ragweed are at sites 2 through 7.

Fig. 202-7
Panels 1 through 5 placed on patient's back after allergen screen is positive.

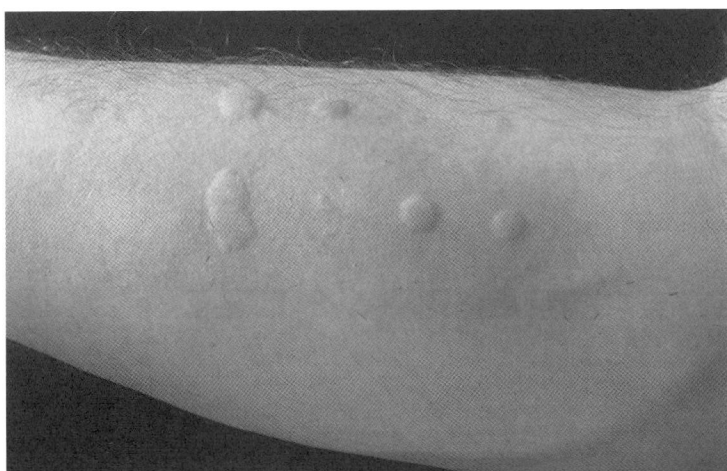

Fig. 202-8
Typical positive response.

BOX 202-1

Scoring the Multi-Test

Multi-Test is scored by comparing the reaction of allergens to the negative (glycerolsaline) and positive (histamine 1 mg/ml) controls applied at the same time and in the same general location. Reaction: no wheal or a wheal no larger than that at the negative control. Wheals of up to 3 mm may occur at the negative control site.

1+   Wheal larger than the negative control, usually 3-4 mm.
2+   Wheal 5-7 mm.
3+   Wheal 7-10 mm (size of the positive control).
4+   Any reaction with a wheal larger than 10 mm or pseudopodia.

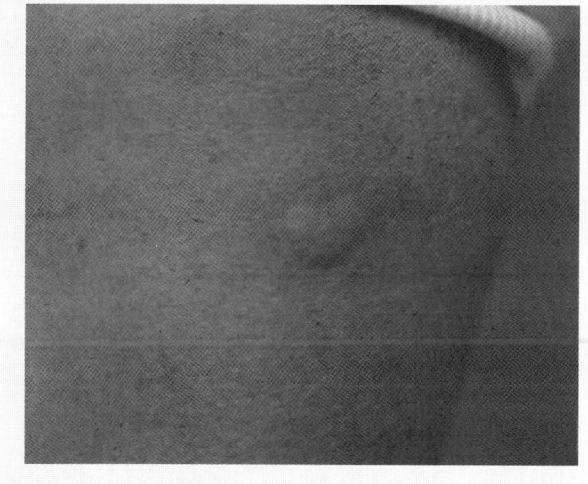

usually surrounded by an area of erythema called a flare (Fig. 202-9). The size and shape of the *wheal* is used in scoring reactions (Box 202-1) and is noted on the recording form.

- The wheal produced by histamine (Fig. 202-9, *A*), usually 7 to 10 mm in an adult and 6 mm in a child, is a 3+ reaction. It should be read and recorded at 10 minutes, since it will begin to fade. Other sites should be read in 15 to 20 minutes.
- Reactions comparable with those at the negative control site (saline or phenolated saline) are negative. It is not unusual to see a small wheal (1 to 3 mm) at the negative control site (Fig. 202-9, *A*).
- Reactions equal to or greater than the positive control (histamine) site correlate best with history. Reactions of 1+ and 2+ may be significant and these allergens should be added to immunotherapy when strongly suggested by history.
- Dermographism (Fig. 202-9, *B*) should be suspected when *all* tests are positive, including the negative control. Such patients must be tested by RAST.
- When all sites are negative (Fig. 202-9, *C*), including the positive control suspect antihistamine or other medication, decreasing the skin response.
- Results of tests are recorded (Fig. 202-1), and a signed

copy is the prescription sent to the laboratory for compounding immunotherapy.

- When house dust mite (Fig. 202-9, *D*) and/or cat are the only positive reactions, avoidance measures are instituted for either or both of these allergens. House dust mite avoidance includes covering pillows and mattresses, dusting regularly, and removing stuffed animals, carpet, and overstuffed furniture. Bedding should be washed weekly with water at 130° F. Lowering humidity to below 50% is helpful. HEPA filtration helps remove small particulate matter. Ideally, cats should be eliminated from the home, but it has been shown that less than 25% of patients or families comply. (At the very least, they should be kept out of the bedroom and off the bed.) Weekly washing will decrease the allergen load. Additional testing and/or immunotherapy can be added if symptoms do not improve within 1 to 2 months.
- When the positive control is positive and all other tests are negative (Fig. 202-9, *E*), nonallergic rhinitis or asthma is present. This occurs 50% of the time.
- Pseudopods (Fig. 202-9, *F*) occur frequently and are recorded as 4+ reactions.

Testing for other nonpollen allergens, such as dog, cockroach, feathers, laboratory and farm animals, may be suggested by history.

COMPLICATIONS

- Itching at the positive test sites is expected. Highly allergic patients may have rapid and large skin responses and will begin to show whealing, erythema, and itching within minutes. These individual reactions should be wiped clean with alcohol, being careful not to contaminate a nearby test site. These will proceed to a 4+ reaction despite wiping and can be treated with oral antihistamines or steroid creams if necessary. They usually resolve in ½ to 2 hours.
- Rarely, systemic symptoms occur that may include hives, urticaria, itching of the roof of the mouth, a sensation of throat closure, shortness of breath, an increase in presenting symptoms (sneezing, rhinorrhea, or wheezing), and anxiety. The remaining allergens should be removed with alcohol. Give 50 to 100 mg of Benadryl PO or IM and observe closely monitoring vital signs. Adrenalin, 0.3 ml (1:1000 dilution) for adults and 0.1 to 0.15 ml for children, should be nearby and used as needed if symptoms proceed to anaphylaxis. This is very rare. In addition to adrenalin, maintenance of the airway, correction of hypotension, and other general measures are used for treatment. Bronchodilation and antihistamines are given as needed. Monitoring of the patient's general condition, including blood pressure and respiration for

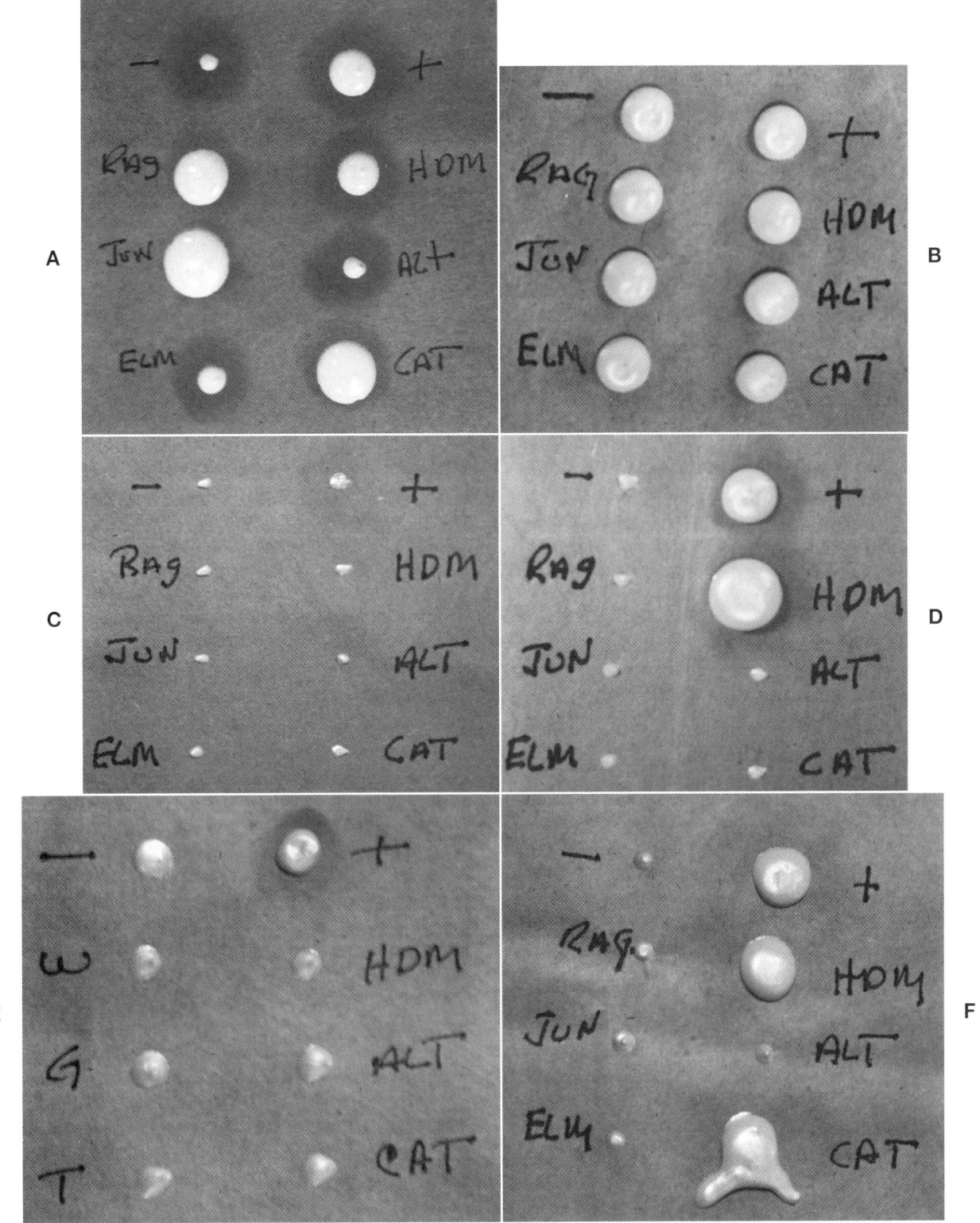

Fig. 202-9
Diameter of the wheal should be measured and recorded. Pseudopods should be noted and recorded by measuring length and width. The tests shown here illustrate results for the following: **A,** Allergic rhinitis with specific allergies noted. **B,** Dermographism with response to all tests, including control. **C,** Antihistamine effect with all tests negative, including positive control (histamine). **D,** House dust mite only. **E,** Nonallergic rhinitis with only a positive control. **F,** Positive test with pseudopod.

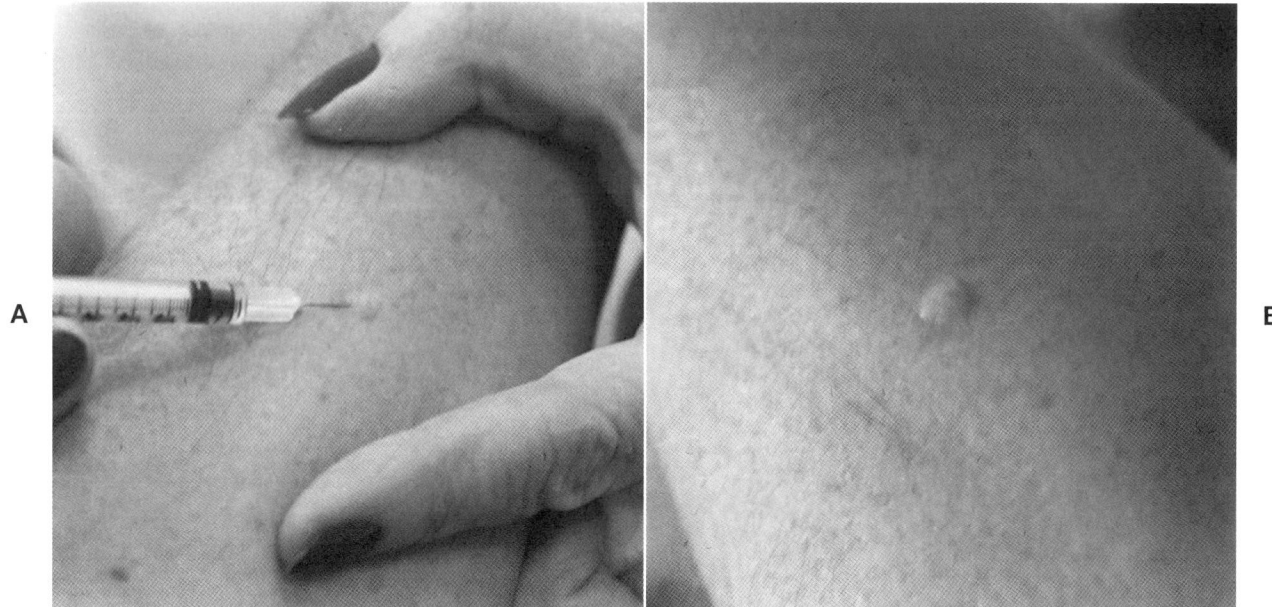

Fig. 202-10
Intradermal "vial" test prior to starting immunotherapy. A 1-ml syringe with 27-gauge needle containing 0.03 to 0.05 ml of allergen is placed intradermally, raising a 4-mm wheal. The needle is inserted (bevel up) just to the point where the hole disappears **(A).** This is intradermal. The bevel is rotated 180 degrees so that it faces down **(B).** Then the allergen is injected into the skin to raise a small wheal. Typical volume necessary to accomplish this is 0.03 ml.

several hours is needed should a delayed reaction occur. Transfer to an emergency room for more intensive help may be indicated. (See Chapter 203, Anaphylaxis.)

- False negatives
- When there is no reaction whatsoever at the positive control site, hypoactive skin caused by antihistamines or steroids should be suspected. The clinician should retest after an appropriate time off medication or consider RAST, which is not affected by any medication.
- Delayed reactions (usually at mold sites) may occur up to hours after testing and last for 2 to 7 days. This is an inflammatory response rather than IgE mediated, and it does not respond to immunotherapy. Local steroids may be helpful.

INTRADERMAL TESTING AND THE VIAL TEST

Historically ID testing has followed negative or equivocal SPT when the history strongly indicates a particular allergen. Recent studies have questioned the presence of clinically significant sensitivity when the SPT is negative and the ID test is positive. The use of positive ID tests after negative prick skin tests may not be an appropriate basis for selecting patients for immunotherapy. An ID test is used for the "vial test" prior to starting immunotherapy. The "vial" test affirms the safety of the

immunotherapy set. It is only needed with the initial vial. The clinician should create a 4-mm ID wheal (Fig. 202-10, *A*, *B*) by injecting about 0.03 ml of the weakest vial (1:100,000 dilution) on the upper outer arm, using a tuberculin syringe and a 26- or 27-gauge needle. The test is read in 15 minutes. Growth of the ID wheal beyond 15 mm indicates increased sensitivity, and a further tenfold dilution (1:1,000,000 dilution) of the vial is necessary. The clinician should take 0.5 ml of the allergen vial and add it to 4.5 ml of phenolated saline (diluting fluid) and repeat the vial test. Rarely, the vial test may cause reproduction of presenting symptoms (e.g., sneezing, rhinorrhea, congestion, or asthma). This indicates increased sensitivity to an allergen in the mix and may occur with pollination of an allergen that has occurred since testing and initiation of immunotherapy. Further dilution of the immunotherapy may be indicated as above.

RADIOALLERGOSORBENT BLOOD TEST

RAST is an in vitro test processed by a reference lab. The same principles of screening apply as for SPT, and most laboratories will provide a geographic screening panel before completing a regional (specific) RAST panel; if not, one can be designed based the allergens in the clinician's local area. A negative RAST screen requires no further testing. RAST is not affected by any medication. Box 202-2 shows indications for RAST testing.

Dermographism
Presence of β-blockers
Unstable or severe asthma
Extensive eczema or other dermatoses
Long-acting antihistamines, steroids
Atrophic or very young skin
History of anaphylaxis
Unstable cardiac patients
Immunodeficiency disorders

In RAST testing, an allergen is coupled to a paper disc or placed in a cellulose suspension to which the patient's serum is added. An antigen-antibody complex is formed which, when tagged with radioactive anti-IgE, forms an antigen-antibody-anti-IgE complex scored by a gamma counter. A grading system provides quantifying levels of IgE antibody on which immunotherapy is based. RAST-based immunotherapy uses either fivefold or tenfold dilutions. RAST laboratories usually provide immunotherapy sets or will suggest an immunotherapy compounding lab. RAST testing is efficacious. Results must be interpreted in light of the clinical history.

RAST is a very good test for allergy and can be used by physicians not wanting to perform skin testing. There are some distinct advantages to skin testing:

- The patient can be tested and results known within minutes.
- The patient sees and experiences the reaction, which reinforces the need for avoidance. This is especially helpful in house dust mite avoidance and cat or dog allergy.
- There is much less hassle with insurance companies over payment for allergy testing. A significant number of HMOs and other insurance carriers will deny payment for RAST.
- RAST testing is more expensive than skin prick testing ($3 to $4 per skin test versus $12 to $15 per RAST).
- RAST results may not be available for a week or longer, depending on the RAST laboratory.

POSTPROCEDURE PATIENT EDUCATION

Avoidance procedures and medications are prescribed where appropriate. Brochures describing general allergen avoidance and specific house dust mite and animal dander measures are readily available. Immunotherapy is considered an adjunct to treatment.

IMMUNOTHERAPY

Immunotherapy is indicated based on the demonstration of immediate hypersensitivity by SPT, Multi-Test, or RAST, and correlation with the patient's history and physical findings. This correlation is imperative for success. When beginning therapy on a patient for the first time, perform ID testing (the "vial test") as noted previously. Increasing amounts of allergen are given subcutaneously until the highest tolerated dose is reached. Generally, immunotherapy based on SPT uses a tenfold dilution system and is started at 0.1 ml of 1:100,000 dilution of each allergen. Shots are graduated—0.1, 0.2, 0.3, 0.4, 0.5 ml—weekly through dilutions of 1:100,000, 1:10,000, 1:1000, and 1:100 until maintenance is reached. The maintenance dose is the highest tolerated dose that can be attained without causing a significant local (painful knot and/or erythema lasting more than 24 hours) or systemic reaction. Using RAST-based immunotherapy and the fivefold dilutional system, the clinician can tailor the starting dose based on the amount of sensitivity to the allergen. The higher the RAST class, the more dilute the starting dose; the lower the RAST class, the more concentrated the starting dose. Immunotherapy is usually started 5 to 25 times weaker than the RAST class, then graduated as with SPT until maintenance is reached.

Based on testing, an allergy laboratory will compound an immunotherapy set consisting of four vials each containing increasing concentrations of all the relevant allergens. If more than 12 allergens are to be included, two sets are needed. As a clinician's allergy practice grows, compounding immunotherapy in the office can be considered. This does require additional space and personnel. By law, immunotherapy sets made by commercial laboratories are "quarantined" for 2 weeks to ensure sterility. This does not apply in office compounding. Phenolated saline with glycerine is used as the diluent in mixing and provides ample sterility and stability.

Escalation of immunotherapy (Box 202-3) proceeds on a weekly schedule with doses adjusted as needed because of local or systemic reactions. Increasing symptoms and skin responses that occur during a pollinating season may require slowing or holding of escalation until pollination ceases. As the season passes, escalation can then proceed with no further problem. Local swelling, whealing, or "knot" formation greater that 2 cm lasting more than 24 hours is considered significant. The subsequent dose should be reduced to one not causing a reaction and escalated at a slower rate for patient comfort. Doses for smaller local reactions of swelling and redness should be repeated or reduced as tolerated. *Immunotherapy should be omitted or delayed* (1) when a febrile illness is present, (2) when the patient is extremely fatigued, (3) following acute exacerbation of allergic symptoms during a pollinating season, (4) or during or following an asthma attack. PEFR should be above 70% of the patient's personal best effort. Some patients can

BOX 202-3

Example of Escalation Schedule for Weekly Immunotherapy

Vial D	
1:100,000 w/v	Green vial
Dose #1	0.05 ml
2	0.10
3	0.20
4	0.30
5	0.40
6	0.50
Vial C	
1:10,000 w/v	Blue vial
7	0.05 ml
8	0.10
9	0.20
10	0.30
11	0.40
12	0.50
Vial B	
1:1,000 w/v	Gold vial
13	0.10 ml
14	0.20
15	0.30
16	0.40
17	0.50
Vial A	
1:100 w/v	Red vial
18	0.05 ml
19	0.10
20	0.15
21	0.20
22	0.25
23	0.30
24	0.35
25	0.40
26	0.45
27	0.50

Maintain for 1 year, then go to every 2 weeks for 3 to 5 years, then try to discontinue.

This is the same antigen mixture in vials A-D but with varying concentrations.

BOX 202-4

Reasons for Allergy Treatment Failures

Inaccurate diagnoses
Incomplete diagnoses (allergic and nonallergic factors)
Development of new allergens
Erratic dosage schedule
Lack of appropriate patient education
Noncompliance with avoidance
Noncompliance with medication
Nonallergic food and chemical sensitivities
Inadequate dose of immunotherapy
Immunotherapy dose beyond the optimal dose
Rhinitis medicamentosa

BOX 202-5

Resuming Immunotherapy After Missed Doses During Escalation

3-10 days	Continue escalation
10-14 days	Repeat last dose
14-21 days	Reduce dose 0.1 ml
Over 21 days	Reduce dose by half and gradually reescalate

BOX 202-6

Resuming Immunotherapy After Missed Doses During Maintenance

1-4 weeks	Continue maintenance dose
4-12 weeks	½ maintenance dose, rebuild to maintenance
3-6 months	Drop full tenfold dilution (i.e., if maintenance is 0.5 ml of A bottle [1:100 dilution], drop back to 0.5 ml of B bottle [1:1000 dilution])

Attempts to discontinue immunotherapy can be made after 3-5 years if the patient is symptom free. The interval between injections can be lengthened from every 2 weeks to 3 or 4 weeks. If there is no exacerbation of symptoms after 6 months to 1 year, immunotherapy may be discontinued. Approximately one third of patients will return within 2 years to restart their allergy program.

produce 120% of their *predicted* value and yet have significant asthma at 70% to 80% of their *predicted* value.

Actions *to prevent untoward reactions and anaphylaxis* during immunotherapy include the following:
- Evaluate the patient's condition prior to injection
- Minimize the chance of errors in dosing and administration
- Use more dilute allergen in highly sensitive patients (by history or testing)
- Observe patients in office for 20 to 30 minutes after injection
- Check the patient and injection site before leaving
- Reduce the first dose of newly prepared extracts by half
- Reduce the dose when local or systemic reactions occur
- Avoid shots to asthmatics whose peak flow is less than 70% of their personal best effort

- Avoid immunotherapy in the presence of a febrile illness
- Avoid giving to patients on beta-blockers

About 80% of allergic patients respond to immunotherapy, whereas some 20% show little or no response (Box 202-4). Maintenance doses should be continued for 3 to 5 years, and the time between doses increased to 2 weeks after the first year, then 2 to 4 weeks after the second year with symptom return used as the guide. The patient will miss doses in the buildup and maintenance phases of immunotherapy. Guidelines for treatment after missed doses are found in Boxes 202-5 and 202-6.

Upon completion and discontinuance of a program after 5 years of therapy, a third of patients may return to restart immunotherapy because of return of symptoms. Reasons for allergy treatment failures are given in Box 202-4.

LABELING AND STORAGE OF EXTRACTS

- Each vial of extract should be labeled with the patient's name, chart number, birthdate, expiration date, and dilution strength.
- Vials are stored in the refrigerator overnight but may be kept out and readily accessible for daily use.
- Dilutions should be discarded and remade after 6 months if not used. Glycerine has been added to ensure stability.
- 2.5-ml vials are used in sets for escalation of doses (five doses will be used in 5 weeks [0.1, 0.2, 0.3, 0.4, 0.5 ml = 1.5 ml]). The remainder may be used to repeat doses if necessary or simply discarded.
- Ten dose vials (number of milliliters [usually 5 ml] will vary depending on the maintenance dose) are formulated for maintenance therapy.

SUMMARY

Studies have shown the beneficial effect on acute allergic disease as well as the long-lasting symptom control after a successful course of immunotherapy. The measurable antiinflammatory influences of immunotherapy do not occur with antihistamines and steroids, suggesting that immunotherapy should be used earlier and more often in the treatment of allergic rhinitis and asthma.

SUPPLIERS

Devices for skin testing
Multi-Test Multiple Antigen Device
Duotip Single Skin Prick Test
Lincoln Diagnostics
P.O. Box 1128
Decatur, IL 62525
Phone: 1-800-537-1336
Website: www.lincolndiagnostics.com

Quintest Multiple Antigen Device
Hollister-Stier Laboratories LLC
3525 North Regal Street
Spokane, WA 99207-5788
Phone: 1-800-992-1120
Website: www.hollister-stier.com

Morrow Brown Needle
Morrow Brown Allergy Diagnostics
Alkaline Corporation Allergy Diagnostics Division
714 West Park Avenue, P.O. Box 306
Oakhurst, NJ 07755-0306
Phone: 1-800-686-6483

Histamine used for positive control
College Pharmacy
3505 Austin Bluffs Parkway
Colorado Springs, CO 80907
Phone: 1-800-888-9358
Website: www.collegepharmacy.com

Allergen extracts, immunotherapy sets, supplies
Allergy Laboratories
P.O. Box 26492
Oklahoma City, OK 73126
Phone: 1-405-235-1451

Antigen Lab, Inc.
30-34 South Main Street
P.O. Box 123
Liberty, MO 64068
Phone: 1-800-821-7013

Center Laboratories
35 Channel Drive
Port Washington, NY 11050-2216
Phone: 1-800-223-6837

Greer Laboratories, Inc.
P.O. Box 800
639 Nuway Circle
Lenoir, NC 28645-0088
Phone: 1-800-438-0088

ALK Laboratory
1700 Royston Lane
Round Rock, TX 78664
Phone: 1-800-252-9778

Miles Allergy Products
Hollister-Stier Laboratories LLC
(See contact information above)

Laboratories providing RAST services
Antigen Laboratories
(See contact information above)

Commonwealth Medical Laboratories
11150 Main Street, Suite 550
Fairfax, VA 22030
Phone: 1-800-222-5775
Website: www.allergytest.com

LabCorp
358 South Main Street
Burlington, NC 27215
Phone: 1-336-584-5171
Website: www.labcorp.com

MRT Laboratories
50 Johnson Avenue
Hackensack, NJ 07601
Phone: 1-800-631-1379
Website: www.mrtlabs.com

Serolab
P.O. Box 3307
Waco, TX 76707-3307
Phone: 1-800-460-4867

SmithKline Beecham Clinical Laboratories
11636 Administration Drive
St. Louis, MO 63146
Phone: 1-800-669-8077

CPT/BILLING CODES

Testing and Immunotherapy

95004	Multiple puncture test, SPT, per test
95024	Intradermal test, per test
86003	RAST per test
86005	RAST multiallergen disc (screen)
95024	Vial test (intradermal)

Allergy Injections

95115	Allergy injection, single (injection only)
95117	Allergy injection, multiple (injection only)
95120	Allergy injection, single antigen (plus antigen if provided)
95125	Allergy injection, multiple antigen (plus antigen if provided)
95165	Allergy extract (specify no. of doses) (vial of antigen)

Other Services

99080	Medical reports
99002	Mailout charge
99071	Educational supplies

ICD-9-CM DIAGNOSTIC CODES FOR COMMON ALLERGY CONDITIONS

372.14	Allergic conjunctivitis
346.20	Allergic headache
381.04	Allergic otitis media
477.8	Allergic rhinitis
477.9	Allergic sinusitis
708.0	Allergic urticaria/hives
558.9	Allergic gastroenteritis
995.0	Anaphylaxis
995.1	Angioedema
493.00	Asthma
786.2	Chronic cough
691.8	Eczema dermatitis

BIBLIOGRAPHY

Altman CA, Becker WB, Williams PV: *Allergy in primary care,* Philadelphia, 2000, WB Saunders.

American Academy of Allergy, Asthma, and Immunology: The allergy report (Volume I: Overview of Allergic Diseases; Volume II: Diseases of the Atopic Diathesis; Volume III: Conditions That May have an Allergic Component), St Louis, 2001, Mosby.

Bierman CW, Pearlman DS, Shapiro GG, Busse WW: *Allergy, asthma, and immunology from infancy to adulthood,* ed 3, Philadelphia, 1996, WB Saunders.

Hedges H, Squillace S: *Asthma, allergic rhinitis, and immunotherapy,* AAFP Home Study Monograph 235, December 1998, Kansas City, Mo, American Academy of Family Physicians.

Immunology and Allergy Clinics of North America, Philadelphia, WB Saunders.

Kaliner MA: *Current review of allergic diseases,* Philadelphia, 2000, Current Medicine.

Kaplan AP: *Allergy,* ed 2, Philadelphia, 1997, WB Saunders.

Kniker WT: Multi-Test skin testing in allergy: a review of published findings, *Ann Allergy* 71:485, 1993.

Mahan C, Spectror S, Siegel S, et al: Validity and reproducibility of multi-test skin test device, *Ann Allergy* 71:25, 1993.

Middleton E Jr, Reed CE, Ellis EF, et al: *Allergy: principles and practice,* ed 5, St Louis, 1998, Mosby.

Nalebuff D: Use of RAST screening in clinical allergy: a cost-effective approach to patient care, *Ear Nose Throat J* 64:107, 1985.

Nelson HS, Oppenheimer J, Buchmeier A, et al: An assessment of the role of intradermal skin testing in the diagnosis of clinically relevant allergy to timothy grass, *J Allergy Clin Immunol* 97(6):1193, 1996.

Nelson HS: Rush immunotherapy: National Jewish Medical and Research Center, *Medical Scientific Update* 13(3):1, 1995.

Ownby DR: Indications and contraindications of allergen immunotherapy. In Creticos PS, Lockey RF, editors: *Immunotherapy: a practical guide to current procedures,* Milwaukee, Wisc, 1994, American Academy of Allergy and Immunology.

Position Paper: Immunotherapy: The European Academy of Allergology and Clinical Immunology, *Allergy* 48(Suppl 14):7, 1993.

Practice parameters for allergen immunotherapy. Joint Task Force on Practice Parameters, representing the American Academy of Allergy, Asthma and Immunology, the American College of Allergy, Asthma and Immunology, and the Joint Council of Allergy, Asthma and Immunology, *J Allergy Clin Immunol* 98(6Pt1):1001, 1996.

Weber R: Aerobiology. In Creticos PS, Lockey RF, editors: *Immunotherapy: a practical guide to current procedures,* Milwaukee, Wisc, 1994, American Academy of Allergy and Immunology.

CHAPTER 203

Anaphylaxis

Daniel J. Derksen

Anaphylaxis is an acute and serious allergic reaction in response to antigen exposure in a previously sensitized patient. It can be encountered after administration of intramuscular (IM) antibiotics; vaccines; contrast material, such as intravenous pyelography (IVP) or computed tomography contrast; local anesthetics; allergy injection in the office setting; or exposure to latex. Patients may also report to the physician's office with a clinical picture of anaphylaxis after being bitten by an insect or snake or exposed to some other allergen (e.g., pollen, latex, certain food products). In some cases the source of the allergic reaction may be unknown to the patient.

Medical procedures frequently require injections or use of foreign materials. The clinician must be prepared to treat the rare but serious complication of anaphylaxis.

DIAGNOSIS

Depending on the severity of reaction, patients may have a variety of symptoms, including swelling, rash, urticaria, pruritus, dyspnea, and decreased blood pressure from baseline. As the anaphylaxis proceeds, respiratory compromise may occur with laryngeal edema, bronchospasm, and hypoxia. The patient may progress into shock as manifested by hypotension, bradycardia, peripheral vasodilation, and mental status changes. If the physician does not take immediate steps to reverse the anaphylactoid reaction in the final stages, vascular collapse and death can occur within minutes.

Vasovagal reactions (e.g., fainting and seizurelike activity) and injection of intravascular anesthetic can cause lightheadedness and ringing in the ears; this may be confused with an anaphylactic response.

EQUIPMENT

As stated previously, physicians and practitioners should be prepared to treat anaphylaxis in the office, especially if any injections are given. A collection of medications and equipment, the "crash cart," can be gathered and placed in one area. Alternatively, a fishing tackle box or medical emergency kit can be made. The simplest and best-organized method is to use commercially available Banyan kits. These kits, similar to suitcases, are stocked with various medications. They vary in size, contents, and cost ($515 to $895). The Banyan Stat Kit 800 is essentially a portable crash cart, lacking only a defibrillator. The Banyan Corporation provides check sheets that can be reviewed regularly to reorder out-of-date stock (see the "Suppliers" section).

Whether the commercially available kits are used or a do-it-yourself collection is assembled, the entire office staff must know where the kit is stored. One person must be in charge of keeping the medications current. Drugs cannot be borrowed from this kit for other purposes.

The physician in charge of office procedures must be prepared for emergencies. Assembling a crash cart or obtaining a Banyan kit may appear expensive, but it is good medicine to have one available and is an inexpensive form of malpractice coverage in the event of an emergency.

The specifics on medications and equipment needed are too extensive to detail in this chapter. Clinicians are encouraged to contact the Banyan Corporation for further information (see the "Suppliers" section).

TECHNIQUE

Patients who exhibit signs and symptoms of anaphylaxis should be treated immediately. In the earliest stages, anxiety, swelling, urticaria, pruritus, and mild dyspnea respond quickly to epinephrine. The dose can be 0.3 to 0.5 ml of a *1:1000* solution, given *subcutaneously* every 20 to 30 minutes as needed (to a maximum of three doses). In the milder reactions, antihistamines such as diphenhydramine hydrochloride (Benadryl), 25 to 50 mg by the intravenous (IV), intramuscular (IM), or oral (PO) route every 6 hours can be given. Systemic steroids can be given as a prednisone taper, beginning with 30 to 60 mg the first day and gradually tapering to nothing over a 2-week period. *In truly emergent situations,* give 100 mg methylprednisolone (Solu-Medrol) IV. For life-threatening reactions, 5 ml of a *1:10,000* solution of epinephrine should be given by IV over 10 minutes and repeated every 5 minutes as needed. In addition, an ambulance should be summoned. Patients on β-blockers may exhibit more severe anaphylactic symptoms and be refractory to epinephrine. Administration of glucagon (1 mg ampule), atropine (1 mg IV), or isoproterenol (0.1 mg/kg initially) may be necessary to stabilize patients on β-blockers that do not respond to epinephrine.

Patients with anaphylaxis or anaphylactoid reactions must be observed for 4 to 6 hours after treatment of a reaction to ensure that there is no recurrence.

Note: A quick way to administer epinephrine is to have a preloaded syringe system of epinephrine (e.g., EpiPen-Epinephrine Auto-Injector, EpiPen-Epinephrine Jr. Auto-Injector, Ana-Kit Anaphylaxis Emergency Treatment Kit) available in the office. This eliminates the delay involved in drawing up epinephrine in a syringe before administration. Appropriate examination or treatment rooms should have one of these injection systems taped to a cabinet door for easy accessibility.

PREVENTION WITH PREVIOUS HISTORY

Some patients may require tests that necessitate the use of known allergens. For example, patients may require a computed tomography scan with contrast material that previously caused urticaria, dyspnea, or other signs of early anaphylaxis. If an alternative contrast agent cannot be used and the test is critical to the diagnostic workup, the patient can be counseled about the risks, asked to sign an informed consent form, and premedicated with Benadryl and steroids to minimize the risk of an anaphylactic reaction. This can be done with 50 to 100 mg of Benadryl PO 1 hour before the procedure and 100 mg hydrocortisone or 50 mg methylprednisolone (Solu-Medrol) IV. The patient should be observed carefully for at least 6 hours after the procedure.

For patients with a history of allergies to local anesthetics, a few simple steps need to be followed. Allergies have been reported to ester drugs (e.g., Novocaine) but not to amide derivatives (e.g., lidocaine [Xylocaine]). If someone is suspected of having an allergy to a local anesthetic, the clinician should use an amide drug from a single-dose vial. Single-dose vials do not contain any preservatives (parabens), which can also be the source of allergy. To date, there have been no reported allergic reactions to amide local anesthetics from single-dose vials. It is still judicious, however, to observe the reaction to a small wheal of injected solution (0.05 ml) for 10 to 15 minutes before injecting a larger volume.

PRECAUTIONS

Procedures and medications that could result in anaphylaxis should not be administered unless the office is equipped to deal with this complication. At a minimum, the office should be able to administer subcutaneous epinephrine, supply supplemental oxygen, and provide ventilation to the patient until emergency services can arrive. In general, procedures and medications that carry a high risk of anaphylaxis should be followed by an appropriate observation period after the procedure to watch for signs and symptoms.

POSTPROCEDURE PATIENT EDUCATION

Sensitized patients should receive detailed patient education. Such patients should be encouraged to wear a medical identification bracelet that identifies the agent that could cause anaphylaxis (e.g., penicillin, bee sting, IVP contrast). Some patients with recurrent, severe anaphylactoid reactions should carry a kit with them (containing 1:1000 epinephrine that can be injected) so that initial treatment can begin without delay. For example, a beekeeper with a known sensitivity to bee stings who refuses to explore a new profession should be encouraged to carry a kit. Patients with previous anaphylaxis should be instructed to seek prompt medical attention for the following symptoms:
- Shortness of breath
- Swelling of eyes, legs, or hands
- Dizziness
- Sensation of swelling in the throat
- Raised, red rashes (urticaria)
- Change in mental status

SUPPLIERS

Banyan kits
Banyan International Corporation
2118 E. Interstate 20
P.O. Box 1779
Abilene, TX 79604-9963
Phone: 1-800-351-4530
Website: www.statkit.com/banyanhome.asp

Ana-Kit anaphylaxis emergency treatment kit
Bayer Corporation
Pharmaceutical Division
Allergy Products
400 Morgan Lane
West Haven, CT 06516
Phone: 1-800-800-5907
Website: www.bayerinstitute.org

EpiPen

Center Laboratories

Division of EM Pharmaceuticals, Inc.

35 Channel Drive

Port Washington, NY 11050

Phone: 1-516-767-1873

BIBLIOGRAPHY

deShazo RD, Kemp SF: Allergic reactions to drugs and biologic agents, *JAMA* 178(22):1895, 1997.

Ewan PW: ABC of allergies: anaphylaxis, *BMJ* 316(7142):1442, 1998.

Fader DJ, Johnson TM: Medical issues and emergencies in the dermatology office, *J Am Acad Dermatol* 36(1):1, 1997.

Hash RB: Intravascular radiographic contrast media: issues for family physicians, *J Am Board Fam Pract* 12(1):32, 1999.

Kemp SF, Lockey RF, Wolf BL, Lieberman P: Anaphylaxis: a review of 266 cases, *Arch Intern Med* 155(16):1749, 1995.

Wyatt R: Anaphylaxis: how to recognize, treat, and prevent potentially fatal attacks, *Postgrad Med* 100(2):87, 1996.

CHAPTER 204

Antibiotic Prophylaxis

John L. Pfenninger

ANTIBIOTIC PROPHYLAXIS FOR BACTERIAL ENDOCARDITIS

The prevention of bacterial endocarditis using prophylactic antibiotics was reviewed in an article in the *Journal of the American Medical Association* by Dajani and associates and last updated in June 1997. The conclusions are summarized in Boxes 204-1 through 204-3 and in Tables 204-1 and 204-2, which are reproduced with permission from the American Heart Association, Committee on Rheumatic Fever, Endocarditis, and Kawasaki Disease of the Council on Cardiovascular Disease in the Young. Fig. 204-1 shows a flow chart to help determine the need for prophylaxis in patients with suspected mitral valve prolapse. Those seeking further discussion are referred to the article in the *Journal of the American Medical Association*.

Conclusions*

Major changes in the updated recommendations include the following:

1. Emphasis that most cases of endocarditis are not attributable to an invasive procedure;
2. Cardiac conditions are stratified into high-, moderate-, and negligible-risk categories based on potential outcome if endocarditis develops;
3. Procedures that may cause bacteremia and for which prophylaxis is recommended are more clearly specified;
4. An algorithm was developed to more clearly define when prophylaxis is recommended for patients with mitral valve prolapse;
5. For oral or dental procedures the initial amoxicillin dose is reduced to 2 g, a follow-up antibiotic dose is no longer recommended, erythromycin is no longer recommended, erythromycin is no longer recommended for penicillin-allergic individuals, but clindamycin and other alternatives are offered; and

*Reprinted from Dajani AS, Taubert KA, Wilson W, et al: *JAMA* 277(22):1794, 1997.

6. For gastrointestinal or genitourinary procedures, the prophylactic regimens have been simplified.

These changes were instituted to more clearly define when prophylaxis is or is not recommended, improve practitioner and patient compliance, reduce cost and potential gastrointestinal adverse effect, and approach more uniform worldwide recommendations.

It is of interest to note that skin procedures, colposcopy, intrauterine contraceptive device (IUD) insertion, flexible sigmoidoscopy, colonoscopy (with or without biopsy), gastroscopy, and most other procedures that would be performed in the office would **NOT** require SBE prophylaxis.

The article notes that those receiving heparin should not receive injections. In addition, if a patient is taking an antibiotic (e.g., penicillin) to prevent the recurrence of acute rheumatic fever, clindamycin, azithromycin, or clarithromycin should be used. Cephalosporins are not adequate.

WOUND PROPHYLAXIS

Although antibiotic prophylaxis can reduce wound infection, the benefits must be weighed against the risks of toxic and allergic reactions; causing resistant bacteria, drug interactions, or superinfections; and possibly unnecessarily increasing the costs of healthcare. Prophylaxis is generally recommended only when involving prosthetic material, for patients for whom infection can be serious consequence, and in major surgeries. The 1999 reference from the *Medical Letter* reviews current recommendations for major surgeries as well.

Patients with prosthetic joints generally do not require antimicrobial prophylaxis even for dental, gastrointestinal (GI), or genitourinary (GU) procedures.

For the outpatient and office practice, the majority of surgeries will involve the skin. For dirty, traumatic wounds, copious irrigation with normal saline or Betadine diluted 1:10 is best. The most common bacteria causing wound infections are *Staphylococcus aureus*, GrA strep, and clostridia. If significant injury exists,

BOX 204-1
Cardiac Conditions Associated with Endocarditis

Endocarditis Prophylaxis Recommended*
High-risk category
- Prosthetic cardiac valves, including bioprosthetic and homograft valves
- Previous bacterial endocarditis
- Complex cyanotic congenital heart disease (e.g., single ventricle states, transposition of the great arteries, Fallot's tetralogy)
- Surgically constructed systemic pulmonary shunts or conduits

Moderate-risk category
- Most other congenital cardiac malformations (other than those listed above and below)
- Acquired valvar dysfunction (e.g., rheumatic heart disease)
- Hypertrophic cardiomyopathy
- Mitral valve prolapse with valvar regurgitation, thickened leaflets, or both*

Endocarditis Prophylaxis NOT Recommended
Negligible-risk category (no greater risk than the general population)
- Isolated secundum atrial septal defect
- Surgical repair of atrial septal defect, ventricular septal defect, or patent ductus arteriosus (without residua beyond 6 months)
- Previous coronary artery bypass graft surgery
- Mitral valve prolapse without valvar regurgitation*
- Physiologic, functional, or innocent heart murmurs*
- Previous Kawasaki disease without valvar dysfunction
- Previous rheumatic fever without valvar dysfunction
- Cardiac pacemakers (intravascular and epicardial) and implanted defibrillators

From Dajani AS, Taubert KA, Wilson W, et al: *JAMA* 277(22):1794, 1997.
*See Fig. 204-1.

BOX 204-2
Dental Procedures and Endocarditis Prophylaxis

Endocarditis Prophylaxis Recommended*
- Dental extractions
- Periodontal procedures including surgery, scaling and root planing, probing, and recall maintenance; dental implant placement and reimplantation of avulsed teeth
- Orthodontic (root canal) instrumentation or surgery only beyond the apex
- Subgingival placement of antibiotic fibers or strips
- Initial placement of orthodontic bands but not brackets
- Intraligamentary local anesthetic injections
- Prophylactic cleaning of teeth or implants where bleeding is anticipated

Endocarditis Prophylaxis NOT Recommended
- Restorative dentistry[†] (operative and prosthodontic with or without retraction cord[‡])
- Local anesthetic injections (nonintraligamentary)
- Intracanal endodontic treatment; after placement and buildup
- Placement of rubber dams
- Postoperative suture removal
- Placement of removable prosthodontic/orthodontic appliances
- Taking of oral impressions
- Fluoride treatments
- Taking of oral radiographs
- Orthodontic appliance adjustment
- Shedding of primary teeth

From Dajani AS, Taubert KA, Wilson W, et al: *JAMA* 277(22):1794, 1997.
*Prophylaxis is recommended for patients with high- and moderate-risk cardiac conditions.
[†]Includes restoring decayed teeth (filling cavities) and replacing missing teeth.
[‡]Clinical judgment may indicate antibiotic use in selected circumstances during which significant bleeding may be created.

BOX 204-3
Other Procedures and Endocarditis Prophylaxis

Endocarditis Prophylaxis Recommended
Respiratory tract
- Tonsillectomy, adenoidectomy, or both
- Surgical operations that involve respiratory mucosa
- Bronchoscopy with a rigid bronchoscope

*Gastrointestinal tract**
- Sclerotherapy for esophageal varices
- Esophageal stricture dilation
- Endoscopic retrograde cholangiography with biliary obstruction
- Biliary tract surgery
- Surgical operations that involve intestinal mucosa

Genitourinary tract
- Prostatic surgery
- Cystoscopy
- Urethral dilation

Endocarditis Prophylaxis NOT Recommended
Respiratory tract
- Endotracheal intubation
- Bronchoscopy with a flexible bronchoscope with or without biopsy[†]
- Tympanostomy tube insertion

Gastrointestinal tract
- Transesophageal echocardiography[†]
- Endoscopy with or without gastrointestinal biopsy[†] (gastroscopy, sigmoidoscopy, colonoscopy)

Genitourinary tract
- Vaginal hysterectomy[†]
- Vaginal delivery[†]
- Cesarean section
- In uninfected tissue:
    Urethral catheterization
    Uterine dilation and curettage
    Therapeutic abortion
    Sterilization procedures
    Insertion or removal of intrauterine contraceptive devices

Other
- Cardiac catheterization, including balloon angioplasty
- Implanted cardiac pacemakers, implanted defibrillators, and coronary stents
- Incision or biopsy of surgically scrubbed skin
- Circumcision

From Dajani AS, Taubert KA, Wilson W, et al: *JAMA* 277(22):1794, 1997.
*Prophylaxis is recommended for high-risk patients; optional for medium-risk patients.
[†]Prophylaxis is optional for high-risk patients.

consider cefazolin, if available, 1 to 2 g intravenous (IV) every 8 hours for one to three doses. For less extensive injuries, oral antibiotics that cover these organisms are also acceptable.

For bite wounds in which likely pathogens may also include oral anaerobes, *Eikenella corrodens* (human) or *Pasteurella multocida* (dog and cat), amoxicillin with clavulanic acid (Augmentin) or ampicillin sulbactam

(Unasyn) are recommended. A 7- to 10-day course may be advisable.

A human bite wound over the metatarsophalangeal joints in the hand can be very serious. If it is suspected that the joint capsule has been entered, IV or intramuscular (IM) antibiotics may be indicated. Close follow-up is essential. This wound is commonly seen after a fistfight.

TABLE 204-1

Prophylactic Regimens for Dental, Oral, Respiratory Tract, or Esophageal Procedures

Situation	Agent	Regimen*
Standard general prophylaxis	Amoxicillin	Adults: 2.0 g Children: 50 mg/kg orally 1 hr before procedure
Unable to take oral medications	Ampicillin	Adults: 2.0 g IM or IV Children: 50 mg/kg IM or IV within 30 min before procedure
Allergic to penicillin	Clindamycin	Adults: 600 mg Children: 20 mg/kg orally 1 hr before procedure
	Cephalexin[†]	Adults: 2.0 g Children: 50 mg/kg or orally 1 hr before procedure
	Cefadroxil[†]	Adults: 500 mg
	Azithromycin or clarithromycin	Children: 15 mg/kg orally 1 hr before procedure
Allergic to penicillin and unable to take oral medications	Clindamycin or	Adults: 600 mg Children: 20 mg/kg IV within 30 min before procedure
	Cefazolin[†]	Adults: 1.0 g Children: 25 mg/kg IM or IV within 30 min before procedure

From Dajani AS, Taubert KA, Wilson W, et al: *JAMA* 277(22):1794, 1997.
IM, Intramuscularly; *IV,* intravenously.
*Total children's dose should not exceed adult dose.
[†]Cephalosporins should not be used in individuals with immediate-type hypersensitivity reaction (urticaria, angioedema, or anaphylaxis) to penicillins.

TABLE 204-2

Prophylactic Regimens for Genitourinary Gastrointestinal (Excluding Esophageal) Procedures

Situation	Agents*	Regimen[†]
High-risk patients	Ampicillin plus gentamicin	Adults: ampicillin 2 g IM) or IV plus gentamicin 1.5 mg/kg (not to exceed 120 mg/kg) within 30 min of starting the procedure; 6 hr later, ampicillin 1 g IM or IV or amoxicillin 1 g orally Children: ampicillin 50 mg/kg IM or IV (not to exceed 2 g) plus gentamicin 1.5 mg/kg within 30 min of starting the procedure; 6 hr later, ampicillin 25 mg/kg IM/IV or amoxicillin 25 mg/kg orally
High-risk patients allergic to ampicillin or amoxicillin	Vancomycin plus gentamicin	Adults: vancomycin 1 g IV over 1-2 hr gentamicin 1.5 mg/kg IV or IM (not to exceed 120 mg); complete injection or infusion within 30 min of starting the procedure Children: vancomycin 20 mg/kg IV over 1-2 hr plus gentamicin 1.5 mg/kg IV/IM; complete injection or infusion within 30 min of starting the procedure
Moderate-risk patients	Amoxicillin or ampicillin	Adults: amoxicillin 2 g orally 1 hr before procedure or ampicillin 2 g IM or IV within 30 min of starting the procedure Children: amoxicillin 50 mg/kg orally 1 hr before procedure or ampicillin 50 mg/kg IM or IV within 30 min of starting the procedure
Moderate-risk patients allergic to ampicillin or amoxicillin	Vancomycin	Adults: vancomycin 1 g IV over 1-2 hr; complete infusion within 30 min of starting the procedure Children: vancomycin 20 mg/kg IV over 1-2 hr; complete infusion within 30 min of starting the procedure

From Dajani AS, Taubert KA, Wilson W, et al: *JAMA* 277(22):1794, 1997.
IM, Intramuscularly; *IV,* intravenously.
*Total children's dose should not exceed adult dose.
[†]No second dose of vancomycin or gentamicin is recommended.

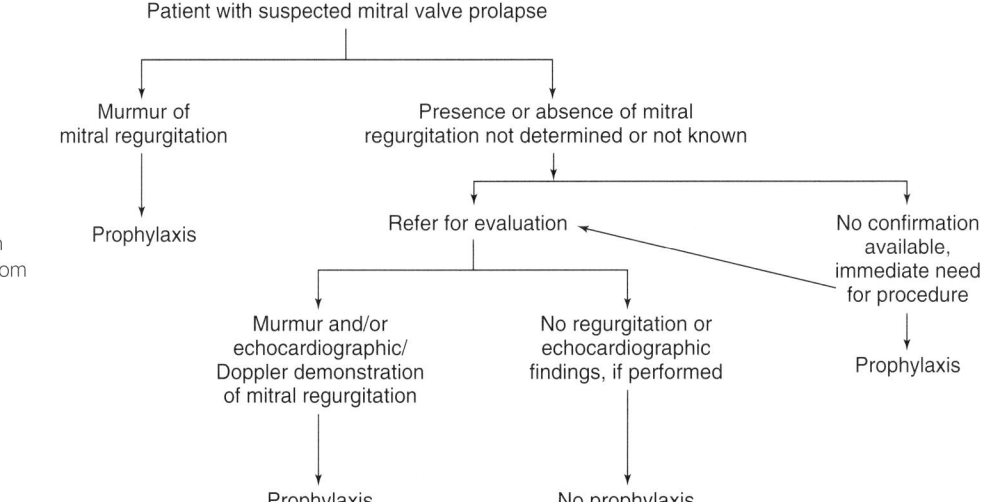

Patient with suspected mitral valve prolapse

Murmur of
mitral regurgitation

Presence or absence of mitral
regurgitation not determined or not known

Prophylaxis

Refer for evaluation

No confirmation
available,
immediate need
for procedure

Murmur and/or
echocardiographic/
Doppler demonstration
of mitral regurgitation

No regurgitation or
echocardiographic
findings, if performed

Prophylaxis

Prophylaxis

No prophylaxis

Fig. 204-1

Clinical approach to determine the need for prophylaxis in patients with suggested mitral valve prolapse. (From Dajani AS, Taubert KA, Wilson W, et al: *JAMA* 277[22]:1794, 1997.)

For other high-risk wounds, such as those obtained in a barnyard, sewer, or meat packing plant, antibiotics are required for 7 to 14 days. Gentamicin and clindamycin IV may be initially needed.

Generally, for most elective dermatologic and plastic surgeries, antibiotic prophylaxis for wound infection is not routinely indicated. The small number of wound infections that would be prevented makes it unwarranted. However, certain groups of patients are at *high risk.* These patients include those with *diabetes mellitus, significant obesity, immunosuppression, vascular insufficiency, malnutrition (i.e., caused by alcoholism, bulimia), chronic steroid use, lymphedema, and older patients,* among others. Depending on the extent of the surgery, prophylaxis should be considered. It is best if the antibiotic is given 1 hour before surgery, but there are benefits up to 4 hours later. There is no benefit to giving it for more than 24 to 48 hours. The cephalosporin group fulfills the requirements of prophylaxis better than any other group; but again, any oral antibiotic that basically covers strep and staph should be sufficient.

Note: The author generally use cephalexin 1000 g PO at the time of surgery followed by 500 mg every 8 hours for two doses. For those who are allergic, erythromycin works well.

Clean, sterile technique is mandatory in the excision and in the repair of any wound in the skin. The 11 most common causes of a wound infection may truly be the naso-oral area and the 10 fingers of the operating physician!

Also see the discussion on wound prophylaxis in Chapter 23, Laceration and Incision Repair. Chapter 148, Intrauterine Device Insertion, discusses the use of antibiotics at the time of insertion to prevent an endometritis or pelvic inflammatory disease (PID).

BIBLIOGRAPHY

Antimicrobial prophylaxis in surgery, *Med Lett* 41(1060):75, 1999.

Dajani AS, Taubert KA, Wilson W, et al: Prevention of bacterial endocarditis: recommendations by the American Heart Association, *JAMA* 277:1794, 1997.

Taubert KA, Dajani AS: Preventing bacterial endocarditis: American Heart Association guidelines, *Am Fam Physician* 57(3):457, 1998.

Weitekamp MR, Caputo GM: Antibiotic prophylaxis: update on common clinical uses, *Am Fam Physician* 48(4):597, 1993.

CHAPTER 205

Biofeedback

David M. Dush

Biofeedback combines physiological monitoring with behavioral conditioning to help patients learn to regulate or control some physical function of the body. Physical functions mediated by the autonomic nervous system, as opposed to those under voluntary control, are usually better candidates for biofeedback. For example, blood pressure, skin temperature (vasodilation), surface EMG activity (muscle tension, muscle strength), heart rate, respiratory rate and volume, volume of blood flow, bowel sounds, and EEG activity are all good candidates for biofeedback. In fact, all of these functions have been studied as applications for biofeedback.

There are three presumed active intervention elements of biofeedback: signal enhancement, reinforcement, and what are called the nonspecific effects. All three elements likely contribute to efficacy; therefore it is advisable for the staff to be trained and experienced in the application of all three elements.

1. *Signal enhancement:* An external device detects and amplifies moment-to-moment variations in a particular physiological function and displays these in a visual or audio signal. Increasing awareness with such a device alone can create a feedback loop, improve sensory discrimination, and enhance control. The device also provides useful monitoring feedback to the clinician.

2. *Reinforcement:* Classical conditioning and operant conditioning systems are often imbedded in the biofeedback session. Dials, video games, meters, beeps, tones, verbal praise, or other audio or visual feedback techniques are designed to reinforce desired signal changes. Such operant conditioning produces changes in physiological function even in lower animals; therefore it presumably does not depend (at least not entirely) on conscious thought.

3. *Nonspecific effects:* Although a variety of biofeedback studies have shown results superior to placebo, it has been difficult to establish that these outcomes are specific to the biofeedback process. Some data and some reviewers suggest that symptom improvement may actually be produced by enhancements in self-awareness, self-regulation, self-confidence, general relaxation skills, or other coping skills that can be a by-product of the biofeedback session.

INDICATIONS

- When conditioning, learning, stress, or other psychological factors seem to play a role in symptom etiology or fluctuations (Table 205-1).
- As a supplement to enhance other medical treatments.
- As an alternative for the patient who cannot tolerate medical treatment.
- When the patient prefers a supplement or alternative to medication for management of symptoms.
- EMG or thermal biofeedback has also been studied for applications with fibromyalgia, chronic fatigue syndrome, irritable bowel syndrome, and tics.
- EEG biofeedback has been used widely in treatment of attention deficit disorder (ADD) and explored for applications with seizures, alcoholism, and other disorders. Sophisticated equipment is now available for selectively reinforcing an increase or decrease of EEG

TABLE 205-1

Biofeedback Applications and Modalities

Application	Common Modalities
Chronic and acute pain	EMG, thermal
Migraine and tension headache	EMG, thermal
Insomnia	EMG, thermal
Hypertension	Thermal
Urinary or fecal incontinence	Internal sensor or catheter
Constipation	Internal catheter
Raynaud's disease	Thermal
Selective muscle retraining (e.g., after stroke)	EMG
Temporomandibular joint pain, bruxism	EMG
Stress management (for any stress-affected disorder)	EMG, thermal

activity within a specified bandwidth, using any conventional brain-monitoring site. Lubar has treated ADD by training children to increase higher-frequency beta-wave EEG activity while simultaneously decreasing slow-wave theta activity. (Although results have been promising, specific effects of the feedback component in these complex EEG applications are not yet well understood.)

- Surface EMG is being used increasingly for diagnostic purposes, most often by physical therapists. With surface EMG, the patient is recorded dynamically across standardized movements and postures. (A large number of symmetrical recording sites are needed to gather the data.)

CONTRAINDICATIONS

- Hypotension (for relaxation applications)
- Delusions, hallucinations, paranoia, or a dissociative disorder
- Disorientation or severe cognitive deficits (i.e., deficits limiting skill acquisition and retention)
- Poor motivation or compliance

Although patients with significant comorbid psychopathology may benefit from biofeedback, optimal efficacy is obtained in patients with intact higher psychological functioning.

EQUIPMENT

Multifunction, sensitive biofeedback devices with flexible application capabilities generally cost $2000 or more. They usually display multiple signals, alone or in combination, derived from various physiological functions. Their displays may use a variety of visual and audio formats. Units may be self-contained or may use a separate personal computer. Less expensive, portable single-function units for EMG or thermal biofeedback may be purchased for as little as $100 to $200. Portable units are useful for patients to take home to practice, but this expense to patients is rarely reimbursable. It should be noted that portable units do not provide the same diagnostic or treatment capabilities as multifunction units. Therefore it would not be advisable to use them as the primary equipment in the office.

PREPROCEDURE
PATIENT PREPARATION

See the sample patient education handout titled "Biofeedback" on page 2011 of Appendix G.

TECHNIQUE

1. The method of attachment varies with the modality, but it is usually straightforward. A medical assistant can perform patient preparation and initial instruction (see the "Training" section). Vascular biofeedback, for instance, requires only attachment of a reusable thermistor to the skin with thin tape. This measures skin temperature changes correlating with vasodilation. EMG biofeedback requires a skin prep, such as cleaning with an alcohol pad, and application of disposable silver-based electrodes prepped with conductive gel. Alignment and spacing of electrodes relative to target muscles easily alters readings and therefore should be standardized. EEG biofeedback electrodes are typically applied with conductive paste in the same standard locations as for diagnostic EEG. Biofeedback for incontinence and constipation requires insertion of a vaginal or anal EMG sensor or an inflatable catheter. With EMG vaginal sensors, patients may be trained to selectively tense (versus relax) appropriate muscles. With anally inserted catheters, the patient is trained to increase sensory discrimination while inflation (volume) levels are varied.

2. The biofeedback session usually follows the same type of format as that used for a physiology research study for a single subject. Once attached and oriented to the session, patients quietly relax while baseline levels and trends are established.

3. Feedback is now introduced in one or more forms, accompanied by a brief explanation to the patient. Any necessary changes in the strategy, activity, patient position, or posture across conditions within the session should be explained to the patient. Patients may be instructed about various relaxation strategies while incorporating feedback as a guide, or the clinician may just give general instructions for the patient to watch the monitor while experimenting for ways to move the signal in the desired direction.

4. Record the final baseline data to complete the session. Changes in levels or trends in functioning can easily be visualized in a graph of data across the session.

5. Following several sessions, these criteria may be helpful for determining whether biofeedback should be continued:
   a. Is there a clear connection between the physiological function being monitored by biofeedback and the patient's symptoms?
   b. Is the benefit for this patient derived from general relaxation training or general support from counseling rather than control of specific physical functions?

c. Were the observations in the first assessment session abnormal? If the readings were nearly optimal at the outset, there are usually few benefits from further training.

d. Across training, has the patient reached target levels (optimal or normal range responses)? Note that some readings, such as nonstandardized surface EMG readings, have no accurate, absolute normal or abnormal levels. Improved control over baseline may be the only target.

e. Is the patient eventually able to reproduce the target levels during monitoring only, without the assistance of feedback from the equipment?

f. Has progress leveled off? If it has, even if target levels have not been reached or the patient's ability to reproduce the change without feedback is limited, treatment is generally discontinued.

Occasionally, benefits are observed after a brief application in the office with limited practice and homework. For example, the author has had patients surprised to know that following a single session they can learn to relax muscles well in normal posture. They also learned that they could not halt climbing muscle tension when they simulated the poor posture they used at work. This knowledge alone may produce definitive behavior or work-site changes and alleviate the need for further training. More often, skill development, generalization, and maintenance require several sessions and considerable home practice.

CPT/BILLING CODES

Most insurers reimburse at low levels for the biofeedback procedure code (90875) when it is used in isolation. Medicare does not reimburse at all for this code, in part because in many regions of the country, biofeedback can be conducted by certified staff trained at a bachelor's level or less. However, as a well-established psychological treatment technique, it seems reasonable to document and include biofeedback training as one of the interventions used within a comprehensive medical or psychological counseling procedure. Such a procedure should be documented as performed by clinicians, nurses, or other ancillary patient care staff. In this manner, it can be billed accordingly under medical psychotherapy or other counseling-related procedure codes.

As part of the overall management of medical disorders typically treated with biofeedback, the implied counseling and behavioral intervention may support the use of time as a determinant for the medical evaluation and management (E & M) codes (e.g., 99202, 99203, 99204, or 99205 for sessions lasting 20, 30, 45, or 60 minutes, respectively). As always, when using time as a criterion for these codes, the practitioner must (1) document total session time, (2) document that more than half of the time was spent counseling or coordinating care, and (3) document the content of the counseling or coordination of care session.

The documented content should include issues related to the prognosis, differential diagnosis, risks, benefits of treatment, instructions, compliance, or risk reduction. For most patients, a medical diagnosis will presumably be the primary concern (e.g., insomnia, fatigue, headaches, etc.). This should be noted and the proper code used (ICD-9-CM), especially since some insurers refuse to reimburse (or assign different criteria) if a psychiatric diagnosis (e.g., depression or anxiety) is identified as the primary problem.

ICD-9-CM DIAGNOSTIC CODES

293.84	Anxiety resulting from or associated with a physical condition
306.8	Bruxism
436.0	Cerebrovascular disease, acute but ill-defined
564.0	Constipation
787.6	Fecal incontinence
346.90	Headache, migraine (not intractable)
307.81	Headache, tension
401.9	Hypertension, unspecified
780.52	Insomnia
724.5	Low back pain, postural
307.89	Low back pain, psychogenic
307.80	Pain, psychogenic, unspecified
307.89	Pain, psychogenic, site specified
443.0	Raynaud's disease
436.0	Stroke
524.60	Temporomandibular joint pain, dysfunction, syndrome
788.30	Urinary incontinence

SUPPLIERS

Thought Technology, Ltd.
2180 Belgrave Avenue
Montreal, Quebec, Canada H4A 2L8
Phone: 1-800-361-3651
Website: www.thoughttechnology.com

Multi Bio Sensors, Inc.
4944 Vista Grande
El Paso, TX 79922
Phone: 1-915-581-9684

Stens Corp.
6451 Oakwood Drive
Oakland, CA 94611
Phone: 1-800-257-8367
Website: www.stens-biofeedback.com

Bio-Medical Instruments, Inc.
2387 East Eight Mile Road
Warren, MI 48091-2486
Phone: 1-800-521-4640
Website: www.bio-medical.com

Stoelting Co.
620 Wheat Lane
Wood Dale, IL 60191
Phone: 1-630-860-9700
Website: www.stoeltingco.com

Neurofeed.com
49 Sprain Valley Road
Scarsdale, NY 10583
Phone: 1-914-472-2292
Website: www.neurofeed.com

Phazx Systems, Inc.
711 North Tejon
Colorado Springs, CO 80903
Phone: 1-800-273-0074
Website: www.phazx.com

TRAINING

Most manufacturers and distributors of biofeedback equipment provide training for use of their equipment. Extensive training is available from the Association for Applied Psychophysiology and Biofeedback. State licensure as a physician, psychologist, or psychotherapist and appropriate training to establish competence in biofeedback are likely sufficient in most states to practice biofeedback, just as a practitioner would use any other psychological intervention. A voluntary certification is available from the Biofeedback Certification Institute of America (BCIA). BCIA certification requires a bachelor's degree in a health profession, extensive coursework, and passing an examination.

Association for Applied Psychophysiology and
    Biofeedback
10200 W. 44th Avenue, Suite 304
Wheat Ridge, CO 80033-2840
Phone: 1-303-422-8436
Website: www.aapb.org

Biofeedback Certification Institute of America
10200 W. 44th Avenue, Suite 310
Wheat Ridge, CO 80033
Phone: 1-303-420-2902
Website: www.bcia.org

ADDITIONAL RESOURCES

- See the sample patient education handout titled "Biofeedback" on page 2011 of Appendix G.

BIBLIOGRAPHY

Krebs DE: Biofeedback in neuromuscular re-education and gait training. In Schwartz MS, editor: *Biofeedback: a practitioner's guide,* New York, 1995, Guilford Press.

Lubar JF: Neocortical dynamics: implications for understanding the role of neurofeedback and related techniques for the enhancement of attention, *Appl Psychophysiol Biofeedback* 22(2):111, 1997.

Schwartz MS, editor: *Biofeedback: a practitioner's guide,* New York, 1995, Guilford Press.

Schwartz MS: What is applied psychophysiology? Toward a definition, *Appl Psychophysiol Biofeedback* 24(1):3, 1999.

Wickramasekera I: How does biofeedback reduce clinical symptoms and do memories and beliefs have biological consequences? Toward a model of mind-body healing, *Appl Psychophysiol Biofeedback* 24(2):91, 1999.

CHAPTER 206

Body Fat Analysis

Arnold M. Ramirez
Russell D. White

Body fat analysis is a useful method for quantitatively assessing obesity and lean body mass, and it is more accurate than the various height-weight ratios. There are several methods of body fat analysis, each with its own advantages and disadvantages (Table 206-1).

Traditional methods such as underwater weighing (the "gold standard") and skinfold measurements are based on the two-compartment model (fat and fat-free mass). Newer methods such as dual energy x-ray absorptiometry (DEXA) and total body electrical conductivity (TOBEC) distinguish four compartments (water, protein, fat, and bone) and may replace underwater weighing as the reference standard. Although some of these methods are impractical and require expensive and bulky instruments, several methods can be performed quickly and easily in the office setting. These include skinfold measurements, bioelectrical impedance, and infrared interactance.

INDICATIONS

- Assessment of conditioning or fitness level
- Assessment of nutritional status
- Obesity
- Risk stratification for disease (e.g., hypertension, diabetes, coronary artery disease)

CONTRAINDICATIONS

- Patient refusal
- Caution in patients with implantable defibrillators or pacemakers using bioelectrical impedance

SKINFOLD MEASUREMENTS

The most widely used and practical method is based on the measurement of skinfold thickness in various predetermined sites.

EQUIPMENT

- Marking pen *(optional)*
- Measuring tape *(optional)*
- Skinfold calipers

TECHNIQUE

1. Although it matters little on which side of the body measurements are taken, by convention, measurements are taken on the right side.
2. Measure the exact same sites for serial comparisons.
3. Be familiar with the skinfold site to be measured, and pull the skinfold once or twice prior to the actual measurement.
4. Grasp the skinfold with the index finger and thumb of one hand and pull a fold away from the body with approximately parallel sides.
5. Visualize a true double fold of skin, and place the caliper heads approximately 0.5 to 1.0 cm away from the fingers holding the skinfold.
6. Ask the patient to contract the underlying muscle to help in grasping only skin and fat.
7. Place the caliper heads perpendicular to the skinfold and measure 4 to 5 seconds after releasing the lever arm of the calipers.
8. Maintain constant pressure with the thumb and index finger throughout the measurement.
9. Take a minimum of two measurements 15 seconds apart at each site until consecutive measurements vary by no more than 1 mm, to ensure consistency.
10. Measuring obese subjects may require both hands to pull a skinfold away with parallel sides. In this case, an assistant is needed to place the caliper heads on the skinfold.
11. Take measurements when the skin is dry and when the subject is not overheated (e.g., after exercise). Vasodilation of the skin in these conditions will inflate normal skinfold size.
12. Proficiency and accuracy require practice.

TABLE 206-1

Comparative Analysis of Methods for Body Fat Analysis

Method	Cost	Difficulty	Accuracy
Skinfold measurements	1	2	3
Bioelectrical impedance	3	1	3*
Infrared interactance	3	1	3*
Underwater weighing	3	4	5
Magnetic resonance	4	3	2
Computerized tomography	4	3	2
Dual-energy x-ray absorptiometry	5	2	5
Total body electrical conductivity test	5	2	5

Range: 1 is low; 5 is high.
*Accuracy diminishes in very lean or very obese subjects.

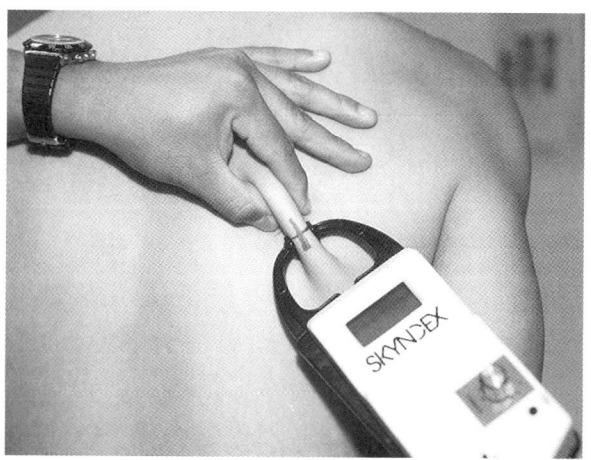

Fig. 206-2
Measurement of the subscapular skinfold.

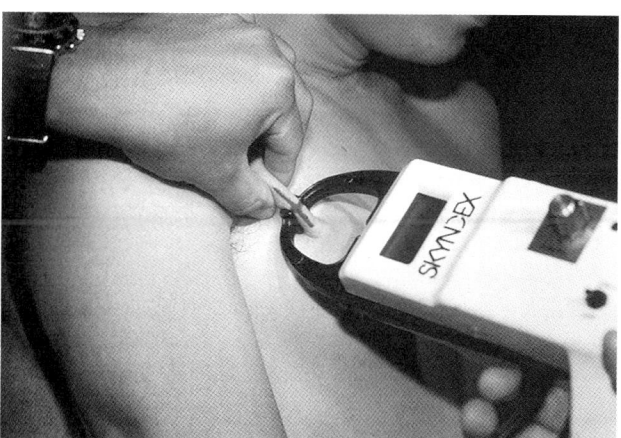

Fig. 206-1
Measurement of the chest or pectoral skinfold.

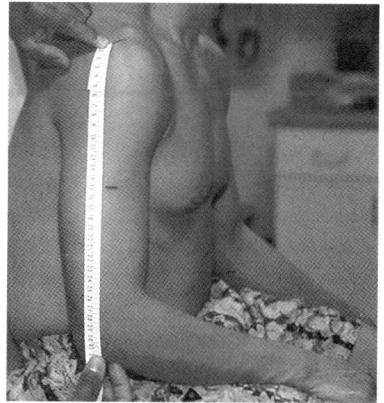

Fig. 206-3
Determining the midpoint between the lateral edge of the acromion and the inferior border of the olecranon.

Seven common sites are described as follows.
- *Chest:* Pick up the pectoral skinfold at the anterior axillary line with the long axis directed to the nipple. Place the skinfold calipers approximately 2 cm anterior to the anterior axillary line (Fig. 206-1).
- *Subscapular:* Lift a diagonal fold parallel to the medial border of the scapula at a point just below the inferior angle of the scapula (Fig. 206-2).
- *Triceps:* Pick up a vertical fold on the posterior arm 1 cm above the midway point between the lateral edge of the acromion and the inferior border of the olecranon. A measuring tape may be helpful in determining the midpoint (Fig. 206-3). Measurements are taken with the arm hanging loosely at the side and with the caliper heads placed precisely at the midpoint (Fig. 206-4).
- *Abdomen:* Pick up a horizontal fold 3 cm lateral to and 1 cm below the navel (Fig. 206-5).
- *Suprailiac:* Pick up a diagonal fold along Langer's lines above the iliac crest just posterior to the midaxillary line, with the calipers placed approximately 1 cm

anterior to the grasping fingers. The arm should hang naturally to the side but can be moved slightly to improve access (Fig. 206-6).
- *Thigh:* Measure a vertical fold midway between the inguinal crease and the superior border of the patella. It may be helpful to use a measuring tape to determine the midpoint of the anterior thigh (Fig. 206-7). Pick up the skinfold 1 cm above this point. The subject should have his or her body weight shifted to the opposite side, with the measured leg in slight knee flexion and the foot flat on the floor (Fig. 206-8).
- *Medial calf:* Measure a vertical fold at the level of the maximum calf circumference on the medial side of the calf. The measured leg should not bear weight and can be measured with the patient in either the standing or the seated position (Fig. 206-9).

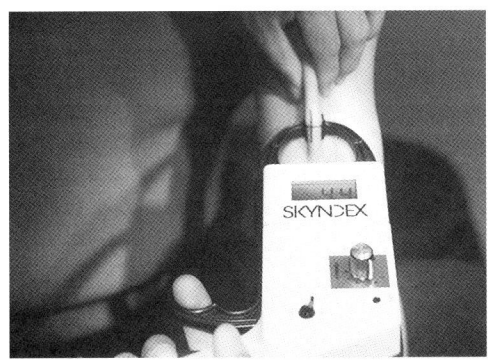

Fig. 206-4
Measurement of the triceps skinfold.

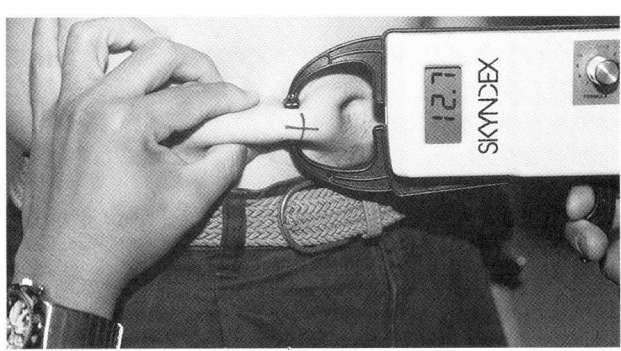

Fig. 206-5
Measurement of the abdominal skinfold.

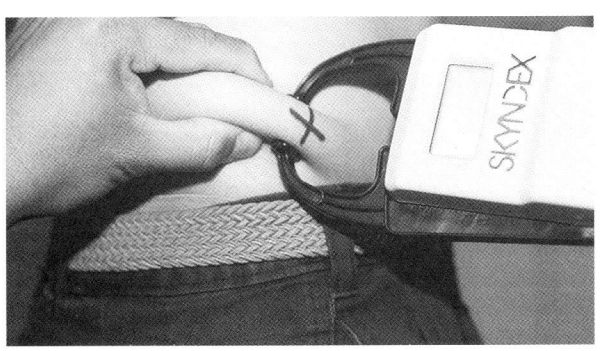

Fig. 206-6
Measurement of the suprailiac skinfold.

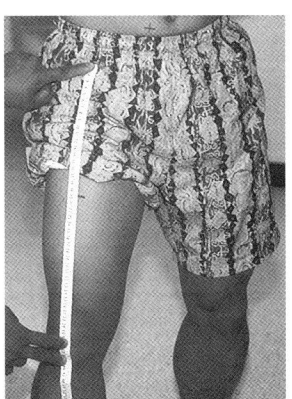

Fig. 206-7
Determining the midpoint of the anterior thigh between the inguinal crease and the superior border of the patella.

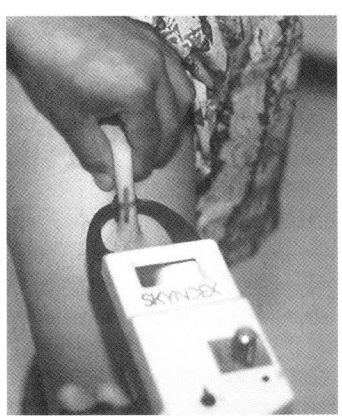

Fig. 206-8
Measurement of the thigh skinfold.

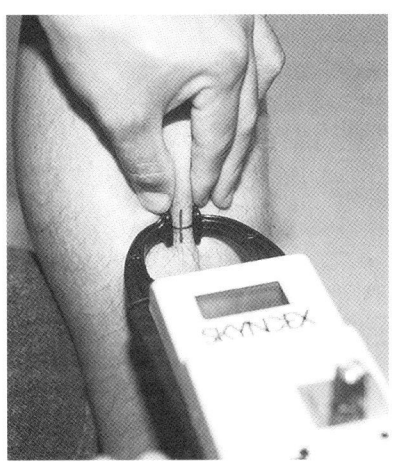

Fig. 206-9
Measurement of the medial calf skinfold.

CALCULATIONS

Numerous regression equations with various anthropometric measurements have been used to calculate body fat percentage. However, the following equations by the American Alliance for Health, Physical Education, Recreation, and Dance (AAHPERD), used in children and youth (ages 6 to 17), and those developed by Jackson and Pollock for adults are among the most widely used and accepted.

- For children and youth, a *two-site* skinfold test is done, using the triceps and medial calf sites:

Males 6 to 17 years:

% body fat = (0.735 × Sum of skinfolds in mm) + 1.0

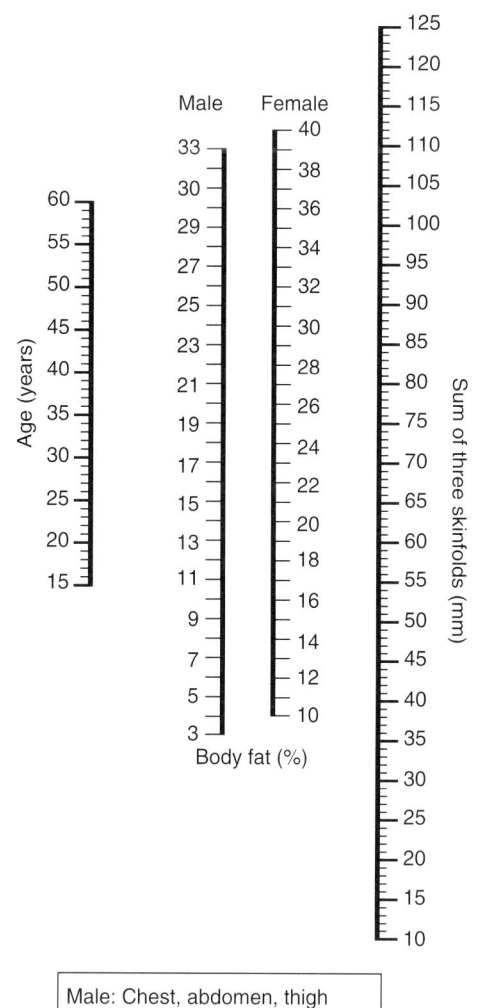

Fig. 206-10
Nomogram for estimating body fat percentage by using the sum of three skinfolds and age. (From Baun WB, Baun MR, Raven PB: *Res Q Exerc Sport* 52[3]:380, 1981.)

Females 6 to 17 years:

% body fat = (0.610 × Sum of skinfolds in mm) + 5.0

- For adults, the *three-site* equations developed by Jackson and Pollock are as follows:

Males:

Body density = 1.1093800 − 0.0008267(x) + 0.0000016(x)^2 − 0.0002574(Age)

(where x = sum of chest, abdomen, and thigh skinfolds in mm)

% body fat = (495/Body density) − 450

or

% body fat = 0.39287(x) − 0.00105(x)^2 + 0.15772(Age) − 5.18845

(where x = sum of abdomen, suprailiac, and triceps skinfolds in mm)

Females:

Body density = 1.0994921 − 0.0009929(x) + 0.0000023(x)^2 − 0.0001392(Age)

(where x = sum of triceps, suprailiac, and thigh skinfolds in mm)

% body fat = (495/Body density) − 450

or

% body fat = 0.41563(x) − 0.00112(x)^2 + 0.03661(Age) + 4.03653

(where x = sum of triceps, abdomen, and suprailiac skinfolds in mm)

Other formulas have been used, such as those developed by Durnin and Womersley. Also, many clinicians have found the nomogram from AAHPERD useful for determining body fat percentage (Fig. 206-10). Table 206-2 shows weight classifications for men and women.

BIOELECTRICAL IMPEDANCE

Bioelectrical impedance is based on differences in electrical conductivity through tissue depending on the amount of fat-free mass. A greater concentration or

TABLE 206-2
Weight Classification (General Body Fat Percentage Categories)

Classification	Women (% of fat)	Men (% of fat)
Essential fat	10%-12%	2%-4%
Athletes	14%-20%	6%-13%
Fitness	21%-24%	14%-17%
Acceptable	25%-31%	18%-25%
Obese	32%+	25%+

From American Council of Exercise.

percentage of fat-free mass increases electrical conductivity and decreases bioelectrical impedance.

EQUIPMENT

- Bioelectrical impedance measuring device (Fig. 206-11)

TECHNIQUE

1. Have the subject lie flat on a table with the limbs *not* touching the body.
2. Electrodes are placed on the right hand and right foot.
3. A harmless 50-kHz current at 800 μA is generated and passed through the subject.
4. Electrical conductance (or impedance) is measured and subsequently percent lean body mass is automatically calculated by the machine.

COMPLICATIONS

Caution must be exercised in using bioelectrical impedance in patients with implantable defibrillators and/or pacemakers; this method should not be used in these patients.

INFRARED INTERACTANCE

Infrared interactance is based on the principles of light absorption and reflection and uses near-infrared spectroscopy. The degree of infrared energy absorption is related to the composition of the substance through which the energy is passing and the particular wavelength of the energy. Hence, lean body mass and fat can be distinguished from each other and a percentage calculated.

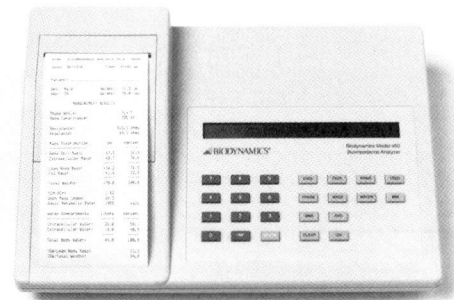

Fig. 206-11
Bioelectrical impedance measuring device. (From Biodynamics Corp., Seattle, Wash.)

EQUIPMENT

- Computerized, near-infrared spectrophotometer with fiberoptic probe, practical for office use (Fig. 206-12).

TECHNIQUE

The fiberoptic probe is placed commonly over the belly of the biceps muscle to gather the near-infrared data. Specific requirements, including anatomic location for probe placement, may differ depending on the individual spectrophotometer (Fig. 206-13).

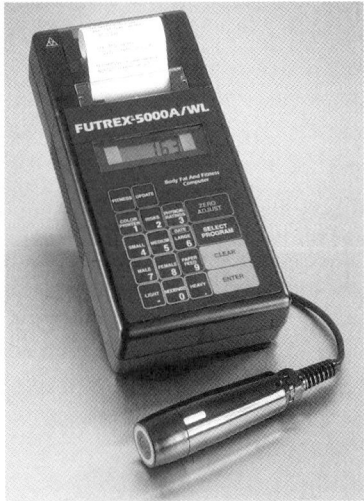

Fig. 206-12
Computerized, near-infrared spectrophotometer with fiberoptic probe. (Courtesy FUTREX, Inc., Gaithersburg, MD.)

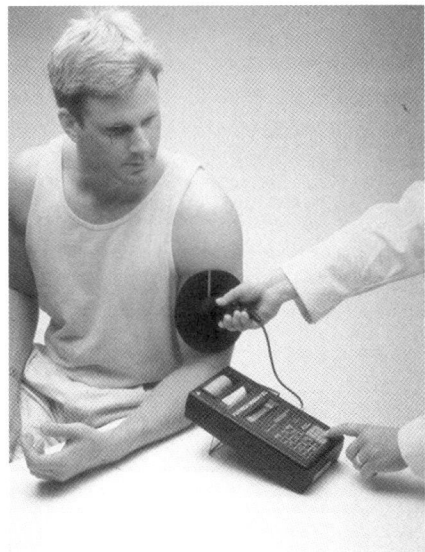

Fig. 206-13
Measurement using infrared interactance. (Courtesy FUTREX, Inc., Gaithersburg, MD.)

COMPLICATIONS

There are no complications.

SUPPLIERS

Skinfold calipers (approximate cost: $250 to $500)

Caldwell, Justiss & Co., Inc.
622 W. Sycamore
P.O. Box 520
Fayetteville, AR 72702
Phone: 1-800-643-4343

Micro Bio-Medics
846 Pelham Parkway
Pelham Manor, NY 10803
Phone: 1-800-431-2743
Website: www.microbiomedics.com

Medco Supply Company
500 Fillmore Avenue
Tonawanda, NY 14150
Phone: 1-800-556-3326
Website: www.medcosupply.com

Bioelectric impedance measuring device (approximate cost: $500 to $2000)

Biodynamics Corporation
3511 NE 45th Street, #2
Seattle, WA 98105
Phone: 1-800-869-6987
Website: www.biodyncorp.com

Near-infrared spectrophotometer (approximate cost: $3000 to $4000)

Futrex Inc.
6 Montgomery Village Avenue, #620
Gaithesburg, MD 20879
Phone: 1-800-255-4206
Website: www.futrex.com

CPT/BILLING CODES

17999   Skinfold measurement
93701   Bioelectrical impedance

ICD-9-CM DIAGNOSTIC CODE

278.00   Skinfold measurement

BIBLIOGRAPHY

American Alliance for Health, Physical Education, Recreation, and Dance: *Technical manual: health-related physical fitness,* Reston, Va, 1984, AAHPERD.

Baun WB, Baun MR, Raven PB: A nomogram for the estimate of percent body fat from generalized equations, *Res Q Exerc Sport* 52(3):380, 1981.

Brodie DA: Techniques of measurement of body composition: parts I and II, *Sports Med* 5:11, 74, 1988.

Durnin JVGA, Womersley J: Body fat assessment from total body density and its estimation from skinfold thickness: measurements on 481 men and women aged 16 to 72 years, *Br J Nutr* 32:77, 1974.

Jackson AS, Pollock ML: Practical assessment of body composition, *Phys Sports Med* 13:76, 1985.

Lukaski HC: Methods for the assessment of human body composition: traditional and new, *Am J Clin Nutr* 46:537, 1987.

Nieman DC: *Fitness and sports medicine: a health-related approach,* ed 3, Mountain View, Calif, 1995, Mayfield.

CHAPTER 207

Bone Marrow Aspiration or Biopsy

Beth A. Choby

Bone marrow aspiration and biopsy are techniques used to obtain marrow needed for evaluation of a variety of disease processes. The procedures obtain two interrelated specimens. The bone marrow aspirate provides a cytological smear for visualization of cell morphology and a count of marrow cellular elements. The bone marrow biopsy evaluates bone marrow cellularity, fibrosis, infection, or infiltrative disease.

Many sites may be used for marrow aspiration, depending on the patient's age and the operator's experience. The posterior iliac crest is the site most commonly used for aspiration and used nearly exclusively for biopsy (Fig. 207-1, *A*). The sternum can be used for aspiration in adults, but its use carries a risk of cardiac tamponade if the posterior sternum is inadvertently penetrated (Fig. 207-1, *B*). The anterior iliac crest is also a possibility, but it has a hard, thick cortical layer that makes sampling difficult. This site is useful when the posterior iliac crest is unavailable (e.g., because the patient has a physical disability, is in a cast, or is obese). The anterior tibia can be used for marrow aspiration in infants younger than 18 months of age.

Techniques for aspiration or biopsy are described for the posterior iliac spine approach. This technique is both easily accessible and safe when performed properly.

INDICATIONS

- Evaluation of anemia or iron metabolism
- Thrombocytopenia
- Leukopenia or leukocytosis
- Pancytopenia
- Unexplained splenomegaly
- Workup of fever of unknown origin
- Diagnosis and staging of leukemia and lymphoma
- Workup of bone marrow transplantation
- Staging for nonhematologic cancers such as neuroblastoma
- Monitoring of chemotherapy- and radiation-induced damage in cancer treatment

- Material for chromosomal studies
- Workup of dysproteinemia or lysosomal storage diseases
- Immunodeficiency states (HIV or AIDS)
- Unusual infections (e.g., tuberculosis, fungal infections)

CONTRAINDICATIONS

Absolute Contraindications

- Hemophilia and related bleeding disorders

Relative Contraindications

- Uncooperative patient
- Severe osteoporosis (risk of bone perforation with injury to underlying tissues)
- Skin infection or osteomyelitis at intended biopsy site
- Previous radiation therapy at biopsy site

Note: Thrombocytopenia is *not* a contraindication for bone marrow aspiration or biopsy. If the patient is on anticoagulation therapy, it *does not* need to be reversed or held prior to the procedure.

EQUIPMENT

Equipment is generally available in prepackaged sterile disposable kits (Fig. 207-2)
- Antiseptic solution (e.g., povidone-iodine)
- Sterile fenestrated drape
- 1% lidocaine
- 3- and 5-ml syringes
- 22-gauge (1½-inch) and 25-gauge (⅝-inch) needle
- No. 11 scalpel
- Bone marrow aspiration needle (Fig. 207-3)
- 11-gauge Jamshidi® Bone Marrow Biopsy needle (Fig. 207-4)

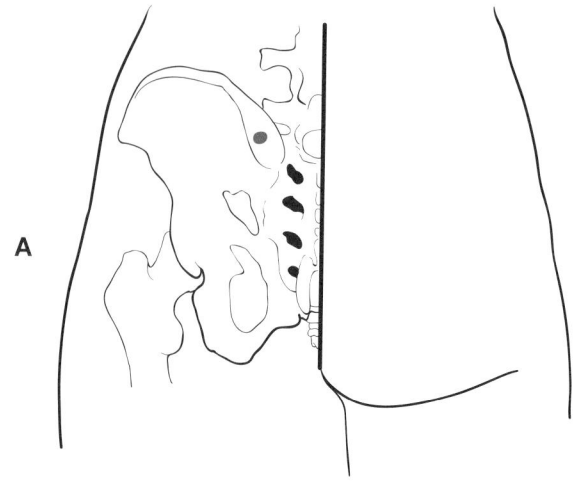

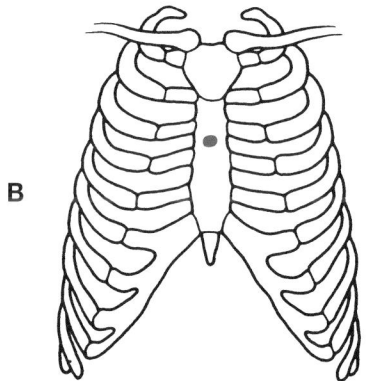

Fig. 207-1
A, Posterior iliac sampling site. **B,** Sternal sampling site.

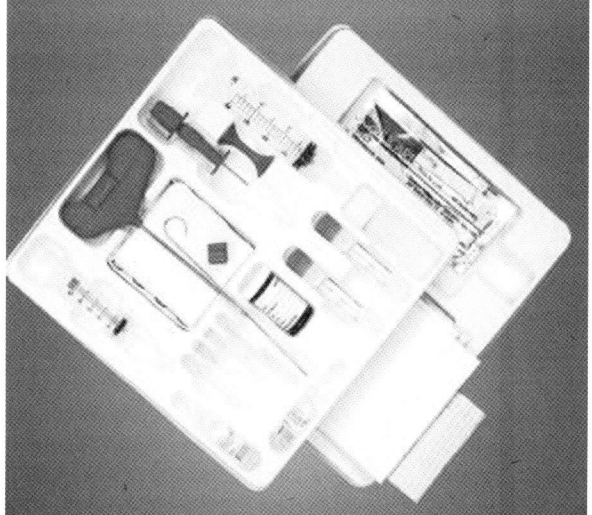

Fig. 207-2
Prepackaged sterile Jamshidi® Bone Marrow Biopsy kit. (Courtesy Cardinal Health, McGaw Park, Ill.)

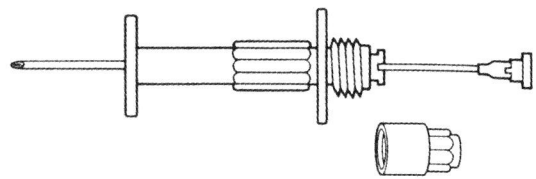

Fig. 207-3
Bone marrow aspiration needle.

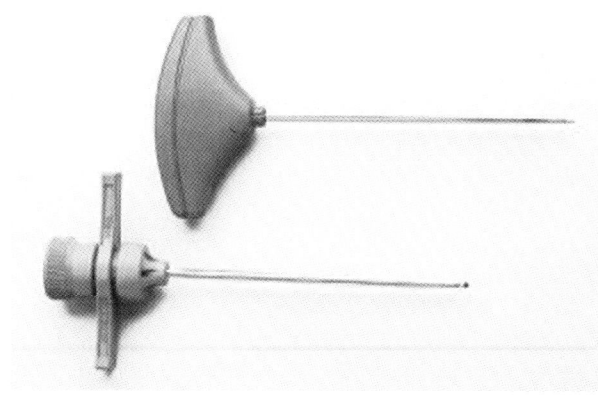

Fig. 207-4
Jamshidi® Bone Marrow Biopsy needle. (Courtesy Cardinal Health, McGaw Park, Ill.)

- 10-ml syringe rinsed with ethylenediamine tetraacetic acid (EDTA)
- EDTA (purple top) tube
- Glass slides (10)
- Bottle or tube with fixative (formalin)
- 4 × 4–inch gauze
- Pressure dressing and tape

PREPROCEDURE PATIENT PREPARATION

A cooperative patient is essential. Discuss indications for the procedure, as well as risks and benefits. Obtain a signed informed consent (see the sample patient consent form titled "Bone Marrow Aspiration/Biopsy" on page 2013 of Appendix G). Inquire about a history of coagulation abnormalities or allergies (i.e., povidone-iodine or lidocaine). A complete blood count with white cell differential, platelet count, and peripheral smear is reviewed before the procedure. Explain that there will be discomfort associated with numbing the skin and periosteum, penetrating the iliac crest, and during the aspiration of marrow. The bladder is emptied before beginning the procedure. If the patient is overly apprehensive, premedication with a mild anxiolytic or analgesic is appropriate. Oral lorazepam (1 to 3 mg) and hydromorphone (1 to 4 mg) given 90 minutes before the biopsy lessen pain and induce varying degrees of amnesia.

TECHNIQUE

It is currently recognized that optimal evaluation of the marrow involves examination of both the marrow aspirate and biopsy (smear preps and sections). Obtaining both aspirate and biopsy simultaneously is better in terms of patient comfort, cost, and diagnostic information gleaned.

The procedures for obtaining bone marrow aspiration and performing a bone marrow biopsy from the posterior iliac crest are described.

Bone Marrow Aspiration

1. Have the patient lie in the right or left lateral decubitus position with knees flexed at the hip. Identify each iliac crest and follow it to its posterior superior spine (Fig. 207-1). Mark the location.

2. Put on sterile gloves and cleanse the biopsy area in a circular pattern with povidone-iodine antiseptic. Drape the site with the fenestrated sterile drape, positioning the biopsy site in the center of the fenestration.

3. Anesthetize the area using 2% lidocaine in the 3-ml syringe. Use a 25-gauge needle to make a skin wheal. Switch to the 22-gauge needle/3-ml syringe for deeper structures. Introduce the needle until the periosteum is reached. Since most of the bone pain fibers are located in the periosteum, it is infiltrated with approximately 1 ml of lidocaine. While removing the needle, inject 2 to 3 ml of anesthetic along the outgoing tract.

4. Make a 2- to 3-mm skin incision with the scalpel to enhance insertion of the aspiration needle.

5. Insert the marrow aspiration needle perpendicularly to the bone, making sure the stylet is locked in place. Insert the needle until it rests against the anesthetized periosteum. Rotate the needle clockwise and counterclockwise using enough force to penetrate the bony cortex. Stop pushing when "give" is felt on entering the marrow cavity. The needle remains stationary without support when placed correctly.

6. Remove the stylet and attach a 10-ml EDTA-rinsed syringe. Warn the patient that he or she will experience pain as the marrow is aspirated. Pull the plunger and rapidly aspirate 0.2 to 2 ml of marrow (higher volumes dilute the specimen with blood).

7. The aspirated material is given to an assistant for slide preparation. The quality of the sample is assessed by the presence of grossly visible marrow spicules. Thin films are prepared quickly with minimal specimen manipulation. Several drops of aspirate are placed on the edge of a glass slide and allowed to run down the surface. The edge of a second slide is then used to spread thinly the aspirate across the slide. Four slides are made and allowed to dry. The slides are stained with either Wright or May-Grünwald-Giemsa stain.

8. The remaining aspirate is placed in a tube with EDTA mixed well and allowed to clot for later fixation and processing by the histologist. If extra material is needed for flow cytometry, culture, cytogenetics, or other special studies, additional aspirations may be performed by withdrawing the needle and repositioning it in a new site.

9. If a "dry tap" is encountered (no aspirate despite seemingly good needle placement), replace the stylet and advance the needle 1 to 2 mm. If still unsuccessful, pull out the needle and reinsert it at another part of anesthetized periosteum near the original site.

10. Once the aspirate sample is deemed adequate, replace the stylet and remove the entire needle using a twisting motion.

11. Place dry gauze over the site and apply pressure until the bleeding stops. Cover the area with an adhesive bandage unless proceeding with a bone marrow biopsy.

Bone Marrow Biopsy

Bone marrow biopsy may be performed directly after aspiration. The sample is obtained from the posterior iliac crest. The steps are identical to bone marrow aspiration. After the bone marrow aspiration needle is removed, the following steps are taken:

1. Confirm that the stylet of the Jamshidi® Biopsy Needle is locked into place with the cap secured (Fig. 207-4). Place the capped end in the palm of your hand with the shaft lying between your index and middle fingers. Introduce the needle inside the puncture wound, pushing the needle through the soft tissue to the periosteum of the posterior iliac spine. Care must be taken to reposition the needle entry site away from the area where the aspiration was performed to avoid collection of a specimen with extensive artifact induced by the aspiration. Using clockwise and counterclockwise rotation with considerable downward pressure, pierce the cortex of the bone to enter the marrow. The cortex is usually around 1 cm thick and entrance into the marrow cavity detected by decreased resistance (Fig. 207-5).

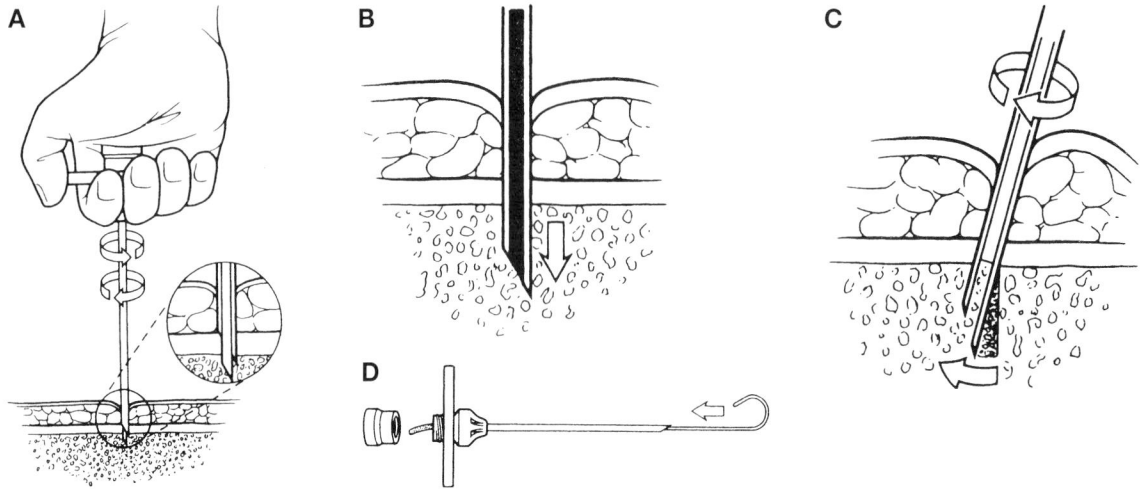

Fig. 207-5
Technique for obtaining a bone marrow biopsy specimen. **A,** The needle is advanced through the cortical bone. **B,** The stylet is removed and the needle advanced an additional 1.5 to 2 cm using downward rotational force. **C,** The needle tip is redirected 15 degrees and rotated to break off the specimen. **D,** The probe is used to push the specimen onto gauze, threaded through the needle tip toward the biopsy needle handle.

2. Unlock the cap and remove the stylet.
3. Slowly and gently advance the needle millimeter by millimeter (1.5 to 2 cm) with an alternating clockwise-counterclockwise motion to obtain an adequate specimen.
4. Pull the needle back 2 to 3 mm and redirect its tip approximately 15 degrees. Advance the needle 2 to 3 mm forward in the new position to break off the specimen.
5. Rotate the biopsy needle 360 degrees four times to the right and then four times to the left.
6. Remove the needle from the patient using rotational movements. The sample should stay in the Jamshidi needle.
7. Remove the biopsy specimen by inserting the blunt probe into the distal end of the needle, pushing the specimen onto sterile gauze. Take care not to injure yourself on the sharp cutting edge (Fig. 207-5, *D*).
8. Prepare the specimens or give the samples to the technician to prepare. Touch preparations (5) are made by gently pressing five glass slides against the biopsy specimen. The slides are generally stained with Wright or Giemsa stain. The remaining biopsy sample is then placed into a container with formalin and sent for sectioning and staining.
9. Cover the biopsy site with gauze and apply pressure until the bleeding stops. Cover the area with gauze and an adhesive bandage to form a pressure dressing. The patient should lie on the biopsy site for 60 minutes.

COMPLICATIONS

Complications of bone marrow aspiration and biopsy are unusual. Adverse outcomes include the following.
- Retroperitoneal hemorrhage or damage to the bowel wall as a result of perforation of the iliac bone in osteoporotic patients
- Hemorrhage at the biopsy site
- Infection at the biopsy site (unusual if sterile technique is followed)
- Dry tap—either marrow is unobtainable or marrow blood is found but no marrow units are present (Although faulty technique or improper needle placement may be responsible, most cases are due to pathology in the marrow such as leukemia or myelofibrosis.)
- Perforation of the lower sternal plate resulting in cardiac tamponade and sudden death
- Pain that usually resolves within a day

POSTPROCEDURE PATIENT EDUCATION

The patient remains recumbent to place pressure on the biopsy site for 1 hour while being observed in the office. If the patient is thrombocytopenic, pressure bandages should be applied and the site checked frequently for prolonged bleeding. The clinician should provide emergency contact numbers and instruct the patient to call in case of bleeding, pain, fever, or erythema at the biopsy site. The pressure dressing may be removed in 12 to 24 hours. Pain medication should be provided as needed.

SUPPLIERS

Illinois sternal/iliac bone marrow aspiration tray
Allegiance Healthcare Corp. (a Cardinal Health company)
1430 Waukegan Road
McGaw Park, IL 60085-6787
Phone: 1-800-964-5227
Website: www.allegiance.net

Jamshidi bone marrow biopsy/aspiration needle
Allegiance Healthcare Corp.
(see above)

CPT/BILLING CODES

85060	Peripheral blood smear interpretation
85095	Bone marrow aspiration
85102	Bone marrow biopsy
85097	Bone marrow interpretation

ADDITIONAL RESOURCES

- See the sample patient education handout titled "Bone Marrow Aspiration/Biopsy" on page 2013 of Appendix G.

- See the sample patient consent form titled "Bone Marrow Aspiration/Biopsy" on page 2015 of Appendix G.

BIBLIOGRAPHY

Aboul-Nasr R, Estey EH, Kantarjian HM, et al: Comparison of touch imprints with aspirate smears for evaluating bone marrow specimens, *Am J Clin Pathol* 111(6):753, 1999.

Bain BJ: Bone marrow aspiration, *J Clin Pathol* 54(9):657, 2001.

Dunlop TJ, Deen C, Lind S, et al: Use of combined oral narcotic and benzodiazepine for control of pain associated with bone marrow examination, *South Med J* 92(5):477, 1999.

Hyun BH, Gulati GL, Ashton JK: Bone marrow examination: techniques and interpretation, *Hem/Onc Clinics North Am* 2:513, 1988.

Hyun BH, Stevenson AJ, Hanau CA. Fundamentals of bone marrow examination, *Hem/Onc Clinics North Am* 4:651, 1994.

Lee GR: Bone marrow examination. In Lee GR, editor: *Wintrobe's clinical hematology*, ed 10, Philadelphia, 1999, Lippincott, Williams & Wilkins.

CHAPTER 208

Drawing Blood Cultures

Theodore X. O'Connell

Bacteremia and septicemia are potentially life-threatening conditions caused by a variety of microorganisms. The successful isolation of microorganisms from blood requires an understanding of the intermittent nature of most bacteremias, the low order of magnitude of most bacteremias, and the great variety of organisms capable of causing septicemia.

Consideration must first be given to the patient's clinical status. Indications for obtaining blood cultures are outlined next. Note that 25% of patients with documented bacteremia have periods without fever. In the elderly population, the proportion is even higher, with 50% of bacteremic patients over the age of 65 years being afebrile.

Most bacteremias are intermittent; ideally, blood collections for culture should be made intermittently during a 24-hour period. Two separate blood culture sets should be collected within a 24-hour period. However, if administration of antibiotics is clinically indicated, two sets of cultures separated by 20 to 30 minutes should be obtained. Each set of culture bottles has one aerobic and one anaerobic bottle.

Most bacteremias are of a very low magnitude; therefore an adequate volume of blood should be collected for each set of cultures. Small children usually have higher numbers of bacteria in the blood than adults, which means that smaller quantities of blood may be obtained from children. Appropriate volumes are noted in Table 208-1.

INDICATIONS

- Fever and unexplained alterations in mental status, functional status, or autonomic status in a previously healthy patient between the ages of 5 and 65 years
- Fever and no source of infection in a patient younger than 2 years of age or older than 65 years of age
- Immunocompromised status with a fever and no source
- All febrile infants younger than 3 months of age
- Persistent rigor, with or without fever
- Fever or no fever in a patient with a toxic or "septic" appearance, including unexplained hypotension, altered mental status, and shock
- Possible infectious endocarditis (changing heart murmur)
- Serious focal infections such as meningitis, septic arthritis, and osteomyelitis
- Patients with pneumonia or pyelonephritis and signs of toxicity

CONTRAINDICATIONS

There are essentially no contraindications to drawing blood cultures. As with any patient, blood should not be drawn through infected skin sites.

EQUIPMENT

- Alcohol pads
- 2% tincture of iodine in 70% alcohol (Alternatively, 2% iodine solution or 10% povidone-iodine may be used.)
- Chlorhexidine (Hibiclens) may be used in the iodine-allergic patient
- Tourniquet
- Sterile gloves
- 21-gauge needle
- 30-ml syringe
- Set of blood culture bottles, aerobic and anaerobic, with labels

PREPROCEDURE PATIENT PREPARATION

Drawing blood for culture does not entail any more risk than drawing blood for any other purpose. Patients should be warned about the needlestick and the potential for bleeding, bruising, and infection. Written consent for this procedure is not necessary.

TECHNIQUE

1. Fill in the laboratory request form and explain the procedure to the patient.
2. Apply the tourniquet and determine the location of the vein to be used for venipuncture (Fig. 208-1, *A*).
3. Cleanse the skin with alcohol swabs three times or until pads are free of surface dirt.
4. Allow the skin to dry.

TABLE 208-1

Optimal Specimen Volumes to be Drawn per Blood Culture Set

Age Group	Ideal Volume per Set (ml)
Neonates	1-2
Infants 5-10 kg	2-4
Children 7-20 kg	3-8
Children 20-40 kg	10
Children over 40 kg	20-30
Adults	20-30

5. Apply iodine three times in centrifugal circles from the anticipated site of venipuncture.
6. After the third swab, allow to dry at least 60 seconds.
7. Remove the protective cap and cleanse the top of the culture bottles with alcohol swabs.
8. Wipe off dry iodine at venipuncture site with alcohol swabs. Do not palpate the vein after disinfecting the site.
9. Obtain the required volume of blood (see Table 208-1 for recommended blood volumes by patient size).
10. Immediately apply pressure to the puncture site after removing needle with a clean cotton sponge.
11. Place up to 10 ml of blood in each culture bottle. (These two bottles constitute one blood culture "set.")
12. Inoculate both bottles without changing needles.
13. Repeat at different sites or different times for the requisite number of blood culture sets.
14. Transport the blood cultures as soon as possible to start incubating or processing.

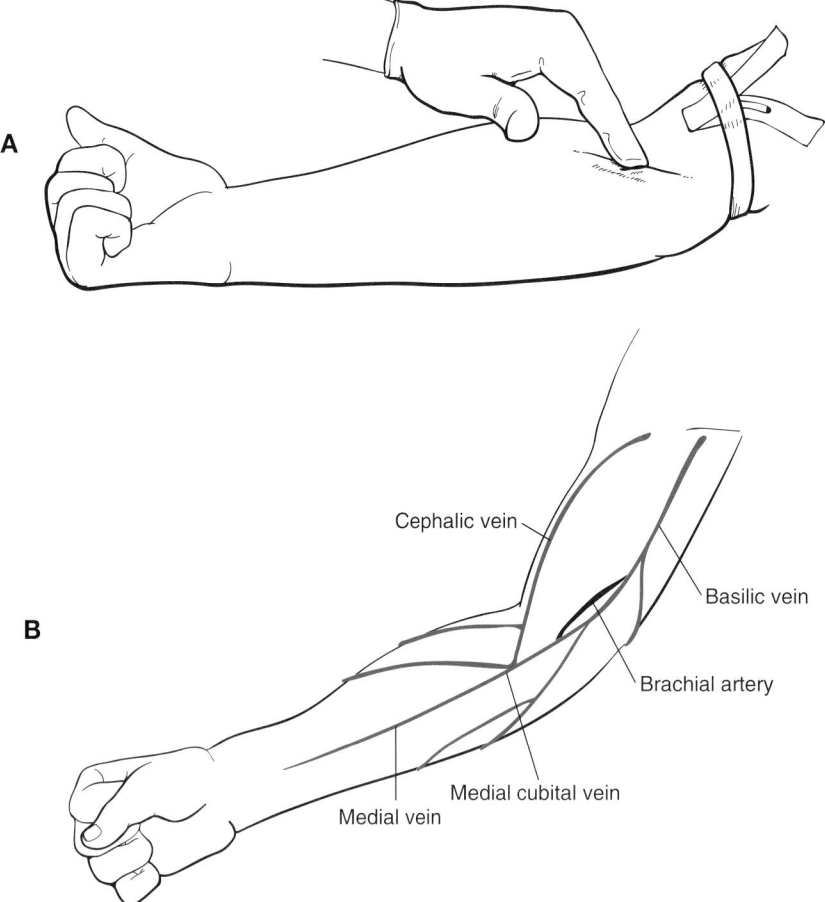

Fig. 208-1
Venipuncture. **A,** After the tourniquet is applied, the vein is located. **B,** Veins in arm.

COMPLICATIONS

- Bleeding
- Bruising
- Infection

INTERPRETATION OF RESULTS

In the case of a positive blood culture, the offending organism or organisms are identified. If sensitivities have been ordered, the antibiotic susceptibility or resistance is reported.

One of the more challenging aspects of interpreting blood culture results is determining which positive blood cultures are actually false-positive results. Features of false-positive blood cultures are outlined next.

- Coagulase-negative staphylococci *(Staphylococcus epidermidis)* and *S. viridans* in a single bottle in patients not suspected of having infectious endocarditis and without chronic indwelling intravenous catheters are usually contaminants.
- *Corynebacterium, Propionibacterium acnes,* and *Bacillus* species are usually contaminants, but they can be pathogens in immunocompromised hosts.
- Multiple organisms in a series suggest contamination.
- Species that grow out after prolonged culture have a greater likelihood of being contaminants.
- The patient's symptoms have resolved or are inconsistent with sepsis. However, special consideration must be given to infectious endocarditis, which can have an indolent course.
- A primary infected source, such as urine, yields a different pathogenic isolate.

SUPPLIERS

BacT/Alert blood culture bottles
Organon Teknika Corp.
100 Akzo Avenue
Durham, NC 27712
Phone: 1-800-682-2666
Website: www.organonteknika.com

CPT BILLING CODES

If cultures done in the office, laboratory codes are as follows.
87040   Culture, bacterial, definitive
87085   with colony count
There is no specific code for drawing blood. Add lab handling fee (99000) to office visit.

ICD-9-CM DIAGNOSTIC CODES

790.7   Bacteremia
771.8   Bacteremia, newborn
038.9   Septicemia

BIBLIOGRAPHY

Little JR, Murray PR, Traynor PS, Spitznagel E: A randomized trial of povidone-iodine compared with iodine tincture for venipuncture site disinfection: effects on rates of blood culture contamination, *Am J Med* 107:119, 1999.

Madell GL, Bennett JE, Dolin R, editors: *Principles and practice of infectious diseases,* ed 5, New York, 2000, Churchill Livingstone.

Mimoz O, Karim A, Mercat A: Chlorhexidine compared with povidone-iodine as skin preparation before blood culture: a randomized, controlled trial, *Ann Intern Med* 131:834, 1999.

Nettina SM, editor: *The Lippincott manual of nursing practice,* Philadelphia, 1996, Lippincott-Raven.

Roberts JR, Hedges JR, editors: *Clinical procedures in emergency medicine,* Philadelphia, 1998, WB Saunders.

Thompson JM, McFarland GK, Hirsh JE, Tucker SM, editors: *Mosby's clinical nursing,* ed 4, St Louis, 2000, Mosby.

CHAPTER 209

Emergency Department and Office Ultrasound

Grant C. Fowler

For many reasons—including more widely available educational programs, high-quality research about applications, and improvements in image quality, portability, and affordability—real-time sonography has become a valuable adjunct to the physical examination in many emergency departments. It is also useful for guiding procedures. Even urgent care centers now often have ultrasound available. The quality of care has been improved and lives have been saved because of immediately available information from real-time ultrasound scanning. Studies continue to document the safety and efficacy of sonography in emergency departments, as well as to clarify the indications. As a result of these developments, the stated policy of the American College of Emergency Physicians (ACEP) is to encourage immediately available ultrasound examination, interpretation, and clinical correlation 24 hours a day for emergency department patients. This policy has been endorsed by the Society for Academic Emergency Medicine (SAEM). SAEM also encourages residency programs to offer ultrasound training. ACEP considers focused, bedside ultrasound imaging to be within the scope of practice of emergency clinicians for at least the following indications: suspected traumatic hemoperitoneum, abdominal aortic aneurysm (AAA), pericardial fluid, ectopic pregnancy, and renal or biliary disease.

Although many of the same applications in emergency medicine are useful in the primary care clinician's office, ultrasound in that setting has not been studied as extensively. However, when the principles of sonography are understood and the equipment is available, certain diagnostic applications (e.g., evaluation of renal colic, right upper quadrant (RUQ) abdominal pain, or pulsatile abdominal mass) can be learned during or after residency. They may improve not only the accuracy of the diagnosis, but also how rapidly the diagnosis is made. Considering ultrasound enhances physical examination skills, it is anticipated that ultrasonically enhanced Periodic Health Evaluations (PHE) will eventually become the norm. Screening asymptomatic patients may find early cancers, carotid artery disease, urinary retention, hydronephrosis, AAAs, etc. One published study (Siepel et al, 2000) of ultrasound-enhanced PHE in the elderly revealed a new diagnosis in 31% of patients that was unsuspected during conventional physical examination. Seven percent of the total patients required prompt treatment for serious unsuspected conditions.

Primary care clinicians already performing obstetric ultrasound are often comfortable with the principles of sonography and are capable of extending its use beyond obstetrics with little additional training. Primary care clinicians who use sonography when covering urgent care centers or emergency departments often extend the use of ultrasound into their office practice. Even for primary care clinicians not comfortable using ultrasound for diagnostic applications, considerable benefit may be found with using ultrasound to facilitate procedures (e.g., ultrasonically directed aspiration of pleural or peritoneal fluid, breast or thyroid cysts; or ultrasonically directed insertion of central lines). Gastroenterologists now use ultrasound to direct liver biopsies to minimize complications and nephrologists use it for renal biopsies for the same reason. The subspecialty of interventional radiology has expanded at a great rate, and physicians in this field frequently use ultrasound to guide procedures formerly performed by surgeons. Primary care clinicians already comfortable performing procedures should be able to readily enhance their skills with ultrasound.

This chapter highlights some of the current diagnostic and procedural applications of ultrasound in both the emergency department and the primary care clinician's office. Obstetric ultrasound is also often performed in the emergency department or primary care clinician's office and is covered in another chapter. (See Chapter 173, Obstetric Ultrasound.)

PRINCIPLES OF ULTRASOUND

Similar to sonar used by submarines and private fishing boats, ultrasound technology analyzes echoes from pulsed sound waves to generate images. Real-time sonography provides continuously updated or "live" images while the patient is being scanned. Live images often allow the clinician to immediately exclude certain diagnoses and to redirect clinical suspicions toward other diagnoses. Live images may also improve the clinician's understanding of a particular patient's underlying anatomy. In addition, the best images are often

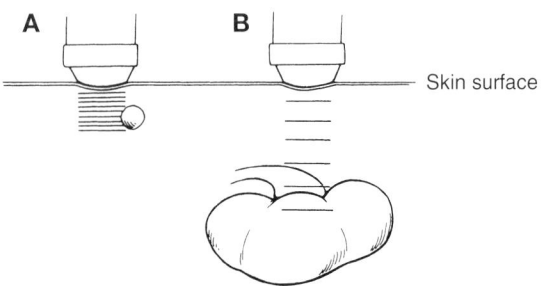

Fig. 209-1
A, High-frequency probe (7.5 to 10 MHz) provides higher resolution images but cannot be used to scan deep organs. This probe is especially useful for organs or structures near the skin surface such as breast or thyroid tissue, veins, or arteries. **B,** Low-frequency probe (3.5 to 5 MHz) for deeper tissue such as abdominal or pelvic organs.

obtained when scanning "live" because the clinician can immediately reposition the patient as necessary to obtain the best images.

One general principle of ultrasound is that the higher the frequency, the sharper the resolution of the image. However, with higher frequencies, there is less depth of penetration into the tissue (Fig. 209-1). The best frequency for a particular scan is often decided by the clinician based on these principles; the probe, or *transducer,* is then chosen to match the desired frequency. High-frequency probes (7.5 to 10 megahertz [MHz]) are useful for scanning tissue close to the skin surface, such as breast or thyroid lumps, testicles, arteries or veins (deep venous thrombosis), or foreign bodies in the skin. Low-frequency probes (3.5 to 5 MHz) are useful for scanning deep internal structures such as those of the abdomen, pelvis, and chest. Linear probes are usually longer probes that use parallel sound waves to produce square or rectangular images (Fig. 209-2, *A*). They require surface contact throughout the length of the probe. Sector probes generally require less surface contact. Sound waves from one point source are

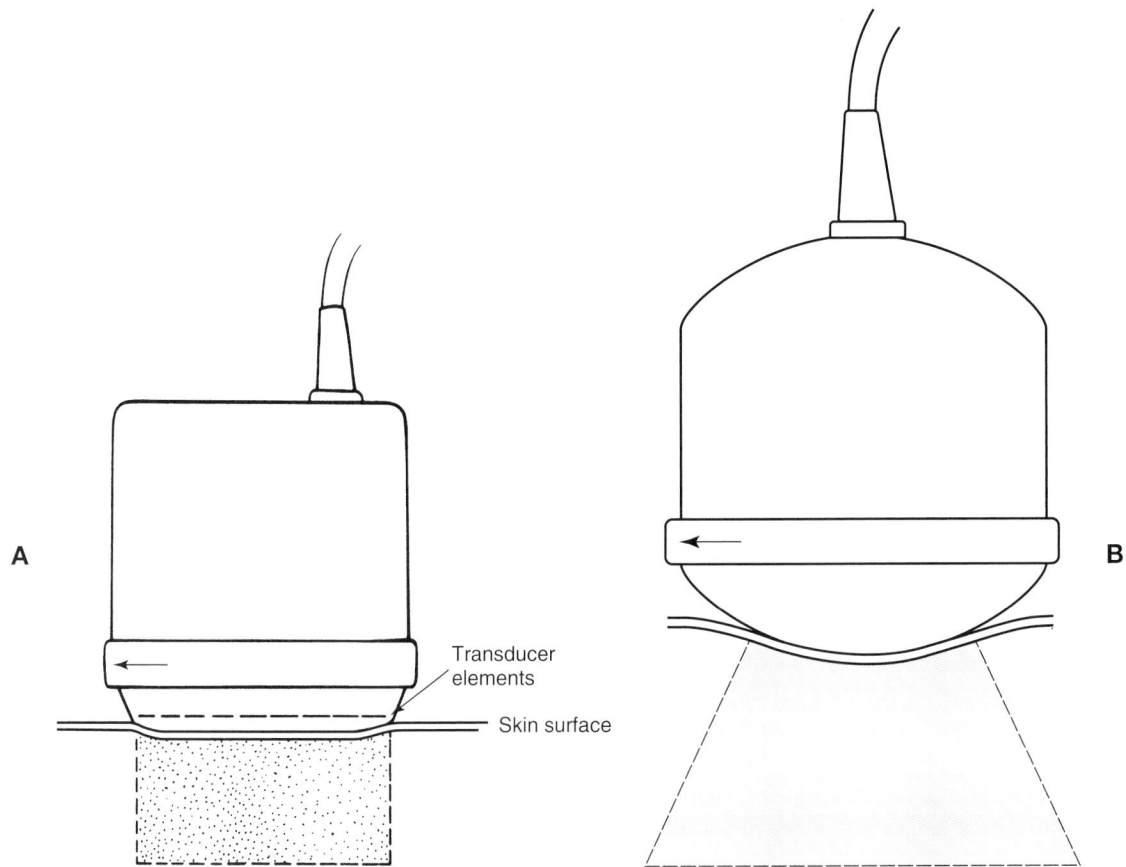

Fig. 209-2
For orientation, either a marker dot or an arrow will be located on one end of the probe. **A,** Linear probe produces a rectangular image and works especially well for obstetrical scans. **B,** Curvilinear probe may be easier to maneuver between ribs. Note wedge-shaped image with curved anterior edge.

directed through a field for sector probes, which produce pie-shaped images (Fig. 209-3). Curvilinear probes are basically linear probes with a curved surface, also requiring less surface contact (Fig. 209-2, *B*). Since less surface contact is required, curvilinear probes make it easier to scan in areas where it would be difficult to maintain good surface contact with a linear probe (e.g., when scanning between ribs).

Another principle of ultrasound is that sound waves travel more readily through solids and liquids than through air; thus acoustic gel must be applied between the body surface and the probe to form an interface. By the same principle, any organs that are predominantly air filled (e.g., lungs or bowel), or any organs posterior to or surrounded by air-filled organs, are difficult to image with sonography. In contrast, the liver, spleen, heart, bladder, and uterus (during pregnancy) are predominantly fluid filled and therefore provide their own excellent "window" for imaging. They also provide "windows" to view surrounding organs or structures. A "window" is an area or organ near the body surface through which sound waves can easily be transmitted to obtain images. For tissue very close to the skin surface such as thyroid, breast masses, and femoral veins, there is very little tissue to be used as a window. In other words, there is little fluid between the probe and the organ. As a result, high-frequency probes often have their own built-in windows.

Note: An after-market standoff or water path can usually be purchased and attached to a low-frequency probe so that, in addition to scanning deep organs, the same probe can be used for scanning near the body surface. If the clinician is not concerned about seeing bubbles, a bag of IV fluid can be used in the same manner, even if it is sometimes awkward to scan through it. Although a higher frequency probe would certainly produce better images in this situation, when first scanning,

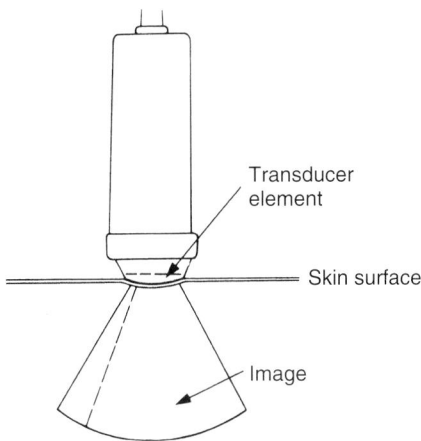

Fig. 209-3
Wedge-shaped image produced by sector scanning probe may be adequate for most applications, depending on width of image.

using a standoff with a low-frequency probe can save the cost of purchasing a high-frequency probe. This allows the primary care clinician to become very proficient with his or her "workhorse" or primary probe, usually a low-frequency 3.5-MHz probe.

Fluid such as amniotic fluid, urine, pus, or blood in the aorta or inferior vena cava appears dark by convention on the ultrasound screen and is "sonolucent" (sound waves pass through). Predominantly fluid-filled organs such as the liver, spleen, or renal cortex appear dark grey on the screen with intermittent, bright echoes within their structure. Solid objects such as polyps, bones, or gallstones are white or "echogenic" (they produce a lot of echoes). If a solid object (calcified or hardened) such as a gallstone is larger than 3 mm, it should cast a well-defined shadow. This type of well-demarcated or "sharp" shadow can be differentiated from shadows cast by air, such as air in the gut. Shadows produced by air are often diffuse or "soft" and change considerably with changes in the placement, angle, or pressure of the probe or with peristalsis.

From an ultrasound perspective, cysts are any fluid-filled structures with smooth walls. Examples include cysts within the ovary, liver, or kidney, but also a full gallbladder, uterus during pregnancy, or urinary bladder. In some ways, the inferior vena cava and abdominal aorta demonstrate cystic properties, such as the following:

- Cysts have smooth walls.
- No echoes or shadows are normally found within cysts.
- There is enhanced visualization of structures or tissue posterior to cysts.
- Cysts demonstrate a penumbra effect.

Due to the third property, cystic structures often serve as excellent windows for tissue being scanned behind or around them. The fourth property is demonstrated as "semi-shadows," or what appear to be shadows, often seen below both sides of a cyst and spreading outward (the penumbra effect). Combined, the appearance of all four acoustic properties may help confirm that whatever is being scanned is a cystic structure. These phenomena may be important after localizing a small mass, especially when trying to determine whether the mass is truly a cyst and might benefit from draining, or whether it is an adenoma.

QUALITY ASSURANCE

For diagnostic purposes, to maximize accuracy and to minimize liability—especially for emergency scans—perhaps only limited, goal-directed studies should be performed instead of complete ultrasound surveys. If the patient is unstable, there may only be time for a limited study. Limited or focused studies can be used to answer a particular clinical question, to improve patient care, or as a follow-up to streamline patient care. Similar to interpreting plain x-rays, the clinician at the bedside knows exactly where the patient is experiencing pain. This information is helpful when interpreting limited studies, especially positive studies. If the patient is stable, complex cases or cases in which portable ultrasound is inconclusive can be referred for a formal study. If the clinical question cannot be answered with certainty, referral or consultation should be obtained. Following these principles, perhaps the rare yet most dreaded error of failure to diagnose can be avoided.

A quality assurance program should be implemented. This could consist of some method of tracking outcomes or comparing results. One method of comparing outcomes while the clinician is learning is to not charge for "learner" scans and to follow-up every scan with a formal scan in the radiology department. Log sheets should be created and used to log the results compared with formal scans. Results should continue to be compared until an acceptable level of clinical accuracy is achieved. Although formal interpretations may differ slightly from "learner" interpretations, the evaluation standard is whether the formal interpretation will lead to a change in clinical management. Having a radiologist overread every scan is another method of ensuring quality; standard images could be obtained with each scan and then reviewed by a radiologist. Internet overreading services by a radiologist are now available (see the "Equipment" section). With either method of quality assurance in place, proof of high-quality clinical data can be maintained and liability can be minimized, especially the liability of failure to diagnose. With these methods of quality assurance, the process of verifying clinician competence can be customized for the individual clinician and documented as well.

As with many procedures in primary care, beginners should develop a relationship with a consultant, either a radiologist or a clinician competent with ultrasound (sonologist). Ultrasound technicians (sonographers) often have extensive skill in multiple areas of ultrasound and can be helpful consultants, especially in rural areas. As the clinician begins performing ultrasound, cases should be discussed and consultation or supervision should be available.

CREDENTIALING

For entire departments adopting ultrasound as a procedure, in addition to quality assurance policies, policies should be in place, regarding credentialing. Without such guidelines, ultrasound can seem quite simplistic, even seductive, and operators may become overconfident. Without guidelines, the risk of failure to diagnose increases with potentially catastrophic outcomes, especially in urgent care or emergency department settings. The author knows of catastrophes in which watchful waiting after failing to diagnose (a leaking abdominal aneurysm and an ectopic pregnancy) was inappropriate management. These catastrophes could have been avoided with appropriate departmental policies, credentialing, and/or a supervision process.

Reasonable guidelines for credentialing nonultrasonographers in an emergency department might require a total of 150 recorded examinations. These examinations should document and demonstrate accuracy with follow-up studies: either formal scans, overreading, or by tracking the clinical outcomes. Experts have suggested documenting 30 examinations of the RUQ; 25 of the pelvis with an abdominal probe and 40 with an endovaginal probe; 25 of the aorta; and 30 trauma examinations, looking for blood in all three of the required locations. At least 50% of the examinations should be abnormal. With these core areas documented, scanning for other diagnoses (pericardial fluid, nephrolithiasis, ultrasonic directed aspiration, etc.) can be managed on a case-by-case basis. Although there is much more to ultrasound that can be learned by performing a certain number of scans, using these numbers merely as guidelines may be helpful when attempting to decide whether a clinician is ready to demonstrate competence. There is also a process where clinicians can be certified as a registered diagnostic medical sonographer (RDMS) after passing certain examinations and being supervised with scanning. It should be noted that the American Academy of Family Physicians does not endorse credentialing for any procedure based on the number of procedures performed or documented.

LIABILITY

When deciding whether performing ultrasound will raise a clinician's liability, the clinician should weigh the liability of failure to diagnose with ultrasound against the risk of not having ultrasound available when certain diagnoses need to be made urgently. If certain diagnoses are not made immediately upon presentation to the office or emergency department (leaking aortic aneurysm, ectopic pregnancy, pericardial effusion, hemoperitoneum, etc.), patients may be endangered and liability may increase. In fact, failure to diagnose ectopic pregnancy has been reported to be the second leading cause (in dollar amounts) of malpractice awards against emergency physicians; ultrasound is the initial procedure of choice to exclude ectopic pregnancy. For these reasons, along with many others, emergency clinicians

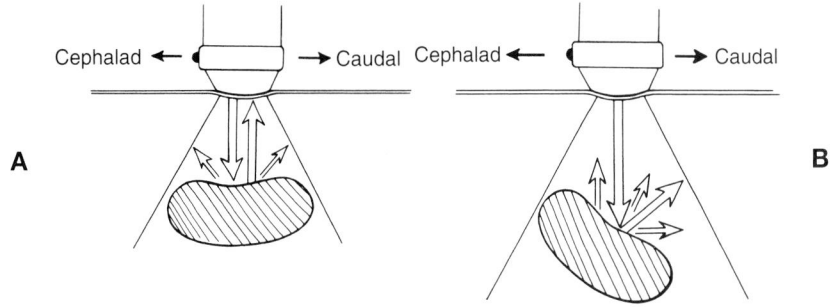

Cephalad ← · → Caudal   Cephalad ← · → Caudal

A   B

Fig. 209-4
A, Best image is produced when the sound beam is perpendicular to the organ interface. **B,** When the sound beam is not perpendicular to the organ interface, scatter is seen, which may cause artifacts.

now perform ultrasound in most large emergency departments. This fact, combined with the fact that ultrasound training is now considered routine for emergency medicine residencies, has led to a change in the standard of care for ultrasound in the emergency department. The standard of care is now considered to be that of a prudent emergency room physician, not a radiologist. Unfortunately, the standard of care in the primary care clinician's office is not as well defined; therefore documentation of competence, absolute certainty of interpretation, or overreading is important.

EQUIPMENT

- Acoustic gel.
- For cardiac and abdominal scanning, a 2.5- to 5.0-MHz sector or curvilinear transducer and scanner is needed. These scanners, or a linear scanner of the same frequency, can also be used for transabdominal obstetric-gynecologic scanning.
- For transvaginal scanning, a 3.5-, 5.0- or 7.5-MHz sector, linear, or curvilinear transducer can be used. Special transvaginal probes are manufactured at those frequencies. Again, the higher the frequency, the higher the resolution and the sharper the image. However, the depth of scanning is decreased with a high-frequency probe, so the transvaginal probe must be applied directly to the cervix. For transvaginal scanning, a probe cover, plain-tipped condom, or examination glove is necessary to place over the probe.
- For pediatric or vascular scans, a 5.0- to 10-MHz sector, curvilinear, or linear scanner can be used.
- For scanning tissue close to the body surface (e.g., thyroid, testicular or breast tissue, veins)—also known as small-parts scanning—a high frequency, 7.5- to 10-MHz, sector, curvilinear, or linear scanner can be used (Box 209-1).

BOX 209-1

Probe Frequencies and Potential Applications (From Low to High Frequency)

3.5 MHz
Cardiac
Abdominal
Pelvic and obstetric
Lumbar puncture in morbidly obese
Pleural effusion

5.0 MHz
Pediatric, including bladder
Transvaginal

7.5-10 MHz
Thyroid mass or cyst
Carotid arteries
Breast mass or cyst
Venous vessels in neck and extremities
Testicular mass
Transvaginal
Pediatric bladder

INITIAL SCANNING

Most clinicians learn human anatomy in three dimensions by dissection. Interpreting ultrasound images requires an ability to translate that knowledge into two dimensions. For proper probe placement and angulation, beginners should understand that the best image is usually generated when the probe is perpendicular to the tissue being studied (Fig. 209-4). Beginners also want to minimize the planes of anatomy with which they must become familiar and should limit their scanning at first to transverse and longitudinal planes. In other words, beginners should keep the transducer marker dot turned toward either the patient's head (longitudinal) or right side (transverse), while holding the probe perpendicular to the organ or tissue being scanned. If the probe can also be held perpendicular to the skin surface, it is easier to scan. Even for the experienced sonographer, using these techniques may be helpful when getting oriented to a particular patient's anatomy at the beginning of any scan.

By convention, when the marker dot is to the patient's right side, it produces a transverse image similar to computed tomography (CT) orientation (Fig. 209-5). The patient's right side will be to the left of the screen. With the marker dot toward the patient's head, the image is what the clinician would see if the patient were dissected longitudinally and viewed looking into the body from the right side with the patient's head to the left of the screen (Fig. 209-6). A

good impression of all of the anatomy and images of most organs can be obtained with longitudinal scanning, alone, at first.

Note: Some European manufacturers reverse the conventional orientation so that the marker dot is found on the right side of the image.

When first getting started, it is important to ask what clinical question(s) can be answered while scanning. Perhaps the answer can be provided with a limited scan rather than an entire ultrasound survey, especially when

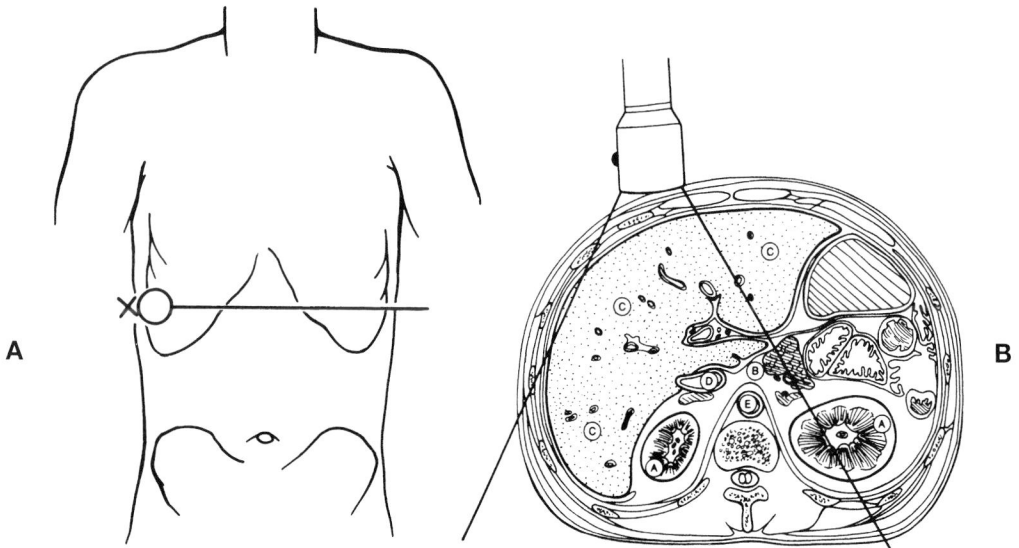

Fig. 209-5
A, Marker dot toward the patient's right side produces a transverse image of the abdomen. **B,** Transverse image: kidneys *(A);* pancreas *(B),* liver *(C);* inferior vena cava *(D);* and aorta *(E).*

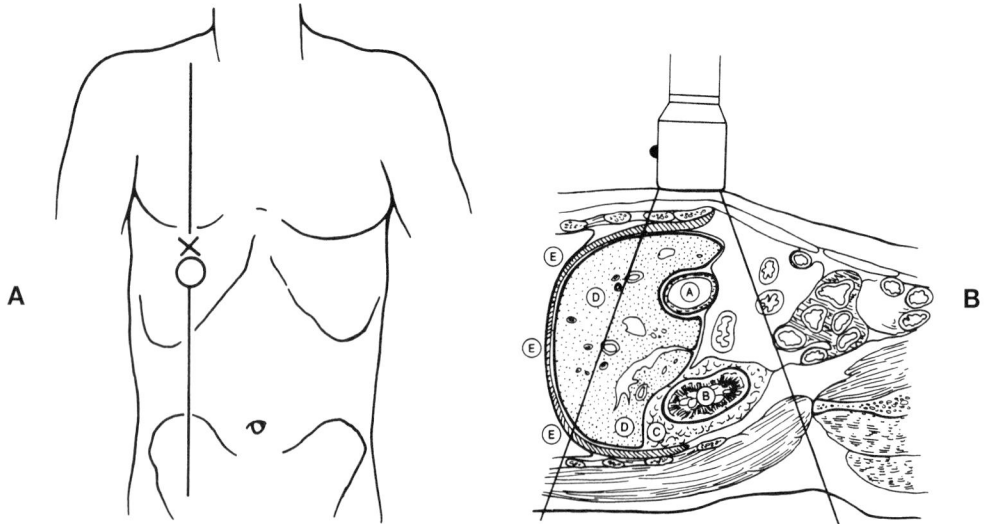

Fig. 209-6
A, Marker dot toward the patient's head produces a longitudinal image of the abdomen. **B,** Longitudinal image: gallbladder *(A);* right kidney *(B);* perirenal fat *(C);* liver *(D);* and diaphragm *(E).*

scanning the abdomen. Again, sonographers and radiologists are trained for formal, complete ultrasound surveys. Emergency department sonography should be brief and goal oriented to answer specific questions raised by the clinical presentation. If a definitive clinical answer cannot be made with portable scanning, a formal study should be ordered or consultation should be obtained.

INDICATIONS

Diagnostic Ultrasound

Cardiac Indications
- Electromechanical dissociation (EMD): narrow electrical complexes on electrocardiogram without measurable blood pressure or clinical evidence of perfusion*
- Suspected pericardial effusion (enlarged cardiac silhouette on chest x-ray, electrical alternans or decreased voltage on ECG)*
- Suspected pericardial tamponade (unexplained hypotension, prominent jugular venous distension, pulsus paradoxus, or EMD)*
- Penetrating wounds to the chest (to exclude hemopericardium)*

Obstetric-Gynecologic Indications
- First trimester vaginal bleeding*
- Suspected ectopic pregnancy*
- Threatened abortion*
- Evaluation of fetal viability (e.g., maternal demise, maternal trauma or inability to auscultate fetal heart tones by Doppler)*
- Misplaced intrauterine device

Abdominal Indications
- RUQ pain*
- Symptoms suggestive of biliary tract disease*
- Suspected acute cholecystitis*
- Obstructive uropathy and renal colic*
- Pulsatile abdominal mass or suspected AAA*
- Suspected hemoperitoneum,* especially when real-time CT is not available or the patient is not stable enough for CT (hemoperitoneum needs to be excluded in a patient with a history of blunt or penetrating trauma to the abdomen or with an altered mental status and an acute abdomen)

---

*These indications have been evaluated thoroughly and are now considered primary applications in emergency medicine. Primary applications are judged to have the greatest potential for bedside use by the emergency clinician in terms of decreasing morbidity or mortality. The remaining indications listed for scanning by nonradiologists have been published, and in many cases studied extensively.

Miscellaneous Indications
- Suspected deep venous thrombosis
- Ultrasonic evaluation of the bladder: prior to suprapubic aspiration (SPA) (e.g., SPA in infants less than 2 years old or in adults) or suprapubic cannulation, or for documentation of postvoiding residual (PVR)
- Subcutaneous foreign bodies
- Testicular mass

Diagnostic-Procedural Ultrasound
- Insertion of central lines
- Lumbar puncture in a morbidly obese individual
- Thyroid or breast mass or cyst, diagnosis and/or aspiration
- Pleural effusion and ultrasonic directed thoracentesis
- Ascites and ultrasonic directed paracentesis

CARDIAC ULTRASOUND

In the unstable hypotensive patient or the patient in shock, if there are narrow QRS ECG complexes, the diagnosis is electro medical dissociation (EMD). The differential includes anything that could cause abrupt cessation of venous return to the heart. Possibilities include: massive pulmonary embolism, tension pneumothorax, acute malfunction of a prosthetic valve, exsanguination, and cardiac tamponade. During resuscitative measures, exclusion of reversible causes is imperative, especially tamponade. Cardiac ultrasound (echocardiography) is the diagnostic procedure of choice for excluding reversible causes of EMD.

A patient with a large pericardial effusion can be completely asymptomatic, can deteriorate rapidly as a result of tamponade, or can be in between. Several scenarios may lead the clinician to suspect a pericardial effusion (e.g., an enlarged cardiac silhouette on chest x-ray, electrical alternans on an ECG), especially in a patient at risk of an effusion. Pericardial tamponade may also result from a penetrating wound to the chest or be the cause of unexplained hypotension, prominent jugular venous distention, or a pulsus paradoxus on physical examination. Echocardiography is also the diagnostic procedure of choice for identifying and quantifying a pericardial effusion. Since rapid intervention is often a necessity in tamponade, ultrasonically directed aspiration of a hemodynamically significant effusion has become the treatment of choice.

Many emergency department clinicians and cardiologists now include a quick portable ultrasound of the heart when evaluating patients with chest pain. By doing this, wall motion abnormalities (suggesting ischemia or a scar) or severe valvular dysfunction can often be noted early in the evaluation. (See Chapter 87, Echocardiography.)

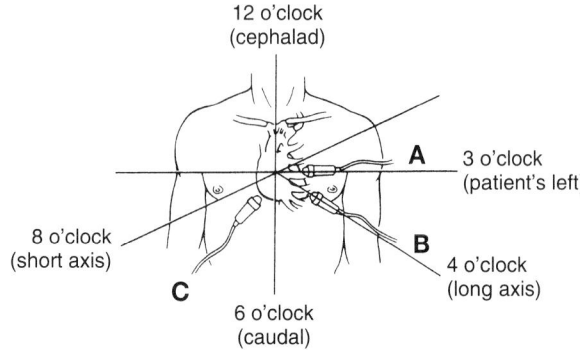

Fig. 209-7
Typical probe positions (placement) for emergency department echocardiogram. **A,** Parasternal position of probe. **B,** Apical position of probe. **C,** Probe in subxiphoid position.

Preprocedure Patient Preparation

Indications for the study and possible findings should be explained to the patient. The patient should be prepared to change positions, if possible during scanning. Adequate gel should be applied to the parasternal, apical, and possibly subxiphoid areas of the chest wall. The patient should be in the supine or left-lateral decubitus position when scanning is initiated.

Technique

While viewing the front of the chest—if the 12 o'clock position is considered cephalad and the 6 o'clock direction caudal—note that the axis of the heart is directed toward the 4 o'clock position. Placing the marker dot of the transducer at about the 4 o'clock position produces the long-axis view of the heart, especially if the probe is located parasternally. The long-axis view is essentially the longitudinal view of the heart, if described in the conventional terminology of ultrasound for the remainder of the body. Rotating the marker dot almost 90 degrees to the 8 o'clock position produces the short-axis view of the heart, which is actually a transverse view of the heart (Fig. 209-7).

1. With the patient in the supine position, place the low-frequency transducer in the parasternal location (third to fourth intercostal space) or apical location (inferolateral to the left nipple at the point of palpated maximal cardiac impulse [PMI]). These are the same two traditional auscultatory points used for a stethoscope.
2. In the parasternal space, the probe or marker dot will be rotated to either the 4 o'clock (long axis) or 8 o'clock (short axis) position. At the apex, the majority of scanning can be performed with the marker dot at the 8 o'clock position.

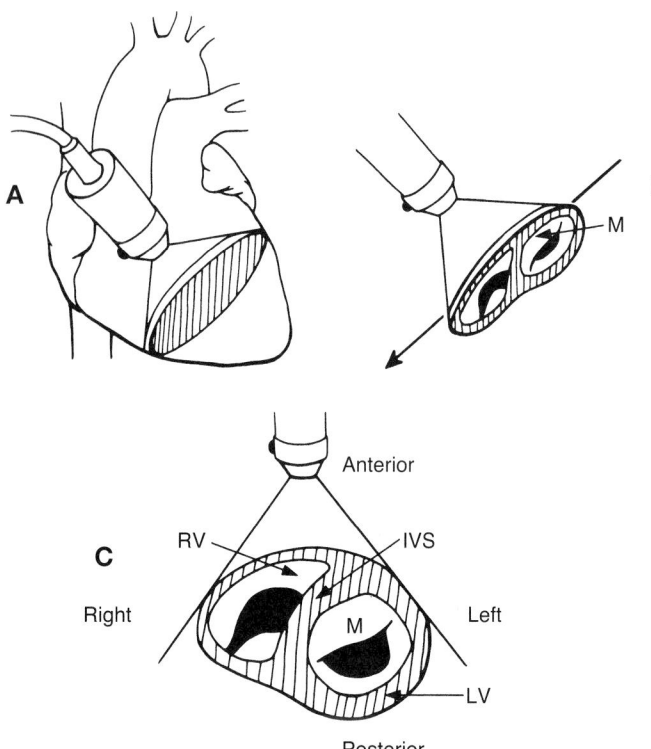

Fig. 209-8
Short axis view at mitral valve level. Probe is in parasternal position with marker dot at the 8 o'clock position. **A,** Ultrasonic plane transects the short axis of the heart at the level of the mitral valve. **B,** Actual endocardiac structures viewed with probe in this position. **C,** Short axis view as it appears on the ultrasound screen. The image is displayed as if it is being viewed from the apex of the heart looking up toward the base. Note "fish mouth" appearance of mitral valve *(M)* as seen from this view. *IVS,* Interventricular septum; *LV,* left ventricle; *RV,* right ventricle.

3. The short-axis view at the level of the mitral valve is often a good view for assessing the adequacy of the window since the mitral valve is usually prominent and easily located. In this view, the mitral valve produces the characteristic "fish-mouth" image (Fig. 209-8), especially if there is any degree of stenosis.
4. If you can change the patient's position easily, place the patient on the left side. This allows the lingula of the lung to fall away from the heart and often provides a better window.

Note: Some ultrasound equipment places the marker dot 180 degrees away from this standard orientation—that is, the 6 o'clock position = what should be the 12 o'clock position. To allow the user to determine the orientation of the probe, the marker on the image should be found. It corresponds with the marker dot on the probe.

For unresponsive patients (those who cannot be moved) or patients with chronic obstructive pulmonary disease (COPD), a subxiphoid view may be needed to obtain a good window. Place the transducer directly below the xiphoid and angle it toward the patient's head with the marker dot toward the patient's right side. A portion of liver will typically be seen at the top of the image.

5. Search for fluid posterior to the heart. If present, it will usually appear at the bottom of the ultrasound screen. If found, quantify the amount of fluid (see Fig. 209-10). For various reasons (including body habitus) up to 10% of patients cannot be scanned adequately for a complete echocardiogram with portable equipment, even under optimal conditions. However, almost all patients with an effusion can be diagnosed, so scan patiently and methodically. With a significant effusion, almost any view is acceptable. If an effusion is not readily apparent, vary the probe angles and amount of pressure applied on the probe for 5 to 10 minutes, if necessary, to find a window. Changing the patient's position may be helpful. All of these maneuvers may be necessary when there is a challenging body habitus or too much air in the lungs (e.g., COPD) obscuring the image. After finding a good window with the parasternal short-axis view, many experts suggest using the parasternal long-axis view to exclude an effusion (Fig. 209-9), because it provides an image of the entire length of the heart. The parasternal long-axis view is obtained after observing the short-axis view by simply rotating the probe about 90 degrees counterclockwise (i.e., marker dot directed toward the 4 o'clock position).

Note: Even large effusions may develop gradually and not cause EMD.

Although the topic is beyond the scope of this chapter, the parasternal long axis view is a great view to qualitatively assess the mitral valve for prolapse. This view cuts the mitral valve lengthwise. The normal anterior leaflet is seen on the superior aspect of the image, and the posterior leaflet is located inferiorly on the image. With real-time scanning, leaflets can be observed opening and closing. In systole, the leaflets should close to about a 90-degree angle from the septal and posterior walls. If the leaflets close and then billow beyond the 90-degree angle, they are prolapsing and a formal echocardiogram may be of benefit to confirm the diagnosis. (See Chapter 87, Echocardiography.)

Interpretation

Electromechanical dissociation. For those patients with EMD, a subjective estimate of the organized cardiac activity is made. Patients with poorly organized or absent cardiac activity when viewed on ultrasound

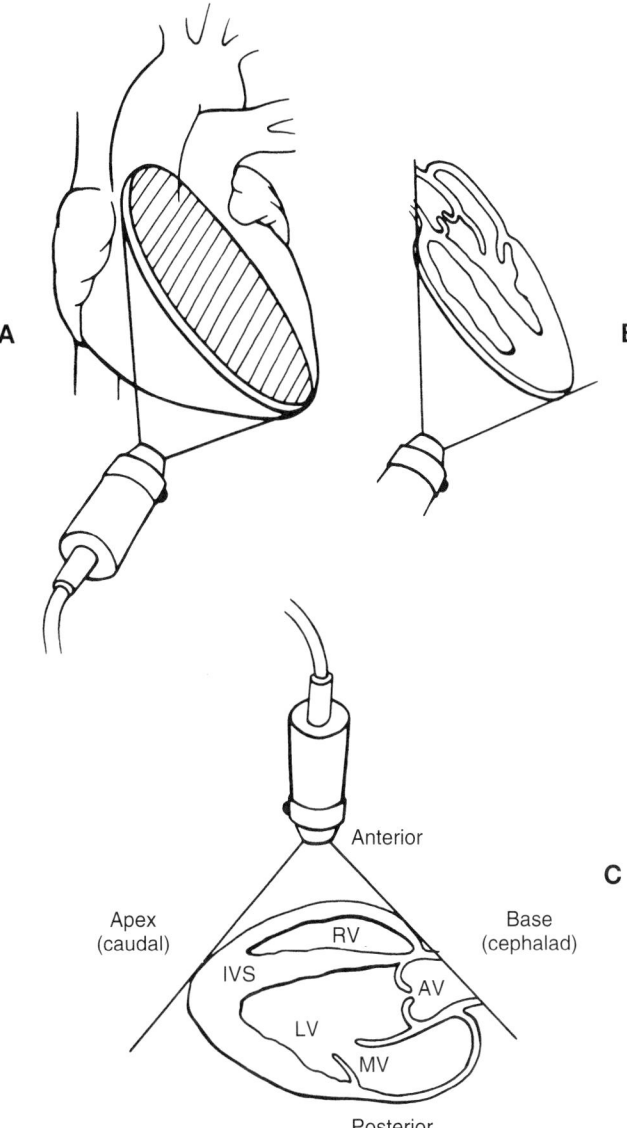

Fig. 209-9
Parasternal long axis view of the heart. Probe is in parasternal position with the marker dot at the 4 o'clock position. **A,** Ultrasonic plane transects heart through the long axis. **B,** Actual endocardial structures viewed. **C,** Image as it appears on ultrasound screen. *AV,* Aortic valve; *IVS,* interventricular septum; *LV,* left ventricle; *MV,* mitral valve; *RV,* right ventricle.

have a prognosis similar to that of patients with the ECG pattern of asystole. Patients with no obtainable blood pressure yet good cardiac contractility appear to carry a better prognosis. An aggressive search for reversible causes of EMD should be carried out in this group. If the EMD is due to pericardial tamponade, a moderate to large pericardial effusion

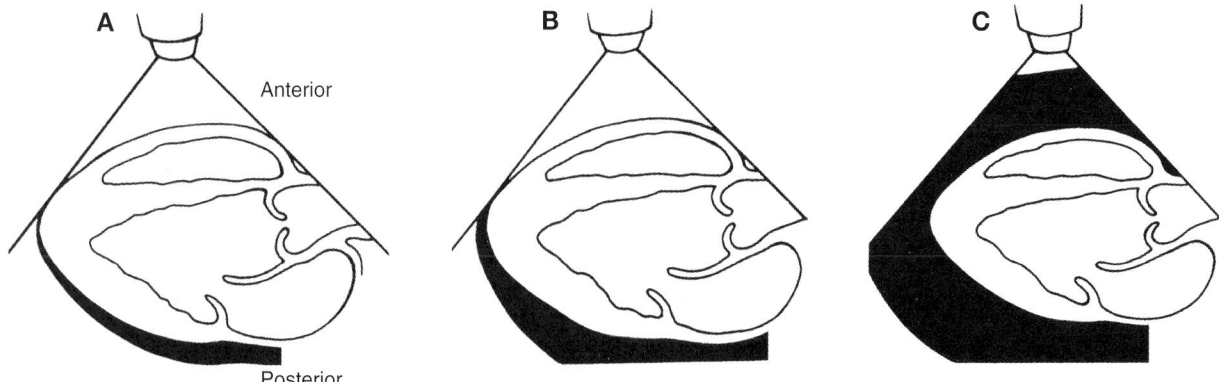

Fig. 209-10
Effusions using a parasternal long axis view. **A,** Small (may be physiologic). **B,** Moderate. **C,** Large.

should be present. The cardiac activity is often well organized with the rhythm regular and the rate tachy. Pericardiocentesis may be life saving. After stabilizing, the findings should be recorded including the size of the effusion.

Effusions *(Fig. 209-10).* A small amount of pericardial fluid may be physiologic. If an effusion is diagnosed, it should be quantified (small, moderate, or large) and recorded. Any hemodynamic compromise should also be noted.

- *Small:* With the patient in the supine position, pericardial fluid is confined posteriorly without anterior, lateral, or apical spread.
- *Moderate:* Effusion more evenly distributed anteriorly, laterally, and apically.
- *Large:* Effusion extends entirely around the heart.

Treatment

Pericardiocentesis should not be performed without sonographic demonstration of an effusion. With experience, the clinician should be able to estimate the amount of fluid that can be aspirated and the depth and angle of penetration necessary for pericardiocentesis. Using this information, a spinal needle can be inserted for pericardiocentesis. Ultrasonic directed pericardiocentesis has replaced blind aspiration as the standard of care in emergency departments.

CPT/Billing Codes

93307	Echocardiography, transthoracic, real-time with image documentation (2D) with or without M-mode recording; complete
93308	Follow-up or limited study
76930	Ultrasonic guidance for pericardiocentesis, imaging supervision and interpretation

ICD-9-CM Diagnostic Codes

423.9	Pericardial effusion, tamponade heart, or unspecified disease of pericardium
420.90	Pericardial effusion, acute
423.0	Hemopericardium
420.99	Pericarditis, acute purulent
420.91	Pericarditis, acute, idiopathic

OBSTETRIC-GYNECOLOGIC ULTRASOUND

I. FIRST-TRIMESTER VAGINAL BLEEDING

Approximately 25% of all diagnosed pregnancies experience bleeding during the first half of pregnancy (see Chapter 173, Obstetric Ultrasound, for differential). Ultrasound is recommended as the first test in patients experiencing bleeding or pain beyond 5 to 7 weeks after their last menstrual period. Two frequent causes of first-trimester vaginal bleeding are ectopic pregnancy and threatened abortion.

Note: If a fetal heartbeat is demonstrated by the less expensive handheld Doppler, pregnancy loss has effectively been ruled out and ectopic pregnancy is much less likely. Doppler heartbeats are not heard until 9 or 10 weeks, and most ectopic pregnancies become symptomatic before that time. With a threatened abortion, demonstrated fetal heartbeats decreases the likelihood of miscarriage to less than 10%. If the Doppler is used during a bimanual pelvic examination and aimed directly at the uterine fundus as it is elevated by the examiner's hand, the likelihood of hearing fetal heart beats is much improved.

A. Suspected Ectopic Pregnancy

Ectopic pregnancies vary in prevalence from 1:28 to 1:200 pregnancies. They account for the majority of first-trimester maternal deaths. The incidence has quadrupled since 1970, and there has been a sevenfold increase in maternal mortality. More than 40% of ectopic pregnancies are misdiagnosed upon first presentation to the healthcare provider.

Emergency department and office sonography coupled with immediately available sensitive radioimmunoassays for human chorionic gonadotropin (HCG) have decreased the morbidity and mortality of ectopic pregnancies. It is important to correlate quantitative HCG levels in your laboratory with the type of equipment available to determine at what level of HCG an intrauterine pregnancy should be visible by sonography. This will vary depending on whether transabdominal or transvaginal scanning is performed.

Risk Factors for Ectopic Pregnancy (in Descending Order of Significance) and Symptoms
* Intrauterine device currently in place or recently used
* Previous tubal, abdominal, or pelvic surgery
* Prior ectopic pregnancy
* Prior sexually transmitted disease, especially pelvic inflammatory disease
* Infertility
* Recent therapeutic abortion

In several large studies, pain (97% to 100% of patients) and amenorrhea (74% to 84%) were more common complaints than vaginal bleeding, although bleeding occurred in the majority of ectopic pregnancies in these studies.

1. Transabdominal Scanning
Preprocedure Patient Preparation
The patient is scanned in the supine position. For an adequate window, the patient's bladder must be full, occasionally to the point of discomfort. If scanning above the pubis does not immediately provide an adequate view, the clinical stability of the patient should be evaluated. If she is stable, either a Foley catheter infusion of fluid (300 to 500 ml) or oral or IV hydration can be used to fill the bladder. If a Foley catheter is used to infuse fluid, the clinician should try to avoid instilling air bubbles into the bladder which can cause echoes and produce a confusing image.

Technique
1. Scanning the bladder first with a low-frequency probe and the marker dot at the patient's right side, determine the shape and orientation of the uterus behind the bladder (Fig. 209-11). Since the bladder is rarely full of floating debris, lower the gain until a minimal number of echoes are demonstrated in the bladder. This will decrease artifact. Confirm that the bladder as opposed to a large ovarian cyst is being used as a window. A large ovarian cyst is usually irregularly shaped, is oval or round, and often

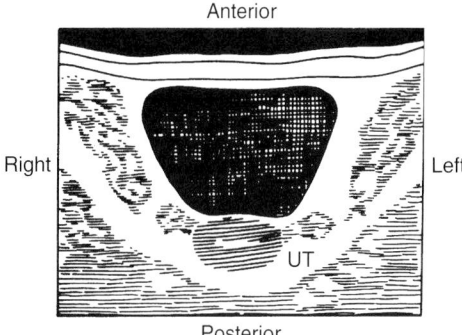

Fig. 209-11
Transverse view of the bladder. Note uterus *(UT),* viewed transversely, is found posterior to the bladder.

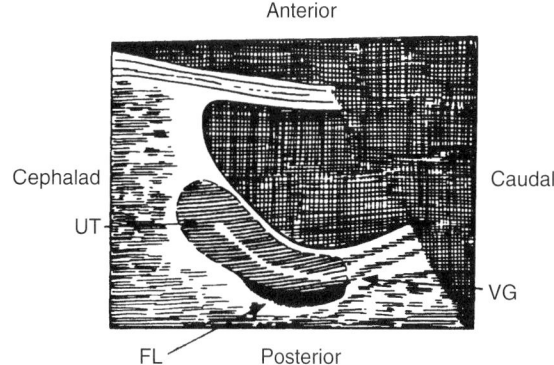

Fig. 209-12
Longitudinal view of the bladder. Note uterus *(UT),* viewed longitudinally, behind the bladder. Fluid in the cul-de-sac *(FL)* is found posterior to the uterus. *VG,* Vagina.

contains complex or echogenic contents. The bladder is basically square in a transverse view.

2. Turn the marker dot cephalad for a longitudinal view (Fig. 209-12). Often the uterus is not quite in the midline, so the probe may need to be rotated slightly out of the midline for a longitudinal image of the uterus. An echogenic line in the midline of the uterus is normal and represents the interface between the anterior and posterior endometria. A pair of dark fluid lines anterior and posterior to the central echogenic line represents endometrium during the proliferative phase. During the secretory phase, the endometrium becomes progressively thicker and echogenic. Occasionally an echogenic line known as the vaginal stripe may be visualized in the vagina, distal to the cervix. It represents another interface.

3. Photograph and document any object or fluid accumulation within the uterus or posterior to the uterus.

4. Scan the adnexa and note any fluid accumulations or abnormalities. Adnexa are usually located by first finding the midline of the uterus. With the probe

producing a longitudinal view of the uterus, rotate it slightly clockwise or counterclockwise so that the marker dot is slightly oblique to the uterus (rotate clockwise to visualize the patient's left adnexa and counterclockwise for her right adnexa). If the adnexa cannot be located with this maneuver, often the probe can be moved laterally off of the midline and while maintaining a longitudinal orientation, the opposite adnexa can be scanned across and through the bladder. In other words, angle the probe about 15 degrees off of the vertical to scan from the patient's left paramedian position. Scan across the midline through the bladder to visualize the patient's right adnexa. The ovary often indents the wall of the bladder.

Interpretation

One technique for excluding ectopic pregnancy is to *rule it out* by *ruling in* an intrauterine pregnancy. With transabdominal scanning, to diagnose ectopic pregnancy by actually visualizing the fetus in a tube or the adnexa is rare (less than 10% of ectopics). Even with higher resolution transvaginal scanning, only occasionally will the ectopic pregnancy be visualized (less than 25% of ectopics).

To confirm an intrauterine pregnancy with ultrasound, a gestational sac with a fetus or fetal pole should be noted. A gestational sac appears as an anechoic (dark) structure within the uterus with highly echogenic borders. The first small echogenic structure seen within the gestational sac is the yolk sac at about 5½ weeks. About a week later, a small collection of echoes may be seen; they constitute the fetal pole. The presence of a gestational sac *with* a fetal pole in the uterus reduces the chance of an ectopic pregnancy to about 1:30,000 cases. This figure represents the likelihood of a concomitant ectopic or "combination" pregnancy during an otherwise low-risk intrauterine pregnancy. Exceptions to this statistic are found in patients undergoing assisted reproduction in which the risk of combination pregnancy may be as high as 1:7000, or in patients taking ovulation stimulating fertility drugs (e.g., clomiphene) in which the incidence may be as high as 1:100. If no fetal pole is seen within what appears to be a gestational sac, the clinician must consider that 10% to 20% of ectopic pregnancies produce pseudogestational sacs in the uterus and that the possibility of an ectopic pregnancy cannot be completely dismissed.

The gold standard for diagnosing an intrauterine pregnancy is the visualization of embryonic cardiac activity. This may be seen as early as 7 weeks after the first day of the patient's last menstrual period or when the mean sac diameter is 12 to 16 mm, depending on the resolution of the equipment and the skill of the examiner. *Mean sac diameter* is determined by measuring a single diameter if the sac is round. It is the average

TABLE 209-1

Dates from Last Menstrual Period Correlated to Findings by Transabdominal Imaging*

Finding	Weeks
Gestational sac	5-6
Yolk sac	5-6
Fetal pole	6-7
Cardiac activity	7-8
Placenta	8-9
Somatic activity	9-10

*Transvaginal imaging can usually locate the same finding 1 week earlier.

of three diameters if the sac is oval. If a fetus is seen, gestational age can also be determined from what else is visualized (Table 209-1). The most accurate estimate of gestational age is at 9 to 11 weeks, using the crown-rump length.

If a normal intrauterine pregnancy is demonstrated, the search for other causes of the patient's symptoms might be facilitated with ultrasound. The clinician should scan for evidence of urolithiasis, adnexal torsion, ruptured ovarian cyst, pelvic inflammatory disease, or appendicitis. Although a description of the ultrasonic findings for most of these situations (except urolithiasis) is beyond the scope of this chapter, the clinician should be aware that each of these diagnoses is associated with particular findings on ultrasound. Urolithiasis is discussed below.

Ovaries are oval-shaped structures of medium echogenicity and lie immediately anterior and medial to the internal iliac arteries, which are pulsatile and have echogenic walls. In women of reproductive age, demonstration of internal follicles often distinguishes ovaries from surrounding structures. Normal ovaries are 2.5 to 5.0 cm long, 1.5 to 3.0 cm wide, and 0.6 to 1.5 cm thick. Evidence of peristalsis on the patient's left side confirms that the colon is being scanned instead of ovary.

If the patient is obese or her bladder is empty, transabdominal ultrasound findings may be limited. Transvaginal scanning may be the only option. In all cases, failure to define an intrauterine pregnancy is interpreted in the proper clinical setting as an ectopic pregnancy until proven otherwise. Eight options exist when an intrauterine pregnancy is not demonstrated by ultrasound (Table 209-2). Correlation with HCG titers may be necessary to complete the interpretation.

With a healthy intrauterine pregnancy, HCG values rise predictably, doubling every 2 to 3 days for the first 8 weeks. In contrast, the HCG titer tends to rise at a slower rate in a patient with an ectopic pregnancy.

Evaluation of the medical literature for quantitative HCG titers correlated with sonographic findings often leads to confusion regarding the standards being used

TABLE 209-2

Possible Diagnoses if an Intrauterine Pregnancy is not Demonstrated by Transabdominal Ultrasound

Diagnosis	Finding	Management
Confirmed ectopic pregnancy	Empty uterus and ectopic fetal heart activity	Surgery or emergent consultation
Highly likely ectopic pregnancy	Empty uterus and echogenic pelvic mass or free pelvic fluid or hemoperitoneum	Surgery, culdocentesis or emergent consultation
Very early normal pregnancy	Serum quantitative HCG <6000 mIU/ml IRP (3000-3250 mIU/ml Second Standard)	Repeat quantitative HCG in 48-72 hr
Occult unruptured ectopic	Empty uterus or may see pseudogestational sac in uterus (seen in 10%-20% of ectopics)	Surgery, consultation, or repeat quantitative HCG in 48-72 hr if stable
Complete or incomplete spontaneous abortion	Empty uterus or atypical echogenic or sonolucent findings in uterus such as a misshapen sac, located low in the uterus or debris in the sac	D & C to treat and/or confirm, consultation, or repeat quantitative HCG. Emergency treatment necessary if cannot exclude ectopic, if patient is unstable or for heavy bleeding.
Dead embryo	Crown-rump length >5 mm and no cardiac motion after continuous observation	Serial quantitative HCGs or repeat ultrasound in a few days; emergency treatment only necessary for heavy bleeding
Embryonic resorption/ blighted ovum	Mean sac diameter of >2.5 cm and no fetal pole or >2.0 cm and no yolk sac (see text for calculating mean sac diameter); also, a misshapen empty sac, located low in uterus or debris in the sac	Emergency treatment only necessary for heavy bleeding.
Hydatidiform mole or trophoblastic disease	Snowstorm appearance of uterine contents	Consultation or D & C

D & C, Dilation and curettage; *HCG,* human chorionic gonadotropin; *IRP,* International Reference Preparation.

TABLE 209-3

Risk of Ectopic Pregnancy in Patients with Positive Human Chorionic Gonadotropin and Empty Uterus on Transabdominal Ultrasound

Ancillary Findings	Risk of Ectopic Pregnancy (%)
Any free fluid	20
Echogenic mass	71
Moderate to large amount of fluid	95
Echogenic mass with fluid	100
No ancillary findings	20

(for a crude conversion, the Second International Standard equals about 50% of the International Reference Preparation [IRP]). Most hospital laboratories are currently using the Second International Standard, whereas much of the early research used IRP. If the IRP standard of HCG quantities is used, transabdominal sonography should detect an intrauterine pregnancy in 94% of cases when the quantitative HCG reaches 6000 to 6500 mIU/ml (3000 to 3250 mIU/ml for Second Standard). This correlates with about 42 days' gestation.

Even if an ectopic pregnancy is not demonstrated by ultrasound, there are associated ultrasonic findings (Table 209-3) that, if seen, significantly increase the likelihood of ectopic pregnancy. In the case of a ruptured ectopic, scanning the upper abdomen may reveal free fluid representing intraabdominal hemorrhage. While a moderate to large amount of fluid is highly correlated with an ectopic pregnancy, any free fluid is significant in the proper clinical situation. A demonstrated echogenic pelvic mass also significantly increases the likelihood of ectopic pregnancy.

2. Transvaginal Scanning

Preprocedure Patient Preparation

The patient is scanned in the supine or lithotomy position. Transvaginal scanning is usually preceded by transabdominal scanning with a full bladder, perhaps allowing the clinician to make the diagnosis, and, if not, to assess the overall anatomy. The bladder can then be emptied; however, some residual urine can serve as a useful marker for locating the bladder.

Technique

1. Prepare the probe by covering with a probe sheath, a plain-ended latex condom, or an examination glove. Adequate gel should be placed on the tip of the transducer before covering. Any bubbles between the cover and transducer should be smoothed out before scanning.

2. Perform a preliminary pelvic examination to relax the vagina as well as to evaluate for palpable masses. Determine the size, shape, and position of the uterus, and define any areas of tenderness. Any tampons should be removed. Counsel the patient about the transvaginal ultrasound examination and obtain verbal consent.

3. While continuing to wear examination gloves, gently insert the probe with posterior vaginal pressure to a position anterior to the cervix.

4. With the marker dot anterior, locate the midline of the uterus in the image.

5. Obtain both longitudinal and coronal scans of the uterus and adnexa by turning the marker dot anterior to the patient or toward her right side. For longitudinal scanning, the image orientation changes slightly (Fig. 209-13), compared with transabdominal scanning. Since the marker dot is pointed toward the anterior abdominal wall of the patient, the left side of the resultant image is actually anterior instead of cephalad. Transverse orientation also changes slightly because true anterior-posterior images of the uterus cannot be obtained by scanning from below. However, various coronal images are obtained that are similar to transverse images. The patient's right side remains on the left side of the image because the marker dot is turned to the patient's right side (Fig. 209-14).

6. Scan the uterus by performing a series of longitudinal, coronal, and oblique scans with the transducer at varying depths of penetration. Oblique views are obtained by rotating the probe with the marker dot in the longitudinal position to either the right or left side of the patient. Oblique views are used to scan the adnexa.

7. Note any evidence of a fetus or fluid accumulations. Any areas of tenderness should be documented along with any other important findings.

Interpretation

The interpretation for transvaginal scanning is the same as for transabdominal scanning, except that with a fetus, everything is visualized approximately 1 week earlier than with transabdominal scanning. The correlations with HCG must also be corrected (Table 209-1). Transvaginal scanning can usually detect an intrauterine gestational sac at 2000 mIU/ml IRP (1000 mIU/ml Second Standard) or about 35 days' gestation. For a patient with a quantitative HCG above this level and no intrauterine pregnancy visualized, ectopic pregnancy must be considered. If there is no vaginal bleeding, ectopic pregnancy becomes almost certain.

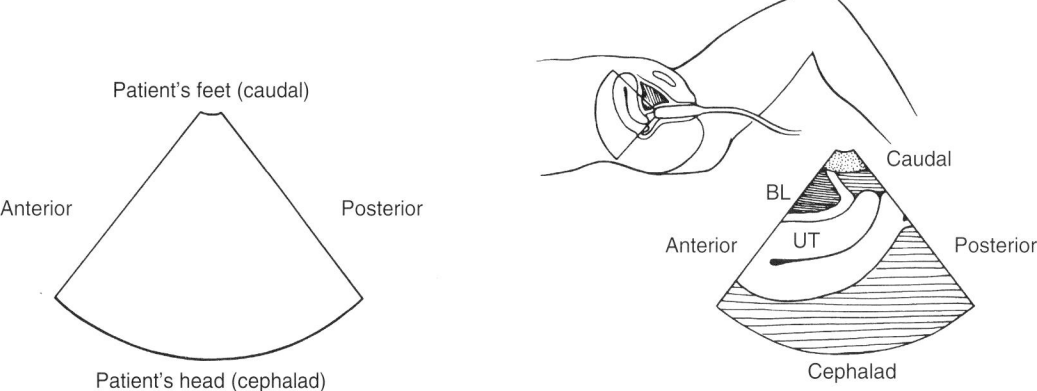

Fig. 209-13
Longitudinal orientation with transvaginal scanning. *BL*, Bladder; *UT*, uterus.

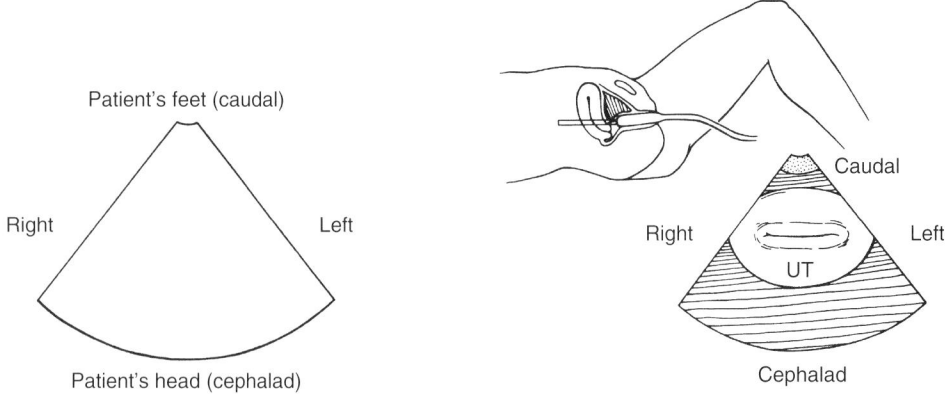

Fig. 209-14
Transverse orientation with transvaginal scanning. *UT*, uterus.

Advantages of transvaginal scanning over transabdominal include the following:

- Higher frequency probe with higher resolution
- Fewer tissue layers through which to scan (nine layers on transabdominal), resulting in less artifact
- Less patient preparation, especially regarding the bladder

These advantages allow an intrauterine pregnancy to be diagnosed by about 5 weeks after the first day of the patient's last menstrual period. Fetal cardiac activity can frequently be seen by 6 weeks. With transvaginal scanning, there is also a greater likelihood of visualizing an ectopic pregnancy in a tube or the adnexa.

Disadvantages include the necessities of an extra probe, a sheath, and additional training. Interpretation is slightly more confusing and the field of imaging is slightly narrower. Despite the fact that patients are becoming more familiar with and accepting of this technology, transvaginal scanning is also slightly more invasive.

ICD-9-CM Diagnostic Codes

623.8	Vaginal bleeding
630	Hydatidiform mole
631	Blighted ovum
632	Missed abortion
633.0	Abdominal pregnancy
633.1	Tubal pregnancy
633.9	Ectopic pregnancy, unspecified
634.91	Abortion or miscarriage, incomplete, without complication
634.92	Abortion or miscarriage, complete, without complication

B. Threatened Abortion

Management of a threatened abortion consists of ruling out possible causes (or treating them), assessing the amount of bleeding, and predicting the prognosis for the pregnancy. If bleeding is minimal and no specific cause is identified, such as infection (e.g., urinary tract or cervix) or anemia, the patient is discharged in most cases with instructions for bed rest, to minimize stress, and to increase hydration. If the evaluation can be completed entirely in the emergency department or the office, treatment goals are more readily accomplished than if the patient must undergo a stressful evaluation in another department. Using specific sonographic criteria, the clinician may also determine which patients need additional ultrasound studies as well as reasonably estimate the prognosis of the early pregnancy. Without ultrasound, the only prediction the clinician can make is that 50% of all threatened abortions will progress to miscarriage.

Preprocedure Patient Preparation and Technique

These are the same as those in the previous "Suspected Ectopic Pregnancy" section. Frequently, the diagnosis of threatened abortion is made after ruling out ectopic pregnancy.

Interpretation and Management

Presence of fetal cardiac activity is an encouraging finding in an early pregnancy, since the risk of spontaneous abortion is less than 2% to 4% if fetal cardiac activity is seen after 12 weeks. The risk of miscarriage is less than 16% if cardiac activity is noted at less than 8 menstrual weeks, which is much lower than the 50% predicted if ultrasound is not available or performed.

With earlier pregnancies (even before the embryo is visible), major and minor criteria are available for evaluating gestational sacs (see Chapter 173, Obstetric Ultrasound). Again, patients with gestational sacs meeting most or all of these criteria by ultrasound are much less likely to miscarry than the 50% rate predicted if the patients are evaluated by clinical means alone.

Failure to meet at least one major criterion is 100% specific in predicting spontaneous abortion. Fifty-three percent of abnormal pregnancies are identified by the same criteria. If there is a question about an abnormal sac, the patient should be scanned 7 to 10 days later. As an additional criterion during that time, the mean sac diameter in normal pregnancies should increase by about 1 mm per day.

Examples of abnormalities include low-lying gestational sacs (sacs in the cervical region) and abnormally shaped sacs. Both of these are worrisome findings and should be followed with a scan a week later. Frequently, low-lying sacs lead to spontaneous abortions, whereas abnormally shaped sacs lead to abnormal pregnancies. Worrisome findings also include failure of the sac to gain 1 cm in mean sac diameter in 1 week or the ability to visualize an embryo when the sac reaches 2.5 cm in mean sac diameter. These findings may assist the clinician in preparing the patient for the possibility of an abnormal pregnancy, such as one resulting in a spontaneous miscarriage.

ICD-9-CM Diagnostic Codes

623.8	Vaginal bleeding
632	Missed abortion
640.03	Threatened abortion, antepartum

II. EVALUATION OF FETAL VIABILITY

Detection of fetal heart activity by the second and third trimester of pregnancy should be reliable by transabdominal scanning. Earlier detection may require transvaginal scanning.

Preprocedure Patient Preparation and Scan Technique

See Chapter 173, Obstetric Ultrasound, for late-trimester scanning. See above for early-trimester scanning.

Interpretation

Absence of fetal movement after scanning for a 5-minute interval in a pregnancy of more than 20 weeks' gestation is said to be 100% reliable for diagnosing a fetal demise. For a first-trimester pregnancy, if uncertainty exists about fetal heart activity, rescanning should be performed in 1 to 2 weeks.

Secondary criteria for fetal demise using ultrasound include fetal anomalies such as hydrops, ascites, and pleural or pericardial effusions. Echogenic gas in the fetal heart and vessels may be early findings. Late findings include morphological changes such as skeletal anomalies and unusual fetal positioning.

Reaction to external stimulation or uterine manipulation should cause brisk reflexes in viable fetuses as opposed to the passive motions seen in a fetal demise. Avoid misinterpreting the passive motions from uterine contractions around a dead fetus as fetal activity.

Since abruptio placenta cannot always be diagnosed with ultrasound (i.e., it is a clinical diagnosis), ultrasound studies should be used in conjunction with maternal-fetal monitoring in the pregnant patient with significant abdominal trauma. A 4-hour monitoring period should be sufficient to identify fetal distress.

ICD-9-CM Diagnostic Codes

655.73   Decreased fetal movements, antepartum
656.43   Intrauterine fetal death, late

III. MISPLACED INTRAUTERINE DEVICE

Certain intrauterine devices (IUDs) are now approved for 10 years of continuous use. This length of time offers many opportunities to lose the string. When a string is not palpable on an IUD, possible causes include a properly positioned IUD in the uterus that has lost its string, an extruded IUD, or an IUD that has perforated the uterus and may even be lying in the abdomen. IUD users who have not lost the string also warrant further evaluation if they are experiencing cramping, pain, or abnormal bleeding. A flat plate radiograph may document the presence of the IUD, but it will not be able to determine whether the IUD is in the uterus. Gynecologic instrumentation is another option, but instrumentation places the patient at risk of infection. It should be reserved for removal of the IUD after the location is documented. In most cases, ultrasound is the diagnostic procedure of choice to determine the location of an IUD. However, the diameter of most IUDs is less than 3 mm; therefore scanning for IUDs in some cases is more difficult than expected.

Preprocedure Patient Preparation and Technique

Preparation and technique are the same as for ectopic pregnancy scanning.

Interpretation

An IUD on ultrasound produces a very straight, sharp-edged, echogenic image. Document the location of the IUD in both longitudinal (Fig. 209-15, *A*) and transverse or coronal views (Fig. 209-15, *B*). If an IUD is not demonstrated and the posterior wall of the uterus is not easily identified, formal scanning may be necessary. IUDs may be difficult to locate when the uterus is retroverted.

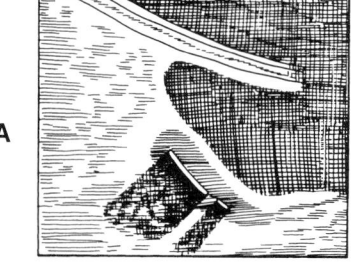 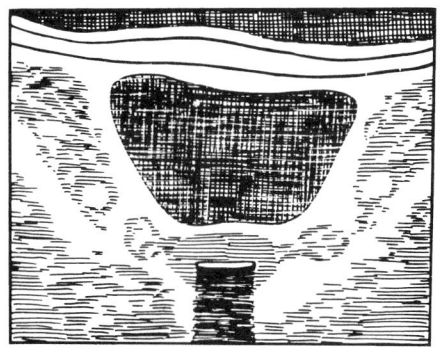

A   **B**

Fig. 209-15
Intrauterine device in, **A,** longitudinal and, **B,** transverse views.

Decidual reaction may mimic an IUD. To differentiate, an IUD should produce shadowing in at least one plane. Echoes from an IUD are typically straighter and sharper-edged than those from a decidual reaction.

A perforation should be recorded as either complete or incomplete. For an incomplete perforation, a portion of the IUD can be demonstrated within the uterine wall. A flat plate x-ray film may be necessary to document the location for a complete perforation if it is not visible by ultrasound.

CPT/Billing Codes

76830   Ultrasound, transvaginal
76856   Ultrasound, pelvic (nonobstetric), B-scan and/or real time with image documentation; complete
76857   Limited or follow-up (e.g., for follicles)

ICD-9-CM Diagnostic Codes

V25.42   Intrauterine device, checking, reinsertion, or removal

See Chapter 173, Obstetric Ultrasound, for coding on gravid uterus.

ABDOMINAL ULTRASOUND

Various tests can be used when deciding whether conditions are good enough to perform a complete abdominal survey, especially if using portable equipment. First, if the bladder is full, the gain on the machine should be set low enough to eliminate echoes from a normally nonechogenic organ. Next, the clinician should attempt to scan the aorta lengthwise. Repositioning may be required, and the liver may be needed as a window. If the aorta is located, the gain should be reset to minimize internal echoes because this organ normally has no echoes. (This gain setting should be used for scanning the majority of the abdomen.)

If the clinician is unable to locate the aorta after several attempts and several minutes of scanning, body habitus or conditions may preclude a complete abdominal survey or scan. The clinician may be restricted to a focused or limited scan. The pelvis with a full bladder and the liver, right kidney, and RUQ structures will probably be easiest to scan. A referral may be necessary for a complete formal scan for other abdominal structures if additional clinical data are needed.

I. BILIARY TRACT DISEASE

Acute cholecystitis in the ambulatory setting results from obstruction of the cystic duct by gallstones in approximately 95% of cases. Unfortunately, the diagnosis of

acute cholecystitis by purely clinical means (without ultrasound) has an accuracy of only 50%, even with a positive "Murphy's sign" (pain over the gallbladder with palpation during inspiration). Therefore real-time ultrasound is the preferred diagnostic test for acute cholecystitis. A "sonographic Murphy's sign" combined with the presence of gallstones increases the diagnostic accuracy for acute cholecystitis to more than 90%. A "sonographic Murphy's sign" is described as pain elicited with probe compression over a gallbladder. Because early surgical management is now the treatment of choice for acute cholecystitis, early diagnosis is also important. Bedside ultrasound is useful in diagnosing most cases of cholelithiasis and acute cholecystitis; however, obscure cases may require additional studies.

Preprocedure Patient Preparation

If possible, the patient should have been in the fasting state for at least 8 hours; this ensures that the gallbladder is fully distended. Early morning scanning may be preferable because bowel gas is usually minimal.

Technique

1. Scan the patient in the supine position, longitudinally, with a low-frequency probe until you locate the gallbladder. It is usually located in about the midclavicular line. The normal gallbladder is a cystic structure; when distended, it demonstrates the properties of cysts elsewhere in the body. The walls are smooth, usually no echogenic matter exists between the walls, and tissue behind the posterior wall is more clearly defined.

Other cystic structures located near the gallbladder that can be confused with the gallbladder include hepatic cysts, hepatic veins, the portal vein, renal cysts, the duodenum, the inferior vena cava, and the abdominal aorta. Hepatic cysts are usually located much deeper in the hepatic parenchyma than the gallbladder. They have very thin walls. Hepatic veins usually run vertically within the liver when the patient is supine. They also have very thin walls, which are compressible with probe pressure. Veins collapse with inspiration and expand with a Valsalva maneuver. If followed posteriorly, the location of where the hepatic veins empty into the inferior vena cava can usually be seen just below the diaphragm. Although the portal vein has echogenic sidewalls similar to the gallbladder, it can usually be viewed coursing horizontally through the liver. Often tributaries to the portal vein, such as the splenic vein, can be traced from where they originate to where they join to form the portal vein near the liver. Renal cysts can usually be demonstrated as very thin walled and contiguous

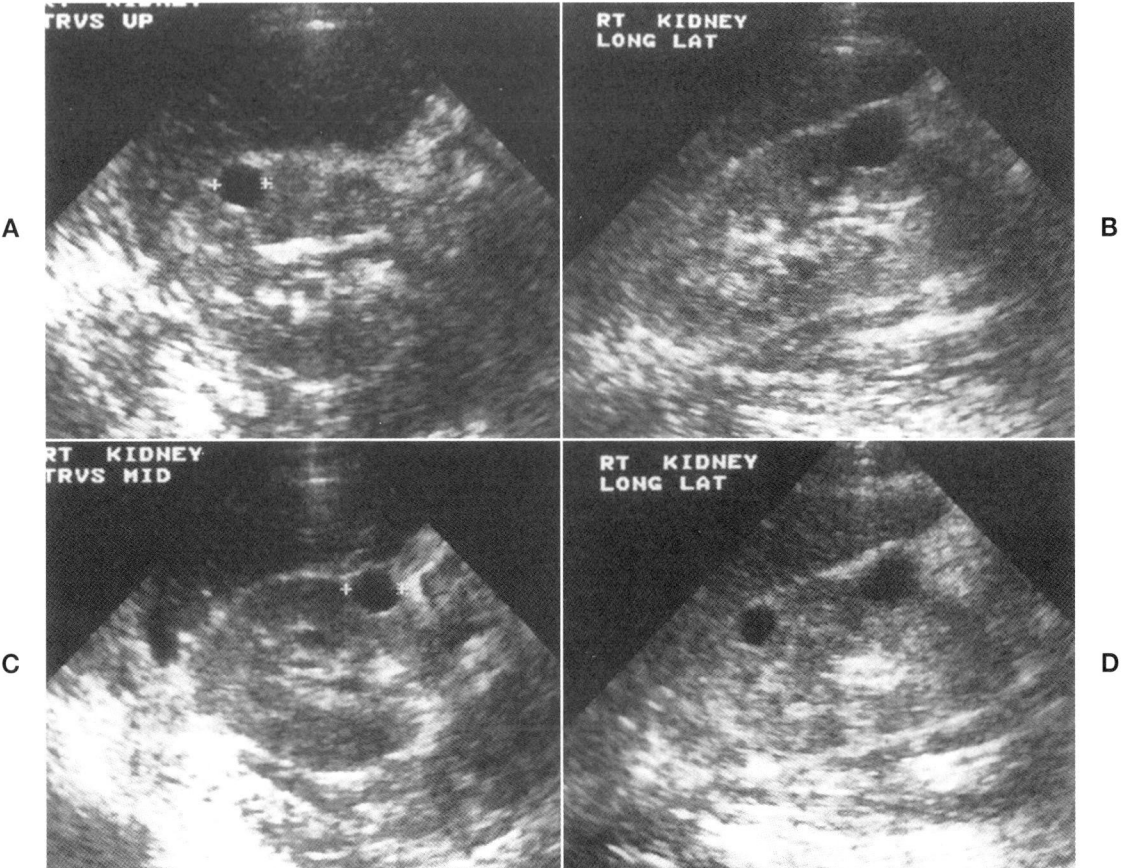

Fig. 209-16
Transverse (**A** and **C**) and longitudinal (**B** and **D**) scans of two small renal cysts along the lateral wall of the kidney. Borders are smooth and well defined. No echoes are present. (From Hagen-Ansert SL: *Textbook of diagnostic ultrasonography,* ed 4, St Louis, 1995, Mosby.)

with renal tissue (Fig. 209-16). They are located much further lateral and posterior than the gallbladder. Although the abdominal aorta has echogenic walls, it demonstrates pulsations and can be followed distally. Pulsations transmitted from the aorta may also be noted in the inferior vena cava. Having the patient take in a large breath should collapse the vena cava; a Valsalva maneuver should cause significant dilation. The duodenum can usually be distinguished from the gallbladder because peristalsis can be observed. Having the patient drink water can stimulate peristalsis in the duodenum. Air in the duodenum usually casts confusing, irregular shadows as opposed to the sharp shadows of gallstones.

Compared with other abdominal organs, the gallbladder usually has a rather superficial location on the inferior edge of the liver. Prolonged deep inspirations by the patient may bring the liver edge down from under the subcostal margin to facilitate locating the gallbladder. Scanning between ribs may also be necessary to obtain a good window through the liver.

2. After locating the gallbladder with the probe in the longitudinal position, obtain a long-axis view of the gallbladder by rotating the probe out of the longitudinal plane of the body until the maximal length of the gallbladder is visualized.
3. Obtain additional views of the gallbladder by moving the patient into one other position: the decubitus (right side up) position or the erect position. Repositioning the patient helps to avoid missing stones that may have rolled into a dependent position out of view.
4. Attempt to identify the source of any local tenderness and scan that area.

Interpretation

An echogenic structure within the gallbladder is a gallstone if it shows prominent posterior shadowing, has circumferential bile visible in at least one view, and has demonstrated mobility when the patient is placed in various positions (Fig. 209-17). When

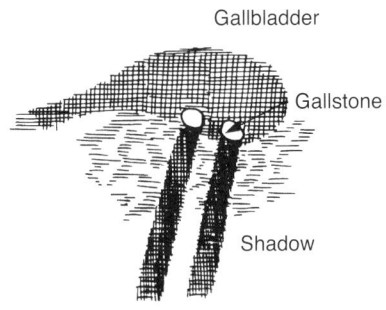

Gallbladder

Gallstone

Shadow

Fig. 209-17
Acoustic shadowing behind two gallstones. Note the "sharpness" of the shadow.

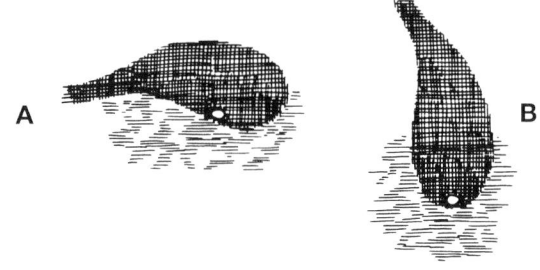

A

B

Fig. 209-18
A, Stone is small and shadowing is not seen. **B,** However, it moves when the patient is repositioned.

coupled with a positive "sonographic Murphy's sign," this is diagnostic of acute cholecystitis. Otherwise, gallstones can have several variations when viewed sonographically:

1. *Nonshadowing:* Gallstones less than 2 to 3 mm in size often do not cast a shadow. In that situation the differential also includes structures such as polyps or folds that can appear echogenic within the gallbladder. In fact, echogenic structures in the gallbladder that are nonshadowing are calculi in only 50% of cases. If, however, an echogenic structure is noted to have gravity-dependent motion it is usually a stone (Fig. 209-18).

2. *Intermittent shadowing:* Multiple small stones may form an irregular layer in the most dependant portion of the gallbladder. They may also cast a variable or intermittent shadow. This may be highly suspicious for cholelithiasis, but further studies are necessary if there is no well-defined shadowing.

3. *Filled gallbladder:* If the gallbladder is entirely filled with stones, bile may not be noted circumferentially around any one stone. Shadowing may be less prominent or hazy. Since a gas-filled duodenum can have this same appearance, it must be carefully eliminated from the differential by studying for other characteristics (e.g., peristalsis).

4. *Adherent stones:* These can appear as echogenic structures that are not gravity dependent. If no shadowing is seen, further studies may be necessary to exclude a polyp, tumor, or fold, which can also be echogenic.

5. *Floating stones:* Stones occasionally float. Either one stone or a collection of stones may appear as an echogenic structure or a line of echoes in a nondependent portion of the gallbladder. If they do not cast a shadow, further studies may be necessary.

6. *Absent gallbladder:* This sonographic finding (absence) may also be noted in a nonfasting patient or in one with chronic cholecystitis and severe scarring preventing expansion of the gall bladder. A patient with a completely stone-filled gallbladder, with a previous cholecystectomy, or with congenital absence of a gallbladder may also have a nonvisible gallbladder. If the gallbladder is not readily imaged and the patient is clinically stable, additional scanning should be performed several hours later with the patient fasting.

Additional possible findings within and around the gallbladder include the following:

1. *Sludge:* Low-level to mixed echogenic material that is slow to layer out after the patient changes positions may be gallbladder sludge. It most commonly represents biliary stasis and may occur in various conditions (e.g., obstructive jaundice, liver disease, sepsis) or in patients receiving hyperalimentation or certain other medications. It may also precede the formation of gallstones by a few years.

2. *Edema:* A thin, dark line of fluid around the gallbladder wall may represent gallbladder edema, which can be found in acute cholecystitis or other conditions such as hypoalbuminemia, hepatitis, or ascites. In the situation where the patient has a "sonographic Murphy's sign," discrete pockets of fluid may represent small abscesses. These abscesses are often near the fundus and are definitive evidence of acute cholecystitis.

3. *Thickening:* Wall thickening is not specific for acute cholecystitis. A rim of diffuse echogenicity greater than 3 mm thick around the gallbladder may represent hepatic dysfunction, congestive heart failure, renal disease, ascites, sepsis, or neoplasms elsewhere (decreased osmotic pressure and elevated portal venous pressures). Patients with AIDS may also have diffuse thickening. Irregular wall thickening is also common with both acute and chronic cholecystitis. If no stone is present, yet the patient has a positive sonographic Murphy's sign, acalculous cholecystitis is a possibility.

ICD-9-CM Diagnostic Codes

575.10	Cholecystitis
575.11	Cholecystitis, chronic
575.12	Cholecystitis, acute and chronic
574.20	Cholelithiasis, without obstruction
574.21	Cholelithiasis, with obstruction
789.0	Pain, abdominal
576.8	Cholestasis
576.9	Pain, bile duct
575.9	Pain, gallbladder

II. OBSTRUCTIVE UROPATHY AND RENAL COLIC

Obstruction of the collecting ducts of the kidney may be acute or chronic, and unilateral or bilateral. As many as 15% of American males will suffer an episode of renal colic severe enough to require emergent medical attention. With flank pain and hematuria being the hallmark signs and symptoms for a stone, no further diagnostics may be necessary if a patient responds to potent analgesics. Expectant management may be adequate. For those in whom further diagnostics are necessary, studies have indicated that plain radiographs (kidney, ureter, and bladder [KUB]) rarely change the clinician's management of renal colic. Intravenous pyelograms (IVPs) can be used when direct imaging of the urinary tract is necessary. Studies comparing sensitivity of ultrasound and IVP have found them to be relatively comparable. However, most studies have found IVP to be somewhat more specific. Nonetheless, in certain situations, ultrasound may be preferred over IVP (Box 209-2). Even if ultrasound does not reveal the diagnosis, at least it is noninvasive and certainly can be followed up with an IVP.

Note: A leaking or dissecting AAA may produce signs and symptoms similar to left-sided renal colic, including hematuria. In fact, left-sided renal colic is the most common misdiagnosis in elderly patients with a symptomatic AAA. In patients over 55 years of age with left-sided renal colic, ultrasound should be considered to exclude this potentially fatal diagnosis which may be missed with an IVP.

BOX 209-2

Conditions in Which Ultrasound May be Preferable to Intravenous Pyelogram (IVP)

Dehydration
Pregnancy
Contrast allergy
Poor venous access
Renal failure or proteinuria
Diabetes mellitus
Differential diagnosis includes dissecting aortic aneurysm or acute cholecystitis
Time constraints
Inadequate abdominal prep for IVP

Preprocedure Patient Preparation

Under optimal conditions, the patient should have been in the fasting state for at least 8 hours to minimize bowel gas. Early morning scanning may be preferable; bowel gas is usually minimal. Understanding that patients do not always come to the emergency department or the office under these conditions, the clinician may need to hydrate the patient to increase the hydronephrosis and enhance the acoustic window. Therefore, administering IV fluids may not only be therapeutic but may also be helpful for making the diagnosis.

Technique

1. Scan the patient in the supine position, longitudinally, with a low-frequency probe until the kidney is located. Kidneys are football shaped with a white stripe (echogenic renal sinus) down the middle. The renal sinus is surrounded by the echolucent renal cortex, which in turn is surrounded by the echogenic renal capsule (Fig. 209-19, *A*). Compared with other abdominal organs, the kidneys are very posterior and lateral organs. On the right, the kidney is located at the posterior, inferior edge of the liver, far lateral to the midclavicular line. Prolonged deep inspiration by the patient should bring the liver edge down from under the subcostal margin to facilitate locating the kidney. Scanning between the ribs may also be necessary to obtain a good window through the liver.

2. The left kidney is located slightly higher than the right. On the left, the same maneuvers may enhance the use of the spleen as an acoustic window. Having the patient turn completely onto their right side to facilitate scanning in the coronal and transverse planes may also be helpful. Even scanning between the ribs from the back may be useful. Occasionally, having the patient sit in the erect position will bring the kidney into view. If no kidney is found on the left side, attempt to locate the kidney by scanning the pelvis for a pelvic kidney or the midline for a horseshoe kidney.

3. After locating each kidney, with the probe in the longitudinal position, obtain a long-axis view. Rotate the probe out of the longitudinal plane of the body until the maximal length of the organ is visualized.

4. Attempt to assess for the presence or absence of hydronephrosis or hydroureter in both kidneys. Also attempt to locate intrarenal or extrarenal calcifications.

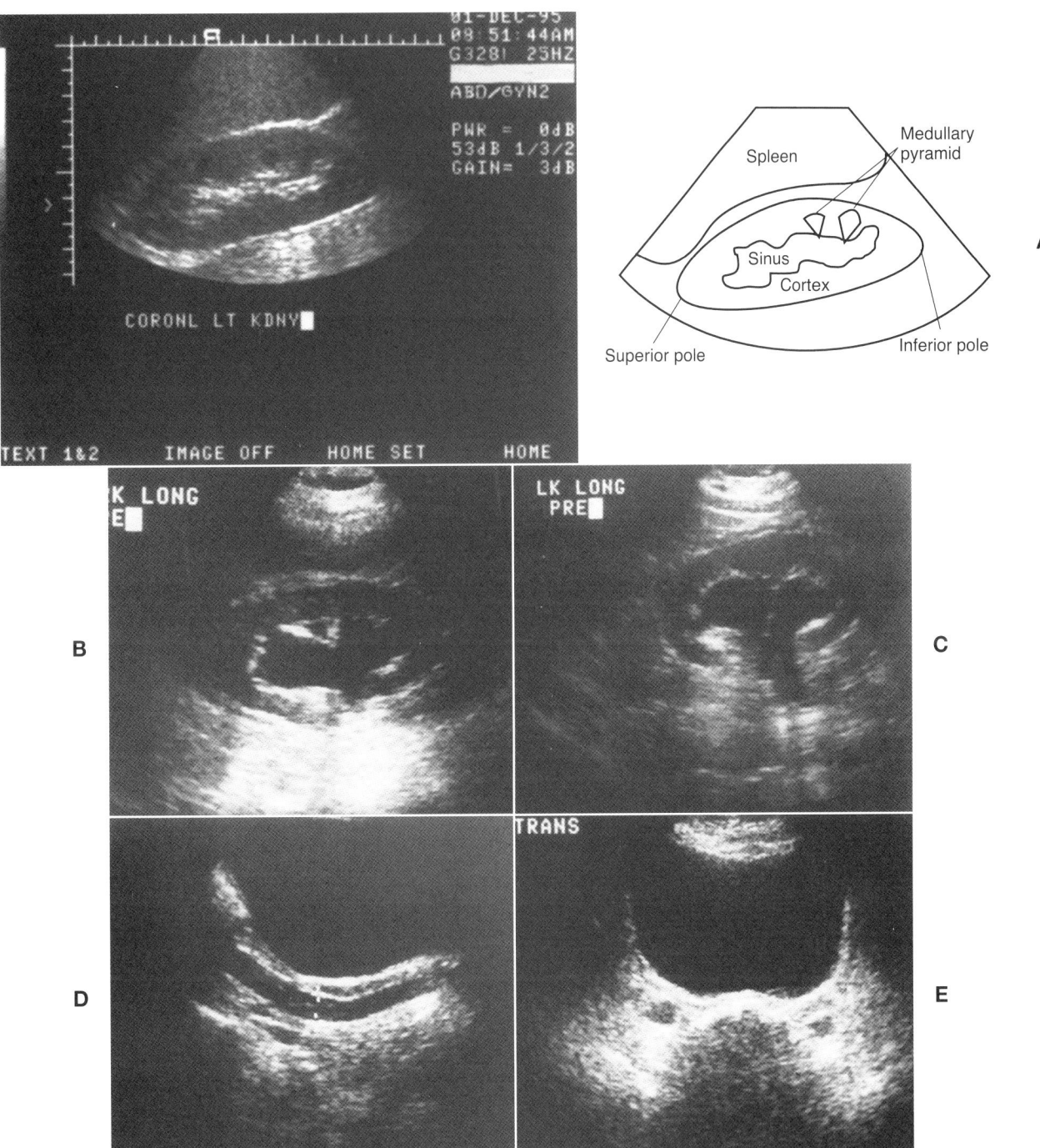

Fig. 209-19
A, Longitudinal view of the left kidney, including inferior and superior poles. Pseudohydronephrosis of both kidneys **(B-C)** and ureters **(D)** associated with a full bladder **(E)**. (**A,** From Simon BC, Snoey ER: *Ultrasound in emergency and ambulatory medicine,* St Louis, 1997, Mosby. **B,** From Hagen-Ansert SL: *Textbook of diagnostic ultrasonography,* ed 4, St Louis, 1995, Mosby.)

Interpretation

Since most episodes of renal colic are caused by small stones (2 to 4 mm), it is uncommon to actually visualize the stone. The confirmation of renal colic is usually made by demonstrating hydronephrosis or hydroureter in the correct clinical setting (flank pain and/or hematuria). Associated intrarenal calcifications further support the diagnosis.

The normal ureter is rarely visualized with the bedside ultrasound examination, so demonstration of a dark, fluid-filled ureter (hydroureter) is usually abnormal. With accumulation of additional fluid, as seen in hydronephrosis, the normal echogenic renal sinus stripe may actually be split by fluid, appearing as an intervening dark stripe. Along with this intervening stripe, the full appearance of hydronephrosis is characterized by increased fluid throughout the kidney, often contiguous with the hydroureter. Make sure the patient has voided before the ultrasound because a very full bladder can cause pseudohydronephrosis, which appears identical to mild or moderate hydronephrosis (Fig. 209-19, *B-C*).

When hydronephrosis is noted, an attempt should be made to follow the hydroureter(s) distally to the source of the obstruction. When associated with hydronephrosis, an echogenic structure found as the source of an obstruction, with or without prominent posterior shadowing, is diagnostic of urolithiasis. A stone larger than 3 mm should be highly echogenic and cast a well-defined shadow. With a good acoustic window and minimal bowel gas, the ureterovesical junction may be visualized and is a common place to find stones. Stones commonly lodge at this level. Occasionally a stone that has passed this junction will be found in the bladder. Even if a stone cannot be located distally, scanning the kidney may reveal intrarenal calcifications. As mentioned previously, intrarenal calcifications associated with a hydroureter support the diagnosis of renal colic.

With chronic hydronephrosis there is thinning of the renal medulla (Fig. 209-20, *A*). With significant, long-standing chronic hydronephrosis, thinning of the renal cortex may also be seen (Fig. 209-20, *B-C*). If bilateral obstructions are found, they are more likely due to an obstruction at the bladder outlet. In this situation, the bladder will be distended and should be easily scanned. The bladder should be scanned carefully for the source of obstruction. If no obstruction is demonstrated, the bladder may simply be overdistended. Hydronephrosis, albeit to a lesser degree, can also be seen with a nonobstructed, overdistended bladder. Hydronephrosis can be a normal finding in pregnancy, especially on the right side.

Renal cysts may mimic hydronephrosis. With ultrasound, simple renal cysts appear like cysts elsewhere in the body. They have smooth borders and no echogenic

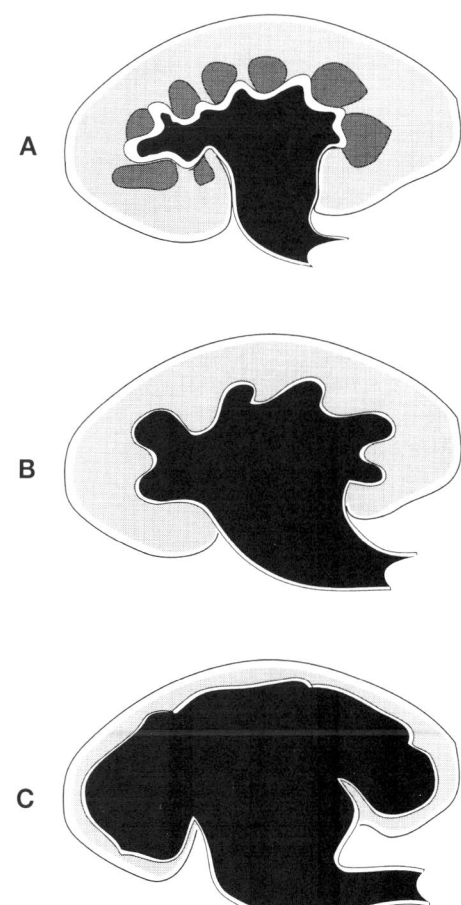

Fig. 209-20
A, Mild hydronephrosis. Note hydroureters. **B,** Moderate hydronephrosis. **C,** Severe hydronephrosis.

material within them. Renal cysts are common, occurring in 50% of individuals over 50 years of age. As opposed to hydronephrosis, renal cysts are well circumscribed and do not communicate with fluid outside the kidney (Fig. 209-16).

ICD-9-CM Diagnostic Codes

591	Hydronephrosis
592.0	Calculus of kidney
592.1	Calculus of ureter
593.5	Hydroureter
594.1	Urinary bladder stone
788.0	Renal colic

III. HEMOPERITONEUM

Many studies indicate that physical examination fails to reveal significant injuries in 25% to 40% of trauma patients. Previously, in the United States, diagnosis of intraabdominal blood was made almost exclusively with diagnostic peritoneal lavage (DPL) or CT. However, with more than two dozen prospective, controlled studies demonstrating the accuracy of ultrasound for detection of hemoperitoneum, diagnostic techniques have changed. In fact, this topic is currently the most heavily researched in the emergency medicine ultrasound literature. Investigators have proven that in the hands of capable, properly trained personnel the sensitivity of ultrasound for diagnosing hemoperitoneum is at least as great as DPL. The indications for ultrasound in suspected hemoperitoneum are therefore the same as for DPL. Many trauma centers in Europe and Japan replaced DPL with ultrasound, long ago, since ultrasound provides immediate results. This is also due in part to the training and comfort level of their general surgeons with ultrasound. The only relative contraindications to assessment with ultrasound include morbid obesity and massive subcutaneous emphysema.

Note: Unfortunately, individuals who already have free fluid on the abdomen (ascites) are often those that are prone to abdominal trauma (e.g., alcoholic cirrhosis). They are also not often the best candidates for surgery. One of the benefits of ultrasound in such a trauma victim is the ability to use serial scans to determine if the fluid is increasing. If increasing abdominal fluid is suspected to be blood, ultrasound can document the true necessity for surgery.

Preprocedure Patient Preparation

If the bladder is about to be emptied, it may be prudent to scan the pelvis before emptying. If the patient is hemodynamically compromised, attempts should be made to stabilize him or her before scanning.

Technique

1. If the bladder is about to be emptied, proceed to step 3. Otherwise, scan the patient longitudinally in the supine position with a low-frequency probe until you locate the right kidney. It is quite lateral and behind the liver, which is used for a window. If the patient is conscious, have him or her inspire and suspend breathing to bring the liver down. This often provides a better window and pushes bowel gas out of the way. The potential space located between the liver and the kidney is Morison's pouch (Fig. 209-21). This is the most important and easiest region to visualize and is usually the most sensitive area for detecting fluid. Factors that may affect the sensitivity include the location of the trauma, the positioning of the patient, and whether there is a history of prior abdominal surgery. If no fluid is seen in the supine position, Trendelenburg positioning may increase the sensitivity.

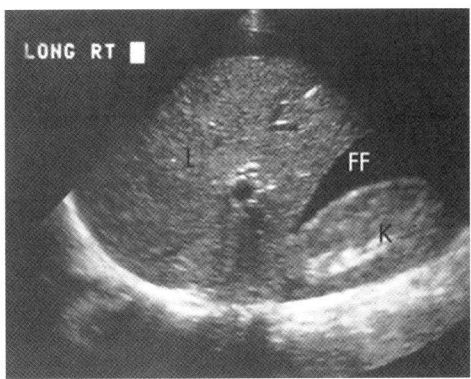

Fig. 209-21
Fluid in Morison's pouch or hemoperitoneum. *FF,* Free fluid; *K,* right kidney; *L,* liver. (From Simon BC, Snoey ER: *Ultrasound in emergency and ambulatory medicine,* St Louis, 1997, Mosby.)

2. If no fluid is seen in Morison's pouch, scan the left upper quadrant (LUQ). Scan it longitudinally and survey the area around the left kidney, the spleen, and the paracolic gutter. Realizing that the spleen is smaller than the liver and often more difficult to locate, use modest inspiration to bring it down to facilitate a window.

Note: Scanning the paracolic gutters requires considerable ultrasonographic experience. While studies have indicated that scanning in this area only minimally improves the sensitivity, such scanning significantly lengthens the time it takes to scan. Clinicians should also be aware that scanning this area frequently increases the number of false positives.

3. If the above scans are negative and the patient remains stable, the region of the pelvic cul de sac can be scanned after placing the patient in reverse Trendelenburg position. If time allows, a full bladder increases the sensitivity of scanning in this area. In women, transvaginal scanning replaces the need for a full bladder and is exquisitely sensitive for free fluid (capable of visualizing as little as 5 ml).

Interpretation

The entire examination can be performed very rapidly, with all three areas being scanned in less than 5 minutes. Fluid above the diaphragm indicates a pleural effusion (see Fig. 209-31). Intraperitoneal blood in small amounts usually accumulates lateral to the right kidney. Fresh, unclotted blood has the same appearance as any free fluid on the abdomen. In the setting of a patient with a possible hemoperitoneum, the appearance of free fluid as a "dark stripe" is diagnostic (Fig. 209-21). As little as 10 ml has been diagnosed in the upper abdomen through transabdominal scanning; however, the threshold for diagnosing hemoperitoneum is probably 250 ml.

A 1-cm fluid stripe roughly corresponds to 1 L of intraabdominal fluid. Again, Morison's pouch in the RUQ is one of the most sensitive areas to find fluid.

In the setting of trauma, the spleen is the most commonly injured abdominal organ. In the LUQ, fluid does not always accumulate between the spleen and the kidney. It may completely surround the spleen or may be located between the spleen and the abdominal wall (Fig. 209-22). Spontaneous rupture of the spleen occurs occasionally, such as in teenagers or individuals in their early twenties following an Epstein-Barr (mononucleosis) infection. In that situation, fluid will usually be found surrounding the spleen.

With large amounts of blood, fluid may be visible from almost anywhere in the abdomen or pelvis. It may accumulate as fluid in the cul-de-sac (Fig. 209-12). As soon as the clotting process begins, blood may produce variable echoes as the fibrin and degenerating cells become more prominent.

Obese patients may have a significant amount of hypoechoic fat around the kidney which can appear to be fluid. However, fat tends to accumulate along the upper and lateral aspect of the kidney, whereas fluid often completely surrounds the kidney. Comparison with the opposite kidney may demonstrate a similar accumulation of fat, confirming the false-positive result. Patients with multiple abdominal surgical scars may accumulate fluid in different patterns and locations because the normal flow of fluid in the abdomen is disrupted (Fig. 209-23).

After examining all three areas for free fluid, the liver, spleen, and kidney capsules and parenchyma should be reexamined for disruption or hematoma. Following a recent hepatic, renal, or splenic contusion an intracapsular hematoma will usually appear cystic with irregular borders. A renal or splenic contusion with a ruptured capsule often appears as fluid surrounding either the kidney or spleen. Keep in mind that it is more difficult to evaluate the spleen for such injuries because the spleen is normally hypoechoic in texture. Consequently, large intraparenchymal and subcapsular splenic injuries can be missed. To avoid missing clinically significant splenic injuries, the ultrasound, along with a hematocrit, should be repeated in 2 to 3 hours or if there is a change in vital signs. Major disruptions of the capsules of all of these organs can be missed by ultrasound.

ICD-9-CM Diagnostic Codes

568.81	Hemoperitoneum
459.0	Hemorrhage, abdomen
866.01	Hematoma, traumatic kidney
865.01	Hematoma, traumatic spleen
573.8	Hematoma, traumatic liver, subcapsular

IV. SUSPECTED ABDOMINAL AORTIC ANEURYSM

While the prevalence of AAA has climbed to as high as 10% in people over the age of 65, ruptured AAA has become the tenth leading cause of death in men more than 55 years old. Unlike coronary artery disease and cerebrovascular disease, the incidence continues to increase; the associated mortality rate is increasing as well. Males are affected three or four times more frequently than females.

The natural history of an AAA is to expand at a rate of 0.21 to 0.4 cm/year. Over 5 years, an AAA of 4 cm has a 10% chance of rupture, a 5-cm aneurysm has an 18% or greater chance, and a 6-cm aneurysm has a 30% or greater likelihood of rupturing. Controlling blood pressure and cessation of smoking may diminish the risk of rupture. Women may have a higher risk of rupture. Elective repair in most large centers has a mortality risk of less than 5%, compared with up to 80% mortality in those patients who live long enough to reach the operating room after rupture. Therefore, elective resection is indicated for low- to moderate-risk patients with aneurysms that measure more than 5 cm in diameter.

Risk Factors

- Male
- 50 years of age or older
- Use of tobacco

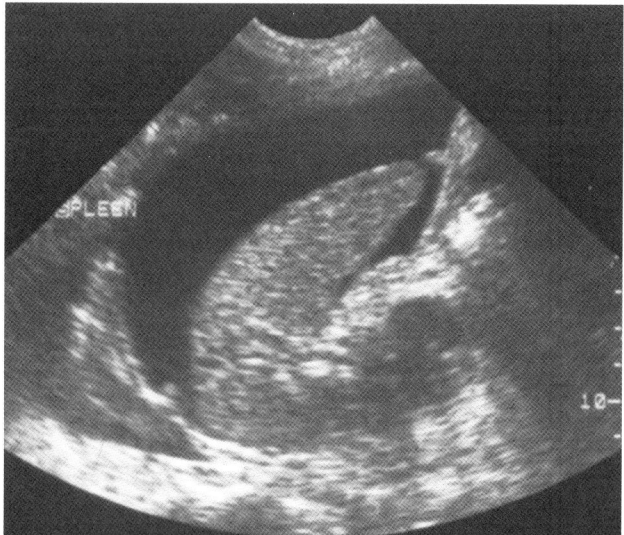

Fig. 209-22
Free fluid in the left upper quadrant. (From Heller M, Jehle D: *Ultrasound in emergency medicine,* Philadelphia, 1995, WB Saunders.)

- Hypertension
- Family history of AAA*
- Other atherosclerotic risk factors may also be AAA risk factors

The classic triad of ruptured AAA is pulsatile abdominal mass; low back, flank, or abdominal pain; and hypotension. Less than 50% of victims, however, possess this triad, and less than 25% are hypotensive on admission. Unfortunately, low back, flank, or abdominal pain is a frequent complaint for patients in the age group at risk for AAA. Patients with a leaking AAA may have many other signs and symptoms as well, including chest pain, hematuria, ecchymoses, and scrotal masses. The most common incorrect diagnosis in an elderly patient with a symptomatic AAA is left-sided renal colic. A leaking AAA may even be associated with hematuria; therefore any elderly patient with left-sided renal colic should be considered to have an AAA until proven otherwise.

Most aortic aneurysms are found in the midabdomen, just above the iliac bifurcation (about the level of the

---

*Family history is most significant when a female relative has been diagnosed. Elastinolytic enzymes, decreased type III collagen, decreased elastin, and other biochemical variants are being studied to determine what is probably a multifactorially inherited etiology.

umbilicus). Physical examination is extremely inaccurate for diagnosing AAA. Aortography may underestimate the size of an aneurysm if it is filled with a thrombus or is dissecting, and lateral radiographs overestimate the possibility and size. For screening, ultrasound is comparable to CT scanning which is the gold standard for both diagnosis and estimation of size. However, ultrasound may be a difficult study if there is a large amount of bowel gas, retained barium, or marked obesity. In addition, CT scanning is better than ultrasound for identifying a leaking aneurysm, although ultrasound may be useful when there is not enough time to perform a CT scan (emergent situation).

Preprocedure Patient Preparation

Under optimal conditions, the patient should have fasted for at least 8 hours to minimize bowel gas. Early morning scanning may also be preferable because bowel gas is usually minimal. Patients do not always come to the emergency department or the office under these conditions; however, if a pulsatile mass is readily palpable through the anterior abdominal wall, it should be readily scannable. The patient should be informed of possible diagnoses and the indication for scanning.

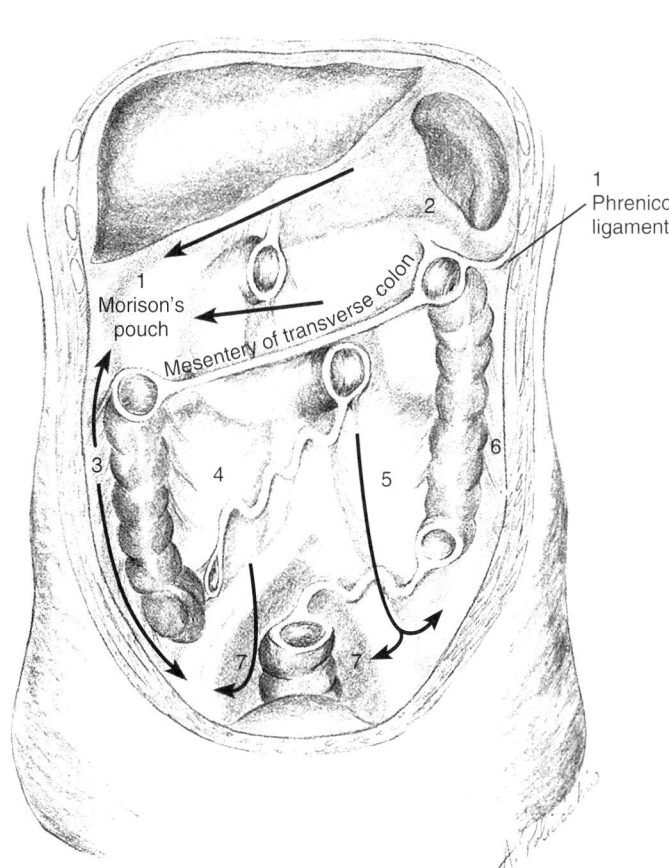

Fig. 209-23
Posterior peritoneum and reflections, indicating potential sites of intraabdominal fluid localization and spread. *1* and *2*, Right and left supramesocolic regions—above the transverse mesocolon and separated by the ridge of the lumbar spine; *3*, right paracolic gutter; *4*, right inframesocolic; *5*, left inframesocolic; *6*, left paracolic gutter; *7*, pelvic cul-de-sac. Arrows indicate movement of free fluid (hemorrhage). (From Simon BC, Snoey ER: *Ultrasound in emergency and ambulatory medicine,* St Louis, 1997, Mosby.)

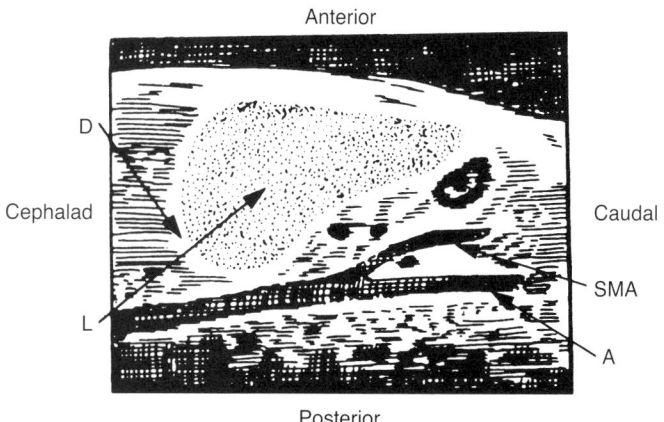

Fig. 209-24
Longitudinal scan slightly to the left of the midline showing normal structures and orientation. *A,* Aorta; *D,* diaphragm; *L,* liver; *SMA,* superior mesenteric artery.

Technique

1. With a low-frequency probe and the patient in the supine position, attempt to define the general outline of the aorta with longitudinal scanning (Fig. 209-24). If a pulsatile mass is palpated, it should not be difficult to determine whether it is contiguous with the abdominal aorta.

2. After defining the general outline, measurements should be taken of the largest anteroposterior (AP) diameter on transverse scanning at 1 to 2 cm increments to a level 3 cm below the umbilicus. Be aware that the transverse diameter of the aorta on a transverse scan may be exaggerated if the aorta is tangentially imaged when it makes a lateral turn. In addition, avoid applying too much probe pressure, which can also distort AP measurements.

3. If there is considerable overlying bowel gas, increased surface pressure with the probe may enhance visualization. Turning the patient to the right or left lateral decubitus position may enhance scanning the aorta in the area of the kidney, although the iliac bifurcation may not be visible unless the liver is enlarged.

Interpretation

With normal anatomy, mean abdominal aortic diameters are approximately equal in males and females during the second decade of life: 12.2 mm and 12.3 mm, respectively. By the eighth decade, the mean diameter increases to 22.8 mm in males and 16.9 mm in females. An AAA is defined by an aortic diameter of greater than 3 cm in a male and greater than 2.5 cm in a female, or an enlargement of greater than 0.5 cm throughout the length of the aorta. The normal aorta tapers in diameter as it descends to its bifurcation.

If an AAA is found (Fig. 209-25) and the patient is hemodynamically stable, the clinician should attempt to determine whether branching vessels are involved. Fluid, usually along the left side of the spine or anterior to a kidney, may indicate a ruptured or leaking aneurysm; surgical consultation should be obtained immediately. If no fluid is visualized and the patient is hemodynamically stable, a CT scan may be useful to check for retroperitoneal hemorrhage. CT angiography or magnetic resonance angiography (MRA) are best for delineating whether other arteries are involved. Surgery should be considered in any patient with persistent abdominal pain and a known AAA. Stents are now offered as an alternative for patients with asymptomatic AAAs.

Echogenic material in the lumen may represent a thrombus or dissection. Alternatively, the clinician should check the gain setting elsewhere on the aorta to make sure it is not artifact.

CPT/Billing Codes

76700	Ultrasound, abdominal, B-Scan and/or real time with image documentation; complete
76705	Limited (e.g., single organ, quadrant, follow-up)
76770	Ultrasound, retroperitoneal (e.g., renal, aorta, nodes), B-scan and/or real time with image documentation; complete
76775	Limited

ICD-9-CM Diagnostic Codes

441.4	Abdominal aortic aneurysm
441.02	dissecting
441.3	ruptured
789.3	Abdominal mass

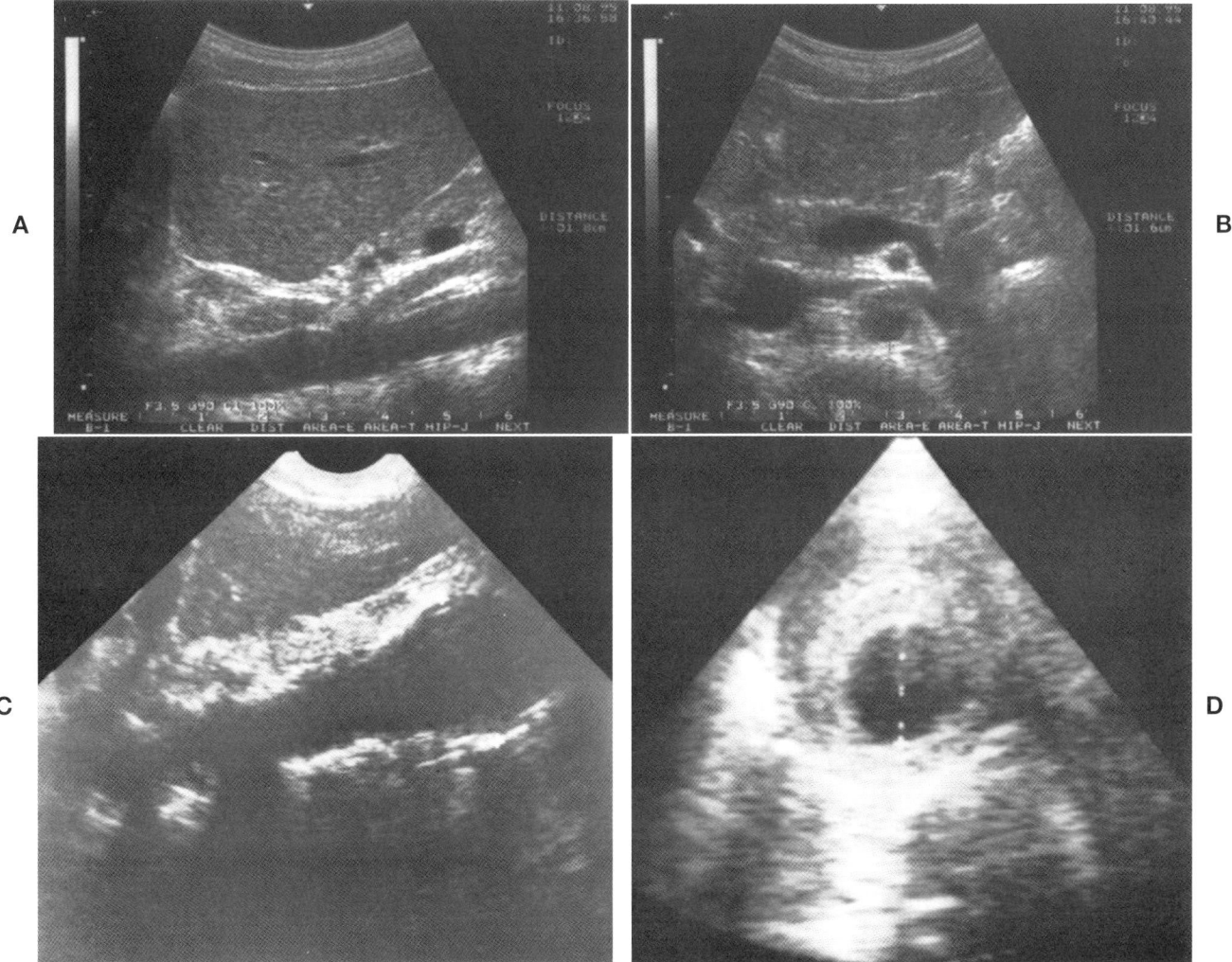

Fig. 209-25
A, Longitudinal view of an abdominal aortic aneurysm (AAA). **B,** Transverse view of an AAA. **C,** Longitudinal view of intrarenal AAA. **D,** Transverse view of a rupturing AAA with thrombus. (**A-B,** From Simon BC, Snoey ER: *Ultrasound in emergency and ambulatory medicine,* St Louis, 1997, Mosby. **C-D,** From Heller M, Jehle D: *Ultrasound in emergency medicine,* Philadelphia, 1995, WB Saunders.)

MISCELLANEOUS

There are many applications being used and further studied for ultrasound in both the emergency department and office settings. For example, one published study found that rib fractures can be accurately diagnosed with ultrasound. The entire outline of affected ribs was scanned with ultrasound, searching for breaks in the normal smooth cortex. Accuracy, in certain situations, was better than that found with radiographs. Ultrasound also spared the patient from radiation. Although the following section is certainly not all-inclusive, it lists some of the indications in the emer-

gency department or office where ultrasound has been either studied or published.

I. SUSPECTED DEEP VENOUS THROMBOSIS

(See Chapter 85, Noninvasive Venous and Arterial Studies of the Lower Extremities.) Even when duplex equipment is available, plain ultrasound scanning using the high-frequency probe for compression should be the initial study performed in most cases.

II. ULTRASONIC EVALUATION OF THE BLADDER PRIOR TO SUPRAPUBIC ASPIRATION (SPA)–CANNULATION OR FOR POSTVOIDING RESIDUAL (PVR)

Up to 8% of infants less than 8 weeks old in the emergency department with a temperature of 100.6° F or higher have a urinary tract infection (UTI). As many as 5% of infants younger than 2 years of age with unexplained fever have UTIs. The rate is 8% in girls and uncircumcised males but less than 1% in circumcised males. White girls have a much higher rate (up to 15%) than black girls. Boys are at the highest risk during the first 3 to 6 months of life.

Using an evidence-based approach, in those infants or children sufficiently ill to warrant immediate antibiotic therapy, the Practice Parameter of the American Academy of Pediatrics (AAP) recommends either SPA or transurethral catheterization to obtain a urine specimen. In those not sufficiently ill to require immediate antibiotics, the same diagnostic approach can be used; however, another option is available. If a urinalysis obtained by the most convenient means indicates a UTI, a sterile urine specimen should then be obtained in the same manner as listed above. These recommendations are based on a summary of the evidence and good clinical judgment; however, whereas a negative culture from a bagged specimen effectively rules out UTI, culture results are not available immediately. Bagged specimen cultures are also rarely negative, and unfortunately culture results cannot be predicted from urinalysis in most cases. Therefore many clinicians opt for SPA or catheterization.

Although catheterization is less invasive than SPA, the process of catheterization may actually cause a UTI. SPA is inherently invasive, yet few serious complications have been reported, and numerous studies have demonstrated the superiority of SPA over alternate techniques. Limiting SPA to patients with proven full bladders further minimizes the risk to the infant (See Chapter 185, Suprapubic Bladder Aspiration).

In adults, there are indications in the emergency department and the office for SPA or suprapubic cannulation. SPA can be useful for obtaining a urine culture whenever a urethral catheter cannot be placed (or is contraindicated) or may be particularly useful in critically ill, potentially septic, or unresponsive adults. Suprapubic cannulation (SPC) is indicated whenever a urethral catheter is indicated yet cannot or should not be placed (e.g., trauma patients who have serious injury to the urethra, patients who recently underwent bladder or gynecologic surgery, or when a sufficiently wide catheter is unable to be passed through the urethra for diagnostic cystometry).

Ultrasound may also be used in adults to measure PVR in order to evaluate the significance or status of urethral obstruction (e.g., significant prostatic hyperplasia) or a neurogenic bladder. PVR can be measured more precisely, albeit more invasively, by inserting a catheter; however, ultrasound provides reasonable estimates of PVR in a much more comfortable manner with less risk of inducing an infection. Considering the fact that recent studies have failed to document an exact level of PVR that would benefit from transurethral resection of the prostate (TURP) as opposed to watchful waiting, PVR estimates from ultrasound may be more than adequate in that situation (considering TURP).

Preprocedure Patient Preparation

The patient (or his or her parents or caregiver) should be informed about the indication for the study. If a suprapubic tap or cannulation is to be performed, counseling should be given for informed consent.

Technique

1. Infants should be placed in the supine, frog-leg position; adults should be supine. Perform the scanning in a transverse manner with a high-frequency transducer in infants. The marker dot should be directed toward the infant's right side, with the transducer placed slightly above the symphysis pubis. The transducer should be directed posteriorly or slightly caudal to locate the bladder. In adults, a low-frequency probe is used with the transducer and marker dot in the same location. The transducer should be angled in more of a caudal direction.

   Note: In infants less than 2 years of age, the bladder is an abdominal organ. As the pelvis grows, the bladder moves into the pelvis; therefore the transducer should be angled more caudal.

2. Move and angle the probe to locate the maximal transverse diameter of the bladder. In infants, this is the probe location and angle to take measurements for determining whether the bladder is full. Take measurements in both the AP and transverse diameters.

3. For aspiration or cannulation, note the angulation of the probe necessary to locate the maximal transverse diameter of the bladder. Note the depth necessary to penetrate the bladder. This same angulation and depth should be used when directing the aspiration needle or trocar.

4. To estimate bladder volume in an adult, including PVR, three diameters should be determined. First, measure and record the greatest transverse measurement (*w* in Fig. 209-26, *A*). Next, turn the marker dot cephalad and find the longest longitudinal plane.

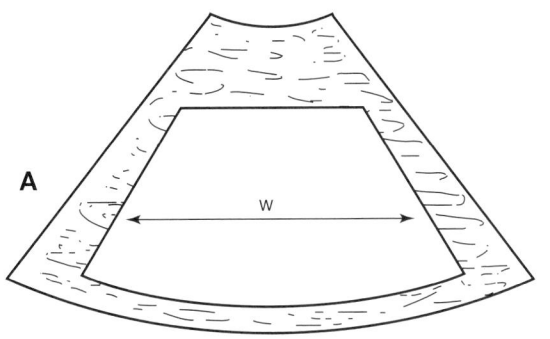
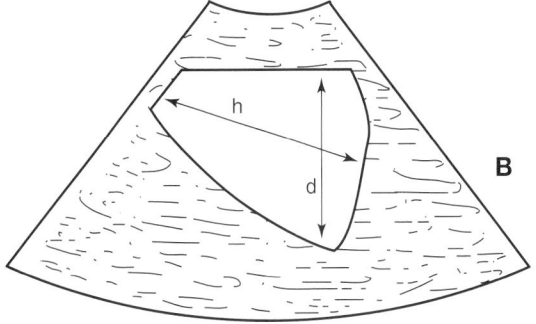

Fig. 209-26
A, Greatest transverse diameter of bladder is shown by *w.* *B,* Maximal supero-infero measurement is shown by *h;* the maximal AP measurement is shown by *d.*

Measure and record the maximal supero-infero measurement (*h* in Fig. 209-26, *B*) in this plane. In the same plane, with that same image, measure and record the maximal AP measurement (*d* in Fig. 209-26, *B*).

Interpretation and Results

In infants, a pocket of fluid larger than 2 cm × 2 cm in the retropubic area measured in the AP and maximal transverse diameters defines a "full" bladder (Fig. 209-27). In adults, the pocket should be much larger in order to reach it with a needle or trocar. Again, SPA or SPC should be attempted at the same angle with which the maximal transverse bladder diameter was measured (Fig. 209-28). One study resulted in obtaining urine in 79% of children meeting these criteria and undergoing aspiration. If the bladder is found to be empty and the patient is clinically stable, repeat scanning to search for a full bladder should be performed 30 minutes to an hour after the initial scan. If a full bladder cannot be found on the repeat scan, bladder catheterization should be considered.

In adults, bladder volume can be calculated with this formula:

$$0.7 \times h \times d \times w$$

This yields a standard error of approximately 21%. Although 21% may seem like a large error, as mentioned above, it is now known that no certain PVR threshold exists where surgery (TURP) ensures success and avoids future morbidity. For that reason, this crude measurement may be more than adequate. If more precise volumes are needed, more sophisticated formulas are available. In addition, software packages are available for more precise estimates using large machines that can take more precise measurements. Portable ultrasound equipment is also available that is used solely for making urologic measurements. Such equipment has been studied extensively and accuracy has been documented.

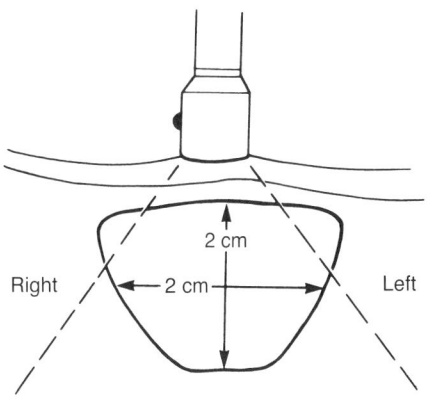

Fig. 209-27
Transverse view of a full infant bladder.

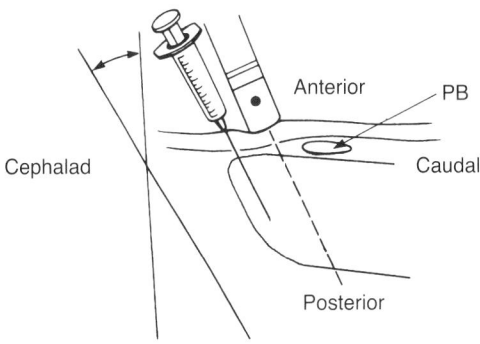

Fig. 209-28
Needle should be inserted next to the probe and parallel to whatever angle demonstrated the fullest diameters of the bladder. *PB,* Pubic bone.

CPT/Billing Codes

76700   Ultrasound, abdominal, B-scan and/or real time with image documentation; complete

76705   Limited (e.g., single organ, quadrant, follow-up)

76942   Ultrasonic guidance for needle placement (e.g., biopsy, aspiration, injection) imaging supervision, and interpretation

ICD-9-CM Diagnostic Codes

788.20   Urinary retention, NEC
788.21   Urinary retention, bladder incomplete
         emptying
599.0   Urinary tract infection, site not specified
595.0   Cystitis, acute

III. SUBCUTANEOUS FOREIGN BODIES

Missed foreign bodies are the second most frequent cause of lawsuits against emergency medicine clinicians. Substances composed of wood, plastic, glass, and vegetable material may not be radiopaque or visible with standard x-ray examinations. Modern military armor is also an example. Most is now fiberglass or cloth and therefore shrapnel is not often visible on routine x-rays. Although fine needles and splinters may be missed, high-frequency ultrasound is usually helpful not only for confirming the presence of a foreign body but also for localization before removal.

Preprocedure Patient Preparation

The patient should be informed about the indication for the study and should understand that not all foreign bodies are visible with either ultrasound or standard x-ray examinations. If a foreign body is located, the patient should decide whether or not he or she wants it removed. They will need an understanding of the possible complications of removing the object as opposed to not removing the object. (See Chapter 19, Foreign Body Removal from Skin or Soft Tissue.)

Technique

1. In most cases, a high-frequency probe is preferred. For objects very near the skin surface, a "stand-off" pad may be needed to raise the probe several millimeters off the skin. Such a device can either be purchased commercially or created using a latex glove filled with water or ultrasound gel. Place the glove or pad on the skin, and scan through it with the transducer.
2. Understanding that layers of normal subcutaneous tissue are not always uniform, scan in the area of the possible foreign body. Scan the contralateral "normal" side if unsure of the diagnosis. Scan both longitudinally and transversely, attempting to clarify the largest dimensions when located.

Interpretation and Results

Foreign bodies may appear as hyperechoic in contrast to the surrounding tissue. If the resolution of the probe is great enough and the foreign body thick enough, an acoustic shadow may also be seen. Metal and glass are more echoic than plastic or wood. Foreign bodies may also be surrounded by a hypoechoic halo representing fluid or inflammation. The exact location of the foreign body should be marked; if it is not round, the predominant direction in which it is lying should be noted. The depth of the object, especially if it is to be removed, should also be noted.

CPT/Billing Codes

76942   Ultrasonic guidance for needle placement (e.g., biopsy, aspiration, injection, localization device), imaging supervision and interpretation

ICD-9-CM Diagnostic Codes

729.6   Residual foreign body in soft tissue

IV. TESTICULAR MASS OR POSSIBLE TORSION

High-frequency ultrasound is helpful in diagnosing testicular cancer as well as for differentiating the four most common causes for a scrotal mass: spermatocele, hydrocele, varicocele, and tumor. Transillumination with a bright penlight can often differentiate a spermatocele or hydrocele from other possible causes of a scrotal mass. When there is still a question following transillumination, ultrasound is the procedure of choice.

Although radioisotope scans are the procedure of choice for diagnosing a torsioned testicle, when the blood supply from a testicle has been interrupted, it is usually less echogenic than the opposite testicle. If radioisotopes are not available, a quick scan may reveal a homogenous loss of the usually sharp intratesticular markings when compared with the opposite side. The texture of a torsioned testicle appears blurry. Since it can be performed fairly rapidly, color Doppler ultrasound may be becoming the procedure of choice for diagnosing torsion.

Preprocedure Patient Preparation

The patient should be informed about the indication for the study. Using a towel, the patient can retract the penis. The testicle and the scrotum are supported by the clinician's hand or by a towel under the scrotum. Either a very cooperative patient or an assistant may be needed to allow the clinician to use both hands for the ultrasound equipment.

Technique

1. Using the same orientation as for the rest of the body, first turn the marker dot toward the patient's head for a longitudinal scan. Parallel longitudinal scans should be made with the high-frequency probe about every 5 mm.
2. Next, turn the marker dot toward the patient's right side for a transverse scan. Transverse scans should also be made approximately every 5 mm.
3. The opposite testicle should be scanned, if indicated, or for a comparison for questionable areas.

Interpretation and Results

Testicles are normally symmetrical in size. A small amount of fluid within the scrotal sac is normal. A normal ultrasonic finding known as the mediastinum testis is seen as an echogenic longitudinal central line within the testicle (Fig. 209-29, *A*). The epididymis usually appears as a slightly sonolucent structure posterior to the testes.

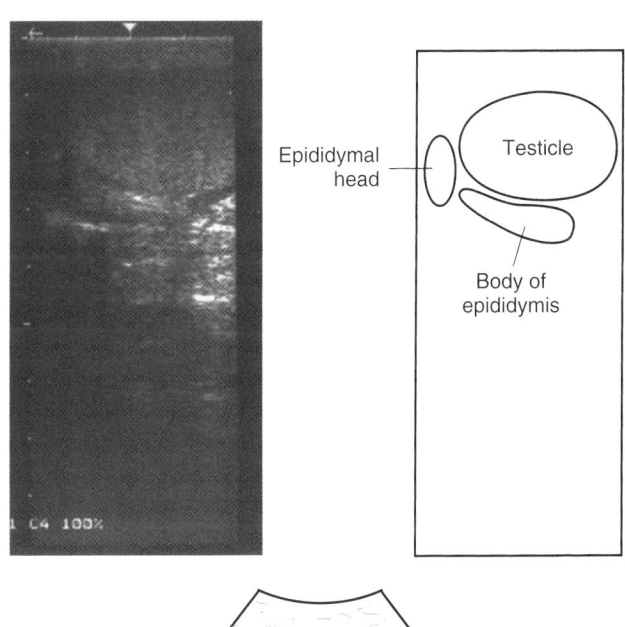

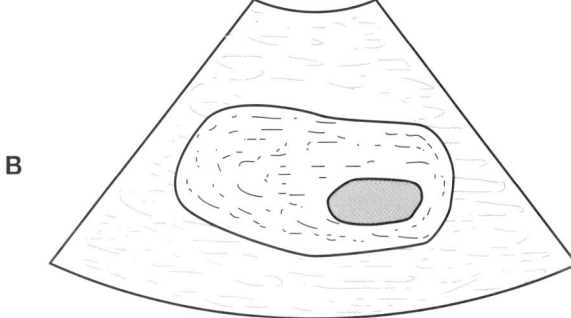

Fig. 209-29
A, Normal testicular tissue with mediastinum testis. **B,** Testicular mass suspicious of cancer. (**A,** From Simon BC, Snoey ER: *Ultrasound in emergency and ambulatory medicine,* St Louis, 1997, Mosby.)

A small mass within the testicle is cancer until proven otherwise, especially in a male less than 40 years of age (Fig. 209-29, *B*). A seminoma, the most common testicular tumor, usually appears as a hypoechoic mass within the testicle. Teratomas and embryonal cell cancers are usually irregularly echogenic.

Hydroceles, spermatoceles, and varicoceles should all be extratesticular. Spermatoceles are usually found superior to the testicle and attached to the vas deferens. Hydroceles may surround the testicle and are predominantly fluid filled. Varicoceles are usually found in the region of the epididymis, extending superiorly. They will often increase considerably in size with a Valsalva maneuver. A torsioned testicle often appears enlarged and less dense when compared with the normal testicle (Fig. 209-30, *C-D*). Texture is often blurry in the torsioned testicle.

CPT/Billing Codes

76870   Ultrasound, scrotum and contents

ICD-9-CM Diagnostic Codes

608.89   Testicular mass
186.9   Primary neoplasm of testicle

DIAGNOSTIC AND/OR PROCEDURAL ULTRASOUND

INSERTION OF CENTRAL LINES

Several studies indicate that the use of ultrasound as an adjunct for inserting central venous catheters not only decreases the failure rate—it also decreases the overall incidence of complications as well as the number of attempts necessary. For these reasons, patient satisfaction should also be improved. A two-person technique is described below. Equipment is now available in many large intensive care units that is portable and dedicated to the insertion of central lines.

Preprocedure Patient Preparation

See Chapter 81, Central Venous Catheter Insertion.

Technique

1. For internal jugular cannulation, the patient is positioned supine, in 15 degrees of Trendelenburg, with the head turned slightly to the opposite side.
2. Perform a preliminary transverse scan with the high-frequency probe just above the clavicle near the insertion of the two heads of the sternocleidomastoid muscle. The pulsatile internal carotid artery should

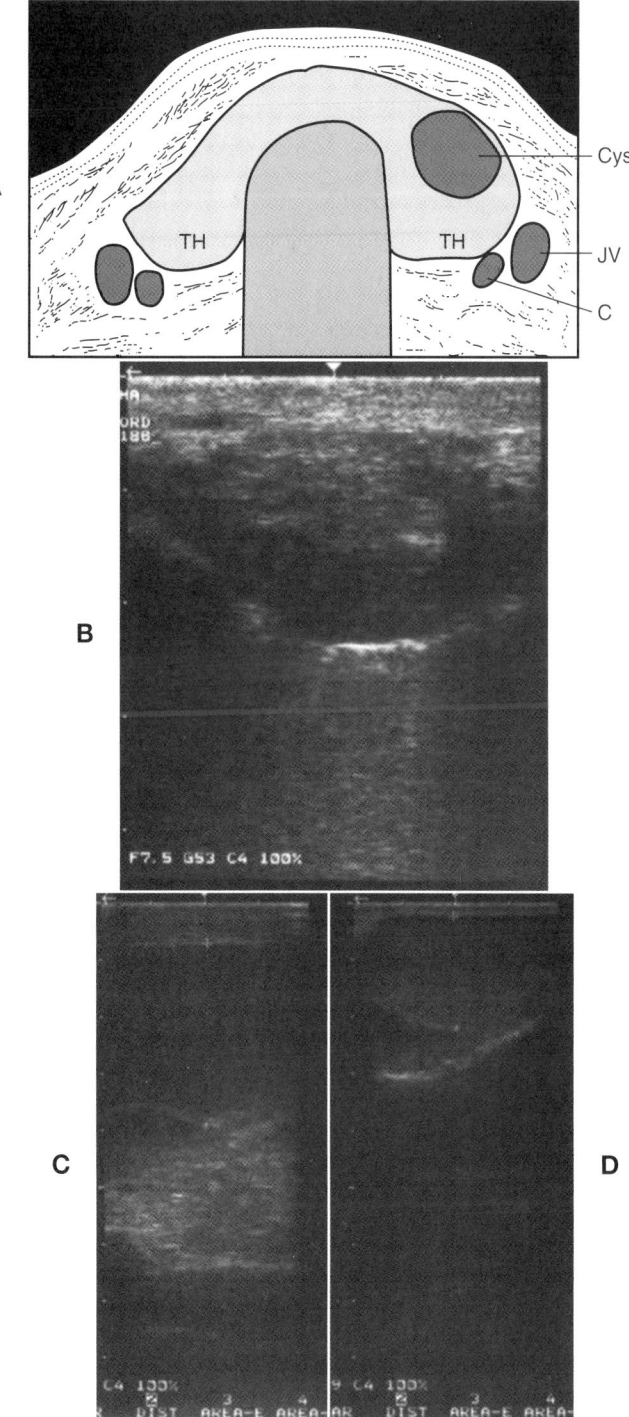

Fig. 209-30
A, Thyroid cyst. **B,** Thyroid mass (adenoma). **C,** Torsion of right testicle demonstrated by an enlarged hypoechoic testicle. **D,** Normal left testicle. *C,* Carotid artery; *JV,* internal jugular vein; *TH,* thyroid. (**B-D,** From Simon BC, Snoey ER: *Ultrasound in emergency and ambulatory medicine,* St Louis, 1997, Mosby.)

appear in cross-sectional view beside and medial to the larger internal jugular vein. With a Valsalva maneuver, the internal jugular will get much larger. Avoid applying too much pressure with the probe, which may temporarily collapse the vein.

3. Cover the probe with a sterile barrier (e.g., a sterile glove). Acoustic gel should have been placed inside the cover with special attention on eliminating all bubbles over the head of the transducer. Prep and drape the patient in the usual sterile fashion.

4. A small amount of sterile acoustic gel is placed on the outside of the probe. The sterilely gowned and gloved ultrasound operator should be located next to the clinician (similarly gowned and gloved) performing the cannulation. They should operate the ultrasound probe beneath the drape to avoid interfering with the cannulation.

5. Position the probe so that the internal jugular vein is centered in the monitor screen. The person performing the cannulation should aim the needle toward the center of the probe. The needle will not always be visualized; if it is, it will appear as a linear, echogenic structure with shadowing. The needle will typically cause slight tenting of the vessel as it enters. The flash of blood in the syringe is often anticipated by the sonographer when they see the tenting of the vein a few seconds before the needle enters. Next, the guidewire can often be visualized as it passes into the vein.

CPT/Billing Codes

76942   Ultrasonic guidance for needle placement (e.g., biopsy, aspiration, injection, localization device), imaging supervision and interpretation

ICD-9-CM Diagnostic Codes

See Chapter 81, Central Venous Catheter Insertion.

LUMBAR PUNCTURE IN MORBIDLY OBESE INDIVIDUAL

In morbidly obese individuals, lumber puncture is often complicated by the inability to palpate the spinous processes. The goal of ultrasound is to locate the midline of the spine.

Preprocedure Patient Preparation

See Chapter 213, Lumbar Puncture.

Technique

1. Ultrasound can be performed either under nonsterile conditions, to mark the midline, or under sterile conditions for ultrasonic guidance of the needle. Usually a low-frequency probe is preferred.
2. With the patient in either the lateral recumbent or sitting position, apply adequate acoustic gel over the midline of the spine. Scan initially in transverse dimensions to locate a vertebra. The L4 spinous process should be noted below a line drawn between the iliac crests. When this vertebra is noted, maneuver the transducer so that the spinous process is centered on the monitor. Next, rotate the probe 90 degrees to scan longitudinally and locate several spinous processes. Mark the location and note the angle necessary to penetrate between the L3 and L4 spinous processes. After local anesthetic is given, insert the spinal needle and follow the remaining technique as described in Chapter 213, Lumbar Puncture.
3. To perform under sterile conditions, cover the probe with a sterile barrier (sterile glove) as noted above for central line insertion. When performing the lumbar puncture, use the same technique as for central line insertion and observe the needle passing over the L4 spinous process.

Interpretation and Results

The spinous process should appear hyperechoic in contrast to surrounding tissue. The vertebral bodies should also be hyperechoic and cast shadows. Spinal fluid is rarely imaged between the spinous processes in adults, but the angles and depths to the vertebral bodes can usually be more clearly defined.

CPT/Billing Codes

76942   Ultrasonic guidance for needle placement, imaging, supervision, and interpretation

ICD-9-CM Diagnostic Codes

047.9   Abacterial or aseptic meningitis
320.9   Bacterial meningitis, NEC

THYROID MASS

Palpable thyroid nodules occur in 3% to 4% of the population. One important goal when scanning a thyroid nodule is to determine whether there is more than one nodule. If multiple nodules are present (40% possibility), the risk of malignancy is very low (1% to 6%), with the exception of those who underwent low-dose irradiation as a child (usually for croup or acne). These patients have a 30% to 40% lifetime risk of malignancy. However, since this type of irradiation has not been performed for many years, most of those individuals who are at risk have already developed their malignancies.

The next goal of scanning a thyroid nodule is to determine whether it is cystic (Fig. 209-30, *A*), solid (Fig. 209-30, *B*), or both (complex). Cold nodules on nuclear studies can be either cystic with low risk of malignancy (20%), malignant (20%), or benign (60%).

If the nodule is cystic, aspiration may be an option and the fluid may be sent for cytology. Fine-needle aspiration is also an option for solid lesions.

Preprocedure Patient Preparation

The patient should be informed about the indication for the study. If an aspiration is to be performed, the patient should be counseled for informed consent.

Technique

1. With the patient in the supine position and their neck slightly hyperextended, apply an adequate amount of acoustic gel. Using a high frequency probe, scan transversely (marker dot to the patient's right side) in a lateral-to-medial fashion on one side. Next, scan the opposite side at the same level from lateral to medial. Apply minimal pressure at the midline to avoid obscuring the texture of the isthmus. Proceed in 5-mm increments throughout the entire gland.
2. Next, scan with longitudinal planes at 5-mm intervals. Observe each plane and then move medially from the carotid artery. Good surface contact is usually obtained at a 10- or 20-degree angle from the vertical. Scan the opposite side in the same manner.
3. For aspiration, see the "Breast Mass Aspiration" section below. If aspiration is to be attempted, mark the location. Note the angle and depth of any nearby structures that need to be avoided.

Interpretation and Results

Carcinomas of the thyroid are usually single nodules with irregular borders, and the majority are hypoechoic. They can be cystic, solid, or both (complex), and they are frequently accompanied by adenopathy. However, there is no pathognomonic feature of cancer of the thyroid. If unsure, the clinician should consider fine-needle aspiration or surgical removal, especially for solitary nodules.

The most common thyroid masses are adenomas. Adenomas almost invariably occur as multiple lesions. They can appear with a halo of hypoechoic tissue surrounding a more echogenic mass, as a solid homogenous mass with few internal echoes, or as a densely echogenic mass. Goiters appear as a diffuse, asymmetrical expansion of the thyroid with a course texture. Multiple nodules are often present. Thyroiditis usually appears as a diffuse enlargement of the thyroid with multiple nodules. Parathyroid glands are rarely seen and usually appear on the posterior aspect of the thyroid near the carotid artery. They are relatively sonolucent; if larger than 5 mm, they are abnormal.

CPT/Billing Codes

76536	Ultrasound, soft tissue of head and neck (e.g., thyroid, parathyroid, parotid), B-scan and/or real time with image documentation
76942	Ultrasonic guidance for needle placement (e.g., biopsy, aspiration, injection, localization device), imaging supervision and interpretation

ICD-9-CM Diagnostic Codes

226	Benign neoplasm of thyroid
246.2	Cyst of thyroid
241.1	Nontoxic multinodular goiter
242.2	Toxic multinodular goiter
193	Primary neoplasm of thyroid gland

BREAST MASS

Ultrasound is very helpful for evaluating breast masses, whether confirming the presence of a palpable mass or locating a nonpalpable mass seen on mammography, evaluating young fibroglandular breasts where mammography is less helpful, or differentiating solid from cystic lesions.

Preprocedure Patient Preparation

The patient should be informed about the indication for the study. She should be aware that this procedure is only being used to evaluate palpable lesions (or lesions noted on mammograms), to localize them, or to determine whether they are cystic or solid. It is not being used solely to exclude cancer. Portable ultrasound may also be used to assist with aspiration of a breast cyst or with fine-needle aspiration of a suspected adenoma. Informed consent should be obtained if aspiration will be attempted.

Technique

1. Place the patient in the supine position. After application of acoustic gel, scan palpable lesions with a high-frequency probe. To locate nonpalpable lesions noted on a mammogram, scan longitudinally in 5-mm parallel increments in the appropriate quadrant. If the lesion is not located, scan in transverse increments through the same quadrant.

2. For cyst aspiration, either a one- or two-person technique can be used. The one-person technique may be adequate for large cysts, especially if they are readily palpable. The ultrasound can be performed under nonsterile conditions. The goal of the ultrasound study is to locate the cyst, note the surrounding structures (especially those that should be avoided), determine the necessary depth for puncture, and mark the puncture site. The transducer can then be set aside and the procedure performed under sterile conditions as noted elsewhere (e.g., suprapubic aspiration, thoracentesis).

3. For smaller or deeper cysts that are difficult to localize, use the two-person technique. Just as with insertion of central lines, one person localizes the cyst with a high-frequency probe and keeps it in the center of the image while maintaining sterile conditions. The second clinician then punctures the cyst also under aseptic conditions. Occasionally the needle can be visualized on the screen as it enters the cyst. The needle usually indents the cyst wall before it punctures.

4. After aspiration, the contents should be sent for cytology. A sample can also be prepared as a smear between two microscope slides that are then pulled apart, sprayed with the same fixative used for Pap smears, allowed to air dry, and sent for cytology.

Interpretation and Results

Breast cysts have the sonographic appearance of cysts elsewhere in the body and are the most common breast masses in women between 35 and 50 years of age. They normally have smooth walls and an absence of internal echoes; therefore they are uniformly hypoechoic. Tissue behind the posterior wall of the cyst is usually more sharply defined than tissue anterior to the cyst. The penumbra affect may be seem.

The cyst should be measured in three dimensions: anteroposterior, longitudinal, and transverse. If aspiration is to be attempted, the depth necessary for penetration should be recorded. Nearby structures should also be noted.

Adenomas are usually ovoid in shape, with lateral diameters larger than anteroposterior diameters. They usually have uniform and regular borders. If the gain is set improperly (too low) and no internal echoes are noted, adenomas may also appear cystic.

In contrast, ductal carcinomas usually have irregular borders and may be dense enough to cast acoustic shadows. Their anteroposterior diameter may be as great or greater than lateral diameters. If they are blocking ducts, the ducts can often be traced to the site of the mass. Medullary carcinoma may be difficult to differentiate from adenomas, with the only differences being a more irregular border and more internal echoes. For this reason, solid solitary breast lesions should either undergo fine-needle aspiration or surgical removal.

Papillary carcinoma is fairly rare, but it can appear as fingerlike projections protruding from a cyst wall. After cyst aspiration, if any tissue remains palpable, it should probably be surgically removed to exclude the possibility of papillary carcinoma. Also after aspiration, air can be reinjected into the cyst and a repeat mammogram performed. The location of the cyst will be marked by the air when the mammogram is repeated. In this manner a mammogram can be used to help exclude papillary carcinoma.

CPT/Billing Codes

76645   Ultrasound, breast(s) (unilateral or bilateral), B-scan and/or real time with image documentation
76942   Ultrasonic guidance for needle placement (e.g., biopsy, aspiration, injection, localization device), imaging supervision and interpretation

ICD-9-CM Diagnostic Codes

174.8   Primary breast neoplasm, upper or lower
610.0   Solitary cyst of breast
610.1   (Fibro) Cystic breast
611.72   Lump or mass in breast

PLEURAL EFFUSION AND ULTRASONIC DIRECTED THORACENTESIS

Ultrasound is an alternative to the use of decubitus x-ray films for confirmation of an effusion (e.g., patient with blunting of costovertebral angles on x-ray). Once the effusion is confirmed, not only can the amount of fluid be quantified, but also the best angle and the depth necessary for inserting the needle can be determined. In patients with a small amount of pleural fluid or a loculated effusion, routine thoracentesis is often unsuccessful and possibly dangerous. Ultrasonically directed thoracentesis should minimize the danger while maximizing the results.

Preprocedure Patient Preparation

The patient should be informed about the indications for the procedure as well as the risks and possible com-

plications. Signed, informal consent should be obtained for thoracentesis. (See Chapter 95, Thoracentesis.)

Technique

1. With the patient in the sitting position, use a low-frequency probe to scan the back intercostally on the appropriate side, just above the liver or spleen. It may be helpful to actually scan the liver or spleen first, and to then move the probe in a cephalad direction to locate the effusion.
2. For large effusions, mark the best location for introduction of the needle. Note the location of the diaphragm, which will appear echogenic and moving with respiration. Also note the location of the spleen or liver, and avoid inserting the needle in that location.

    Effusions may move with respiration, so note where to direct the needle relative to each phase of respiration. Plan to perform the insertion during the optimal phase. Note the depth necessary to reach fluid, especially for large or obese patients; an extra-long needle may be necessary for these patients. A needle stop, set to the appropriate depth, may be helpful for preventing penetration of lung tissue and causing a pneumothorax.
3. For smaller or loculated effusions, the thoracentesis is best performed under ultrasonic guidance. Cover the probe with a sterile barrier (sterile glove) as noted above for central line insertion. This procedure may also require two persons: one to hold the transducer while the other performs the aspiration. When performing ultrasonically directed thoracentesis, use the same technique as for central line insertion. With the probe held scanning longitudinally, the top of the rib over which the thoracentesis is to be performed should be highlighted by the transducer. If a curvilinear or sector scanner is being used, the transducer should be held at the same optimal angle as that needed to reach the effusion. The thoracentesis needle should then be advanced to the appropriate depth at the same angle as the transducer. Again, a properly set needle stop may prevent penetrating lung tissue and causing a pneumothorax. Occasionally the echogenic needle will be observed passing over the rib. Once fluid is obtained, complete the procedure in the same manner as if it were done without ultrasonic guidance.

Interpretation and Results

Pleural effusions that are predominantly fluid appear dark or hypoechoic on ultrasound. They are located above the echogenic diaphragm, which moves with respiration (Fig. 209-31). An empyema may demonstrate echogenic objects within the fluid. Loculations and the

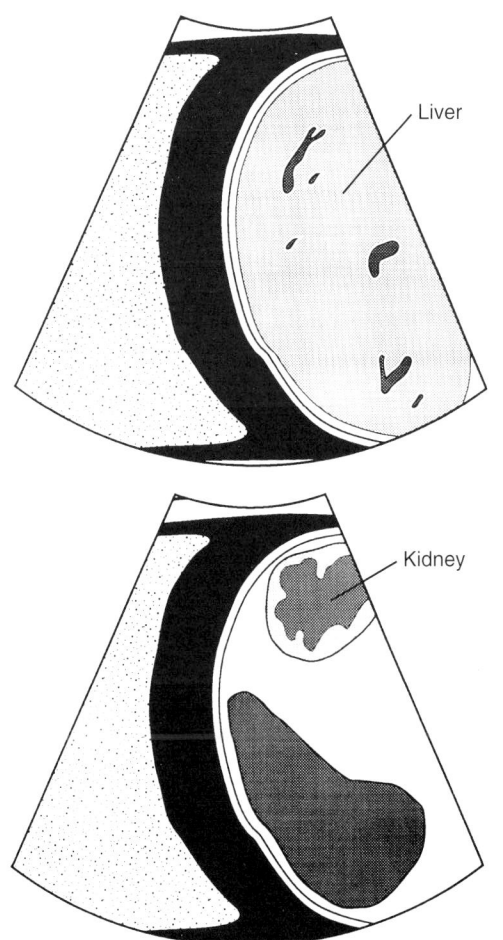

Fig. 209-31
Pleural effusion. Note the fluid is above the diaphragm. (From Heller M, Jehle D: *Ultrasound in emergency medicine,* Philadelphia, 1995, WB Saunders.)

diaphragm appear as echogenic borders to the fluid. Fluid located below the diaphragm (and not within an organ) is ascites.

CPT/Billing Codes

76942   Ultrasonic guidance for needle placement (e.g., biopsy, aspiration, injection, localization device), imaging supervision and interpretation

ICD-9-CM Diagnostic Codes

511.9	Pleural effusion
197.2	Pleural effusion, malignant
511.1	Bacterial, nontuberculous pleural effusion
012.0	Tuberculous pleural effusion
862.29	Traumatic pleural effusion

ASCITES AND ULTRASONIC DIRECTED PARACENTESIS

As discussed in the "Hemoperitoneum" section, the presence of abdominal fluid is not always obvious on physical examination. Ultrasound can be used to confirm the presence of ascites and to determine the best location for diagnostic paracentesis. Although routine paracentesis may be contraindicated in certain situations (such as in patients with adhesions from prior abdominal surgery), paracentesis directed by ultrasound may remain an option for those patients.

Preprocedure Patient Preparation

The patient should be informed about the indications for the procedure as well as the risks and possible complications. If there is a relative contraindication, the patient should be informed of the increased risk. (See Chapter 97, Abdominal Paracentesis.)

Technique

1. With the patient in the supine position, use a low-frequency probe to scan the usual location for performing paracentesis (in the midline, approximately one third the distance from the umbilicus to the symphysis). Confirm that there is adequate fluid in this location for a successful paracentesis. Also, confirm absence of bowel and whether the bladder has been emptied adequately. If these conditions are met, perform the procedure in the usual manner.
2. For small amounts of fluid, or if there is need for stereotactic paracentesis, perform it under ultrasonic guidance. Cover the probe with a sterile barrier (sterile glove) as noted above for central line insertion. When performing the paracentesis, use the same technique as for central line insertion or thoracentesis. In some cases, the echogenic needle may be observed passing into the fluid.

Interpretation and Results

Peritoneal fluid appears dark or hypoechoic on ultrasound. Bowel or bladder wall is relatively echogenic. With peritonitis, echogenic objects will occasionally be seen floating in the fluid.

CPT/Billing Codes

76942   Ultrasonic guidance for needle placement (e.g., biopsy, aspiration, injection, localization device), imaging supervision and interpretation

ICD-9-CM Diagnostic Codes

789.5	Ascites
567.2	Suppurative peritonitis
998.7	Chemical peritonitis

SUPPLIERS (see Suppliers in Chapter 173, Obstetric Ultrasound)

Overreading services

Overread.com
3037 Hopyard Road, Suite I
Pleasanton, CA 94588
Phone: 1-888-426-6331
Website: www.overread.com

ADDITIONAL RESOURCES

- See the sample patient consent form titled "Breast Mass Aspiration/Thyroid Mass Aspiration" on page 2016 of Appendix G.

BIBLIOGRAPHY

American College of Emergency Physicians: Use of ultrasound imaging by emergency physicians. *Ann Emerg Med* 30(3):364, 1997.

Deutchman M: The problematic first-trimester pregnancy, *Am Fam Physician* 39(1):185, 1989.

Gochman RF, Karasic RB, Heller MB: Use of portable ultrasound to assist urine collection by suprapubic aspiration, *Ann Emerg Med* 20:631, 1991.

Heller M, Jehle D: *Ultrasound in emergency medicine,* Philadelphia, 1995, WB Saunders.

Jehle D, Davis E, Evans T, et al: Emergency department sonography by emergency physicians, *Am J Emerg Med* 7(6):605, 1989.

Mahoney BS, Filly RA, Nyberg DA, Callen PW: Sonographic evaluation of ectopic pregnancy, *J Ultrasound Med* 4:221, 1985.

Mortality results for randomized controlled trial of early elective surgery or ultrasonographic surveillance for small abdominal aortic aneurysms: the UK small aneurysm trial participants, *Lancet* 352(9141):1649, 1998.

Roberts KB: The AAP practice parameter on urinary tract infections in febrile infants and young children, *Am Fam Physician* 62(8):1815, 2000.

Sanders RC, Miner NS, editors: *Clinical sonography: a practical guide,* ed 3, Boston, 1998, Little, Brown.

Schlager D, Lazzaresch G, Whitten D, et al: A prospective study of ultrasonography in the ED by emergency physicians, *Am J Emerg Med* 12(2):185, 1994.

Siepel T, Clifford DS, James PA, Cowan TM: The ultrasound-assisted physical examination in the periodic health evaluation of the elderly, *J Fam Pract* 49(7):628, 2000.

Simon B, Snoey E: *Ultrasound in emergency and ambulatory medicine,* St Louis, 1997, Mosby.

CHAPTER 210

Fine-Needle Aspiration Cytology and Biopsy

Lee A. Green

Fine-needle aspiration (FNA) and biopsy is a rapid, safe, relatively painless method of sampling solid and cystic masses in a variety of anatomic sites for cytologic examination. Both benign and suspected malignant conditions can be diagnosed with FNA.

Although the procedure is successfully used to sample lesions of the prostate, salivary glands, and intraabdominal and intrathoracic organs, the primary care physician will find FNA most useful for masses in the *breast* and *thyroid,* and for *lymph nodes.* For tumors of these sites, positive and negative predictive values for malignancy are typically in the 92% to 98% range, with overall diagnostic accuracy of greater than 70%. However, these rates are highly dependent on the skill of the clinician. It is clear from the literature that FNA should be performed by clinicians who are skilled at technical procedures and well-trained in FNA in order to obtain adequate diagnostic accuracy. Proper preparation of the smears is as important as the aspiration technique, as is the availability of a cytopathologist skilled in reading FNA specimens.

As implied by the overall diagnostic accuracy rate, as many as one fourth of specimens will return with nondiagnostic results, necessitating repeat aspiration or open biopsy. However, FNA will provide diagnosis in most cases with a procedure that is safer, more comfortable, less invasive, and less costly than open biopsy. These same advantages allow FNA to be used with less hesitation than would open biopsy. For example, many samples can be drawn over time from breast lesions in a patient with fibrocystic disease, whereas repeated open biopsy with subsequent scarring would be unacceptable.

Although false-negative results are generally more common than false-positives with FNA, the reverse is true for breast aspirations among young women; more than half of all "suspicious" FNAs of palpable breast masses among women under 30 prove to be benign on excisional biopsy. Fibroadenomas can show cellular atypia, nuclear overlapping, hyperchromasia, and epithelial clustering, and are thus easily overinterpreted. Some authors advocate use of FNA of breast lesions as one component of a "triple test," comprising clinical examination, mammography or ultrasound, and FNA. When all three elements are concordant for malignancy or nonmalignancy, the predictive value of the triple test approaches 100%. The majority of the predictive use of the triple test is the FNA result, but discordance—suspicious clinical and imaging findings with a negative or nonspecific FNA—may help the clinician identify potential false-negative FNAs for further workup. In the breast, any palpable mass that is new and questionable must be removed if fluid cannot be aspirated, regardless of other test findings.

In all breast complaints, FNA provides significant information. If a mass is palpable, FNA is carried out. If nonbloody cystic fluid is retrieved and the mass is gone, the woman can be reassured of the extremely low likelihood of cancer if the mass does not recur at 6 to 8 weeks. If it does recur, repeat aspiration should be performed. If it recurs a third time, it should be excised. Mammograms are usually done for baseline or confirmation a week after the aspiration.

INDICATIONS

- Presence of a palpable suspicious mass in the breast
- Thyroid nodule
- Clinically suspicious lymph node or group of nodes
- Any palpable, superficial, nonpulsating mass

The primary care physician ordinarily does not perform x-ray, ultrasound, or computed tomography–guided FNA of nonpalpable lesions. FNA is probably the procedure of first choice, even over imaging studies, of evaluating thyroid nodules and detecting the rare parathyroid tumor.

CONTRAINDICATIONS

- Unskilled clinician *(relative)*
- Absence of a cytopathologist capable of proper interpretation of the resulting slides

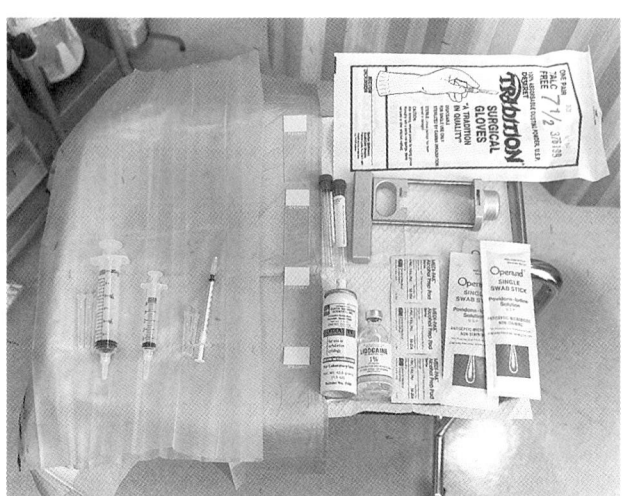

Fig. 210-1
Setup tray for fine-needle aspiration when using Comeco syringe.

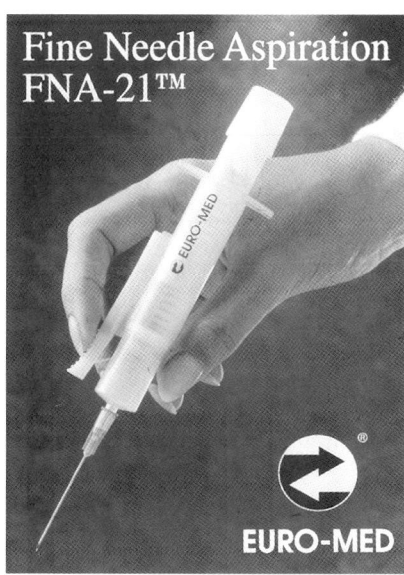

Fig. 210-2
Cooper Surgical FNA-21. (Courtesy CooperSurgical, Trumbull, Conn.)

- Sites of active pyogenic infection, although suspected granulomatous infection (fungal or mycobacterial) of a node does not contraindicate FNA
- Nonpalpable lesion

FNA may be performed safely in the anticoagulated patient if studies are in the therapeutic range, with proper attention to compression of the site afterwards to avoid hematoma. It may be performed in all but the most severely immunocompromised patients.

EQUIPMENT

- The Cameco syringe pistol (Fig. 210-1) is available in various sizes from Precision Dynamics Corporation (Van Nuys, Calif.), *or*
- A disposable, spring-loaded syringe (FNA-21) is now available from Cooper Surgical (Shelton, Conn.) (Fig. 210-2), *or*
- Milex supplies a breast aspiration biopsy needle (Fig. 210-3), which is unique because of its separate cutting port near the tip, *or*
- A 21-gauge needle can be used on the end of a regular 3-, 5-, or 10-ml syringe, *or*
- A 21-gauge butterfly can be connected to a syringe. The assistant aspirates the syringe while the clinician manipulates the needle.

Note: The first four of the above will allow a single-handed aspiration technique, which frees the other hand for better isolation and stabilization of the mass.

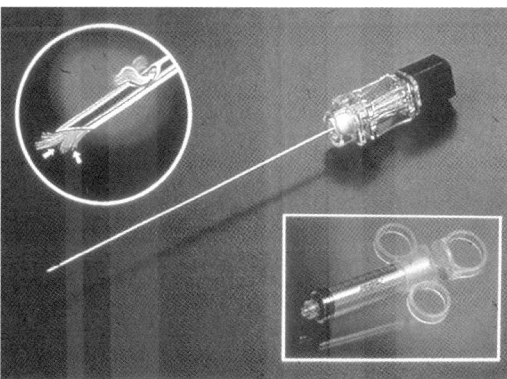

Fig. 210-3
Milex needle used for needle biopsy. Note the special extra side port to sample more tissue. (Courtesy Milex, Chicago, Ill.)

- Two sterile, plain (nonanticoagulant), evacuated blood tubes
- 21-, 22-, or 23-gauge needle
- Syringe of appropriate size
- Slides with frosted ends (three to four)
- Containers with fixative if necessary. Pap smear fixative is generally used and all that is needed, but check with the pathologist for his or her preferences and preferred technique.
- Glass cover slips or extra slides for smearing the specimens
- 4 × 4–inch gauze pads
- Sterile gloves
- Isopropyl alcohol pads or povidone-iodine swabs
- 1-ml syringe with 30-gauge half-inch needle and 1% plain lidocaine for anesthesia of skin *(optional)*

PREPROCEDURE PATIENT PREPARATION

Advise patients of the risks and benefits of the procedure, the indications, the alternatives, and the comparative risks and benefits of the alternatives. (See the sample patient education handout titled "Fine-Needle Aspiration (FNA)" on page 2017 of Appendix G and the sample patient consent form titled "Fine-Needle Aspiration (FNA)" on page 2019 of Appendix G.) Significant complications of FNA are rare. A small hematoma or ecchymosis for a few days (especially from thyroid FNA), and some mild soreness are to be expected. The patient must understand that nondiagnostic results occur commonly and may require repeat FNA or open biopsy, and that false-negative and false-positive results are possible. Patients undergoing FNA of breast lesions should wear a supportive brassiere.

TECHNIQUE

Setup and Preparation

1. Prophylaxis for bacterial endocarditis is not required.
2. Prep the skin with 70% isopropyl alcohol. Povidone-iodine preparation may be used but is not required for FNA. Sterile draping is not required, although neither the needle nor the skin entry site should be touched except with a sterile glove after the skin is prepared.
3. Fig. 210-1 illustrates the typical equipment set up for FNA. The sterile tray contains both a 5-ml syringe for freehand aspiration and a 20-ml syringe for use with the Cameco aspirator handle; ordinarily one or the other is used, not both. Both 21- and 23-gauge needles are illustrated; either size may be used, though 23-gauge may be preferred in the thyroid and 21-gauge for dense masses and the breast. The 1-ml syringe with a 30-gauge, ½-inch needle may be used for skin anesthesia, if desired. The slides on which the smears will be made have one frosted end, allowing easy labeling with sequence numbers. The sterile plain (nonanticoagulant) blood specimen tubes are for cyst fluid, if obtained. Alternatively, the fluid can just be placed in the formalin jars. If breast fluid is nonbloody (urine colored or green), it does *not* need to be sent to pathology (for cell block, cytology, or anything else) and should just be discarded. The spray fixative is that ordinarily used for Pap smears. Not illustrated are 4 × 4–inch gauze pads, which should also be ready, and a saline or formalin jar for a solid-core specimen, if obtained.
4. Skin anesthesia is often not necessary for FNA, since the needles are small and not painful. If desired,

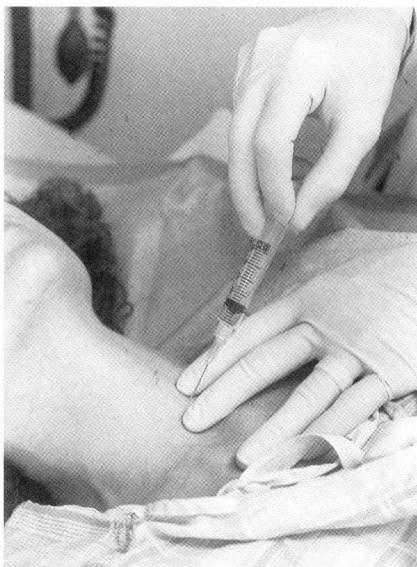

Fig. 210-4
Thyroid fine-needle aspiration using ordinary syringe. (Courtesy CooperSurgical, Trumbull, Conn.)

however, excellent anesthesia can be obtained with 1% plain lidocaine by using a 30-gauge needle on a 1-ml syringe. If the lidocaine is injected slowly and in small volume (approximately 0.5 ml) into the subcutaneous tissues without raising a skin wheal, and then allowed to remain for 5 minutes, anesthesia can be achieved painlessly and without obscuring the lesion to be aspirated.

Sampling

Pneumothorax has been reported with needle aspiration and needle biopsy of the breast. To prevent this, aspirate with the mass positioned over a rib or at a tangential angle as opposed to perpendicular to the body. If the person is thin or the lesion is deep, it may be prudent to have the patient hold her breath while sampling. Fig. 210-2 shows the proper way to hold the FNA-21.

Fig. 210-4 illustrates the aspiration of a thyroid nodule using one-handed manual withdrawal of the syringe plunger to create vacuum. The fingers hold the plunger while the thumb exerts pressure on the syringe top flange.

Fig. 210-5 illustrates aspiration of a breast cyst using the Cameco syringe holder to withdraw the plunger.

Whatever technique is used, the fingers of the nondominant hand stabilize the lesion to be aspirated and provide tactile feedback when the needle has been placed in the lesion.

Before the puncture is made, draw air into the syringe, filling approximately one fifth of its volume. The purpose of this is to have the air to flush out the needle

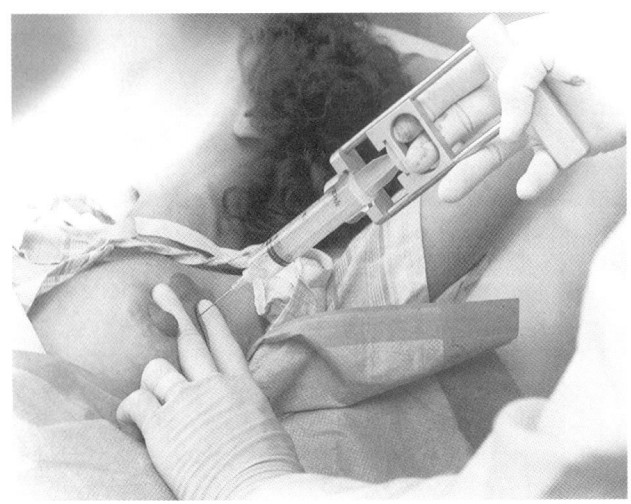

Fig. 210-5
Breast fine-needle aspiration using Comeco syringe holder.

and its contents onto a slide. Without the air, there is no good way to empty the needle. (*Do not* aspirate air after withdrawing the needle from the mass, since this will spread the sparse contents all over the inside of the syringe, making it hard to retrieve. Also note that this step is not needed with the FNA-21, since it will create a vacuum using the spring mechanism.) Carefully note the position of the plunger against the syringe markings. Then introduce the needle into the lesion, and withdraw the plunger to create vacuum.

Fig. 210-6 illustrates the technique of sampling a solid lesion or a cyst that remains palpable after fluid has been drained. Make several (10 to 20) passes into the lesion, filling the needle with cells and sampling all areas of the lesion (Fig. 210-7). Return the plunger to its previously noted resting position *before withdrawing the needle from the mass* to avoid aspirating the cells up into the syringe when the needle is withdrawn. Withdraw the needle from the lesion and skin, and use the air that was in the syringe to express

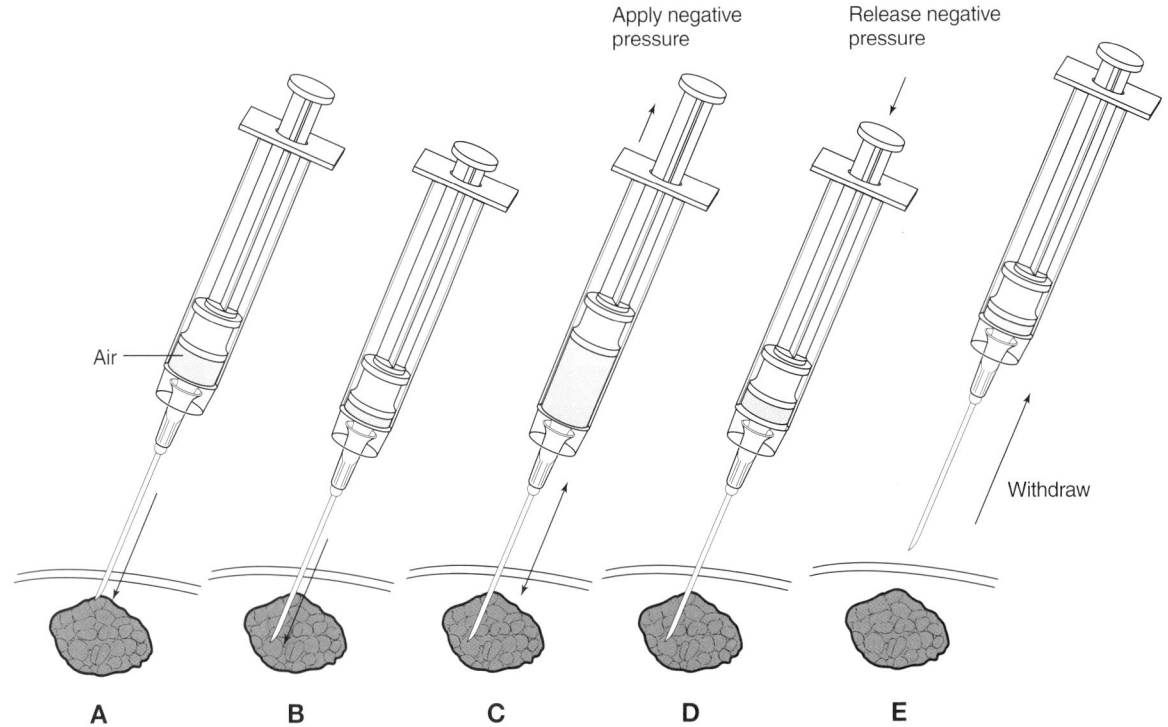

Fig. 210-6
Fine-needle aspiration technique of a solid lesion or cyst (a palpable breast mass, in this case) that remains palpable after fluid has been drained. **A,** Aspirate 1 to 2 ml of air into syringe before inserting needle. **B,** Insert the needle into the mass and aspirate. If cystic fluid is not obtained or the mass does not resolve, the mass is solid. **C,** Maintain negative pressure in the syringe and move the needle back and forth through the tissue 15 to 20 times to collect cells for analysis (see Fig. 210-7). **D,** Release the plunger. **E,** Withdraw needle and spread contents on a slide, which is immediately fixed.

the sample from the needle onto the slide. Handle the specimen as described below. Repeat the procedure if necessary.

If a lesion is cystic and fluid is obtained, draw as much as possible into the syringe. Withdraw the needle and empty the syringe, then perform another aspiration if more fluid remains. Alternatively, detach the needle from the syringe and leave the needle in place, empty the syringe and reattach it, and withdraw more fluid. As noted, for nonbloody cystic masses of the breast, the fluid can be discarded and there is no need to send it to pathology.

Specimen Handling

Preparation of the smears to be submitted for cytologic analysis is of crucial importance in obtaining accurate results. The technique is similar to making a blood or bone marrow smear and may be performed in several ways. Clinicians, especially if not well practiced in slide preparation, are strongly urged to make practice slides under the direction of the cytopathologist until good results are consistently obtained, or to have a skilled technician attend FNAs to prepare the slides. The nurse or office assistant who is to prepare slides should be directly and formally trained by the cytopathologist or experienced medical technician. Slides may be stained by the Papanicolaou or the May-Grünwald-Giemsa method; slides destined for the former must be alcohol-fixed within 5 to 10 seconds of smearing to prevent drying, and slides destined for the latter should be allowed to air-dry completely. The choice of procedure will be determined by the pathologist who will read the slides.

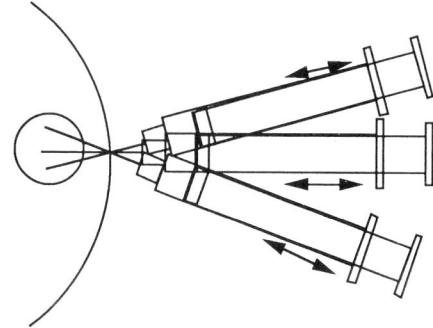

Fig. 210-7
Depiction of how to carry out step C in Fig. 210-6. The needle is passed multiple times into the mass to obtain adequate sampling.

Alternatively, some cytology laboratories prefer to receive specimens in cytologic fixative fluid (e.g., Cytolyt) for examination with the ThinPrep automated method. The role of ThinPrep in FNA is currently unclear; it may yield more cells but fewer elements of background (e.g., stroma). The reader is advised to consult her or his pathologist regarding the decision to submit using fixative fluid. If done, the typical method is to aspirate the lesion in the usual fashion, then place the needle into the solution and aspirate and express the fluid, to wash the cells into the fluid container. The fluid container is then submitted in its entirety.

If a solid-core specimen is expressed from the needle, it can be washed from the slide into a vial of saline or formalin and submitted for histologic examination. Consult a pathologist regarding whether to submit cores intact and which solution to use. Fluid obtained from cysts can be smeared on a slide, as noted above, or submitted in bulk in a sterile tube. (Standard evacuated blood tubes are sterile; those without anticoagulant should be used.) When a breast cyst is aspirated, the fluid should be submitted for pathologic evaluation only if tinged with blood. Yellow or green fluid is diagnostic of benign cysts, and cytology is unnecessary. A sterile tube can also be used to submit semisolid material such as that obtained from a lymph node for culture. If infection is suspected, fluid and solid specimens can be submitted in transport media as well.

POSTPROCEDURE CARE

Compression of the site with a gauze pad for 5 to 15 minutes will minimize bruising, especially of the highly vascular thyroid area. A compression dressing of folded gauze pads under Elastoplast tape can be applied on suitable sites. In breast biopsies, placement of a stack of folded gauze pads under a snug brassiere forms an effective compression dressing that may be left in place for several hours to prevent hematoma formation. Some physicians apply a small ice pack to the FNA site for 15 to 60 minutes after the procedure.

COMPLICATIONS

Complications of FNA are limited primarily to diagnostic failure or to false-negative and false-positive results. The incidence of failures is strongly dependent on the operator. Minor hematoma formation is a frequent occurrence but is seldom of clinical significance. Pneumothorax has been reported in rare instances. Before the widespread use of FNA, concern was often expressed about the possibility of seeding the needle track with malignant cells or releasing malignant cells to spread through lymphatics. Neither of these theoretical complications has been documented to occur, and they should not be considered complications of FNA. Damage to local anatomic structures (e.g., recurrent laryngeal nerve injury with thyroid FNA) is possible but occurs rarely, if at all; large case series have not reported such injuries. The lack of complications is probably due to the small diameter of the needles used for FNA, in contrast to cutting-needle biopsies, which do cause injury with some frequency.

SUPPLIERS

FNA-21
CooperSurgical
95 Corporate Drive
Trumbull, CT 06611
Phone: 1-203-601-4741
Website: www.coopersurgical.com

Special syringe
Milex Products, Inc.
4311 N. Normandy
Chicago, IL 60634
Phone: 1-800-621-1278
Website: www.milexproducts.com

Comeco syringe
Precision Dynamics Corp.
P.O. Box 9043
Van Nuys, CA 91409
Phone: 1-800-847-0670
Website: www.pdcorp.com

CPT/BILLING CODES

10021	Fine-needle biopsy w/o imaging
19000	Aspiration drainage of a breast cyst; one cyst
19001	Aspiration drainage of a breast cyst; additional cyst
19100	Core needle biopsy breast

ICD-9-CM DIAGNOSTIC CODES

217	Benign lesion breast
610.0	Solitary cyst of breast
610.1	Fibrocystic breast disease
610.2	Fibroadenosis of breast
611.72	Breast lump
174.1	Cancer breast central
174.0	Cancer breast areola
174.4	Cancer breast upper/outer quadrant
174.6	Cancer breast, axillary fold

ADDITIONAL RESOURCES

- See the sample patient education handout titled "Fine-Needle Aspiration (FNA)" on page 2017 of Appendix G.
- See the sample patient consent form titled "Fine-Needle Aspiration (FNA)" on page 2019 of Appendix G.

BIBLIOGRAPHY

Bottles K, Miller TR, Cohen MB, Ljung BM: Fine-needle aspiration biopsy: has its time come? *Am J Med* 81:525, 1986.

Cady B, Steele GD Jr, Morrow M, et al: Evaluation of common breast problems: guidance for primary care providers, *CA Cancer J Clin* 48:49, 1998.

Caruso DR, Mazzaferri EL: Practical evaluation of thyroid nodules, *Hosp Med* January:46, 1992.

Conry C: Evaluation of a breast complaint: is it cancer? *Am Fam Physician* 49(2):445, 1994.

Donnegan WL: Evaluation of a palpable breast mass, *N Engl J Med* 327:937, 1992.

Erickson R, Shank JC, Gratton C: Fine-needle breast aspiration biopsy, *J Fam Physician* 28(3):306, 1989.

Frable W: Thin-needle aspiration biopsy, *Am J Clin Pathol* 6(5):168, 1976.

Hamburger JI: Needle aspiration for thyroid nodules: skip ultrasound—do initial assessment in the office, *Postgrad Med* 84(8):61, 1988.

Hammond S, Keyhani-Rofagha S, O'Toole RV: Statistical analysis of fine-needle aspiration cytology of the breast, *Acta Cytol* 3(1):276, 1987.

Kopicki MT: Management of the palpable breast mass, *Female Pat* 23:45, 1998.

Layfield LJ, Chrischilles EA, Cohen MB, Bottles K: The palpable breast nodule: a cost-effectiveness analysis of alternate diagnostic approaches, *Cancer* 72:1642, 1993.

Lee KR, Foster RS, Papillo JL: Fine-needle aspiration of the breast: importance of the aspirator, *Acta Cytol* 3(1):281, 1987.

Lever JV, Trott PA, Webb AJ: Fine-needle aspiration cytology, *J Clin Pathol* 3(8):1, 1985.

Lieu D: Fine-needle aspiration: technique and smear preparation, *Am Fam Physician* 55(3):839, 1997.

Perez-Reyes N, Mulford DK, Rutkowski MA, et al: Breast fine-needle aspiration: a comparison of thin-layer and conventional preparation, *Am J Clin Pathol* 102(3):349, 1994.

Stanley MW: Fine-needle aspiration biopsy: diagnosis of cancerous masses in the office, *Postgrad Med* 85(1):163, 1989.

CHAPTER 211

Heimlich Maneuver

Raymond F. Jarris, Jr.
Timothy J. Downs

Each year in the United States, 3000 people die from swallowing or aspirating objects. When a patient displays the distress signal for choking (i.e., clutching the neck) or becomes cyanotic, unconscious, or unable to effectively cough or breathe (suggesting complete obstruction), efforts to clear the obstruction are warranted. The Heimlich maneuver causes a sudden increase in intrathoracic pressure, forcing an obstructing object from the glottis (Fig. 211-1).

Note: In the event of partial foreign-body aspiration, if the patient is able to breathe and speak, the Heimlich maneuver and probing of the oropharynx should be avoided and the patient should be transported to a source of medical care.

INDICATIONS

* Asphyxiation from foreign-body obstruction of the upper airway

CONTRAINDICATIONS

* Infants, small children, and pregnant women (abdominal thrusts inappropriate)

TECHNIQUE

Adults and Children Greater than 1 Year of Age

Sitting or Standing

Apply three to five abdominal or chest thrusts (Fig. 211-2, *A*).

Lying

1. Place the patient in the supine position.
2. Place one hand on top of the other, with the heel of the bottom hand positioned in the midline of the patient, between the umbilicus and xiphoid.

3. Lean forward with shoulders over the patient's abdomen and quickly press inward and upward three to five times (Fig. 211-2, *B*).
4. In pregnant or obese patients, use chest thrusts delivered in the same fashion as Step 3, but place hands over the sternum.
5. Clear material from the oropharynx with a finger sweep or Magill forceps.

Infants to 1 Year of Age

1. Place the child face down on your arm with head directed downward, supporting head and neck with knee and one hand (Fig. 211-3).
2. Deliver three to five gentle back blows between the scapulae with the palm of the hand.
3. If obstruction is still present, roll the child over, lower his or her head, and deliver chest thrusts gently with two to three fingers as in cardiopulmonary resuscitation.
4. Repeat Steps 2 and 3 until the object is cleared or surgical intervention is required (Chapter 72, Cricothyroidotomy, Transtracheal Catheter Insertion and Tracheostomy).

COMPLICATIONS

* Abdominal aortic aneurysm thrombosis
* Esophageal rupture
* Gastric rupture
* Jejunal rupture
* Liver, spleen, or pancreas injury
* Pneumomediastinum
* Regurgitation
* Rib fracture

The Heimlich maneuver is usually performed outside of medical facilities. Although complications are rare, most of the complications are severe and can be life threatening. For example, gastric rupture has a high mortality rate. A physician should evaluate all persons

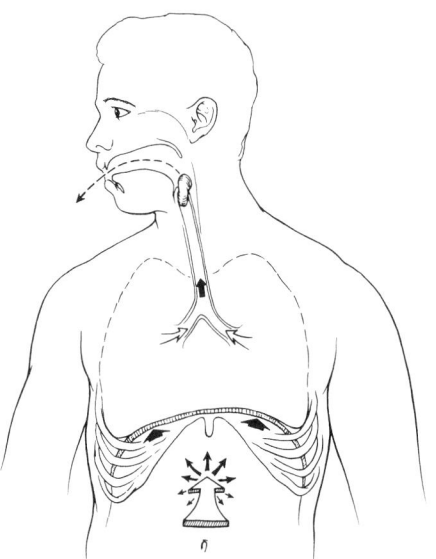

Fig. 211-1
If the patient is sitting or standing, the physician should stand behind the patient and wrap his or her arms around the patient's waist. The physician's fist should be placed with the thumb side against the patient's abdomen, above the umbilicus but below the rib cage.

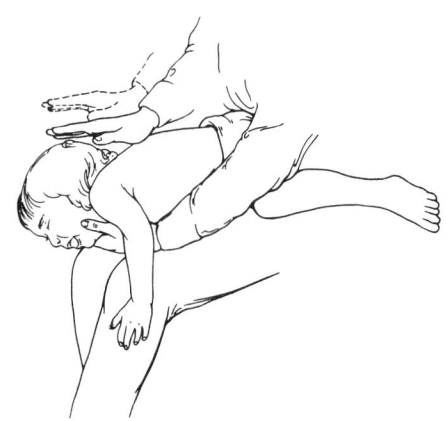

Fig. 211-3
Back blows for infants and small children. See text for details.

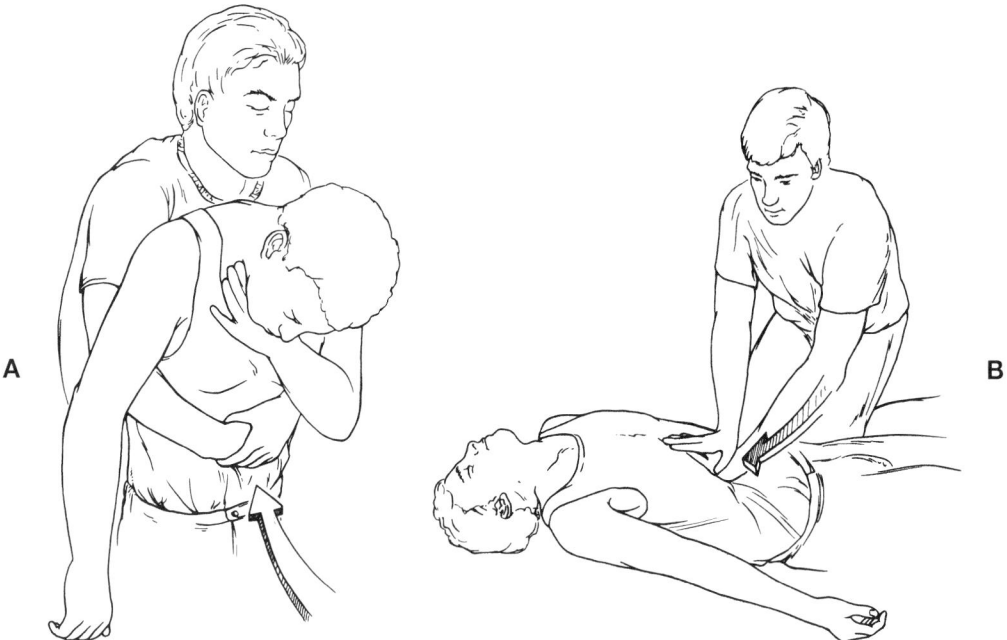

Fig. 211-2
Abdominal thrusts. **A,** If the patient is sitting or standing, the physician should stand behind the patient, wrap his or her arms around the patient's waist, grasp the fist or wrist of one hand with the other, place the hands against the patient's abdomen between the navel and rib cage, and press the fist into the patient's abdomen with a quick thrust upward. This should be repeated up to three to five times. **B,** If the patient has collapsed or is unable to be lifted, he or she should be placed in the supine position and the physician should kneel beside the patient's abdomen or straddle it. The physician should place one hand on top of the other, with the heel of the bottom hand in the midline between the patient's navel and rib cage. He or she should lean forward so that the shoulders are over the patient's abdomen and press toward the diaphragm with a quick thrust, inward and upward. The physician should not press to the right or left of the midline. This should be repeated up to three to five times if necessary.

who have been subjected to the Heimlich maneuver. Focused evaluation by the physician should include history and physical examination of the respiratory and gastrointestinal system. Early intervention may reduce the morbidity and mortality associated with these complications.

BIBLIOGRAPHY

Bintz M, Cogbill TH: Gastric rupture after the Heimlich maneuver, *J Trauma* 40:159, 1996.

Haynes DE, Haynes BE, Yong YV: Esophageal rupture complicating Heimlich maneuver, *Am J Emerg Med* 2:507, 1984.

Hedges R: *Clinical procedures in emergency medicine,* Philadelphia, 1991, WB Saunders.

Kirschner RL, Green RM: Acute thrombosis of abdominal aortic aneurysm subsequent to Heimlich maneuver: a case report, *J Vasc Surg* 2:594, 1985.

Majumdar A, Sedman PC: Gastric rupture secondary to successful Heimlich maneuver, *Postgrad Med J* 74:609, 1998.

Razaboni RM, Brathwaite CE, Dwyer WA Jr: Ruptured jejunum following Heimlich maneuver, *J Emerg Med* 4:95, 1986.

Schwartz GR: *Principles and practice of emergency medicine,* Philadelphia, 1986, WB Saunders.

CHAPTER 212

Medical Hypnosis

Daniel A. Zelling

The use of hypnosis dates to ancient times. Found in the earliest writings in China, India, Tibet, Greece, and Egypt are descriptions of this "strange" phenomenon. The Ebers Papers, dated approximately 3000 BC, describe sleep temples for the ill and infirm, where they were placed in trance and supposedly visited by the gods to cure their diseases. Despite what some authorities suggest, hypnosis was not invented some 200 years ago by Franz Anton Mesmer. Hypnosis is not a new medical treatment, nor is it a New Age phenomenon. Indeed, healing in the trance state is one of the oldest medical arts. In certain areas of medicine, it is also used on a daily basis. Lamaze developed his technique to assist with childbirth after studying with a hypnotherapist in Russia. Note that throughout this chapter, when the word *hypnosis* is used, it refers to medical hypnosis as opposed to stage hypnosis, forensic hypnosis, sports hypnosis, and so forth.

Medical hypnosis is the art and science of suggestive therapy. Acceptance of suggestions is enhanced when the patient is in a receptive mood. Hypnosis can be viewed as a left- to right-brain shift, in which the critical left-brain thinking is diminished and the right-brain creative-imaginative thinking is increased, thereby enhancing receptiveness. Although the word *hypnosis* is derived from the Greek *hypnos,* which means sleep, the patient is not really asleep. The experience of formally induced hypnosis may resemble sleep, but the patient remains alert while being relaxed. Despite this reality, confusion between physical sleep and the hypnotic trance has persisted and grown in magnitude. In part, this is because the subject's eyes are closed during hypnosis. In addition, the word *sleep* is frequently used in the induction procedure. However, the patient in hypnosis never loses consciousness, unless of course the subject goes to sleep, in which case he or she is no longer in hypnosis.

One way to understand the hypnotic state is to think of it as the semiaware state into and out of which we drift when we daydream. For example, everyone has experienced being spoken to while daydreaming. With the mind distracted by the daydream, often none of the conversation registers, even though there is complete consciousness. In fact, hypnosis can be defined as concentrated and directed daydreaming. Under hypnosis, most surrounding noises, conversations, and thoughts do not register.

In 1958, the American Medical Association (AMA) officially approved the use of hypnosis in medicine and dentistry. Before that, the medical profession generally had condemned hypnosis for being unscientific and bordering on charlatanism and quackery. The extravagant and unsubstantiated claims of cures by unqualified operators led to great skepticism that has persisted to the present day. This skepticism is no longer valid because of the amount of scientific work and valuable research that has been carried out over the past four decades. In fact, now that the medical value of hypnosis has been recognized, it has provoked legislation in several states, including New York, California, Illinois, and Florida. In the Florida Hypnosis Law, Section 656-31, hypnosis has attained the status of a medical intervention for illness, both mental and physical. For that reason, it should be restricted to therapeutic purposes and to certain practitioners of the healing arts who are qualified by professional training. Such practitioners must have within the scope of their competence the ability to diagnose and treat human illness, disease, or injury that is appropriate for the use of hypnosis.

Although there is a great need for legislation and controls, most of all there is a need for greater public understanding of medical hypnosis. Unfortunately, some patients think of stage hypnosis when they hear the term *hypnosis.* However, they must be reassured that stage hypnosis is only one, insignificant phase of this broad area of psychological phenomena and that as an example, it fails to reflect the potential of hypnosis. In fact, the British Medical Association and the AMA are unalterably opposed to stage hypnotism and to hypnotism by amateurs or poorly qualified individuals.

For primary care clinicians, a better understanding has gradually developed that there is nothing magical or even remarkable about hypnotic treatment. Used like other procedures in medicine, with care, good judgment and skill, hypnosis has proved valuable not only as a primary procedure but also as an adjunct to other procedures. This chapter discusses the basic principles behind hypnosis and the techniques of both guided hypnosis, or hetero-hypnosis, and self-hypnosis. Examples of both are provided. For thorough discussions of the indications listed below as well as others, comprehensive textbooks are listed in the "Bibliography" section.

INDICATIONS

The following is a sample of indications and is not all inclusive.

- Alcoholism and addiction*
- Allergies*
- Amnesia*
- Anxiety disorders and phobias
- Bashful bladder*
- Bruxism
- Cancer treatment: adverse affects*
- Childbirth, including hyperemesis gravidarum*
- Depression
- Dyspareunia
- Eating disorders
- Ego strengthening (see "Technique: Guided Hypnosis or Hetero-Hypnosis" section)*
- Enuresis
- Fear of flying
- Fear of public speaking
- Gagging
- Headaches (both tension and migraine)*
- Hiccups
- Insomnia
- Nailbiting*
- Pain management*
- Painful procedures*
- Smoking*
- Test anxiety
- Thumb sucking
- Trichotillomania

CONTRAINDICATIONS

- Diagnoses for which another form of therapy would be more appropriate
- Unwilling or uncooperative patient or lack of informed consent
- Language barrier
- Lack of practitioner experience
- Inability to understand verbal instructions (e.g., young

*These topics are discussed in this chapter.

age [under 5 years old] or mental retardation with equivalent young mental age)
- Frank paranoid schizophrenia
- Decompensated personality disorder (e.g., schizoid with psychosis)

Note: A relative contraindication is a litigious patient. Although this class of individuals is difficult to define, common sense should be used with certain patients. If a procedure is performed under hypnosis and there is a complication, the patient may become even more litigious.

EQUIPMENT

- A quiet room with comfortable chairs is necessary. Attempts should be made to minimize interruptions. Soft, classical music in the background can be helpful.
- Props, as needed (e.g., pen, pencil, or card with yellow and blue rectangles).

PREPROCEDURE PATIENT PREPARATION

Before a patient undergoes hypnosis, certain misconceptions should be discussed and the patient should be aware of certain facts. It is also important to discuss the patient's beliefs about hypnosis and his or her expectations. The clinician should know if the patient has experienced hypnosis in the past, whether it was successful, who induced the hypnosis (professional or nonprofessional), and the nature of the experience, including how the patient felt about it. Entertainment media have given the false impression that the patient will lose control. They have also given the false impression that hypnosis takes place because of some "magical power" the hypnotist possesses. The patient should be aware that in reality all hypnosis is self-hypnosis and that the clinician is merely the guide or the catalyst to help the patient do what he or she wants to do. Using hypnosis, the clinician can aid the patient in accepting suggestions and guide the patient through a particular experience. The patient remains in control. A useful analogy for patients is that the clinician is like an orchestra conductor and the patient a musician. For the conductor to do his or her job, the musician must be willing to play the music.

Another misconception is that only certain people can be hypnotized; the fact is that anyone who wants to be hypnotized can be hypnotized. The reverse is also true; anyone who does not want to be hypnotized cannot be hypnotized. In 35 years of practice, the author has not seen a single patient who wanted to be hypnotized who was unsuccessful. In addition, the ability to be hypnotized has nothing to do with will power or lack thereof, and nothing to do with intelligence, although it might be more difficult to hypnotize a severely retarded person. In general, the higher the person's intelligence, the easier he or she can be hypnotized. (This can be a good motivator for many skeptics!) Another misconception is that some people are not able to come out of hypnosis. There is no record of this *ever* happening. Hypnosis is a state of focused attention controlled by the patient; therefore the patient allows the trance to start and to end. The patient should be reassured that hypnosis will never cause harm, embarrassment, or loss of dignity.

The patient should recognize that hypnosis is not a cure-all or a panacea. It is excellent in the treatment of some diseases, and it is absolutely of no value in the treatment of others. Just as penicillin is the treatment of choice for some infections, it is useless in the treatment of others. Sometimes the results of hypnosis are so outstanding and rapid that they seem miraculous or magical. However, this is actually only because hypnosis, when properly used by a qualified clinician, is more effective than similar but outmoded or alternative forms of therapy.

The patient should be aware of the 10 facts shown in the patient education handout titled "Medical Hypnosis: 10 Frequently Asked Questions" (on page 2020 of Appendix G) before he or she is hypnotized.

TECHNIQUE: GUIDED HYPNOSIS OR HETERO-HYPNOSIS

Hypnosis is a normal psychologically altered state of consciousness that is similar to, but not the same as, being awake and similar to, but not the same as, being asleep. It is produced by the presence of two conditions: (1) a central focus of attention and (2) surrounding areas of inhibition. The state of hypnosis in turn produces three things: (1) an increased relaxation of the body, (2) an increased concentration of the mind, and (3) an increased susceptibility to suggestion.

There are basically eight steps per induction:

1. Prehypnosis patient education
2. Induction of trance
3. Progressive relaxation
4. Deepening of relaxation
5. Protective suggestions
6. Reinduction suggestions (first time only)
7. Diagnostic or therapeutic suggestions
8. Wake-up

An example of a hypnotic session is used below to demonstrate the eight steps (for the indication of ego strengthening).

1. *Prehypnosis patient education.* Before any attempt is made to produce a trance state, all misconceptions about hypnosis must be removed. After the patient is asked what he or she knows about hypnosis and

what he or she may have seen, heard, or read about hypnosis, the following explanation is made:

Hypnosis is a state of consciousness. The patient is not "out" or "under." Hypnosis is not an anesthetic. It is an altered state of consciousness, very similar to daydreaming. While a person is in a daydream, the body is relaxed and the mind is concentrated on the daydream. In hypnosis, the person is at least 10 times more relaxed and is concentrated on what is going on. You (the patient) have been hypnotized many, many times. For example, when it was really important to you to get up at an unusual time, you awakened 10 minutes before the alarm went off. A woman with a small, ill child can sleep through a thunderstorm, but if that child whimpers she is wide awake. Many times you may have pulled your car into the driveway and not known how you got there, driving perfectly well in trance. So it's not magical, and I have no power over you. Anyone who wants to be hypnotized can be, and anyone who does not want to be hypnotized cannot be. This is because hypnosis is really self-hypnosis. The patient does the hypnosis, and the clinician is merely a catalyst or orchestra conductor. It is the patient who makes hypnosis happen.

At this point, having the patient read the facts from the patient education handout titled "Medical Hypnosis: 10 Frequently Asked Questions" (on page 2020 of Appendix G) may be helpful. Any questions should be answered.

Note: Just as the patient needs to know that he or she can be hypnotized, the clinician doing the hypnotic induction needs to be sure of his or her ability to induce the trance state. It therefore behooves the clinician to practice this skill under competent supervision. One reason hypnosis can fail is if the clinician panics. Practice makes this highly unlikely.

2. *Induction of trance.* There are probably more than 40 different techniques for inducing the trance state. The practitioner needs only two or three that fit the personality of the clinician and the patient. In the past, many inductions were authoritarian, using phrases like "your eyes will close" and "you cannot move a muscle even if you try." These phrases give the impression that the clinician has a certain power over the patient. Modern hypnotherapy uses more permissive inductions, which puts the ability to enter trance where it belongs—with the patient.

A very commonly used technique is the *eye fixation* induction (see below for alternative techniques). After the patient is seated in a comfortable chair, legs uncrossed and hands resting comfortably on midthigh, the patient is asked to stare at the tip of a pencil or pen that the clinician is holding, approximately 30 cm away from the patient's eyes. The pen should be above eye level to induce eye muscle fatigue and enhance the desire to eventually let the eyelids close. With the clinician holding the pen at a

45-degree angle and speaking in a slow, monotonous tone, the wording goes something like this:

Just breathe slowly and evenly and stare at the tip of my pen. Keep staring at the tip of my pen. Next, I'd like you to take a deep, deep breath in; now breathe it out slowly while staring at the pen. And as you continue to breathe slowly and evenly, you will find that in a few moments your eyes will begin to blink, and as they begin to blink you may find that they begin to close. Just stare, breathe slowly, and very soon your eyes begin to blink, and as they begin to blink they begin to close. Blinking and closing, blinking and closing, blinking and closing, blinking and closing, closing, closing, closing.

After enough repetition, when the patient closes his or her eyes, proceed to the next step.

3. *Progressive relaxation.* Next, the patient is more progressively relaxed:

Good! Now relax the muscles of your forehead and face. Relax the muscles of your forehead and face, and down your neck, and from your neck on down. Relax on down to your shoulders, down your upper arms to your elbows and from your elbows on down. Relax down your forearms to your wrists and from your wrists on down, down your hands. Feel all the tension now just dripping out from your fingers. [Notice the repetition of the word *down*. It suggests a deeper trance for the patient. However, the word "down" should be avoided in terminally ill patients.] Now relax the muscles inside your chest as your breathing becomes more and more regular, and the relaxation goes down your abdomen and from your abdomen on down. Relax on down your hips and pelvis, and from your hips on down your upper legs to your knees, and from your knees on down. Relax on down your lower legs to your ankles and from your ankles on down. Relax on down your feet and feel all the tension now dripping out from the tips of your toes and the tips of your fingers. Observe how still and relaxed you have become.

4. *Deepening of relaxation.* After the induction and progressive relaxation, proceed with deepening, the wording for which can be as simple as:

In a few moments I am going to count to five, and as I count to five you will become five times more relaxed than you are now. One, becoming more and more relaxed. Two, peaceful, calm and tranquil. Three, letting go as you become more and more completely relaxed. Four, breathing slowly, breathing evenly, and with each breath becoming more and more deeply relaxed. Five, way down. Good.

5. *Protective suggestions.* After the deepening, during a patient's first hypnotic session, he or she should be given the following protective suggestions:

You can never be taken advantage of while in the state of hypnosis. You can never be hypnotized unless you want to be hypnotized. You cannot be hypnotized against your will or without your consent. You cannot be hypnotized while holding the steering wheel of an automobile in your hands or in any situation that might be dangerous to you. You will always awaken from the state of hypnosis, wide awake, clear headed, and refreshed. Should an emergency situation arise while you are in the state of hypnosis, you will become immediately wide awake, clear headed, refreshed, and alert. You will be able to handle that situation as capably and effectively as you normally would.

6. *Reinduction suggestions.* In addition to these protective suggestions, this is the time to give the reinduction suggestions, as simple as follows:

From this moment on, when I say the words "relax deeply," you will be able to immediately go into a deep, deep hypnotic trance—even deeper than the one you are in now. Your eyes can close, and all your muscles can just give way, and you sink deeper and deeper, relaxed with every breath you take. The words "relax deeply" will never cause you to be hypnotized unless I say "relax deeply," and only when you want to be hypnotized. You can never be hypnotized by accident.

Of course, this last set of suggestions is given only during a patient's first hypnotic induction. These suggestions enable future trance inductions to go more quickly.

7. *Subsequent inductions.* After a brief discussion of how the patient is doing and any concerns the patient may have, the wording can go like this:

At the count of three you will be deeply hypnotized. One, take a nice deep breath in. Now breathe it out, and feel all the tension leaving your body and your mind. Two, allow your muscles to go loose and limber. Three, relax *deeply*, becoming more and more relaxed with every breath you take.

8. *Diagnostic or therapeutic suggestions.* After induction and deepening comes the diagnostic or therapeutic stage. Different than the trances induced with meditation, Zen, or Yoga, with medical hypnosis there is a diagnostic or therapeutic intervention.

As an example of a therapeutic suggestion for an anxious person with low self-esteem, ego strengthening might be performed as follows:

You have now become so pleasantly relaxed that your mind has become totally concentrated on what feels good and what is good. What is good is that you have survived all these years. And as you grow older, you grow stronger in mind, body, and spirit. No matter what happened to you in the past, you are in the now and you can relax with every treatment that I give you. You can become even more relaxed. There were things that bothered you in the past, but they are not in the now. Now you are learning to relax and feel better about yourself, not just when you are with me in this room, but later today and every day, no matter where you are, you remain more relaxed and at ease in every way. Every day you are able to see things in their *true* perspective, without magnifying your difficulties or ever allowing them to get the better of you. And since you are becoming more relaxed, you will be able to concentrate better, which makes you more effective and efficient at home, at work, and no matter where you are. You begin to accept yourself *just as* you are, for you really *are* unique. There is no one on the planet exactly like you. You have talents and abilities you haven't even explored yet. Now, relax as you let all these suggestions reinforce themselves in the few moments of silence that begin now.

Note: In today's age of global competition, suggestions of ego strengthening may be of benefit to most patients. In addition to whatever was the intended therapeutic intervention, ego strengthening suggestions can be included in almost any session as a bonus.

After several hypnosis sessions, when the patient is capable of performing self-hypnosis, there are certain reinforcements that can be given before wake-up to enhance patient compliance. Tell the patient to induce self-hypnotic trances frequently. Reassure the patient that after a certain amount of training, he or she will be able to induce a trance on his or her own. Many patients respond to the invitation to "take my voice with you."

9. *Wake-up.* The session ends with a wake-up (actually a poor choice of words because the patient is not asleep; "coming out of trance" or "coming back to a state of full awareness" is probably better; however, for some reason people prefer to hear "wake-up"). The "wake up" wording is something like this:

Now, in a few moments, I am going to wake you up, and when you are awakened you will be wide awake, clear headed and refreshed, calm and comfortable. Now at the count of three, wide awake, clear headed, and refreshed. One, beginning to come up now. Two, almost awake and, three, wide awake, clear headed, and refreshed. You can open your eyes, stretch vigorously, and I will see you next week (or appropriate time).

At this point, the author gives one more suggestion. Instead of asking "Do you feel better?" he says "Feel better," shakes hands, and tells the patient when he wants to see him or her again. Both clinicians and staff should be aware that statements made *right after* a trance state may have significant power as well.

Note that while a patient is under hypnosis, his or her ability to think critically is somewhat diminished. The left brain thinks more literal than the right brain. Therefore the clinician should keep the suggestions simple and literal and say only what is intended (e.g., if an error is made, don't say "shoot"). Think carefully before making every statement. The patient also listens very carefully, so do not be surprised if,

when you ask the patient to raise his or her right hand, he or she does not raise the right arm as most of us would do from having been conditioned in classrooms but instead raises just the right hand. In addition, the patient is in a more suggestible state, and any words spoken, whether in the room or by someone else outside the room, may have an impact on the patient (e.g., if someone passing in the hallway says "I hate having to wait," it might be taken as a suggestion). Clinic staff should be aware of the importance of minimizing distractions, and attempts should be taken to keep the environment quiet. If disruptions are unavoidable, during deepening of the trance, suggestions can be made to counteract the effect of disruptions: "You concentrate on the sound of my voice only. . . . you may notice certain sounds in the background like a telephone ringing, a typewriter running, or a door closing, but they will fade away and have no meaning to you as you concentrate on the sound of my voice only."

Alternative Induction Techniques

1. *Body focus technique.*

I would like you to close your eyes and concentrate your mind on the sound of my voice. . . . let your mind go blank as I ask you to concentrate on *one* part of your body. . . . I would like you to focus your attention on your right big toe, and as you concentrate your attention to your right big toe, you may begin to feel a pleasant, warm sensation in that right big toe. . . . and you will find that this pleasant, warm sensation begins to spread to your next toe, and as you breathe slowly you will feel it spreading to your middle toe. . . . (describe other toes, etc.). . . . now it is beginning to spread around the bottom and the top of your foot. . . .

You feel warm, safe, and comfortable, and your breathing is easy and relaxed, and as you breathe comfortably and relaxed, you can feel this pleasant, warm, soothing sensation spreading up your legs and into your thighs, up to your hips, and on into your abdomen, etc.

You find yourself sinking deeper and deeper into a pleasant state of relaxation. . . . your muscles becoming completely limp and relaxed; with every breath you take you will sink deeper and deeper into a deeper state of relaxation. . . .

2. *Double-bind technique.*

In a few moments I want you to close your eyes and let your little eye muscles relax completely until you are certain they won't work . . . . test them to be certain they don't work. . . . don't test them to find out that they will work, but test them to make certain they won't work. . . . when you are certain they won't work, close them and relax completely. . . . now relax the other muscles of your face. . . . the muscles around your scalp and on down your neck, etc.

Note: If the clinician learns one induction technique very well, most patients (95%) will respond. Knowledge of one or two other induction techniques may be of value for the other 5%.

3. *Color contrast technique.* Based on the normal tiring of the rods and cones in the retina, if someone stares at the blank space between a yellow and a blue rectangle, both the clinician and patient will observe the same phenomena. As you stand close and behind the patient, describe what you see, but phrase it as follows:

As you breathe slowly and evenly, stare at the space between the yellow and the blue rectangle. Notice that the blue next to the white space gets darker blue and yellow next the white space gets more yellow, and outside the blue rectangle yellow begins to appear. You will also notice that outside the yellow rectangle, a blue line begins to appear. Your eyes get so tired that you just want to close them. Go ahead and close them. Let the card slip out of your fingers as you relax completely.

HYPNOTIC STRATEGIES AND SUGGESTIONS FOR OTHER INDICATIONS

Suggestions should be kept positive whenever possible.

1. *Alcoholism and addiction.* With or without a 12-step program, hypnosis can help improve patients' self-esteem and increase their resolve to remain alcohol or substance free. These are the goals of the suggestions under hypnosis. Most alcoholics and addicts seem to have one thing in common, and that is shame. Shame is different from guilt. If a child does something wrong, breaks something, or spills something, he or she may feel guilty, but that goes away. If a person grows up in an environment in which the person feels that he or she cannot do anything right, then he or she may develop permanent shame, a feeling that "I must be rotten to the core." That is a spiritual problem that requires re-parenting of self and the ability to say "I love me." This break in humanity and divinity that I call a "hole in the soul" is found in nearly every addiction: morphine, heroin, cannabis, and even gambling. Direct suggestions can be helpful in overcoming any addiction once the "hole in the soul" has been repaired. Multiple sessions may be necessary to work on repairing the "hole in the soul." In addition to repairing the soul, hypnosis can be helpful in most cases for determining specifically why the person drinks or abuses drugs.

2. *Allergies.* If a patient has not been successful with standard immunotherapy or desensitization treatment, hypnotherapy may be of value. It is important for the patient to understand the basic aspects of the antigen-antibody principle of allergies. The patient should know that the antibodies are formed to get rid of a noxious substance. This should be explained as a normal and healthy reaction, but hypnosis helps the patient to understand that he or she no longer needs to defend against strawberries, wheat, grass, pollen, ragweed, or cats. By visualizing himself or herself without symptoms several times in the trance state, the patient may show remarkable improvement.

3. *Amnesia.* Amnesia can be neurophysiological, such as seen with head trauma, or, more frequently, psychophysiological. If a psychologically traumatic event is overwhelming, a person may withdraw (disassociate). Withdrawal can be so severe that the patient may not even know his or her name or where he or she lives. In trance, the traumatic event can be released. A return to normality can take place in just a few sessions in the hands of a qualified practitioner. However, an inexperienced hypnotist may be very challenged with this indication, so it may be wise to refer to an experienced medical hypnotist.

4. *Anxiety disorders and phobias.* All fear is learned; it is not just a chemical imbalance. With agoraphobia, for example, it is hard to explain that a patient can function well inside the home, and yet when he or she leaves the house, chemical changes occur suddenly in the brain. Through appropriate regression, the original cause of the fear can be located and removed. A short period of reeducation and rehabilitation has freed many patients from benzodiazepines and other anxiolytic medications.

5. *Bashful bladder.* The bashful bladder is a condition in which the patient, usually a male, is able to urinate when he is by himself in his own bathroom, but is totally unable to urinate in a public facility where other people might be present. Analytically, the reason for the inability to urinate in public is shame. Someone at some time has shamed the patient about penis size, or he was shamed during his upbringing about genitals and bodily functions, or he has been shamed by the sound of the urine hitting the toilet. The patient is desensitized as follows: ask him to imagine, when he is urinating normally all by himself, that a very important person has entered the bathroom while he is urinating. If the patient practices this, he will find that as soon as he imagines a very important person entering his private bathroom while he is urinating, his muscles will tighten up and

the flow of urine will be interrupted. If he then tells himself that this is utter nonsense, there is no person in his bathroom, especially since the door is locked, the flow of urine will return. This technique gives the patient the insight that he is in control. Under hypnosis, reinforcement assists the patient to understand that nobody cares about him urinating. With a gradual desensitization process, most people are able to use public bathrooms after approximately 10 sessions of therapy. The author knows of no other modality that can cure the bashful bladder.

6. *Cancer: side effects of chemotherapy and radiation.* When a patient is vomiting after chemotherapy, certainly the vomiting may be a side effect of the drug being used. However, many patients begin vomiting upon arrival at the parking lot of the oncologist, much too early for true side effects. During hypnosis, the patient learns that drugs like penicillin are poison, but a stronger poison for the bacteria than for the patient. In this manner, he or she can welcome and accept the penicillin to overcome an infection. Patients can also learn to welcome the chemotherapeutic agent as a poison to the cancer cells, but far less of a poison to normal cells. With radiation oncology the patient can be taught that the radiation is like tiny silver bullets, aimed at the tumor. In this manner, the patient can be helped to accept the radiotherapy with far less severe complications.

For the hair loss caused by chemotherapeutic agents, the author suggests that the patient shave his or her head completely. To find a plug of hair on the pillow in the morning is a very depressing thing. If the patient shaves his or her head, then the return of hair growth is a very positive thing.

Psychoneuroimmunology is a very helpful adjunct to cancer treatment. Patients should see themselves getting well, see themselves already well, and visualize their immune systems as defending armies doing battle for them. Such suggestions and visualization may not only change the outcome of the therapy, but may also change the patients' outlook, and may even help them to enjoy living again instead of merely surviving.

7. *Childbirth.* The use of hypnosis during childbirth has been popularized by the Frenchman Lamaze, who studied under Bykov in Russia. Lamaze techniques are actually fractionated hypnotic techniques. The goal is for the patient to accept that every contraction is a feeling that she welcomes because every contraction brings her closer to holding her baby, finally, in her arms. Words like *labor, hard labor,* or *pain* should never be used; in fact, the woman should forget anything she has been told regarding unpleasant experiences related to delivery. She should

understand that through the process of being able to relax completely, all that she has done to prepare for the baby will be successful and she will have a wonderful baby. As she relaxes completely, the perineum can stretch with greater ease and an episiotomy may not even be necessary. The patient should not let any worries or fears of *any* kind distract her from her focus on her pleasant contractions. She should look forward to each contraction, which she can learn to perceive as pressure and warmth.

For hyperemesis gravidarum, the patient is told during hypnosis that when she comes out of trance she will feel relaxed, comfortable, and pleasantly hungry. Hunger and nausea cannot exist at the same time, and the positive suggestion of feeling pleasantly hungry can eliminate the excessive vomiting of pregnancy. Also, under hypnosis, the patient can be asked what is the problem with the pregnancy. Occasionally, hyperemesis is a form of subconscious rejection of the pregnancy. All emesis basins should be thrown away to remove the suggestion of vomiting that they evoke.

8. *Headaches.*
   a. *Tension headaches.* Tension headaches frequently are associated with anger, and it is usually anger from the past (father, mother, etc.). Hypnotists experienced with regression techniques can often regress the patient to the time when he or she had the first headache.

For those who say, "My head is on fire," say the following:

Pretend that you are in California, it is a hot summer, everything is very dry. . . . a spark plunges the forest into fire. . . . visualize the Coast Guard deluging the fire with massive amounts of water. . . . it puts the fire out. . . . new growth happens in an area of old fire. . . . sweet blackberries first. . . .

An alternative is as follows:

Make a tight fist in your nondominant hand. . . . make it so tight that it holds all the anger and tension. . . . once it contains all the anger it can hold, open your hand and feel the anger harmlessly dissipate as it falls to the floor. . . .

   b. *Migraines.* Have the patient visualize a brain blood vessel spasm. This spasm cannot last forever, and when it relaxes, the headache occurs. The patient can be taught to avoid the spasm under certain conditions. After the headache has occurred, visualizing the remainder of the body relaxing, more than the blood vessel, may take some of the blood (pain) away from the headache.

9. *Nailbiting*. Nailbiting is a common compulsive disorder that is more frequent in males than in females. A recent survey of eighth-grade students showed that 8% of the boys and 3% of the girls admitted to involuntary nailbiting, especially when anxious. For high school seniors, the percentages are 3% of the males and 1% of the females. Although no numbers are available for adults, the author sees in his private practice at least five adult nailbiters (age range, 21 to 69) every year.

Consider the following example: Even if everyone is telling you not to do something (parents, teachers, siblings, and, yes, yourself), telling a person or yourself not to do something does not really work. Why? As an example, what happens when you give a little boy a full glass of milk and tell him not to spill it? Usually, as soon as this is said, the milk is on the floor. This is called a *counternegative* suggestion. As in a digital computer, "don't" goes in one way, does not register, and "spill the milk" goes in the other way and registers. When this is all that registers, the child does what he was told to do; he spills the milk. If you want a child to be careful, just tell the child to be careful, and chances are he or she will. If you want your little daughter to stay in the backyard, tell her to stay in the backyard; if you tell her not to leave, chances are that in just a few moments she will be gone. Under hypnosis, the subconscious is very literal, and handles a counternegative suggestion as a child would in the example with the milk.

In or out of hypnosis, telling a child not to bite his or her nails only makes things worse. What makes sense to the nailbiter are the following suggestions, given while the patient is in trance:

I am *not* going to prohibit you from biting your nails. You know that nailbiting is an unconscious habit, and we are going to make it conscious. From this moment on, when your hand moves in the direction of your mouth for you to bite your nails, when your hand is about 6 inches from your mouth, you will become aware of your hand. Since you will be aware of your hand, you can make the decision. If you decide to bite your nails, go right ahead and enjoy it. Chances are, however, that once you are aware of your hand, you will decide not to bite your nails and you can just drop your hand down. Remember, however, that you are not prohibited from biting your nails. If you decide to do it, go ahead and enjoy it, and if you decide not to do it, you can just drop your hand down and take a deep breath to relax.

These suggestions are repeated three or four times during each of four weekly sessions. On each subsequent session, the patient is complimented on how well he or she is doing. The patient is reminded about how much he or she will enjoy having the nails filed and how good it feels to have smooth, normal nails. Most patients are cured in four or five sessions. The occasional patient needs one or two extra sessions, a situation that usually

is due to parents "helping the clinician" by reminding the child not to bite his or her nails. The essence of this very successful treatment is that the patient wants to overcome the problem. Helping a motivated patient overcome a habit markedly improves the chance for success.

Note: The author's son was a nailbiter until, at age 17, he asked if he could be helped. Not until he asked for help to stop nailbiting was any hypnotherapy done. The likelihood for success is much higher when the patient is motivated enough to ask for help.

10. *Pain management*. No oral medications can completely alleviate pain; however, most can increase comfort. So avoid prescribing medications for "pain"; rather, prescribe medications and treatment (prn) for comfort. For guided therapy, have the patient imagine playing with children in a snowball fight, losing one glove, and the hand without the glove getting colder and colder, colder and colder, colder and number, colder and numb, number and number, number, number. After the patient agrees that the hand is feeling cold and numb, have him or her place the hand against the affected area and allow the anesthesia to drift out of the hand into the affected area. This should result in a more comfortable feeling.

11. *Painful procedures*. Make sure to avoid counternegative suggestions with hypnosis for painful procedures. We all know the response to a statement like "Don't think of an elephant": It is almost impossible to avoid thinking about an elephant, even if only very briefly. Therefore the strategy for painful procedures has to be considered carefully and planned in advance.

The following statements should be compared with the second set of statements:

Hold still and it won't bother you. . . . don't move or it's gonna hurt. . . . please don't move and you'll be all right. . . . if you just hold still, you'll be all right.

Just make yourself limp as a ragdoll; the more relaxed you become, the less tense you are. . . . tension frequently causes and always aggravates pain, and therefore the more relaxed you become, the less discomfort you will have. . . . to concentrate your mind, it is easier if you just allow your eyes to close. . . . you can concentrate better on the sound of my voice when your eyes are closed. . . . after all, a blind man can hear better than a seeing person. . . . so go ahead and close your eyes. . . . now focus your attention on what I have to say. . . . I would like you to visualize in your mind the best time that you have ever had at (a baseball game, football game, play, TV show, etc). . . . and just let your body go limp, limp as a ragdoll. . . . see that very special time in your life. . . . tell me what it was. . . . feel the joy. . . . now while you concentrate with the front of your mind on that very special time, you listen to me with the back of your mind. . . . if anything annoys you, just say to yourself: "This is a little annoying, but I'm not going to let it bother me a bit. . . . I just concentrate on my (ball game, play, TV show, etc.)."

These latter statements are more positive and avoid the counternegative suggestions. If discomfort is evident, the clinician can add: "You'll remember only those things that were pleasant and helpful to you."

Even if hypnotherapy is not utilized for an uncomfortable, painful, or anxiety-provoking procedure, recalling the principles of hypnotherapy may be beneficial. If the clinician uses a low, monotonous voice when talking, and the staff is trained to not make loud interruptions during a procedure, patient tolerance tends to improve.

Children over the age of five respond to hypnosis very well, especially for painful procedures. In fact, there are reported cases in which a previously hypnotized child was confronted with an unexpected painful situation (auto or bicycle accident with a fracture), and immediately put himself or herself into trance. In trance, the child remained calm and safe, with minimal or manageable pain, until help arrived.

For injections in children, the trance induction could be something like this:

Would you like to have a Magic Spot on your arm for injections? The Magic Spot is amazing. . . . can you raise your sleeve a little bit? This Magic Spot works for adults and children, but it is very special for children. . . . I want you to open your eyes wide. . . . now, I'm going to pull your eyes shut. . . . all you have to do is to pretend that you can't open your eyes and keep on pretending that you can't open your eyes. . . . so much so that when you try to open your eyes, they just won't open. . . . now let me see you try to open them while you're pretending. . . . that's right. . . . now stay like that and keep on pretending you can't open your eyes, and the most amazing thing is going to happen. . . . you're going to have a Magic Spot put on your arm. . . . once this Magic Spot is put on you, never again will you have to feel an injection or a poke. . . . your doctor or the nurse is working there, but nothing will disturb you and nothing will bother you. . . . you'll never have any discomfort from an injection, either before, during, or afterward. . . . now, notice that I take this area, and I paint a Magic Spot with wet stuff (alcohol), like that. . . . whenever an injection is given in that area, you will be able to point out to the doctor or nurse your Magic Spot. . . . nothing will be felt at all except that you'll know they're doing something there. . . . but you'll feel nothing. . . . (give the injection) now, isn't that beautiful?. . . . you've already had your injection, and you know you didn't feel a thing. . . . from now on, you will always be able to have injections this easily. . . . after a while, that Magic Spot I painted on your arm will no longer be visible to you or anyone else, except for one important thing. . . . you will know exactly where it is, so any time you must receive an injection, you will be able to point out the spot to your

doctor or nurse. . . . all right, open your eyes. . . . what did you feel?

12. *Smoking.* Every psychopharmacologist will agree that nicotine is a stimulant. However, 99% of all people who smoke cigarettes do so in order to relax. There is the rare four-pack-a-day smoker who smokes in order to remain alert. The nicotine patch, nicotine gum, and nicotine nasal spray are only about 15% to 17% percent effective, the same as placebo.

The principle of the counternegative suggestion applies (see the "Nailbiting" section): if a person is told not to smoke, he or she will smoke more. However, a suggestion like "More oxygen in my lungs means more oxygen in my tissues and my brain, and I will live longer and be happier" is a suggestion that the subconscious can accept easily and comfortably. Harping on the negatives of smoking, the nicotine, the tars and the phenanthrenes, is certainly less helpful than increasing the motivation of being able to breathe better, to sleep better, and to have more stamina and energy.

Self-hypnosis can also help with smoking. Patients who smoke for the sense of relaxation (pacifier) can repeat to themselves "I am more relaxed" whenever they have the urge to smoke. This has the effect of not needing the cigarette to relax, especially if they repeat that phrase approximately 20 times whenever the urge to smoke bothers them. By the time they have repeated the phrase 20 times, the urge will be gone. If they say the phrase while counting on each of their fingers, by the time they have counted each of their fingers twice (20 times), the urge will be gone. This also gives them something to do with their hands while they are having the urge.

13. *Other indications.* Other indications for hypnosis include bruxism, depression, dyspareunia, eating disorders, enuresis, fear of flying, fear of public speaking, gagging, hiccups, insomnia, trichotillomania, thumb sucking, and test anxieties. Comprehensive textbooks are available for more thorough discussions of the topics covered in this chapter as well as these indications.

TECHNIQUE: SELF-HYPNOSIS

For optimal self-hypnosis, it is best for the patient to have experienced guided hypnosis, or hetero-hypnosis, first. Patients may experience various types of phenomena during hypnosis. If these phenomena occur during hetero-hypnosis, they may be helpful for convincing a person that he or she has been in trance. Sometimes patients experience phenomena like a floating feeling, either up like a balloon, or down like a feather, or just floating along like a leaf on a pond. Other patients experience a heavy feeling. Many patients experience time distortion. When a patient is awakened after his or her first hypnotic session, I frequently ask, "How long do you think you have been in this room?" Most patients will guess 10 or 15 minutes, whereas they may have been in trance for half an hour to an hour. After the time distortion is pointed out to the patient, another hypnotic phenomenon that should be brought to the patient's attention is the fact that he or she was able to sit absolutely still for that length of time without any body movement. When these phenomena occur, they can be very useful for convincing patients that they have been in trance.

After patients have experienced hetero-hypnosis one or more times, self-hypnosis can be taught. Patients should be aware that for self-hypnosis to work, it must be applied appropriately and they must practice it on a regular basis. The patient should find a place where he or she will not be disturbed. The patient should take the phone off the hook, and if there are family members present, they should be instructed that the patient does not want to be disturbed for the next 10 minutes or so. The patient then sits down or lies down and gets comfortable. The wording goes something like this:

Start out by taking a huge, deep, deep breath. Close your eyes and just breathe slowly and evenly, concentrating on relaxing your forehead, face, neck, shoulders, upper arms, forearms, wrists, hands, and fingers. Then, focusing on the gentle rising and falling of the abdomen, tuning into the gentle breathing, relaxing the muscles in the chest as the breathing becomes more even and regular, allow that relaxed feeling to drift down your abdomen, hips and pelvis, upper legs, lower legs, ankles, and feet. As you breathe slowly and evenly, on each breath out, repeat the word "one." Keep repeating the word "one" over and over for a couple of minutes or however long you like (do not set a timer). If other thoughts come in, just let the thoughts pass through and say something to yourself ("oh, well") and return right back to repeating "one," After your body has been stilled by using the progressive relaxation and your mind has been stilled by repeating "one" for two or three minutes, begin visualization. See, feel, and sense yourself in a place where you can be comfortable. Now, this might be out on a beach on a cool summer morning; it could be lying in a hammock under a tree or out in the woods or lying in a meadow, whatever visualization suits you. Repeat whatever suggestion you feel you need while in that meadow or on that beach (e.g., "I am calm and I am confident in any and all situations"). The suggestion you give yourself has to be a positive suggestion. Suggestions like "I'm not nervous" actually make you more nervous, and if it is for anxiety or

nervousness that you are using the hypnosis, then repeat the suggestion "I am calm and I am confident." Whatever suggestion you use at this point is either a suggestion that was given to you or it can be your own. It should have been written down and read at least 20 times before you begin your self-hypnosis. Another possible suggestion could be "I eat slowly. I enjoy my food, and I stop eating the moment I am the least bit satisfied." Again. remember that the suggestion has to be phrased positively and affirmatively and in the present tense. If you choose, you may enhance the effectiveness of the self-hypnosis by playing some slow classical music in the background. After having repeated your suggestions several times while in your place of comfort, you can easily awaken yourself by counting up from one to three, telling yourself that at the count of three you will be wide awake, clear headed, and refreshed, and then you begin to count. One, beginning to come up now. Two, almost awake, and, three, wide awake. You then stretch a bit and go on your way.

The author highly recommends the use of self-hypnosis a minimum of twice a day, using the same suggestion for several weeks. Benefits of self-hypnosis include the fact that it is as effective as many therapeutic agents, and the patient learns to have control at all times. Another advantage is that a patient can induce a trance whenever he or she needs it, with no side effects. Few medications have such benefits.

Box 212-1 lists samples of self-hypnosis suggestions that patients can use. It is recommended to use only four or five suggestions that are applicable to a particular patient. More important, clinicians can write their own suggestions, but the suggestions should be phrased positively.

COMPLICATIONS

With hypnosis, there are no complications when it is used by a qualified practitioner. It is possible during any hypnotic session for the patient to spontaneously age regress, and he or she may start crying as he or she relives a painful episode. If the clinician feels comfortable, he or she can work the patient through that episode. If the clinician is not comfortable, it is better to reorient the patient and awaken him or her. To reorient, tell the patient that he or she is not 5 years old (or whatever the patient has told the clinician), and give the patient his or her correct age. Next tell the patient that he or she is in your office and is deeply hypnotized. You can state that you realize that the patient has a problem related to that particular episode in his or her life and that he or she will be referred to a clinician who can easily help the patient through that emotion. After reorienting the patient to the correct place and time, guide the patient out of trance.

BOX 212-1

Self-Hypnosis Suggestions

The following are self-hypnosis suggestions that can be given to the patient. Only four or five suggestions that are applicable to that particular patient should be used. More importantly, practitioners can write their own, making certain that the suggestions are phrased positively.

- My eating habits are in keeping with my best interests.
- My goals are realistic and attainable.
- I am balanced in my mind and emotions.
- I am a very confident person.
- My memory improves daily.
- My physical condition improves rapidly.
- I am happy and outgoing.
- I am a very patient person.
- I accept those things over which I have no control.
- I always wake up energetic and refreshed.
- I eat only at mealtime and then sparingly.
- I enjoy abundant health and energy.
- I experience complete, restful, revitalizing sleep.
- I feel invincible during competition.
- I listen with interest and absorb rapidly.
- I meet new people with ease and comfort.
- I praise others freely and sincerely.
- I place facts in order of importance.
- I am successful in positive thought and action.
- I anticipate a comfortable delivery.
- I have the incentive and the will to succeed.
- During examinations, I'm always calm, serene, and composed.
- My self-esteem and positive self-image grow steadily every day.
- I feel and enjoy the surge and inner power of self-control.
- Positive thinking brings me the results I desire.
- Fresh clean air invigorates me.
- More oxygen in my lungs means more oxygen in my tissues. My brain and I will live longer, and I will be happier.
- I am aware that the longer I abstain, the easier it will be to give up smoking permanently.

CPT/BILLING CODES

90801	Psychiatric diagnostic interview examination
90802	Interactive psychiatric diagnostic interview examination using play equipment, physical devices, language interpreter, or other mechanisms of communication
90804	Individual psychotherapy, insight oriented, behavior modifying and/or supportive, in an office or outpatient facility, approximately 20 to 30 minutes face-to-face with the patient;
90805	Individual psychotherapy, insight oriented, behavior modifying and/or supportive, in an office or outpatient facility, approximately 20 to 30 minutes face-to-face with the patient; with medical evaluation and management services
90806	Approximately 45 to 50 minutes
90807	With medical evaluation and management services
90808	75 to 80 minutes
90810	Individual psychotherapy, interactive, using play equipment, physical devices, language interpreter, or other mechanisms of nonverbal communication, in an office or outpatient facility, approximately 20 to 30 minutes face-to-face with the patient
90811	With medical evaluation and management services
90812	Approximately 45 to 50 minutes
90880	Medical hypnotherapy

ICD-9-CM DIAGNOSTIC CODES

303.9	Alcoholism, chronic, NOS
300.12	Amnesia, psychogenic
300	Anxiety disorder
314	Attention deficit disorder
311	Depression, NOS
346.9	Headache, migraine (not intractable)
307.81	Headache, tension
643.03	Hyperemesis gravidarum, antepartum
995.3	Hypersensitivity
780.52	Insomnia
307.9	Nailbiting
787.02	Nausea
787.01	Nausea with vomiting
307.8	Pain, psychogenic, unspecified
307.89	Pain, psychogenic, site specified
V22.2	Pregnant state, NOS
305.1	Tobacco abuse, nondependent
788.2	Urinary retention, unspecified

ADDITIONAL TRAINING OPPORTUNITIES AND RESOURCES

The National Procedures Institute
4909 Hedgewood Drive
Midland, MI 48640
Phone: 1-800-462-2492
Website: www.npinstitute.com

The Ohio Institute of Medical Hypnosis
2708 Crawfis Boulevard
Akron, OH 44333
Phone: 1-330-867-6677
Website: www.mdhypnosis.com

American Society of Clinical Hypnosis
130 E. Elm Court, Suite 201
Roselle, IL 60172-2000
Phone: 1-630-980-4740
Website: www.asch.net

Australian Society of Hypnosis
Royal Talbot Hospital
Yarra Boulevard KEW VIC 3101
Phone: +61 3 9496 4548
Website: www.ozhypnosis.com.au

Canadian Society for Clinical Hypnosis
Suite 200, 10050—112 Street
Edmonton, AB T5K 2JI
Phone: 1-800-386-7230
Website: www.csch.org

Society for Clinical and Experimental Hypnosis
Central Office
Washington State University
P.O. Box 642114
Pullman, WA 99164-2114
Fax: 1-509-335-2097
Website: www.sunsite.utk.edu/IJCEH/scehframe.htm

ADDITIONAL RESOURCES

- See the sample patient education handout titled "Medical Hypnosis: 10 Frequently Asked Questions" on page 2020 of Appendix G.

BIBLIOGRAPHY

Cousins N: *Head first,* New York, 1989, EP Dutton.

Crasilneck HB, Hall JA: *Clinical hypnosis: principle & applications,* New York, 1985, Norton.

Elman D: *Hypnotherapy,* Glendale, Calif, 1970, Westwood Publishing. (This reference is still available and contains excellent examples.)

Gardner GC, Olness K: *Hypnosis in hypnotherapy with children,* New York, 1981, Grune & Stratton.

Hammond DC: *Hypnotic suggestions and metaphors,* New York, 1990, Norton.

Hartland J: *Medical and dental hypnosis,* Baltimore, 1973, Williams & Wilkins.

Hilgard ER, Hilgard JR: *Hypnosis in the relief of pain,* New York, 1994, Brunner/Mazel.

Kroger WS: *Clinical and experimental hypnosis,* Philadelphia, 1963, JB Lippincott.

Yapko MD: *Essentials of hypnosis,* New York, 1995, Brunner/Mazel.

Zelling DA: Migraine: symptom or disease? *J Med Hypnoanalysis* 1(1):38, February 1981.

Zelling DA: Premenstrual syndrome, *Enigma J Am Acad Med Hypnoanalysts* 2(3):38, September 1986.

Zelling DA: The triple allergenic theory, *Med Hypnoanalysis J* 3(2):58, June 1988.

CHAPTER 213

Lumbar Puncture

Jeffrey A. German
John O'Brien

Lumbar puncture is performed to obtain cerebrospinal fluid (CSF) and is vital for making many neurologic diagnoses. Examination of the CSF remains the most direct and accurate method of determining if there is a central nervous system infection. Whereas computed tomography (CT) and magnetic resonance imaging have somewhat superseded lumbar puncture for making various other diagnoses, they have also increased the safety of performing a lumbar puncture. Although lumbar puncture is generally a diagnostic procedure, it can also have therapeutic applications (e.g., pseudotumor cerebri, elevated CSF pressure).

INDICATIONS

- Suspected central nervous system infection (e.g., meningitis, encephalitis)
- Suspected subarachnoid hemorrhage (If available, a CT scan should be done first. It will exclude increased intracranial pressure. However, CT has a false-negative rate of up to 25% for blood. With a bleed, xanthochromic color of CSF and an abnormal red blood cell (RBC) count [>1000/mm^3] should be noted.)
- Pseudotumor cerebri (therapeutic) or normal hydrocephalus (NPH) (diagnostic)
- Guillain-Barré syndrome (very high protein level [>200 mg/100 ml])
- Multiple sclerosis (Usually the IgG level is elevated and oligoclonal banding is present on electrophoresis.)
- Spinal analgesia
- Systemic lupus erythematosus
- Acute demyelinating disorders (e.g., encephalomyelitis, transverse myelitis)
- Dementia (However, the geriatric literature indicates little benefit of performing lumbar puncture in demented elderly patients.)

- Meningeal carcinomatosis
- Unexplained neurologic disorders if CT is negative (e.g., altered level of consciousness, polyneuropathy)
- Intrathecal antibiotics or chemotherapeutics
- Imaging procedures (myelography or cisternography)

CONTRAINDICATIONS

- Local skin infection (*absolute contraindication*)
- Raised intracranial pressure (all right for pseudotumor cerebri or suspected normal pressure hydrocephalus)
- Supratentorial mass lesions (should be evaluated by CT scan first)
- Severe bleeding diathesis, coagulopathy, or anticoagulated patient *(relative contraindication)*
- Platelet count less than 50,000/mm^3

PREPROCEDURE PATIENT PREPARATION

Indications, alternatives, risks, potential benefits, and expected results should be discussed with the patient (see the sample patient education handout titled "Lumbar Puncture" on page 2021 of Appendix G), and he or she should sign an informed consent form (see the sample patient consent form titled "Lumbar Puncture" on page 2022 of Appendix G).

EQUIPMENT

Spinal tray (Fig. 213-1) containing the following:
- Povidone-iodine skin swabs
- Alcohol swab
- Fenestrated drape and sterile gloves
- Manometer, three-way stopcock

- 1% lidocaine
- 3-ml syringe with 20- to 23-gauge needle (for drawing up anesthetic)
- 25- to 27-gauge skin needle
- 20- to 22-gauge spinal needle plus a spare*
- Four numbered, capped test tubes
- Sterile dressing (Band-Aid)

TECHNIQUE

1. Position the patient near the edge of the bed (or the examination table) in the lateral recumbent or sitting position. Slightly flex the neck anteriorly. If the

---

*Atraumatic spinal needles have been shown to reduce the complication of spinal headache (i.e., less risk of a CSF leak).

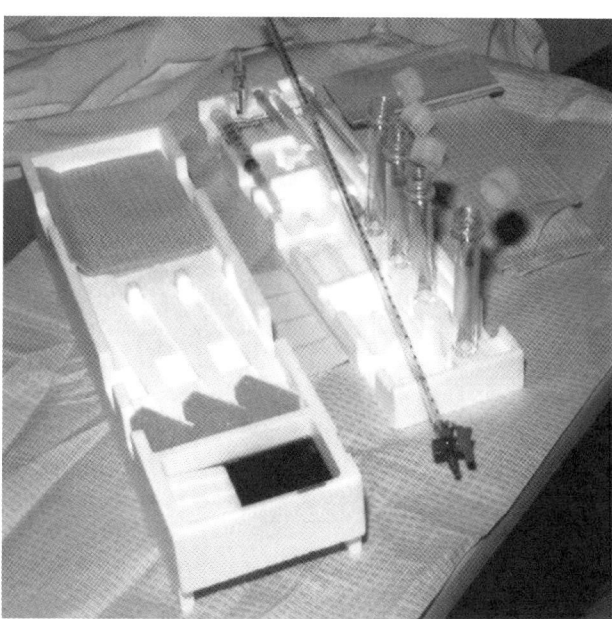

Fig. 213-1
Lumbar puncture equipment tray.

patient is lying, ask him or her to "roll up into a ball" with the knees drawn up to the abdomen (Fig. 213-2). The shoulders and pelvis should be aligned vertically without forward or backward tilt. Identify the L3-L4 interspace (a line drawn between the superior aspect of the iliac crests intersects the body of L4). If necessary, the L2-L3 or L4-L5 interspaces can be used (Fig. 213-3).

2. Open the spinal tray in a sterile manner. Put on sterile gloves and preassemble the manometer. Attach the three-way stopcock and set this assembly to the side on the sterile field. Next, open the numbered test tubes. Place them upright, in order, in the slots provided in the plastic tray.

3. Prepare the skin at the selected interspace, plus the one above and below, with an antiseptic solution such as povidone-iodine. Cover the area with a fenestrated drape.

4. Draw 3 ml of 1% lidocaine into the syringe with the 20- to 23-gauge needle. Administer local anesthetic with the skin needle and raise a wheal over the L3-L4 interspace. Inject a small amount deeper into the posterior spinous region, in the direction that the spinal needle will follow.

5. Palpate the posterior spinous process. Using this and the umbilicus as landmarks, insert a 20- or 22-gauge spinal needle through the skin. Angle the needle about 15 degrees cephalad, toward the umbilicus, keeping it level with the sagittal midplane of the body (Figs. 213-4 and 213-5). Keep the bevel of the needle parallel to the longitudinal axis of the spine. If bone is encountered, withdraw the needle slightly and change its angle. Depending on the size of the patient, after the needle has advanced about 3 to 4 cm, stop, withdraw the stylus, and check the hub for fluid. If there is no fluid, replace the stylus and advance another fraction before repeating this again. Usually a slight "pop" is felt as the spinal needle penetrates the dura. Advance the needle 1 to

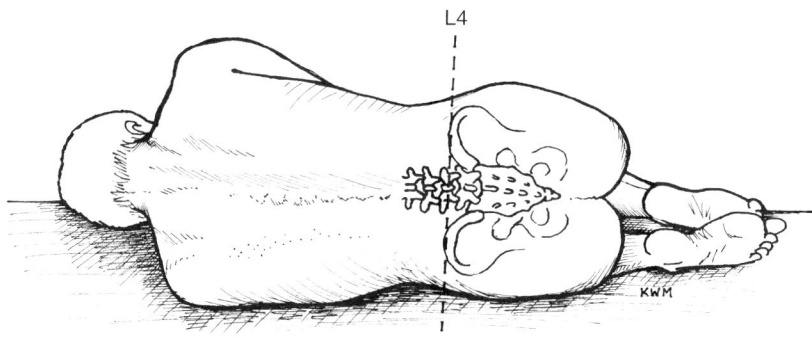

Fig. 213-2
Location of anatomic landmarks.

2 mm farther and withdraw the stylus. Rotating the needle 90 to 180 degrees is sometimes helpful if no fluid returns. If the patient experiences pain radiating down one leg or the tap is "dry," remove the needle completely and make an attempt at a different interspace. A "dry" tap is more often due to a poorly positioned patient or an improperly placed needle than to an obliterated subarachnoid space. Reposition the patient from lying to sitting or vice versa.

Note: For very large or obese patients, it may be impossible to palpate the spinous process for use as a landmark. Ultrasound may help locate the bone in the spinous process. (See Chapter 209, Emergency Department and Office Ultrasound.)

6. Once fluid is obtained, place the end of the stopcock with the attached manometer onto the hub of the needle. Have the patient straighten their legs and relax their position so that the opening pressure is not artificially elevated. The cerebrospinal fluid should rise in the manometer to the level of the opening pressure. Note the color of the fluid and the opening pressure. CSF pressure should oscillate slightly with the pulse and with respiration.

7. In case the fluid is bloody and does not clear after the first few drops of fluid (bloody tap), replace the stylus and remove the spinal needle. Select an alternative lumbar interspace above or below the current level and reattempt lumbar puncture as described in steps 4 and 5. Note: Bloody

CSF due to subarachnoid hemorrhage will *not* clot. Also, after spinning in a centrifuge, the supernatant is xanthochromic.

8. Turn the stopcock to allow the cerebrospinal fluid to flow into the test tubes. Keep track of the order in which they are filled. Fill at least three test tubes

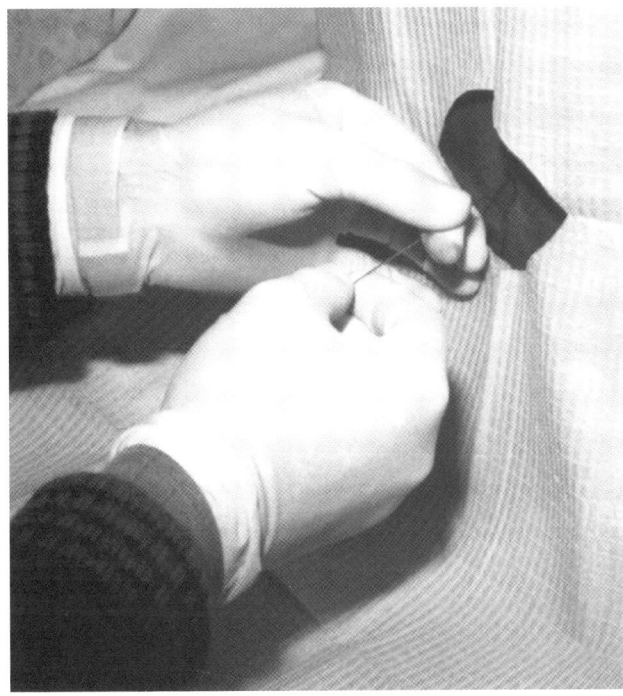

Fig. 213-4
Proper angle for entering spinal canal (with patient seated). Needle is directed cephalad.

Fig. 213-3
Line across the iliac crests intersects the body of L4.

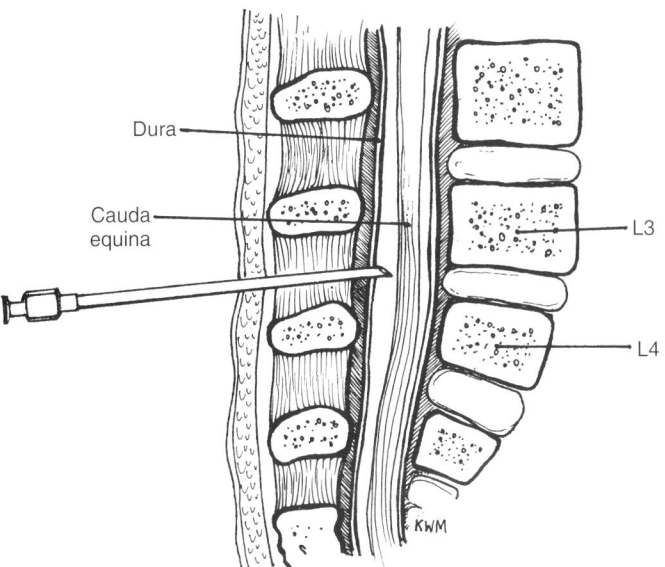

Fig. 213-5
Drop in resistance will be felt as the needle penetrates the dura.

with 2 to 3 ml of cerebrospinal fluid each. Label each tube in the order it was collected. A fourth tube can be filled and frozen in case further studies are needed. Box 213-1 shows normal cerebrospinal fluid values, and Table 213-1 lists recommended cerebrospinal fluid tests. Tube 1 is most likely to be contaminated with blood from the needle insertion. Therefore tube 3 should be tested for the cell count and differential. Minor blood contamination usually clears by the third tube.

9. Once you have obtained enough cerebrospinal fluid, replace the stylus and withdraw the needle.

10. Cover the puncture site with a sterile dressing. Have the patient turn to the supine position and remain there for the next 2 hours.

11. For a therapeutic lumbar puncture (i.e., for pseudotumor cerebri), remove enough spinal fluid to reduce the closing pressure to 100 mm H_2O or less (usually 25 to 35 ml of CSF). For a diagnostic tap, removal of 35 to 50 ml may result in transient improvement in gait or cognition for suspected NPH.

TECHNIQUE FOR PEDIATRIC PATIENTS

The preferred position for infants (especially premature infants and neonates) is with the infant seated with the head only slightly flexed. Overflexion of the head can lead to respiratory arrest in young infants. Draping should be done conservatively to avoid interfering with the infant monitor. The skin should be anesthetized initially with a patch containing a eutectic mixture of local anesthetic (EMLA), if it is available, followed by an injection with lidocaine. The spinal needle is directed slightly cephalad. In young infants a "pop" or change in resistance may not be felt as the needle penetrates the dura. Use a 20- to 22-gauge, 1½-inch needle for infants. A 3½-inch spinal needle can be used in children over the age of 12 years.

COMPLICATIONS

- *Post–lumbar puncture headache* occurs in 10% to 25% of patients and is usually self-limited. The headache usually lasts for only a few days, but may last longer than a week and can be debilitating. Spinal headache usually occurs within 48 hours following dural puncture, but it may occur up to 12 days later. It is exacerbated by sitting upright and is relieved by lying down. The incidence is reduced by using a 20-gauge or smaller needle; by keeping the bevel of the needle oriented parallel to the long axis of the patient's spine, thereby spreading rather than cutting the fibers of the ligamenta flava; and by telling the patient to remain at bed rest following the procedure. Oral and intravenous caffeine benzoate can be used to treat refractory headaches. Intravenous doses of 500 mg are given over a few minutes. A repeat dose can be given in an hour for an 85% chance of alleviation of symptoms. Epidural blood patch can be performed for those refractory to caffeine. This is performed by injecting 15 ml of autologous blood into the dural space. Although the mechanism of action is not known, it usually provides immediate relief.

BOX 213-1
Normal Cerebrospinal Fluid Values

Opening pressure	50-200 mm H_2O
White blood cell count	<5/mm^3
Neutrophils	None
Glucose level	60% to 70% of blood glucose
Protein level	15 to 45 mg/100 ml

TABLE 213-1
Recommended Cerebrospinal Fluid Tests

Tube 1	Tube 2	Tube 3	Tube 4
Bacteriology	**Biochemistry**	**Hematology**	**Optional**
Gram stain	Glucose	Cell count	VDRL*
Culture	Protein	Differential	India ink*
Bacteria	Protein electrophoresis (need		Cryptococcal antigen*
Fungal*	concurrent serum study)		Cytology*
TB*			Oligoclonal bands*
Viral*			Myelin basic protein*
			Countercurrent
			immunoelectrophoresis*
			Serologic and genetic tests
			for other microorganisms*

TB, Tuberculosis; *VDRL,* Veneral Disease Research Laboratory.
*If clinically indicated.

- *Epidermoid tumors* have been associated with lumbar punctures performed in the neonatal period, when needles are used without a stylus.
- *Seizures* have been reported in a small percentage of patients with post–dural puncture headaches.
- *A traumatic or "bloody" tap* from inadvertent puncture of the spinal venous plexuses is possible. This is self-limiting in the majority of patients, but could lead to a spinal hematoma in patients with bleeding disorders. Some authorities recommend sending the first and fourth tubes for cell count (RBCs and WBCs with a differential) if a traumatic tap is suspected. The RBC count will decrease from tube one to tube four in the case of a traumatic tap. A correction can be made for CSF leukocytes and CSF protein if the tap is traumatic. For each 700 RBCs, CSF leukocytes increase by one and CSF protein rises 1 mg/100 ml.
- *Brain herniation* from a supratentorial mass or increased intracranial pressure is another complication. Always check the fundi for papilledema before performing lumbar puncture. If a tumor, an intracranial bleed, or marked increased pressure is suspected, an emergency CT scan should be obtained before a lumbar puncture is done, to reduce the chance of herniation.
- *Paresthesias* in the lower extremities are usually transient, but in rare cases can last for more than a year.
- *Local pain* in the back may be due to injury of the periosteum or the spinal ligaments.
- *Nerve root aspiration* is a possible complication. Replacing the stylus before withdrawing the needle may prevent aspiration of nerve roots. Very rarely, nerve root diverticula can rupture as a result of lumbar puncture, causing a brief CSF leak and a spinal headache.
- *Meningitis* resulting from the procedure is a theoretical complication.

CPT/BILLING CODES

62270   Spinal puncture, lumbar, diagnostic
62272   Spinal puncture, therapeutic, for drainage of spinal fluid

62274   Injection of diagnostic or therapeutic anesthetic or antispasmodic substance; subarachnoid or subdural, single

ICD-9-CM DIAGNOSTIC CODES

322.9   Suspected meningitis
852.00   Subarachnoid hemorrhage
348.2   Pseudotumor cerebri
357.0   Guillain-Barré syndrome
340   Multiple sclerosis
710.0   SLE
239.7   Meningeal carcinoma

ADDITIONAL RESOURCES

- See the sample patient education handout titled "Lumbar Puncture" on page 2021 of Appendix G. See the sample patient consent form titled "Lumbar Puncture" on page 2022 of Appendix G.

BIBLIOGRAPHY

Behrman RE, Kliegman RM, Jenson HB: *Nelson textbook of pediatrics,* ed 16, Philadelphia, 2000, WB Saunders.
Eng RHK, Seligman SJ: Lumbar puncture induced meningitis, *JAMA* 245:1456, 1981.
Raskin NH: Lumbar puncture headache: a review, *Headache* 30:197, 1990.
Siberry GK, Iannone R: *The Harriet Lane handbook,* St Louis, 2000, Mosby.
Thomas SR et al: Randomized controlled trial of atraumatic versus standard needles for diagnostic lumbar puncture, *BMJ* 321:986, 2000.
Tohmo H, Vuorinen E, Muuronen A: Prolonged impairment in activities of daily living due to postdural puncture headache after diagnostic lumbar puncture, *Anaesthesia* 53:299, 1998.

CHAPTER 214

Muscle Biopsy

James R. Shepich

Many disorders of the motor unit can be identified by clinical presentation, but occasionally a muscle biopsy is necessary for diagnosis. Muscle biopsy is a relatively straightforward procedure, which may be performed under local anesthesia. However, many authorities contend that a superior sample can be obtained under general anesthesia, because nonjudicious local infiltration can affect the specimen. The site of biopsy and the type of biopsy (open versus core needle) vary with the patient and disease. The muscle of choice should show the effects of the disease process. However, the most severely affected muscles should be avoided, as the muscle mass may be replaced by scar tissue or fat, and an adequate pathologic diagnosis may not be possible. Some commonly biopsied muscles include the lateral aspect of quadriceps femoris, deltoid, biceps brachii, tibialis anterior, and gastrocnemius. The biopsy method depends on clinical judgment. Core needle biopsy is less invasive and causes less pain and scarring than open biopsy. It is easier to perform, especially in children, and allows repeat biopsy of the same muscle if necessary. Open biopsy allows a larger specimen to be taken, which increases the chance of definitive diagnosis and allows multiple modalities of pathologic preparation of the specimen if needed, including electron microscopy. Open biopsy is also ideal if disease of the motor end plate is suspected. With either approach the muscle to be biopsied should be placed in an extended, relaxed position. Muscles with recent trauma, including EMG or infection, should not be biopsied. Muscle in areas of tendinous transition should be avoided, because the increased connective tissue may be mistaken for fibrosis during pathologic assessment.

INDICATIONS

A muscle biopsy is performed to identify syndromes of muscle weakness that do not present with classical findings. Several diseases, such as Duchenne's muscular dystrophy, Werdnig-Hoffmann disease, and myasthenia gravis, have classic presentations and muscle biopsy is not necessary. Muscle biopsy can be used to distinguish between neurogenic and myopathic processes, identify congenital myopathies, and diagnose connective tissue disorders and muscle infections, such as trichinosis and toxoplasmosis. Metabolic disorders of the muscle may also be found by biopsy. Biopsy is also indicated in the identification and indexing of hereditary disorders.

CONTRAINDICATIONS

- Anticoagulation and bleeding disorders
- Recent trauma of the muscle including EMG
- Clinical appearance of Duchenne's muscular dystrophy (biopsy can cause scarring and contracture of muscle)
- Infection in region of proposed biopsy

EQUIPMENT

Open Biopsy

- Sterile drapes
- Povidone-iodine
- Local anesthesia (1% lidocaine without epinephrine)
- Scalpel with no. 11 or no. 15 blade
- Forceps, iris scissors, suture scissors
- 3-0 vicryl or Monocryl sutures
- 4-0 vicryl or Monocryl sutures
- Electrocautery or diathermy (not to be used until after biopsy sample is procured)
- Gauze sponges, 4 × 4 inch
- Tongue blade, cut into 6- to 7-cm lengths, with V-groove in ends, or 22-gauge needles to pin specimen
- 3-0 nylon or prolene suture
- Steri-Strips, Tegaderm, Op-Site, or dressing of choice

Core Needle Biopsy

- Sterile drape
- Povidone-iodine

- Local anesthesia
- Tru-Cut, Biopty, Conchotome, or equivalent needle
- Band-Aid

PREPROCEDURE PATIENT PREPARATION

The patient should be informed that the procedure is relatively painless, but that the biopsy site may be sore for several days. Many patients experience a sensation of muscle bruising and occasionally a pulling sensation. The patient does not need to restrict food and fluids before the procedure, but he or she should be instructed to wear loose-fitting clothes that readily allow access to the intended biopsy site. Little postprocedural disability or recovery time is expected and the patient may return to usual activity immediately. Analgesic medication is rarely needed, and when it is necessary, it is usually only for 24 to 48 hours. Risks, benefits, and potential complications should be discussed with the patient before the procedure (see the sample patient education handout titled "Muscle Biopsy" on page 2023 of Appendix G).

TECHNIQUE

Open Biopsy

The patient should be prepared and draped, with the muscle in an extended, relaxed position. To prevent a vasovagal episode, the patient should be lying down. The skin overlying the muscle to be biopsied is infiltrated with local anesthesia. Care should be taken to avoid infiltration of the muscle itself. A 3 to 4 cm incision is made over the muscle belly, in an axial orientation to the muscle. The skin and subcutaneous tissue is retracted and the fascia exposed. The fascia is opened sharply in a longitudinal fashion, and the muscle is exposed. Care should be taken to avoid injuring cutaneous nerve branches, which often lie on the fascia. A portion of muscle approximately 3 to 4 cm in length and 5 mm in diameter is excised after a nonabsorbable suture is placed at each end. The excisional sites are "outside" of the sutures. The specimen is maintained in an extended state and transferred to the tongue depressor, where the suture can be placed in a V-groove on either end or pinned to the surface with 22-gauge needles (Fig. 214-1). Hemostasis is achieved with diathermy or electrocautery. The fascia is then closed with 3-0 vicryl sutures to prevent muscle herniation. The skin is then closed with a running subcuticular stitch. Steri-Strips and a sterile dressing are applied.

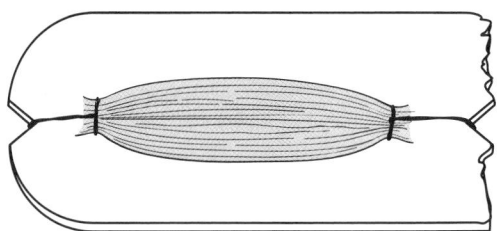

Fig. 214-1
Muscle biopsy specimen mounted on tongue blade and secured with suture tied behind blade.

Core Needle Biopsy

The patient is prepared, draped, and anesthetized as previously described for an open biopsy. A small nick is made in the skin with a no. 11 blade, and the bioptome is introduced. Care should be taken that the throw of the needle does not carry it into vital structures or bone. The bioptome is then activated. Multiple passes may be taken through the muscle in different areas, and usually three cores of tissue are obtained. Pressure is held at the site for 2 to 3 minutes, and a Band-Aid is then applied.

COMPLICATIONS

Potential complications include bleeding, hematoma, or bruising at site of biopsy. The wound may become infected or be slow to heal, especially in patients with connective tissue disorders who have been on steroids. In some conditions biopsy may lead to fibrosis and contracture of the muscle. Mild postprocedural discomfort is usual, and prolonged paresthesia can be experienced if a sensory nerve is injured. Also, the biopsy may be nondiagnostic, requiring a repeat biopsy.

HANDLING OF TISSUE AND INTERPRETATION OF RESULTS

Muscle biopsy should be performed in coordination with a pathologist, as the specimen should never be placed in a fixative and should be processed within 30 minutes of its removal. A longer interval will cause specimen desiccation and architectural distortion. Standard pathologic assessment includes sectioning after cryostat freezing of the specimen, electron microscopy, and immunohistochemical analysis. The pathologic diagnosis is based on the architecture of the muscle group, the characteristics of the individual fibers, and the presence of increased connective tissue or inflammatory cells. Electron microscopy will reveal abnormalities of the mitochondria and other cellular infrastructure. Special staining for oxidative, glycolytic, and hydrolytic enzymes will add information about enzyme deficiency, inflammation, and mitochondrial and lysosomal abnormalities. Stains with periodic acid–Schiff reagent and Oil Red O will help diagnose glycogen and lipid storage disorders. Immunohistochemical assay will add information regarding dystrophin, MHC receptors, and autoimmune disorders.

Note the muscle biopsied for the pathologist. (The deltoid muscle has an unusual connective tissue pattern that may be misinterpreted.) Other information supplied to the pathologist should include a clinical summary of symptoms and their distribution and duration. The results of EMG, nerve conduction velocity, and pertinent laboratory studies should also be included.

POSTPROCEDURE PATIENT EDUCATION

The patient should be instructed to monitor the area of biopsy for signs or symptoms of infection, excessive bleeding, or hematoma formation. A small amount of serosanguineous fluid may accumulate beneath the dressing. The outer dressing should be maintained for at least 48 hours and then removed. The Steri-Strips may be removed between the fifth and seventh day after the biopsy (see the sample patient education handout titled "Muscle Biopsy" on page 2023 of Appendix G).

CPT/BILLING CODE

20200   Muscle biopsy

ICD-9-CM DIAGNOSTIC CODES

728.9   Muscle weakness
710.3   Dermatomyositis
710.4   Polymyositis
335.0   Werdnig-Hoffmann syndrome (muscular atrophy)
728.2   Muscular atrophy (NOS or idiopathy)
359.9   Myopathy
359.89   Myopathy, primary

Also, see numerous specific conditions.

ADDITIONAL RESOURCES

- See the sample patient education handout titled "Muscle Biopsy" on page 2023 of Appendix G.
- See the sample patient consent form titled "Muscle Biopsy" on page 2024 of Appendix G.

BIBLIOGRAPHY

Crago L: Muscle biopsy. In Pfenninger JL, editor: *Procedures for primary care,* ed 1, St Louis, 1994, Mosby.

Rubin E, Farber J, editors: *Pathology,* Philadelphia, 1988, JB Lippincott.

WEBSITES

www.neuro.wustl.edu/neuromuscularlab/mbiopsy.htm
www.biomed2.man.ac.uk/ns/mm/musbiop.htm
www.medicine.uiowa.edu/path_handbook/Appendix/Anatomicpath/ex_muscle_biopsy.html

CHAPTER 215

Transcutaneous Electrical Nerve Stimulation, Phonophoresis, and Iontophoresis

Russell D. White

Mary Beth Shaw

The procedures described in this chapter—transcutaneous electrical nerve stimulation (TENS), phonophoresis, and iontophoresis—can be performed either by primary care clinicians in their office or by physical therapists when ordered by a clinician. The procedures are often used in conjunction with other physical therapy modalities such as manual therapy or therapeutic exercise. The choice of procedure depends upon the size (localized vs. diffuse) and depth (superficial vs. deep) of the proposed treatment area as well as the specific pathology.

EQUIPMENT

- Scissors to trim hair
- Isopropyl alcohol 70% to cleanse skin
- TENS: TENS unit with either disposable or reusable electrodes and gel
- Phonophoresis: therapeutic ultrasound unit, appropriate medication, and coupling gel
- Iontophoresis: direct current generator with constant current output (calibrated in milliamperes), electrodes, and appropriate medications

PREPROCEDURE PATIENT PREPARATION

After discussing the patient's diagnosis, the risks and benefits of the selected treatment should be explained, along with any treatment options. Oral or written consent should be obtained from the patient. Patients should be aware that their skin will be cleansed and that their hair may be trimmed. The anticipated treatment plan and total number of treatments should also be discussed.

TRANSCUTANEOUS ELECTRICAL NERVE STIMULATION UNIT THERAPY

TENS uses low-voltage electrical pulses and applies them to the nervous system for the treatment of pain syndromes. Skin surface electrodes are used to pass the electricity into the affected area. TENS units are Class II, FDA-approved devices and are typically selected for larger, generalized areas of pain, for chronic joint pains, or for persistent myalgias. This procedure can be performed in the clinician's office and is reimbursable if performed by the clinician. However, TENS therapy is usually prescribed by a clinician and performed by the physical therapist. When prescribed for home use, the patient must be competent in operating a TENS unit.

TENS therapy is based on the *gate theory of pain*. According to this theory, nociperception (injury information) is transmitted through (T) cells that convey information to the higher brain centers. This information is presynaptically inhibited by interneurons in the substantia gelatinosa. TENS therapy bombards these interneurons, attempting to modulate or decrease the pain transmission. Other theories suggest that TENS therapy achieves its result by an acupuncture effect, by release of natural opiates, or by direct local vasodilation, which may reduce relative ischemia.

The goal of TENS therapy is to reduce or relieve pain and discomfort. This result may be either short lived or prolonged. TENS therapy may slowly break the *pain-spasm-pain cycle* and reduce perceived discomfort. Unfortunately, TENS therapy is not effective for pain of central origin (e.g., headache).

Treatment parameters are chosen based upon several factors:

Intensity. Small unmyelinated fibers require more current than large myelinated fibers.

Pulse rate. Small unmyelinated fibers respond better to a low-frequency rate (less than 100 Hz), whereas large myelinated fibers respond better to a high-frequency rate (greater than 100 Hz).

Wave characteristics. These characteristics are either monophasic (positive rectangular pattern) or biphasic (negative spike pattern).

Pulse width. Small unmyelinated fibers respond to a long pulse (200 msec), whereas large myelinated fibers respond to a short pulse (50 msec).

Modulation. Modulation allows gradual variation of the frequency or pulse width and retards accommodation of the nervous tissue.

INDICATIONS

- Chronic pain
- Acute pain
- Musculoskeletal pain
- Neurologic pain (*Herpes zoster*)
- Phantom limb pain
- Prior to another procedure to elevate the pain threshold and to decrease patient discomfort following the procedure
- Postoperative pain
- Obstetric pain (after the first trimester)

CONTRAINDICATIONS

- Patients with demand-type pacemakers (Newer pacemakers with improved shielding are not affected by TENS units. Check with a cardiologist or the manufacturer.)
- Patients in first-trimester pregnancy
- Patients with known cardiac dysrhythmias
- Mentally incompetent patients, uncooperative patients, those with paranoid disorders, or pediatric patients without adult supervision

TENS therapy is also contraindicated over the following areas:

- Undiagnosed pain syndromes without established etiology
- Carotid sinuses
- Chest areas in patients with a cardiac history
- Head or neck area of patients with an epileptic history
- Laryngeal or pharyngeal muscles
- Local areas of skin irritation or loss of skin integrity
- Mucosal surfaces
- Eyes

TECHNIQUE

1. Before initiating therapy, organize the necessary materials (Fig. 215-1) and prepare the skin area to which the electrodes will be attached. Trimming hair and cleansing the skin with 70% isopropyl alcohol will promote the adhesiveness and conductivity of the electrodes.

2. Select the proper electrodes. For 24 hours or more of use, select either a carbon-impregnated rubber electrode with gel or a carbon-filled silicone electrode.

3. Attach electrodes to the selected treatment site, whether isolated trigger points, individual dermatomes or myotomes, or in the distribution of a specific nerve. Position the electrodes so that a paresthesia will be felt in the area of pain or dysfunction (Fig. 215-2). If the electrodes are secured poorly to the skin, they may cause a burning sensation instead of a paresthesia. In addition, electrodes should be placed at least 2 inches apart. Placing electrodes closer together can cause a burning sensation. The electrodes should also be placed so that the perimeter of the painful area is entirely surrounded by the electrodes.

4. Select the treatment parameters. Conventional set-

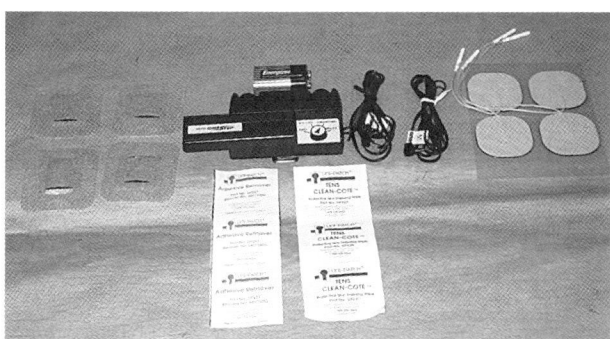

Fig. 215-1
TENS unit (generator) with supplies for skin preparation, disposable and reusable electrodes and electrode wires.

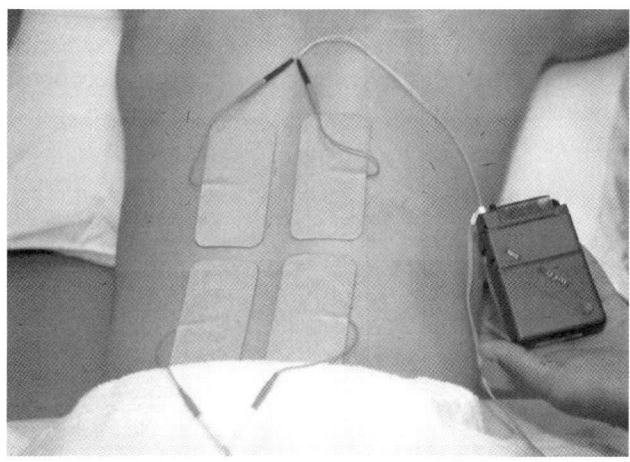

Fig. 215-2
Placement of TENS unit electrodes.

tings use a high-frequency rate with a narrow pulse width. The intensity level is less than that which results in muscle stimulation.

5. With the amplitude control in the *off* position, attach wires to the TENS unit. Turn on the generator unit and increase the amplitude slowly, up to the patient's comfort level. Again, paresthesia should be felt by the patient before the threshold for motor stimulation.

6. If desired results are not achieved, change the stimulation sites or adjust the treatment settings.

7. When the treatment is completed, turn off the unit, return the settings to zero, and remove the electrodes.

8. Typically, patients are treated once or twice daily for a duration of 30 to 60 minutes. Some patients may benefit from more frequent treatments and may require a home unit for therapy.

9. Avoid using TENS within one meter of a transmitting two-way radio or a cellular (wireless) phone.

COMPLICATIONS

- Skin irritation from electrode placement
- Contact dermatitis resulting from electrode gels
- Pacemaker malfunction (typically an older pacemaker)

PHONOPHORESIS

Phonophoresis uses therapeutic ultrasound to enhance the diffusion of medications across the skin and into body tissues. Commonly used medications include dexamethasone, hydrocortisone, and lidocaine. While phonophoresis is usually performed by the physical therapist, some clinicians provide this modality in the office setting. Clinicians can be reimbursed for phonophoresis, even if not performed by a physical therapist.

The dual action of phonophoresis—thermal and mechanical—counteracts the inflammatory response by a process called *acoustic streaming,* which increases cell membrane permeability. This effect also facilitates the passage of medications into body tissue. With *acute* inflammation, using pulse mode ultrasound avoids an increase in tissue temperature. In addition to the alteration of tissue permeability, beneficial effects are obtained through nonthermal changes (e.g., stimulation of fibroblasts). With *chronic* inflammation, using continuous or nonpulsed ultrasound can produce thermal changes that counteract or prevent the chronic changes of scarring and tissue edema.

Ultrasound dose is measured in intensity (intensity = W/cm^2), which is the acoustic energy delivered through the surface area of the head of the transducer. Areas of inflammation are usually treated with 1 to 2 W/cm^2 for 5 to 10 minutes. Results are measured by the improvement

(either immediate or gradual) in pain or function of the treated area.

INDICATIONS

- Muscular strains, fibrosis, spasm, myositis
- Superficial periarticular disorders: bursitis, tendonitis, ligament sprains
- Contracture of joint capsules or adhesive scars
- Reflex sympathetic dystrophy
- Plantar warts
- Neuromas

CONTRAINDICATIONS

- Allergy to medications being used
- Tumors
- Thrombophlebitis
- Pregnancy (*Therapeutic* ultrasound is contraindicated over the abdomen and pelvis.)
- Hemorrhagic or infected areas
- Cardiac disease (*Therapeutic* ultrasound over the cervical ganglia, cardiac area, or an implanted pacemaker may produce a detrimental cardiac reflex.)
- Unhealed fracture sites
  Phonophoresis should also be avoided over the following areas:
- Epiphyseal plate in growing bones
- Spinal cord
- Area of previous radiation therapy (wait 6 months before applying ultrasound)
- Eyes

TECHNIQUE

1. A clinician's prescription is required for the medications when phonophoresis is administered by a physical therapist.

2. Select an area of inflammation for treatment that is no greater than twice the surface area of the sound head.

3. Select the proper ultrasound equipment (Figs. 215-3 and 215-4).

4. Cleanse the general area to be treated. Inspect the skin for excessive dryness and trim excess hair. Skin areas may be pre-treated with moist heat packs to facilitate drug absorption by dilating the hair follicles.

5. Since the chosen agent can affect ultrasound transmissivity, select only topical agents that transmit ultrasound. (Hydrocortisone 10% in an aqueous base is a commonly used medication for phonophoresis.) Apply the medication followed by the coupling gel.

6. Apply phonophoresis through the sound head in a moving pattern of overlapping strokes or circles (Fig. 215-5).

7. Recommended *intensities* of 1 to 2 W/cm^2 usually provide effective results. Use *frequencies* of 3 MHz for superficial tissues and 1 MHz for deeper tissues.

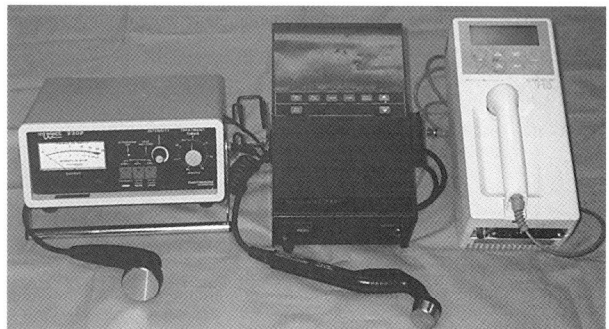

Fig. 215-3
Ultrasound units used for phonophoresis.

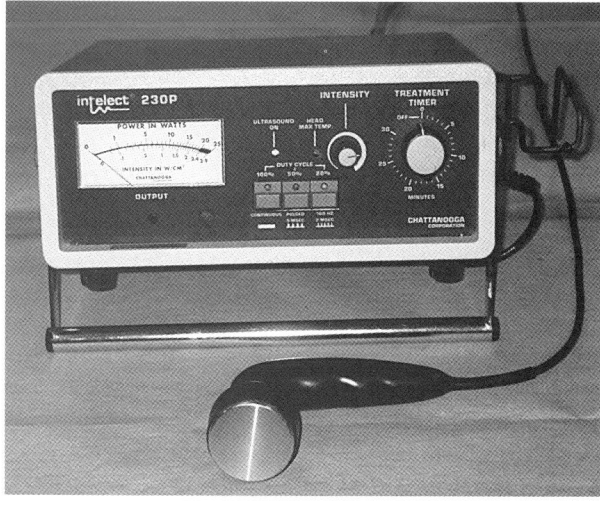

Fig. 215-4
Ultrasound unit showing treatment settings.

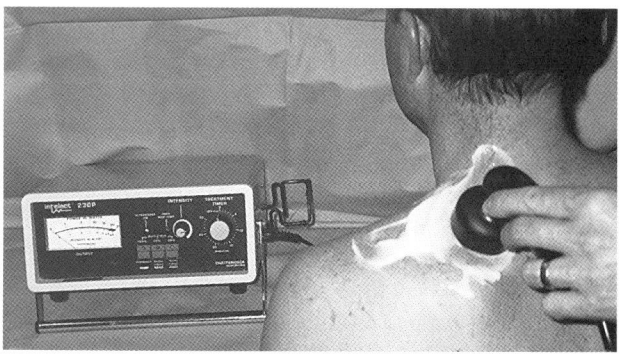

Fig. 215-5
Phonophoresis treatment.

Apply for 5 to 10 minutes. Treatment for greater than 10 minutes increases the risk of a negative effect (e.g., periosteal burn).

8. When finished, remove the coupling gel but leave the topical medication on the skin. Cover this with an occlusive dressing to promote continued absorption.

COMPLICATIONS

- Previously unknown allergy or sensitivity to medication
- Systemic side effects from excessive absorption of applied medication
- Damage to susceptible areas (listed in "Contraindications" section)

IONTOPHORESIS

Iontophoresis uses direct electrical current to enhance the diffusion of ionically charged medications across the skin and mucous membranes. With this technique, medicinal ions can penetrate tissue for 0.2 to 1.5 cm, depending on the drug used and the characteristics of the local tissue. This technique is based on repulsion of similarly charged ions; charged ions in solution are driven from like-charged electrodes.

Iontophoresis works best when the pathology is superficial and localized. This treatment is usually performed in an outpatient rehabilitation setting or in the clinician's office. Primary care clinicians can be reimbursed for the procedure, even if it is not performed by a physical therapist.

The most common *medications* utilized are dexamethasone or lidocaine and the amount depends on the size of the treatment area. The amount used also depends on the electrode size and the volume it takes to fill it. Electrode size varies from 1.5 to 3.5 cm^3. Dexamethasone is the primary agent indicated for inflammatory lesions. Lidocaine is the agent typically used for preoperative topical anesthesia.

The *electrical* dose for administration is expressed in milliampere minutes (mA minutes) and is the product of the *intensity* (milliamperes) and *duration* (minutes). Most treatments last 10 to 20 minutes each and are repeated three to eight times (depending on patient response).

INDICATIONS

- Same indications as for a superficial injection of a therapeutic agent (superficial, since the medications only *penetrate* up to 1.5 cm with iontophoresis)
- Inflammation

— Bursitis
— Tendonitis
— Fasciitis
— Sprain
— Strain
— Trigger points
— Carpal tunnel syndrome
— de Quervain's disease
• Analgesia
— Neuritis
— Local anesthesia for invasive procedures, such as dermatological procedures
• Other (limited case reports) (Table 215-1)
— Ganglion
— Hyperhidrosis of feet or palms
— Ischemic ulcer
— Neuroma
— Post-traumatic edema
— Scar tissue
— Tinea pedis
— Turf toe
— Warts
— Wound healing

CONTRAINDICATIONS

• Allergy or sensitivity to therapeutic agent
• Patients with pacemakers, since electric current could interfere with sensitive implanted devices

Iontophoresis should also be avoided over the following areas:

• Areas of abnormal skin sensation (Patients must be able to give feedback so that the intensity can be set correctly.)
• Superficial abrasions, cuts, and bruises
• Areas of recent bleeding
• Areas surrounding or superficial to an implanted or embedded wire, screws, staples, or other metallic objects
• Recent scars or skin graft
• Area over heart
• Area over carotid sinus

Areas of abnormal sensation or a loss of skin integrity have decreased skin resistance; this raises the risk that an increased current dose may be given. Such a dose may lead to undesired skin reactions. Areas of increased vascularity or those near metal objects can also be subjected to enhanced current dosage.

TECHNIQUE

1. A clinician's prescription is required for the medications administered by a physical therapist using iontophoresis.
2. Position the patient to obtain good exposure for the area to be treated. Inspect the skin of the treatment area for any recent injury or any contraindications previously listed.
3. Clip excessive hair but do not shave. Clean the skin treatment area with 70% isopropyl alcohol to remove surface oils and skin cells.
4. Before initiating therapy, the clinician should organize the equipment and select a direct-current generator (Fig. 215-6). Next, inject the premeasured medication into the electrode reservoir according to the manufacturer's recommendations. (Properly filling electrodes to specified volumes decreases skin irritation.)
5. The *active* electrode (*drug containment electrode*) should be attached over the treatment area. It should

TABLE 215-1

Indications and Dosages for Common Iontophoresis Agents

Ion (Dose)	Polarity	Therapeutic Use
Acetic acid (3-4 mA × 10-20 min)	Negative	Calcified tendonitis, calcium deposit
Chloride, sodium (4 mA × 20-45 min)	Negative	Keloids, scar tissue
Copper sulfate (4 mA × 20-30 min)	Positive	Fungal infection
Dexamethasone (1-4 mA × 15-20 min)	Negative	Tendonitis, tenosynovitis, bursitis, arthritis
Hyaluronidase (1-2 mA × 20-40 min)	Positive	Edema, lymphedema, scleroderma
Iodine (2 mA × 1 min; then 4 mA × 5 min)	Negative	Fibrosis, scar tissue, "trigger finger"
Lidocaine 4% (4 mA × 20-30 min)	Positive	Skin anesthesia
Methylprednisolone (1-4 mA × 15-20 min)	Negative	Postherpetic neuralgia
Salicylate (4 mA × 45 min)	Negative	Analgesia, myalgia, plantar warts
Zinc (4 mA × 15 min)	Positive	Wound healing, ulcers

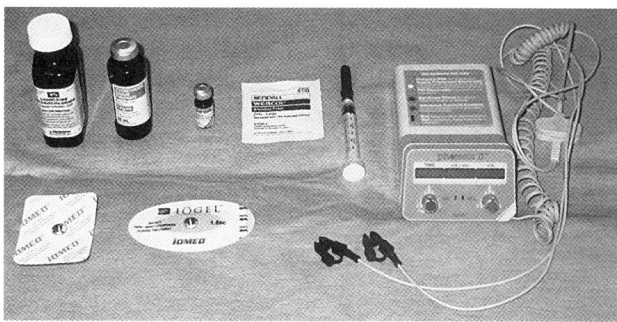

Fig. 215-6
Iontophoresis current generator with dexamethasone, 4% lidocaine, measuring syringe, electrodes, and electrode leads.

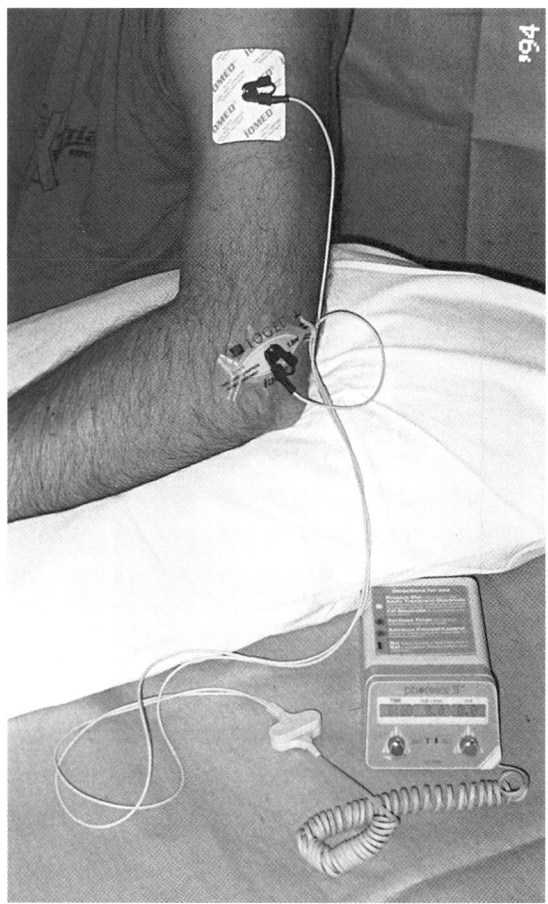

Fig. 215-7
Iontophoresis treatment with proper electrode separation.

have the same polarity as the medication to be used. Attach the larger *dispersive* electrode (*indifferent electrode*) over an area that is at least 3 inches distant (Fig. 215-7) from the active electrode.

6. Connect the electrode leads to the current generator. Current settings should range from 0.1 to 4.0 mA.

7. Determine the current dosage on the basis of the diagnosis and treatment. The recommended dosage for dexamethasone or lidocaine is listed in Table 215-1 and measured in mA × min. (milliamps [current] × minutes [time] = mA × min [dosage])

8. *Gradually* increase the current until the patient barely feels it. Any *sudden* change in current may produce burning, stinging, or a twitch response. With most units, the treatment time is automatically set by the device once the intensity (current) and dosage are determined and entered.

9. During and after the procedure, ask the patient every 2 to 4 minutes if he or she is experiencing any adverse effects.

10. When the procedure is completed, remove the attached electrodes. Instruct the patient to report

any delayed adverse effects. (Note: Post-treatment erythema is common, resulting from either changes in skin pH or a histamine reaction.)

COMPLICATIONS

- Previously unknown drug allergy or sensitivity to medications
- Galvanic rash: hypersensitivity reaction to the direct current that develops within 5 minutes of initiating the electrical stimulation
- "Twitch" response secondary to stimulation of a nerve in the treatment area by inappropriate current
- "Negative electrode burn": skin burn resulting from a decrease in skin resistance and an alkaline reaction when the negative electrode (cathode) is the active electrode. (Newer electrodes stabilize the pH better and cause less skin irritation.)
- Local immunologic inhibition from the steroid. (Dexamethasone is not detected in the bloodstream after treatment.)

POSTPROCEDURE PATIENT CARE AND EDUCATION

The patient's results are evaluated by determining the decrease in pain or inflammation following treatment(s). Treatment(s) can be terminated when the patient has reached the desired clinical goal. The number or frequency of treatments can be increased to improve the results, as long as no adverse effects have been noted. On the contrary, after five treatments with any of these modalities, if there are no results, another type of therapy should be considered.

The patient should know to report any delayed adverse reactions to the clinician. He or she should also know when to make a follow-up appointment.

SUPPLIERS

TENS units
AliMed, Inc.
297 High Street
Dedham, MA 02026
Phone: 1-800-225-2610
Website: www.alimed.com

Electro-Med Health Industries
11601 Biscayne Boulevard, Suite 200-A
North Miami, FL 33181
Phone: 1-800-232-3644
Website: www.emhi.com

Thera-Tronics, Inc.
623 Mamaroneck Avenue
Mamaroneck, NY 10543
Phone: 1-914-698-9802

EMPI, Inc.
599 Cardigan Road
St. Paul, MN 55126-4099
Phone: 1-88-FOR-EMPI
Website: www.empi.com

Phonophoresis
AliMed, Inc.
(see contact information above)

Chattanooga Group, Inc.
4717 Adams Road
Hixson, TN 37343
Phone: 1-800-592-7329
Website: www.chattgroup.com

Dynatronics
7030 Park Centre Drive
Salt Lake City, UT 84121
Phone: 1-800-874-6251
Website: www.dynatronics.com

DynaWave Corporation
2520 Kaneville Court
Geneva, IL 60134
Phone: 1-630-232-4945
Website: my.inil.com/~dynawave/

Iontophoresis
EMPI, Inc.
(see contact information above)

IOMED, Inc.
2441 West 3850 South, Suite A
Salt Lake City, Utah 84120
Phone: 1-800-621-3347
Website: www.iomed.com

Smith & Nephew
N104 W13400 Donges Bay Road
P.O. Box 1005
Germantown, WI 53022-8205
Phone: 1-800-558-8633
Website: www.smith-nephew.com/us/rehab

CPT/BILLING CODES

Note: Healthcare Common Procedure Coding System (HCPCS) codes are used for procedures and supplies when there is no CPT code. They are the alphanumeric codes listed below and reimbursement is variable.

TENS

64550	Application of surface transcutaneous neuro-stimulator (TENS)

TENS unit

E0720	TENS, two lead localized stimulation*
E0730	TENS, four lead, larger/multiple nerve stimulation*

*Prior authorization is required by Medicare for this item.

Phonophoresis

97035	Ultrasound Therapy
A4558	Conductive paste or gel supplies

Iontophoresis

97033	Iontophoresis, each 15 minutes

Medication/Supplies

J2000	Lidocaine 4%
J1100	Dexamethasone sodium phosphate, 4 mg/ml
J1020	Methylprednisolone acetate, 20 mg
J1030	Methylprednisolone acetate, 40 mg
J1040	Methylprednisolone acetate, 80 mg
A4556	Electrodes

ICD-9-CM DIAGNOSTIC CODES

718.5	Adhesions
715.17	Arthritis(osteo), ankle and foot
715.10	Arthritis(osteo), site unspecified
715.16	Arthritis(osteo), lower leg
726.10	Bursitis of shoulder
726.5	Bursitis of hip
726.60	Bursitis of knee
727.82	Calcific tendonitis
354.0	Carpal tunnel syndrome
727.04	de Quervain's disease
782.0	Dermal pain
782.3	Edema
728.71	Fasciitis, plantar
727.42	Ganglion, tendon sheath
924.9	Hematoma, muscle
780.8	Hyperhidrosis
959.7	Injury, knee, leg, ankle, and foot
959.1	Injury, trunk

959.2	Injury, shoulder and upper arm
707.9	Ischemic ulcer, bacterial
701.4	Keloids
726.32	Lateral epicondylitis
848.9	Ligament sprain, unspecified site
724.2	Low back pain
457.1	Lymphedema
728.2	Muscle fibrosis
728.85	Muscle spasm
848.9	Muscular strain, unspecified site
729.1	Myalgias and myositis, unspecified
729.2	Neuritis
355.6	Neuroma, Morton's
625.9	Pain, obstetric (by site)
	Pain, postoperative
353.6	Phantom limb pain
078.19	Plantar warts
053.9	Postherpetic neuralgia
355.0	Pyriformis syndrome
337.20	Reflex sympathetic dystrophy
728.89	Scar tissue
524.60	Temporomandibular syndrome
726.71	Tendonitis, Achilles
726.64	Tendonitis, patellar
726.5	Tendonitis, hip
726.11	Tendonitis, shoulder (calcifying)
727.00	Tenosynovitis and synovitis, unspecified
110.4	Tinea pedis
350.1	Trigeminal neuralgia
727.03	"Trigger finger"
726.90	"Turf toe"
707.1	Ulcer, wound lower extremity

BIBLIOGRAPHY

Abram SE: Advances in chronic pain management since gate control, *Reg Anesth* 18:66, 1993.

Arvidsson I, Eriksson E: Postoperative TENS pain relief after knee surgery: objective evaluation, *Orthopedics* 9:1346, 1986.

Byl NN: The use of ultrasound as an enhancer for transcutaneous drug delivery: phonophoresis, *Phys Ther* 75:539, 1995.

Costello CT, Jeske AH: Iontophoresis: applications in transdermal medication delivery, *Phys Ther* 75:554, 1995.

Deyo RA et al: A controlled trial of transcutaneous electrical nerve stimulation (TENS) and exercise for low back pain, *N Engl J Med* 322:1627, 1990.

Glass JM, Stephen RL, Jacobsen SC: The quantity and distribution of radiolabeled dexamethasone delivered to tissues by iontophoresis, *Int J Dermatol* 19:519, 1980.

Gudeman SC, Eisele SA, Heidt RS Jr, et al: Treatment of plantar fasciitis by iontophoresis of 0.4% dexamethasone: a randomized, double-blind, placebo-controlled study, *Am J Sports Med* 25:312, 1997.

Guillot M: Urinary leak of salicylic acid after topical application, *J Physiol* (Paris) 46:31-37, 1954.

Guy RH, Hadgraft J: The effect of penetration enhancers on the kinetics of percutaneous absorption, *J Control Rel* 5:43, 1987.

Klaiman MD, Shrader JA, Danoff JV, et al: Phonophoresis versus ultrasound in the treatment of common musculoskeletal conditions, *Med Sci Sports Exerc* 30:1349, 1998.

Mehreteab TA: Iontophoresis. In Hecox B, Mehreteab TA, Weisberg J, editors: *Physical agents: a comprehensive text for physical therapists*, East Norwalk, Conn, 1994, Appleton & Lange.

Moll MJ: A new approach to pain: lidocaine and Decadron with ultrasound, *USAF Med Serv Digest* 8-11, 1997.

Petelenz TJ, Buttke JA, Bonds C, et al: Iontophoresis of dexamethasone: laboratory studies, *Journal of Controlled Release* 20:55, 1992.

Robinson AJ: Transcutaneous electrical nerve stimulation for the control of pain in musculoskeletal disorders, *J Orthop Sports Phys Ther* 24:208, 1996.

Russo J Jr, Lipman AG, Comstock AJ, et al: Lidocaine anesthesia: comparison of iontophoresis, injection, and swabbing, *Am J Hosp Pharm* 37:843, 1980.

Spielholz NI, Nolan MF: Conventional TENS and the phenomena of accommodation, adaption, habituation, and electrode polarization, *J Clin Electrophysiol* 7:16, 1995.

Sweitzer RW: Ultrasound. In Hecox B, Mehreteab TA, Weisberg J, editors: *Physical agents: a comprehensive text for physical therapists*, East Norwalk, Conn, 1994, Appleton & Lange.

Venous Methylene Blue Therapy

Timothy J. Downs

Methylene blue is a water-soluble thiazine dye used therapeutically to treat, among other things, toxic levels of methemoglobin (i.e., the oxidized form of hemoglobin). This chapter will describe the diagnosis of methemoglobinemia and its treatment with methylene blue.

Methemoglobinemia has been a serious and common occupational hazard in the United States. Between 1935 and 1965 numerous cases of methemoglobinemia caused by exposure to 2-chloronitrobenzene were reported in the United States; most of these cases were the result of exposure in the dye-manufacturing industry. The condition was so common that fellow workers were usually the first to recognize a toxic exposure to this methemoglobin-forming agent. Because of occupational safety measures, occupational exposure is much less common. However, cases caused by recreational drug use and exposure to normal and high doses of both prescription and over-the-counter medications are still reported.

The naturally occurring physiologic level of methemoglobin is approximately 1% of the total hemoglobin. Normally the enzyme methemoglobin reductase (NADH), which converts methemoglobin back to hemoglobin, prevents toxic levels of methemoglobin. Exposure of hemoglobin to oxidizing substances (Box 216-1) can increase methemoglobin levels. Cyanosis becomes clinically obvious when methemoglobin levels exceed 10% of total hemoglobin (1.5 g/dl). This cyanosis, which may have a grayish-brown hue, can be indistinguishable from the more common cardiac and pulmonary causes of cyanosis. When more than 20% of hemoglobin is oxidized to methemoglobin, symptoms can occur. The symptoms result from hypoxia and include headache, fatigue, dyspnea, or tachycardia. Severe toxic symptoms occur at methemoglobin concentrations of 50%. Stupor, cardiac arrhythmias, seizures, and even coma are symptoms of severe toxic methemoglobin levels. When the levels of methemoglobin are in excess of 70%, the hypoxic effects are usually lethal.

Cyanosis is the most clinically obvious sign of methemoglobinemia. However, because cyanosis is more commonly caused by cardiac or pulmonary disorders, the differential diagnosis usually does not include methemoglobinemia until the more common causes are ruled out. One clue should be that *the cyanosis does not respond to initial therapy with oxygen*. Acquired toxic methemoglobinemia, the most serious form of methemoglobinemia, is caused by exposure to various chemicals or medications. This form of methemoglobinemia can be life threatening; thus prompt and appropriate treatment can be life saving. The other two causes of methemoglobinemia, hereditary hemoglobin M (Hgb-M) and NADH deficiency, are inherited and generally clinically mild.

Methemoglobin binds oxygen so tightly that oxygen is not released as it reaches the end organs. This "shift to the left" of the oxyhemoglobin dissociation curve is

---

BOX 216-1

Causes of Severe Acquired Toxic Methemoglobinemia

Occupational Exposure
Dyes, explosives, rubber
Aniline
o-Anisidine
Dinitrotoluene and trinitrotoluene
Nitroglycerin
2-Chloronitrobenzene
o-Toluidine
Other aromatic amino and nitro compounds

Recreational and Therapeutic Drug Use
Amyl nitrate
Butyl nitrate (i.e., "poppers")
Methamphetamines
Medications
Benzocaine (common in over-the-counter topical anesthetics)
Dapsone (long half-life)
Lidocaine
Nitric oxide
Phenazopyridine
Prilocaine
Primaquine and related antimalarials
Silver nitrate
Sodium nitroprusside
Sulfonamides
Valproate

similar to the changes caused by carbon monoxide poisoning. The oxidation of hemoglobin causes a color change from red to chocolate brown, which can be a diagnostic clue.

DIAGNOSIS OF METHEMOGLOBINEMIA

Three common clinical scenarios can lead to acquired toxic methemoglobinemia:

1. Occupational exposure
2. Recreational drug use
3. Use of medications known to cause methemoglobinemia

The key to diagnosis is suspicion of methemoglobinemia so that the level can be determined and the appropriate level of aggressive therapy can be initiated.

For occupational exposure, removing contaminated clothing and washing skin to remove residues of the offending agent are necessary to prevent further absorption. The scalp, hair, nostrils, ear canals, toenails, and fingernails are potential sites for the toxic agents to escape detection. Hospitalization is recommended for patients with methemoglobin levels greater than 20% or who are symptomatic. With time and supportive care, patients with mild methemoglobinemia will spontaneously return to normal. Supplemental oxygen helps relieve general malaise and headache. For patients with stupor, status epilepticus, or coma, intravenous (IV) methylene blue is indicated. In addition, patients with severe symptoms may need exchange transfusions.

Clues to the Diagnosis of Acquired Toxic Methemoglobinemia

1. The patient has clinical hypoxia, but arterial oxygen levels do not respond to 100% oxygen.
2. The patient has no history of cardiac or pulmonary disease. (Comorbid conditions can be worsened dramatically by methemoglobinemia.)
3. The patient has a history of occupational exposure, uses illicit drugs, or takes a medication known to be a methemoglobin former (Box 216-1). (The patient or observers should be questioned about exposure to these agents.)
4. Chocolate-brown blood sent for laboratory analysis is suspicious for methemoglobinemia. (Sulfhemoglobin may look similar but does not respond to methylene blue.)
5. An anticoagulated blood sample at bedside tests positive. (The top of the vacuum tube should be opened to allow air inside; then the tube should be closed and inverted rapidly several times. If cyano-

sis is caused by hypoxia, the dark purple blood will turn red. If cyanosis is caused by toxic methemoglobinemia, the chocolate brown blood will remain unchanged.)
6. Laboratory testing has confirmed methemoglobinemia quantitatively.
7. The failure of methylene blue to reduce the level of methemoglobinemia may indicate Hgb-M or NADH deficiency, the testing of which is not normally available on an immediate basis.
8. Pulse oximeters do not accurately register the patient's oxygenation levels, and arterial blood gases are needed to accurately assess the patient and his or her response to treatment.

METHYLENE BLUE PHARMACOKINETICS

Methylene blue is reduced to leukomethylene blue in the tissues shortly after IV injection. Approximately 70% is excreted in the urine as leukomethylene blue. Some of the drug is excreted in the bile, and a small portion is excreted as unchanged drug in the urine. Leukomethylene blue is colorless. However, when the urine is exposed to air, it is oxidized to methylene azure and the urine turns green or blue.

General Supportive Measures

1. High-flow oxygen
2. Decontamination of the patient

Note: For external exposure, contaminated clothing should be removed and the skin washed with soap and water. For toxic ingestions, gastric lavage and administration of activated charcoal may be indicated (see Chapter 105, Gastric Lavage).

INDICATIONS

- Methemoglobinemia, severe symptoms
- Gastrointestinal fistula diagnosis
- Patency evaluation of fallopian tubes
- Ifosfamide encephalopathy

Some texts recommend limiting IV use of methylene blue to patients with severe symptoms, such as stupor, arrhythmias, seizures, or coma caused by potential adverse affects. Comorbid conditions, such as angina or emphysema, may be exacerbated and require treatment with methylene blue. Ifosfamide, a chemotherapy agent, is known to be neurotoxic by an oxidation process. Treatment and pretreatment with methylene blue has been helpful in reversing and preventing the encephalopathy associated with ifosfamide treatment.

CONTRAINDICATIONS

- Cyanide poisoning
- Complete glucose-6-phosphate dehydrogenase (G6PD) deficiency
- Intrathecal administration
- Subcutaneous administration

Methylene blue should not be used to treat methemoglobinemia associated with cyanide poisoning. Methylene blue increases the release of cyanide from methemoglobin, increasing the cyanide concentration in the blood. Sodium nitrite is considered a safer and more effective alternative. Methylene blue requires reduced nicotinamide adenine dinucleotide phosphate (NADPH) and is not effective in the treatment of methemoglobinemia resulting from G6PD deficiency. Administration of the drug can precipitate an acute hemolytic episode in these patients. Methylene blue can be administered either IV or orally (PO) and has been used by the intraosseous route. *Intrathecal administration* can cause neural damage and should not be used. *Subcutaneous administration* or extravasation can produce necrotic abscesses.

PRECAUTIONS

- Renal insufficiency
- Severe anemia
- Chronic use (orally)
- Pregnancy
- Phototherapy

Methylene blue's primary route of elimination is through the kidneys. It should be used with caution in patients with renal impairment. Dosage adjustment may be needed. Methylene blue destroys erythroblasts. Prolonged administration (for the cosmetic treatment of Hgb-M or NADH deficiency) can cause *anemia*. Hemoglobin levels should be determined regularly in patients receiving *chronic* methylene blue therapy. Patients with preexisting anemia should be treated with caution. Methylene blue is classified as *pregnancy category C.* Adequate evaluations have not been performed for safe use during pregnancy, so the potential risks to the fetus must be weighed against the potential benefits to the mother. Methylene blue has been reported to cause a severe *photosensitivity reaction* after treatment with bilirubin lights in a premature neonate exposed to methylene blue prenatally.

EQUIPMENT

- Arterial blood gas analysis
- Methylene blue (injectable) USP 1% solution in saline
- Syringe and needles
- IV access (intraosseous access optional)
- Near-patient (bedside) methemoglobin analyzer (optional)

TECHNIQUE

1. Calculate dose: Adults and children should receive 1 to 2 mg/kg (0.1 to 0.2 ml/kg of 1% solution) or 25 to 50 mg/M^2.
2. Draw up calculated dose of methylene blue 1% solution into syringe.
3. Infuse methylene blue IV slowly over 5 to 10 minutes.

Note: Ensure that extravasation does not occur.

4. The dose of 2 mg/kg may be repeated after 1 hour, if the cyanosis has not completely resolved.
5. Recheck methemoglobin levels every 3 to 6 hours for the next 24 hours.
6. For skin contamination, repeat skin cleansing if the methemoglobin levels rise after 3 to 4 hours. For recent ingestions, repeat administration of activated charcoal may be indicated (see Chapter 105, Gastric Lavage).
7. Confirm oxygenation status by arterial blood gases if the oxygen saturation deteriorates by pulse oximetry.

Caution: To avoid toxic side effects, the total dose should not exceed 7 mg/kg.
Note: Intraosseous administration of methylene blue in an infant has been successfully used when IV access was not available (see Chapter 181, Intraosseous Venous Access).

COMPLICATIONS

Toxic effects include the following:
- Dyspnea
- Precordial pain
- Restlessness
- Apprehension
- Hemolytic crisis in patients with G6PD deficiency
- Blue staining of skin, nails, or clothing
- Tissue necrosis because of extravasation
- Anemia because of chronic use (from oral administration)

Note: Administration of methylene blue may worsen cyanide poisoning (see Contraindications). There are no known drug interactions or adequate evaluations concerning the use of methylene blue in pregnancy.

INTERPRETATION OF RESULTS AND FINDINGS

Methylene blue IV in doses 1 to 2 mg/kg (0.1 to 0.2 ml/kg of 1% solution) or 25 to 50 mg/M^2 is expected to rapidly reduce methemoglobin levels of 40% to approximately 20% in 1 to 2 hours. The dose may be repeated after 1 hour if needed. Some reports recommend observation for 24 hours in the hospital because further absorption or metabolization of the oxidizing substances has caused methemoglobinemia to worsen after initial improvements.

Patients who do not respond to methylene blue injection should be evaluated for Hgb-M or NADH deficiency or sulfhemoglobinemia.

Commonly used pulse oximeters may give false low oxygen–saturation readings after administration of methylene blue because the blue color is misinterpreted as nonoxygenated hemoglobin. Arterial blood gas analysis will give accurate oxygen saturation.

Methemoglobinemia is a known complication of therapeutic use of nitric oxide in intensive care situations (especially after cardiopulmonary bypass surgery). Several commercial devices make near-patient measurements of methemoglobin possible. However, methylene blue interferes colorometrically with the methemoglobin measurements in a dose-dependent manner for these instruments, leading to falsely lowered measurements up to 15%. Because the methylene blue has been found to reduce the methemoglobin by less than 2% within 2 minutes of treatment, it has been suggested that the methemoglobin levels be measured before and immediately after the administration of methylene blue. Then calculations of the error coefficient caused by the color interference can be calculated for the particular instrument. Repeat infusions would require repeat calculations because higher concentrations of methylene blue produce more interference.

CONCLUSION

The diagnosis of acute toxic methemoglobinemia as the cause of cyanosis is the critical step in starting effective therapy. Methemoglobinemia should be considered in any cyanotic patient who has no evidence of heart or lung disease. Most patients with methemoglobinemia improve after removal of the offending agent, supportive care, supplemental oxygen, and time to allow the body to spontaneously reduce the methemoglobin. Methylene blue IV injection should be reserved for toxic patients with stupor or coma or where comorbid conditions, such as angina, are worsened by the methemoglobine-

mia. Exchange transfusions have been used in the most severely ill patients.

SUPPLIERS

Methylene blue injection USP 1% solution is available from several suppliers and is a standard stock item in most hospital pharmacies.

CPT/BILLING CODE

90784   IV injection, diagnostic or therapeutic

ICD-9-CM DIAGNOSTIC CODES

289.7	Methemoglobinemia, acquired, toxic, Hgb-M disease, hereditary
E931.9	Methylene blue, therapeutic use
983	Aniline poisoning
972.4	Nitrates, poisoning
972.4	Nitrite, amyl poisoning
E858.3	Nitroglycerin, accidental poisoning
972.4	Nitroglycerin, poisoning
983	Nitrobenzene, poisoning
983	Nitrotoluene, poisoning
E855.2	Drug, topical anesthetics, accidental
969.7	Amphetamine, poisoning

BIBLIOGRAPHY

Braunwald E, Fauci AS, Kasper DL, et al: *Harrison's principles of internal medicine,* ed 14, New York, 1996, McGraw-Hill.

Coleman MD, Coleman NA: Drug-induced methemoglobinemia: treatment issues, *Drug Saf* 14(6):394, 1996.

Herman MI, Chyka PA, Butler AY, Rieger SE: Methylene blue by intraosseous infusion for methemoglobinemia, *Ann Emerg Med* 33(1):111, 1999.

McCunney RJ: *A practical approach to occupational and environmental medicine,* ed 2, Boston, 1994, Little, Brown.

Malhotra R, Hughes G: Methaemoglobinaemia presenting with status epilepticus, *J Accid Emerg Med* 13(6):427, 1996.

Rudlof B, Lampert B et al: The use of pulse oximetry in prilocaine induced methemoglobinemia, *Anaesthesist* 44 (12):887, 1995.

Tierney LM, McPhee SJ, Papadakis MA: *Current medical diagnosis and treatment 2001,* ed 40, New York, 2000, McGraw-Hill.

Verzosa JD: Methemoglobinemia: cyanosis and street methamphetamines, *J Am Board Fam Pract* 10(2):137, 1997.

Commonly Used Instruments/Equipment

John L. Pfenninger

Listed below are the most commonly used instruments in a primary care physician's office. This list at least provides a basic beginning for ordering equipment for the office. A physician can alter the equipment depending on the procedures performed.

Biopsy instruments

- Skin: 2-, 3-, 4-, 5-mm disposable punches or a set of Keyes reusable punches (Fig. A-1)

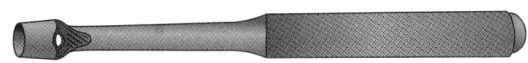

Fig. A-1
Keyes cutaneous punch, 4 mm.

- Cervical: Mini-Townsend, Baby Tischler, Kevorkian (see Chapter 139, Colposcopic Examination, Fig. 139-3)
- Endometrial: reusable, Novak; disposable: Endocell (Wallach), PipetCuret (Milex), Pipelle (Unimar, CooperSurgical) (see Chapter 146, Endometrial Biopsy, Figs. 146-3 and 146-6)
- For flexible sigmoidoscopy, colonoscopy, EGD procedures (see Chapter 104, Flexible Sigmoidoscopy, Fig. 104-6)
- Breast: FNA-21 (CooperSurgical), Milex breast biopsy needle Comeco syringe, 21-gauge butterfly needle (see Figs. 210-1 through 210-3)

Dermal curettes

- Fox type (3-, 4-, 5-, 6-mm reusable; 3-, 4-, 5-mm disposable) (Fig. A-2)

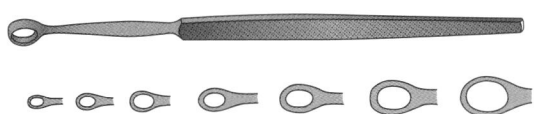

Fig. A-2
Fox dermal curette.

Forceps

- Adsons with and without teeth, 4¾ inches (Fig. A-3)

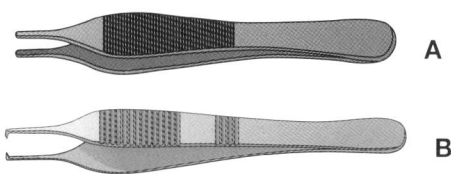

Fig. A-3
Adson forceps. **A,** Serrated jaws. **B,** With teeth.

- Splinter (Fig. A-4)

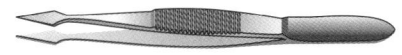

Fig. A-4
Carmalt splinter.

- Allis (Fig. A-5)

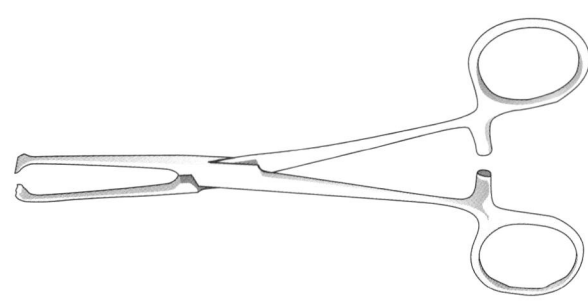

Fig. A-5
Allis tissue forceps.

- Uterine packing (look like long, large hemostats)
- Norgrasp (removal of Norplants)
- Ring (sponge)

Can grasp tissue or clot during gynecologic procedures, and are useful for holding gauze or cotton to apply solutions (such as antiseptics or acetic acid to the cervix during colposcopy) or to stop blood (Fig. A-6).

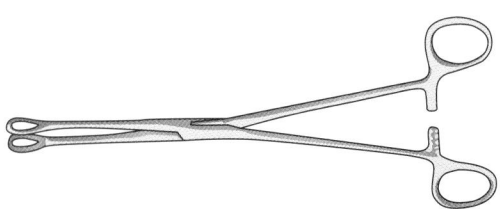

Fig. A-6
Foerster sponge/ring forceps.

Hemostats/Clamps
- Mosquito: 5-inch straight, 5-inch curved (for fine application) (Fig. A-7)

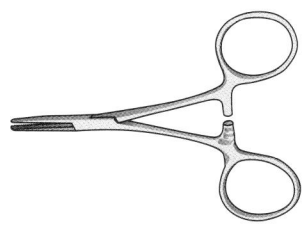

Fig. A-7
Pedifine Hartman mosquito hemostats.

- Kelly: 5½-inch straight, 5½-inch curved (for larger application) (Fig. A-8)

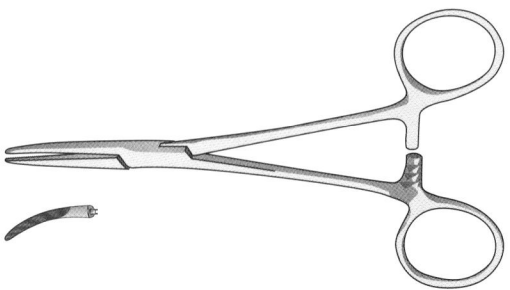

Fig. A-8
Kelly straight and curved (inset) hemostats.

- Towel clips (Fig. A-9)

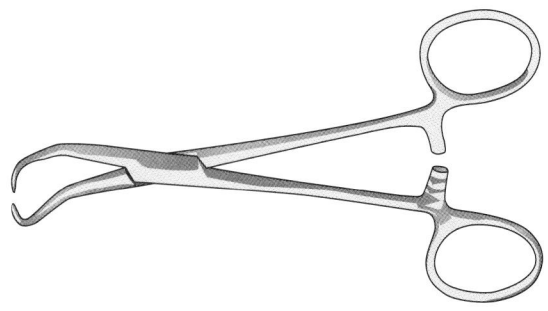

Fig. A-9
Backhaus towel clamps.

Scissors
- Suture removal (Spencer 3½-inch) (Fig. A-10)

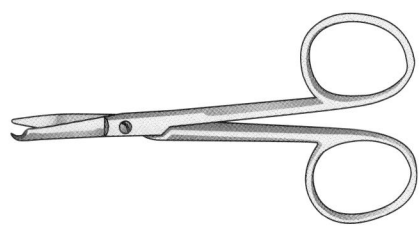

Fig. A-10
Spencer 3½-inch suture removal scissors.

- Suture (William 4½-inch) (Fig. A-11)

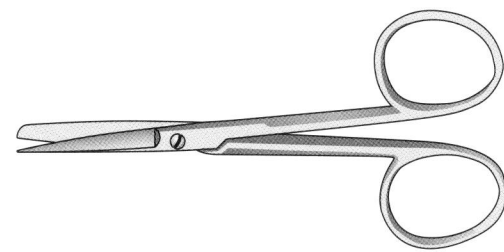

Fig. A-11
William 4½-inch suture applying scissors.

- Tissue
  - Mayo 6¾-inch (Fig. A-12)

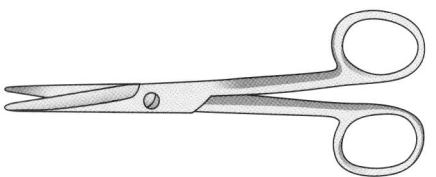

Fig. A-12
Mayo 6¾-inch operating scissors.

–Curved Metzenbaum 5-inch, 7-inch (Fig. A-13)

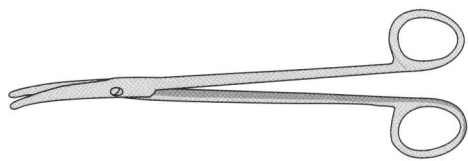

Fig. A-13
Curved Metzenbaum 5- and 7-inch operating scissors.

–Fine Tissue (iris) 4⅛-inch (Fig. A-14)

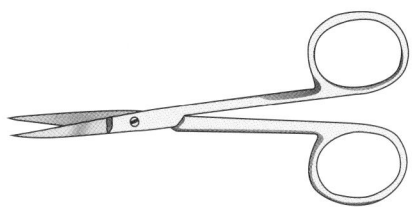

Fig. A-14
Fine tissue (iris) 4⅛-inch scissors.

• Bandage 5½-inch (Fig. A-15)

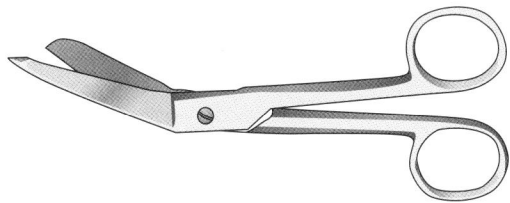

Fig. A-15
Bandage removal scissors.

Needle driver 5-inch (9-inch for vaginal/uterine procedures)
• Webster serrated jaws

Note: This is not the place to save a few pennies. Buy the best needle holders (Fig. A-16).

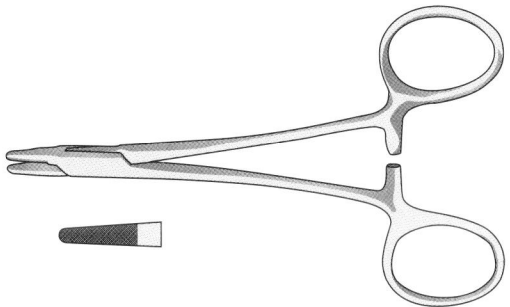

Fig. A-16
Webster serrated jaw needle holder.

Minor surgery pack
• Scalpel handle with metric ruler inscribed on it (Fig. A-17)

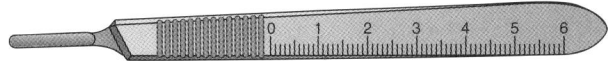

Fig. A-17
Scalpel handle with metric rule.

• Fine hemostats (2), curved and straight
• 5-inch curved Metzenbaum scissors
• Pick-ups with teeth
• Pick-ups without teeth
• Disposable skin markers
• Suture scissors
• Stainless steel basin
• 4 × 4s
• Glass jar for specimen
• Needle driver

Vasectomy set-up (no-scalpel)
• Small curved hemostats (2)
• Hemoclip applicator (medium) and clips
• Vas dissecting forceps
• Vas clamp (Wilson or Li)
• Sharp tissue scissors
• Battery-powered cautery unit
• Medicine cup
• 4 × 4s, large pack

Skin hooks
• Useful for nontraumatic skin or wound edge retraction (Fig. A-18)

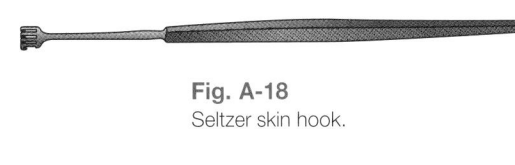

Fig. A-18
Seltzer skin hook.

Staple applicator

Staple remover
• Removes surgical stainless steel skin staples. Removers are sold as disposable, and many patients have staples, especially after being treated in the emergency room.

Staple removers may be reused, however, with appropriate sterilization (Fig. A-19).

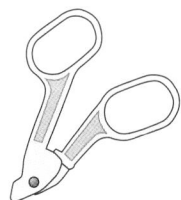

Fig. A-19
Davis & Geck appose staple remover.

Syringes

• Clinicians need mostly 1 ml for skin procedures as well as some 3 ml, a few 5 ml, and even fewer than 10 ml. Two 25-ml syringes may also come in handy for thoracenteses, knee aspirations, etc.

Needles

• Note: The larger the number, the smaller the needle! Clinicians need mostly 1½-inch, 25-gauge and ½-inch, 30-gauge needles for skin. Clinicians will need some 21 gauge and 18 gauge. The latter are used to aspirate viscous fluid (e.g., ganglions) or large amounts of fluid (e.g., knee aspiration). Eighteen-guage needles are also used to draw up anesthetic; it goes much more quickly than using needles that are smaller.

5-inch needle extender

• After twisting the extender on a syringe, the practitioner then locks the needle to this "extender." It is reusable and can be used to reach deep areas like the cervix, posterior pharynx, anus, etc. (See Chapter 150, Loop Electrosurgical Excision Procedure [LEEP] for Treating Cervical Intraepithelial Neoplasia.)

Suture

• Use cutting needles for the majority of patients.
— Skin: 3-0, 4-0, 5-0, and 6-0 nylon (for most interrupted procedures)
— 4-0 and 5-0 Prolene (for subcuticular procedures)
— Deep inverted: 3-0, 4-0, and 5-0 Vicryl

Sterile drapes, fenestrated and nonfenestrated

• The polyurethane type is very helpful and stays in place much better than the paper one, since central portion has a self-adhesive backing.

Mayo stand with tray to hold instruments

Magnification loupes

• Welch Allyn: 2.5× to 3×; has light with battery pack

Comedone extractor

• Saalfield or Unna types (Fig. A-20)

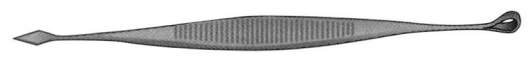

Fig. A-20
Saalfield comedone extractor.

Ear loop

• For cerumen removal: Sklar #67-2513

For ingrown toenails

• Locke periosteal nail elevator (Fig. A-21)

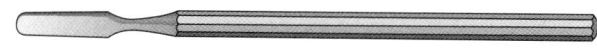

Fig. A-21
Locke elevator.

• Nail splitter (Fig. A-22)

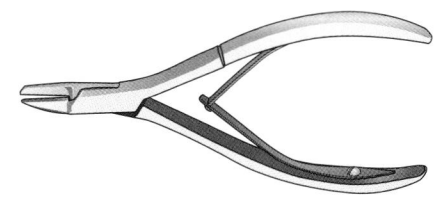

Fig. A-22
Nail splitter.

Chalazion clamp (small) with curette

(Figs. A-23 and A-24)

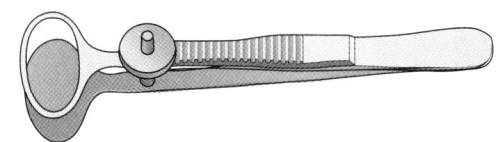

Fig. A-23
Desmarres chalazion clamp.

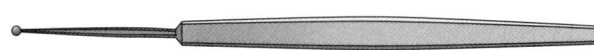

Fig. A-24
Skeele chalazion curette.

Vaginal Speculum

• Small, medium, large Grave's
• Nonconductive, vented for LEEP
• Extra long (Snowman; CooperSurgical) for obese patients; very helpful for difficult cases

Endocervical curette (Kevorkian, without a basket)

Endocervical speculum (small, large)
- For colposcopy and removal of cervical polyps (see Chapter 139, Colposcopic Examination)

Cervical dilators (including silver probe)
- For endometrial biopsy, cervical stenosis, and D & Cs (see appropriate chapters)

Dilateria (thin, medium thick, thick)
- For cervical stenosis
- Used to dilate a cervix atraumatically

Word Bartholin cyst catheter

Uterine sound
- Malleable rod is used to determine the depth of the uterus (from external os to back wall). Such information decreases the likelihood of uterine perforation during procedures.

Vaginal sidewall retractors
(Cryotherapy of cervix, LEEP; see Chapter 150, Loop Electrosurgical Excision Procedure [LEEP] for Treating Cervical Intraepithelial Neoplasia)

Single tooth tenaculum for cervix
- Used to stabilize the cervix for IUD placement, endometrial biopsy, laminaria insertion, or dilation, or to perform colpocentesis (see Chapter 130, First-Trimester Abortion and Emergency Oral Contraceptives; Fig. 130-9)

IUD remover
(see Chapter 149, Intrauterine Device Removal)

Anoscope
- Ive's slotted (see Chapter 100, Anoscopy; Fig. 100-1)
- Plastic, disposable
- Pediatric

McGivney hemorrhoid ligator (see Chapter 108, Office Treatment of Hemorrhoids; Fig. 108-6)

Infrared coagulator (Redfield) (see Chapter 108, Office Treatment of Hemorrhoids; Fig. 108-10)
- Used for hemorrhoids, warts, tattoos, nasal turbinates, and bleeders.

Liquid nitrogen cryogun and Dewar (Brymill, Wallach) for skin (see Chapter 15, Cryosurgery)

Nitrous oxide cryotherapy unit (see Chapter 141, Cryotherapy of the Cervix; Fig. 141-1)

- Tips: 19- and 25-mm flat and slight conical for cervix
  — Slanted end tips for skin
  — Hemorrhoid tip (multifunctional for skin lesions; virtually never used for hemorrhoids!)

Casting supplies

Wall blood pressure cuff with stethoscope

Glucose monitor

Oxygen tank on mobile cart

ECG machine

Pulse oximeter/Vital Signs monitor (Welch Allyn)

Defibrillator

Stress ECG unit (see Chapter 92, Exercise [Stress] Testing)

Banyon Emergency Kit (see Chapter 203, Anaphylaxis)

Electrosurgical/coagulation unit (ESU) (see Chapter 31, Radiofrequency Surgery [Modern Electrosurgery]; Fig. 31-1)
- Spend a little more and purchase a high-frequency unit for cutting (Ellman, Wallach, CooperSurgical)

Smoke evacuator for electrosurgical application (see Chapter 31, Radiofrequency Surgery; Fig. 31-1)

Cart for ESU unit and smoke evacuator

Colposcope (see Chapter 139, Colposcopic Examination; Fig. 139-6)

Flexible sigmoidoscope with suction pump and light source, cart (see Chapter 104, Flexible Sigmoidoscopy; Fig. 104-1)

Nasopharyngoscope (see Chapter 69, Flexible Fiberoptic Nasolaryngoscopy)

Colonoscope (see Chapter 101, Colonoscopy)

Gastroscope (see Chapter 102, Esophagogastroduodenoscopy)

Otoscope/Ophthalmoscope

Binocular microscope

Air purifier

Sharps containers

Hands-free anesthetic bottle holder (AMI)
- Saves time; holds multidose vials of anesthetic; inexpensive.

Safety goggles

IV pole

Halogen flexible floor light or mobile high-intensity ceiling surgical light

Exam tables, powered
- A matter of an inch or two makes a big difference. (Twenty-four inches is the ideal height when the table is as low as it can go. It cannot be higher.)

Exam stools

Refrigerator for medications
- Must be separate unit from the one used to store lunches!

Autoclave

TV for patient education videos

APPENDIX B

Informed Consent

Julie Graves Moy

Before the performance of any procedure, the patient and the physician must discuss the reasons for performing the procedure, the treatment options, the possible complications from the procedure, and the possible complications from not having the procedure. Informed consent is often considered to be just a signature on a form before beginning the procedure, and many physicians believe (or hope) that a signed consent form will prevent a malpractice lawsuit. However, as it is currently interpreted by many courts, a consent form is not sufficient to protect a physician from litigation.

There is no single doctrine of informed consent across the country, and different court decisions have used different standards. Before 1957, physicians accused of not informing patients of potential risk were charged on grounds of battery. In 1957, the emphasis changed to that of deviation from the standard of conduct of a reasonable and prudent physician; a physician was negligent in informing the patient only if the process used was different from that used by most other physicians. The current, most common standard, introduced in 1972, is the "reasonable man" standard of material risk. Under this standard, physicians must tell a patient what a reasonable person in the patient's position would want to know, and that risks that are not serious or are unlikely are not considered material. *Most courts expect the disclosure before a procedure to include diagnosis, the nature of the proposed procedure, risks and benefits of the procedure, available alternatives and their risks and benefits, and the consequences of not having the procedure.* Courts usually do not require the physician to disclose the risks the patient is already aware of or which an average patient is likely to know. The courts have been criticized for setting standards that do not actually reflect medical practice and may interfere with the doctor-patient relationship. The problem may lie in the implementation, not in the actual concept. The ethical concept of informed consent includes the concepts from the courts, but it goes further: the patient must be a partner in the decision-making process (Box B-1).

The legal development of medical informed consent has not been uniform across states, and some states have codified certain procedures, clarifying the responsibility of the physician. Texas, for example, established panels of doctors and lawyers who together write rules for informed consent for many surgical procedures. Michigan mandates that all women receive a state-approved booklet before mastectomy for breast cancer. All physicians should be aware of the law in their own state, both legislative efforts and court decisions. Most state medical societies can provide lists of such procedures and the specific forms that must be used.

In cases that do not require specific forms, a general consent form that allows identification of the patient, the procedure, the indications, and the risks can be used (Fig. B-1). Most states require a witness to sign the consent; many offices ask nurses or other office staff to witness, but there are possible conflict-of-interest issues if litigation ensues. *If possible, a family member or friend of the patient should serve as a witness to the consent process in addition to office staff.*

Just as the laws have evolved in clarifying informed consent, the transition toward involving the patient more in the process has also changed. There are basically four models of medical decision making:

1. Traditional model: The physician decides whether to perform a procedure and which procedure to perform; the patient's trust and confidence in the doctor replace the need for consent.
2. Traditional informed consent: The physician decides whether to perform a procedure and which procedure to perform with the patient's informed consent.
3. Collaboration: The physician and the patient work together to make a joint decision about the procedure.
4. Patient choice: The patient decides with the physician's counsel.

Some patients will choose the traditional model if given the option of one of the four, and a few will choose the last model. Most patients and physicians are more comfortable with either traditional informed consent or collaboration, and physicians should learn to use both of these models as well as how to determine which to use for a specific patient.

All office procedures should be preceded by a discussion that allows the patient to participate in, and perhaps even lead, the decision about whether to have the procedure. The patient should sign a document that summarizes the process. Some states have laws that specify certain language on consent forms for certain procedures. There is rarely an exception to the rule that *all procedures should be preceded by the patient's consent*. It may be permissible in some cases to obtain verbal consent, but this should be documented explicitly by the physician in the medical record summarizing all the essential points (risks, benefits, possible complications, alternative therapies) and expected outcomes.

Minor children and adults who are not competent to make decisions about their own health may not give consent. For these patients, consent must be obtained from a parent or legal guardian. *In emergencies*, it is permissible to perform procedures without patient consent, but state law determines the appropriate guidelines such as having two physicians not involved in the case sign the form. Some states also allow the suspension of the *informed consent process for reason of therapeutic privilege*, the principle under which the physician is excused from disclosure if information given to the patient might have a detrimental effect on

BOX B-1

Elements of Informed Consent

Disclosure of information
Competency (the patient is not a minor, unconscious, intoxicated, or incapable of participating in the process)
Understanding
Voluntarism
Decision-making
Patient participation

Patient Consent Form

I came to the office of Dr. _____ on _____ (date) for evaluation and treatment of the following condition:

(description of diagnosis, etiology, and differential diagnosis)

We discussed the different treatments possible, and discussed the risks of not treating the condition. Based on the advice given by Dr. _____ and my own judgment, I agree to undergo the following procedure:

(description of anesthetic, procedure, and dressing)

We discussed the different outcomes that could occur, and most of the possible complications. I am aware that other complications could occur that we could not foresee. I agree to follow the instructions for self-care after the procedure, and to return for follow-up care on: _____.
I will call the office or answering service if any problems arise before the scheduled follow-up visit.

_____   _____
Patient's signature   Date/time

_____   _____
Witness' signature   Physician's signature

One copy for chart, one copy for patient.

Fig. B-1
Sample of patient consent form

the physical or psychological well-being of the patient. This situation can be interpreted differently by different courts, and physicians should use caution before using the privilege.

The process of discussing the procedure with the patient or guardian and providing education about the procedure itself, the possible complications, and after-care responsibilities of the patient should all be considered part of the consent process. The consent form can be used as a patient education tool, with a copy containing the patient's signature to be given to the patient for reference. Patients can be educated during the consent process about the legal requirements for the signed form and the fact that results of medical procedures are not guaranteed. However, bringing the form out at the last minute for signature is thought to produce some patient anxiety and suspicion. A better strategy may be to start the process by giving the patient the consent form to read, then using the form to guide the discussion. For office procedures such as vasectomy, the form can be sent out before the consultation visit or given at the time of the consultation. The patient can read it, think about it, then return it before surgery. The consent form can include postprocedure instructions as well as instructions for contacting the physician or an associate if complications occur after hours.

Many liability insurance companies are beginning to advise that patients view videotapes discussing the proposed procedure. This ensures that the patient has an opportunity to consider all the pertinent information and serves as a record for defense of a lawsuit.

The actual process of informed consent can be summarized as follows:
1. Establish responsibility.
   a. The doctor's role.
   b. The patient's role.
2. Establish expected duration of responsibility.
3. Define the problem in negotiation with patient.
4. Set goals for treatment and establish whether cure is a reasonable expectation.
5. Select an approach to treatment; during this step the informed consent form is signed.
6. Perform extended treatment and follow-up.

COMPLICATIONS

Surgical complications, which are at the core of most lawsuits, are either a surprise or deep disappointment.

Physicians must not rely solely on a signed form for protection in court in the case of a malpractice lawsuit. Courts have imposed a duty-to-warn on physicians, and they do not always consider the patient's role in decision making or causation of injury. The usual method of bringing out a highly technical consent form to be

signed at the last minute is not looked upon well by the courts and does not satisfy the condition of "informed consent." Courts consider consent documents as only one form of evidence, and in lawsuits other evidence is examined as well. The form itself cannot substitute for candid discussion with the patient about the procedure and inclusion of the patient in the decision-making process, or for documentation (in the medical record) of the discussion before signing the form. For some patients, particularly uninformed or anxious patients, knowledge of the risk can dissuade them from undergoing a needed procedure.

Similarly, courts do not consider a signed form as evidence that consent was "informed." Many forms use language that is too technical; the forms are often too long to read and interpret during an office visit; consent forms are often handed to patients during hospital registration by nonprofessional personnel; and some patients are unable to comprehend the procedure even after explanation. *In order to provide the type of documentation most useful in a court case, the physician should include in the patient's chart a narrative of the discussion between doctor and patient during the decision-making process, in addition to the actual consent form.*

Clinicians should always *be careful not to "over-promise"* what a procedure can do. Honesty is best. "Never say never and never say always!" There are always exceptions. If someone asks about a rare complication, the clinician should not say it *won't* happen! It could. An example should be given instead. If the patient plays the lotto, the clinician should ask if he or she if likely to win. The answer is usually "No." But could the patient win? Is it possible? The answer is usually "Yes." So it goes with complications. Will it happen? "Most likely not. But, in rare instances, it could."

It goes without saying that *no consent form will cover anyone from true malpractice.* Competence and keeping up-to-date educationally are essential. Seeking expert advice and second opinions is encouraged, and knowing one's limits is essential. Especially in primary care, clinicians must be sure to inform the patient of their training and background; they should not pretend to be an orthopedist, or obstetrician, or plastic surgeon. The patient should get another opinion if he or she is at all uncomfortable.

As many have said before, the best way to avoid a lawsuit is to *have an excellent doctor-patient relationship, with both the patient and the family.* Patients are different. Some have a lot of questions that need to be addressed and answered. Some have been let down by the medical system in the past and are fearful. Some have extreme anxiety and no amount of reassurance helps them. Some want absolute assurances that are impossible. *When the "vibes are bad," clinicians should not try to make things work.* The "other experts" should deal with the problem. Clinicians should not try to be everything to everyone all the time.

CPT/BILLING CODES

98900   Medical conference by physician regarding medical management with patient and/or relative or guardian; 30 minutes

98902   Medical conference by physician regarding medical management with patient and/or relative or guardian; 60 minutes

BIBLIOGRAPHY

Caterine JM, Miller B: Informed consent: procedure specific, *Iowa Med* 79(5):231, 1989.

Green JA: Minimizing malpractice risk by role clarification: the confusing transition from tort to contract, *Ann Intern Med* 109(3)234, 1988.

Hansson MO: Balancing the quality of consent, *J Med Ethics* 24:182, 1998.

Lidz CW, Appelbaum PS, Meisel A: Two models of implementing informed consent, *Ann Intern Med* 148(6):1385, 1988.

Loewy EH: *Textbook of healthcare ethics,* New York, 1996, Plenum Press.

Mazur DJ: What should patients be told prior to a medical procedure? Ethical and legal perspectives on medical informed consent, *Am J Med* 81(6):1051, 1986.

Savulescu J, Momeyer RW: Should informed consent be based on rational beliefs? *J Med Ethics* 23:282, 1997.

Sprung CL, Winick BJ: Informed consent in theory and practice: legal and medical perspectives on the informed consent doctrine and a proposed reconceptualization, *Crit Care Med* 17(12):1346, 1989.

WEBSITES

www.rnabc.bc.ca/pdf/359.pdf (Registered Nurses association of British Columbia statement on informed consent)

www.tsbme.state.tx.us (Texas State Board of Medical Examiners)

Latex Allergy Guidelines

Sumana Reddy

Sensitivity to natural rubber latex (NRL) has been gaining increasing prominence over the last decade. Although NRL has been in widespread use for over a century, multiple factors, including a dramatic increase in use and changes in production time and production quality, have led to recent reports of severe reactions. In 1991, 16 deaths associated with a latex barium enema tip were reported to the Food and Drug Administration (FDA), which led to recall of the tips. In 1997, the National Institute for Occupational Safety and Health (NIOSH) issued an advisory recommending that latex gloves be used only by those workers exposed to blood or body fluids, and not by food handlers, hobbyists and those performing many housekeeping activities. NIOSH also recommends that if NRL gloves are to be used, they should be low protein and powder free.

SYMPTOMS OF LATEX ALLERGY

Reactions to NRL are Type I, immediate hypersensitivity reactions. They can cause local or systemic urticaria, symptoms of rhinoconjunctivitis or bronchospasm, and anaphylaxis. The proteins of NRL have been described as unique in that an unpredictable course may occur in the progression from no or mild symptoms to anaphylaxis. The sensitization begins and is perpetuated both as a contact allergen and as an inhalant. The greatest degree of sensitization occurs in areas where powdered latex gloves with a high NRL protein content are used. In these situations, the cornstarch powder particles appear to adsorb latex to the surface. These latex-cornstarch powder particles have been demonstrated to aerosolize, especially when gloves are removed. Prolonged exposure through the lungs appears to cause high rates of sensitization. Those who are sensitized may cross-react to certain foods such as banana, kiwi, chestnut, or avocado. NRL gloves may also cause an irritant contact dermatitis from occlusion and frequent hand washing, or a delayed hypersensitivity reaction from chemicals used in processing. These are not reactions to latex itself (Box C-1).

RISK GROUPS

Those at greatest risk of sensitization are all those groups with cumulatively prolonged exposure to latex. The greatest prevalence appears to be in those who have undergone repeated surgeries, especially children with spina bifida or urogenital abnormalities. Others at risk include workers in the latex manufacturing industry and healthcare workers. Studies indicate 10% to 17% of healthcare workers have already become sensitized, and over 2% have occupational asthma as a result of latex exposure. In addition, over 50% of persons who are sensitive to latex have a history of atopic illness, or hay fever (Box C-2).

NONLATEX MATERIALS

The establishment of universal precautions in 1985 has led to an increased use of latex gloves through the spectrum of health services from phlebotomy to nursing home care. This use should be reevaluated in light of our new and growing understanding of the process of sensitization. As recommended by NIOSH, all healthcare providers should make purchasing decisions avoiding the use of powdered, high-protein latex gloves, in favor of powder-free, low-protein gloves. Where possible, nonlatex gloves should be used.

There is a range of surgical and nonsurgical gloves available in nonlatex materials. These have been ASTM (American Society for Testing and Materials) tested for barrier integrity and are expected to provide protection against viral particles such as HIV when used as recommended. Vinyl gloves are not as effective against viral penetration. Where exposure to body fluids is not an issue, vinyl gloves are cost-effective.

DIAGNOSIS

In performing procedures, there are issues of identifying the patient who may be latex allergic, and avoiding

BOX C-1
Symptoms Associated with Latex Glove Use

Irritant Contact Dermatitis (Nonimmune)
Gradual onset, over days, caused by hand washing, occlusion, antiseptics, and glove chemicals
Redness
Cracks, fissures
Scaling

Allergic Contact Dermatitis or Type LV (Delayed Hypersensitivity)
Onset 6-48 hours after contact, caused by chemicals
Erythema
Vesicles
Papules
Pruritus
Blisters
Crusting

Immediate Hypersensitivity, or Type I
Local and generalized urticaria onset within minutes, very rarely longer than 2 hours; caused by latex
Feeling of faintness
Feeling of impending doom
Angioedema
Nausea, vomiting, abdominal cramps
Rhinoconjunctivitis
Bronchospasm
Anaphylactic shock

BOX C-2
Risk Groups for Latex Allergy

Occupational Latex Exposure
Healthcare workers
Rubber industry workers

Medical Patient Exposure
Spina bifida
Urogenital abnormalities
Other repeated or prolonged surgeries or mucous membrane exposure to latex devices, especially early in life

Atopic History or Food Allergy (especially bananas, avocados, kiwis, and chestnuts) (Cross-Reacting Protein Epitopes)

Low Risk: No Identifiable Risk Factors

BOX C-3
Screening Questionnaire for Latex Sensitivity

I. Allergies
Have you had a history of hayfever, asthma, eczema, allergies, or problems with rashes?
Are you allergic (rash, oral itching, swelling, or wheezing) to any foods, especially bananas, avocados, kiwi, or chestnuts?

II. Job-Related Symptoms
Does your work involve any exposure to latex products, including latex gloves? Have you ever had allergic reactions to something in your work environment?
If you have had a rash on your hands after wearing latex gloves, how long after putting on the gloves did the rash develop? What did it look like?

III. Hidden Reactions to Latex
Have you ever had swelling, itching, hives, shortness of breath, cough, or other allergic symptoms during or after blowing up a balloon, undergoing a dental procedure, using condoms or diaphragms, or following a vaginal or rectal examination?
Have you ever had an allergic reaction of unknown cause, especially during a medical or dental procedure?

IV. Surgical History
Have you ever had surgeries, and if so, what?
Do you have spina bifida or any urinary tract problem requiring surgery or catheterizations?

exposure, through inadvertent use of a product containing latex. Use of a standardized questionnaire is recommended where any suspicion may exist (Box C-3). It is also important to prevent the development of latex sensitization in the healthcare workers performing and assisting in the procedure.

The diagnosis of latex sensitivity is not straightforward. It is made through a combination of thorough medical history and immunologic testing. Because symptoms can be generalized and nonspecific, the sensitized individual often remains unaware. Standardized extracts for prick testing are not available in the United States. Therefore such skin testing should be carried out only by centers with experience in preparing extracts and may cause a high incidence of anaphylaxis. FDA-approved in vitro tests to measure latex-specific IgE are available (Pharmacia CAP, Pharmacia-UpJohn Diagnostics Inc. Kalamazoo, Mich; AIaSTAT, Diagnostic Products Corp., Los Angeles, Calif). The low specificity of these tests, with at least 20% false-negative results and unclear positive predictive value, give them limitations. Negative serologic testing with a strongly positive history would suggest the value of skin prick testing in experienced hands to confirm the diagnosis. Since individuals with no risk factors or prior symptoms have had anaphylactic reactions, those who are asymptomatic with positive tests should be advised to exercise caution.

If in doubt at the time of performing a procedure, it is best to avoid use of latex-containing medical devices and products. Especially prone to cause reactions are gloves and urinary catheters placed in direct contact with mucosal surfaces (e.g., during pelvic examinations).

The task of identifying latex-containing medical devices has been simplified by recent FDA requirements indicating on packaging whether latex is contained in a product. Lists of latex-containing and latex-free devices may be obtained both directly from individual manufacturers and from the Spina Bifida Association of America. As Box C-4 shows, many medical and household items contain latex. To a sensitized person, all of these may be

BOX C-4
Sources of Possible Latex Exposure

Medical Devices with Potential Latex Content

Gloves
Urinary catheters
Face masks
Tourniquets
Adhesive tape
Bandages
Wound drains
Injection ports
Electrode pads
Rubber syringe stoppers and medication vial stoppers
Bulb syringes
Mattresses on stretchers
Dental devices
Stethoscope and BP cuff tubing
Ambu-bags
PCA syringes

Household Items with Potential Latex Content

Balloons
Condoms and diaphragms
Rubber bands
Shoe soles
Erasers
Many toys
Sports equipment
Carpet backing
Feeding nipples and pacifiers
Clothing, including elastic on underwear
Food handled with powdered latex gloves
Handles on racquets, tools
Diapers, sanitary and incontinence pads
Computer mouse pads
Buttons on electronic equipment

A more detailed and periodically updated list of latex-containing products and nonlatex substitutes by brand name is available from the Spina Bifida Association of America (1-800-621-3141 or http://www.sbaa.org/html/sbaa_latex.html).

BOX C-5
Latex Allergy Management Guidelines for the Hospital Setting

Ask all patients about latex sensitivity, using a screening questionnaire if relevant.
Place latex allergy identification bracelet on patient in admitting area.
Label room as latex safe and enter in all relevant areas of signage, notes, and databases.
Disseminate latex allergy protocol and lists of nonlatex substitutes for latex-containing materials that may contact the patient.
Remove all latex products that would contact the patient and remove all latex gloves. Use PVC tubing or wrap cotton gauze over the extremity if using latex cuffs and tubing or tourniquets.
Ensure that adhesives and tapes, including ECG electrodes and dressing supplies, are checked for latex content.
Have a latex-free crash cart available to follow the patient through his or her stay.
Notify Pharmacy and Central Supply that the patient is latex sensitive so latex contact can be eliminated when preparing materials or drugs for the patient.
Notify Dietary of relevant food allergies to avoid handling food with powdered latex gloves.

---

contact with latex. For the most part, then, extreme measures (e.g., only using medication from glass ampules or glass syringes) are not recommended. The hospital guidelines provided may be adapted as applicable for an outpatient setting (Box C-5).

Premedication with antihistamines or steroids is not helpful. It may only mask symptoms leading to anaphylaxis without preventing anaphylactic reactions. Persons with latex hypersensitivity should carry an epinephrine auto-injection kit and wear MedicAlert identification. In the medical office it is always advisable to have available sterile nonlatex gloves for use.

INFORMATION AND PATIENT EDUCATION

Patient education and additional information are available through the following groups:

Latex Allergy News: The Information Sharing Vehicle of ELASTIC (Education for Latex Allergy Support Team and Information Coalition)
Phone:1-860-482-6869
Website: www.latex-allergy.org

ALERT (Allergy to Latex Education and Resource Team, Inc).
Phone: 1-888-97-ALERT
Website: www.latexallergyresources.org

Spina Bifida Association of America
Phone: 1-800-621-3141
Website: www.sbaa.org

problematic. To an unsensitized person, the thin stretchy rubber of gloves, condoms, and balloons provides the greatest source of rubber particles leaching from the surface. Solid, molded rubber objects are less likely to leach proteins from their surfaces.

MANAGEMENT

A history of Type 1, immediate hypersensitivity reactions necessitates a latex-safe environment.

Patient records should be identified clearly for latex allergy, and at no time in treatment should latex gloves, tourniquets, catheters, or other materials come in direct contact with the patient. If blood pressure cuffs and tubing are made of latex, the patient's extremities should be wrapped to prevent contact. Although rubber medication vial and syringe stoppers are listed, to date there have been only rare reactions to medication in

TABLE C-1

Hypoallergenic Nonlatex Gloves

Type of Glove	Material	Company/Phone Number	Cost vs. Latex
Surgical Gloves			
Dermaprene	Neoprene (polychloroprene polymer)	Ansell (1-800-327-8659)	6×
Neolon	Neoprene (polychloroprene polymer)	Maxxim (1-800-346-8849)	6×
Elastyren	Styrene butadiene block polymer	Center Labs (1-800-437-6251)	5×
Tactylite	Styrene ethylene butadiene co-polymer	Smartpractice (1-800-822-8956)	10×
Pure Advantage	Nitrile* (butadiene co-polymer)	Tillotson (1-800-445-6830)	2×
Examination Gloves			
Royal Shield	Polyvinyl chloride	Smartpractice (1-800-822-8956)	
Sensicare and Trutouch	Polyvinyl chloride	Maxxim (1-800-346-8849)	
Allerderm	Polyvinyl chloride and nitrile	Allerderm (1-800-365-6868)	
Triflex	Polyvinyl chloride	Allegiance (1-800-327-7503)	
Allergard	Styrene butadiene block polymer	Allergard (1-800-255-2500)	
N-DEX	Nitrile* (butadiene co-polymer)	Best Glove (1-800-241-0323)	

*Gloves made from nitrile are produced with the same accelerator (mercaptobenzathiazole) as some latex gloves. Those with suspected irritant or allergic contact dermatitis to latex gloves may also react to nitrile.
Kits containing everything needed for one latex-safe surgical procedure are obtainable from DeRoyal Surgical (1-800-251-9864).
Other nonlatex supplies besides gloves may be obtained by contacting suppliers or manufacturers directly. Contact the Spina Bifida Association for its list of suppliers.

Comprehensive Internet Site, Latex Allergy Links
Website: http://pw2.netcom.com/~nam l/latex_allergy. html

SUPPLIERS

See Table C-1 for a list of suppliers of hypoallergenic nonlatex gloves.

CONCLUSION

For those who have been sensitized, avoidance is the cornerstone of management. In all settings where gloves are heavily used, avoiding sensitization through purchase of powder-free gloves is recommended. Many hospitals are banning powdered gloves altogether. This will both help to safely treat the patient with latex allergy and prevent sensitization in the healthcare worker. Ironically, with this condition, it is the healthcare worker who is often the patient.

ICD-9-CM DIAGNOSTIC CODE

989.82   Latex allergy

BIBLIOGRAPHY

Arellano R, Bradley J, Sussman G: Prevalence of latex sensitization among hospital physicians occupationally exposed to latex gloves, *Anesthesiology* 77:905, 1992.

Beezhold DH, Beck WC: Surgical glove powders bind latex antigens, *Arch Surg* 127:1354, 1992.

Blanco C, Carrillo T, Castillo R, et al: Latex allergy: clinical features and cross-reactivity with fruits, *Ann Allergy* 73:309, 1994.

Cheng L, Lee D: Review of latex allergy, *J Am Board Fam Pract* 12(4):285, 1999.

Food and Drug Administration: *Latex-containing devices: user labeling,* Fed Regist 61:122, 32618-3262, June 24, 1996.

Kwittken PL, Becker J, Oyefara B, et al: Latex hypersensitivity reactions despite prophylaxis, *Allergy Proc* 13:123, 1992.

Kwittken P, Sweinberg S: Childhood latex allergy: an overview, *Am J Asthma Allergy Pediatr 6:27, 1992.*

Turjanmaa K: Incidence of immediate allergy to latex gloves in hospital personnel, *Contact Dermatitis* 17:270, 1987.

United States Department of Health and Human Services, Public Health Service, Centers for Disease Control and Prevention, National Institute for Occupational Safety and Health: *Preventing allergic reactions to natural rubber latex in the workplace,* NIOSH pub no 97-135, Cincinnati, 1997, Government Printing Office.

Supplier Information

3Gen
23801 Salvador Bay
Dana Point, CA 92629
Phone: 1-949-481-6384
Website: www.3genllc.com
(DermLite, for dermoscopy [epiluminescence
   microscopy])

3M Abrasive Systems Division
3M Center, Building 223-6N-01
St. Paul, MN 55144-1000
Phone: 1-800-742-9546
Website: www.3m.com
(Silicone carbide wet or dry sandpaper, for
   dermasanding; skin stapling)

3M Health Care Corporation
3M Center Bldg. 275-4E-01
P.O. Box 33275
St. Paul, MN 55133-3275
Phone: 1-800-228-3957
Website: www.3m.com (Wound dressing; casting and
   splinting materials)

ACMI Corporation (Circon)
136 Turnpike Road
Southborough, MA 01772-2104
Phone: 1-888-524-7266
Website: www.circoncorp.com
(Endoscopes, for cystourethroscopy; endometrial
   ablation; hysteroscopy; and cryosurgery)

Accuscope/Vineland Medical Products, Inc.
P.O. Box 575
1471 E. Chestnut Avenue
Vineland, NJ 08360-0575
Phone: 1-609-692-5140
(For colposcopies)

Acuderm, Inc.
5370 NW 35 Terrace
Fort Lauderdale, FL 33309
Phone: (800) 327-0015
Website: www.acuderm.com
(Disposable and reusable punches and curettes, for
   skin biopsy)

Acuson (owned by Siemens)
1220 Charleston Road
P.O. Box 7393
Mountain View, CA 94039-7393
Phone: 1-800-422-8766
Website: www.acuson.com
(For obstetric ultrasound)

Ackrad Laboratories, Inc.
70 Jackson Drive
Cranford, NJ 07016
Phone: 1-800-684-4252
Website: www.ackrad.com
(For hysterosalpingography/
   sonohysterosalpingography)

Advanced Diagnostics and Interventions (ADI)
216 Via Linda Vista
Redondo Beach, CA 90277
Phone: 1-310-373-6769
(For diagnostic needle arthroscopy, lavage (DNAL),
   and biopsy of the knee)

Advanced Medical Products, Inc.
111 Research Drive
Columbia, SC 29203
Phone: 1-800-443-3816
(For ambulatory blood pressure monitoring)

Advanced Medical Systems, Inc.
440 E. Cheyenne Mountain Boulevard, #26
Colorado Springs, CO 80906
Phone: 1-800-876-7145
Website: www.amsintl.com
(Prenatal care record and patient education system, for
   pregnancy)

Advanced Meditech International (AMI)
86-20 53rd Avenue, Suite 100
Flushing, NY 11373
Phone: 1-800-635-2452
Website: www.ameditech.com
(Norgrasp forceps for contraceptive implant [Norplant] removal; no-scalpel vasectomy instruments; AMI Battery Cautery, for vasectomy and subungual hematoma evacuation; written patient education handouts, technique videotapes for physicians, for no-scalpel vasectomy; and teaching models, for vasectomy)

Advanced Technology Laboratories (ATL) (owned by Phillips)
22100 Bothell Everett Highway
P.O. Box 3003
Bothell, WA 98041-3003
Phone: 1-800-526-4963
Website: www.atl.com
(For obstetric ultrasound)

Aesculap
3773 Corporate Parkway
Center Valley, PA 18034
Phone: 1-800-282-9000
Website: www.aesculap-usa.com
(Phlebectomy hooks for ambulatory phlebectomy)

Aesculap–Meditec
2525 McGan Avenue
Irvine, CA 92623
Phone: 1-949-660-2770
Website: www.asclepion.com
(For laser hair removal)

Aesthetic Technologies, Inc.
2150 W. Sixth Avenue
Bloomfield, CO 80020
Phone: 1-800-262-4412
Website: www.parisianpeel.com
(Parisian Peel for microdermabrasion)

Agilent Technology (formerly Hewlett-Packard)
3000 Minuteman Road
Andover, MA 01810
Phone: 1-800-934-7372
Website: www.agilent.com
(For obstetric ultrasound)

Aircast, Inc.
92 River Road
Summit, NJ 07901
Phone: 1-800-526-8785
Website: www.aircast.com
(Splints and braces, for Ankle and Foot Splinting)

Air-Tite Products Company
565 Central Drive
Virginia Beach, VA 23455
Phone: 1-800-231-7762
Website: www.air-tite.com
(Syringes and needles for sclerotherapy)

Alderm N.A., LLC
17951 Skypark Circle, Suite G
Irvine, CA 92614
Phone: 1-800-254-8505
Website: www.aldermna.com
(For laser therapy)

Alexerin Productions Inc.
P.O. Box 3477
Pinedale, CA 93650
Phone: 1-800-635-5340
(Educational videos for ambulatory phlebectomy)

AliMed, Inc.
297 High Street
Dedham, MA 02026
Phone: 1-800-225-2610
Website: www.alimed.com
(TENS units, for transcutaneous electrical nerve stimulation, phonophoresis, and iontophoresis; high-tensile strength adhesive tape [Nocturnal splints, Freedom PF Night Splint II] for ankle and foot splinting)

ALK Laboratory
1700 Royston Lane
Round Rock, TX 78664
Phone: 1-800-252-9778
(Allergen extracts, immunotherapy sets, supplies, for allergy testing and immunotherapy)

Alkaline Corporation Allergy Diagnostics Division
Morrow Brown Allergy Diagnostics
714 West Park Avenue, P.O. Box 306
Oakhurst, NJ 07775-0306
Phone: 1-800-686-6483
Website: www.lincolndiagnostics.com
(Devices for skin testing [Morrow Brown needle], for allergy testing)

Allegiance Healthcare Corp. (a Cardinal Health
   Company)
1430 Waukegan Road
McGaw Park, IL 60085-6787
Phone: 1-800-964-5227
Website: www.allegiance.net
(Thoracentesis tray with catheter and needle, for chest
   tube insertion and removal; thoracentesis; anal retractors, for anal fissure/lateral sphincterotomy; used
   or refurbished equipment for colonoscopy; Illinois
   sternal/iliac bone marrow aspiration tray, Jamshidi
   bone marrow biopsy/aspiration needle, for bone
   marrow aspiration or biopsy)

Allergan, Inc.
2525 Dupont Drive
P.O. Box 19534
Irvine, CA 92623-9534
Phone: 1-800-553-6783
Website: www.allergan.com/profpath/js_ind.htm
(MD Forte, for skin peels; Botox [and information
   on it])

Allergy Laboratories
P.O. Box 26492
Oklahoma City, OK 73126
Phone: 1-405-235-1451
(Allergen extracts, immunotherapy sets, supplies, for
   allergy testing and immunotherapy)

Allermed Laboratories
7203 Convoy Court
San Diego, CA 92111
Phone: 1-800-221-2748
(*Candida* antigen [Candin], for wart [verruca]
   treatment)

Allied Biomedical Corp.
3850 Ramada Drive, C-2
Paso Robles, CA 93446
Phone: 1-800-276-1322
Website: www.alliedbiomedical.com
(Silastic topical gel Kelokote, for hypertrophic scars
   and keloids)

Allied Healthcare Products, Inc.
Gomco Division
1720 Sublette Avenue
St. Louis, MO 63110
Phone: 1-800-444-3940
Website: www.alliedhpi.com
(Gomco circumcision clamps, for newborn
   circumcision)

Aloka
10 Fairfield Boulevard
Wallinford, CT 06492
Phone: 1-203-269-5088
Website: www.aloka.com
(For obstetric ultrasound)

Altus Medical
821 Cowan Road
Burlingame, CA 94010
Phone: 1-650-552-9700
Website: www.altusmedical.com
(For laser therapy)

American Academy of Dermatology Association
930 North Meacham Road
P.O. Box 4014
Schaumburg, IL 60168-4014
Phone: 1-847-330-0230
Website: www.aadassociation.org
(For patient education information)

American Academy of Family Physicians
11400 Tomahawk Creek Parkway
Leawood, KS 66211-2672
Phone: 1-913-906-6000 or 1-800-274-2237, ext. 4148
Website: www.aafp.org
(Patient education materials; procedure training
   courses; training videotapes for clinicians; practice
   management information)

American Academy of Osteopathy
3500 DePauw Blvd., Suite 1080
Indianapolis, IN 46268-1136
Phone: 1-317-879-1881
Website: www.academyofosteopathy.org
(For manipulative medicine)

American Academy of Pediatrics (AAP)
Division of Publications
141 Northwest Point Boulevard
Elk Grove Village, IL 60007-1098
Phone: 1-800-433-9016
Website: www.aap.org
(Patient education brochures)

American Chiropractic Association
1701 Clarendon Boulevard
Arlington, VA 22209
Phone: 1-800-986-4636
Website: www.amerchiro.org
(For manipulative medicine)

American College of Obstetricians and Gynecologists
  (ACOG)
409 12th St., S.W., P.O. Box 96920
Washington, D. C. 20090-6920
Phone: 1-800-762-2264
Website: www.acog.org
(Patient education materials, physician training)

American College of Phlebology
100 Webster Street, Suit 101
Oakland, CA 94607-3724
Phone: 1-510-834-6500
Website: www.phlebology.org
(Patient education, physician training in sclerotherapy)

American Massage Therapy Association
820 Davis Street, Suite 100
Evanston, IL 60201-4444
Phone: 1-847-864-0123
Website: www.amtamassage.org
(For manipulative medicine)

American Osteopathic Association
142 E. Ontario Street
Chicago Illinois 60611
Phone: 1-800-621-1773
Website: www.aoa-net.org

American Social Health Association
P.O. Box 13827
Research Triangle Park, NC 27709
Phone: 1-919-361-8400
Website: www.ashastd.org
(Patient education brochures and support groups, for
  patients with STDs)

American Society for Colposcopy and Cervical
  Pathology (ASCCP)
20 West Washington Street, Suite 1
Hagerstown, MD 21740
Phone: 1-800-787-7227
Website: www.asccp.org
(National society for promotion of quality education
  and patient care for cervical/vaginal disease; for
  colposcopy training, videos, slides, and patient
  brochures)

American Society for Gastrointestinal Endoscopy
  (ASGE)
13 Elm Street
Manchester, MA 01944
Phone: 1-505-526-8330
Website: www.asge.org
(Patient education materials, physician training)

American Society of Phlebectomy
2425 Westown Parkway
West Des Moines, IA 50266-1425
Phone: 1-515-221-1500
Fax: 1-515-222-0472
Website: www.phlebectomy.org
(Physician training, patient education brochures)

American Urological Association
1120 North Charles Street
Baltimore, MD 21201
Phone: 1-800-908-9414
Website: www.auanet.com
(Written patient education handouts)

America's Endoscopy Corporation
24865 Five Mile Road, Suite 2
Redford, MI 48239
Phone: 1-800-845-8863
(For GI endoscopes)

Anatometal
411 Ingalls Street
Santa Cruz, CA 95060
Phone: 1-888-262-8663
Website: www.anatometal.com
(For body piercing)

Antigen Laboratories, Inc.
P.O. Box 123
Liberty, MO 64069
Phone: 1-800-821-7013
Website: www.antigenlab.com
(*Candida* antigen [generic], for wart [verruca] treat-
  ment; allergen extracts, immunotherapy sets, sup-
  plies, for allergy testing and immunotherapy; RAST
  services, for allergy testing and immunotherapy)

Arlington Scientific Inc (ASI)
1840 North Technology Drive
Springville, UT 84663
Phone: 1-800-654-0146
Website: www.arlingtonscientific.com
(Nasal smear kit and allergy detection for nasal turbi-
  nate injection and reduction)

Arrow International
2400 Bernville Road
Reading, PA 19605
Phone: 1-800-233-3187
Website: www.arrowintl.com
(For Swan-Ganz [pulmonary artery] catherization,
  abdominal paracentesis, and peritoneal lavage kits)

Asclepion-Meditec AG
Goeschwitzer Strasse 51-52
07745 Jena
Germany
Phone: +49 (0) 36 41 / 2 20 — 0
Website: www.asclepion.com
(For laser therapy)

Aspen Labs
952 S. Zephr Court
Lakewood, CO 80226
Phone: 1-303-699-9854
(Equipment, for loop electrosurgical excision proce-
dure [LEEP])

Atrium Medical Corporation
5 Wentworth Drive
Hudson, NH 03051
Phone: 1-800-528-7486
Website: www.atriummed.com
(Atrium Ocean Water Seal Chest Drain System and
Thoracostomy Tubes)

B. Braun Medical Inc.
824 12th Avenue
Bethlehem, PA 18018
Phone: 1-800-854-6851
Website: www.bbraunusa.com
(Disposable trays, infusion pumps, needles, etc.
for saddle block anesthesia and epidural anesthesia;
Banyan kits)

B-Met Endoscopic, Inc.
72 South Wyoming Avenue
Edwardsville, PA 18704
Phone: 1-877-498-2638
(For GI scopes)

Banyan International
2118 E. Interstate 20
P.O. Box 1779
Abilene, TX 79604-1779
Phone: 1-800-782-8548
Website: www.statkit.com
(Banyan kit ["crash cart" in a suitcase])

Bard
730 Central Avenue
Murray Hill, NJ 07974
Phone: 1-800-367-2273
Website: www.bard.com
(Wound dressings)

Bard Access Systems, Inc.
5425 West Amelia Earnhart Drive
Salt Lake City, UT 84116
Phone: 1-800-545-0890
Website: www.bardaccess.com
(For vascular access products)

Bard Peripheral Technologies
13183 Harland Drive NE
Covington, GA 30014
Phone: 1-770-385-2300
Website: www.bard.com
(Bard Biopty cut instruments and needle, for prostate
biopsy)

Bartor Pharmacal Co.
70 High Street
Rye, NY 10580
Phone: 1-914-967-4219
(Implantable hormone pellets, for testosterone
deficiency)

Baxter Healthcare Corporation
Anesthesia & Critical Care
Pharmaceuticals
95 Spring Street
New Providence, NJ 07974
Phone: 1-908-286-7000
Website: www.baxter.com
(Disposable trays, infusion pumps, needles, etc., for
saddle block and epidural anesthesia and analgesia)

Bayer Corporation
Pharmaceutical Division
Allergy Products
400 Morgan Lane
West Haven, CT 06516
Phone: 1-800-800-5907
Website: www.bayerinstitute.org
(Ana-Kit anaphylaxis emergency treatment kit)

Becton, Dickinson and Co.
1 Becton Drive
Franklin Lakes, NJ 07417
Phone: 1-201-847-6800 or 1-888-237-2762
Website: www.bd.com
(Bonnano catheter kit, for Suprapubic Catheter
Insertion; 60-ml syringe with catheter tip [Toomey
syringe], for nasogastric tube and Salem sump
insertion; disposable trays, infusion pumps, needles,
etc., for saddle block and epidural anesthesia)

BEI Medical Systems Company, Inc.
100 Hollister Road
Teterboro, NJ 07608
Phone: 1-210-727-4900
Website: www.beimedical.com
(Hydrothermablation for endometrial ablation)

Beiersdorf
P.O. Box 5529
Norwalk, CT 06856-5529
Phone: 1-203-853-8008
Website: www.beiersdorf.com
(Aquaphor gauze for unna paste boot)

Beiersdorf-Jobst, Inc.
Wilton Corporate Center
187 Danbury Road
Wilton, CT 06897
Phone: 1-203-563-5800
(Compression stockings, for ambulatory phlebectomy
    and sclerotherapy; Leukotape-P high-tensile strength
    adhesive tape, for ankle and foot splinting)

Bella Products, Inc.
27136 Burbank
Foothill Ranch, CA 92610
Phone: 1-877-550-5655
Website: www.bellaproducts.com
(Bellamed for microdermabrasion)

Benefoot, Inc.
1507 Executive Drive
Edgewood, NY 11717
Phone: 1-800-554-3668
Website: www.benefoot.com
(Orthotics for corns, calluses, and plantar warts)

Bergen Brunswig Medical Corp.
5301 Peoria, Unit B
Denver, CO 80239
Phone: 1-800-727-3877, ext. 104
(Medical and surgical supplies for skin grafting)

Berkeley Medevices, Inc.
1330 South 51st Street
Richmond, CA 94804
Phone: 1-800-227-2388
(Special equipment, suction machines, hosing curettes,
    dilators, laminaria, Vabra aspirator and ancillary
    instruments for endometrial biopsy and uterine
    evacuation)

Berlex Laboratories
300 Fairfield Road
Wayne, NJ 07470-7358
Phone: 1-973-694-4100
Website: www.berlex.com
(Mirena Intrauterine System [IUS])

Bernsco
25 Plant Avenue
Hauppauge, NY 11788-3804
Phone: 1-800-843-6266
Website: www.bernsco.com
(Eye protection, books and supplies for laser therapy)

Bernsco Surgical Supply, Inc. (now a subsidiary of
    George Tiemann & Co.)
4055 23rd Avenue W
Seattle, WA 98199-1208
Phone: 1-800-231-8409
Website: www.bernsco.com
(VHS videos narrated by John Arlette, MD: a 3½-
    minute one for patient information and a 20-minute
    one for physician training)

Beutlich LP Pharmaceuticals
1541 Shields Drive
Waukegan, IL 60085
Phone: 1-800-238-8542
Website: www.beutlich.com
(Hurricane syrup spray, gel for mucosal anesthesia)

Biodermis
3078 East Sunset Road, Suite #1
Las Vegas, NV 89120
Phone: 1-800-322-3729
Website: www.biodermis.com
(Silastic gel sheeting and topical products for hyper-
    trophic scars and keloids)

Biodynamics Corporation
3511 NE 45th Street, #2
Seattle, WA 98105
Phone: 1-800-869-6987
Website: www.biodyncorp.com
(Bioelectric impedance measuring device for body fat
    analysis)

Bioglan
7 Great Valley Parkway
Malvern, PA 19355
Phone: 1-888-246-4526
Website: www.bioglan.com
(Beta lift 2-0 (20%) and 3-0 (30%), salicylic acid for
    skin peels)

BioMedic
4602 East Hammond Lane
Phoenix, AZ 85034
Phone: 1-800-736-5155
Website: www.biomedic.com
(MicroDelivery Peel II for microdermabrasion)

Bio-Medical Instruments, Inc.
2387 East Eight Mile Road
Warrenten, MI 48091-2486
Phone: 1-800-521-4640
Website: www.bio-medical.com
(For biofeedback)

Biomedix
4205 White Bear Parkway
Vadnais Heights, MN 55110
Phone: 1-877-854-0012
Website: www.biomedix.com
(Portable vascular equipment, including duplex ultra-
    sound, for noninvasive venous and arterial studies
    of the lower extremities)

Bionix Corporation
757 Warehouse Road
Toledo, OH 43615
Phone: 1-800-551-7096
Website: www.bionix.com
(For cerumen impaction removal devices and various
    unique medical instruments)

Bionix Development Corp.
5154 Enterprise Boulevard
Toledo, OH 43612
Phone: 1-419-727-8421
(Wound closure forceps for tissue glues)

Biosense Webster
3333 Diamond Canyon Road
Diamond Bar, CA 91765
Phone: 1-800-729-9010
Website: www.biosensewebster.com
(For temporary cardiac pacing)

Biosound Esaote, Inc. (IPIE Medical)
8000 Castleway Drive
Indianapolis, IN 46250
Phone: 1-800-428-4374
Website: www.biosound.com
(For obstetric ultrasound; James L. Scheffer [10234
    Marion St, Lenexa, KS, 66220; iit-jim@msn.com] is a
    helpful resource)

Bio-Vision, Inc.
350 Fifth Avenue, Suite 3304
New York, NY 10118
Phone: 1-800-665-VIRUS (8478)
Website: www.bio-v.com
(Physician teaching slides and tapes, for Coloscopy
    and LEEP)

Birtcher Medical Systems, Inc.
1435 Henry Brennan Drive, #J
El Paso, TX 79936
Phone: 1-915-858-1895
(Hyfrecator Plus for subungual hematoma evacuation,
    cautery for skin)

Bivona Medical Technologies
5700 West 23rd Avenue
Gary, IN 46406
Phone: 1-800-348-6064
Website: www.bivona.com
(For cricothyroidotomy and tracheostomy supplies)

Bledsoe Brace Systems
2601 Pinewood Drive
Grand Prairie, TX 75051
Phone: 1-888-253-3763
Website: www.bledsoebrace.com
(For knee braces)

Body Circle Designs
P.O. Box 68249
Seattle, WA 98168
Phone: 1-800-244-8430
Website: www.bodycircle.com
(For body piercing)

Body Vision
220 West Fifth Street, Suite 802
Los Angeles, CA 90013
Phone: 1-888-991-2639
(For body piercing)

Brymill Corporation (Cryogun/CRYAC-3)
105 Windemere Avenue
Ellington, CT 06029
Phone: 1-860-875-2460
Website: http://www.brymill.com
(For liquid nitrogen cryosurgery supplies)

BSN-Jobst Institute, Inc.
Rutherford College
100 Beiersdorf Drive
P.O. Box 390
Rutherford College, NC 28671
Phone: 1-828-879-5100
Website: www.jobst.com
(For compression hose)

Burton Medical Products Corp.
21100 Lassen Street
Chatsworth, CA 91311
Phone: 1-800-444-9909
(For Wood's Light)

Byron Medical Corp.
602 W. Rillito
Tucson, AZ 85705
Phone: 1-800-777-3434
Website: www.byronmedical.com
(For tattoo removal: infrared light obliteration method;
    Mepiform [self-adherent silicone dressing] for hyper-
    trophic scars and keloids)

Caldwell, Justiss & Co., Inc.
622 W. Sycamore
P.O. Box 520
Fayetteville, AR 72702
Phone: 1-800-643-4343
(Skinfold callipers for body fat analysis)

CanDerm Pharma Inc.
5353 Thimens
St. Laurent, Quebec, Canada
H4R 2H4
Phone: 1-877-278-3265
Website: www.canderm.com
(Wound dressings)

Candela Corp.
530 Boston Post Road
Wayland, MA 01778
Phone: 1-508-358-7637
Website: www.clzr.com
(For laser hair removal: photoepilation; lasers)

Carruthers, Alistair MD and Jean Carruthers, MD
Website: www.carruthers.net
(Teaching videos for clinicians and patients, for
    Botox)

Center Laboratories
Division of EM Pharmaceuticals, Inc
35 Channel Drive
Port Washington, NY 11050
Phone: 1-516-767-1873 or 1-800-223-6837
(EpiPen, for anaphylaxis; allergen extracts,
    immunotherapy sets, supplies, for allergy testing and
    immunotherapy)

Cervical Cap Ltd
430 Monterey Ave, Suite 1B
Los Gatos, CA 95030
Phone: 1-408-395-2100
Website: www.cervcap.com
(Cervical caps)

Cetacaine
Cetylite Industries, Inc.
9051 River Road
Pennsauken, NJ 08110
Phone: 1-800-257-7740
Website: www.cetylite.com
(Topical anesthetic for mucosa)

Chattanooga Group, Inc.
4717 Adams Road
Hixson, TN 37343
Phone: 1-800-592-7329
Website: www.chattgroup.com
(For transcutaneous electrical nerve stimulation,
    phonophoresis, and iontophoresis)

Coherent Medical Group
2400 Condensa Street
Santa Clara, CA
Phone: 1-408-764-3757
Website: www.coherentmedical.com
(For laser hair removal, lasers)

Cold Steel
45-46 Millmead Industrial Centre
Tottenham Hale N17 9QU
London, England
Phone: +44 (020) 8880 3334
Website: www.coldsteel.co.uk
(For body piercing)

College Pharmacy
3505 Austin Bluffs Parkway
Colorado Springs, CO 80907
Phone: 1-800-888-9358
Website: www.collegepharmacy.com
(Devices for skin testing and immunotherapy)

Commonwealth Medical Laboratories
11150 Main Street, Suite 550
Fairfax, VA 22030
Phone: 1-800-222-5775
Website: www.allergytest.com
(RAST services for allergy testing and immunotherapy)

Computerized Imaging Reference Systems, Inc.
2428 Almeda Avenue, Suite 212
Norfolk, VA 23513
Website: www.cirsinc.com
(For osteoporosis screening)

Conceptus, Inc.
1021 Howard Avenue
San Carlos, CA 94070
Phone: 1-650-628-4900
For training information: 1-877-377-8732
Website: www.essure.com
(Essure for permanent female sterilization)

Contemporary Health Communications
16714 Benton Taylor Drive
Chesterfield, MO 63005
Phone: 1-800-234-1742
Website: www.patient-info.com
(Customizable patient education brochures for various
aesthetic procedures)

Continuum Biomedical
3150 Central Expressway
Santa Clara, CA 95051
Phone: 1-800-956-7757
Website: www.continuumlasers.com/mainswf.html
(For laser hair removal, lasers)

Convatec (division of Bristol-Myers Squibb)
P.O. Box 5254
Princeton, NJ 08543-5254
Phone: 1-800-422-8811
Website: www.convatec.com
(Unna-Flex bandage for unna paste boot)

Convergent Laser Technologies
900 Alice Street
Oakland, CA 94607
Phone: 1-510-832-2130
Website: www.convergentlaser.com
(For laser hair removal, lasers)

Cook, Inc.
925 South Curry Pike
P.O. Box 489
Bloomington, IN 47402-0489
Phone: 1-800-457-4500
Website: www.cookingcorporated.com
(For tracheal [endotracheal and nasotracheal] intuba-
tion; nasogastric tube, nasoenteric tube, and Salem
Sump insertion; for intraosseous venous access);
emergency pneumothorax kits for chest tube inser-
tion and removal

Cook Ob/Gyn
1100 W. Morgan Street
P.O. Box 271
Spencer, IN 47460
Phone: 1-800-541-5591
Website: www.cookobgyn.com
(Tao brush for endometrial biopsy; hysterosalpingog-
raphy/sonohysterosalpingography equipment)

Cook Urological
1100 West Morgan Street
P.O. Box 227
Spencer, IN 47460
Phone: 1-800-457-4448
Website: www.cookurological.com
(Stamey percutaneous suprapubic catheter kit)

CooperSurgical
95 Corporate Drive
Trumbull, CT 06611
Phone: 1-800-645-3760
Website: www.coopersurgical.com
(Mechanical dilators and os locators; colposcopes, hysterosalpingography/sonohysterosalpingography equipment; intrauterine device removers; endometrial ablation supplies; FNA-21, for fine-needle aspiration cytology and biopsy of breast; nitrous oxide; cryosurgery supplies; disposable punch biopsy units; Pipelle for endometrial biopsy; no-scalpel vasectomy instruments; equipment for Loop Electrosurgical Excision Procedure [LEEP]; most instruments for Ob/Gyn procedures)

Corometrics (General Electric Medical Systems, Inc.)
P.O. Box 414
Milwaukee, WI 53201
Phone: 1-800-433-5566
Website: www.gemedicalsystems.com
(For fetal-movement counting, nonstress test, and contraction stress test equipment)

Corpak MedSystems/VIASYS Healthcare
100 Chaddick Drive
Wheeling, IL 60090
Phone: 1-800-323-6305
Website: www.corpakmedsystems.com
(Feeding tubes)

Corthel, Inc.
1202 Technology Drive
Aberdeen, MD 21001
Phone: 1-410-297-6512
Website: www.corthelinc.com
(For GI endoscopes)

Cosmetic Surgery Center and Spa
109 Gallery Circle #127
San Antonio, TX 78528
Phone: 1-210-495-8825
(TOBIL System for tattoo removal: infrared light obliteration method)

Cosmos Medical Technology, Inc.
42230 Zevo Drive
Temecula, CA 92590
Phone: 1-800-634-7921
Website: www.cosmosmed.com
(Europeel, for Microdermabrasion; lasers)

The Cranial Academy
8202 Clearvista Parkway #9D
Indianapolis, IN 46256
Website: www.cranialacademy.org
(For manipulative medicine)

Creative Health Communications
4675 South Portsmouth Road
Bridgeport, MI 48722
Phone: 1-800-462-2492
Patient education videotapes (HPV, vasectomy, Botox, sclerotherapy, more); physician training tapes (no-scalpel vasectomy, suturing, coding dermatologic procedures, radiofrequency surgery, Botox, sclerotherapy, casting, more)

Cryogen, Inc.
11065 Sorrento Valley Ct.
San Diego, CA 92121
Phone: 1-888-634-0444
Website: www.cryogen-inc.com
(Cryoablation for endometrial ablation)

Cryosurgery, Inc.
P.O. Box 50035
Nashville, TN 37205
Phone: 1-800-729-1624
Website: www.cryosurgeryinc.com
(Verruca-Freeze [canister kits], for cutaneous cryosurgery)

Crystal Focus
19 rue Ampere
91302 Massy, France
Phone: +33-1-69-20-84-54
(For laser hair removal)

Custom Steel
13 Custom Steel Drive
Paguate, NM 87040
Phone: 1-800-877-5855
Website: www.customsteel.com
(For body piercing)

Cynosure Inc
10 Elizabeth Drive
Chelmsford, MA 01824
Phone: 1-800-886-2966
Website: www.cynosurelaser.com
(For laser hair removal)

CYTYC Corp.
85 Swanson Road
Boxborough, MA 01719
Phone: 1-800-442-9892
Website: www.cytyc.com
(For Pap smear, thin prep procedures)

DS Vasconelles
19260 NE 22nd Road
North Miami Beach, FL 33179
Phone: 1-800-933-0009
Website: www.dfv.com.br
(For colposcopy equipment)

Danco Laboratories
P.O. Box 4816
New York, NY 10185
Phone: 1-877-432-7596
Website: www.dancolaboratories.com
(Mifeprex for abortion)

Davol, Inc.
100 Sockanossett Crossroad
P.O. Box 8500
Cranston, RI 02920
Phone: 1-401-463-7000
Website: www.davol.com
(For anal fissure treatment)

Del Mar Medical Systems
1621 Alton Parkway
Irvine, CA 92606-4878
Phone: 1-949-250-3200
Website: www.delmarmedical.com
(For ambulatory electrocardiogram-Holter
   monitoring)

Delasco
608 13th Avenue
Council Bluffs, IA 51501-6401
Phone: 1-800-831-6273
Website: www.delasco.com
(Hypertonic saline/Sotradecol for sclerotherapy; tri-
   chloroacetic acid [TCA], glycolic acid [GA] for skin
   peels; KOH solutions for KOH Micro Preps [20%
   KOH with Dimethyl Sulfoxide; Chlorazol Black E
   Fungal Stain]; Madajet injector for hypertrophic scars
   and keloids; the complete supplies for dermatologic
   surgery needs)

DermaMed, Inc.
394 Parkmount Rd.
P.O. Box 198
Lenni, PA 19052-0198
Phone: 1-877-789-MEGA
Website: www.megapeel.com
(Megapeel for microdermabrasion)

Diamond Medical Aesthetics
One Madison St., Building C
East Rutherford, NJ 07073
Phone: 1-877-754-6749
Website: www.slimtoneusa.com
(Diamond peel for microdermabrasion)

Digene Corp.
1201 Clopper Road
Gaithersburg, MD 20878
Phone: 1-800-344-3631
Website: www.digene.com
(For human papillomavirus DNA typing)

Diomed, Inc
1 Dundee Park
Andover, MA 01810
Phone: 1-978-475-7771
Website: www.diomed-lasers.com
(For laser hair removal, lasers)

dj Orthopedics
2985 Scott Street
Vista, CA 92083
Phone: 1-800-321-9549
Website: www.donjoy.com
(DonJoy Products Knee Guard [unilateral support] or
   Playmaker [bilateral supports], Donjoy Legend, or
   Defiance, DonJoy OnTrack, for Knee Braces; splints
   and braces, and high-tensile strength adhesive tape,
   for ankle and foot splinting)

DunnAmics, Inc.
3502 Fairview Way
West Linn, OR 97068
Phone: 1-800-690-8824
Website: www.dunnamics.com
(For GI endoscopes)

Dynatronics
7030 Park Centre Drive
Salt Lake City, UT 84121
Phone: 1-800-874-6251
Website: www.dynatronics.com
(Equipment for transcutaneous electrical nerve stimulation, phonophoresis, and iontophoresis)

DynaWave Corporation
2520 Kaneville Court
Geneva, IL 60134
Phone: 1-630-232-4945
Website: my.inil.com/~dynawave/
(Equipment for transcutaneous electrical nerve stimulation, phonophoresis, and iontophoresis)

Edwards Lifesciences Corp (formerly a division of Baxter)
One Edwards Way
Irvine, CA 92614
Phone: 1-800-424-3278
Website: www.edwards.com
(For Swan-Ganz [pulmonary artery] catherization)

Electro-Med Health Industries
11601 Biscayne Boulevard, Suite 200-A
North Miami, FL 33181
Phone: 1-800-232-3644
Website: www.emhi.com
(Equipment for transcutaneous electrical nerve stimulation, phonophoresis, and iontophoresis)

Ellman, Inc.
1135 Railroad Avenue
Hewlett, NY 11577
Phone: 1-800-835-5355
Website: www.ellman.com
(Radiofrequency units [both unipolar and bipolar] for nasal turbinate reduction; sclerotherapy; for skin surgery/blepharoplasty, and varicose vein treatment; for LEEP procedures; IsoDent for tissue glue; battery-operated cautery for vasectomy smoke evacuators; MediFrig for cryotherapy agent)

Emed, Inc.
31320 Via Colinas, Suite 112
Westlake Village, CA 91362
Phone: 1-888-848-3633
Website: www.4emed.com
(MD Peel for microdermabrasion)

EMPI, Inc.
599 Cardigan Road
St. Paul, MN 55126-4099
Phone: 1-88-FOR-EMPI
Website: www.empi.com
(TENS units for transcutaneous electrical nerve stimulation, phonophoresis, and iontophoresis)

Endoscopy Support Services, Inc.
2 Fallsview Lane
Brewster, NY 10509
Phone: 1-845-277-1700
Website: www.endoscopy.com
(For endoscopes and repair)

EngenderHealth (formerly Association for Voluntary Surgical Contraception [AVSC])
440 Ninth Avenue
New York, NY 10001
Phone: 1-212-561-8000
Vasectomy information line: 1-888-VASEC-4-U
Website: www.engenderhealth.org
(Videotapes for patient education, written patient education handouts, and technique videotapes for physicians for vasectomy preceptor matching program; national listing service for physicians)

ERBE USA, Inc.
2225 Northwest Parkway
Marietta, GA 30067
Phone: 1-770-955-4400
(Equipment, for Loop Electrosurgical Excision Procedure [LEEP])

ESC Medical Systems
250 First Avenue, Suite 300
Needham, MA 02194
Phone: 1-781-444-8446
Website: www.escmed.com
(For laser hair removal, lasers)

Estring
Pharmacia Corp.
100 Route 206 North
Peapack, NJ 07977
Phone: 1-888-768-5501
Website: www.pharmacia.com
(For pessaries)

Ethicon, Inc.
P.O. Box 151
Sommerville, NJ 08876-0151
Phone: 1-800-255-2500
Website: www.ethiconinc.com
(Suturing supplies, knot tying manual and practice
board, hemoclips and clip applicators for
vasectomy)

Ethicon Inc.
249 Vanderbilt Avenue
Norwood, MA 02062
Phone: 1-800-356-4835
Website: www.ethicon.com
(Dermabond tissue glue)

Ethox Corp.
251 Seneca Street
Buffalo, NY 14204
Phone: 1-800-521-1022
Website: www.ethoxcorp.com
(TUM-E-VAC for gastric lavage)

Factory Authorized Medical Scope Repair, Inc.
2859 West McNab Road
Pompano Beach, FL 33069
Phone: 1-954-984-1844
Website: www.famsr.com
(For used endoscopes and repair)

FLA Orthopedics
2881 Corporate Way
Miramar, FL 33025
Phone: 1-800-327-4110
Website: www.clinitex.com

Focus Medical LLC
23 Francis J. Clarke Circle
Bethel, CT 06801
Phone: 1-866-633-5273
Website: www.focusmedical.com
(NaturaLase, lasers)

Franklin Medical
1320 Airport Road
Montrose, CO 81401
Phone: 1-800-255-1196
Website: www.franklinmedical.com
(Silastic suprapubic catheter)

Fredricks-Jobst Institute Inc.
P.O. Box 653
Toledo, OH 43697-0653
(Jobst postoperative brassiere, breast surgery)

Fujinon Medical
10 High Point Drive
Wayne, NJ 07470
Phone: 1-800-872-0196
Website: www.fujinon.com
(Flexible fiberoptic nasolaryngoscope, colonoscopes,
gastroscopes, sigmoidoscopes, light sources and
supplies)

Futrex Inc.
6 Montgomery Village Avenue, #620
Gaithesburg, MD 20879
Phone: 1-800-255-4206
Website: www.futrex.com
(Near-infrared spectrophotometer for body fat analysis)

Galderma Laboratories, L.P.
14501 North Freeway
Fort Worth, TX 76177
Phone: 1-817-961-5000
Website: www.galderma.com

Gastroccult (formerly from Smith-Kline Diagnostics)
Beckman Coulter, Inc.
4300 N. Harbor Boulevard
P.O. Box 3100
Fullerton, CA 92834-3100
Phone: 1-800-877-6242
Website: www.beckmancoulter.com
(Hemoccult Guaiac cards)

GE Medical Systems
P.O. Box 414
Milwaukee, WI 53201
Phone: 1-800-558-5102
Website: www.gemedicalsystems.com
(For obstetric ultrasound)

GE Medical Systems, Clinical Services
5020 Campbell Boulevard
Baltimore, MD 21236
Phone: 1-410-931-4411
Website: www.gemedicalsystems.com
(For colonoscopy)

Genzyme Biosurgery
One Kendall Square
Cambridge, MA 02139
Phone: 1-800-367-7874
Website: www.genzymebiosurgery.com
(Pleur-Evac Water Seal chest drain system and thoracos-
tomy tubes)

George Tiemann and Co.
25 Plant Avenue
Hauppauge, NY 11788-3804
Phone: 1-800-843-6266
Website: www.atozsurgical.com
(Botulinum exotoxin supplies)

Gieserlab Equipment and Supply
P.O. Box 659
Chestertown, MD 21620
Phone: 1-888-778-7829
Website: www.gieserlab.com
(Sexual assault evidence collection kit)

Gill Podiatry Supply & Equipment Co.
7803 Freeway Circle
Middleburg Heights, OH 44130-6399
Phone: 1-800-321-1348
(Shower bag cover, casts, splints)

Good Art, LLC
1420 Fourth Street
Santa Monica, CA 90401
Phone: 1-310-395-4663
Website: www.goodart.com
(For body piercing)

GPT Glendale, Inc.
5300 Region Court
Lakeland, FL 33815
Phone: 1-800-500-4739
Website: www.glendale-laser.com
(Derm-Aid non-laser disposable eye shields)

Graham-Field, Inc.
400 Rabro Drive
East Hauppauge, NY 11788
Phone: 1-516-582-5900
(Medicopaste bandage for unna paste boot)

Grason-Stadler, Inc.
1 Westchester Drive
Milford, NH 03055-3056
Phone: 1-800-700-2282
Website: www.grasonstadler.com
(For audiometry, tympanometry equipment)

Greer Laboratories, Inc.
P.O. Box 800
639 Nuway Circle
Lenoir, NC 28645-0088
Phone: 1-800-438-0088
(Allergen extracts, immunotherapy sets, supplies for
   allergy testing and immunotherapy)

Gyne-Tech Instrument Co.
1115 Chestnut Street
Burbank, CA 91506
Phone: 1-323-849-1512
(For colposcopy equipment)

Gynecare, Inc. (Division of Ethicon, Inc.)
P.O. Box 151
Somersville, NJ 08876-0151
Phone: 1-800-255-2500
Website: www.gynecare.com
(Thermal balloon for endometrial ablation)

Handtronix
P.O. Box 21081
Salt Lake City, UT 84121
Phone: 1-800-832-7715
Website: www.handtronix.com
(For audiometry, tympanometry supplies)

Hardwood Products Co.
P.O. Box 149
Gulliford, ME 04443
Phone: 1-800-321-2313
Website: www.hwppuritan.com

Health Sciences Center for Educational Resources
University of Washington
T-252 Health Sciences Bldg, Box 357161
Seattle, WA 98195-7161
Phone: 1-206-685-1158
Website: www.hscer.washington.edu/hscer
(Technique videotapes for physicians for vasectomy)

Healwell Night Splint
FLA Orthopedics
2881 Corporate Way
Miramar, FL 33025
Phone: 1-800-327-4110
Website: www.clinitex.com
(High-tensile strength adhesive tape for ankle and foot
   splinting)

Heine USA
1 Washington Street, Suite 555
Dover, NH 03820-3851
Phone: 1-800-367-4872
Website: www.heine.com
(Dermatoscope, for dermoscopy [epiluminescence
   microscopy])

Henry Schein Co.
135 Duryea Road
Melville, NY 11747
Phone: 1-800- 772-4346
Website: www.henryschein.com
(Instrument for trimming nail plate and various derma-
    tologic equipment and supplies)

Hitachi Medical Corp.
660 White Plains Road
Tarrytown, NY 10591-5107
Phone: 1-800-852-2080
Website: www.hitachiultrasound.com
(For obstetric ultrasound)

Hollister Inc.
2000 Hollister Drive
Libertyville, IL 60048
Phone: 1-800-323-4060
Website: www.hollister.com
(Plastibell device)

Hollister-Stier Labs
3525 North Regal
Spokane, WA 99207-5788
Phone: 1-800-992-1120
Website: www.hollister-stier.com
(*Candida* antigen for wart [verruca] treatment; devices
    for skin testing [Quintest Multiple Antigen Device];
    allergen extracts, immunotherapy sets, supplies
    [Miles Allergy Products])

Hologic Inc.
35 Crosby Drive
Bedford, MA 01730
Phone: 1-781-999-7300
Website: www.hologic.com
(DXA, QUS, for osteoporosis screening)

Hy-Tape International
P.O. Box 540
Patterson, NY 12563-0540
Phone: 1-800-248-0101
Website: www.hytape.com
(Latex-free, zinc oxide tape)

ICN Pharmaceuticals
3300 Hyland Drive
Costa Mesa, CA 92626
Phone: 1-800-556-1937
Website: www.icnpharm.com
(Glycolic acid and other skin care products and skin
    peel supplies)

Image Analysis, Inc
1380 Burkesville Street
Columbia, KY 42728
Phone: 1-800-548-4849
Website: www.image-analysis.com
(For osteoporosis screening)

INAMED Aesthetics (formerly McGann Medical)
5540 Ekwill Street
Santa Barbara, CA 93111
Phone: 1-800-766-0171
Website: www.inamedaesthetics.com
(For collagen injection)

Industrial Strength
1945 Martin Luther King, Jr. Way
Berkeley, CA 94704
Phone: 1-510-644-0968
Website: www.isbodyjewelry.com
(For body piercing)

Instrument Specialists, Inc.
32390 IH-10 West
Boeme, TX 78006
Phone: 1-800-537-1945
(For endoscopy equipment)

Integrated Medical Systems, Inc.
1823 27th Avenue South
Birmingham, AL 35209
Phone: 1-800-783-9251
Website: www.imsservices.com
(For colonoscopy)

IOMED, Inc.
2441 West 3850 South, Suite A
Salt Lake City, UT 84120
Phone: 1-800-621-3347
Website: www.iomed.com
(For iontophoresis equipment/supplies)

Iriderm
1212 Terra Bella Avenue
Mountain View, CA 94043
Phone: 1-650-940-4700
Website: www.iriderm.com
(For laser hair removal, lasers)

J. Hewitt Incorporated
6 Faraday, Unit B
Irvine, CA 92618
Phone: 1-800-543-9488
Website: www.medi-system.com
(Professional ear piercing kit for ear piercing)

Jedmed Instruments Co.
5416 Jedmed Court
St Louis, MO 63129
Phone: 1-314-845-3770
Website: www.jedmed.com
(For colposcopy equipment)

Johnson & Johnson Medical Inc.
2500 East Arbrook Boulevard
Arlington, TX 76014-3631
Phone: 1-800-255-2500
Website: www.johnsonandjohnson.com
(Wound dressings)

Johnson & Johnson Professional, Inc.
325 Paramount Drive
Raynham, MA 02767-0350
Phone: 1-800-526-2459
Website: www.johnsonandjohnson.com
(Casting and splinting materials)

Juzo, Inc
80 Chart Road
P.O. Box 1088
Cuyahoga Falls, OH 44223
Phone: 1-800-222-4999
Website: www.juzo.com
(Support hose)

Karl Storz Endoscopy—America
600 Corporate Pointe
Culver City, CA 90230
Phone: 1-310-338-8100
Website: www.karlstorz.com
(For GI and GU endoscopes; endometrial ablation
    equipment)

The Kendall Company
15 Hampshire Street
Mansfield, MA 02048
Phone: 1-800-962-9888
Website: www.kendallhq.com
(Water Seal Chest Drain Systems, Argyle Edlich gastric
    lavage tray; Salem sump and feeding tubes; epidural
    and saddle block needles; wound dressings)

Kendall LTP
The Ludlow Company LP
Two Ludlow Park Drive
Chicopee, MA 01022
Phone: 1-800-962-9888
Website: www.kendall-ltp.com
(Softrans intrauterine pressure catheter)

Kimberly-Clark/Ballard Medical Products
12050 Lone Peak Parkway
Draper, UT 84020
Phone: 1-800-528-5591
Website: www.kchealthcare.com
(Easi-Lav for gastric lavage)

Krames Communications
1100 Grundy Lane
San Bruno, CA 94066
Phone: 1-800-333-3032
Website: www.krames.com
(Written patient education handouts for vasectomy,
    LEEP, and many other procedures and conditions)

LabCorp
358 South Main Street
Burlington, NC 27215
Phone: 1-336-584-5171
Website: www.labcorp.com
(RAST services for allergy testing and immunotherapy)

Laborie Medical Technologies
310 Hurricane Lane # 2
Williston, VT 05495
Phone: 1-802-878-1110
Website: www.laborie.com
(For urodynamic testing [multichannel])

Laserscope
3070 Orchard Drive
San Jose, CA 95134-2011
Phone: 1-408-943-0636
Website: www.laserscope.com
(For laser hair removal, lasers)

Leisegang Medical
95 Corporate Drive
Trumbull, CT 06611
Phone: 1-203-601-5200
Website: www.leisegang.com
(Equipment for loop electrosurgical excision procedure
[LEEP] and colposcopy)

Lhasa Medical, Inc.
539 Accord Station
Accord, MA 02018-0539
Phone: 1-800-722-8775
Website: www.lhasamedical.com
(Acupuncture needles and related equipment)

Life-Tech, Inc.
4235 Greenbriar Drive
Stafford, TX 77477-3995
Phone: 1-281-491-6600
Website: www.life-tech.com
(For urodynamic testing [multichannel])

Lincoln Diagnostics
P.O. Box 1128
Decatur, IL 62525
Phone: 1-800-537-1336
Website: www.lincolndiagnostics.com
(Devices for skin testing [Multi-Test Multiple Antigen
Device, Duotip Single Skin Prick Test], for allergies
and for immunotherapy)

Lumenis, Inc. (formerly ESC Medical Systems)
2400 Condensa Street
Santa Clara, CA 95051
Phone: 1-800-562-5916
Website: www.lumenis.com
(PhotoDerm and lasers of all wavelengths, for hair re-
moval and other applications)

Lunar Corporation (GE Medical Systems)
726 Heartland Trail
Madison, WI 53717-1915
Phone: 1-800-445-8627
Website: www.gemedicalsystems.com
(Peripheral DXA for osteoporosis screening)

Luxtec
99 Hartwell Street
West Boylston, MA 01583
Phone: 1-800-325-8966
Website: www.luxtec.com
(Head lamp for sclerotherapy and other procedures)

MADA Medical Products, Inc.
625 Washington Avenue
Carlstadt, NJ 07072
Phone: 1-800-526-6370
Website: www.madamedical.com
(MadaJet gun for subcutaneous injections)

Maico Diagnostics
9675 W. 76th Street
Eden Prairie, MN 55344
Phone: 1-888-941-4201
Website: www.maico-diagnostics.com
(For audiometry; for tympanometry devices)

Mallinckrodt Medical
675 McDonnell Boulevard
Hazelwood, MO 63042
Phone: 1-800-635-5267 or 1-888-744-1414
Website: www.mallinckrodt.com
(Shiley tracheostomy products)

Matlock Endoscopic
2969 Armory Drive, Suite 400
Nashville, TN 37204
Phone: 1-800-394-9822
Website: www.matlockendo.com
(Endoscopes)

McDavid Sports Medical Products
10305 Argonne Drive
Woodridge, IL 60517
Phone: 1-800-237-8254
Website: www.mcdavidinc.com
(McDavid Products Knee Guard [unilateral support] or
Pro Stabilizer [bilateral supports])

McKesson HBOC Inc.
12555 West Jefferson Blvd., Suite 101
Los Angeles, CA 90066
Phone: 1-800-523-9626
(Laminaria, mechanical dilators for cervical stenosis;
complete medical needs supplier with regional locations throughout the United States)

MD, Inc.
408 State of Franklin Road, Suite 43
Johnson City, TN 37604
Phone: 1-800-35-MDINC
(Sodium bicarbonate [Neutracaine] in 5-ml vials, for
reducing sting in local anesthetics)

MedAmicus, Inc.
15301 Highway 55 West
Plymouth, MN 55447
Phone: 1-800-559-2613
Website: www.medamicus.com
(For urodynamic testing [multichannel])

Medasonics (CooperSurgical)
38875 Cherry Street
Newark, CA 94560
Phone: 1-800-227-8076
Website: www.coopersurgical.com
(Pocket Dopplers for noninvasive venous and arterial
    studies)

Medco Supply Company
500 Fillmore Avenue
Tonawanda, NY 14150
Phone: 1-800-556-3326
Website: www.medcosupply.com
(For body fat analysis)

MedGyn
328 N. Eisenhower Lane
Lombard, IL 60148
Phone: 1-800-451-9667
Website: www.medgyn.com
(Laminaria and Lamicel, mechanical dilators, os locator,
    and canal finder; loop electrosurgical excision pro-
    cedure [LEEP] and colposcopy supplies)

Medi USA
6481 Franz Warner Parkway
Whitsett, NC 27377
Phone: 1-800-633-6334
Website: www.mediusa.com
(Compression hose)

Medical Center Pharmacy
4600 N. Habana Avenue
Tampa, FL 33614
Phone: 1-800-226-7094
(Betacaine and Bleacheze for skin peels: Betacaine LA
    and Betacaine Plus)

Medical Graphics
350 Oak Grove Parkway
St. Paul, MN 55127
Phone: 1-800-950-5597
Website: www.medgraph.com
(Expired gas analysis with cardiopulmonary exercise
    testing)

Medical Optics
559 Sawgrass Corporate Parkway
Sunrise, FL 33325
Phone: 1-800-286-9542
Website: www.medicaloptics.com
(For endoscopes)

Medical Replacement Parts LLC
6302 Manatee Avenue West, Suite F1
Bradenton, FL 34209
Phone: 1-800-363-6726
Website: www.endoscopepartsplus.com
(Endoscope repair)

Medical Systems International Corp.
6414 Northwest 82nd Avenue
Miami, FL 33166
Phone: 1-305-597-0322
Website: www.medicalsystems.com
(For pulmonary function testing equipment)

Medison USA
6616 Owens Drive
Pleasanton, CA 94588
Phone: 1-800-829-7666
Website: www.medisonusa.com
(For obstetric ultrasound)

Medsurge Medical, Inc.
210-828 Harbourside Drive
North Vancouver, BC V7P 3R9
Phone: 1-888-287-1958
Website: www.medsurgemedical.com
(O'Regan Hemorrhoid Banding Kit)

Medscand (Cytobrush)
CooperSurgical
95 Corporate Drive
Trumbull, CT 06611
Phone: 1-800-645-3760
Website: www.medscand.se
(For Pap smears)

MedTech International
P.O. Box 162992
Altamonte Springs, FL 32716-2992
Phone: 1-800-447-0014
Website: www.1ivenue.com/medtechinternational/
    item123593.ctlg
(Sexual assault evidence collection kit)

Medtronic
710 Medtronic Parkway NE
Minneapolis, MN 55432-5604
Phone: 1-763-514-4000
Website: www.medtronic.com
(For temporary pacing)

Medtronic Functional Diagnostics
3850 Victoria Street, MS V215
Shoreview, MN 55126-2978
Phone: 1-612-514-1700
Website: www.medtronic.com
(For urodynamic testing [multichannel])

Medtronic Xomed Surgical Products, Inc.
(Manufacturer of nasal balloons and packing kits,
    including the Merocel Park and the Pope Pak)
6743 Southpoint Drive North
Jacksonville, FL 32216-0980
Phone: 1-800-874-5797
Website: www.xomed.com
(Xomed Epistat I and Epistat II for management of
    epistaxis)

Mentor Corporation
201 Mentor Drive
Santa Barbara, CA 93111
Phone: 1-805-879-6000
Website: www.mentorcorp.com
(For pessaries)

Merz Pharmaceuticals
4215 Tudor Lane
Greensboro, NC 27410
Phone: 1-888-925-8989
Website: www.mederma.com
(Mederma gel for hypertrophic scars and keloids)

Micro Audiometrics
655 Keller Road
Murphy, NC 28906
Phone: 1-800-729-9509
Website: www.microaud.com
(For audiometry; for tympanometry equipment)

Micro Bio-Medics
846 Pellham Parkway
Pelham Manor, NY 10803
Phone: 1-800-431-2743
Website: www.microbiomedics.com
(For body fat analysis)

Miles Inc. (Pharmaceutical Division)
1127 Myrtle Street
Elkhart, IN 46514
Phone: 1-800-800-4793
(Dome-Paste medicated bandage [4-inch × 10-yard], for
    unna paste boot)

Milex Products, Inc.
4311 N. Normandy
Chicago, IL 60634
Phone: 1-800-621-1278
Website: www.milexproducts.com
(Amino Cerv Crème, pap supplies; Kegel Kones, Kegel
    Exersizer, and related pessary products; special sy-
    ringe, for fine-needle aspiration cytology and bi-
    opsy; Pipet Curet and Tis-u-Trap sampler device for
    endometrial biopsy; Word Bartholin's gland catheter
    for Bartholin's cyst/abscess; other gynecologic
    supplies

Miltex, Inc.
700 Hicksville Road
Bethpage, NY 11714
Phone: 1-800-645-8000
Website: www.miltex.com
(For skin biopsy, skin grafting and other dermatologic
    and medical instruments)

Minogue Medical
180 Dundas St. West, Suite 1507
Toronto, Onterio, Canada M5G 1Z8
(For skin stapling)

Mission Pharmacal Co.
10999 IH-10 West Suite 1000
San Antonio, Texas 78230
Phone: 1-800-531-3333
Website: www.missionpharmacal.com
(Vacuum Erection Device [VED] for impotence)

MJD Patient Communications
4915 St. Elmo Ave., Suite 306
Bethesda, MD 20814
Phone: 1-301-657-8010
Website: www.mjdpc.com
(Patient education materials, for hair removal, Botox,
    microdermabrasion, and other cosmetic procedures)

Mobile Instrument Service
333 Water Avenue
Bellefontaine, OH 43311
Phone: 1-800-722-3675
Website: www.mobileinstrument.com
(Endoscopes)

Mogen Instrument Co.
437 Crown Street
Brooklyn, NY 11225
Phone: 1-718-604-8833
(Mogen clamp for newborn circumcision)

Moore Medical Corporation
P.O. Box 1500
New Britain, CT 06050-1500
Phone: 1-800-234-1464
Website: www.mooremedical.com
(Supplies for orthotics, corns, calluses, and plantar
  warts; for flaps and plasties; and for laser therapy)

Mortara
7865 N. 86th Street
Milwaukee, WI 53224
Phone: 1-800-231-7437
Website: www.mortara.com
(For exercise [stress] testing)

M-Pact
1040 OCL Parkway
Eudora, KS 66025
Phone: 1-800-255-4152
Website: www.m-pactmed.com
(Casting and splinting materials, saws, and cast
  splitters)

MRT Laboratories
50 Johnson Avenue
Hackensack, NJ 07601
Phone: 1-800-631-1379
Website: www.mrtlabs.com
(RAST services for allergy testing and immunotherapy)

Multi Bio Sensors, Inc.
4944 Vista Grande
El Paso, TX 79922
Phone: 1-915-581-9684
(For biofeedback)

Myriad Ultrasound Systems, Ltd
Rehovot, Israel
Phone: 1-888-722-6994
(For osteoporosis screening)

The National Procedures Institute, Inc. (NPI)
4909 Hedgewood Drive
Midland, MI 48640
Phone: 1-800-462-2492 or 1-866-NPICMEI
Website: www.npinstitute.com
E-mail: info@NPInstitute.com
(Over 150 procedural skills courses offered each year,
  videotapes for patient education, technique videotapes for physicians, and teaching models for various procedures; NPI Reimbursement Manual comes
  out annually, updates the current fees being charged
  for various procedures performed by primary care
  physicians [approx. 55 pages])

National Testing Laboratories
400 Biltmore Drive, Suite 407
Fenton, MO 63026
Phone: 1-800-842-7135
Website: www.ntlworldwide.com
(Cerviscopes for cervicography)

Neurofeed.com
49 Sprain Valley Road
Scarsdale, NY 10583
Phone: 1-914-472-2292
Website: www.neurofeed.com
(Biofeedback)

Nicolet Vascular
6355 Joyce Drive
Golden, CO 80403
Phone: 1-800-525-2519
Website: www.nicoletvascular.com
(For noninvasive venous and arterial studies of the
  lower extremities)

Norland Medical Systems, Inc.
106 Corporate Park Drive, Suite 106
White Plains, NY 10604
Phone: 1-914-694-2285
Website: www.norland.com
(SXA, Peripheral QCT for osteoporosis screening)

Novacept, Inc.
1047 Elwell Court
Palo Alto, CA 94303
Phone: 1-650-428-0300
Website: www.novacept.com
(Bipolar cautery equipment/mesh, for endometrial
  ablation)

Norton Construction Products (Construction Products
    Division, North America)
P.O. Box 2898
Gainesville, GA 30503-2898
Phone: 1-770-967-3954
Website: www.nortonabrasive.com
(Norton silicon carbide paper for dermasanding)

Nuell, Inc.
P.O. Box 55
Warsaw, IN 46581-0055
Phone: 1-800-829-7694
Website: www.nuell.com
(Endoscopes)

Oculo-Plastik
200 Sauve West
Montreal (Quebec) Canada
H3L 1YD
Phone: 1-888-381-3292
Website: www.oculoplastik.com
(Equipment for laser therapy)

Olympus Corp.
Medical Instrument Division
8370 Dow Circle
Strongsville, OH 44136
Phone: 1-800-627-6264
Website: www.olmpusamerica.com
(For colonoscopy)

Olympus America Corp.
2 Corporate Center Drive
Melville, NY 11747
Phone: 1-800-548-5515
Website: www.olympusamerica.com
(For flexible fiberoptic nasolaryngoscopes,
    gastroscopes, sigmoidoscopes, cystourethroscopes,
    colposcopes, hysteroscopes)

Olympic Medical Corp.
5900 1st Avenue South
Seattle, WA 98108
Phone: 1-800-426-0353
Website: www.olymed.com
(Circumstraint for dorsal penile and subcutaneous ring
    block for newborn circumcision)

OMS Medical Supplies
1950 Washington Street
Braintree, MA 02184
Phone: 1-800-323-1839
Website: www.omsmedical.com
(For acupuncture)

ONYX Body Jewelry
22817 Ventura Boulevard, #495
Woodland Hills, CA 91364
Phone: 1-818-999-2540
Website: www.onyxbodyjewelry.com
(For body piercing)

OraSure Technologies
150 Webster Street
Bethlehem, PA18015
Phone: 1-800-869-3538
Website: www.stctech.com
(Histofreezer for cryosurgery)

Organon Teknika Corp.
100 Akzo Avenue
Durham, NC 27712
Phone: 1-800-682-2666
Website: www.organonteknika.com
(BacT/Alert blood culture bottles)

Ortho-Care
11911 East 83rd Street
Raytown, MO 64138
Phone: 1-800-821-1303
Website: www.ortho-care.com
(Ortho-Care Body Flex for knee braces)

Ortho-McNeil Pharmaceutical Company
1000 Route 202 South
Raritan, NJ 08869-0602
Phone: 1-800-682-6532
Website: www.ortho-mcneil.com
(Diaphragms)

Ortho-McNeil Pharmaceutical Company
P.O. Box 300
Raritan, NJ 08869-0602
Phone: 1-800-682-6532
Website: www.paragardiud.com
(ParaGard T380A IUD)

Osteometer MediTech, Inc.
12515 Chadron Avenue
Hawthorne, CA 90250
Phone: 1-310-978-3073
Website: www.osteometer.com
(For osteoporosis screening)

Overread Corp.
3037 Hopyard Road, Suite I
Pleasanton, CA 94588
Phone: 1-888-426-6331
Website: www.overread.com
(Overreading services for emergency department and office ultrasound)

Padgett Instruments, Inc.
1730 Walnut Street
Kansas City, MO 64108-1384
Phone: 1-800-842-1029
(Pressure earrings for ear piercing)

Palomar Medical Technologies, Inc.
82 Cambridge Street
Burlington, MA 01803
Phone: 1-800-725-6627
Website: www.palmed.com
(For laser hair removal, lasers)

Palumbo Orthopedics
8206 Leesburg Pike, Suite 404
Vienna, VA 22182
Phone: 1-800-292-7223
Website: www.palumbobrace.com
(Palumbo Tracker knee braces)

Parks Medical Electronics
19460 SW Shaw
Aloha, OR 97006
Phone: 1-800-547-6427
Website: www.parksmed.com
(Vascular equipment, including duplex [also pocket Dopplers], for noninvasive venous and arterial studies)

Person and Covey Dermatologicals
616 Allen Avenue
Glendale, CA 91221-5018
Phone: 1-800-423-2341
(Aquanil for dermasanding)

Pentax Precision Instruments Corporation
30 Ramland Road
Orangeburg, NY 10962-2699
Phone: 1-800-431-5880
Website: www.pentaxmedical.com
(For flexible fiberoptic nasolaryngoscopes, colonoscopes, gastroscopes, and flexible sigmoidoscopes)

Pharmacy Specialists (Sam Pratt, RPh)
650 Maitland Avenue
Altemonte Springs, FL 32701
Phone: 1-800-224-7711
(Polidocanol for sclerotherapy and other compounding pharmaceutical needs)

Pharmagen Inc.
155 Knickerbocker Avenue
Bohemia, NY 11716
Phone: 1-800-445-2595
(Dermatopics or Pharmatopix for skin peels)

Phazx Systems, Inc.
711 North Tejon
Colorado Springs, CO 80903
Phone: 1-800-273-0074
Website: www.phazx.com
(For biofeedback)

Philips Medical Systems
Cardiac and Monitoring Systems Headquarters
3000 Minuteman Road
Andover, MA 01810
Phone: 1-800-934-7372
Website: www.medical.philips.com
(For ambulatory electrocardiography: Holter and event monitoring; for fetal-movement counting, nonstress test, and contraction stress test equipment)

Phillips Medical Systems of North America, Inc. (also owners of ATL)
20 Center Point Drive, Suite 110
La Palma, CA 90623
Phone: 1-800-843-7572
Website: www.medical.philips.com
(For obstetrics ultrasound)

Phillips Medical Systems
Heartstream Operation
2401 4th Ave, Suite 500
Seattle, WA 98121-1436
Phone 1-800-263-3342
Website: www.medical.philips.com
(Heartstream semiautomatic defibrillator)

Physicians Learning Unlimited Seminars (The Course Seminars)
7209 South Mount Holy Cross
Littleton, CO 80127-3202
Phone: 1-800-916-7587
(Training and materials for radiofrequency sclerotherapy)

Physicians Office Lab Supplies (POLS)
1913 East Lincoln Road
Royal Oak, MI 48067
Phone: 1-248-336-8075
(Mycosel fungal culture media, tight-seal Petri dishes,
    for fungal studies)

Pie Medical (also see Biosound)
8000 Castleway Drive
Indianapolis, IN 46250-1943
Phone: 1-800-927-0708
Website: www.piemedicalusa.com
(For obstetric ultrasound)

Power Peel
530 College Parkway
Annapolis, MD 21401
Phone: 1-800-925-5022
Website: www.powerpeel.com
(Power Peel for microdermabrasion)

Precision Dynamics Corp.
13880 Del Sur Street
San Fernando, CA 91340-3490
or
P.O. Box 9043
Van Nuys, CA 91409
Website: www.pdcorp.com
(Comeco syringe for fine-needle aspiration cytology
    and biopsy)
Phone: 1-800-847-0670
(Cameco syringe pistol for peritonsillar abscess
    drainage)

Premier Medical Products
1710 Romano Drive, Box 4500
Plymouth Meeting, PA 19462
Phone: 1-888-773-6872
Website: www.premusa.com
(Equipment for loop electrosurgical excision procedure
    [LEEP])

Procter & Gamble Pharmaceuticals
1 or 2, Procter & Gamble Plaza
Cincinnati, OH 45201
Phone: 1-513-983-1100
Website: www.pgpharma.com
(Written patient education handouts for vasectomy)

Pro Orthopedic Devices, Inc.
2884 E. Ganley Road
Tucson, AZ 85706
Phone: 1-800-523-5611
Website: www.proorthopedic.com
(Pro 50 KS 5 ACL Brace [prefabricated], PRProPro 180
    Dr. "M-U" Universal Patella Support)

Puritan Bennett (Tyco Healthcare)
4280 Hacienda Drive
Pleasanton, CA 94588
Phone: 1-800-635-5267
Website: www.puritanbennett.com
(For pulmonary function testing)

Quinton Instrument Co.
3303 Monte Villa Parkway
Bothell, WA 98121
Phone: 1-888-784-6866
Website: www.quinton.com
(For exercise [stress] testing)

Reality Female Condom
Female Health Company
515 North State Street, Suite 2225
Chicago, IL 60610
Phone: 1-312-595-9123
Website: www.femalehealth.com
(Vaginal condoms)

Redfield Corp.
336 West Passaic Street
Rochelle Park, NJ 07662
Phone: 1-201-845-3990
Website: www.IRC2100.com
(Infrared coagulator [IRC] for nasal turbinate reduction,
    tattoo removal, internal hemorrhoid, and condyloma
    treatment; hemorrhoid band ligator; Ive's slotted
    anoscope)

Redwing Book Company
44 Linden Street
Brookline, MA 02445
1-800-873-3946
Website: www.redwingbooks.com
(Books and references on acupuncture)

Rejuvi Laboratory Inc.
360 Swift Avenue, Suite 38
South San Francisco, CA 94080
Phone: 1-800-588-2279
Website: www.rejuvilab.com
(Alternative tattoo removal system)

ReJuveness, Inc.
Phone: 1-800-588-7455
Website: www.rejuveness.com
(ReJuveness silicone sheets for hypertrophic scars and
    keloids)

RF Scleroneedles, Ltd.
7209 South Mount Holy Cross
Littleton, CO 80127-3202
Phone: 1-800-916-7587
(Scleroneedle for sclerotherapy)

Richard Wolf Medical Instruments
353 Corporate Woods Parkway
Vernon Hills, IL 60061-3110
Phone: 1-800-323-9653
Website: www.richardwolf.com
(For endometrial ablation, cystoscopy, hysteroscopy
    equipment)

Roche Biomedical Labs (Viral Typing)
1447 York Court
Burlington, NC 27215
Phone: 1-800-334-5161
(For DNA typing information)

Roman Research, Inc.
430 Court Street
Plymouth, MA 02360
Phone: 1-800-451-5700
Website: www.romanresearch.com
(Hypoallergenic jewelry)

Rusch Inc.
2450 Meadowbrook Parkway
Duluth, GA 30096
Phone: 1-770-623-0816
Website: www.ruschinc.com
(Lawrence Supra Foley suprapubic catheter introducer;
    tracheal [endotracheal and nasotracheal] intubation
    supplies; disposable trays, infusion pumps, needles,
    etc. for saddle block anesthesia, epidural anesthesia,
    Word Bartholin's gland catheter for Bartholin's cyst/
    abscess)

Sam Wagner
P.O. Box 431
202 Dodd Street
Middlebourne, WV 26149
Phone: 1-304-758-2370
(Venous noninvasive diagnostic equipment [e.g., PPG,
    Doppler] and assistance with all sclerotherapy sup-
    plies; editor's note: Sam will have or help you find
    whatever you need for evaluation and treatment of
    venous disease)

Saratoga Diagnostics
12619 Paseo Olivos
Saratoga, CA 95070
Phone: 1-800-998-1555
Website: www.saratogadiagnostics.com
(Ultrapeel for microdermabrasion)

SB Office Diagnostics, Inc.
10 Hampden Drive
Easton, MA 02375
Phone: 1-800-678-5782
(For pulmonary function testing)

Schick Technologies, Inc.
30-00 47th Avenue
Long Island City, NY 11101
Phone: 1-718-937-5765
Website: www.schicktech.com
(For osteoporosis screening)

The Scope Exchange
4210 Tudor Lane
Greensboro, NC 27410
Phone: 1-888-299-3977
Website: www.scopex.com
(For endoscopes)

Seattle Orthopedic Group, Inc.
26296 Twelve Trees Lane NW, Building One
Poulsbo, WA 98370
Phone: 1-800-248-6463
Website: www.soginc.com/SOGI
(Lenox Hill Precision Fit [prefabricated] or Spectra
    Light [custom] knee braces)

Serolab
P.O. Box 3307
Waco, TX 76707-3307
Phone: 1-800-460-4867
(RAST services for allergy testing and
    immunotherapy)

Shippert Medical Technologies
7002 South Revere Parkway, Suite 60
Englewood, CO 80112-6703
Phone: 1-800-888-8663
Website: www.shippertmedical.com
(Rhino Rocket for management of epistaxis; company
    also manufactures nasal packing kits and balloons,
    with and without airways)

Sigvaris
1119 Highway 74
Peachtree City, GA 30269
or
P.O. Box 570
Branford, CT 06405
Phone: 1-800-322-7744
Website: www.sigvaris.com
(Compression hose for sclerotherapy)

Siemens Medical Solutions, Inc. (also owners of
    Acuson)
22010 SE 51st Street
Issaquah, WA 98029
Phone: 1-800-367-3569
Website: www.siemansmedical.com
(For obstetric ultrasound)

Sims Portex
Hythe, Kent CT21 6JL
United Kingdom
Phone: +44(0) 1303 260551
Website: www.portex.com
(For tracheal [endotracheal and nasotracheal] supplies)

Sims Portex Inc.
10 Bowman Drive
Keene, NH 03431
Phone: 1-800-258-5361
Website: www.portexusa.com
(Disposable trays, infusion pumps, needles, etc., for
    saddle block and epidural anesthesia)

Sirchie Fingerprint Laboratories, Inc.
100 Hunter Place
Youngsville, NC 27596
Phone: 1-800-356-7311
Website: www.sirchie.com
(Sexual assault evidence collection kit)

Smith & Nephew, Inc.
Wound Management Division
11775 Starkey Road
P.O. Box 1970
Largo, FL 33779-1970
Phone: 1-800-876-1261
Website: www.snwmd.com
(Wound dressing; Hypafix dressing retention sheet
    (skin tape) for splinting, casting, and taping)

Smith & Nephew
N104 W13400 Donges Bay Road
P.O. Box 1005
Germantown, WI 53022-8205
Phone: 1-800-558-8633
Website: www.smith-nephew.com

Smithers Bio-Medical Systems
P.O. Box 118
Kent, OH 44240
Phone: 1-800-321-8286
(Orthotics)

SmithKline Beecham Clinical Laboratories
11636 Administration Drive
St. Louis, MO 63146
Phone: 1-800-669-8077
(RAST services for allergy testing and
    immunotherapy)

SOS Medical
740 East Arrow Highway
Covina, CA 91722
Phone: 1-888-592-5550
Website: www.sos-medical.com
(For endoscopes)

SoundSkin Corp.
429 Main Street
Oswego, IL 60543
Phone: 1-888-596-5277
Website: www.soundskin.com
(Smartpeel for microdermabrasion)

Space Labs Burdick
500 Burdick Parkway
Deerfield, WI 53531
Phone: 1-800-777-1777
Website: www.burdick.com
(Ambulatory electrocardiography for Holter and event
    monitoring exercise [stress] testing)

Spectrum Surgical Instruments
4575 Hudson Drive
Stow, OH 44224
Phone: 1-800-444-5644
Website: www.spectrumsugical.com
(For endoscopes)

SSR Surgical Instruments
P.O. Box 537, 5 Shore Avenue
Oyster Bay, NY 11771
Phone: 1-800-932-7364
Website: www.ssrsurgical.com
(Surgical dermatologic equipment)

St. Jude Medical
One Lillehei Plaza
St Paul, MN 55117-9913
Phone: 1-800-328-9634
Website: www.sjm.com
(For temporary pacing)

STD Pharmaceutical
Fields Yard, Plough Lane
Hereford HR4 OEL, England
Phone: +44 (0)1432 353684
Website: www.stdpharm.co.uk
(Compression wraps for ambulatory phlebectomy,
    sclerotherapy)

Stens Corp.
6451 Oakwood Drive
Oakland, CA 94611
Phone: 1-800-257-8367
Website: www.stens-biofeedback.com
(For biofeedback)

Steris Corp.
5960 Heisley Road
Mentor, OH 44060-1834
Phone: 1-800-989-7575
Website: www.steris.com

Stoelting Co.
620 Wheat Lane
Wood Dale, IL 60191
Phone: 1-630-860-9700
Website: www.stoeltingo.com
(For biofeedback)

Stryker Instruments
4100 E. Milham
Kalamazoo, MI 49001
Phone: 1-800-253-3210
Website: www.inst.strykercorp.com
(Pressure transducer for compartment syndrome
    evaluation)

Sunlight Medical, Inc
100 Davidson Avenue, Suite 108
Somerset, NJ 08873
Phone: 1-800-750-6011
Website: www.sunlightmedical.com
(Office ultrasound for osteoporosis screening)

Suntech Medical Instruments, Inc.
8917 Glenwood Avenue
Raleigh, NC 27612
Phone: 1-919-782-3005
Website: www.suntechmed.com
(For ambulatory blood pressure monitoring)

Surgical Optics LLC
1900 Wyatt Drive, Suite 7
Santa Clara, CA 95054
Phone: 1-888-884-6887
Website: www.surgical-optics.com
(For endoscopes)

Surgical Repair Technologies
930 Blue Gentian Road, Suite 1400
Eagan, MN 55121
Phone: 1-800-495-0297
Website: www.sohniks.com
(Endoscopes)

Sutherland Cranial Teaching Foundation
4116 Hartwood Drive
Ft. Worth, TX 76109
Phone: 1-817-926-7705
(For manipulative medicine)

Swede-O, Inc.
611 Ash St.
P.O. Box 610 North Branch, MN 55056
Phone: 1-800-525-9339
Website: www.swedeo.com
(Braces for ankle and foot splinting)

Thera-Tronics, Inc.
623 Mamaroneck Avenue
Mamaroneck, NY 10543
Phone: 1-914-698-9802
(TENS units for transcutaneous electrical nerve
    stimulation)

Thermolase Corp. (Thermo Electron Corp.)
81 Wyman Street
Waltham, MA 02454-9046
Phone: 1-781-622-1000
Website: www.thermo.com
(For laser hair removal)

Thomas Medical, Inc.
4100-C Nine McFarland Drive
Alpharetta, GA 30004
Phone: 1-800-556-0349
Website: www.thomasmedical.com/vbmproducts2.htm
(Double-cuff Pneumatic Tourniquet for bier block)

Thought Technology, Ltd.
2180 Belgrave Avenue
Montreal Quebec, Canada H4A 2L8
Phone: 1-800-361-3651
Website: www.thoughttechnology.com
(For biofeedback)

TIMM Medical Technologies
6585 City West Parkway
Eden Prairie, MN 55344
Phone: 1-800-438-8592
Website: www.timmmedical.com
(ErecAid vacuum device for erectile dysfunction)

Toshiba America Medical Systems
2441 Michelle Drive
Tustin, CA 92780
Phone: 1-800-421-1968
Website: www.medical.toshiba.com
(For obstetric ultrasound)

Townsend Design
4615 Shepard Street
Bakersfield, CA 93313
Phone: 1-800-432-3466
Website: www.townsenddesign.com
(Townsend Design Rebel 99 [prefabricated] or Air
   [custom] knee braces)

Transtracheal Systems
109 Inverness Drive East, Suite J
Englewood, CO 80112-5105
Phone: 1-800-527-2667
Website: www.TTO2.com
(Indwelling transtracheal catheter)

Trylon Corporation
970 West 190th Street, Suite 850
Torrance, CA 90502
Phone: 1-800-486-8979
Website: www.tryloncorp.com
(PapSure system for cervical cancer screening
   [speculoscopy])

Unimax Supply Company
365 Canal Street
New York, NY 10013
Phone: 1-800-986-4629
Website: www.unimaxsupply.com
(For body piercing)

United Endoscopy
10405 San Sevaine Way, Suite B
Mira Lorma, CA 91752-1150
Phone: 1-800-899-4847
Website: www.endoscope.com
(Endoscopes)

Universal Endoscopic Services
6861 SW 196th Avenue, Suite 402
Pembroke Pines, FL 33332
Phone: 1-800-266-1464
Website: www.ues1.com
(Endoscopes)

The Upledger Institute
11211 Prosperity Farms Road, Suite D-325
Palm Beach Gardens, FL 33410
Phone: 1-561-622-4334
Website: www.upledger.com
(For manipulative medicine)

U.S. Medical Inc.
4601 DTC Boulevard, 7th Floor
Denver, CO 80237
Phone: 1-800-607-7455
(Endoscopes)

Used Medical Equipment and Devices Medline
278 S. Lincoln Street
Minster, OH 45865
Phone: 1-888-355-9692
Website: www.1-medical-equipment.com
(Endoscopes)

Utah Medical Products, Inc. (United States)
7043 South 300 West
Midvale, UT 84047-1048
Phone: 1-800-548-8667 *or* 1-800-533-4984
Website: www.utahmed.com
(Intran Plus IUP-400, intrauterine pressure catheter
   equipment for loop electrosurgical excision proce-
   dure [LEEP])

Valleylab, Inc.
5920 Longbow Drive
Boulder, CO 80301-3209
Phone: 1-800-255-8522
(Equipment for loop electrosurgical excision proce-
   dure [LEEP])

VBM Medical, Inc.
15013 Herriman Boulevard
Noblesville, IN 46060
Phone 1-800-580-7117
Website: www.vbm-medical.de/set2.html
(Equipment for bier block)

Venosan
718 Industrial Park Avenue
P.O. Box 1067
Asheboro, NC 27204-1067
Phone: 1-888-250-7617
Website: www.venosanonline.com
(Compression hose)

Venoscan
1617 N. Fayetteville Street
P.O. Box 4068
Asheboro, NC 27204-4068
Phone: 1-910-672-6062
(Phlebectomy vein hooks)

Vision-Sciences, Inc.
(Manufactures a scope as well as disposable sheath
    covers for various brands of scopes)
9 Strathmore Road
Natick, MA 01760
Phone: 1-800-874-9975
Website: www.visionsciences.com
(For flexible fiberoptic nasolaryngoscopy)

Vitalograph
8347 Quivira
Lenexa, KS 66215
Phone: 1-800-255-6626
Website: www.vitalograph.com
(For pulmonary function testing)

Wagner Medical
P.O. Box 431
202 Dodd Street
Middlebourne, WV 26149
Phone: 1-304-758-2370
(An excellent general resource for all sclerotherapy
    and phlebectomy instruments and equipment; this
    source will have it or know where to find it)

Wallach Surgical
235 Edison Road
Orange, CT 06477
Phone: 1-800-243-2463
Website: www.wallachsurgical.com
(Papette for Pap smears; for colposcopes; for
    nitrous oxide cryosurgical units; liquid nitrogen
    cryoguns; Endocell endometrial sampler; loop elec-
    trosurgical excision procedure [LEEP] equipment and
    supplies)

Weck Closure Systems
2917 Weck Drive
P.O. Box 12600
Research Triangle Park, NC 27709
Phone: 1-800-234-9325
Website: www.weckclosure.com
(Skin stapling; hemoclips and clip applicators)

Welch Allyn, Inc.
4341 State Street Road
P.O. Box 220
Skaneateles Falls, NY 13153-0220
Phone: 1-800-535-6663
Website: www.welchallyn.com
(Audiometry and tympanometry supplies; headlamp
    and ocular loupes; pulmonary function testing; for
    colposcopes; vital signs monitors; EpiScope for der-
    moscopy; for cryotherapy unit; equipment for loop
    electrosurgical excision procedure [LEEP]; many
    other varied pieces of equipment)

Weslee Medical, Inc.
1187 Wilmette Ave. PMB 149
Wilmette, IL 60091-2719
Phone: 1-877-624-6681
Website: www.wesleemedical.com

Dr. Charles Wilson
The Vasectomy Clinic
5402 47th Avenue NE
Seattle, WA 98105
Phone: 1-206-525-4090
Website: www.thevasectomyclinic.org
(Technique videotapes for physicians and teaching
    models for vasectomy)

Wyeth Laboratories
Philadelphia, PA
Phone: 1-800-922-0877
(Norplant System professional assistance, including patient educational supplies, training, and free Norgrasp removal forceps)

Zeiss
One Zeiss Drive
Thornwood, NY 10594
Phone: 1-800-442-4020
Website: www.zeiss.com
(For colposcopes)

Zerowet
P.O. Box 4375
Palos Verdes Penninsula, CA 90274
Phone: 1-800-438-0938
(Zerowet Splash Shields and Klenzalac Wound Irrigation Systems)

Zimmer, Inc.
727 North Detroit Street
Warsaw, IN 46580
Phone: 1-800-613-6131
Website: www.zimmer.com

Zimmer Orthopaedic Surgical Products
P.O. Box 10
200 West Avenue
Dover, OH 44622
Phone: 1-330-343-8801
(Adjustable Dermatomes for skin grafting)

Resources for Learning Procedures

Stephen J. Wetmore

The well-rounded primary care physician includes a variety of medical and surgical procedures in his or her practice. The procedures included in any practice depend strongly on the training that one has received in performing those procedures. Advancing technology and changing practice patterns lead primary care physicians to add new procedures to their practice and/or update their skills in procedures that they already perform. Regardless of whether the clinician is learning a procedure for the first time or wishing to update skills, it is helpful to have a good understanding of the resources that are available to facilitate learning.

This appendix provides information about the variety of resources available for learning procedures and how these can be accessed. This is also of considerable interest to teachers of procedural skills. It is beyond the scope of this appendix to include every possible resource, but each section will have examples and provide ideas about where to search for other similar resources. Approximate costs will be provided where appropriate.

COURSES IN PROCEDURES FOR PRIMARY CARE PHYSICIANS

In both Canada and the United States, national medical associations such as the College of Family Physicians of Canada and the American Academy of Family Physicians provide opportunities to learn and update procedure skills. National and state or provincial meetings of these bodies often have seminars or workshops on common procedures in primary care. Seminars or workshops are excellent starting points for physicians hoping to learn procedures because they will include the pertinent background knowledge for each procedure, including indications, contraindications, technical details, and complications. Many of these workshops also include an opportunities for "hands-on" experience, which allows physicians to become familiar with equipment and techniques. These sessions are suitable as updates for physicians already familiar with the procedures but do not provide enough practical experience in some procedures for new learners to commence performing them right away. They are, nevertheless, good starting points.

The National Procedures Institute in Michigan provides a variety of courses in procedure skills that are well publicized on its website (www.npinstitute.com). The range of procedures covered in these courses is extensive, and readers are referred to the course outlines on the website for details.

GAINING PRACTICAL EXPERIENCE IN PROCEDURES

Although formal courses or workshops such as those described above are suitable for learning information about procedures, equipment, and techniques, it may not be possible for the clinician to gain enough experience in this way to begin performing the procedure. Practice and supervised practice are necessary to gain confidence in skills for many procedures. There are no clear guidelines as to how many supervised procedures are necessary to achieve competence. For example, it has been suggested that 25 to 30 supervised flexible sigmoidoscopies are necessary to achieve competence in that procedure and 10 to 15 supervised no-scalpel vasectomies for the vasectomy procedure. There is no consensus on numbers necessary to achieve competence and therefore no reliable standards for competence in most procedures. The number of supervised procedures necessary to achieve competence for any given procedure depends on the complexity of the procedure, and the confidence and physical dexterity of the operator, among other things. Clinicians should consider performing procedures with a supportive colleague, in a supervised setting, until comfortable with carrying on in his or her own practice. Supportive colleagues can be a major resource toward getting started in procedures and providing backup and support when difficulties arise. As an example, in the author's local community, several family physicians who perform no-scalpel vasectomy have formed an interest group. The group holds meetings periodically, which may include videotape review, and discussion of techniques and complications. This same model could afford support for primary care physician proceduralists in many communities. EngenderHealth (New York, NY; formerly the Association for Voluntary Surgical Contraception) has a program to match preceptors with those learning the no-scalpel vasectomy technique. Once a course has been attended, the organization will provide the name of a preceptor in a certain area and help the clinician with the hands-on technique. There is no charge for the matching service. The National Procedures Institute also has a limited number of physicians available for preceptors.

BOOKS ON PROCEDURES IN PRIMARY CARE

Despite the rise in technology and increasing use of CD-ROMs, computer animations, and virtual reality, books are still a major resource for many of the things we do in practice. A good book on procedural skills is an essential part of the primary care physician's library. This book, *Pfenninger and Fowler's Primary Care Procedures,* is one example of an ideal resource book because of its comprehensive nature, inclusion of background material, patient education, description of technique, helpful illustrations, company names and addresses for obtaining equipment, and billing and coding information.

Some of the more recent texts on procedures, in addition to this book, are listed in Box E-1. The Clinics Atlas of Office Procedures series (WB Saunders) reviews various topics in depth, including many of the topics in this book. This series is excellent for those truly interested in development of procedural skills. New subjects are published quarterly.

Also, many clinicians are searching for an excellent book on dermatology, since many of the procedures do include the skin. There is no better source than Habif's *Clinical Dermatology,* ed 4 (WB Saunders, 2003).

CD-ROM RESOURCES FOR PROCEDURES IN PRIMARY CARE

CD-ROMs are useful resources for learning procedures because the technology allows the integration of text with voice, pictures, computer animation, and videotape. These can be searched easily to focus on specific details of any given procedure. Like textbooks, CD-ROMs can provide all the relevant background information necessary to perform the procedure. One strength of this technology is the capacity to incorporate video

footage, since the visual presentation of the technique is a powerful learning aid. CD-ROMs are portable and can be used in a variety of settings, including the office, clinic, or even the home.

More CD-ROMs in procedure skills are becoming available all the time. Some of the recent releases are listed in Box E-2.

WEBSITES

PD × MD is an informative website that is constantly being updated. It will have a discussion of 25 procedure topics online by the end of 2003. Each will include a short videoclip of the procedure reviewed.

VIDEOTAPE RESOURCES FOR PROCEDURES IN PRIMARY CARE

Like CD-ROMs, videotapes have the advantage of providing a visual image for the learner of the procedure being performed. They are also portable, but the requirement of a video player and monitor for viewing may limit their usefulness. In spite of this, when the equipment is available, videotapes are excellent resources for group learning of procedures. Recent videotape releases on procedures in primary care are listed in Box E-3.

Videotapes are a perfect patient education resource. They not only reduce clinicians' time while performing a more comprehensive discussion, but they also help document facts should legal problems arise.

ARTIFICIAL MODELS AND LEARNING PROCEDURES

A major problem with learning procedures in primary care is the lack of opportunities for enough practice of the technical skill involved to learn the procedure adequately or to maintain a previously learned skill. Books, videotapes, and CD-ROMs are all valuable for background information and presenting a visual image of the skill, but the opportunity to practice must also be present. Models and simulations can provide this opportunity to practice skills repeatedly without endangering patients or learners. They are widely used in courses and workshops for teaching procedures. Research has shown that artificial models can be effective for learning and retaining technical skills. They can also be helpful directly in the practice setting for rehearsal of procedures before performing the skill in clinical care.

Many physicians are familiar with the mannequins and models used for skills teaching in such courses as

Text continued on p. 1725

BOX E-1

Recent Textbooks and Material on Procedures Pertinent to Primary Care Physicians

GENERAL TEXTBOOKS	
TITLE:	Procedures in Practice, ed 3
AUTHOR:	Scott N
PUBLISHER:	BMJ Publishing Group, 1994
COST (US):	$27.00
COMMENT:	Includes adult resuscitation skills, chest tubes, lumbar puncture, liver biopsy, suturing, ear syringing
TITLE:	Procedures in Women's Health
AUTHOR:	Smith RP
PUBLISHER:	Williams & Wilkins, 1997
COST (US):	$69.00
COMMENT:	Covers procedures in most systems including dermatology, orthopedics, urology, ENT, ophthalmology
TITLE:	Essential Medical Procedures
AUTHOR:	Toghill PJ
PUBLISHER:	Little, Brown & Co., 1997
COST (US):	$29.50
COMMENT:	Includes skin procedures, pleural tap, cervical smears, lumbar puncture, joint aspiration
TITLE:	Procedural Skills for Internal Medicine: Reference Manual
AUTHOR:	Wigton RS
PUBLISHER:	Mosby, 1996
COST (US):	$22.50
TITLE:	Practical Procedures in the Emergency Department, ed 1
AUTHOR:	Bache J
PUBLISHER:	Mosby, 1998
COST (US):	$34.95
COMMENT:	Covers many orthopedic procedures, wound care, foreign bodies, pediatric problems
TITLE:	Office and Bedside Procedures
AUTHOR:	Chesnutt MS
PUBLISHER:	Appleton & Lange, 1999
COST (US):	N/A
COMMENT:	Illustrated guide to many office and bedside procedures
TITLE:	Emergency Procedures and Techniques, ed 3
AUTHOR:	Simon RR; Brenner BE
PUBLISHER:	Williams & Wilkins, 1994
COST (US):	$70.00
COMMENT:	Wide variety of procedures covered, both emergency and office-based, with illustrations
TITLE:	Office Procedures
AUTHOR:	Zuber TJ
PUBLISHER:	Williams & Wilkins, 1999
COMMENT:	Limited number of procedures included in text
TITLE:	Office and Bedside Procedures
AUTHOR:	Chesnutt MS, Dewar TN, Locksley RM, Tureen JH
PUBLISHER:	Appleton & Lange, 1992
TITLE:	Atlas of Outpatient and Office Surgery
AUTHOR:	Benjamin RB
PUBLISHER:	Lea & Febiger, 1994
TITLE:	Primary Care: Clinics in Office Practice
AUTHOR:	Ferris DG
PUBLISHER:	WB Saunders, Vol. 24, No. 2, 1997
TITLE:	Field Guide to Urgent and Ambulatory Care Procedures
AUTHOR:	James DM
PUBLISHER:	Lippincott, Williams & Wilkins, 2001
TITLE:	Minor Surgery in Practice
AUTHOR:	Sodera VK
PUBLISHER:	Cambridge University Press, 1994

Continued

BOX E-1—cont'd

Recent Textbooks and Material on Procedures Pertinent to Primary Care Physicians

GENERAL TEXTBOOKS—cont'd	
TITLE:	Patient Care Procedures for Your Practice
AUTHOR:	Driscoll CE, Rakel RE
PUBLISHER:	Practice Management Information Corporation, 1991
TITLE:	Office Surgery for Family Physicians
AUTHOR:	Pories WJ
PUBLISHER:	Butterworth Publishers, 1984
TITLE:	Manual of Common Bedside Surgical Procedures by the Halsted Residents of the Johns Hopkins Hospital
AUTHOR:	Chen H, Sola JE, Lillemoe KD
PUBLISHER:	Williams & Wilkins, 1995
TITLE:	Procedures for the Primary Care Practitioner, ed 2
AUTHOR:	Edmunds MW, Mayhew MS
PUBLISHER:	Mosby, 2003
TITLE:	Minor Surgery: a Text and Atlas, ed 3
AUTHOR:	Brown JS
PUBLISHER:	Chapman & Hall, 1997
TITLE:	Procedures in Practice
AUTHOR:	Scott NA
PUBLISHER:	BMJ Publishing Group, 1994
TITLE:	Minor Surgery: A Text and Atlas, ed 4
AUTHOR:	Brown JS
PUBLISHER:	Arnold, 2000
TITLE:	Manual of Medical Procedures
AUTHOR:	Suratt PM, Gibson RS
PUBLISHER:	Mosby, 1982
TITLE:	Pfenninger and Fowler's Procedures for Primary Care, ed 2
PUBLISHER:	Mosby, 2003
COMMENT:	JAMA said the first edition was "the most comprehensive text available anywhere on medical procedures."
CODING AND BILLING	
TITLE:	Medicode's 2003 Publications & Software for Coders
PUBLISHER:	Ingenix St. Anthony Medicode, 2525 Lake Park Blvd, West Valley City, UT 84120; 1-801-982-3000
COMMENT:	Updated annually
TITLE:	2003 Physicians Fee & Coding Guide
PUBLISHER:	MAG Mutual Healthcare Solutions, Inc., 1054 Claussen Rd, Suite 307, Augusta, GA 30907; 1-706-738-2078
COMMENT:	A comprehensive coding and fee reference, updated annually
TITLE:	Physicians' Fee Reference 2003
PUBLISHER:	Yale Wasserman, D.M.D. Medical Publishers, P.O. Box 510949, Milwaukee, WI 53203; 1-800-669-3337
COMMENT:	Updated annually
TITLE:	NPI Reimbursement Manual for Office Procedures, 2003
AUTHOR:	Pfenniger JL
PUBLISHER:	The National Procedures Institute
COST (US):	$69.95, inserts only $49.95
COMMENT:	The fee guides listed above contain every CPT code available and a range of fees charged in the United States. The NPI Reimbursement Manual is smaller and more specific. It lists the most common office surgery and procedure codes (CPTs). For each CPT code, there is a comparison of RVUs, BCBS rates, average national Medicare reimbursement, Michigan Medicaid fee, and an estimated 50th percentile charge in the country. Pertinent ICD-9 codes are listed on the same page. Updated annually.
	Every office needs the current ICD-9 and CPT coding book available from the American Medical Association. If one of the fee guides is purchased (higher cost but helpful to have at least one), all the CPT codes are listed so another CPT code book would not be necessary.

BOX E-1—cont'd

Recent Textbooks and Material on Procedures Pertinent to Primary Care Physicians

<u>COLPOSCOPY</u>

TITLE:	Basic and Advanced Colposcopy
AUTHOR:	Burke L, Antonioli DA, Ducatman BS
PUBLISHER:	Appleton & Lange, 1991

TITLE:	Basic and Advanced Colposcopy: a Practical Handbook for Diagnosis and Treatment
AUTHOR:	Wright VC, Lickrish GM
PUBLISHER:	Biomedical Communications, Inc., 1989

TITLE:	Colposcopy Principles and Practice: An Integrated Textbook and Atlas
AUTHOR:	Apgar BS, Brotzman GL, Spitzer M
PUBLISHER:	WB Saunders, 2002

TITLE:	Practical Colposcopy, ed 2
AUTHOR:	Cartier R
PUBLISHER:	Gustav Fischer Verlag, 1984
COMMENT:	810 color figures

TITLE:	Handbook of Colposcopy: Diagnosis and Treatment of Lower Genital Tract Neoplasia and HPV Infections
AUTHOR:	Hatch KD
PUBLISHER:	Little, Brown, 1989

TITLE:	Colposcopy Syllabus and Videotape
PUBLISHER:	American Academy of Family Physicians
COST (US):	$225 (members); $275 (nonmembers); $185 (residents)
COMMENT:	Provides evaluation and therapy for women with preneoplastic changes of the genital system; includes a color photo atlas. Currently in revision.

<u>ENDOSCOPY</u>

TITLE:	Primary Care Clinics in Office Practice: Colonoscopy
AUTHOR:	Varma JR
PUBLISHER:	WB Saunders, Vol. 22, No. 3, 1995

TITLE:	The Clinics Atlas of Office Procedures: Gastrointestinal Procedures
AUTHOR:	Merli GJ, DiMarino Jr AJ
PUBLISHER:	WB Saunders, Vol. 2, No. 2, June, 1999

TITLE:	Endoscopy of the Colon, Rectum, and Anus
AUTHOR:	Church JM
PUBLISHER:	Igaku-Shoin Medical Publishers, 1995

TITLE:	Gastroenterologic Endoscopy
AUTHOR:	Sivak Jr MV
PUBLISHER:	WB Saunders, 1987

TITLE:	Atlas of Clinical Gastrointestinal Endoscopy
AUTHOR:	Wilcox CM
PUBLISHER:	WB Saunders, 1995
COMMENT:	Companion to Sleisenger and Fordtran's Gastrointestinal Disease

TITLE:	Gastrointestinal Endoscopy, ed 3
AUTHOR:	Silverstein FE, Tytgat GNJ
PUBLISHER:	Mosby, 1996

TITLE:	Planning an Endoscopy Suite for Office and Hospital
AUTHOR:	Waye, JD, Rich, ME
PUBLISHER:	Igaku-Shoin Medical Publishers, 1990

TITLE:	Practical Flexible Sigmoidoscopy
AUTHOR:	Cohen LB, Basuk P, Wayne JD
PUBLISHER:	Igaku-Shoin Medical Publishers, 1995

TITLE:	EGD Syllabus
PUBLISHER:	American Academy of Family Physicians
COST (US):	$100 (members); $140 (nonmembers); $85 (residents)
COMMENT:	Comprehensive overview of diagnostic EGD.

Continued

BOX E-1—cont'd
Recent Textbooks and Material on Procedures Pertinent to Primary Care Physicians

MISCELLANEOUS	
TITLE:	Clinics Atlas of Office Procedures: Joint Injection Techniques
AUTHOR:	Pfenninger JL
PUBLISHER:	WB Saunders, Vol. 5, No. 4, 2002
TITLE:	Rheumatology Examination and Injection Techniques, ed 2
AUTHOR:	Doherty M, Hazleman BL, Hutton CW, *et al.*
PUBLISHER:	WB Saunders, 1999
COMMENT:	Excellent, concise, practical text
TITLE:	Chemical Peeling and Resurfacing, ed 2
AUTHOR:	Brody HJ
PUBLISHER:	Mosby, 1997
TITLE:	Sclerotherapy: Treatment of Varicose and Telangiectatic Leg Veins, ed 3
AUTHOR:	Goldman MP, Bergan JJ
PUBLISHER:	Mosby, 2001
TITLE:	Manual of Sclerotherapy
AUTHOR:	Sadick NS
PUBLISHER:	Lippincott, Williams & Wilkins, 2000
TITLE:	Atlas of Interventional Pain Management
AUTHOR:	Waldman SD
PUBLISHER:	WB Saunders, 1998
TITLE:	The Acupuncture Treatment of Pain
AUTHOR:	Chaitow L
PUBLISHER:	Healing Arts Press, 1990
TITLE:	Office Hysteroscopy
AUTHOR:	Isaacson KB
PUBLISHER:	Mosby, 1996
TITLE:	Common Foot Problems in Primary Care
AUTHOR:	Birrer RB, DellaCorte MP, Grisafi PJ
PUBLISHER:	Hanley & Belfus, 1992
TITLE:	Primary Care: Clinics in Office Practice: Exercise Testing
AUTHOR:	Evans CH
PUBLISHER:	WB Saunders, Vol. 28, No. 1, 2001
TITLE:	No-Scalpel Vasectomy: an Illustrated Guide for Surgeons
AUTHOR:	Gonzales B, Marston-Ainley S, Vansintejan G, Li PS
PUBLISHER:	EngenderHealth, 1992
TITLE:	Handbook of Fractures, ed 2
AUTHOR:	Koval KJ, Zuckerman JD
PUBLISHER:	Lippincott, Williams & Wilkins, 2002
TITLE:	Office Orthopedics for Primary Care: Diagnosis and Treatment
AUTHOR:	Anderson CB
PUBLISHER:	WB Saunders, 1995
TITLE:	Procedures in Women's Health
AUTHOR:	Smith RP, Ling FW
PUBLISHER:	Williams & Wilkins, 1997
TITLE:	Office Gynecology, ed 4
AUTHOR:	Glass RH
PUBLISHER:	Williams & Wilkins, 1993
TITLE:	Emergency Procedures and Techniques, ed 3
AUTHOR:	Simon RR, Brenner BE
PUBLISHER:	Williams & Wilkins, 1994
TITLE:	Emergency Medicine: a Comprehensive Study Guide, ed 4
AUTHOR:	Tintinalli JE, Ruiz E, Krome RL
PUBLISHER:	The American College of Emergency Physicians, 1996

BOX E-1—cont'd

Recent Textbooks and Material on Procedures Pertinent to Primary Care Physicians

MISCELLANEOUS—Cont'd	
TITLE:	Patient Education and Procedure Forms
AUTHOR:	Pfenninger JL
PUBLISHER:	NPI
COST (US):	$100.00
COMMENT:	A complete set of patient education handouts and the forms used to document procedures in Dr. Pfenninger's office.
TITLE:	Procedural Skills Quiz Sets
	Quiz Set I: Flexible sigmoidoscopy, hemorrhoid procedures, colonoscopy, upper endoscopy (EGD)
	Quiz Set II: Skin excisional surgery, radiofrequency skin surgery, skin cryosurgery, skin cancer management
	Quiz Set III: Intrauterine device (IUD), contraceptive implants (Norplant), no-scalpel vasectomy, sclerotherapy
	Quiz Set IV: Colposcopy, LEEP procedure, endometrial biopsy, breast biopsy
	Quiz Set V: Joint and soft tissue injection, exercise treadmill testing, nasolaryngoscopy, fracture management
PUBLISHER:	NPI
COST (US):	$29.95 each
COMMENT:	20 different procedural skills topics help to enhance learning and give both learner and instructor feedback.
TITLE:	Flexible Sigmoidoscopy/Colonoscopy Syllabus
PUBLISHER:	American Academy of Family Physicians
COST (US):	$120 (members); $160 (nonmembers); $95 (residents)
COMMENT:	Offers a comprehensive overview, including techniques of scope manipulation.
TITLE:	Nasolaryngoscopy: a Self-Study Program for the Family Physician Interested in Nasolaryngoscopy
PUBLISHER:	American Academy of Family Physicians
COST (US):	$75 (members); $95 (nonmembers); $65 (residents)
COMMENT:	Covers upper airway endoscopy; includes a color photo atlas.
TITLE:	Soft-tissue Surgery: Illustrated Manuals and Videotapes
PUBLISHER:	American Academy of Family Physicians
COST (US):	Complete Set (19 hrs of CME): $230 (members); $265 (nonmembers); $190 (residents)
	Book 1 w/videotape (7 hrs of CME): $105 (members); $120 (nonmembers); $85 (residents)
	Book 2 w/videotape (6 hrs of CME): $90 (members); $105 (nonmembers); $75 (residents)
	Book 3 w/videotape (6 hrs of CME): $90 (members); $105 (nonmembers); $75 (residents)
COMMENT:	Offers a 3-volume set of illustrated text plus video to enhance ability to perform office skin surgery.
PATIENT EDUCATION	
TITLE:	Patient Education: Literature
PUBLISHER:	Staywell Krames
COMMENT:	Large assortment of brochures on various topics
TITLE:	Patient Education: Literature
PUBLISHER:	American Social Health Association
COMMENT:	Sexually transmitted disease topics
TITLE:	Patient Education Videotapes (30 minutes each):
	Genital Warts and Cervical Cancer: The Woman's Side
	Genital Warts and Cancer: The Man's Side
	Vasectomy (this tape can be personalized with your introduction)
	Microdermabrasion, colonoscopy, Botox, LEEP, sclerotherapy, others
PUBLISHER:	NPI
COST (US):	$49.95 each
TITLE:	Various and extensive handouts on dermatologic topics
PUBLISHER:	American Academy of Dermatology, National Skin Foundation
SKIN	
TITLE:	Minor Injuries and Repairs
AUTHOR:	Grossman JA
PUBLISHER:	Gower Medical Publishing, 1993
TITLE:	Atlas of Cutaneous Surgery
AUTHOR:	Robinson JK
PUBLISHER:	WB Saunders, 1996
TITLE:	Regional Anesthesia: An Atlas of Anatomy and Techniques
AUTHOR:	Hahn, MB, McQuillan, PM, Sheplock, GJ
PUBLISHER:	Mosby, 1995

Continued

BOX E-1—cont'd

Recent Textbooks and Material on Procedures Pertinent to Primary Care Physicians

SKIN—Cont'd	
TITLE:	Illustrated Atlas of Cutaneous Surgery
AUTHOR:	Fewkes JL, Pollack SV, Cheney ML
PUBLISHER:	Gower Medical Publishing, 1992
TITLE:	Skin Surgery: a Practical Guide
AUTHOR:	Usatine RP, Tobinick EL, Moy RL, Siegel DM
PUBLISHER:	Mosby, 1998
COMMENT:	Excellent comprehensive text
TITLE:	Wounds and Lacerations: Emergency Care and Closure
AUTHOR:	Trott A
PUBLISHER:	Mosby, 1991
TITLE:	Atlas of Cutaneous Surgery
AUTHOR:	Swanson NA
PUBLISHER:	Little, Brown & Company, 1987
TITLE:	Electrosurgery of the Skin
AUTHOR:	Pollack, SV
PUBLISHER:	Churchill Livingstone, 1991
TITLE:	Clinics Atlas of Office Procedures: Dermatologic Procedures
AUTHOR:	Alguire PC, Mather BM
PUBLISHER:	WB Saunders, March, Vol. 2, No. 1, 1999
TITLE:	Management of Facial Lines and Wrinkles
AUTHOR:	Blitzer A
PUBLISHER:	Lippincott, Williams & Wilkins, 2000
TITLE:	Principles and Techniques of Cutaneous Surgery
AUTHOR:	Lask G, Moy RL
PUBLISHER:	The McGraw-Hill Companies, 1996
TITLE:	Cosmetic Surgery of the Skin: Principles and Practice
AUTHOR:	Coleman III WP, Hanke CW, Alt TH, Asken S
PUBLISHER:	Mosby, 1997
TITLE:	Lasers in Cutaneous Medicine and Surgery
AUTHOR:	Ratz JL
PUBLISHER:	Mosby, 1986
TITLE:	Skin Lesions: a Practical Guide to Diagnosis, Management and Minor Surgery
AUTHOR:	Schofield J, Kneebone R
PUBLISHER:	Chapman & Hall Medical, 1996
TITLE:	Clinical Dermatology: a Color Guide to Diagnosis and Therapy, ed 3
AUTHOR:	Habif, TP
PUBLISHER:	Mosby, 1996
TITLE:	Cutaneous Cryosurgery: Principles and Clinical Practice, ed 2
AUTHOR:	Dawber R, Colver G, Jackson A, Pringle F
PUBLISHER:	Mosby, 1997
TITLE:	Manual of Skin Surgery: a Practical Guide to Dermatologic Procedures
AUTHOR:	Leffell DJ, Brown MD
PUBLISHER:	John Wiley & Sons, 1997
COST (US):	$49.95
COMMENT:	Includes common skin procedures, cryosurgery, electrosurgery, curettage, nail surgery
TITLE:	Clinics Atlas of Office Procedures: Respiratory Procedures
AUTHOR:	Elliott CG
PUBLISHER:	WB Saunders, Sept, Vol. 2, No. 3, 1999
TITLE:	Clinics Atlas of Office Procedures: Ear, Nose, and Throat Problems
AUTHOR:	Doyle G
PUBLISHER:	WB Saunders, Dec, Vol. 2, No. 4, 1999

BOX E-2

CD-ROM Resources for Procedures In Primary Care

TITLE:	Colposcopy Image Library Exercises in Pattern Recognition
AUTHOR:	Brotzman G, Spitzer M, Apgar B
PUBLISHER:	SABK Inc.; order from NPI
COST:	$250.00
COMMENT:	Over 800 cervical images demonstrating 3000+ features
TITLE:	Minor Surgery & Skin Lesions
AUTHOR:	Kneebone R, Schofield J.
PUBLISHER:	Primal Medical Information Ltd., 1998
COST (US):	$135.00
COMMENT:	Includes suture and excision techniques, computer animation, stills, and video with realistic models
TITLE:	CD-ROM Series for Primary Care Practitioners: Volume 1, Arthrocentesis (and other topics)
AUTHOR:	Tape TG, Moore GF
PUBLISHER:	Mosby, 1998
COST (US):	$99.00
COMMENT:	Multimedia components including video of techniques. Other discs expected in this series include gynecologic procedures, GI procedures, and geriatric procedures.
TITLE:	Procedural Skills for Internal Medicine
AUTHOR:	Wigton RS.
PUBLISHER:	Mosby, 1998
COST (US):	$200.00
COMMENT:	Includes central venous lines, thoracentesis, joint aspiration, lumbar puncture, abdominal paracentesis, arterial puncture for blood gas analysis, NG tube intubation
TITLE:	Clinical Dermatology Illustrated
PUBLISHER:	CMEA (Continuing Medical Education Associates)
COST (US):	$200.00
COMMENT:	Includes videotaped procedures, biopsy, cryosurgery, and electrodesiccation.
TITLE:	Comprehensive Review of Colposcopy
AUTHOR:	Developed by the American College of Obstetricians and Gynecologists and the American Society of Colposcopy and Cervical Pathology.
COST (US):	$180.00
COMMENT:	Interactive patient presentations and tutorials; includes 3-D animation.
TITLE:	Colposcopy CD-ROM for the Family Physician
PUBLISHER:	American Academy of Family Physicians
COST (US):	$110 (members); $140 (nonmembers); $90 (residents)
COMMENT:	Includes video and audio instructions, an extensive color photo atlas, searchable text documents, and an interactive test.
TITLE:	Nasolaryngoscopy for the Family Physician: a Self-Study CD-ROM Program
AUTHOR:	
PUBLISHER:	American Academy of Family Physicians
COST (US):	$50 (members); $75 (nonmembers); $45 (residents)
COMMENT:	Includes video and audio instructions, an extensive color photo atlas, searchable text documents, and an interactive test.
TITLE:	Soft-tissue Surgery: CD-ROM Program
PUBLISHER:	American Academy of Family Physicians
COST (US):	Complete Set (19 hrs of CME): $140 (members); $165 (nonmembers); $115 (residents)
	Basic Techniques CD (7 hrs of CME): $70 (members); $90 (nonmembers); $60 (residents)
	Advanced Techniques CD (6 hrs of CME): $60 (members); $85 (nonmembers); $50 (residents)
	Skin Biopsy Techniques CD (6 hrs of CME): $60 (members); $85 (nonmembers); $50 (residents)
COMMENT:	Includes the soft-tissue video, text and illustrations, and an interactive posttest
TITLE:	Colposcopy and LEEP CDs
PUBLISHER:	BioVision
TITLE:	Anatomy CDs
PUBLISHER:	Anatomical Chart Company
COMMENT:	Also charts, books, and models

Continued

BOX E-3
Videotape Resources for Procedures in Primary Care*

TITLE:	Echocardiography videotapes
PUBLISHER:	Mayo Clinic (200 First St, SW, Rochester, MN 55905; 1-507-266-6703; echome@mayo.edu)
COMMENT:	Over 50 tapes averaging $30.00 each on various echocardiographic findings
TITLE:	Dermatology Procedures for the Primary Care Physician
AUTHOR:	Presented by RS Scheinberg.
PUBLISHER:	CMEA (Continuing Medical Education Associates)
COST (US):	$149.00
COMMENT:	Covers wide variety of skin procedures
TITLE:	Gynecology Essentials I: Pelvic and Breast Exam
AUTHOR:	Presented by AL Nelson
PUBLISHER:	CMEA
COST (US):	$149.00
COMMENT:	Includes breast cyst aspiration technique
TITLE:	Gynecology Essentials II: Procedures
AUTHOR:	Presented by JH Liu, MA Thomas
PUBLISHER:	CMEA
COST (US):	$149.00
COMMENT:	Includes IUD insertion, diaphragm fitting, colposcopy, Norplant insertion and removal
TITLE:	Office Orthopedics: Essentials I.
PUBLISHER:	CMEA
COST (US):	$149.00
COMMENT:	Includes splinting and casting techniques, shoulder injections
TITLE:	Office Orthopedics: Essentials II.
PUBLISHER:	CMEA
COST (US):	$149.00
COMMENT:	Includes hip, knee, and ankle injections and other procedures
TITLE:	Cardiac Stress Testing for the Primary Care Physician
AUTHOR:	Presented by J Hizon, VF Froelicher
PUBLISHER:	CMEA
COST (US):	$149.00
TITLE:	Joint and Fracture Care Videos
	Office Evaluation & Treatment of the Joint/Fractures (3)
	The Knee, The Foot & Ankle, The Elbow, The Hip, The Wrist & Hand, The Shoulder, Joint Injection Syllabus(4), Set of Six Videotapes and Syllabus(5), Upper Extremities—Fractures(6), Lower Extremities—Fractures(7)
	Also Botox, sclerotherapy, microdermabrasion, radiofrequency techniques, skin biopsy, coding and reimbursement for skin lesion removal
AUTHOR:	Presented by RL Kalb
PUBLISHER:	National Procedures Institute (NPI)
COST (US):	$124.95(1); $114.95(2); $80.00(3); $40.00(4); $400.00(5); $80.00 (6&7)
COMMENT:	Includes six different tapes and syllabi that cover office evaluation and injections and joints; two tapes on fractures.
TITLE:	Vasectomy Video
AUTHOR:	Presented by CL Wilson
PUBLISHER:	The National Procedures Institute
COST (US):	$79.95
COMMENT:	Offers surgical footage of the no-scalpel vasectomy, including variations, pitfalls, and tips for success
TITLE:	Colposcopy Syllabus and Videotape
PUBLISHER:	American Academy of Family Physicians
COST (US):	$225 (members); $275 (nonmembers); $185 (residents)
COMMENT:	Provides evaluation and therapy for women presenting with preneoplastic changes of the genital system; includes a color photo atlas.

*Most companies that sell equipment will have videotapes or CDs available for instruction. Be sure to ask for them before completion of the sale.

BOX E-3—cont'd

Videotape Resources for Procedures in Primary Care

TITLE:	Soft-Tissue Surgery: Illustrated Manuals and Videotapes
PUBLISHER:	American Academy of Family Physicians
COST (US):	Complete Set (19 hrs of CME): $230 (members); $265 (nonmembers); $190 (residents)
	Book 1 w/videotape (7 hrs of CME): $105 (members); $120 (nonmembers); $85 (residents)
	Book 2 w/videotape (6 hrs of CME): $90 (members); $105 (nonmembers); $75 (residents)
	Book 3 w/videotape (6 hrs of CME): $90 (members); $105 (nonmembers); $75 (residents)
COMMENT:	Designed to enhance physician's ability to perform office skin surgery techniques
TITLE:	No-Scalpel Vasectomy Procedural Learning Package
PUBLISHER:	American Academy of Family Physicians
COST (US):	$75 (members); $95 (nonmembers); $65 (residents)
COMMENT:	Video and text
TITLE:	Nasolaryngoscopy: A Self-study Program for the Family Physician Interested in Nasolaryngoscopy
PUBLISHER:	American Academy of Family Physicians
COST (US):	$75 (members); $95 (nonmembers); $65 (residents)
COMMENT:	Covers upper airway endoscopy; includes a color photo atlas.
TITLE:	Patient Education Videotapes
	Genital Warts and Cervical Cancer: The Woman's Side; Genital Warts and Cancer: The Man's Side; vasectomy (emphasizing the no-scalpel technique); colonoscopy; microdermabrasion; Botox; LEEP; sclerotherapy; etc.
PUBLISHER:	NPI
COST (US):	$49.95 each video; $89.95 per set; $79.95 per vasectomy video
TITLE:	Physician Learning Tapes
	Suturing Techniques (1)
	No-Scalpel Vasectomy Demonstration Video (2)
	Office Evaluation & Treatment of the Joint/Fractures (3)
	The Knee, The Foot & Ankle, The Elbow, The Hip, The Wrist & Hand, The Shoulder, Joint Injection Syllabus(4), Set of Six Videotapes and Syllabus(5), Upper Extremities—Fractures(6), Lower Extremities—Fractures(7)
	Also Botox, sclerotherapy, microdermabrasion, radiofrequency techniques, skin biopsy, coding and reimbursement for skin lesion removal
PUBLISHER:	NPI
TITLE:	Colposcopy and LEEP Videos
PUBLISHER:	BioVision
COMMENT:	Also CDs, reference materials, and slides
TITLE:	Treatment of Hemorrhoids, Using the Infrared Coagulation
PUBLISHER:	Redfield Corp.
TITLE:	Liquid Nitrogen Cryotherapy
PUBLISHER:	Brymill Corp.
TITLE:	Gastroenterology Topics
PUBLISHER:	Glaxo Video Library

Advanced Cardiac Life Support (ACLS), Advanced Trauma Life Support (ATLS), and neonatal resuscitation (NRP). The principles of practicing and learning with models are evident to all who have taken part in these courses. The mannequins and models used for advanced course teaching are not described any further in this appendix; the focus is on other models available for learning individual procedures in primary care.

Realism is important in models for learning skills, but it comes with a high price tag. Companies such as Medisim Corp. and Limbs & Things Ltd. have developed highly realistic models for learning and practicing medical and surgical procedures.

Fig. E-1 shows the artificial breast model developed by Medisim Corp. The texture and feel of the skin and breast tissue is highly lifelike. With this model a breast cyst can be palpated and aspirated. The cyst will actually disappear when aspirated properly in a very real simulation of a clinical situation.

Fig. E-2 shows the simulated skin model produced by Limbs & Things Ltd. Once again the skin is very lifelike when handled with instruments. Modifications of this model can be used to practice cyst or lipoma excision in a realistic fashion. The skin simulator can be adapted for different features as is illustrated in Fig. E-3, which shows the skin with a sebaceous cyst for practice excision.

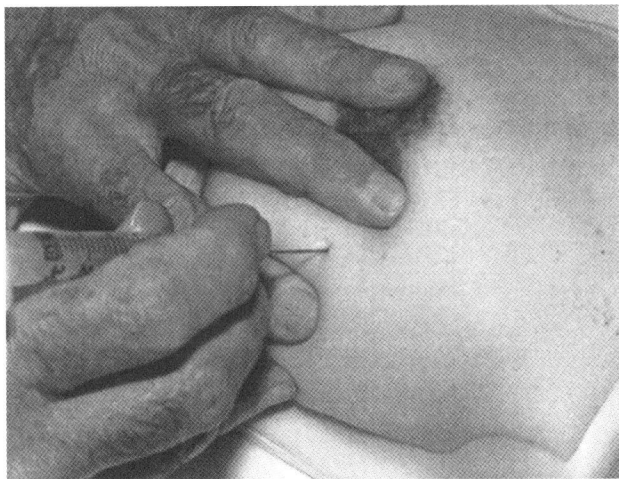

Fig. E-1
Artificial breast model. This lifelike model contains a cyst that can be aspirated as shown to simulate aspiration in a real clinical situation. (Courtesy Medisim Corp., Canada.)

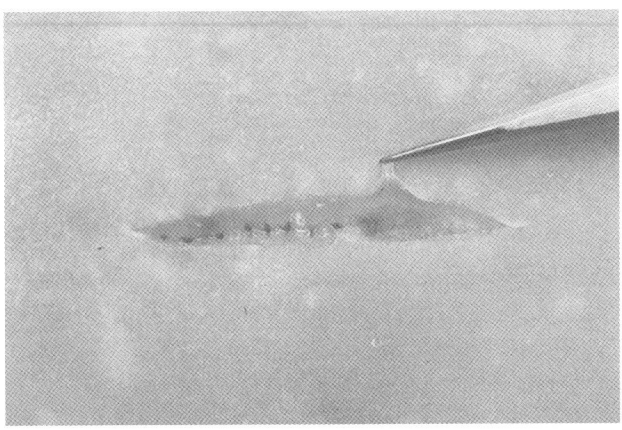

Fig. E-2
Skin Simulator model. The artificial skin is very lifelike and feels realistic when using a scalpel or other instruments. It can be used to practice incisions and suture techniques. (Courtesy Limbs & Things Ltd., United Kingdom.)

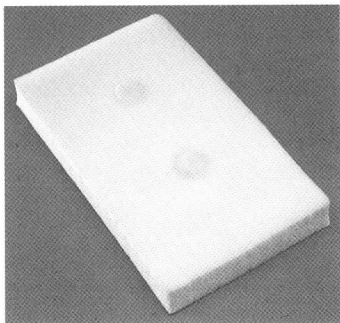

Fig. E-3
Adaptation of the skin simulator model, showing a sebaceous cyst that can be excised by the operator. The texture of the artificial skin and cyst are very lifelike and produce a realistic cyst excision procedure. (Courtesy Limbs & Things Ltd., United Kingdom.)

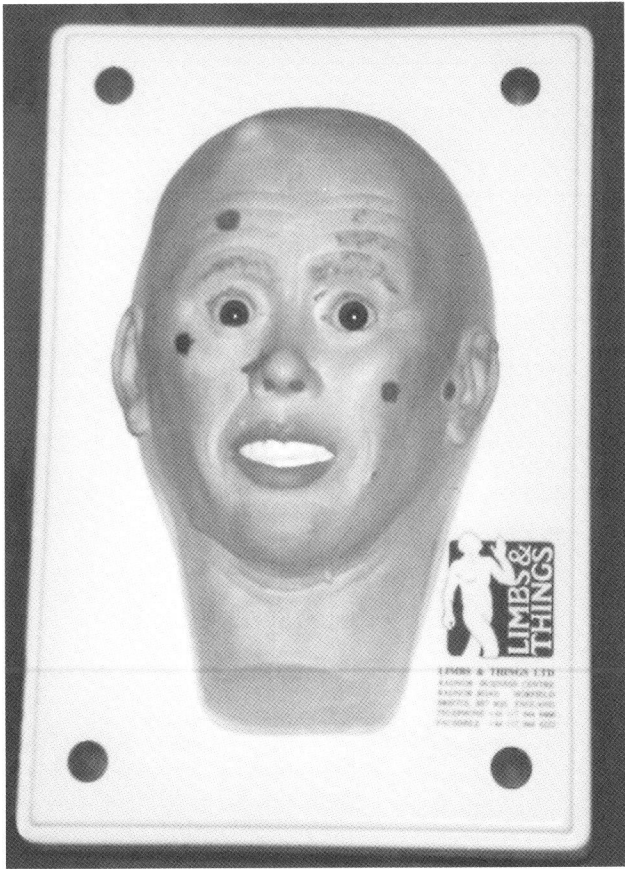

Fig. E-4
The Face with Lesions model has realistic skin lesions for diagnosis. Some lesions can be excised and the skin repaired to practice the fine surgical techniques necessary for the face. (Courtesy Limbs & Things Ltd., United Kingdom.)

Fig. E-4 shows the Face with Lesions, produced by Limbs & Things. Some of these lesions can be excised, creating a realistic simulation of skin surgery of the face, where scar orientation, lines of tension, etc. have to be considered.

Fig. E-5 shows the NPI Down's Cervical Model, which can be biopsied, frozen, and used for performing an endocervical curettage. Fig. E-6 illustrates a simple model that can be used to practice endometrial aspiration biopsy.

Fig. E-7 shows the very realistic NPI vasectomy model.

Table E-1 contains examples of several commercially available artificial models useful for learning procedures.

The cost of realistic, commercially available models for practicing procedure skills can be considerable, as the figures in Table E-1 illustrate. There is always the possibility of using less expensive, less realistic models for learning procedures. Some of these have been developed in ingenious fashions. For example, Cain *et al*

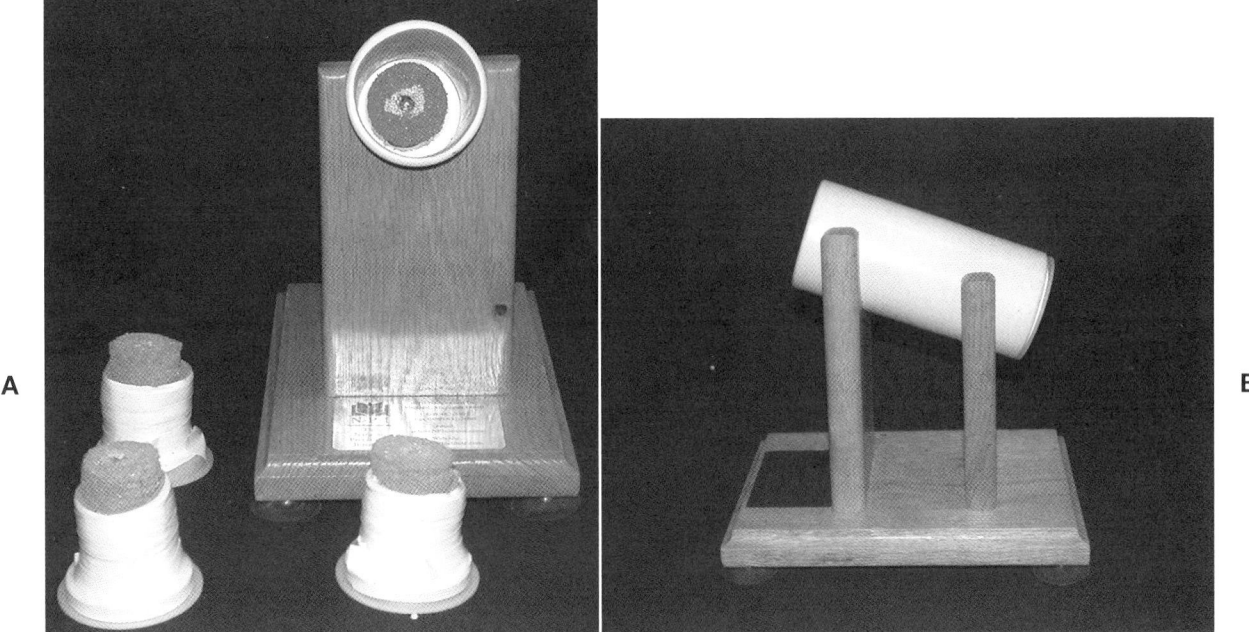

Fig. E-5
NPI Down's Cervical Model. This cervical model is unique because biopsies can be performed, endocervical curettage (ECC) can be practiced, and it can be frozen. **A,** With replaceable inserts. **B,** Side view. (Courtesy The National Procedures Institute, Midland, Mich.)

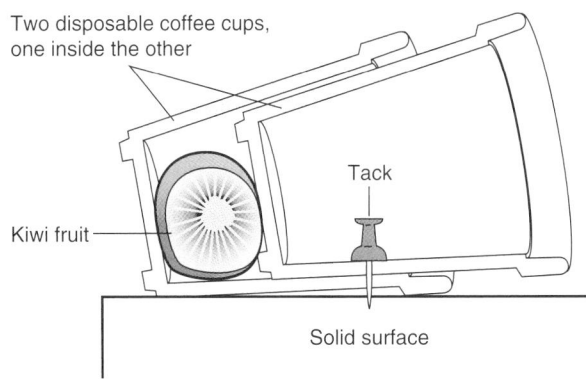

Fig. E-6
Simple model for practicing endometrial aspiration biopsy. The model is made from two disposable coffee cups, one fitted inside the other, with a kiwi fruit trapped between their bases. The aspiration catheter is passed through a hole in the bottom of the inner cup into the fruit. Aspiration of the fruit pulp simulates aspiration of endometrial tissue.

have shown that a simple model made from a face cloth can be effective for teaching episiotomy repair skills. Fig. E-6 illustrates a simple model made from coffee cups and kiwi fruit to create a simulation suitable for practicing endometrial aspiration techniques using the Pipelle catheter.

In addition, many biological materials are readily available at low cost and are somewhat effective for practicing techniques for a variety of procedures. These are often used in workshops and seminars. There is no reason these would not also be useful for the individual clinician to practice skills. Examples of these materials are listed in Table E-2.

COMPUTER SIMULATION AND VIRTUAL REALITY IN LEARNING PROCEDURES

Simulation as a teaching technique has played a significant role in the training of pilots. The advent of virtual reality means that there is now the capability to combine 3-D visual imagery with the ability to interact. This can create very realistic simulations, which are useful for training surgeons. The use of this has been demonstrated for laparoscopic and neurosurgical procedures and will be valuable for such techniques as sigmoidoscopy, colonoscopy, and hysteroscopy, among others. The advantage of this technology for procedures learning is that repeated realistic practice can be performed with the simulator, therefore reducing the requirement for supervised practice in a clinical setting. Although such virtual simulations are very expensive to develop, they can be reused indefinitely without deterioration and may be available, in part or in total, for long-distance learning over the Internet. There is currently an excellent computer simulator available from Immersion Medical to teach flexible sigmoidoscopy, colonoscopy, and EGD.

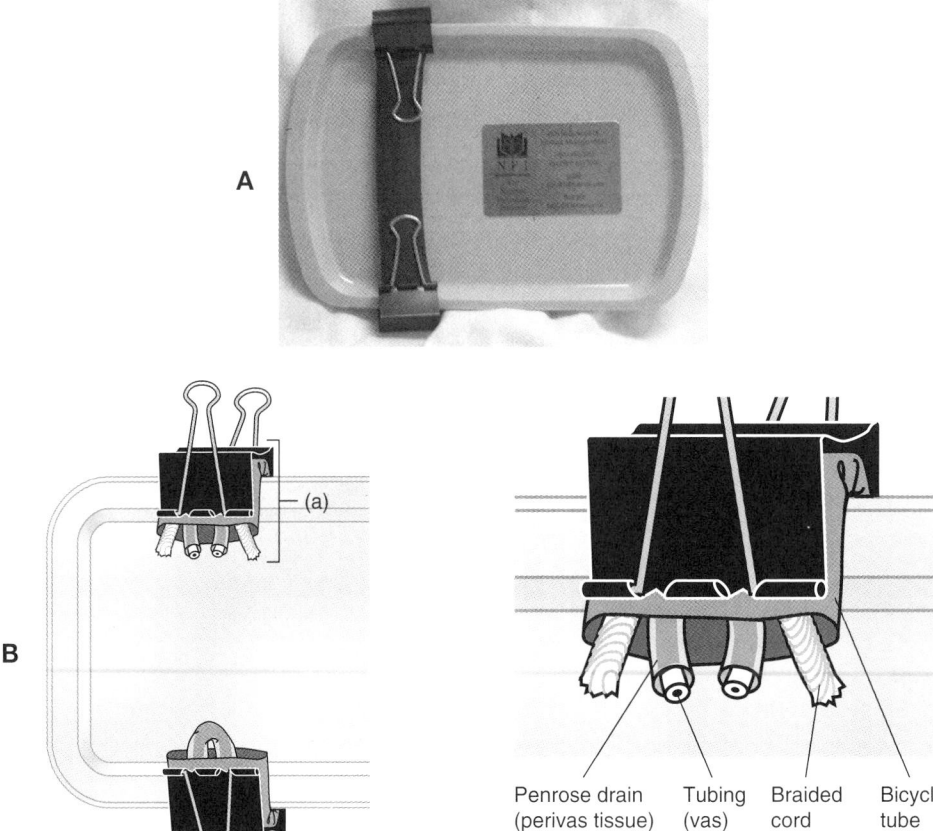

A

B

Penrose drain | Tubing | Braided | Bicycle
(perivas tissue) | (vas) | cord | tube

Close-up of (a)

Fig. E-7
NPI vasectomy model. **A,** Model. **B,** Illustration detailing the make-up of the model (underside) and what each material represents. The model is very realistic and provides a lifelike experience. (Courtesy The National Procedures Institute, Midland, Mich.)

Although expensive, this unit comes as close to the real-life experience as possible.

At the moment, virtual reality teaching is being used for the more complex surgical procedures. Eventually these techniques will prove valuable for training in many primary care procedures as well.

PRODUCERS AND SUPPLIERS

American Academy of Dermatology
930 E. Woodfield Road
Schaumburg, IL 60168-4014
Phone: 1-847-330-0230
Website: www.aad.org

American Academy of Family Physicians
11400 Tomahawk Creek Parkway
Leawood, KS 66211-2672
Phone: 1-800-274-2237
Website: www.aafp.org

American College of Emergency Physicians
1125 Executive Circle
Irving, TX 75038-2522
Phone: 1-800-798-1822
Website: www.acep.org

American Social Health Association (ASHA)
P.O. Box 13827
Research Triangle Park, NC 27709
Phone: 1-919-361-8400
Website: www.ashastd.org

American Society of Gastrointestinal Endoscopy
1520 Kensington Road, Suite 202
Oak Brook, IL 60523
Phone: 1-630-573-0600
Website: www.asge.org

TABLE E-1

Examples of Artificial Models Available for Learning and Practicing Procedures in Primary Care

Skill type and Model(s) Available	Producer(s)	Cost (US)*
Suturing		
Life/form suture arm	NASCO	$105.00
Skin Simulator Kit	Limbs & Things Ltd.	$85.00
Skin Lesion Excision		
Skin Simulator Kit	Limbs & Things Ltd.	$136.00
The Face with Lesions	Limbs & Things Ltd.	$430.00
Joint Models		
Excellent teaching models; lights up when needle is inserted correctly	Pacific Research Laboratories	
Joint Aspiration		
Knee	Limbs & Things Ltd.	$1450
Shoulder	Limbs & Things Ltd.	$1450
Wrist and hand	Limbs & Things Ltd.	$885
Breast Cyst Aspiration		
Breast model with cyst	Limbs & Things Ltd.	$325.00
Breast model with cyst	Medisim Corp.	$1000
Gynecology Procedures		
Gynecology simulator—IUD	NASCO	$605.00
Life/form episiotomy repair	NASCO	$94.00
Sigmoidoscopy/ Colonoscopy		
Life/form sigmoidoscopy model	NASCO	$470.00
Ingrown Toenail Surgery		
Ingrown toenail model	Limbs & Things Ltd.	$200.00
NPI Down's Cervical Model		
Biopsy and freeze	NPI	$145.95
Six replaceable inserts		$29.95
Vasectomy Model		
Simulates real life situation and helps prepare for the "first one"	NPI	$34.95
Models for Colonoscopy/Flexsigmoidoscopy, Gastroscopy, Obstetrical and Gynecologic Procedures, Injections, Catheterizations, Blood Drawing, and CPR Procedures		
These are the most extensive types and kinds of training models	Koken Company, Ltd.–International Dept	
Models for Injections/IVs, Venipuncture, Catheterization, Central Lines, Ostomy Care, Colonoscopy/Flexsigmoidoscopy, Wound Care/Suturing, Complete Patient Care (Adult /Child/Infant), Obstetrical and Gynecologic Procedures, Trauma Treatment, CPR Skills		
Also training videos and CDs, charts, and books	NASCO (Life/form)	
Models for Complete Care, CPR Skills, IVs and Injections (Adult and Infant), ALS (Adult/Child/Infant), Intubation, Trauma Treatment (Burn/Crushes/Amputations), Skeletons, Joint Models, Internal Organs		
Also, training videos and CDs, charts, and books	Medical Plastics Laboratory	
Anatomy Models		
Skin, organs, bones, circulatory system, and digestive system	Anatomical Chart Company	

*Costs are approximate and may vary depending on location.

TABLE E-2

Examples of Low-Cost Biological Materials Useful for Procedures Practice and Teaching

Model Type	Practice Use	Comments
Pig's feet	Suture techniques Minor surgery	Readily available at local butcher shops
Pig abdominal skin	Suture techniques Minor surgery	Readily available; quite thick and tough
Chicken breast	Cryosurgery Electrosurgery	
Chicken or turkey skin	Suture techniques Hemorrhoid banding	
Chicken legs	Tendon repair	
Beefsteak	Cryosurgery Electrosurgery	
Liver, beef, or kidney	Fine needle aspiration of lumps	Place inside surgical glove
Cow's eye	Corneal foreign body removal	
Kiwi fruit	Endometrial aspiration biopsy	Using pipelle
Bovine cervix[3]	Electrosurgical loop excision	

Anatomical Chart Company
8221 Kimball Ave.
Skokie, IL 60076
Phone: 1-800-ANATOMY
Website: www.anatomical.com

Association for Voluntary Surgical Contraception (see EngenderHealth)

BioVision, Inc.
63 Springgrove
Outremont, Quebec, Canada, H2V 3J1
Phone: 1-800-665-VIRUS
Website: www.bio-v.com

Brymill
105 Windmere Avenue
Ellington, CT 06029
Phone: 1-800-777-2796

CMEinfo.com
1008 Astoria Blvd, Suite A
Cherry Hill, NJ 08003
Phone: 1-856-874-0010
Website: www.cmeinfo.com

Continuing Medical Education, Inc. (CME Inc.)
1436 West Randolph St.
Chicago, IL 60607
Phone: 1-800-227-CMEA
Website: www.cmeinc.com

Creative Health Communications, Inc.
803 Elm St.
Essexville, MI 48734
Phone: 1-989-892-7614

EngenderHealth
440 Ninth Avenue
New York, NY 10001
Phone: 1-212-561-8000
Website: www.engenderhealth.org

Immersion Medical
55 West Watkins Mill Road
Gaithersburg, MD 20878
Phone: 1-301-984-3706
Website: www.immersion.com

Koken Company, Ltd. (International Dept.)
3-14-3 Mejiro
Toshima-Ku
Tokyo, Japan 171-0031
Phone: 81-3-3950-7622
Website: www.kokenmpc.co.jp

Limbs & Things Ltd.
Sussex Street, St Philips
Bristol, BS2 0RA, UK
Phone: +44 (0)117 311 0500
Website: www.limbsandthings.com

Medical Plastics Laboratory
P.O. Box 38
Gatesville, TX 76528
Phone: 1-800-433-5539
Website: www.medicalplastics.com

Medisim Corp.
RR 1 261804 concession 18
Hanover, Ontario
Canada N4N 3B8
Phone: 1-519-364-5855
Website: www.medisim.ca

NASCO (Lifeform): Health Care and Health Education Materials

901 Janesville Ave.

P.O. Box 901Fort Atkinson, WI 53538

Phone: 1-800-558-9595 (Canada: 1-800-668-0600

Website: www.enasco.com

The National Procedures Institute (NPI)

John Pfenninger, MD, Medical Director

4909 Hedgewood Dr.

Midland, MI 48642

Phone: 1-800-462-2492 or 1-800-866-NPICMEI

Website: www.npinstitute.com

Network for Continuing Medical Education

1 Harmon Plaza

Secaucus, NJ 07094

Phone: 1-800-223-0433

Website: www.ncme.com

Pacific Research Laboratories

10221 SW 188th Street

P.O. Box 409

Vashon, WA 98070

Phone: 1-206-463-5551

Website: www.sawbones.com

Redfield Corp.

336 W. Passaic Street

Rochelle Park, NJ 07662

Phone: 1-800-678-4472

The Skin Cancer Foundation

Box 561

New York, NY 10156

Phone: 1-800-SKIN-490

Website: www.skincancer.org

Staywell Krames

1100 Grundy Lane

San Bruno, CA 94066

Phone: 1-800-333-3032

Website: www.staywell.com *or* www.krames.com

CONCLUSION

In conclusion, the resources necessary for learning procedures range from courses at medical association meetings to books, CD-ROMs, artificial models, and simulations all the way to virtual reality.

Clinicians can learn the background for each procedure, indications, contraindications, complica-

tions, and techniques from books, CD-ROMs, and videotapes. However, the ability to practice psychomotor skills is crucial to gaining confidence. Suitable practice can be achieved by using appropriate artificial models, biological models, and simulations to develop psychomotor skills. Such practice will facilitate learning in the clinical setting and skill maintenance.

Primary care physicians should remember that their colleagues and specialist colleagues are valuable resources for learning procedures through their teaching, encouragement, and support during skill learning.

The listing of resources provided in this chapter should be helpful for teachers and learners in developing the skills and the support necessary to provide our patients with quality care in primary care procedures.

The National Procedures Institute (NPI) has agreed to become a "clearing house" and catalogue all procedural teaching aids available. Should the reader have information or resources that are helpful for the learner, they can be submitted to NPI. They will be catalogued and listed for those interested.

BIBLIOGRAPHY

Al-Turk M, Susman J: Perceived core procedural skills for Nebraska family physicians, *Fam Pract Res J* 12:297, 1992.

Cain JJ, Shirar E: A new method for teaching the repair of perineal trauma of birth, *Fam Med* 28:107, 1996.

Ferris DG, Waxman AG, Miller MD: Colposcopy and cervical biopsy educational training models, *Fam Med* 26(1):30, 1994.

Hawes R, Lehman GA, Hast J, et al: Training resident physicians in fiberoptic sigmoidoscopy: how many supervised examinations are required to achieve competence? *Am J Med* 80:465, 1986.

Moser DK, Coleman S: Recommendations for improving cardiopulmonary resuscitation skills retention, *Heart Lung* 21(4):372, 1992.

Pringle M, Hasler J, De Marco P: Training for minor surgery in general practice during preregistration surgical posts, *BMJ* 302:830, 1991.

Reynolds JL: Trends in vasectomy: analysis of one teaching practice, *Can Fam Physician* 44:552, 1998.

Satava RM. Virtual reality surgical simulator: the first steps, *Surg Endosc* 7:203, 1993.

The National Procedures Institute, Midland, Mich (website: www.npinstitute.com).

Wigton RS: Measuring procedural skills, *Ann Intern Med* 125:1003, 1996.

Universal Precautions

Madelyn Pollock

In discussion of universal precautions, it is important to understand the terminology used by the entities that promulgate the guidelines: primarily the Centers for Disease Control and Prevention (CDC) and the Occupational Safety and Health Administration (OSHA). Before 1983, the recommendations of public health agencies in handling blood and body fluids centered on special precautions taken with individuals known or suspected of being infected with bloodborne pathogens. These guidelines were known in the healthcare industry as "Blood and Body Fluid Precautions." With the increasing prevalence of HIV and HBV infections and the possibility that these diseases could be undiagnosed in patients, the CDC published "universal precautions" in 1983, recommending that blood and body fluids from *all patients* be considered potentially infectious and that rigorous infection control precautions be taken to minimize the risk of exposure to healthcare workers.

In 1996, the CDC modified its recommendations for infection control in the hospital setting introducing the terminology "standard precautions." To quote the CDC in *Guideline for Isolation Precautions in Hospitals,* "Standard Precautions synthesize the major features of Universal (Blood and Body Fluid) Precautions (designed to reduce the risk of transmission of bloodborne pathogens) and Body Substance Isolation (designed to reduce the risk of transmission of pathogens from moist body substances). Standard Precautions apply to (1) blood; (2) all body fluids, secretions, and excretions except sweat, regardless of whether or not they contain visible blood; (3) nonintact skin; and, (4) mucous membranes."

In 1991, OSHA, a federal agency within the Department of Labor, issued a separate standard. OSHA's Bloodborne Pathogen Standards is based on the concept of universal precautions. It is intended to protect employees who might be exposed to blood or body fluids on the job. (See references for complete statute.)

A physician or other administrator managing a healthcare facility must attend to both the practical matters of reducing risk to people as well as satisfying regulatory agencies through appropriate documentation and follow-through. This appendix focuses on the procedures, policies, and equipment recommended for reducing risk to healthcare workers (HCWs) and patients as well as meeting statutory regulations, especially as they apply to office procedures. It also outlines the requirements of an "Exposure Control Plan" as required for all healthcare employers by OSHA. Be aware that OSHA focuses only on employee protection.

Infection Prevention Strategy: Workers

Recommended guidelines for prevention of infections in HCWs encompass four domains: (1) formulation and implementation of site-specific policies in infection control (an "Exposure Control Plan"), (2) HCW screening and education at time of employment, (3) HCW immunization at the time of entry into an employment situation with risk, and (4) HCW use of barrier protection at time of risk of exposure. **All aspects of the prevention strategy require regular reevaluation and updating** as well as ongoing education of all workers.

The elements of an OSHA-compliant "Exposure Control Plan" are detailed in the statute and must be adapted to each individual site. In general, the plan must include common policies (Table F-1) as well as documentation of orientation and ongoing training of personnel. It must also delineate policies for record keeping (employee health screen information, records of training, records of any incidents or injuries, etc.). The plan must be in written form and available to all employees. There should be evidence of periodic review of the plan for currency and accuracy. Proprietary agencies, including some medical supply marketers, sell "kits" for preparation of a site's "Exposure Control Plan" that include templates customizable to a site. Federal regulations require that all HCWs be evaluated initially with a health inventory. This should include determination of suitability for a position at risk for infectious exposure as well as determination of the worker's immune status for vaccine-preventable ill-

TABLE F-1

Infection Control Policies for a Typical Physician's Office

Area	Specific Details to Include
Handwashing	Rules for both areas with and without running water available. Handwashing *before and after* eating, drinking, smoking, applying cosmetics, handling contact lenses, or using the restroom as well as between patients.
Contaminated sharps	Both disposable and reusable sharps; no recapping of needles or use one-handed recapping technique; disposal of filled sharps containers.
Areas for eating, drinking, smoking, and applying cosmetics	Application of lip balm should be mentioned specifically.
Contaminated equipment	Follow manufacturers' guidelines for disinfection.
Personal Protection Equipment (PPE)	Use of gloves, gowns, masks, goggles, and impervious aprons.
Cleaning/disposal of PPE	Method of documentation of cleaning.
Contaminated spills	Choice of cleaning agent.
Contaminated laundry	Bagging in room of use; use of closed bags for transport.
Employee HBV vaccination	Hepatitis B vaccine declination form (OSHA Regulation 1910.1030 App. A).
Postexposure evaluation and follow-up	Procedure to document details of injury; testing of both employee and source individual; document counseling; procedure for administration of antiretroviral agents.
Employee training	Initial and ongoing training schedule.
Specimen handling	Separation of food items and specimens; use of gloves when handling specimens.
Triage of patients	Carefully screen patients for communicable diseases at check-in so that susceptible workers can avoid contact, and infectious patients can be removed promptly from contact with other waiting patients.

TABLE F-2

Summary of Advisory Committee on Immunization Practices (ACIP) Recommendations for Healthcare Workers Including Special Conditions

Worker status	Hepatitis B Recombinant Vaccine	Influenza Vaccine	Measles/Mumps/Rubella Live-Virus Vaccine	Varicella Zoster Live-Virus Vaccine
Healthy, non-pregnant	R	R	R	R
Pregnant	R	R	C	C
HIV-positive	R	R	R*	C
Severe immunosuppression	R	R	C	C
Asplenia	R	R	R	R
Renal failure	R	R	R	R
Diabetes	R	R	R	R
Alcoholism and cirrhosis	R	R	R	R

Adapted from Centers for Disease Control and Prevention. Immunization of Health-Care Workers: Recommendations of the Advisory Committee on Immunization Practices (ACIP) and the Hospital Infection Control Practices Advisory Committee (HICPAC), *MMWR* 46(No. RR-18):36, 1997.
C, Contraindicated; *R,* recommended.
*Contraindicated in persons with HIV infection and severe immunosuppression.

nesses (OSHA's only *required* immunization policy is for hepatitis B vaccine). These health screens must be recorded in written form, and workers must be reevaluated periodically. Each employee in the facility should have a health record available and updated with the necessary information. This health record should be maintained separately from the employee's other employment record and must be maintained for 30 years by OSHA regulations. At this initial evaluation, a determination of the need for additional vaccination should be made. Current CDC recommendations are listed in Table F-2.

After initial assessment, infection control in HCWs continues with education. Simple hand washing is the most important activity in reducing transmission of infections in the workplace. Education about policies such as sharps disposal, no recapping of needles, and prompt reporting of injury is crucial. Healthcare facilities should take steps to ensure initial orientation to infection control policies for all employees and periodic reinstruction of all established personnel. Policies should be written clearly and include supporting information so that employees can understand the rationale for the policies. Employees should be evaluated for the specific risk associated with their particular job and special education for risk reduction implemented and documented.

An often overlooked aspect of an infection control strategy is the immunization of HCWs who are at risk for vaccine-preventable diseases. Appropriate use of vaccines in susceptible individuals cannot only help prevent nosocomial infections in HCWs, but also reduce loss of workdays because of isolation following potential exposures. In addition, prevention of infection through optimal use of vaccinations and/or laboratory determination of immune status is much more cost effective than case management following an exposure in a nonimmunized HCW. Immune status of all healthcare facility personnel should be recorded at initiation of employment, and the Hepatitis B vaccination series should be made available to all susceptible employees (OSHA 1910.1030). An employee who declines the vaccine should sign the Hepatitis B Vaccine Declination Form (Fig. F-1). Barrier protection using personal protection equipment (PPE) is the last line of prevention for HCW exposure to potentially infectious material. All HCWs must use appropriate personal protective equipment (PPE) for the task at hand. In summary:

- Gloves should be worn when contact with any blood, body fluids, mucous membranes, or broken skin is anticipated or possible; this includes contact with soiled items or surfaces and for venipuncture.
- Masks and eye shields should be worn when splashes of blood or body fluids are possible or during procedures in which blood, body fluids, or tissue could be aerosolized.
- Gowns or impervious aprons should be worn in situations in which blood or body fluids could contaminate the HCW's clothing.

Hepatitis B Vaccine Declination Form

I understand that due to my occupational exposure to blood or other potentially infectious materials I may be at risk of acquiring hepatitis B virus (HBV) infection. I have been given the opportunity to be vaccinated with hepatitis B vaccine, at no charge to myself. However, I decline hepatitis B vaccination at this time. I understand that by declining this vaccine, I continue to be at risk of acquiring hepatitis B, a serious disease. If in the future I continue to have occupational exposure to blood or other potentially infectious materials and I want to be vaccinated with hepatitis B vaccine, I can receive the vaccination series at no charge to me.

_____   _____
Signature of employee   Date

Fig. F-1
Hepatitis B Vaccine Declination (Mandatory): 1910.1030 App A (From OSHA Regulations (Standards – 29 CFR) [56 FR 64004, Dec. 06, 1991, as amended at 57 FR 12717, April 13, 1992; 57 FR 29206, July 1, 1992; 61 FR 5507, Feb, 1996].)

- Gowns, aprons, and gloves must be changed and discarded between patients.
- Mouth-to-mouth ventilation should be performed using a "mouth-to-mask" ventilation device with no direct contact between the patient's mouth and the HCW's.

See Table F-1 for an example of an office guideline, and consult the OSHA statute for a detailed discussion of the regulations.

Environmental Considerations

Environmental considerations for prevention of infection from the HCW to the patient (or between patients) can be defined in three areas: (1) surface disinfection, (2) instrument sterilization/disinfection, and (3) policies regarding function of actively infected HCWs in the healthcare facility.

A full discussion of all the issues in the choice and use of agents for disinfection of surfaces and instruments is beyond of the scope of this appendix. The Association for Professionals in Infection Control and Epidemiology, Inc. (APIC) has published a comprehensive guideline that can serve as a reference for further details. In general, it is important to know some of the history of this area in order to understand some of the terminology. A classification developed in the 1960s by E. H. Spaulding is still used today to determine appropriate levels of decontamination of medical surfaces and equipment. In general, Spaulding divided devices into three levels of decontamination. The first level is *"critical,"* meaning that the device enters sterile tissue or the vascular system. These devices must be *sterilized,* that is, devoid of microbial life, including spores. This can be accomplished by heat, ethylene oxide gas, and a number of immersion techniques. For many physicians' offices, a small autoclave accomplishes the task of rendering reusable devices and instruments sterile between patients. For critical instruments that cannot be subjected to heat or for facilities in which use of heat or ethylene oxide sterilization is not available, several immersion fluids are available. Manufacturers' recommendations for use of these solutions, with special attention to treatment time, should be followed closely.

The second level is *"semi-critical"* for devices that touch mucous membranes. These include endoscopes, endotracheal tubes, and laryngoscopes as well as thermometers. These devices must be subjected to *high-level disinfection.* Since many of these devices cannot be subjected to heat, special cleaning devices and fluids must be used for disinfection of these instruments. It is important to follow manufacturers' recommendations completely to avoid incomplete disinfection as well as damage to the instruments. Again, thorough cleaning of instruments prior to disinfection is important. Routine changing of fluids and cleaning tools is an important part of an effective routine.

The third level of decontamination according to Spaulding is *"non-critical"* and includes stethoscopes, examination room surfaces, and bedpans. These items should be cleansed appropriately with agents that are known to kill most surface microbes without significant corrosion of the items or without being excessively toxic to the HCW. Typical agents in this category include alcohols (ethyl and isopropyl), household bleach (5.2% sodium hypochlorite), phenols, iodophors, and quaternary ammonium compounds. These agents are commonly sold by medical supply companies for use on surfaces. Manufacturers' guidelines must be understood and followed. Be aware of the corrosive nature of some of these products on certain surfaces, and follow instructions for protection of HCWs from any potentially toxic fumes.

An important concept in the handling of reusable instruments is the direction of workflow. It is important that "clean" and "soiled" areas are separated and policies are established so that item flow does not risk contamination of "clean" items. There should be clearly defined areas for the receipt of contaminated items with physical barriers preventing accidental contamination. Policies for maintaining these processing standards should be clear to all workers.

Use and maintenance of autoclaves in an office should be governed by policies and routine, reflecting good infection control practices. The first step in sterilization of instruments is thorough cleaning (removal of surface debris) of all instruments to be sterilized. Biological and chemical indicators for use in heat sterilizers should be used and checked consistently. Temperature and pressure and results of indicators should be recorded in a log form. Remember, biological indicators require use of a manufacturer-recommended incubator for proper use.

Regarding transmission of disease from the ill or potentially ill HCW to the patient, the healthcare facility's administration is responsible for development and implementation of policies to address this issue. At times, such policies may result in restriction of HCWs from patient contact, therefore it is important that policies be designed to encourage reporting of exposures and illnesses protecting wages, benefits, and job status if possible. The policies should reflect exclusions resulting from both acute infection and known exposure. The policies should be clear regarding who in the facility is responsible for making isolation exclusions.

The decision-making falls into two broad categories that require quite different management and follow-through. For chronic bloodborne communicable diseases such as HIV and Hepatitis B, the CDC recommends the HCW ". . .not perform exposure-prone invasive procedures until counsel from an expert review panel has been sought, which will determine under what circumstances the worker may or may not perform exposure-prone, invasive procedures." Exposure-prone invasive procedures include those that involve manipulating a needle inside the body or placing the fingers and a needle or other sharp instrument in a poorly visualized or highly confined anatomic site. The CDC recommends no restrictions for workers with chronic hepatitis B if hepatitis B e antigen becomes negative and currently recommends no restriction regarding workers with hepatitis C. Each facility should develop its own policy regarding HIV and hepatitis B– and C–infected workers.

For more acute disease entities, the CDC has developed guidelines that can be adapted for most facilities (see Table F-3). The guidelines summarize recommended work restrictions including duration. These guidelines apply to both exposure and infection with the disease. They should always be compared with any local or state guidelines that may apply in your area. Consideration of your facility's patient population and the worker's level of patient exposure is important. In jobs in which close contact with patients is unlikely, a worker might be able to remain on the job but could use certain precautions (such as wearing a mask) and still not jeopardize patients or co-workers.

Conclusion

It is important that the leadership of every healthcare facility, regardless of size, become familiar with the standards and regulations regarding infection control in the workplace. The facility must formulate and implement policies to protect healthcare workers as well as patients from communicable diseases. These policies should reflect current guidelines from the CDC and comply with regulations promulgated by OSHA. In addition to this appendix, the infection control officer of your local hospital should be considered as an ally and information source in development or review of policies and procedures for your particular site.

General Resources

Centers for Disease Control and Prevention
1600 Clifton Road, NE
Atlanta, GA 30333
Phone: 1-404-639-3311
Division of AIDS/HIV Prevention: 1-800-843-6356
Website: www.cdc.gov

U.S. Department of Labor
Occupational Safety and Health Administration
200 Constitution Avenue, NW
Washington, DC 20210
Website: www.osha.gov

TABLE F-3

Summary of Suggested Work Restrictions for Healthcare Workers Exposed to or Infected with the Most Common Acute Communicable Diseases of Importance in the Ambulatory Setting*

Disease/Problem	Work Restriction	Duration
Conjunctivitis	Restrict from patient contact and contact with the patient's environment.	Until discharge ceases
CMV infection	No restriction	
Diarrheal diseases		
Acute stage	Restrict from patient contact, contact with the patient's environment and food handling	Until symptoms resolve
Convalescent stage (*Salmonella spp.*)	Restrict from care of high-risk patients	Until symptoms resolve; consult with local health agencies regarding need for negative cultures
Enteroviral infections	Restrict from care of infants, neonates, and immunocompromised patients and their environments	Until symptoms resolve
Hepatitis A	Restrict from patient contact, contact with the patient's environment, and food handling	Until 7 days after onset of jaundice
Herpes simplex		
Genital	No restriction	
Hands (Whitlow)	Restrict from patient contact and contact with the patient's environment	Until lesions heal
Orofacial	Evaluate for need to restrict from care of high-risk patients	
Measles		
Active	Exclude from duty	Until 7 days after rash appears
Post-exposure (susceptible)	Exclude from duty	From 5th day after first exposure through 21st day after last exposure and/or 4 days after rash appears
Meningococcal infection	Exclude from duty	Until 24 hours after start of effective therapy
Mumps		
Active	Exclude from duty	Until 9 days after onset of parotitis
Post-exposure (susceptible)	Exclude from duty	From 12th day after first exposure through 26th day after last exposure or until 9 days after onset of parotitis
Pediculosis	Restrict from patient contact	Until treated and observed to be free of adult and immature lice
Rubella		
Active	Exclude from duty	Until 5 days after rash appears
Post-exposure (susceptible)	Exclude from duty	From 7th day after first exposure through the 21st day after last exposure
Scabies	Restrict from patient contact	Until cleared by medical evaluation
S. aureus infection		
Active, still draining lesions	Restrict from patient contact, contact with patient's environment, and food handling	Until lesions have resolved
Carrier state	No restriction unless personnel are epidemiologically linked to transmission of the organisms	
Streptococcal, group A infection	Restrict from patient contact, contact with patient's environment, and food handling	Until 24 hr after adequate treatment started
Tuberculosis		
Active disease	Exclude from duty	Exclude from duty until proven noninfectious
PPD converter	No restriction	
Varicella		
Active		Until all lesions dry and crusted
Post-exposure (susceptible)	Exclude from duty	From 10th day after first exposure through the 21st day (28th day if VZIG given) after last exposure
Zoster		
Localized in healthy person	Cover lesions, restrict from care of high-risk patients	Until all lesions dry and crusted
Generalized or localized in the immunocompromised person	Restrict from patient contact	Until all lesions dry and crusted
Post-exposure (susceptible)	Restrict from patient contact	From 10th day after first exposure through the 21st day (28th day if VZIG given) after last exposure, or if varicella occurs, until all lesions dry and crusted
Viral URI, acute febrile	Consider excluding from the care of high-risk patients or contact with their environment during community outbreak of RSV and influenza	Until acute symptoms resolve

*Current Post-Exposure Prophylaxis Recommendations, *MMWR Recomm Rep* 47(RR-7):1, 1998. Available at www.cdc.gov/ncidod/hip/guide/phspep.htm.
CMV, Cytomegalovirus; *RSV,* respiratory syncytial virus; *VZIG,* varicella zoster immunoglobulin.

Association for Professionals in Infection Control and Epidemiology, Inc.
1275 K Street, NW, Suite 1000
Washington, DC 20005-4006
Phone: 1-202-789-1890
Website: www.apic.org

SPECIFIC RESOURCES

OSHA Regulation: Exposure Control Plan. Occupational Safety and Health Administration, Department of Labor. 29 CFR Part 1910.1030, Occupational exposure to blood-borne pathogens; final rule. Federal Register 1991;56:64004-182. Available at www.osha-slc.gov/pls/oshaweb/owadisp.show_document?p_table=STANDARDS&p_id=10051.

Current Post-Exposure Prophylaxis Recommendations, *MMWR Recomm Rep* 47(RR-7):1, 1998. Available at www.cdc.gov/ncidod/hip/guide/phspep.htm.

BIBLIOGRAPHY

Bolyard EA, Tablan OC, Williams WW, et al: The Hospital Infection Control Practices Advisory Committee: Special article: guideline for infection control in healthcare personnel, 1998, *Am J Infect Control* 26:289, 1998.

Centers for Disease Control and Prevention: Public Health Service guidelines for the management of health-care worker exposures to HIV and recommendations for postexposure prophylaxis, *MMWR Recomm Rep* 47(RR-7):1, 1998.

Centers for Disease Control and Prevention: Recommendations for preventing transmission of human immunodeficiency virus and hepatitis B virus to patients during exposure-prone invasive procedures, *MMWR Recomm Rep* 40(RR-8):1, 1991.

Garner JS and the Hospital Infection Control Practices Advisory Committee: Guidelines for isolation precautions in hospitals, CDC Guidelines, published Jan 1, 1996.

Rutala WA: APIC guideline for selection and use of disinfectants: 1994, 1995, and 1996 APIC Guidelines Committee: Association for Professionals in Infection Control and Epidemiology, Inc, *Am J Infect Control* 24:313, 1996.

Patient Education Handouts and Consent Forms

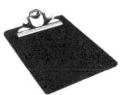 *Patient Education Handout*

CONSCIOUS SEDATION

Conscious sedation is used by your doctor to prevent or reduce pain and anxiety during medical, surgical, diagnostic, or therapeutic procedures. It is achieved by the intravenous administration of sedative, amnesic (so you will forget), and analgesic (pain killing) drugs. The goal of conscious sedation is to place you in a state where you are still conscious but are relaxed and comfortable while the clinician performs the procedure.

You should be aware that there are certain risks with any medical, surgical, or diagnostic procedure, including conscious sedation. The medications used in conscious sedation may include potent narcotics, tranquilizers, hypnotic, and sedative drugs. This is why you will be closely monitored during the procedure. There is always a risk of oversedation, which may result in decreased or absent breathing, decreased blood pressure, and other problems. If undiagnosed or left untreated, these complications are serious and can result in death. Your clinician has remedies for these problems immediately available and will use them if necessary.

There are certain preparations you must take in order to have conscious sedation. A history and physical examination must be performed, and occasionally laboratory tests, to make sure you are in suitable health to have conscious sedation. These preparations also include having nothing to eat or drink for a few hours prior to the procedure (your clinician will tell you specifically how many hours, depending on your medical history). This is important because it is both dangerous and uncomfortable to vomit while under conscious sedation. You must also arrange for a responsible adult to transport you home and to be with you overnight. You will need to sign a consent form for both the medical/surgical procedure and for conscious sedation.

Just before beginning the procedure, your clinician will apply several monitoring devices to you. These will monitor your blood pressure, pulse rate, and blood oxygen levels. Other monitors may also be connected. An IV will also be started. Supplemental oxygen may also be administered through a nasal tube or mask. Once these preparations are underway, your clinician will give you sedation medication through your IV. When you are properly sedated, your clinician will begin the procedure. His or her assistant will monitor your condition throughout the procedure.

There will be a period of monitoring your vital signs and oxygen levels after your clinician has completed the procedure. This is because the medications do not wear off immediately afterward. You should report any pain, nausea, anxiety, or other symptoms or concerns to your clinician or to the person in charge of monitoring your condition. When your clinician has determined that you are able to go home, you will be discharged in the company of a responsible adult. You will be given a list of instructions to follow at home, as well as a telephone number to call if you experience any problems, such as difficulty breathing, bleeding, severe pain, or other complications.

Do not operate a motor vehicle or other dangerous equipment for 24 hours after conscious sedation. Do not make any important decisions or sign any legal documents for 24 hours. Also, ask your clinician what medications you should or may take, and what to specifically avoid. You should specifically avoid alcohol, sedatives, and other depressant drugs for 24 hours. Call your clinician's office if you have questions, concerns, or new symptoms.

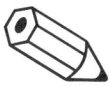 *Patient Consent Form*

CONSCIOUS SEDATION

My clinician, _____ , has informed me that I may receive conscious sedation for relief of pain, anxiety, or discomfort during my scheduled medical, surgical, or diagnostic procedure. I understand that the medications used for conscious sedation may cause side effects, including but not limited to, problems with breathing, oversedation, pain or discomfort with injection, muscle stiffness, nausea, vomiting, temporary amnesia, difficulty voiding, constipation, allergic reactions, or infection.

Less common complications include, but are not limited to, injury to teeth, pneumonia, nerve injury, heart problems, stroke, brain damage, respiratory arrest, cardiac arrest, and death.

My questions regarding conscious sedation have been answered. I understand the benefits and risks of conscious sedation, and I wish to proceed. If a complication should develop, I give permission for my clinician to take the necessary corrective action.

_____   _____
Patient's signature   *Date/Time*

_____   _____
Witness' signature   *Date/Time*

One copy for chart; one copy for patient.

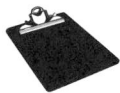

Patient Education Handout

EPIDURAL ANESTHESIA

Your clinician may offer a choice of techniques to increase your comfort during the birth of a child or during or after surgery, including epidural anesthesia or epidural analgesia. If used with childbirth, you should know that these procedures are optional and do carry certain risks. Although there is general agreement that epidural anesthesia is the most successful method for improving comfort during labor and delivery, it is not necessary to have any procedure for analgesia or anesthesia to have a healthy baby.

Epidural procedures involve injecting doses of a local anesthetic and/or a narcotic through a needle or through a catheter (i.e., a long, small-diameter plastic tube) into the epidural space (i.e., the space just outside the spinal cord). Epidural anesthesia may be administered while you are in the sitting position or with you lying on the side with your back arched toward the clinician. An assistant will help you obtain the proper position and stay with you during the performance of the procedure.

Your clinician will start by pressing on your lower back to determine the exact area for the injection. Then an antibacterial solution will be applied to the area to prevent infection. This will be followed by the injection of a local anesthetic into your skin to numb the area in preparation for insertion of a needle into the epidural space. After inserting the needle, a test dose of the medication will be injected. You will then be asked to remain in the same position for several minutes.

There is always the risk of bruising, bleeding, or infection at the site with such a procedure. Although most patients do not experience any side effects, several others can occur. Blood pressure (BP) and pulse rate may rise or drop, you may feel nervous (or unusual) or may start to feel numbness and tingling sensations in your legs, feet, or other parts of your body. You should inform the clinician immediately if any unusual symptoms appear after the test injection. The clinician is prepared to treat any of these side effects promptly and safely.

If your clinician is going to use a catheter, he or she will carefully insert it through the needle into the epidural space. The clinician will then remove the needle. The catheter may be left in place for additional injections to prolong anesthesia. In addition, the catheter may be hooked to a pump for automatic injections of the medication.

Studies do not agree as to whether epidurals increase the risk for cesarean section. However, there is consensus among studies that epidurals prolong labor, especially the second stage, which begins when you start pushing. There is also consensus that epidurals increase the need for assisted delivery and the likelihood of maternal fever. The cause of the fever is unknown.

Fetal heart rate changes are common with epidurals. Using extra IV fluids before performing the procedure may minimize this risk. However, these extra fluids must be used very cautiously if you have problems with high blood pressure.

A possible postoperative complication is a headache. It may occur if the epidural needle is inadvertently advanced into the space in the spinal canal where the spinal fluid is contained. Occasionally the headache will be severe and require treatment by an injection of blood into the area where the epidural needle was originally inserted. Rarely, more serious or permanent complications may occur, including paralysis, infection, or bleeding.

If you are being treated for postoperative pain, your clinician may attach the epidural catheter to an infusion pump or a patient-controlled epidural (PCEA) pump. The epidural catheter may be left in place for several days. If no further surgical procedures are expected (e.g., tubal ligation) or you no longer requires pain relief, the catheter will be removed.

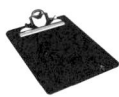

Patient Education Handout

PEDIATRIC SEDATION

In order to perform the medical or surgical procedure on your child, it is necessary to use sedation. Please read this handout carefully. We will be glad to answer any questions that you may have.

Pediatric sedation simply means that medication is given to cause sleepiness (sedation) in your child. Once your child is sleepy, the surgical or medical procedure becomes easier and safer. The medicine may be given by mouth, dropped into the nose, or by injection.

Although pediatric sedation is very safe, occasional temporary problems are possible. Most common are problems that would occur in any sleepy child. These include difficulty walking and eating or drinking until fully awake. Less common are reactions to one of the medications given. These include being fearful while waking up and prolonged sedation. If the medicine was injected, local irritation at the injection site is possible.

If your child has any unusual or worrisome problems afterwards, please call this office immediately.

Special Precautions

Your child may remain sleepy for up to 2 hours after the procedure. During this time, it is okay to allow your child to rest where he or she can be observed. Provide help in standing or walking if needed and do not give any food or drink until fully awake. Finally, give no medicines during this time unless you were specifically instructed to do so.

Additional Instructions

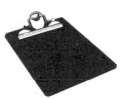 *Patient Education Handout*

PERIPHERAL NERVE BLOCKS AND FIELD BLOCKS

What is a Peripheral Nerve Block?

A technique for placing local anesthetics (numbing medicine) around a nerve so that the area that the nerve supplies will not feel pain.

What is a Field Block?

A technique for anesthetizing (numbing) an area so that surgery can be performed or stitches can be placed without you feeling pain.

Why Do I Need This Procedure?

You need surgery that is painful, and the block will allow you to have it without feeling pain.

How Do I Prepare for a Peripheral Nerve Block or Field Block?

Tell your doctor if you have had any injury to the area, and if you feel numbness or tingling there.

What Happens During the Procedure?

The doctor cleans the area, then injects the local anesthetics (numbing medicine) with a small needle. You will feel a stick and a burn as the medicine goes in.

What Happens After the Procedure?

Your skin will get numb.

What are the Benefits of This Procedure?

You will not feel pain during your surgical procedure.

What Do I Need to do Following the Procedure to Prevent Infection?

Keep the skin clean.

When Should I Call My Healthcare Provider?

If there is bleeding or excess pain. Numbness, tingling, or weakness that lasts more than 3 hours should be reported.

Websites That May be of Interest to You:

www.sambahq.org (The Society for Ambulatory Anesthesia)

www.soba.org (Society for Office Based Anesthesia)

www.oyston.com/anaes/local.html (A patient's guide to local and regional anesthesia)

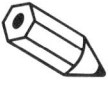

Patient Consent Form

PERIPHERAL NERVE BLOCKS AND FIELD BLOCKS

I came to the office of my clinician, _____, on _____ (date) for the following condition (description of diagnosis, etiology, and differential diagnosis):

We discussed the different treatments possible and the risks of not treating the condition. Based on the advice given by my clinician, _____, and my own judgment, I agree to undergo the following procedure (description of anesthetic, procedure, and dressing):

We discussed the different outcomes that could occur and most of the possible complications. I know that anytime an incision (cut) is made in the skin that pain, scarring, bleeding, infection, and recurrence of the lesion can occur. I am aware that other complications could occur that we could not foresee. I agree to follow the instructions for self-care after the procedure and to return for follow-up care on _____ (date).

I will call the office or answering service at _____ if any problems arise before the scheduled follow-up visit.

_____
Patient's signature

_____
Date/Time

_____
Witness' signature

_____
Date/Time

One copy for chart; one copy for patient.

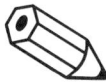 *Patient Consent Form*

TRIGGER-POINT INJECTION

Tender areas or nodules under the skin are referred to as "trigger points." Injection of these tender points with medication may alleviate or greatly relieve the discomfort. At times the trigger points may produce pain in an area distant from the site of origin. The physician performing the procedure will palpate the various muscle groups to locate the trigger points and the most tender areas. An antiseptic solution will be applied to the skin as the initial step. Next the medication will be injected into one or more painful areas. You should feel immediate relief; however, the pain may return with even greater intensity than the original pain. Several follow-up injections may be necessary.

In some cases, complications may occur, which include the following:

1. Dizziness or fainting
2. Skin infection
3. Reactions to the local anesthetic
4. Bruising
5. Inflammation or nerve injury
6. Temporary worsening of the pain if the injections are around the chest or back
7. Collapsed lung

By my signature, I certify that I have read and understand the procedure as outlined above, including the possibility of complications, and I hereby authorize the physician to perform the procedure.

_____   _____
Patient's signature   *Date/Time*

_____   _____
Witness' signature   *Date/Time*

One copy for chart; one copy for patient.

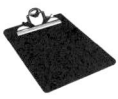

Patient Education Handout

MOIST HEALING AFTER SKIN SURGERY

1. For the next 7 to 14 days, gently wash the treated areas with soap and water, at least four times per day. DO NOT USE PEROXIDE. For some treatments like skin cancers, we go quite deep. Keep washing and follow steps 2 and 3 until it looks like there is a good layer of skin growing over the treated area. That may take up to 4 weeks.

2. If any scab forms, remove it. Gently washing with a washcloth should do this. *The objective is to prevent a scab from forming.* Scabs impair healing and actually cause more scarring.

3. After washing, keep a thin layer of an antibiotic ointment on the wound. This will not only be soothing, but will also help the areas heal. The ointment can be obtained over the counter at most stores that sell medications. If you already have another antibiotic ointment, it is okay to use it. It is probably best, however, to use something without neosporin. Even Vaseline works well. The objective is to keep the area moist. Apply the ointment 10 times per day, if necessary, to keep the area moist.

4. It is best not to cover treated areas, especially the neck and face, if possible. However, apply Band-Aids if the area is under clothing so things don't get soiled. Also, cover all treated areas at night so they don't dry out when the ointment rubs off on the bed sheets.

5. You will note an area of redness around the place where the lesion was removed. This is to be expected. However, if you see streaks of red leading away from the area, this could signal infection or an allergy to the antibiotic. If small water blisters and itching develop, STOP THE ANTIBIOTIC AT ONCE. You are allergic to it. Just use Vaseline instead and keep the area moist or ask your pharmacist for an antibiotic ointment *without neosporin* (e.g., Bacitracin, Polysporin).

6. Any pain can be controlled with ice, Tylenol, or ibuprofen. Take three (3) 200-mg ibuprofen pills four times per day as necessary. Avoid aspirin since it may cause bleeding.

7. Remember that any lesions can return. If an abnormality was removed and appears to come back or the area looks changed or different, please call our office for a follow-up appointment. You never know when cancer can start.

8. If you haven't heard from us in 2 weeks after your biopsy was taken, please call us for the report.

Please note: Band-Aid has just introduced a new Band-Aid called "Advanced Care." This has material in it that keeps the wound moist. It can be placed over the area and left there 3 or 4 days so all washing and antibiotic ointment recommended above would not be necessary. The only wounds this will not work for are those that are oozing a lot. The fluid will lift the Band-Aid off the skin.

(Used with permission of The National Procedures Institute, Midland, Mich.)

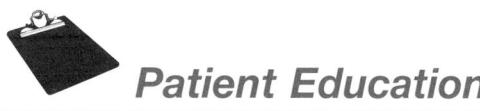

HOME BURN CARE

Leave the burn dressing on your burn until tomorrow. Depending on the size and seriousness of your burn, your provider may want you to return for a wound check. Your healthcare provider will remove and replace the dressing when you come back in for follow-up or give you instructions on how and when to change your dressing.

You may want to take a dose of your pain medication about 30 minutes before your follow-up appointment because removing and replacing the dressing on a burn can be uncomfortable until it heals more. If you are taking a narcotic pain reliever, do not drive; have a friend or relative drive you to your appointment.

If the burn appears to be stable, you may be taught how to change your own dressings. For burns that do not need hospitalization, wash with tap water and mild soap, and then apply an antibiotic ointment or cream, a nonstick dressing, and gauze to hold the dressing in place. Topical antibiotics are not needed on areas with only superficial injury (red areas without blisters or open skin).

Do not apply ointment, butter, ice, medications, fluffy cotton dressing, adhesive bandages, cream, oil spray, or any household remedy to a burn at this time. This can interfere with proper healing. Only use what the doctor has approved

Do not let the burn get dirty. Keep the dressings clean and dry. Avoid sneezing or coughing on the burn area.

Do not open any blisters or remove the dead skin. If any of the blisters break at home, change the dressing as described above and call your healthcare provider during the next office hours for advice.

Do not scratch the burn. The chances of infection and scarring increase with scratching.

Loose cotton clothing may be the most comfortable to wear early after a burn. Do not wear clothing with constricting elastic bands directly over the burn areas.

Watch for signs of infection. These include increasing pain, pus, fever, or redness spreading from the edges of the burn. Call your healthcare provider immediately if you notice these symptoms.

Watch for development of an allergy to the topical antibiotic. Symptoms can include increasing redness and itching that seem to worsen each time the antibiotic is applied. The development of pinpoint water blisters with itching is one of the most consistent signs of a new topical allergy. Call your healthcare provider if this develops.

Most minor burns heal within 2 weeks. If the burn is not healing properly or if the deep area of the burn is greater than 2 inches in diameter, call your healthcare provider.

After the skin has healed over the burn, pink or red skin may be present for a number of months (the deeper the burn, the longer the time to get pigmentation back). Protect the new skin with sunscreen (SPF 15 or greater).

A deeper burn can damage the nerve endings and cause the area to be itchy or hypersensitive. Fragrance-free moisturizing lotions can help relieve the itching. Antihistamines can also be helpful. Massaging the scar daily until it no longer appears red can decrease discomfort and the risk of thick scars.

Superficial burns (e.g., sunburn) do not need covering. You may apply aloe vera cream or gel, topical anesthetics such as Solarcaine, or 1% hydrocortisone cream.

Keep your follow-up appointments. Talk to your healthcare provider if you have further questions.

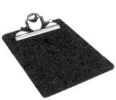

Patient Education Handout

WART REMOVAL

The removal of warts in certain locations can be difficult, especially if they are on the bottom of the feet or fingertips. With your help, a combination of acid and cryosurgery (freezing) can be used to more effectively remove these viral infections without much disability during treatment and without damage to the surrounding skin.

Every night for about 2 weeks, clean the lesion, and apply some Compound W (17% salicylic acid gel) on the wart and cover with a Band-Aid, or cover the wart with Mediplast (40% salicylic acid pads with adhesive backing) so that the pad slightly overlaps the wart.

Leave the pads on as long as possible. Remove them each evening, bathe, and then reapply. The treated wart should turn white and look fluffy. If the area becomes very sore or red, stop treatment for a day or two. If the pad moves excessively during the day because of your activity, apply it in the evening when you come home or when you do not have to move around as much and then remove it in the morning.

Once you have prepared the area well, it will be easy for the physician to remove the layer that covers the wart and to freeze the base where the root is. Cryosurgery leaves little or no scar, and usually only leaves the skin lighter in color, which diminishes with time. Most people can continue to do all their daily activities, including swimming and bathing, during treatment. No anesthesia is needed if the warts are few and small.

The freezing employed with cryosurgery can kill hair follicles, so it's not appropriate for treating large areas of the scalp. If you have an intense skin reaction to cold, please tell the doctor *before* the warts are removed.

Treating skin warts usually requires several visits (3 to 5) over a few months, 1 to 3 weeks apart. After each 3-week visit, leave the treated area alone for 2 weeks and then use the acid applications described above for 1 week before returning to the office. If you see no wart tissue remaining after the 2-week recovery period, do not use the acid treatments, and return to the office to confirm eradication of the warts and to determine whether further treatment is needed.

A new technique using duct tape can also be tried. Cut the tape to the size of the wart and apply it over the area. Leave it on for 7 days. Remove it overnight and then reapply. This is done for 6 to 8 weeks. It can also be used for the 2 weeks before seeing the doctor to soften up the wart before freezing it.

Good luck! Together we should be able to clear these invaders from your skin.

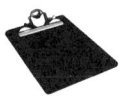 *Patient Education Handout*

CRYOTHERAPY (FREEZING)

Cryotherapy means treatment with extreme cold. The area that is treated actually freezes and then falls off. There are several different ways that the treatment can be carried out.

Liquid nitrogen has a temperature of –196° C. It can be either poured out into a Styrofoam cup and applied with a cotton-tipped applicator or sprayed onto the wound with a special thermos-like gun.

Another method is to use *nitrous oxide* in a blue tank. This gas has a temperature of –89° C and has an effect similar to that of liquid nitrogen. It is less cold so it may take a little longer to achieve the proper effect. A special unit with different types of tips is used to freeze the tissue.

A third method is to use refrigerants that are *compressed gas* in a small can. These are around –40° to –50° C, and the area to be treated is sprayed with this gas.

Advantages of Cryotherapy

Cryotherapy is very *effective*. Both benign and malignant (cancer) changes can be treated. One of the advantages of using cryotherapy is that the final results are generally *cosmetically excellent*. There is minimal or *no scarring*. It is very *quick*, and if there are only a few lesions, *relatively painless*. If there are large lesions or numerous lesions, the doctor may want to numb the area first. Infection is extremely rare, and there is no bleeding. *Postoperative care is minimal* except for washing the area three to four times a day with soap and water and applying antibiotic ointment. Generally, patients can bathe and go about their usual daily activities.

Disadvantages of Cryotherapy

The freezing does have *some discomfort* associated with it as does the thawing. That's why we will numb the area if there are large lesions or multiple lesions present. Many times the treated area will not completely resolve and will need a second a third treatment. It is difficult to treat areas where there is hair growth, such as around the eyebrows and eyelashes, because hair may not grow back in the treated areas. Probably the most significant "hassle factor" is that a *blister* often will form. When this blister breaks, there may be a very heavy *watery discharge*. You may need to return to the doctor's office so that the area can be treated to stop this discharge. Also, if the area treated is under clothing, the discharge may stick to the clothes and cause discomfort. Apply antibiotic ointment and keep it covered to prevent this. If you are a light-skinned individual, cryotherapy is ideal for you. However, if you are dark-skinned, the area treated *may heal with a lighter color*. This may not be of concern if the area usually is covered, but if it is around the face or some other cosmetic area, then it may be best not to do cryotherapy.

Preparation for the Office Visit

No real preparation is necessary for the office visit. You may want to take Tylenol or 600 to 800 mg of ibuprofen just to help decrease the swelling afterwards. Let the doctor know if you prefer to have an injection to numb the area.

Continued

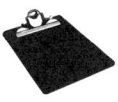

Patient Education Handout—cont'd

CRYOTHERAPY (FREEZING)—cont'd

Who Should Not Have Cryotherapy

If you have any type of arthritis condition, cancer, ulcerative colitis, glomerulonephritis, heart valve infection, syphilis, mononucleosis, cytomegalovirus infection, hepatitis, diabetes, peripheral vascular disease, Burger's disease, are on steroids, or are known to have high levels of cryoglobulins, be sure that your doctor knows. You may be much more sensitive to the freezing.

As stated above, if you are dark-skinned, you may want to choose another method of treatment because of possible loss of color in the area treated.

Care After Treatment

See the patient education handout titled "Wound Care After Cryosurgery."

(Modified from The National Procedures Institute, Midland, Mich.)

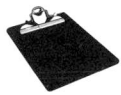 *Patient Education Handout*

WHAT TO EXPECT AFTER CRYOSURGERY

Physicians use freezing agents to treat certain skin growths such as warts, skin tags, age spots, and a variety of other skin growths. These skin growths are destroyed by the freezing action.

From a few hours to a few days after treatment, the area may blister, turn black, or form a scab. This is a desirable result. In some patients, no reaction is apparent.

1. You are allowed to get the area wet even immediately after treatment.

2. If the area is painful within the first few hours after treatment, soaking the area in warm water and taking aspirin will give pain relief. Most persons have little or no pain from this treatment.

3. It is not necessary to cover the area with a bandage. In fact, this is undesirable. Treated areas heal better if left open to the air. You should protect the area from injury as much as possible.

4. Painful large blisters (even blisters filled with blood) can occur at times. These can be opened and the fluid drained to relieve the pain. If such painful blisters occur and you feel uncomfortable removing them, or if you have any other trouble with the treated area, contact your physician.

5. As the treated area heals, the unwanted skin growth will fall off. This will take several days to weeks depending on the size and nature of the growth treated, the location, and the way your body heals.

6. Allow the growth to fall off by itself; do not pick at it or pull it off.

7. Once the blister comes off, wash the area three to four times a day with mild soap and water. Do not use peroxide. Keep it covered if it is under clothes; otherwise it can be left open. Cover it at night with a Band-Aid to keep it moist.

8. When the growth does come off, the skin underneath will be reddish. As time passes, it will assume the color of normal skin. The area may be sensitive to touch and temperature, and it may be itchy as it heals. This is normal and it may take some time before it is exactly like the skin around it once more.

(Used with permission of The Medical Procedures Center, PC, Midland, Mich.)

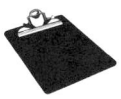

Patient Education Handout

WOUND CARE AFTER CRYOSURGERY

Wound Care

A lesion treated with cryosurgery freezing should be kept clean and protected from irritation and injury. Bandages are necessary only to protect from repetitive irritation or if exposure to dirt is likely. Avoid exposure to sun because the new skin forming is very sensitive to injury. On occasion the wound may ooze clear fluid requiring a bandage.

Often there will be a blister. Leave it in place. If the blister ruptures, cut away the excess skin to avoid the unlikely chance of infection. Then wash the area 3 to 4 times a day with mild soap and water. *Do not use peroxide.* Apply an ointment with or without antibiotic and keep the wound moist. Cover the wound with a bandage if it is under clothing. At night while you are sleeping, all wounds may need to be covered to prevent drying and rubbing on bed covers.

Activity

Activity is not restricted other than avoiding excessive irritation of the wound site.

Bathing and Showering

There are no limits on bathing, swimming, or showering.

Pain Control

Aspirin, acetaminophen, ibuprofen, and other similar medications can be used for pain.

Infection

Infection is extremely rare, but certainly possible because even normal skin can get infected. If you see any redness with streaks adjacent to the wound, yellow or creamy thick drainage, if you have a fever, have increased pain, or get dirt in the wound, please call or come in to be seen.

Other Things to Watch

Although some blister formation is normal, rarely treated areas will swell excessively or form large blisters. If this occurs, it means you are extremely sensitive to cryosurgery. Please come in to be checked if you believe excessive blister formation has occurred.

Tetanus Immunizations

Everyone should have a tetanus booster every 10 years. Having cryosurgery does not require more frequent immunizations.

Suture Removal

One big advantage of cryosurgery is that *no sutures* are needed.

Continued

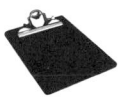 *Patient Education Handout—cont'd*

WOUND CARE AFTER CRYOSURGERY—cont'd

Follow-Up

Cryosurgery does not change the lesion immediately. The abnormal cells slowly die over a period of 2 to 4 weeks depending on the lesion. Consequently, several treatments may be required to carefully remove the lesion without causing damage to the surrounding normal tissue. The hassle of sutures and wound care are virtually nonexistent, but depending on the abnormality, more than two visits may be required to achieve the final desired result.

An advantage of cryotherapy is that if the final result is not sufficient, surgery can still be used to remove the lesion. And, usually, the lesion is at least made smaller by the cryotherapy, which makes surgery easier than it would have been before cryotherapy.

Side Effects

Freezing lesions does not produce scars, but pigment changes (lightening) of the skin can occur. Over time, the lighter tone in skin color decreases and blends in with normal skin. If you are dark-skinned or the lesion is in a location where a lightening of the skin is not acceptable, then cryosurgery should not be selected for treatment. It is best not to freeze areas where hair growth is important. Although hair often grows back, it sometimes does not.

Tissue Diagnosis

Cryosurgery does not produce a tissue specimen for microscopic analysis, so if the lesion is worrisome for cancer, a surgical biopsy is preferred. Lesions that do not respond to cryosurgery (especially after several attempts) should be considered for biopsy.

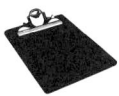
Patient Education Handout

HOME WOUND CARE INSTRUCTIONS

The following instructions will help you in caring for your wound after surgery in order to achieve the best results. Your repair was more complicated and involved than usual, so special attention should be paid to these instructions.

- **Rest.** Do not exert yourself or do any bending, lifting, or exercising until the sutures are removed. Avoid heating pads, saunas, ice packs, or other extreme temperature exposure to the wound area, which may be unusually sensitive to heat or cold while healing.
- Keep the wound clean and dry.
- After 24 hours you may wash around the wound or allow clean shower water to run over it. Pat dry.
- Do not drink alcohol or take aspirin for 24 hours after the surgery. If you have pain, take an aspirin-free pain medicine such as acetaminophen (Tylenol) or ibuprofen (Motrin).
- After 24 hours, remove the top bandage. If a thin plastic dressing has been applied to the wound, leave it in place until the sutures are removed. If Steri-Strips have been placed, these will be removed by your doctor or allowed to fall off on their own. Do not pull them off unless instructed to do so.
- If the thin dressing becomes wet from wound drainage, you may cover it with a second dressing. If the dressing becomes loose, reinforce it with tape or see the doctor. If neither a plastic dressing nor Steri-Strips have been used, you may remove the soiled dressing and gently wash around the wound area with a mild soap and water three to four times a day. Apply an antibiotic ointment to keep the area moist and protected. Any over-the-counter antibiotic ointment will work. Cover the wound with gauze or other bandage, wear loose clothing, and avoid excessive rubbing and irritation to the wound site.
- If the wound begins to bleed significantly, apply firm pressure for 15 minutes. If the bleeding continues, call your physician.
- If you notice pus coming from the wound site, redness, increased pain, swelling, or breakdown of the wound, or if you develop a fever, call your physician or go to the emergency room.
- If the surgery was on the face, avoid sleeping on the same side as the wound. Keep your head slightly elevated for the first two nights, and avoid bending over with your head lower than heart level for the first 48 hours.
- Return for a wound check and/or suture removal in _____ days.

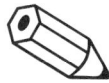 *Patient Consent Form*

SKIN SURGERY

I came to the office today to see Dr. _____ on _____ (date) for evaluation and treatment of the following condition:

_____

_____

We discussed the different treatments possible and the risk of not treating the condition. Based on the advice given by Dr. _____ and my own judgment, I agree to undergo the following procedure(s):

☐ Scar revision
☐ Skin biopsy
☐ Removal of lesion or tumor
☐ Other _____

We discussed the different outcomes that could occur and most of the possible complications, including the following:

- Pain
- Bleeding
- Infection
- Scar formation
- Recurrence of the lesion

- Persistent redness
- Increase or decrease of skin pigmentation
- Local nerve damage or numbness
- Allergic reaction to the anesthetic, dressing, or other medications
- Possible need for further surgery if the entire lesion is not removed

I am aware that other unforeseeable complications could occur. I understand the risks and benefits of the procedure and have had the opportunity to have all of my questions answered.

I agree to follow the instructions for self-care after the procedure and to return for follow-up care on _____.

I will call the office or answering service if any problems arise before the scheduled follow-up visit.

_____   _____
Patient's signature   *Date/Time*

_____   _____
Witness' signature   *Clinician's signature*

One copy for chart; one copy for patient.

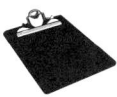

Patient Education Handout

FOREIGN BODY REMOVAL FROM SKIN AND SOFT TISSUE

Not all foreign bodies, even pencil lead, need to be removed. Most are safe to leave in place for quite a while, especially if they are not infected or causing symptoms. In fact, removal may cause more trauma than leaving the object alone. Although it may take days, weeks, or decades for the object to work its way to the surface, in many cases this is a better way to locate an object. It is safe to let the object "rest" in the skin until this happens. If infection occurs, it will be treated with an antibiotic. Often a cyst forms as a result of infection, making it easier to locate and remove the object.

However, after a discussion with a clinician, you may decide that you want him or her to remove the foreign body in your skin. Success in removal requires relaxation and cooperation. You may be given a sedative, a local anesthetic, or an injection. The clinician will use special instruments and techniques to carefully remove the object. One attempt will be made, not lasting more than 15 to 20 minutes, to avoid damaging too much tissue.

In certain situations, it may be necessary to attempt removal without an anesthetic. For small objects it may be easier to locate the object using your sense of feel while the clinician probes, rather than for the clinician to probe blindly under skin distorted by local anesthetic. If the object is moderately sized, local anesthetic may be applied before removal as soon as the object is grasped and stabilized. If an incision is necessary, local anesthetic definitely will be used.

Complications may occur, including damage to the skin or to local structures such as arteries, veins, nerves, or tendons. Bleeding may also occur. Infection or scarring may occur as a result of the original injury, a necessary incision to remove the object, or the application of sutures. If the object is not able to be removed or is incompletely removed, you may be referred to a different specialist.

After removal, a dull ache or stretching sensation is normal for up to a day, especially if sutures were placed. Itching is a normal sign of healing. An appointment should be made with the clinician in 2 days and again in the appropriate number of days (typically 7 days) for suture removal if sutures were placed.

Your clinician may give you antibiotics to take by mouth or to apply locally. You may also use over-the-counter bacitracin or Polysporin ointment. The dressing should remain over the wound for 48 hours. It should be changed if it gets wet during that time. After the first 48 hours, a dressing should be used only if the wound continues to drain or if it could get dirty. After the first 48 hours, the wound may be washed with soap and water.

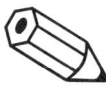 *Patient Consent Form*

FOREIGN BODY REMOVAL FROM SKIN AND SOFT TISSUE

I came to the office of my clinician, _____, on_____ (date) for a foreign body to be removed from skin and soft tissue. We discussed the different treatment methods and the risks involved.

Based on that discussion and my own judgement, I agree to allow my clinician to remove the foreign body using whatever means necessary. This may involve anesthesia with an injection of lidocaine and use of a metal instrument to probe for, extract, or grasp the foreign body. An incision may need to be made and x-rays taken or ultrasound images made. The wound may also be irrigated, and perhaps stitches will be placed.

I understand that there will be some discomfort with this procedure and that in certain situations, no anesthesia will be used while the clinician attempts to precisely locate the object.

We discussed the different outcomes that could occur and most of the possible complications, including failure to remove the foreign body, bleeding, infection, scarring, and damage to local structures such as nerves, tendons, arteries, or veins. I am aware that there are other rare, unforeseeable complications. I have read and understand the patient teaching guide. I agree to follow the instructions for self-care after the procedure and to return for follow-up care on _____.

I will call the office or answering service if any problems occur.

_____
Patient's signature

_____
Date/Time

_____
Witness' signature

_____
Clinician's signature

One copy for chart; one copy for patient.

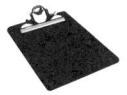
Patient Education Handout

SUTURE CARE

1. For the first 24 hours, keep the wound as clean and dry as possible. If there is bleeding or the area does get wet, remove the dressing, pat the stitches dry, and apply a clean bandage. It is okay to shower after 24 hours.

2. It is normal for the wound to bleed slightly for several hours after stitches are placed. After 72 hours, you can leave off the bandage unless you will be doing dirty or dusty work. Cover the wound while sleeping. If the wound gets crusted, dirty, or grimy, you can clean it with soap and water.

3. After the first 24 hours, wash the incision gently with soap and water two to three times a day. After washing, apply an antibiotic ointment. Some people are allergic to Neosporin, so we advise avoiding it. Bacitracin or Polysporin is fine. If the area becomes very red and itchy, or if it develops small blisters, stop the ointment immediately, because you are probably allergic to it. Even Vaseline alone will help the healing process. Keep an ointment on for 4 to 5 days or until you can see that the skin is sealed over well.

4. Use Tylenol (two every 4 hours) or ibuprofen (three 200-mg pills four times per day) for pain as needed. Avoid aspirin, since it may cause bleeding.

5. Whenever there is a break in the skin, germs can get underneath and cause infection. If a wound infection does occur, it usually starts 2 to 4 days after the sutures were placed. Signs of infection include the following:
   a. Increased redness
   b. Increased swelling
   c. Increased tenderness
   d. Increased pain
   e. Yellow drainage or pus
   f. Red streaks leading from the wound
   g. Fever or chills

   If you think you might have an infection, call the doctor or seek medical care promptly. You may have been given an antibiotic already. The drug was _____, _____ mg. Take the rest of the medicine as follows: _____.

6. Be careful not to put excessive pressure on the sutured area. Ask your doctor what kind of activities you can do.

7. If Steri-Strips were applied, leave them on until they drop off by themselves. If the edges curl up, cut them off with scissors. It's okay to get them wet, but don't scrub over them. Also, if Steri-Strips or glue were used, do **not** apply the antibiotic ointment as directed above.

8. The sutures should be removed in _____ days.

9. Generally any sutured wound will have some scarring. Wound healing takes time, so you won't know the final results for at least 10 to 12 months.

10. If you had a tissue sample sent to lab, call us for results if we haven't called you in 14 days.

11. **If Durabond ("super glue") was used on your wound, keep it dry for 24 hours, but after that showering is allowed. Do not apply too much pressure to the wound, which can cause it to break open. Don't use the antibiotic ointment if super glue is used.**

(Used with permission of The National Procedures Institute, Midland, Mich.)

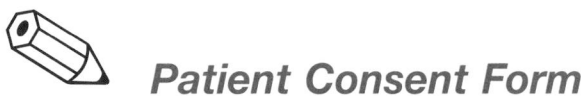

Patient Consent Form

SKIN LESION EXCISION (ELECTIVE)

Your physician _____ has decided that the best care for your skin lesion would be to have it removed. There are certain things that you need to know about this surgery. It is intended to remove your lesion by _____.

You need to know that there are always some complications involved with the surgery. **Pain** is generally minimal but at times can be a concern. Your wound could **bleed,** and **further surgery may be indicated. Bruising** and **swelling** are very common and will go away. Sometimes wounds get **infected,** and they may actually break apart. In severe infections, the wound may have to be left open and allowed to heal in on its own. A later surgery may be required to actually improve the appearance. **Scarring** is always present to some degree. We will try to minimize this using special techniques. The scars, however, sometimes become thick and raised up. This is called hypertrophic scarring or keloids. Further treatment may be needed for this also. The area of removal may become **more pigmented** (darker) or **lighter pigmented.** If **hair** is in the area, it may not grow back through the treated site. At times, unanticipated **nerve damage** can occur. This would mean there would be an area of **numbness** around the area of the operation. When the skin is put back together, at times it will be somewhat **distorted and irregular.** It may be "humped up" or tighter than the area on the opposite side. This is especially common when large areas of skin have to be removed. At times a **deep stitch may come to the surface** and actually cause a small abscess. Sometimes if the surgery involves the area around the eye, eyelids may be turned out a bit or eyebrows lifted up. The lip may also be pulled down or pushed up. It is also **impossible to know absolutely that the entire lesion has been removed** until the specimen comes back from pathology. It is possible that the abnormality will regrow if all of it wasn't removed.

To obtain the best outcome, it will be important for you to follow the instructions given after surgery very closely. If you are concerned about anything prior to surgery, the doctor will help you find a second opinion or refer you to another physician.

By signing this permit form, I acknowledge that all of these conditions are possible. The doctor and staff have answered all of my questions and have explained the alternative methods of care. I agree to proceed with the surgery as planned.

_____   _____
Patient's signature   *Date/Time*

_____   _____
Witness' signature   *Date/Time*

_____   _____
Responsible party (for minors)   *Relationship to patient*

One copy for chart; one copy for patient.

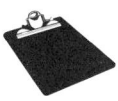

Patient Education Handout

COOLTOUCH LASER SKIN REJUVENATION

This handout is intended to provide you with the information you need to make a decision whether or not to undergo CoolTouch Laser treatment. If you have any questions or concerns, please do not hesitate to ask before your treatments.

What is CoolTouch Laser Skin Rejuvenation?

CoolTouch is a revolutionary way to combat the signs of aging. This noninvasive procedure stimulates smoother, healthier-looking skin. An infrared laser is used with a cooling process to rejuvenate your skin from the inside out. There are no harsh chemicals and no long recovery times, just younger-looking skin.

A cooling spray combined with an invisible 1320-nanometer (wavelength), neodymium:YAG laser is used to give you optimal results with the least inconvenience. The protective cooling spray is applied to the skin, allowing the CoolTouch laser light to pass harmlessly through the upper layers of your skin and stimulate the cells deep below the surface to produce natural collagen. The collagen and elastin fibers continue to multiply after your treatment. At first you may see little result. Over several months and multiple treatments, you will see gradual improvement and softening of fine wrinkles.

What are the Potential Benefits of This Treatment?

The most obvious benefit is a simple, relatively painless treatment to create younger-looking skin. The CoolTouch laser treatment can be performed on any facial area—around the eyes, mouth, cheek, and chin—with minimal discomfort. A topical anesthetic cream can be used on extremely sensitive areas, but it is seldom needed.

Other benefits include almost immediate recovery with virtually no postoperative care and gradual, perceptible improvement over time. (Fine line, wrinkle, and acne scar reduction are cosmetic in nature and are not medically necessary. They are treated as a cosmetic condition and are not eligible for any medical insurance consideration.)

How Long does a Treatment Take? And How Many Will I Need?

The CoolTouch treatment is so quick and easy, many patients come in during their lunch hour. The treatment takes from 15 to 30 minutes, with virtually no side effects. You can reapply your makeup right away and carry on with your day. No one will even know you had anything done.

Clinical studies suggest that an average of three to five treatments are needed to stimulate new collagen growth. We also recommend regular maintenance treatment to sustain the continued growth of new collagen two to four times per year, depending on the degree of sun aging.

How is This Different From Other Resurfacing Treatments?

This treatment is unlike any other resurfacing treatment. Your skin is not subjected to harsh chemicals or the intense superficial trauma caused by CO_2 and erbium lasers. The CoolTouch laser protects the sensitive surface layers of your skin, allowing the laser light to penetrate to a deeper level and stimulate new collagen growth.

Continued

Patient Education Handouts and Consent Forms

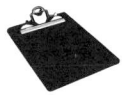 *Patient Education Handout—cont'd*

COOLTOUCH LASER SKIN REJUVENATION—cont'd

Are My Results Guaranteed?

No. Most patients, as noted, require multiple sessions. Some patients may be resistant to treatment, and optimal results may not include complete wrinkle reduction. However, according to recent histological studies and clinical research, the results of CoolTouch laser are permanent and effective.

What are the Possible Side Effects?

Side effects are rare, but the following may occur.

- *Discomfort:* Some people feel discomfort during treatments. Patients typically report feeling a very short, mild sting on the treated area. In some patients this may range from moderate to minimal, but it does not last long. Topical anesthetic cream may be used on some patients.
- Redness or swelling: Immediately after treatment, especially in sensitive areas, tissue may swell. This is temporary and not harmful. Swelling usually subsides over several hours (rarely, several days) and may require topical ice.
- Fragile skin: The skin in or near the treatment site may become fragile. This area should not be rubbed because this activity could cause the skin to tear.
- Open wound: In a small number of patients, a wound may occur. This could take 3 to 5 days to heal and could possibly leave a scar.
- Other: There is a remote possibility of increased or decreased pigmentation in the treatment area.

Please contact the office with any questions or concerns you may have following your treatment.

Please initial this sheet as an indication that you have read and understand this information. _____

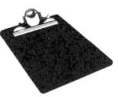

Patient Education Handout

SKIN CARE INSTRUCTIONS AFTER LASER TREATMENT

Apply a thin layer of antibiotic ointment (Polysporin or Bacitracin) to the laser-treated areas twice daily until the skin surface is healed. *Do not use any products containing Neosporin or neomycin.*

Laser-treated areas can be protected with a bandage, gauze, or Telfa dressing, if desired, for the first 10 days. Protection of the area is strongly recommended for children, for areas of the body likely to be rubbed or scratched such as the side of the face, and for individuals who are working in dusty or contaminated areas or participating in contact sports.

You may shower or bathe, but do not soak. Gently pat the treated area dry. Do not rub with a towel or washcloth because the skin is tender for the first 2 weeks after treatment.

When areas on the face have been treated, please keep your head elevated and apply ice packs gently over the laser-treated area for 20 minutes each hour for the first 4 to 6 hours after treatment. This significantly reduces swelling in the area. Sleep with the head elevated on several pillows for the first few nights after laser surgery of the face. Oral prednisone may be prescribed, if needed, to decrease swelling.

Do not rub, scratch, or put pressure on the laser-treated areas until obvious skin changes such as crusting have disappeared. Your laser-treated skin is very delicate for 10 to 14 days after treatment. Picking off crusts or scabs can cause scarring and pitting.

Do not apply makeup to the treated areas if any scabbing, blistering, oozing, or crusting of the skin is present.

Do not use aspirin or products containing aspirin for at least a week following laser treatment.

Do not drink alcohol while you are taking narcotic pain medication or anxiety medication.

Keep all areas previously treated or scheduled for future laser treatments protected with sunscreen at all times. Tanning, either from natural sunlight or tanning booths, can interfere with laser treatment.

Physical exercise is permitted, but do not swim or soak until the skin is healed.

If your neck is treated, do not wear a turtleneck or tight-fitting clothing around the neck for 2 weeks. Do not wear jewelry for 2 weeks.

Remember, after all the bruising disappears, it takes an additional 6 to 8 weeks (sometimes more) for the skin to return to a more normal appearance and redness can last weeks or even months. For this reason, it is important to return to this office in 6 to 8 weeks so that we may assess the improvement and determine if further treatments are needed at the treated site or at untreated sites.

Please call immediately if there is any suggestion of infection such as redness, tenderness, or purulent drainage. Some swelling occurs after any surgery and is normal during the first few days.

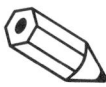 *Patient Consent Form*

CARBON DIOXIDE LASER TREATMENT

Patient name: _____

Dr. _____ has recommended (check one):

      ☐ Biopsy   ☐ Excision and/or destruction   ☐ Repair

of a (check one):

☐ Suspicious, changing, growing, infected, or traumatized skin lesion(s)

☐ Benign, cosmetic skin lesion(s) at my request

☐ Other: _____

on my _____.

1. The procedure starts with cleansing the skin. Anesthetic is then applied or injected around and into the surgical site. There is a rare risk of allergic reaction to the anesthetic or cleansing solutions.
2. Next, minimally invasive surgery is performed. Stitches are/are not required. A specimen will/will not be sent to a pathologist for evaluation.
3. The risks with this procedure are very small. They include local infection, prolonged redness and scarring. A skin lesion may be removed incompletely, recur, or require further treatment.
4. The treated area may heal either lighter or darker than the surrounding skin. This is usually temporary.
5. There will be some postoperative discomfort. Temporary bruising, bleeding, and swelling are expected.
6. I consent to photographs or videos being taken for medical records, education, and advertising. If used for education or advertising, I will not be identified by name.

I agree to follow a specific postoperative treatment plan as provided by my practitioner.

Alternatives to this procedure have been discussed and any questions have been answered to my satisfaction.

I have explained the above information: _____ MD/agent.

I understand the information contained in these sheets and consent to the procedure. This consent is effective for the duration of the laser sessions that are needed to treat the condition(s) named above.

*Patient's signature:*_____ *Date:* _____

One copy for chart; one copy for patient.

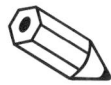

Patient Consent Form

INTENSE PULSED LIGHT TREATMENT

The intense pulsed light (IPL) treatment machine combines an intense pulsed light device and near infra-red pulsed laser energy to treat benign blood vessels, pigmented lesions, facial aging, tattoos, and unwanted hair. The purpose of the IPL procedure is to lighten, fade, or remove benign blood vessels, birthmarks, sun damage or pigmentation spots, leg veins, hair, or stretch marks. The IPL machine is set to destroy the unwanted changes yet causes minimal damage to the surrounding skin.

The damaged blood vessel, pigmented lesion, tattoo pigment, or hair follicle is gradually absorbed or rejected by the body as part of the normal healing process. Depending on the target and how your body handles the treatments, multiple treatments over several months are usually required to obtain the best results. Sun exposure may cause prolonged darkening or irregular pigmentation at treatment sites.

The clinical results of the treatments may vary. The best results are obtained when the pigment in the "target" abnormalities (hair, blood vessels, tattoos, etc.) contrasts greatly with the surrounding skin. Patients who have light skin, sunburn easily, and have little tan, but who have dark "targets," usually obtain good results more easily. Darker-skinned patients whose skin color is closer to the target pigment may experience partial or, rarely, no improvement at all. For best results, do not tan before being treated for at least 4 weeks.

Contraindications to procedures with IPL include being pregnant, using medications that increase sensitivity to sunlight, having a history of keloid scarring, and having a bleeding disorder.

There is a possibility of temporary side effects that resolve in days to weeks. These side effects include reddening, mild burning, swelling, bruising, blistering, and temporary discoloring. Scarring and permanent discoloration of the skin are *very* rare if the posttreatment instructions are followed.

Injections, electric needles, single- and multi-wavelength lasers, dermabrasion, and freezing are some of the other methods that have been used to lighten, fade, or remove benign blood vessels, birthmarks, sun damage or pigmentation spots, leg veins, hair, or stretch marks. These methods are generally not as effective, are less comfortable, and may be more expensive than IPL.

Treatment by IPL usually involves multiple treatments. Hair and vascular lesions (veins) may require periodic treatments—perhaps once or twice per year—to maintain the results obtained. Often, we start therapy with several "test spots" after reviewing your history and performing an examination. The charge for test spots is applied toward the cost of any treatments you have.

Continued

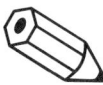 *Patient Consent Form—cont'd*

INTENSE PULSED LIGHT TREATMENT—cont'd
Patient Consent

I, _____, understand that this is considered cosmetic surgery; therefore I am responsible for the bill because insurance does not cover these treatments.

I have read and understand this consent form. My questions have been addressed and answered to my satisfaction. I freely agree to the above terms and indicate so with my signature below.

_____   _____
Patient's signature   *Date/Time*

_____   _____
Witness' signature   *Physician's signature*

One copy for chart; one copy for patient.

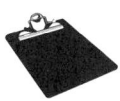

Patient Education Handout

MUCOCELE TREATMENT

1. Mucoceles are benign lesions of the inside lining of the mouth. A mucocele is basically a cyst that formed after injury or obstruction of a minor saliva gland. Usually, mucoceles occur on the inside surface of the lower lip.

2. Mucoceles are frequently bothersome and tend to require treatment to cure them.

3. A relatively simple treatment is to make an opening in the cyst, drain it, and then destroy it by freezing or electrical cauterization.

4. Complications of the procedure are uncommon but would include bleeding, infection, or an allergic reaction to the anesthetic given.

5. You may experience minor discomfort for a few days after the treatment. You should rinse your mouth with diluted salt water, or hydrogen peroxide mixed half and half with water, three to four times a day for 5 days. Also, a mild anesthetic such as Orajel can be applied on the irritated area if needed.

6. Occasionally mucoceles come back, requiring repeat treatment.

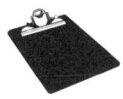 *Patient Education Handout*

NAIL PLATE AND NAIL BED BIOPSY

A biopsy of unusually pigmented skin under the nail is necessary to confirm the presence or absence of cancer.

The toe or finger will be anesthetized by injecting small amounts of medication around the nerves at the base. Part of the nail will be removed from the underlying tissue and a small round piece (biopsy) of the pigmented skin will be obtained. The opening may be closed with several small stitches.

For several days there may be mild pain and swelling; elevation will minimize these symptoms. It is okay to take Tylenol or ibuprofen (up to 1600 mg per day). Wash the wound three or four times per day and apply an antibiotic ointment until it heals.

It is possible to experience infection of the skin, bleeding, and pain after this procedure. If pain increases rather than decreases over the first 2 days, or if fever and/or red streaks develop from the affected site, seek your healthcare provider.

Unfortunately, any time the nail bed is biopsied, the nail can be deformed when it grows out. Also, even though we biopsy the area, we could miss the diagnosis. If the area continues to grow or comes back after removal, let us see it again. Call in 2 weeks if you have not heard from us about the pathology report.

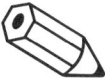 *Patient Consent Form*

NAIL PLATE AND NAIL BED BIOPSY

I came to the office of Dr. _____ on _____ (date) for evaluation and treatment of the following condition: unusually pigmented streak in or under fingernail or toenail. Such discolored streaks can be the result of previous injury, infection, or cancer of the skin.

We discussed the different treatments possible and the risks of not treating the condition. Based on the advice given by Dr. _____ and my own judgment, I agree to undergo the following procedure: removal of a portion of the nail and biopsy of a portion of the pigmented lesion for pathologic evaluation.

Local-digital anesthesia will be used, sterile techniques followed in obtaining the biopsy, and topical antibiotic ointment and gauze dressing applied.

We discussed the different outcomes that could occur and most of the possible complications, including pain, bleeding, infection, and deformity of the nail when it regrows. I am aware that other complications could occur that we could not foresee. I agree to follow the instructions for self-care after the procedure and to return for follow-up care on _____.

I will call the office or answering service if any problems arise before the scheduled follow-up visit.

_____
Patient's signature

_____
Date/Time

_____
Witness' signature

_____
Physician's signature

One copy for chart; one copy for patient.

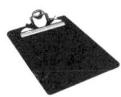 *Patient Education Handout*

SKIN GRAFT POSTPROCEDURE INSTRUCTIONS

1. You have just received a skin graft to cover the area of skin that you lost. It is very important that you keep your dressings clean and dry.
2. You should not take aspirin or herbal medication without the advice of the doctor.
3. Your pain may be worse in the site from which the skin was taken than to where it was transplanted.
4. Movement of the bandage over the skin graft will injure it and not allow it to heal properly.
5. Do not attempt to change the bandage yourself unless instructed to do so by your doctor.
6. Report any bleeding or odor from the dressing.
7. Return for a dressing check if pain worsens.
8. Do not worry if the graft turns dark blue or even black on the surface. This is common and does not mean the graft is dead. One or two deeper layers of cells may be alive and germinating, much like a scab on an abrasion. Let the dead dry skin fall off on its own.
9. Let the dressing on the site where the skin was taken fall off on its own, because pulling it off will injure the remaining cells and prevent healing.
10. After the dressings are off, do not put creams, lotions, or vitamin oils on the graft sites without the consent of your physician. Harsh oils and creams may injure the new skin.

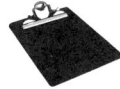

Patient Education Handout

PINCH (PATCH) GRAFTING

What Is Pinch Grafting?

Pinch grafting is the removal of small pieces of skin from a healthy part of your body (usually your thigh). These pieces of skin are then placed on your leg ulcer(s) to help it heal.

Why Do I Need This Procedure?

This procedure may speed the healing of your ulcer and may help keep it from coming back.

How Do I Prepare for Pinch Grafting?

Keep the area around the ulcer and the skin of your inner thighs clean and dry. Try to elevate your leg with the ulcer(s) to keep the swelling down. Follow any special instructions from your doctor.

What Happens During the Procedure?

The skin around your leg ulcer(s) and the skin of your inner thigh will be cleaned. Local anesthetic will be injected into the skin of your thigh in several small areas. Small pieces ("pinches") of skin will be taken from your thigh and placed on the ulcer. Dressings will be put on your leg to cover the spots where skin was removed and on your leg ulcer(s).

What Happens After the Procedure?

After the grafts are put on your ulcer, you **must** be in bed with your leg elevated higher than your heart for 7 days. (You will be able to get up to use the toilet.) Your doctor will need to check your dressings from time to time. If you cannot be in bed for 7 days after this procedure, please notify your doctor.

What Are the Benefits of This Procedure?

Pinch grafting may help your ulcer to heal faster and come back less often than with some other forms of treatment.

What Are the Risks Associated With This Procedure?

You may have light bleeding in the area where skin is removed. There is a very small risk of skin infection and of blood clots in your legs. There will be some scarring where the graft was taken. The graft may not grow, so the procedure may need to be repeated. There may be some scarring on your thigh where the skin was removed. Generally the procedure is not very painful. Tylenol or ibuprofen can be used for pain.

What Do I Need to Do After the Procedure to Prevent Infection?

Follow all instructions given by your doctor. In general, do not touch the dressings applied by your doctor. It is important to stay in bed for 7 days, as noted previously.

When Should I Call My Healthcare Provider?

Call if the following occur:
- Bleeding that soaks through your dressings or if your leg becomes red, swollen, painful, or warm.
- Bad-smelling drainage from the ulcer or the area where skin was removed.
- A temperature greater than 100° F (37.5° C) (or if you have fever and chills).
- Pain in your leg that is not controlled by over-the-counter pain medicine.

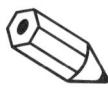 *Patient Consent Form*

PINCH (PATCH) GRAFTING

I came to the office of Dr. _____ on _____ (date) for evaluation and treatment of leg ulcer(s) caused by problems with circulation or injury.
(Description of diagnosis, etiology, and differential diagnosis can be added here.)

We discussed the different treatments possible, and discussed the risks of not treating the condition. Based on the advice given by Dr. _____ and my own judgment, I agree to undergo pinch grafting. This procedure involves the injection of local anesthetic into the skin of my thigh, removal of small pieces of skin from my thigh (or other area), and then placement of these pieces of skin on my leg ulcer(s). The ulcer and graft sites will then be bandaged. This procedure is called *pinch grafting.*

We discussed the different outcomes that could occur and most of the possible complications. I understand the graft may get infected or not grow. Since I will be on bedrest for 7 days, I may experience blood clots in my legs. There may be some scarring where the graft was taken from and over the ulcer. I am aware that other complications could occur that we could not foresee. I agree to follow the instructions for self-care after the procedure and to return for follow-up care on _____.

I will call the office or answering service if any problems arise before the scheduled follow-up visit.

_____
Patient's signature

_____
Date/Time

_____
Witness' signature

_____
Physician's signature

One copy for chart; one copy for patient.

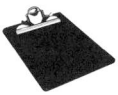

Patient Education Handout

SUBUNGUAL HEMATOMA EVACUATION

Why Do I Need This Procedure?
To relieve painful pressure caused by bleeding and swelling under the nail as a result of trauma.

What Happens During the Procedure?
After gentle cleansing of the nail, a pointed heated instrument is applied to the nail creating an opening for release of the underlying blood and pressure.

What are the Benefits of This Procedure?
Immediate relief of painful pressure should be expected.

What are the Risks Associated With This Procedure?
It is possible to experience infection of the underlying blood collection.

What Do I Need to Do After the Procedure to Prevent Infection?
Elevation of the affected hand or foot for the first 24 hours can help prevent swelling and pain.

When Should I Call My Healthcare Provider?
If pain, swelling or bleeding increase from the affected site, seek your healthcare provider.

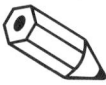 *Patient Consent Form*

SUBUNGUAL HEMATOMA EVACUATION

I came to the office of Dr. _____ on _____ for evaluation and treatment of the following condition: painful bleeding beneath a fingernail or toenail injury.

We discussed the different treatments possible and discussed the risks of not treating the condition. Based on the advice given by Dr. _____ and my own judgment, I agree to undergo the following procedure: creation of a small opening through the injured nail to allow release of pressure and blood.

The affected nail will be cleaned carefully, and a pointed, heated instrument will create a small opening in the nail, allowing the trapped blood to escape and pressure to be relieved.

We discussed the different outcomes that could occur and most of the possible complications. I am aware that other complications could occur that we could not foresee. I agree to follow the instructions for self-care after the procedure and to return for follow-up care on _____.

I will call the office or answering service if any problems arise before the scheduled follow-up visit.

_____   _____
Patient's signature   *Date/Time*

_____   _____
Witness' signature   *Physician's signature*

One copy for chart; one copy for patient.

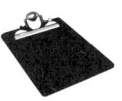

Patient Education Handout

TICK REMOVAL AND PREVENTION OF INFECTION

You are about to have a surgical removal of a tick by punch biopsy.

Your physician has determined that the risk of an infection (e.g., Lyme disease) by the tick is high. Routine removal would increase the possibility of pushing the tick's gut contents into your skin.

Your physician will cleanse the area, introduce a local anesthetic, and then use a tiny circular blade to "cut out" the bite area. The wound then might be closed with a suture, which will be removed in 5 to 7 days. The tick or its parts may be sent to the lab for analysis.

You may also be given a prescription for antibiotics, and you should warn your physician of any allergies or signs of infection.

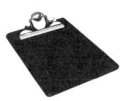 *Patient Education Handout*

TICKBORNE DISEASES: WHAT YOU SHOULD KNOW

What are Tickborne Diseases?

Tickborne diseases are a group of illnesses that people get from tick bites. They occur in all areas of the United States and affect people of all ages. These diseases are more common in the spring and summer months when tick bites are more common. Some of the common tick-borne diseases in the United States are Lyme disease, ehrlichiosis, Rocky Mountain spotted fever, and tularemia.

Who Gets Tickborne Diseases?

People who spend time in areas where tick bites are common, either through work or recreation, are at higher risk of getting tickborne diseases. Ticks usually wait near the top of grassy plants and low bushes for people or animals to brush up against their perch. Ticks will often crawl upward on a person's clothes or body for up to several hours or more before attaching to the skin.

How Would I Know if I Have a Tickborne Disease?

You may first have flulike symptoms. Often, you will have fever, chills, and body aches. You may also have a rash. You may not recall being bitten by a tick.

How are Tickborne Diseases Treated?

Most tickborne diseases respond well to treatment with antibiotics. You will get better more quickly if you see a doctor and begin treatment right away.

How Can I Prevent Tickborne Diseases?

The best way to prevent tickborne diseases is to avoid being bitten by ticks. Use tick repellents according to their instructions to help prevent bites. Tick repellents that contain DEET can be put directly on your skin or on your clothing before going into tick-infested areas. Repellents containing permethrin should only be put on clothing.

Wear tops with long sleeves and wear long pants to prevent ticks from getting into the skin. Tuck pant legs into socks to help you see ticks before they get on your skin and bite. Check the entire body for ticks after you have been in tick-infested areas as soon as possible to help prevent illness.

To remove an attached tick, use fine tweezers to grab the tick firmly by the head or as close to the head as possible and pull. Do not use heat, petroleum jelly, or other things on the tick to try to make it "back out" on its own.

(Courtesy the American Academy of Family Physicians, Washington, DC.)

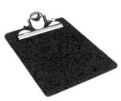

Patient Education Handout

WOUND CARE AFTER TREATMENT WITH TOPICAL SKIN ADHESIVE (TISSUE GLUE)

Tissue glue is a liquid skin adhesive that holds wound edges together. The film usually remains in place for 5 to 10 days before naturally sloughing (falling) off your skin.

The following answers some of your questions and provides instructions for proper care for your wound while it is healing:

Wound Appearance

Some swelling, redness, and pain is common with all wounds and normally goes away as the wound heals. Contact a doctor if swelling, redness, or pain increases; if the wound feels warm to touch; or if you note some pus. If the wound edges reopen or separate, contact a doctor.

Bandaging

- Keep the bandage dry if you have one.
- Replace the dressing twice a day or as directed by the doctor until the adhesive film has fallen off. If the dressing becomes wet, replace it.
- Do not scratch, rub, or pick at the adhesive film. This may loosen the glue before your wound is healed.
- Do not place tape directly over the adhesive film because removing the tape may also remove the glue.
- Protect the wound from prolonged exposure to sunlight or tanning lamps while the film is in place.

Topical Medications

- *Do not* apply liquid or ointment medications or any other product to your wound while the adhesive film is in place. This may loosen the film before your wound is healed.

Keep Wound Dry and Protected

- Protect your wound from repeated injury until the skin has had sufficient time to heal. Do not stretch the skin over the area, especially during the first few days, since it may pull the edges apart.
- You may occasionally and briefly wet your wound in the shower or bath. Do not soak or scrub your wound or swim, and avoid periods of heavy perspiration until the adhesive has fallen off naturally. If a protective dressing is being used, remove it before showering. After showering or bathing, gently blot your wound dry with a soft towel. Apply a clean, dry bandage over the wound if necessary to protect the wound.

If you have any questions or concerns about this product, please consult your doctor.

(Adapted from package insert supplied with Dermabond adhesive. From Ethicon, Inc.)

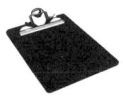 *Patient Education Handout*

INGROWN TOENAILS

Why Do I Have Ingrown Toenails?

Usually ingrown toenails are from improper trimming of the nails into a curved instead of flat shape, tearing of the nail into the skin instead of clipping the nail properly, and from shoes that don't fit right.

What is Ingrown Toenail Removal?

Part or all of the toenail that is causing pain, swelling, and infection of the skin along the edge of the toenail will be removed. It will grow back over 6 to 12 months unless the doctor performs a procedure to permanently remove it.

Why Do I Need This Procedure?

To relieve the pain and swelling and allow resumption of usual activities. Without removal, a significant infection could occur.

What Happens During the Procedure?

The toe will be anesthetized, and the nail or a portion of the nail will be separated and removed gently from the surrounding tissue.

Are There Complications After the Procedure?

For several days there may be pain and swelling. Elevation of the foot will minimize these symptoms. It is possible to experience infection of the skin, bleeding, and pain after this procedure. The nail may be deformed if it regrows. Although extremely rare, the bone under the nail could become infected when permanent nail removal is performed. This would require antibiotics for several weeks.

What Should I Do After the Procedure to Prevent Infection?

Elevation and rest of the affected foot for the first 24 hours is helpful. Soak the toe in warm water if needed for comfort. After 12 hours, begin washing the toe with soap and water three to four times a day for 4 to 5 days.

When Should I Call My Healthcare Provider?

If pain, swelling, or bleeding increases rather than decreases over the first 2 days, or if fever or red streaks develop from the toe, call your healthcare provider.

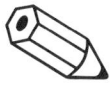 *Patient Consent Form*

INGROWN TOENAILS

I came to the office of Dr. _____ on _____ for evaluation and treatment of the following condition: chronic pain, swelling, or infection resulting from an ingrown toenail.

We discussed the different treatments possible and the risks of not treating the condition. Based on the advice given by Dr. _____ and my own judgment, I agree to undergo the following procedure: removal of the offending portion of the toenail or permanent destruction of a portion or all of the toenail growth center.

Local/digital anesthesia will be used, sterile techniques followed, and topical antibiotic ointment and gauze dressing applied.

We discussed the different outcomes that could occur and most of the possible complications. I am aware that other complications could occur that we could not foresee. I agree to follow the instructions for self-care after the procedure and to return for follow-up care on _____.

I will call the office or answering service if any problems arise before the scheduled follow-up visit.

_____
Patient's signature

_____
Date/Time

_____
Witness' signature

_____
Clinician's signature

One copy for chart; one copy for patient.

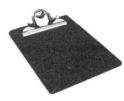

WART (VERRUCA) TREATMENT

The treatment of warts remains difficult and frustrating, for both the patient and the physician. Under the best of circumstances, failure rates are in the range of 30%, even after several treatments. Unfortunately, recurrences are common and frustrating. This is not the fault of your physician, but rather the nature of the disease process itself.

Warts are quite contagious and *caused by a virus.* All of us are probably exposed to the wart virus every day. Some people's immune systems resist the warts; others do not. We are not as yet sure of all the factors that may make the warts grow. In other words, we have not answered why some people get them while others do not, if we indeed are all exposed to the virus.

There are over 80 different varieties of the human papillomavirus (HPV) *virus that causes warts.* The most common warts evaluated in the office are those that occur on the *bottom of the feet (plantar warts), on the hands,* and *in the genital area (condyloma).* When numerous warts come out in small clumps, they are called *mosaic warts.* When they occur under a fingernail or toenail, they are called *periungual warts.* Those that occur on the front of the lower legs are usually very flat and known as *planar warts.*

We know that smoking causes genital warts to grow more rapidly and makes them more difficult to treat. We are not aware of any research showing what happens to the more common hand and foot warts if you smoke, but since *smoking depresses the immune system, it is best not to smoke.* A poor diet may also play a role in patient's exhibiting warts. In patients with low folic acid levels, genital warts that can cause cancer are much more common. Again, although the research does not draw any conclusions with regard to warts on the hands and feet with relationship to diet, it would be prudent to eat five helpings a day of fruits and vegetables and to take a multivitamin with folic acid. Stress, immune disorders (like AIDS), the use of cortisone, and other similar conditions do increase the possibility of having warts, and they are hard to treat in these cases.

Over-the-counter treatments are very common and very effective if the patient is persistent and compliant in using the medication. Duofilm is a liquid that is now available over the counter. A small drop is applied to the wart nightly and the area covered. The macerated or dead tissue is rubbed off each evening (a pumice stone helps) before a new application is made. Generally, 4 to 6 weeks of this type of therapy for hand and plantar warts resolve the lesions. If this does not work, it is time to see your physician.

Your physician can offer several methods for treating your warts: cryosurgery *(freezing with very low temperatures),* surgery, electrocautery, and injection therapy. *With the first three methods, the patient is left with an open sore for 7 to 10 days. Often there can be scarring, and there will be significant discomfort. As noted previously, failure rates can be as high as 30%. Sometimes, however, there are no better options, and one of these forms of therapy will be needed.*

Since 1990 a new method of treating warts by *injection therapy with* Candida *antigen* has been developed. *Candida* is actually a yeast that causes vaginal infections in women. To prepare the solution for injection, the yeast is killed. Since all of us have been exposed to this yeast in our daily living, if the yeast is injected into the superficial skin, it will cause a red reaction much like a mosquito bite.

Physicians have used the solution for over 40 years to check a patient's immune system. When injected the skin should turn red in a few days. If it does not, then the immune system is impaired. Injection of this material into a wart causes the immune system to become very active in that area.

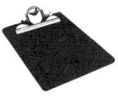

Patient Education Handout—cont'd

WART (VERRUCA) TREATMENT—cont'd

In removing the injected yeast from the body, the immune system generally also identifies the wart tissue and removes that as well. The *advantages of injection therapy* is that it is quick and relatively painless, and there is no scarring or open sore. The patient can immediately return to full activity, including swimming, sports, jazzercise, etc. No special care is needed.

The side effects of injection therapy with Candida have been rare. Occasionally someone develops a *rash (hives)*. This means that the patient can no longer receive any further injections. In general, the less time the warts have been present and the younger the patient, the better the response. However, we have treated patients in their 70s who have failed numerous other modes of therapy but have responded. Generally, there will be some *itching*. Rarely, there is some mild *blistering*. Often the warts turn somewhat black and the crust falls off. About one third of the time a *second injection* will be needed 1 month later, and half of these respond. In the remaining 15% who have not responded to the first or second injection, a third injection another month later can be tried. Approximately 50% of these respond. We do not normally give more than three injections but at times have given five. If all three injections have failed, then one of the previously mentioned older treatments is needed.

The *Candida* therapy for treatment of warts *has not been approved by the Food and Drug Administration (FDA)*. However, it was approved to test immune system competence and activity. Subsequently, we "check the immune system at the site of the warts" using the injection. It is not recommended that those who are pregnant have any injections, although it probably has no adverse effect.

Because of the ease of treatment, the lack of side effects, and the excellent results it provides, in most instances we start our treatment of warts using the *Candida* antigen. If you have any questions whatsoever, please discuss them with us before treatment. If you notice a rash after treatment, please call our office as soon as possible. If you develop hives, take 50 to 100 mg of Benadryl immediately (for older child and adult, respectively) and call us. For children younger than 5 years old, check with us about the dosage.

Generally a follow-up visit is scheduled for 1 month later. If you are *absolutely sure your wart is gone, cancel the visit.* If you are not absolutely sure it is gone, keep your visit. Let us decide if further treatment is necessary.

Recurrences have been rare. Good luck!

Note: Regarding Candin, the medicine used for injection. For your first visit the medication (Candin) used for injection of warts is taken from our supplies. However, if further injections are needed, you will need to pick up a bottle from a pharmacist and bring it with you to the second visit. On your first visit, the doctor will write a prescription for you. Do not purchase the material until you find out if it will be needed. Many times, one injection is all that is needed. If it appears that the wart is not going to go away with the first injection, then about 2 or 3 days before your next scheduled visit, go to the pharmacist with the prescription and pick up the material. Just keep it refrigerated until your office visit. No further purchases will be necessary, even if a third visit is required. *If it appears that the warts have resolved after the first visit, call and cancel your scheduled appointment at least 72 hours in advance.*

Candida antigen (Candin) is not carried by most pharmacies. Go to a hospital pharmacy to obtain it. Call beforehand to be sure they have it for you. Other pharmacies will usually get it for you if you call them a few days in advance.

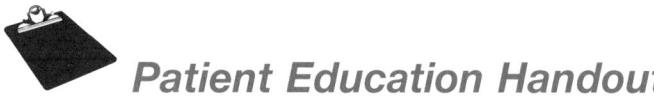

BODY PIERCING

The first and most important rule is to take care of your new piercing so that it can heal properly. Follow these guidelines to ensure your piercing remains healthy.

1. Always wash your hands with antibacterial soap before touching the piercing.
2. Some crusts will form around the jewelry; these are normal and should be removed by soaking the piercing site with a warm sea salt solution (¼ teaspoon of sea salt in 8 ounces of distilled water) using a soft cloth, gauze, or an inverted glass for 5 to 10 minutes. Then gently wipe off the crust using a clean, damp cloth or cotton applicators before gently twisting the jewelry in the moistened area to ensure it is not trapped. Crust will be present until the piercing has completely healed.
3. Wash the piercing with an antibacterial soap that does not contain irritating fragrances. A good choice is Provon (GOJO Laboratories), which contains chloroxylenol. An alternative would be an antibacterial soap containing triclosan, such as Softsoap, Lever 2000, or Septicare. Gently lather and work the suds into the piercing and over the jewelry. Rotate the jewelry carefully to make sure it can move freely, but do not move it forcefully. Rinse the area with warm water to remove the soap residue.
4. Avoid using antibiotic ointments. Prolonged use of antibacterial ointment may irritate the skin and prevent it from healing normally. Only use these products when told to do so by a physician.
5. Avoid applying topical alcohol, which will dry out your skin.
6. Avoid povidone-iodine (Betadine) and hydrogen peroxide because they are toxic to healing tissue.
7. Make sure your clothing does not rub or irritate your new piercing. Also, try not to touch your piercing. The more a piercing is left alone and does not move, the faster it will heal.
8. Avoid changing jewelry until the piercing has completely healed (when the crusts have stopped forming).
9. A water-based lubricant such as K-Y Jelly can be applied, if needed. Petroleum-based products should not be used because they affect healing.
10. For a tongue piercing, rinse your mouth three to four times per day (after meals and after smoking) with antibacterial mouthwash that does not contain alcohol. Replace your toothbrush every 30 days.
11. If something does not look right, do not take out the jewelry! Look at the list below and call your physician. If you take out the jewelry the hole will close.

Please let your physician know if you begin to notice any of the following:

1. New or increasing redness, swelling, or pain around the piercing. Use a warm compress three to four times a day if you notice these symptoms.
2. Pus draining out of the piercing (pus is more "milky" in consistency than the normal fluid that can occur).
3. A piercing that is starting to move or "migrate."
4. Jewelry that becomes "stuck."
5. Abnormal tissue or a scar is forming around the jewelry.

Recommended Websites

www.safepiercing.org (Association of Professional Piercers)
www.piercinglinks.com (Almost Complete Body Piercing Links)
www.bme.freeq.com/index.html (BME: Body Modification Ezine)
www.cs.uu.nl/wais/html/na-dir/bodyart/piercing-faq/.html (Bodyart Newsgroup FAQ on Piercing)
dir.yahoo.com/Arts/Visual_Arts/Body_Art/ (Yahoo! Body Art)

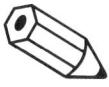

Patient Consent Form

BODY PIERCING

I, _____, the undersigned, request that Dr. _____ and the doctor's assistants perform the following body piercing procedure on me: _____.

I understand that body piercing is an elective procedure that is not medically indicated and is of cosmetic value only. I further understand that my cosmetic outcome and satisfaction with this procedure are not guaranteed.

The piercing procedure has been explained to me in detail and I have asked all the questions I have about the piercing. My doctor has answered all of my questions and has explained the risks of this elective body piercing procedure to me.

I understand that the risks include, but are not limited to, the following: pain, bleeding, infection, and scarring (including keloid formation), along with possible adverse reactions to the jewelry. Further, I am aware that there may be a negative social stigma based on the appearance of body piercing. I understand that this procedure will leave a hole, scar, mark, or other damage to the area pierced even after the removal of the jewelry. Piercing may interfere with anatomic function or damage surrounding structures. The pierced track may migrate or change shape over time.

I have received a detailed explanation of this piercing both in general to piercing and specific to the site that I have selected. I understand that other complications could also occur that may not be foreseen or may not have been discussed.

I agree to follow the instructions given for self-care after the piercing, and I will contact my physician immediately if any problems arise.

I understand that this piercing will take _____ or longer to heal.

I have read and understand this information. I understand the risks of this procedure, and I choose freely to go ahead with this piercing. I have had all of my questions answered to my satisfaction, and I give my consent to proceed with this body piercing.

_____   _____
Patient's signature   *Date/Time*

_____   _____
Legal Guardian's signature   *Witness' signature*

One copy for chart; one copy for patient.

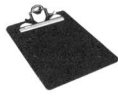

Patient Education Handout

BOTOX INJECTIONS: COSMETIC DENERVATION OF FROWN, FOREHEAD, AND EYE EXPRESSION LINES

What is Cosmetic Denervation?

Cosmetic denervation is a procedure used to improve the appearance of "worry lines," "frown lines," "crow's feet," and other so-called "dynamic" or aging wrinkles. "Dynamic" wrinkles occur when we smile, laugh, or frown and the delicate muscles underlying the skin contract. In cosmetic denervation, botulinum toxin ("Botox") is injected into these muscles. Botulinum toxin works by weakening these tiny facial muscles. By weakening these tiny muscles, the overlying skin will smooth out, whereas untreated facial muscles contract normally, allowing facial expression to be unaffected. Hence, those severe frown lines between the eyes, forehead creases, and crow's feet around the eyes can be smoothed out.

Although cosmetic denervation is a relatively new treatment for wrinkles, botulinum toxin injections were FDA approved in 1989 and have been used safely and effectively used for over a decade for many neurologic disorders. No irreversible clinical effects have been reported. Today the use of Botox has emerged as an exciting new treatment for erasing the visible consequences of aging skin.

How is Cosmetic Denervation Performed?

Cosmetic denervation is a simple and safe procedure. A small amount of diluted Botox is injected with a very fine needle into several locations of the muscles of the face (particularly the area of the frown creases of the forehead and the crow's feet lateral to the eyes). Because the needle is so fine and only a tiny amount of liquid is used, the pain associated with the injections is usually tolerable without anesthesia. We try to minimize the discomfort by applying cold compresses before each area is treated. The medicine stings during the injection and has been compared to the sting on an insect bite, but it clears rapidly within minutes. You will be able to drive and engage in your normal daily activities immediately after your injections. A small number of people will have some temporary bruising of the skin at some injection sites, which fades over several days. Foundation can be applied immediately if this occurs. Otherwise there will be no visible signs of your treatment.

What are the Contraindications? Who Should Not be Treated With Botox?

Botox is not recommended for the following:
- Persons allergic to human albumin or botulinum toxin
- Pregnant or breastfeeding women
- Those with neuromuscular disease such as myasthenia gravis
- Those being treated at the same time with tissue fillers (collagen)

Are There any Side Effects?

Mild, temporary bruising may occur. Very slight droopiness of the upper eyelid occurs in about 2% of people who have their frown lines injected. About 5% of people who have their forehead injected immediately above the eyebrows may notice this effect. A much smaller number of people will notice slight asymmetry of the lower face after injections of the crow's feet muscles. These effects are not usually noticeable by others and fully recover after 3 to 5 weeks. An extremely rare side effect—temporary double vision—has been reported in the literature. To minimize the possibility of such rare effects, please be sure to follow the posttreatment instructions.

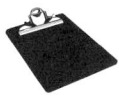

Patient Education Handout—cont'd

BOTOX INJECTIONS: COSMETIC DENERVATION OF FROWN, FOREHEAD, AND EYE EXPRESSION LINES—cont'd

A very small percentage of people do not have much effect from the treatment. A rare patient may even develop antibodies against Botox and develop resistance to response over time. Usually, just the opposite occurs; they respond more to the same dose as time goes on.

What Kind of Results Can I Expect?

If dynamic wrinkles are making you look older and more "serious," cosmetic denervation can smooth these out and give you a more youthful and rested appearance. However, this treatment will not improve the more common "static" wrinkles that are unrelated to facial muscle contraction, nor does it improve loose or sagging skin. Results are typically seen within 2 to 10 days of the treatment and last for 6 weeks to 6 months (typically 3 to 4 months). Occasionally, there is a muscle that does not respond, and a "touch-up" may be needed in 2 to 3 weeks.

How Long Do the Results Last?

Initially, most people require a repeat injection every 3 months to maintain the effect. However, after three to five injections, the effect may last longer and a repeat injection may only be required every 6 to 12 months.

What Instructions Should I Follow After Treatment?

Do not rub the injection sites for 4 hours, since this may spread the solution to adjacent muscles. Do not lie down for 4 hours, for the same reason. Exercise the muscles by doing the full range of animated facial expressions (raise your brows, furrow your brows and frown deeply, smile, etc.) every 15 minutes for 1 to 2 hours. Botulinum toxin attaches better to active muscles. A small number of people will require a higher dose than that given with the first treatment to obtain an effect. If you have seen no improvement after 2 weeks, please call us to schedule a "touch-up."

How Much Will it Cost?

Botox is very expensive. The cost per treatment will be $_____. The majority of insurance policies, including Medicaid and Medicare, refuse to pay for "cosmetic" medical care and will not, therefore, pay for Botox therapy. Our office will request fee-for-service at the time of your visit, payable by cash, check, or charge.

(Modified from O'Hanlon KO, MD, Marshall University School of Medicine.)

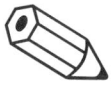

Patient Consent Form

BOTULINUM TOXIN TYPE A *(BOTOX COSMETIC)*

Botox is made from Botulinum Toxin Type A, a protein produced by the bacterium *Clostridium botulinum.* For the purpose of improving the appearance of wrinkles, small doses of the toxin are injected into the affected muscles blocking the release of a chemical that would otherwise signal the muscle to contract. The toxin thus paralyzes or weakens the injected muscle. The treatment usually begins to work within 24 to 48 hours and can last up to 4 months. The Food and Drug Administration (FDA) approved the cosmetic use of Botulinum Toxin Type A for the temporary relief of moderate to severe frown lines between the brow and recommends that the procedure be performed no more frequently than once every 3 months.

It is not known whether Botulinum A Toxin can cause fetal harm when administered to pregnant women or can affect reproductive capabilities. It is also not known if Botulinum A Toxin is excreted in human milk. For these reasons, Botulinum A Toxin should not be used on pregnant or lactating women.

I authorize and direct _____, with associates or assistants of his or her choice, to perform the following procedure of Botulinum A Toxin injection(s) on _____ (patient name) for the treatment of _____ (e.g., brow, forehead, crow's feet).

_____ The details of the procedure have been explained to me in terms I understand.

_____ Alternative methods and their benefits and disadvantages have been explained to me.

_____ I understand that the FDA has only approved the cosmetic use of Botulinum A Toxin for frown lines between the brow. Any other cosmetic use is considered off label.

_____ I understand and accept the most likely risks and complications of Botulinum A Toxin injection(s) include but are not limited to:
  • Paralysis of a nearby muscle that could interfere with opening the eye(s)
  • Local numbness
  • Headache, nausea, or flulike symptoms
  • Swallowing, speech, or respiratory disorders
  • Swelling, bruising, or redness at injection site
  • Disorientation or double vision
  • Temporary asymmetrical appearance
  • Abnormal or lack of facial expression
  • Inability to smile when injected in the lower face
  • Facial pain
  • Product ineffectiveness

_____ I understand and accept that the long-term effects of repeated use of Botox Cosmetic are as yet unknown. Possible risks and complications that have been identified include but are not limited to:
  • Muscle atrophy (weakness)
  • Nerve irritability
  • Production of antibodies with unknown effect to general health

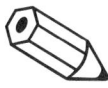

Patient Consent Form

BOTULINUM TOXIN TYPE A *(BOTOX COSMETIC)—cont'd*

_____ I understand and accept the less common complications, including the remote risk of death or serious disability, that exist with this procedure.

_____ I am aware that smoking during the pre- and postoperative periods could increase chances of complications.

_____ I have informed the doctor of all my known allergies.

_____ I have informed the doctor of all medications I am currently taking, including prescriptions, over-the-counter remedies, herbal therapies, and any others.

_____ I have been advised whether I should take any or all of these medications on the days surrounding the procedure.

_____ I am aware and accept that no guarantees about the results of the procedure have been made or applied.

_____ I have been informed of what to expect post-treatment, including but not limited to: estimated recovery time, anticipated activity level, and the necessity of additional procedures if I wish to maintain the appearance this procedure provides me.

_____ I am not currently pregnant or nursing, and I understand that should I become pregnant while using this drug there are potential risks, including fetal malformation.

_____ If pre- and postoperative photos and/or videos are taken of the treatment for record purposes, I understand that these photos will be the property of the attending physician.

_____ I understand that these photos may only be used for scientific or record keeping purposes.

_____ The doctor has answered all of my questions regarding this procedure.

_____ I have been advised to seek immediate medical attention if swallowing, speech, or respiratory disorders arise.

Patient Consent

I certify that I have read and understand this treatment agreement and that all blanks were filled in prior to my signature.

_____   _____

Patient's Signature/Date   *Witness' Signature/Date*

_____   _____

Print Patient Name   *Print Witness name*

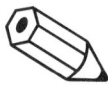 *Patient Consent Form*

BOTULINUM TOXIN TYPE A *(BOTOX COSMETIC)—cont'd*
Physician Certification

I certify that I have explained the nature, purpose, benefits, risks, complications, and alternatives to the proposed procedure to the patient. I have answered all questions fully, and I believe that the patient fully understands what I have explained.

_____   _____
Physician's Signature   *Date*

Copy was given to patient: _____   _____
                                                    Date   *Initials*

Original was placed in chart: _____   _____
                                                    Date   *Initials*

One copy for chart; one copy for patient.

(Courtesy Allergan, Inc., Irvine, Calif.)

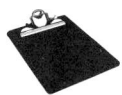

Patient Education Handout

COLLAGEN REPLACEMENT THERAPY

What is Collagen Replacement Therapy?

Collagen replacement therapy (CRT) is a simple, nonsurgical cosmetic treatment of facial lines, wrinkles, and scars. Collagen is a connective tissue, which forms support for our skin. It can be placed around the eyes, cheeks, mouth, and chin, as well as on the forehead. It is also used to augment lips. A purified collagen extract from beef is used. It is very similar to that produced by humans.

Who Should Undergo CRT?

Anyone who is concerned about his or her appearance. The typical patient is usually female (although males also have it done) and usually 35 to 55. Anyone who has acne scars, has lines from sun damage or heredity, or desires fuller lips is a candidate.

What Preparation is Required?

You'll need to meet with the doctor to review your medical history and discuss the procedure. Usually one skin test is required, and this can be done on the first visit. If there is no adverse reaction in 4 weeks, CRT may proceed.

How is the Procedure Performed?

Collagen is injected (into facial wrinkles, scars, or the lips) with a syringe using a small, short needle. Numbing medicine is mixed in the collagen. Some people have it performed during their lunch hour. No other time off work is needed.

How Long Do the Results Last?

Results should be considered permanent, although that rarely happens. Like any beauty or fitness routine, CRT requires a maintenance program. Patients may need touch-up treatments every 3 to 6 months for optimal results. Sometimes, however, results last 2 years or more.

Does it Hurt?

Collagen is injected with a fine, short needle. Lidocaine, a numbing medicine, is incorporated into the product, but some people still feel discomfort, usually described as a stinging. It only lasts a few moments.

How Much Does it Cost?

In a recent survey of collagen patients, most reported spending on the average of $175 per month for personal care (hair, nails, exercise, skin care, cosmetics, etc.). As a comparison, biannual collagen treatments (every 6 months) cost, on average, approximately $80 per month, or about $550 per injection. Insurances do not cover this procedure, so you will need to pay on the day of injection.

Continued

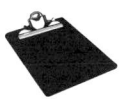 *Patient Education Handout—cont'd*

COLLAGEN REPLACEMENT THERAPY—cont'd

Who Should Not Have the Injections?

This procedure has been performed safely in thousands of men and women. However, some safety issues should be noted. Collagen injections may not be right for you if have any of the following conditions:

- A reaction to the required skin test
- Known allergy to injected collagen or lidocaine or a history of serious allergic reactions
- A connective tissue disease (e.g., lupus, rheumatoid arthritis), or area immunosuppressed

What are Some Possible Complications?

- Slight discomfort
- Bruising
- Allergic reactions
- Overcorrection of intended problem with distortion of facial features

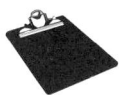 *Patient Education Handout*

PHOTOEPILATION/LASER HAIR REMOVAL
What is Photoepilation?
Epilation is hair removal. Photoepilation is the newest technology to provide permanent hair reduction. Specific wavelengths of laser light or intense pulsed light are used to destroy hair roots. Most authorities feel this is better than any other current technology. It is faster, and it has fewer complications than other methods. Some hair loss occurs initially, but maximum hair loss may not be seen for several weeks after each treatment. In general, multiple treatments will be needed depending on the site.

What Do You Mean by Permanent Hair Reduction?
Permanent hair reduction is defined as a long-term, stable reduction in the number of hairs regrowing after treatment. Permanent hair reduction is not equivalent to complete hair loss. A certain percentage of the hairs treated will not regrow after each treatment. Based on findings from recent studies, the average patient will experience a minimum of 60% to 80% permanent hair reduction with virtually no adverse side effects. Different cycles in follicle (hair root) growth make it impossible to destroy all hair in one treatment. Only hair that is in the growing phase can be destroyed; this is why it usually takes six to ten sessions to achieve a good result. Removal of all hair may never be accomplished, but there should be permanent reduction.

How Many Treatments are Needed?
It varies with the area being treated and on what percentage of the hair is actively growing. Darker hair has more melanin and is more easily removed. People with dark skin and light hair are difficult to treat. The average number of treatments can vary anywhere from six to ten treatments and varies from person to person. The treatments are usually scheduled every 5 to 6 weeks to allow optimal hair growth in the area being treated.

Does it Hurt?
Relative to waxing, electrolysis, plucking, and ripping, laser hair removal does not hurt to that degree. But it has been described as stinging, or like a rubber band snapping against the skin when a light pulse is triggered. This stinging or snapping sensation should not last more than 5 seconds after the light flash.

What are the Side Effects?
Fortunately, there are few side effects. In the first hour, treated skin may develop redness, burning, and swelling around the hair shaft. This responds quickly to a cool ice pack and aloe vera lotion. Rarely, blistering will occur, but this also responds to ice and aloe vera. Permanent scarring is rare. Very dark skin can become hypopigmented (turn lighter), and lighter shades can become hyperpigmented (darker). Hyperpigmentation usually fades in 3 to 6 months. Excessive swelling can occur but subsides in 3 to 7 days. If skin becomes fragile at the treatment site, avoid makeup and rubbing the area. Of course, lack of hair removal could be called an unwanted side effect.

Continued

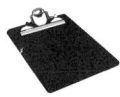

Patient Education Handout—cont'd

PHOTOEPILATION/LASER HAIR REMOVAL—cont'd

What Should I Do Before the Visit?

For the best result, avoid sun or tanning 4 to 6 weeks before treatment. If you have tanned recently, you cannot undergo photoepilation. There is a danger of overheating the treatment area because of darker pigment in the skin. Let your hair grow for 1 to 2 days in the place you want treatment. This helps conduct the energy to the follicle for effective hair destruction. If you usually shave the hair you want removed, let it grow for several days. Remove your makeup before treatment and keep your skin clean. Tell the doctor if you start any medications; some can make you more susceptible to burning with treatment.

What Will be Done at the Visits?

At the first visit the doctor will evaluate you and determine the correct light setting for your treatments. This will take about 30 minutes. The cost will be _____, of which _____ will be applied to your first treatment fee. You will receive some small "test spot" treatments. The first treatment can be scheduled with the receptionist after your consultation visit. Payment will need to be made at the time of your treatments. Fees will be charged based on the size and location of the area treated.

How Should I Care for Treated Skin?

Gentle washing and the use of an aloe vera gel are generally sufficient.

(Used with permission of The National Procedures Institute, Midland, Mich.)

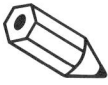

Patient Consent Form

PHOTOEPILATION/LASER HAIR REMOVAL

I understand that the _____ is intended for epilation (hair removal) and that clinical results may vary with different skin types, hair color, and location. I understand that there is a possibility of rare side effects, such as scarring and permanent discoloration, as well as short-term effects such as reddening, mild burning, temporary bruising, and temporary discoloration. These effects have all been fully explained to me. _____ *(please initial)*

I understand that the number of visits required for optimal results may vary considerably from patient to patient, depending on skin type, hair color, and hair texture. Patients with gray, white, or lightly colored hair will experience partial results and some may experience no improvement at all. I understand there is no guarantee that all hair will be removed.

I understand that the treatment by the _____ system is not covered by insurance. The fee structure has been fully explained to me, and I will need to pay for each treatment on the day I am seen.

I also understand that other options such as electrolysis, waxing, and chemical preparations are available. _____ *(please initial)*

I understand that a photograph of the area to be treated may be taken at the first visit, and follow-up pictures may be taken intermittently throughout the course of the treatments.

I have read and understand this agreement, and all my questions have been addressed and answered to my satisfaction. I agree to the terms of this agreement. I fully understand the risks, benefits, and possible complications.

Patient's name: _____ *Signature:* _____

Date: _____

Witness' signature: _____

One copy for chart; one copy for patient.

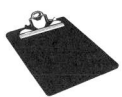 *Patient Education Handout*

MICRODERMABRASION PREPARATION

You will be having a light peel or microdermabrasion treatment on the day of your next appointment. Please follow the outline below to prepare:

1. Please refrain from the following activities within 14 days of your appointment:
   - Chemical peel
   - Tanning in a tanning booth
   - "Wax" treatment
   - Collagen injections
   - Microdermabrasion treatments
2. Be sure to inform us if you are pregnant or think you may be pregnant.
3. Please refrain from sun exposure for 10 days before your appointment. Do not come to the appointment with a sunburn. (Please let us know if you are unable to keep your appointment.)
4. Delay use of Retin-A, Renova, Differin, and high percentage glycolic products for approximately 5 days before your appointment. (Any of these will take the treatment deeper and make your results less predictable.)

These superficial peels will result in little to no downtime. Treatments may include slight redness, tightness, peeling, flaking, or temporary dryness. Make-up use can be resumed the day after the treatment.

(Used with permission of The Medical Procedures Center, P.C., Midland, Mich. Adapted from various sources.)

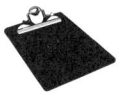

Patient Education Handout

CHEMICAL PEEL/MICRODERMABRASION POSTTREATMENT INSTRUCTIONS

You have just had a chemical peel or microdermabrasion skin treatment. Due to the nature of these treatments, you should not necessarily expect to "peel." However, you may have light flaking for a few days. Most patients who undergo these treatments have only residual redness for anywhere from 1 to 12 hours.

It is recommended that you do not apply make-up the day of the treatment. It is ideal to allow the skin to stabilize and rest overnight. However, make-up *can* be applied, if necessary. Tonight your skin will feel tight and "pulled." Apply moisturizer as frequently as needed. Although you may or may not actually "peel," it is likely that you will experience a light "exfoliation." It may take two or more treatments for the surface skin to loosen and "peel." Everyone responds differently, and most patients look quite normal the day after their treatment. Unless recommended by your esthetician, do not apply other medications or AHA products to your skin, since they may be too irritating.

- *Avoid direct sun exposure and excessive heat. Use your daily sunscreen protection.*
- Do not pick at or pull on any loosening or exfoliating skin. This could potentially cause hyperpigmentation.
- *ABSOLUTELY do not go to a tanning booth for at least 3 weeks before or after treatment.*
- Discontinue use of Retin-A/Renova/Differin for 7 days after treatment.
- Do not have electrolysis, collagen injections, and facial waxing, and do not use depilatories, for approximately 5 days.

(Used with permission of The Medical Products Center, P.C. Adapted from various sources.)

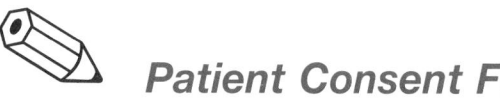

Patient Consent Form

MICRODERMABRASION

My signature acknowledges that I have read the following and agree to receive the treatments or series of treatments listed below.

I, _____, consent to authorize _____, or members of his or her staff, to perform microdermabrasion skin exfoliation and other services.

Areas to be treated:

Number of treatments estimated: _____

- The nature and purpose of the treatment has been explained to me, and any questions I have regarding this procedure have been explained to my satisfaction. _____ (initial)
- I understand that, with any treatment, certain risks are involved and that any complications or side effects from known or unknown causes could occur. I freely assume these risks. _____ (initial)
- Possible side effects include, but are not limited to: Mild redness, extreme redness, bruising, local swelling, stinging, tenderness, dry skin, flaking, lightening or darkening of the skin, infections, pimples, bumpy appearance, and cold sores. Most side effects are temporary and generally subside within 72 hours. _____ (initial)
- If I am prone to herpes outbreaks, I agree to use a prescription medication to prevent an outbreak during the time of treatments. _____ (initial)
- I have been advised to discontinue all AHA's, glycolics, Retin-A, Renova, or any exfoliating products for up to 72 hours after the procedure. I understand that I must use hydrating and soothing antioxidants for healing, and ice for swelling and inflammation reduction. Also, I understand there should be no sun exposure for 72 hours and that the use of an SPF 30 at all times during treatment duration is advised. _____ (initial)
- I have been advised to avoid collagen injections for 10 to 14 days before any microdermabrasion treatment and agree to these restrictions. _____ (initial)
- I have been advised to avoid Botox injections for up to at least 24 hours before any microdermabrasion treatment, and I agree to these restrictions. _____ (initial)
- I agree to adhere to all safety precautions and home skin care program as recommended by my practitioner. _____ (initial)
- I am over 18 years of age or I have parental consent co-signed below. _____ (initial)
- I will call to inform the office of any complications or concerns I may have as soon as they occur. _____ (initial)

_____   _____
Client/Patient's signature   *Date/Time*

_____   _____
Parent's signature   *Witness' signature*

One copy for chart; one copy for patient.

(Used with permission of The Medical Procedures Center, P.C., Midland, Mich. Adapted from various sources.)

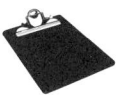

Patient Education Handout

SKIN PEELS

Individuals likely to benefit the most from chemical skin peels are from 25 to 50 years of age with photodamage (e.g., sun spots, age spots, fine wrinkles, irregular skin texture) on the face and hands. Fair-skinned, light-eyed individuals with a lot of sun damage or wrinkles at rest also benefit the most from peels. It is very unusual to see significant photodamage before 25 years of age. After 50 years of age, other skin aging factors decrease the benefit of peels.

In addition, chemical peels are often useful for patients with acne or actinic keratoses; however, the acne or any kind of dermatitis should be treated and under control before undergoing a peel. Chemical peels are sometimes helpful for mild scars from acne. Patients that fail certain other topical therapies may also benefit from a peel.

Fine wrinkles with skin motion, such as smiling, may respond to a peel but usually not as well as fine wrinkles seen only at rest. Deep wrinkles at rest such as those seen with intrinsically aging skin may require deeper peels or plastic surgery interventions. Deeper wrinkles that are muscle or motion induced will probably not respond to any peeling or resurfacing technique.

To produce peeling, a chemical such as glycolic acid (GA) or another α-hydroxy acid (AHA), salicylic acid (SA), or trichloroacetic acid (TCA) is applied directly to the skin. Dermatologic or plastic surgeons also use phenol occasionally. These chemicals change the composition of the skin, delivering a controlled type of shallow or superficial tissue destruction or wound. As the wound heals, the outer layers of the skin peel or slough off. Deeper peels can also affect the lower collagen and elastin layers of the skin to remove deeper wrinkles.

The minimal scabbing associated with a peel usually clears within 3 to 7 days. As the scabbing clears, the pigmentation of the skin is often removed. When the skin heals, the pigmentation should be more uniform, the texture should be smoother and the skin should be more youthful in appearance.

Some mild GA, SA, or TCA peels may be repeated, whereas the deeper peels (e.g., phenol) usually do not require repeat treatment. Multiple applications of superficial-depth peels will usually produce the same results as the deeper peels, and it will not be as obvious to friends and family that you have had a peel. Multiple shallow peels may also be safer because each superficial-depth peel is better controlled than a single deep peel. Superficial-depth peels can be applied near the end of the week so that most of the peeling occurs over the weekend. By the next week, there is usually little or no sign that you have had a peel.

Whenever the skin is peeled or wounded, there is a risk of scarring and infection. There is also a risk of pigmentary augmentation that is both short term (which almost always resolves) and long term and a slight risk of permanent pigmentary augmentation. Medium and deep peels increase the risk of all of these side effects and complications. Although rare, persistent hyperpigmentation is often adequately treated with prescribed bleaching agents. If you are $\frac{1}{32}$ Native American or more, you have a higher risk of a skin reaction and resulting hyperpigmentation with this procedure; therefore you need to inform the clinician of your heritage so that he or she can use precautions.

If you are a smoker, have frequent fever blisters (e.g., herpes outbreaks), have had prior radiation therapy to the skin, or are taking hormones or using isotretinoin (Accutane), inform your clinician because you may not be a good candidate for a chemical peel. Chemical peels are not really effective against the damage of persistent smoking.

Continued

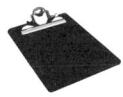 *Patient Education Handout—cont'd*

SKIN PEELS—cont'd

For GA (AHA), SA 20% to 30%, and TCA 10% superficial-depth peels, you can wear make-up the day of the peel and it will be removed in the office.

For superficial-depth peels, Renova or Retin-A should be stopped 3 days before the procedure.

To ensure even skin penetration for medium and deep peels, the skin should be washed the evening before the procedure to remove all cosmetics and again the next morning. Often you will be asked to prepare the skin with topical Renova or Retin-A for several weeks to months before the peel. Benefits of pretreatment include accelerated new skin growth and reduced healing time. If you develop bothersome or severe flaking, itching, redness, or irritation with these medications, discontinue for several days and resume application on alternate days.

When the peel is performed, after the face is prepped with petrolatum, it usually takes less than 1 minute to apply the solution for superficial- to medium-depth peels. Deep peels may take longer, even requiring several hours to prepare the face, apply the chemical, and complete the peel.

For superficial-depth peels, you may experience a stinging or burning sensation during application of the peel, which increases for 2 minutes after the application, reaches a peak at 3 minutes, and then goes away over the following minute. The chemicals themselves will cause slight anesthesia.

For superficial-depth peels you will often sense a slight tightness and smoothness of the skin immediately after the peel. Several days later, some patients experience slight skin crusting, swelling, and occasionally what looks like a slight "black eye" in the lower eyelid areas. These resolve rapidly. Actual peeling usually begins 2 days after the peel and can last for up to 7 days. Most patients peel in the central part of the face more heavily than peripherally, and only lightly on the forehead. Some patients peel in fine sheets, but most peel in flakes.

For superficial-depth peels, the effect is maximal at 48 hours, so you should avoid the sun completely for at least 3 days. The skin is most vulnerable to damage during this time, and sun exposure can cause many problems (including a deepening of the peel or postinflammatory hyperpigmentation).

The effect of a medium-depth peel is maximal at 48 hours, usually subsides within the first week, and is gone by the third month after the procedure. Crusts or scabs usually appear and some swelling may occur. The clinician may prescribe a mild pain medication to relieve any tingling or throbbing. In about 1 week to 10 days, new skin will be apparent and you should be healed sufficiently to return to normal activities. However, you should avoid the sun for several months.

For all depth of peels, sunburn may occur at lower doses of sunlight and result in hyperpigmentation or hypopigmentation. Preservatives, scents, or the chemicals used in sunblock may provoke a sensitivity reaction and cause persistent erythema; therefore a hypoallergenic, nonscented, complete sunblock (SPF 20 or greater) for sensitive skin should be used.

Even after healing, the skin is thinner after a peel; therefore it is more susceptible to sun damage and sunburn.

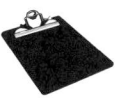

Patient Education Handout—cont'd

SKIN PEELS—cont'd

Thinner or irritated skin is also more susceptible to drying out, so a moisturizer should be applied daily.

Note: Disappointment from a chemical peel is often the result of overly high expectations. This patient education sheet should be read carefully. Superficial-depth peels often produce only modest clinical effects. Multiple peels may be necessary for appreciable benefits. A medium-depth peel is not comparable to a face-lift.

Websites That May be of Interest to You:

The following websites provide information regarding chemical peels and alternatives to chemical peels:

www.plasticsurgery.org/surgery/chempeel.htm

www.plastic-surgery.net (Plastic Surgery Network)

www.plastic-surgery.net/procedures/chemical.html (Plastic Surgery Network: Chemical peels)

www.plastic-surgery.net/procedures/dermabrasion.html (Plastic Surgery Network: Dermabrasion and dermaplaning)

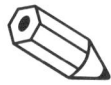

Patient Consent Form

TATTOO TREATMENT USING THE INFRARED LIGHT OBLITERATION METHOD

The infrared coagulator (IRC) has been widely used in Europe for tattoo treatment and has now been introduced in the United States. It is a simple unit that uses infrared light to remove the tattoo. The treated area will blister up and take several weeks to heal. The results and complications are similar to laser.

All current methods of tattoo obliteration are costly, and insurances will not cover the cost of removal. Each has advantages and disadvantages. With all methods, including IRC, there will be some degree of skin scarring, lack of skin pigment (lightening of the skin), and other problems. *No tattoo can be removed without a trace! All tattoo treatments leave scars and often treatments must be repeated to remove residual pigment.* Current treatments include the following:
• Salt abrasion
• Dermabrasion
• Surgical excision (cutting it out)
• Pulsed laser/dye laser
• IRC (infrared light)
• Skin grafting
• Tattooing over the area to make it look different
• Injections

The U.S. FDA approved IRC for treatment of tattoos in 1991. Healing of the skin often requires 4 to 6 weeks. The quality of the healed areas are comparable to laser treatments. The heat of IRC delivered into the skin is painful in some cases despite the use of local anesthesia. Ink may be visible after treatment but will frequently go away during healing.

The blisters that occur after each IRC treatment are followed by "crusts." Scars slowly lose their red color over many months. Skin pigment (color) will be decreased to some degree after any type of tattoo treatment!

The major concern after treatment is excessive scarring. It is very important to follow the instructions the doctor gives to reduce this complication.

Please answer the following questions:
I (have/have not) been treated for mental illness.
I (have/have not) had problems with local anesthetic (numbing shots) in the past.
I (have/have not) formed heavy, wide, or thick scars in the past.

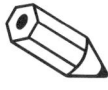

Patient Consent Form—cont'd

TATTOO TREATMENT USING THE INFRARED LIGHT OBLITERATION METHOD—cont'd

My tattoo(s) were done in the year _____. The colors are _____.
My tattoos are (professional/amateur). They are located:

_____

_____

Describe any previous attempts to "remove" or obliterate your tattoos:

_____

_____

By signing and initialing below, I give my permission for Dr. _____ and his staff to treat my tattoo or tattoos with the infrared coagulation method. I further agree to be photographed and know that these photographs will be used for both professional and patient education. I understand there will be some scarring and have seen pictures of what to expect. I know the insurance company will not cover these treatments and I will pay on the date of service. I have discussed other methods of treatment and have no further questions.

_____   _____
Patient's signature   *Date/Time*

_____
Parent/legal guardian's signature

_____
Witness' signature

1. I understand that I may have pain, blistering, and scars of some degree.
2. I am aware that two or more treatments may be required.
3. I am aware that I may be uncomfortable or dissatisfied with my scarring or other result of this infrared light treatment.
4. I am aware that some tattoos cannot be completely obliterated.
5. I am aware that I must follow directions for aftercare and return for an evaluation in 60 days.
6. I am aware that there will be additional charges for subsequent treatments.
7. I am aware that certain areas of the body (back, chest, shoulder) are considered "worst scar areas."
8. I am aware that people with certain skin types scar more than others, and that the degree of scarring or pigment change cannot be predicted.

Continued

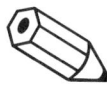 *Patient Consent Form—cont'd*

TATTOO TREATMENT USING THE INFRARED LIGHT OBLITERATION METHOD—cont'd

9. I am aware of the risks and complications of surgery and skin treatments and understand the explanations of the procedure and risks that were explained to me.
10. I am aware that treatment of a tattoo by any method may leave the tattoo areas worse than before treatment. I accept this risk.
11. My questions have been answered to my satisfaction regarding treatment, results, complications, etc.

_____   _____

Patient's signature   *Date/Time*

_____

Parent/legal guardian's signature

_____

Witness' signature

One copy for chart; one copy for patient.

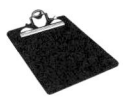

Patient Education Handout

CHALAZION/HORDEOLUM

CHALAZION

What is Chalazion Excision?

A chalazion (commonly called a "stye") is an inflamed oil gland within the eyelid, which results in an annoying lump that can last for many months. Chalazion excision is a minor surgical procedure to remove the inflamed tissue and get rid of the lump.

Why Do I Need This Procedure?

If the chalazion does not go away with medical treatments, and you would like to be rid of the lump, chalazion excision is an effective treatment. Without treatment, it may continue to grow or become unsightly.

How Do I Prepare for Chalazion Excision?

You should stop taking aspirin for 1 week in order to prevent excessive bleeding. You should inform your doctor if you are taking any blood-thinner medication, if you bleed or bruise easily, or if you have had a reaction to anesthetic injections.

What Happens During the Procedure?

You will receive a shot to numb the eyelid. An instrument will be placed on the eyelid, and you will feel some pressure while the chalazion is being removed. Afterwards, a patch will be placed on the eye.

What Happens After the Procedure?

You will go home with a patch on your eye. You may remove the patch in the evening. The eye will be bloody and mattered, and the eyelid will be swollen and bruised. This is normal. You may gently clean the eyelid. If it begins to bleed, put pressure on the eyelid until it stops, which may take several minutes. If the bleeding does not stop after 20 minutes, call your doctor.

You will be given a prescription for an eye ointment, which you should put inside the eye twice a day starting the morning after the procedure, until the eye seems back to normal.

What are the Risks Associated With the Procedure?

It is possible that you may need stitches in the skin, and you could have a small scar on the outside of the eyelid. Sometimes a part of the chalazion remains after the procedure, or it may recur. Occasionally you may need to have the procedure repeated. You may have excessive bleeding, and there is a small chance that you could develop an infection. Rarely, the tear drainage system could be damaged, causing permanent watering of the eye that could be corrected by surgery.

What Do I Need to Do Following the Procedure to Prevent Infection?

It is important to use the antibiotic eye ointment as prescribed. Infection is very uncommon because of the good blood supply in the eyelid.

Continued

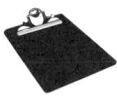 *Patient Education Handout—cont'd*

CHALAZION/HORDEOLUM—cont'd

CHALAZION—cont'd
When Should I Call my Healthcare Provider?
If the eyelid becomes more swollen, red, and painful as time passes, you should call your doctor. Also call if the eyelid begins to bleed and you are unable to stop the bleeding after applying pressure for 20 minutes.

Websites That May be of Interest to You:
www.rxmed.com/illnesses/chalazion.html
www.inform.umd.edu/UHC/Library/Handouts/chalaz.html
www.eyenet.org

HORDEOLUM
What is Incision and Drainage of a Hordeolum?
A hordeolum (commonly called a "stye") is an abscess (infection with a collection of pus) within the eyelid, which results in a painful lump. Incision and drainage of the hordeolum is a minor surgical procedure to remove the pus and get rid of the infection and lump.

Why Do I Need This Procedure?
Without treatment, the infection may spread to the surrounding skin and become more serious. In addition, pus may build up and become more painful, although it may eventually drain on its own.

How Do I Prepare for Incision and Drainage of a Hordeolum?
You should stop taking aspirin before the procedure in order to prevent excessive bleeding. You should inform your doctor if you are taking any blood-thinner medication, if you bleed or bruise easily, or if you have had a reaction to anesthetic injections.

What Happens During the Procedure?
You will receive a shot to numb the eyelid. A scalpel will be used to make a small cut in your eyelid to allow the pus to escape. You may feel some pressure while the hordeolum is being incised, but you are likely to have relief of your pain when the pus is released.

What Happens After the Procedure?
You may go home. The eye may be bloody and mattered, and the eyelid may be swollen and bruised. This is normal. You may gently clean the eyelid. If it begins to bleed, put pressure on the eye until it stops, which may take several minutes. If the bleeding does not stop after 20 minutes, call your doctor.

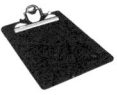

Patient Education Handout—cont'd

CHALAZION/HORDEOLUM—cont'd

HORDEOLUM—cont'd

What are the Risks Associated With the Procedure?

You may have a small scar on the outside of the eyelid. Sometimes a part of the hordeolum remains after the procedure, or it may recur. You may need to have the procedure repeated. You may have excessive bleeding, and there is a chance that the infection could spread to nearby tissues. Rarely, the tear drainage system could be damaged, causing permanent watering of the eye (which is correctable by surgery.)

What Do I Need to Do Following the Procedure to Prevent Infection?

It is important to use the antibiotic medication as prescribed.

When Should I Call My Healthcare Provider?

If the eyelid becomes more swollen, red, and painful as time passes, or if pus forms under the skin, you should call your doctor. Also call if the eyelid begins to bleed and you are unable to stop the bleeding after applying pressure for 20 minutes.

Websites That May be of Interest to You:

www.inform.umd.edu/UHC/Library/Handouts/chalaz.html
www.eyenet.org

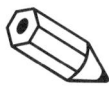 *Patient Consent Form*

CHALAZION/HORDEOLUM (STYE) EXCISION

I came to the office of Dr. _____ on _____ (date) for evaluation and treatment of the following condition: chalazion/hordeolum (stye) of the eyelid.

We discussed the different treatments possible and discussed the risks of not treating the condition. Based on the advice given by Dr. _____ and my own judgement, I agree to undergo the following procedure: excision of chalazion of my _____ (right/left, upper/lower) eyelid. I understand that this involves a local anesthetic injection, an incision into my eyelid with removal of tissue, and placement of a bandage over the eye.

I have read over the handouts provided, and the physician and I discussed the different outcomes that could occur and most of the possible complications. I am aware that other complications could occur that we could not foresee. I agree to follow the instructions for self-care after the procedure and to return for follow-up care on: _____.

I will call the office or answering service if any problems arise before the scheduled follow-up visit.

_____
Patient's signature

_____
Date/Time

_____
Witness' signature

_____
Physician's signature

One copy for chart; one copy for patient.

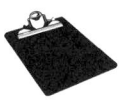 *Patient Education Handout*

TONOMETRY

What is Glaucoma?

Glaucoma is a group of conditions with various causes that, if not detected early, can lead to the loss of visual function and complete blindness. It is the third-leading cause of blindness in the United States, estimated to have caused some degree of blindness in 1.6 million Americans. Early glaucoma can be asymptomatic, so over half of individuals with glaucoma do not know they have it.

What are the Risk Factors for the Development of Glaucoma?

- Age over 45 years
- Family history of glaucoma
- African Americans
- Myopia or hyperopia (nearsightedness or farsightedness)

What is Tonometry?

Tonometry is used to detect increased intraocular (eye) pressure, which could help in the early diagnosis of glaucoma.

How Do I Prepare for Tonometry?

There is no specific preparation needed before going to your clinician's office for this procedure.

What Happens During Tonometry?

Your clinician will use eyedrops to numb the eye and then use an instrument to measure the eye pressure. The numbing medicine may sting a little until your eye goes numb. The instrument will momentarily touch the eyeball, but you will not feel it. It is very important to remain calm and relaxed during this procedure. You should concentrate on staring at the distant object recommended by your clinician.

What Precautions Do I Have to Take After the Procedure?

Since your eyes will be numb, your clinician will advise you not to rub or touch your eyes for about 1 to 2 hours after the procedure. Contact lens should not be worn until the eyes have feeling again. As long as your eye is numb, you are at risk of scratching your cornea. Use eye protection and avoid dusty environments.

What Happens if the Pressure in the Eye is High?

Your clinician will tell you the results of the test when it is completed. If the pressure is high, you may need further testing to detect glaucoma. Even if the pressure in your eye is not high, if you have risk factors for glaucoma, it may be prudent to see an ophthalmologist yearly for additional eye tests.

Continued

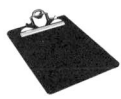 *Patient Education Handout—cont'd*

TONOMETRY—cont'd

What are the Advantages of Tonometry?

This test is probably the least expensive and easiest way to identify increased eye pressure, which is a high-risk factor for the development of glaucoma. If left untreated the condition could lead to complete blindness.

What are the Risks Associated With the Test and When Should I Call My Clinician?

The risks are redness of the eye with minimal pain, occasional blurry vision, and eye infection. Sometimes there can be false-positive or false-negative test results. The eye pain and redness should last for less than 24 hours; if it persists or is unbearable, you should call your clinician to make sure you have not had a complication. It is extremely unusual to scratch your eye during the procedure, but your eye will be at risk of being scratched if you rub it afterwards.

Websites That May be of Interest to You:

www.eyecare.org (New Jersey's Eyecare Organization)
www.glaucomafoundation.org (The Glaucoma Foundation)

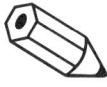 *Patient Consent Form*

TONOMETRY

I came to the office of my clinician, _____, on _____ (date) with an eye problem or a need for glaucoma screening. The cause, risk factors, complications, and techniques of screening for glaucoma were discussed in detail with me.

My clinician discussed tonometry with me, which is a procedure used to test for the presence of increased eye pressure. It was explained that if the eye pressure is elevated, glaucoma could be diagnosed or ruled out with further tests. I was also told that glaucoma cannot be ruled out completely in the face of a normal intraocular pressure and that, in the presence of risk factors for the disease, additional tests or a referral may be needed. The complications of the procedure were described to me and are as follows:
1. Corneal trauma, corneal abrasion
2. Conjunctival redness
3. Eye infection, visual function abnormalities
4. Unable to obtain a correct reading
5. False positives and false negatives
6. Rarely other complications could occur which are not foreseen

Preprocedure and postprocedure care and preparation of the eye were explained to me.

Should any problems arise before the scheduled follow-up, I was also instructed to call the office.

I understand the procedure to be used and the risks associated with it, and I believe that I have sufficient information to give this informed consent.

I certify that this form has been fully explained to me and that I have read it or have had it read to me, that the blank spaces have been filled in, and that I understand its contents.

_____   _____
Patient's signature   *Date/Time*

_____   _____
Witness' signature   *Clinician's signature*

One copy for chart; one copy for patient.

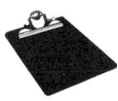

Patient Education Handout

BIFID EARLOBE REPAIR

Why Do I Need This Procedure?

Occasionally, forceful or repeated pulling on an earring may lead to a split earlobe. The edges within the split are often healed over by the time a physician is consulted for possible repair. It is still possible to have the earlobe repaired to wear pierced earrings again. The surgery is relatively minor and can be performed in your physician's office.

What Happens During the Procedure?

To perform the repair, the area is first cleansed with an antiseptic. Next, an anesthetic is injected around the ear. The healed-over skin in the inside part of the tear in the lobe is shaved off and then the two parts of the earlobe can be stitched back together.

What Happens After the Procedure?

After the repair is complete, your physician will apply a dressing to the wound. Keep the dressing clean and dry. Your physician will give you instructions for caring for the wound until the stitches are removed, usually about 5 days after the repair. After the stitches are out, surgical tapes may be placed to give the earlobe extra support for a few more days. In 6 to 8 weeks you may return to your physician for a recheck and to discuss possible repiercing of the earlobe.

What are the Risks Associated With This Procedure?

Risks of the surgery are rare but include bleeding, infection, scarring, and allergic reaction to the anesthetic or to other substances used along with the surgery. There is little pain. Of course, new earrings could always pull through the lobe again.

What Do I Need to Do After the Procedure?

To prevent this problem in the future, avoid pulling on the earlobes and do not wear heavy, dangling, or hoop earrings.

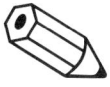 *Patient Consent Form*

MYRINGECTOMY/TYMPANOCENTESIS

I came to the office of Dr. _____ on _____ (date) for evaluation and treatment of the following condition: Ear pain, middle ear fluid, or infection that is severe or continuous.

We discussed the different treatments possible and the risks of not treating the condition. Based on the advice given by Dr. _____ and my own judgement, I agree to undergo the following procedure(s):

Instillation of anesthetic/antibiotic drops followed by tympanocentesis (a sterile needle is used to perforate my eardrum to obtain a culture) and/or myringotomy (a sterile surgical knife is used to cut a slit in my eardrum to relieve pressure and for possible suction of fluid). Both maneuvers should provide relief of pain and/or allow a culture to be obtained. Anesthetic/antibiotic drops will be instilled after the procedure.

We discussed the different outcomes that could occur and most of the possible complications. I am aware that other complications could occur that we could not foresee. I agree to follow the instructions for self-care after the procedure and to return for follow-up care on _____.

I will call the office or answering service if any problems arise before the scheduled follow-up visit.

_____
Patient's signature

_____
Date/Time

_____
Witness' signature

_____
Physician's signature

One copy for chart; one copy for patient.

Patient Education Handouts and Consent Forms

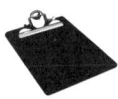 *Patient Education Handout*

FOREIGN BODY REMOVAL FROM NOSE OR EAR

Foreign bodies that obstruct the nose or ear must be removed to prevent further damage to the airway or to hearing. Success in removal requires relaxation and cooperation. You may be given sedation, a local anesthetic, or an injection. You may also be required to inhale a medication, which will decrease swelling. The clinician will then use special instruments and techniques to carefully remove the object.

Complications may occur, including damage to the skin and membranes, perforation of the ear drum, or bleeding. A severe nosebleed may also occur. If the foreign body is dislodged into the back of the nose, choking and aspiration may occur. If the obstruction is complicated, you may be referred to another specialist.

The ear canal and nasal passageways are very sensitive and may become quite swollen for several days after removal. Bleeding and infection are very common. Your clinician may give you antibiotics. You should alert your clinician for any specific allergies to antibiotics. In addition, you should report any headaches, sinusitis, fever, nasal, or ear drainage. After removal of nasal foreign bodies, you need to perform saline washes two to three times per day for 2 to 3 days.

Call your healthcare provider for any further obstruction, bleeding, or pain.

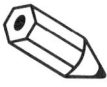 *Patient Consent Form*

FOREIGN BODY REMOVAL FROM NOSE OR EAR

I came to the office of my clinician, _____, on _____ (date) for removal of a foreign body in the nose or ear canal. We discussed the different treatment methods and the risks involved.

Based on that discussion and my own judgement, I agree to allow my clinician, _____, to remove the foreign body using whatever means necessary to do so. This may involve anesthesia with an injection of lidocaine, use of a metal or plastic instrument to extract or grasp the foreign body, use of suction or salt water irrigation, inhalation of epinephrine, and/or the use of "Super Glue."

We discussed the different outcomes that could occur and most of the possible complications, including bleeding, infection, aspiration, and damage to the mucous membranes or eardrum. I am aware that other rare complications could occur that we could not foresee. I have read and understand the patient education handout. I agree to follow the instructions for self-care after the procedure and to return for follow-up care on _____. I will call the office or answering service if any problems occur.

_____
Patient's signature

_____
Date/Time

_____
Witness' signature

_____
Physician's signature

One copy for chart; one copy for patient.

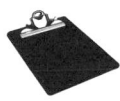 *Patient Education Handout*

EPISTAXIS (NOSEBLEED)

What is Epistaxis?

Epistaxis is the medical name for a nosebleed. Most of the time, a nosebleed can be stopped by simply pinching the nose. Ice can also be applied to the bridge of the nose. However, there are times when a clinician needs to perform a procedure to stop the bleeding.

Why Do I Need This Procedure?

You need this procedure to avoid the loss of too much blood. If the nosebleed persists or comes back, you need to return to the clinic for further assistance and to stop the bleeding before too much blood is lost.

How Do I Prepare for the Treatment of Epistaxis?

All that is required is for you to simply sit on the examination table or bed. Usually you will be given an examination gown or will be draped with protective sheets. Try to relax and remain calm. The more relaxed you are, the better your experience will be and the quicker the procedure will be finished.

What Happens During the Procedure?

Depending on the severity of the nosebleed, there are several types of procedures that can be performed. Most commonly, your nasal passages will be cleaned out and cotton-tipped swabs (Q-Tips) will be used to dab the area of bleeding. Some numbing medicine and other medicines may be applied with cotton-tipped swabs to slow the bleeding. Silver nitrate sticks or other types of instruments may be used to stop the bleeding.

With severe nosebleeds, the nasal passage may need to be packed by a clinician to stop the bleeding.

What Happens After the Procedure?

If it is not necessary to place a packing, you will be instructed to keep the inside of your nose moist with either Vaseline or A & D ointment. This is important, especially at night. You may also be asked to keep tissue paper in that nostril to prevent breathing through it and drying out your nose.

If a packing is left in your nose, you will be asked to return to the office in a day or two to be evaluated. You may also be placed on antibiotics.

What are the Benefits of This Procedure?

It can allow your clinician to stop the nosebleed and prevent more serious problems.

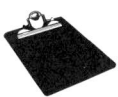

Patient Education Handout—cont'd

EPISTAXIS (NOSEBLEED)—cont'd

What are the Risks Associated With this Procedure?

It may feel uncomfortable to have your nose packed or to have the bleeding stopped. Packing your nose may decrease your breathing or irritate your heart and require observation in a hospital. During an attempt to stop the bleeding, a hole could be placed through the nasal septum (inside wall). In addition, you could develop an infection in your ears, sinuses, or lungs. There is always a chance of having an allergic reaction to the materials and medicines that are to be used.

Special Instructions:

Websites That May be of Interest to You:

www.entmanual.com (A private ENT specialist's educational web site)

www.nosebleeds.com (A commercial product to help with simple nose bleeds)

www.entnet.org/nosebleeds.htlml (Patient education from ENT specialist society)

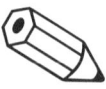 *Patient Consent Form*

TREATMENT OF EPISTAXIS (NOSEBLEED)

I came to the office of my clinician _____ on _____ (date) for evaluation and treatment of a nose bleed (medically called "Epistaxis").

We discussed the various procedures possible and discussed the risks of not treating the condition. Based on the advice given by my clinician, _____, and my own judgement, I agree to undergo nasal cauterization, nasal packing, or _____.

We discussed the different possible outcomes and most of the possible complications including bleeding, discomfort, permanent damage to my nose, and respiratory difficulty. I am aware that other complications could occur that we could not foresee. Alternatives have been discussed, and all of my questions have been answered. In addition, I have been told the risk of severe problems, including death, if I fail to follow instructions or to return to the clinic if instructed. I agree to follow the instructions for self-care after the procedure and to return for follow up care on _____ (date).

I will call the office or answering service if any problems arise before the scheduled follow-up visit.

_____   _____
Patient's signature   *Date/Time*

_____   _____
Witness' signature   *Clinician's signature*

One copy for chart; one copy for patient.

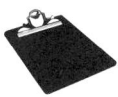

Patient Education Handout

TRACHEOSTOMY

Your clinician has recommended a surgical procedure called a tracheostomy. Medical conditions for which this surgery is commonly performed include: obstruction of the airway that limits breathing, the need for ventilator assistance when you cannot breath on your own, and the need to suction the lungs to remove infected, accumulated, or aspirated secretions. Your clinician believes that this procedure will help heal or manage your specific medical condition.

Tracheostomy is performed in an operating room under local or general anesthesia. Sedation may be given to relieve anxiety. You lie on your back and an incision is made in the center of the lower neck just above the collarbone. A second incision is made in the windpipe that lies beneath the skin. A tube is used to connect the windpipe to the skin so that you now breathe through the tube instead of the nose or mouth.

After the procedure, you will be hospitalized for at least several days until healing can occur and self-care can be taught. Although swallowing is usually not compromised, your ability to talk can be impaired, since exhaled air no longer passes between the vocal cords to produce a sound.

The major benefit of this procedure is the improved ability to manage the illness requiring it. Risks include bleeding, infection, scarring, or introduction of air around the lungs, which may deflate them. (This condition can be corrected but may require further surgery.) The tube itself requires attention to keep it positioned properly and to keep it clean and unobstructed. Scarring can injure the vocal cords and the windpipe and may compromise your voice or breathing. The tracheotomy tube can be used temporarily or permanently, and no further surgery is usually required to remove it.

After the procedure, you or your caregiver must learn how to clean up secretions, the tube, and the skin of your neck. Mucus must be suctioned from the tube if you cannot cough it out. Proper care will prevent infection. Diet and activity are not limited except for swimming (because you will not be able to hold your breath). Visiting nurses are usually available to ease your transition from hospital to home care.

You or your caregiver should call your clinician for any difficulty breathing, for bleeding from the tube, or if the tube has become displaced. If the tube is displaced, the surgically created opening will narrow over several hours, often complicating the reinsertion of the tube. Do not delay in notifying your clinician or in going to the emergency department if you feel this has occurred. Please call during office hours for routine questions or to reorder supplies.

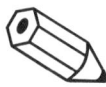 *Patient Consent Form*

TRACHEOSTOMY

I am in the office/hospital where my clinician, _____, practices on _____ (date) for evaluation and treatment of respiratory failure requiring prolonged ventilation or an obstructed airway.

We discussed the different treatments possible and the risks of not treating the condition. Based on the advice given by my clinician, _____, and my own judgment, I agree to undergo tracheostomy under general anesthesia.

We discussed the different outcomes that could occur and most of the possible complications. I am aware that other complications could occur that we could not foresee. I agree to follow the instructions for self-care after the procedure and to return for follow-up care on _____ (date).

I will call the office or answering service if any problems arise before the scheduled follow-up visit.

_____
Patient's signature

_____
Date/Time

_____
Witness' signature

_____
Clinician's signature

One copy for chart; one copy for patient.

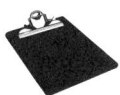

Patient Education Handout

PERITONSILLAR ABSCESS DRAINAGE

What is a Peritonsillar Abscess?

A peritonsillar abscess is a collection of pus in the upper throat just above the tonsil.

Why Do I Need This Treated?

If a peritonsillar abscess is not treated, it can cause death by blocking the airway. It can also cause infection to spread throughout the bloodstream.

What are the Options for Treatment?

Your clinician may choose either to remove the pus with a needle and syringe or to make a small incision to drain the pus. This can usually be done in the office. If there have been a lot of infections, the tonsil and abscess cavity may need to be removed. If this is necessary, it would be performed in an operating room under general anesthesia.

What Happens During the Needle Procedure?

Your clinician will use a syringe and needle to withdraw the pus from the peritonsillar abscess. Usually this gives immediate relief of most of your symptoms. If your clinician chooses to make an incision, the pus will be suctioned out after the incision is made.

What Happens After the Procedure?

If the procedure is successful, your clinician will send you home with antibiotics and pain medications. Because the symptoms might return, your clinician will want to see you in the next few days. You will probably be advised to use saltwater gargles to help with the discomfort. If the pus cannot be removed, you may need to be hospitalized.

What are the Benefits of This Procedure?

Because this procedure can be performed in the office or the emergency room, you will likely not need to be hospitalized.

What are the Risks Associated With This Procedure?

The major risk of this procedure is bleeding. It is possible to injure an artery that might require surgery to repair.

When Should I Call My Healthcare Provider?

If the symptoms reappear, you should return to see your clinician. If you experience shortness of breath, trouble swallowing, fever higher than 101° F, or bleeding, call your clinician immediately.

Special Instructions:

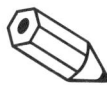 *Patient Consent Form*

PERITONSILLAR ABSCESS DRAINAGE

I, _____, am under the care of my clinician
_____ on _____ (date) for evaluation and treatment of
the following condition: peritonsillar abscess. This is a collection of pus in the upper back of the
throat above the tonsil.

We discussed the different treatments possible and the risks of not treating the condition. Based on
the advice given by my clinician and my own judgment, I agree to undergo the following procedure:
needle aspiration and/or incision and drainage. I understand my clinician will use a local anesthetic
to numb the area and either will use a needle to remove the pus or will make a small incision at the
back of my throat near the tonsil to allow the pus to drain out.

We discussed the different outcomes that could occur. We also discussed most of the possible
complications, including infection, aspiration, pneumonia, hemorrhage, and recurrence of the
abscess. I am aware that these complications, or worse, can occur if we *do not* perform the
procedure. I am aware that other complications can occur that we cannot foresee. I agree to follow
the instructions for self-care after the procedure and to return for follow-up care on
_____.

I will call the office or answering service if any problems arise before the scheduled follow-up visit.

_____   _____
Patient's signature   *Date/Time*

_____   _____
Witness' signature   *Clinician's signature*

One copy for chart; one copy for patient.

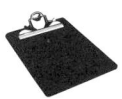

Patient Education Handout

AMBULATORY BLOOD PRESSURE MONTIORING

Your provider has recommended that your blood pressure be measured for the next 24 hours or longer. Because your blood pressure will be measured while you are doing your normal daily activities, a more accurate idea of what your blood pressure is actually averaging should result. However, there are some things you can do during this time for more accurate results.

1. Do not move or talk while the cuff is deflating. Movement and talking while the cuff is deflating (during the measurement cycle) can interfere with the measurement and cause inaccurate blood pressure readings. Try to let the arm with the cuff rest by your side when you feel the cuff start to deflate until the cuff is completely deflated.

2. Avoid activities that make it difficult to relax your arm during measurements, such as lawn mowing, golfing, running, and racquet sports.

3. Record your activities in the 24-hour diary provided. Your blood pressure will normally change with your activity level. Blood pressure is normally higher while you are awake and lower when you sleep. The machine cannot tell us what you are doing or when you take medications. The 24-hour diary is as important as the blood pressure measurements themselves. Please write down the times and a brief description of when you start and finish work and home activities, take medications, drive, eat, begin to sleep, and wake up.

4. Please do not wet or immerse the blood pressure monitoring equipment in the shower or bathtub. We recommend washing with a moistened washcloth, but it should not drip water onto the equipment.

5. The equipment can sometimes cause minor discomfort. If you notice swelling, you can elevate your hand and arm above your heart by resting them on a pillow over your chest. Some patients are aroused during sleep by the inflating cuff. To help with this, the machine is set to take fewer measurements during your normal sleep hours. A minor rash can occur under the cuff. If this happens, notify the technician or nurse when they remove the equipment tomorrow so it can be examined. A soothing cream may be prescribed. Although it is rare, you may experience a persistent discomfort. If you experience persistent discomfort in the arm with the cuff, call the number provided below for instructions.

6. Your test results will be analyzed and a report given to your provider within _____ days. You should schedule a follow-up visit with your provider to review the results or follow your provider's instructions for follow-up.

   The phone number to call if you experience problems during normal business hours is (_____) _____. After normal business hours, call (_____) _____ for instructions.

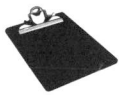

Patient Education Handout

AMBULATORY PHLEBECTOMY (PREPROCEDURE)

Varicose veins are a chronic and recurrent condition. Injection sclerotherapy and surgery will not offer a cure but rather a control of the condition. The hereditary tendency of developing new veins will not be corrected by this or any other form of treatment. Your treatment options for large veins are (1) classical "stripping" or the removal of the entire large superficial vein in your leg(s), (2) ambulatory phlebectomy, (3) ultrasound-guided and regular repeated sclerotherapy, and (4) conservative therapy with only elastic compression hosiery.

Classical "stripping" is performed in the hospital under general anesthesia. Recovery is prolonged, and considerable pain may be encountered. There will also be substantial scars at the incision sites.

Ultrasound-guided injections of various medications (sclerotherapy) can be performed under certain situations. Recurrence is very low if the veins are 6 mm or less, but the recurrence rate for large varicose veins (greater than 7 mm) is very high with sclerotherapy.

Ambulatory phlebectomy—excision and removal of varicose veins with multiple small incisions—is a surgical alternative to the classical stripping in the treatment of varicose veins. However, unlike stripping, no general anesthesia is required, no hospitalization is needed, and there is no need for prolonged recovery and subsequent loss of income. Moreover, the customary long incisions used for the excision of the varicose vein, which result in unacceptable scarring, are not needed. In contrast, ambulatory phlebectomy uses small 1 to 2 mm (1/16 inch) stab wounds, which, in the majority of cases, leave no scars or only minimal scars. It is an office procedure performed completely under local anesthesia, and it consists of one to three parts:

1. Surgical ligation or clipping. We will identify the area where the vein valve problems first start and where the bad valves allow the blood to back up in the lower veins (reflux). In the majority of cases this will be either in the groin (at the saphenofemoral junction), or behind the knee (at the saphenopopliteal junction). If these areas need treatment, we will tie off and clip the abnormal vessels. These major vessels, however, may not need treatment.

2. Ligation of perforator veins. A perforator vein is a vein that connects the deep veins to the superficial veins. When it is not working correctly, the direction of blood flow reverses. Instead of blood going back to the heart, it goes into the surface veins of the leg. These abnormal veins are tied off using a 1- to 2-mm incision at the site of the bulging perforator.

3. Removal of visible varicose veins. Using the ambulatory phlebectomy technique, the physician carefully places multiple small incisions of 1 to 2 mm (1/16 inch) in length along the varicose veins that have been identified and anesthetized previously. With the aid of specially designed hooks, the veins are brought through the skin incisions, clamped, cut, and separately removed. Special dressings that help prevent bleeding are then placed on the leg.

Ambulatory phlebectomy is an office procedure that permits most patients to resume their regular activities the same day. Compression hose need to be worn for 10 to 14 days. Occasionally, knee-level stockings will be used for an additional 3 to 4 weeks. The results are not immediate, and sometimes several weeks are needed for the desired level of improvement to occur.

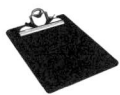

Patient Education Handout—cont'd

AMBULATORY PHLEBECTOMY (PREPROCEDURE)—cont'd

Expectations After Surgery

- Mild leg pain or discomfort: The pain is rarely ever severe enough to warrant strong pain medication, even the first evening after the procedure. If you do not have any contraindications, two or three ibuprofen (200 mg) every 8 hours will be sufficient.
- Bruising and discoloration of the skin of the leg: Some people bruise more, and some bruise less. Overall, this is a normal occurrence that will disappear in 1 to 2 weeks.
- Slight bleeding into the dressing: This is a normal occurrence after any minor surgical procedure. If you take aspirin regularly, please notify the doctor. Aspirin will increase your bleeding and bruising.

Risks of Vein Ligation and/or Ambulatory Phlebectomy

- Wound infection: Increasing pain, fever, and redness around the wounds may indicate an infection. Please call the doctor, because you may need an antibiotic. Be sure the doctor is aware of any allergies to medications.
- Residual varicose veins: Occasionally, a few varicose veins may have been missed and left behind. They may or may not need further surgery or treatment.
- Allergic reaction: The only medication typically used during ambulatory phlebectomy is the local anesthetic. Please notify the doctor if you have ever had any problems during local anesthesia, such as during dental treatments.
- Bleeding after surgery
- Other complications: As with any surgical procedure, other complications can occur, although they are rare. These would include: persistent swelling of the leg; damage to a nerve, causing numbness; inflammation of the venous system; a blood clot in the surface veins (which can be removed with a needle); or a blood clot in deep veins of the leg (which would increase the risk of a clot reaching the lungs).

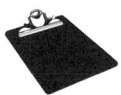 *Patient Education Handout*

AMBULATORY PHLEBECTOMY (POSTPROCEDURE)

This information is for patients who have had an ambulatory phlebectomy:

1. Immediately after surgery (before you get in your car) we request that you walk about one-half mile. Thereafter we would like you to walk between 1 and 3 miles per day for 2 weeks after surgery.
2. If there are no contraindications, we would like you to take Advil, Aleve, or Orudis as directed on the bottle for 1 week after surgery.
3. Please take one aspirin, 12 to 16 hours after surgery and then one every day for the next 2 weeks.
4. Unless there is discomfort (please call us if there is), leave all dressings on for 1 week. You have been fit with a compression stocking that is to remain on over the dressings until your next appointment.
5. The shower bag you received has directions with it. Please do not modify the directions, because the bags really do work when applied properly. This will allow you to shower and keep your dressing dry. Cool showers are best for keeping your blood vessels from dilating.
6. We will remove your bandage at your follow-up appointment in 1 week. The outer stocking will be worn during the day for an additional week.
7. Please avoid any strenuous workouts or heavy lifting for 2 weeks.
8. A small spot of blood may seep through the dressing. Do not get alarmed. Call us if you have any problems.
9. Please avoid sunbathing and tanning beds for 30 days after surgery.

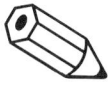 *Patient Consent Form*

AMBULATORY PHLEBECTOMY

I have read and understand the information provided and know the potential complications with ambulatory phlebectomy, ligation of perforator veins, and surgical ligation of veins. I also understand my other options for treatment of my varicose veins. I hereby authorize _____ and/or associates, to surgically remove, tie off, or inject diseased veins for the purpose of attempting to improve the symptoms and/or appearance of my legs.

_____

Patient's signature

_____

Date/Time

_____

Witness' signature

_____

Date/Time

One copy for chart; one copy for patient.

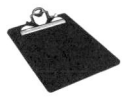 *Patient Education Handout*

ARTERIAL LINE

Arteries carry blood with oxygen away from your heart to the organs, tissue and cells of your body. An arterial line (catheter or cannula) can be used to obtain frequent arterial blood samples without having to puncture an artery every time. It is also one of the most accurate methods for continuously measuring or monitoring your true blood pressure. You will need this procedure because you have a disorder in either the gases in your body (e.g., oxygen or carbon dioxide), the acid-base balance in your blood (pH), your blood pressure, or the output of your heart. These problems could potentially harm the cells in your body, resulting in organ, cell or tissue death. By doing this procedure, we will be able to determine the severity of the problem as well as to monitor the problem. In certain cases, we may also be able to determine the cause.

The most important thing for you to do during this procedure is to try and relax and to remain calm, and to not move the chosen arm or leg.

During this procedure, your clinician will place your arm, leg or foot into a certain position and may do some tests to determine which artery is the best to use. They may give you an injection to numb the skin over the artery. The skin will be cleansed before any injections. The clinician will then use a needle to puncture the artery and insert a catheter (plastic tube). You may experience some discomfort with any of the injections or the puncture.

After the procedure, a line will be connected from your artery to some instruments. The benefits of this procedure include the ability to obtain frequent arterial samples, to determine the amount of oxygen and carbon dioxide in your body, the pH of your blood, your blood pressure, and possibly your cardiac output. Treatment decisions may be based on these results. When the catheter is removed, pressure will be placed over the artery. Then a bandage will be placed.

The risks associated with the procedure are few but must be discussed. Possible complications include: bleeding, infection, scarring and blood clots (large or small). The artery could become temporarily or permanently narrowed or blocked. Local structures such as nerves, tendons, arteries, or veins as well as structures downstream from the artery could be damaged. If the line gets disconnected, you are at a much higher risk of hemorrhage than with a routine intravenous line. There are also other rare complications that could occur that we could not foresee. In order to minimize complications, it is important for you to notify the clinician or nursing staff at the earliest sign of a possible complication.

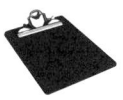 *Patient Education Handout*

ARTERIAL PUNCTURE

Arteries carry blood with oxygen away from your heart and to the organs, tissue, and cells of your body. Arterial puncture is a procedure in which we use a syringe to obtain blood from one of your arteries. You need this procedure because you have a disorder in either the gases in your blood (e.g., oxygen or carbon dioxide) or the acid-base balance in your blood (pH). These blood gas problems could harm the cells in your body, causing organ, cell, or tissue death. By performing this procedure, we will be able to determine the severity of the problem. In certain cases, we may also be able to determine the cause.

The most important thing for you to do during this procedure is to relax and remain calm.

During this procedure, your clinician will put your arm or leg into a certain position and may do some tests to determine which artery is the best to use. He or she may give you an injection to numb the skin over the artery. The skin will be cleansed before any injections. The clinician will then use a needle to puncture the artery and obtain blood. You may experience some discomfort with any of the injections or the puncture.

After the procedure, pressure will be placed over the artery, followed by placement of a bandage. The benefits of this procedure include the ability to determine the amount of oxygen and carbon dioxide in your body as well as the pH of your blood. There may also be other blood tests to be run on this blood. Treatment decisions may be based on all of these results.

The risks associated with the procedure are few but must be discussed. Possible complications include bleeding, infection, scarring, and blood clots (large or small). Local structures (e.g., nerves, tendons, arteries, or veins) as well as structures downstream from the artery could be damaged. There are also other rare and unforeseeable complications that could occur. In order to minimize complications, it is important for you to notify the clinician or nursing staff at the earliest sign of a possible complication.

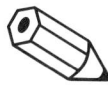 *Patient Consent Form*

ARTERIAL LINE (CANNULATION)

I am under the care of my clinician _____ on _____ (date) for treatment of an abnormality with the gases in my blood (oxygen or carbon dioxide), the acid-base balance of my blood, my blood pressure, and/or possibly my cardiac output. We discussed the different evaluation and monitoring methods and the risks involved.

Based on that discussion and my own judgment, I agree to allow my clinician, _____, to use a needle to insert a catheter into my artery. This may involve local anesthesia with an injection of lidocaine.

I understand that there will be some discomfort with this procedure and that in certain situations, no anesthesia will be utilized while the clinician attempts to insert the line.

We discussed the different outcomes that could occur and most of the possible complications including bleeding, infection, scarring and large or small blood clots. My artery could become temporarily or permanently blocked. Local structures such as nerves, tendons, arteries, or veins as well as structures downstream from the artery could be damaged. I am aware that there are other rare complications that could occur that we could not foresee. I have read and understand the Patient Education Handout. I agree to follow the instructions for self-care after the procedure and to return for follow-up care on _____. All of my questions have been answered.

I will call the office or answering service if any problems occur.

_____

Patient's signature

_____

Witness' signature

_____

Date/Time

_____

Clinician's signature

One copy for chart; one copy for patient.

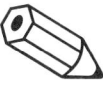 *Patient Consent Form*

ARTERIAL PUNCTURE

I am under the care of my clinician, _____, on _____ (date) for treatment of an abnormality with the gases in my blood (oxygen or carbon dioxide) or with the acid-base balance of my blood. We discussed the different evaluation methods and the risks involved.

Based on that discussion and my own judgement, I agree to allow my clinician, _____, to use a needle to obtain a sample of my arterial blood. This may involve local anesthesia with an injection of lidocaine.

I understand that there will be some discomfort with this procedure and that in certain situations, no anesthetic will be administered while the clinician attempts to obtain the blood sample.

We discussed the different outcomes that could occur and most of the possible complications, including bleeding, infection, scarring, and large or small blood clots. Local structures (e.g., nerves, tendons, arteries, or veins) as well as structures downstream from the artery could be damaged. I am aware that there are other rare and unforeseeable complications that could occur. I have read and understand the patient teaching guide. I agree to follow the instructions for self-care after the procedure and to return for follow-up care on _____. All of my questions have been answered.

I will call the office or answering service if any problems occur.

_____
Patient's signature

_____
Date/Time

_____
Witness' signature

_____
Clinician's signature

One copy for chart; one copy for patient.

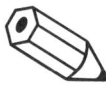 *Patient Consent Form*

CARDIAC PROCEDURE–CARDIOVERSION

State law guarantees that you have both the *right* and *obligation* to make decisions concerning your health care. Your doctor can provide you with the necessary information and advice, but as a member of the health care team, you must enter into the decision making process. This form has been designed to acknowledge your acceptance of treatment recommended by your doctor.

The information that follows is a description of the procedure, a list of complications that could occur from the procedure, and text from a standardized consent form. This consent form is used for the most minor of procedures and the most complicated and serious ones. It is not meant to frighten you but rather to inform you that *all* cardiac procedures carry some risks. This form hopefully will allow you to better understand your upcoming cardiac procedure. If you don't understand something, *ask.*

I hereby authorize _____ and/or assistants selected by my doctor to diagnose and/or treat, in this case, atrial fibrillation, an irregular heart rhythm resulting from disorganized electrical activity in the top chambers of the heart (atria).

The cardiac procedure(s) planned for the treatment of my condition(s) have been explained to me by my physician and is listed below:

Electrical Cardioversion
This procedure helps to restore your heart to normal rhythm. After you are sedated with intravenous medications, an electrical shock is administered. This restores the normal electrical rhythm to your heart. Because you are sedated for the procedure, you will not feel the shock. You will be monitored throughout, including an automatic blood pressure cuff and a device to measure the oxygen in your blood.

Possible Risks Associated with this Procedure Include the Following:
Failure to restore normal rhythm: The cardioversion procedure may be unsuccessful. The procedure may fail to restore normal rhythm or may do so only temporarily.

Medications: There may be allergic reactions or side effects to one or more medications administered before, during, or after the procedure.

Heart: The heart's performance can be affected by the procedure, causing low blood pressure or shock. Heart rhythm disturbances may occur. These might require medications, temporary pacemaker insertion, additional electrical shocks, or resuscitation (CPR). Rarely, death may occur as a complication of this procedure.

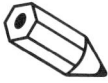

Patient Consent Form—cont'd

CARDIAC PROCEDURE–CARDIOVERSION—cont'd

Other: Atrial fibrillation and atrial flutter can cause small blood clots to form inside your heart. When the heart rhythm is restored to normal, it is possible that a blood clot could dislodge and travel out to the brain, which could cause a stroke. To prevent this, your doctor will administer blood thinners. If you have been in atrial fibrillation or flutter for less than 48 hours, clots are unlikely and blood thinners may not be used. The shock(s) administered can cause redness to the skin where the paddles are applied. There may even be a superficial burn.

Possible Alternatives to This Procedure Include the Following:
- Observation
- Treatment with Medications

I certify that this form has been explained to me and that I have read it, or have had it read to me, and that I understand its contents.

_____

Patient's or guardian's signature

_____

Date/Time

_____

Name (print)

_____

Witness' signature

I recognize that, during the course of the procedure, postprocedure care, medical treatment, anesthesia administration, or other procedures, unforeseen conditions may necessitate additional or different procedures than those set forth. *I therefore authorize my above doctor, and the doctor's assistants or designees, to perform such procedures that, in the exercise of their professional judgment, are deemed necessary and desirable.* The authority granted under this paragraph shall extend to the treatment of all conditions that require treatment and are not known to my physician at the time the cardiac procedure is commenced.

I have been informed that there are significant risks such as cardiac arrest that can lead to death or permanent or partial disability, which may be attendant to the performance of any procedure.

I realize that the list of risks and complications on this form may not include all possible or known risks of the intended cardiac procedure but is a list of the more common or severe ones. I realize that other or new risks may exist or may be found in the future that are not mentioned on this consent form.

Continued

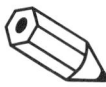 *Patient Consent Form—cont'd*

CARDIAC PROCEDURE–CARDIOVERSION—cont'd

I acknowledge that no warranty or guarantee has been made to me as to the results of my procedure, including the cure of my condition.

I understand that any aspect of this consent form that I do not understand can be explained to me in further detail by asking my physician(s) or their associates.

I certify that my physician has informed me of the nature and character of the proposed treatment, of the anticipated results of the proposed treatment, of the possible alternative forms of treatment including nontreatment; and the recognized serious possible risks, complications, and the anticipated benefits involved in the proposed treatment.

Patient or guardian initials _____

The cardiac procedure stated on this form, including the possible risks and complications was explained by me to the patient or his or her representative before the patient or his or her representatives consented.

Physician's signature _____ *Date* _____

One copy for chart; one copy for patient.

(Adapted from iMed Consent, LLC [www.dialogmedical.com].)

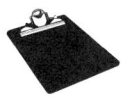

Patient Education Handout

CENTRAL VENOUS CATHETER INSERTION

Central vein catheterization is a procedure in which we place a catheter into one of the large veins that empties into your heart. You need this procedure to enable us to inject medications or because we are having difficulty managing the fluids in your body. Your peripheral veins may not be adequate to inject medications or needed fluid. With a catheter inside this large vein, we will be able to make certain measurements, including blood pressure on the right side of the heart. From these measurements, we are able to estimate the blood pressures inside your lungs. We may be able to tell if or why you have too much fluid in your lungs. In addition, we may need a catheter in a large cardiac vein for dialysis, for diagnostic purposes, or for preparing the insertion of other cardiac monitoring or pacing devices.

During this procedure, we will insert the catheter into a large vein in the neck or near the clavicle. You should not feel this catheter going into your heart. Except for our gowns, mask, goggles or glasses, and the drapes we place on you, you should not know that this procedure is occurring.

The most important thing for you to do during this procedure is to try to relax and remain calm. We may ask you to help us by taking deep breaths or by changing positions at a certain stage of the procedure. You will feel some discomfort when we inject the local anesthetic and occasionally when we advance the catheter through the anesthetized area.

The benefits of this procedure depend on why we are inserting the catheter. It can include being better able to manage your fluids, medications, dialysis, or heart rhythm. We may also be better able to make the correct diagnosis. All of these should result in better care for you.

The risks associated with this procedure include pain, infection, bleeding, pneumothorax (punctured lung), perforation of vital organs, and blood clots. There is also a slight risk of a rhythm problem with your heart (irregular heart beat). If the catheter is left in place more than 3 days, there is an increased risk of infection.

After the procedure, the catheter will be connected to a monitor for us to watch. Periodically it will be flushed and checked for accuracy. You should report symptoms or signs of local or system-wide infection, or swelling. If the catheter becomes disconnected, pressure should be placed immediately over the site and you should ask for help. Since this is a large vein, bleeding from the area can result in a serious or life-threatening hemorrhage.

You will undergo formal training for management of the catheter unless another trained individual is going to provide the catheter care. After the catheter is removed, you should notify a nurse or clinician if pain, swelling, or signs of infection occur at the insertion site. You should also notify the nurse or clinician for any related chest symptoms, such as chest pain (including when taking a big breath), shortness of breath, or coughing up blood.

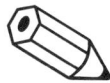 *Patient Consent Form*

CENTRAL VENOUS CATHETER INSERTION

Name of Patient :_____

1. My clinician, _____, has recommended the following procedure: central vein catheter insertion.
2. Upon my authorization and consent, I understand this procedure will be performed on me.
3. My clinician has explained the benefits of the procedure and that the procedure may involve risk of complications, injury, or even death, from both known and unknown causes. No warranty or guarantee as to the results has been made. I recognize that I have the right to consent to or to refuse the proposed procedure at any time before its performance.
4. I have received a detailed explanation of this procedure from my clinician including limitations, alternatives and possible risks that include but are not limited to pain, infection, bleeding, pneumothorax (punctured lung), perforation of vital organs, blood clots, and cardiac dysrhythmias (abnormal heart beat).
5. I understand that the procedure may fail and/or possible complications may require additional procedures (chest tube placement), surgery, or electrical shock cardioversion (to restore a normal heart rhythm) on an emergent basis.
6. I understand that during the procedure I will be placed in a position lying with the head tilted down, and that if I am on a ventilator, it will be stopped (15 to 30 seconds) momentarily during the procedure (introducer needle insertion).
7. My signature on this form indicates the following:
   - I have read and understand the information provided in this form.
   - The procedure set forth above has been adequately explained to me by my clinician.
   - I have had the chance to ask questions and they have all been answered.
   - I have received all the information that I desire concerning the procedure and alternatives.
   - I authorize and consent to the performance of the procedure.

Date: _____ *Time:* _____

Signature: _____
                (Patient/Parent/Guardian: indicate if other than patient)

Witness: _____

If the patient is unable to sign, indicate the reason:

One copy for chart; one copy for patient.

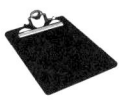 *Patient Education Handout*

ENDOTRACHEAL INTUBATION

Endotracheal intubation is a procedure in which we place a tube into the voice box in your throat (larynx) to assist your breathing. You will need this procedure because you are unable to breath adequately in order to keep the blood oxygenated in your body. Lack of oxygen could potentially harm the cells in your body, resulting in cell and tissue death. By performing this procedure and placing you on a ventilator, we can control your respirations and the amount of oxygen you breathe.

The most important thing for you to do during this procedure is to try and relax and remain calm.

During this procedure, your clinician will position your neck and give you medicine to numb your throat. Any materials that happen to be in the back of your throat will be suctioned away. A tube will then be passed through your mouth or nose and into your larynx. It will also pass across your vocal cords. This tube will be hooked up to a machine to help you breathe.

The major benefits of this procedure are to allow your body to get plenty of oxygen, to have plenty of carbon dioxide removed, and to protect your lungs from aspiration

After the procedure, we will secure the tube in place with tape. You will not be able to talk; however, your breathing will be managed safely by us. In general, there are no serious side effects. You will probably have a sore throat after the tube is removed.

Additional risks associated with the procedure are few but must be discussed. The tube could be placed down the "wrong pipe." We could conceivably hurt your larynx or your breathing apparatus. We could also break a tooth or cause a little tear in your mouth. You will not be able to call the healthcare provider with the tube in place, but if there seems to be a problem, please feel free to summon the nurse with the call button. If we place the tube through your nose, you may develop a nosebleed or have a sinus infection.

In order to prevent infection following this procedure, we will ask you to take deep breaths once the tube is removed and to cough up any phlegm that might be present.

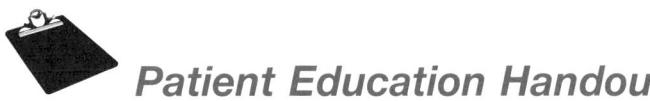

Patient Education Handout

OFFICE ELECTROCARDIOGRAMS (ECG OR EKG)

What is an ECG?

This is a very common test performed in your clinician's office. It detects certain heart functions by gathering the tiny electrical impulses that the heart creates.

Why Do I Need This Procedure?

The ECG can detect certain abnormal changes in the heart, possibly allowing your clinician to diagnosis heart problems or damage.

How Do I Prepare for an ECG?

Simply rest on the examination table or bed. Usually you will have your shirt off (male) or an examination gown will be given to you (females). It will be important for you to remain still, breathe normally, and not talk during the procedure.

What Happens During the Procedure?

Small electrodes (plastic sticker-like objects) will be put on your chest. The electrodes may tickle but certainly do not hurt. Wires from the ECG machine are connected to the electrodes in order to record the electrical activity of your heart. THEY DO NOT SHOCK YOU!

What Happens After the Procedure?

The electrodes are removed, and usually you will need to wipe off the small amount of electrode gel that may remain on your skin. You can then get dressed.

What are the Benefits of This Procedure?

It can allow your clinician to detect certain abnormal changes in your heart. Over time, serial ECGs can monitor your heart to see if it is developing problems.

What are the Risks Associated With This Procedure?

This test is very safe. In rare cases there is skin irritation from the electrode gel and some redness that usually goes away rapidly. Occasionally an ECG will fail to detect an abnormality.

Special Instructions:

Websites That May be of Interest to You:

www.cardiology.org (Dr. Victor Froelicher, Stanford Medical University/VAH, Cardiology)

www.kg-ekgpress.com (Dr. Ken Grauer, family physician in Gainesville, Fla)

www.ACC.org (American College of Cardiology)

www.americanheart.org (American Heart Association)

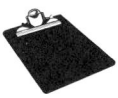

Patient Education Handout

PERICARDIOCENTESIS

What Procedure is Being Performed?

Your clinician will perform a pericardiocentesis. This is a procedure that is designed to remove fluid from the sac around the heart. The sac, called the *pericardium,* normally contains only a few tablespoons of fluid. If too much fluid accumulates, it can interfere with the pumping action of your heart. Using pericardiocentesis, your clinician will be able to remove fluid to improve your heart's function and to help determine what caused the fluid to accumulate.

How is This Procedure Performed?

You will be asked to lay on a table, and your head may be elevated. Your clinician may elect to give you a mild sedative. An ultrasound machine, an x ray, or an ECG is used to help your clinician guide the needle to an appropriate target. An area of your lower chest and upper abdomen is cleaned with an antiseptic solution, and a sterile drape will be placed in that area. You should not touch the drape or the cleansed area, because that would increase your risk of infection. A small area of skin is numbed with a needle and syringe—this will be slightly uncomfortable. After your skin is numb, a longer needle is passed through the skin toward the heart. Be careful not to move at this time. When the needle enters the pericardium, you may feel a sharp, brief chest pain. Once the pericardial space has been entered, your clinician will withdraw some fluid for testing. If there is a lot of fluid or the fluid seems likely to rapidly reaccumulate, a small plastic drainage tube may be left in place temporarily to prevent further fluid buildup around the heart.

What are the Risks?

The most common risk is that no fluid will be obtained. This may be because the pericardial space was not entered, or the fluid may be in pockets in other areas of the pericardial space, or that possibly the fluid is too thick to flow through a fine needle. Because the needle used to puncture the pericardium has a sharp tip that is brought close to your constantly moving heart, there is also the risk of puncturing or cutting the surface of the heart or some of the blood vessels of the heart. Ultrasound, x-ray, or ECG guidance has helped minimize this risk. There is an even smaller risk of death from bleeding or heart rhythm problems. As with any invasive procedure, there is a small chance of infection and pain. Generally the risk that the fluid will continue to build up around your heart and stop it from pumping effectively is greater than the risks from having this procedure performed.

What are the Alternatives?

If you have accumulated fluid around your heart, there are few alternatives to pericardiocentesis. Some surgeons have relied on a surgical procedure called a *pericardial window,* which may have a lower complication rate but involves general anesthetic and cutting open the front of your chest. It is more invasive than a simple needle puncture. As in many medical conditions, a "watchful waiting" alternative may be considered, although very few causes of pericardial fluid will go away without treatment.

Continued

 *Patient Education Handout—cont'd*

PERICARDIOCENTESIS—cont'd

What Should the Patient Expect After the Procedure?

Normally, your vital signs will be monitored as a precaution while a chest radiograph is obtained. The chest radiograph will ensure that your lungs have not been injured. Laboratory testing will be performed on the fluid that was removed. If a specific cause for the fluid buildup is determined, specific treatment can then be started. Your provider will notify you of the test results or explain how they can be obtained.

Most of the time, there are no complications from this procedure. Most patients notice that they feel better after the fluid around the heart has been removed. You should notify your provider if you notice increasing discomfort, lightheadedness, fever, chills, palpitations or rapid heart rate, or if your original symptoms return or seem to worsen.

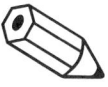 *Patient Consent Form*

PERICARDIOCENTESIS

I, _____, authorize my clinician, _____, and any assistants that they select, to perform a pericardiocentesis on _____ (date). I have received and reviewed information on the nature and purpose of this procedure, possible alternative methods of treatment, the risks involved, and the possibility of complications.

I further consent to the administration of such local anesthetics or injections as may be considered necessary or advisable by my clinician to complete the procedure, except as follows:

_____

_____

I have also been informed that in the performance of any invasive medical procedure, there are risks such as loss of blood, infection, etc. I am aware that medicine and surgery are not exact sciences. I acknowledge that no guarantees have been made to me concerning the results of the procedure and that I could even die as a result of the procedure.

_____   _____
Patient's signature   *Date/Time*

_____   _____
Parent's or legal guardian's signature   *Date/Time*

If parent or legal guardian is signing, relationship to patient: _____

_____   _____
Witness' signature   *Date/Time*
In my opinion, this is an informed consent.

_____   _____
Clinician's signature   *Date/Time*

One copy for chart; one copy for patient.

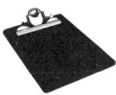 *Patient Education Handout*

SCLEROTHERAPY BILLING PROCEDURES

The purpose of this communication is to discuss the cost and payment mechanism, should you desire to have sclerotherapy (vein injections) performed.

For the *first visit,* we will spend approximately 30 minutes discussing your problem and conducting an examination. In addition, a test called a photoplethysmogram (PPG) will be conducted to determine if there are any problems deeper in your veins that would prevent the use of sclerotherapy. For this first visit, we will essentially accept what your insurance company allows as the "reasonable and customary" fee, provided the insurance company covers these services. You are responsible for any copay or deductible. If these services are not covered by your insurance, payment is expected at the time of service.

If you decide to proceed with sclerotherapy, you will usually need to purchase compression (special support) stockings at the first visit. Most patients will need to wear panty hose (but occasionally below-the-knee hose, single-leg hose, thigh-high hose, or even Ace wraps will be used) after the injections. We will order them for you at a reduced rate. *However, these items will need to be paid for before they are ordered. The cost is $_____ for panty hose, $_____ for knee-high hose, $_____ for thigh-high hose, and $_____ for single-leg hose. Compression hose can be purchased elsewhere. MediUSA, Sigvaris, or Jobst brands are recommended.*

Unfortunately, most insurance companies feel sclerotherapy injections are "cosmetic" and do *not* cover such procedures. When we first began performing vein injections, we tried to bill insurance companies directly. However, so many claims were rejected that this became impossible. Thus you will be responsible for the cost of injections on the date of service (cash, credit card, or check). The fee is $_____ for approximately 30 to 40 injections, which take approximately 30 minutes. You may submit the bill to your insurance company, which may reimburse you directly. *Medicaid and Medicare are particularly difficult to deal with regarding vein injections and they consider nearly all sclerotherapy injections cosmetic.* Therefore, although we accept Medicare and Medicaid patients, this may not be a covered benefit; you will be responsible for payment *on the date of service.* We will try to help you with documentation for reimbursement.

If you belong to an HMO and they have approved sclerotherapy for you, you are responsible for obtaining any referrals from the primary care doctor. We will only be able to do 15-minute sessions because they reimburse at such low rates, so you will need to return more times than other patients. Some "regular" insurance companies also require preapproval for sclerotherapy. Depending on reimbursement fees, even if the patient is preapproved for this procedure, sclerotherapy may only be done in 15-minute sessions for reimbursement purposes. If your insurance does not cover sclerotherapy at all and you have decided to pay for the procedure directly, 30-minute sessions are generally scheduled. *You will be responsible for payment of the entire bill at each session.*

Please call in advance with any questions regarding billing and fees. In addition, read all handouts and fill out all forms before your counseling and evaluation visit.

(Used by permission from The Medical Procedures Center, Midland, Mich.)

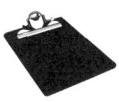

Patient Education Handout

SCLEROTHERAPY: POSTPROCEDURE INSTRUCTIONS

After leaving the office: It is best to walk for 15 to 30 minutes after leaving the office. This will help reduce the chances of getting a blood clot in the deeper veins.

Days 1 to 3: The stockings should remain in place for 3 days (no bathing; wear them to bed). The compression stockings are an important part of the treatment because they minimize the amount of blood reentering the injected vein. Elevate your legs as much as possible. No jogging or high-impact aerobics are allowed at this time. At the end of the 3 days, you may remove the stockings and discard the gauze pads. (You may find that standing in the shower is a convenient way to loosen the tape that holds the gauze pads; this also reduces the irritation to sensitive skin.) Do not be surprised if injected areas appear bruised. This is normal! You will look worse before you look better. You may resume normal activity if only small veins were injected.

Days 4 to 30: Continue to wear the compression stockings daily, but remove them at night to sleep. You may resume daily cool showers. Avoid jogging or high-impact aerobics for 1 week during this time if large veins were injected. Do not life weights for 1 week regardless of the vein size. Your doctor will tell you when you can return to these activities.

Days 30 forward: Continue to wear the compression stockings whenever possible to reduce the rate of recurrence of spider and varicose veins.

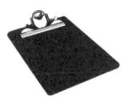

Patient Education Handout

SCLEROTHERAPY (VEIN INJECTION)

Spider veins are known medically as "telangiectasias" and are small, dilated blood vessels. These may become unsightly with time and may also lead to dull aching, itching, or stinging of the legs after prolonged standing. *Varicose veins* are the large veins you see.

Sclerotherapy is the technique of injecting a solution into these vessels using a small needle. The solution (_____) irritates and destroys the inner lining of the blood vessel so that it collapses and scars shut. *This does not harm the circulation—it improves it by eliminating the abnormal, unnecessary vessel.* Several injections may be needed to totally eliminate the vessels. The procedure is virtually painless. Fading of the vessels is a slow process that takes *1 to 6 months.* The goal is to produce a 75% to 90% improvement in both appearance and symptoms.

A *consultation appointment* is required in advance of the injection visit. The doctor examines the patient and explains the procedure. Any testing that may be required is done, and the patient is custom measured for support hose. Jobst, Sigvaris, or MediUSA brand support hose are recommended. These stockings are available in several colors, are washable, and will last 6 months with proper care. They are specially made so they create more pressure at the foot and less as they go up the leg, which helps push blood back to the heart. In addition to this handout, the patient should receive a color brochure on injection therapy before the visit. *The patient should wear a skirt or bring loose, comfortable shorts to the visit. Lotion should not be used on the lower legs the day of the consultation or for treatment sessions.*

Charges relate to the amount of time spent injecting. Because billing, reimbursement, and insurance policies are complicated for this procedure, *the patient should review the special billing information sheet carefully.*

Results of treatment cannot be guaranteed, but most patients are very pleased with the cosmetic and functional improvement.

Some commonly asked questions include the following:

What Causes Spider Veins?

No one is completely sure. Certain families are predisposed to this condition, so it is in part genetic. Estrogens (i.e., female hormones), pregnancy, birth control pills, tight girdles and garter belts, prolonged standing or sitting, and trauma make spider and varicose veins worse.

How Does Sclerotherapy Work?

The solution destroys the tiny cells that line the blood vessels, without damage to the surrounding tissues.

How Soon Will the Vessels Disappear?

Each vessel usually requires one to three treatments. The vessels disappear over a period of 2 weeks to 3 months. Recurrences may occur over a period of 1 to 5 years, but this is rare. However, this treatment does not prevent new vessels from developing.

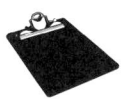

Patient Education Handout—cont'd

SCLEROTHERAPY (VEIN INJECTION)—cont'd

Are There Certain Vessels That Tend to Recur More Commonly?

Yes. They are the type of vessels that occur in a mat of very fine radiating vessels. This can occur on its own or may even come on after the injection itself. Large veins also may not respond well to injections.

How Often Can Treatments be Administered?

The same area should not be injected for 3 to 4 weeks to allow for complete healing. Different areas may be treated every week if necessary.

How Many Times Do Injections Have to be Done?

This varies with the number of areas that have to be injected, how numerous the veins are, their size, as well as the response to each injection. It usually takes one to three injections to obliterate any vessel; 10 to 40 vessels may be treated in any one session.

Are There Certain Kinds of Veins That Cannot be Treated?

Certain types of large varicose veins may not respond readily to sclerotherapy alone. These vessels may require a minor surgical procedure to remove them with follow-up sclerotherapy for the smaller vessels at a later time. The patient may be referred to a vascular surgeon for complete or partial treatment of these specific types of large varicose veins. Some of the extremely small vessels may require treatment with a pulsed dye laser or a new method called PhotoDerm therapy. Vessels on the face do better with treatments other than sclerotherapy.

Are There Other Methods of Treating These Vessels?

Five other methods are used:

1. Laser surgery: To date, this method has only been effective for tiny blood vessels. The present laser systems tend to produce a greater risk of scarring. The laser is an expensive device; thus treatment is more costly.
2. Electrodesiccation or cautery: This method produces a nonspecific destruction of both the vessel and overlying skin, which results in a greater incidence of scarring. This method works well on the face but not the legs.
3. Surgical ligation and stripping: This operative procedure is carried out in an operating room. It is best reserved for large varicose veins.
4. PhotoDerm treatment: This method is new and expensive, but it does work for some patients.
5. Endovascular vein ablation with a radiofrequency or laser catheter. There are a lot of big words here, but this is a fairly simple new procedure that is being developed for large veins. A small tube or wire is actually placed inside the vein, and it is then cauterized.

Continued

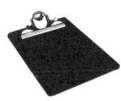 *Patient Education Handout—cont'd*

SCLEROTHERAPY (VEIN INJECTION)—cont'd
Is There any Way to Prevent Spider Veins?

The use of support hose may be helpful. Reducing weight and exercising regularly may also be of help.

What are the Side Effects to Injection Treatments?

• Slight *stinging or burning* may occur with injection of certain types and concentrations of solutions in certain areas.

• Sometimes a *clot* develops at the injection site (especially if the recommended pressure stockings are not worn for the proper amount of time or if large veins are injected). This clot will not generally cause internal problems, but its removal within 2 weeks of the injection will speed the healing process and decrease the incidence of discoloration. Removal is simple and only requires a small incision.

• *Swelling and bruising* over the injection site may occur, but it is rare. It is particularly common when patients have jobs at which they stand for long periods of time or when vessels in the ankles are injected. The swelling is rarely dangerous but occasionally must be treated with elevation and compression dressings.

• Superficial *thrombophlebitis,* an irritation of the injected vessel, occurs in less than 1 per 1000 patients. The area around the vein turns red and becomes tender. It may have to be treated with antiinflammatory agents and compression stockings.

• Some patients (10% to 30%) develop a small frecklelike *tan to brown spot* around the injected vessel. This usually resolves in 80% of patients within 3 to 6 months. However, a few patients will have a persistent discoloration for up to 1 year.

• A small superficial *ulceration* of the skin overlying the injected vessel may occur. This does not usually leave a scar but needs to be seen as soon as possible by the doctor. It can take 6 to 8 weeks to heal.

• Sometimes the body replaces the injected vessel with a *"mat" of very fine vessels,* causing an apparent darkened area. This may need follow-up injections.

   Note: The injected sites will definitely look worse for a few weeks before they look better!

What Should the Patient Do Before Treatment?

• Discontinue aspirin 1 week before the appointment. If you are taking blood thinners, talk to your doctor to be sure he or she can tell you what to do.

• Do not shave the legs for 2 days before the appointment and *do not apply any creams or lotions on the day of injection.*

• Eat a light breakfast or lunch 1 hour or so before the appointment.

• Bring loose shorts to wear during the procedure and slacks to wear out of the office to allow for bulky bandages.

• Call the office 2 or 3 days before the appointment to be sure support hose have arrived.

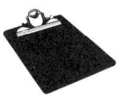

Patient Education Handout—cont'd

SCLEROTHERAPY (VEIN INJECTION)—cont'd
What Should the Patient Do After the Procedure?

- Walk for 30 minutes immediately after the injections.
- While riding home, keep legs moving and tense and relax the leg muscles. If it is a long drive, make frequent stops for walking (every 20 minutes).
- Maintain normal daytime activities and walk at least 1 hour per day—the more the better.
- Avoid hot baths for 2 weeks.
- Avoid standing without moving about. If it is necessary to stand in one place, feet and toes should be moved frequently.
- If the legs become painful after the injection, walk.
- Stockings should not be removed at all for 3 days and 2 nights. For large veins, the physician may request that they be worn longer.
- Avoid strenuous physical activity (e.g., aerobics) for the first 72 hours. Avoid weight-lifting for a week.
- After the first 2 days the patient may remove the stockings at night, but it is recommended that they be worn for at least 3 weeks whenever the patient is not reclining. Ideally the patient will use support hose the rest of his or her life.

Note: The patient should remember that injection therapy only treats the symptoms. Whatever has caused the patient's abnormal veins is still there after the injection. New abnormal veins can form and may recur, requiring future treatments in 1 to 2 years. Wearing support hose regularly may reduce the need for repeat follow-up treatments.

Patients should review the handout on billing procedures before the visit. In most instances patients are expected to pay on the day of the visit.

(Modified from Dermatology Associates of San Diego County, Inc.)

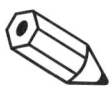 *Patient Consent Form*

SCLEROTHERAPY

I acknowledge that I have received a copy of this sclerotherapy informed consent form. I have read and understand the numerous handouts given to me.

I acknowledge that I have read the this informed consent form and that the doctor has adequately informed me of the risks of sclerotherapy treatment, alternative methods of treatment, and the risks of not treating my condition. I hereby consent to sclerotherapy treatment performed by my clinician, _____.

I also understand there are many problems with insurance covering my injections. I agree to pay at the time of service, and I assume all financial responsibility (even if my insurance company does not reimburse me).

_____	_____
Patient's signature	*Date/Time*
_____	_____
Witness' signature	*Relationship to patient*

One copy for chart; one copy for patient.

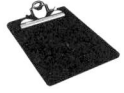

Patient Education Handout

RADIOFREQUENCY SCLEROTHERAPY

Why Do I Need This Procedure?

Radiofrequency sclerotherapy is designed to eliminate varicose veins, which produce swelling and pain in the feet and legs.

How Do I Prepare for This Procedure?

You do not need to do anything special for radiofrequency sclerotherapy. You should be well rested and you should not shave your legs for 2 days before or 7 days after the procedure. Do not apply lotions or creams for 24 hours before your appointment.

What Happens During This Procedure?

A needle will be inserted into the enlarged vein, similar to having blood drawn. The area around the needle will be numbed and the tissue inside of the vein will be treated. The outer wall of the vein will remain intact but the vein collapses.

What Happens After the Procedure?

Because of compression hose worn after the procedure, the injured inner aspect of the vein walls will heal together and close off. This will block any further blood flow and therefore swelling of the vein.

What are the Benefits of This Procedure?

The varicose vein will disappear immediately. If proper compression is applied with the special hose and no complicating circumstances exist the puncture wound will heal with little or no residual evidence of treatment. The veins will be gone.

What are the Risks Associated With This Procedure?

The most common finding is a visible discoloration at the spot of the needle puncture. This usually occurs in patients with very sensitive skin. Most patients will observe some black and blue discoloration around the treated area, which disappears quickly when compression stockings are used. Other rare complications may include ulcerations of the skin, blood clots, and areas of swelling, with or without infection, at or near the treatment site.

When Should I Call My Physician?

Your doctor will give you an appointment for follow-up evaluation. If you experience pain, swelling, or discoloration of the skin above or below the pads applied, call your doctor. Some minor irritation around the treatment site is to be expected. Most patients may have an itching sensation; however, sharp burning sensations should be reported to your doctor immediately.

Special Instructions:

Gradient compression hose are the key to successful results. They are important to keep the vein collapsed as the walls heal together. You will need to wear them at least 48 hours continuously and then while up for another 1 to 4 weeks.

Website That May be of Interest to You:

www.veinsaway.com
www.vnus.com

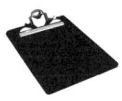 *Patient Education Handout*

POSTSCLEROTHERAPY TREATMENT INSTRUCTIONS: INJECTION AND RADIOFREQUENCY SCLEROTHERAPY

First 2 Days (48 Hours)

Keep all pads and compression hose on for 48 hours when you are wearing panty hose and need to go to the bathroom, pull them down only as far as necessary.

Walk at least 1 hour after your treatment! Then walk for 30 minutes every 2 hours during the first 8 hours after your treatment.

Keep your feet elevated with your legs slightly bent while sitting. Elevation is not necessary when lying.

Do not participate in heavy aerobics or jogging.

Day 3 Through 7

You may remove your pads and hose while sleeping. Make sure you put them on *before* getting out of bed or immediately after a brief, cool shower.

Walk as much as you can. Try to avoid standing in one place for more than 2 straight minutes without moving.

You may return to your normal gym, aerobics, or jogging as long as you wear your hose and pads.

Weeks 2 Through 4

Discontinue the use of the pads.

Keep wearing your hose anytime you are not lying down.

Continue walking as much as possible.

General Instructions:

Always be alert for signs of swelling, itching, burning, or pain at the treatment site.

Do not take aspirin or antiinflammatories (Motrin, etc.) during the first week. It is best to avoid antiinflammatories during your entire course of treatment. Tylenol may be used for mild pain or headache.

Contact your physician if you suspect any unusual events.

Gradient compression hose, used properly, are the foundation of your treatment. Even the smallest spider veins require compression and in fact require more compression than larger veins. *Wear your hose as instructed!*

ALWAYS CONSULT YOUR PHYSICIAN IF YOU ARE UNCLEAR WITH THESE INSTRUCTIONS OR WITH ANY PHASE OF YOUR TREATMENT.

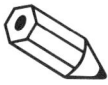

Patient Consent Form

RADIOFREQUENCY TREATMENT OF VARICOSE VEINS

I came to the office of Dr. _____ on _____ (date) for evaluation and treatment of the following condition:

(Description of diagnosis, etiology and differential diagnosis)

We discussed the different treatments possible and discussed the risks of not treating the condition. Based on my interpretation of the advice given by Dr. _____ and my own judgment, I request that radiofrequency sclerotherapy be performed upon me.

I understand that certain drugs may be necessary and that local anesthesia will be necessary for my comfort. I request and consent to the use of all and any drugs or medications as determined medically advisable for my health and safety. I further direct Dr. _____ to use any measures deemed advisable to improve my outcome or for my personal safety and well being.

Special dressings will be used to improve the effectiveness of the procedure, and I understand that for maximum benefit, I must adhere to all instructions and comply with directions to the best of my ability. Photographs taken before, during, and after the procedure will document my progress. I request that such photographs be taken upon the discretion of Dr. _____.

I understand that anything can happen during or after this procedure, which has nothing to do with the care or treatment rendered. I have been advised that this may be considered a cosmetic procedure and that I assume all risks associated with it. I also understand that the advantages of this procedure are normally less scaring, minimal or no post treatment recuperation, little anesthetic, and minimal tissue damage. Despite all these advantages I am completely aware that I may experience untoward reactions or outcomes and I *have not* been promised or given any *assurance* as to the good or the aesthetic results I may have.

The more possible risks of this treatment are as follows:
a. Scab formation at or over the treatment area
b. Increased skin pigmentation (discoloration)
c. Burns or ulcers at the treatment site
d. Inflammation (with or without) swelling of the skin
e. Scar formation
f. Cellulitis (infection) of the skin or other structures
g. Incomplete obliteration or recurrence of the vein condition requiring retreatment
h. Formation of blood clots, phlebitis and deep vein thrombosis
i. Blood clots can travel to the lungs or body parts and cause injury or death.

Continued

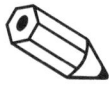 *Patient Consent Form—cont'd*

RADIOFREQUENCY TREATMENT OF VARICOSE VEINS—cont'd

I request radiofrequency sclerotherapy and assume all risks whether or not stated above. I understand medicine is an art and a science, and I feel the beneficial outcomes outweigh the risks.

I will call the office if any problems arise before my scheduled follow-up and will carry out all posttreatment instructions, including wearing compression hose as advised. I will return for all follow-up appointments or reschedule upon the recommendations given.

THIS IS A LEGAL DOCUMENT—DO NOT SIGN IT UNTIL YOU HAVE FULLY READ IT AND UNDERSTAND IT

I understand and have fully read this consent form. I request that radiofrequency sclerotherapy be performed as recommended. My signature is proof that I will hold Dr. _____ liable only for reasonable and normal medical care.

_____   _____
Patient's signature   *Date/Time*

_____   _____
Witness' signature   *Date/Time*

I, Dr. _____, have personally consulted with _____ and have discussed fully the ramifications of the proposed treatment. I have not given any assurances as to outcomes and will provide this treatment according to normally established guidelines.

_____   _____
Physician's signature   *Date*

One copy for chart; one copy for patient.

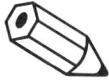

Patient Consent Form

CARDIAC EXERCISE TESTING

Your clinician has decided that an exercise test will be helpful in the diagnosis or management of your medical condition. Exercise testing is designed to evaluate the function of the heart, lungs, and blood vessels, especially the coronary arteries. Before the test, the clinician, will need to screen you for certain contraindications and to perform a resting electrocardiogram. You will then be asked to walk faster and faster on a treadmill (or pedal a bicycle or exercise on some other device) until the increasing fatigue, breathlessness, chest pain, or other symptoms are too much and you feel it is time to stop. If you feel that the test should be stopped, notify the medical personnel in the room immediately.

Your blood pressure (BP), heart rate, level of exertion, symptoms, overall condition, and electrocardiogram will be monitored during the test.

Risks of exercise testing include occasional changes in the rhythm of the heart and the possibility of very high BP. There is a rare chance of fainting and an even rarer chance of a heart attack or sudden cardiac death (about 1 in 10,000).

Benefits of testing include learning how much exercise you can do safely and determining if there are any serious problems with your heart. Your maximal heart rate will usually be determined, which can be used to customize your exercise prescription. The knowledge gained from the exercise test allows a better diagnosis of your medical condition and a more accurate treatment.

Consent

Your signature on the form indicates that (1) you have read, understood, and agreed to all of the previous statements; (2) you have had an opportunity to ask questions about the exercise test; (3) the test has been adequately explained to you, and you have been given sufficient information regarding the test, its risks, and its benefits; and (4) your consent to take the exercise test is given voluntarily (because you have the right to refuse to take the test).

I hereby consent to undergo the performance of the cardiac exercise test under the supervision of _____.

_____   _____
Patient's signature   *Date/Time*

_____   _____
Patient's name   *Witness' signature*

One copy for chart; one copy for patient.

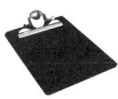 *Patient Education Handout*

PULMONARY ARTERY CATHETERIZATION

Pulmonary artery (Swan-Ganz) catheterization is a procedure in which we place a catheter into one of the large veins that empties into your heart. It is then advanced into the right side of your heart, and eventually into the artery going to your lungs. You need this procedure because we are having difficulty managing the fluids in your body or in making a diagnosis. With a catheter inside your heart, we will be able to make certain measurements, including the blood gases (oxygen), blood flow, and pressures on the right side of the heart. From these measurements, we are able to estimate the blood pressure inside your lungs. We may be able to tell if or why you have too much fluid in your lungs.

During this procedure, we will insert a catheter that is approximately 2 feet long. It will be inserted through another catheter that is already in your vein. You should not feel this catheter going into your heart. Except for our gowns, mask, goggles or glasses, and the drapes we place on you, you should not know that we are performing this procedure.

The most important thing for you to do during this procedure is to relax and remain calm. We may ask you to help us by taking deep breaths or by changing positions at a certain stage of the procedure. The benefits of this procedure include better management of your fluids and, in some cases, your medications. It should improve our ability to make a diagnosis. This should lead to better care for you.

The risks associated with this procedure include those for central venous catheter insertion. There is also a slight risk of a rhythm problem with your heart, blood clots, and damage to your lungs. If the catheter is left in place more than 3 days, there is an increased risk of infection.

After the procedure is performed, the catheter will be connected to another monitor for us to watch. Periodically it will be flushed and checked for accuracy.

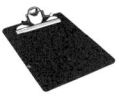

Patient Education Handout

TEMPORARY PACING

Occasionally a heart will fail to keep up its pace or to beat fast enough or strong enough to generate sufficient blood pressure. In that situation, a temporary pacemaker is needed.

There are two possible methods of providing a temporary pacemaker: externally (across your chest through electrodes) and internally (through the vein that leads into your heart).

If you need a pacemaker across your chest (external pacemaker), two large electrodes will be applied to your skin. One will be placed on your chest and the other on your back. We will then apply electricity through the electrodes and attempt to speed up your heart.

You will feel some of the electricity and notice some muscle twitching. You may experience some cramping and discomfort. If the symptoms are too strong, we can give you a sedative. There is no way to prepare for such a procedure except to remain calm.

The benefits of this procedure are that your heart will beat stronger and faster, and you may not need as many medications to maintain your blood pressure. Risks of this procedure include failure to pace your heart and the possibility of slight burns to the skin.

If you need an internal pacemaker, we will insert a 1- or 2-foot-long catheter. It will have a pacemaker attached to it and will be inserted through another catheter that is already in your vein. You should not feel this catheter going into your heart, but you will notice the drapes we place on you.

The most important thing for you to do during this procedure is to relax and remain calm. We may ask you to help us by taking deep breaths or by changing positions at a certain stage of the procedure.

After the internal pacemaker is placed, we will apply electricity to it. It is low-dose electricity, and you should not feel it.

The benefits of this procedure are that your heart will beat stronger and faster, and you may not need as many medications to maintain your blood pressure. The risks associated with this procedure include those for central venous catheter insertion as well as failure to pace your heart and potential rupture of your heart wall. If the pacemaker is left in place more than three days, there is an increased risk of infection.

The nurse will drape and dress the area to prevent infection. You will not be discharged with a temporary pacer; a permanent pacemaker may need to be inserted. Call the nurse or clinician if you have any questions.

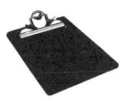 *Patient Education Handout*

THORACENTESIS

What is Thoracentesis?

Thoracentesis is the removal of air or fluid from the area around the lung.

Why is a Thoracentesis Performed?

It is not normal to have fluid or air in the area around your lung. Sometimes the only way to figure out why someone has this fluid is to take a sample. Fluid or air around the lung can make breathing difficult. Removing it may make you feel better.

How is a Thoracentesis Performed?

An area on your chest or back will be washed off, and numbing medicine will be injected. Then a needle will be inserted between your ribs and the air or fluid removed.

Does it Hurt?

Yes, but most people say it is not much worse than having blood drawn.

What Sort of Things Can Go Wrong?

The most common problem that occurs from thoracentesis is for more air to get into the area around the lung, causing the lung to "collapse." This happens 5% to 20% of the time. Most often the collapsed lung gets better on its own, but sometimes a tube has to be put in to get the air out. This tube would stay in for several days, and you would have to stay in the hospital.

You may feel short of breath right after the procedure, but this should get better. Very rarely, the needle goes through an organ, causing bleeding. Sometimes the needle can cause an infection. The goal of thoracentesis is to gain important information and to make you feel better, but there is always the chance it could make you worse.

What Can I Do to Make Things Go Smoothly?

The most important thing during the procedure is to lie or sit still. Let the doctor know if you are having any chest pain or shortness of breath. After the procedure, you will have to lie quietly and may need to breathe oxygen for a while. You can take off the bandage 24 hours after the procedure and wash the area. Tell the doctor if you have a hard time breathing, develop a new fever or chills, or develop redness at the puncture site.

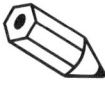 *Patient Consent Form*

THORACENTESIS

I, _____, authorize Dr. _____ or an assistant to perform a thoracentesis. I have read the patient education handout and have had the procedure explained to me. All of my questions have been answered. I understand that every procedure has risks and that not all of the risks may be listed here. I know I have other choices, but I choose freely to have the thoracentesis. I agree to return for follow-up care and will call the office or answering service if any problems arise.

_____   _____

Patient's signature   *Date/Time*

_____   _____

Witness' signature   *Date/Time*

One copy for chart; one copy for patient.

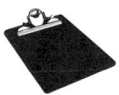 *Patient Education Handout*

VENOUS CUTDOWN

Veins carry blood from the organs, tissue, and cells of your body to your heart. The oxygen in the blood in your veins has been used by the organs, tissue, and cells and must be returned through the heart to the lungs to obtain more oxygen. A certain amount of blood in veins is necessary to keep the organs, tissue, and cells working. Venous cutdown is a procedure in which we make a small incision near a vein to isolate it so that a catheter (plastic tube) can be inserted into the vein. You will need this procedure because you have a suspected disorder in the amount of your blood volume (dehydration or volume depletion) or your blood pressure is too low (shock) or certain fluids or medications need to be given immediately. Low blood volume or blood pressure or the lack of certain fluids or medications could result in harm to the cells in your body, resulting in organ, cell, or tissue death. By doing this procedure, we will be able to minimize the severity of the problem. A routine intravenous (IV) catheter cannot be obtained at this point.

The most important thing for you to do during this procedure is to try and relax and remain calm.

During this procedure, your clinician will put your arm or leg into a certain position while they determine the best location for the procedure. They may give you an injection to numb the skin over the vein. The skin will be cleansed before any injections. The clinician will then make a small incision, isolate the vein, and use a catheter to puncture the vein. You may experience some discomfort with any of the injections.

After the procedure, the incision will be closed with stitches. Then it will be covered with a bandage. The benefits of this procedure include the ability to start an IV.

The risks associated with the procedure are few but must be discussed. Possible complications include bleeding, infection, scarring, and blood clots. Local structures near the incision such as nerves, tendons, or arteries could be damaged. There are also other rare complications that could occur that we could not foresee. In order to minimize complications, it is important for you to notify the clinician or nursing staff at the earliest sign of a possible complication.

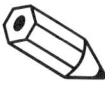 *Patient Consent Form*

VENOUS CUTDOWN

I am under the care of my clinician, _____, on _____ (date) for treatment of an abnormality with my blood pressure, blood volume, or access to my blood vessels. We discussed the different treatment options and the risks involved.

Based on that discussion and my own judgment, I agree to allow my clinician, _____, to make an incision, isolate a vein, and then start an IV. This may involve local anesthesia with an injection of lidocaine.

I understand that there will be some discomfort with this procedure.

We discussed the different outcomes that could occur and most of the possible complications, including bleeding, infection, scarring, and blood clots. Local structures near the incision such as nerves, tendons, arteries, or veins could be damaged. I am aware that there are other rare complications that could occur that we could not foresee. I have read and understand the patient education handout. I agree to follow the instructions for self-care after the procedure and to return for follow-up care on: _____. All of my questions have been answered.

I will call the office or answering service if any problems occur.

_____   _____

Patient's signature   *Date/Time*

_____   _____

Witness' signature   *Clinician's signature*

One copy for chart; one copy for patient.

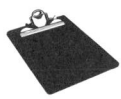 *Patient Education Handout*

FINE ANAL FISSURES AND PRURITIS ANI ("ITCHY ANAL AREA")

Many patients come to our office with symptoms of severe itching around the anus. Others come thinking they have hemorrhoids because they have experienced bright red rectal bleeding. On physical examination, physicians often find an area that is very sore and irritated with very fine cracks in the skin. These cracks are called *fissures*. Some fissures are more external on the skin and readily visible. Other fissures are situated more deeply inside. Your physician will be able to determine at the time of the examination which type of fissure you have and what the best treatment is.

Many people feel that their itching is due to being "dirty down there." Almost always, itching and irritation is actually caused by keeping the anal area *too clean.*

Do not wash after a bowel movement. *Do not* scrub the anal area when showering or bathing. Just rinse with plain water.

It is important to use hypoallergenic soaps and shampoos. Many people with this condition have fair skin. They are very sensitive to perfumes and dyes. Aveeno, Oilatum, or Lever 2000 soaps are recommended. Any product that states that it is hypoallergenic would probably suffice. Those who really have problems will also need to get a hypoallergenic shampoo.

Cotton underwear is essential. If you have very sensitive skin, an extra rinse cycle may be necessary when washing underwear.

The immune system should be helped as much as possible to resolve the situation. A good multivitamin, a total of 1000 mg of vitamin C per day, and 400 IU of vitamin E are recommended. In addition, the herb Echinacea (available at grocery stores and health food stores) taken two to three times per day is also helpful.

You should really avoid any offending foods. Common items are coffee, anything spicy, and acidic items. Try eliminating foods to see if it makes things better. If it does not, you can go back to them later.

At times, a hydrocortisone cream or suppositories may also be prescribed. The patient has to be careful not to overuse these since they will thin out the skin and actually make the problem worse. At times xylocaine ointment can also be prescribed. This merely numbs up the area. It does not treat the condition, but it helps to avoid the itch-scratch cycle, which can often make things persist and get worse.

The final means of managing this problem is a prescription of Atarax. It is actually a strong antihistamine, and its only side effect is that it can cause drowsiness. Subsequently, patients should take 25 to 50 mg an hour before bedtime. Many times, the scratching of the anal area makes the problem worse. It often occurs at night. If the nighttime scratching could just be eliminated, things often improve. Patients can actually take up to 100 mg of Atarax at bedtime. Men with prostate problems should go very slowly because this can sometimes make that worse.

For those fissures that are deeper inside, your physician may suggest that you try suppositories and other ointments. If the fissures do not resolve within 3 months, surgery may be indicated, so keep us informed if you do not feel improvement.

Your physician will tell you which, if any, of these approaches he or she wants you to take. Generally, a follow-up visit is required 1 month after beginning treatment.

(Adapted from The Medical Procedures Center, PC, Midland, Mich.)

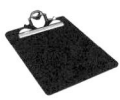

Patient Education Handout

ANESTHESIA FOR COLONOSCOPY

There are many new ways that physicians can assist patients undergoing colonoscopy examination. In the past, these examinations were performed in a hospital setting. Anesthesia was always performed by placing a needle in the patient's arm, and an intravenous medication was given to make patients sleepy and more comfortable.

We now know that these examinations can generally be safely performed in the office setting. The cost savings of performing this examination in the office can be great.

Normally you should not eat or drink anything the day of the procedure. You should take your routine medications with water first thing in the morning. If your procedure is scheduled in the afternoon, we prefer that you drink some liquids early that morning. Then only take your Halcion tablets if needed as described below.

The risk of a colonoscopy examination is influenced by the method of anesthesia chosen. Intravenous medications can carry a slightly higher risk of heart or lung complications. They can also be the best method to make the examination comfortable. We can provide intravenous medications for our patients, but can also offer alternate methods for making the examination comfortable for you. Up to 25% or 30% of patients can have a full colonoscopic examination without any anesthesia. Discuss with your doctor what may be the best method of anesthesia for you.

Some patients may prefer oral medications. This method of sedation is safe, effective, and often much cheaper for patients. Patients should take two 0.25-mg triazolam (Halcion) tablets 1 hour before the scheduled procedure. Please take these tablets with a small amount of water. This medication is a benzodiazepine, the same type that is given intravenously. The medication is safe and helps patients to relax for the procedure.

Just before the procedure the nurse will spray your nose with a medication called butorphanol (Stadol). Some women received Stadol during labor. This medication relieves pain and makes patients sleepy for the procedure. It is safe and effective, and administration in the nose is less uncomfortable than having an injection or IV placed. Of course, you can always choose to have intravenous sedation, which would include starting an IV for a sedative and pain reliever. Whether you choose the oral or IV routes, you will be clinically monitored at all times.

Someone must drive you to and from the office if sedating medication of any form is used for the procedure. When you arrive for your procedure, immediately tell our staff if you have eaten anything, and if you have taken your medication. If you choose the oral/nasal medication and find you need extra medication during the procedure, we can give you an injection in your arm or place a needle into your veins. However, most patients do very well with just the oral medication and nasal spray.

We look forward to serving you, and in assisting you to make the procedure as comfortable and as safe as possible. If you experience any problems after the procedure like prolonged pain, bleeding, fever, vomiting, or anything else, please call us.

(Used by permission of The Medical Procedures Center, Midland, Mich.)

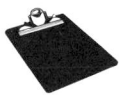 *Patient Education Handout*

COLONOSCOPY

What is Colonoscopy?

Colonoscopy is a special test that allows your physician to examine the lining of the colon (large bowel) for abnormal growths, such as polyps or cancer. A long tube about the size of your little finger will be passed into your bowel. A light on the end allows the examiner to see the inside of the bowel. This is where polyps, then cancer, grow.

Who Should Have a Colonoscopy?

Your physician may recommend a colonoscopy for the following:

- A change in bowel habits
- Rectal bleeding
- Unexpected abdominal pain
- Inflammatory bowel disease (i.e., colitis)
- When polyps or tumors are found on a barium enema x-ray
- A past or family history of colorectal polyps or cancer
- Over 50 years of age and require routine screening (every 10 years)
- As an evaluation prior to some other surgeries

What Preparation is Required?

The colon must be completely clean for the procedure to be accurate and complete. Your physician will give you detailed instructions regarding the dietary restrictions to be followed and the cleansing routine to be used. Most medications may be continued as usual, but some medications can interfere with the preparation or the examination. Therefore it is best to inform your physician of your current medications and any allergies to medications.

How is the Procedure Performed?

Your doctor will usually give you medication intravenously to help you relax during the procedure. During the colonoscopy, the bowel will be examined. If an abnormal area is found, a small biopsy will be done. In addition, polyps or growths may be removed. You will not feel the biopsies if they are done.

What are Polyps and Why are They Removed?

Polyps are abnormal growths from the lining of the colon. They vary in size from a tiny dot to several inches. The majority of polyps are benign (noncancerous), but the doctor cannot always tell a benign from a malignant (cancerous) polyp by its outer appearance alone. For this reason, polyps are removed by passing special instruments through the colonoscope. They are then sent for tissue analysis. Removal of colon polyps is an important means of preventing colorectal cancer.

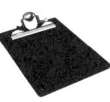 *Patient Education Handout—cont'd*

COLONOSCOPY—cont'd

What Happens After Colonoscopy?

The examination usually takes less than 1 hour. After colonoscopy, your physician will explain the results to you. If you have been given medications during the procedure, you will be observed until most of the effects of sedation have worn off (for 30 minutes to 2 hours). You will need someone to drive you home after the procedure. You may not remember anything that happened since the medications used often cause you to forget everything.

What are Possible Complications of Colonoscopy?

Although complications after colonoscopy are uncommon, it is important for you to recognize early signs of any possible complications. Contact the physician who performed the colonoscopy if you notice any of the following symptoms: severe abdominal pain, fever and chills, or rectal bleeding of more than one-half cup. Bleeding can even occur several days after the removal of a polyp.

In addition to excessive bleeding, possible complications include infection and a perforation or tear through the bowel wall. (The latter may require hospitalization and surgery to repair it.) You could have a reaction or oversedation from the drugs, especially if you already have lung disease. With the stress, you could experience heart problems, just like with any other surgery. It is important to understand that although it is very helpful, colonoscopy can miss lesions too or the entire abnormality may not be removed. So, if you continue to have symptoms, be sure to see your doctor again to discuss them. Also, be sure to keep any follow-up visits or examinations that your doctor recommends.

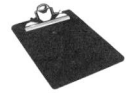 *Patient Education Handout*

COLONOSCOPY PREPARATION

Patient name: _____ DOB: _____

Arrival time: _____ Appointment date: _____ Procedure time: _____

Preparation

1. Please purchase the following supplies, which are available over-the-counter (no prescription needed):

   2 bottles magnesium citrate (plain)

   6 tablets Dulcolax

   1 Phospho-Soda Fleet's enema (green and white box)

2. Clear liquid diet 36 hours before examination. Drink at least 3 to 4 quarts of liquid a day. Start diet after lunch on _____ (2 days before your appointment, with lunch about noon).

   Food allowed: Clear broth, hard candy, Jell-O, coffee, tea, soft drinks, clear fruit juices, fruit-flavored drinks, plain or vanilla yogurt, milk, sugar, Popsicles, plain vanilla ice cream, and sherbet. **Note: Avoid the red products of Jell-O, Popsicles, and drinks.** A fast-food vanilla or chocolate milk shake is allowed (not homemade). **Call with any questions regarding diet.**

3. Drink 10 oz of magnesium citrate (preferably chilled over ice) at 2 pm on _____ (2 days before your appointment) and _____ (1 day before your appointment).

4. Take 3 Dulcolax tablets (oral) at bedtime on _____ (2 days before your appointment) and _____ (1 day before your appointment).

5. Use a Fleet enema (green and white box) on the morning of the examination (about one [1] hour before you leave the house).

6. Nothing to eat or drink 3 hours before your colonoscopy.

7. If you wish sedation, you must have someone with you to drive you home.

Special Instructions Regarding Medications

1. Blood thinners such as Coumadin, Persantine, and *all aspirin products* such as Advil, Ecotrin, Bufferin, and arthritis medications *must be stopped* 7 days before the procedure. Check with your doctor to be sure it's okay to stop the Coumadin.

2. Your regular morning medications (heart, hypertension, etc.) may be taken as directed on the morning of the procedure.

3. Do not take any antidiarrhea medication such as Lomotil, Kaopectate, Imodium, or iron supplements while taking this preparation.

   Diabetics: Diabetics may use Ensure to supplement their caloric intake. Diabetics on insulin should check with their physician regarding insulin dosage on day of colonoscopy.

4. Please bring with you a list of medications you are currently taking along with any medication allergies you have.

After Your Procedure

1. If you have any problems after the procedure, such as pain, bleeding, fever, or vomiting, please call us.

2. Call us for biopsy results 2 weeks after your procedure.

3. No driving for at least 8 hours if you received any sedation

(Used by permission of The Medical Procedures Center, Midland, Mich.)

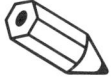 *Patient Consent Form*

COLONOSCOPY, BIOPSY, AND POLYPECTOMY

All of these procedures apply to looking into your large intestine with a flexible tube and removing small amounts of abnormal tissue. The tissue is sent to the laboratory for further analysis and there will be a separate charge from the hospital for this. The procedures being planned for you are: (a) Colonoscopy (looking in large bowel), (b) Endoscopic biopsy (sampling tissue), and (c) Polypectomy (removing abnormal tissue)

The benefits to you are the early diagnosis and potential cure of disease—cancer would be one example, but there are others. The procedure may also allow proper diagnosis and appropriate treatment (e.g., ulcerative colitis). There are risks. We believe the procedures are safe and that the potential benefits are greater than the risks. Please read and understand that the risks are as follows:

1. **Infection** can occur rarely. You might need antibiotics after the procedure.
2. **Bleeding** is rare. You could have some spotting or even enough bleeding to need a transfusion.
3. **Perforation** is a hole or small tear in the intestine or stomach caused by the tube. When this occurs, you would need to go to the hospital and you may need an operation.
4. The **medications** we give to prevent pain can cause a reaction. One rare side effect is a swelling and redness in the arm. Another might be a severe allergic reaction. Too much sedation can also cause heart and breathing problems. We use precautions to minimize these risks.
5. **Pain** from the procedure itself.
6. Even with our best efforts, an abnormality could be missed and further procedures may be necessary, especially if symptoms persist.

What are the Alternatives?
1. You can request more time to think about this or have an x-ray examination.
2. You can refuse to have the procedure done, but you are subject to the risk of delayed diagnosis. In the case of cancer, this could allow a cancer to spread and even lead to death.
3. If there are other alternatives that you, your family, friends, or other doctors have discussed with you, we are happy to discuss these as well. Please mention them if you wish.

Informed Consent
Having read and understood the above, I feel that the benefits of this procedure outweigh its risks. I have also read and understand the other patient education materials given to me.

I agree to allow Drs. _____ and _____ to perform the procedure.

_____

Patient's signature

_____

Witness' signature

_____

Printed name

_____

Date

One copy for chart; one copy for patient.

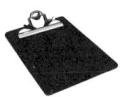 *Patient Education Handout*

ANESTHESIA FOR UPPER ENDOSCOPY

There are many new ways that physicians can assist patients undergoing an upper endoscopy (EGD) examination. In the past, these examinations were performed in a hospital setting. Anesthetic was administered by placing a needle in the patient's arm, and an intravenous (IV) medication was given to make patients sleepy.

We now know that these brief examinations can be safely performed in the office setting. The cost savings of performing this examination in the office can be great.

The risk of an EGD examination is greatly influenced by the method of anesthesia chosen. Many IV medications may carry a higher risk of heart or lung complications. We can provide IV medications for our patients, but we prefer to use alternative methods.

We prefer to give patients oral medications when possible. This method of conscious anesthesia is safe, effective, and often much cheaper for patients. Patients should take two 0.25 mg triazolam (Halcion) tablets *1 hour* before the scheduled procedure. Please take these tablets with a small amount of water. This medication is a benzodiazepine—the same type that is given intravenously. The medication is safe and helps patients relax for the procedure.

A full stomach can result in vomiting during the procedure. Normally you should not eat or drink anything the day of the procedure. You should take your routine medications with water first thing in the morning. If your procedure is scheduled in the afternoon, we prefer that you drink some liquids early that morning. Then, only take your Halcion tablets 1 hour before your scheduled procedure.

Just before the procedure the nurse will spray your nose with a medication called butorphanol (Stadol). Some women receive Stadol during labor. This medication relieves pain and makes patients sleepy for the procedure. It is safe and effective, and administration in the nose is less uncomfortable than having an injection or IV placed.

Just before the examination, we will spray a local anesthetic into your throat. This medication may taste bitter initially, but it makes the examination much more comfortable. This medicine will keep your throat numb for an hour or two after the procedure, so do not eat or drink until the effect wears off. You may also experience a mild sore throat from the procedure after this medication wears off.

Someone must drive you to and from the office for the procedure. When you arrive for your procedure, immediately tell our staff if you have eaten anything and if you have taken your medication. If you need extra medication during the procedure, we may give you an injection in your arm or place a needle into your veins. However, most patients do very well with just the oral medication, nasal spray, and topical anesthetic. Your driver can expect to take you home about 1 to 1½ hours after the start of your procedure.

We look forward to serving you, and in assisting you to make the procedure as comfortable and as safe as possible.

(Used by permission of The National Procedures Institute, Midland, Mich.)

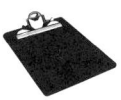

Patient Education Handout

ESOPHAGOGASTRODUODENOSCOPY (EGD)

What is an EGD?

EGD stands for esophagogastroduodenoscopy. This short procedure allows the physician to directly view the lining of the esophagus (swallowing tube), the stomach, and the first part of the small intestine (the duodenum.

Why Do I Need This Test?

An EGD gives the physician specific information about the upper digestive tract that x-rays and other tests do not provide. This test helps the doctor diagnose the problem so that the right treatment may be started.

How is EGD Done?

During the EGD, a flexible tube connected to a light source (a "flexible fiberoptic endoscope" or "gastroscope") is inserted into the mouth and advanced through the esophagus into the stomach. As the tube is slowly withdrawn, the physician will carefully examine the lining of the duodenum, stomach, and esophagus. If anything abnormal is seen, a biopsy will be done. This will not be felt. Another test, called the rapid urease test (CLO) test, that checks for a special bacteria may also be performed.

Is it Uncomfortable?

In most cases little or no pain is associated with a performance of an EGD. There may be a full feeling in the throat. A sedative is given before the examination to ensure comfort during the procedure. A local anesthetic is also sprayed in the throat before the tube is inserted in the mouth. This numbs the gag reflex and enables the tube to be swallowed comfortably. Once the tube is in the back of the throat, the physician will ask the patient to swallow the instrument. The instrument may not be felt, but the physician will gently guide the tube from the throat into the esophagus. Even if the tube is felt in the back of the throat, breathing and swallowing will still be comfortable during the test.

How Long does the Test Take?

The examination usually takes 10 to 15 minutes. You may actually be in the procedure room for approximately 30 minutes, including the time it takes to prepare for the examination and provide the appropriate sedation to make the test comfortable. However, plan to be in the office approximately 2 hours. This includes the preprocedure time, the examination time, the recovery period, and the conference time with the doctor after EGD is completed.

Are Medications Given?

Medications are given. The physician will provide a sedative before the examination to ensure comfort. Some medications are given by mouth, whereas others are given with a needle through an IV site.

Continued

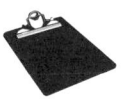 *Patient Education Handout—cont'd*

ESOPHAGOGASTRODUODENOSCOPY (EGD)—cont'd

What are the Possible Complications?

Complications are quite rare but include oversedation; bleeding from biopsies or trauma; missing the abnormality because there is food, excessive mucus, blood, or lack of patient cooperation; or, very rarely, a tear through the esophagus or stomach. Of course, mechanical and technical problems can also occur anytime.

Do I Have to Do Anything Special After the Test?

Typically, you can eat immediately after the test unless otherwise advised by the physician. The freezing sensation or numb feeling in the back of the throat will usually wear off about 30 minutes after the procedure. You may not drive on the day of the procedure or drink alcohol because of the residual effect of the medications given during the procedure. However, you can begin taking usual medications approximately 1 hour after arriving home.

When Will I Get the Results?

After the test the doctor will discuss the examination with you and your family. It takes approximately 7 to 10 days to get biopsy results from the laboratory. If you do not hear from the office within 2 weeks, it is advisable to call.

If there are any questions about the test or instructions, please call the doctor.

(Modified from Tom E. Norris, MD, Associate Dean for Primary Care Education, University of Washington, Seattle, Wash.)

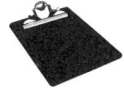
Patient Education Handout

ESOPHAGOGASTRODUODENOSCOPY (EGD) PREPARATION

Do not eat or drink anything for 8 hours before the procedure.

If you are taking a medication, such as aspirin or another arthritis medication, notify your physician before the examination is scheduled. Do not take aspirin or the common arthritis medications within 7 days of the test day. In addition, ask the physician whether you should take your other regular medications on the day of the procedure.

If you have any of the following conditions, notify the physician:
• Diabetes (controlled with insulin or prescription drugs)
• Any history of heart disease or strokes
• History of bleeding tendencies or bleeding problems
• History of heart infection
• History of artificial heart valve
• History of joint replacement
• Drug therapy with any blood-thinning medications, aspirin, or arthritis medications
• Drug therapy with tranquilizers or sleeping pills

Get a good night's sleep before the performance of the procedure and do not worry about the EGD. Most patients have little discomfort.

It is essential to arrange for a responsible adult to be present in the office to drive you home after the completion of the procedure. It is wise to have that individual remain at home with you for a few hours after the procedure to ensure that you have recovered sufficiently from the effects of the conscious sedation.

This person *must* drive you home after the test. You should not drive for the rest of the day.

You should avoid alcohol and any other mind-altering drugs because they can interact with the medications given during the test.

Call immediately if any of the following symptoms develop after the procedure:
• Dizziness
• Chest pain
• Neck pain
• Painful or difficult swallowing
• "Coffee ground" vomit
• Black or bloody stools
• Any temperature above 99° F

If biopsies were completed during the performance of the procedure, call the office within 2 weeks to get the results if they have not been received.

These instructions have been discussed with me.

_____   _____
Patient's signature   *Date/Time*

_____
Nurse's/physician's signature

One copy for chart; one copy for patient.

(Modified from Tom E. Norris, MD, Associate Dean for Primary Care Education, University of Washington, Seattle, Wash.)

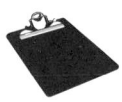 *Patient Education Handout*

ESOPHAGOGASTRODUODENOSCOPY (EGD): POSTPROCEDURE INSTRUCTIONS

Esophagogastroduodenoscopy (EGD) procedure: You have just completed a valuable diagnostic procedure intended to help with your diagnosis and treatment. The procedure is usually well tolerated so you should expect little to no effects. If you have significant side effects, please call.

Diagnosis: The following diagnoses were discovered during your procedure:

_____

_____

IV medication: If you were given IV sedative medication, you should expect to be drowsy for up to 8 hours. Most patients sleep for a few hours and are then fine. You should avoid driving or doing anything delicate or dangerous for the rest of the day. Do not drink any alcoholic beverages for 8 hours after this procedure. Please notify the staff if you are taking any tranquilizers and if we did not discuss when to resume your medication.

Topical anesthetic: If you had anesthetic sprayed in your throat, you may have some numbness for up to 2 hours. The anesthetic affects the sensory nerves, not the motor nerves. Therefore you may have some minor problems for a short period coordinating swallowing. Wait until the effect has completely worn off before eating or drinking. Start slow and chew carefully to avoid problems.

Diet: If you had IV sedation/analgesia, we recommend you eat small meals today and resume your normal diet tomorrow. Avoid alcohol, coffee, caffeine, and spicy foods for today.

Avoid: Smoking   Alcohol   Coffee   Spicy Foods   Milk   NSAIDs

Treatment:

_____

_____

Prophylactic antibiotics: If you were given preprocedure prophylactic antibiotics, please complete your postprocedure dosing.

Follow-up: Please call the office today for an appointment in _____. In-office rapid urease (CLO) test results for *H. pylori* are available in 24 hours. Biopsy results are usually available in 8 to 10 days. Call our office if you have not received a call from us in 2 weeks.

Call immediately for the following: Severe dizziness or any alarming physical symptom. These symptoms are extremely rare and are not expected, but please call should any occur. You should expect belching for a few hours; if you feel bloated or have bleeding, fever, vomiting, or an inability to clear the gas, please call the office.

Follow-up with your family physician: _____

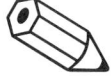

Patient Consent Form

ESOPHAGOGASTRODUODENOSCOPY (EGD)

EGD is a procedure in which the physician looks into the esophagus (swallowing tube), stomach, and duodenum (the first portion of the small intestine) with a flexible lighted tube. A small amount of tissue (a biopsy) may be removed for examination in the laboratory under a microscope.

The benefits of the EGD include the early diagnosis of gastrointestinal problems. It will also enable the physician to better treat the diseases from which the patient may suffer. Causes of gastrointestinal problems include ulcers and cancer.

Although certain rare risks are associated with EGD, the potential benefits of this procedure outweigh the potential risks. However, it is important to understand the following:
- Infection occurs very rarely, and antibiotic medication may be necessary.
- Bleeding is extremely rare, but it is possible. With severe bleeding a blood transfusion, hospitalization, or even surgery may be required.
- Perforation (causing a hole in the esophagus, stomach, or duodenum) is extremely rare. However, if it happens, it could require hospitalization or surgery.
- The medications that are provided during the course of the procedure to prevent pain and discomfort can cause adverse reactions. If the medications are injected, they can cause redness and swelling of the arm. Any medication can cause an allergic reaction or excessive sedation. They can also cause heart or breathing problems.

The many alternatives to EGD include x-ray studies. However, they do not allow clinicians to see inside the upper GI tract directly or to take biopsies or samples.

If there are any questions about the procedure, ask the physician. If more time to consider the procedure is needed, do not hesitate to inform the physician. However, the longer the procedure is delayed, the greater the risk of a delayed diagnosis (especially of cancer).

If there are any questions, please ask.

Physician's name: _____

Office address/phone number: _____

Having read and understood the previous statements, I feel that the benefits of this procedure outweigh the risks. I have read and understood the patient teaching guides. I agree to allow Dr. _____ to perform an EGD procedure with biopsy, if needed.

_____   _____
Patient's signature   *Date/Time*

_____
Witness' signature

One copy for chart; one copy for patient.

(Modified from Tom E. Norris, MD, Associate Dean for Primary Care Education, University of Washington, Seattle, Wash.)

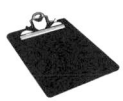

Patient Education Handout

BOWEL PREPARATION FOR SIGMOIDOSCOPY

1. Stay on a clear liquid diet after the evening meal the day before your examination. If you have an afternoon appointment, you may eat breakfast, but stay on clear liquids after breakfast until your examination.
2. One-and-a-half hours before the scheduled time of the examination, administer a Fleet enema (which can be obtained at any local pharmacy). Follow the instructions provided in the box.
3. One-half hour before the scheduled time of the examination, administer another Fleet enema.
4. The return from the last enema should be clear. If it is not, it may be necessary to administer a third enema.
5. If you have a problem with chronic constipation, you may take a laxative the night before.
6. You may take your usual medicines. If you have diabetes, talk to the doctor for special instructions.

CLEAR LIQUID DIET

Only the following foods are allowed; avoid *all* others.

    Beverages: Carbonated beverages, coffee, Kool-Aid, and tea
    Desserts: Gelatin dessert (Jell-O), clear Popsicles
    Fruit: Apple juice, cranberry juice, and grape juice
    Soups: Beef bouillon or clear broth
    Sweets: Hard candies or sugar

(Used with permission of The Medical Procedures Center, P.C., Midland, Mich.)

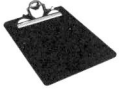

Patient Education Handout

FLEXIBLE SIGMOIDOSCOPY

This sheet of information is to help you become informed about a procedure called flexible sigmoidoscopy. Should you have any questions after reading this sheet, please feel free to discuss them with your physician. In 1995, the United States Preventive Services Task Force, which has very stringent guidelines for approval of screening tests, agreed with the recommendation below. All other organizations essentially promoted this test long ago. In 1998, Medicare began paying for flexible sigmoidoscopy even if it was done only for screening.

Purpose
- To identify and diagnose growths of the bowel (polyps) to prevent cancer
- To find cancer that may already be developed in earlier stages so that it might be more beneficially treated.

Who Needs a Colon Examination (Flexible Sigmoidoscopy or Colonoscopy)?
- Any person 50 years of age and older. Flexible sigmoidoscopy is performed every 5 years along with cards that check for blood in the stool every year. (If a colonoscopy is done, it is repeated in 10 years.)
- Those who experience a change in bowel habits (constipation or diarrhea that persists).
- Those with rectal bleeding of any sort.
- Those who have a stool specimen that tests positive for blood (positive "guaiac" or "hemoccult").
- Those with unexplained weight loss or fevers.
- Those who are anemic.
- Those who need follow-up of previous polyps or cancers.
- Those in high-risk groups who may need to be screened before 50 (previous cancer, history of ulcerative colitis or Crohn's disease, history of female genital cancer, family history of cancer, history of multiple polyps, history of a family member diagnosed with colon polyps or colon cancer before age 60). High-risk groups should begin screening at 35 to 40 years of age and will most likely require colonoscopy or an x-ray (barium enema) along with the flexible sigmoidoscopy.

What are the Benefits of Screening?
Colon cancer is the second most common cause of cancer death in the United States, being surpassed only by lung cancer. Approximately 35,000 lives per year could be saved by early diagnosis. It has now been fairly well documented that cancers begin as small polyps or growths in the colon. It takes approximately 10 years before these benign polyps become cancerous. If these polyps can be detected early and removed, cancer can be prevented. If polyps are found in the lower part of the bowel, this can indicate an association with polyps higher up in the bowel, or with other cancers. Therefore a screening procedure can identify those patients who need a more extensive procedure called colonoscopy. If all polyps are removed and a vigorous screening program is initiated, the chance of colon cancer is decreased to only 15% of what is predicted for an unscreened population. Of the patients who are found to have colon cancer on a screening examination (i.e., no symptoms), 90% are alive 5 years later. Compare this to 30% to 40% of patients who are alive in 5 years if they develop symptoms first.

Continued

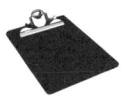 *Patient Education Handout—cont'd*

FLEXIBLE SIGMOIDOSCOPY—cont'd

There is a debate as to what the best screening method is in someone who is not at risk and has no symptoms. In our office, we do the flexible sigmoidoscopy at 50 and 55 years of age, followed by colonoscopies after 60.

What Is Done?

The procedure of "flexible sigmoidoscopy" is easily performed in a physician's office. The appointment is scheduled for 30 minutes, but the procedure itself only takes 5 to 10 minutes. You generally lie on a flat table on your left side. The physician performs a rectal examination with a finger, trying to feel for any growths, and then inserts the instrument called a flexible sigmoidoscope. This consists of a small tube approximately one-half inch in diameter. It is about 28 inches (70 cm) long and is actually quite movable, like a small piece of rubber tubing. The physician can control the movement with dials at one end. He can make the scope go up and down and to the right or left. The end of the tubing has a small hole for lighting, another for sucking up any fluid that might be left in the bowel, another for inserting air, and a final one to pass biopsy forceps. By gently manipulating this tubing, the physician can insert it into the rectum and look at the lower part of the bowel (the "sigmoid colon") and the left descending colon.

How Much Pain Is Involved?

The discomfort is generally quite minimal. It will feel like you are having gas cramps, because the physician does need to inflate the colon with air so that he or she can see the inside. Most people compare it to a slightly uncomfortable bowel movement. Occasionally, if the bowel really has a lot of loops, there will be added pain, but this is unusual. Women who have had a hysterectomy may be a little more uncomfortable. No medication is generally needed before or after the procedure, unless a patient feels particularly anxious and requests it. Many prefer to take four (4) 200-mg ibuprofen (Advil, Nuprin, Motrin) 1½ to 2 hours before the procedure. This is acceptable. Most patients can come straight from work and return to work after the procedure.

How Do I Prepare for the Procedure?

Usually, one or two cleansing (Fleet) enemas 30 to 90 minutes before the procedure should be sufficient. If you notice that the fluid is not clear, occasionally a third enema is needed. Inactive, elderly, or laxative-dependent patients may require 24 hours of clear liquids, as well as four Dulcolax tablets or Milk of Magnesia, the night before. This is rarely recommended, but if you think this may be needed, use it. If at all possible, no aspirin should be taken for the 2 weeks before the procedure. If you have taken aspirin, or if you are on any medication, please notify the doctor. Generally medications can be taken as usual.

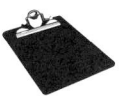

Patient Education Handout—cont'd

FLEXIBLE SIGMOIDOSCOPY—cont'd

When Should the Procedure not Be Done?

In some instances, if you are having severe enough abdominal pain to be admitted to the hospital, the procedure should not be performed. Your physician will need to be the guide for this. Likewise, if you are pregnant, have had a recent heart attack, or have some other significant medical disease, you should let your physician evaluate this before proceeding with the procedure. If you have an artificial heart valve or an artificial joint, you should receive antibiotics before the procedure. Some heart murmurs also require antibiotics. Please alert the physician at the time of the visit and discuss these issues with him. Some patients also need the longer study (colonoscopy).

What Are Possible Complications?

The procedure of flexible sigmoidoscopy is relatively safe. In approximately 1 out of 10,000 procedures, a tear could be made in the bowel wall. This may require further surgery. Very rarely, there may be some bleeding. Generally, there is little discomfort, but occasionally this is a little more bothersome. In some people who get lightheaded when they see blood or are under stress, fainting is a possibility. (If you are one of these, inform your physician; he or she can prescribe medicine to prevent this.)

Possible Biopsy

In instances where your physician sees a lesion, he or she may want to take a small sample of the tissue (biopsy). This will be sent to the pathologist to look at under the microscope and define what it is. This increases your chance of bleeding a small amount, but, again, it is usually negligible. You cannot feel this, and it will not hurt. There are four types of polyps. One type (hyperplastic) is like a skin tag and has no association with cancer. The other three are associated with cancer (adenomatous types) and further diagnostic intervention will be needed.

Costs

The charge for flexible sigmoidoscopy alone is $_____ plus an office charge if you are a new patient. If it is done totally for the purpose of screening, your insurance company may not cover the charge. However, if you have any symptoms at all, insurance companies generally will provide coverage. Medicare will now also cover screening.

If a biopsy is taken and sent to the pathologist, you will receive a separate bill directly from the laboratory for analyzing this specimen. Be sure to call the office if you have not received the results by 2 weeks after the procedure.

Additional questions and/or concerns can be answered by your physician. Please discuss them with him or her.

(Used with permission of The Medical Procedures Center, P.C., Midland, Mich.)

Patient Education Handouts and Consent Forms

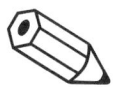 *Patient Consent Form*

FLEXIBLE SIGMOIDOSCOPY

I, _____, consent of my own free will and request that
Dr. _____ and the doctor's assistants perform the procedure of
flexible sigmoidoscopy on me.

If any unforeseen conditions arise in the course of this operation that, in the physician's judgment, require procedures in addition to or different from those now considered, I further request and authorize the physician to do whatever is advisable.

I understand that flexible sigmoidoscopy involves the insertion of a tube into my rectum. This tube can be inserted up to 70 cm (28 inches) for the purpose of evaluating the condition of my colon either to help diagnose a symptom I have or to screen for problems. I understand that, in some instances, a biopsy specimen may be taken. This means taking a small piece of tissue for further analysis.

I understand the procedure is not without complications, such as (but not limited to) pain and cramping, bleeding, and possible perforation (causing a small hole in the bowel). I also understand that at times some lesions are not visible to the physician and may be missed. The risks involved and the possibility of complications have been fully explained to me.

I have read the information provided and agree to the terms and conditions. I understand the risks, the benefits, the procedure itself, and the alternatives. I hereby release the physician performing the procedure from all and any liability arising from, or connected with, the performance of the procedure.

_____   _____
Patient's signature   *Date/Time*

_____   _____
Witness' signature   *Date/Time*

One copy for chart; one copy for patient.

(Used by permission of The Medical Procedures Center, P.C., Midland, Mich.)

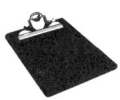

Patient Education Handout

GASTRIC LAVAGE

What is Gastric Lavage?

Gastric lavage is performed to evacuate undesirable stomach contents through a large-bore flexible catheter (tube). Large syringes are used to literally flush the stomach of its contents. The gastric lavage is quite effective for treating ingested toxic substances. It can also be used to treat an upper gastrointestinal hemorrhage.

Why Do I Need to Do This Procedure?

This procedure prevents the absorption of poisons and empties the stomach of undesirable contents.

What Happens During the Procedure?

A large tube will be inserted through your mouth or nose and down to the stomach. Solutions will be flushed into the stomach and then the stomach contents will be suctioned out. Charcoal may also be injected to absorb poisons.

What are the Potential Risks Associated With This Procedure?

Although serious complications are rare, there is the possibility of injury to the stomach or esophageal ("food-pipe") lining or perforation of the upper gastrointestinal tract with this procedure. It is also possible for a patient to aspirate food or chemicals into his or her lungs. Occasionally a patient develops a fluid or electrolyte disturbance or hypothermia (low body temperature). A patient can suffer from low oxygen or spasms in their larynx ("wind-pipe") because of this procedure. He or she can also choke or have difficulty breathing. Rarely, a patient can develop a cardiac rhythm problem. The tube can also be placed incorrectly down the "wind-pipe" instead of the "food-pipe." Precautions will be taken to minimize the risk of any of these complications.

Special Instructions:

Irritation of the esophagus and throat may persist for weeks after the procedure. Discomfort can be relieved by either antacids or a viscous lidocaine solution. Contact your healthcare provider for any problems with breathing, swallowing, or eating.

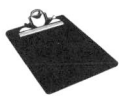 *Patient Education Handout*

HEMORRHOIDS

What are Hemorrhoids?

Hemorrhoids are a very common problem. Hemorrhoids are nothing more than enlarged veins. When they occur in the lower legs, we call them *varicose veins.* When they occur in the rectum, they are called hemorrhoids or "piles." There are many ways to treat hemorrhoids.

What are the Different Types of Hemorrhoids?

Internal hemorrhoids: Hemorrhoids that start above the pectinate line. These hemorrhoids are easy to treat because they start in an area where there are no pain fibers. The "line" is visible to the physician during the examination.

External hemorrhoids: Hemorrhoids that start below the pectinate line. These hemorrhoids are more difficult to treat because they start in an area that has pain fibers.

Mixed hemorrhoids: Hemorrhoids that are actually a combination of the previous two types.

Thrombosed hemorrhoids: Hemorrhoids that have developed a small blood clot inside the vein. These clots do not cause any major problems and are not dangerous. Rather, these small clots just cause severe pain. If you develop very severe discomfort, then you probably have a small clotted hemorrhoid. These are easily treated in the office by simply removing the clot. Some discomfort is involved.

Prolapsed hemorrhoids: Many times a hemorrhoid will protrude through the anus. Many people call these external hemorrhoids, but that is not technically correct. Hemorrhoids are classified as internal or external, based on where they start. Usually hemorrhoids that protrude out through the anus have their base above the pectinate line, so they actually are internal hemorrhoids. Sometimes these prolapsed hemorrhoids come down and then go back up; other times, they stay down.

Skin tags: Oftentimes even after the hemorrhoid or vein is gone, the stretched skin that was over it will remain as a skin tag, or an accumulation of loose, stretched-out skin. Many people are bothered by skin tags, which are not painful but make it difficult to keep the area clean.

Each type of hemorrhoid problem requires a different type of approach. After the physician evaluates you, he will tell you what he thinks is best for the treatment of your condition.

Types of Treatment

In the past, people would simply tolerate most hemorrhoids until they became so bad that surgery was needed. Modern techniques have eliminated the need for surgical excision (cutting out) of hemorrhoids except in the most advanced cases. You may have heard of the "Barron ligation" or rubber band technique, which involves placing a small rubber band around the hemorrhoids. This method has been used for many years. It is less painful than surgery and can be performed in the physician's office. Laser techniques have also been used. More advanced techniques using infrared coagulation, and radiofrequency are available. They frequently provide excellent results with even less pain and less complications.

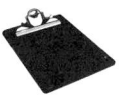

Patient Education Handout—cont'd

HEMORRHOIDS—cont'd

Surgery is reserved for only the most advanced cases of hemorrhoids. Surgery is performed in the hospital operating room with the patient under general anesthesia.

Rubber-band ligation is still used frequently by many physicians to treat many types of internal hemorrhoids. It is also known as *Baron ligation.*

Infrared coagulation involves the application of infrared *light* to the base of the hemorrhoid, which clots the hemorrhoid. There are usually three different areas inside the rectum where hemorrhoids occur, and they are referred to as *complexes.* One area, or complex, is treated at each office visit. Although the patient will occasionally feel a little warmth, there generally is minimal pain or discomfort. The patient may return to work the same or next day. Occasionally a little bleeding will occur between the fourth and tenth day after treatment. The patient returns in approximately 1 month for follow-up treatment.

Radiofrequency surgery involves the application of a very high–frequency current to remove external skin tags. The frequency is the same as that of an AM radio. The advantage of this technique is that it will prevent the bleeding that is frequently associated with excision of these tags. Also, little other tissue is damaged using this technique. It is similar to a laser procedure. Because skin is removed, the patient will experience tenderness in the area for a longer period (1 to 3 weeks) until the wound is healed. A local anesthetic (to numb the area) is injected before the procedure to minimize pain.

How Do I Prepare for Treatment of Hemorrhoids?

If the infrared coagulator is used, you probably will not need to take time off from work; however, it might be best if you could take it easy for a couple of days after the procedure. Before coming in for the procedure, administer an enema (Fleet enemas are available without a prescription) approximately an hour before the planned surgery. Hold the contents of the enema for 5 to 10 minutes, and then expel it. After the procedure, expect some weeping from the area and some soreness for up to several weeks. You should be able to do most normal activities within a few days. Often little or no pain medication is needed.

Continued

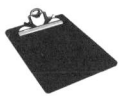

Patient Education Handout—cont'd

HEMORRHOIDS—cont'd

If you would like to play it safe, you may take three 200-mg ibuprofen tablets about an hour before coming to the office. You might want to schedule the procedure later in the day so that you do not have to go back to work. You may want to take a stool softener such as Colace, or a bulk laxative such as Metamucil, Citrucel, or Benefiber for a few days before the procedure. You just need enough to keep the stool soft. Also remember to drink plenty of water. You will probably want to continue this regimen for a week or so after the procedure.

What Do I Do After Hemorrhoid Treatment?

After any hemorrhoid procedure, it is important that you maintain a high bulk diet (a lot of fruits, vegetables, bran, etc.) so that your stool remains soft. Drink at least four to five glasses of water per day. You may use suppositories, if desired. Sitz baths are beneficial; simply sit in a hot bath for 20 to 30 minutes three or four times per day. It may help to apply an ointment such as Preparation H after bathing to keep the areas from rubbing together. Your doctor may prescribe some Silvadene cream, benzocaine, or lidocaine ointment. Use them as directed. Ice bags may also help relieve the discomfort.

What are the Risks Associated With Treatment of Hemorrhoids?

Complications include pain, bleeding, infection, return of the hemorrhoids, and failure of the treatment itself so that the hemorrhoids persist.

When Should I Call My Healthcare Provider?

After any of these procedures, if you have extreme pain, excessive bleeding, or difficulty urinating—or if you develop fevers, chills, or sweats—call your physician immediately. You should make an appointment for a follow-up visit in 4 weeks.

Special Note

Sometimes hemorrhoids can be caused by a tumor in the bowel. Your physician may suggest a screening test with a flexible sigmoidoscopy either before or after treatment. Be sure to discuss this with the physician.

(Used with permission of The Medical Procedures Center, Midland, Mich.)

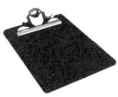

Patient Education Handout

AFTER HEMORRHOID TREATMENT

1. Take a sitz bath (soaking in a tub) for 20 to 30 minutes three or four times a day for the next 2 or 3 days if needed for tenderness.

2. You may apply witch hazel or Balneol cream to the rectal area between baths as needed for dryness or local irritation.

3. After you have a bowel movement, clean the area with a moistened tissue or with a Tucks pad. Baby wipes (without alcohol) are cheaper and probably just as effective. Blot the area dry, and apply a small amount of Balneol with a tissue.

4. Eat a high-fiber diet (bran, fresh fruit, and vegetables). Continue this habit forever. Drink lots of fluids.

5. Until the rectal area is completely healed, use a stool bulking agent or a stool softener daily to keep your bowel movements very soft. Examples include Metamucil, Perdiem Plain, Fibermed, Naturacil, Konsyl, Colace 100-mg capsules, or Surfak 240-mg capsules. Follow the directions on the package.

6. You may have some swelling and weeping of the tissues that have been treated. You can use a sanitary pad to absorb the drainage.

7. Note that slight blood-tinged drainage is normal. You may actually have some bleeding for 3 to 7 days after the procedure. Unless bleeding is severe, there should really be no worry. Call your physician if you are concerned. More bleeding may occur 7 to 14 days after the treatment when the scab comes off.

8. Call if you begin running a fever or notice redness or swelling past the rectum anytime after the procedure is done. Also call if you are unable to urinate.

9. The swollen tissue inside the rectum can often cause a false sensation and an urge to move the bowels. Avoid prolonged straining and do not take enemas for at least 10 days after the procedure. The enema tube could damage the tissue and cause bleeding.

10. Use acetaminophen 1000 mg (two Extra Strength Tylenol, 500 mg) or ibuprofen 600 mg (three Advil, 200 mg) every 6 hours as needed for pain. Avoid aspirin.

11. Please make a follow-up appointment for approximately 4 to 6 weeks from the day your procedure was performed.

(Used with permission of The Medical Procedures Center, Midland, Mich.)

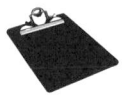 *Patient Education Handout*

URINARY CATHETER CARE

A urinary catheter is a hollow tube, measuring approximately 17 inches in length. It is placed through the opening you urinate through (urethra) into your bladder and connected to a drainage bag. Once inserted, a balloon on the end of the catheter is inflated to keep the catheter in place. To remove the catheter, air is removed from the balloon.

You may take a shower with the catheter in place, but should not take a bath or swim.

The catheter will be connected to a drainage bag. The bag will either be a leg bag or an overnight bag. The former is placed around your thigh and held in place by rubber or Velcro straps. This bag usually will hold up to 500 ml (1 pint). It is emptied by twisting a spigot or turning a clamp at the bottom of the bag. This is best done as you stand over a toilet bowl. The overnight bag will usually hold up to 2000 ml (2 quarts). This is emptied in the same manner as the leg bag. The overnight bag should be placed below your waist for proper drainage.

The bags may be washed out with warm soap and water on a daily or every other day basis. This is to keep them clean and to reduce the odor from the urine. To reduce the urine odor further, you may rinse the bags with tap water and vinegar, using 1 part vinegar to four parts water.

You may experience irritation where the catheter enters the urethra (or urinary tube.) This may be reduced by washing this area once or twice daily with soap and water, and afterwards applying Vaseline or an antibiotic ointment.

Potential Problems

1. You may experience some blood in the urine, especially if physically active. This will normally subside with rest and increased fluids. If it does not, you should contact your physician.

2. If the urine becomes cloudy, and does not clear with increased fluids, this may be a sign of a bladder infection. You should contact your physician, if this persists.

3. If you experience a temperature above 101° F, especially if you have cloudy urine, you may have an infection. Please contact your physician.

4. If the catheter becomes plugged and there is no urine output, despite increasing your fluid consumption, you should contact your physician or go to the nearest emergency room to have it cleared.

5. You may experience leakage around the catheter as it exits the urethra. If the catheter is draining well, and the leakage persists, this may indicate a bladder infection or bladder spasms. You should contact your physician for treatment.

6. If the catheter is draining well, it will usually be changed by a nurse or your physician, every six weeks. Occasionally, it may need to be changed more often.

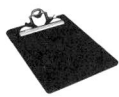

Patient Education Handout

URODYNAMIC TESTING

What Is Urodynamic Testing?

Urodynamic testing is special testing that evaluates the storage of urine in the bladder and also what happens with the flow of urine as it leaves the bladder and goes through the urethra (bladder outlet). Urodynamic testing helps to isolate problems with the nerves and muscles of the lower urinary tract and pelvis.

Why Is Urodynamic Testing Ordered?

Your provider may want to obtain this testing if you have symptoms that suggest problems of incontinence (loss or leakage of urine). Sometimes these symptoms occur unexpectedly during normal everyday activities or when there is greater stress on the system, such as when you exercise, cough, sneeze or laugh. Sometimes the bladder does not seem to hold as much as it used to, and this testing helps determine why. You may have had previous testing of the urinary system that suggested a mixture of problems, or your previous treatment may have failed to give you symptom relief. Other reasons for testing include medical conditions that cause problems with the nervous system, such as diabetes after pelvic radiation or surgery. This test may be ordered prior to urinary tract or pelvic floor surgery to help the surgeon determine the best surgery for you.

What Do I Have to Do to Prepare for Urodynamic Testing?

You should drink enough fluid to have a full bladder when you arrive for your testing. Testing cannot be performed if you have an untreated bladder infection or see blood in your urine that has not been evaluated. You should contact your primary provider to be evaluated and treated for either of these.

What Does Urodynamic Testing Involve?

Urodynamic testing will measure the urine flow and the bladder muscle contractions during filling and emptying of the bladder. The first test involves measuring the flow of urine as you empty the full bladder. Arriving with a full bladder will allow complete testing during your appointment time. Then a small tube (catheter) with pressure sensors will be inserted into the bladder through your urethra. Another small tube will be placed in the rectum or vagina to measure the pressure inside the abdomen as you cough or strain. The bladder will be filled, usually with water, and the pressure measurements will help determine what is normal and what is abnormal. The bladder is emptied at the end of testing. The testing takes about an hour.

Is This Testing Painful?

No, testing is not painful, but you may briefly experience the discomfort of a full bladder during the testing. Your sensations will be correlated with the actual amount of fluid in the bladder and how the nerves and muscles respond.

Continued

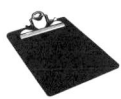

Patient Education Handout—cont'd

URODYNAMIC TESTING—cont'd
What Can I Expect After the Testing Is Done?

You should be able to go about your normal activities after your appointment. Antibiotics are routinely prescribed after this procedure to help prevent a bladder infection. Be sure to notify the testing personnel if you have any drug allergies. Phenazopyridine is also routinely prescribed for up to 2 days to prevent discomfort after the procedure. This may cause your urine to turn bright orange while you are taking it, but will resolve after you stop it. Wearing a pad while taking this medication is recommended to prevent staining of your underwear. If you experience discomfort after 48 hours, or if it worsens you should contact us at _____ (phone number) or obtain other medical attention. You may notice some blood in the urine for up to 48 hours after the procedure, especially if there was difficulty inserting the catheter. If this persists or you see blood clots, notify us right away. If you develop fever, flank pain, or difficulty voiding, notify us or seek medical attention immediately.

You will be told when you can expect your test results before you go home. If you do not receive your results as expected, please call us at the above phone number. The results will help us design an individualized treatment plan or determine if further testing is needed.

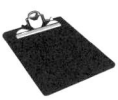

Patient Education Handout

ADULT CIRCUMCISION

What Is Adult Circumcision?
Adult circumcision is an operation performed to remove the foreskin of the penis.

Why Do I Need This Procedure?
This operation is performed for repeated infections or tightening of the foreskin. It may also be done at your request for your own personal reasons.

How Do I Prepare for Adult Circumcision?
No special preparation is needed except to take your usual prescription medications as directed by your doctor. If you are likely to be quite anxious, a pill can be given to help relax you. If you have a tendency to faint with procedures, tell the doctor. Do not take any aspirin or herbal pills for 1 week before the surgery. These drugs can increase the risk of bleeding.

What Happens During the Procedure?
After numbing the area, your doctor will remove the foreskin and stitch the skin edges together again.

What Are the Benefits of This Procedure?
Circumcision can prevent infections of the foreskin and relieve pain from a foreskin that is too tight.

What Are the Risks Associated With This Procedure?
Bleeding, pain, and infection are the most common. Injury to the tube that carries urine from the bladder (urethra) is possible though rare. Scarring could cause discomfort with intercourse for a few months, but this usually passes.

What Do I Need to Do After the Procedure?
Replace the dressing two to three times a day, after washing with soap and water, for the first week. Avoid sexual stimulation for 1 month. It is advisable to take 3 to 4 days off work. Take three 200-mg ibuprofen tablets four times a day for 3 to 4 days. Keep ice over the area for at least 12 hours.

When Should I Call My Healthcare Provider?
Call your doctor for severe pain, active bleeding, or signs of infection (e.g., redness, drainage of pus).

Special Instructions

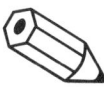 *Patient Consent Form*

CIRCUMCISION/DORSAL PENILE NERVE BLOCK

I came to the office of Dr. _____ on _____ (date) for evaluation and treatment of the following conditions: problems with my foreskin including balanitis (infections), phimosis, paraphimosis (tightening), pain during intercourse, or other (_____).

We discussed the different treatments possible, and discussed the risks of not treating the condition. Based on the advice given by Dr. _____ and my own judgment, I agree to undergo the following procedure: local anesthesia and/or dorsal penile nerve block and circumcision (surgical removal of the penile foreskin)

I have read over and understand the information given to me. We discussed the different outcomes that could occur and most of the possible complications. I am aware that other complications could occur that we could not foresee. I agree to follow the instructions for self-care after the procedure and to return for follow-up care on _____.

I will call the office or answering service if any problems arise before the scheduled follow-up visit.

_____
Patient's signature

_____
Date/Time

_____
Witness' signature

_____
Physician's signature

One copy for chart; one copy for patient.

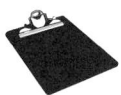

Patient Education Handout

ANDROSCOPY

Androscopy is a procedure for examining the male genitals in a very detailed and thorough fashion. This is done by using a special microscope (the colposcope) and is carried out in the office.

Androscopy is done specifically to identify signs of genital warts. The medical term for these warts is condyloma acuminata. They are caused by the human papilloma virus. These lesions are very contagious and are passed readily by sexual intercourse. There is an 80% chance of getting the wart virus with just one sexual contact with an infected person. Condoms are not very effective in preventing transmission. There is now evidence that they can occasionally be picked up without sex, but this is very rare. The wart virus may lie dormant or inactive for up to 20 years after infection before the warts show up.

Long-term effects on males are not totally certain, although there is a rare chance that condyloma may cause penile cancer. Recent studies suggest a possible link to rectal cancer. It is more clear that infection with this virus is the primary cause of cancer of the cervix in females. If there is evidence of infection in the female, which is often picked up on a Pap smear, the male sexual partner may also need to be examined. We now know, however, that it is almost impossible to totally "cure" a person of the infection. The cervix can be treated and cancer prevented 99% of the time, but it is difficult to completely eradicate the virus from the penis, vagina and rectal areas. Indications to treat the male include symptoms (visible lesions, itching, or a large number of lesions seen on staining). Even with treatment, the warts, whether visible or not, frequently come back and the man must assume he is contagious for the rest of his life.

Although many warts are visible to the naked eye, many others are too small to be seen and require examination with great magnification to identify or confirm their warty nature. During the procedure, vinegar will be sprayed on the penis. This causes the warty tissues to turn whiter than the surrounding skin, thus making it easier to identify and examine. Men can have the virus and look totally normal before staining and examination. Thus they can be spreading warts—and cervical cancer—without knowing it.

Men who are infected are advised to be monogamous so as not to spread the disease further. Condoms make sex safer but not totally safe. Previous partners should be advised to be sure they get their Pap smears regularly and possibly have a colposcopic examination, since the Pap smear alone is known to miss 25% of lesions. You have the legal liability to tell any future partners that you have the wart virus.

Women who smoke have twice the risk of cervical cancer. *Even if you smoke,* your partner's risk for cervical cancer increases. It is recommended that you stop smoking.

Description of the Procedure

The procedure itself will take approximately 15 to 20 minutes. You will be asked to undress from the waist down and will be draped appropriately. You will be placed in a lying position with your feet in stirrups, similar to the position for doing pelvic examinations on females. The penis and entire genital area will be soaked with vinegar for at least 5 minutes.

Continued

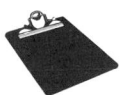 *Patient Education Handout—cont'd*

ANDROSCOPY—cont'd

You will then be examined first with the naked eye to detect any visible lesions, and then examined again with the colposcope (a special microscope) at 5 and 10 power to confirm the nature of the lesions.

Once warty lesions have been identified, they may be biopsied to confirm their diagnosis. Larger lesions may be treated by excision, strong acid, cryocautery, or laser vaporization. All these modalities are quite simple, and no time off work (other than for the office visit) is necessary. You may also be prescribed a cream called Efudex to treat these warts. See a special handout on this if it is used. Some medications can be applied at home and require a prescription.

Follow-up examinations with the microscope may be needed to confirm resolution of all lesions treated and to identify any recurrent or new lesion. Times for these rechecks will vary, depending on the treatment used. You will be advised by your doctor.

Videotapes

Videotapes that discuss the above information in more detail are available in our office for your viewing at home. Ask the receptionist for details. It often helps to review the tapes before your examination.

Reminders

- Be monogamous (same sexual partner).
- Do not smoke.
- Be sure your partner has a Pap smear at least every year.
- Tell your doctor you've had or been exposed to genital warts when you have your general physicals.
- Report any nonhealing sores on your penis or rectum.
- Inform any new partners about your condition. If you still decide to have sex, use condoms and nonoxynol-9 jelly, even though we're unsure of the benefits in preventing transmission of genital warts.
- Multivitamins with folic acid may help the body's immune system control the wart virus.
- Eat at least five helpings of fruits and vegetables to boost the immune system.

(Used with permission of The Medical Procedures Center, P.C., Midland, Mich.)

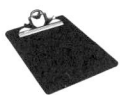 *Patient Education Handout*

GENITAL CONDYLOMA (WART) REMOVAL

The area that was treated will be quite sore for the next 4 to 5 days. Minimal scarring or decreased pigmentation (lightening) of the treated skin may occur, but usually the results of the procedure—removal of the warts—are far superior to having the warts themselves. To obtain the best results, please follow these directions:

1. For the first 7 days, *shower or bathe* two or three times per day. Wash all treated areas with soap and water.
2. After bathing, apply a thin layer of an antibiotic ointment, which can be obtained over the counter. This aids the healing process, decreases scarring, and is soothing. Your doctor may also prescribe Silvadene. If so, use the Silvadene instead of the other ointments.
3. Taking three 200-mg ibuprofen tablets four times per day will minimize any pain or discomfort that you might experience. Do not take them if your stomach is easily upset by this medication or if you are taking aspirin.
4. If you continue to have discomfort, a benzocaine ointment can often provide some relief. This can be mixed with the antibiotic ointment. Benzocaine ointment can be purchased without a prescription at your local pharmacy.
5. *Warm tea bags* can be applied on the wounds and may provide significant relief. *Ice packs* may also help.
6. If you have significant redness or discharge, or if the pain has not decreased after 48 hours, please call your physician.
7. Schedule a *follow-up appointment* about 4 weeks after the procedure.
8. One third of the time, the warts will return. If the warts return, see your physician immediately, rather than waiting until they multiply and enlarge. The smaller the lesions, the easier they are to treat and the less likely you are to have any scars.
9. If you had warts that were treated around the rectal area, keep your stools soft. Use stool softeners for 2 to 3 weeks. You may also find that *benzocaine* or *lidocaine* ointment applied to the rectal area about 10 to 15 minutes before a bowel movement will help ease pain.
10. Stop smoking, and your partner should stop too.
11. Eat 5 helpings of *fruits and vegetables* per day.
12. Take a *multivitamin with folic acid* each day to help the immune system.
13. *Be monogamous.* It's safer for you and you don't spread the warts.
14. Women must obtain *regular Pap smears* the rest of their lives.
15. Call for lab results in 2 weeks if any biopsies were taken.
16. Return or call if there is excessive pain, bleeding, signs of infection, or recurrence of any lesions.
17. A *return checkup* is recommended in 4 to 6 weeks.

Please feel free to ask any questions.

(Used with permission of the Medical Procedures Center, P.C., Midland, Mich.)

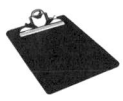 *Patient Education Handout*

DORSAL SLIT FOR PHIMOSIS

What Is a Dorsal Slit?

Dorsal slit is a simple procedure involving a single cut along the top of the foreskin that permits easy retraction of the foreskin. The procedure takes about 10 minutes. A local anesthetic will be used so that you do not feel pain from the procedure.

Why Do I Need This Procedure?

A dorsal slit is used when the foreskin cannot be pulled back because of infection or inflammation and causes symptoms of pain or retention of urine. The procedure is performed so that the foreskin can be pulled back and the infected area can be cleaned, or urine can be drained from the bladder with a catheter.

How Do I Prepare for Dorsal Slit?

There are no special preparations for this procedure.

What Happens During the Procedure?

The penis will be cleansed with an antiseptic solution, and a local anesthetic will be used at the base of the penis to prevent pain during the procedure. A cut will then be made in the top of the foreskin to allow the foreskin to be pulled back easily so that the head of the penis can be cleansed or a catheter can be placed into the bladder. Stitches may then be placed to control bleeding from the cut edges of the foreskin.

What Happens After the Procedure?

You will be instructed to keep the wound clean and dry. Some swelling of the foreskin is normal. A clear to light-yellow crust will probably form over the area. Wear loose briefs so that the wound does not get irritated. You may notice a small amount of dried blood from the incision site. Follow up with your doctor to check the wound under his or her advice.

What Are the Benefits of the Procedure?

When a dorsal slit is completed, the foreskin can be pulled back easily to improve hygiene. This will reduce the risk of infection and urinary retention resulting from swelling and scarring of the foreskin.

What Are the Risks of the Procedure?

As with any surgical procedure, bleeding, infection, and pain are the most common problems. Medication will be provided for pain control following the procedure. Bleeding and infection should be monitored and brought to the attention of your doctor if they occur. With infection, there will be increased discharge, redness, and tenderness. At times patients are not satisfied with the appearance of the dorsal slit. If this should occur, discuss this with your healthcare provider.

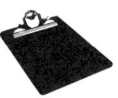

Patient Education Handout—cont'd

DORSAL SLIT FOR PHIMOSIS—cont'd

What Do I Need to Do to Prevent Infection?

Gently cleanse the wound with soap and water three to four times a day. Apply an over-the-counter antibiotic ointment afterwards. Avoid intercourse for 4 to 6 weeks to prevent infection and bleeding.

When Should I Call My Healthcare Provider?

Call if the following occurs:

- Bleeding of more than a few drops from the incision that doesn't stop after 5 minutes of pressure.
- The head of the penis turns blue or black.
- You develop a fever, or red streaks coming up the penis develop.
- You are unable to urinate.
- You have other concerns or questions.

Special Instructions:

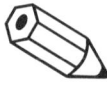 *Patient Consent Form*

DORSAL SLIT FOR PHIMOSIS

I came to the office of Dr. _____ on _____ (date) for evaluation and treatment of the following condition: phimosis of the foreskin of the penis.

We discussed the different treatments possible and discussed the risks of not treating the condition. Based on the advice given by Dr. _____ and my own judgment, I agree undergo the following procedure: Dorsal slit for phimosis using local penile nerve block anesthesia.

The penis will be cleansed with antiseptic solution and draped with sterile drapes. A cut will be made to loosen the foreskin so that it can slide easily over the penis. Bleeding will be controlled with sutures as needed. Risks include bleeding, pain, infection, poor cosmetic result, and reaction to anesthetic. Benefits include improved hygiene, decreased infection, and decreased urinary retention.

We discussed the outcomes that could occur and most of the possible complications. I am aware that other complications could occur that we could not foresee. I agree to follow the instructions for self-care after the procedure and to return for follow-up care on _____.

I will call the office or answering service if any problems arise before the scheduled follow-up visit.

_____   _____
Patient's signature   *Date/Time*

_____   _____
Witness' signature   *Physician's signature*

One copy for chart; one copy for patient.

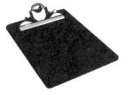

Patient Education Handout

PROSTATE ULTRASOUND AND BIOPSY

Why Do You Need This Test?

If a potential prostate problem is identified through a digital rectal examination or a prostate-specific antigen (PSA) blood test, your clinician may suggest that you have an ultrasound. It is an imaging technique that uses high-frequency sound waves to create an image of the prostate. Ultrasound, along with a possible biopsy (tissue sample), may help your clinician discover cancer early, when it is more likely to be treatable.

How Do I Prepare for This Procedure?

The ultrasound test is simple and often performed in your clinician's office. It usually takes less than 15 minutes. You may need to use an enema or suppository on the morning of your examination to clear your rectum (only if you have not moved your bowels). You may eat breakfast on the day of the examination and a light lunch. If you are taking *any* of the following medications, you will be asked to stop taking them 7 *days* before your appointment:

- *Aspirin,* or any aspirin-containing products (such as Ecotrin)
- *Ibuprofen* or similar products (such as Motrin, Advil, Nuprin, Aleve)
- *Antiarthritis medication* (such as Indocin, Feldene, Voltaren, Clinoril)
- *Persantine* (dipyridamole)
- *Coumadin, clopidogrel* (Plavix), or any other blood thinners

If a biopsy is to be performed, you will be given antibiotics both before and after the test.

What Happens During the Ultrasound Procedure?

You will lie on your side or with your feet in stirrups. A tubelike probe barely bigger than a thumb is covered with a condom and gently inserted into your rectum. The probe emits sound waves, which you cannot feel, and creates an image of your prostate on a video screen. Your doctor views the image, looking at the size, shape, and structure of your prostate.

When Is a Biopsy Needed?

If your clinician finds suspicious areas in your prostate or if your PSA blood test is abnormal, a biopsy may be recommended. A biopsy is often done during the ultrasound test.

What Happens During a Biopsy?

The small tip of the biopsy needle is inserted through the rectum into your prostate. One or more tissue samples are taken from the prostate (this is only slightly uncomfortable). Your tissue samples are sent to a lab for examination.

What Happens After the Procedure?

You may notice some rectal bleeding or blood in your urine for a few days, and some blood in your semen for 2 to 3 weeks. Ask your clinician if you should limit exercise or sexual intercourse after your biopsy. Make sure you finish all of your antibiotics.

When Should I Call My Healthcare Provider?

Call your clinician if you have a fever, excessive urinary or rectal bleeding, muscle aches, fatigue, or difficulty urinating.

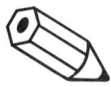 *Patient Consent Form*

TRANSRECTAL ULTRASOUND OF THE PROSTATE WITH OR WITHOUT BIOPSY

Patient name: _____

Complications for transrectal ultrasound of the prostate (with or without biopsy), include bleeding, infection, urinary retention, and injury to the rectum.

_____ Has taken antibiotic   BP _____

_____ Has followed instructions

_____ Patient denies taking any aspirin, aspirin products, NSAIDs, or blood thinners for 7 days before the procedure

The procedure was explained to me. All of my questions were answered. I have followed the instructions given to me to prepare for this procedure. My signature below confirms my consent for this procedure.

_____   _____
Patient's signature   *Date/Time*

_____   _____
Witness' signature   *Date/Time*

_____   _____
Clinician's signature   *Date/Time*

One copy for chart; one copy for patient.

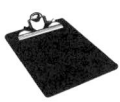

Patient Education Handout

SELF-INJECTION THERAPY FOR IMPOTENCE

The self-injection of a medication (usually alprostadil) into the penis to produce an erection is usually a safe, well tolerated, and effective treatment option for erectile dysfunction. This guide will outline the technique you should use and the potential risks and management of possible, but generally infrequent, complications.

The medication, when injected properly, should produce an erection within 15 minutes and will normally last 30 to 120 minutes, with a goal of 60 minutes. This medication allows more blood to go into the penis and less blood to leave, resulting in the desired, normal erection. (Blood filling the penis is what causes an erection. Just like air in a balloon makes it firm, it is blood that makes the penis firm and erect.)

Most men experience minimal pain during the injection process and minor pain afterwards. However, mild to moderate pain does occur in up to 11% of men. In up to 3%, the pain will be severe enough that they will not want to use the medication again.

At first the doctor will try different dosages of the medication to see what works best for you. During the time period that you and your physician are determining the correct dose, the risk of developing a prolonged, painful erection (priapism) is 4 out of 100. If the erection lasts longer than 4 hours, you should contact your physician. You may require additional medications injected into the penis, surgery, or both to eliminate the prolonged erection. If the erection continues too long, you may develop damage to the vascular tissue within the shaft of your penis, which may prevent you from having an erection in the future.

Medical conditions that might predispose you to a prolonged erection include sickle cell anemia, leukemia, and multiple myeloma. Injection therapy should not be used in patients with these conditions. In addition, if you have a penile prosthesis or implant in place, or have scar tissue in your penis that causes pain or curvature with an erection, you should not use this form of therapy to treat your erectile dysfunction.

If you are taking blood thinners, such as aspirin, warfarin (Coumadin) or clopidogrel (Plavix), you should discuss this with your physician. As a result of the blood thinner, you may bleed more than normal after the injection and, consequently, may need to apply pressure to the injection site for 5 minutes or until the bleeding ceases. You are also more likely to bruise at or around the injection site. With the above precautions, patients who are taking blood thinners usually do not have problems using penile injections.

You will need assistance in performing self-injection therapy if you have difficulty seeing, have impaired use of your hands, or if you cannot see your penis because of a protruding lower abdomen. In the latter case a mirror may be useful to you. If you need assistance in injection therapy, your assistant should come with you to your physician's office to receive the appropriate instructions.

Instructions for Injection Therapy

1. You should disrobe from the waist down or slide your pants and underwear down to your mid-thigh. This should be done in the standing or sitting position.

Continued

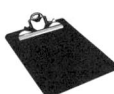

Patient Education Handout—cont'd

SELF-INJECTION THERAPY FOR IMPOTENCE—cont'd

2. If you are not circumcised, you will need to retract the foreskin back over the head of the penis. Otherwise, take the thumb of your nondominant hand and place it on top of the penis at the 12 o'clock position. Place your second and third fingers onto the head of the penis to stabilize it. The nerves of the penis are at the 12 o'clock position and the urinary tube is at the 6 o'clock position. YOU DO NOT WANT TO INJECT THESE SITES. Do not insert the needle in the half inch along the top of the middle and on the bottom. When you inject the medication into the side of the penis, you should do so anywhere along the shaft of the penis from the attachment to just before the head of the penis. The shaft of the penis contains two cylinders or erectile bodies called the corpora cavernosa. One is on each side. You will insert the needle through the skin and into the center of the erectile tissue. Only one injection is needed, since the medication will then pass from one side to the other, causing an erection to occur.

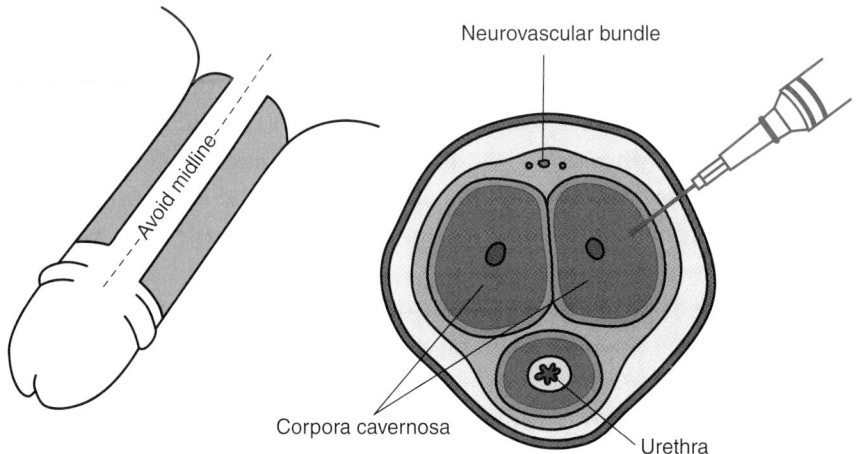

Intracavernous injection site. The clinician grasps the glans and pulls firmly outward to tense penis without rotating.

Before preparing the medication, carefully inspect the shaft of the penis to determine where you will be inserting the needle. There are usually several veins of various sizes just below the skin. These should be avoided. If you hit one of them, it should not cause any harm but may result in more bleeding than usual. In that case, you should apply pressure to the injection site for a longer time period than normal. Do not put the needle through any area that may be infected or red.

Now that you have an understanding of the anatomy of the penis and where you are going to inject yourself, you are ready to prepare the medication.

3. If you are preparing alprostadil (Caverject, Edex), you need to inject the liquid in the syringe into the vial containing the powder. Remove the top of the vial and wipe it with an alcohol swab. Then remove the needle cover from the syringe and insert the needle into the middle of the

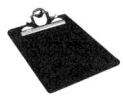

Patient Education Handout—cont'd

SELF-INJECTION THERAPY FOR IMPOTENCE—cont'd

rubber top of the vial. Inject all of the fluid into the vial, and swirl the vial until all the medication has dissolved. Now slowly withdraw the plunger so that the proper amount of medication is in the syringe. Your physician will tell you how much of the medication should be injected. Never inject more than the advised amount. **You should use the medication no more than three times a week and never within 24 hours of the last injection.** Remove the air and excess drug by holding the needle up in the air and slowly advance the plunger until all of the air has been removed from the barrel of the syringe. Place the needle cover back on the syringe and lay the syringe in a convenient place. Rotate or vary the injection sites to reduce the chance of scar tissue developing in the shaft of the penis. Both sides of the penis can be used.

4. You are now ready to prepare the shaft of the penis for the injection. As previously described, use your nondominant hand to pull your penis gently toward the thigh. Wipe the predetermined injection site with an alcohol swab. Remove the needle cover and place the barrel of the syringe between your second and third fingers of your dominant hand with the thumb on the plunger. Place the tip of the needle above the injection site at a 90-degree angle to the skin. To prevent twisting of the penis, remember to keep the thumb of your other hand on the head of the penis at the 12 o'clock position. Recheck the position of the penis and injection site. You are now ready to proceed.

   Advance the tip of the needle through the skin and the wall of the penis (corpus cavernosa). Surprisingly most men feel little or no discomfort during the injection process because the needle is so small. The needle should be advanced its full length into the shaft of the penis, perpendicular to the skin. Now use your thumb on top of the plunger and push it downward until the syringe is empty. This usually occurs in less than 15 seconds. If you meet resistance as you are injecting the medicine, withdraw or pull the syringe back 0.25 inch. This will move the tip of the needle and allow the medication to flow into the center of the erectile body without resistance. When the syringe is empty, withdraw the needle from the penis and then apply an alcohol swab to the injection site for 30 to 60 seconds. If the bleeding continues, reapply this swab for an additional 5 minutes or until the bleeding stops. Apply the needle cover to the syringe and dispose of your supplies as advised by your physician.

5. Normally, an erection will occur within 15 minutes of the injection. You may begin your planned sexual activities at any time. The erection will usually occur during foreplay and last for 30 to 120 minutes.

Remember to follow the above instructions carefully. If you have any questions or problems, please contact your physician promptly.

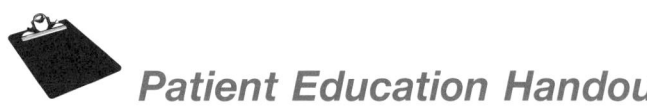

Patient Education Handout

VACUUM DEVICES FOR ERECTILE DYSFUNCTION

What Are Vacuum Devices?

Vacuum devices are used to produce an erection-like state, making the penis hard enough for sexual intercourse.

Why Do I Need This Device?

Men who are unable to have an erection naturally can use vacuum devices to have sex.

What Happens During the Procedure?

The vacuum tube is placed over the penis and a vacuum is created with a small hand pump or battery device. This draws blood into the penis. Blood is trapped in the penis, and this is what makes it hard. A constriction band is placed at the base of the penis next to the body to keep the blood in the penis. This will keep the penis hard once the vacuum tube is removed. An erection will be maintained only beyond the band, so the penis will still be able to pivot at its base. You may need to hold the penis for insertion into the vagina and for intercourse. The constriction band should not be left in place for longer than 30 minutes.

What Are the Risks Associated With This Procedure?

You may occasionally notice penile pain and numbness when the constriction band is in place. The secretions (semen) may not come out when you reach ejaculation and will sometimes feel uncomfortable, since the constriction band blocks the urethra. Once the constriction band is removed, the semen will drain out. Because of the suction, you may notice small areas of bruising on the penis. With prolonged use over 30 minutes, the penis will continue to swell and turn blue. You should avoid wearing the constriction band for longer than 30 minutes.

When Should I Call My Healthcare Provider?

Contact your healthcare provider if you have continuous swelling of the penis, persistent pain in the penis, or sores and ulcers after using the vacuum device. These could be serious problems and may signify a need to modify the technique when using the vacuum device.

Websites That May Be of Interest to You:

www.urologychannel.com (Urology Channel)
www.missionpharmacal.com (Mission Pharmacal)
www.timmmedical.com (Timm Medical Technologies)

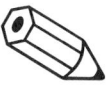

Patient Consent Form

VACUUM DEVICES FOR ERECTILE DYSFUNCTION

I came to the office of Dr. _____ on _____ (date) for evaluation and treatment of erectile dysfunction.

We discussed the different treatments possible and their risks. Based on the advice given by Dr. _____ and my own judgment, I agree to undergo the following procedure: use of vacuum device on the penis to produce an erection-like state.

We discussed the different outcomes that could occur and most of the possible complications. I am aware that other complications could occur that we could not foresee. I agree to follow the instructions for self-care after the procedure and return or call for follow-up care should abnormalities arise.

_____   _____
Patient's signature   *Date/Time*

_____   _____
Witness' signature   *Physician's signature*

One copy for chart; one copy for patient.

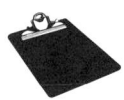 *Patient Education Handout*

VASECTOMY (PERMANENT MALE STERILIZATION)

Because vasectomy is designed to be permanent, the patient should think about it carefully before undergoing the procedure. *Vasectomy is a small procedure, but a large decision.* When children are definitely not wanted in the future, vasectomy removes the fear of pregnancy.

Vasectomy simply blocks the travel of sperm to the penis; it prevents the sperm from getting out of the man's body. Male hormones are *not* affected by vasectomy, and they continue to circulate normally. Vasectomy does not cause voice changes, hair loss, impotence, or loss of sexual desire.

How Is the Procedure Performed?

Usually the doctor gives an injection of local anesthetic into the skin of the scrotum (i.e., the sac holding the testicles). This may feel like a brief pinch for 30 seconds. The anesthetic will numb the area for about 2 hours. The doctor then makes one or two small, half-inch openings in the skin, gently pulls up each tube (i.e., vas deferens), cuts them, burns or ties them shut, and places a barrier between the cut ends. The procedure takes about 30 minutes to complete.

What Is the "No-Scalpel" Vasectomy Technique?

The *no-scalpel technique* is a method developed by Dr. Li, a Chinese physician. In this method the doctor uses a special instrument instead of a scalpel to enter the scrotum. This instrument has a sharp point and spreads the skin instead of cutting it. This makes a smaller opening and may cause less bleeding and less pain afterwards. Many patients ask about the possibility of undergoing a "laser vasectomy," but this technique does not exist. Although the doctor could use a laser to cut into the scrotum, there would be no benefit over using the no-scalpel surgical equipment.

When Can I Return to Work?

Patients need 1 or 2 days of rest after the vasectomy. They should avoid heavy lifting, jogging, and other sustained strenuous activities for at least 1 week. Usually if the vasectomy is performed on a Friday, patients return to work on Monday.

Is There Much Pain After Vasectomy?

No. Patients may experience a few days of mild discomfort, such as a pulling or an aching feeling in the groin. This discomfort can usually be relieved with ibuprofen (Motrin, Advil, or Nuprin) and good support with tight underwear. On a scale of 1 to 10, most men say the pain is a 2 to 3. Some bruising may occur, but this is perfectly normal. A very small number of men have more serious side effects, such as significant bleeding, infection, or painful sperm leakage (i.e., sperm granuloma).

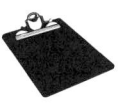

Patient Education Handout—cont'd

VASECTOMY (PERMANENT MALE STERILIZATION)—cont'd

Does Vasectomy Affect Sex Life?

That depends: If a couple has been worried about pregnancy, their sex life could improve, especially as they come to trust the vasectomy. The procedure does not change anything, except that there will no longer be sperm in the semen. Sex, orgasm, and ejaculation are not affected. However, if the patient does not truly want a vasectomy but is having one to please a wife or partner, some resentment may be felt after the procedure (which may affect the patient's sexual relationship negatively). In addition, if there are conditions affecting the patient's sex life negatively before the procedure, chances are that a vasectomy will not improve those conditions. Therefore patients should expect that their sex lives will remain about the same after vasectomy.

When Can I Have Sex Again?

Patients should wait 1 week until some healing has taken place, and they should *use another form of birth control until examination shows sperm are no longer present.*

When Is the Vasectomy Effective?

It is effective when the semen has been tested and has been found to be free of sperm. A sperm check is done about 6 weeks after the procedure (after at least 15 ejaculations). Many physicians will request a second check at 12 weeks to be sure the tubes have not reconnected.

What Happens if the Vasectomy Is Not Successful?

In the rare cases where the sperm can still get through, a repeat vasectomy may be required (this is the case in just 1 out of 1200 surgeries).

Is it Possible to Ejaculate After a Vasectomy?

Yes. The testicles produce the sperm, which make up only 5% of the semen (the fluid that is produced with ejaculation). The other 95% of semen is produced by other glands that continue to function normally. Unless the semen is placed under a microscope, it is impossible to tell whether or not sperm are present. Ejaculation feels the same.

What Happens to Sperm After a Vasectomy?

The sperm continue to be produced by the testicles, but their passage to the penis is blocked. Therefore the sperm cells break down in the body and are recycled. This process is normal and occurs even in men who have not had a vasectomy, especially if there is a long time between ejaculations.

What are the Complications?

Only 5% or less of patients experience complications. In a few cases a small blood vessel may continue to bleed inside the scrotum, causing *bruising* or even a larger accumulation of blood. *Infection* in the scrotum may also occur. *Pain* after a vasectomy is minimal; on a scale of 1 to 10, it

Continued

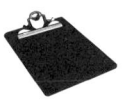 *Patient Education Handout—cont'd*

VASECTOMY (PERMANENT MALE STERILIZATION)—cont'd

is rated a 3. *Failure* rates vary between 1 per 500 and 1 per 1500 vasectomies. Failures can be found by obtaining a semen check. Some concerns were raised that having a vasectomy could increase the chances of getting *prostate cancer.* After careful review of all the data, several major organizations, including the American Cancer Society and the National Institute of Health, have found no increase. Similarly there do not appear to be any increased risks of any other diseases. Although rare, some patients can experience an ongoing chronic discomfort in the sacks and groin after vasectomy. No one knows why this happens. It is intermittent and more of a nuisance than a true problem. Very rarely does it need any special treatment.

Is Vasectomy Reversible?

Vasectomy should always be considered permanent; therefore patients should not undergo a vasectomy until they are completely sure that it is what they want. In patients who undergo reversal operations, 20% to 30% are unsuccessful in getting a woman pregnant. Occasionally a patient may want to save his sperm before the procedure and have it frozen (the doctor can answer questions about this process).

What Are the Other Options for Contraception?

Many other temporary and reversible options for contraception exist: condoms, spermicides, diaphragms, IUDs, Norplant, hormone injections, contraceptive sponges, birth control pills, and patches. Patients should ask for information if they have any questions about these other methods.

Is Vasectomy Anything Like Castration?

No. Castration means removal of the testicles. Vasectomy does not touch the testicles and does not reduce the production of male sex hormones.

Are There Men Who Should Not Have Vasectomies?

Perhaps. Some examples are men who feel masculine only when they can cause a pregnancy, men or partners who change their minds frequently, men who may get divorced and then marry someone else who wants children, and men who think they might want children later. Clinicians will consider performing a vasectomy for any man who has seriously thought about the implications and who wants no more children. This applies equally to men who are single, married, divorced, widowed, childless, or with families, regardless of age.

Why Is it Best to Use Local Anesthesia?

General anesthesia (being put to sleep) poses certain well-established health risks. Because vasectomy is such a simple and quick procedure, it is unwise to subject patients to the unnecessary risks of general anesthesia. Although some doctors use general anesthesia, the vast majority of vasectomies in the United States are performed using local anesthesia (just numbing injection in the area).

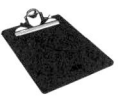

Patient Education Handout—cont'd

VASECTOMY (PERMANENT MALE STERILIZATION)—cont'd

Do I Need the Consent of My Wife or Partner?

Only the patient's written consent is required, although it is wise for the patient to discuss this decision with the wife or partner. It is advised that the wife or partner be present during counseling, if possible.

What Can I Expect After Vasectomy?

After the procedure the patient will need to remain in the office for a short time. After arriving home the patient should relax for the rest of the day. It is a good idea to take 2 days off of work. Patients may shower the day after surgery. For adequate support, *tight* briefs or, even better, an athletic supporter should be worn for the next week. Some men experience bruising that can be extensive. This is harmless and is caused by leakage of blood under the skin. It fades slowly. Some men ache about 6 hours after the procedure. Others may begin to ache about 5 days after the procedure. If swelling or pain persists or if the incision looks infected, the patient should call the physician. If the area is allowed to heal for 7 days before the patient has an ejaculation, the result is more likely to be a success.

What Should I Do to Prepare for the Day of Surgery?

- No aspirin should be taken for 2 weeks before surgery; however, acetaminophen (Tylenol) is permitted.
- Hair in front of the scrotum should be clipped with scissors just before coming to the office (a razor should not be used because it can cut the skin and lead to infection).
- A shower (washing well with soap and water) should be taken before coming into the office.
- Three or four 200 mg ibuprofen tablets (Advil or Nuprin) should be taken 2 hours before surgery (in addition to any other medicine the doctor prescribes).
- A jock strap or tight, snug-fitting underwear should be brought to the office.

(Used with permission of The Medical Procedures Center, P.C., Midland, Mich.)

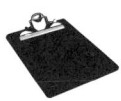 *Patient Education Handout*

NOW THAT YOU HAVE HAD YOUR VASECTOMY

There are a few routines and instructions you can use to ensure the greatest degree of comfort possible. The counseling session you had provides an opportunity to ask any and all questions and to prepare you for your vasectomy. To remind you of suggestions given on the videotape, during the private interview, and in the previous reading materials, *keep this instruction sheet handy.* Please feel free to call if you have any further questions.

After Your Vasectomy
Activity

Day 1: This is the day of surgery. Put your feet up in an easy chair with an ice bag on your groin to reduce the swelling and bleeding. Wear a jock strap. Get up only to go to the bathroom and to eat. Take ibuprofen (up to 2400 mg/day). If you still experience pain, it is okay to also take Tylenol (but not aspirin). See the "Pain" section for the correct dose.

Day 2: Shower and walk around but avoid heavy lifting or vigorous physical exercise. If swelling increases, sit down and relax. Wear a jock strap and take the ibuprofen (three tablets four times a day).

Day 3: Increase activity but hold back on vigorous activity. Continue wearing the athletic supporter for comfort, if needed. Take ibuprofen up to 2400 mg/day for any pain.

Day 4: Resume normal activity. Return to work but limit jogging and weight-lifting for at least 1 week.

Pain

Take three 200-mg ibuprofen four times per day for the first 2 days, whether you need it or not. If you feel you need something more, take two or three Tylenol up to four times per day, 2 hours after each dose of ibuprofen. After 2 days use it only as needed.

Bandage

Day 1: You will wear an athletic supporter filled with gauze when you leave the office. This is fine for day 1. Replace the gauze with a washcloth if necessary after a few hours or after going to the bathroom. You can use an antibiotic ointment over the wound if you want to do so.

Day 2: Wear an athletic supporter.

Day 3: Wear an athletic supporter until you are comfortable without it.

Sexual Activity

Week 1: You may engage in sexual activity once after 5 to 6 days, if comfortable.*

Week 2: You may engage in sexual activity two times.*

Week 3: You may engage in sexual activity as desired.

*This is the maximum recommended (another form of contraception is required until semen checks are negative).

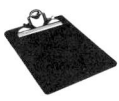

Patient Education Handout—cont'd

NOW THAT YOU HAVE HAD YOUR VASECTOMY—cont'd

Possible Reactions

Infections: Call the physician if excessive redness, swelling, tenderness, fever, or oozing of pus from incision occurs. Although rare, this usually will occur after the second day. It is permissible to apply antibiotic ointment to the opening if you want to do so.

Bruising: This is normal for up to about 2 weeks (over the scrotum).

Swelling: A small amount is not uncommon. Anything more should be reported. You will feel a small "lump" inside where the surgery was done for a few weeks. However, it will go away.

Granuloma: Some men get a small nodule where the vas was cut. Usually it is not painful and will go away. If it is larger than ½ inch, call the physician and medication will be prescribed to shrink it. This can start a few months or even years after a vasectomy. (Remember, a small lump can usually be felt after surgery for up to 3 months in most cases.)

Failure: This is always a possibility. You should use contraception until you have two semen checks without sperm in them.

Bloody Ejaculate: Although rare, it is possible for up to 6 months.

Pain: Like an old fracture, a few men can have a long-term ache in the scrotum (or even in the groin) where the surgery was done. Rarely is any treatment even needed.

Long-term effects: No other long-term side effects are caused by a vasectomy. (There is no reported increase in problems such as prostate cancer, high blood pressure, or high cholesterol.)

Semen Checks

Two semen checks are done to confirm sterilization. Although no appointment is needed, be sure that the office is open. The first will be done at 6 weeks or after 15 ejaculations (whichever is later). The second will be done at 3 months. *There is no charge for this.* Bring a semen sample in a clean jar or the container provided within 1 or 2 hours after ejaculation. If ever you are concerned or want reassurance of sterilization, the office will examine your semen anytime in the future (at no charge for the first year). Be sure your name is on the container.

Note: Another form of contraception should be used until the second semen sample is clear of sperm. The vasectomy is not successful until two negative samples have been documented.

(Used with permission of The Medical Procedures Center, P.C., Midland, Mich.)

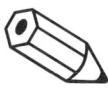 *Patient Consent Form*

REQUEST FOR VASECTOMY

I, _____, the undersigned, request that Dr. _____ and the doctor's assistants perform a vasectomy on me.

It has been explained that this operation is intended to result in sterility, and I understand that a sterile person is not capable of becoming a parent. I also understand that the operation may not result in the intended sterility and that no guarantee of sterility has been given to me.

I have been told that the operation has possible complications, the most common of which are infection, pain, hematoma (i.e., bleeding and bruising), sperm granuloma (i.e., a reaction to sperm in the scrotum), reuniting of the channels (i.e., failure), and reaction to the local anesthetic.

I voluntarily request the operation; I understand that if it proves successful, the results will be permanent. If they are, it will be impossible for me to father children.

I have been advised that because of the supply of sperm in the reservoir beyond the vasectomy site, I will remain fertile after the procedure until this reservoir is empty. I have been advised to bring a semen sample after at least 15 ejaculations and that a sperm count will be performed on it. If necessary, repeat counts may be advised.

I have read this entire statement and agree to its terms and conditions. I understand the risks, the benefits, the procedure, and the alternatives to this operation. I have been given a chance to have all my questions answered.

_____

Patient's signature

_____

Date/Time

_____

Wife's or partner's signature (optional)

_____

Withness' signature

One copy for chart; one copy for patient.

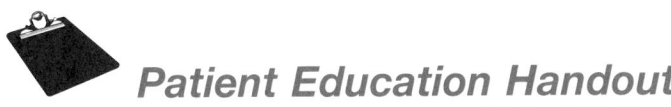

INSTRUCTIONS AFTER TERMINATION OF PREGNANCY

Resuming Normal Activities

On the day of the procedure you may wish to rest, avoid school or work and refrain from vigorous physical activity. On the next day you may return to most normal activities, including work, school, and exercise. Do not place anything in your vagina for 10 days. You may bathe or shower any time.

Bleeding

Bleeding is common after abortion and may even last for a few weeks. Take one Methergine pill four times a day starting when you get home from the surgery to help reduce this. Take the medication for 3 days. Light bleeding (lighter than a menstrual period) is normal and will eventually stop. If bleeding becomes heavy—if you are soaking a pad in less than a hour or passing large clots—you should notify your physician or go to the hospital emergency room. You may be given medication to reduce bleeding. Some women will notice small fragments of placental tissue in the blood after an abortion. This is normal and does not require a visit to the doctor or hospital. Your first period should occur in 4 to 6 weeks. If you do not have your period, notify your physician.

Antibiotics

Your physician may have given you antibiotic pills to treat or prevent any infection. Take them until they are gone. If you cannot tolerate the pills for any reason, please call before you stop taking them.

Cramping

There will be some cramping for a couple of days. You may take three 200-mg ibuprofen tablets four times a day for the cramping.

Sex and Fertility

You should avoid intercourse for 10 days after an abortion. When you do resume sexual activity, you should use a method of birth control, because you can become pregnant again 2 weeks after an abortion. The physician can give you a prescription for birth control pills. Start them the Sunday following the abortion. Other methods of birth control may be discussed with your physician. An uncomplicated suction abortion should have no effect on your ability to have children in the future.

Danger Signs

If any of these following signs occur, please notify your physician promptly.
- Fever of 100.4° F (38° C) or higher
- Increasing or severe pain in the lower abdomen
- Excessive bleeding
- Foul-smelling vaginal discharge

If you believe that there is any other serious problem after your abortion, please call your physician or report to the emergency room at the hospital immediately.

Follow-Up Visit

You should see your physician in 2 weeks. Your appointment is _____ (date/time). There is no additional charge for this visit. If you are unable to see your physician, you should have a follow-up visit with another physician. The follow-up visit is important to make sure everything has returned to normal, and to see that you are comfortable with your birth control method.

Dr. _____   Phone # _____

Answering Service # _____   Hospital Emergency Room # _____

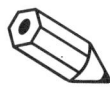 *Patient Consent Form*

TERMINATION OF PREGNANCY

You have requested that Dr. _____ terminate your pregnancy. This will be done by removing the contents of the uterus by suction, a procedure commonly called a *suction curettage* or *suction abortion.* The procedure consists of two steps:

1. The evening before the actual procedure, a small fiber cylinder will be inserted into the cervix (opening of the womb). This cylinder is called a *laminaria,* and it is about the size of a wooden match. It is used to dilate the opening to the uterus. It gradually expands by absorbing water, and although it is very small when it goes in, it comes out much larger—about the size of a pencil or more.
2. In the morning, the suction abortion will be performed. First, the physician will inject a local anesthetic into the cervix, which freezes and numbs the opening to the uterus. Then the doctor will insert a plastic tube through the opening of the cervix and into the uterus and suction will be applied by a machine to empty the uterus. The whole procedure will take only a few minutes. You can expect some cramping during the procedure, but this usually subsides within 5 to 10 minutes. If no complications occur, you may leave within 1 hour.

Complications of suction curettage are uncommon, but they may occur.

Complications from laminaria insertion include the following:
- *Infection* may occur if the laminaria is left in place for more than 24 hours.
- The laminaria may *perforate* (poke a hole through) the cervix.
- The laminaria may *fall out, break into pieces, or be difficult to remove.*
- A spontaneous abortion or *miscarriage* may occur after the laminaria is inserted.
- The laminaria may cause *painful cramps* as the cervix is dilating.

Complications from local anesthesia include the following:
- An *allergic reaction* may occur.
- If the anesthetic enters the bloodstream, you may feel its effects: buzzing in the ears, taste in the mouth, etc. This is common and not dangerous.

Complications from the suction abortion itself include the following:
- *Bleeding* may occur. This can usually be controlled with medication; however, rarely it may be severe, and you may need to have the procedure repeated, be admitted to the hospital, or have a blood transfusion.
- *Infection* may occur. This can usually be treated with oral antibiotics; but, rarely, intravenous antibiotics, hospital admission, or surgery may be necessary.
- *Perforation* of the uterus (poking a hole in the wall of the womb) is rare. This may require admission to the hospital and further surgery.

Continued

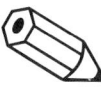

Patient Consent Form—cont'd

TERMINATION OF PREGNANCY—cont'd

- The *abortion may fail* to interrupt the pregnancy. If this occurs, the suction curettage will have to be repeated.
- *Other very rare complications* may occur, including blood clots in the veins which can travel to the lungs, hysterectomy (removal of the womb), or even death. It is impossible to mention every possible complication of this procedure. Serious complications occur very rarely.

I have read this form and I understand how suction abortion is performed, its risks, and its possible complications. I understand the other options of treatment and managing this pregnancy. All of my questions have been answered.

_____
Patient's signature

_____
Date/Time

_____
Witness' signature

_____
Relative or Legal Guardian

One copy for chart; one copy for patient.

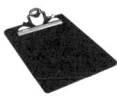 *Patient Education Handout*

CERVICAL CAP: USE FOR CONTRACEPTION

- Before use, one third of the inner side of the dome should be filled with spermicidal jelly.
- The jelly should not be applied to the inner surface of the rim. The cap may be inserted anytime, from immediately before intercourse up to 40 hours before intercourse. It is most easily inserted in a squatting or semireclining position.
- The cap should be left in place for at least 8 hours after intercourse.
- The cap may be left in place for up to 72 hours, but it should be removed within 48 hours after the last episode of intercourse.
- If intercourse occurs more than once while the cap is in place, no additional spermicide is needed. However, the wearer should check for correct positioning of the cap before each episode.
- An additional contraceptive method should be used the first 3 times the cap is worn during intercourse (to ensure protection should the cap become dislodged). If dislodgement occurs, cap use should be discontinued and the cap should be refitted.
- The cap should not be used during menses.
- Refitting is necessary after abortion or childbirth.
- The cap should not be used in the presence of vaginal infection, discharge, pain, or odor. If these occur, medical evaluation is necessary.
- If lubrication is needed for intercourse, only water-based lubricants should be used. (Spermicide works well for this purpose.)
- The cap should be washed carefully after use with soap and water. If an odor develops, it can be soaked in vinegar or a cup of water with a teaspoon of lemon juice. Alternatively, the cap can be cleaned with a 25% bleach solution for 20 minutes; then it should be rinsed thoroughly.
- A Pap smear should be taken 3 months after beginning use of the cap. If this is normal, then obtain your Pap smear every year thereafter.
- The cap should be replaced yearly (sooner if thin spots or tears occur). Make an appointment so your doctor can check if it still fits adequately.
- If used properly, 6% of women will become pregnant after using the cervical cap for a year.
- If left in too long, infections can occur so be sure to follow guidelines listed above.

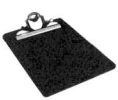

Patient Education Handout

HOW TO USE CONDOMS FOR CONTRACEPTION AND DISEASE PREVENTION

- Only latex- or polyurethane-based condoms should be used to prevent disease transmission. Animal membrane (i.e., natural) condoms do not protect against transmission of hepatitis B or human immunodeficiency virus (HIV). No condom prevents the risk of wart virus (HPV) transmission.
- Condoms with spermicide already applied may provide additional protection against STD. Simultaneous use of spermicidal jellies or foams that contain nonoxynol-9 or octoxynol-9 provides even more protection.
- A male condom should be applied to the penis or female condom into the vagina **before** any genital contact occurs.
- Space must be left at the tip of the male condom for collection of ejaculate.
- After intercourse, **the base of the male condom must be held** onto the erect penis while the penis is withdrawn from the vagina. This will prevent the condom from slipping off the penis.
- Condoms should **never** be reused.
- For latex condoms, lubrication (if necessary) should be accomplished only with water-soluble lubricants or spermicidal jellies. Oil-based lubricants will damage the latex, making it more likely to rupture (see box below).
- Condoms should be stored in a cool, dry place out of the sun and should not be used if they appear discolored or stiff.
- Condoms should be handled carefully to prevent punctures.
- When using these contraceptive methods, the possibility of failure must be considered. Condom breakage occurs in roughly one out of every 100 episodes of intercourse. Also, one of the most common ways a women gets pregnant is that the condom simply isn't used as it is supposed to be. Ask your doctor about emergency contraception when a barrier method is selected. Obtaining a prescription for emergency contraception should be considered.
- After reviewing the package insert provided with the condom, please ask the doctor about any questions you still have.

Continued

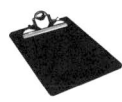 *Patient Education Handout—cont'd*

HOW TO USE CONDOMS FOR CONTRACEPTION AND DISEASE PREVENTION—cont'd
Common Oil-Based Preparations That Should Not Be Used with Condoms (Male or Female)

Medications
Butoconazole (Femstat); conjugated estrogens (Premarin), estradiol (Estrace); miconazole (Monistat); tioconazole (Vagistat-1)

Lubricants
Baby oil, butter, cocoa butter, cold cream, mineral oil, hand lotion, petroleum jelly, shortening, suntan oil, vegetable oil

If there are any questions about the lubricant you are using, ask the pharmacist for some safe suggestions.

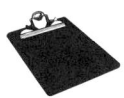

Patient Education Handout

HOW TO INSERT AND USE A DIAPHRAGM

- The diaphragm is an effective birth control method when used correctly. The following provides guidelines for its proper insertion:
- The diaphragm can be inserted up to 2 hours before intercourse. If it is in place for longer than 2 hours, you must reapply contraceptive jelly or cream, taking care not to move it.
- Place about 1 tablespoon (15 ml) of contraceptive jelly or cream in the dome (the hollow area of the thin rubber) of the diaphragm and spread it around the inside of the dome. Place a thin layer on the rim of the diaphragm to ease its insertion.
- Find a comfortable position, such as squatting, standing with one leg raised, or lying down. With one hand, spread the outer lips of the outer part of the *vagina,* or birth canal.
- With your other hand, fold the diaphragm (dome side down) with your thumb and finger and insert it into the vagina. Push the diaphragm as far back into the vagina as possible, pointing down and to the back (see illustration). Slip the other "end" under the pubic bone.

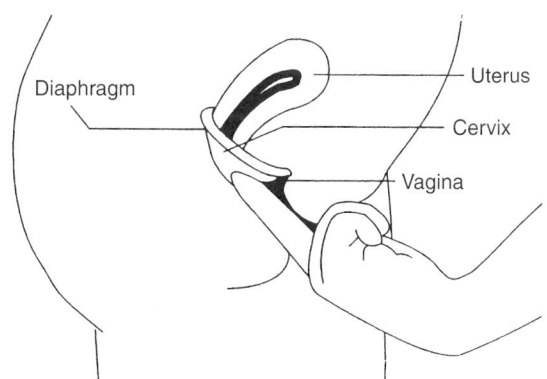

- You can make sure the diaphragm is placed properly by inserting one finger into your vagina and feeling for the cervix. The cervix is the narrow lower end of the uterus that feels similar to the tip of a nose. The cervix must be covered if the diaphragm is going to work properly. If the diaphragm covers the cervix and the outer edge is behind the pubic bone, it is in the correct position. *Neither you nor your partner should notice the diaphragm during intercourse.*
- After intercourse, leave the diaphragm in place for at least 6 hours. Do *not* douche during this time. If you have intercourse more than once, you must reapply more contraceptive jelly or cream. Use the plastic applicator to reapply the cream. If you find that this is too messy, you may want to ask your partner to use a condom. Do *not* remove the diaphragm, however.
- Remove the diaphragm 6 hours or longer after intercourse. *Do not leave it in place for more than 24 hours.*
- To remove the diaphragm, insert your finger into your vagina and slide it under the rim of the diaphragm that is tucked under the pelvic bone. Pull the diaphragm down and out.

Continued

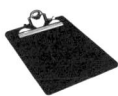

HOW TO INSERT AND USE A DIAPHRAGM—cont'd

- Wash the diaphragm with mild soap and warm water after use, and it should be rinsed well and patted dry, especially around the edges where water might remain. You may dust it lightly with cornstarch. However, other powders or creams should not be used.
- Place the diaphragm in its container (sunlight and air can weaken the rubber latex).
- Check your diaphragm for holes and tears each time before use by filling it with water or holding it up to a light and gently stretching it. Never use a diaphragm with tears or holes.
- At each annual checkup, have your doctor check the diaphragm and its fit. Also, you may need a diaphragm of a different size, especially if you have lost or gained 10 lb, been pregnant, recently had a baby, or had pelvic surgery.
- Be sure to call your doctor if you experience any of the following: signs of allergy to the rubber latex or the contraceptive cream or jelly (i.e., itching, discomfort) or signs of bladder infection (i.e., difficulty urinating when the diaphragm is in place, frequent need to urinate, burning during urination).
- Ask your doctor or nurse for help if you have trouble inserting or removing the diaphragm.
- Pap smears must continue to be done every year even if the diaphragm is used with every sexual encounter.

(Adapted from Attico NB: *Fam Pract Recert* 14[1]:65, 1992.)

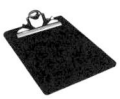 *Patient Education Handout*

BREAST BIOPSY

What Is a Breast Biopsy?

A breast biopsy is a procedure performed by a doctor to remove a lump or small piece of a lump from your breast. The tissue is then sent to a pathologist for a diagnosis. A pathologist is a physician who specializes in identifying tissue under a microscope. Most breast biopsies are performed in a physician's office or outpatient surgery center.

There are two types of breast biopsies. The type of abnormality in your breast determines which type of biopsy will be performed.

The first type is a *needle biopsy*. For this procedure a physician uses a special needle to draw fluid or a small piece of tissue from a breast lump. The goal of a needle biopsy is to obtain tissue or fluid for a diagnosis. The entire lump will not be removed, only sampled.

The second type of biopsy is an *excisional biopsy*. The physician will remove the entire lump during this procedure and obtain a definite diagnosis.

Why Do I Need This Procedure?

A breast biopsy is performed when a physician feels a worrisome lump or the patient detects a new lump. Sometimes breast lumps cannot be felt by a physician and are seen only on a mammogram (a breast x-ray). A biopsy will then also be recommended if a mammogram or ultrasound identifies a suspicious lump or area in the breast.

How Do I Prepare for a Breast Biopsy?

You should avoid taking aspirin-containing medications as well as nonsteroidal medications for 1 week before surgery. Examples of nonsteroidal medications include ibuprofen (Advil, Motrin, Nuprin) and Aleve. You should shower or bathe as usual on the day of the biopsy. Do not use any deodorant, powder, or lotion on the breast, which will be biopsied.

If the biopsy is to be performed in an operating room, you may be given special instructions about eating and drinking before the procedure.

What Happens During This Procedure?

The breast biopsy is usually an outpatient procedure, and hospitalization is not required. You will be given a time to report to the physician's office or the surgery center. You should bring a tight-fitting, supportive bra to the procedure (even if you do not usually wear one).

An incisional biopsy is performed after the breast area is numbed with an anesthetic (a *local anesthetic*). No other type of anesthesia is usually necessary. Patients may receive a relaxing or sleep-inducing type of anesthesia in addition to a local or numbing type of anesthesia for an excisional biopsy.

The breast area is first cleansed with a disinfectant solution. The doctor will then remove the lump or fluid and send it to the pathologist. An excisional (removal) biopsy may take an hour, and the patient may then spend 1 to 2 hours in a recovery room. If performed in the office, the

Continued

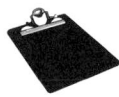 *Patient Education Handout—cont'd*

BREAST BIOPSY—cont'd

procedure usually takes only 30 minutes. The doctor will follow the natural shape of your breast when making the cut, or *incision*, in the breast skin. The incision will be different for each patient. You should review this with your doctor before the procedure.

The doctor usually uses an absorbable type of suture to close the skin incision. There will be no sutures to remove later. Occasionally a dressing is placed over the biopsy site.

You can return home after the procedure. You should wear a supportive bra for comfort after the procedure. The weight of your breast may pull on the biopsy site, and a bra will help prevent this. Some women sleep with their bra on the first night or two after a biopsy. Many women return to work and their normal activity the day after surgery. You should avoid vigorous exercise and lifting of any heavy items until the biopsy site is healed (approximately 7 to 10 days).

Generally, showering after the biopsy is allowed. If a dressing is placed over the site, you should ask your doctor for approval. Women should avoid sitting in water up to the biopsy site (e.g., a bathtub, swimming pool, hot tub) for 7 to 10 days after the procedure.

The pathologist will provide your diagnosis to your doctor in 3 to 5 business days. Call the office if you have not heard from us in 5 days.

What Are the Risks of This Procedure?

Bleeding and infection are common risks of any surgical procedure. Many women notice bruising around the area of a biopsy. This is common and should not alarm you; the bruising will fade. Pain is usually minimal. Tylenol as needed is permitted.

A breast biopsy may become infected. If this happens, you may notice a fever, or have redness, pain, or drainage at the biopsy site.

It is possible, especially with needle biopsy, that the abnormal cells will be missed. Your doctor will need to follow up with you to be sure the diagnosis is correct.

There will always be a scar. Usually it is minor. However, at times, they can stretch and become unsightly. Also, if an infection occurs, they may be worse.

What Do I Need to Do After the Procedure to Prevent Infections?

You should avoid exposing the area to water such as bathtubs, pools, lakes, and hot tubs. Showering should be the only time the area is exposed to water.

The biopsy site should be kept clean. Your doctor will tell you how to do this after the procedure.

When Should I Call My Healthcare Provider?

You should notify your doctor immediately if you have any of the following symptoms or problems:
- A fever of 100° F or higher
- A change in the amount of drainage from the biopsy or if the drainage changes
- The pain from the procedure suddenly changes or worsens
- The biopsy site opens up
- The breast begins swelling, feels hot, or becomes reddened

You should call your doctor or healthcare provider if you develop any symptom that worries you.

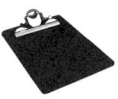

Patient Education Handout—cont'd

BREAST BIOPSY—cont'd

Special Instructions

Follow any special instructions given to you by your doctor.

Websites That May Be of Interest to You:

www.noah.cuny.edu (NOAH: New York Online Access to Health describes numerous health-related topics in both English and Spanish)

www.cancernet.nci.nih.gov (CancerNet [National Cancer Institute]: an online guide to Understanding Breast Changes)

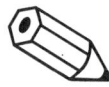 *Patient Consent Form*

BREAST BIOPSY

I came to the office of Dr. _____ on _____ (date) for evaluation and treatment of the following condition: a right / left breast lump (circle the appropriate side)

We discussed the different treatments possible and discussed the risks of not treating the condition. Based on the advice given by Dr. _____ and my own judgment, I agree to undergo a right/left excisional biopsy.

I understand that this procedure will be performed in an outpatient day surgery/the physician's office setting. I may be given a relaxing type of medication called a *light sedative.* My breast will be cleansed with a disinfectant solution, and a numbing medication (a *local anesthetic*) will be administered into the breast area. The doctor will then make a cut *(incision)* into the breast and remove the breast lump. I understand the incision will be stitched or sutured closed. I may have a dressing placed over the area.

We discussed the different outcomes that could occur and most of the possible complications, including pain, bleeding, infection, missing the lesion, and scarring. I am aware that other complications could also occur that we could not foresee. I agree to follow the instructions for self-care after the procedure and to return for follow-up care on _____.

I will call the office or answering service if any problems arise before the scheduled follow-up visit.

_____
Patient's signature

_____
Date/Time

_____
Witness' signature

_____
Physician's signature

One copy for chart; one copy for patient.

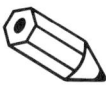

Patient Consent Form

McDONALD'S CERCLAGE

The procedure recommended for you is called a McDonald cervical cerclage. This technique is used to avoid the consequences of incompetent cervix and the loss of your pregnancy. It involves placing a nonabsorbable suture (stitch) around your cervix to keep it from dilating open.

Complications arising from this procedure can include infection, hemorrhage, pregnancy loss (miscarriage), and scarring to your cervix. Most patients will also require an anesthetic, which carries with it risks that will be discussed by the anesthesia personnel. Having this cerclage placed also requires that it be removed either at term or earlier if you should go into premature labor.

Failure to have this surgery could lead to the loss of your pregnancy, but this may also happen even if it is placed. The surgery does not cause any health defects in the baby.

I understand the risks, benefits, and possible complications. I have been given the opportunity to ask questions and obtain another opinion. I desire to proceed with the surgery.

_____   _____
Patient's signature   *Date/Time*

_____   _____
Witness' signature   *Date/Time*

One copy for chart; one copy for patient.

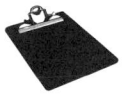 *Patient Education Handout*

COLD-KNIFE CONIZATION OF THE CERVIX (CONE BIOPSY)

What Is a "Cone Biopsy" of the Cervix?

This procedure involves cutting out a cone-shaped piece of tissue from the cervix using a surgical knife. You will be given either heavy sedation, a spinal, or general anesthesia in the operating room.

Why Is This Procedure Necessary?

This procedure is being done to either find or treat abnormal, possibly precancerous, cells of the cervix and to rule out cancer.

How Do I Prepare for a Cone Biopsy of the Cervix?

You should have nothing to eat after midnight the night before surgery. There should also be *no* chance of pregnancy (unless otherwise advised by the physician in special situations).

What Happens After the Procedure?

You will be monitored for a couple of hours after the procedure and then discharged with special instructions (see following discussion of postprocedure instructions).

What Are the Benefits of This Procedure?

This procedure gives the pathologist a large piece of tissue to look at under the microscope to aid in diagnosing abnormal cervical cells. It also provides the possibility of completely removing the abnormal cells of the cervix, which will prevent progression to cancer.

What Are the Risks Associated With This Procedure?

Risks include *bleeding, pain, infection, problems with anesthesia, cervical scarring or stenosis* (narrowing of the opening to the uterus), and *cervical weakening* during pregnancy, making miscarriage more likely. *Stenosis* means the opening to the uterus scars shut. Other procedures may need to be done to dilate or open the canal. This is necessary to have periods and obtain Pap smears. Another complication is called a *perforation* of the uterus. When the instruments to do the surgery are inserted, they can unknowingly be pushed right through the uterus muscle, causing a small hole. Usually it heals on its own, but it could cause bleeding, infection, damage to the bladder, the bowel, or intraabdominal organs. Finally, even though a large piece of tissue is obtained, the doctor can still *miss removing the abnormality.*

What Do I Need to Do After the Procedure to Prevent Complications?

You should abstain from intercourse, swimming, weight lifting, vaginal douching, and tampon use for 4 weeks. Tylenol or ibuprofen (600 mg) can be taken four times a day for pain and cramping.

When Should I Call the Healthcare Provider?

You should call the healthcare provider in the event of heavy bleeding, abdominal or pelvic pain, abnormal vaginal discharge, or fever.

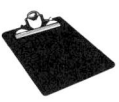

Patient Education Handout—cont'd

COLD-KNIFE CONIZATION OF THE CERVIX (CONE BIOPSY)—cont'd

Special Instructions:

You should do no heavy lifting or excessive bouncing and jarring-type activities (e.g., jogging) for 4 weeks. Avoid intercourse until after your postoperative appointment in 4 weeks. In most cases a follow-up Pap smear will be required at 4, 8, and 12 months after the procedure, as well as each year thereafter for the rest of your life. The doctor may even want to perform another colposcopy in 8 or 12 months as well. Avoid smoking because it increases the chance of recurrence. Also eat five helpings of fruits and vegetables a day and remain monogamous.

Websites That May Be of Interest to You Include the Following:

www.healthanswers.com (Health Answers)

www.merck.com (Merck)

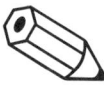 *Patient Consent Form*

CERVICAL CONIZATION

I came to the office of Dr. _____ on _____ (date) for evaluation and treatment of the following condition:

_____

We discussed the different treatments possible and discussed the risks of not treating the condition. Based upon the advice given by Dr. _____ and my own judgment, I agree to undergo cold-knife conization of the cervix.

I understand that this procedure involves removing a cone-shaped piece of tissue from my cervix with a surgical knife while I am under anesthesia.

We discussed the different possible outcomes and most of the possible complications, including pain, bleeding, infection, scarring, problems with future pregnancies, perforation, and recurrences. I have read over the information given to me and understand it. I am aware that other complications could occur that we could not foresee. I agree to follow the instructions for self-care after the procedure and to return for a follow-up check in 4 to 6 weeks. I understand the need for follow-up Pap smears and that I should receive a Pap smear every year for the rest of my life.

I will call the office or answering service if any problems arise before the scheduled follow-up visit.

_____   _____
Patient's signature   *Date/Time*

_____   _____
Witness' signature   *Physician's signature*

One copy for chart; one copy for patient.

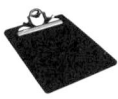

Patient Education Handout

CERVICAL STENOSIS AND CERVICAL DILATION

What Is Cervical Stenosis?
Cervical stenosis is a narrowing of the cervix (the opening to the uterus).

What Is Cervical Dilation?
Cervical dilation widens the narrowing of your cervix.

Why Do I Need This Procedure?
Cervical stenosis needs to be treated if it is painful and blood or fluid builds up in the uterus. Sometimes the opening is so small that menstrual products cannot escape. This can cause severe pain at the time of your period. You may need this procedure to allow the clinician to perform other procedures, such as dilation and curettage (D & C), abortion, endometrial biopsy, Pap smear, or insertion of an IUD.

How Do I Prepare for Cervical Dilation?
If your doctor is planning to sedate you during the procedure, you should not eat or drink at least 6 hours before the procedure. There is no other special preparation before the procedure. Take four 200 mg ibuprofen pills 1 hour before the procedure to lessen cramping.

What Happens During Cervical Dilation?
The doctor may numb your cervix and will then dilate the opening by one of two methods. With the first method, a thin metal probe is inserted, followed by a larger probe. This will be repeated until the opening is large enough for the planned procedure. With the second method your doctor would place a laminaria tent in the cervix. A laminaria tent is a dried piece of seaweed molded in the shape of a small stick. This material absorbs fluid and swells overnight. It is removed the next day before the procedure.

What Happens After the Procedure?
If you receive sedation during the procedure, you may feel sleepy after the procedure. You may also feel some cramping. If you do, take ibuprofen 600 mg every 4 to 6 hours. There may also be some spotting for a few days.

What Are the Benefits of This Procedure?
Cervical dilation is very safe and can relieve pelvic menstrual pain or allow for a good Pap smear to be obtained. It will also allow the other needed procedures to be performed.

Continued

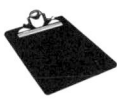 *Patient Education Handout—cont'd*

CERVICAL STENOSIS AND CERVICAL DILATION—cont'd
What Are the Risks Associated With This Procedure?
In rare cases there can be severe bleeding from the cervix or trauma to the uterus with the instrument. Rarely, the probe can penetrate through the uterus muscle (a perforation), which could cause pain, bleeding, or infection. Usually nothing will happen, but you will need to keep the doctor informed of your progress. After this perforation heals, another attempt at the procedure can be made in 6 to 8 weeks.

What Do I Need to Do After the Procedure to Prevent Infection?
If a laminaria is placed, sexual intercourse should be avoided until it is removed. You may want to continue taking ibuprofen (three 200-mg tablets) every 6 hours for the next 24 to 48 hours, depending on the cramping. A reexamination will be required in 4 to 6 weeks.

When Should I Call My Healthcare Provider?
You should call your doctor if you develop severe pain, bleeding, or fever.

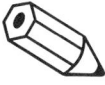

Patient Consent Form

CERVICAL STENOSIS AND CERVICAL DILATION

I came to the office of Dr._____ on _____ (date) for evaluation and treatment of cervical stenosis. Cervical stenosis is a narrowing of the cervical opening that can lead to pelvic pain, endometriosis, and collection of fluid in the uterus. In some instances it may also prevent obtaining an adequate Pap smear.

We discussed the different treatments possible and the risks of not treating the condition. Based on the advice given by Dr. _____ and my own judgment, I agree to undergo the following procedure (check the appropriate boxes):

☐ Intravenous sedation

☐ Paracervical or local block (numbing of the cervix with local anesthetic)

☐ Dilation of the cervix using dilators

☐ Dilation of the cervix using a laminaria tent (dried seaweed shaped like a small stick)

☐ Curettage (scraping) of the inner surface of the uterus

We discussed the different outcomes that could occur and most of the possible complications. These most commonly include pain, bleeding, infection, recurrence of the narrowing, and perforation (or putting a small opening) in the uterus. I am aware that other complications could occur that we could not foresee. I agree to follow the instructions for self-care after the procedure and to return for follow-up care on _____.

I will call the office or answering service if any problems arise before the scheduled follow-up visit.

_____   _____
Patient's signature   *Date/Time*

_____   _____
Witness' signature   *Physician's signature*

One copy for chart; one copy for patient.

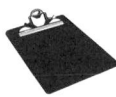 *Patient Education Handout*

COLPOSCOPY

Colposcopy is a relatively painless 30-minute office procedure for examining the female cervix when an abnormal Pap smear has been detected or when there has been exposure to genital warts. This is done using a special microscope called the *colposcope,* which we have in our office. It usually cannot be done if you are flowing heavily on your period, *but if you are only spotting, keep your appointment.*

Colposcopy identifies areas on the cervix which might be causing the abnormality on the Pap smear and which may be considered premalignant (precancerous). The changes may vary from mild to severe. If left alone, these changes may revert to normal, may stay the same, or may progress to malignancy (cancer) over a period of years. After proper evaluation, these abnormal cells can usually be treated with a freezing technique called cryocautery or with surgical removal. In certain cases laser therapy may be recommended. In this way cancer can usually be prevented. As with any procedure, *there is no guarantee* that the doctor can always eliminate the precancerous area. Therefore *close follow-up is always needed.* If you are found to have a premalignant lesion, there is about a 1% lifetime chance of developing cancer even after treatment. *Please follow your doctor's recommendations for follow-up.*

Research has shown that infection with the human papilloma virus is closely associated with cancer of the cervix. *This is the same virus that causes warts in the genital areas,* including inside the vagina and on the cervix. The medical term for these warts is *condyloma acuminata.* These lesions are *very contagious* and are passed readily by sexual intercourse. It is rare that people can be infected in other ways than through sexual contact. These wart viruses can remain dormant or inactive for up to 20 years after initial infection. If there is evidence of infection in the female (seen by an abnormal Pap smear or obvious warts around the genitals), then *the male sexual partner(s) is also infected.* In some instances it may be advised that the man be examined. That procedure is called *androscopy.* A separate handout is available that describes androscopy. Men may need to be treated if they have warts or have symptoms. If you have already had unprotected sex with your partner, a condom (rubber) is not necessary for future sex with the same person.

Description of Procedure (Colposcopy)

This procedure will take 30 minutes. You will be asked to undress from the waist down and will be draped appropriately. You will be asked to lie back and put your feet in stirrups, just like when you had the Pap smear taken. You may want to take *four (4) 200-mg ibuprofen (Advil, Nuprin, etc.) 2 hours before your appointment time, but do not take any aspirin for a week before the procedure.*

The speculum will be inserted and the Pap smear may be repeated.

The doctor will then look through the fancy microscope (colposcope) at the cervix and note if there are any abnormalities (see diagram). He will next stain the cervix with a vinegar douche. This makes abnormal cells turn white. If such changes are seen, the doctor will take a small biopsy of these areas. This is generally not painful. (The biopsies are very small, about 2 to 3 mm [⅛ inch].) If a biopsy is taken, *it does not mean you have cancer.* It only means there are abnormal cells that

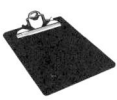

Patient Education Handout—cont'd

COLPOSCOPY—cont'd

need closer inspection. The biopsies will be sent to the hospital laboratory for further evaluation. *The hospital laboratory will bill you separately for looking at those biopsies.* Because the biopsies are so small, there are very few complications from this procedure except possibly some spotting.

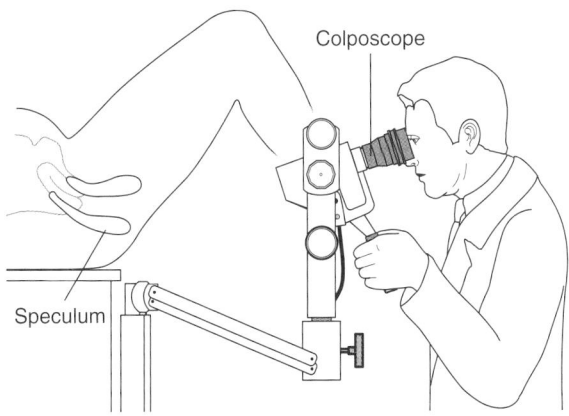

The final step is to do a scraping inside the cervix. This is called an endocervical curettage (ECC). This will cause cramping but lasts only 15 to 20 seconds. Many women find it helpful to take four (4) 200-mg ibuprofen (Advil, Nuprin, etc.) 2 hours before the procedure to decrease this cramping. Occasionally there will be some spotting afterwards for several days. Bring a sanitary pad with you to the office.

No time off work is needed except for the time in the doctor's office. Normal activities, including sex, may be resumed. As long as you are with the same partner, condoms are *not* needed.

Depending on the results of the biopsies and the ECC, which take about a week to return, your physician will advise you on the treatment of your condition. If we do not call you within 2 weeks, please call our office for results.

Other Information

About 90 different types of wart virus have been identified. They are all numbered, and types 6, 11, 16, and 18 are the most common ones in the genital area. Patients often ask if these viruses can be transmitted to the hands, feet, etc. Generally this does not happen. Genital warts for some reason stay in the genital area and usually are not transmitted to other parts of the body. Only 20% of these warts can be seen with the naked eye. The remaining 80% need to be stained to be seen and properly evaluated.

Unfortunately, once someone has the wart virus in the vagina or rectum or on the penis, it is almost impossible to totally eliminate it. Treatment can put them in "remission," but they can come back anytime. *The cervix is at very high risk of developing cancer if exposed to the wart virus so it must be evaluated, and then treated if there are significant changes there. There is a 99% chance of cure/prevention if the cervix is treated in time.* Since the warts can come back into the vagina

Continued

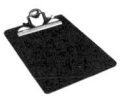 *Patient Education Handout—cont'd*

COLPOSCOPY—cont'd

anytime, you can spread the disease around anytime. Experts strongly recommend that *you remain monogamous.* This means that you have intercourse with only one partner—the same partner—the rest of your life. As long as you are with the same partner, you do not need to use condoms; you already have whatever he has. Using condoms does not cut down on reinfection if you are with the same partner. However, if you have a new partner, you can "catch" new and different types of viruses, so *a condom is necessary.* Remember, although a condom provides protection, it never makes sex "totally safe."

We now know, too, that if you smoke your chance of developing cervical cancer is markedly increased. Even if your partner smokes, *your risks go up! You must stop smoking* and your sexual partner should too. Also, *diet is very important.* You should eat at least five servings of vegetables and fruits every day. A handout is available from the receptionist regarding this. Many authorities now also suggest extra vitamins with folic acid and antioxidants.

Remember that even after you are treated, you will need three or four Pap smears during the next 12 months, and then Pap smears at least every year for the rest of your life. Your doctor may also recommend periodic colposcopy, since we know that *the Pap smear may miss up to 25% of lesions on the cervix.* You should notify any new sexual partners that you have been treated for condyloma.

Videotapes

If you like, you can obtain videotapes that discuss these issues from our office to view before or after the procedure. The woman's tape is 35 minutes long and the man's tape is 25 minutes long. Both explain much of the above information in more detail.

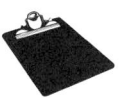

Patient Education Handout

AFTER COLPOSCOPY AND BIOPSY INFORMATION

As your clinician has explained, colposcopy and biopsy is a procedure to help evaluate precancerous conditions of the cervix or vagina. During this testing procedure, the cervix or vagina is magnified, cleansed, and treated with solutions to direct actual biopsy of the cervix or vagina. During the biopsy, a small piece of tissue is removed and sent for analysis by a specialist to determine the presence or absence of possible precancerous conditions. Your doctors would like you to be aware of the following instructions regarding the immediate time period after your colposcopy and biopsy.

1. *Bleeding.* It is normal to have some spotting after colposcopy. Normally this spotting would taper off in the immediate 12-hour period following biopsy. Other than minor spotting or sometimes a blackish discharge, any fresh clotting or bright red bleeding is abnormal. Should this occur, you are asked to call the office to arrange for an examination.

2. *Infection.* Ordinarily the cervix is highly resistant to infection. Occasionally, however, the cervix will become infected after biopsy. Infection usually will take 1 to 3 days after your biopsy to develop. Infection may show up as a thick cloudy vaginal discharge that will often have a bad odor. Furthermore, pain in the vagina or the low pelvic area may signify infection, as may fever or chills. Should any of these symptoms occur within several days of your cervical biopsy, call the office immediately so that an examination may be arranged.

3. *Pelvic pain.* During and immediately after cervical biopsy, some patients may notice menstrual-like cramps. These pains are usually gone by the day following biopsy. Any persistent symptoms should prompt a call to the office.

4. *Intercourse.* Normally the cervix or vagina heals very quickly after a small biopsy. To allow the cervix to heal completely and to become resistant to local irritation and infection, you are asked to abstain from intercourse for 5 days after the biopsy. Beyond the 5 days, unless there is a complication, intercourse can be resumed without problems.

5. *Discharge.* Ordinarily the discharge after colposcopy and biopsy is fairly heavy for the first day or two. The discharge is often dark, occasionally slightly bloody, but usually without a bad odor. During the biopsy procedure, medicine is applied to the cervix to control bleeding, which will eventually fall out and be black and grainy. This is normal for the first day or two after your biopsy but would be abnormal after that. Should your discharge become very heavy or remain bloody, especially with a bad odor, please call the clinic so that an appointment may be set up.

Notify the office should you change your phone number or address. This will allow the clinician or nurse the ability to find you for follow-up testing and reporting of your biopsy results. Remember, colposcopy and biopsy is not treatment of your condition and it will be mandatory that you return to the clinic for definitive treatment or recommendations for referral.

Please feel free to call the office should you have any questions regarding this information sheet or any complications or concerns that may arise after your colposcopy and biopsy.

(Courtesy Gary Newkirk, MD, Spokane, Wash.)

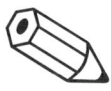 *Patient Consent Form*

CLINICAL PHOTOGRAPHY AND/OR VIDEOTAPING

I hereby authorize the clinician, _____, to take photographs and/or to videotape or to permit others to take photographs and/or videotape me in connection with my diagnosis, care, and treatment (including surgical procedures) and to use the negatives or prints for purposes of medical study, teaching, and research. I also authorize the use of such photographs and/or videotape in medical publications, unless I specifically state otherwise.

_____
Patient's signature

_____
Date/Time

_____
Other Responsible Person (Parent or Guardian)

_____
Relationship

_____
Witness' signature

One copy for chart; one copy for patient.

(Courtesy Family Medicine Spokane, Spokane, Wash.)

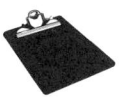

Patient Education Handout

NORPLANT SYSTEM

The purpose of this handout is to discuss with you the Norplant System. As you may have heard, the Norplant was used for years in Europe and was introduced in 1991 in the United States. The "system" consists of six thin, flexible capsules or Silastic tubes that are sealed at each end with silicone. Each capsule contains a type of hormone called progesterone. This is the same hormone used in "Depo shots." This hormone slowly leaks from the capsule, which measures about 1¼ inches long and ⅒ of an inch wide. These capsules are placed under the skin and can remain there for up to 5 years.

The Norplant System is particularly good for those who:
- Are considering surgical sterilization but are not ready to make the final decision
- Want long-term, reversible contraception
- Want to avoid daily contraceptive use or methods that have to be used with each intercourse
- Want to avoid estrogen containing contraceptives that may have more adverse effects
- Cannot use an IUD

The Norplant System may be contraindicated in women who:
- Have had problems with blood clots or strokes
- Have undiagnosed abnormal genital bleeding
- May be pregnant
- Have liver disease of any sort
- Have a history of cancer of the breast or a family history of breast cancer

Methods of Insertion

Insertion of the capsules usually takes 10 to 15 minutes, as does the removal. A local anesthetic (just like you receive in a dentist's office) is administered in the skin over the inner aspect of the upper arm. A small incision just big enough to allow the capsule to enter (2 mm or ⅒ of an inch) is made. The six capsules are then placed one at a time just under the skin. The incision site is covered with a small "butterfly." Stitches or sutures are not needed.

Effectiveness

A blood level of hormone sufficient to prevent contraception is reached within 24 hours. The effectiveness may last for as long as 5 years, but then the capsules must be removed. Of course, they can be removed at any time should the user so desire.

The Norplant System is one of the most effective forms of reversible contraception ever developed. The average annual pregnancy rate over 5 years is less than 1%. This compares favorably with the use of birth control pills as well as IUDs and sterilization.

Benefits

The Norplant System has a number of distinct benefits. It is very **effective.** It provides continuous, long-term protection for as long as 5 years, if so desired. It is **estrogen free** and delivers one of the lowest doses of hormone. It is very convenient and very comfortable. It is completely **reversible.** Upon removal, a woman returns to her previous level of fertility. There is nothing a woman must do after they are once inserted **except for annual Pap and pelvic examinations.**

Continued

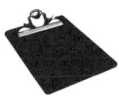

Patient Education Handout—cont'd

NORPLANT SYSTEM—cont'd

Side Effects

The most frequent side effect experienced is a **change in the menstrual bleeding pattern.** This may include more frequent bleeding, heavier bleeding, spotting, and even a lack of periods. Approximately 6% of women experience one of these conditions. Irregular and prolonged bleeding is more likely to occur during the first year of use and with less or no bleeding in subsequent years. Most women can expect to become more regular within 9 to 12 months.

Other than the bleeding, the most frequently reported side effects after the menstrual changes include **headache, nervousness, nausea,** and **dizziness.**

Infection at the insertion site can occur but is very rare. Rarely the ovaries can develop **cysts** but they will usually go away on their own.

Overall, after one year, 81% of all patients continued using the Norplant System. Despite the high rate of bleeding changes, only 9% of women had the Norplant removed because of this. Basically, it is well liked. Women can play tennis, lift weights, golf, run, and resume any other activity that they may have been involved in prior to the insertion.

Even though the Norplant System is extremely effective, there are some groups of women such as those **over 150 lb** who are more likely to get pregnant. If there are any other questions about Norplant side effects, please ask the doctor.

Breast Feeding

The Norplant System may be inserted six weeks after delivery and will have no effects on the child.

When to Schedule Your Appointment

Generally you will need to have an initial counseling appointment of about 15 minutes to discuss the issues about the Norplant. You will be able to either view the videotape available in the office or take it home for your viewing. If there are no contraindications to inserting the Norplant, an appointment will be scheduled during the first **seven days of your cycle.** (Day 1 of your cycle is the first day of bleeding.) You can return to work immediately afterwards if you so desire. **You must have a breast exam, pelvic exam, and Pap smear within the previous 6 months.** It is suggested that you have this done by your family doctor or gynecologist prior to the visit so the results can be discussed with the doctor.

Payment for the Implant:

It is expected that you pay for the implant on the day of insertion unless you can provide evidence that is will be covered by your insurance company. Please call them if you have questions. The fee for insertion is _____. The cost of the device is _____.

Should you have any questions whatsoever, please feel free to discuss them with the doctor at the time of the counseling visit.

Remember: You still must get regular Pap smears every year. The Norplant prevents pregnancy but has no effect on cervical cancers.

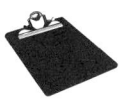

Patient Education Handout

CRYOTHERAPY OF THE CERVIX

Cryotherapy of the cervix is a procedure used to treat certain abnormalities on the cervix, such as chronic inflammation, an abnormal Pap smear, or genital warts. The outer layers of cells of the cervix are frozen using a special instrument with a tip about the size of a quarter that gets very cold. This procedure is quick and you generally do not experience much pain. (The cervix is the opening to the uterus.)

This freezing procedure is done in our office. You should plan on 20 minutes of time. You will be asked to lie back in the usual Pap and pelvic position. It is *best* to have the procedure done during the 5 days *after* your period. We *cannot* do it *5 days before or during your period.*

When the doctor turns the instrument on, you will hear a small hissing sound. Then you may feel some cramping as if you were having a menstrual period. The freezing lasts for only about 3 minutes. The cervical tissue is allowed to thaw, then is frozen for a second time. There is no cutting, burning, or bleeding of any sort. *Taking four (4) 200-mg ibuprofen (Advil or Nuprin) 1-2 hours before the procedure* will help prevent the discomfort of the cramps.

After cryotherapy you can expect a rather profuse watery vaginal discharge for 2 to 3 weeks. THIS IS NORMAL. You will want to wear a mini-pad. Your doctor may recommend using a vaginal cream (Amino-Cerv Vaginal Creme) to help reduce this discharge. If you bring the tube to the office, the first application will be given right after the freezing. You'll then need to insert one application in the vagina at bedtime until the tube is gone.

You may resume normal activity, including sex, when you feel comfortable, but it is probably best to wait at least 2 weeks to allow adequate healing. You may also have some spotting when you resume intercourse or use tampons.

Fortunately there are only rare complications with this procedure. You may experience cramping as already mentioned. If the cramping persists, you may take 400 to 600 mg of ibuprofen four times per day if there are no contraindications. Very rarely cryotherapy may cause scarring and narrowing of the cervical canal to the degree that it actually blocks the opening (stenosis). This could potentially cause problems in getting pregnant. Cryotherapy is best avoided during pregnancy if possible. Tell the doctor if you think you might be pregnant. Infection could occur, so if your discharge lasts more than three weeks and is not getting better, call the office. Also, no treatment is 100% effective, so the abnormalities could come back.

It is recommended that you have a *follow-up Pap smear at 4, 8, and 12 months, then every year for the rest of your life.* If any of these Pap smears return as abnormal, your physician will give you specific instructions as to what to do next. Many times a colposcopy will be done at 8 months.

It is very important to note that cryotherapy is effective 85% to 95% of the time, depending on the lesion. That means *5% to 15% of patients will need to be retreated.* Sometimes cryotherapy is used again or your doctor may recommend other treatments. This emphasizes why follow-up is so important. After two treatments, the cervix is protected in 99% of the cases.

Continued

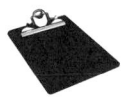 *Patient Education Handout—cont'd*

CRYOTHERAPY OF THE CERVIX—cont'd

The wart or human papilloma virus (HPV) that causes cervical cell changes and cervical cancer is contagious. Most of the time the virus is not visible. However, if your partner has any obvious genital lesions, he should see his physician for possible treatment. Decrease your risk of developing cervical cancer by not smoking and follow a diet high in fruits and vegetables with adequate vitamin intake. Remain monogamous. THE MOST IMPORTANT THING TO HELP PREVENT CERVICAL CANCER, HOWEVER, IS TO CONTINUE TO HAVE REGULAR PAP SMEARS AS RECOMMENDED BY YOUR PHYSICIAN. CLOSE FOLLOW-UP IS ESSENTIAL.

These are only general guidelines and may be modified depending on your particular situation. Should you have any questions or concerns, please feel free to discuss these with your physician.

Adapted with permission from The National Procedures Institute, Midland, Mich.

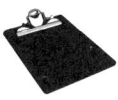

Patient Education Handout

AFTER CRYOTHERAPY OF THE CERVIX

1. You will have a heavy watery vaginal discharge for 2 to 4 weeks after this procedure.
2. The discharge may have an odor and may be tinged with blood; this is normal.
3. You may need to wear a sanitary pad, especially the first few days. Be sure to change the pads frequently.
4. Avoid putting anything into your vagina for 2 to 3 weeks after cryotherapy unless instructed by your doctor. This includes avoiding tampons, sexual intercourse, and douching.
5. Your doctor may prescribe some vaginal cream to help decrease the odor from the discharge. Use as directed.
6. Avoid excessive and heavy exercise for the first 2 or 3 days after this treatment; this could cause vaginal bleeding.
7. Showering, bathing, and swimming are allowed.
8. You will need a repeat pelvic examination and Pap smear in 4 months. Please schedule that appointment today before you leave. You will also need a Pap smear at 8 and 12 months after the treatment to be sure there is no return of any cervical abnormality. If all repeat Pap tests are normal after that time, then you can return to having yearly Pap smears for the rest of your life. Close follow-up is essential to protect against any further problems.
9. Please call your doctor if you experience any severe pain, heavy bleeding, fever, or if the vaginal discharge lasts longer than 4 weeks.

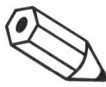 *Patient Consent Form*

DIAGNOSTIC HYSTEROSCOPY

1. I hereby authorize and request Dr. _____ and/or his/her associates or assistants to perform a diagnostic hysteroscopy on me (mechanically open the cervix, insert a tube into the uterus, and attempt to evaluate and possibly treat my problem). If during the course of the operation, unanticipated conditions are revealed that require more surgery than planned, this authorization shall extend to correcting such additional conditions that are considered necessary and advisable to my physician's professional judgment.

2. I consent to the administration of such anesthetics/analgesics as may be considered necessary and advisable by the doctor responsible for this service.

3. The operation and the significant potential risks and complications have been explained satisfactorily to me by my physician. These risks and complications may reasonably include, but are not limited to, the following:
   - Mild uterine cramps and some bleeding (a common problem)
   - Infection or more severe bleeding
   - Injury (mechanical and/or thermal) to the uterine cervix, corpus, and surrounding structures
   - Complications associated with the use of the fluid to open the uterus, which includes, but is not limited to, fluid in the lungs, blood clotting problems, seizures, and allergic reactions including shock
   - Air embolism (passage of air into the blood stream, leading to serious injury or death)
   - Inability to introduce the hysteroscope into the uterine cavity, requiring further surgery
   - Difficulties with anesthesia/analgesia
   - Missing, or incomplete removal of, a lesion

Any of these occurrences may require additional hospitalization or further surgery to repair either immediately or in the future.

I understand that the explanation that I have received is not exhaustive and that other more remote risks and complications may arise, including the remote possibility of death, that are inherent in the performance of any operation or procedure.

4. In connection with the medical services that I am receiving, I authorize photographs to be taken of me or parts of my body, provided the photographs shall be used for medical record purposes only, unless in the judgment of my physician, medical research, education, or science will benefit by their use. In that event, my photographs may be published for such purposes, provided that I shall not be identified by name.

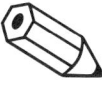

Patient Consent Form—cont'd

DIAGNOSTIC HYSTEROSCOPY—cont'd

5. I have also had explained to me the risks and benefits of the alternative medical and surgical modes of treatment, if any, plus the results likely if my present medical condition remains untreated.
6. I acknowledge that no guarantees have been made to me concerning the results of the operation or procedure.

_____

Patient's signature

_____

Witness' signature

_____

Date/Time

_____

Patient or person authorized to consent for patient (relationship)

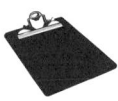 *Patient Education Handout*

DILATION AND CURETTAGE (D & C)

What Is a D & C?

A D & C is a procedure where the opening of the uterus or womb is opened with metal instruments and then the contents of the uterus or womb are removed.

Why Do I Need This Procedure?

Because a D & C can be done for various reasons, the doctor will discuss the reasons for the procedure with you. It may be needed to remove excessive uterine tissue that can lead to cancer, to remove a partial miscarriage, to diagnose other problems such as polyps or fibroids, or to find the cause of abnormal uterine bleeding. Most of the time, abnormal bleeding occurs because of a hormone imbalance. However, until known for sure, the physician must be sure there is no cancer. This rarely occurs before age 40 but must be considered after this age.

How Do I Prepare for a D & C?

Empty your bladder before coming to the office or hospital. Avoid use of any vaginal creams for 48 hours before the procedure. Someone should be available to drive you home after the procedure (in the event that sedation is required). It is best not to eat or drink anything for at least 8 hours before coming to the office.

What Happens During the Procedure?

You are placed on an examination table on your back, and your legs are placed in stirrups. A vaginal examination is performed and a speculum is placed into your vagina (just like for a Pap smear). The vagina and cervix are then cleaned with an antiseptic solution. An IV may be started to provide fluids and medications to make you drowsy. The cervix or opening of the uterus (i.e., womb) is numbed with medication. An instrument is then inserted to scrape out the tissue inside the uterus. The material that was obtained is then checked in a laboratory.

What Happens After the Procedure?

If sedation is used, you are allowed to wake up. After an appropriate time, you are released. Some medication may be prescribed to slow down bleeding, prevent infection, and decrease pain.

What Are the Benefits of This Procedure?

This procedure is performed to help rule out or diagnose cancer, decrease vaginal bleeding if heavy bleeding is occurring, or remove an incomplete miscarriage.

What Are the Risks Associated With This Procedure?

The risks are excessive bleeding, infection requiring antibiotics, or perforation. A perforation is a hole in the uterus caused by one of the instruments. Should this happen, you may require observation at home or hospitalization with or without surgery. Even with all attempts to scrape the entire lining of the uterus, it is still possible to miss some of the tissue and leave it behind. Therefore

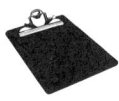

Patient Education Handout

DILATION AND CURETTAGE (D & C)—cont'd

missing the proper diagnosis or not treating the situation appropriately could also be considered a complication.

Will There Be Much Pain?

Although most patients experience very little pain, some cramping is possible. Use ibuprofen (Advil, Nuprin, Motrin) to control this.

What Should Be Done to Prevent Infection After the Procedure?

Avoid tampons, douching, having sex, or placing anything in the vagina for at least 2 weeks after procedure. Showering and bathing is allowed.

When Should the Patient Call the Healthcare Provider?

Call if excessive vaginal bleeding (i.e., bleeding that soaks more than one regular sanitary napkin per hour) is experienced or if large clots are seen. If you experience moderate to severe abdominal pain or cramping, fever, or foul-smelling and puslike vaginal discharge, notify the doctor. If you have not received the lab results 2 weeks after the procedure, contact the office.

Special Instructions:

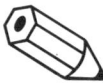 *Patient Consent Form*

DILATION AND CURETTAGE (D & C) REQUEST

I came to the office of Dr. _____ on _____ (date) for evaluation and treatment of the following condition:
- Abnormal uterine bleeding
- Uncontrollable uterine bleeding
- Incomplete miscarriage
- Other: _____

The different treatment options and the risks of not treating this condition were discussed. Based on the advice given by Dr. _____ and my own judgment, I agree to undergo the following procedures:
- Starting venous access
- Injecting medicine for pain control and sedation into my veins
- Scraping out the lining of my uterus
- Sending all removed products for analysis

We discussed the different outcomes that could occur and most of the possible complications, including pain, bleeding, infection, perforation, scarring, and missing the true diagnosis. There can also be complications from any anesthetic used. I am aware that other complications could occur that we cannot foresee. I agree to follow the instructions for self-care after the procedure and to return for follow-up care on _____.

I understand the procedure will be performed in the indicated location:

    ☐ Office   ☐ Day Surgery Center   ☐ Hospital

I have reviewed the benefits of each location, have read over the patient teaching guide the doctor has provided, and have no further questions. I will call the office or answering service if any problems arise before the scheduled follow-up visit.

_____
Patient's signature

_____
Date/Time

_____
Witness' signature

_____
Physician's signature

One copy for chart; one copy for patient.

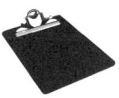
Patient Education Handout

ENDOMETRIAL BIOPSY

This procedure is relatively simple. However, to make this test as comfortable and useful as possible, we want you to have the following information.

An endometrial biopsy takes a sample from the tissue that lines the uterus (womb). This tissue is then examined under the pathologist's microscope to assist in making a diagnosis and to check for cancer. The sample is taken by means of a thin tube about the size of a ballpoint pen refill, which is passed into the uterine cavity through the opening in the cervix. A small amount of tissue from each portion of the uterus is then sampled by a gentle scraping technique. The procedure will take approximately 10 to 20 minutes. The endometrial biopsy may be sufficient to avoid a "D & C" in the hospital.

The following instructions are important to help provide the best results.

1. *Timing of the test is critical.* The best time to perform an endometrial biopsy is before your menstrual period. Thus your appointment should be made on day 22 following the first day of your last menstrual period. If your periods are unpredictable, the biopsy can usually be performed if it has been at least 3 weeks since your last period. Your appointment needs to be rescheduled if your period begins.

   If you will be having your menstrual period on the day of your appointment, please call our office as soon as possible to reschedule.

2. The discomfort during the test is usually mild. If you can, take three 200-mg ibuprofen (Advil, Nuprin, Motrin) an hour before your appointment. This should make you more comfortable. Please let us know if you think a stronger medication is needed. If we suggested something else to you when we talked about this procedure, then follow those directions.

3. You should be able to drive yourself to and from the office and return to work immediately after the procedure. Other than the cramping you may feel when we do the procedure, side effects are usually minimal.

4. You may have a small amount of spotting afterwards; this usually disappears within 1 to 2 days. Cramping similar to menstrual cramps is uncommon but may be treated with ibuprofen. Those who cannot tolerate ibuprofen may take acetaminophen (Tylenol).

5. You may resume sex when you feel comfortable (usually in 2 to 3 days).

6. *Significant complications* from an endometrial biopsy are extremely rare, but, as with any surgery, they are always a possibility. The possible complications would be bleeding, infection, and uterine perforation (causing a small hole in the uterus). Pain is usually minimal but if you experience pelvic pain for more than 24 hours, excessive bleeding more than your usual period, or begin running a temperature after the procedure, please call our office. If your symptoms persist, call the doctor. It is also possible that the endometrial biopsy will miss the diagnosis and further studies may be needed.

7. If you don't hear from our office about the test results in 10 days, please call us.

If you have any questions about a possible complication, please call.

(Used with permission from The National Procedures Institute, Midland, Mich.)

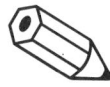 *Patient Consent Form*

ENDOMETRIAL BIOPSY

Patient name _____ ID# _____ Date of birth _____

My clinician, _____, has explained the procedure and anesthesia necessary to diagnose or treat my condition.

I understand the nature of the procedure summarized below. I request and authorize the performance of endometrial biopsy.

I have been informed and understand that the following are risks associated with this procedure:
- *Perforation* of uterus, which may require hospitalization (rare)
- *Infection* (rare)
- *Pain* during procedure and cramping afterwards for 1 to 2 days
- *Bleeding* (slight or severe), which may be controlled with outpatient treatment or may require hospitalization
- A *missed abnormality* by biopsy (rare)

I have been informed of the following benefits of this procedure:
- It helps to plan future therapy.
- Obtaining tissue from inside the uterus will generally help make a diagnosis of my condition.

I have been informed of the alternative(s) to diagnose or treat my condition. (I also understand that the cause of my symptoms may not be found so further studies may be necessary).

I have been given an explanation of the procedures, read and understand this information, and have had all questions answered to my satisfaction.

_____   _____
Patient's signature   *Date/Time*

_____   _____
Witness' signature   *Date/Time*

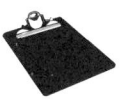

Patient Education Handout

LOOP ELECTROSURGICAL EXCISION PROCEDURE (LEEP)

In 1991 a new treatment was found to remove precancerous conditions of the cervix, vulva (i.e., lips), vagina, and anus. This procedure uses high frequency electrical waves to remove tissue. The waves are similar to the AM radio and cause less destruction of tissue than older techniques used in the past. This procedure is replacing most operating room surgical and laser surgeries.

As you know, you have an abnormality on your cervix. In the past, many of these were treated with freezing (i.e., cryosurgery) or conization (a way of cutting out the abnormality) in the hospital. Many of your friends have probably told you about that. The advantage of the loop electrosurgical excision procedure (LEEP) procedure is that it can be done in the office. The same equipment can also be used to remove growths in the genital areas.

When you come in for the LEEP procedure, you will be placed in stirrups (just as you are for a Pap smear). The vaginal speculum will be placed. You will be stained with vinegar and looked at with the colposcope (essentially a magnifying glass). Iodine will be placed on the cervix to help identify the abnormal tissue. The cervix will then be numbed with Xylocaine, just like you receive in the dentist's office. Using a thin wire loop, the doctor will remove the abnormal tissue. You can think of it like an ice cream scoop taking a very tiny piece of tissue. You will hear a lot of noise from a vacuum that removes the smoke. Although 30 minutes are reserved for your appointment, the procedure itself only takes 8 to 10 minutes.

The complications from LEEP are rare. Only 2% or 3% of patients have significant problems such as the following:

- *Pain and discomfort.* This is minimal. On a scale of 1 to 10, with 10 representing severe pain, women only rate the pain a 2 (not bad at all). Some patients complain that they did not like the feeling of the speculum in the vagina or the shot to numb the area. However, you should not feel much else. After the procedure there may be slight cramping for 24 hours, but that is minimal. Take four (4) 200-mg ibuprofen 1 hour before coming in, and take three (3) 4 hours later. That may be all you need. Do not take any aspirin products; they may cause bleeding complications.
- *Bleeding.* You'll have some spotting for 8 to 10 days. When the "scab" comes off in 10 to 14 days, you may notice a little more bleeding. If you pass large clots (more than you have with your periods) or are concerned, call the office. You may also pass some "black stuff" that looks like tissue; however, it is the medicine we used to control bleeding. Do not worry about that.
- *Infection.* This is rare, but it can happen. You may have a slight discharge. If it lasts over 2 weeks, call the office. You should also call if you have a fever or experience severe pain in the lower abdominal area.
- *Recurrence.* Some of the abnormality may be missed, or it may come back on its own. Be sure to keep your follow-up appointments for rechecks and Pap smears.
- *Stenosis.* This means the opening of the cervix scars shut. We must keep it open in order for you to obtain Pap smears, to have periods, and to get pregnant. There is no way to know if stenosis happens unless the doctor rechecks you. Keep your appointment in 4 to 6 weeks for this examination. If stenosis is found early, it is easy for the doctor to insert a small probe and reopen the cervix.

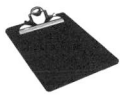 *Patient Education Handout—cont'd*

LOOP ELECTROSURGICAL EXCISION PROCEDURE (LEEP)—cont'd

Take four (4) 200-mg ibuprofen (Advil, Nuprin, Motrin, etc.) 1 hour before your appointment to help ease any discomfort. Schedule your appointment anytime after your period but at least 5 days *before* your next expected period. Tell the doctor if you think you could be pregnant.

The real *advantages* of LEEP are that it is quick, has a high cure rate with the first treatment, and is much cheaper than laser or operating room procedures. In fact, it has almost replaced all the other procedures completely. Studies show that it does not interfere with getting pregnant or having a baby unless repeat procedures are needed.

After the LEEP is carried out, please follow these instructions:

- Refrain from sex for 4 weeks.
- Avoid lifting heavy weights for 3 weeks (limit to less than 20 lb).
- A brownish-black vaginal discharge for a few days to 2 weeks is normal. However, if a malodorous (i.e., smelly) discharge develops or if the odor or discharge persists, please call the office.
- If spotting or bleeding persists longer than 2 weeks, call the office.
- If you develop bleeding with clots, call the office anytime.
- Return to the office in 4 weeks for a brief check. In 6 and 12 months you will need follow-up Pap smears (either in this office or your doctor's office).

Remember that even though you have been treated, you still have an increased lifetime risk of developing cervical, vaginal, and vulvar cancer. You and your partner *must refrain from smoking.* To prevent the wart virus from spreading, all major authorities recommend monogamy—having sex with the same partner for the rest of your life. Although condoms and nonoxynol-9 spermicidal jelly may help prevent the spread of warts, they are not completely protective. Even after the two Pap smears mentioned previously are normal, you must obtain a Pap smear at least once a year for the rest of your life to screen for cervical cancer. A healthy diet that includes at least five portions of fruits or vegetables each day is essential. It may also be beneficial to take a good multivitamin with folic acid each day.

Please feel free to ask if you have further questions or desire further information. Videotapes discussing many of these issues are available for your home viewing.

(Used with permission of The Medical Procedure Center, P.C., Midland, Mich.)

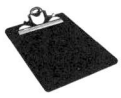

Patient Education Handout

PAP SMEAR INFORMATION

The frequency at which Pap smears should be performed depends on individual considerations. Rarely do I ever recommend going longer than 1 year between examinations. We now know the Pap can miss up to 25% of lesions even when done correctly. Some women may have risk factors that necessitate Pap smears every 4 or 6 months.

In the past, Pap smears were reported to our office according to a system based on "classes" and were graded Class I through Class V. You may be more familiar with this old system.

In 1988, a new system was adopted. They *do not report classes* as before, but rather describe more of what they see. This new way of giving reports is called the Bethesda System. In 2001, updated recommendations came out from the Bethesda Group. The following are the various reports possible:

Terminology/Reports

1. **Negative (previously Class I):** This is a *negative smear* with no abnormal or unusual cells seen. The smear is clean and clear of any inflammatory cells and is easy for the pathologist to read as not having any evidence of malignancy (cancer).
2. **Atypical (previously Class II):** This is further broken down into two terms: atypical squamous cells, cannot exclude high-grade lesion (ASC-H) and atypical squamous cells of uncertain significance (ASC-US). With these smears, it is more difficult for the pathologist to unequivocally say that it is negative. There may be evidence of regeneration of cells on the cervix or changes in the cells related to infections or the trauma of childbirth. Depending on other descriptions the pathologist uses, you may need treatment for infection, a repeat Pap smear, special DNA testing, observation, or further diagnostic testing with colposcopy. Your doctor will tell you what steps to take. Some type of follow-up is needed.
3. **Low-grade squamous intraepithelial lesion (previously Class III, mild dysplasia):** This classification is for abnormal cells, which may be considered to have mild "premalignant" potential. This same category would be used if there is any sign of the human papilloma (wart) virus. *Dysplasia* is a precancerous change and this finding requires further evaluation. If left alone, these changes may revert to normal, may stay the same, or may progress to malignancy over a period of years. The interval for the development of malignancy from dysplasia is variable, but commonly felt to be as little as 3 or most likely as long as 10 years. Office colposcopy, a special technique using a microscope to look at the cervix, will probably be recommended. Biopsies will be performed. If only mild changes are confirmed, usually no treatment is required. However, more frequent Pap smears will be needed. In some instances of large lesions or persistent changes, treatment will be recommended.
4. **High-grade squamous intraepithelial lesion (previously Class III, moderate to severe and Class IV):** This classification is indicative of a more advanced precancerous change. The changes in the cells are severe enough to warrant very prompt and complete evaluation with colposcopy. Treatment with freezing or excision of the abnormality is usually needed.

Continued

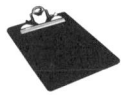

Patient Education Handout—cont'd

PAP SMEAR INFORMATION—cont'd

5. **Cancer (previously Class V):** This classification indicates a high probability of cancer and again, warrants prompt and complete evaluation to determine the extent of the problem. A plan of treatment for best results can be determined.

Modern research has now shown that the genital wart virus (human papilloma virus, also called condyloma) causes cervical cancer. This virus is very contagious—with just one sexual contact there is an 80% chance of becoming infected. Be sure to tell your physician if you or your partner has or did have genital warts. Unfortunately, only about 20% of genital warts can be seen without using special techniques. The remaining 80% must be stained with vinegar and properly evaluated to be seen. If a woman has warts in her vagina or around the external genitals, there is a 75% to 80% chance she has changes on her cervix.

It takes 10 days to 2 weeks to get the Pap results back. Please call our office if you have not heard from us in 2 weeks' time.

High-Risk Factors for Developing Cervical Cancer
You are in a higher risk group for developing cancer of the cervix if:
- You have had more then three sexual partners in your lifetime
- You first had sexual intercourse before the age of 18
- You have had genital warts (papilloma virus) or other venereal diseases
- A sexual partners of yours has had intercourse with a women who developed cervical cancer or abnormal Pap smears, or had genital warts
- You smoke or your partner smokes
- Your mother took DES (diethylstilbestrol) during pregnancy with you
- You have had a previous Pap smear that showed abnormal or suspicious cells
- You have a poor diet (less than five helpings of fruits and vegetables per day)
- You have AIDS or other conditions that suppress your immune system

Only a small percentage of women are classified as low risk. The vast majority of women have one or more of the above and are therefore considered at much greater risk for developing cancer of the cervix. Due to this trend, most women should be screened at least once a year, as a general rule, to ensure early diagnosis of the disease.

The wart virus is spreading rapidly. New cases of genital warts now outnumber new cases of gonorrhea and chlamydia combined. Discuss any concerns you might have with your doctor.

To Improve Your Pap Smears
1. Do not douche for 3 days prior to your appointment.
2. Do not have intercourse for 3 days before your appointment.
3. Schedule your appointment when you are not bleeding.
4. If you have an unusual discharge, tell your doctor so this can be treated before your Pap.
5. Tell your doctor of any risk factors you may have.
6. If you are on Depo-Provera shots, have the Norplant in, or are no longer menstruating (and are not taking estrogens), you may need to take estrogens before your visit. Discuss this with your doctor.

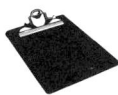

Patient Education Handout—cont'd

PAP SMEAR INFORMATION—cont'd

To Prevent Cervical Cancer

1. Be monogamous (stay with one partner)
2. Don't smoke (your partner either)
3. Eat five helpings of fruits and vegetables per day (the more green, red, orange, yellow the better)
4. Take multivitamins with folic acid
5. Get regular Pap smears every year
6. Wait until at least age 21 before having sex

(Used with permission of The Medical Procedures Center, P.C., Midland, Mich.)

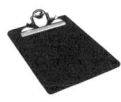 *Patient Education Handout*

PERMANENT FEMALE STERILIZATION (TUBAL LIGATION)

Permanent female sterilization is a surgical procedure that women can undergo to permanently prevent pregnancy. A small incision is made in the abdomen, the fallopian tubes are cut, and a small portion of the tube is removed. This surgery prevents the egg from becoming fertilized by the male's sperm. Minilaparotomy is the name of the procedure that your doctor offers for performing permanent sterilization on an outpatient or same-day-surgery basis. The surgery is usually performed while you are under general anesthesia (asleep); therefore you must come to the hospital early on the day following a complete 8-hour fast (nothing taken by mouth). Generally, you will be able to go home within 3 or 4 hours after surgery. A friend or family member is required to drive you home. You must return for a follow-up visit 2 weeks after your surgery, or at any time a complication develops. Minilaparotomy is a safe, common, and popular way to perform permanent sterilization. You should realize that sterilization, or tubal ligation as it is sometimes called, is permanent. You should not have this surgery unless you are certain that you do not wish to have any more children. The decision must be made by you. You and your partner must agree that you will never want any more children. Even though reversal is possible for some women, that surgery is expensive and frequently does not work.

You should understand that there are a number of alternatives to permanent female sterilization, such as barrier methods (condoms, diaphragm); natural family planning; spermicide gels; cervical cap; birth control pills; the Norplant System, which is placed under the skin and lasts for 5 years; intrauterine devices (IUDs), which are effective for 5 to 10 years; hormone patches; and Depo-Provera shots. Men can also undergo permanent sterilization, called *vasectomy*, which is less expensive and safer. It is also possible to check the man after surgery to be sure the surgery was successful. There is no way to do this in the woman. Failure rates for vasectomy are about 1 in 1200—only one fifth or one sixth that of tubal ligation. Before having your tubal ligation, you are free to ask questions and express your desires and concerns. You may change your mind about your surgery at any time. You should be aware of the following major risks regarding these procedures:

Pain

All women experience pain from their sterilization surgery. It is felt in the incision, as well as deeper around the fallopian tubes. In general, this pain can be controlled with oral medications, but you should not expect to return to work any sooner than several days after the procedure. Many women prefer to take a week off or to schedule surgery during a vacation. Lifting or twisting will be uncomfortable to some extent for at least 2 weeks. You will benefit from arranging your schedule so that you can take it easy for a reasonable period after your surgery, and at least until you have your follow-up appointment in the office in 2 weeks.

Infection

There is a small chance, less than 1 out of 100, that you may experience an abdominal infection in the fallopian tubes or the skin incision. Inner abdominal infections are very rare; however, they are always serious and may require hospitalization. Skin incision infections are more common, and treatment usually involves skin cleansing, oral antibiotics, and, rarely, a stay in the hospital.

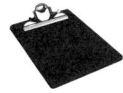

Patient Education Handout—cont'd

PERMANENT FEMALE STERILIZATION (TUBAL LIGATION)—cont'd

Bleeding

Bleeding in the abdomen from your tubal surgery is uncommon. Most bleeding is controlled during surgery. Bleeding may develop in the skin incision and require drainage. It is unlikely that you would ever require a blood transfusion to correct the bleeding experienced during or after your surgery.

Injury

Other organs—most commonly the urinary bladder, the tissues next to the uterus, or the bowel—are very rarely (less than 1 chance in 100) injured during sterilization surgery. Prior pelvic or abdominal surgery or infection increases the likelihood of injury to other abdominal organs during sterilization surgery. These injuries may require repair during surgery, and hospitalization may be necessary for initial treatment. In rare instances, the uterus may be injured from the instruments that are used to move or control its position.

Failure

Although tubal ligation is highly successful at preventing future pregnancies, it is not perfect. In other words, there is a small chance (approximately 1 in 100 to 250) that the tubes may grow back together and that you may become pregnant. Furthermore, if you do become pregnant after tubal ligation, there is an increased chance that your pregnancy would *not* be in the uterus, but rather in the tube around the scar. These are called *ectopic* or *tubal pregnancies,* and they can require emergency surgery.

Regret

Approximately 1% to 2% of women who undergo tubal ligation change their minds and seek reversal surgery so that they can become pregnant again. Only 50% of these will be successful and it is expensive. Women seeking permanent sterilization should make their decision freely. You should be aware of alternatives for birth control and your questions should be answered. If you are not sure about your decision, wait before having surgery.

Other Complications

Other complications of tubal ligation are possible, but these are very rare. Death has occurred from sterilization surgery (3 to 11 out of 100,000). However, far more women die from complications of pregnancy than from complications of sterilization surgery. Reactions to the drugs given during surgery are possible. Risks of general anesthesia include allergic reactions, pneumonia, blood clots (pulmonary embolism), heart attacks, and other very rare events. In some instances, your doctor or the anesthesia specialist may advise alternative forms of pain control for your surgery depending on your medical condition and desires.

Summary

In conclusion, tubal ligation (permanent sterilization) is a safe, effective form of birth control. It is impossible to discuss every possible risk or complication from this surgery. You should feel comfortable with your decision, and feel free to raise questions you may have.

Note: Permanent sterilization does not eliminate the need for Pap smears, nor does it prevent you from getting sexually transmitted diseases. Please consult your physician about the recommended frequency as well as other disease-screening recommendations.

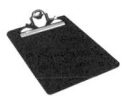

Patient Education Handout

AFTER TUBAL LIGATION

Your sterilization surgery was accomplished by entering the tissues of the abdominal wall. This small opening was sutured together by both deep and surface stitches. These stitches will eventually dissolve; you do not need to see the physician to have them removed. The surgery site is normally most painful the first several days after surgery. You may also experience a deeper pelvic discomfort as the tubes themselves begin to heal. The discomfort at both places should gradually improve over 2 weeks. Certain activities such as lifting or bearing down will cause discomfort and should be avoided. It is extremely unlikely that your stitches will come loose, but it is best if you avoid lifting or any activity that causes pain. Acetaminophen or ibuprofen will help reduce the discomfort (unless you are allergic to or cannot tolerate this medication).

Bandages have been placed over the surgery site. It is normal for them to become stained with a small amount of blood and tissue fluids. On the day after your surgery, you may remove these bandages and replace them with sterile gauze and paper tape. By the third day after surgery, you may shower without bandages (however, do not soak the area by taking a tub bath). You should keep the surgery site covered for about 7 days to reduce irritation by clothing or bedding that may rub this area, but you may want to change the dressing two to three times a day. It is normal for the skin to itch as healing begins.

Your tubal ligation is immediately effective. You will be able to have intercourse without concern for pregnancy. Most women prefer to wait at least 2 weeks before having intercourse in order to allow their surgery to heal and to become more comfortable. It is also important to remember that your tubal ligation prevents pregnancy but in no way protects you from infections that can be transmitted from sexual intercourse. If at any time you feel you may be exposing yourself to sexually transmitted disease (gonorrhea, AIDS, chlamydia, syphilis, HPV-warts, or herpes) you should avoid intercourse, or at least insist that your partner wear a condom. Also, permanent sterilization does not eliminate the need for Pap smears. Your physician will recommend how frequently you need to have a Pap smear and other disease-screening procedures.

Finally, you should call the doctor's office if you feel you are having problems. Signs of infection include discharge, pus, redness, increasing pain in this area, fever, aches, muscle pains (flu-like symptoms), and abdominal pain. Let your doctor know if you experience burning with urination, which may indicate a bladder infection.

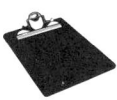

Patient Education Handout

POSTPARTUM TUBAL LIGATION

Please review the information about permanent sterilization surgery. The postpartum (after delivery) time has become popular for sterilization surgery, which is generally performed within 48 hours of delivery. Postpartum tubal ligation by minilaparotomy is similar to the sterilization procedure performed on women who have not recently delivered. However, there are some important differences. Often the same anesthetic (epidural, caudal) that you had to deliver your baby can be extended to provide anesthesia for your tubal ligation. Another popular way to undergo postpartum sterilization is by general anesthesia (be put to sleep) the day after delivery.

Remember that although you may plan to undergo postpartum sterilization, a number of things can happen during and after labor to postpone or delay this surgery, such as infection, fever, excessive blood loss, and high blood pressure. If any of these complications occur, sterilization surgery will need to be postponed until at least 6 weeks after delivery. Furthermore, if your newborn is ill, you may wish to wait until you are confident that your baby is healthy.

After delivery, minilaparotomy surgery requires that the abdomen be entered at or near the umbilicus (belly button). The abdominal incision (cut) is usually at the pubic hair line if the surgery is performed at other times. Most women recover quickly after postpartum sterilization surgery, and only rarely is it necessary to stay in the hospital longer than the normal amount of time you would stay for a simple delivery (1 to 2 days). Having help at home is always a good idea with a newborn, but this is especially true if you have undergone postpartum sterilization. Lifting your newborn baby may be quite uncomfortable for at least a week. Finally, if your baby is born by cesarean section, tubal sterilization surgery can easily be performed if desired; but remember, how and when you have your permanent sterilization surgery should be determined by your desires and commitment, not simply because it is convenient.

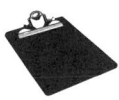 *Patient Education Handout*

PATIENT EDUCATION FOR YOUR PESSARY

Your pessary is designed to restore your anatomy to a more normal and comfortable position. Proper care of the pessary will lengthen its useful life and help prevent complications and discomfort. Follow the manufacturer's instructions on removing, washing, and reinserting the pessary. Use warm water and mild soap. Do not use detergents or bleach.

Call your healthcare provider immediately if you experience the following: persistent pain or discomfort, difficulty with emptying your bladder or having a bowel movement, vaginal bleeding, vaginal odor, or irritation. The amount of vaginal discharge may increase but should not have an odor and should not be irritating to you. If your pessary comes out and you cannot reinsert it, call your provider.

If you are postmenopausal or have had your ovaries removed and are not on estrogen replacement, use of estrogen is very important to keep your vaginal lining healthy and to prevent sores or irritation. Follow your provider's instructions on estrogen use.

Use only water-soluble lubricants such as K-Y Jelly or Surgilube to aid in inserting your pessary. Petroleum-based products will increase the chance of infection or irritation and reduce the life of the pessary.

Practicing the Kegel (pelvic tightening) exercises daily will increase the effectiveness of the pessary and decrease the need to be refit for a different size or style of pessary.

You should remove your pessary before sexual intercourse. If you will be sexually active, be sure to inform your clinician so proper devices can be selected.

Return for follow-up with your healthcare provider as directed for follow-up checks and replacement of the device.

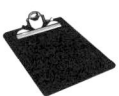

Patient Education Handout

PAPSURE

Your Health Is Important

The Pap smear is the most common screening examination used to find abnormal cell changes in the cervix that may lead to cancer. This procedure has saved thousands of lives. Unfortunately, the Pap smear does not always find those important abnormal changes.

As a result, doctors developed a new visual screening examination called speculoscopy. This quick and painless new examination is done at the same time as the Pap smear, and the combined screening test is known as PapSure. Clinical studies in the United States and around the world have shown that combining these examinations can increase the doctor's ability to detect problems of the cervix. In fact, the studies show that more than twice as many abnormal changes of the cervix are found with PapSure than with the Pap smear test alone. A negative PapSure establishes cervical health (no disease present).

With the PapSure examination, you can be assured that you are receiving one of the most reliable gynecological screening exams available today for finding cervical abnormalities and reassuring women regarding the health of their cervix.

What Should I Know About the PPS Examination?

PapSure is a simple, fast, and painless examination. Your doctor begins by taking a routine Pap smear. Your Pap smear is sent to a laboratory selected by your doctor, where it is evaluated under a microscope as it is usually done. Next comes the speculoscopy examination. During this part of the examination, your doctor washes your cervix with a diluted vinegar solution. Then, with magnification and a special lighting device called Speculite, your doctor closely examines your cervix and is able to see potential abnormal changes on the cervix.

Why Is This Examination Important?

If an abnormal condition of the cervix exists, your doctor must find it as soon as possible. PapSure can assist your doctor or healthcare professional in finding potential problems earlier. With any questionable problems, the appropriate follow-up diagnostic tests or monitoring can be performed. If the test is negative, you can more reliably trust that the risk of missing disease on your cervix is less than if the Pap smear alone was performed.

How Reliable Is PapSure?

Although no screening test is 100% reliable, the combination of PapSure with the Pap smear is more reliable than the Pap smear alone for the detection of cervical abnormalities. If both the Pap test and the speculoscopy are negative, it is very unlikely that you have an abnormality on the cervix.

Is There Anything Else That I Should Know?

Yes. In order for your doctor or healthcare provider to see any possible cervical abnormalities, the room lights will be dimmed or turned off during the speculoscopy portion of your examination.

Continued

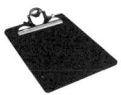 *Patient Education Handout—cont'd*

PAPSURE—cont'd

With the Speculite, any changes of the cervix are best seen with low-level lighting. To obtain the best results, do not put anything in the vagina for 3 days before the examination and avoid intercourse. You should not be on your period during the examination. If you have an infection in the vagina, it may have to be treated before speculoscopy is performed. If you are postmenopausal and not on estrogen, you may need to take some for a few weeks before the examination. Be sure to let your doctor know several weeks *before* you are seen.

How Long Will the Examination Take?

The time required to perform PapSure is usually no more than 5 minutes longer than your routine Pap smear examination.

What About Costs of the Procedure?

There will be a small additional fee for PapSure. However, the additional cost is well worth the peace of mind women feel knowing they have received one of the most reliable cervical screening examinations available today. Check with your insurance provider regarding coverage for this procedure.

How Do I Get PapSure?

Ask your nurse, doctor, or healthcare provider if he or she offers PapSure. If not, visit the manufacturer's website at www.papsure.com. The company may make this information available to your physician. You can also call PapSure at 1-800-486-8979 for more information.

How Do I Get Further Information?

Simply ask your nurse or doctor. He or she will be happy to answer questions you may have. You may obtain general information at www.papsure.com.

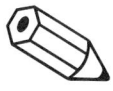

Patient Consent Form

PAPSURE

The Pap smear has been widely used for the detection of cervical cancer for the past 50 years. However, the Pap smear has limitations. The Pap smear is not as good at finding problems before they become cancer, when they are most easily and successfully treated.

PapSure is a new visual test, cleared by the FDA, that we can do along with your normal Pap smear. The new visual test gives us the best possible chance to find any cervical problems you may have, at the earliest possible stage.

Because most insurance companies are slow to look at new technologies, like PapSure, this examination is not yet covered by insurance. For now, there is a fee of $25 for a PapSure examination.

For our records, please indicate below whether or not you wish to have the PapSure examination:

YES please, I authorize my clinician to do the more accurate PapSure examination along with my normal Pap smear, and I accept financial responsibility for the visual examination, as noted above.

Print name: _____

Signature: _____ Date: _____

NO thank you, I would prefer not to have the PapSure examination:

Print name: _____

Signature: _____ Date: _____

(From Trylon Corp., Torrance, Calif.)

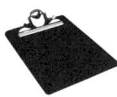 *Patient Education Handout*

EFUDEX PROTOCOL

As your doctor has explained, it is important to treat genital warts. Recent research indicates they are associated with cervical cancer in women. Women also have an increased risk of vaginal cancer and vulvar cancer, especially if they smoke. In men, there may be a slightly increased incidence of penile cancer and rectal cancer. Treatment with freezing or surgery can protect the cervix 97% of the time. Treatment of warts in other areas is difficult, and they can recur anytime no matter which of many treatments is used.

One of the drugs that has been used for your condition is Efudex. It is a cream that has been approved for use on the skin for several different precancerous lesions. However, the Food and Drug Administration has not approved Efudex for the treatment of genital warts. Even though many leaders in the field have used it for 15 years or more, it still must be considered somewhat experimental.

Both you and your partner should be evaluated with possible treatment afterward. There is approximately a 75% chance of the visible warts going away after this protocol. Approximately 4 to 8 weeks after starting Efudex, you will need to be reexamined. If you are found to be free of warts at the repeat examination, you will then need to use the Efudex once a month for 6 months. Other topical medicines, including Condylox and Aldara, are also available and may be used for you. The doctor may also recommend a variety of surgical procedures.

For Women

If there are warts in the vagina, you will need to use one third of a vaginal applicator of 5% Efudex cream (1.5 g) in the vagina at bedtime once a week for 10 weeks. You may notice that 5 to 6 days after using it, there will be some irritation, redness, swelling, and even some discharge. Nothing need be done unless you are extremely uncomfortable. You may want to put on some Vaseline ointment or Cortaid cream (over-the-counter) and apply it around the irritated areas on the outside of the vagina. If this does not help, you can call our office for further instructions. It is probably best to wear a pad to bed at night on the nights that you use Efudex cream in the vagina. You may want to douche it out the following morning. You can shower or bathe as usual. Intercourse is permitted when you are comfortable, but not on the night that you use it. Be sure to immediately wash off any cream that you may get on your hands or it will also cause irritation. If your doctor has indicated, you may want to put a very slight amount of the cream around external warts also. Two to four weeks after stopping the medication (three months after starting), you will need to be rechecked by your doctor. *Do not use the cream if you are pregnant.* If you had cryocautery (freezing), begin applying Efudex four weeks after having it done. *Do not use this cream more than once per week unless instructed to do so.*

For Men

If you have warts, they are most likely on the penis or around the rectum. Your doctor will describe exactly where he wants you to put the cream. You will also be using 5% Efudex cream, *applying it only once a week for 10 weeks.* Use very little cream, since this will cause a lot of irritation in some

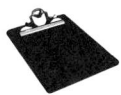

Patient Education Handout—cont'd

EFUDEX PROTOCOL—cont'd

people. If you do not have a severe reaction, it is okay to apply the cream on the penis and the rectum all on the same night. *If a reaction occurs, it usually does so on the fifth or sixth day after application.* You can use Vaseline or Cortaid cream or ointment to lessen this. It is also permissible to use ibuprofen to control the pain. If there is little reaction when using the cream every 7 days, try using it every 6 days.

The scrotum is extremely sensitive to this medication and must be protected. Either apply Vaseline first, or use an athletic supporter to cover the scrotum (cut out a hole for the penis).

After using the medication for 10 weeks, you will need to wait 2 to 4 weeks before being rechecked by the doctor. If he or she does not find any residual warts, you will need to use this cream in the same manner once a month for 6 months. If warts are found, your doctor will instruct you as to what to do next. If you and your partner are being treated at the same time, you do not need to use a condom. If your partner is not being treated, use a condom to protect her.

Summary of Instructions for Use of 5-FU (Efudex) Cream
- Do not use the 5-FU cream if you are pregnant.
- Use adequate birth control to prevent pregnancy!
- Avoid sex during nights of treatment.
- Have your sexual partner wear a condom during intercourse while being treated.
- If the treated area is irritated, postpone further applications of 5-FU until the irritation has subsided.
- If you experience severe irritation, please call your healthcare provider.
- Your condition is contagious. Examination of your sexual partner *may* be beneficial.
- Please call your healthcare provider if you need any of the prescription medications mentioned below.
- Stop smoking.
- Eat five helpings of fruit and vegetables per day.
- Take a good multivitamin with folic acid.
- Be monogamous.
- Women should have regular Pap smears.
- Call in 2 weeks for results of any biopsies.

Vaginal Lesions
- Insert an Ortho estrogen cream applicator one third full of 5-FU cream deeply into the vagina once a week at bedtime for 10 weeks.
- Anticipate a watery discharge during the time of treatment.

Continued

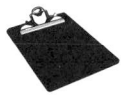

Patient Education Handout—cont'd

EFUDEX PROTOCOL—cont'd

Urethral Lesions (Opening Where the Urine Comes Out)

- Apply a small amount of 5-FU cream (just a dab will do) with a cotton-tipped applicator to the urethral opening and (if instructed) into the urethra once weekly at bedtime for 10 weeks. The urethra is the opening where urine comes out. Men may need to do this twice a day for a week.
- Anticipate irritation or burning during urination. If troublesome, apply 2% lidocaine jelly with a cotton-tipped applicator every 1 to 2 hours as necessary.

Vulvar (Lips) and Penile Skin/Scrotal Lesions

- Cleanse and dry the vulva (genital lips) carefully. Use a hair dryer to ensure dryness.
- Apply a small amount of 5-FU cream (¼ to ½ inch out of the tube) and massage into affected skin at bedtime once a week for 10 weeks.
- Cleanse and dry the treated area the next morning.
- Anticipate some irritation. If troublesome, take sitz baths three times a day and after each urination; apply Tucks pads to the irritated area as needed.

Perianal and Anorectal Lesions

- Cleanse and dry the anus carefully.
- Apply a small amount of 5-FU cream (¼ to ½ inch out of the tube) and massage into affected skin at bedtime once a week for 10 weeks.
- Cleanse and dry the treated area the next morning.
- Take Doxidan capsules 100 mg orally twice a day to keep stools soft.
- Anticipate anal/rectal irritation. If troublesome, apply Proctofoam HC or Anusol HC suppositories or cream and/or take sitz baths three times a day and after each bowel movement.

(Used with permission of The National Procedures Institute, Midland, Mich.)

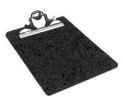 *Patient Education Handout*

SEXUAL ASSAULT

One out of every four women will be sexually assaulted in her lifetime. In the United States, one out of ten women will be assaulted each year. And it is not only women; almost 10 percent of sexual assault victims are male. As a victim of sexual assault, you are certainly not alone. Although every victim will have a unique response to the assault, there are feelings and reactions that are common for victims, and many of them are listed below. There are also stages most victims go through before reaching a stage where they can move forward with their life. Progressing through these stages can take from months to years. Obtaining help from an advocate or a professional counselor within the first 72 hours following an assault is one of the best ways to ensure recovery. You will also need a follow-up appointment with your clinician in the first 72 hours and again in about 1 or 2 weeks. Working as an advocate yourself and counseling other victims after you are through some of the first stages of this process can be very therapeutic for you.

Fear. Not only were you afraid during the assault, but you may also have persistent fears, including a fear of going out in public, a fear for your safety, a fear of being around men, a fear of being alone, and a fear of reporting the crime. Your fear may be especially strong if you know the assailant and are afraid of this happening again or of any retribution for reporting the crime. You may even have a fear for the assailant about what will happen to them. Talking about these fears will help, whether it is to your advocate, the law enforcement officer, someone you trust, your counselor, or your clinician. Don't ignore these fears; the more that you talk about them to a trained and trusted listener, the faster some of these feelings will subside.

Flashbacks, anxiety, and nightmares. Similar to individuals with posttraumatic stress disorder, you may have flashbacks of painful memories whenever you are exposed to even small reminders of the assault. You may be anxious, startle easily, and have recurrent nightmares about the assault. Counseling and medications can help with these symptoms and also improve your sleep.

Moodiness. For some time, your feelings and emotions may go through dramatic swings with little warning. It may be difficult to control these emotions. This is normal after any assault, especially a sexual assault. Part of you is grieving the loss of the sense of safety and security in your life. You have been violated. Talking about these feelings will help.

Anger. Rage and anger are common emotions following sexual assault. When you are able to feel them, it may actually be a sign that you are healing. The anger and rage may be toward the attacker, toward anyone involved in the situation, or even toward yourself. If you have strong feelings of wanting to hurt someone or yourself, tell your clinician or seek help from a counselor. Talking to someone you trust may help you to uncover these feelings as well as to experience them safely.

Guilt or shame. You may have feelings that in some way the assault was your fault, that you may have done something to provoke it, or that you should have done more to prevent it. However, keep in mind that sexual assault is an assault crime like any other violent assault crime. It just happens to be a crime where some of the weapons used are the sex organs. Also, it is important to know that certain of your body's responses are uncontrollable with physical contact. You should not feel guilty or ashamed if part of your body responded or became physically aroused during the assault.

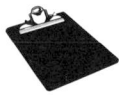

Patient Education Handout—cont'd

SEXUAL ASSAULT—cont'd

Sexual difficulties. After a sexual assault, you may have a loss of interest in sex, strong feelings of fear during sex, difficulty becoming aroused, discomfort during sex, and difficulty achieving orgasm, even with a trusted, supportive partner. Counseling will help with these problems. Time will also help. Remember it is normal to not be interested in sex immediately after a sexual assault. You must feel safe to have a satisfying sex life following an assault. When you feel like being active again, make sure that you are with someone you trust and someone you can talk to about any difficulties with sex.

Physical symptoms. After a sexual assault, you may fatigue very easily for months. It is not unusual to have headaches, body aches, or abdominal or pelvic symptoms or pain. Insomnia is common and depression may occur. After time, these symptoms will get better. Again, counseling is very important and helpful. Medications may be useful. Your clinician can reassure you against any dangerous medical problems.

To find out more about sexual assault or to talk to a counselor, talk to your clinician or call the Rape Abuse and Incest National Network Hotline (RAINN) at 1-800-656-HOPE. Information is also available online at www.rainn.org.

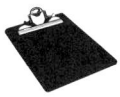

General Patient Consent Form/Forensic Evaluation

I am under the care of my clinician, _____, on _____ (date). I hereby authorize him or her to perform a medical forensic examination, collection of evidence, and treatment. We have discussed the different steps of the evaluation and the limitations involved. I further permit the photographic documentation and release of copies, as well as the complete report, to the law enforcement agency. In addition to my clinician, someone else will be in the room at all times during the evaluation.

I understand that there may be some discomfort with this evaluation. For women, it may include a Pap smear and a pelvic examination, an evaluation with a colposcope, a rectal examination, and a proctoscopic examination. We have discussed the different outcomes that could occur and most of the possible complications, including failure to obtain evidence that will be useful in court or adequate to convict someone, and failure to diagnose an injury or a sexually transmitted disease (or pregnancy in women). I may have some bleeding from any lacerations or trauma that happened during the assault, and I am aware that there are other rare complications that could occur that we could not foresee.

I have read and understand the patient education handout. I agree to follow the instructions for self-care after the procedure and to return for follow-up care on _____. All of my questions have been answered.

My signature below releases _____ (name of clinic or hospital) and its representatives from legal responsibility or liability for the release of this information. I also authorize a request for payment for this forensic evidence examination from the law enforcement jurisdiction to which the crime is reported.

I will call the office or answering service if any problems occur.

_____   _____
Patient's signature   *Date/Time*

_____   _____
Witness' signature   *Clinician's signature*

One copy for chart; one copy for patient.

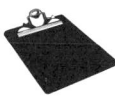 *Patient Education Handout*

SEXUAL ABUSE

How Does a Sexual Abuse Investigation Take Place?

The examination performed on your child will be part of an evaluation for possible sexual abuse. The other portions of the sexual abuse evaluation include interviews by a Protective Services worker and/or a law enforcement officer.

It is usually not possible to be certain whether sexual abuse has occurred until all portions of the evaluation are complete. Usually the physical examination takes place early in the evaluation so that what is found at the physical examination can assist in the remainder of the evaluation. We strongly recommend that you fully cooperate with the other investigating professionals for the remainder of the evaluation.

Today's findings will be made available to the Protective Services worker or the law enforcement officer when all results have returned from the laboratory. Although those results are usually sent via written report, we sometimes call the investigating professional immediately. Many states require this by law.

It is the responsibility of Protective Services or law enforcement to put all available evidence together and then decide whether to recommend to the judge that prosecution be pursued. Although you may have a very strong opinion about prosecution, the available evidence must be so strong that it would stand up in a court of law. If you have questions about this process and decision, please contact a Protective Services worker or a law enforcement officer.

Will Additional Treatment or Medical Examinations Be Necessary?

This office will contact you if your child requires any additional treatment or evaluation based upon the history, examination and lab results.

Will There Be Any Complications from Today's Examination?

It is unlikely that your child will complain of any problems resulting from the examination today. If any concerns arise, please feel free to call this office.

Other Services Available

Counseling for you or your child is often available through the Protective Services worker or law enforcement officer who is working with your child.

Special Instructions: An Examination with Sedation

If your child will be sedated during the examination, please make certain that you understand instructions for her care until she is completely awake.

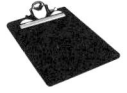

Patient Education Handout

VULVAR BIOPSY

What Is the Name of the Procedure?

The procedure is vulvar biopsy. The vulva are tissues around the vagina that many people call "the lips."

Why Do I Need This Procedure?

There is an abnormal growth or rash of the skin in the genital area.

What Are the Benefits of This Procedure?

The procedure can be done in the office, helps to clarify the diagnosis, and helps plan future therapy. Actually the biopsy may remove the entire growth if it is small.

How Do I Prepare for a Vulvar Biopsy?

No specific preparation is needed. You may want to take two Tylenol or 600 mg of ibuprofen just before coming to the doctor's office (do not take if you are allergic).

What Happens During the Procedure?

Your doctor will look at the skin of the vulvar area and clean the area off with some soap. Your doctor will then numb skin and remove a piece of the skin with a biopsy instrument or with a scalpel, depending on how big the area is. There should be very little pain.

What Happens After the Procedure?

You will have some mild discomfort that can be treated with over-the-counter pain medications, warm-water sitz baths, or sometimes ointments. You will need to wear a panty liner since the materials used to stop any bleeding can stain your underwear.

What Are the Risks Associated with This Procedure?

Light bleeding, heavy bleeding (rare) that may require a stitch, pain during the procedure or afterwards, infection of biopsy site, bleeding, bruising, pigment changes at the biopsy site (lightened or darkened skin), and scar formation. If the entire growth is not removed, it's also possible the worst area won't be biopsied, leading to more treatment later.

What Do I Need to Do Following the Procedure to Prevent Infection?

Avoid intercourse for about 3 days. Keep the area clean. Apply a topical antibiotic ointment two times a day until healed.

When Should I Call My Healthcare Provider?

Call if signs of infection occur, such as redness, swelling, increased pain, or foul-smelling discharge. Also call if the growths come back. If you are diagnosed with genital warts, be sure to have a Pap smear at least once a year.

Special Instructions:

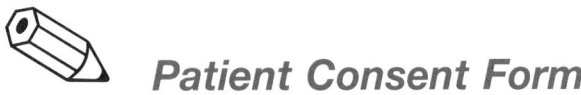 *Patient Consent Form*

VULVAR BIOPSY

I came to the office today to see Dr._____ for a vulvar biopsy for the following condition(s):

☐ Pigmented lesion ☐ Rash of the vulva ☐ Other (specify) _____

I understand that it can be difficult to tell the difference between normal and abnormal skin changes in the vulvar area. My doctor feels that a biopsy is necessary to help determine whether the lesion noted above is normal or abnormal. A biopsy can help determine the correct diagnosis.

We discussed the different treatments possible, and discussed the risks of not treating the condition. Based on the advice given by Dr. _____ and my own judgment, I agree to undergo a vulvar biopsy.

I understand that the skin will be cleaned with a soap solution and then may be anesthetized with an anesthetic gel and an injection of Xylocaine to make the skin numb. A piece of skin will be removed with a biopsy instrument. Stitches may be needed to close the skin. Bleeding will be controlled with a thickened iron solution or with chemical tipped sticks as needed. I will need to keep the area clean and apply antibiotic ointment (unless allergic) twice a day until healing is complete, usually about 7 days.

I have been informed and understand that the following are possible risks associated with the procedure: light bleeding, heavy bleeding (rare) that may require a stitch; pain during the procedure or afterwards; infection of biopsy site; pigment changes at the biopsy site (lightened or darkened skin); scar formation; and not obtaining an accurate diagnosis unless all the abnormal area was removed.

I have been informed that the procedure helps to clarify the diagnosis and to plan future therapy and follow-up.

We have discussed the different risks and benefits of vulva biopsy, and I am aware that other complications could occur that we could not foresee. I agree to follow the instructions for self-care after the procedure and to return for follow-up care on _____. I will call the office or answering service if any problems arise before the scheduled follow-up visit. I have read and understand this information, and I have had all questions and consent to having a vulvar biopsy.

_____
Patient's signature

_____
Witness' signature

_____
Date/Time

_____
Clinician's signature

One copy for chart; one copy for patient.

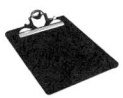

Patient Education Handout

FOLLOWING AMNIOCENTESIS

Rest as much as possible and avoid heavy lifting or prolonged standing for the rest of the day. Normal light activities are permitted, but avoid more strenuous tasks such as using a vacuum cleaner or wet mop or moving furniture. Also avoid heavy yard or garden work. You should not have intercourse for 24 hours.

Report any of the following problems to your clinician immediately:

- Abdominal pain or bleeding from the needle mark
- Vaginal bleeding
- Leaking of fluid from the vagina
- Fever or chills
- Feeling of weakness or faintness
- Baby not moving when stimulated
- Labor pains or contractions

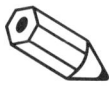 *Patient Consent Form*

AMNIOCENTESIS

I, _____, agree to the performance of an amniocentesis by my clinician, _____, and his or her associates. I understand that amniocentesis involves inserting a needle through my abdominal wall into the fluid that surrounds my baby and taking a sample of that fluid.

Although amniocentesis is a common procedure, complications can occur. I understand that although the clinician will use the utmost care when performing the amniocentesis, I (or the baby) could be harmed. Although unlikely, it is possible to introduce infection into the uterus (i.e., womb), to puncture the umbilical cord and cause bleeding from the cord, to cause premature rupture of membranes or premature labor or both, and to cause the afterbirth (i.e., placenta) to separate prematurely (possibly causing my death or the death of my baby). I realize that there are other possible complications that we could not foresee. The alternatives for care have been explained to me and all of my questions have been answered.

I am having the amniocentesis because _____.

_____   _____
Patient's signature   *Date/Time*

_____
Witness' signature

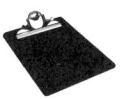 *Patient Education Handout*

CONTRACTION STRESS TEST

Your clinician has recommended a test to evaluate your baby's health. This test, the contraction stress test, monitors your baby's response to contractions of your uterus. A normal contraction stress test provides some reassurance that your baby is currently healthy. The results of this test will help guide your treatment plan.

The uterine contractions associated with this test may occur spontaneously or it may be necessary to stimulate your nipples to produce a natural hormone. This hormone should cause contractions. If there are still no contractions, a small amount of a synthetic hormone may need to be administered into one of your veins. This medicine, oxytocin, resembles the natural hormone in your body. A pumping device may be used with the IV to carefully control the amount of medicine you receive. Your baby's heart rate will be followed on a monitor while you have the contractions. Your contractions will also be monitored.

It is advisable to not eat a large meal for 2 to 3 hours before this procedure in the event that your clinician needs to induce your labor following this test. After completion of this test, you should receive not only the results, but also some instructions regarding follow-up plans or appointments.

A "negative" or normal contraction stress test occurs if your baby does not experience any slowing of its heartbeat following contractions of your uterus. The test will be regarded as "positive" or "suspicious" if your baby's heartbeat becomes slower after some or all of the contractions of your uterus. There is one pattern of slow heartbeats that is of more concern than others. Your clinician will monitor closely for this pattern.

Please tell your medical provider, before undergoing the test, if you are ill or experiencing any symptoms, because this could lead to a false-positive or abnormal test result. There is a small risk (about 1 to 3 out of 100 tests) that your uterus will contract too frequently or too strongly. If that happens, we may need to give you an injection to slow down these contractions. Very rarely, the contractions will not be able to be stopped, so you and your baby will need an intervention (e.g., cesarean section) or you will progress into labor and deliver your baby.

Special Instructions

Please contact your medical provider for any concerns that may arise out of this test or your pregnancy in general.

Website That May Be of Interest to You:

www.nlm.nih.gov/medlineplus/ency/article/003405.htm (fetal heart monitoring)
www.med.umich.edu/1libr/crs/strstst.htm (contraction stress test)

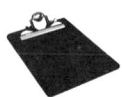 *Patient Education Handout*

FETAL-MOVEMENT COUNTING

A large medical study has shown that mothers may be able to protect their baby's health by spending some time each day counting the number of times the baby moves. This simple process is called *fetal-movement counting.*

Find a comfortable position on your left side. Count every time your baby moves, which may be felt as a kick, flutter, swish, or roll. If the baby rolls, kicks, and punches all in the same motion, it should be counted as three fetal movements. *Continue counting until you have felt your baby move 10 times and then record the time it took for this to happen.* Although this may take up to 1 hour, often it will occur within 20 minutes.

Note: If you have counted six movements in 15 minutes, you can quit counting. In that situation, you will almost always note 10 movements in less than an hour.

We would like for you to perform this count perhaps two to three times a week. Your clinician will tell you at what point during the pregnancy to start the counting. They will also tell you if you should do it more frequently than two to three times a week. *Make a chart and note the date, time of day, and amount of time* it took you to count the 10 movements. Try to start this at the same time each day, when the baby is usually most active. For many pregnancies, this is during the evening.

If 2 hours go by without the baby moving 10 times, please contact your clinician or go to your hospital's labor suite for further evaluation.

When you follow these instructions, it may result in a visit to your hospital labor suite. It may even result in an unnecessary intervention. However, your clinician will do everything possible to avoid that. In addition, by checking your baby's movements, you may be given an increased sense of security as well as an early alert for you and your clinician to possible problems. Bring your fetal-movement counting chart with you at each office visit.

Website That May Be of Interest to You:

uuhsc.utah.edu/pated/handouts/pdfs/handout728.pdf (fetal movement counts)

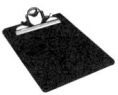

Patient Education Handout

NONSTRESS TEST

Your clinician has recommended a nonstress test to check on your baby's health. This test is accomplished by using a special monitor to measure and record your baby's heart rate. Performing the test will not hurt you, and it will not harm your baby.

You will be asked to let the nurse know when you feel your baby move, or you may be asked to push a button with each movement. If your baby's heart rate becomes faster shortly after you feel your baby move, this will be regarded as a normal, reassuring nonstress test. Your clinician will then determine whether additional nonstress tests are needed.

If your baby's heart rate does not increase shortly after you feel movements, it may mean that your baby is asleep or hungry. For this reason, you should not take any type of pain or sleeping medication for at least 6 hours before this test. Make sure you eat within at least 4 hours before this test. Your clinician should be told about all prescription or over-the-counter medications you are taking. Tell your clinician if you have had an ultrasound during this pregnancy, especially if it was abnormal. You may be asked to drink sweetened fruit juice or to extend the time of testing to reach a conclusion that provides you and your clinician with accurate, reassuring information. Your clinician may also use a buzzer to wake up the baby. It will not harm your baby. Please do not smoke for at least 2 hours before arriving. The whole test may only take 30 to 40 minutes, but sometimes it may last up to 2 hours.

If the nonstress test does not provide the reassurance the clinician is seeking about your baby's health, your clinician will discuss additional options, and possibly further testing, to learn more about your baby's health.

Website That May Be of Interest to You:

www.madonnaperinatal.com/mps-fetaleval.html (fetal evaluations)

www.med.umich.edu/1libr/tests/testn05.htm (non-stress test, amniotic fluid index biophysical profile)

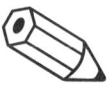 *Patient Consent Form*

CONTRACTION STRESS TEST

I came to the office of my clinician, _____, or to _____ (hospital) on _____ (date) for evaluation and treatment of the following condition(s):

We discussed the different evaluation and treatment methods available as well as the risks of not evaluating or treating the condition. Based on the advice given by my clinician, _____, and my own judgment, I agree to undergo a contraction stress test (CST).

Using either breast self-stimulation or an intravenous administration of oxytocin, I will begin to have regular uterine contractions (about three per 10 minutes). I will undergo continuous monitoring of these contractions and my baby's heartbeats. The purpose of this test is to see how my baby responds and tolerates these contractions.

We discussed the different outcomes that could occur and most of the possible complications. The most common complication is excessive uterine stimulation, which occurs in about 1 to 3 of every 100 tests. Medicine is available to treat this complication if it were to arise. Very rarely, the contractions will not be able to be stopped and I will need an intervention (e.g., cesarean section) or I will deliver my baby. One other possible complication is a falsely abnormal test resulting in unnecessary interventions. However, your clinician will use every effort to avoid this complication. The CST is the most commonly used technique to evaluate the function of the placenta and it has been used the longest. I am aware that other complications could occur that we could not foresee. As with all tests during pregnancy, this test, even if normal, cannot guarantee that everything is all right with my baby. I agree to follow the instructions for self-care after the test and to return for follow-up care on _____.

I will call the office or answering service if any problems arise before or after the scheduled follow-up visit.

_____
Patient's signature

_____
Date/Time

_____
Witness' signature

_____
Clinician's signature

One copy for chart; one copy for patient.

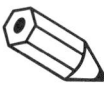 *Patient Consent Form*

FETAL-MOVEMENT COUNTING

As recommended by my clinician, I have agreed to periodically evaluate how frequently my baby is moving. This can be done on my own time and in my own home. This evaluation is called fetal-movement counting (FMC) and is being done for the following indication(s):

My clinician(s) and I have discussed the usefulness of this evaluation. I agree to follow the recommendations set forth on the attached paper to perform FMC. If I have not felt my baby move at least 10 times during a 2-hour period, I will either contact my clinician or go to the labor and delivery area for further evaluation of my baby.

We discussed the different outcomes that could occur and most of the possible complications. One possible complication is a falsely abnormal test resulting in unnecessary interventions. Your clinician will make every effort to avoid this complication. I am aware that other complications could occur that we could not foresee. As with all tests during pregnancy, this test, even if normal, cannot guarantee that everything is all right with my baby. I agree to follow the instructions for self-care after the procedure, to write down my results, and to return with the results for follow-up care on _____ (date).

All of my questions have been answered and I will call the office or answering service if any problems arise before the scheduled follow-up visit.

_____
Patient's signature

_____
Date/Time

_____
Witness' signature

_____
Clinician's signature

One copy for chart, one copy for patient.

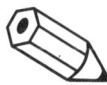 *Patient Consent Form*

NONSTRESS TEST

I came to the office or labor and delivery unit of my clinician, on _____ (date) for evaluation and treatment of the following condition:

We discussed the different evaluation and treatment methods available as well as the risks of not evaluating or treating the condition. Based on the advice given by my clinician, and my own judgment, I agree to undergo a nonstress test.

During this test, my baby will be evaluated using a machine called an electronic fetal monitor. Every time I feel my baby move, I should notify the nursing staff in the manner that they suggest. This usually means pushing a button. This test may take a short time if my baby is moving a lot or it may take up to 1 or 2 hours.

We discussed the different outcomes that could occur and most of the possible complications. One possible complication is a falsely abnormal test resulting in unnecessary interventions. Your clinician will use every effort to avoid this complication. (However, if the test result is normal, it is very reassuring [997 out of 1000] that the baby is getting enough oxygen.) The accuracy of the test is somewhat variable, depending on the reason the test is being used. For that reason an accuracy is not stated. I am aware that other complications could occur that we could not foresee. As with all tests during pregnancy, this test, even if normal, cannot guarantee that everything is all right with my baby. I agree to follow the instructions for self-care after the procedure and to return for follow-up care on _____ (date). I will call the office or answering service if any problems arise before the scheduled follow-up visit.

_____   _____
Patient's signature   *Date/Time*

_____   _____
Witness' signature   *Clinician's signature*

One copy for chart, one copy for patient.

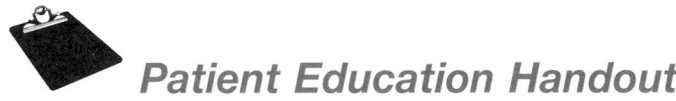
Patient Education Handout

EXTERNAL CEPHALIC VERSION (ECV)

What is External Cephalic Version (ECV)?

ECV is a way to try to turn a baby from breech position (i.e., buttocks down instead of head down) to vertex position (i.e., head down) while it is still in the mother's uterus (womb).

Why Do I Need This Procedure?

Before birth, most babies are in a head-down position in the mother's uterus. However, sometimes the baby's position is reversed; this is called a breech baby or breech birth. Many obstetric providers believe that the vaginal delivery of a breech baby can lead to more complications. As a result, a cesarean section is often recommended to avoid these complications. If the ECV procedure is tried and the baby is turned to the normal head-down position, a cesarean section may not be needed.

How Do I Prepare for ECV?

Avoid eating any heavy foods for 3 hours before the procedure.

What Happens During the Procedure?

ECV is usually performed in the hospital. Before the procedure, you will have an ultrasound to confirm that the baby is breech. The clinician will also do a nonstress test (monitor the baby's heart rate) to make sure it is normal. A tube of blood will be drawn, and an anesthesiologist will be notified in case an emergency cesarean delivery is required. Next, you will be given medicine through a vein in the arm to relax the uterus. This medicine is very safe, with almost no risk to you or your baby. You will be asked to lie down, and your abdomen will be coated with ultrasound gel. Then the clinician will place his or her hands on the outside of the abdomen. After locating the baby's head, the clinician will gently try to turn the baby to the vertex position.

What Happens After the Procedure?

When the procedure is completed, the clinician will perform another nonstress test and ultrasound. If everything is normal, there is no need to stay in the hospital. The clinician will show you how to check daily for reversion to breech.

If the procedure is not successful or the baby reverts, the clinician may suggest repeating the ECV at another time. The clinician may also talk to you about the possibility of having a vaginal delivery or a cesarean section.

What Are the Benefits of This Procedure?

If ECV is successful a cesarean section can be avoided in many cases.

What Are the Risks Associated With This Procedure?

The chance of a complication is very small (about 1%). However, the following are possible:
- Premature labor
- Premature rupture of the membranes
- Fetal distress leading to an emergency cesarean section
- Baby might turn back to the breech position after the ECV

When Should I Call My Healthcare Provider?

- If there is premature rupture of membranes (leaking of fluid from your vagina)
- If labor begins
- If your daily check reveals that the baby has turned back to a breech position

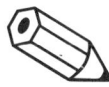 *Patient Consent Form*

EXTERNAL CEPHALIC VERSION (ECV)

I came to the office of my clinician, _____, on _____ (date) for evaluation and treatment of breech presentation.

We discussed the different treatments possible, and discussed the risks of not treating the condition. Based on the advice given my clinician, _____, and my own judgment, I agree to undergo external cephalic version (ECV). The clinician, using his or her hands on the outside of my abdomen, will attempt to turn the fetus from a breech presentation to a vertex presentation. The procedure will be monitored with an ultrasound machine.

We discussed the different outcomes that could occur and most of the possible complications. I am aware that other complications could occur that we could not foresee. I agree to follow the instructions for self-care after the procedure and to return for follow-up care on _____.

I will call the office or answering service if any problems arise before the scheduled follow-up visit.

_____   _____
Patient's signature   *Date/Time*

_____   _____
Witness' signature   *Clinician's signature*

One copy for chart, one copy for patient.

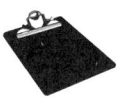

Patient Education Handout

INTRATHECAL NARCOTIC ANALGESIA

Your clinician may offer intrathecal narcotic analgesia to improve your comfort during labor. The procedure involves administering pain medication into the spinal canal with a needle. Because the medication acts directly on pain receptors in the spinal canal, less medication is needed than when it is given through your blood stream (intravenously) or muscles (intramuscularly). The low dose of medication is almost always safe for you and your baby. However, you should know that any analgesic/anesthesia during labor is optional and does have certain risks. It is not necessary to have any procedure for analgesia/anesthesia in order to have a healthy baby.

In preparation for this procedure, you will be either lying on your left side or sitting, with your back arched toward your clinician. A cleansing solution will then be used on your back to prevent infection. Next, your clinician will use a local anesthetic to numb the skin of your lower back. A long, narrow needle will then be inserted into the spinal canal to inject the medication.

When your clinician removes the needle, you will be asked to remain on your left side, or move to your left side if initially sitting. You will be in this position for up to 15 minutes to facilitate blood flow to the baby. After this time, you will be able to move to a more comfortable position.

You can expect pain relief in 5 to 10 minutes. Depending on the medications used, you will have some pain relief for 2 to 6 hours. Once you are fully dilated and are able to push, the medicine gradually loses its effectiveness.

The most common side effect of this procedure is itching, which occurs in over 90% of patients. This can be treated with IV medication if desired. Less common side effects include nausea and vomiting, which can also be treated with IV medication. Occasionally patients will need to have a urinary catheter placed. Approximately 5% of patients experience headaches. This, too, is treatable. Your nurse will be monitoring your breathing, since this can be affected (rarely [<1%]) by the medication; if affected, it will be treated.

After delivery, you will be given a pill to reverse the effects of the medication, also preventing further side effects.

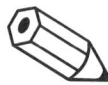 *Patient Consent Form*

INTRATHECAL ANALGESIA

1. Upon my authorization and consent, I understand this procedure may be performed on me by my clinician and/or his or her assistants.

2. My clinician has explained to me the potential benefits of the procedure and that it may involve risk of complications, injury or even death of myself (or the baby if pregnant), from both known and unknown causes. No warranty or guarantee as to the results has been made. I recognize that I have the right to consent to or refuse the proposed procedure at any time prior to its performance. I have received and read a patient education handout about intrathecal analgesia.

3. I have received a detailed explanation of this procedure from my clinician, including limitations, alternatives, and possible risks that include but are not limited to toxicity from the medication, pain, infection, bleeding, blood clots, nausea, vomiting, aspiration, urinary retention and cardiac dysrhythmias (abnormal heart beat) for myself or my baby if I'm pregnant. The most common side effect is itching, which can be treated with medications, if desired. Other complications may occur that are not foreseen.

4. I understand that the procedure may fail and/or possible complications may require additional procedures.

5. I understand that during the procedure I will be either sitting up or lying down on my left side.

6. My signature on this form indicates that:
   - I have read and understand the information provided in this form and in the handout
   - The procedure set forth above has been adequately explained to me by my clinician
   - I have had the chance to ask questions and they have all been answered
   - I have received all the information I desire concerning the procedure and alternatives
   - I authorize and consent to the performance of the procedure

_____   _____

Patient's signature   *Date/Time*
(or parent/guardian; indicate if other than patient)

_____   _____

Witness' signature   *Clinician's signature*

If patient is unable to sign, indicate reason:

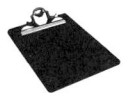

Patient Education Handout

OBSTETRIC ULTRASOUND

Why Do I Need an Obstetric Ultrasound?

Your clinician has recommended an ultrasound examination. There are many reasons why pregnant women undergo sonography. Most often, sonograms are performed at the request of a woman's clinician because the clinician would like to answer a question regarding your pregnancy. If you have questions at any time during the procedure, please feel free to ask.

How Do I Prepare for the Procedure?

Occasionally, the clinician or sonographer will require you to have a full bladder before a sonogram is performed. A full bladder is usually needed for scanning during the first 3 months of pregnancy but not after this time.

What Happens During a Sonogram?

The obstetric ultrasound procedure involves placing a gel on your skin and scanning the abdomen with a device to visualize the uterus and your baby. The ultrasound emits sound waves that will enter your body and be reflected back to form an image of the pregnancy. Occasionally, a probe with a sheath on it will be inserted into your vagina. This allows for clearer pictures to be obtained, especially early in pregnancy.

What Happens After the Procedure?

Because the test is noninvasive and requires no medication, usually you may go home as soon as the procedure is completed. A report of the findings will be sent to your clinician, who will discuss the findings with you.

What Are the Benefits of the Procedure?

Sonography is a completely noninvasive procedure that allows the clinician or sonographer to visualize your pregnancy. In most studies, the following information about your pregnancy is gathered: (1) dating of the pregnancy, (2) growth, (3) presence of a fetal heart beat, (4) fetal number (single baby vs twins, etc.), (5) the amount of amniotic fluid, (6) the location of the placenta and fetal head, and (7) whether there are any gross fetal problems or anomalies (large birth defects). A normal basic scan performed today is not intended to guarantee the absence of birth defects. A 2% to 5% risk for birth defects is still present (as in the general population) despite a normal basic scan.

What Are the Risks Associated With This Procedure?

Currently, there are no known harmful effects from sonography to either the mother or to the fetus.

Will I Know the Sex of the Baby?

National guidelines for ultrasound do not list determining the baby's sex as an indication for ultrasound.

Continued

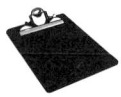 *Patient Education Handout—cont'd*

OBSTETRIC ULTRASOUND—cont'd

What Do I Need to Do Related to This Procedure to Prevent Infection?

There is no risk of infection associated with this procedure.

When Should I Call My Healthcare Provider Regarding This Study?

Generally, your healthcare provider will contact you or discuss the results at your next visit following an ultrasound. However, if you have not heard from your clinician within 1 week of the examination or if you do not have an appointment scheduled within 3 weeks, contact the office.

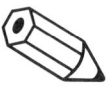 *Patient Consent Form*

OBSTETRIC ULTRASOUND

Your clinician has recommended that you undergo an ultrasound examination. The obstetric ultrasound procedure involves placing a gel on your skin and scanning the abdomen with a device to visualize your uterus and baby. Occasionally, a probe with a sheath on it will be inserted into your vagina to obtain clearer pictures. The ultrasound device emits sound waves that will enter your body and be reflected back to form an image of the pregnancy.

The test is noninvasive and requires no medication. Currently, there are no known harmful effects from sonography to either you or your fetus.

Sonography allows the clinician or sonographer to visualize your pregnancy, as well as some of the organs around it. In most studies, the following information about your pregnancy is gathered: (1) dating of the pregnancy, (2) growth, (3) presence of a fetal heart beat, (4) fetal number (single baby vs twins, etc.), (5) the amount of amniotic fluid, (6) the location of the placenta and fetal head, and (7) whether there are any gross fetal problems or anomalies (large birth defects). A normal basic scan performed today is not intended to guarantee the absence of birth defects. A 2% to 5% risk for birth defects is still present (as in the general population) despite a normal basic scan.

I have read and understand the above information. Based on the recommendation of my clinician, _____, and my own judgment, I agree to undergo the procedure.

_____   _____
Patient's signature   *Date/Time*

_____   _____
Witness' signature   *Clinician's signature*

One copy for chart; one copy for patient.

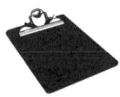 *Patient Education Handout*

PARACERVICAL BLOCK

Your clinician may offer a choice of techniques to increase your comfort during the birth of your child or during or after your surgery, including a paracervical block. If this procedure is used with childbirth, you should know that it is an optional procedure and does carry certain risks. It is not necessary to have any procedure for analgesia/anesthesia in order to have a healthy baby.

A paracervical block involves injecting a dose(s) of local anesthetic through the skin inside the vagina where it meets the cervix (opening of the womb). If effective, this anesthesia will decrease the sensations you would normally experience during your surgery or, if you are in labor, the contractions as your cervix dilates.

You will be put into the same position as for a Pap smear (in stirrups). Next, the area will be cleansed with an antibacterial solution (e.g., Betadine) to prevent infection.

If you are pregnant, your clinician will then insert two fingers into your vagina, just like when he or she examines your cervix and ovaries during a well-woman examination after the speculum has been removed. This will be followed by the injection of a local anesthetic into the skin high inside the vagina where it meets the cervix. An injection(s) will then be made slightly deeper to anesthetize the cervix for the procedure or for labor. You will then be allowed to get out of the stirrups.

If you are not pregnant, a speculum may be inserted, just like for a Pap smear, and the injection may be made with the speculum in place.

Although most patients do not have any side effects from the injection, several side effects can occur. Your blood pressure and pulse rate may rise or drop, you may feel nervous or unusual, or you may start to feel numbness and tingling sensations in your legs, feet, or other parts of your body. This is extremely rare, but be sure to inform your clinician immediately if you notice any unusual symptoms after the injection. Your clinician is prepared to treat any of these side effects, promptly and safely.

During pregnancy, fetal heart rate changes can occur with a paracervical block. However, there is generally no adverse outcome unless the infant is delivered while the heart rate is abnormal. There is the slight risk of injecting the infant, but the clinician will do everything possible to prevent this from happening. There is also a slight risk of prolonging labor.

Whenever a patient undergoes an injection, there is also the possibility of local infection and bleeding. There is also the possibility of nerve damage from pressure on a nerve.

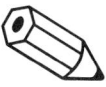 *Patient Consent Form*

PARACERVICAL BLOCK

1. My clinician, _____, has offered the paracervical block.
2. Upon my authorization and consent, I understand this procedure will be performed on me.
3. My clinician has explained the potential benefits of the procedure and that it may involve risk of complications, injury, or even death, from both known and unknown causes. No warranty or guarantee as to the results has been made. I recognize that I have the right to consent to or to refuse the proposed procedure at any time before its performance. I have received and read the patient education handout about paracervical block.
4. I have received a detailed explanation of this procedure from my clinician including limitations, alternatives, and possible risks that include but are not limited to toxicity from the medication, pain, infection, bleeding, blood clots, and cardiac dysrhythmias (abnormal heart beat) for myself or my baby if I am pregnant.
5. I understand that the procedure may fail and/or possible complications may require additional procedures.
6. I understand that during the procedure I will be placed in a lying down position, in stirrups.
7. My signature on this form indicates the following:
• I have read and understand the information provided with this form
• The procedure set forth above has been adequately explained to me by my clinician
• I have had the chance to ask questions and they have all been answered
• I have received all the information I desire concerning the procedure and alternatives
• I authorize and consent to the performance of the procedure by my clinician and/or his or her assistants

_____
Patient's signature
(or parent/guardian; indicate if other than patient)

_____
Witness' signature

If patient is unable to sign, indicate reason:

_____
Date/Time

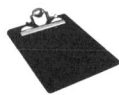 *Patient Education Handout*

SADDLE BLOCK ANESTHESIA

Your clinician may offer a choice of procedures to increase your comfort during the birth of your child or your surgery. If used with childbirth, you should know that these procedures are optional and do carry certain risks. It is not necessary to have these procedures to have a healthy baby.

In obstetrics, saddle block anesthesia is administered only during the final stages of labor, just before the baby's birth. The procedure is performed by injecting a small dose of local anesthetic into the spinal canal. If you are very uncomfortable earlier in labor, you should consider other procedures to minimize the discomfort (continuous spinal or epidural analgesia).

Saddle block anesthesia is administered while you are in the sitting position. Your back should be arched toward the clinician. An assistant will help you get positioned and stay with you during the performance of the procedure.

At the beginning of the procedure, your clinician will press on your lower back to determine the exact location for the injection. An anti-bacterial solution is then applied to prevent infection. Next, a local anesthetic is injected into the skin to numb the area for insertion of the saddle block needle. The saddle block needle is then inserted and directed into the spinal canal. When that needle is in the canal, the clinician will inject the medication and ask you to remain in the sitting position for several minutes.

Shortly after the medication is injected, as the anesthesia moves down the spinal cord, you will feel numbness and tingling and then total loss of sensation in the genital area. You will then be placed in the stirrups in preparation for surgery or delivery of your baby. While the anesthetic is working, you may not be able to move your legs; however, this effect will wear off soon.

There is always the risk of bruising, bleeding, or infection at the site of such a procedure. Several side effects can also occur as a result of this procedure. Your blood pressure may drop, you may become nauseated and vomit, or the anesthesia may extend beyond the saddle block area. On rare occasions, the anesthesia has been reported to extend considerably higher and interfere with the ability to breathe. Allergic reactions are unusual, and problems with heart rhythms are very rare. Your clinician is prepared to treat any of these side effects promptly and safely.

Postoperative side effects include (1) headache and (2) inability to urinate voluntarily. Headaches are usually treated successfully with medication, fluid intake, and rest. Occasionally headaches are severe and require another injection into the area where the spinal (saddle block) needle was originally inserted. Urinary retention may require temporary placement of a urinary catheter. On rare occasions, more serious, permanent effects may occur, including inflammation of the lining of the spinal cord. Permanent paralysis and other complications are extremely rare but may occur.

The effects of the saddle block will usually wear off within several hours.

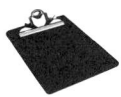

Patient Education Handout

TRANSCERVICAL AMNIOINFUSION

What Is Transcervical Amnioinfusion?

Transcervical amnioinfusion is a simple procedure that can be performed when a patient is in labor. When your bag of water breaks, fluid is lost from around your baby. Sometimes it could be helpful if the fluid were to be replaced during labor. To replace the fluid, a small plastic tube (catheter) about the size of a straw is put into the uterus (womb) through the cervix (opening to the womb). Intravenous (IV) fluid then runs through this tube to replace your water.

Why Do I Need This Procedure?

Sometimes the loss of the fluid around the baby prevents the umbilical cord from floating. If the cord is squeezed between the baby and your uterus when you have contractions, the baby's heart rate could slow down too much. Before your bag of water broke, the fluid around the baby acted like a cushion. Putting fluid back allows the cord to float again, and the baby can get more oxygen from the cord if it needs it. Without this procedure, you might have to have a cesarean section to deliver the baby.

    The other reason you might need this procedure is if there is meconium in the fluid around the baby. Meconium is found in the baby's first bowel movements. If the baby has a bowel movement before delivery, it may cause the fluid around the baby to become thick. Putting fluid back into the womb may thin this fluid and decrease the risk that the baby will get meconium into its lungs.

What Happens During the Procedure?

During the procedure, fluid is run through the tube into your uterus. It then surrounds the baby. After the uterus is full of fluid again, you will feel some of it leak out of your vagina.

What Happens After the Procedure?

If the problem with the baby's heart rate is corrected, labor will be allowed to proceed. If the heart rate does not correct, a cesarean section may be needed.

    If the problem is with meconium, after the fluid is diluted, the fluid will be continued until the baby delivers.

What Are the Benefits of This Procedure?

- Less risk of slow heart rate (fetal heart rate decelerations) for the baby
- Less need for cesarean delivery
- Possibly less risk of infection for you
- Less risk of thick meconium in the baby's lungs

Continued

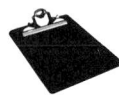 *Patient Education Handout—cont'd*

TRANSCERVICAL AMNIOINFUSION—cont'd
What Are the Risks of This Procedure?

- Damage to the uterus (uterine perforation)
- Damage to the umbilical cord
- Damage to the placenta (abruption or separation from uterus)
- Too much fluid around the baby (hydramnios)
- Fetal distress
- Amniotic fluid embolism (amniotic fluid gets into your blood stream); very rare, but can be serious
- If infusion is needed for too long, there may be a slight risk of infection for you
- Other problems may occur that we cannot foresee

Special Instructions:

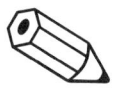 *Patient Consent Form*

TRANSCERVICAL AMNIOINFUSION

During the course of my labor on _____, my clinician _____ noted severe repetitive variable decelerations and/or thick meconium-stained amniotic fluid.

We discussed the different treatments possible and discussed the risks of not intervening in this condition(s). Based upon the advice given by my clinician _____ and my own judgment, I agree to undergo transcervical amnioinfusion. We also discussed the potential benefits of performing this procedure. The procedure requires passing an intrauterine pressure catheter through the cervix into my uterine cavity (womb). The catheter tip will then lie next to the fetus. Fluid will be infused through this catheter and into the uterus.

We discussed the different outcomes that could occur. I understand the possible complications and risks of placing this intrauterine pressure catheter and then infusing fluid (e.g., uterine perforation, umbilical cord trauma, uterine abruption [separation of placenta], hydramnios [too much fluid], fetal distress, possible infection, a fluid embolism). I am aware that this procedure could fail and that there are other possible complications that we could not foresee.

All of my questions have been answered, and I wish to proceed with the procedure.

_____
Patient's signature

_____
Date/Time

_____
Witness' signature

_____
Clinician's signature

One copy for chart; one copy for patient.

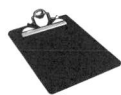 *Patient Education Handout*

CARE FOLLOWING A VAGINAL DELIVERY

Your medicines are: _____

- Keep a written list of what medicines you take and when and why you take them. Bring the list of your medicines or the pill bottles when you see your clinician. Learn why you take each medicine. Ask your clinician for information about your medicines.
- Always take your medicine as directed by the clinician. Call your clinician if you think your medicines are not helping or if you feel that you are having side effects. Do not quit taking the medicine until you discuss it with your clinician. If you are taking antibiotics, take them until they are all gone, even if you feel better.
- Medicine like acetaminophen may be helpful for comfort. If you are taking medicine that makes you drowsy, do not drive or use heavy equipment. Let your clinician know if you have any problems or questions.

Check the amount and color of the discharge coming out of your vagina several times a day. If it is decreasing, it shows how fast you are healing. Wear peri-pads in your underwear to catch the blood and discharge. Change your pads often to keep from getting an infection.

- For the first 2 to 3 days after you have your baby, blood flow will be heavy and dark red. Some women pass clots and blood for 3 to 5 days.
- From the third to tenth day, the amount of discharge should slow down and become pink. After that, you will have a creamy or yellowish discharge for another 1 or 2 weeks.

The perineum is the area between your vagina and your rectum. To care for this area, rinse your perineum with water after you use the toilet and before you put on a new perineal pad. Caregivers will show you how to use a peri-bottle (handheld squirt bottle). Squirting warm tap water on your perineum will keep it clean and help the pain.

- While you are sitting on the toilet, rinse your perineum for at least 2 minutes. Aim the bottle opening at your perineum and spray so that the water moves from front to back.
- Pat the area dry with toilet paper or cotton wipes, from front to back.
- Put on a fresh perineal pad.
- Stand before flushing the toilet to keep from being sprayed with the water from the toilet.

Caregivers may tell you about other ways to help your perineum feel better as it heals.

- Take sitz baths during the first week after having your baby. Fill the bath tub with warm water. Sit for 10 minutes, twice a day. Put on a fresh perineal pad after the bath.
- An ice pack may be helpful for comfort. Fill a plastic bag with crushed ice. Wrap the ice pack in a washcloth. Gently place the ice bag between your legs for 15 to 20 minutes out of each hour. Continue this treatment as long as needed.
- Caregivers may also give you a medicine spray or wipes soaked with a numbing medicine to increase your comfort. You also may be given a medicine to soften your bowel movements.
- Begin Kegel exercises as tolerated. Your caregiver will explain how to do these exercises.
- Pelvic rest for 1 month: Refrain from using tampons and from intercourse for 1 month.

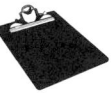

Patient Education Handout—cont'd

CARE FOLLOWING A VAGINAL DELIVERY—cont'd

Call your caregiver if any of the following occur:

- The discharge coming out of your vagina gets heavier (soaks more than 1 pad every 1 to 2 hours), turns bright red, or starts to smell bad.
- You develop significant swelling
- You develop a fever, chills, nausea, vomiting or start to feel bad.
- You have abdominal pain.
- You have any questions.

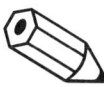 *Patient Consent Form*

VAGINAL DELIVERY

My treating clinician has explained my medical condition to my satisfaction, and all of my questions have been answered.

My proposed treatment, its purpose, and its alternatives have been explained to me. I have been given information about the risks of having any medical procedures, including those listed below or of choosing no treatment. In hopes of obtaining the desired benefit, I accept the risk of substantial and serious harm, if any. I am also aware that there are possible complications that we did not discuss or could not foresee.

My signature below indicates that I accept the proposed treatment.

Proposed medical procedures:

_____ Pitocin induction or augmentation
_____ Vaginal delivery with episiotomy
_____ Vaginal delivery following cesarean
_____ Forceps or vacuum delivery
_____ Cesarean section

_____

Patient's signature

_____

Signature of witness, next of kin or legal guardian

_____

Date/Time

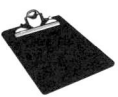

Patient Education Handout

INTRAOSSEOUS VENOUS ACCESS (IOVA)

Veins carry blood from the organs, tissue, and cells of the body to the heart. The oxygen in the blood in the veins has been used by the organs, tissue, and cells, and the blood must be returned through the heart to the lungs to obtain more oxygen. A certain amount of blood in the veins is necessary to keep the organs, tissue, and cells working. Intraosseous venous access (IOVA) is a procedure in which we insert a needle through a child's thin bones to use the bone like a catheter (plastic tube) in order to increase the amount of fluid in the veins. This procedure is needed because of suspected inadequate blood volume (dehydration or volume depletion) or the blood pressure is too low (shock) or certain fluids or medications need to be given immediately. A routine intravenous (IV) catheter cannot be obtained at this point. Low blood volume or blood pressure or the lack of certain fluids or medications could harm the cells in your child, resulting in organ, cell, or tissue death. By doing this procedure, we will be able to minimize the severity of the problem.

The most important thing for your child to do during this procedure is to try and relax and remain calm.

During this procedure, your clinician will put your child's leg into a certain position while they determine the best location for the procedure. They may give an injection to numb the skin over the bone. The skin will be cleansed before any injections. The clinician will then insert a needle into the bone marrow (center of the bone). Your child may experience some discomfort with any of the injections.

After the procedure, the needle will be covered with a dressing. Then a bandage will be placed. The benefits of this procedure include the ability to infuse fluids and medications until an IV can be started.

The risks associated with the procedure are few but must be discussed. Possible complications include: bleeding, infection, scarring, blood clots, and leakage of fluid or medications from the site. The procedure may fail to provide access to your child's blood vessels. Local structures near the IOVA site such as nerves, tendons, or arteries could be damaged. Fractures have been reported, but they are very rare. There are also other rare complications that can occur that we could not foresee. In order to minimize complications, it is important for you to notify the clinician or nursing staff at the earliest sign of a possible complication.

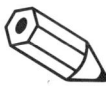 *Patient Consent Form*

INTRAOSSEOUS VENOUS ACCESS (IOVA)

My child is under the care of a clinician, _____, on _____ (date) for treatment of an abnormality with his or her blood pressure, blood volume, or access to the blood stream. We discussed the different treatment methods and the risks involved.

Based on that discussion and my own judgment, I agree to allow the clinician, _____, to insert a needle into my child's bone marrow in order to infuse fluid until an IV can be started. This may involve local anesthesia with an injection of lidocaine.

I understand that there will be some discomfort with this procedure.

We discussed the different outcomes that could occur and most of the possible complications, including bleeding, infection, scarring, blood clots, and leakage of fluid or medications from the site. The procedure may fail to provide access to my child's blood vessels. Local structures near the IOVA site such as nerves, tendons, arteries, or veins could be damaged. Fractures have been reported, but they are very rare. I am aware that there are other rare complications that could occur that we could not foresee. I have read and understand the patient education handout. I agree to follow the instructions for care after the procedure and to bring my child back for follow-up care on _____. All of my questions have been answered.

I will call the office or answering service if any problems occur.

_____
Patient's signature

_____
Date/Time

_____
Witness' signature

_____
Clinician's signature

One copy for chart; one copy for patient.

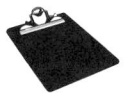

Patient Education Handout

NEWBORN CIRCUMCISION

What Is Circumcision?

Circumcision is the surgical removal of the portion of the foreskin that normally covers the tip of the penis. It usually takes 5 to 10 minutes. The infant does experience some pain during the operation, but a simple nerve block can minimize this pain. Healing takes 5 to 7 days.

Is Circumcision Necessary?

Although circumcision is commonly performed on male infants in the United States, it is an entirely elective procedure. There is no law or requirement that a baby boy must be circumcised. Parents must carefully consider the risks and benefits before deciding to have their baby circumcised. The American Academy of Pediatrics (AAP) issued a statement in 1999 concluding that there is existing scientific evidence demonstrating potential medical benefits of newborn male circumcision. However, the AAP determined that the data is insufficient to recommend routine neonatal circumcision.

The existing scientific evidence of potential medical benefits include the fact that circumcision can decrease the chance of getting cancer of the penis. There is also some evidence that the risk of urinary tract infections and some sexually transmitted diseases may be lower in circumcised males. Their partners may also have a lower risk of abnormal Pap smears, but more research is needed in this area before a recommendation can be made.

If My Son Is Not Circumcised, How Will I Care for My Son's Penis?

In the first few months, your baby's uncircumcised penis is simply cleaned and bathed with soap and water like the rest of the diaper area. Initially, the foreskin is connected to the glans (head) of the penis, so do not try to pull back the foreskin. It is not necessary to cleanse the penis with Q-Tips or antiseptics, but watch your baby urinate occasionally to make sure that the hole in the foreskin is large enough to permit a normal urine stream. If the stream is consistently no more than a trickle or if your baby seems to have some discomfort while urinating, consult his clinician. The American Academy of Pediatrics (1-847-434-4000, or www.aap.org) has a helpful brochure on taking care of a baby with an uncircumcised penis.

Your clinician will tell you when the foreskin has separated and can be retracted safely. This will not be for several years. After this separation occurs, retract the foreskin occasionally to cleanse the tip of the penis underneath. Once your son is bathing himself, you will need to teach him how to do this himself.

Are There Times When an Infant Should Not Be Circumcised?

Circumcision should not be performed if there is any abnormality of the penis. This is especially true when the urinary opening is at some point on the penis other than the tip. The tissue of the foreskin is often used for surgical correction of penile defects. Removing the foreskin could make such a repair much more difficult or even impossible. If there is a family history of bleeding problems, circumcision should not be performed until laboratory tests show that the baby's blood clotting is normal.

Continued

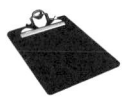 *Patient Education Handout—cont'd*

NEWBORN CIRCUMCISION—cont'd

What Are the Risks of Circumcision?

Overall, complications from circumcision are rare. As with any surgical procedure, bleeding and infection are possible. On rare occasions, damage to the tip or shaft of the penis may occur.

When Is Circumcision Done?

Newborn circumcision is usually performed a day or two after delivery and must be performed before 6 to 8 weeks of age, depending on your clinician's preference and the condition of the baby. If the baby is ill in any way, circumcision is delayed until he is well. Note that some insurance plans will cover circumcision if it is performed on a newborn, but they will not cover it once the baby has been released from the hospital. Others will not cover circumcision for babies over 8 weeks of age.

What Does the Penis Look Like After Circumcision?

After circumcision, the tip of the penis is red and moist, and it often becomes covered with a yellowish mucus-like substance. This is part of the normal process of healing and may last for a week. Petroleum jelly gauze is applied to the penis to prevent it from sticking to the diaper. This gauze is removed when it becomes soiled.

Is There Anything Special That Should Be Done After We Go Home?

Take care to keep the circumcision area as clean as possible. Use a soft wash cloth and warm water for cleaning. (Diaper wipes may irritate the healing area.) At each diaper change for the first week, gently pull back the penile shaft skin and apply petroleum jelly to the groove between the back of the tip of the penis and the shaft skin. Also apply petroleum jelly to the front of the diaper until healing is complete to prevent the penis from sticking to the diaper.

Very rarely, a narrowing of the urinary opening will occur. The opening may begin to look like a pinhole, and the urinary stream will become very strong and may squirt out at an angle. This rarely occurs before age 1 year. It can be corrected in the office, so tell your clinician if you find that this narrowing has developed.

A Website That May Be of Interest

www.aap.org/visit/circumcision.htm (circumcision information)

If you have any further questions regarding circumcision or anything related to the procedure, please discuss them with your clinician. This is a decision which you, the parents, should discuss completely before deciding to have the procedure done.

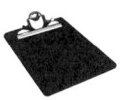 *Patient Education Handout*

CAST CARE

Why Do I Need a Cast?

You have been given a cast to help your broken bone or torn ligaments heal. A cast can help keep the injured area from moving so you can heal faster without risk of repeated injury. How long you'll need to wear your cast depends on the type of injury you have and how serious it is. Your doctor may want to check your cast 1 to 3 days after putting it on to be sure that the cast isn't too tight and that your broken bone or torn ligament is starting to heal.

Will the Broken Bone Hurt?

Almost all broken bones cause pain. The cast should relieve some pain by limiting your movements. Your pain should become less severe each day. Call your doctor immediately if the pain in the casted area gets worse after the cast has been applied. You should also call your doctor right away if you have new pain that develops in another area (for example, pain in your fingers or forearm if you have a wrist or thumb injury, or pain in your toes or calf if you have an ankle or foot injury). New pain that you didn't have before the injury may mean that the cast is too tight. If you have this symptom, raise your cast. This may reduce pain and swelling. Your doctor will probably want to see you right away to check the cast.

Is It Okay to Get the Cast Wet?

With some fiberglass casts, you can swim and bathe. However, most casts shouldn't get wet. If you get one of these casts wet, irritation and infection of the skin could develop. Talk to your doctor about how to care for your cast.

To avoid getting the cast wet during bathing, you can put a plastic bag over the cast and hold it with a rubber band. If the cast does get wet, you may be able to dry out the inside padding with a blow dryer. (Use a low setting and blow the air through the outside of the cast.) Ask your doctor about using a blow dryer before trying this.

What Can I Do About Itching?

If your skin itches underneath the cast, don't slip anything inside the cast, since it may damage your skin and you could get an infection. Instead, try tapping the cast or blowing air from a blow-dryer down into the cast.

(Reprinted with permission from American Family Physician, 1999, Copyright American Academy of Family Physicians.)

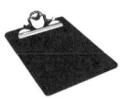 *Patient Education Handout*

CARE OF CASTS AND SPLINTS

Why Splints and Casts?

Splints and casts support and protect injured bones and soft tissue, reducing pain, swelling, and muscle spasm. In some cases, splints and casts are applied following surgery.

Splints or "half casts" provide less support than casts. However, splints can be adjusted to accommodate swelling from injuries easier than enclosed casts. Your doctor will decide which type of support will be best for you.

Types of Splints and Casts

Casts are custom-made and applied by your doctor or an assistant. Casts can be made of plaster or fiberglass. Splints or half casts also can be custom-made, especially if an exact fit is necessary. Other times, a ready-made splint will be used. These off-the-shelf splints are made in a variety of shapes and sizes and are much easier and faster to use. They have Velcro straps that make the splints easy to adjust and to put on and take off. Your doctor will explain both how to use your injured arm or leg while it is healing and how to adjust your splint to accommodate swelling.

What Materials Are Used in Splints and Casts?

Fiberglass or plaster materials form the hard supportive layer in splints and casts. Fiberglass is lighter in weight, is longer wearing, and "breathes" better than plaster. Plaster is less expensive than fiberglass and for some uses shapes better than fiberglass. Both materials come in strips or rolls, which are dipped in water and applied over a layer of cotton or synthetic padding covering the injured area. X-rays to check the healing process of an arm or leg within a splint or cast penetrate or "see through" fiberglass better than plaster.

How Are Splints and Casts Applied?

Both fiberglass and plaster splints and casts use padding, usually cotton, as a protective layer next to the skin. The splint or cast must fit the shape of the injured arm or leg correctly to provide the best possible support. Generally, the joint above and below the fractured bone is also covered by the splint or cast. Frequently, a splint is applied to a fresh injury first, and, as swelling subsides, a full cast may be used to replace the splint. Sometimes, it may be necessary to replace a cast as swelling decreases and the cast "gets too big." Often as a fracture heals, a splint may be applied again to allow easy removal for therapy.

Getting Used to the Splint or Cast

If your treatment is to be successful, you must follow your doctor's instructions carefully. *The following information provides general guidelines only and is not a substitute for your doctor's advice. Swelling due to your injury may cause pressure in your splint or cast for the first 48 to 72 hours. This may cause your injured arm or leg to feel snug or tight in the splint or cast. To reduce the swelling:*

• Elevate your injured arm or leg above your heart by propping it up on pillows or some other support. You will have to recline if the splint or cast is on your leg. Elevation allows clear fluid and blood to drain "downhill" to your heart.

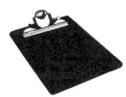

Patient Education Handout—cont'd

CARE OF CASTS AND SPLINTS—cont'd

- Move your uninjured and possibly swollen fingers or toes gently and often.
- Apply ice to the splint or cast. Place the ice in a dry plastic bag or ice pack and loosely wrap it around the splint or cast at the level of the injury. Ice that is packed in a rigid container and touches the cast at only one point will not be effective.

Warning Signs Following Splint or Cast Application

After application of a splint or cast, it is very important to elevate your injured arm or leg for 24 to 72 hours. The injured area should be elevated well above the heart. Rest and elevation greatly reduce pain and speed the healing process by minimizing early swelling. If you experience any of the following warning signs, contact your doctor's office immediately for advice.

- Increased pain, which may be caused by swelling, and the feeling that the splint or cast is too tight.
- Numbness and tingling in your hand or foot, which may be caused by too much pressure on the nerves.
- Burning and stinging, which may be caused by too much pressure on the skin.
- Excessive swelling below the cast, which may mean the cast is slowing your blood circulation.
- Loss of active movement of toes or fingers, which requires an urgent evaluation by your doctor.

Taking Care of Your Splint or Cast

After you have adjusted to your splint or cast for a few days, it is important to keep it in good condition. This will help your recovery.

- Keep your splint or cast dry. Moisture weakens plaster and damp padding next to the skin can cause irritation. Use two layers of plastic or purchase waterproof shields to keep your splint or cast dry while you shower or bathe.
- Do not walk on a "walking cast" until it is completely dry and hard. It takes about 1 hour for fiberglass, and 2 to 3 days for plaster to become hard enough to walk on.
- Keep dirt, sand, and powder away from the inside of your splint or cast.
- Do not pull out the padding from your splint or cast.
- Do not stick objects such as coat hangers inside the splint or cast to scratch itching skin. Do not apply powders or deodorants to itching skin.
- If itching persists, contact your doctor.
- Do not break off rough edges of the cast or trim the cast before asking your doctor.
- Inspect the skin around the cast. If your skin becomes red or raw around the cast, contact your doctor.
- Inspect the cast regularly. If it becomes cracked or develops soft spots, contact your doctor's office.

Continued

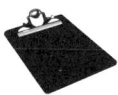 *Patient Education Handout—cont'd*

CARE OF CASTS AND SPLINTS—cont'd

Proper Cast Removal

Never remove the cast yourself. You may cut your skin or prevent proper healing of your injury. Your doctor will use a cast saw to remove your cast. The saw vibrates but does not rotate. If the blade of the saw touches the padding inside the hard shell of the cast, the padding will vibrate with the blade and will protect your skin. Cast saws make noise and may feel "hot" from friction, but will not harm you—their "bark is worse than their bite."

Use common sense. You have a serious injury and you must protect your cast from damage so it can protect your injury while it heals. After initial swelling has subsided, proper splint or cast support will usually allow you to continue your daily activities with a minimum of inconvenience.

Take care of your cast and it will take care of you.

Your doctor has extensive training in the diagnosis and nonsurgical and surgical treatment of the musculoskeletal system, including bones, joints, ligaments, tendons, muscles, and nerves. This information has been prepared by the American Academy of Orthopaedic Surgeons and is intended to contain current information on the subject from recognized authorities. However, it does not represent official policy of the Academy and its text should not be construed as excluding other acceptable viewpoints.

(Courtesy American Academy of Orthopaedic Surgeons. Accessed at http://www.aaos.org/wordhtml/pat_educ/castcare.htm on October 28, 2002.)

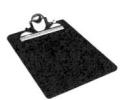 *Patient Education Handout*

CRUTCH USE

What Are Crutches?

Crutches are supports that help you walk when you have an injured leg or foot.

How Do I Use Crutches?

Walking: Bring the crutches forward evenly, keeping your injured leg off the ground. Lean forward, putting your weight on your hands against the grips of the crutches. Don't rest your armpits on the crutches. This can cause damage to a nerve that passes through the armpit. Swing your good leg forward, placing your foot just in front of the crutches. Repeat. (Note: In some cases your clinician may allow you to put some weight on your injured leg while you are using crutches.)

Getting up from a chair or bed: Hold both crutches by the grips in the hand on the side of the injured leg. Push up from the chair or bed with the other hand while pushing down on the crutches. Use your good leg to bring you to a standing position. Get your balance and bring your crutches into position before starting to walk.

Sitting down: Hold your crutches by the grips in the hand on the injured side. Hold onto the chair or bed with the other hand and lower yourself slowly. Unless you are allowed to put some weight on your injured leg, keep your injured leg off the ground and keep your weight on the good leg.

Stairs: Going up, get close to the stairs. Step up with the good leg, then bring the crutches and the injured leg up to the stair that the good leg is on. Repeat. Going down, first bring the crutches and the injured leg down to the lower step. Then step down with the good leg. Repeat. If there is a handrail, put both crutches under the opposite arm and use the rail for support. Remember: "Up with the good, down with the bad."

Going through doorways: Be sure to give yourself enough room to allow your feet and crutches to clear the door. After opening the door, block it from swinging closed with a crutch tip. Walk through the doorway.

How Can I Take Care of Myself While I'm Using Crutches?

- Be careful not to slip on water or ice.
- Sometimes crutches rub against the skin between your arm and chest. You may want to use body lotion or talcum powder to prevent skin chafing.
- If your hands get sore or tired, you may want to put extra padding on the crutch grips.
- Be sure not to lean on the crutches and put pressure on your armpits. If there is pressure on your armpits even when you use the crutches correctly, they are too long and need to be shortened.

(From Pierre Rouzier, MD: The Sports Medicine Advisor, McKesson Health Solutions LLC, Broomfield, Colo, copyright 2003.)

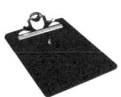 *Patient Education Handout*

TRAUMA TO EXTREMITIES AND AVOIDANCE OF THE COMPARTMENT SYNDROME

You have suffered a significant injury to your arm or leg. Even if there was not a fracture, the tissue can swell quite dramatically. When this happens, there can be so much pressure that the heart cannot pump blood strong enough to keep the tissues alive. Muscles, nerves, and tendons can die. If this happens, you may suffer a significant disability and require even further surgeries.

When damaged tissues swell and the blood supply is cut off, it is called a "compartment syndrome." The muscle layers of your legs and arms are wrapped in tubes of tissue to hold them in place. These "tubes" are like the casings around hot dogs and do not give with the swelling. If the pressure inside "the tubes" becomes high enough, the "tubes" have to be cut open to relieve the excessive pressure that has built up. (This is similar to a hot dog bursting open on the grill to relieve all the pressure inside.) Thus surgery is required to save the injured tissues.

Anytime you have a cast or splint placed, you are more susceptible to a compartment syndrome. Just like the casings around muscles, the cast prevents the muscles from stretching so the pressure builds up inside. Sometimes the casts have to be removed or replaced.

There are several things you can do to prevent or lessen your chances of having a compartment syndrome. First of all, it is important that you elevate the affected limb above your heart. If you have an arm injury, it is best to actually place your arm on your head! If you have a leg injury, the leg should be elevated above the level of the heart. It is not enough just to lay back in an easy chair or to have the leg up on a couch. The leg **must be higher than the heart.** It may be necessary to lie flat in bed with the hip flexed forward and the knee on a stack of blankets.

For patients who have borderline injuries and insist on going to work, it will be necessary to prop the leg up on the desk with pillows beneath it and lean back in a chair to keep the leg as high as possible.

Ice will lessen the swelling. On the contrary, heat may increase bleeding and swelling and make the condition worse. It is best not to take hot baths and not put any heat over the area for at least 4 to 5 days. Pain medications that help prevent swelling (nonsteroidal antiinflammatory drugs like ibuprofen, Naprosyn, and others) can help both the pain and the swelling.

Signs of compartment syndrome include extreme pain, tingling of the fingers or toes in the affected extremity, or poor color in the tissue from decreased circulation. If any of these happen, call the doctor immediately. Sometimes an infection with swelling can cause a similar problem. Check too for excessive pain with movement of the thumbs or great toes. If pain is severe and seems to be worsening, it is important that you be examined.

It is often difficult even for physicians to diagnose a compartment syndrome. It must be recognized early to prevent serious complications. If you have any questions whatsoever, it is best to call the doctor to be sure that everything is okay.

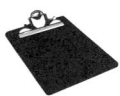

Patient Education Handout

DIAGNOSTIC ARTHROSCOPY AND LAVAGE PATIENT INFORMATION AND INSTRUCTIONS

This information sheet will remind you of some of the many things discussed during your visit regarding diagnostic arthroscopy and arthroscopic lavage.

Arthroscopy (looking into a joint) and lavage (washing out of a joint) is performed with a fiberoptic scope of small diameter. The entire combined procedure takes about 60 minutes.

Arthroscopy allows the physician to directly visualize (see) almost every portion of the knee joint and provides an opportunity to improve the accuracy of diagnosis even beyond the best imaging studies available to date (e.g., MRI). The general intended purpose is to diagnose joint disease and to remove any debris from the joint spaces. There will be no surgical repair of any damaged structure found on arthroscopy.

Because of advances in technology, the procedure is now easily capable of being performed in the office setting. Upon your arrival to the office, nursing assistants will ask for your written permission to perform these two procedures. After that, you will be given a small oral dose of a medication to help you relax. After changing from your "street clothes" into a hospital type of gown, you will be taken to the arthroscopy room where your leg will be scrubbed and painted with a cool brown antiseptic solution. You will then be covered with a sterile sheet from below your chin, to over and down below you toes.

The next step is when you will experience some pain with the numbing or "freezing" of the knee. The medicine used is either lidocaine (Xylocaine) or bupivacaine (Marcaine), and this renders the two injection sites and the knee painless. You may experience a feeling of distention, fullness, or pressure without pain. You may also hear clicking or snapping sounds coming from the knee, but these will also be non-painful.

There are complications with any procedure, including arthroscopy. There is less than a 1% chance of any complication with diagnostic arthroscopy and arthroscopic lavage. The known problems include, but are not limited to, allergy or unusual reactions to the medications used; reaction to the antiseptic cleanser; infection; bleeding; damage to the joint surface, ligament, and/or tendons; enlargement or rupture of the cysts (pouches) of the joint; and instrument breakage. These are rare events, and we take measures to prevent them from occurring.

1. You will be called the day prior to confirm the date and time of your arthroscopic lavage, which will be: _____
2. Have nothing to eat or drink, except your prescription medications with a small sip of water, four (4) hours before your appointment.
3. Shower or bathe before the arthroscopy, but do not use lotion on your legs.
4. Bring a list of any known allergies to medications.
5. Have a family member or a friend pick you up 2 hours after your arrival to your appointment.
6. Your follow-up appointment will be: _____

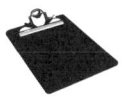 *Patient Education Handout*

AFTER ARTHROSCOPY AND LAVAGE INFORMATION AND CARE

1. DRESSINGS: A small adhesive gauze has been applied to your knee. No stitches were used, since the entry site is very small. The adhesive gauze may be removed safely at any time and reapplied over the next 2 to 3 days if needed.

2. WOUNDS: The small points of entry may be sore and develop bruising over the subsequent 1 to 2 days. This bruising will eventually disappear and does not require any special care.

3. BATHING: The Betadine solution (the brown antiseptic liquid) may be removed with soap and water, but bathing or soaking the leg should be delayed for 2 or more days. You may shower after 24 hours.

4. PAIN: You may resume all your medications, except as follows: _____
You may have also been given an additional pain medication, and if so the name and directions are as follows _____
Finally, application of an ice pack to the knee, 20 minutes every hour if needed, will decrease swelling and discomfort in the first 48 hours.

5. ACTIVITY: The knee may feel wonderful or normal following the procedure. You may be tempted to increase your activity to get things done that you have been putting off for some time. Resist that temptation! Minimal activity (e.g., trips to the bathroom, couch/chair, or kitchen table) is allowed, but no chores for the first 12 to 24 hours. You may then progressively increase your activity over the following 2 days to your normal level.

6. COMPLICATIONS: If you develop a temperature greater than 101.0° F, redness around the knee, joint swelling, or pain in excess of what you would consider "usual" or "normal" following the lavage, please call the office.

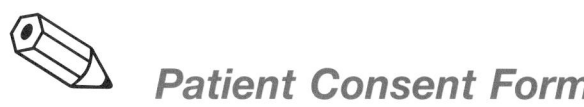

Patient Consent Form

CONSENT TO DIAGNOSTIC OR THERAPEUTIC PROCEDURES AND ADMINISTRATION OF ANESTHESIA

I authorize and direct _____ to perform the following:

These operations and procedures may all involve risks, or unsuccessful results, complications, injury of the knee both from known and unknown causes, and no warranty or guarantee is made as to result or care.

You have the right to be informed of such risks as well as the nature of the operation or procedure, the expected benefits of such operation or procedure, and the available alternative methods of treatment and their expected risks and benefits. Except in cases of emergency, operations or procedures are not performed until you have had the opportunity to receive the information and have given your consent. You have the right to consent to or refuse any proposed operation or procedure at any time prior to its performance.

To make sure that you fully understand the operation or procedure your physician will fully explain the operation or procedure to you before you decide whether or not to give consent. If you have any questions, you are encouraged to ask them.

I understand that the above named physician and his/her associates or assistants will be occupied solely with performing such procedure.

I hereby authorize the pathologist to use his discretion in the disposition or use of any severed tissue.

Your signature on the form will (1) indicate that you have read and understood the information provided in this form, (2) that you have had a chance to ask questions, (3) that you have received all of the information you desire concerning the operation or procedure, and (4) that you authorize and consent to the performance of the operation or procedure.

_____   _____
Patient's signature   *Date/Time*

_____   _____
Signature of Parent, Conservator, Guardian   *Date/Time*

If signed by other than patient, indicate relationship: _____

_____   _____
Witness' signature   *Date/Time*

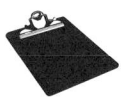 *Patient Education Handout*

REPAIR OF EXTENSOR TENDON(S) INJURY

The anticipated procedure that you are considering is repair of your torn extensor tendon of the hand/foot. The goal of this operation is to restore function. Without this repair, the tendon(s) will not allow full function of your hand/finger/foot/toe.

Your doctor may require that you fast for a certain time before your anticipated operation. Certain medications and herbal formulas may need to be discontinued before surgery. Your nutritional status and associated illnesses (e.g. diabetes, connective tissue disease such as rheumatoid arthritis) will affect healing of your injury. Tobacco use of any form *will delay* and *may even prevent* complete healing of your injury.

During your operation, the surgical site will be anesthetized with a local anesthetic or you may need more substantial anesthesia depending on your circumstances. After sterile preparation, the wound will be cleaned up as much as possible. Repair or reconstruction of the damaged tendon(s) will require sutures. Associated structures may also need repair. Typically a sterile dressing with some form of splint immobilization will be necessary after surgery. This may be needed for 6 to 8 weeks. Eventually therapy and progressive use will be encouraged.

Risks associated with this operation include failure of the repair, rupture of the tendon later when the hand is used for work, deformity, stiffness/scarring, weakness, need of further surgery, residual pain, and infection. It is also possible that once the wound is fully seen and evaluated, the tendon will not be able to be brought together. You then may need a referral to a specialist hand surgeon. Furthermore, any other tissue damage such as to the nerve, artery, or skin may contribute to a poorer outcome. You will need to keep the wound clean until the tissues have healed. Keep the wound dry until you are told it is okay to get it wet. To obtain optimal results, you likely will need to complete a physical therapy program.

After the repair, call the doctor if there is increased pain, increased swelling, or increased redness around the wound, especially if it goes up the arm. Also notify the physician if there is drainage or a fever greater than 100.5° F. If the dressings or splints feel too tight and/or there is tingling in the fingers/toes, call immediately. The doctor will tell you when to have the sutures out and what medication to use for pain. Antibiotics may also be used.

Websites That May Be of Interest to You:

www.aaos.org (American Academy of Orthopaedic Surgeons website for patient education on tendon injuries)

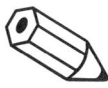 *Patient Consent Form*

REPAIR OF EXTENSOR TENDON(S) INJURY

I came to the office of Dr. _____ on _____ (date) for evaluation and treatment of repair of extensor tendon(s) injury.

We discussed the different treatments possible and discussed the risks of not treating the condition. I understand that I could request a different specialist to carry out the procedure or be referred to another center. Based on the advice given by Dr. _____ and my own judgment, I agree to undergo repair of extensor tendon(s) injury.

We discussed the different outcomes that could occur and most of the possible complications. I am aware that other complications could occur that we could not foresee. I have read over the information provided. I agree to follow the instructions for self-care after the procedure and to return for follow-up care on _____.

I will call the office or answering service if any problems arise before the scheduled follow-up visit.

_____
Patient's signature

_____
Date/Time

_____
Witness' signature

_____
Physician's signature

One copy for chart, one copy for patient.

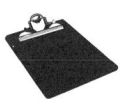 *Patient Education Handout*

KNEE BRACES

What Are Knee Braces?

Knee braces are external knee supports that are used to prevent or treat knee injuries. They are designed for different uses and are constructed from various materials such as metal, plastic, and foam. Some braces are prefabricated to fit standard sized legs, but others are customized to fit your leg exactly.

Why Should I Wear a Knee Brace?

Knee braces come in several different types. Your physician may recommend a knee brace to help prevent a knee injury during contact activities. A brace may also be used after you have had a ligament injury or knee surgery. Some people use knee braces for pain or swelling in the front of the knee.

How Do I Prepare for Knee Bracing?

After your doctor has determined that you need a knee brace and selected the correct type of brace, you will need to be sized for a brace. This process is easily performed and is not painful. In general, you should wait until the swelling subsides after an acute injury before being fit for a knee brace.

What Happens During the Knee Brace Sizing?

You will need to wear shorts in order to fit the brace accurately to your leg. Your physician will take several measurements of your leg to determine the correct brace size. In some cases, both of your legs will be measured if you will be using a brace on each leg.

What Happens After the Knee Brace Sizing?

The brace will be ordered in the correct size after the measurements have been obtained. Some braces are presized and readily available. Custom braces take longer to be manufactured but may be better for certain people. Your physician may request that you limit activities until you have your knee brace.

What Are the Benefits of Knee Braces?

Some knee braces may prevent or minimize knee injuries. Some also seem to support your knee if the ligaments are torn or damaged. Knee braces may minimize pain and swelling in your knee and allow you to return to activities more quickly. Some people may get more benefit from knee braces than others. It is not clear that knee braces are helpful for all knee disorders.

What Are the Risks of Knee Braces?

In general, knee braces are fairly safe when used as directed by your physician. Wearing a knee brace may actually increase the likelihood of your having a knee or other injury under some conditions. A knee brace may also irritate or damage the skin under the brace. Knee braces may cause injuries to others during contact activities. Other potential risks may include increased leg fatigue or decreased athletic ability during brace wear.

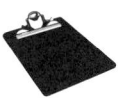

Patient Education Handout—cont'd

KNEE BRACES—cont'd

When Should I Call My Healthcare Provider?

Contact your provider if you are concerned that the knee brace does not fit well or moves easily during activities. You should also report a broken or damaged brace in order to have it repaired or replaced. If your knee pain or symptoms worsen while using the brace, you should limit your activities and check with your provider.

Websites That May Be of Interest to You:

www.proorthopedic.com (Pro Orthopedic Devices, Inc.)

www.donjoy.com (dj Orthopedics, Inc.)

www.bledsoebrace.com (Bledsoe Brace Systems)

www.orthocare.com (Ortho-Care)

www.townsenddesign.com (Townsend Design)

www.palumbobrace.com (Palumbo Orthopaedics)

www.soginc.com/SOGI (Seattle Orthopedic Group, Inc.)

www.mcdavidinc.com

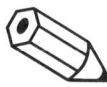 *Patient Consent Form*

KNEE BRACES

I came to the office of Dr. _____ on _____ (date) for evaluation and treatment of the following condition(s): knee pain and/or ligament damage that may be related to the knee joint, collateral ligaments, cruciate ligaments, or the patella. Structures involved may include bones, muscles, tendons, or ligaments of the knee.

We discussed the different treatments possible and discussed the risks of not treating the condition. Based on the advice given by Dr. _____ and my own judgment, I agree to undergo fitting and application of an appropriate knee brace.

I will call the office or answering service if any problems arise before the scheduled follow-up visit.

_____

Patient's signature

_____

Date/Time

_____

Witness' signature

_____

Physician's signature

One copy for chart; one copy for patient.

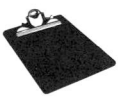

Patient Education Handout

CORNS AND CALLUSES OF THE FEET

Corns and calluses of the feet are caused by mechanical stress and pressure on the skin. They are not diseases of the skin but rather a result of excess pressure. The body attempts to protect itself against trauma by building up a thick layer of skin. However, the more the area is rubbed, the thicker the skin becomes. As this cycle continues, the increased pressure leads to the formation of what's called a "corn" or "callus." Any bony prominence can develop one of these lesions. If the bone protrudes more, pressure changes are more likely to occur. Hammertoes are very likely to develop corns and calluses. Tight shoes and vigorous exercise also predispose to their development.

A *callus* is rather broad based. There is no central core. It usually occurs under the ball of the foot. Most are not very discrete, but some can be more focal and have a thickened center much like a corn.

A *corn* is also a thickened area of skin but it has a central plug of keratin. Keratin is the same material that makes the fingernails and toenails, hair, and the outer surface of the skin. In a corn, the area of keratin buildup causes pain and inflammation because it acts like a small stone.

There are two types of corns: the *hard corn* and the *soft corn. Hard corns* are dry with the central core as mentioned. They most commonly occur on the tops of the toes or on the lateral part of the fifth toe. The *soft corn* usually develops between the fourth and fifth toe and is extremely painful. It, too, is due to pressure, but it remains soft because of the moisture between the toes. It absorbs fluid from perspiration and looks like a small ulceration.

Patients often think that calluses and corns are plantar warts. When *true warts* are scraped away, they will usually bleed and pinpoint dots of blood vessels can be seen. Calluses and corns do not have this type of bleeding. Rather, there will just be the thickened skin (and, for corns, that central "plug").

The treatment for these problems is to remove the pressure. The built-up dry skin should be pared away and the core of the corn or the thickened callus removed. Various pads can be used to keep the pressure off the skin. If it still builds up, soaking and paring or filing with a pumice stone can reduce the excess tissue. Acid plasters (used for warts) can actually harm surrounding skin and make things worse but sometimes are needed to soften hardened skin so it can be scraped away. Acid plasters must be used carefully. Soft corns located between the toes can also be shaved off, but the use of protective padding is even more important.

Women more commonly have these pressure lesions because of poorly fitting shoes. It is important to wear low-heeled shoes with a soft upper portion with plenty of room for the toes. If the toes have a tendency to be curled up (hammertoes), even bigger and wider shoes may be needed. The inside of shoes must be examined for irregularities or pressure points.

In some instances where there is a bony deformity, surgery may be required. This should be done only after all other conservative treatments have failed.

Pain from calluses and corns can cause an irregular gait and then cause pain in the knees, hips, and back. It's important to consider corns and calluses as a potential source of these problems.

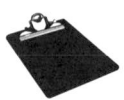 *Patient Education Handout*

OSTEOPOROSIS SCREENING INFORMATION

Osteoporosis is a condition in which bones become fragile and are more likely to break. Osteoporosis is painless and, if undetected or untreated, can progress until a bone breaks. Broken bones, or fractures, caused by osteoporosis most commonly occur in the hip, spine, and wrist.

A physician recommends a bone density test when the patient appears to be at risk for osteoporosis. This is a screening test, much like a Pap smear. It is totally painless. If the results indicate that bone density is low, the physician may recommend a different or more complete evaluation of the patient's bones.

Assessment of the risk of having bone fractures secondary to osteoporosis is based on the patient's T-score result. The T-score reveals the density of bones compared with the bones of young adults of the patient's gender. If the T-score is above 0, bone density is higher than average for a young adult. If the T-score is less than –1, the bones are considered osteopenic, which means that the patient may be at risk for developing osteoporosis. If the T-score is less than –2.5, the bones are affected with osteoporosis.

If the T-score comes back low, it does not mean that the patient definitely has bone fractures or any other problems. What it means is that the risk of fracturing bones, such as the hip or spine, is higher than that of others without osteoporosis. Because of this, the physician may recommend preventive measures, prescribe medications, or both to treat or prevent osteoporosis. These medications can slow or stop bone loss, increase bone density, and reduce the risk of fracturing bones.

One of the best things that the patient can do to prevent further weakening of the bones is to do weight-bearing exercise, such as walking, dancing, jogging, or hiking. It is also important to eat a balanced diet that is rich in calcium and vitamin D. An appropriate calcium intake is approximately 1200 mg per day. If the patient finds it difficult to get enough calcium from the diet, calcium supplements are recommended. For vitamin-D intake most experts recommend between 400 and 800 mg per day, which can be found in fortified dairy products, egg yolks, many types of fish, as well as in dietary supplements. If the patient smokes, quitting smoking is probably the best way to protect the bones and general health. Excessive alcohol drinking should also be avoided because it increases the risk of developing weak bones.

If the doctor recommends a medication to treat or prevent osteoporosis and the patient decides to take it, another bone density test will need to be performed in approximately 2 years to evaluate how well the medication is working.

For more information about osteoporosis, the patient may contact the National Osteoporosis Foundation (NOF) at 202-223-2226 or on the Internet at www.nof.org.

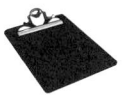

Patient Education Handout

OSTEOPOROSIS AND BONE DENSITY SCREENING TESTS

What Is Osteoporosis?

Osteoporosis is a condition in which the bones become fragile and are more likely to break. Osteoporosis is painless and, if undetected or untreated, can progress until a bone breaks. Broken bones, or fractures, caused by osteoporosis most commonly occur in the hip, spine, and wrist.

What Is Bone Mineral Density (BMD) Testing?

BMD testing, performed by a number of different methods such as dual-energy x-ray absorptiometry (DXA) or quantitative ultrasound (QUS), is a simple, noninvasive, and inexpensive method of estimating the fragility of bones to screen for osteoporosis. BMD testing is done on an outpatient basis and takes anywhere from 5 to 15 minutes, depending on the method used.

Why Is This Procedure Necessary?

This procedure is used to determine whether or not the patient has osteoporosis, because there are usually no signs or symptoms of osteoporosis until a person's bones become so fragile that they break. If osteoporosis can be detected by BMD testing before a bone fractures, different preventive measures, including medicines, can be prescribed that can prevent and treat osteoporosis.

How Does a Patient Prepare for BMD Testing?

No preparation is needed. The patient remains dressed during the procedure and must only lie still for several minutes during the measurement process. The procedure is absolutely painless.

What Happens During the Procedure?

A BMD device will take measurements of the patient's bones. Some devices require the patient to lie on a table while the device moves around the body much like a mobile x-ray machine (but with much less radiation exposure to the patient). Other devices, such as ultrasound devices, move a small probe over different bones to measure bone density (with no radiation exposure to the patient).

What Are the Benefits of the Procedure?

Determining whether or not the BMD is low provides information that can help the physician decide if the patient may benefit from certain medications that can prevent and treat osteoporosis.

What Are the Risks Associated With the Procedure?

One of the types of BMD testing, the DXA scan, exposes the patient to a small amount of radiation (less than one tenth of the radiation exposure of a chest x-ray).

Continued

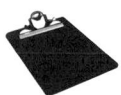 *Patient Education Handout—cont'd*

OSTEOPOROSIS AND BONE DENSITY SCREENING TESTS—cont'd

How Can the Chances of Developing Osteoporosis Be Reduced?

One of the best things that patients can do to prevent further weakening of bones is to do weight-bearing exercise, such as walking, dancing, jogging, or hiking. Eating a balanced diet that is rich in calcium and vitamin D is also important. An appropriate calcium intake is approximately 1200 mg per day. If the patient finds it difficult to get enough calcium from the diet, calcium supplements are recommended. For vitamin-D intake, most experts recommend between 400 and 800 mg per day, which can be found in fortified dairy products, egg yolks, many types of fish, as well as in dietary supplements. If the patient smokes, quitting smoking is probably the best way to protect the bones and general health. Excessive alcohol drinking should also be avoided because it increases the risk of developing weak bones.

For more information about osteoporosis, the patient may contact the National Osteoporosis Foundation (NOF) at 1-202-223-2226 or on the Internet at www.nof.org.

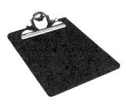 *Patient Education Handout*

SHOULDER REDUCTION OR PUTTING DISLOCATED SHOULDER BACK INTO PLACE

What Is Shoulder Reduction?

Your arm is out of its socket at the shoulder joint. The physician should put it back where it belongs.

Why Do I Need This Procedure?

The longer your shoulder is out of socket, the harder it is to replace it, and nerve and blood vessel damage may occur. Problems related to arthritis can also ensue.

What Happens During the Procedure?

The physician can use any one of a number of techniques to get your shoulder joint back into place. The arm and shoulder usually feel better immediately after the "reduction."

What Happens After the Procedure?

Your arm should be kept in the "sling and swatch" device until directed to do otherwise by your physician. He or she will most likely instruct you to remove it several times daily to exercise your elbow (first) and shoulder joints so they do not become stiff. A typical exercise for the elbow is just to straighten the joint several times a day. The shoulder is kept from "getting too stiff" by exercising the muscles around the joint. With the arm hanging down at the side, start with the palm of the hand facing backward. The arm is then raised until it finally faces forward during the exercises, and the arm is gradually raised more and more until it moves in a complete circle. These exercises can be instituted from 6 weeks to 3 months after the injury, at which time your physician may recommend more strenuous motion. They should never cause pain.

What Are the Risks of This Procedure?

There is a small chance that a bone fracture or nerve or blood vessel damage may occur during this procedure.

When Should I Call My Healthcare Provider?

You should notify your healthcare provider if pain returns, if you think your shoulder has come out of its socket again, if you have trouble moving your arm or hand, if you have trouble feeling with your arm or hand, or if your arm or hand seems cooler or has a grey or dusky color.

Special Instructions:

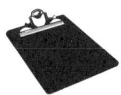 *Patient Education Handout*

ACUPUNCTURE

Acupuncture is a useful treatment for many chronic and acute conditions. It is helpful when you have either not responded to conventional medical therapy or prefer a safe alternative. The benefits of acupuncture are many, including relief of pain and improvement for chronic or acute illness. Common examples of conditions treated are headache, backache, arthritis, addictions such as tobacco, and many other medical and musculoskeletal problems.

No special preparation is needed for this procedure. During the procedure, several fine needles the size of a human hair are inserted into the body. These may be attached to a small electrical stimulation device or heated with an herb called moxa. The treatment usually takes from 20 to 30 minutes.

The most common question that people ask about acupuncture is, "Does it hurt?" The very fine needles and their location of insertion may cause a mild and brief sensation of aching, but most people feel no pain.

Although rare, some risks are present, and they include fainting during the procedure, infection if nonsterile needles are used, puncture of an organ, damage to a nerve, or bleeding. In our practice, all needles are sterile, single-use, and disposable. Aftereffects of acupuncture are rare, though some people report a slight "high" or relaxed feeling due to the release of painkilling chemicals from the brain. This feeling is self-limited and passes in a few hours. To maximize the benefit of your treatment and to allow the body to balance itself after a treatment, we recommend you avoid the following for at least 8 hours after the treatment: (1) strenuous physical or sexual activity, (2) heavy meals, and (3) alcohol or recreational drugs. Although no harm should occur if you do any of these things, the benefit of the treatment may be lessened. Some patients experience a temporary worsening of their condition before improvement occurs. If you have any questions about how you feel, or if you experience any discomfort that seems out of the ordinary, please call our office.

Web sites that may be of interest to you can be found on the Internet by searching for the keyword *acupuncture.* The American Academy of Medical Acupuncture has a useful site at www.medicalacupuncture.org

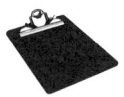
Patient Education Handout

BIOFEEDBACK

Biofeedback uses sensitive equipment to train you and your body for better control of particular physical functions or symptoms. It is based on hooking up a meter to the body, which works the same as hooking up a meter to just about anything: it allows you to monitor what is happening. With muscles, for example, most people can generally tell whether their muscles are tight or relaxed. However, by using a meter, different levels of tenseness can be monitored more precisely. Similarly, if you are running a fever, you probably have a general sense of whether you are just a little feverish, quite feverish, or very hot. A thermometer, however, gives you more accurate information. Similarly, a biofeedback meter provides precise information from moment to moment. When you can easily see such tiny changes in your body, you can more easily learn to control those changes. The meter acts as a guide, and eventually most people can produce larger and larger changes that actually affect their physical functions, symptoms, or concerns.

Biofeedback began with the idea that the body's ability to control a physical function is limited by the amount of information it has about that function. The biofeedback device is a means of artificially increasing that information and providing this information to the brain. A biofeedback device does not do anything *to* you, any more than a thermometer under your tongue changes your temperature. It works by giving you more information about what is going on inside the body. This information may be combined with a training program. The goal is to learn to change the readings in order to change the body functions or symptoms. Eventually you learn what to do to make the signal change the most, and then the biofeedback signal is no longer needed.

Procedure

Biofeedback is painless. You are attached to a sensor that monitors information from your body, much like a thermometer or an ECG. After some initial readings at rest, you work with the machine and the clinician to find strategies that will help you control the readings.

Effectiveness

There is a limit to how much control you can get with biofeedback training, but it is often enough to produce a change in functions or symptoms. For example, the patient with high blood pressure may be able to drop blood pressure by 10 to 20 points through relaxation or biofeedback training. A patient with Raynaud's phenomena and painfully cold fingers and toes may be able to warm them by 10 to 20 degrees. The patient with urinary incontinence may be able to increase pelvic muscle tone and contraction strength enough to reduce or completely eliminate incontinence. For chronic neck tightness, the patient may be able to reduce muscle tension enough to ease pain. You should know that biofeedback takes time for you to develop skills, and it does not work for all persons. However, early indications of benefit should be seen within four to eight sessions for most applications. The total number of sessions required may be as high as 50 for some applications, but usually a full course of biofeedback training can be completed in 4 to 12 sessions. With longer training programs, there should always be continued improvement if the training is to be continued.

Continued

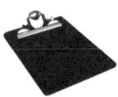 *Patient Education Handout—cont'd*

BIOFEEDBACK—cont'd
Side Effects
There are no known permanent side effects of biofeedback training. A small number of patients may experience discomfort from lowering blood pressure too much or may feel odd or out of control if they become too relaxed. If any discomfort develops, the procedure can be altered or discontinued. Biofeedback should not be practiced while driving or operating dangerous equipment unless the training program has been designed to help with symptoms that occur at such times (e.g., attention deficit disorder).

Scheduling and Time Commitment
Training generally requires frequent home practice. Even after new skills are learned, deliberate practice may be required during day-to-day life to maintain them. In fact, the results of biofeedback may have little usefulness unless these new skills are practiced on a day-to-day basis. It is never the device itself that causes the change, but rather what you learn to do to make the readings change. Therefore whatever is learned must be practiced to maintain the skill.

Occasionally people have difficulty producing the same results when not attached to the machine, but usually reproducing the effect is not particularly difficult with some practice. What may be difficult, however, is the ability to find the time to practice often enough, to remember to do it from day to day, and to not drift away from the new habits over weeks or months.

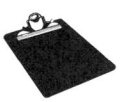 *Patient Education Handout*

BONE MARROW ASPIRATION/BIOPSY

What Is Bone Marrow Aspiration/Biopsy?

This is a procedure used to obtain blood and bone samples from the spongy inside of a hollow bone. The edge of the pelvic bone is usually sampled. The procedure is performed in the office, emergency room, or your hospital bed.

Why Do I Need This Procedure?

Your physician needs to examine what is going on with your body's blood-producing system and infection-fighting cells. Bone marrow sampling also is useful in managing treatment in people with cancer and other blood diseases such as anemia and HIV (the virus that causes AIDS).

How Do I Prepare for Bone Marrow Aspiration/Biopsy?

Do not eat after midnight the night before your procedure. You may take your morning medicines. Empty your bladder. You will need to lie still for approximately 30 minutes. If this will be difficult, inform your physician before the procedure. If you are overly anxious, a small dose of anti-anxiety or pain medication may be given in the office or hospital 90 minutes before the procedure.

What Happens During the Procedure?

You lie on one side. Cleaning solution is used to disinfect your skin. A sterile towel is used to cover the area. Numbing medicine is injected to anesthetize your skin. A needle is used to touch the pelvic bone, and the needle is twisted until the spongy inner bone is reached. Mild pain is felt when the marrow sample is collected. A second needle is used to get a tissue sample from the same area. Tell your physician if you are in too much pain.

What Happens After the Procedure?

The skin over the needle puncture is covered with a tight dressing. You lie on your side to put pressure on the area for 1 hour. You should be able to go home the same day. If you receive anxiety or pain medicine, someone should drive you home.

What Are the Benefits of This Procedure?

The tissue will be examined microscopically to look for diseases or abnormalities in your body's blood and infection-fighting cells. This may help your physician diagnose and treat your health problems more effectively.

What Are the Risks Associated With This Procedure?

An allergic reaction to the numbing, cleaning, or pain medicine is possible. Tell your physician if you have any allergies. The most dangerous risk is that the needle can go through both sides of the pelvic bone and damage organs such on the other side (e.g., bowel).

Continued

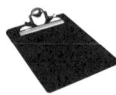 *Patient Education Handout—cont'd*

BONE MARROW ASPIRATION/BIOPSY—cont'd

What Do I Need to Do Following the Procedure to Prevent Infection?

Keep the pressure dressing on for 12 to 24 hours. Take the rest of the day off work to rest. Keep the biopsy site clean and dry.

When Should I Call My Healthcare Provider?

Call your provider for significant bleeding or drainage from the biopsy area. Call if you have severe pain, fever, chills, or redness or warmth at the site.

Special Instructions:

Please write down the telephone number of your physician's office in case there are problems.

Websites That May Interest You

www.health.sa.gov.au/cancare/TREATS/TESTS/bmbiop.HTM (CanCareSA Bone Marrow Biopsy)
www.nlm.nih.gov/medlineplus/ency/article/003934.htm#visualfile (Medline plus health information)

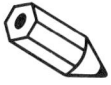 *Patient Consent Form*

BONE MARROW ASPIRATION/BIOPSY

I came to the office of my clinician, _____, on _____ (date) for evaluation and treatment of the following condition: abnormalities of the blood and infection-fighting cells of the body (too numerous or not enough).

I have read the patient education handout the clinician has given me and I understand the risks, benefits, and possible complications. I also understand the risks of not obtaining these samples. Based upon the advice given by my clinician, _____ and my own judgment, I agree to undergo the following procedure: bone marrow aspiration/biopsy from the posterior iliac crest.

I am aware that other complications could occur that we could not foresee. I agree to follow the instructions for self-care after the procedure and to return for follow-up care on _____.

I will call the office or answering service if any problems arise before the scheduled follow-up visit.

_____

Patient's signature

_____

Date/Time

_____

Witness' signature

_____

Relationship to patient

_____

Clinician's signature

One copy to chart; one copy to patient.

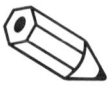 *Patient Consent Form*

BREAST MASS ASPIRATION/THYROID MASS ASPIRATION

I came to the office of my clinician, _____, on _____ (date) for diagnosis of a breast or thyroid mass. We discussed the different treatment methods and the risks involved. Based on that discussion and my own judgment, I agree to allow my clinician, _____, to aspirate either fluid or tissue from the mass.

Using ultrasound, we will determine whether the mass is a solid mass or a cyst. It could also be a combination of the two (mixed). Before aspiration, an injection of lidocaine will be used for anesthesia. A needle will then be inserted into the area to drain fluid or to aspirate some tissue.

I understand that there will be some discomfort with this procedure. We discussed the different outcomes that could occur and most of the possible complications including bleeding, infection, scarring, and damage to local structures such as nerves, tendons, arteries, or veins. There is also a slight risk of failure to make the correct diagnosis. In addition, cysts will frequently reoccur.

I am aware that there are other rare complications that could occur that we could not foresee. All of my questions have been answered. I agree to follow the instructions for self-care after the procedure and to return for follow-up care on _____.

I will call the office or answering service if any problems occur.

_____   _____
Patient's signature   *Date/Time*

_____   _____
Witness' signature   *Clinician's signature*

One copy for chart; one copy for patient.

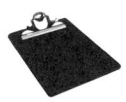

Patient Education Handout

FINE-NEEDLE ASPIRATION (FNA)

What Is Fine-Needle Aspiration (FNA)?

FNA is a way to obtain cells from a lump to diagnose what the lump is. The doctor puts a small needle into the lump and draws up some cells. Those cells are sent to the laboratory, where a pathologist can analyze them to tell what the lump is and whether it is cancerous.

Why Do I Need an FNA?

Either you or your doctor has felt a lump where one should not be and is worried about what it might be. FNA is used for breast lumps, thyroid nodules, swollen lymph nodes ("glands"), and other lumps. FNA is a way to find out what the lump is without more extensive surgery.

How Do I Prepare for FNA?

No special preparation is necessary. If the lump is in your breast, it is helpful to bring a snug brassiere, preferably a sports bra, to wear afterwards.

What Happens During an FNA?

The doctor will clean the skin over the lump with alcohol or iodine and may inject a tiny bit of local anesthetic there. He or she will use a syringe (like that used for a "shot") and take several samples from the lump. Those samples will be smeared out on a slide or put in a special container to go to the lab. If the lump is a cyst, the fluid in the cyst will be drawn out with the syringe, and the lump may disappear entirely. FNA usually hurts very little, although it may feel somewhat bruised, like getting a tetanus or flu shot. A simple bandage is all that is usually required afterward.

What Happens After an FNA?

The cells drawn up in the syringe are sent to the laboratory for analysis. The results take from 3 to 10 days to come back. Your doctor will discuss the results with you when they are available.

How Accurate Is FNA?

It depends. However, a good estimate considering all things is that it is about 90% accurate. If it says cancer is there, it usually is. However, it may miss a cancer and further tests would be needed.

What Are the Benefits of FNA?

The main benefit is to diagnose the lump. If it is a simple cyst, FNA can also remove the fluid and make the lump disappear. Usually a surgical biopsy can then be avoided.

What Are the Risks Associated With FNA?

The main risk is not getting enough cells and so not knowing for sure what the lump is. About a quarter of all FNAs come back "indeterminate," which means the laboratory cannot tell for sure what it is, or whether it is good or bad news. If that happens, the FNA can be redone, or surgery can be performed instead.

Continued

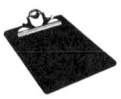

Patient Education Handout—cont'd

FINE-NEEDLE ASPIRATION (FNA)—cont'd

It is possible to hit a blood vessel or nerve with the needle used for FNA. Since the needle is so small, that usually causes no permanent harm. In fact, the needle is the same kind used to draw blood from blood vessels. However, just as with any blood draw, you can get a bruise from hitting a vessel.

Can the Needle Biopsy Spread Cancer?
Studies show it does not.

When Should I Call My Healthcare Provider?
If you have swelling or more than just mild soreness after FNA, you should call to ask about it. It is also important to call your doctor if the lump comes back or you feel the lump is growing. Tests can be wrong. If the lump persists, no matter what the tests say, it must be removed.

Is Any Follow-Up Needed?
Yes. Usually your doctor will want to recheck the area in 6 weeks to 3 months. It is important to make sure the lump is gone or has not changed.

Special Instructions:

Websites That May Be of Interest to You:
home.aafp.org/afp/970215ap/970215a.html (fine needle aspiration biopsy)
www.health.harvard.edu/fhg/diagnostics/FNA/FNA.shtml
www.thyroid-cancer.net/topics/35
www.endocrineweb.com/fna.html (thyroid nodule diagnosis)

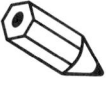 *Patient Consent Form*

FINE-NEEDLE ASPIRATION (FNA)

I came to the office of Dr. _____ on _____ (date) for evaluation
of a lump or nodule in my: (location)

which could be: (differential diagnosis)

We discussed the different ways to diagnose this lump and the risks of not evaluating it. Based on the
advice given by Dr. _____ and my own judgment, I request and agree to
undergo fine-needle aspiration (FNA) biopsy of this lump. I understand that FNA means putting a
needle, like those used for blood tests or shots, into the lump and drawing out cells to send to the
laboratory. I understand that it takes several days to get a report from the laboratory. I understand
that sometimes the results are not clear, in which case the FNA may need to be performed again (or
other tests performed).

We discussed the different outcomes of the test. I understand that the spot may bruise afterwards,
and that unforeseeable complications can arise from any medical procedure. I agree to follow the
instructions for bandaging, and I will return for follow-up care and discussion of the results on
_____ (date).

I will call the office or the answering service if any problems arise before the scheduled follow-up
visit.

_____   _____
Patient's or guardian's signature   *Date/Time*

_____   _____
Witness' signature   *Physician's signature*

One copy for chart; one copy for patient.

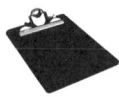 *Patient Education Handout*

MEDICAL HYPNOSIS: 10 FREQUENTLY ASKED QUESTIONS

1. Doesn't the Hypnotist Have Control Over His Subject?

No, a hypnotized person is not under the control of the hypnotist and will not do or say anything that they do not want to do or say.

2. Is the Hypnotized Person Asleep or Unconscious?

No, a hypnotized person, even in a trance, is not unconscious or asleep.

3. I Thought You Had to Be Slow or Dull Mentally to Be Able to Be Hypnotized?

No, actually the person of above-average intelligence makes the best subject.

4. Isn't it True That Most People Cannot Be Hypnotized?

No, 95% of people can be hypnotized. The 5% who cannot be hypnotized include the very young (under 5 years of age). With the very young, there may not be enough language ability to follow certain suggestions. Also included in the 5% are the feeble-minded (mental age less than 5 years) and a limited number of patients suffering from psychosis.

5. I Heard That It Can Be Dangerous to Be Hypnotized. Is That True?

No, there are no dangers from hypnosis in the hands of a qualified medical hypnotist.

6. Can People Get "Hooked" on Hypnosis?

No, hypnosis is not habit forming.

7. Can the Hypnotist Make a Hypnotized Person Tell a Secret He or She Does Not Want to Tell?

No, the hypnotized person will not tell any secrets he or she wishes to retain.

8. Can a Hypnotized Patient Get "Stuck" in the Hypnotic Trance?

No, the patient will awaken from a hypnotic trance quickly and easily.

9. What if the Hypnotist Wanted to Keep the Patient in a Trance for Some Reason?

Actually, the hypnotized person is in control and can come out of trance anytime he or she wishes. It is similar to an orchestra conductor (hypnotist) and musician (hypnotized patient). The conductor directs the musician, but if the musician wants to stop playing for any reason, the musician could stop at any time. The hypnotized patient, like the musician, is in control.

10. Aren't There After-Effects of Being Hypnotized, Like Feeling Tired or Drugged?

No, there are no after-effects from hypnosis, unlike chemical anesthetics and tranquilizers. Generally, the patient comes out of the hypnotic trance alert and rested.

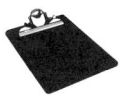 *Patient Education Handout*

LUMBAR PUNCTURE

What Is Lumbar Puncture?

A lumbar puncture is performed to diagnose and treat many disorders of the central nervous system.

Why Do I Need This Procedure?

Your clinician is trying to diagnose, treat, or exclude a condition of your central nervous system, and lumbar puncture is usually the best way to accomplish this.

How Do I Prepare for a Lumbar Puncture?

No preparation is necessary, but your clinician should discuss the procedure beforehand and have you sign a consent form before the procedure is done.

What Happens During the Procedure?

First, an area of skin on the back is cleaned with a sterile soap solution. Then a small amount of local anesthesia is used to numb the skin. A needle is then placed into the back to withdraw fluid from around the spinal cord. This fluid is collected and sent to the lab for analysis.

What Are the Risks Associated With This Procedure?

The procedure is very safe, and serious side effects are rare; but some complications can occur. You will feel some discomfort as the anesthesia is injected over the site. Another common side effect is a temporary headache, and your clinician may have you lie on your back for 1 to 2 hours after the procedure, to lessen the chance of getting this side effect.

Other possible complications are very rare and include infection, bleeding, the formation of a blood clot around the spinal cord, seizures, or even death.

What Do I Need to Do Following the Procedure to Prevent Infection?

Your clinician will place a Band-Aid on the spot where the needle was placed to help prevent infection.

Special Instructions:

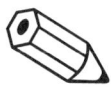 *Patient Consent Form*

LUMBAR PUNCTURE

I came to the office of my clinician, _____, on _____(date) for evaluation and/or treatment of the following condition:

We discussed the different treatments/evaluations possible, and discussed the risks of not treating the condition. Based on the advice given by my clinician, _____, and my own judgment, I agree to undergo a lumbar puncture.

Description of the procedure: Local anesthesia is used to numb an area of skin on the lower back. A needle is then used to obtain fluid from around the spinal cord for diagnosis and/or treatment. A sterile bandage is placed over the puncture site, and I will then be asked to lie on my back for 2 hours.

We discussed the different outcomes that could occur and most of the possible complications. I am aware that other complications could occur that we could not foresee. I agree to follow the instructions for self care after the procedure and to return for follow-up care on _____.

I will call the office or answering service if any problems arise before the scheduled follow-up visit.

_____   _____
Patient's signature   *Date/Time*

_____   _____
Witness' signature   *Clinician's signature*

One copy for chart; one copy for patient.

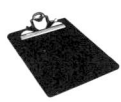 *Patient Education Handout*

MUSCLE BIOPSY

Muscle biopsy is a procedure in which a piece of muscle tissue is removed for examination. The test is performed to help diagnose diseases of the muscles that may cause pain or weakness.

No fasting is necessary to prepare for the procedure. Loose clothing should be worn on the day of the procedure, and a consent form must be signed.

In the first step of the biopsy, the skin over the muscle intended for biopsy is numbed with a local anesthetic. A small incision is made in the skin, and a piece of muscle about 2 inches long is removed. There may be a pulling and pinching sensation during the removal of the muscle tissue. The incision is then closed under the skin with a stitch that will later dissolve. Pulling and pressure sensations may be felt, and the amount of pain should be minimal.

Possible complications of this procedure include bleeding, infection, and excessive scarring of the muscle, all of which happen rarely. There is also a chance that the biopsy will not provide adequate information and a diagnosis cannot be made. If this occurs, a second biopsy may be needed.

After the biopsy there is little activity restriction. The area of biopsy may feel bruised, and some pulling sensation is normal. Pain medication may or may not be necessary and is supplied if needed. The dressing should stay in place for at least 48 hours and then may be removed. The paper-tape strips under the dressing should stay in place for 5 to 7 days. A shower can be taken immediately with the outer dressing in place. Soaking the incision should be avoided for 7 to 10 days.

The area of the biopsy should be watched for signs of bleeding. A small amount of red to pink fluid may accumulate under the dressing. This is normal. If excessive drainage, pain, swelling, or bruising is noted, the physician should be contacted. The area should also be monitored for signs of infection. If increasing redness, worsening pain, or drainage that looks like pus develops, the physician should be contacted.

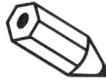

Patient Consent Form

MUSCLE BIOPSY

1. I hereby authorize the clinician, _____, and whomever he or she may designate as his or her assistant to perform a muscle biopsy.

2. If an unforeseen condition arises in the course of the procedure, I further request and authorize the clinician to do procedures in addition to or different from those now contemplated if, in the clinician's judgment, he or she deems it advisable.

3. I acknowledge that the contemplated procedure, possible procedures in addition to the contemplated operation, and possible complications have been explained to me by the clinician to my satisfaction.

4. I acknowledge that no guarantee or assurance has been made as to the results that may be obtained. I understand that I am to have the usual and ordinary care practiced by clinicians and surgeons and furnished in this community and that no other promise or representation written or implied is made, nor is any employee or representative of the medical center authorized to make any other promise or representation.

5. I consent to the administration of anesthesia prescribed or chosen by the attending physician, surgeon, and/or anesthesiologist.

6. I consent to photographing or videotaping the operation to be performed, including appropriate portions of my body, for medical, scientific, or educational purposes.

7. I hereby authorize the medical center to retain, preserve, and use for scientific or teaching purposes any specimen or tissue taken from my body.

8. I consent to the disposal by authorities of the medical center of any tissue or parts that may be removed.

9. I consent to the admittance of medical observers to the surgical department for the purpose of advancing medical science.

10. **I acknowledge that I have read and fully understand the above consent to procedure.**

_____   _____
Patient's signature   *Date/Time*

_____   _____
Witness' signature   *Date/Time*

_____
Relationship, if parent or guardian

Patient unable to sign because: _____

Additional remarks: _____

(Adapted from MidMichigan Regional Medical Center, Midland, Mich.)

Neoplasm, Skin: ICD-9 Codes

	Malignant			Benign	Uncertain Behavior	Unspecified
	Primary	Secondary	Ca in situ			
Skin NEC	173.9	198.2	232.9	216.9	238.2	239.2
Abdominal wall	173.5	198.2	232.5	216.5	238.2	239.2
Ala nasi	173.3	198.2	232.3	216.3	238.2	239.2
Ankle	173.7	198.2	232.7	216.7	238.2	239.2
Antecubital space	173.6	198.2	232.6	216.6	238.2	239.2
Anus	173.5	198.2	232.5	216.5	238.2	239.2
Arm	173.6	198.2	232.6	216.6	238.2	239.2
Auditory canal (external)	173.2	198.2	232.2	216.2	238.2	239.2
Auricle (ear)	173.2	198.2	232.2	216.2	238.2	239.2
Auricular canal (external)	173.2	198.2	232.2	216.2	238.2	239.2
Axilla, axillary fold	173.5	198.2	232.5	216.5	238.2	239.2
Back	173.5	198.2	232.5	216.5	216.5	239.2
Breast	173.5	198.2	232.5	216.5	238.2	239.2
Brow	173.3	198.2	232.3	216.3	238.2	239.2
Buttock	173.5	198.2	232.5	216.5	238.2	239.2
Calf	173.7	198.2	232.7	216.7	238.2	239.2
Canthus (eye) (inner) (outer)	173.1	198.2	232.1	216.1	238.2	239.2
Cervical region	173.4	198.2	232.4	216.4	238.2	239.2
Cheek (external)	173.3	198.2	232.3	216.3	238.2	239.2
Chest (wall)	173.5	198.2	232.5	216.5	238.2	239.2
Chin	173.3	198.2	232.3	216.3	238.2	239.2
Clavicular area	173.5	198.2	232.5	216.5	238.2	239.2
Clitoris	184.3	198.82	232.3	221.2	236.3	239.5
Columnella	173.3	198.2	232.3	216.3	238.2	239.2
Concha	173.2	198.2	232.2	216.2	238.2	239.2
Contiguous sites	173.8					
Ear (external)	173.2	198.2	232.2	216.2	238.2	239.2
Elbow	173.6	198.2	232.6	216.6	238.2	239.2
Eyebrow	173.3	198.2	232.3	216.3	238.2	239.2
Eyelid	173.1	198.2	232.1	216.1	238.2	239.2
Face NEC	173.3	198.2	232.3	216.3	238.2	239.2
Female genital organs (external)	184.4	198.82	233.3	221.2	236.3	239.5
Clitoris	184.3	198.82	233.3	221.2	236.3	239.5
Labium NEC	184.4	198.82	233.3	221.2	236.3	239.5
Majus	184.1	198.82	233.3	221.2	236.3	239.5
Minus	184.2	198.82	233.3	221.2	236.3	239.5
Pudendum	184.4	198.82	233.3	221.2	236.3	239.5
Vulva	184.4	198.82	233.3	221.2	236.3	239.5
Finger	173.6	198.2	232.6	216.6	238.2	239.2
Flank	173.5	198.2	232.5	216.5	238.2	239.2
Foot	173.7	198.2	232.7	216.7	238.2	239.2
Forearm	173.6	198.2	232.6	216.6	238.2	239.2
Forehead	173.3	198.1	232.3	216.3	238.2	239.2
Glabella	173.3	198.2	232.3	216.3	238.2	239.2
Gluteal region	173.5	198.2	232.5	216.5	238.2	239.2
Groin	173.5	198.2	232.5	216.5	238.2	239.2
Hand	173.6	198.2	232.6	216.6	238.2	239.2
Head NEC	173.4	198.2	232.4	216.4	238.2	239.2
Heel	173.7	198.2	232.7	216.7	238.2	239.2

International Classification of Diseases, rev 9: ICD-9-CM 2003, ed 6, 2003, Ingenix/St. Anthony Publishing.

Continued

| | Malignant | | | | Uncertain | |
	Primary	Secondary	Ca in situ	Benign	Behavior	Unspecified
Helix	173.2	198.2	232.2	216.2	238.2	239.2
Hip	173.7	198.2	232.7	216.7	238.2	239.2
Infraclavicular region	173.5	198.2	232.5	216.5	238.2	239.2
Inguinal region	173.5	198.2	232.5	216.5	238.2	239.2
Jaw	173.3	198.2	232.3	216.3	238.2	239.2
Knee	173.7	198.2	232.7	216.7	238.2	239.2
Labia						
Majora	184.1	198.82	233.3	221.2	236.3	239.5
Minora	184.2	198.82	233.3	221.2	236.3	239.5
Leg	173.7	198.2	232.7	216.7	238.2	239.2
Lid (lower) (upper)	173.1	198.2	232.1	216.1	238.2	239.2
Limb NEC	173.9	198.2	232.9	216.9	238.2	239.2
Lower	173.7	198.2	232.7	216.7	238.2	239.2
Upper	173.6	198.2	232.6	216.6	238.2	239.2
Lip (upper) (lower)	173.0	198.2	232.0	216.0	238.2	239.2
Male genital organs	187.9	198.82	232.6	222.9	236.6	239.5
Penis	187.4	198.82	232.5	222.1	236.6	239.5
Prepuce	187.1	198.82	232.5	222.1	236.6	239.5
Scrotum	187.7	198.82	232.6	222.4	236.6	239.5
Mastectomy site	173.5	198.2				
Specified as breast tissue	174.8	198.81				
Meatus, acoustic (external)	173.2	198.2	232.2	216.2	238.2	239.2
Melanoma (see Melanoma)						
Nates	173.5	198.2	232.5	216.5	238.2	239.0
Neck	173.4	198.2	232.4	216.4	238.2	239.2
Nose (external)	173.3	198.2	232.3	216.3	238.2	239.2
Palm	173.6	198.2	232.6	216.6	238.2	239.2
Palpebra	173.1	198.2	232.1	216.1	238.2	239.2
Penis NEC	187.4	198.82	233.5	222.1	236.6	239.5
Perianal	173.5	198.2	232.5	216.5	238.2	239.2
Perineum	173.5	198.2	232.5	216.5	238.2	239.2
Pinna	173.2	198.2	232.2	216.2	238.2	239.2
Plantar	173.7	198.2	232.7	216.7	238.2	239.2
Popliteal fossa or space	173.7	198.2	232.7	216.7	238.2	239.2
Prepuce	187.7	198.82	233.5	222.1	236.6	239.5
Pubes	173.6	198.2	232.5	216.5	238.2	239.2
Sacrococcygeal region	173.7	198.2	232.5	216.5	238.2	239.2
Scalp	173.8	198.2	232.4	216.4	238.2	239.2
Scapular region	173.5	198.2	232.5	216.5	238.2	239.2
Scrotum	187.7	198.82	233.6	222.4	236.6	239.5
Shoulder	173.6	198.2	232.6	216.6	238.2	239.2
Sole (foot)	173.7	198.2	232.7	216.7	238.2	239.2
Specified sites NEC	173.8	198.2	232.8	216.8	232.8	239.2
Submammary fold	173.5	198.2	232.5	216.5	238.2	239.2
Supraclavicular region	173.4	198.2	232.4	216.4	238.2	239.2
Temple	173.3	198.2	232.3	216.3	238.2	239.2
Thigh	173.7	198.2	232.7	216.7	238.2	239.2
Thoracic wall	173.5	198.2	232.5	216.5	238.2	239.2
Thumb	173.6	198.2	232.6	216.6	238.2	239.2
Toe	173.7	198.2	232.7	216.7	238.2	239.2
Tragus	173.2	198.2	232.2	216.2	238.2	239.2
Trunk	173.5	198.2	232.5	216.5	238.2	239.2
Umbilicus	173.5	198.2	232.5	216.5	238.2	239.2
Vulva	184.4	198.8	233.3	221.2	236.3	239.5
Wrist	173.6	198.2	232.6	216.6	238.2	239.2

Pearls of Practice

John L. Pfenninger
Grant C. Fowler
Chapter authors

1. When repairing or removing **scalp lesions,** remember that patients do not like to have their hair shaved unless it is absolutely necessary. **Remove minor lesions without shaving.** To keep the hair from continually falling into the operative field, use antibiotic ointment to flatten it down. Apply it after performing the usual prep.

2. The majority of **skin lesion removals** are performed either with a shave technique or with cautery and curettement. The **key** to an excellent long-term outcome with **minimal scarring is moist healing.** Eschars (scabs) impair the normal healing process. Healing tissue is much like a new lawn: It needs to be kept moist. Unless under clothes, wounds should remain uncovered when possible. If under clothes, they will obviously need to be covered. Likewise, facial areas need to be covered at night. Basically, the patient just washes the area three to four times a day with mild soap and water and applies an ointment afterwards. It does not necessarily have to be an antibacterial ointment; even Vaseline will do. In fact, avoid neomycin, hydrogen peroxide, or Betadine after the first day. The key is to keep the area moist. The deeper the wound, the longer this will be necessary (generally 7 to 14 days).

   Even with sutures, have the patient gently wash the area within 12 hours and apply antibiotic ointment three or four times a day (unless tissue glue or Steri-Strips have been applied).

   See the patient education handout titled "Moist Healing After Skin Surgery" on page 1747 of Appendix G.

3. There is **no need to stop Coumadin or aspirin for routine dermatologic procedures.** Several articles have been published documenting that embolic events occur during the period of stopping and restarting the Coumadin. Meticulous attention must be paid to hemostasis. Clotting parameters should be checked before significant excisional surgery. However, for shaves, curettements, and most excisions, it is not necessary to stop coumadin or to check lab results. (From Alcalay J: *Dermatol Surg* 27:756, 2001; Schanbacher CF, Bennett RG: *Dermatol Surg* 26:785, 2000.)

4. **"Bridge therapy" is for patients on chronic anticoagulation** who need elective surgery. It is defined as protected periprocedural discontinuation of warfarin (Coumadin) 3 to 4 days before performing procedures in patients at high risk for thromboembolism. The first step is initiation of low-molecular-weight heparin (LMWH) at full therapeutic dose on the day after warfarin is stopped (e.g., no warfarin Monday, begin LMWH on Tuesday morning). The patient receives the last dose of LMWH the morning of the day before the procedure. Then the invasive procedure or surgery occurs. Warfarin and LMWH are reintroduced later that day if deemed safe and hemostasis has been achieved. Subsequently, LMWH is discontinued after discharge once the INR has been therapeutic for 3 or 4 days.

   Bridge therapy is for patients with a high risk of atrial fibrillation (i.e., for CVA prevention), prosthetic valves, indications for prolonged warfarin therapy, a recent (last 3 months) thromboembolic event, or a history of a hypercoagulable state.

   This therapy avoids prolonged hospitalization, changing of anticoagulation while preparing for surgery, vitamin K administration, and a prolonged period without anticoagulation with the attendant risk for thromboembolism.

   The disadvantages are cost of LMWH, self-injection, and a relative lack of reversibility. (Submitted by James Lile, pharmacist, MidMichigan Regional Medical Center, Midland, Mich.)

5. For those who want to **diminish the pain with anesthetic injections,** add a little bicarb to the anesthetic (1 part bicarb to 9 parts of anesthetic).

Anesthetics sting with injection because of a low pH; this supposedly inhibits bacterial growth but at the same time is uncomfortable. The bicarb takes the "sting" out of the injection. Also, use a small needle (27 or 30 gauge), use warm solutions, and inject slowly. Injecting deeper into the dermis will cause less pain, but it takes longer for the anesthetic to work. Injecting more superficially will hurt a little more, but the anesthetic will work faster. Do not add sodium bicarb to Marcaine since Marcaine will precipitate in a neutral pH.

6. When **injecting lidocaine** into an area where you have to be able to palpate later (foreign body removal, vasectomy, etc.), you can massage the lidocaine into the skin so it does not obstruct your fine touch.

7. Melman and Siegel (1999) have shown that it is perfectly okay to **draw up anesthetic solutions in syringes up to 7 days before use.** There is no increased bacterial contamination or growth, and the anesthetic still functions. We used to pull up our syringes at the beginning of the day and then discard them at the end of the day, but there is no need to do this. We now fill numerous 1-ml syringes, date them, and continue to use them throughout the week. It is much more efficient for the nurse to pull up multiple syringes than to do just one at a time. It is not efficient for the physician to spend time pulling up anesthetic! (Melman D, Siegel DM: *Dermatol Surg* 25:492, 1999.)

8. Consider using the **MadaJet for local injections.** It is a small handheld "gun" that "injects" medications without a needle. It is only for superficial type injections but can be used to treat keloids and hypertrophic scars with steroids, etc. It has even been used for vasectomies! (See Wilson CL: No-needle anesthetic for no-scalpel vasectomy, *Am Fam Physician* 63:1295, 2001.) It is available from Delasco at 1-800-831-6273 (website: www.delasco.com).

9. When someone complains of an **allergy to local anesthetics,** they have usually received an *ester.* This includes novocaine. To date, there have been no reported allergic reactions to the *amides* such as lidocaine (Xylocaine). Some patients still report that they have had a reaction to lidocaine or to "all local anesthetics." In these instances, they have usually had medication drawn from a multidose vial, which has preservatives (parabens) in it. If someone does complain of having a history of local anesthetic reaction, use single-dose vials of Xylocaine and they will be able to tolerate it without incident. It is inexpensive and helpful to have around. (Also see no. 43.)

10. Advanced Meditech International (AMI) has designed **a small anesthetic bottle holder that mounts on the wall** (VE-11 Handzfree Anesthetic Bottle Holder). The cost is only around $40, but in our office, it is indispensable. It holds the anesthetic where it is readily available and makes filling syringes an easy task. It also allows the entire staff to see how much anesthetic is left in the bottle. There is nothing more frustrating than pulling out the drawer with the anesthetic solution and finding that the bottle is empty! Contact AMI at 1-800-635-2452 (website: www. ameditech.com).

11. Physicians must **maximize the time in the office.** Inefficiency has to be eliminated. I (JLP) literally try to **find 30 seconds to save on every patient.** Having the syringes prefilled (see no. 7) saves time! When I discuss this at our courses, there are often chuckles about "the 30 seconds." However, I am usually able to see 20 to 25 patients in a day. If I save 30 seconds on each one, this is 10 to 12 minutes per day, which actually allows an extra office visit or procedure in a day. If you work 4 days a week, that is four extra visits a week. Working 45 weeks out of the year, this amounts to 180 visits. If you average $100 per visit, that is an extra $18,000 per year. At $150 per visit, that is an extra $27,000 a year. . . just for saving 30 seconds per patient! If you see more than 20 to 25 patients per day, even more can be earned. **Efficiency is essential.**

12. OSHA has numerous requirements for a safe office practice. One of them is the use of **fluid-resistant coats when performing procedures.** My (JLP's) staff ordered these coats for me. They made an error and actually selected the coats with the **knit sleeves**—how fortuitous! As residents rotate through the office, they frequently have the large sleeves that look like the old nuns' habits! The sleeves hang down 8 to 10 inches from the wrist. Subsequently when they reach for an instrument, the sleeve often drags across the sterile field. Knit cuffs help protect a sterile field and I highly recommend them. The fluid-resistant coats are also beneficial in that any fluid that gets on them is easily wiped off, and the coats last a long time. And remember, not using them could make you liable for a $25,000 OSHA fine!

13. I (JLP) have found that a **good way to explain the risk of complications** to patients is to use the example of a lottery. In medicine, you "never say 'never' and never say 'always'." And yet, the likelihood of some things happening are almost "never." So I ask the patients if they play the lotto.

Most of them do sometimes. I then ask them if they will ever win. Most of them say, "No." Then I reply, "But you could, right?" and they say, "Yes." I then explain that many complications are just like that. It is not going to happen, but if you play "the lotto," it could. This really helps them understand the risk of complications. (So one day, a patient called up and said that he had won the lotto. A resident who was working with me got excited. I had to tell him that that wasn't good!)

14. I (JLP) have always liked to explain to patients how the particular surgery or procedure went. I try to be very honest. I will often say, "Technically, things went well," or "Technically, this case was quite difficult and we had a few problems." **Patients appreciate honesty.** They know things cannot go perfectly all the time. I never tell patients that it was "an easy case"; should complications arise, they think you have done something wrong. If you tell them, however, that the case was difficult, you are not looked on so negatively if complications do arise. Also, if there are no complications with tough cases, they think you have done a better job. The point of this tip: *Never overstate how well something went.* Just say that technically things went well, but complications can still occur.

15. I (JLP) have done perhaps 125 or 130 medical legal cases as an expert witness. A **brief tip to avoid litigation:** When a patient comes in to the office, always review the last note to see what the complaint was. Ask the patient if the problem has resolved. Just jot a little note (e.g., "breast mass resolved" with the date, or "rectal bleeding gone" with the date, or perhaps "cough cleared"). Many times patients come into the office for a new complaint and the physician forgets about a significant old complaint, but the patient thinks that you remember. Just looking back at the record and asking that simple question could have cleared many physicians from later malpractice suits. You would also be amazed how many problems persist that the patients don't complain about and physicians subsequently overlook.

16. The **height of your exam table** is extremely important. When I (JLP) opened a new office, I purchased a table that was only 2 inches higher than my current one. Old folks had a difficult time getting up on the table. I found that the lowest height can be no more than 24 inches. A **power table is essential** if you are going to be doing procedures.

17. There are really few **medical emergencies** in a physician's office. However, one of them can be **anaphylaxis** (see Chapter 203). In addition to

the **Banyan Kit** that is mentioned there ("a crash cart in a suitcase"), I keep an **EpiPen** taped to one of our cupboard doors. Right beside it is a vial of **atropine** and some **ammonia salts.** I have only had occasion to use the EpiPen once after an injection with candida. However, people were not rushing around looking for the proper dose of epinephrine, or the syringe, or even trying to find the epi! We just opened the cupboard door where it was taped, and gave the injection. Consider having these three medications readily available in your office, especially if you perform a significant number of procedures or injections. The Banyan Kit is the most cost efficient and safe, practical way to maintain resuscitation capabilities in your office.

18. I (JLP) have developed a simple **method for determining whether or not a patient is likely to faint during a procedure.** I think vasovagal symptoms have occurred more with vasectomy than with any other procedure I do. Subsequently, I ask the patient how well they tolerate pain. The options are "well," "okay," and "poorly." I also ask them if they have a tendency to faint or if they faint when they see blood. If the answer is that they tolerate pain well, I just use a local anesthetic. If they tolerate pain "okay", I'll give them 10 mg of diazepam an hour before significant procedures. If they tolerate pain poorly or if they say they have a tendency to faint, in addition to the 10 mg of diazepam orally, I'll give 0.5 of atropine IM on arrival to the office. (I'll often listen to the wife's answers, too, as opposed to just a man's response!) Since using this approach, I haven't had a single patient have a vasovagal episode while on the table during a vasectomy or any other procedure.

19. It is important that your office staff know that **epinephrine should not be used in fingers, nose, penis, and toes.** These are end-arterial and the vessels can go into spasm. Interestingly, these very same areas are very sensitive to anesthetic injections. In addition to the "fingers, nose, penis, toes," I (JPL) add genitals and anorectal area for sensitivity. Warn patients that injections in these areas are very uncomfortable.

20. Now that I (JLP) receive numerous referrals from primary care physicians, I think the **single largest error that I see involves anal complaints.** Frequently patients are sent to me for "hemorrhoids" and I have found fissures, fistulas, cancers, polyps, warts, and solitary anal ulcers. It seems that for both physicians and patients, when there is any rectal bleeding, it is automatically assumed to be "hemorrhoids." My only plea

would be to look. Many times just spreading the glutei will give you the diagnosis. If nothing else, **perform a digital examination and a good anoscopy.** In my opinion, the only anoscope to use is an **Ive's slotted anoscope.** The long cylindrical scopes just do not allow adequate visualization for anorectal complaints. If you as a clinician do not feel comfortable evaluating anorectal complaints, then don't treat them; but don't make a diagnosis for the patient. Just send them to a clinician who is willing to evaluate them.

21. It always amazes me (JLP) that when patients have anal complaints, one of the first things they are treated with is **hydrocortisone cream for presumed hemorrhoids.** I ask at many of my courses how many physicians treat varicosities of the lower extremities with steroids. Not surprisingly, no one does. Then why does everyone treat "hemorrhoids," which are engorged veins, with steroids? It is an appropriate thing to do if the hemorrhoids are inflamed, but probably less than 10% of those with rectal bleeding truly have inflammation. Again, **a caveat would be to examine the patient first before making the diagnosis of hemorrhoids** and to use hydrocortisone preparations only if inflammation is present.

22. A study was performed that looked at **absorbable vs. nonabsorbable sutures after a punch biopsy.** The study found that the cosmetic results after the sutures were pulled and 3 months later were equal.

23. When performing a **punch biopsy of the skin,** use a 3-mm punch. The advantage is that it provides enough tissue for diagnosis but will not need suture closure. A 4-mm punch often requires a suture, and a 5-mm punch definitely does. However, when you close a circular lesion that is 5 mm with suture, you will end up with dog ears on each side. A 2-mm punch is generally adequate for diagnosis, but the tissue is often macerated and it is difficult to give the pathologist a good specimen. If a 3-mm punch defect is not closed, there will usually be no visible scar remaining. At the very worst, the patient may end up with a small acne pockmark-like lesion.

24. Performing a **needle biopsy does not spread malignant cells** in the needle track. It is safe even with nodes that contain metastatic melanoma. Similarly, shaving a nevus does not lead to malignant transformation.

25. **The work-up for abnormal uterine bleeding** is now generally managed with an endometrial biopsy (see Chapter 146). In the past, when

D & Cs were performed, a "fractional" D & C was recommended. This meant that an endocervical curettage preceded the D & C. When the studies confirmed that endometrial biopsies alone were an adequate method of evaluating abnormal uterine bleeding, many dropped the endocervical curettage (ECC). However, an ACOG Bulletin recommends that the **evaluation for abnormal uterine bleeding includes an ECC along with the endometrial biopsy.** If these studies are negative and symptoms resolve, no further work-up is necessary. Although many of us have jumped to performing **vaginal ultrasounds to evaluate abnormal uterine bleeding, there is an ethnic variance.** Although the safe cut-off quoted is 5 mm of endometrial stripe, cancers have been found with only 3 mm of stripe in Japanese patients. Endometrial biopsy with ECC is still, in my (JLP's) estimation, the best way to evaluate abnormal uterine bleeding. The caveat is to be sure that it is "uterine" and that other potential causes are not overlooked.

26. Unless extensive stitching is to be done, **sterile gloves are not needed for routine biopsies and most skin procedures.**

27. A potential **pitfall in interpreting Pap smear results** is to confuse atypical squamous cells of uncertain significance (ASCUS) with atypical glandular cells of uncertain significance (AGUS). The new Bethesda 2001 terminology divides ASCUS into ASC-US (atypical squamous cells of undetermined significance) and ASC-H (atypical squamous cells, high-grade lesion cannot be ruled out). In addition, atypical glandular cells are now identified as just "AGC"; it is no longer "of undetermined significance." Should a Pap smear come back with either ASC-H or atypical glandular cells, it is imperative that the patient undergo a complete work-up, beginning with colposcopy. A consensus of studies shows that approximately 10% of patients with atypical glandular cells will have a cancer somewhere in the genital tract if indeed the cells are glandular and atypical. Another 10% to 15% will have high-grade dysplastic lesions. **Be careful not to confuse atypical squamous cells with atypical glandular cells.**

28. I (JLP) have found that using the **medium titanium hemoclips for performing vasectomies for fascial occlusion** has been a real timesaver and reduces the amount of bleeding present during the procedure. When introduced to the clips 12 years ago, I was resistant because I was going to have to incur another cost for the applicators. However, when suture material is

used to perform the purse string around the fascia, the suture material also adds to the cost. In addition, bleeding often occurs with the insertion of the needle and it takes more time. Now, if there is bleeding in the fascial tissues around the vas, the titanium clip will readily and quickly control it. Patients often ask if the clips set off metal detectors. Since they are nonmagnetic, they do not. After a vas there will often be a slight palpable nodule, but by 3 months, patients are unable to detect any sign of the clip. If the patient continues to be worried, I just tell him to think about all the men who have fought in various battles during war. They have shrapnel everywhere and it does not cause a problem. This usually eases their mind.

29. In regard to billing, **consider billing a handling fee (99000)** when any labs are sent out to the hospital or other laboratory. Although many HMOs, Medicare, and Medicaid may not reimburse it, a good portion of private insurances do. This covers your costs for documenting that the labs were sent out, for receiving the labs back, and for calling the patient. Even if only a small percentage of these fees is paid, it is still worthwhile charging for them.

30. **"Insurance only" statements on your bills may get you into trouble.** If you write "insurance only," it negates the insurance company's obligation to pay you. Treating certain patients such as physicians and friends for free is a medical tradition, but be careful. The changes in the law have made it a bad idea. The courts ruled in 1991 that physicians cannot charge insurance companies if they make this statement! (Don't you just love how everyone else tells us what to do? My suggestion: Be creative and be the doctor you want to be. You can figure out a way around this bureaucratic hassle.)

31. **If you write off the patient portion of a Medicare bill,** document well why it is a hardship case. Otherwise, Medicare can sue you and reclaim many of the fees they have paid you.

32. **For Medicare, you cannot bill for treating your families,** which include husband, wife, parents (even if adopted), children, siblings, step-relatives, grandparents, and domestic employees. It is okay for your partner to treat them, but they cannot do it for insurance only. See above.

33. For those of you who are audited and your CPT coding is questioned, see the following article: King MS, Lipsky MS, Sharp L: **Current procedural terminology coding: do the experts agree?** *J Am Board Fam Pract* 13(2):144, 2000.

They found that giving the same procedure to various coding experts resulted in various methods of coding out the procedure. Their conclusion was that CPT coding is not objective. This may help you in court!

34. I (GCF) suggest that you spend some quality time on coding and that you **buy a good book on coding.** While writing the foreign body removal chapter, I found that "10120" is the routine code for general removal of a subcutaneous foreign body. However, if the foreign body is located in the area of the shoulder, and is subcutaneous, the code is 23330 and the RVUs for this code are almost three times that for 10120! Knowing your coding and billing can markedly increase reimbursement. Consider the National Procedure Institute's *Reimbursement Manual,* which is updated annually (Phone: 1-800-462-2492; website: www.npinstitute.com).

35. It is difficult for us to know exactly **what to charge for each procedure.** There are three books to which I (JLP) commonly refer: *Yale Wasserman DMD Medical Publishers Ltd. Physicians' Fee Reference* (2003); *The Health Care Consultants of America, Inc. 2003 Physicians Fee & Coding Guide;* and the *Medicode National Fee Analyzer* (2003). Over the past 7 years, the National Procedures Institute has developed a 53-page manual that is especially helpful for office practices. It lists all the common procedures normally performed by primary care physicians. For each CPT code, the HCFA RVUs and Medicare, Medicaid, Michigan Blue Cross/ Blue Shield and 50th percentile fees are listed. The three above references list fees based on national surveys of what physicians charge. We take the 50th percentile from each book and average those three values to come up with the 50th percentile charge. This would give at least a starting point to determine what to charge patients. For instance, what is reasonable for removing an ingrown toenail? A vasectomy? Sclerotherapy? Incision of a thrombosed hemorrhoid? Many physicians are undercharging. This manual, which is updated annually, does a lot of the work for you and is available for $69.95 from The National Procedures Institute, 4909 Hedgewood Drive, Midland, MI 48640 (phone: 1-800-462-2492).

36. Medicare did have a list of procedures in which they would reimburse a surgical tray. However, as of 2003, a **surgical tray fee** is not allowed. They apparently incorporated the cost of the tray into the reimbursement for the procedure (in other words, a nice way to cut reimbursement

without admitting that they've done it!). However, a surgical tray can still be charged to other insurances with the procedures that require more medical supplies (e.g., LEEP). A surgical tray should never be charged for routine laceration repair or lesion removal, since it is indeed incorporated into the usual reimbursement fee.

37. With **coding and billing multiple procedures** performed on the same day, always have the biller code out the highest reimbursed procedure first. The procedures listed second, third, fourth, and fifth will be reduced by 50%. Those listed after that will be reduced to only 25% of the routine charge. **When seeing a new patient,** it is essential to obtain a past medical history and evaluate the patient for other medical problems before performing the procedure. Proper coding and billing (current procedural terminology [CPT]) allows for payment of an initial office visit along with the procedure that same day. However, if the patient has been seen in the practice within the last 3 years, only the procedure can be charged. If the procedure is performed and another separate identifiable service has been provided (e.g., treatment for diabetes), a **modifier 25** is used to receive reimbursement for both the procedure and the visit.

38. Some patients are sensitive to **nonsteroidal antiinflammatory drugs** (NSAIDs) and will have **increased bleeding** when using them. A simple way to check this out is just to obtain a bleeding time on and off the drug. If the bleeding time is prolonged while on the drug, patients are indeed sensitive. **Bleeding can be minimized by using rofecoxib (Vioxx) or any other COX-2 inhibitor.** Rofecoxib has been found to be comparable to codeine and hydrocodone for dental pain (wisdom teeth extraction), and yet the patient is not too sedated to drive home after a procedure. This medication will provide the nonsteroidal antiinflammatory pain relief desired but has minimal to no effect on platelets.

39. It is amazing to us that more physicians are not **incorporating ultrasound into the office practice.** The newer units are cheaper and smaller, and the definition has really been improved. Ultrasound is the modern stethoscope. If the stethoscope were developed today, we would call the HMO and get approval before we listen to someone's lungs to rule out pneumonia or congestive heart failure. Of course, approval for this procedure ("auscultation of the lungs") would probably cost $24.99! Physicians should be embracing ultrasound technology as a means to enhance diagnostic capabilities, reduce delay in diagnosis, and actually bring down healthcare costs. It reimbursed better than colonoscopy. After a 6-year review, one academic family medicine department found that a complete abdominal ultrasound was the best reimbursed procedure for the amount of time it took to perform it.

40. It concerns me (JLP) that so many physicians are **jumping to the LEEP procedure** to treat every dysplastic lesion on the cervix. **Cryotherapy has worked** for 30 years, and the documentation is excellent on efficacy and lack of complications. Cryotherapy only fails when there is a large extensive lesion or if the lesion goes into the os. It treats small CIN III lesions as well as conization (whether it be by laser, cold knife, or the LEEP procedure). Appropriate treatment with cryotherapy removes approximately 3 to 4 mm of cervix. Treatment with LEEP not only costs four to six times more (don't forget about the pathology fee to interpret the sample), but removes a minimum of 8 mm of cervix and often 15 mm. Every study that has been done shows that in properly selected patients, cryotherapy of the cervix has the same cure rate as the LEEP procedure. Some OB/GYN residency programs do not even teach cryotherapy anymore! I have a difficult time understanding the lack of science in medicine. (See Mitchell MF, Tortolero-Luna G, Cook E, et al: A randomized clinical trial of cryotherapy, laser vaporization, and loop electrosurgical excision for treatment of squamous intraepithelial lesions of the cervix, *Obstet Gynecol* 92:737, 1998; and Pfenninger JL: Good things still come in old packages: cryosurgery vs LEEP. Loop electrosurgical excision procedure, *J Am Board Fam Pract* 12:416, 1999.) (Could it be physicians choose the procedure that reimburses the most? No, we're above that, right?)

41. A fantastic **buying resource for dermatologic equipment** is Delasco (available at 1-800-831-6273 or www.delasco.com).

42. Now do you want to read something really interesting? See Harris WS, Gowda M, Kolb JW, et al: **A randomized, controlled trial of the effects of remote, intercessory prayer on outcomes in patients admitted to the coronary care unit,** *Arch Intern Med* 159:2273, 1999; and Cha KY, Wirth DP, Lobo RA: **Does prayer influence the success of in vitro fertilization-embryo transfer? Report of a masked, randomized trial,** *J Reprod Med* 46:9, 2001. When treating patients, always try to emphasize treating the "whole" patient. We need to include surgery, medicines, x-rays, faith, and the person in the healing process. The second reference is fascinating. Women attending an infertility clinic in South Korea were placed in the study to

evaluate the effects of prayer. Half of the group was prayed for in the United States; the other half was treated routinely. The average fertility rate for the clinic was 27% for the previous 2 years. For the control group, the average rate of pregnancy was 28%. For the group that was prayed for, the average pregnancy rate was 56%! And the rest of the story: None of these patients or their doctors even knew that they were enrolled in a study, let alone that they were being prayed for in the United States (while they were in South Korea)! I don't think we understand ESP, clairvoyance, or the power of prayer. But just because we don't understand it doesn't mean we shouldn't use it!

43. When **injecting steroids** into joints, many of the steroids will precipitate when mixed with multi-dose vials of anesthetic. (See Chapter 194, Joint and Soft Tissue Aspiration and Injection [Arthrocentesis].) When the steroids precipitate, small crystals are then injected into the joint space. Some have postulated that this may be one of the causes for the **postinjection flare** some people experience. To avoid this, use single-dose vials of the anesthetic that lack parabens, and the steroid will remain in solution. It is the reaction with the parabens that causes the precipitation.

44. Many people have asked how to obtain excellent **quality clinical photographs.** For 35 mm slides, I (JLP) have used the Yashica Dental Eye II camera, which in my estimation is unsurpassed for quality. There is a built-in flash, which always seems to have the appropriate exposure. It is available from Canfield Clinical Systems (1-800-815-4330 or www.canfieldsci.com) and costs around $1000. For those who are into digital, Olympus just came out with the new Camedia, which is 3 megapixels. A unique feature on this camera is that it has **8X Optical Zoom** as well as 3X Digital. The Optical Zoom gives you much clearer definition. It was introduced in June 2002 at a price of $600.

45. For those who have to treat **umbilical stump granulomas,** an article by Lotan G et al (Lotan G, Klin B, Efrati Y: Double-ligature: a treatment for pedunculated umbilical granulomas in children, *Am Fam Physician* 65:2067, 2002) suggests using two ligatures rather than silver nitrate or other methods. The first ligature is tied to hold the stump and pull it up while a deeper ligature is placed to necrose the entire stump. It will fall off in 7 to 14 days and apparently has a better outcome than using silver nitrate.

46. Many people think that **taking photographs of pathology** (e.g., colposcopic findings) is beneficial and will help in a suit situation. However, if you draw out the findings, you are the expert. In a photograph, an expert can contest what you identify. Drawing out your findings may indeed be more protective than photographing them.

47. **Hypnotherapy** can be a remarkable aid for controlling pain. Even if full hypnosis is not used, several relaxation techniques can be used. Use a low monotone voice during painful or uncomfortable procedures. Avoid noisy interruptions by the staff or too much noise in the hallways and around the room. Soft, soothing music helps. Engaging the patient to help relax is important.

48. **Compounding pharmacists** are now making a comeback. They can make lollipops with lidocaine for anesthesia for oral procedures for children and with nicotine for those trying to stop smoking. "Rectal rockets" can make treatment of inflamed hemorrhoids easier. It is beneficial to learn what a compounding pharmacist can do.

49. Consider using a **skin hook for vasectomies** if you do not have the no-scalpel vasectomy instruments. It not only helps to stabilize the vas but it is reassuring that the vas is isolated, since fascia will flatten out or tear with pressure or tension. The skin hook can also be used for the minimally invasive sebaceous cyst removal. It can fixate the cyst sac, making it easier to invert and remove the sac itself.

50. **Aesthetic procedures** are really "hot" at this time. Not only are patients demanding them, but reimbursement is reasonable! A 15- or 30-minute therapy may reimburse as much as 3 hours in the intensive care unit working on someone with diabetic ketoacidosis or cardiogenic shock. Caution: Many of the new instruments being offered are very expensive. Be sure to do your homework and determine what the maintenance fees will be per year. They can often run $5000 to $10,000! Also, check on cost for supplies. Be cautious about the salesman's pitch that "everyone will be running to your office." Many of us have been caught with equipment that generates cash—not for the doctor, but for the salesman and the company!

51. **The correct suture removal scissors** can make a tough job much easier. Fine, close sutures are often difficult to remove. It is worth the money to obtain Shortbent Stitch Scissors (3½ inch), curved, delicate (Miltex no. 9-101).

52. **Good 2.5× to 3× optical loops** do help to evaluate lesions, treat telangiectasias, and remove foreign bodies and sutures. Consider the Welch Allyn LumiView Portable Binocular Microscope or Flat Surface Magnifier (Welch Allyn, Inc., 4341 State Street Rd., Skaneateles Falls, NY 13153-0220; phone: 1-800-535-6663; website: www.welchallyn.com) or Keeler Loupes (Keeler, Clewer Hill Road,

Windsor, Berkshire, SL4 4AA; phone: +44 (0)1753 857177; website: www.keeler.co.uk).

53. If you are having difficulty **passing the sigmoidoscope or colonoscope** at 25 cm, roll the patient all the way onto his or her back. This opens up the rectosigmoid junction and allows the scope to pass more easily (GCF).

54. Pay critical attention to proper patient positioning for the **slit-lamp examination,** since this will greatly facilitate obtaining a good examination. Most ocular pathology can be visualized appropriately under low magnification. Use of high magnification causes many users to miss the forests for the trees (Christopher J. Bigelow, Midland, Mich).

55. The extensor tendons have a significant excursion over the metacarpophalangeal joints. When lacerations occur in this area, carefully explore the underlying joint capsule for penetration throughout the entire arc of motion. **Unrecognized open joint injuries** can lead to significant infection if not treated appropriately. However, bites or tooth lacerations are especially bad and occur during fistfights. Use a low index of suspicion to start broad-spectrum antibiotics.

   A sizeable **ganglion will typically transilluminate,** thereby providing affirmation of the diagnosis (David T. Bortel, Midland, Mich).

56. Take a lot of time to establish rapport with your young female patient. The pelvic-genital examination itself takes no more than 5 minutes if the fearful patient trusts you long enough to be cooperative.

   Don't expect the **child** who has just received **nasal midazolam** to sleep through your procedure. However, he or she will be cooperative.

   Do not be tempted to use **DeLee suctioning** to clear the airway of particulate meconium in a newborn. Use an appropriately sized endotracheal tube (David B. Bosscher, Knoxville, Tenn).

57. Since fewer elective vaginal breech deliveries are being attempted, **external cephalic version** often provides the only option in attempting to avoid a cesarean section for breech presentation. If the initial attempt is unsuccessful, it is safe and cost-effective to repeat the procedure in 1 week (Andrew Coco, Hershey, Penn).

58. **Topical anesthesia** is an efficacious adjunct or substitute for local anesthesia, but you must anticipate the need 1 to 2 hours in advance (William H. Dery, Midland, Mich).

59. Practice is the key to master laceration and incision repair. Begin with easy procedures and work up to larger excisions and skin flaps.

Remember, it is okay to cut a suture that is incorrect and replace it (William Jackson Epperson, Murrells Inlet, SC).

60. Consider **event monitoring rather than Holter monitoring** if the patient's symptoms are infrequent (Dave Feller, Gainesville, Fla).

61. **Infarction q-waves** can be normal in limb leads III, AVL, and precordial lead V_1.

   ST elevation can be normal in healthy people but is ominous in the patient with chest pain (Victor F. Froelicher, Stanford, Calif).

62. The **cesarean section** is a lifesaving procedure that can be performed competently by Family Physicians with adequate training. Hospital privileges should be granted on the basis of experience with the operation and expertise of the surgeon.

   The evaluation and selection of the patient for cesarean section is the most important step in the procedure. Knowledge of risk factors and indications for cesarean section is essential to proper patient care (Rebecca H. Gladu, Houston, Tex).

63. **Allergy screening** with only six to ten allergens can separate your allergic patient from nonallergic patients in a cost-effective way.

   Immunotherapy is the patient's only "cure" for allergic rhinitis (Harold Hedges, Little Rock, Ark).

64. Every **spider vein,** no matter how small, comes from venous incompetence that can be traced back to a perforator. Always try to inject the vein that is closest to the source of this incompetence.

   The longer **postinjection compression** (up to 3 weeks) is used, the better the result (Stanley A. Hirsch, Pittsburgh, Penn).

65. Many **paracentesis** kits have a 16- or 18-gauge needle for the paracentesis. This is generally too large. A smaller needle can limit the amount of "leakage" of ascitic fluid from the entry site after the procedure is completed (Kenneth Hu, Santa Monica, Calif).

66. **Knee braces** should be used only in conjunction with a rehabilitation program incorporating strength training, flexibility, activity modification, and technique refinement (Scott A. Paluska, Seattle, Wash).

67. A tissue diagnosis is required for any dominant breast mass, even if the mammogram and/or ultrasound are negative.

   Plan incisions carefully to achieve optimal cosmesis while preserving future surgical options if the lesion proves unexpectedly malignant (Helen A. Pass, Royal Oak, Mich).

68. **Electrical cardioversion,** unlike defibrillation, is administration of DC current synchronized with the R wave of the QRS complex.

Adequate anticoagulation of 3 weeks' duration and performance of an echocardiogram to evaluate left atrial diameter are generally considered necessary before **cardioversion of atrial fibrillation** of longer than 48 hours' duration (David V. Power, Minneapolis, Minn).

69. Send **thoracocentesis** fluid for protein, pH, and LDH. Do not order other tests unless the fluid is an exudate (Terry S. Ruhl, Altoona, Penn).

70. When injecting a **trigger point,** inject directly into the area and then fan the needle to each side along the lines of the skin for best results. Trigger points are usually not round, but are oblong and amenable to fanning (Gary E. Ruoff, East Lansing, Mich).

71. To best visualize the sides and top of the bladder, the **cystoscope** should be rotated around the long axis of the scope rather than levered from side to side. This minimizes patient discomfort (Andrew C. Steele, Travis AFB, Calif).

72. **Endometrial ablation** significantly improves PMS, moodiness, and dysmenorrhea.

    Postmenopausal bleeding resulting from hormone replacement therapy can be controlled completely by **endometrial ablation** (Duane E. Townsend, Park City, Utah).

73. **When performing a punch biopsy, it is not necessary to obtain normal skin.** The only time normal tissue is needed is with vesicular and bullous disease. Perform this biopsy on a new, fresh lesion right at the edge where is lifts up off the epidermis. This will afford the pathologist a better chance of making the diagnosis.

74. When using the **plastic endometrial aspirators** for endometrial biopsy, it may be difficult to insert the unit into the os because of the flexibility of the tube. The aspirator can be "stiffened" by placing it in a freezer for a few minutes. When cold it may easily enter the os. A full bladder often pushes the fundus posteriorly, opening the internal os if traction with a tenaculum has not succeeded in doing the same thing. Alternatively, a metal cervical dilator can be used.

75. Recently, the Centers for Disease Control and Prevention and other organizations have made the recommendation that rather than frequent hand-washing with soap and water, medical caretakers should use an **antimicrobial hand gel.** Various brands are available. In our office (JLP), we use **Prevacare** (Johnson & Johnson). It's hypoallergenic and has moisturizers. Several of my staff have eczema, and frequent hand-washing was really exacerbating symptoms. Using the new gels without any water improved their symptoms while producing a better compliance and efficacy rate than soap and water. We get the hand pump container and feel it's well worth the cost.

76. Some patients are indeed **allergic to iodine,** even in topical preparations (e.g., Betadine). We use Techni-Care Surgical Scrub (Care-Tech Laboratories, Inc., St Louis, MO [phone: 1-800-325-9681]). It's a broad-spectrum topical antiseptic microbicide with a 99.99% bacterial reduction in 30 seconds of contact. There is minimal to no dermal irritation. It's nonstinging and also safe on mucous membranes. The only difficulty is its tendency to foam up.

77. Children undergoing surgery develop more postsurgical scarring than adults. This is probably due to increased elasticity of the skin as well as an inability to get the children to limit activity. A report in the Family Practice News (Sept. 15, 2002, p. 30) gives several pearls to limit the scarring:

    - Use more subcutaneous sutures and place them deeper. They suggest that if you normally would use four sutures, then use eight for children! If the wound is fairly deep, consider using clear nylon for buried sutures, which will give permanent strength to the wound.
    - Leave in nondissolving running subcuticular stitches. If not visible, they won't hurt anything. If the stitch begins to work out, remove it later.
    - Place bulky dressings over the wound. This will inhibit some movement and help the child remember that surgery has occurred.
    - Immobilize the joints if there are any incisions over them.
    - Provide written instructions and emphasize the necessity of limiting activity.

"I don't think I'm unique. Anybody can do quite a lot by refusing to give in to limitations."
Christopher Reeves

Index

Index for Appendix G
Patient Education Handouts and Consent Forms, pp. 1739-2024

Continued on next page

Patient Consent Forms